BRENNER & RECTOR'S

The Kidney

BRENNER & RECTOR'S
The Kidney

Volume 2

Seventh Edition

Barry M. Brenner,
**M.D., A.M. (Hon.), D.Sc. (Hon.),
D.M.Sc. (Hon.), M.D. (Hon.), Dipl. (Hon.),
F.R.C.P. (Lond., Hon.)**

Samuel A. Levine Professor of Medicine
Harvard Medical School
Director Emeritus, Renal Division, and Senior Physician,
Department of Medicine
Brigham and Women's Hospital
Boston, Massachusetts

SAUNDERS
An Imprint of Elsevier

SAUNDERS
An Imprint of Elsevier

The Curtis Center
Independence Square West
Philadelphia, Pennsylvania 19106

Volume 1: Part no. 9997637097
Volume 2: Part no. 9997637100
Two-volume set ISBN 0-7216-0164-2

BRENNER & RECTOR'S THE KIDNEY

NOTICE

Nephrology is an ever-changing field. Standard safety precautions must be followed, but as new research and clinical experience broaden our knowledge, changes in treatment and drug therapy may become necessary or appropriate. Readers are advised to check the most current product information provided by the manufacturer of each drug to be administered to verify the recommended dose, the method and duration of administration, and contraindications. It is the responsibility of the treating physician, relying on experience and knowledge of the patient, to determine dosages and the best treatment for each individual patient. Neither the Publisher nor the editor assumes any liability for any injury and/or damage to persons or property arising from this publication.

The Publisher

Library of Congress Cataloging-in-Publication Data

Brenner & Rector's the kidney / editor, Barry M. Brenner—7th ed.
    p. cm.
    Includes bibliographical references and index.
    ISBN 0-7216-0164-2
    1. Kidneys—Diseases. 2. Kidneys. I. Title: Kidney. II. Brenner, Barry M. III. Rector, Floyd C.

RC902.K53 2004
616.6′1—dc21

2003042846

Acquisitions Editor	Susan Pioli
Developmental Editor	Jennifer Ehlers
Project Manager	Lee Ann Draud
Cover Design	Steven Stave

Printed in the United States of America

Last digit is the print number: 9   8   7   6   5   4   3   2   1

Jane and I
dedicate this edition
to our mothers
Beatrice and Sally
our children
Rob, Jen, and Ron
and our wonderful grandson
Sam

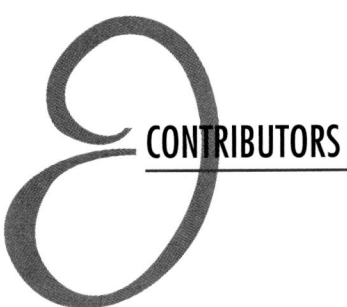

CONTRIBUTORS

Zaid A. Abassi, Ph.D.
Senior Lecturer, Faculty of Medicine, Technion, Israeli Institute of Technology; Principal Investigator, Laboratory of Vascular Biology and Renal Physiology, Rambam Medical Center, Haifa, Israel
Control of Extracellular Fluid Volume and the Pathophysiology of Edema Formation

Sharon Anderson, M.D.
Professor of Medicine, Oregon Health Sciences University School of Medicine, Portland, Oregon
Renal and Systemic Manifestations of Glomerular Disease

Gerald B. Appel, M.D.
Professor of Clinical Medicine, Columbia University College of Physicians and Surgeons; Director of Clinical Nephrology, Presbyterian Hospital Division of the New York–Presbyterian Hospital, New York, New York
Secondary Glomerular Disease

Raymond Ardaillou, M.D.
Emeritus Professor of Physiology, Faculty of Medicine, University of Paris 6—Saint-Antoine, Paris, France
Biology of Renal Cells in Culture

Allen I. Arieff, M.D.
Emeritus Professor of Medicine, University of California, San Francisco, School of Medicine, San Francisco; Attending Physician, Cedars-Sinai Medical Center, Los Angeles, California
Neurologic Complications of Renal Insufficiency

George R. Aronoff, M.D.
Professor of Medicine, Pharmacology, and Toxicology, University of Louisville School of Medicine, Louisville, Kentucky
Prescribing Drugs in Renal Disease

John R. Asplin, M.D.
Clinical Associate, University of Chicago Pritzker School of Medicine; Medical Director, Litholink Corporation, Chicago, Illinois
Nephrolithiasis

Michael B. Atkins, M.D.
Professor of Medicine, Harvard Medical School; Physician, Beth Israel Deaconess Medical Center, Boston, Massachusetts
Renal Neoplasia

Kamal F. Badr, M.D.
Professor and Chair, Department of Medicine, American University of Beirut; Attending Physician, American University of Beirut Medical Center, Beirut, Lebanon
Microvascular Diseases of the Kidney

James L. Bailey, M.D.
Professor of Medicine, Emory University School of Medicine; Attending Physician, Grady Memorial Hospital and Emory University Hospital, Atlanta, Georgia
Pathophysiology of Uremia

Matthew A. Bailey, Ph.D.
Postdoctoral Fellow, Department of Cellular and Molecular Physiology, Yale University School of Medicine, New Haven, Connecticut
Control of Renal Potassium Excretion

Laurent Baud, M.D., Ph.D.
Professor of Physiology, Faculty of Medicine, University of Paris 6—Saint-Antoine; Director, Department of Physiology, Hôpital Tenon, Paris, France
Biology of Renal Cells in Culture

Michel Baum, M.D.
Professor of Pediatrics and Internal Medicine, Department of Pediatrics, University of Texas Southwestern Medical Center at Dallas, Dallas, Texas
Renal Transport of Glucose, Amino Acids, Sodium, Chloride, and Water

Bradford C. Berk, M.D., Ph.D.
Faculty, GEBS Cell Regulation and Molecular Pharmacology, University of Rochester School of Medicine and Dentistry; Physician-in-Chief, Strong Memorial Hospital, University of Rochester Medical Center, Rochester, New York
Biology of the Vascular Wall in Hypertension

Tomas Berl, M.D.
Professor of Medicine and Head, Division of Renal Diseases and Hypertension, University of Colorado School of Medicine, Denver, Colorado
Pathophysiology of Water Metabolism

Christine A. Berry, Ph.D.
Professor Emeritus, Department of Medicine,
University of California, San Francisco, School of Medicine,
San Francisco, California
Renal Transport of Glucose, Amino Acids, Sodium,
  Chloride, and Water

Daniel G. Bichet, M.D.
Professor of Medicine, Université de Montréal; Director,
Clinical Research Unit, Centre de Recherche,
Hôpital du Sacré-Cœur de Montréal, Montréal, Québec,
Canada
Inherited Disorders of the Renal Tubule

Jon D. Blumenfeld, M.D.
Associate Professor of Medicine, Weill Medical College of
Cornell University; Associate Attending Physician in Medicine,
Rogosin Institute, New York–Presbyterian Hospital, New York,
New York
Essential Hypertension

Alain Bonnardeaux, M.D., Ph.D.
Associate Professor of Medicine, Université de Montréal;
Scientific Director, Centre de Recherche Guy-Bernier,
Hôpital Maisonneuve-Rosemont, Montréal, Québec,
Canada
Inherited Disorders of the Renal Tubule

Hugh Redmond Brady, M.D., Ph.D.
Professor of Medicine and Therapeutics, Conway Institute of
Biomolecular and Biomedical Research, University College
Dublin; Attending Physician, Mater Misericordiae University
Hospital, Dublin, Ireland
Cell-Cell and Cell-Matrix Interactions; Acute Renal Failure

Barry M. Brenner, M.D.
Samuel A. Levine Professor of Medicine,
Harvard Medical School; Director Emeritus, Renal Division, and
Senior Physician, Department of Medicine, Brigham and
Women's Hospital, Boston, Massachusetts
The Renal Circulations; Glomerular Ultrafiltration;
  Renal and Systemic Manifestations of Glomerular Disease;
  Adaptation to Nephron Loss

Matthew D. Breyer, M.D.
Division of Nephrology and Hypertension, Vanderbilt University
School of Medicine, Nashville, Tennessee
Arachidonic Acid Metabolites and the Kidney

Michael E. Brier, M.D.
Professor of Medicine, University of Louisville School of
Medicine; Kidney Disease Program, Division of Nephrology,
Department of Veterans Affairs, Louisville, Kentucky
Prescribing Drugs in Renal Disease

Dennis Brown, Ph.D.
Professor of Medicine, Harvard Medical School; Associate Chief,
Renal Unit, Massachusetts General Hospital, Boston,
Massachusetts
The Cell Biology of Vasopressin Action

John M. Burkart, M.D.
Professor of Internal Medicine and Nephrology, Wake Forest
University School of Medicine, Winston-Salem, North Carolina
Peritoneal Dialysis

Louise M. Burrell, M.D.
Associate Professor of Medicine, University of Melbourne,
Melbourne, Australia
Vasoactive Peptides and the Kidney

Kevin T. Bush, Ph.D.
Assistant Project Scientist, Department of Medicine,
University of California, San Diego, School of Medicine,
La Jolla, California
Developmental Biology of the Kidney

Vito M. Campese, M.D.
Professor of Medicine, Keck School of Medicine of USC;
Chief, Division of Nephrology, The Hypertension Center,
Los Angeles, California
Hypertension and Renal Disease

Riccardo Candido, M.D.
Physician, Department of Medicine and Neurology,
University of Trieste, Trieste, Italy
Vasoactive Peptides and the Kidney

Charles B. Carpenter, M.D.
Professor of Medicine, Harvard Medical School; Senior
Physician, Laboratory of Immunogenetics and Transplantation,
Brigham and Women's Hospital, Boston, Massachusetts
Transplantation Immunobiology

Anil Chandraker, M.D.
Instructor of Medicine, Harvard Medical School; Director,
Renal Transplant Clinics, Brigham and Women's Hospital,
Boston, Massachusetts
Transplantation Immunobiology

Ingrid J. Chang, M.D.
Fellow, Division of Nephrology, Vanderbilt University Medical
Center, Nashville, Tennessee
Extracorporeal Treatment of Poisoning

Devasmita Choudhury, M.D.
Associate Professor of Internal Medicine, University of Texas
Southwestern Medical Center at Dallas; Director of Dialysis,
Dallas Veterans Affairs Medical Center, Dallas, Texas
Effect of Aging on Renal Function and Disease

Michael R. Clarkson, M.B.
Fellow in Nephrology, Renal Division, Brigham and Women's
Hospital, Boston, Massachusetts
Acute Renal Failure

Fredric L. Coe, M.D.
Professor of Medicine and Physiology, University of Chicago
Pritzker School of Medicine; Director of Kidney Stone Program,
University of Chicago Hospitals, Chicago, Illinois
Nephrolithiasis

Jeffrey J. Connaire, M.D.
Assistant Professor of Medicine, University of Minnesota
Medical School—Minneapolis; Staff Nephrologist, Minneapolis
Veterans Affairs Medical Center, Minneapolis, Minnesota
The Kidney and Hypertension in Pregnancy

Mark E. Cooper, M.D., Ph.D.
Professor of Medicine, Monash University; Head, Vascular
Division, Baker Heart Research Institute, Melbourne, Australia
Vasoactive Peptides and the Kidney

Ramzi S. Cotran, M.D.*
Former Frank B. Mallory Professor of Pathology,
Harvard Medical School; Former Chair, Department of Pathology,
Brigham and Women's Hospital and Children's Hospital,
Boston, Massachusetts
Urinary Tract Infection, Pyelonephritis, and Reflux Nephropathy
*Deceased

John K. Crean, Ph.D.
Lecturer, University College Dublin, Dublin, Ireland
Cell-Cell and Cell-Matrix Interactions

Pirouz Daeihagh, M.D.
Assistant Professor, Department of Internal Medicine and
Nephrology, Wake Forest University School of Medicine,
Winston-Salem, North Carolina
Peritoneal Dialysis

Vivette D. D'Agati, M.D.
Professor of Pathology and Director, Renal Pathology Laboratory,
Columbia University College of Physicians and Surgeons;
Attending Physician in Pathology, Columbia Presbyterian
Medical Center, New York, New York
Secondary Glomerular Disease

Mogamat Razeen Davids, M.D.
Associate Professor, University of Stellenbosch, Cape Town;
Senior Specialist, Tygerberg Hospital, Tygerberg, South Africa
Interpretation of Urine Electrolyte and Acid-Base Parameters

Paul E. de Jong, M.D., Ph.D.
Professor of Nephrology, University of Groningen; Head,
Division of Nephrology, University Hospital Groningen,
Groningen, The Netherlands
Specific Pharmacologic Approaches to Clinical Renoprotection

Dick de Zeeuw, M.D., Ph.D.
Professor and Head, Department of Clinical Pharmacology,
University Hospital Groningen, Groningen, The Netherlands
Specific Pharmacologic Approaches to Clinical Renoprotection

Matthew Dollins, M.D.
Assistant Professor of Clinical Medicine, Division of Nephrology,
Indiana University School of Medicine; Attending Physician,
University Hospital, Indianapolis, Indiana
Intensive Care Nephrology

Thomas D. DuBose, Jr., M.D.
Professor and Chair, Department of Internal Medicine,
Wake Forest University Health Sciences; Chief of Internal
Medicine Service, North Carolina Baptist Hospital,
Winston-Salem, North Carolina
Acid-Base Disorders

Lance D. Dworkin, M.D.
Professor of Medicine and Director, Division of Renal Diseases,
Brown University School of Medicine; Director, Division of
Renal Diseases, Rhode Island Hospital, Providence, Rhode Island
The Renal Circulations

Ronald J. Falk, M.D.
Chief, Division of Nephrology and Hypertension, and Professor
of Medicine, University of North Carolina at Chapel Hill School
of Medicine, Chapel Hill, North Carolina
Primary Glomerular Disease

Murray J. Favus, M.D.
Professor of Medicine, University of Chicago Pritzker School of
Medicine; Director, Bone Program, University of Chicago
Hospital, Chicago, Illinois
Nephrolithiasis

Bernard V. Fishbach, M.D.
Clinical Fellow, Division of Nephrology, Vanderbilt University
Medical Center, Nashville, Tennessee
Extracorporeal Treatment of Poisoning

Steven Fishbane, M.D.
Associate Professor of Medicine, State University of New York
at Stony Brook School of Medicine, Stony Brook;
Vice Chairman, Department of Medicine, Winthrop-University
Hospital, Mineola, New York
Erythropoietin Therapy in Renal Disease and Renal Failure

Gerard Friedlander, M.D., Ph.D.
Professor of Physiology, Faculty of Medicine of Xavier Bichat,
University of Paris 7; Director, Inserm Unit 426, Paris, France
Biology of Renal Cells in Culture

Gerardo Gamba, M.D., Ph.D.
Professor, Biomedical Research Institute, Faculty of Medicine,
National University of Mexico; Department of Nephrology,
Instituto Nacional de Ciencias Mèdicas y Nutriciòn Salvador
Zubiràn, Instituto de Investigaciones Biomèdicas, Mexico City,
Mexico
Urine Concentration and Dilution

Daniel J. George, M.D.
Associate Professor of Medicine, Harvard Medical School;
Dana Farber Cancer Institute, Boston, Massachusetts
Renal Neoplasia

Gerhard Giebisch, M.D.
Sterling Professor of Cellular and Molecular Physiology, Yale
University School of Medicine, New Haven, Connecticut
Control of Renal Potassium Excretion

Thomas A. Golper, M.D.
Professor of Medicine and Medical Director, Medical
Specialties Patient Care Center, Division of Nephrology,
Vanderbilt University Medical Center, Nashville,
Tennessee
Extracorporeal Treatment of Poisoning

Esther A. González, M.D.
Associate Professor of Medicine, St. Louis University School of
Medicine; Attending Physician, Division of Nephrology,
St. Louis University Hospital, St. Louis, Missouri
Renal Osteodystrophy

Jared J. Grantham, M.D.
University Distinguished Professor, University of Kansas Medical
Center, Kansas City, Kansas
Cystic Diseases of the Kidney

Mitchell L. Halperin, M.D.
Professor of Medicine, University of Toronto Faculty of
Medicine; Staff Nephrologist, St. Michael's Hospital, Toronto,
Ontario, Canada
*Interpretation of Urine Electrolyte and Acid-Base
Parameters*

L. Lee Hamm, M.D.
Professor of Medicine and Chief, Section of Nephrology and Hypertension, Tulane University School of Medicine; Vice Chairman, Department of Medicine, Tulane University Health Sciences Center, New Orleans, Louisiana
Renal Acidification Mechanisms

Donna S. Hanes, M.D.
Assistant Professor, Division of Nephrology, University of Maryland School of Medicine; Attending Physician, University of Maryland Hospital, Baltimore, Maryland
Antihypertensive Drugs

Raymond C. Harris, M.D.
Professor of Medicine and Director, Division of Nephrology and Hypertension, Vanderbilt University School of Medicine, Nashville, Tennessee
Arachidonic Acid Metabolites and the Kidney

Matthias A. Hediger, Ph.D.
Associate Professor, Harvard Medical School; Director, Membrane Biology Program, Renal Division, Brigham and Women's Hospital, Boston, Massachusetts
The Molecular Basis of Solute Transport

William L. Henrich, M.D.
Professor of Medicine, University of Maryland School of Medicine; Chairman, Department of Medicine, University of Maryland Medical Center, Baltimore, Maryland
Toxic Nephropathy

Jonathan Himmelfarb, M.D.
Clinical Professor of Medicine, University of Vermont College of Medicine, Burlington, Vermont; Director, Division of Nephrology and Transplantation, Maine Medical Center, Portland, Maine
Hemodialysis

Hedvig Hricak, M.D., Ph.D.
Professor of Radiology, Weill Medical College of Cornell University; Chairman, Department of Radiology, Memorial Sloan-Kettering Cancer Center, New York, New York
Radiologic Assessment of the Kidney

Joseph E. Izzo, Jr., M.D.
Professor, Department of Medicine, Clinical Pharmacology Division, State University of New York at Buffalo School of Medicine and Biomedical Sciences, Buffalo, New York
Hypertension and Renal Disease

Karin A. Jandeleit-Dahm, M.D., Ph.D.
Senior Lecturer, Department of Medicine, Monash University; Physician, Alfred Hospital, Melbourne, Australia
Vasoactive Peptides and the Kidney

J. Charles Jennette, M.D.
Professor and Chair, Department of Pathology and Laboratory Medicine, University of North Carolina at Chapel Hill School of Medicine, Chapel Hill, North Carolina
Primary Glomerular Disease

Eric Jonasch, M.D.
Assistant Professor of Medicine, University of Texas—Houston Medical School; Attending Physician, M. D. Anderson Cancer Center, Houston, Texas
Renal Neoplasia

Kamel S. Kamel, M.D.
Assistant Professor of Medicine, University of Toronto Faculty of Medicine; Staff Nephrologist, St. Michael's Hospital, Toronto, Ontario, Canada
Interpretation of Urine Electrolyte and Acid-Base Parameters

Hussein H. Karnib, M.D.
Senior Fellow, Division of Nephrology, Department of Internal Medicine, American University of Beirut Medical Center, Beirut, Lebanon
Microvascular Diseases of the Kidney

Bertram L. Kasiske, M.D.
Professor, University of Minnesota Medical School—Minneapolis; Director, Division of Nephrology, Hennepin County Medical Center, Minneapolis, Minnesota
Laboratory Assessment of Kidney Disease: Clearance, Urinalysis, and Kidney Biopsy

Carolyn J. Kelly, M.D.
Professor of Medicine, University of California, San Diego, School of Medicine, La Jolla; Associate Chief of Staff, Veterans Affairs San Diego Health Care System, San Diego, California
Tubulointerstitial Diseases

Andrew J. King, M.D.
Clinical Professor, University of California, San Diego, School of Medicine; Head, Division of Nephrology, Scripps Clinic, La Jolla, California
Donor and Recipient Issues in Renal Transplantation

David K. Klassen, M.D.
Professor of Medicine, Division of Nephrology, University of Maryland School of Medicine; Attending Physician, University of Maryland Hospital, Baltimore, Maryland
Antihypertensive Drugs

Mark A. Knepper, M.D., Ph.D.
Chief, Laboratory of Kidney and Electrolyte Metabolism, National Heart, Lung, and Blood Institute, National Institutes of Health, Bethesda, Maryland
Urine Concentration and Dilution

Radko Komers, M.D., Ph.D.
Research Assistant Professor, Division of Nephrology and Hypertension, Oregon Health Sciences University School of Medicine, Portland, Oregon; Deputy Head, Diabetes Center, Institute of Clinical and Experimental Medicine, Prague, Czech Republic
Renal and Systemic Manifestations of Glomerular Disease

Bruce C. Kone, M.D.
Vice Chairman, Department of Medicine, and Director, Division of Renal Diseases and Hypertension, University of Texas—Houston Medical School; Chief of Nephrology, Memorial Hermann Hospital, Houston, Texas
The Metabolic Basis of Solute Transport

Michael A. Kraus, M.D.
Associate Professor of Clinical Medicine, Division of Nephrology, Indiana University School of Medicine University Hospital, Indianapolis, Indiana
Intensive Care Nephrology

John H. Laragh, M.D.
Professor of Medicine, Weill Medical College of Cornell
University; Attending Physician in Medicine,
New York–Presbyterian Hospital, New York, New York
Essential Hypertension

Moshe Levi, M.D.
Professor of Medicine, Physiology, and Biophysics and Head,
Division of Renal Diseases and Hypertension, University of
Colorado Health Sciences Center, Denver, Colorado
Effect of Aging on Renal Function and Disease

Wilfred Lieberthal, M.D.
Professor, Department of Medicine, Division of Nephrology,
Boston University School of Medicine, Boston, Massachusetts
Acute Renal Failure

Francisco Llach, M.D.
Division of Nephrology and Hypertension, Georgetown
University Hospital, Washington, D.C.
Disorders of the Renal Arteries and Veins

Valerie A. Luyckx, M.B., B.Ch.
Instructor in Medicine, Harvard Medical School; Associate
Physician, Renal Division, Brigham and Women's Hospital,
Boston, Massachusetts
Adaptation to Nephron Loss

David A. Maddox, Ph.D.
Professor of Internal Medicine, University of South Dakota
School of Medicine; Director of Basic Research, Avera Research
Institute, Sioux Falls, South Dakota
Glomerular Ultrafiltration

Kirsten M. Madsen, M.D., Ph.D.
Associate Professor of Medicine, Division of Nephrology,
Hypertension, and Transplantation, University of Florida College
of Medicine, Gainesville, Florida
Anatomy of the Kidney

Colm C. Magee, M.D.
Instructor in Medicine, Harvard Medical School; Attending
Physician, Renal Division, Brigham and Women's Hospital,
Boston, Massachusetts
Clinical Aspects of Renal Transplantation

Gerhard Malnic, M.D.
Professor, Department of Physiology and Biophysics, Instituto de
Ciências Biomédicas, Universidade de São Paulo, São Paulo, Brazil
Control of Renal Potassium Excretion

Kevin J. Martin, M.B., B.Ch.
Professor of Medicine, St. Louis University School of Medicine;
Director, Division of Nephrology, St. Louis University Hospital,
St. Louis, Missouri
Renal Osteodystrophy

Michael Mauer, M.D.
Department of Pediatric Nephrology, University of Minnesota
Hospital and Clinic, Minneapolis, Minnesota
Diabetic Nephropathy

Dianne B. McKay, M.D.
Assistant Member, Scripps Research Institute; Director of
Research, Division of Nephrology, Scripps Clinic, La Jolla,
California
Donor and Recipient Issues in Renal Transplantation

Lawrence P. McMahon, M.D.
Senior Lecturer, University of Melbourne; Director, Department
of Nephrology, Western Hospital, Melbourne, Australia
Cardiovascular Aspects of Chronic Kidney Disease

Maya Meux, M.D.
Assistant Clinical Professor of Radiology, University of California,
San Francisco, School of Medicine, San Francisco, California
Radiologic Assessment of the Kidney

Edgar L. Milford, M.D.
Associate Professor of Medicine, Harvard Medical School;
Laboratory of Immunogenetics and Transplantation, Renal
Division, Brigham and Women's Hospital, Boston, Massachusetts
Clinical Aspects of Renal Transplantation

Luigi Minetti, M.D.
Professor of Nephrology, Clinical Research Center for Rare
Diseases, Ranica, Italy
Hematologic Consequences of Renal Failure

William E. Mitch, M.D.
Professor and Chair, Department of Internal Medicine, University
of Texas Medical Branch, University of Texas Medical School at
Galveston, Galveston, Texas
*Pathophysiology of Uremia; Nutritional Therapy
   in Renal Disease*

Orson W. Moe, M.D.
Associate Professor of Internal Medicine, Department of Internal
Medicine and Center of Mineral Metabolism and Clinical
Research, University of Texas Southwestern Medical Center at
Dallas, Dallas, Texas
*Renal Transport of Glucose, Amino Acids, Sodium,
   Chloride, and Water*

Bruce A. Molitoris, M.D.
Professor of Medicine and Director, Nephrology Division,
Indiana University School of Medicine, Indianapolis, Indiana
Intensive Care Nephrology

David B. Mount, M.D.
Assistant Professor of Medicine, Harvard Medical School;
Attending Physician, Renal Division, Brigham and Women's
Hospital, Boston, Massachusetts
*The Molecular Basis of Solute Transport; Disorders of
   Potassium Balance*

Patrick H. Nachman, M.D.
Associate Professor of Medicine, Division of Nephrology,
University of North Carolina at Chapel Hill School of Medicine,
Chapel Hill, North Carolina
Primary Glomerular Disease

Gerjan Navis, M.D.
Professor of Experimental Nephrology and Renal
Pharmacology, University Hospital Groningen, Groningen,
The Netherlands
Specific Pharmacologic Approaches to Clinical Renoprotection

Eric G. Neilson, M.D.
Hugh Jackson Morgan Professor of Medicine and Chair,
Department of Medicine, Vanderbilt University School of
Medicine; Physician-in-Chief, Vanderbilt University Hospital,
Vanderbilt University Medical Center, Nashville, Tennessee
Tubulointerstitial Diseases

Soren Nielsen, M.D., Ph.D.
Professor of Cell Biology and Pathophysiology,
Institute of Anatomy, Water and Salt Research Center,
University of Aarhus, Denmark
The Cell Biology of Vasopressin Action

Sanjay K. Nigam, M.D.
Professor, Departments of Pediatrics, Medicine, and Cellular and
Molecular Medicine, and Nancy Kaehr Chair in Pediatric
Research, University of California, San Diego, School of
Medicine, La Jolla, California
Developmental Biology of the Kidney

Allen R. Nissenson, M.D.
Professor of Medicine, David Geffen School of Medicine at
UCLA; Director, Dialysis Program, UCLA Medical Center,
Los Angeles, California
Erythropoietin Therapy in Renal Disease and Renal Failure

Mark S. Paller, M.D.
Professor of Medicine, University of Minnesota Medical
School—Minneapolis, Minneapolis, Minnesota
The Kidney and Hypertension in Pregnancy

Biff F. Palmer, M.D.
Professor of Internal Medicine and Director, Nephrology
Fellowship Program, University of Texas Southwestern Medical
School, Dallas, Texas
Toxic Nephropathy

Patrick S. Parfrey, M.D.
University Research Professor, Health Sciences Center;
Staff Nephrologist and Director, Patient Research Centre,
Health Care Corporation of St. John's, St. John's,
Newfoundland, Canada
Cardiovascular Aspects of Chronic Kidney Disease

Hans-Henrik Parving, M.D.
Steno Diabetes Center, Gentofte, Denmark
Diabetic Nephropathy

David L. Perkins, M.D.
Associate Professor, Harvard Medical School; Laboratory of
Molecular Immunology, Department of Medicine, Brigham and
Women's Hospital, Boston, Massachusetts
Transplantation Immunobiology

Georgi Pirtskhalaishvili, M.D., Ph.D.
Fellow and AFUD Scholar, Department of Urology,
University of Pittsburgh School of Medicine, Pittsburgh,
Pennsylvania
Urinary Tract Obstruction

Martin R. Pollak, M.D.
Assistant Professor of Medicine, Harvard Medical School;
Attending Physician, Brigham and Women's Hospital, Boston,
Massachusetts
*Clinical Disturbances of Calcium, Magnesium, and Phosphate
    Metabolism*

Hamid Rabb, M.D.
Associate Professor of Medicine, Johns Hopkins
University School of Medicine; Physician Director, Kidney
Transplant Program, Johns Hopkins Hospital, Baltimore,
Maryland
Cell-Cell and Cell-Matrix Interactions

Jai Radhakrishnan, M.D.
Assistant Professor of Medicine, Columbia University College of
Physicians and Surgeons; Program Director, Nephrology
Fellowship, New York–Presbyterian Hospital, New York,
New York
Secondary Glomerular Disease

Dominic S. C. Raj, M.D.
Assistant Professor, Division of Nephrology, University of
New Mexico Health Sciences Center, Albuquerque, New Mexico
Effect of Aging on Renal Function and Disease

Floyd C. Rector, Jr., M.D.
Professor Emeritus, Department of Medicine, University of
California, San Francisco, School of Medicine, San Francisco,
California
*Renal Transport of Glucose, Amino Acids, Sodium,
    Chloride, and Water*

Gautham Reddy, M.D., M.P.H.
Assistant Professor of Radiology and Associate Director of
Diagnostic Radiology Residency Program, University of
California, San Francisco, School of Medicine, San Francisco,
California
Radiologic Assessment of the Kidney

Giuseppe Remuzzi, M.D.
Professor of Nephrology, Mario Negri Institute for
Pharmacological Research, Negri Bergamo Laboratories,
Division of Nephrology and Dialysis, Bergamo, Italy
Hematologic Consequences of Renal Failure

Eberhard Ritz, M.D.
Nephrology, Dialysis, and Transplantation, Sektion Nephrologie,
Med. Universitätsklinik, Heidelberg, Germany
Diabetic Nephropathy

Michael V. Rocco, M.D.
Professor, Internal Medicine and Nephrology, Wake Forest
University School of Medicine, Winston-Salem, North Carolina
Peritoneal Dialysis

Andreas Rolfs, Ph.D.
Department of Biochemistry and Molecular Pharmacology,
Harvard Medical School, Boston; Harvard Institute of
Proteomics, Cambridge, Massachusetts
The Molecular Basis of Solute Transport

Michael F. Romero, Ph.D.
Associate Professor, Department of Physiology and Biophysics,
Case Western Reserve University School of Medicine,
Cleveland, Ohio
The Molecular Basis of Solute Transport

Pierre Ronco, M.D., Ph.D.
Professor of Renal Medicine, Faculty of Medicine, University of
Paris 6—Saint-Antoine; Director, Department of Nephrology and
Inserm Unit 489, Hôpital Tenon, Paris, France
Biology of Renal Cells in Culture

Robert H. Rubin, M.D.
Professor of Medicine, Harvard Medical School; Associate
Director, Division of Infectious Diseases, Brigham and Women's
Hospital, Boston, Massachusetts
*Urinary Tract Infections, Pyelonephritis, and
    Reflux Nephropathy*

Mohamed H. Sayegh, M.D.
Associate Professor of Medicine, Harvard Medical School;
Research Director, Laboratory of Immunogenetics and
Transplantation, Brigham and Women's Hospital, Boston,
Massachusetts
Transplantation Immunobiology

Arrigo Schieppati, M.D.
Associate Professor of Nephrology, Mario Negri Institute for
Pharmacological Research, Negri Bergamo Laboratories,
Division of Nephrology and Dialysis, Bergamo, Italy
Hematologic Consequences of Renal Failure

Anton C. Schoolwerth, M.D.
Visiting Professor, Dartmouth Medical School, Hanover;
Visiting Professor, Dartmouth-Hitchcock Medical Center,
Lebanon, New Hampshire
*Renal Handling of Organic Anions and Cations: Excretion of
Uric Acid*

Gerald Schulman, M.D.
Professor of Medicine, Vanderbilt University
School of Medicine; Director, End-Stage Renal
Disease Program, Vanderbilt University Medical Center,
Nashville, Tennessee
Hemodialysis

Domenic A. Sica, M.D.
Professor of Medicine, Virginia Commonwealth University
School of Medicine; Chairman, Section of Clinical Pharmacology
and Hypertension, Virginia Commonwealth University Health
System, Richmond, Virginia
*Renal Handling of Organic Anions and Cations: Excretion of
Uric Acid*

Saba Silé, M.D.
Fellow in Nephrology, Vanderbilt University School of Medicine,
Nashville, Tennessee
Extracorporeal Treatment of Poisoning

John R. Silkensen, M.D.
Assistant Professor, University of Minnesota Medical
School—Minneapolis; Staff Nephrologist, Division of
Nephrology, Hennepin County Medical Center, Minneapolis,
Minnesota
*Laboratory Assessment of Kidney Disease: Clearance, Urinalysis,
and Kidney Biopsy*

Karl L. Skorecki, M.D.
Professor, Bruce Rappaport Faculty of Medicine, Technion,
Israeli Institute of Technology; Director, Department of
Nephrology and Molecular Medicine, Rambam Medical Center,
Haifa, Israel
*Control of Extracellular Fluid Volume and the Pathophysiology of
Edema Formation*

Eduardo Slatopolsky, M.D.
Professor of Medicine and Joseph Friedman Professor of
Renal Diseases in Medicine, Washington University School
of Medicine; Attending Physician, Barnes-Jewish Hospital,
St. Louis, Missouri
Renal Osteodystrophy

John C. Stivelman, M.D.
Associate Professor of Medicine, Division of Nephrology,
University of Washington School of Medicine; Chief Medical
Officer, Northwest Kidney Centers, Seattle, Washington
Erythropoietin Therapy in Renal Disease and Renal Failure

Robert O. Stuart, M.D.
Assistant Professor of Medicine, University of California,
San Diego, School of Medicine, La Jolla; Physician,
Veterans Affairs San Diego Healthcare System, San Diego,
California
Developmental Biology of the Kidney

Maarten W. Taal, M.B., Ch.B.
Consultant Renal Physician, Derby City General Hospital,
Derby, United Kingdom
Adaptation to Nephron Loss

Stephen C. Textor, M.D.
Professor of Medicine, Divisions of Hypertension and
Nephrology, Mayo Medical School; Consultant, Divisions of
Hypertension and Nephrology/Transplant, Mayo Clinic,
Rochester, Minnesota
Renovascular Hypertension and Ischemic Nephropathy

C. Craig Tisher, M.D.
Professor, Departments of Medicine, Pathology, and
Anatomy and Cell Biology, and Dean, University of Florida
College of Medicine, Gainesville, Florida
Anatomy of the Kidney

Nina E. Tolkoff-Rubin, M.D.
Associate Professor of Medicine, Harvard Medical School;
Director, Hemodialysis and Continuous Ambulatory
Peritoneal Dialysis Units, Massachusetts General Hospital,
Boston, Massachusetts
*Urinary Tract Infections, Pyelonephritis, and
Reflux Nephropathy*

Robert D. Toto, M.D.
Professor of Medicine, University of Texas Southwestern Medical
Center at Dallas, Dallas, Texas
Approach to the Patient with Kidney Disease

Joseph Verbalis, M.D.
Professor of Medicine, Georgetown University School of
Medicine; Chief, Endocrinology and Metabolism, Georgetown
University Hospital, Washington, D.C.
Pathophysiology of Water Metabolism

Mackenzie Walser, M.D.
Professor of Pharmacology and Medicine,
Johns Hopkins University School of Medicine;
Attending Physician, Johns Hopkins Hospital, Baltimore,
Maryland
Nutritional Therapy in Renal Disease

Matthew R. Weir, M.D.
Professor of Medicine and Director, Division of Nephrology,
University of Maryland School of Medicine; Attending Physician,
Renal Division, University of Maryland Medical System,
Baltimore, Maryland
Antihypertensive Drugs

Christopher S. Wilcox, M.D., Ph.D.
George E. Schreiner Professor of Nephrology and Chief,
Division of Nephrology and Hypertension, Georgetown
University School of Medicine, Washington, D.C.
Diuretics

Joseph Winaver, M.D.
Associate Professor, Faculty of Medicine, and Head,
Renal Laboratory, Department of Physiology and Biophysics,
Technion, Israeli Institute of Technology, Haifa, Israel
*Control of Extracellular Fluid Volume and the Pathophysiology
of Edema Formation*

Franz Winklhofer, M.D.
Assistant Professor of Medicine, University of Kansas Medical
Center, Kansas City, Kansas
Cystic Diseases of the Kidney

Alan S. L. Yu, M.B., B.Ch.
Assistant Professor of Medicine, Division of Nephrology,
Keck School of Medicine of USC, Los Angeles, California
*Renal Transport of Calcium, Magnesium, and Phosphate;
Clinical Disturbances of Calcium, Magnesium, and Phosphate
Metabolism*

Michael Yudd, M.D.
Assistant Professor, Department of Clinical Medicine,
UMDNJ—New Jersey Medical School; Medical Director,
Dialysis Unit, Department of Veterans Affairs, New Jersey Health
Care System, Newark, New Jersey
Disorders of the Renal Arteries and Veins

Kambiz Zandi-Nejad, M.D.
Clinical/Research Fellow in Nephrology, Renal Division,
Brigham and Women's Hospital, Boston, Massachusetts
Disorders of Potassium Balance

Mark L. Zeidel, M.D.
Professor of Medicine, Cell Biology, and Physiology,
University of Pittsburgh School of Medicine;
Chairman, Department of Medicine, UPMC Health
System—University of Pittsburgh, Pittsburgh, Pennsylvania
Urinary Tract Obstruction

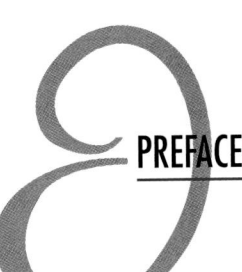

PREFACE

In the twenty-eight-year period from the first edition of *The Kidney* (1976) to the present seventh edition (2004), the knowledge base of nephrology has expanded remarkably. Progressing in logical order from the study of whole kidney function in intact organisms to the investigation of the individual nephron unit—discrete glomerulus and tubule segments and epithelial, endothelial, mesangial, or other renal-specific cell types—the basic thrust in nephrology research now extends to the level of cellular organelles, membrane channels, transporters, and exchangers and to the myriad genes that govern renal cell protein expression and regulation. At each of these levels of the reductive cascade, specific derangements are increasingly implicated as causes of the disorders of renal structure and function that lead to organ-specific injury and to the generalized disturbances of body fluid volume and composition—the panoply of syndromes that constitutes the oeuvre of clinical nephrology.

In 1976, the largest annual meeting of nephrology, the American Society of Nephrology, received approximately 500 abstracts. In 2003, this number exceeded 4000. Such explosive growth in the fruits of research in the basic renal sciences, pathophysiology, and clinical nephrology challenges our individual abilities to receive, store, assimilate, and synthesize this ever-increasing fund of new knowledge. In keeping with previous editions, the seventh edition once again strives to confront these challenges by expanding the scope of topics covered, in particular by adding 10 new chapter headings in addition to the many already added to the fifth and sixth editions. To ensure a fresh perspective in the formidable task of assimilating and synthesizing new information, we have continued the approach taken in previous editions, namely, to rewrite chapters, sometimes partially but more often completely, by inviting internationally recognized new authorities as contributors. Their challenge, as well as mine, has been to accomplish our stated goals without adding further bulk to an already formidable two-volume tome and to ensure the inclusion of thousands of references that accurately reflect the progress that has been made since the previous edition 4 years ago.

To further address the needs and interests of clinicians treating renal disease, we are pleased to continue to update and expand our library of companion volumes to *Brenner & Rector's The Kidney*. These books represent highly current, comprehensive, and integrated content and focus on the significant advances made in the diagnosis and management of acute and chronic kidney disease and hypertension.

We are pleased to have just published the second edition of *Therapy in Nephrology and Hypertension*, edited by Hugh Brady and Christopher Wilcox. To be published in the fall of 2004 will be the second editions of *Hypertension*, edited by Suzanne Oparil and Michael Weber, and *Chronic Kidney Disease: Dialysis and Transplantation*, edited by Brian Pereira, Mohamed Sayegh, and Peter Blake. In addition, we remain delighted with the success of our current volumes: *Acute Renal Failure*, edited by Bruce Molitoris and William Finn, and *Acid-Base and Electrolyte Disorders*, edited by Thomas DuBose and Lee Hamm. In the near future we will also add to the companion library an *Atlas of Renal Pathology, The Molecular and Genetic Basis of Renal Disease*, a new concise *Pocket Companion to Brenner & Rector's The Kidney*, and a board-review workbook. A most exciting part of our future planning is an e-edition, a web site based on the entire library, which will include updates and other multimedia not possible in print form.

I continue to be indebted to our authors for their unrivaled scholarship, splendid cooperation, and timeliness in meeting austere deadlines. I also wish to express my sincere gratitude to my very able editorial assistant, Francesca Quinn, and to the many dedicated professionals at Elsevier—in particular Susan Pioli, Jennifer Ehlers, Lee Ann Draud, and Steven Stave—for their enthusiasm, guidance, and unrelenting support.

Barry M. Brenner

FOREWORD

The publication of the seventh edition of *The Kidney* is a momentous occasion in nephrology as it reflects three decades of extraordinary advances in our understanding of kidney function in health and disease. This gain in scientific understanding has been the result of remarkable and unprecedented discoveries in biomedical science. Such developments depend on the simultaneous emergence of new ideas, as well as new technologies and methods to rigorously test these ideas. The techniques and methods that were referred to in the early editions, such as micropuncture and immunofluorescence, have been superseded with advances in molecular and cellular biology, including those that have resulted from the explosion in information related to molecular genetics in the genome-proteomics era. Nephrologists have rapidly improved their knowledge based on such fundamental discoveries as the three-dimensional structure of ion channels, gene transcription, signal transduction, apoptosis, angiogenesis, intracellular protein trafficking, cell growth and differentiation, and intricacies of immune cell function, to name a few. Now, at the beginning of the 21st century, there is a depth of understanding of nephrology that could not have been envisioned in the 1970s. There is now specificity to diagnosis, which was then unimagined, as, for example, in genotyping for polycystic kidney disease and a host of other genetic glomerular and tubuler disorders and hypertension.

Clinical nephrology has matured in step with basic science. Highly developed training programs have yielded thousands of expertly trained, informed, and articulate physicians of high caliber. Sophisticated nephrology centers with research and training exist not only in North America, Europe, and Japan but also in emerging countries. Renal care is at a substantially elevated level. An effective armamentarium of therapeutic nephrology has resulted from basic university and pharmaceutical corporate research, yielding powerful immunosuppressives, erythropoietin, selective antihypertensives, effective vitamin D metabolites, and other modern therapeutics, all of which give the nephrologist of today advantages unimagined by the physician in the 1970s.

The treatment of chronic renal failure has mushroomed into a global industry. In 2003, more than 1 million patients in more than 100 countries are receiving hemodialysis or peritoneal dialysis, and 350,000 others have had renal transplants with a high survival rate. However, despite major advances, the field of dialysis continues to be faced with questions about quality and adequacy, as well as the reasons for the intractable loss of one tenth of dialysis patients annually, mostly through fatal complications of cardiovascular disease. The total cost of dialysis has skyrocketed, and continuing efforts to deal with the increasing demand remain a challenge for even the most affluent nations. Renal transplantation is well established, but here again many questions remain, and the field suffers from insufficient donors and organ availability in many parts of the world. There is also an urgent need for more transplant centers in less developed societies.

Prevention of clinical kidney disease has clearly been placed on the renal agenda in the last decade. In his Foreword to the first edition of *Brenner & Rector's The Kidney*, the late Dr. Robert W. Berliner referred to the "half-way technology" of renal replacement therapy when he stated, "This burden [of kidney disease] will be reduced only when we have improved our understanding of the initiating factors in chronic renal disease and the nature of the processes that perpetuate the progressive damage and have learned how to prevent or interrupt them." Barry Brenner has been the leader in the fulfillment of this major challenge posed by Dr. Berliner, who was an early mentor of Dr. Brenner, of whom he was justly proud. The challenge of the accelerating increase in the number of patients with kidney failure can be met only with the strategies of primary and secondary prevention emphasized in the seventh edition. Reduction in glomerular hypertension and proteinuria retards the relentless progression of renal disease. Now, important measures of renoprotection to delay renal disease progression have been proved in extensive, multicenter clinical trials—another new development in clinical nephrology. Such progress allows for more comprehensive clinical strategies in which the emphasis is on prevention, in addition to the therapy of active disease. If all measures fail, renal replacement therapy is the eventual treatment. Regrettably, the number of patients with clinical renal failure requiring dialysis and transplantation continues to grow in the developed and—even more rapidly—in the developing world. It is currently predicted that there will be 300 million people with diabetes in 2020, one third of whom will be at risk of developing kidney failure.

Finally, modern nephrology is truly global. Hardly a nation is without a nephrologist and at least minimal access to dialysis. Postgraduate medical education is taking place regularly in more than 100 countries. In an attempt to deal with the epidemic of kidney diseases due to diabetes mellitus and hypertension, the issues of kidney disease in the developing world are increasingly on the agenda of professional societies, world health agencies, and national governments. Barry Brenner and I, along with many devoted colleagues, are involved in this global mission and have expended our educational and counseling efforts in many lands. It is noteworthy that *Brenner & Rector's The Kidney* is often the only book about renal disease on the shelf of the local university or hospital library, and the electronic version has proved to be particularly useful in enhancing accessibility and regular usage.

The seventh edition of *Brenner & Rector's The Kidney* brings together a unique survey of nephrology at the cutting edge in 2003. Established and young nephrologists from 16 countries are authors of the chapters in this edition, ensuring international diversity of opinion and experience. As a lifelong friend and colleague of Barry Brenner, I congratulate him and the contributors on this monumental endeavor. It will be fascinating to anticipate the even greater advances that will be heralded in future editions of what has deservedly been recognized as the leading textbook in the field.

John H. Dirks, M.D.

CONTENTS

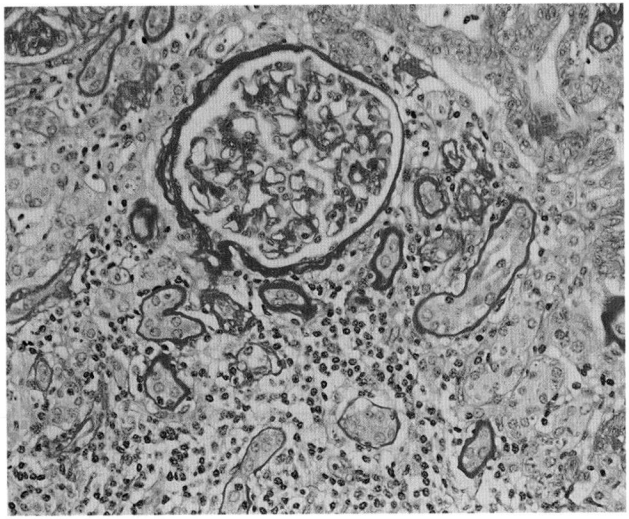

A

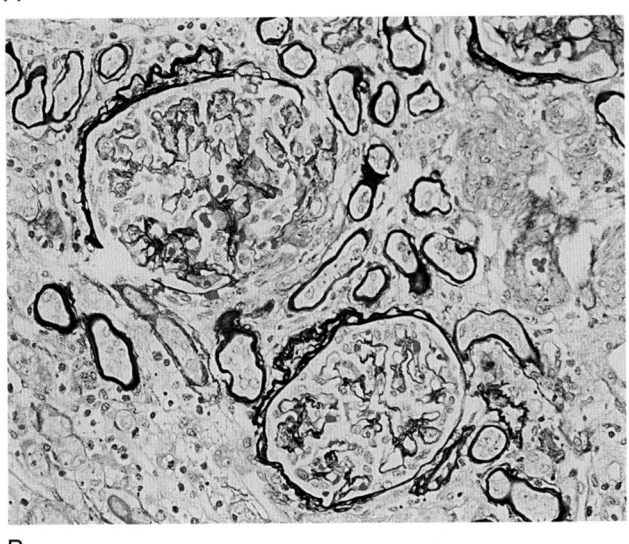

B

FIGURE 46-10. A and **B**, Photomicrographs obtained from a kidney beyond an occlusive renal artery lesion. The glomerular volume is small, with tubular atrophy and interstitcil fibrosis with patchy areas of inflammatory cellular infiltrate (From Textor SC, Wilcox, CS: Renal artery stenosis: A common, treatable cause of renal failure? Annu Rev Med 52: 421-442, 2001.)

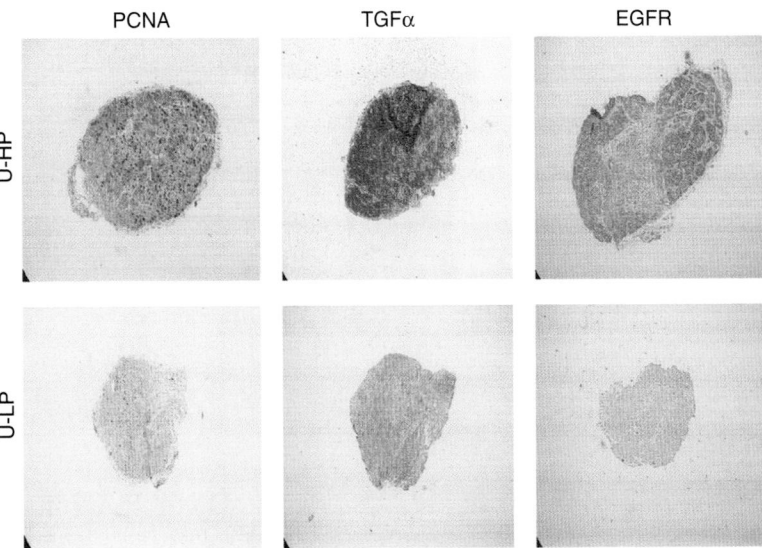

FIGURE 52-7. Dietary phosphorus regulation of parathyroid growth directly correlates with expression of transforming growth factor-α (TGFα) and epidermal growth factor receptor (EGFR). High dietary phosphorus (HP) induces, and low dietary phosphorus (LP) prevents, increases in the expression of proliferating cell nuclear antigen (PCNA) as well as that of TGFα and EGFR in uremic (U) rats.

Uremia = 7 days

COLOR PLATE I

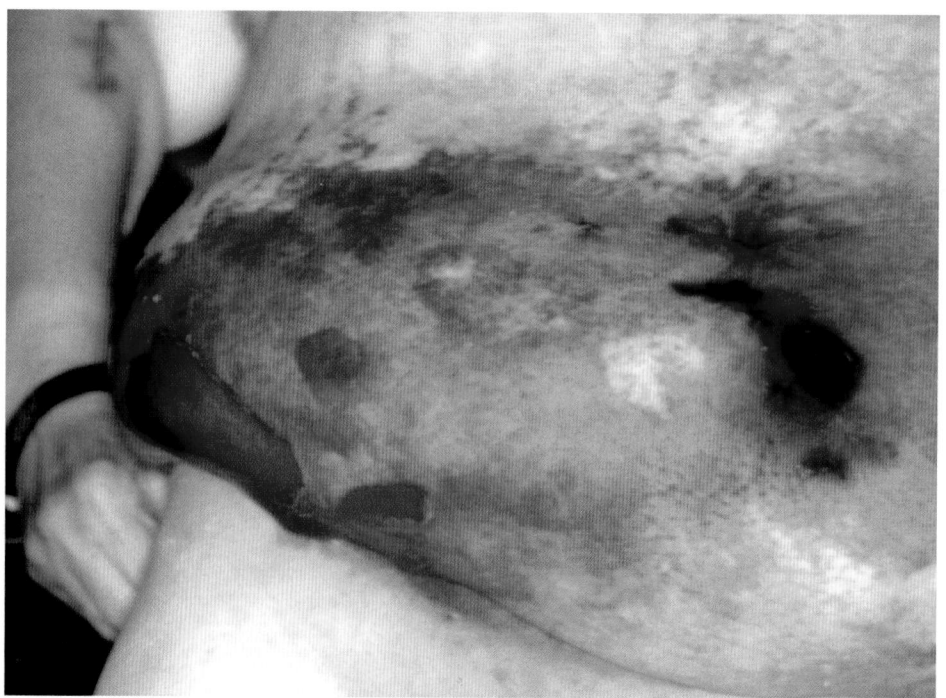

A

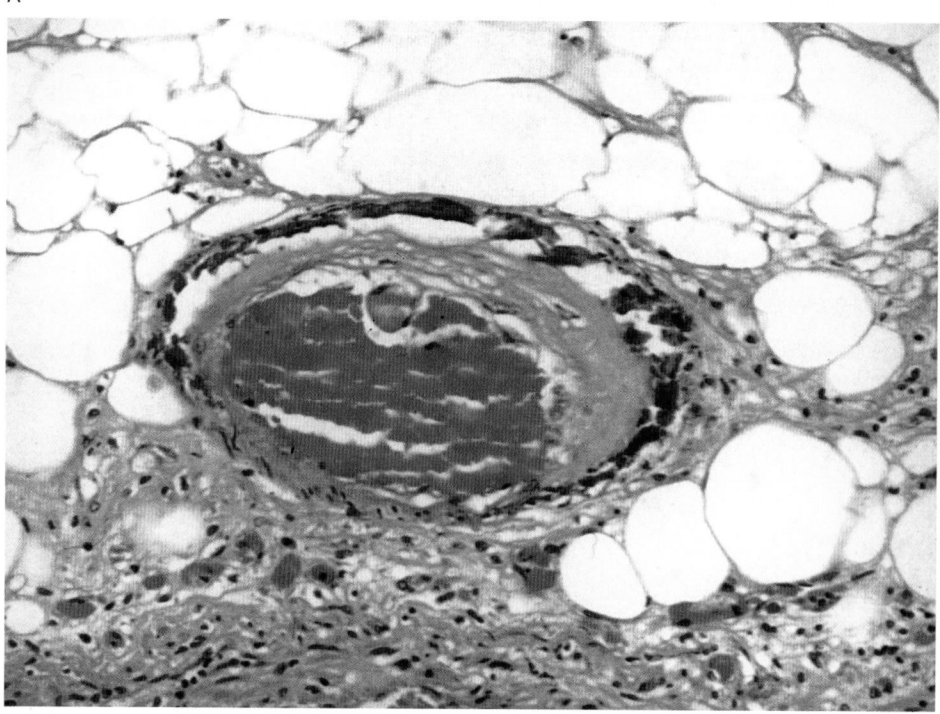

FIGURE 52-13. Calciphylaxis. **A,**
Ulceration of the abdominal wall
with a characteristic violaceous rash.
B, Skin biopsy specimen with thrombosis of a calcified blood vessel.
(From Gonzalez EA, Martin KJ: Bone
and mineral metabolism in chronic
renal failure. *In* Johnson J, Feehally
RJ [eds]: Comprehensive Clinical
Nephrology. London, Mosby, 2000,
pp 69.1-69.11, with permission.)

B

COLOR PLATE II

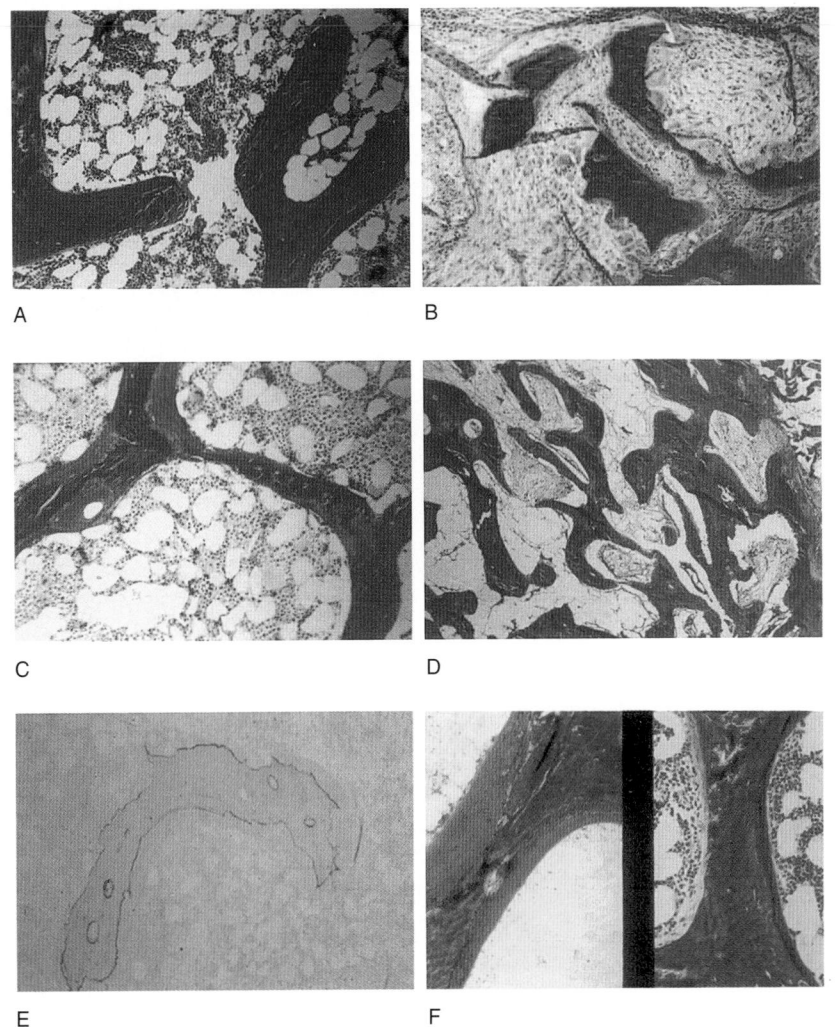

A

B

C

D

E

F

FIGURE 52-24. The characteristic histologic features of renal osteodystrophy. **A,** Normal trabecular bone. Modified Masson stain results in the mineralized matrix staining blue. The is little osteoid present. **B,** Osteitis fibrosa. There is excess osteoid (stained red) lined by osteoblasts surrounding the trabeculae (stained blue). There are numerous multinucleated osteoclasts, and there is marrow fibrosis. **C,** Osteomalacia. There is excess osteoid (stained red) and little osteoblast activity. **D,** Osteosclerosis. There is loss of distinction between cortical and trabecular bone, and wide osteoid seams are evident. **E,** Staining for aluminum, demonstrating a red band at the junction of the trabecular bone and the wide osteoid seams (the mineralization front). **F,** A higher-power view of the findings in aluminum-induced osteomalacia *(left)* and resolution of the findings after therapy with deferoxamine *(right)*. (**A-D** and **F,** Courtesy of S. L. Teitelbaum, M.D.; **E,** courtesy of D. J. Sherrard, M.D.)

COLOR PLATE III

CHAPTER 30

Tubulointerstitial Diseases

Carolyn J. Kelly and Eric G. Neilson

HISTORICAL PERSPECTIVE

The tubulointerstitial compartment comprises everything that is not glomerular.[1] It is formed first during embryogenesis and its structures quickly become the principal mass of the mature kidney.[2] The understanding of its function is deeply rooted in the study of its structure. That the kidney is comprised of tubules has been known since the 16th century.[3] Bowman's[4] report in 1842 that malpighian bodies were connected to tubules forged the basis of the filtration theory of urine. By 1852 the interstitium had received anatomic recognition as a separate compartment of its own.[5] Biermer, in 1860, first observed interstitial infiltrates in the absence of infection[6]; at the same time, Taylor and Pavy[7] introduced a model of experimental interstitial injury following exposure to mercury bichloride. This was soon followed by an early description of lead nephropathy.[8] By 1868 Dickinson[9] had devoted an entire chapter of his book on albuminuria to diseases of tubular nephritis. Ponfick's[10] description in 1869 of stiletto fibroblast-like cells in the interstitium of the kidney led to the suggestion that interstitial alterations in Bright disease may be responsible for the contracted kidneys of end-stage renal failure.[11] In 1898 Councilman[12] provided the first comprehensive report on the cause and effect of acute interstitial nephritis. This work led in 1910, to Pearce's[13] critical discussion of different models of tubulointerstitial injury, and set the stage for Vollhard and Fahr[14] to assign interstitial nephritis a place in their 1914 classification of renal diseases.

Longcope[15] in 1913 began injecting rabbits with heterologous proteins to produce lymphocyte infiltration and fibrosis in the renal interstitium, which led to a century of study of immune-mediated interstitial nephritis.[16] In 1943 Melnick[17] reported that antibiotics would produce interstitial nephritis in humans, and Spühler and Zollinger[18] later suggested the same for analgesics, starting an expansive catalog of drugs that could inflict injury on the interstitial compartment. In 1966 Unanue and colleagues[19] described interstitial nephritis in rabbits developing glomerulonephritis. This observation refocused attention on the immunologic basis of interstitial injury, with the suggestion that glomerular and interstitial processes may be related. In 1971, Steblay and Rudofsky[20] produced anti-tubular basement membrane (anti-TBM) disease in guinea pigs, and in 1976 Lehman and Wilson[21] demonstrated such diseases could be transferred with immune lymphocytes in rats. In 1984 an inheritable model of spontaneous interstitial nephritis was described in mice.[22] This work, through to the present era, has stimulated an intense study of immunologic and cell-mediated mechanisms of interstitial nephritis using the tools of cellular and molecular biology.[16, 23]

Progressive inflammation or injury to the renal interstitium typically destroys extensive amounts of kidney tissue and, as a result, usually produces a considerable decrement in renal function. Interstitial inflammation can begin either from within the interstitial compartment or as a secondary event following glomerular or vascular injury. The clinical distinction between acute and chronic interstitial inflammation can be confirmed at a pathologic or tissue level, but these distinctions are not very useful in biochemical or immunologic terms because these processes are time-sensitive. It is also difficult to make useful comparisons of the pathogenesis of interstitial lesions between experimental animals and humans because nearly all we know about this process in humans comes from work in experimental systems.

Although some forms of injury to the tubulointerstitial compartment are the result of toxic insult or exposure to infection and drugs, much of the inflammatory process is immunologic. The mononuclear infiltrates which appear as part of tubulointerstitial disease lead to the release of paracrine cytokines which collectively create a microenvironment impaired in function and appearance.[23, 24] Knowledge of such events has also led to an examination of immune effects on somatic epithelium expressing renal target antigens. That the immune system is capable of signaling somatic cells directly, as well as just destroying them in phenotypically distinct ways, is one of the more interesting outgrowths of current research.[25] More recently, studying the transition between interstitial nephritis and fibrosis has become intensely rewarding.[26, 27]

STRUCTURE-FUNCTION RELATIONSHIPS

Simple correlations between disturbances in glomerular structure and functional impairment of the kidney are, surprisingly, imperfect.[28, 29] Glomerular disease is only one aspect of the anatomic representation in renal dysfunction. Damage to the tubulointerstitial compartment is another and, perhaps, a more accurate gauge of renal performance (Fig. 30-1).

The concept of tubulointerstitial damage mediating impaired renal function is not new.[18] Many studies have pointed to the guarded prognostic significance of severe interstitial disease in lupus nephritis,[30, 31] membranous nephropathy,[32] and chronic glomerulonephritis.[33] Functional comparative parameters such as inulin clearance, maximal concentrating ability, and Na_4^+ excretion are often best correlated with a semiquantitative scoring of tubulointerstitial disease and inflammation.[29]

The analyses of this topic by Bohle and co-workers[34, 35] have employed quantitative morphometric comparisons between tubulointerstitial damage and renal function. Tubulointerstitial changes were studied in a wide variety of glomerulopathies arising from disparate pathogenic mechanisms, and decreasing maximal urine osmolality was correlated best with increasing interstitial volume, decreasing cross-sectional area of proximal tubular epithelium, and decreasing cross-sectional area of epithelium from the thick segment of the loop of Henle. T lymphocytes near or among epithelial cells were also evident in these cases. Other key morphologic components of tubulointerstitial nephritis include the presence of edema, activated fibroblasts, collagen, proteoglycans, lymphocytes, monocytes, antibody, and complement as imaged by light microscopy, immunofluorescence, or histochemistry. Some of these reports suggest that such interstitial changes may also predict the long-term prognosis in chronic glomerulonephritis.[34, 35]

The structure-function relationship between tubulointerstitial disease and renal function can be understood at a hypothetical level by several mechanisms that are not mutually exclusive. The first and simplest explanation for this relationship is that urinary flow is impeded by tubular obstruction on an anatomic basis as a result of inflammation.[24, 34] Interstitial inflammation and fibrosis may also occlude the tubules and cause increased intratubular pressure. In the absence of direct measurements, an analogy may be found in rats that, after unilateral ureteral ligation, develop retrograde Tamm-Horsfall casts in the proximal nephron.[36] Tubular atrophy or debris within tubules would therefore essentially represent a clogged drain.

A second hypothetical mechanism implicates an increase in vascular resistance with progressive tubular injury and fibrosis.[34] The volume of peritubular capillaries is decreased in areas of interstitial inflammation, edema, or fibrosis.[37]

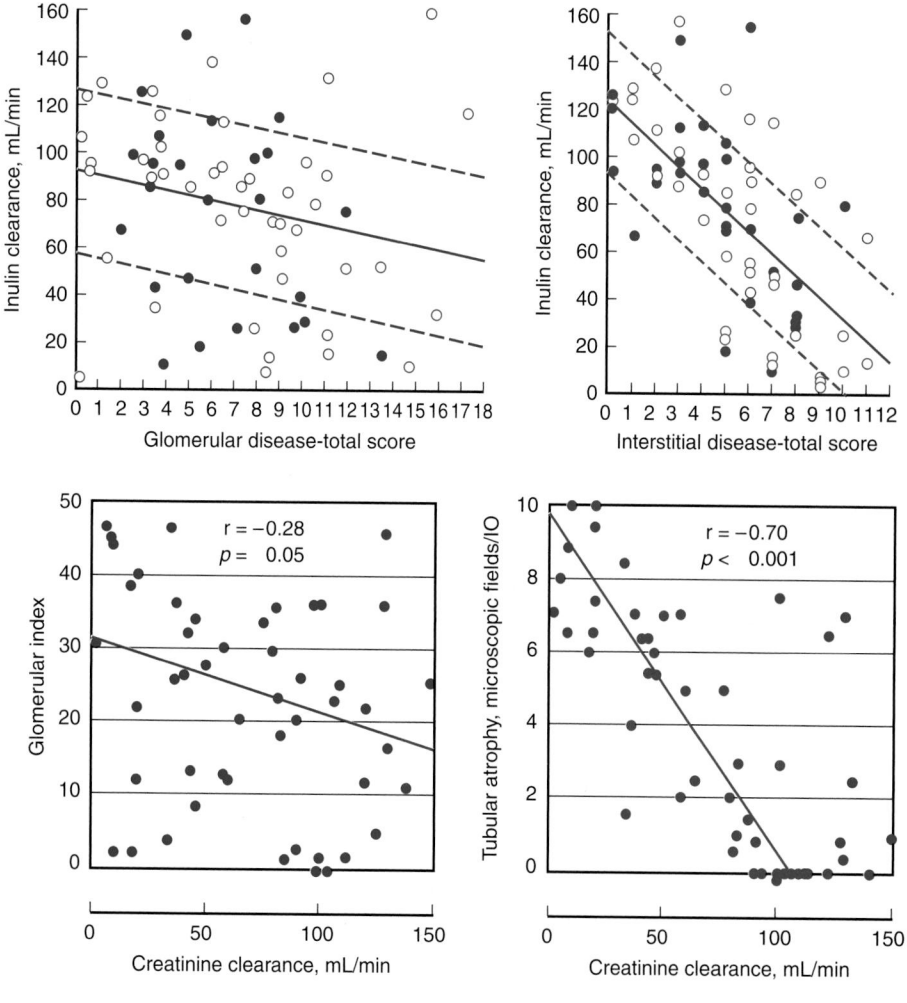

FIGURE 30-1. Structure-function relationships. **A,** Grading scale evaluations of patient biopsies are correlated with inulin clearance (acute glomerulonephritis, chronic glomerulonephritis, interstitial nephritis, nephrosclerosis, miscellaneous); $y = 92-0.02X$ for glomerular disease and $y = 122-8.8X$ for interstitial disease. **B,** Comparisons also are made between biopsies graded for degrees of normal architecture (glomerular index and tubular atrophy scores) plotted against creatinine clearance. The findings in these two studies indicate that falling glomerular filtration correlates better with progressive interstitial changes than with changes in the glomerular tuft. (**A,** from Schainuck LI, Striker GE, Cutler RE, Benditt EP: Structural-functional correlations in renal disease. Hum Pathol 1:631-641, 1970; **B,** from Risdon RA, Sloper JC, deWardener HE: Relationship between renal function and histological changes found in renal-biopsy specimens from patients with persistent glomerular nephritis. Lancet 2:363-366, 1968.)

The number and cross-sectional area of the postglomerular capillaries diminish with increasing interstitial width.[38] These studies demonstrate that tubulointerstitial processes may render this compartment relatively avascular, and therefore somewhat ischemic. Impairment of glomerular arteriolar outflow may also lead to increased intraglomerular hypertension. An increased cross-sectional area of the glomerular capillary tuft has been observed in cases of membranous and membranoproliferative glomerulonephritis with chronic sclerosing interstitial nephritis.[39] Increased intracapillary pressures within the glomerulus may be reflected in this change. Intraglomerular hypertension may also lead to mesangial sclerosis and glomerular damage.[40] These mechanisms are most applicable when injury is still relatively mild. For this second mechanism to achieve a credible level of effect, however, the net reduction in cross-sectional area of peritubular vessels must increase postglomerular resistance sufficiently such that the compensatory increase in glomerular hydrostatic pressure cannot fully restore filtration to normal levels. Tubuloglomerular feedback can also assume increasing importance in the transition from acute to chronic glomerulonephritis when autoregulation of renal blood flow is disrupted by permanent structural change,[41] such as after tubulointerstitial fibrosis. Loss of autoregulation here, as a third hypothesis, could indicate insensitivity of the afferent arteriole to a tubuloglomerular feedback signal, or alternatively, to a loss of the signal. Perhaps more significant is the effect of interstitial pressure on the sensitivity of the feedback mechanism.[42] Such modulation may be transmitted through the local renin-angiotensin system or by alterations in local prostaglandin production.

In slightly damaged tubules, as a fourth explanation, there can be atrophy of interstitial regions, and attenuation of epithelium along the proximal tubules and thick ascending limbs of the loops of Henle. The normal renal osmotic gradient is diminished consequently by a decrease in Na^+ transport in the thick ascending loop. This leads to a diminution in the abstraction of water from the filtrate and results in hyposthenuria and polyuria. Such an increase in solute content and water within the tubular fluid decreases glomerular filtration by adaptively regulating the filtering process in the face of tubular insufficiency.[43-46] Such adaptations include reductions in glomerular capillary pressure and filtration coefficient.[43, 47] Feedback also occurs in cortical and juxtamedullary nephrons and results in a reduction of renin output from the juxtaglomerular apparatus.[43, 48] Consequently, the vasoconstrictive influence of angiotensin II (AII) on the vas efferens decreases, and filtration drops from the decrease in arteriolar tone.[24]

In summary, these collective effects likely contribute to the structure-function interactions relating interstitial damage to progressive deterioration in renal function. Whereas active and acute elements of tubulointerstitial disease correspond to potentially recoverable renal function, tubular atrophy and fibrosis probably represent function lost permanently.

MECHANISMS OF TUBULOINTERSTITIAL INJURY

Tubulointerstitial Antigens

Nephritogenic antigens are derived from surrounding interstitial cells and their extracellular structures, or they are added to this microenvironment by extraction and implantation from the circulation.[24, 49] Some renal structures may also mimic other nonrenal moieties, and become antigenic based on sequence or conformational similarity. The extent of known renal antigens can be arbitrarily divided into several categories.[49]

ANTIGENS FROM RENAL CELLS AND TUBULAR BASEMENT MEMBRANES. Antibodies that react to cellular brush border have been observed in Heymann nephritis[50-53] and although the membranous lesion stands out as an early feature of this disease, interstitial infiltrates and injury are also seen with time.[54-56] The antigen complex goes by several names, including Fx1A, gp 330, megalin, and Heymann nephritis antigen complex.[57-60] The antigen system seems multimeric and involves more than one gene. Tamm-Horsfall protein is also on the tubule cell surface, and can be secreted into tubule fluid by cells of the ascending limb of Henle. Tamm-Horsfall protein, or uromodulin, is a glycoprotein that has been sequenced and studied biochemically.[61-63] The protein can also form immune deposits along the base of the tubule cells and to some extent in the lymphatic drainage of the ascending limb.[64-65] These deposits are associated with mild interstitial inflammation[65-67] and are most noticeable after lower tract obstruction.[68, 69] In another system, *kdkd* mice spontaneously develop interstitial nephritis.[22, 70, 71] The antigen has been partially identified using functional properties of the T cell repertoire. A 56 kD protein produces a delayed-type hypersensitivity (DTH) response in the CD8+ cell population from *kdkd* spleen cells.[71] (C. Kelly, unpublished information). Human autoantibodies in some forms of tubulointerstitial nephritis recognize a 58-kD basement membrane glycoprotein.[72] This glycoprotein exhibits restricted expression to renal tubular basement membranes. It is developmentally regulated, and interacts with type IV collagen and laminin to promote cell adhesion. It also serves as a ligand for $\alpha_3\beta_1$ and $\alpha_v\beta_3$ integrins.[73] Finally, the antigen of anti-TBM disease is called 3M-1.[74, 75] It has an observed molecular mass of 48 to 54 kD in humans down to 30 kD in mice.[49, 75-78] There is polymorphism of expression in rats and human, and allotypic differences in its expression among humans may occasionally result in anti-TBM disease following renal transplantation.[79-83] The gene in rats is inherited as a dominant trait and maps to linkage groups I and IV.[84, 85] The antibody-binding site has some protein sequence homology with intermediate filament-associated proteins.[86]

DRUG-HAPTEN CONJUGATES AS NEPHRITOGENIC ANTIGENS. Extrarenal antigens that form interstitial immune deposits producing inflammation either develop locally in situ, or precipitate as a circulating complex.[87-89] The antigen in that deposit, however, does not have to be chemically linked to the tubular basement membrane as a conjugate for interstitial nephritis to ensue. This has been observed with members of the penicillin family,[89] with cephalosporins,[87] following treatment with phenytoin,[88] and after prolonged exposure to aurothiomalate or mercuric chloride.[90, 91] Sulfamethoxazole may be presented to T cells in a major histocompatibility complex (MHC)-restricted fashion that is independent of antigen processing.[92] Antibodies and inflammatory cells then find these new antigens, and interstitial disease ensues in the susceptible host.

ANTIGENS BASED ON MOLECULAR MIMICRY. Mimicry has always held a special place in the thinking regarding the origins of autoimmunity and inflammation.[93]

The universe of epitopes, while theoretically limitless, nevertheless presents some shared redundancies among self-proteins and the external environment.[94-96] Some antibodies to nephritogenic streptococci cross-react with type IV collagen,[95] for example, and some antibodies to *Escherichia coli* cross-react with Tamm-Horsfall protein.[94] The role of virus-infected tubulointerstitial cells presenting new or modified antigen is not yet fully explored, although interstitial nephritis can appear after viral exposure.[97-100] Whereas most examples of shared epitope expression are derived from infectious agents,[93] work in the autoimmunity of DNA has also provided examples in which anti-DNA antibodies also equally recognize extracellular matrix components such as laminin[101] or heparan sulfate.[102]

EXTRARENAL ANTIGENS IN PREFORMED OR IN SITU IMMUNE DEPOSITS. Immune deposit formation in the tubulointerstitium can result in interstitial nephritis. Rabbits with chronic serum sickness provide a good example of this process,[103] as does systemic lupus with DNA deposits, IgA nephropathy, Sjögren's nephropathy, cryoglobulinemia, and occasionally chronic idiopathic interstitial nephritis in humans.[49, 104] The localization of such deposits depends on the charge and structure of the antigen and antibody, renal flow mechanics, the presence of Fc receptors, the effectiveness of clearance from the circulation, the receptivity of the vasculature, and many other unknown factors.[49, 105]

Immune Response Genes

Currently it is fair to state that most forms of tubulointerstitial disease are mediated by an immunologic process. Target antigens are incapable of inciting an immune response by themselves. Rather, antigen must be processed by antigen-presenting cells (most commonly a macrophage or dendritic cell) and presented on the surface of that cell in association with class I or class II MHC antigens.[106] As a general rule, helper T cells, which induce antibody-producing B cells and effector T cells, recognize processed antigen in the context of class II MHC determinants (in humans, these are human leukocyte antigen–D [HLA-D] region antigens; in mice, they are H-2 $A_\alpha A_\beta / E_\alpha E_\beta$), whereas cytotoxic T cells respond to antigen in the context of class I MHC molecules (in humans, HLA-A, HLA-B, and HLA-C antigens; in mice, H2 K/D).

The ability to mount an immune response to antigen is furthermore known to be a genetic trait, which often maps to the major histocompatibility locus. These immune response genes are associated with susceptibility to disease. Decades of intensive investigation have resulted in the suggestion that the ability to respond to antigen may depend on any of four distinct processes.[16] These processes are illustrated by various experimental models. The first model requires the proper association of antigen and MHC molecules. In this determinant selection theory,[107] tolerance or unresponsiveness is explained by evidence that some self-antigens and the available major histocompatibility determinants of a host do not constitute an effective stimulatory event. Hence the appropriate activation of T cells is impossible. This is illustrated in mice with interstitial nephritis in which antigen associated with MHC genes of one haplotype leads to autoimmune interstitial injury, but not in others.[108] The second model predicts that the presence of T cells with receptors complementary to self-antigen plus MHC product might lead to autoimmunity. Some cases of nonresponsiveness may be explained, therefore, by a lack of T cells that react to antigen in the context of MHC determinants. Such findings form the basis of the clonal deletion theory,[109] and probably reflect the failure of some strains of rats to develop acute interstitial nephritis.[110] Third, in certain individuals, the lack of interference by suppressor or regulatory T cells that act to specifically repress an immune response to self-antigen might facilitate the expression of disease. Regulatory T cell function is restricted by genes in the MHC. Susceptibility to interstitial injury may depend on the selective absence of these regulatory programs in some individuals.[111] Finally, T cell contact with antigen expressed on epithelium lacking appropriate costimulators may produce anergy.[112, 113] The immune basis for tubulointerstitial disease, in its simplest terms, probably represents the abrogation of tolerance to self-determinants in the kidney.[114] In other words, it is implicit that an autoimmune process must ignore or bypass the protective mechanisms that exist to preclude a response to autologous tissues.

Antibody-Mediated Immunity

Most forms of interstitial nephritis in humans are not associated with antibody deposition. In lesions in which immunofluorescence demonstrates deposited antibody, it is seen in association with tubulointerstitial cells, along the tubule basement membranes, or as immune complexes. Anti-TBM antibodies are observed in several different clinical settings. Seventy percent of patients with anti-glomerular basement membrane (anti-GBM) disease, for example, also display a linear deposition of anti-TBM antibodies.[115] It is not known whether these antibodies recognize the NC1 domain of type 3(IV) collagen as do the anti-GBM antibodies.[116] Some cases of drug-associated interstitial nephritis show linear anti-TBM antibodies staining, but the majority do not.[24, 89] Tubular basement membrane staining occasionally occurs as a primary renal disease in the absence of anti-GBM antibodies, and in this case, the antigen recognition appears to be the same as in experimental anti-TBM disease (see earlier).[74, 75] Anti-TBM antibodies also appear commonly in the setting of renal transplantation.[83, 117, 118] Most of these antibodies probably result from antigenic polymorphisms when an antigen-expressing kidney is transplanted into a nonexpressing recipient.[83, 117, 118] Anti-TBM antibodies do not predictably modify the length of successful engraftment.

Primary immune deposit-mediated interstitial nephritis is quite uncommon.[24] Such deposits are probably formed in situ because circulating immune complexes would be more likely to be deposited in the glomeruli. Indeed, interstitial immune deposits are observed more regularly after glomerular inflammation.[119, 120] The best example of spontaneous immune-deposit interstitial nephritis is in the setting of lupus in mice and humans.[50, 121] Other renal lesions like cryoglobulinemia, IgA nephropathy, Sjögren's syndrome, and membranous disease, can also produce similar lesions on occasion.[49] In such cases, pre-existent proteinuria probably facilitates delivery of immune reactants to the tubulointerstitial compartment.[54, 55, 122-124] Even though hypersensitivity reactions can be part of the clinical picture of interstitial nephritis, IgE has only rarely been seen among tubulointerstitial immune deposits.

Because mononuclear interstitial infiltration often occurs in the absence of any antibodies, the pathologic role of antibody can be uncertain. This role can be directly assessed only in experimental models after passive transfer into a naive host.[125, 128] In a few but not all species or strains of experimental animal, this is sufficient to engage an inflammatory process. This selective expression of disease after antibody transfer suggests the additional need for cellular immune response genes for the full measure of injury to be seen.

The nephritogenic antibody response has been most extensively studied in experimental anti-TBM disease. The role of these anti-TBM antibodies (anti-TBM antibodies/anti-3M-1antibodies) varies, depending on the species under study.[126, 129-132] The antibody responses in rats and mice have provided a great deal of insight into the requirements for immune response genes in this disease.[84, 110] All mice are 3M-1+, and all strains tested make anti-3M-1 antibodies, but only selected strains like SJL, SWR, and BALB/c develop disease following immunization, which suggests, as in guinea pigs, that other immune response or susceptibility genes are required for the expressing of cellular lesions.[108, 133] Anti-3M-1 antibodies eluted from the tubules of susceptible and nonsusceptible mice have a similar epitope binding pattern, express a similar spectrum of idiotypes, have broad class representation, and are of similar titer.[128] Anti-3M-1 antibodies may even subserve a protective function in immunized mice, because they decrease MHC class II expression by tubule epithelium expressing 3M-1.[134]

The 3M-1-reactive B cell repertoire has been quantitatively assessed in BN rats.[74] These studies indicated the presence of approximately 58 distinct B cell clones involved in the anti-3M-1 antibody response and also demonstrated some biased V_H gene usage among these autoantibodies. Epitopic recognition of 3M-1 by these antibodies was strikingly similar despite their considerable variability in affinity. Many of these antibodies also expressed a disease-protective cross-reactive idiotype. This cross-reactive idiotype localizes to the CDR3 region of the heavy chain. Computer modeling of the idiotype suggests a conformational structure largely dependent on hydroxyl groups within the CDR3 region of V_H.[135]

The idiotypes on the T and B cell repertoires in anti-TBM disease can also be recognized by the immune system. This recognition induces anti-idiotypic antibodies that often have immunoregulatory properties.[136-139] The B and T cell repertoires in anti-TBM disease broadly express a cross-reactive idiotype.[140] Heterologous antisera to this cross-reactive determinant were effective both as a prophylactic regimen to abrogate disease and as therapeutic modality to arrest progression of disease.

Other antibody responses that have been experimentally studied and shown to produce immune deposits and experimental interstitial lesions include those to the Heyman nephritis antigen complex in brush border[50, 52, 53, 58, 121] and to Tamm-Horsfall protein.[64, 66]

Cell-Mediated Immunity

Cell-mediated immune responses were historically implicated in the pathogenesis of interstitial nephritis because of both in vivo (delayed-type hypersensitivity) and in vitro (lymphoblast transformation) evidence of hypersensitivity

to specific inciting antigens.[141] Phenotypic analysis of infiltrating mononuclear cells in human interstitial nephritis of different causes has demonstrated that, in most cases, the majority (> 50%) of infiltrating mononuclear cells are T lymphocytes.[142-146] The remaining cells are predominantly monocytes. Significant numbers of B cells, plasma cells, or natural killer cells are only occasionally seen. In most cases the CD4/CD8 ratio of the interstitial infiltrate is approximately 1, and usually greater than 1. Several studies have observed lower CD4/CD8 ratios in nonsteroidal anti-inflammatory drug–associated interstitial nephritis than in interstitial nephritis related to metabolic derangements, granulomatous diseases, or autoimmune diseases.[145, 147] Such observations do not have direct functional implications: experimental work has shown that T cell phenotype correlates poorly with classically assigned functions in interstitial disease.[148, 149] The predominant T cell population may also be altered by immunosuppressive therapy before biopsy or the stage of disease at the time of biopsy. Corticosteroids can markedly deplete the number of lymphocytes seen in interstitial nephritis. Other phenotypic characteristics of interstitial nephritis include augmented expression of class II MHC antigens on T cells and tubular epithelial cells,[146, 147] and augmented tubular cell expression of adhesion molecules, such as intracellular adhesion molecule-1 (ICAM-1). Expression of class II MHC is seen in fewer than 5% of tubular cells from normal kidneys. Augmented class II MHC and adhesion molecule expression on tubular cells may facilitate their ability to serve as antigen-presenting cells (see later).

It is difficult in human interstitial nephritis to define the antigenic-specificity, antigen-recognition requirements, or cytokine expression profiles of infiltrating cells. Insight into such issues has been facilitated by work in experimental models. CD4+ helper T cells become activated by antigen-presenting cells expressing class II MHC antigens and other costimulatory molecules.[150, 151] This process may occur in the peripheral lymphoid system or locally within the kidney by tissue-associated macrophages or other antigen-presenting cells, such as dendritic cells. When priming occurs in the periphery, the processed antigenic peptides expressed by antigen-presenting cells, in conjunction with class II MHC molecules, may either be additionally expressed in the kidney or be cross-reactive with renal antigens. Experimental work supports the notion that renal parenchymal cells (including proximal tubular epithelial cells, glomerular epithelial cells, and mesangial cells) can be antigen-presenting cells.[113, 150-155] Antigen-presenting function by renal parenchymal cells extends to both endogenous and exogenous antigens. For a tubular-specific antigen (the target antigen of anti-TBM disease), presentation by tubular epithelial cells can be inhibited by antibodies to the target antigen,[153] an effect probably mediated through transcriptional inhibition of class II MHC antigen expression by such antibodies.[134] Tubular epithelial cells typically do not express costimulatory molecules such as CD80 and CD86, an absence that likely limits their ability to present antigen under physiologic conditions.[156] Normal human kidneys demonstrate constitutive expression of B7RP-1, a B7-related protein that serves as a ligand for the inducible costimulator, ICOS.[157] B7RP-1 is expressed in distal tubules, collecting ducts, and urothelium. Expression of B7RP-1 may negatively regulate T cell activation upon MHC class II–restricted antigen presentation by tubular epithelial cells.[157] Therefore either diminished expression of B7RP-1, or up-regulated expression of CD80 and CD86 or other potential costimulators (such as ICAM-1 and CD40) may facilitate antigen presentation by tubular epithelial cells under pathologic conditions.[158, 159]

Although the antigenic specificity of kidney-infiltrating T cells has been difficult to decipher in human interstitial nephritis, presumptive evidence of antigen-driven clonal expansion of T cells can be obtained by examining the DNA sequence of T cell receptor hypervariable junctional sequences from infiltrating cells. In the interstitial nephritis associated with Sjögren syndrome, such an analysis suggests that the repertoire of the T cell receptor β chain expressed on kidney-infiltrating T cells is restricted to several variable regions, with evidence of polyclonal expansion of T cells.[160] In experimental models of interstitial nephritis, the T cell receptor variable regions utilized by the earliest infiltrating T cells are heterogeneous.[161]

The histologic appearance of human interstitial disease can vary from granulomatous interstitial nephritis with an intense cellular infiltrate to sparse infiltrates with striking microcystic change. Whereas this kind of variable appearance may reflect different stages of an immune-mediated lesion or different target antigens, it may also reflect the biologic activity of discrete populations of stimulated T cells. Some experimental interstitial lesions are histologically analogous to a cutaneous delayed-type hypersensitivity reaction. This type of lesion is frequently seen in experimental anti-TBM disease. The kidneys of these immunized animals display focal aggregates of mononuclear cells, including T cells, B cells, natural killer cells, and macrophages.[126] More intensive infiltration is sometimes associated with granuloma formation. Impressive granuloma formation in the interstitium is consistently seen when Lewis rats are immunized with a renal tubular antigen preparation derived from BN rats, emulsified with tuberculin and pertussis.[162] In murine anti-TBM disease, the aforementioned histologic appearance can be largely reproduced after adoptive transfer of a T cell clone which mediates both delayed-type hypersensitivity to the target antigen and cytotoxic injury to renal tubule cells.[163] Whereas injury induced by a T cell clone confirms that a single cell can initiate a lesion, it does not imply that other cells are not involved. The resultant damage to interstitial and tubular cells and the architecture is the end result of interactions between many cell types. A number of cytokines and enzymes elaborated by activated macrophages and T cells have the potential to alter renal parenchymal cell biology. These biologically active products include matrix-degrading enzymes such as collagenases and elastases,[164] as well as cytokines such as transforming growth factor–β (TGF-β), tumor necrosis factor-α, and interleukin-1 (IL-1), which may lead to the pathologic overexpression of extracellular matrix.[165-169]

The cytotoxic activity of renal antigen-reactive T cell clones may well account for tubule cell destruction and resultant tubule atrophy. Cultured cytotoxic T cells synthesize proteins with serine esterase activity[170, 171] as well as pore-forming proteins, which can effect membrane damage much like the activated membrane attack complex of the complement cascade.[172-174] Such enzymatic activity provides a cogent structural explanation for target cell lysis. In experimental model systems of interstitial nephritis, T cell clones which express pore-forming proteins, such as perforin, and serine esterase granzymes elicit interstitial nephritis following adoptive transfer, and maneuvers that decrease the expression of these mediators abrogate the ability to mediate interstitial inflammatory lesions.[175-177] Whereas cytotoxicity provides a direct explanation for tubular cell dropout, cytotoxic T lymphocytes may also injure renal parenchymal cells by noncytotoxic mechanisms, largely through cytokine release, leading to changes in basement membrane synthesis, altered tubule cell function, or proliferation of interstitial fibroblasts. Whether the relative expression of functionally distinct types of T cell clones varies within the course of a spontaneous interstitial lesion or whether certain antigens predominantly activate clones of discrete function remains to be determined.

Cytokine and Amplification Processes

The term "amplification process" refers to events resulting from the deposition of specific antibody, deposition of immune complexes, or infiltration of T cells, which augment inflammation and injury. These processes include the activation of the complement cascade; the release of a wide array of cytokines and proteases from T cells; and the attraction and activation of a number of nonspecific immune effector cells, including macrophages and eosinophils,[164] both of which have a wide array of secretory products. Although these events have traditionally been viewed as amplifying damage, secondary events may also serve to quench further tissue injury.

Complement is only variably present in both human and experimental interstitial nephritis. When complement components are demonstrable by immunofluorescence, they are seen in association with deposition of IgG and immune complexes,[103, 120, 178] or IgE and eosinophils.[103, 120, 178, 179] Complement can also be activated through the alternative pathway by ammonia, in the absence of antibody.[180] This reaction, triggered by amidated C3, may be an important one for progressive localized injury because it occurs as a secondary event in several nonimmune models of renal injury.[181, 182] Experimental work suggests that C3 expression is markedly up-regulated in tubular epithelium of rodents with acute glomerulonephritis. The absence of C5a receptor in such models markedly attenuates interstitial injury, strongly implicating complement in the pathogenesis of the interstitial injury.[183] Complement activation can be proinflammatory, through the release of chemotactic components, but may also contribute to the clearance of immune complexes and thereby to tissue healing.[105] Parenchymal cells and infiltrating cells can also express proinflammatory molecules, such as chemokines, which act in an attractive capacity.[184] These chemokines include IL-8, RANTES, and monocyte chemotactic peptide-1.[159, 185-187] Their expression by infiltrating cells, as well as tubular epithelial cells, likely plays an important role as an amplification mechanism in both primary interstitial nephritis and the interstitial nephritis associated with glomerular disease.[187, 188]

T cell–related amplification mechanisms influence renal parenchymal cell biology through the release of cytokines. Among CD4+ T cells, discrete subsets express different profiles of cytokines (Th1 cells express IL-2 and interferon-γ (IFN-γ); Th2 cells express IL-4 and IL-10).[189]

This distinction has been widely studied in mice but also has relevance to humans. The relative expression of one subset versus another in situ may have profound effects on the expression of an immune response. Infiltration of T cells expressing IL-2, INF-γ, and tumor necrosis factor-α, for example, might be expected to clonally expand (the IL-2 effect) and induce the expression of adhesion molecules and class II MHC molecules on organ parenchymal cells. INF-γ and tumor necrosis factor–α will activate macrophages and lead to the release of cytotoxic mediators, including oxygen radicals and nitric oxide.[190] However, experimental work is now emerging which suggests that the initial paradigm of Th1-like responses as injurious and Th2-like responses as protective is an oversimplification.[191] Both INF-γ and nitric oxide, for example, can have host-protective rather than injurious effects in models of immune-mediated injury.[192-194] In addition, therapies which elicit immune deviation to Th2-like responses can ultimately result in other forms of tissue injury.[195]

Fibrogenesis and Atrophy

The ubiquitous appearance of extracellular matrix during embryogenesis is essential to the successful development of a complex body plan. Fibroblasts, and to a lesser extent epithelium or vascular cells, provide additional tissue matrix in response to wounding or inflammation in adult life. Although many details of this complex process remain unclear—particularly in kidney—several general features are shared with paradigms in other organ systems, such as liver, lung, and skin.[196-198]

In the kidney there are several interstitial cell types (tubulointerstitial fibroblasts, tubular epithelium, and vascular endothelium) that may act as targets for inflammatory mediators and whose activation is directly responsible for new or modified synthesis of extracellular matrix.[199] Some of these cells probably change phenotype once they are activated by inflammation.[200-203] Although wound repairs are usually self-limited and tightly controlled by homeostatic mechanisms that regulate fibrosis, these regulatory processes tend to deteriorate during episodes of persistent inflammation like interstitial nephritis. In this latter circumstance fibrosis is progressive, pathologic, and often detrimental to the host.

Most interstitial fibrosis is secondary to inflammation or injury that began in another renal compartment. There may be nonspecific drivers for the spreading of this interstitial fibrosis in a variety of nephritic conditions. Two emerging as most important are glomerular proteinuria or the presence of inflammatory cells in interstitial spaces.[24, 204-206] Both proteinuria and cellular infiltration can induce a local cytokine bath that is complex and transforms interstitial epithelium into fibroblasts, induces their proliferation, and activates matrix synthesis or proteolysis, or both.[207] The fibrogenesis that ensues perniciously disturbs normal morphogenic cues as well as the physiologic harmony between structure and function.[198, 208] As fibrosis consumes the tubulointerstitium, renal function deteriorates and scarification in its advanced stages becomes acellular through apoptosis.[209, 210]

Tubulointerstitial scars are comprised principally of fibronectin, collagen types I and III, and tenascin,[211-216] but other glycoproteins such as thrombospondin,[217] SPARC,[218] osteopontin[219] and proteoglycan[220] may be involved. The early

stages of a tissue scar also contain mononuclear cells (lymphocytes and macrophages), tubular cells, and fibroblasts.[204, 221] Fibroblasts are a heterogeneous population of cells that are particularly sensitive to growth factors elaborated by monocytes.[197, 199] Many of these lymphoid cells initiate a local cytokine bath that is either proinflammatory or counterinflammatory.[197] The phenotype of the fibroblast response also seems to depend on the microenvironment from which they were harvested originally.[197, 200] Tubulointerstitial fibroblasts, for example, are less repressed in their secretion of collagen types I, III, IV, and V in response to TGF-β, epidermal growth factor (EGF), and IL-2 than are dermal fibroblasts.[200] Cytokine-induced responses for collagen types I and III in tubulointerstitial fibroblasts tend to be discordant; and for collagen types I and IV, IFN-γ and EGF inhibit, while TGF-β stimulates, the secretory process. T cells from guinea pigs with anti-TBM disease recognizing the 3M-1 antigen, for example, secrete cytokines which will activate fibroblast growth and collagen expression in renal cells.[204, 216, 222] Cytokines from these cells contribute to the local signaling cascade that modulates the fibrogenic process.

AII,[27, 223] TGF-β,[224, 225] hepatocyte growth factor (HGF),[226-228] platelet-derived growth factor (PDGF),[203] EGF,[229] Wnt-4[230] and endothelin-1[215, 231] are important cytokines with mitogenic or morphogenic effects on interstitial cells. Emerging data now suggest that AII is a critical morphogenic cytokine and may be a principal, proximal driver of the fibrogenic process in kidneys.[27, 223, 232-235] AII activates a variety of fibrogenic cytokines,[232, 236] induces plasminogen activator inhibitor–1 (PAI-1),[233] and engages interstitial collagen biosynthesis.[237-239] Fibroblasts, in some hands, are thought to have special properties related to location, complement binding capacity, synthesis of prostaglandin E_2, ecto-5'-nucleotides, antigen expression, expression of PDGF, lipid metabolism, or their ability to differentially respond to cytokines in culture.[200] Residing in the kidney they have little in the way of distinguishing anatomic features. When harvested from normal or diseased kidneys, however, fibroblasts grown from fibrotic tissues seen to proliferate faster and look different, suggesting they may undergo phenotypic change during fibrosis.[201, 202] Fibroblasts activated during fibrogenesis also demonstrate some structural features of smooth muscle cells and express α-smooth muscle actin.[240] This later activation marker, however, does not identify resting fibroblasts or distinguish between myofibroblasts and smooth muscle cells.[241] Therefore, it and other suggested proteins do not have much to recommend them as compelling lineage markers for fibroblasts.[207]

A new protein, called fibroblast-specific protein 1 (FSP1), has recently been reported to express near exclusivity in fibroblasts from nontumor tissue in mice.[26, 229] FSP1 belongs to the S100 superfamily of intracellular calcium-binding proteins. The members of the S100 superfamily are implicated in microtubule dynamics, cytoskeletal-membrane interactions, calcium signal transduction, p53 and cell cycle regulation, and cellular growth and differentiation.[207] Although the precise function of FSP1 and its homologs is not entirely clear, their interaction with nonmuscle myosin II, nonmuscle tropomyosin, actin, or tubulin, and the inducibility of a migratory or metastatic phenotype when transfected into nonmetastatic tumor cells in vitro suggests that FSP1 plays a role in mesenchymal cell shape and motility.[26, 229] There are cis-acting elements in its promoter that are found in the regulatory regions of other promoters encoding fibrogenic proteins, suggesting there may be a regulatory program for fibrogenesis at a transcriptional level.[207, 242]

Although fibroblasts have been characterized by microscopy in vitro, the absence of specific markers in resting cells has hampered the investigation of their origin and in vivo behavior. One school of thought is that interstitial and periadventitial fibroblasts derive from metanephric mesenchyme not used in the formation of the nephron. Other than the fact that mesenchymal cells have a shape that resembles FSP1+ fibroblasts, and like fibroblasts express fibronectin and fibrillar collagens, there is no evidence that they are of direct mesenchymal lineage.[207] In fact, using FSP1 as a probe for fibroblasts suggests there may be other, alternative precursors. First, metanephric mesenchyme does not express FSP1 in vivo (unpublished observations). Second, aside from transient expression of FSP1 by early S- and comma-shaped epithelium, FSP1+ interstitial cells do not appear until late in renal development (unpublished observations). Third, time course analysis of fibrosis during renal injury indicates it often begins in the periadventitial spaces around medium-sized blood vessels or near periglomerular interstitial compartments, and later spreads to the broad hinder regions of the kidney mass.[243] Since this spreading becomes diffuse and remote from initial perivascular sites, resident fibroblasts would have to migrate significant distances into new areas of injury using chemotaxis or hapotaxis, and then divide. This is a cumbersome notion. We now know that kidney fibroblasts mainly arise from local resident cells like tubular epithelium,[244] and to a lesser extent from bone marrow,[244] through a phenomenon called epithelial-mesenchymal transition (EMT).[26, 229, 240] Although such transitions are well accepted as a mechanism of plasticity in developing tissue,[198, 245] for them to occur in mature organs is relatively novel. Recent evidence for EMT in renal fibrosis has been reported following the onset of experimental ureteral obstruction,[244] five-sixths nephrectomy,[240, 246] polycystic kidney disease,[241] glomerulonephritis,[246, 247] and diabetic nephropathy,[248] and in human renal disease.[249]

Tubular epithelium in culture can lose polarity and adherence to adjacent cells and the basal lamina, convert into elongated fusiform shapes, and gain mesenchymal properties, including motility.[200, 207] To do this the basement membrane structure upon which they sit must disrupt and attenuate,[250, 251] and profibrotic cytokines like AII, TGF-β, EGF, PDGF, and fibroblast growth factor–2 (FGF-2) engage.[207] Moieties like tissue plasminogen activator (t-PA) will accelerate fibrogenesis by inducing metalloproteinases and PAI-1,[252, 253] while IFN-γ attenuates remodeling.[200] Antigen-binding cytokines secreted by T lymphocytes in the kidney can also specifically repress the cellular transcription and secretion of basement membrane type IV collagen.[169] This immune-mediated repression of transcription of type IV collagen may modulate the remodeling of the interstitial infrastructure and contribute to the process of tubular atrophy attendant to prolonged renal inflammation.

When tubular epithelium are transfected with complementary DNA (cDNA) encoding FSP1, they undergo mesenchymal transition,[229] demonstrate a loss of cell adhesion and cytokeratin, and begin expressing new quantities of vimentin and FSP1.[26] Growth factors, oncogenes, and cell-surface adhesion molecules can modulate EMT.[207] EMT in tubular epithelium is shaped by a combination of several cytokines and enzymes, TGF-β, EGF, FGF-2 and t-PA,[229, 252, 254] whereas HGF opposes the transition.[226-228] Furthermore, the transition can be attenuated if epithelium stimulated toward EMT is concomitantly exposed to antisense oligomers to messenger RNA (mRNA) encoding FSP1,[229] suggesting that the appearance of FSP1 is an important early event in transition.

The process of EMT during interstitial nephritis parsimoniously satisfies at once four conditions representative of renal fibrosis.[207] First, it explains how tubular atrophy occurs, hand in hand, with increasing numbers of fibroblasts at sites of fibrosis. Second, it clarifies why fibroblasts harvested from one microenvironment, like the kidney, have different synthetic responses or cytokine reactivities when compared to fibroblasts harvested from other tissues—they likely retain a small residuum of their previous epithelial phenotype, harboring selected receptors or interactional programs that modulate based on this imprinted experience. Third, it explains why angiotension receptor-rich tubular epithelium at the site of fibrogenic reactions begins expressing fibrosis-related proteins osteopontin, thrombospondin-1, PDGF, and FSP1. And fourth, it avoids developing a complex notion to explain how remote fibroblasts travel great distances to participate in fibrogenesis.[244]

Fibroblast progeny from EMT would be expected to proliferate and locally migrate based on the cytokine composition of their microenvironment. PDGF appears to play a significant role in fibroblast cell division.[203, 255-257] PDGF and TGF-β also act as powerful, local fibroblast chemoattractants, as does a cleavage fragment of complement C5.[258-260] Cleavage of fibronectin and collagen types I and II can also enhance cell motility.[190, 261] Movement of fibroblasts through the extracellular matrix is further facilitated by the secretion of metalloproteinases released by macrophages or by fibroblasts themselves.[262] Countering these attractants are the inhibitory fibroblastic growth effects of IL-1 and tumor necrosis factor–α.[263, 264] Finally, fibroblasts themselves can secrete TGF-β, thereby amplifying the process.[265]

Although tubular epithelium[266, 267] is capable of synthesizing type I and type III collagen and is modulated by a variety of growth factors,[200] these epithelia attenuate through tubular atrophy, leaving the fibroblast as a significant contributor to matrix production in fibrogenesis. After fibroblasts acquire a synthetic phenotype, expand their population,[26] and locally migrate around residential areas of inflammation, they begin to deposit a fibronectin matrix that provides a scaffold for the association of interstitial collagens.[212, 268] In the initial stages of collagen deposition and fibril formation, type III collagen appears in greater amounts than type I. As fibrogenesis progresses, however, there is a proportional decrease in type III collagen.[269] The local regulators of collagen and fibronectin synthesis are not really known, but both moieties are stimulated by the action of TGF-β and IL-1, whereas IFN-γ tends to inhibit the transcription of type I collagen.[212, 268, 270, 271] The synthesis of collagenase and stromelysin is also inhibited by TGF-β, whereas the synthesis of a metalloproteinase inhibitor is stimulated.[271] This reciprocal effect produces a net increase in the amount of interstitial collagen. Specific mechanisms which reduce or block the fibrogenic response in the tubulointerstitium remain speculative. Therapy directed to decorin,[272] PDGF,[203] or FSP1[273] may be important in the future.

ACUTE INTERSTITIAL NEPHRITIS

In walking healthy populations who have a renal biopsy during a workup for hematuria or proteinuria about 1% will have primary interstitial nephritis.[274] This problem also exists in the elderly.[275] Furthermore, significant interstitial nephritis has been observed in a series of 8000 autopsies, and 1% to 15% of all renal biopsies in patients with apparent renal disease will have acute interstitial nephritis.[276, 277] The figure is somewhat consistent with chart review data indicating that chronic interstitial nephritis accounts for approximately 25% of cases leading to permanent renal failure.[277] Primary acute interstitial nephritis is now recognized as a frequent renal ailment.

Pathology

The hallmark of acute primary interstitial nephritis is the infiltration of inflammatory cells into the interstitial compartment with sparing of glomeruli. Lesions that reduce renal function are usually diffuse, but it is said that drug-induced interstitial injury is often patchy, beginning deep in the cortex.[278] Glomerular involvement producing a nil lesion in association with interstitial nephritis is frequently observed with use of nonsteroidal anti-inflammatory drugs.[279] The infiltrating cell population in acute interstitial nephritis is comprised mainly of T cells and monocytes, but plasma cells and eosinophils may be seen.[23, 280-282] The T cells are of a mixed phenotype with a distinct preference for $CD4^+$ lymphocytes.[126, 146, 282-284]

Together with interstitial edema, this infiltrate causes the tubules to be pushed away from one another, rather than lying in close apposition. The TBM may be disrupted in more severe cases.[281] Staining of the TBM for IgG, IgM, or complement may occasionally be seen by immunofluorescence, with both linear and granular patterns having been reported. Most forms of acute interstitial nephritis do not have immune deposits present.[23, 34] In nearly all cases, the tubular epithelium involved in the inflammatory process will aberrantly express MHC class II antigens and adhesion molecules like ICAM-1.[155, 285] Both of these determinants are important for the engagement of T cells. In some instances this engagement will enhance inflammation; in others it will attenuate the process.[113]

In the chronic lesion, the cellular infiltrate is largely replaced by interstitial fibrosis, which accounts for the irregular and contracted gross appearance of the kidney. The tubular epithelial cells are atrophied and the tubular lumens are dilated. "Chronic" is a relative term, because fibrotic changes can be seen within 7 to 10 days of initiation of an inflammatory process. Chronic vascular and glomerular changes, consisting of nephrosclerosis and glomerulosclerosis, are often present at later stages of the disease, so that pathologic determination of the primary cause may be impossible.

A third pathologic category can be seen in either the acute or chronic setting, namely, that of granuloma formation.[286] In acute granulomatous interstitial nephritis, the granulomas are sparse and non-necrotic, giant cells are rare, and an accompanying interstitial infiltrate is common. The granulomas of the chronic lesion contain more giant cells, and if due to tuberculosis, may become necrotic.[287] Drugs are a common cause of this lesion in the acute setting, and most of the drugs associated with acute interstitial nephritis have been reported to cause granuloma formation.[288] Sarcoidosis[289, 290] or tuberculosis[291] should be considered when granulomas are seen in chronic disease. When renal granulomas are seen in Wegener granulomatosis, they are almost always accompanied by glomerular and vascular pathology.[292]

Clinical Features

The characteristic features of acute interstitial nephritis are both clinical and pathologic. The typical presentation of acute tubulointerstitial disease is that of a sudden decrement in renal function, most commonly in an asymptomatic patient who has experienced an intervening illness or who was begun on a new medication. Occasionally, the nephritis is severe enough to result in total renal failure. It is important, consequently, to consider this diagnosis in any patient with an unexplained precipitous diminution in renal function. Several features of acute interstitial nephritis may help in distinguishing it from acute tubular necrosis or glomerulonephritis. Some predisposing factors are usually identifiable in both acute tubular necrosis and acute interstitial nephritis. Furthermore, in the case of infection, there often will be fever and localizing signs, and with drug-induced acute tubulointerstitial disease, the patient commonly exhibits an allergic process, such as a maculopapular skin rash, fever, or eosinophilia. The frequency of such signs has been evaluated in patients with acute interstitial nephritis taking penicillin-like drugs. In these patients skin rash was present in fewer than 50%, whereas fever occurred in 75% and eosinophilia in 80%. The entire triad, however, was present in fewer than 33% of patients.[293, 294] IgE levels are occasionally increased in these patients.[295] Such signs, however, seem to be uncommon when acute interstitial nephritis is caused by the nonsteroidal anti-inflammatory drugs.[279] Lumbar pain, and occasionally unilateral lumbar pain, can be seen in either acute interstitial nephritis or acute tubular necrosis.[296, 297] This is possibly due to distention of the renal capsule from diffuse swelling of the kidney.

The course of renal failure in acute interstitial nephritis is most commonly several days to weeks. Interestingly, this appears to parallel, in the majority of cases, the kinetics of a primary immune response, with immune reactivity peaking at approximately 2 weeks. However, on occasion, renal failure can be precipitous, especially in those patients re-exposed to a nephropathic agent[298]; conversely, it can be protracted, with a steadily declining glomerular filtration rate over months. This protracted course is more common with diuretic-induced interstitial nephritis.[299] The onset of drug-induced nephritis ranges from days to weeks following initiation of drug therapy. A previous allergic history is only rarely obtained. A classic setting for a drug reaction is a febrile patient with an infectious process who defervesces on appropriate antibiotic therapy and in whom recrudescent fever occurs several days later.

Valuable information can also be obtained from the urinalysis because several features may strongly speak for or against the diagnosis of acute interstitial nephritis. The cumulative experience from several different studies suggests that a chemical and microscopic evaluation will reveal mild to moderate proteinuria and hematuria in over 75% of cases of tubulointerstitial disease.[278, 300, 301] Gross hematuria has been reported in 44% of cases, but that seems high to us. The sediment, also in approximately 75% of patients, will show red and white blood cells. White blood cell casts are occasionally observed. Red blood cell casts have been reported in primary acute interstitial nephritis,[302] but are so infrequent that they should suggest a glomerular diagnosis. The finding of eosinophils in the urine is suggestive of allergic interstitial nephritis. This is optimally observed by using a Hansel stain on the sediment from a urine specimen.[303, 304] Although two reports[278, 300] indicate that eosinophiluria is a common concomitant of acute tubulointerstitial disease due to drug allergy, this has not been a uniform experience.[305] The absence of eosinophiluria should never discourage the diagnostic pursuit of acute interstitial nephritis.

Serum creatinine levels are usually elevated and often first draw attention to the renal failure. The magnitude of proteinuria in acute tubulointerstitial disease is usually modest and nearly always less than 2 g/24 hours.[298] Nephrotic-range proteinuria is not usually seen in acute interstitial nephritis unless there is a coexisting glomerular lesion after exposure to nonsteroidal anti-inflammatory drugs.[279] Many patients with acute interstitial nephritis also have a fractional excretion of Na^+ greater than 1.[306] They are often oliguric, but nonoliguric renal failure also occurs.[278, 300, 307] Oliguria may be related to interstitial inflammation severe enough to cause tubular obstruction and impede urine flow. Actual compromise of the ureteral lumen has also been documented in severe acute interstitial nephritis with marked edema and cellular infiltration of the ureteral submucosa and muscularis.[308] Tubular defects and tubular syndromes such as Fanconi syndrome and renal tubular acidosis are rarely observed in acute interstitial nephritis and are more common with chronic tubulointerstitial diseases. There are some electrolyte complications occasionally associated with various antibiotic therapies.[309]

Some imaging procedures may provide helpful diagnostic information. The kidney in acute interstitial nephritis is usually normal or slightly increased in size by echographic or pyelographic criteria.[298] This finding can have practical implications; for example, the patient who presents with presumed end-stage renal disease but normal-sized kidneys may have acute interstitial nephritis or another acute process. Interestingly, some reports have correlated markedly increased cortical echogenicity with diffuse interstitial infiltrates on renal biopsy,[310] although no correlation exists between echogenicity and specific lesions.[311] Acute interstitial nephritis may be suggested by such a finding in a patient with acute renal failure. Gallium scanning has also been suggested as a useful diagnostic tool.[278, 312, 313] Unfortunately, because a variety of other renal processes can similarly result in gallium uptake (including minimal-change glomerulonephritis, cortical necrosis, and acute tubular necrosis),[314, 315] and because biopsy-proven acute tubulointerstitial disease can be associated with a negative gallium scan,[313] the predictive value of this test may be limited.

Many features of the patient's history, presentation, urinalysis, and laboratory evaluation may suggest the diagnosis of acute interstitial nephritis. Unfortunately, none of these findings are pathognomonic, and ultimately the diagnosis can only be established with certainty by renal biopsy.[316] Occasionally intersititial nephritis has even presented as a nil lesion.[317] A biopsy should be performed in patients with

acute renal failure who present with suggestive signs or symptoms of an interstitial process or who, alternatively, lack a typical clinical picture for glomerulonephritis and acute tubular necrosis and in whom obstructive nephropathy and prerenal azotemia have been excluded. Algorithms for this decision process are available.[318]

Etiology

The causative factors leading to acute interstitial nephritis are usually limited to a few broad categories. In our experience drugs are the predominant etiologic agents today, followed by infection, particularly in children, and then the autoimmune idiopathic lesions.

Drugs

A list of potentially offending pharmacologic agents is presented in Table 30-1. Although a multitude of agents have been reported to cause acute interstitial nephritis, far fewer are implicated commonly.[319-321] The β-lactam antibiotics (including the cephalosporins[322]) are the best-studied group because of methicillin, a drug no longer in common use.[278, 293] Autopsy studies reveal that penicillin moieties can bind to the TBM in patients treated with penicillin-related antibiotics who do not have associated interstitial pathology,[89, 323] which suggests that immune response genes are also necessary for pathogenesis. After methicillin, generic penicillin and ampicillin have been commonly implicated in acute tubulointerstitial disease.[324] Nafcillin has only rarely been observed to produce such disease,[325] nor has piperacillin.[326] It should be remembered that recurrent acute interstitial nephritis, after an initial insult with one penicillin derivative, has occurred with the use of a different penicillin, or even with a cephalosporin.[298]

In addition to the penicillin-like antibiotics, many other antimicrobials have been associated with acute interstitial nephritis. Prominent among these are the sulfonamides[300] and rifampin.[327-329] Trimethoprim-sulfamethoxazole[330] and the quinolones[331] are additional offenders. The sulfonamides have also been reported to cause a vasculitis, and rifampin appears to be most often associated with acute tubulointerstitial disease in conjunction with intermittent or discontinuous dosing. Drugs other than antibiotics have also been reported to cause acute interstitial nephritis. These include phenindione,[332] phenytoin,[333] allopurinol,[334, 335] thiazides,[336] furosemide,[337] ranitidine,[338] and cimetidine.[339]

In the past decade the nonsteroidal anti-inflammatory drugs have also been observed to produce serious nephrologic injury,[279] including over-the-counter nonsteroidal preparations.[340] It has become evident with more experience that at least four types of renal injury are associated with nonsteroidal anti-inflammatory drugs: acute renal ischemic renal insufficiency, analgesic-associated nephropathy, a flank pain–renal failure syndrome, and acute interstitial nephritis. Acute interstitial nephritis appears in two forms. The first is an occasional pure lesion, with or without papillary necrosis, but without any glomerular disease. Its counterpart in 86% of cases, however, is a combined lesion of minimal-change glomerulonephritis and interstitial infiltrates.[341] This has recently also been described with selective cyclooxygenase-2 inhibitors, such as celecoxib.[342-344] Patients with the combined lesion can present with nephrotic-range

TABLE 30-1

Acute Interstitial Nephritis

Drugs[319]	All-*trans* retinoic acid[543]
Antibiotics	Wasp stings[544]
Penicillins[324-326]	Nicergoline[545]
Rifampin[327-329]	
Sulfa drugs[300, 518, 519]	**Infection**
Vancomycin[520, 521]	Bacteria
Ciprofloxacin[331, 522]	Legionella[353]
Cephalosporins[322]	Brucella[354]
Erythromycin[523]	Diphtheria[305]
Minocycline[524-526]	Streptococcus[355]
Trimethoprim-sulfamethoxazole[330]	Staphylococcus[356]
Acyclovir[527]	Yersinia[357]
Ethambutol[528]	Salmonella[358]
Nonsteroidal anti-inflammatory drugs[279, 345]	*Escherichia coli*[359]
Selective COX-2 inhibitors[342-344]	Campylobacter[360]
Mesalazine[529]	Viruses
Diuretics[530]	Epstein-Barr virus[361, 362]
Thiazides[336]	Cytomegalovirus[99]
Furosemide[337]	*Hantavirus*[100]
Triamterene[531]	HIV[97]
Miscellaneous	Herpes simplex[363]
Captopril[532]	*Polyomavirus*[364, 378, 546]
Cimetidine[339]	Hepatitis B virus[365]
Ranitidine[338]	Other
Omeprazole[533]	Mycoplasma[366]
Phenobarbital[534]	Rickettsia[367, 368]
Nitrofurantoin[535]	Leptospira[370]
Phenindione[332]	Tuberculosis[369]
Phenytoin[333]	*Schistosoma mekongi*[371]
Sodium valproate[536]	Toxoplasmosis[373]
Carbamazepine[537]	Chlamydia[372]
Allopurinol[334, 335]	
Interferon[538, 539]	**Idiopathic**
Interleukin-2[540, 541]	Anti-TBM disease[24, 115]
Anti-CD4 antibody[542]	TINU syndrome[547, 548]
	Kawasaki disease[549]

COX-2, cyclooxygenase-2; HIV, human immunodeficiency virus; anti-TBM, anti–tubular basement membrane; TINU, tubulointerstitial nephritis and uveitis.

proteinuria, nephrotic syndrome, and renal failure. Thus, the nonsteroidal anti-inflammatory drugs, particularly fenoprofen,[345] must be added to diabetes mellitus and amyloidosis as considerations in the differential diagnosis of advanced renal failure with massive proteinuria. A further basis of distinction in regard to nonsteroidal anti-inflammatory drug–induced acute tubulointerstitial disease is the observation that signs of a hypersensitivity reaction are frequently missing.[279] The interstitial lesion can appear as early as 1 week after medication is begun, but more commonly is seen after several months to a year of use.[345] Most patients respond to removal of the offending nonsteroidal agent after a few months without steroid therapy.[345, 346]

Finally, alternative medicines, particularly some Chinese herb preparations, idiosyncratically produce renal failure.[347, 348] Some of this has been rapidly progressive (or subacute) interstitial nephritis, but occasional patients appear with acute renal failure.[349] A link to aristolochic acid is suspected but as yet has not received rigorous experimental proof.[350]

Infection

Acute pyelonephritis is frequently associated with transient interstitial infiltrates containing polymorphonuclear leukocytes. In the patient who presents with acute pyelonephritis and renal compromise, serious consideration should be given to the presence of reflux, obstruction, papillary necrosis, volume depletion, or urosepsis with acute tubular necrosis as an explanation for diminished glomerular filtration rate. It has also become clear that invasive pyelonephritis is closely associated with bacterial virulence.[351]

Acute interstitial nephritis and renal failure, however, can frequently be seen in the setting of systemic infection.[23, 24] Whereas drugs are clearly the most common etiologic agent in acute interstitial nephritis in adults, studies from the pediatric literature would suggest that infections, particularly streptococcal, are preeminent.[305, 352] The interstitial lesion, as indicated by Councilman,[12] seems to be a response to disseminated infection, and not simply a matter of hematogenous seeding of the kidney with bacteria. This view is supported by the mononuclear character of the interstitial infiltrate and by the observation of a low rate of bacterial isolation from the involved kidney. The possibility of an idiosyncratic (or genetically restricted) response to a microbial antigen that is cross-reactive with renal parenchymal tissue is a provocative one.[94, 95] In addition to streptococcal infection, acute interstitial nephritis has been associated with the infectious diseases of legionella,[353] brucella,[354] diphtheria,[305] streptococcus,[355] staphylococcus,[356] yersinia,[357] salmonella,[358] *Escherichia coli*,[359] campylobacter,[360] Epstein-Barr virus,[361, 362] cytomegalovirus,[99] *Hantavirus*,[100] human immunodeficiency virus (HIV),[97] herpes simplex,[363] polyomavirus,[364] hepatitis B virus,[365] myco-plasma,[366] rickettsia,[367, 368] tuberculosis,[369] leptospira,[370] *Schistosoma mekongi*,[371] chlamydia,[372] and toxoplasmosis.[373] The definitive distinction between all infectious entities causing interstitial nephritis is ultimately made by culture or molecular identification, or, in some cases, by serology or biopsy. Renal failure from infection-related acute interstitial nephritis generally resolves with treatment of the underlying infection, and steroid therapy, although sometimes advo-cated, is often not needed.[374]

HIV has not been shown to directly cause an isolated interstitial nephritis; however, it has been emphasized recently that tubulointerstitial lesions are common with this infection for a variety of factors.[375, 376] These include oppor-tunistic infections with cytomegalovirus, cryptococcus or histoplasmosis, nephrocalcinosis, and sulfa derivatives. Similarly, renal allograft recipients may be susceptible to such Epstein-Barr virus and cytomegalovirus.[377] Polyomavirus is increasingly recognized as a cause of renal insufficiency in immunosuppressed patients with renal allografts. Renal biopsies typically demonstrate viral intranuclear inclusions within tubular epithelium. Current clinical approaches to this entity include diminution of immunosuppression and antiviral therapy.[378] The various forms of *Hantavirus* infec-tion, particularly through airborne transmission from dis-persing rodent dander, have also been growing in frequency in western Europe and North America.[100, 379, 380] Finally, it has been recently suggested that in the absence of drug exposure or autoimmune disease, acute to chronic interstitial nephritis might be mediated by persistent Epstein-Barr virus in tubular epithelium.[362, 381]

Idiopathic Acute Interstitial Nephritis

Idiopathic interstitial nephritis is said to be an uncommon lesion. Interestingly, however, in one series of 30 patients with acute interstitial nephritis, no etiologic factor could be demonstrated in 30% of the group.[296] The predominance of mononuclear cells in the interstitial infiltrate, the presence of constitutional symptoms, and the spontaneous nature of the lesion all suggest a possible immunologic basis. In humans anti-3M-1 antibodies have been observed in several different clinical settings. As discussed before, linear deposition of anti-TBM antibodies have been observed in 70% of patients with anti-GBM disease,[115] and they probably include several specificities. For example, although anti-GBM antibodies principally recognize the NC1 domain of type 3(IV) collagen as the Goodpasture antigen,[116, 382] it is not known for sure whether this is the same specificity for the anti-TBM anti-bodies in that serum. Several cases of drug-associated inter-stitial nephritis have been reported to show linear anti-TBM antibody staining, but the majority of patients with drug-associated interstitial nephritis do not have these deposits.[24] Anti-TBM staining occurs without anti-GBM antibodies occasionally as a primary renal disease, and in this case the antigen recognition appears to be 3M-1.[86] Most commonly, however, anti-TBM antibodies appear in the setting of renal transplantation.[83, 117, 118] Most of these antibodies probably result from 3M-1 polymorphisms where a 3M-1+ trans-planted kidney is placed in a 3M-1–recipient.[110, 383] Anti-TBM antibodies do not appear to cause predictable changes in the length of successful engraftment.[384] Unlike drug-induced

lesions, the idiopathic forms of interstitial nephritis are infrequently associated with rash or eosinophilia, although fever, is common.[296] The absence of obvious predisposing factors for acute interstitial nephritis should not bias one against consideration of this diagnosis in an otherwise appropriate clinical setting. Its potentially subtle nature forms the basis for many diagnostic renal biopsies.

One particular category of idiopathic patient has received special attention: patients with tubulointerstitial nephritis and uveitis (the so-called TINU syndrome).[385-388] These patients are usually adolescent girls, or occasionally adults, who pre-sent with constitutional symptoms, reduced renal function and tubule dysfunction, bone marrow or lymphoid granulomas, and uveitis during some point in the course of disease. On renal biospy there is interstitial nephritis, sometimes fibrosis (particularly in adults) and no evidence or acidosis, tubercu-losis, toxoplasmosis, Wegener granulomatosis, or Sjögren syndrome. In some patients nephritis can occur quickly.[389] The cause is unknown, but a report has suggested an associ-ation with chlamydia infection.[372, 386] The prognosis in chil-dren seems to be excellent with or without treatment with steroids, whereas the course is more guarded in adults. Adult patients are generally treated with corticosteroids, and partial recovery of renal function may occur over several weeks.

Course and Treatment

As a general rule many cases of acute interstitial nephritis resolve with removal of the offending agent. The likelihood of complete recovery, however, appears to be inversely proportional to the duration of renal failure; in one study serum creatinine levels averaged approximately 1.0 mg/dL in patients with acute renal failure of less than 2 weeks' duration compared with an average value of 3.0 mg/dL in those who were diagnosed and treated after 3 weeks of acute renal failure.[296, 390] Prolonged and active tubulointerstitial injury and a subsequent lack of total resolution have their pathologic correlate in irreversible interstitial fibrosis. An additional prognostic factor appears to be the extent to which the interstitium is involved with mononuclear cell infiltrates. Scattered infiltrates are associated with return of impairment.[296] Unless an offending agent can be identified and removed, progression to end-stage renal disease is more likely. In the case of idiopathic acute interstitial nephritis, although spontaneous resolution occurs, more that 50% of patients are left with residual renal dysfunction. The pres-ence of anti-TBM antibodies in spontaneous disease may occasionally portend especially severe injury.

The primary therapeutic principle in acute interstitial nephritis is to identify the likely inciting factor and remove or treat it.[391] An algorithm for offering therapy for this family of lesions has been devised.[318] Withdrawal of the drug or offending agent often results in improvement in renal func-tion within several days in many patients. In the absence of a prompt response, early institution of chemotherapy may be appropriate. For example, we believe a time frame exists for the use of steroids in acute interstitial disease. This trial of corticosteroids consists of a dose equivalent to 1 mg/kg/day of prednisone in patients with absent infection. Improvement in renal function should begin within 1 to 2 weeks of initiation of treatment, in which case the course can be discontinued after 4 to 6 weeks. If no improvement is seen within the first

2 weeks, the addition of a second agent such as cyclophosphamide (2 mg/kg/day) may be considered; if successful, this treatment should be continued for up to 1 year with appropriate monitoring of the white blood cell count. Lack of any evidence of improvement after 6 weeks of combined therapy consititutes grounds for discontinuation of both agents. In our experience this program has been particularly effective in the setting of sarcoidosis. Three points are worth mentioning, however. First, no prospective, randomized, well-controlled trials assessing the value of chemotherapy in this setting in humans are available. Anecdotal case reports provide provocative temporal relationships between the institution of steroid therapy and improvement in renal function. Two reports [278, 392] looking at such treatment in a series of patients with acute interstitial nephritis similarly indicate its likely value. Second, although there are rare reports of improvement in renal function after prolonged renal failure secondary to acute tubulointerstitial disease, the presence of marked interstitial fibrosis on renal biopsy specimens suggests a more appropriate diagnosis of chronic interstitial nephritis, and mitigates against the use of chemotherapy. [199, 285] Finally, the case report of rifampin-related acute interstitial nephritis in a patient receiving 40 mg/day of prednisone suggests that this drug may not always prove efficacious. [393] Anecdotal reports have supported the use of cytotoxic therapy in some patients; such effect has been demonstrated in the experimental literature. [394, 395] Up to one third of patients with drug-induced acute interstitial nephritis (and more in the case of rifampin) also require dialytic therapy before resolution of the disease. Plasmapheresis, specifically, may be reasonable to consider in patients with anti-TBM antibodies. [318]

CHRONIC INTERSTITIAL NEPHRITIS

Pathology

The pathologic features of chronic tubulointerstitial nephritis are remarkably conserved among a wide variety of presumed causes. These include tubular cell atrophy with flattened epithelial cells and tubule dilation, interstitial fibrosis, and areas of mononuclear cell infiltration within the interstitial compartment between tubules. Tubular basement membranes are frequently thickened. Neutrophils or lymphocytes may also be seen adjacent to tubular epithelium ("tubulitis") with resulting cellular luminal casts; these findings are typically seen with acute interstitial disease but are not inconsistent with pathologic or clinical chronic intestitial nephritis. [396] The cellular infiltrate in chronic interstitial disease is composed of lymphocytes with only occasional neutrophils, plasma cells, or eosinophils. Rare cases may demonstrate interstitial edema, hemorrhage, and a cellular infiltrate with predominant neutrophils. Immunofluorescent evaluation of biopsy specimens from chronic interstitial disease occasionally reveals the presence of C3 or immunoglobulin along the TBM, typically in a linear distribution.

In chronic interstitial disease, the glomeruli can remain remarkably normal by light microscopy, even when a lowered glomerular filtration rate demonstrates marked functional impairment. As chronic interstitial injury progresses, glomerular abnormalities are more evident and consist of periglomerular fibrosis, segmental sclerosis, and ultimately global sclerosis. Progressive glomerular sclerosis also occurs with aging, and this must be considered in interpretation of a biopsy specimen. By immunofluorescence studies, the response of glomeruli to staining is usually negative, with only occasional faint segmental mesangial staining for C3 and IgM. [396] Small arteries and arterioles typically show fibrointimal thickening of variable severity, but vasculitis is not a feature of chronic interstitial disease.

Clinical Features

Unless a patient is found to have an abnormal urinalysis or elevated serum creatinine level from a screening test, patients with chronic interstitial disease present either because of systemic symptoms of a primary disease (see later) or because of nonspecific symptoms of renal failure. These nonspecific symptoms depend on the severity of the renal failure, but may include lassitude, weakness, nausea, nocturia, and sleep disturbances. In a series of patients with biopsy-documented chronic interstitial disease, the creatinine clearance at presentation was below 50 mL/minute in 75% of cases and below 15 mL/minute in roughly 33% of them. Typical laboratory findings in these patients included non-nephrotic-range proteinuria, microscopic hematuria and pyuria, glycosuria (25% of cases), and, surprisingly, positive urine cultures in 28% of patients. [396] Acidifying and concentrating defects are common. Some causes of chronic interstitial disease display characteristic patterns of tubular dysfunction (proximal or distal renal tubular acidosis) or marked early concentrating defects (primary medullary dysfunction). [397] More often, the pattern of tubular dysfunction is not highly restricted. Serum uric acid levels are usually lower than expected for the degree of renal failure, presumably because of tubular defects in the reabsorption of uric acid. Anemia occurs relatively early in the course of certain forms of chronic interstitial disease, presumably because of early destruction of erythropoietin-producing interstitial cells. Approximately 50% of patients presenting with chronic interstitial disease have hypertension. This figure is unrelated to the degree of renal failure, and persists at glomerular filtration rates lower than 15 mL/minute. [396]

Etiology

The pathologic and clinical scenarios we have described can occur in association with a number of diseases of diverse etiology. Distinguishing features of many of these are discussed individually in the paragraphs that follow. For many of these entities, biopsies are infrequently performed, which limits clinicopathologic correlations. Table 30-2 provides a more exhaustive list of common and rare causes of chronic interstitial disease. Some causes, which are discussed fully in other chapters, are additionally listed here. A number of drugs are also associated with chronic interstitial nephritis.

Endemic Nephropathy

Balkan nephropathy is a form of chronic interstitial disease endemic to areas of Bulgaria, the former Yugoslavia, and Romania. Its cause remains unknown, although it has been attributed over the years to long-term lead exposure, infection,

TABLE 30-2

Chronic Interstitial Nephritis

Hereditary diseases

Autosomal dominant polycystic kidney disease[550]
Medullary cystic disease–juvenile nephronophthisis[551]
Mitochondrial mutation[552]

Metabolic disturbances

Hypercalcemia/nephrocalcinosis[553]
Hyperoxaluria[554]
Hypokalemia[478]
Hyperuricemia[277, 475]
Cystinosis[555]
Methylmalonic acidemia[556]

Drugs and toxins

Analgesics[557]
Cadmium[512]
Lead[512]
Nitrosoureas[561]
Herbs[350, 562]
Germanium lactate citrate[563]
Lithium[558]
Cyclosporine[559]
Cisplatin[560]
Slimming regimens with Chinese herbs[350, 562]

Immune-mediated

Renal allograft rejection[564, 565]
Wegener granulomatosis[567]
Sjögren syndrome[569]
Systemic lupus erythematosus[566]
Vasculitis[568]
Sarcoidosis[570, 571]

Hematologic disturbances

Multiple myeloma[415]
Light chain deposition disease[420]
Sickle cell disease[574]
Paroxysmal nocturnal hemoglobinuria[572]
Lymphoma[573]

Infection

Direct infection[575]
Malacoplakia[576]
Xanthogranulomatous pyelonephritis[577]

Obstructive and mechanical disorders

Tumors[578]
Stones[277]
Outlet obstruction[487, 493]
Vesicoureteral reflux[579]

Miscellaneous

Endemic nephropathy[400]
Radiation nephritis[436]
Progressive glomerular disease[497]
Extracorporeal shock wave lithotripsy[583]
Aging[580]
Hypertension[581]
Ischemia[582]

environmental agents (including fungus-contaminated food-stuffs), and genetic factors, alone or in combination.[398, 399] The disease typically manifests clinically in the fourth or fifth decade of life, and is only rarely seen in individuals under the age of 20 years.[400] Initial pathologic abnormalities may occur decades before the development of end-stage renal disease: the consensus is that this is a slowly progressive disease. There is no specific diagnostic test for Balkan nephropathy,

which makes early diagnosis difficult. Asymptomatic patients typically have elevated excretion of "tubule" proteins (lysozyme, light chains, beta$_2$-microglobulin, retinal binding protein), increased enzymuria (N-acetyl-β-D-glucosaminidase), and submaximal urinary concentrating ability.[400] Excretion of beta$_2$-microglobulin is a sensitive indicator of early damage.[401] Serum complement values are typically normal, as is the serum protein electrophoresis, and there are no detectable anti-GBM or anti-TBM antibodies. The kidneys are normal in size in the latent stages of the disease and become small with progressive disease. Various series have reported that anywhere from 2% to 47% of patients with Balkan nephropathy have uroepithelial tumors.[400]

Sarcoidosis

Sarcoidosis most commonly affects the kidney through disordered Ca^{2+} metabolism.[402] Approximately 10% to 15% of patients with sarcoidosis have hypercalcemia (even more have normocalcemic hypercalciuria), which can lead to concentrating defects, depress glomerular filtration, or result in nephrocalcinosis or nephrolithiasis.

Although autopsy series have demonstrated that non-caseating granulomas are present within the renal interstitium in 15% to 30% of patients with sarcoidosis,[403] it is unusual for these pathologic abnormalities to result in clinically apparent renal dysfunction. Granulomatous interstitial nephritis can also coexist with hypercalcemia, and in some cases renal insufficiency is improved or corrected simply by volume expansion and treatment of hypercalcemia. Despite these qualifications, there clearly is a small subset of patients with sarcoidosis who develop granulomatous interstitial nephritis that leads to renal insufficiency. Some reports have also emphasized the tubular defects present in such patients, including glycosuria, concentrating defects, and renal tubular acidosis.[404] It is unusual to see renal sarcoidosis without other apparent organ involvement.[402] The population at risk for granulomatous interstitial nephritis appears to be a distinct subset of all patients with sarcoidosis. Reported cases are predominantly in men,[404, 405] whereas at least 50% (and in the African-American population >50%) of patients with sarcoidosis are women.[406] One series has emphasized that patients with sarcoidosis and granulomatous interstitial nephritis may also present atypically, lacking skin, eye, and pulmonary imvolvement.[405] In this series, patients presented with systemic symptoms and hypercalcemia, which suggest malignant neoplasm or infection.

The pathologic findings in renal sarcoidosis consist of interstitial noncaseating granulomas, composed of giant cells, histiocytes, and lymphocytes. The extent of such granulomas is variable, but in some cases they may virtually replace the majority of the cortical volume, severely distorting the tubular architecture.[404] Focal areas of lymphocytic infiltrate and periglomerular fibrosis are commonly seen in addition to granulomas. Immunofluorescent and electron microscopic studies typically show no immune deposits.[404, 407]

These patients often have an impressive therapeutic response to corticosteroid therapy, with improvement in glomerular filtration[405] and, on repeat biopsy, loss of granulomas and lymphocytic infiltrate. The often concomitant hypercalcemia is also corticosteroid-responsive.[408] Healing of this lesion may result in interstitial fibrosis. Cyclophosphamide is occasionally used in patients refractory to or intolerant of corticosteroids.

Rarely, patients with sarcoidosis have primary glomerular disease, including focal glomerulosclerosis and membranous nephropathy. Arteritis has also been described.[409] Other diseases characterized by granuloma formation, including tuberculosis, silicosis, and histoplasmosis, can cause hypercalcemia and renal insufficiency on that basis. They do not appear to frequently cause granulomatous interstitial nephritis, although case reports exist.[291]

Multiple Myeloma

Acute and chronic renal failure is common in patients with multiple myeloma and can be attributable to multiple interacting mechanisms, including cast nephropathy ("myeloma kidney"), and coexistent volume depletion, hypercalcemia, nephrocalcinosis, and uric acid nephropathy.

The classic pathologic changes in myeloma kidney include the presence of proteinaceous casts in dilated, atrophic distal nephron segments with surrounding multinucleated giant cells, probably of monocyte-macrophage origin.[410] The casts typically contain both Tamm-Horsfall protein and the pathologic light chain.[411, 412] Coexisting abnormalities may include plasma cell and mononuclear cell infiltration of the interstitium, calcifications in the interstitium, and amyloid deposits in the vessels and glomeruli. Immunofluorescent staining may reveal light chain deposition along both the glomerular and tubular basement membranes.[413]

The pathogenesis of cast nephropathy has been an area of investigative interest for many years. Attention has focused on the role of filtered light chains for the following reasons: (1) the majority of myeloma patients with renal failure have Bence Jones proteinuria[414]; (2) patients with plasma cell dyscrasias without Bence Jones proteinuria do not typically develop renal failure[415]; and (3) light chains are an integral part of the intraluminal proteinaceous casts.[411, 412] The current consensus is that light chains are nephrotoxic both through their ability to directly injure tubular epithelial cells and through intrarenal obstruction from cast formation.[416] Light chains are normally synthesized by plasma cells in excess of heavy chains and, as low-molecular-weight proteins (approximately 22kD) they are filtered at the glomerulus. Light chains are normally reabsorbed by the proximal tubule, probably by receptor-mediated endocytosis through low-affinity, high-capacity binding sites on the apical membrane of proximal tubular cells.[417] This process is saturable, so that in the setting of excess light chain production, the proximal tubule reabsorptive capacity is overwhelmed, which leads to eventual urinary excretion of light chains as "Bence Jones" proteins.[416, 418-420] Hemodynamic studies have suggested that elevated intratubular pressures account for the decline in glomerular filtration in experimental case nephropathy.[421]

The observation that there is no consistent relationship between quantitative excretion of pathologic light chains and glomerular filtration[422, 423] has led to extensive physicochemical analysis of light chain properties that correlate with tubular toxic effects or the propensity to precipitate intraluminally. The physicochemical factors important for light chain precipitation include light chain concentration,[424] perhaps isoelectric point[421, 425-427]; the acidic intraluminal pH of the distal nephron[428]; tubular flow rate[424]; and the

presence of Tamm-Horsfall protein.[419] In addition, elevated intratubular concentrations of Na^+ and Ca^{2+} augment light chain aggregation with Tamm-Horsfall protein.[419] Experimental work has demonstrated that colchicine can prevent obstruction from cast-forming light chains. The mechanism underlying this effect may be due to an alteration in Tamm-Horsfall glycoprotein, because Tamm-Horsfall protein purified from colchicine-treated rats does not aggregate with potentially toxic light chains, and possesses less carbohydrate than does Tamm-Horsfall glycoprotein from control rats.[424]

Based on these findings, appropriate therapy for presumed cast nephropathy in multiple myeloma includes chemotherapy to ameliorate excess light chain production; treatment of hypercalcemia; alkalinization of the urine in conjunction with induction of polyuria by hypotonic fluids (if tolerated); and avoidance of radiocontrast agents, which may enhance the nephrotoxicity of light chains.[415, 428] Because furosemide can increase distal tubular Na^+ and Ca^{2+} concentrations, loop diuretics should be used with caution, particularly in the setting of volume depletion.[424] Colchicine is effective in familial Mediterranean fever in preventing amyloidosis,[429] and, based on experimental studies, may be effective in ameliorating cast nephropathy as well.

Radiation Nephritis

It is uncommon to see patients with radiation nephritis any longer because recognition of radiation-induced renal damage has altered protocols for the administration of therapeutic radiation. Radiation nephritis can present in several forms.[430] An acute form is usually seen within a year following radiation and presents with hypertension, anemia, and edema. A more insidious chronic form presents primarily with diminished glomerular filtration, hypertension, and occasionally proteinuria.[431] There is another subset of patients who may develop hypertension within several years following radiation but have no significant azotemia.[430] A small fraction of this latter group can develop malignant hypertension with accelerated loss of renal function. A final pattern of less severe renal injury following radiation is that of isolated proteinuria. This can first occur more than a decade after radiation and may be persistent or intermittent.[431] The common pathologic finding in those patients with chronic radiation nephritis is interstitial fibrosis.[431, 432] Because hypertension so commonly accompanies radiation nephritis, it is difficult to separate the effects of the radiation and hypertension on the fibrotic process.

Experimental models of radiation nephritis have helped to elucidate the pathogenesis of radiation injury. The initial injury is to endothelial cells and results in endothelial cell swelling. Subsequent vascular occlusion develops with resultant tubular atrophy.[433] Irradiated renal parenchymal cells display impaired proliferation and are highly susceptible to multiple forms of injury.[434] At the organ level, the irradiated kidney initially undergoes a period of augmented blood flow, which is followed by a fall in renal blood flow and glomerular filtration rate.[435-437] It is possible that the fall in renal blood flow is accompanied by augmented renin release and, secondarily, AII-dependent hypertension.[438] Hypertension in some patients with radiation nephritis has been reversible with removal of a unilaterally irradiated kidney.[439, 440]

Radiation nephritis is dose-dependent, affecting the majority of those exposed to more than 2300 rad.[431, 441] It can be prevented by kidney shielding, or, alternatively, by fractionating doses which increase renal tolerance to the damaging effects of radiation.[442] Even with fractionated schedules, patients exposed to other nephrotoxins (chemotherapeutic agents, antibiotics, radioconstrast agents) are at an increased risk for toxicity.

Analgesic Nephropathy

Long-term ingestion of large quantities of analgesics has been associated in epidemiologic studies with chronic interstitial nephritis and papillary necrosis.[443] Because discontinuation of heavy analgesic use can slow or arrest progression of the renal disease,[444] this is an important diagnosis to make. The incidence of analgesic nephropathy varies among different countries and among different geographic areas of the United States.[445] It is a relatively common cause of chronic renal failure in Scotland, Belgium, and Australia, accounting for 10% to 20% of patients with end-stage renal disease in those countries.[446-448] In the United States, case-control studies from the Philadelphia area did not detect an excess risk of renal disease in daily users of analgesics,[449] whereas this was apparent in North Carolina.[450] These two populations differed markedly by the degree of regular analgesis use, consistent with previous suggestions that variations in the frequency of analgesic nephropathy track closely with patterns of analgesic use.

Analgesic nephropathy is recognized more frequently (five to seven times) in women than men. Patients typically take analgesics for chronic headaches, abdominal discomfort, or non-specific joint pain. The caffeine component of certain over-the-counter analgesics may encourage dependence. Because over-the-counter analgesics are widely available, the typical patient may not come to medical attention until renal failure is quite advanced. On presentation, patients frequently have nocturia (decreased concentrating ability), sterile pyuria, and hypertension. The hypertension may be exacerbated by volume depletion, which suggests it is rennin-dependent.[451]Anemia is frequently seen, attributable to both the renal failure and chronic blood loss from peptic ulcer disease. Uroepithelial malignancies occur with increased frequency in these patients.[452, 453] Current clinical practice is to screen patients annually with urine cytology. A new onset of hematuria in such a patient warrants an aggressive workup.

Several generalities have emerged from the epidemiologic study of analgesic nephropathy. One is that its development requires prolonged regular ingestion of combination analgesics (six tablets daily for more than 3 years).[454] It has been frequently stated that analgesic nephropathy requires ingestion of combinations of analgesics, including aspirin, acetaminophen, phenacetin, caffeine, or codeine. A recent case-control study of analgesic use in North Carolina, however, demonstrated an increased odds risk for those patients with excessive ingestion of only acetaminophen.[450] Several case reports of chronic interstitial disease and end-stage renal disease after long-term heavy ingestion of nonsteroidal anti-inflammatory agents increase this concern over the toxicity of single agents.[455, 456] Whether chronic interstitial disease related to nonsteroidal anti-inflammatory drugs is an immune-mediated extension of the well-defined acute lesion or toxic nephropathy is unclear.

The pathologic abnormalities in analgesic nephropathy are nonspecific and typical of chronic interstitial disease with papillary necrosis. At the time of clinical presentation, the kidneys are typically small. Papillary necrosis is usually present but not required for the diagnosis. At a light microscopic level the interstitium is fibrotic with tubule atrophy and occasional mononuclear cell infiltration.[457] There may be concomitant focal glomerular sclerosis and interstitial calcifications as well. Recent studies have emphasized that gross pathologic changes in kidneys affected by analgesic nephropathy may be recognized by noncontrast computed tomography.[458] Such abnormalities include papillary calcification, decrease in renal volume, and bumpy renal contours. These abnormalities may additionally be useful diagnostic tests in individuals with chronic renal insufficiency due to analgesic nephropathy.[459] Papillary calcification, in particular, has a high sensitivity and specificity in the latter population.

Acetaminophen (a hepatic metabolite of phenacetin) is highly concentrated in the papillary tip, especially during antidiuresis. It is further metabolized in the kidney to a number of reactive metabolites.[460, 461] The toxicity of these metabolites may be exacerbated by the actions of other analgesics, such as aspirin or other nonsteroidal anti-inflammatory agents, which inhibit the activity of the hexose monophosphate shunt, thereby diminishing the intracellular supply of glutathione and reducing potential.[277, 462] In addition, the inhibition of prostaglandin synthesis can exacerbate medullary damage from ischemia.[463]

Uric Acid Nephropathy

Although it is widely accepted that overproduction of uric acid and hyperuricemia (especially in acutely treated myeloproliferative disease) can cause acute renal failure,[464, 465] it is less clear that chronic hyperuricemia independently results in chronic interstitial nephritis and progressive renal failure. Historically, chronic hyperuricemia associated with chronic interstitial disease was called "gouty nephropathy." In a review of the causes of chronic interstitial nephritis in the late 1970s, Murray and Goldberg[277] attributed 11% of chronic interstitial disease primarily to disorders of uric acid metabolism and cited uric acid as a contributing factor in an additional 7% of cases. This association was challenged in the early 1980s by Yu and Berger[466] who could not demonstrate an association of hyperuricemia with chronic interstitial disease that could not be attributed to hypertension, vascular disease, stones, or aging. The existence of gouty nephropathy received another challenge by the finding that infusion of ethylenediaminetetraacetic acid (EDTA) into patients with gout and interstitial disease elicited an abnormal increase in lead excretion, which suggests that heavy metal intoxication may be the primary event resulting in hypertension, interstitial disease, and hyperuricemia.[467]

Despite the clear associations between lead intoxication and hyperuricemia, it is still controversial whether chronic hyperuricemia alone can lead to interstitial disease. It is an important question, especially as many patients with chronic renal failure have serum uric acid levels above 10 mg/dL, attributable to diminished glomerular filtration and the effects of diuretics.[468] Although underexcretion of uric acid is often clinically assumed to not be harmful to the kidney, this assumption may not be true. If hyperuricemia in chronic renal failure can accelerate progression, then it is an important metabolic abnormality to specifically treat. Lowering to the serum uric acid in chronic renal failure can be most safely accomplished through protein and purine restriction.[468]

Hypercalcemia

Disorders of Ca^{2+} metabolism leading to hypercalcemia or increased Ca^{2+} turnover have a multiplicity of effects on the kidney. Hypercalcemia can decrease glomerular filtration through renal vasoconstriction,[469] a decrease in the glomerular ultrafiltration coefficient,[470] and volume contraction due to the vasopressin-resistant concentrating defect.[471] Disorders of Ca^{2+} metabolism may also lead to nephrocalcinosis, with deposition of Ca^{2+} in the kidney, around the TBMs and especially around distal tubules and collecting ducts. Such deposition secondarily lead to mononuclear cell infiltration and tubular necrosis.

Ca^{2+} deposition begins in the medullary tubules, followed by the cortical proximal and distal tubules and within the interstitial space.[472, 473] In addition to frank hypercalcemia, nephrocalcinosis can occur in normocalcemic disorders of augmented gut absorption of Ca^{2+} (sarcoidosis, vitamin D intoxication), skeletal breakdown (neoplasms or multiple myeloma), or classic distal renal tubular acidosis. Therapy is directed toward the primary disease, in addition to measures aimed at reducing the serum Ca^{2+} and correcting acid-base disturbances.

Hypokalemic Nephropathy

It is rare for sustained hypokalemia to cause chronic interstitial nephritis. There are both inherited and acquired forms of hypokalemic nephropathy.[474-476] The inherited form is HLA-linked and characterized by primary renal wasting of K^+, normal blood pressure, but elevated renin, aldosterone, and urinary prostaglandin E excretion. These patients have an interstitial nephritis with progressive renal failure. A pathologic characteristic of both acquired and inherited forms is the finding of vacuoles in the proximal convoluted tubules,[477, 478] the composition of which is unknown. An insight into the possible pathogenesis of hypokalemic nephropathy comes from studies of experimental hypokalemia in the rat.[181] In this setting hypokalemia stimulates ammoniogenesis (because of the associated intracellular acidosis) which then elicits complement activation, initiating the influx of immune cells into the interstitium.

Oxaloses

Hyperoxaluria occurs in the setting of inborn errors of metabolism,[479] increased bowel absorption of oxalate,[480] or acute massive oxalate loads.[481] In all three settings, renal dysfunction can occur. Primary hyperoxaluria is due to a defect in either the 2-oxoglutarate:glyoxylate carboligase (type I) or the 2-glyceric dehydrogenase (type II). These patients develop chronic renal failure typically before reaching adulthood.[479] Patients with inflammatory bowel disease or ileal-jejunal bypass surgery have increased bowel absorption of oxalate and can develop chronic renal insufficiency, which can be progressive. Ethylene glycol ingestion or ascorbic acid overdoses result in acute massive oxalate loads and acute renal failure associated with intrarenal obstruction by intratubular precipitation of oxalic acid crystals.[481] In each setting the pathogenesis appears to be intraluminal obstruction by oxalate crystals, followed by progressive tubule atrophy and fibrosis.

Obstructive Nephropathy

The etiology and pathophysiology of urinary tract obstruction is discussed in detail elsewhere. Complete or partial urinary tract obstruction is accompanied by a decline in glomerular filtration and a plethora of tubule abnormalities, including diminished reabsorption of solutes,[482-484] impaired excretion of H^+ and K^+,[485] and a vasopressin-resistant concentrating defect (nephrogenic diabetes insipidus).[486] These functional alterations are accompanied by pathologic changes in both the tubulointerstitium and glomeruli consisting of interstitial fibrosis, tubular atrophy, and occasionally focal glomerular sclerosis.

The pathophysiology of urinary tract obstruction has been studied extensively. In models of both unilateral and bilateral ureteral obstruction, there is a fall in the glomerular filtration rate attributable to both a fall in the single-nephron glomerular filtration rate (SNGFR) and a decrease in the number of filtering nephrons. The fall in SNGFR occurs because of diminished plasma flow, diminished net hydraulic pressure, and a depressed filtration coefficient.[487] Mediators that have been identified as relevant to the diminished SNGFR include AII,[488, 489] thromboxane A_2,[488] antidiuretic hormone,[490] and leukotrienes.[491] Diminished production of nitric oxide may also play a role, because dietary arginine can augment glomerular filtration in postobstructed kidneys.

In both chronic and acute ureteral obstruction, there are mononuclear cells in the interstitium.[492, 493] They are most evident surrounding distal tubular cells but are present throughout the cortex and medulla. In experimental models of obstruction, the majority of these cells are macrophages or CD8+ lymphocytes.[493] The cells disappear following release of obstruction. Whereas the relationship of these cells to renal functional abnormalities has not been fully elucidated, manipulations which diminish the cellular infiltrate (such as irradiation) are associated with a less marked decrement in glomerular filtration after obstruction.[494] Because AII[495] and thromboxane A_2 can be expressed by such infiltrating cells,[494] the infiltrate may be of functional significance. Insight into why leukocytes migrate into a kidney experiencing elevated intratubular pressures comes from the observation that a lipid chemoattractant is released by the obstructed kidney.[496] Growth factors, such as TGF-β, released by infiltrating cells may, in addition, contribute to the interstitial fibrosis[497] and glomerular sclerosis[498] accompanying chronic urinary tract obstruction.

Lead Nephropathy

Occupational exposure to lead in the United States is currently restricted by governmental regulations. Continuing sources of exposure occur, though, from old water pipes, pottery, crystal, and lead-based paint in older dwellings. Several epidemiologic analyses support the association of excess lead burden with chronic renal failure.[499] Lead nephropathy is underdiagnosed because no simple blood test is diagnostic. The diagnosis is suggested by an augmented (> 0.6 mg)

24-hour urinary excretion of lead after two 1-g doses of disodium EDTA.[500] EDTA is not nephrotoxic at these doses. Because the lead content in bones of patients with chronic renal failure unrelated to lead intoxication is not elevated, this test can also be used in patients with chronic renal insufficiency.[501] The correlation between chelatable lead and bone lead concentration determined by atomic absorption spectroscopy is excellent.[501] For those patients with low urine output, the collection times following EDTA administration can be prolonged up to several days. X-ray fluorescent measurements of in vivo skeletal lead stores correlate well with the results of EDTA chelation tests and have the advantage of being rapid and noninvasive.[502] Blood lead levels only reflect recent, not chronic, exposure and can be normal in patients with multisystem damage from lead.[500] Despite this, epidemiologic studies have additionally documented a correlation between blood lead concentrations and diastolic blood pressure,[503] as well as blood lead concentrations, zinc protoporphyrin, and creatinine clearance.[499]

Lead preferentially deposits in the S3 portion of the proximal tubule.[504] Nuclear inclusions within proximal tubular cells are characteristic of lead nephropathy.[505] The pathophysiologic correlate of this is that lead exposure can result in proximal tubular dysfunction (especially in children), with either isolated tubule defects or a full Fanconi syndrome.[506] These defects are potentially reversible. It is unusual to see chronic renal failure from lead in children.

In adults, lead nephropathy is pathologically a chronic interstitial nephritis, with interstitial fibrosis, atrophy, and nephrosclerosis.[507] Patients frequently have recurrent gout,[508] and the majority of patients have hyperuricemia and hypertension. Ingestion of moonshine liquor with its high lead content, is an important historical clue to the diagnosis.[509, 510] EDTA has been advocated as therapy, in addition to a diagnostic test.[500] The goal of chelation therapy is to normalize the EDTA mobilization test. In some patients this may arrest or reverse progression of renal failure.

Cadmium Nephropathy

Cadmium nephropathy can develop in individuals with prolonged low-level exposure to excess cadmium. Such persons are likely to be employed in smelters. Cadmium is bound to metallothionein and these complexes are pinocytosed by proximal tubular cells.[511] The liver and kidney are the two major organs in which cadmium accumulates. Its half-life in the body is more than 10 years.

Like blood levels of lead, the blood levels of cadmium fall after an acute exposure because of extensive tissue deposition.[512] Once a threshold of renal deposition is exceeded, excess cadmium will be excreted in the urine.[513] Cadmium intoxication also produces proximal tubule dysfunction, hypercalciuria, and a high frequency of metabolic bone disease and nephrolithiases. The major clinical manifestation of an unfortunate massive environmental exposure to cadmium (through contaminated water and rice in Japan) was bone pain (called Itai-Itai ("ouch-ouch") disease).[514] The tubular dysfunction seen with cadmium is not reversible. Epidemiologic studies have documented an excess mortality from chronic renal failure in areas contaminated by cadmium.[515]

The mechanism by which cadmium and lead elicits chronic inflammation and fibrosis is relatively unstudied.

Some work has suggested that exogenous agents such as cadmium, which markedly augments expression of inducible heat shock proteins, can lead to interstitial renal damage initiated by T cells reactive to an immunodominant peptide of such inducible heat shock proteins.[516]

Course and Therapy

Most forms of chronic interstitial nephritis display slowly progressive renal deterioration. General therapeutic principles include treating the primary diseases and identifying and eliminating any exogenous agents (drugs, heavy metals) or conditions (obstruction, infection) associated with the chronic interstitial lesion. Other prudent maneuvers include good control of blood pressure[517] (particularly angiotensin-converting enzyme inhibition) and treatment of electrolyte disturbances (particularly metabolic acidosis, hyperuricemia, and hyperphosphatemia). More specific therapies, such as chelation in lead nephropathy and corticosteroids in sarcoidosis, have been discussed before. Many of the discussed entities present with moderate to advanced renal failure and have no specific therapy. For these reasons, renal biopsy is often not indicated when chronic interstitial nephritis is suspected because the pathologic diagnosis will not affect therapy. With the exception of sarcoidosis, there are as yet no strong indications for immunosuppressive therapies in chronic interstitial nephritis.

ACKNOWLEDGMENTS

This work was supported, in part, by grants from the National Institutes of Health (DK-46282 and DK-45346). The authors thank Dr. Gunter Wolf for identifying some of the early non-English literature.

REFERENCES

1. Lemley KV, Kriz W: Anatomy of the renal interstitium. Kidney Int 39:370-381, 1991.
2. Ekblom P: Developmentally regulated conversion of mesenchyme to epithelium. FASEB J 3:2141-2150, 1989.
3. Eustachio E (ed). Opuscula Anatomica: Luchinus, Vincent; 1564.
4. Bowman W: On the structure and use of malpighian bodies of the kidney, with observations on the circulation through the gland. Philos Trans R Soc Lond 4:57-80, 1842.
5. Kolliker A: Mikroskopische Anatomie oder Gewebelehre des Menschen. Berlin, Wilhelm Engelmann, 1852.
6. Biermer A: Ein ungewöhnlicher Fall von Scharlach. Virchows Arch 19:537-584, 1860.
7. Pavy FW, Taylor AS: Poisoning by white precipitate: Physiological effects of this substance on animals. Guys Hosp Rep 6:504-511, 1860.
8. Lancereaux E: Néphrite et arthrite saturnines: Coïncidence de ces affections: Parallèle avec la néphrite el l'arthrite goutteuses. Arch Gen Med Paris 6:641, 1881.
9. Dickinson WH (ed): On the Pathology and Treatment of Albuminuria. New York, William Wood, 1868.
10. Ponfick E: Studien über die Schicksale körniger Farbstoffe im Organismus. Virch Arch 48:1-55, 1869.
11. Traube L: Zur Pathologie der Nierenkrankheiten. Ges Beiträge 2:996, 1870.
12. Councilman WT: Acute interstitial nephritis. J Exp Med 3:393-418, 1898.
13. Pearce RM: The problems of experimental nephritis. Arch Intern Med 5:133-167, 1910.
14. Vollhard F, Fahr TH (eds): Die Bright'sche Nierenkrankheiten. Berlin, Springer-Verlag, 1914.
15. Longcope WT: The production of experimental nephritis by repeated protein intoxication. J Exp Med 18:678-703, 1913.

16. Danoff TM, Neilson EG: Immunologic mechanisms of interstitial disease. *In* Seldin DW, Giebisch G (ed): The Kidney: Physiology and Pathophysiology. Philadelphia, Lippincott Williams and Wilkins, 2000.

17. Melnick PJ: Acute interstitial nephritis with uremia. Arch Pathol 36: 499-504, 1943.

18. Spühler O, Zollinger HU: Die chronische interstitielle Nephritis. Z Klin Med 131: 1-50, 1953.

19. Unanue ER, Dixon FJ, Feldman JD: Experimental allergic glomerulonephritis induced in the rabbit with homologous renal antigens. J Exp Med 125:163-175, 1966.

20. Steblay RW, Rudofsky U: Renal tubular disease and autoantibodies against basement membrane induced in guinea pigs. J Immunol 107: 589-594, 1971.

21. Lehman DH, Wilson CB: Role of sensitized cells in antitubular basement membrane interstitial nephritis. Int Arch Allergy Immunol 51: 168-174, 1976.

22. Neilson EG, McCafferty E, Feldman A, et al: Spontaneous interstitial nephritis in kdkd mice. I. An experimental model of autoimmune renal disease. J Immunol 133:2560-2565, 1984.

23. Kelly CJ, Tomaszewski J, Neilson EG: Immunopathogeneic mechanisms of tubulointerstitial injury. *In* Tisher CC, Brenner BM (eds): Renal Pathology, 3rd ed. Philadelphia, WB Saunders, 1994, pp. 699-722.

24. Neilson EG: Pathogenesis and therapy of interstitial nephritis. Kidney Int 35:1257-1270, 1989.

25. Yee J, Neilson EG: The immune modulation of biologic systems in renal cells. Kidney Int 43:128-134, 1993.

26. Strutz F, Okada H, Lo CW, et al: Identification and characterization of a fibroblast marker: FSP1. J Cell Biol 130:393-405, 1995.

27. Matsusaka T, Hymes J, Ichikawa I: Angiotensin in progressive renal disease: Theory and practice. J Am Soc Nephrol 7:2025-2043, 1996.

28. Brenner BM: Nephron adaptation to renal injury of ablation. Am J Physiol 249:F334-F337, 1985.

29. Schainuck LI, Striker GE, Cutler RE, Benditt EP: Structural-functional correlations in renal disease. Hum Pathol 1:631-641, 1970.

30. Schwartz MM, Fennell JS, Lewis EJ: Pathologic changes in the renal tubule in systemic lupus erythematosus. Hum Pathol 13:534-547, 1982.

31. Muehrcke RC, Kark RM, Pirani CL, Pollak VE: Lupus nephritis: A clinical and pathologic study based on renal biopsies. Medicine (Baltimore) 36:1-145, 1957.

32. Andropoulos E, Seron D, Hartley RB, et al: Immune mechanisms in idiopathic membranous nephropathy: The role of the interstitial infiltrates. Am J Kidney Dis 13:404-412, 1989.

33. Risdon RA, Sloper JC, deWardener HE: Relationship between renal function and histological changes found in renal-biopsy specimens from patients with persistent glomerular nephritis. Lancet 2:363-366, 1968.

34. Bohle A, Mackensen-Haen S, von-Gise H: Significance of tubulointerstitial changes in the renal cortex for the excretory function and concentration ability of the kidney: A morphometric contribution. Am J Nephrol 7:421-433, 1987.

35. Bohle A, Mackensen-Haen S, von Gise H, et al: The consequences of tubulo-interstitial changes for renal function in glomerulopathies. Pathol Res Pract 186:135-144, 1990.

36. Dziukas LJ, Sterzel RB, Hodson CJ, Hoyer JR: Renal localization of Tamm-Horsfall protein in unilateral obstructive uropathy in rats. Lab Invest 47:185-193, 1982.

37. Ljungquist A: The intrarenal arterial pattern in the normal and diseased human kidney. Acta Med Scand (suppl 5) 174:5-36, 1963.

38. Bohle A, von Gise H, Mackensen-Haen S, Stark-Jakob B: The obliteration of the postglomerular capillaries and its influence upon the function of both glomeruli and tubuli. Functional interpretation of morphologic findings. Klin Wochenschr 59:1043-1051, 1981.

39. Mackensen S, Grund KE, Sindjic M, Bohle A: Influence of the renal cortical interstitium on the serum creatinine concentration and creatinine clearance in different chronic sclerosing interstitial nephritides. Nephron 24:30-34, 1979.

40. Brod J, Benesova D: A comparative study of functional and morphological renal changes in glomerulonephritis. Acta Med Scand 157: 23-32, 1957.

41. Iversen BM, Ofstad J: Loss of renal blood flow autoregulation in chronic glomerulonephritic rats. Am J Physiol 23:F284-F290, 1990.

42. Persson AEG, Boberg U, Hahne B et al: Interstitial pressure as a modulator of tubuloglomerular feedback control. Kidney Int Suppl 22: S122-S128, 1982.

43. Persson AEG, Gushwa LC, Blantz RC: Feedback pressure-flow responses in normal and angiotensin-prostaglandin-blocked rats. Kidney Int 247:F925-F931, 1984.

44. Peterson OW, Gushwa LC, Wilson CB, et al: Tubuloglomerular feedback activity after glomerular injury. Am J Physiol 26:F67-F71, 1989.

45. Thurau K, Boylan JW: Acute renal success: The unexpected logic of oliguria in acute renal failure. Am J Med 61:308-315, 1976.

46. Wright FS, Okusa MD: Functional role of tubuloglomerular feedback control of glomerular filtration. Adv Nephrol 19:119-134, 1990.

47. Ichikawa I: Hemodynamic influence of altered distal salt delivery on glomerular microcirculation. Kidney Int Suppl 22:S109-S113, 1982.

48. Muller-Suur R, Persson AEG, Ulfendahl HR: Tubuloglomerular feedback in juxtamedullary nephrons. Kidney Int Suppl 22:S104-S108, 1982.

49. Wilson CB: Nephritogenic tubulointerstitial antigens. Kidney Int 39: 501-517, 1991.

50. Salant D, Cybulsky A: Experimental glomerulonephritis. Methods Enzymol 162:421-461, 1988.

51. Klassen J, Sugisaki T, Milgrom F, McCluskey RT: Studies on multiple renal lesions in Heymann nephritis. Lab Invest 25:577-585, 1971.

52. Couser W: Mediation of immune glomerular injury. J Am Soc Nephrol 1:13-29, 1990.

53. Brown D, McCluskey RT, Ausiello DA: The cell biology of Heymann nephritis: A model of human membranous glomerulonephritis. Am J Kidney Dis 10:74-76, 1987.

54. Noble B, Mendrick DL, Brentjens JR, Andres GA: Antibody-mediated injury to proximal tubules in the rat kidney induced by passive transfer of homologous anti-brush border serum. Clin Immunol Immunopathol 19:289-301, 1981.

55. Noble B, Andres GA, Brentjens JR: Passively transferred anti-brush border antibodies induce injury of proximal tubules in the absence of complement. Clin Exp Immunol 56:281-288, 1983.

56. Gronhagen-Riska C, von-Willebrand E, Honkanen E, et al: Interstitial cellular infiltration detected by fine-needle aspiration biopsy in nephritis. Clin Nephrol 34:189-196, 1990.

57. Kerjaschki D, Farquhar MG: The pathogenic antigen of Heymann nephritis is a membrane glycoprotein of the renal proximal tubule brush border. Proc Natl Acad Sci U S A 79:5557-5561, 1982.

58. Kerjaschki D, Farquhar MG: Immunocytochemical localization of the Heymann nephritis antigen (GP330) in glomerular epithelial cells of normal Lewis rats. J Exp Med 157:667-686, 1983.

59. Pietromonaco S, Kerjaschki D, Binder S, et al: Molecular cloning of a cDNA encoding a major pathogenic domain of the Heymann nephritis antigen gp330. Proc Natl Acad Sci U S A 87:1811-1815, 1990.

60. Raychowdhury R, Niles JL, McCluskey RT, Smith JA: Autoimmune target in Heymann nephritis is a glycoprotein with homology to the LDL receptor. Science 244:1163-1165, 1989.

61. Ronco P, Brunisholz M, Geniteau-Legendre M, et al: Physiopathologic aspects of Tamm-Horsfall protein: A phylogenetically conserved marker of the thick ascending limb of Henle's loop. Adv Nephrol 16:231-250, 1987.

62. Hoyer JR, Seiler MW: Pathophysiology of Tamm-Horsfall protein. Kidney Int 16:279-289, 1979.

63. Hession C, Decker JM, Sherblom AP, et al: Uromodulin (Tamm-Horsfall glycoprotein): A renal ligand for lymphokines. Science 237: 1479-1484, 1987.

64. Seiler MW, Hoyer JR: Ultrastructural studies of tubulointerstitial immune complex nephritis in rats immunized with Tamm-Horsfall protein. Lab Invest 45:321-327, 1981.

65. Fasth A, Hoyer JR, Seiler MW: Renal tubular immune complex formation in mice immunized with Tamm-Horsfall protein. Am J Pathol 125:555-562, 1986.

66. Hoyer JR: Tubulointerstitial immune complex nephritis in rats immunized with Tamm-Horsfall protein. Kidney Int 17:284-292, 1980.

67. Mayrer AR, Kashgarian M, Ruddle NH, et al: Tubulointerstitial nephritis and immunologic responses to Tamm-Horsfall protein in rabbits challenged with homologous urine or Tamm-Horsfall protein. J Immunol 128:2634-2642, 1982.

68. Fasth AL, Hoyer JR, Seiler MW: Extratubular Tamm-Horsfall protein deposits induced by ureteral obstruction in mice. Clin Immunol Immunopathol 47:47-61, 1988.

69. Thomas DBL, Davies M, Williams JD: Tamm-Horsfall protein: An aetiological agent in tubulointerstitial disease? Exp Nephrol 1: 281-284, 1993.

70. Kelly CJ, Korngold R, Mann R, et al: Spontaneous interstitial nephritis in kdkd mice. II. Characterization of a tubular antigen-specific,

H-2K-restricted Lyt-2+ effector T cell that mediates destructive tubulointerstitial injury. J Immunol 136:526-531, 1986.

71. Kelly CJ, Neilson EG: Contrasuppression in autoimmunity. Abnormal contrasuppression facilitates expression of nephritogenic effector T cells and interstitial nephritis in kdkd mice. J Exp Med 165:107-123, 1987.

72. Nelson TR, Charonis AS, McIvor RS, Butkowski RJ: Identification of a cDNA encoding tubulointerstitial nephritis antigen. J Biol Chem 270:16265-16270, 1995.

73. Kanwar YS, Kumar A, Yang Q, et al: Tubulointerstitial nephritis antigen: An extracellular matrix protein that selectively regulates tubulogenesis vs. glomerulogenesis during mammalian renal development. Proc Natl Acad Sci U S A 96:11323-11328, 1999.

74. Clayman MD, Martinez-Hernandez A, Michaud L, et al: Isolation and characterization of the nephritogenic antigen producing anti-tubular basement membrane disease. J Exp Med 161:290-305, 1985.

75. Clayman MD, Michaud L, Brentjens J, et al: Isolation of the target antigen of human anti-tubular basement membrane antibody-associated interstitial nephritis. J Clin Invest 77:1143-1147, 1986.

76. Butkowski RJ, Kleppel MM, Katz A, et al: Distribution of tubulointerstitial nephritis antigen and evidence of multiple forms. Kidney Int 40:838-846, 1991.

77. Yoshioka K, Hino S, Takemura T, et al: Isolation and characterization of the tubular basement membrane antigen associated with human tubulo-interstitial nephritis. Clin Exp Immunol 90:319-325, 1992.

78. Miyazato H, Yoshioka K, Hino S, et al: The target antigen of anti-tubular basement membrane antibody-mediated interstitial nephritis. Autoimmunity 18:259-265, 1994.

79. Wilson CB: Individual and strain differences in renal basement membrane antigens. Transplant Proc 12 (suppl 1): 69-73, 1980.

80. Hart DNJ, Fabre JW: Kidney-specific alloantigen system in the rat. Characterization and role in transplantation. J Exp Med 151:651-666, 1980.

81. Paul LC, Carpenter CB: Antigenic determinants of tubular basement membranes and Bowman's capsule in rats. Kidney Int 21:800-807, 1982.

82. Sugisaki T, Kano K, Andres G, Milgrom F: Antibodies to tubular basement membrane elicited by stimulation with allogeneic kidney. Kidney Int 21:557-564, 1982.

83. Lehman DH, Lee S, Wilson CB, Dixon FJ: Induction of antitubular basement membrane antibodies in rats by renal transplantation. Transplantation 17:429-431, 1974.

84. Matsumoto AK, McCafferty E, Neilson EG, Gasser DL: Mapping of the genes for tubular basement membrane antigen and a submaxillary gland protease in the rat. Immunogenetics 20:117-123, 1984.

85. Guery C-J, Hedrick HJ, Mercier P, et al: Mapping of a gene for the M 48000 tubular basement membrane antigen in the rat. Immunogenetics 29:350-354, 1989.

86. Neilson EG, Sun MJ, Kelly CJ, et al: Molecular characterization of a major nephritogenic domain in the autoantigen of anti-tubular basement membrane disease. Proc Natl Acad Sci U S A 88:2006-2010, 1991.

87. Joh K, Shibasaki T, Azuma T, et al: Experimental drug-induced allergic nephritis mediated by antihapten antibody. Int Arch Allergy Immunol 88:337-344, 1989.

88. Hyman LR, Ballow M, Knieser MR: Diphenylhydantoin interstitial nephritis. Roles of cellular and humoral immunologic injury. J Pediatr 92:915-920, 1978.

89. Border WA, Lehman DH, Egan JD, et al: Antitubular basement-membrane antibodies in methicillin-associated interstitial nephritis. N Engl J Med 291:381-384, 1974.

90. Druet E, Sapin C, Gunther E, et al: Mercuric chloride-induced anti-glomerular basement membrane antibodies in the rat. Genetic control. Eur J Immunol 7:348-351, 1977.

91. Ueda S, Wakashin M, Wakashin Y, et al: Experimental gold nephropathy in guinea pigs: Detection of autoantibodies to renal tubular antigens. Kidney Int 29:539-548, 1986.

92. Schnyder B, Mauri-Hellweg D, Zanni M, et al: Direct, MHC-dependent presentation of the drug sulfamethoxazole to human alphabeta T cell clones. J Clin Invest 100:136-141, 1997.

93. Oldstone MBA: Molecular mimicry and autoimmune disease. Cell 80:819-820, 1987.

94. Fasth A, Ahlstedt S, Hanson LA, et al: Cross-reactions between the Tamm-Horsfall glycoprotein and *Echerichia coli*. Int Arch Allergy Immunol 63:303-311, 1980.

95. Fitzsimons EJJ, Weber M, Lange CF: The isolation of cross-reactive monoclonal antibodies: Hybridomas to streptococcal antigens cross-reactive with mammalian basement membrane. Hybridoma 6:61-69, 1987.

96. Kraus W, Beachey EH: Renal autoimmune epitope of a group A streptococci specified by M protein tetrapeptide Lle-Arg-Leu-Arg. Proc Natl Acad Sci U S A 85:4516-4520, 1988.

97. Bourgoignie JJ, Pardo V: The nephropathology in human immuno-deficiency virus (HIV-1) infection. Kidney Int Suppl 35:S19-S23, 1991.

98. Woodroffe AJ, Row PA, Meadows R, Lawrence JR: Nephritis in infectious mononucleosis. Q J Med 43:451-460, 1974.

99. Platt JL, Sibley RK, Michael AF: Interstitial nephritis associated with cytomegalovirus infection. Kidney Int 28:550-552, 1985.

100. van-Ypersele-de-Strihou C, Mery JP: *Hantavirus*-related acute interstitial nephritis in western Europe. Expansion of world-wide zoonosis. Q J Med 73:941-950, 1989.

101. Madaio MP, Carlson J, Cataldo J, et al: Murine monoclonal anti-DNA antibodies bind directly to glomerular antigens and form immune deposits. J Immunol 138:2883-2889, 1987.

102. Faaber P, Rijke TPM, Van de Putte LBA, et al: Cross-reactivity of human and murine anti-DNA antibodies with heparan sulfate. J Clin Invest 77:1824-1830, 1986.

103. Brentjens JR, O'Connell DW, Pawlowski IB, Andres GA: Extraglomerular lesions associated with deposition of circulating antigen-antibody complexes in kidneys of rabbits with chronic serum sickness. Clin Immunol Immunopathol 3:112-126, 1974.

104. Makker SP: Tubular basement membrane antibody-induced interstitial nephritis in systemic lupus erythematosus. Am J Med 69:949-952, 1980.

105. Neilson EG, Phillips SM: The immunobiology of nephritis. Prog Allergy 27:167-249, 1980.

106. Germain RN, Margulies DH: The biochemistry and cell biology of antigen processing and presentation. Annu Rev Immunol 11:403-450, 1993.

107. Schwartz RH: T-lymphocyte recognition of antigen in association with gene products of the major histocompatibility complex. Annu Rev Immunol 3:237-261, 1985.

108. Neilson EG, Phillips, SM: Murine interstitial nephritis. I. Analysis of disease susceptibility and its relationship of pleomorphic gene products defining both immune-response genes and a restrictive requirement for cytotoxic T cells at H-2K. J Exp Med 155:1075-1085, 1982.

109. Kappler JW, Roehm N, Marrack N: T cell tolerance by clonal elimination in the thymus. Cell 49:273-280, 1987.

110. Neilson EG, Gasser DL, McCafferty E, et al: Polymorphism of genes involved in anti-tubular basement membrane disease in rats. Immunogenetics 17:55-65, 1983.

111. Kelly CJ, Silvers WK, Neilson EG: Tolerance to parenchymal self. Regulatory role of major histocompatibility complex-restricted, OX8+ suppressor T cells specific for autologous renal tubular antigen in experimental interstitial nephritis. J Exp Med 162:1892-1903, 1985.

112. Singer GG, Yokoyama H, Bloom RD, et al: Stimulated renal tubular epithelial cells induce anergy in CD4+ T cells. Kidney Int 44:1030-1035, 1993.

113. Neilson EG: Is immunologic tolerance of self modulated through antigen presentation by parenchymal epithelium? Kidney Int 44:927-931, 1993.

114. Heeger PS, Neilson EG: Overcoming tolerance in autoimmune renal disease. Curr Opin Nephrol Hypertens 3:123-132, 1994.

115. Andres G, Brentjens J, Kohli R, et al: Histology of human tubulo-interstitial nephritis associated with antibodies to renal basement membranes. Kidney Int 13:480-491, 1978.

116. Kalluri IR, Gunwar S, Reeders S, et al: Goodpasture syndrome. Localization of the epitope for the autoantibodies to the carboxyl-terminal region of the alpha 3(IV) chain of basement membrane collagen. J Biol Chem 266:24018-24024, 1991.

117. Klassen J, Kano K, Milgrom F, et al: Tubular lesions produced by autoantibodies to tubular basement membrane in human renal allografts. Int Arch Allergy Immunol 45:675-682, 1973.

118. Wilson CB, Lehman DH, McCoy RC, et al: Antitubular basement membrane antibodies after renal transplantation. Transplantation 18:447-452, 1974.

119. Andrews BS, Eisenberg RA, Theofilopoulos AN, et al: Spontaneous murine lupus-like syndromes. Clinical and immunopathological manifestations in several strains. J Exp Med 148:1198-1215, 1978.

120. Lehman DH, Wilson CB, Dixon FJ: Extraglomerular immunoglobulin deposits in human nephritis. Am J Med 58:765-796, 1975.

121. Salant DJ, Quigg RJ, Cybulsky AV: Heymann nephritis: Mechanisms of renal injury. Kidney Int 35:976-984, 1989.

122. Mendrick DL, Noble B, Brentjens JR, et al: Antibody-mediated injury to proximal tubules in Heymann's nephritis. Kidney Int 18:328-343, 1980.

123. Brentjens JR, Matsuo S, Fukatsu A, et al: Immunologic studies in two patients with antitubular basement membrane nephritis. Am J Med 86:603-608, 1989.

124. Brentjens JR, Andres G: Lesions of the kidney caused by the interaction of antibodies with antigens on the surface of renal cells, Kidney Int 35:954-968, 1989.

125. Steblay RW, Rudofsky U: Transfer of experimental autoimmune renal cortical tubular and interstitial disease in guinea pigs by serum. Science 180:966-968, 1973.

126. Zakheim B, McCafferty E, Phillips SM, et al: Murine interstitial nephritis. II. The adoptive transfer of disease with immune T lymphocytes produces a phenotypically complex interstitial lesion. J Immunol 133:234-239, 1984.

127. Hall CL, Colvin RB, Carey K, McCluskey R: Passive transfer of autoimmune disease with isologous IgG1 and IgG2 antibodies to the tubular basement membrane in strain XIII guinea pigs. J Exp Med 146:1246-1260, 1977.

128. Clayman MD, Michaud L, Neilson EG: Murine interstitial nephritis. VI. Characterization of the B cell response in anti-tubular basement membrane disease. J Immunol 139:2242-2249, 1987.

129. Zanetti M, Wilson CB: Characterization of anti-tubular basement membrane antibodies in rats. J Immunol 130:2173-2179, 1983.

130. Ulich TR, Bannister KM, Wilson CB: Tubulointerstitial nephritis induced in the Brown Norway rat with chaotropically solubilized bovine tubular basement membrane: The model and the humoral and cellular responses. Clin Immunol Immunopathol 36:187-200, 1985.

131. Hyman LR, Colvin RB, Steinberg AD: Immunopathogenesis of autoimmune tubulointerstitial nephritis. I. Demonstration of differential susceptibility in strain II and strain XIII guinea pigs. J Immunol 116:327-335, 1976.

132. Bannister KM, Wilson CB: Transfer of tubulointerstitial nephritis in the Brown Norway rat with anti-tubular basement membrane antibody: Quantitation and kinetics of binding and effect of decomplementation. J Immunol 135:3911-3917, 1995.

133. Rudofsky UH, Dilwith RL, Tung KS: Susceptibility differences of inbred mice to induction of autoimmune renal tubulointerstitial lesions. Lab Invest 43:463-470, 1980.

134. Haverty TP, Watanabe M, Neilson EG, Kelly CJ: Protective modulation of class II MHC gene expression in tubular epithelium by target antigen-specific antibodies. Cell-surface directed down-regulation of transcription can influence susceptibility to murine tubulointerstitial nephritis. J Immunol 143:1133-1141, 1989.

135. Karp SL, Kieber-Emmons T, Sun MJ, et al: The molecular structure of a cross-reacting idiotype on autoantibodies recognizing parenchymal self. J Immunol 150:867-879, 1993.

136. Brown CA, Carey K, Colvin RB: Inhibition of autoimmune tubulointerstitial nephritis in guinea pigs by heterologous antisera containing anti-idiotype antibodies. J Immunol 123:2102-2107, 1979.

137. Neilson EG, Phillips M: Suppression of interstitial nephritis by auto-anti-idiotypic immunity. J Exp Med 155:179-189, 1982.

138. Neilson EG, McCafferty E, Phillips SM, et al: Antiidiotypic immunity in interstitial nephritis. II. Rats developing anti-tubular basement membrane disease fail to make an antiidiotypic regulatory response: The modulatory role of an RT7.1+,OX8-suppressor T cell mechanism. J Exp Med 159:1009-1026, 1984.

139. Zanetti M, Mampaso F, Wilson CB: Anti-idiotype as a probe in the analysis of autoimmune tubulointerstitial nephritis in the Brown-Norway rats. J Immunol 131:1268-1273, 1983.

140. Clayman MD, Sun MJ, Michaud L, et al: Clonotypic heterogeneity in experimental interstitial nephritis. Restricted specificity of the anti-tubular basement membrane B cell repertoire is associated with a disease-modifying crossreactive idiotype. J Exp Med 167:1296-1312, 1988.

141. McLeish KR, Sentizer D, Gohara AF: Acute interstitial nephritis in a patient with aspirin hypersensitivity. Clin Immunol Immunopathol 14:64-69, 1979.

142. Rosenberg ME, Schendel PB, McCurdy FA, Platt JL: Characterization of immune cells in kidneys from patients with Sjögren's syndrome. Am J Kidney Dis 11:20-22, 1988.

143. Stachura I, Si L, Madan E, Whiteside T: Mononuclear cell subsets in human renal disease. Enumeration in tissue sections with monoclonal antibodies. Clin Immunol Immunopathol 30:362-373, 1984.

144. Husby G, Tung KS, Williams RC Jr: Characterization of renal tissue lymphocytes in patients with interstitial nephritis. Am J Med 70:31-38, 1981.

145. Bender WL, Whelton A, Beschorner WE, et al: Interstitial nephritis, proteinuria, and renal failure caused by nonsteroidal anti-inflammatory drugs. Immunologic characterization of the inflammatory infiltrate. Am J Med 76:1006-1012, 1984.

146. Boucher A, Droz D, Adafer E, Noel LH: Characterization of mononuclear cell subsets in renal cellular interstitial infiltrates. Kidney Int 29:1043-1049, 1986.

147. Cheng HF, Nolasco F, Cameron JS, et al: HLA-DR display by renal tubular epithelium and phenotype of infiltrate in interstitial nephritis. Nephrol Dial Transplant 4:205-215, 1989.

148. Neilson EG, McCafferty E, Mann R, et al: Murine interstitial nephritis. III. The selection of phenotypic (Lyt and L3T4) and idiotypic (RE-Id) T cell preferences by genes in Igh-1 and H-2K characterizes the cell-mediated potential for disease expression: Susceptible mice provide a unique effector T cell repertoire in response to tubular antigen. J Immunol 134:2375-2382, 1985.

149. Kelly CJ, Clayman MD, Neilson EG: Immunoregulation in experimental interstitial nephritis: Immunization with renal tubular antigen in incomplete Freund's adjuvant induces major histocompatibility complex-restricted, OX8+ suppressor T cells which are antigen-specific and inhibit the expression of disease. J Immunol 136:903-907, 1986.

150. Babbitt BP, Allen PM, Matsueda G, et al: Binding of immunogenic peptides to Ia histocompatibility molecules. Nature 317:359-361, 1985.

151. Unanue ER, Allen PM: The basis for the immunoregulatory role of macrophages and other accessory cells. Science 236:551-557, 1987.

152. Hagerty DT, Allen PM: Processing and presentation of self and foreign antigens by the renal proximal tubule. J Immunol 148:2324-2330, 1992.

153. Hines WH, Haverty TP, Elias JA, et al: T cell recognition of epithelial self. Autoimmunity 5:37-47, 1989.

154. Mendrick DL, Kelly DM, Rennke HG: Antigen processing and presentation by glomerular visceral epithelium in vitro. Kidney Int 39:71-78, 1991.

155. Rubin Kelley VR, Singer GG: The antigen presentation function of renal tubular epithelial cells. Exp Nephrol 1:102-111, 1993.

156. Hagerty DT, Evavold BD, Allen PM: Regulation of the costimulator B7, not class II major histocompatibility complex, restricts the ability of murine kidney tubule cells to stimulate CD4+ T cells. J Clin Invest 93:1208-1215, 1994.

157. Wahl P, Schoop R, Bilic G, et al: Renal tubular epithelial expression of the costimulatory molecule B7RP-1 (inducible costimulatory ligand). J Am Soc Nephrol 13:1517-1526, 2002.

158. Hagerty DT: Intercellular adhesion molecule-1 is necessary but not sufficient to activate CD4+ T cells. Discovery of a novel costimulator on kidney cells. J Immunol 156:3652-3659, 1996.

159. Deckers JG, De Haij S, van der Woude FJ, et al: IL-4 and IL-13 augment cytokine- and CD40-induced RANTES production by human renal tubular epithelial cells in vitro. J Am Soc Nephrol 9:1187-1193, 1998.

160. Murata H, Kita Y, Sakamoto A, et al: Limited TCR repertoire of infiltrating T cells in the kidneys of Sjögren's syndrome patients with interstitial nephritis. J Immunol 155:4084-4089, 1995.

161. Heeger PS, Smoyer WE, Jones M, et al: Heterogeneous T cell receptor V beta gene repertoire in murine interstitial nephritis. Kidney Int 49:1222-1230, 1996.

162. Bannister KM, Ulich TR, Wilson CB: Induction, characterization, and cell transfer of autoimmune tubulointerstitial nephritis in the Lewis rat. Kidney Int 32:642-651, 1987.

163. Meyers CM, Kelly CJ: Effector mechanisms in organ-specific autoimmunity. I. Characterization of a CD8+ T cell line that mediates murine interstitial nephritis. J Clin Invest 88:408-416, 1991.

164. Nathan C: Secretory products of macrophages. J Clin Invest 79:319-326, 1987.

165. Mizel SB, Dayer J-M, Krane SM, Mergenhagen SE: Stimulation of rheumatoid synovial cell collagenase and prostaglandin production by partially purified lymphocyte activating factor (interleukin 1). Proc Natl Acad Sci U S A 78:2474-2477, 1981.

166. Roberts AB, Sporn MB, Assoian RK, et al: Transforming growth factor type β: Rapid induction of fibrosis and angiogenesis *in vivo* and stimulation of collagen formation *in vitro*. Proc Natl Acad Sci U S A 83:4167-4171, 1986.

167. Sporn MB, Roberts AB: Peptide growth factors are multifunctional. Nature 332:217-219, 1988.

168. Beutle B, Cerami A: Cachectin and tumour necrosis factor as two sides of the same biological coin. Nature 320:584-588, 1986.

169. Haverty TP, Kelly CJ, Hoyer JR, et al: Tubular antigen-binding proteins repress transcription of type IV collagen in the autoimmune target epithelium of experimental interstitial nephritis. J Clin Invest 89:517-523, 1992.

170. Masson D, Tschopp J: A family of serine esterases in lytic granules of cytoltyic T lymphocytes. Cell 49:679-685, 1987.

171. Gershenfeld HK, Weissman IL: Cloning of a cDNA for a T cell-specific serine protease from a cytotoxic T lymphocyte. Science 232:854-858, 1986.

172. Lowrey DM, Aebischer T, Olsen K, et al: Cloning, analysis, and expression of murine perforin 1 cDNA, a component of cytolytic T cell granules with homology to complement component C9. Proc Natl Acad Sci U S A 86:247-251, 1989.

173. Podack ER, Young JD-E, Cohn ZA: Isolation and biochemical and functional characterization of perforin 1 from cytolytic T cell granules. Proc Natl Acad Sci U S A 82:8629-8633, 1985.

174. Zalman LS, Martin DE, Jung G, Muller-Eberhard HJ: The cytolytic protein of human lymphocytes related to the ninth component (c9) of human complement: Isolation from anti-CD3 activated peripheral blood mononuclear cells. Proc Natl Acad Sci U S A 84:2426-2429, 1987.

175. Meyers CM, Kelly CJ: Immunoregulation and TGF-beta 1. Suppression of a nephritogenic murine T cell clone. Kidney Int 46:1295-1301, 1994.

176. Meyers CM, Kelly CJ: Inhibition of murine nephritogenic effector T cells by a clone-specific suppressor factor. J Clin Invest 94:2093-2104, 1994.

177. Bailey NC, Kelly CJ: Nephritogenic T cells use granzyme C as a cytotoxic mediator. Eur J Immunol 27:2302-2309, 1997.

178. Couser WG: Mechanisms of glomerular injury: An overview. Semin Nephrol 11:254-258, 1991.

179. Hyun J, Galen MA: Acute interstitial nephritis. A case characterized by increase in serum IgG, IgM, and IgE concentrations. Eosinophilia, and IgE deposition in renal tubules. Arch Intern Med 141:679-681, 1981.

180. Nath KA, Hostetter MK, Hostetter TH: Pathophysiology of chronic tubulo-interstitial disease in rats. Interactions of dietary acid load, ammonia, and complement C3. J Clin Invest 76:667-675, 1985.

181. Tolins JP, Hostetter MK, Hostetter TH: Hypokalemic nephropathy in the rat: Role of ammonia in chronic tubular injury. J Clin Invest 79:1447, 1987.

182. Clark EC, Nath KA, Hostetter MK, Hostetter TH: Role of ammonia in tubulointerstitial injury. Miner Electrolyte Metab 16:315-321, 1990.

183. Welch TR, Frenzke M, Witte D, Davis AE: C5a is important in the tubulointerstitial component of experimental immune complex glomerulonephritis. Clin Exp Immunol 130:43-48, 2002.

184. Heeger P, Wolf G, Sun MJ, Meyers C, et al: Isolation and characterization of cDNA from renal tubular cells encoding murine RANTES, a small cytokine from the Scy superfamily. Kidney Int 41:220-225, 1992.

185. Deckers JG, Van Der Woude FJ, Van Der Kooij SW, Daha MR: Synergistic effect of IL-1, IFN-γ, and TNF-α on RANTES production by human renal tubular epithelial cells in vitro. J Am Soc Nephrol 9:194-202, 1998.

186. Gerritsma JS, Hiemstra PS, Gerritsen AF, et al: Regulation and production of IL-8 by human proximal tubular epithelial cells in vitro. Clin Exp Immunol 103:289-294, 1996.

187. Grandaliano G, Gesualdo L, Ranieri E, et al: Monocyte chemotactic peptide-1 expression in acute and chronic human nephrites: A pathogenetic role in interstitial monocytes recruitment. J Am Soc Nephrol 7:906-913, 1996.

188. Lloyd CM, Minto AW, Dorf ME, et al: RANTES and monocyte chemoattractant protein-1 (MCP-1) play an important role in the inflammatory phase of crescentic nephritis, but only MCP-1 is involved in crescent formation and interstitial fibrosis. J Exp Med 185:1371-1380, 1997.

189. Mossman TR, Coffman RL: TH1 and TH2 cells: Different patterns of lymphokine secretion lead to different functional properties. Annu Rev Immunol 7:145-173, 1989.

190. Nathan C: Nitric oxide as a secretory product of mammalian cells. FASEB J 6:3051-3064, 1992.

191. Kelly CJ, Frishberg Y, Gold DP: An appraisal of T cell subsets and the potential for autoimmune injury. Kidney Int 53:1574-1584, 1998.

192. Gabbai FB, Boggiano C, Peter T, et al: Inhibition of inducible nitric oxide synthase intensifies injury and functional deterioration in autoimmune interstitial nephritis. J Immunol 159:6266-6275, 1997.

193. Gold DP, Schroder K, Powell HC, Kelly CJ: Nitric oxide and the immunomodulation of experimental allergic encephalomyelitis. Eur J Immunol 27:2863-2869, 1997.

194. Bogdan C: The multiplex function of nitric oxide in (auto)immunity. J Exp Med 187:1361-1365, 1998.

195. Genain CP, Abel K, Belmar N, et al: Late complications of immune deviation therapy in a nonhuman primate. Science 274:2054-2057, 1996.

196. Libby P, Fiedman GB, Saloman RN: Cytokines as modulators of cell proliferation in fibrotic diseases. Am Rev Respir Dis 140:1114-1117, 1989.

197. Freundlich B, Bomalaski JS, Neilson EG, Jimenez SA: Immune regulation of fibroblast proliferation and collagen synthesis by soluble factors from mononuclear cells. Immunol Today 7:303-307, 1986.

198. Strutz F, Neilson EG: Transdifferentiation: A new angle on renal fibrosis. Exp Nephrol 4:267-270, 1996.

199. Kuncio GS, Neilson EG, Haverty TP: Mechanisms of tubulointerstitial fibrosis. Kidney Int 39:550-556, 1992.

200. Alvarez RJ, Haverty TP, Watanabe M, et al: Biosynthetic and proliferative heterogeneity of anatomically distinct fibroblasts probed with paracine cytokines. Kidney Int 41:14-23, 1992.

201. Muller GA, Rodemann HP: Characterization of human renal fibroblasts in health and disease. I. Immunophenotyping of cultured tubular epithelial cells and fibroblasts derived form kidneys with histologically proven interstitial fibrosis. Am J Kidney Dis 17:680-683, 1991.

202. Rodemann HP, Muller GA: Characterization of human renal fibroblasts in health and disease: II. In vitro growth, differentiation, and collagen synthesis of fibroblasts from kidneys with interstitial fibrosis. Am J Kidney Dis 17:R684-R686, 1991.

203. Tang WW, Ulich TR, Lacey DL, et al: Platelet-derived growth factor-BB induces renal tubulointerstitial myofibroblast formation and tubulointerstitial fibrosis. Am J Pathol 148:1169-1180, 1996.

204. Strutz F, Neilson EG: The role of lymphocytes in the progression of interstitial disease. Kidney Int Suppl 45:S106-S110, 1994.

205. Remuzzi G, Bertani T: Pathophysiology of progressive nephropathies. N Engl J Med 339:1448-1456, 1998.

206. Tang S, Leung JC, Abe K, et al: Albumin stimulates interleukin-8 expression in proximal tubular epithelial cells in vitro and in vivo. J Clin Invest 111:515-527, 2003.

207. Neilson EG, Plieth D, Venkov C: Epithelial-mesenchymal transitions and the intersecting cell fate of fibroblasts and metastatic cancer cells. Trans Am Clin Climatol Assoc 114:87-100, 2003.

208. Okada H, Strutz F, Danoff TM, et al: Possible mechanisms of renal fibrosis. Contrib Nephrol 118:147-154, 1996.

209. Yang CW, Faulkner GR, Wahba IM, et al: Expression of apoptosis-related genes in chronic cyclosporine nephrotoxicity in mice. Am J Transplant 2:391-399, 2002.

210. Razzaque MS, Ahsan N, Taguchi T: Role apoptosis in fibrogenesis. Nephron 90:365-372, 2002.

211. Keller F, Rehbein C, Schwarz A, et al: Increased procollagen III production in patients with kidney disease. Nephron 50:332-337, 1988.

212. Bornstein P, Sage H: Regulation of collagen gene expression. Prog Nucleic Acid Res Mol Biol 37:67-106, 1989.

213. Truong LD, Foster SV, Barrios R, et al: Tenascin is an ubiquitous extracellular matrix protein of human renal interstitium in normal and pathologic conditions. Nephron 72:579-586, 1996.

214. Tang WW, Van GY, Qi M: Myofibroblasts and alpha 1(III) collagen expression in experimental tubulointerstitial nephritis. Kidney Int 51:926-931, 1997.

215. Ruiz-Ortega M, Gomez-Garre D, Alcazar R, et al: Involvement of angiotensin II and endothelin in matrix protein production and renal sclerosis. J Hypertens Suppl 12:S51-S58, 1994.

216. Neilson EG, Jimenez SA, Phillips SM: Cell-mediated immunity in interstitial nephritis. III. T lymphocyte-mediated fibroblast proliferation and collagen synthesis: An immune mechanism for renal fibrogenesis. J Immunol 125:1708-1714, 1980.

217. Hugo C, Pichler R, Shackland S, et al: Thrombospondin 1 (TSP1) precedes and predicts tubulointerstitial fibrosis in glomerular disease [abstract]. J Am Soc Nephrol 8:A897, 1996.

218. Pichler RH, Bassuck JA, Hugo C, et al: SPARC is expressed by mesangial cells in experimental mesangial proliferative nephritis and inhibits platelet-derived-growth-factor–mediated mesangial cell proliferation in vitro. Am J Pathol 148:1153-1167, 1994.

219. Giachelli CM, Pichler R, Lombardi D, et al: Osteopontin expression in angiotensin II-induced tubulointerstitial nephritis. Kidney Int 45:515-524, 1994.

220. Sibalic V, Fan X, Loffing J, Wuthrich RP: Upregulated renal tubular CD44, hyaluronan, and osteopontin in kdkd mice with interstitial nephritis. Nephrol Dial Transplant 12:1344-1353, 1997.

221. Strutz F, Neilson EG: New insights into mechanisms of fibrosis in immune renal injury. Semin Immunol Immunopathol 24:459-476, 2003.

222. Neilson EG, Phillips SM, Jimenez S: Lymphokine modulation of fibroblast proliferation. J Immunol 128:1484-1486, 1982.

223. Ishidoya S, Morrissey J, McCraken R, et al: Angiotensin II receptor antagonist ameliorates renal tubulointerstitial fibrosis caused by unilateral ureteral obstruction. Kidney Int 47:1285-1294, 1995.

224. Pimentel JL Jr, Sundell CL, Wang S, et al: Role of angiotensin II in the expression and regulation of transforming growth factor-beta in obstructive nephropathy. Kidney Int 48:1233-1246, 1995.

225. Noble NA, Border WA: Angiotensin II in renal fibrosis: Should TGFβ rather than blood pressure be the therapeutic target? Semin Nephrol 17:455-466, 1997.

226. Yang J, Liu Y: Blockage of tubular epithelial to myofibroblast transition by hepatocyte growth factor prevents renal interstitial fibrosis. J Am Soc Nephrol 13:96-107, 2002.

227. Yang J, Dai C, Liu Y: Hepatocyte growth factor gene therapy and angiotensin II blockade synergistically attenuate renal interstitial fibrosis in mice. J Am Soc Nephrol 13:2464-2477, 2002.

228. Inoue T, Okada H, Kobayashi T, et al: Hepatocyte growth factor counteracts transforming growth factor-beta 1, through attenuation of connective tissue growth factor induction, and prevents renal fibrogenesis in 5/6 nephrectomized mice. FASEB J 17:268-270, 2003.

229. Okada H, Danoff TM, Kalluri R, Neilson EG: An early role for FSP1 in epithelial-mesenchymal transformation. Am J Physiol 273:563-574, 1997.

230. Surendran K, McCaul SP, Simon TC: A role for Wnt-4 in renal fibrosis. Am J Physiol 282:F431-F441, 2002.

231. Hocher B, Thöne-Reineke C, Rohmeiss P, et al: Endothelin transgenic mice develop glomerulosclerosis, interstitial fibrosis, and renal cysts but not hypertension. J Clin Invest 99:1380-1389, 1997.

232. Mezzano SA, Ruiz-Ortega M, Egido J: Angiotensin II and renal fibrosis. Hypertension 38:635-638, 2001.

233. Brown NJ, Vaughan DE, Fogo AB: Aldosterone and PAI-1: Implications for renal injury. J Nephrol 15:230-235, 2002.

234. Brown NJ, Vaughan DE, Fogo AB: The renin-angiotensin-aldosterone system and fibrinolysis in progressive renal disease. Semin Nephrol 22:399-406, 2002.

235. Okada H, Inoue T, Kanno Y, et al: Interstitial fibroblast-like cells express renin-angiotensin system components in a fibrosing murine kidney. Am J Pathol 160:765-772, 2002.

236. Wolf G, Neilson EG: Angiotensin II as a renal growth factor. J Am Soc Nephrol 3:1531-1540, 1993.

237. Wolf G, Haberstroh U, Neilson EG: Angiotensin II stimulates the proliferation and biosynthesis of type I collagen in cultured murine mesangial cells. Am J Pathol 140:95-107, 1992.

238. Tharaux PL, Chatziantoniou C, Fakhouri F, Dussaule JC: Angiotensin II activates collagen I gene through a mechanism involving the MAP/ER kinase pathway. Hypertension 36:330-336, 2000.

239. Fakhouri F, Placier S, Ardaillou R, et al: Angiotensin II activates collagen type I gene in the renal cortex and aorta of transgenic mice through interaction with endothelin and TGF-beta. J Am Soc Nephrol 12:2701-2710, 2001.

240. Ng Y-Y, Huang T-P, Yang W-C, et al: Tubular epithelial-myofibroblast transdifferentiation in progressive tubulointerstitial fibrosis in 5/6 nephrectomized rats. Kidney Int 54:864-877, 1998.

241. Okada H, Ban S, Nagao S, et al: Progressive renal fibrosis in murine polycystic kidney disease: An immunohistochemical observation. Kidney Int 58:587-597, 2000.

242. Okada H, Danoff TM, Strutz F, et al: Novel cis-acting elements in the *FSP1* gene regulate fibroblast-specific transcription. Am J Physiol 44:306-311, 1998.

243. Wiggins R, Goyal M, Merritt S, Killen PD: Vascular adventitial cell expression of collagen I messenger ribonucleic acid in anti-glomerular basement membrane antibody-induced crescentic nephritis in the rabbit. A cellular source for interstitial collagen synthesis in inflammatory renal disease. Lab Invest 68:557-565, 1993.

244. Iwano M, Plieth D, Danoff TM, et al: Evidence that fibroblasts derive from epithelium during tissue fibrosis. J Clin Invest 110:341-350, 2002.

245. Hay ED, Zuk A: Transformations between epithelium and mesenchyme: Normal, pathological, and experimentally induced. Am J Kidney Dis 26:678-690, 1995.

246. Ng YY, Fan JM, Mu W, et al: Glomerular epithelial-myofibroblast transdifferentiation in the evolution of glomerular crescent formation. Nephrol Dial Transplant 14:2860-2872, 1999.

247. Fujigaki Y, Sun DF, Fujimoto T, et al: Mechanisms and kinetics of Bowman's epithelial-myofibroblast transdifferentiation in the formation of glomerular crescents. Nephron 92:203-212, 2002.

248. Ina K, Kitamura H, Tatsukawa S, et al: Transformation of interstitial fibroblasts and tubulointerstitial fibrosis in diabetic nephropathy. Med Electron Microsc 35:87-95, 2002.

249. Jinde K, Nikolic-Paterson DJ, Huang XR, et al: Tubular phenotypic change in progressive tubulointerstitial fibrosis in human glomerulonephritis. Am J Kidney Dis 38:761-769, 2001.

250. Zeisberg M, Bonner G, Maeshima Y, et al: Renal fibrosis: collagen composition and assembly regulates epithelial-mesenchymal transdifferentiation. Am J Pathol 159:1313-1321, 2001.

251. Zeisberg M, Maeshima Y, Mosterman B, Kalluri R: Renal fibrosis. Extracellular matrix microenvironment regulates migratory behavior of activated tubular epithelial cells. Am J Pathol 160:2001-2008, 2002.

252. Yang J, Shultz RW, Mars WM, et al: Disruption of tissue-type plasminogen activator gene in mice reduces renal interstitial fibrosis in obstructive nephropathy. J Clin Invest 110:1525-1538, 2002.

253. Oda T, Jung YO, Kim HS, et al: PAI-1 deficiency attenuates the fibrogenic response to ureteral obstruction. Kidney Int 60:587-596, 2001.

254. Strutz F, Zeisberg M, Ziyadeh FN, et al: Role of basic fibroblast growth factor-2 in epithelial-mesenchymal transformation. Kidney Int 61:1714-1728, 2002.

255. Alpers CE, Seifert RA, Hudkins KL, et al: PDGF-receptors localize to mesangial, parietal epithelial and interstitial cells in human and primate kidneys. Kidney Int 43:286-294, 1993.

256. Fellström B, Klareskog L, Heldin CH, et al: Platelet-derived growth factor receptors in the kidney—Upregulated expression in inflammation. Kidney Int 36:1099-1102, 1989.

257. Lindahl P, Johansson BR, Levéen P, Betsholtz C: Pericyte loss and microaneurysm formation in PDGF-β-deficient mice. Science 277:242-245, 1997.

258. Shimokado K, Raines EW, Madtes DK, et al: A significant part of macrophage-derived growth factor consists of at least two forms of PDGF. Cell 43:277-286, 1985.

259. Wahl S, Hunt D, Wakefield L, et al: Transforming growth factor beta (TGF-β) induces monocyte chemotaxis and growth factor production. Proc Natl Acad Sci U S A 84:5788-5792, 1987.

260. Postlethwaite AE, Synderman R, Kang AH: Generation of a fibroblast chemotactic factor in serum by activation of complement. J Clin Invest 64:1379-1385, 1979.

261. Postlethwaite AE, Seyer JM, Kang AH: Chemotactic attraction of human fibroblasts to type I, II, III collagens and collagen-derived peptides. Proc Natl Acad Sci U S A 75:871-875, 1978.

262. Wahl LM, Winter CC: Regulation of guinea pig macrophage collagenase production by dexamethasone and colchicine. Arch Biochem Biophys 230:661-667, 1984.

263. Schmidt JA, Mizel SB, Cohen D, Green I: Interleukin-1, a potential regulator of fibroblast proliferation. J Immunol 128:2177-2181, 1982.

264. Vilcek J, Palombell VJ, Hinriksen-DeStefano D, et al: Fibroblast growth enhancing activity of tumor necrosis factor and its relationship to other polypeptide growth factors. J Exp Med 163:632-643, 1986.

265. Roberts A, Flanders KC, Kondaiah P, et al: Transforming growth factor β: Biochemistry and roles in embryogenesis, tissue repair and remodeling, and carcinogenesis. Recent Prog Horm Res 44:57-197, 1988.

266. Haverty TP, Kelly CJ, Hines WH, et al: Characterization of a renal tubular epithelial cell line which secretes the autologous target antigen of autoimmune experimental interstitial nephritis. J Cell Biol 107:1359-1368, 1988.

267. Creely JJ, Commers PA, Haralson MA: Synthesis of type III collagen by cultured kidney epithelial cells. Connect Tissue Res 18:107-122, 1988.

268. Vaheri A, Salonen E-M, Varito T: Fibronectin in formation and degradation of the pericellular matrix. Ciba Found Symp 114:111-126, 1985.

269. Wahl SM: Fibrosis: Bacterial-cell-wall-induced hepatic granulomas. *In* Gallin JI, Goldstein IM, Snyderman R. (eds): Inflammation: Basic Principles and Clinical Correlates. New York, Raven Press, 1988, pp. 841-859.

270. Dean DC, Newby RF, Bourgeois J: Regulation of fibronectin biosynthesis by dexamethasone, transforming growth factor β, cAMP in human cell lines. J Cell Biol 106:2159-2170, 1988.

271. Kerr LD, Miller DB: TGFβ-1 inhibition of transin/stromelysin gene expression is mediated through a fos binding sequence. Cell 61:267-278, 1990.

272. Schaefer L, Macakova K, Raslik I, et al: Absence of decorin adversely influences tubulointerstitial fibrosis of the obstructed kidney by enhanced apoptosis and increased inflammatory reaction. Am J Pathol 160:1181-1191, 2002.

273. Iwano M, Fischer A, Okada H, et al: Conditional abatement of tissue fibrosis using nucleoside analogs to selectively corrupt DNA replication in transgenic fibroblasts. Mol Ther 3:149-159, 2001.

274. Pettersson E, von-Bonsdorff M, Tornroth T, Lindholm H: Nephritis among young Finnish men. Clin Nephrol 22:217-222, 1984.

275. Davison AM, et al: Acute interstitial nephritis in the elderly: A report from the UK MRC Glomerulonephritis Register and a review of the literature. Nephrol Dial Transplant 13(suppl 7):12-16, 1998.

276. Wilson DB: Value of renal biopsy in acute intrinsic renal failure. BMJ 2:447-459, 1978.

277. Murray T, Goldberg M: Chronic interstitial nephritis: Etiologic factors. Ann Intern Med 82:453-459, 1975.

278. Galpin JE, Shinaberger JH, Stanley TM, et al: Acute interstitial nephritis due to methicillin. Am J Med 65:756-765, 1978.

279. Murray MD, Brater DC: Renal toxicity of the nonsteroidal anti-inflammatory drugs. Annu Rev Pharmacol Toxicol 33:435-465, 1993.

280. Cameron JS: Tubular and interstitial factors in the progression of glomerulonephritis. Pediatr Nephrol 6:292-303, 1992.

281. Olsen TS, Wassef NF, Olsen HS, Hansen HE: Ultrastructure of the kidney in acute interstitial nephritis. Ultrastruct Pathol 10:1-16, 1986.

282. Muller GA, Muller CA, Markovic LJ, et al: Renal major histocompatibility complex antigens and cellular components in rapidly progressive glomerulonephritis identified by monoclonal antibodies. Nephron 49:132-139, 1988.

283. Patel R, Connor G, Patel DR, et al: T cell subsets in idiopathic glomerulonephritis. Int Arch Allergy Immunol 79:182-187, 1986.

284. Saito T, Atkins RC: Contribution of mononuclear leucocytes to the progression of experimental focal glomerular sclerosis. Kidney Int 37:1076-1083, 1990.

285. Muller GA, Markovic-Lipkovski J, Rodemann HP: The progression of renal diseases: On the pathogenesis of renal interstitial fibrosis. Klin Wochenschr 69:576-586, 1991.

286. Langer KH, Thoenes W: Characterization of cells involved in the formation of granuloma. An ultrastructural study on macrophages, epithelioid cells, and giant cells in experimental tubulointerstitial nephritis. Virchows Arch 36:177-194, 1981.

287. Mignon F, Mery JP, Mougenot B, et al: Granulomatous interstitial nephritis. Adv Nephrol Necker Hosp 13:219-245, 1984.

288. Singer DR, Simpson JG, Catto GR, Johnston AW: Drug hypersensitivity causing granulomatous interstitial nephritis. Am J Kidney Dis 11:357-359, 1988.

289. van-Dorp WT, Jie K, Lobatto S, et al: Renal failure due to granulomatous interstitial nephritis after pulmonary sarcoidosis. Nephrol Dial Transplant 2:573-575, 1987.

290. Hannedouche T, Grateau G, Noel LH, et al: Renal granulomatous sarcoidosis: Report of six cases. Nephrol Dial Transplant 5:18-24, 1990.

291. Somvanshi PP, Patni PD, Khan MA: Renal involvement in chronic pulmonary tuberculosis. Indian J Med Sci 43:55-58, 1989.

292. Fannin SW, Hagley MT, Seibert JD, Koenig TJ: Bronchocentric granulomatosis, acute renal failure, and high titer antineutrophil cytoplasmic antibodies: Possible variants of Wegener's granulomatosis. J Rheumatol 20:507-509, 1993.

293. Ditlove J, Werdmann P, Bernstein M, Massry SG: Methicillin nephritis. Medicine (Baltimore) 56:483-505, 1977.

294. Appel GB, Garvey G, Silva F, et al: Acute intestinal nephritis due to amoxicillin therapy. Nephron 27:313-315, 1981.

295. Ooi BS, Pesce AJ, First MR, et al: IgE levels in interstitial nephritis. Lancet 1:1254-1256, 1974.

296. Laberke HG, Bohle A: Acute interstitial nephritis: Correlations between clinical and morphological findings. Clin Nephrol 14:263-273, 1980.

297. van Ypersele de Strihou C: Aucte oliguric interstitial nephritis. Kidney Int 16:751-760, 1979.

298. Appel GB, Kunis CL: Acute tubulointerstitial nephritis. *In* Cotran RS, Brenner BM, Stein JH (eds): Contemporary Issues in Nephrology. New York, Churchill Livingstone, 1983, pp 151-185.

299. Lyons H, Pinn VW, Cortell S, et al: Allergic interstitial nephritis causing reversible renal failure in four patients with idiopathic nephrotic syndrome. N Engl J Med 288:124-128, 1973.

300. Linton AL, Clark WF, Driedger AA, et al: Acute interstitial nephritis due to drugs: Review of the literature with a report of nine cases. Ann Intern Med 93:735-741, 1980.

301. Ooi BS, Jao W, First MR, et al: Acute interstitial nephritis. A clinical and pathologic study based on renal biopsies. Am J Med 59:614-628, 1975.

302. Sigala JF, Biava CG, Hulter HN: Red blood cell casts in acute interstitial nephritis. Arch Intern Med 138:1419-1421, 1978.

303. Corwin HL, Bray RA, Haber MH: The detection and interpretation of urinary eosinophils. Arch Pathol Lab Med 113:1256-1258, 1989.

304. Nolan CR, Anger MS, Kelleher SP: Eosinophiluria—a new method of detection and definition of the clinical spectrum. N Engl J Med 315:1516-1519, 1986.

305. Ellis D, Fried WA, Yunis EJ, Blau EB: Acute interstitial nephritis in children: A report of 13 cases and review of the literature. Pediatrics 67:862-870, 1981.

306. Lins RL, Verpooten GA, De-Clerck DS, De-Broe ME: Urinary indices in acute interstitial nephritis. Clin Nephrol 26:131-133, 1986.

307. van-Ypersele-de-Strihou C, Vandenbroucke JM, Levy M, et al: Diagnosis of epidemic and sporadic interstitial nephritis due to Hantaan-like virus in Belgium. Lancet 2:1493, 1983.

308. Simenhoff ML, Guild WR, Dammin GJ: Acute diffuse interstitial nephritis. Review of the literature and case report. Am J Med 44:618-625, 1968.

309. Kasama R, Sorbello A: Renal and electrolyte complications associated with antibiotic therapy. Am Fam Physician 53:227-232, 1996.

310. Rosenfield AT, Siegel NJ: Renal parenchymal disease: Histopathologic-sonographic correlation. Am J Radiol 137:793, 1981.

311. Patel PJ: Renal parenchymal disease: Histopathologic-sonographic correlation. Urol Int 41:289-291, 1986.

312. Wood BC, Sharma JN, Germann DR, et al: Gallium citrate Ga 67 imaging in noninfectious interstitial nephritis. Arch Intern Med 138:1665-1666, 1978.

313. Graham GD, Lundy MM, Moreno AJ: Failure of gallium-67 scintigraphy to identify reliably noninfectious interstitial nephritis: Concise communication. J Nucl Med 24:568-570, 1983.

314. Kumar B: Significance of delayed 67-gallium localization in the kidneys. J Nucl Med 17:872, 1976.

315. Linton AL, Richmond JM, Clark WF, et al: Gallium-67 scintigraphy in the diagnosis of acute renal disease. Clin Nephrol 24:84-87, 1985.

316. Bhaumik SK, Kher V, Arora P, et al: Evaluation of clinical and histological prognostic markers in drug-induced acute interstitial nephritis. Ren Fail 18:97-104, 1996.

317. Dharnidharka VR, Rosen S, Somers MJ, et al: Acute interstitial nephritis presenting as presumed minimal change nephrotic syndrome. Pediatr Nephrol 12: 576-578, 1998.

318. Fisher M, Nielson EG: Treatment of acute interstitial nephritis. *In* Brady H, Wilcox C (eds): Therapy in Nephrology and Hypertension, 2nd ed. Philadelphia, Saunders, 2003, pp 297-304.

319. Murry KM, Keane WR: Review of drug-induced acute interstitial nephritis. Pharmacotherapy 12:462-467, 1992.

320. Paller MS: Drug-induced nephropathies. Med Clin North Am 74:909-917, 1990.

321. Jorkasky DK, Singer I: Drug-induced tubulo-interstitial nephritis: Special cases. Semin Nephrol 8:62-71, 1988.

322. Quin JD: The nephrotoxicity of cephalosporins. Adverse Drug React Toxicol Rev 8:63-72, 1989.

323. Colvin RB, Burton JR, Hyslop NE Jr, et al: Penicillin-associated interstitial nephritis [letter]. Ann Intern Med 81:404-405, 1974.

324. Appel GB: A decade of penicillin related acute interstitial nephritis—more questions than answers. Clin Nephrol 13:151-154, 1980.

325. Guharoy SR, Kar S, McGalliard J: Suspected nafcillin-induced interstitial nephritis. Ann Pharmacother 27:170-173, 1993.

326. Pill MW, O'Neill CV, Chapman MM, Singh AK: Suspected acute interstitial nephritis induced by piperacillin-tazobactam. Pharmacotherapy 17:166-169, 1997.

327. Gabow PA, Lacher JW, Neff TA: Tubulointerstitial and glomerular nephritis associated with rifampin. Report of a case. JAMA 235: 2517-2518, 1976.

328. Katz MD, Lor E: Acute interstitial nephritis associated with intermittent rifampin use. Drug Intell Clin Pharm 20:789-792, 1986.

329. Neugarten J, Gallo GR, Baldwin DS: Rifampin-induced nephrotic syndrome and acute interstitial nephritis. Am J Nephrol 3:38-42, 1983.

330. Smith EJ, Light JA, Filo RS, Yum MN: Interstitial nephritis caused by trimethoprim-sulfamethoxazole in renal transplant recipients. JAMA 244:360-361, 1980.

331. Hadimeri H, Almroth G, Cederbrant K, et al: Allergic nephropathy associated with norfloxacin and ciprofloxcin therapy. Report of two cases and review of the literature. Scand J Urol Nephrol 31:481-485, 1997.

332. Storck D, Christmann D, Vetter JM, et al: Acute nephritis and allergic vasculitis due to phenindione [in French]. Semin Hop Paris 55:1330-1334, 1979.

333. Hoffman EW: Phenytoin-induced interstitial nephritis. South Med J 74:1160-1161, 1981.

334. Arellano F, Sacristan JA: Allopurinol hypersensitivity syndrome: A review. Ann Pharmacother 27:337-343, 1993.

335. Magner P, Sweet J, Bear RA: Granulomatous interstitial nephritis associated with allopurinol therapy. Can Med Assoc J 135:496-497, 1986.

336. Magil AB, Ballon HS, Cameron EC, Rae A: Acute interstitial nephritis associated with thiazide diuretics. Clinical and pathologic observations in three cases. Am J Med 69:939-943, 1980.

337. Jennings M, Shortland JR, Maddocks JL: Interstitial nephritis associated with furosemide. J R Soc Med 79:239-240, 1986.

338. Gaughan WJ, Sheth VR, Francos GC, et al: Ranitidine-induced acute interstitial nephritis with epithelial cell foot process fusion. Am J Kidney Dis 22:337-340, 1993.

339. Ozawa TT, Smith P Jr, Vance D, et al: Acute interstitial nephritis induced by cimetidine. J Tenn Med Assoc 80:411-413, 1987.

340. Stoves J, Rosenberg K, Harden P, Turney JH: Acute interstitial nephritis due to over-the-counter ibuprofen in a renal transplant recipient. Nephrol Dial Transplant 13:227-228, 1998.

341. Pirani CL, Valeri A, D'Agati V, Appel GB: Renal toxicity of non-steroidal anti-inflammatory drugs. Contrib Nephrol 55:159-175, 1987.

342. Henao J, Hisamuddin I, Nzerue CM, et al: Celecoxib-induced interstitial nephritis. Am J Kidney Dis 39:1313-1317, 2002.

343. Rocha JL, Fernandez-Alonso J: Acute tubulointerstitial nephritis associated with the selective COX-2 enzyme inhibitor, rofecoxib. Lancet 357:1946-1947, 2001.

344. Alper AB, Meleg-Smith S, Krane NK: Nephrotic syndrome and interstitial nephritis associated with celecoxib. Am J Kidney Dis 40:1086-1090, 2002.

345. Porile JL, Bakris GL, Garella S: Acute interstitial nephritis with glomerulopathy due to nonsteroidal anti-inflammatory agents: A review of its clinical spectrum and effects of steroid therapy. J Clin Pharmacol 30:468-475, 1990.

346. Brezin JH, Katz SM, Schwartz AB, Chinitz JL: Reversible renal failure and nephrotic syndrome associated with non-steroidal anti-inflammatory drugs. N Engl J Med 310:1271-1273, 1979.

347. Vanhaelen M, Vanhaelen-Fastre RJ, But P, Vanherweghem JL: Identification of aristolochic acid in Chinese herbs. Lancet 343:174, 1994.

348. Reginster F, Jadoul M, van Ypersele de Strihou C: Chinese herbs nephropathy presentation, natural history and fate after transplantation. Nephrol Dial Transplant 12:81-86, 1997.

349. Abt AB, Oh JY, Huntington RA, Burkhart KK: Chinese herbal medicine induced acute renal failure. Arch Inter Med 155:211-212, 1995.

350. Chang CH, Wang YM, Yang AH, Chiang SS: Rapidly progressive interstitial renal fibrosis associated with Chinese herbal medications. Am J Nephrol 21:441-448, 2001.

351. Svanborg C, de Man P, Sandberg T: Renal involvement in urinary tract infection. Kidney Int 39:541-550, 1991.

352. Brughard R, Brandis M, Hoyer PF, et al: Acute interstitial nephritis in childhood. Eur J Pediatr 142:103-110, 1984.

353. Haines JD Jr, Calhoon H: Interstitial nephritis in a patient with Legionnaires' disease. Postgrad Med 81:77-79, 1987.

354. Patino R, Blanco J, Yubero B: Interstitial nephritis caused by *Brucella*. Rev Clin Esp 129:93-96, 1973.

355. Haddow JE, Robotham JL: Acute interstitial nephritis in children—a process produced by streptococcal infection and by chemotherapeutic agents. A review. J Maine Med Assoc 69:1-6, 1978.

356. Martinez-Costa X, Ribera E, Segarra A, et al: Acute interstitial nephritis secondary to tricuspid endocarditis caused by *Staphylococcus aureus*. An Med Interna 6:595-597, 1989.

357. Sato T: Acute renal failure due to interstitial nephritis associated with *Yersinia pseudotuberculosis* infection. Pediatr Nephrol 7:327, 1993.

358. Laing RB, Nathwani D, Adamson DJ: *Salmonella typhimurium* infection leading to acute interstitial nephritis. Infection 19:254, 1991.

359. Singhal PC, Horowitz B, Molho L: Acute interstitial nephritis following Enterobacteriaceae sepsis. Ann Allergy 61:205-208, 1988.

360. Rautelin HI, Outinen AV, Kosunen TW: Tubulointerstitial nephritis as a complication of *Campylobacter jejuni* enteritis. Scand J Nephrol 21:151, 1987.

361. Kopolovic J, Pinkus G, Rosen S: Interstitial nephritis in infectious mononucleosis. Am J Kidney Dis 12:76-77, 1988.

362. Becker JL, Miller F, Nuovo GJ, et al: Epstein-Barr virus infection of renal proximal tubule cells: Possible role in chronic interstitial nephritis. J Clin Invest 104:1673-1681, 1999.

363. Silbert PL, Matz LR, Christiansen K, et al: Herpes simplex virus interstitial nephritis in a renal allograft. Clin Nephrol 33:264-268, 1990.

364. Rosen S, Harmon W, Krensky AM, et al: Tubulointerstitial nephritis associated with polyomavirus (BK type) infection. N Engl J Med 308:1192-1196, 1983.

365. Boulton J, Davison AM: Persistent infection as a cause of renal disease in patients submitted to renal biopsy: A report from the Glomerulonephritis Registry of the United Kindom MRC. Am J Med 58:123, 1986.

366. Pasterneck A, Helin H, Vanttinen T: Acute tubulointerstitial nephritis in a patient with *Mycoplasma pneumoniae* infection. Scand J Infect Dis 11:85, 1979.

367. Walker DH, Mattern WD: Acute renal failure in Rocky Mountain spotted fever. Arch Intern Med 139:443-448, 1979.

368. Schumann V, Fritschka E, Helmchen U, et al: Interstitial nephritis in typhus. Dtsch Med Wochenschr 118:893-897, 1993.

369. al-Sulaiman MH, Dhar JM, al-Hasani MK, et al: Tuberculous interstitial nephritis after kidney transplantation. Transplantation 50: 162-164, 1990.

370. Lai KN, Aarons I, Woodroffe AJ, Clarkson AR: Renal lesions in leptospirosis. Aust N Z J Med 12:276-279, 1982.

371. Byram JE, von Lichtenberg F: Experimental infection with *Schistosoma mekongi* in laboratory animals: Parasitological and pathological findings. Malacol Rev 2:125-159, 1980.

372. Branley P, Speed B: Acute interstitial nephritis due to *Chlamydia psittaci*. Aus N Z J Med 25:365, 1995.

373. Guignard JP, Torrado A: Interstitial nephritis with toxoplasmosis. J Pediatr 85:381, 1974.

374. Schwarz A, Perez-Canto A: Nephrotoxicity of antiinfective drugs. Int J Clin Pharmacol Ther 36:164-167, 1998.

375. D'Agati V, Appel GB: Renal pathology of human immunodeficiency virus infection. Semin Nephrol 18:406-421, 1998.

376. Kopp JB: Renal dysfunction in HIV-1-infected patients. Curr Infect Dis Rep 4:449-460, 2002.

377. Rubin RH, Wolfson JS, Cosimi AB, Tolkoff-Rubin NE: Infection in the renal transplant recipient. Am J Med 70:405, 1981.

378. Ramos E, Drachenberg CB, Papadimitrious JC, et al: Clinical course of polyoma virus nephropathy in 67 renal transplant patients. J Am Soc Nephrol 13:2145-2151, 2002.

379. Grcevska L, Polenakovic M, Oncevski A, et al: Different pathohistological presentations of acute renal involvement in Hantaan virus infection: Report of two cases. Clin Nephrol 34:197-201, 1990.

380. Bren AF, Pavlovcic SK, Koselj M, et al: Acute renal failure due to hemorrhagic fever with renal syndrome. Ren Fail 18:635-638, 1996.

381. Neilson EG: Interstitial nephritis: Another kissing disease? J Clin Invest 104:1671-1672, 1999.

382. Neilson EG, Kalluri R, Sun MJ, et al: Specificity of Goodpasture antibodies for the recombinant noncollagenous (NC1) domains of type IV collagen. J Biol Chem 268:8402-8405, 1993.

383. Butkowski RJ, Langwald JPM, Wieslander J, et al: Characterization of a tubular basement membrane component reactive with autoantibodies associated with tubulointersitital nephritis. J Biol Chem 265:21091-21098, 1990.

384. Kelly CJ, Roth DA, Meyers CM: Immune recognition and response to the renal interstitium. Kidney Int 39:518-531, 1991.

385. Riminton S, O'Donnell J: Tubulo-interstitial nephritis and uveitis (TINU) syndrome in an adult. Aust N Z J Med 23:57, 1993.

386. Stupp R, Mihatsch MJ, Matter L, Streuli RA: Acute tubulo-interstitial nephritis with uveitis (TINU syndrome) in a patient with serologic evidence for *Chlamydia* infection. Klin Wochenschr 68: 971-975, 1990.

387. van-Leusen R, Assmann KJ: Acute tubulo-interstitial nephritis with uveitis and favourable outcome after five months of continuous ambulatory peritoneal dialysis (CAPD). Neth J Med 33:133-139, 1988.

388. Okada K, Okamoto Y, Kagami S, et al: Acute interstitial nephritis and uveitis with bone marrow granulomas and anti-neutrophil cytoplasmic antibodies. Am J Nephrol 15:337-342, 1995.

389. Navarro JF, Gallego E, Gil J, et al: Idiopathic acute interstitial nephritis and uveitis associated with deafness. Nephrol Dial Transplant 12:781-784, 1997.

390. Muller GA, Markovic-Lipkovski J, Frank J, Rodemann HP: The role of interstitial cells in the progression of renal diseases. J Am Soc Nephrol 2:S198-S205, 1992.

391. Aradhye S, Neilson EG: Treatment of acute interstitial nephritis. *In* Brady H, Wilcox C (eds): Therapy in Nephrology and Hypertension. Philadelphia, WB Saunders, 1999, pp 232-235.

392. Laberke HG: Treatment of acute interstitial nephritis. Klin Wochenschr 58:531-532, 1980.

393. Qunibi WY, Godwin J, Eknoyan G: Toxic nephropathy during continuous rifampin therapy. South Med J 73:791-792, 1980.

394. Agus D, Mann R, Clayman M, et al: The effects of daily cyclophosphamide administration on the development and extent of primary experimental interstitial nephritis in rats. Kidney Int 29:635-640, 1986.

395. Shih W, Hines WH, Neilson EG: Effects of cyclosporin A on the development of immune-mediated interstitial nephritis. Kidney Int 33:1113-1118, 1988.

396. Eknoyan G, McDonald MA, Appel D, Truong LD: Chronic tubulo-interstitial nephritis: Correlation between structural and functional findings. Kidney Int 38:736-743, 1990.

397. Cogan MG: Tubulointerstitial nephropathies: A pathophysiological approach. West J Med 132:134, 1980.

398. Schaaf GJ, Nijmeijer SM, Maas RF, et al: The role of oxidative stress in the ochratoxin A–mediated toxicity in proximal tubular cells. Biochim Biophys Acta 1588:149-158, 2002.

399. Nenov VD, Nenov DS: Balkan nephropathy: A disorder of renal embryogenesis? Am J Nephrol 22:260-265, 2002.

400. Radonic M, Radosevic Z: Clinical features of Balkan endemic nephropathy. Food Chem Toxicol 3:189-192, 1992.

401. Karlsson FA, Lenkei R: Urinary excretion of albumin and beta-2-microglobulin in a population from an area where Balkan nephrology is endemic. Scand J Clin Lab Invest 37:169, 1977.

402. Muther RS, McCarron DA, Bennett WM: Renal manifestations of sarcoidosis. Arch Intern Med 141:643, 1981.

403. Lebacq E, Verhaegen H, Desmet V: Renal involvement in sarcoidosis. Postgrad Med J 46:526, 1970.

404. Muther RS, McCarron DA, Bennett WM: Granulomatous sarcoid nephritis: A cause of multiple renal tubular abnormalities. Clin Nephrol 14:190, 1980.

405. McCurley T, Salter J, Glick A: Renal insufficiency in sarcoidosis. Arch Pathol Lab Med 114:488-492, 1990.

406. Mayock AL, Bertrand P, Morrison CE, Scott JH: Manifestations of sarcoidosis: Analysis of 145 patients with a review of nine series selected from the literature. Am J Med 35:67, 1963.

407. Simonsen O, Thysell H: Sarcoidosis with normocalcemic granulomatous nephritis. Nephron 40:411, 1985.

408. Korzets Z, Schneider M, Taragan R, et al: Acute renal failure due to sarcoid granulomatous infiltration of the renal parenchyma. Am J Kidney Dis 6:250, 1986.

409. Coburn PW, Hobbs C, Johnston GS, et al: Granulomatous sarcoid nephritis. Am J Med 42:273-283, 1967.

410. Sedmak DD, Tubbs RR: The macrophagic origin of multinucleated giant cells in myeloma kidney: An immunohistologic study. Hum Pathol 18:304-306, 1987.

411. Rota S, Mougenot B, Baudouin B, et al: Multiple myeloma and severe renal failure: A clinicopathologic study of outcome and prognosis in 34 patients. Medicine (Baltimore) 66:126-137, 1987.

412. Cohen AH, Border WA: An immunomorphogenetic study of renal biopsies. Lab Invest 42:248-256, 1980.

413. Koss MN, Pirani CL, Osserman EF: Experimental Bence Jones cast nephropathy. Lab Invest 35:579, 1976.

414. DeFronzo RA, Cooke CR, Wright JR, et al: Renal function in patients with multiple myeloma. Medicine (Baltimore) 57:151, 1978.

415. Smolens P: The kidney in dysproteinemic states. AKF Nephrol Lett 4:27-42, 1987.

416. Sanders PW, Herrera GA, Lott RL, Galla JH: Morphologic alterations of the proximal tubules in light chain-related renal disease. Kidney Int 33:881-889, 1988.

417. Batuman V, Dreisbach AW, Cyran J: Light chain binding sites on renal brush border membranes. Am J Physiol 258:F1259-F1265, 1990.

418. Sanders PW, Herrera GA, Galla JH: Human Bence Jones protein toxicity in rat proximal tubule epithelium in vivo. Kidney Int 32:851-861, 1987.

419. Sanders PW, Booker BB, Bishop JB, Cheung HC: Mechanisms of intranephronal proteinaceous cast formation by low molecular weight proteins. J Clin Invest 85:570-576, 1990.

420. Sanders PW, Herrera GA, Kirk KA, et al: Spectrum of glomerular and tubulointerstitial renal lesions associated with monotypical immunoglobulin light chain deposition. Lab Invest 64:527-537, 1991.

421. Weiss JH, Williams RH, Galla JH, et al: Pathophysiology of acute Bence Jones protein nephrotoxicity in the rat. Kidney Int 20:198, 1981.

422. Kapadis SB: Multiple myeloma: A clinicopathologic study of 62 consecutively autopsied cases. Medicine (Baltimore) 59:380, 1980.

423. Kyle RA: Multiple myeloma: Review of 869 cases. Mayo Clin Proc 50:29, 1975.

424. Sanders PW, Booker BB: Pathobiology of cast nephropathy from human Bence Jones proteins. J Clin Invest 89:630-639, 1992.

425. Smolens P, Venkatachalam M, Stein JH: Myeloma kidney cast nephropathy in a rat model of multiple myeloma. Kidney Int 24:192, 1983.

426. Cline DH, Pesce AJ, Thomson RE: Nephrotoxicity of Bence Jones protein in the rat: Importance of protein isoelectric point. Kidney Int 16:345, 1979.

427. Coward RA, Delamore IW, Mallick NP, et al: The importance of urinary immunoglobulin light chain isoelectric point (pI) in nephrotoxity in multiple myeloma. Clin Sci (Colch) 66:229, 1984.

428. Holland MD, Galla JH, Sanders PW, Luke RG: Effect of urinary pH and diatrizoate on Bence Jones protein nephrotoxicity in the rat. Kidney Int 27:46-50, 1985.

429. Zemer D, Pras M, Sohar E, et al: Colchicine in the prevention and treatment of the amyloidosis of familial Mediterranean fever. N Engl J Med 314:1001-1005, 1986.

430. Luxton RW: Radiation nephritis: A long-term study of 54 patients. Lancet 2:1221, 1961.

431. Redd BL Jr: Radiation nephritis: Review, case report and animal study. AJR Am J Roentgenol 83:88, 1960.

432. Grossman BJ: Radiation nephritis. J Paediatr 47:424, 1955.

433. Scanlon GT: Vascular alteration in the irradiated rabbit kidney: A microangiographic study. Radiology 94:401, 1970.

434. Withers HR, Mason KA, Thomas HD Jr: Late radiation response of kidney assayed by tubule-cell survival. Br J Radiol 59:587, 1986.

435. Robbins MEC, Hopewell JW, Gunn Y: Effects of single doses of x-rays on renal function in unilaterally irradiated pigs. Radiother Oncol 4:143, 1985.

436. Gup AK, Schlegel JV, Caldwell T, Schlosser J: Effect of irradiation on renal function. J Urol 97:36, 1967.

437. Concannon JP, Summers RE, Brewer R et al: High oxygen tension and radiation effect on the kidney. Radiology 82:508, 1964.

438. Bloomfield DK, Schneider DH, Vertes V: Renin and angiotensin II: Studies in malignant hypertension after X-irradiation for seminoma. Ann Intern Med 68:146, 1968.

439. Ljungvist A, Unge G, Lagergren C, Notter G: The intrarenal vascular alterations in radiation nephritis and their relationship to the development of hypertension. Acta Pathol Microbiol Scand 79:629, 1971.

440. Wacholz BW, Casarett GW: Radiation hypertension and nephrosclerosis. Radiat Res 41:39, 1970.

441. Kunkler PB, Farr RF, Luxton RW: Limits of renal tolerance to x-rays. Br J Radiol 25:190, 1952.

442. Thames HD, Withers HR, Peters LJ, Fletcher GH: Changes in early and late radiation responses with altered dose fractionation: Implications for dose-survival relationships. Int J Radiat Oncol 8:219, 1982.

443. Dubach UC, Rosner B, Pfister E: Epidemiologic study of abuse of analgesics containing phenacetin: Renal morbidity and mortality (1968-1979). N Engl J Med 308:357-362, 1983.

444. Gonwa TA, Hamilton RW, Buckalew VM Jr: Chronic renal failure and end-stage renal disease in northwest North Carolina: Importance of analgesic-associated nephropathy. Arch Intern Med 141:462-465, 1981.

445. McAnally JF, Winchester JF, Schreiner GE: Analgesic nephropathy: An uncommon cause of end-stage renal disease. Arch Intern Med 143:1897, 1983.

446. Kincaid-Smith P: Analgesic nephropathy. Ann Intern Med 68:949, 1968.

447. Pommer W, Glaeske G, Molzahn M: The analgesic problem in the Federal Republic of Germany: Analgesic consumption, frequency of analgesic nephropathy and regional differences. Clin Nephrol 26:273-278, 1986.

448. Prescott LF: Analgesic nephropathy: A reassessment of the role of phenacetin and other analgesics. Drugs 23:75, 1982.

449. Murray T, Stolley PD, Anthony JC, et al: Epidemiologic study of regular analgesic use and end-stage renal disease. Arch Intern Med 143:1687-1693, 1983.

450. Sandler PD, Smith JC, Weinberg CR, et al: Analgesic use and chronic renal disease. N Engl J Med 320:1238-1243, 1989.

451. Nanra RS, Taylor JS, Deleon AH, White KH: Analgesic nephropathy: Etiology, clinical syndrome and clinicopathologic correlations in Australia. Kidney Int 13:79, 1978.

452. Lornoy W, Becaus I, De Vleeschouwer M, et al: Renal cell carcinoma, a new complication of analgesic nephropathy. Lancet 1:1271, 1986.

453. Bach PH, Bridges JW: Chemically induced renal papillary necrosis and upper urothelial carcinoma. Crit Rev Toxicol 15:331-441, 1986.

454. Murray TG: Analgesic use and kidney disease. Arch Intern Med 141:423-424, 1981.

455. Griffiths ML: End-stage renal failure caused by regular use of anti-inflammatory analgesic medication for minor sports injuries. A case report. S Afr Med J 81:377-378, 1992.

456. Boletis J, Williams AJ, Shortland JR, Brown CB: Irreversible renal failure following mefenamic acid. Nephron 51:575-576, 1989.

457. Gault MH, Blennerhassett J, Muehrcke RC: Analgesic nephropathy: A clinicopathologic study using electron microscopy. Am J Med 51:740-756, 1971.

458. Elseviers MM, Waller I, Nenoy D, et al: Evaluation of diagnostic criteria for analgesic nephropathy in patients with end-stage renal failure: Results of the ANNE study. Analgesic Nephropathy Network of Europe. Nephrol Dial Transplant 10:808-814, 1995.

459. Elseviers MM, De Schepper A, Corthouts R, et al: High diagnostic performance of CT scan for analgesic nephropathy in patients with incipient to severe renal failure. Kidney Int 48:1316-1323, 1995.

460. Mudge GH, Gemborys MW, Duggins GG: Covalent binding of metabolics of acetaminophen to kidney protein and depletion of renal glutathione. J Pharmacol Exp Ther 206:218, 1978.

461. McMurtry RJ, Snodgrass WR, Mitchell JR: Renal necrosis, glutathione depletion and covalent binding after acetaminophen. J Toxicol Appl Pharmacol 46:87, 1978.

462. Walker RJ, Duggin GG: Drug nephrotoxicity. Annu Rev Pharmacol Toxicol 28:331-345, 1988.

463. Brezis M, Rosen S, Epstein FH: The pathophysiological implications of medullary hypoxia. Am J Kidney Dis 13:253-258, 1989.

464. Kjellstrand CM, Campbell DD, von Hartitzsch B, et al: Hyperuricemic acute renal failure. Arch Intern Med 133:349, 1974.

465. Passwell J, Boichis H, Cohen BE: Hyperuricemic nephropathy. Am J Dis Child 120:154, 1970.

466. Yu TA-F, Berger L: Impaired renal function in gout: Its association in hypertensive vascular disease and intrinsic renal disease. Am J Med 72:95-100, 1982.

467. Batuman V, Maesaka JK, Haddad B, et al: The role of lead in gout nephropathy. N Engl J Med 304:520-523, 1981.

468. Porter GA: Uric acid nephropathy. *In* Bennett WM (ed): Drugs and Renal Disease. New York, Churchill-Livingstone, 1986, p 142.

469. Edvall CA: Renal function in hyperparathyroidism: A clinical study of 30 cases with special reference to selective renal clearance and renal vein catheterization. Acta Chir Scand 229(suppl):1, 1958.

470. Humes HD, Ichikawa I, Troy JL, Brenner BM: Evidence for a parathyroid hormone–dependent influence of calcium on the glomerular filtration. J Clin Invest 61:32, 1978.

471. Beck N, Singh H, Reed SW: Pathogenic role of cyclic AMP in the impairment of urinary concentrating ability in acute hypercalcemia. J Clin Invest 54:1049, 1974.

472. Ganote CE, Philipshorn DS, Chen E: Acute calcium nephrotoxicity: An electron microscopic and semiquantitative light microscopic study. Arch Pathol Lab Med 99:650, 1975.

473. Nguyen HT, Wodward JD: Intranephronic calculosis in rats. Am J Pathol 100:39, 1980.

474. Wallace MR, Bruton D, North A, Wild DJ: End-stage renal failure due to familial hypokalaemic interstitial nephritis with identical HLA tissue types. N Z Med J 98:5-7, 1985.

475. Kraikitpanitch S, Lindeman RD, Mandal AK: Severe hyperuricemia, hypokalemic alkalosis and tubulointerstitial nephritis. Am J Med Sci 271:77, 1976.

476. Gullner HG, Bartter FC, Gill JR Jr, et al: A sibship with hypokalemic alkalosis and renal proximal tubulopathy. Arch Intern Med 143:1534, 1983.

477. Biava GG, Dyrda I, Genest J, et al: Kaliopenic nephropathy: A correlated light and electron microscopy study. Lab Invest 12:443, 1963.

478. Cremer W, Bock KD: Symptoms and course of chronic hypokalemic nephropathy in man. Clin Nephrol 7:112-119, 1977.

479. Williams HE: Oxalic acid and the hyperoxaluric syndromes. Kidney Int 13:410, 1978.

480. Cryer PE, Garber AJ, Hoffsten P, et al: Renal failure after small intestinal bypass for obesity. Arch Intern Med 135:1610, 1975.

481. Collins JM, Hennes DM, Halzgauz CR, et al: Recovery after prolonged oliguria due to ethylene glycol intoxication: The prognostic value of several percutaneous renal biopsies. Arch Intern Med 125:1059, 1970.

482. Hanley MJ, Davidson K: Isolated nephron segments from rabbit models of obstructive nephropathy. J Clin Invest 69:165-174, 1982.

483. Buerkert J, Head M, Klahr S: Effects of acute bilateral ureteral obstruction on deep nephron and terminal collecting duct function in the young rat. J Clin Invest 59:1055-1065, 1977.

484. Buerkert J, Martin D, Head M, et al: Deep nephron function after release of acute unilateral ureteral obstruction in the young rat. J Clin Invest 62:1228-1239, 1978.

485. Batlle DC, Arruda JAL, Kurtzman NA: Hyperkalemic distal renal tubular acidosis associated with obstructive uropathy. N Engl J Med 304:373-380, 1981.

486. Campbell HT, Bello-Reuss E, Klahr S: Hydraulic water permeability and transepithelial voltage in the isolated perfused rabbit cortical collecting tubule following unilateral ureteral obstruction. J Clin Invest 75:219-225, 1985.

487. Klahr S, Harris KPG, Purkerson ML: Effects of obstruction on renal function. Pediatr Nephrol 2:34-42, 1988.

488. Purkerson ML, Klahr S: Prior inhibition of vasoconstriction normalizes GFR in postobstructed kidneys. Kidney Int 35:1305-1314, 1989.

489. Yarger WE, Schockein DD, Harris RH: Obstructive nephropathy in the rat: Possible roles for the renin-angiotensin system, prostaglandins, and thromboxanes in postobstructive renal function. J Clin Invest 65:400-412, 1980.

490. Reyes AA, Robertson G, Klahr S: Role of vasopressin in rats with bilateral ureteral obstruction. Proc Soc Exp Biol Med 197:49-55, 1991.

491. Klahr S: New insights into the consequences and mechanisms of renal impairment in obstructive nephropathy. Am J Kidney Dis 18:689-699, 1991.

492. Nagle RB, Johnson ME, Jervis HR: Proliferation of renal interstitial cells following injury induced by ureteral obstruction. Lab Invest 35:18-22, 1976.

493. Schreiner G, Harris KPG, Pukerson ML, et al: The immunological aspects of acute ureteral obstruction: Immune cell infiltrate in the kidney. Kidney Int 34:487-493, 1988.

494. Harris KP, Schreiner GF, Klahr S: Effect of leukocyte depletion on the function of the postobstructed kidney in the rat. Kidney Int 36:210-215, 1989.

495. Costerousse O, Allegrini J, Lopez M, Alhenc-Gelas F: Angiotensin I-converting enzyme in human circulating mononuclear cells: Genetic polymorphism of expression in T-lymphocytes. Biochem J 290:33-40, 1993.

496. Rovin BH, Harris KP, Morrison A, et al: Renal cortical release of a specific macrophage chemoattractant in response to ureteral obstruction. Lab Invest 63:213-220, 1990.

497. Yee J, Kuncio GS, Neilson EG: Tubulointerstitial nephritis following glomerulonephritis. Semin Nephrol 11:361-366, 1991.

498. Border WA, Noble NA, Yamamoto T, et al: Natural inhibitor of transforming growth factor-β protects against scarring in experimental kidney disease. Nature 360:361-364, 1992.

499. Staessen JA, Lauwerys RR, Buchet J-P, et al: Impairment of renal function with increasing blood lead concentrations in the general population. N Engl J Med 327:151-156, 1992.

500. Wedeen RP, Malik DK, Batuman V: Detection and treatment of occupational lead nephropathy. Arch Intern Med 139:53-57, 1979.

501. Van de Vyver FL, D'Haese PC, Visser WJ, et al: Bone lead in dialysis patients. Kidney Int 33:601-607, 1988.

502. Sokas R, Besarab A, McDiarmid M, et al: Sensitivity of in vivo X-ray fluorescence determination of skeletal lead stores. Arch Environ Health 45:268-272, 1990.

503. Harlan WR, Landis JR, Schmouder RL: Relationship of blood lead and blood pressure in the adolescent and adult U.S. population. JAMA 253:530, 1985.

504. Cramer K, Goyer RA, Jagenburg R, Wilson MH: Renal ultrastructure, renal function, and parameters of lead toxicity in workers with different periods of lead exposure. Br J Ind Med 31:113-127, 1974.

505. Mistry P, Lucier GW, Fowler BA: High-affinity lead-binding proteins in rat kidney cytosol mediate cell-free nuclear translocation of lead. J Pharmacol Exp Ther 232:462, 1985.

506. Chisolm JJ, Baltrop D: Recognition and management of children with increased lead absorption. Arch Dis Child 54:249, 1979.

507. Emmerson BT: Chronic lead nephropathy. Kidney Int 4:1, 1973.

508. Craswell PW, Price J, Boyle PD, et al: Chronic renal failure with gout: A marker of chronic lead poisoning. Kidney Int 26:319, 1984.

509. Crutcher JC: Clinical manifestations and therapy of acute lead intoxication due to the ingestion of illicitly distilled alcohol. Ann Intern Med 59:707, 1963.

510. Wedeen RP: The role of lead in renal failure. Clin Exp Dial Apheresis 6:113-146, 1982.

511. Suzuki CA, Cherian G: Renal toxicity of cadmium metallothionein and enzymuria in rats. J Pharmacol Exp Ther 240:314, 1987.

512. Wedeen RP: Environmental renal disease: Lead, cadmium, and Balkan endemic nephropathy. Kidney Int Suppl 404:S4-S8, 1991.

513. Roels HA, Lauwerys R, Buchet JP: In vivo measurement of liver and kidney cadmium in workers exposed to this metal: Its significance with respect to cadmium in blood and urine. Environ Res 26:217, 1981.

514. Nogawa K: Biologic indicators of cadmium nephrotoxicity in persons with low-level cadmium exposure. Environ Health Perspect 54:163, 1984.

515. Lauwerys R, DeWals P: Environmental pollution by cadmium and mortality from renal diseases. Lancet 1:383, 1981.

516. Weiss RA, Kelly CJ, Madaio MP: Heat shock protein–reactive T cells eluted from the kidneys of nephritis mice are nephritogenic and cytotoxic to stressed renal tubular cells. J Am Soc Nephrol 4:641, 1993.

517. Hannedouche T, Albouze G, Chauveau P, et al: Effects of blood pressure and antihypertensive treatment on progression of advanced chronic renal failure. Am J Kidney Dis 21:131-137, 1993.

518. Robson M, Levi J, Dolberg L, Rosenfeld JB: Acute tubulo-interstitial nephritis following sulfadiazine therapy. Isr J Med Sci 6:561-566, 1970.

519. Segasothy M, Pang KS: Acute interstitial nephritis due to endosulfan. Nephron 62:118, 1992.

520. Codding CE, Ramseyer L, Allon M, et al: Tubulointerstitial nephritis due to vancomycin. Am J Kidney Dis 14:512-515, 1989.

521. Hsu SI: Biopsy-proved acute tubulointerstitial nephritis and toxic epidermal necrolysis associated with vancomycin. Pharmacotherapy 21:1233-1239, 2001.

522. Gaut PL, Carron WC, Ching WT, Meyer RD: Intravenous/oral ciprofloxacin therapy versus intravenous ceftazidime therapy for selected bacterial infections. Am J Med 87:169S-175S, 1989.

523. Rosenfeld J, Gura V, Boner G, et al: Interstitial nephritis with acute renal failure after erythromycin. BMJ 286:938-939, 1983.

524. Wilkinson SP, Stewart WK, Spiers EM, Pears J: Protracted systemic illness and interstitial nephritis due to minocycline. Postgrad Med J 65:53-56, 1989.

525. Walker RG, Thomson NM, Dowling JP, Ogg CS: Minocycline-induced acute interstitial nephritis. BMJ 1:524, 1979.

526. Kiessling S, Forrest K, Moscow J, et al: Interstitial nephritis, hepatic failure, and systemic eosinophilia after minocycline treatment. Am J Kidney Dis 38:E36, 2001.

527. Rashed A, Azadeh B, Abu-Romeh SH: Acyclovir-induced acute tubulo-interstitial nephritis. Nephron 56:436-438, 1990.

528. Garcia-Martin F, Mampaso F, de-Arriba G, et al: Acute interstitial nephritis induced by ethambutol. Nephron 59:679-680, 1991.

529. Frandsen NE, Saugmann S, Marcussen N: Acute interstitial nephritis associated with the use of mesalazine in inflammatory bowel disease. Nephron 92:200-202, 2002.

530. Prichard BN, Owens CW, Woolf AS: Adverse reactions to diuretics. Eur Heart J 13:96-103, 1992.

531. Sica DA, Gehr TW: Triamterene and the kidney. Nephron 51:454-461, 1989.

532. Smith WR, Neill J, Cushman WC, Butkus DE: Captopril-associated acute interstitial nephritis. Am J Nephrol 9:230-235, 1989.

533. Myers RP, McLaughlin K, Hollomby DJ: Acute interstitial nephritis due to omeprazole. Am J Gastroenterol 96:3428-3431, 2001.

534. Sawaishi Y, Komatsu K, Takeda O, et al: A case of tubulo-interstitial nephritis with exfoliative dermatitis and hepatitis due to phenobarbital hypersensitivity. Eur J Pediatr 151:69-72, 1992.

535. Kahn SR: Acute interstitial nephritis associated with nitrofurantoin. Lancet 348:1177-1178, 1996.

536. Yoshikawa H, Watanabe T, Abe T: Tubulo-interstitial nephritis caused by sodium valproate. Brain Dev 24:102-105, 2002.

537. Moutard ML, Bavoux F, Mensire A, et al: Immunoallergic tubulo-interstitial nephritis following ingestion of carbamazepine. Arch Fr Pediatr 44:191-193, 1987.

538. Averbuch SD, Austin HA, Sherwin SA, et al: Acute interstitial nephritis with the nephrotic syndrome following recombinant leukocyte α interferon therapy for mycosis fungoides. N Engl J Med 310:32-35, 1984.

539. Nishimura, S, Miura H, Yamada H, et al: Acute onset of nephrotic syndrome during interferon-alpha retreatment for chronic active hepatitis C. J Gastroenterol 37:854-858, 2002.

540. Diekman MJ, Vlasveld LT, Krediet RT, et al: Acute interstitial nephritis during continuous intravenous administration of low-dose interleukin-2. Nephron 60:122-123, 1992.

541. Vlasveld LT, van-de-Wiel-van-Kemenade E, de-Boer AJ, et al: Possible role for cytotoxic lymphocytes in the pathogenesis of acute interstitial nephritis after recombinant interleukin-2 treatment for renal cell cancer. Cancer Immunol Immunother 36:210-213, 1993.

542. Choy EH, Kingsley GH, Panayi GS: Treatment with anti-CD4 monoclonal antibody and acute interstitial nephritis. Arthritis Rheum 36:723-724, 1993.

543. Tomita N, Kanamori H, Fujita H, et al: Granulomatous tubulointerstitial nephritis induced by all-trans retinoic acid. Anticancer Drugs 12:677-680, 2001.

544. Zhang R, Meleg-Smith S, Batuman V: Acute tubulointerstitial nephritis after wasp stings. Am J Kidney Dis 38:E33, 2001.

545. Kim MJ, Chang JH, Lee SK, et al: Acute interstitial nephritis due to nicergoline (Sermion). Nephron 92:676-679, 2002.

546. Boucek P, Voska L, Saudek F: Successful retransplantation after renal allograft loss to polyoma virus interstitial nephritis. Transplantation 74:1478, 2002.

547. Yoshioka K, Takemura T, Kanasaki M, et al: Acute interstitial nephritis and uveitis syndrome: Activated immune cell infiltration in the kidney. Pediatr Nephrol 5:232-234, 1991.

548. Rosenbaum JT: Bilateral anterior uveitis and interstitial nephritis. Am J Ophthalmol 105:534-537, 1988.

549. Veiga PA, Pieroni D, Baier W, Feld LG: Association of Kawasaki disease and interstitial nephritis. Pediatr Nephrol 6:421-423, 1992.

550. Kelly CJ, Neilson EG: The interstitium in cystic kidney disease. In: Gardner KD, Bernstein J (eds): The Cystic Kidney. Dordrecht, Netherlands, Kluwer Academic, 1989, pp 43-54.

551. Kelly CJ, Neilson EG: Medullary cystic disease: An inherited form of autoimmune interstitial nephritis? Am J Kidney Dis 10:389-395, 1987.

552. Tzen CY, Tsai JD, Wu TY, et al: Tubulointerstitial nephritis associated with a novel mitochondrial point mutation. Kidney Int 59:846-854, 2001.

553. Adams ND, Rowe JC: Nephrocalcinosis. Clin Perinatol 19:179-195, 1992.

554. Wandzilak TR, Williams HE: The hyperoxaluric syndromes. Endocrinol Metab Clin North Am 19:851-867, 1990.

555. Broyer M, Guillot M, Gubler MC, Habib R: Infantile cystinosis: A reappraisal of early and late symptoms. Adv Nephrol 10:137, 1981.

556. Rutledge SL, Geraghty M, Mroczek E, et al: Tubulointerstitial nephritis in methylmalonic acidemia. Pediatr Nephrol 7:81-82, 1993.

557. Fillastre JP, Moulin B, Josse S: Aetiology of nephrotoxic damage to the renal interstitium and tubuli. Toxicol Lett 46: 45-54, 1989.

558. Walker RG, Bennet WM, Davies BM, Kincaid-Smith P: Structural and functional effects of long-term lithium therapy. Kidney Int Suppl 11:S13, 1982.

559. Myers BD, Ross J, Newton L, et al: Cyclosporine-associated chronic nephropathy. N Engl J Med 311:699, 1984.

560. Gonzalez-Vitale JC, Hayes DM, Cvitkovic E, et al: The renal pathology in clinical trials for cis-platinum (II) diaminedichloride. Cancer 39:1362, 1977.

561. Schacht RG, Baldwin DS: Chronic interstitial nephritis and renal failure due to nitrosourea therapy. Kidney Int 14:661, 1978.

562. Vanherweghem JL, Depierreux M, Tielemans C, et al: Rapidly progressive interstitial renal fibrosis in young women. Association with slimming regimen including Chinese herbs. Lancet 341:387-391, 1993.

563. Hess B, Raisin J, Zimmermann A, et al: Tubulointerstitial nephropathy persisting 20 months after discontinuation of chronic intake of germanium lactate citrate. Am J Kidney Dis 21:548-552, 1993.

564. Faull RJ, Russ GR: Tubular expression of intercellular adhesion molecule-1 during renal allograft rejection. Transplantation 48:226-230, 1989.

565. Cosimi AB, Conti D, Delmonico FL, et al: In vivo effects of monoclonal antibody to ICAM-1 (CD54) in nonhuman primates with renal allografts. J Immunol 144:4604-4612, 1990.

566. Schwartz MM: Lupus vasculitis. Contrib Nephrol 99:35-45, 1992.

567. Jennette JC, Falk RJ: Antineutrophil cytoplasmic autoantibodies and associated diseases: A review. Am J Kidney Dis 15:517-529, 1990.

568. Matsutani H, Mizusawa J, Shimoda M, et al: Severe glomerulonephritis and tubulo-interstitial nephritis accompanied with urticaria and vasculitis. Child Nephrol Urol 10: 214-217, 1990.

569. Siamopoulos KC, Mavridis AK, Elisaf M, et al: Kidney involvement in primary Sjögren's syndrome. Scand J Rheumatol Suppl 61: 156-160, 1986.

570. Casella FJ, Allon M: The kidney in sarcoidosis. J Am Soc Nephrol 3:1555-1562, 1993.

571. Brause M, Magnusson K, Degenhardt S, et al: Renal involvement in sarcoidosis—a report of 6 cases. Clin Nephrol 57:142-148, 2002.

572. Zachee P, Henckens M, Van-Damme B, et al: Chronic renal failure due to renal hemosiderosis in a patient with paroxysmal nocturnal hemoglobinuria. Clin Nephrol 39:28-31, 1993.

573. Srinivasa NS, McGovern CH, Solez K, et al: Progressive renal failure due to renal invasion and parenchymal destruction by adult T-cell lymphoma. Am J Kidney Dis 16:70-72, 1990.

574. Falk RJ, Scheinman J, Phillips G, et al: Prevalence and pathologic features of sickle cell nephropathy and response to inhibition of angiotensin-converting enzyme. N Engl J Med 326:910-915, 1992.

575. Meyrier A, Condamin MC, Fernet M, et al: Frequency of development of early cortical scarring in acute primary pyelonephritis. Kidney Int 35: 696-703, 1989.

576. Dobyan DC, Truong LD, Eknoyan G: Renal malacoplakia reappraised. Am J Kidney Dis 22:243-252, 1993.

577. Goodman M, Curry T, Russell T: Xanthogranulomatous pyelonephritis: A local disease with systemic manifestations. Report of 23 cases and review of the literature. Medicine (Baltimore) 58:171, 1979.

578. Petkovic SD: Treatment of bilateral renal pelvic and ureteral tumors. A review of 45 cases. Eur Urol 4:397-400, 1978.

579. Stickler GB, Kelalis PP, Burke EC, Segar WE: Primary interstitial nephritis with reflux. Am J Dis Child 122:144-148, 1971.

580. Preston RA, Stemmer CL, Materson BJ, et al: Renal biopsy in patients 65 years of age or older. An analysis of the results of 334 biopsies. J Am Geriatr Soc 38:669-674, 1990.

581. Farrington K, Levison DA, Greenwood RN, et al: Renal biopsy in patients with unexplained renal impairment and normal kidney size. Q J Med 70:221-233, 1989.

582. Truong LD, Farhood A, Tasby J, Gillum D: Experimental chronic renal ischemia: Morphologic and immunologic studies. Kidney Int 41:1676-1689, 1992.

583. Karalezli G, Gogus O, Beduk Y, et al: Histopathologic effects of extracorporeal shock wave lithotripsy on rabbit kidney. Urol Res 21:67-70, 1993.

CHAPTER 31

Urinary Tract Infection, Pyelonephritis, and Reflux Nephropathy

Nina E. Tolkoff-Rubin, Ramzi S. Cotran, and Robert H. Rubin*

Urinary tract infection (UTI) is the most common of all bacterial infections, affecting humans throughout their life span. UTI occurs in all populations, from the neonate to the geriatric patient, but it has a particular impact on females of all ages (especially during pregnancy), males at the two extremes of life, kidney transplant recipients, and anyone with functional or structural abnormalities of the urinary tract. Not only is UTI common, but the range of possible clinical syndromes it can produce is exceptionally broad, including pyelonephritis with gram-negative sepsis, asymptomatic bacteriuria, and even so-called symptomatic abacteriuria. In approaching this complex entity, there are three issues that must be kept in mind:

1. What is the pathogenesis of UTI, and how can such pathogenetic events be interrupted? In particular, are there specific clones of bacteria that possess genetically encoded virulence properties that are required for ascending, invasive infection of the urinary tract?
2. How does one best diagnose, prevent, and treat the infectious disease aspects of UTI?
3. Does UTI have any long-term effects on the individual other than the direct inflammatory effects of microbial replication and invasion? In particular, what are the contributions of UTI to the development of chronic renal disease, hypertension, or both; its effects on longevity and survival; and, finally, does it have significant effects on the outcome of pregnancy?

PROBLEMS IN DEFINITION

Generally, "pyelonephritis" means inflammation of the kidney and its pelvis, but from a historical point of view and through

common usage, the term has come to designate a disorder of the kidney resulting from bacterial invasion. This is certainly true in the case of acute pyelonephritis, with its relatively simple histopathologic features—acute interstitial inflammation and tubular cell necrosis. The role of active bacterial infection in chronic pyelonephritis is more complex. Based on careful radiologic and pathologic studies,[1-3] there is now general agreement that the term "chronic pyelonephritis" should be restricted to cases that manifest unequivocal evidence of pelvocaliceal inflammation, fibrosis, and deformity. When these criteria are employed, three observations emerge:

1. In most patients with chronic pyelonephritis, bacterial infection of the urinary tract is superimposed on an anatomic urinary tract anomaly—urinary obstruction or, most commonly, vesicoureteral reflux (VUR).
2. UTI in the absence of obstruction or VUR is an uncommon cause of significant chronic pyelonephritis.
3. In contrast, chronic tubulointerstitial disease without pyelocaliceal involvement can be caused by a host of factors, including toxins, metabolic disorders, vascular diseases, and autoimmune disorders.

The term "reflux nephropathy" is used to categorize the renal scarring associated with VUR[4]; although this is frequently caused or accompanied by bacterial infection, some patients are free from bacteriuria when the condition is discovered.

BACTERIOLOGY OF URINARY TRACT INFECTION

General Considerations: The Urine Culture and Urinalysis

The cornerstone of the approach to patients with possible UTI is the evaluation of the results of a quantitative urine

*Deceased.

culture and urinalysis. This evaluation is complicated by two factors. First, there is an incomplete correlation between the clinical symptoms of urinary tract inflammation and the presence of true UTI, so objective evidence of the presence and the type of infection is of great importance. Second, there is frequently great difficulty in obtaining a spontaneously voided urine specimen that is uncontaminated by the normal flora of the distal urethra, vagina, or skin. Therefore, certain guidelines are necessary for evaluating the results of urine cultures.

The first clue to the importance of a positive urine culture report comes from the nature of the organism or organisms isolated on culture. In more than 95% of UTIs, the infecting organism is a gram-negative bacillus, *Enterococcus faecalis*, or, in the case of reproductive-age women who are sexually active, *Staphylococcus saprophyticus* (Table 31-1).[5] In contrast, the organisms that commonly colonize the distal urethra and skin of both men and women and the vagina of women rarely cause UTI. These include *Staphylococcus epidermidis*, *Corynebacteria*, lactobacilli, *Gardnerella vaginalis*, and a variety of anaerobes (Table 31-2). Similarly, the search for such fastidious organisms as *Ureaplasma urealyticum* and *Mycoplasma hominis* as causes of UTI is not justified.[5-8]

A more difficult problem in interpreting urine cultures is vaginal contamination because 5% to 20% of women may harbor gram-negative bacilli at this site in the absence of UTI. In these situations, further information can be gained from the number of different bacterial species identified in a particular urine specimen. In more than 95% of true UTIs, a single bacterial species is responsible for the infection. True polymicrobial UTI occurs uncommonly and is observed in very few clinical situations: when a long-term urinary catheter or another "foreign body" (e.g., calculi, necrotic tumors) is in place; when the patient has a stagnant pool of urine

because of inadequate emptying of the bladder, particularly when repeated instrumentation is necessary; or when there is a fistulous communication between the urinary tract and the gastrointestinal or female genital tracts. Otherwise, the isolation of two or more bacterial species on urine culture usually signifies a contaminated specimen.[8-10]

The second major criterion for determining the validity of culture results is based on the quantification of the number of colony-forming units (CFUs) in the urine; this number reflects the number of viable bacteria present. Since the early studies of Kass,[11, 12] it has been apparent that quantitative urine cultures can prove useful in determining whether or not true infection is present: those individuals with urine cultures that revealed at least 10^5 CFU/mL (often termed "significant bacteriuria") had a high probability of true infection; those with lesser numbers of CFUs ("insignificant bacteriuria") had a high probability of being free of infection, with those bacteria isolated being probable contaminants. This approach was particularly useful in the performance of population-based epidemiologic studies, the setting in which Kass formulated this concept.

Unfortunately, the direct application of these quantitative criteria in clinical practice has led to significant confusion. It is now apparent that patients with symptoms referable to the urinary tract may have treatable bacteriuria (and the awkward designation of "true but less than significant bacteriuria") with as few as 10^2 CFU/mL on quantitative culture. As a result, new criteria have been established to ensure adequate sensitivity and specificity: Women who present with symptoms of acute, uncomplicated UTI (dysuria, frequency, suprapubic discomfort) are thought to have true infection when at least 10^3 CFU/mL of a single species of uropathogen are found on quantitative culture (sensitivity of 80% and specificity of 90%). In patients with symptoms of acute, uncomplicated pyelonephritis (fever, rigors, flank pain, with or without dysuria or frequency), the cutoff is at least 10^4 CFU/mL (sensitivity and specificity of 95%).[5, 9, 10]

Examination of a gram-stained specimen of urine has been traditionally used as a screening test for significant bacteriuria because the finding of at least one organism per oil immersion field has a 95% sensitivity for detecting bacteriuria at a level of 10^5 CFU/mL or greater, whereas the finding of at least five organisms confers a specificity of 95%.[13] Given the present recognition that lesser numbers of bacteria can be clinically important, this approach has fallen out of favor. Perhaps its greatest use today is in patients with pyelonephritis, in whom the demonstration of gram-positive or gram-negative bacteria can be useful in choosing initial antimicrobial therapy.

TABLE 31-1

Bacteriologic Findings among 250 Outpatients and 150 Inpatients with Urinary Tract Infection

BACTERIAL SPECIES	OUTPATIENTS (%)	INPATIENTS (%)
Escherichia coli	89.2	52.7
Proteus mirabilis	3.2	12.7
Klebsiella pneumoniae		
Enterococci		
Enterobacter aerogenes		
Pseudomonas aeruginosa		
Proteus spp (excluding *P. mirabilis*)	2.4	
	2.0	
	0.8	
	0.4	
	0.4	9.3
	7.3	
	4.0	
	6.0	
	3.3	
Serratia marcescens	0.0	3.3
Staphylococcus epidermidis*	1.6	0.7
Staphylococcus aureus	0.0	0.7

*It is likely that most of the outpatient *S. epidermidis* strains in healthy, sexually active young women were *S. saprophyticus*.

Modified from Rubin RH: Infections of the urinary tract. *In* Dale DC, Federman DD (eds): Scientific American Medicine, sec 7, subsec 23. New York, Scientific American, 1996, pp 1-10. Copyright © [1996] Scientific American, Inc. All rights reserved.

TABLE 31-2

Common Bacterial Contaminants of Urine Cultures That Are Unlikely Causes of True Urinary Tract Infections

Staphylococcus epidermidis
Corynebacteria (diphtheroids)
Lactobacillus
Gardnerella vaginalis
Anaerobic bacteria

Circumstances associated with lower densities of bacteria in the urine when the patient has true infection include acute urethral syndrome, infection with *S. saprophyticus* and *Candida* species, prior administration of antimicrobial therapy, rapid diuresis, extreme acidification of the urine, obstruction of the urinary tract, and extraluminal infection.[5, 9, 10]

Examination of the urine for leukocytes is the final validation test that can be applied in the evaluation of patients with possible UTI. When a randomly collected urine sample is examined in a hemocytometer and at least 10 leukocytes per cubic millimeter are found, there is a high probability of clinical infection:

1. More than 96% of symptomatic men and women with significant bacteriuria have at least this level of pyuria; fewer than 1% of asymptomatic, nonbacteriuric individuals have this level of pyuria.
2. Most symptomatic women with pyuria but without significant bacteriuria have urinary infection with either bacterial uropathogens present in colony counts of less than 10^5 CFU/mL (which will respond to appropriate antimicrobial therapy) or with some other condition (pyuria always requires an explanation). In reproductive-age, sexually active women, *Chlamydia trachomatis* is a common cause of this problem. Other causes of "sterile pyuria" include interstitial cystitis, genitourinary tuberculosis, systemic mycotic infection, and contiguous infection resting on the ureter or bladder and inducing "sympathetic inflammation" in the urine. This last usually occurs in the setting of colonic or gynecologic pathology (e.g., diverticular abscess or cancer).
3. One situation in which the finding of pyuria does not add significantly to the diagnostic evaluation is in patients with indwelling urinary catheters. In these individuals, the finding of pyuria does not necessarily indicate infection.[14]

Although assessing pyuria has utility, a reliable technique must be employed. The traditional method of counting the number of white blood cells present per high-power field in the resuspended sediment of a centrifuged aliquot of urine is notoriously inaccurate in this regard. In contrast, the leukocyte esterase test is a useful screening test for pyuria, with a reported sensitivity of 75% to 96% and a specificity of 94% to 98%.[5, 9, 13]

Etiologic Agents
Bacterial Pathogens

The usual mechanism by which bacteria invade the urinary tract is via the ascending route, with the gastrointestinal tract being the reservoir from which the bacteria emerge. Reflecting this, the Enterobacteriaceae and *E. faecalis* are the most important causes of UTI in all population groups, accounting for more than 95% of all UTIs. Of the Enterobacteriaceae, *Escherichia coli* is by far the most common invader, causing some 90% of UTIs in outpatients and approximately 50% in hospitalized patients (see Table 31-1). The likelihood of a non–*E. coli* UTI or the possibility that the bacterial isolate will be antibiotic-resistant is influenced by three major factors: whether the flora of the gastrointestinal tract reservoir has been modified by previous antimicrobial therapy, whether the urinary tract has been subjected to instrumentation, and whether structural or functional obstruction of the urinary tract is present.

Clearly, hospitalized patients are most likely to have been subjected to one or more of these factors: environmental exposure to such organisms as *Serratia marcescens* and *Pseudomonas aeruginosa* and frequent treatment with broad-spectrum antimicrobial agents. In addition, they may have been subjected to urinary tract instrumentation (e.g., an indwelling bladder catheter) at a relatively high rate, thus increasing the chances of introduction of this modified gastrointestinal flora into the urinary tract.

Certain bacterial pathogens are especially associated with UTI in a particular population group. One notable example is the recognition that *S. saprophyticus* is an important cause of symptomatic UTI in young, sexually active women,[15-17] while being an uncommon cause of infection in men.[18] Other reported associations include an increased frequency of *Proteus* infections in boys aged 1 to 12 years, particularly if uncircumcised, and *E. faecalis* infection in elderly men with prostatism.[19-21]

Anaerobic bacteria play a minor role in the occurrence of UTI, becoming clinically important only in complicated infections in which malignancy is present, with anaerobic infection of necrotic tumor being the source of such infections.[22] The tumor may be present in the urinary tract, the gut, or the genital tract, with a fistulous tract being a common means of introducing these organisms into the urine in the case of gastrointestinal or gynecologic tumors.

In more than 95% of instances, UTI develops through the ascending route, from urethra to bladder to kidney. However, if bacteremia occurs from some other site, seeding of the urinary tract, particularly the kidney, can occur, with the most common manifestation being a positive urine culture. The incidence of hematogenous seeding is determined by the virulence of the organism present in the blood, with *Staphylococcus aureus*, *P. aeruginosa*, and *Salmonella* species accounting for virtually all hematogenously derived UTI. Indeed, a positive urine culture may be the first laboratory evidence of disseminated infection due to these organisms.[23]

Hematogenously derived infection of the urinary tract is particularly common in instances of *Salmonella* sepsis. Thus, approximately 25% of patients with *Salmonella typhi* infection have positive urine cultures. An unusual example of this phenomenon occurs in areas of the world where urinary tract schistosomiasis due to *Schistosoma haematobium* is common. In such patients, bacteremic seeding of the urinary tract with *Salmonella* species results in infection of the schistosomes and in chronic *Salmonella* bacteriuria. Reentry to the bloodstream by the salmonellae from the seeded urinary tract can then occur on a regular basis. Interestingly, such infections can be controlled only by eradicating the schistosomal infection first.[24]

Other bacteria that have been unusual causes of hematogenous UTI include *Brucella*,[25] *Nocardia*,[26] and *Actinomyces* species.[27] Far more important are cases of urinary tract tuberculosis. The kidney is the most common extrapulmonary site of tuberculosis; the tubercle bacilli reach the kidney from the lung by the hematogenous route, usually with later spread down the urinary tract to the ureter, bladder, and, in the male patient, prostate, seminal vesicle, and epididymis.[28]

Fungal Pathogens

By far the most common form of fungal infection of the urinary tract is that caused by *Candida* species. Most such infections occur in patients with indwelling Foley catheters who have been receiving broad-spectrum antibacterial therapy, particularly if diabetes mellitus is also present or corticosteroids are being administered. Although most of these infections remain limited to the bladder and clear with removal of the catheter, cessation of the antibacterial therapy, and control of the diabetes, the urinary tract is the source of approximately 10% of episodes of candidemia—usually in association with urinary tract manipulation or obstruction.[29, 30] Spontaneously occurring lower UTI caused by *Candida* species is far less common, although papillary necrosis, caliceal invasion, and fungal ball obstruction have all been described as resulting from ascending candidal UTI that is not related to catheterization. Candidal obstructive uropathy is particularly important in children with congenital anatomic abnormalities of the urinary tract and in kidney transplant recipients.[31-34] In the transplant patient, obstructive uropathy due to candiduria is a particularly dangerous situation, being associated with a high risk of systemic dissemination from the urinary tract.[34]

The urinary tract is more commonly the site of metastatic spread in cases of disseminated candidiasis than the portal of entry from which dissemination spreads. Indeed, as with hematogenously spread bacterial infection, the appearance of *Candida* species, particularly *Candida albicans* or *Candida tropicalis*, in the urine of a nonpregnant, nondiabetic, noncatheterized individual can be an early warning of disseminated candidiasis.[35] Other *Candida* species are less invasive for the urinary tract but can on occasion cause catheter-related UTI and, less commonly, focal pyelonephritis or disseminated infection.[30]

Hematogenous spread to the kidney and other sites within the genitourinary tract may be seen in any systemic fungal infection, but it occurs particularly in coccidioidomycosis and blastomycosis.[36, 37] In coccidioidomycosis, renal seeding is more common; in blastomycosis, lower genitourinary tract involvement is the rule.[38] In immunosuppressed patients, a common hallmark of disseminated cryptococcal infection is the appearance of this organism in the urine. *Cryptococcus neoformans* commonly seeds the prostate and, far less commonly, may cause a syndrome of papillary necrosis, pyelonephritis, and pyuria akin to that seen in tuberculosis.[39, 40] Thus, in the appropriate clinical and epidemiologic settings, the possibility of hematogenous seeding with a variety of fungal organisms in addition to tuberculosis and chlamydial infection (see later) should be considered in patients with bacteriologically sterile pyuria.

Other Pathogens

Several other classes of microorganisms, most notably *Chlamydia trachomatis*, the genital mycoplasmas, and certain viruses, can invade the urinary tract. *C. trachomatis* has been clearly shown to be an important cause of the acute

urethral syndrome.[5] Whether this organism could have an impact on the upper urinary tract remains to be demonstrated.

The two genital mycoplasmas are *Ureaplasma urealyticum* (formerly called T-strain mycoplasma) and *Mycoplasma hominis*. Both have been associated more with genital infection than with UTI, but *U. urealyticum* does cause a significant number of cases of urethritis (albeit fewer than *C. trachomatis*),[41] and both have been implicated as causes of chronic pyelonephritis, although this remains controversial.[5] Perhaps the best argument that these organisms may play a role in upper UTI is the report of the association of *U. urealyticum* with renal stones.[44]

Viruses have received far less attention in terms of their pathogenicity for the urinary tract. In normal persons, the most convincing case for virally induced disease can be made for adenoviruses. Thus, adenovirus types 11 and 21, particularly type 11, have been shown to cause between one fourth and one half of cases of hemorrhagic cystitis in schoolchildren, with sporadic cases also occurring in immunologically normal adults.[45] In such immunosuppressed patients as organ transplant and bone marrow transplant recipients, hemorrhagic cystitis, interstitial nephritis, and disseminated infection caused by adenoviruses are far more common.[36, 46] Similarly, tubulointerstitial nephritis due to papovaviruses, cytomegalovirus, and other agents can occur in these immunosuppressed individuals but are quite uncommon in other populations.[36, 47-50]

PATHOGENESIS

The first consideration in discussing the pathogenesis of UTI is the route by which microbes, especially bacteria, reach the urinary tract in general and the kidney in particular. Two potential routes have been noted: (1) the hematogenous route, with seeding of the kidney as a consequence of bloodstream infection, and (2) the ascending route, with microorganisms introduced from the urethra to the bladder, and then ascending to affect the kidney(s).

Hematogenous Infection

In humans, blood-borne infection of the urinary tract accounts for fewer than 3% of cases of UTI. The organisms responsible for such infection are very different from the usual causes of UTI (as outlined in Table 31-1). The major causes of hematogenous infection are *S. aureus*, *Salmonella* species, *P. aeruginosa*, and *Candida* species.[4]

Although *E. coli* accounts for the vast majority of UTIs, it is a rare cause of infection of the urinary tract as a consequence of bacteremia, unless some other factor is introduced. The inability of most *E. coli* strains to cause infection via the hematogenous route is related not only to their intrinsic non-pathogenicity by this route of infection but also to the small proportion of circulating bacteria that are actually deposited in the kidney. In addition, intrinsic bacterial clearing mechanisms within the renal tissue are able to clear the kidneys of these small numbers of organisms without sequelae. In sum, the level of *E. coli* infection required to accomplish seeding of the kidneys via the bloodstream will have lethal consequences for the individual long before infection can be established in the kidneys.[51-53] In contrast, *S. aureus* can cause suppurative infection of the kidney in the face of a low level of organisms in the bloodstream, a level that is compatible with life—the exact opposite situation as is obtained with *E. coli*.[51, 54]

Although the intact kidney is resistant to hematogenous *E. coli* infection, various processes affecting renal structure and function can increase the susceptibility of the kidney and can favor the initiation of pyelonephritis by the hematogenous route (and, presumably, via the ascending route as well). These processes include obstruction of urine flow (even for relatively short periods of time)[51, 55, 56]; intratubular chemical injury from drugs[58]; vascular factors, such as renal vein constriction[58] or arterial constriction[59]; hemorrhagic hypotension[51]; hypertension[60, 61]; K^+ depletion[62]; analgesics[63]; renal massage[64]; polycystic kidney disease[65]; experimentally induced diabetes mellitus[66-68]; and administration of estrogens.[69]

The mechanism by which obstruction increases the susceptibility of the kidney to infection is not entirely clear. The leading hypothesis is that increased tissue pressure in the kidney could be interfering with the renal microcirculation during the obstructive phase, interfering with the innate ability of the kidney to clear infection.[70, 71]

These experimental observations offer several important insights that are relevant to human infection:

1. In patients with normal urinary tract anatomy, the simultaneous demonstration of *E. coli* in the urine and the blood strongly suggests the kidney as a portal of entry for the bacteremia. In contrast, the simultaneous demonstration of *S. aureus*, *Candida*, or *Salmonella* infection in the blood and urine suggests a portal of entry outside the urinary tract with spread to the kidney and underscores the need for a careful search for the primary source of the infection. *P. aeruginosa* and *Proteus* infection can manifest either pattern.

2. Patients with increased intrarenal pressures resulting from urinary tract obstruction may be at risk for metastatic infection with various organisms, including those like *E. coli* that are usually not pathogenic for the kidney when bacteremia is present.

3. A kidney subjected to trauma may be at particular risk for the development of pyelonephritis. This observation may be especially relevant to patients who have undergone kidney transplantation and those experiencing physical trauma.

Ascending Infection

There is overwhelming clinical evidence that most infections of the kidney result from the inoculation of bacteria derived from the gastrointestinal tract into the urethra, from there to the bladder, and finally to the kidney. What has emerged since the 1980s is that there are specific virulence factors that are required to accomplish this task in the anatomically and functionally normal urinary tract, which has intrinsic host defenses to prevent this occurrence.[4, 72, 73]

Initiation of Ascending Urinary Tract Infection

The reservoir from which urinary tract pathogens emerge is the gastrointestinal tract. This observation has several profound implications:

- Females, because of the proximity of the anus to the urethra, are at increased risk for UTI (just as male homosexuals who engage in rectal intercourse are at increased risk for such infection[74]).
- Modification of the normal gastrointestinal flora caused by exposure to antibiotics or by residence within a nursing home or hospital markedly changes the microbial cause of UTIs that occur in these settings—the antibiotic-susceptible *E. coli* is less likely to be the cause in these cases; instead, the typical responsible organism is relatively antibiotic-resistant gram-negative species, including *P. aeruginosa*, *Proteus* species, and *S. marcescens*.
- Among the characteristics that render a particular clone of *E. coli* uropathogenic is the ability to maintain stable residence in the colon, from which it can then be introduced into the urinary tract.

As is discussed subsequently, the same bacterial surface ligands that mediate attachment to the uroepithelium and the same mucosal receptors that interact with these bacterial ligands in the urinary tract are present in the gastrointestinal tract and play a significant role in the maintenance of stable colonization by the uropathogens.[72, 75, 76] The crucial next step in the pathogenesis of UTI is the colonization of the distal urethra, the periurethral tissues, and, in the female patient, the vaginal vestibule with potential urinary tract pathogens. Although an effort has been made to correlate the occurrence of this initial step with personal hygiene habits, methods of menstrual protection, and types of intimate clothing, no clear-cut relationship has emerged.[77]

In contrast, a major host defense against this first step in the pathogenesis of UTI is the presence of the normal vaginal flora, particularly the lactobacilli. Stapleton and Stamm[77] have defined several mechanisms by which the lactobacilli, alone or in combination with other constituents of the normal vaginal flora, could protect against the initiation of UTI: (1) by contribution to the maintenance of an acid vaginal environment, which diminishes *E. coli* colonization; (2) by interference with the adherence of uropathogens, such as *E. coli*, by way of steric hindrance or other mechanisms; (3) by production of hydrogen peroxide, which interacts with peroxidase and halides in the vagina to kill *E. coli*; and, perhaps, (4) by elaboration of other antimicrobial substances that have not yet been defined. The clinical importance of this natural defense mechanism is demonstrated by the following observations:

1. Postmenopausal women, because of the lack of estrogens, have a higher pH in their vagina, have lost their lactobacilli, and, in many cases, are subject to recurrent UTI; estrogen replacement, topically or systemically, corrects these defects and is associated with a significantly decreased incidence of UTI.

2. Reproductive-age women, using spermicides containing nonoxynol-9, whether in conjunction with a diaphragm or another contraceptive strategy, have an increased risk of UTI associated with the antilactobacillus effect of the spermicide that is introduced into the vagina; repopulation of the vagina with the lactobacilli and other constituents of the normal flora by switching to alternative contraceptive strategies decreases

the subsequent risk of both vaginal colonization and UTI.[77, 78]

Whether sustained bacteriuria results from the colonization of the vaginal vestibule and distal urethra depends on the interaction of several factors: whether the colonizing species possesses surface adhesins that promote the *attachment* of the organisms to the epithelial surface (see later); whether the mucosal cells of a particular woman have a particularly high affinity for these bacterial adhesins; whether the subject secretes blood group antigens that block adhesin-receptor interaction (see later); and whether the bacteria are physically translocated into the bladder. Periurethral and vaginal mucosal cells derived from women who experience recurrent UTIs adhere to uropathogenic *E. coli* strains to a much greater extent than do cells derived from women who are free of this problem. Women who do not secrete AB blood group antigens in their body fluids (nonsecretors) are particularly susceptible to recurrent UTI (with a risk three to four times that of secretors). Binding of bacteria to the cells is accomplished through specific bacterial ligand–epithelial cell receptor interaction, which is physically blocked by the presence of secreted ABH blood group antigens in the urine and vaginal secretions of individuals who are secretors (approximately two thirds of the general population). Nonsecretors do not have this protective mechanism and hence are at increased risk for UTI. The secretor gene encodes glycosyltransferases that act on cell surface glycoproteins and glycosphingolipids, resulting in the release of ABH antigens into bodily secretions. One consequence of this process is that the vaginal epithelium of nonsecretors expresses unique glycosphingolipids that bind uropathogenic *E. coli*; these glycosphingolipids are not expressed on the epithelial cells of secretors. In sum, two genetically determined characteristics play a key role in the initiation of UTI: the genetic constitution of the bacterial strain that is colonizing (i.e., whether it possesses adhesins that mediate attachment) and the woman's own genetic constitution. Studies in mice have confirmed the role of specific genes in determining the susceptibility to *E. coli* UTI.[72, 76-86]

Men are normally protected against the initiation of UTI because of the anatomic separation of the urethral meatus and the anus, the length of the male urethra, and the bactericidal activity of prostatic secretions. Lack of circumcision has been linked to an increased risk of UTI, as have homosexual activity that involves anal intercourse and, rarely, heterosexual vaginal intercourse with a partner colonized with a uropathogen (a virulent strain, as opposed to a commensal strain, is far more efficient in transmitting infection to the male partner). However, because sustained colonization of the distal urethra in the male is difficult to accomplish, even in these circumstances, bacteriuria is unusual in the absence of prostatic dysfunction or other urogenital abnormalities. When isolates from men with prostatitis are compared with those from women with cystitis or pyelonephritis, the isolates from men exhibit far more virulence than do those from women.[74, 87-93]

Entry of Pathogens into the Bladder

The processes by which bacteria ascend from the urethra into the bladder are incompletely understood. One clearly demonstrated mechanism by which bacteria are introduced into the bladder is by instrumentation of the urethra and bladder, such as occurs with cystoscopy, urologic surgery, and the Foley catheter. In situations where no instrumentation is involved, manual manipulation of the urethra results in the introduction of bacteria into the bladder.[94]

A more common mechanism for introducing bacteria into the bladder is through sexual intercourse. A large number of studies have established this mechanism: the frequency of bacteriuria in the general female population was 12.8 times greater than among nuns of a similar age[95]; in another study it was shown that the frequency of bacteriuria was inversely related to the interval since last intercourse in a population of women attending a clinic for sexually transmitted diseases.[96] Nicolle and associates[97] reported a high association between the development of significant bacteriuria in women and intercourse in the previous 24 hours and noted that the frequency of intercourse was higher in infected women than in uninfected women. In this study, 75% of the episodes of UTI in women with a history of recurrent UTIs occurred within 24 hours of intercourse.

If intercourse is an important pathogenetic event in the development of UTI, then therapy directed at the immediate postintercourse period should be effective. Indeed, Vosti[98] noted that a single dose of antibiotic taken after intercourse is effective in preventing UTI in a group of women susceptible to recurrent UTI. Perhaps the most compelling data come from a study that showed that bacteria are routinely introduced during intercourse but that in most instances these bacteria are components of the normal flora of the vagina and distal urethra (*Staphylococcus epidermidis*, diphtheroids, and lactobacilli), which rarely cause UTI and are promptly cleared by voiding. However, if the vaginal vestibule is colonized with a uropathogenic strain of *E. coli*, then sustained bacteriuria can be established by intercourse. Once the vaginal vestibule is so colonized, the risk of UTI is approximately 10% in sexually active women.[23, 99]

On balance, it appears that sexual intercourse alone does not establish bacteriuria and that bacteriuria can occur in the absence of intercourse, but if intercourse is coupled with the presence of virulent bacteria in the vagina, it leads to an increased frequency of infection. Other factors that have been suggested as contributing to the entry of bacteria into the bladder include the following: urodynamic considerations (the frequency and timing of voiding, the volume of residual urine left in the bladder), hormonal changes, variations in the toxicity and antibacterial properties of the urine, personal hygiene habits, patterns of masturbation, and virulence properties of the resident bacterial flora.[100]

Bacterial Multiplication in the Bladder and Bladder Defense Mechanisms

Whatever the mode of entry of bacteria into the bladder, it has long been known that the normal bladder is capable of clearing itself of organisms within 2 to 3 days of their introduction. This property of the normal bladder represents an important defense mechanism against urinary infection and appears to depend on the combined effects of three factors: (1) the elimination of bacteria by voiding, (2) the antibacterial properties of urine and its constituents, and (3) the intrinsic mucosal bladder defense mechanisms.

Perhaps the most effective way of eliminating bacteria from the bladder is by voiding, which eliminates approximately 99% of bacteria present. This hydrokinetic defense mechanism is supplemented by constant dilution of the bladder urine by the constant inflow of urine from the kidneys, as well as the ability of the bladder mucosa to eliminate the small number of residual organisms that persist.[101-103]

The net effect of urine on bacterial growth in the bladder represents an integration of the influences of a variety of physicochemical entities. Urea, organic acids, salts, and low-molecular-weight polyamines in the urine, as well as conditions of low pH and high or low osmolality, inhibit bacterial growth. Both low pH and high osmolality adversely affect polymorphonuclear leukocyte function. In addition, such urinary osmoprotective substances as glycine and proline betaine protect *E. coli* against the effects of hypertonic urine. The inherent antibacterial activity of the bladder mucosa also plays a role in blocking the establishment of infection. Such activity appears to be due, at least in part, to the production of bactericidal molecules by the uroepithelium, with UTI-prone individuals producing fewer of these factors than healthy control subjects. Finally, inhibition of bacterial adherence to mucosal receptors acts as a useful defense against infection. These inhibitors include the layer of glycosaminoglycan that overlies the epithelial cell layer of the bladder and blocks bacterial attachment to the bladder mucosa. Adherence to the uroepithelium itself, through the adenylate cyclase signal transduction pathway, triggers the antibacterial activity mediated directly by uroepithelial cells.[72, 103-113]

Clinically, clearing of bacteriuria does not occur in the presence of frank residual urine, inadequate micturition, foreign bodies or stones in the bladder, increased vesical pressure, or previous inflammation of the bladder mucosa. The role of residual urine, foreign bodies, and preexisting inflammatory lesions is readily recognized. Residual urine not only increases the number of bacteria remaining in the bladder but also lowers the ratio between the surface area of the bladder mucosa and the volume of urine exposed to it, thus reducing the effectiveness of potential antibacterial

mucosal factors. Distention of the bladder and increased hydrostatic pressure inhibit clearance of bacteria.[114, 115]

The efficacy of bladder bacterial clearance mechanisms is demonstrated not only by experimental studies but also by clinical observation. A group of Swedish women with acute, uncomplicated UTI had a 70% clearance rate over a 1-month period, despite treatment only with a placebo.[116]

Vesicoureteral Reflux

An important host defense against ascending infection from the bladder to the kidneys is the competency of the vesicoureteral valve. Indeed, the combination of VUR and infected urine is the most common factor predisposing to chronic pyelonephritic scarring, particularly in infants and children.[117]

In the normal adult, the vesicoureteral valve is competent despite the high bladder pressures generated during micturition. VUR is prevented by virtue of the length of the intramural segment of the ureter; the ureter is obliquely inserted into a tunnel in the bladder wall (Fig. 31-1), so the intravesical portion of the ureter is compressed by the bladder musculature during micturition.[118, 119] Failure of this valve mechanism is most commonly due to shortening of the intravesical portion of the ureter (primary VUR).[120, 121] This shortening is thought to be caused by abnormal embryologic development of an ectopically located ureteric bud, so the ureteral orifices are displaced laterally. The intravesical portion of the ureter lengthens with growth, increasing the competence of the valve mechanisms and rendering it less susceptible to reflux.[121] The temporal aspects of the normal development of the vesicoureteral valve are, at present, incompletely delineated. One epidemiologic study[122] suggests, however, that two thirds of healthy infants younger than 6 months of age have at least mild to moderate reflux, with a rapid decrease thereafter. In the absence of infection, even antenatally demonstrated gross reflux improves or, in some cases, resolves by 2 years of age—a pattern of maturation of the vesicoureteral valve mechanism that has been well documented in nonhuman primates.[123-126]

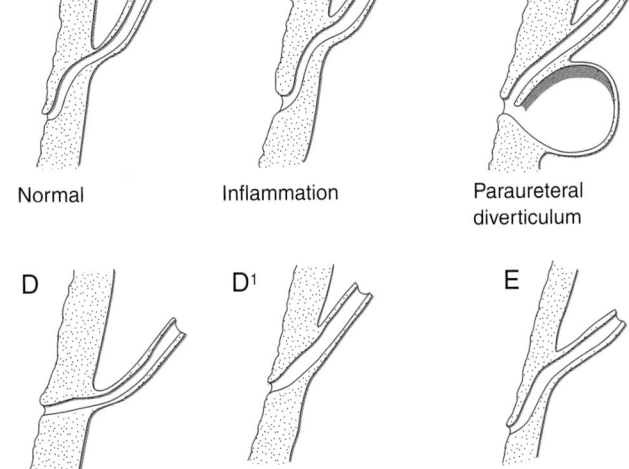

FIGURE 31-1. Intravesical position of the ureter in the normal person (**A**) and in patients with vesicoureteral reflux. Types **D** and **D**¹ are by far the most common in children and infants. **A** to **E**, From King LR, Surian MA, Wendel RM, Burden JJ: Vesicoureteral reflux: A classification based on cause and the results of treatment. JAMA 203:169-174, 1968. Copyright 1968, American Medical Association.)

Normal

Inflammation

Paraureteral diverticulum

Absence of intravesical ureter

Partial absence of intravesical ureter

Flaccid neurogenic bladder wall

In children, VUR may also be secondary, occurring in association with other anomalies and usually manifested by obstruction.[117] Neonates with neurogenic bladder disorders, such as myelodysplasia, in which high-pressure obstruction occurs, have no demonstrable VUR but eventually experience secondary VUR with typical ureteral "golf-hole" orifices as well as ureteral dilation and tortuosity. VUR develops in 45% of patients with meningomyelocele by the age of 5 years, sometimes with renal scarring.[127]

Bladder-sphincter dysfunctional disturbances in toddlers and children are associated with high-pressure VUR.[127-130] The elevated pressures apparently result from uninhibited bladder contractions followed by voluntary constriction of perineal musculature. In a study of 458 children with bladder dysfunction, Griffiths and Scholtmeiger[131] identified two different types of reflux and dysfunction complexes with contrasting urodynamic characteristics. In one, the bladder contracted poorly during voiding, and overactivity of the urethral closure mechanism was present. In this group, VUR was bilateral and was associated with upper urinary tract anomalies and renal scarring. In the second type, there was bladder instability and powerful voiding contractions of the bladder; this type was associated with unilateral reflux and rare renal scarring.

Of the congenital anatomic anomalies, VUR occurs commonly in the presence of a paraurethral diverticulum[132]; in 25% to 50% of boys with posterior urethral valves[132, 133]; in 10% of those with ureteropelvic junction obstruction[134]; and in patients with ureteral duplications, hypospadias, and ureteroceles. With the increasing application of ultrasound techniques to examine the fetus during pregnancy, numerous studies have now addressed the cause and the long-term implications of a dilated urinary tract, specifically hydronephrosis, identified antenatally. Although obstructive uropathy is assumed to be the cause of fetal hydronephrosis, VUR is found to be present in 10% to 40% of these infants studied postnatally, often with advanced grades of reflux. The hope would be that the aggressive treatment of these neonates, 75% to 80% of whom are boys, would help preserve renal function and facilitate kidney growth.[135-138]

Congenital VUR is five times more common in boys than in girls and tends to occur in families. When asymptomatic siblings of children with VUR are studied with sensitive radiologic procedures, approximately 40% have been shown to also have reflux, some with evidence of clinically silent scarring. Approximately two thirds of the offspring of parents with known VUR have evidence of reflux as well when they are studied by voiding cystourethrogram.[139-141] On the basis of segregation analysis of 88 affected families, Chapman and colleagues[142] concluded that the best model was that of a single dominant gene acting together with a random environmental effect. Computer modeling indicated that the gene frequency was 1 in 600 and that mutation was uncommon.

VUR occurs in 18% of adults who have spinal cord injuries and in a variable percentage of adults with bladder tumors, prostatic hypertrophy, and urinary tract stones.[143] It can also follow fulguration of lesions in the area of the orifice or simple trauma, such as extraction of a ureteral calculus by means of a "basket."[117]

Still unresolved is the question of whether bladder infection can precede and, in a way, cause VUR. Bladder infection can cause reflux in some experimental animals, but studies in adult primates with chronic cystitis demonstrate no reflux.[143] A series of studies on renal infection and reflux in monkeys by Roberts and co-workers[143, 144] suggests, however, that bladder infection increases the duration of reflux and renders a partially competent ureterovesical junction that is overtly refluxing. The clinical evidence suggests that infection is not a necessary cause of reflux but that it can precipitate reflux in a ureterovesical junction that is congenitally defective or, indeed, can increase the grade of reflux.[145] E. coli infection has been shown to inhibit cell division in the baby rat, an effect that is apparently mediated by endotoxin.[146] Presumably, because cell multiplication is required for the maturation of the vesicoureteral junction, this is the mechanism for the link between infection and reflux and is the explanation for the beneficial effects of long-term antibiotic therapy in the management of these patients (see later).

VUR, which can be unilateral or bilateral, may vary considerably in severity. Severity of reflux is graded by means of voiding cystourethrography in numerous ways.[147] The grading system adopted by the International Reflux Study Committee is as follows (Fig. 31-2)[148]:

Grade I: reflux partly up the ureter
Grade II: reflux up to the pelvis and calices without dilation; normal caliceal fornices
Grade III: same as grade II, but with mild or moderate dilation and tortuosity of the ureter and no blunting of the fornices
Grade IV: moderate dilation and tortuosity of the ureters, pelvis, and calices; complete blunting of fornices
Grade V: gross dilation and tortuosity of the ureter, pelvis, and calices; absent papillary impressions in the calices

Many technical and clinical factors can influence the grade of the reflux as seen on the voiding cystogram, however, and few attempts have been made to standardize this procedure.[147-149] Despite this, it is clear that there is a correlation between the severity of the reflux and the extent of renal scarring.[150, 151]

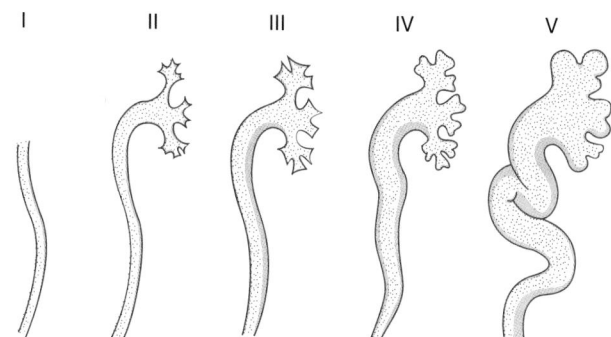

FIGURE 31-2. Grades of reflux. International Reflux Study classification. I. Ureter only. II. Ureter, pelvis, and calices. No dilation, normal caliceal fornices. III. Mild or moderate dilation or tortuosity of ureter or both, and mild or moderate dilation of renal pelvis but no or slight blunting of fornices. IV. Moderate dilation or tortuosity of ureter or both, and moderate dilation of renal pelvis and calices. Complete obliteration of sharp angle of fornices but maintenance of papillary impressions in majority of calices. V. Gross dilation and tortuosity of ureter. Gross dilation of renal pelvis and calices. Papillary impressions are no longer visible in majority of calices.

Radionuclide cystography is emerging as an alternative and, in many ways, superior technique for evaluating VUR.[152] Indirect radionuclide cystography, in which the radionuclide is injected intravenously, is noninvasive but detects only high-pressure gross VUR and requires good renal function. Conversely, cystography after direct instillation of radionuclide (technetium 99m pertechnetate) has proved to be a sensitive, quantitative, and safe procedure that also serves as a test for evaluating functional bladder disorders.[152]

Although the significance of VUR was appreciated as early as 1903 by Sampson, it was Hodson and Edwards who demonstrated renal pyelonephritic scarring by radiographic means.[153] Since then, a great deal of evidence linking VUR, renal infection, and renal scarring has accumulated,[117, 154-157] and the findings can be summarized as follows:

1. In various series, VUR can be demonstrated by voiding cystourethrography in 30% to 50% of children with recurrent infection and in 85% to 100% of children and 50% of adults with chronic pyelonephritic scarring.[126, 132, 155] Furthermore, even in children and adults with renal scars who do not exhibit reflux, anatomic abnormalities of the ureteral orifices (lateral ectopia and abnormal configuration) are seen cystoscopically, which suggests that reflux had been present in the past.[120]
2. Alternatively, between 30% and 60% of children with VUR exhibit pyelonephritic scarring, the higher figure being derived from surgical clinics and the lower from medical studies.[158]
3. Renal scarring of the pyelonephritic type is found in up to 25% of children with UTI, and as mentioned, about 30% to 50% of these have VUR.[126, 159-170]
4. Several studies have documented the progressive development of clubbing of the calices and renal scarring after discovery of VUR in previously normal kidneys.[126, 171-177] Progressive scarring appears in the severer forms of reflux and almost always in the presence of infected urine. It must be stressed, however, that in many infants and children with VUR, pyelonephritic scarring never develops, and VUR may disappear either spontaneously or with antibacterial therapy in up to 80% of ureters after long follow-up.[159] Even severe reflux associated with scarring may disappear, although reflux is more likely to cease if it is mild or moderate and if the kidneys are unscarred. Among adults, about 90% with severe VUR have renal scars.[177, 178]
5. All stages of pyelonephritis, from acute suppurative inflammation to typical chronic pyelonephritic scarring, can be produced in experimental animals by inducing VUR and concomitant lower UTI.[179, 180]

Intrarenal Reflux

Whereas VUR is responsible for the ascent of bacteria into the renal pelvis, considerable evidence now suggests that the spread of infection from the pelvis into the cortex occurs by virtue of a phenomenon known as intrarenal reflux. Brodeur and associates,[181] Amat,[182] and Rolleston and colleagues[183] found that in some children with urinary infection, contrast medium instilled into the bladder during voiding cystourethrography permeated the renal parenchyma as far as the renal capsule. Intrarenal reflux occurred with the severer grades of VUR (Fig. 31-3). Curiously, intrarenal reflux

was focal in distribution and affected predominantly the two polar regions of the kidney, areas that are frequently the site of chronic scars. It was suggested that such intrarenal reflux could form the basis of the spread and distribution of infection. Intrarenal reflux has since been reported by others,[184-187] although, for a number of reasons, conventional techniques may fail to demonstrate it.

The importance of intrarenal reflux in the pathogenesis of pyelonephritic scarring has been confirmed by two series of elegant experimental studies. Hodson and associates[154, 179] induced VUR in piglets by incising the anterior wall of the intramural ureter. When bladder pressures were raised in these animals by placement of a silver ring around the proximal urethra, intrarenal reflux could be readily demonstrated (Fig. 31-4). Particularly in the presence of infected urine, the precise foci that exhibited intrarenal reflux developed acute inflammation and subsequent scarring (Figs. 31-5 and 31-6), and the distribution of intrarenal scars was remarkably similar to that occurring in human kidneys in that it affected mainly the lower and upper poles.

Ransley and Risdon[188-190] confirmed and extended these studies and made the observation that intrarenal reflux in the multipapillary kidneys of both human infants and young pigs occurred only in renal papillae with particular morphologic characteristics. They found two basic forms of renal papillae:

1. Nonrefluxing papillae are conic, and their papillary ducts open obliquely near the tip of the papilla onto a

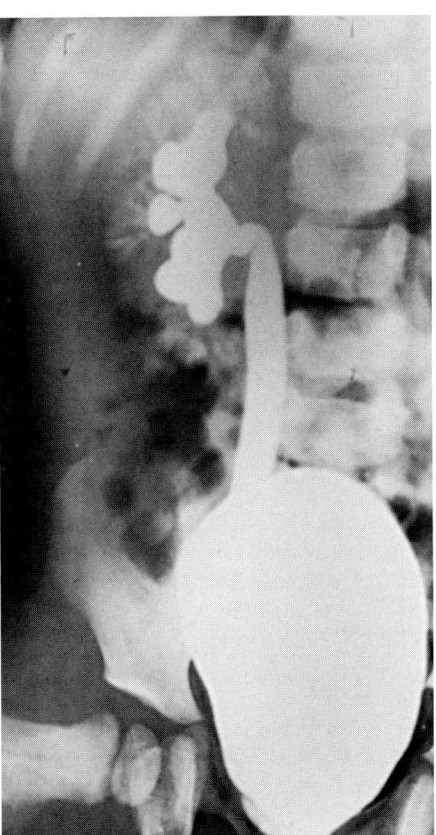

FIGURE 31-3. Cystogram showing severe grade of vesicoureteral reflux (grade IV) with scattered intrarenal reflux into all zones of the kidney. (From Hodson CJ: Reflux nephropathy. Med Clin North Am 62:1201, 1978.)

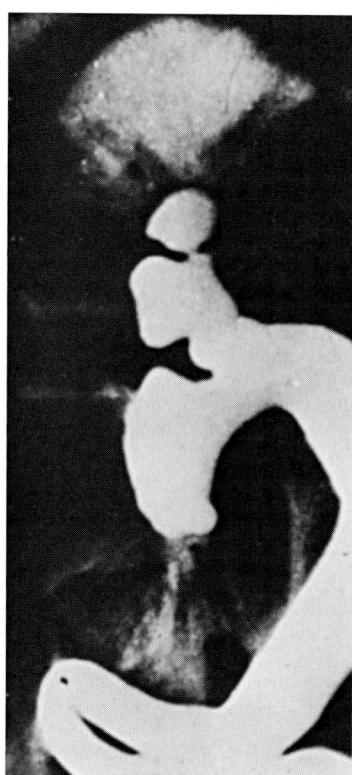

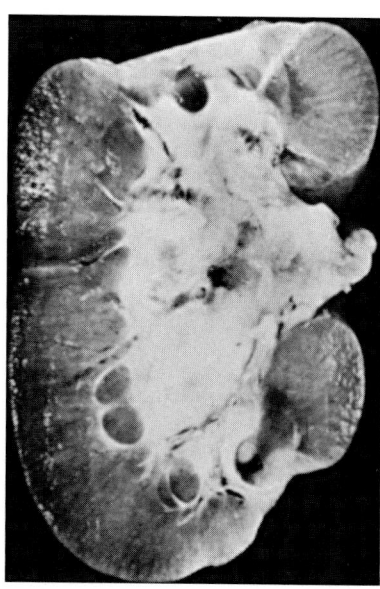

FIGURE 31-6. Typical polar scars 3 months after infected intrarenal reflux in the pig. Note dilation of the calyx underlying the scars. (From Hodson CJ, Maling RM, McManamon PJ, Lewis MJ: The pathogenesis of reflux nephropathy [chronic atrophic pyelonephritis]. Br J Radiol 13:1, 1975.)

FIGURE 31-4. Intrarenal reflux in the pig. Note that there is major involvement of the upper pole but somewhat less involvement of the lower pole. Compare the distribution of polar intrarenal reflux with that of acute inflammation (see Fig. 31–5) and scarring (see Fig. 31–6). (From Hodson CJ, Maling RM, McManamon PJ, Lewis MJ: The pathogenesis of reflux nephropathy [chronic atrophic pyelonephritis]. Br J Radiol 13:1, 1975).

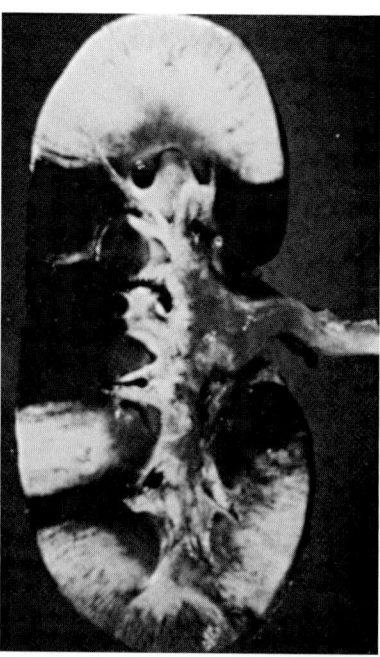

FIGURE 31-5. Large acute lesions of acute bacterial inflammation from infected intrarenal reflux in the pig. The subsequent contraction of these lesions gives rise to focal scars (see Fig. 31–6). (From Hodson CJ: Reflux nephropathy. Med Clin North Am 62:1201, 1978.)

convex surface through slitlike orifices (Fig. 31-7A). These papillae may be simple, representing a single renal reniculus, or compound, in which two or more reniculi have fused. Such papillae are never associated with intrarenal reflux, because even in the presence of VUR, their orifices are closed by the rise of pressure within the calyx.

2. Refluxing papillae are larger as a result of fusion of several adjacent reniculi (see Fig. 31-7B). They have concave rather than convex tips, and the papillary ducts open with gaping orifices that cannot be closed by an increase in intracaliceal pressure. Of great significance is that both in infants and in young pigs, refluxing papillae are present predominantly in the upper and lower poles (which are more susceptible to renal scarring); the simple and compound types are present mostly in the midzones (Table 31-3). In addition, although the number of refluxing papillae is less in the human than in the pig, approximately two thirds of human kidneys contained at least one potentially refluxing papilla, and in one fifth of the kidneys, the percentage of nonconvex papillae was 30% or more. Tamminen and Kaprio[191] reported similar findings in the kidneys of infants and children dying of nonrenal causes.

In summary, there are two main determinants for the progression of ascending infection from the bladder into the renal parenchyma:

1. VUR most commonly is apparently due to a congenital anatomic abnormality of the insertion of the ureter into the bladder.
2. Intrarenal reflux is determined by the presence of morphologically distinct papillae with open ducts, which

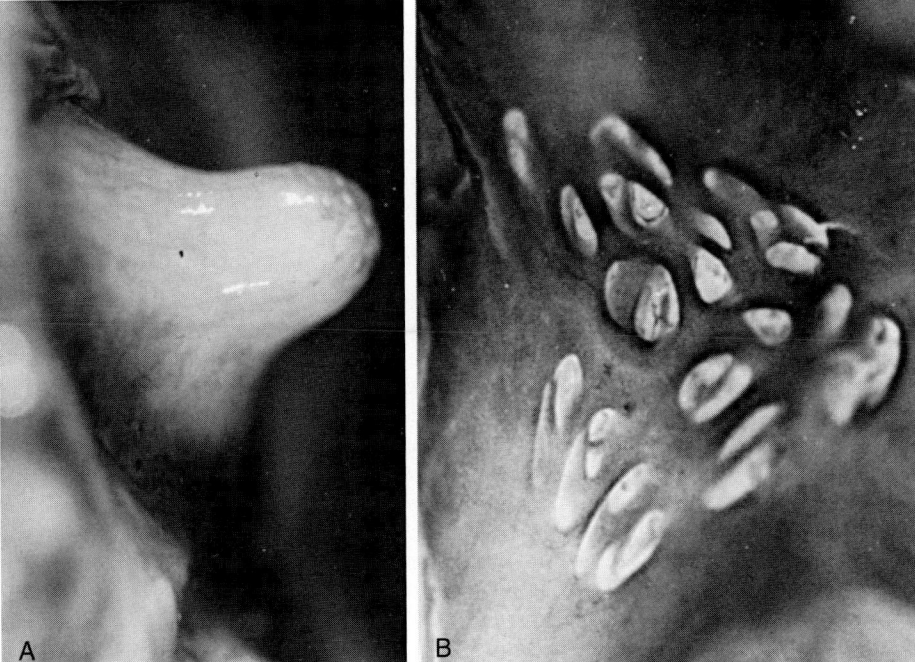

FIGURE 31-7. A, A simple, nonrefluxing papilla from pig kidney. Note the conic form, with papillary ducts opening near the tip onto a convex surface. **B,** A compound refluxing papilla with a concave surface and wide-open papillary duct orifices. (From Ransley PG, Risdon RA: The pathogenesis of reflux nephropathy. Br J Radiol 14:1, 1978.)

TABLE 31-3

Distribution of Compound Type II and III (Refluxing) Papillae in Normal Young Human and Porcine Kidneys

SPECIES	NONE	BOTH UPPER AND LOWER POLES	UPPER POLE ONLY	LOWER POLE ONLY
Human* (*n* = 33)	6 (18%)	14 (42%)	4 (12%)	9 (27%)
Pig (*n* = 25)	24 (96%)	1 (4%)	0 (0%)	0 (0%)

*Only one kidney showed a refluxing papilla in the midzone.

From Ransley PG, Risdon RA: Renal papillary morphology in infants and young children. Urol Res 3:111, 1977.

allows spread of organisms into the renal parenchyma in the presence of high intracaliceal pressure. VUR and intrarenal reflux, in combination, are almost certainly the major mechanisms responsible for the renal inflammation and scarring characteristic of chronic pyelonephritis.

These findings of VUR, intrarenal reflux, and papillary morphologic characteristics can also explain some perplexing clinical observations in children. It has been amply shown that in most children with VUR who have renal scars, scarring is already evident at the initial radiologic investigation, which is usually performed because of recurrent UTI. Scarring thus appears to occur early in life, possibly even in utero. For example, Rolleston and associates[149] found that 147 (42%) of 350 infants (age range, 3 days to 12 months; mean age, 3 months) had VUR, 49 with gross reflux. Twenty-nine of the 49 infants with gross VUR (59%) had kidneys that were already damaged by 12 months of age. No damage associated with the lesser degrees of VUR was found. Bailey[155] noted that 10 infants presenting with UTI and

VUR from 9 days to 7 weeks of life already had evidence of renal scarring. Indeed, the development of new scars in children is unusual beyond the age of 5 years (and possibly the age of 2 years), regardless of proven episodes of UTI.[192] Ransley and Risdon[190] proposed the "big bang" theory of scar formation to account for such findings: in the presence of gross VUR, the first few episodes of clinical or subclinical UTI in infants and children affect potentially refluxing papillae, leaving nonrefluxing papillae intact. The nonrefluxing papillae are resistant to damage by further episodes of UTI. Normal kidney parenchyma drained by nonrefluxing papillae continue to resist the challenge of UTI and VUR. These findings also point to the importance of early detection of UTI and the gross forms of VUR if renal scarring is to be prevented.

Sterile Reflux

Although the association between VUR in the infected child and renal scarring is unequivocal, the question of whether reflux results in renal damage in the absence of bacterial infection (sterile reflux) deserves consideration. This is a particularly attractive notion because VUR can disappear from one or both involved ureters; sterile reflux would then account for those cases of pyelonephritic scarring not associated with infection and not exhibiting obvious signs of reflux when they are discovered (see later). It has been shown that renal inflammation and scarring can result from high-pressure VUR in the total absence of infection, particularly if there is sustained bladder decompensation (i.e., if bladder pressure does not return to normal between micturitions in the presence of outflow obstruction).[179, 193-195] However, there is still considerable controversy as to the frequency with which such damage occurs clinically.

Several authors have reported progressive renal dysfunction or end-stage kidney disease apparently associated with sterile reflux.[149, 196-202] Others have found no consistent correlation between the frequency of UTI and the occurrence of progressive damage in patients with VUR. Unfortunately, it is difficult to acquire clinical evidence on both these points. Most patients with reflux nephropathy already have renal scars when they are first seen, and the finding of sterile urine at this time does not mean that infection has never occurred. Progression of an established scar may simply reflect contraction of the scar with hypertrophy of the surrounding parenchyma from a previous infection rather than progression in the presence of sterile urine.[202] Furthermore, a large group of children with reflux who were observed for up to 15 years had no new renal scars when a sterile urine was maintained by prophylactic antibacterial therapy.[203, 204] On the basis of their review of the clinical literature, Ransley and Risdon[189] contended that the occurrence of a completely new scar in a previously normal kidney with continuously sterile urine has not been reported. However, infected reflux may so modify the morphologic features of some apparently nonrefluxing papillae as to allow intrarenal reflux and progressive scarring but only in the presence of reinfection. In addition, the development of hypertension or glomerular injury in some patients with reflux nephropathy may be responsible for functional deterioration unrelated to the direct effects of VUR.

Hodson and Cotran[117] and others have suggested that high-pressure obstructed situations, which occur in children with reflux associated with congenital obstruction (i.e., posterior urethral valves), may lead to sterile renal damage akin to that in the experimental models described earlier. Ransley and colleagues,[193] however, argued that the renal scarring in these patients is more probably due to coexistent renal dysplasia or unrecognized UTI.

The balance of evidence on this issue suggests that renal involvement in reflux nephropathy occurs early in childhood, before age 5 years, largely as a result of superimposition of bacterial UTI on VUR and intrarenal reflux.[205] Because most potentially refluxing papillae are thus affected early on, additional progressive scarring occurs rarely, owing to the transformation of papillae from nonrefluxing to refluxing types. This accounts for the occurrence of new segmental scars or sequential scarring of an already scarred kidney, but such progression is rare. If sterile intrarenal reflux induces renal damage, it does so in the presence of severe obstructive uropathy with high intrapelvic pressures. Such may be the case in children with posterior urethral valves or other obstructive congenital anomalies.

Before this discussion of the significance of VUR in the pathogenesis of renal pyelonephritic scarring is concluded, a few points regarding VUR and renal disease should be emphasized. First, most cases of VUR are detected during investigations for UTI, the most common marker for this disorder. The actual frequency of VUR in the general population, and in particular in patients with other renal manifestations, such as proteinuria and hypertension, is unknown. Second, there is evidence that VUR, when sought, may be detected in patients with nonpyelonephritic forms of chronic renal disease, including chronic glomerulonephritis and nephrosclerosis.[206-209] Bishop and colleagues,[208] for example, found VUR in 12 of 40 patients with chronic glomerulonephritis who were maintained on long-term hemodialysis. In all but one ureter, reflux was mild or moderate. In four of these patients, reflux occurred after long-term dialysis, which suggests that hemodialysis may in some way provoke VUR. In 85 consecutive adult patients with end-stage renal disease, Huland and associates[209] found 11 patients with chronic glomerulonephritis or nephrosclerosis who had VUR (grades I and II). Third, in addition to renal scarring, VUR in children is associated with reduced renal growth, and there is some question as to whether VUR or UTI or both play a role in such growth retardation.[210-212] Finally, in patients with VUR, renal function may deteriorate for reasons other than UTI, particularly hypertension, an associated glomerulopathy, urinary obstruction, or analgesic abuse. All these points emphasize the complexity of assessing the interrelationships among VUR, UTI, and chronic renal disease.[213-223]

Bacterial Virulence Factors Influencing Infection
Escherichia coli

Perhaps the most important advance in the study of UTI has been the recognition that a limited number of clones of *E. coli* are responsible for the great majority of UTIs occurring in healthy women. These virulent clones possess a variety of virulence factors that facilitate the accomplishment of the tasks involved in the pathogenesis of ascending UTI and acute pyelonephritis. These tasks include the following: prolonged intestinal carriage, persistence in the vaginal vestibule, and then ascension and invasion of the anatomically normal urinary tract. In the presence of foreign bodies, VUR, or obstruction, ascending UTI can be caused by nonvirulent strains of *E. coli* (and other bacteria).[224-227] There is abundant clinical evidence of this pathogenesis, perhaps most notably in outbreaks of UTI in which the same clone was found in the patients so affected.[228, 229]

The first evidence that *E. coli* strains causing pyelonephritis were different from other isolates came from serotyping studies, in which the O (somatic or surface cell wall) antigen, H (flagellar) antigen, and K (capsular) antigen of isolates from well-defined clinical populations were determined. Whereas the serotypes associated with asymptomatic bacteriuria do not differ from those present in the fecal reservoir,[230] strains from symptomatic patients are significantly different both when serotyping is carried out and when molecular genetic analyses are performed.[225] Thus, a small minority of *E. coli* strains, as determined by their O antigens (O1, O2, O4, O6, O7, O8, O9, O11, O16, O18, O22, O25, O39, O50, O62, O75, and O78), account for more than 80% of the cases of pyelonephritis caused by *E. coli*. Similarly, a small number of K antigens (K1, K2, K3, K5, K12, and K13 or K51) are identifiable on more than 70% of the pyelonephritis isolates. In contrast, the H antigens appear not to be independently associated with virulence.[230-236]

It is likely that these O antigens are not themselves responsible for the uropathogenicity of these strains of *E. coli*; rather, the genes that determine the O antigen structure are closely linked to other genes that are responsible for the pathogenicity of these isolates.[237, 238] In contrast, the acidic polysaccharide capsular K antigens do appear to be directly pathogenic by inhibiting both phagocytosis and complement-mediated bactericidal activity. The amount of K antigen expressed appears to be especially important because strains of *E. coli* that are particularly rich in K antigen appear to be more successful both in reaching the bladder and in ascending to and invading the kidney than are strains with low amounts of K antigen.[233, 236, 239-244]

A variety of additional factors have been defined that are believed to contribute to the virulence of a particular isolate. These include surface adhesins that mediate attachment to specific receptors on the uroepithelium; molecules that preferentially capture metabolites and growth factors that enhance growth and proliferation (e.g., iron); and toxins that injure the tissue of the urinary tract and induce a brisk inflammatory response. The term *pathogenicity-associated islands (PAIs)* is used to describe the clustering of virulence genes on the chromosome; these stretches of DNA are not found in nonuropathogenic organisms, such as routine isolates of *E. coli* of fecal origin from uninfected individuals. PAI sequences are found in the great majority of uropathogenic strains, are uncommonly found in fecal isolates, and are sometimes demonstrable in other gram-negative UTI isolates. The genes found in these PAIs encode the following virulence traits: P fimbriae and other adhesins (surface structures of bacteria that attach to particular receptors on the uroepithelium that results in sustained attachment of the bacteria—an essential step in the pathogenesis of UTI and pyelonephritis), hemolysin, the iron-binding protein aerobactin, toxins (e.g., cytotoxin necrotizing factor type 1), and resistance to the bactericidal effect of normal human serum.[229, 245-250]

Type 1, or common, fimbriae were the first of the bacterial adhesins identified. They were defined on the basis of the ability of mannose to inhibit agglutination of red blood cells. Similarly, mannose will inhibit the adherence of the bacteria to uroepithelial cells. These structures are widely distributed in gram-negative bacteria and are present on approximately 75% of *E. coli*. These adhesins mediate binding to mannose residues on the Tamm-Horsfall protein in the urine (thus preventing ligand-receptor interaction and sustained attachment of the bacteria to the uroepithelium), to the carbohydrate portion of secretory IgA, and to phagocytic cells. Given the ubiquity of type 1 fimbriae, it has been difficult to define their role. It has been suggested that type 1 fimbriae may be important in the injury to kidney that bacteria can produce by the release of free oxygen radicals and other tissue-destroying enzymes that are products of an enhanced inflammatory response; similarly, renal scarring has been associated with the presence of type 1 fimbriae on the invading bacteria. Type 1 fimbriae have been particularly associated with bacterial isolates from patients with cystitis. Studies in mice suggest an even greater role for type 1 fimbriae: bacterial

mutants lacking the tip adhesion (FimH) of the type 1 fimbriae fail to colonize the urinary tract of mice, whereas restoration of FimH restores virulence and the ability to cause UTI. Of particular interest is that a FimH-based vaccine had provided significant protection against UTI in both mice and monkeys.[227, 231, 233, 251-264]

In contrast to the situation with type 1 fimbriae in which the precise role these adhesins play in the pathogenesis of UTI has not been established, type 2 pili (P fimbriae) are intimately involved in the pathogenesis of pyelonephritis in individuals with normal urinary tract anatomy and physiology. The P fimbriae are not only the most important of the adhesin-receptor systems thus far identified but also the most important uropathogenic virulence factors that have been defined. These adhesins, whose binding is resistant to the effects of mannose, have been given a variety of names reflecting their association with pyelonephritis and a particular receptor: P pili, P fimbriae, Pap pili (pyelonephritis-associated pili), and Gal-Gal pili. Their binding-specificity is to the globoseries of glycolipid receptors that have a common disaccharide, αGal(1-4)-βGal. These receptors are identical to the glycosphingolipids of the P blood group system and are found on the epithelial tissues of the urinary tract, kidneys, and large intestine, but not on phagocytic cells. This provides a mechanism for sustained colonization of the large intestine by uropathogenic clones, colonization of the vaginal vestibule, and the ability to ascend the urinary tract, even in the absence of an anatomic abnormality. In addition, the absence of these receptors on granulocytes provides protection to these uropathogens. Essentially all *E. coli* blood isolates from normal individuals with pyelonephritis express P fimbriae; non–P-piliated isolates are isolated from individuals with compromised host defenses, especially defects in leukocyte number or function.[227, 229, 231, 235, 249, 250, 252, 265]

An additional binding site for piliated *E. coli* is fibronectin, thus providing a mechanism for attachment of the bacteria to the extracellular matrix. The presence of P fimbriae on uropathogenic *E. coli* clones is maintained stably, presumably related to the chromosomal localization (usually as a component of a pathogenicity island with other virulence genes). The operon for these fimbriae, known as Pap, consists of 11 genes.[265-271] Expression of these pili is under a phase variation control mechanism in which individual bacterial cells alternate between being phenotypically pilus-positive and pilus-negative through a process involving DNA methylation by deoxyadenosine methylase.[272] Phase variation can be extremely rapid and appears to be dependent on both the growth phase of the bacterial cell and the growth conditions present. Although the genetic mechanisms by which this occurs are still unclear, there is no question that phase variation occurs in vivo and has an important effect on the pathogenesis and consequences of UTI.[235]

Other, less well-characterized, adhesins have been reported to be present on uropathogenic strains of *E. coli*: S fimbriae, which bind to terminal sialic acid residues on both epithelial cells and phagocytes; adhesins that bind to the blood group M antigen (specifically the NH_2-terminal portion of glycophorin A); and X fimbriae, whose binding is sensitive to neuraminidase. In addition, several nonfimbrial adhesins have been defined that bind to a variety of commonly expressed human tissue antigens. Perhaps the most important of these are the Dr family of adhesins, which bind to the

CD55 antigen (so-called decay-accelerating factor), which is expressed on tissues throughout the body, including the uroepithelium and the kidney. At present, it is fair to say that the major determinant of uropathogenicity is the sum of the adhesive interactions between the invading strain of bacteria and the uroepithelium, although that mediated by the P fimbriae appears to be quantitatively the most important.[75, 235, 273-293]

In addition to surface adhesins, which are clearly associated with uropathogenicity, other characteristics have been linked with virulence. These include the production of hemolysin, the presence of the iron-binding protein aerobactin, the ability of the bacteria to resist the bactericidal effect of normal human serum, the production of colicin V and other colicins, the ability to ferment salicin and perhaps other substrates, and the ability to induce an inflammatory response (see later). Perhaps the most completely studied of these additional virulence factors are hemolysin production and the presence of aerobactin. Hemolysin is present in most P pili–positive isolates, and has been shown to kill cultured human renal proximal tubule epithelial cells, which could be important in the pathogenesis of renal injury. It is also possible that bacterial growth is promoted by the induction of hemolysis, thus freeing erythrocyte iron, an important growth factor for bacteria. Not surprisingly, then, aerobactin, which would facilitate the uptake of iron by bacteria, is also associated with virulence.[226, 231, 235, 273, 294-299]

A critical determinant of the effects of UTI on the host is the inflammatory response to the presence of replicating bacteria. Thus far, the virulence characteristics of uropathogenic *E. coli* clones have been defined in terms of colonization of the large intestine and the vaginal vestibule, the ability to adhere to the relevant epithelial surface, and ascension from the bladder to the kidneys, with subsequent invasion and entry into the bloodstream. It is quite clear that such events can lead to an inflammatory response, with certain aspects of this response qualifying as a virulence factor that helps to determine both the short-term (inflammatory and "septic" events) and long-term (renal scarring) consequences of this particular host-microbial interaction. There is abundant clinical evidence of this inflammatory response: elevated temperature; an increased erythrocyte sedimentation rate; an acute cytokine response involving interleukin-1 (IL-1), IL-6, IL-8 (which acts as a chemotactic factor to attract polymorphonuclear leukocytes to the involved mucosa), and tumor necrosis factor (TNF); and an increased level of C-reactive protein. Soluble receptors for TNF, IL-6, IL-8, and other proinflammatory cytokines are also elaborated into the urine in response to these infections. This response is due primarily to the mobilization of nonspecific innate immunity, rather than a specific immune response. Central to this response are such chemokines as CXC, CXCR1, and others.[300-303]

P fimbriae and endotoxin play a significant role in initiating the inflammatory response to the replicating bacteria. A toxin termed cytotoxic necrotizing factor 1, produced by uropathogenic *E. coli*, appears to contribute to the inflammatory events by inducing the killing of uroepithelial cells with the exfoliation of these cells from the mucosa and by interfering with neutrophilic killing of the bacteria.[277, 300-307]

Not surprisingly, the inflammatory response is greater, and pyelonephritis more common in women who are nonsecretors of blood group antigens.[307, 308] Studies in animal models have emphasized the importance of proinflammatory mediators

in the pathogenesis of pyelonephritis. Chemokine receptors such as CXC play a key role in directing transepithelial neutrophil migration. This neutrophilic response is modulated by IL-8, the IL-8 receptor, TNF, and IL-6. IL-8 receptor deficiency increases the susceptibility to pyelonephritis and, at least in animal models, is associated with renal scarring.[309-316] The genetically determined nature of the cytokine response in humans appears to play an important role here as well. For example, TNF-β gene polymorphisms dictate the extent of TNF response to a particular inflammatory stimulus: low producers of TNF have a higher incidence of UTI than high producers, particularly in the face of exogenous immunosuppressive therapy (e.g., after renal transplantation).[317, 318] An impaired IL-6 response in mice is associated with an increase in the extent of pyelonephritis. There also appears to be a linkage between early inflammatory events and later consequences. Transforming growth factor-β (TGF-β) and, perhaps, platelet-derived growth factor are stimulated by the preceding inflammatory response and play a significant role in repair and scarring of the kidney as a consequence of pyelonephritis. In this regard, it is likely that genetic polymorphisms that control these events also help to determine the long-term outcome of these episodes of inflammation and infection. Of potential interest, an angiotensin II type 1 receptor antagonist (losartan) down-regulates TGF-β production, perhaps providing a new therapeutic tool for preventing renal scarring.[319-323]

Virtually all the data presented on urovirulence factors and pathogenesis were derived from studies of women and girls. Although much less complete, it is of interest that *E. coli* strains isolated from men with prostatitis and from patients with spinal cord injury with inflammatory manifestations of UTI have the same virulence factor profile as those isolated from females.[324-326]

Other Bacterial Species

Information is beginning to accumulate as to the pathogenetic mechanisms involved when non–*E. coli* bacteria invade the urinary tract. Reflecting its position as the most common non–*E. coli* cause of UTI, *Proteus mirabilis* is the other bacterial species that has received the most attention. Flagellae and so-called mannose-resistant *Proteus*-like fimbriae have been identified on strains isolated from patients with UTI. These are expressed preferentially on isolates from patients with pyelonephritis. Flagellae appear to mediate penetration of renal epithelial cells, whereas the fimbriae appear to be responsible for binding to the uroepithelium. There is considerable structural homology between these fimbriae and the P pili of *E. coli*. The possibility that other surface structures of *P. mirabilis* are important is suggested by the observation that an outer membrane protein vaccine prepared from a uropathogenic strain offered considerable protection in a murine model of pyelonephritis.[327-332]

After attachment to the uroepithelium, three *P. mirabilis* enzymes have been linked to virulence: urease, hemolysin, and a protease. Elegant studies in a mouse model of ascending infection, using isogeneic mutant strains as well as the wild-type UTI isolate, have shown that the presence of urease greatly lowered the infecting inoculum necessary to produce sustained infection, was associated with a far more virulent form of pyelonephritis, and resulted in the formation of urinary tract calculi. Both urease and, even more, hemolysin are cytotoxic for renal proximal tubule cells. Finally, an IgA protease elaborated by this organism, which destroys IgA normally present in the urine, may play a role in promoting the occurrence of ascending infection.[333-337]

Klebsiella isolates from patients with pyelonephritis were serum-resistant and were more likely to be aerobactin-positive and to possess type 1 fimbriae than were isolates from patients with asymptomatic bacteriuria or cystitis. The presence of intact O antigen has been correlated with uropathogenicity, which, in the case of these bacteria, includes the ability to invade the uroepithelium.[338-340]

Studies of entercoccal strains have suggested that urinary tract isolates are notable for their ability to adhere to the uroepithelium. If they enter the bloodstream from this site, they undergo a change that can be reproduced by the presence of human serum that renders them better able to adhere to the endocardium, thus producing endocarditis.[341] With the advent of antibiotic-resistant enterococci, particularly vancomycin-resistant enterococci, this phenomenon will undoubtedly become of growing importance clinically.

Host Factors Influencing Infection
Factors Predisposing to Pyelonephritis

Several factors are important clinically in predisposing the kidney to infection.

URINARY TRACT OBSTRUCTION. Reference has already been made to the role of obstruction in hematogenous and ascending pyelonephritis. Clinically, renal infections are associated with a variety of obstructive lesions (see Chapter 41). Experimentally, even temporary obstruction markedly increases susceptibility to infection; indeed, almost 100% of rats become infected after ligation of the ureter followed by intravenous injection of *E. coli*. Obstruction at the level of the urinary bladder interferes with the mechanisms by which the normal bladder eradicates bacteria in at least three ways: first, the increase in residual urine volume raises the number of bacteria remaining in the bladder after voiding; second, bladder distention decreases the surface area of the mucosa relative to the total volume of the bladder and thus decreases the effect of the postulated mucosal bactericidal factors; and finally, there is some experimental evidence that bladder wall distention diminishes the flow of blood to the bladder mucosa and hence the delivery of leukocytes and antibacterial factors. The net result is that even "nonuropathogenic" strains can cause ascending infection and bacteremic pyelonephritis.

Whereas complete ureteral obstruction markedly increases the susceptibility of the kidney to infection and also results in reactivation of healing lesions, gradual or partial ureteral obstruction induced either surgically or by irradiation of ureters affects renal susceptibility to hematogenous infection to only a slight degree.[51] It is probable, therefore, that the association between partial obstruction and pyelonephritis in humans is due to an effect on the ascending mechanism of infection, either by interfering with ureteral urodynamics or by accentuating the effect of VUR.

VESICOURETERAL REFLUX. The role of vesicoureteral and intrarenal reflux in predisposing to ascending infection was discussed earlier.

INSTRUMENTATION OF THE URINARY TRACT. Any instrumentation of the urinary tract increases the possibility of infection. The following risk factors have been shown to play a role in the pathogenesis of catheter-associated infection: duration of catheterization, absence of use of a urinometer, microbial colonization of the drainage bag, diabetes mellitus, absence of antibiotic use, female sex, complex urologic problem (i.e., a requirement for a catheter other than to passively drain the urine perioperatively or to monitor urine output), abnormal renal function, and errors in catheter care. Once a urethral catheter is in place, even with closed drainage systems, the daily frequency of bacteriuria is 3% to 10%, with the great majority of patients becoming bacteriuric by the end of 1 month.[342]

PREGNANCY. The interrelationships among pregnancy, bacteriuria, and pyelonephritis are described later.

DIABETES MELLITUS. Bacteriuria and clinical UTI are three to four times more common in diabetic women than in nondiabetic ones. However, there is no evidence that diabetic men are at increased risk of UTI. Further, studies of school-girls and pregnant women with and those without diabetes have shown no difference in the incidence of UTI. These epidemiologic observations suggest that the metabolic derangements of diabetes are not the primary factors involved in the increased incidence of UTI in diabetic patients. Rather, the important effects of diabetes in this context are mediated by the end-organ damage produced by long-standing diabetes. First, diabetic neuropathy affecting the bladder can have profound effects on bladder emptying, thus increasing the risk of UTI. This is probably the most important single factor in the pathogenesis of UTI in diabetic patients, both directly and because of the increased rate of instrumentation that occurs in such patients.[343]

There is, in addition, an increased rate of both pyelonephritis and such complications of pyelonephritis as renal papillary necrosis in diabetic patients with UTI. Presumably, this increase is due to the combined effects of diabetes-induced vascular disease, increased pressures within the urinary tract resulting from poor bladder emptying, and, perhaps, the effects of hyperglycemia on subtle aspects of host defense. In this last category, for example, both complement components and immunoglobulins of diabetic patients are glycosylated, and leukocyte function may be modified.[343]

Finally, an unusual form of necrotizing, tissue-invasive infection, usually caused by *E. coli*, occurs in diabetic patients (indeed, 70% to 90% of such cases occur in diabetic patients)— emphysematous pyelonephritis or cystitis or both.[344-347] Other Enterobacteriaceae and, on occasion, streptococci and *Candida* species can cause this same entity.[348-350] The pathogenesis of these entities is incompletely understood, but three factors seem to be necessary: (1) invasion by gas-forming bacteria, (2) high local tissue glucose levels, (3) and impaired tissue perfusion.[343]

Noninfectious Renal Disorders

Various forms of glomerular, tubule, and vascular renal diseases have been reported to show an increased frequency of secondary pyelonephritis. Most reports are based on pathologic studies, without bacteriologic confirmation. It seems probable that in some cases the high frequency represents noninfectious interstitial nephritis rather than infection.

In the case of analgesic nephropathy, however, it is well recognized that many patients have bouts of proven urinary infection.

DIFFERENTIAL SUSCEPTIBILITY OF RENAL CORTEX VERSUS MEDULLA. Experimental studies of hematogenous pyelonephritis have revealed a distinct difference in susceptibility to bacterial infection between the renal medulla and the cortex. Gorrill[351] first demonstrated that after intravenous inoculation of *E. coli* in animals with ligated ureters, the number of organisms rose logarithmically with time in the medulla, but there was a lag before the increase began in the cortex. Rocha and Fekety[352] then induced localized foci of injury by electrocautery in the cortex and medulla of rabbits; subsequent intravenous injection of bacteria resulted in infection in more than 85% of instances after injury to the medulla, whereas no infection occurred after cortical injury. The most critical experiments were those of Freedman and Beeson,[353] which showed that as few as 10 bacteria injected into the medulla could produce infection, whereas 10^5 organisms were required in the cortex. Immunofluorescence studies confirmed that in some models of pyelonephritis, bacterial multiplication occurred first in the interstitium of the medulla and then spread to the cortex.[354] However, this vulnerability of the medulla is not a universal finding in all models of pyelonephritis: in some species, both cortical and medullary lesions can be found at the same time; in others, the first lesions are clearly in the cortex.

Although older evidence implicated the anticomplementary action of ammonia as the cause of the exquisite susceptibility of the medulla, more probable explanations are reduced blood flow to the medulla, delayed mobilization of leukocytes, and medullary hypertonicity.[355, 356] In addition to affecting granulocyte mobilization and bacterial multiplication, medullary hypertonicity also interferes with antigen-antibody reactions, serum bactericidal effect,[357] and phagocytosis by leukocytes.

Immunologic Reactions

Interest in the immunologic reactions occurring in the course of pyelonephritis has focused on two events:

1. The possible role of acquired immunity directed against bacterial antigens in determining the outcome of infection. Theoretically, these reactions could be protective, serving to eliminate bacteria from renal tissue; conversely, they could enhance establishment of the infection or cause progression of the tissue damage.
2. The possibility that bacterial infection may somehow stimulate an autoimmune reaction against renal tissue, thus accounting for the progression of renal lesions after infection has been eradicated.[358]

ANTIBODY PRODUCTION IN PYELONEPHRITIS. Bacterial infection of the urinary tract regularly induces a specific antibody response directed against the infecting organism, which can be demonstrated in both urine and serum. The level of antibody response is proportional to the degree of tissue invasion that has occurred. Thus, antibody levels produced in response to pyelonephritis and prostatitis are far higher than those seen in most patients with cystitis. Indeed, attempts have been made to diagnose silent renal infection on the basis of this antibody response—both the serum level measurement and the antibody-coated bacteria assay (see later). Although the concept is correct, there is so much overlap clinically that such approaches have been largely abandoned. The bacterial antigens that induce most of the antibody response are the O antigen, fimbriae, and, to a much lesser extent, the K antigen. The serum response is primarily IgG and IgM, whereas the urinary response is largely secretory IgA, emphasizing the presence of antibody-producing cells throughout the urinary tract.[72, 359-361]

Despite the abundance of data demonstrating the occurrence of a specific antibody response to bacterial invasion, the protective effects of such antibody remain somewhat unclear. In some animal models, antibody clearly plays a protective role against both hematogenous and ascending infection. Immunization with antibodies to O antigen reduces the frequency of infection and abscesses in both hematogenous and ascending *E. coli* pyelonephritis in rats, and K antibodies are even more efficiently protective. Transfer of urine from animals immunized intravesically with killed *E. coli* protects against ascending pyelonephritis, and this immunity is diminished by absorption of the urine with K antigen. Antibodies against bacterial pili also afford protection from experimental ascending pyelonephritis.[72, 359, 361-365] In humans, reduced levels of secretory IgA in the urine have been associated with an increased risk of UTI. Thus, it may be important that certain bacteria produce proteases that cleave IgA, thus obviating any protective benefit.[72, 366, 367]

At most, however, antibody synthesis should be regarded as only one of the factors that protect against further bacterial growth and tissue damage. In some experimental models, passively administered antibodies do not afford protection, or infection may disappear despite a lack of antibody response.[72] The major argument that can be mustered against a significant protective effect for specific humoral immunity comes from studies of hypogammaglobulinemic individuals, both mouse and human. Mouse strains with profound B cell deficiency (CBA/N) are able to clear pyelonephritis equally as well as normal mice. Humans with hypogammaglobulinemia have neither a higher incidence of UTI than the general population nor a more complicated course with infections that do occur.[72, 368] Thus, the role of antibody remains obscure in the pathogenesis of events that follow urinary tract invasion.

CELL-MEDIATED IMMUNITY IN PYELONEPHRITIS. A role for cell-mediated immunity against bacterial antigens in either the pathogenesis of pyelonephritis or the protection against bacterial invasion has not been clearly defined. T cells are present in interstitial tissue and submucosa of biopsies from patients with acute bacterial invasion. However, studies in athymic, T cell–depleted, and cyclosporine-treated animal models failed to demonstrate a role for T cells in either the susceptibility to infection or the recovery from established infection. The finding, however, that a specific T cell response against bacterial peptides can be demonstrated suggests that this issue should be reopened. Further, an indirect role of T cells in the production of proinflammatory cytokines warrants attention. However, at present, any role for T cells in the pathogenesis of UTI and pyelonephritis has to be regarded as speculative.[72, 359, 369, 370]

POSSIBLE AUTOIMMUNE MECHANISMS IN PYELONEPHRITIS. There has been considerable interest in the possibility that renal infection can stimulate an autoimmune reaction against renal antigens, which could contribute to the perpetuation of renal damage in the absence of continued bacterial proliferation.[358] It is theoretically possible, for example, that the tubule injury in acute pyelonephritis may release tubule antigens into the circulation and initiate an antibody-mediated tubulointerstitial disease. However, several studies failed to demonstrate antikidney antibodies in the serum of patients or animals with bacterial pyelonephritis or locally synthesized IgG and IgM in experimental pyelonephritis. Further, neither granular staining for IgG and complement (suggesting immune complex tubule disease) nor linear deposition (suggesting anti–tubular basement membrane disease) has been demonstrated by immunofluorescence microscopy in experimental or human pyelonephritis.[371-373] However, studies have found antibodies directed against an antigenic determinant of *E. coli* in rabbit experimental pyelonephritis that also reacted against antigens derived from kidney and liver tissue. A telling argument against an antibody-mediated autoimmune reaction to pyelonephritis is that pyelonephritis can remain localized to one kidney, often leading to its complete destruction, whereas the contralateral kidney remains normal. This occurs in patients with unilateral obstruction and has been repeatedly demonstrated in experimental animals.

The profound mononuclear cell infiltrate characteristic of chronic pyelonephritis has also raised the question of whether cell-mediated immune reactions to renal antigens may be involved in the progression of the renal lesions. Indeed, Kalmanson and associates[374] reported a number of experiments supporting such a possibility. Histologic lesions resembling chronic pyelonephritis were found to develop in normal rats joined by parabiosis to rats with chronic enterococcal pyelonephritis after bacteria had been eliminated from the infected rats by means of antibiotic therapy. In addition, peritoneal lymphocytes from animals with chronic enterococcal pyelonephritis produced inhibition of macrophage migration when they were incubated with homologous renal antigen. However, using the same experimental model, Cotran and Galvanek[372] found that whereas significant stimulation of pyelonephritic lymphocytes occurred after exposure to the bacterial antigen (*E. faecalis* cell wall), there was little stimulation after incubation with renal antigen. Although this discrepancy with regard to cell-mediated immunity to renal antigen cannot be resolved, the presence of cell-mediated immunity to bacterial antigen is interesting in light of experiments by van Zwieten and colleagues.[375] These workers induced mononuclear cell infiltrates in sensitized guinea pigs and rats by intracortical injections of aggregated but not soluble bovine gamma globulin. The reactivity could be transferred with lymph node cells but not with serum, which suggests that delayed hypersensitivity reactions occur in the kidney if the antigen is in a particulate form. It is possible, therefore, that the mononuclear infiltrate in chronic pyelonephritis may in part reflect a delayed hypersensitivity reaction to particulate bacterial antigen.

One variant of the persistent bacterial antigen hypothesis that has received attention over the years is what might be termed the "L-form hypothesis." L-forms are osmotically fragile bacterial variants that are cell wall–deficient and can be induced experimentally by exposure to cell wall–active antibiotics, particularly penicillins. *Proteus* rather than *E. coli* strains appear to be more likely to form these variants.

In theory, the high osmolarity of the renal medulla would protect L-forms both by exerting a direct osmotic protective effect and by inhibiting the killing effects of complement, to which L-forms are susceptible. According to this theory, L-forms would persist despite antimicrobial therapy or would revert to the fully virulent form once antimicrobial pressures are removed. This would provide a continuing source of bacterial antigen for a host response that could result in chronic renal injury. Indeed, consistent with this hypothesis, L-forms have been isolated from sites of chronic pyelonephritis. However, this hypothesis has not been confirmed and has fallen out of fashion, although, admittedly, it has not been totally refuted.[376]

On balance, however, it is doubtful that T cell– or B cell–mediated immune reactions have an important bearing on the establishment or the course of pyelonephritis. The ablation of 99% of T lymphocytes by thymectomy and serial sublethal irradiation did not perceptibly alter the bacteriologic or pathologic course of experimental pyelonephritis. In these experiments, the response to both O and K antigens appeared to be T cell–independent.[377] Asscher and associates[378] also concluded that delayed hypersensitivity reactions do not play a role in the pathogenesis of kidney scarring associated with *E. coli* infection of rat kidney.

There has been interest in the possibility that immune reactions to Tamm-Horsfall protein may play a role in renal damage. Tamm-Horsfall protein is a urinary mucoprotein formed by the cells of the ascending thick limb and the distal convoluted tubule and is normally restricted largely to renal tubule cells, urine itself beyond the distal convoluted tubule, and renal casts.[379] It has been shown to leak into the interstitium in human and experimental reflux nephropathy, obstructive uropathy, and some other tubulointerstitial disorders.[380, 381] The first evidence was of a humoral reaction to Tamm-Horsfall protein developing within 3 weeks of the onset of either VUR or ureteral obstruction in pigs[382]; this finding has since been corroborated.[383] A further protocol involved rabbits "immunized" by rabbit urine. A focal interstitial nephritis developed in 19 of 23 animals killed between 16 and 48 weeks after the commencement of the study. A similar response followed challenge by isolated rabbit Tamm-Horsfall protein, whereas there was no response to a challenge by Tamm-Horsfall protein–depleted urine. However, no relationship was demonstrable between cellular Tamm-Horsfall protein extravasation and interstitial fibrosis in another study of rats subjected to unilateral ureteral obstruction for periods varying from 6 hours to 3 weeks,[384, 385] which can be regarded as a short-term study of this problem. Serum autoantibodies to Tamm-Horsfall protein have been detected in patients with acute pyelonephritis and VUR,[386, 387] but their relationship to renal damage is unclear. Thus, the pathogenetic role of Tamm-Horsfall protein in immunologic renal injury must be judged an unproven hypothesis.[388]

EVOLUTION OF THE RENAL LESION. The usual course of uncomplicated *E. coli* acute pyelonephritis in both experimental animals and humans is one of healing rather than of progressive damage. In most experimental models of *E. coli* pyelonephritis, the phase of acute suppurative inflammation in the kidney lasts 1 to 3 weeks. The tissue destruction is largely the result of bacterial multiplication and inflammation. With healing, an increase in the number of mononuclear cells, a decrease in neutrophils in the interstitium, and a replacement of necrotic tubules by fibrous tissue and foci of tubule atrophy occur. These changes are accompanied by a decrease in the number of bacteria cultured from the kidneys; by the 6th to the 10th week, the kidneys are sterile, and the resultant renal lesion is a triangular, depressed scar extending from the cortex, with its apex in the medulla and pelvis. However, a variety of bacterial and host factors can modify this sequence of events and can lead to progressive damage. Although *Staphylococcus* infections may eventually heal, they tend to remain active for longer periods and to result in considerable tissue destruction. In *Klebsiella* infection, the original infecting strain persists in the kidney for at least 24 weeks. *Proteus* infections do not heal as a consequence of the urinary obstruction resulting from the deposition of magnesium ammonium phosphate calculi.[389]

In human pyelonephritis, persistence of the original infecting organism is more likely to occur with unusual organisms, such as *Proteus* and *Klebsiella*, and is frequently associated with obstructive uropathy, renal calculi, renal carbuncle, or bacterial prostatitis. However, bacterial persistence within the renal parenchyma as a cause of progressive damage has been difficult to demonstrate convincingly in humans. It is probable that most instances of recurrences of UTI with the same pathogen (defined as "relapse") are caused by its persistence in the lower urinary tract (bladder, periurethral tissues, and prostate) rather than in the kidney. Indeed, serologic studies of UTI suggest that most recurrences are actually reinfections with a different strain of the same bacterial species or with a pathogen of a different species. This is particularly true in young women with uncomplicated recurrent cystitis. Most of these infections do not lead to renal damage except in the presence of obstruction or VUR.

Because a variable but small number of patients with the typical morphologic lesion of chronic pyelonephritis have no evidence of bacterial infection, the question has arisen whether progression of renal lesions can still occur after the bacteria have been totally eradicated. Several mechanisms have been postulated to explain such events[358, 390]:

1. The role of autoimmune mechanisms was discussed in detail earlier. Suffice it to say that there is no conclusive evidence that either antibody or cell-mediated autoimmune reactions play a major role in progressive renal damage in chronic pyelonephritis.[356]
2. Vascular changes caused by the initial inflammation with consequent ischemia may conceivably produce progressive tissue destruction, even when bacteria disappear. This explanation derives credence from the frequency with which vascular thickening and angiographic abnormalities are seen in human chronic pyelonephritis and the similarity between lesions induced by ischemia and infection.[391, 392] However, interpretation of human data is hampered by the frequent occurrence of hypertensive vascular changes, which contribute to renal parenchymal atrophy, and by our inability to determine whether the vascular changes precede the parenchymal damage or are merely an expression of it. Kincaid-Smith and Hodson[393] reported on remarkable myointimal as well as perivascular thickening in a study in which VUR and urinary infection were maintained in four pigs for more than 2 years. They suggested that these lesions may contribute to both the hypertension and the parenchymal atrophy that developed in these pigs. (Vascular lesions, however, were not present in noninfected animals with VUR.) Both clinical and experimental evidence suggests that superimposition of secondary hypertension in the course of chronic pyelonephritis measurably hastens deterioration of renal function and reduction of renal mass.[394-396] It is possible, therefore, that progressive renal insufficiency in some cases of chronic pyelonephritis may be due to vascular disease rather than pyelonephritic scarring.
3. The possibility that sterile reflux may induce progressive renal damage was discussed earlier. Granted that sterile reflux may be harmful, how is the damage induced? Urodynamic factors (water-hammer effect),[393] vascular narrowing and ischemia, and leakage of urinary constituents (e.g., Tamm-Horsfall protein) into the interstitium[381, 383, 384] have all been implicated as possible mechanisms but, to date, without conclusive proof.
4. It has been discussed previously that the ability of bacteria to survive in the kidney as bacterial variants that lack part or all of their cell wall (spheroplasts, protoplasts, or L-forms) may account for persistent or progressive renal infection. Such variants may remain viable in the hypertonic environment of the renal medulla and may induce pathologic changes either as variants or after reversion to bacterial forms. However, despite scattered clinical studies reporting the presence of such forms in the urine after UTI and in renal biopsy specimens of patients with sterile pyuria, other studies have failed to detect such forms. Experimentally, protoplasts can indeed produce renal lesions but only after they have reverted to the parent bacterial form. More than 2 decades after the suggestion was first made, the role of bacterial variants is still unclear.[376, 377, 397]

In concluding this discussion of factors affecting the evolution of renal lesions in pyelonephritis, the work of Glauser and associates[398] should be noted. These authors evaluated the importance of suppuration, persistent infection, and scar formation in the evolution of *E. coli* chronic pyelonephritis by treating rats with different antibiotic regimens at different stages of the disease. They found that the magnitude of the suppuration in the acute phase of pyelonephritis was the most significant factor in predicting the eventual development of small, chronically scarred kidneys. Persistent low-grade infection did not lead to chronic pyelonephritis if the acute suppuration was suppressed; antigen load and antibody- or cell-dependent autoimmune processes did not appear to play a significant role in the progression of infection. Essentially similar conclusions were reached by Ransley and Risdon,[399] based on experiments in pigs. The clinical evidence summarized is for the most part consistent with these conclusions and further emphasizes the need for prompt and effective antibiotic treatment of the earliest pyelonephritic lesions, particularly in infants with VUR.

PATHOLOGY

Acute Pyelonephritis

Typical descriptions of the pathologic changes in acute pyelonephritis in humans are based on severely affected kidneys from patients dying with sepsis. Changes in uncomplicated acute pyelonephritis, such as occur in pregnancy or after single attacks of obstructive acute pyelonephritis, are less well known. However, from studies on experimental animals with ascending pyelonephritis, it is clear that the acute lesions can vary considerably in severity, from some that affect only the pelvic mucosa (pyelitis) to others that involve entire lobules of the medulla and cortex.

On macroscopic examination, kidneys from patients with severe acute pyelonephritis are enlarged and contain a variable number of abscesses on the capsular surface and on cut sections of the cortex and medulla. Tissue between infected areas appears normal. Occasionally, areas of inflammation extend from the cortex into the medulla in the shape of a wedge. In the presence of obstruction, the calices are enlarged, the papillae are blunted, and the pelvic mucosa is sometimes congested and thickened. The papillae may be completely normal in some cases or may show outright papillary necrosis in others.

Histologic changes are characterized by involvement of the tubules and the interstitium. The interstitium is edematous and infiltrated by a variety of inflammatory cells, predominantly neutrophils. Within abscesses, the tubules show necrosis, and many tubules contain polymorphonuclear leukocytes. The patchiness of the inflammation is particularly striking. Thus, completely normal tubules and interstitium may lie adjacent to a large necrotizing renal abscess. Even in areas of the most severe inflammation, normal glomeruli can be seen, and indeed, intraglomerular inflammation is rare except in some forms of monilial glomerulonephritis. In the presence of total ureteral obstruction, the inflammatory reaction sometimes affects the entire kidney.

The morphologic appearance of acute renal infections associated with reflux in children has, to our knowledge, rarely been described. In experimental acute reflux nephropathy in the pig, large acute inflammatory lesions corresponding to zones of intrarenal reflux have been referred to as "acute lobar nephronia" by Hodson and Cotran[117] (see Fig. 31-5).

The sequence of events in the healing of acute pyelonephritis has been deduced from experimental studies. The neutrophilic exudate is rapidly replaced by one that is predominantly mononuclear, with macrophages and plasma cells and, later, lymphocytes. There are formation of granulation tissue, deposition of collagen, and eventual replacement of abscesses by scars that can be seen on the cortical surface as fibrous depressions. Such scars are characterized microscopically by atrophy of tubules, interstitial fibrosis, and lymphocyte infiltration. Progressive scarring has also been documented radiologically in children with reflux nephropathy and in reflux nephropathy in the pig. Such scars have a characteristically depressed cortical surface associated with a blunt and often deformed calyx (see Fig. 31-6).

Chronic Pyelonephritis and Reflux Nephropathy
Terminology and Frequency

Despite the long-standing controversy over the use of the term *chronic pyelonephritis*, there is now reasonable agreement as to the morphologic changes sufficient to distinguish this condition from the many other tubulointerstitial diseases (see earlier discussion).

Radiologic studies demonstrated the relatively specific anatomic features used in the diagnosis of chronic pyelonephritis. Hodson[2] drew attention to the association between cortical scarring and a corresponding deformity of the underlying calyx as a diagnostic feature that differentiated pyelonephritic from other types of renal scarring. This suggestion was confirmed in a morphologic study by Smith.[3] The requirement for caliceal deformity for the diagnosis of chronic pyelonephritis, subsequently expounded by Heptinstall,[1] measurably limits the differential diagnosis and the possible causes for the renal scarring. Only a limited number of conditions can lead to a morphologic picture of chronic corticomedullary tubulointerstitial damage coupled with caliceal abnormality, and they are as follows:

1. *Vesicoureteral reflux.* As detailed earlier, renal damage in VUR is associated with intrarenal reflux and is most frequently caused by infected reflux. This is the most common cause of entities referred to as "chronic atrophic" or chronic nonobstructive pyelonephritis. The term "reflux nephropathy" is slowly replacing chronic pyelonephritis to describe this condition. Besides emphasizing the role of VUR, the term has the virtue of including two types of changes associated with VUR: (a) the more common and widely recognizable focal scarring, which is attributed to scarring at the site of compound papillae with intrarenal reflux, and (b) the diffuse renal damage affecting all papillae and usually associated with high-pressure obstructive reflux. Whereas most children with chronic pyelonephritic scars demonstrate VUR, only about half of adults do. However, up to 89% of adults have abnormal ureteral orifices, which suggests (but by no means proves) that ureteral reflux may have occurred in the past.[400-402]

2. *Urinary obstruction.* It is frequently difficult to differentiate an uninfected obstruction from a combination of obstruction and infection, but discrete parenchymal scars usually indicate the coexistence of infection.

3. *Analgesic nephropathy,* with or without bacterial infection. This is usually readily distinguished by the widespread papillary necrosis (see Chapter 34).

4. *Unusual forms of noninfectious acute papillary necrosis.* Included in this category are acute papillary necrosis due to such conditions as sickle cell disease and dehydration in infants. Chrispin and associates[403,404] described infants with severe acute gastroenteritis who had papillary necrosis and subsequent corticopapillary scarring that resembled chronic pyelonephritis.

5. *Segmental hypoplasia* (the Ask-Upmark kidney). This condition, previously considered a developmental anomaly, is now also thought to be caused by VUR in most cases.[405,406]

A small number of patients exhibit corticomedullary scarring and caliceal deformity in the apparent absence of the aforementioned conditions or of bacterial infection. The more diligently one looks for a recognized cause, the fewer of these cases are reported. Such cases were described more frequently before the widespread use of voiding cystourethrography to exclude reflux and before caliceal deformity was appreciated as the diagnostic criterion for chronic pyelonephritis.[407] In children with urinary tract anomalies, some scars show histologic evidence of renal dysplasia (e.g., dysplastic tubules, embryonic cartilage) and are almost certainly coexistent developmental abnormalities of the renal parenchyma. Nonetheless, a few cases with no apparent cause still appear in most series.[408-410]

For these reasons, chronic pyelonephritis can be subdivided into three types: (1) chronic pyelonephritis with reflux (reflux nephropathy), (2) chronic pyelonephritis with obstruction (chronic obstructive pyelonephritis), and (3) idiopathic chronic pyelonephritis.

If the morphologic criteria are adhered to, we have found the incidence of chronic pyelonephritic scarring at autopsy to be 1.85% in two series of patients examined at the Boston City Hospital between 1965 and 1972. This figure is remarkably close to that of Farmer and Heptinstall.[409] Admittedly, the numbers may be somewhat larger or smaller in hospitals serving other population groups.

The frequency of chronic pyelonephritis as a cause of end-stage kidney disease is also variable. The Human Renal Transplant Registry reports a frequency of about 13%, and data from the European Dialysis and Transplant Association show that 22% of adults with end-stage kidney disease have chronic pyelonephritis. Unfortunately, the criteria for diagnosis of chronic pyelonephritis in these series are not certain. Chronic pyelonephritis was found in 10 (11%) of 95 consecutive pretransplant nephrectomy specimens examined grossly, microscopically, and bacteriologically by Schwartz

and Cotran.[408] A series from New South Wales lists the diagnoses etiologically.[410] Of 317 histologically studied cases of adult end-stage renal disease, 8% had reflux nephropathy; 1%, idiopathic chronic pyelonephritis; and 6%, obstruction, congenital malformations, or renal calculi. In Kincaid-Smith's series[400] of 147 pretransplant nephrectomy specimens, 30 (20%) of the patients had chronic pyelonephritis; of these, about half had demonstrable reflux. In a later account of her series, 15.3% of patients with end-stage renal failure had clinical and radiologic features of reflux nephropathy.[411] In Christchurch Hospital, 12% of a patients who entered dialysis and transplant programs had reflux nephropathy.[412] In children younger than 16 years, reflux nephropathy accounts for 19% to 34% of patients entering renal replacement programs.[413]

Gross Pathology

The most characteristic changes are seen on gross rather than microscopic examination. The most common morphologic appearance of chronic pyelonephritis and reflux nephropathy is that referred to as coarse renal scarring or focal scarring, consisting of corticopapillary scars overlying dilated, blunted, or deformed calices (Fig. 31-8). The remarkable pelvocaliceal deformity is not easy to visualize grossly on pathologic examination but is particularly obvious in tracings of the calices made on excretory urograms (Fig. 31-9).

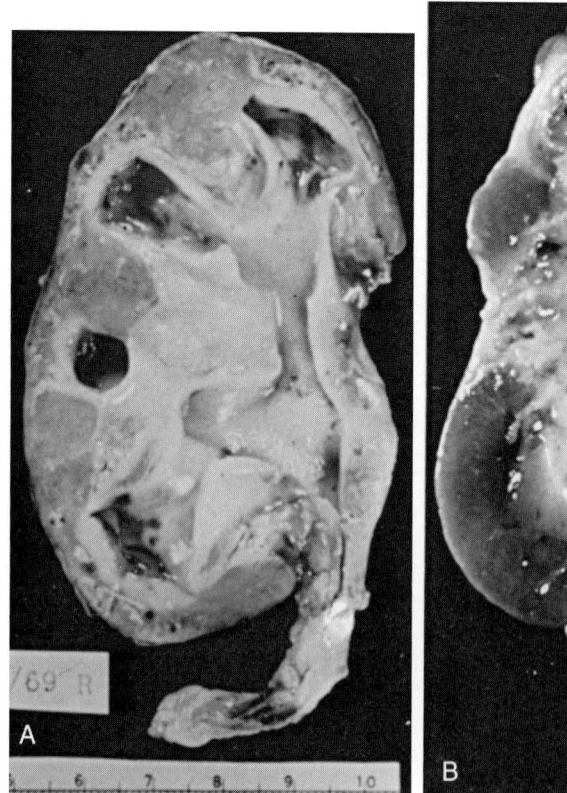 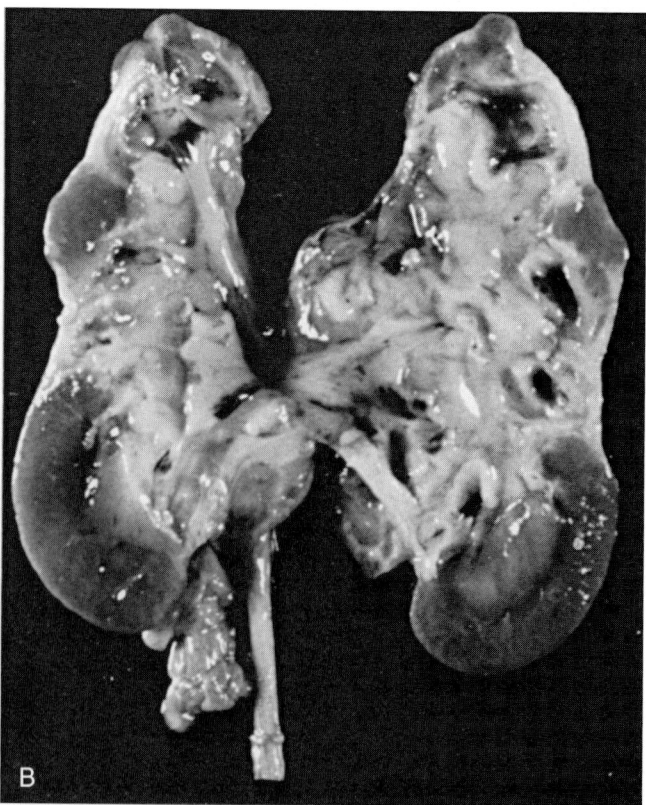

FIGURE 31-8. A, Chronic pyelonephritis. Note irregularly scarred kidney, dilated and blunted calices, and a thickened ureter that suggests chronic vesicoureteral reflux. **B,** Typical pyelonephritic broad scars in a patient with reflux nephropathy. The scars involve entire lobes. Note prominent underlying caliceal dilatation. (**B,** From Bhathena DB, Holland NH, Weiss JH, et al: Morphology of coarse renal scars in reflux-associated nephropathy in man. *In* Hodson CJ, Kincaid-Smith P [eds]: Reflux Nephropathy. New York, Masson, 1979, p 243.)

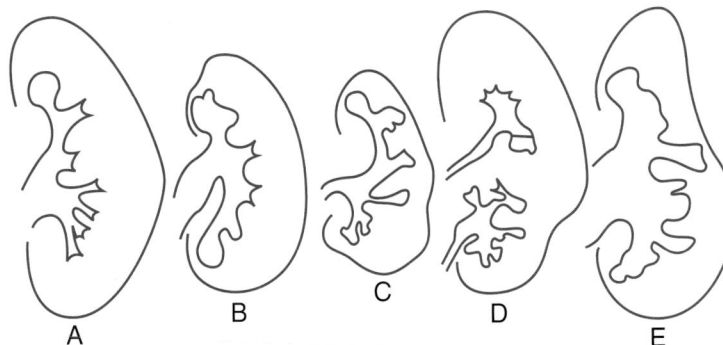

FIGURE 31-9. Tracings of urograms showing common patterns of scarring and caliceal deformities in reflux nephropathy. **A**, Upper pole. **B**, Severe bipolar. **C**, Generalized, with one lower pole lobe spared. **D**, Duplex kidney, with severe deformities in the lower pole. **E**, Generalized diffuse caliceal involvement. (From Hodson CJ: Reflux nephropathy. Med Clin North Am 62:1201, 1978.)

The kidneys are usually smaller than normal, and extreme reductions in size of one of the two kidneys are not unusual. Involvement can be bilateral or unilateral, depending on whether reflux or obstruction has occurred on one or both sides; with bilateral involvement, the kidneys are usually asymmetrically scarred. The scars vary in size but are usually broad, involve a whole lobe, are rather shallow, and have a flatter surface than do healed infarcts (see Fig. 31-8B). The areas between scars may be smooth but are usually finely granular, reflecting hypertrophic changes. Although any part of the kidney may be involved, most scars are in the upper and lower poles, consistent with the frequency of intrarenal reflux in these areas. The medulla is distorted, and affected papillae are flattened. In cases with obstruction, the pelvis and calices are distinctly dilated, but they may be of normal caliber in the absence of obstruction (in late cases) or after obstruction has been relieved. The pelvic and caliceal mucosa can be thickened and granular, particularly in cases of chronic reflux. Kincaid-Smith and colleagues[411] emphasized the importance of examining the ureters because thickening of the ureteral wall with or without dilation is a reliable sign of the preexistence of VUR (Fig. 31-10).

A second morphologic variety, referred to as diffuse or generalized reflux nephropathy by radiologists, occurs in patients with severe VUR together with obstruction (e.g., children with posterior urethral valves).[414] The scarring is so generalized that the cortical surface appears to be relatively smooth or finely granular. In these cases, the pelvis and calices are diffusely dilated, and the renal parenchyma shows widespread atrophy resembling postobstructive atrophy (see Fig. 31-10). In these kidneys, the presence of a thickened pelvic and ureteral wall (or the cystoscopic appearance of ureteral orifices) suggests previous VUR. Lying somewhere between those with coarse scars and those with generalized damage are kidneys in which two or more areas of coarse scarring are associated with generalized dilation of calices and overall reduction in kidney size, labeled "mixed damage" by Hodson.[414]

Microscopic Findings

The histologic appearance is one of tubule damage and interstitial inflammation and scarring, and it varies according to the evolutionary stage of the lesion. Old, extensive scars can be composed almost entirely of atrophic or dilated tubules, separated by fibrous tissue, with remaining large blood vessels (Fig. 31-11). More recent scars show variable

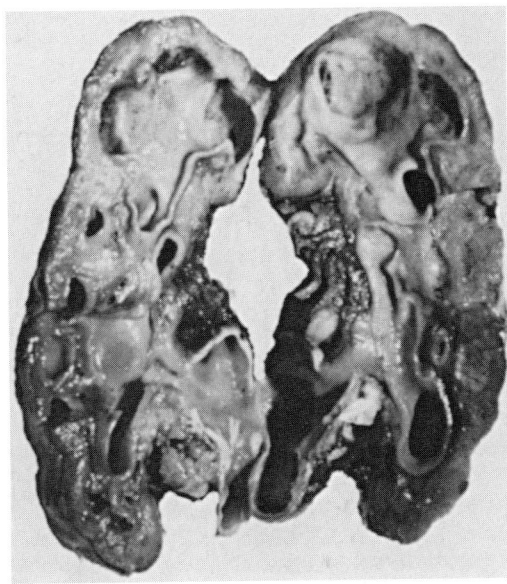

FIGURE 31-10. Kidney showing the "generalized" or diffuse form of reflux nephropathy. There is more or less uniform dilation of calices and thinning of renal parenchyma. Note thickening of the pelvis and base of the ureter. (From Hodson CJ: Formation of renal scars with special reference to reflux nephropathy. Contrib Nephrol 16:83, 1979, by permission of S Karger AG, Basel.)

amounts of interstitial mononuclear inflammation, tubule atrophy and necrosis, increase in interstitial fibrous tissue, and periglomerular fibrosis. Many tubules are dilated, lined by flattened epithelium, and filled with colloid casts (thyroidization). The inflammatory infiltrate is variable. Lymphocytes and monocytes predominate, but occasionally one can see large foci of plasma cells; in the presence of active inflammation, neutrophils can be plentiful. Pus casts are also frequently present, particularly when there is active infection. However, pus casts can also be present in the absence of bacteriuria, presumably owing to ischemic damage.

Vascular changes within the scars can be either mild or more severe. Both arteries and arterioles may show medial and intimal thickening; the intimal thickening is of the fine, concentric cellular type. In some cases, there is clear-cut elastic reduplication. Vascular changes within the scarred areas are present even in patients who are not hypertensive, although they become more severe in the presence of hypertension. In the nonscarred areas, hyaline

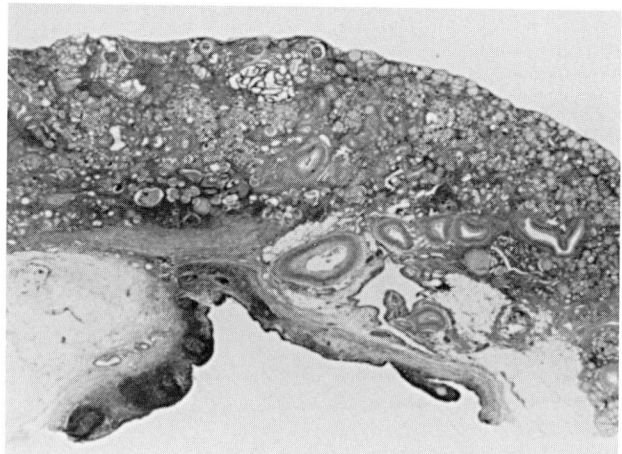

FIGURE 31-11. Pyelonephritic scar composed of atrophic or dilated tubules, a few sclerosed or sclerosing glomeruli, and thickened vessels. Note the dilated calyx with prominent lymphoid infiltrate beneath the mucosa.

arteriolar changes are limited to those patients with secondary hypertension.

The pelvis and calices are universally affected. Usually, there is infiltration of the subendothelial connective tissue by inflammatory cells, which often form large masses or lymphoid follicles (see Fig. 31-11). Neutrophils, eosinophils, and occasionally giant cells may also be present. The mucosal epithelium may be severely thickened and infiltrated with inflammatory cells. The amount of collagen in the underlying connective tissue is usually also increased.

Of interest is the presence of interstitial deposits of Tamm-Horsfall protein precipitates in the kidneys with chronic pyelonephritis associated with reflux or obstruction. Tamm-Horsfall protein can be localized specifically by immunofluorescence microscopy, but its presence in casts and in interstitial tissue can be suspected by histologic examination as a strongly periodic acid–Schiff (PAS) reaction-positive amorphous or fibrillar material. Interstitial deposits of Tamm-Horsfall protein have been detected in kidneys from patients with chronic pyelonephritis, reflux nephropathy, urinary tract obstruction, and other interstitial diseases.[380, 415] These deposits are sometimes surrounded by an intense inflammatory infiltrate consisting of mononuclear cells, occasional neutrophils, and even giant cells. Deposits probably result from tubule disruption, with discharge of urinary contents into the interstitium. Tamm-Horsfall protein has also been seen in thin-walled renal veins and lymphatics, possibly from pyelovenous or pyelolymphatic ruptures.[416, 417] Interstitial Tamm-Horsfall protein deposits have also been demonstrated in experimental reflux nephropathy,[381] and the question has been raised about whether they may play a role in inducing tissue damage and fibrosis either by direct toxic effects or by inducing an immunologic reaction in the interstitium. At present, as mentioned earlier, there is little evidence supporting this hypothesis.[418]

In a careful morphologic study of 23 cases of coarse renal scarring associated with VUR, Bhathena and associates[419] detected histologic evidence of renal dysplasia, including immature medullary segments and islands of cartilage, in nine scars. Whether this type of scar represents an intrinsic

embryologic anomaly of the ureteric bud or whether intrauterine VUR plays a role in its genesis is unknown.

Although glomeruli may be entirely normal or may show only periglomerular fibrosis, a variety of glomerular changes may be present. These have been well described and illustrated by Heptinstall.[420] Ischemic changes, consisting of solidification of glomerular tufts and deposition of collagen within the Bowman space, are frequent, as are small shrunken glomeruli. Focal or diffuse proliferation and necrosis can also be present; these have been considered secondary to hypertension. Kincaid-Smith[421, 422] has drawn attention to the association of chronic pyelonephritis and reflux nephropathy with a glomerular lesion best described as focal segmental sclerosis and hyalinosis, similar to that seen in some patients with focal sclerosis and the nephrotic syndrome. She noted that in patients with reflux nephropathy, those with proteinuria were more likely to progress to renal failure, even in the absence of hypertension, overt infection, or persistent VUR. Renal biopsy specimens showed focal and segmental hyalinosis and sclerosis in most of these patients. Similar findings have since been described by numerous other investigators. The pathogenesis and clinical significance of these glomerular lesions are discussed in detail later.

NATURAL HISTORY OF BACTERIURIA AND PYELONEPHRITIS

Frequency and Epidemiology of Urinary Tract Infection

The frequency of UTI and its clinical impact are different for the two sexes at different stages of life (Fig. 31-12). Approximately 1% of neonates ate bacteriuric, with a twofold to fourfold higher frequency among boys, presumably because of an increased occurrence of urogenital congenital anomalies in male infants.[423, 424] Equally striking is a fourfold increase in bacteriuria among premature infants (2.9% vs. 0.7% among full-term infants)[425]; approximately half of these premature infants demonstrate VUR.[424]

Uncircumcised male infants are at increased risk for UTI and pyelonephritis in the neonatal period, with some of this increased risk continuing into adulthood. The presence of a foreskin has been shown to be associated with a markedly increased risk of colonization of the preputial space with potential uropathogens, the reservoir from which UTI is derived in these individuals. Once circumcision has taken place, and healing has occurred, such carriage no longer occurs.[426-429]

After infancy and until age 55 years, when prostatic hypertrophy starts becoming apparent in men, UTI is predominantly a female disease. From infancy until age 10 years, the frequency of UTI in girls is about 1.2%, with approximately one third of these infections being symptomatic. After an initial episode of bacteriuria, approximately 80% of schoolgirls have one or more recurrences; 80% of these recurrences are due to reinfections rather than relapses of sequestered deep tissue infection. It has been estimated that a minimum of 5% to 6% of schoolgirls have at least one episode of UTI between the ages of 5 and 18 years. Approximately 20% of schoolgirls with bacteriuria have demonstrable VUR.[424, 430, 431]

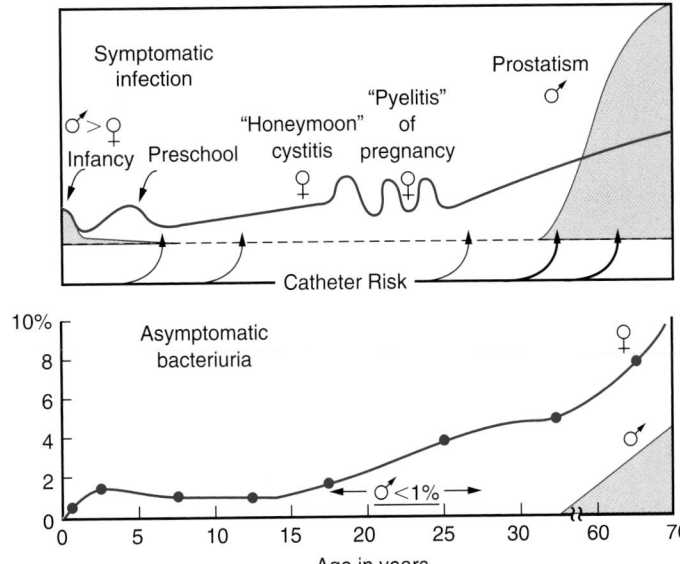

FIGURE 31-12. Overview of the frequency of symptomatic urinary tract infection and of asymptomatic bacteriuria according to age and sex (modified from the original concept of Jawetz). (From Kunin CM: Detection, Prevention and Management of Urinary Tract Infections, 3rd ed. Philadelphia, Lea & Febiger, 1979.)

When cohorts of schoolgirls with and without bacteriuria are observed for periods as long as 18 years, some important observations emerge. Although the urine may have remained sterile for long periods in many of these bacteriuric schoolgirls, bacteriuria usually redeveloped shortly after marriage or during the first pregnancy. There is an increase in the number of episodes of bacteriuria and the number of hospitalizations for UTI over the 1 to 2 decades of follow-up among the initially bacteriuric schoolgirls. This increase is most marked during pregnancy, with a 63.8% frequency of pregnancy-associated bacteriuria in women who were bacteriuric as schoolgirls, as opposed to a 26.7% frequency for those who were not. Of potentially great clinical and pathogenetic importance is the observation that 10.8% of the children of the bacteriuric schoolgirls who were studied became bacteriuric themselves, as opposed to none of the children of the nonbacteriuric control patients. Persistence of bacteriuria appears to be more common in children with VUR than in those with normal urinary tracts.[432-434]

Among adult women, the incidence and prevalence of bacteriuria are related to age, degree of sexual activity, and form of contraception employed. Approximately 1% to 3% of women between the ages of 15 and 24 years have bacteriuria; the incidence increases by 1% to 2% for each decade thereafter up to a level of about 10% to 15% by the sixth or seventh decades. Approximately 40% to 50% of women will have at least one UTI in their lifetimes. College women who have a first episode of *E. coli* UTI are three times as likely to have a second UTI in the next 6 months than those with other forms of UTI. In noninstitutionalized elderly patients, UTIs cause one fourth of all infections. The estimated annual cost of community-acquired UTI is $1.6 billion.[424, 435, 436]

There is an incomplete correlation between the presence of bacteriuria and the occurrence of clinical symptoms. Dysuria occurs each year in approximately 20% of women between the ages of 24 and 64 years, half of whom come to medical attention. Of the group seeking medical care, one third have the acute urethral syndrome (see later), and two

thirds (approximately 6% of the adult female population) have significant bacteriuria in association with clinical symptoms referrable to the urinary tract.[437-439]

Bacteriuria, whether asymptomatic or clinically overt, is unusual in males before they reach their 50s in the absence of urinary tract instrumentation. The frequency of bacteriuria among schoolboys is between 0.04% and 0.14%. Although the frequency of structural and neurologic defects of the urinary tract is much higher in boys than in girls with UTI, such abnormalities are not invariable. Indeed, if the first episode of bacteriuria in boys is delayed until after the age of 10 years, the frequency of structural abnormalities is low, the prognosis is excellent, and the recurrence is infrequent after an adequate course of antimicrobial therapy. One male population that appears to be at an increased risk for UTI is sexually active male homosexuals, who become infected with the same uropathogenic *E. coli* clones that infect women. Human immunodeficiency virus infection does not increase the incidence of UTI, but once UTI occurs, the higher the viral load the greater the inflammatory consequences of the UTI. Heterosexual transmission of virulent strains of *E. coli* from infected women to their sexual partners has been clearly documented. Several investigators have noted a high frequency of *Proteus* infection, as opposed to *E. coli* infection, among boys with UTI, perhaps related to a high rate of colonization of the preputial sac with *Proteus* species.[405, 406, 424, 440-446]

As the aging process progresses and prostatic disease becomes more common, the frequency of UTI in men rises dramatically. By age 70 years, the frequency of bacteriuria reaches a level of 3.5% in otherwise healthy men and a level of greater than 15% in hospitalized men. With the onset of chronic debilitating illness and long-term institutionalization, bacteriuria rates in both sexes reach levels of 25% to 50%, with the frequency in women now only slightly greater than that in men.[446-449]

Certain populations of patients are at increased risk for UTI. This risk is most marked in pregnant women, who have a 4% to 10% frequency of bacteriuria—a rate at least twice that for similarly aged nonpregnant women.[450, 451] Symptomatic infection develops in as many as 60% of pregnant women with asymptomatic bacteriuria early in pregnancy if it is untreated, with symptomatic pyelonephritis developing in approximately one fourth to one third.[450, 451] The profound physiologic changes associated with pregnancy are responsible for these events: beginning at the end of the first trimester, hydroureter develops, more as a result of hormonal effects on ureteral smooth muscle than the mechanical effects of the enlarging uterus (these changes return to normal by 2 months post partum). Although urinary flow rates initially are increased during pregnancy, eventually relative urinary stasis develops. Both a decrease in the concentrating ability of the kidney during pregnancy and gestational diabetes (when it occurs) also contribute to the susceptibility of the urinary tract, particularly for pyelonephritis, during pregnancy.[450, 451]

About 25% to 33% of women with pregnancy-associated bacteriuria have infection at postpartum follow-up, even if this follow-up occurs as many as 10 to 14 years post partum, as opposed to 5% of similarly aged women who never had pregnancy-associated bacteriuria. Approximately 30% of women with a history of bacteriuria of pregnancy have changes on the excretory urogram that suggest chronic pyelonephritis. This is not to say, however, that bacteriuria of pregnancy is responsible for these changes. Currently available data would suggest that the kidneys of the women with postpartum infection after pregnancy-associated infection were probably damaged during childhood, with recurrent infection being exacerbated by the hormonal and mechanical changes induced by pregnancy. There is little evidence that infection developing for the first time during pregnancy is responsible for long-term effects.[4, 450-453] Indeed, the frequency of bacteriuria during pregnancy is significantly higher in women with a history of past childhood UTI.[453] As in other populations, the occurrence of pyelonephritis among pregnant women is particularly associated with infection with uropathogenic strains possessing P pili to mediate adherence to the uroepithelium.[454]

Epidemics of pyelonephritis have been reported in newborn infants being provided care on neonatal wards. These have been shown to be due to the patient-to-patient spread of P-fimbriated *E. coli* strains on the ward, resulting in intestinal colonization of these children. Once such intestinal colonization with uropathogenic strains occurs, invasion of the urinary tract can then develop.[455-457]

Patients with anatomic or neurologic disorders of the urinary tract of any type that result in obstruction or incomplete voiding have an increased frequency of UTI and pyelonephritis. A particularly important group of such patients are those rendered paraplegic or quadriplegic as a result of spinal cord injury. Bacteriuria, urosepsis, and the eventual development of VUR and progressive renal scarring are common in these individuals. It is of great interest that the organisms causing UTI in these patients are the same nonuropathogenic strains of bacteria associated with scarring in children with VUR. Risk factors associated with the development of UTI in these patients include overdistention of the bladder, VUR, high-pressure voiding, large postvoid residuals, presence of stones in the urinary tract, bladder outlet obstruction, indwelling catheterization, and urinary diversion.[458, 459]

Recipients of kidney transplants are another population at particular risk for UTI, with a reported frequency of 35% to 79% of such infections if no antimicrobial prophylaxis is administered. The major factors associated with the occurrence of UTI in this population include the technical complications associated with the ureteral anastomosis, a UTI present before transplantation that has not been eradicated (by antibiotics or native nephrectomy before or at the time of transplantation), the postoperative urinary catheter, the physical and immunologic trauma that the kidney suffers, and the immunosuppressive therapy that is administered. The first two of these have been largely eliminated because of advances in the preparation of the patient for transplantation and in the technical aspects of the operation. However, the requirement for bladder catheters for 1 to 7 days after transplantation provides a reservoir from which infection is derived. In animal models, the combination of bacteria inoculated into the bladder and trauma to the kidney results in pyelonephritis, whereas bladder infection without renal trauma results only in a transient cystitis. It is reasonable to postulate that the kidney is rendered susceptible to invasive infection as a result of the physical trauma of the transplant procedure as well as the immunologic trauma. Once infection develops, its impact can be greatly amplified by the effects of immunosuppressive therapy.[460, 461]

UTI occurring in the first 3 months after transplantation is frequently associated with invasion of the allograft, bacteremia, and high rate of relapse when it is treated with a conventional course of antibiotics. In contrast, UTI occurring at a later time is usually benign, can be managed with a conventional 10- to 14-day course of antibiotics, is rarely associated with bacteremia or requires hospitalization, and has an excellent prognosis. Exceptions to this general pattern should be evaluated for functional or anatomic abnormalities of the urinary tract, such as a stone, an obstructive uropathy, or a poorly functioning bladder. Pancreatic transplantation for diabetes in which exocrine drainage is accomplished through a bladder (as opposed to an enteric) anastomosis is associated with a relatively high rate of urologic complications and UTI, including that due to *Candida* species.[460, 461]

Clinical Impact of Urinary Tract Infection

The most important issues regarding UTI have to do with whether there are long-term consequences of bacteriuria over and above the direct infectious disease morbidity and mortality these infections cause. The particular questions that have received the most attention are the following:

1. Does UTI, particularly when it is chronic or recurrent, lead to significant loss of renal function, to hypertension, or to both? If it does, is there a particular subset of patients at special risk for these complications?
2. Does UTI have an adverse effect on the outcome of pregnancy—on the mother, the fetus, or both?
3. Is UTI associated with an increased mortality? If it is, is it a causative factor or just a marker for poor health, and will effective therapy decrease the mortality rate?

Urinary Tract Infection, Renal Failure, and Hypertension

As previously discussed, it is now clear that in the past, the diagnosis of pyelonephritis was loosely applied to a wide variety of tubulointerstitial inflammatory conditions. With more stringent criteria for pathologic diagnosis, several workers in the 1960s began to question the hypothesis that uncomplicated UTI could lead to progressive renal injury.[462, 463] Murray and Goldberg[464] reported the results of a retrospective review of all the cases of chronic renal disease seen at the Hospital of the University of Pennsylvania between 1969 and 1972. They identified 101 patients with chronic interstitial nephritis, approximately one third of the patients with chronic renal disease—a figure similar to that attributed previously to chronic pyelonephritis.[465, 466] However, in none of these 101 cases of chronic interstitial nephritis was infection the primary cause of the renal disease; instead, analgesic abuse and anatomic abnormalities of the urinary tract accounted for most cases. It was suggested, however, that in approximately one third of these patients, infection played an important secondary role, but only when it was superimposed on such primary problems as anatomic abnormalities, calculous disease, or analgesic abuse.[464]

These concepts have since been confirmed in several prospective, long-term studies of bacteriuria in adults. Freedman and Andriole[465] observed 250 women with UTI for periods up to 12 years and found no evidence of deterioration in renal function or blood pressure elevation. Similarly, Asscher and associates[466] studied 107 women with bacteriuria and 88 matched control subjects for a period of 5 years and found that untreated bacteriuria, in the absence of hypertension or obstructive uropathy, was not associated with progressive renal dysfunction. Freeman and colleagues[467] prospectively studied 249 men with bacteriuria for periods up to 10 years and again found no deterioration in renal function in the absence of severe urologic disease or concomitant noninfectious renal disease. Even in a particularly high-risk group of adult patients, the 25% of adult patients with asymptomatic bacteriuria who had renal scars demonstrable by urography at the time of entry into the study, renal damage did not seem to progress, and no new scars developed unless such complicating factors as obstruction, hypertension, analgesic abuse, or diabetes mellitus were present concurrently.[465-467]

Thus, in adults, there is little evidence that UTI beginning in adult life, by itself, leads to progressive chronic renal injury. It is still possible that bacteriuria, when superimposed on other urinary tract lesions, could accelerate the development of renal damage. There is no justification at this time, then, to advocate mass screening of adults for asymptomatic bacteriuria; bacteriuria screening in the adult population should be restricted to pregnant women and to patients with urinary tract or renal disease of other primary causes or to patients with a history of recurrent symptomatic infection (see later).

In contrast to the experience in adults, bacteriuria may have a significant impact on children. As discussed in detail earlier, current information suggests that most renal damage caused by UTI develops in childhood, usually in association with an anatomic or functional abnormality, particularly VUR. Studies of children between the ages of 5 and 15 years have demonstrated that if scarring has not occurred by the age of 5 years, the kidneys, sometimes in the face of continued bacteriuria and VUR, remain unscarred and renal growth remains unimpaired. It is primarily the children who have pyelonephritis before the age of 5 years who manifest not only renal scarring but also a decreased glomerular

filtration rate and a failure of compensatory renal growth. Experimental studies in young rats have confirmed that ascending pyelonephritis inhibits renal growth.[468-471]

Edwards and associates[472] have reported extremely encouraging results with long-term continuous low-dose antimicrobial prophylaxis in children who initially presented with symptomatic UTI and were found to have VUR. Whereas Lenaghan and colleagues[473] noted a 20% frequency of fresh scarring and a 66% frequency of increased scarring in children treated with intermittent antimicrobial therapy, Edwards and associates,[472] in an apparently similar population of children, found only one new scar and only one extension among 75 children treated continuously for a 7- to 15-year period.

Thus, there is little question that the combination of VUR and UTI can have potentially disastrous consequences, which might be amenable to early recognition and prolonged therapy. Long-term studies of these children have shown that once scarring has occurred, the prognosis depends on the severity of initial damage and the presence of proteinuria, which is a measure of the degree of secondary glomerulosclerosis. As discussed elsewhere in this book, secondary glomerulosclerosis is thought to be due to glomerular hyperfiltration and hypertension in remnant nephrons, causing changes in permselectivity to macromolecules that are delivered to the kidney. Progressive damage to the remaining glomeruli then ensues, with progression of the degree of proteinuria from microalbuminuria to frank nephrotic syndrome and progressive azotemia.[470, 471, 474-476]

Chronic pyelonephritis appears to be the most common cause of hypertension in children, accounting for some 30% of childhood hypertension, and is also a frequent cause of secondary hypertension in adults.[470, 471, 476] Hypertension as a complication of chronic pyelonephritis is discussed in detail later.

Urinary Tract Infection and the Outcome of Pregnancy

The clearest demonstration that untreated, asymptomatic bacteriuria has an adverse effect on the human host comes from studies carried out in the pregnant woman. As previously discussed, approximately half of such untreated women subsequently have symptomatic UTI, and 25% to 30% have acute pyelonephritis. Such pyelonephritis may be associated with the development of the adult respiratory distress syndrome and disseminated intravascular coagulation. An association of pregnancy bacteriuria with anemia, hypertension, decreased glomerular filtration rate, and decreased urinary concentration ability, which is alleviated by therapy, has also been noted.[450-453, 477,478] There also appears to be an increased risk of preeclampsia in pregnant women with UTI, with this being most marked among primiparous women (a fivefold increase in risk).[479]

More controversial has been the question of an increased risk of maternal toxemia and neonatal prematurity, low birth weight, and perinatal mortality in pregnancies complicated by bacteriuria. Kincaid-Smith[480] and McFadyen[478] both have reported an increased rate of spontaneous abortion in pregnancies complicated by bacteriuria. In addition, there appears to be a higher frequency of low-birth-weight-for-date infants born to bacteriuric mothers, particularly those with hypertension or those in whom treatment programs have failed to eradicate the bacteria.[478-481] In addition to the increase in low-birth-weight infants, acute UTI is associated with an increased fetal mortality rate.[482]

Most compelling are two reports derived from data generated in a multicenter study of more than 55,000 pregnant women.[483, 484] Sever and colleagues[483] noted a higher frequency of low birth weights and stillbirths resulting from the pregnancies of the 3.5% of women with symptomatic UTI. From the same database, Naeye[484] reported a frequency of perinatal death of 42 per 1000 when the mothers were bacteriuric as opposed to 21 per 1000 when they were not. In this study, virtually all the excess mortality occurred when the UTI was present within 15 days of delivery, with the highest death rates occurring when UTI coexisted with maternal hypertension and acetonuria. Women who had pyuria and bacteriuria close to the time of delivery had a 24% greater frequency of amniotic fluid infection than did women without pyuria. Hypertension was 88% more common in mothers who had pyuria and bacteriuria than in those who did not have pyuria. In addition, bacteriuria was associated with growth-retarded placentas. The mechanisms by which bacteriuria exerts its effects on the outcome of pregnancy are unclear, although it has been suggested that an adverse effect of bacterial endotoxin on the placental circulation plays an important role.[485]

However, proof that eradication of the bacteriuria prevents fetal complications (as opposed to the maternal complications, which are clearly benefited) is incomplete. In addition, an alternative explanation for these associations is available: bacteriuria, hypertension, fetal wastage, and prematurity are all far more common in pregnancies of women from lower socioeconomic groups. The question can be fairly asked, then, as to whether these associations are not linked as cause and effect but rather represent a series of unrelated phenomena that are common in a particular population—pregnant women of lower socioeconomic backgrounds.[486]

On balance, however, we believe that routine screening for, and treatment of, bacteriuria of pregnancy are indicated for both the mother's and the child's health. Although complete evidence that treatment prevents all of the complications of pregnancy-associated bacteriuria will probably never become available, the withholding of therapy for such bacteriuria, whether symptomatic or asymptomatic, must be regarded as both ethically wrong and medically insupportable.[487, 488]

Long-term studies of schoolgirls with previously diagnosed bacteriuria and renal scarring have shown that when they reach adulthood and become pregnant, they have a greater than threefold increased risk of hypertension and a greater than sevenfold risk of preeclampsia. Despite these findings, with skilled obstetric management, the outcome of the pregnancy in terms of the health of both the mother and the child should be satisfactory.[489]

Urinary Tract Infection and Survival of the Patient

The final question regarding the biologic impact of UTI has to do with the patient's survival. Although it is absolutely clear that gram-negative sepsis originating in the urinary tract can have lethal consequences, occasionally even with the best of treatment, the question has been raised whether survival of the patient can be adversely influenced outside of the direct infectious disease effects of UTI. Several reports have

suggested that bacteriuria, particularly in the elderly, is associated with an increased risk of subsequent mortality.[448, 490-492] Although a cause-and-effect relationship between bacteriuria and death was usually postulated, some data have led investigators to question this relationship. It would now appear that the occurrence of bacteriuria is related to the degree of functional impairment present and is a marker for how seriously ill the individual is. Bacteriuria is not an independent variable that evolves with mortality. It is not surprising, then, that antimicrobial therapy aimed at bacteriuria has no effect on subsequent mortality rates. Indeed, in the elderly patient, antimicrobial therapy has little long-term benefit in terms of the occurrence of the bacteriuria itself. Therefore, there appears to be little justification for either screening adult patients, particularly elderly patients, for asymptomatic bacteriuria or treating them with antimicrobial agents.[450, 493-497]

CLINICAL PRESENTATIONS

The clinical evaluation of the patient with UTI can be surprisingly difficult because the range of clinical illness is remarkably broad: from the dysuria-frequency syndrome to full-blown pyelonephritis, from symptomatic to asymptomatic bacteriuria (the acute urethral syndrome). It is also clear that the ability of the clinician to accurately define the cause of the urinary tract symptoms or the anatomic site of involvement is limited. On the one hand, the patient who presents with frank rigors, a temperature of 104° F, exquisite loin pain, and signs suggesting gram-negative sepsis clearly has acute pyelonephritis. On the other hand, the absence of such findings does not rule out the presence of renal involvement, that is, covert pyelonephritis. In dealing with the patient who presents with possible UTI, the tasks of the clinician are the following:

1. To define the microbial etiologic agent of the symptoms and the ideal form of antimicrobial management.
2. To make a judgment as to the anatomic site within the urinary tract that is the site of infection. That is, does infection involve the kidney as well as the lower urinary tract, or is it restricted to the lower urinary tract? In the male patient, does it involve the prostate as well as the bladder?
3. To ascertain the risk of complicating structural or functional disease of the urinary tract that might alter clinical management and, when indicated, carry out such diagnostic tests as cystoscopy, voiding cystourethrography, ultrasonography, radioscintigraphy, or excretory urography.

The next sections are devoted to an approach designed to allow fulfillment of these tasks in each category of patients who present with possible UTI.

Acute Urinary Tract Infection
Acute Uncomplicated Cystitis

By far the most common clinical symptoms associated with UTI that bring patients to medical attention are those referable to the lower urinary tract: dysuria (burning or discomfort on urination), frequency, nocturia, and suprapubic discomfort. Approximately 10% of women of reproductive age come to medical attention each year with these symptoms.[439] Of these, two thirds have significant bacteriuria, whereas one third (those with the acute urethral syndrome) do not. Of the patients with significant bacteriuria, 50% to 70% have infection restricted to the bladder, but fully 30% to 50% have covert infection of the upper urinary tract as well.[4, 439,498-500] As demonstrated in Table 31-4, patients with and patients without covert renal involvement cannot be differentiated on clinical grounds alone. This lack of sensitivity of clinical evaluation in delineating the anatomic site of UTI has led to two practices: (1) treatment of most forms of UTI with identical therapeutic regimens, and (2) intensive effort by many investigators to develop noninvasive techniques for localizing the anatomic site of infection. However, as described subsequently, such techniques have proved to be too insensitive to be useful in the clinical management of the individual patient. Therefore, treatment of the patient with the dysuria-frequency syndrome has to be based on the recognition of the possibility that infection more serious than simple cystitis may be present (see later).[4, 498-500]

The greatest advances in this area have come from the partial unraveling of the causes of the acute urethral syndrome. Women with the acute urethral syndrome can be divided into two groups. Approximately 70% have pyuria on urinalysis and have true infection. An occasional patient in this category has tuberculosis, fungal disease of the urinary tract, or, rarely, an intra-abdominal or pelvic abscess adjoining the urinary tract, causing "sympathetic inflammation." For the most part, however, these patients have infection with *C. trachomatis* or with the usual bacterial uropathogens (e.g., *E. coli, S. saprophyticus*) but in "less than significant" numbers (10^2-10^4/mL). The remaining 30% of patients with the acute urethral syndrome, but no pyuria, have no known microbial etiologic agent for their symptoms. Presumably, these symptoms result from trauma related to intercourse, local irritation or allergy, or some other as yet undefined process.[498-501]

Confirmation of these microbiologic results comes from treatment data. Stamm and colleagues[501] reported on a double-blind, randomized study of doxycycline (100 mg given twice daily by mouth for 10 days) versus placebo in the treatment of patients with the acute urethral syndrome. The results were striking: 11 of 12 women with the acute urethral syndrome due to "true but less than significant bacteriuria" with coliform organisms or *S. saprophyticus* became asymptomatic with therapy, whereas only 4 of 10 women given placebo responded; all five women with documented *C. trachomatis* infection responded to doxycycline, whereas only two of six responded to placebo. In contrast, doxycycline failed to have any discernible clinical effect on patients with the acute urethral syndrome without pyuria. Although less well documented bacteriologically, a similar experience was reported by Tolkoff-Rubin and associates[502] with trimethoprim-sulfamethoxazole; this drug and doxycycline are active against both bacterial uropathogens and *C. trachomatis*.

Recurrent Cystitis

Recurrent symptoms of lower urinary tract inflammation may be due to either relapsing infection or reinfection. Relapse occurring in either sex is caused by reappearance of the same organism from a sequestered focus, usually within the kidney or prostate, shortly after completion of therapy. In reinfection, the course of therapy has successfully eradicated the infection, and there is no sequestered focus, but organisms are reintroduced from the fecal reservoir. More than 80% of all recurrences are due to reinfection.[499, 500]

Among schoolgirls with symptomatic UTI, about 20% remain infection-free after each course of treatment, with 25% having repeated bouts of infection.[424] Among the group of adult women susceptible to recurrent UTIs (defined as three or more infections in a calendar year), the attack rate over several years is approximately 0.15 infection per month, with virtually all such infections being symptomatic. Approximately one third of such infections are followed by an infection-free interval of at least 6 months, the average infection-free interval being approximately 1 year.

TABLE 31-4

Relationship among Clinical Syndromes, Presence of Significant Bacteriuria, and Anatomic Site of Urinary Tract Infection (UTI) in a General Practice Population (% with Symptoms)

	INSIGNIFICANT OR ABSENT BACTERIURIA (ACUTE URETHRAL SYNDROME)	RENAL BACTERIURIA	BLADDER BACTERIURIA
Symptoms suggesting lower UTI			
Frequency	95	98	70
Burning	70	68	70
Suprapubic pain	70	68	51
Symptoms suggesting upper UTI			
Loin pain	50	48	19
Fever	35	44	4
Rigors	15	32	15
Nausea and vomiting	25	24	8
Macroscopic hematuria	25	20	12

Modified from Fairley F, Carson NE, Gutch RC, et al: Site of infection in acute urinary tract infection in general practice. Lancet 2:615, 1971. Copyright by The Lancet Ltd., 1971.

Unfortunately, even prolonged remission in these individuals does not mean cure because infections tend to recur even after an infection-free interval of a year or longer.[503]

The most important cause of recurrent symptoms of lower urinary tract inflammation in adult men is prostatitis caused by either *E. coli* or the other bacterial uropathogens seen in women. Acute bacterial prostatitis is a febrile illness associated with chills; perineal, back, or pelvic pain; dysuria; and urinary frequency and urgency. There may be bladder outlet obstruction; on physical examination, the prostate is enlarged, tender, and indurated. Chronic prostatitis, in contrast, may be more occult; asymptomatic infection is manifested as recurrent bacteriuria or variable low-grade fever with back or pelvic discomfort. Urinary symptoms are usually due to reintroduction of infection into the bladder from a chronic prostatic focus that has been inadequately treated and only temporarily suppressed by a previous course of antimicrobial therapy.[4, 5, 88, 424]

Acute Pyelonephritis

The clinical findings associated with full-blown acute pyelonephritis are familiar: recurrent rigors and fever, back and loin pain (with exquisite tenderness or percussion of the costovertebral angle), often with colicky abdominal pain, nausea and vomiting, dysuria, frequency, and nocturia. Although bacteremia may complicate the course of symptomatic pyelonephritis in any patient, such bacteremias are seldom associated with the more serious sequelae of gram-negative sepsis, that is, the triggering of the complement, clotting, and kinin systems, which may lead to septic shock, disseminated intravascular coagulation, or both. When shock or disseminated intravascular coagulation occurs in the setting of pyelonephritis, the possibility of complicating obstruction must be ruled out. In one particularly important form of obstructive uropathy, which is associated with acute papillary necrosis, the sloughed papilla may obstruct the ureter. This form should be particularly suspected in diabetic patients with severe pyelonephritis and high-grade bacteremia, especially if the response to therapy is delayed.

In children younger than 2 years, fever, vomiting, nonspecific abdominal complaints, or failure to thrive may be the only manifestations of significant acute pyelonephritis. Indeed, UTI accounts for approximately 10% of these febrile episodes. In older children, clinical manifestations resemble more closely those seen in the adult, although the reappearance of enuresis may be a marker for the decreased urinary concentrating ability that is sometimes associated with renal infection (see later).[504-506]

Complicated Urinary Tract Infection

The term "complicated UTI" encompasses a wide range of clinical syndromes that include asymptomatic bacteriuria, cystitis, pyelonephritis, and frank urosepsis. The common element is the presence of bacterial infection of the urinary tract in patients with structurally abnormal (e.g., ureteral and bladder neck obstruction—including that due to prostatic enlargement, polycystic kidney disease, obstructing stones, or the presence of a catheter or some other foreign body) or functionally abnormal (e.g., a neurogenic bladder from spinal cord injury, diabetes mellitus, and multiple sclerosis)

urinary tracts, intrinsic renal disease, or a systemic process that renders the patient particularly susceptible to bacterial invasion. The range of organisms causing such infections is far broader than that noted in patients with uncomplicated infection, and the level of antibiotic resistance of these bacteria is also greater than that seen in isolates from the general population. Because the therapeutic requirements and management strategies for complicated UTI are different from those for uncomplicated infection (see later), this differentiation is clinically important.[88, 499]

Two unusual forms of renal infection are macroscopic renal and perinephric abscesses. In the past, most such abscesses were secondary to hematogenous infection with *S. aureus* or, less commonly, group A streptococci. These were primarily located in the renal cortex. Today, most are secondary to UTI with the usual Enterobacteriaceae, complicated by renal calculi and obstruction of urine flow from either the kidney or the ureter. Such abscesses are typically located at the corticomedullary junction. Less commonly, preexisting renal cysts may become infected and develop into abscesses; rarely, there may be contiguous spread from neighboring sites of suppuration, such as the colon and overlying rib. Renal abscesses may extend into the perinephric space or further. The usual presentation of renal and perinephric abscesses is insidious, with chronic symptoms of fever, weight loss, night sweats, and anorexia, often associated with flank or back pain. At times, when infection is under pressure, usually because of obstruction, a more acute presentation occurs with associated bacteremia. Symptoms specific to the urinary tract, such as dysuria, hematuria, and urinary retention, are sometimes noted. On physical examination, costovertebral angle tenderness or even a palpable mass may be found, but in 30% to 50% of patients, the examination results are normal. Routine laboratory tests are of variable value: leukocytosis may be present, anemia is not unusual, and urinalysis may reflect signs of inflammation, such as pyuria, proteinuria, or both. In more than half of patients, the same organism may be isolated on urine culture as that present in the abscess. Definitive diagnosis, however, is dependent on the demonstration of a mass lesion, as by excretory urography with nephrotomograms. Gallium and ultrasonographic scans and computed tomography may also yield evidence of an inflammatory mass lesion in and around the kidney. If prompt drainage and therapy with antibiotics is not carried out, such abscesses may be complicated by extension to the peritoneal cavity, the chest, or the skin.[507-509]

An unusual form of "complicated infection" occurs when the *E. coli* invading the urinary tract carries the genes for certain toxins. For example, UTI with Shiga toxin producing *E. coli* causing hemolytic-uremic syndrome has been reported.[510, 511]

Chronic Pyelonephritis and Reflux Nephropathy

Unlike the dramatic clinical presentation of many patients with acute pyelonephritis, chronic disease typically has a more insidious course. Clinical signs and symptoms may be divided into two categories: (1) those related directly to infection and (2) those related to the degree and the location of injury within the kidney. Surprisingly, the infectious aspects of the disease may be minor. Although intermittent episodes of full-blown pyelonephritis may occur, these are the exception. More common is asymptomatic bacteriuria, symptoms referable to the lower urinary tract (dysuria and frequency), vague complaints of flank or abdominal discomfort, and intermittent low-grade fevers.

Much more striking than the infectious or inflammatory symptoms are the physiologic derangements that result from the long-standing tubulointerstitial injury. These derangements include hypertension, inability to conserve Na^+, decreased concentrating ability, and tendency to develop hyperkalemia and acidosis. Although all of these are seen to some extent in all forms of renal disease, in patients with tubulointerstitial nephropathy such as this, the degree of physiologic derangement is out of proportion to the degree of renal failure (or serum creatinine elevation). Thus, in other forms of renal disease, physiologic derangements are minimal at serum creatinine levels of 2 to 3 mg/dL; in the patient with chronic pyelonephritis and reflux nephropathy with serum creatinine at this level, polyuria, nocturia, hyperkalemia, and acidosis may all be observed. Clinically, it is particularly important to recognize that such patients are especially susceptible to dehydration because of their inability to excrete a concentrated urine.

The diagnosis of chronic pyelonephritis is either a pathologic one or one based on specific radiologic findings of excretory urography. As defined by Hodson,[2, 414] these consist of focal, coarse cortical scarring with underlying retraction of the papillae and blunting and dilation of the calices. Scars are most frequently observed in the upper and lower poles. In patients with diffuse injury related to the presence of significant VUR, there are usually more marked cortical thinning and generalized caliceal dilation (see Fig. 31-10). Renal cortical scintigraphy with use of technetium Tc 99m–labeled dimercaptosuccinic acid has emerged as the most sensitive means of detecting renal changes caused by acute pyelonephritis, as well as the most sensitive way of detecting renal scarring. This is particularly true if tomographic imaging (so-called single-photon emission computed tomography) is employed as part of the scan. What is less clear, however, is the clinical importance of detecting small areas of renal abnormality by radioscintigraphy (which can be confirmed pathologically and thus are not artifacts) that are not demonstrable by excretory urography. Our practice is to regard such findings as "an early warning of potential danger" and to observe such individuals closely with intensive medical therapy (see later).[512-521]

The laboratory findings are as nonspecific as the clinical findings. Although pyuria is usually present, it may be absent, particularly if no active infection is present. Less common is the presence of white blood cell casts on urinalysis. Bacteriuria may or may not be demonstrable.

The determination of 24-hour protein excretion may be an important prognostic indicator in patients with chronic pyelonephritis and reflux nephropathy. Most patients with this condition excrete less than 1 g/day of protein. Alt and associates[522] reported an average 24-hour protein excretion of 1.12 g in patients with creatinine clearances of less than 40 mL/minute, with minimal proteinuria in those whose creatinine clearances exceeded 65 mL/minute. However, heavy proteinuria, including the nephrotic syndrome, may develop in a subset of patients. Renal biopsies in such patients reveal the superimposition of focal and segmental glomerulosclerosis on the basic tubulointerstitial injury. These patients

have a particularly poor prognosis and progress to end-stage renal disease (see later).

Natural History of Vesicoureteral Reflux and Reflux Nephropathy

The natural history of VUR and reflux nephropathy is variable, depending on the severity of the VUR, the concurrence of other congenital anomalies or obstruction, the age at presentation, the surgical or antibacterial intervention, and the development of such complications as hypertension and glomerulosclerosis.

It is useful in discussing the natural history to separate the issue of coarse scar formation in the kidney from the progressive deterioration of renal function not related to new scar formation; although coarse scar formation is closely linked to VUR and infection, the progressive deterioration of renal function can result from numerous secondary mechanisms.

Formation of Scars

The two main conclusions of the studies summarized earlier are that (1) scar development usually represents the combined effects of infection, VUR, and intrarenal reflux, and (2) the severity of VUR is the single most important determinant of whether renal demage will occur. The importance of infection in the development of new scars was shown by Smellie and associates,[203, 204] who found only two fresh scars developing among 75 compliant children observed for 15 years and given low-dose prophylactic antibacterial therapy. It has been suggested that infection and high pressure may alter some borderline papillae to the refluxing state. Children who have UTI but unscarred kidneys after age 3 years have an estimated risk of developing new scars of 2% to 3%.[523-527]

Progressive Renal Failure

The progressive renal failure seen in patients with reflux nephropathy is frequently caused not by infection nor by continued VUR but by other complicating or related conditions. These include (1) retardation of renal growth, (2) obstruction or other congenital anomalies, (3) hypertension, and (4) progressive glomerulosclerosis.

RETARDATION OF RENAL GROWTH. The effect of VUR on renal growth is important because normal renal growth is an indication of a healthy kidney and has a linear relationship with the child's height.[528] Earlier studies had reported retardation or arrest of renal growth in children with UTI with or without VUR.[210] Several studies have examined this issue in some detail. Winberg and colleagues[529] observed 22 infants with acute pyelonephritis who had no visible scarring at first presentation. No scars developed after 9 years of follow-up, but there was a significant reduction in the parenchymal thickness of the patients' kidneys compared with that of control subjects, regardless of the presence of VUR. Claesson and associates[530] studied renal growth profiles in 26 patients with unilateral scarring and found that renal tissue loss was compensated for almost completely by hypertrophy of the contralateral kidney, which took place even in the presence of VUR. The glomerular filtration rate was normal in these patients after 10 to 15 years of follow-up.

A renal growth spurt eventually follows growth impairment, but this may be postponed until puberty in both scarred and unscarred kidneys for unknown reasons. Winberg and colleagues' conclusion was that focal scarring and growth impairment are two different consequences of renal infection.

Smellie and colleagues[203] reported the effects of VUR on renal growth in 70 children with initial UTI and VUR managed with continuous antibacterial prophylaxis. Renal growth was abnormal in 11 of 11 kidneys drained by refluxing ureters, and 10 of these 11 kidneys were exposed to recurrence of urinary infection. In pairs of kidneys with unilateral VUR, there was a significant difference in growth only if the refluxing ureter drained a scarred kidney. Seven kidneys that grew least well had established severe scarring associated with persisting gross VUR, and each had a period of infection during observation. It was concluded that the prognosis of renal growth is generally excellent with VUR, particularly if the kidneys are unscarred and there is no recurrence of infection. The prognosis for growth is poorest for patients with gross, persistent VUR; severe generalized scarring; and increased tendency toward recurrent infection.

In the report of the Newcastle Covert Bacteriuria Research Group,[531] schoolgirls 4 to 18 years of age with covert bacteriuria who were observed for 5 years had below-average renal growth only when the kidneys were scarred, regardless of whether they had received antibacterial therapy. However, none of the girls in this group became hypertensive or had abnormal blood chemistry profiles during the follow-up.

The balance of the evidence suggests that renal growth may be transiently impaired in children with VUR, but mainly in those with renal scarring and usually in the presence of infection. However, this reduction in renal growth does not seem to be a major determinant of the later progressive deterioration of renal function in patients with reflux nephropathy.[468, 469,523-531]

OBSTRUCTION AND OTHER CONGENITAL ANOMALIES. Children with UTI with or without VUR may have a variety of renal and lower urinary tract anomalies that contribute to renal damage. These include duplex kidneys, cysts, hydronephrosis due to ureteropelvic obstruction, renal calculi, vesicoureteral or urethral obstruction, and bladder diverticula.[204] These anomalies predispose to repeated renal infection. The coexistence of VUR and an obstructive anomaly, such as posterior urethral valves, is particularly harmful, and it is under these conditions that sterile reflux may cause renal damage.

HYPERTENSION. The association between chronic pyelonephritis or reflux nephropathy and hypertension is well documented; the frequency of the hypertension varies with both age and severity of disease.[476] In Bengtsson's series,[532] more than 90% of the patients observed to terminal uremia became hypertensive, but Gower[533] found hypertension in only 12% of patients with unilateral pyelonephritis and in 28% of those with bilateral pyelonephritis whose renal function was normal. Kincaid-Smith and associates[411] found hypertension in 27% of 145 adults with reflux nephropathy. The degree of the hypertension was related to the severity of the reflux nephropathy.

Reflux nephropathy is one of the most common causes of hypertension in children. Gill and colleagues[534] found that 83% of 100 severely hypertensive children had associated renal disease and that 14% of these had reflux nephropathy.

Most of Holland and colleagues' 177 children with malignant hypertension and scarred atropic kidneys had reflux nephropathy,[535, 536] and Rance and associates[537] found that 29 (30%) of 96 children with persistent hypertension had chronic pyelonephritis, making it the most common etiologic factor in the group. About 10% of children with renal scarring become hypertensive, and 15% of patients with reflux nephropathy who reach adulthood have hypertension.[538-540] Reflux nephropathy diagnosed for the first time in adulthood is highly associated with UTI, proteinuria, back pain, and renal calculi, in addition to hypertension.[541]

The pathogenesis of hypertension in reflux nephropathy is unclear. In humans, there is some evidence both for and against a role for hyperreninemia.[542-545] Although it has been difficult to produce hypertension in rats and rabbits that have been made pyelonephritic, studies in pigs show that hypertension develops in some animals 1 to 2 years after the induction of VUR with scarring and that such hypertension is associated with pronounced arterial lesions and activation of the renin-angiotensin system (C.J. Hodson, unpublished data). Hypertension also occurs in unilateral reflux nephropathy, but there is uncertainty about whether such hypertension can be prevented or ameliorated by unilateral nephrectomy.[544]

PROTEINURIA AND PROGRESSIVE GLOMERULOSCLEROSIS. There is a prognostically important association among the development of proteinuria, focal segmental glomerulosclerosis, and progressive renal insufficiency in patients with reflux nephropathy.[474-476, 546] Although several authors had reported occasional severe proteinuria or overt nephrotic syndrome in patients diagnosed as having chronic pyelonephritis,[547, 548] it was Kincaid-Smith[411, 421, 422, 549] who first stressed the occurrence of proteinuria and glomerulosclerosis in patients with chronic pyelonephritis and reflux nephropathy. In 55 adult patients with reflux nephropathy, she found that 19 had proteinuria. All but 1 of 11 patients whose renal function subsequently declined had significant proteinuria, with the mean being 2.36 g/24 hours, whereas all patients whose serum creatinine level remained stable had either no proteinuria (seven patients) or proteinuria of less than 1 g/24 hours (two patients). The degree of proteinuria correlated well with the presence and the extent of glomerular lesions, most of which consisted of focal and segmental glomerulosclerosis and hyalinosis. Microalbuminuria (a urinary albumin excretion rate of 20-200 μg/minute) may be the first sign of glomerular injury in these patients, as it is in diabetic patients.[550]

Other studies have confirmed the association of proteinuria, glomerulosclerosis, and reflux nephropathy.[551-555] In the study of Bhathena and colleagues[555] of 23 patients with end-stage reflux nephropathy, all had focal glomerulosclerosis, and their average protein excretion ranged from 1.2 to 5.8 g/24 hours. In 29 of the 54 patients described by Torres and associates,[553] the 24-hour urinary protein excretion ranged from 0.5 to 10.4 g. There was a significant positive correlation between the 24-hour protein excretion and the simultaneous determination of creatinine clearance. The clinical course to end-stage renal disease was not appreciably altered by late surgical correction of the VUR, by infection, or by hypertension. In our series of patients with chronic pyelonephritis or reflux nephropathy, half of those with focal glomerulosclerosis had radiologic or morphologic evidence of bilateral renal disease and a serum creatinine level of more than

2.5 mg/dL, and 63% had a 24-hour urinary protein excretion of greater than 1 g.[388, 556] In contrast, patients without focal sclerosis had normal serum creatinine levels, minimal proteinuria, and unilateral disease.

The precise mechanism responsible for the development of proteinuria and glomerulosclerosis in patients with reflux nephropathy is still unclear. Immunologic injury by circulating immune complexes was suggested by the presence of IgM and C3 in the mesangium and in sclerotic areas in more than half of the patients reported.[553, 557] However, the search for bacterial products as antigens within the glomeruli has proved negative.[525] Autologous antigens, such as brush border antigen and Tamm-Horsfall protein, have also been incriminated as antigens causing autoimmune glomerular injury, but we and others[555] have failed to localize this protein in the mesangium of patients with focal sclerosis and reflux nephropathy. The presence of the membrane attack complex of complement in sclerotic areas[558] and evidence of alternative complement pathway activation suggest a role for complement in the glomerular injury, but it is improbable that this is the primary event. A second possible explanation for the development of focal sclerosis is mesangial dysfunction occurring as a result of the hydrodynamic changes consequent to VUR and resembling the changes occurring with ureteral obstruction in experimental animals.[558, 559] Alternatively, the glomerular changes could represent local responses to growth factor and cytokine elaboration in response to the tissue injury engendered by infection and reflux.

Vascular changes consisting of intimal hyperplasia and medial hypertrophy are found in most patients with focal sclerosis and reflux nephropathy and may well play a role in the development of focal sclerosis. However, these vascular changes occur in the absence of hypertension or before the development of hypertension in patients with reflux nephropathy and proteinuria.

The most attractive explanation for glomerulosclerosis in reflux nephropathy is that it results from the adaptive changes occurring in glomeruli because of reductions in renal mass (see Chapter 44).[560, 561] With certain exceptions, the clinical data are consistent with this hypothesis. In most series, proteinuria and glomerulosclerosis are most prominent in patients with bilateral disease and impaired renal function, although they have occasionally been reported in patients with unilateral disease and those with normal renal function. In patients with normal renal function, it is probable that the adapted glomeruli have maintained normal function and that this continues until progressive sclerosis of the remaining glomeruli leads to reduction of the glomerular filtration rate. Occasionally, proteinuria occurs in patients with unilateral reflux nephropathy,[178, 562] and the glomerulosclerosis is present in the normal hypertrophied kidney. Although this has been cited as evidence against the hemodynamic mechanism, it is consistent with it because hemodynamic changes have been well documented in uninvolved kidneys of patients with unilateral scars.[563] Finally, morphometric studies confirm the hypertrophy of glomeruli in biopsy specimens of patients with reflux nephropathy and show a relationship between renal size, glomerular size, and renal function in these patients.[564]

Whatever the mechanisms, it is now clear that progressive glomerulosclerosis is a major determinant of the development of chronic renal failure in reflux nephropathy.

DIAGNOSTIC EVALUATION

History and Physical Examination

Despite the incomplete relationship between clinical symptoms and presence of infection at various sites in the urinary tract, useful information can be gained from a skillfully obtained history. When a patient with a single acute episode of symptomatic UTI is examined, the first consideration is whether there are signs or symptoms suggesting the presence or imminent development of systemic sepsis: spiking fevers, rigors, tachypnea, colicky abdominal pain, and exquisite loin pain. Such patients require immediate attention and probably parenteral therapy in a hospital setting. If the patient is not acutely septic, attention turns to such concerns as previous history of UTIs, renal disease, and such conditions as diabetes mellitus, multiple sclerosis, other neurologic conditions, history of renal stones, and previous genitourinary tract manipulation—conditions that could predispose to UTI and could affect the efficacy of therapy. A careful neurologic examination can be particularly important in suggesting the possibility of a neurogenic bladder.

The patient with a history of recurrent UTIs merits special attention in terms of obtaining a clear history of sexual activity, response to therapy, and temporal relationships of recurrences to the cessation of therapy. Thus, women with recurrent bacterial UTIs temporally related to intercourse could benefit from the administration of antibiotics after each sexual exposure (see later).[98] The woman with the acute urethral syndrome due to *C. trachomatis* infection may respond only temporarily to antichlamydial therapy because of reinfection from the untreated sexual partner (so-called ping-ponging infection); cure occurs when both individuals are treated simultaneously. Women with recurrent UTIs who have relapsing infection as opposed to reinfection often give a different history of the temporal relationship between the end of therapy and the onset of new symptoms. The majority of women with relapsing infection relapse within 4 to 7 days of completing a course of therapy of 14 days or less, whereas those with recurrent reinfection usually have a longer interval between episodes unless bladder dysfunction or some other disturbance of urinary tract function is present. Similarly, men with persistent prostatic foci of infection often relapse promptly after a similar conventional course of therapy.[15, 86] In addition, a history of prostatic obstruction to urine flow should be sought (e.g., narrowing of the urine stream, hesitancy, nocturia, and dribbling).

When the patient with possible chronic pyelonephritis and reflux nephropathy is examined, two types of information should be sought: the history of UTI in childhood and during pregnancy, and the possible presence of such pathophysiologic consequences as hypertension, proteinuria, polyuria, nocturia, and frequency.

Urine Tests

The criteria used to evaluate the presence of infection by culture and the presence of pyuria on microscopic examination have been described previously. Because of the ubiquity of UTIs in all age groups, the expense of culturing urine by conventional techniques, and the emphasis on attempting to diagnose UTI in the home or in the physician's office (as opposed to the hospital setting), a great deal of attention has been paid to the development of simple tests for bacteriuria that require a minimum of expertise and equipment. These are summarized in the following sections.

Chemical Tests for the Presence of Bacteriuria

Four major chemical tests have been evaluated as rapid diagnostic tools. By far the most commonly used is the Griess nitrate reduction test, which is dependent on the bacterial reduction of nitrate in the urine to nitrite, with a variety of commercially available tapes or dipsticks employed to measure the presence of nitrites. This test is most accurate on first–morning urine specimens and is reasonably effective in identifying infection due to Enterobacteriaceae but fails to detect infection due to gram-positive organisms and *Pseudomonas*. False-negative results may also be caused by lack of dietary nitrate or diuresis because bladder incubation time is necessary for bacteria to reduce the nitrates. Because of its simplicity, this test is best used as part of a home or epidemiologic screening program, particularly if multiple specimens can be evaluated from a single individual.[424, 565-567]

The combination of the nitrate test with a test for leukocyte esterase on a single, inexpensive dipstick that can be read in less than 2 minutes has greatly increased the utility of this approach. This system provides a useful assessment for the presence of more than 10^5 Enterobacteriaceae per milliliter of urine and of pyuria. A negative test result has a predictive value of 97%. False-negative test results can be caused by proteinuria and the presence of gentamicin or cephalexin in the urine. Overall, this test has an 87% sensitivity and a 67% specificity (false-positive results usually result from vaginal contamination). This approach is far more effective in screening urine specimens from patients with symptoms as opposed to screening asymptomatic patients, such as occurs in obstetric practice.[13, 567-571]

The other commonly employed chemical test is the reduction of triphenyltetrazolium chloride to triphenylformazan (which has a red color) by bacteria. False-positive test results are caused by the ingestion of large amounts of vitamin C or a urine pH of less than 6.5. False-negative test results are due to deterioration of the reagent (common) and infection with staphylococci, some enterococci, and *Pseudomonas* species. Other tests that have been employed are a glucose oxidase test (bacteria consume the small amount of glucose present in the nondiabetic urine) and an assay for urinary catalase (which most uropathogens possess, but so do inflammatory cells of any cause). Unfortunately, these are even less accurate than the first two methods.[422, 566, 567]

DIP-SLIDE METHODS

Far more useful are a variety of dip-slide methods in which plastic paddles with agar on their surfaces are immersed in the urine, drained, and incubated. An agar medium selective for gram-negative organisms (e.g., MacConkey agar) is usually present on one side of the paddle or slide, and a nonselective medium that supports the growth of most bacterial species, including gram-positive organisms, is present on the other side. After overnight incubation, the number of colonies on both agar surfaces is then compared with standardized pictures of inoculated dip slides to achieve a semiquantitative

estimation of the number of organisms present. Positive slides can then be sent to a reference laboratory for species identification and antibiotic susceptibility testing. The technique is useful for office or home screening.[422, 566, 567, 572]

INFECTION-LOCALIZING TESTS

Although there may be great similarity in the clinical presentation of patients with upper and lower UTIs, there can be vast differences in the response to therapy and the type of pathologic process. Bladder infection is a superficial mucosal infection at an anatomic site to which high concentrations of antibiotics can be easily delivered, whereas renal infection (and prostatic infection in men) is a deep parenchymal infection at a tissue site where natural host defenses are rendered less effective by a hostile physicochemical environment and to which antimicrobial delivery may be limited. One would predict that the type of antimicrobial therapy necessary to eradicate infection from the urinary tract would be different for these two anatomic sites, with renal infection (and prostatic infection) requiring a more intensive or prolonged course of therapy, or both, than bladder infection.[5, 573]

The problem has been to develop a means of assessing the anatomic site of infection, given the 30% to 50% frequency of covert renal infection in patients with symptoms referable only to the lower urinary tract.[5, 573, 574] The only direct method of localizing the infection site is bilateral ureteral catheterization. Although too invasive for general use, it remains the standard against which all other methods of localization are compared. A less invasive procedure is the bladder washout procedure introduced by Fairley and colleagues.[574] In this procedure, a Foley catheter is introduced into the bladder, the bladder is irrigated with an antibiotic solution (usually neomycin or neomycin and polymyxin), and several urine samples are collected. Patients with lower UTI have sterile urine during the collection period after the washout, whereas patients with renal infection have bacteria in all of the samples after the washout. The major drawback with this technique is its inability to distinguish between unilateral and bilateral renal infection. However, because it is easy to perform, safe, and inexpensive and does not require an expert cystoscopist, it has replaced the ureteral catheterization studies as the method against which all noninvasive techniques are compared.

Three types of noninvasive techniques have been employed in an attempt to differentiate between renal and bladder infection: (1) assay of renal medullary function by measurement of maximal urinary concentrating capacity,[575-578] (2) measurement of urinary enzymes as an index of tissue injury and inflammation,[579-580] (3) and measurement of the immunologic response to infection.[581-585] The basis for each of these tests is the pathologic differences between upper and lower tract infections: renal medullary infection occurs at a site where critical aspects of urine formation are taking place and where inflammatory and immunologic responses are brisk and extensive; bladder infection occurs in the superficial mucosa, where little is occurring functionally and where both inflammatory and immunologic responses are limited.[586]

Urinary Concentrating Ability

As previously observed, acute or chronic tubulointerstitial inflammation of the kidney is commonly associated with a defect in concentrating ability, best measured by a maximal urinary concentrating test.[574-576] The defect in urinary concentrating ability in pyelonephritis appears to be due to the elaboration of prostaglandins in the renal medulla associated with inflammation because it can be blocked by the administration of the prostaglandin synthetase inhibitor indomethacin.[576-579] A typical result was reported by Ronald and associates[577] in a group of 38 patients whose site of infection was directly localized by ureteral catheterization. They demonstrated that renal but not bladder bacteriuria was associated with a decreased concentrating ability and that bilateral renal infection was associated with a greater defect than unilateral infection. In patients with unilateral infection, they were able to show a defect in the involved kidney and normal concentrating ability in the uninfected kidney. Eradication of infection was associated with return of concentrating ability. This approach to infection localization is flawed by frequent overlap in values in patients with bladder, unilateral renal, and bilateral renal infection. Thus, in addition to being inconvenient to perform, such tests are too insensitive to be useful in the routine management of patients.[573]

Measurement of C-Reactive Protein

Jodal and colleagues[580, 581] reported that consistently elevated levels of C-reactive protein in serum, as detected by an immunodiffusion technique, were seen in children with pyelonephritis. Children with acute cystitis, conversely, did not have elevated C-reactive protein levels. Sequential determination of C-reactive protein values in children with pyelonephritis showed that effective therapy led to a progressive decrease in these levels. However, localization of infection in these studies was made primarily on clinical grounds, and the assigned diagnosis did not correlate with bladder washout studies in 5 of 25 patients studied. The C-reactive protein level may also be elevated in other inflammatory conditions, and false-positive values may be observed.[582] Hellerstein and associates,[583] in a study of children in whom infection was localized by the bladder washout technique, failed to show any correlation with the C-reactive protein determination. In our experience, this test is even less sensitive in evaluating adult UTI.

Measurement of Antibody Responses to Bacteria

Renal infection is associated with the net synthesis of specific antibody directed against antigens of the infecting organism.[584] Various investigators have attempted to apply immunologic techniques to the problems of UTI anatomic localization. Percival and colleagues,[585] using a bacterial agglutination test, found elevated serum antibody levels in patients with symptoms of acute pyelonephritis, with these titers falling in response to antimicrobial therapy. Patients with clinically inapparent pyelonephritis also had high antibody levels, whereas patients with bladder infections had normal titers. Clark and associates[586] localized the site of infection by ureteral catheterization, examined the hemagglutinating antibody response, and confirmed that some patients with renal infection had higher hemagglutinating andibody titers than those of patients with bladder bacteriuria. However, a wide range of titers and a considerable overlap between the two groups of patients was once again observed, so that such serum studies are of limited use in the individual patient.[13]

The most widely used infection-localizing technique employed in more recent years has been the assay for antibody-coated bacteria (ACB assay) in the urine. Thomas and co-workers[587] and Jones and co-workers,[588] using an immunofluorescence assay, showed that bacteria originating from the kidney were coated with antibody, whereas bacteria associated with lower UTIs were antibody negative. Their work was confirmed by several investigators,[589-591] although some problems have emerged as the assay has been used more widely. The following appears to be a fair summary[5, 573] of the current status of this assay.

1. False-positive test results occur if vaginal or rectal flora contaminate a urine specimen; if heavy proteinuria appears, as in patients with the nephrotic syndrome; and if infection invades the uroepithelium outside the kidney (prostatitis, hemorrhagic cystitis, or bladder infections in the presence of bladder tumors or catheters).[591-593]
2. False-negative ACB test results have been noted in 16% to 38% of adult patients with acute pyelonephritis[594] and in most children.[595] In contrast, the ACB assay appears to have an accuracy of 95% or better in patients with chronic pyelonephritis.[588] This difference is presumably related to the 10- to 15-day lag with first infections between initiation of renal bacterial invasion and the ACB test result's turning positive[596]; lesser amounts of time are required with repeated infection because of an anamnestic antibody response.
3. The frequency of positive ACB test results in women with acute uncomplicated UTI appears to vary among different populations of patients. These differences may be related to the ease of access to medical care and the amount of time that elapses between the onset of symptoms and the initiation of medical care.[573]
4. The ACB-positive population is heterogeneous in its response to single-dose antimicrobial therapy; 50% to 60% of women with acute uncomplicated UTI who are ACB-positive respond to such therapy, as opposed to approximately 95% of those with ACB-negative infection.[5, 596, 597]

Because of these observations, the ACB test is not recommended for routine management of patients. Clearly, continuing efforts to develop better noninvasive tests for UTI localization are indicated.

Radiologic and Urologic Evaluations

The primary objective of radiologic and urologic evaluations in UTI is to delineate abnormalities that would lead to changes in the medical or surgical management of the patient. Such studies are particularly useful in the evaluation of children and adult men. In women, there is more controversy regarding their appropriate deployment. The following guidelines[4] would appear to be reasonable:

1. Either an excretory urogram or an ultrasound study is indicated to rule out obstruction in patients requiring hospital admission for bacteremic pyelonephritis,

particularly if the infection is slow to respond to appropriate therapy. Patients with septic shock in the setting require such procedures on an emergency basis because such patients often cannot be effectively resuscitated unless their "pus under pressure" is relieved by some form of drainage procedure that bypasses the obstruction.

2. Children with first or second UTIs, particularly those younger than 5 years, merit both excretory urography and voiding cystourethrography for detection of obstruction, VUR, and renal scarring. Dimercaptosuccinic acid scanning is a sensitive technique for detecting scars, and serial studies can be useful in assessing the course of scarring and the success of preventive regimens. However, this approach does not delineate anomalies in the pyelocaliceal system or the ureters. This imaging effort in children is aimed at identifying those who might benefit from intensive medical evaluation, particularly from prolonged antimicrobial prophylaxis. Because active infection by itself can produce VUR, it is usually recommended that the radiologic procedures be delayed until 4 to 8 weeks after the eradication of infection, although some groups perform these studies as early as 1 week after infection.[598-603]

   This approach is not ideal in that the results of 60% to 90% of the studies that are undertaken are negative, the cost is relatively high, and the exposure of young children to both radiation and bladder catheterization is undesirable. However, there have been few other parameters available for delineating the pediatric population at highest risk for anatomic abnormalities of the urinary tract. In particular, the noninvasive infection-localizing techniques have been of little diagnostic value in this population of patients.

3. Most men with bacterial UTI have some anatomic abnormality of the urinary tract, most commonly bladder neck obstruction secondary to prostatic enlargement. Therefore, anatomic investigation, starting with a good prostatic examination and then proceeding to excretory urography or urinary tract ultrasound studies with postvoiding views, should be seriously considered in all male patients with UTI.

4. Although there is general agreement that first UTIs in women do not merit radiologic or urologic study, the management of recurrent infection is more controversial. In such women, the once routine cystoscopic study with urethral dilation has fallen out of fashion. In addition, several studies have demonstrated the lack of cost-effectiveness of radiologic and urologic studies in the evaluation of women with recurrent UTIs. Fair and co-workers[604] reviewed the results of urograms in 164 women with histories of UTI, finding a 5.5% frequency of abnormalities but with none of these having an impact on clinical management. Engel and colleagues[605] reviewed the records of 153 women who had undergone urography and cystoscopy for the evaluation of infection. Abnormalities were observed in 11%; only one abnormality, a colovesical fistula, influenced clinical management. Fowler and Pulaski[606] studied 126 women with recurrent UTIs by use of urography, cystography, and cystoscopy and found only three instances (all patients with urethral diverticula) in which the results

of the studies influenced the clinical management of the patients' UTIs. Similar findings have been reported by others.[607]

Therefore, it would appear that the routine anatomic evaluation of women with recurrent UTIs cannot be recommended. This is not to say that a few patients might not benefit from such studies. Characteristics of a population of women who might benefit from such anatomic studies include patients who fail to respond to appropriate antimicrobial therapy or who rapidly relapse after such therapy; patients with continuing hematuria; patients with infection with urea-splitting bacteria; patients with symptoms of continuing inflammation, such as night sweats; and patients with symptoms of possible obstruction, such as back or pelvic pain that persists despite adequate antimicrobial therapy.[608, 609] In our experience, a disappointing response to antimicrobial therapy has been the most useful indicator for the need for radiologic and urologic evaluation.

TREATMENT

General Principles of Antimicrobial Therapy

The rational deployment of antimicrobial agents in the management of UTI is based on certain important clinical pharmacologic principles. Superficial mucosal infection, such as bladder infection, can be easily cured by the delivery of effective concentrations of antibiotic into the urine, with serum levels being of less importance. Therapy of deep tissue infection, such as that involving the kidney or the prostate, likewise requires delivery of effective concentrations of drug to the site of involvement. In addition, effective serum concentrations would seem to be advantageous.

The goals of treatment of UTI are to prevent or treat systemic sepsis, to relieve symptoms, to eradicate sequestered infection, to eliminate uropathogenic bacterial strains from fecal and vaginal reservoirs, and to prevent long-term sequelae—all at minimal cost, with the lowest rate of side effects, and with the least selection of an antibiotic-resistant bacterial flora. These goals can be best achieved by prescribing different forms of therapy for different types of UTIs.[610]

Specific Recommendations
Acute Uncomplicated Cystitis in Young Women

Therapy for healthy women of reproductive age who present with symptoms of lower urinary tract inflammation (dysuria, frequency, urgency, nocturia, and suprapubic discomfort) in the absence of signs and symptoms of vaginitis (vaginal discharge or odor, pruritus, dyspareunia, external dysuria without frequency, and vulvovaginitis on examination) should be approached with two objectives in mind: (1) eradication of superficial mucosal infection of the lower urinary tract, and (2) eradication of uropathogenic clones from the vagina and the lower gastrointestinal tract. Since the 1990s, the treatment of choice has been short-course therapy with trimethoprim-sulfamethoxazole or a fluoroquinolone; both of these are superior to β-lactam in the treatment of UTI. Both these drugs achieve high concentrations in vaginal secretions that are more than sufficient to eradicate the usual *E. coli* and other major uropathogens (with the notable exception of enterococci). At the same time, the antibacterial spectrum of activity of these drugs is such that the normal anaerobic and microaerophilic vaginal flora, which provides colonization resistance against the major uropathogens, is left intact. In contrast, β-lactam drugs, such as amoxicillin, appear to promote vaginal colonization with uropathogenic *E. coli*.[5, 89, 499, 610, 611]

Unfortunately, antimicrobial resistance has increased significantly since the early 1990s, particularly to trimethoprim-sulfamethoxazole, which has been the primary choice for treatment of acute uncomplicated cystitis because of cost and efficacy. Widespread distribution of a uropathogenic clone of *E. coli* that has acquired resistance to trimethoprim-sulfamethoxazole has been documented in several geographic areas of the United States. When trimethoprim-sulfamethoxazole is prescribed for a resistant organism, a failure rate higher than 50% is expected. Isolates from women younger than 50 years are more likely to be resistant than are those from older women. There is wide variation in different geographic areas in terms of the incidence of trimethoprim-sulfamethoxazole resistance, and the prescribing physician is obligated to obtain such information for his or her community of practice. If the incidence is higher than 20%, then it is recommended that a fluoroquinoline be prescribed as the drug of choice. However, it must be emphasized that monitoring of resistance to this class of drugs will be important as well, as it is likely that resistance will slowly develop to these drugs as well.[612-616]

There are two forms of short-course therapy: single-dose therapy and a 3-day course of therapy. There is now compelling evidence that a 3-day course of therapy is superior to a single dose, with either trimethoprim-sulfamethoxazole or a fluoroquinolone, provided the infecting organism is susceptible. Both forms of short-course therapy are probably equally efficacious in eradicating bladder infection in women. However, single-dose therapy is not as effective in

eradicating the uropathogenic clones from the vaginal or intestinal reservoir. As a result, early recurrence, predominantly resulting from reinfection from these reservoirs, is significantly more common with single-dose therapy.[617-634]

However, short-course therapy is specifically designed for the treatment of superficial mucosal infection and to serve as a guide for those with unsuspected deep tissue infection who would benefit from a more extended course of therapy (e.g., women with occult pyelonephritis). Short-course therapy should therefore never be given to individuals who fall into the following categories of patients with a high probability of deep tissue infection: any man with UTI (in whom tissue invasion of at least the prostate should be assumed), anyone with overt pyelonephritis, patients with symptoms of longer than 7 days' duration, patients with underlying structural or functional defects of the urinary system, immunosuppressed individuals, patients with indwelling catheters, and patients with a high probability of infection with antibiotic-resistant organisms.[5, 620, 639-642]

Acute uncomplicated UTI in otherwise healthy women is so common, the range of organisms causing the infection is so well defined, the susceptibility of these organisms to the antimicrobial agents recommended is so uniform, and the efficacy and lack of side effects of short-course therapy are now so well established that all have combined to lead to a cost-effective approach that minimizes both laboratory studies and the need for visits to the physician (Fig. 31-13). The first step is to initiate short-course therapy in response to the compliant of dysuria and frequency without evidence of vaginitis. If a urine specimen is readily available, a leukocyte esterase dipstick test can be carried out (which has a reported sensitivity of 75% to 96% in this situation)[635]; urine culture and microscopic examination of the urine are reserved for the patient with atypical presentations. Alternatively, a reliable patient who reports a typical clinical presentation by telephone could have short-course therapy prescribed without initial examination of the urine. Because short-course

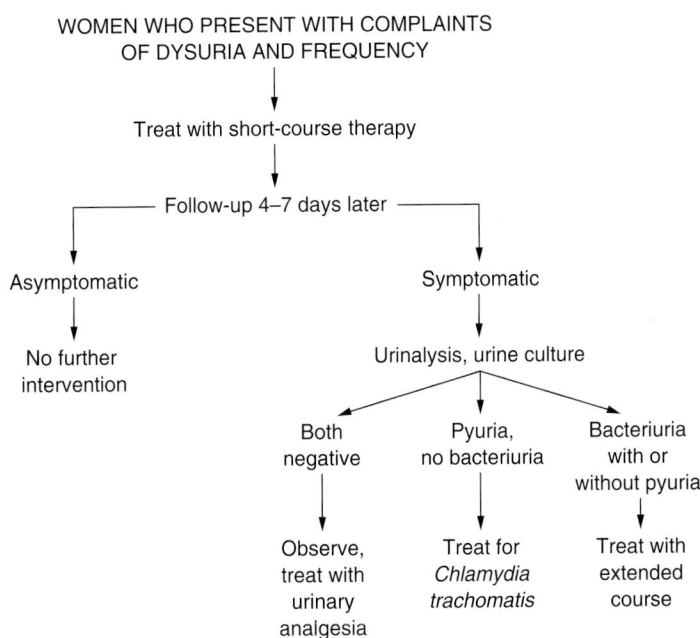

WOMEN WHO PRESENT WITH COMPLAINTS
OF DYSURIA AND FREQUENCY

Treat with short-course therapy

Follow-up 4–7 days later

Asymptomatic

No further
intervention

Symptomatic

Urinalysis, urine culture

Both
negative

Observe,
treat with
urinary
analgesia

Pyuria,
no bacteriuria

Treat for
*Chlamydia
trachomatis*

Bacteriuria
with or
without pyuria

Treat with
extended
course

FIGURE 31-13. Clinical approach to the woman with dysuria and frequency. (Modified from Tolkoff-Rubin NE, Wilson ME, Zuromskis P, et al: Single-dose amoxicillin therapy of acute uncomplicated urinary tract infections in women. Antimicrob Agents Chemother 25:626, 1984.)

therapy is both safe and inexpensive, and because most practitioners begin therapy on the basis of symptoms before culture data are available, this approach appears to be cost-effective.[620, 629, 636]

The critical practitioner-patient interaction comes after the completion of therapy: if the patient is asymptomatic, nothing further needs to be done. If the patient is still symptomatic, both urinalysis and urine culture are necessary. If the symptomatic patient has a negative urinalysis and bacterial culture, no clear microbial etiologic agent is present, and the physician's attention should be directed toward analgesia and concerns about trauma, personal hygiene, allergy to clothing dyes, or primary gynecologic conditions. If the patient is pyuric but not bacteriuric, the possibility of *C. trachomatis* urethritis should be considered, particularly if the woman is sexually active with multiple partners. Optimal therapy for *C. trachomatis* infection consists of a 7- to 14-day regimen of a tetracycline or sulfonamide for the patient and her sexual partner. Finally, patients with symptomatic bacteriuria due to an organism susceptible to the antibiotic that had been prescribed in a short-course regimen should be regarded as having covert renal infection. A more prolonged course of therapy should be administered, initially 14 days, with the potential for a more extended course if needed. Again, either a fluoroquinolone or trimethoprim-sulfamethoxazole (assuming the isolate is sensitive) would be the most effective drug in this circumstance.[620, 629, 636]

Recurrent Urinary Tract Infection in Young Women

Recurrent bacterial UTI is common in women, accounting for more than 5 million visits to physicians in the United States each year.[637] Approximately 20% of young women with a first episode of UTI will have recurrent infection.[89] Various regimens have been designed to prevent repeated reinfections, which account for more than 90% of UTI recurrences. Before the physician embarks on these antimicrobial approaches, however, such simple interventions as voiding immediately after sexual intercourse and switching from a diaphragm and spermicide-based contraceptive strategy to some other approach should be implemented. If these measures are not effective, it is then time to consider which of a variety of preventive strategies is most appropriate for a particular patient. For such preventive regimens to be acceptable, they should be effective at low doses, have minimal side effects, and should have minimal impact on the makeup and antibiotic susceptibility of the bowel flora, the reservoir from which UTIs are derived.

One strategy that is moderately efficacious in treating recurrent bacterial UTI is to acidify the urine with either methenamine mandelate or methenamine hippurate plus ascorbic acid, which results in the release of formaldehyde when the urine pH is maintained at 5.5 or lower. An extremely high rate of compliance by the patient and frequent checks of the urine pH are necessary for such a regimen to succeed. In the one direct comparison of this regimen with a placebo or low-dose trimethoprim-sulfamethoxazole regimen, the frequency of UTI per patient-year in a population of women susceptible to recurrent reinfections was 3.4 for placebo treatment, 1.6 for the methenamine mandelate plus ascorbic acid regimen, and 0.15 for the trimethoprim-sulfamethoxazole program.[650]

Several prospective studies have now demonstrated the efficacy of either nitrofurantoin, 50 mg, or nitrofurantoin macrocrystals, 100 mg, at bedtime for prophylaxis against recurrent reinfection of the urinary tract. Such a regimen has little if any effect on the fecal flora and presumably acts by providing intermittent urinary antibacterial activity.[637] Although this regimen is effective, a report from Sweden[639] has suggested that long-term nitrofurantoin prophylaxis against UTI is associated with an alarming rate of adverse side effects. These adverse effects include chronic interstitial pneumonitis, acute pulmonary hypersensitivity reactions, liver damage, blood dyscrasias, skin reactions, and neuropathy. In addition, nitrofurantoin should not be used in patients with renal impairment.

Perhaps the most popular prophylactic regimen currently used in women susceptible to recurrent UTI is low-dose trimethoprim-sulfamethoxazole; as little as half a tablet (trimethoprim, 40 mg; sulfamethoxazole, 200 mg) three times weekly at bedtime is associated with an infection frequency of less than 0.2 per patient-year. The efficacy of this prophylactic regimen appears to remain unimpaired even after several years. This regimen would be cost-effective in most practice settings for women who have more than two UTIs per year. Like trimethoprim-sulfamethoxazole, the fluoroquinolones may be used in a low-dose prophylactic regimen. The efficacy of these prophylactic regimens is further delineated by their potency in preventing UTI in the far more challenging population of kidney transplant recipients. A variation on these efficacious continuous prophylaxis programs is to use a fluoroquinolone or trimethoprim-sulfamethoxazole as postcoital prophylaxis.[638-642]

An important unanswered question is the duration of prophylactic therapy against recurrent UTI: Our practice has been to continue such therapy for 6 months and then to discontinue it. If infection then recurs, prophylaxis is reinstituted for periods of 1 to 2 years or longer. Although obvious side effects of such a program have not been apparent, more subtle long-term adverse effects on otherwise healthy women remain a concern. In particular, Freeman and co-workers,[467] in a study of men with chronic UTIs treated with a sulfonamide for 25 months, observed a significantly increased rate of cardiovascular mortality compared with that seen in patients treated with placebo, nitrofurantoin, or methenamine mandelate. Because of concerns regarding long-term adverse effects, compliance, and cost in the long-term prophylaxis of recurrent UTI, one final approach has been taken to this problem: to provide women having histories of recurrent infections with a supply of trimethoprim-sulfamethoxazole, a fluoroquinolone, or another effective single-dose regimen drug. The patient is then instructed to initiate single-dose therapy with the onset of symptoms; further medical attention is sought only when the symptoms do not abate or the number of treated episodes exceeds four in a 6-month period.[89, 643-645]

A nonantibiotic approach to preventing recurrent infection is cranberry juice. Apparently, proanthocyanidins derived from cranberry juice block bacterial adhesion at the epithelial level, presumably through binding to and blocking access to the mucosal receptor. In our experience, this has been moderately effective, and we advocate a trial of such an intervention before one of the antimicrobial approaches detailed previously is prescribed.[646-648]

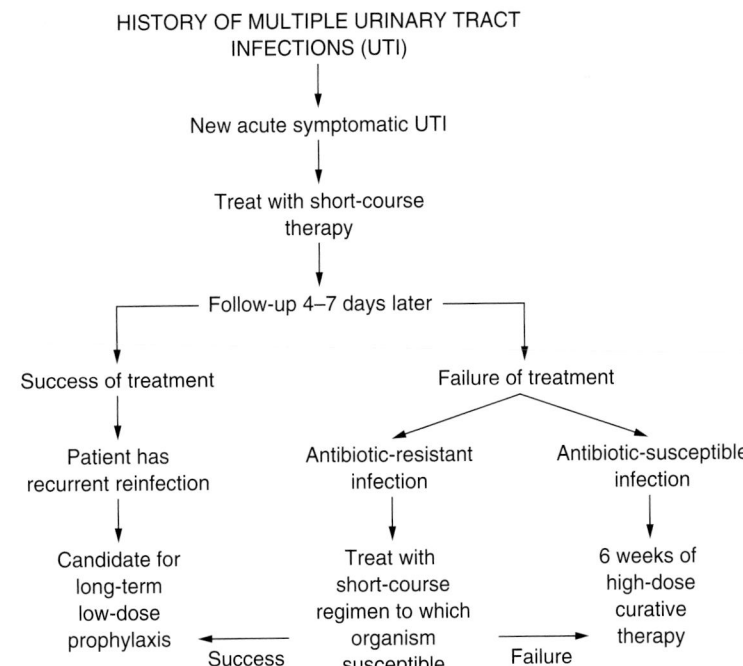

FIGURE 31-14. Clinical approach to the woman with recurrent urinary tract infections.

The approach to the minority of patients with relapsing infection is different. Two factors may contribute to the pathogenesis of relapsing infection in women: (1) deep tissue infection of the kidney that is suppressed but not eradicated by a 14-day course of antibiotics, and (2) structural abnormality of the urinary tract (e.g., calculi). At least some of these patients respond to a 6-week course of therapy.[649, 650] Because the strategy in dealing with relapsing infection and repeated reinfection is so different, the critical decision to be made by the clinician concerns the form of recurrent infection present in the individual patient. Certain clues to this are available from the past history and bacteriologic information. Most relapses occur within 1 week of the cessation of antimicrobial therapy, and virtually all occur within 1 month, so information concerning the timing of the recurrences can be helpful. Knowledge of the bacterial species isolated and the antibiotic susceptibility pattern of the species can help in deciding whether it is the same organism or different from the original pathogen. However, this kind of information is too often either unavailable or inadequate for this assessment to be made. We have found that the response to short-course therapy in such women is helpful in making the management decision: if the patient responds to short-course therapy, it is likely that she has been having recurrent reinfection and is thus a candidate for long-term prophylaxis; if the patient does not respond to short-course therapy, it is probable that she has been having relapsing infection and is thus a candidate for an intensive course of prolonged therapy. Thus, one can more exactly delineate those patients in whom the greatest clinical benefit would compensate for the increased costs and side effects of prolonged treatment (Fig. 31-14).

Acute Uncomplicated Cystitis in Older Women

Several aspects of UTI in postmenopausal women merit special attention. The frequency of both symptomatic and asymptomatic bacteriuria is considerably higher than in younger age groups, probably as a result of at least two factors: (1) many postmenopausal women have significant amounts of residual urine in their bladders after voiding as a consequence of childbirth and loss of pelvic tone, and (2) the lack of estrogens causes a marked change in the susceptibility of the uroepithelium and vagina to pathogens. This is at least partly due to such changes in the vaginal microflora as the loss of lactobacilli, which causes a rise in vaginal pH.[89, 650-653] Whereas symptoms referable to the lower urinary tract in younger women are almost invariably due to uropathogens and *C. trachomatis* (see earlier), other possibilities exist in older women. In particular, in symptomatic women with pyuria and negative cultures, the possibility of genitourinary tuberculosis, systemic fungal infection, and diverticulitis or a diverticular abscess impinging on the bladder or ureters merits consideration, rather than the chlamydial infection that represents a major cause of such infections in younger women.

The antimicrobial strategies discussed before for the management of acute cystitis in younger women are applicable in postmenopausal women as well. In addition, however, other interventions have an important role in this population. Several studies have now shown that estrogen replacement therapy, either locally by use of a vaginal cream or systemically with oral therapy, restores the atrophic genitourinary tract mucosa of the postmenopausal woman, is associated with a reappearance of lactobacilli in the vaginal flora and a fall in vaginal pH, and decreases vaginal colonization by Enterobacteriaceae.[653-655] In a carefully controlled study, Raz and Stamm[653] demonstrated unequivocally that these physiologic effects were translated into significant protection against recurrent UTI in postmenopausal women.

In a study that may be applicable to other populations as well, Avorn and co-workers[656] have reported that the regular intake of cranberry juice significantly reduced the frequency of both bacteriuria and pyuria in a population of elderly women. Although the possibility of this effect has been postulated for many years, it has in the past been linked to urinary acidification. Because consistent acidification with oral intake of cranberry juice requires the consistent ingestion of prodigious volumes, this approach had fallen out of favor. What is noteworthy in this study is that the therapeutic effect was clearly independent of any changes in urine pH. Rather than an acidification effect, it has been postulated that cranberry and blueberry juice contain materials that are excreted in the urine that inhibit the attachment of bacterial adhesins to the uroepithelium (see later).[656-658]

Asymptomatic bacteriuria is particularly common in elderly women, especially those not receiving hormonal replacement therapy. It is now clear that treatment of this serves no purpose, and thus screening for asymptomatic bacteriuria in this population is not indicated.[659]

Acute Uncomplicated Pyelonephritis in Women

Patients with clear-cut symptomatic pyelonephritis have deep tissue infection, have or are at risk for bacteremia, and merit intensive antimicrobial therapy. The key principle in the management of these patients is the immediate delivery to the bloodstream and to the urinary tract of effective concentrations of an antimicrobial agent to which the invading organism is susceptible. A variety of strategies are available to accomplish this; the following general principles are a useful guide.[89, 499]

1. There are three goals in the antimicrobial therapy of symptomatic pyelonephritis: control or prevention of the development of urosepsis (i.e., the consequences of bloodstream invasion), eradication of the invading organism, and prevention of recurrences.
2. It is useful to divide the therapeutic program to accomplish these aims into two parts: the immediate control of systemic sepsis, which often requires parenteral therapy; and the eradication of the infecting organism (and prevention of early recurrence) with an oral agent, after initial control of the systemic sepsis and acute inflammatory consequences of pyelonephritis.
3. Initial antimicrobial programs to obtain control of systemic sepsis are prescribed to fulfill two objectives: the infecting organism has a greater than 99% probability of being sensitive to the regimen chosen, and adequate blood levels of the drugs can be reliably achieved promptly in the particular patient. At present, there is no evidence to suggest that one antibiotic or program is inherently superior to another for control of systemic sepsis provided that these two requirements are fulfilled. Thus, the objection to ampicillin, amoxicillin, or first-generation cephalosporins as initial therapy for pyelonephritis when the nature and the susceptibility of the infecting organism are unknown (as is usually the case) is due to the fact that 20% to 30% of isolates are now resistant to these drugs. Similarly, the merits of intravenous therapy have to do with the reliability of drug delivery, rather than something inherently more desirable about intravenous drugs (indeed, as is well recognized, vascular access devices have their own infectious disease complications). In patients with milder disease, who are free of nausea and vomiting, advantage can be taken of the excellent antimicrobial spectrum

and bioavailability (with the easy achievement of high blood levels with oral administration provided that the gastrointestinal tract is functioning adequately) of such drugs as trimethoprim-sulfamethoxazole and the fluoroquinolones to prescribe oral therapy for the entire therapeutic course.

4. Once the patient has been afebrile for 24 hours (usually within 72 hours of initiation of therapy), there is no inherent benefit to maintaining parenteral therapy. At this point, prescription of trimethoprim-sulfamethoxazole or a fluoroquinolone to complete a 14-day course of therapy appears to be the most effective means of eradicating both tissue infection and residual clones of uropathogen present in the gastrointestinal tract that could cause early recurrence if left in place. One important point that bears emphasis in this regard: parenteral trimethoprim-sulfamethoxazole and fluoroquinolones are effective drugs for the initial control of systemic sepsis, but there is no special benefit of initiating therapy with one of these to be able to continue the same drug orally. Initial control with any effective parenteral regimen, followed by oral trimethoprim-sulfamethoxazole or fluoroquinolone for eradication, is the cornerstone of the therapeutic strategy. For example, a single large intravenous dose of gentamicin (10 mg/kg) followed by oral ciprofloxacin has been shown to be a cost-effective program for acute pyelonephritis.[660] As previously discussed, antimicrobial susceptibility of the isolate will be an important guide to therapy.

With these principles in mind, what, then, should be used as initial parenteral therapy? If possible, a Gram stain of the urine should be performed to establish whether enterococcal infection could be present. If gram-positive cocci are present, or if that information is not available, initial therapy should include intravenous ampicillin (or vancomycin) plus gentamicin to provide adequate coverage of both enterococci and the more common gram-negative uropathogens. If only gram-negative bacilli are present, there are a large number of choices ranging from parenteral trimethoprim-sulfamethoxazole and fluoroquinolones to gentamicin; such broad-spectrum cephalosporins as ceftriaxone, aztreonam, the β-lactam–β-lactamase inhibitor combinations (ampicillin-sulbactam, ticarcillin-clavulanate, and piperacillin-tazobactam); and imipenem-cilastatin. In general, these last agents on the list (beginning with aztreonam) are reserved for patients with more complicated histories, previous episodes of pyelonephritis, and recent urinary tract manipulations.[89, 503]

Urinary Tract Infection in Pregnancy

As previously discussed, pregnant women are the one population in whom screening for asymptomatic bacteriuria is not only cost-effective but also obligatory to prevent consequences for the developing fetus and the mother. Treatment of pregnant women with asymptomatic bacteriuria or symptoms of lower urinary tract inflammation (dysuria and frequency, akin to acute uncomplicated cystitis in the nonpregnant woman of reproductive age) is similar to that in nonpregnant women: short-course therapy.[89, 661] Although studies comparing single-dose with 3-day regimens are not available, and both have been effective in pregnant women, our preference is for a 3-day regimen. There are two major differences, however, in the approach to pregnant women with UTI: the drugs that can be safely used are far more limited, and intensive follow-up with the institution of prophylaxis for the duration of the pregnancy is an important management consideration.

Sulfonamides, nitrofurantoin, ampicillin, and cephalexin have been considered relatively safe for use in early pregnancy; sulfonamides are avoided near term because of a possible role in the development of kernicterus. Trimethoprim is usually avoided because of evidence of toxic effects in the fetus at high doses in experimental animals, although it has been used successfully in humans during pregnancy without evidence of toxicity or teratogenicity. Fluoroquinolones are avoided because of possible adverse effects on fetal cartilage development. Our preference is the use of nitrofurantoin, ampicillin, or cephalosporins—the drugs that have been used most extensively in pregnancy—in pregnant women with asymptomatic or minimally symptomatic UTI whenever possible. In pregnant women with overt pyelonephritis, admission to the hospital for parenteral therapy should be the standard of care; β-lactam drugs, aminoglycosides, or both are the cornerstone of therapy.[89, 661-663]

Effective prevention of UTI, including pyelonephritis, can be accomplished during pregnancy with postcoital prophylaxis with nitrofurantoin, cephalexin, or ampicillin. Alternatively, these drugs may be given at bedtime without relation to coitus. Patients who should be considered for such prophylaxis during pregnancy include patients with histories of acute pyelonephritis during pregnancy, patients with bacteriuria during pregnancy who have had a recurrence after a treatment course, and patients with a history of recurrent UTI before pregnancy that has required a prophylaxis program outside the added stresses of pregnancy.[664, 665]

Urinary Tract Infections in Men

UTI is uncommon in men younger than 50 years, although UTI without associated urologic abnormalities can occur under the following circumstances: in homosexual men, in men having intercourse with women colonized with uropathogens, and in men with the acquired immunodeficiency syndrome with a CD4+ lymphocyte count of less than 200/mm^3. Such individuals should never be treated with short-course therapy; rather, 10- to 14-day regimens of trimethoprim-sulfamethoxazole or a fluoroquinolone should be regarded as standard therapy unless antimicrobial intolerance or an unusual pathogen requires an alternative approach.[89, 666-668]

In men older than 50 years with UTI, tissue invasion of the prostate, the kidneys, or both should be assumed, even in the absence of overt signs of infection at these sites. Because of the inflammation usually present, acute bacterial prostatitis initially responds well to the same array of antimicrobial agents used to treat UTIs in other populations. However, after a conventional course of therapy of 10 to 14 days, relapse is common. Recurrent infection in men usually connotes a sustained focus within the prostate that has not been eradicated by previous courses of therapy. Several factors at work here make the eradication of prostatic foci so difficult:

- Many antimicrobial agents do not diffuse well across the prostatic epithelium into the prostatic fluid, where the infection lies.
- The prostate may harbor calculi, which can serve to block drainage of portions of the prostate gland or act as foreign bodies around which persistent infection can be hidden.
- An enlarged (and inflamed) prostate gland can cause bladder outlet obstruction, resulting in pools of stagnant urine in the bladder that are difficult to sterilize.[88, 89, 669-672]

As a result of these factors, it is now recognized that intensive therapy for at least 4 to 6 weeks and as many as 12 weeks is required to sterilize the urinary tract in many of these men. The drugs of choice for this purpose, assuming that the invading organisms are susceptible, are trimethoprim-sulfamethoxazole, trimethoprim (in the individual allergic to sulfonamide), and the fluoroquinolones. Prolonged treatment with each of these has a greater than 60% chance of eradicating infection. Most of the failures are due to one of two factors: the anatomic factors listed before are too abnormal to permit cure, and the infection that is present is a result of *E. faecalis* or *P. aeruginosa*, two organisms with a particularly high rate of relapse after treatment with antimicrobial agents. When relapse occurs, a choice then has to be made among three therapeutic approaches: (1) long-term antimicrobial suppression, (2) repeated treatment courses for each relapse, and (3) surgical removal of the infected prostate gland under coverage of systemic antimicrobial therapy. The choice from among these approaches depends on the age, sexual activity, and general condition of the patient; the degree of bladder outlet obstruction present; and the level of suspicion that prostate cancer could be present.[88, 89, 669-672]

In addition to the usual uropathogens that cause a UTI in men, one additional entity merits attention. After instrumentation of the urinary tract, most commonly after repeated insertion of a Foley catheter, infection with *S. aureus* may occur; the use of antistaphylococcal therapy and the removal of the foreign body are required for cure.

Treatment of Childhood Urinary Tract Infection

The treatment of full-blown pyelonephritis in the child is similar to that in the adult: broad-spectrum parenteral therapy until the antimicrobial susceptibility pattern of the infecting organism is known, followed by narrow-spectrum, least-toxic therapy parenterally until the patient is afebrile for 24 to 48 hours. A prolonged 1- to 3-month course of oral therapy is then instituted. Follow-up urine cultures within a week of completion of therapy and at frequent intervals for the next year are indicated. In children with acute, uncomplicated UTI, conventional 7- to 14-day regimens appear to be preferable, although many respond to short-course therapy. One potential exception to this observation is adolescent girls, for whom the increased compliance associated with short-course therapy can be a significant advantage. The one major difference in the approach to children as opposed to adults is that fluoroquinolones are not used in children because of possible adverse effects on developing cartilage.[673-678]

Recurrent UTI in children, particularly in those with renal scarring or demonstrable VUR, is dealt with by long-term prophylaxis with such agents as trimethoprim-sulfamethoxazole (2 mg/kg per dose once or twice per day of the trimethoprim component, which gives 10 mg/kg per dose of the sulfamethoxazole component), nitrofurantoin (2 mg/kg/day as single dose), or methenamine mandelate (50 mg/kg/day in three divided doses). Sulfonamides are less effective because of the emergence of resistance. Trimethoprim-sulfamethoxazole and nitrofurantoin macrocrystals have been particularly effective in this regard.[677-681] An auxiliary intervention that can be effective in some children with recurrent UTI is the aggressive treatment of constipation, particularly if this is present in conjunction with urinary incontinence.[682]

Results of trials comparing medical therapy with surgical correction of VUR in children have failed to show significant benefit from the surgical approach in terms of renal function, progressive scarring, or renal growth, despite the fact that the technical aspects of the surgical repair could be accomplished satisfactorily. As a result, current views are to aggressively prevent scarring with prolonged antimicrobial therapy and close monitoring as primary therapy. Surgical correction is reserved for the child who, in a 2- to 4-year period, appears to not be responding to medical therapy.[683-693]

Complicated Urinary Tract Infection

The term "complicated UTI," by its nature, encompasses a heterogeneous group of patients with a wide variety of structural and functional abnormalities of the urinary tract and kidney. In addition, the range of organisms causing infection in these patients is particularly broad, with a high percentage of these organisms being resistant to one or more of the antimicrobial agents frequently used in other populations of patients with UTI. Having said this, the following general principles appear to be reasonable in approaching patients with complicated UTI[88, 89, 502]:

1. Therapy should be aimed primarily at symptomatic UTI because there is little evidence that treatment of asymptomatic bacteriuria in this population of patients either alters the clinical condition of the patient or is likely to be successful. The one exception to this rule is if the asymptomatic patient is scheduled for instrumentation of the urinary tract. In this instance, sterilization of the urine before manipulation and continuation of antimicrobial therapy for 3 to 7 days after manipulation can prevent serious morbidity and even mortality from urosepsis.
2. Because of the broad range of infecting pathogens and their varying sensitivity patterns, culture data are essential in prescribing therapy for symptomatic patients. If therapy should be needed before such information is available, initial therapy must encompass a far broader spectrum than in other groups of patients. Thus, in a patient with apparent pyelonephritis or urosepsis in a complicated setting, initial therapy with such regimens as ampicillin plus gentamicin, imipenem-cilastatin, and piperacillin-tazobactam is indicated. In the patient who is more subacutely ill, trimethoprim-sulfamethoxazole or a fluoroquinolone appears to be a reasonable first choice.

3. Every effort should be made to correct the underlying complicating factor, whenever possible, in conjunction with the antimicrobial therapy. If this is possible, a prolonged 4- to 6-week "curative" course of therapy in conjunction with the surgical manipulation is appropriate. If such correction is not possible, shorter courses of therapy (7-14 days), aimed at controlling symptoms, appear to be more appropriate. Frequent symptomatic relapses are worth an attempt at long-term suppressive therapy.

A particular subgroup of patients susceptible to complicated UTI are patients with neurogenic bladders secondary to spinal cord injury. In these, intermittent self-catheterization with clean catheters and methenamine prophylaxis have been shown to decrease the morbidity associated with UTI.[458, 694-696]

Catheter-Associated Urinary Tract Infection

Infections of the urinary tract are by far the most common cause of hospital-acquired infection. Most such nosocomial UTIs are due to the use of bladder catheters. More than 900,000 episodes of catheter-associated bacteriuria occur in acute care hospitals in the United States each year. Approximately 2% to 4% of these patients develop gram-negative sepsis, and such events can contribute to the mortality of patients.[89, 697, 698]

The development of a biofilm on the surface of the catheter is important in determining the effectiveness of antibiotic treatment of catheter-associated UTI. Bacteria adhering to the surface of the catheter initiate the formation of a complex biologic structure containing the bacteria, bacterial glycocalices, Tamm-Horsfall protein, apatite, struvite, and other constituents. This structure protects bacteria from antimicrobial therapy, which leads to prompt relapse once therapy is stopped. Thus, replacement of the bladder catheter should be part of the treatment of catheter-associated UTI, when treatment is thought to be indicated.[89, 698-700]

Although bacteriuria is inevitable with long-term catheterization, certain guidelines can be employed to delay the onset of such infections and to minimize the rate of acquisition of antibiotic-resistant pathogens (Table 31-5). Critically important in this regard are sterile insertion and care of the catheter, use of a closed drainage system, and prompt removal. Isolation of patients with catheter-associated bacteriuria from other patients with indwelling bladder catheters will also decrease the spread of infection. Whether such additions as silver ion–coated catheters, the use of disinfectants in collecting bags, and other local strategies offer additional benefit is still unclear, although topical meatal care with povidone-iodine may be especially useful. Systemic antimicrobial therapy can delay the onset of bacteriuria and can be useful in those clinical situations in which the time of catheterization is clearly limited (e.g., in association with gynecologic or vascular surgery and kidney transplantation).[89, 698, 701-704]

Treatment of catheter-associated UTI requires good clinical judgment. In any patient symptomatic from the infection (e.g., exhibiting fever, chills, dyspnea, and hypotension), immediate therapy with effective antibiotics is indicated, with use of the same antimicrobial strategies described before for other forms of complicated UTI. In an asymptomatic

TABLE 31-5

Guidelines for Bladder Catheter Care to Prevent Infection

1. Use catheter only when absolutely necessary; remove as soon as possible.
2. Insert catheters aseptically and maintain by trained personnel only; the use of "catheter teams" is preferable.
3. A sterile closed drainage system is mandatory. The catheter and drainage tube must never be disconnected except when irrigation is necessary to relieve obstruction. Strict aseptic technique is employed under these circumstances.
4. Urine for culture should be obtained by aspirating the catheter with a 21-gauge needle after the catheter is prepared with povidone-iodine.
5. Maintain downhill, unobstructed flow, with the collection bag always below the level of the bladder and emptied at frequent intervals.
6. Replace indwelling catheters when obstruction or concretions are demonstrated.
7. Separate catheterized patients whenever possible; in particular, a patient with a sterile bladder catheter system should always be kept separate from patients with infected urine, and strict hand-washing procedures should be observed by staff caring for these patients.

Modified from Kaye D, Santoro J: Urinary tract infection. *In* Mandell GL, Douglas RG Jr, Bennett JE (eds): Principles and Practice of Infectious Diseases. New York, John Wiley & Sons, 1979, p. Copyright 1979 John Wiley & Sons. Reprinted by permission of John Wiley & Sons, Inc.

patient, no therapy is indicated. Patients with long-term indwelling catheters rarely become symptomatic unless the catheter is obstructed or is eroding through the bladder mucosa. In those patients who do become symptomatic, antibiotics should be given and close attention should be directed to changing the catheter or changing the type of urinary drainage.

Candidal Infection of the Urinary Tract

Clear-cut guidelines for the treatment of candidal infection of the urinary tract are not available, particularly because there are no criteria that are generally accepted to distinguish between colonization and infection.[705] Until more information is available, the following approach is the one that we currently advocate:

1. In patients with catheter-associated candidal UTI, removal of the preceding catheter, insertion of a three-way catheter, and infusion of an amphotericin rinse for a period of 3 to 5 days appear to have a greater than 75% success rate in eradicating this infection. Success is increased if such contributing factors as hyperglycemia, corticosteroid use, and antibacterial therapy can be eliminated.[706]
2. In patients with candiduria without an indwelling catheter, insertion of a catheter for an amphotericin rinse appears to introduce another hazard, the risk of bacteriuria. Our preference is to treat such patients with fluconazole, 200 to 400 mg/day for 10 to 14 days. Oral fluconazole therapy is at least as effective as amphotericin rinses in the management of candiduria.[707, 708] In a population of organ transplant patients, such an approach has been successful in more than 75% of patients with candiduria.[709-711]
3. Any patient with candiduria who is to undergo instrumentation of the urinary tract requires systemic therapy with amphotericin or fluconazole to prevent the consequences of transient candidemia.

SPECIAL FORMS OF PYELONEPHRITIS

Renal Tuberculosis

Approximately 10% of the new cases of tuberculosis reported annually are extrapulmonary, with the genitourinary tract being the most common site of extrapulmonary tuberculosis.[28, 712-715] Unfortunately, many cases of renal tuberculosis remain clinically silent for years while irreversible renal destruction takes place. Thus, unexplained "sterile" pyuria or hematuria should prompt the clinician to undertake an evaluation for renal tuberculosis.[28]

Genitourinary tuberculosis usually results from "silent" bacillemia accompanying pulmonary tuberculosis. However, active lesions in the kidney may not become manifest clinically for many years, often at a time when little evidence of active pulmonary disease exists. If routine screening of urine specimens for tubercle bacilli is undertaken in a group of patients hospitalized specifically for active pulmonary infection, a number of silent urinary infections are detected.[30] In the general population, symptoms referable to the urinary tract rather than the lung are those most likely to cause the patient with renal tuberculosis to visit the physician. In one series describing 41 cases of genitourinary tuberculosis observed from 1962 through 1974, concomitant pulmonary findings were present in only 66% of newly diagnosed cases of genitourinary tuberculosis.[712] In the same series, dysuria (34%), hematuria (27%), flank pain (10%), and pyuria (5%) were the most frequent presenting symptoms for active urinary tuberculosis. Constitutional symptoms occurred in only 14% of cases, and no symptoms attributable to tuberculosis could be elicited in 20% of patients. An abnormal urinalysis was found in well over half these cases. A positive skin test result (purified protein derivative) was present in 95% of cases, and urine cultures grew *Mycobacterium tuberculosis* in 90%. Excretory urograms were abnormal in 93% of patients examined. Thus, genitourinary tuberculosis should not be a difficult diagnosis to make if patients with localizing urinary symptoms plus abnormal urinalyses are screened for tuberculosis after routine urine cultures have been found to be negative. The pathologic changes—granulomatous inflammation and caseous necrosis—often (but not always) begin in the medulla and papilla, causing papillary necrosis, but soon involve the cortex and occasionally the perirenal tissues. Coalescence of the lesions sometimes leads to large caseous cavities.

Radiographic examinations are rarely pathognomonic for renal tuberculosis, but the intravenous urogram and computed tomographic scan may be helpful in the differential diagnosis of tuberculosis from other infectious and granulomatous entities.[716] The gross strictures, cavities, and calcifications of advanced renal tuberculosis are distinctive.[28]

Recommendations for the treatment of genitourinary tuberculosis are as follows[28]:

1. Uncomplicated urinary tract tuberculosis, likely to be due to drug-sensitive organisms, is well treated with an initial 2 months of daily rifampin, isoniazid, and pyrazinamide followed by 4 months of daily rifampin and isoniazid. Such a regimen is particularly useful in women. In men, in whom concern regarding sequestered foci within the prostate is an issue, we prefer to continue such a program for an additional 3 to 6 months. If pyrazinamide is not tolerated, rifampin and isoniazid therapy for 9 months is recommended for women, with a preference for an additional 3 to 6 months in men.

2. There is little published experience with these relatively short regimens in patients with caseating destruction of the kidneys or in men with overt genital disease. In such instances, we would prefer to prolong the isoniazid and rifampin components so that a minimum of 12 to 18 months of therapy with at least two bactericidal agents is delivered.

3. Anyone with possible drug-resistant tuberculosis should have therapy instituted with isoniazid, rifampin, and pyrazinamide to ensure the use of at least two bactericidal agents, plus one of the following: ethambutol, ofloxacin, or streptomycin. Once drug sensitivity results are available, the regimen can be modified accordingly. If two bactericidal agents can be employed, we prefer a minimum of 12 months of therapy in patients with drug-resistant disease. If only one bactericidal agent plus ethambutol is possible, a minimum of 24 months of therapy is recommended.

4. Preliminary experience with the treatment of tuberculosis in the setting of acquired immunodeficiency syndrome suggests that 9 to 12 months of therapy may be adequate, particularly with the initial 2 months of isoniazid, rifampin, and pyrazinamide being part of this regimen. However, the possibility of relapse in this population of immunocompromised patients must be considered. In selected patients with progressive acquired immunodeficiency syndrome, longer courses of therapy or reinstitution of therapy should be considered.

5. In patients who cannot tolerate at least two of the three primary bactericidal agents because of side effects, one bactericidal agent plus a second agent such as ethambutol should be used for a period of 24 months.

Additional issues that should be addressed include the following: antimicrobial sensitivity testing should be carried out on all primary isolates (owing to the increase in drug-resistant tuberculosis in more recent years); proof of cure must be documented by culture; and follow-up urograms or ultrasound examinations must be performed to rule out the development of obstructive uropathy as a consequence of the healing process. Such a development would obligate surgical correction to salvage renal function.[30]

Xanthogranulomatous Pyelonephritis

Xanthogranulomatous pyelonephritis is a form of chronic bacterial pyelonephritis characterized by the destruction of renal parenchyma and the presence of granulomas, abscesses, and collections of lipid-filled macrophages (foam cells).[717-722]

Although the disease remains uncommon, accounting for 6 in 1000 surgically proven cases of chronic pyelonephritis,[718] it has apparently increased in frequency in more recent years.[717] It occurs at any age, from 11 months to 89 years, but is most common in adults in the fifth through seventh decades. Women are affected more often than men (2:1), and except in a rare patient with bilateral disease,[723] the lesions affect only one kidney. Most patients present with renal pain, recurrent UTI, fever (of undetermined nature), malaise, anorexia, weight loss, and constipation. Duration of treatment before diagnosis is between 3 months and 9 years. Seventy-three percent of patients have a history of previous calculous disease, obstructive uropathy, or diabetes mellitus, and 38% have undergone urologic procedures. A renal mass is present in 60% of cases and hypertension in about 40%.[721, 724]

In gross appearance, the kidney is usually enlarged, and the capsule and perirenal tissue are often thickened and adherent. The process may be localized to one tumor mass involving one pole of the kidney or may be diffuse and multifocal. On section, the pelvis and calices are dilated and contain either purulent fluid or calculi (often staghorn calculi) or both. The renal parenchyma, particularly surrounding the dilated calices, is replaced by orange-yellow, soft inflammatory tissue, often with surrounding small abscesses. The tumor can be mistaken grossly for renal cell carcinoma, but the presence of calculi, obstruction, abscesses, and purulent material and the localization of yellow tissue adjacent to the pelvis and calices points to an inflammatory disorder (Fig. 31-15). However, there have been reports of coexistent renal cell carcinoma in the same or contralateral kidney, as well as a transitional cell carcinoma of the renal pelvis.[725-730]

On microscopic examination, the orange-yellow areas are made up of inflammatory tissue consisting of an admixture of large foamy macrophages, smaller macrophages with granular cytoplasm, neutrophils, lymphocytes, plasma cells, and fibroblasts. Neutrophils and necrotic debris are particularly abundant surrounding the pelvic mucosa. An occasional foreign body giant cell may be present. The cytoplasm of the foamy macrophages and particularly of the small granular monocytes stains strongly with PAS.[721]

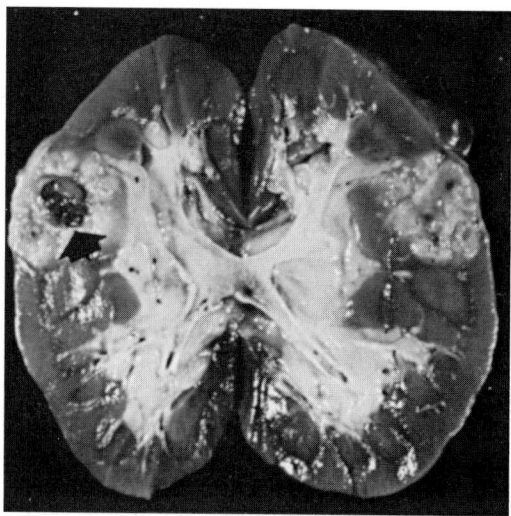

FIGURE 31-15. Xanthogranulomatous pyelonephritis, localized form. The orange-yellow granulomatous mass surrounds a black calculus (*arrow*) in a caliceal diverticulum. Note resemblance to renal cell carcinoma.

The radiographic picture is varied.[731, 732] The heterogeneous pattern is due to diverse combinations of localized or diffuse lesions; the radiologic appearance depends on the presence of obstruction, calculi, or other anomalies. On excretory urograms, a stone-bearing, nonfunctioning kidney is present in about 80% of cases. Caliceal deformity and irregularity are also common, particularly in the diffuse type. The localized lesions appear as cystic or cavitary masses that show no "puddling" of contrast medium. On angiograms, most xanthogranulomatous renal masses are hypovascular or avascular. There is spreading of intrarenal arteries without peripheral arborization, but usually there are no pathologic vessels; however, some cases have shown increased vascularity. Furthermore, the avascular solitary mass of xanthogranulomatous pyelonephritis cannot be definitively distinguished from necrotic avascular adenocarcinoma by angiography alone. Computed tomography is helpful in the diagnosis and particularly in identifying extension of the inflammation to the perirenal fat. Magnetic resonance imaging may also aid in the diagnosis.[731-736]

The diagnosis of xanthogranulomatous pyelonephritis should be considered in patients with a history of chronic infection and certain radiologic features.[732] The radiologic findings include unilateral renal enlargement; a nonfunctioning kidney on intravenous urogram; the presence of renal calculi, ureteral calculi, or both; angiographic demonstration of an avascular mass or masses with stretched attenuated intrarenal vessels, prominent capsular periureteric vessels, and an irregular impaired nephrogram with prominent avascular areas; and suggestive changes by computed tomography or magnetic resonance imaging. With these features, some 40% of cases can be diagnosed or suspected preoperatively.[735, 736]

Bacterial cultures of the urine are almost invariably positive. *P. mirabilis* and *E. coli* are the organisms that are most commonly cultured.[737] Series reporting a high frequency of *E. coli* also showed a low frequency of staghorn calculi. Methicillin-resistant *S. aureus* can also cause the condition.[738]

The pathogenesis of xanthogranulomatous pyelonephritis is unclear, although it seems certain that the condition is caused by bacterial infection and accentuated by urinary obstruction. Similar cells with PAS reaction–positive granules have been produced by *Proteus*, *E. coli*, and staphylococcal infection in rats. Electron microscopy shows that the foamy macrophages initially contain bacteria and subsequently contain numerous phagolysosomes filled with myelin figures and amorphous material.[739] The presence of these phagolysosomes has suggested that there may be a lysosomal defect of macrophages that interferes with the digestion of bacterial products.[739]

Most kidneys with xanthogranulomatous pyelonephritis are removed surgically, largely because a correct preoperative diagnosis is made infrequently, but studies suggest that diagnosis by a combination of clinical and radiologic features is possible in 40% of cases.[735] In the focal disease, unnecessary radical surgery may be prevented in the poor-risk patient. Recurrences in the other kidney have not been reported after surgery.[740-742] The disease has also been reported in transplant recipients.[743]

Malakoplakia

Malakoplakia is a rare, histologically distinct inflammatory reaction usually caused by enteric bacteria and affecting many organs but most commonly the urinary tract. In most cases, the condition is confined to the urinary bladder mucosa, where it appears as soft, yellow, slightly raised, often confluent plaques 3 to 4 cm in diameter. It is most common in middle-aged women with chronic UTI. The microscopic picture is typical. Plaques are composed of closely packed, large macrophages with occasional lymphocytes and multinucleate giant cells. The macrophages have abundant, foamy, PAS reaction–positive cytoplasm; in addition, laminated mineralized concretions, known as Michaelis-Gutmann bodies, are typically present within macrophages and in the interstitial tissue. The Michaelis-Gutmann bodies measure 4 to 10 fm in diameter, stain strongly with PAS, and contain calcium (Fig. 31-16). On electron microscopic studies, they show a typical crystalline structure with a central dense core, an intermediate halo, and a peripheral lamellated ring.[744] Intracellular bacteria and giant phagolysosomes can be demonstrated within macrophages.[744-746]

Identical lesions have been discovered in the prostate, ureteral and pelvic mucosa, bones, lungs, testes, gastrointestinal tract, skin, and kidneys. Renal malakoplakia occurs in the same clinical setting as xanthogranulomatous pyelonephritis—chronic infection and obstruction—and indeed, except for the presence of Michaelis-Gutmann bodies, there is considerable overlap in the gross histologic features of both conditions.[747] *E. coli* is the most common organism cultured from urine. Clinical findings usually include flank pain and signs of active renal infection. Bilateral involvement has been reported, as has a clinical presentation simulating acute renal failure.[748, 749]

The pathogenesis of malakoplakia is unclear, but about half of the cases are associated with immunodeficiency or

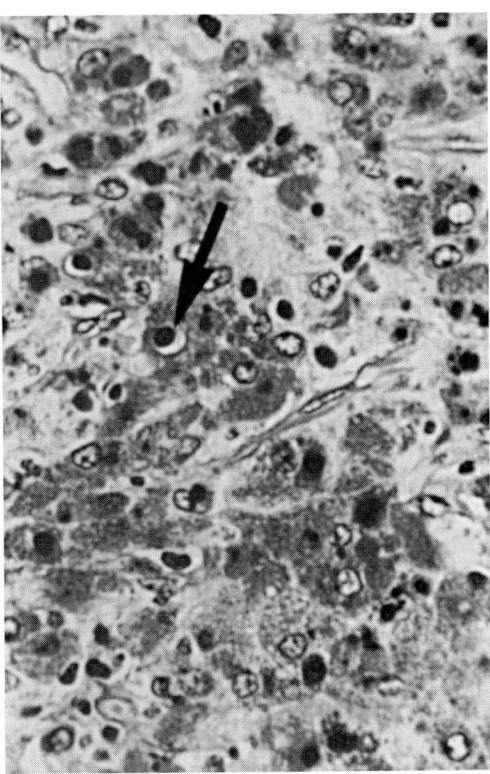

FIGURE 31-16. Michaelis-Gutmann bodies of malakoplakia (*arrow*).

autoimmune disorders, including hypogammaglobulinemia, therapeutic immunosuppression, malignant neoplasms, chronic debilitating disorder, rheumatoid arthritis, and acquired immunodeficiency syndrome.[745] One scenario is that the lesions result from a defect in macrophage function that blocks the lysosomal enzymatic degradation of engulfed bacteria and overloads the cytoplasm with undigested bacterial debris. Microtubule defects impairing the movement of lysosomes to phagocytic vacuoles and decreased lysosomal enzyme release within phagocytes have been postulated.[750-752] The Michaelis-Gutmann bodies are thought to result from the deposition of calcium phosphate and other minerals on these overloaded phagosomes.

Another histologic entity that overlaps with both malakoplakia and xanthogranulomatous pyelonephritis is so-called megalocytic interstitial nephritis; in this variant, the interstitial infiltrate is polymorphous with predominance of histiocytes containing crystalloid material.[752]

REFERENCES

1. Heptinstall RH: The enigma of chronic pyelonephritis. J Infect Dis 120:104, 1969.
2. Hodson CJ: Radiological diagnosis of pyelonephritis. Proc R Soc Med 52:669, 1959.
3. Smith JF: The diagnosis of the scars of chronic pyelonephritis. J Clin Pathol 15:522, 1962.
4. Risdon RA: Pyelonephritis and reflux nephropathy. In Tisher C, Brenner B (eds): Renal Pathology. Philadelphia, JB Lippincott, 1989, pp 775-808.
5. Hooton TM, Stamm WE: Diagnosis and treatment of uncomplicated urinary tract infection. Infect Dis Clin North Am 11:551, 1997.
6. Vosti KL: Infections of the urinary tract in women. Medicine (Baltimore) 81:369, 2002.
7. Ronald AR, Conway B: An approach to urinary tract infections in ambulatory women. Curr Clin Top Infect Dis 9:76, 1988.
8. Lifshitz E, Kramer L: Outpatient urine culture. Arch Intern Med 160:2537, 2000.
9. Stamm WE: Measurement of pyuria and its relation to bacteriuria. Am J Med 75:53, 1983.
10. Stamm WE: Diagnosis of coliform infection in acutely dysuric women. N Engl J Med 307:463, 1982.
11. Kass EH: Asymptomatic infections of the urinary tract. Trans Assoc Am Physicians 69:56, 1956.
12. Kass EH: Bacteriuria and the diagnosis of infections of the urinary tract, with observations on the use of methenamine as a urinary antiseptic. Arch Intern Med 100:709, 1957.
13. Morgan MG, McKenzie H: Controversies in the laboratory diagnosis of community-acquired urinary tract infection. Eur J Clin Microbiol Infect Dis 12:491, 1993.
14. Tambyah PA, Maki DG: The relationship between pyuria and infection in patients with indwelling urinary catheters. Arch Intern Med 160:673, 2000.
15. Latham RH, Running K, Stamm WE: Urinary tract infections in young women caused by *Staphylococcus saprophyticus.* JAMA 250:3063, 1983.
16. Pead L, Marshall R, Morris J: *Staphylococcus saprophyticus* as a urinary pathogen: A six-year perspective survey. BMJ 291:1157, 1985.
17. Marrie TJ, Kwan C, Noble MA, et al: *Staphylococcus saprophyticus* as a cause of urinary tract infections. J Clin Microbiol 16:427, 1982.
18. Kaufman CA, Hertz CS, Sheagren IN: *Staphylococcus saprophyticus:* Role in urinary infections in men. J Urol 130:493, 1983.
19. Maskell R, Pead L, Hollett RJ: Urinary pathogens in the male. Br J Urol 47:691, 1975.
20. Cascio S, Colhoun E, Puri P: Bacterial colonization of the prepuce in boys with vesicoureteral reflux who receive antibiotic prophylaxis. J Pediatr 139:160, 2001.
21. Schoen EJ, Colby CJ, Ray GT: Newborn circumcision decreases incidence and costs of urinary infections during the first year of life. Pediatrics 105:441, 2000.
22. Marrie TJ, Swantee CA, Harlen M: Aerobic and anaerobic urethral flora of healthy females in various physiological age groups and of females with urinary tract infections. J Clin Microbiol 11:654, 1980.
23. Foxman B, Brown P: Epidemiology of urinary tract infections. Transmission and risk factors, incidence and cost. Infect Dis Clin North Am 17:227, 2003.
24. Rubin RH, Weinstein L: Salmonellosis: Microbiologic, Pathologic and Clinical Features. New York, Stratton Intercontinental, 1977.
25. Abernathy RS, Price WE, Spink WW: Chronic brucellar pyelonephritis simulating tuberculosis. JAMA 159:1534, 1955.
26. Cruz PT, Clancy CF: Nocardiosis: Nocardial osteomyelitis and septicemia. Am J Pathol 28:607, 1952.
27. Rosenblum PS: Renal actinomycosis: A case report. Urol Cutan Rev 53:329, 1949.
28. Pasternack MS, Rubin RH: Urinary tract tuberculosis. In Schrier RW, Gottschalk CW (eds): Diseases of the Kidney, 6th ed. Boston, Little, Brown (in press).
29. Goldberg PK, Kozinn PJ, Wise GJ, et al: Incidence and significance of candiduria. JAMA 241:582, 1979.
30. Ang BSP, Telenti A, King B, et al: Candidemia from a urinary tract source: Microbiological aspects and clinical significance. Clin Infect Dis 17:662, 1993.
31. Scerpella EG, Alhalel R: An unusual cause of acute renal failure: Bilateral ureteral obstruction due to *Candida tropicalis* fungus balls. Clin Infect Dis 18:440, 1994.
32. Guze LB, Haley LD: Fungus infections of the urinary tract. Yale J Biol Med 30:292, 1958.
33. Guziel LP, Stone WJ, Schaffner W, et al: Case report: Primary renal candidiasis with renal granulomata and salt-losing nephropathy. Am J Med Sci 269:123, 1975.
34. Rubin RH: Infection in the organ transplant patient. In Rubin RH, Young LS (eds): Clinical Approach to Infection in the Compromised Host, 4th ed. New York, Kluwer/Academic/Plenum, 2002, p 629.
35. Edwards JE Jr, Lehrer RI, Stiehm ER, et al: Severe candidal infections: Clinical perspective, immune defense mechanisms, and current concepts of therapy. Ann Intern Med 89:91, 1978.
36. Petersen EA, Friedman BA, Crowder ED, et al: Coccidioido-uria: Clinical significance. Ann Intern Med 85:34, 1976.
37. Rubin RH: Mycotic infections. In Dale DC (ed): The Scientific American Textbook of Medicine. New York, Scientific American, sec 7, chap 9, 2000, pp 1-5.
38. Bissada NK, Finkbeiner AE, Redman JF: Prostatic mycosis: Nonsurgical diagnosis and management. Urology 9:427, 1977.
39. Randall RE Jr, Story WK, Toone EC, et al: Cryptococcal pyelonephritis. N Engl J Med 279:60, 1968.
40. Rubin RH: Infection in the immunosuppressed host. In Dale DC (ed): The Scientific American Textbook of Medicine. New York, Scientific American, sec 7, chap 9, 2000, pp 1-19.
41. Bowie WR, Wang SP, Alexander ER, et al: Etiology of nongonococcal urethritis. J Clin Invest 59:735, 1977.
42. Pettersson S, Brorson JE, Grenabo L, Hedelin H: *Ureaplasma urealyticum* in infectious urinary tract stones. Lancet 1:526, 1983.
43. Nufson MA, Belske RB: A review of adenovirus in the etiology of acute hemorrhagic cystitis. J Urol 115:191, 1976.
44. Walter EA, Bowden RA: Infection in the bone marrow transplant recipient. Infect Dis Clin North Am 9:823, 1995.
45. Rosen S, Harmon W, Krensky AM, et al: Tubulo-interstitial nephritis associated with polyomavirus (BK type) infection. N Engl J Med 308:1192, 1983.
46. Coleman DV, MacKenzie EFD, Gardner SD, et al: Human polyomavirus (BK) infection and ureteric stenosis in renal allograft recipients. J Clin Pathol 31:338, 1978.
47. Hashida Y, Gaffney PC, Yunis EJ: Acute hemorrhagic cystitis of childhood and papovavirus-like particles. J Pediatr 89:85, 1976.
48. Rubin RH, Colvin RB: Impact of cytomegalovirus infection on renal transplantation. In Burdick JF, Racusen LC, Solez K (eds): Kidney Transplant Rejection: Diagnosis and Treatment, 3rd ed. New York, Marcel Dekker, 1998, pp 605-625.
49. Beeson PB: Factors in the pathogenesis of pyelonephritis. Yale J Biol Med 28:81, 1955.
50. Rubin RH: Infection in organ transplant recipients. In Rubin RH, Young LS (eds): Clinical Approach to Infection in the Immunocompromised Host, 4th ed. New York, Kluwer/Academic/Plenum, 2002, p 573.
51. Cotran RS: Experimental pyelonephritis In Rouiller C, Miller AF (eds): The Kidney, vol 2. New York, Academic Press, 1969, pp 269-345.

52. Gorrill RH, Klyhn LM, McNeil EM: The initiation of infection in the mouse kidney after intravenous injection of bacteria. J Pathol Bacteriol 91:157, 1966.
53. Gorrill RH: The fate of *Pseudomonas aeruginosa, Proteus mirabilis* and *Escherichia coli* in the mouse kidney. J Pathol Bacteriol 89:81, 1975.
54. Freedman LR: Experimental pyelonephritis: VI. Observations on susceptibility of the rabbit kidney to infection by a virulent strain of *Staphylococcus aureus.* Yale J Biol Med 32:272, 1960.
55. DeNavasquez S: Further studies in experimental pyelonephritis produced by various bacteria, with special reference for renal scarring as a factor in pathogenesis. J Pathol Bacteriol 71:27, 1956.
56. Rocha H, Guze LB, Freedman LR, Beeson PB: Experimental pyelonephritis: III. The influence of localized injury in different parts of the kidney on susceptibility to bacillary infection. Yale J Biol Med 30:341, 1958.
57. Rocha H, Guze LB, Beeson PB: Experimental pyelonephritis: V. Susceptibility of rats for hematogenous pyelonephritis following chemical injury to the kidneys. Yale J Biol Med 32:120, 1959.
58. Brumfitt W, Heptinstall RH: Experimental pyelonephritis: The effects of renal vein constriction on bacterial localization and multiplication in the rat kidney. Br J Exp Pathol 40:145, 1959.
59. Godley JA, Freedman LR: Experimental pyelonephritis: XI. A comparison of temporary occlusion of renal artery and vein on susceptibility of rat kidney for infection. Yale J Biol Med 36:268, 1964.
60. Jones RK, Shapiro AP: Increased susceptibility to pyelonephritis during acute hypertension by angiotensin II and norepinephrine. J Clin Invest 42:179, 1963.
61. Shapiro AP, Kobernick JL: Susceptibility of rats with renal hypertension for pyelonephritis and predisposition of rats with chronic pyelonephritis to hormonal hypertension. Circ Res 9:869, 1961.
62. Woods JW, Welt LG, Hollander WJ: Susceptibility of rats for experimental pyelonephritis during potassium depletion. J Clin Invest 40:599, 1961.
63. Miescher P, Schnyder V, Kresh V: Zur Pathogenese der "interstitiellen Nephritis" bei Abusus phenacetin-haltigen Analgetica. Tierexperimentelle Untersuchungen. Schweiz Med Wochenschr 88:432, 1958.
64. Braude AI, Shapiro AP, Siemienski J: Hematogenous pyelonephritis in rats: I. Its pathogenesis when produced by a simple new method. J Clin Invest 34:1489, 1955.
65. Kime SW Jr, McNamara JJ, Lu Se S, et al: Experimental polypeptic renal disease in rats: Electron microscopy, function, and susceptibility to pyelonephritis. J Lab Clin Med 60:64, 1962.
66. Boschell BR, Hunter EO Jr, Warren TL, Lipton CH Jr: Experimental pyelonephritis in the alloxan diabetic animal. Diabetes 12:56, 1963.
67. Browder AA, Petersdorf RG: Experimental pyelonephritis in rats with alloxan diabetes. Proc Soc Exp Biol Med 115:332, 1961.
68. Cod JA, Davis JH: Altered host response to experimental pyelonephritis in alloxan diabetic rats. J Surg Res 7:1, 1967.
69. Andriole VT, Cohn GL: The effect of diethylstilbestrol on the susceptibility of rats to hematogenous pyelonephritis. J Clin Invest 43:1136, 1964.
70. Freedman LR, Kaminskas R, Beeson PB: Experimental pyelonephritis: VII. Evidence on the mechanisms by which obstruction of urine flow enhances susceptibility to pyelonephritis. Yale J Biol Med 33:65, 1960.
71. Schwartz MM, Venkatachalam MA, Cotran RS: Reversible inner medullary vascular obstruction in acute unilateral hydronephrosis in the rat. Am J Pathol 86:425, 1977.
72. Sobel JD: Pathogenesis of urinary tract infection: Role of host defenses. Infect Dis Clin North Am 11:531, 1997.
73. O'Hanley P, Lark P, Falkow S, Schoolnik G: Molecular basis of *Escherichia coli* colonization of the upper urinary tract in BALB/c mice. J Clin Invest 75:347, 1985.
74. Barnes RC, Diafuku R, Roddy RE, et al: Urinary tract infection in sexually active homosexual men. Lancet 1:171, 1986.
75. Johnson JR: Microbial virulence determinants and the pathogenesis of urinary tract infection. Infect Dis Clin North Am 17:261, 2003.
76. Svanborg C, Jodal U: Host-parasite interaction in urinary tract infection. *In* Brumfitt W, Hamilton-Miller JMT, Bailey RR (eds): Urinary Tract Infections. London, Chapman & Hall, 1998, p 87.
77. Stapleton A, Stamm WE: Prevention of urinary tract infection. Infect Dis Clin North Am 11:719, 1997.
78. Hooten TM, Scholes D, Stapleton AE, et al: A perspective study of asymptomatic bacteriuria in sexually active women. N Engl J Med 343:1037, 2000.
79. Schaeffer AJ, Jones JM, Dunn JK: Association of in vitro *Escherichia coli* adherence to vaginal and buccal epithelial cells with susceptibility of women to recurrent urinary tract infections. N Engl J Med 304:1062, 1981.
80. Sheinfeld J, Schaeffer AJ, Cordon-Cardo C, et al: Association of the Lewis blood-group phenotype with recurrent urinary tract infections in women. N Engl J Med 320:773, 1989.
81. Stapleton A, Nudelman E, Clausen H, et al: Binding of uropathogenic *Escherichia coli* R45 to glycolipids extracted from vaginal epithelial cells is dependent on histo–blood group secretor status. J Clin Invest 90:965, 1992.
82. Kinane DF, Blackwell CC, Brettle RF, et al: ABO blood group, secretor state and susceptibility to recurrent urinary tract infection in women. BMJ 285:7, 1981.
83. Lomberg H, Hellstrom M, Jodal U, Svangorg-Eden C: Secretor state and renal scarring in girls with recurrent pyelonephritis. FEMS Immunol Med Microbiol 47:371, 1989.
84. Scholes D, Hooten TM, Roberts PL, et al: Risk factors for recurrent urinary tract infection in young women. J Infect Dis 182:1177, 2000.
85. Hopkins WJ, Elkahawaji JE, Heisey DM, Ott CJ: Inheritance of susceptibility to induced *Escherichia coli* bladder and kidney infections in female C3H/HeJ mice. J Infect Dis 187:418, 2003.
86. Hooten TM: Pathogenesis of urinary tract infection: An update. J Antimicrob Chemother 46:Suppl A1, 2000.
87. Spach DH, Stapleton AE, Stamm WE: Lack of circumcision increases the risk of urinary tract infection in young men. JAMA 267:679, 1992.
88. Lipsky BA: Urinary tract infections in men: Epidemiology, pathophysiology, diagnosis, and treatment. Ann Intern Med 110:138, 1989.
89. Stamm WE, Hooton TM: Management of urinary tract infections in adults. N Engl J Med 329:1328, 1993.
90. Ulleryd P, Lincoln K, Scheutz F, Sandberg T: Virulence characteristics of *Escherichia coli* in relation to host response in men with symptomatic urinary tract infection. Clin Infect Dis 18:579, 1994.
91. Fair WR, Timothy MM, Churg HD: Antibacterial nature of prostatic fluid. Nature 218:444, 1968.
92. Foxman B, Manning SD, Tallman P, et al: Uropathogenic *Escherichia coli* are more likely than commensal strains to be shared between heterosexual sex partners. Am J Epidemiol 156:1133, 2002.
93. Ruiz J, Simon K, Horcajada JP, et al: Differences in virulence factors among clinical isolates of *Escherichia coli* causing cystitis and pyelonephritis in women and prostatitis in men. J Clin Microbiol 40:4445, 2002.
94. Bran JL, Levinson ME, Kaye D: Entrance of bacteria in the female urinary bladder. N Engl J Med 286:626, 1972.
95. Kunin CM, McCormack RC: An epidemiologic study of bacteriuria and blood pressure among nuns and working women. N Engl J Med 278:635, 1968.
96. Kelsey MC, Mead MG, Gruneberg RN, Oriel JD: Relationship between sexual intercourse and urinary tract infection in women attending a clinic for sexually transmitted diseases. J Med Microbiol 12:511, 1979.
97. Nicolle LE, Harding GKM, Preiksaitis J, Ronald AR: The association of urinary tract infection with sexual intercourse. J Infect Dis 146:579, 1982.
98. Vosti KL: Recurrent urinary tract infections: Prevention by prophylactic antibodies after sexual intercourse. JAMA 231:934, 1975.
99. Stamm WE: An epidemic of urinary tract infection? N Engl J Med 345:1055, 2001.
100. Kunin CM: Sexual intercourse and urinary infections. N Engl J Med 298:336, 1978.
101. Cox CE, Hinman F: Experiments with induced bacteriuria, vesical emptying and bacterial growth on the mechanisms of bladder defense to infection. J Urol 86:739, 1961.
102. Hinman FJ, Cox CE: Residual urine volume in normal male subjects. J Urol 97:641, 1967.
103. Norden CW, Green GM, Kass EH: Antibacterial mechanisms of the urinary bladder. J Clin Invest 47:2689, 1968.
104. Svanborg C, Bergsten G, Fischer H, et al: The "innate" host response protects and damages the infected urinary tract. Ann Med 33:563, 2001.
105. Bodel P, Cotran RS, Kass EH: Cranberry juice and the antibacterial action of hippuric acid. J Lab Clin Med 54:881, 1959.
106. Cicmanec JF, Shank RA, Evans T: Overnight concentration of urine: Natural defense mechanism against urinary tract infection. Urology 26:157, 1985.

107. Gargan RA, Hamilton-Miller JMT, Brumfitt W: Effect of alkalinisation and increased fluid intake on bacterial phagocytosis and killing in urine. Eur J Clin Microbiol Infect Dis 12:534, 1993.

108. Aronson M, Medalia O, Schori L: Prevention of colonization of the urinary tract of mice with *Escherichia coli* by blocking of bacterial adherence with methyl-alpha D-mannopyranoside. J Infect Dis 139:329, 1979.

109. Parsons CL, Stauffer C, Schmidt J: Bladder surface glycosaminoglycans: An efficient mechanism of environmental adaptation. Science 208:605, 1980.

110. Schulte-Wissermann H, Mannhardt W, Schwarz J, et al: Comparison of the antibacterial effect of uroepithelial cells from healthy donors and children with asymptomatic bacteriuria. Eur J Pediatr 144:230, 1985.

111. Wold AE, Mestecky J, Svanborg C: Agglutination of *Escherichia coli* by secretory IgA: A result of interaction between bacterial mannose-specific adhesins and immunoglobulin carbohydrate. Monogr Allergy 24:307, 1988.

112. Mannhardt W, Becker A, Putzer M, et al: Host defense within the urinary tract: I. Bacterial adhesion initiates a uroepithelial defense mechanism. Pediatr Nephrol 10:568, 1996.

113. Mannhardt W, Putzer M, Zepp F, Schulte-Wissermann H: Host defense within the urinary tract: II. Signal transducing events activate the uroepithelial defense. Pediatr Nephrol 10:573, 1996.

114. Lapides J: Role of hydrostatic pressure and distention in urinary tract infection. *In* Kass EH (ed): Progress in Pyelonephritis. Philadelphia, FA Davis, 1965, pp 578-580.

115. Fiveash JG, Foster EA, Paquin AJ: Experimental *Escherichia coli* bacteriuria in the rabbit. *In* Kass EH (ed): Progress in Pyelonephritis. Philadelphia, FA Davis, 1965, pp 581-590.

116. Mabeck CE: Treatment of uncomplicated urinary tract infection in nonpregnant women. Postgrad Med 48:69, 1972.

117. Hodson CJ, Cotran RS: Vesicoureteral reflux, reflux nephropathy, and chronic pyelonephritis. *In* Cotran RS (ed): Contemporary Issues in Nephrology. Vol 10, Tubulointerstitial Nephropathies. New York, Churchill Livingstone, 1983, pp 83-120.

118. Castro JE, Fine H: Passive antireflux mechanisms in the human and cadaver. Br J Urol 41:559, 1969.

119. Retik AB: Vesicoureteral reflux. *In* Edelmann CM Jr (ed): Pediatric Kidney Disease. Boston, Little, Brown, 1978.

120. Stephens FD: Cytoscopic appearance of the ureteric orifices associated with reflux nephropathy. *In* Hodson CJ, Kincaid-Smith P (eds): Reflux Nephropathy. New York, Masson, 1979, p 119.

121. Risdon RA: Reflux nephropathy. Diagn Histopathol 4:61, 1981.

122. Kollerman MW, Ludwig H: Über den vesico-ureteralen Reflux beim mormalen Kind im Säuglings- und Kleinkindalter. Z Kinderheilkd 100:185, 1967.

123. Roberts JA: Studies of vesicoureteral reflux: A review of work in a primate model. South Med J 71:28, 1978.

124. Steele B, Robtaille P, DeMaria J, Grignon A: Follow-up evaluation of a prenatally recognized vesicoureteric reflux. J Pediatr 115:95, 1989.

125. Burge DM, Griffiths MD, Malone PS, Atwell JD: Fetal vesicoureteral reflux: Outcome following conservative postnatal management. J Urol 148:1743, 1992.

126. Tullus K, Winberg J: Urinary tract infections in children. *In* Brumfitt W, Hamilton-Miller JMT, Bailey RR (eds): Urinary Tract Infections. London, Chapman & Hall, 1998, p 175.

127. Koff SA, Lapides J, Piazza DH: Association of urinary tract infection and reflux with uninhibited bladder contractions and voluntary sphincteric obstruction. J Urol 122:373, 1979.

128. van Gool JD, Kuitjen RH, Donckerwolcke RA, et al: Bladder-sphincter dysfunction, urinary infection and vesico-ureteral reflux with special reference to cognitive bladder training. Contrib Nephrol 39:190, 1984.

129. Koff SA, Muttagh D: The uninhibited bladder in children: Effect of treatment on vesicoureteral reflux resolution. Contrib Nephrol 39:211, 1984.

130. Noe HN: The role of dysfunctional voiding in failure or complication of ureteral implantation for primary reflux. J Urol 134:1172, 1985.

131. Griffiths JD, Scholtmeiger RJ: Vesicoureteral reflux and lower urinary tract dysfunction: Evidence for 2 different reflux/dysfunction complexes. J Urol 137:240, 1987.

132. Fowler R: The many faces of vesicoureteral reflux: Factors contributing to renal damage. Aust N Z J Surg 54:417, 1984.

133. Parkhouse HF, Barratt TM, Dillon MJ, et al: Long-term outcome of boys with posterior urethral valves. Br J Urol 62:59, 1988.

134. Lebowitz RL, Blickman JG: The coexistence of ureteropelvic function, obstruction and reflux. Am J Radiol 140:231, 1983.

135. Dejter SW Jr, Gibbons MD: The fate of infant kidneys with fetal hydronephrosis but initially normal postnatal sonography. J Urol 142:661, 1989.

136. Elder JS: Commentary: Importance of antenatal diagnosis of vesicoureteral reflux. J Urol 148:1750, 1992.

137. Ring E, Petritsch P, Riccabona M, et al: Primary vesicoureteral reflux in infants with a dilated fetal urinary tract. Eur J Pediatr 152:523, 1993.

138. Zerin JM, Ritchey ML, Chang AC: Incidental vesicoureteral reflux in neonates with antenatally detected hydronephrosis and other renal abnormalities. Radiology 187:157, 1993.

139. Eccles MR, Bailey RR, Abbott GD, Sullivan MJ: Unravelling the genetics of vesicoureteric reflux: A common familial disorder. Hum Mol Genet 5(special number):1425, 1996.

140. Vesicoureteric reflux: All in the genes? Report of a meeting of physicians at the Hospital for Sick Children, Great Ormond Street, London (clinical conference). Lancet 348:725, 1996.

141. Buonomo C, Treves ST, Jones B, et al: Silent renal damage in symptom-free siblings of children with vesicoureteral reflux: Assessment with technetiun Tc 99m dimercaptosuccinic acid scintigraphy. J Pediatr 122:721, 1993.

142. Chapman CJ, Bailey RR, Janus ED: Vesicoureteral reflux: Segregation analysis. Am J Med Genet 20:577, 1985.

143. Roberts JA: The monkey as a model of urinary tract infection and reflux nephropathy in man. *In* Davison AM (ed): Nephrology, vol 2. Philadelphia, WB Saunders, 1988, pp 844-853.

144. Roberts J, Kaack B, Morvant A: Vesicoureteral reflux in the primate: IV. Infection as cause of prolonged high-grade reflux. Pediatrics 82:91, 1988.

145. King LR, Levitt SB: Vesicoureteral reflux. *In* Walsh PC, Perlmutter AD, Gittes RF, Stamey TA (eds): Campbell's Urology, 5th ed. Philadelphia, WB Saunders, 1986, p 251.

146. Hannertz L, Celsi G, Eklot AC, et al: Ascending pyelonephritis in young rats retards kidney growth. Kidney Int 35:1133, 1989.

147. Friedland GW: The voiding cystourethrogram: An unreliable examination. *In* Hodson CJ, Kincaid-Smith P (eds): Reflux Nephropathy. New York, Masson, 1979, p 91.

148. International Reflux Study Committee: Medical versus surgical treatment of primary vesicoureteral reflux: Prospective International Reflux Study in Children. J Urol 125:277, 1981.

149. Rolleston GL, Shannon FT, Utley WL: Follow-up of vesicoureteral reflux in the newborn. Kidney Int 8:S59, 1975.

150. Smellie JM, Edwards D, Hunter N, et al: Vesico-ureteric reflux and renal scarring. Kidney Int 8:S65, 1975.

151. Shah KJ, Robins DG, White RHR: Renal scarring and vesicoureteric reflux. Arch Dis Child 53:210, 1978.

152. Chapman SG, Chantler G, Haycock GB, et al: Radionuclide cystography in vesicoureteric reflux. Arch Dis Child 63:650, 1988.

153. Hodson CJ, Edwards D: Chronic pyelonephritis and vesicoureteral reflux. Clin Radiol 2:19, 1960.

154. Hodson CJ: Reflux nephropathy. Med Clin North Am 62:1201, 1978.

155. Bailey RR: An overview of reflux nephropathy. *In* Hodson CJ, Kincaid-Smith P (eds): Reflux Nephropathy. New York, Masson, 1979, p 3.

156. Lerner GR, Fleischman LE, Perlmutter AD: Reflux nephropathy. Pediatr Clin North Am 34:747, 1987.

157. Williams DI: Vesicoureteral reflux. *In* Williams DI (ed): Urology in Childhood. Basel, Springer-Verlag, 1974, p 357.

158. Smellie JM, Normand ICS: Bacteriuria, reflux and renal scarring. Arch Dis Child 50:581, 1975.

159. Smellie JM, Normand ICS: Reflux nephropathy in childhood. *In* Hodson CJ, Kincaid-Smith P (eds): Reflux Nephropathy. New York, Masson, 1978, p 14.

160. Smellie JM, Hodson CJ, Edwards D, Normand ICS: Clinical and urological features of urinary infection in childhood. BMJ 2:1222, 1964.

161. Savage DCL, Wilson MI, McHardy, et al: Covert bacteriuria of childhood. Arch Dis Child 48:8, 1973.

162. Asscher AW, McLachlan MSF, Jones RV, et al: Screening for asymptomatic urinary tract infection in schoolgirls. Lancet 2:1, 1973.

163. Newcastle Asymptomatic Bacteriuria Group: Asymptomatic bacteriuria in schoolchildren in Newcastle-upon-Tyne. Arch Dis Child 50:902, 1975.

164. Lindberg U, Claesson I, Hanson LA, Jodal U: Asymptomatic bacteriuria in school girls. Acta Paediatr Scand 64:425, 1975.

165. Edwards B, White RHR, Maxted H, et al: Screening methods for covert bacteriuria in school girls. BMJ 1:463, 1975.

166. Smellie JM, Normand ICS: Experience of follow-up of children with urinary tract infections. *In* O'Grady F, Brumfitt W (eds): Urinary Tract Infection. London, Oxford University Press, 1968, p 297.

167. Wein J, Schoenberg HW: A review of 402 girls with recurrent urinary tract infection. J Urol 107:329, 1972.

168. Winberg J, Andersen HJ, Bergstrom TB, et al: Epidemiology of symptomatic urinary tract infection in childhood. Acta Paediatr Scand Suppl 252:1, 1974.

169. Shannon FT: Urinary tract infection in infancy. N Z Med J 75:282, 1972.

170. Drew JH, Acton CM: Radiological findings in newborn infants with urinary infection. Arch Dis Child 51:628, 1976.

171. Penn IA, Briedahl PD: Ureteric reflux and renal damage. Aust N Z J Surg 37:163, 1967.

172. Bergstrom T, Larson H, Lincoln K, Winberg J: Studies of urinary tract infection in infancy and childhood: 1280 patients with neonatal infection. J Pediatr 80:858, 1972.

173. Rolleston GL, Maling TMJ, Hodson CJ: Intrarenal reflux and the scarred kidney. Arch Dis Child 49:531, 1974.

174. Filly R, Friedland GW, Govan DE, Fair WR: Development and progression of clubbing and scarring in children with recurrent urinary tract infection. Radiology 113:145, 1974.

175. Lenaghan D, Whitaker JG, Hensen F, Stephens FD: The natural history of reflux and long-term effects of reflux on the kidney. J Urol 115:728, 1976.

176. Shah KJ, Robins DG, White RHR: Renal scarring and vesico-ureteric reflux. Arch Dis Child 53:210, 1978.

177. Kincaid-Smith P, Becker GJ: Reflux nephropathy in the adult. *In* Hodson CJ, Kincaid-Smith P (eds): Reflux Nephropathy. New York, Masson, 1979, p 21.

178. Zuchelli P, Gaggi R: Vesicoureteral reflux and reflux nephropathy in adults. Contrib Nephrol 61:220, 1987.

179. Hodson CJ, Maling RM, McManamon PJ, Lewis MJ: The pathogenesis of reflux nephropathy (chronic atrophic pyelonephritis). Br J Radiol 13(suppl):1, 1975.

180. Ransley PG, Risdon RA: The pathogenesis of reflux nephropathy. Br J Radiol 14(suppl):1, 1978.

181. Brodeur AE, Goyer RA, Melick W: A potential hazard of barium cystography. Radiology 85:1080, 1965.

181. Amat AD: Calicotubular backflow with vesico-ureteral reflux. JAMA 213:293, 1970.

183. Rolleston GL, Shannon FT, Utley WLF: Relationship of infantile vesico-ureteric reflux to renal damage. BMJ 1:460, 1970.

184. Bourne HR, Condon NR, Hoyt TS, Nixon GW: Intrarenal reflux and renal damage. J Urol 110:255, 1976.

185. Rose JS, Glassberg KI, Waterhouse K: Intrarenal reflux and its relationship to renal scarring. J Urol 113:400, 1975.

186. Ransley PF: Intrarenal reflux: Anatomical, dynamic and radiological studies (part I). Urol Res 5:61, 1977.

187. Maling RMJ, Rolleston GL: Intrarenal reflux in children demonstrated by micturating angiography. Clin Radiol 25:81, 1974.

188. Ransley PG, Risdon RA: Renal papillary morphology in infants and young children. Urol Res 3:111, 1977.

189. Ransley PG, Risdon RA: The pathogenesis of reflux nephropathy. Contrib Nephrol 16:90, 1979.

190. Ransley PG, Risdon RA: The renal papilla, intrarenal reflux, and chronic pyelonephritis. *In* Hodson CJ, Kincaid-Smith P (eds): Reflux Nephropathy. New York, Masson, 1979, p 126.

191. Tamminen TE, Kaprio EA: The relation of the shape of the renal papilla and of collecting duct openings to intrarenal reflux. Br J Urol 49:345, 1977.

192. Bailey RR: Long-term follow-up of infants with gross vesicoureteric reflux. Contrib Nephrol 39:146, 1984.

193. Ransley PG, Risdon RA, Godley ML: High-pressure sterile vesicoureteral reflux and renal scarring: An experimental study in the pig and minipig. Contrib Nephrol 39:320, 1984.

194. Heptinstall RH, Hodson CJ: Pathology of sterile reflux in the pig. Contrib Nephrol 39:344, 1984.

195. Jorgensen TM, Olsen S, Djurhuus JC, Norgaard JP: Renal morphology in experimental vesicoureteric reflux in pigs. Scand J Urol Nephrol 18:49, 1984.

196. Hutch JA, Smith DR: Sterile reflux: Report of 24 cases. Urol Int 24:460, 1969.

197. Stephens FD: Urologic aspects of recurrent urinary tract infection in children. J Pediatr 80:725, 1972.

198. Bakshandeh K, Lynne C, Carrion H: Vesicoureteral reflux and end-stage renal disease. J Urol 116:557, 1976.

199. Bailey RR: Sterile reflux: Is it harmless? *In* Hodson CJ, Kincaid-Smith P (eds): Reflux Nephropathy. New York, Masson, 1979, p 334.

200. Stickler BG, Kelalis PP, Burke EC, Segar WE: Primary interstitial nephritis with reflux: A cause of hypertension. Am J Dis Child 122:144, 1971.

201. Salvatierra O Jr, Tanagho EA: Reflux as a cause of end-stage kidney disease: Report of 32 cases. J Urol 117:441, 1977.

202. (VUR + IRR) + UTI = CPN [editorial] Lancet 2:301, 1978.

203. Smellie JM, Edwards D, Normand ICS, Prescod N: Effect of VUR on renal growth in children with urinary tract infection. Arch Dis Child 56:593, 1981.

204. Smellie JM, Normand ICM, Katz G: Children with urinary infection: A comparison of those with and without VUR. Kidney Int 20:717, 1981.

205. Holland NH, Jackson EC, Kazee M, et al: Relation of urinary tract infection and vesicoureteral reflux to scars: Follow-up of thirty eight patients. J Pediatr 116:S65, 1990.

206. Mosconi CEV, Ianhez LE, Borrelli M, et al: Vesicoureteral reflux in patients in end-stage chronic renal failure. Urol Int 4:357, 1975.

207. Mosconi CEV, Ianhez LE, Borrelli M, Campos Friere JG: Bladder dysfunction in uremic patients. Acta Urol Belg 42:418, 1974.

208. Bishop MC, Moss SW, Oliver O, et al: The significance of vesicoureteral reflux in non-pyelonephritic patients supported by long-term hemodialysis. Clin Nephrol 8:354, 1977.

209. Huland R, Buchard P, Kollerman M, Augustin I: Vesicoureteral reflux in end-stage renal disease. J Urol 121:10, 1979.

210. McCrae CV, Shannon FT, Utley WLF: Effect on renal growth or reimplantation of refluxing ureters. Lancet 1:1310, 1974.

211. Willscher MK, Bauer SB, Zammuto PJ, Retik AB: Renal growth and urinary infection following anti-reflux surgery in infants and children. J Urol 115:722, 1976.

212. Ransley PG, Risdon RA, Godley ML: Effects of vesicoureteric reflux on renal growth and function. Br J Urol 60:193, 1987.

213. Maskell R: Broadening the concept of urinary tract infection. Br J Urol 76:2, 1995.

214. Fairley KF, Birch DF: Detection of bladder bacteriuria in patients with acute urinary symptoms. J Infect Dis 159:226, 1989.

215. Rubin RH, Shapiro ED, Andriole VT, et al: Evaluation of new anti-infective drugs for the treatment of urinary tract infection. Clin Infect Dis 15:216, 1972.

216. Rubin RH: Infection of the urinary tract. *In* Dale DC (ed): Scientific American Textbook of Medicine. New York, Scientific American, 1998, pp 1-13.

217. Vermeulen CW, Goetz RL: Experimental urolithiasis: VIII. Furadantin in treatment of experimental proteus infection with stone formation. J Urol 72:99, 1954.

218. Bowie WR, Potlock HM, Forsyth PS, et al: Bacteriology of the urethra in normal men and men with nongonococcal urethritis. J Clin Microbiol 6:482, 1977.

219. Singer C, Kaplan MH, Armstrong D: Bacteremia and fungemia complicating neoplastic disease. Am J Med 62:731, 1977.

220. Dembry LM, Andriole VT: Renal and perirenal abscesses. Infect Dis Clin North Am 11:663, 1997.

221. Beeson PB: Factors in the pathogenesis of pyelonephritis. Yale J Biol Med 28:81, 1955.

222. Kleeman CR, Hewitt WL, Guze LB: Pyelonephritis. Medicine (Baltimore) 39:3, 1960.

223. Teplitz C, Raultson GL, Walker HL, et al: Spontaneous hematogenous *Pseudomonas* pyelonephritis in rats. J Infect Dis 114:75, 1964.

224. Mabeck CE, Orskov R, Orskov I: *Escherichia coli* serotypes and renal involvement. Lancet 1:1312, 1971.

225. Cougant DA, Levin BR, Lidin-Javson G, et al: Genetic diversity and relationship among strains of *Escherichia coli* in the intestine and those causing urinary tract infections. Prog Allergy 33:203, 1983.

226. Schoolnik GK, O'Hanley P, Lark D, et al: Uropathogenic *Escherichia coli*: Molecular mechanisms of adherence. Adv Exp Med Biol 224: 53, 1987.

227. Svanborg-Eden C, Hausson S, Jodal Y, et al: Host-parasite interaction in the urinary tract. J Infect Dis 157:421, 1988.

228. Phillips T, Eykyn S, King A, et al: Epidemic multiresistant *Escherichia coli* infection in West Lambeth health district. Lancet 1:1038, 1988.

229. Tullus K, Korlin K, Svenson SB, et al: Epidemic outbreak of acute pyelonephritis caused by nosocomial spread of P fimbriated *Escherichia coli* in children. J Infect Dis 150:728, 1984.

230. Liden-Jenson F, Hanson LA, Kaijsen B, et al: Comparison of *Escherichia coli* from bacteriuric patients with those from feces of healthy school children. J Infect Dis 136:346, 1977.

231. Svanborg-Eden C, de Man P: Bacterial virulence in urinary tract infection. Infect Dis Clin North Am 1:731, 1987.

232. Olling S, Hanson LA, Holmgren J, et al: The bactericidal effect of normal human serum on *E. coli* strains from normals and from patients with urinary tract infection. Infection 1:24, 1973.

233. Kaijser B, Hanson LA, Jodal U, et al: Frequency of *E. coli* K antigens in urinary tract infections in children. Lancet 1:663, 1977.

234. Achtman M, Mercer A, Kusecek B, et al: Six widespread bacterial clones among *Escherichia coli* K1 isolates. Infect Immun 39:315, 1983.

235. Steadman R, Topley N: The virulence of *Escherichia coli* in the urinary tract. *In* Brumfitt W, Hamilton-Miller JMT, Bailey RR (eds): Urinary Tract Infections. London, Chapman & Hall, 1998, p 37.

236. Sandberg T, Stenquist K, Svanborg-Eden C, et al: Host-parasite relationship in urinary tract infections during pregnancy. Prog Allergy 33:228, 1983.

237. Vosti KL, Goldberg LN, Monto AS, Pantz LA: Host-parasite interactions in patients with infections due to *Escherichia coli*: I. The serogrouping of *E. coli* from intestinal and extraintestinal sources. J Clin Invest 43:2377, 1964.

238. Van den Bosch JF, Postima P, Koopman PAR, et al: Virulence of urinary and fecal *Escherichia coli* in relation to serotype, haemolysis and haemagglutination. J Hyg 88:567, 1982.

239. Guze LB, Montgomerie JZ, Potter CS, Kalmanson GM: Pyelonephritis: XVI. Correlates of parasite virulence in acute ascending *Escherichia coli* pyelonephritis in mice undergoing diuresis. Yale J Biol Med 46:203, 1973.

240. Howard CJ, Glynn AA: The virulence for mice of strains of *Escherichia coli* related to the effects of K antigens on their resistance for phagocytosis and killing by complement. Immunology 20:767, 1971.

241. Jann K, Jann B: Cell surface components and virulence: *Escherichia coli* O and K antigens in relation to virulence and pathogenicity. *In* Sussman M (ed): The Virulence of *Escherichia coli*: Reviews and Methods. London, Academic Press, 1985, p 157.

242. Svanborg-Eden C, Hagberg L, Hull R, et al: Bacterial virulence versus host resistance in the urinary tracts of mice. Infect Immun 55:1224, 1987.

243. Kaijser B, Vatilne G: *Escherichia coli* K antigen. Bakt Hyg 243:271, 1979.

244. Hanson LA, Fasth A, Jodal Y, et al: Biology and pathology of uninary tract infections. J Clin Pathol 34:695, 1981.

245. Falkow S: Molecular Koch's postulates applied to microbial pathogenesis. Rev Infect Dis 10:5274, 1988.

246. Kao JS, Stucker DM, Warren JW, et al: Pathogenicity island sequences of pyelonephritogenic *Escherichia coli* CFT073 are associated with virulent uropathogenic strains. Infect Immun 65:2812, 1997.

247. Swanson DL, Bukanov NO, Berg DE, et al: Two pathogenicity islands in uropathogenic *Escherichia coli* J96: Cosmid cloning and sample sequencing. Infect Immun 64:3736, 1996.

248. Guyer DM, Kao JS, Mobley HLT: Genomic analysis of a pathogenicity island in uropathogenic *Escherichia coli* CFT073. Infect Immun 66:4471, 1998.

249. Lee CA: Pathogenicity islands and the evaluation of bacterial pathogens. Infect Agents Dis 5:1, 1996.

250. Oelschlager TA, Dobrindt U, Hecker J: Pathogenicity islands of uropathic *Escherichia coli* and the evolution of virulence. Int J Antimicrob Agents 19:517, 2002.

251. Hagberg L, Jodal U, Karhonen TK, et al: Adhesion, hemagglutination and virulence of *E. coli* causing urinary tract infections. Infect Immun 31:564, 1981.

252. Dyguid JP, Old DC: Adhesive properties of Enterobacteriaceae. *In* Brachay EH (ed): Bacterial Adherence. London, Chapman & Hall, 1988, p 187.

253. Orskov O, Ferencz A, Orskov F: Tamm-Horsfall protein or uromucoid is the normal urinary slime that binds type I fimbriated *E. coli*. Lancet 1:887, 1980.

254. Bar-Shavit Z, Ofek I, Goldman R, et al: Mannose residues on phagocytes as receptors for the attachment of *Escherichia coli* and *Salmonella* typhi. Biochem Biophys Res Commun 78:455, 1977.

255. Svanborg C, de Man P, Sandberg T: Renal involvement in urinary tract infection. Kidney Int 39:541, 1991.

256. Topley N, Steadman R, Mackenzie R, et al: Type 1 fimbriate strains of *Escherichia coli* initiate renal parenchymal scarring. Kidney Int 36:609, 1989.

257. Mundi H, Bjorkseten B, Svanborg C, et al: Extracellular release of reactive oxygen species from human neutrophils upon interaction with *Escherichia coli* strains causing renal scarring. Infect Immun 59:4168, 1991.

258. Connell I, Agace W, Klemm P, et al: Type 1 fimbrial expression enhances *Escherichia coli* virulence for the urinary tract. Proc Natl Acad Sci U S A 93:9827, 1996.

259. Mizunoe Y, Matsumoto T, Sakumoto M, et al: Renal scarring by mannose-sensitive adhesin of *Escherichia coli* type 1 pili. Nephron 77:412, 1997.

260. Thankavel K, Madison B, Ikeda T, et al: Localization of a domain in the FimH adhesin of *Escherichia coli* type 1 fimbriae capable of receptor recognition and use of a domain-specific antibody to confer protection against experimental urinary tract infection. J Clin Invest 100:1123, 1997.

261. Sokurenko EV, Chesnokova V, Doyle RJ, Hasty DL: Diversity of the *Escherichia coli* type 1 fimbrial lectin: Differential binding to mannosides and uroepithelial cells. J Biol Chem 272:17880, 1997.

262. Gunther NW, Lockatell V, Johnson DE, Mobley HL: In vivo dynamics of type 1 fimbria regulation in uropathogenic *Escherichia coli* during experimental urinary tract infection. Infect Immun 69:2838, 2001.

263. Pak J, Pu Y, Zhang ZT, et al: Tamm-Horsfall protein binds to type 1 fimbriated *Escherichia coli* and prevents *Escherichia coli* from binding to uroplakin Ia and Ib receptors. J Biol Chem 276:9924, 2001.

264. Bahrani-Mougeot FK, Buckler EL: Type 1 fimbriae and extracellular polysaccharides are preeminent *Escherichia coli* virulence determinants in the murine urinary tract. Mol Microbiol 45:1079, 2002.

265. Bjorksten B, Knigsen B: Interaction of human serum and neutrophils with *Escherichia coli* chains: Differences between strains isolated from urine of patients with pyelonephritis or asymptomatic bacteriuria. Infect Immun 22:308, 1978.

266. Leffler H, Svanborg-Eden C: Chemical definition of a glycosphingolipid receptor for *Escherichia coli* attaching to human urinary tract epithelial cells and agglutinating erythrocytes. FEMS Microbiol Lett 8:127, 1980.

267. Svanborg-Eden C, Hagberg L, Hanson LA, et al: Bacterial adherence: A pathogenetic mechanism in urinary tract infections caused by *Escherichia coli*. Prog Allergy 33:175, 1983.

268. Lindberg FP, Lund B, Normark S: Genes of pyelonephritogenic *E. coli* required for digalactoside-specific agglutination of human cells. EMBO J 3:1167, 1984.

269. Klemm P, Orskov I, Orskov F: F7 and type 1-like fimbriae from three *Escherichia coli* strains isolated from urinary tract infections: Protein and immunological aspects. Infect Immun 36:462, 1982.

270. Johnson JR, O'Bryan TT, Delavari P, et al: Clonal relationships and extended virulence genotypes among *Escherichia coli* isolated from women with a first or recurrent episode of cystitis. J Infect Dis 183:1508, 2001.

271. Rasko DA, Phillips JA, Li X, Mobley HL: Identification of DNA sequences from a second pathogenicity island from uropathogenic *Escherichia coli* CFT073. J Infect Dis 184:1041, 2001.

272. Nou X, Skinner B, Braaten B, et al: Regulation of pyelonephritis-associated pili phase-variation in *Escherichia coli*: Binding of the PapI and the Lrp regulatory proteins is controlled by DNA methylation. Mol Microbiol 7:545, 1993.

273. Warren JW, Mobley HLT, Donnenberg MS: Host-parasite interactions and host defense mechanisms. *In* Schrier RW (ed): Diseases of the Kidney and Urinary Tract, 7th ed. Philadelphia, Lippincott Williams & Wilkins, 2001, p 903.

274. Svanborg-Eden C, Eriksson B, Hanson LA, et al: Adhesion to normal human non-epithelial cells of *Escherichia coli* from children with various forms of urinary tract infections. J Pediatr 93:398, 1978.

275. Blanco M, Blanco JE, Alonso MP, Blanco J: Virulence factors and O groups of *Escherichia coli* isolates from patients with acute pyelonephritis, cystitis and symptomatic bacteriuria. Eur J Epidemiol 12:191, 1996.

276. Leffler H, Svanborg-Eden C, Schoolnick G, Wastrom T: Glycosphingolipids as receptors for bacterial adhesion, host glycolipid diversity. *In* Boedekke ED (ed): Adherence of Organisms in the Gut Mucosa, vol 2. Boca Raton, FL, CRC Press, 1984, p 177.

277. Svanborg-Eden C, Hanson LA, Jodal U, et al: Variable adherence to normal human urinary tract epithelial cells of *Escherichia coli* strains associated with various forms of urinary tract infection. Lancet 2:490, 1976.

278. Svanborg-Eden C, Hanson HA: *E. coli* pili as mediators of attachment for human urinary tract epithelial cells. Infect Immun 21:229, 1978.

279. Svanborg-Eden C, Gotschlich EC, Korhonen TK, et al: Aspects of structure and function of pili on *Escherichia coli.* Prog Allergy 33:189, 1983.

280. Svanborg-Eden C, Bjursten LM, Hull R, et al: Influence of adhesion in the interaction of *Escherichia coli* with human phagocytes. Infect Immun 44:407, 1984.

281. Otto G, Sandberg T, Marklund BI, et al: Virulence factors and pap genotype in *Escherichia coli* isolates from women with acute pyelonephritis, with or without bacteremia. Clin Infect Dis 17:448, 1993.

282. Lomberg H, Eden CS: Influence of P blood group phenotype on susceptibility to urinary tract infection. FEMS Microbiol Immunol 1:363, 1989.

283. Korhonen TK, Vaisanen-Rhen V, Rhen M, et al: *Escherichia coli* fimbriae recognize sialyl galactosides. J Bacteriol 159:76, 1984.

284. Vaisanen-Rhen V, Korhonen T, Jokinen M, et al: Blood group M specific haemagglutination in pyelonephritogenic *Escherichia coli.* Lancet 1:119, 198.

285. Labigne-Roussel A, Falkow S: Distribution and degree of heterogeneity of the afimbrial adhesion encoding operon (afa) among uropathogenic *Escherichia coli* isolates. Infect Immun 56:640, 1988.

286. Le Bouguenec C, Garcia MI, Ouin V, et al: Characterization of plasmid-borne afa-3 gene clusters encoding afimbrial adhesins expressed by *Escherichia coli* strains associated with intestinal or urinary tract infections. Infect Immun 61:5106, 1993.

287. Parkkinen J, Finne J, Achtman M, et al: *Escherichia coli* strains binding to neuroaminyl alpha-2-3 galactosides. Biochem Biophys Res Commun 11:456, 1983.

288. Johnson JR: Virulence factors in *Escherichia coli* urinary tract infection. Clin Microbiol Rev 4:80, 1991.

289. Nowicki B, Truong L, Moulds J, Hull R: Presence of the Dr receptor in normal human tissues and the possible role in pathogenesis of ascending urinary tract infection. Am J Pathol 133:11, 1988.

290. Pham TQ, Goluszko P, Popov V, et al: Molecular cloning and characterization of Dr-II, a nonfimbrial adhesin-I-like adhesin isolated from gestational pyelonephritis-associated *Escherichia coli* that binds to decay-accelerating factor. Infect Immun 65:4309, 1997.

291. Goluszko P, Moseley SL, Truong LD, et al: Development of experimental model of chronic pyelonephritis with *Escherichia coli* O75:K5:H-bearing Dr fimbriae: Mutation in the dra region prevented tubulointerstitial nephritis. J Clin Invest 99:1662, 1997.

292. Goluszko P, Popov V, Selvarangan R, et al: Dr fimbriae operon of uropathogenic *Escherichia coli* mediate microtubule-dependent invasion to the HeLa epithelial cell line. J Infect Dis 176:158, 1997.

293. Yamamoto S, Nakata K, Yuri K, et al: Assessment of the significance of virulence factors of uropathogenic *Escherichia coli* in experimental urinary tract infection in mice. Microbiol Immunol 40:607, 1996.

294. Connell H, de Man P, Jodal U, et al: Lack of association between hemolysin production and acute inflammation in human urinary tract infection. Microb Pathog 14:463, 1993.

295. Arthur M, Johnson CE, Rubin RH, et al: Molecular epidemiology of adhesin and hemolysin virulence factors among uropathogenic *Escherichia coli.* Infect Immun 57:303, 1989.

296. Mobley HL, Green DM, Trifillis AL, et al: Pyelonephritogenic *Escherichia coli* and killing of cultured human renal proximal tubular epithelial cells: Role of hemolysin in some strains. Infect Immun 58:181, 1990.

297. O'Hanley P, Lalonde G, Ji G: Alpha hemolysin contributes to the pathogenicity of piliated digalactoside-binding *Escherichia coli* in the kidney: Efficacy of an alpha hemolysin vaccine in preventing renal injury in the BALB/c mouse model of pyelonephritis. Infect Immun 59:1153, 1991.

298. O'Hanley P, Low D, Romero I, et al: Gal-Gal binding and hemolysin phenotypes and genotype associated with uropathogenic *E. coli.* N Engl J Med 313:414, 1985.

299. Svanborg C, Jodal U: Host-parasite interaction in urinary tract infection. *In* Brumfitt W, Hamilton-Miller JMT, Bailey RR (eds): Urinary Tract Infections. London, Chapman & Hall, 1998, p 87.

300. Wullt B, Bergsten G, Connell H, et al: P. fimbriae trigger mucosal response to *Escherichia coli* in the urinary tract. Cell Microbiol 3:255, 2001.

301. Mills M, Meysick KC, O'Brien AD: Cytotoxic necrotizing factor type 1 of uropathogenic *Escherichia coli* kills cultured human uroepithelial 5637 cells by an apoptotic mechanism. Infect Immun 68:5869, 2000.

302. Rippere-Lampe KE, O'Brien AD, Conran R, Lockman HA: Mutation of the gene encoding cytotoxic necrotizing factor type (1) attenuates the virulence of uropathogenic *Escherichia coli.* Infect Immun 69:3954, 2001.

303. Svanborg C, Bergsten G, Fischer H, et al: The "innate" host response protects and damages the infected urinary tract. Ann Med 33:563, 2001.

304. Hedges S, Stenqvist K, Lidin-Janson G, et al: Comparison of urine and serum concentrations of interleukin-6 in women with acute pyelonephritis or asymptomatic bacteriuria. J Infect Dis 166:653, 1992.

305. de Man P, Jodal U, Svanborg C: Dependence among host response parameters used to diagnose urinary tract infection. J Infect Dis 163:331, 1991.

306. Rugo HS, O'Hanley P, Bishop AG, et al: Local cytokine production in a murine model of *Escherichia coli* pyelonephritis. J Clin Invest 89:103, 199.

307. Lomberg H, Jodal U, Leffler H, et al: Blood group non-secretors have an increased inflammatory response to urinary tract infection. Scand J Infect Dis 4:77, 199.

308. Ishitoya S, Yamamoto S, Mitsumore K, et al: Non-secretor status is associated with female acute uncomplicated pyelonephritis. BJU Int 56:851, 2002.

309. Frendeus B, Godaly G, Hang L, et al: Interleukin 8 receptor deficiency confers susceptibility to acute experimental pyelonephritis and may have a human counterpart. J Exp Med 192:881, 2000.

310. Hang L, Frendeus B, Godaly G, Svanborg C: Interleukin 8 receptor knockout mice have subepithelial neutrophil entrapment and renal scarring following acute pyelonephritis. J Infect Dis 182:1738, 2002.

311. Olszyna DP, Lorquin S, Sewnath M, et al: CXC chemokine receptor 2 contributes to host defense in murine urinary tract infection. J Infect Dis 184:301, 2001.

312. Roberts JA, Kaack MB, Martin LN: Cytokine and lymphocyte activation during experimental acute pyelonephritis. Urol Res 23:33, 1995.

313. Tullus K, Wang JA, Lu Y, et al: Interleukin-1α and interleukin-6 in the urine, kidney, and bladder of mice inoculated with *Escherichia coli.* Pediatr Nephrol 10:453, 1996.

314. Tullus K, Escobar-Billing R, Fituri O, et al: Interleukin-1α and interleukin-1 receptor antagonist in the urine of children with acute pyelonephritis and relation to renal scarring. Acta Paediatr 85:158, 1996.

315. Svanborg C, Hedlund M, Connell H, et al: Bacterial adherence and mucosal cytokine responses: Receptors and transmembrane signaling. Ann N Y Acad Sci 797:177, 1996.

316. Benson M, Jodal U, Agace W, et al: Interleukin (IL)-6 and IL-8 in children with febrile urinary tract infection and asymptomatic bacteriuria. J Infect Dis 174:1080, 1996.

317. Tullus K, Escobar-Billing R, Fituri O, et al: Soluble receptors to tumour necrosis factor and interleukin-6 in urine during acute pyelonephritis. Acta Paediatr 86:1198, 1997.

318. Kimball P, Reid F: Tumor necrosis factor β gene polymorphisms associated with urinary tract infections after renal transplantation. Transplantation 73:1110, 2002.

319. Godaly G, Bergsten G, Hang L, et al: Neutrophil recruitment, chemokine receptors, and resistance to mucosal infection. J Leukocyte Biol 69:899, 2001.

320. Jantausch BA, O'Donnell R, Wiedermann BL: Urinary interleukin 6 and interleukin 8 in children with urinary infection. Pediatr Nephrol 15:236, 2000.

321. Khalil A, Tullus K, Bartfai T, et al: Renal cytokine responses in acute *Escherichia coli* pyelonephritis in Il-6 deficient mice. Clin Exp Immunol 122:200, 2000.

322. Cotton SA, Gbadegsin RA, Williams S, et al: Role of TGF-β 1 in renal parenchymal scarring following childhood urinary tract infection. Kidney Int 61:61, 2002.

323. Khalil A, Tullus K, Bakhiet M, et al: Angiotensin II type 1 receptor antagonist (losartan) down-regulates transforming growth factor β in experimental acute pyelonephritis. J Urol 164:186, 2000.

324. Andreu A, Stapleton AE, Fennell C, et al: Urovirulence determinants in *Escherichia coli* strains causing prostatitis. J Infect Dis 176:464, 1997.

325. Terrai A, Yamamoto S, Mitsumori K, et al: *Escherichia coli* virulence factors and serotypes in acute bacterial prostatitis. Int J Urol 4:289, 1997.

326. Hull RA, Rudy DC, Wieser IE, Donovan WH: Virulence factors of *Escherichia coli* isolates from patients with symptomatic and asymptomatic bacteriuria and neuropathic bladders due to spinal cord and brain injuries. J Clin Microbiol 36:115, 1998.

327. Bahrani FK, Johnson DE, Robbins D, Mobley HL: *Proteus mirabilis* flagella and MR/P fimbriae: Isolation, purification, N-terminal analysis, and serum antibody response following experimental urinary tract infection. Infect Immun 59:3574, 1991.

328. Bahrani FK, Mobley HL: *Proteus mirabilis* MR/P fimbriae: Molecular cloning, expression, and nucleotide sequence of the major fimbrial subunit gene. J Bacteriol 175:457, 1993.

329. Massad G, Lockatell CV, Johnson DE, Mobley HL: *Proteus mirabilis* fimbriae: Construction of an isogenic *pmfA* mutant and analysis of virulence in a CBA mouse model of ascending urinary tract infection. Infect Immun 6:536, 1994.

330. Moayeri N, Collins CM, O'Hanley P: Efficacy of a *Proteus mirabilis* outer membrane protein vaccine in preventing experimental *Proteus* pyelonephritis in a BALB/c mouse model. Infect Immun 59:3778, 1991.

331. Li X, Zhao H, Geymonat L, et al: *Proteus mirabilis* mannose-resistant, *Proteus*-like fimbriae: MrpG is located at the fimbrial tip and is required for fimbrial assembly. Infect Immun 65:1327, 1997.

332. Zhao H, Li X, Johnson DE, et al: In vivo phase variation of MR/P fimbrial gene expression in *Proteus mirabilis* infecting the urinary tract. Mol Microbiol 23:1009, 1997.

333. Mobley HL, Belas R, Lockatell V, et al: Construction of a flagellum-negative mutant of *Proteus mirabilis*: Effect on internalization by human renal epithelial cells and virulence in a mouse model of ascending urinary tract infection. Infect Immun 64:5332, 1996.

334. Johnson DE, Russell RG, Lockatell CV, et al: Contribution of *Proteus mirabilis* urease to persistence, urolithiasis, and acute pyelonephritis in a mouse model of ascending urinary tract infection. Infect Immun 61:748, 1993.

335. Mobley HL, Chippendale GR: Hemagglutinin, urease, and hemolysin production by *Proteus mirabilis* from clinical sources. J Infect Dis 161:55, 1990.

336. Mobley HL, Chippendale GR, Swihart KG, Welch RA: Cytotoxicity of the HpmA hemolysin and urease of *Proteus mirabilis* and *Proteus vulgaris* against cultured human renal proximal tubular epithelial cells. Infect Immun 59:036, 1991.

337. Senior BW, Loomes LM, Kerr MA: The production and activity in vivo of *Proteus mirabilis* IgA protease in infections of the urinary tract. J Med Microbiol 35:03, 1991.

338. Podschun R, Sievers D, Fischer A, Ullmann U: Serotypes, hemagglutinins, siderophore synthesis, and serum resistance of *Klebsiella* isolates causing human urinary tract infections. J Infect Dis 168:1415, 1993.

339. Camprubi S, Merino S, Benedi V-J, Tomas JM: The role of O-antigen lipopolysaccharide and capsule on an experimental *Klebsiella pneumoniae* infection of the rat urinary tract. FEMS Microbiol Lett 111:9, 1993.

340. Oelschlaeger TA, Tall BD: Invasion of cultured human epithelial cells by *Klebsiella pneumoniae* isolated from the urinary tract. Infect Immun 65:2950, 1997.

341. Guzman CA, Pruzzo C, LiPira G, Calegari L: Role of adherence in pathogenesis of *Enterococcus faecalis* urinary tract infection and endocarditis. Infect Immun 57:1834, 1989.

342. Platt R, Polk BF, Murdock B, et al: Risk factors for nosocomial urinary tract infection. Am J Epidemiol 14:977, 1986.

343. Patterson JE, Andriole VT: Bacterial urinary tract infections in diabetes. Infect Dis Clin North Am 11:735, 1997.

344. Geerlings SE, Meiland R, Hoepelman AI: Pathogenesis of bacteriuria in women with diabetes mellitus. Int J Antimicrob Agents 19:539, 2002.

345. Harding GK, Zhanel GG, Nicolle LE, et al: Antimicrobial treatment in diabetic women with asymptomatic bacteriuria. N Engl J Med 347:1576, 2002.

346. Goswami R, Bal CS, Tejaswi S, et al: Prevalence of urinary tract infection and renal scars in patients with diabetes mellitus. Diabetes Res Clin Pract 53:181, 2001.

347. Geerlings SE, Stolk RP, Camps MJ, et al: Consequences of asymptomatic bacteriuria in women with diabetes mellitus. Arch Intern Med 161:1421, 2001.

348. McDermid KP, Watterson J, van Eiden SF: Emphysematous pyelonephritis: Case report and review of the literature. Diabetes Res Clin Pract 44:71, 1999.

349. Huang JJ, Tseng CC: Emphysematous pyelonephritis: Clinicoradiological classification, management, prognosis, and pathogenesis. Arch Intern Med 160:797, 2000.

350. Hildebrand TS, Nibbe L, Frei U, Schindler R: Bilateral ephysematous pyelonephritis caused by *Candida* infection. Am J Kidney Dis 33:E10, 1999.

351. Gorrill RH: The effect of obstruction of the ureter on the renal localization of bacteria. J Pathol Bacteriol 7:59, 1956.

352. Rocha H, Fekety FR Jr: Delayed granulocyte mobilization in the renal medulla. *In* Kass EH (ed): Progress in Pyelonephritis. Philadelphia, FA Davis, 1964, p 11.

353. Freedman LR, Beeson PB: Experimental pyelonephritis: IV. Observations on infections resulting from direct inoculation of bacteria in different zones of the kidney. Yale J Biol Med 30:406, 1958.

354. Cotran RS, Vivaldi E, Zangwill DP, Kass EH: Retrograde *Proteus* pyelonephritis in rats: Bacteriologic, pathologic, and fluorescent antibody studies. Am J Pathol 43:1, 1963.

355. Rocha H, Fekety FR: Acute inflammation in the renal cortex and medulla following thermal injury. J Exp Med 119:131, 1964.

356. Andriole VT: Acceleration of the inflammatory response of the renal medulla by water diuresis. J Clin Invest 45:847, 1966.

357. Hubert EG, Montgomerie JZ, Kalmanson GM, Guze LB: Effect of renal physicochemical milieu on serum bactericidal activity. Am J Med Sci 53:5, 1967.

358. Mayrer AR, Miniter P, Andriole VT: Immunopathogenesis of chronic pyelonephritis. Am J Med 75:59, 1983.

359. Svanborg-Eden C, Kulhavy R, Marild S, et al: Urinary immunoglobulins in healthy individuals and children with acute pyelonephritis. Scand J Immunol 21:305, 1985.

360. Rene P, Silverblatt FJ: Serological response to *Escherichia coli* pili in pyelonephritis. Infect Immun 37:749, 1982.

361. Kantele A, Papunes R, Virtahen E, et al: Antibody secreting cells in acute urinary tract infection as indicators of local immunoresponse. J Infect Dis 169:1023, 1994.

362. Kaijser B, Larsson P, Olling S, et al: Protection against acute, ascending pyelonephritis caused by *Escherichia coli* in rats, using isolated capsular antigen conjugated to bovine serum albumin. Infect Immun 39:142, 1983.

363. Roberts JA, Hardaway K, Kaack B, et al: Prevention of pyelonephritis by immunization with p-fimbriae. J Urol 131:602, 1984.

364. O'Hanley P, Lark D, Falkow S, et al: Molecular basis of *Escherichia coli* colonization of the upper urinary tract in BALB/c mice: Gal-Gal pili immunization prevents *Escherichia coli* pyelonephritis in the BALB/c mouse model of human pyelonephritis. J Clin Invest 75:347, 1985.

365. Svanborg-Eden C, Svennerholm AM: Secretory IgA and IgG antibodies prevent adhesion of *Escherichia coli* to human urinary tract epithelial cells. Infect Immun 22:790, 1997.

366. Reidasch G, Heck P, Rautenberg E, et al: Does low urinary SIgA predispose to urinary tract infection? Kidney Int 23:579, 1983.

367. Miliazzo FH, Delisle GJ: Immunoglobulin A proteases in gram-negative bacteria isolated from human urinary tract infections. Infect Immun 43:11, 1984.

368. Svanborg-Eden C, Briles D, Hagberg L, et al: Genetic factors in host resistance to urinary tract infection. Infection 12:118, 1984.

369. Kurnick J, McCluskey R, Bhat A, et al: *Escherichia coli*–specific T lymphocytes in experimental pyelonephritis. J Immunol 141:3220, 1988.

370. Wilz SW, Kurnick JT, Pandolfi F, et al: T lymphocyte response to antigens of gram negative bacteria in pyelonephritis. Clin Immunol Immunopathol 69:36, 1993.

371. Cotran RS, Piessens WF: Pathogenesis of chronic pyelonephritis: The role of humoral and cell-mediated reactions to bacterial and renal antigen. *In* Giovannetti S, Bonomini V, D'Amico G (eds): Proceedings of the 6th International Congress on Nephrology (Florence). Basel, S Karger, 1976, p 311.

372. Cotran RS, Galvanek EG: Immunopathology of human tubular interstitial diseases: Localization of immunoglobulins and Tamm-Horsfall protein. Contrib Nephrol 16:16, 1979.

373. McCluskey RT, Colvin RG: Immunologic aspects of renal, tubular and interstitial disease. Annu Rev Med 9:191, 1978.

374. Kalmanson GM, Glassock RJ, Harwick HJ, Guze MB: Cellular immunity in experimental pyelonephritis. Kidney Int 8(suppl 4):S35, 1975.

375. van Zwieten MJ, Leber PD, Bhan AK, McCluskey RT: Experimental and cell-mediated interstitial nephritis induced with exogenous antigens. J Immunol 118:589, 1977.

376. Gutman LT, Schaller J, Wedgwood RJ: Bacterial L-forms in relapsing urinary tract infection. Lancet 1:464, 1967.

377. Miller TE, Burnham S, Simpson G: Selective deficiency of thymus-derived lymphocytes in experimental pyelonephritis. Kidney Int 8:88, 1975.

378. Asscher AW, Jones BM, MacKenzie R: Delayed hypersensitivity to *E. coli* in the rat: A study of its possible relevance to the pathogenesis of kidney scars. Br J Exp Pathol 58:549, 1977.

379. Hoyer JR, Seiler MW: Tamm-Horsfall protein. Kidney Int 16:79, 1979.

380. Zager RA, Cotran RS, Hoyer JR: Histological localization of Tamm-Horsfall protein in interstitial deposits in renal disease. Lab Invest 38:5, 1978.

381. Cotran RS, Hodson CJ: Extratubular localization of Tamm-Horsfall protein in experimental reflux nephropathy in the pig. *In* Hodson CJ, Kincaid-Smith P (eds): Reflux Nephropathy. New York, Masson, 1979, p 13.

382. Hodson CJ, Davies A, Prescod A: Renal parenchymal radiographic measurement in infants and children. Pediatr Radiol 3:16, 1975.

383. Mayrer AR, Dziukas LJ, Hodson CJ, Andriole VT: Antibody to Tamm-Horsfall protein in porcine reflux nephropathy. Kidney Int 19:187, 1981.

384. Mayrer AR, Kashgarian M, Ruddle NH, et al: Tubulointerstitial nephritis and immunologic responses to Tamm-Horsfall protein in rabbits' challenged homologous urine or Tamm-Horsfall protein. J Immunol 18:634, 1983.

385. Dziukas LJ, Sterzel RB, Hoyer JR, Hodson CJ: Unilateral ureteric obstruction in rats. J Lab Invest 47:185, 1983.

386. Fasth A, Bjure J, Hjalmas K, et al: Serum autoantibodies to Tamm-Horsfall protein and their relation to renal damage and glomerular filtration rate in children with urinary tract malformations. Contrib Nephrol 39:85, 1984.

387. Lynn KI, Bailey RR, Groufsky A, et al: Antibodies to Tamm-Horsfall urinary glycoprotein in patients with urinary tract infection, reflux nephropathy, urinary obstruction and paraplegia. Contrib Nephrol 39:96, 1984.

388. Cotran RS: Pathogenetic mechanisms in the progress of reflux nephropathy: The roles of glomerulosclerosis and extravasation of Tamm-Horsfall protein. *In* Zurukzoglu W, Papadimitriou M, Pyrpasopoulous M, Sion M, Zamboulis C (eds): Advances in Basic and Clinical Nephrology. Basel, S Karger, 1981, p 368.

389. Sanford JP, Hunter BW, Akins LL, Barnett JA: Immunity and obstructive uropathy as determinants in the pathogenesis of experimental pyelonephritis with observations in the distribution of antibody in hydronephrotic kidneys. *In* Kass EH (ed): Progress in Pyelonephritis. Philadelphia, FA Davis, 1965, pp 255-271.

390. Cotran RS: Interstitial nephritis. *In* Churg J, Spargo BH, Mostofi FK, Abell MR (eds): Kidney Disease: Present Status. Baltimore, Williams & Wilkins, 1979, p 254.

391. Gill M, Pudvan WR: The angiographic diagnosis of renal parenchymal diseases. Radiology 96:81, 1970.

392. Hodson CJ: Radiology and the kidney. Contrib Nephrol 5:41, 1977.

393. Kincaid-Smith P, Hodson CJ:, Lesions in the pig kidney with chronic reflux nephropathy. *In* Hodson CJ, Kincaid-Smith P (eds): Reflux Nephropathy. New York, Masson, 1979, pp 197-212.

394. Gill DG, Mendes da Costa B, Cameron JS, et al: Analysis of 100 children with severe and persistent hypertension. Arch Dis Child 51:951, 1976.

395. Holland NH, Kotchen T, Bhathena D: Hypertension in children with chronic pyelonephritis. Kidney Int 8:S43, 1975.

396. Holland NH: Reflux nephropathy and hypertension. *In* Hodson CJ, Kincaid-Smith P (eds): Reflux Nephropathy. New York, Masson, 1970, p 57.

397. Gutman LT, Turck M, Petersdorf RG, Wedgwood RJ: Significance of bacterial variants in urine of patients with chronic bacteriuria. J Clin Invest 44:1945, 1965.

398. Glauser MP, Lyons JM, Braude AI: Prevention of chronic experimental pyelonephritis by suppression of acute suppuration. J Clin Invest 61:403, 1978.

399. Ransley PG, Risdon RA: Reflux nephropathy: Effects of antimicrobial therapy on the evolution of early pyelonephritic scar. Kidney Int 20:733, 1981.

400. Kincaid-Smith P: The Kidney: A Clinicopathologic Study. Oxford, Blackwell Scientific, 1975.

401. Vermillion CD, Heale CD: Ureteral reflux in infancy: Relation to pyelonephritic scarring in adults. Rocky Mt Med J 7:200-204, 1975.

402. Blomjous EM, Meijer CJLM: Pathology of urinary tract infections. *In* Brumfitt W, Hamilton-Miller JMT, Bailey RR (eds): Urinary Tract Infections. London, Chapman & Hall, 1998, p 17.

403. Chrispin AR, Hull D, Lillie JG, Risdon RA: Renal tubular necrosis and papillary necrosis after gastroenteritis in infants. BMJ 1:410, 1970.

404. Chrispin AR: Medullary necrosis in infancy. Br Med Bull 8:33, 1972.

405. Benz G, Willich E, Scharer K: Segmental renal hypoplasia in childhood. Pediatr Radiol 5:86, 1976.

406. Arant BS Jr, Sotelo-Avila C, Bernstein J: Segmental hypoplasia of the kidney (Ask-Upmark). J Pediatr 95:931, 1979.

407. Angell ME, Relman AS, Robbins SL: "Active" chronic pyelonephritis without evidence of bacterial infection. N Engl J Med 78:1303, 1968.

408. Schwartz MM, Cotran RS: Primary renal disease in transplant recipients. Hum Pathol 7:455, 1976.

409. Farmer EF, Heptinstall RH: Chronic non-obstructive pyelonephritis: A reappraisal. *In* Kincaid-Smith P, Fairley KF (eds): Renal Infection and Renal Scarring. Melbourne, Mercedes, 1970.

410. Stewart JF, McCarthy SW, Storey BG, et al: Diseases causing end-stage renal failure in New South Wales. BMJ 1:440, 1975.

411. Kincaid-Smith PS, Bastos MG, Becker GJ: Reflux nephropathy in the adult. Contrib Nephrol 39:94, 1984.

412. Bailey RR: Clinical presentations and diagnosis of vesicoureteric reflux and reflux nephropathy. *In* Davison A (ed): Nephropathy II. Philadelphia, WB Saunders, 1988, pp 835-843.

413. Bailey RR, Lynn KL: End-stage reflux nephropathy. Contrib Nephrol 39:10, 1984.

414. Hodson CJ: Reflux nephropathy: Scoring the damage. *In* Hodson CJ, Kincaid-Smith P (eds): Reflux Nephropathy. New York, Masson, 1979, p 29.

415. Resnick JS, Sisson S, Vernier RL: Tamm-Horsfall protein: Abnormal localization in renal disease. Lab Invest 38:550, 1978.

416. Solez K, Heptinstall RH: Intra-renal urinary extravasation with formation of venous polyps containing Tamm-Horsfall protein. J Urol 119:180, 1977.

417. Heptinstall RH, Bhagavan BS, Solez K: Urinary deposits in veins and interstitium of the kidney: Their possible role in causing renal damage. Contrib Nephrol 16:70, 1979.

418. Papanikolaou G, Arnold AJ, Howie AJ: Tamm-Horsfall protein in reflux nephropathy. Scand J Urol Nephrol 29:141, 1995.

419. Bhathena DB, Holland NH, Weiss JH, et al: Morphology of coarse renal scars in reflux-associated nephropathy in man. *In* Hodson CJ, Kincaid-Smith P (eds): Reflux Nephropathy. New York, Masson, 1979, p 40.

420. Heptinstall RH: Pathology of the Kidney. Boston, Little, Brown, 1983.

421. Kincaid-Smith P: Glomerular lesions in atrophic PN and reflux nephropathy. Kidney Int 8:S81, 1975.

422. Kincaid-Smith P: Glomerular and vascular lesions in chronic atrophic PN and reflux nephropathy. Adv Nephrol 5:3, 1975.

423. Abbott GD: Neonatal bacteriuria: A prospective study in 1,460 infants. BMJ 1:67, 197.

424. Kunin CM: Detection, Prevention and Management of Urinary Tract Infections, 3rd ed. Philadelphia, Lea & Febiger, 1979.

425. Edelman CM Jr, Ogwo JE, Fine BP, Martinez AB: The prevalence of bacteriuria in full-term and premature newborn infants. J Pediatr 8:15, 1973.

426. Rushton Hg, Majd M: Pyelonephritis in male infants: How important is the foreskin? J Urol 148:733, 1992.
427. Spach DH, Stapleton AE, Stamm WE: Lack of circumcision increases the risk of urinary tract infection in young men. JAMA 67:679, 1992.
428. Serour F, Samra Z, Kushel Z, et al: Comparative periurethral bacteriology of uncircumcised and circumcised males. Genitourin Med 73:288, 1997.
429. Wijesinha SS, Atkins BL, Dudley NE, Tam PK: Dose circumcision alter the periurethral bacterial flora? Pediatr Surg Int 13:146, 1998.
430. Kunin CM: The natural history of recurrent bacteriuria in school girls. N Engl J Med 8:1443, 1970.
431. Kunin CM: Epidemiology and natural history of urinary tract infection in school age children. Pediatr Clin North Am 18:50, 1971.
432. Kunin CM: Emergence of bacteriuria, proteinuria and symptomatic urinary tract infections among a population of school girls followed for 7 years. Pediatrics 41:968, 1968.
433. Gillenwater JW, Harrison RB, Kunin CM: Natural history of bacteriuria in school girls: A long-term case control study. N Engl J Med 301:396, 1979.
434. Jones ERV, Miller ST, McLachlan MSF, et al: Treatment of bacteriuria in school girls. Kidney Int Suppl 8:585, 1975.
435. Foxman B: Epidemiology of urinary tract infections—incidence, morbidity, and economic costs. Am J Med 113:55, 2002.
436. Foxman B, Gillespie B, Koopman J, et al: Risk factors for second urinary tract infections among college women. Am J Epidemiol 151:1194, 2000.
437. Waters WE, Elwood PC, Asscher AW, et al: Clinical significance of dysuria. BMJ 2:754, 1970.
438. Freedman LR, Phair JP, Saki M, et al: The epidemiology of urinary tract infections in Hiroshima. Yale J Biol Med 37:262, 1975.
439. Sanford JP: Urinary tract symptoms and infections. Annu Rev Med 26:485, 1976.
440. Silverberg DS: City-wide screening for urinary abnormalities in school boys. Can Med Assoc J 111:410, 1974.
441. Cohen M: The first urinary tract infection in male children. Am J Dis Child 130:810, 1976.
442. Baines RC, Daifuku R, Roddy RE, Stamm WE: Urinary tract infection in sexually active homosexual men. Lancet 1:171, 1986.
443. Foxman B, Zhang L, Tallman P, et al: Transmission of uropathogens between sex partners. J Infect Dis 175:989, 1997.
444. Saxena DR, Bassett DCJ: Sex-related incidence in *Proteus* infection of the urinary tract in childhood. Arch Dis Child 50:899, 1975.
445. Hallet RJ, Pead L, Maskell R: Urinary infection in boys. Lancet 2:1107, 1976.
446. Park J, Buono D, Smith DK, et al: Urinary tract infections in women with or at risk for human immunodeficiency virus infection. Am J Obstet Gynecol 187:581, 2002.
447. Freedman LR: Urinary tract infections in the elderly. N Engl J Med 309:1451, 1983.
448. Dontas AS, Kasviki-Charvati P, Papanayiotou PC, Marketos SG: Bacteriuria and survival in old age. N Engl J Med 304:939, 1981.
449. Nicolle LE: Urinary tract infection in geriatric and institutionalized patients. Curr Opin Urol 12:51, 2002.
450. Millar LK, Cox SM: Urinary tract infections complicating pregnancy. Infect Dis Clin North Am 11:13, 1997.
451. Patterson TF, Andriole VT: Detection, significance, and therapy of bacteriuria in pregnancy: Update in the managed health care era. Infect Dis Clin North Am 11:593, 1997.
452. Zinner SH, Kass EH: Long-term (10 to 14 years) follow-up of bacteriuria of pregnancy. N Engl J Med 285:820, 1971.
453. Martinell J, Jodal U, Lidin-Janson G: Pregnancies in women with and without renal scarring after urinary infections in childhood. BMJ 300:840, 1990.
454. Stenqvist K, Lidin-Janson G, Sandberg T, Eden CS: Bacterial adhesion as an indicator of renal involvement in bacteriuria of pregnancy. Scand J Infect Dis 21:193, 1989.
455. Tullus K, Horlin K, Svenson SB, Kallenius G: Epidemic outbreaks of acute pyelonephritis caused by nosocomial spread of P fimbriated E. coli in children. J Infect Dis 150:728, 1984.
456. Tullus K, Kuhn I, Kallenius G, et al: Fecal colonization with pyelonephrogenic E. coli in neonates as a major factor for pyelonephritis. Eur J Clin Microbiol 5:643, 1986.
457. Tullus K, Kallenius G: Epidemiological aspects of p-fimbriated E. coli: IV. Extraintestinal E. coli infections before the age of

one year and their relation to fecal colonization with p-fimbriated E. coli. Acta paediatr Scand 76:463, 1987.
458. The prevention and management of urinary tract infections among people with spinal cord injuries. National Institute on Disability and Rehabilitation Research Consensus Statement. J Am Paraplegia Soc 15:194, 1992.
459. Montgomerie JZ: Infections in patients with spinal cord injuries. Clin Infect Dis 25:1285, 1997.
460. Rubin RH: Infection in the organ transplant recipient. In Rubin RH, Young LS (eds): Clinical Approach to Infection in the Immunocompromised Host, 4th ed. New York, Kluwer/Academic/Plenum, 2002, p 573.
461. Tolkoff-Rubin NE, Rubin RH: Urinary tract infection in the immunocompromised host: Lessons from kidney transplantation and the AIDS epidemic. Infect Dis Clin North Am 11:707, 1997.
462. Pawlowski J, Blosdoric J, Kimmelstiel P: Chronic pyelonephritis: A morphologic and bacteriologic study. N Engl J Med 286:965, 1960.
463. Freedman L: Chronic pyelonephritis at autopsy. Ann Intern Med 66:697, 1967.
464. Murray T, Goldberg MJ: Chronic interstitial nephritis: Etiologic factors. Ann Intern Med 82:453, 1975.
465. Freedman LR, Andriole V: The long-term follow-up of women with urinary tract infections. In Villarreal H (ed): Proceedings of the 5th International Congress of Nephrology. Basel, S Karger, 1972, p 230.
466. Asscher AW, Chick S, Radfors N, et al: Natural history of asymptomatic bacteriuria in non-pregnant women. In Brumfitt W, Asscher AW (eds): Urinary Tract Infection. London, Oxford University Press, 1973, p 51.
467. Freeman RB, Smith WM, Richardson JA, et al: Long-term therapy for chronic bacteriuria in men: US Public Health Service Cooperative Study. Ann Intern Med 83:133, 1975.
468. Berg UB: Long-term follow-up of renal morphology and function in children with recurrent pyelonephritis. J Urol 148:1715, 1992.
469. Hannerz L, Celsi G, Eklof AC, et al: Ascending pyelonephritis in young rats retards kidney growth. Kidney Int 35:1133, 1989.
470. Hansson S, Martinell J, Stokland E, Jodal U: The natural history of bacteriuria in childhood. Infect Dis Clin North Am 11:499, 1997.
471. Tullus K, Winberg J: Urinary tract infections in childhood. In Brumfitt W, Hamilton-Miller JMT, Bailey RR (eds): Urinary Tract Infections. London, Chapman & Hall, 1998, p 175.
472. Edwards D, Normand ICS, Prescott N, Smellie JM: Disappearance of reflux during long-term prophylaxis of urinary tract infection in children. BMJ 2:285, 1977.
473. Lenaghan D, Whitaber JG, Jemsen F, Stephens FD: The natural history of reflux and long-term effects of reflux on the kidney. J Urol 115:728, 1976.
474. Becker GJ, Kincaid-Smith P: Reflux nephropathy: The glomerular lesion and progression of renal failure. Pediatr Nephrol 7:365, 1993.
475. Coppo R, Porcellini MG, Gianoglio B, et al: Glomerular permselectivity to macromolecules in reflux nephropathy: Microalbuminuria during acute hyperfiltration due to amino acid infusion. Clin Nephrol 40:299, 1993.
476. Jacobson SH, Eklof O, Eriksson CG, et al: Development of hypertension and uraemia after pyelonephritis in childhood: 27 year follow up. BMJ 299:703, 1989.
477. Cunningham FG, Luca MJ, Hankins GD: Pulmonary injury complicating antepartum pyelonephritis. Am J Obstet Gynecol 156:797, 1987.
478. McFadyen IR: Pregnancy bacteriuria and *Escherichia coli*. J R Soc Med 73:227, 1980.
479. Mittendorf R, Lain KY, Williams MA, Walker CK: Preeclampsia: A nested, case-control study of risk factors and their interactions. J Reprod Med 41:491, 1996.
480. Kincaid-Smith P: Bacteriuria and urinary infection in pregnancy. Clin Obstet Gynecol 11:533, 1968.
481. Harris RE, Thomas VL, Shelokov A: Asymptomatic bacteriuria in pregnancy: Antibody-coated bacteria, renal function, and intrauterine growth retardation. Am J Obstet Gynecol 126:20, 1976.
482. McGrady GA, Daling JR, Peterson DR: Maternal urinary tract infection and adverse fetal outcomes. Am J Epidemiol 121:377, 1985.
483. Sever JL, Ellenberg JH, Edmonds D: Urinary tract infection during pregnancy: Maternal and pediatric findings. In Kass EH, Brumfitt W (eds): Infections of the Urinary Tract. Chicago, University of Chicago Press, 1979, p 12.

484. Naeye RL: Cause of the excessive rates of perinatal mortality and prematurity in pregnancies complicated by maternal urinary tract infections. N Engl J Med 300:819, 1979.

485. Coid CR, Landsoun ABG, McFadyen IR: Urinary tract infection in pregnancy. *In* Coid CR (ed): Infections in Pregnancy. London, Academic Press, 1977, p 289.

486. Gilstrap LC III, Whalley PJ: Asymptomatic bacteriuria during pregnancy. *In* Brumfitt W, Hamilton-Miller JMT, Bailey RR (eds): Urinary Tract Infections. London, Chapman & Hall, 1998, p 199.

487. Zinner SH: Bacteriuria and babies revisited. N Engl J Med 300:853, 1979.

488. Gilstrap LC, Leveno KJ, Cunningham FG, et al: Renal infection and pregnancy outcome. Am J Obstet Gynecol 141:709, 1981.

489. McGladdery SL, Aparicio S, Verrier-Jones K, et al: Outcome of pregnancy in an Oxford-Cardiff cohort of women with previous becteriuria. Q J Med 83:533, 1992.

490. Evans DA, Kass EH, Hennekens CH, et al: Bacteriuria and subsequent mortality in women. Lancet 1:156, 1982.

491. Sourander LB, Kasnanen A: A 5 year follow-up of bacteriuria in the aged. Gerontol Clin 14:274, 1972.

492. Platt R, Polk BF, Murdock B, Rosner B: Mortality associated nosocomial urinary tract infection. N Engl J Med 307:637, 1982.

493. Nordenstam GR, Brandberg CA, Oden AS, et al: Bacteriuria and mortality in an elderly population. N Engl J Med 314:1152, 1986.

494. Nicolle LE, Mayhew WJ, Bryan L: Prospective randomized comparison of therapy and no therapy for asymptomatic bacteriuria in institutionalized elderly women. Am J Med 83:27, 1987.

495. Nicolle LE, Henderson E, Bjornsen J, et al: The association of bacteriuria with resident characteristics and survival in elderly institutionalized men. Ann Intern Med 106:682, 1987.

496. Abrutyn E, Mossey J, Berlin JA, et al: Does asymptomatic bacteriuria predict mortailty and does antimicrobial treatment reduce mortality in elderly ambulatory women? Ann Intern Med 120:827, 1994.

497. Nicolle LE: Asymptomatic bacteriuria in the elderly. Infect Dis Clin North Am 11:647, 1997.

498. Johnson JR, Stamm WE: Diagnosis and treatment of acute urinary tract infections. Infect Dis Clin North Am 1:773, 1987.

499. Rubin RH, Shapiro ED, Andriole VT, et al: Evaluation of new anti-infective drugs for the treatment of urinary tract infection. Clin Infect Dis 15(suppl 1): S216, 1992.

500. Stamm WE, Running K, McKevitt M, et al: Treatment of acute urethral syndrome. N Engl J Med 304:956, 1981.

501. Stamm WE, Wagner KF, Amsel R, et al: Causes of the acute urethral syndrome. N Engl J Med 303:409, 1980.

502. Tolkoff-Rubin NE, Weber D, Fang LST, et al: Single-dose therapy with trimethoprim-sulfamethoxazole for urinary tract infection in women. Rev Infect Dis 4:444, 1982.

503. Kraft JA, Stamey TA: The natural history of symptomatic recurrent bacteriuria in women. Medicine (Baltimore) 56:55, 1977.

504. Hoberman A, Chao HP, Keller DM, et al: Prevalence of urinary tract infection in febrile infants. J Pediatr 123:17, 1993.

505. Hoberman A, Wald ER: Urinary tract infections in young febrile children. Pediatr Infect Dis J 16:11, 1997.

506. Rushton HG: Urinary tract infections in children: Epidemiology, evaluation, and management. Pediatr Clin North Am 44:1133, 1997.

507. Thorley JD, Jones SR, Sanford JP: Perinephric abscesses. Medicine (Baltimore) 53:441, 1974.

508. Dembry LM, Andriole VT: Renal and perirenal abscesses. Infect Dis Clin North Am 11:663, 1997.

509. O'Brien JD, Ettinger NA: Nephrobronchial fistula and lung abscess resulting from nephrolithiasis and pyelonephritis. Chest 108:1166, 1995.

510. Miedouge M, Hacini J, Grimont F, Wattine J: Shigatoxin producing *Escherichia coli* urinary tract infections associated with hemolytic-uremic syndrome in an adult and possible adverse effect of ofloxacin therapy. Clin Infect Dis 30:395, 2000.

511. Scheutz F, Olesen B, Norgaard A: Two cases of human urinary tract infection complicated by hemolytic uremic syndrome caused by verotoxin-producing *Escherichia coli*. Clin Infect Dis 31:815, 2000.

512. Rushton HG, Majd M, Jantausch B, et al: Renal scarring following reflux and nonreflux pyelonephritis in children: Evaluation with ^{99m}technetium-dimercaptosuccinic acid scintigraphy. J Urol 147:1372, 1992.

513. Rushton HG, Majd M: Dimercaptosuccinic acid renal scintigraphy for the evaluation of pyelonephritis and scarring: A review of experimental and clinical studies. J Urol 148:1726, 1992.

514. Majd M, Rushton HG: Renal cortical scintigraphy in the diagnosis of acute pyelonephritis. Semin Nucl Med 22:98, 1992.

515. Kass EJ, Fink-Bennett D, Cacciarelli AA, et al: The sensitivity of renal scintigraphy and sonography in detecting nonobstructive acute pyelonephritis. J Urol 148:606, 1992.

516. Jakobsson B, Nolstedt L, Svensson L, et al: ^{99m}Technetium-dimercaptosuccinic acid scan in the diagnosis of acute pyelonephritis in children: Relation to clinical and radiological findings. Pediatr Nephrol 6:328, 1992.

517. Shanon A, Feldman W, McDonald P, et al: Evaluation of renal scars by technetium-labeled dimercaptosuccinic acid scan, intravenous urography, and ultrasonography: A comparative study. J Pediatr 120:399, 1992.

518. Eggli DF, Tulchinsky M: Scintigraphic evaluation of pediatric urinary tract infection. Semin Nucl Med 23:199, 1993.

519. Benador D, Benador N, Slosman DO, et al: Cortical scintigraphy in the evaluation of renal parenchymal changes in children with pyelonephritis. J Pediatr 124:17, 1994.

520. Goldraich NP, Goldraich IH: Update on dimercaptosuccinic acid renal scanning in children with urinary tract infection. Pediatr Nephrol 9:221, 1995.

521. Webb JAW: Imaging in the investigation of urinary tract infections. *In* Brumfitt W, Hamilton-Miller JMT, Bailey RR (eds): Urinary Tract Infections. London, Chapman & Hall, 1998, p 117.

522. Alt JM, Janig H, Schrurek HJ, Stollet H: Study of renal protein excretion in chronic pyelonephritis. Contrib Nephrol 16:37, 1939.

523. Torres VE, Neves JR, Svensson J: Vesicoureteral reflux in the adult: II. Pathogenesis. J Urol 130:10, 1983.

524. Greenfield SP, Ng M, Wan J: Experience with vesicoureteral reflux in children: Clinical characteristics. J Urol 158:574, 1997.

525. Vernon SJ, Coulthard MG, Lambert HJ, et al: New renal scarring in children who at age 3 and 4 years had had normal scans with dimercaptosuccinic acid: Follow up study. BMJ 315:905, 1997.

526. Benador D, Benador N, Slosman D, et al: Are younger children at highest risk of renal sequelae after pyelonephritis? Lancet 349:17, 1997.

527. Martinell J, Claesson I, Lidin-Janson G, Jodal U: Urinary infection, reflux and renal scarring in females continuously followed for 13–38 years. Pediatr Nephrol 9:131, 1995.

528. Hodson CJ: The 1980 Neuhauser Lecture. Am J Radiol 137:451, 1981.

529. Winberg J, Claesson I, Jacobsson B, et al: Renal growth after acute pyelonephritis in childhood: An epidemiological approach. *In* Hodson CJ, Kincaid-Smith P (eds): Reflux Nephropathy. New York, Masson, 1979, p 309.

530. Claesson I, Jacobsson B, Jodal V, Winberg J: Compensatory kidney growth in children with urinary tract infection and unilateral renal scarring: An epidemiological study. Kidney Int 20:759, 1981.

531. Newcastle Covert Bacteriuria Research Group: Covert bacteria in schoolgirls in Newcastle-upon-Tyne: A 5-year follow-up study. Arch Dis Child 56:585, 1981.

532. Bengtsson U: Long-term pattern in chronic pyelonephritis. Contrib Nephrol 16:31, 1979.

533. Gower PE: A prospective study of patients with radiological pyelonephritis, papillary necrosis and obstructive atrophy. Q J Med 45:315, 1976.

534. Gill DG, Mendes da Costa B, Cameron JS, et al: Analysis of 100 children with severe and persistent hypertension. Arch Dis Child 51:951, 1976.

535. Holland NH, Kotchen T, Bhathena D: Hypertension in children with chronic pyelonephritis. Kidney Int 8:S243, 1975.

536. Holland NH: Reflux nephropathy and hypertension. *In* Hodson CJ, Kincaid-Smith P (eds): Reflux Nephropathy. New York, Masson, 1979, p 257.

537. Rance CP, Arbus GS, Balfe JW, Kooh SW: Persistent systematic hypertension in infants and children. Pediatr Clin North Am 21:735, 1976.

538. Wallace DMA, Rothwell DL, Williams DI: The long-term followup of surgically-treated vesicoureteral reflux. Br J Urol 50:479, 1978.

539. Martinell J, Lidin-Janson G, Jagenburg R, et al: Girls prone to urinary infections followed into adulthood: Indices of renal disease. Pediatr Nephrol 10:139, 1996.

540. Goonasekera CED, Shah V, Wade AM, et al: 15-year follow-up of renin and blood pressure in reflux nephropathy. Lancet 347:640, 1996.

541. Kohler J, Tencer J, Thysell H, Forsberg L: Vesicoureteral reflux diagnosed in adulthood: Incidence of urinary tract infections, hypertension, proteinuria, back pain and renal calculi. Nephrol Dial Transplant 12:2580, 1997.

542. Bailey RR, McRae CU, Mailing TMJ, et al: Renal vein renin concentration in the hypertension of unilateral reflux nephropathy. J Urol 120:21, 1978.

543. Savage JM, Shah V, Dillon MJ, et al: Renin and blood pressure in children with renal scarring and vesicoureteral reflux. Lancet 2:441, 1978.

544. Bailey RR, Lynn KL, McRae CU: Unilateral reflux nephropathy and hypertension. Contrib Nephrol 39:116, 1984.

545. Savage JM, Koh CT, Shah V, et al: Five-year prospective study of plasma renin activity and blood pressure in patients with corresponding reflux nephropathy. Arch Dis Child 62:678, 1987.

546. Cotran RS: Glomerulosclerosis in reflux nephropathy. Kidney Int 21:528, 198.

547. Delano BG, Goodwin NJ, Thomson GE, et al: Chronic pyelonephritis as a cause of massive proteinuria of nephrotic syndrome. Arch Intern Med 129:73, 1972.

548. Woods HF, Walls J: Nephrotic syndrome in vesicoureteral reflux. BMJ 2:917, 1976.

549. Kincaid-Smith P: Clinical implications of reflux in the adult. In Zurukzoglu W, et al (eds): Advances in Basic and Clinical Nephrology. Basel, S Karger, 1981, p 359.

550. Karlen J, Linne T, Wikstad I, Aperia A: Incidence of microalbuminuria in children with pyelonephritic scarring. Pediatr Nephrol 10:705, 1996.

551. Senekjian HO, Stinebaugh BJ, Mattioli CA, Suki WN: Irreversible renal failure following vesicoureteral reflux. JAMA 241:160, 1979.

552. Aladjem M, Schoeneman JJ, Bennett B, et al: Focal segmental glomerulosclerosis with proteinuria and chronic interstitial nephritis. N Y State J Med 78:579, 1978.

553. Torres VE, Velosa JA, Holley KE, et al: The progression of vesicoureteral reflux nephropathy. Ann Intern Med 92:776, 1980.

554. Zimmerman SW, Uehling DT, Burkholder PM: Vesicoureteral reflux nephropathy: Evidence for immunologically mediated glomerular injury. Urology 2:531, 1973.

555. Bhathena DB, Weiss JH, Holland NH, et al: Focal and segmental glomerular sclerosis in reflux nephropathy (chronic pyelonephritis). Am J Med 68:886, 1980.

556. Schwartz MM, Cotran RS: Primary renal disease in transplant recipients. Hum Pathol 7:455, 1976.

557. Velosa J, Miller K, Michael AF: Immunopathology of end-stage kidney: Immunoglobulin and complement deposition in nonimmune disease. Am J Pathol 84:149, 1976.

558. Yoshioka K, Takemura T, Matsubara K, et al: Immunohistochemical studies of reflux nephropathy: The role of extracellular matrix, membrane, attack complex, and immune cells in glomerulosclerosis. Am J Pathol 129:223, 1987.

559. Raij L, Keane WF, Osswald H, Michael AF: Mesangial function in ureteral obstruction in the rat: Blockade of the efferent limb. J Clin Invest 64:1204, 1979.

560. Hostetter RH, Olson JL, Rennke HG, et al: Hyperfiltration in remnant nephrons: A potentially adverse response to renal ablation. Am J Physiol 241:F85, 1981.

561. Olson JL, Hostetter TH, Rennke HG, et al: Altered charge and size-selective properties of the glomerular wall: A response to reduced renal mass. Kidney Int 22:112, 1982.

562. Bailey RR, Swainson CP, Lynn KL, Burry AF: Glomerular lesions in the "normal" kidney in patients with unilateral reflux nephropathy. Contrib Nephrol 39:126, 1984.

563. Verrier Jones K, Asscher W, Verrier Jones R, et al: Renal functional changes in schoolgirls with covert asymptomatic bacteriuria. Contrib Nephrol 39:152, 1984.

564. Khatib ML, Becker GJ, Kincaid-Smith P: Morphometric aspects of reflux nephropathy. Kidney Int 32:261, 1987.

565. Bartlett RC, O'Neill D, McLaughlin JC: Detection of bacteriuria by leukocyte esterase, nitrate, and the automicrobic system. Am J Clin Pathol 82:683, 1984.

566. Pollack HM: Laboratory techniques for detection of urinary tract infection and assessment of value. Am J Med 75:79, 1983.

567. Sanderson PJ: Laboratory methods. In Brumfitt W, Hamilton-Miller JMT, Bailey RR (eds): Urinary Tract Infection. London, Chapman & Hall, 1998, p 1.

568. Guignard JP, Torrado N: Nitrite indicator strip test for bacteriuria. Lancet 1:47, 1978.

569. Lejeune B, Baron R, Guillois B, Mayeux D: Evaluation of a screening test for detecting urinary tract infection in newborns and infants. J Clin Pathol 44:1029, 1991.

570. Evans PJ, Leaker BR, McNabb WR, Lewis RR: Accuracy of reagent strip testing for urinary tract infection in the elderly. J R Soc Med 84:598, 1991.

571. Lachs MS, Nachamkin I, Edelstein PH, et al: Spectrum bias in the evaluation of diagnostic tests: Lessons from the rapid dipstick test for urinary tract infection. Ann Intern Med 117:135, 1992.

572. Bachman JW, Heise RH, Naessens JM, Timmerman MG: A study of various tests to detect asymptomatic urinary tract infections in an obstetric population. JAMA 270:1971, 1993.

573. Fang LST, Tolkoff-Rubin NE, Rubin RH: Efficacy of single-dose and conventional amoxicillin therapy in urinary tract infection localized by the antibody-coated bacteria technique. N Engl J Med 298:413, 1979.

574. Fairley KF, Carson NE, Gutch RC, et al: Site of infection in acute urinary tract infection in general practice. Lancet 2:615, 1971.

575. Norden CW, Levy PS, Kass EH: Predictive effect of urinary concentrating ability and hemagglutinizing antibody taken upon response to antimicrobial therapy in bacteriuria of pregnancy. J Infect Dis 121:588, 1970.

576. Clark H, Ronald AR, Cutler RE, Turck M: The correlation between site of infection and maximal concentrating ability in bacteriuria. J Infect Dis 120:47, 1969.

577. Ronald AR, Cutler RE, Turck M: Effect of bacteriuria on the renal concentrating mechanism. Ann Intern Med 70:723, 1969.

578. Levison SP, Levison ME: Effect of indomethacin and sodium meclofenamate on the renal concentrating defect in experimental enterococcal pyelonephritis in rats. J Lab Clin Med 88:958, 1976.

579. Levison SP, Levison ME: Papillary plasma flow in experimental pyelonephritis in rats: Effect of antibiotic therapy and indomethacin. J Lab Clin Med 92:570, 1978.

580. Jodal U, Lindberg U, Lincoln K: Level diagnosis of symptomatic urinary tract infections in childhood. Acta Paediatr Scand 64:201, 1975.

581. Jodal U, Hanson LA: Sequential determination of C-reactive protein in acute childhood pyelonephritis. Acta Paediatr Scand 65:319, 1976.

582. Sabel KG, Hanson LA: The clinical usefulness of C-reactive protein (CRP) determinations in bacterial meningitis and septicemia in infancy. Acta Paediatr Scand 63:381, 1974.

583. Hellerstein S, Duggan E, Welchert E, Mansour F: Serum C-reactive protein and the site of urinary tract infections. J Pediatr 100:21, 1982.

584. Rubin RH, Cotran RS: Immunological aspects of pyelonephritis with a critical survey of antibody-coated bacteria test. In Losse H, Asscher AW (eds): Pyelonephritis, Vol 4. Urinary Tract Infections. Stuttgart, Georg Thieme Verlag, 1980, p 124.

585. Percival A, Brumfitt W, DeLouvois J: Serum antibody levels as an indication of clinically apparent pyelonephritis. Lancet 2:1027, 1964.

586. Clark H, Ronald AR, Turck M: Serum antibody response in renal versus bladder bacteriuria. J Infect Dis 123:539, 1971.

587. Thomas V, Shelokov A, Forland M: Antibody-coated bacteria in the urine and the site of urinary tract infection. N Engl J Med 290:588, 1974.

588. Jones SR, Smith JW, Sanford JP: Localization of urinary tract infections by detection of antibody-coated bacteria in urine sediment. N Engl J Med 290:591, 1974.

589. Montplaisir S, Cote PA, Martineau B, et al: Localisation du site de l'infection urinaire chez l'enfant par la recherche de bactéries découvertes d'anticorps. Can Med Assoc J 115:1096, 1976.

590. Thomas VL, Harris RE, Gilstrap LC III: Antibody-coated bacteria in the urine of hospitalized patients with acute pyelonephritis. J Infect Dis 131(suppl): S57, 1975.

591. Montplaisir S, Courteau C, Roche AJ: Antibody-coated bacteria in contaminated urine specimens. N Engl J Med 296:758, 1977.

592. Braude R, Block C: Proteinuria and antibody-coated bacteria in the urine. N Engl J Med 297:617, 1977.

593. Riedasch F, Ritz E, Mohring K, Bommer J: Antibody coating of urinary bacteria: Relation to site of infection and invasion of uroepithelium. Clin Nephrol 10:239, 1978.

594. Rumans LW, Vosti KL: The relationship of antibody-coated bacteria to clinical syndromes, as found in unselected populations with bacteriuria. Arch Intern Med 138:1077, 1978.

595. Hellerstein S, Kennedy E, Nussbaum L, Rice K: Localization of the site of urinary tract infections by means of antibody-coated bacteria in the urinary sediments. J Pediatr 92:188, 1978.

596. Smith JW, Jones SR, Kaijser B: Significance of antibody-coated bacteria in urinary sediment in experimental pyelonephritis. J Infect Dis 135:577, 1977.

597. Savard-Fenton M, Fenton BW, Roller LB, et al: Single-dose amoxicillin therapy with follow-up urine culture: Effective initial management for acute uncomplicated urinary tract infections. Am J Med 73: 808, 1982.

598. Smellie JM, Rigden SP: Pitfalls in the investigation of children with urinary tract infection. Arch Dis Child 72:251, 1995.

599. Clarke SE, Smellie JM, Prescod N, et al: Technetium-99m-DMSA studies in pediatric urinary infection. J Nucl Med 37:823, 1996.

600. Stokland E, Hellstrom M, Jacobsson B, et al: Renal damage one year after first urinary tract infection: Role of dimercaptosuccinic acid scintigraphy. J Pediatr 129:815, 1996.

601. Lavocat MP, Granjon D, Allard D, et al: Imaging of pyelonephritis. Pediatr Radiol 27:159, 1997.

602. Craig JC, Knight JF, Sureshkumar P, et al: Vesicoureteric reflux and timing of micturating cystourethrography after urinary tract infection. Arch Dis Child 76:275, 1997.

603. Stark H: Urinary tract infections in girls: The cost-effectiveness of currently recommended investigative routines. Pediatr Nephrol 11: 174, 1997.

604. Fair WR, McClennan BL, Jost RG: Are excretory urograms necessary in evaluating women with urinary tract infection? J Urol 121: 313, 1979.

605. Engel G, Schaeffer AJ, Grayback JT, Wendel EF: The role of excretory urography and cystoscopy in the evaluation and management of women with recurrent urinary tract infection. J Urol 123:190, 1980.

606. Fowler JE Jr, Pulaski ET: Excretory urography, cystography and cystoscopy in the evaluation of women with urinary tract infection: A prospective study. N Engl J Med 304:462, 1981.

607. Delange EE, Jones B: Unnecessary intravenous urography in young women with recurrent urinary tract infections. Clin Radiol 34:551, 1983.

608. Sandberg T, Stokland E, Brolin I, et al: Selective use of excretory urography in women with acute pyelonephritis. J Urol 141:1290, 1989.

609. Nickel JC, Wilson J, Morales A, Heaton J: Value of urologic investigation in a targeted group of women with recurrent urinary tract infections. Can J Surg 34:591, 1991.

610. Warren JW, Abrutyn E, Hebel JR, et al: Guidelines for antimicrobial treatment of uncomplicated acute bacterial cystitis and acute pyelonephritis in women. Infectious Diseases Society of America (IDSA). Clin Infect Dis 29:745, 1999.

611. Herthelius M, Mollby R, Nord CE, Winberg J: Amoxicillin promotes vaginal colonization with adhering *Escherichia coli* present in faeces. Pediatr Nephrol 3:443, 1989.

612. Manges AR, Johnson JR, Foxman B, et al: Widespread distribution of urinary tract infection caused by a multiresistant *Escherichia coli* clonal group. N Engl J Med 345:1007, 2001.

613. Raz R, Chazen B, Kenner Y, et al: Empiric use of trimethoprim-sulfamethoxazole in the treatment of women with uncomplicated urinary tract infections in a geographic area with a high prevalence of TMP-SMX-resistant uropathogens. Clin Infect Dis 34:1165, 2002.

614. Karlowsky JA, Kelly LJ, Thornsberry C, et al: Trends in antimicrobial resistance among urinary tract infection isolates of *Escherichia coli* from female outpatients in the United States. Antimicrob Agents Chemother 46:2540, 2002.

615. Gupta K, Stamm WE: Outcomes associated with trimethoprim/sulphamethoxazole (TMP/SMX) therapy in TMP/SMX resistant community-acquired urinary tract infection. Int J Antimicrob Agents 19:554, 2002.

616. Gupta K, Sahm DF, Mayfield D, Stamm WE: Antimicrobial resistance among uropathogens that cause community acquired urinary tract infections in women: A nationwide analysis. Clin Infect Dis 33:89, 2001.

617. Ronald AR, Boutros P, Mourtoda H: Bacteriuria localization and response to single-dose therapy in women. JAMA 235:1854, 1976.

618. Nicolle LE, Ronald AR: Recurrent urinary tract infections in adult women: Diagnosis and treatment. Infect Dis Clin North Am 1:793, 1987.

619. Bailey RR: Single-Dose Therapy of Urinary Tract Infection. Sydney, ADIS Health Science Press, 1983.

620. Tolkoff-Rubin NE, Wilson ME, Zuromskis P, et al: Single-dose amoxicillin therapy of acute uncomplicated urinary tract infection in women. Antimicrob Agents Chemother 25:626, 1984.

621. Harbord RB, Gruneborg RN: Treatment of urinary tract infection with a single dose of amoxicillin, co-trimoxazole, or trimethoprim. BMJ 303:409, 1981.

622. Ludwig P, Buckwold F, Harding G, et al: Single-dose therapy of acute cystitis is adult females: Prospective randomized comparison of four regimes. *In* Nelson JD, Grass C (eds): Current Chemotherapy and Infectious Disease–1980. Washington, DC, American Society for Microbiology, 1980, p 1297.

623. Counts GW, Stamm WE, McKevitt M, et al: Treatment of cystitis in women with a single-dose of trimethoprim-sulfamethoxazole. Rev Infect Dis 4:484, 1982.

624. Fairley KF, Whitworth JA, Kincaid-Smith P, Durman O: Single-dose therapy in management of urinary tract infection. Med J Aust 2:75, 1978.

625. Kallenius F, Winberg J: Urinary tract infections treated with a single dose of short-acting sulfonamide. BMJ 1:1175, 1979.

626. Johnson JR, Stamm WE: Diagnosis and treatment of acute urinary tract infections. Infect Dis Clin North Am 1:773, 1987.

627. Greenberg RN, Reilly PM, Luppen KL, et al: Randomized study of single-dose three-day, and seven-day treatment of cystitis in women. J Infect Dis 153:277, 1986.

628. Fihn SD, Johnson C, Roberts PL, et al: Trimethoprim-sulfamethoxazole for acute dysuria in women: A single-dose or 10-day course. A double-blind, randomized trial. Ann Intern Med 108:350, 1988.

629. Tolkoff-Rubin NE, Rubin RH: New approaches to the treatment of urinary tract infection. Am J Med 82(suppl 4A):270, 1987.

630. Johnson JR, Stamm WE: Urinary tract infections in women: Diagnosis and treatment. Ann Intern Med 111:906, 1989.

631. Inter-Nordic Urinary Tract Infection Study Group: Double-blind comparison of 3-day versus 7-day treatment with norfloxacin in symptomatic urinary tract infections. Scand J Infect Dis 20:619, 1988.

632. Hooton TM, Johnson C, Winter C, et al: Single dose and three day regimens of ofloxacin versus trimethoprim-sulfamethoxazole for acute cystitis in women. Antimicrob Agents Chemother 35:1479, 1991.

633. Norrby SR: Short term treatment of uncomplicated lower urinary tract infections in women. Rev Infect Dis 12:458, 1990.

634. Hooton TM, Stamm WE: Management of acute uncomplicated urinary tract infection in adults. Med Clin North Am 75:339, 1991.

635. Pappas PG: Laboratory in the diagnosis and management of urinary tract infections. Med Clin North Am 75:313, 1991.

636. Carlson KJ, Mulley AG: Management of acute dysuria: A decision-analysis model of alternative strategies. Ann Intern Med 102:244, 1985.

637. Harding GKM, Ronald AR: A controlled study of antimicrobial prophylaxis of recurrent urinary infection in women. N Engl J Med 291:597, 1974.

638. Ronald AR, Harding GKM: Urinary infection prophylaxis in women. Ann Intern Med 9:268, 1981.

639. Holmber L, Boman G, Bottinger LE, et al: Adverse reactions to nitrofurantoin: Analysis of 921 reports. Am J Med 69:733, 1980.

640. Harding GKM, Buckwald FJ, Marrie TJ, et al: Prophylaxis of recurrent urinary tract infection in female patients: Efficacy of low dose, thrice weekly therapy with trimethoprim-sulfamethoxazole. JAMA 224:1975, 1979.

641. Tolkoff-Rubin NE, Rubin RH: Ciprofloxacin in the management of urinary tract infection. Urology 31:359, 1988.

642. Stapleton A, Latham RH, Johnson C, Stamm WE: Postcoital antimicrobial prophylaxis for recurrent urinary tract infection: A randomized, double-blind, placebo-controlled trial. JAMA 264:703, 1990.

643. Wong-Beringer A, Jacobs RA, Guglielmo BJ: Treatment of funguria. JAMA 207:2780, 1992.

644. Wong ES, McKevitt M, Running K, et al: Management of recurrent urinary tract infections with patient-administered single dose therapy. Ann Intern Med 102:302, 1985.

645. Gupta K, Hooton TM, Roberts PL, Stamm WE: Patient-initiated treatment of uncomplicated recurrent urinary tract infections in young women. Ann Intern Med 135:9, 2001.

646. Stathers L: A randomized trial to evaluate effectiveness and cost-effectiveness of naturopathic cranberry products as prophylaxis against urinary tract infections in women. Can J Urol 9:1558, 2002.

647. Kontiokari T, Sundquist K, Nuutinen M, et al: Randomized trial of cranberry-lingonberry juice and lactobacillus drink for the prevention of urinary tract infection in women. BMJ 322:1571, 2001.

648. Howell AB: Cranberry proanthocyanidins and the maintenance of urinary tract health. Crit Rev Food Sci Nutr 42:273, 2002.

649. Turck M, Anderson KN, Petersdorf RG: Relapse and reinfection in chronic bacteriuria. N Engl J Med 275:70, 1966.

650. Sobel JD, Muller G: Pathogenesis of bacteriuria in elderly women: The role of *Escherichia coli* adherence to vaginal epithelial cells. J Gerontol 39:682, 1984.

651. Romano JM, Kaye D: UTI in the elderly: Common yet atypical. Geriatrics 36:113, 1981.

652. Molander U, Milson I, Ekelund P, et al: Effect of oral oestriol on vaginal flora and cytology and urogenital symptoms in the postmenopause. Maturitas 12:113, 1990.

653. Raz R, Stamm WE: A controlled trial of intravaginal estriol in postmenopausal women with recurrent urinary tract infections. N Engl J Med 329:753, 1993.

654. Parsons CL, Schmitd JD: Control of recurrent lower urinary tract infection in postmenopausal women. J Urol 12:1224, 1982.

655. Brandberg A, Mellstrom D, Samside G: Low dose oral estriol treatment in elderly women with urogenital infections. Acta Obstet Gynecol Scand Suppl 140:33, 1987.

656. Avorn J, Monane M, Gurwitz JH, et al: Reduction of bacteriuria and pyuria after ingestion of cranberry juice. JAMA 271:751, 1994.

657. Zafriri D, Ofek I, Adar R, et al: Inhibitory activity of cranberry juice on adherence of type 1 and P fimbriated *Escherichia coli* to eukaryotic cells. Antimicrob Agents Chemother 33:92, 1989.

658. Ofek I, Goldhar J, Zafriri D, et al: Anti-*Escherichia* adhesin activity of cranberry and blueberry juices. N Engl J Med 324:1599, 1991.

659. Abrutyn E, Berlin J, Mossey J, et al: Does treatment of asymptomatic bacteriuria in older ambulatory women reduce subsequent symptoms of urinary tract infection? J Am Geriatr Soc 44:293, 1996.

660. Bailey RR, Begg EJ, Smith AH, et al: Prospective, randomized, controlled study comparing two dosing regimens of gentamicin/oral ciprofloxacin switch therapy for acute pyelonephritis. Clin Nephrol 46:183, 1996.

661. Zinner SH: Management of urinary tract infections in pregnancy: A review with comments on single dose therapy. Infection 20(suppl 4): S280, 1992.

662. Sanchez-Ramos L, McAlpine KJ, Adair CD, et al: Pyelonephritis in pregnancy: Once-a-day ceftriaxone versus multiple doses of cefazolin. A randomized, double-blind trial. Am J Obstet Gynecol 172:129, 1995.

663. Millar LK, Wing DA, Paul RH, Grimes DA: Outpatient treatment of pyelonephritis in pregnancy: A randomized controlled trial. Obstet Gynecol 86:560, 1995.

664. Pfau A, Sacks TG: Effective prophylaxis for recurrent urinary tract infections during pregnancy. Clin Infect Dis 14:810, 1992.

665. Sandberg T, Brorson JE: Efficacy of long term antimicrobial prophylaxis after acute pyelonephritis in pregnancy. Scand J Infect Dis 23:221, 1991.

666. Wong ES, Stamm WE: Sexual acquisition of urinary tract infection in a man. JAMA 250:3087, 1983.

667. Hoepelman AI, van Buren M, van den Broek J, Borleffs JC: Bacteriuria in men infected with HIV-1 is related to their immune status (CD4+ cell count). AIDS 6:179, 1992.

668. Tolkoff-Rubin NE, Rubin RH: Urinary tract infection in the immunocompromised host: Lessons from kidney transplantation and the AIDS epidemic. Infect Dis Clin North Am 11:707, 1997.

669. Meares EM Jr: Acute and chronic prostatitis: Diagnosis and treatment. Infect Dis Clin North Am 1:855, 1987.

670. Gleckman R, Crowley M, Natsios GA: Therapy of recurrent invasive urinary tract infections of men. N Engl J Med 301:878, 1979.

671. Smith JW, Jones SR, Reed WP, et al: Recurrent urinary tract infection in men: Characteristics and response to therapy. Am Intern Med 91:544, 1979.

672. Pewitt EB, Schaeffer AJ: Urinary tract infection in urology, including acute and chronic prostatitis. Infect Dis Clin North Am 11:623, 1997.

673. Avner ED, Ingelfinger JR, Herrin JT, et al: Single-dose amoxicillin therapy of uncomplicated pediatric urinary tract infections. J Pediatr 102:63, 1983.

674. Mofatt M, Embrec J, Grimm P, Law B: Short-course antibiotic therapy for urinary tract infections in children: A methodological review of the literature. Am J Dis Child 142:57, 1988.

675. Madrigal G, Odio CM, Mohs E, et al: Single-dose antibiotic therapy is not as effective as conventional regimens for management of acute urinary tract infections in children. Pediatr Infect Dis J 7:316, 1988.

676. Fine JS, Jacobsen MS: Single-dose versus conventional therapy of urinary tract infections in female adolescents. Pediatrics 75:916, 1985.

677. Durbin WA Jr, Peter G: Management of urinary tract infections in infants and children. Pediatr Infect Dis 3:564, 1984.

678. McCracken GH Jr: Options in antimicrobial management of urinary tract infections in infants and children. Pediatr Infect Dis J 8:552, 1989.

679. Smellie JM, Gruneberg RN, Leahey A, et al: Long-term low-dose co-trimoxazole in prophylaxis of childhood urinary tract infection: Clinical aspects. BMJ 2:203, 1976.

680. Marks MI: Cystitis. *In* Feigin RD, Cherry JD (eds): Textbook of Pediatric Infectious Diseases. Philadelphia, WB Saunders, 1981, p 352.

681. Belman AB, Skoog SJ: Nonsurgical approach to the management of vesicoureteral reflux in children. Pediatr Infect Dis J 8:556, 1989.

682. Loening-Baucke V: Urinary incontinence and urinary tract infection and their resolution with treatment of chronic constipation of childhood. Pediatrics 100:228, 1997.

683. Birmingham Reflux Study Group: Prospective trial of operative versus non-operative treatment of severe vesicoureteric reflux in children: Five years' observation. BMJ 295:237, 1987.

684. Duckett JW, Walker RD, Weiss R: Surgical results: International Reflux Study in Children—United States branch. J Urol 148:1674, 1992.

685. Weiss R, Duckett J, Spitzer A: Results of a randomized clinical trial of medical versus surgical management of infants and children with grades III and IV primary vesicoureteral reflux (United States). The International Reflux Study in Children. J Urol 148:1667, 1992.

686. Tamminen-Mobius T, Brunier E, Ebel KD, et al: Cessation of vesicoureteral reflux for 5 years in infants and children allocated to medical treatment: The International Reflux Study in Children. J Urol 148:1662, 1992.

687. Hjalmas K, Lohr G, Tamminen-Mobius T, et al: Surgical results in the International Reflux Study in Children (Europe). J Urol 148:1657, 1992.

688. Olbing H, Claesson I, Ebel KD, et al: Renal scars and parenchymal thinning in children with vesicoureteral reflux: A 5-year report of the International Reflux Study in Children (European branch). J Urol 148:1653, 1992.

689. Jodal U, Koskimies O, Hanson E, et al: Infection pattern in children with vesicoureteral reflux randomly allocated to operation or long term antibacterial prophylaxis. The International Reflux Study in Children. J Urol 148:1650, 1992.

690. Arant BS Jr: Medical management of mild and moderate vesicoureteral reflux: Followup studies of infants and young children. A preliminary report of the Southwest Pediatric Nephrology Study Group. J Urol 148:1683, 1992.

691. McLorie GA, McKenna PH, Jumper BM, et al: High grade vesicoureteral reflux: Analysis of observational therapy. J Urol 144:537, 1990.

692. Smellie JM: Commentary: Management of children with severe vesicoureteral reflux. J Urol 148:1676, 1992.

693. Elder JS, Peters CA, Arant BS Jr, et al: Pediatric Vesicoureteral Reflux Guidelines Panel summary report on the management of primary vesicoureteral reflux in children. J Urol 157:1846, 1997.

694. Banovac K, Wade N, Gonzalez F, et al: Decreased incidence of urinary tract infections in patients with spinal cord injury: Effect of methenamine. J Am Paraplegia Soc 14:52, 1991.

695. Perrouin-Verbe B, Labat JJ, Richard I, et al: Clean intermittent catheterisation from the acute period in spinal cord injury patients: Long term evaluation of urethral and genital tolerance, Paraplegia 33:619, 1995.

696. Larsen KDM, Chamberlin DA, Khonsari F, Ahlering TE: Retrospective analysis of urologic complications in male patients with spinal cord injury managed with and without indwelling urinary catheters. Urology 50:418, 1997.

697. Kreger BE, Craven DE, Carling PC, McCabe WR: Gram-negative bacteremia: III. Reassessment of etiology, epidemiology and ecology in 612 patients. Am J Med 68:332, 1980.

698. Warren JW: Catheter-associated urinary tract infections. Infect Dis Clin North Am 11:609, 1997.

699. Nickel JC, Gristina AG, Costerton JW: Electron microscopic study of an infected Foley catheter. Can J Surg 28:50, 1985.

700. Nickel JC, Ruseka I, Wright JB, Costerton JW: Tobramycin resistance of *Pseudomonas aeruginosa* cells growing as a biofilm on urinary catheter material. Antimicrob Agents Chemother 27:619, 1985.

701. Platt R, Polk BF, Murdock B, Rosner B: Risk factors for nosocomial urinary tract infection. Am J Epidemiol 124:977, 1986.

702. Johnson JR, Roberts PL, Olsen RJ, et al: Prevention of catheter-associated urinary tract infection with a silver oxide–coated urinary catheter. Clinical and microbiologic correlates. J Infect Dis 162:1145, 1990.

703. Fryjkybd B, Haeggman S, Burman LG: Transmission of urinary bacterial strains between patients with indwelling catheters: Nursing in the same room and in separate rooms compared. J Hosp Infect 36:147, 1997.

704. Matsumoto T, Sakumoto M, Takahashi K, Kumazawa J: Prevention of catheter-associated urinary tract infection by meatal disinfection. Dermatology 195(suppl 2):73, 1997.

705. Wong-Beringer A, Jacobs RA, Guglielmo BJ: Treatment of funguria. JAMA 267:2780, 1992.

706. Jacobs LG, Skidmore EA, Cardoso LA, Ziv F: Bladder irrigation with amphotericin B for treatment of fungal urinary tract infections. Clin Infect Dis 18:313, 1994.

707. Potasman I, Castin A, Moskovitz B, et al: Oral fluconazole for *Candida* urinary tract infection. Urol Int 59:252, 1997.

708. Jacobs LG, Skidmore EA, Freeman K, et al: Oral fluconazole compared with bladder irrigation with amphotericin B for treatment of fungal urinary tract infections in elderly patients. Clin Infect Dis 22:30, 1996.

709. Hibberd PH, Rubin PH: Clinical aspects of fungal infection in organ transplant recipients. Clin Infect Dis 19(suppl 1):533, 1994.

710. Lundstrom T, Sobel J: Nosocomial candiduria: A review. Clin Infect Dis 32:1602, 2001.

711. Sobel JD, Kauffman CA, McKinsey D, et al: Candiduria: A randomized, double-blind study of treatment with fluconzaole and placebo. The National Institute of Allergy and Infectious Disease (NIAID) Mycosis Study Group. Clin Infect Dis 30:19, 2000.

712. Simon HB, Weinstein AJ, Pasternak MS, et al: Genitourinary tuberculosis: Clinical features in a general hospital population. Am J Med 63:410, 1977.

713. Garcia-Rodriguez JA, Garcia Sanchez JE, Munoz Bellido JL, et al: Genitourinary tuberculosis in Spain: Review of 81 cases. Clin Infect Dis 18:557, 1994.

714. Christiansen WJ: Genitourinary tuberculosis: Review of 102 cases. Medicine (Baltimore) 53:377, 1974.

715. Narayana AS: Overview of renal tuberculosis. Urology 19:231, 1982.

716. Hartman DS: Radiologic-pathologic correlation of the infectious granulomatous diseases of the kidney. Monogr Urol 6:3, 1985.

717. Malek RS, Eza S, Elder JS: Xanthogranulomatous pyelonephritis: A critical analysis of 26 cases and of the literature. J Urol 119:589, 1978.

718. Parson MA, Harris SC, Longstaff AJ, Grainger RG: Xanthogranulomatous pyelonephritis: A pathological, clinical and etiological analysis of 87 cases. Diagn Histopathol 6:203, 1983.

719. Goodman M, Curry T, Russell T: Xanthogranulomatous pyelonephritis: A local disease with systemic manifestations. Report of 23 cases and review of the literature. Medicine (Baltimore) 58:171, 1979.

720. Braun G, Moussali L, Balamzar JL: Xanthogranulomatous pyelonephritis in children. J Urol 133:326, 1985.

721. Clapton WK, Boucat HA, Dewan PA, et al: Clinicopathological features of xanthogranulomatous pyelonephritis in infancy. Pathology 25:110, 1993.

722. Hammadeh MY, Nicholls G, Calder CJ, et al: Xanthogranulomatous pyelonephritis in childhood: Preoperative diagnosis is possible. Br J Urol 73:83, 1994.

723. Rossi P, Myers DH, Furey R, Bonfils-Roberts EA: Angiography in bilateral xanthogranulomatous pyelonephritis. Radiology 93:20, 1968.

724. Nataluk EA, McCullough DL, Scharling EO: Xanthogranulomatous pyelonephritis, the gatekeepers' dilemma: A contemporary look at an old problem. Urology 45:377, 1995.

725. Cowley JP, Connolly CE, Hehir M, O'Brien SF: Renal carcinoma with staghorn calculus, perinephritic abscess, and xanthogranulomatous pyelonephritis in same kidney. Urology 21:635, 1983.

726. Piscioli F, Luciani L: Association of xanthogranulomatous pyelonephritis with small renal cell carcinoma: Case report and review of the literature. Eur Urol 10:62, 1984.

727. List AR, Johansson SL, Nilson AE, Pettersson S: Xanthogranulomatous pyelonephritis and renocolic fistula and coexistent contralateral renal carcinoma. Scand J Urol Nephrol 17:139, 1983.

728. Lopez-Medina A, Ereno MJ, Fernandez-Canton G, Zuazo A: Focal xanthogranulomatous pyelonephritis simulating malignancy in children. Abdom Imaging 20:270, 1995.

729. Marteinsson VT, Due J, Aagenaes I: Focal xanthogranulomatous pyelonephritis presenting as renal tumour in children: Case report with a review of the literature. Scand J Urol Nephrol 30:235, 1996.

730. Val-Bernal JF, Castro F: Xanthogranulomatous pyelonephritis associated with transitional cell carcinoma of the renal pelvis. Urol Int 57:240, 1996.

731. Crane LM, McClellan L: Xanthogranulomatous pyelonephritis. J Can Assoc Radiol 27:45, 1976.

732. Gammill S, Rabinowitz JG, Peace R, et al: New thoughts concerning xanthogranulomatous pyelonephritis. AJR Am J Roentgenol 125:154, 1975.

733. Subramanyam BR, Megibow AJ, Rashavendra BN, Bosniak MA: Diffuse xanthogranulomatous pyelonephritis: Analysis by computed tomography and sonography. Urol Radiol 4:5, 1982.

734. Solomon A, Braf Z, Papo J, Merimsky E: Computerized tomography in xanthogranulomatous pyelonephritis. J Urol 130:323, 1983.

735. Goldman SM, Hartman DS, Fishman EK: Computerized tomography of xanthogranulomatous PN: Radiological-pathological correlations. Am J Radiol 141:963, 1984.

736. Mulapulos GP, Patel SK, Pessis D: MR imaging of xanthogranulomatous PN. J Comput Assist Tomogr 10:154, 1986.

737. Oosterhof G, Delacre K: Xanthogranulomatous pyelonephritis. Urol Int 41:180, 1986.

738. Treadwall TL, Craven DC, Delfin H, et al: Xanthogranulomatous pyelonephritis caused by methicillin-resistant *Staphylococcus aureus*. Am J Med 76:533, 1984.

739. Khalyl-Mawad J, Greco MA, Schinella RA: Ultrastructural demonstration of intracellular bacteria in xanthogranulomatous pyelonephritis. Hum Pathol 13:41, 1982.

740. Brown PS Jr, Dodson M, Weintrub PS: Xanthogranulomatous pyelonephritis: Report of nonsurgical management of a case and review of the literature. Clin Infect Dis 22:308, 1996.

741. Rodo J, Martin ME, Salarich J: Xanthogranulomatous pyelonephritis in children: Conservative management. Eur Urol 30:498, 1996.

742. Raziel A, Steinberg R, Kornreich L, et al: Xanthogranulomatous pyelonephritis mimicking malignant disease: Is preservation of the kidney possible? Pediatr Surg Int 12:535, 1997.

743. Carson CC, Weinerth JL: Xanthogranulomatous pyelonephritis in renal transplant recipient. Urology 23:50, 1984.

744. Lambrid PA, Yardley JH: Urinary tract malakoplakia: Report of a fatal case with ultrastructural observations of Michaelis-Gutmann bodies. Johns Hopkins Med J 216:1, 1970.

745. Stanton MJ, Maxted W: Malakoplakia: A study of the literature and current concepts of pathogenesis, diagnosis, and treatment. J Urol 125:139, 1981.

746. McClurg FR, D'Agostino AN, Martin JH, Race GJ: Ultrastructural demonstration of intracellular bacteria in three cases of malakoplakia of the bladder. Am J Clin Pathol 60:780, 1973.

747. Schwartz DT, Mascatello VJ, David-Nelson MA: Malakoplakia of the kidney. South Med J 76:11427, 1983.

748. Bowers JH, Cathey WJ: Malakoplakia of the kidney with renal failure. Am J Clin Pathol 55:765, 1971.

749. Cadnapaphornchai P, Rosenberg BF, Taber S, et al: Renal parenchymal malakoplakia: An unusual cause of renal failure. N Engl J Med 299:1110, 1978.

750. Lou TY, Teplitz C: Malakoplakia: Pathogenesis and ultrastructural morphogenesis. A problem of altered macrophage (phagolysosomal) response. Hum Pathol 5:191, 1974.

751. Malfunctioning microtubules [editorial]. Lancet 1:697, 1978.

752. Abdou NI, NaPombejara C, Sagawa A, et al: Malakoplakia: Evidence for monocyte lysosomal abnormality correctable by cholinergic agonist in vitro and in vivo. N Engl J Med 297:1413, 1977.

CHAPTER 32

Disorders of the Renal Arteries and Veins

Michael Yudd and Francisco Llach

Vascular complications of the main renal arteries and veins are complex and varied. This chapter focuses on (1) acute thrombosis of the renal artery, (2) thromboembolism of the renal artery, (3) renal artery aneurysms, (4) dissecting aneurysms of the renal artery, (5) atheroembolic disease, and (6) acute and chronic renal vein thrombosis, which occurs primarily in patients with the nephrotic syndrome. Thromboembolic phenomena associated with the nephrotic syndrome are also discussed. Other conditions, such as fibromuscular dysplasia and atherosclerosis of renal arteries, that usually cause renovascular hypertension are not considered in this chapter.

ACUTE OCCLUSION OF THE RENAL ARTERY

Traumatic Renal Artery Thrombosis

Blunt abdominal trauma is a major cause of acute renal artery thrombosis. Car accidents, athletic activities, and street fights are typical settings. The main renal artery, renal vein, or branch vessels may be injured in trauma, resulting in lacerations, contusions, or thrombosis.[1, 2] Thrombosis, the most common injury, is usually unilateral and more commonly left-sided, but it may be bilateral.[3] Renal artery thrombosis may occur in 1% to 3% of cases of severe blunt abdominal trauma.[4, 5] In a review of 250 patients who underwent surgery for traumatic renal artery injury,[6] the following lesions were found: thrombosis (52%), avulsion of the renal pedicle (12%), branch injury (4%), and laceration (3%), among others. Renal lesions were bilateral in 22% of the cases and were accompanied by extrarenal abdominal injuries in 45%. Besides blunt trauma, stab wounds and iatrogenic surgical or endovascular manipulation from percutaneous transcatheter procedures may be complicated by renal artery thrombosis.[7]

The major concern of acute thrombosis is severe renal ischemia and the rapid progression to renal infarction. From early studies, it is known that the maximal warm ischemic time tolerated by a human kidney before the onset of irreversible damage is about 60 to 90 minutes, although the precise time is uncertain.[8] Incomplete occlusions and occlusions to kidneys with previous stenosis and collateral circulation are viable for longer periods. In experimental occlusion studies in animals, 1 hour of complete occlusion was followed by irreversible renal damage, whereas partial occlusions for longer periods had better outcomes.[9]

Common clinical signs and symptoms associated with renal artery thrombosis and impending renal infarction include flank and abdominal pain, nausea, vomiting, and fever. New-onset renin-mediated hypertension may be severe. The finding of anuria should raise the suspicion of bilateral thrombosis or thrombosis of a solitary functioning kidney. Gross or microscopic hematuria is common but may be absent in one quarter of the cases, and mild proteinuria is often present.[1] Elevations of lactate dehydrogenase (LDH) in particular, but also of creatinine phosphatase (CPK), serum transaminases, and alkaline phosphatase, may be noted.

A rapid diagnosis is critical if attempts at revascularization are considered. Spiral computed tomography (CT) with contrast is the preferred diagnostic study for suspected renal trauma, especially when other abdominal injuries are suspected. The key findings of main renal artery thrombosis are the absence of renal parenchymal enhancement with contrast (CT nephrogram) and the lack of contrast excretion (CT pyelogram).[5] In some cases, there may be enhancement of the peripheral renal cortex ("cortical rim sign"), which is presumably the result of capsular or collateral perfusion to the cortex (Fig. 32-1).[5, 10] In addition to these findings of poor renal perfusion, CT can also identify other injuries including intrarenal and perinephric hematomas, renal vascular lacerations with extravasation of the contrast agent, and traumatic injury to other organs. Magnetic resonance imaging (MRI) and the time-honored intravenous pyelography (IVP) can furnish useful information, but spiral CT is preferred for its speed and accuracy. If the diagnosis is uncertain, renal angiography can provide the definitive diagnosis. With arteriography, the precise location and the extent of the occlusion, as well as individual variations of the vascular anatomy, are visualized, all providing important information for the surgeon.

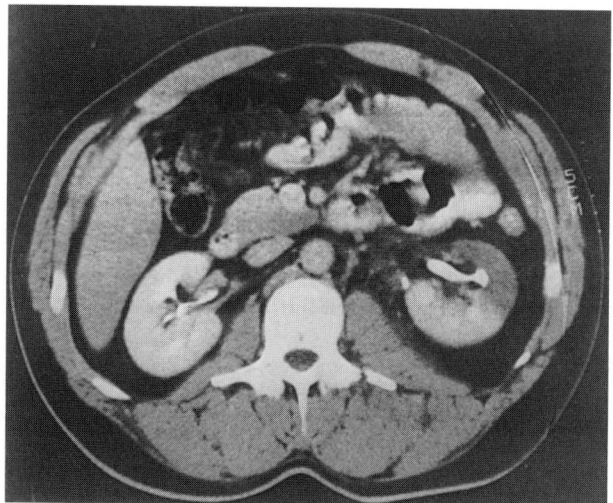

FIGURE 32-1. Acute focal infarct. A 32-year-old man suffered blunt abdominal trauma. This computed tomographic scan with contrast, taken 6 hours after the incident, shows an acute focal infarct in the midpole of the left kidney. (From Davidson AJ: Radiology of Kidneys. Philadelphia, WB Saunders, 1985, pp 525-581.)

With current digital subtraction technology, angiography can be performed using very little iodinated contrast material, and carbon dioxide or gadolinium (or one of its derivatives) can be substituted to further decrease the dose of contrast agent. This decreases concerns of contrast-induced renal failure (RF) in unstable patients who are considered to be at high risk for this complication. If a trauma patient is too unstable to undergo these diagnostic procedures, a simple intravenous bolus injection of contrast material followed by a "one-shot" excretory urogram may furnish valuable information to the surgeon preoperatively. A normal urogram would exclude the presence of major trauma to that kidney.

Prompt revascularization has been attempted to avoid renal infarction. However, the surgical outcomes for renal salvage in acute renal artery thrombosis have been mixed,[1, 11-13] and many unsuccessful cases may require later nephrectomy. The ischemic time is a crucial factor; most successful outcomes have occurred with a presumed renal ischemic time of less than 12 hours.[11-13] Maggio and Brosman[14] noted an 80% success rate for kidneys repaired within 12 hours, 57% for those repaired between 12 and 18 hours, and 0% (0/13) for later attempts. Other factors that influence outcome are the extent of renal injury, the presence of collateral renal circulation, the technical difficulty of the surgical procedure, and the injury to other organs. In general, all attempts should be made to revascularize the kidneys of patients with bilateral arterial thrombosis or with thrombosis to a solitary functioning kidney, because of the risk of severe irreversible RF. However, in patients with a unilateral thrombosis and a functional contralateral kidney, the outcomes with surgery may not be better than those of observation and medical management,[15] so the indication for surgery in this setting is uncertain.[11-13]

Despite the concerns regarding ischemic time, there have been rare cases of successful revascularization long after the presumed onset of traumatic renal artery thrombosis.[16-20] Late revascularization may be considered if the kidney size is normal on imaging studies and if preserved glomerular architecture is noted on renal biopsy.[16]

Several surgical procedures can be performed for the repair of a renal pedicle injury: thrombectomy, resection of the injured arterial segment and replacement with a venous or graft bypass, and autotransplantation with ex vivo repair of the vascular lesions.[21, 22] Endovascular stent placements for traumatic intimal tears have been described.[23-26] Nephrectomy is required at times to control renal hemorrhage.

Nontraumatic Renal Artery Thrombosis

Nontraumatic renal artery thrombosis occurs infrequently, and often it is unsuspected early in the clinical presentation, even by astute clinicians. Table 32-1 lists the settings for renal artery thrombosis. Most of this information has been collected from small series of patients or from case reports.

Arterial thrombi are composed primarily of platelets, with relatively little fibrin. The thrombi develop at sites of vessel wall injury in the presence of high-velocity blood flow. Thrombosis of preexisting atherosclerotic plaques is the most common setting for arterial thrombosis. Venous thrombi, on the other hand, have different characteristics: they are composed predominantly of thrombin and trapped red blood cells, with few platelets, and they form in areas of stasis after activation of the blood coagulation system. Inherited disorders of the anticoagulant pathways (e.g., factor V Leiden mutation, protein C and protein S deficiencies) play a major role in the formation of venous thrombosis, but not arterial thrombosis.[27] Screening for these defects usually produces a low yield in arterial thrombosis.[28, 29]

Damage or disruption of the endothelial surface of the renal arterial vasculature promotes platelet adhesion and aggregation, which leads to thrombosis. In addition to the setting of atherosclerosis, arterial thrombosis develops in the damaged endothelial surfaces associated with fibromuscular dysplasia, in renal artery aneurysms and dissecting aneurysms, and in infectious and inflammatory states, including the various vasculitides (see Table 32-1).

Renal artery thrombosis has been described in the acquired hypercoagulable states, in the antiphospholipid syndrome (APS),[30-40] and in heparin-induced thrombocytopenia.[41, 42] Severe cases of catastrophic diffuse arterial and venous thromboses can occur in both diseases. In APS, thrombosis may be localized at any location within the renal vasculature, from the renal artery trunk to the renal veins. Renal artery thrombosis has been noted in primary APS and also in secondary APS associated with systemic lupus erythematosus.[30-40] Factor V Leiden mutation has been implicated as the cause of renal artery thrombosis in native kidneys and in renal allografts.[28, 29] Arterial thrombosis has also been observed rarely in patients with the nephrotic syndrome[43-45] and in those with hyperhomocysteinemia.[46]

Acute renal artery occlusion in the renal transplantation patient usually occurs within several weeks after surgery, with consequent graft loss.[47-53] Thrombosis is responsible for one third to one half of early graft losses.[50] Early renal artery thrombosis in the transplant is usually attributed to technical factors of the surgical anastomoses, the presence of multiple donor vessels, kidneys from pediatric donors, and severe hyperacute rejection.[50, 51] Transplant renal artery thrombosis has also been attributed to APS. In a retrospective review of 96 consecutive patients with systemic lupus nephritis who underwent transplantation, 29% were found

TABLE 32-1

Nontraumatic Causes of Renal Artery Thrombosis

CAUSE	REF. NO.
Causes associated with endothelial damage or disruption	
Atherosclerosis	—
Renal artery aneurysms	27
Dissecting aneurysms	28
Fibromuscular dysplasia	—
Cocaine	63–65
Vascular inflammation	
Polyarteritis nodosa	66, 67
Takayasu arteritis	68, 69
Behçet disease	70–73
Infection-related causes	
Syphilis	72
Phycomatosis	73, 74
Hypercoagulable states	
Acquired causes	
Anti-phospholipid antibodies	30–40
Heparin-induced thrombocytopenia	41, 42
Hyperhomocysteinemia	46
Nephrotic syndrome	43–45
Hereditary causes	
Factor V Leiden mutation	28, 29
Miscellaneous causes	
Sickle cell anemia	75
Umbilical artery catheters in neonates	58–62
Urothelial carcinoma of renal pelvis	76
Strenuous aerobic exercise	77
Automobile seat belt pressure	78

TABLE 32-2

Diseases Associated with Thromboemboli to the Renal Arteries

Cardiac causes
  Arrhythmias, especially atrial fibrillation
  Myocardial infarction
  Congestive cardiomyopathy
  Rheumatic valvular disease
  Prosthetic heart valves
  Bacterial endocarditis
  Paradoxic thromboemboli
Aortic and renal aneurysms and dissecting aneurysms
Complications of intra-arterial catheterization
Tumor emboli
Fat emboli

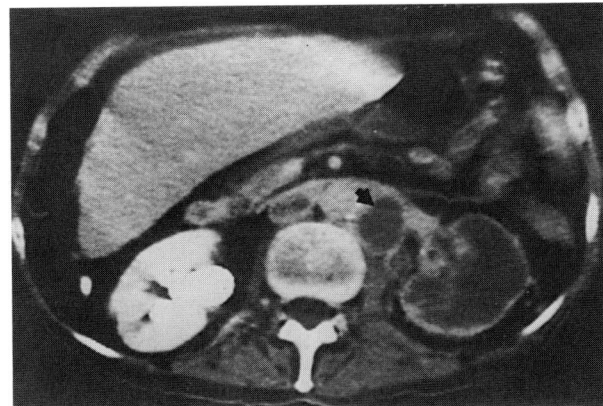

FIGURE 32-2. Occlusion of the left main renal artery by a metastatic deposit from lung carcinoma, causing renal infarction. The low-density metastasis *(arrow)* has occluded the left renal artery. Collateral circulation continues to perfuse the cortex of the left kidney (cortical rim sign). Computed tomogram, contrast material enhanced. (From Davidson AJ: Radiology of Kidneys. Philadelphia, WB Saunders, 1985, pp 525-581.)

to have laboratory evidence for APS, and 4 patients had renal arterial or venous thrombosis in their transplants.[40]

Earlier studies suggested that cyclosporine therapy may predispose to renal artery thrombosis, but later studies did not find this association.[54-57] Cyclosporine can cause a microangiopathic hemolytic anemia with RF. There are scattered reports of renal artery thrombosis following closely after rejection therapy with OKT3.[49]

In neonates, renal artery thrombosis has been a complication of umbilical artery catheterization.[58-61] Urokinase therapy has been successfully employed in these neonates.[59, 62]

Thromboembolism of the Renal Artery

Thromboemboli to the renal arteries usually originate from the heart. Various cardiac diseases and arrhythmias, in particular atrial fibrillation,[79-81] are associated with thromboemboli. These conditions are listed in Table 32-2. The greatest risk of thromboemboli originating from the heart is in the cerebral circulation. The risk of renal artery thromboembolism is relatively low. A large Danish study reported the incidence of peripheral arterial thromboembolism (i.e., not involving the cerebral circulation) in 30,000 patients with atrial fibrillation.[81] The relative risk for a peripheral thromboembolism in this population was fourfold higher in men and almost sixfold higher in women with atrial fibrillation, compared to the population without atrial fibrillation. Only 2% of these peripheral thromboemboli involved the renal arteries; the circulatory vessels of the upper and lower extremities (61% of peripheral emboli) and the mesenteric arteries (29%) had a much higher incidence of thromboembolism than the renal arteries did.

Thrombi may form in the heart after a myocardial infarction as a mural thrombus over the infarct site, in a dyskinetic ventricle, or from the atrium. Endocarditis, rheumatic vascular disease, or a prosthetic heart valve may be the source for thrombi. Paradoxical renal emboli have been rarely described. These originate in the venous circulation, traverse a patent cardiac septal defect, and gain access to the arterial circulation. Tumors may be the source of thromboemboli (Fig. 32-2). Thrombi may also develop in the aorta or renal artery walls on atherosclerotic lesions or in aneurysms, and they may embolize distally to the kidney.[82-85]

Renal thrombosis and thromboembolism sometimes occur as complications of endovascular repair of aortic aneurysms or of renal artery stenoses.[86-90] Among 174 patients who underwent endovascular repair of aneurysms of the thoracic or abdominal aorta using a variety of endografts, follow-up CT scans showed newly recognized perfusion defects and infarctions in 9%, with most occurring in the kidneys. Most of these were small infarctions and asymptomatic, but a few were serious.[86] Clinically significant renal complications of endovascular stent placement in renal artery stenosis is reported to be approximately 9%.[86, 88] These complications include renal artery thrombosis, dissection, and hemorrhage.

Pathology of Renal Infarction

Renal infarction is an infrequent clinical diagnosis, but it is not an uncommon autopsy finding. In a review of more than 14,000 autopsies, renal infarctions of various sizes were noted in 1.4% of the cases, and most of these were postmortem diagnoses of conditions asymptomatic during life.[91] Renal infarctions occur when the main renal artery, branch artery, or interlobar and arcuate arteries are occluded acutely. Infarction may also result from renal vein occlusion, but this is much less likely than infarction from arterial occlusions.[92]

The gross appearance of the infarct depends on the size of the occluded artery, the age of the infarct, and the presence of infection. In the first hour, the infarct is red and pyramidal in shape; within hours, the infarcted area becomes gray and has a narrow red rim of congested parenchyma. The necrotic area is eventually replaced by collagen. The area shrinks, forming a V-shaped scar with the wide base toward the surface of the kidney. Infarctions involve only the renal cortex; the medulla usually is spared.[83] The scarring can give the kidney an irregular, bumpy surface.

The microscopic picture of sterile infarctions is the classic image of coagulative necrosis. The initial findings of marked congestion are followed by cytoplasmic and nuclear degenerative changes and gradual loss of viable cytologic structure. The cytoplasm becomes homogeneous and eosinophilic, and the nuclei undergo condensation and karyorrhexis. Surrounding this necrotic area is a transitional zone of sublethal injury with findings similar to those of acute tubular necrosis. This peripheral area becomes infiltrated with polymorphonuclear leukocytes. The central necrotic area becomes smaller and eventually collapses, being replaced by a collagenous scar[92] (Fig. 32-3).

Clinical Features of Renal Thromboembolism

The clinical features of renal artery embolization are variable and depend on the size and extent of the emboli.[93] Bilateral artery emboli or an embolism to a solitary functioning kidney would be more likely to produce acute renal failure (ARF) and anuria than would a unilateral embolism with a normal contralateral kidney. However, in the latter case, anuria or marked oliguria may occur, presumably because of arterial spasm of the contralateral renal vasculature.[33]

Patients commonly experience some degree of abdominal or flank pain, often with nausea and vomiting. The pain is often dull and unrelenting, but it may be absent, particularly with small infarcts. Gross hematuria may be present. Some patients may have had prior embolic events in one or both kidneys or in other organs.

Abdominal or flank tenderness is usually present on physical examination, and signs of peritoneal irritation may be noted. Fever is common, and chills may occur. Hypertension can be severe, and it is the prominent clinical problem in some cases. Other organs, especially the brain or extremities, should be evaluated for signs of arterial embolization. Cardiac arrhythmias, particularly atrial fibrillation, the presence of valvular disease, or a recent myocardial infarction,

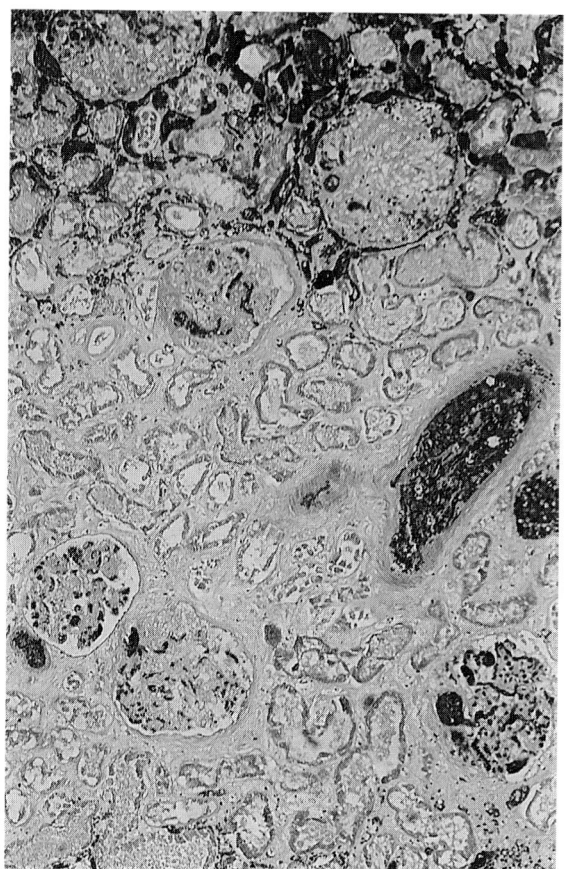

FIGURE 32-3. Renal infarction. A white/pale infarct with ischemic coagulative necrosis surrounded by marked congestion and hemorrhage is shown. The basic outlines of the renal tubules are preserved, but there is loss of nuclei in the epithelial cells. (Hematoxylin and eosin stain.) (Compliments of Shahida Ahmed, M.D.)

should alert the clinician to the possibility of a cardiac source of the emboli.

Early diagnosis of acute arterial occlusion is often difficult, because the initial diagnostic considerations are usually directed toward other, more common diseases such as nephrolithiasis, pyelonephritis, acute myocardial infarction, acute cholecystitis, and acute tubular necrosis.

A common laboratory abnormality is an elevated LDH concentration, which may rise to 2000 IU/L in cases of large infarctions. Most patients have microscopic hematuria, and mild proteinuria. Leukocytosis may develop. A low urinary sodium concentration has been noted, which suggests the presence of a renal hypoperfusion state.[94] Serum aspartate aminotransferase and alanine aminotransferase levels may be increased, but not to the same extent as the LDH. The urinary excretion of alanine aminopeptidase (AAP) and N-acetyl-D-glucosaminidase (NAG), expressed per milligram of creatinine excreted, is increased as much as 7 to 10 times above the normal range, and the augmented excretion persists for 2 to 3 weeks or longer.[95]

A rapid diagnosis is critical if acute intervention with thrombolysis or surgery is contemplated in the hope of preserving renal function. Several imaging studies are useful, and the choice is often determined by which study is readily available. The helical CT with contrast can furnish a rapid and accurate diagnosis and is considered the best rapid test[96] (see earlier discussion). Contrast is essential, and a noncontrast study is useless for studying renal perfusion. Contrast-enhanced three-dimensional magnetic resonance angiography (MRA) can show sharp images of the renal arteries and renal perfusion abnormalities. It may be considered a better alternative to helical CT if RF is present and it is preferable to avoid the use of iodinated contrast material.[97] Isotopic flow

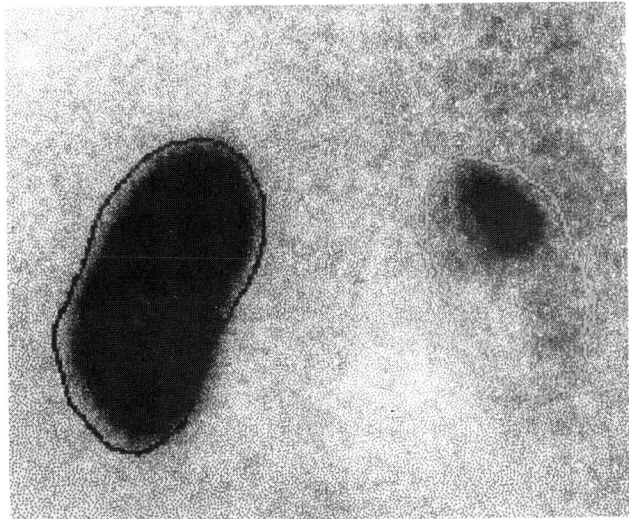

FIGURE 32-4. Thromboembolism and poor function of the right kidney. ^{99m}Tc-Glucoheptonate renal scan shows that only the upper third of the right kidney is functioning. The left kidney appears to be normal. This 69-year-old man presented with severe flank pain. Workup revealed left atrial thrombi, the source of the thromboemboli. (Courtesy of Anthony Reda, M.D., Northport, NY.)

scans, typically with a technetium 99m (^{99m}Tc)-labeled agent such as dimethylenetriamine pentaacetic acid (DTPA), show absent or markedly reduced perfusion of the affected kidney (Fig. 32-4). Ultrasound of the renal vessels using color and power-Doppler techniques is of limited value because it is technically difficult to image the entire renal arteries, and the quality of the studies are operator dependent.[98]

Renal arteriography, the "gold standard" study, is the definitive method for diagnosis of renal artery occlusion (Fig. 32-5). Angiography has the added advantage that thrombolysis can be administered right away if a thrombosis or embolus is found. With the use of carbon dioxide and gadolinium, iodinated contrast can be avoided during arteriography in patients with ARF associated with renal embolism or thrombosis.[99]

Therapy for Acute Occlusive Renal Arterial Disease

Intra-arterial thrombolysis and vascular surgical procedures have been used to lyse or remove renal artery thromboses or thromboemboli. Most of the reports on this issue involve small series of patients or case reports, so it is difficult to draw firm conclusions from them. The duration of warm ischemic time, the degree of occlusion (complete or partial), and the size of the occluded artery or arteries (main, branch, or interlobar) are all factors determining whether renal function can be preserved through an intervention. In the surgical literature dealing with traumatic renal artery thrombosis, the duration of warm ischemia was a critical factor in the development of renal infarction. Surgical success in preserving renal function was inversely proportional to the period of renal ischemia, and most interventions were successful when revascularization was performed within 12 hours after the presumed onset of renal ischemia.[1, 11-13] Outcomes were poor with longer periods of ischemia (see earlier discussion).

FIGURE 32-5. Segmental renal artery occlusions. This 70-year-old man presented with severe flank pain and microscopic hematuria. This digital subtraction left renal angiogram shows a large, wedge-shaped defect in the superior pole, along with multiple smaller peripheral defects involving the middle and inferior pole of the kidney. The diagnosis was multiple thromboemboli with segmental renal infarctions. The emboli originated from left atrial thrombi and from a large thoracic aortic thrombus. (Courtesy of Anthony Reda, M.D., Northport, NY.)

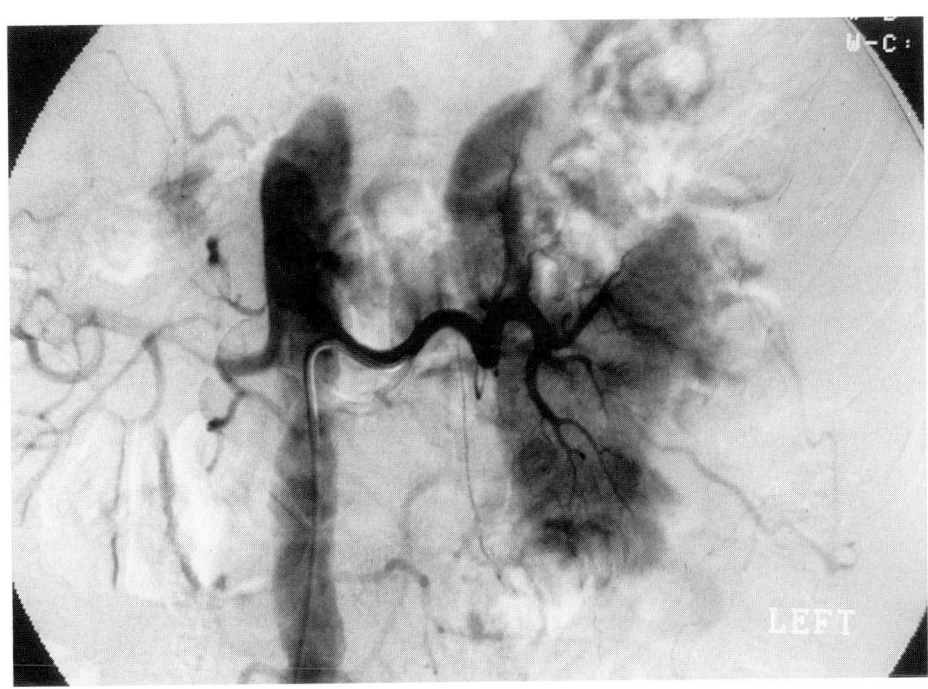

Blum and associates[100] described 14 patients with acute embolic renal artery occlusion who were treated with thrombolytic therapy, either with intra-arterial streptokinase, urokinase, or tissue-type plasminogen activator. The estimated ischemic time from onset of symptoms to therapy varied from 12 hours to 8 days. Recanalization and adequate renal perfusion was achieved in 13 of the 14 patients. Nevertheless, renal function did not improve in any patient with complete occlusion, but it did stabilize in those patients with partial occlusions. Infarction had developed before the successful recanalization in many of the cases. There are a number of case reports that describe successful outcomes of intra-arterial thrombolysis even in cases of prolonged renal ischemia (20 to 72 hours), and in renal transplants as well.[101-109] In some of these cases, anuria and severe ARF were present before thrombolytic therapy and were reversed after the procedure. Similar successful outcomes despite prolonged ischemic times have also been described in neonates.[110-112]

Surgical outcomes for preserving renal function in acute nontraumatic obstructions are mixed. Lacomb[113] showed very good surgical results in preserving renal function, but the mortality rate was high. Twenty patients with acute obstruction of the main renal arteries (25 kidneys at risk), 5 from acute embolism and 15 from acute thrombosis, underwent revascularization 18 hours to 68 days after the obstruction. The kidney salvage rate was 64%, but the postoperative mortality rate was 15%. It is unclear whether some of these cases were caused by thrombosis associated with atherosclerosis with collateral circulation, which may carry a better prognosis for renal salvage than an acute occlusion without collateral circulation; other studies do not show such optimistic outcomes. Surgical embolectomy failed to restore renal function in 13 patients with acute renal artery embolism.[114]

Intra-arterial thrombolysis is preferable to a surgical procedure, but it has its own risks, mainly hemorrhage and distal embolization. An aggressive approach with either means should be attempted in bilateral occlusions or occlusions to solitary functioning kidneys, in the hope of preserving adequate renal function and avoiding the need for dialysis. For unilateral occlusions with normal contralateral kidneys, clinical judgment is required regarding whether to intervene. Either therapy is probably futile if complete occlusion of the renal artery has been present for a prolonged period. On the other hand, intervention may be successful for shorter ischemic durations, and the shorter the period the better. If the obstruction is incomplete, the kidney may remain viable longer. If the perfusion defects are small and renal function is good, anticoagulation alone may be the best therapy.

Many reports describe the relief of severe pain during thrombolytic intervention. Severe pain, which suggests ongoing ischemia, is probably a good indication for thrombolytic intervention regardless of the presumed duration of ischemia.

In patients with embolic disease, particular attention should be paid to the source of embolization. Some patients (e.g., those with atrial fibrillation) require long-term anticoagulation to avoid future recurrences of embolization to the kidneys or other vital organs.

RENAL ARTERY ANEURYSMS

Renal artery aneurysms (RAAs) are uncommon in the general population. Large autopsy studies suggest the incidence of RAAs to be 0.01% in the general population.[115] In selected patients who undergo renal arteriography, this incidence is higher. In a large series of patients undergoing renal arteriography primarily for the evaluation of renovascular hypertension, RAAs were observed in 1%.[116] Many RAAs remain asymptomatic. However, the clinical concerns of RAAs are their potential to rupture, thrombose, cause distal embolization, or lead to renovascular hypertension. Intrarenal aneurysms may erode into adjacent veins to produce arteriovenous fistulae.

RAAs are classified as saccular, fusiform, dissecting, or intrarenal. They may be located anywhere along the vascular tree, but most of them are found at the bifurcation of the renal artery or in the first-order branch arteries.[117] Anatomic and clinical characteristics of RAAs that were described in five series are listed in Table 32-3.[117-121]

TABLE 32-3

Renal Artery Aneurysms (RAAs)—Anatomic and Clinical Characteristics from Five Recent Studies

PARAMETER	HENKE[117]	LUMSDEN[118]	DZSINICH[119]	BULBUL[120]	HUPP[121]
Number of patients	168	28	32	56	23
RAA anatomy					
Saccular/fusiform (%)	79/21	80/20	84/9	70/23	32/68
Mean size (range, cm)	1.5	2.1 (0.5–8)	1.7 (0.7–9)	?	?
Right-left-bilateral (%)	60/40/19	43-36-21	65-31-3	?	?
Clinical characteristics					
Mean age (range, yr)	51	58 (24–76)	48 (15–83)	63 (20–75)	49.9 (16–74)
Female/male (%)	64/36	64/36	53/47	61/39	65/35
Hypertension history (%)	73	79	88	55	91
Etiology of RAA					
Atherosclerosis (%)	25	75	31	?	34
Fibromuscular dysplasia (%)	34	21	56	20	26
Clinical outcome					
Spontaneous rupture	3	1	0	1 (pregnant)	2
Treated surgically (%)	72	36	100	30	78

Saccular aneurysms, the most common type, constitute 60% to 90% of RAAs. They are diagnosed typically at about 50 years of age, but the range is large, 13 to 78 years of age. There may be a slightly greater tendency for right-sided aneurysms, and in approximately 20% of cases the RAAs are bilateral. Extrarenal aneurysms are not commonly associated with RAAs. Concomitant aortic, splenic, or mesenteric aneurysms were observed in only 6.5% of 168 patients with RAAs.[117] Renal artery stenosis may be associated with RAAs.

RAAs are sometimes attributed to atherosclerosis, but marked atherosclerotic changes were found in only 16% of the excised aneurysm walls of 56 RAAs in a recent study.[117] Atherosclerotic changes may be a secondary development rather than the cause of RAAs. The primary cause may be a congenital weakness in the internal elastic lamina of the artery, although this is uncertain.[122]

Fusiform aneurysms are often seen in medial fibromuscular dysplasia.[123-128] These aneurysms usually arise distal to a focal stenotic segment, giving the image of a poststenotic dilatation (Fig. 32-6). Occasionally, several small aneurysms in sequence give the "string of beads" appearance seen in fibromuscular dysplasia. Fusiform aneurysms are typically found in young hypertensive patients who undergo renal angiography for the evaluation of renovascular hypertension. As with fibromuscular dysplasia, fusiform aneurysms are more common in women.

RAAs have been described in polyarteritis nodosa,[129, 130] Takayasu arteritis,[131-133] Behçet disease,[70-72] the Ehlers-Danlos syndrome,[133-135] and mycotic aneurysms.[136-138]

Intraparenchymal renal aneurysms make up 10% to 15% of RAAs, and are frequently multiple. They may be congenital, post-traumatic (e.g., after renal biopsy), or associated with polyarteritis nodosa.

Clinical Manifestations of Renal Artery Aneurysms

Many patients with RAAs are asymptomatic; they are diagnosed with RAA when the kidneys are imaged as part of a workup for renovascular hypertension. Occasionally, such patients have flank pain. Flank pain should raise the concern of an expanding aneurysm, rupture and hemorrhage, thrombosis or thromboemboli with impending renal infarction, or dissection.

The majority of patients in whom RAAs are diagnosed have hypertension. In several recent series that included more than 300 patients with RAAs, hypertension was present in 55% to 91% (see Table 32-3).[117-121] This incidence of hypertension may be inaccurately high, because the diagnosis of RAA is often made in patients undergoing angiography for the evaluation of hypertension. Hypertension may contribute to the formation and expansion of RAAs, and, conversely, RAAs may contribute to the development of renovascular hypertension. It has been suggested that RAAs may cause regional renal hypoperfusion and ischemia and consequent renin-mediated hypertension through several mechanisms: compression or kinking of adjacent branch arteries by the aneurysm; thrombosis or distal embolization; altered blood flow through the aneurysm; and formation of arteriovenous fistulae.[122] The topic of renovascular hypertension is reviewed in Chapter 47. Repair of the aneurysm may result in significant improvement in hypertension.[120, 121, 139-141]

A patient with rupture of an RAA, a potentially catastrophic event, may present with vascular collapse and hemorrhagic shock. Aneurysm size is a factor in the potential for rupture. The risk of rupture of small RAAs, those less than 2.0 cm in diameter, appears to be low, based on data from several studies that followed the natural history of RAAs. Large aneurysms, especially those larger than 4.0 cm in diameter, have a greater tendency to rupture and usually require surgical intervention.[122] The older literature suggested that aneurysms without calcified walls also had a greater tendency to rupture, but this may not be true. In a recent study, 63% of 252 RAAs were noncalcified, and the incidence of rupture was very low.[117] Six studies described the natural history of small aneurysms in almost 300 patients with small aneurysms who were monitored conservatively without surgery for up to 17 years.[116, 117, 142-145] Most of these aneurysms were smaller than 2.0 cm in diameter. During follow-up, none of the aneurysms ruptured, and very few caused symptoms or increased considerably in size (Table 32-4). Henriksson and associates[144] described 34 patients with RAAs who had repeat angiographic studies; 28 patients exhibited no change in RAA size on follow-up, and 5 had slight enlargement, thrombosis, or calcification. One patient had worrisome dilatation of the RAA and underwent surgical repair. These studies suggest that in nonpregnant patients small aneurysms (less than 2.0 cm in diameter) are unlikely to rupture, enlarge, or cause symptoms. It appears safe to monitor such RAAs conservatively with periodic imaging studies.

Pregnant women make up a disproportionate number of cases of RAA rupture. In a review of 43 cases of rupture, 18 (42%) occurred in pregnant women.[145] Most of these occurred

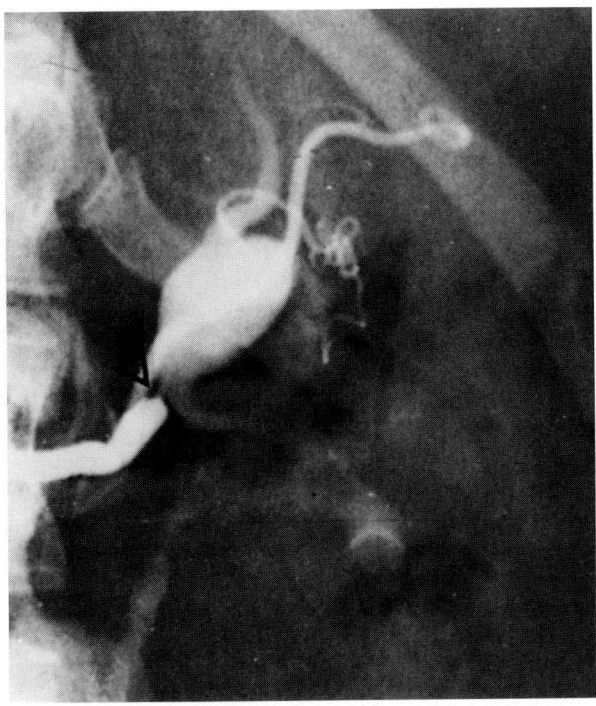

FIGURE 32-6. Poststenotic fusiform aneurysm caused by intimal fibroplasia. Renal arteriogram shows a narrow annular band *(arrow)* followed by the fusiform aneurysm. (From Davidson AJ: Radiology of Kidneys. Philadelphia, WB Saunders, 1985, pp 525-581.)

TABLE 32-4

Major Studies with Surgery and Conservative Management of Renal Artery Aneurysms (RAAs)

STUDY	NO. OF PATIENTS	NO. RAAs OPERATED	NO. RAAs RUPTURED ON PRESENTATION	RAAs MONITORED CONSERVATIVELY	RAA SIZE (cm)
Henke[117]	168	121	3	86	1.3
Hageman[142]	29	10	1	25	<2.0
Hubert[143]	67	5	0	62	1.0–3.0
Tham[116]	83	14	0	69	<2.0
Henriksson[144]	56	15	4	34	0.3–2.5
Martin[145]	39	18	3	18	0.6–2.6

during the last trimester of pregnancy, but rupture and hemorrhage also occurred earlier in pregnancy and during the postpartum period.[146-152] Renal artery rupture during pregnancy has also been described in a renal transplant recipient.[153] Many of the pregnant women who suffered RAA rupture did not have hypertension before or during their pregnancy. The reason for the increased incidence of rupture in pregnancy is not certain. Pathogenic considerations include increased renal blood flow particularly during the last trimester, the effect of female hormones on the vasculature, and increased intra-abdominal pressure.[154] Emergency nephrectomy is usually required in this setting to control the hemorrhage. In recent years, maternal mortality has decreased to 6% and fetal mortality to 25% if the pregnancy had reached the third trimester.[122, 155] If rupture occurred before the third trimester, fetal mortality approached 100%.

The clinical presentation of rupture of an RAA includes flank pain, vascular collapse, and shock. Abdominal distention or a flank mass may be detected. Hematuria may be a helpful finding in some patients, but its absence does not exclude this diagnosis. Renal angiography and MRA will diagnose RAA; CT and radionuclide scanning may be useful screening techniques.

Various authors have attempted to provide criteria for elective surgical intervention in RAA.[113, 116, 117, 119, 156] There is considerable uncertainty inherent in these criteria. A conservative approach, based on the previous discussion, would incorporate a number of factors in deciding about elective surgical intervention. First is the absolute size of the aneurysm. Many authorities agree that an aneurysm larger than 4.0 cm in diameter should be resected, and one less than 2.0 cm in diameter can be safely followed with periodic imaging studies. There is uncertainty about the mid-sized aneurysms, those between 2.1 and 4.0 cm. It may be prudent to recommend repair of RAAs greater than 3.0 cm in diameter in patients with surgical risks if there is reasonable certainty that nephrectomy will not be required.[156] Besides (1) large size of the aneurysm, the following factors are considered in the choice for elective surgical intervention: (2) aneurysms with lobulations, which may have a greater tendency to rupture; (3) any aneurysm showing significant expansion during follow-up imaging studies; (4) aneurysms causing clinical signs and symptoms, which may include abdominal or flank pain, an abdominal mass, or symptoms associated with distal embolization; (5) aneurysms of any size in young women of child-bearing age, because the risk of rupture is increased with pregnancy; (6) the presence of

an aneurysm to a solitary kidney with the potential for embolization from a thrombus or a risk of dissection; and (7) renovascular hypertension, particularly with lateralization of renal renin levels. Henke and associates,[117] authors of the largest study of patients with RAAs, recommend a more aggressive surgical approach to patients with RAAs.

Several surgical techniques for treatment of RAAs have been described, but the most commonly used approach is in situ aneurysmectomy and revascularization. Henke and colleagues[117] used this technique in all but one of their 168 RAA repairs. When carefully done, this surgery carries the least risk of damage to the kidney and ureter. Given the technically demanding nature of RAA surgery, this intervention should be performed by surgeons with demonstrated expertise in renal artery reconstructive procedures. Even with the vast experience of Henke's group, almost 5% of their patients had to undergo unplanned nephrectomy because of technical complications encountered during attempted revascularization. The renal vasculature can be unforgiving terrain. The most distal RAAs and the more complex cases might best be treated by ex vivo repair, but the risks are greater for this technically demanding surgery.

Catheter-based interventions of stent grafts and embolization techniques using microcoils and Gelfoam have been used to treat RAAs as an alternative to surgery (Fig. 32-7).[157-166] Many RAAs are not technically amenable to these interventions. Exceptions are the saccular aneurysms with narrow necks, which have been treated successfully with these endovascular techniques. Possible complications include occlusion of the renal artery by maldeployed or migrated coils or by thromboemboli dislodged during catheter manipulation. These complications appear to be greater in the saccular aneurysms with wide necks.[162] Long-term outcomes of these procedures are not known.

Endovascular embolization techniques are also used to treat distal renal artery branch aneurysms. Here, the therapeutic goal is occlusion of the branch artery feeding the aneurysm, with consequent elimination of the aneurysm and limited renal infarction.

Dissecting Aneurysms of the Renal Artery

Dissecting aneurysms of the renal artery are uncommon, and they can cause acute or chronic occlusion of the artery. Acute dissections may manifest in an explosive manner, with malignant hypertension, flank pain, and renal infarction. Chronic dissection most commonly manifests as renovascular

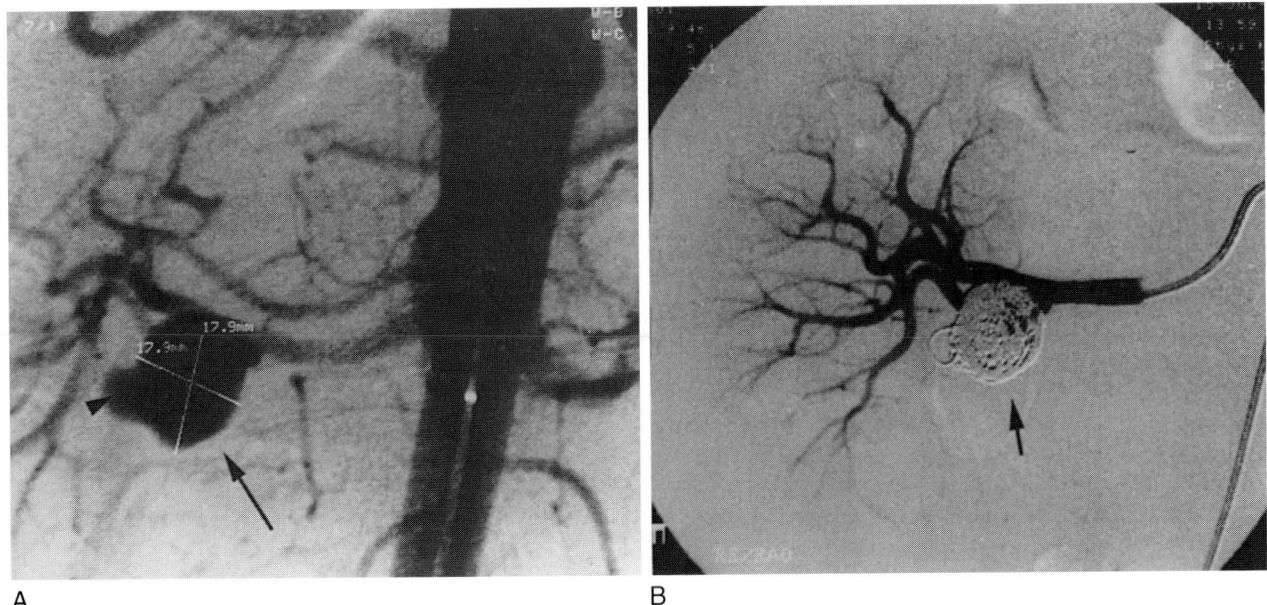

A   B

FIGURE 32-7. Successful embolization of a large right renal artery aneurysm with microcoils. **A,** Abdominal aortic angiogram shows a large saccular aneurysm *(arrow)* with a small daughter aneurysm *(arrowhead).* **B,** Selective renal artery angiogram. After placement of microcoils, there is complete occlusion of the aneurysm *(arrow).* (From Klein GE, Brien LE, Raith J, Schreyer HH: Endovascular treatment of renal aneurysms with conventional non-detachable microcoils and Guglielmi detachable coils. Br J Urol 79:852-860, 1997.)

hypertension.[124] Renovascular hypertension is discussed in Chapter 46. Acute dissection can occur spontaneously, and it can be precipitated by strenuous physical activity or trauma.[167] Fibromuscular dysplasia and atherosclerosis are common predisposing factors that lead to intimal tears, medial necrosis of the artery wall, and dissection. Iatrogenic dissection due to angiographic procedures may occur from trauma induced by guide wires, catheters, or angioplasty balloons.[168] Dissections have also been found as incidental autopsy findings, apparently without clinical symptoms during life.[168]

Renal artery dissections are about three times more common in men, and there is a predilection toward involvement of the right side. Approximately 20% to 30% are bilateral. Dissection is most common in 40- to 60-year-olds, although younger patients with fibromuscular dysplasia may be affected.

With acute dissection, patients may present with new-onset, accelerated, or worsening hypertension.[169-172] Flank pain is frequent, and headache may occur, perhaps as a result of hypertension. In some cases, especially with lesions that develop from an angiographic procedure, the patient may be asymptomatic except for worsening hypertension. Mild proteinuria may be detected, and hematuria is noted in only 20% to 35% of the patients.[167] Impaired renal function with serum creatinine greater than 1.5 mg/dL was present in only 9% and 33% of patients in two series.[167, 173] Intravenous urography may show decreased renal function, reduced renal size, and delayed appearance, or it may be normal. Selective angiography is necessary for the diagnosis. Dissection on arteriography appears as an abrupt narrowing of the arterial lumen, which is caused by the unfilled false lumen (Fig. 32-8). Less commonly, both true and false lumens fill with contrast material, giving the appearance of a double lumen separated by an intimal flap. The dissection may extend distally to the

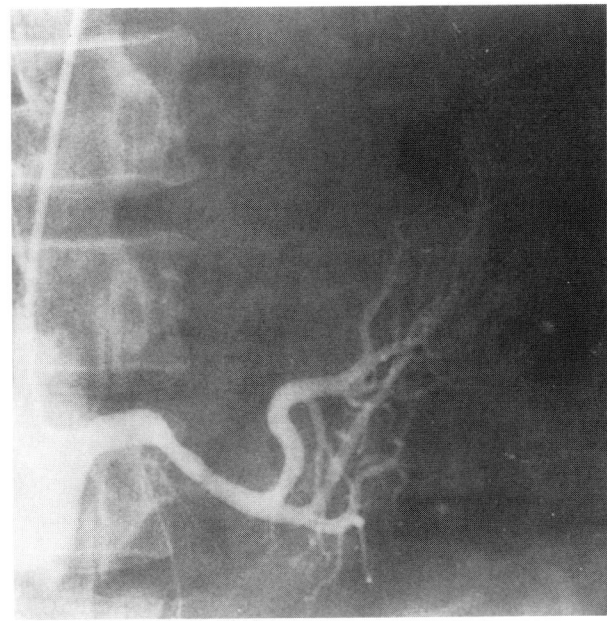

FIGURE 32-8. Dissecting aneurysm of the right renal artery. Arteriogram shows uniform narrowing of the main artery, starting approximately 1 cm distal to the arterial origin. (From Alamir A, Middendorf DF, Baker P, et al: Renal artery dissection causing renal infarction in otherwise healthy men. Am J Kidney Dis 30:851-855, 1997.)

first bifurcation and then to the branches, and there may be cuffing at the branches. In approximately 50% of cases, there is lateralization of renal vein renin levels, and the isotope renogram shows unilateral abnormalities in a similar fraction.[167]

The clinical outcome appears to be variable. Some patients have persistent severe renovascular hypertension that may be resistant to medical therapy. These patients may benefit from revascularization or nephrectomy if they suffered renal infarction, and many show improvement or complete resolution of hypertension after these procedures.[172, 173] Endovascular interventions have also been reported.[174-176]

Other patients present similarly with new-onset severe hypertension and flank pain, but with conservative medical management their hypertension is controlled and may even resolve with time. These patients may remain normotensive after long-term follow-up. Furthermore, repeat angiographic studies may show complete resolution of the dissection.[169, 170, 176] The appropriate therapy depends on the severity of the hypertension and its response to antihypertensive therapy. Edwards and colleagues[167] noted adequate responses to medical management in the majority of patients. Others have emphasized the importance of vascular reconstruction, which may require autotransplantation.[177-179]

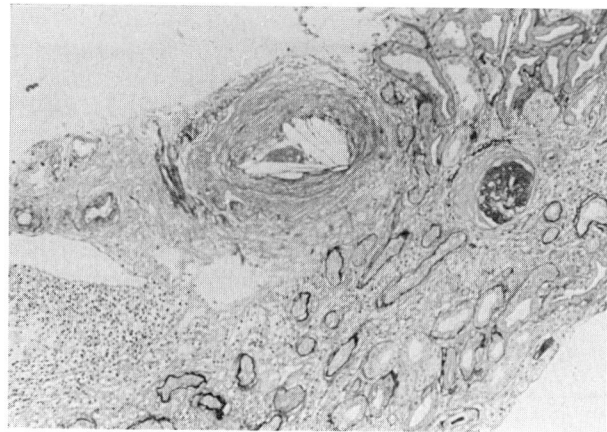

FIGURE 32-9. Cholesterol clefts are shown completely occluding the lumen of an arcuate artery. (Hematoxylin and eosin stain.) (Courtesy of Surya Seshan, M.D., New York, NY.)

ATHEROEMBOLIC RENAL DISEASE

Atheroembolic disease (AED), also known as cholesterol embolization, can have a wide range of clinical manifestations due to showering of cholesterol crystals from the aorta or other major arteries. It is a disease of the elderly, especially those with evidence of diffuse atherosclerosis. Atheromatous plaques may slough off the walls of the great vessels, travel downstream, and become lodged in the lumen of small arteries, arterioles, and capillaries. Local ischemia and inflammatory reactions ensue. Clinical findings depend on the location, severity, and duration of the atheromatous showering. Virtually every organ may be involved, but most commonly the skin, kidneys, gastrointestinal tract, and central nervous system are the sites of cholesterol showering. AED is usually precipitated by surgical or interventional manipulation of the arterial tree or by treatment with anticoagulants or thrombolytic agents. Less commonly, it occurs spontaneously without any precipitating factors. The severity of disease varies from mild to life-threatening.

Pathologic Features

Cholesterol-containing microemboli occluding the renal vasculature is not an uncommon pathologic finding. Autopsy studies report the incidence of AED as 5% in men and 3% in women older than 50 years of age.[180] This is far higher than the clinically apparent disease, which suggests that only the more severe cases of AED have clinical manifestations, whereas mild cases are asymptomatic. In autopsy studies of patients with AED, the kidney is the most commonly involved internal organ. Seventy-five percent of 173 autopsy cases of AED had renal involvement.[181] Cholesterol emboli were widespread, and each autopsy averaged 3.4 organs with emboli. Besides renal involvement, other common organ sites for atheroemboli were the spleen, pancreas, and gastrointestinal tract.[181]

In AED, renal injury arises from the occlusion of multiple small arteries, typically with diameters of 150 to 200 μm. The arcuate and interlobular arteries, terminal arterioles, and glomerular capillaries are most commonly involved.[182, 183]

Pathologic examination reveals characteristic biconvex, needle-shaped clefts that occlude the lumen of the vessels. The cholesterol crystals within the emboli dissolve during tissue fixation, leaving in their place the clefts (Fig. 32-9). Complete obstruction of the small arteries or arterioles leads to distal areas of small infarction and necrosis; in incomplete obstruction, distal areas exhibit ischemic atrophy.

In the acute period after atheroembolization, cholesterol crystals may be surrounded by eosinophilic material with little inflammatory reaction in the surrounding interstitium. Subsequently, intimal thickening appears, and macrophages and multinucleated giant cells of the foreign-body type become evident. Later, marked intimal thickening with concentric fibrosis develops. Necrosis of the arterial wall does not occur despite this inflammation.

The occlusion of multiple small vessels produces patchy areas of renal ischemia. Atrophy is usually predominant, and small areas of infarction can occur. Glomeruli appear ischemic and may become hyalinized; occasionally, cholesterol crystals are noted in glomerular capillaries. The tubules become atrophic. Grossly, the kidney may be reduced in size with a rough granular surface and scars. Similar lesions produced in experimental animals closely resemble the pathologic features observed in human tissue.[184-186]

The internal surface of the aorta is commonly covered with atheromatous plaques that are shaggy and ulcerating, and with fibrin and platelet thrombi (Fig. 32-10).[187-190] These thrombi are pliable and soft, and they can easily be dislodged. The intima may be completely eroded, revealing direct communication between an atheroma and the lumen of the aorta.[183, 190-192]

Focal glomerulosclerosis may be associated with AED. In a report of 24 patients with renal biopsy evidence of AED, focal glomerulosclerosis was also found in the majority of patients.[193] Among those with nephrotic-range proteinuria, the collapsing variant of focal glomerulosclerosis was common. The authors speculated that the progressive loss of the remnant glomeruli to hyperfiltration or chronic ischemia could lead to focal glomerulosclerosis and glomerular collapse.

Clinical Manifestations

Elderly patients with evidence of diffuse atherosclerosis are most at risk for development of AED. Table 32-5 lists the baseline clinical features of patients who later developed AED. These data were gathered from 350 patients who were described in three of the largest series of patients with AED[194-196] and from a large review on the subject.[197] The typical patients were elderly, in their 60s, predominantly male, and overwhelmingly Caucasian. Hypertension was present in 60% to 100%, and a significant history of past or current cigarette smoking was noted in 80% to 90%. A history of vascular disease was very common; coronary artery, peripheral vascular, and cerebrovascular disease, often concomitantly present, were noted in one half to three fourths of the patients, and abdominal aortic aneurysms were seen in one fourth to two thirds. Baseline renal function was frequently depressed; from three series[195, 196, 198] that reported baseline serum creatinine concentrations in almost 150 patients, the mean value approximated 2.0 mg/dL. The cause of the underlying chronic renal insufficiency was probably multifactorial, but ischemic nephropathy from atherosclerotic renovascular disease may have been a factor in some cases.[199] One fourth to one half of the patients were hypercholesterolemic, and fewer were diabetic.

The precipitating causes of AED—invasive procedures, vascular surgery, or medical therapy with anticoagulants and thrombolytic agents—were implicated to varying degrees (see Table 32-5). Invasive angiographic studies (usually coronary, carotid, or aortic studies) were considered to be the precipitating cause in 18% to 96% of the cases, and cardiovascular or aortic surgery in about 10%.[200-202] Anticoagulants with heparin or warfarin and thrombolytic therapy were considered to be contributing factors in 14% to 37% of the

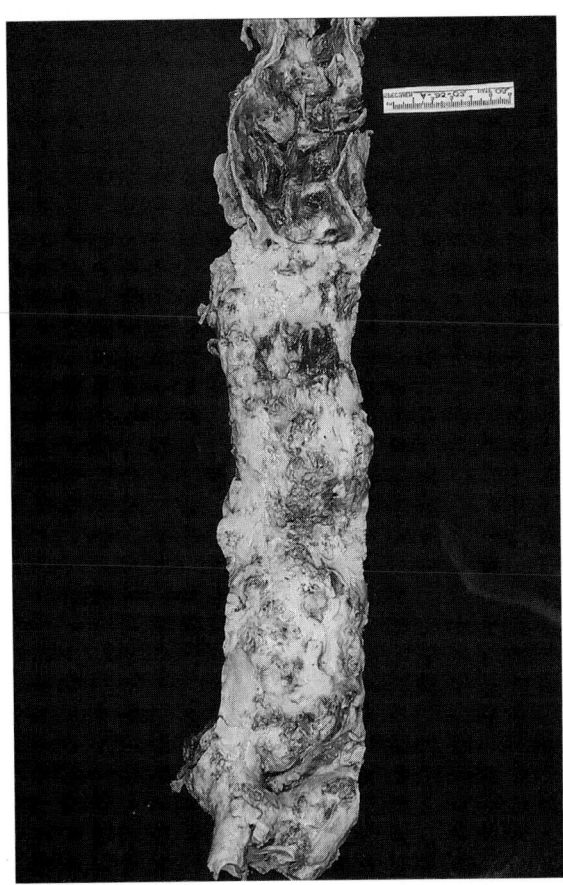

FIGURE 32-10. Severe atherosclerosis of the aorta with aneurysmal dilatation containing atheromatous plaques. Autopsy specimen from a 70-year-old man with atheroemboli found throughout the gastrointestinal tract and spleen. (Compliments of Shahida Ahmed, M.D.)

TABLE 32-5

Atheroembolic Disease—Clinical Characteristics from Three Series and One Large Review

PARAMETER	BELENFANT[194]	THADHANI[195]	VIDT[196]	FINE[197a]
Demographics				
Number of patients	67	52	24	221
Mean age (range, yr)	69 ± 8	69 ± 7	62 (45–75)	66 (26–90)
Male (%)	96	75	80	77
White race (%)	100[b]	100	?	94
Clinical Characteristics				
Cigarette smoking history (%)	79	90	92	?
Hypertension (%)	91	81	100	61
Baseline mean serum creatinine (mg/dL)	2.0 ± 0.9	1.67 ± 0.59	2.0 (1.0–6.5)	?
Baseline medical problems (%)				
Hypercholesterolemia	?	49	29	?
Diabetes mellitus	?	33	8.3	?
Coronary artery disease	54	73	67	44
Peripheral vascular disease	57	69	75	?
Cerebrovascular disease	32	46	62	?
Abdominal aortic aneurysm	67	48	29	25
Precipitating factors (%)				
Angiography	85	96	?	18
Vascular surgery	36	8	?	9
Anticoagulation or thrombolytics	76	37	?	14

[a]Review of clinical cases.
[b]This study was from France.

cases.[203-208] AED has also been attributed to blunt abdominal trauma,[209] intra-aortic balloon placement, cardiopulmonary resuscitation,[202] and percutaneous renal angioplasty.[208] In a minority of cases, no precipitating factors are evident and AED is considered to have occurred spontaneously. In a 1999 study, only 3 of 67 patients with AED did not have an identifiable precipitating cause.[194]

The time to onset of clinically apparent AED after a precipitating event is extremely variable. Clinical signs and symptoms of AED may be obvious within 1 day after a precipitating event, or they may follow the event by days, weeks, or a few months.[194, 200, 209, 210] In 52 patients with AED and RF, clinical manifestations were noted within 1 day in half of the patients.[195] In another recent study, Belenfant and colleagues[194] reported a long interval—2 months—between the precipitating event and the recognition of worsening of renal function due to AED.

The array of presenting signs and symptoms of AED is vast and variable and can mimic other diseases. The onset of symptoms may be abrupt and severe, or there may be gradual worsening or development of new symptoms coinciding with recurrent showering of cholesterol emboli. Skin manifestations, seen in 35% to 50% of cases, are the most common presentation.[195, 211, 212] These include livedo reticularis, gangrene, ulcers, violaceous mottling of the toes ("purple toe syndrome"), nodules, purpura, and petechiae (Fig. 32-11). These are frequently bilateral and usually limited to the lower extremities, although other parts of the skin also may be involved. Severe cases of scrotal and penile necrosis have been described.[213]

The RF frequently is severe and often is the most critical manifestation of AED. The incidence of RF in AED cannot be determined from the retrospective studies, but it appears to be common. In 52 patients with histologically proven AED, serum creatinine rose to more than 2 mg/dL in 83% of the patients, and to more than 5 mg/dL in 25% of them.[197] An autopsy review of 121 cases of AED noted the kidney to be the most commonly involved internal organ, with 75% of the cases showing evidence of cholesterol emboli (Table 32-6).[199]

TABLE 32-6

Location of Cholesterol Emboli Found at Autopsy on Patients with Atheroembolic Disease

ORGANS INVOLVED (%)	VIDT[199] (N = 173*)	THADHANI[195] (N = 33)
Kidney	75	100†
Spleen	95	70
Pancreas	52	—
Gastrointestinal tract	31	70
Adrenals	20	17
Liver	17	—
Brain	14	43
Testes	11	—
Muscle	9	—
Prostate	9	—
Thyroid	7	—
Skin	6	—
Bone marrow	5	—
Heart	4	—
Vasa vasorum	3	—
Gallbladder	3	—
Bone	3	—
Urinary bladder	3	—
Coronary arteries	2	—
Lungs	1	—

*Of these 173 patients, autopsy was the sole means of diagnosis in 153; in the other 20, cholesterol embolization was diagnosed before death and confirmed on autopsy.

†To enter this study, all patients had to have acute renal failure due to atheroembolic disease.

Table courtesy of Vidt.[199]

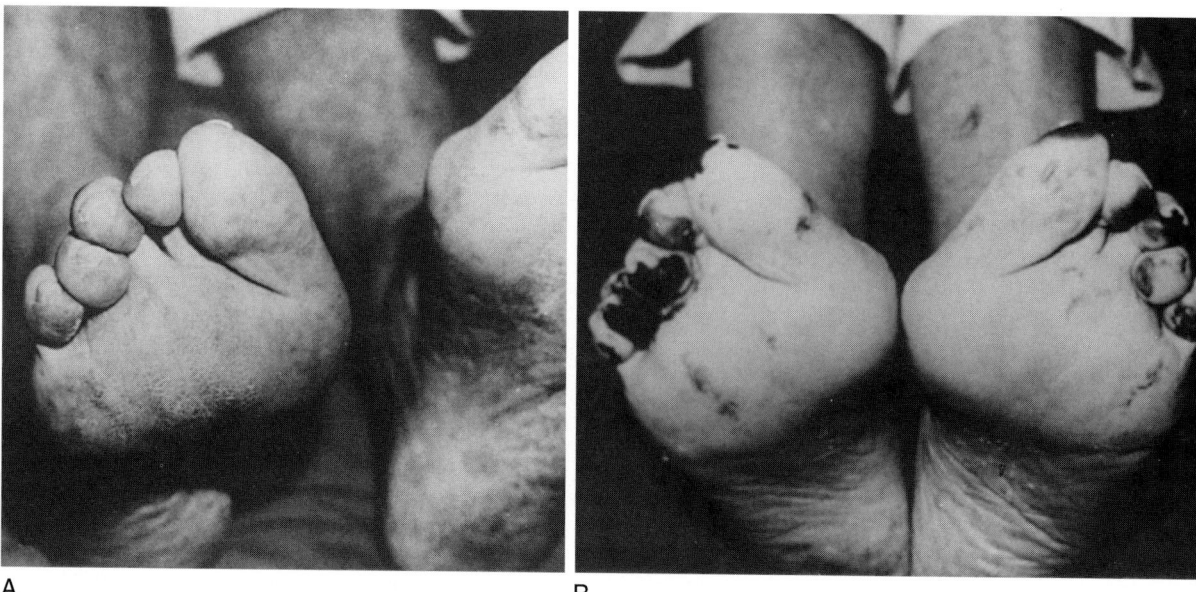

A   B

FIGURE 32-11. Peripheral manifestations of atheroembolic disease. **A,** Mottling of both feet (livedo reticularis). **B,** Gangrenous lesions of several toes, which was preceded by violaceous mottling ("purple toe syndrome"). (From Siemons L, Van Den Heuvel P, Parizel G, et al: Peritoneal dialysis in acute renal failure due to cholesterol embolization: Two cases of recovery of renal function and extended survival. Clin Nephrol 28: 205-209, 1987.)

RF can have multiple presentations, including acute oliguric or nonoliguric RF or a more insidious and prolonged progression. There may be an intermittent and stepwise progression of azotemia, possibly coinciding with recurrent waves of atheroemboli.[200] These presentations are often superimposed on mild chronic renal insufficiency, as noted previously. From recent reports of patients with ARF due to AED, severe RF requiring dialysis developed in 17% to 61% of them.[195, 196, 198] The clinical course of RF is variable. In some cases, it resolves partially or completely, but many patients are left with some degree of chronic RF. Of patients requiring dialysis because of AED, approximately 20% to 30% regain function adequate to stop the dialysis.[214] The time course for this improvement is variable, but it may be prolonged. Thadhani and co-workers[195] noted that the time to renal recovery once severe RF developed ranged from 42 to 122 days.

Gastrointestinal manifestations of AED are common and occur in 18% to 48% of the patients.[215, 216] Abdominal pain and gastrointestinal hemorrhage from mucosal ulcerations or infarcts are the usual presentations, but diarrhea, bowel obstruction, postprandial pain, and, rarely, small bowel perforation have been described.[216, 217] Pancreatitis, acalculous necrotizing cholecystitis, pseudopolyps, splenic infarcts, and angiodysplastic lesions have been noted.[217, 218]

Cerebrovascular involvement may manifest as confusion, obtundation, or focal neurologic deficits.[197] Visual defects may be noted, and small retinal atheroembolic plaques (Hollenhorst plaques), an important physical finding in AED, may be seen on funduscopic examination.[219, 220] Nonspecific findings include fever, myalgias, and weight loss. A few case reports documented histologic evidence of pulmonary involvement of AED, with clinical findings of hemoptysis and respiratory distress.[221-223] This pulmonary-renal presentation is rare.

The urinalysis, like much of the laboratory work, is often abnormal but not specific. Proteinuria is typically mild, but a few cases of new-onset nephrotic-range proteinuria, coincident with the AED, have been documented.[194, 195, 224] Three of 67 patients with ARF and AED developed nephrotic-range proteinuria.[194] The urine sediment may be inactive, or hematuria, pyuria, and granular casts may be present. Rarely, the sediment may have a nephritic appearance, with dysmorphic erythrocytes and red blood cell casts.

Eosinophilia and eosinophiluria have been variably noted.[225-227] In a review of 80 patients with RF due to AED, 71% had transient eosinophilia.[226] Conflicting reports of the incidence of eosinophilia were found in two studies: eosinophilia was noted in 10 of 13 patients with ARF from AED in one study,[198] but in only 14% of 37 patients in another study.[195] The transient nature of the eosinophilia and the retrospective analysis of these reports may have contributed to these discrepancies. Reports of eosinophiluria in AED are also contradictory: eosinophiluria, demonstrated by the Hansel stain, was found in 8 of 9 patients,[227] but in another study it was found in only 5% of 37 patients with use of the Wright stain.[195] Other abnormal laboratory findings include a normochromic normocytic anemia, leukocytosis, an elevated sedimentation rate, elevated C-reactive protein, and hypocomplementemia.[195, 228] Depending on the organs involved, elevations of amylase, lipase, CPK, and liver enzymes may be noted.

Most reported mortality rates of patients with RF due to AED are disturbingly high. Because these rates are obtained from retrospective studies and case reports, they are probably biased toward the more severe cases. Two studies of ARF and AED reported mortality rates of 65% at 6 months among 52 patients, and 30% at 1 year among 15 patients.[195, 198] Death was frequently attributed to multifactorial causes, commonly congestive heart failure, sepsis, and hypotension. Belenfant and colleagues[194] had better outcomes among their 67 patients: the in-hospital mortality rate during the first 3 months was 16%, and at 4 years the long-term survival rate was 50%.

The diagnosis may be clear-cut on clinical grounds if the constellation of clinical and laboratory findings of AED is present and there is a close temporal relation with the precipitating event. However, in other cases the diagnosis may be difficult, particularly when AED occurs spontaneously. A strong index of suspicion for AED and a search for extrarenal manifestations are needed when unexplained RF develops in an elderly patient with evidence of atherosclerosis. In such cases, a definitive diagnosis may require histologic confirmation. Biopsies of involved areas of skin, muscle, or kidney are likely to yield the diagnosis. When cutaneous manifestations are present, biopsies of the affected skin are diagnostic in 90% of the cases.[197] Percutaneous renal biopsies may miss the cholesterol clefts, given their patchy presence. A histologic diagnosis of AED has been made from such varied tissue specimens as bone marrow aspirates, prostatic curettage, and gastric and lung biopsy specimens.[221, 222, 229] Given the multisystemic presentation of many cases of AED, the differential diagnosis includes the various vasculitides, bacterial endocarditis, Schönlein-Henoch purpura, rhabdomyolysis, and, rarely, the pulmonary-renal syndromes. When ARF closely follows an interventional radiologic procedure, it may be difficult to differentiate AED from contrast-mediated acute tubular necrosis. Extrarenal manifestations and the subsequent clinical course of RF are often helpful in this regard. Not infrequently, the diagnosis is made after death. Table 32-6 shows the location of cholesterol emboli found at autopsy.[199]

There is no specific therapy for AED. Once AED develops, good supportive care and avoidance of precipitating factors that would cause further devastating atheroemboli appear to be critical for a successful outcome. Belenfant and co-workers[194] attributed the relatively low mortality rates in their large group of patients with AED and severe RF, noted previously, to this approach. To prevent recurrent disease, they withdrew all anticoagulant therapy regardless of the indication, and they canceled all further diagnostic and therapeutic aortic catheterizations. Supportive care measures include aggressive treatment of hypertension and of cardiac failure, nutritional support, and renal replacement therapy with minimal or no heparin.

Corticosteroids, statins, prostaglandin analogs, and plasmapheresis have been described as beneficial in small, uncontrolled series or in case reports. From the scarcity of data, no recommendations can be made regarding their use in AED. These treatments have been recently reviewed.[209, 210, 230]

Some patients with concomitant AED and atherosclerotic renal artery stenosis may improve renal function with correction of the renal artery stenosis.[149, 152, 196, 199] In the reported cases, renal function was allowed to stabilize for a few months after the initial episode of atheroemboli before interventions, either surgical bypass or intra-arterial stent placement, were attempted.

Surgical benefit has also been described in AED, mainly for limb salvage.[231] In a study of 100 patients with AED, surgery was attempted to remove the source of the atheroemboli. Surgical outcome and long-term prognosis, especially limb salvage, were good in the patients in whom the infrarenal aorta or iliac artery was the source of the atheroemboli. However, clinical outcomes were poor and mortality rates were high in patients who underwent suprarenal aortic surgery.[216] In another study, 42 patients with AED underwent bypass surgery or endarterectomy, most of them at the level of the infrarenal aorta or more distally. The authors reported good limb salvage, low operative mortality, and excellent long-term relief of embolization.[232] Surgical candidates among this elderly population, many with comorbid conditions, must be chosen carefully.

RENAL VEIN THROMBOSIS

Thrombosis of the renal vein was originally thought to be a relatively uncommon vascular complication of the kidney. Although the first description of thrombosis of the renal vein was made by Hunter,[233] it was Rayer who in 1840 was the first to make an association between renal vein thrombosis (RVT) and the nephrotic syndrome.[234] Much later, Abeshouse[235] extensively reviewed the medical literature in regard to thrombotic disease of the renal vein. Among the most important causes cited were infectious suppuration, malignancy, and trauma. In all of these patients, the diagnosis of RVT was made post mortem. Later, with the development of more advanced radiographic techniques and selective catheterization, antemortem diagnosis of RVT was made possible, and the number of patients in the adult population diagnosed with RVT increased. Although RVT may be caused by trauma or tumor, it has become apparent that it occurs most commonly in the nephrotic patient.

Because of the early descriptions, emphasis was placed on the presence of lumbar pain with flank tenderness, edema, and the appearance of a lumbar mass. As a consequence, the early reports focused attention on these symptoms, and it was generally assumed that RVT always manifested suddenly and with florid symptomatology. However, Harrison and colleagues,[236]

in 1956, described two groups of patients with RVT. Those with complete acute thrombosis of the renal vein characteristically had severe lumbar or abdominal pain, enlargement of the affected kidney, proteinuria, edema, and deterioration of renal function. A second group patients, however, had only the nephrotic syndrome and absence of acute symptomatology.

Etiology

The incidence of RVT in the adult population is difficult to establish. A review of 29,280 necropsy studies performed at the Mayo Clinic from 1920 to 1961 revealed 17 cases of bilateral RVT in adults, an incidence of approximately 0.6 per 1000 necropsies.[237] Only 2 of these 17 patients had the nephrotic syndrome, however. More recently, prospective studies have evaluated the incidence of RVT in the nephrotic patient and found it to be significant, although variable. In Table 32-7 are displayed various prospective studies evaluating the incidence of RVT in patients with nephrotic syndrome and membranous nephropathy.[237-245] This table includes data only from prospective studies evaluating patients undergoing routine renal venograms, regardless of the presence or absence of symptoms suggestive of RVT. It can be appreciated that the overall incidence of RVT in both the nephrotic syndrome and membranous nephropathy is significant; however, there are marked differences, ranging from 5% to 62%. The reason for such differences is not clear. One possibility, in light of current immunologic advances, is that membranous nephropathy may include different immunologic entities, some of which may be more prone to develop RVT than others. Another possibility is that the duration of the nephrotic syndrome and the persistence and magnitude of the hypoalbuminemia may have varied in these studies. It is generally agreed that the most common underlying nephropathy associated with RVT is membranous nephropathy. A review of all our patients with nephrotic syndrome is shown in Table 32-8. Of 151 patients with the syndrome, 33 had RVT, and 20 of those had membranous nephropathy.[246] However, it can be appreciated that there are other causes, such as membranoproliferative glomerulonephritis, lipoid nephrosis, and amyloidosis, that may be associated with RVT. It should be emphasized that, of our 33 patients with RVT, only 4 had an acute mode of presentation.

The concept of the relationship between RVT and the nephrotic syndrome has changed in the last three decades.[247]

TABLE 32-7

Prospective Studies Evaluating the Incidence of Renal Vein Thrombosis (RVT) in Patients with Nephrotic Syndrome (NS) and Membranous Glomerulopathy (MGN)

STUDY	PATIENTS WITH RVT IN NS	INCIDENCE (%)	PATIENTS WITH RVT IN MGN	INCIDENCE (%)
Bennett[238]	—	—	5/10	50
Noel et al[242]	—	—	5/16	31
Wagoner et al[245]	—	—	14/27	52
Cameron et al[239]	—	—	2/15	13
Pohl et al[243]	1/54	2	1/20	9
Llach et al[246]	33/151	22	20/69	29
Monteon et al[241]	15/53	28	15/24	62
Vosnides et al[347]	7/44	16	5/30	17
Velazquez-Forero et al[244]	8/39	42	3/5	60

Modified from Llach, F: The hypercoagulability and thrombotic complication of nephrotic syndrome. Editorial review. Kidney Int 28:429, 1985.

TABLE 32-8

Etiology of the Nephrotic Syndrome in 151 Patients

RENAL DIAGNOSIS	PATIENTS WITH RENAL VEIN THROMBOSIS (NO.)	PATIENTS WITHOUT RENAL VEIN THROMBOSIS (NO.)	TOTAL
Membranous nephropathy	20	49	69
Membranoproliferative GN	6	21	27
Lipoid nephrosis	2	8	10
Rapidly progressive GN	1	1	2
Amyloidosis	1	5	6
Focal sclerosis	1	3	4
Renal sarcoidosis	1	0	1
Lupus nephritis	1	10	11
Diabetic nephropathy	0	15	15
Focal GN	0	3	3
Acute poststreptococcal GN	0	2	2
End-stage renal disease	0	1	1
Total	33	118	151

GN, glomerulonephritis.

From Llach F, Koffler A, Massry SG: Renal vein thrombosis and the nephrotic syndrome. Nephron 19:65, 1977, with permission.

For many years, it was thought that RVT was the cause of the nephrotic syndrome, a belief that is no longer held. Several lines of evidence have seriously questioned this hypothesis. First, experimentally induced RVT causes only mild proteinuria, and the renal histology as demonstrated by immunofluorescent findings in these cases does not resemble that of membranous nephropathy.[248-251] Second, RVT has been reported in the surgical literature in the absence of the nephrotic syndrome.[252, 253] Moreover, in autopsy studies of patients with RVT, nephrotic syndrome is present antemortem in only a few patients.[235] Third, most patients with RVT and nephrotic syndrome who have been subjected to renal morphologic study have exhibited an identifiable glomerulopathy most of the time: membranous nephropathy, which is responsible for the nephrotic syndrome.[254] Finally, it has been shown that RVT occurs after the onset of the nephrotic syndrome.[255, 256] Therefore, the general view today is that the nephrotic syndrome provides a favorable milieu for the development of RVT.

Pathophysiology

An important factor in the causation of RVT in patients with the nephrotic syndrome is the presence of a hypercoagulable state. Profound clotting factor abnormalities have been noted in the nephrotic syndrome by various investigators. There are five major functional classes of coagulation components: (1) zymogens (factors II, V, IX, XI, and XII), which are activated by enzymes and cofactors (factors V and VIII) whose major role is to accelerate the role of enzymes; (2) fibrinogen and products from the conversion of fibrinogen to fibrin; (3) the fibrinolytic system; (4) clotting inhibitors; and (5) components of the platelet reaction and thrombogenesis. Alterations in all of these coagulation components have been observed in the nephrotic patient.

Alterations in zymogens and cofactors include a decrease in the levels of factors IX, XI, and XII. The low levels of these proteins most likely are the result of urinary loss secondary to their small molecular size rather than to impaired protein synthesis. An increase in the levels of factor II and combined factors VII and X has also been described.[257] In general, most of these zymogen abnormalities tend to normalize with clinical remission of the nephrotic syndrome. Most consistently, increased levels of cofactors (factors V and VIII) have been noted in the nephrotic syndrome.[258-260] A number of studies have shown a correlation between increases in factors V and VIII and a fall in serum albumin.[258-261] It appears that the alterations in cofactors result from increased synthesis of these proteins by the liver: the mitochondria of the liver cells are the final sites of production for most of these proteins. A decrease in plasma oncotic pressure or a decrease in serum albumin concentration, or both, may be sensed by these liver cells, leading in response to an increased production of various proteins.[262]

During the earlier description of the hypercoagulable state of the nephrotic syndrome, the hypothesis was advanced that an increase in cofactors may lead to hypercoagulability and may explain the high incidence of thrombosis in these patients. However, two important points must be made regarding this hypothesis. First, all of these factors are normally present in great excess in the circulation, with only a small amount of any given factor being activated during thrombus formation. Therefore, it seems unlikely that high levels of any of these zymogens would lead to thrombosis or that reduced levels of some coagulation factors would be a sensitive marker of the presence of thrombosis. Second, there is no evidence to suggest that the increased level of cofactors may lead to thromboembolic phenomena. High levels of these factors are usually present during acute inflammatory responses, because they are an acute phase reactant protein. There is no current evidence that these conditions are associated with an increased risk of thrombosis.

An elevation of the plasma fibrinogen concentration is a consistent and significant abnormality observed in nephrotic patients.[256, 263-265] With the use of iodine 131 (^{131}I)-labeled fibrinogen, the rate of fibrinogen catabolism was found to be normal in these patients, and the observed increase in plasma fibrinogen was found to be caused by an increased liver synthesis that is proportional to the urinary protein loss.[265] In addition, there is a significant correlation between fibrinogen and cholesterol levels, and both are inversely related to the levels of serum albumin. The concentration of fibrinogen in nephrotic patients may be as high as 1 g/dL and has been shown to alter plasma viscosity considerably.[264] Therefore, increased plasma fibrinogen reflects increased hepatic synthesis of fibrinogen; contracted intravascular distribution may be present, and there is a normal degradation rate of fibrinogen in the nephrotic patient. It is likely that the high fibrinogen levels, by significantly increasing blood viscosity, are important in the hypercoagulable state of nephrotic syndrome.

Various tests for determination of the products of fibrinogen to fibrin conversion have been developed for diagnosis of a prethrombotic state. An increase in the plasma concentration of fibrinogen degradation products (FDP) is not commonly observed in nephrotic patients but has been observed in the urine of patients with glomerulonephritis.[266] Some nephrotic patients have been found to have increased urinary levels of FDP.[267] However, these findings should not be taken as definite evidence for increased fibrinolysis in the systemic or renal vasculature, because in patients with nonselective proteinuria fibrinogen is filtered at the glomerulus and may undergo proteolytic degradation by protease. In this regard, gel chromatography clearly shows that material that has in the past been interpreted as FDP is actually filtered fibrinogen that has been degraded in the tubules.[264, 268]

Alterations in the fibrinolytic system have also been observed in nephrotic patients.[269] The basic reaction of the fibrinolytic system is the conversion by plasminogen activators of a β-globulin, plasminogen, to an active serum protease, plasmin. This system is modulated by inhibitors of both plasminogen and plasmin. A number of clinical studies have reported an association between defective fibrinolysis and thrombosis; the association has included oral contraceptive ingestion,[270] pregnancy,[271] postoperative states,[272] malignant disease,[273] obesity,[274] and the nephrotic syndrome.[275] The data in regard to the fibrinolytic abnormalities in nephrotic patients have shown in general a decrease in plasma plasminogen concentration[275-277] that is correlated with a low serum albumin and the magnitude of the proteinuria.[275, 278-280] The clinical significance of this abnormality is not known, and a cause-effect relationship between these abnormalities and RVT has not been made. However, Du and associates[279] identified a plasmin inhibitor to be identical with α_2-antiplasmin. They evaluated 14 nephrotic patients with RVT and 30 nephrotic patients without RVT. In both groups, the level of total fibrinolytic activity was normal and that of the plasma inhibitor (α_2-antiplasmin) of plasminogen activation was elevated. However, the plasmin inhibitor was elevated in 13 of 14 patients with RVT and only in 12 of 30 patients without RVT. The authors suggested that the increased level of α_2-antiplasmin may be a factor in determining susceptibility to the development and persistence of RVT in the nephrotic patients. Further studies are needed to confirm the importance of these observations.

Alterations in coagulation inhibitors have been observed in nephrotic patients. The components of the coagulation system exist in the circulation as zymogens, and they are cleaved to form proteolytic enzymes. Activated clotting factors are inhibited by naturally occurring coagulation inhibitors.[281, 282] The most important physiology of these inhibitors is antithrombin-III (AT-III). This is an α_2-globulin that is the main inhibitor of thrombin and also inhibits activated factors XII, IX, X, XI, and plasmin.[283-288] The

rate of inhibition of these enzymes by AT-III is markedly increased in the presence of heparin. In patients from families with an inherited deficiency of AT-III, an increased incidence of thromboembolic complications is generally observed when AT-III levels are less than 75% of normal.[283, 285] Kauffman and associates[289] studied AT-III levels in 48 patients with proteinuria and their relationship to the occurrence of thromboembolic phenomena. Nine patients had evidence of thrombosis, including four with RVT. In eight of these nine patients, the serum AT-III levels were less than 70% of normal. There was a significant correlation between AT-III concentration and the urine protein excretion. Only 6 of the 32 patients who excreted less than 10 g per 24 hours showed depressed AT-III levels (less than 85% of normal), whereas 13 of 16 patients with a proteinuria higher than 10 g per 24 hours showed depressed AT-III levels. Because the molecular weight of AT-III is relatively low, excretion in the urine would be expected in patients with proteinuria. Because of similar molecular weights, renal clearance rates of AT-III and of albumin were compared. A significant correlation was noted between the plasma concentrations of these two proteins. In addition, there was a significant correlation between the renal AT-III clearance rate and the degree of AT-III deficiency. It was concluded that thrombosis in nephrotic patients may be associated with deficiency of AT-III caused by increased urinary loss and that low levels of AT-III may be insufficient to inactivate procoagulant factors, resulting in the development of thrombosis. These results are in apparent conflict with studies showing normal or increased antithrombin activity in nephrotic children.[290-294] This latter finding may have resulted from the nonspecific in vitro inhibition of thrombin by α_2-globulin and α_2-antitrypsin (two other clotting inhibitors), and therefore the apparent increment in AT-III activity may not have reflected a true increase in AT-III levels. In addition, AT-III deficiency was generally reported by other investigators in association with a serum albumin concentration lower than 2 g/dL,[264, 289-290] whereas in the earlier studies only a few patients had severe hypoalbuminemia. Panicucci and colleagues[292] reported normal levels of AT-III despite high urinary AT-III levels. They suggested that increased AT-III synthesis compensated for its renal loss. Later, Vaziri and associates[293] observed a significant decrease in AT-III plasma concentration and activity in 20 nephrotic patients compared with normal subjects. Also, substantial urinary losses of AT-III were demonstrated in nephrotic patients.

Thus, although the rate of synthesis and degradation of AT-III and its distribution have not been determined, it is likely that renal losses of AT-III in nephrotic patients contribute to AT-III deficiency. It is possible that the danger of thromboembolic phenomena may arise with sudden changes in the activity of the renal disease, resulting in abrupt renal losses of AT-III while hepatic synthesis of AT-III has not yet increased. An interesting observation is the increase in AT-III levels in nephrotic children after steroid therapy.[292] Also of interest is the observation of a healthy, non-nephrotic 13-year-old girl presenting with acute flank pain and anuria due to RVT.[291] The patient was noted to have a marked familial deficiency of AT-III levels. Urgent surgical thrombectomy and anticoagulation resulted in recovery of renal function.

An early diagnosis of this familial condition therefore may lead to the use of preventive measures or acute specific therapeutic interventions at the onset of the acute thrombosis.

Important data about the role of coagulation inhibitors in the development of thrombosis have been reported. Protein C and protein S have been identified as potent anticoagulants. Protein C is a vitamin K–dependent serum protease zymogen that is homologous with other known vitamin K–dependent serum proteases.[295, 296] This protein is an anticoagulant because it prolongs the clotting time of plasma in various clotting assays.[296] The clinical role of protein C as an important antithrombotic regulatory molecule has been demonstrated by identifying a familial thrombotic disease that is associated with an inherited partial deficiency of protein C.[297] Families with a deficiency in plasma protein C have recurrent thrombosis. It appears that protein C levels lower than 50% of normal result in thrombosis. Whereas AT-III appears to be a major regulatory protein limiting the activity of procoagulant plasma enzymes, activated protein C may represent a major regulatory protein limiting the activity of activated procoagulant factor (factors V and VIII). In this respect, the anticoagulant properties of activated protein C and AT-III are complementary.

The rate of inactivation of factor V by activated protein C has been found to be stimulated by another vitamin K–dependent protein, protein S.[298, 299] Protein S has no effect on factor V activity in the absence of activated protein C, indicating that it is not a protease. In a protein S–deficient plasma, the anticoagulant activity of protein C is restored. It appears that the complex between protein S and activated protein C is formed only in the presence of phospholipids.[300, 301] Because protein S is required for the expression of the anticoagulant activity of activated protein C, it is not surprising that a deficiency of protein S has been found to predispose to recurrent thrombosis.[302] Comp and Esmon[301] identified six unrelated persons with severe, recurrent venous thrombosis who were deficient in protein S, with levels between 15% and 37% of normal.

Early high levels of protein C and protein S were observed in nephrotic patients.[303] Later, other investigators noted normal protein C concentration in nephrotic patients.[304] However, still later, it was observed that the functional levels of protein S did not correlate with the immunologic levels. Further, protein S was noted in two forms in plasma, as free and functionally active protein S and as protein S complexed to C4b-binding protein. When compared with control subjects, nephrotic patients had reduced functional levels of protein S despite having increased levels of total protein S antigen.[305] Decreased total protein S activity was caused by significant reductions in free (active) protein S due to selective urinary loss of free protein S and increased levels of C4b-binding protein, which favors complex formation. The authors also observed that the specific activity of protein C (activity-antigen ratio) was lower in nephrotic patients than in control subjects. They concluded that acquired protein S deficiency occurs in nephrotic syndrome and may be a risk factor for the development of the thromboembolic complications.

Platelet abnormalities have also been observed in nephrotic patients. Thrombocytosis often is present,[258-260] and an increased platelet aggregation with adenosine diphosphate (ADP) and collagen, but not with epinephrine, has been observed.[264, 306] Remuzzi and colleagues[306] observed that the degree of platelet function abnormalities correlates with the degree of hypoalbuminemia and the severity of the proteinuria.[306] The levels of β-thromboglobulin, a specific protein released by platelets on aggregation, are significantly increased in nephrotic patients, and they return to normal with clinical remission.[262-264] This suggests that nephrotic patients have an increase in platelet aggregation. However, normal β-thromboglobulin levels have also been reported in nephrotic patients.[307, 308] A study of nephrotic patients demonstrated that thrombotic complications occurred only in patients with increased platelet aggregation and an elevated β-thromboglobulin concentration.[309] In addition, these complications occurred primarily in patients with a serum albumin level of less than 2 g/dL.

In summary, the hypercoagulable state of the nephrotic syndrome is characterized by low zymogen factors, a marked increase in cofactors, an increase in plasma fibrinogen levels, decreased levels of AT-III and antiplasmin activity, thrombocytosis, increased plasma aggregation, and increased levels of β-thromboglobulin. The high concentrations of fibrinogen leading to increased plasma viscosity may be an important factor in the hypercoagulable state. A convincing relationship has been found between low AT-III and thrombosis, and it is likely that increased platelet aggregation may also be an important factor in hypercoagulability; the increased levels of β-thromboglobulin may be a reliable marker of platelet aggregation. The severity of the hypoalbuminemia, by increasing hepatic synthesis of fibrinogen and platelet aggregation, may play a pivotal role in the generation and maintenance of these abnormalities.

In regard to the role of a protein S deficiency in the hypercoagulable state, additional studies in nephrotic patients with thrombosis are necessary to reach any conclusion. However, inasmuch as protein S deficiency is an acquired problem, it should be assayed in patients with thromboembolic complications.

In addition to hypercoagulability, other factors may be important in the pathogenesis of RVT. A persistent reduction in plasma volume, which is an important feature in some patients with the nephrotic syndrome, especially in those with membranous nephropathy, may provide a milieu favorable to RVT. Theoretically, a sustained reduction in blood volume could lead to decreased renal venous flow, thereby favoring the development of RVT. In this regard, we have been impressed by the marked decrease in washout time in renal venograms in patients with membranous nephropathy who do not have RVT.[254] Diuretics may enhance volume depletion and thus contribute to the thromboembolic phenomena of the nephrotic syndrome. Data presented by Cheng and associates,[310] in their evaluation of 97 nephrotic patients, strongly suggest that intensive diuretic therapy is associated with a high incidence of RVT. The nature of the immunologic injury may also be important. A study investigating the relationship between membranous nephropathy and RVT separated a subpopulation of patients with both conditions.[311] It is attractive to speculate that such complexes may be the triggering factor in the coagulation process. The presence of factor XII and prekallikrein in subepithelial deposits was observed in 29 patients with membranous nephropathy.[311, 312] It is tempting to relate the high incidence of RVT in membranous nephropathy to activation of factor XII, a factor that is at the crossroads of important proteolytic pathways. Clinically, it has been shown that patients with nephrotic syndrome and membranous nephropathy have a high incidence of other thromboembolic phenomena in addition to RVT.[254] Also, greater disturbances of hypercoagulability were noted in patients with membranous nephropathy than in those nephrotic patients with minimal change disease.[301, 303] An underestimated factor predisposing to acute peripheral vascular thrombosis and even RVT may be arterial diagnostic puncture as well as placement of central catheters.[313] Finally, the role of steroids in the pathogenesis of RVT has not yet been defined. Steroids have been shown to aggravate the hypercoagulable state,[314, 315] and historically the advent of steroid therapy coincided with an increase in thromboembolic complications.[315, 316] The previously mentioned study by Cheng and co-workers[310] indicated that steroid therapy was associated with a high incidence of RVT. Therefore, these agents should be used cautiously in the treatment of nephrotic syndrome.

In summary, the pathogenesis of RVT in patients with nephrotic syndrome may be multifactorial. A general integrated scheme of the pathogenetic factors leading to RVT and other thromboembolic complications of nephrotic syndrome is displayed in Figure 32-12.

Clinical Manifestations: Acute versus Chronic Disease

The pattern and mode of clinical presentation of the nephrotic syndrome and RVT may differ from those mentioned in the early literature. Rayer's description of RVT included lumbar pain with tenderness, swelling, and the appearance of a lumbar mass.[234] Subsequent reports stressed the presence of flank pain and macroscopic hematuria in the clinical presentation of RVT.[317] However, as more cases were described, it was noted that in many instances RVT did not have any local symptoms or signs. The clinical spectrum of RVT varies from patient to patient. The rapidity of venous occlusion and the development of venous collateral circulation determine the clinical presentation and subsequent renal

function; however, in general, patients with RVT usually have two modes of clinical presentation: acute and chronic. The chronic presentation of RVT is observed most frequently and in general is asymptomatic. Acute RVT is characterized by sudden onset and usually occurs in younger patients, who complain of persistent acute flank pain, which may be colicky at times; marked costovertebral angle tenderness and macroscopic hematuria are usually present.

The following case is a representative example of acute RVT.[318] A 25-year-old white man came to the hospital with a year-long history of proteinuria and ankle swelling. Physical examination revealed no acute distress with normal blood pressure. The only physical finding was ankle edema. Urinary sediment demonstrated 3+ proteinuria. Biochemical data were consistent with the presence of nephrotic syndrome and normal renal function. Renal biopsy revealed early membranous nephropathy. Lung scan and IVP were within normal limits. An inferior venacavogram and a left renal venogram were within normal limits. At the time the left renal venogram was performed, the patient experienced an acute left flank pain that lasted 4 to 5 hours and was accompanied by macroscopic hematuria and marked tenderness in the left costovertebral angle. The procedure was terminated, and the patient was returned to the ward. A second IVP was obtained, and it showed marked enlargement of the left kidney with poor visualization of the pelvocalyceal system (Fig. 32-13). A selective left renal venogram obtained 1 week later revealed complete obstruction of the main renal vein. Creatinine clearance was reduced, and the patient was anticoagulated. In 2 days the flank pain resolved completely, and after 6 months of anticoagulant therapy, the creatinine clearance rate had increased from 40 to 90 mL/minute.

On occasion, acute RVT is bilateral, resulting in marked oliguric ARF and flank pain. The severity of the symptomatology and oliguria and the magnitude of renal function deterioration depend on various factors. Previously compromised renal function, absence of collateral circulation, and a large thrombus involving both renal veins may result in a florid clinical presentation as well as rapid renal function deterioration.

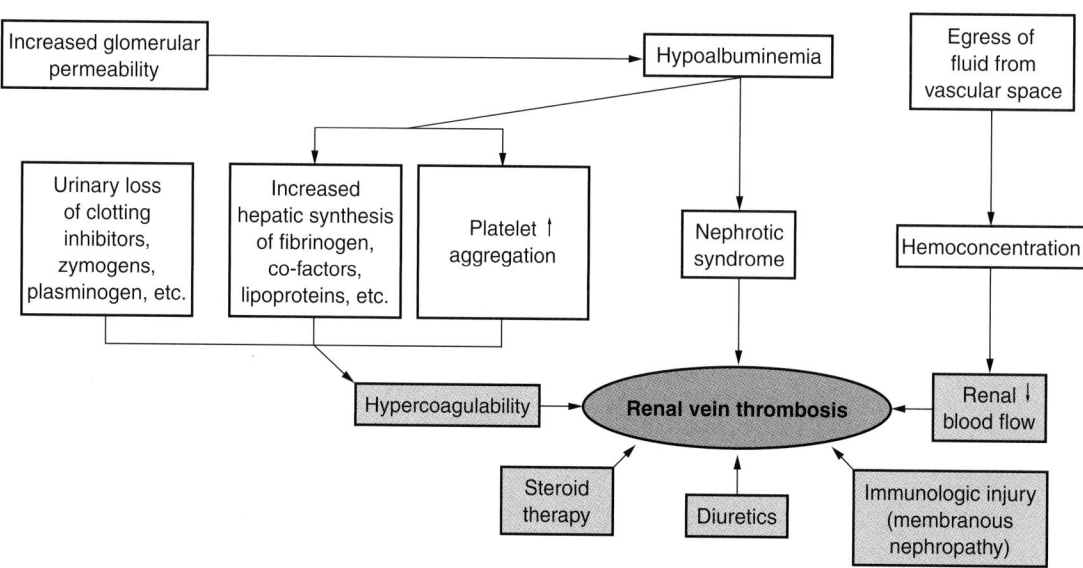

FIGURE 32-12. Schematic representation of pathogenetic factors leading to renal vein thrombosis in nephrotic syndrome.

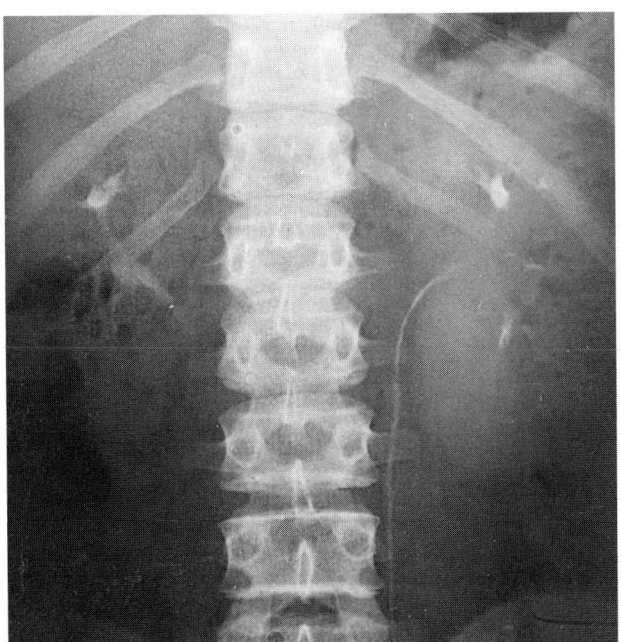

FIGURE 32-13. Intravenous pyelogram of a patient with acute renal vein thrombosis. Note blurring and irregularities of the left pelvicalyceal system as well as marked enlargement of the left kidney. (Courtesy of Dr. Llach.)

Other causes of acute RVT with or without the nephrotic syndrome are trauma, ingestion of oral contraceptive agents, dehydration (mostly in infants), and steroid administration.

RVT secondary to trauma is usually accompanied by renal artery thrombosis. The history of the trauma, the severe acute flank pain, and a palpable mass are usually suggestive of this condition.

The use of oral contraceptives has been implicated occasionally as a cause of RVT. A young woman who was taking oral contraceptives and had no history of nephrotic syndrome or any traumatic event developed acute RVT with florid clinical manifestations.[319] Whether there was a cause-and-effect relationship between the contraceptive agents and the RVT was not clear.

Dehydration has been clearly associated with RVT in infants.[320] In this condition, thrombosis develops in the small renal veins, predominantly the arcuate or intralobular vein. The majority of these infants do not have nephrotic syndrome or even significant proteinuria. This syndrome develops initially in the clinical setting of diarrhea, vomiting, and often shock. Oliguria and hematuria rapidly ensue. Contributing factors are a history of maternal diabetes, congenital heart disease, and performance of angiocardiography. An enlarged, palpable kidney may be found in 60% of cases. The common clinical presentation is a hyperosmolar hypovolemic syndrome. The mortality rate of RVT in infants is high. Fortunately, the frequency of this syndrome has diminished with earlier therapy and control of volume-depleting events.

Steroid administration has been clearly associated with acute and chronic RVT as well as other thrombotic complications[315, 316]; however, the causative role of these agents in RVT remains to be established. The role of steroids cannot be appraised until other factors influencing thrombus formation

are understood. As mentioned earlier, Cheng and associates[310] presented preliminary data in 97 nephrotic patients prospectively evaluated. Of these, 44 patients were found to have RVT by routine renal venogram. Multivariate regression analysis revealed that steroid therapy was associated with a high tendency to develop RVT ($P < .01$).

Acute RVT has been noted with increasing frequency in the transplanted kidney,[321-323] which unlike the native kidney has a single drainage system. In this setting, RVT may be accompanied by thrombosis of extrarenal sites.[324] Recently, Bakir and associates[324] reviewed the number of episodes of RVT in 558 consecutive cadaveric kidney transplants. They noted a 6% incidence of RVT, which accounted for one third of all early (90 days) graft failures. In the transplanted kidney RVT usually leads to permanent damage of the graft within hours. Predisposing factors are the use of OKT3 and cyclosporine therapy.[322-323, 325] The available evidence suggests that cyclosporine may predispose to vascular thrombosis by exacerbating the hypercoagulability.[326] In fact, rupture of a renal allograft, an uncommon complication, usually is an early manifestation of acute RVT, which often is attributable to cyclosporine therapy.[323]

Finally, abdominal tumors, especially hypernephroma, are a common cause of RVT; however, in the majority of these cases chronic rather than acute RVT is the common clinical presentation.

The radiologic manifestations of acute RVT are well defined and characteristic, in contrast to those of chronic RVT, which often are minimal. Experimentally, with complete occlusion of the renal vein, the kidney increases rapidly in size within the first 24 hours, reaching a peak within 1 week after renal vein occlusion.[327] Thereafter, there is a progressive decrease in renal size over the next 2 months, resulting in a small, atrophic kidney. A progressive decrease in the caliber and length of the renal artery occurs after the occlusion.

Clinically, in a patient with acute RVT, the renal ultrasound initially reveals an enlarged kidney. With IVP, if the obstruction is sudden and complete, there may not be any visualization of the collecting system. However, in most patients, due to the presence of some collateral circulation, there is renal enlargement and opacification of varying degree with some visualization of the kidney. Often the renal pelvis can be visualized, and usually it is stretched, distorted, and blurred (see Fig. 32-13). This may be the result of severe interstitial edema and swelling of the pelvocalyceal system. At this stage, the radiographic appearance has been compared to that observed in polycystic kidney disease, and on occasion it has led to this mistaken diagnosis. The acute symptomatology of RVT in association with this radiologic appearance establishes the diagnosis. Ureteral edema may progress to the point at which the collecting system is completely obliterated; there have been cases of complete ureteral obstruction in which, during retrograde pyelography, the catheter could not be advanced into the pelvis.

A characteristic radiographic finding of RVT is notching of the ureter, which usually occurs when collateral veins in close relation to the ureters become tortuous as they dilate to form an alternative drainage route. Originally, the notching of the ureters was interpreted as representing mucosal edema; however, more detailed radiographic studies showed indentation of the ureters by the collateral venous circulation.[328, 329] Notching of the ureter is a very infrequent finding in nephrotic patients with RVT and usually occurs only in a minority of patients with chronic rather than acute RVT.[246]

Retrograde pyelography may be useful in the patient with complete RVT who does not excrete the contrast material. In such instances, retrograde pyelography may demonstrate a rectangular, linear mucosal pattern with irregular renal pelvic outlines similar to those described earlier with the IVP.

Inferior venacavography with selective catheterization of the renal vein establishes the diagnosis of RVT. If the inferior vena cava is patent and free of filling defects, and if a good streaming of unopacified renal blood is demonstrated to wash out contrast from the vena cava, a diagnosis of RVT is unlikely. The Valsalva maneuver is useful during venacavography; when the intra-abdominal pressure is increased, the transit of contrast agent and blood from the inferior vena cava is slowed, the proximal part of the main renal vein may be opacified, and the patency of the lumen or even the outline of the thrombus may be demonstrated. On occasion, a lack of washout in the area of the renal vein may be suggestive of RVT; sometimes partial defects in the area of the renal vein, characteristic of renal venous thrombus extending into the inferior vena cava, may be demonstrated. In the presence of complete inferior vena cava obstruction below the renal vein, it is desirable to demonstrate the proximal extent of the thrombus, and this can readily be accomplished by transbrachial catheterization with passage of the catheter into the inferior vena cava via the subclavian vein.

Often the inferior venacavogram is not diagnostic, and selective catheterization of the renal vein must be performed. A normal renal venogram demonstrates the entire intralobular venous system to the level of the arcuate vein. In general, the use of epinephrine for better visualization of the smaller vessels is not necessary. However, in the presence of normal renal blood flow, all contrast material is washed out of the renal vein within 3 seconds or less, and occasionally only the main renal vein and major branches are visualized. In this situation there may be uncertainty about thrombi in major or smaller branches. Then the use of intrarenal arterial epinephrine, by decreasing blood flow, enhances retrograde venous filling and allows later visualization of the smaller intrarenal veins. An abnormal renal venogram usually demonstrates a thrombus within the lumen as a filling defect surrounded by contrast material (Fig. 32-14). In the presence of partial thrombosis, extensive collateral circulation can be demonstrated. The presence of such collaterals usually reflects the chronicity of the RVT and may explain the lack of renal functional deterioration.

Renal arteriography was considered originally by many investigators to be preferable to renal venography for the diagnosis of RVT. With renal arteriography, important information is obtained about the status of the renal parenchyma. In addition, the theoretical danger of dislodging the clot material from the renal vein during renal venography and precipitating a pulmonary embolism is avoided. However, this complication has not occurred after renal venography in several extensive radiographic series of patients with RVT.[246, 250] Renal arteriography may be useful in patients being evaluated for RVT associated with renal trauma or tumor because of the common involvement of the renal artery phase; deviation and stretching of the interlobular

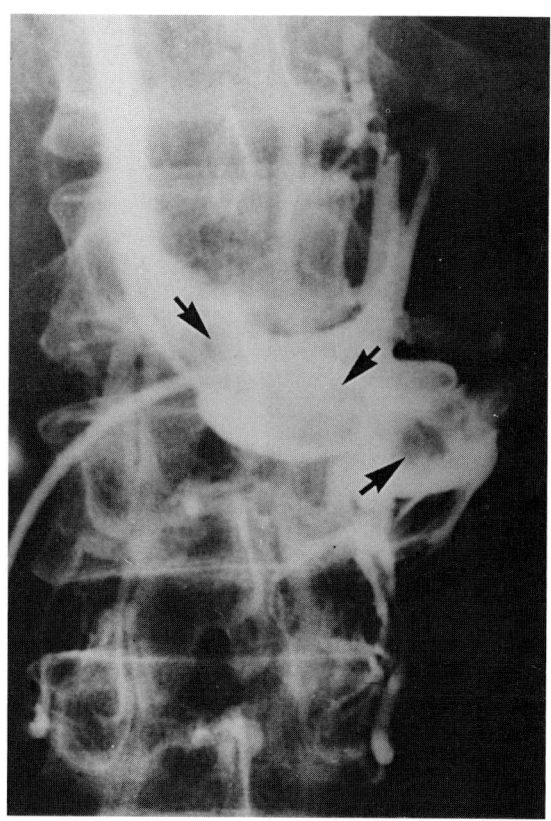

FIGURE 32-14. Left renal venography from a patient with renal venous thrombosis. Note the arrows indicating filling defects, which reflect accumulation of thrombotic material surrounded by contrast material. There is complete obstruction of the main renal vein as well as of collateral circulation. (Courtesy of Dr. Llach.)

arteries are usually observed in these conditions. In the nephrographic phase, the medullary pyramids are more densely opacified than the cortex, and instead of presenting the usual triangular appearance, they appear to bulge and sometimes are even ovoid in appearance.

Renal ultrasonography may be a useful potential diagnostic procedure for the diagnosis of RVT.[330] The sonographic diagnosis of RVT is based on direct visualization of thrombi within the renal vein and inferior vena cava, demonstration of renal vein dilatation proximal to the point of occlusion, loss of normal renal structure, and increase in renal size during the acute phase. These ultrasonography findings, however, usually need to be confirmed by other diagnostic procedures.

Combined ultrasonic scanning and Doppler ultrasonography for the diagnosis of RVT may be useful. This is a noninvasive technique that essentially measures the renal venous flow velocity. However, Doppler ultrasonography has a high incidence of false-negative findings in the diagnosis of RVT.

CT is the procedure of choice for the noninvasive evaluation of acute RVT. Lower attenuation density shows a thrombus that may be identified within the renal vein and inferior vena cava, or the venous diameter may be enlarged owing to obstruction. In general, intravenous infusion of contrast material, together with CT, may help to visualize the thrombus. The radiographic findings include enlargement and distention of the affected renal vein, with visualization of the clots within the vein and sometimes extension into the inferior vena cava.[250]

Persistent parenchymal opacification with kidney enlargement is usually observed. Capsular venous collaterals, thickening of Gerota's fascia, and pericapsular "whiskering" are often observed.

Preliminary observations of isolated cases suggest that MRI may be, in the future, the diagnostic procedure of choice in the noninvasive diagnosis of RVT.[331] Because MRI produces highly contrasting images of flowing blood, vascular walls, and surrounding tissues, vascular patency may be best determined by this technique. A major potential advantage in using this method is the avoidance of the use of contrast material. Also, because both the arterial and the venous phase are imaged, occult renal artery stenosis can be disclosed as well.[332, 333]

Clinical Course and Treatment

The experience to date on the course, prognosis, and treatment of RVT in nephrotic patients is limited. In 1963, Kowal and co-workers reviewed 65 patients with RVT.[328] Only 14 of these patients were alive after 2 years of follow-up. Unfortunately, clinical data and literature references were given only for the 14 surviving patients. Ten of these patients seemed to have acute RVT. Recurrent thromboembolic phenomena were cited as the most common cause of death. Later, Rosenmann and associates observed 11 of 15 nephrotic patients with RVT over a period of 24 to 115 months.[318] Only 4 of these patients had symptoms suggestive of acute RVT. The incidence of thromboembolic phenomena was high, and thromboembolism was fatal in 7 patients. One or more episodes of pulmonary embolism occurred in 7 patients, and 4 had evidence of repeated episodes of thrombosis involving the renal venous system. Three patients received anticoagulant therapy and had no new episodes of pulmonary emboli. These data suggest that the prognosis for nephrotic patients with RVT may be poor and is determined by the presence or absence of recurrent thrombotic complications.

In 1970, Richet and Meyrier reviewed 112 cases of RVT reported in the literature; 72 of the patients had died, constituting a 64% mortality rate.[334] Earlier, McCarthy and colleagues estimated the average survival period after onset of RVT to be 9 months.[237] These data, however, may not be representative of the present prognosis of this entity. First, because most of the earlier data about the course and prognosis of RVT were obtained from autopsy studies, the mortality rate may have been overestimated. Second, renal insufficiency secondary to RVT was a common cause of death in these patients, and dialysis therapy has now reduced uremic death considerably. Third, the new diagnostic techniques and

better understanding of this entity, together with better use of anticoagulant therapy, have contributed to better management of these patients. Nevertheless, a serious complication in patients with RVT is still thromboembolic phenomena, most often pulmonary embolism.

More recently, Lavelle and associates[335] reevaluated 27 nephrotic patients with RVT, 10 of whom had acute lumbar pain and ARF. Eleven patients died within the first 6 months. Survivors were observed for 6 months to 19 years. Nephrotic syndrome improved or even disappeared in 12 patients, and renal function did not worsen throughout the follow-up period. The main prognostic factors were initial renal function and type of nephropathy; that is, patients with membranous nephropathy had significantly better renal function and a lower mortality rate than did patients with other nephropathies. Initial renal insufficiency was significantly associated with a poor prognosis. In fact, six of the eight patients with ARF died; hemorrhagic complications were the major cause of death in these patients.

Renal function may dramatically improve in patients with acute RVT treated with anticoagulant therapy. Table 32-9 shows the follow-up data on patients with nephrotic syndrome and acute or chronic RVT who were treated with anticoagulant therapy. Those with acute RVT had significant improvement in renal function during the follow-up period, and it is recommended that such patients be maintained on long-term anticoagulant therapy. Convincing evidence has been gathered suggesting that anticoagulant therapy reduces the incidence of new thromboembolic episodes and often reverses the deterioration of renal function that occurs with acute RVT. Patients treated with anticoagulant therapy may have recanalization of the renal vein, and in some instances a total dissolution of the clot may occur.[336] Heparin is the initial therapy of choice. In patients with a large renal vein thrombus and pulmonary embolism, the clearance of heparin is increased; and such patients may need higher doses of heparin in the early stages of therapy. Although the dosage of heparin varies from patient to patient, the aim is to maintain the clotting time at 2 to 2.5 times normal. In general, because of fewer complications, continued infusion of heparin is preferable to intermittent intravenous administration. Warfarin therapy is instituted after the patient has been treated with heparin for 5 to 7 days and the partial thromboplastin time is within the desired range. Warfarin is started orally with small loading doses. A common clinical problem with warfarin therapy is drug interactions related to the kinetics of warfarin, such as drug absorption, protein binding, metabolism, and excretion. These drug interactions are very

TABLE 32-9

Follow-up Data on Nephrotic Patients with Acute or Chronic Renal Vein Thrombosis (RVT)

PATIENTS	URINE PROTEIN (g/24 h)	CREATININE CLEARANCE (mL/min)	SERUM ALBUMIN (g/dL)	SERUM CHOLESTEROL (g/dL)	NO. OF PATIENTS UNDERGOING DIALYSIS
29 with chronic RVT	5.9 ± 3.9* (4.8 ± 2.3)	71 ± 25* (65 ± 29)	2.4 ± 0.7* (2.9 ± 0.7)	370 ± 110* (360 ± 88)	4
4 with acute RVT	5.2 ± 1.2* (5.0 ± 1.2)	76 ± 19* (98 ± 8)†	2.1 ± 0.2* (2.3 ± 0.2)	347 ± 19* (332 ± 26)	0

*Initial laboratory data (mean ± SD). Data obtained after anticoagulant therapy are shown in parentheses.
†*P* < .05.

common and may play an important role in enhancement of, or decrease in, the anticoagulant effect of heparin. It should also be remembered that drugs such as aspirin and indomethacin may increase the risk of bleeding in these patients owing to their effect on the gastrointestinal mucosa and platelet aggregation. From all these observations, it is obvious that individualization of warfarin therapy is essential, and the clinical status, patient sensitivity, metabolism, and possible drug interactions must all be taken into consideration.

Once oral anticoagulant therapy is established, the prothrombin time should be kept at about 1.5 to 2 times normal. The recommended duration of anticoagulant therapy in these patients is difficult to establish. The severity of the hypoalbuminemia is a good indicator of the magnitude of the hypercoagulability. The nephrotic patient should probably be treated with anticoagulants so long as the serum albumin concentration is less than 2.5 g/L. Relapses with new episodes of acute RVT have been observed after cessation of anticoagulant therapy.[337] It is our belief that in general these patients should continue receiving anticoagulation therapy as long as they have the nephrotic syndrome.

Early resolution of the acute RVT has been reported with the use of either streptokinase or urokinase, either systemically or with selective infusion.[338-341] However, it appears that selective infusion of these agents is also successful in the RVT of the transplanted kidney.[340, 341]

Surgical treatment for RVT is rarely used today, because the role of thrombectomy in the treatment of RVT has not been established as beneficial. Although marked improvement in renal function has been occasionally observed after thrombectomy, the majority of these patients do not improve with surgery. This modality of therapy may be theoretically useful in patients with acute bilateral RVT who are not otherwise expected to survive the acute episode, especially if recurrent pulmonary emboli occur despite anticoagulation therapy.

THROMBOEMBOLIC COMPLICATIONS OTHER THAN RENAL VEIN THROMBOSIS

The high cumulative risks of thromboembolic complications in the nephrotic patient have been recognized only recently.[247, 259, 263] These complications have been observed in the pulmonary arteries,[342] in the axillary and subclavian veins,[343] and in femoral, coronary, and mesenteric arteries.[343-345] However, the most common observation may be deep vein thrombosis of the extremities. A summary of thromboembolic complication studies is shown in Andrassy and Ritz studied 84 nephrotic patients and observed 37 episodes of thromboembolic complication in 30 patients during a period of 3 years.[346] There were 23 episodes of deep vein thrombosis, an incidence of 44%, and among the highest number encountered in medical patients. Kanfer and colleagues observed arterial and vein thrombosis in five of eight children and in 10 of 29 adult nephrotic patients during a period of 7 years.[258] Although the percentage of patients affected was lower (27%), this is still a significant incidence. Four other investigators have observed a 17% incidence of mostly deep vein thrombosis. In our prospective studies,[246] 26 episodes of thromboembolic complications other than RVT were noted in 151 nephrotic patients (17%). Of note, Pohl and colleagues[243] reported only 1 patient with RVT out of 54, but they observed three episodes of thrombosis, an 8.5% incidence, which is still high; as shown in Table 32-10 the incidence of thromboembolic complications does range from 8.5% to 44%.[347] Peripheral venous thrombosis and pulmonary embolism were the most frequent complications, but arterial thrombosis also occurred.

In our prospective study, ventilation-perfusion lung scanning was performed in 94 nephrotic patients, 24 with and 70 without RVT.[254] Asymptomatic perfusion defects in the presence of normal chest radiographs were observed in 12 patients, including 5 with and 7 without RVT. Because no pulmonary angiographic studies were done in these patients, a definitive interpretation of this defect is not possible. However, these data suggest a significant incidence of pulmonary embolism in the nephrotic patients. Similar observations were made by Cameron and colleagues,[348] who reported that 7 (19%) of 37 nephrotic patients had abnormal ventilation-perfusion lung scans and only 1 had RVT.[348]

Clearly, there is a significant incidence of thromboembolic phenomena other than RVT in nephrotic patients, but the morbidity and mortality of these complications are not well defined. Prospective longitudinal studies are needed to elucidate both the magnitude of this problem and the use of appropriate prophylaxis and therapy in patients at high risk for thrombosis.

TABLE 32-10

Summary of Published Studies Evaluating Thromboembolic Complications in the Nephrotic Syndrome

STUDY	NO. OF PTS.	NO. OF PTS. WITH THROMBOSIS (%)	LOCATION OF THROMBOSIS						TOTAL NO. OF EPISODES OTHER THAN DVT (%)
			Renal	Pulm	Extremities	Coronary	Cerebral	Peripheral	
Andrassy[308]	84	30 (38)	6	7	23	3	1	3	37 (44)
Kauffman[289]	48	9 (19)	4	4	3	—	—	1	8 (17)
Kanfer[258]	45	13 (29)	3	3	6	—	2	1	12 (27)
Pohl[243]	59	5 (10)	1	2	3	—	—	—	5 (8.5)
Kuhlmann[309]	17	4 (23)	1	2	1	—	—	—	3 (17)
Velazquez Forero[244]	19	8 (42)	8	1	2	—	—	—	3 (16)
Llach[255]	151	41 (26)	33	18	3	2	2	1	26 (17)
Kendall[257]	35	4 (23)	1	3	—	1	1	1	6 (17)

DVT, deep vein thrombosis; Pts, patients; Pulm, pulmonary.

ACKNOWLEDGMENTS

We thank Ms. Gale MacArthur for her secretarial assistance. Also, we thank Drs. Shahida Ahmed and Anthony Reda for their contributions of medical images.

REFERENCES

1. Stables DP, Pouches RF, De Villera Van Nierkerk J: Traumatic renal artery occlusion: 21 cases. J Urol 115:229-235, 1974.
2. Dinchman KH, Spirnak JP: Traumatic renal artery thrombosis. Semin Urol 13:90-93, 1995.
3. Barlow B, Gandhi R: Renal artery thrombosis following blunt trauma. J Trauma 20:614-618, 1980.
4. Bretan PN, McAnineh JW, Federle MP, Jeffrey RB: Computerized tomographic staging of renal trauma: 85 consecutive cases. J Urol 136: 561-565, 1986.
5. Lupetin AR, Mainwaring BL, Daffner RH: CT diagnosis of renal artery injury caused by blunt abdominal trauma. Am J Radiol 153:1065-1068, 1989.
6. Clark DE, Georgitis JW, Ray FS: Renal artery injuries caused by blunt trauma. Surgery 90:87-96, 1981.
7. Martin LG, Casarella WJ, Alspaugh JP, Chuang VP: Renal artery angioplasty: Increased technical success and decreased complications in the second 100 patients. Radiology 159:631-634, 1986.
8. Vollmar J, Helmstadter D, Hallwacks O: Complete occlusion of the renal artery. J Cardiovasc Surg 12:441-446, 1971.
9. Lang EK, Sullivan J, Frentz G: Renal trauma: Radiological studies. Comparison of urographic, computed tomography, angiography, and radionuclide studies. Radiology 154:159, 1985.
10. Kamel IR, Berkowitz JF: Assessment of the cortical rim sign in post-traumatic renal infarction. J Comput Assist Tomogr 20:803-806, 1996.
11. Spirnak JP, Resnick MI: Revascularization of traumatic thrombosis of the renal artery. Surg Gynecol Obstet 164:229, 1987.
12. Brunetti DR, Sasaki TM, Friedlander G, et al: Successful renal auto-transplantation in a patient with bilateral renal artery thrombosis. Urology 43:235-237, 1994.
13. Cass AS: Renovascular injuries from external trauma: Diagnosis, treatment and outcome. Urol Clin North Am 16:213-220, 1989.
14. Maggio AJ, Brosman S: Renal artery trauma. Urology 11:125-131, 1978.
15. Elkik F, Corvol P, Idatte J, Menard J: Renal segmental infarction: A cause of reversible malignant hypertension. J Hypertens 2:149-156, 1984.
16. Weimann S, Flora G, Dittrich P, et al: Traumatic renal artery occlusion: Is late reconstruction advisable? J Urol 137:727-729, 1987.
17. Fort J, Camps J, Ruiz P, et al: Renal artery embolism successfully revascularized by surgery after 5 days anuria: Is it never too late? Nephrol Dial Transplant 11:1843-1845, 1996.
18. Crosby RB, Miller PD, Schrier RW: Traumatic renal artery thrombosis. Am J Med 81:890-894, 1986.
19. Adovaso R, Pancrazio F: Acute thrombosis of renal artery: Restoration of renal function after late revascularization. Vasa 18: 239-246, 1989.
20. Fay R, Brosman SA, Lindstrom R, et al: Renal artery thrombosis: A successful revascularization by autotransplantation. J Urol 111: 572-577, 1974.
21. Peterson NE: Review article: Traumatic bilateral infarction. Trauma 29:158-167, 1989.
22. Lohhse JR, Botham RJ, Waters RF: Traumatic bilateral renal artery thrombosis: Case report and review of literature. J Urol 127:522-526, 1982.
22. Pineo GF, Thorndyke WC, Steed BL: Spontaneous renal artery thrombosis: Successful lysis with streptokinase. J Urol 138:1223-1228, 1987.
24. Goodman NF, Saibil EA, Kodama RT: Traumatic intimal tear of the renal artery treated by insertion of a Palmaz stent. Cardiovasc Intervent Radiol 21:69-72, 1998.
25. Elen P, Ozlu E, Sakalihassan N, et al: Renal artery occlusion following blunt abdominal trauma. Acta Chir Belg 100:107-110, 2000.
26. Whigham CJ, Bodehaner JR, Miller JK: Use of the Palmaz stent in primary treatment of renal artery intimal injury secondary to blunt trauma. J Vasc Interv Radiol 6:175-178, 1995.
27. Thomas DP, Roberts HR: Hypercoagulability in venous and arterial thrombosis. Ann Intern Med 126:638-644, 1997.
28. Guirguis N, Budisavljevic MN, Rajagopalan PR, et al: Acute renal artery and vein thrombosis after renal transplant, associated with a short partial thomboplastin time and factor V Leiden mutation. Ann Clin Lab Sci 30:75-78, 2000.
29. Klein O, Bernheim J, Strahilevitz J, et al: Renal colic in a patient with anti-phospholipid antibodies and factor V Leiden mutation. Nephrol Dial Transplant 14:2502-2504, 1999.
30. Ostuni PA, Lazzarin P, Pengo V, et al: Renal artery thrombosis and hypertension in a 13 year old girl with antiphospholipid syndrome. Ann Rheum Dis 49:184-187, 1990.
31. Poux JM, Boudet R, Lacroix P, Levoux-Robert C: Renal infarction and thrombosis of the infrarenal aorta in a 35 year old man with primary antiphospholipid syndrome. Am J Kidney Dis 27:712-725, 1996.
32. Sonpal GM, Sharma A, Miller A: Primary antiphospholipid antibody syndrome, renal infarction and hypertension. J Rheumatol 7:1221-1223, 1993.
33. Hernandez D, Dominguez ML, Diaz F, et al: Renal infarction in a severely hypertensive patient with lupus erythematosus and antiphospholipid antibodies. Nephron 72:298-301, 1996.
34. Kleinknecht D, Bobric G, Meyer O, et al: Recurrent thrombosis and renal vascular disease in patients with a lupus anticoagulant. Nephrol Dial Transplant 4:854-858, 1989.
35. Arnold MH, Schrieber L: Splenic and renal infarction in systemic lupus erythematosus: Association with anti-cardiolipin antibodies. Clin Rheumatol 7:406-410, 1988.
36. Dasgupta B, Almond MK, Tanqeray A: Polyarteritis nodosa and the antiphospholipid syndrome. Br J Rheumatol 36:1210-1212, 1997.
37. Chitalia VC, Kolhe N, Kothari J, Almeida AF: Acute renal failure in a renal transplant donor due to primary antiphospholipid syndrome. Am J Nephrol 21:55-57, 2001.
38. Remondino GI, Mysler E, Pissano MN, et al: A reversible bilateral renal artery stenosis in association with anti-phospholipid syndrome. Lupus 9:65-67, 2000.
39. Riccialdelli L, Arnaldi G, Giacchetti G, et al: Hypertension due to renal artery occlusion in a patient with antiphospholipid syndrome. Am J Hypertens 14:62-65, 2001.
40. Stone JH, Amend WJ, Criswell LA: Antiphospholipid antibody syndrome in renal transplantation: Occurrence of clinical events in 96 consecutive patients with systemic lupus erythematosus. Am J Kidney Dis 34:1040-1047, 1999.
41. Aird WC: Case records of the Massachusetts General Hospital: Case 15-2002. N Engl J Med 346:1562-1570, 2002.
42. Warkentin TE: Heparin-induced thrombocytopenia: A ten-year retrospective. Annu Rev Med 50:129-147, 1999.
43. Pochet JM, Bobrie G, Basile C, et al: Renal arterial thrombosis complicating nephrotic syndrome. Presse Med 17:2139-2146, 1988.
44. Nakamura M, Ohnishi T, Okamoto S: Abdominal aortic thrombosis in a patient with nephritic syndrome. Am J Nephrol 18:64-67, 1998.
45. Temes M, Montes XL, Jimenez A: Renal artery thrombosis occurring in an adult with the idiopathic nephrotic syndrome: Results of local treatment with streptokinase. Clin Nephrol 12:90-93, 1979.
46. Queffeulou G, Michel C, Vrtovsnik F, et al: Hyperhomocysteinemia, low folate status, homozygous C667 T mutation of the methylene tetrahydrofolate reductase and renal arterial thrombosis. Clin Nephrol 57:158-162, 2002.
47. Rouviere O, Berger P, Beziat C, Garnier JL: Acute thrombosis of renal transplant artery: Graft salvage by means of intra-arterial fibrinolysis. Transplantation 73:403-409, 2002.
48. Humar A, Key N, Ramcharan T, et al: Kidney retransplants after initial graft loss to vascular thrombosis. Clin Transplant 15:6-10, 2001.
49. Deira J, Alberca I, Lerma JL, et al: Changes in coagulation and fibrinolysis in the postoperative period immediately after kidney transplantation in patients receiving OKT3 or cyclosporine A as induction therapy. Am J Kidney Dis 32:575-581, 1998.
50. Groggel GC: Acute thrombosis of the renal transplant artery: A case report and review of the literature. Clin Nephrol 36:42-45, 1991.
51. Plainfosse MC, Calonge VM, Beyloune-Mainardi C, et al: Vascular complications in the adult kidney transplant recipient. J Clin Urol 20:517-527, 1992.
52. Bakir N, Sluiter WJ, Ploeg RJ: Primary renal graft thrombosis. Nephrol Dial Transplant 11:40-44, 1996.
53. Penny MJ, Nankivell BJ, Disney AP: Renal graft thrombosis. Transplantation 58:565-569, 1994.
54. Samara EN, Voss BL, Pederson JA: Renal artery thrombosis associated with elevated cyclosporine levels: A case report and review of the literature. Transplant Proc 10:119-122, 1990.

55. Rigotti P, Flechner SM, Van Buren CT: Increased incidence of renal allograft thrombosis under cyclosporine immunosuppression. Int Surg 71:38-41, 1986.

56. Dodhia N, Rodby RA, Jensik SC: Renal transplant arterial thrombosis: Association with cyclosporine. Am J Kidney Dis 17:532-537, 1991.

57. Remuzzi G, Bertani T: Renal vascular and thrombotic effects of cyclosporine. Am J Kidney Dis 13:261-266, 1989.

58. Kavalier E, Hensle TW: Renal artery thrombosis in the newborn infant. Urology 50:282-284, 1997.

59. Siebert JJ, Lindley DG, Corbitt SS, et al: Clot formation in the renal artery in the neonate demonstrated by ultrasound. J Clin Ultrasound 14:470-473, 1986.

60. Ellis D, Kaye RD, Bontempo FA: Aortic and renal artery thrombosis in a neonate: Recovery with thrombolytic therapy. Pediatr Nephrol 11:641-644, 1997.

61. Molteni KH, George J, Messersmith R, et al: Intrathrombic urokinase reverses neonatal renal artery thrombosis. Pediatr Nephrol 7:413-415, 1993.

62. Greenberg R, Waldman K, Brooks C: Endovascular treatment of renal artery thrombosis caused by umbilical artery catheterization. J Vasc Surg 28:949-953, 1998.

63. Heng MC, Haberfield G: Thrombotic phenomena associated with intravenous cocaine. J Am Acad Dermatol 16:462-466, 1987.

64. Goodman PE, Rennie WP: Renal infarction secondary to nasal insufflation of cocaine. Am J Emerg Med 13:421-423, 1995.

65. Kramer RK, Turner RC: Renal infarction associated with cocaine use and latent protein C deficiency. South Med J 86:1436-1438, 1993.

66. Hoover LA: Polyarteritis involving only the main renal arteries. Am J Kidney Dis 11:66-69, 1988.

67. Templeton PA, Pats SO: Renal artery occlusion in polyarteritis nodosum. Radiology 156:308-309, 1985.

68. Teoh MK: Takayasu's arteritis with renovascular hypertension: Results of surgical treatment. Cardiovasc Surg 7:626-633, 1999.

69. Dardik A, Ballermann BJ, Williams GM: Successful delayed bilateral renal revascularization during active phase of Takayasu's arteritis. J Vasc Surg 27:552-557, 1998.

70. Akpolat T, Akkoyunu M, Akpolat I, Dilek M: Renal Behçet's disease: A cumulative analysis. Semin Arthritis Rheum 31:317-337, 2002.

71. Sherif A, Stewart P, Mendes DM: The repetitive vascular catastrophies of Behçet's disease: A case report with review of the literature. Ann Vasc Surg 6:85-89, 1992.

72. Price RK, Skelton R: Hypertension due to syphilitic occlusion of the main renal arteries. Br Heart J 10:29-35, 1948.

73. Sane SY, Deshmukh SS: Total renal infarct and peri-renal abscess caused by phycomycosis. Case report. J Postgrad Med 34:448-450, 1998.

74. Vesa J, Bielsa O, Arango O, et al: Massive renal infarction due to mucormycosis in an AIDS patient. Infection 20:234-236, 1992.

75. Granfortuna J, Zamkoff K, Urrutia E: Acute renal infarction in sickle cell disease. Am J Hematol 23:59-62, 1986.

76. Hitti IF, Celmer EJ, Rapuano J: Hemorrhagic infarction of the kidney: An uncommon presentation of infiltrating urothelial carcinoma of the renal pelvis. Urol Int 41:212-217, 1986.

77. Montgomery JH, Moinuddin M, Buchignani JS: Renal infarction after aerobics. Clin Nucl Med 9:664-667, 1984.

78. Coulshed SJ, Caterson RJ, Mahony JF: Traumatic infarct at the lower pole of a renal transplant secondary to seat belt compression. Nephrol Dial Transplant 10:1464-1465, 1995.

79. Moris D, Kisly A, Stoyka CG, Provenzano R: Spontaneous bilateral renal artery occlusion associated with chronic atrial fibrillation. Clin Nephrol 39:257-259, 1993.

80. Argiris A: Splenic and renal infarctions complicating atrial fibrillation. Mt Sinai J Med 64:342-349, 1992.

81. Frost L, Engholm G, Johnsen S, et al: Incident thromboembolism in the aorta and the renal, mesenteric, pelvic, and extremity arteries after discharge from the hospital with a diagnosis of atrial fibrillation. Arch Intern Med 161;272-276, 2001.

82. Delalu P, Ferretti GR, Bricault I, et al: Paradoxical emboli: Demonstration using helical computed tomography of the pulmonary artery associated with abdominal computed tomography. Eur Radiol 10:384-386, 2000.

83. Sternbergh WC, Ramee SR, DeVun DA, Money SR: Endovascular treatment of multiple visceral artery paradoxical emboli with mechanical and pharmacologic thrombolysis. J Endovasc Ther 7:155-160, 2000.

84. Carey HB, Boltax R, Dickey KW, Finkelstein FO: Bilateral renal infarction secondary to paradoxical embolism. Am J Kidney Dis 34:752-755, 1992.

85. Martin DC: Renal artery aneurysm with peripheral embolization of kidney. Urology 15:590-598, 1980.

86. Gorich J, Kramer S, Tomczak R, et al: Thomboembolic complications after endovascular aortic aneurysm repair. J Endovasc Ther 9:180-184, 2002.

87. Kramer SC, Seifarth H, Pamler R, et al: Renal infarction following endovascular aortic aneurysm repair: Incidence and clinical consequences. J Endovasc Ther 9:98-102, 2002.

88. Bush RL, Najibi S, MacDonald J, et al: Endovascular revascularization of renal artery stenosis: Technical and clinical results. J Vasc Surg 33:1041-1049, 2001.

89. Beek FJ, Kaatee R, Beutler JJ, et al: Complications during renal artery stent placement for atherosclerotic ostial stenosis. Cardiovasc Intervent Radiol 20:184-190, 1997.

90. Kitchens C, Jordan W, Wirthlin D, Whitley D: Vascular compications arising from maldeployed stents. Vasc Endovasc Surg 36:145-154, 2002.

91. Hoxie HJ, Coggin CB: Renal infarction: Statistical study of two hundred and five cases and detailed report of an unusual case. Arch Intern Med 65:587-593, 1940.

92. Jennette JC, Olson JL, Schwartz MM: Heptinstall's Pathology of the Kidney, 5th ed. New York, Lippincott-Raven, 1998.

93. Lessman RK, Johnson SF, Coburn JW, Kaufman JJ: Renal artery embolism: Clinical features and long-term follow-up of 17 cases. Ann Intern Med 89:477-482, 1978.

94. Miller TR, Anderson RJ, Linas SL: Urinary diagnostic indices in acute renal failure. Ann Intern Med 89:47-52, 1978.

95. Gault MH, Steiner G: Serum and urinary enzyme activity after renal infarction. Can Med Assoc J 93:1101-1108, 1965.

96. Kawashima A, Sandler CM, Ernst RD, et al: CT evaluation of renovascular disease. Radiographics 20:1321-1340, 2000.

97. Vosshenrich R, Fischer U: Contrast-enhanced MR angiography of abdominal vessels: Is there still a role for angiography? Eur Radiol 12:218-230, 2002.

98. Zubarev AV. Ultrasound of renal vessels. Eur Radiol 11:1902-1915, 2001.

99. Spinosa DJ, Matsumoto AH, Angle JF, et al: Renal insufficiency: Usefulness of gadodiamide-enhanced renal angiography to supplement CO$_2$-enhanced renal angiography for diagnosis and percutaneous treatment. Radiology 210:663-672, 1999.

100. Blum U, Billmann P, Krause T: Effect of local low-dose thrombolysis on clinical outcome in acute embolic renal artery occlusion. Radiology 189:549-557, 1993.

101. Pilmore HL, Walker RJ, Solomon C: Acute bilateral renal artery occlusion: Successful revascularization with streptokinase. Am J Nephrol 15:90-94, 1995.

102. Skinner RE, Hefty T, Long TD: Recovery of function in a solitary kidney after intra-arterial thrombolytic therapy. J Urol 141:108-110, 1989.

103. Marron B, Ubeda I, Gallego J: Functional renal recovery after spontaneous renal embolization in a sole kidney. Nephrol Dial Transplant 12:2417-2420, 1997.

104. Hirota S, Matsumoto S, Yoshikawa T, et al: Simultaneous thrombolysis of superior mesenteric artery and bilateral renal artery thromboembolisms with three transfemoral catheters. Cardiovasc Intervent Radiol 20:397-400, 1997.

105. Wilms G, Vermylen J, Baert A: Intra-arterial low-dose streptokinase infusion in the treatment of acute renal thromboembolism. Eur J Radiol 7:72-76, 1987.

106. Campieri C, Raimondi C, Fatone F: Normalization of renal function and blood pressure after dissolution with intra-arterial fibrinolytics of a massive renal artery embolism to a solitary functioning kidney. Nephron 52:399-402, 1989.

107. Gluck G, Croitoru M, Deleanu D, Platon P: Local thrombolytic treatment for renal arterial embolism. Eur Urol 38:339-343, 2000.

108. Roufiere O, Berger P, Beziat C, et al: Acute thrombosis of renal transplant artery-graft salvage by means of intraarterial fibrinolysis. Transplantation 73:403-409, 2002.

109. Levin M, Nakhoul F, Keidar Z, Green J: Acute oliguric renal failure associated with unilateral renal embolism: A successful treatment with iloprost. Am J Nephrol 18:444-447, 1998.

110. Molteni KH, George J, Messersmith R, et al: Intrathrombic urokinase reverses neonatal renal artery thrombosis. Pediatr Nephrol 7:413-415, 1993.

111. Kaye ED, Bontempo FA: Aortic and renal artery thrombosis in a neonate: Recovery with thrombolytic therapy. Pediatr Nephrol 11: 641-644, 1997.

112. Gunnarsson B, Heard CM, Martin DJ, et al: Successful lysis of an obstructive aortic and renal artery thrombus in a neonate on extracorporeal membrane oxygenation. J Perinatol 20:555-557, 2000.

113. Lacombe M: Acute nontraumatic obstructions of the renal artery. J Cardiovasc Surg 33:163-170, 1992.

114. Ouriel K, Andrus CH, Ricotta JJ, et al: Acute renal artery occlusion: When is revascularization justified? J Vasc Surg 5:348-355, 1987.

115. Cummings KB, Lecky JW, Kaufman JJ: Renal artery aneurysms and hypertension. J Urol 109:144-148, 1973.

116. Tham G, Ekelund L, Herrlin K, et al: Renal artery aneurysms: Natural history and prognosis. Ann Surg 197:348-352, 1983.

117. Henke PK, Cardneau J, Welling TH, et al: Renal artery aneurysms: A 35-year clinical experience with 252 aneurysms in 168 patients. Ann Surg 234:454-463, 2001.

118. Lumsden AB, Salam TA, Walton KG: Renal artery aneurysm: A report of 28 cases. Cardiovasc Surg 4:185-189, 1996.

119. Dzsinich C, Gloviczki P, McKusick MA, et al: Surgical management of renal artery aneurysm. Cardiovasc Surg 1:243-247, 1993.

120. Bulbul MA, Farrow GA: Renal artery aneurysms. Urology 40: 124-126, 1992.

121. Hupp T, Allenberg JR, Post K, et al: Renal artery aneurysms: Surgical indications and results. Eur J Vasc Surg 6:477-486, 1992.

122. Cinat M, Yoon P, Wilson SE: Management of renal artery aneurysms. Semin Vasc Surg 9:236-244, 1996.

123. Kincaid OW, Davis GD, Hallermann FJ, Hunt JC: Fibromuscular dysplasia of the renal arteries: Arteriographic features, classification and observations on natural history of the disease. AJR Am J Roentgenol 104:271-278, 1968.

124. Barth RA: Fibromuscular dysplasia with clotted renal artery aneurysm. Pediatr Radiol 23:296-297, 1993.

125. Siegelbaum MH, Weiss JP: Renal infarction secondary to fibrous dysplasia and aneurysm formation of renal artery. Urology 35: 73-75, 1990.

126. Stinchcombe SJ, Manhire AR, Bishop MC, Gregson RH: Renal arterial fibromuscular dysplasia: Acute renal failure in 3 patients with angiographic evidence of medial fibroplasia. Br J Radiol 65:81-84, 1992.

127. Heller RM, Hernanz-Schulman M, Johnson J, et al: Pediatric case: Fibromuscular dysplasia with aneurysm. Am J Radiol 158: 1372-1377, 1992.

128. Bisschops RH, Popma JJ, Meyerovitz MF: Treatment of fibromuscular dysplasia and renal artery aneurysm with use of a stent-graft. J Vasc Interv Radiol 12:757-760, 2001.

129. Smith DL, Vernick R: Spontaneous rupure of a renal artery aneurysm in polyarteritis nodosa: Critical review of the literature and report of a case. Am J Med 87:464-467, 1989.

130. Brogan PA, Davies R, Gordon I, Dillon MJ: Renal angiography in children with polyarteritis nodosa. Pediatr Nephrol 17:277-283, 2002.

131. Yamamoto S, Ogawa S, Kitano T, Shima K: Complete evaluation of the cardiovascular lesions in 24 patients with Takayasu's aortitis using four-image intravenous digital subtraction angiography. Am Heart J 114:1426-1431, 1987.

132. Chugh KS, Jain S, Sakhuja V, et al: Renovascular hypertension due to Takayasu's arteritis among Indian patients. Q J Med 85:833-843, 1992.

133. Millar AJ, Gilbert RD, Brown RA, et al: Abdominal aortic aneurysms in children. J Pediatr Surg 31:1624-1628, 1996.

134. Mattar SG, Kumar AG, Lumsden AB: Vascular complications in Ehlers-Danlos syndrome. Am Surg 60:827-831, 1994.

135. Witz M, Lehmann JM: Aneurysmal arterial disease in a patient with Ehlers-Danlos syndrome: Case report and literature review. J Cardiovasc Surg 38:161-163, 1997.

136. Garbino J, Morel P, Pittet D, Romand JA: Arterial mycotic aneurysm rupture following kidney-pancreas transplantation with exocrine pancreatic drainage into the bladder. Ann Vasc Surg 15:393-395, 2001.

137. Potti A, Danielson B, Sen K: True mycotic aneurysm of a renal artery allograft. Am J Kidney Dis 31:E3, 1998.

138. Millar AJ, Gilbert RD, Brown RA, Immelman EJ: Abdominal aortic aneurysms in children. J Pediatr Surg 31:1624-1628, 1996.

139. Bastounis E, Pioulis E, Georgopoulos S, et al: Surgery for renal artery aneurysms: A combined series of two large centers. Eur Urol 33:22-27, 1998.

140. Seki T, Koyanagi T, Togashi M, et al: Experience with revascularizing renal artery aneurysms: Is it feasible, safe and worth attempting? J Urol 158:357-362, 1997.

141. Murray SP, Kent C, Salvatierra O, Stoney RJ: Complex branch renovascular disease: Management options and late results. J Vasc Surg 20:338-346, 1994.

142. Hageman JH, Smith RF, Szilagyi DE: Aneurysms of the renal artery: Problems of prognosis and surgical management. Surgery 84:563-572, 1978.

143. Hubert JP Jr, Pairolera PC, Kazmier FJ: Solitary renal artery aneurysm. Surgery 88:557-565, 1980.

144. Henriksson C, Lukes P, Nilson A: Angiographically discovered non-operated renal artery aneurysms. Scand J Urol Nephrol 18:59-62, 1984.

145. Martin RS, Meacitam PW, Ditesheim JA: Renal artery aneurysm: Selective treatment for hypertension and prevention of rupture. J Vasc Surg 9:26-34, 1989.

146. Hidai H, Kindshita Y, Murayama T: Rupture of renal artery aneurysm. Eur Urol 11:249-253, 1985.

147. Cohen JR, Shamash FS: Ruptured renal artery aneurysms during pregnancy. J Vasc Surg 16:51-59, 1987.

148. Schoon I, Seeman T, Niemand D, et al: Rupture of renal arterial aneurysm in pregnancy: Case report. Acta Chir Scand 154:593-598, 1988.

149. Smith JA, Cacleish DG: Postpartum rupture of a renal artery aneurysm to a solitary kidney. Aust N Z J Surg 55:299-305, 1985.

150. Pliskin MJ, Dressner ML, Hassell LH, et al: A giant renal artery aneurysm diagnosed post-partum. J Urol 144:1459-1461, 1990.

151. Meabed AH, Onuora VC, Al Turki M, et al: Rupture of a renal artery aneurysm in pregnancy. Urol Int 69:72-74, 2002.

152. Lacroix H, Bernaerts P, Nevelsteen A, Hanssens M: Ruptured renal artery aneurysm during pregnancy: Successful ex situ repair and autotransplantation. J Vasc Surg 33:188-190, 2001.

153. Richardson AJ, Liddington M, Jaskowski A: Pregnancy in a renal transplant recipient complicated by rupture of a transplant renal artery aneurysm. Br J Surg 77:228, 1990.

154. Milsom I, Forssman L: Factors influencing aortocaval compression in late pregnancy. Am J Obstet Gynecol 148:764-771, 1984.

155. Yang JC, Hye RJ: Ruptured renal artery aneurysm during pregnancy. Ann Vasc Surg 10:370-372, 1996.

156. Calligaro KD, Dougherty MJ: Renal artery aneurysms and arteriovenous fistulae. *In* Rutherford JM (ed): Vascular Surgery, 2nd ed. Philadelphia, WB Saunders, 2000, pp 1697-1712.

157. Klein GE, Brien LE, Raith J, Schreyer HH: Endovascular treatment of renal aneurysms with conventional non-detachable microcoils and Guglielmi detachable coils. Br J Urol 79:852-860, 1997.

158. Ligouri G, Trombetta C, Bucci S: Percutaneous management of renal artery aneurysm with a stent graft. J Urol 167:2518-2519, 2002.

159. Rikimaru H, Sato A, Hashizume E, et al: Saccular renal artery aneurysm treated with an autologous vein-covered stent. J Vasc Surg 34:169-171, 2001.

160. Majwal TK, Ismail A, Alaqily R: Intervention in peripheral vascular disease: Renal artery stenosis associated with saccular aneurysm and arteriovenous fistula. J Invas Cardiol 14:411-413, 2002.

161. Bruce M, Kuan Y: Endoluminal stent-graft repair of a renal artery aneurysm. J Endovasc Ther 9:359-362, 2002.

162. Tshomba Y, Deleo G, Ferrari S, et al: Renal artery aneurysm: Improved renal function after coil embolization. J Endovasc Ther 9: 54-58, 2002.

163. Halloul Z, Buerger T, Grote R, Meyer F: Selective embolization of a renal artery aneurysm. Vasa 29:285-287, 2000.

164. Mounayer C, Aymard A, Saint-Maurice JP, et al: Balloon-assisted coil embolization for large-necked renal artery aneurysms. Cardiovasc Intervent Radiol 23:228-230, 2000.

165. Karkos CD, D'Souza SP, Thomson GJ, et al: Renal artery aneurysm: Endovascular treatment by coil embolisation with preservation of renal blood flow. Eur J Vasc Endovasc Surg 19:214-216, 2000.

166. Planer D, Verstandig A, Chajek-Shaul T: Transcatheter embolization of renal artery aneurysm in Behçet's disease. Vasc Med 6:109-112, 2001.

167. Edwards BS, Stanson AW, Holley KE: Isolated renal artery dissection: Presentation, evaluation, management and pathology. Mayo Clin Proc 57:564-569, 1982.

168. Smith B, Holcomb GW, Richie R: Renal artery dissection. Ann Surg 200:134, 1984.

169. Alamir A, Middendorf DF, Baker P, et al: Renal artery dissection causing renal infarction in otherwise healthy men. Am J Kidney Dis 30:851-855, 1997.

170. Mori H, Hayashi K, Tasaki T, et al: Spontaneous resolution of bilateral renal artery dissection: A case report. J Urol 135:114-116, 1986.

171. Goldfarb R, Pool JL, Wheeler T: Isolated renal artery dissection secondary to medial degeneration. J Urol 139:346-347, 1988.

172. Esayag-Tendler B, Yamase H, Ramsey G, White WB: Accelerated hypertension with encephalopathy due to an isolated dissection of a renal artery branch vessel. Am J Kidney Dis 23:869-873, 1994.

173. Reilly LM, Cummingham CG, Maggisano R, et al: The role of arterial reconstruction in spontaneous renal artery dissection. J Vasc Surg 14:468-479, 1991.

174. Starnes BW, O'Donnell SD, Gillespie DL, et al: Endovascular management of renal ischemia in a patient with acute aortic dissection and renovascular hypertension. Ann Vasc Surg 16:368-374, 2002.

175. Gewertz BL, Stanley JC, Fry WJ: Renal artery dissection. Arch Surg 122:409-416, 1977.

176. Ramamoorthy SL, Vasquez JC, Taft PM, et al: Nonoperative management of acute spontaneous renal artery dissection. Ann Vasc Surg 16:157-162, 2002.

177. Mokri B, Stanson AW, Houser OW: Spontaneous dissections of the renal arteries in a patient with previous spontaneous dissections of the internal carotid arteries. Stroke 16:959-963, 1985.

178. Lauterbach SR, Cambria RP, Brewster DC, et al: Contemporary management of aortic branch compromise resulting from acute aortic dissection. J Vasc Surg 33:1185-1192, 2002.

179. Lacombe M: Isolated spontaneous dissection of the renal artery. J Vasc Surg 33:385-391, 2001.

180. Handler FP: Clinical and pathologic significance of atheromatous embolization with emphasis on the etiology of renal hypertension. Am J Med 20:366-372, 1956.

181. Chomette G, Auriol M, Trambaloc P: Cholesterol emboli: Anatomic locations and clinical manifestation. Ann Med Interne (Paris) 131: 17-25, 1980.

182. Eliot RS, Kanjuh VI, Edwards JE: Atheromatous embolism. Circulation 30:611-615, 1964.

183. Handler FP: Clinical and pathologic significance of atheromatous embolization, with emphasis on the aetiology of renal hypertension. Am J Med 20:366-373, 1956.

184. Gore I, Collins DP: Spontaneous atheromatous embolization: Review of the literature and report of 16 additional cases. Am J Clin Pathol 33:416-421, 1960.

185. Otken LB Jr: Experimental production of atheromatous embolization. Arch Pathol 68:685-693, 1959.

186. Snyder HE, Shapiro JL: Correlative study of atheromatous embolism in human beings and experimental animals. Surgery 49:195, 1961.

187. Flory CM: Arterial occlusions produced by emboli from eroded aortic atheromatous plaques. Am J Pathol 21:549, 1945.

188. Sayre GP, Campbell DC: Multiple peripheral emboli in atherosclerosis of the aorta. Arch Intern Med 103:799-807, 1959.

189. Thurleck WM, Castleman B: Atheromatous emboli to the kidneys after aortic surgery. N Engl J Med 257:442-448, 1957.

190. Moldveen-Geronimus M, Merriam JC Jr: Cholesterol embolization from pathological curiosity to clinical entity. Circulation 35:946-954, 1967.

191. Harrington JT, Sommers SC, Kassirer JP: Atheromatous emboli with progressive renal failure: Renal arteriography as the probable inciting factor. Ann Intern Med 68:152-157, 1968.

192. Kaplan K, Miller JD, Cancilla PA: "Spontaneous" atheroembolic renal failure. Arch Intern Med 110:218-225, 1962.

193. Greenberg A, Bastacky SI, Iqbal A: Focal segmental glomerulosclerosis associated with nephrotic syndrome in cholesterol atheroembolism: Clinicopathological correlations. Am J Kidney Dis 29: 334-340, 1997.

194. Belenfant X, Meyrier A, Jacquot C: Supportive treatment improves survival in multivisceral cholesterol crystal embolism. Am J Kidney Dis 33:840-850, 1999.

195. Thadhani RI, Camargo CA, Xavier RJ, et al: Atheroembolic renal failure after invasive procedures. Medicine (Baltimore) 74:350-358, 1995.

196. Vidt DG, Eisele G, Gephardt GN, et al: Atheroembolic renal disease: Association with renal artery stenosis. Cleve Clin J Med 56:407-413, 1989.

197. Fine MJ, Kapoor W, Falanga V: Cholesterol crystal embolization: A review of 221 cases in the English literature. Angiology 22:769-784, 1987.

198. Scolari F, Bracchi M, Valzorio B, et al: Cholesterol atheromatous embolism: An increasingly recognized cause of acute renal failure. Nephrol Dial Transplant 11:1607-1612, 1996.

199. Vidt DG: Cholesterol emboli: A common cause of renal failure. Annu Rev Med 48:375-385, 1997.

200. Rudnick MR, Berns JS, Cohen RM, Goldfarb S: Nephrotoxic risks of renal angiography: Contrast media-associated nephrotoxicity and atheroembolism—A critical review. Am J Kidney Dis 24:713-727, 1994.

201. Mashiah A, Pasik S, Hurwitz N: Massive atheromatous emboli to both kidneys: A fatal complication following aortic surgery. J Cardiovasc Surg 29:60-62, 1988.

202. Dahlberg PJ, Frecentese DR, Cogbill TH: Cholesterol embolism: Experience with 22 histologically proven cases. Surgery 105:737-746, 1989.

203. Wong FK, Chan SK, Ing TS, Li CS: Acute renal failure after streptokinase therapy in a patient with acute myocardial infarction. Am J Kidney Dis 26:508-510, 1995.

204. Larry JA, Falkenhain ME, Mazzaferr EL: Acute renal failure in an elderly man taking warfarin. Hosp Pract 52:119-124, 1996.

205. Schwartz MW, McDonald G: Cholesterol embolization syndrome: Occurrence after intravenous streptokinase therapy for myocardial infarction. JAMA 258:1934, 1987.

206. Queen M, Blem HJ, Moe GW: Development of cholesterol embolization after intravenous streptokinase for acute myocardial infarction. Am J Cardiol 65:1042-1055, 1990.

207. Hyman B, Landas S, Ashman R, et al: Warfarin-related purple toes syndrome and cholesterol microembolization. Am J Med 82: 1233-1239, 1987.

208. Tilley WS, Harston WE, Siami G: Renal failure due to cholesterol emboli following PTCA. Am Heart J 110:1301-1302, 1985.

209. Scolari F, Tardanico R, Zani R, et al: Cholesterol crystal embolism: A recognizable cause of renal disease. Am J Kidney Dis 36:1089-1109, 2000.

210. Modi KS, Rao M, Rao VK: Atheroembolic renal disease. J Am Soc Nephrol 12:1781-1787, 2001.

211. Pennington M, Yeager J, Skelton H, Smith KJ: Cholesterol embolization syndrome: Cutaneous histopathological features and the variable onset of symptoms in patients with different risk factors. Br J Dermatol 146:511-517, 2002.

212. Falanga V, Fine MJ, Kapoor WN: The cutaneous manifestations of cholesterol crystal embolization. Arch Dermatol 122:1194-1198, 1986.

213. Quintart C, Treille S, Lefebvre P, Pontus T: Penile necrosis following cholesterol embolism. Br J Urol 80:347-348, 1997.

214. Lye WC, Cheah JS, Sinniah R: Renal cholesterol embolic disease. Am J Nephrol 13:489-493, 1993.

215. Jiminez-Heffernan JA, Martinez-Garcia M, Burgos E: Small bowel perforation due to cholesterol atheromatous embolism. Dig Dis Sci 40:481-484, 1995.

216. Mollenaar W, Lamers CB: Cholesterol crystal embolization and the digestive system. Scand J Gastroenterol 188:69-72, 1991.

217. Socindki MA, Frankel JP, Morow PL, Krawitt EL: Painless diarrhea secondary to intestinal ischemia: Diagnosis of atheromatous emboli by jejunal biopsy. Dig Dis Sci 51:674-677, 1984.

218. Probstein JG, Joshi RA, Blumenthan HT: Atheromatous embolism: An etiology of acute pancreatitis. Arch Surg 75:566-572, 1957.

219. David MJ, Klintworth GK, Friedbert SG, et al: Fatal atheromatous cerebral embolism associated with bright plaques in retinal arterioles: Report of a case. Neurology 13:708-711, 1963.

220. Hollenhorst RW: Significance of bright plaques in the retinal arterioles. Trans Am Ophthalmol Soc 59:252-256, 1961.

221. Sabatine MS, Oelberg DA, Mark EJ, Kanarek D: Pulmonary cholesterol crystal embolization. Chest 112:1687-1692, 1997.

222. Vacher CH, Pache X, Dussol B, Berland Y: Pulmonary-renal syndrome responding to corticosteroids: Consider cholesterol embolization. Nephrol Dial Transplant 12:1977-1979, 1997.

223. Stanton RC: Case records of ten Massachusetts General Hospital. N Engl J Med 334:973-979, 1996.

224. Williams HH, Wall BM, Cooke CR: Reversible nephrotic range proteinuria and renal failure in atheroembolic renal disease. Am J Med Sci 299:58-65, 1990.

225. Kasinath BS, Lewis EJ: Eosinophils as a clue to the diagnosis of atheroembolic renal disease. Arch Intern Med 147:1384-1388, 1987.

226. Kasinath BS, Corwin HL, Bidani AK, et al: Eosinophilia in the diagnosis of atheroembolic renal disease. Am J Med 7:173-177, 1987.

227. Wilson DM, Salazer TL, Farkooh ME: Eosinophiluria in atheroembolic renal disease. Am J Med 91:186-189, 1991.

228. Cosio F, Zager R, Sharma H: Atheroembolic renal disease causes hypocomplementemia. Lancet 2:118-120, 1985.

229. Knechtges TC, Defever BA: Cholesterol emboli in transurethral curettings: Report of 4 cases. J Urol 114:102-104, 1975.

230. Smyth JS, Scoble JE: Atheroembolism. Curr Treat Options Cardiovasc Med 4:255-265, 2002.

231. Keen RR, McCarthy WJ, Shireman PK, Fineglass J: Surgical management of atheroembolization. J Vasc Surg 21:773-781, 1995.

232. Baumann DS, McGraw D, Rubin BG, Allen BT: An institutional experience with arterial atheroembolism. Ann Vasc Surg 8:258-265, 1994.

233. Hunter J: Guide to the Hunterian Collection, Part 1: Pathological Series in the Hunterian Museum. Specimen p. 389. A Case of Renal Vein Thrombosis (Lady Beauchamp). Edinburgh, Livingstone, 1966, p 267.

234. Rayer PR: O. Traite des Maladies des Reins et des Alterations de la Secretions Urinaire, Vol 2. Paris, JB Bailiere, 1840, pp 590-599.

235. Abeshouse BS: Thrombosis and thrombophlebitis of the renal veins. Urol Cutan Rev 49:661-672, 1945.

236. Harrison CV, Milne MD, Steiner RE: Clinical aspects of renal vein thrombosis. Q J Med 25:285-301, 1956.

237. McCarthy LJ, Titus JL, Daugherty GW: Bilateral renal vein thrombosis and the nephrotic syndrome in adults. Ann Intern Med 58:837-849, 1963.

238. Bennett WM: Renal vein thrombosis and nephrotic syndrome. Ann Intern Med 83:577-586, 1975.

239. Cameron JS, Ogg CS, Wass V: The complications of the nephrotic syndrome. *In* Cameron JS, Glassock RJ (eds): The Nephrotic Syndrome. New York, Marcel Dekker, 1988, pp 925-949.

240. Llach F, Koffler A, Massry SG: Renal vein thrombosis and the nephrotic syndrome. Nephron 19:65-72, 1977.

241. Monteon F, Trevino A, Exaire E, et al: Nephrotic syndrome with renal vein thrombosis treated with thrombectomy and anticoagulants. 8th International Congress of Nephrology, Athens, 1981. Abstracts, p 82.

242. Noel LH, Zannetti M, Droz D, et al: Long-term prognosis of idiopathic membranous glomerulonephritis: Study of 116 untreated patients. Am J Med 66:82-93, 1979.

243. Pohl MA, MacLaurin JP, Alfidi RJ: Renal vein thrombosis and the nephrotic syndrome. 10th Annual Meeting of the American Society of Nephrology, Washington, DC, 1977. Abstracts, p 20A.

244. Velazquez-Forero F, Garcia-Prugue N, Ruiz-Morales N: Idiopathic nephrotic syndrome of the adult with asymptomatic thrombosis of the renal vein. Am J Nephrol 8:457-462, 1988.

245. Wagoner RD, Stanson AW, Holley K, et al: Renal vein thrombosis in idiopathic membranous glomerulopathy and the nephrotic syndrome: Incidence and significance. Kidney Int 23:368-376, 1983.

246. Llach F, Papper S, Massry SG: The clinical spectrum of renal vein thrombosis: Acute and chronic. Am J Med 69:819-829, 1980.

247. Llach R: Nephrotic syndrome: Hypercoagulability, renal vein thrombosis, and other thromboembolic complications. *In* Brenner B, Stein J (eds): Contemporary Issues in Nephrology, Vol 9. New York, Churchill-Livingstone, 1982, pp 121-144.

248. Cornog JL, Rawson AJ, Karp LA, et al: Immunofluorescent and ultrastructural study of the renal lesions observed in human renal vein thrombosis and the nephrotic syndrome. Lab Invest 18:689-694, 1968.

249. Fisher ER, Sharkey D, Pardo V, et al: Experimental renal constriction: Its relation to renal lesions observed in human renal vein thrombosis and the nephrotic syndrome. Lab Invest 18:689-692, 1968.

250. Gatewood OM, Siegelman SS, Fishman EK, et al: Renal vein thrombosis in patients with nephrotic syndrome: CT diagnosis. Radiology 159:117-120, 1986.

251. Hruby MA, Honig GR, Shapiro E: Immunoquantitation of Hageman factor in the urine and plasma of children with nephrotic syndrome. J Lab Clin Med 96:501-506, 1980.

252. Deodhar KP, Bharlerao RA, Kelkar MD, et al: Inferior vena cava obstruction. J Postgrad Med 25:64-72, 1969.

253. Jackson BT, Thomas ML: Post-thrombotic inferior vena cava obstruction: A review of 24 patients. Br Med J 1:18-20, 1970.

254. Llach F, Koffler A, Finck E, et al: On the incidence of renal vein thrombosis in the nephrotic syndrome. Arch Intern Med 137:33-36, 1977.

255. Llach F, Arieff AI, Massry SG: Renal vein thrombosis and nephrotic syndrome: A prospective study of 36 adult patients. Ann Intern Med 83:8-15, 1975.

256. Trew P, Biava C, Jacobs R, et al: Renal vein thrombosis in membranous glomerulopathy: Incidence and association. Medicine (Baltimore) 57:69-88, 1978.

257. Kendall AG, Lohmann RE, Dossetor JB: Nephrotic syndrome: A hypercoagulable state. Arch Intern Med 127:1021-1027, 1971.

258. Kanfer A, Kleinknecht D, Broyer M, et al: Coagulation studies in 45 cases of nephrotic syndrome without uremia. Thromb Diathes Haemorrh 24:562-568, 1970.

259. Thompson C, Forbes CD, Prentice CRM, et al: Changes in blood coagulation and fibrinolysis in the nephrotic syndrome. Q J Med 43:399-412, 1974.

260. Earley LE, Haule RJ, Hopper J, et al: Nephrotic syndrome. Calif Med 115:123, 1971.

261. Green D, Arruda J, Honig G, et al: Urinary loss of clotting factor due to hereditary membranous nephropathy. Am J Clin Pathol 65:376-382, 1976.

262. Llach F: Renal vein thrombosis and the nephrotic syndrome. *In* Llach F (ed): Renal Vein Thrombosis. Mount Kisco, NY, Futura, 1983, p 155.

263. Andrassy K, Ritz E, Bommer J: Hypercoagulability in the nephrotic syndrome. Klin Wochenschr 58:1029-1038, 1980.

264. Takeda Y, Chen A: Fibrinogen metabolism and distribution in patients with the nephrotic syndrome. J Lab Clin Med 70:678-689, 1967.

265. Clarkson A, MacDonald M, Petrie J, et al: Serum and urinary fibrinogen/fibrin degradation products in glomerulonephritis. Br Med J 3:447-454, 1971.

266. Cade R, Spooner G, Juncos L, et al: Chronic renal vein thrombosis. Am J Med 63:387-399, 1977.

267. Hall C, Pejhan N, Terry J, et al: Urinary fibrin/fibrinogen degradation products in nephrotic syndrome. Br Med J 1:419-425, 1975.

268. Wu KK, Hoak JC: Urinary plasminogen and chronic glomerulonephritis. Am J Clin Pathol 60:915-921, 1973.

269. Astedt B, Issacson S, Milsson IM: Thrombosis and oral contraceptives: Possible predisposition. Br Med J 4:631-633, 1973.

270. Bonnar J, McNichol GP, Douglas AS: Fibrinolytic enzyme system and pregnancy. Br Med J 3:387-389, 1969.

271. Ygge J: Changes in blood coagulation and fibrinolysis during the postoperative period. Am J Surg 119:225-234, 1970.

272. Rennie J, Ogston D: Fibrinolytic activity in malignant disease. J Clin Pathol 28:872-879, 1975.

273. Almer LO, Janzon L: Low vascular fibrinolytic activity in obesity. Thromb Res 6:171-179, 1975.

274. Edward N, Young DPG, Macleod M: Fibrinolytic activity in plasma and urine in chronic renal disease. J Clin Pathol 17:365-372, 1961.

275. Hedner U, Nilsson IM: Antithrombin III in a clinical material. Thromb Res 3:631-642, 1973.

276. Scheinman JI, Stiehm ER: Fibrinolytic studies on the nephrotic syndrome. Pediatr Res 5:206-212, 1971.

277. Lau SO, Tkachuk JY, Hasegawa DK, et al: Plasminogen and antithrombin III deficiencies in the childhood nephrotic syndrome associated with plasminogenuria and antithrombinuria. J Pediatr 96:390-402, 1980.

278. Llach F: The hypercoagulability and thrombotic complications of nephrotic syndrome. Editorial review. Kidney Int 28:429-442, 1985.

279. Du XH, Glass-Greenwalt P, Kank KS, et al: Nephrotic syndrome with renal vein thrombosis: Pathogenetic importance of a plasmin inhibitor. IX International Congress of Nephrology, Los Angeles, June, 1984. Abstracts, p 84A.

280. Honig GR, Lindley A: Deficiency of Hageman factor (factor XII) in patients with nephrotic syndrome. J Pediatr 78:633-642, 1971.

281. Lange LG III, Carvalho A, Bagdasarian A, et al: Activation of Hageman factor in the nephrotic syndrome. Am J Med 56:565-569, 1974.

282. Natelson EA, Lynch EC, Hettig RA, et al: Acquired factor IX deficiency in the nephrotic syndrome. Ann Intern Med 73:373-382, 1970.

283. Godal HC, Rygh M, Laake K: Progressive inactivation of purified factor VIII by heparin and antithrombin III. Thromb Res 5:773, 1974.

284. Marciniak E, Farley CH, Desimone PA: Familial thrombosis due to antithrombin III deficiency. Blood 43:219-228, 1974.

285. Rosenberg JS, McKeena P, Rosenberg RD: The inhibition of human factor IXa by human antithrombin. J Biol Chem 250:8883-8891, 1975.

286. Rosenberg RD: Actions and interactions of antithrombin and heparin. N Engl J Med 292:146-154, 1975.

287. Yin ET, Wessler S, Stroll PJ: Identity of plasma-activated factor X inhibitor with antithrombin III and heparin cofactor. J Biol Chem 246:3712-3719, 1971.

288. Kauffman RH, Veltkamp JJ, Van Tilburg NH, et al: Acquired antithrombin III deficiency and thrombosis in the nephrotic syndrome. Am J Med 65:607-619, 1978.

289. Kauffman RH, De Graeff J, Brutel De La Rivierre G, et al: Unilateral renal vein thrombosis and nephrotic syndrome. Am J Med 60:1048-1056, 1976.

290. Thaler E, Blazar E, Kopsa H, et al: Acquired antithrombin III deficiency in patients with glomerular proteinuria. Hemostasis 7:257-262, 1978.

291. Ellis D: Recurrent renal vein thrombosis and renal failure associated with antithrombin-III deficiency. Pediatr Nephrol 6:131-134, 1992.

292. Panicucci R, Sagripanti A, Pinori E, et al: Comprehensive study of haemostasis in nephrotic syndrome. Nephron 33:9-21, 1983.

293. Vaziri ND, Paule P, Toohey J, et al: Acquired deficiency and urinary excretion of antithrombin III in nephrotic syndrome. Arch Intern Med 144:1802-1812, 1984.

294. Egebert O: Inherited antithrombin deficiency causing thrombophilia. Thromb Haemost 13:516-523, 1974.

295. Stenflo J: A new vitamin K-dependent protein: Purification from bovine plasma and preliminary characterization. J Biol Chem 251:355-364, 1976.

296. Kisiel W, Canfield W, Ericsson L, Davie E: Anticoagulation properties of bovine plasma protein C following activation by thrombin. Biochemistry 16:5824-5831, 1977.

297. Griffin JH, Evatt B, Zimmerman TS, et al: Deficiency of protein C in congenital thrombotic disease. J Clin Invest 68:1370-1379, 1981.

298. Walker FJ: Regulation of activated protein C by protein S. J Biol Chem 256:1128-1135, 1981.

299. Walker FJ: Regulation of activated protein C by a new protein. J Biol Chem 255:5521-5529, 1980.

300. Wardle EN, Memom IS, Ratogi SP: Study of proteins and fibrinolysis in patients with glomerulonephritis. Br Med J 2:260-261, 1970.

301. Comp P, Esmon CT: Recurrent venous thromboembolism in patients with a partial deficiency of protein S. N Engl J Med 311:1525-1532, 1984.

302. Cosio FG, Harker C, Batard MA, et al: Plasma concentrations of the natural anticoagulants protein C and protein S in patients with proteinuria. J Lab Clin Med 106:218-225, 1985.

303. Sorenson PJ, Knudsen F, Nielsen AH, Dyerberg T: Protein C activity in renal disease. Thromb Res 38:243-248, 1985.

304. Vigano-D'Angelo S, D'Angelo A, Kauffman CE, et al: Protein S deficiency occurs in the nephrotic syndrome. Ann Intern Med 107:42-51, 1987.

305. Bang N, Tygstad C, Schroeder J: Enhanced platelet function in glomerular renal disease. J Lab Clin Med 81:651-659, 1973.

306. Remuzzi G, Mecca G, Marchest D, et al: Platelet hyperaggregability and the nephrotic syndrome. Thromb Res 16:345-351, 1979.

307. Alder AJ, Jundin AP, Feinroth AP, et al: B-thrombo-globulin levels in the nephrotic syndrome. Am J Med 69:551-558, 1980.

308. Andrassy K, Depperman D, Walter E, et al: Is beta thromboglobulin a useful indicator of thrombosis in nephrotic syndrome? Thromb Haemost 42:486-493, 1979.

309. Kuhlmann U, Stevrer J, Rhyner K, et al: Platelet aggregation and β-thromboglobulin levels in nephrotic patients with and without thrombosis. Clin Nephrol 15:229-238, 1981.

310. Cheng HF, Liu YG, Pan JS, et al: A prospective study of renal vein thrombosis. XI International Congress of Nephrology, Tokyo, Japan, 1990. Abstracts, p 6A.

311. Ooi BS, Ooi YM, Pollak VE: Circulating immune complexes in renal vein thrombosis. 11th Annual Meeting of the American Society of Nephrology, New Orleans, 1978. Abstracts, p 24A.

312. Andrassy K, Depperman D, Walter E, et al: Is beta-thromboglobulin a useful indicator of thrombosis in nephrotic syndrome? Throm Haemost 42:483-493, 1979.

313. Lohman RC, Kendal AG, Dossetor JB, et al: The fibrinolytic system in the nephrotic syndrome. Clin Res 17:333, 1969.

314. Harms K, Speer CP: Thrombosis: An underestimated complication of central catheters. Subclavian vein and renal vein thrombosis after Silastic catheters. Monatsschr Kinderheilkd 141:21-25, 1993.

315. Mukherjee AP, Tog BH, Chan GL: Vascular complications in nephrotic syndrome: Relationship to steroid therapy and accelerated thromboplastin generation. Br Med J 4:273-282, 1970.

316. Luetscher JA, Deming QB: Treatment of nephrotics with cortisone. J Clin Invest 29:1576-1585, 1950.

317. Cosgriff SW, Diefenbach AF, Vogt W Jr: Hypercoagulability of the blood associated with ACTH and cortisone therapy. Am J Med 9:752-761, 1950.

318. Rosenmann E, Pollak VE, Pirani CL: Renal vein thrombosis in the adult: A clinical and pathological study based on renal biopsies. Medicine (Baltimore) 47:269-292, 1968.

319. Slick GL, Schnetzler DE, Koloyanides GJ: Hypertension, renal vein thrombosis and renal failure occurring in a patient on an oral contraceptive agent. Clin Nephrol 3:70-78, 1975.

320. Arneil GC, MacDonald AM, Murphy AV, et al: Renal venous thrombosis. Clin Nephrol 1:119-126, 1973.

321. Hay CRM, McEvoy P: Main graft vessel thromboses due to conventional dose OKT3 in renal transplantation. Lancet 339:1612-1613, 1992.

322. Hollenbeck M, Westhoff A, Dieter B, et al: Doppler sonography and renal graft vessel thromboses after OKT3 treatment. Lancet 340:619-620, 1992.

323. Richardson AJ, Higgins RM, Jaskowski AJ, et al: Spontaneous rupture of renal allografts: The importance of renal vein thrombosis in the cyclosporin era. Br J Surg 77:558-560, 1990.

324. Bakir N, Sluiter WJ, Ploeg RJ, et al: Primary renal graft thrombosis. Nephrol Dial Transplant 11:140-147, 1996.

325. Brown Z, Neild GH, Willoghby JJ, et al: Increased factor VIII as an index of vascular injury in cyclosporin nephrotoxicity. Transplantation 42:150-153, 1986.

326. Brown Z, Neild GH: Cyclosporin inhibits prostaglandin production by cultured human endothelial cells. Transplant Proc 19:1170-1180, 1987.

327. Koehler PR, Bowles WT, McAlister WH: Renal arteriography in experimental renal vein occlusion. Radiology 86:851-872, 1966.

328. Kowal J, Figur A, Hitzig WM: Renal vein thrombosis and the nephrotic syndrome with complete remission. J Mt Sinai Hosp 30:47-53, 1963.

329. Scanlon GT: Radiographic changes in renal vein thrombosis. Radiology 80:208-219, 1963.

330. MacLennan AC, Baxter BM, Harden P, Rowe PA: Renal transplant vein occlusions: An early diagnostic sign? Clin Radiol 50:251-253, 1995.

331. Rahmouni A, Jazaerli N, Radier C: Evaluation of magnetic resonance imaging for the assessment of renal vein thrombosis in the nephrotic syndrome. Clin Nephrol 68:271-272, 1994.

332. Prince MR, Narasimham DL, Stanley JC: Breath-hold gadolinium-enhanced MR angiography of the abdominal aorta and its major branches. Radiology 197:785-792, 1995.

333. Kanagasundaraman NS, Bandyopadhyay D, Brownjorlan AM, Meaney JFM: The diagnosis of renal vein thrombosis by magnetic resonance angiography. Nephrol Dial Transplant 13:200-202, 1998.

334. Richet G, Meyrier A (eds): Liposclerose Retroperitoneal: Thrombose des Veines Renales. Deux Syndromes Retroperitoneaux. Paris, Masson, 1970.

335. Lavelle M, Aguilera D, Maillet PJ, et al: The prognosis of renal vein thrombosis: A reevaluation of 27 cases. Nephrol Dial Transplant 3:247-261, 1988.

336. Vogelsang RL, Moel DI, Cohn RA: Acute renal vein thrombosis: Successful treatment with intraarterial urokinase. Radiology 169:681-682, 1988.

337. Briefel GR, Manis T, Gordon DH: Recurrent renal vein thrombosis consequent to membranous nephropathy. Clin Nephrol 10:32-39, 1978.

338. Kennedy JS, Gerety BM, Silverman R, et al: Simultaneous renal arterial and venous thrombosis associated with idiopathic nephrotic syndrome: Treatment with intra-arterial urokinase. Am J Med 90:124-133, 1991.

339. Monte XLT, Jimenez AA, Aguilar L: Renal arterial thrombosis occurring in an adult with idiopathic nephrotic syndrome: Results of local treatment with streptokinase. Clin Nephrol 12:90-92, 1979.

340. Chiu AS, Ladsberg DN: Successful treatment of acute renal vein thrombosis with selective streptokinase infusion. Transplant Proc 23:2297-2300, 1991.

341. Schwieger J, Reiss R, Cohen JL, et al: Acute renal allograft dysfunction in the setting of deep venous thrombosis: A case of successful urokinase thrombolysis and a review of the literature. Am J Kidney Dis 22:345-350, 1993.

342. Gootman M, Groo J, Mensch A: Pulmonary artery thrombosis. Pediatrics 34:861-868, 1964.

343. Coon WW, Willis PW: Thrombosis of axillary and subclavian vein. Arch Surg 94:622-657, 1967.

344. Mukherjee AP, Toh BH, Chan GL, et al: Vascular complications in nephrotic syndrome: Relationship to steroid therapy and accelerated thromboplastin generation. Br Med J 4:273-276, 1970.

345. Berlyne GM, Mallick NP: Ischemic heart as a complication of nephrotic syndrome. Lancet 2:392-399, 1969.

346. Andrassy K, Ritz R: Biochemie und klinische Bedeutung von Urokinase. Dtsch Med Wochenschr 24:1015-1026, 1978.

347. Vosnides GR, Nicoloupoulon N, Spanos H, et al: Renal vein thrombosis in patients with nephrotic syndrome. IX International Congress of Nephrology, Los Angeles, June, 1984. Abstracts, p 138A.

348. Cameron JS, Ogg CS, Wass V: The complications of the nephrotic syndrome. *In* Cameron JS, Glassock RJ (eds): The Nephrotic Syndrome. New York, Marcel Dekker, 1985.

CHAPTER 33

Microvascular Diseases of the Kidney

Hussein H. Karnib and Kamal F. Badr

The kidney is involved in a number of discreet clinico-pathologic conditions that affect systemic and renal microvasculature. Certain of these entities are characterized by primary injury to endothelial cells, such as the spectrum of hemolytic-uremic syndrome (HUS)–thrombotic thrombocytopenic purpura (TTP) and radiation nephritis. In others, the microvasculature of the kidney is involved in autoimmune disorders, such as systemic sclerosis (scleroderma). The renal microcirculation can also be affected in sickle cell disease, to which the kidney is particularly susceptible because of the low oxygen tension attained in the deep vessels of the renal medulla as a result of countercurrent transfer of oxygen along the vasa recta. The smaller renal arteries and arterioles can also be the site of thromboembolic injury from cholesterol-containing material dislodged from the walls of the large vessels. These conditions are considered jointly in this chapter.

Taken as a group, diseases that cause transient or permanent occlusion of renal microvasculature uniformly result in disruption of glomerular perfusion, and hence of the glomerular filtration rate, thereby constituting a serious threat to systemic homeostasis. Early recognition and aggressive management of these disorders is therefore crucial for the long-term preservation of renal function.

HEMOLYTIC-UREMIC SYNDROME AND THROMBOTIC THROMBOCYTOPENIC PURPURA

HUS and TTP are closely related diseases characterized by microangiopathic hemolytic anemia and variable organ impairment Traditionally, the diagnosis of HUS is made when renal failure is a predominant feature of the syndrome, as is common in children.[1] In adults, neurologic impairment frequently predominates and the syndrome is then referred to as TTP.[2, 3] Thrombotic microangiopathy is the underlying pathologic lesion in both syndromes,[4] and the clinical and laboratory findings in patients with either HUS or TTP overlap to a large extent.[5] This has prompted several investigators to regard the two syndromes as a continuum of a single disease entity.[5, 6]

Clinical Features

A report by Moschcowitz[7] in 1925 described a 16-year-old girl who developed fever, anemia, petechiae, renal failure, and neurologic impairment. In 1936, Baehr and colleagues[8] described the presence of thrombocytopenia and reticulocytosis in a similar case. In both reports, the term TTP was used to describe the syndrome. Several large series of patients have been reported since that time.[9-15] TTP is usually a sporadic disease, with an incidence of approximately 1 case per 1 million population.[15] It is more common in women (female:male ratio, 3:2 to 5:2) and in whites (white:black ratio, 3:1).[9, 10] Although the peak incidence is in the third and fourth decades of life, TTP can affect any age group.[13, 16]

TTP is an acute illness that is often accompanied by non-specific constitutional symptoms, such as malaise, nausea, and vomiting.[10] The classic triad of microangiopathic hemolytic anemia, thrombocytopenia, and neurologic symptoms occurs in approximately 75% of patients.[10] Hemorrhagic manifestations (83% to 96% of the cases) occur anywhere on the body and manifest as petechiae, purpura, ecchymoses, or bleeding.[9] Neurologic symptoms (84% to 92% of cases) are common at presentation and include headache, altered mental status, paresis, aphasia, dysphasia, paresthesias, visual problems, seizures, and coma.[9, 16, 17] Fever occurs in 98% of patients during the course of illness and is the most common symptom in TTP.[10] Renal involvement in TTP (80% to 90% of patients) is usually mild but can range from abnormal urinalysis to severe renal insufficiency that requires dialysis therapy (see later discussion).[18] Severe acute renal failure (ARF) or anuria occurs in fewer than 10% of the cases.[10]

The term HUS was introduced in 1955 by Gasser and co-workers[19] in their description of an acute fatal syndrome in children that is characterized by hemolytic anemia, thrombocytopenia, and severe renal failure. Gastrointestinal prodromes (vomiting, diarrhea, and abdominal pain) commonly occur a few days to a few weeks before the onset of HUS.[2, 19-21] Hemolytic anemia and renal involvement are uniformly present.[1] ARF is detected in 90% of patients, and anuria occurs in one third (see later discussion).[22] Neurologic symptoms and signs are similar to those of TTP but occur less often (40% of patients).[23, 24] As with TTP, purpura and fever are frequently present.[1] The source of bleeding is most commonly the gastrointestinal tract. HUS is characteristically a disease of young children. The average annual incidence is 2.65 cases per 100,000 population for ages 5 years and younger and 0.97 per 100,000 for ages 18 years and younger.[25] Both sporadic and epidemic HUS occur in children.[1] There are some reports that the incidence of HUS parallels the seasonal fluctuation of *Escherichia coli* O157:H7 infections, with peaks between June and September, affecting mainly young children and the elderly.[26, 27] The epidemic form is the typical presentation and is characteristically preceded by diarrhea.[28]

Additional clinical findings in either TTP or HUS result from microvascular thromboses in the intestines, pancreas, skeletal muscle, and heart. Gastrointestinal involvement may lead to symptoms of acute abdomen with occasional perforation.[15, 29, 30] Microinfarcts in the pancreas can cause pancreatitis[31] and, rarely, insulin-dependent diabetes mellitus.[32, 33] Acute rhabdomyolysis has been reported in association with HUS.[34] Cardiac manifestations include congestive heart failure and arrhythmias.[35] Ocular involvement presenting as retinal, choroidal, or vitreous hemorrhage is also observed in patients with HUS or TTP.[36, 37]

Despite the historical distinction between HUS and TTP,[4] the two syndromes overlap to a large extent and may indeed represent a spectrum of a single disease.[6, 38] Occurrence of HUS is not restricted to children,[39, 40] and neither is TTP limited to adults.[13, 16] An epidemic form of HUS, similar to the one seen in children, has been described in adult nursing home patients.[41] The underlying pathologic process, thrombotic microangiopathy, is identical in both syndromes and can affect multiple organs.[4] Renal damage does not reliably differentiate HUS from TTP, because 80% to 90% of TTP patients have some evidence of renal involvement,[18] and 40% to 80% have depressed renal function.[15, 42] Similarly, neurologic involvement is not characteristic of TTP, because it is frequently observed in patients with the clinical diagnosis of HUS.[23, 24] These observations suggest that the two syndromes are variable presentations of the same disease and have prompted the use of the term HUS/TTP to describe patients with thrombotic microangiopathy.[38] However, recent studies suggest that TTP and HUS may now often be distinguished on a biochemical basis by measuring the plasma von Willebrand factor (VWF)–cleaving metalloprotease activity, which has been shown to be deficient in most patients with TTP but not in those with HUS (see later discussion). Because in some cases TTP and HUS are still not easily distinguished,[43] the broader term TTP/HUS remains in use.

Laboratory Findings

The hallmark laboratory finding, essential for the diagnosis of HUS/TTP, is microangiopathic hemolytic anemia.

The peripheral smear reveals increased schistocyte number (burr cells, helmet cells, and other erythrocyte fragments).[44] In adults, hemoglobin levels are less than 10 mg/dL in 99% of the cases and less than 6.5 mg/dL in 40%.[45] Reticulocyte counts are uniformly elevated. Other indicators of intravascular hemolysis include elevated lactate dehydrogenase (LDH), increased indirect bilirubin, and low haptoglobin level.[17] The Coombs test is negative, indicating that the anemia is not immunologically mediated. Moderate leukocytosis may accompany the hemolytic anemia, but white cell counts rarely exceed 20,000/mm³.[10] Thrombocytopenia is uniformly present in HUS/TTP, and the platelet counts are usually less than 60,000/mm³.[12, 13, 15] The presence of giant platelets in the peripheral smear and reduced platelet survival time are consistent with peripheral consumption or destruction of platelets, or both.[46] In children, the duration of thrombocytopenia is variable and does not correlate with the course of renal disease.[47] Bone marrow biopsy specimens usually show erythroid hyperplasia and an increased number of megakaryocytes. Prothrombin time (PT), partial thromboplastin time (PTT), fibrinogen level, and coagulation factors are normal, thus differentiating HUS/TTP from disseminated intravascular coagulation (DIC).[17, 48] Mild fibrinolysis with minimal elevation in fibrin degradation products, however, may be observed. Complement levels are decreased in some patients.[49] Diagnostic central nervous system studies in HUS/TTP have not been extensively evaluated. Punctate lesions in the white matter were detected by magnetic resonance imaging (MRI), but not by computed tomography (CT), in two patients with classic TTP presentation.[50, 51]

Renal Involvement

Evidence of renal involvement is present in the majority of patients with HUS/TTP.[1, 15, 18, 22] Microscopic hematuria and subnephrotic proteinuria are the most consistent findings. Male sex, hypertension, prolonged anuria, and hemoglobin levels greater than 10 g/L at onset are associated with a higher risk of renal sequelae in children.[52] In a retrospective study of 216 patients with a clinical picture of TTP, hematuria was detected in 78% and proteinuria in 75% of the patients.[18] Sterile pyuria and casts were present in 31% and 24% of the patients, respectively.[18] Gross hematuria is rare.[18] More than 90% of patients with HUS presentation have significant renal failure, one third of whom are anuric.[22] Dialysis is required in a large percentage of these patients.[53] The mean duration of renal failure is 2 weeks.[22] Severe ARF or anuria occurs in fewer than 10% of cases of classic TTP.[10] The degree of elevation of blood urea nitrogen (BUN) on presentation may be a prognostic indicator in patients with HUS/TTP.[18]

Pathology

The characteristic lesion in HUS/TTP is thrombotic microangiopathy.[4, 54] Microthrombi have been demonstrated in arterioles and capillaries of the kidney, brain, skin, pancreas, heart, spleen, and adrenals.[17] In TTP, microthrombi are composed predominantly of platelet aggregates and a thin layer of fibrin.[17, 55] The platelet thrombi stain strongly for VWF,[56] which has been implicated in the pathogenesis of TTP (see later discussion). In contrast, immunohistochemical studies on microthrombi in HUS showed prominent fibrin.[17, 43] Subendothelial hyaline deposits and endothelial cell swelling also contribute to the occlusion of the lumens of arterioles and capillaries.[17, 56] Venules rarely are affected, and vasculitis usually is absent.[17]

Three patterns of renal lesions have been described in HUS/TTP: glomerular, arterial, and a combination of both.[57] In younger children, the pathology is confined mainly to the glomeruli. On light microscopy, it is characterized by thickening of capillary walls, endothelial cell swelling, and narrowing or obliteration of capillary lumens. Widening of the subendothelial space may result in a double contour or double-track appearance of the glomerular capillary walls. Clumps of red blood cells, platelets, or thrombi may be seen in the glomerular capillaries. Widening of the mesangium may be present without evidence of mesangial cell proliferation.[58]

Arterial involvement in children with HUS usually is minimal. In older children and in adults, significant arterial changes coexist with glomerular lesions.[57, 59] Thrombi are present in the interlobular arteries, which also demonstrate intimal edema and myointimal cell proliferation.[59] This process may result in arterial fibroplasia.

The glomerular lesions in these patients are ischemic in origin.[57] The glomerular capillary walls are wrinkled, the glomerular tuft may be atrophied, and the Bowman capsule is thickened. In some patients, the glomerular changes described in younger children coexist with the pattern of arterial injury.[60] Acute cortical or tubular necrosis may occur in patients with HUS/TTP.[57]

Immunofluorescence studies performed on renal biopsy specimens of patients with HUS/TTP invariably demonstrate fibrinogen along the glomerular capillary walls and in the arterial thrombi.[61] Granular deposits of C3 and immunoglobulin M (IgM) may be observed in the vessel walls and in glomeruli.[62] Electron microscopic studies demonstrate swelling of the glomerular endothelial cells and detachment from the glomerular basement membrane.[38]

Electron-lucent, "fluffy" material fills the space between the glomerular basement membrane and the detached endothelium. The basement membrane itself remains intact. Similar findings are present in arteries and arterioles.[63]

Etiology

Epidemiologic and laboratory data suggest that bacterial cytotoxins may be causative agents in HUS/TTP.[64, 65] Outbreaks of hemorrhagic colitis in children have led to the isolation of a new *E. coli* strain (serotype O157:H7) that produces shiga-like cytotoxins.[66, 67] Because of the cytotoxic activity of these toxins on Vero cells, they are referred to as verotoxins.[67, 68] Currently, four main toxins have been isolated from verotoxin-producing *E. coli*. These are referred to as shiga-like toxins (SLT-I, SLT-II, SLT-IIc, and SLT-IIe) or verotoxins (VT-1, VT-2, VT-2c, and VT-2e).[65, 69] Strong epidemiologic evidence links cytotoxin-producing *E. coli*, serotype O157:H7 in particular, to sporadic cases and outbreaks of HUS[41, 68, 70, 71] and TTP.[72, 73]

Transmission of *E. coli* O157:H7 appears to be caused by contaminated food, such as ground beef and other cattle products.[74] Contaminated lamb, fish, poultry, pork, and unpasteurized milk may also be involved.[26, 75]

Moreover, person-to-person contact and municipal water supplies are reported as sources of contamination.[26, 75]

Gastrointestinal symptoms were shown to be clinically present after exposure to fewer than 70 viable *E. coli* O157:H7 bacteria.[76] In an epidemic of diarrhea caused by cytotoxin-producing *E. coli* O157:H7, 4 of 37 patients (ages 1 to 78 years) developed HUS, and 4 others developed TTP.[72, 73, 77] In HUS outbreaks, 75% of patients show greater than fourfold increases in verotoxin-neutralizing antibodies.[41, 69] Less commonly, HUS/TTP is associated with gastrointestinal and respiratory infections caused by other cytotoxin-producing bacteria, such as *Shigella dysenteriae* type I,[78] *Salmonella typhi*,[79] *Campylobacter jejuni*,[80] and *Streptococcus pneumoniae*.[81] HUS/TTP accompanying viral infections has also been described.[82-85] Furthermore, TTP syndrome has been reported in association with the acquired immunodeficiency syndrome (AIDS).[86, 87]

Drug-induced HUS/TTP is well recognized.[17] It was most commonly diagnosed in patients receiving chemotherapeutic agents,[88, 89] the majority of whom were treated with mitomycin C.[90] HUS occurred in 5% to 15% of patients who had received a cumulative dose of 20 to 30 mg/m^2 or greater. The onset of hemolytic anemia and renal failure is usually sudden, and the mortality rate is high despite supportive therapy.[90] Treatment with plasma exchange, however, was successful in some cases.[91] HUS/TTP has also been reported after chemotherapy with other agents (Table 33-1). Thrombotic microangiopathy, unrelated to chemotherapy, has been described in conjunction with vascular tumors, acute promyelocytic leukemia, and prostatic, gastric, and pancreatic carcinomas.[92] Sporadic cases of HUS/TTP have been reported in bone marrow and solid organ transplantation patients who received immunosuppressive treatment with either cyclosporine[93-97] or FK-506.[98, 99] Ticlopidine, an antiplatelet agent, was associated with the development of TTP with an estimated incidence of 1 case per 1600 to 9000 patients treated.[100] Clopidogrel, a new antiplatelet drug that has achieved widespread clinical acceptance because it has a more favorable safety profile than ticlopidine, has also been associated with the disease, and 11 cases were reported recently.[101] In renal allograft recipients, cyclosporine-induced HUS occurs during the first week after transplantation, and renal failure reverses with the cessation of cyclosporine.[102, 103] HUS/TTP may occur after bone marrow transplantation independent of prior radiation or cyclosporine therapy.[104] Tacrolimus (FK-506)-induced HUS/TTP is reported in 1% to 4.7% of treated patients, and it is more frequently diagnosed during the first year after transplantation.[105] Other drugs[106-110] and toxins[111-114] less commonly associated with HUS/TTP are listed in Table 33-1.

The association between HUS/TTP and pregnancy is also well recognized.[115] Neurologic involvement predominates in the prepartum form, whereas severe renal failure is more typical in postpartum HUS/TTP.[116]

The fetal mortality rate from pregnancy-associated TTP approaches 80%, but successful plasma exchange treatment that permits near-term delivery has been reported.[117, 118] Like pre-eclampsia, pregnancy-associated TTP usually resolves with delivery.[115] It is possible that these two syndromes are a continuum of the microvascular abnormalities that occur during gestation. They differ, however, in that consumptive coagulopathy is present in severe pre-eclampsia but is characteristically absent in HUS/TTP.[119, 120] The etiologic agents in pregnancy-associated HUS/TTP are not established. The absence of thrombocytopenia or other manifestations of

TABLE 33-1

Hemolytic-Uremic Syndrome/Thrombotic Thrombocytopenic Purpura: Causes and Associations

Infectious agents
  Bacteria
    Escherichia coli O157:H7 (verotoxin-producing)[68-74]
    Shigella dysenteriae type I[77]
    Salmonella typhi[78]
    Streptococcus pneumoniae[81]
    Campylobacter jejuni[79]
    Yersinia pseudotuberculosis[81]
    Pseudomonas species
    Bacteroides[80]
    Mycobacterium tuberculosis
  Viruses
    Togavirus (rubella)[84]
    Coxsackievirus[82]
    Echoviruses[83]
    Influenza virus[82]
    Epstein-Barr virus[85]
    Rotaviruses[82]
    Cytomegalovirus
    Human immunodeficiency virus[86, 87]
Drugs
  Immunosuppressants
    Cyclosporine[93-97]
    FK-506[98, 99, 105]
    OKT3
  Chemotherapeutics
    Mitomycin C[91]
    Cisplatin[89, 90]
    Daunorubicin[89]
    Cytosine arabinoside[89]
    Methyl CCNU[89]
    Chlorozotocin[89]
    Zinostatin[89]
    Deoxycoformycin[89]
  Others
    Oral contraceptives
    Quinine[107]
    Penicillin[108]
    Penicillamine[109]
    Metronidazole[110]
    Ticlopidine[100]
    Clopidogrel[101]
Toxins
  Carbon monoxide[111]
    Bee sting[112]
    Arsenic[113]
    Iodine[114]
Pregnancy[115-120]
  Prepartum
  Postpartum
Disorders
  Malignant neoplasm[92]
  Transplantation[104]
  Systemic lupus erythematosus
  Polyarteritis nodosa
  Primary glomerulopathies

HUS/TTP in surviving infants excludes the possibility of an etiologic agent that crosses the placenta.[115]

Several case reports have suggested a genetic predisposition for pregnancy-associated HUS/TTP.[121-123]

A hereditary form of recurrent HUS/TTP has also been described in children and adults.[20, 124] Sheth and co-workers[125] described an increased incidence of human leukocyte antigen (HLA)-B40 group antigens in children with HUS/TTP.

Several investigators have reported a genetic deficiency of factor H, a regulatory protein of the alternative complement pathway, leading to low levels of complement C3 in patients with familial or recurrent HUS.[125-127]

Other diseases associated with HUS/TTP, such as primary glomerular and autoimmune disorders, are listed in Table 33-1.

In 1984, Boccia and co-workers[128] reported a case of HUS in a patient with AIDS. Since then, more than 40 cases of human immunodeficiency virus (HIV)–related HUS/TTP have been reported in patients with known HIV infection or AIDS. The predominant presenting features are those of TTP, although some patients presented with HUS. More recently, HUS has been reported as the initial presentation of HIV infection.[129]

Although the etiologic mechanisms in HUS/TTP are not completely defined, the available data suggest that environmental factors (infection, drugs, toxins), combined with genetic predisposition in some patients, are responsible for initiation of thrombotic microangiopathy. The link between bacterial toxins and HUS offers the strongest etiologic evidence.[64, 65]

Pathogenesis

Experimental data strongly suggest that endothelial cell injury is the primary event in the pathogenesis of HUS/TTP.[3, 38, 130] Endothelial damage triggers a cascade of events that includes local intravascular coagulation, fibrin deposition, and platelet activation and aggregation. The end result is the histopathologic finding of thrombotic microangiopathy common to the different forms of the HUS/TTP syndrome. This section describes the various mediators and events involved in the pathogenesis of HUS/TTP.

Endothelial Injury

Many of the infectious agents and drugs implicated in the etiology of HUS/TTP are toxic to the vascular endothelium. The shiga-like toxins, which include the verocytotoxins produced by *E. coli* O157:H7, inhibit eukaryotic protein synthesis and directly damage human vascular endothelial cells.[131, 132] The glycolipid receptor for verotoxins is present on the membranes of endothelial cells[127] and has been shown to be more prevalent in the renal cortex than in the medulla.[133] Although measurement of circulating shiga-like toxins in humans after intestinal infection has not been reported, it is plausible that small amounts may enter the bloodstream.[130] The extreme potency of these toxins in inhibiting protein synthesis (50% inhibitory concentration [IC_{50}] in the picomolar range)[131] supports the concept that even minute amounts of toxin entering the circulation could initiate endothelial cell injury in HUS/TTP. Injection of purified VT-1 (SLT-I) in rabbits showed specific binding of the toxin to endothelial cells, as well as histopathologic findings of thrombotic microangiopathy.[134] VT-1 has been shown to mediate leukocyte adhesion by up-regulating adhesive proteins on the endothelial surface membrane.[135] Te Loo and co-workers[136] recently showed that, during in vitro co-cultures, polymorphonuclear leukocytes (PMNs) loaded with shiga toxin (sTx) transferred the ligands to the higher-affinity receptors on the glomerular endothelial cells which promote cell death. Should this occur in vivo, it would explain the rapid clearance of sTx from the circulation and its release to target organs, where the toxin exerts its cytopathic effect.[137]

Bacterial and viral neuraminidases have indirect toxic effects on endothelial cells.[2, 130] *S. pneumoniae*–derived neuraminidase removes sialic acid from the membranes of erythrocytes, platelets, and glomerular capillary endothelial cells, thus exposing a cryptic antigen known as Thomsen-Friedenreich antigen. It is postulated that exposure of this antigen leads to the formation of IgM antibodies, which in turn could cause platelet aggregation and possibly endothelial damage.[138-140]

Complement-fixing antibodies to endothelial antigens have been detected in the plasma of HUS/TTP patients but not in normal subjects, further suggesting a role for immunologic mechanisms in endothelial injury.[141, 142] Anti-endothelial antibodies are also present in patients with various autoimmune diseases, which could explain the occurrence of HUS/TTP in patients with systemic lupus erythematosus and polyarteritis nodosa.[142] One study suggested that plasma from patients with idiopathic or HIV-associated TTP induces the apoptosis of cultured microvascular endothelial cells.[143] Endothelial cells from larger vessels were resistant to apoptosis induced by plasma from these patients. The mechanism of apoptosis was independent of secretion of tumor necrosis factor-α (TNF-α) but appeared to be linked to induction of Fas molecules. In fact, the addition of anti-Fas antibody has been shown to suppress TTP plasma-mediated microvascular endothelial cell apoptosis.[142]

Drugs associated with HUS/TTP have also been shown to cause endothelial damage. These include mitomycin[144] and cyclosporine.[145] Cancer or chemotherapy-induced endothelial lesions in the kidney could result from the generation of small, soluble circulating immune complexes (CIC) and autoantibodies that damage endothelial cells directly and trigger aggregation and deposition of platelets around the lesions.[146]

Local Thrombosis and Fibrin Deposition

Microthrombi and fibrin deposits are characteristically found in the glomerular capillaries of patients with HUS/TTP.[17, 57] Fibrinolytic mechanisms in the glomerulus mediated by tissue plasminogen activator (tPA) and urokinase may play a role in the removal of such deposits.[147]

Bergstein and associates[148] demonstrated the presence of an inhibitor of glomerular fibrinolysis (plasminogen-activator inhibitor 1 [PAI-1]) in plasma from 17 children with HUS. More recently, these investigators demonstrated that increased circulating levels of PAI-1 correlate with poor outcome in HUS.[149] Moreover, removal of PAI-1 by peritoneal dialysis correlated with improvement in renal function.[151]

Chandler and co-workers[150] showed that, in HUS induced by *E. coli* O157:H7, thrombin generation and inhibition of fibrinolysis precede renal injury and may be the cause of such injury. Increased plasma levels of tPA inhibitors have also been measured in patients with TTP.[151] The sources of inhibitors of fibrinolysis are the platelets and the endothelial cells.[152] Primary endothelial injury could also cause decreased production of physiologic anticoagulants, such as thrombomodulin, and lead to thrombosis at the site of injury.[153]

Von Willebrand Factor, Prostacyclin, and Platelet Aggregation

Platelet aggregates are a major constituent of microthrombi found in HUS/TTP.[17] Controversy exists as to whether platelet aggregation is a consequence of endothelial damage or a primary platelet abnormality.[154] Because higher-molecular-weight polymers of VWF support platelet adhesion to the subendothelium and promote platelet aggregation, VWF was suspected of playing a pathogenetic role in HUS/TTP.[155, 156] Patients with relapsing TTP have very large circulating polymers of VWF during remissions, but not during relapses.[157] A specific protease responsible for cleavage of VWF multimers was isolated from normal human plasma and was originally found to be deficient in patients with chronic relapsing TTP.[158] These findings suggested that acquired as well as constitutional deficiency of the VWF-cleaving protease may predispose to TTP.

More recently, Furlan and colleagues[159] and Tsai and Lia[160] independently showed that plasma from patients with acute TTP had deficiency in VWF-cleaving protease activity that returned to normal on recovery. Moreover, the plasma of these patients contained inhibitors of VWF-cleaving protease activity that were found to be IgG autoantibodies probably directed against components of the enzyme.[159, 160] The VWF-cleaving protease deficiency and the presence of circulating autoantibodies were also reported in patients who developed TTP after treatment with the antiplatelet drugs ticlopidine or clopidogrel.[100, 101] It is postulated, therefore, that inefficient clearance of VWF polymers leads to microvascular thrombosis. The polymers are consumed during TTP relapse, so their levels decrease. In HUS patients, VWF antigens are elevated and the largest polymers are decreased during acute illness.[161] This pattern returns to normal with clinical improvement, but it persists in patients with progressive renal disease.[162] No abnormalities in VWF-cleaving protease have been found in children with diarrhea-induced HUS.[159, 163] Moreover, a decrease in VWF size was accompanied by an increase in VWF proteolytic fragments, presumably caused by enhanced proteolysis from abnormal shear stress in the microcirculation.[163] A platelet-aggregating factor (PAF p00) has been detected in the plasma of HUS[164] and TTP[165] patients, but its pathogenetic role is not clear. Circulating antibodies to the Thomsen-Friedenreich antigen 1[138-140] or cancer- and chemotherapy-related immune complexes[146] could also enhance platelet aggregation in HUS/TTP. Recently, it was shown that sTx, through its binding subunits, can directly interact with platelets, leading to aggregation and binding to endothelium.[166]

The discovery that endothelial cells produce a potent inhibitor of platelet aggregation, prostacyclin (PGI$_2$), led to the investigation of its role in HUS/TTP.[2, 38] Several groups have demonstrated decreased endothelial production of prostacyclin in HUS and TTP patients.[167, 168] The presence of a circulating inhibitor of endothelial cell production of PGI$_2$ was reported in patients with HUS.[169] Interestingly, patients with pre-eclampsia do not have the increase in PGI$_2$ observed in normal pregnancies, suggesting that this could contribute to the thrombocytopenia and microangiopathic hemolytic anemia of severe pre-eclampsia.[170, 171] It is not clear, however, whether reduced prostacyclin production is a primary pathogenetic event in HUS/TTP or an epiphenomenon of microangiopathic hemolysis. Moreover, clinical trials of PGI$_2$ infusion in HUS/TTP patients gave equivocal results (see later discussion).[172]

Cytokines

Bacterial lipopolysaccharides activate neutrophils, leading to endothelial cell injury by release of TNF-α, interleukin-1 (IL-1), elastase, and free radicals.[173, 174] Because IL-1 and TNF-α mediate endothelial injury in septic shock,[175] their role in HUS/TTP has been examined.

Kaplan and co-workers[130] demonstrated that IL-1 and TNF-α synergize with the cytotoxic action of shiga toxin on umbilical vein endothelial cells. Furthermore, IL-1, TNF-α, and lipopolysaccharide up-regulate the receptors for verocytotoxin on the surface of endothelial cells by approximately 100-fold.[176] Increased plasma levels of IL-1b and TNF-α were demonstrated in 13 patients with acute TTP and were found to decrease as the patients went into remission.[177] Increased levels of soluble IL-2 receptor and of IL-6 correlated with poorer prognosis in these patients. The data suggest that monocyte-derived cytokines (IL-1, IL-6, and TNF-α) may contribute to the pathogenesis of HUS/TTP. Several studies indicate that IL-6 levels are elevated in patients with extrarenal manifestations of HUS.[178, 179] Moreover, increased formation of nitric oxide has been observed in patients with acute HUS/TTP.[180]

Fitzpatrick and associates[174] demonstrated increased levels of IL-8, a chemokine that attracts and activates neutrophils, in children with HUS. IL-8 was not detected in the 17 normal children, but was significantly elevated in 20 of 25 children with diarrhea-associated HUS and in 3 of 9 with non–diarrhea-associated HUS. IL-8 levels correlated with PMN counts and with circulating α_1-antitrypsin–complexed elastase, a marker of neutrophil degranulation. The highest values of IL-8 were seen in children who died in the acute phase of the disease. Antineutrophil cytoplasmic antibody (ANCA) was not detected in any of the patients, and TNF-α was increased in only one patient. Direct evidence of the role of these cytokines in the pathogenesis of HUS/TTP remains to be determined.

Prognosis and Treatment

If HUS/TTP is left untreated, the mortality rate approaches 90%.[10] A study of the outcome of 678 patients with HUS by Gianantonio and colleagues[22] showed a trend toward better survival between the late 1950s and 1972. The mortality rate in children dropped from approximately 47% to 6.25%. A more recent analysis of 108 HUS/TTP patients (ages 16 to 77 years) treated between 1979 and 1990 revealed a 9% mortality rate.[11] Survival has significantly increased because of improved management of HUS/TTP complications and because of the treatment modalities used (see later discussion).

Several prognostic factors have been postulated to predict the outcome in patients with HUS/TTP. Younger children who present during the summer with the "typical" diarrheal prodrome have a better prognosis than older children with HUS that occurs in the colder months of the year and is not heralded by diarrhea.[181] A high blood PMN count at the time of onset of the disease in children is associated with a higher probability of a poor outcome.[182, 183] A retrospective, 10-year

follow-up study of 73 children with HUS demonstrated that severe renal involvement, determined by duration of oliguria or anuria, is associated with a higher incidence of long-term complications such as hypertension, reduced renal function, and proteinuria.[184] Adults presenting with HUS tend to have a poorer prognosis than do children. In a study of 43 adults with HUS, the overall mortality rate was 14%, and approximately 70% of the patients required hemodialysis.[185] The same study suggested that HUS occurring secondary to an underlying disease, such as scleroderma or cancer, carries a poorer prognosis. The degree of renal dysfunction and the severity of vascular lesions in renal biopsy specimens are also indicators of poor outcome in HUS/TTP.[18, 60]

Supportive therapy—including dialysis, antihypertensive medications, blood transfusions, and management of neurologic complications—contributes to the improved survival of patients with HUS/TTP.[2, 11] Adequate fluid balance and bowel rest are important in treating typical HUS associated with diarrhea.

Antibiotics given to treat infection caused by sTx-producing *E. coli* O157:H7 have been found to increase the risk of overt HUS by 17-fold,[186] probably by favoring the acute release of large amounts of preformed toxin after the injury to the bacterial cell membrane, or by giving a selective advantage to *E. coli* O157:H7 if these organisms are not as readily eliminated from the bowels as other normal intestinal flora are.[105] Moreover, several antimicrobial drugs, particularly the quinolones, trimethoprim, and furazolidone, are potent inducers of the expression of the sTx gene and may increase the level of toxin in the intestine.[187] On the other hand, in developing countries where hemorrhagic colitis is precipitated by *E. coli* strains other than O157:H7 or more commonly by *S. dysenteriae* type I,[188] early and empiric antibiotic therapy has been shown to shorten the duration of diarrhea and decrease the incidence of complications and therefore should be started early, even before the involved pathogen is identified.[188]

New agents targeted to prevent organ exposure to sTx are currently under evaluation.[105] Preliminary analysis of an ongoing trial in Canada found that early treatment (within 2 days after the onset of diarrhea) with Synsorb-pk, a resin that binds sTx, decreased the risk of HUS from 17% to 7%.[189] Platelet transfusions are avoided because of the risk of precipitous worsening of the patient's clinical status.[9, 11, 190, 191] It is postulated that transfused platelets, in combination with high circulating levels of von Willebrand multimers, induce further organ damage.[11]

Among the therapeutic modalities used to treat patients with HUS/TTP, plasma exchange (plasmapheresis combined with fresh-frozen plasma replacement) is currently the treatment of choice. Significant benefit from plasma exchange was observed in 1977 in adults with acute TTP.[192] Several reports have since confirmed the efficacy of this treatment modality in both children[193, 194] and adults[195-197] with HUS/TTP. Response rates vary between 60% and 80%.[197] Although significant benefit has also been observed with plasma infusion alone,[198-200] one randomized prospective trial demonstrated that plasma exchange is more effective than plasma infusion for the treatment of TTP.[197] After a 6-month follow-up period, patients treated with plasma exchange had a 78% response rate and a 22% mortality rate, compared with 49% and 37%, respectively, among patients receiving plasma infusions only. Plasmapheresis could have the advantage of removing the recently identified inhibitory autoantibodies against VWF protease from the circulation and supplying larger amounts of the protease enzyme.[160] No unanimous protocol has been established regarding the frequency and duration of plasma exchange. Usually plasma exchange is performed once a day and replaces one plasma volume (40 mL/kg).[201] For patients with poor initial response to treatment, plasma exchange may be intensified by increasing the volume of plasma replaced or, preferably, by initiating twice-daily exchange to minimize recycling of infused plasma.[201] A theoretical benefit for cryosupernatant over plasma was suggested because it is depleted of large VWF multimers, and a retrospective survey suggested greater efficacy.[202] However, findings from a small randomized trial suggested equivalent outcomes with both products.[203]

Plasma exchange should be performed daily until remission is achieved, remission being normalization of platelet count, or resolution of neurologic symptoms, or both.[200] Hemoglobin level, percent schistocytosis, reticulocyte count, and renal indices do not appear to be determinants of initial response to therapy, because they may be abnormal for an undefined period after remission.[196] (Continuation of plasma exchange for several sessions after remission has been advocated to prevent relapses.[11, 196]) TTP relapses occur between 1 and 140 months (median, 20 months) after the initial episode in as many as 40% of the patients.[204] Because 85% of children with HUS recover with supportive therapy alone, plasma exchange is generally reserved for patients with poor prognostic indicators.[1, 205]

When administered alone, corticosteroids induce remission in fewer than 30% of patients with TTP.[11] Inconclusive data suggest that corticosteroids used in combination with plasma therapy decrease relapse rates and may improve survival in some patients.[9, 11] Other immunosuppressive agents have been used to treat TTP, either alone or in combination with plasma therapy. These include vincristine,[206, 207] azathioprine,[208] and cyclophosphamide.[209] Recently, the presence in the circulation of autoantibodies against VWF-cleaving protease has been claimed to help identify patients who may benefit from such therapy.[159]

Although platelet thrombi are invariably present in the thrombotic angiopathies, therapy with aspirin and dipyridamole has proved ineffective.[11, 210] Antiplatelet agents, however, may induce a more rapid recovery of the platelet count.[2, 211] Some investigators recommend their use in combination with plasma exchange, based on inconclusive evidence that the relapse rate is lower in patients receiving antiplatelet agents.[197, 204, 211] Increased incidence of bleeding complications should, however, be kept in mind.[197] Fibrinolytic therapy with either streptokinase or urokinase is ineffective and increases the risk of bleeding.[212, 213] Prospective studies of heparin treatment in HUS/TTP patients also failed to demonstrate any benefit.[214]

Intravenous immunoglobulins as a means of neutralizing the platelet aggregation factor or factors have been tried in TTP patients.[215-217] Controlled studies, however, are required to establish whether benefits from this treatment outweigh its disadvantages (anaphylaxis and infections).[218]

Splenectomy performed on patients with TTP to reduce platelet consumption can be associated with fatal complications.[11] In the absence of solid evidence that splenectomy is beneficial, its use is not recommended for the treatment of HUS/TTP.[11, 44] Experimental evidence indicating reduced bioavailability of prostacyclin in thrombotic microangiopathies suggested the use of PGI_2 infusions. Data on patient outcomes are contradictory, however.[2] Reports of dramatic remission in intractable TTP are available,[219, 220] but PGI_2 infusions have proved ineffective in other patients.[221] Moreover, the hypotensive effects of PGI_2 limit its usefulness.[2]

Based on the findings of decreased serum levels of vitamin E and the reduced antioxidant potential of erythrocytes, oral vitamin E supplements have been administered to children with HUS. In a series of 16 patients treated with vitamin E, 100% survival and complete recovery of renal function were attained despite the presence of poor prognostic features.[222] However, a controlled trial is needed to confirm this observation.

Patients with refractory HUS/TTP who do not respond to plasma exchange therapy may benefit from therapy with vincristine[223-225] or cyclosporine, which may induce an immediate and sustained response.[226]

Cancer- and/or chemotherapy-induced HUS/TTP carries a poor prognosis despite treatment. Snyder and co-workers[146] reported improved survival in this group of patients using extracorporeal immunoadsorption with protein A columns to remove circulating immune complexes. Patients whose malignant neoplasms were in complete or partial remission at the time of development of HUS/TTP had a significantly higher estimated 1-year survival rate (74%), compared with a historical control group of patients receiving other treatments (22%).

Treatment of Renal Failure in HUS/TTP

Severe renal insufficiency resulting from HUS/TTP often requires dialysis. Renal transplantation has also been performed. Regardless of the etiologic agent, HUS/TTP may recur in the renal allograft independent of cyclosporine use.[227, 228] The risk of recurrence of HUS after renal transplantation in one study was as high as 16.6%,[229] and higher recurrence rates have been reported for familial HUS.[230] Kaplan and colleagues[230] reported that six of seven patients with familial HUS had recurrence after renal transplantation. Similarly, the risk of cyclosporine-induced HUS is not a deterrent to the use of this essential immunosuppressive agent.[2]

SYSTEMIC SCLEROSIS

Clinical Features

Systemic sclerosis is a rare disease, with a reported incidence of 2 and 19 new cases per 1 million population in the United States.[231, 232] It characteristically affects women between the ages of 30 and 50 years.[233] The overall incidence in females is three times that in males, and the female-to-male ratio increases to 15:1 during the child-bearing years.[234] Children and younger men rarely are affected.[234] Although there is no overall racial predilection, young black women have a 10-fold higher incidence of systemic sclerosis than do young white women.[234]

Involvement of the skin and subcutaneous tissue is the predominant feature of systemic sclerosis.[235] This explains the use of the traditional term "scleroderma" to describe the disease.[236] In the diffuse cutaneous, or classic, form of the disease, thickening of the skin is observed on the face, trunk, and distal and proximal extremities. This phase is followed by sclerosis, which leads to a taut, shiny appearance of the skin and tapering of the fingertips (sclerodactyly). Rapid progression of the cutaneous induration with extension into the underlying tendon sheaths and joints is a harbinger of visceral involvement.[237] Among other extrarenal manifestations of systemic sclerosis,[235, 236, 238] Raynaud phenomenon[239] is the most prevalent (93% to 97% of patients) and is usually the first symptom in patients with limited cutaneous disease. Telangiectasias on the skin of the face and upper torso are commonly present in patients with either diffuse or limited cutaneous sclerosis. Arthralgias or arthritis occurs in most of the patients. Myopathy presenting as muscle atrophy and fibrosis occurs in approximately 20% of these patients and usually involves the shoulder and pelvic girdle muscles.[240] Esophageal hypomotility or diminished tone of the lower esophageal sphincter (or both) is present in 75% of systemic sclerosis cases.[235] Diffuse pulmonary fibrosis occurs in 45% of the patients, causing restrictive lung disease. Myocardial fibroses in systemic sclerosis manifest as conduction disturbances and, occasionally, refractory congestive heart failure.[241, 242]

Laboratory Findings

The most common serologic abnormality in systemic sclerosis is a positive antinuclear antibody titer (ANA ≥ 1:16), which occurs in 70% of the patients.[235, 243, 244] The specificity of the ANA test is increased if the immunofluorescence pattern is speckled or nucleolar. Although antibodies to DNA topoisomerase I (anti-Scl-70)[245] are more specific, they are found in only 30% of patients with diffuse cutaneous involvement and in only 15% of those with the limited form. Anticentromere antibodies[245] are present in half of the patients, most of whom have limited systemic sclerosis. Approximately 30% of the patients have positive tests for rheumatoid factor.[235] Antibodies to double-stranded DNA are rarely noted.[235]

Renal Involvement

Kidney involvement in systemic sclerosis manifests as a slowly progressing chronic renal disease or as scleroderma renal crisis (SRC), which is characterized by malignant hypertension and acute azotemia.[238] The two presentations are not mutually exclusive. Based on autopsy studies, the incidence of renal disease in systemic sclerosis approaches 80%.[246] Clinical indicators of chronic renal involvement in systemic sclerosis include proteinuria, hypertension, and decreased glomerular filtration rate (GFR). The proteinuria is usually subnephrotic and occurs in 15% to 36% of the patients.[233, 247] Hypertension is present in 24%, and elevated BUN in 19%.[247] Estimates of the incidence of chronic renal disease in systemic sclerosis vary, depending on which markers of disease are employed.[238] Renal manifestations rarely antedate the other features of systemic sclerosis.

SRC is defined by the sudden onset of accelerated or malignant arterial hypertension, followed by rapidly progressive oliguric renal failure.[238, 248] The reported incidence of SRC varies between 5% and 15%.[249-251] It occurs most commonly during the first 5 years after diagnosis, but in 5% to 10% of cases there is no prior history of systemic sclerosis.[237] Patients with the diffuse cutaneous form are at much higher risk for development of SRC than are those with limited cutaneous systemic sclerosis. The symptomatology is predominantly that of accelerated/malignant hypertension.[238, 248] Presenting complaints include severe headaches, blurring of vision, encephalopathy, convulsions, and acute left ventricular failure. Grade III or IV retinopathy is present in most of the cases. Oliguria and a rapidly rising serum creatinine concentration follow shortly thereafter.[238, 248] Proteinuria is universal but is rarely nephrotic. The urinalysis reveals microscopic hematuria and granular casts. Plasma renin activity is markedly elevated during SRC, but it is unclear whether this is a primary phenomenon or a result of renal ischemia.[247, 248] SRC progresses rapidly to severe renal failure that requires dialysis. Before the advent of angiotensin-converting enzyme (ACE) inhibitors, the majority of patients died from hypertensive complications within 1 to 3 months.[247, 248, 250, 251] Renal function may recover spontaneously even after 18 months of dialysis.[252] Other clinical manifestations of SRC include microangiopathic hemolytic anemia with thrombocytopenia,[253] which also occurs in association with other forms of malignant hypertension.[254] HUS was reported in a patient with mixed connective tissue disease who had combined features of systemic sclerosis and systemic lupus erythematosus.[255]

No reliable predictors of the advent of SRC exist. The prior presence of proteinuria, renal insufficiency, or hypertension in a patient with diffuse systemic sclerosis does not necessarily portend progression to SRC.[237] A rise in plasma renin activity does not seem to herald the onset of SRC, either.[237, 248] A higher frequency of SRC and hypertension has been noted among blacks with systemic sclerosis.[248] It is not clear, however, whether this observation is simply a reflection of the overall increased incidence of essential and malignant hypertension in the black population.

Pathology

Autopsy studies demonstrate renal histopathologic changes in the majority of patients with systemic sclerosis in whom SRC has not developed.[256] Subintimal proliferation and luminal narrowing of small and medium-sized arteries in the kidney is the most prominent finding. The arterial changes coexist with varying degrees of tubule atrophy, interstitial fibrosis, and glomerular obsolescence. These histopathologic findings have been described in patients with systemic sclerosis even before the onset of hypertension.[247]

Arterial changes also characterize the SRC kidney.[246, 247] Microscopically, small and medium-sized arteries (interlobular and arcuate arteries in the renal cortex) show intimal edema and intimal cell proliferation. Accumulation of mucoid substance, composed of glycoproteins and mucopolysaccharides, may separate the endothelium from the internal elastic lamina. Myointimal cells, absent from normal arteries, possibly participate in the intimal thickening seen in systemic sclerosis. The common end point of these vascular changes is luminal narrowing and subsequent tissue ischemia (Fig. 33-1). The presence of adventitial and periadventitial fibrosis differentiates the renovascular lesions of systemic sclerosis from those of other forms of malignant

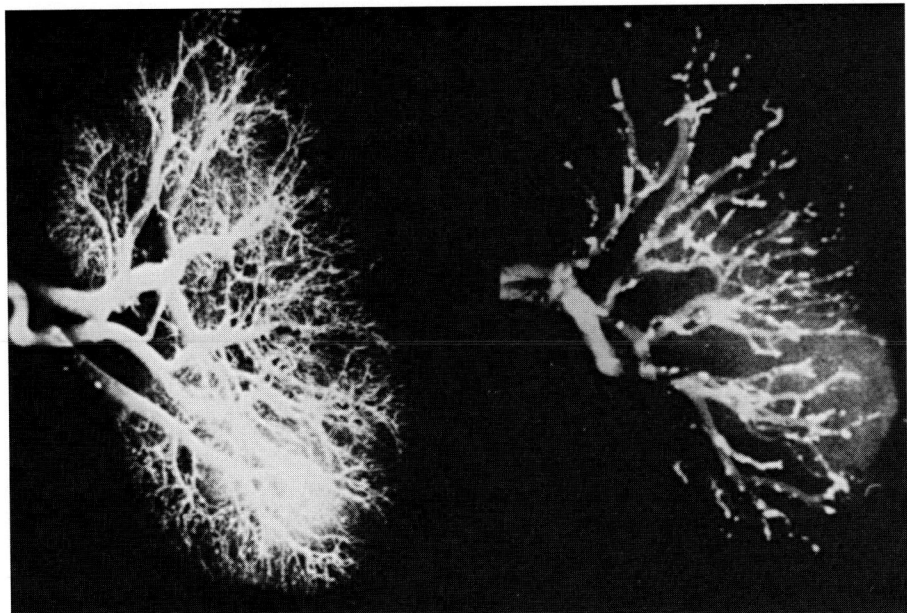

FIGURE 33-1. Latex injection of postmortem normal kidney *(left)* and kidney from a patient with scleroderma renal crisis *(right)*. Note obstruction to flow at the level of the medium-sized interlobular arteries.

hypertension.[246, 257] The typical lesion in smaller renal arteries and afferent arterioles in systemic sclerosis is fibrinoid necrosis.[258] Interestingly, these changes can be seen in patients who do not have hypertension or SRC.[246, 257] Lymphocytes and inflammatory cells are typically absent from the vascular lesions.

Glomerular pathology in SRC is probably ischemic in origin and consists of basement membrane thickening, obliteration of the capillary loops, and glomerulosclerosis.[256, 258] Hyperplasia of the juxtaglomerular apparatus has been observed but is not specific for SRC.[259] Tubule epithelial degeneration and scattered interstitial fibrosis are also present. Immunofluorescence findings are generally nonspecific and may reveal IgM, complement, and fibrin deposits in small renal arteries.[260] In a few cases, ANAs have been eluted from renal biopsy tissue.[260, 261]

Pathogenesis
Vasospasm

Abnormal vasomotor control is a dominant feature of systemic sclerosis, as evidenced by the presence of Raynaud phenomenon in the vast majority of the patients.[233] In addition to vasospasm of the digital arteries, a cold stimulus has been shown to decrease renal,[247, 257] coronary,[262, 263] and pulmonary perfusion.[264] The cause of abnormal vasomotor control is not known. Increased circulating levels of catecholamines do not seem to be a significant mediator of Raynaud phenomenon.[265] Renin and angiotensin II levels in systemic sclerosis increase after cold exposure and could possibly contribute to arterial vasospasm.[257] In addition to the juxtaglomerular apparatus, vascular smooth muscle cells produce renin.[266] In a vessel "primed" by renin-angiotensin, severe vasospasm can be precipitated by cold exposure, physical stress, caffeine, or nicotine.[238] Knock and co-workers[267]

demonstrated significantly increased endothelin-binding density in microvessels of skin from patients with systemic sclerosis and primary Raynaud phenomenon, compared with normal controls.

Increased Collagen Production

Fibroblast secretion of collagen, the main extracellular matrix component of connective tissue, is markedly increased in systemic sclerosis.[268] Several investigators have provided evidence that transforming growth factor-β (TGF-β) can mediate increased collagen production in systemic sclerosis.[269-271] Gabrielli and associates[271] demonstrated increased immunostaining for TGF-β in the vascular endothelium and dermal fibroblasts of patients with systemic sclerosis. Impaired production of interferon-γ (IFN-γ) by T lymphocytes isolated from patients with systemic sclerosis and fibrosing alveolitis has been observed.[272] This defect could contribute to fibrosis, because IFN-γ is known to suppress collagen synthesis by fibroblasts.[273] Other investigators have provided evidence of the production of abnormal collagen in patients with systemic sclerosis.[274, 275] Douvas[274] demonstrated that Scl-70 (DNA topoisomerase I) binds to collagen genes from scleroderma tissue, but not to genes from normal tissue. The pathogenetic significance of this observation is unclear.

Endothelial Cell Abnormalities

Damage to the endothelial cell has been postulated to be a primary event in the pathogenesis of systemic sclerosis.[276] Cytotoxicity of patient serum to cultured endothelial cells has been demonstrated.[276, 277] It is possible that platelet aggregation at the site of endothelial denudement could lead to the release of platelet-derived growth factor (PDGF) and TGF-β. Both cytokines are mitogenic to smooth muscle cells and fibroblasts, in addition to stimulating collagen production. Theoretically, this would account for the subintimal cell proliferation and the fibrosis seen in systemic sclerosis. Increased PDGF levels and circulating platelet aggregates have been demonstrated in patients with systemic sclerosis.[278, 279] Antiplatelet therapy, however, failed to provide any clinical benefit.[238]

Immunologic Mediators

Although several antinuclear autoantibodies have been detected in patients with systemic sclerosis, their contribution to the disease process is not established. Indirect evidence of immunologic mechanisms in systemic sclerosis has been reported.[280] γ-δ T lymphocytes, activated helper T cells, tissue macrophages, mast cells, and fibroblasts are activated,[281] leading to increased production of extracellular matrix proteins, fibronectin, and proteoglycans.[281] Cytokines such as IL-1, IL-2, IL-8, TNF-α, PDGF, TGF-β, IFN-γ, and endothelin are increased.[281, 282] Moreover, intercellular adhesion molecules and soluble IL-2 receptors have been demonstrated in patients.[280, 283-286] Fibroblasts cultured from the skin of patients with systemic sclerosis produce much higher levels of IL-6 than normal fibroblasts do and may contribute to T cell activation.[287] More recently, IL-6 and PDGF-A were shown to be elevated through the action of endogenous IL-1α in fibroblasts from patients with systemic sclerosis.[288] It is unclear whether these immunologic changes constitute primary events in systemic sclerosis or are epiphenomena.

Microchimerism

Because of its clinical similarities to chronic graft-versus-host disease and its occurrence more often after child-bearing years in women, scleroderma has been proposed as a variant of such a disease. Studies have demonstrated increased frequency of persistent fetal cells among women with scleroderma and a history of pregnancy and the presence of fetal cells in the involved skin of such patients.[289, 290] These associations, however, do not necessarily prove causality.[291]

Pathogenesis of Scleroderma Renal Crisis

It is postulated that SRC is caused by a Raynaud-like phenomenon in the kidney.[248] Severe vasospasm leads to cortical ischemia and enhanced production of renin and angiotensin II, which in turn perpetuate renal vasoconstriction. Hormonal changes (pregnancy),[292] physical and emotional stress, or cold temperature[247] may trigger the Raynaud-like arterial vasospasm. The role of the renin-angiotensin system in perpetuating renal ischemia is underscored by the significant benefit of ACE inhibitors in treating SRC (see later discussion).

Management of Renal Complications

The one form of therapy that appears to have made a major difference in the prognosis of SRC is aggressive treatment of hypertension with ACE inhibitors.[248, 252, 293] In one study, the 1-year survival rate was only 18% for patients treated before the availability of ACE inhibitors, compared with 76% for those treated with such drugs.[251] Progression to severe renal failure that required dialysis was observed in

only half of the patients treated with ACE inhibitors. This suggests that ACE inhibition can forestall progression of SRC in some, but not all, of the patients.[294] Recently, a prospective cohort study on short- and long-term outcomes of SRC in 154 patients who received ACE inhibitors showed that 61% of the patients had good outcomes (no dialysis or temporary dialysis), with a survival rate at 8 years of 80% to 85%, similar to that of patients with diffuse scleroderma without SRC.[295] Diuretics are best avoided because of their ability to stimulate renin release.[238]

In patients with SRC who progress to severe renal insufficiency despite antihypertensive treatment, dialysis becomes a necessity. Both peritoneal dialysis and hemodialysis have been employed.[296, 297] The End-Stage Renal Disease (ESRD) Network report on 311 patients with systemic sclerosis–induced ESRD dialyzed between 1983 and 1985[296] revealed a 33% survival rate at 3 years. On the bright side, recovery of renal function sufficient to render the patient independent of dialysis occurred in 6.8% of the cases in this series. Other reports have documented reversal of SRC-induced renal failure with ACE inhibitors even after dialysis was initiated.[251, 298] In a recent report, more than half of patients with SRC who initially required dialysis and were treated aggressively with ACE inhibitors were able to discontinue dialysis 3 to 18 months later, suggesting that patients should continue to take ACE inhibitors even after beginning dialysis, in the hope of being able to discontinue it later.[295] Interestingly, Raynaud phenomenon of the hands and Raynaud-type vasospasm of peritoneal blood vessels (manifesting as decreased peritoneal clearance) was observed in systemic sclerosis patients using unheated peritoneal dialysate fluid.[297]

Renal transplantation for systemic SRC–induced ESRD has been performed successfully,[296, 299, 300] and recurrence of systemic sclerosis in the transplanted kidney was documented in one case.[261]

The various agents used for treatment of the nonrenal complications of systemic sclerosis are reviewed elsewhere.[301, 302] In a study of 143 patients with diffuse systemic sclerosis, treatment with high-dose D-penicillamine was compared with low-dose therapy. No statistical difference was found between the groups regarding skin thickness scores, incidence of SRC, or overall mortality during a mean follow-up of 3.8 years.[303]

More recently, a retrospective case-control study showed a significant association between antecedent high-dose corticosteroid therapy and the development of SRC, discouraging the use of high-dose corticosteroids in patients with early diffuse scleroderma who are at increased risk for development of SRC.[304] Cytokine therapy with IFN-α has been unsuccessful.[305] Several authors have investigated the role of IFN-γ in the treatment of systemic sclerosis.[306-308] Although some moderate improvement of skin involvement was reported, significant adverse effects, such as digital infarction and renal failure, may limit its clinical usefulness.

RADIATION NEPHRITIS

Clinical Features

The long-term consequences of renal irradiation in excess of 2500 rad can be divided into five clinical syndromes.[309, 310] *Acute radiation nephritis* occurs in approximately 40% of patients after a latency period of 6 to 13 months. It is characterized clinically by abrupt onset of hypertension, proteinuria, edema, and progressive renal failure. The proteinuria is generally mild but can occasionally result in nephrotic syndrome.[311] The urinalysis may also demonstrate microscopic hematuria.[309] In most cases, the progressive renal failure results in end-stage kidneys.[309] Acute radiation nephritis may be accompanied by intravascular hemolysis.[312] *Chronic radiation nephritis,* conversely, has a latency period that varies between 18 months and 14 years after the initial insult. It is insidious in onset and is characterized by hypertension, proteinuria, and gradual loss of renal function.[309] The third syndrome manifests 5 to 19 years after exposure to radiation as *benign proteinuria* with normal renal function.[309] A fourth group of patients exhibits only *benign hypertension* 2 to 5 years later and may have variable proteinuria.[309] *Late malignant hypertension* arises 18 months to 11 years after irradiation in patients with either chronic radiation nephritis or benign hypertension.[309] High-renin hypertension resulting from irradiation of one kidney has been described.[313] Removal of the affected kidney reversed the hypertension. Radiation-induced damage to the renal arteries with subsequent renovascular hypertension has been reported.[314]

A syndrome of renal insufficiency analogous to acute radiation nephritis has been observed in bone marrow transplantation (BMT) patients who were treated with total-body irradiation (TBI).[315-318] In a long-term study of 103 adult survivors of BMT, Lawton and associates[315] reported late renal dysfunction in 14 patients. The syndrome developed at a median of 9 months (range, 4.5 to 26 months) after transplantation and was characterized by progressive decline in GFR, hypertension, and anemia. Eight of the 14 patients had non–nephrotic-range proteinuria and microscopic hematuria. Renal biopsies performed on seven of these patients revealed changes consistent with those of acute radiation nephritis (see later discussion). All of the affected patients had received 1400 rad TBI prior to BMT, whereas none of the patients receiving lower doses of irradiation developed late hypertension or decreased GFR. Chemotherapy administered as part of the preparative regimen could potentiate the effects of irradiation on the kidneys.[319, 320] Increased sensitivity of the kidney to radiation injury has been observed with the use of actinomycin-D,[320] bleomycin-vinblastine,[321] and cyclophosphamide.[317] The incidence of radiation nephritis after TBI and BMT in children is higher than that observed in adults, and it is associated with severe hemolytic anemia.[316] Clinically, the presentation may be indistinguishable from that of HUS.

Radiographic studies may aid in the diagnosis of acute radiation nephritis. CT with contrast enhancement demonstrates sharply demarcated, dense, persistent nephrograms corresponding to the irradiated areas.[322, 323] Increased uptake of technetium-99m in the damaged areas of the kidneys is also observed after renal irradiation.[324]

Pathology

The pathologic hallmark of acute radiation nephritis is glomerular capillary endothelial injury.[325] Because inflammatory cells are not observed in the renal parenchyma, the term "nephritis" is actually a misnomer. Keane and colleagues[325] analyzed renal biopsies obtained from two patients who developed renal insufficiency within 1 year after abdominal irradiation. On light microscopy, mild endothelial cell swelling and basement membrane splitting were consistently observed in the glomerular capillaries. Electron microscopic examination revealed marked subendothelial expansion with deposition of basement membrane–like material adjacent to the endothelial cells. The endothelial cell lining was absent in some capillary loops. Immunofluorescence studies were negative. Similar pathologic findings were also noted in a biopsy specimen from a patient who had received 4500 rad to the kidney 3 months earlier.[311] Similar glomerular endothelial injury was observed in kidney biopsy specimens from patients who developed renal insufficiency and hypertension after TBI and BMT.[315, 316] Some of these biopsies also revealed arteriolar intimal thickening and tubule atrophy. Glomerular capillary endothelial cell loss and mesangiolysis is observed within weeks after irradiation.[326] It appears that the endothelial injury resolves but mesangial lesions progress, as evidenced by increased mesangial matrix, mesangial sclerosis, and, finally, glomerulosclerosis.[326]

Pathogenesis

Sequential morphologic studies performed on rat kidneys after exposure to irradiation suggest that injury begins in the glomerular endothelium and the tubule epithelium.[327, 328] It has been reported that irradiation causes endothelial dysfunction but spares vascular smooth muscle cells in the early postradiation phase.[329] Radiation could directly damage DNA, leading to decreased regeneration of these cells and denudement of the basement membrane in the glomerular capillaries and tubules. How this initial insult eventually leads to glomerulosclerosis, tubule atrophy, and interstitial fibrosis is unclear. It is postulated that degeneration of the endothelial cell layer may result in intravascular thrombosis in capillaries and smaller arterioles.[312, 330] This intrarenal angiopathy would then explain the progressive renal fibrosis and the hypertension that characterize radiation nephritis. A recent study of irradiated mouse kidneys showed a dose-dependent increase in leukocytes in the renal cortex, suggesting a role for inflammatory processes in radiation-induced nephritis.[331]

Treatment

Aggressive treatment of hypertension in patients with radiation nephritis may slow the progression of disease. Evidence in experimental animals suggests that ACE inhibitors may have a renoprotective effect on radiation nephritis independent of their antihypertensive action.[332] In fact, a marked reduction of glomerular, tubule, vascular, and interstitial damage was observed in ACE inhibitor–treated rats after irradiation.[333] Moreover, therapy with ACE inhibitors may be effective in limiting radiation-induced renal injury, even if given for a short course of 3 to 10 weeks, after irradiation of experimental animals.[334] There is evidence that angiotensin II receptor antagonists alone are sufficient for the prophylaxis of radiation nephropathy.[335] It was recently shown in irradiated rats that this protective effect of ACE inhibitors and angiotensin II receptor blockers occurs in the absence of increased activity of the renin-angiotensin system (RAS), suggesting that normal activity of the RAS may be deleterious to the irradiated kidney.[336] Data in experimental rats suggest that radiation nephropathy is ameliorated by postradiation treatment with corticosteroids.[337] This regimen appears to be as effective as ACE inhibitors alone. The same study suggested that there may be an additive effect when ACE inhibitors and corticosteroids are combined.[337] Hypertension due to unilateral disease may respond to nephrectomy.[313] Radiation-induced renovascular hypertension may require angioplasty or surgical repair.[314] Uncontrolled hypertension in patients with radiation nephritis who progress to ESRD warrants bilateral nephrectomies.[338] Because radiation nephritis is generally an irreversible process, preventive measures should be observed during the administration of radiation therapy. These include selective shielding of the kidneys and the use of minimum effective doses of fractionated radiation when possible.[339] The use of radioprotectors such as glutathione or cysteine concomitant with irradiation is still in the experimental phase.[340]

ATHEROEMBOLIC RENAL DISEASE

Atheroembolic renal disease is part of a systemic syndrome of cholesterol crystal embolization. Renal damage results from embolization of cholesterol crystals from atherosclerotic plaques present in large arteries, such as the aorta, to small arteries in the renal vasculature. Atheroembolic renal disease is an increasingly common and often underdiagnosed cause of renal insufficiency in the elderly.[341] A review of 372 autopsies identified cholesterol emboli in 2.4% of renal tissue samples.[342] Male gender, older age, hypertension, and diabetes mellitus are important predisposing factors.[343-345] Patients with cholesterol embolization syndrome often have a history of ischemic cardiovascular disease, aortic aneurysm, cerebrovascular disease, congestive heart failure, or renal insufficiency.[343-345] A significant association between renal artery stenosis and atheroembolic renal disease has also been reported.[346] Precipitating factors, which include vascular surgery, arteriography, angioplasty, anticoagulation with heparin, and thrombolytic therapy, can be identified in about 50% of cases.[343, 345, 347, 348] Arteriographic procedures constitute the most common intervention reported to incite cholesterol embolization.[343, 345] An estimated 15% of patients with atheroembolism do not have any of the known risk factors, and about 50% do not have antecedent precipitating events (referred to as spontaneous cholesterol embolization).[343, 345]

Clinical Features

Clinical manifestations usually appear 1 to 14 days after an inciting event, but their onset can be more insidious.[344, 349] General systemic manifestations occur in fewer than half of the patients and include fever, myalgias, headaches, and weight loss.[345] Cutaneous manifestations such as livedo reticularis, "purple" toes, and toe gangrene occur in 40% to 50% of patients with cholesterol crystal embolization and constitute the most common extrarenal findings.[343, 350] A greater incidence of cutaneous lesions (more than 90%) was reported in two recent series, probably due to closer monitoring.[351, 352] Cholesterol emboli affect mainly the lower limbs, causing the so-called purple-toe syndrome. Other parts of the body, such as the eyes, musculoskeletal system, nervous system, and abdominal organs, can be targets of cholesterol crystal emboli.

The kidneys are affected in approximately 50% of patients.[343, 345] Accelerated or labile hypertension, the most common manifestation, is present in 48% of patients.[343] Malignant hypertension has been described.[353] Renal insufficiency is usually subacute and advances in a stepwise fashion over a period of several weeks. However, renal failure can be acute and oliguric.[343, 354-357] Lye and co-workers[343] reported in a series of 129 patients that uremic signs and symptoms requiring dialysis therapy occur in 40% of cases. Only half of these patients recovered sufficient renal function to stop dialysis over a period of 1 year. More recent data suggest less inexorable deterioration, with a possibility of recovery of renal function in about one third of patients even after variable periods of dialysis support.[351] Renal infarction secondary to cholesterol embolization is rare. Cholesterol embolic disease in renal allografts has been reported.[358-361] Cholesterol emboli can be of donor as well as recipient origin.[361] In 10 of 15 cases of biopsy-proven cholesterol emboli to renal allografts, atheroemboli were believed to originate from the donor arteries, with poor prognosis for the graft.[351]

A high degree of suspicion is required to diagnose atheroembolic renal disease.[362] The differential diagnosis includes systemic vasculitis, subacute bacterial endocarditis, polymyositis, myoglobinuric renal failure, drug-induced interstitial nephritis, and renal artery thrombosis or thromboembolism.[341] The time course of decline in renal function may aid in the diagnosis of atheroembolic renal disease. Renal failure due to procedure-induced atheroembolic renal disease is characterized by a decline in renal function over 3 to 8 weeks. Radiocontrast-induced nephropathy, conversely, usually manifests earlier and often resolves within 2 to 3 weeks after appropriate intervention.[363] Histologic demonstration of cholesterol crystals in small arteries and arterioles of target organs is the most definitive method of diagnosing atheroembolic renal disease. Kidney, muscle, and skin biopsy specimens are the most likely to yield a positive diagnosis.[343, 345]

Laboratory Findings

Renal involvement in the cholesterol crystal embolization syndrome is manifested by increased serum creatinine and BUN levels.[343, 345] At the time of diagnosis, as many as 25% of patients have a serum creatinine concentration higher than 5 mg/dL, and in about 80% it is higher than 2 mg/dL.[345] Although the urinary sediment is abnormal in more than half of cases, it is nondiagnostic. Fine and associates[345] reported 1+ proteinuria by dipstick in 53% of the patients; when quantitated, it was found to be mostly in the non-nephrotic range. However, Haqqie and colleagues[364] reported four patients with cholesterol embolic disease that reached nephrotic-range proteinuria. In a more recent report,[365] 8 of 24 patients with cholesterol embolism had nephrotic-range proteinuria with histologic features of focal segmental or global glomerulosclerosis, indicating that focal segmental glomerulosclerosis can be a presenting feature of renal cholesterol embolism.[365] Granular and hyaline casts occur in approximately 40% of cases, whereas microscopic hematuria or pyuria are observed in fewer than 30%.[345] Eosinophiluria was observed in one third of patients with renal biopsy–proven atheroembolic renal disease.[366] Urinary fractional excretion of Na$^+$ is usually greater than 1%.[367]

Several studies have noted eosinophilia in cholesterol crystal embolic disease.[343, 345, 368] Lye and co-workers[343] reported a 71% incidence of eosinophilia, defined as at least 500 eosinophils per milliliter of blood. Other investigators also reported a 73% to 80% incidence.[345, 368] Belenfant and colleagues[352] and Scolari and associates[351] reported eosinophilia in 59% and 62%, respectively. Eosinophilia ranges between 5% and 42% of the total white blood cell count and is usually transient,[343] although persistent eosinophilia has been reported.[343, 369] Increased erythrocyte sedimentation rate, leukocytosis, and anemia are also commonly present.[345] Hypocomplementemia and thrombocytopenia have been described in six patients.[370] Based on experimental models, the investigators postulated that hypocomplementemia could result from complement activation by denuded atheromas. Lye and co-workers[343] found hypocomplementemia in 39% of their patients in whom complement levels were measured. In two recent series, hypocomplementemia was not observed.[351, 352]

Pathology

The pathologic hallmark of atheroembolic renal disease is the demonstration of cholesterol crystals in the renal microvasculature. The renal vessels most commonly involved are the arcuate, interlobular, and terminal arterioles, which are approximately 150 to 200 nm in diameter.[371, 372] Histologic examination of the occluded vessels reveals biconvex, needle-shaped clefts of cholesterol crystals present in the

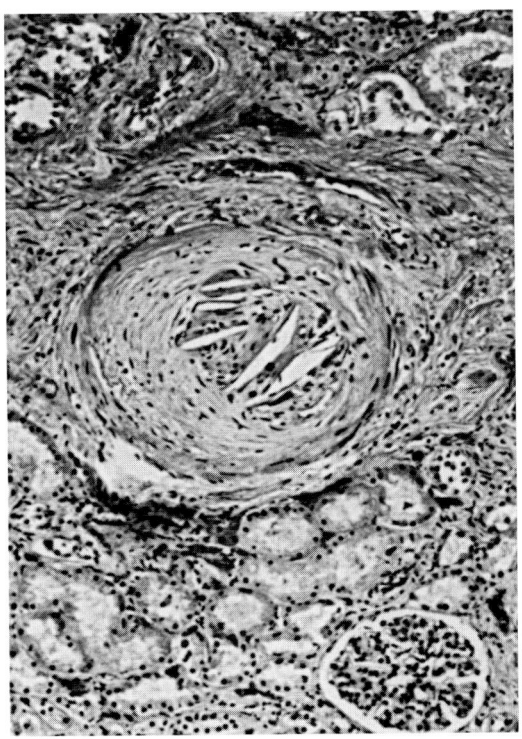

FIGURE 33-2. Atheroemboli lodged in an interlobular artery of a kidney obtained postmortem. The elongated clefts are actually voids where cholesterol crystals were located before fixation and staining. Note the exuberant intimal thickening and the cellular proliferation, which completely occlude the lumen. (Courtesy of W. Margaretten.)

lumen (Fig. 33-2). Cholesterol crystals are birefringent under polarized light. The subsequent intravascular inflammatory reaction has been studied in experimental models of atheroembolism and in human biopsy and autopsy samples.[373-376] The early phase is characterized by a variable PMN and eosinophil infiltrate, followed by the appearance of macrophages and multinucleated giant cells in the lumens of affected vessels within 24 to 48 hours after atheroembolism. In the chronic phase, tissue ischemia is perpetuated by marked endothelial proliferation, intimal thickening, concentric fibrosis of the vessel wall, and persistence of cholesterol crystals and giant cells in the lumens of affected arteries. Hyalinization of glomeruli, atrophy of renal tubules, and multiple wedge-shaped infarcts in the kidney result in reduced kidney size.[371, 377]

Outcome

Atheroembolic renal disease is associated with high morbidity and mortality. A 64% to 81% mortality rate has been reported in the literature.[343, 345] The most significant morbidity associated with atheroembolic renal disease is severe renal insufficiency that requires dialysis. This occurs in approximately 40% of patients, only half of whom recover sufficient renal function to stop dialysis.[343] Mortality is significantly higher in patients who progress to ESRD than in those who recover renal function: 75% versus 17%, respectively.[344]

Treatment

No effective therapy for atheroembolic renal disease has been reported. Unsuccessful medical treatments that have been attempted include plasma expanders, vasodilators, sympathetic blockade, anticoagulants, and corticosteroids.[345, 371] Anticoagulants should be avoided because of the risk of precipitating more atheroembolization.[343, 345] In fact, withdrawal of anticoagulation may be beneficial.[378] Surgical excision of atheromatous plaques in the suprarenal region of the aorta is not advocated because of significant postoperative mortality, worsening renal function, and lower limb loss.[379]

Despite high mortality and the absence of effective therapy, several reports have shown a favorable clinical outcome in patients with atheroembolic renal disease.[344, 380] In many cases, kidney function improved significantly even after a prolonged period of renal insufficiency. Cholesterol-lowering agents have been reported in some cases to lead to improved outcome.[381, 382] In a recent report by Belenfant and colleagues,[352] meticulous care and "aggressive" therapeutic protocols in 67 patients monitored for up to 74 months after diagnosis of multivisceral cholesterol embolism with ARF resulted in a 1-year survival rate of 87%, which compares favorably with that found in the literature. The regimen is characterized by immediate withdrawal of anticoagulants, postponement of aortic procedures, control of blood pressure (lower than 140/80 mm Hg), control of heart failure, dialysis therapy, and adequate nutritional support. Scolari and associates,[351] in their series of 52 patients with a diagnosis of atheroembolic renal disease and a similar general therapeutic approach, observed a 1-year survival rate of 69%. The data from these two recent studies suggest that an aggressive therapeutic approach with patient-tailored supportive measures may be associated with favorable clinical outcome.

RENAL INVOLVEMENT IN SICKLE CELL DISEASE

Clinical Manifestations

Sickle cell anemia, and occasionally the heterozygous forms of sickle cell disease, can lead to multiple renal abnormalities, which include tubular, medullary, and glomerular dysfunction or a combination of these. Gross hematuria is not an uncommon feature of sickle cell anemia, sickle cell trait (Hb-AS disease), and Hb-SC disease.[383, 384] The hematuria is usually painless and self-limited. A total of 15% to 36% of patients with sickle cell disease develop renal papillary necrosis (Fig. 33-3), which could manifest as an episode of gross hematuria. Papillary necrosis occurs in both the homozygous and the heterozygous forms of sickle cell disease and is best diagnosed by intravenous pyelography (see Fig. 33-3). Renal vein thrombosis is an occasional cause of hematuria in patients with Hb-SS disease. Microscopic hematuria is present in most patients with sickle cell anemia.

Proteinuria is also a common finding in patients with sickle cell disease.[385, 386] In a series of 381 patients (71% of whom had sickle cell anemia), Falk and co-workers[387] found that 26% had proteinuria. Proteinuria was twice as common in patients with sickle cell anemia as in patients with heterozygous forms of sickle cell disease (31% versus 16%, respectively). Other investigators have observed a 40% incidence of albuminuria in sickle cell disease.[388] Although

it is mainly in the non-nephrotic range, nephrotic-range proteinuria and the nephrotic syndrome are observed in approximately 3% of all patients.[385, 387] Patients with sickle cell disease who are nephrotic have a poorer prognosis and tend to progress to renal failure.[389]

Powars and colleagues[390] reported that chronic renal failure develops in 4.2% of patients with sickle cell anemia and 2.4% of those with Hb-SC disease. The onset is usually in the third and fourth decades of life, respectively. It is important to note, however, that the GFR in most patients with Hb-SS who are younger than 30 years of age is either normal or increased. Others have reported up to 18% prevalence of chronic renal failure in patients with sickle cell anemia. The vast majority of patients with sickle cell disease and chronic renal insufficiency have proteinuria. They also have more episodes of sickle cell pain crises and poorer prognosis. Progression to ESRD occurs within 2 years in 50% of these patients,[389] and survival time is approximately 4 years, even with dialysis therapy.[390] The cause of progressive renal failure in patients with sickle cell disease is not entirely clear. Although ARF is uncommon, it has been reported in the setting of sickle cell pain crisis.[391] Frequently, concomitant infection or rhabdomyolysis is detected with renal failure. Less often, renal vein thrombosis and intravascular hemolysis have been reported as causes of acute renal insufficiency in patients with sickle cell disease.[392]

The inability to maximally concentrate the urine is a consistent finding in both the homozygous and the heterozygous forms of sickle cell disease.[393-395] This defect results from sickling in the medullary microcirculation, with resultant medullary ischemia.[395] Patients with sickle cell anemia are capable of diluting their urine normally. Another renal

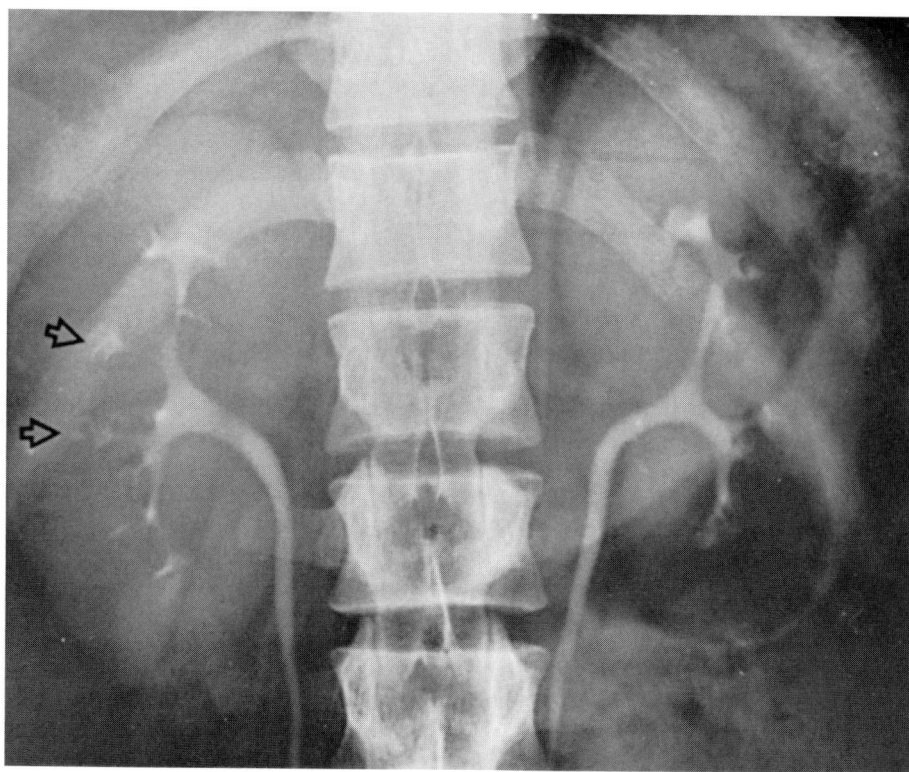

FIGURE 33-3. Renal papillary necrosis with various forms of cavitation in a 33-year-old man with sickle cell hemoglobinopathy and hematuria. Kidneys are normal size and smooth in contour. Central cavitation is present in many papillae, particularly in right interpolar areas *(arrows)*. (From Davidson AJ, Hartman DS: Radiology of the Kidney and Urinary Tract, 2nd ed. Philadelphia, WB Saunders, 1994, p 184.)

defect seen in patients with sickle cell disease, particularly those with the Hb-SS or Hb-SC phenotype, is an incomplete form of distal renal tubule acidosis characterized by the inability to achieve minimal urinary pH during acid loading because of impairment of titratable acid excretion. This defect, however, is not severe enough to cause systemic acidosis. Patients with sickle cell trait (Hb-AS) do not have evidence of impaired urinary acidification. Other tubule defects in sickle cell anemia include increased fractional excretion of creatinine that necessitates the use of inulin clearance to measure GFR accurately, mild impairment of K^+ excretion that does not lead to clinical hyperkalemia, and increased PO_4^{3-} reabsorption in the proximal tubule. The latter could account for the hyperphosphatemia observed in these patients. Renal cell carcinoma has been described in some patients with sickle cell disease. Davis and co-workers[396] reported a cohort of 33 patients who had hematuria and flank pain as frequent clinical symptoms; survival from the time of surgery was 15 weeks, demonstrating the aggressive nature of the tumor.

Pathology

In 1923, Sydenstricker and colleagues[397] described enlarged glomeruli distended with blood in the kidneys of patients with sickle cell disease. Necrosis and pigmentation of tubular cells was also observed. Medullary lesions are the most prominent finding in the kidneys of these patients. Edema, focal scarring, interstitial fibrosis, and tubule atrophy are observed. Cortical infarction has also been reported in patients with sickle cell disease or sickle cell trait.[398, 399] In Hb-SS patients without renal insufficiency, renal pathology includes glomerular hypertrophy characterized by open, dilated glomerular capillary loops.[400] Enlarged glomeruli are most commonly found in the juxtamedullary region of the kidney. In patients with proteinuria and mild renal insufficiency, Falk and co-workers[387] reported glomerular hypertrophy and focal segmental glomerulosclerosis. Tejani and co-workers[401] found that 8 of 13 children with sickle cell anemia who underwent a renal biopsy for persistent proteinuria had focal segmental or global glomerulosclerosis. The remaining five children had mesangial proliferation. In a study of 240 adult patients with sickle cell anemia and the nephrotic syndrome, Bakir and associates[389] reported the presence of mesangial expansion and glomerular basement membrane duplication by electron microscopy. Effacement of epithelial cell foot processes was also observed. These changes suggest hyperfiltration injury and often are referred to in these patients as sickle cell glomerulopathy. Others have reported granular immune deposits consisting of immunoglobulin, complement, and renal tubular epithelial antigens along the glomerular basement membrane in a small group of patients with either sickle cell anemia or sickle cell trait.[402, 403] Membranoproliferative pathology was observed in these patients.

Pathogenesis

The underlying biologic defect in sickle cell disease is a single amino acid substitution of valine for glutamic acid at the sixth position in the hemoglobin beta-chain.[404] This alteration leads to aggregation of deoxygenated sickle cell hemoglobin (Hb-SS) molecules, resulting in deformation of the shape and decreased flexibility of red blood cells.[405] Hb-SS polymer formation is promoted by higher degrees of deoxygenation, increased intracellular hemoglobin concentration,[406] and the absence of hemoglobin F.[405] As red blood cells from sickle cell patients flow through arterioles and capillaries, Hb-SS polymerization may occur. However, the transit time of red blood cells in the microcirculation is usually shorter than the time required for polymerization of sickle hemoglobin.[407] Therefore, factors that increase the microcirculatory transit time may lead to vaso-occlusion in sickle cell disease. Increased adherence of Hb-SS erythrocytes to the vascular endothelium has been described recently. Gee and Platt[408] found that sickle reticulocytes adhere to the endothelium via vascular cell adhesion molecule-1 (VCAM-1). Kumar and co-workers[409] reported that increased sickle erythrocyte adherence to the endothelium involves $\alpha 4\beta 1$-integrin receptors. Platelet activation has also been suggested to play a role in sickle cell–mediated vaso-occlusion.[410] Thrombospondin from activated platelets promotes sickle erythrocyte adherence to the microvascular endothelium.[410, 411] Increased concentration of intracellular sickle hemoglobin may promote polymerization and trigger the sickling process. Drugs that induce hyponatremia may lead to osmotic swelling of erythrocytes and decrease intracellular sickle hemoglobin concentration.[412] The studies of Brugnara and colleagues[413] indicate that there is a reduction of red blood cell dehydration in patients with sickle cell disease treated with the antifungal clotrimazole. It has been suggested that hemoglobin F acts as an inhibitor of the polymerization of deoxyhemoglobin S. Platt and co-workers[414] showed that there is an inverse correlation between the frequency of pain crises and hemoglobin F concentration. Certain drugs, such as 5-azacitidine, hydroxyurea, and sodium phenylbutyrate, have been found to increase the hemoglobin F concentration in patients with sickle cell anemia.[415-417]

The pathogenesis of medullary renal lesions in sickle cell disease is attributed largely to microvascular occlusion by erythrocytes that carry the mutant hemoglobin beta-chain. Erythrocytes passing through the vessels of the inner renal medulla and the renal papillae are most vulnerable to sickling because of the high osmolality of the blood, which leads to cell shrinkage and increased hemoglobin concentration. The pathogenesis of sickle cell glomerulopathy is generally attributed to hyperfiltration. In children with sickle cell disease, renal function is characterized by glomerular hyperperfusion.[418] Later in life, the GFR often declines, despite persistent high renal blood flow rates.[419] Guasch and associates[420, 421] described a distinct pattern of glomerular dysfunction in patients with sickle cell anemia that consists of a generalized increase in permeability to dextrans secondary to increased pore radius in the glomerular basement membrane. With progression to chronic renal failure, the number of pores is reduced and a size-selectivity defect occurs.[420] This abnormality may account for the proteinuria observed in patients with sickle cell glomerulopathy.

Recently, genetic studies of sickle cell anemia have suggested that the coinheritance of microdeletions in one of the four α-globin genes (α-thalassemia) may be renoprotective, because they are associated with a lower prevalence of macroalbuminuria and lower mean arterial pressure, compared with intact α-globin genes.[422]

Treatment

The management of patients with sickle cell disease is targeted at limiting sickle cell crises and end-organ damage. Factors that trigger sickling, such as infection and dehydration, should be treated aggressively. Exposure to hypoxia, cold, or medications that may induce sickle cell crisis should be avoided. Treatment options include transfusion therapy and, more recently, BMT.[423] Interestingly, multiple transfusions may restore urinary concentrating capacity in very young children with sickle cell anemia.[394] Novel approaches that target pathogenetic mechanisms have been proposed. In a double-blind, randomized clinical trial, treatment with hydroxyurea, which increases the hemoglobin F concentration, resulted in a 44% reduction in the median annual rate of pain crises.[424] It is not known whether a reduction in the frequency of sickle cell crises translates to a lower incidence of renal disease. ACE inhibitors such as captopril or enalapril reduce the albuminuria observed in patients with sickle cell disease.[387, 425, 426] The effect of these agents on the rate of progression of sickle cell glomerulopathy remains to be studied.

Patients with sickle cell disease who reach ESRD have a 60% survival rate at 2 years after the administration of renal replacement therapy.[388] Dialysis is the most common form of renal replacement therapy employed. Kidney transplantation as a possible alternative to dialysis has been attempted with reported success.[427] However, most patients experience further episodes of pain crises after renal transplantation.[428, 429] Moreover, sickle cell nephropathy may recur after transplantation.[430] Ojo and colleagues[431] recently reported the largest series of African Americans with end-stage sickle cell nephropathy who received kidney transplants between 1984 and 1996. The 1-year graft survival rate in recipients with end-stage sickle cell nephropathy was similar to that in age-matched recipients with other causes of ESRD (78% versus 77%). However, the 3-year graft survival rate and the patients' survival were diminished in recipients with sickle cell nephropathy compared to those with other causes of renal disease (48% and 78% versus 60% and 90%, respectively). Nevertheless, there was a trend toward better patient survival with renal transplantation compared with maintenance hemodialysis, suggesting that these encouraging results should be taken into consideration when offering renal replacement therapy to patients with end-stage sickle cell nephropathy.

REFERENCES

1. Stewart CL, Tina LU: Hemolytic uremic syndrome. Pediatr Rev 14:218, 1993.
2. Ruggenenti P, Remuzzi G: Thrombotic thrombocytopenic purpura and related disorders. Hematol Oncol Clin North Am 4:219, 1990.
3. Nalabandian RM, Henry RL, Bick RL: Thrombotic thrombocytopenic purpura: An extended editorial. Semin Thromb Hemost 5:216, 1979.
4. Symmers W: Thrombotic microangiopathic haemolytic anaemia (thrombotic microangiopathy). BMJ 2:897, 1952.
5. Remuzzi G, Ruggenenti P: The hemolytic uremic syndrome (Perspectives in Clinical Nephrology). Kidney Int 47:2, 1995.
6. Kaplan BS, Drummond KN: The hemolytic-uremic syndrome is a syndrome. N Engl J Med 298:964, 1978.
7. Moschcowitz E: Acute febrile pleiochromic anemia with hyaline thrombosis of the terminal arterioles and capillaries: An undescribed disease. Arch Intern Med 36:89, 1925.
8. Baehr G, Klemperer P, Schifrin A: An acute febrile anemia and thrombocytopenic purpura with diffuse platelet thrombosis of capillaries and arterioles. Trans Assoc Am Physicians 51:43, 1936.
9. Ridolfi RL, Bell WR: Thrombotic thrombocytopenic purpura: Report of 25 cases and review of the literature. Medicine (Baltimore) 60:413, 1981.
10. Amorosi EL, Ultmann JE: Thrombotic thrombocytopenic purpura: Report of 16 cases and review of the literature. Medicine (Baltimore) 45:139, 1966.
11. Bell WR, Braine HG, Ness PL, et al: Improved survival in thrombotic thrombocytopenic purpura-hemolytic uremic syndrome: Clinical experience in 108 patients. N Engl J Med 325:398, 1991.
12. Cuttner J: Thrombotic thrombocytopenic purpura: A ten-year experience. Blood 56:302, 1980.
13. Kennedy SS, Zacharski LR, Beck JR: Thrombotic thrombocytopenic purpura: Analysis of 48 unselected cases. Semin Thromb Hemost 6:341, 1980.
14. Melnyk AMS, Solez K, Kjellstrand CM: Adult hemolytic-uremic syndrome: A review of 37 cases. Arch Intern Med 155:2077, 1995.
15. Petitt RM: Thrombotic thrombocytopenic purpura: A thirty-year review. Semin Thromb Hemost 6:350, 1980.
16. Monnens LAH, Retera RJM: Thrombotic thrombocytopenic purpura in a neonatal infant. J Pediatr 71:118, 1967.
17. Kwaan HC: Clinicopathologic features of thrombotic thrombocytopenic purpura. Semin Hematol 24:71, 1987.
18. Eknoyan G, Riggs SA: Renal involvement in patients with thrombotic thrombocytopenic purpura. Am J Nephrol 6:117, 1986.
19. Gasser C, Gautier E, Steck A, et al: Haemolytisch-uraemische Syndrome: Bilaterale Nierenrindennekrosen bei akuten erworbenen haemolytischen Anaemien. Schweiz Med Wochenschr 85:905, 1955.
20. Drummond KN: Hemolyic uremic syndrome: Then and now. N Engl J Med 312:116, 1985.
21. Kibel M, Barnard PJ: The haemolytic-uremic syndrome: A survey in South Africa. S Afr Med J 42:692, 1966.
22. Gianantonio CA, Vitacco M, Mendilaharzu F, et al: The hemolytic uremic syndrome. Nephron 11:174, 1973.
23. Rooney JC, Anderson RM, Hopkins IJ: Clinical and pathological aspects of central nervous system involvement in the haemolytic uraemic syndrome. Aust Paediatr J 7:28, 1971.
24. Sheth KJ, Swick HM, Haworth N: Neurological involvement in hemolytic-uremic syndrome. Ann Neurol 19:90, 1986.
25. Rogers MF, Rutherford GW, Alexander SR, et al: A population-based study of hemolytic uremic syndrome in Oregon, 1979-1982. Am J Epidemiol 123:137, 1986.
26. Su C, Brandt LJ: Escherichia coli O157:H7 infections in humans. Ann Intern Med 123:698, 1995.
27. Boyce TG, Swerdlow DL, Griffin PM: Escherichia coli O157:H7 and the hemolytic uremic syndrome. N Engl J Med 333:364, 1995.
28. Spika JS, Parsons JE, Nordenberg D, et al: Hemolytic uremic syndrome and diarrhea associated with Escherichia coli O157:H7 in a day-care center. J Pediatr 109:287, 1986.
29. Hellstrom HR, Nash EC, Fischer ER: Thrombotic thrombocytopenic purpura as a cause of massive gastrointestinal hemorrhage: Report of a case. Gastroenterology 36:132, 1959.
30. Whitington PF, Friedman AL, Chesney RW: Gastrointestinal disease in the hemolytic uremic syndrome. Gastroenterology 76:278, 1979.
31. Jackson B, Files JC, Morrison FS, et al: Thrombotic thrombocytopenic purpura and pancreatitis. Am J Gastroenterol 84:667, 1989.
32. Andreoli SP, Bergstein JM: Development of insulin-dependent diabetes mellitus during the hemolytic-uremic syndrome. J Pediatr 100:541, 1982.
33. Andreoli SP, Bergstein JM: Exocrine and endocrine pancreatic insufficiency and calcinosis after uremic syndrome. J Pediatr 110:816, 1987.
34. Andreoli SP, Bergstein JM: Acute rhabdomyolysis associated with hemolytic-uremic syndrome. J Pediatr 103:78, 1983.
35. Ridolfi RL, Hutchins GM, Bell WR: The heart and conduction system in thrombotic thrombocytopenic purpura. Ann Intern Med 91:357, 1979.
36. Percival SPB: Ocular findings in thrombotic thrombocytopenic purpura (Moschcowitz's disease). Br J Ophthalmol 54:73, 1970.
37. Siegler RL, Brewer ED, Swartz M: Ocular involvement in hemolytic-uremic syndrome. J Pediatr 112:594, 1988.
38. Remuzzi G: HUS and TTP: Variable expression of a single entity. Kidney Int 32:292, 1987.
39. Karlsberg RP, Lacher JW, Bartecchi C: Adult hemolytic-uremic syndrome: Familial variant. Arch Intern Med 137:1155, 1977.
40. Shapiro CM, Kanter A, Lopas H, et al: Hemolytic-uremic syndrome in adults. JAMA 213:567, 1970.

41. Carter AO, Borczyk AA, Carlson JA, et al: A severe outbreak of *Escherichia coli* O157:H7-associated hemorrhagic colitis in a nursing home. N Engl J Med 317:1496, 1987.

42. Dunea G, Muehrcke RC, Nakamato S, et al: Thrombotic thrombocytopenic purpura with acute renal failure. Am J Med 41:1000, 1966.

43. Grabowski EF: The hemolytic uremic syndrome: Toxin, thrombin, and thrombosis. N Engl J Med 346:58, 2002.

44. Symmers WC: Thrombotic microangiopathy: Histological diagnosis during life. Lancet 1:592, 1956.

45. Bukowski RM: Thrombotic thrombocytopenic purpura: A review. *In* Spaet TH (ed): Progress in Hemostasis and Thrombosis. New York, Grune & Stratton, 1982, pp 287-337.

46. Berberich FR, Cuene SA, Chard RL, et al: Thrombotic thrombocytopenic purpura: Three cases with platelet and fibrinogen survival studies. J Pediatr 84:503, 1974.

47. Kaplan BS, Proesmans W: The hemolytic uremic syndrome of childhood and its variants. Semin Hematol 24:148, 1987.

48. Harker LA, Slichter SJ: Platelet and fibrinogen consumption in man. N Engl J Med 287:999, 1972.

49. Kaplan BS, Thompson PC, MacNab GM: Serum complement levels in haemolytic-uraemic syndrome. Lancet 2:1505, 1973.

50. Tardy B, Page Y, Convers P, et al: Thrombotic thrombocytopenic purpura: MR findings. AJNR Am J Neuroradiol 14:489, 1993.

51. De la Sayette V, Gallet E, Le Doze F, et al: Thrombotic thrombocytopenic purpura: A case diagnosed by MRI. Rev Neurol (Paris) 147:314, 1991.

52. Toenshoff B, Sammet A, Sanden I, et al: Outcome and prognostic determinants in the hemolytic uremic syndrome of children. Nephron 68:63, 1995.

53. Ekberg M, Holmberg L, Denneberg T: Hemolytic uremic syndrome: Results of treatment with hemodialysis. Acta Pediatr Scand 66:693, 1977.

54. Habib R, Mathieu H, Royer P: Le syndrome hemolytique et uremique de l'enfant. Nephron 4:139, 1967.

55. Nishioka GJ, Chilcoat CC, Aufdemorte TB, et al: The gingival biopsy in the diagnosis of thrombotic thrombocytopenic purpura. Oral Surg Oral Med Oral Pathol 65:580, 1988.

56. Asada Y, Sumiyoshi A, Hayashi T, et al: Immunohistochemistry of vascular lesion in thrombotic thrombocytopenic purpura, with special reference to factor VIII-related antigen. Thromb Res 38:469, 1985.

57. Levy M, Gagnadoux MF, Habib R: Pathology of hemolytic uremic syndrome in children. *In* Remuzzi G, Mecca G, De Gaetano G (eds): Hemostasis, Prostaglandins and Renal Disease. New York, Raven Press, 1980, pp 383-397.

58. Shigematsu H, Dikman SH, Churg J, et al: Mesangial involvement in hemolytic uremic syndrome. Am J Pathol 85:349, 1976.

59. Kanfer A, Morel-Maroger L, Solez K, et al: The value of renal biopsy in hemolytic-uremic syndrome in adults. *In* Remuzzi G, Mecca G, De Gaetano G (eds): Hemostasis, Prostaglandins, and Renal Disease. New York, Raven Press, 1980, pp 399-406.

60. Morel-Maroger L, Kanfer A, Solez K, et al: Prognostic importance of vascular lesions in acute renal failure with microangiopathic hemolytic anemia (hemolytic-uremic syndrome): Clinicopathologic study in 20 adults. Kidney Int 15:548, 1979.

61. Koffler D, Paronetto F: Fibrinogen deposition in acute renal failure. Am J Pathol 49:383, 1966.

62. Gonzalo A, Mampaso F, Gallego N, et al: Hemolytic-uremic syndrome with hypocomplementemia and deposits of IgM and C3 in the involved renal tissue. Clin Nephrol 16:193, 1981.

63. Feldman JD, Mardiney MR, Unanue ER, et al: The vascular pathology of thrombotic thrombocytopenic purpura: An immunohistochemical and ultrastructural study. Lab Invest 15:927, 1966.

64. Ashkenazi S: Role of bacterial cytotoxins in hemolytic uremic syndrome and thrombotic thrombocytopenic purpura. Annu Rev Med 44:11, 1993.

65. Kaplan BS, Meyers KE, Schulman SL: The pathogenesis and treatment of hemolytic uremic syndrome. J Am Soc Nephrol 9:1126, 1998.

66. Riley LW, Remis RS, Helgerson SD, et al: Hemorrhagic colitis associated with a rare *E. coli* serotype. N Engl J Med 308:681, 1983.

67. Konowalchuk J, Speirs JI, Stavric S: Vero response to a cytotoxin of *E. coli*. Infect Immun 18:775, 1977.

68. Karmali MA, Steele BT, Petric M, et al: Sporadic cases of haemolytic uraemic syndrome associated with fecal cytotoxin and cytotoxin-producing *E. coli*. Lancet 1:619, 1983.

69. Arbus GS: Association of verotoxin-producing *E. coli* and verotoxin with hemolytic uremic syndrome. Kidney Int 51:S91-S96, 1997.

70. Karmali MA, Petric M, Lim C, et al: The association between hemolytic uremic syndrome and infection by verotoxin-producing *E. coli*. J Infect Dis 151:775, 1985.

71. Morrison DM, Tyrell DLJ, Jewell LD: Colonic biopsy in verotoxin-induced hemorrhagic colitis and thrombotic thrombocytopenic purpura (TTP). Am J Clin Pathol 86:108, 1985.

72. Kovacs MJ, Roddy J, Gregoire S, et al: Thrombotic thrombocytopenic purpura following hemorrhagic colitis due to *E. coli* O157:H7. Am J Med 88:177, 1990.

73. Griffin PM, Ostroff SM, Tauxe RV, et al: Illness associated with *E. coli* O157:H7 infections. Ann Intern Med 109:705, 1988.

74. Bell BP, Goldoft M, Griffin PM, et al: A multistate outbreak of *Escherichia coli* O157:H7-associated bloody diarrhea and hemolytic uremic syndrome from hamburgers: The Washington experience. JAMA 272:1349, 1994.

75. Samadpour M, Ongerth JE, Liston J, et al: Occurrence of Shiga-like toxin producing *Escherichia coli* in retail fresh seafood, beef, lamb, pork, and poultry from grocery stores in Seattle, Washington. Appl Environ Microbiol 160:1038, 1994.

76. Robins-Browne RM: Enterohaemorrhagic *Escherichia coli*: An emerging food-borne pathogen with serious consequences. Med J Aust 162:511, 1995.

77. Raghupathy P, Date A, Shastry JCM, et al: Haemolytic-uremic syndrome complicating shigella dysentery in South Indian children. BMJ 1:1518, 1978.

78. Baker NM, Mills AE, Rachman I, et al: Hemolytic uremic syndrome in typhoid fever. BMJ 2:84, 1974.

79. Denneberg TM, Friedberg M, Homberg L, et al: Combined plasmapheresis and hemodialysis treatment for severe hemolytic uremic syndrome following campylobacter colitis. Acta Pediatr Scand 71:243, 1982.

80. Morel-Maroger L: Adult hemolytic-uremic syndrome. Kidney Int 18:125, 1983.

81. Prober CG, Tune B, Hoder L: *Yersinia pseudotuberculosis* septicemia. Am J Dis Child 133:623, 1979.

82. Ray CH, Tucker VL, Harris DJ, et al: Enteroviruses associated with hemolytic-uremic syndrome. Pediatrics 46:378, 1970.

83. O'Regan S, Robitaille P, Mongeau JB, et al: The hemolytic uremic syndrome associated with ECHO 22 infection. Clin Pediatr 19:125, 1980.

84. Ueda K, Shingaki Y, Sato T, et al: Hemolytic anemia following postnatally acquired rubella during the 1975-1977 rubella epidemic in Japan. Clin Pediatr 24:155, 1985.

85. Shashaty GC, Atamaer MA: Hemolytic uremic syndrome associated with infectious mononucleosis. Am J Dis Child 127:720, 1974.

86. Segal GH, Tubbs RR, Ratliff NB, et al: Thrombotic thrombocytopenic purpura in a patient with AIDS. Cleve Clin J Med 57:360, 1990.

87. Nair JM, Bellevue R, Bertoni M, et al: Thrombotic thrombocytopenic purpura in patients with the acquired immunodeficiency syndrome (AIDS)-related complex: A report of two cases. Ann Intern Med 109:209, 1988.

88. Madrazo A, Suzuki Y, Churg J: Radiation nephritis: Acute changes following high dose of radiation. Am J Pathol 54:507, 1969.

89. Murgo AJ: Thrombotic microangiopathy in cancer patients including those induced by chemotherapeutical agents. Semin Hematol 24:161, 1987.

90. Weinblatt ME, Kahn E, Scimeca PG, et al: Hemolytic uremic syndrome associated with cisplatin therapy. Am J Pediatr Hematol Oncol 9:295, 1987.

91. Verweij J, van der Burg ME, Pinedo HM: Mitomycin C-induced hemolytic uremic syndrome: Six case reports and review of the literature on renal, pulmonary and cardiac side effects of the drug. Radiother Oncol 8:33, 1987.

92. Garibotto G, Acquarone N, Saffioti S, et al: Successful treatment of mitomycin C-associated hemolytic uremic syndrome by plasmapheresis. Nephron 51:409, 1989.

93. Galli FC, Damon LE, Tomlanovich SJ, et al: Cyclosporine-induced hemolytic uremic syndrome in a heart transplant recipient. Heart Lung Transplant 12:440, 1993.

94. Noel C, Saunier P, Hazzan M, et al: Incidence and clinical profile of microvascular complications in renal allografted patients treated with cyclosporine. Ann Med Interne (Paris) 143:33, 1992.

95. Butkus DE, Herrera GA, Raju SS: Successful renal transplantation after cyclosporine-associated hemolytic-uremic syndrome following bilateral lung transplantation. Transplantation 54:159, 1992.

96. Atkinson K, Biggs JC, Hayes J, et al: Cyclosporin A-associated nephrotoxicity in the first 100 days after allogeneic bone marrow transplantation: Three distinct syndromes. Br J Haematol 54:59, 1983.

97. Bonser RS, Adu D, Franklin I, et al: Cyclosporin-induced haemolytic uraemic syndrome in liver allograft recipient. Lancet 2:1337, 1984.

98. Randhawa PS, Shapiro R, Jordan ML, et al: The histopathological changes associated with allograft rejection and drug toxicity in renal transplant recipients maintained on FK506: Clinical significance and comparison with cyclosporine. Am J Surg Pathol 17:60, 1993.

99. Holman MJ, Gonwa TA, Cooper B, et al: FK506-associated thrombotic thrombocytopenic purpura. Transplantation 55:205, 1993.

100. Tsai HM, Rice L, Sarode R, et al: Antibody inhibitors to Von Willebrand factor metalloprotease and increased Von Willebrand factor-platelet binding in ticlopidine-associated thrombotic thrombocytopenic purpura. Ann Intern Med 132:794, 2000.

101. Bennett CH, Connors JM, Carwile JM, et al: Thrombotic thrombocytopenic purpura associated with clopidogel. N Engl J Med 342:1773, 2000.

102. Giroux L, Smeesters C, Corman J, et al: Hemolytic uremic syndrome in renal allografted patients treated with cyclosporin. Can J Physiol Pharmacol 65:1125, 1987.

103. Wolfe JA, McCann RL, San Filippo F: Cycloporin-associated microangiopathy in renal transplantation: A severe but potentially reversible form of early graft injury. Transplantation 41:541, 1986.

104. Oursler DP, Holley KE, Wagoner RD: Hemolytic uremic syndrome after bone marrow transplantation without total body irradiation. Am J Nephrol 13:167, 1993.

105. Trimarchi HM, Truona LD, Brennan S, et al: FK 506-associated thrombotic microangiopathy. Transplantation 67:539, 1999.

106. Schoolwerth AC, Sandler RS, Klahr S, et al: Nephrosclerosis postpartum in women taking oral contraceptives. Arch Intern Med 136:178, 1976.

107. Gottschall JL, Elliot W, Liano E, et al: Quinidine-induced immune thrombocytopenia associated with hemolytic uremic syndrome: A new clinical entity. Blood 77:306, 1991.

108. Parker JC, Barrett DA: Microangiopathic hemolysis and thrombocytopenia related to penicillin drugs. Arch Intern Med 127:474, 1971.

109. Ahmed R, Sumalnop V, Spain DM, et al: Thrombohemolytic thrombocytopenic purpura during penicillamine therapy. Arch Intern Med 138:1292, 1983.

110. Powell HR, Davidson PM, McCredie DA, et al: Haemolytic-uremic syndrome after treatment with metronidazole. Med J Aust 149:222, 1988.

111. Stonesifer LD, Bone RC, Hiller FC: Thrombotic thrombocytopenic purpura in carbon monoxide poisoning. Arch Intern Med 140:104, 1980.

112. Jones AM, Armitage JO, Stone DV: Self-limited TTP-like syndrome after bee sting. JAMA 242:2212, 1979.

113. Symmers WC: Thrombotic microangiopathy (TTP) associated with acute haemorrhagic leukoencephalitis and sensitivity to oxophenarsine. Brain 79:511, 1956.

114. Ehrich WE, Seifter J: Thrombotic thrombocytopenic purpura caused by iodine. Arch Pathol 47:446, 1949.

115. Miller JMJ, Pastorek JG: Thrombotic thrombocytopenic purpura and hemolytic syndrome in pregnancy. Clin Obstet Gynecol 34:64, 1991.

116. Hayslett JP: Current concepts: Postpartum renal failure. N Engl J Med 312:1556, 1985.

117. Rozdzinski E, Hertenstein B, Schmeiser T, et al: Thrombotic thrombocytopenic purpura in early pregnancy with maternal and fetal survival. Ann Hematol 64:245, 1992.

118. Maina A, Donvito V, Giachino O, et al: Thrombotic thrombocytopenic purpura in pregnancy with maternal and fetal survival: Case report. Br J Obstet Gynaecol 97:443, 1992.

119. Krane NK: Acute renal failure in pregnancy. Arch Intern Med 148:2347, 1988.

120. Inglis TCM, Steward J, George JJ: Haemostatic and rheological changes in normal pregnancy and preeclampsia. Br J Haematol 50:461, 1982.

121. Wiznitzer A, Mazor M, Leiberman JR, et al: Familial occurrence of thrombotic thrombocytopenic purpura in two sisters during pregnancy. Am J Obstet Gynecol 166:20, 1992.

122. Wallace DC, Loveric A, Clubb JS, et al: Thrombotic thrombocytopenic purpura in four siblings. Am J Med 58:724, 1975.

123. Fuchs WE, George JN, Dotin LN, et al: Thrombotic thrombocytopenic purpura occurrence two years apart during late pregnancy in two sisters. JAMA 19:235, 1976.

124. Berns JS, Kaplan BS, Mackow RC, et al: Inherited hemolytic uremic syndrome in adults. Am J Kidney Dis 19:331, 1992.

125. Sheth KJ, Gill JC, Leichter HE, et al: Increased incidence of HLA-B40 group antigens in children with hemolytic-uremic syndrome. Nephron 68:433, 1994.

126. Pichette V, Querin S, Schurch W, et al: Familial haemolytic-uraemic syndrome and homozygous factor H deficiency. Am J Kidney Dis 24:936, 1994.

127. Roodhooft AM, McLean RH, Elst E, et al: Recurrent hemolytic uremic syndrome and acquired hypomorphic variant of the third component of complement. Pediatr Nephrol 4:597, 1990.

128. Boccia RV, Gelmann EP, Baker CC, et al: A hemolytic-uremic syndrome with the acquired immunodeficiency syndrome. Ann Intern Med 101:716, 1984.

129. Badesha PS, Saklayen MG: Hemolytic uremic syndrome as a presenting form of HIV infection. Nephron 72:472, 1996.

130. Kaplan BS, Cleary TG, Obrig TG: Recent advances in understanding the pathogenesis of the hemolytic uremic syndromes. Pediatr Nephrol 4:276, 1990.

131. Obrig TG, Vecchio PHD, Brown EJ, et al: Direct cytotoxic action of Shigatoxin on human vascular endothelial cells. Infect Immun 56:2372, 1988.

132. Tesh VL, Samuel JE, Perera L, et al: Evaluation of the role of Shiga-like toxins in remediating direct damage to human vascular endothelial cells. J Infect Dis 164:344, 1991.

133. Boyd B, Lingwood C: Verotoxin receptor glycolipid in human renal tissue. Nephron 51:207, 1989.

134. Richardson SE, Rotman TA, Jay V, et al: Experimental verocytotoxemia in rabbits. Infect Immun 60:4154, 1992.

135. Morigi M, Micheletti G, Figliuzzi M, et al: Verotoxin-1 promotes leukocyte adhesion to cultured endothelial cells under physiologic flow conditions. Blood 86:4553, 1995.

136. Te Loo DM, Monnens LA, van Der Velden TJ, et al: Binding and transfer of verotoxin by polymorphonuclear leukocytes in hemolytic uremic syndrome. Blood 95:3396, 2000.

137. Ruggenenti P, Noris M, Remuzzi G: Thrombotic microangiopathy, hemolytic uremic syndrome, and thrombotic thrombocytopenic purpura. Kidney Int 60:831, 2001.

138. Klein PJ, Bulla M, Newman RA, et al: Thomsen-Friedenreich antigen in haemolytic-uraemic syndrome. Lancet 2:1024, 1977.

139. Novak RW, Martin CR, Orsini EN: Hemolytic-uremic syndrome and T-cryptantigen exposure by neuraminidase-producing pneumococci: An emerging problem? Pediatr Pathol 1:409, 1983.

140. McGraw ME, Lendon M, Stevens RF, et al: Haemolytic uraemic syndrome and the Thomsen-Friedenreich antigen. Paediatr Nephrol 3:135, 1989.

141. Leung DYM, Moake JL, Havens PL, et al: Lytic anti-endothelial cell antibodies in haemolytic-uraemic syndrome. Lancet 2:183, 1988.

142. Dillon MJ, Tizard EJ: Anti-neutrophil cytoplasmic antibodies and anti-endothelial cell antibodies. Pediatr Nephrol 5:256, 1991.

143. Laurence J, Mitra D, Steiner M, et al: Plasma from patients with idiopathic and human immunodeficiency virus-associated thrombotic thrombocytopenic purpura induces apoptosis in microvascular endothelial cells. Blood 87:3245, 1996.

144. Cattell V: Mitomycin-induced hemolytic uremic kidney: An experimental model in the rat. Am J Pathol 121:88, 1985.

145. Zoja C, Furci L, Ghilardi F, et al: Cyclosporin induced endothelial cell injury. Lab Invest 55:455, 1986.

146. Snyder HWJ, Mittelman A, Oral A, et al: Treatment of cancer chemotherapy-associated thrombotic thrombocytopenic purpura/hemolytic uremic syndrome by protein A immunoadsorption of plasma. Cancer 71:1882, 1993.

147. Bergstein JM, Riley M, Bang NU: Analysis of the plasminogen activator activity of the human glomerulus. Kidney Int 33:868, 1988.

148. Bergstein JM, Kuederli U, Bang NU: Plasma inhibitor of glomerular fibrinolysis in the hemolytic-uremic syndrome. Am J Med 73:322, 1982.

149. Bergstein JM, Riley M, Bang NU: Role of plasminogen-activator inhibitor type 1 in the pathogenesis and outcome of the hemolytic uremic syndrome. N Engl J Med 327:755, 1992.

150. Chandler WL, Jelacic S, Boster DR, et al: Prothrombotic coagulation abnormalities preceding the hemolytic-uremic syndrome. N Engl J Med 346:23, 2002.

151. Glas-Greenwald P, Hall JM, Panke TW, et al: Fibrinolysis in health and disease: Abnormal levels of plasminogen activator, plasminogen activator inhibitor, and protein C in thrombotic thrombocytopenic purpura. J Lab Clin Med 108:415, 1986.

152. Hekman CM, Loskutoff DJ: Fibrinolytic pathways and the endothelium. Semin Thromb Hemost 13:514, 1987.

153. Esmon CT: Protein C: Biochemistry, physiology and clinical implications. Blood 62:1155, 1983.

154. Lian EC-Y: Pathogenesis of thrombotic thrombocytopenic purpura. Semin Hematol 24:82, 1987.

155. Bloom AL: von Willebrand factor: Clinical features of inherited and acquired disorders. Mayo Clin Proc 66:743, 1991.

156. Moake JL, McPherson PD: von Willebrand factor in thrombotic thrombocytopenic purpura and the hemolytic-uremic syndrome. Transfus Med Rev 4:163, 1990.

157. Moake JL, Rudy CK, Troll JH, et al: Unusually large plasma factor VIII: von Willebrand factor multimers in chronic relapsing thrombotic thrombocytopenic purpura. N Engl J Med 307:1432-1435, 1982.

158. Furlan M, Robles R, Solenthaler M, et al: Acquired deficiency of von Willebrand factor-cleaving protease in a patient with thrombotic thrombocytopenic purpura. Blood 91:2839, 1998.

159. Furlan M, Robles R, Galbusera M, et al: Von Willebrand factor-cleaving protease in thrombotic thrombocytopenic purpura and the hemolytic-uremic syndrome. N Engl J Med 339:1578, 1998.

160. Tsai HM, Lia ECX: Antibodies to Von Willebrand factor-cleaving protease in acute thrombotic thrombocytopenic purpura. N Engl J Med 339:1585, 1998.

161. Moake JL, Byrnes JJ, Troll JH, et al: Abnormal factor VIII: von Willebrand factor patterns in plasma of patients with the hemolytic-uremic syndrome. Blood 64:592, 1984.

162. Rose PE, Enayat SM, Sunderland R, et al: Abnormalities of factor VIII related protein multimers in the haemolytic uraemic syndrome. Arch Dis Child 59:1135, 1984.

163. Tsai HM, Chandler WL, Sarode R, et al: Von Willebrand factor and Von Willebrand factor-cleaving metalloprotease activity in *Escherichia coli* O157:H7-associated hemolytic uremic syndrome. Pediatr Research 49:653, 2001.

164. Monnens L, Van De Meer W, Langenhuysen C, et al: Platelet aggregating factor in the epidemic form of hemolytic uremic syndrome in childhood. Clin Nephrol 24:135, 1985.

165. Siddiqui FA, Lian ECY: Novel platelet-agglutinating protein from a thrombotic thrombocytopenic purpura patient. J Clin Invest 76:1330, 1985.

166. Karpman D, Papadopoulou D, Nilsson K, et al: Platelet activation by Shiga toxin and circulatory factors as a pathogenetic mechanism in the hemolytic uremic syndrome. Blood 97:3100, 2001.

167. Remuzzi G, Misiani R, Mecca G, et al: Thrombotic thrombocytopenic purpura: A deficiency of plasma factor regulating platelet-vessel wall interaction. N Engl J Med 299:311, 1978.

168. Walters S, Levin M, Smith C, et al: Intravascular platelet activation in the hemolytic uremic syndrome. Kidney Int 33:107, 1988.

169. Levin M, Elkon KB, Nokes TJC, et al: Inhibitor of prostacyclin production in sporadic haemolytic uraemic syndrome. Arch Dis Child 58:703, 1983.

170. Ylikorkala O, Makila UM, Viinikka L: Amniotic fluid prostacyclin and thromboxane in normal, preeclamptic, and some other complicated pregnancies. Am J Obstet Gynecol 141:487, 1981.

171. Goodman RP, Killiam AP, Brash AR, et al: Prostacyclin production during pregnancy: Comparison of production during normal pregnancy and pregnancy complicated by hypertension. Am J Obstet Gynecol 142:817, 1982.

172. Defreyn G, Prosemans W, Machin SJ, et al: Abnormal prostacyclin metabolism in the hemolytic uremic syndrome: Equivocal effects of prostacyclin infusions. Clin Nephrol 18:43, 1982.

173. Forsyth KD, Simpson AC, Fitzpatrick MM, et al: Neutrophil-mediated endothelial injury in haemolytic uraemic syndrome. Lancet 2:213, 1989.

174. Fitzpatrick MM, Shah V, Trompeter RS, et al: Interleukin-8 and polymorphoneutrophil leucocyte activation in hemolytic uremic syndrome of childhood. Kidney Int 42:951, 1992.

175. Abbas AK, Lichtman AH, Pober JS: Cellular and Molecular Immunology. Philadelphia, WB Saunders, 1997, p 235.

176. van de Kar NC, Monnens LA, Karmali MA, et al: Tumor necrosis factor and interleukin-1 induce expression of the verocytotoxin receptor globotriaosylceramide on human endothelial cells: Implications for the pathogenesis of the hemolytic uremic syndrome. Blood 80:2755, 1992.

177. Wada H, Kaneko T, Ohiwa M, et al: Plasma cytokine levels in thrombotic thrombocytopenic purpura. Am J Hematol 40:167, 1992.

178. Karpman D, Andreasson A, Thysell H, et al: Cytokines in childhood hemolytic uremic syndrome and thrombocytopenic purpura. Pediatr Nephrol 9:694, 1995.

179. van de Kar NC, Sauerwein RW, Demacker PN, et al: Plasma cytokine levels in hemolytic uremic syndrome. Nephron 71:309, 1995.

180. Noris M, Ruggenenti P, Todeschini M, et al: Increased nitric oxide formation in recurrent thrombotic microangiopathies: A possible mediator of microvascular injury. Am J Kidney Dis 27:790, 1996.

181. Trompeter RS, Schwartz R, Chantler C, et al: An analysis of prognostic features. Arch Dis Child 58:101, 1983.

182. Walters MDS, Matthei IU, Kay R, et al: The polymorphonuclear leukocyte count in childhood haemolytic uraemic syndrome. Pediatr Nephrol 3:130, 1989.

183. Martin DL, MacDonald KL, White KE, et al: The epidemiology and clinical aspects of the hemolytic uremic syndrome in Minnesota. N Engl J Med 323:1161, 1990.

184. DeJong M, Monnens L: Haemolytic-uraemic syndrome: A 10-year follow-up study of 73 patients. Nephrol Dial Transplant 3:379, 1988.

185. Schieppati A, Ruggenenti P, Plata R, et al: Renal function at hospital admission as prognostic factor in adult haemolytic uraemic syndrome. J Am Soc Nephrol 2:1640, 1992.

186. Wong CS, Jelacic S, Habeeb RL, et al: The risk of hemolytic uremic syndrome after antibiotic treatment of *Escherichia coli* O157:H7 infections. N Engl J Med 342:1930, 2000.

187. Zimmerhackl LB: *E. coli*, antibiotics, and the hemolytic uremic syndrome. N Engl J Med 342:1990, 2000.

188. Oryan MM, Prado V: Risk of the hemolytic uremic syndrome after antibiotic treatment of *Escherichia coli* O157:H7 infections. N Engl J Med 343:1271, 2000.

189. Donnelly JJ, Rappuoli R: Blocking bacterial enterotoxins. Nat Med 6:257, 2000.

190. Harkness DR, Brynes JJ, Lian ECY, et al: Hazard of platelet transfusion in thrombotic thrombocytopenic purpura. JAMA 246:1931, 1981.

191. Gordon LI, Kwaan HC, Rossi EC: Deleterious effects of platelet transfusions and recovery thrombocytosis in patients with thrombotic microangiopathy. Semin Hematol 24:194, 1987.

192. Bukowski RM, King JW, Hewlett JS: Plasmapheresis in the treatment of thrombotic thrombocytopenic purpura. Blood 50:413, 1977.

193. Beattie TJ, Murphy AV, Willoughby MLN, et al: Plasmapheresis in the haemolytic-uraemic syndrome in children. BMJ 282:1667, 1981.

194. Gillor A, Bulla M, Roth B, et al: Plasmapheresis as a therapeutic measure in hemolytic-uremic syndrome in children. Klin Wochenschr 61:363, 1983.

195. Hakim R, Schulman G, Churchill WH, et al: Successful management of thrombocytopenia, microangiopathic anemia, and acute renal failure by plasmapheresis. Am J Kidney Dis 5:170, 1985.

196. Blitzer JB, Granfortuna JM, Gottlieb AJ, et al: Thrombotic thrombocytopenic purpura: Treatment with plasmapheresis. Am J Hematol 24:329, 1987.

197. Rock GA, Shumak KH, Buskard NA, et al: Comparison of plasma infusion in the treatment of thrombotic thrombocytopenic purpura. N Engl J Med 325:393, 1991.

198. Byrnes JJ, Khurana M: Treatment of thrombotic thrombocytopenic purpura with plasma. N Engl J Med 297:1386, 1977.

199. Misiani R, Appiani AC, Edefonti A, et al: Haemolytic uraemic syndrome: Therapeutic effect of plasma infusion. BMJ 285:1304, 1982.

200. Shepard KV, Bukowski RM: The treatment of thrombotic thrombocytopenic purpura with exchange transfusions, plasma infusions and plasma exchange. Semin Hematol 24:178, 1987.

201. George JN: How I treat patients with thrombotic thrombocytopenic purpura–hemolytic uremic syndrome. Blood 96:1223, 2000.

202. Rock G, Shumak KH, Sutton DMC, et al: Cryosupernatant as replacement fluid for plasma exchange in thrombotic thrombocytopenic purpura. Br J Haematol 94:383, 1996.

203. North America TTP Group, Ziegler Z, Gryn JF, et al: Cryopoor plasma does not improve early response in primary adult thrombotic thrombocytopenic purpura (TTP). Blood 92:707, 1998.

204. Rose M, Eldor A: High incidence of relapses in thrombotic thrombocytopenic purpura. Am J Med 83:437, 1987.

205. Siegler RL: Management of hemolytic-uremic syndrome. J Pediatr 112:1019, 1988.

206. Gutterman LA, Stevenson TD: Treatment of thrombotic thrombocytopenic purpura with vincristine. JAMA 247:1433, 1982.

207. Schreeder MT, Prchal JT: Successful treatment of thrombotic thrombocytopenic purpura by vincristine. Am J Hematol 14:75, 1983.

208. Moake LJ, Rudy CK, Troll JH, et al: Therapy of chronic relapsing thrombotic thrombocytopenic purpura with prednisone and azathioprine. Am J Hematol 20:73, 1985.

209. Wallach HW, Oren ME, Herskowitz A: Treatment of thrombotic thrombocytopenic purpura with plasma infusion and cyclophosphamide. South Med J 72:1346, 1979.

210. Rosove MH, Ho WG, Goldfinger D: Ineffectiveness of aspirin and dipyridamole in the treatment of thrombotic thrombocytopenic purpura. Ann Intern Med 96:27, 1981.

211. del-Zoppo GJ: Antiplatelet therapy in thrombotic thrombocytopenic purpura. Semin Hematol 24:130, 1987.

212. Diekmann L: Treatment of the hemolytic-uremic syndrome with streptokinase and heparin. Klin Pediatr 192:430, 1980.

213. Loirat C, Beaufils F, Sonsino E, et al: Urokinase treatment for hemolytic uremic syndrome in childhood: A multicenter controlled trial from the French Society of Pediatric Nephrology. Abstract. Int J Pediatr Nephrol 3:46, 1982.

214. Proesmans W, Ki Muaka B, Van Damme B, et al: The use of heparin in childhood hemolytic uremic syndrome. In Remuzzi G, Mecca G, De Gaetano G (eds): Hemostasis, Prostaglandins, and Renal Disease. New York, Raven Press, 1980, p 407.

215. Wong P, Itoh K, Yoshida S: Treatment of thrombotic thrombocytopenic purpura with intravenous gamma globulin. N Engl J Med 314:385, 1986.

216. Chin D, Chyczij H, Etches W, et al: Treatment of thrombotic thrombocytopenic purpura with intravenous gamma globulin. Transfusion 27:115, 1987.

217. Gilcher RO, Goldman SN: Refractory TTP responding to IV gamma globulin. Blood 64:237, 1987.

218. Berkman SA, Lee ME, Gale RP: Clinical uses of intravenous immunoglobulins. Ann Intern Med 112:278, 1990.

219. Guelpa G, Trono D, Audetat F, et al: Purpura thrombotique thrombocytopénique traité par la prostacycline. Schweiz Med Wochenschr 116:647, 1986.

220. Payton CD, Belch JJF, Boulton Jones JM: Successful treatment of thrombotic thrombocytopenic purpura by epoprostenol infusion. Lancet 1:927, 1985.

221. Johnson JE, Mills GM, Batson AG, et al: Ineffective epoprostenol therapy for thrombotic thrombocytopenic purpura. JAMA 250:3089, 1983.

222. Powell HR, McCredie DA, Taylor CM, et al: Vitamin E treatment of haemolytic uraemic syndrome. Arch Dis Child 59:401, 1984.

223. Van Gool S, Brock P, Van Laer P, et al: Successful treatment of recurrent thrombotic thrombocytopenic purpura with plasmapheresis and vincristine. Eur J Pediatr 153:517, 1994.

224. Wolf G, Thaiss F, Duhrsen U, et al: Treatment of thrombotic thrombocytopenic purpura (Moschcowitz's disease) with vincristine. Deutsch Med Wochenschr 120:442, 1995.

225. Bobbio-Pallavicini E, Porta C, Centurioni R, et al: Vincristine sulfate for the treatment of thrombotic thrombocytopenic purpura refractory to plasma-exchange. The Italian Cooperative Group for TTP. Eur J Haematol 52:222, 1994.

226. Hand JP, Lawlor ER, Yong CK, et al: Successful use of cyclosporine A in the treatment of refractory thrombotic thrombocytopenic purpura. Br J Haematol 100:597, 1998.

227. Grino JM, Caralps JM, Carreras L, et al: Apparent recurrence of hemolytic uremic syndrome in azathioprine-treated allograft recipients. Nephron 49:301, 1988.

228. Hebert D, Sibley RK, Mauer SM: Recurrence of hemolytic uremic syndrome in renal transplant recipients. Kidney Int 19:S51, 1986.

229. Muller T, Sikora P, Offner G, et al: Recurrence of renal disease after kidney transplantation in children: 24 years of experience in a single center. Clin Nephrol 49:82, 1998.

230. Kaplan BS, Papadimitriou M, Brezin JH, et al: Renal transplantation in adults with autosomal recessive inheritance of hemolytic uremic syndrome. Am J Kidney Dis 30:760, 1997.

231. Steen VD, Conte C, Santoro D, et al: Twenty-year incidence survey of systemic sclerosis. Abstract. Arthritis Rheum 31:S21, 1988.

232. Medsger TA, Masi AT: Epidemiology of systemic sclerosis (scleroderma). Ann Intern Med 74:714, 1971.

233. Tuffanelli DL, Winkelmann RK: Systemic scleroderma: A clinical study of 727 cases. Arch Dermatol 84:359, 1961.

234. Steen VD, Medsger TAJ: Epidemiology and natural history of systemic sclerosis. Rheum Dis Clin North Am 16:1, 1990.

235. Medsger TA: Systemic sclerosis and localized scleroderma. In Schumacher HR (ed): Primer on the Rheumatic Diseases. Atlanta, Arthritis Foundation, 1988, pp 111-117.

236. Steen VD: Clinical manifestations of systemic sclerosis. Semin Cutan Med Surg 17:48, 1998.

237. Steen VD, Medsger TA, Osial TAJ, et al: Factors predicting development of renal involvement in progressive systemic sclerosis. Am J Med 76:779, 1984.

238. Donohoe JF: Scleroderma and the kidney. Kidney Int 41:462, 1992.

239. Raynaud M: De la Gangrene Symetrique des Extremites. Paris, Universite de Paris, 1862.

240. Clements PJ, Furst DE, Campion DS, et al: Muscle disease in progressive systemic sclerosis: Diagnostic and therapeutic considerations. Arthritis Rheum 21:62, 1978.

241. Ridolfi RL, Bulkley BH, Hutchins GM: The cardiac conduction system in progressive systemic sclerosis: Clinical and pathological features of 35 patients. Am J Med 61:361, 1976.

242. Follansbee WP, Curtiss EI, Medsger TA, et al: Physiologic abnormalities of cardiac function in progressive systemic sclerosis with diffuse scleroderma. N Engl J Med 310:142, 1984.

243. Steen VD: Systemic sclerosis. Rheum Dis Clin North Am 16:641, 1990.

244. Okano Y: Antinuclear antibodies in systemic sclerosis. Rheum Dis Clin North Am 22:709, 1996.

245. Sturgess A: Recently characterised autoantibodies and their clinical significance. Aust N Z J Med 22:279, 1992.

246. D'Angelo WA, Fries JF, Masi AT, et al: Pathologic observations in systemic sclerosis. Am J Med 46:428, 1969.

247. Cannon PJ, Hassar M, Case DB, et al: The relationship of hypertension and renal failure in scleroderma (progressive systemic sclerosis) to structural and functional abnormalities of the renal cortical circulation. Medicine (Baltimore) 41:1, 1974.

248. Traub YM, Shapiro AP, Rodnan GP, et al: Hypertension and renal failure (scleroderma renal crisis) in progressive systemic sclerosis. Review of a 25-year experience with 68 cases. Medicine (Baltimore) 62:335, 1983.

249. Eason RJ, Tan PL, Gow PJ: Progressive systemic sclerosis in Auckland: A ten year review with emphasis on prognostic features. Aust N Z J Med 11:657, 1981.

250. Medsger TA, Masi AT, Rodnan GP, et al: Survival with systemic sclerosis (scleroderma): A life-table analysis of clinical and demographic factors in 309 patients. Ann Intern Med 75:369, 1971.

251. Steen VD, Constantino JP, Shapiro AP, et al: Outcome of renal crisis in systemic sclerosis: Relation to availability of angiotensin converting enzyme (ACE) inhibitors. Ann Intern Med 113:352, 1990.

252. Steen VD: Scleroderma renal crisis. Rheum Dis Clin North Am 22:861, 1996.

253. Salyer WR, Salyer DC, Heptinstall RH: Scleroderma and microangiopathic hemolytic anemia. Ann Intern Med 87:895, 1973.

254. Kincaid-Smith P: Participation of intravascular coagulation in the pathogenesis of glomerular and vascular lesions. Kidney Int 7:242, 1975.

255. Braun J, Sieper J, Schwarz A, et al: Widespread vasculopathy with hemolytic uremic syndrome, perimyocarditis, and cystic pancreatitis in a young woman with mixed connective tissue disease. Case report and review of the literature. Rheumatol Int 13:31, 1993.

256. Trostle DC, Bedetti CD, Steen VD, et al: Renal vascular histology and morphometry in systemic sclerosis: A case-control autopsy study. Arthritis Rheum 31:393, 1988.

257. Kovalchik MT, Guggenheim SJ, Silverman MH, et al: The kidney in progressive systemic sclerosis: A prospective study. Ann Intern Med 89:881, 1978.

258. McCoy RC, Tisher CC, Pepe PF, et al: The kidney in progressive systemic sclerosis. Lab Invest 35:124, 1976.

259. Stone RA, Tisher CC, Hawkins HK, et al: Juxtaglomerular hyperplasia and hyperreninemia in progressive systemic sclerosis complicated by acute renal failure. Am J Med 36:119, 1974.

260. Lapenas D, Rodnan GP, Cavallo T: Immunopathology of the renal vascular lesion of progressive systemic sclerosis (scleroderma). Am J Pathol 91:243, 1978.

261. Woodhall PB, McCoy RC, Gunnells JC, et al: Apparent recurrence of progressive systemic sclerosis in a renal allograft. JAMA 236:1032, 1976.

262. Miller D, Waters DD, Warmca W, et al: Is variant angina the coronary manifestation of a generalized vasospastic disorder? N Engl J Med 304:763, 1981.

263. Kahan A, Deveaux JY, Amor B, et al: Nifedipine and thallium-201 myocardial perfusion in progressive systemic sclerosis. N Engl J Med 314:1397, 1986.

264. Fahey PJ, Utell MJ, Condemi JJ, et al: Raynaud's phenomenon of the lung. Am J Med 76:263, 1984.

265. Sapira JD, Rodnan GP, Scheib ET, et al: Studies of endogenous catecholamines in patients with Raynaud's phenomenon secondary to progressive systemic sclerosis (scleroderma). Am J Med 52:330, 1972.

266. Dzau VJ: Significance of the vascular renin-angiotensin pathway. Hypertension 8:553, 1986.

267. Knock GA, Terenghi G, Bunker CB, et al: Characterization of endothelin-binding sites in human skin and their regulation in primary Raynaud's phenomenon and systemic sclerosis. J Invest Dermatol 101:73, 1993.

268. LeRoy EC: Increased collagen synthesis by scleroderma skin fibroblasts in vitro. J Clin Invest 54:880, 1974.

269. Smith EA, LeRoy EC: A possible role for transforming growth factor-beta in systemic sclerosis. J Invest Dermatol 95:125S, 1990.

270. Falanga V, Gerhardt CO, Dasch JR, et al: Skin distribution and differential expression of transforming growth factor beta 1 and beta 2. J Dermatol Sci 3:131, 1992.

271. Gabrielli A, Di-Loreto C, Taborro R, et al: Immunohistochemical localization of intracellular and extracellular associated TGF beta in the skin of patients with systemic sclerosis (scleroderma) and primary Raynaud's phenomenon. Clin Immunol Immunopathol 68:340, 1993.

272. Prior C, Haslam PL: In vivo levels and in vitro production of interferon-gamma in fibrosing interstitial lung diseases. Clin Exp Immunol 88:280, 1992.

273. Rosenbloom J, Feldman G, Freundlich B, et al: Inhibition of excessive scleroderma fibroblast collagen production by recombinant gamma-interferon. Arthritis Rheum 29:851, 1986.

274. Douvas A: Does Scl-70 modulate collagen production in systemic sclerosis? Lancet 2:475, 1988.

275. Bashey RI, Jimenez SA, Perlish JS: Characterization of secreted collagen from normal and scleroderma fibroblasts in culture. J Mol Med 2:153, 1977.

276. Kahaleh MB, Sherer GK, LeRoy EC: Endothelial injury in scleroderma. J Exp Med 149:1326, 1979.

277. Meyer O, Haim T, Dryll A, et al: Vascular endothelial cell injury in progressive systemic sclerosis and other connective tissue diseases. Clin Exp Rheumatol 1:29, 1983.

278. Kahaleh MB, Osborn I, LeRoy EC: Elevated levels of circulating platelet aggregates and beta-thromboglobulin in scleroderma. Ann Intern Med 96:610, 1982.

279. Pandolfi A, Florita M, Altomare G, et al: Increased plasma levels of platelet-derived growth factor activity in patients with progressive systemic sclerosis. Proc Soc Exp Biol Med 191:1, 1989.

280. Sfikakis PP, Tesar J, Baraf H, et al: Circulating intercellular adhesion molecule-1 in patients with systemic sclerosis. Clin Immunol Immunopathol 68:88, 1993.

281. Varga J, Jimenez SA: Pathogenesis of scleroderma: Cellular aspects. *In* Clements PJ, Furst DE (eds): Systemic Sclerosis. Baltimore, Williams & Wilkins, 1996, pp 123-152.

282. Kinsella MB, Smith EA, Miller KS, et al: Spontaneous production of fibronectin by alveolar macrophages in patients with scleroderma. Arthritis Rheum 32:577, 1989.

283. Needleman BW: Immunologic aspects of scleroderma. Curr Opin Rheumatol 4:862, 1992.

284. Kahaleh MB, Yin TG: Enhanced expression of high-affinity interleukin-2 receptors in scleroderma: Possible role for IL-6. Clin Immunol Immunopathol 62:97, 1992.

285. LeRoy EC: A brief overview of the pathogenesis of scleroderma (systemic sclerosis). Ann Rheum Dis 51:286, 1992.

286. Sollberg S, Peltonen J, Uitto J, et al: Elevated expression of beta 1 and beta 2 integrins, intercellular adhesion molecule 1, and endothelial leukocyte adhesion molecule 1 in the skin of patients with systemic sclerosis of recent onset. Arthritis Rheum 35:290, 1992.

287. Feghali CA, Bost KL, Boulware DW, et al: Mechanisms of pathogenesis in scleroderma: I. Overproduction of IL-6 by fibroblasts cultured from affected skin sites of patients with scleroderma. J Rheumatol 19:1207, 1992.

288. Kawaguchi Y, Hara M, Wright TM: Endogenous IL-1alpha from systemic sclerosis fibroblasts induces IL-6 and PDGF-A. J Clin Invest 103:1253, 1999.

289. Artlett CM, Smith JB, Jimenez SA: Identification of fetal DNA and cells in skin lesions from women with systemic sclerosis. N Engl J Med 338:1186, 1998.

290. Nelson JL, Furst DE, Maloney S, et al: Microchimerism and HLA-compatible relationships of pregnancy in scleroderma. Lancet 351:559, 1998.

291. Nelson JL: Microchimerism and autoimmune disease. N Engl J Med 338:1224, 1998.

292. Silman AJ: Pregnancy and scleroderma. Am J Reprod Immunol 28:238, 1992.

293. Lopez-Ovejero JA, Saal SD, D'Angelo WA, et al: Reversal of vascular and renal crisis of scleroderma by oral angiotensin-converting enzyme blockade. N Engl J Med 300:1417, 1979.

294. Whitman HHI, Case DB, Laragh JH, et al: Variable response to oral angiotensin-converting enzyme blockade in hypertensive scleroderma patients. Arthritis Rheum 25:241, 1982.

295. Steen VD, Medsger TA: Long term outcomes of scleroderma renal crisis. Ann Intern Med 133:600, 2000.

296. Nissenson AR, Port FK: Outcome of end-stage renal disease in patients with rare causes of renal failure: III. Systemic/vascular disorders. Q J Med 273:63, 1990.

297. Copley JB, Smith BJ: Continuous ambulatory peritoneal dialysis and scleroderma. Nephron 40:353, 1985.

298. London RD, Dikman SH, Spiera H: Recovery of renal function in undifferentiated connective tissue disease after treatment with angiotensin-converting enzyme inhibitors. Am J Kidney Dis 18:716, 1991.

299. Richardson JA: Hemodialysis and kidney transplantation for renal failure from scleroderma. Arthritis Rheum 16:265, 1973.

300. Merino GE, Sutherland DER, Kjellstrand CM, et al: Renal transplantation for progressive systemic sclerosis with renal failure. Am J Surg 133:745, 1977.

301. Steen V: Treatment of systemic sclerosis. Curr Opin Rheumatol 3:979, 1991.

302. Medsger TAJ: Treatment of systemic sclerosis. Ann Rheum Dis 50(suppl 4):877, 1991.

303. Clements PJ, Wong WK, Seibold JR, et al: High-dose vs low-dose penicillamine in early diffuse systemic sclerosis (SSc) trial. Arthritis Rheum 40:S558, 1997.

304. Steen VD, Medsger TA: Case-control study of corticosteroids and other drugs that either precipitate or protect from the development of scleroderma renal crisis. Arthritis Rheum 41:1623, 1998.

305. Silman A, Herrick A, Denton C, et al: Alpha interferon does not improve patient outcome in early diffuse scleroderma. Arthritis Rheum 40:S556, 1997.

306. Kahan A, Amor B, Menkes CJ, et al: Recombinant interferon-gamma in the treatment of systemic sclerosis. Am J Med 87:273, 1989.

307. Hunzelmann N, Anders S, Fierlbeck G, et al: Systemic scleroderma: Multicenter trial of 1 year of treatment with recombinant interferon gamma. Arch Dermatol 133:609, 1997.

308. Freundlich B, Jimenez SA, Steen VD, et al: Treatment of systemic sclerosis with recombinant interferon-gamma. Arthritis Rheum 35:1134, 1992.

309. Luxton RW: Radiation nephritis: A long-term study of fifty-four patients. Lancet 2:1221, 1961.

310. Luxton RW: Radiation nephritis. Acta Radiol 2:169, 1964.

311. Jennette JC, Ordonez NG: Radiation nephritis causing nephrotic syndrome. Urology 22:631, 1983.

312. Steele BT, Lirenman DS: Acute radiation nephritis and the hemolytic uremic syndrome. Clin Nephrol 11:272, 1979.

313. Shapiro A, Cavallo T, Cooper W, et al: Hypertension in radiation nephritis: Report of a patient with unilateral disease, elevated renin activity levels, and reversal after unilateral nephrectomy. Arch Intern Med 137:848, 1977.

314. Staab GE, Tegtmeyer J, Constable WC: Radiation-induced renovascular hypertension. AJR Am J Roentgenol 126:634, 1976.

315. Lawton CA, Cohen EP, Barber-Derus SW, et al: Late renal dysfunction in adult survivors of bone marrow transplantation. Cancer 67:2795, 1991.

316. Guinan EC, Tarbell NJ, Niemeyer CM, et al: Intravascular hemolysis and renal insufficiency after bone marrow transplantation. Blood 72:451, 1988.

317. Bergstein J, Andreoli SP, Provisor AJ, et al: Radiation nephritis following total-body irradiation and cyclophosphamide in preparation for bone marrow transplantation. Transplantation 41:63, 1984.

318. Tarbell NJ, Guinan EC, Niemeyer C, et al: Late onset of renal dysfunction in survivors of bone marrow transplantation. Int J Radiat Oncol Biol Phys 15:99, 1988.

319. Arneil GC, Emmanuel IG, Flatman GE, et al: Nephritis in two children after irradiation and chemotherapy for nephroblastoma. Lancet 1:960, 1974.

320. Phillips TL, Fu KK: Quantification of combined radiation therapy and chemotherapy effects on critical normal tissues. Cancer 37:1186, 1976.

321. Churchill DN, Hong K, Gault MH: Radiation nephritis following combined abdominal radiation and chemotherapy (bleomycin-vinblastine). Cancer 41:2162, 1978.

322. Anderson BL, Lauver JW, Ross P, et al: Demonstration of radiation nephritis by computed tomography. Comput Radiol 6:187, 1982.

323. Moore L, Curry NS, Jenrette JM: Computed tomography of acute radiation nephritis. Urol Radiol 8:89, 1986.

324. Desai A: Renal imaging after partial renal irradiation. Clin Nucl Med 7:113, 1982.

325. Keane WF, Crosson JT, Staley NA, et al: Radiation-induced renal disease: A clinicopathologic study. Am J Med 60:127, 1976.

326. Robbins ME, Bonsib SM: Radiation nephropathy: A review. Scanning Microsc 9:535, 1995.

327. Madrazo A, Suzuki Y, Churg J: Radiation nephritis: Chronic changes after high doses of radiation. Am J Pathol 61:37, 1970.

328. Madrazo A, Churg J: Radiation nephritis: Chronic changes following moderate doses of radiation. Lab Invest 34:283, 1976.

329. Juncos LI, Cornejo JC, Gomes J, et al: Abnormal endothelium-dependent responses in early radiation nephropathy. Hypertension 30:672, 1997.

330. Cogan MG, Arieff AI: Radiation nephritis and intravascular coagulation. Clin Nephrol 10:74, 1978.

331. Stewart FA, Te Poele JA, Van der Wal AF, et al: Radiation nephropathy: The link between functional damage and vascular mediated inflammatory and thrombotic changes. Acta Oncol 40:952, 2001.

332. Juncos LI, Carrasco-Duenas S, Cornejo JC, et al: Long-term enalapril and hydrochlorothiazide in radiation nephritis. Nephron 64:249, 1993.

333. Cohen EP, Molteni A, Hill P, et al: Captopril preserves function and ultrastructure in experimental radiation nephropathy. Lab Invest 75:349, 1996.

334. Cohen EP, Fish BL, Moulder JE: Successful brief captopril treatment in experimental radiation nephropathy. J Lab Clin Med 129:536, 1997.

335. Moulder JE, Fish BL, Cohen EP, et al: Angiotensin II receptor antagonists in the prevention of radiation nephropathy. Radiat Res 146:106, 1996.

336. Cohen EP, Fish BL, Moulder JE: The renin-angiotensin system in experimental radiation nephropathy. J Lab Clin Med 139:251, 2002.

337. Geraci JP, Sun MC, Mariano MS: Amelioration of radiation nephropathy in rats by postirradiation treatment with dexamethasone and/or captopril. Radiat Res 143:58, 1995.

338. Luscher TF, Wanner C, Hauri D, et al: Curable renal parenchymal hypertension: Current diagnosis and management. Cardiology 72(suppl):33, 1985.

339. Maisin JR: Chemical protection against long-term effects in mice exposed to supralethal doses of X rays. C R Seances Soc Biol Fils Paris 176:68, 1982.

340. Coia LR, Hanks GE: Complications from large field intermediate dose infradiaphragmatic radiation: An analysis of the patterns of care outcomes for Hodgkin's disease and seminoma. Int J Radiat Oncol Biol Phys 15:29, 1988.

341. Saleem S, Lakkis FG, Martinez-Maldonaldo M: Atheroembolic renal disease. Semin Nephrol 16:309, 1996.

342. Cross SS: How common is cholesterol embolism? J Clin Pathol 44:859, 1991.

343. Lye WC, Cheah JS, Sinniah R: Renal cholesterol embolic disease. Am J Nephrol 13:489, 1993.

344. Frock J, Bierman M, Hammeke M, et al: Atheroembolic renal disease: Experience with 22 patients. Nebr Med J 79:317, 1994.

345. Fine M, Kapoor W, Falanga V: Cholesterol crystal embolization: A review of 221 cases in the English literature. Angiology 38:769, 1987.

346. Vidt DG, Eisele JS, Gephardt GN, et al: Atheroembolic renal disease: Association with renal artery stenosis. Cleve Clin J Med 56:407, 1989.

347. Schwartz MW, McDonald G: Cholesterol embolization syndrome: Occurrence after intravenous streptokinase therapy for myocardial infarction. JAMA 258:1934, 1987.

348. Belenfant X, d'Auzac C, Bariety J, et al: Cholesterol crystal embolism during treatment with low-molecular-weight heparin. Presse Med 26:1236, 1997.

349. Dahlberg PJ, Frecentese DF, Cogbill TH: Cholesterol embolization: Experience with 22 histologically proven cases. Surgery 105:737, 1989.

350. Falanga V, Fine MJ, Kapoor WN: The cutaneous manifestations of cholesterol crystal embolization. Arch Dermatol 122:1194, 1986.

351. Scolari F, Tardanico R, Zani R, et al: Cholesterol crystal embolism: A recognizable cause of renal disease. Am J Kidney Dis 36:1089, 2000.

352. Belenfant X, Meyrier A, Jacquot C, et al: Supportive treatment improves survival in multivisceral cholesterol crystal embolism. Am J Kidney Dis 33:840, 1999.

353. Dalakos TG, Streeten DPH, Jones D, et al: "Malignant" hypertension resulting from atheromatous embolization predominantly of one kidney. Am J Med 57:135, 1974.

354. Fraser I, Ihle B, Kincaid-Smith P: Renal failure due to cholesterol emboli. Aust N Z J Med 21:418, 1991.

355. Goldman M, Thoua Y, Dhaene M, et al: Necrotising glomerulonephritis associated with cholesterol microemboli. BMJ 290:205, 1985.

356. Remy P, Jacquot C, Nochy D, et al: Cholesterol atheroembolic renal disease with necrotizing glomerulonephritis. Am J Nephrol 7:164, 1987.

357. Wong FK, Chan SK, Ing TS, et al: Acute renal failure after streptokinase therapy in a patient with acute myocardial infarction. Am J Kidney Dis 26:508, 1995.

358. Singh I, Killen PD, Leichtman AB: Cholesterol emboli presenting as acute allograft dysfunction after renal transplantation. J Am Soc Nephrol 6:165, 1994.

359. Pirson Y, Honhon B, Cosyns JP, et al: Cholesterol embolism in a renal allograft after treatment with streptokinase. BMJ 296:394, 1988.

360. Jennings WC, Smith J, Cory RJ: Atheromatous embolization as a cause of increasing creatinine levels in a renal transplant patient. Transplant Proc 22:279, 1990.

361. Aujla N, Greenberg A, Banner F, et al: Atheroembolic involvement of renal allografts. Am J Kidney Dis 13:329, 1989.

362. Robson MG, Scoble JE: Atheroembolic disease. Br J Hosp Med 55:648, 1996.

363. Thadhani RI, Camargo CA Jr, Xavier RJ, et al: Atheroembolic renal failure after invasive procedures: Natural history based on 52 histologically proven cases. Medicine (Baltimore) 74:350, 1995.

364. Haqqie SS, Urizar RE, Singh J: Nephrotic-range proteinuria in renal atheroembolic disease: Report of four cases. Am J Kidney Dis 28:493, 1996.

365. Greenberg A, Bastacky SI, Iqubal A, et al: Focal segmental glomerulosclerosis associated with nephrotic syndrome in cholesterol atheroembolism: Clinicopathological correlations. Am J Kidney Dis 29:334, 1997.

366. Wilson DM, Salazer TL, Farkouh ME: Eosinophiluria in atheroembolic renal disease. Am J Med 91:186, 1991.

367. Case Records of the Massachusetts General Hospital (Case 4-1984). N Engl J Med 310:244, 1984.

368. Kasinath BS, Corwin HL, Bidani AK, et al: Eosinophilia in the diagnosis of atheroembolic renal disease. Am J Nephrol 7:173, 1987.

369. Levine J, Rennke HG, Idelson BA: Profound persistent eosinophilia in a patient with spontaneous renal atheroembolic disease. Am J Nephrol 12:377, 1992.

370. Cosio FG, Zager RA, Sharma HM: Atheroembolic renal disease causes hypocomplementaemia. Lancet 2:118, 1985.

371. Kassirer JP: Atheroembolic renal disease. N Engl J Med 280:812, 1969.

372. Eliot RS, Kanjuh VI, Edwards JE: Atheromatous embolism. Circulation 30:611, 1964.

373. Snyder HE, Shapiro JL: A correlative study of atheroembolism in human and experimental animals. Surgery 49:195, 1961.

374. Gore I, McComb HL, Lindquist RI: Observations on the fate of cholesterol emboli. J Atheroscler Res 4:527, 1964.

375. Otken LB: Experimental production of atheromatous embolization. Arch Pathol 68:685, 1959.

376. Warren BA, Vales O: The ultrastructure of the reaction of arterial walls to cholesterol crystals in atheroembolism. Br J Exp Pathol 57:67, 1976.

377. Coburn JW, Agre KL: Renal thromboembolism, atheroembolism, and other acute diseases of renal arteries. *In* Schrier RW, Gottschalk CW (eds): Diseases of the Kidney, 5th ed. Boston, Little, Brown, 1993, pp 2119-2135.

378. Bruns FJ, Segel DP, Adler S: Control of cholesterol embolization by discontinuation of anticoagulation therapy. Am J Med Sci 275:105, 1978.

379. Keen RR, McCarthy WJ, Shireman PK, et al: Surgical management of atheroembolism. J Vasc Surg 21:773, 1995.

380. McGowan JA, Greenberg A: Cholesterol atheroembolic renal disease: Report of 3 cases with emphasis on diagnosis by skin biopsy and extended survival. Am J Nephrol 6:135, 1986.

381. Kawakami Y: Management of multiple cholesterol embolization syndrome: A case report. Angiology 41:248, 1990.

382. Woolfson RG, Lachmann H: Improvement in renal cholesterol emboli syndrome after simvastatin. Lancet 351:1331, 1998.

383. Chapman ZA, Reeder PS, Friedman IA, et al: Gross hematuria in sickle cell trait and sickle cell hemoglobin C disease. Am J Med 19:773, 1955.

384. Allen TD: Sickle cell disease and hematuria: A report of 29 cases. J Urol 91:177, 1964.

385. Sweeney MJ, Dobbins WT, Etteldorf JN: Renal disease with elements of the nephrotic syndrome associated with sickle cell anemia. J Pediatr 60:42, 1962.

386. Berman LB, Tublin I: The nephropathies of sickle cell disease. Arch Intern Med 103:602, 1959.

387. Falk RJ, Scheinman J, Phillips G, et al: Prevalence and pathologic features of sickle cell nephropathy and response to inhibition of angiotensin-converting enzyme. N Engl J Med 326:910, 1992.

388. Aoki RY, Saad ST: Microalbuminuria in sickle cell disease. Braz J Med Biol Res 23:1103, 1990.

389. Bakir AA, Hathiwala SC, Ainis H, et al: Prognosis of the nephrotic syndrome in sickle cell glomerulopathy: A retrospective study. Am J Nephrol 7:110, 1987.

390. Powars DR, Elliot-Mills DD, Chan L, et al: Chronic renal failure in sickle cell disease: Risks factors, clinical course and mortality. Ann Intern Med 115:614, 1991.

391. Devereux S, Knowles SM: Rhabdomyolysis and acute renal failure in sickle cell anemia. BMJ 290:1707, 1985.

392. Saborio P, Scheinman J: Sickle cell nephropathy. J Am Soc Nephrol 10:187, 1999.

393. Hatch FE, Culbertson JW, Diggs LW: Nature of renal concentrating defect in sickle cell disease. J Clin Invest 46:336, 1967.

394. Keitel HG, Thompson D, Itano HA: Hyposthenuria in sickle cell anemia: A reversible defect. J Clin Invest 35:998, 1956.

395. Statius van Eps LW, Pinedo-Veels C, de Vries GH, et al: Nature of the concentrating defect in sickle cell nephropathy. Lancet 1:450, 1970.

396. Davis CJ Jr, Mostofi FK, Sesterhenn IA: Renal medullary carcinoma: The seventh sickle cell nephropathy. Am J Surg Pathol 19:1, 1995.

397. Sydenstricker VP, Mulherin WA, Houseal RW: Sickle cell anemia: Report of two cases in children with necropsy in one case. Am J Dis Child 26:132, 1923.

398. Femi-Pearse D, Odunjo EO: Renal cortical infarcts in sickle cell trait. BMJ 3:34, 1968.

399. Kimmelstiel P: Vascular occlusion and ischemic infarction in sickle cell disease. Am J Med Sci 216:11, 1948.

400. Bhathena DB, Sondheimer JH: The glomerulopathy of homozygous sickle hemoglobin (SS) disease: Morphology and pathogenesis. J Am Soc Nephrol 1:1241, 1991.

401. Tejani A, Phadke K, Adamson O, et al: Renal lesions in sickle cell nephropathy in children. Nephron 39:352, 1985.

402. Pardo V, Strauss J, Kramer H, et al: Nephropathy associated with sickle cell anemia: An autologous autoimmune complex nephritis. II: Clinicopathologic study of seven patients. Am J Med 59:650, 1975.

403. Ozawa T, Mass MF, Guggenheim S, et al: Autologous immune complex nephritis associated with sickle cell trait: Diagnosis of the hemoglobinopathy after renal structural and immunological studies. BMJ (Clin Res) 1:369, 1976.

404. Ingram VM: Gene mutations in human hemoglobin: The chemical difference between normal and sickle cell hemoglobin. Nature 180:326, 1959.

405. Bunn HF: Pathogenesis and treatment of sickle cell disease. N Engl J Med 337:762, 1997.

406. Hofrichter J, Ross PD, Eaton WA: Kinetics and mechanisms of deoxyhemoglobin S gelation: A new approach to understanding sickle cell disease. Proc Natl Acad Sci U S A 71:4864, 1974.

407. Mozzarelli A, Hofrichter J, Eaton WA: Delay time of hemoglobin S polymerization prevents most cells from sickling in vivo. Science 237:500, 1987.

408. Gee BE, Platt OS: Sickle reticulocytes adhere to VCAM-1. Blood 85:268, 1995.

409. Kumar A, Eckmann JR, Swerlick RA, et al: Phorbol ester stimulation increases sickle erythrocyte adherence to endothelium: A novel pathway involving a4b1 integrin receptor on sickle reticulocytes and fibronectin. Blood 88:4348, 1996.

410. Sugihara K, Sugihara T, Mohandas N, et al: Thrombospondin mediates adherence of CD36+ sickle reticulocytes to endothelial cells. Blood 80:2634, 1992.

411. Brittain HA, Eckman JR, Swerlick RA, et al: Thrombospondin from activated platelets promotes sickle erythrocyte adherence to human microvascular endothelium under physiologic flow: A potential role for activation in sickle cell vaso-occlusion. Blood 81:2137, 1993.

412. Rosa RM, Bierer BE, Thomas R, et al: A study of induced hyponatremia in the prevention and treatment of sickle-cell crisis. N Engl J Med 303:1138, 1980.

413. Brugnara C, Gee B, Armsby CC, et al: Therapy with oral clotrimazole induces inhibition of the Gardos channel and reduction of erythrocyte dehydration in patients with sickle cell disease. J Clin Invest 97:1227, 1996.

414. Platt OS, Thorington BD, Brambilla DJ, et al: Pain in sickle cell disease: Rates and risk factors. N Engl J Med 325:11, 1991.

415. Platt OS, Orkin SH, Dover G, et al: Hydroxyurea enhances fetal hemoglobin production in sickle cell anemia. J Clin Invest 74:652, 1984.

416. Ley TJ, DeSimone J, Noguchi CT, et al: 5-Azacytidine increases gamma-globin synthesis and reduces the proportion of dense cells in patients with sickle cell anemia. Blood 62:370, 1983.

417. Dover GJ, Brusilow S, Charache S: Induction of fetal hemoglobin production in subjects with sickle cell anemia by oral sodium phenylbutyrate. Blood 84:339, 1994.

418. Etteldorf JN, Tuttle AH, Clayton GW: Renal hemodynamics in children with sickle cell anemia. Am J Dis Child 83:185, 1952.

419. Etteldorf JN, Smith JD, Tuttle AH, et al: Renal hemodynamic studies in adults with sickle cell anemia. Am J Med 18:243, 1955.

420. Guasch A, Millicent C, You W, et al: Sickle cell anemia causes a distinct pattern of glomerular dysfunction. Kidney Int 51:826, 1997.

421. Guasch A, Cua M, Mitch WE: Early detection and the course of glomerular injury in patients with sickle cell anemia. Kidney Int 49:786, 1996.

422. Guasch A, Zayas CF, Eckman JR, et al: Evidence that microdeletions in the alpha globulin gene protect against the development of sickle cell glomerulopathy in humans. J Am Soc Nephrol 10:1014, 1999.

423. Platt OS, Guinan EC: Bone marrow transplantation in sickle cell anemia: The dilemma of choice. N Engl J Med 335:426, 1996.

424. Charache S, Terrin ML, Moore RD, et al: Effect of hydroxyurea on the frequency of painful crises in sickle cell anemia. N Engl J Med 332:1317, 1995.

425. Aoki RY, Saad STO: Enalapril reduces the albuminuria of patients with sickle cell disease. Am J Med 98:432, 1995.

426. Foucan L, Bourhis V, Bangou J, et al: A randomized trial of captopril for microalbuminuria in normotensive adults with sickle cell disease. Am J Med 104:339, 1998.

427. Chatterjee SN: National study in natural history of renal allografts in sickle cell disease or trait: A second report. Transplant Proc 21:33, 1987.

428. Spector D, Zachary JB, Sterioff S, et al: Painful crises following renal transplantation in sickle cell anemia. Am J Med 64:835, 1978.

429. Barber WH, Deierhoi MH, Julian BA, et al: Renal transplantation in sickle cell anemia and sickle cell disease. Clin Transplant 1:169, 1987.

430. Miner DJ, Jorkasky DK, Perloff LJ, et al: Recurrent sickle cell nephropathy in a transplanted kidney. Am J Kidney Dis 10:306, 1987.

431. Ojo AO, Govaerts TC, Schmouder RL, et al: Renal transplantation in end stage sickle cell nephropathy. Transplantation 67:291, 1999.

CHAPTER 34

Toxic Nephropathy

Biff F. Palmer and William L. Henrich

ANTIBACTERIAL AGENTS
Aminoglycoside Antibiotics
Penicillins and Cephalosporins
Vancomycin
Sulfonamides
Amphotericin
ANTIVIRAL AND
ANTIPROTOZOAL AGENTS
Acyclovir and Ganciclovir
Pentamidine
Foscarnet
Antiretroviral Therapy
RADIOCONTRAST AGENTS
DRUGS USED IN
TRANSPLANTATION
Cyclosporine
FK-506

ANTINEOPLASTIC DRUGS
Cisplatin
Carboplatin
Cyclophosphamide
Streptozotocin
Semustine and Carmustine
Ifosfamide
Mitomycin C
Plicamycin
Methotrexate
Cytarabine
6-Thioguanine
5-Fluorouracil
Interleukin-2
NEPHROTOXICITY SECONDARY
TO TUMOR CELL LYSIS
IMMUNOGLOBULIN THERAPY

HEAVY METALS
Lead
Cadmium
Mercury
Uranium
Other Heavy Metals
ALTERNATIVE MEDICINE
ANTIRHEUMATIC AGENTS
Penicillamine
Gold
Nonsteroidal Anti-inflammatory Drugs
DRUGS USED IN INFLAMMATORY
BOWEL DISEASE
Mesalazine and Olsalazine
ANGIOTENSIN-CONVERTING
ENZYME INHIBITORS
HYDROCARBONS

As the kidney concentrates and excretes metabolic waste, chemicals, and drugs, it is often exposed to toxic concentrations of these substances. The term "toxic nephropathy" encompasses renal disorders produced by a wide array of drugs, diagnostic agents, and chemicals. Nephrotoxins induce a variety of clinical syndromes that are related, in large part, to the specific nephron segment affected by the agent. The following section discusses the nephrotoxic syndromes related to specific therapeutic and diagnostic agents.

ANTIBACTERIAL AGENTS

Aminoglycoside Antibiotics

The aminoglycoside antibiotics (neomycin, gentamicin, tobramycin, amikacin, netilmicin) are bactericidal agents that have nephrotoxicity as their major adverse effect. The incidence of nephrotoxicity from these aminoglycosides has increased since their introduction in 1969, when the reported incidence of nephrotoxicity was 2% to 3%. In 1993, the incidence was reported to be 20%, a figure that has changed little in the past decade, despite the proliferation of nomograms and pharmacokinetic programs devised to prevent renal toxicity.[1] The percentage of patients who develop nephrotoxicity rises with the duration of therapy, reaching almost 50% with 14 days or more of therapy.

Aminoglycosides penetrate the cytoplasmic membrane of bacteria and act on ribosomes, causing misreading of the genetic code and, ultimately, death of the microorganism. Aminoglycosides are polycations, a property that is responsible for their poor oral absorption, poor penetration into the cerebrospinal fluid, and rapid renal excretion. The polycationic charge also appears to contribute to nephrotoxicity.

Clinical Features

The most common clinical presentation of aminoglycoside nephrotoxicity is nonoliguric acute renal failure (Table 34-1). The onset of renal failure is usually slower and the daily rise in serum creatinine tends to be lower than that observed in acute renal failure from other causes. In greater than 50% of patients with nephrotoxicity, the decline in renal function occurs only after therapy has been completed.[1] Recovery from aminoglycoside nephrotoxicity is usually slow, often requiring 4 to 6 weeks. In some patients, particularly those with prior renal insufficiency, recovery to baseline renal

TABLE 34-1

Clinical Features of Aminoglycoside Antibiotic–Induced Nephrotoxicity

Nonoliguric acute renal failure
Slow recovery of renal function over
    several weeks
Proximal tubular dysfunction
    Enzymuria
    Low-grade proteinuria
    Glucosuria
Hypomagnesemia
Hypocalcemia
Hypokalemia

function may be incomplete.[2] The explanation for incomplete recovery to baseline function is probably permanent loss of nephrons. Supporting this explanation are animal models of aminoglycoside nephrotoxicity that show residual areas of interstitial fibrosis in the renal cortex.[3, 4] In addition to reducing the glomerular filtration rate (GFR), aminoglycoside administration can cause enzymuria, proteinuria, aminoaciduria, glucosuria, and a variety of electrolyte disorders, including hypomagnesemia, hypocalcemia, and hypokalemia.[5-9]

Pathophysiology

The mechanisms involved in aminoglycoside nephrotoxicity are well studied. Because of their highly basic charge, aminoglycosides penetrate cell membranes poorly. However, to impair bacterial growth, and presumably to damage kidney cells, at least a small fraction of the administered aminoglycoside must gain access to the cell interior. Serum protein binding of aminoglycosides is minimal, and the renal clearance of gentamicin is very close to that of insulin, indicating little secretion or reabsorption.[10, 11] Of all the tissues in the body, the renal cortex stands alone in its ability to concentrate aminoglycosides several-fold greater than plasma. The relatively non-nephrotoxic streptomycin is the only exception to this rule. The proximal, but not distal, tubular cells concentrate aminoglycosides and are the cells that demonstrate significant injury in experimental nephrotoxicity in the rat.[12] Changes in proximal tubular cell morphology can be detected within hours of drug administration.[13] Gentamicin gains access to proximal tubular cells through pinocytosis occurring at the brush border membrane on the luminal surface of the cell. Studies of renal cortical tissue slices (in which gentamicin presumably cannot gain access to the tubule from the luminal side) also demonstrate tissue uptake of gentamicin, indicating uptake at the basolateral (contraluminal) surface as well.[14] Although transtubular secretion of gentamicin and netilmicin can be demonstrated by micropuncture techniques, glomerular filtration is quantitatively the most important route of aminoglycoside elimination.[15]

Once inside the cell, gentamicin binds to subcellular organelles or is taken up into lysosomes. The typical electron microscopic findings following the administration of gentamicin are an increase in the number of secondary lysosomes and the presence within them of myeloid bodies.[16] Aminoglycosides induce a lysosomal phospholipidosis.[17, 18] This probably occurs because the electrostatic attachment of aminoglycosides to anionic membrane phospholipids interferes with the normal action of phospholipases.[19, 20] How aminoglycoside-induced lysosomal dysfunction leads to cell injury and death is unclear. Release of aminoglycosides into the cytoplasm through permeabilized lysosomes could interfere with the phosphatidylinositol cascade and stimulation by agonists, as has been shown in cell culture.[21] The findings of this study are consistent with the possibility that aminoglycosides bind to phosphatidylinositol 4, 5-biphosphate (PIP_2) and prevent the hydrolysis of phospholipase C upon stimulation by agonists. The lysosomal system is not the only subcellular organelle affected by aminoglycosides. Measurement of fluorescent gentamicin uptake and movement within LLC-PK1 cells revealed the expected lysosomal uptake, but also showed early localization in the Golgi complex.[22] No uptake was

detected in endoplasmic reticulum, a likely target site for aminoglycosides to impair protein synthesis, but the detection methods may not have been sufficiently sensitive.

The role of free radicals in the pathogenesis of aminoglycoside nephrotoxicity is unsettled. In vivo and in vitro models of gentamicin nephrotoxicity show evidence supporting the production of free radicals, but studies designed to assess whether free radical scavengers protect against gentamicin nephrotoxicity are conflicting.[23-26] Tissue accumulation of aminoglycoside is an important factor in the generation of nephrotoxicity. In the rat, a subcutaneous injection of gentamicin, tobramycin, or kanamycin accumulates in high concentrations in the renal cortex, but streptomycin, an aminoglycoside with no nephrotoxicity, disappears rapidly. The half-life of gentamicin in renal tissue is 109 hours and, once concentrated in renal tissues, may take several months to be excreted.[27] The transport and accumulation of aminoglycosides in the renal cortex is mediated by a low-affinity, high-capacity system that is not easily saturable.[28, 29] The tissue accumulation of gentamicin and netilmicin is different, with a lower renal cortical accumulation noted for netilmicin. These findings are consistent with the observation that netilmicin has a lower absorptive flux and a higher secretory flux in the proximal tubule as compared with gentamicin.[28, 29] Thus, while both the apical and basolateral membranes of proximal tubular cells participate in aminoglycoside uptake, quantitatively the apical membrane is far more important.[30, 31] Other aminoglycosides and organic polycations appear to compete for the same transport system with a relative affinity that is directly related to the net cationic charge of the molecule.[28]

The membrane binding sites for aminoglycosides appear to be anionic phospholipids, PIP_2 being one of the most important.[32, 33] The epithelial glycoprotein (GP) 330/megalin is an endocytic receptor found in renal proximal tubules and is capable of binding gentamicin.[34] Anionic phospholipids and the GP 330 receptor may work in concert to bind and internalize aminoglycosides and other polybasic drugs.[34] Ischemia enhances apical membrane binding and internalization of gentamicin, an effect that is paralleled by a marked increase in the membrane content of phosphatidylinositol.[35]

The risk of developing aminoglycoside nephrotoxicity is affected by a number of factors (Table 34-2). The method of administration of aminoglycosides has a marked effect on

TABLE 34-2

Risk Factors for Development of Aminoglycoside Nephrotoxicity

INCREASED RISK	DECREASED RISK
Decreased absolute or effective circulatory volume	Organic polycations
Potassium deficiency	Urinary alkalinization
Endotoxemia	Thyroid hormone
Obesity	Potassium loading
Renal ischemia	Experimental diabetes
Liver disease	
Advanced age	
Coadministration of other nephrotoxins	

renal cortical uptake. Multiple injections cause greater tissue accumulation and nephrotoxicity than the same total dose on a weight basis given as a single bolus.[36] Other risk factors for nephrotoxicity that are associated with increased tissue accumulation of aminoglycosides are male sex, sodium depletion, potassium depletion, endotoxemia, obesity, and ischemia.[37-41] In contrast, a number of factors and interventions are associated with reduced renal tissue accumulation aminoglycosides and reduced nephrotoxicity, including administration of organic polycations, alkalinization of the urine, thyroid hormone administration, potassium chloride loading, and experimental diabetes mellitus.[28, 29, 42-44] Polyaspartic acid protects the rat against gentamicin nephrotoxicity through an effect that does not depend on decreased renal cortical uptake of the drug.[45-47] The protective effect appears to depend on polyaspartic acid preventing gentamicin from interacting with anionic phospholipids and is present even when gentamicin is administered in a dose three times higher than what normally is a nephrotoxic dose.[48, 49] The essential biochemical event that leads to protection may be that polyaspartic acid, by complexing to the aminoglycoside, prevents aminoglycoside inhibition of lysosomal phospholipases.[50] In the rat model, kallikrein gene delivery begun simultaneously with gentamicin administration leads to a threefold increase in GFr and renal blood flow and protection against nephrotoxicity.[51] The mechanism whereby the kallikrein gene, or possibly the enhanced renal hemodynamics, protected against nephrotoxicity, and specifically whether renal tissue accumulation of gentamicin was reduced, was not explored.

Although the intracellular concentration of aminoglycosides correlates roughly with nephrotoxicity, other factors also are involved. Administration of gentamicin to rats for 6 weeks leads to renal failure followed by recovery in spite of continued administration of the drug.[52] Although recovery of renal function occurs, the renal cortical concentration of gentamicin remains high. In a similar experimental model of aminoglycoside tolerance, proximal tubular cells that have recovered after 19 days of gentamicin administration show a reduced height and number of apical microvilli, have increased apical membrane binding of gentamicin, but have selected inhibition of uptake across the apical membrane.[53] Thus, increased binding but reduced internalization could explain renal functional recovery occurring in the presence of high tissue aminoglycoside levels.

How the aminoglycosides cause cell injury and cell death is unknown, but interactions with the cell membrane, as well as with intracellular structures such as lysosomes, mitochondria, and microsomes, are likely to be involved.[54-58] Bennett and associates demonstrated in the rat that organic acid transport (*p*-aminohippuric acid, PAH) is stimulated prior to development of overt renal failure, an effect possibly reflecting an early change in membrane permeability.[59] The reported effects of gentamicin on membrane fluidity are conflicting, with several indicating a decrease, but another reporting an increase.[60-62] The timing of the measurement may be important inasmuch as the report showing increased fluidity examined the brush border vesicles prior to a reduction in GFR.[62] In addition, this study detected a gentamicin-induced decrease in the V_{max} of Na^+/Pi cotransport and Na^+/H^+ exchange activity without an effect on $Na^+/glucose$ or $Na^+/$ proline cotransport activity, suggesting that the gentamicin

effects within the apical membrane are highly selective. In addition to tubular changes induced by gentamicin, at least one glomerular defect has been reported. Baylis and colleagues, using micropuncture techniques, demonstrated in the rat that gentamicin caused a marked decline in the glomerular capillary ultrafiltration coefficient (K_f) at a time when both whole-kidney GFR and single-nephron GFR had fallen by 30% to 50%.[63] Neither tubule obstruction nor renal ischemia appeared to be involved in the reduction of GFR.

Combining an aminoglycoside with a known nephrotoxin, such as amphotericin, cisplatin, and possibly x-ray contrast material, can enhance nephrotoxicity.[64-66] The combined use of aminoglycosides with cephalosporin or penicillin antibiotics does not seem to lead to enhanced nephrotoxicity. The combined use of aminoglycosides with vancomycin may be associated with a slightly greater incidence of nephrotoxicity (see later). Advanced age, shock, use of furosemide, liver disease, volume depletion, and prior renal insufficiency enhance aminoglycoside nephrotoxicity.[1, 67]

The specific aminoglycoside preparation utilized might also be an important factor in the frequency of nephrotoxicity. Laboratory and clinical studies demonstrate a direct relationship between the number of free amino groups on the aminoglycoside molecule and the risk of nephrotoxicity. In a prospective clinical study, nephrotoxicity developed in 19 (26%) of 72 patients given gentamicin and in 9 (12%) of 74 patients given tobramycin.[68] However, ototoxicity developed in 10% of patients receiving both drugs.

Aminoglycosides will continue to be valuable agents for the treatment of serious gram-negative infections. The nomograms and formulas designed to estimate the aminoglycoside dosage in patients with renal failure may be helpful in planning the initial dose of drug. For accurate determination of subsequent doses, peak levels (drawn 1 hour after injection) and trough levels (drawn immediately before the next calculated dose) are useful to ensure that adequate bactericidal serum levels are achieved. Individualized pharmacokinetic dosing programs for aminoglycosides are available in many hospitals, often in cooperation with the pharmacy service. Although these dosing programs appear to decrease the number of treatment failures, there is little indication that their use reduces nephrotoxicity.[1, 69, 70] Leehey and associates compared the incidence of aminoglycoside nephrotoxicity in a group of patients given drug dosages based on an estimate of creatinine clearance versus two groups given doses based on a bayesian pharmacokinetic computer program.[1] The incidence of nephrotoxicity did not differ between the groups and averaged 20%. Peak and trough aminoglycoside blood levels have been proposed as indicators of aminoglycoside nephrotoxicity.[67, 71, 72] However, there is little evidence to support the belief that the blood level of these agents is an important risk factor for, or indicator of, nephrotoxicity. When prospectively followed, mean peak and trough levels were not associated with nephrotoxicity.[1] Bennett and associates have shown in the rat that a single large dose of gentamicin producing a high peak blood level was less nephrotoxic than the same amount given in divided doses in which the resulting peak blood levels were much lower.[73] A rising trough level, rather than indicating impending nephrotoxicity, represents drug retention due to an already reduced GFR.

Prevention

In attempting to minimize clinical nephrotoxicity, several points should be emphasized. Aminoglycoside nephrotoxicity is directly dependent on the dose and duration of drug administration.[1] Thus, nephrotoxicity is more likely to be apparent when large doses of aminoglycosides are given over prolonged periods, or when usual doses are given to individuals with renal impairment who have diminished capacity to excrete the drugs. The goal of treatment should be the lowest dose and shortest course of therapy compatible with clinical cure. The recent clinical success of once-daily aminoglycoside dosing schedules indicates that the efficacy of these valuable agents can be retained while the cost of managing toxicity is reduced, and toxicity is no worse and possibly reduced.[74-80]

When aminoglycoside therapy is empirically begun for an infection subsequently proved to be due to an aerobic gram-negative bacillus, therapy should be changed to a less toxic agent, even if the patient is responding satisfactorily during the initial aminoglycoside therapy. Empiric aminoglycoside therapy in a patient with presumed sepsis or other serious infection must be re-evaluated when culture results are available. A "clinical response" in the absence of positive cultures is not usually sufficient justification for prolonged treatment with an empirically started aminoglycoside. It is appropriate to think of aminoglycosides as nephrotoxins for all patients who receive them. In most patients, nephrotoxicity is subclinical and beyond detection with the usual tests (e.g., serum creatinine, creatinine clearance). Nevertheless, serial monitoring of renal function (e.g., serum creatinine every other day) should be carried out in patients receiving these aminoglycosides.

Concomitant administration of other potential nephrotoxins (radiographic contrast material, amphotericin, cisplatin, diuretics) should be avoided. Extracellular fluid volume and renal perfusion should be optimized during aminoglycoside therapy, inasmuch as renal tissue accumulation of aminoglycosides is enhanced during states of volume depletion. Dosing should be based on the best index of GFR available. A steady-state serum creatinine concentration often suffices. However, in elderly patients or patients with diminished renal function, a creatinine clearance is preferable. When the clinical response to aminoglycoside treatment is inadequate, assessment of plasma drug levels is often helpful, particularly when impaired renal function is present.

Penicillins and Cephalosporins

True nephrotoxic reactions with penicillins and cephalosporins are rare. The only agent with a clear potential to cause nephrotoxicity is cephaloridine, an antibiotic that has not been used for more than 15 years. More often, acute interstitial nephritis is the cause of altered renal function with these agents.

Vancomycin

Vancomycin is valuable for the treatment of gram-positive infections, particularly methicillin-resistant staphylococcal infections, *Staphylococcus epidermidis* infections, and *Clostridium difficile* diarrhea. It is particularly useful in patients on hemodialysis where weekly or twice-weekly intravenous injections may be all the drug that is required. The early formulations of this drug carried a substantial nephrotoxic potential, but current preparations are largely free of this adverse effect. Used alone, the incidence of vancomycin nephrotoxicity is reported to be 5%, defined as a rise in serum creatinine level of 0.5 mg/dL.[81] Whether aminoglycoside administration with vancomycin has a synergistic nephrotoxic effect is unclear. Retrospective and prospective studies report that 5% to 35% of patients given this combination experience nephrotoxicity.[81-85] Without knowing the incidence of aminoglycoside nephrotoxicity in a separate control group given only aminoglycosides, it is impossible to determine whether these incidence figures represent synergy or simply the nephrotoxicity of the aminoglycoside alone.

Sulfonamides

Most cases of sulfonamide-induced renal disease represent acute interstitial nephritis. However, in the presence of an acid urine (pH < 5.5), several of these agents are capable of precipitating in tubule urine, causing an acute intratubular obstructive nephropathy. The recent use of high doses of sulfadiazine and sulfamethoxazole for aquired immunodeficiency syndrome (AIDS)–related diseases has led to a resurgence of this form of acute renal failure.[86-89] The crystals caused by sulfadiazine resemble shocks of wheat and are formed by its primary metabolite, acetylsulfadiazine.[87] Renal failure can be prevented by increasing fluid intake during therapy and by maintaining an alkaline urine, which increases the solubility of these drugs in the urine.

Amphotericin

Amphotericin B is a polyene antibiotic containing a hydrophilic backbone as well as a lipophilic region. These characteristics allow the drug to complex with sterol moieties in cell membranes, disrupt them, and increase their permeability.[90] Amphotericin also causes renal vasoconstriction leading to renal ischemia, and may be the cause of structural injury.[91-93] Amphotericin B use has increased with the rise in the number of fungal infections in patients with AIDS and the increasing number of immunosuppressed organ transplant recipients.

Nephrotoxicity with amphotericin B is initially a distal tubular phenomenon characterized by a loss of urinary concentration, distal renal tubule acidosis, and wasting of potassium and magnesium.[94] However, chronic administration of amphotericin in the rat also leads to medullary injury, an effect that appears to be due to hypoxia. Chronic amphotericin nephrotoxicity may in part be mediated by elevated endothelin levels.[95] Nearly all patients receiving amphotericin will experience a rise serum creatinine. Fortunately, azotemia is rarely severe and a small dosage reduction or short-term interruption of therapy is usually sufficient to reverse the azotemia such that drug administration can be started. The most important risk factor for nephrotoxicity is salt depletion.[96-98] This has led to the common practice of saline loading prior to and during drug administration.[99-100] Newer preparations, including liposome-encapsulated amphotericin B and lipid complex formulations of the drug, are less nephrotoxic in experimental animals and in humans.[101-103]

ANTIVIRAL AND ANTIPROTOZOAL AGENTS

Acyclovir and Ganciclovir

Acyclovir is an antiviral agent used in the treatment of herpes infections. When given by the intravenous route in doses of 500 mg/m^2, it can cause both nephrotoxicity and neurotoxicity.[104, 105] Acyclovir is excreted by the kidney through the processes of glomerular filtration and tubular secretion; it has a low solubility in urine. Nephrotoxicity results from intratubular precipitation leading to tubular obstruction. Clinical signs of nephrotoxicity include nausea, flank pain, and hematuria.[106] Urinalysis may show needle-shaped crystals under polarizing light. Interstitial inflammation may be seen adjacent to areas of intratubular obstruction.[106] Although an occasional patient may require hemodialysis, most experience nonoliguric acute renal failure.[105] Withdrawal of therapy usually leads to recovery of near-normal renal function within several days.[107] Patients who experience nephrotoxicity may be rechallenged with a lower dose, usually less than 250 mg/m^2.[105] Volume depletion predisposes to nephrotoxicity and most cases can probably be prevented by vigorous hydration before and during infusion.[108] Ganciclovir, an antiviral related structurally to acyclovir and used in the treatment of chorioretinitis, does not seem to be nephrotoxic.

Pentamidine

Intravenous pentamidine is commonly used to treat *Pneumocystis carinii* pneumonia, but nephrotoxicity occurs in 25% to 65% of patients.[109, 110] Nephrotoxicity following nebulized pentamidine is a rarity.[111] Pharmacokinetic studies indicate that the intravenous half-life of pentamidine is approximately 6.5 hours.[112] The apparent volume of distribution of pentamidine is very large, averaging 205 L in five adults with normal renal function (creatinine clearance > 80 mL/minute). The kidney accounts for less than 5% of plasma clearance of pentamidine and, not unexpectedly, dialysis removes little drug.[112]

Like aminoglycoside antibiotics, accumulation of pentamidine in real tissue occurs following multiple doses and the drug can be detected in plasma and urine weeks after completion of therapy.[113, 114] Although the mechanism of nephrotoxicity is incompletely understood, pentamidine is clearly a tubular toxin. Hypocalcemia, hypomagnesemia with an inappropriately high fractional excretion of magnesium, and hyperkalemia occur with prolonged therapy.[113, 114] The simultaneous use of amphotericin with pentamidine appears to be synergistic in causing nephrotoxicity.[115]

Foscarnet

Foscarnet is a pyrophosphate analog, which acts by inhibiting DNA polymerase, RNA polymerase, and reverse transcriptase, depending on the viral species.[116, 117] Intravenous foscarnet is used in the management of cytomegalovirus infection in transplant recipients, and more recently in patients with human immunodeficiency virus (HIV) infection and clinical AIDS. It is used topically for genital herpes. The kidney is the only apparent organ of excretion and the drug is not biotransformed. Nephrotoxicity occurs in up to 66% of patients.[118, 119] Postmortem histopathology showed proximal tubular necrosis in one patient dying with acute renal failure following foscarnet treatment.[118] In a group of 27 patients receiving foscarnet, intravenous saline administration before and during drug administration (2.5 L/24 hours) virtually eliminated nephrotoxicity.[118]

Hypocalcemia, hyperphosphatemia, and increased serum parathyroid hormone developed in some patients during foscarnet treatment.[118-120] The etiology of hyperphosphatemia is not certain, but suggested possibilities include foscarnet deposition in bone with release of stored phosphorus or inhibition of Na$^+$/Pi cotransport in the proximal tubule by foscarnet.[119] Hypocalcemia and elevated serum parathyroid hormone levels suggest bony resistance to the effect of parathyroid hormone. Foscarnet can be successfully administered to patients on hemodialysis.[121]

Antiretroviral Therapy

INDINAVIR. Indinavir is a protease inhibitor that can result in crystalluria and nephrolithiasis due to the precipitation of indinavir monohydrate in the tubules. Asymtomatic crystalluria occurs in approximately 4% to 10% of treated patients.[122] Fewer than 5% of patients develop symptoms of loin pain and hematuria. In some cases intratubular obstruction with crystals can incite a local interstitial inflammatory reaction giving rise to granuloma formation. This process can lead to interstitial fibrosis and tubular atrophy, eventually causing irreversible renal failure in some patients.[123]

ADEFOVIR. Adefovir is a nucleoside reverse transcriptase inhibitor that is primarily excreted unchanged in the urine. Adefovir is associated with proximal tubular injury characterized by phosphaturia, low-grade proteinuria, and a rise in the serum creatinine concentration. Proximal tubular dysfunction has been noted in more that 35% of patients within the first year of therapy. Discontinuation of therapy usually results in recovery of renal function. Adefovir-induced nephrotoxicity is mediated by a direct toxic effect on the replication of mitochondrial DNA responsible for the synthesis of cytochrome-*c* oxidase.[124] Inhibition of this oxidase leads to the accumulation of free oxygen radicals that can then result in tubular injury. Mitochondrial toxicity may also explain the association between use of nucleoside analogs and the development of lactic acidosis.[125]

RADIOCONTRAST AGENTS

Radiocontrast acute renal failure is more likely to occur in the presence of advanced age, renal insufficiency, diabetes mellitus, severe congestive heart failure, multiple myeloma, volume depletion, low cardiac output states, and high-dose contrast studies (> 125 mL)[126, 127] (Table 34-3). The incidence of nephrotoxicity varies depending on the underlying risk factors and the sensitivity of the measure used to determine nephrotoxicity. Using a rather sensitive index of renal dysfunction (an increase in the level of serum creatinine > 0.3 mg/dL and > 20% on day 1, 2, or 3 and day 5, 6, or 7), the incidence of nephrotoxicity was 2% in nondiabetic, nonazotemic patients and 16% in diabetic, nonazotemic patients.[128] Diabetic patients with azotemia had a 38% incidence of nephrotoxicity. In another study of 59 diabetic

TABLE 34-3

Risk Factors for Radiocontrast Nephrotoxicity

Advanced age
Renal insufficiency
Decreased absolute and effective circulatory volume
Diabetes mellitus
Multiple myeloma
Coadministration of other nephrotoxic agents

patients with advanced azotemia (mean serum creatinine of 5.9 mg/dL) undergoing coronary angiography, 30 (51%) developed contrast nephrotoxicity as defined by a serum creatinine that was 25% above baseline 48 hours after angiography. Nine patients (15%) required hemodialysis.[129]

The warning against using radiocontrast in the presence of multiple myeloma appears to be relative rather than absolute. In a retrospective review of 476 patients with multiple myeloma undergoing radiocontrast studies, the incidence of acute renal failure was 0.6% to 1.25%, substantially higher than the reported incidence of 0.15% in the general population as reported by Byrd and Sherman,[130] yet not so prohibitive that contrast could not be used if the clinical indications are compelling.[130-131]

Renal failure may be oliguric or nonoliguric, with nonoliguric renal failure being more common in patients with near-normal prior renal function. Most episodes of contrast nephrotoxicity are mild, characterized by a reversible 1 to 3 mg/dL rise in serum creatinine; dialysis therapy is rarely needed and usually only in those patients whose baseline serum creatinine is high, for example, greater than 3 mg/dL.[128, 132-136] Many episodes of radiocontrast nephrotoxicity are probably not clinically apparent, characterized by an episode of nonoliguric acute renal failure with a 0.5 to 3.0 mg/dL rise in the serum creatinine. Unlike ischemia-induced acute renal failure, where the urinary sodium valve is characteristically high, radiocontrast nephrotoxicity may be associated with a low urinary sodium concentration (<10 mEq/L).[137, 138] The effect of radiocontrast on the urinalysis is variable. Renal tubular epithelial cell casts or coarsely granular casts may or may not be present in the presence or absence of functional deterioration.[133, 139] A persistent nephrogram during the 24 to 48 hours following the administration of radiocontrast is a characteristic and sensitive indicator of contrast nephropathy, but there are many false positives, giving it a low predictive value of 19%.[134]

Pathologic findings are restricted to the proximal tubule. The characteristic finding is an intense vacuolization of the proximal tubule called osmotic nephrosis but the origin of the vacuoles is uncertain and they have not been shown to contain iodine.[140, 141] Heyman and colleagues have suggested that endocytosis is not the cause, but rather the vacuoles represent invaginations of the lateral cell membrane of the proximal tubules.[142]

The pathogenesis of radiocontrast nephrotoxicity has been elusive. A healthy kidney is very resistant to radiocontrast injury. Most animal models require that renal function be compromised in some way before exposure to contrast impairs function.[142, 143] One study correlated renal functional injury with damage to the more distal and highly

oxygen-dependent medullary thick ascending limb (MTAL), an effect that may result from damage to Na^+,K^+-ATPase in the basolateral membrane.[142] The vasodilator properties of nitric oxide and prostanoids also appear to be important in protecting this segment of the nephron from radiocontrast nephrotoxicity.[144] Renal vasoconstriction develops transiently following administration of radiocontrast and could play a role in the pathogenesis of contrast nephrotoxicity. The vasoconstriction appears to be a calcium-dependent effect because it can be blocked with calcium channel blockers, but not α-blockers.[145, 146] In vitro and in vivo studies show that both ionic and nonionic contrast agents induce release of the potent vasoconstrictor endothelin, suggesting a possible local mediator of contrast-induced vasoconstriction.[147] However, ioversol, a nonionic, low-molecular-weight contrast medium, is less nephrotoxic that iothalamate and has a reduced tendency to stimulate release of endothelin, both in vivo and in vitro. This finding lends support to the idea that radiocontrast toxicity is linked to endothelin release.[148] Rats fed a high-cholesterol diet have a lower insulin clearance and renal blood flow following radiocontrast, presumably related to an effect of hypercholesterolemia to impair endothelium-dependent vasodilation.[149] The ability of L-arginine, a precursor of nitric oxide formation, to attenuate nephrotoxicity upon exposure to radiocontrast in hypercholesterolemic rats suggested to the authors that nitric oxide was important in the pathogenesis of renal hemodynamic changes. Evidence against the role of renal vasoconstriction as an important element of radiocontrast nephrotoxicity is the observation that intracardiac injection of radiocontrast is not associated with a fall in total renal blood flow in most patients with chronic renal failure.[150] In addition, the clinical use of dopamine, a potent renal vasodilator, in high-risk patients with chronic renal failure, before and during angiography does not reduce the incidence of nephrotoxicity.[151]

Prevention of radiocontrast nephrotoxicity includes cautious volume expansion with saline before the procedure and the use of the lowest possible dose of contrast. Addition of mannitol or furosemide to saline expansion adds no additional protection, and furosemide may enhance toxicity.[152] Although the nonionic contrast agents cause fewer allergic, cardiovascular, and endothelial reactions than the ionic agents, there is still uncertainty about whether their use leads to reduced nephrotoxicity.[153] In vitro studies suggest that cellular injury is less likely from nonionic agents.[154] However, clinical studies are in the disagreement on this point, with some showing no benefit of nonionic agents in lowering the incidence of nephrotoxicity in high-risk patients and others showing less nephrotoxicity.[155-160] A meta-analysis of 45 trials dealing with this question indicates that low-osmolality contrast material is associated with reduced nephrotoxicity.[161]

DRUGS USED IN TRANSPLANTATION

Cyclosporine

Cyclosporine causes acute reversible nephrotoxicity, as well as a chronic, largely irreversible nephrotoxicity. During the early phase of cyclosporine treatment in humans, vasoconstriction develops in the systemic circulation, leading to arterial hypertension.[162, 163] In the kidney, cyclosporine causes vasoconstriction of both the afferent and efferent glomerular arterioles.[164] This leads to a reduction in glomerular plasma flow and GFR and the rapidly reversible prerenal azotemia seen with large doses. However, tubular reabsorption and secretion remain largely intact.[165] Cyclosporine appears to enhance the renal vascular reactivity to certain vasoconstrictors while also diminishing the responsivity to certain vasodilators, possibly mediated by a reduced endothelial capacity to produce nitric oxide.[164, 166] Activation of the renin-angiotensin and sympathetic nervous systems, although present, seems not to play an important role in this vasoconstriction. However, increased intracellular calcium, endothelial injury with release of endothelin, and reduced vasodilator prostaglandins appear to be prominently involved.[167-169] In vitro studies show that the afferent and efferent glomerular arterioles vasoconstrict in a concentration-dependent way following exposure to cyclosporine, with the afferent arteriole being more sensitive.[170] A receptor antagonist for endothelin was able to block cyclsporine afferent arteriole vasoconstriction, but not that in the efferent arteriole. In another study, afferent arteriole vasoconstriction, but not efferent arteriole vasoconstriction, was blocked by a cyclooxygenase inhibitor, indicating that locally released cyclooxygenase products mediated sustained cyclosporine vasoconstriction.[171]

Within hours of each oral dose of cyclosporine in renal transplant recipients, there is a reduction in renal plasma flow and GFR. Calcium channel blockers can provide some protection against early cyclosporine nephrotoxicity in laboratory animals and humans.[172-176] In addition, several reports of long-term transplant recipients receiving cyclosporine suggest that calcium channel blockers improve graft survival and diminish long-term cyclosporine nephrotoxicity, but other studies have not found a beneficial effect.[177-180] Cyclosporine influences the production of several prostaglandins in vitro and in vivo.[181-185] Misoprostol, a prostaglandin E analog, can largely reverse the acute vasoconstrctive effects of cyclosporine in experimental animals and can reduce the incidence of acute rejection in renal transplant recipients treated with cyclosporine.[185, 186] However, another prostaglandin E analog, enisoprost, failed to improve renal function when given to human renal allograft recipients acutely or chronically exposed to cyclosporine.[187, 188] In addition, blockade of thromboxane A_2 in experimental animals affords some protection against the vasoconstriction.[189]

Chronic cyclosporine nephrotoxicity, as described in cardiac transplant recipients and patients with autoimmune disease with initially normal renal function, is characterized by a 35% to 45% reduction in GFR compared with patients not treated with cyclosporine. End-stage renal disease requiring chronic hemodialysis was reported in 6.5% of cardiac transplant recipients.[190] In addition, the ability of cyclosporine to reduce acute renal allograft loss, but not to improve chronic allograft survival, suggests that a similar nephrotoxic effect is occurring in renal transplant recipients as well.

Chronic cyclosporine administration causes an obliterative arteriolopathy that results in a form of interstitial nephritis and a progressive, largely irreversible decline in renal function. A peculiar form of tubulointerstitial damage called striped interstitial fibrosis is probably due to tubular collapse induced by constriction of the afferent arteriole. Cyclosporine nephropathy is associated with increased apoptosis of tubular and interstitial cells and appears to be partly mediated by the vasoconstrictor angiotensin II and the

inhibition of the vasodilator properties of nitric oxide.[191] An analog of cyclosporine, cyclosporin G, appears to be less nephrotoxic in the rat model.[192] Cyclosporine also is a direct cellular toxin, causing hyperkalemia, hypophosphatemia, impaired urinary concentration, and a hyperchloremic acidosis.

FK-506

FK-506 (tacrolimas), a potent immunosuppressive agent, is similar to cyclosporine in its effect on T cell function; it binds to an immunophilin, FK-506–binding protein, and prevents signal transduction pathways in the lymphocyte.[193] It has been used primarily in liver transplant recipients, but it has also found a use in kidney and heart transplant recipients. Early use of this drug was confined initially to one center and, although nephrotoxicity was reported as an adverse consequence, details about its effect on kidney function and comparisons with other immunosuppressive agents were scant. In two groups of liver transplant recipients 4 weeks after transplant, FK-506 caused less systemic hypertension than cyclosporine, but had quite similar effects on the kidney, that is, a significant reduction in renal blood flow and GFR.[194] FK-506 and cyclosporine have similar depressing effects on the level of urinary thromboxane B_2, plasma renin activity, and plasma aldosterone; FK-506 had a significantly greater effect in reducing the urinary excretion of 6-keto-$PGF_{1\alpha}$, the stable arachidonate of prostacyclin, a renal vasodilator. A subsequent study from these same investigators of liver transplant recipients demonstrates a significantly lower GFR at 12 months in the FK-506 group compared with the cyclosporine group (45 ± 4 vs. 64 ± 6 mL/minute per body surface area, $P < .05$). Severe early nephrotoxic reactions were seen only in some patients who received FK-506.[195] Renal tubular damage from FK-506 results in a 50% incidence of hyperkalemia.[196] Like cyclosporine, long-term administration of FK-506 produces striped interstitial fibrosis in the renal cortex, suggesting that, despite their chemical dissimilarity, they probably share a common pathway in producing nephrotoxicity.[197]

ANTINEOPLASTIC DRUGS

Cisplatin

Cisplatin (*cis*-diamminedichloroplatinum) is a highly effective antineoplastic agent with a very broad spetrum of antitumor activity.[198-203] The drug has been shown to be effective in several different types of cancer, particularly testicular, ovarian, small cell of the lung, and head, neck, and bladder cancers.[198-203] In addition to being useful against primary solid tumors, cisplatin has also been helpful in improving the outlook for patients who suffer from metastatic testicular and ovarian carcinomas.[204] The major toxicity of cisplatin therapy has been the nephrotoxicity that occurs with successive treatments of the drug. The toxicity observed in patients was predicted by early studies that showed renal injury as a major problem.[205] An unusual feature of cisplating nephrotoxicity is that in many cases the renal damage is irreversible.

The usual pattern of cisplatin nephrotoxicity is that of a dose-related and cumulative form of renal failure noted after one or more doses of the drug. This toxicity may be gradual and subtle or, on occasion, abrupt. The renal damage incurred by cisplatin is often irreversible. The hallmark of the nephrotoxicity is a tubulointerstitial pattern of injury without heavy proteinuria. Tubular proteinuria and prominent tubular casts may be a particularly impressive feature of the clinical presentation.[206] Beta$_2$-microglobulin excretion has also been demonstrated to antedate renal failure, suggesting that renal tubular damage may occur on a subclinical level before an increase in the serum creatinine concentration.[207] A recent study suggested retinol-binding protein was a valuable marker for assessing early cisplatin nephrotoxicity.[208] The pathology of the lesion is one of tubular damage with impressive light and electron microscopic changes that show hyaline droplets in the proximal tubular cells, degeneration of the tubular basement membrane, and areas of final tubular necrosis.[209] The glomeruli and blood vessels are largely spared these processes.

As might be expected, a variety of clinically apparent tubular defects occur in the presence of cisplatin nephrotoxicity: renal magnesium wasting, hyperphosphaturia, and disorders of renal calcium and amino acid handling have all been reported.[210-212] The renal magnesium wasting associated with cisplatin is particularly notable, mainly because the hypomagnesemia that results may be severe and be accompanied by hypocalcemia and tetany. In a particularly large series of patients who received 70 mg/m^2 cisplatin every 3 weeks, 52% of patients were hypomagnesemic.[213] The peak incidence of hypomagnesemia occurred 3 weeks following therapy; it should be noted that the hypomagnesemia associated with cisplatin has been observed to be exacerbated by the concomitant use of other drugs, particularly the aminoglycoside antibiotics.[214-216] This defect in renal magnesium handling usually abates after a period of weeks and is easily treated with oral magnesium supplementation. There are exceptions to this pattern, however, as some patients have had persistent hypomagnesemia lasting for years.[217]

The exact mechanism of cisplatin nephrotoxicity is unclear. Experimental studies have shown that there is an abrupt fall in the effective renal plasma flow within 3 hours of the first dose of cisplatin.[218] Cisplatin in known to be filtered by the glomeruli and concentrated in the glomerular filtrate from which it gains entrance into proximal tubular cells. It is activated in the presence of a low intracellular chloride concentration and the aquated or activated agent forms intrastrand and interstrand cross-links between DNA molecules.[219] [Renal damage is seen in the S3 portion of the proximal tubule, the distal tubule, and the collecting duct.[219-220]] Glomeruli are relatively well preserved despite the extensive damage to tubular elements.[221] More research is needed to clarify the effects of cisplatin on potent oxidative (cytochrome P-450 oxidase) and reducing substances (glutathione transferase) that are well known to be abundant in renal tubular cells. A recent study by Matushima and colleagues found that cisplatin-induced proximal tubule injury in rats could be ameliorated by the administration of hydroxyl radical scavengers.[222] In these studies in rats, cisplatin (5 mg/kg body weight) caused lipid peroxidation; the hydroxyl radical scavenger prevented acute renal failure by attenuating tubule damage and enhancing the regenerative response of damaged tubule cells, and a superoxide anion scavenger had a similar effect by preserving renal

blood flow.[222] This proposed mechanism of hydroxyl radical–induced injury is supported by data that iron may be released from cells upon exposure to cisplatin and cause oxidant damage.[223] The S3 portion of the proximal tubule may be more vulnerable to oxidant injury and mitochondrial dysfunction occurs by inhibition of complexes I to IV of the respiratory chain.[224, 225] The precise mechanism by which the respiratory chain is affected by generated reactive oxygen species is unclear.[225]

Some investigators have postulated a role for the renin-angiotensin system in the pathogenesis of cisplatin nephrotoxicity, but studies testing the effects of angiotensin receptor blockade on toxicity suggest acute toxicity is not ameliorated.[226] Protection from cisplatin toxicity has generally focused on providing free radical scavengers, N-acetylcysteine, and methylprednisolone.[227-229] Other strategies to reduce nephrotoxicity have included reducing the dose and giving it over a longer period, and volume expansion (see later).[230-232] As mentioned earlier, renal tubule dysfunction may persist well after cisplatin therapy has been completed, and, if this occurs, hypocalcemia may be a common feature of the clinical presentation.[233] A worrisome feature of cisplatin toxicity is that, despite measures to avoid toxicity, silently progressive renal tubulointerstitial damage leading to a gradual decline in GFR can occur both experimentally and in humans.[234, 235]

The first step in preventing cisplatin nephrotoxicity is to avoid the concomitant use of other agents that are known to induce nephrotoxicity, such as aminoglycoside antibiotics. In addition, given the relationship of the toxicity to the dose administered, careful attention to the necessary dose is of key importance. Doses of cisplatin exceeding 25 to 33 mg/m^2/week predispose to nephrotoxicity and other toxicities, including ototoxicity and myelosuppression.[236] It is clear that a significant reduction in the incidence of cisplatin nephrotoxicity can be achieved by induction of a brisk diuresis. A urine output of at least 100 mL/hour for several hours before and after a dose of cisplatin reduces the nephrotoxicity.[237] Several studies have shown that the use of mannitol or furosemide to produce a natriuresis allows doses of cisplatin of up to 100 to 120 mg/m^2 without toxicity.[238] The administration of cisplatin is also better tolerated if the dose is administered in hypertonic saline, which does not alter the pharmacokinetics of cisplatin.[239-241] Some authors now suggest that the saline infusion precede the dose of cisplatin by 12 hours and be extended for another 12 hours following the completion of the cisplatin dose.[241] These protective maneuvers have recently been summarized.[242]

Additional renal protective measures that may be undertaken to prevent cisplatin nephrotoxicity include the concomitant administration of sodium thiosulfate, which is recommended in patients who are to receive in excess of 200 mg/m^2 cisplatin. Sodium thiosulfate alters the pharmacokinetics of cisplatin, resulting in a reduction in the fall in the white blood cell count, platelet count, and also less neurotoxicity and vomiting. In one recent study, the concomitant use of sodium thiosulfate allowed for a significant dose intensification of cisplatin chemotherapy in patients receiving biweekly administration of the antineoplastic drug.[236] In this study, although sodium thiosulfate was effective in reducing nephrotoxicity, other types of toxicity, including myelosuppression, were not reduced. The therapeutic goal of this therapy is to shorten the cycle intervals of cisplatin therapy and thereby increase dosage intensity.

In addition to sodium thiosulfate as a drug to reduce the toxicity of cisplatin, other protective agents have undergone testing recently, including amifostine (WR-2721), diethyl-dithiocarbamate (DDTC), ORG-2766, free radical scavengers, *N*-acetylcysteine, and methylprednisolone.[227-229] These drugs require further testing to determine whether they reduce nephrotoxicity. Strategies to reduce the accumulation of cisplatin in the kidney include the use of probenecid, but this approach has not been tested extensively.[243] Finally, new platinum compounds are expected to reduce the dependence of the oncologist on cisplatin, including carboplatin (*cis*-diamminecyclobutane dicarboxylatoplatinum II). A list of several antineoplastic agents and the type of toxicity caused is provided in Table 34-4.

Carboplatin

Carboplatin was approved for clinical use in 1989 and has less nephrotoxicity than cisplatin; however, myelosuppression and thrombocytopenia remain as features of carboplatin toxicity.[244-246] This drug was synthesized to be a nonnephrotoxic platinum analog.[247] Carboplatin is available for use as chemotherapy for ovarian, small cell of the lung, and head and neck cancers. The usual dose of carboplatin is 400 to 500 mg/m² every 4 weeks when used as a single agent.[248] When used in combination with other chemotherapy, carboplatin doses of 250 mg/m² have been very well tolerated.[249] Several dose escalation studies have shown that nephrotoxicity is detectable in increasing frequency at doses greater than 900 mg/m².[250, 251] However most of this nephrotoxicity occurred in patients who had received cisplatin previously or who were receiving other nephrotoxic drugs during preparation for autologous bone marrow transplantation. As to specific nephrotoxicity with carboplatin, hypomagnesemia

appears to be the most common manifestation.[252] Combination of carboplatin, etoposide, and ifosfamide for solid tumor and lymphoma treatment results in nephrotoxicity in as many as 29% of patients[253]; the nephrotoxicity is usually reversible. Efforts to reduce nephrotoxicity include careful attention to dose optimization and the area under the curve in the drug's pharmacokinetics.[254] In addition, free radical scavengers such as amifostine may be useful in reducing carboplatin toxicity.[227] Finally, although hypermagnesuria is the most common clinical manifestation of carboplatin administration, recurrent salt wasting has been reported in at least one instance.[255]

Cyclophosphamide

Cyclophosphamide is a highly useful antineoplastic agent with significant antitumor activity against lymphomas and hematologic malignancies. Primary side effects of the drug include a myelosuppressive effect, gastrointestinal symptoms, and hemorrhagic cystitis. The primary renal effect of cyclophosphamide has been that of hyponatremia, which has been observed with doses of 50 mg/kg.[256] The hyponatremia involves impaired water excretion because urine osmolality is high in the face of a decreased plasma osmolality. This effect is dissipated by approximately 24 hours after the drug has been discontinued and is caused via a direct antidiuretic effect in the distal nephron and not through increased levels of vasopressin.[257]

Streptozotocin

Streptozotocin is a nonmyelosuppressive nitrosourea that is utilized in the management of patients with metastatic carcinoma of the pancreas and carcinoid tumors.[258] Some kidney dysfunction occurs in approximately 65% of patients who are exposed to this drug.[259-261] In most cases,

TABLE 34-4

Nephrotoxicity of Chemotherapeutic Drugs

DRUG	REPORTED TOXICITY
Alkylating Agents	
Cisplatin	Tubulointerstitial nephritis (TIN) occasionally irreversible; often acute renal failure
Carboplatin	Less nephrotoxic than cisplatin; can cause acute renal failure secondary to TIN
Cyclophosphamide	Associated with hyponatremia; also causes hemorrhagic cystitis
Streptozocin	Nitrosourea compound; renal dysfunction in 65% of patients; acute renal failure secondary to TIN
Semustine, carmustine	Nitrosourea compounds that can lead to chronic deterioration in renal function 3 yr after therapy; semustine is more nephrotoxic than carmustine
Ifosfamide	Nephrogenic diabetes insipidus and direct toxic injury to proximal and distal tubule
Antibiotics	
Mitomycin C	Hemolytic-uremic syndrome
Plicamycin	Nephrotoxic injury in as many as 40% of patients with long-term treatment; causes proximal and distal tubule damage
Antimetabolites	
Methotrexate	Volume expansion reduces nephrotoxic risk; intratubule deposition of 7-hydroxymethotrexate a factor in toxicity; also causes direct tubule damage; associated with nonoliguric acute renal failure
Cytarabine	Associated with TIN
6-Thioguanine	Parenteral administration and high doses associated with azotemia and acute renal failure syndrome
5-Fluorouracil	Associated with acute renal failure, often in combination with other drugs; less nephrotoxic than methotrexate
Interleukin-2	High doses cause acute renal failure in ~ 90%; avoid use with nonsteroidal anti-inflammatory drugs

proteinuria antedates the development of azotemia. It appears that the rate of streptozotocin administration plays a larger role in the development of nephrotoxicity than the total cumulative dose. A total weekly dose of 1.0 to 1.5 g/m^2 is safe and effective. However, a cumulative dose of greater than 4 g/m^2 has been associated with a higher incidence of toxicity.

Semustine and Carmustine

Semustine is a nitrosourea useful in the therapy of malignant melanoma and some lymphomas. This drug is lipid-soluble and therefore has also been used as a chemotherapeutic agent in the treatment of malignant brain tumors because it crosses the blood-brain barrier easily. High-dose therapy (1500 mg/m^2) in children with brain tumors resulted in a pattern of insidious renal failure leading to renal insufficiency some 3 to 5 years after the onset of therapy.[262] The renal pathology in these patients included a modest lymphocytic infiltrate accompanied by interstitial fibrosis. Doses greater than 1400 mg/m^2 for therapy of malignant melanoma in adults have resulted in a similar interstitial nephritis in these patients.[263] However, doses less than 1400 mg/m^2 are not typically associated with nephrotoxicity in adults. Multiple doses of nitrosoureas have previously been associated with a very high incidence of interstitial and glomerular scarring.[264]

Carmustine is another nitrosourea compound that has been associated with a very mild interstitial infiltrate and tubular changes. The main side effect of this drug is a proclivity to cause an interstitial pneumonitis.

Ifosfamide

Ifosfamide is an alkylating agent that has as its major side effect hemorrhagic cystitis, but it has also been associated with renal tubular toxicity. The incidence of clinical nephrotoxicity is believed to be less than 10%, but some cases of irreversible renal failure have been noted. Damage induced by ifosfamide is typically concentrated in the proximal tubule in experimental animals, and Fanconi syndrome has been observed following therapy.[265] Patients with preexisting renal dysfunction may be more vulnerable to the nephrotoxic effects of ifosfamide.[266, 267] Doses of 6 g/m^2 of ifosfamide result in detectable increases in both proximal and distal tubular enzymes in the urine; recently β_2-microglobulin and Tamm-Horsfall protein have been suggested as markers useful in predicting toxicity.[268-270] Clinically, the occurrence of nephrogenic diabetes insipidus has been linked to therapy with ifosfamide.[266-272] In addition, Elias and associates have reported that 72% of patients administered doses of ifosfamide of 8 to 18 g/m^2 (given over 4 days) developed renal tubular acidosis and 24% of the patients went on to develop serum creatinine levels greater than 2.0 mg/dL.[273] The pathogenesis of these lesions is difficult to determine because of the frequent combination of ifosfamide with other chemotherapeutic agents such as cisplatin.[274] Renal metabolism of ifosfamide may produce other toxic metabolites of ifosfamide.[275] Recently, uninephrectomy has been suggested to be a risk factor for toxicity, but dose remains the main predictive factor for toxicity. Nephrotoxicity is reversible in most patients.[276-278]

Mitomycin C

Nephrotoxicity from mitomycin C is unusual with cumulative doses of less than 30 mg/m^2. The drug is useful in the therapy of gastrointestinal carcinomas when used in combination with 5-fluorouracil. A cancer-associated hemolytic-uremic syndrome has been reported in the majority of patients who were treated with mitomycin C in excess of 60 mg/m^2.[279-282] In one large study in which the incidence of mitomycin C nephrotoxicity was assessed, fewer than 1% of patients developed a dose-related renal dysfunction.

There appear to be no predictive laboratory tests to prospectively identify those patients at risk of mitomycin C–induced hemolysis and uremia. Renal biopsy changes that have been reported with mitomycin C toxicity include glomerular sclerosis and marked interstitial scarring. Fibrin deposits have been noted within glomeruli and small blood vessels. These findings coupled with the clinical observations of a hemolytic process suggest that in certain circumstances mitomycin C may precipitate a microangiopathic hemolytic anemia. In one case, plasma exchange therapy resulted in improvement of thrombocythemia and microangiopathic hemolytic anemia but not renal function.[283]

Plicamycin

Plicamycin (mithramycin) is an antitumor antibiotic with activity against testicular cancers and glioblastomas.[284] The drug is usually administered daily for several consecutive days or via a three-times weekly schedule in a dose between 15 and 50 mg/kg. Renal toxicity from the drug may approach an incidence of 40% of patients when given on a daily schedule.[285] Plicamycin-induced inhibition of RNA in neoplastic cells persists for 48 hours, whereas inhibition of RNA in normal cells was reversed within this period of time.[286] This study also demonstrated that nephrotoxicity was reduced by the use of alternate-day dosing. However, nephrotoxicity was not eliminated inasmuch as 6 of 54 patients died of azotemia while on the alternate-day dosing schedule.[287] In the further evaluation of patients on the alternate-day schedule, Kennedy and associates reported trace to 1+ proteinuria in 78% of patients and some evidence of chronic renal dysfunction in all of the patients tested.[287] However, there are no correlations available between the type of kidney damage incurred and the clinical syndrome of plicamycin toxicity. Several other types of toxicity have been observed with plicamycin, including liver dysfunction, thrombocytopenia, and hypocalcemia.[288-290]

The mechanism for the nephrotoxicity observed with plicamycin is unknown. This drug forms a complex with DNA and inhibits DNA-dependent RNA synthesis.[291] Moreover, the proximal tubule concentration of plicamycin is believed to be high.[286] The short half-life of the drug is due to the fact that it is not extensively metabolized and has a relatively rapid appearance in urine, presumably favoring a high concentration of plicamycin in proximal tubular cells. Both proximal and distal tubular necrosis and tubular atrophy have been observed following plicamycin administration; as with cisplatin, glomeruli are usually not involved.

Plicamycin is widely used as an agent to treat the hypercalcemia of malignancy. In this setting, a single infusion of 25 mg/kg has been shown to decrease bone absorption and improve serum calcium in about 90% of patients. When used in the setting of hypercalcemia, mithramycin is usually not nephrotoxic, although exceptions exist.[292, 293] It is therefore recommended that renal function be monitored whenever mithramycin is utilized.

Methotrexate

Methotrexate is an antimetabolite that has been proved to be an effective chemotherapeutic agent in combination regimens for choriocarcinoma, acute lymphocytic leukemia, bladder cancers, squamous cell cancers of the head and neck, osteogenic sarcoma, breast carcinoma, and non-Hodgkin's lymphoma. Standard doses of methotrexate are not associated with nephrotoxicity unless the patient has some elements of underlying renal dysfunction.[294] However, high-dose therapy given without concomitant volume expansion or urinary alkylinization, or both, is associated with nephrotoxicity in at least 10% of treated patients.[295, 296] The intratubular deposition of 7-hydroxymethotrexate is believed to be at least partly responsible for the nephrotoxicity.[296, 297]

Evidence for the importance of intratubular hydroxy-methotrexate deposition is provided by the fact that the prophylactic use of volume expansion and an adequate urine output (> 3 L/day) and of urinary alkylinization appears to have reduced the nephrotoxicity from methotrexate.[298] Another possibility for methotrexate toxicity is direct tubular toxicity; hence, proximal tubular necrosis has been documented without the presence of intratubular deposits.[299] Finally, it is not clear whether methotrexate has a consistent effect on the afferent arteriole to cause vasoconstriction, although this has been suspected in some instances in which methotrexate has been administered to children for osteogenic sarcoma.

The clinical course of methotrexate toxicity is usually that of nonoliguric renal failure. It is important to recognize this early because any reduction in GFR may result in very high levels of methotrexate, thereby incurring risk for other toxicities of the drug. There are also reports of methotrexate causing nephrotoxicity when combined with other agents: This has been true for the use of methotrexate with nonsteroidal anti-inflammatory drugs (NSAIDs) and procarbazine.[300, 301] Tubular atrophy and interstitial fibrosis are the lesions most often described in association with streptozotocin administration. The proximal tubular cells are more commonly affected, and there often is an exuberant interstitial infiltrate.

The avoidance of nephrotoxicity with streptozotocin involves using the drug in a dosage schedule in which less than 1.5 g/m^2/week (or 0.5 g/m^2/day for 5 days) is employed. Repeat courses may be given every 3 to 4 weeks. Patients who receive the drug should be monitored for the appearance of proteinuria or other renal tubular defects. A general rule is that if these abnormalities are detected early, discontinuance of the drug will result in resolution of the toxicity. In patients who develop nephrotoxicity, anion-binding resins and hemoperfusion have been proposed as therapies; more research is needed before this therapy is recommended.[302] High doses of folinic acid have been thought to be helpful in reducing nephrotoxicity, but more clinical experience is required before this therapy is shown to be clinically reliable.[303]

Cytarabine

Cytarabine (cytosine arabinoside) is an antimetabolite with antitumor activity against non-Hodgkin's lymphoma and acute leukemia. Interstitial nephritis has been reported with the use of this drug in combination with other drugs.[304] However, the precise contribution of cytarabine to the interstitial nephritis observed is unclear. In a recent study of long-term survivors of bone marrow transplantation treated with high-dose cytarabine renal functional abnormalities were limited to hyperfiltration in 10 of 17, with 2 of 17 (11%) having hypertension, glucosuria, and hematuria.[305]

6-Thioguanine

Intravenous doses of 6-thioguanine exceeding 800 mg/m^2 have been associated with an increase in blood urea nitrogen (BUN) and creatinine. The use of oral 6-thioguanine has not been shown to be nephrotoxic. The development of acute renal failure following intravenous 6-thioguanine is usually reversible within several weeks of discontinuing therapy.[306]

5-Fluorouracil

5-Fluorouracil is a mainstay of tumor therapy for cancers of the gastrointestinal tract. Nephrotoxicity has been reported in approximately 10% of patients who receive 5-fluorouracil in combination with other agents, including mitomycin C.[307] Some of these patients with acute renal failure appear to have a microangiopathic hemolytic anemia, whereas others follow a more insidious course to renal failure. A high percentage of fatalities have occurred with either type of renal failure, however. Necropsy studies revealed evidence for fibrin deposition in the smaller arterioles of the kidneys.

Interleukin-2

Interleukin-2 is a glucoprotein that possesses killer cell function. The drug is now commercially available due to the large production made possible through recombinant DNA technology. High-dose parenteral interleukin-2 infusions result in acute renal failure in approximately 90% of patients subject to such therapy.[308] This hemodynamic effect on the GFR is rapidly reversible, however. Patients with preexistent renal failure subjected to such therapy were observed to have a prolonged course of acute renal failure. Because the effect of interleukin-2 given as an acute bolus appears to be mediated through a vasoconstrictor mechanism in the kidney, it is recommended that the drug not be given in the context of NSAIDs. Presently, constant infusions of interleukin-2 are being used to avoid the high incidence of toxicity.[309, 310]

NEPHROTOXICITY SECONDARY TO TUMOR CELL LYSIS

The rapid lysis of tumor cells can lead to either an acute renal failure that is characterized by acute hypocalcemia or marked hyperphosphatemia and hyperkalemia in addition to hypercalcemia.[311] First, acute uric acid nephropathy is an acute renal failure syndrome characterized by acute oliguria secondary to uric acid precipitation within the tubules.[312]

This syndrome is usually due to the overproduction and overexcretion of uric acid in patients with lymphoma or myeloproliferative disease, and follows the initiation of chemotherapy or radiation. Less frequent causes of uric acid nephropathy are tissue catabolism due to seizure activity or due to the treatment of solid tumors, overproduction of uric acid due to the rare syndrome of hypoxanthine-guanine phophoribosyl transferase deficiency, or hyperuricosuria due to decreased uric acid reabsorption of the proximal tubule.[312-313] Although flank pain may occur in the syndrome, more often there are no symptoms referable to the urinary tract. The uric acid concentration is typically above 15 mg/dL; urinalysis may or may not show uric acid crystals. Overexcretion of uric acid is proved by obtaining a uric acid-to-cretinine ratio on a spot urine specimen; a ratio of greater than 1 suggests overexcretion of uric acid, whereas a value below 0.6 to 0.75 is more typical of other forms of acute renal failure.[314] The therapy of acute uric acid nephropathy begins with prophylaxis with allopurinol in higher than normal doses (500-600 mg/day). Fluid loading to maintain a urine output of 2.5 to 3.0 L/day is also suggested; sodium bicarbonate may also be administered to yield a more alkaline urine (urine pH of ~ 6.5). Once renal failure occurs in this syndrome, therapy consists of allopurinol and administration of fluids and loop diuretics. Hemodialysis has been used in those patients in whom a diuresis cannot be induced.

The second common clinical syndrome resulting from tumor lysis is characterized by hyperphosphatemia, hyperkalemia, hypocalcemia, and hyperuricemia.[315] In this syndrome, the release of cellular contents from tumor cells leads to several metabolic derangements and acute renal failure. This illness is most often associated with treatment of Burkitts lymphoma but has also been described following therapy for ductal carcinoma of the breast and metastatic seminoma.[316, 317] This disease may be particularly devastating in patients with preexistent renal dysfunction. It is worth noting that if the patient has been hypercalcemic as a consequence of the tumor before treatment, the sudden increase in serum phosphate levels may result in marked metastatic calcification. In fact, the intrarenal precipitation of calcium phosphate has been suggested as the cause of acute renal failure in this setting.[318] Therapy is directed at vigorous diuresis, allopurinol administration, and dialysis if necessary to reduce the serum phosphate level.[319]

IMMUNOGLOBULIN THERAPY

Intravenous immunoglobulin preparations are now being used in the treatment of an increasing number of immunodeficiency and immune-related disorders. In order to minimize the formation of immunoglobulin aggregates, many preparations contain sugar additives such as glucose, maltose, or sucrose to serve as stabilizing agents. Intravenous infusion of immunoglobulin preparations that contain these sugars can result in acute renal failure accompanied by vacuolization and swelling of renal proximal tubular cells.[320] This effect is thought to be due to osmotic-induced renal tubular injury and is often referred to as osmotic nephrosis. The majority of reported cases have been with preparations that contain sucrose but cases have been described with

other sugars. Risk factors for this lesion include advancing age, underlying diabetes mellitus, and preexisting chronic renal failure.

HEAVY METALS

Lead

Lead toxicity is an ancient disease with a fascinating history. The Greek poet, grammarian, priest, and physician Nicander (fl. 185-135) was the first to note the syndrome of lead toxicity.[321] The first reports of nephrotoxicity associated with exposure to lead were provided by Lancereaux in 1862. Other early descriptions of lead poisoning were provided by Ramazzini, who in 1700 described classic lead poisoning in potters and portrait painters, and by Thackrah, who associated chronic lead exposure in plumbers and lead manufacturers with clinical disease.[321, 322] Finally, Legge proposed in 1934 that absorption of lead occurred via several routes, most notably inhalation of lead particles and from the skin.[323] The clinical syndrome associated with acute and sometimes chronic lead intoxication includes gastrointestinal colic, paralysis, visual disturbances, and encephalopathy.

As far as the kidney is concerned, acute lead nephropathy has most often been observed in children, with resultant damage to the proximal tubule and aminoaciduria, phosphaturia, and glycosuria.[324, 325] This constellation of findings is consistent with Fanconi syndrome and appears to be rapidly reversible by chelation therapy. The renal pathology in this case typically shows intranuclear inclusions in proximal tubule cells, as well as several mitochondrial defects.[326] The proximal tubule is a major site of lead damage, and markers of tubular damage may prove to be useful markers of toxicity.[327, 328] Perhaps the largest study on the effects of childhood exposure to lead was performed by Nye in 1928.[329] This study was carried out in Australia, and consisted of a series of observations made on children who had been exposed to household lead-based paint. This and later studies made the association of prior lead intoxication with renal failure, hypertension, and gout.[329-331] At tissue in these investigations was whether or not chronic sequelae of exposure to lead as a child could result in chronic renal failure later.

In experimental animals, prenatal exposure to lead may contribute to nephrotoxicity if exposure is repeated.[332] Gender does not seem to be a risk factor for lead nephrotoxicity.[333] A prospective analysis of 62 subjects with significant lead poisoning (plasma lead level > 100 mg/dL) was undertaken with a control group consisting of eight control siblings (plasma lead level < 40 mg/dL).[334] Multiple regression analysis failed to demonstrate a significant influence of the presence of plumbism on blood pressure. Moreover, only 4 of the 62 study subjects had an elevated serum creatinine value. There were no significant differences in renal function or blood pressure between the study subjects and the controls. Another review concluded that definitive proof that chronic renal failure may be a consequence of lead exposure was lacking,[335] although, chronic lead exposure had been associated with a high prevalence of renal dysfunction in earlier studies.[336-340] In another study, Hu reported on 192 subjects with well-documented lead poisoning who had a follow-up of 50 years.[341] These patients were carefully matched to a control group. The result showed that the patients with prior lead exposure had a sevenfold greater chance of developing hypertension; in addition, these patients had a lower hematocrit than controls. Interestingly, creatinine clearances were similar in the patients with lead exposure and their controls. Thus, the exact relationship between early lead exposure and chronic renal failure remains unresolved in the setting of childhood exposure. There are a number of studies that have provided evidence for excess mortality from renal disease in adults who have been exposed to lead.[342-345] Most of these exposures are industrial exposures in lead smelters or in battery assembly plants. Another common route of exposure is in the preparation of moonshine whiskey.

The classic clinical presentation of lead nephropathy is that of a benign urinary sediment, less than 2 g/day of urinary protein excretion, hyperuricemia, and hypertension. Gouty arthritis affects about half of the patients with lead nephropathy.[346] The association between gout and chronic renal failure is strong enough to merit a lead chelation screening test with ethylenediaminetetraacetic acid (EDTA) in patients with chronic renal failure who develop gout. The combination of hypertension with prior lead exposure limits the ability of clinicians to determine which disorder is responsible for renal dysfunction. The renal pathology in lead exposure includes a nonspecific tubular atrophy and an element of interstitial fibrosis with minimal inflammatory infiltrates; there also may be lysosomal dense bodies in the proximal tubule.[347, 348] Inclusion bodies may be less prominent in far-advanced interstitial damage from lead. The kidneys are usually small and contracted and have irregular cortical surfaces. The initial primary insult to the kidney appears to occur via damage to the proximal tubule, a finding that has been confirmed in animal models of this disease.[349]

The diagnosis of lead nephropathy may be quite difficult. In one recent study of workers exposed to lead pollutants in a battery factory, there were no noninvasive simple tests that distinguished the exposed workers from unexposed controls.[350] The main finding of this study was that the renal excretion of 6-keto-$PGF_{1\alpha}$ was reduced in patients who had been exposed to lead. In addition, these workers also had enhanced excretion of thromboxane. The significance of these observations is unclear, but it does suggest that the kidney may be more vulnerable to the effects of drugs that reduce the synthesis of locally produced vasodilaters such as NSAIDs. Another study of workers exposed to lead postulated that some hyperfiltration may be involved in many cases; what this observation implies for long-term renal function is not clear.[351] The blood lead concentration is relatively insensitive in assessing cumulative body stores that have been acquired over many years of exposure. This is the case because blood lead levels tend to fall quite rapidly after acute exposure is completed. The main repository of lead in the body is bone; however, high blood levels (> 80 mg/dL) suggest an increased body burden of lead. Levels above 40 mg/dL are considered high in children. Of note is the fact that sustained blood lead levels greater than 10 mg/dL may be associated with lead-induced disease.[352, 353] The best available method of screening for lead toxicity is the use of two 1-g doses of sodium calcium edetate.[354] After the injections, a 24-hour urine sample is collected. Adults excrete up to 650 mg of lead-chelate in the urine; patients with a serum creatinine greater than 1.5 mg/dL should have a 48- or 72-hour urine collection performed because the excretion of lead may be delayed in these individuals. In all collections, creatinine must also be measured to verify an accurate collection. The chelatable lead found in the urine correlates very well with bone lead stores.[355, 356] Another method that may be used in the future to quantitate the amount of lead in the body is x-ray fluorescence.[357]

The therapy of lead nephropathy consists of three weekly 1-g treatments of sodium calcium edetate intramuscularly. The end point of therapy is a lead-chelate product that is normal. Studies that have tested the utility of 2, 3-dimercaptosuccinic acid and iron and a chelator have produced promising results, although no major improvement in renal function has been documented.[358] Chelation therapy is effective in reversing acute lead nephropathy, but there is no evidence that it reverses the established interstitial disease. Failure to demonstrate an improvement in renal function in these patients does not mean that the therapy has not been effective; on the contrary, Koster and associates documented a high mobilization of lead in patients with high renal failure.[359] Finally, it is important for the physician to realize that repeated exposure of the patient to the EDTA chelator may create a separate toxicity.[360] However, this is believed to be an unusual occurrence and does not warrant discontinuing the practice of lead chelation as the mainstay of therapy.

Cadmium

Cadmium is a metal with a wide variety of industrial uses, including the manufacture of glass, metal alloys, and electrical equipment. The first cases of acute poisoning by cadmium were reported in 1958 by Sovet, but the first recognition of cadmium as a definite industrial toxin was made in 1948 by Fryberg and colleagues.[361] Chronic exposure to cadmium reaches a plateau in the blood after about 4 months.[362] The relation between urinary excretion of cadmium and urinary creatinine is a reliable indicator of the total body cadmium burden.[362] A progressive increase in cadmium excretion is observed in both humans and experimental animals with increasing dosage of cadmium. In one recent study of exposed workers, the average concentration of blood cadmium was 5.5 mg/dL and urinary cadmium was per gram of 5.4 mg creatinine.[363] Based on the sampling of a number of workers exposed to cadmium in Belgium, Roels and colleagues estimated a threshold for cadmium toxicity as follows: individuals with 2 mg of cadmium per gram creatinine were noted to have mainly biochemical alterations; individuals excreting 4 mg of cadmium per gram creatinine were noted to excrete some high-molecular-weight proteins and some antigens or enzymes; and individuals who excreted 10 mg of cadmium per gram creatinine also were noted to excrete low-molecular-weight proteins in the urine.[363] The recommendation of the American Conference of Governmental Industrial Hygienists was that a value of 5 mg of cadmium per gram of creatinine in the urine is the occupational exposure limit to cadmium.[363] In studies by Kido and associates, the appearance of metallothionein in the urine was used as an index of renal toxicity.[364, 365] These investigators found that the prevalence rate for metallothioneinuria was calculated to be 4.2 mg/g creatinine for men and 4.8 mg/g creatinine for women. If the appearance of β_2-microglobulin in the urine is used as an index of tubular damage from cadmium, cadmium valves of 3.8 mg/g creatinine for men and 4.1 mg/g creatinine for women could be used as predictors of toxicity.[365]

The reason that cadmium toxicity has been linked to metallothionein is because cadmium accumulation in proximal tubule cells is linked to binding to metallothionein; metallothionein is synthesized in the liver and transfers bound cadmium to the kidney via the blood.[366] This cadmium-metallothionein complex is nephrotoxic because it stored in lysosomes of proximal tubule cells. Recent studies have emphasized the importance of cadmium-binding protein in nephrotoxicity.[367] The concentration of cadmium in renal biopsies has been estimated at approximately 8.7 mg/g protein; in this study the highest concentrations of cadmium were associated with the most pronounced tubular interstitial changes.[368] Other methods of diagnosing cadmium toxicity in the kidney have been used; Jung and colleagues have suggested that the combination of α_1-microglobulin and N-acetyl-β-D-glucosaminidase be utilized to determine the amount of nephrotoxicity from cadmium.[369] Induction of metallothionein by streptozotocin or zinc and copper may serve to reduce nephrotoxicity.[370, 371]

The chronic effects of exposure to cadmium are often subtle. Toffoletto and colleagues found that urinary cadmium excretion greater than 10 mg/g creatinine was associated with evidence of renal tubular damage at a prevalence rate of about 8.4% in 105 workers exposed to cadmium for over 10 years.[372] In 16 workers previously exposed to cadmium, Jarup and associates noted that all had evidence of persistent tubular damage as documented by increased excretion of β_2-microglobin in the urine.[373] Moreover, the GFR was reduced from about 77 to 72 mL/minute over a 5-year period. This reduction in GFR exceeds the usual rate of reduction in the GFR that could be accounted for by age alone. Other studies have documented similar changes in renal function over time.[374-376] Clinical nephrotoxicity is manifested by aminoaciduria, glycosuria, renal tubular acidosis, and, as mentioned above, the excretion of metallothionein and β_2-microglobin. Given the deposition of cadmium in bone as well as kidney, it is not surprising that many patients have a combination of renal failure and severe osteopenia that may lead to fractures.[377] Tsuchiya and associates described an outbreak of cadmium toxicity in Japan; there the disease is known as *itai-itai* ("ouch-ouch") because of the painful fractures associated with the renal dysfunction.[378] Renal involvement in the disease is characterized by a prominent tubular interstitial infiltrate with very little involvement with glomeruli.

If cadmium exposure is eliminated, the usual trend is for renal function to stabilize, but continued deterioration is not usual. The general consensus is that in most instances cadmium-induced tubular interstitial disease is not reversible. In this regard, the treatment of cadmium toxicity with sodium calcium edetate has not improved renal function dramatically. This is believed to be so because the binding of cadmium with metallothionein in the proximal tubule is the event that produces damage. New therapies with other chelating agents have been reported but the efficacy of these treatments is at present uncertain.[379, 380] Nephrolithiasis may be a limiting factor in treating the bone disorders associated with cadmium. The presence of hypercalcuria is the main factor that leads to the development of osteopenia. It is interesting to note that the presence of overt chronic renal failure is relatively unusual given the fact that the disorder causes so much in the way of proximal tubule dysfunction.

Mercury

Mercury toxicity usually occurs as a result of accidental exposure to mercury vapor. Mercury is present in alloy and mirror manufacturing plants, and in some batteries.[381] If ingested in the elemental form, mercury is harmless. However, transformation to the organic salt produces toxicity. The major site of mercury damage in the kidney is the proximal tubule; acute mercury exposure leads to frank tubular necrosis, which is reversible in most cases.[382] Lower exposures to mercury may affect the S3 segment of the proximal tubule; higher doses may affect the S1 and S2 segments. Mercury-induced release of hydrogen peroxide from proximal tubular cells in vitro suggests that oxidant stress may contribute to renal injury.[383, 384] In patients with acute mercury intoxication, the administration of 2,3-dimercaprol leads to some improvement in the natural history of the disease.[366] Intracellular mercury has an affinity for sulfhydryl groups in lysosomes and may produce toxicity in this location.[366, 385] A blood mercury level greater than 3 mg/dL or a urine level above 50 mg/g creatinine are considered abnormal, but the relationship of these values to overt disease is not always clear.[386]

The consequences of endemic methyl mercury poisoning were reported from Japan and revealed that neurologic sequelae of mercury ingestion dominated the clinical picture.[387] This outbreak of mercury intoxication occurred as a result of industrial pollution in a bay that was heavily fished. In this group of patients, the renal disease was surprisingly benign, consisting only of tubular proteinuria and no changes in serum creatinine or significant albuminuria. Postmortem evaluation revealed few overt changes in renal histology. Thus, the nephrotoxicity of mercury appears to be an acute poisoning syndrome in which proximal tubular necrosis occurs. The evidence for a progressive decline in renal function with chronic ingestion is not impressive.

Uranium

Uranium is used as an investigational agent to produce experimental acute renal failure in laboratory animals. Human exposure is limited to very low-level industrial sources. In one recent study, the evaluation of uranium workers revealed modest tubular dysfunction characterized by an increased excretion of amino acids and β_2-microglobulin in uranium workers versus controls. In addition, acute tubular necrosis was reported in atom bomb workers during the Manhattan Project in the 1940s, but chronic renal failure due to uranium exposure has not been reported.[388] If suspicion of uranium exposure exists, then screening of the urine for β_2-microglobulin and renal function tests should be undertaken. In general, uranium levels in excess of 30 mg/L in the urine suggest an overabundance of uranium. New studies on uranium nephrotoxicity are needed to delineate the pathogenesis and course of the disease.[389, 390]

Other Heavy Metals

Arsenic and arsine gas have been shown to cause acute renal failure, but this may be a result of the amylases that also accompany the ingestion of these substances, as well as the severe hypotension.[391] Proximal and distal necrosis have been observed after arsenic exposure in animals.[392] Other metals that have been associated with renal toxicity include thallium, copper, nickel, antimony, and silver; however, reports of these substances causing nephrotoxicity are unusual.[393] Chromium has also been associated with proximal renal tubular damage in acute renal failure, but this is also very unusual.[394]

ALTERNATIVE MEDICINE

ARISTOLOCHIC ACID NEPHROPATHY. Aristolochic acid nephropathy, also referred to as Chinese herb nephropathy, is a subacute form of renal failure first described in Belgium women taking a herbal preparation as part of a weight reduction program[395] (Table 34-5). The cause of the disorder has been linked to the nephrotoxin *Aristolochia fangchi* in the herbal powder. The typical clinical syndrome occurs in young women with severe anemia, proteinuria, and renal failure progressing to end-stage renal failure over several months. Blood pressure and kidney size are normal. Histopathologic findings are typical of chronic interstitial nephritis with interstitial fibrosis and tubular atrophy with little in the way of a cellular infiltrate.

Aristolochic acid nephropathy has also been reported to present with features of Fanconi syndrome.[396] Most of these cases have originated in Asia. The reason for different clinical manifestations between cases in Belgium and Asia is not known but may relate to differences in dose or varying mutagenic potential of the aristolochic acid in different races.

There is also an increased incidence of uroepithelial tumors in patients who develop end-stage renal disease due to aristolochic acid nephropathy.[397] The pathophysiology of this disorder is not known but aristolochic acid DNA adducts have been found in malignant tissue samples.

EPHEDRA *(MA HUANG).* Ephedra is commonly used for a variety of reasons: asthma, flu symptoms, weight reduction, euphoria, and sexual enhancement, among others. Ephedra stimulates α-adrenergic receptors and has been reported to cause hypertension, palpitations, seizures, and strokes. Use of this supplement is associated with an increased risk of kidney stones that contain ephedrine and its metabolites.[398]

STAR FRUIT JUICE. Star fruit is used to produce carambola juice, which is a popular beverage in Asia. Commercially prepared carambola juice is prepared in such a way that the oxalate content is reduced. By contrast, pure fresh juice ingested for traditional remedies contains high quantities of oxalate and has been reported to cause acute oxalate nephropathy.[399] Fatal cases have been reported in dialysis patients who ingested star fruit juice.

VITAMIN C. Vitamin C is normally metabolized to oxalic acid and is not associated with renal toxicity when ingested at therapeutic doses. There have been several reports of patients with acute renal failure due to acute oxalate nephropathy related to large doses of vitamin C used as a nonprescription vitamin supplement.[400]

OTHERS. Creatine is used as a dietary supplement in weightlifters and has occasionally been reported to cause tubulointerstitial nephritis.[401] Renal toxicity has also been reported in experimental animals. Cat's claw (uno de gato) has been reported to cause acute interstitial nephritis when used to treat various rheumatic complaints.[402] Ingestion of the gallbladder of the Rohu or Indian carp (*Labeo rohita*), used to treat various chronic diseases, has been reported to cause acute renal failure.

ANTIRHEUMATIC AGENTS

Penicillamine

Penicillamine has been used to treat rheumatoid arthritis, scleroderma, and cystinuria. If therapy is prolonged, as it commonly is in rheumatoid arthritis, renal complications from the drug are not uncommon. In one large series of patients receiving penicillamine, 7% developed a nephrotic syndrome secondary to membranous nephropathy.[403, 404] Proteinuria usually develops within the first 6 to 8 months of therapy, but the onset of proteinuria may be delayed up to 6 years. Proteinuria disappeared in these patients when the drug was stopped; in four of seven patients who were administered the drug again, proteinuria returned.[405]

The usual pathologic finding in patients treated with penicillamine who developed nephrotic syndrome is membranous nephropathy.[404-406] Deposits of immunoglobulins have been identified in the glomerular basement membrane, and circulating antibodies to penicillamine have been demonstrated.[407]

TABLE 34-5

Nephrotoxicity of Alternative Medicine Preparations

PREPARATION	REPORTED TOXICITY
Aristolochic acid	Chronic tubulointerstitial nephritis (TIN) with rapid course to end-stage renal disease, Fanconi syndrome, increased risk of uroepithelial cancer
Ephedra (ma huang)	Hypertension, increased risk of nephrolithiasis consisting of ephedra and its metabolites
St. John's wort	Induces liver microsomal enzymes with increased degradation of drugs such as cyclosporine
Star fruit juice (carambola juice)	Acute oxalate nephropathy
Vitamin C	Oxalate nephropathy
Creatine	Acute TIN
Noni juice (*Morinda citrofolia*)	High potassium content leading to hyperkalemia in chronic renal failure patients
Rohu or Indian Carp (*Labeo rohita*)	Acute renal failure
Cat's claw (uno de gato)	Acute TIN

A genetic predisposition of patients with human leukocyte antigen HLA-B8 and HLA-DRw3 to gold-induced proteinuria is also true of penicillamine.[408] A more serious but less common complication of penicillamine is the development of acute renal failure due to a crescentic, rapidly progressive glomerulonephritis.[408, 409] Pulse prednisone, cyclophosphamide, and plasmapheresis have all been used to treat this disorder with some success.[409] In one study the effect of continuing penicillamine or gold treatment was examined in 53 patients with biopsy-proven penicillamine (32 patients) or gold (21 patients) nephropathy.[410] Thirty-two of the patients stopped penicillamine or gold therapy as soon as proteinuria was detected while 21 patients continued therapy between the periods of 2 and 11 months. There were no significant differences observed in the initial or maximal proteinuria, the duration of the proteinuria, or in the initial or latest creatinine clearances between the two groups. The results suggest that penicillamine and gold may be continued for short periods without causing permanent renal damage. However, despite the fact that there appears to be little impact of continued therapy on the GFR, it is not recommended that this strategy be undertaken except in cases in which gold or penicillamine is absolutely essential for therapeutic control.

Gold

The prevalence of proteinuria in therapeutic gold administration is approximately 30%. The magnitude of proteinuria in patients treated with gold is usually less than 3.5 g/day. Renal biopsy findings in patients who have been treated with gold for a long period of time typically reveal membranous glomerulopathy. Minimal-change pathology and biopsy-demonstrated mesangial and subendothelial electron-dense deposits have also been described.[411] A decline in the GFR is unusual in gold-treated patients, but both severe renal failure and nephrotic syndrome have been reported.[412] Of interest is the fact that parenteral gold administration is more likely to be associated with proteinuria than oral administration.[413] The cause of gold nephropathy is unknown; particles of gold have been detected in proximal tubular endothelium, and tubular proteinuria and β_2-microglobulinuria have also been reported. There does not seem to be a close relationship between the dose of gold and the renal lesion that develops. Animals receiving gold therapy develop an autoimmune tubulointerstitial nephritis and an immune complex glomerulopathy. As mentioned above, gold toxicity and penicillamine toxicity are associated with the histocompatibility antigens HLA-DRw3 and HLA-B8. Of note is the fact that idiopathic membranous nephropathy is also associated with the same HLA haplotype.[414]

Nonsteroidal Anti-inflammatory Drugs

The incidence of nephrotoxicity secondary to NSAIDs is low, and generally the drugs are regarded to be safe and well tolerated. The most common overall side effect from the use of NSAIDs involves toxicity of the gastrointestinal tract, where ulcer disease and gastrointestinal bleeding result from the use of the drugs. However, the growing use of these agents (and the fact that between 30 and 40 million people consume NSAIDs daily in the United States) means that even with a relatively low incidence rate, nephrotoxicity will be seen commonly. There are several forms of NSAID nephrotoxicity, including a syndrome with acute renal failure related to hemodynamic changes in the kidney, tubulointerstitial nephritis often associated with nephrotic-range proteinuria, salt and water retention, and hyperkalemia (Table 34-6).

Several of the effects of NSAIDs on the kidney are linked to the inhibition of renal prostaglandin synthesis. Prostaglandins (PGs) are derivatives of arachidonic acid, a 20-carbon tetraenoic acid that is acetylated to membrane phospholipids. Species of prostaglandins produced in the kidney are varied; the main categories include prostacyclin (PGI_2), thromboxane (TXA_2), and PGE_2 (Table 34-7). Prostaglandins exert physiologic actions at the location where they are synthesized; thus, they are really autocoids rather than hormones because they are made to act locally rather than at distant loci. PGE_2 and PGF_2 are synthesized primarily by interstitial cells, whereas prostacyclin is synthesized by cortical arterioles and glomeruli. PGE_2 an TXA_2 are also produced in the renal cortex by glomerul[415, 416] (see Table 34-7).

NSAID-Induced Hemodynamically Mediated Acute Renal Failure

The basic concept regarding the hemodynamic role of prostaglandins in the kidney has evolved to the following scheme: (1) Under euvolemic conditions there is typically a

TABLE 34-6

Renal Syndromes Associated with Use of Nonsteroidal Anti-inflammatory Drugs

Vasomotor acute renal failure
Nephrotic syndrome with tubulointerstitial nephritis
Chronic renal failure
Salt retention
Hyponatremia
Hyperkalemia

TABLE 34-7

Compartmentalization and Function of Renal Prostaglandins

SITE	EICOSANOID	ACTION
Arterioles	Prostacyclin (PGI_2), PGE_2	Vasodilation
Glomeruli	Prostacyclin, > PGE_2 (human), PGE_2 > prostacyclin (rat)	Maintain glomerular filtration rate
	Thromboxane A_2	Vasoconstriction
Tubules	PGE_2, $PGF_{2\alpha}$	Enhance NaCl and water excretion
Interstitial cells	PGE_2	Enhances NaCl and water excretion; influences regional blood flow
Juxtaglomerular apparatus	PGE_2, prostacyclin	Stimulate renin release

very low rate of prostaglandin synthesis, thereby making it difficult to demonstrate that prostaglandins exert any maintenance role on renal function; (2) when prostaglandin synthesis is stimulated, it is usually in circumstances in which the systemic circulation has become destabilized. Under these conditions, prostaglandins have been shown to exert a moderating influence on renal physiology by exposing the stimulus to prostaglandin synthesis. For example, vasopressin stimulates prostaglandin synthesis and release, but prostaglandins antagonize the hydro-osmotic effects of vasopressin on collecting tubular epithelium. Similarly, angiotensin II and norepinephrine (both renal vasoconstrictors) are potent stimulators of prostacyclin12 and PGE_2 formation. Prostacyclin12 and PGE_2 are renal vasodilators that then attenuate any vasoconstrictor response to angiotensin II.[416] Hence, prostaglandins have a number of important roles to play in the renal circulation, including renal vasodilation, renin secretion, and sodium and water excretion.

The consequences of inhibiting prostaglandin synthesis with powerful nonsteroidal drugs include an increase in vascular tone, an antinatriuretic affect, an antirenin effect, and an antidiuretic effect. This interplay between vasoconstrictor and vasodilator forces in the kidney is dynamic and has been shown to exist in vivo in several models.[417-420] In addition to opposing the vasoconstrictive effects of circulating hormones, prostaglandins also oppose the vasoconstrictive influence in the renal sympathetic nervous system.[421-423] Thus, there is a balance between the vasodilator and vasoconstrictor forces that influence renal circulation. In the presence of NSAIDs, compensatory vasodilation is inhibited and the vasoconstrictive forces dominate, leading to a decline in renal blood flow and renal insufficiency.

The patients at greatest risk for this complication are those in whom blood volume or effective arterial blood volume is compromised.[424-431] These patients include those with congestive heart failure, cirrhosis (particularly with ascites), underlying renal disease, advanced age (> 65 years old), volume depletion or shock, septicemia, hypertension, concomitant diuretic therapy, and postoperative patients with "third space" fluid sequestration.[432] Usually the urinalysis is unremarkable in the majority of patients during the acute deterioration of acute function. In addition, the fractional excretion of sodium may be low (< 1%) in some of these patients who experience this form of renal failure.[433] If recognized early, the renal failure is reversible with discontinuation of NSAIDs. In one survey of 27 patients with NSAID-induced vasoconstrictive renal failure, only three patients required dialysis, and only one required permanent dialysis.[434] Hyperkalemia may be a pronounced feature of this disorder, occurring in about 25% of cases. The unifying antecedent state for the patients who develop this form of NSAID-related disease is that of a high-renin, high-angiotensin state[435-442] (Table 34-8).

Of particular note are two groups of patients who are susceptible to this form of renal failure. Patients with underlying renal disease have been shown to be particularly susceptible, given the fact that up to 30% of the patients may develop worsening of renal function when exposed to an NSAID.[443-445] Renal disease may lead to increased prostaglandin production and therefore make renal function dependent in part upon prostaglandins to maintain renal blood flow and glomerular filtration.[446-448] Another group

that may be more vulnerable is the elderly, and this is so for several reasons:(1) The elderly often have lower albumin levels, which reduce protein binding of the NSAID and result in higher free drug levels; (2) they have reduced total body water, which leads to an increased concentration of the NSAID; and (3) they have decreased hepatic metabolism of the NSAID, an effect that would lead to increased drug levels. All of these factors may summate to cause increased toxicity from NSAIDs[449](Table 34-9).

Two additional points should be made regarding this form of NSAID-induced acute renal failure. First, the question has arisen as to whether some NSAIDs are "renal protective." This issue has been discussed in the context of sulindac, a drug that requires a hepatic conversion from the inactive sulindac sulfoxide to an active sulfide.[450] Although there appears to be some reduced risk of vasoconstriction-induced renal insufficiency in patients who take sulindac versus other NSAIDs,[451-456] the kidney can activate the prodrug, leading to vasoconstrictive renal failure or hyperkalemia.[457-463] In addition, Schlondorff has pointed out that sulindac has a long half-life, and because of this the active sulindac sulfide can accumulate in the plasma over several days to weeks, eventually reaching levels that are two to four times higher than those observed in patients with normal hepatic and renal function.[442] Another recent debate regarding the risk of nephrotoxicity with parenteral ketorolac exposure resulted in a retrospective cohort study that such

TABLE 34-8

Risk Factors for NSAID-Induced Acute Vasomotor Renal Failure

DECREASED EABV	NORMAL OR INCREASED EABV
Congestive heart failure	Chronic renal failure
Cirrhosis	Glomerulonephritis
Nephrotic syndrome	Advanced age
Sepsis	Contrast-induced nephropathy
Hemorrhage	Obstructive uropathy
Diuretic therapy	Cyclosporine
Postoperative patients with "third space" fluid	
Volume depletion/hypotension	

EABV, effective arterial blood volume; NSAID, nonsteroidal anti-inflammatory drug.

TABLE 34-9

Predisposing Factors for NSAID-Induced Nephrotoxicity in the Elderly

Age-related changes in renal function
  ↓Glomerular filtration rate
  ↓Renal blood flow
  ↑Renal vascular resistance
Age-related changes in pharmacokinetics
  ↑Free drug concentration
    Hypoalbuminemia
    Retained metabolites
  ↓Total body water
  ↓Hepatic metabolism with longer drug half-life

exposure did not result in an increased risk of toxicity if exposure was limited to less than 5 days.[464-466] The other question that has been raised is whether the cyclooxygenase-inhibitors have renal sparing properties. This issue is discussed in the following section.

Cyclooxygenase-2 Inhibitors and Nephrotoxicity

It has been widely anticipated that specific cyclooxygenase-2 (COX-2) inhibitors would provide a means to treat inflammatory and pain syndromes without the development of renal complications. This anticipation is based on the belief that COX-2 is primarily an inducible enzyme confined to sites of inflammation and plays little to no role in maintenace of normal renal homeostasis. However, evidence now suggests that COX-2 is constitutively expressed in renal tissue and may play an important role in maintaining renal function in states of prostaglandin dependency (Table 34-10). In experimental animals COX-2 is known to be constitutively expressed in the macula densa, epithelial cells of the thick ascending limb, and intercalated cells in the cortical collecting duct.[467-469] Salt depletion has been shown to up-regulate the expression of COX-2 in both the macula densa and thick limb, suggesting a role for this enzyme in the regulation of rennin.[468] Salt loading in rats has been shown to increase COX-2 messenger RNA (mRNA) and protein expression in the inner medulla where increased prostaglandins may play a role in facilitating a natriuretic response to help protect against volume overload.[468] Both angiotensin II and endothelin induce and up-regulate COX-2 and prostaglandin synthesis in vascular smooth muscle cells and rat glomerular mesangial cells, respectively.[470, 471] The COX-2 enzyme also plays an important role in the process of nephrogenesis. COX-2–deficient mice generated in gene knockout studies or mice administered a specific COX-2 inhibitor exhibit renal dysgenesis associated with hypoplastic glomeruli.[472]

Constitutive expression of COX-2 has also been demonstrated in human renal tissue, primarily in endothelial and smooth muscle cells of arteries, arterioles, and veins, and visceral epithelial cells of cortical glomeruli but not the macula densa.[473] Clinical studies examining the specific COX-2 inhibitors celecoxib and rofecoxib suggest that the risk of renal toxicity is similar to traditional NSAIDs in high-risk patients. In data presented to the Food and Drug Administration (FDA) advisory committee, celecoxib was

reported to increase blood pressure and decrease urinary sodium excretion similar to traditional NSAIDs.[474] A similar antinatriuretic effect has also been reported with rofecoxib in a study of elderly patients on a high-sodium intake.[475] In salt-depleted normal subjects, celecoxib and naproxen were found to produce similar reductions in GFR, urine output, and sodium and potassium excretion.[476] Celecoxib has also been found to reduce urinary excretion of the prostacyclin metabolite 2,3-dinor-6-keto-PGF$_{1\alpha}$ comparably to indomethacin.[477] In a preliminary report involving elderly patients with a creatinine clearance ranging from 30 to 80 mL/minute, administration of rofecoxib or indomethacin reduced GFR to an extent that was significantly greater than placebo.[478] Three cases were recently reported in which celecoxib and refecoxib were linked to the development of reversible acute renal failure complicated by hyperkalemia and volume overload.[479]

Thus, the nephrotoxicity patterns for specific COX-2 inhibitors continue to evolve. At present, both experimental and clinical studies suggest that the specific COX-2 inhibitors are associated with renal toxicity similar to that associated with traditional NSAID use.[480] As with other NSAIDs, these agents need to be used with caution and require close monitoring of renal function in patients at high risk for adverse renal outcomes (Table 34-11).

NSAID-Induced Sodium Retention

Prostaglandins are normally natriuretic and affect sodium excretion by both direct and indirect mechanisms. Acting as renal vasodilators, prostaglandins may cause an increase in the filtered load of sodium. In addition, prostaglandins augment medullary blood flow to the kidney, thereby reducing hypertonicity of the medullary interstitium and leading to a decrease in water reabsorption in the descending limb of the loop of Henle.[481, 482] Because of this effect, the sodium concentration at the loop is reduced, leading to a reduction in passive sodium reabsorption along the water-impermeable thin ascending limb.[483-486] In addition, prostaglandins exert a vasodilator effect at the efferent arteriolar site of the glomerular capillary, and this leads to a reduction in the filtration fraction and peritubular oncotic pressure. Peritubular hydraulic pressure is increased, and the sum of the changes in Starling forces causes a decrease in tubular sodium reabsorption.[480, 487] In addition to these effects on Starling forces, there is some evidence that prostaglandins act directly to inhibit sodium reabsorption. A number of in vivo and in vitro studies have shown that prostaglandins have a natriuretic effect by the inhibition of sodium transport in the loop

---

TABLE 34-10

Evidence Suggesting a Role for Cyclooxygenase-2 (COX-2) in Normal Renal Homeostasis

Constitutive expression in
  Macula densa (rat and not human)
  Epithelial cells in thick ascending limb of loop of Henle
  Intercalated cells of collecting duct
  Endothelial and smooth muscle cells of renal arteries, arterioles, veins
  Visceral epithelial cells of glomerulus
Increased expression in macula densa and thick limb with salt depletion
Increased expression in inner medulla with salt loading
Angiotensin II–mediated increased expression in vascular smooth muscle
Endothelin-mediated increased expression in mesangial cells
Specific COX-2 inhibitors resulting in renal dysgenesis

TABLE 34-11

Clinical Features of NSAID-Induced Vasomotor Renal Failure

Oliguria
Usually occurs within a few days of beginning medicine
Hyperkalemia out of proportion to renal failure
Low fractional excretion of sodium
Usually does not require dialysis
Usually reversible

of Henle, distal nephron, and collecting tubule.[488-492] Other studies show that prostaglandins may play a key permissive role in the sodium excretion that follows volume expansion and an increase in renal perfusion pressure.[493-495] NSAIDs also are able to partially blunt the natriuretic effect of some diuretics, mainly working through an effect on renal vasomotor tone.[495] This resistance to the natriuretic effects of diuretics has been seen in several circumstances and has been confirmed in a study using the model of head-out water immersion following indomethacin administration in salt-depleted subjects.[496-501]

An important consequence of NSAID-induced salt retention is the development of hypertension. When the effect of NSAIDs was examined in a large patient population, the following points emerged: First, in controlled studies, an average increase of between 6 and 8 mm Hg of mean blood pressure is seen in patients treated with NSAIDs. This increase in blood pressure appears to be most pronounced in patients who are already hypertensive, and less pronounced in patients who are normotensive when they begin therapy. Second, patients who take diuretics or β-blockers seem to be more vulnerable to the hypertensive effect of NSAIDs than of other agents. In this regard, it is particularly interesting to note that propranolol has been shown to increase prostacyclin formation and thus make the drug more susceptible to the antihypertensive effects of NSAIDs.[502] Third, calcium channel blockers, direct vasodilators, and clonidine appear to be less vulnerable to the effects of NSAIDs on blood pressure. Angiotensin-converting enzyme (ACE) inhibitors are also relatively unaffected by the use of NSAIDs, but there have been a few case reports of the deterioration of renal function that can follow the concominant use of an ACE inhibitor and an NSAID.[503] Fourth, the patients who appear to be most at risk for developing an NSAID-related increase in blood pressure appear to be those with low-renin hypertension, that is, the elderly and blacks. Physicians should be cognizant of this interaction, and be particularly mindful of the effects of NSAIDs on blood pressure in patients who are already taking antihypertensive medicines and who require an NSAID temporarily.[504] The pathogenesis of NSAID-induced hypertension is not known with certainty, but, the elimination of the vasodilator prostacyclin from the resistance of blood vessels is believed to play some role in the development of hypertension in these individuals.[505-512] The large reviews that have examined this subject have shown only a modest but usually significant effect of NSAIDs on blood pressure.[513-515]

NSAID-Induced Water Retention

Prostaglandins impair the ability of the kidney to concentrate the urine maximally, and NSAIDs impair urinary dilution. Both in vivo and in vitro experiments have shown that prostaglandins oppose the hydro-osmotic effects of vasopressin.[516, 517] This serves to limit free water reabsorption by the collecting duct. Vasopressin also stimulates PGE_2 synthesis in the epithelial cells, thereby inducing its own antagonist. Thus, the antidiuretic effect is modulated by having vasopressin and PGE_2 play opposing roles in the collecting duct epithelium. The clinical importance of this effect is that NSAIDs would be expected to impair renal water excretion, and in so doing lead to a tendency toward water retention and hyponatremia.

NSAID-Induced Hyperkalemia

PGE_2 and prostacyclin12 are known to be renin agonists, likely working through an increase in cyclic adenosine monophosphate in the juxtaglomerular cell.[518, 519] In addition, prostaglandins appear to be important in the normal functioning of the arterial baroreceptor that governs renin release and in macula densa renin release as well.[520-523] By contrast, the β-adrenergic pathway to renin release appears to operate normally despite prostaglandin synthesis inhibition.[522-526] The practical clinical point made by these experiments in renin release is that in the presence of NSAID administration, positive potassium balance may occur via the effect of the NSAID to cause hyporeninemia and hypoaldosteronism. This endogenous hyporenin-hypoaldosterone state could thereby favor the retention of potassium and lead to hyperkalemia. There also may be an effect of the NSAIDs to reduce sodium delivery to distal exchange sites in the nephron, and this would also favor positive potassium balance. Monitoring should be performed in patients who require an NSAID and who have borderline high potassium concentrations (i.e., >5.0 mEq/L). Hyperkalemia has been observed to follow NSAID administration in patients with both normal and abnormal renal function.[432]

NSAID-Induced Tubulointerstitial Disease

Another form of NSAID-induced kidney disease is interstitial nephritis (Table 34-12). The NSAID that is most often associated with this lesion is fenoprofen, but all NSAIDs have been linked to at least one case of this syndrome.[527-529] The key features of this syndrome are that the time to develop the syndrome is variable, with a mean of 5.4 months; only 19% of patients have a fever, rash, or eosinophilia; and 83% of patients have the nephrotic syndrome. The renal biopsy findings in this disorder typically include a focal interstitial infiltrate with some fibrosis. Immunofluorescence studies are usually not remarkable, but in some cases weak and variable staining for IgG, IgA, IgM, and C3 are seen in interstitial membranes. The most common glomerular lesion is that of minimal-change disease. There have also been reports of membranous histologic changes.[530, 531] Electron-dense deposits have been noted in the mesangium in three patients.[528] The pathogenesis of this disorder is not known. A delayed hypersensitivity response to the NSAID appears to

TABLE 34-12

Clinical Characteristics of NSAID-Induced Tubulointerstitial Nephritis (TIN) vs. Typical Drug-Induced TIN

CHARACTERISTIC	NSAID-INDUCED TIN	TYPICAL DRUG-INDUCED TIN
Duration of exposure	5 days to >1 yr	5–26 days
Hypersensitivity symptoms	7%–8%	80%
Eosinophilia	17%–18%	75%–80%
Proteinuria > 3.5 g/24 hours	> 90%	< 10%
Eosinophiluria	0%–5%	80%–85%
Peak serum creatinine	1.5%-> 10 mg/dL	3.7%-> 10 mg/dL

be a tenable hypothesis, but the involvement of the glomeruli to cause nephrotic syndrome without a lesion is unclear. Another possibility is the fact that inhibition of cyclooxygenase will shunt arachidonic acid metabolites to the lipooxygenase pathway and produce leukotrienes.[532, 533] Leukotrienes mediate inflammation and increase vascular permeability and are chemotactic for white blood cells, including T lymphocytes and eosinophils.[534, 535] Torres has summarized this scheme in detail.[536] Finally, a recent study has offered the hypothesis that underlying renal insufficiency is necessary for ibuprofen-induced interstitial disease to occur.[537]

NSAID-Induced Chronic Renal Failure and Analgesic Nephropathy

The most common form of drug-induced chronic renal failure is analgesic nephropathy. This lesion has most commonly been linked to the chronic ingestion of compound analgesics containing aspirin, phenacetin, and caffeine.[538] A still unresolved question is whether long-term use of NSAIDs alone can similarly result in a progressive and irreversible form of chronic renal failure. In this regard, a number of observations have emerged that would appear to substantiate the belief that long-term use of NSAIDs can lead to a chronic form of renal injury. Furthermore, the clinical characterstics of NSAID-induced chronic renal failure are sufficiently different from those in analgesic nephropathy to suggest that this is a distinct clinical entity. Before reviewing the data linking chronic NSAID use and renal insufficiency, a brief description of analgesic nephropathy is provided.

Analgesic nephropathy is a chronic renal disease characterized by renal papillary necrosis and chronic interstitial nephritis.[538-540] The early reports linking analgesics and renal disease were generally found in patients who consumed combination products containing phenacetin. This finding focused attention on phenacetin as the primary cause of the syndrome and prompted many countries to officially remove the drug from nonprescription analgesics. Significantly, the removal of phenacetin has not been uniformly followed by the expected reduction in the incidence of the syndrome.[541] Given that other agents such as acetaminophen or salicylamide have been substituted for phenacetin in many combination products, the lack of decline in incidence of analgesic nephropathy suggests that the use of combination products is as important as whether the compound contains phenacetin.[541, 542] This conclusion is further supported by experience in Belgium where a strong geographic correlation exists between the prevalence of analgesic nephropathy and sales of analgesic mixtures containing a minimum of two analgesic components.[543, 544]

Numerous epidemiologic studies performed in the past demonstrated a wide variation in the geographic incidence of analgesic nephropathy.[541, 542, 545-548] Much of this variability could be explained by differences in the annual per capita consumption of phenacetin.[540, 541] In countries with the highest consumption, such as Australia and Sweden, analgesic nephropathy was found responsible for up to 20% of cases of end-stage renal disease. In Canada, which had the lowest per capita consumption, analgesic nephropathy accounted for only 2% to 5% of end-stage renal disease patients. It has been estimated that between 2% and 4% of all end-stage renal disease cases in the United States can be attributed to habitual analgesic consumption. Within the United States, there are also regional differences in the reported incidence of analgesic nephropathy, which are though to reflect differences in analgesic consumption.[541, 542, 545, 546] For example, the use of combination analgesics is more common in the southeastern United States, and the incidence of analgesic nephropathy is three to five times more common as a cause of end-stage renal disease in North Carolina compared to Philadelphia.[541, 542, 545, 546]

The development of analgesic nephropathy is associated with a number of well-defined clinical characteristics.[549] The disease is more common in women by a factor of two to six and has a peak incidence at age 53 years. Patients typically consume compound analgesics on a daily basis, often for chronic complaints such as headache, dyspepsia, or to improve work productivity. It has been estimated that nephropathy occurs after the cumulative ingestion of 2 to 3 kg of the index drug. Often patients will exhibit a typical psychiatric profile characterized by addictive behavior. Gastrointestinal complication such as peptic ulcer disease are common. The patients are frequently anemic as a result of gastrointestinal blood loss as well as renal insufficiency. Ischemic heart disease and renal artery stenosis have both been reported to occur with higher frequency in these patients.[540] In fact, regular use of analgesic drugs containing phenacetin is associated with an increased risk of hypertension of mortality and morbidity due to cardiovascular disease.[548, 550] Finally, long-term use of analgesics is known to be a risk factor for the subsequent generation of uroepithelial tumors.[551]

Patients with analgesic nephropathy have predominantly tubulomedullary dysfunction characterized by impaired concentrating ability, acidification defects, and occasionally a salt-losing state. Proteinuria tends to be low to moderate in quantity. Interestingly, the pattern of proteinuria is typically a mixture of glomerular and tubular origin. Pyuria is common and is often sterile. Occasionally hematuria is noted, but if persistent should raise the possibility of a uroepithelial tumor.

There are several features of analgesic nephropathy that make it difficult to diagnose. The disease is slowly progressive and the symptoms and signs are nonspecific. Patients are often reluctant to admit to heavy usage of analgesics and therefore are either misdiagnosed or not diagnosed at all until the renal failure is far advanced. In addition, the lack of a simple and noninvasive test that reliably implicates analgesics as the cause of the renal injury has been an important limiting factor. Noncontrast abdominal computed tomography may emerge as a useful diagnostic tool in this setting given its usefulness in the diagnosis of papillary necrosis.[552]

As mentioned earlier, there are a number of reports that suggest that chronic use of NSAIDs alone may also lead to renal injury. In this regard, several NSAIDs have been associated with the development of papillary necrosis either when administered alone or in combination with aspirin.[553] In addition to inhibiting prostaglandin synthesis, the ability of these agents to redistribute blood flow to the cortex, rendering the renal medulla ischemic, may underlie this association.[432] While the reports linking papillary necrosis and NSAIDs are predominantly anecdotal, more recent observations suggest that chronic renal failure resulting from long-term use of NSAIDs may be more prevalent than once thought.[554, 555] In a multicenter case-control study, Sandler and colleagues found a twofold increase in the risk for chronic renal failure associated with the previous daily used of NSAIDs.[554] Chronic renal failure was newly diagnosed and was defined as a serum creatinine concentration of 1.5 mg/dL or greater. This increased risk was primarily limited to older men. An additional report linking chronic use of NSAIDs with development of chronic renal failure described 56 patients from Australia.[540] These patients had taken only NSAIDs over a period of 10 to 20 years for treatment of various rheumatic diseases. In 19 patients (34%), radiographic evidence of papillary necrosis was found. In 37 patients, renal biopsy material was available that disclosed evidence of chronic interstitial nephritis. The clinical characteristics of these patients were quite different from those with analgesic nephropathy, suggesting that NSAID-induced chronic renal failure is indeed a distinct entity. In particular, patients with NSAID-associated renal disease were older, had an equal female-to-male ratio, had a lower incidence of papillary necrosis, had less severe renal insufficiency, and had a lower incidence of urinary tract infections.[540] In addition, an increased risk of uroepithelial tumors has not been described in these patients.

Further evidence of chronic toxicity has been reported in a preliminary communication in which patients treated with NSAIDs for rheumatoid arthritis and osteoarthritis were compared to a matched control arthritis population.[556] In this study, the NSAID-treated patients had a rise in serum creatinine concentration from 1.28 mg/dL to 2.58 mg/dL over a mean period of 47.5 months. The control group not taking NSAIDs had stable renal function. Finally, Segasothy and co-workers reported on the risk of chronic renal disease in a prospective study of 259 heavy analgesic abusers.[555] In this study, 69 patients developed radiographic evidence of papillary necrosis. Of these, 29 used NSAIDs either alone (17 patients) or in combination with another NSAID (12 patients). Another 9 patients used NSAIDs in combination with paracetamol, aspirin, caffeine, or a traditional herbal medicine. Renal insufficiency (serum creatinine concentration 126–778 μ/mol/L) was noted in 26 of the 38 patients who had used an NSAID chronically. Similar to the patients from Australia,[540] this disorder was more common in males (1.9:1), distinguishing it from classic analgesic nephropathy, which typically occurs in females. Similarly, these patients did not exhibit the usual psychological profile associated with analgesic abuse.

Thus, although further studies are needed to definitively assess the question of cumulative toxicity, it appears that some chronically treated patients may develop a change in renal function over the long term. Given the abuse potential of powerful NSAIDs and the fact that ibuprofen, naproxen, and ketoprofen are now available on an over-the-counter basis, it is possible that chronic NSAID abuse may become a more common cause of chronic renal failure in the future. In considering the association of compound analgesic abuse and the possible linkage of chronic NSAID use with the development of chronic renal failure, it has become common clinical practice to recommend acetaminophen whenever possible for analgesia. In this regard, a recent case-control study examining the use of over-the-counter analgesics as a risk factor for end-stage renal disease found that acetaminophen may also cause chronic renal injury when used on a

continual basis.[557] In this study, heavy use of acetaminophen (more than one pill per day) and medium to high cumulative intake (1000 or more pills in a lifetime) each doubled the odds of end-stage renal disease. These authors concluded that reduced consumption of acetaminophen could decrease the overall incidence of end-stage renal disease by approximately 8% to 10%. The findings in this study confirmed an earlier report that also concluded that long-term daily use of acetaminophen is associated with an increased risk of chronic renal disease.[545] While these studies do not establish a cause-and-effect relationship between acetaminophen ingestion and chronic renal disease, the data do suggest that ingestion of acetaminophen on a continual and chronic basis should be discouraged. A potential flaw in this study was the problem of confounding by indication, a complication of studying a condition (renal disease) that may result in the use of a drug to ameliorate the condition.

Two recent studies have further elucidated the relationship between chronic ingestion of analgesics and chronic kidney disease. One study performed in the Untied States used the Physician Health Study Database to define the relationship between analgesic use over time and renal insufficiency as measured by a reduced creatinine clearance or an elevated serum creatinine concentration.[558] This study had the virtue of examining a large number of subjects (> 11,000), but was limited to men and did not query individuals with the heaviest analgesic consumption; the greatest consumption category was 2500 tablets over the years of the study, or fewer than 200 tablets per year. The study concluded that this moderate intake of analgesics was not associated with a detectable reduction in renal function.

A second study, by Fored and colleagues [559] from Sweden was a case-control study of over 900 newly identified individuals with a serum creatine of 2.8 mg/dL or greater. When compared to age- and gender-matched controls, these subjects had substantially greater ingestion of acetaminophen and aspirin in their medical histories. A lagged time analysis was performed in the study to be certain to query patients regarding analgesic consumption in the somewhat distant past (10 and 15 years before presentation) so that confounding by indication could be avoided. The study concluded that cumulative ingestion of analgesics of over 500 g was associated with chronic kidney disease.

An organized review by a consensus panel of the National Kidney Foundation surveyed over 600 articles and studied the implications of several different kinds of analgesic ingestion and renal failure risks.[560, 561] The highlights of the recommendations were that ingestion of aspirin and non-steroidal combinations should not be encouraged because of an increased risk of renal failure; that habitual consumption of analgesics should be discouraged, and monitoring is recommended when such use is mandatory; that combination analgesics should be available by prescription only with an explicit warning to physicians that the habitual consumption of these combination products could lead to the insidious development of chronic renal failure; and that there should be an explicit warning to consumers regarding NSAID ingestion. New studies to define the scope of the problem in the United States are underway. For the present, renal function should be monitored in a serial fashion in patients who require long-term use of NSAIDs.

DRUGS USED IN INFLAMMATORY BOWEL DISEASE

Mesalazine and Olsalazine

Sulfasalazine is used in the treatment of inflammatory bowel disease. New formulations of this drug such as mesalazine and olsalazine are free of sulfhapyridine and improve the delivery of 5-aminosalicylic acid (5-ASA) to the small bowel. 5-ASA is converted to acetyl-5-ASA in the bowel epithelium. Free 5-ASA has been reported to cause renal tubular damage and acute interstitial renal disease in rodents. Early tubular injury in humans is characterized by increased excretion of tubular proteins such as β_2-microglobulin, alanine aminopeptidase, and N-acetyl-D-glucoseamidase.[562] Patients who receive these agents on a chronic basis should have renal function monitored closely.

ANGIOTENSIN-CONVERTING ENZYME INHIBITORS

ACE inhibitors have been observed to cause reversible acute renal failure in the setting of hypertension and congestive heart failure. The reason for this phenomenon appears to be related to the role angiotension II (AII) plays in sustaining the renal circulation under conditions of hypoperfusion.[563] GFR is largely governed by the relative tone of the afferent and efferent arterioles. When renal perfusion pressure declines, the afferent arteriole dilates and total renal vascular resistance declines. This vasorelaxation is a compensatory myogenic reflex to the decline in renal perfusion pressure. In addition, depending upon the level to which renal perfusion declines, an increase in efferent arteriole resistance may be required to maintain the intracapillary glomerular pressure at a level sufficiently high to sustain glomerular filtration. The net effect of this increase in efferent resistance is to sustain GFR in the context of some increase in renal vascular resistance, thereby increasing the filtration fraction.[563, 564] The increase in efferent vascular tone that occurs under renal hypoperfusion conditions is in large part secondary to the vasoconstrictive effect of AII. What emerges from the number of studies that have been performed to examine this question is that the renal autoregulatory adjustments required to maintain GFR in prerenal conditions are highly dependent upon a sustained efferent resistance that is, in turn, dependent upon AII. It is under these conditions that the administration of an ACE inhibitor could lead to a fall in GFR. What appears to occur is that ACE inhibitors blunt the vasoconstrictive effect of AII at the efferent arteriole and therefore lead to a decline in efferent arteriolar resistance. This decline in efferent arteriole resistance leads to a fall in glomerular capillary pressure, and then to a fall in GFR.[563]

The clinical settings in which this physiology become important are as follows: First, in a setting of significant (usually > 70%) obstruction of both renal arteries, efferent tone is increased to maximize the GFR. Second, in a setting of unilateral obstruction to a solitary functioning kidney, efferent tone again sustains the GFR necessary to maintain homeostasis. In both of these examples, there is ischemia to the whole renal mass, thereby making the kidney and GFR dependent upon efferent resistance to sustain blood flow. Third, under circumstances in which cardiac output is low or in which there is an intense prerenal vasoconstriction, perfusion pressure may be low enough to mimic the conditions in which there is actual physical obstruction of the renal arteries. Such an occurrence would be in a setting of moderate to severe congestive heart failure. Under these circumstances, efferent arteriolar tone again sustains GFR, and the use of an ACE inhibitor would result in loss of efferent tone and a consequent decline in the GFR. A fourth circumstance in which this physiologic construct holds is in severe small-vessel disease of the kidney, as might be seen in severe nephrosclerosis. Even though the main renal arteries are patent, the obstruction to renal perfusion occurs more distally in arcuate and interlobular vessels, leading to another type of functional renal ischemia.

These complex interrelationships between AII and efferent tone have made the use of ACE inhibitors more complicated than other antihypertensive or unloading agents. Furthermore, the proliferation of these agents on the market and their widespread use has brought the problem of silent ischemic disease of the kidney to greater attention.[565] It is estimated that approximately 10% to 15% of patients with end-stage renal disease may have occlusive renal artery obstruction or partial obstruction as a cofactor in the cause of the renal failure.[566] Similarly, it is common to observe a decline in renal function in the setting of ACE inhibitor therapy and heart failure.[567] This is more pronounced if cardiac filling pressures decline during the course of therapy.

The sum of all these interrelationships is that if renal insufficiency or a decline in renal function follows the use of an ACE inhibitor, underlying obstructive renal artery disease should be suspected. In fact, it has been proposed that ACE inhibitor challenge be used to screen for renal transplant artery stenosis and other types of renin-mediated hypertension in transplant patients.[567, 568] It is also clear that in the severely hypertensive patients who come to medical attention when renal pressure declines too far, renal insufficiency may ensue. This was pointed out in studies by Ying and colleagues[569] and by Textor and associates[570] who showed that bilateral renal artery stenosis or unilateral stenosis in patients with one functioning kidney could lead to acute renal insufficiency if renal perfusion pressure was lowered below the autoregulatory threshold by drugs other than ACE inhibitors. In both of these studies, revascularization or angioplasty of the renal artery reversed the effect.

When a decline in renal function follows the use of an ACE inhibitor, suspicion of obstructive renal artery disease should be raised.[571] If the decline in renal function occurs upon exposure to an ACE inhibitor in the context of congestive heart failure, then a reduction in the dose of the drug, liberalization of the salt diet of the patient, or a decrease in diuretic therapy may improve renal function without obviating the effect of the drug on afterload. Screening tests for renal artery obstruction include captopril scintigraphy using orthohippurate or EDTA.[572-577] Some investigators have advocated the use of the peripheral plasma renin activity test as a screening test for this lesion, but the test may lose its value in patients with bilateral artery stenosis, renal parenchymal disease, or essential hypertension.[578] These patients may have very high values that are affected by ACE inhibitor therapy.[579] The use of duplex scanning to diagnose obstructive renal artery disease is promising, but remains impractical for many patients with obesity or prior abdominal surgery.[580]

TABLE 34-13

Risk Factors for Acute Renal Dysfunction Associated with Angiotensin-Converting Enzyme Inhibitors and Angiotensin Receptor Blockers

Bilateral renal artery stenosis or stenosis in solitary kidney
Polycystic kidney disease
Decreased absolute or effective circulatory volume
Nonsteroidal anti-inflammatory agents
Sepsis

The best diagnostic test is renal artery arteriography. Other renal complications of ACE inhibitor therapy are provided in Table 34-13. Acute tubular necrosis is unusual but has been reported.[581-584] A few cases of membranous nephropathy have been reported, but the overall incidence of this complication and that of tubulointerstitial nephritis are believed to be low.[585, 586]

HYDROCARBONS

A large body of literature suggests that chronic hydrocarbon exposure may predispose individuals to the development of several different types of renal disease.[587] Acute tubular necrosis, chronic interstitial nephritis, and glomerulonephritis have all been described.[588-595] In a 1992 study, three groups of healthy men working in separate areas of a manufacturing plant were evaluated.[596] Group 1 was exposed to paint-based hydrocarbons; a second group of 101 volunteers worked in the transmission assembly area of the plant and was exposed to petroleum-base mineral oils; group 3 was comprised of 92 automated press operators with minimal exposure to lubricants or solvents. The group 1 workers had a significantly higher prevalence of elevated serum creatinine and a higher prevalence of abnormal urinary total protein, *N*-acetylglucosaminidase, γ-glutamyltransferase, and leucineaminopeptidase than groups 2 or 3. Group 2 had a normal serum creatinine but a significantly higher prevalence of abnormal total urinary proteins, transferrin-binding protein, *N*-acetylglucosaminidase, and leucineaminopeptidase than group 3. Blood pressures were similar in all three groups. The elevation in serum creatinine seen in group 1 was mild and the elevation of urinary proteins observed in group 2 was also modest.

The pathogenesis of hydrocarbon-induced renal disease is not known with certainty; but, the possibility that solvents cause renal damage and thereby release a tubular antigen that results in an autoimmune reaction is a theory that is held in some regard. Animal studies that suggest that the tubulointerstitial nephritis that follows chronic hydrocarbon exposure can be ameliorated by the pretreatment with radiation support an autoimmune mechanism for this disease.[596] Another hypothesis is that potentially toxic immune factors arise independently of hydrocarbon exposure and that hydrocarbons facilitate the deposit of these mediators in renal tissue.[597] Alternatively, the immune system could be damaged by hydrocarbons, leading to impaired clearance of antigen material, which then lodges in glomerular capillary loops and incites an inflammatory response.[598]

REFERENCES

1. Leehey DJ, Braun BI, Tholl DA, et al: Can pharmacokinetic dosing decrease nephrotoxicity associated with aminoglycoside therapy? J Am Soc Nephrol 4:81-90, 1993.
2. Luft FC: Clinical significance of renal changes engendered by aminoglycosides in man. J Antimicrob Chemother 13(suppl A):23-30, 1984.
3. Houghton DC, English J, Bennett WM: Chronic tubulointerstitial nephritis and renal insufficiency associated with long-term "subtherapeutic" gentamicin. J Lab Clin Med 112:694-703, 1988.
4. Cronin RE, Bulger RE, Southern P, et al: Natural history of aminoglycoside nephrotoxicity in the dog. J Lab Clin Med 95:463-474, 1980.
5. Schwartz JH, Schein P: Fanconi syndrome associated with cephalothin and gentamicin therapy. Cancer 41:769-772, 1978.
6. Melnick JZ, Baum M, Thompson JR: Aminoglycoside-induced Fanconi's syndrome. Am J Kidney Dis 23:118-122, 1994.
7. Bar RJ, Wilson HE, Mazzaferri EL: Hypomagnesemic hypocalcemia secondary to renal magnesium wasting: A possible consequence of high dose gentamicin therapy. Ann Intern Med 82:646-649, 1975.
8. Patel R, Savage A: Symptomatic hypomagnesemia associated with gentamicin therapy. Nephron 23:50-52, 1979.
9. Brinker KR, Bulger RE, Dobyan DC, et al: Effect of potassium depletion on gentamicin nephrotoxicity. J Lab Clin Med 98:292-301, 1981.
10. Pastoiza-Munoz E, Timmerman D, Feldman S, et al: Ultrafiltration of gentamicin and netilmicin in vivo. J Pharmacol Exp ther 220: 604-608, 1982.
11. Senekjian HO, Knight TF, Weinman EJ: Micropuncture study of the handling of gentamicin by the rat kidney. Kidney Int 19:416-423, 1981.
12. Pastoriza-Munoz E, Bowman RL, Kaloyanides GJ: Renal tubular transport of gentamicin in the rat. Kidney Int 15:440-450, 1979.
13. Silverblatt FJ, Kuehn C: Autoradiography of gentamicin uptake by the rat proximal tubule cell. Kidney Int 15:335-345, 1979.
14. Kluwe WM, Hook JB: Analysis of gentamicin uptake by rat renal cortical slices. Toxicol Appl Pharmacol 45:531-539, 1978.
15. Sheth AU, Senekjian HO, Babion H, et al: Renal handling of gentamicin by the Munich-Wister rat. Am J Physiol 241:F645-F648, 1981.
16. Kosek JC, Mazze RI, Cousins MJ: Nephrotoxicity of gentamicin. Lab Invest 30:48-57, 1974.
17. Feldman S, Wang M, Kaloyanides GJ: Aminoglycosides induce a phospholipidosis in the renal cortex of the rat: An early manifestation of nephrotoxicity. J Pharmacol Exp Ther 220:514-520, 1982.
18. Josepovitz C, Farruggella T, Levine R, et al: Effect of netilmicin on the phospholipid composition of subcellular fractions of rat renal cortex. J Pharmacol Exp Ther 235:810-819, 1985.
19. Carlier MD, Laurent G, Claes PJ, et al: Inhibition of lysosomal phospholipases by aminoglycoside antibiotics: In vitro comparative studies. Antimicrob Agents Chemother 23:440-449, 1983.
20. Hostetler KY, Hall LB: Inhibition of kidney lysosomal phospholipases A and C by aminoglycoside antibiotics: Possible mechanism of aminoglycoside toxicity. Proc Natl Acad Sci U S A 79:1663-1667, 1982.
21. Ramsammy LS, Josepovitz C, Kaloyanides GJ: Gentamicin inhibits agonist stimulation of the phosphatidylinositol cascade in primary cultures of rabbit proximal tubular cells and in rat renal cortex. J Pharmacol Exp Ther 247: 989-996, 1988.
22. Sandoval R, Leiser J, Molitoris, BA: Aminoglycoside antibiotics traffic to the Golgi complex in LLC-PK1 cells. J Am soc Nephrol 9: 167-174, 1998.
23. Ramsammy L, Ling KY, Josepovitz C, et al: Effect of gentamicin on lipid peroxidation in rat renal cortex. Biochem Pharmacol 34: 3895-3900, 1985.
24. Kaloyanides GJ, Ramsammy L, Josepovitz C: Assessment of three therapeutic interventions for modifying gentamicin nephrotoxicity in the rat. *In* Bach PH, Delacruz L, Gregg NJ, Wilks MF (eds): Proceedings of the Fourth International Symposium of Nephrotoxicity. New York, Marcel Dekker, 1990, p 103.
25. Walker PD, Shah SV: Gentamicin enhanced production of hydrogen peroxide by renal cortical mitochondria. Am J Physiol 253: C495-C499, 1987.
26. Walker PD, Shah SV: Evidence suggesting a role for hydroxyl radical in gentamicin-induced acute renal failure in rats. J Clin Invest 91: 334-341, 1988.
27. Luft FC, Kleit SA: Renal parnechymal accumulation of aminoglycoside antibiotics in rats. J Infect Dis 130:656-659, 1974.

28. Josepovitz C, Pastorize-Munoz E, Timmerman D, et al: Inhibition of gentamicin uptake in rat renal cortex in vivo by aminoglycosides and organic polycations. J Pharmacol Exp Ther 223:314-321, 1982.

29. Pastoriza-Munoz E, Josepovitz C, Ramsammy L, et al: Renal handling of netilmicin in the rat with streptozotocin-induced diabetes mellitus. J Pharmacol Exp Ther 241:166-173, 1987.

30. Collier VU, Lietman PS, Mitch WE: Evidence for luminal uptake of gentamicin in the perfused rat kidney. J Pharmacol Exp Ther 210:247-251, 1979.

31. Chiu PJS, Long JF: Urinary excretion and tissue accumulation of gentamicin and para-aminohippurate in post-ischemic kidneys. Kidney Int 15:618-623, 1979.

32. Ramsammy LS, Kaloyanides GJ: Effect of gentamicin on the transition temperature and permeability to glycerol of phosphatidylinositol-containing liposomes. Biochem Pharmacol 36:1179-1181, 1987.

33. Sastrasinh M, Knauss TC, Weinberg JM, et al: Identification of the aminoglycoside binding site in rat renal brush border membranes. J Pharmacol Exp Ther 222:350-358, 1982.

34. Moestrup SK, Cui S, Vorum H, et al: Evidence that epithelial glycoprotein 330/megalin mediates uptake of polybasic drugs. J Clin Invest 96:1404-1413, 1995.

35. Molitoris BA, Meyer C, Dahl R, et al: Mechanism of ischemia-enhanced aminoglycoside binding and uptake by proximal tubule cells. Am J Physiol 264:F907-F916, 1993.

36. Benett WM, Plamp C, Gilbert DN, et al: The effects of dosage regimen on experimental gentamicin nephrotoxicity: Dissociation of peak serum levels from renal failure. J Infect Dis 140:576-580,1979.

37. Bennett WM, Parker RA, Elliot WC, et al: Sex-related differences in the susceptibility of rats to gentamicin nephrotoxicity. J Infect Dis 45;370-373, 1982.

38. Bennett WM, Hartnett MN, Gilbert D, et al: Effect of sodium intake on gentamicin nephrotoxicity in the rat. Proc Soc Exp Biol Med 151:736-738, 1976.

39. Tardif D, Beauchamp D, Bergeron MG: Influence of endotoxin on the intracortical accumulation kinetics of gentamicin in rats. Antimicrob Agents Chemother 34:576-580, 1990.

40. Corcoran GB, Salazar DE, Schentag JJ: Excessive aminoglycoside nephrotoxicity in obese patients. Am J Med 85:279, 1988.

41. Spiegel DM, Shanley PF, Molitoris BA: Mild ischemia predisposes the S3 segment to gentamicin toxicity. Kidney Int 38:459-464, 1990.

42. Chiu PJS, Miller GH, Long JF, et al: Renal uptake and nephrotoxicity of gentamicin during urinary alkalinization in rats. Clin Exp Pharmacol Physiol 6:317-326, 1979.

43. Cronin R, Inman L, Eche T, et al: Effect of thyroid hormone on gentamicin accumulation in rat proximal tubule lysosomes. Am J Physiol 257:F86-F91, 1989.

44. Thompson JR, Simonsen R, Spindler MA, et al: Protective effect of KCl loading in gentamicin nephrotoxicity. Am J Kidney Dis 15:583-591,1990.

45. Williams PD, Hottendorf GH: Inhibition of renal membrane binding and nephrotoxicity of gentamicin by polyasparangine and polyaspartic acid in the rat. Res Commun Chem Pathol Pharmacol 47:317-320, 1985.

46. Gilbert DN, Wood CA, Kohlhepp SJ, et al: Polyaspartic acid prevents experimental aminoglycoside nephrotoxicity. J Infect Dios 159: 945-953, 1989.

47. Ramsammy LS, Josepovitz C, Lane BP, et al: Polyaspartic acid protects against gentamicin nephrotoxicity in the rat. J Pharmacol Exp Ther 250:149-153, 1989.

48. Ramsammy L, Josepovitz C, Lane B, et al: Polyaspartic acid inhibits gentamicin-induced perturbations of phospholipid metabolism. Am J Physiol 258:C1141-C1149, 1990.

49. Swan SK, Gilbert DN, Kohlhepp SJ, et al: Pharmacologic limits of the protective effect of polyaspartic acid on experimental gentamicin nephrotoxicity. Antimicrob Agents Chemother 37:347-348, 1993.

50. Kishore BK, Kallay Z, Lambricht P, et al: Mechanism of protection afforded by polyaspartic acid against gentamicin-induced phospholipidosis. 1. Polyaspartic acid binds gentamicin and displaces it from negatively charged phospholipid layers in vitro. J Pharmacol Exp Ther 255:867-874, 1990.

51. Murakami H, Yayama K, Chao L, et al: Human kallikrein gene delivery protects against gentamycin-induced nephrotoxicity in rats. Kidney Int 53:1305-1313, 1998.

52. Gilbert DN, Houghton DC, Bennett WL, et al: Reversibility of gentamicin nephrotoxicity in rats: Recovery during continuous drug administration. Proc Soc Exp Biol Med 160:99-103, 1979.

53. Sundin DP, Meyer C, Dahl R, et al: Cellular mechanism of aminoglycoside tolerance in long-term gentamicin treatment. Am J Physiol 272:C1309-C1318, 1997.

54. Simmons CF, Bogusky RT, Humes HD: Inhibitory effects of gentamicin on renal mitochondrial oxidative phosphorylation. J Pharmacol Exp Ther 214:709-715, 1980.

55. Mela-Riker LM, Widener LL, Houghton DC, et al: Renal mitochondrial integrity during continuous gentamicin treatment. Biochem Pharmacol 35:979-984, 1986.

56. Buss WC, Piatt MK, Kauten R: Inhibition of mammalian microsomal protein synthesis by aminoglycoside antibiotics. J Antimicrob Chemother 14:231-241, 1984.

57. Buss WC, Piatt MK: Gentamicin administered in vivo reduces protein synthesis in microsomes subsequently isolated from rat kidneys but not from rat brains. J Antimicrob Chemother 15: 715-721,1985.

58. Bennett WM, Mela-Riker LM, Houghton DC, et al: Microsomal protein synthesis inhibition: An early manifestation of gentamicin nephrotoxicity. Am J Physiol 255:F265-F269, 1988.

59. Bennett WM, Plamp CE, Parker RA, et al: Alterations in organic ion transport induced by gentamicin nephroxicity in the rat. J Lab Clin Med 95: 32-39, 1980.

60. Kirschbaum BB: Interactions between renal brush border membranes and polyamines. J Pharmacol Exp Ther 229:409-416, 1984.

61. Morigama T, Nakahama H, Fukahara Y, et al: Decrease in the fluidity of brush-border membrane vesicles induced by gentamicin. A spin-labelling study. Biochem Pharmacol 48:1169-1174, 1989.

62. Levi M, Cronin RE: Early selective effects of gentamicin on renal brush-border membrane Na-Pi cotransport and Na-H exchange. Am J Physiol 258:1379-1387, 1990.

63. Baylis C, Rennke HR, Brenner BM: Mechanisms of the defect in glomerular ultrafiltration associated with gentamicin administration. Kidney Int 12:344-353, 1977.

64. Barshay ME, Kaye JH, Goldman R, et al: Acute renal failure in diabetic patients after intravenous infusion pyelography. Clin Nephrol 1:35-39, 1973.

65. Churchill DN, Seely J: Nephrotoxicity associated with combined gentamicin-amphotericin B therapy. Nephron 19:176-181, 1977.

66. Dentino ME, Luft FC, Yum MN, et al: Long term effect of cis-diaminedichloride platinum(CDDP) on renal function and structure in man. Cancer 41:1274-1281, 1978.

67. Moore RD, Smith CR, Lipsky JJ, et al: Risk factors for nephrotoxicity in patients treated with aminoglycosides. Ann Intern Med 100: 352-357, 1984.

68. Smith CR, Lipsky JJ, Laskin OL, et al: Double-blind comparison of the nephrotoxicity and auditory toxicity of gentamicin and tobramycin. N Engl J Med 302:1106-1109, 1980.

69. Dillon KR, Dougherty SH, Casner P, et al: Individualized pharmacokinetic versus standard dosing of amikacin: Comparison of therapeutic outcomes. J Antimicrob Chemother 24:581-589, 1989.

70. Burton ME, Ash CL, Hill DP Jr, et al: A controlled trial of the cost benefit of computerized bayesian aminoglycoside administration. Clin Pharmacol Ther 49:685-694, 1991.

71. Sawyers CL, Moore RD, Lerner SA, et al: A Model for predicting nephrotoxicity in patients treated with aminoglycosides. J Infect Dis 153:1062-1068, 1986.

72. Dahlgren JG, Anderson ET, Hewitt WL: Gentamicin blood levels: A guide to nephrotoxicity. Antimicrob Agents Chemother 8:58-62, 1975.

73. Bennett WM, Plamp CE, Gilbert DN, et al: The influence of dosage regimen on experimental nephrotoxicity: Dissociation of peak serum levels from renal failure. J Infect Dis 140:576-579, 1979.

74. Hitt CM, Klepser ME, Nightingale CH, et al: Pharmacoeconomic impact of once-daily aminoglycoside administration. Pharmacotherapy 17:810-814, 1997.

75. Gilbert DN: Once-daily aminoglycoside therapy. Antimicrob Agents Chemother 35:399-405, 1991.

76. Levison ME: New dosing regimens for aminoglycoside antibiotics. Ann Intern Med 117:693-694, 1992.

77. Prins JM, Buller HR, Kuijper EJ, et al: Once versus thrice daily gentamicin in patients with serious infections. Lancet 341:335-339, 1993.

78. Maller R, Ahrne H, Holmen C, et al: Once- versus twice-daily amikacin regimen: Efficacy and safety in systemic gram-negative infections. Scandinavian Amikacin Once Daily Study Group. J Antimicrob Chemother 31:939-948, 1993.

79. Nicolau DP, Freeman CD, Belliveau PP, et al: Experience with once-daily aminoglycoside program administered to 2184 adult patients. Antimicrob Agents Chemother 39:650-655, 1995.

80. Koo J, Tight R, Rajkumar V, et al: Comparison of once-daily versus pharmacokinetic dosing of aminoglycosides in elderly patients. Am J Med 101:177-183, 1996.

81. Farber BF, Moellering RC: Retrospective study of the toxicity of preparations of vancomycin form 1974 to 1981. Antimicrob Agents Chemother 23:138-141, 1983.

82. Sorrell TC, Collignon PJ: A prospective study of adverse reactions associated with vancomycin therapy. J Antimicrob Chemother 16:235-241, 1985.

83. Mellor JA, Kindgom J, Cafferkey M, et al: Vancomycin toxicity: A prospective study. J Antimicrob Chemother 15:773-780, 1985.

84. Downs NJ, Neihart RE, Dolezal JM, et al: Mild nephrotoxicity associated with vancomycin use. Arch Intern Med 149:1777-1781, 1989.

85. Rybak MJ, Albrecht LM, Burke SC, et al: Nephrotoxicity of vancomycin, alone and with an aminoglycoside. J Antimicrob Chemother 25:679-687, 1990.

86. Carbone LG, Bendixen B, Appel GB: Sulfadiazine-associated obstructive nephropathy occurring in a patients with the acquired immune deficiency syndrome. Am J Kidney Dis 12:72-75, 1988.

87. Simon DI, Brosius FC III, Rothstein DM: Sulfadiazine-induced crystalluria revisited. The treatment of *Toxoplasma* encephalitis in patients with acquired immune deficiency syndrome. Arch Intern Med 150:2379-2384, 1990.

88. Sasson JP, Dratch PL, Shortsleeve MJ: Renal US findings in sulfadiazine-induced crystalluria. Radiology 185:739-740, 1992.

89. Becker K, Jablonowski H, Haussinger D: Sulfadiazine-associated nephrotoxicity in patients with the acquired immunodeficiency syndrome. Medicine (Baltimore) 75:185-194, 1996.

90. Andreoli TE, Monahan M: The interaction of polyeneantibiotics with thin lipid membranes. J Gen Physiol 52:300-325, 1968.

91. Cheng JT, Witty RT, Robinson RR, et al: Amphotericin B nephrotoxicity: Increased renal resistance and tubule permeability. Kidney Int 22:626-633,1982.

92. Sawaya BP, Weihprecht H, Campbell WR, et al: Direct vasoconstriction as a possible cause for amphotericin B–induced nephrotoxicity in rats. J Clin Invest 87:2097-2107, 1991.

93. Sawaya BP, Briggs JP, Schnerman J: Amphotericin B nephrotoxicity: The adverse consequences of altered membrane properties. J Am Soc Nephrol 6:154-164, 1995.

94. Douglas JB, Healy JK: Nephrotoxicity effect of amphotericin B, including renal tubular acidosis. Am J Med 46: 154-162, 1969.

95. Heyman SN, Clark BA, Kaiser N, et al: In-vivo and in-vitro studies on the effect of amphotericin B on endothelin release. J Antimicrob Chemother 29:69-77, 1992.

96. Heyman SN, Stillman IE, Brezis M, et al: Chronic amphotericin nephropathy: Morphometric, electron microscopic, functional studies. J Am Soc Nephrol 4:69-80, 1993.

97. Gerkens JF, Branch RA: The influence of sodium status and furosemide on canine acute amphotericin nephrotoxicity. J Pharmacol Exp Ther 214:306-311, 1980.

98. Tolins JP, Raij L: Chronic amphotericin B nephrotoxicity in the rat, protective effects of prophylactic salt loading. Am J Kidney Dis 11:313-317, 1988.

99. Heidemann HTH, Gerkens JF, Spickard WA, et al: Amphotericin B nephrotoxicity in humans decreased by salt repletion. Am J Med 75:476-481, 1983.

100. Fisher MA, Talbot GH, Maislin G, et al: Risk factors for amphotericin B–associated nephrotoxicity. Am J Med 87:547-552, 1989.

101. Dorea EL, Yu L, De Castro I, et al: Nephrotoxicity of amphotericin B is attenuated by solubilizing with lipid emulsion. J Am Soc Nephrol 8:1415-1422, 1997.

102. Sorkine P, Nagar H, Weinbroum A, et al: Administration of amphotericin B in lipid emulsion decreases nephrotoxicity: Results of a prospective, randomized, controlled study in critically ill patients. Crit Care Med 24:1311-1315, 1996.

103. Moreau P, Milpied N, Fayette N, et al: Reduced renal toxicity and improved clinical tolerance of amphotericin B mixed with intralipid compared with conventional amphotericin B in neutropenic patients. J Antimicrob Chemother 30:535-541, 1992.

104. Berns JS, Cohen RM, Stumacher RJ, et al: Renal aspects of therapy for human immunodeficiency virus and associated opportunistic infections. J Am Soc Nephrol 1:1061-1080, 1991.

105. Krieble BF, Ruby DW, Glick MR, et al: Case report: acyclovir neuroxicity and nephrotoxicity—a role for hemodialysis. Am J Med Sci 305:36-39, 1993.

106. Sawyer MH, Webb DE, Balow JE, et al: Acyclovir-induced renal failure. Clinical course and histology. Am J Med 84:1067-1071, 1988.

107. Bianchetti MG, Roduit C, Oetliker OH: Acyclovir-induced renal failure: Course and risk factors. Pediatr Nephrol 5:238-239, 1991.

108. Dos Santos M de F, Dos Santos OF, Boim MA, et al: Nephrotoxicity of acyclovir and ganciclovir in rats: Evaluation of glomerular hemodynamics. J Am Soc Nephrol 8:361-367, 1997.

109. Wharton JM, Coleman DL, Wofsy CB, et al: Trimethoprim-sulfamethoxazole or pentamidine for *Pneumocystis carinii* pneumonia in the acquired immunodeficiency syndrome. Ann Intern Med 105: 37-44, 1986.

110. Sattler FR, Cowan R, Nielsen DM, et al: Trimethoprim-sulfamethoxazole compared with pentamidine for treatment of *Pneumocystis carinii* pneumonia in the acquired immunodeficiency syndrome. Ann Intern Med 109;280-287, 1988.

111. Miller RF, Delany S, Semple SJG: Acute renal failure after nebulised pentamidine. Lancet 1:1271-1272, 1989.

112. Conte JE, Upton RA, Lin ET: Pentamidine pharmacokinetics in patients with AIDS with impaired renal function. J Infect Dis 156:885-890, 1987.

113. Lachaal M, Venuto RC: Nephrotoxicity and hyperkalemia in patients with acquired immunodeficiency syndrome treated with pentamidine. Am J Med 87:260-263, 1989.

114. Shah GM, Alvarado P, Kirschenbaum MA: Symptomatic hypocalcemia and hypomagnesemia with renal magnesium wasting associated with pentamidine therapy in a patient with AIDS. Am J Med 89:380-382, 1990.

115. Antoniskis D, Larsen RA: Acute, rapidly progressive renal failure with simultaneous use of amphotericin B and pentamidine. Antimicrob Agents Chemother 34:470-472, 1990.

116. Oberg B: Antiviral effects of phosphonoformate (PFA, foscarnet sodium). Pharmacol Ther 19:387-415, 1983.

117. Sundquist B, Oberg B: Phosphonoformate inhibits reverse transcriptase. J Gen Virol 45:273-281, 1979.

118. Deray G, Martinez F, Katlama C, et al: Foscarnet nephrotoxicity: Mechanism, incidence and prevention. Am J Nephrol 9:316-321, 1989.

119. Jacobson MA, O'Donnell JJ, Mills J: Foscarnet treatment of cytomegalovirus retinitis in patients with AIDS. Antimicrob Agents Chemother 33;736-741, 1989.

120. Cacoub P, Deray G, Baumelou A, et al: Acute renal failure induced by foscarnet:4 cases. Clin Nephrol 29:315-318, 1988.

121. MacGregor RR, Graziani AL, Weiss R, et al: Successful foscarnet therapy for cytomegalovirus retinitis in an AIDS patient undergoing hemodialysis: Rationale for empiric dosing and plasma level monitoring. J Infect Dis 164:785-787, 1991.

122. Olyaei A, De Mattos A, Bennett W: Renal toxicity of protease inhibitors. Curr Opin Nephrol Hypertens 9:473-476, 2000.

123. Sarcletti M, Petter A, Roamni N, et al: Pyuria in patients treated with indinavir is associated with renal dysfunction. Clin Nephrol 54: 261-270, 2000.

124. Tanji N, Tanji K, Kambham N, et al: Adefovir nephrotoxicity: Possible role of mitochondrial DNA depletion. Hum Pathol 32:734-740, 2001.

125. Cote H, Brumme Z, Criab K, et al: Changes in mitochondrial DNA as a marker of nucleoside toxicity in HIV-infected patients. N Engl J Med 346:811-820, 2002.

126. Cronin RE: Renal failure following radiologic procedures. Am J Med Sci 296: 342-356, 1989.

127. Rich MW, Crecelius CA: Incidence, risk factors, clinical course of acute renal insufficiency after cardiac catheterization in patients 70 years of age or older. A prospective study. Arch Intern Med 150:1237-1242, 1990.

128. Lautin EM, Freeman NJ, Schoenfeld AH, et al: Radiocontrast-associated renal dysfunction: Incidence and risk factors. AJR Am J Roentgenol 157: 49-58, 1991.

129. Manske CL, Sprafka JM, Strony JT, et al: Contrast nephropathy in azotemic diabetic patients undergoing coronary angiography. Am J Med 89:615-620, 1990.

130. Byrd L, Sherman RL: Radiocontrast-induced acute renal failure: A clinical and pathophysiologic review. Medicine (Baltimore) 58: 270-279, 1979.

131. McCarthy CS, Becker JA: Multiple myeloma and contrast media. Radiology 183:519-521, 1992.

132. Harkonen S, Kjellstrand CM: Exacerbation of diabetic renal failure following intravenous pyelography. Am J Med 63: 939-946, 1977.

133. Weinrauch LA, Healy RW, Leland OS, et al: Coronary angiography and acute renal failure in diabetic azotemic nephropathy. Ann Intern Med 86:56-59, 1977.

134. D'Elia JA, Gleason RE, Alday M, et al: Nephrotoxicity from angiographic contrast material. A prospective study. Am J Med 72: 719-725, 1982.

135. Martin-Paredero V, Dixon SM, Baker JD, et al: Risk for renal failure after major angiography. Arch Surg 118:1417-1420, 1983.

136. Taliercio CP, Vlietstra RE, Fisher LD, et al: Risk of renal dysfunction with cardiac angiography. Ann Intern Med.104:501-504, 1986.

137. Fang LS, Sirota RA, Ebert TH, et al: Low fractional excretion of sodium with contrast media-induced acute renal failure. Arch Intern Med 140:531-533, 1980.

138. D'Elia JA, Kaldany A, Weinbrauch LA, et al: Inadequacy of fractional excretion of sodium test [letter]. Arch Intern Med 141:818, 1981.

139. Gelman ML, Rowe JW, Coggins CH, et al: Effects of an angiographic contrast agent on renal function. Cardiovasc Med 4:313-320, 1979.

140. Moreau JF, Droz D, Sabto J, et al: Osmotic nephrosis induced by water-soluble tri-iodinated contrast media in man. Radiology 115: 329-336, 1975.

141. Moreau JF, Droz D, Noel LH, et al: Tubular nephrotoxicity of water-soluble iodonated contrast media. Invest Radiol 15:S54-S60, 1980.

142. Heyman SN, Brezis M, Reubinoff CA, et al: Acute renal failure with selective medullary injury in the rat. J Clin Invest 82:401-412, 1988.

143. Vari RC, Natarajan LA, Whitescarver SA, et al; Induction, prevention and mechanisms of contrast media–induced acute renal failure. Kidney Int 33:699-707, 1988.

144. Agmon Y, Peleg H, Greenfeld Z, et al: Nitric oxide and prostanoids protect the renal outer medulla from radiocontrast toxicity in the rat. J Clin Invest 94:1069-1075, 1994.

145. Bakris GL, Burnett JC, Jr: A role for calcium in radiocontrast-induced reductions in renal hemodynamics. Kidney Int 27:465-468, 1985.

146. Caldicott WJH, Hollenberg NK, Abrams HL: Characteristics of response of renal vascular bed to contrast media. Evidence of vasoconstriction induced by renin-angiotensin system. Invest Radiol 5: 539-547, 1970.

147. Heyman SN, Clark BA, Kaiser N, et al: Radiocontrast agents induce endothelin release in vivo and in vitro. J Am Soc Nephrol 3:58-65, 1992.

148. Heyman SN, Clark BA, Cantley L, et al: Effects of ioversol versus iothalamate on endothelin release and radiocontrast nephropathy. Invest Radiol 28:313-318, 1993.

149. Andrade L, Campos SB, Seguro AC: Hypercholesterolemia aggravates radiocontrast nephrotoxicity: Protective role of L-arginine, Kidney Int 53:1736-1742, 1998.

150. Weisberg. LD, Kurnik PB, Kurnik BR: Radiocontrast-induced nephropathy in humans: Role of renal vasoconstriction. Kidney Int 41:1408-1415, 1992.

151. Weiberg LS, Kurnick PB, Kurnick BR: Dopamine and renal blood flow in radiocontrast-induced nephropathy in humans. Ren Fail 15:61-68, 1993.

152. Solomon R, Werner C, Mann D, et al: Effects of saline, mannitol, furosemide on acute decreases in renal function induced by radiocontrast agents. N Engl J Med 331:1416-1420, 1994.

153. Bettmann MA: Angiographic contrast agents: Conventional and new media compared. AJR Am J Roentgenol 139:787-794, 1982.

154. Messana JM, Cieslinski DA, Nguyen VD, et al: Comparison of the toxicity of the radiocontrast agents, iopamidol and diatrizoate, to rabbit renal proximal tubule cells in vitro. J Pharmacol Exp Ther 244:1139-1144, 1988.

155. Schwab SJ, Hlatky MA, Pieper KS; Contrast nephotoxicity: A randomized controlled trial of a nonionic and an ionic radiographic contrast agent. N Engl J Med 320:149-153, 1989.

156. Parfrey PS, Groffiths SM, Barrett BJ, et al: Contrast material–included renal failure in patients with diabetes mellitus, renal insufficiency, or both. N Engl J Med 320: 143-149, 1989.

157. Barrett BJ, Parfrey PS, Vavasour HM, et al: Contrast nephropathy in patients with impaired renal function: High versus low osmolar media. Kidney Int 41:1274-1279, 1992.

158. Moore RD, Steinberg EP, Powe NR, et al: Nephrotoxicity of high-osmolality versus low-osmolity contrast media: Randomized clinical trail. Riodiology 182:649-655, 1992.

159. Lautin EM, Freeman NJ, Schoenfeld AH, et al: Radiocontrast-associated renal dysfunction: A comparison of lower-osmolality and conventional high-osmolality contrast media. AJR Am J Roentgenol 157:59-65, 1991.

160. Rudnick MR, Goldfarb S, Wexler L, et al: Nephrotoxicity of ionic and nonionic contrast media in 1196 patients: A randomized trial. Kidney Int 47:254-261, 1995.

161. Barrett BJ, Carlisle EJ: Meta-analysis of the relative nephrotoxicity of high and low-osmolality iodinated contrast media. Radiology 188:171-178, 1993.

162. Kopp JB, Klotman PE: Cellular and molecular mechanisms of cyclosporin nephrotoxicity. J Am Soc Nephrol 1:162-179, 1990.

163. Cutis JJ: Hypertension after renal transplantation: Cyclosporine increases the diagnostic and therapeutic considerations. AmJ Kidney Dis 13(suppl):28-32, 1989.

164. Takenaka T, Hashimoto Y, Epstein M: Diminished acetylcholine-induced vasodilation in renal microvessels of cyclosporine-treated rats. J Am Soc Nephrol 4:42-50, 1992.

165. English J, Evan A, Houghton DC, et al: Cyclosporine-induced acute renal dysfunction in rats: Evidence of arteriolar vasoconstriction with preservation of tubular function. Transplantation 44:135-141, 1987.

166. Garr MD, Paller MS: Cyclosporine augments renal but not systemic vascular reactivity. Am J Physiol 258:F211-F217, 1990.

167. Zoja C, Furci L, Ghilardi F, et al: Cyclosporin-induce endothelial cell injury. Lab Invest 55:455-462, 1986.

168. Lau DCW, Wong K, Hwang WS: Cyclosporine toxicity on cultured rat microvascular endothelial cells. Kidney Int 35:604-613, 1989.

169. Kon V, Sugiura M, Inagami T, et al: Role of endothelin in cyclosporine-induced glomerular dysfunction. Kidney Int 47: 1487-1491, 1990.

170. Lanese DM, Conger JD: Effects of endothelin receptor antagonist on cyclosporine-induced vasoconstriction in isolated rat renal arterioles. J Clin Invest 91:2144-2149, 1993.

171. Munger KA, Takahashi K, Awazu M, et al: Maintenance of endothelin-induced renal arteriolar constriction in rats is cyclooxygenase dependent. Am J Physiol 264:F637-644, 1993.

172. Rooth P, Dawidson I, Diller et al: Protection against cyclosporine-induced impairment of renal microcirculation by verapamil in mice. Transplantation 45:433-437, 1988.

173. Wagner K, Henkel M, Heinemeyer G, et al: Interaction of calcium blockers and cyclosporine. Transplant Proc 20(suppl 2): 561-568, 1988.

174. Dawidson I, Rooth P, Fry WR, et al: Prevention of acute cyclosporine-induced renal blood flow inhibition and improved immunosuppression with verapamil. Transplantation 48:575-580, 1989.

175. Dawidson I, Rooth P, Alway C, et al: Verapamil prevents post-transplant delayed function and cyclosporine A nephrotoxicity. Transplant Proc 22:1379-1380, 1990.

176. Weir MR, Klassen DK, Shen SY, et al: Acute effects of intravenous cyclosporine on blood pressure, renal hemodynamics, urine prostaglandin production of healthy humans. Transplantation 49: 41-47, 1990.

177. Feehally J, Walls J, Mistry N, et al: Does nifedipine ameliorate cyclosporin A nephrotoxicity? BMJ 295:310,1987.

178. Hauser AC, Derfler K, Stockenhuber F, et al: Effect of calcium-channel blockers on renal function in renal-graft recipients treated with cyclosporine [letter]. N Engl J Med 324:1517, 1991.

179. Palmer BF, Dawidson, I, Sagalowsky A, et al: Improved outcome of cadaveric renal transplantation due to calcium channel blockers. Transplantation 52:640-645, 1991.

180. Pirsh JD, D'Alessandro AM, Roecker EB, et al: A controlled, double-blind, randomized trial of verapamil and cyclosporine in cadaver renal transplant patients. Am J Kidney Dis 21:189-195, 1993.

181. Kawaguchi A, Goldman MH, Shapiro R, et al: Increase in urinary thromboxane B_2 in rats caused by cyclosporine. Transplantation 40:214-216, 1985.

182. Perico N, Benigni A, Zoja C, et al: Functional significance of exaggerated renal thromboxane A_2 synthesis induced by cyclosporine A. Am J Physiol 251: F581-F587, 1986.

183. Coffman TM, Carr DR, Yarger WE, et al: Evidence that renal prostaglandin and thromboxane production is stimulated in chronic cyclosporine nephrotoxicity. Transplantation 43:282-285, 1987.

184. Voss BL, Hamilton KK, Samara S, et al: Cyclosporine suppression of endothelial prostacyclin generation. Transplantation 45:793-796, 1988.

185. Paller MS: Effects of the prostaglandin E$_1$ analog misoprostol in cyclosporine nephrotoxicity. Transplantation 45:1126-1131, 1988.

186. Moran M, Mozes MF, Maddux MS, et al: Prevention of acute graft rejection by the prostaglandin E$_1$ analogue misoprostol in renal-transplant recipients treated with cyclosporine and prednisone. N Engl J Med 322:1183-1188, 1990.

187. Adams MB: Enisoprost in renal transplantation. Transplantation 53:338-345, 1992.

188. Pollak R, Knight R, Mozes MF, et al: A trial of the prostaglandin E$_1$ analogue, enisoprost, to reverse chronic cyclosporine-associated renal dysfunction. Am J Kidney Dis 20:336-341, 1992.

189. Perico N, Rossini M, Imberti O, et al: Thromboxane receptor blockade attenuates chronic cyclosporine nephrotoxicity and improves survival in rats with renal isograft. J Am Soc Nephrol 2:1398-1404, 1992.

190. Goldstein DJ, Zuech N, Sehgal V, et al: Cyclosporine-associated end-stage nephropathy after cardiac tranplantation: Incidence and progression. Transplantation 63:664-668, 1997.

191. Thomas SE, Andoh TF, Pichler RH, et al: Accelerated apoptosis characterizes cyclosporine–associated interstitial fibrosis. Kidney Int 53; 897-908, 1998.

192. Henry ML, Elkhammas EA, Davies EA, et al: A clinical trial of cyclosporine G in cadaveric renal transplantation. Pediatr Nephrol 9(suppl): S49-S51,1995.

193. Van Duyne GD, Standaert RF, Karplus PA, et al: Atomic structure of FKBP FK-506, an immunophilin-immunosuppressant complex. Science 252:839-842, 1991.

194. Textor SC, Wiesner R, Wilson DJ, et al: Systemic and renal hemodynamic differences between FK-506 and cyclosporine in liver transplant recipients. Transplantation 55:1332-1339, 1993.

195. Porayko MK, Textor SC, Krom RAF, et al: Nephrotoxic effects of primary immunosuppression with FK-506 and cyclosporine regimens after liver transplantation. Mayo Clin Proc 69:105-111, 1994.

196. Fung JJ, Alessiani M, Aub-Elmagd, M, et al: Adverse effects associated with the use of FK-506. Transplant Proc 23:3105-3108, 1991.

197. Randhawa PS, Shapiro R, Jordan ML, et al: The histopathological changes associated with allograft rejection and drug toxicity in renal transplant recipients maintained on FK-506. Am J Surg Pathol 17: 60-68, 1993.

198. Levin L, Hryniuk W: The application of dose intensity to problems in chemotherapy of ovarian and endometrial cancer, Semin Oncol 14:12-19, 1987.

199. Samson MK, Rivkin SE, Jones SE, et al: Dose-respone and dose-survival advantage for high versus low dose cisplatin combined with vinblastine and bleomycin in disseminated testicular cancer. Cancer 53:1029-1035,1984.

200. Nichols CR, Williams SD, Loehrer PJ, et al: Randomized study of cisplatin dose intensity in poor-risk germ cell tumors: A Southeastern Cancer Study Group and Southwest Oncology Group Protocol. J Clin Oncol 9: 1163-1172, 1991.

201. Wiernik PH, Yeap B, Vogl SE, et al: Hexamethylmelamine and low or moderate dose cisplatin with or without pyridoxine for treatment of advanced ovarian carcinoma: A Study of the Eastern Cooperative Oncology Group. Cancer Invest 10:1-9, 1992.

202. McGuire WP, Hoskins WJ, Brady MF, et al: A phase III trial of dose intense versus standard dose cisplatin and cytoxan in advanced ovarian cancer. Proc Am Soc Clin Oncol 11:718-722, 1992.

203. Kaye SB, Lewis CR, Paul J, et al: Ramadized study of two doses of cisplatin with cyclophosphamide in epithelial ovarian cancer. Lancet 340:329-333, 1992.

204. Einhorn LH, Williams SD: The role of *cis*-platinum in solid tumor therapy. N Engl J Med 300:289-293, 1979.

205. Schaeppi U, Heyman IA, Fleischman RW, et al: *Cis*-diamminedichloroplatinum (II) (NSC-119875): Preclinical toxicologic evaluation of intravenous injection in dogs, monkeys and mice. Toxicol Appl Pharmacol 25:230, 1973.

206. Hardaker WT, Stone RA, McCoy R: Platinum nephrotoxicity. Cancer 34:1030-1034, 1974.

207. Fleming J, Collis C, Peckham MJ: Renal damage after *cis*-platinum. Lancet 2:960-963, 1979.

208. Verplanke AJ, Herber RF, de Wit R, Veenhof CH: Comparison of renal function parameters in the assessment of cisplatin induced nephrotoxicity. Nephron 66:267-272, 1994.

209. Weiner MW, Jacobs C: Mechanism of cisplatin nephrotoxicity. Fed Proc 42:2974-2977, 1983.

210. Schilsky RL, Barlock A, Ozols RF: Persistent hypomagnesemia following cisplatin chemotherapy for testicular cancer. Cancer Treat Rep 66;1767-1769, 1982.

211. Bitran JD, Desser RK, Billings M, et al: Acute nephrotoxicity following cis-dichlorodiammine-platinum. Cancer 49:1874-1888, 1982.

212. Vogelzang NJ, Torkelson JL, Kennedy BJ: Hypomagnesemia, renal dysfunction and Raynaud's phenomenon in patients treated with cisplatin, vinblastine and bleomycin. Cancer 56:2765-2770, 1985.

213. Buckley JE, Clark VL, Meyer TJ, Pearlman NW: Hypomagnesemia after cisplatin combination chemotherapy. Arch Intern Med 144: 2347-2348, 1984.

214. Lerner SA, Seligsohn R, Mak GJ: Comparative clinical studies of ototoxicity and nephrotoxicity of amikacin and gentamicin, Am J Med 62:919, 1977.

215. Aso Y, Ohtawara YU, Suzuki K, et al: The effect of gentamicin and mercuric chloride on cyclic AMP and lipoperoxide in rat kidneys. Nippon Jinzo Gakkai Shi 6:583, 1982.

216. Levi M, Cronin RE: Early selective effects of gentamicin on renal brush-border membrane Na-Pi contransport and Na-H exchange. Am J Physiol 258:F1379, 1990.

217. Ariceta G, Rodriguez-Soriano J, Vallo A, Navajas A: Acute and chronic effects of cisplatin therapy on renal magnesium homeostasis. Med Pediatr Oncol 28:35-40,1997.

218. Offerman JJG, Meijer S, Sleijfer DT, et al: Acute effects on cis-dichlorodiammine-platinum (CDDP) on renal function. Cancer Chemother Pharmacol 12:36, 1984.

219. Walker EM, Fazekas-May MA, Bowen WR: Nephrotoxic and ototoxic agents. Clin Toxicol 10:323, 1990.

220. Wolf W, Manaka RC: Synthesis and distribution of ^{195m}Pt *cis*-dichlorodiammine platinum (II). J Clin Hematol Oncol 7:79, 1976.

221. Marcussen N: Atubular glomeruli in cisplatin-induced chronic interstitial nephropathy: An experimental stereological investigation.APMIS 98:1087-1097, 1990.

222. Matushima H, Yonemura K, Ohishi K, Hishida A: The role of oxygen free radicals in cisplatin-induced acute renal failure in rats. J Lab Clin Med 131:518-526, 1998.

223. Baliga R., Zhang Z, Baliga M, Ueda N, Shah SV: In vitro and in vivo evidence suggesting a role for iron cisplatin–induced nephrotoxicity. Kidney Int, 53:394-401, 1998.

224. Tsutsumishita Y, Onda T, Okada K, et al: Involvement of H_2O_2 production in cisplatin-induced nephrotoxicity. Biochem Biophys Res Commun 242:310-312,1998.

225. Kruidering M, Van de Water B, de Heer, E, et al: Cisplatin-induced nephrotoxicity in porcine proximal tubular cells: Mitochondrial dysfunction by inhibition of complexes in I to IV of the respiratory chain. J Pharmacol Exp Ther 280:638-649, 1997.

226. Deegan PM, Nolan C, Ryan MP, et al: The role of the renin-angiotensin system in cisplatin nephrotoxicity. Ren Fail 17:665-674, 1995.

227. Foster-Nora JA, Siden R: Amifostine for protection from antineoplastic drug toxicity. Am J Health Ayst Pharm 54:787-800, 1997.

228. Sheikh-Hamad D, Timmins K, Jalali Z: Cisplatin-induced renal toxicity:Possible reversal by *N*-acetylcysteine treatment. J Am Soc Nephrol 8:1640-1644, 1997.

229. Uozumi J, Koikawa Y, Yasumasu T, et al: The protective effect of methylprednisolone against cisplatin-induced nephrotoxicity in patients with urothelial tumors. Int J Urol 3:343-347, 1996.

230. Donadio C, Lucchesi A, Gadducci A: Prevention of *cis*-platium nephrotoxicity in a high-risk patient. Ren Fail 18:691-695, 1996.

231. Cornelison TL, Reed E: Nephrotoxity and hydration management for cisplatin, carboplatin, ormaplatin. Gynecol Oncol 50: 147-158, 1993.

232. Meyer KB, Madias NE: Cisplatin nephrotoxicity. Miner Electrolyte Metab 20:201-213, 1994.

233. Bianchetti MG, Kanaka C, Ridolfi-Luthy A, et al: Persisting renotubular sequelae after cisplatin in children and adolescents. Am J Nephrol 11:127-130, 1991.

234. Guinee DG, Van Zee B, Houghton DC: Clinically silent progressive renal tubulointerstitial disease during cisplatin chemotherapy. Cancer 71:4050-4054, 1993.

235. Brillet G, Deray G, Dubois M, et al: Chronic cisplatin nephropathy in rats. Nephrol Dial Transplant 8:206-212, 1993.

236. Kim S, Howell SB, McClay E, et al: Dose intensification of cisplatin chemotherapy through biweekly administration. Ann Oncol 4: 221-227, 1993.

237. Vogelzang NJ, Torkelson JL, Kennedy BJ: Hypomagnesemia, renal dysfunction and Raynaud's phenomenon in patients treated with cisplatin, vinblastine and bleomycin. Cancer 56:2765-2770, 1985.

238. Hayes DM: High-dose cis-platinum diammine dichloride: Amelioration of renal toxicity by mannitol diuresis. Cancer 39: 1372-1376, 1977.

239. Ozols RF, Corden BJ, Jacob J, et al: High dose cisplatin in hypertonic saline. Ann Intern Med 100:19-24, 1984.

240. Bajorin DF, Bosl GJ, Jacob J, et al: Pharmacokinetics of cis-diamminedichloroplatinum (II) after administration in hypertonic saline. Cancer Res 46:5969-5972, 1986.

241. Ozols RF, Young RC: High-dose cisplatin therapy in ovarian cancer. Semin Oncol 12 (suppl 6):21-30, 1985.

242. Gandara DR, Perez EA, Weibe V, De Gregorio MW: Cisplatin chemoprotection and rescue: Pharmacologic modulation of toxicity. Semin Oncol 18 (suppl 3):49-55, 1991.

243. Ross RD, Gale CR: Reduction of the renal toxicity of cis-dichlorodiammine-platinum (II) by probenecid. Cancer Treat Rep 63:781, 1979.

244. Edmonson JH, McCormack GW, Krook JE, et al: Pilot study of cyclophosphamide plus in advanced ovarion carcinoma. Cancer Treat Rep 71:199-204, 1987.

245. Foster BJ, Claggett-Carr K, Leyland-Jones B, Hoth D: Results of NCI-sponsored phase I trials with carboplatin. Cancer Treat Rev 12 (suppl A):43-49, 1985.

246. Rozencweig M, Nicaise C, Beer M, et al: Phase I study of carboplatin given on a five-day intravenous schedule. J Clin Oncol 1: 621-626, 1983.

247. Christian MC: Carboplatin. In De Vita VT Jr, Hellman S, Rosenberg SA (eds): Principles and Practice of Oncology. Updates. Philadelphia, JB Lippincott, 1989, pp 1-16.

248. Van Echo DA, Egorin MJ, Whitacre MY, et al: A phase I clinical and pharmacologic trial of carboplatin daily for 5 days. Cancer Treat Rep 65:1103-1107, 1984.

249. Egorin MJ, Van Echo DA, Tipping SJ, et al: Pharmacokinetics and dosage reduction of cis-diammine(1,1-cyclobutanedicarboxylato) platinum in patients with impaired renal function. Cancer Res 44:5432-5438, 1984.

250. Gore ME, Calvert AH, Smith IE: High dose carboplatin in the treatment of lung cancer and mesothelioma: A phase I dose escalation study. Eur J Cancer Clin Oncol 23:1391, 1987.

251. Shea TC, Flaherty M, Elias A, et al: A phase I clinical and pharmacokinetic study of carboplatin and autologous bone marrow support. J Clin Oncol 7:651,1989.

252. Vogelzang NJ: Nephrotoxicity from chemotherapy: Prevention and management. Oncology 5:97-102, 1991.

253. Beyer J, Rick O, Weinknecht S, et al: Nephrotoxicity after high-dose carboplatin, etoposide and ifosfamide in germ-cell tumors: Incidence and implications for hematologic recovery and clinical outcome. Bone Marrow Transplant 20:813-819, 1997.

254. Duffull SB, Roninson BA: Clinical pharmacokinetics and dose optimisation of carboplatin. Clin Pharmacokinet 33:161-183, 1997.

255. Tscherning C, Rubie H, Chancholle A, et al: Recurrent renal salt wasting in a child treated with carboplatin and etoposide. Cancer 73:1761-1763, 1994.

256. DeFronzo RA, et al: Cyclophosphamide and the kidney. Cancer 33:483, 1974.

257. Bode U, Seif SM, Levine AS: Studies on the antidiuretic effect on cyclophosphamide: Vasopressin release and sodium excretion. Med Pediatr Oncol 8:295, 1980.

258. Weiss RB: Streptozocin: A review of its pharmacology, efficacy and toxicity. Cancer Treat Rep 66:427, 1982.

259. Sadoff L: Nephrotoxicity of streptozocin (NSC 85988). Cancer Chemother Rep 54:457-459, 1970.

260. Meyerowik RL, Sartiano GP, Cavallo T: Nephrotoxic and cytoproliferative effects of streptozocin. Cancer 38:1550-1555, 1976.

261. Hricik DE, Goldsmith GH: Uric acid nephrolithiasis and acute renal failure secondary to streptozocin nephrotoxicity. Am J Med 84: 153-156, 1988.

262. Schacht RG, Feiner HD, Gallo GR, et al: Nephrotoxicity of nitrosoureas. Cancer 48:1328, 1981.

263. Micetich KC, Jensen-Akula M, Mandard JC, et al: Nephrotoxicity of semustine (methyl-CCNU) in patients with malignant melanoma receiving adjuvant chemotherapy. Am J Med 71:967, 1981.

264. Schacht RG, Feiner HD, Gallo GR, et al: Nephrotoxicity of nitrosoureas. Cancer 48:1328-1334, 1981.

265. Springate JE, Van Liew JB: Nephrotoxicity of ifosfamide in rats. J Appl Toxicol 15:399-402, 1995.

266. Goren MP, Wright RK, Pratt CB, et al: Potentiation of ifosfamide neurotoxicity, hematotoxicity, tubular nephrotoxicity by prior cis-diamminedichloroplatinum (II) therapy. Cancer Res 47:1457-1460, 1987.

267. Goren MP, Wright RK, Horowitz ME, et al: Ifosfamide-induced subclinical tubular nephrotoxicity. Cancer Treat Rep 71:127-130, 1987.

268. Zalupski M, Baker LH: Ifosfamide. J Natl Cancer Inst 80:556-566, 1988.

269. Tokuc G, Yalciner A, Kebudi R, et al: Renal dysfunctions secondary to ifosfamide treatment in children. J Exp Clin Cancer Res 16: 227-230, 1997.

270. MacLean FR, Skinner R, Hall AG, et al: Acute changes in urine protein excretion may predict chronic ifosfamide nephrotoxicity: A preliminary observation. Cancer Chemother Pharmacol 41:413-416, 1998.

271. Skinner R, Pearson AD, Price L, et al: Nephrotoxicity after ifosfamide. Arch Dis Child 65:732-738, 1990.

272. Burk CD, Restaino I, Kaplan BS, et al: Ifosfamide induced renal tubular dysfunction and rickets in children with Wilms tumor. J Pediatr 117:331-335, 1990.

273. Elias AD, Eder JP, shea T, et al: High dose ifosfamide with mesna uroprotection: A phase I study. J Clin Oncol 8:170-178, 1990.

274. Rossi R, Danzebrink S, Hillebrand D, et al: Ifosfamide-induced subclinical nephrotoxicity and its potentiation by cisplatinum. Med Pediatr Oncol 22:27-32, 1994.

275. Springate J, Zamlauski-Tucker MJ, Lu H, Chan KK: Renal clearance of ifosfamide. Drug Metab Dispos 25:1081-1082, 1997.

276. Rossi R, Godde A, Kleinebrand A, et al; Unilateral nephroctomy and cisplatin as risk factors of ifosfamide-induced nephrotoxicity: Analysis of 120 patients. J Clin Oncol 12:159-165, 1994.

277. Loebstein R, Koren G: Ifosfamide-induced nephrotoxicity in children: Critical review of predictive risk factors. Pediatrics 101:E8, 1998.

278. Beyer J, Rick O, Weinknecht S, et al: Nephrotoxicity after high-dose carboplatin, etoposide and ifosfamide in germ-cell tumors: Incidence and implications for hematologic recovery and clinical outcome. Bone Marrow Transplant 20:813-819, 1997.

279. Lesesne JB, Rothschild N, Erickson B, et al: Cancer associated hemolytic-uremic syndrome: Analysis of 85 cases from a national registry. J Clin Onal 7:781-789, 1989.

280. Valavaara R, Nordman E: Renal compliations of mitomycin C therapy with special reference to the total dose. Cancer 55:47-50, 1985.

281. Cattell V: Mitomycin-induced hemolytic uremic kidney: An experimental model in the rat. Am J Pathol 121:88-95, 1985.

282. Verwey J, de Vries J, Pinedo HM: Mitomycin C–induced renal failure a dose dependent side effect? Eur J Clin Oncol 23: 795-799,1987.

283. Price TM, Murgo AJ, Keveney JJ, et al: Renal failure and hemolytic anemia associated with mitomycin C. Cancer 55:51, 1985.

284. Kennedy BJ, Brown JH, Yarbro JW: Mithramycin (NSC-24559) therapy for primary glioblastomas. Cancer Chemother Rep 48:34, 1979.

285. Kennedy BJ: Metabolic and toxic effects of mithramycin during therapy. Am J Med 49:494, 1970.

286. Kennedy BJ, Sandberg-Wolheim M, Loken M, et al: Studies with tritiated mithromycin in C3H mice. Cancer Res 27:1534, 1967.

287. Kennedy BJ: Metabolic and toxic effects during mithramycin therapy. Am J Med 49: 494-503, 1970.

288. Green L, Donehower RC: Hepatic toxicity of low doses of mithramycin in hypocalcemia. Cancer Treat Rep 68:1379-1381, 1984.

289. Perlia CP, Gubish NJ, Wolter J, et al: Mithramycin treatment of hypercalcemia. Cancer 25:389-394, 1970.

290. Kiag DT, Lokien MK, Kennedy BJ: Mechanism of the hypocalcemic effect of mithramycin. J Clin Endocrinol Metab 48:341-344, 1979.

291. Chabner BA, Meyers CD: Clinical pharmacology of cancer chemotherapy. In De Vita VT Jr, Hellman S, Rosenberg SA (eds): Principles and Practice of Oncology, 3rd ed. Philadelphia, JB Lippincott, 1989, pp 349-388.

292. Singer FR, Neer RM, Murray TM, et al: Mithramycin treatment of intractable hypercalcemia due to parathyroid cariicinoma. N Engl J Med 283:634, 1970.

293. Benedetti RG, Heilman KJ III, Gabow PA: Nephrotoxicity following single dose mithramycin therapy. Am J Nephrol 3:277-278, 1983.

294. Bleyer WA: The clinical pharmacology of methotrexate. Cancer 41:36-51, 1978.

295. Ackland SP, Schilsky RL: High-dose methotrexate: A critical reappraisal. J Clin Oncol 5:2017, 1987.

296. Jacobs SA, Stoller RG, Chabner BA, et al: 7-Hydroxymethotrexate as a urinary metabolite in human subjects and rhesus monkeys receiving high-dose methotrexate. J Clin Invest 57:534-538, 1976.

297. Glode LM, Pitman SW, Ensminger WD, et al: A phase I study of high-dose aminopterin with leucovorin rescue in patients with advance metastatic tumor. Cancer Res 39:3707-3714, 1979.

298. Pitman SW, Frei E III: Weekly methotrexate calcium leukovorin rescue: Effect of alkalinization on nephrotoxicity; pharmacokinetics in the CNS, use in CNS non-Hodgkin's lymphoma. Cancer Treat Rep 61:695, 1977.

299. Abelson HT, Garnick MB: Renal failure induced by cancer chemotherapy. *In* Rieselbach RE, Garnick MB (eds): Cancer and the Kidney. Philadelphia, Lea & Febiger, 1982.

300. Thyss A, Milano G, Kubar J, et al: Clinical and pharmacokinetic evidence of a life-threatening interaction between methotrexate and ketoprofen. Lancet 1:256-258, 1988.

301. Price P, Thompson H, Bessell EM, et al: Renal impairment following the combined use of high dose methotrexate and procarbazine. Cancer Chemother Pharmacol 21:265-267, 1988.

302. Giardino R, Fini M, Giavaresi G, et al: In vitro and ex vivo evaluation of methotrexate removal by different sorbents haemoperfusion. Biomater Artif Cells Immobilization Biotechnol 21:447-454, 1993.

303. Kepka L, De Lassence A, Ribrag V, et al: Successful rescue in a patient with high dose methotrexate-induced nephrotoxicity and acute renal failure. Leuk Lymphoma 29:205-209, 1998.

304. Slavin RE, Dias MA, Saral R: Cytosin arabinoside induced gastrointestinal toxic alteration in sequential chemotherapeutic protocols. A clinical pathological study of 33 patients. Cancer 42:1747, 1978.

305. Kumar M, Kedar A, Neiberger RE: kidney function in long-term pediatric survivors of acute lymphoblastic leukemia following allogeneic bone marrow transplantation. Pediatr Hematol Oncol 13: 375-379, 1996.

306. Presant CA, Denes AE, Klein L, et al: Phase I and preliminary phase II observations of high-dose intermittent 6-thioguanine. Cancer Treat Rep 64:1109, 1980.

307. Hanna WT, Krauss S, Regester RF, et al: Renal disease after mitomycin C therapy. Cancer 48:2583, 1981.

308. Belldegrun A, Webb DE, Austin HA, et al: Effects of interleukin-2 on renal function in patients receiving immunotherapy for advanced cancer. Ann Intern Med 106:817, 1987.

309. Sosman JA, Kohler PC, Hank J, et al: Repetitive weekly cycles of recombinant human interleukin-2: Responses of renal carcinoma with acceptable toxicity. J Natl Cancer Inst 80:60, 1988.

310. West WH, Tauer KW, Yannelli JR, et al: Constant-infusion recombinant interleukin-2 in adoptive immunotherapy of advanced cancer. N Engl J Med 316:898, 1987.

311. Zusman J, Brown DM, Nesbit ME: Hyperphosphataemia, hyperphosphaturia and hypocalcaemia in acute lymphoblastic leukemia. N Engl J Med 289:1335, 1973.

312. Kjellstrand CM, Campbell DC, von Hartikch B, Buselmeier TJ: Hyperuricemic acute renal failure. Arch Intern Med 133:349, 1974.

313. Hricik DE, Goldsmith GH: Uric acid nephrolithiasis and acute renal failure due to streptozotocin nephrotoxicity. Am J Med 84: 153, 1988.

314. Kelton J, Kelley WN, Holmes EW: A rapid method for the detection of acute uric acid nephropathy. Arch Intern Med 138:612, 1978.

315. Chastyl RC, Liu-Yin JA: Acute tumor lysis syndrome. Br J Hosp Med 49:488-492, 1993.

316. Hande KR, Garrow GC: Acute tumor lysis syndrome in patients with high grade non–Hodgkin's lymphoma. Am J Med 94:133-138, 1993.

317. Barton JC: Tumor lysis syndrome in nonhematopoietic neoplasms. Cancer 64:738-740, 1989.

318. Cadman E, Lundberg W, Bertino J: Hyperphosphatemia and hypocalcemia accompanying rapid cell lysis in a patients with Burkitt's cell leukemia. Am J Med 62:283, 1977.

319. Ettinger DS, Harker WG, Gerry HW, et al: Hyperphosphatemia, hypocalcemia, transient renal failure: Results of cytotoxic treatment of acute lymphoblastic leukemia. JAMA 239:2472, 1978.

320. Ahsan N, Palmer BF, Wheeler DD, Greenlee R, Toto RD. Intravenous immonoglubulin induced osmotic nephrosis. Arch Intern Med 152:1985-1987, 1994.

321. Ramazzini B: De Morbis Artificum Diatriba, Wright WC (trans). Chicago, University of Chicago Press, 1913.

322. Thackrah CT: The Effects of Arts, Trades, and Professions and of Civic States and Habits of Living, on Health and Longevity with Suggesstions for the Removal of Many of the Agents Which Produce Disease and Shorten the Duration of Life, 2nd ed. London, Longman, Rees, Orme, Brown, Green & Longman, 1832.

323. Legge Sir T: Industrial Maladies. London, Oxford University Press, 1934.

324. Bariety J, Druet P, Laliberte F: Glomerulonephritis with α- and β globulin deposits induced in rats by mercuric chloride. Am J Pathol 65:293,1971.

325. Barry PSI: A comparison of concentrations of lead in human tissues. Br J Ind Med 32:119, 1975.

326. Goyer RA, Wilson MH: Lead-induced inclusion bodies. Results of ethylenediaminetetraacetic acid treatment. Lab Invest 32;149, 1975.

327. Fels LM, Herbort C, Pergande M, et al: Nephron target sites in chronic exposure to lead. Nephrol Dial Transplant 9:1740-1746, 1994.

328. Chia KS, Jeyaratnam J, Lee J, et al: Lead-induced nephropathy: Relationship between various biological exposure indices and early markers of nephrotoxicity. Am J Ind Med 27: 883-895, 1995.

329. Nye LJJ: An investigation of the extraordinary incidence of chronic nephritis in young people in Queensland, Med J Aust 2;145-159, 1929.

330. Lilis R, Gavirlescu N, Nestorescu B, et al: Nephropathy in chronic renal lead poisoning. Br J Ind Med 25: 196-202, 1968.

331. Inglis JA, Henderson DA, Emmerson BT: The pathology and pathogenesis of chronic nephropathy occurring in Queensland. J Pathal 124:55-76, 1978.

332. Vyskocil A, Cizkova M, Tejnorova I: Effect of prenatal and postnatal exposure to lead on kidney function in male and female rats. J Appl Toxicol 15:327-328, 1995.

333. Vyskocil A, Semecky V, Fiala Z, et al: Renal alterations in female rats following subchronic lead exposure. J Appl Toxical 15:257-262, 1995.

334. Moel DI, Sachs HK: Renal function 17 to 23 years after chelation therapy for childhood plumbism. Kidney Int 42:1226-1231, 1992.

335. Nuyts GD, Daelemans RA, Jorens G, et al: Does lead play a role in the development of chronic renal disease? Nephrol Dial Transplant 6:307-315, 1991.

336. Pinto de Almeida AR, Carvalho FM, Spinola AG, et al: Renal dysfunction in Brazilian lead workers. Am J Nephrol 7:455-458. 1987.

337. Behringer D, Craswell P, Mohl C, et al: Urinary lead excretion in uremic patients. Nephron 42:323-329, 1986.

338. Koster J, Erhardt A, Stoeppler M, et al: Mobilizable lead in patients with chronic renal failure. Eur J Clin Invest 19:228-233, 1989.

339. Cooper WC, Wong O, Kheifets L: Mortality among employees of lead battery plants and lead producing plants, 1947-1980. Scand J Work Environ Health 11:331-345, 1985.

340. Searle J, Craswell P, Boyle P, et al: The current status of chronic lead nephropathy in Queensland. Aust N Z J Med Oct: 600-601, 1981.

341. Hu H: A 50-year follow-up of childhood plumbism. Am J Dis Child 145:681-687, 1991.

342. Cooper WC, Gaffey WR: Mortality of lead workers. J Occup Environ Med 17:100-107, 1975.

343. Malcolm D, Barnett HAR: A mortality study of lead workers, 1925–76. Br J Ind Med 39:402-404, 1982.

344. McMichael AJ, Johnson HM: Long-term mortality profile of heavily-exposed lead smelter workers. J Occup Environ Med 24: 375-378, 1982.

345. Selevan SG, Landrigan PJ, Stern FB, et al: Mortality of lead smelter workers. Am J Epidemiol 122:673-683, 1985.

346. Craswell PW, Price J, Boyle PD, et al: Chronic renal failure with gout: A marker of chronic lead poisoning. Kidney Int 26:319, 1979.

347. Coffman TM, Yarger WE, Klotman PE: Functional role of thromboxane production by acutely rejecting renal allografts in rats. J Clin Invest 75:1242, 1985.

348. Warren GV, Korbet SM, Schwartz MM, et al: Minimal change glomerulopathy associated with non-steroidal anti-inflammatory drugs. Am J Kidney Dis 13:127, 1989.

349. Vyskocil A, Pancl J, Tusl M, et al: Dose-related proximal tubular dysfunction in male rats chronically exposed to lead. J App Toxicol 9:395-399, 1989.

350. Cardenas A, Roels H, Bernard AM, et al: Markers of early renal changes induced by industrial pollutants. II. Application to workers exposed to lead. Br J Ind Med 50:28-36, 1993.

351. Roels H, Lauwerys R, Konings J, et al: Renal funtion and hypertension capacity in lead smelter workers with high bone lead. Occup Environ Med 51:505-512, 1994.

352. Piomelli A, Seaman C, Zullow D, et al: Threshold for lead damage to heme synthesis in urban children. Proc Natl Acad Sci U S A 79:3335, 1982.

353. Wedeen RP: Blood lead levels, dietary calcium, hypertension. Ann Intern Med 102:403, 1985.

354. Wedeen RP, Mallik DK, Batumen V: Detection and treatment of occupational lead nephropathy. Arch Intern Med 139:53, 1979.

355. Inglis JA, Henderson DA, Emmerson BT: The pathology and pathogenesis of chronic lead nephropathy occurring in Queensland. J Pathol 124:65, 1978.

356. Van de Vyber FL, D'Hase PC, Visser WJ: Bone lead in dialysis patients. Kidney Int 33:601, 1988.

357. Craswell P: Chronic lead nephropathy. Annu Rev Med 38:169, 1987.

358. Haust H, Inwood M, Spence JD, et al: Intramuscular administration of iron during long-term chelation therapy with 2,3-dimercaptosuccinic acid in a man with severe lead poisoning. Clin Biochem 22:189-196, 1989.

359. Koster J, Erhardt A, Stoeppler M, et al: Mobilizable lead in patients with chronic renal failure. Eur J Clin Invest 19:228-233, 1989.

360. Yver L, Marechaud R, Picaud D, et al: Insuffisance rénate aiguë au cours d'un saturnisme professionel. Nouvelle Presse Med 7: 1541,1978.

361. Bernard A, Lauwerys R: Cadmium in the human population. Experientia 40:143-151, 1984.

362. Bernard A, Roels A, Buchet JP, et al: Cadmium and health: The Belgian experience. In Nordberg GF, Herber RFM (eds): Cadmium in the Human Environment: Toxicity and Carcinogenicity. Lyon, France, IARC, 1992, pp 15-33.

363. Roels H, Bernard AM, Cardenas A, et al: Markers of early renal changes induced by industrial pollutants. III. Application to workers exposed to cadmium. Br J Ind Med 50:37-48, 1993.

364. Shaikh ZA, Kido T, Kito H, et al: Prevalence of metallothioneinuria among the population living in the Kakehashi River basin in Japan: An epidemiological study. Toxicology 64:59-69, 1990.

365. Nogawa K, Kido T, Shaikh ZA: Dose-response relationship for renal dysfunction in a population environmentally exposed to cadmium. In Nordberg OF, Herber RFM (eds): Cadmium in the Human Environment: Toxicity and Carcinogenicity. 1992, 311-318.

366. Wedeen RP: Occupational renal disease. Am J Kidney Dis 3:241, 1984.

367. Nordberg GF, Jin T, Nordberg M: Subcellular targets of cadmium nephrotoxicity: Cadmium binding to renal membrane proteins in animals with or without protective metallothionein synthesis. Environ Health Perspect 102 (suppl 3):191-194, 1994.

368. Lindqvist K, Nystrom K, Stegmayr B, et al: Cadmium concentration in human kidney biopsies. Scand J Urol Nephrol 23:213-217, 1989.

369. Jung E, Pergande M, Graubaum HJ, et al: Urinary proteins and enzymes as early indicators of renal dysfunction in chronic exposure in cadmium. Clin Chem 39: 757-765, 1993.

370. Jin T, Nordbert G, Sehlin J, Vesterberg O: Protection against cadmium-metallothionein nephrotoxicity in streptozotocin-induced diabetic rats: Role of increased metallothionein synthesis induced by streptozotocin. Toxicology 106:55-63, 1996.

371. Liu X, Jin T, Nordberg GF, et al: Influence of zinc and copper administration on metal disposition in rats with cadmium-metallothionein–induced nephrotoxicity. Toxicol Appl Pharmacol 126:84-90, 1994.

372. Toffoletto F, Apostoli P, Ghezzi I, et al: Ten-year follow-up of biological monitoring of cadmium-exposed workers. In Nordberg GF, Herber RFM (eds): Cadmium in the Human Environment: Toxicity and Carcinogenicity. Lyon, France, IARC, 1992, pp 107-111.

373. Jarup L, Persson B, Edling C, Elinder CG: Renal function impairment in workers previously exposed to cadmium. Nephron 63:75-81, 1993.

374. Kahan E, Derazne E, Rosenboim J, Ashkenazi R: Adverse health effects in workers exposed to cadmium. Am J Ind Med 21:527-537, 1992.

375. Mueller P, Paschal DC, Hammel RR, et al: Chronic renal effects in three studies of men and women occupationally exposed to cadmium. Arch Environ Contam Toxicol 23:125-136, 1992.

376. Shibuya Y: A long-term surveillance of occupational health hazards faced by cadmium workers. Kissato Arch Exp Med 63: 37-48, 1990.

377. Kido R, Nogawa K, Hochi Y, et al: The renal handling of calcium and phosphorus in environmental cadmium-exposed subjects with renal dysfunction J Appl Toxicol 13:43-47, 1993.

378. Tsuchiya K: Health effects of cadmium with special references to studies in Japan. In Nordberg GF, Herber RFM (eds): Cadmium in the Human Environment: Toxicity and Carcinogenicity. Lyon, France, IARC, 1992, pp 35-49.

379. Shimada H, Kamenosono T, Kawagoe M, et al: Mobilization of renal and hepatic cadmium by dithiocarbamates in rats. J Pharmacobiodyn 14:555-560, 1991.

380. Jones MM, Gale GR, Singh PK, et al: The rate of the in vivo dithiocarbamate-induced mobilization of hepatic and renal cadmium deposits. Toxicology 48:313-323, 1989.

381. Landrigan PJ: Occupational and community exposures to toxic metals: Lead, cadmium, mercury and arsenic. West J Med 137:531, 1982.

382. Gerstner HB, Huff JE: Selected case histories and epidemiologic examples and human mercury poisoning. Clin Toxicol 11:131, 1977.

383. Diamond GL, Zalups RK: Understanding renal toxicity of heavy metals. Toxicol Pathol 26:92-103, 1998.

384. Nath KA, Croatt AJ, Likely S, et al: Renal oxidant injury and oxidant response induced by mercury. Kidney Int 50:1032-1043, 1996.

385. Wedeen RP: Occupational and environmental renal diseases. Curr Nephrol 11:65, 1988.

386. Kazantzis G: Mercury. In Waldron HA (ed): Metals in the Environment. New York, Academic Press, 1980.

387. Nomiyama K: Recent progress and perspectives in cadmium health effects studies. Sci Total Environ 14:199, 1980.

388. Dounce AL: The mechanism of action of uranium compounds in the animal body. In Voegtlin C, Hodge HC (eds): Pharmacology and Toxicology of Uranium Compounds. Div VI, Vol 1. New York, McGraw-Hill, 1949, chap 15.

389. Leggett RW: The behavior and chemical toxicity of U in the kidney: A reassessment. Health Phys 57:365-383, 1989.

390. Domingo JL, de la Torre A, Belles M, et al: Comparative effects of the chelators sodium 4,5-dihydroxybenzene-1,3-disulfonate (Tiron) and diethylenetriaminepentaacetic acid (DTPA) on acute uranium nephrotoxicity in rats. Toxicology 118:49-59, 1997.

391. Fowler BA, Weissberg JB: Arsine poisoning. N Engl Med 291:1171, 1972.

392. Tsukamoto H, Parker HR, Gribble DH, et al: Nephrotoxicity of sodium arsenate in dogs. Am J Vet Res 44:2324-2330, 1983.

393. Lilis R, Valciukas JA, Weber JP, et al: Epidemiologic study of renal function in copper smelter workers. Environ Health Perspect 54: 181-192, 1984.

394. Kaufman DB, DiNickola W, McIntosh R: Acute potassium dichromate poisoning. Am J Dis Child 119:374, 1970.

395. Vanherweghem J, Depierreux M, Tielmans C, et al: Rapidly progressive interstitial fibrosis in young women: Association with slimming regimen including Chinese herbs. Lancet 341:387-391, 1993.

396. Tanaka A, Nishida R, Maeda K, et al: Chinese herb nephropathy in Japan presents adult-onset Fanconi syndrome: Could different components of aristolochic acids cause a different type of Chinese herb nephropathy? Clin Nephrol 53:301-306, 2000.

397. Nortier J, Martinez M, Schmeiser H, et al: Urothelial carcinoma associated with use of Chinese herb. N Engl J Med 342:1686-1692, 2000.

398. Mansoor G: Herbs and alternative therapies in the hypertension clinic. Am J Hypertens 14: 971-975, 2001.

399. Chen C, Fang H, Chou K, Wang J, et al: Acute oxalate nephropathy after ingestion of star fruit. Am J Kidney Dis 37:418-422, 2001.

400. Mashour S, Turner J, Merrel R: Acute renal failure, oxalosis, and vitamin C supplementation. Chest 118:561-563, 2000.

401. Koshy K, Griswold E, Schneeberger E: Interstitial nephritis in a patient taking creatine. N Engl J Med 340:814-815, 1999.

402. Hilepo J, Belluci A, Mossey R: Acute renal failure caused by "cats claw" herbal remedy in a patient with systemic lupus erythematosus. Nephron 77:361, 1997.

403. Stein HB, Patterson AC, Offer RC, et al: Adverse effects of D-pencillamine in rheumatoid arthritis. Ann Intern Med 92:24, 1980.

404. Bacon PA, Tribe CR, Mackenzie JC, et al: Penicillamine nephropathy in rheumatoid arthritis—a clinical pathological and immunological study. Q J Med 55:661, 1976.

405. Chisolm JJ, Baltrop D: Recognition and management of children with increased lead absorption. Arch Dis Child 54:249, 1979.

406. Lachmann PJ: Nephrotic syndrome from pencillamine. Postgrad Med J 23:44, 1968.

407. Verroust PJ: Kinetics of immune deposits in membranous nephropathy. Kidney Int 35:1418, 1989.

408. Wooley PH, Griffin JK, Panayi GS, et al: HLA-DR antigens and toxic reaction to sodium aurothiomalate and D-penicillamine in patients with rheumatoid arthritis. N Engl J Med 303:300, 1980.

409. Adu Ntoso K, Tomazewski JE, Jimenez SA, et al: Penicillamine-induced rapidly progressive glomerulonephritis in patients with primary systemic sclerosis: Successful treatment of two patients and a review of the literature. Am J Kidney Dis 8:159, 1986.

410. Hall OL: The natural course of gold and penicillamine nephropathy: A long-term study of 54 patients. Adv Exp Biol. 252:247-256, 1989.

411. Francis KL, Jenis EH, Hensen GE, et al: Gold-associated nephropathy. Arch Pathol Lab Med 108:234, 1984.

412. Blum M, Liron M, Aviram A: Nephrotic syndrome with reversible severe renal failure after gold therapy. Int J Clin Pharmacol Ther Toxicol 22:562, 1984.

413. Katz WA, Blodgett RC, Pietrusko RG: Proteinuria in gold-treated rheumatoid arthritis. Ann Intern Med 101:176, 1984.

414. Wooley PH, Griffin J, Panayi GS, et al: HLA-DR antigens and toxic reaction to sodium aurothiomalate and D-penicillamine in patients with rheumatoid arthritis. N Engl J Med 303:300, 1980.

415. Dunn MJ, Howe D: Prostaglandins lack a direct inhibitory action on electrolyte and water transport in the kidney and the erythrocyte. Prostaglandins 13:417-429, 1977.

416. Palmer BF, Henrich WL. Nephrotoxicity of non-steroidal anti-inflammatory agents, analgesics, and angiotensin converting enzyme inhibitors. In Schrier R (ed), Diseases of the Kidney, 7th ed. Philadelphia, WB Saunders, 2001, pp 1189-1209.

417. Aiken JW, Vane JR: Intrarenal prostaglandin release attenuates the renal vasoconstrictor activity of angiotensin. J Pharmacol Exp Ther 184:678-687, 1973.

418. Finn W, Arendshorst WJ: Effect of prostaglandin synthetase inhibitors on renal blood flow in the rat. Am J Physiol 231:1541-1545, 1976.

419. Satoh S, Zimmerman BG: Influence of the renin-angiotensin system on the effect of prostaglandin synthesis inhibitors in the renal vasculature. Circ Res 36(suppl 1):89, 1975.

420. Swain JA, Heyndricks GR, Boettcher DR, Vatner SF: Prostaglandin control of renal circulation in the unanesthetized dog and baboon. Am J Physiol 229:826-830, 1975.

421. Lonigro AJ, Itsokovitz HD, Crowshaw K, McGiff JC: Dependency of renal blood flow on prostaglandin synthesis in the dog. Circ Res 32:712-717, 1973.

422. Needleman P, Marshall GR, Johnson EM Jr: Determinants and modification of adrenergic and vascular resistance in the kidney. Am J Physiol 227:665-669, 1974.

423. Susic H, Malik KU: Prostacyclin and prostaglandin E$_2$ effects on adrenergic transmission in the kidney of the anesthetized dog. J Pharmacol Exp Ther 218:588-592, 1981.

424. Clive DM, Stoff JS: Renal syndromes associated with nonsteroidal antiinflammatory drugs. N Engl J Med 310:563-572, 1984.

425. Stillman MT, Schleisinger PA: Nonsteroidal anti-inflammatory drug nephrotoxicity. Arch Intern Med 150:268-270, 1990.

426. Unsworth J, Sturman S, Lunec J, et al: Renal impairment associated with non-steroidal anti-inflammatory drugs. J Rheum Dis 46: 233-236, 1987.

427. Patrono C, Dunn MJ: The clinical significance of inhibition of renal prostaglandin synthesis. Kidney Int 32:1-12, 1987.

428. Carmichael J, Shankel SW: Effects of nonsteroidal anti-inflammatory drugs on prostaglandins and renal function. Am J Med 78: 992-1000, 1985.

429. Adams DH, Michael J, Bacon PA, et al: Non-steroidal anti-inflammatory drugs and renal failure. Lancet 1:57-59, 1986.

430. Murray MD, Brater DC: Adverse effects of nonsteroidal anti-inflammatory drugs on renal function. Ann Intern Med 112:559-560, 1990.

431. Leehey DJ, Uckerman MT, Rahman MA: Role of prostaglandins and thromboxane in the control of renal hemodynamics in experimental liver cirrhosis. J Lab Clin Med 113:309-315, 1989.

432. Palmer BF: Renal complications associated with use of non-steroidal antiinflammatory agents. J Invest Med 43:516-533, 1995.

433. Galler M, Folkert VW, Schlondorf D: Reversible acute renal insufficiency and hyperkalemia following indomethacin therapy. JAMA 246:154, 1981.

434. Garella S, Matarese RA: Renal effects of prostaglandins and clinical adverse effects of nonsteroidal anti-inflammatory agents. Medicine (Baltimore) 63:165-181, 1984.

435. Kimberly RP, Bowden RE, Keiser HR, et al: Reduction of renal function by newer nonsteroidal anti-inflammatory drugs. Am J Med 64:804-807, 1978.

436. Kimberly RP, Plotz PH: Aspirin-induced depression of renal function. N Engl J Med 296:418-424, 1977.

437. Lipsett MB, Goldman R: Phenylbutazone toxicity: Report of a case of acute renal failure. Ann Intern Med 41:1075, 1954.

438. McCarthy JT, Torres VE, Romero JC, et al: Acute intrinsic renal failure induced by indomethacin. Role of prostaglandin synthetase inhibition. Mayo Clin Proc 57:289, 1982.

439. Pawaz-Estrup F, Ho G Jr: Reversible acute renal failure induced by indomethacin. Arch Intern Med 141: 1670, 1981.

440. Tan SY, Franco R, Stockard H, et al: Indomethacin-induced prostaglandin inhibition with hyperkalemia. A reversible cause of hyporeninemic hypoaldosteronism. Ann Intern Med 90:783, 1979.

441. Zisper RD, Hoefs JC, Speckart PF, et al: Prostaglandins: Modulators of renal function and presser resistance in chronic liver disease. J Endocrinol Metab 48:89S-900, 1979.

442. Schlondorff D: Renal complications of nonsteroidal anti-inflammatory drugs. Kidney Int 44:643-653, 1993.

443. Gurwitz JH, Avorn J, Ross-Deghan D, et al: Nonsteroidal anti-inflammatory drug-associated azotemia in the very old. JAMA 264: 471-475, 1990.

444. Simon LS, Basch CM, Youny DY, et al: Effects of naproxen on renal function in older patients with mild to moderate renal dysfunction. Br J Rheumatol 31:163-168, 1992.

445. Whelton A, Stout RL, Spilman PS, et al: Renal effects of ibuprofen, piroxicam and sulindac in patients with asymptomatic renal failure. Ann Intern Med 112:568-576, 1990.

446. Marasco WA, Gikas PW, Aziz-Baumgartner R, et al: Ibuprofen-associated renal dysfunction. Pathophysiologic mechanisms of acute renal failure hyperkalemia, tubular necrosis, proteinuria. Arch Intern Med 147:2107-2116, 1987.

447. Patrono C, Pierucci A: Renal effects of nonsteroidal antiinflammatory drugs in chronic glomerular disease. Am J Med 81(suppl 2B): 71-83, 1986.

448. Laxer RM, Silverman E, Balfe D, et al: Indomethacin and ibuprofen-induced reversible acute renal failure in a patient with systemic lupus erythematosus. Neth J Med 30:181-186, 1987.

449. Blankshear JL, Davidman M, Stillman MT: Identification of risk for renal insufficiency from non-steroidal anti-inflammatory drugs. Arch Intern Med 43:1130-1134, 1983.

450. Bunning RD, Barth WF: Sulindac. A potentially renal-sparing nonsteroidal anti-inflammatory drug. JAMA 248:2864-2867, 1982.

451. Whelton A, Stout RL, Spilman PS, et al: Renal effects of ibuprofen, piroxicam and sulindac in patients with asymptomatic renal failure. Ann Intern Med 112:568-576, 1992.

452. Daskalopoulos G, Kronborg I, Katkov W, et al: Sulindac and indomethacin suppress the diuretic action of furosemide in patients with cirrhosis and ascites: Evidence that sulindac affects renal prostaglandins. Am J Kidney Dis 6:217-222, 1985.

453. Dixey JJ, Noormohamed FH, Lant AF: The effects of naproxen and sulindac on renal function and their interaction with hydrochlorothiazide and piretanide in man. Br J Clin Pharmacol 23:55-63, 1987.

454. Swainson CP, Griffiths P: Acute and chronic effects of sulindac on renal function in chronic renal disease. Clin Pharmacol Ther 37: 298-300, 1985.

455. Klassen DK, Stout RL, Spilman PS, et al: Sulindac kinetics and effects on renal function and prostaglandin excretion in renal insufficiency. J Clin Pharmacol 29:1037-1042, 1989.

456. Eriksson L-O, Sturfelt G, Thysell H, et al: Effects on sulindac and naproxen on prostaglandin excretion in patients with impaired renal function and rheumatoid arthritis. Am J Med 89:313-321, 1990.

457. Brater MJS, Bednar MM, McGiff JC: Renal metabolism of ibuprofen, naproxen and sulindac on prostaglandins in men. Kidney Int 27: 66-72, 1985.

458. Miller MJS, Bednar MM, McGiff JC: Renal metabolism of sulindac: Functional implications. J Pharmacol Exp Ther 231:449-456, 1984.

459. Cibattoni G, Cinotti GA, Pierucci A: Effects of sulindac and ibuprofen in patients with chronic glomerular disease: Evidence for the dependence of renal function on prostacyclin. N Engl J Med 310:279-288, 1984.

460. Laffi G, Daskalopoulos G, Kronborg I, et al: Effects of sulindac and ibuprofen in patients with cirrhosis and ascites. An explanation for the renal-sparing effect of sulindac. Gastroenterology 90:182-187, 1986.

461. Zipser RD, Hoefs JC, Speckart PF, et al: Prostaglandins: Modulators of renal function and pressor resistance in chronic liver disease. J Clin Endocrinol Metab 48:895-900, 1979.

462. Quintero E, Gines P, Arroyo V: Sulindac reduces the urinary excretion of prostaglandins and impairs renal function in cirrhosis with ascites. Nephron 42:298-303, 1986.

463. Husserl FE, Lange RK, Kantrow CM Jr: Renal papillary necrosis and pyelonephritis accompanying fenoprofen therapy. JAMA 242:1896-1898, 1979.

464. Pearce CJ, Gonzalez FM, Wallin JD: Renal failure and hyperkalemia associated with ketorolac tromethamine. Arch Intern Med 153:1000-1002, 1993.

465. Corelli RL, Gericke KR: Renal insufficiency associated with intramuscular administration of ketorolac tromethamine. Ann Pharmacother 27:1055-1057, 1993.

466. Feldman HI, Kinman JL, Berlin JA, et al: Parenteral ketorolac: The risk for acute renal failure. Ann Intern Med 126:193-199, 1997.

467. Ferguson S, Hebert R, Laneuville O: NS-398 upregulates constitutive cyclooxygenase-2 expression in the M-1 cortical collecting duct cell line. J Am Soc Nephrol 10:2261-2271, 1999.

468. Yang T, Singh I, Pham H, et al: Regulation of cyclooxygenase expression in the kidney by dietary salt intake. Am J Physiol 274:F481-F489, 1998.

469. Harris R, McKanna J, Akai Y, et al: Cyclooxygenase-2 is associated with the macula densa of rat kidney and increases with salt restriction. J Clin Invest 94:2504-2510, 1994.

470. Kester M, Coroneos E, Thomas P, Dunn M: Endothelin stimulates prostaglandin endoperoxide synthase-2 mRNA expression and protein synthesis through a tyrosine kinase–signaling pathway in rat mesangial cells. J Biol Chem 269:22574-22580, 1994.

471. Ohnaka K, Numaguchi K, Yamakawa T, Inagami T: Induction of cyclooxygenase-2 by angiotensin II in cultured rat vascular smooth muscle cells. Hypertension 35:68-75, 2000.

472. Komhoff M, Wang J, Cheng H, et al: Cyclooxygenase-2–selective inhibitors impair glomerulogenesis and renal cortical development. Kidney. Int. 57:414-422, 2000.

473. Komhoff M, Grone H, Klein T, et al: Localization of cyclooxygenase-1 and -2 in adult and fetal human kidney: Implication for renal function. Am J Physiol. 272:F460-F468, 1997.

474. Brater C: Effects of nonsteroidal anti-inflammatory drugs on renal function: Focus on cyclooxygenase-2-selective inhibition. Am J Med. 107(suppl 6A)65S-71S, 1999.

475. Catella-Lawson F, McAdam B, Morrison B, et al: Effects of specific inhibition of cyclooxygenase-2 on sodium balance, hemodynamics, vasoactive eicosanoids. J Pharmacol Exp Ther 289:735-741, 1999.

476. Rossat J, Maillard M, Nussberger J, et al: Renal effects of selective cyclooxygenase-2 inhibition in normotensive salt-depleted subjects. Clin Pharmacol Ther 66:76-84, 1999.

477. McAdam B, Catella-Lawson F, Mardini I, et al: Systemic biosynthesis of prostacyclin by cyclooxygenase (COX)-2: The human pharmacology of a selective inhibitor of COX-2. Proc Natl Acad Sci U S A. 96:272-277, 1999.

478. Swan S, Lasseter K, Ryan C, et al: Renal effects of multiple dose rofecoxib, a COX-2 inhibitor in elderly subjects [abstract]. J Am Soc Nephrol 10:641A, 1999.

479. Perazella M, Eras J: Are selective COX-2 inhibitors nephrotoxic? Am J Kidney Dis 35:937-940, 2000.

480. Dunn M: Are COX-2 selective inhibitors nephrotoxic? Am J Kidney Dis 35:976-977, 2000.

481. Dunn MJ, Zambrask E: Renal effects of drugs that inhibit prostaglandin synthesis. Kidney Int 18:609-617, 1980.

482. Levenson DJ, Simmons CE Jr, Brenner BM: Arachidonic acid metabolism, prostaglandins and the kidney. Am J Med 72:354, 1979.

483. Fulgraff G, Meiforth A: Effects of prostaglandin E$_2$ on excretion and reabsorption of sodium and fluid in rat kidneys (micropuncture studies). Plfugers Arch 330:243, 1971.

484. Ganguli M, Tobian L, Azar S, et al: Evidence that prostaglandin synthesis inhibitors increase the concentration of sodium and chloride in rat renal medulla. Circ Res 40:135, 1977.

485. Shimizu K, Kurosawa T, Maeda T, et al: Free water excretion and washout of renal medullary urea by prostaglandin E. Jpn Heart J 10:437, 1969.

486. Ichicawa I, Brenner BM: Mechanism of inhibition of proximal tubule fluid reabsorption after exposure of the rat kidney to the physical effects of expansion of extracellular fluid volume. J Clin Invest 64:1466, 1979.

487. Ichicawa I, Brenner BM: Importance of efferent arteriolar vascular tone in regulation of proximal tubular fluid reabsorption and glomerulotubular balance in the rat. J Clin Invest 65:1192, 1980.

488. Higashihara E, Stokes JB, Kokko JP, et al: Cortical and papillary micro-puncture examination of chloride transport in segments in the rat kidney during inhibition of prostaglandin production. J Clin Invest 64:1277-1287, 1979.

489. Iino Y, Imai M: Effects of prostaglandins on Na transport in isolated collecting tubules. Pflugers Arch 373:125-133, 1978.

490. Roman RJ, Kauker ML: Renal effect of prostaglandin synthetase inhibition in rats: Micropuncture studies. Am J Physiol Renal Fluid Electrolyte Physiol, 235:F111-F118, 1978.

491. Stokes J, Kokko JP: Inhibition of sodium transport by prostaglandin E$_2$ across the isolated, perfused rabbit collecting tubule. J Clin Invest 49:1099-1104, 1977.

492. Work J, Baehler TR, Kotchen A, et al: Effect of prostaglandin inhibition on sodium chloride reabsorption in the diluting segment of the conscious dog. Kidney Int 17:24-30, 1980.

493. Carmines PK, Bell DP, Roman RJ, et al: Prostaglandins in the sodium excretory response to altered renal arterial pressure in dogs. Am J Physiol Renal Fluid Electrolyte Physiol, 248: F8-F14, 1985.

494. Wilson DR, Honrath U, Sonnenberg H: Prostaglandin synthesis inhibition during volume expansion: Collecting duct function. Kidney Int 22:1-7, 1982.

495. Nies AS, Gal J, Fadul S, et al: Indomethacin-furosemide interaction: The importance of renal blood flow. J Pharmacol Exp Ther 226:27-32, 1983.

496. Berg XJ: Acute effects of acetylsalicylate acid in patients with chronic renal insufficiency. Eur J Clin Pharmacol 11:111, 1977.

497. Mirouze D, Zisper RD, Reynolds TB: Effect of inhibitors of prostaglandin synthesis on induced cirrhosis. Hepatology 3:50, 1983.

498. Patak RV, Moorkejeree BK, Bentzel CJ, et al: Antagonism of the effects of furosemide by indomethacin in normal and hypertensive man. Prostaglandins 10:649, 1975.

499. Tiggeler RG, Koene RA, Wijdeveld PG: Inhibition of furosemide-induced natriuresis by indomethacin in patients with nephrotic syndrome. Clin Sci Mol Med 2:149, 1977.

500. Williamson HE, Bourland UA, Marchand GR: Inhibition of furosemide-induced increase in renal blood flow by indomethacin. Proc Soc Exp Biol Med 148:164, 1975.

501. Epstein M, Lifschitz MD, Hoffman DS, et al: Relationship between renal prostaglandin E and renal sodium handling during water immersion in normal man. Circ Res 45:71-80, 1979.

502. Beckman ML, Gerber JG, Byyny RL, et al: Propranolol increases prostacyclin synthesis in patients with hypertension. Hypertension 12:582, 1988.

503. Seelig CB, Maloley PA, Campbell JR: Nephrotoxicity associated with concomitant ACE inhibitor and NSAID therapy. South Med J 83:1144, 1990.

504. Houston MC: Nonsteroidal anti-inflammatory drugs and antihypertensives. Am J Med 90:42S-47S, 1991.

505. Diederich D, Yang Z, Buhler FR, et al: Impaired endothelium-dependent relaxations in hypertensive resistance arteries involve cyclooxygenase pathway. Am J Physiol Heart Circ Physiol 258: H445-H451, 1990.

506. Panzer JA, Quyyumi AA, Brush JE, et al: Abnormal endothelium-dependent vascular relaxation in patients with essential hypertension. N Engl J Med 323:22-27, 1990.

507. Vane JR, Anggard EE, Botting RM: Regulatory functions of the vascular endothelium. N Engl J Medi 323:27-35, 1990.

508. Linder L, Wolfgang K, Buhler FR, et al: Indirect evidence for release of endothelium-derived relaxing factor in human forearm circulation in vivo. Circulation 81:1762-1767, 1990.

509. Kato T, Iwama Y, Okumura K, et al: Prostaglandin H$_2$ may be the endothelium-derived contracting factor released by acetylcholine in the aorta of the rat. Hypertension 15:475-481, 1990.

510. Minuz P, Barrow SE, Crockcroft JR, et al: Prostacyclin and thromboxane biosynthesis in mild essential hypertension. Hypertension 15:469-474, 1990.

511. Luscher TF: Imbalance of endothelium-derived relaxing and contracting factors. Am J Hypertens 3:317-330, 1990.

512. Houston MC: Nonsteroidal anti-inflammatory drugs and antihypertensives. Am J Med 90:425-430, 1991.

513. Minuz P, Barrow SE, Crockcroft JR, et al: Effects of non-steroidal anti-inflammatory drugs on prostacyclin and thromboxane biosynthesis in patients with mild essential hypertension. Br J Clin Pharmacol 30:519-526, 1990.

514. Abe K, Sato M, Takeuchi K, et al: The roles of renal prostaglandin in the regulatory mechanism of renal excretory function and blood pressure in hypertension. Adv Prostaglandin Thromboxane Leukot Res 19:216-220, 1989.

515. Pope JE, Anderson JJ, Felson DT: A meta-analysis of the effects of nonsteroidal anti-inflammatory drugs on blood pressure. Arch Intern Med 153:477-484, 1993.

516. Dunn MJ, Hood VL: Prostaglandins and the kidney. Am J Physiol 233:F169, 1977.

517. Dunn MJ, Zambraski E: Renal effects of drugs that inhibit prostaglandin synthesis. Kidney Int 18:609-622, 1980.

518. Henrich WL, Campbell WB: Importance of intracellular calcium in tissue renin release [abstract]. Clin Res 32:242A, 1984.

519. Henrich WL, Campbell WB: Relationship between prostaglandins and the β-adrenergic pathway to renin secretion. An in vitro study. Am J Physiol 247:E343-E348, 1984.

520. Berl T, Henrich W, Erickson AL, et al: Prostaglandins in the beta adrenergic and baroreceptor-mediated secretion of renin. Am J Physiol 236:F472-F477, 1979.

521. Blackshear JL, Spielman WS, Knox FG, et al: Dissociation of renin release and renal vasodilatation by prostaglandin synthesis inhibitions. Am J Physiol 237:F20-F27, 1979.

522. Gerber JG, Olson RD, Nies AS: Control of canine renin release: Macula dense requires prostaglandin synthesis. J Physiol (Lond) 319:419-429, 1981.

523. Henrich WL: Prostaglandins in renin secretion. Kidney Int 19:822-830, 1981.

524. Henrich WL, Anderson RJ, Berl T, et al: Role of angiotension II and prostaglandins in renal response to hypotensive hemorrhage. Am J Physiol 235:F48-F51, 1978.

525. Henrich WL, Anderson RJ, Berns AS, et al: Role of renal nerves and prostaglandins in control of renal hemodynamics and plasma renin activity during hypotensive hemorrhage in the dog. J Clin Invest 61:744-750, 1978.

526. Henrich WL, Campbell WB: The β-adrenergic pathway to renin release: Relations with the prostaglandin system. Endocrinology 113:2247-2254, 1983.

527. Gokal R, Matthews DR: Renal papillary necrosis after aspirin and alclofenac. BMJ 2:1517-1518, 1977.

528. Finklestein A, Fraley D, Stachura I, et al: Fenoprofen nephropathy: Lipoid nephrosis and interstitial nephritis. A possible T-lymphocyte disorder. Am J Med 72:81-87, 1982.

529. Karz S, Capaldo R, Everts E, et al: Association with reversible renal failure and acute interstitial nephritis. JAMA 246:243-245, 1981.

530. Morgenstern SJ, Burns FJ, Fraley DS, et al: Ibuprofen-associated lipid nephrosis without interstitial nephritis. Am J Kidney Dis 16:50-52, 1989.

531. Schwartzman M, Dagati V: Spontaneous relapse of naproxen-related nephrotic syndrome. Am J Med 82:329-332, 1987.

532. Goetzl E: Selective feed-back inhibition of the 5 lipoxygenation of the arachidonic acid in human T-lymphocytes. Biochem Biophys Res Commun 101:344-350, 1981.

533. Siegl M, McConnell R, Porter N, et al: Arachidonate metabolism via lipoxygenase and 12-L-hydroperoxy-5,8,10,14-eicosatetraenoic acid peroxidase sensitive to anti-inflammatory drugs. Proc Natl Acad Sci U S A 77:308-312, 1980.

534. Bokoch F, Boeynaems J, Hubbard W: Chemotactic and chemokinetic activity of products of mammalian lipoxygenases. Pick Lymphokines 4:271-295, 1981.

535. Goetzl E: Mediators of immediate hypersensitivity derived from arachidonic acid. N Engl J Med 303:822-825, 1980.

536. Torres VE: Present and future of the nonsteroidal antiinflammatory drugs in nephrology. Mayo Clin Proc 57:389-393, 1982.

537. Chen CY, Pang VF, Chen CS: Pathological and biochemical modifications of renal function in ibuprofen-induced interstitial nephritis. Ren Fail 18:31-40, 1996.

538. Duggin GG: Mechanisms in the development of analgesic nephropathy: Kidney Int 18:553, 1980.

539. Sabatini S: Analgesic-induced papillary necrosis. Semin Nephrol 8:41, 1988.

540. Nanra RS: Analgesic nephropathy in the 1990's: An Australian perspective. Kidney Int 44 (suppl 42):86, 1993.

541. Buckalew VM, Schey HM: Renal disease from habitual antipyretic analgesic consumption: An assessment of the epidemiologic evidence. Medicine, (Baltimore) 11:291, 1986.

542. Pommer W, Bronder E, Greiser E, et al: Regular analgesic intake and the risk of end-stage renal disease. Am J Nephrol 9:403, 1989.

543. Elseviers M, De Broe M: Analgesic nephropathy in Belgium is related to the sales of particular analgesic mixtures. Nephrol Dial Transplant 9:41-46, 1994.

544. De Broe M, Elseviers M, Bengtsson U, et al: Analgesic nephropathy. Nephrol Dial Transplant 11:2407-2408, 1996.

545. Sandler DP, Smith J, Weinberg C, et al: Analgesic use and chronic renal disease. N Engl J Med 320:1238, 1989.

546. Murray TG, Stolley P, Anthony J, et al: Epidemiologic study of regular analgesic use and end-stage renal disease. Arch Intern Med 143:1687, 1983.

547. Morlans M, Laporte J, Vidal X, et al: End-stage renal disease and non-narcotic analgesics: A case control study. Br. J. Clin. Pharmacol 30:717, 1990.

548. Dubach UC, Rosner B, Pfister E: Epidemiologic study of analgesics containing phenacetin. N Engl J Med 308:357, 1983.

549. Elseviers M, De Broe M: A long-term prospective controlled study of analgesic abuse in Belgium. Kidney Int 48:1912-1919, 1995.

550. Dubach UC, Rosner B, Stumer T: An epidemiologic study of abuse of analgesic drugs. N Engl J Med 324:155, 1991.

551. Piper JM, Tonascia J, Matanoski GM: Heavy phenacetin use and bladder cancer in women aged 20 to 49 years. N Engl J Med 313:292, 1985.

552. Elseviers M, De Schepper A, Corthouts B, et al: High diagnostic performance of CT scan for analgesic nephropathy in patients with incipient to severe renal failure. Kidney Int 48:1316-1323, 1995.

553. Carmichael J, Shankel SW: Effects of nonsteroidal anti-inflammatory drugs on prostaglandins and renal function. Am J Med 78:992, 1985.

554. Sandler DP, Burr R, Weinburg CR: Nonsteroidal anti-inflammatory drugs and the risk for chronic renal disease. Ann Intern Med 115:165, 1991.

555. Segasothy M, Samad SA, Zulfigar A, Bennett WM: Chronic renal disease and papillary necrosis associated with the long-term use of nonsteroidal anti-inflammatory drugs as the sole or predominant analgesic. Am J Kidney Dis 24:17, 1994.

556. Rice D: Renal failure in patients with rheumatoid arthritis and osteoarthritis on nonsteroidal anti-inflammatory drugs. Fed Proc 43:1100, 1984.

557. Perneger TV, Whelton PK, Klag MJ: Risk of kidney failure associated with the use of acetaminophen, aspirin, and nonsteroidal anti-inflammatory drugs. N Engl J Med 331:1675, 1994.

558. Rexrode KM, Buring JE, Glynn RJ, et al: Analgesic use and renal function in men. JAMA 286:315-321, 2001.

559. Fored CM, Ejerblad E, Lindblad P, et al: Acetaminophen, aspirin, and chronic renal failure. N Engl J Med 345:1801-1803, 2001.

560. Henrich W, Agodoa L, Barrett B, et al: Analgesics and the kidney: Summary and recommendations to the scientific advisory board of the NKF from an ad hoc committee of the NKF. Am J Kidney Dis. 27:162-165, 1996.

561. Henrich W: Analgesic nephropathy. Trans Am Clin Climatol Assoc 109:147-159, 1998.

562. De Broe M, Stolear J, Nouwen E, Elseviers M: 5-Aminosalicylic acid (5-ASA) and chronic tubulointerstitial nephritis in patients with chronic inflammatory bowel disease, Is there a link? Nephrol Dial Transplant 12:1839-1841, 1997.

563. Henrich WL: Functional and organic ischemic renal disease. In Seldin DG, Giebisch GH (eds): The Kidney, 2nd ed. New York, Raven Press, 1992, pp 3289-3304.

564. Badr KF, Ichikawa K: Prerenal failure: A deleterious shift from renal compensation to decompensation. N Engl J Med 319:623-629, 1988.

565. Curtis JJ, Luke RG, Whelchel JD, et al: Inhibition of angiotensin-converting enzyme is renal transplant recipients with hypertension. N Engl J Med 308:377, 1983.

566. Jacobson HR: Ischemic renal disease: An overlooked clinical entity? Kidney Int 34:729-743, 1988.

567. Packer M, Lee WH, Medina N, et al: Influence of diabetes mellitus on changes in left ventricular performance and renal function produced by converting enzyme inhibition in patients with severe chronic renal failure. Am J Med 823:1119-1126, 1987.

568. Nath KA, Crumbley AJ, Murray BM, et al: [Letter]. N Engl J Med 309:546-547, 1983.

569. Ying CY, Tifft CP, Gavras H, et al: Renal revascularization in the azotemic hypertensive patient resistant to therapy. N Engl J Med 311:1070-1075, 1984.

570. Textor SC, Novick AC, Tarazi RC, et al: Critical perfusion pressure for renal function in patients with bilateral atherosclerotic renal vascular renal disease. Ann Intern Med 102:308-314, 1985.

571. Van de Ven PJ, Beutler JJ, Kaatee R, et al: Angiotensin converting enzyme inhibitor–induced renal dysfunction in atherosclerotic renovascular disease. Kidney Int 53:986-993, 1998.

572. Bender W, LaFrance N, Walter WG: Mechanism of deterioration in renal function in patients with renovascular hypertension treated with enalapril. Hypertension 6:I193-I197, 1984.

573. Fommei E, Ghione S, Palla L: Renal scintigraphic captopril test in the diagnosis of renovascular hypertension. Hypertension 10:212-220, 1987.

574. Gruenewald SM, Collins LT: Renovascular hypertension: Quantitative renography as a screening test. Radiology 149: 287-291, 1983.

575. Jackson B, McGrath BP, Matthews G, et al: Differential renal function during angiotensin converting enzyme inhibition in renovascular hypertension. Hypertension 8:650-654, 1986.

576. Miyanmori I, Yasuhara S, Takeda Y, et al: Effects of converting inhibition on split renal function in renovascular hypertension. Hypertension 8:415-421, 1986.

577. Nally JV Jr: Renal scintigraphy in the evaluation of renovascular hypertension: A note of optimism yet caution. J Nucl Med 28: 1501-1505, 1987.

578. Schohn DC, Jahn HA, Schmitt RL: Predictability of a standardization captopril-test in hypertension in end-stage renal failure. Kidney Int 34:S145-S148, 1988.

579. Thibonnier M, Joseph A, Sassano P: Diagnostic value of a single dose of captopril in renin and aldosterone-dependent surgically curable hypertension. Cardiovasc Rev Rep 3:165-168, 1982.

580. Kohler TR, Zierler RE, Martin RL: Non-invasive diagnosis of renal artery stenosis by ultrasonic duplex scanning. J Vasc Surg 4: 450-456, 1986.

581. Garcia TM, Da Costa JA, Costa RS, Ferraz AS: Acute tubular necrosis in kidney transplant patients treated with enalapril. Ren Fail 16:419-423, 1994.

582. Dussol B, Nicolino F, Brunet P, et al: Acute transplant artery thrombosis induced by angiotension-converting inhibitor in a patient with renovascular hypertension. Nephron 66:102-104, 1994.

583. Mandal AK, Markert RJ, Saklayen MG, et al: Diuretics potentiate angiotensin converting enzyme inhibitor–induced acute renal failure. Clin Nephrol 42:170-174, 1994.

584. Nakhoul F, Better OS: Acute renal failure following massive mannitol infusion and enalapril treatment. Clin Nephrol 44:118-120, 1995.

585. Donker AJM: Nephrotoxicity of angiotensin converting enzyme inhibition. Kidney Int 31:S132, 1987.

586. Cleland JGF, Dargie HJ, Gillen G, et al: Captopril in heart failure: A double-blind study of the effects on renal function. J Cardiovasc Pharmacol 8:700, 1986.

587. Yaqoob M, Bell GM, Stevenson A, et al: Renal impairment with chronic hydrocarbon exposure. Q J Med 86:165-174, 1993.

588. Barrientos A, Ortuno MT, Morales JM, et al: Acute renal failure after use of diesel fuel as shampoo. Arch Intern Med 137:1217, 1977.

589. Crisp AJ, Balla AK, Hoffbrand BI: Acute tubular necrosis after exposure to diesel oil. BMJ 2:177, 1979.

590. Narvarte J, Saba SR, Ramirez G: Occupational exposure to organic solvents causing chronic tubulointerstitial nephritis. Arch Intern Med 149:154-159, 1989.

591. Anderson K: Acute nephritis due to turpentine absorbed by the skin. BMJ 3:881, 1912.

592. Cagnoli I, Cassanova S, Pasquali S, Zuccheli P: Relationship between hydrocarbon exposure and the nephrotic syndrome. BMJ 280:1068-1069, 1980.

593. Beirne GJ, Brennan JT: Glomerulonephritis associated with hydrocarbon solvents. Arch Environ Health 25:365-369, 1972.

594. Daniell WE, Couser WG, Rosenstock L: Occupational solvent exposure and glomerulonephritis. JAMA 259:2280-2283, 1988.

595. Klavis G, Drommer W: Goodpasture's syndrome and the effects of benzene. Arch Toxicol 26:40-55, 1970.

596. Ogawa M, Moti T, Mori Y, et al: Study on chronic renal injuries induced by carbon tetrachloride: Selective inhibition of the nephrotoxicity by irradiation. Nephron 60:68-73, 1992.

597. Yamamoto T, Wilson CB: Binding of anti–basement membrane after intratracheal gasoline instillation in rabbits. Am J Pathol 126: 497-505, 1987.

598. Ravnskov U: Possible mechanisms of hydrocarbon-associated glomerulonephritis. Clin Nephrol 23:294, 1985.

CHAPTER 35

The Kidney and Hypertension in Pregnancy

Mark S. Paller and Jeffrey J. Connaire

Nephrologists have long been interested in the care of pregnant women because pre-eclampsia, the most common cause of hypertension in pregnancy, leads to renal disease. In addition, the extraordinary changes in cardiovascular and renal function that occur during pregnancy have fascinated clinical investigators. An appreciation of these dramatic changes in renal function and hemodynamics is needed in the care of the pregnant woman, and understanding the changes brought about by pregnancy gives insight into physiologic mechanisms in the nonpregnant state. This chapter covers the changes in cardiovascular and renal function during pregnancy, with particular attention to the changes that occur with the development of hypertension and pre-eclampsia. Also, improvements in the care of women with underlying renal disease have resulted in more of these women becoming pregnant. The effect of pregnancy on the mother and fetus when underlying renal disease is present is examined.

RENAL ANATOMY AND FUNCTION DURING PREGNANCY

Anatomic Changes

The kidney increases 1 cm in length during pregnancy. This increase in renal size results from an increase in renal vascular volume and capacity of the collecting system as well as hypertrophy of the kidney. In experimental animals, the length of the proximal tubules of the kidney increased by 20% in the first trimester.[1] Kidney volume (excluding the

renal pelvis) increased by up to 30% when it was assessed by ultrasonography in 24 pregnant women.[2] Kidney volume decreased to normal values within 1 week after delivery.

A more remarkable change is the increased capacity of the dilated renal collecting system, known as physiologic hydronephrosis of pregnancy. Hormonal influence is one likely cause of the dilatation of the urinary collecting system, because it can be reproduced in animals by the administration of estrogen and progesterone and may be seen in women taking oral contraceptives.[3] Pregnancy also induces increased synthesis of prostaglandin E_2 (PGE_2), which inhibits ureteral peristalsis in dogs and may be responsible for ureteral hypomotility and distention in pregnant women as well.[4] In addition, mechanical obstruction can at times contribute to ureteral distention, particularly on the right side, where intraureteral pressures are higher above than below the pelvic brim. Smooth muscle relaxation also contributes to an increased occurrence of vesicoureteral reflux during pregnancy.[5] Although dilatation of the renal pelvis and ureters begins in the first trimester, it may persist for as long as 12 weeks after delivery.

CARDIOVASCULAR AND RENAL PHYSIOLOGY IN PREGNANCY

Blood Pressure

One of the most striking features of pregnancy is that blood pressure and peripheral vascular resistance fall soon after conception. Peripheral vasodilatation is evident in the palmar erythema and spider telangiectases that frequently develop during pregnancy. The fall in vascular resistance is thought to be caused by increased synthesis of vasodilating prostaglandins, particularly prostacyclin (PGI$_2$), which causes resistance to circulating vasoconstrictors such as angiotensin II and norepinephrine. The effectors of vasodilatation are apparently the voltage-dependent calcium channels because, in the rat model, specifically stimulating these channels to open results in a loss of the normal decrease in blood pressure seen in pregnancy.[6]

MacGillivray and co-workers[7] found in 226 primigravid women on their first visit to an obstetric clinic that blood pressure was 103 ± 11 mm Hg systolic and 56 ± 10 mm Hg diastolic sitting, 113 ± 10 mm Hg systolic and 57 ± 10 mm Hg diastolic supine. Although a rise in both systolic and diastolic pressures occurs after the 28th week of gestation, blood pressure at term remained 109 ± 12 mm Hg systolic and 69 ± 9 mm Hg diastolic sitting and 116 ± 10 mm Hg systolic and 71 ± 12 mm Hg diastolic supine.

Cardiac Output

Cardiac output increases in the first trimester of pregnancy, reaching a maximum of 30% to 40% above the nonpregnant level by the 24th week of gestation.[8] Despite the rise in cardiac output, blood pressure falls because of the decrease in vascular resistance. When hypertension occurs in pregnancy, cardiac output tends to fall in response to reflex activation of the parasympathetic nervous system, but it usually remains higher than in the nonpregnant state.[9]

Blood Volume

Blood volume increases by approximately 50% in pregnancy, beginning in the first trimester with a rise in both plasma volume and red blood cell volume. A greater increase in plasma than in red blood cell volume causes the "physiologic anemia" of pregnancy. Expansion of maternal extracellular volume continues throughout pregnancy, with a cumulative Na$^+$ retention of between 500 and 900 mEq.[10] Na$^+$ retention proceeds at the rate of approximately 20 to 30 mEq/week, which results in a mean weight gain of 12.5 kg. The major stimulus for the kidney to retain Na$^+$ is the decrease in peripheral vascular resistance, a recognized stimulus for Na$^+$ retention. When pregnant baboons were studied serially with Swan-Ganz catheters from the onset of pregnancy, decreases in right atrial, systemic, and pulmonary vascular resistance were found by the fourth week of gestation.[11] Plasma volume was not observed to be expanded until 8 weeks later.

The expanded extracellular volume may cause edema, which is present in 35% to 83% of healthy pregnant women, the frequency depending on the effort made to detect it.[12] Edema is benign, because pregnant women with edema have fewer infants of low birth weight and there is no association of edema with increased perinatal mortality or poor fetal development.[13] In contrast, inadequate maternal weight gain is associated with increased frequency of low birth weight and stillbirth. The edema in pregnancy is usually localized to the legs, whereas involvement of the face and hands with an angioneurotic appearance is more characteristic of preeclampsia. In late pregnancy, other factors contributing to leg edema may be compression of the inferior vena cava by the enlarged uterus and a reduction in colloid osmotic pressure. Limiting the time a pregnant woman spends standing and sleeping in a lateral recumbent position usually minimizes the edema.

Renal Blood Flow and Glomerular Filtration Rate

Early in pregnancy, substantial increases in renal blood flow (RBF) occur (Fig. 35-1). In one case studied prospectively, renal plasma flow had increased 45% by the ninth week of pregnancy.[14] When renal plasma flow was estimated from *p*-aminohippuric acid clearance studies, the mean renal plasma flow was 809 mL/min in the first trimester, 695 mL/min in the last 10 weeks of pregnancy, and 482 mL/min after delivery.[14–18] The increase in RBF is caused by an increase in cardiac output and a decrease in renal vascular resistance. The increase in cardiac output is probably less important than renal vasodilatation, because cardiac output, which increases approximately 40%, does not increase blood flow uniformly to all regional beds. In contrast to the large increase in RBF, there is no increase in cerebral or hepatic blood flow during pregnancy.

Studies in pregnant rats, in which precise micropuncture determinations of glomerular filtration rate (GFR) and RBF can be performed, have demonstrated proportional reductions in afferent and efferent arteriolar resistance causing the decrease in renal vascular resistance and the increase in RBF.[19] Conscious, chronically instrumented rats demonstrate similar changes in GFR and renal plasma flow in midpregnancy, averaging 26% and 20%, respectively.[20] Estimates of renal vascular resistance have suggested a 50% decrease by the end of the first trimester of pregnancy.

Despite significant renal vasodilatation, the renal response to both volume expansion and hemorrhage is maintained in pregnant rats and rabbits.[21–23] Tubuloglomerular feedback activity is also as vigorous in pregnant rats as in nonpregnant rats.[24] These renal responses suggest that the kidneys react to and sense the expanded plasma volume normally. In addition, pregnant rats retain the ability to respond to an amino acid

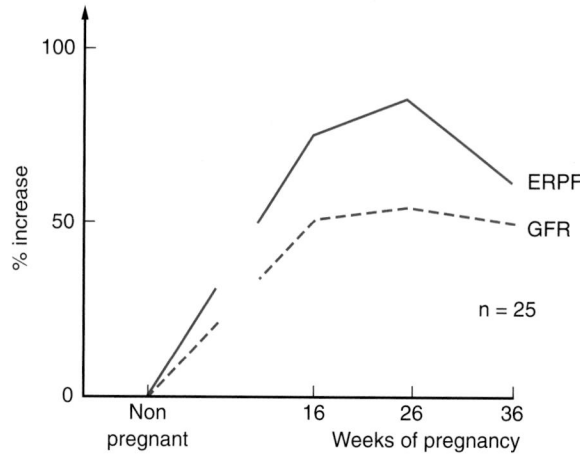

FIGURE 35-1. Effect of pregnancy on glomerular filtration rate (GFR) and effective renal plasma flow (ERPF). (From Davison JM: Overview: Kidney function in pregnant women. Am J Kidney Dis 9:248, 1987.)

infusion, with a further increase in RBF and GFR that is proportionately as great as that in nonpregnant rats.[25]

The cause of pregnancy-induced renal vasodilatation is not known. Pregnancy results in large increases in the urinary excretion of PGE_2 and PGI_2.[26–29] Exogenous administration of PGE_2 and PGI_2 results in renal vasodilatation and an increase in RBF. However, several investigators have demonstrated that the increase in RBF in pregnant rats is not reversed by the administration of cyclooxygenase inhibitors, which prevents synthesis of all prostaglandins, both vasodilators and vasoconstrictors.[30, 31] Mechanisms other than the production of prostaglandins may contribute to renal vasodilatation during pregnancy. Prolactin may be a hormonal mediator of renal vasodilatation, because the pattern of prolactin excretion during pregnancy parallels that of RBF. When rats were made pseudopregnant by prolactin injection, they developed an increase in GFR and RBF similar to that seen in early pregnancy.[32, 33] Hyperprolactinemia can also induce renal vasodilatation and an increase in RBF in male rats.[34] However, the ability of prolactin to stimulate RBF and GFR has not been universally observed.[35] Pseudopregnancy, like prolactin administration, stimulates renal PGE_2 production similar to that observed during true pregnancy.[36] Therefore, the renal vasodilatory effects of prolactin could be mediated through increased renal prostaglandin synthesis. Chapman and colleagues[37] found that in the luteal phase of the menstrual cycle there is a decrease in systemic vascular resistance and mean arterial pressure (MAP), an increase in cardiac output, and an increase in RBF and GFR that correlate with increased urinary cyclic adenosine monophosphate (cAMP) excretion and activation of the renin-angiotensin system without increased urinary cyclic guanosine monophosphate (cGMP) or nitrite/nitrate excretion.[37] These changes closely parallel the systemic and renal hemodynamic changes of early pregnancy.

The most important consequence of the increase in RBF during pregnancy is an increase in glomerular filtration. The pattern of the change in GFR is similar to that observed for RBF, with an early increase of approximately 45%. GFR determinations by inulin clearance revealed a mean GFR of 96 mL/min in nonpregnant women that increased to 143 mL/min in the first trimester of pregnancy.[18] Bucht and Werko[38] reported that inulin clearance increased from 122 ± 24 to 170 ± 23 mL/min from the 8th to the 32nd week of pregnancy. Unlike renal plasma flow, which tends to decrease toward nonpregnant levels in the last few weeks of pregnancy, GFR remains elevated until term (see Fig. 35-1). The level of dietary protein correlates positively with GFR in pregnancy, as it does in the nonpregnant state.[39]

Micropuncture studies of pregnant rats suggest that the increase in GFR is solely a consequence of the increase in RBF.[40] Comparison of superficial single-nephron GFR and glomerular plasma flow rate (Q_A) with whole-kidney values revealed proportional increases, suggesting that the renal vasodilatation was uniformly distributed throughout the kidney.[40] When Baylis[40] studied euvolemic Munich-Wistar rats on day 12 of a 21-day gestation, she found these rats to be in filtration pressure equilibrium. Values for mean glomerular hydraulic pressure gradient (ΔP) and for afferent and efferent arteriolar oncotic pressure were no different from those measured in nonpregnant rats. There were also no major changes in the glomerular capillary ultrafiltration

coefficient (K_f), because the estimated minimal value was similar in gravid and virgin rats.[40] At some disagreement with these findings are those of Dal Canton and colleagues,[41] who studied hydropenic, 15-day-pregnant Munich-Wistar rats. In their studies, the increase in GFR was dependent on a small increase in glomerular capillary hydraulic pressure as well as an increase in glomerular plasma flow. These rats were in filtration pressure disequilibrium and had a decrease in mean K_f of 14%. A possible explanation for these discrepant results is that the former study was performed in euvolemic rats, whereas the latter was performed in hydropenic rats, and that there were substantial differences in volume status of these animals. In either case, however, the major determinant of the pregnancy-induced increase in GFR was an increase in RBF.

The practical consequences of these changes in RBF and GFR are that normal laboratory values change in the healthy pregnant woman. For example, blood urea nitrogen values in normal pregnancy average 8.7 ± 1.5 mg/dL, and serum creatinine levels average 0.46 ± 0.13 mg/dL.[14]

The Renin-Angiotensin-Aldosterone System in Pregnancy

The level of plasma angiotensin II is dependent on several factors: the renin concentration in plasma, the concentration of its substrate angiotensinogen, the activity of the converting enzyme, and tissue angiotensinase activity. Under most circumstances, the concentration of renin in plasma is the most important determinant of plasma angiotensin II concentration, but in pregnancy there is an increase in both plasma renin and angiotensinogen. There is a threefold to fourfold increase in angiotensinogen concentration, and plasma renin concentration is approximately eight times higher than in nonpregnant women.[42–45] With the combined rise in renin and substrate concentration, plasma renin activity, which measures the amount of angiotensin generated with incubation of plasma, is approximately 15 times higher than in nonpregnant women.

The paradox of pregnancy is that high renin secretion occurs during expansion of the extracellular volume and increased delivery of filtered Na^+ to the distal tubule, both of which should cause renin secretion to fall by baroreceptor and macula densa mechanisms. The increased renin secretion is probably largely a result of the increase in PGI_2 synthesis, which directly increases renal renin secretion and causes resistance to angiotensin II in the peripheral vasculature. The suggestion that the elevated renin secretion in pregnancy is caused by a salt-losing tendency of pregnancy resulting from increased GFR and elevated secretion of progesterone, which acts as an antagonist to aldosterone at the renal tubule, has not proved to be the case: A 300 mEq sodium intake for 7 days, intravenous saline, or prolonged mineralocorticoid administration does not suppress renin or aldosterone secretion to the levels seen in nonpregnant subjects.[27] The elevation in plasma angiotensin II in pregnancy maintains arterial blood pressure, because angiotensin blockade with saralasin or with an angiotensin I–converting enzyme inhibitor causes a reduction in arterial pressure.[27]

The molecular precursor of renin, prorenin, which circulates in plasma and constitutes 80% to 90% of potential human plasma renin activity, is elevated throughout pregnancy.[42, 43]

Prorenin is converted to active renin by acid, storage in the cold, and incubation with proteolytic enzymes. The role of prorenin, except as a precursor of renin, is unknown, because there is no evidence of conversion of plasma prorenin to renin under physiologic conditions.[42, 46, 47] The uterus, placenta, and ovaries synthesize prorenin in high concentration, and release of prorenin from the uterus occurs with reduction in uterine blood flow.[48, 49]

Uterine prorenin may function as a local hormone controlling blood flow to the uterus and placenta by maintaining a high uterine angiotensin II concentration. Unlike its vasoconstrictor effect on most vascular beds, angiotensin II increases uterine blood flow in the pregnant dog, rabbit, and monkey.[50, 51] Because angiotensin II increases uterine PGE_2 synthesis, the increase in blood flow with angiotensin may be caused by concomitant increase in prostaglandin synthesis. Sealey and co-workers[52] suggested that the presence of prorenin in the afferent arteriole of the kidney and in the uterus might result in tachyphylaxis to angiotensin II, because a high local concentration of angiotensin II would cause resistance to circulating angiotensin II. It is interesting that the sheep uterus does not contain prorenin, and angiotensin II does not increase uterine blood flow in that species.[53, 54]

Angiotensin II is also an angiogenesis factor, inducing new blood vessel growth in experimental circumstances.[55] Uterine prorenin may be involved in the extensive neovascularization that occurs in the uterus and placenta during pregnancy. Inhibitors of both prostaglandin and angiotensin II synthesis decrease uterine blood flow in pregnant rabbits.[50, 56, 57] Therefore, uterine prostaglandin synthesis depends not only on the cyclooxygenase enzyme necessary for prostaglandin synthesis but also on the angiotensin-converting enzyme.

Prostaglandin Synthesis in Pregnancy

Pregnancy is associated with increases in both PGI_2 and thromboxane synthesis. Placental tissues are capable of generating PGI_2, and the umbilical artery has a 10- to 100-fold greater capacity to synthesize PGI_2 than other arteries do.[58–62] A reduction in PGI_2 synthesis has been demonstrated in umbilical artery specimens from women with pre-eclampsia.[59–62] The concentration of the major urinary metabolite of PGI_2, 2,3-dinor-6-keto-PGF_1, was found by Fitzgerald and co-workers[63] to be 1321 ± 160 ng/g creatinine in pregnant women, compared with 254 ± 31 ng/g creatinine in nonpregnant women. Thromboxane synthesis was also elevated, with increased urinary excretion of 2,3-dinor-thromboxane B_2 and 11-dehydro-thromboxane B_2 in the last trimester.[64]

The stimulus for the increase in prostaglandin synthesis during pregnancy is not known. In pregnant animals, resistance to angiotensin II, norepinephrine, and arginine vasopressin (AVP) occurs early in pregnancy and has been found to be caused by the increased synthesis of prostaglandins.[36, 65] Pseudopregnancy, induced by mating female rats with sterile males, increases urinary PGE_2 excretion for up to 10 days, with a fall in peripheral vascular resistance and resistance to angiotensin II and norepinephrine.[36] The findings in pseudopregnancy indicate that conception is not needed to increase prostaglandin synthesis and suggest that a hormonal change triggered by the central nervous system (CNS) occurs. It is curious that pregnancy has many similarities to

Bartter syndrome, a disorder characterized by insensitivity to angiotensin II, high plasma renin and angiotensin II concentrations, low to normal blood pressure, and increased prostaglandin synthesis.[66] In both conditions, prostaglandin synthesis inhibitors increase angiotensin II sensitivity and reduce renin secretion.[66, 67]

Relaxin, a 6-kD peptide produced by the corpus luteum, appears to have a role in the changes in renal hemodynamics and osmoregulation seen in pregnancy.[68] Neutralization of relaxin by either a blocking antibody or ovariectomy resulted in attenuation of the normal pregnancy-associated increase in GFR and decrease in plasma sodium and osmolality.[68] This result may be due to downstream effects on nitric oxide (NO) and cGMP metabolism,[69] because inhibition of nitric oxide synthase counteracts the increases in GFR found in normal pregnancy.[70]

Endothelin has a similar effect on renal hemodynamics, and its role in relation to relaxin remains to be determined.[71] Another peptide, neurokinin B, a tachykinin related to substance P, is expressed in syncytiotrophoblasts in normal human placenta, is elevated in the circulation in pregnancy-induced hypertension, and causes a pressor response when in used in pregnant rats.[72]

Renal Tubule Function

Pregnancy is the most striking example in humans of the need for glomerular-tubule balance to prevent extraordinary losses of Na^+. A 50% increase in GFR during pregnancy necessitates an equal increase in Na^+ reabsorption by the renal tubules. For an Na^+ concentration of 140 mEq/L in glomerular filtrate and a GFR of 100 mL/min, the daily filtered Na^+ equals 140 mEq/L × 0.1 L/min × 1440 min/day, or 20,160 mEq. An increase of 50% in GFR increases daily Na^+ filtration to 30,240 mEq, which necessitates that the renal tubules absorb 10,080 mEq more Na^+ than in the nonpregnant state to avoid Na^+ wasting. Most of the increase in Na^+ reabsorption occurs in the proximal tubule, but all segments of the nephron are involved. Physical factors such as capillary hydraulic pressure and oncotic pressure in the renal interstitial space alter proximal Na^+ reabsorption, whereas many hormonal factors are involved in distal portions of the nephron.

Most evidence suggests that pregnant women maintain Na^+ balance normally when sodium intake is either increased or decreased. With a sodium intake of 10 mEq, pregnant women reduced urinary Na^+ excretion as readily as nonpregnant women did without excessive weight loss.[26] Conversely, when pregnant women had a sodium intake of 300 mEq, they came into balance after 4 days, and the excretion of a short-term intravenous Na^+ load was as rapid in pregnant as in nonpregnant women.[26, 73] Therefore, despite changes in extracellular fluid volume and the renal demands of increased Na^+ reabsorption, Na^+ balance is maintained in a normal manner.

Pregnant women also maintain normal water balance and retain the ability to produce a maximally concentrated and maximally dilute urine. In a study of 75 normotensive pregnant women, the maximal urine osmolality after water deprivation was 900 mOsm/kg H_2O, a value not different from that in nonpregnant women.[74] The ability to concentrate the urine is surprising, because pregnant women have two features that would limit urine concentrating ability: an increase in RBF and increased renal production of PGE_2, an antagonist of AVP in the collecting tubule. Renal diluting ability is also normal during pregnancy. After a water load, urine osmolalities in pregnant women ranged between 25 and 88 mOsm/kg H_2O, values similar to those observed in nonpregnant women.[75] The 24-hour urine volumes tend to be similar in nonpregnant and pregnant women early and late in pregnancy, although some studies have found an increase in urine volume of up to 25% in midpregnancy.[76, 77] Because there is no abnormality in renal water handling, an increase in urine volume would suggest an increase in water intake mediated by increased thirst.

Despite unaltered renal water handling, pregnant women have a decrease in serum Na^+ of approximately 5 mEq/L and a decrease in plasma osmolality of approximately 10 mOsm/kg H_2O.[78] Pregnant women have a decrease in the osmotic threshold for AVP secretion, although the sensitivity for AVP release is not altered (Fig. 35-2).[79] Nonpregnant women secrete AVP when plasma osmolality exceeds 285 mOsm/kg H_2O, whereas pregnant women secrete AVP when plasma osmolality exceeds 276 to 278 mOsm/kg H_2O.[76, 77] They respond in a quantitatively normal manner to increases or limitations in water availability, except that their set point is reduced by approximately 10 mOsm/kg H_2O. Nonosmotic release of AVP is not altered by pregnancy in either rats or women.[80, 81]

Although a change in the osmotic threshold for AVP release is one factor that contributes to the hypo-osmolality in pregnancy, other factors also exist, because pregnant Brattleboro rats, which have congenital lack of AVP, also develop hypo-osmolality.[82] To maintain hypo-osmolality, thirst would also have to be altered. Whereas nonpregnant women have an osmotic thirst threshold (derived from analog scales relating the desire to drink water to plasma osmolality) of 290 mOsm/kg H_2O and perceive thirst (the conscious desire to drink) at 298 mOsm/kg H_2O, pregnant women have an osmotic thirst threshold of 280 mOsm/kg H_2O and perceive thirst at 288 mOsm/kg H_2O.[77] The decrease in thirst threshold may actually precede the change in threshold for AVP release. Thirst threshold reaches its minimal value within 5 to 8 weeks of gestation, whereas the decreased threshold for AVP release reaches its minimum at 10 to 12 weeks.

The mechanism of the resetting of thirst and of AVP osmoreceptors is not entirely clear, but changes in the concentration of chorionic gonadotropin may be involved. Infusion of human chorionic gonadotropin into nonpregnant women lowered the osmotic thresholds for AVP release and for thirst by 3 and 4 mOsm/kg H_2O, respectively.[77] In addition, in a patient with a hydatidiform mole and elevated serum chorionic gonadotropin concentration, abnormalities in the thresholds for AVP release and for thirst paralleled the serum chorionic gonadotropin levels.[77] Although pregnant rats show similar changes in resetting of osmotic thresholds, pseudopregnant rats do not manifest these changes.[83] This contrasts to the previously cited findings of alterations in RBF, GFR, and renal prostaglandin production that

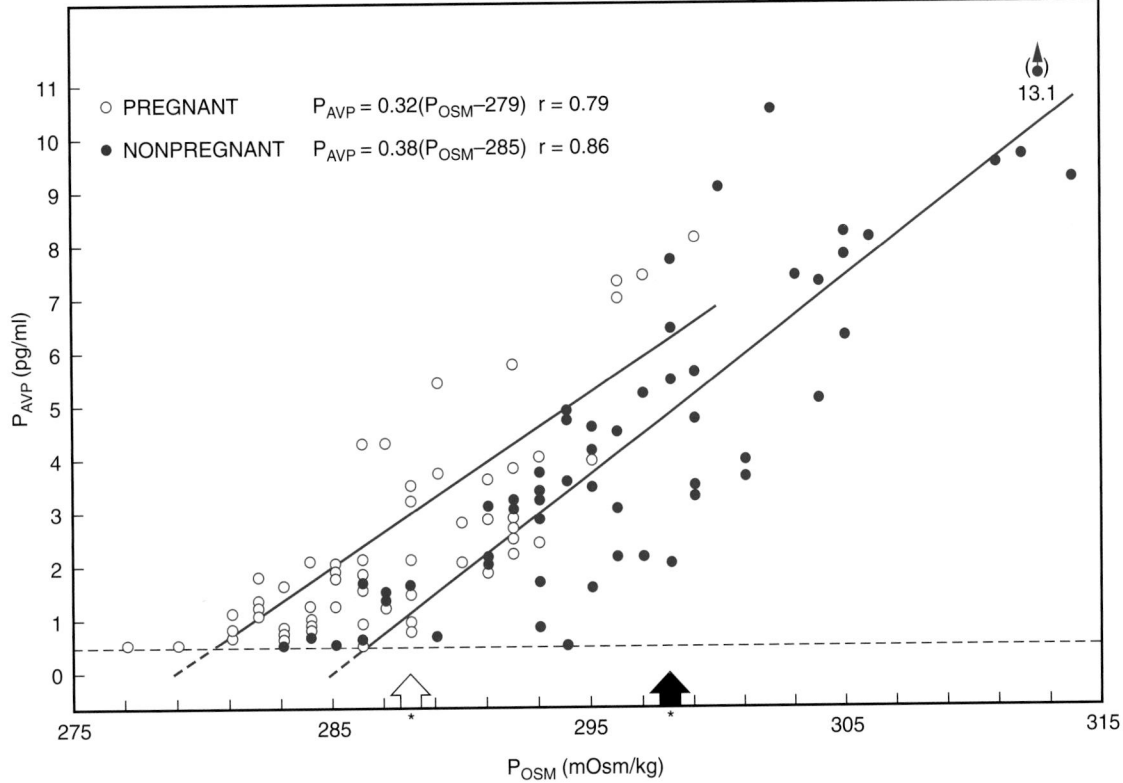

FIGURE 35-2. Relationship between plasma osmolality (P_{OSM}) and plasma arginine vasopressin (P_{AVP}) when osmolality was altered by infusion of 5% saline in pregnant and nonpregnant women. Arrows represent thirst thresholds. (From Davison JM, Gilmore EA, Durr J, et al: Altered osmotic thresholds for vasopressin secretion and thirst in human pregnancy. Am J Physiol 246:F105, 1984.)

have been seen in pseudopregnant as well as pregnant rats.[32, 33] Therefore, the fetal-placental unit apparently is not necessary to induce changes in renal hemodynamics, but it is a necessary component of the osmoregulatory changes of pregnancy.

K^+ metabolism during pregnancy is generally unchanged, although the cumulative retention of approximately 350 mEq of K^+ is necessary for fetal-placental development and for expansion of maternal red blood cell mass.[10] Although plasma aldosterone levels are increased in pregnancy, renal K^+ wasting does not occur.[26, 84, 85] This may be because elevated plasma progesterone in pregnancy inhibits the kaliuretic effect of mineralocorticoids.[86] On the other hand, pregnant women receiving high doses of the mineralocorticoid deoxycorticosterone acetate develop Na^+ retention.[86] Although some women with primary hyperaldosteronism may have a reversal of K^+ wasting, this is not a universal finding, and hypertension may remain severe during pregnancy.[87–90]

An interesting consequence of the pregnancy-induced antagonism of mineralocorticoid action is the occasional unmasking of otherwise insignificant defects in K^+ excretion. Two women with sickle cell anemia, a disease known to occasionally produce hyperkalemia by defective renal K^+ excretion, were reported to have developed life-threatening hyperkalemia during pregnancy.[91] Other conditions that potentially predispose to the development of hyperkalemia during pregnancy include diabetes mellitus, renal insufficiency, and use of β-adrenergic antagonists. However, although these cases are interesting in terms of their pathophysiology, they are rare.

Pregnancy causes a compensated respiratory alkalosis. The arterial partial pressure of carbon dioxide (Pco_2) decreases by approximately 10 mm Hg, and arterial pH increases slightly to 7.44.[92, 93] Progesterone is a major factor in stimulating the respiratory center of the CNS.[94] Chronic respiratory alkalosis is accompanied by a decrease in plasma HCO_3^- to 18 to 20 mEq/L. This reduction in total buffering capacity predisposes pregnant women to more severe acidosis with the development of either ketoacidosis or lactic acidosis. On the other hand, acid excretion by the kidney is unchanged during pregnancy. After the administration of an acid (ammonium chloride) load, pregnant women excreted normal amounts of both titratable acid and NH_4^+.[95]

The changes in renal hemodynamics during pregnancy also result in changes in the excretion of uric acid, glucose, and amino acids. Urate synthesis remains constant during pregnancy, but urate clearance increases, resulting in a decrease in serum uric acid to between 2.5 and 4 mg/dL early in pregnancy.[96] Late in pregnancy, uric acid clearance decreases in parallel with RBF so that the serum uric acid level rises.

Glucosuria is common during pregnancy. The combination of an increase in the filtered load of glucose and a tendency to less efficient tubule reabsorption of glucose is the cause of glucosuria. Women with the least efficient tubule glucose reabsorption (determined before pregnancy) are the ones who develop glucosuria during pregnancy.[97–99]

The urinary excretion of some, but not all, amino acids is increased with diminished fractional amino acid reabsorption. In particular, excretion of glycine, histidine, threonine, serine, and alanine is increased.[100–102]

HYPERTENSION AND PRE-ECLAMPSIA

Hypertension is the most common medical complication of pregnancy; blood pressure of 140/90 mm Hg or higher occurs in approximately 10% of pregnant women. It has a bimodal frequency, being more common in young women in their first pregnancy and in older multiparous women. A rise in blood pressure in pregnancy virtually always indicates the presence of one of four conditions: (1) pre-eclampsia (toxemia), (2) pre-eclampsia superimposed on chronic hypertension or renal disease, (3) chronic essential hypertension, or (4) gestational hypertension.[103]

The decrease in blood pressure observed in pregnancy makes the upper limit of normal blood pressure in nonpregnant women, 140/90 mm Hg, of little significance. The upper limit of blood pressure is determined in the nonpregnant population on epidemiologic evidence of subsequent development of vascular disease; this criterion has no relevance in pregnancy, in which hypertension is short-lived and virtually always disappears after delivery. One relevant criterion is the level of blood pressure that adversely affects fetal survival. Data from a study of more than 24,000 pregnancies demonstrated that blood pressure in excess of 125/75 mm Hg before the 32nd week of gestation and 125/85 mm Hg thereafter was associated with a significant increase in fetal risk (Fig. 35-3).[104] In another report of 15,000 pregnant women, the perinatal mortality rate rose progressively with each 5 mm Hg rise in MAP, and those with a MAP of 90 mm Hg or higher during the second trimester had a higher risk of stillbirth, fetal growth retardation, and progression to pre-eclampsia.[105] A trend toward increased perinatal mortality is found when the MAP is greater than 82 mm Hg at midpregnancy or greater than 92 mm Hg at the beginning of the third trimester. Because a blood pressure of 120/80 mm Hg indicates an MAP of 93 mm Hg, one can appreciate how values of blood pressure must be viewed differently in pregnancy.

Blood pressure in early pregnancy has value in the detection of women in whom pre-eclampsia will ultimately develop in late pregnancy. The frequency of pre-eclampsia increases linearly with increase in systolic pressure in the first trimester from 100 to 134 mm Hg, and pre-eclampsia develops in late pregnancy in one third of women with a MAP higher than 90 mm Hg in the second trimester, compared with only 2% of those with a lower MAP.[106, 107] Blood pressure that is considered normal in nonpregnant women must be of concern in pregnancy.

Ambulatory blood pressure monitoring has also revealed early changes in cardiovascular function. Heart rate and blood pressure variability are increased.[108] One group has developed a "hyperbaric index" to quantitate circadian variability during ambulatory blood pressure monitoring and to prospectively identify women who will eventually develop pre-eclampsia.[109] Moreover, "white-coat" hypertension occurs in up to 60% of women with elevated office blood pressure.[110] However, several trials have suggested that ambulatory blood pressure monitoring does not have sufficient predictive value to be employed as a clinical test in early pregnancy to identify women who will subsequently develop pre-eclampsia.[111–113]

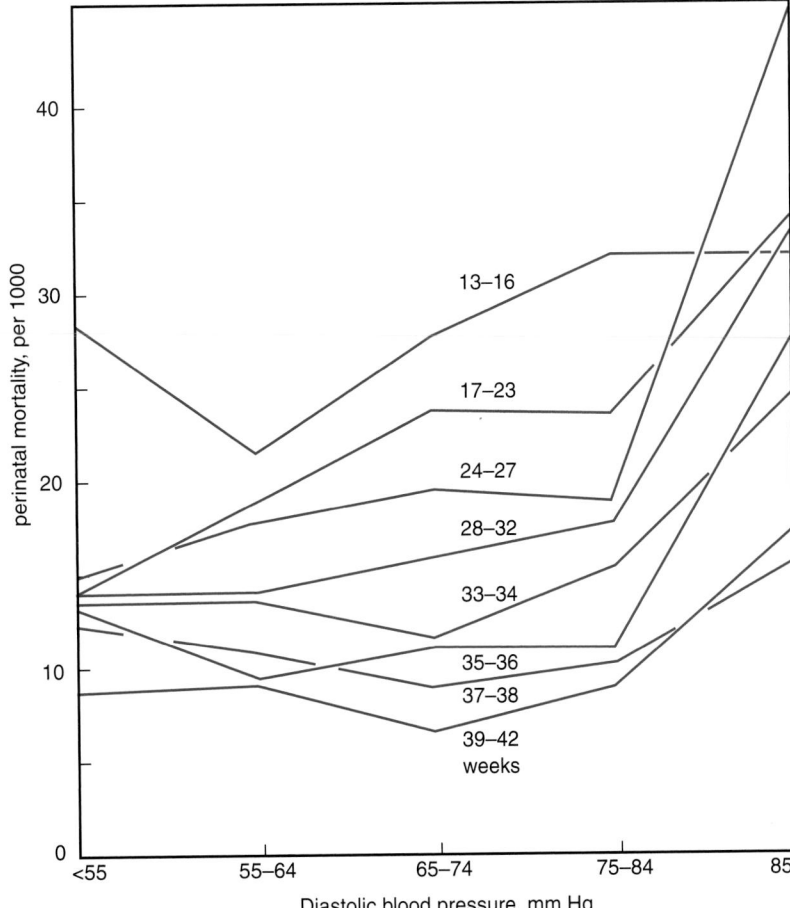

FIGURE 35-3. Relationship between blood pressure and perinatal mortality. Diastolic blood pressure is grouped by gestational age epochs. Note the uniformly increased mortality rate associated with pressures exceeding 84 mm Hg. (From Friedman EA, Neff RK: Pregnancy Hypertension: A Systemic Evaluation of Clinical Diagnostic Criteria. Littleton, MA, PSG Publishing, 1977, p 64. By permission of Mosby–Year Book.)

Etiology of Pre-eclampsia

The term *pre-eclampsia*, which implies that eclampsia is the ultimate manifestation of the disease, is commonly used to describe the disease unique to pregnancy that is manifested by hypertension and multiple organ involvement. Historically, convulsions have been the most dramatic expression of the disease, but life-threatening pre-eclampsia can occur without seizures. The disease is not unique to humans; gorillas in the wild and in captivity may have convulsions in late pregnancy, and reducing uterine blood flow in monkeys causes hypertension with glomerular disease similar to pre-eclampsia.[114, 115]

Two characteristic pathophysiologic abnormalities of pre-eclampsia, impaired placentation and diffuse endothelial cell dysfunction, are presumed to be causal in its development. Impaired placentation may even be a localized manifestation of abnormal endothelial cell behavior. During pregnancy, trophoblast cells from the embryo invade the uterine wall and vasculature. Columns of cytotrophoblastic cells invade the decidua of the endometrium by secretion of proteolytic enzymes and aggressive migration and proliferation. To establish the fetal-maternal circulation, cytotrophoblasts invade the spiral arteries in the inner third of the myometrium. Uteroplacental hypoperfusion caused by inadequate trophoblastic invasion of the uterus with failure of normal development of the spiral arteries is a feature of pre-eclampsia and has been suggested to be pathogenetic.[116, 117]

However, abnormal placentation is also a feature of intrauterine growth retardation that occurs without pre-eclampsia.[118]

Zhou and colleagues[119] found that the cytotrophoblastic invasion of the uterus is characterized by a conversion of cellular characteristics from epithelial to endothelial. This conversion requires a transformation of cell adhesion molecules to an endothelial phenotype. The same authors also demonstrated that in placentas from women with pre-eclampsia the cytotrophoblasts did not express the integrins and cadherins characteristic of endothelial cells.[120] In culture, cytotrophoblasts from preeclamptic placentas failed to properly modulate the expression of cell adhesion molecule (α_1 integrin) or matrix metalloproteinase-9.[121] Therefore, in pre-eclampsia there was a failure of cytotrophoblast epithelial-to-endothelial transformation. If this were to cause inadequate vascularization of the placenta, fetal ischemia could ensue.

Apoptosis of syncytiotrophoblast cells, a normal feature in placentation,[122] has been putatively linked to normal placental development and aging of the placenta. Apoptosis has been observed to be increased in the trophoblasts of women affected by pre-eclampsia.[123, 124] Although microscopic evidence of increased apoptosis is reproducible, the molecular details in regard to the expression of the *Fas* and *Bcl-2* genes have varied.[123, 124] The phenomenon of placental apoptosis is unlikely to be etiologic, because it has also been detected in placentas of infants with intrauterine growth retardation in the absence of pre-eclampsia.[124]

There is also evidence of generalized endothelial cell dysfunction in pre-eclampsia. Manifestations of endothelial cell dysfunction are systemic vasoconstriction and coagulopathy.[125–128] Pre-eclampsia has been associated with increased synthesis of the vasoconstrictor substances thromboxane and endothelin and decreased synthesis of the vasodilators prostacyclin and NO. Endothelin, the endothelium-derived peptide with vasoconstricting and platelet-aggregating properties, is a potential factor in pre-eclampsia. Although measurements of plasma endothelin in pre-eclampsia have been conflicting, as for all autacoids, plasma endothelin levels do not necessarily reflect concentration at the site of synthesis.[129–134] Infusion of endothelin-1 in pregnant sheep produced hemodynamic and vascular changes similar to those observed in pre-eclampsia.[135]

The endothelium-derived vasodilating factor, NO, normally plays a role in the regulation of vascular resistance. Decreased synthesis of endothelium-derived relaxing factor in response to bradykinin has been demonstrated in umbilical vessels from women with pre-eclampsia.[136] Flow-mediated vasodilatation, a NO-mediated phenomenon, is also impaired in small arteries from preeclamptic women.[137] Inhibition of NO synthesis in pregnant animals produces hemodynamic changes similar to those observed in pre-eclampsia.[138] Pregnant women and animals have decreased plasma L-arginine resulting, in part, from increased renal excretion of L-arginine during pregnancy. This may reduce the capacity of endothelial cells to synthesize NO during pregnancy and may play a role in the propensity of pregnant animals to develop the Shwartzman reaction after administration of endotoxin.[139] The ischemia and subsequent release of inflammatory mediators may inhibit the ability of the endothelium to facilitate vasodilation, because infusion of tumor necrosis factor-α leads to impaired endothelium-dependent vasodilation in the pregnant rat.[140]

Because a balance exists in pregnancy between the increased synthesis in platelets of thromboxane and the endothelial cell synthesis of PGI_2, the rise in peripheral vascular resistance causing hypertension may be due to an imbalance in synthesis of these counteracting prostaglandins. Consistent with this hypothesis is the finding that, in contrast to the fall in urinary PGI_2 metabolites with pre-eclampsia, urinary excretion of thromboxane metabolites increases.[141]

Serum from preeclamptic women demonstrates several effects on cultured endothelial cells. A cytotoxic effect occurs, as evidenced by radioactive chromate release from endothelial cells, but the cells maintain viability and show no defect in attachment, spreading behavior, or proliferation during incubation. Also, preeclamptic serum reduces endothelin and PGI_2 synthesis and causes lipid accumulation within the cells, similar to changes noted in glomerular and myocardial endothelial cells in pre-eclampsia.[125, 142, 143] Serum from preeclamptic women also induces expression of intercellular adhesion molecule-1 (ICAM-1) and increases intercellular calcium in cultured endothelial cells.[144] The factors in preeclamptic sera that cause these changes are unknown but may be released from the uterus and placenta in response to ischemia.

Because the uterus and placenta are rich sources of prorenin, which in experimental animals is released into the circulation with uterine hypoperfusion, one might speculate about its potential role in pre-eclampsia.[49, 50] Although the plasma prorenin concentration does not increase with the development of pre-eclampsia, it does not fall as does plasma renin.[42] The presence of a high concentration of prorenin in the uterus makes renin release an attractive as an etiologic factor in hypertension, but plasma renin, angiotensin II, and aldosterone levels fall with the development of pre-eclampsia. However, the concomitant reduction in PGI_2 synthesis increases sensitivity to angiotensin II, and pregnancy-associated insensitivity to angiotensin and norepinephrine disappears with the development of pre-eclampsia. A fall in urinary 6-keto-$PGF_{1\alpha}$ precedes the development of hypertension, coinciding with the increased sensitivity to angiotensin II, which can also be demonstrated before hypertension.[63] Angiotensin insensitivity in human pregnancy is detectable as early as the 10th week of gestation, with a decrease occurring as early as the 18th week in women in whom pre-eclampsia is destined to develop. In contrast, normotensive women maintain insensitivity to angiotensin throughout pregnancy, with a slight increase in sensitivity after the 32nd week (Fig. 35-4).[145]

Increased sensitivity to angiotensin is probably the cause of the positive rollover test, in which pregnant women in whom pre-eclampsia ultimately develops are found to have an excessive rise in blood pressure when they turn from a lateral recumbent to a supine position.[146] Lying supine in pregnancy compresses the inferior vena cava and reduces cardiac output. The consequent fall in RBF would increase renin secretion and serve as an endogenous test of angiotensin sensitivity. Although the clinical reliability of the test as a predictor of pre-eclampsia has not been validated in all studies, it probably does reflect angiotensin II sensitivity. A hint at the molecular basis for angiotensin sensitivity is the discovery of increased numbers of heterodimers of the angiotensin type 1 (AT_1) and bradykinin 2 receptors in preeclamptic women.[147] Not only were increased heterodimers discovered in the placentas of women with pre-eclampsia, but omental vessels obtained at the time of cesarean section also exhibited evidence of increased angiotensin II sensitivity.[147]

Striking changes in coagulation occur in pregnancy, with an increase in most clotting factors and diminished fibrinolysin activity. Plasma fibrinogen and factors VII, VIII, X, and XIII increase with pregnancy, accompanied by a progressive decrease in plasminogen activator. Pregnancy is associated with a change in the balance of clotting toward a state of enhanced coagulability. Pre-eclampsia may be associated with thrombocytopenia, fibrin deposits in the kidney and liver, microangiopathic hemolytic anemia, and fulminant consumptive coagulopathy, all features of endothelial cell injury. Although overt evidence of a consumptive coagulopathy with reduction in clotting factors occurs in a minority of women with the disease, a great deal of evidence suggests mild intravascular coagulation.[148, 149] Studies of factor VIII consumption, estimated by the difference between the level of factor VIII–related antigen and factor VIII clotting activity, show a high correlation with the severity of pre-eclampsia.[127] Studies of platelet function in pre-eclampsia reveal significantly lower maximal aggregation rates in response to collagen, AVP, and arachidonic acid, which may indicate that these platelets have undergone

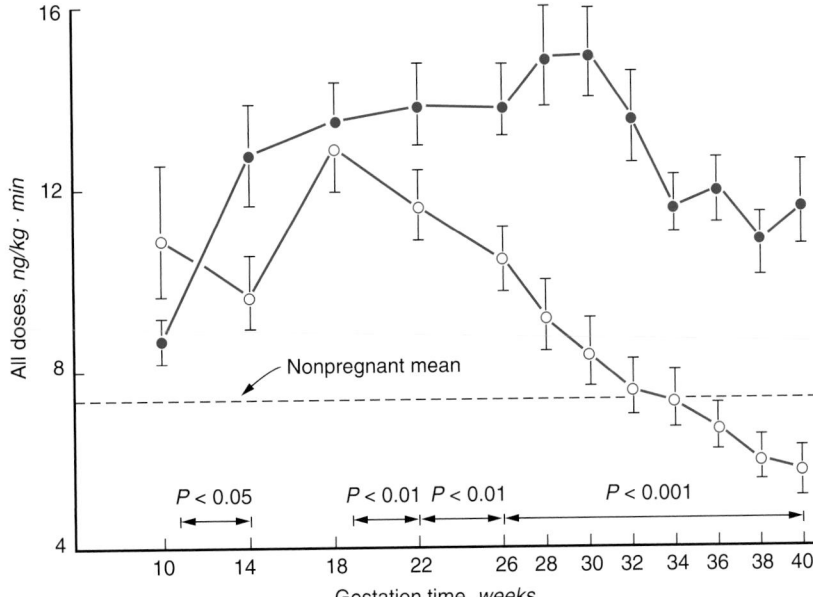

FIGURE 35-4. Effect of pregnancy on sensitivity to the pressor effects of angiotensin II. The ordinate displays the dose of angiotensin II needed to raise diastolic blood pressure 20 mm Hg. In normal pregnancy (*closed circles*; n = 120), a higher dose was required than for nonpregnant women (*dashed line*); in women in whom preeclampsia ultimately developed (*open circles*; n = 72), insensitivity to angiotensin II was lost. (From Gant NF, Daley GL, Chand S, et al: A study of angiotensin II pressor response throughout primigravid pregnancy. Reproduced from the Journal of Clinical Investigation, 1973, vol 52, pp 2682-2689, by copyright permission of the American Society for Clinical Investigation.)

aggregation and disaggregation in the circulation. In one study, a fall in platelet count occurred as early as the 22nd week in women in whom pre-eclampsia developed.[150] Flow cytometric analyses of platelets from women with pre-eclampsia demonstrate increase expression of activation markers, including cell adhesion molecules such as endothelial cell adhesion molecule-1.[151, 152] The AT_1 receptor heterodimerism noted in women with pre-eclampsia also confers an increase in calcium flux in platelets, implying increased platelet sensitivity to angiotensin II.[147] Increased circulating levels of soluble adhesion molecules are also consistent with endothelial injury and may identify women at risk for pre-eclampsia.[153, 154] Urinary and serum fibrin degradation products are elevated in pre-eclampsia and can remain elevated in the urine for up to 7 days after delivery. Recent recognition of an association of pregnancy complications, including pre-eclampsia, with genetic thrombophilia may imply that imbalances of thrombolysis homeostasis have a role in pre-eclampsia.[155]

A decrease in PGI_2 synthesis in endothelial cells without concomitant reduction in thromboxane synthesis in platelets would predispose to widespread platelet aggregation and intravascular clotting. Urinary excretion of thromboxane metabolites increases in pre-eclampsia, which probably reflects platelet aggregation, because it can be partially prevented with aspirin.[64] Several postpartum complications, such as renal failure, cardiomyopathy, and pituitary failure, may be caused by endothelial dysfunction with small-vessel thrombosis.

Oxidative stress has been posited as having a role in the pathogenesis of pre-eclampsia. The plasma of pre-eclamptic women induced neutrophil activation[156] and contained increased levels of proteins damaged by reactive oxygen species[157] and increased levels of the vasoconstrictive prostaglandin metabolite 8-isoprostane.[158, 159] Levels of the antioxidants α-tocopherol and ascorbic acid were decreased in these women as well.[160] Studies implicating excessive lipid peroxidation have been published,[157–168] but negative

studies have been reported as well.[169] A randomized, controlled trial of ascorbic acid and α-tocopherol in 283 women believed to be at risk for pre-eclampsia on the basis of abnormal uterine artery waveform or history of pre-eclampsia showed a decrease in the risk of pre-eclampsia.[170] This finding may suggest antioxidant therapy as a useful area of further clinical inquiry.

Although changes in coagulation can be explained by diffuse endothelial injury, the link between diminished uteroplacental blood flow and the systemic endothelium remains enigmatic. However, the link between abnormal endothelial function and the cardiovascular manifestations of pre-eclampsia are easier to understand. The hypertension that develops with pre-eclampsia is caused by an increase in peripheral vascular resistance. Cardiac output measurements, on the other hand, are variable, depending on the level of blood pressure. Both increased synthesis of vasoconstrictor substances and decreased synthesis of endothelial vasorelaxants conspire to sensitize the vasculature to vasoconstrictors (e.g., angiotensin II) and to produce an increase in peripheral vascular tone. Indeed, omental arteries from preeclamptic women demonstrated augmented contraction and impaired relaxation when studied in vitro.[171] Venous distensibility is similarly impaired in pre-eclampsia.[172] In addition, there is evidence of increased sympathetic nervous activity in pre-eclampsia.[173] Sympathetic hyperactivity is a likely contributor to the hypertension of pre-eclampsia, but it is difficult to directly link this observation with endothelial cell injury.

In pre-eclampsia, the RBF and GFR fall by 62% to 84%.[9] Plasma urate rises, frequently before a measurable rise in the serum creatinine or urea nitrogen level.[96, 174, 175] Because there is no increase in urate production in pre-eclampsia, hyperuricemia indicates decreased renal clearance. Urate clearance is more dependent on plasma flow to the tubule secretory site than on glomerular filtration. When the filtration fraction increases (i.e., renal plasma flow is diminished more than GFR is), urate clearance decreases.[176] Hyperuricemia occurs with essential hypertension and volume depletion, both of which are associated with high filtration fraction.[177, 178] If increased sensitivity of the efferent arteriole to angiotensin II were present in pre-eclampsia, a similar change in renal hemodynamics would occur. Measurements of filtration fraction in pre-eclampsia have been difficult because of small urine volumes. The decrease in urate clearance that occurs with volume depletion can be corrected by increasing sodium intake, whereas in pre-eclampsia, saline loading does not increase urate clearance.[179, 180] Hyperuricemia is a valuable marker to differentiate pre-eclampsia from other causes of hypertension in pregnancy when a decrease in urate clearance does not occur. A serum urate level greater than 5.5 mg/100 mL is a strong indicator of the presence of pre-eclampsia, and when it exceeds 6.0 mg/100 mL, the disease is usually severe. Hyperuricemia correlates well with the clinical severity of pre-eclampsia, with the histologic lesion found on renal biopsy, and with fetal survival.[175]

The majority of women with pre-eclampsia have sudden weight gain with development of edema, particularly of the face and upper extremities. The edema of pre-eclampsia has similarities to angioneurotic edema and probably has a different etiology from the common peripheral edema of pregnancy. There is evidence of a change in capillary permeability to protein in pre-eclampsia, with increased disappearance of Evans blue dye and higher concentration of protein in edema fluid.[181–183] Although salt retention in pregnancy does not increase blood pressure, swelling with an increase in blood pressure suggests pre-eclampsia. Salt retention in the presence of hypertension increases blood pressure through several mechanisms, including increased sensitivity to angiotensin and altered arteriolar Na$^+$ and Ca^{2+} concentrations. It is imperative for physicians to appreciate the difference between benign peripheral edema and edema with a rise in blood pressure, which heralds the onset of pre-eclampsia. Because up to 83% of healthy pregnant women develop localized edema, and about 10% develop generalized edema, this finding has no diagnostic value for pre-eclampsia.

Na$^+$ retention with pre-eclampsia is probably caused by the reduction in GFR that occurs. The urinary Ca^{2+} level also falls, consistent with the reduction in GFR.[184, 185] In spite of Na$^+$ retention, plasma volume in pre-eclampsia is frequently, although not always, diminished when compared with that in normotensive pregnancy.[186] In all hypertension, extracellular volume is preferentially shifted from the vascular to the interstitial space because of loss of venous capacitance and increase in capillary hydraulic pressure. Severe volume depletion may occur with renal artery stenosis, pheochromocytoma, and malignant hypertension, and mild volume contraction is present in essential hypertension.[187, 188] The average contraction of plasma volume in pre-eclampsia is approximately 9%, which is the same as that reported in nonpregnant patients with essential hypertension.[188] However, in contrast to in other hypertensive states, the volume contraction in pre-eclampsia may precede the onset of hypertension, and plasma volume contraction correlates better with stillbirths and small-for-gestational-age infants than the severity of hypertension does.[180, 189] If plasma volume expansion in pregnancy is caused by vasodilatation, diminished plasma volume may be caused by decreased PGI$_2$ synthesis. An intriguing feature of pre-eclampsia is the greater antagonism to insulin that occurs compared with normal pregnancy.[190] Because insulin antagonism may occur

with essential hypertension, the effect of insulin resistance on endothelial cell function is of obvious importance. It is known that hyperglycemia reduces endothelial cell PGI$_2$ synthesis and promotes generation of vasoconstrictor prostanoids in rabbit aortas.[191, 192] It is of interest that diabetic patients do not synthesize PGI$_2$ as well as nondiabetic patients do, and diabetic women have less volume expansion during pregnancy.[191, 192] Increased urinary thromboxane excretion occurs in diabetic patients, which may also be a factor in the increased incidence of pre-eclampsia in diabetic women.[193]

The decrease in plasma volume with pre-eclampsia should not be treated with volume expansion, which can lead to pulmonary edema. Although plasma volume is reduced, pre-eclampsia is accompanied by increased total exchangeable Na$^+$, normal venous pressure, and either a normal or a high pulmonary capillary wedge pressure (PCWP).[194] In one study of 49 women with severe pre-eclampsia, 8 had high PCWP, and the rest had normal left ventricular filling pressure.[195] Cardiac output and peripheral vascular resistance were elevated in most patients. When pulmonary edema occurs in women with pre-eclampsia, it is usually the result of administration of large volumes of fluid before and during delivery.[196] Plasma oncotic pressure falls after delivery because of rapid mobilization of fluid from the interstitial space; when combined with elevated PCWP, it can also be a factor leading to pulmonary edema.[197]

Figure 35-5 depicts a hypothetical sequence of events occurring with pre-eclampsia based on the hypothesis that hypoperfusion of the uterus and placenta is the proximate cause of the disease. The increased occurrence of pre-eclampsia with twin pregnancies with a large placenta and with a hydatidiform mole suggests ischemia, and measurements of uterine blood flow in pre-eclampsia demonstrate reduction in flow.[198] Experimentally, reduction of uterine blood flow in pregnant monkeys causes hypertension with changes in the kidney similar to those observed in women with pre-eclampsia.[115]

Pathology of Pre-eclampsia
Kidney

Significant changes in the glomeruli in pre-eclampsia were first described in 1918 by Lohlein,[199] and in 1920 Fahr[200] called attention to the swelling of the capillary wall. The first electron microscopic study of the glomerulus in pre-eclampsia was reported in 1959 by Farquhar,[201] who demonstrated pronounced swelling of the glomerular endothelial cells and deposits of fibrin-like material within and under the endothelial cells. Spargo and co-workers[202] confirmed this report and called the lesion glomerular capillary endotheliosis (Fig. 35-6A), because of the lipid accumulation within endothelial cells (see Fig. 35-6B). In 1963, Pirani and colleagues[203] demonstrated with immunofluorescence staining that the deposits in the glomeruli were fibrinogen or one of its derivatives. Light microscopic studies of renal biopsy specimens demonstrated that the capillary lumen is bloodless and endothelial and mesangial cells are swollen. The lesion is generalized, involving all glomeruli. The basement membrane is not thickened, but there is proliferation of mesangial cells.[204] Complete resolution of these glomerular changes has been reported to occur

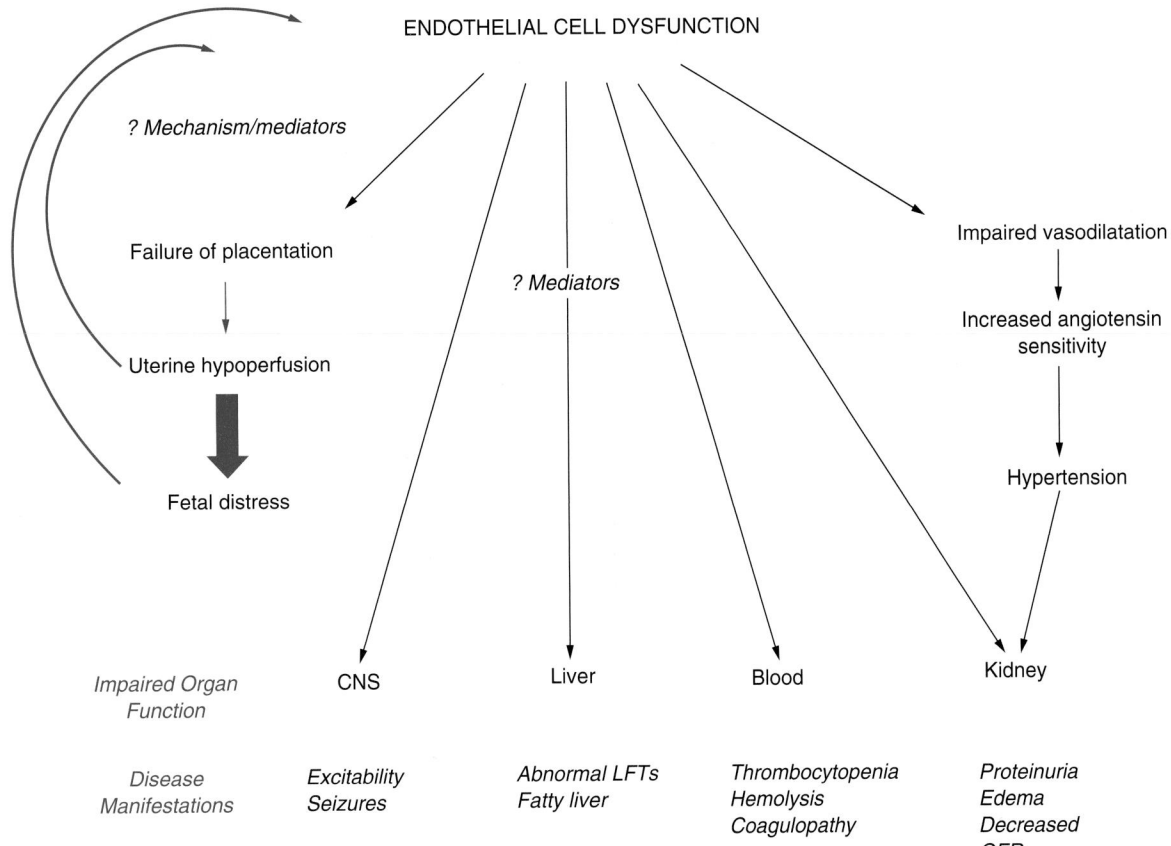

FIGURE 35-5. Pathogenesis of pre-eclampsia. Central to this hypothesis are uterine hypoperfusion and diffuse endothelial cell injury. Failure of cytotrophoblasts to develop an endothelial phenotype may be the initiating factor in pre-eclampsia. CNS, central nervous system; GFR, glomerular filtration rate; LFTs, liver function tests.

as early as 4 weeks after delivery. Kincaid-Smith[205] emphasized the need for biopsy during pregnancy or immediately postpartum to demonstrate the fibrin deposits that disappear quickly after delivery. Hypertension is not the cause of the glomerular disease; similar changes are seen in ovine toxemia, a disease similar to pre-eclampsia in which convulsions, proteinuria, and decreased GFR occur in the absence of hypertension.[53]

There is no evidence of immunologically mediated damage to the glomerulus. The swollen endothelial cells point to endothelial cell injury with resultant local activation of intravascular coagulation. When immunoglobulins have been noted by immunofluorescence in the glomeruli of patients with pre-eclampsia, they represent nonspecific trapping in injured glomeruli.

Liver

Before the advent of liver biopsy, studies of hepatic disease in pre-eclampsia were limited to patients with fatal disease. In these patients, large subcapsular hematomas were found, some of which had ruptured into the peritoneal cavity. The subcapsular hematomas arise either from deep within the liver or from the capsule.[206, 207] Sheehan and Lynch[208] postulated that the hemorrhagic changes in the liver were caused by intense spasm of hepatic arterioles and not by fibrin deposits. However, studies of percutaneous liver

biopsy specimens from patients with toxemia have demonstrated patchy areas of necrosis with fibrin deposits.[209] Of 12 preeclamptic women, 2 had focal areas of fibrinoid necrosis with either patchy or extensive necrosis of the liver cells. Immunofluorescence studies of all 12 biopsy specimens showed diffuse sinusoidal staining with antiserum to fibrinogen. In biopsy specimens from normal pregnant women, fibrin deposits were not demonstrated. Abnormalities in liver function with pre-eclampsia are usually manifested by elevations in lactate dehydrogenase and aspartate aminotransferase. In several patients with pre-eclampsia, histologic evidence of microvesicular fat, necrosis, and cholestasis has been found; these are the typical findings of acute fatty liver of pregnancy, a disease now thought to be a hepatic manifestation of pre-eclampsia.[210-214]

Placenta

At 16 weeks' gestation in normal human pregnancy, the spiral arteries in the placental bed progressively lose their musculoelastic tissue and widen, thereby allowing the increase in blood supply required by the pregnant uterus. In pre-eclampsia, in infants born small for gestational age, and in women with chronic hypertension, necrosis and infiltration of these spiral vessels produce the picture of acute atherosis.[119, 215] The cause of these changes was discussed earlier.

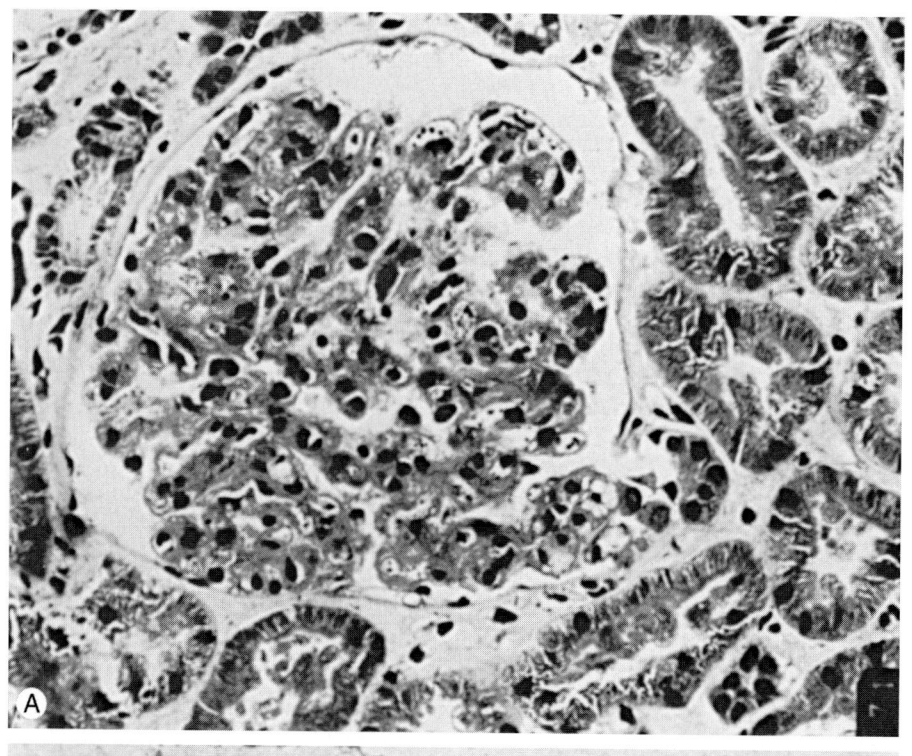

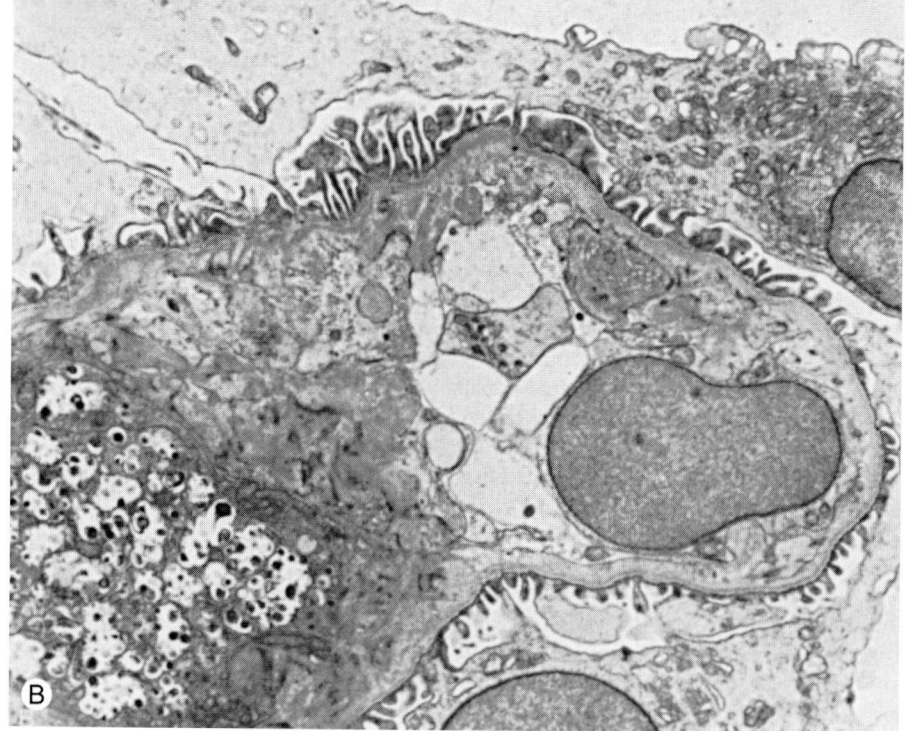

FIGURE 35-6. Renal histologic findings in pre-eclampsia. **A,** Light microscopic findings of glomerular endotheliosis (magnification ×500). **B,** Electron micrograph of a glomerulus in pre-eclampsia. Note the swollen intracapillary cells with lipid-containing lysosomes in the mesangial cell. The endothelial cell contains vacuoles, and there is a trapped platelet (magnification ×10,000). (Photomicrographs courtesy of Dr. B. Spargo.)

Central Nervous System

A common cause of death in pre-eclampsia is cerebral hemorrhage, which occurs in about 60% of patients who die after eclampsia. The hemorrhages are petechial as well as large hematomas.[208] Frequently, a large hemorrhage occurs in the white matter and may extend into the subarachnoid space or ventricles. Cerebral edema is frequently detected by computed tomography or magnetic resonance imaging in women with CNS symptoms.[216] Cerebral edema occurs with malignant hypertension, but hypertension in pre-eclampsia seldom reaches the levels seen in malignant hypertension. Hypertension does not account for the CNS manifestations of pre-eclampsia, which are more likely to be related to endothelial cell dysfunction with platelet aggregation and fibrin deposition similar to that seen in glomeruli, liver, and heart. Fibrin deposits have been described in the brain in some patients dying of pre-eclampsia, but because some of these patients had a consumptive coagulopathy, it is difficult to ascertain whether the cerebral disease was primary or secondary to the coagulopathy.

An unusual cause of postpartum headache and convulsion is central venous thrombosis. Thrombosis most commonly occurs in a vein over the parietal cortex and causes convulsions that may be indistinguishable from those of eclampsia. There are more than 396 recorded causes of postpartum central venous thrombosis, with a mortality rate of approximately 40%.[217] Occasionally, central venous thrombosis may occur during pregnancy and mimic eclampsia. The absence of hypertension and proteinuria argues against pre-eclampsia in these women. Central venous thrombosis may be caused by the hypercoagulable state that occurs after delivery.

Heart

In 12 of 34 patients dying of eclampsia, postmortem examination revealed contraction band necrosis on myocardial sections.[218] In one woman with pre-eclampsia who underwent cardiac catheterization, an endocardial biopsy revealed narrowed capillary lumens. On electron microscopic studies, endothelial cell swelling and lipid accumulation similar to those noted in the glomeruli of preeclamptic women were seen.[219]

Clinical Features and Epidemiology of Pre-eclampsia

The clinical onset of pre-eclampsia may be insidious and not accompanied by overt symptoms. Headache, visual disturbances, epigastric pain, and apprehension may occur. The usual sequence is rapid weight gain with edema, particularly of the hands and face, with increased blood pressure and proteinuria. Rarely, proteinuria precedes the hypertension. Proteinuria in pre-eclampsia can range from minimal levels (500 mg/24 hours) to levels seen in the nephrotic syndrome, but pre-eclampsia does not cause microscopic hematuria.[220] Measurement of 24-hour protein excretion is not required, because measurement of the ratio of protein to creatinine in the urine has been validated in pregnant, proteinuric women.[221] Some patients with pre-eclampsia have severe proteinuria with minimal hypertension, and in others the hypertension is prominent. Pre-eclampsia usually begins after the 32nd week of pregnancy, but it may begin earlier, particularly in women with preexisting renal disease or hypertension. When it occurs in the first trimester, it is pathognomonic of a hydatidiform mole. The disease may be seen postpartum, with hypertension and convulsions occurring within 24 to 48 hours after delivery, and it has been reported as late as 7 days postpartum.[222] Pre-eclampsia usually resolves within 10 days after delivery.[223]

The disease has a bimodal frequency, being more common in young primiparous and older multiparous women (>40 years of age).[224] Primiparous women are three to eight times more susceptible to pre-eclampsia than are multiparous women. This fact, in combination with the observation that a change in partner is a risk factor for subsequent pre-eclampsia, has led to the belief that immunologic incongruity and subsequent tolerance play a role in pre-eclampsia.[225, 226] Although this hypothesis may be true, it appears that it may be the interval between pregnancies,

rather than the change in partners, that confers the risk. A change in partner may simply be an indicator of a long interpartum period.[227] The presence of underlying essential hypertension, diabetes mellitus, or renal disease increases the risk of pre-eclampsia. Other risk factors for pre-eclampsia are twin pregnancies, the antiphospholipid syndrome, fetal hydrops, insulin resistance,[228] and hydatidiform mole. Pre-eclampsia has a familial prevalence.[229] In one series, the frequency of hypertension during pregnancy was 28% in daughters of preeclamptic mothers, compared with 13% in daughters of normotensive mothers.[230] In another, a population-based study, the incidence of pre-eclampsia in primiparous women who had a sister with pre-eclampsia was 20%.[231] The role of a paternal contribution to the pathogenesis of pre-eclampsia was suggested by examination of a large Utah database.[232] Men who were themselves the product of a preeclamptic pregnancy were 2.1 times more likely than control subjects to father a pregnancy complicated by pre-eclampsia.[232] Consistent with previous observations, women who were the product of a preeclamptic pregnancy were 3.3 times more likely than controls to have a pregnancy complicated by pre-eclampsia.[232] These increased risks were noted after controlling for sex, gestational weight, gestational age, and parity.

The genetic basis of pre-eclampsia remains obscure. Using restriction fragment length polymorphisms, Lachmeijer and colleagues[233] showed that pre-eclampsia and the so-called HELLP syndrome have different allelic associations on linkage analysis. A variant of the nitric oxide synthase-3 gene was noted to be a risk factor for pregnancy-induced hypertension,[234] and an activating mutation of the mineralocorticoid receptor was also associated with a worsening of early-onset hypertension in pregnancy.[235]

Whether pre-eclampsia is more common in black women is unclear. The higher frequency of essential hypertension in black women makes pre-eclampsia more common in multiparous women but probably not in primiparous black women.[236] In Chesley's[236] follow-up study of 270 white women with eclampsia, 26% of the daughters had pre-eclampsia in their first pregnancy, compared with 8% of the daughters-in-law. A possible genetic explanation for the familial incidence of pre-eclampsia is the suggested association of pre-eclampsia with a molecular variant of the angiotensinogen gene or a gene located close to the gene encoding eNOS (epithelial nitric oxide synthetase).[237, 238] Women who smoke have smaller infants compared with nonsmokers, and the frequency of toxemia is lower in smokers.[239] However, the adverse effect of smoking on fetal size outweighs the protective effect on the development of pre-eclampsia. Epidemiologic studies have also noted an association between certain types of antigenic exposures and the risk of developing pre-eclampsia. Women who received heterologous blood transfusions, practiced oral sex, had a long period of cohabitation before conception, or were inseminated by partner sperm rather than donor sperm have been observed to have a lower incidence of pre-eclampsia.[240, 241] These observations have not yet been supported by a demonstrable immunologic explanation for the etiology of pre-eclampsia.

The physical examination reveals puffy edema of the face and hands. Diastolic hypertension is prominent, with the systolic pressure usually lower than 160 mm Hg. Systolic blood pressure greater than 200 mm Hg points to pre-eclampsia superimposed on underlying chronic hypertension. Ophthalmoscopic examination shows segmental arteriolar narrowing with a wet, glistening appearance indicative of retinal edema; hemorrhages and exudates are rare. Detachment of the retina may occur, with spontaneous reattachment occurring after diuresis and control of the hypertension.[242] Pulmonary edema is a common complication of pre-eclampsia and is usually caused by left ventricular failure. It may occur with normal PCWP because of change in pulmonary capillary permeability.[9, 196, 243] CNS excitability measures the severity of neurologic involvement, which is assessed by examination of the spinal reflexes.

Because pre-eclampsia is a multisystem disease, its presentation frequently mimics that of other diseases.[244] Thrombocytopenia may be prominent and may suggest idiopathic thrombocytopenic purpura; when accompanied by neurologic features, it is reminiscent of thrombotic thrombocytopenic purpura. A microangiopathic anemia with hemolysis is frequent. Abdominal pain and elevated serum amylase concentration may suggest acute pancreatitis. The HELLP syndrome comprises severe pre-eclampsia with hemolysis, elevated liver enzymes, and low platelet count.[245] Jaundice, which may be severe particularly when hemolysis occurs, and abnormalities of liver function tests suggest hepatitis.[212, 246] In some patients, hepatic abnormalities are more prominent than either hypertension or proteinuria.

Acute fatty liver of pregnancy, which occurs in 1 in 13,000 pregnancies, may be an extreme hepatic manifestation of pre-eclampsia.[247] More than 90% of cases occur in the third trimester (isolated cases occur in the second trimester or after delivery).[248, 249] Nonspecific symptoms related to hepatic insufficiency (e.g., fatigue, malaise, nausea, vomiting), are found; abdominal pain is often severe but is not invariably present. Laboratory findings suggest hepatic failure (marked elevation of bilirubin, lesser elevation of hepatic enzymes). A microangiopathic hemolytic anemia with thrombocytopenia and prolonged clotting times may develop.[250] In a review of 49 cases of acute fatty liver of pregnancy, 22% had evidence of pre-eclampsia preceding the onset of hepatic disease.[211] This may be an underestimation of the true occurrence of pre-eclampsia, because for many patients available information concerning blood pressure was not given. Liver biopsy results in pre-eclampsia show mild fatty infiltration of the liver even when hepatic involvement is not clinically apparent.[213, 251]

In as many as 60% of women with acute fatty liver of pregnancy, acute renal failure develops.[252] This has often been diagnosed clinically as acute tubule necrosis (ATN) and has occasionally been confirmed by renal biopsy.[253] In other cases, renal biopsy has revealed no abnormalities or fatty infiltration.[211, 254] Therefore, the possibility that this is a form of hepatorenal syndrome should be considered. There is no specific treatment for this disease, and the prognosis appears to depend on the quality of supportive obstetric care, because the mortality rate has decreased from more than 80% to approximately 20%.[255]

A fascinating feature of a few patients with pre-eclampsia and hepatic involvement is the development of transient diabetes insipidus.[256, 257] Of the 16 cases reported in the literature, 12 patients had hypertension, and all had severe hyperuricemia and abnormal liver function. Vasopressinase activity, which is thought to be of placental origin, increases in pregnancy.[258] Whether higher vasopressinase activity occurs in pre-eclampsia is not known. The severe hepatic involvement present in most of these patients suggests a combination of hepatic disease and increased vasopressinase activity as the cause of the diabetes insipidus. It can be treated with the synthetic AVP analog, desmopressin (DDAVP), which is not metabolized by vasopressinase. Remission occurs after delivery.

Treatment of Pre-eclampsia

The first objective in the treatment of pre-eclampsia is its prevention. Proper prenatal care with attention to adequate but not excessive weight gain and careful monitoring of blood pressure and urinary protein concentration during pregnancy reduce the frequency and severity of the disease. There is no evidence of a nutritional basis for the disease, but in many countries there is a higher frequency of pre-eclampsia among the poor. In Jerusalem, pre-eclampsia in illiterate women was twice that in control subjects, and in the United States a higher frequency was reported among the poor.[259]

In an attempt to correct a potential imbalance in endothelial PGI_2 and platelet thromboxane synthesis, low-dose aspirin has been administered to women at high risk for pre-eclampsia. Low-dose aspirin inhibits platelet thromboxane synthesis more than endothelial PGI_2 synthesis. A meta-analysis of six published trials of low-dose aspirin up to 1992 demonstrated a significant reduction in pre-eclampsia but not in hypertension in the aspirin-treated group.[260] In a National Institutes of Health study of 3135 healthy, nulliparous women randomly assigned to receive either 60 mg aspirin or a placebo daily throughout pregnancy, the incidence of pre-eclampsia was lower (4.7% versus 6.3%) in the treated group but there was no significant difference in gestational hypertension (6.7% versus 5.9%).[106] In women with a greater risk for pre-eclampsia (i.e., those with an initial systolic blood pressure of 120 to 134 mm Hg), aspirin reduced the incidence of pre-eclampsia from 11.9% to 5.6%. In the CLASP study of 9364 women, low-dose aspirin was not beneficial overall.[261] However, for women with premature delivery and for those who began taking aspirin before the 20th week of pregnancy, there was a significant trend toward prevention of pre-eclampsia. Other studies have failed to demonstrate a beneficial effect of low-dose aspirin.[262, 263] The most disappointing result so far has been a National Institutes of Health study focussing on 2539 high-risk women.[264] Low-dose aspirin did not reduce the incidence of pre-eclampsia or improve perinatal outcomes. Several studies have, however, confirmed the safety of low-dose aspirin when employed to prevent pre-eclampsia.[265, 266] Perhaps the only remaining consideration about the use of low-dose aspirin that remains to be resolved before finally dismissing it is the possibility that time-dependent effects were not considered in some of these large studies. Hermida and associates[267] found that low-dose aspirin did not lower blood pressure in pregnant women when given in the morning but had a significant effect when given 8 hours after awakening or at bedtime. A systematic review of the literature including more than 32,000 women in randomized, controlled trials found a reduction in pre-eclampsia of 15%;

the number of women that needed to be treated with an antiplatelet agent to prevent one case of pre-eclampsia was 89, regardless of risk status at entry.[268] A reduced risk of preterm birth (8%) and of infant death (14%), but no difference in intrauterine growth retardation, was also observed in the studies that reported these outcomes.[268]

Calcium supplementation, 2 g daily, has been shown to lower blood pressure in most studies of nonpregnant hypertensive women.[269] Several studies found that calcium supplementation also reduced the frequency of hypertension in pregnancy.[270–273] However, a large study of 4589 pregnant women revealed no benefit of calcium supplementation in terms of pre-eclampsia, hypertension, or pregnancy outcome.[273] In that trial, some of the effect of supplemental calcium may have been masked by the fact that the control group received low-dose normal supplementary calcium (50 mg/day), while the treatment group received doses of calcium similar to those seen in other trials (2 g/day).[273] The administration of calcium to pregnant women is not without potential risk, because urinary excretion of Ca^{2+} in pregnant women is about 300 mg/day, compared with 100 mg/day in nonpregnant women. When the results of 11 properly randomized trials were systematically reviewed, the overall incidence of hypertension was decreased (relative risk [RR], 0.68), but the beneficial effects were greater in those women at high risk for pre-eclampsia (RR, 0.47) and greatest in those with low baseline calcium intake (RR, 0.38).[274] The reduction in risk for pre-eclampsia followed a similar pattern.[274] Criticism has been raised regarding that review of the literature on the basis of a high degree of heterogeneity of published trials, and a meta-analysis of the literature by the authors who leveled the criticism reached no conclusion regarding calcium supplementation in pregnancy.[275] The hypercalciuria is caused by increased intestinal absorption of Ca^{2+} induced by high plasma vitamin D levels.[276] The addition of 2 g of calcium to the diet increases urinary Ca^{2+} excretion and might increase the risk of renal calculi, which occur in about 1 in 2000 pregnancies.

The physician must carefully evaluate all women who have a rise in blood pressure in late pregnancy for evidence of pre-eclampsia, because it is the most frequent cause of maternal mortality. Hypertension with clinical or laboratory evidence of systemic disease must be presumed to represent pre-eclampsia. Although all hypertension in pregnancy poses a risk to mother and child, pre-eclampsia poses a far greater risk. If the presumptive diagnosis is pre-eclampsia, hospitalization is indicated, whereas a rise in blood pressure without evidence of pre-eclampsia can be treated on an outpatient basis.

If the disease is mild (blood pressure <140/90 mm Hg, proteinuria <500 mg/24 hours, normal renal function, serum urate level <4.5 mg/100 mL, normal platelet count, and no evidence of hemolysis or hepatic involvement), bed rest is usually sufficient therapy to lower the blood pressure and allow time for estimation of fetal size and maturity. If fetal size and maturation are thought to be adequate, delivery is the definitive treatment. If fetal size and maturation are of concern, management by an obstetrician and a physician with expertise in the treatment of hypertension is required. If there is no evidence of worsening of pre-eclampsia, the pregnancy can be continued. Any sign of worsening of the disease should be an indication for delivery, particularly if

the pregnancy is of 32 weeks' duration or longer, because fetal survival at that age in neonatal units is now close to 100%.

If the blood pressure is greater than 140/95 mm Hg with decreased renal function, hyperuricemia, or proteinuria greater than 500 mg/24 hr, delivery is indicated in pregnancies thought to be more than 32 weeks' duration. Blood pressure should be lowered to 140/90 mm Hg before delivery. Antihypertensive therapy lessens the likelihood of a rise in blood pressure during delivery with potential complications of congestive heart failure or cerebral hemorrhage. Methyldopa, the β-adrenergic antagonists atenolol or pindolol, or the α/β-adrenergic antagonist labetalol can be given orally.[223, 277–281] There may be some advantage to pindolol because of its intrinsic sympathomimetic property, which prevents the development of fetal bradycardia.[279] Atenolol was demonstrated to reduce proteinuria and to reduce the need for hospitalization in a group of women with pre-eclampsia.[280] Hydrochlorothiazide is not usually employed as a first-line antihypertensive medication because of the reduction in plasma volume that can occur with pre-eclampsia. However, thiazides have been used in pregnancy more extensively than any other antihypertensive drug. A meta-analysis of nine randomized trials comprising more than 11,000 pregnant women given diuretics throughout pregnancy revealed a decrease in the frequency of hypertension without adverse effects on the fetus.[281] Diuretics also potentiate the effect of all other antihypertensive drugs.

If the blood pressure is greater than 160/100 mm Hg, parenteral therapy may be needed. Although intravenous hydralazine has been used extensively in pregnancy, its rapid duration of action and the reflex tachycardia it induces make it less effective than labetalol.[249–253] Although sodium nitroprusside, a vasodilator, is frequently used for hypertensive emergencies in the nonpregnant patient, the possibility of fetal cyanide toxicity, which has been demonstrated in pregnant ewes, argues against its prolonged use in pregnancy.[282] Whether treatment of hypertension in pre-eclampsia affects the underlying disease is less clear, but it is not unreasonable to assume that hypertension is a factor adversely affecting endothelial cell function. Antihypertensive therapy can prevent pulmonary edema and cerebral hemorrhage, two severe complications of pre-eclampsia. However, the presence of convulsions (eclampsia) or the HELLP syndrome is always an indication for delivery.[283]

Obstetricians in the United States have relied on magnesium sulfate, a mild vasodilator, for the treatment of pre-eclampsia. At therapeutic serum levels of 4 to 6 mEq/L, Mg^{2+} increases PGI_2 synthesis in cultured endothelial cells,[284] which may account for its efficacy. However, at therapeutic serum Mg^{2+} levels, there is suppression of myoneuronal transmission, which can cause respiratory paralysis leading to maternal death.[285, 286] Vital capacity and maximal inspiratory and expiratory pressures fall in pregnant women receiving magnesium sulfate.[287] Nevertheless, in two prospective studies comparing magnesium sulfate to phenytoin in 1089 women, and to placebo in more than 10,000 women,[288] magnesium sulfate was superior in preventing seizures, and it remains the drug of choice.[289]

If pre-eclampsia occurs in the second trimester, when delivery of the infant is not compatible with fetal survival, a difficult decision must be made by the mother and physician. In 109 preeclamptic women presenting in the second trimester, Sibai and co-workers[290] recommended termination of pregnancy if the pregnancy was less than 24 weeks' duration. Fifteen of the 25 women in this category refused termination, and there was only one surviving infant. The HELLP syndrome developed in three women, one woman had eclampsia, and two women had abruptio placentae. There were no maternal deaths, but all of the women were hospitalized in intensive care units. Of the 84 preeclamptic women thought to have pregnancies of longer duration than 24 weeks, 30 were delivered immediately; there were 20 fetal deaths, and the 10 living infants spent an average of 115 days in the neonatal intensive care unit. The 54 women not delivered immediately were treated with antihypertensive medications to maintain diastolic pressure lower than 100 mm Hg. There were 13 perinatal deaths. Pregnancy was prolonged in this group an average of 13 days, and there were 42 live infants who spent an average of 70 days in the neonatal intensive care unit. Therefore, in women with pre-eclampsia in the second trimester whose pregnancy is longer than 24 weeks' duration, fetal survival was increased by prolonging the pregnancy with treatment of the hypertension. Measurements of uterine blood flow in women with preeclampsia and in hypertensive pregnant animals usually demonstrate an increase in blood flow with antihypertensive therapy.[278, 279, 291, 293, 295, 296] Although there is an appropriate reluctance to administer any drug during pregnancy, the burden of proof today is on the physician who does not treat severe hypertension during pregnancy.

ESSENTIAL HYPERTENSION IN PREGNANCY

There has been some reluctance to treat hypertension in pregnant women with essential hypertension. Although antihypertensive therapy may result in fewer exacerbations of hypertension, a lower frequency of proteinuria, and improved perinatal outcome,[280, 297–302] the overall benefit in women with mild to moderate hypertension may be small.[303, 304] The specific drug used to control hypertension reflects the experience of the physician caring for the patient.

Most physicians would continue current therapy throughout pregnancy.[224, 305] An important exception to this rule is the use of angiotensin-converting enzyme inhibitors (ACEIs). ACEIs have been associated with increased fetal loss in experimental animals and with fetal renal tubular dysplasia, perinatal acute renal failure, and other congenital anomalies.[306] The mothers of these infants all consumed ACEIs in the second or third trimester of pregnancy (or both). A recent postmarketing survey of ACEIs in the United States, Canada, and Israel revealed no adverse fetal outcomes resulting from the use of ACEIs in the first trimester only.[307] Therefore, if a woman receiving ACEIs becomes pregnant, other antihypertensive agents should be substituted. However, if exposure is limited to the first trimester, it does appear necessary to intentionally terminate the pregnancy. AT_2 receptors are certainly involved in development of the fetal kidney, but adverse fetal outcomes from the AT_1 receptor blocker losartan[308–310] and from valsartan in combination with atenolol have also been reported.[311] Considering the large number of acceptable alternatives, these agents should not be employed.

With the number of effective agents available, it is possible to normalize blood pressure in the pregnant woman without undesirable side effects and without risk to the fetus. A meta-analysis of randomized trials of various antihypertensive drugs showed a lower risk of fetal or neonatal death in the treated group.[312] As in the nonpregnant population, the beneficial effect of antihypertensive therapy is demonstrated best at higher levels of pressure. In one study of 44 pregnant women with severe essential hypertension primarily controlled by β-blockers and diuretics, all antihypertensive drugs and diuretics were stopped, and only methyldopa was given throughout pregnancy.[300] Pre-eclampsia developed in 52% of these women, 45% had a decrease in renal function, and malignant hypertension with encephalopathy developed in one woman. The perinatal mortality rate was 25%, and the surviving children spent an average of 39 days in the neonatal intensive care unit. These results are reminiscent of the experience of pregnant women with hypertension in the era before the availability of antihypertensive therapy. For instance, in 1937, John P. Peters[313] reported a 13% maternal mortality rate in 203 women with hypertension in pregnancy. The evidence today indicates that maternal mortality from hypertensive complications can be eliminated in women with essential hypertension, provided that the hypertension is treated throughout pregnancy.

The optimal management of mild to moderate hypertension in pregnancy, defined as a systolic blood pressure between 140 and 169 mm Hg and a diastolic blood pressure between 90 and 109 mm Hg, is not well defined. Although the risk of developing severe hypertension is decreased with treatment,[303, 314] other outcomes, such as perinatal mortality and the incidence of pre-eclampsia, do not appear to be reduced.[303, 304, 314]

Before the availability of effective antihypertensive therapy, two thirds of women with chronic hypertension had a rise in blood pressure in late pregnancy, with proteinuria developing in half.[315] The hesitancy to treat maternal hypertension in the past has been based on unfounded assumptions concerning the beneficial effect of hypertension on uterine blood flow. The view that hypertension might increase perfusion of the uterus failed to recognize that an increase in pressure causes vasoconstriction in all vascular beds—the phenomenon of autoregulation. Pregnant rabbits autoregulate uterine blood flow over a wide range of blood pressures,[48] and when pregnant rats are made hypertensive by clipping the renal artery, uteroplacental blood flow is reduced to 68% of that in normotensive pregnant rats.[316]

Pregnant women with chronic essential hypertension have an increased risk of pre-eclampsia, abruptio placentae, intrauterine growth retardation, and second-trimester fetal death. However, those without proteinuria do well during pregnancy, provided that their blood pressure is controlled.[317–319] Approximately half of women with essential hypertension have a spontaneous reduction in pressure during the second trimester, which may allow lowering of the dose or discontinuation of their antihypertensive medication. If blood pressure is taken for the first time in the second trimester, a subsequent rise in pressure in the third trimester is often diagnosed as gestational hypertension. Persistence of gestational hypertension after delivery frequently indicates that chronic hypertension was present before the pregnancy. Because these women usually are taking antihypertensive medication before pregnancy, it is important to maintain whatever therapy has controlled their hypertension, with the exception of ACEIs and the angiotensin receptor blockers. Thiazides may be continued throughout pregnancy. Although in one study plasma volume increased only 18% in women taking diuretics, compared with 36% in hypertensive women not receiving diuretics, there was no difference in fetal survival or birth weight.[320]

The optimal degree of blood pressure control in the woman with mild to moderate hypertension is matter of conjecture. A meta-analysis of 14 randomized, controlled trials comparing the decrease in maternal MAP with indicators of fetal growth revealed that a greater lowering in MAP was associated with a higher proportion of small-for-gestational-age infants.[321] This finding must be tempered by the fact that a decreased incidence of respiratory distress syndrome in infants, and decreased severe hypertension and hospitalization before delivery in mothers, was observed in a separate review by the same authors.[304] Another systematic review only found an increased risk of being born small for gestational age in those infants whose mothers had been treated with β-blockers (compared with no treatment).[322] The retrospective nature of these observations and the weaknesses inherent in meta-analysis are reasons to pursue the answer to the question of what level of blood pressure control is optimal for the mother and fetus in a prospective fashion.

Many women with chronic hypertension have been treated with β-adrenergic blockers throughout pregnancy.[323, 324] In randomized trials comparing atenolol and metoprolol, no adverse fetal effects were demonstrated with either drug.[280] One trial of atenolol given throughout pregnancy to a group of women with essential hypertension reported smaller infants in the treated group, although fetal survival was unchanged.[325] This finding was also noted in a retrospective review of the use of atenolol.[326] Although these findings have not been confirmed prospectively, the American College of Obstetrics and Gynecology does not recommend atenolol for use in pregnancy.[327]

The central α-adrenergic agonist, methyldopa, has been used extensively in pregnancy and has been shown to diminish second-trimester stillbirths with no untoward effects in the children who have been observed for up to 7 years of age.[328] Birth weights and fetal maturation with methyldopa treatment were similar to those of the control group. However, methyldopa causes somnolence, a frequent problem in pregnant women. Randomized trials comparing the use of β-blockers with methyldopa throughout pregnancy did not demonstrate significant differences in blood pressure control or in the occurrence of pre-eclampsia with either agent.[301] Labetalol was better tolerated than methyldopa in one study, and methyldopa was not as effective in treating severe hypertension as were the β-blockers or Ca^{2+} channel blockers.[322]

Clonidine, another central α-adrenergic agonist, has been used throughout pregnancy in women with chronic hypertension.[330] Evidence of embryotoxicity in pregnant rats given low doses of clonidine and a report of behavioral changes in the offspring of women treated with clonidine make consideration of another agent during pregnancy reasonable.[331] Clonidine should not be stopped abruptly, because severe hypertension may ensue; it should be gradually withdrawn over a period of 7 to 10 days.

The α-adrenergic receptor antagonist prazosin has also been used throughout pregnancy, and no untoward effects were reported.[332]

The Ca^{2+} channel blockers merit mention from the standpoint of their common use for hypertension and because of interest in their potential to exert tocolytic effects on the uterus.[333, 334] Meta-analysis of trials involving 685 women comparing nifedipine with β-blockers found the odds ratios for not delivering in 48 hours and in 1 week to be 0.68 and 0.69, respectively.[335] One study of 100 normotensive, pregnant smokers with impaired fetal growth found that the Ca^{2+} channel blocker flunarizine increased birth weight by 380 g.[336, 337] In hypertensive pregnancies, nifedipine decreased blood pressure to a greater degree than placebo[338] and was equivalent to[339] or better than[340] hydralazine; nifedipine was also found to be equivalent to prazosin[341] and to labetalol.[342] A comparison of atenolol and nifedipine reported no differences.[343] Birth weights, fetoplacental hemodynamics, and Apgar scores were similar in the two groups.

Ketanserin, a selective antagonist of the type 2 serotonin receptor that is not currently approved for use in the United States, has been studied in hypertensive pregnancies[344–349] and in combination with aspirin for the prevention of pre-eclampsia.[350] It appears to reduce diastolic blood pressure more than placebo does,[345] and may it be equivalent to dihydralazine in antihypertensive potency.[348–350] One randomized, double-blind, placebo-controlled trial of 138 women showed that, among women receiving aspirin whose diastolic blood pressure was greater than 80 mm Hg, those treated with oral ketanserin had a decreased risk of pre-eclampsia and severe hypertension, compared with women taking placebo.[350]

GESTATIONAL HYPERTENSION

Hypertension that appears in late pregnancy, is not associated with signs of pre-eclampsia, and disappears after delivery is termed *gestational hypertension.* Women with gestational hypertension are usually multiparous, are frequently overweight, and have a positive family history of hypertension; essential hypertension ultimately develops in many of them. For reasons not understood, pregnancy is a hypertensionogenic stress in susceptible women. The diabetogenic and hypertensionogenic effects of pregnancy may be related, because although insulin resistance occurs in all pregnant women, greater insulin antagonism occurs in hypertensive pregnant women.[190] There is a genetic link among obesity, insulin resistance, and hypertension in many hypertensive populations. Chesley,[236] in his follow-up of white women with eclampsia, found no higher frequency of hypertension in later life but a sevenfold higher occurrence of diabetes.

If gestational hypertension occurs in late pregnancy, the patient can be observed at weekly intervals as an outpatient. A β-adrenergic blocker such as atenolol or labetalol, methyldopa, nifedipine, or hydrochlorothiazide often controls the blood pressure. Frequently, obstetricians recommend bed rest for these women, which lowers blood pressure but is an inconvenience, particularly for a working woman or one with household responsibilities. Studies of women who were hospitalized or placed in a day care facility for treatment of gestational hypertension have not demonstrated advantages to either form of treatment.[351, 352]

PRE-ECLAMPSIA SUPERIMPOSED ON CHRONIC HYPERTENSION

Chronic essential hypertension may be associated with nephrosclerosis, particularly in multiparous black women. Because proteinuria in nephrosclerosis is minimal, it is often overlooked in routine urinalyses. With nephrosclerosis, as with all renal diseases, autoregulation of glomerular pressure is compromised, so that any increase in blood pressure during pregnancy increases the glomerular pressure, which may cause or worsen proteinuria (see later discussion). When this occurs, the distinction between pre-eclampsia and increased proteinuria induced by glomerular hypertension is difficult.[212] Hyperuricemia or a rise in serum creatinine suggests pre-eclampsia.

SECONDARY HYPERTENSION AND PREGNANCY

Renal Artery Stenosis

Superimposed pre-eclampsia frequently develops in women with renal artery stenosis who become pregnant. Of the nine patients in the series of Landesman and co-workers,[353] five had exacerbation of hypertension during pregnancy, and pre-eclampsia developed in four. Interestingly, in one group of women with renal artery stenosis observed during pregnancy, plasma renin fell with the development of pre-eclampsia.[42] The presence of renal artery stenosis should be suspected in any woman with severe hypertension early in pregnancy, particularly if an abdominal bruit is present and there is no family history of hypertension. Because ACEIs are contraindicated in pregnancy, medical treatment for renal hypertension is complicated. Angioplasty has been carried out successfully in pregnant women to correct renal artery stenosis.[354, 355] If hypertension is refractory to other drugs and the lesion is not amenable to angioplasty, use of an ACEI can be considered. Women have been carried through pregnancy successfully with the use of converting enzyme inhibitors despite their potential to adversely affect the fetus.[356, 357]

Primary Aldosteronism in Pregnancy

The original report of primary aldosteronism by Biglieri and Slaton[87] noted disappearance of hypokalemia and amelioration of hypertension in pregnancy, but these have not been uniform findings. Although increased progesterone secretion in pregnancy antagonizes the effect of aldosterone on the renal tubule, some pregnant patients have severe hypertension and hypokalemia.[358] The diagnosis can be difficult to make in pregnancy, because plasma renin activity is not suppressed as it is in nonpregnant patients, and plasma aldosterone levels are high in all pregnant women. Treatment with spironolactone has been successful in some pregnant patients, but if an adenoma is identified in the first or second trimester, surgical therapy can be accomplished. One woman with hyperaldosteronism due to adrenal hyperplasia was treated with enalapril, which controlled blood pressure, but fetal distress necessitated early delivery.[90]

Coarctation of the Aorta in Pregnancy

Coarctation of the aorta is a rare cause of hypertension and can be associated with pre-eclampsia. Of 10 patients requiring surgical repair for this condition during pregnancy, 9 underwent uncomplicated deliveries of live infants.[359] One patient died in her seventh month of pregnancy from an aneurysm of the aorta at the anastomotic site. The major danger to the pregnant woman with an aortic coarctation is aortic rupture from the cystic medial necrosis that often is present in the aortic wall. These pathologic changes may be put under stress by the increase in cardiac output of pregnancy, the increase in blood pressure during pre-eclampsia, or the strain of labor.

Pheochromocytoma

Although pheochromocytoma is a rare cause of hypertension, it is potentially lethal during pregnancy. The maternal mortality rate in pregnant women is 17% and fetal loss is 26% if the diagnosis is not made.[360–363] The cause of maternal mortality is usually pulmonary edema, cerebral hemorrhage, or cardiovascular collapse. Treatment with α- and β-adrenergic blockers has eliminated maternal mortality, although fetal loss remains high (15%). Women with characteristic symptoms of paroxysmal hypertension, palpitations, diaphoresis, and headache should be evaluated with measurements of urinary catecholamine excretion. If catecholamine excretion is elevated, either a computed tomographic scan or magnetic resonance imaging should be done to localize the tumor. In the first or second trimester of pregnancy, most physicians would recommend surgical treatment, although some patients have been treated medically throughout pregnancy with surgical removal of the tumor after delivery.[364]

RENAL DISEASE COMPLICATING PREGNANCY

Bacteriuria

Urinary tract infection (UTI) occurs with the same frequency in pregnant as in nonpregnant women. However, the consequences of infection are far more serious during pregnancy, warranting the prompt diagnosis and treatment of infection. Women with diabetes or sickle cell trait or disease, as well as those from lower socioeconomic groups, have a higher prevalence of UTI in pregnancy.[365] If left untreated, bacteriuria becomes symptomatic or evolves into pyelonephritis in approximately 30% of cases.[366] The increased capacity of the urinary collecting system combined with slowed emptying and vesicoureteral reflux is a major factor accounting for the increased occurrence of serious UTI in pregnancy. Glucosuria and aminoaciduria also aid bacterial growth.

Maternal risks associated with UTI are the development of bacteremia, septic shock, and decreases in renal function. Risks to the fetus may be even greater. Bacteriuria has been linked to an increased risk of midtrimester abortions and to a twofold increase in perinatal mortality when UTI occurs within 2 weeks of delivery.[367] Acute pyelonephritis has been associated with an increased frequency of intrauterine growth retardation and prematurity.[368] Only half of pregnant women with bacteriuria are symptomatic,[365] which is the rationale for obtaining a screening urine culture at the initial prenatal visit. On the other hand, many pregnant women with symptoms suggestive of bacteriuria are not infected, because nocturia, polyuria, and stress incontinence are common complaints during uncomplicated pregnancy.

Women with a history of asymptomatic bacteriuria during childhood also have an increased frequency of complications during pregnancy. These women have a significantly greater frequency of bacteriuria and pyelonephritis in pregnancy, compared with pregnant women with no previous history of bacteriuria.[369] The possibility that asymptomatic bacteriuria during childhood results in subtle renal damage that can be unmasked during pregnancy is suggested by the finding that GFR and fractional reabsorption of glucose increased less in such women during pregnancy.[370] Those who were known to have sustained renal injury during childhood, as evidenced by the presence of renal scars on intravenous pyelograms, had an increased frequency of pre-eclampsia compared with normal pregnant women or women with a history of bacteriuria but no scars.[369] Women with subtle renal damage (but normal renal function) because of previous infection are more likely to require induction of labor or operative delivery than are those without such a history.[369] Apgar scores were also reported to be lower in children of women with a history of bacteriuria during childhood, regardless of the presence or absence of renal scars.[369] Nevertheless, fetal outcome is generally satisfactory.

Because of the potential for fetal and maternal morbidity as a consequence of bacteriuria, infection, even if asymptomatic, should be treated. Treatment of asymptomatic bacteriuria is supported by systematic review of the literature.[371] Short courses of therapy for 5 to 10 days result in long-term cure rates of approximately 65%.[372, 373] Single-dose therapy may be an effective alternative means of treating bacteriuria, although some studies suggest that the results with 3 days of therapy are superior to those achieved with single-dose regimens.[373–375] Women in whom pyelonephritis develops usually require more prolonged therapy for eradication of the infection. In all women with UTI, close follow-up during the remainder of the pregnancy is essential. UTI in pregnant women usually develops in the absence of underlying structural abnormalities. Only when UTI is difficult to eradicate or the history is suggestive of underlying disease should evidence of structural abnormalities be sought. As noted earlier, vesicoureteral reflux is seen in otherwise uncomplicated pregnancy and does not in itself indicate a urinary tract pathophysiologic process.

Asymptomatic Urinary Abnormalities: Proteinuria and Hematuria

The development of proteinuria during pregnancy may be an indicator of unmasked kidney disease, worsening of preexisting renal disease, the de novo development of renal disease, or the development of pre-eclampsia in which renal involvement is part of a systemic disorder. In normal pregnancy, both because of the increase in GFR and because of an increase in glomerular capillary permeability to albumin, there is increased urinary excretion of albumin. When corrected for GFR, fractional albumin excretion increases by approximately 80%.[376] Nevertheless, in otherwise healthy

pregnant women, this should not result in a 24-hour urinary excretion of protein of greater than 200 to 250 mg, a value lower than that considered to represent microalbuminuria.[377, 378] Urinary protein electrophoresis in normal pregnant women reveals that urinary proteins are not different from those observed in nonpregnant women.[379] When urinary protein is evaluated by dipstick testing of a concentrated urine specimen, trace-positive results can be seen despite quantitatively normal protein excretion. Whenever one is in doubt, a 24-hour quantitation of urinary protein should be performed. A random urine protein-creatinine ratio is probably also a valid tool to detect significant proteinuria in pregnancy.[380] As is true for renal disease in general, urinary protein excretion of greater than 2 g/day is suggestive of a glomerular process, whereas tubulointerstitial disease may produce less proteinuria. Although pregnancy does not predispose to the development of renal disease, the de novo development of glomerulonephritis, membranous nephropathy, focal glomerulosclerosis, minimal change nephropathy, diabetic nephropathy, systemic lupus erythematosus (SLE), and other renal diseases may occasionally occur in pregnant women.

The presence of red blood cells in the urine is almost always the result by an organic process. Although pre-eclampsia causes glomerular lesions and proteinuria, it does not cause hematuria. Therefore, the finding of hematuria, particularly with red blood cell casts, in a patient with pre-eclampsia suggests the presence of underlying renal disease.[220]

If a pregnancy becomes complicated by the apparent development of glomerulonephritis or other renal disease, a biopsy of the kidney is often contemplated. The necessity of renal biopsies has been debated for years, because most renal diseases have no specific therapy.[381, 382] Empirical trials of steroids have been recommended for patients with uncomplicated nephrotic syndrome by some clinicians, because minimal-change nephropathy readily responds to that treatment.[382] For the rare case of rapidly progressive glomerulonephritis with onset during pregnancy, a renal biopsy can be diagnostic and can suggest appropriate therapy (e.g., pulse methylprednisolone, cytotoxic agents, plasmapheresis). In these cases, pregnancy is not likely to succeed. In most cases in which renal disease is first recognized during pregnancy, a renal biopsy can be postponed until after delivery. However, when a specific diagnosis is required immediately, renal biopsy can be safely performed in a pregnant patient. If the usual guidelines for renal biopsy are followed (i.e., control hypertension, avoid aspirin for 7 to 10 days before biopsy), complications are no more frequent than in nongravid patients.[383, 384]

Acute Renal Failure

Acute renal failure is defined as impairment of renal function and reduction in urine output developing over a period of hours to days. Acute renal failure during pregnancy usually takes the form of one of three renal diseases—ATN, renal cortical necrosis, or postpartum acute renal failure. Rarely, fatty liver of pregnancy or obstructive uropathy causes acute renal failure. Acute renal failure occurring during pregnancy should be approached in the same manner as in the nonpregnant patient.[385] When acute renal failure develops, there are often clues as to which renal disease is responsible (see later discussion). However, if diagnostic clues are not available and the history does not suggest the underlying process, a systematic approach should be taken. This approach requires evaluating the patient for the possibility of prerenal azotemia by a careful physical examination to observe for signs of volume depletion, evaluation of the urinary tract collecting system to rule out obstructive uropathy, and then careful physical and laboratory evaluation. If urinary tract obstruction is suspected, abdominal ultrasonography can be performed to rule out hydronephrosis. However, because of the physiologic hydronephrosis of pregnancy, this diagnosis can be difficult (see later discussion).

Acute Tubule Necrosis

ATN occurs as a complication of many conditions, most commonly sepsis or hypotension. This condition has become rare in industrialized nations as the frequency of septic abortion has dramatically diminished and now occurs in about 1 in 20,000 pregnancies.[386] A variety of nephrotoxins can cause ATN (see Chapter 27), but exposure of pregnant women to these agents is limited. In the first trimester, septic abortion accounts for the majority of patients with acute renal failure. Septic abortion is particularly likely to cause ATN when shock develops. Sepsis caused by any gram-negative organism, most commonly *Escherichia coli*, can result in hypotension leading to acute renal failure. When *Clostridium perfringens* is the responsible bacterium, toxin-induced hemolysis is an additional factor predisposing to ATN. *Clostridium*-induced myonecrosis of the uterus is a source of myoglobin, which is also a nephrotoxin, particularly in the setting of impaired renal perfusion, as would occur during hypotension. Profound or prolonged volume depletion can also cause ATN. This may be the result of hemorrhage complicating spontaneous abortion or, rarely, a consequence of hyperemesis gravidarum.

In late pregnancy, acute renal failure is a complication of pre-eclampsia or of uterine bleeding in abruptio placentae. ATN is a rare complication of pre-eclampsia, occurring in 1% to 2% of cases.[387] It is not exactly clear how ATN develops in this condition, but the diffuse endothelial cell swelling is postulated to produce renal ischemia and ATN. The HELLP syndrome is a complication of pre-eclampsia, occurring in 2% to 12% of cases of pre-eclampsia.[387] In the largest series of patients with HELLP syndrome, reported by Sibai and Ramadan,[387] acute renal failure occurred in 32 of 435 cases (7.4%). One case was caused by renal cortical necrosis, and the rest were caused by ATN. In this series, there were four maternal deaths (13%); disseminated intravascular coagulation was seen in 84% of the patients, and pulmonary edema complicated 44% of cases. Dialysis was required in one third of these cases of ATN. Fetal complications were also high: perinatal mortality occurred in 34%, and premature delivery in 72%. Nevertheless, at follow-up averaging 4.5 years, maternal renal function and blood pressure were normal.

Abruptio placentae can cause ATN, but it is also the most common cause of renal cortical necrosis. Severe volume depletion due to hemorrhage resulting in renal ischemia is presumed to be the cause of ATN in this setting. The occurrence of oliguria and a rising creatinine level suggest ATN. Physical findings are usually not diagnostic, but the urinalysis can be. In ATN, the urine contains renal tubule epithelial cells, debris derived from necrotic epithelial cells, and numerous dark or "muddy brown" granular casts.

Renal Cortical Necrosis

Many of the risk factors for ATN are also risk factors for the development of renal cortical necrosis. The majority of cases of acute cortical necrosis are caused by abruptio placentae, but other obstetric complications, including septic abortion, severe pre-eclampsia, amniotic fluid embolism, and retained fetus, are also associated with the development of renal cortical necrosis.[388, 389] Initially, it may be difficult to distinguish renal cortical necrosis from ATN, although anuria suggests the former. Renal cortical necrosis should also be suspected when oliguria or anuria persists for longer than 1 week. In addition, hematuria is more likely in renal cortical necrosis than in ATN. Definitive diagnosis may be made by renal biopsy or, preferably, by renal arteriogram. The renal arteriogram shows patchy blood flow or an absent nephrogram. The diagnosis has also been made by computed tomographic scan, on which a radiolucent rim in the cortex parallel to the capsule represents the ischemic zone.[390]

Activation of the coagulation system has been proposed as a predisposing factor in the development of renal cortical necrosis. Postpartum rats have markedly increased sensitivity to endotoxin infusion, which causes a generalized Shwartzman reaction with renal effects similar to those of postpartum hemolytic-uremic syndrome. Postpartum rats more readily develop glomerular hemodynamic changes and intraglomerular capillary deposition of fibrin.[391] However, increases in clotting factors V, VIII, and X are also seen in uncomplicated pregnancy.[392] In one study comparing ATN with renal cortical necrosis, only plasma fibrinogen level was lower in the latter group; there were no differences in platelet count, thrombin, or fibrin degradation productions between the two conditions.[389]

It is not clear why ATN develops in some women whereas renal cortical necrosis develops in others during obstetric emergencies. In addition to obstetric complications, cortical necrosis is more frequently seen in older women and multigravidas, although these may not be independent risk factors but merely factors associated with the development of obstetric complications.[389] In some series, maternal mortality in cortical necrosis was high because of the severity of the underlying disease.[393] A large number of patients with cortical necrosis never recover renal function or recover renal function transiently with later development of end-stage renal disease.[389]

Postpartum Acute Renal Failure

Postpartum acute renal failure is also known as postpartum hemolytic-uremic syndrome. This disease is characterized by hypertension and coagulation abnormalities, particularly microangiopathic hemolytic anemia.[394] It occurs in otherwise uncomplicated pregnancies anywhere from 1 to 2 days to several months after delivery. A history of a preceding viral illness is often obtained. Symptoms are those related to renal insufficiency, such as headache, nausea, and vomiting. The signs include oliguria or anuria, evidence of a bleeding diathesis, and, in many cases, hypertension. The examination of the peripheral blood smear is remarkable for the presence of schistocytes and burr cells. Thrombocytopenia is usual. Bleeding times are not usually prolonged, although fibrin degradation products may be increased.[394] Neurologic symptoms, when present, suggest thrombotic thrombocytopenic purpura. Many believe that hemolytic-uremic syndrome and thrombotic thrombocytopenic purpura are different manifestations of the same general disease process (see Chapter 33). Indeed, endothelial injury is central to a number of pregnancy-related diseases, including preeclampsia, the HELLP syndrome, postpartum acute renal failure, and acute fatty liver of pregnancy, suggesting a continuum of disease.

Although the precise etiology of postpartum hemolytic-uremic syndrome is not known, the findings in this systemic disease are suggestive of diffuse vascular endothelial cell injury. A similar form of hemolytic-uremic syndrome has occurred in women taking oral contraceptives, which suggests a link with the hormonal changes of pregnancy.[395] Evidence of endothelial cell injury in the kidney, obtained by renal biopsy, includes glomerular thromboses and fibrin deposition as well as fibrinoid necrosis within arterioles.[360] Interstitial fibrosis becomes more prominent with chronicity of the disease.

Supportive therapy usually requires dialysis. Other therapies employed have derived from experience with thrombotic thrombocytopenic purpura in nonpregnant patients. In attempts to reduce intravascular clotting, anticoagulants, antiplatelet agents, and PGI_2 have all been administered. Because uncontrolled trials in thrombotic thrombocytopenic purpura have suggested beneficial effects of plasma exchange or the infusion of fresh-frozen plasma, these therapies have also been tried.[396] However, there has not been substantial experience with any one of these therapies for a general recommendation to be provided for their use. Plasma exchange is most frequently employed currently, despite the imperfections in our database.

Obstructive Uropathy

Fewer than 20 cases of acute renal failure due to bilateral ureteral obstruction from a gravid uterus have been reported.[397–399] Although no specific predisposing cause has been identified, approximately one third of these cases were multiple gestations, and one third were complicated by polyhydramnios.[397] Three quarters of the cases occurred in primigravidas. Amniotomy was a successful therapy in a patient with polyhydramnios.[397] Alternatively, several cases have been successfully treated by ureteral stenting.[400] The diagnosis of obstructive uropathy due to ureteral obstruction by the gravid uterus is suggested by the finding of oliguria or anuria in the setting of moderate or severe dilatation of the urinary collecting system, particularly on the left. Ultrasound evaluation in uncomplicated pregnancy revealed moderate dilatation on the left in 14% of cases and severe dilatation on the left in only 1% of cases.[401] As noted previously, dilatation on the right side is far more common.

Nephrolithiasis

Urinary calculi occur in pregnant women with the same frequency as in nonpregnant women.[402] This is perhaps surprising, because urinary Ca^{2+} excretion increases in pregnancy as a consequence of increased gut Ca^{2+} absorption and intake.[403, 404] However, urinary calculi are probably the most common cause of hospitalization for abdominal pain during pregnancy.[405] In most series, more than 90% of women diagnosed as having urinary calculi during pregnancy presented with flank or abdominal pain.[406, 407] More than 95% also had microscopic or gross hematuria to suggest the cause of the pain. Ultrasonography is the recommended procedure for detection of urinary calculi to avoid the low risk of radiation required by intravenous pyelography. However, when it is essential for diagnosis and therapy, limited intravenous pyelography can be safely performed.

The effects of pregnancy on stone formation in women with a history of chronic stone formation have been assessed. In 78 women, only UTI appeared to be a serious complication of chronic nephrolithiasis in pregnancy.[402] Pregnancy did not increase the rate of stone formation or the frequency of complications related to stones.[402] In 20 pregnancies in stone formers, urologic instrumentation and operations were not necessary.[402] On the other hand, selected reports of experiences with urinary tract calculi during pregnancy have suggested a higher rate of complications and need for intervention. This suggests that case reports collect only the most serious problems. In the past, there was a high frequency of a need for surgical intervention. However, in those patients unable to pass a ureteral calculus spontaneously, it is possible to place an internal ureteral stent safely and efficaciously in a pregnant woman.[408] The presence of a ureteral stent does not present complications for subsequent vaginal delivery.[408] Inadvertent extracorporeal shock wave lithotripsy has been performed in the first month of pregnancy.[409] The six women reported all went on to deliver healthy babies. Although lithotripsy cannot be recommended on this basis, should it be performed on a woman in the first month of pregnancy it is unlikely to affect the pregnancy.

Renal Disease in the Fetus

It is beyond the scope of this chapter to discuss renal abnormalities of the fetus. However, there are rare instances when maternal renal disease may have a direct or indirect impact on fetal or neonatal renal function. One example is the effects of medications administered to the mother that affect fetal renal function after transplacental passage of the drug. ACEIs, which are now contraindicated for use in pregnancy, provide one such example. When these drugs were administered to pregnant women near term, there were several reports of neonatal acute renal failure or hyperkalemia.[410, 411] It was postulated that the immature neonatal kidney, which has impaired RBF autoregulation in early life, was dependent on angiotensin II to maintain renal perfusion. Fetal accumulation of the ACEIs resulted in a form of reversible but severe and sometimes prolonged prerenal azotemia. Several neonatal deaths were attributed to this complication. Infants exposed to ACEIs in the second or third trimester also had renal tubular dysplasia.[411] As discussed previously, fetal abnormalities have not been noted when exposure to ACEIs occurred only in the first trimester, before pregnancy was identified and the drug was discontinued.[307]

An unlikely occurrence is the transmission of nonhereditary renal disease from mother to infant. However, there is at least one carefully evaluated report of the development of membranous nephropathy in a neonate due to transplacental passage of maternal immunoglobulin G resulting in neonatal glomerulopathy with anuria.[412] The rarity of such reports suggests that this phenomenon, although of great pathophysiologic interest, is not a major clinical consideration.

PREGNANCY IN WOMEN WITH RENAL DISEASE

There are several considerations relevant to the interaction between pregnancy and renal disease, whether the disease is preexisting or develops during pregnancy. Renal disease can have significant and serious consequences for both maternal health and fetal outcome. On the other hand, there is the risk that pregnancy will have an adverse effect on renal function that might be permanent. Although these topics are discussed individually, when the physician is counseling the patient with renal disease as to the advisability and risks of pregnancy, no simple recommendations can be given to a particular patient. Any pregnancy with underlying renal disease should be managed jointly by an obstetrician experienced in high-risk pregnancies and by a nephrologist.[413]

Effects of Renal Disease on Fetal Outcome

Fertility is greatly diminished by renal insufficiency, particularly when the GFR is less than 50% of normal.[414] Nevertheless, pregnancy occasionally occurs in patients with severe renal insufficiency and even in patients receiving chronic dialysis therapy. In one report of 907 women treated with chronic hemodialysis in Saudi Arabia, 7% of married women younger than 50 years of age experienced at least one pregnancy between 1 month and 5 years after beginning hemodialysis.[415] Although a successful outcome was observed in only one third of pregnancies (see later discussion), it is apparent that pregnancy occasionally occurs even in women with marginal renal function. In Belgium, pregnancy proceeding beyond the first trimester in dialysis patients had an incidence of 0.3 per 100 patient-years.[416] In the United States, 2% of hemodialysis patients of childbearing age became pregnant over a 4-year period.[417] Conception in women undergoing peritoneal dialysis is even less frequent than in hemodialysis patients, occurring at a rate of approximately one-half of the hemodialysis rate.[417]

The important consequences of maternal renal disease include an increased frequency of fetal loss, intrauterine growth retardation, and prematurity. The major risk factor for these undesirable outcomes is hypertension. Renal insufficiency and the presence of the nephrotic syndrome are additional fetal risk factors. In 1962, Rauramo and colleagues[418] noted an inverse relationship between the interval between the onset of renal disease (when known) and pregnancy on the one hand, and the frequency of pre-eclampsia, perinatal mortality, and premature birth on the other. Those women with a more chronic and stable course (i.e., a longer interval between disease onset and pregnancy) had a lower risk of adverse outcome. Mackay[419] prospectively studied 150 women with renal disease complicating pregnancy during a 10-year period and observed that the overall rate of fetal wastage was 34%. However, in women with proteinuria and normal renal function, fetal loss depended on whether

pre-eclampsia was superimposed on the pregnancy. Fetal loss was 10% in women in whom pre-eclampsia did not develop and 29% in those with superimposed pre-eclampsia. Among women who had impaired renal function when they became pregnant, fetal outcome was worse: When renal function was impaired, fetal loss was approximately 40%. In pregnancies in which renal insufficiency was accompanied by severe hypertension (blood pressure >175/110 mm Hg), fetal loss was 60%.[419] It is often difficult to measure the severity of maternal renal disease other than by GFR. When Barceló and co-workers[420] analyzed their experience using the 24-hour excretion of protein as one indicator of the extent of renal disease in women with glomerulonephritis, they found an inverse relationship with birth weight (Fig. 35-7). In women with autosomal dominant polycystic kidney disease studied by Chapman and associates,[421] only those with preexisting hypertension had fetal complications, largely because of the development of pre-eclampsia.

Katz and colleagues[422] reported the outcome of 121 pregnancies in 89 women with a variety of renal disorders treated at three medical centers. In their series, renal function was good in all women (serum creatinine level ≤1.4 mg/dL), hypertension was present before pregnancy in only 20%, and nephrotic syndrome was present in only four women. Superimposed pre-eclampsia developed in 12% of the pregnancies. The perinatal mortality rate was 9%, three to four times greater than the usual rate for the participating hospitals. Preterm deliveries occurred in 20% of the pregnancies, and infants were small for gestational age in 24% (a fourfold increase). Therefore, in women with a variety of glomerular diseases but preservation of renal function, there was still a considerable increase in the frequency of fetal morbidity and mortality.

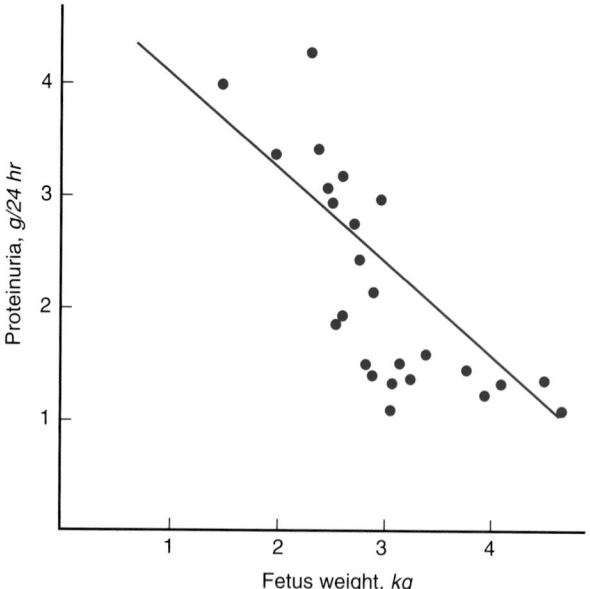

FIGURE 35-7. Inverse relationship between extent of proteinuria and fetal weight in women with primary glomerular disease ($r = .71$, $P < .01$). (From Barceló P, López-Lillo J, Cabero L, Del Río G: Successful pregnancy in primary glomerular disease. Used with permission from Kidney International, volume 30, p 914, 1986.)

In a retrospective review of 25 years' experience of pregnancy (398 pregnancies) in 238 Australian women with glomerulonephritis, Packham and associates[423] reported a fetal loss rate of 20%, with three quarters of these losses occurring in the second half of pregnancy. Twenty-four percent of infants were premature; only 50% of pregnancies resulted in live births at term. Infants were small for gestational age in 15% of live births. The presence of impaired renal function, preexisting hypertension (or development of severe hypertension), or the nephrotic syndrome resulted in a perinatal mortality rate of 30%, whereas women without any of these features had only a 5% perinatal mortality. Surian and co-workers[424] reported the course of 123 pregnancies in 86 patients with biopsy-proven glomerular disease. Their results were somewhat better: The perinatal death rate was 9%; 5.7% of infants were small for gestational age; and 14% were premature.

One of the difficulties of evaluating the available literature is that obstetric outcomes in general have improved dramatically in recent decades. This makes it difficult to compare newer studies to older ones or to use historical control outcomes for comparisons. For example, Hou and colleagues[425] reported on the outcomes of 25 pregnancies in women with moderate renal insufficiency (creatinine level ≥1.4 mg/dL, a value that in earlier studies was associated with worse outcome). The fetal mortality rate was 16%, and 61% of live births were premature. Imbasciati and co-workers[426] reported their experience with a similar group of women in Italy. Fetal loss occurred in 21% of pregnancies, and 54% of the live births were preterm. Jungers and associates[427] retrospectively reviewed outcome of 148 pregnancies in women with a variety of biopsy-proven glomerulonephritides. As was seen in other studies, poor fetal outcome was associated with the presence of uncontrolled hypertension, nephrotic range proteinuria, or renal insufficiency (creatinine level >1.8 mg/dL). Similarly, in a report of 240 pregnancies in 166 Japanese women with renal disease, the rate of live birth was 86%; perinatal death, 6%; and spontaneous abortion, 8%.[428] Perinatal loss occurred with greater frequency in women who had hypertension or a GFR of less than 70 mL/min. In 1996, Holley and colleagues[429] reviewed their experience of pregnancy in 40 women with renal disease. Women with renal disease had a fetal loss rate of 32% and a higher rate of prematurity than controls, representing no improvement in fetal outcome relative to the authors' experience in the 1970s and 1980s. In women with moderate to severe renal insufficiency reported by Jones and Hayslett,[430] the fetal survival rate was 93%, although prematurity was present in 59% of births and intrauterine growth retardation complicated 37% of pregnancies.

The signs and symptoms of renal disease influence the outcome of pregnancy, rather than the specific renal diagnosis. Stettler and Cunningham[319] evaluated the outcome of 65 pregnancies in 53 women with proteinuria greater than 500 mg/24 hours but no previously documented renal disease and normal renal function at the onset of pregnancy. Forty percent of the women had chronic hypertension, which suggests established but merely undiagnosed renal disease. Although the live birth rate was 93%, 45% of infants were preterm, and 23% had intrauterine growth retardation. Two thirds of the women had superimposed pre-eclampsia. Twenty-one of these women eventually underwent renal biopsy and were found to have histologic evidence for renal disease.

Leppert and co-workers[431] assessed the outcome of pregnancy in women who had a history of childhood renal disease (pyelonephritis or acute glomerulonephritis) that had apparently resolved. The frequency of spontaneous abortion and perinatal mortality was not different between these women and concurrent control groups. However, the frequency of small-for-gestational-age infants was increased from 1.5% to 5.5%. Women in whom childhood renal disease resulted in sustained renal insufficiency (creatinine level >1.5 mg/dL) had, not unexpectedly, greater fetal mortality and a higher frequency of superimposed pre-eclampsia. In summary, even a history of previous renal disease represents a small but real risk factor for unfavorable fetal outcome. Renal insufficiency, hypertension, and heavy proteinuria are much more serious risk factors for an unfavorable pregnancy outcome.

As noted, the risk of developing superimposed pre-eclampsia during pregnancy varies between 20% and 40% in women with some form of underlying renal disease. When pre-eclampsia is associated with renal disease, multiparous as well as nulliparous women are affected, and the disease may manifest earlier than 32 weeks. In one study, 25% of all cases of pre-eclampsia had onset before 37 weeks of gestation. Ninety percent of these women had chronic renal disease or essential hypertension.[432] Because the chances for the development of superimposed pre-eclampsia are so great in women with renal disease, this high-risk group would seem to be most appropriate for intervention with therapeutic agents, such as low-dose aspirin or calcium. Most such trials have specifically excluded women with known or suspected renal disease. In the Italian study of aspirin in 1106 pregnant women, 232 had either chronic hypertension or nephropathy.[262] Low-dose aspirin therapy resulted in a nonsignificant increase in birth weight and decrease in percentage of infants below the 10th percentile for birth weight, but this subgroup was too small for any firm conclusions to be made regarding the benefit of aspirin therapy. The effects of aspirin therapy on blood pressure were not reported for this subgroup. Although the earlier reported studies suggested overall that the greater the risk for the development of pre-eclampsia or intrauterine growth retardation, the greater the likelihood of benefit of low-dose aspirin therapy, more recent studies do not necessarily support that concept. Even women who are at higher risk for the development of pre-eclampsia (i.e., those with diabetes, chronic hypertension, or multifetal gestations) were not benefited by low-dose aspirin.[264] Patients with renal disease were not specifically studied, although 5% of the subjects had proteinuria at baseline. Most physicians wait until a specific trial in a group of patients with renal disease has been performed. One could not fault those physicians who, with a more aggressive approach, prescribe low-dose aspirin for pregnant patients with renal disease, because the risk of aspirin is relatively low and the potential benefits may be great.[433–436]

Risk of Progression of Renal Disease in Pregnancy

Most renal diseases enter an inexorably deteriorating course once a threshold of initial renal injury has been reached, even if the initiating process resolves.[437, 438] In the last decade, there has been an explosion of interest in and generation of information about this process, in large part deriving from work in experimental renal disease. Brenner and Hostetter and their colleagues[437–439] proposed that the common feature in all chronic progressive renal disease is an increase in glomerular capillary blood flow and intraglomerular capillary pressure. Intraglomerular hypertension leads to progressive damage that is manifested by the histologic findings of glomerulosclerosis and subsequent interstitial fibrosis. Indeed, these are the features of chronic renal disease regardless of the initiating form of injury (see Chapter 43 for a more complete discussion of this subject).

The potential implication of pregnancy in women with chronic renal disease is that the development or worsening of hypertension during pregnancy will have a particularly detrimental effect on the disease. Because pregnancy, like chronic renal disease, is characterized by dilatation of the afferent arteriole of the glomerulus, systemic blood pressure would be more completely transmitted into the glomerulus, and systemic hypertension would potentially be more damaging to the kidney, than if chronic renal disease or pregnancy did not exist. Animal studies suggest that, in normotensive rats, afferent arteriolar dilatation results in increases in glomerular blood flow but no change in intraglomerular pressure and consequently no renal damage despite repeated pregnancy.[19] Spontaneously hypertensive rats might be expected to develop accelerated renal injury when pregnant. However, of great interest, these rats have been observed not to develop afferent arteriolar relaxation during pregnancy and, therefore, there is no pregnancy-induced increase in GFR.[440] On the other hand, the absence of the normal renal vasodilatory response to pregnancy means that the kidneys of spontaneously hypertensive rats were not subjected to increased intraglomerular pressure during pregnancy, and repetitive pregnancies in spontaneously hypertensive rats did not lead to progressive renal insufficiency.[441] In a normotensive model of mild glomerulonephritis produced by injection of anti–glomerular basement membrane antibody, glomerular capillary hydraulic pressure did not increase during the first half of pregnancy, and there was no pregnancy-related worsening of proteinuria or glomerular morphologic features.[442] However, in another model of experimental glomerulonephritis produced by injection of rats with doxorubicin, pregnancy was associated with systemic hypertension and a marked increase in urinary protein excretion that presumably reflected an early adverse effect on the kidney.[443]

From these experiments, it is hard to predict what the effect of pregnancy would be in a woman with chronic renal disease, except that hypertension might adversely affect renal outcome. Women with mild renal insufficiency respond in a qualitatively normal way to pregnancy, with an increase in GFR and RBF in a pattern similar to that shown in Figure 35-1. When renal function is more severely impaired, the magnitude of the pregnancy-induced hyperfiltration is diminished.[422]

Risk Factors for Progression of Renal Disease

Studies of the effects of pregnancy on renal outcome in women with renal disease in general bear out these predictions. For the most part, women with renal disease who become pregnant when renal function is normal or minimally depressed tolerate pregnancy without permanent deleterious effects on renal function. Conversely, as many as one third of women with moderate renal insufficiency experience a more rapid decline in renal function after pregnancy than would have been predicted on the basis of the natural history of their disease. The majority of observations of the effects of pregnancy on the course of renal disease were made before there was a complete understanding of the importance of systemic hypertension to the course of renal disease. For this reason, there has not been an adequate trial of vigorous control of hypertension during pregnancy in women with moderate renal insufficiency to see whether this would prevent an accelerated downhill course in some of these women.

In the study by Katz and colleagues[422] of pregnancy effects on renal disease in women with a variety of glomerulonephritides but normal renal function before conception, permanent impairment of renal function as a result of pregnancy was rare. Sixteen percent of women developed transient decrements in renal function during pregnancy. In three patients, pregnancy occurred while glomerular filtration was already falling, but gestation did not appear to alter the time course. In 57 of the 121 pregnancies observed, there was severe or substantially increased proteinuria; in 68% of these cases, proteinuria was in the nephrotic range. As noted previously, superimposed pre-eclampsia developed in 12% of the women. However, after pregnancy, pre-eclampsia, by definition, resolved. Renal function returned to its previous level, except as noted, and proteinuria tended to return to prepartum levels. Other investigators studying several different populations have come to similar conclusions—that in women with prepartum renal disease but preserved renal function, pregnancy does not appear to adversely affect the underlying renal disease.[420, 427, 428] Abe and colleagues[428] suggested that, as long as the GFR was greater than 70 mL/min and blood pressure remained below 140/90 mm Hg, the underlying glomerular disease was not adversely affected in 244 pregnancies. In another group of 148 women with chronic glomerulonephritis who became pregnant, the overall course of renal disease was not different from that in a control cohort of 172 women with the same types of glomerulonephritis who did not become pregnant.[427] Barceló and co-workers[420] evaluated 66 pregnancies in 48 women with glomerular disease. Although most patients had mild renal dysfunction, several had greater impairment of renal function, severe hypertension, or nephrotic-range proteinuria. As a group, these women, evaluated 1 and 5 years after pregnancy, fared no worse in terms of their renal disease than did a control group of women who had not become pregnant. Individually, there were cases of apparent worsening of renal function in two women and the development of irreversible proteinuria in four, but these effects could not be differentiated from chance alone.[420] With 2 years of follow-up of 70 pregnancies in 62 women with primary renal disease or diabetic nephropathy, Bar and colleagues[444] found that only two of these women had an increase in creatinine of greater than 1 mg/dL. Jungers and colleagues[445] reported that there was no pregnancy-related acceleration of the progression of renal disease in 360 women with glomerulonephritis who had normal renal function during pregnancy.

Several studies do suggest, however, that if women become pregnant when they have moderate impairment of renal function, there is a greater chance of permanent deterioration in renal function as a consequence of pregnancy. Hou and associates[425] studied the effects of 25 pregnancies in 23 women with renal insufficiency before pregnancy (serum creatinine level ≥1.4 mg/dL). In seven of these women, whose baseline creatinine level was between 1.7 and 2.7 mg/dL, pregnancy resulted in a decline in renal function that was greater than expected. In more than half of these pregnancies, hypertension developed or worsened; in 36% of the pregnancies, the diastolic blood pressure exceeded 110 mm Hg. Imbasciati and co-workers[426] studied a similar group of 18 women. In 14 pregnancies, there were sufficient data to plot reciprocal plasma creatinine values versus time before and after pregnancy. In 5 of these 14 women, there was an apparent acceleration in the rate of progression after pregnancy. These two studies found a remarkably similar frequency (approximately 33%) of women with renal insufficiency that developed an accelerated course during pregnancy. In 1996, Jones and Hayslett reported the outcomes of pregnancy in 67 women with moderate to severe renal insufficiency.[430] Pregnancy resulted in a doubling of the prevalence of hypertension and proteinuria. Forty-three percent of these women suffered a pregnancy-related decline in renal function, which persisted after pregnancy in 31%. In 10% of women, the decrease in renal function was rapid, resulting in end-stage renal disease.

Proteinuria may be an independent risk factor for pregnancy-related declines in renal function. In a small group of women with glomerular disease, Hemmelder and associates[446] found that the degree of proteinuria (greater or less than 2.0 g/day) better predicted which 10 of 30 pregnancies would result in worsening of renal function than did blood pressure or initial level of renal function.

Progression in Specific Renal Diseases

In most studies, the number of women evaluated has been too small for conclusions to be drawn about the chance of progression of renal disease during pregnancy for a specific renal diagnosis. However, there is a suggestion that women with membranoproliferative glomerulonephritis, immunoglobulin A nephropathy, focal sclerosis, or reflux nephropathy have a greater risk for the development of irreversible renal failure than do those with other diagnoses of renal disease. For example, although Barceló and colleagues[420] observed that pregnancy did not, in general, adversely affect renal disease, the few cases of renal deterioration they observed occurred in women with membranoproliferative glomerulonephritis. Similarly, Abe and colleagues[428] reported that the highest frequency of development of hypertension or decreased renal function in pregnant women with glomerular disease occurred in those with membranoproliferative glomerulonephritis. Jungers and associates[427] noted that several patients with membranoproliferative glomerulonephritis were among those who suffered deterioration in renal function during pregnancy, but these women also had impaired renal function before pregnancy.

Reflux nephropathy has been suggested as a specific diagnosis imparting increased risk for renal deterioration during pregnancy. Becker and co-workers[447] observed 20 women with reflux nephropathy and plasma creatinine levels between 2.3 and 4.5 mg/dL. Six of these women had a pregnancy lasting longer than 12 weeks. All six experienced a

rapid deterioration in renal function, and four reached end-stage renal failure within 2 years of pregnancy. In the women who never became pregnant, renal function deteriorated slowly, and no patient reached end-stage renal failure within 7 years. By contrast, in women with reflux nephropathy and a serum creatinine level less than 2 mg/dL renal deterioration was not observed.[447, 448] Hypertension complicated fewer than 10% of pregnancies when the serum creatinine concentration was lower than 1 mg/dL. El-Khatib and colleagues[449] reported similar findings of worse fetal and maternal outcomes when renal insufficiency complicated reflux nephropathy. They further noted that bilateral renal scarring portended worse fetal and maternal outcome than did unilateral scarring.

Immunoglobulin A nephropathy is a common form of primary glomerulonephritis. In Japan, Abe[450] studied 168 pregnancies in 118 women with immunoglobulin A nephropathy during an 18-year period. Overall, the rate of spontaneous abortion was 9%, the live birth rate 87%, and the perinatal death rate 4%. When results were stratified by maternal renal function, if the GFR was lower than 70 mL/min before conception, the perinatal mortality rate was 14%, versus 3% if the GFR was higher than 70 mL/min. Similarly, if the baseline blood pressure was consistently greater than 140/90 mm Hg, the perinatal mortality was 33%, versus 1% if the pressure was lower. When the results were stratified by year of diagnosis, it was found that the perinatal death rate was 9% during the 1970s but 0% during the 1980s. More than half of the women were observed for 3 years or longer, and it was judged that their course was not different from the natural history of immunoglobulin A nephropathy. This study suggests that, with the current excellent standards of obstetric care, complications should be minimal if renal function is preserved and hypertension is controlled before pregnancy. A more recent series of 60 women reached similar conclusions.[451]

One feature that seemed to predict a poor outcome was the presence on renal biopsy specimens of lesions in the arterioles, tubules, and interstitium, in addition to glomerular lesions.[404] This is of interest because Packham and colleagues[423] noted that the presence of vascular lesions on renal biopsy specimens from patients with glomerulonephritis also predicted a higher rate of fetal loss during pregnancy. In other series evaluating the outcome of pregnancy in women with glomerulonephritis, women with immunoglobulin A nephropathy have usually fared better than the mean. This was true in the series reported by Packham and colleagues[423] and by Barceló and co-workers.[420] Jungers and co-workers[427] found no effect of pregnancy on the course of immunoglobulin A nephropathy in 48 women who experienced at least one pregnancy, compared with 44 who did not become pregnant.

SLE is a not uncommon disease affecting women of childbearing age. Historically, there were concerns that pregnancy induced exacerbations of SLE and that fetal wastage was extremely high in this disease.[452] Modern studies have not generally borne out these fears. Clinical exacerbations or relapses have been reported in between 9% and 60% of pregnancies.[452–454] However, the rate of disease exacerbation is not different in concurrent control groups and nonpregnant patients.[454] The major factor determining whether pregnancy results in an exacerbation of lupus is the stability of the disease before the pregnancy. When SLE has been in remission or well controlled for a period of more than 6 months, the chance of a clinical flare during pregnancy is low.[452, 453] On the other hand, when pregnancy occurs in close temporal association with an exacerbation of SLE, exacerbations are also frequently seen during or shortly after pregnancy.

Fetal survival is also closely related to the clinical status of SLE before conception. Hayslett and Lynn[455] reported a fetal survival rate of 88% in women in remission at the onset of pregnancy, compared with 64% when SLE was active at the beginning of pregnancy. Several other reports document a similar differential effect of lupus activity on fetal outcome in pregnancy.[453, 456] In a prospective study of planned pregnancy in women with inactive SLE, the live birth rate was 96%.[457] Nevertheless, prematurity was common. The presence of anticardiolipin antibodies is certainly related to an increased likelihood of spontaneous abortion.[458] However, it is controversial whether fetal outcome beyond the first trimester is adversely affected by the presence of antiphospholipid antibody. Le Huong and colleagues[457] did find severe prematurity to be more common in women with SLE and antiphospholipid syndrome. Permanent adverse effects on renal function are rare in women with lupus who have become pregnant. Packham and co-workers[459] found a 19% occurrence of reversible renal function deterioration during pregnancy, but in only 1 of 64 pregnancies was there irreversible deterioration in renal function. As is true for all women with renal disease, hypertension may worsen during pregnancy. Packham and colleagues[459] observed the development of hypertension in 28% of their cases. The hypertension was severe in 13%. Similarly, proteinuria increased in 48% of pregnancies, but this increase was irreversible in only 5%. In the report of Bobrie and co-workers[453] on 213 pregnancies in 73 patients, irreversible deterioration in renal function was observed in 4 of the 53 pregnancies that occurred in women whose SLE was not active at conception.

The effects of diabetes mellitus on fetal outcome are well known and include prematurity, congenital abnormalities, large-for-gestational-age infants, and the respiratory distress syndrome. Kitzmiller and associates[460] observed the effects of pregnancy on diabetic nephropathy. They studied 35 women with diabetes and nephropathy (defined as 24-hour urinary protein excretion >400 mg) who became pregnant. Of 26 women whose pregnancy reached 24 weeks' gestation, the nephrotic syndrome developed in 69% in the third trimester (58% had urinary protein excretion in excess of 6 g/24 hours). Fifty-seven percent of the 14 initially normotensive women became hypertensive. Despite these pregnancy-induced exacerbations in proteinuria and hypertension, proteinuria decreased postpartum in 60%, and the rate of decline of the GFR was not accelerated by pregnancy.

Researchers at Yale[461] studied a group of women with 31 pregnancies. One fourth of the patients had nephrotic syndrome at the beginning of pregnancy, and renal function was reduced in half of the pregnancies. One third of the pregnancies were complicated by further deterioration in renal function, and nephrotic syndrome was present in three fourths by the third trimester. Hypertension developed or worsened in two thirds of the pregnancies. Nevertheless, fetal survival was 94%; after delivery, renal function, proteinuria, and hypertension returned to baseline levels. Purdy and colleagues[462]

identified 11 diabetic women with serum creatinine levels greater than 1.4 mg/dL who became pregnant.[462] Forty-five percent had a permanent decline in renal function as a result of pregnancy. Almost 80% had transient worsening of hypertension or developed superimposed pre-eclampsia.

Pregnancy appears to have a similar effect on nonglomerular renal disease, although this has been less well studied. In autosomal dominant polycystic kidney disease, pregnancy was frequently complicated by hypertension or pre-eclampsia (18%, versus 1.6% in control subjects), although changes in renal function were not immediately apparent.[463] Despite the association of polycystic kidney diseases and infection, pregnancy did not increase the frequency of UTI.[463] On the other hand, in their broad survey of the risk factors associated with progression of renal disease in polycystic kidney disease, Gabow and co-workers[464] noted a positive association a history of three or more pregnancies and worse renal function. However, because the number of pregnancies was not treated as a continuous variable in that study, it is not clear whether a smaller number of pregnancies also has an adverse consequence on polycystic kidney disease. This is one of the best available studies for evaluating the consequences of pregnancy in a renal disease that has a sufficiently slow and stable course to determine whether pregnancy represents an independent risk factor for renal disease progression. In this instance, pregnancy had the small but discernible effect of accelerating chronic renal injury.

Although it is often difficult to compare series of patients from different hospitals and different eras, it seems that differences in outcome are more heavily affected by the severity of the renal disease than by the histologic diagnosis or type of renal disease. Regardless of the specific type of glomerulonephritis or other renal disease, almost every study has demonstrated that the presence of renal insufficiency, heavy proteinuria or nephrotic syndrome, or severe or uncontrollable hypertension represents an important risk factor for worsening of renal function during and after pregnancy.[465] Knowing the importance of these three risk factors for an adverse outcome in pregnancy associated with renal disease permits the counseling physician to relate this information to women who are contemplating pregnancy.

Preventing Progression of Renal Disease

For many renal diseases, there is little that can be done therapeutically to restore renal function or to dramatically reduce proteinuria that is chronically present (two obvious exceptions are disease exacerbations in minimal-change glomerulopathy and SLE). On the other hand, hypertension is treatable. Although prospective data are not available, it is probable that strict control of hypertension during pregnancy would have protective effects on the kidney, as has been demonstrated in nonpregnant women and in men. An increase in proteinuria, even in the absence of increasing blood pressure, suggests the need for more aggressive blood pressure control. What is more controversial is the precise blood pressure goal for pregnant women. Recalling that pregnancy is a condition associated with afferent arteriolar vasodilatation and greater transmission of systemic blood pressure into the glomerulus, a nephrologist would generally recommend aggressive blood pressure control. However, this goal must be balanced with concerns for fetal well-being.

High levels of dietary protein intake are also associated with an adverse renal outcome in chronic progressive renal disease.[466] Dietary protein increases the RBF and stimulates renin secretion, factors that would lead to increased glomerular capillary flow and pressure.[467] In a prospective study of protein supplementation in pregnant women *without* renal disease, there was an increase in the frequency of premature birth, neonatal death, and intrauterine growth retardation.[468] Therefore, protein supplementation is not advisable for any pregnant woman and certainly not for women with renal disease. Women with renal disease who become pregnant should follow a normal or modestly restricted dietary protein intake rather than a high one.

TREATMENT OF RENAL FAILURE IN PREGNANCY

Dialysis

Although women undergoing chronic hemodialysis do occasionally become pregnant, as noted earlier, most experience in the treatment of pregnant patients by hemodialysis has accrued with women who became pregnant with moderate renal insufficiency and progressed to end-stage renal disease during pregnancy. The general principle for treatment of chronic hemodialysis patients is that more dialysis is usually better.[469] This dictum has been empirically employed in cases complicated by pregnancy. This course of action has included instituting dialysis early (e.g., when the GFR is approximately 10 mL/min, rather than waiting until it falls further) and treating with more frequent and longer hemodialysis sessions.[415, 470, 471] In Belgium, the dose of dialysis during pregnancy correlated with birth weight.[416] Among dialysis patients, the therapeutic abortion rate is higher than for the general population, which makes an unbiased assessment of the literature difficult. Most studies of dialysis in pregnancy consist of collections of case reports from several medical centers. It is not known whether the general trend to report only successful cases or those in which longer dialysis sessions were performed has biased these reports. The European Dialysis and Transplant Association reported on pregnancy in 115 women. Of those not electively terminating pregnancy, 23% of pregnancies resulted in live birth.[472] Redrow and co-workers[470] reported cases of 13 pregnant women treated with hemodialysis. During pregnancy, hypertension worsened in most patients (77%). Premature labor complicated all but two pregnancies. Ninety percent of the infants were small for gestational age, but neither respiratory distress nor fetal abnormalities were a problem during delivery. Souqiyyeh and colleagues[415] reported on 8 live births in 27 cases of pregnancy in women receiving hemodialysis. Their patients did not have uncontrollable hypertension during pregnancy. In most reports of successful pregnancies, hemodialysis sessions were lengthened or their frequency was increased from three times to five or more times per week. Anemia has been more aggressively treated, and this is now an easier task with the availability of erythropoietin, which has been successfully used in pregnant hemodialysis patients.[473] In addition, hypotension has been carefully avoided to lessen the chance of fetal hypoperfusion. Recent experience has been more favorable. A successful outcome was observed in Belgium in 40% of women on hemodialysis before pregnancy and 74% in pregnancies in which dialysis was initiated after conception. Nevertheless, prematurity and low birth weight occurred in every pregnancy, and 66% of infants were delivered by cesarean section.[416]

In the United States, infant survival rate was 40% and 74%, respectively.[417] Fetal survival rates were similar for hemodialysis and peritoneal dialysis. Eighty-four percent of the infants were premature. In 1981, a nationwide survey of dialysis patients in Japan reported 9% live births; when this survey was undertaken again in 1996, the percentage was 49%. This occurred despite a much lower rate of elective abortion (64% versus 19% in the respective series). In the same survey, there was no difference in pregnancies between women who had been receiving dialysis for less than, versus longer than, 10 years; all patients were on maintenance hemodialysis. Dialysis treatments occurred a mean of 4.5 times per week (22 hours per week).[474]

As an alternative modality to provide continuous dialysis and to avoid the risks of intermittent hypotension and anticoagulation, chronic peritoneal dialysis has been employed. Both continuous ambulatory peritoneal dialysis and continuous cycling peritoneal dialysis have been reported to produce modest success.[471, 475] Interestingly, continuous ambulatory peritoneal dialysis was not technically difficult, and catheter leaks and inadequate peritoneal cavity volume were not problems. Most patients could tolerate exchanges of at least 1500 mL. If abdominal discomfort with drainage occurs, tidal peritoneal dialysis may be beneficial in reducing pain.[476] Problems unique to peritoneal dialysis include hypokalemia and peritonitis due to an increase in dialysis intensity.[477] Blood in the dialysate should prompt the clinician to consider abortion or abruption.[477]

In some cases of pregnancy occurring in women with advanced renal insufficiency (GFR <10 mL/min), prophylactic dialysis has been employed. The reasoning is that in normal pregnancy the GFR increases substantially to meet the needs of the mother and developing fetus, whereas in women with far-advanced renal disease this is not possible. Successful reports of this strategy are available, but controlled studies have not been performed.[478] It should be pointed out that there also exist a small number of case reports of pregnancy in women with advanced renal failure treated conservatively or with dietary protein restriction.[479, 480] These results apparently were not different from those reported for women who were treated more aggressively with hemodialysis. However, it is unlikely that such a conservative approach will gain wide acceptance or be subjected to a controlled trial.

Transplantation

Kidney transplantation restores fertility in women with chronic kidney disease,[481, 482] and outcomes of pregnancies that occur in women who are recipients of kidney transplants are dramatically different from those experienced by hemodialysis patients. Davison[483] surveyed 2309 pregnancies in 1594 women who had previously received a kidney transplant. After therapeutic abortions and the 13% of pregnancies that ended in spontaneous abortion were accounted for, pregnancies were successful in 92%. When specifically evaluated, renal function was found to be increased in the transplanted kidney in a manner consistent with that observed in normal native kidneys.[484] Acute rejection episodes were seen in 9% of the patients, a frequency believed to be no greater than that in nonpregnant women.[483] Hypertension or preeclampsia developed in approximately 30% of pregnancies, representing the most important maternal complication. Anemia caused by inadequate erythropoiesis despite normal iron stores has been shown to occur in women with well-functioning grafts.[485] As in the pregnant hemodialysis patient, erythropoietin has been used and is believed to be safe.[486] The most significant fetal complication was preterm delivery, which occurred in 45% to 60% of cases. Between 20% and 30% of infants were small for gestational age. Vaginal delivery was not made difficult by the presence of the pelvic kidney. Therefore, cesarean sections should be reserved for the usual obstetric indications.

Although much of the experience with pregnancy in transplant recipients occurred before the general availability of cyclosporine, results in women treated with cyclosporine are similar. Muirhead and co-workers[487] reported their experience at a single transplantation center and were able to compare results in women receiving versus not receiving cyclosporine. In infants whose mothers received cyclosporine, mean birth weight was 2.1 kg, versus 2.6 kg without cyclosporine. The mean gestational age was 34 versus 36 weeks, respectively, and the frequency of preterm delivery was 79% versus 50%. A report by the National Transplantation Pregnancy Registry of 947 pregnancies revealed similar outcomes in women treated with or without cyclosporine.[488] Live birth rates were 78% and 82% in the cyclosporine and non-calcineurin inhibitor–based regimens, respectively.[489] Birth weight was lower when cyclosporine was used, 2.5 kg versus 2.7 kg. In women who had received transplants longer than 5 years before pregnancy, outcomes were also favorable.[490] Live births resulted from 76% of pregnancies, and prematurity (31%), low birth weight (15%), and very low birth rate (7.7%) were tolerable. Two-year graft survival was 100%. In addition to the effects on birth weight, maternal cyclosporine treatment has been noted to have negative effects on B, T and natural killer lymphocytes in human infants, and these effects can be seen at up to 1 year of age.[491] None of the six infants studied had clinical evidence of immunodeficiency. Cyclosporine levels usually decline during pregnancy and should be monitored closely.[492]

The experience with tacrolimus in pregnancy is limited. Twenty-eight pregnancies in women treated with tacrolimus were reported with the registry data; the live birth rate was 69%, and the mean birth weight was 2100 g.[489] Hypertension occurred in 46% of the tacrolimus pregnancies, compared with 63% of the cyclosporine pregnancies, and gestational diabetes occurred in 19% and 12%, respectively.[489] The level of statistical significance was not reported, but these differences may imply clinically important differences between the regimens.

Not all drugs used for the prevention of allograft rejection are acceptable in pregnancy. Tacrolimus is believed to be safe in pregnancy, and experience with solid organ transplantation has revealed a low rate of congenital defects.[493] Mycophenolate mofetil and sirolimus are embryotoxic in animals,[494, 495] and it is recommended that these drugs not be used during pregnancy or while attempting to conceive,[496]

TABLE 35-1

Guidelines for Considering Pregnancy in Renal Transplant Recipients

Good general health for approximately 2 years after transplantation
Stable allograft function (serum creatinine <2 mg/dL, preferably <1.5 g/dL)
No recent episodes of acute rejection or evidence of ongoing rejection
Normal blood pressure or minimal antihypertensive regimen (only one drug)
Absence of or minimal proteinuria (<0.5 g/day)
Normal allograft ultrasound (absence of pelvicalyceal distension)
Recommended immunosuppression:
   Prednisone <15 mg/day
   Azathioprine ≤2 mg/kg/day
   Cyclosporine or tacrolimus at therapeutic levels
   Mycophenolate mofetil and sirolimus are contraindicated
   Mycophenolate mofetil and sirolimus should be stopped 6 wk before conception is attempted

Adapted from Pregnancy in renal transplant recipients. Nephrol Dial Transplant 17 (suppl 4):50, 2002.

although successful pregnancies with mycophenolate have been described.[497]

Pregnancy in the renal transplant recipient has become a common enough occurrence that guidelines have emerged to direct the treating transplantation team (Table 35-1).[496] Contraception counseling should be a part of post-transplantation care in women of childbearing age.

Kidney allografts appear to tolerate pregnancy well. There was a fear that pregnancy-induced hyperfiltration could adversely affect long-term survival of allografts. Sturgiss and Davison[498] performed a case-control study of women who had transplanted kidneys when they became pregnant and monitored these women for a mean follow-up period of 12 years. At the end of that time, the GFR was similar whether pregnancy had occurred or not. Graft loss, chronic rejection, and death occurred with equal frequency, regardless of whether pregnancy had occurred. In an extension of their study for an additional 3 years, no adverse effects of pregnancy became apparent.[499] Although this study encompassed only 36 patients, it suggests that there is no adverse effect of pregnancy on long-term outcome in kidney allograft recipients. A retrospective single-center review from Cincinnati revealed no adverse effect of pregnancy on graft survival or function.[500] The registry of the European Dialysis and Transplant Association also reported no adverse effect of successful pregnancy on graft function.[501] Renal function deteriorated in 18% of women experiencing a successful pregnancy and in 24% of control subjects during a similar period. Repeated pregnancies in kidney transplant recipients were similarly not detrimental to graft function.[502]

REFERENCES

1. Garland HO, Green R, Moriarty RJ: Changes in body weight, kidney weight and proximal tubule length during pregnancy in the rat. Renal Physiol 1:42, 1978.
2. Christensen T, Klebe JG, Bertelsen V, et al: Changes in renal volume during normal pregnancy. Acta Obstet Gynecol Scand 68:541, 1989.
3. Guyer PB, Delany D: Urinary tract dilation and oral contraceptives. BMJ 4:488, 1970.
4. Bozarki S, Lebay P, Gerber C: Prostaglandin inhibition of ureteral peristalsis. Invest Urol 4:9, 1966.

5. Sala NL, Rubi RA: Ureteral function in pregnant women: V. Incidence of vesicoureteral reflux and its effect upon ureteral contractility. Am J Obstet Gynecol 112:871, 1972.

6. Simaan M, Cadoretter C, Poterek M, et al: Calcium channels contribute to the decrease in blood pressure of pregnant rats. Am J Physiol Heart Circ Physiol 282:H665, 2002.

7. MacGillivray I, Rose GA, Rowe B: Blood pressure survey in pregnancy. Clin Sci 37:395, 1969.

8. DeSwiet M: The cardiovascular system. *In* Hytten FE, Chamberlain GVP (eds): Clinical Physiology in Obstetrics. Oxford, Blackwell Scientific Publications, 1980, p 3.

9. Visser W, Wallenburg HCS: Central hemodynamic observations in untreated pre-eclamptic patients. Hypertension 17:1072, 1991.

10. Hytten FE, Leitch I: The Physiology of Human Pregnancy, 2nd ed. Oxford, Blackwell Scientific Publications, 1971.

11. Phippard AF, Horvath JS, Glynn EM, et al: Circulatory adaptation to pregnancy: Serial studies of hemodynamics, blood volume, renin and aldosterone in the baboon *(Papio hamadryas)*. J Hypertens 4:773, 1986.

12. Robertson EG: The natural history of oedema during pregnancy. J Obstet Gynaecol Br Commonw 78:520, 1971.

13. Thompson AM, Hytten RE, Billewecz WZ: The epidemiology of oedema during pregnancy. J Obstet Gynaecol Br Commonw 74:1, 1967.

14. Sims EAH, Krantz KE: Serial studies of renal function during pregnancy and the puerperium in normal women. J Clin Invest 37: 1764, 1958.

15. Assali NS, Dignam WJ, Dasgupta K: Renal function in human pregnancy: Effects of venous pooling on renal hemodynamics and water, electrolyte and aldosterone excretion during normal gestation. J Lab Clin Med 54:394, 1959.

16. DeAlvarez RR: Renal glomerulotubular mechanisms during normal pregnancy: I. Glomerular filtration rate, renal plasma flow and creatinine clearance. Am J Obstet Gynecol 75:931, 1958.

17. Dunlop W: Renal physiology in pregnancy. Postgrad Med J 55:329, 1979.

18. Davison JM, Dunlop W: Renal hemodynamics and tubular function in normal human pregnancy. Kidney Int 18:152, 1980.

19. Baylis C, Reckelhoff JF: Renal hemodynamics in normal and hypertensive pregnancy: Lessons from micropuncture. Am J Kidney Dis 17: 98, 1991.

20. Conrad KP: Renal hemodynamics during pregnancy in chronically catheterized, conscious rats. Kidney Int 26:24, 1984.

21. Baylis C, Brango C, Engels K: Renal effects of moderate hemorrhage in the conscious pregnant rat. Am J Physiol 259:F945, 1990.

22. Reckelhoff J, Samsell L, Baylis C: Dissociation between plasma volume expansion (PVE) and increases in GFR during pregnancy in the rat. Kidney Int 35:472, 1989.

23. Woods LL, Mizelle HL, Hall JE: Autoregulation of renal blood flow and glomerular filtration rate in the pregnant rabbit. Am J Physiol 252:R69, 1987.

24. Baylis C, Blantz RC: Tubuloglomerular feedback activity in virgin and 12 day pregnant rats. Am J Physiol 249:F169, 1985.

25. Baylis C: Effect of amino acid infusion as an index of renal vasodilatory capacity in pregnant rats. Am J Physiol 254:F650, 1988.

26. Bay WH, Ferris TF: Factors controlling plasma renin and aldosterone during pregnancy. Hypertension 1:410, 1979.

27. Lewis PJ, Boylan P, Friedman LA, et al: Prostacyclin in pregnancy. BMJ 280:1581, 1980.

28. Brown GP, Venuto RE: In vitro renal eicosanoid production during pregnancy in rabbits. Am J Physiol 254:E687, 1988.

29. Conrad KP, Dunn MJ: Renal synthesis and urinary excretion of eicosanoids during pregnancy in rats. Am J Physiol 253:F1197, 1987.

30. Baylis C: Renal effects of cyclooxygenase inhibition in the pregnant rat. Am J Physiol 253:F158, 1987.

31. Conrad KP, Colpoys MC: Evidence against the hypothesis that prostaglandins are the vasodepressor agents of pregnancy: Serial studies in chronically instrumented, conscious rats. J Clin Invest 77: 236, 1986.

32. Baylis C: Glomerular ultrafiltration in the pseudopregnant rat. Am J Physiol 243:F300, 1982.

33. Walker J, Garland HO: Single nephron function during prolactin-induced pseudopregnancy in the rat. J Endocrinol 107:127, 1985.

34. Conrad KP: Possible mechanisms for changes in renal hemodynamics during pregnancy: Studies from animal models. Am J Kidney Dis 9:253, 1987.

35. Baylis C, Badr K, Collins R: Effects of chronic prolactin administration on renal hemodynamics in the rat. Endocrinology 117:722, 1985.

36. Paller MS, Gregorini G, Ferris TF: Pressor responsiveness in pseudo-pregnant and pregnant rats. Am J Physiol 257:R866, 1989.

37. Chapman AB, Zamudio S, Woodmansee W, et al: Systemic and renal hemodynamic changes in the luteal phase of the menstrual cycle mimic early pregnancy. Am J Physiol 273:F777, 1997.

38. Bucht H, Werko L: Glomerular filtration rate and renal blood flow in hypertensive toxaemia of pregnancy. J Obstet Gynaecol Br Commonw 60:157, 1953.

39. Shiffman RL, Tejani N, Verma U, et al: Effect of dietary protein on glomerular filtration rate in pregnancy. Obstet Gynecol 73:47, 1989.

40. Baylis C: The determinants of renal hemodynamics in pregnancy. Am J Kidney Dis 9:260, 1987.

41. Dal Canton A, Conte G, Esposito C, et al: Effects of pregnancy on glomerular dynamics: Micropuncture study in the rat. Kidney Int 22:608, 1982.

42. August P, Levy T, Ales KL, et al: Longitudinal study of the renin-angiotensin-aldosterone system in hypertensive pregnant women. Am J Obstet Gynecol 163:1612, 1990.

43. Brown MA, Zammit VC, Adsett D: Stimulation of active renin release in normal and hypertensive pregnancy. Clin Sci 79:505, 1990.

44. Hanssens M, Keirse MJ, Spitz B: Angiotensin II levels in pregnancy. Br J Obstet Gynaecol 98:155, 1991.

45. Weir RJ, Brown JJ, Fraser R, et al: Plasma renin, renin substrate, angiotensin II and aldosterone in hypertensive disease of pregnancy. Lancet 1:291, 1973.

46. Lenz T, Sealey JE, Happe RW, et al: Infusion of recombinant human pro-renin into rhesus monkeys. Am J Hypertens 3:257, 1990.

47. Sealey JE, Von Lutterotte N, Rubattu S, et al: The greater renin system: Its pro-renin directed vasodilator limb. Am J Hypertens 4:972, 1991.

48. Venuto R, Cox JW, Stein JH, et al: Regulation of uterine blood flow in the pregnant rabbit. J Clin Invest 57:938, 1976.

49. Woods LL, Brooks VL: Role of the renin-angiotensin system in hypertension during reduced uteroplacental perfusion pressure. Am J Physiol 251:R204, 1989.

50. Ferris TF, Stein JH, Kauffman J: Uterine blood flow and uterine renin secretion. J Clin Invest 51:2828, 1972.

51. Franklin GO, Dowd AJ, Caldwell BV, et al: The effect of angiotensin II intravenous infusion on plasma renin activity and prostaglandins A_1, E, and F levels in the uterine vein of the pregnant monkey. Prostaglandins 6:271, 1974.

52. Sealey JE, Atlas SA, Laragh JH: Plasma pro-renin: Physiological and biochemical characteristics. Clin Sci 63:133, 1981.

53. Ferris TF, Herdson PB, Dunnill MS, et al: Toxemia of pregnancy in sheep: A clinical physiological and pathological study. J Clin Invest 48:1643, 1969.

54. Lardner CN, Brinkman CR III, Weston PV: Dynamics of uterine circulation in pregnant and non-pregnant sheep. Am J Physiol 218: 257, 1970.

55. Fernandez LA, Twickler J, Mead A: Neovascularization produced by angiotensin II. J Lab Clin Med 105:141, 1985.

56. Broughton Pipkin F, Symonds EM, Turner SR: The effect of captopril (SQ14,225) upon mother and fetus in the chronically canulated ewe and in the pregnant rabbit. J Physiol (Lond) 323:415, 1982.

57. Ferris TF, Weir EK: The effect of captopril on uterine blood flow and prostaglandin synthesis in the rabbit. J Clin Invest 71:80, 1983.

58. Kawano M, Mori N: Prostacyclin producing activity of human umbilical, placental and uterine vessels. Prostaglandins 26:645, 1983.

59. Bussolino F, Benedetto C, Massobrio M, et al: Maternal vascular prostacyclin activity in pre-eclampsia. Lancet 2:702, 1980.

60. Dadak C, Kefalides A, Singinger H, et al: Reduced umbilical artery prostacyclin formation in complicated pregnancies. Am J Obstet Gynecol 144:792, 1982.

61. Koullapis EN, Nicolaides KH, Collins WP, et al: Plasma prostanoids in pregnancy-induced hypertension. Br J Obstet Gynaecol 89:617, 1982.

62. Remuzzi G, Marchesi D, Mecca G, et al: Reduction of fetal vascular prostacyclin activity in pre-eclampsia [letter]. Lancet 2:310, 1980.

63. Fitzgerald DJ, Entmann SS, Mulloy K, et al: Decreased prostacyclin biosynthesis preceding the clinical manifestations of pregnancy induced hypertension. Circulation 75:956, 1987.

64. Fitzgerald DJ, FitzGerald GA: Eicosanoids in pre-eclampsia. *In* Laragh JH, Brenner BM (eds): Hypertension: Pathophysiology and Diagnosis and Management. New York, Raven Press, 1990, p 1789.

65. Paller MS: Mechanism of decreased pressor responsiveness to Ang II, NE, and vasopressin in pregnant rats. Am J Physiol 247:H100, 1984.

66. Gill JR: Bartter's syndrome. Annu Rev Med 31:405, 1980.
67. Everett RB, Worley RJ, MacDonald PC, et al: Effect of prostaglandin synthesis inhibitors on pressor response to angiotensin II in human pregnancy. J Clin Endocrinol Metab 46:1007, 1978.
68. Novak J, Danielson LA, Kerchner LJ, et al: Relaxin is essential for renal vasodilation during pregnancy in conscious rats. J Clin Invest 107:1469, 2001.
69. Danielson LA, Sherwood OD, Conrad KP: Relaxin is a potent renal vasodilator in consious rats. J Clin Invest 103:525, 1999.
70. Abram SR, Alexander BT, Bennett WA, et al: Role of neuronal nitric oxide synthase in mediating renal hemodynamic changes during pregnancy. Am J Physiol Regul Integr Comp Physiol 281:1390, 2001.
71. Conrad KP, Gandley RE, Ogawa T, et al: Endothelin mediates renal vasodilation and hyperfiltration during pregnancy in chronically instrumented conscious rats. Am J Physiol 276:F767, 1999.
72. Page NM, Woods RJ, Gardiner SM, et al: Excessive placental secretion of neurokinin B during the third trimester causes pre-eclampsia. Nature 405:797, 2000.
73. Chesley LC, Valenti C, Rein H: Excretion of sodium loads by nonpregnant and pregnant normal, hypertensive and pre-eclamptic women. Metabolism 7:575, 1958.
74. Katz AL: Urinary concentrating ability in pregnant women with asymptomatic bacteriuria. J Clin Invest 40:1331, 1961.
75. Lindheimer MD, Weston PV: Effect of hypotonic expansion on sodium, water and urea excretion in late pregnancy: The influence of posture on these results. J Clin Invest 48:947, 1969.
76. Davison JM, Gilmore EA, Durr J, et al: Altered osmotic thresholds for vasopressin secretion and thirst in human pregnancy. Am J Physiol 246:F105, 1984.
77. Davison JM, Shiells EA, Philips PR, et al: Serial evaluation of vasopressin release and thirst in human pregnancy: Role of human chorionic gonadotrophin in the osmoregulatory changes of gestation. J Clin Invest 81:798, 1988.
78. MacDonald HN, Good W: The effect of parity on plasma sodium, potassium, chloride and osmolality levels during pregnancy. Br J Obstet Gynaecol 72:173, 1972.
79. Lindheimer MD, Barron WM, Davison JM: Osmotic and volume control of vasopressin release in pregnancy. Am J Kidney Dis 17:105, 1991.
80. Barron WM, Stamoutsos BA, Lindheimer MD: Role of volume in the regulation of vasopressin secretion during pregnancy in the rat. J Clin Invest 73:923, 1984.
81. Davison JM, Shiells EA, Philips PR, et al: Influence of humoral and volume factors on altered osmoregulation of normal human pregnancy. Am J Physiol 258:F900, 1990.
82. Durr JA, Stamoutsos B, Lindheimer MD: Osmoregulation during pregnancy in the rat. J Clin Invest 68:337, 1981.
83. Barron WM, Lindheimer MD: Osmoregulation in pseudopregnant and prolactin-treated rats: Comparison with normal gestation. Am J Physiol 254:R478, 1988.
84. Ehrlich EN, Nolten WE, Oparil S, et al: Mineralocorticoids in normal pregnancy. In Lindheimer MD, Katz AL, Zuspan FP (eds): Hypertension in Pregnancy. New York, John Wiley & Sons, 1976, p 217.
85. Brown MA, Sinosich MJ, Saunders DM, et al: Potassium regulation and progesterone-aldosterone interrelationships in human pregnancy: A prospective study. Am J Obstet Gynecol 155:349, 1986.
86. Ehrlich EN, Lindheimer MD: Effect of administered mineralocorticoid or ACTH in pregnant women: Attenuation of kaliuretic influence of mineralocorticoids during pregnancy. J Clin Invest 51:1301, 1972.
87. Biglieri EG, Slaton PE Jr: Pregnancy and primary aldosteronism. J Clin Endocrinol 27:1628, 1967.
88. Hammond TG, Buchanan JD, Scoggins BA, et al: Primary hyperaldosteronism in pregnancy. Aust N Z J Med 2:537, 1982.
89. Lotgering FR, Derks FM, Wallenburg HC: Primary hyperaldosteronism in pregnancy. Am J Obstet Gynecol 155:986, 1986.
90. Merrill RH, Dombroski R, Mackenna JM: Primary hyperaldosteronism during pregnancy. Am J Obstet Gynecol 150:786, 1984.
91. Lindheimer MD, Richardson DA, Ehrlich EN, et al: Potassium homeostasis in pregnancy. J Reprod Med 32:517, 1987.
92. Lim VS, Katz AI, Lindheimer MD: Acid-base metabolism in pregnancy. Am J Physiol 231:1764, 1976.
93. Blechner JN, Cotter JR, Stenger VG, et al: Oxygen, carbon dioxide and hydrogen ion concentration in arterial blood during pregnancy. Am J Obstet Gynecol 100:1, 1968.
94. Lyons HA, Antonio R: The sensitivity of the respiratory center in pregnancy and after the administration of progesterone. Trans Assoc Am Physicians 72:173, 1959.

95. Assali NS, Herzig D, Singh BP: Renal responses to ammonium chloride acidosis in normal and toxemic pregnancies. J Appl Physiol 7:367, 1955.
96. Dunlop W, Davison JM: The effect of normal pregnancy upon the renal handling of uric acid. Br J Obstet Gynaecol 84:13, 1977.
97. Christensen PJ: Tubular reabsorption of glucose during pregnancy. Scand J Clin Lab Invest 10:364, 1958.
98. Welsh GW, Sims EAH: The mechanisms of renal glucosuria in pregnancy. Diabetes 9:363, 1960.
99. Davison JM, Hytten FE: The effect of pregnancy on the renal handling of glucose. Br J Obstet Gynaecol 82:374, 1975.
100. Christensen PJ, Date JW, Sconheyder F, et al: Amino acids in blood plasma and urine during pregnancy. Scand J Clin Lab Invest 9:54, 1957.
101. Wallraff EB, Brodie EC, Borden AL: Urinary excretion of amino acids in pregnancy. J Clin Invest 29:1542, 1950.
102. Hytten FE, Cheyne GA: The aminoaciduria of pregnancy. J Obstet Gynaecol Br Commonw 79:424, 1972.
103. National High Blood Pressure Education Program Working Group report on high blood pressure in pregnancy. Am J Obstet Gynecol 163:1691, 1990.
104. Friedman EA, Neff RK: Pregnancy Hypertension: A Systemic Evaluation of Clinical Diagnostic Criteria. Littleton, MA, PSG Publishing, 1977.
105. Page EW, Christianson R: The impact of mean arterial pressure in the middle trimester upon the outcome of pregnancy. Am J Obstet Gynecol 125:740, 1976.
106. Sibai BM, Caritis S, Thom E, et al: Prevention of pre-eclampsia with low dose aspirin in healthy, nulliparous pregnant women. N Engl J Med 329:1213, 1993.
107. Oney T, Kaulhausen H: The value of the mean arterial blood pressure in the second trimester as a predictor of pregnancy-induced hypertension and pre-eclampsia: A preliminary report. Clin Exp Hypertens 2:211, 1983.
108. Ekholm EM, Tahvanainen KU, Metsala T: Heart rate and blood pressure variabilities are increased in pregnancy-induced hypertension. Am J Obstet Gynecol 177:1208, 1997.
109. Hermida RC, Ayala DE, Mojon A, et al: Blood pressure excess for the early identification of gestational hypertension and pre-eclampsia. Hypertension 31:83, 1998.
110. Biswas A, Choolani MA, Anandakumar C, Arulkumaran S: Ambulatory blood pressure monitoring in pregnancy induced hypertension. Acta Obstet Gynecol Scand 76:829, 1997.
111. Kyle PM, Clark SJ, Buckley D, et al: Second trimester ambulatory blood pressure in nulliparous pregnancy: A useful screening test for pre-eclampsia? Br J Obstet Gynecol 100:914, 1993.
112. Higgins JR, Walshe JJ, Halligan A, et al: Can 24-hour ambulatory blood pressure measurement predict the development of hypertension in primigravidae? Br J Obstet Gynecol 104:356, 1997.
113. Hermida RC, Ayala DE: Diagnosing gestational hypertension and pre-eclampsia with the 24-hour mean of blood pressure. Hypertension 30:1531, 1997.
114. Thornton JG, Onerude MB: Convulsions in pregnancy in related gorillas. Am J Obstet Gynecol 167:240, 1992.
115. Combs CA, Katz MA, Kitzmiller JL, et al: Experimental pre-eclampsia produced by chronic constriction of the aorta in conscious rhesus monkeys. Am J Obstet Gynecol 169:215, 1993.
116. Pijnenborg R, Anthony J, Davey DA, et al: Placental bed spiral arteries in the hypertensive disorders of pregnancy. Br J Obstet Gynaecol 98:648, 1991.
117. Roberts JM, Redman CWG: Pre-eclampsia: More than pregnancy-induced hypertension. Lancet 341:1447, 1993.
118. Khong TY: Acute atherosis in pregnancies complicated by hypertension, small-for-gestational-age infants and diabetes mellitus. Arch Pathol Lab Med 115:722, 1991.
119. Zhou Y, Fisher SJ, Janatpour M, et al: Human cytotrophoblasts adopt a vascular phenotype as they differentiate: A strategy for successful endovascular invasion? J Clin Invest 99:2139, 1997.
120. Zhou Y, Damsky CH, Fisher SJ: Pre-eclampsia is associated with failure of human cytotrophoblasts to mimic a vascular adhesion phenotype: One cause of defective endovascular invasion in this syndrome? J Clin Invest 99:2152, 1997.
121. Lim KH, Zhou Y, Janatpour M, et al: Human cytotrophoblast differentiation/invasion is abnormal in pre-eclampsia. Am J Path 151:1809, 1997.
122. Smith SC, Baker PN, Symonds EM: Placental apoptosis in normal human pregnancy. Am J Obstet Gynecol 177:57, 1997.

123. Allaire AD, Ballenger KA, Wells SR, et al: Placental apoptosis in pre-eclampsia. Obstet Gynecol 96:271, 2000.

124. Ishihara N Matsuo H, Murakoshi H, et al: Increased apoptosis in the syncytiotrophoblast in human term placentas complicated by either pre-eclampsia or intrauterine growth retardation. Am J Obstet Gynecol 186:158, 2002.

125. Downing I, Shepherd GL, Lewis PJ: Reduced prostacyclin production in pre-eclampsia. Lancet 2:1374, 1980.

126. Roberts JM, Taylor RM, Goldfein A: Clinical and biochemical evidence of endothelial cell dysfunction in pre-eclampsia. Am J Hypertens 4:700, 1991.

127. Redman CWG, Denson KW, Bellin LJ, et al: Factor-VII consumption in pre-eclampsia. Lancet 2:1249, 1977.

128. Taylor RN, Crombleholme WR, Friedman SA, et al: High plasma cellular fibronectin levels correlate with biochemical and clinical features of pre-eclampsia but cannot be attributed to hypertension alone. Am J Obstet Gynecol 165:895, 1991.

129. Benigni A, Orisio S, Gaspari F, et al: Evidence against a pathogenetic role for endothelin in pre-eclampsia. Br J Obstet Gynaecol 99: 798, 1992.

130. Branch DW, Dudley DJ, Nutchell MD: Preliminary evidence for homeostatic mechanism regulating endothelin production in pre-eclampsia. Lancet 337:443, 1991.

131. Florijn KW, Derkx FH, Visser W, et al: Elevated plasma levels of endothelin in pre-eclampsia. J Hypertens 9:S166, 1991.

132. Ihara Y, Sagawa N, Hasegawa M, et al: Concentrations of endothelin-1 in maternal and umbilical cord blood at various stages of pregnancy. Cardiovasc Pharmacol 17:S443, 1991.

133. Taylor RN, Varma M, Teng NN, et al: Women with pre-eclampsia have higher plasma endothelin levels than women with normal pregnancies. J Clin Endocrinol Metab 71:1675, 1990.

134. Tsunoda K, Abe K, Yoshinaga K, et al: Maternal and umbilical venous levels of endothelin in women with pre-eclampsia. Hypertension 6:61, 1992.

135. Greenberg SG, Baker RS, Yang D, Clark KE: Effects of continuous infusion of endothelin-1 in pregnant sheep. Hypertension 30:1585, 1997.

136. Pinto A, Sorrentino R, Sorrentino P: EDRF (NO) released by endothelial cells of human umbilical vessels. Am J Obstet Gynecol 164:507, 1991.

137. Cockell AP, Poston L: Flow-mediated vasodilatation is enhanced in normal pregnancy but reduced in pre-eclampsia. Hypertension 30:247, 1997.

138. Deng A, Engels K, Baylis C: Impact of nitric oxide deficiency on blood pressure and glomerular hemodynamic adaptations to pregnancy in the rat. Kidney Int 50:1132, 1996.

139. Raij L: Glomerular thrombosis in pregnancy: Role of the L-arginine-nitric oxide pathway. Kidney Int 45:775, 1994.

140. Davis JR, Giardina JB, Green GM, et al: Reduced endothelial NO-cGMP vascular relaxation pathway during TNF-alpha-induced hypertension in pregnant rats. Am J Physiol Regul Integr Comp Physiol 282:R390, 2002.

141. Fitzgerald DJ, Rocki W, Murray R, et al: Thromboxane A_2 synthesis in pregnancy-induced hypertension. Lancet 335:751, 1990.

142. Lorentzen B, Endresen MJ, Hovig T, et al: Effect of sera from pre-eclampsia in PGI_2 synthesis. Thromb Res 63:363, 1991.

143. Zammit VC, Whitworth JA, Brown MA: Endothelium-derived prostacyclin: Effect of serum from women with normal and hypertensive pregnancy. Clin Sci 82:383, 1992.

144. Haller H, Ziegler EM, Homuth V, et al: Endothelial adhesion molecules and leukocyte integrins in preeclamptic patients. Hypertension 29:291, 1997.

145. Gant NF, Daley GL, Chand S, et al: A study of angiotensin II pressor response throughout primigravid pregnancy. J Clin Invest 52:2682, 1973.

146. Gant NF, Chand S, Worley RJ, et al: A clinical test useful for predicting the development of acute hypertension in pregnancy. Am J Obstet Gynecol 120:1, 1974.

147. AbdAlla S, Lother H, el Massiery A, et al: Increased AT(1) receptor heterodimers in pre-eclampsia mediate enhanced angiotensin II responsiveness. Nat Med 7:999, 2001.

148. Leduc L, Wheeler JM, Kirshon B, et al: Coagulation profile in severe pre-eclampsia. Obstet Gynecol 79:14, 1992.

149. Schrocksnadel H, Sitte B, Steckel-Berger G, et al: Hemolysis in hypertensive disorders of pregnancy. Gynecol Obstet Invest 34:211, 1992.

150. Redman CWG, Bonnar J, Beilin L: Early platelet consumption in pre-eclampsia. BMJ 1:467, 1978.

151. Konijnenberg A, van der Post JA, Mol BW, et al: Can flow cytometric detection of platelet activation early in pregnancy predict the occurrence of pre-eclampsia? A prospective study. Am J Obstet Gynecol 177:434, 1997.

152. Konijnenberg A, Stokkers EW, van der Post JA, et al: Extensive platelet activation in pre-eclampsia compared with normal pregnancy: Enhanced expression of cell adhesion molecules. Am J Obstet Gynecol 176:461, 1997.

153. Austgulen R, Lien E, Vince G, Redman CW: Increased maternal plasma levels of soluble adhesion molecules (ICAM-1 VCAM-1, E-selectin) in pre-eclampsia. Eur J Obstet Gynecol Reprod Biol 71: 53, 1997.

154. Krauss T, Kuhn W, Lakoma C, Augustin HG: Circulating endothelial cell adhesion molecules as diagnostic markers for the early identification of pregnant women at risk for development of pre-eclampsia. Am J Obstet Gynecol 177:443, 1997.

155. Kupferminc MJ, Eldor A, Steinman N, et al: Increased frequency of genetic thrombophilia in women with complications of pregnancy. N Engl J Med 340:9, 1999.

156. Barden A, Ritchie J, Walters B, et al: Study of plasma factors associated with neutrophil activation and lipid peroxidation in pre-eclampsia. Hypertension 38:803, 2001.

157. Zusterzeel PL, Mulder TP, Peters WH, et al: Plasma protein carbonyls in nonpregnant, healthy pregnant and preeclamptic women. Free Radic Res 33:471, 2000.

158. McKinney ET, Shouri R, Hunt RS, et al: Plasma, urinary, and salivary 8-epi-prostaglandin f2alpha levels in normotensive and preeclamptic pregnancies. Am J Obstet Gynecol 183:874, 2000.

159. Barden A, Beilin LJ, Ritchie J, et al: Plasma and urinary 8-isoprostane as an indicator of lipid peroxidation in pre-eclampsia and normal pregnancy. Clin Sci (Lond) 91:711, 1996.

160. Kharb S: Vitamin E and C in pre-eclampsia. Eur J Obstet Gynecol Reprod Biol 93:37, 2000.

161. Bowen RS, Moodley J, Dutton MF, et al: Oxidative stress in pre-eclampsia. Acta Obstet Gynecol Scand 80:719, 2001.

162. Raijmakers MT, Zusterzeel PL, Roes EM, et al: Oxidized and free whole blood thiols in pre-eclampsia. Obstet Gynecol 97:272, 2001.

163. Walsh SW, Vaughan JE, Wang Y: Placental isoprostane is significantly increased in pre-eclampsia. FASEB J 14:1289, 2000.

164. Little RE, Gladen BC: Levels of lipid peroxides in uncomplicated pregnancy: Reprod Toxicol 13:347, 1999.

165. Schiff E, Friedman SA, Stapfer M, et al: Dietary consumption and plasma concentrations of vitamin E in pregnancies complicated by pre-eclampsia. Am J Obstet Gynecol 177:484, 1996.

166. Jain SK, Wise R: Relationship between elevated lipid peroxides, vitamin E deficiency and hypertension in pre-eclampsia. Mol Cell Biochem 151:33, 1995.

167. Uotila JF, Tuimala RJ, Aarnio TM, et al: Findings on lipid peroxidation and antioxidant function in hypertensive complications of pregnancy. Br J Obstet Gynaecol 100:270, 1993.

168. Hubel CA, Kozlov AV, Kagan VE, et al: Decreased transferrin and increased transferrin saturation in sera of women with pre-eclampsia: Implications for oxidative stress. Am J Obstet Gynecol 175:692, 1996.

169. Regan CL, Levine RJ, Baird DD, et al: No evidence for lipid peroxidation in severe pre-eclampsia. Am J Obstet Gynecol 185:572, 2001.

170. Chappell LC, Seed PT, Briley AL, et al: Effect of antioxidants on the occurrence of pre-eclampsia in women at increased risk: A randomised trial. Lancet 357,131, 1999.

171. Pascoal, Istenio F, Lindheimer, et al: Pre-eclampsia selectively impairs endothelium-dependent relaxation and leads to oscillatory activity in small omental arteries. J Clin Invest 101:464, 1998.

172. Sakai K, Imaizumi T, Maeda H, et al: Venous distensibility during pregnancy: Comparisons between normal pregnancy and pre-eclampsia. Hypertension 24:461, 1994.

173. Schobel H, Fischer T, Heuszer K, et al: Pre-eclampsia: A state of sympathetic overactivity. N Engl J Med 335:1480, 1996.

174. Hill LM: Metabolism of uric acid in normal and toxemic pregnancy. Mayo Clin Proc 53:743, 1978.

175. Redman CWG, Bonnar J: Plasma urate changes in pre-eclampsia. Br Med J 1:484, 1978.

176. Ferris TF, Gorden P: The effect of angiotensin and norepinephrine upon urate clearance in man. Am J Med 4:359, 1968.

177. Stander HJ, Cadden JF: Blood chemistry in pre-eclampsia and eclampsia. Am J Obstet Gynecol 28:856, 1934.

178. Steele TH: Evidence for altered renal urate reabsorption during changes in volume of the extracellular fluid. J Lab Clin Med 74:288, 1969.

179. Fadel HE, Northrop G, Misenheimer HR: Hyperuricemia in pre-eclampsia: A reappraisal. Am J Obstet Gynecol 125:640, 1976.
180. Gallery EDM: Volume homeostasis in normal and hypertensive human pregnancy. Semin Nephrol 4:221, 1984.
181. Brown MA, Zammit VC, Lowe SA: Capillary permeability and extracellular fluid volumes in pregnancy-induced hypertension. Clin Sci 77:599, 1989.
182. Brown MA, Zammit VC, Mitar DM: Extracellular fluid volume in pregnancy-induced hypertension. Hypertension 10:61, 1992.
183. Fadnes HO, Oian P: Transcapillary fluid balance and plasma volume regulation: A review. Obstet Gynecol Surv 44:769, 1989.
184. August P, Marcaccio B, Gertner JM, et al: Abnormal 1,25-dihydroxy-vitamin D metabolism in pre-eclampsia. Am J Obstet Gynecol 166:1295, 1992.
185. Tanfield PA, Ales KL, Resnick LM, et al: Hypocalciuria in pre-eclampsia. N Engl J Med 316:715, 1989.
186. Hays PM, Cruikshank DP, Dunn LJ: Plasma volume determination in normal and pre-eclamptic pregnancies. Am J Obstet Gynecol 151:958, 1985.
187. Cohn JN: Relationship of plasma volume changes to resistance and capacitance vessel effects of sympathomimetic amine and angiotensin in man. Clin Sci 30:267, 1966.
188. Tarazi RC, Dustan HP, Frohlich ED: Relation of plasma to intersti-tial fluid volume in essential hypertension. Circulation 40:357, 1969.
189. Arias F: Expansion of intravascular volume and fetal outcome in patients with chronic hypertension and pregnancy. Am J Obstet Gynecol 123:610, 1975.
190. Bauman WA, Maimen M, Langer O: An association between hyper-insulinemia and hypertension during the third trimester of preg-nancy. Am J Obstet Gynecol 159:446, 1988.
191. Ono H, Umeda F, Inoguch T, et al: Glucose inhibits prostacyclin production by cultured aortic endothelial cells. Thromb Haemost 60:174, 1988.
192. Tesformarian B, Brown ML, Deyhin D, et al: Elevated glucose pro-motes generation of endothelium derived vasoconstrictor prostanoids in rabbit aorta. J Clin Invest 85:929, 1990.
193. Van Assche FA, Spitz B, Hanssens M, et al: Increased thromboxane formation in diabetic pregnancy as a possible contribution to pre-eclampsia. Am J Obstet Gynecol 168:84, 1993.
194. Lang RM, Pridjian G, Feldman T: Left ventricular mechanics in pre-eclampsia. Am Heart J 121:1768, 1991.
195. Mabie WC, Ratts TE, Sibai BM: The central hemodynamics of severe pre-eclampsia. Am J Obstet Gynecol 161:1443, 1989.
196. Sibai BM, Mabie BC, Harvey CJ: Pulmonary edema in pre-eclamp-sia. Am J Obstet Gynecol 156:1174, 1987.
197. Zinaman M, Rubin J, Lindheimer MD: Serial plasma oncotic pres-sure levels during and after delivery in severe pre-eclampsia. Lancet 1:1245, 1985.
198. Lunell NO, Nylund L, Lewander R, et al: Uteroplacental blood flow in pre-eclampsia in measurements with indium 113. Clin Exp Hypertens 1:105, 1982.
199. Lohlein M: Zur Pathogenese der Nierenkrankheiten Nephritis und Nephrose mit besonderer Besichtigung der Nephropathia gravi-darum. Dtsch Med Wochenschr 44:1187, 1918.
200. Fahr T: Über Marenveranderungen bei Eklampsie. Zentralbl Gynaekol 44:991, 1920.
201. Farquhar MG: Review of normal and pathologic glomerular ultra-structure. In Metcalf J (ed): Proceedings of the Tenth Annual Conference on the Nephrotic Syndrome. New York, National Kidney Disease Foundation, 1959.
202. Spargo B, McCartney CO, Winemiller R: Glomerular capillary endotheliosis in toxemia of pregnancy. Arch Pathol 68:593, 1959.
203. Pirani CL, Pollak VE, Lannigan R, et al: The renal glomerular lesions of pre-eclampsia. Am J Obstet Gynecol 87:1047, 1963.
204. Altchek A: Electron microscopy of renal biopsies in toxemia of pregnancy. JAMA 175:791, 1961.
205. Kincaid-Smith P: The renal lesion of pre-eclampsia revisited. Am J Kidney Dis 17:144, 1991.
206. Bis KA, Waxman B: Rupture of the liver associated with pregnancy: A review of the literature and report of 2 cases. Obstet Gynecol Surv 31:763, 1976.
207. Browne CH, Hanson GC, DeJude LR, et al: Rupture of sub-capsular haematoma of the liver in a case of eclampsia. Br J Surg 62:237, 1975.
208. Sheehan HL, Lynch JB: Pathology of Toxemia of Pregnancy. New York, Longman, 1973.
209. Arias F, Mancilla-Jimenez R: Hepatic fibrinogen deposits in pre-eclampsia. N Engl J Med 295:578, 1976.
210. Amon E, Allen SR, Petrie RH, et al: Acute fatty liver of pregnancy associated with pre-eclampsia. Am J Perinatol 8:278, 1991.
211. Hatfield AK, Stein JH, Greenberger NJ, et al: Idiopathic acute fatty liver of pregnancy: Death from extrahepatic manifestations. Am J Dig Dis 17:167, 1972.
212. Killam AP, Dillard SH, Patton RC, et al: Pregnancy induced hypertension complicated by acute liver disease and dissemi-nated intravascular coagulation. Am J Obstet Gynecol 123:823, 1975.
213. Minakami H, Oha N, Sato T, et al: Pre-eclampsia: A microvascular fat disease of the liver? Am J Obstet Gynecol 159:1043, 1988.
214. Riely CA, Lathan PS, Romero R: Acute fatty liver of pregnancy. Ann Intern Med 106:703, 1987.
215. Robertson WB, Khong TY, Brosens I, et al: The placental bed biopsy: A review of three European Centers. Am J Obstet Gynecol 155:401, 1986.
216. Brown CEL, Purdy P, Cunningham FG: Head computed tomo-graphic scan in women with eclampsia. Am J Obstet Gynecol 159:915, 1988.
217. Donaldson JO: Neurologic complications. In Burrow GN, Ferris TF (eds): Medical Complications During Pregnancy, 3d ed. Philadelphia, WB Saunders, 1988, p 485.
218. Bauer TW, Moore GW, Hutchins GM: Morphologic evidence for coronary artery spasm in eclampsia. Circulation 65:255, 1982.
219. Barton JR, Hiett AK, O'Connor WN, et al: Endomyocardial ultra-structural findings in pre-eclampsia. Am J Obstet Gynecol 165:389, 1991.
220. Gallery ED, Ross M, Gyory AZ: Urinary red blood cell and cast excretion in normal and hypertensive human pregnancy. Am J Obstet Gynecol 168:67, 1993.
221. Ramos JG, Martins-Costa SH, Mathias MM, et al: Urinary pro-tein/creatinine ratio in hypertensive pregnant women. Hypertens Pregnancy 18:209, 1999.
222. Miles JF, Martin JN, Blake PG: Postpartum eclampsia a recurring perinatal dilemma. Obstet Gynecol 76:328, 1990.
223. National High Blood Pressure Education Program Working Group: Report on high blood pressure in pregnancy. Am J Obstet Gynecol 163:1691, 1990.
224. ACOG Technical Bulletin: Hypertension in pregnancy. Int J Gynecol Obstet 53:175, 1996.
225. Trupin LS, Simon LP, Eskenazi B: Change in paternity: A risk factor for pre-eclampsia in multiparas. Epidemiology 7:240, 1996.
226. Robillard PY, Hulsey TC, Alexander GR, et al: Paternity patterns and risk of pre-eclampsia in the last pregnancy in multiparas. J Reprod Immunol 24:1, 1993.
227. Skjaerven R, Wilcox AF, Lie RT: The interval between pregnancies and the risk of pre-eclampsia. N Engl J Med 346:33, 2002.
228. Innes KE, Wimsatt JH, McDuffie R: Relative glucose tolerance and subsequent development of hypertension pregnancy. Obstet Gynecol 97:905, 2001.
229. Chesley LC, Cooper DW: Genetics of hypertension in pregnancy. Br J Obstet Gynaecol 93:898, 1986.
230. Humphries J: Occurrence of hypertensive toxemia of pregnancy in mother-daughter pairs. Bull Johns Hopkins Hosp 107:271, 1960.
231. Dawson LM, Parfrey PS, Hefferton D: Familial risk of pre-eclamp-sia in Newfoundland: A population-based study. J Am Soc Nephrol 13:1901, 2002.
232. Esplin MS, Fausett MB, Fraser A, et al: Paternal and maternal com-ponents of the predisposition to pre-eclampsia. N Engl J Med 344:867, 2001.
233. Lachmeijer AM, Arngrimsson R, Bastiaans EJ, et al: A genome-wide scan for pre-eclampsia in the Netherlands. Eur J Hum Genet 9:758, 2001.
234. Kobashi G, Yamada H, Ohta K, et al: Endothelial nitric oxide syn-thase gene (NOS3) variant and hypertension in pregnancy. Am J Med Genet 103:241, 2002.
235. Geller DS, Farhi A, Pinderton N, et al: Activating mineralocorticoid receptor mutation in hypertension exacerbated by pregnancy. Science 289:119, 2000.
236. Chesley LC: The remote prognosis of eclamptic women. Am Heart J 93:407, 1977.
237. Ward K, Hata A, Jeunemartre X, et al: A molecular variant of angiotensinogen associated with pre-eclampsia. Nat Genet 4:59, 1993.

238. Arngrimsson R, Hayward C, Nadaud S, et al: Evidence for a familial pregnancy-induced hypertension locus in the eNOS-gene region. Am J Hum Gen 61:354, 1997.

239. Marcoux S, Brisson J, Fabia J: The effect of cigarette smoking on the risk of pre-eclampsia and gestational hypertension. Am J Epidemiol 130:950, 1989.

240. Taylor RN: Review: Immunobiology of pre-eclampsia. Am J Reprod Immunol 37:79, 1997.

241. Smith GN, Walker M, Tessier JL, Millar KG: Increased incidence of pre-eclampsia in women conceiving by intrauterine insemination with donor versus partner sperm for treatment of primary infertility. Am J Obstet Gynecol 177:455, 1997.

242. Arulkumaran S, Gibb DM, Rauff M, et al: Transient blindness associated with pregnancy-induced hypertension: Case reports. Br J Obstet Gynaecol 92:847, 1985.

243. Hankins GDV, Wendel GD, Cunningham FG, et al: Longitudinal evaluation of hemodynamic changes in eclampsia. Am J Obstet Gynecol 150:506, 1984.

244. Goodlin RC: Pre-eclampsia as the great imposter. Am J Obstet Gynecol 164:1577, 1991.

245. Martin JN, Blake PG, Perry KG, et al: The natural history of HELLP syndrome. Am J Obstet Gynecol 164:1500, 1991.

246. Long RG, Scheuer PJ, Sherlock S: Pre-eclampsia presenting with deep jaundice. J Clin Pathol 30:212, 1977.

247. Dani R, Mendes GS, Medeiros JL, et al: Study of the liver changes occurring in pre-eclampsia and their possible pathogenetic connection with acute fatty liver of pregnancy. Am J Gastroent 91:292, 1996.

248. Holzbach RT: Jaundice in pregnancy. Am J Med 61:367, 1976.

249. Grunfeld JP, Ganeval D, Bournerias F: Acute renal failure in pregnancy. Kidney Int 18:179, 1980.

250. Kaplan MM: Acute fatty liver of pregnancy. N Engl J Med 313:367, 1985.

251. Mabie WC: Acute fatty liver of pregnancy. Gastroenterol Clin North Am 21:951, 1992.

252. Burroughs AK, Seong NGH, Dojcinov DM, et al: Idiopathic acute fatty liver of pregnancy in 12 patients. Q J Med 51:481, 1982.

253. Recant L, Lacy P: Clinicopathologic conference: Fulminating liver disease in a pregnant woman. Am J Med 35:231, 1963.

254. Ober WB, LeCompte PM: Acute fatty metamorphosis of the liver associated with pregnancy: A distinctive lesion. Am J Med 19:743, 1955.

255. Hou SH, Levin S, Ahola S, et al: Acute fatty liver of pregnancy: Survival with early cesarean section. Dig Dis Sci 29:449, 1984.

256. Durr JA, Haggard JG, Hunt JM, et al: Diabetes insipidus in pregnancy associated with high vasopressinase activity. N Engl J Med 316:1070, 1987.

257. Kreg J, Katz VL, Bower WA: Transient diabetes insipidus of pregnancy. Obstet Gynecol Surv 44:789, 1989.

258. Davison JM, Shiells EA, Barron WM: Changes in the metabolic clearance of AVP and plasma vasopressinase throughout human pregnancy. J Clin Invest 83:1313, 1989.

259. Davies AM: Geographical epidemiology of the toxemias of pregnancy. Isr J Med Sci 7:753, 1971.

260. Imperiale TF, Petrulis AS: A meta-analysis of low-dose aspirin for the prevention of pregnancy-induced hypertensive disease. JAMA 266:260, 1991.

261. CLASP Collaborative Group: CLASP: A randomized trial of low-dose aspirin for the prevention and treatment of pre-eclampsia among 9364 pregnant women. Lancet 343:619, 1994.

262. Italian Study of Asprin in Pregnancy: Low-dose aspirin in prevention and treatment of intrauterine growth retardation and pregnancy-induced hypertension. Lancet 341:396, 1993.

263. ECPPA: Randomized trial of low dose aspirin for the prevention of maternal and fetal complications in high risk pregnant women. Br J Obstet Gynaecol 103:39, 1996.

264. Caritis S, Sibai B, Hauth J, et al: Low dose aspirin to prevent pre-eclampsia in women at high risk. N Engl J Med 338:701, 1998.

265. CLASP Collaborative Group: Low dose aspirin in pregnancy and early childhood development: Follow up of the Collaborative Low Dose Aspirin Study in Pregnancy. Br J Obstet Gynecol 102:861, 1995.

266. Sibai BM, Caritis SN, Thom E, et al: Low-dose aspirin in nulliparous women: Safety of continuous epidural block and correlation between bleeding time and maternal-neonatal bleeding complications. National Institute of Child Health and Human Developmental Maternal-Fetal Medicine Network. Am J Obstet Gynecol 172:1553, 1995.

267. Hermida RC, Ayala DE, Iglesias M, et al: Hypertension 30:589, 1997.

268. Knight M, Duley L, Henderson-Smart DJ, et al: Antiplatelet agents for preventing and treating pre-eclampsia. Cochrane Database Syst Rev 2:CD000492, 2000.

269. McCarron DA: Calcium metabolism and hypertension. Kidney Int 35:717, 1989.

270. Belizan JM, Villar J, Gonzalez L, et al: Calcium supplementation to prevent hypertension disorders of pregnancy. N Engl J Med 325:1399, 1991.

271. Kawasaki N, Matsui K, Ito M: Effect of calcium supplementation on the vascular sensitivity to angiotensin II in pregnant women. Am J Obstet Gynecol 153:576, 1985.

272. Bucher HC, Guyatt GH, Cook RJ, et al: Effect of calcium supplementation on pregnancy-induced hypertension and pre-eclampsia: A meta-analysis of randomized controlled trials. JAMA 275:1113, 1996.

273. Levine RJ, Hauth JC, Curet LB, et al: Trial of calcium to prevent pre-eclampsia. N Engl J Med 337:69, 1997.

274. Atallah AN, Hofmeyr GJ, Duley L: Calcium supplementation during pregnancy for preventing hypertensive disorders and relate problems. Cochrane Database Syst Rev 1:CD001059, 2002.

275. Der Simonian R, Levine RJ: Resolving discrepancies between a meta-analysis and a subsequent large controlled trial. JAMA 282:664, 1999.

276. Gertner JM, Coustan DR, Kliger AS, et al: Pregnancy as a state of physiologic absorptive hypercalciuria. Am J Med 81:451, 1986.

277. Rey E, LeLorier J, Burgess E, et al: Report of the Canadian Hypertension Society Consensus Conference: 3. Pharmacologic treatment of hypertension disorders in pregnancy. Can Med Assoc J 157:1245, 1997.

278. Moretti MM, Fairlie FM, Akl S: The effect of nifedipine on fetal and placental doppler wave forms in pre-eclampsia. Am J Obstet Gynecol 163:1844, 1990.

279. Montan S, Ingemarsson I, Marsal K, Sjoberg NO: Randomised controlled trial of atenolol and pindolol in human pregnancy: Effects on fetal haemodynamics. BMJ 304:946, 1992.

280. Rubin PC, Butters L, Clark DM, et al: Placebo-controlled trial of atenolol in treatment of pregnancy associated hypertension. Lancet 1:431, 1983.

281. Collins R, Yusuf S, Peto R: Overview of randomised trials of diuretics in pregnancy. BMJ 290:17, 1985.

282. Shoemaker CT, Meyers M: Sodium nitroprusside for control of severe hypertensive disease of pregnancy: Case report and discussion of potential toxicity. Am J Obstet Gynecol 149:171, 1984.

283. Sibai BM: Eclampsia. VI. Maternal-perinatal outcome in 254 consecutive cases. Am J Obstet Gynecol 163:1049, 1990.

284. Watson KV, Moldow CF, Ogburn PL, et al: Magnesium sulfate: Rationale for its use in pre-eclampsia. Proc Natl Acad Sci U S A 83:1075, 1986.

285. McCubbin JM, Sibai BM, Ardella TN, Anderson GD: Cardiopulmonary arrest due to acute maternal hypermagnesaemia [letter]. Lancet 1:1058, 1981.

286. Richards A, Stather-Dunn L, Moodley J: Cardiopulmonary arrest after administration of $MgSO_4$. S Afr Med J 67:145, 1985.

287. Herpolsteimer A, Brady R, Yancey MK, et al: Pulmonary function of pre-eclamptic women receiving intravenous $MgSO_4$ for seizure prophylaxis. Obstet Gynecol 78:241, 1991.

288. The Magpie Trial Collaborative Group: Do women with pre-eclampsia, and their babies, benefit from magnesium sulphate? The Magpie Trial: A randomised placebo-controlled trial. Lancet 359:1877, 2002.

289. Lucas MJ, Leveno KJ, Cunningham FG: A comparison of magnesium sulfate with phenytoin for the prevention of eclampsia. N Engl J Med 333:201, 1995.

290. Sibai BM, Ald S, Fairlie F: Management of severe pre-eclampsia in the second trimester. Am J Obstet Gynecol 163:773, 1990.

291. Ahoha RA, Mabie WC, Sibai BM, et al: Labetalol does not decrease placental perfusion in the hypertensive term pregnant rat. Am J Obstet Gynecol 160:480, 1989.

292. Ashe RG, Moodley J, Richards AM: Comparison of labetalol and hydralazine in hypertensive emergencies of pregnancy. S Afr Med J 7:384, 1987.

293. Eisenach JC, Mandell G, Dervas DM: Maternal and fetal effects of labetalol in pregnant ewes. Anesthesiology 74:292, 1991.

294. Jouppila P, Kirkinen P, Koivula A, Ylikorkala O: Labetalol does not alter the placental and fetal blood flow or maternal prostanoids in pre-eclampsia. Br J Obstet Gynaecol 93:543, 1986.

295. Morgan MA, Silavrin SL, Donner KJ, et al: Effect of labetalol on uterine blood flow and cardiovascular hemodynamics in the hypertensive baboon. Am J Obstet Gynecol 168:1504, 1993.

296. Pirkonen JP, Eskhole RV: Labetalol in pre-eclampsia: Effect on maternal hemodynamics and uterine and fetal flow velocity waveforms. J Perinat Med 19:167, 1991.

297. Blake S, MacDonald D: The prevention of the maternal manifestations of pre-eclampsia by intensive antihypertensive treatment. Br J Obstet Gynaecol 98:244, 1991.

298. Odendaal H, Pattinson RC, Dutoit R: Aggressive or expectant management with severe pre-eclampsia between 28–34 weeks. Obstet Gynecol 76:1070, 1991.

299. Phippard AF, Fischer WE, Horvath JS, et al: Early blood pressure control improves pregnancy outcome in primigravida women with mild hypertension. Med J Aust 154:378, 1991.

300. Sibai BM, Anderson GD: Pregnancy outcome of intensive therapy in severe hypertension in the first trimester. Obstet Gynecol 67:517, 1986.

301. Sibai BM, Mabie BC, Shamsa F, et al: A comparison of no medication versus methyldopa or labetalol in chronic hypertension during pregnancy. Am J Obstet Gynecol 62:960, 1990.

302. Wichman K, Ryden G, Karlberg BE: A placebo controlled trial of metoprolol in the treatment of hypertension in pregnancy. Scand J Clin Lab Invest 169:80, 1984.

303. Ferrer RL, Sibai BM, Chiquette E, et al: Evidence report on management of chronic hypertension during pregnancy. Evidence Report/Technology Assessment No. 14. AHRQ Publication no. 00-E11. Rockville, MD: Department of Health and Human Services, Agency for Health Care Research and Quality, 2000.

304. Magee LA, Ornstein MP, von Dadelszen P: Fortnightly review: Management of hypertension in pregnancy. BMJ 318:1332, 1999.

305. Sibai BM: Treatment of hypertension in pregnant women. N Engl J Med 335:257, 1996.

306. Buttar HS: An overview of the influence of ACE inhibitors on fetal-placental circulation and perinatal development. Mol Cell Biochem 176:61, 1997.

307. Post-marketing surveillance for angiotensin-converting enzyme inhibitor use during the first trimester of pregnancy—United States, Canada, and Israel, 1987–1995. MMWR Morb Mortal Wkly Rep 46:240, 1997.

308. Saji H, Yamanaka M, Hagiwara A, et al: Losartan and fetal toxic effects. Lancet 357:363, 2001.

309. Martinovic J, Benachi A, Laurent N, et al: Fetal toxic effects and angiotensin-II-receptor antagonists. Lancet 358:241, 2001.

310. Chung NA, Lip GY, Beevers M, et al: Angiotensin-II-receptor inhibitors in pregnancy. Lancet 357:1620, 2001.

311. Briggs GG, Nageotee MP: Fatal fetal outcome with the combined use of valsartan and atenolol. Ann Pharmacother 35:859, 2001.

312. Collins R, Wallenburg HCS: Pharmacological prevention and treatment of hypertensive disorders of pregnancy. In Chalmers I, Enkin M, Keirse MJ (eds): Effective Care in Pregnancy and Childbirth. Oxford, Oxford University Press, 1989, p 512.

313. Peters JP: Toxemias of pregnancy. Yale J Biol Med 9:311, 1937.

314. Abalos E, Duley L, Steyn DW, et al: Antihypertensive therapy for mild to moderate hypertension during pregnancy. Cochrane Database Syst Rev 2:CD0002252, 2001.

315. Chesley LC, Annitto JE: Pregnancy in a patient with hypertensive disease. Am J Obstet Gynecol 53:372, 1947.

316. Karlson K, Ljungblad U, Lundgren Y: Blood flow of the reproductive system in renal hypertensive rats during pregnancy. Am J Obstet Gynecol 142:1039, 1982.

317. Chia S, Redman CWG: Prognosis for pre-eclampsia complicated by 5 gms or more of proteinuria/24 hrs. Eur J Obstet Gynecol Reprod Biol 43:9, 1992.

318. Ferrazzani S, Caruso A, DeCarolis S, et al: Proteinuria and outcome of 444 pregnancies complicated by hypertension. Am J Obstet Gynecol 162:366, 1990.

319. Stettler RW, Cunningham FG: Natural history of chronic proteinuria complicating pregnancy. Am J Obstet Gynecol 167:1219, 1992.

320. Sibai BM, Grossman RA, Grossman HG: Effects of diuretics on plasma volume in pregnancies with hypertension. Am J Obstet Gynecol 150:831, 1984.

321. von Dadelszen P, Ornstein MP, Bull SB, et al: Fall in mean arterial pressure and fetal growth restriction in pregnancy hypertension: A meta-analysis. Lancet 355:87, 2000.

322. Magee LA, Duley L: Oral beta-blockers for mild to moderate hypertension during pregnancy. Cochrane Database Syst Rev 4: CD0002863, 2000.

323. Fabregues G, Alvarez L, Varas-Juri P, et al: Effectiveness of atenolol in the treatment of hypertension during pregnancy. Hypertension 19:II-129, 1992.

324. Lunell NO, Persson B, Aaron G, et al: Circulatory and metabolic effects of acute beta 1-blockade in severe pre-eclampsia. Acta Obstet Gynecol Scand 58:443, 1979.

325. Butters L, Kennedy S, Rubin PC: Atenolol in essential hypertension during pregnancy. Br Med J 301:587, 1990.

326. Lip GY, Beevers M, Churchill D, et al: Effect of atenolol on birth weight. Am J Cardiol 79:1436, 1997.

327. ACOG Practice Bulletin No. 29: Chronic hypertension in pregnancy. Obstet Gynecol 98:177, 2001.

328. Ounsted M, Cockburn J, Moar VA, et al: Maternal hypertension with superimposed pre-eclampsia: Effects on child development at 7 1/2 years. Br J Obstet Gynaecol 90:644, 1983.

329. el-Qarmalawi AM, Morsy AH, al-Fadly A, et al: Labetalol vs. methyldopa in the treatment of pregnancy-induced hypertension. Int J Gynaecol Obstet 49:125, 1995.

330. Horvath JS, Phippard A, Karda A: Clonidine: A safe and effective antihypertensive agent in pregnancy. Obstet Gynecol 66: 634, 1985.

331. Huisjes HJ, Hadders-Algra M, Towwen BCI: Is clonidine a behavioral teratogen in the human? Early Hum Dev 14:43, 1986.

332. Rubin PC, Butters L, Low RA: Clinical pharmacological studies with prazosin during pregnancy complicated by hypertension. Br J Clin Pharmacol 16:543, 1983.

333. Harake B, Gilbert RD, Ashwal S, et al: Nifedipine: Effects on fetal and maternal hemodynamics in pregnant sheep. Am J Obstet Gynecol 157:1003, 1987.

334. Golichowski AM, Tzeng DY: Binding of the calcium antagonist nitrendipine to human myometrial plasmalemma. Biol Reprod 33:1105, 1985.

335. Papatsonis DN, Lok CA, Bos JM, et al: Calcium channel blockers in the management of preterm labor and hypertension in pregnancy. J Obstet Gynecol Reprod Biol 97:122, 2001.

336. Gulmezoglu AM, Hofmey GJ: Calcium channel blockers for potential impaired fetal growth. Cochrane Database Syst Rev 2:CD000049, 2000.

337. Janssens D. Prevention of low birth weight by flunarizine given to smoking mothers. In Proceedings of 11th World Congress of Gynecology and Obstetrics, Berlin, September 15–20, 1985. Springer Verlag, 1986, p 397.

338. Ismail AA, Medhat I, Tawfic TA, et al : Evaluation of calcium-antagonist (nifedipine) in the treatment of pre-eclampsia. Int J Gynaecol Obstet 40:39, 1993.

339. Jegasothy R, Paranthaman S: Sublingual nifedipine compared with intravenous hydralazine in the acute treatment of severe hypertension in pregnancy: Potential for use in rural practice. J Obstet Gynaecol Res 22:21, 1996.

340. Fenakel K, Fenakel G, Appelman Z, et al: Nifedipine in the treatment of severe pre-eclampsia 77:331, 1991.

341. Hall DR, Odendaal HJ, Steyn DW, et al: Nifedipine or prazosin as a second agent to control early severe hypertension in pregnancy: A randomised controlled trial. Br J Obstet Gynaecol 107:759, 2000.

342. Scardo JA, Vermillion ST, Newman RB, et al: A randomized, double-blind, hemodynamic evaluation of nifedipine and labetalol in preeclamptic hypertensive emergencies. Am J Obstet Gynecol 181: 862, 1999.

343. Ciraru-Vigneron C, Pruna A, Minta PH, et al: Comparison of nifedipine and atenolol in treatment of moderate pregnancy-hypertension. Perugia, Italy, VII World Congress of Hypertension in Pregnancy, 1990.

344. van Schie DL, de Jeu RM, Steyn DW, et al: The optimal dosage of ketanserin for patients with severe hypertension in pregnancy. Eur J Obstet Gynecol Reprod Biol 102:161, 2002.

345. Steyn DW, Odendaal JH: Blood pressure patterns in pregnant patients on oral ketanserin. Cardiovasc J S Afr 12:82, 2001.

346. Bolte AC, van Eyck J, Gaffar SF, et al: Ketanserin for the treatment of pre-eclampsia. J Perinat Med 29:14, 2001.

347. Bolte AC, van Eyck J, Kanhai HH, et al: Ketanserin versus dihydralazine in the management of severe early-onset pre-eclampsia: Maternal outcome. Am J Obstet Gynecol 180:371, 1999.

348. Bolte AC, van Eyck J, Strack van Schijndel RJ, et al: The haemodynamic effects of ketanserin versus dihydralazine in severe early-onset hypertension in pregnancy. Br J Obstet Gynaecol 105:723, 1998.

349. Rossouw HJ, Howarth G, Odendaal HJ: Ketanserin and hydralazine in hypertension in pregnancy: A randomised double-blind trial. S Afr Med J 85:525, 1995.

350. Steyn DW, Odendaal HJ: Randomised controlled trial of ketanserin and aspirin in prevention of pre-eclampsia. Lancet 350:1267, 1997.

351. Crowther CA, Boumeester AM, Ashurst NM: Does admission to hospital for bed rest prevent disease progression or improve fetal outcome in pregnancy complicated by nonproteinuric hypertension? Br J Obstet Gynaecol 99:13, 1991.

352. Tuffnell DJ, Lilford RJ, Buchan PC, et al: Randomised controlled trial of day care for hypertension in pregnancy. Lancet 339:224, 1992.

353. Landesman R, Halpern M, Knapp RC: Renal artery lesions associated with the toxemias of pregnancy. Obstet Gynecol 18:645, 1961.

354. Heyborne KD, Schultz MF, Goodlin RC, et al: Renal artery stenosis during pregnancy. Obstet Gynecol Surv 46:509, 1991.

355. Sellors L, Siamopoulous K, Wilkenson R: Prognosis for pregnancy after correction of renovascular hypertension. Nephron 39:280, 1985.

356. Coen G, Cugini P, Gerlini G, et al: Successful treatment of long-standing severe hypertension and captopril during a twin pregnancy. Nephron 40:498, 1985.

357. Millar JA, Wilson PD, Morrison N: Management of severe hypertension in pregnancy by a combined drug regimen including captopril: Case report. N Z Med J 96:796, 1983.

358. Neerhof MG, Shlossman PA, Poll DS, et al: Idiopathic aldosteronism in pregnancy. Obstet Gynecol 78:489, 1991.

359. Hillestad L: Aortic coarctation and pregnancy. Acta Obstet Gynecol Scand 51:95, 1972.

360. Easterling TR, Carlson K, Benedette TJ, et al: Hemodynamics associated with the diagnosis and treatment of pheochromocytoma in pregnancy. Am J Perinatol 9:462, 1992.

361. Feldman JM: Adult respiratory distress syndrome in a pregnant patient with a pheochromocytoma. J Surg Oncol 29:5, 1985.

362. Harper MA, Murnaghen GA, Kennedy L, et al: Pheochromocytoma in pregnancy. Br J Obstet Gynaecol 96:594, 1989.

363. Lyons CW, Colmargen GH: Medical management of pheochromocytoma in pregnancy. Obstet Gynecol 72:450, 1988.

364. Venuto R, Burnstein P, Schneider R: Pheochromocytoma: Antepartum diagnosis and management with tumor resection in the puerperium. Am J Obstet Gynecol 150:431, 1984.

365. Cunningham FG: Urinary tract infections complicating pregnancy. Baillieres Clin Obstet Gynaecol 1:891, 1987.

366. Whalley PJ: Bacteriuria of pregnancy. Am J Obstet Gynecol 47:723, 1967.

367. Kass EH: Infectious diseases and perinatal morbidity. Yale J Biol Med 55:231, 1982.

368. Gilstrap LC, Leveno KJ, Cunningham FG, et al: Renal infection and pregnancy outcome. Am J Obstet Gynecol 141:709, 1981.

369. Sacks SH, Jones KV, Roberts R, et al: Effect of symptomless bacteriuria in childhood on subsequent pregnancy. Lancet 2:991, 1987.

370. Davison JM, Sprott MS, Selkon JB: The effect of covert bacteriuria in schoolgirls on renal function at 18 years and during pregnancy. Lancet 2:651, 1984.

371. Smaill F: Antibiotics for asymptomatic bacteriuria in pregnancy. Cochrane Database Syst Rev 2:CD000490, 2001.

372. Hanis RE, Gilstcap LC: Cystitis during pregnancy: A distinct clinical entity. Obstet Gynecol 57:578, 1981.

373. Bailey RR, Peddie BA, Bishop V: Comparison of single dose with a five-day course of trimethoprim for asymptomatic (correct) bacteriuria of pregnancy. N Z Med J 99:501, 1986.

374. Olsen L, Nielsen IK, Zachariassen A, et al: Single-dose versus six-day therapy with sulfamethizole for asymptomatic bacteriuria during pregnancy: A prospective randomized study. Dan Med Bull 36:486, 1989.

375. Vercaigne LM, Zhanel GG: Recommended treatment for urinary tract infection in pregnancy. Ann Pharmacother 28:248, 1994.

376. Wright A, Steele P, Bennett JR, et al: Urinary excretion of albumin in normal pregnancy. Br J Obstet Gynecol 94:408, 1987.

377. Kuo VS, Koumantakis G, Gallery ED: Proteinuria and its assessment in normal and hypertensive pregnancy. Am J Obstet Gynecol 167:723, 1992.

378. Higby K, Suiter CR, Phelps JY, et al: Normal values of urinary albumin and total protein excretion during pregnancy. Am J Obstet Gynecol 171:984, 1994.

379. Nesselhut T, Rath W, Grospietsch G, et al: Urinary protein electrophoresis profile in normal and hypertensive pregnancies. Arch Gynecol Obstet 246:97, 1989.

380. Robert M, Sepandj F, Liston RM, Dooley KC: Random protein-creatinine ratio for the quantitation of proteinuria in pregnancy. Obstet Gynecol 90:893, 1997.

381. Kassirer JP: Is renal biopsy necessary for optimal management of the idiopathic nephrotic syndrome? Kidney Int 24:561, 1983.

382. Levey AS, Lau J, Pauker SG, et al: Idiopathic nephrotic syndrome: Puncturing the biopsy myth. Ann Intern Med 107:697, 1987.

383. Packham D, Fairley KF: Renal biopsy: Indications and complications in pregnancy. Br J Obstet Gynaecol 94:935, 1987.

384. Lindheimer JD, Katz AI: Gestation in women with kidney disease: Prognosis and management. Baillieres Clin Obstet Gynaecol 1:921, 1987.

385. Paller MS: Pathophysiology of acute renal failure. *In* Greenberg A (ed): National Kidney Foundation Kidney Diseases Primer. Orlando, FL, National Kidney Foundation, 1994, p 126.

386. Stratta P, Besso L, Canavese C, et al: Is pregnancy-related acute renal failure a disappearing clinical entity? Renal Fail 18:575, 1996.

387. Sibai BM, Ramadan MK: Acute renal failure in pregnancies complicated by hemolysis, elevated liver enzymes, and low platelets. Am J Obstet Gynecol 168:1682, 1993.

388. Kelleher SP, Berl T: Acute renal failure in pregnancy. Semin Nephrol 1:61, 1981.

389. Kleinknecht D, Grunfeld JP, Cia Gomez P, et al: Diagnostic procedures and long-term prognosis in bilateral renal cortical necrosis. Kidney Int 4:390, 1973.

390. Papo J, Aviram A, Peer G, et al: Acute renal cortical necrosis as revealed by computerized tomography. Isr J Med Sci 21:862, 1985.

391. Conger JD, Falk SA, Guggenheim SJ: Glomerular dynamics and morphologic changes in the generalized Shwartzman reaction in postpartum rats. J Clin Invest 67:1334, 1981.

392. Bonar J: Blood coagulation and fibrinolytic systems during pregnancy. Clin Obstet Gynecol 2:321, 1975.

393. Chugh KS, Singhal PC, Kher VK, et al: Spectrum of acute cortical necrosis in Indian patients. Am J Med Sci 286:10, 1983.

394. Hayslett JP: Postpartum renal failure. N Engl J Med 312:1556, 1985.

395. Brown CB, Clarkson AR, Robson JS, et al: Haemolytic uraemic syndrome in women taking oral contraceptives. Lancet 1:1479, 1973.

396. Rock GA, Shumak KH, Buskard NA, et al: Comparison of plasma exchange with plasma infusion in the treatment of thrombotic thrombocytopenic purpura. N Engl J Med 325:393, 1991.

397. Brandes JC, Fritsche C: Obstructive acute renal failure by a gravid uterus: A case report and review. Am J Kidney Dis 18:398, 1991.

398. Homans DC, Blake GD, Harrington JT, et al: Acute renal failure caused by ureteral obstruction by a gravid uterus. JAMA 246:1230, 1981.

399. Jena M, Mitch WE: Rapidly reversible acute renal failure from ureteral obstruction in pregnancy. Am J Kidney Dis 28:457, 1996.

400. LaPata RE, McElin TW, Adelson BH: Ureteral obstruction due to compression by the gravid uterus. Am J Obstet Gynecol 106:941, 1970.

401. Peake SL, Roxburgh HB, Langlois SL: Ultrasonic assessment of hydronephrosis of pregnancy. Radiology 146:167, 1983.

401. Coe FL, Parks JH, Lindheimer MD: Nephrolithiasis during pregnancy. N Engl J Med 298:322, 1978.

403. Kumar R, Cohen WR, Epstein FH: Vitamin D and calcium hormones in pregnancy. N Engl J Med 302:1143, 1980.

404. Pitkin RM: Calcium metabolism in pregnancy and the perinatal period: A review. Am J Obstet Gynecol 151:99, 1985.

405. Folger GK: Pain and pregnancy. Obstet Gynecol 5:513, 1955.

406. Maikranz P, Coe FL, Parks J, et al: Nephrolithiasis in pregnancy. Am J Kidney Dis 9:354, 1987.

407. Stothers L, Lee LM: Renal colic in pregnancy. J Urol 148:1383, 1992.

408. Loughlin KR, Bailey RB Jr: Internal ureteral stents for conservative management of ureteral calculi during pregnancy. N Engl J Med 315:1647, 1986.

409. Asgari MA, Safarinejad MR, Hosseini SY, et al: Extracorporeal shock wave lithotripsy of renal calculi during early pregnancy. Br J Urol Int 84:615, 1999.

410. Schubiger G, Flury G, Nussberger J: Enalapril for pregnancy-induced hypertension: Acute renal failure in a neonate. Ann Intern Med 108:215, 1988.

411. Pryde PG, Sedman AB, Nugent CE, et al: Angiotensin-converting enzyme inhibitor fetopathy. J Am Soc Nephrol 3:1575, 1993.

412. Nanta J, de Heer E, Baldwin WM, et al: Transplacental induction of membranous nephropathy in a neonate. Pediatr Nephrol 4:111, 1990.

413. Jungers P, Chauveau D: Pregnancy in renal disease. Kidney Int 52:871, 1997.

414. Lim VS: Reproductive function in patients with renal insufficiency. Am J Kidney Dis 9:363, 1987.

415. Souqiyyeh MZ, Huraib SO, Mohd AG, et al: Pregnancy in chronic hemodialysis patients in the kingdom of Saudia Arabia. Am J Kidney Dis 19:235, 1992.

416. Bagon JA, Vernaeve H, deMuylder X, et al: Pregnancy and dialysis. Am J Kidney Dis 31:756, 1998.

417. Okundaye I, Abrinko P, Hou S: Registry of pregnancy in dialysis patients. Am J Kidney Dis 31:766, 1998.

418. Rauramo L, Kasanen A, Elfving K, et al: Fertility, pregnancy and labour in women with a history of nephritis or pyelonephritis. Acta Obstet Gynecol Scand 41:357, 1962.

419. Mackay EV: Pregnancy and renal disease: A ten-year survey. Aust N Z J Obstet Gynaecol 3:21, 1963.

420. Barceló P, López-Lillo J, Cabero L, Del Río G: Successful pregnancy in primary glomerular disease. Kidney Int 30:914, 1986.

421. Chapman AB, Johnson AM, Gabow PA: Pregnancy outcome and its relationship to progression of renal failure in autosomal dominant polycystic kidney disease. J Am Soc Nephrol 5:1178, 1994.

422. Katz AI, Davison JM, Hayslett JP, et al: Pregnancy in women with kidney disease. Kidney Int 18:192, 1980.

423. Packham DK, North RA, Fairley KF, et al: Primary glomerulonephritis and pregnancy. Q J Med 71:537, 1989.

424. Surian M, Imbasciati E, Cosci P: Glomerular disease and pregnancy: A study of 123 pregnancies in patients with primary and secondary glomerular diseases. Nephron 36:101, 1984.

425. Hou SH, Grossman SD, Madias NE: Pregnancy in women with renal disease and moderate renal insufficiency. Am J Med 78:185, 1985.

426. Imbasciati E, Pardi G, Capetta P, et al: Pregnancy in women with chronic renal failure. Am J Nephrol 6:193, 1986.

427. Jungers P, Houillier P, Forget D, et al: Specific controversies concerning the natural history of renal disease in pregnancy. Am J Kidney Dis 17:116, 1991.

428. Abe S, Amagasaki Y, Konishi K, et al: The influence of antecedent renal disease on pregnancy. Am J Obstet Gynecol 153:508, 1985.

429. Holley JL, Bernardini J, Quadri KH, et al: Pregnancy outcomes in a prospective matched control study of pregnancy and renal disease. Clin Nephrol 45:77, 1996.

430. Jones DC, Hayslett JP: Outcome of pregnancy in women with moderate or several renal insufficiency. N Engl J Med 335:226, 1996.

431. Leppert P, Risher CC, Cheng SS, et al: Antecedent renal disease and the outcome of pregnancy. Ann Intern Med 90:747, 1979.

432. Ihle BU, Long P, Oats J: Early onset pre-eclampsia: Recognition of underlying renal disease. BMJ 294:79, 1987.

433. Slone D, Siskind V, Heinonen OP, et al: Aspirin and congenital malformations. Lancet 1:1373, 1976.

434. Shapiro S, Siskind V, Monson RR: Perinatal mortality and birth-weight in relation to aspirin taken during pregnancy. Lancet 1:1375, 1976.

435. Werler MM, Mitchell AA, Shapiro S: The relation of aspirin use during the first trimester of pregnancy to congenital cardiac defects. N Engl J Med 321:1639, 1989.

436. Benigni A, Gregorini G, Frusca T, et al: Effect of low-dose aspirin on fetal and maternal generation of thromboxane by platelets in women at risk for pregnancy-induced hypertension. N Engl J Med 321:357, 1989.

437. Brenner BM, Meyer TW, Hostetter TH: Dietary protein intake and the progressive nature of kidney disease: The role of hemodynamically mediated glomerular injury in the pathogenesis of progressive glomerular sclerosis in aging, renal ablation, and intrinsic renal disease. N Engl J Med 307:652, 1982.

438. Hostetter TH, Rennke HG, Brenner BM: The case for intrarenal hypertension in the initiation and progression of diabetic and other glomerulopathies. Am J Med 72:375, 1982.

439. Neuringer JR, Brenner BM: Hemodynamic theory of progressive renal disease: A 10-year update in brief review. Am J Kidney Dis 22:98, 1993.

440. Baylis C: Immediate and long-term effects of pregnancy on glomerular function in the SHR. Am J Physiol 257:F1140, 1989.

441. Baylis C, Rennke HG: Renal hemodynamics and glomerular morphology in repetitively pregnant aging rats. Kidney Int 28:140, 1985.

442. Baylis C, Reese K, Wilson CB: Glomerular effects of pregnancy in a model of glomerulonephritis in the rat. Am J Kidney Dis 14:452, 1989.

443. Podjarny E, Bernheim J, Rathaus M, et al: Adriamycin nephropathy: A model to study effects of pregnancy on renal disease in rats. Am J Physiol 263:F711, 1992.

444. Bar J, Ben Rafael Z, Padoa A: Prediction of pregnancy outcome in subgroups of women with renal disease. Clin Nephrol 53:437, 2000.

445. Jungers P, Houillier P, Forget D, et al: Influence of pregnancy on the course of primary chronic glomerulonephritis. Lancet 346:1122, 1995.

446. Hemmelder MH, de Zeeuw D, Fidler V, et al: Proteinuria: A risk factor for pregnancy-related renal function decline in primary glomerular disease? Am J Kidney Dis 26:187, 1995.

447. Becker GJ, Ihle BU, Fairley KF: Effect of pregnancy on moderate renal failure in reflux nephropathy. BMJ 292:796, 1986.

448. Jungers P, Houillier P, Chauveau D, et al: Pregnancy in women with reflux nephropathy. Kidney Int 50:593, 1996.

449. el-Khatib M, Packham DK, Becker GJ, et al: Pregnancy-related complications in women with reflux nephropathy. Clin Nephrol 41:50, 1994.

450. Abe S: Pregnancy in IgA nephropathy. Kidney Int 40:1098, 1991.

451. Koido S, Makino H, Iwazaki K, et al: IgA nephropathy and pregnancy. Tokai J Exp Clin Med 23:31, 1998.

452. Hayslett JP: Maternal and fetal complications in pregnant women with systemic lupus erythematosus. Am J Kidney Dis 17:123, 1991.

453. Bobrie G, Liote F, Houillier P: Pregnancy in lupus nephritis and related disorders. Am J Kidney Dis 9:339, 1987.

454. Mintz G, Rodriguez-Alvarez E: Systemic lupus erythematosus. Rheum Dis Clin North Am 15:255, 1989.

455. Hayslett JP, Lynn RI: Effect of pregnancy in patients with lupus nephropathy. Kidney Int 18:207, 1980.

456. Houser NT, Fish AJ, Tagatz GE, et al: Pregnancy and systemic lupus erythematosus. Am J Obstet Gynecol 138:409, 1980.

457. Le Huong D, Wechsler B, Vauthier-Brouzes D, et al: Outcome of planned pregnancies in systemic lupus erythematosus: A prospective study on 62 pregnancies. Br J Rheumatol 36:772, 1997.

458. Branch DW, Scott JR, Kochenour NK, et al: Obstetric complications associated with the lupus anticoagulant. N Engl J Med 313:1322, 1985.

459. Packham DK, Lam SS, Nicolls K, et al: Lupus nephritis and pregnancy. Q J Med 83:315, 1992.

460. Kitzmiller JL, Brown ER, Phillippe M, et al: Diabetic nephropathy and perinatal outcome. Am J Obstet Gynecol 141:741, 1981.

461. Reece EA, Coustan DR, Hayslett JP, et al: Diabetic nephropathy: Pregnancy performance and feto-maternal outcome. Am J Obstet Gynecol 159:56, 1988.

462. Purdy LP, Hantsch CE, Molitch ME, et al: Effect of pregnancy on renal function in patients with moderate-to-severe diabetic renal insufficiency. Diabetes Care 19:1067, 1996.

463. Milutinovic J, Fialkow PJ, Agodoa LY, et al: Fertility and pregnancy complications in women with autosomal dominant polycystic kidney disease. Obstet Gynecol 61:566, 1983.

464. Gabow PA, Johnson AM, Kaehny WD, et al: Factors affecting the progression of renal disease in autosomal-dominant polycystic kidney disease. Kidney Int 41:1311, 1992.

465. Imbasciati E, Ponticelli C: Pregnancy and renal disease: Predictors for fetal and maternal outcome. Am J Nephrol 11:353, 1991.

466. Fouque D, Laville M, Boissel JP, et al: Controlled low protein diets in chronic renal insufficiency: Meta-analysis. BMJ 304:214, 1992.

467. Hostetter TH, Olson JL, Rennke HG, et al: Hyperfiltration in remnant nephrons: A potentially adverse response to renal ablation. Am J Physiol 241:F85, 1981.

468. Rush D, Stein Z, Susser M: A randomized controlled trial of prenatal nutritional supplementation in New York City. Pediatrics 65:683, 1980.

469. Hakim RM, Depner TA, Parker TF III: Adequacy of hemodialysis. Am J Kidney Dis 20:107, 1992.

470. Redrow M, Cherem L, Elliott J, et al: Dialysis in the management of pregnant patients with renal insufficiency. Medicine (Baltimore) 67:199, 1988.

471. Hou S: Peritoneal dialysis and hemodialysis in pregnancy. Baillieres Clin Obstet Gynaecol 1:1009, 1987.

472. Registration Committee of EDTA: Successful pregnancies in women treated by dialysis and kidney transplantation. Br J Obstet Gynecol 87:839, 1980.

473. Hou S, Orlowski J, Pahl M, et al: Pregnancy in women with end-stage renal disease: Treatment of anemia and premature labor. Am J Kidney Dis 21:16, 1993.

474. Toma H, Tanabe K, Tokumoto T, et al: Pregnancy in women receiving renal dialysis or transplantation in Japan: A nationwide survey. Nephrol Dial Transplant 14:1511, 1999.

475. Gadallah MF, Ahmad B, Karubian F, et al: Pregnancy in patients on chronic ambulatory peritoneal dialysis. Am J Kidney Dis 20:407, 1992.

476. Chang H, Miller M, Bruns F: Tidal peritoneal dialysis during pregnancy improves clearance and abdominal symptoms. Perit Dial Int 22: 272, 2002.

477. Hou S: Conception and pregnancy in peritoneal dialysis patients. Perit Dial Int 21:S290, 2001.

478. Alcalay M, Blau A, Barkai G, et al: Successful pregnancy in a patient with polycystic kidney disease and advanced renal failure: The use of prophylactic dialysis. Am J Kidney Dis 19:382, 1992.

479. Vogt K, Keusch G, Baumann U, et al: Successful pregnancy in advanced renal failure without dialysis. Pediatr Nephrol 3:189, 1989.

480. Frohling PT: Successful pregnancy of a woman with advanced renal failure on nutritional treatment. Nephron 44:195, 1986.

481. Abramovici H, Brandes JM, Better OS, et al: Menstrual cycle and reproductive potential after kidney transplantation: Report of 2 patients. Obstet Gynecol 37:121, 1971.

482. Schover LR, Novick AC, Steinmuller DR, et al: Sexuality, fertility and renal transplantation: A survey of survivors. J Sex Marital Ther 16:3, 1990.

483. Davison JM: Dialysis, transplantation, and pregnancy. Am J Kidney Dis 17:127, 1991.

484. Davison JM: The effect of pregnancy on kidney function in renal allograft recipients. Kidney Int 27:74, 1985.

485. Magee LA, von Dadelszen P, Darley J, et al: Erythropoiesis and renal transplant pregnancy. Cin Transplant 14:127, 2000.

486. Zeidan BS, Waltzer BC, Monheit AG, et al: Anemia associated with pregnancy in a cyclosporine-treated renal allograft recipient. Transplant Proc 23:2301, 1991.

487. Muirhead N, Sabharwal AR, Rieder MJ, et al: The outcome of pregnancy following renal transplantation: The experience of a single center. Transplantation 54:429, 1992.

488. Armenti VT, Ahlswede KM, Ahlswede BA, et al: National Transplant Pregnancy Registry Outcomes of 154 pregnancies in cyclosporine-treated female kidney transplant recipients. Transplantation 57:502, 1994.

489. Armenti VT, Radomski JS, Moritz MJ et al: Report from the National Transplantation Pregnancy Registry (NTPR): Outcomes of Pregnancy after Transplantation. Clin Transpl nv:123, 2000.

490. Gaughan WJ, Moritz MJ, Radomski JS, et al: National Transplantation Pregnancy Registry: Report on outcomes in cyclosporine-treated female kidney transplant recipients with an interval from transplant to pregnancy of greater than five years. Am J Kidney Dis 28:266, 1996.

491. Di Paolo S, Schena A, Morrone LF, et al: Immunologic evaluation during the first year of life of infants born to cyclosporine-treated female kidney transplant recipients: Analysis of lymphocyte sub-populations and immunoglobulin serum levels. Transplantation 69:2049, 2000.

492. Thomas AJ, Burrows L, Knight R, et al: The effect of pregnancy on cyclosporine levels in renal allograft patients. Obstet Gynecol 90:916, 1997.

493. Kainz A, Harabacz I, Cowlrick IS, et al: Analysis of 100 pregnancy outcomes in women treated systemically with tacrolimus. Transpl Int 13:S299, 2000.

494. CellCept package insert. Basel, Switzerland, Roche Pharmaceuticals, 2002.

495. Rapamune package insert. Collegeville, PA, Wyeth Pharmaceuticals, 2002.

496. Pregnancy in renal transplant recipients. Nephrol Dial Transplant 17(suppl 4):50, 2002.

497. Armenti VT, Wilson GA, Radomski JS, et al: Report from the National Transplantation Pregnancy Registry (NTPR): Outcomes of Pregnancy after Transplantation. Clin Transpl nv:111, 1999.

498. Sturgiss SN, Davison JM: Effect of pregnancy on long-term function of renal allografts. Am J Kidney Dis 19:167, 1992.

499. Sturgiss SN, Davison JM: Effect of pregnancy on the long-term function of renal allografts: An update. Am J Kidney Dis 26:65, 1995.

500. First MR, Combs CA, Weiskittel P, Miodovnik M: Lack of effect of pregnancy on renal allograft survival or function. Transplantation 59:472, 1995.

501. Rizzoni G, Ehrich JH, Broyen M, et al: Successful pregnancies in women on renal replacement therapy: Report from the EDTA registry. Nephrol Dial Transplant 7:279, 1992.

502. Ehrich JH, Loirat C, Davison JM, Rizzoni G, et al: Repeated successful pregnancies after kidney transplantation in 102 women. Nephrol Dial Transplant 11:1314, 1996.

CHAPTER 36

Inherited Disorders of the Renal Tubule

Alain Bonnardeaux and Daniel G. Bichet

INHERITED DISORDERS ASSOCIATED WITH GENERALIZED DYSFUNCTION OF THE PROXIMAL TUBULE (RENAL FANCONI SYNDROME)
Dent Disease, X-Linked Recessive Hypophosphatemic Rickets, X-Linked Recessive Nephrolithiasis
Idiopathic Causes of the Renal Fanconi Syndrome
Cystinosis
Glycogenosis Type 1 (von Gierke Disease)
Tyrosinemia
Galactosemia
Lowe Oculocerebrorenal Syndrome
Wilson Disease
Hereditary Fructose Intolerance
INHERITED DISORDERS OF RENAL AMINO ACID TRANSPORT
Cystinuria
Lysinuric Protein Intolerance
Hartnup Disease
Iminoglycinuria
INHERITED DISORDERS OF RENAL PHOSPHATE TRANSPORT
Renal Phosphate Excretion

Adaptation to States of Altered Phosphate Metabolism
X-Linked Hypophosphatemic Rickets
Hereditary Hypophosphatemic Rickets with Hypercalciuria
Hereditary Selective Deficiency of $1\alpha,25(OH)_2D_3$
Hereditary Generalized Resistance to $1\alpha,25(OH)_2D_3$
INHERITED DISORDERS OF RENAL GLUCOSE TRANSPORT
Normal Glucose Reabsorption by the Kidney
Renal Glucosuria
Glucose-Galactose Malabsorption
INHERITED DISORDERS OF ACID-BASE TRANSPORTERS
Mechanisms of Renal Acidification
Proximal Renal Tubular Acidosis
Distal Renal Tubular Acidosis
INHERITED HYPOKALEMIC HYPOTENSIVE DISORDERS
Bartter Syndrome
Gitelman Syndrome
INHERITED HYPOKALEMIC HYPERTENSIVE DISORDERS

Congenital Adrenal Hyperplasia
Liddle Syndrome
Apparent Mineralocorticoid Excess
Autosomal Dominant Early-Onset Hypertension with Severe Exacerbation During Pregnancy
Glucocorticoid-Remediable Hyperaldosteronism
Familial Hyperaldosteronism Type II
INHERITED HYPERKALEMIC HYPOTENSIVE DISORDERS
Pseudohypoaldosteronism Type I
INHERITED HYPERKALEMIC HYPERTENSIVE DISORDERS
Pseudohypoaldosteronism Type II
INHERITED DISORDERS OF RENAL MAGNESIUM HANDLING
Familial Hypomagnesemia with Hypercalciuria and Nephrocalcinosis
Familial Hypomagnesemia with Secondary Hypocalcemia
Isolated Dominant Hypomagnesemia with Hypocalciuria
Calcium/Magnesium-Sensing Receptor–Associated Disorders
DIABETES INSIPIDUS

Considerable progress has been achieved in the last few years in understanding the molecular basis of several inherited renal tubule disorders. These advances have served several purposes. First, they have allowed the identification of genes expressed in the renal tubule that encode proteins whose function has been investigated (Table 36-1). Second, by providing natural variations in gene function, they have increased our knowledge of basic renal physiology. Third, they have increased our understanding of the diseases themselves and allowed us to make phenotype-genotype correlations. Fourth, it is now possible to offer natal and prenatal diagnosis and initiate research on gene therapy.

Most transport disorders discussed in this chapter are inherited as autosomal recessive traits. Thus, "private" mutations frequently produce the disease in each kindred and the frequency of the disease increases in populations with a high frequency of consanguineous matings. Although such diseases are rare and previously restricted to *pediatric* nephrology, recent progress in therapy is increasing longevity for many patients, thus confronting the *adult* nephrologist with new clinical challenges. Each disorder is referenced with its OMIM (Online Mendelian Inheritance in Man) number.

OMIM is a database containing a catalog of human genes and genetic disorders.

INHERITED DISORDERS ASSOCIATED WITH GENERALIZED DYSFUNCTION OF THE PROXIMAL TUBULE (RENAL FANCONI SYNDROME)

The renal Fanconi syndrome is a generalized dysfunction of the proximal tubule with no primary glomerular involvement. It is usually characterized by variable degrees of phosphate, glucose, amino acid, and bicarbonate wasting by the proximal tubule. The clinical presentation in children is usually rickets and impaired growth. In adults, bone disease is manifested as osteomalacia and osteoporosis. In addition, polyuria, renal salt wasting, hypokalemia, acidosis, hypercalciuria, and low-molecular-weight proteinuria can be part of the clinical spectrum.

There are hereditary and acquired forms of the Fanconi syndrome (see review in reference 1). Acquired forms in adults are usually associated with abnormal proteinurias such as the paraproteinemias or the nephrotic syndrome, with

TABLE 36-1

Impact of DNA Variation on Protein Function

Loss-of-function:	a mutation that reduces or abolishes a normal physiologic function (likely to be recessive)
Gain-of-function:	a mutation that increases the function of a protein (likely to be dominant)
Dominant negative:	a mutation that dominantly affects the phenotype by means of a defective protein or RNA molecule that interferes with the function of the normal gene product in the same cell

TABLE 36-2

Causes of Inherited and Acquired Fanconi Syndrome

Inherited
  Idiopathic (AD)
  Dent disease (X-linked hypophosphatemic rickets, X-linked recessive nephrolithiasis)
  "Sporadic"
  Cystinosis (AR)
  Tyrosinemia type I (AR)
  Galactosemia (AR)
  Glycogen storage disease
  Wilson disease (AR)
  Mitochondrial diseases (cytochrome-*c* oxidase deficiency)
  Oculocerebrorenal syndrome of Lowe
  Hereditary fructose intolerance
Acquired
  Paraproteinemias (multiple myeloma)
  Nephrotic syndrome
  Chronic tubulointerstitial nephritis
  Renal transplantation
  Malignancy
Exogenous factors
  Heavy metals (cadmium, mercury, lead, uranium, platinum)
  Drugs (cisplatin, aminoglycosides, 6-mercaptopurine, valproate, outdated tetracyclines, methyl-3-chrome, ifosfamide)
  Chemical compounds (toluene, maleate, paraquat, Lysol)

AD, autosomal dominant; AR, autosomal recessive.

residual cases being secondary to tubular damage caused by toxic (reviewed in reference 2) or immunologic factors. Most hereditary forms of the Fanconi syndrome occur as part of the manifestations of readily identifiable inborn errors of metabolism or as sporadic or rare familial forms. Inherited disorders are classified into forms that primarily affect the proximal renal tubule (idiopathic) and forms that derive from the accumulation of toxic metabolic products in the kidneys (secondary) (Table 36-2). Such metabolic disorders give rise to the renal Fanconi syndrome as part of a particular clinical spectrum.

Other inherited disorders of the proximal tubule can result in isolated anomalies of transport. Isolated or partial defects of the proximal tubule result in the selective wasting of amino acids, phosphate, bicarbonate, or glucose, and are described in other sections of this chapter.

Pathogenesis

The proximal tubule is responsible for reclaiming almost all the filtered load of bicarbonate, glucose, and amino acids, as well as most of the filtered load of sodium, fluid, chloride, and phosphate. The renal proximal tubule exhibits a very extensive apical endocytic apparatus consisting of an elaborate network of coated pits and small coated and noncoated endosomes (see Chapter 1). In addition, the cells contain a large number of late endosomes or prelysosomes, lysosomes, and so-called dense apical tubules involved in receptor recycling from the endosomes to the apical plasma membrane. This endocytic apparatus is involved in the reabsorption of molecules filtered in the glomeruli. The process is very effective as demonstrated by the fact that although several grams of protein are filtered daily in the human glomeruli, human urine is virtually devoid of proteins under physiologic conditions. Reabsorption of solutes by proximal tubule cells is achieved by transport systems at the brush border membrane that are directly or indirectly coupled to sodium movement, by energy production and transport from the mitochondria, and by the Na^+,K^+-ATPase at the basolateral membrane. The Na^+,K^+-ATPase lowers intracellular Na^+ concentration and provides the electrochemical gradient that allows Na^+-coupled solute entry into the cell. A second pathway, the paracellular route, is responsible for reclaiming up to one half of the sodium and most of the water through tight junctions.

Multiple transport anomalies characterize the renal Fanconi syndrome. In addition, amino acids, glucose, phosphate, and bicarbonate are transported by multiple carriers. Therefore, defects responsible for the Fanconi syndrome lead to a general dysfunction of the proximal tubule cell. Examples of genetic defects associated with the renal Fanconi syndrome are storage diseases thought to affect proximal tubule cells in addition to other cells (hepatocytes). Specific organelle dysfunction of proximal tubule cells is thought to explain cystinosis (lysosomes) and Dent disease (endosomes).

The Fanconi syndrome, even when genetically transmitted, can be reversible, occurring following prolonged exposure to the noxious substance. For example, the defect is reversed after dietary restriction of tyrosine and phenylalanine in tyrosinemia,[3] fructose in hereditary fructose intolerance,[4] and galactose in galactosemia.[5] The duration of exposure is also important for the disorder to be expressed and is protracted in cadmium intoxication,[6] or short in fructose intolerance following a fructose load.[7]

Clinical Presentation

AMINOACIDURIA

All amino acids are filtered by the glomerulus, and more than 98% are subsequently reabsorbed by the proximal tubule. Multiple transporters are responsible for the reabsorption. In the renal Fanconi syndrome, all amino acids are excreted in excess. Amino acids in the urine are usually quantified by one of several chromatographic methods at specialized centers. The excretion of amino acids parallels the physiologic excretion but to an elevated degree, particularly for the amino acids that have the highest levels of excretion physiologically (histidine, serine, cystine, lysine, and glycine). Clinically, amino acid losses are relatively modest, do not lead to specific deficiencies, and there is no need to supplement affected patients.

PHOSPHATURIA AND BONE DISEASE

Phosphate wasting is a cardinal manifestation of the Fanconi syndrome. Serum phosphate levels are usually decreased and tubular reabsorption of phosphate (TRP and TmP/GFR) is systematically reduced. Rickets and osteomalacia are produced by the increased urinary losses of phosphate as well as by impaired 1α-hydroxylation of 25-hydroxy vitamin D_3 by proximal tubule cells. Rickets manifests itself by a bowing deformity of the lower limbs with metaphyseal widening of the proximal and distal tibia, distal femur, the ulna, and the radius. Bone manifestations in patients with adult-onset renal Fanconi syndrome are severe bone pain and spontaneous fractures.

RENAL TUBULAR ACIDOSIS

Acidosis is a frequent finding and is caused by defective bicarbonate reabsorption by the proximal tubule. Hence, renal acidification by the distal tubule is normal, as demonstrated by the ability to acidify urines at a pH below 5.5 when plasma bicarbonate is below the threshold. The metabolic acidosis is hyperchloremic and is also known as type II. Large doses of alkali may be necessary to correct serum bicarbonate levels.

GLUCOSURIA

Glucosuria is the fourth manifestation of the renal Fanconi syndrome. Serum glucose is normal and the amount of glucose lost in the urine varies from 0.5 to 10 g/24 hours. Massive glucosuria (and hypoglycemia) may be seen in glycogenosis type I.[8]

SODIUM AND POTASSIUM WASTING

Renal sodium losses can be important in the Fanconi syndrome and lead to hypotension, hyponatremia, and metabolic alkalosis. Supplementation with sodium chloride is indicated and leads to improvement of symptoms. Potassium losses are secondary to increased delivery of sodium to the distal tubule and activation of the renin-angiotensin system secondary to hypovolemia. Potassium supplementation is indicated to correct serum potassium levels.

POLYURIA

Polyuria, polydipsia, and dehydration can be prominent features of the Fanconi syndrome. There is a decreased concentrating ability of the kidney that could be related to abnormal tubule function of the distal tubule and collecting duct, possibly caused by hypokalemia.

PROTEINURIA

Low-molecular-weight proteinuria is almost always present in patients with the renal Fanconi syndrome, and is usually low to moderate in amounts. The dipstick test is frequently positive because of the presence of albuminuria. Beta$_2$-microglobulin excretion rates can be measured to identify "tubular proteinuria."

HYPERCALCIURIA

Hypercalciuria is a frequent finding in patients with the renal Fanconi syndrome. The pathogenesis is not known or multifactorial, but could be attributed to abnormal recycling of proteins involved in calcium reabsorption by the proximal tubule. Hypercalciuria is rarely associated with nephrolithiasis in the Fanconi syndrome, possibly because of the polyuric syndrome that frequently occurs.

Dent Disease, X-Linked Recessive Hypophosphatemic Rickets, X-Linked Recessive Nephrolithiasis
Pathogenesis

Dent disease, X-linked recessive hypophosphatemic rickets, and X-linked recessive nephrolithiasis (OMIM 300009) represent the same inherited disorder caused by mutations in the *Clcn5* gene (chromosome Xp11.22) encoding a renal chloride channel, ClC-5.[10, 11] This X-linked recessive disease is associated with a primary renal Fanconi syndrome. ClC-5 function is not at the plasma membrane but rather in intracellular compartments, subapical endosomes of the proximal tubule, where it colocalizes with the V-type H^+-ATPase and with reabsorbed proteins. Because several hormones or their precursors are endocytosed from the primary urine, loss-of-function of the *Clcn5* gene leads to secondary changes in calciotropic hormones and changes in phosphate excretion. The clinical spectrum includes varying degrees of low-molecular-weight proteinuria, hypercalciuria with calcium nephrolithiasis, rickets, nephrocalcinosis, and renal failure. The molecular basis for Dent disease offers important mechanistic insight into the role of organelle dysfunction (Fig. 36-1).

In the proximal tubule, endocytosis of many proteins is mediated by megalin, a recycling receptor of the low-density lipoprotein (LDL) family. After internalization, acidification of the endosomes is required for receptor-ligand interactions and cell-sorting events.[12] Inhibition of the acidification interferes with cell-surface receptor recycling.[12] ClC-5 may play a role in proximal tubular (early) endocytosis, probably by providing an electrical shunt to enable efficient pumping of the H^+-ATPase (reviewed in reference 13). ClC channels are believed to be dimers that have two largely independent pores (reviewed in reference 13). These pores can be gated individually or can be closed together by a common gate. ClC-5 is an endosomal chloride channel of 746 amino acids that spans approximately 12 transmembrane domains (see Fig. 36-1). It is weakly homologous to other CLC channels, but is more homologous to ClC-3.[14] ClC-5 messenger RNA (mRNA) is predominantly expressed in the kidney, but is also present in liver, brain, testis, and intestine and colon. ClC-5 is highly expressed in all three segments (S1-S3) of the proximal tubule and in α-intercalated cells of the distal tubule of the rat kidney.[15] ClC-5 expression is highest below the brush border membrane in a region rich in endocytotic vesicles and colocalizes with the proton pump and with internalized proteins early after uptake.[15] In vivo endocytosis of a fluorescently labeled filtered protein revealed that ClC-5 colocalizes with the internalized protein at early (2 minutes), but not late (13 minutes), time points of uptake. ClC-5 was present in human kidney membrane fractions that also

PROXIMAL TUBULE

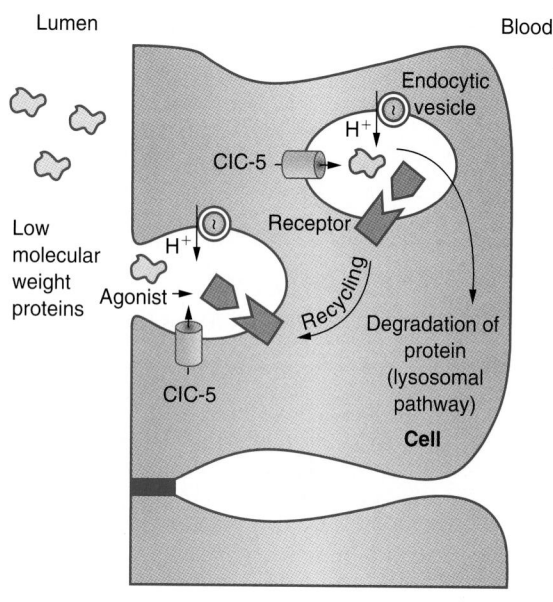

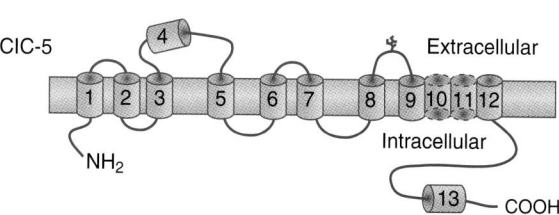

FIGURE 36-1. Schematic representation of ClC-5 with 12 putative membrane-spanning helices and its colocalization with the proton pump and with endocytosed low-molecular-weight proteins at the proximal tubular level. Expression of ClC-5 is highest below the brush border membrane in a region rich in endocytic vesicles. ClC-5 may be essential for proximal endocytosis by providing an electrical shunt necessary for the efficient acidification of vesicles in the endocytic pathway, explaining the proteinuria observed in Dent disease.[15] Dent disease, X-linked recessive hypophosphatemic rickets, and X-linked recessive nephrolithiasis are caused by inactivating mutations of the renal chloride channel ClC-5. In mice with targeted inactivation of *Clcn5*, there is a substantial impairment in proximal tubule protein absorption that correlated with reduced receptor-mediated and fluid-phase endocytosis in proximal tubular epithelial cells. Parathyroid hormone (PTH) is reabsorbed from glomerular filtrate by the proximal tubule and therefore is predicted to be more concentrated in tubular fluid when ClC-5 is inactive. Stimulation of luminal PTH receptors may increase conversion of $25(OH)D_3$ to the active compound $1,25(OH)D_3$, which in turn promotes intestinal calcium absorption, increases circulating calcium levels, and increases renal calcium excretion (absorptive hypercalciuria). Abnormal recycling of the proximal tubular Na^+/Pi cotransporter and associated urinary phosphate loss is also observed in *Clcn5* null mice and this may also contribute to metabolic derangements.[457]

contained rab5, rab4, and the 31-kDa subunit of the H^+-ATPase.[16] In transfection studies with ClC-5, the cells induce outwardly rectifying Cl^- currents on whole-cell configuration that are measurable only at voltages greater than +20 mV. Because these positive voltages seem unphysiologic, it is unclear whether there is an additional, unknown β-subunit or another regulatory mechanism that may alter the voltage dependence. As a first step to identify sorting signals in ClC-5, a PY motif was found to be important for the internalization from the plasma membrane.[17] This was ascribed to an interaction with the WW domain containing ubiquitin protein ligases.

This resembles the model proposed for the regulation of the epithelial Na^+ channel (ENaC), whose internalization and degradation is triggered by the PY motif–dependent ubiquitination by a WW domain containing ubiquitin protein ligase.[18]

Piwon and colleagues[19] disrupted the *Clcn5* gene by homologous recombination. The complete loss of functional ClC-5 channels led to proteinuria and secondary changes of calciotropic hormone levels that entailed significant hyperphosphaturia. No hypercalciuria was detected. Several proteins, including retinol binding protein and vitamin D binding protein, were drastically increased in urine. The defect in proximal tubular endocytosis affected receptor-mediated endocytosis of proteins, fluid-phase endocytosis, and the retrieval of plasma membrane proteins. Endocytosis was not abolished completely, but reduced to less than 30% of normal. Within the proximal tubule, cells expressing ClC-5 endocytosed more efficiently than neighboring cells that lacked ClC-5. Megalin was reduced about twofold in $Clcn5^-$ cells in a cell-autonomous manner, possibly suggesting that recycling was more affected than onward transport to lysosomes. This decrease in megalin expression likely reduces renal endocytosis even further.

Like patients with Dent disease, $Clcn5^-$ mice have elevated urinary phosphate excretion.[19] The proximal tubule reabsorbs phosphate predominantly through the Na^+-coupled phosphate transporter NPT2a. Defective endocytosis in $Clcn5^-$ mice should have predicted increased, not decreased, NPT2a expression at the plasma membrane. However, and consistent with the observed phosphaturia, NPT2a was internalized in most segments of $Clcn5^-$ mice. This suggested that the increased internalization of NPT2a and the ensuing phosphaturia was due to a rise in luminal parathyroid hormone (PTH) in $Clcn5^-$ mice. Proximal tubule cells express functional PTH receptors also apically, and PTH is endocytosed in a megalin-dependent process.[20] Thus, PTH increases phosphate excretion by stimulating the endocytosis of NPT2a from the plasma membrane and targeting it to lysosomes. As predicted, urinary PTH excretion was increased in the $Clcn5^-$ mice, and NPT2a was predominantly apical in early segments of the tubule where a lack of endocytosis has a negligible impact on luminal PTH. Furthermore, PTH-induced endocytosis of NPT2a was still possible, albeit it occurred at drastically slower rates. These findings suggest that phosphaturia in Dent disease might be secondary to increased luminal PTH concentrations that are caused by a defect in endocytosis.

The causes of hypercalciuria and renal stones are not well understood. The proximal tubule metabolizes $25(OH)D_3$ to the active form, 1,25-dihydroxyvitamin D_3. The transcription of the responsible enzyme, α-hydroxylase, is induced by PTH. As a consequence, the ratio of serum $1,25(OH)_2D_3$ to $25(OH)D_3$ was elevated in $Clcn5^-$ mice.[19] However, the concentration of both forms of vitamin D_3 was reduced in serum, as there was significant loss of $25(OH)D_3$ and its binding protein into the urine. This is consistent with findings in knockout mice lacking the endocytic receptor megalin who lose $25(OH)D_3$ in the urine and develop bone disease. Similar results have been found with cubilin, a membrane-associated protein colocalizing with megalin, which facilitates the endocytic process by sequestering steroid-carrier complexes on the cellular surface.[21, 22] Hence, disrupting *Clcn5* has two opposing effects on $1,25(OH)_2D_3$. The impairment of endocytosis increases luminal PTH concentrations, which in turn leads to increased α-hydroxylase activity and $1,25(OH)_2D_3$ production. At the same time, however, the defective endocytosis also leads to a decreased availability of the precursor. The balance between these effects determines whether there is an increase in serum $1,25(OH)_2D_3$, which may then cause hypercalciuria by stimulating intestinal Ca^{2+} reabsorption. Indeed, $1,25(OH)_2D_3$ is slightly elevated in many patients with Dent disease.[23] Wang and co-workers reported another *Clcn5* knockout mouse that surprisingly displayed both low-molecular-weight proteinuria and an approximate twofold increase in urinary Ca^{2+}.[24] No calciotropic hormone levels were reported.[24] Given the similarity in strategies and genetic backgrounds, it is unclear why these two models differ in the extent of urinary Ca^{2+} excretion.

Clinical Presentation

The clinical spectrum of Clcn5 mutations includes hypercalciuria with calcium phosphate nephrolithiasis, rickets, nephrocalcinosis, low-molecular-weight proteinuria, and renal failure (see reviews in references 23, 25). The same mutation can induce different phenotypes in different families,[26] probably because of genetic or environmental modifiers or both.[27] The disease affects males predominantly but females frequently have an attenuated phenotype. However, only males develop renal failure.[26]

The excretion of low-molecular-weight proteins in the urine, such as albumin, beta$_2$-microglobulin, and alpha$_1$-microglobulin, is thought to be the most reliable marker for the disease. It is not a specific finding as it can be seen in tubulointerstitial diseases as well. It is much more pronounced in males (frequently above 1g/day) and sufficient to give a positive Labstix test. The degree of proteinuria is relatively constant and amounts to 0.5 to 2.0 g/ day in adults and up to 1 g/ day in children.[25, 28, 29] The nephrotic syndrome does not occur and albumin excretion represents less than half of the proteins excreted. Affected males usually excrete β$_2$-microglobulin in amounts that are more than 100-fold the upper limit of normal. Female carriers can also have low-molecular-weight proteinuria, but this is usually less pronounced than in males, and sometimes absent. Several studies have suggested that an attenuated form of the disease with low-molecular-weight proteinuria as the only or predominant feature might be prevalent in Japan.[30] Further clinical studies have shown that these patients have most of the features of Dent disease, with hypercalciuria and declining renal function,[29] and carry inactivating mutations in the *Clcn5* gene.[31]

Hypercalciuria is also a hallmark of this disorder and is present in most cases, beginning in childhood. It is usually overt and predominant in males (>7.5 mmol/day in males). Females are also frequently hypercalciuric but the values are usually closer to the upper limit of the normal range. Kidney stones are present in 50% of males investigated in several pedigrees, and are composed of calcium phosphate or a mixture of calcium phosphate and oxalate.[25] Multiple episodes starting during the teenage years are frequent. Radiologic nephrocalcinosis of the medullary type is seen in most affected males and occasionally females. Serum phosphate levels are usually below normal values or at the lower limit of the normal range. TmP/GFR is decreased, indicating defective reabsorption by the proximal tubule. Rickets is

also a frequent event in children. It is cured by the administration of pharmacologic doses of vitamin D. Osteomalacia occurs in adults, and is also corrected following administration of vitamin D. Serum levels of $1,25(OH)D_3$ are normal or slightly raised, whereas $25(OH)D$ levels are normal.

Systemic acidosis is usually not seen before renal function deteriorates significantly. Males have urinary acidification defects detectable by an ammonium chloride load but renal acidification abnormalities are not a consistent feature of the phenotype. Spontaneous hypokalemia is common in males and there is an inability to concentrate urine maximally following vasopressin injection. Aminoaciduria and glucosuria are also frequent. Half the males of four pedigrees had raised serum creatinine with progressive renal failure. End-stage renal failure occurred at 47 ± 13 years. Renal biopsy specimens show a pattern of a chronic interstitial nephritis with scattered calcium deposits.[25, 28] The glomeruli are normal or hyalinized; there is prominent tubular atrophy with diffuse inflammatory infiltrate composed of lymphocytes, and foci of calcification around and within epithelial cells.

Treatment

Treatment is largely supportive. Renal stones and hypercalciuria are treated with supportive measures (and in particular, increasing fluid intake). Dietary restriction of calcium reduces calcium excretion but is not recommended because it might contribute to the bone disease.[23] Thiazide diuretics may be given in small doses, but it is important to remember that these patients tend to have a salt-losing nephropathy and seem to respond with an excessive diuresis and decrease in blood pressure following the administration of diuretics.[25] Rickets is treated with small doses of vitamin D, but this treatment should be given with caution as it might increase urine calcium excretion and the risk of nephrolithiasis. Verifying urine calcium excretion before and after vitamin D therapy might be appropriate.[23]

Idiopathic Causes of the Renal Fanconi Syndrome

Idiopathic renal Fanconi syndrome occurs in the absence of known inborn errors of metabolism or acquired causes of the Fanconi syndrome (see Table 36-2). Most cases are sporadic, although familial cases associated with progressive renal failure have been reported and transmitted as an autosomal dominant trait.[32-34] No specific loci or genes have been discovered.

Cystinosis
Pathogenesis

Cystinosis is a rare autosomal recessive disease due to defective transport of the disulfide amino acid cystine across the lysosomal membrane. The transport of cystine out of the lysosome is impaired, with consequent cellular accumulation and crystallization that destroys tissues, causing renal failure at 10 years of age, and a variety of other complications (reviewed in reference 35). The incidence of the disease in North America is 1 in 160,000 and is caused by inactivating mutations in *CTNS*, encoding an integral lysosomal membrane protein termed *cystinosin*.[36] *CTNS* has 12 exons and a 2.6-kb mRNA encoding a 367–amino acid putative cystine transporter with seven transmembrane domains. Recent studies have suggested that cystinosin represents a novel H[+]-driven transporter that is responsible for cystine export from lysosomes.[37] In cystinosis, free cystine accumulates and forms crystals within the lysosomes in various tissues and at variable rates.

Clinical Presentation

Cystinosis is the most frequent cause of the renal Fanconi syndrome in children (see Table 36-2). The clinical presentation of cystinosis is variable (reviewed in references 35, 38) and each variant is part of a clinical spectrum that encompasses classic nephropathic cystinosis, a rare "adolescent" variant, and a mild adult-onset variant.[39] Nephropathic cystinosis usually presents in the first year of life with failure to thrive, increased thirst, excessive urination (polyuria), poor feeding, and hypophosphatemic rickets (Table 36-3). In whites, affected subjects frequently have blond hair and blue eyes, and are more lightly pigmented. Renal wasting of sodium, calcium, and magnesium is frequently seen, as well as tubular proteinuria. Progressive renal damage usually culminates in end-stage renal failure by the end of the first decade. The disease does not recur in the donor kidney. However, photophobia, hypothyroidism, and continued accumulation in tissues resulting in retinal blindness, corneal erosions, diabetes mellitus, distal myopathy, swallowing difficulties, decreased pulmonary function, pancreatic failure, primary hypogonadism in males, and neurologic deterioration in a significant number of renal transplant recipients occur (reviewed in reference 35).

Cystinosis can affect most of the structures of the eye, with variable rates of progression. In the cornea, crystal deposits are absent at birth and appear by the end of the first year of life. They can be seen by slit-lamp examination as pathognomonic fusiform crystals involving the anterior third of the central cornea and the full thickness of the peripheral

cornea. Eventually these deposits progress to develop a characteristic haziness. Deposits can also be found in the iridis and conjunctiva, as well as in the retina, with consequent development of a characteristic peripheral retinopathy.

Other features of cystinosis include hypothyroidism from cystine crystallization in the follicular cells of the thyroid gland. It is present in more than 70% of patients after age 10 years.[40] Insulin-dependent diabetes mellitus can result from pancreatic long-standing cystine crystal accumulation, particularly after renal transplantation.[41] Hepatomegaly and splenomegaly with little clinical impact occur in more than 40% of patients after age 10.[40] A distal vacuolar myopathy is also a frequent late finding in 25% of cystinotic patients, with wasting in the small hand muscles, with or without facial weakness and dysphagia. In a previous study, muscle biopsies revealed marked variability in fiber size, prominent acid phosphatase–positive vacuoles, and absence of fiber-type grouping or inflammatory cells. Crystals of cystine were detected in perimysial cells but not within the muscle cell vacuoles. The muscle cystine content of clinically affected muscles was markedly elevated.[42] Central nervous system involvement has been described in the late stages of the disease (reviewed in reference 38), and cystine crystal accumulation has been reported.

The diagnosis is usually made by measuring the cystine content of peripheral leukocytes or cultured fibroblasts. Cystinotic patients usually have values higher than 2 nmol of half-cystine per milligram of protein (normal <0.2 nmol of half-cystine per milligram of protein). Alternatively, the diagnosis can be made by recognizing the characteristic corneal crystals on slit-lamp examination. Cystinosis can be diagnosed in utero by cystine measurements in amniocytes or chorionic villi, or at birth cystine measurements on the placenta.

Treatment

Early diagnosis, and appropriate treatment with dialysis and renal transplantation has improved the outcome of patients with nephropathic cystinosis, and patients are now reaching adulthood. Symptomatic treatment involves rehydration, particularly during episodes of gastroenteritis. Replacement of bicarbonate losses with citrate or bicarbonate-containing salts is frequently indicated. Phosphate losses are replaced with phosphate salts and oral vitamin D therapy. Indomethacin has been used for decreasing the renal salt- and water-wasting syndrome. Dialysis has to be initiated at age 10 on average. Recombinant human growth hormone can also be given to increase growth and does not increase the rate of progression of renal failure.[43]

The cystine-leting drug cysteamine is now widely used for cystinosis (Fig. 36-2). It has been shown to slow the rate of progression of renal failure, and increase growth in affected patients.[43-45] Kidney function stabilizes upon initiation of therapy and even allows glomerular function to improve if begun in the first year or two of life.[45] The growth rate becomes normal, but there is no catching up. It is expected that cystinotic patients treated at an early age will reach adulthood without end-stage renal failure. Topical cysteamine eye drops can be used to treat ocular complications of cystinosis, and results in dissolution of corneal crystals.[46]

Transplantation is now routinely performed in cystinotic patients, and most do well.[47] Kidneys from heterozygous

TABLE 36-3

Age-Related Clinical Characteristics of Untreated Nephropathic Cystinosis

AGE (YR)	SYMPTOM OR SIGN	PREVALENCE OF AFFECTED PATIENTS (%)
6-12 mo	Renal Fanconi syndrome (polyuria, polydipsia, electrolyte imbalance, dehydration, rickets, growth failure)	95
5-10	Hypothyroidism	50
8-12	Photophobia	50
8-12	Chronic renal failure	95
12-40	Myopathy, difficulty swallowing	20
13-40	Retinal blindness	10-15
18-40	Diabetes mellitus	5
18-40	Male hypogonadism	70
21-40	Pulmonary dysfunction	100
21-40	Central venous system calcifications	15
21-40	Central venous system symptomatic deterioration	2

Data from Gahl WA, Thoene JG, Schneider JA: Cystinosis. N Engl J Med 347:111-112, 2002.

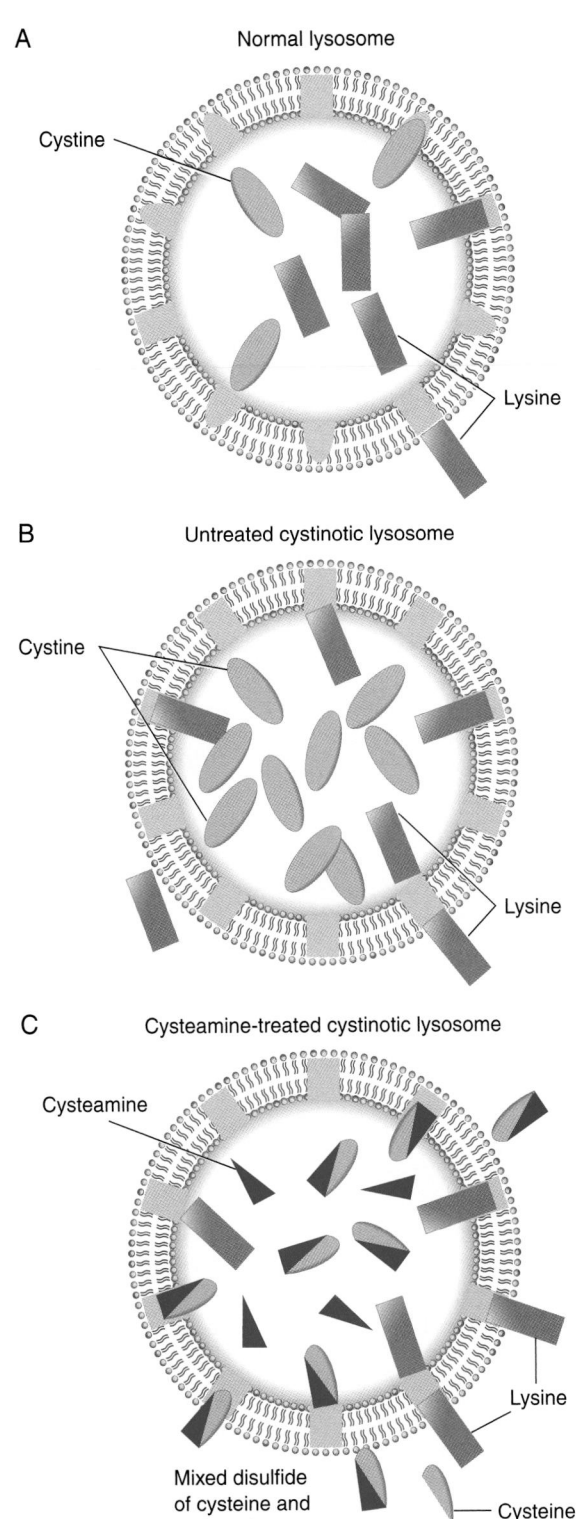

A Normal lysosome

Cystine

Lysine

B Untreated cystinotic lysosome

Cystine

Lysine

C Cysteamine-treated cystinotic lysosome

Cysteamine

Lysine

Mixed disulfide of cysteine and cysteamine

Cysteine

FIGURE 36-2. Mechanism of cystine depletion by cysteamine. **A,** In normal lysosomes, cystine and lysine freely traverse the lysosomal membrane through specific transporters (rectangular shape for the lysine transporter, cup shape for the cystine transporter). **B,** In cystinotic lysosomes (note the absence of specific cystine transporters), lysine can freely traverse, through specific transporters, the lysosomal membrane, but cystine cannot, and it therefore accumulates inside the lysosome. **C,** In cysteamine-treated lysosomes, cysteamine combines with half-cystine (i.e., cysteine) to form the mixed disulfide cysteine-cysteamine, which uses the lysine transporter to exit the lysosome. (Modified from Gahl WA, Thoene JG, Schneider JA: Cystinosis. N Engl J Med 347:111-121, 2002. Copyright © 2002 Massachusetts Medical Society. All rights reserved.)

donors are widely accepted because there is no evidence of cystine accumulation in kidney transplants.

Glycogenosis Type 1 (von Gierke Disease)

Type 1 glycogen storage disease is the only glycogenosis associated with primary renal involvement. Type 1a glycogenosis is the most frequent, and other forms (types 1b, 1c, and 1d) are extremely rare. Type 5 glycogen storage disease (McArdle disease), as well as other rare glycogenoses, can be associated with acute tubular necrosis from rhabdomyolysis and myoglobinuria, but will not be discussed further here.

Pathogenesis

Glycogen storage disease type 1, also known as von Gierke disease, refers to a group of autosomal recessive metabolic disorders caused by deficiencies in the activity of the glucose-6-phosphatase (G6Pase) system that consists of at least two membrane proteins, glucose 6-phosphate transporter (G6PT) and G6Pase (reviewed in reference 48). Mutations in the gene encoding G6Pase on chromosome 17 have been identified and shown to cause type 1a,[49-51] whereas type 1b is caused by a deficiency in a microsomal G6PT on chromosome 11.[52, 53] Other variants include types 1c and 1d (defect in microsomal glucose transport), but the molecular basis remains to be identified.[54]

G6PT translocates glucose 6-phosphate from cytoplasm to the lumen of the endoplasmic reticulum and G6Pase catalyzes the hydrolysis of glucose 6-phosphate to produce glucose and phosphate (Fig. 36-3). Therefore, G6PT and G6Pase work in concert to maintain glucose homeostasis. Whereas G6Pase is exclusively expressed in gluconeogenic cells, G6PT is ubiquitously expressed and its deficiency generally causes a more severe phenotype. Liver and muscle store important quantities of glycogen, and are primarily affected in glycogen storage diseases.

Hypoglycemia occurs because of impaired gluconeogenesis, glycogenolysis, and recycling of glucose through the glucose 6-phosphate-to-glucose system. Accumulation of glucose 6-phosphate leads to increased glycolysis and lactic acidosis. Hyperuricemia and gout are a consequence of increased activity of hepatic adenosine monophosphate (AMP)–deaminase and adenine nucleotide production, thus increasing uric acid production. Hyperuricemia also results from decreased renal excretion because urate competes with lactate for secretion. Dyslipidemia is caused by increased synthesis of very low-density lipoprotein (VLDL), and LDL, and decreased lipolysis. Fatty infiltration of the liver is a frequent finding.

Clinical Presentation

In the first year of life, glycogenosis type 1 presents with hepatomegaly or hypoglycemic seizures, or both, with lactic acidosis. An enlarged abdomen from hepatomegaly, short stature from impaired growth, and skin manifestations from dyslipidemia (xanthomas) are frequent findings. Hypoglycemia can cause seizures. Easy bruising and epistaxis result from prolonged bleeding time as a consequence of impaired platelet adhesion and aggregation. Gout is seen in adults, but rarely in children. Muscle cramps and weakness, exercise

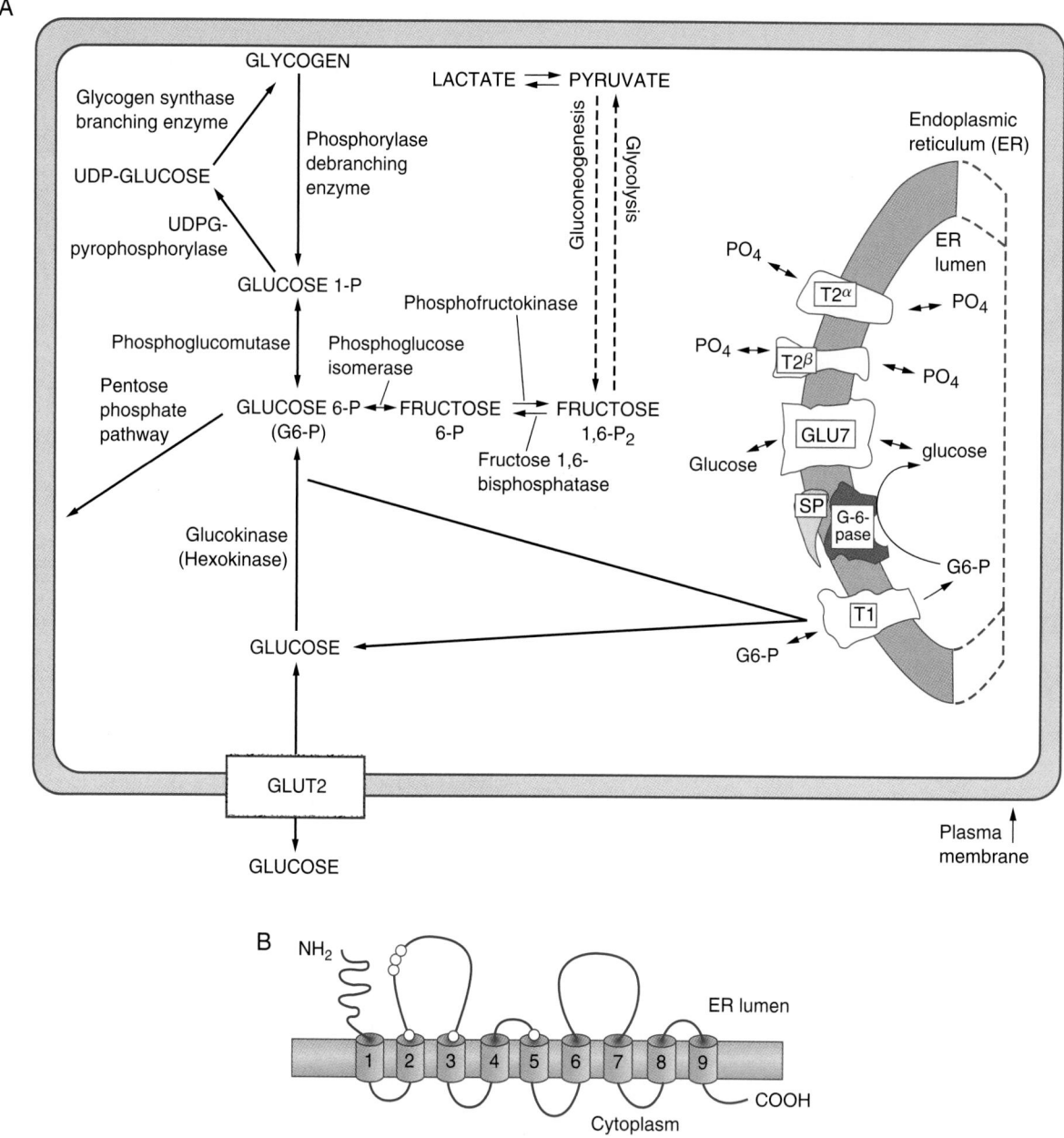

FIGURE 36-3. A, Left part of the figure: major pathways of synthesis and breakdown of glycogen in liver. The broken line indicates that several enzymes have been omitted between pyruvate and fructose-1,6-P₂. GLUT, glucose transport protein; UDP, uridine diphosphate; UDPG, uridine diphosphate glucose. Right part of the figure: schematic working model of the hepatic microsomal glucose-6-phosphatase system; E, the catalytic subunit of glucose-6-phosphatase; ER, endoplasmic reticulum; GLUT7, the microsomal glucose transport protein; SP, the stabilizing protein, and regulatory Ca²⁺-binding protein; T1, a microsomal glucose-6-phosphate transport protein; T2α, a microsomal Pi transport protein; T2β, a microsomal series: Pi, PPi, and carbamoylphosphate transport protein. This model is not meant to represent the actual topology of the six proteins in the membrane. **B,** Glucose-6-phosphatase is anchored in the endoplasmic reticulum (ER) by nine transmembrane helices. The NH₂ terminus faces the ER lumen and the COOH terminus faces the cytoplasm. (**A,** Modified with permission from Chen WM, Deng HW: A general and accurate approach for computing the statistical power of the transmission disequilibrium test for complex disease genes. Genet Epidemiol 21:53-67, 2001; **B,** modified with permission from Pan C-J, Lei K-J, Chen H, et al: Ontogeny of the murine glucose-6-phosphate system. Arch Biochem Biopys 358:17-24, 1998.)

intolerance, and fatigue are other clinical manifestations of glycogen storage diseases.

Adults usually present with hypoglycemic symptoms exacerbated by exercise and relieved by food. However, 48-hour fasting blood glucose levels are frequently normal.[55] Hepatomegaly is a usual finding. Renal disease is common (reviewed in references 56, 57) with untreated glycogenosis.

In children, increased kidney size, hyperfiltration, and moderate proteinuria are common.[58] Renal failure evolves slowly. Renal stones containing calcium can occur as distal renal tubular acidosis, hypocitraturia, and hypercalciuria, and nephrocalcinosis can be variably associated. Virtually all patients studied have impaired distal tubular acidification.[59] This might be secondary to decreased ammonia excretion.

A renal Fanconi syndrome with aminoaciduria, low-molecular-weight proteinuria, phosphaturia, and bicarbonaturia can be present.[60, 61] The most common histologic finding in type 1 glycogenosis is focal and segmental glomerulosclerosis with tubulointerstitial atrophy. Glomerular changes include thickening, lamellation, and glycogen deposition in the glomerular basement membrane.[62]

A glucagon test with 1 mg given intramuscularly can be used to screen for glycogenosis and is frequently abnormal (rise in blood glucose <4 mmol/L, usually at 30 minutes). The definitive diagnosis of glycogenosis type 1 requires a liver biopsy with measurement of G6Pase activity or one of the three microsomal translocase systems. The liver histology is characterized by hepatocyte distention from glycogen and fat with large lipid vacuoles. There is no fibrosis. Abnormally high glycogen levels are noted in liver biopsy samples. Electron microscopy shows moderate to large excesses of glycogen in the cytoplasm, often displacing the organelles in the hepatocytes. Sequencing of the defective gene can be used to avoid liver biopsy.

Treatment

The objective of treatment is to maintain normoglycemia to avoid metabolic complications and lactic acidosis. Normoglycemia can be accomplished at night with nasogastric feeding of glucose[63] or with orally administered uncooked cornstarch. A single dose (1.75-2.5 g/kg) of the latter at bedtime will maintain serum glucose concentrations higher than 3.9 mmol/L for 7 hours or longer in most young adults.[64] Because hypoglycemia and lactic acidosis occur in adults as well, treatment might also be indicated after growth.[65] Kidney transplantation has been successfully performed, but it does not correct the hypoglycemia.

Tyrosinemia
Pathogenesis

Hepatorenal tyrosinemia (tyrosinemia type 1) is a rare autosomal recessive disorder (reviewed in reference 66) affecting principally the liver, kidney, and peripheral nerves. Mutations in the gene encoding fumarylacetoacetate hydrolase on chromosome 15q23-q25 are responsible for tyrosinemia type 1.[67-72] The hepatic toxicity is caused by fumarylacetoacetate accumulation, apparently inducing the release of cytochrome *c*, which in turn triggers activation of the caspase cascade in hepatocytes of affected animal models.[73] It is unlikely that tryrosine accumulation leads to the hepatic and renal manifestations of the disease because hypertyrosinemia has been described in other settings without renal and liver involvement.

Clinical Presentation

Tyrosinemia is characterized by severe liver disease, which either causes liver failure in infancy or may take a more protracted course, with death often occurring during childhood or adolescence because of hepatoma development. It is particularly prevalent in the genetically isolated region of Saguenay-Lac-Saint-Jean in Quebec where the carrier rate is 1 in 20 and the incidence is 1 in 2000, and where nearly 80% of the gene pool comes from founders who settled in the 17th century.[68] Worldwide, the incidence is 1 in 100,000. Initially, liver dysfunction often affects coagulation factors, even before other signs of liver failure appear. In fact, jaundice and elevated liver enzymes are rare in the early stages of tyrosinemia. A common presentation mode is the "acute hepatic crisis" in which ascites, jaundice, and gastrointestinal bleeding are precipitated by an acute event such as an infection. Acute hepatic crises usually resolve spontaneously, but on occasion progress to complete liver failure and encephalopathy. Cirrhosis eventually develops in most patients with the disease and hepatocellular carcinoma is frequent in tyrosinemic subjects with chronic liver disease.[74] It is believed that the toxic metabolites that accumulate in tyrosinemia, such as fumarylacetoacetate, are mutagenic and contribute to the elevated rate of liver carcinoma.[75] Serial ultrasounds and computed tomography (CT) scans are indicated. Neurologic crises are acute episodes of peripheral neuropathy with painful paresthesias and eventually autonomic dysfunction.[66, 76] Renal involvement is almost always present in tyrosinemic subjects[66] and is probably caused by succinylacetone toxicity.[77, 78] It ranges from mild tubular dysfunction to renal failure.

Hypophosphatemic rickets is the principal sign of tubular dysfunction, and acute decompensation can exacerbate the dysfunction. Generalized aminoaciduria is frequent. Nephrocalcinosis and nephromegaly can often be seen on renal ultrasounds.[79] Glucosuria and proteinuria are usually mild. The glomerular filtration rate (GFR) is frequently decreased. Tubular defects respond to diet but may be irreversible in chronic cases.

Treatment

Orthotopic liver transplantation has been used for several years (see review on management in references 66, 80). The decision to perform liver transplantation depends on the patient's liver status and neurologic symptoms. Stable patients with adequate liver function and the absence of nodules on CT scan can be managed conservatively with a low-phenylalanine, low-tyrosine diet. The renal dysfunction may persist following transplantation as the renal enzyme is still defective.[81]

Galactosemia
Pathogenesis

Galactosemia is an inherited metabolic disorder in which there is an inability to metabolize lactose. Three inherited disorders of galactose metabolism resulting in galactosemia have been described and are transmitted by an autosomal recessive mode (reviewed in references 82, 83). Clinical manifestations appear following exposure to galactose and can produce failure to thrive, vomiting, inanition, liver disease, cataracts, and developmental delay. The genetic defects responsible for galactosemia can be a deficiency of galactose 1-phosphate uridyltransferase,[84] galactokinase, or uridine diphosphate galactose 4'-epimerase. These enzymes catalyze the reactions in the unique pathway converting galactose to glucose.

Clinical Presentation

The clinical manifestations of galactosemia range from cataracts for galactokinase deficiency, to important toxicity syndromes resulting from galactose exposure in galactose 1-phosphate uridyltransferase and uridine diphosphate galactose 4′-epimerase deficiency. Vomiting, diarrhea, jaundice, hepatomegaly, and ascites occur in transferase deficiency. Tubular proteinuria, generalized aminoaciduria, and bicarbonaturia may occur and can quickly disappear following withdrawal of galactose.

The diagnosis is suggested by galactose or galactose 1-phosphate in serum, or galactose in the urine. The definitive diagnosis is made by the demonstration of the enzyme deficiency in blood cells, cultured skin fibroblasts, or other tissues.[82, 83]

Treatment

Elimination of dietary lactose from the diet is the mainstay of therapy for galactosemia.[83, 85]

Lowe Oculocerebrorenal Syndrome

The oculocerebrorenal syndrome of Lowe (OMIM 309000) is an X-linked recessive multisystem disorder characterized by congenital cataracts, mental retardation, and renal Fanconi syndrome (reviewed in reference 86). The *OCRL1* gene, which, when mutated, is responsible for OCRL,[87, 88] encodes a 105-kDa Golgi protein with phosphatidylinositol (4,5) bisphosphate 5-phosphatase activity. Therefore, OCRL is mainly a lipid phosphatase that may control cellular levels of a critical metabolite, phosphatidylinositol 4,5-bisphosphate,[89] and is involved in the inositol phosphate signaling pathway. The mechanism whereby this enzyme leads to the abnormalities remains obscure.

Renal dysfunction (Fanconi syndrome) is a major feature and occurs in the first year of life, but the severity and age of onset vary. It is characterized by proteinuria (0.5-2.0 g of urinary protein per square meter of body surface area per day), generalized aminoaciduria (100-1000 μmol of urinary amino acid per kilogram of body weight per day), carnitine wasting (mean fractional excretion, 0.05-0.15), phosphaturia, and bicarbonaturia.[90] Glucosuria is usually not present. Linear growth decreases after 1 year of age. Glomerular function also falls with age, with renal failure predicted between the second and fourth decade of life. Neurologic findings include infantile hypotonia, mental retardation, and areflexia. Prenatal development of cataracts is universal and other ocular anomalies include glaucoma, microphthalmos, and corneal keloid formation. Visual acuity is frequently decreased. Mental retardation is very common but not universal. Cranial magnetic resonance imaging (MRI) shows mild ventriculomegaly and cysts in the periventricular regions. Status epilepticus is also frequent. Death usually occurs in the second or third decade from renal failure or infection.

In the absence of reliable biochemical tests or a confirmed family history, the diagnosis is made clinically. It depends on the cardinal ocular, renal, and neurologic manifestations. Carrier detection by slit-lamp examination has high but not absolute sensitivity. Concentrations of the muscle enzymes creatine kinase, aspartate aminotransferase, and lactate dehydrogenase, as well as of total serum protein, serum α_2-globulin, and high-density lipoprotein (HDL) cholesterol, are elevated. Carrier detection can be performed by slit-lamp examination or by mutation detection or linkage analysis of markers when the mutation is unknown.

Treatment is supportive and includes taking care of ocular (cataract extraction, treatment of glaucoma), neurologic (anticonvulsants, speech therapy), and renal complications. Bicarbonate therapy is usually given at a dose of 2 to 3 mmol/kg/day every 6 to 8 hours. Sodium or potassium phosphate can be given in amounts of 1 to 4 g/day for phosphate depletion and if unsuccessful, vitamin D may be added.

Wilson Disease
Pathogenesis

Wilson disease (OMIM 277900) is an autosomal recessive disorder in which biliary excretion of copper and incorporation into ceruloplasmin is impaired, leading to liver damage and neuronal degeneration from accumulation of copper (reviewed in reference 91). Accumulation in the brain, kidney, and eyes leads to loss of coordination, proximal tubular dysfunction, and the characteristic corneal rings. The frequency of the disease is approximately 1 in 100,000 births. Biliary excretion of copper and incorporation into ceruloplasmin are both severely impaired. This causes accumulation in the liver, and eventually in the brain. The disease-associated gene encodes a copper-transporting P-type adenosine triphosphatase (ATPase), the WND protein,[92-95] that is targeted to the mitochondria. This suggests that its role in copper-dependent processes takes place in this organelle.[96]

Clinical Presentation

Affected adults often show most features of the Fanconi syndrome with aminoaciduria, bicarbonaturia, phosphaturia, glucosuria, and low-molecular-weight proteinuria.[97] Hypercalciuria is frequent, and kidney stones and nephrocalcinosis have been described in several cases.[98-101] Children usually do not have renal manifestations. Renal tubular dysfunction is probably caused by copper accumulation. Ultrastructural findings on renal biopsy include electron-dense deposits in the tubular cytoplasm.[102] Most patients with Wilson disease present with liver dysfunction, neurologic symptoms, or a combination. Liver symptoms can take multiple forms, that is, chronic and acute liver failure. The biliary excretion defect leads to accumulation of copper in the liver, with progressive damage, and overflow to the brain. This causes accumulation of copper in the central nervous system, frequently manifested as dysarthria and coordination defects of voluntary movements. This is frequently accompanied by involuntary movements. Pseudobulbar palsy is frequent and a common mode of death in unrecognized cases. The Kayser-Fleischer ring is the most important sign of Wilson disease. It is a yellow-brown (dull copper-colored) granular deposit on the Descemet membrane at the limbus of the cornea, usually seen earliest at the upper and lower poles.[103] Wilson disease should be suspected in all patients with acute or chronic liver dysfunction. The diagnosis of Wilson disease can be made by identifying Kayser-Fleischer rings, or by finding increased levels of serum or urine copper and reduced serum ceruloplasmin levels. Increased liver copper (>300 μg/g dry weight) is a reliable finding. Lack of incorporation of ^{64}Cu or ^{67}Cu into ceruloplasmin over 48 hours is the most definitive test available.

Treatment

Chelation of copper with D-penicillamine, the treatment of choice for Wilson disease, is very effective and has dramatically changed the course of the liver disease.[104] Adults usually require 1 g/day of D-penicillamine given in two doses. In patients, 24-hour urinary excretion of copper should be monitored to achieve copper losses of 2 mg/day. Doses of D-penicillamine can be decreased after 1 or 2 years to achieve urinary losses of 1 mg/day. There are several problems with D-penicillamine, including toxicity and increased serum copper levels initially, that can worsen the neurologic symptoms. Alternative treatments include zinc salts, which block intestinal copper absorption by inducing metallothionein synthesis in the mucosal intestinal cells. Tetrathiomolybdate appears to be an excellent form of initial treatment in patients who present with neurologic symptoms and signs. In contrast to penicillamine therapy, initial treatment with tetrathiomolybdate rarely allows further neurologic deterioration.[105] Orthotopic liver transplantation can be used in cases with severe hepatic decompensation.[106]

Hereditary Fructose Intolerance

There are several disorders of fructose metabolism secondary to deficiencies in aldolase B, fructose 1-phosphate aldolase, and fructokinase, respectively (reviewed in reference 107). Hereditary fructose intolerance (OMIM 229600), caused by aldolase B deficiency (fructose-1,6-bisphosphate aldolase, EC 4.1.2.13), is an autosomal recessive disorder characterized by severe hypoglycemia and vomiting shortly after the intake of fructose.[107, 108] The disease can be associated with proximal tubule dysfunction with aminoaciduria, bicarbonaturia and phosphaturia, and lactic acidosis. Kidney biopsy shows discrete findings. Liver dysfunction, hepatomegaly, cirrhosis, and jaundice appear from prolonged exposure. Hypoglycemia is, unfortunately, frequently absent. Continued ingestion of noxious sugars leads to hepatic and renal injury and growth retardation. The most common mutation has a prevalence of 1.3%, suggesting a frequency of 1 in 23,000 homozygotes.[109]

The pathophysiology of the renal Fanconi syndrome is not clear, but could be related to vacuolar proton pump dysfunction in the proximal tubule, as a direct binding interaction between V-ATPase and aldolase was demonstrated for the regulation of the V-ATPase.[110] This study, showed that aldolase B was abundant in endocytosis zones of the proximal tubule, a subcellular domain also abundant in V-ATPase.[110] V-H$^+$-ATPases are essential for acidification of intracellular compartments and for proton secretion from the plasma membrane in kidney epithelial cells and osteoclasts. Perhaps the release of nonfunctional aldolase B in response to fructose ingestion impairs the coupling of the V-ATPase to glycolysis. Thus, mechanistic similarities in organelle dysfunction between Dent disease and hereditary fructose intolerance are apparent.

The treatment of hereditary fructose intolerance involves withdrawal of sucrose, fructose, and sorbitol from the diet.

INHERITED DISORDERS OF RENAL AMINO ACID TRANSPORT

Because amino acids are not significantly bound to proteins in the plasma (except for tryptophan, which is 60%-90% bound), they are freely filtered by the glomerulus. However, the proximal tubule will reabsorb 95% to 99.9% of the filtered load; thus the excretion of more than 5% of the filtered load of an amino acid is significant. Aminoaciduria occurs when a renal transport defect of the proximal tubule decreases the reabsorptive capacity for one or several amino acids, or when the threshold for reabsorbing an amino acid is exceeded by elevated plasma levels as a result of a metabolic defect ("overflow aminoaciduria"). Such inherited diseases of amino acid metabolism will not be discussed in this section, and the reader is invited to consult recent reviews.[111] Theoretically, renal aminoacidurias (Table 36-4) can be secondary to defects in brush border or basolateral transporters and intracellular trafficking of amino acids. They are usually detected by newborn urine screening programs in several Western countries, and the most frequent abnormalities identified (apart from phenylketonuria, now normally detected by blood screening) are cystinuria, histidinemia, Hartnup disease, and iminoglycinuria.[112] Clinically, the most significant renal aminoaciduria is cystinuria. Most of the other disorders are rarely symptomatic.

Proteins ingested in the regular diet and degraded in the intestine are absorbed by the intestinal mucosa as amino acids and small oligopeptides. Apical and basolateral transporters carry the amino acids into the blood, where they are used for metabolic needs, but are also freely filtered by the kidneys. Renal amino acid reabsorption occurs in the proximal tubule through a variety of transporters. Most amino acids are reabsorbed by more than one transporter and almost completely reclaimed, except for histidine which has a fractional excretion of 5% (reviewed in reference 113). Most amino acids are probably reabsorbed by a transporter that is shared by several amino acids and has a low affinity but high transport capacity, and one that is specific for one amino acid and has a high affinity and low maximal transport capacity. Because most amino acid carriers have not been cloned, a more detailed discussion is not possible at this stage. Common carriers have been divided into five groups and transport neutral and cyclic amino acids, glycine

TABLE 36-4

Classification of the Aminoacidurias

DISEASE	AMINO ACIDS
	Basic amino acids
Cystinuria	Cystine, lysine, ornithine, arginine
Lysinuric protein intolerance	Lysine, arginine, ornithine
Isolated cystinuria	Cystine
Lysinuria	Lysine
	Neutral amino acids
Hartnup disease	Alanine, asparagine, glutamine, histidine, isoleucine, leucine, phenylalanine, serine, threonine, tryptophan, tyrosine, valine
Blue diaper syndrome	Tryptophan
Iminoglycinuria	Glycine, proline, hydroxyproline
Glycinuria	Glycine
Methioninuria	Methionine

and imino acids, cystine and dibasic amino acids, dicarboxylic amino acids, and β-amino acids (reviewed in reference 3). The transport of amino acids is coupled to the sodium gradient established by the basolateral Na^+,K^+-ATPase.

Cystinuria

Cystinuria (OMIM 220200) is the most frequent and best known of the aminoacidurias. It is an autosomal recessive disorder associated with defective transport of cystine and the dibasic amino acids ornithine, lysine, and arginine. It involves the epithelial cells of the renal tubule and gastrointestinal tract (Fig. 36-4). The formation of cystine calculi in the urinary tract, potentially leading to infection and renal failure, is the hallmark of the disorder. Cystine is the least soluble of the naturally occurring amino acids, particularly at low pH. Worldwide, the prevalence is approximately 1 in 7000. Thus, it is one of the most frequent mendelian disorders. The prevalence varies according to geographic location and has been estimated at 1 in 15,000 in the United States,[114] 1 in 2000 in England,[115] 1 in 4000 in Australia,[116] and 1 in 2500 in Jews of Libyan origin.[117] Newborn screening programs worldwide now help identify cases.

Pathogenesis

GENETICS

Cystinuria is genetically heterogeneous and caused by mutations in either of two genes implicated in dibasic amino acid

transport by the proximal tubule: *SLC3A1* (solute carrier family 3, member 1) and *SLC7A9*.*SLC3A1* encodes rBAT, and *SLC7A9* encodes $b^{o,+}$AT, a subunit that associates with rBAT to form the active transporter (reviewed in reference 118). Each cystinuria subtype is characterized by the amounts of cystine excreted by the parents (who are usually asymptomatic heterozygotes). Based on recent developments in the genetics and physiology of cystinuria, the traditional classification, which was based on the excretion of cystine and dibasic amino acids in obligate heterozygotes, is no longer supported.[119] By itself, the subunit $b^{o,+}$AT is sufficient to catalyze transmembrane amino acid exchange, that is, the exchange of dibasic amino acids for neutral amino acids.[120] A model for the reabsorption of different amino acids in the proximal tubule is represented in Figure 36-4.

Type A cystinuria is caused by mutations in both alleles of *SLC3A1* (chromosome 2). It is a completely recessive disease in which both parents excrete normal amounts of cystine (0-100 μmol/g creatinine). Jejunal uptake of cystine and dibasic amino acids is absent and there is no plasma response to an oral cystine load. The risk of nephrolithiasis is very high. The disorder is due to mutations in the *SLC3A1* gene, which encodes the renal proximal tubule S3 segment and intestinal dibasic amino acid transporter (Fig. 36-5).[121] Over 40 different mutations have been reported to date. The most common point mutation, the M467T and its relative M467K, have been expressed in vitro in oocytes.[122] The amount of rBAT protein was similar in normal and mutant-injected oocytes. The K_m and the voltage dependence for transport of

PROXIMAL TUBULE

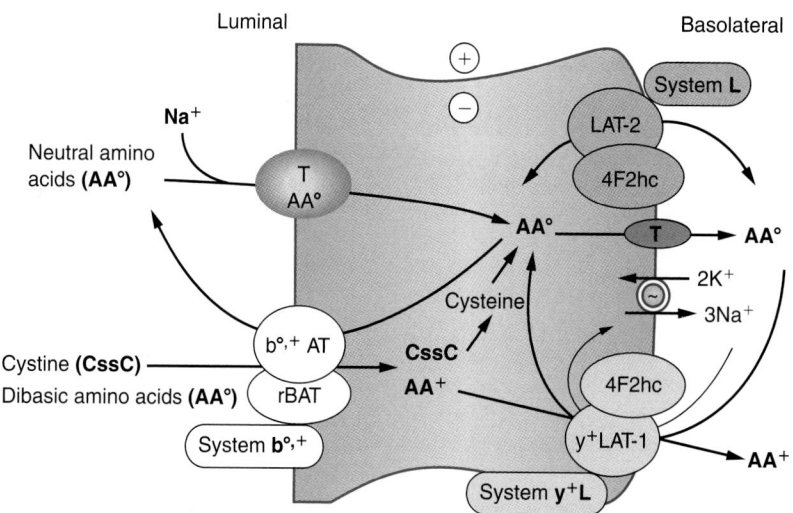

FIGURE 36-4. Model for the reabsorption of different amino acids in the opossum kidney proximal tubule cell. Transepithelial flux of amino acids through the cell is ensured by the presence of different transport systems at the apical and basolateral membrane. A tertiary active transport mechanism accounts for the reabsorption of dibasic amino acids (AA⁺) and cystine (CssC); an apical Na⁺-dependent neutral amino acid transport system (T AA⁰) accounts for the high accumulation of neutral amino acids (AA⁰) in the cell, which provide the driving force for the entry of cystine and dibasic amino acids through system $b^{o,+}$ (rBAT-$b^{o,+}$AT). Dibasic amino acid and cysteine influx is favored by the negative membrane potential and the rapid reduction of cystine to cystine, respectively. Net efflux of dibasic amino acids is accounted for by exchange with neutral amino acids plus sodium via system y+L (4F2hc-y+LAT-1) at the basolateral membrane. The pool of intracellular neutral amino acids (including cysteine) can be exchanged with the extracellular neutral amino acid pool via the basolateral system L (4F2hc-LAT-2). As long as this exchange is 1:1, the neutral amino acid individual pools, but not the total pool, will change depending on the concentrations of the different amino acids at either side of the basolateral membrane and on the intrinsic asymmetry of the transporter. Therefore, a facilitative neutral amino acid transporter (T) must be present at the basolateral membrane to explain net transport of the these amino acids. (Modified from Chillaron J, Roca R, Valencia A, et al: Heteromeric amino acid transporters: Biochemistry, genetics, and physiology. Am J Physiol Renal Physiol 281:F995-F1018, 2001.)

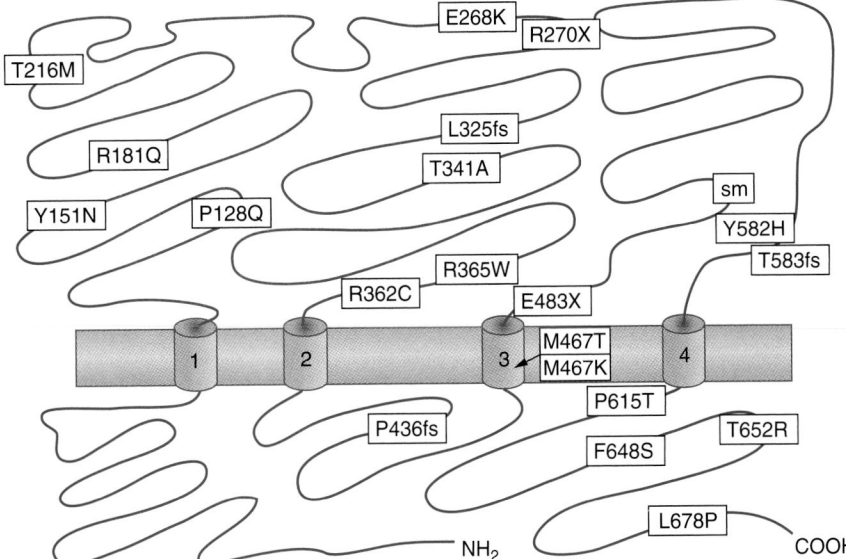

FIGURE 36-5. A four-transmembrane domain topology model of the human rBAT protein. Twenty-one cystinuria-specific mutations are indicated by arrows. fs, frameshift mutations, sm, splice site mutation. (Modified with permission from Palacín M, Estévez P, Běrtran J, et al: Molecular biology of mammalian plasma membrane amino acid transporters, Physiol Rev 78:969-1054, 1998.)

the different substrates were the same in both M467T and wild-type injected oocytes. The M467K mutant displayed a normal K_m, but the V_{max} was between 5% and 35% of the wild type. Most of the M467T and M467K proteins were located in an intracellular compartment, contrary to the wild-type protein, and were endoglycosidase H–sensitive, suggesting longer residence time in the endoplasmic reticulum. These data indicate impaired maturation and transport to the plasma membrane of the M467T and M467K mutants.

Type B cystinuria (see Figure 36-5) is an incompletely recessive form in which both parents excrete intermediate amounts of cystine (100-600 μmol/g creatinine). Parents may also have a normal pattern as demonstrated in 14% of cases.[119] In 1999, the *SLC7A9* gene encoding BAT1 was located on chromosome 19q13.[123] BAT1 is a subunit linked to the rBAT via a disulfide bond. It belongs to a family of light subunits of amino acid transporters, expressed in the kidney, liver, small intestine, and placenta. Cotransfection of b[o, +]AT and rBAT brings the latter to the plasma membrane, and results in the uptake of L-arginine in vitro. Several mutations in non-type I cystinuria have been identified.[123]

Type AB cystinuria is caused by one mutation in *SLC3A1* and one mutation in *SLC7A9*. This type would involve the offspring of one parent carrier of a mutation on chromosome 2 and of another parent with a mutation on chromosome 19. Interestingly, the observed prevalence of AB patients is much lower than expected. Considering a similar frequency of mutations in *SLC7A9* and *SLC3A1*, we would expect one third of the patients to suffer from type A disease, one third from B disease, and one third from AB disease. Indeed, the prevalence of type A disease is similar to that of type B disease; however, type AB is extremely rare.[119] Two explanations could account for this low prevalence. The first is that type AB patients may suffer from a mild phenotype and therefore, in most cases, escape detection. Alternatively, these patients may actually represent type B (two mutations in *SLC7A9*, one of which was detected, the other yet to be defined) and a coincidental carrier state for an *SLC3A1* mutation.[119]

Renal transport defect. The existence of cystinuria has been recognized since 1810, first suspected from two patients with bladder stones, hence the name cystic oxide and cystine to characterize the chemical composition of the stones.[124, 125] Garrod later suspected that the disorder was due to a defect of cystine metabolism.[126] This turned out not to be the case as cystinuria is caused by a transporter defect. Reabsorption of cystine and dibasic amino acids across the proximal brush border membrane occurs via a common carrier that has been identified in several species, including the rat,[127] rabbit,[128] and human.[129]

Intestinal transport defect. Cystinuria also presents with a defective intestinal absorption of dibasic amino acids, which implies that there is a transporter defect in the gut similar to renal proximal tubule cells. This was first suggested from the increased urinary excretion of decarboxylation products such as putrescine and cadaverine,[130] which originate from the bacterial degradation of lysine and arginine, respectively. Following feeding with such amino acids, Milne and colleagues noted increases in the urinary excretion of these polyamines.[131, 132] Direct measurement of defective intestinal uptake of cystine was demonstrated in 1964 by Thier and co-workers on biopsy specimens.[133]

Subsequently, it was shown that the transporter was also expressed in the intestine.[134] Why an intestinal amino acid transport defect does not lead to more serious metabolic problems is not known, but could be explained by the ability of the intestine to absorb small (di- and tri-) peptides.[135, 136] It is also likely that there are other transporters of dibasic amino acids, as isolated cystinuria without lysinuria, argininuria, and ornithinuria[137] and dibasic amino aciduria without cystinuria have been described.[138]

Clinical Presentation

The only known manifestation of cystinuria is nephrolithiasis. Clinical expression of the disease frequently starts during the first to third decade but may occur from the first year of life up to the ninth decade. The disease occurs equally in both sexes but males tend to be more severely affected than females. Cystine stones are made of yellow-brown substance, are very hard, and appear radiopaque on roentgenograms. Radiopacity is due to sulfur molecules, but is lower than calcium stones. Stones are frequently multiple, staghorn, and tend to be smoother than calcium stones. Magnesium ammonium phosphate and calcium stones can also form as a result of infection.

Type A patients can be readily identified because their parents excrete normal amounts of cystine. More than 50% of type I patients will form one or more stones within the first decade of life. These patients are also more likely to exceed the solubility threshold for cystine than other groups.[139] Type B heterozygotes show the highest levels of urinary cystine excretion (990-1740 µmol/g creatinine).

Diagnosis can be made by the analysis of a simple urine sample wherein typical hexagonal crystals appear. Acidification of concentrated urine with acetic acid can also precipitate crystals not visible initially. Diagnosis is ultimately made by measurement of cystine excretion in the urine. This is usually performed in specialized centers using chromatographic methods. Quantitative ion-exchange chromatography is a frequently used method.[140] Quantitation of cystine can also be easily performed using a colorimetric method after reduction to the thiol.[141] Methods based on spectrophotometry, involving oxidation of cysteine by thallium, have been described.[142] High-performance liquid chromatography methods are also used.[143] The cyanide-nitroprusside test has been widely applied as a qualitative screening procedure. This method is particularly useful for the detection of homozygotes.[144] False positives include homocystinuria and patients with acetonuria.

Treatment

A recent study shows that a regularly followed medical program based on high diuresis and alkalization with second-line addition of thiols slows down or markedly decreases stone formation, and precludes the need for urologic procedures in more than half of the patients.[145] Patients poorly compliant with hyperdiuresis remain at risk for recurrence.

DIET

The primary treatment of cystinuria is based either on decreasing cystine supersaturation in the urine to prevent formation of crystals, or on the reduction of cystine excretion. Cystine production arises from the metabolism of methionine. Attempts at reducing methionine in the diet are uncomfortable and have been tried in the past with resulting limited usefulness.[146, 147] Reducing sodium in the diet results in lower urine cystine.[148-150]

DECREASING URINE CYSTINE SATURATION. This is usually accomplished with a combination of increased fluid intake and increasing urine pH. Increasing fluid intake should ideally reach 4 L/day because many patients excrete 1 g or more of cystine daily. At the least, daily urine output of 3 L seems necessary.[145] It is also important that the patient drink at bedtime and during sleep to prevent supersaturation during periods of reduced urine output.[151] Cystine solubility can also be increased by alkalinization of the urine with potassium citrate or bicarbonate, but the solubility of cystine

does not increase until the pH reaches 7.0 to 7.5. Citrate is the preferred method as alkalinization lasts longer. The requirements for alkali often reach 3 to 4 mmol/kg.

PENICILLAMINE

Patients who are unable to comply with a regimen of high-fluid intake and urine alkalinization or who fail despite adequate treatment can be given D-penicillamine in doses of 30 mg/kg up to a maximum of 2 g/day. Through a disulfide exchange reaction, D-penicillamine can form the disulfide cysteine-penicillamine which is much more soluble than cystine.[152] The usual doses vary between 1 and 2 g/day and lead to a reduction in urine cystine excretion and stone formation. This drug is variably tolerated and has frequent side effects such as rash, fever, and more rarely, arthralgias and medullary aplasia (reviewed in references 153, 154). Other reactions include proteinuria and membranous nephropathy, epidermolysis, and loss of taste. Inhibition of pyridoxine by D-penicillamine is also a potential side effect.[155] However, several studies have found that D-penicillamine is generally well tolerated in cystinurics.[156, 157] Another drug that may be useful in cystinuria is mercaptopropionylglycine.[158-161] The mechanism of action of mercaptopropionylglycine is identical to that of D-penicillamine. This drug is as effective as D-penicillamine in reducing urine cystine excretion but also has substantial side effects. These include skin rash, fever, nausea, proteinuria, and membranous nephropathy. However, it has been suggested that mercaptopropionylglycine might have fewer side effects and be better tolerated, particularly by patients who have had adverse effects from D-penicillamine.[162] Therefore, it may substitute for D-penicillamine in the treatment of cystinuria. Captopril has been advocated as a potential treatment for cystinuria, but its efficacy is controversial.

SURGICAL MANAGEMENT

Symptomatic stones that do not pass spontaneously often require surgical treatment.[163] The introduciton of extracorporeal shock wave lithotripsy has not been of great benefit to cystinuric patients. Cystine stones are hard and have proved difficult to pulverize. Consequently, percutaneous lithotripsy is more effective. Recent progress in urologic treatment of kidney stones has decreased the need for open surgery.[164] Urinary alkalinization, as well as direct irrigation of the urinary tract with D-penicillamine, N-acetylpenicillamine, or tromethamine to form disulfide compounds, has resulted in the dissolution of stones. This approach often requires irrigation for several weeks with a risk for potential complications of catheterization.

Transplantation is sometimes necessary for patients with terminal renal failure from chronic obstruction or infection. A kidney from an unaffected donor will not form cystine stones.

Lysinuric Protein Intolerance

Lysinuric protein intolerance (LPI; OMIM 222700) is a very rare recessively inherited dibasic amino acid transport disorder, mostly reported in Finland (reviewed in reference 165). The disease is caused by defective basolateral membrane efflux of the cationic amino acids lysine, arginine, and ornithine in the intestinal, hepatic, and renal tubular epithelia. The amino acid deficiency leads to an impaired urea cycle and postprandial hyperammonemia. Clinical findings include protein aversion, nausea, jaundice, hyperammonemia, coma, and metabolic acidosis. Micronodular cirrhosis of the liver occurs from protein malnutrition, and pulmonary alveolar proteinosis is an occasional finding.[166] Hyperammonemia is induced by low levels of ornithine, which provides the carbon skeleton for the urea cycle.[167] Affected subjects are symptom-free while on breast feeding but fail to thrive on weaning. Various renal disorders, including IgA nephropathy, have been described.[168, 169] LPI can also present as childhood osteoporosis.[170] The urinary excretion of lysine and all cationic amino acids is increased and the plasma levels are decreased.

Inactivating mutations in a novel transcript, *SCL7A7*, have been found in several families with LPI.[171-173] *SCL7A7* complementary DNA (cDNA) encodes a 511–amino acid protein, y⁺LAT-1, predicted to harbor 12 membrane-spanning domains, with both NH_2 and COOH termini located intracellularly. This protein is thought to be part of the y⁺L multimeric unit. Cationic amino acid transport occurs through five different systems: y⁺, y⁺L, b⁺, b⁰,⁺, and B⁰,⁺ (reviewed in reference 174). Defective system y⁺L transport explains the abnormality in cationic amino acid transport. System y⁺L mediates sodium-independent high-affinity transport of cationic amino acids and the transport of zwitterionic amino acids with low affinity. It is responsible for renal reabsorption and intestinal absorption of dibasic amino acids at the basolateral membranes. y⁺L transport is induced by a cell surface glycoprotein heavy chain (4F2hc) that represents the heavy chain subunit of a disulfide-linked heterodimer.[175]

The defect also appears to be expressed in skin fibroblasts.[176] Various immunologic abnormalities have been described,[177] and are possibly secondary to low arginine levels, the substrate for nitric oxide synthase and NO production.[178] The current treatment of lysinuric protein intolerance involves moderate protein restriction with supplementation with 3 to 8 g of citrulline daily during meals and lysine.[179, 180] Citrulline is transported by a different pathway than are dibasic amino acids and can be converted to ornithine and arginine in the liver. Lysine cannot be made from citrulline.

Hartnup Disease

Described initially in 1956 in the Hartnup family,[181] Hartnup disease (OMIM 234500) is an autosomal recessive, and usually benign, condition, consisting in excessive urinary excretion of the monoamino, monocarboxylic (neutral) amino acids alanine, asparagine, glutamine, histidine, isoleucine, leucine, methionine, phenylalanine, serine, threonine, tryptophan, tyrosine, and valine (reviewed in reference 182). Its incidence has been estimated in newborn screening programs at 1 in 26,000.[183] Although it is suspected that it is an amino acid carrier, the gene that encodes the defective protein responsible for Hartnup disease has not been cloned. Most newborns identified prospectively by genetic screening programs have been completely asymptomatic.[184, 185] In most affected individuals there is also a decreased intestinal absorption of neutral amino acids, particularly tryptophan.[186]

The clinical features of this disorder, if any, are due to nicotinamide deficiency, which is partly derived from tryptophan. These include a photosensitive erythematous skin rash

(pellagra-like) clinically identical with niacin deficiency, intermittent cerebellar ataxia, and rarely mental retardation. Emotional instability, psychosis, and depression have been noted rarely, particularly during episodes of ataxia. Although the Hartnup family had several cases with mental retardation,[181] most affected subjects described subsequently have not had mental retardation. Hartnup disease should be suspected in all subjects with pellagra and unexplained intermittent ataxia. Siblings of affected patients should be screened as well. Clinical manifestations can be triggered by periods of inadequate dietary intake or increased metabolic needs. For example, a young woman presenting with pellagra precipitated by prolonged lactation and increased activity[187] was diagnosed with Hartnup disease.

The diagnosis is easily made by performing a urinary aminogram and shows increased excretion of neutral amino acids, but not glycine, cystine, dibasic, dicarboxylic, and imino amino acids. Thus, any confusion with the renal Fanconi syndrome is avoided by performing a complete evaluation of amino acids in the urine using one of several chromatographic methods. The pattern of amino acid excretion, rather than the total amount, is the determining factor.[182] The reabsorption defect involves 12 amino acids and most patients with Hartnup disease have the same pattern of aminoaciduria. The levels of amino acids in the monoamino, dicarboxylic group (such as glutamic acid and aspartic acid), and basic group (lysine, ornithine, arginine) are normal or slightly increased. The excretion of proline, hydroxyproline, and cystine is also normal. Thus, Hartnup disease can be easily differentiated from the generalized aminoaciduria of Fanconi syndrome. Despite the defect, substantial renal tubular transport of the involved amino acids remains. Renal clearances are inferior to GFR, which suggests that amino acids are transported by other systems or that the defect is incomplete. Because amino acids might be reabsorbed by high-capacity low-affinity and low-capacity highly specific transporters, residual renal reabsorption of neutral amino acids might occur through specific transporters, passive diffusion, and partial activity of the defective transporter.[182]

Treatment of symptomatic cases involves the administration of nicotinamide in doses of 50 to 300 mg/day. The value of treating asymptomatic cases is not known, but given the harmlessness of the treatment, this might be a rational choice.

Iminoglycinuria

Familial iminoglycinuria (OMIM 242600) is a benign autosomal recessive disorder with no clinical symptoms whose main interest is that it suggests the presence of a common carrier for the imino acids proline and hydroxyproline, as well as glycine.[188] It was discovered after the application of chromatographic methods to the investigation of disorders of amino acid metabolism. The diagnosis is usually suggested by an increased urinary excretion of imino acids and glycine. Newborns and infants usually excrete detectable amounts of imino acids and glycine for up to 3 months (see review in reference 189). Thus, the presence of increased urinary excretion of imino acids and glycine after 6 months can be considered abnormal. It can be part of a generalized defect of the proximal tubule (the Fanconi syndrome) or a selective defect.

INHERITED DISORDERS OF RENAL PHOSPHATE TRANSPORT

Inherited disorders of renal phosphate transport have in common persisting hypophosphatemia caused by a reduction in renal tubule reabsorption of inorganic phosphate (reviewed in reference 190). Each disorder is characterized by an increased fractional excretion of Pi (or decreased TmP/GFR) with frequent metabolic bone disease presenting as rickets in childhood and osteomalacia in adults. Each differs biochemically and in its response to treatment.

Renal Phosphate Excretion

The determinants of phosphate homeostasis are phosphate ingestion, intestinal absorption, and renal excretion (see also Chapter 12). The normal phosphate intake in adults varies from 800 to 1600 mg/day and the average serum phosphate levels remain normal over a wide range of intake. Contrary to active calcium absorption, which is greatest in the duodenum with a lower rate in the jejunum, ileum, and colon, active Pi absorption is highest in the jejunum and ileum with a lower rate in the duodenum and colon.[191] Intestinal phosphate absorption is regulated by active vitamin D metabolites,[192] and vitamin D supplementation results in increased intestinal phosphate absorption in renal failure patients.[193] Pi is filtered by the glomerulus and reabsorbed in the proximal tubule. The difference between the amounts of Pi filtered and reabsorbed determine the net appearance of Pi in the urine. Phosphate reabsorption by the proximal tubule occurs by a Tm-limited active process. The fractional reabsorption of filtered phosphate is usually estimated by the tubular reabsorption of Pi (TRP), and is a simple equation to assess the renal tubular phosphate transport:

$$TRP = \left(1 - \frac{Up \times Pcr}{Ucr \times Pp}\right)$$

Given a normal renal function and a normal diet, the TRP is usually above 85%. A more precise way of estimating the tubular reabsorption of Pi is to calculate the theoretical threshold:

$$TmP / GFR = Pp - \frac{(Up \times Pcr)}{Ucr}$$

Adaptation to States of Altered Phosphate Metabolism

In the normal state, moderate phosphate deprivation that leads to a marginal decrease in serum phosphate levels induces a reduction in urine excretion of phosphate and an increase in 1,25(OH)$_2$D$_3$ levels.[194] Further reduction that leads to moderate decreases in serum phosphate levels induces a virtual disappearance of urine Pi.[195] This occurs by an increase in Pi reabsorption by the proximal tubule as demonstrated by animal and vesicle studies (reviewed in reference 196). Renal proximal tubular reabsorption of Pi is determined by an Na/Pi-cotransporter system.[197] Several Na/Pi cotransporters have been identified (see also Chapter 12). The Na/Pi type II cotransporter appears to be the most important brush border membrane Na/Pi cotransporter. It is down-regulated

by PTH and phosphate overload and up-regulated by phosphate deprivation (reviewed in reference 197). A reduction in serum phosphate levels also leads to increased 1,25(OH)$_2$D$_3$ levels[198, 199] from increased activity of the rate-limiting enzyme for the synthesis of 1,25(OH)$_2$D$_3$, the 1α-hydroxylase. This mitochondrial enzyme is a member of the P-450 family[200] and is located in the proximal tubule principal cells. The mechanism by which decreased phosphate levels lead to increased 1α-hydroxylase enzymatic activity is not known but is not related to phosphate transport in the proximal tubule cell mitochondria.[201] The fall in serum phosphate levels also inhibits bone deposition, and the increase in serum 1,25(OH)$_2$D$_3$ increases bone resorption, thus favoring a net shift of phosphate from bone. Higher serum levels of 1,25(OH)$_2$D$_3$ also increase intestinal phosphate and calcium absorption. As a consequence, serum calcium levels increase and inhibit PTH secretion. The reduction in PTH levels does not lead to a further increase in phosphate reabsorption by the kidney because the proximal tubule is insensitive to the action of PTH in states of phosphate deprivation. As a result, one should predict that a renal phosphate leak will lead to raised serum 1,25(OH)$_2$D$_3$ levels, decreased PTH, and consequent hypercalciuria.

X-Linked Hypophosphatemic Rickets
Pathogenesis

X-linked hypophosphatemic rickets (OMIM 307800) is an X-linked dominant disorder characterized by hypophosphatemia with reduced TmP/GFR, normal serum calcium and PTH levels, normal to low serum 1,25(OH)$_2$D$_3$ levels, and elevated levels of serum alkaline phosphatase. Because serum 1,25(OH)$_2$D$_3$ levels are decreased in the face of hypophosphatemia, the regulation of 1α-hydroxylase must be altered. Although the defective gene is known, the pathogenesis of the disease is poorly understood. The mutated gene, *PHEX* (formerly known as *PEX*), encodes a large protein of 749 amino acids[202] that has similarities with neutral endopeptidases, and is composed of intracellular, transmembrane, and extracellular domains.[203] *PHEX* expression is high in osteoblasts[204, 205] and in tumor tissue associated with the paraneoplastic syndrome of renal phosphate wasting. The wide range of mutations that align with regions required for protease activity suggests that *PHEX* might function as an osteoblast protease, and may act by processing factor(s) involved in mineral metabolism.[202, 206, 207] For example, cell membranes from cultured COS cells transiently expressing *PHEX*, degrade exogenously added PTH-derived peptides, demonstrating endopeptidase activity.[203] However, the substrate for the enzyme has yet to be identified, and the renal defect responsible for phosphaturia is still not understood.

Familial X-linked hypophosphatemic rickets has a murine model termed the *Hyp* mouse. In this model, a large deletion in the 3′ region of the *Pex* gene (the mouse homolog of human *PHEX*) was found, thus proving that both disorders are genetically similar.[208] In parabiotic experiments in which normal and *Hyp* mice are surgically joined, normal mice develop renal phosphate wasting.[209] Furthermore, a *Hyp* kidney cross-transplanted in a normal mouse handles phosphate normally.[210] Conversely, a normal kidney transplanted in a *Hyp* mouse does not handle phosphate normally. The cellular

PROXIMAL TUBULE

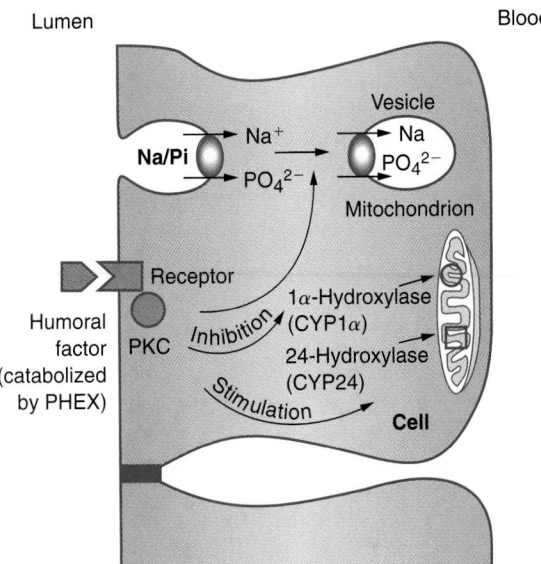

FIGURE 36-6. Schematic representation of the molecular genetic basis of three inherited forms of rickets. Vitamin D–dependent rickets type 1 is secondary to mutations in the 1α-hydroxylase gene. This gene is responsible for the 1α-hydroxylation of 25-hydroxyvitamin D(25-OH) that occurs in the convoluted and straight portions of the renal proximal tubule. This 1α-hydroxylation is catalyzed by 25-hydroxyvitamin D–1α-hydroxylase (1α-hydroxylase), a mitochondrial cytochrome P-450 enzyme that is subject to complex regulation by parathyroid hormone, calcium, phosphorus, and 1,25-dihydroxyvitamin D itself. This disorder is characterized by failure to thrive, muscle weakness, hypocalcemia, secondary hyperparathyroidism, and the bony changes of rickets. The hallmarks of the disease are the findings of greatly reduced serum concentrations of $1,25(OH)_2D$ despite normal or increased concentrations of 25(OH)D, and the reversal of clinical and laboratory abnormalities by administration of physiologic amounts of $1,25(OH)_2D_3$.[460] Vitamin D–dependent rickets type 2, also termed hereditary vitamin D–resistant rickets, is due to mutations in the gene for the vitamin D receptor. X-linked hypophosphatemic rickets results from loss-of-function mutations in the *PHEX* gene (phosphate-regulating gene with homologies to endopeptidases, on the X chromosome). In this disease, serum concentrations of $1,25(OH)_2D$ are inappropriately low despite the hypophosphatemia.

transduction mechanism responsible for this phenomenon is thought to be mediated by protein kinase C (PKC).[211, 212] PKC activity is increased in the kidney of the *Hyp* mouse.[213] PKC activation in the proximal tubule leads both to decreased phosphate transport by the Na/phosphate cotransporter,[214] decreased $1,25(OH)_2D_3$ synthesis, and increased 24-hydroxylase activity.[215] Thus, a circulating factor is thought to bind to an unidentified receptor at the apical membrane of the proximal tubule, activate PKC, and decrease Na/phosphate cotransporter content in the apical membrane. Activation of PKC is also thought to inhibit 1α-hydroxylase activity and stimulate 24-hydroxylase activity (Fig. 36-6).

Clinical Presentation

X-linked hypophosphatemic rickets is the most frequent type of hereditary disorder of renal phosphate metabolism (reviewed in reference 216). Its hallmark is "inappropriately" normal $1,25(OH)_2D_3$ levels in the presence of hypophosphatemia

and rickets.[217, 218] There is no renal wasting of amino acids and glucose. The patients demonstrate short stature (growth retardation), femoral or tibial bowing presenting early in life, and histomorphometric evidence of rickets and osteomalacia. Males are usually more severely affected than females and there is variable penetrance. X chromosome inactivation patterns in peripheral lymphocytes are normal in affected females, but the X-inactivation pattern in renal tubule cells has not been investigated.[219] Serum phosphate levels are usually lower than 2.5 mg/dL (0.8 mmol/L) and the TmP/GFR is lower than 1.8 mg/dL (0.56 mmol/L). A report of 116 pediatric patients failed to show any evidence for genetic heterogeneity or for gender, race, anticipation, or parent-of-origin effects on XLH expression.[220] There is apparently no correlation between the serum level of phosphate and the severity of the disease. Affected children tend to have higher serum phosphate and TmP/GFR levels compared to affected adults, as is the case with normal subjects. The earliest sign of the disease in children can be increased serum alkaline phosphatase levels.

Treatment

Early therapy with $1,25(OH)_2D_3$ (1.0-3.0 μg/day) and phosphate (1-2 g/day in divided doses) has a beneficial effect on growth, bone density, and deformations.[221] Nephrocalcinosis due to vitamin D and phosphate therapy can lead to deterioration of renal function.

Hereditary Hypophosphatemic Rickets with Hypercalciuria

Hereditary hypophosphatemic rickets associated with hypercalciuria (OMIM 241530) is a very rare and apparently autosomal recessive disease initially described in a Bedouin family with multiple consanguineous matings.[222] A second pedigree of Jewish Yemenites has also been described.[223] The genetic defect responsible for this disease is not known and genetic mapping efforts have not been successful. Affected subjects appear to have a chronic renal phosphate leak with an appropriate response to hypophosphatemia. The characteristic features are rickets, short stature, increased renal phosphate clearance, hypercalciuria, normal serum calcium levels, increased gastrointestinal absorption of calcium and phosphorus, elevated serum concentration of $1,25(OH)_2D_3$, and suppressed parathyroid function. There appears to be two degrees of severity, one that corresponds to the full-blown syndrome, and the other with an attenuated form compatible with a heterozygote carrier with reduced penetrance (see reference 216 for review). The defect in phosphate reabsorption is presumed to be in the proximal tubule. Phosphate deprivation leads to an appropriate increase in $1,25(OH)_2D_3$ production and increased intestinal absorption of calcium and phosphate leading to hypercalciuria. As a result, PTH is suppressed, and chronic hypophosphatemia leads to a reduction in bone mineralization and growth. Patients respond to administration of daily oral phosphate (1.0-2.5 g/day). This leads to an increase in serum phosphate levels and decreased serum $1,25(OH)_2D_3$, calcium, and alkaline phosphatase levels. Growth rate is increased, and the clinical manifestations of rickets and osteomalacia (bone pain, muscle weakness) disappear.

Hereditary Selective Deficiency of $1\alpha,25(OH)_2D_3$

This rare form of autosomal recessive vitamin D–responsive rickets (OMIM 264700) is not a disease of tubule transport per se, but a 1α-hydroxylation deficiency, and is described in this chapter because the enzyme is specifically expressed in the proximal tubule (see Fig. 36-6). It results from inactivating mutations in the P-450 enzyme 1α-hydroxylase.[224, 225] Vitamin D is metabolized by sequential hydroxylations in the liver (25-hydroxylation) and kidney (1α-hydroxylation). Hydroxylation of $25(OH)D_3$ is mediated by $25(OH)D_3$ 1α-hydroxylase in the proximal tubule of the kidney. Using a kidney cDNA expression library from genetically engineered mice lacking the vitamin D receptor expressed in cells also containing a reporter chimeric vitamin D receptor gene, Takeyama and colleagues cloned the P-450 component of the enzyme 1α-hydroxylase.[200] The human gene maps to chromosome 12q14 and the structure has been subsequently determined.[226, 227] Patients usually appear normal at birth and develop muscle weakness, tetany, convulsions, and rickets starting at 2 months of age. Serum calcium levels are low, PTH levels are high, with low to undetectable $1,25(OH)_2D_3$.[228] Serum levels of $25(OH)D_3$ are normal or slightly increased. Once recognized, this rare disorder is easily treated with physiologic doses of $1,25(OH)_2D_3$ and results in healing of rickets and restoring of the plasma calcium, phosphate, and PTH levels.

Hereditary Generalized Resistance to $1\alpha,25(OH)_2D_3$

This rare autosomal recessive disorder (OMIM 277400) is similar to selective deficiency of $1\alpha,25(OH)_2D_3$ with the salient features that serum levels of $25(OH)D_3$ and $1\alpha,25(OH)_2D_3$ are increased and the disease does not respond to doses of $1\alpha,25(OH)_2D_3$ and $1\alpha,(OH)D_3$. In addition, approximately half of the cases described have associated alopecia. In a subset of affected kindreds, the disease is due to mutations in the vitamin D receptor gene. Premature stop codons in the vitamin D receptor gene are responsible for the phenotype, resulting in the absence of the ligand-binding domain.[229, 230]

INHERITED DISORDERS OF RENAL GLUCOSE TRANSPORT

Under normal conditions, glucose is almost completely reabsorbed by the proximal tubule. Thus, very small amounts of glucose are present in the urine of most normal people. The appearance of a significant amount of glucose in the urine (500 mg/day or 2.75 mmol/day in adults) is most often due to hyperglycemia (overload glucosuria), and, rarely, to abnormal handling of glucose by the kidney (Table 36-5). Renal glucosuria may be part of a generalized defect of the proximal tubule (Fanconi syndrome), or present as an isolated defect.

Normal Glucose Reabsorption by the Kidney

Glucose is freely filtered by the glomerulus, and is reabsorbed in the proximal tubule by a Na^+-coupled active transport located in the brush border membrane (Fig. 36-7, see also Chapter 9). There is no evidence for glucose transport in the

loop of Henle and the distal tubule. A small fraction of glucose may be reabsorbed in the collecting duct. Glucose reabsorption involves several transporters at the apical and basolateral membranes of the proximal tubule principal cells (reviewed in reference 231). The driving force for D-glucose reabsorption is provided by the electrochemical gradient for sodium maintained by the Na^+,K^+-ATPase in the plasma membrane. Glucose absorption along the proximal tubule is heterogeneous.[232] Active reabsorption of glucose was found

TABLE 36-5

Causes of Glucosuria

Hyperglycemia
  Diabetes mellitus
  Iatrogenic
    Glucocorticoids
    Catecholamines
    Angiotensin I–converting enzymes inhibitors[456]
    Intravenous dextrose solutions
    Total parenteral nutrition
Renal glucosuria
Idiopathic renal glucosuria
Glucose-galactose malabsorption
Fanconi syndrome
Pregnancy

PROXIMAL TUBULE

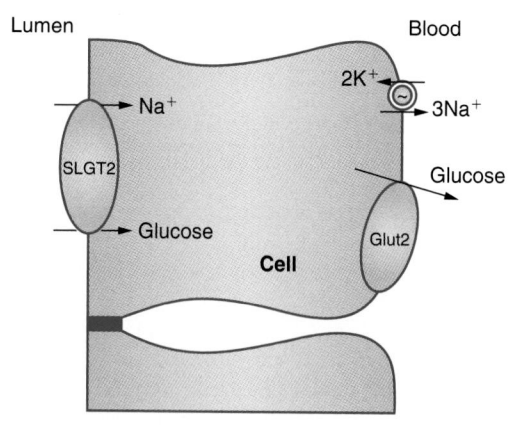

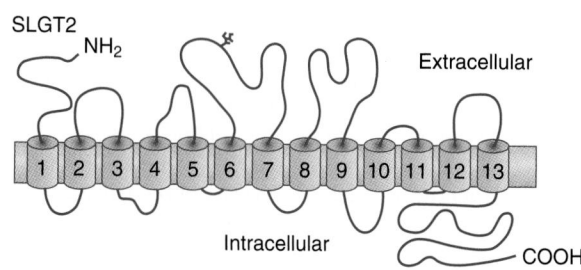

FIGURE 36-7. Schematic representation of glucose transport across a proximal tubular cell from the S1 segment. A low-affinity high-capacity system in the S1 segment (SLGT2) is represented. The low-capacity high-affinity system in the S3 segment is not represented. Congenital glucose-galactose malabsorption is secondary to loss-of-function mutations of SLGT1 expressed in both the intestine and the kidney. (Modified with permission from Wright EM: Genetic disorders of membrane transport. I. Glucose galactose malabsorption. Am J Physiol Gastrointest Liver Physiol 275:G879-G882, 1998.)

to occur via a low-affinity, high-capacity system in the S1 segment (SGLT2), and a low-capacity high-affinity system in the S3 segment (SGLT1). These characteristics of a high-transport capacity with moderate leak in the proximal convoluted tubule (PCT) and lower transport capacity with a low leak in the proximal straight tubule allow the establishment of steep glucose concentration gradients in the PCT that are maintained and augmented in the late proximal nephron.[232] Studies that have compared glucose transport from the outer cortex (thought to contain S1 and S2 segments) with the outer medulla (thought to contain S3 segments) have found evidence for a high-capacity low-affinity transport in the S1 and S2 segments, and a low-capacity high-affinity transport in the S3 segments.[233] It was suggested that the sodium glucose stoichiometry was 1:1 in the S1-S2 segment, and 2:1 in the pars recta (S3 segment).

The high-capacity low-affinity transporter was cloned from a kidney cDNA library and is termed SGLT2.[234] It comprises 672 amino acids and has 59% identity with the high-affinity Na^+ glucose cotransporter (SGLT1).[235] Contrary to SGLT1, SGLT2 is not expressed in the intestine. It is strongly and exclusively expressed in proximal tubule S1 segments.[236] All family members of the SGLT family share a common core of 13 transmembrane helices, but some, like SGLT1 itself, have one additional span appended to the COOH terminus, and others have two such spans (reviewed in reference 237). Conformational changes are responsible for the coupling of Na^+ and sugar transport for these transporters. SGLT1 forms a pore that allows the transmembrane passage of water and glucose. Extracellular Na^+ is required to maintain patency of this transporter's water-permeable transmembrane pore. Expression studies in *Xenopus* oocytes have shown that SGLT1 carries 260 molecules of water for each molecule of sugar (glucose or galactose) reabsorbed.[238] From this, it has been estimated that SGLT1 could account for almost half (5 L) the daily reuptake of water from the small intestine in humans.[238]

Facilitative glucose transport at the basolateral membrane is mediated by GLUT2 and to a lesser extent by GLUT1, GLUT protein family that belongs to a much larger superfamily of 12 transmembrane segment transporters (reviewed in reference 239). Six members of the GLUT family have been described thus far. These proteins are expressed in a tissue- and cell-specific manner and exhibit distinct kinetic and regulatory properties that reflect their specific functional roles (see also Chapter 9). GLUT2 is a high-K_m isoform, also expressed in hepatocytes and pancreatic beta cells, in addition to the basolateral membranes of intestinal and renal epithelial cells. It acts as a high-capacity transport system to allow the uninhibited (non–rate-limiting) flux of glucose into or out of these cell types. GLUT2 is only expressed in the proximal convoluted tubule, whereas GLUT1 is present in glomeruli, proximal convoluted, and straight tubules.[240] Thus, GLUT1 and GLUT2 are responsible for glucose efflux in the early proximal tubule. In the lateral proximal tubule, where transcellular glucose flux is lower, only GLUT1 mediates glucose efflux.[240]

Renal Glucosuria

Initial studies by Shannon and Fisher[241] and by Smith and colleagues[242] have provided glucose titration curves. These showed that the renal Tm for glucose varies in normal persons and in diabetics.[243] Renal glucosuria (OMIM 233100) is

generally a benign clinical condition that denotes a renal tubular abnormality characterized by variable amounts of glucose in the urine of affected individuals with normal serum glucose levels (reviewed in reference 244). Some cases have been associated with *selective* aminoaciduria,[245] unlike the generalized aminoaciduria seen in the Fanconi syndrome. Renal glucosuria is a rare occurrence when strict diagnostic criteria are applied.[246, 247] The definition of glucosuria is arbitrary and different investigators have proposed different guidelines to define abnormal from normal glucosuria. A currently accepted stringent definition of glucosuria proposes the following criteria:

1. The oral glucose tolerance test, levels of plasma insulin and free fatty acids, and glycosylated hemoglobin levels should all be normal.
2. The amount of glucose in the urine (10-100 g/day) should be relatively stable except during pregnancy when it may increase.
3. The degree of glucosuria should be largely independent of diet but may fluctuate according to the amount of carbohydrates ingested. All specimens of urine should contain glucose.
4. The carbohydrate excreted should be glucose. Other sugars are not found (fructose, pentoses, galactose, lactose, sucrose, maltose, heptulose).
5. Subjects with renal glucosuria should be able to store and utilize carbohydrates normally.

Glucose reabsorption curves in glucosuric patients have allowed the identification of subtypes (Fig. 36-8). In type A, there is an abnormally low TmG/GFR, although the shape of the curve is normal. In type B glucosuria, the TmG/GFR is normal, but the splay is increased. Type O glucosuria is characterized by a severe or complete reduction in the reabsorption of glucose, and the curve is flat. Type A glucosuria might be a mutation in a glucose transporter present in all nephrons with a reduction in the capacity of the transport system. Type B glucosuria might be caused by a mutation that decreases the affinity of the transporter for glucose, or a consequence of functional or anatomic nephron heterogeneity. Type O glucosuria might be caused by genetic events that render the transporter absent or inactive.

All cases of renal glucosuria are benign, except type O glucosuria in which dehydration and ketosis may develop during pregnancy and starvation.[248] For example, a proband whose parents had respectively 1.1 and 2.7 g/day/1.73 m² had enuresis, polyuria, and polydipsia with episodes of polyphagia. He excreted 136 to 163 g/day/m² of glucose. A similar family has been described with type O glucosuria in a boy whose mother and brother both had type A glucosuria and whose father was normal.[249]

The genetics of renal glucosuria is unknown and this could be due to the fact that different definitions have been used in family studies. In 1937, Hjarne performed a very large study of a pedigree and observed that glucosuria occurred in both male and female members of the family.[250] When both parents were unaffected, offspring were also unaffected. When one of the parents had the defect, some children also had glucosuria. A later study also supported the view that glucosuria was inherited as an autosomal dominant trait.[251] Another study suggested that heavy continuous glucosuria appears to be transmitted as an autosomal recessive trait,[252] with some

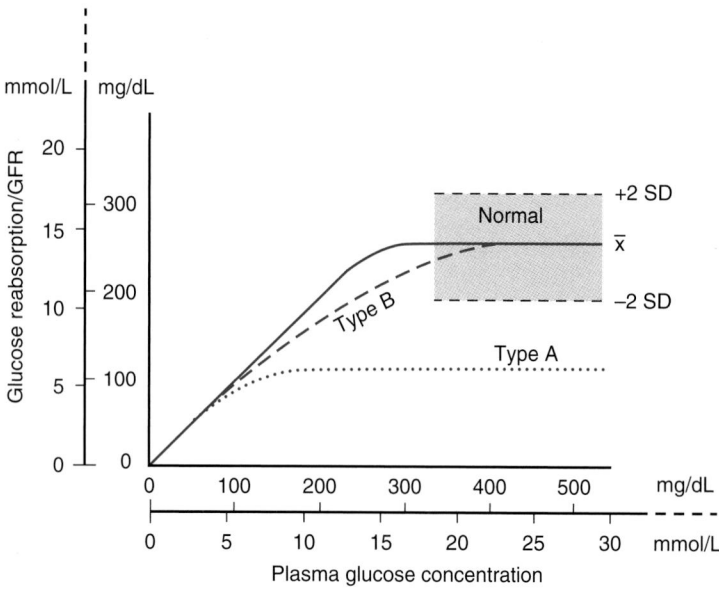

FIGURE 36-8. Glucose reabsorption curves for normal subjects and patients with two main types of renal glycosuria. (Reprinted with permission from Haycock GB: Isolated defects of tubular function. *In* Davison AM, Cameron JS, Grünfeld J-P. et al (eds): Oxford Textbook of Clinical Nephrology, 2nd ed. New York, Oxford University Press, 1998, pp 1039-1069.)

abnormalities detectable in heterozygotes. Genetic defects for idiopathic renal glucosuria have yet to be described with certainty. A study of three Japanese patients found that heterozygotes for two mutations (L389P and V423E) of the GLUT2 glucose transporter showed renal glucosuria.[253] This was apparently not found in another study.[254] A patient with isolated renal glucosuria was recently found to bear a mutation in the sodium glucose cotransporter gene *SGLT2*.[255] The disease might also be linked to the HLA locus on chromosome 6p.[251] Renal glucosuria has been described in the X-linked hypophosphatemic mice.[256]

Glucose-Galactose Malabsorption

Initially described in 1962, glucose-galactose malabsorption (OMIM 606824) is a rare congenital disease resulting from a selective defect in the intestinal transport of glucose and galactose.[257, 258] It is inherited as an autosomal recessive trait and is characterized by the neonatal onset of severe watery and acidic diarrhea that results in death unless these sugars are removed from the diet. Normally, lactose in milk is broken down into glucose and galactose by lactase, an ectoenzyme on the brush border, and the hexoses are transported into the cell by the Na+/glucose cotransporter SGLT1. The disease can occasionally be diagnosed in adults. The acidic diarrhea results from bacterial metabolism of sugar in the stools and can be improved with antibacterial treatment. Important weight losses from hyperosmolar dehydration and metabolic acidosis are frequent. The disease is usually suspected from the clinical history and the presence of glucosuria despite normal serum glucose levels. Dramatic improvement occurs after withdrawal of glucose and galactose from the diet.

The disease is caused by mutations in the glucose/galactose transporter SGLT1[259] located on chromosome 22q13.1.[260] This results in the absence of the transporter in the intestine and the kidney. Most mutations expressed in vitro result in a complete loss of Na+-dependent glucose transport because

of decreased cotransporter trafficking to the plasma membrane.[259, 261, 262] Subjects with glucose-galactose malabsorption have type B glucosuria.

INHERITED DISORDERS OF ACID-BASE TRANSPORTERS

Renal tubular acidosis (RTA) is a clinical syndrome characterized by hyperchloremic (normal anion gap) metabolic acidosis secondary to abnormal urine acidification. This can be identified by inappropriately high urine pH, bicarbonaturia, and reduced net acid excretion. Proximal and distal forms of RTA are frequently accompanied by hypokalemia. Proximal RTA generally occurs as part of the renal Fanconi syndrome. In contrast, distal RTA is mostly associated with an acquired systemic illness. Rare cases of hereditary proximal and distal RTA have been described (reviewed in references 263, 264), and are discussed here.

Mechanisms of Renal Acidification

A typical Western diet generates an acid load of approximately 1 mmol of mineral acid per kilogram of body weight, which must be excreted by the kidney. In addition, the kidney filters approximately 4000 mmol of bicarbonate daily and must reclaim most of the filtered load to maintain acid-base balance. Excretion of the ingested acid load and reabsorption of filtered bicarbonate are accomplished by complex processes requiring coordinated actions of transport and enzymatic activities in the apical and basolateral membranes (Figs. 36-9 and 36-10). Proximal tubule cells secrete H+ across the apical membrane via the NHE3 Na+/H+ exchanger and the H+-ATPase. The H+ is made available for secretion by intracellular generation through hydration of CO_2 by carbonic anhydrase II. Carbonic anhydrases are zinc metalloenzymes

PROXIMAL TUBULE

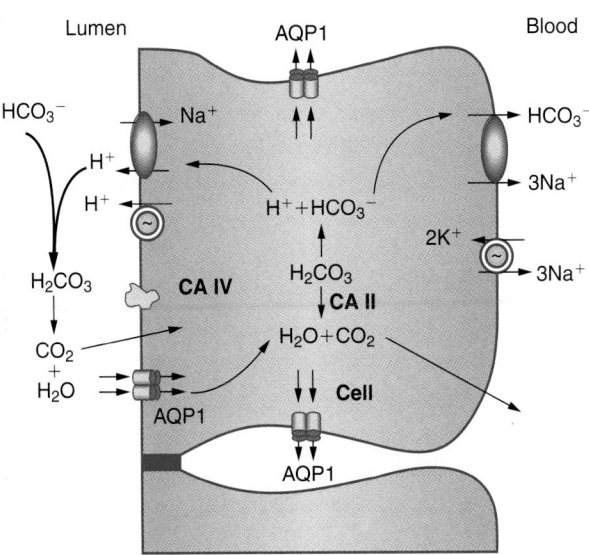

FIGURE 36-9. Mechanisms of renal acidification.

that catalyze the reversible hydration of CO_2 to form HCO_3^- and protons, according to the following reaction:

$$CO_2 + H_2O \leftrightarrow H_2CO_3 \leftrightarrow H^+ + HCO_3^-$$

The first reaction is catalyzed by carbonic anhydrase and the second reaction occurs instantaneously. Carbonic anhydrase IV is a membrane-associated enzyme anchored to plasma membrane surfaces by a phosphatidylinositol glycan linkage. It accelerates the formation of CO_2 and H_2O from $H_2CO_3^-$.

Eighty-five per cent of the filtered load of HCO_3^- is reabsorbed in the *proximal tubule* (see Fig. 36-9). The main driving force for the reabsorption of HCO_3^- is the lumen-to-cell sodium gradient provided by the basolateral Na^+,K^+-ATPase. The transepithelial HCO_3^- flux is accomplished by an apical membrane Na^+/H^+ exchanger and a basolateral Na^+/HCO_3^- cotransporter (NBC; encoded by *SLC4A4*) (reviewed in reference 265).

In the *connecting segment* and *collecting duct* (see Fig. 36-10), type A intercalated cells secrete H^+ into the lumen via a vacuolar Mg^{2+}-dependent H^+-ATPase. The generation of H^+ is catalyzed by carbonic anhydrase II and HCO_3^- is transported across the basolateral membrane through

COLLECTING TUBULE

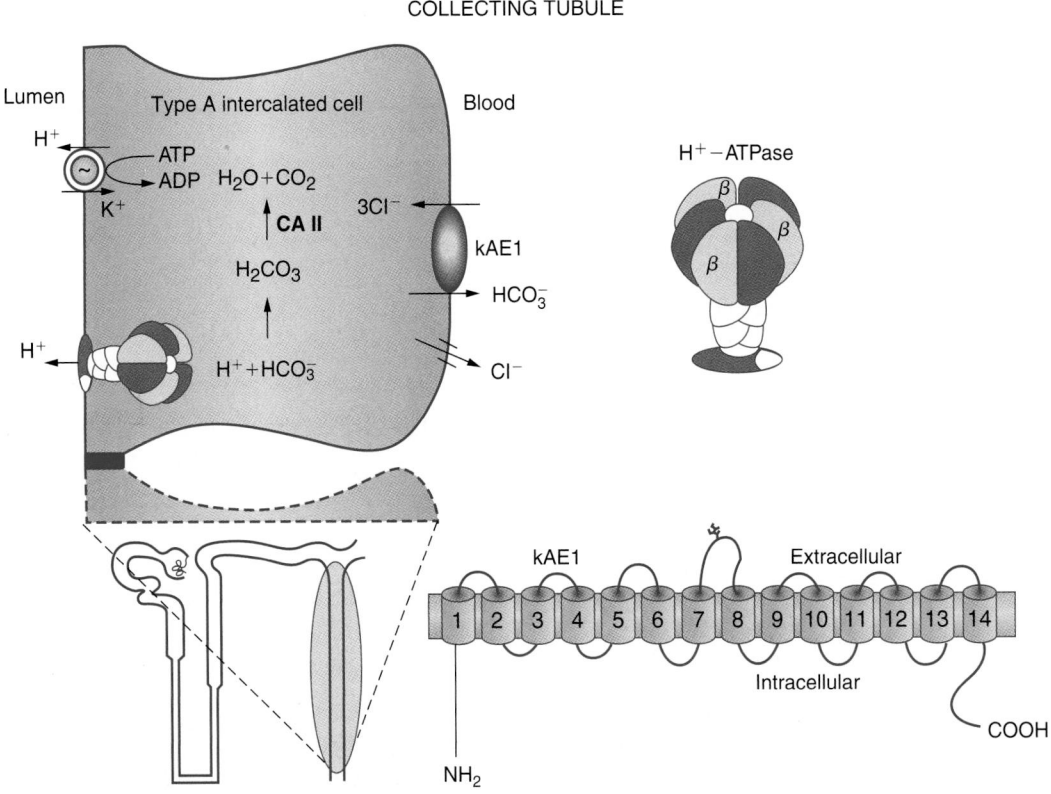

FIGURE 36-10. Autosomal dominant and autosomal recessive distal renal tubular acidosis (dRTA). dRTA is due to mutations in the gene *SLC4A1* encoding the Na^+/HCO_3^- exchanger AE1.[277, 279] The *AE1* gene (chromosome 17) encodes both the erythroid (eAE1) and the kidney (kAE1) isoforms of the band 3 protein.[463] Mutations in the gene (*ATP6V1B1*, 2p13) encoding the β_1-subunit of H^+-ATPase cause recessive dRTA with sensorineural deafness.[282] dRTA with preserved hearing is secondary to mutations in *AIP6V0A4*, which encodes the a4 subunit of the proton pump.[276] Both H^+ and H^+/K^+-ATPases are represented. The H^+-ATPase is schematically represented according to the proposed structure of the F_1-ATPase of the inner mitochondrial membrane.[464] F_1 is represented as a flattened sphere 80 Å high and 100 Å across. The three α- and three β-subunits are arranged alternately like the segments of an orange around a central α-helix 90 Å long. Mutations in the β-subunit cause autosomal recessive dRTA. Autosomal recessive dRTA has also been found, in a small kindred, for the *SLC4A1* mutation G701D.[281]

the AE1 HCO_3^-/Cl^- exchanger. Luminal H^+ is trapped by urinary buffers, including ammonium secreted by the proximal tubule and phosphate.

Proximal Renal Tubular Acidosis

Primary, isolated hereditary proximal RTA (type II RTA) is an extremely rare disorder. Proximal RTA usually occurs as part of the spectrum of the Fanconi syndrome in which excretion of glucose, amino acids, and phosphate is increased. The diagnosis of proximal RTA rests on an appropriately acid urine pH (pH <5.5) in acidotic patients and a high fractional excretion of HCO_3^- (>10%-15%) in subjects with normal or near-normal serum HCO_3^- concentrations. An additional clue to the diagnosis are the large amounts of HCO_3^- that have to be given to correct the serum HCO_3^- levels.

Sodium-Bicarbonate Symporter Mutations

Inactivating mutations in *SLC4A4*, the gene coding for the Na^+/HCO_3^- symporter (OMIM 604278), cause permanent isolated proximal RTA with various ocular abnormalities such as band keratopathy, glaucoma, and cataracts.[266] The Na^+/HCO_3^- symporter has been found to be expressed in multiple ocular tissues,[267] thus explaining abnormalities.

Carbonic Anhydrase II Deficiency

Recessive mixed proximal-distal RTA accompanied by osteopetrosis and mental retardation is caused by inactivating mutations in the cytoplasmic carbonic anhydrase II gene (OMIM 259730).[268-272] The pathogenesis of the mental subnormality and cerebral calcification is poorly understood. More than 50 cases have been described, predominantly from the Middle East and Mediterranean region. The disorder is discovered late in infancy or early in childhood through developmental delay, short stature, fracture, weakness, cranial nerve compression, dental malocclusion, or mental subnormality, individually or severally. Typical radiographic features of osteopetrosis are present, and histopathologic study of the iliac crest reveals unresorbed calcified primary spongiosa. The radiographic findings are unusual, however, in that cerebral calcification appears by early childhood and the osteosclerosis and skeletal modeling defects may gradually resolve by adulthood. Patients are usually not anemic. A hyperchloremic metabolic acidosis, sometimes with hypokalemia, is caused by renal tubular acidosis that may be a proximal, distal, or combined type.[273] Bilateral recurrent renal stones, hypercalciuria, and medullary nephrocalcinosis have been described.[274] There is no established medical therapy, and the long-term outcome remains to be characterized. There is a mouse model for carbonic anhydrase II deficiency for which gene therapy has been transiently successful, using retrograde injections in the renal pelvis.[275]

Distal Renal Tubular Acidosis

Hereditary distal RTA (dRTA) is a genetically heterogeneous disorder with dominant and recessive forms. It is characterized by reduced ability to acidify urine, variable hyperchloremic, hypokalemic metabolic acidosis, hypercalciuria, nephrocalcinosis, and nephrolithiasis. Patients with recessive dRTA present with either acute illness or growth failure at a young age, sometimes accompanied by deafness. Dominant dRTA is usually a milder disease and involves no hearing loss. These disorders are caused by the dysfunction of type A intercalated cells (reviewed in references 264, 276). Affected transporters include the AE1 Cl^-/HCO_3^- exchanger of the basolateral membrane and at least two subunits of the apical membrane V-H^+-ATPase, the V1 (head) subunit B1 (associated with deafness), and the V0 (stalk) subunit a4.

Chloride/Bicarbonate Exchanger Mutations

Inactivating mutations in the gene encoding the Na^+/HCO_3^- exchanger AE1 can lead to dominant or recessive distal RTA. The *AE1* gene encodes Cl^-/HCO_3^- exchangers that are expressed in the erythrocyte and in type A intercalated cells of the kidney. The renal AE1 contributes to urinary acidification by providing the major exit route for HCO_3^- across the basolateral membrane.

Autosomal dominant RTA caused by *SLC4A1* mutations encoding AE1 (OMIM 179800)[9] is usually a mild disorder that can be discovered incidentally after a kidney stone episode.[277-279] In a previous study of four kindreds, affected subjects had serum HCO_3^- concentrations between 14 and 25 mmol/L,[277] and serum potassium levels between 2.1 and 4.2 mmol/L. Minimum urine pH following an acid load varied from 5.95 to 6.8 (normal <5.30). Nephrocalcinosis and kidney stones were present in approximately 50% of patients. Deafness was absent. Recent results indicate that autosomal dominant dRTA results from aberrant targeting of AE1 to the luminal membrane.[280]

The recessive form of RTA (OMIM 109270)[9] caused by *AE1* mutations is usually diagnosed at a younger age, often before 1 year. It is found in Southeast Asia (Thailand, Papua New Guinea, and Malaysia) where it is associated with ovalocytosis.[281] Affected individuals present with vomiting, dehydration, failure to thrive, or delayed growth. Nephrocalcinosis, kidney stones, or both are frequent, and rickets can be present. Severe metabolic acidosis with serum pH less than 7.30 and serum HCO_3^- less than 15 mmol/L is frequent. Serum potassium levels are also lower than autosomal dominant dRTA, being below 3.5 in a majority of cases.

Proton ATPase Subunit Mutations

Mutations in *ATP6V1B1*, the B1-subunit of the apical proton pump mediating distal nephron acid secretion (OMIM 267300), cause dRTA with sensorineural deafness in a significant proportion of families.[282, 283] In type A intercalated cells, the H^+-ATPase pumps protons against an electrochemical gradient. Active proton secretion is also necessary to maintain proper endolymph pH. These findings implicate ATP6B1 in endolymph pH homeostasis and in normal auditory function, as nearly all patients with ATP6B1 mutations also have sensorineural hearing loss.[279]

Mutations in the *ATP6V0A4* gene (OMIM 602722) also give rise to recessive dRTA,[284] but hearing is preserved.[276, 283, 285] The gene *ATP6V0A4* on chromosome 7 encodes a newly identified kidney-specific a4 isoform of the proton pump's 116-kDa accessory a subunit.[284]

Correction of dehydration and alkali replacement results in correction of electrolyte abnormalities and improvement of symptoms. In adults, administration of 1 to 3 mmol alkali/kg body weight usually corrects the metabolic abnormality. In children, up to 5 mmol/kg may be required. Potassium supplementation may be required even after correction of the acidosis.

INHERITED HYPOKALEMIC HYPOTENSIVE DISORDERS

In 1962, Bartter and colleagues described two patients with hypokalemic metabolic alkalosis, hyperreninemic hyperaldosteronism, and normal blood pressure, as well as hyperplasia and hypertrophy of the juxtaglomerular apparatus.[286] Since then, it has been recognized that familial hypokalemic, hypochloremic metabolic alkalosis is not a single entity but rather a set of closely related disorders (reviewed in references 287, 288). This has created a tremendous amount of confusion regarding the various subtypes. Authors have interchangeably used Bartter syndrome with hyperprostaglandin syndrome in newborns and infants, and Bartter syndrome with Gitelman syndrome in adults, to characterize the various forms of the disorder. The recent molecular characterization

of the subtypes has answered many questions and largely dissipated this confusion. Bartter syndrome is a genetically heterogeneous disorder affecting the loop of Henle, typically presenting during the neonatal period, and associated with hypercalciuria and nephrocalcinosis[289-291] (Fig. 36-11). In contrast, Gitelman syndrome (Fig. 36-12) is a disorder affecting the distal tubule,[292] is usually diagnosed at a later stage, and is associated with hypocalciuria and hypomagnesemia, with predominant muscular signs and symptoms.[293]

Bartter Syndrome
Pathogenesis

Bartter syndrome (OMIM 241200) is a group of of autosomal recessive disorders affecting the function of the thick ascending limb of the loop of Henle, giving a clinical picture of salt-wasting and hypokalemic metabolic alkalosis. It is caused by inactivating mutations in one of at least four genes encoding membrane proteins of this nephron segment,[294-297] namely, the $Na^+/K^+/2Cl^-$ cotransporter (NKCC2), the apical inward-rectifying potassium channel (ROMK), and a basolateral chloride channel (ClC-Kb) or Barttin, a protein that acts

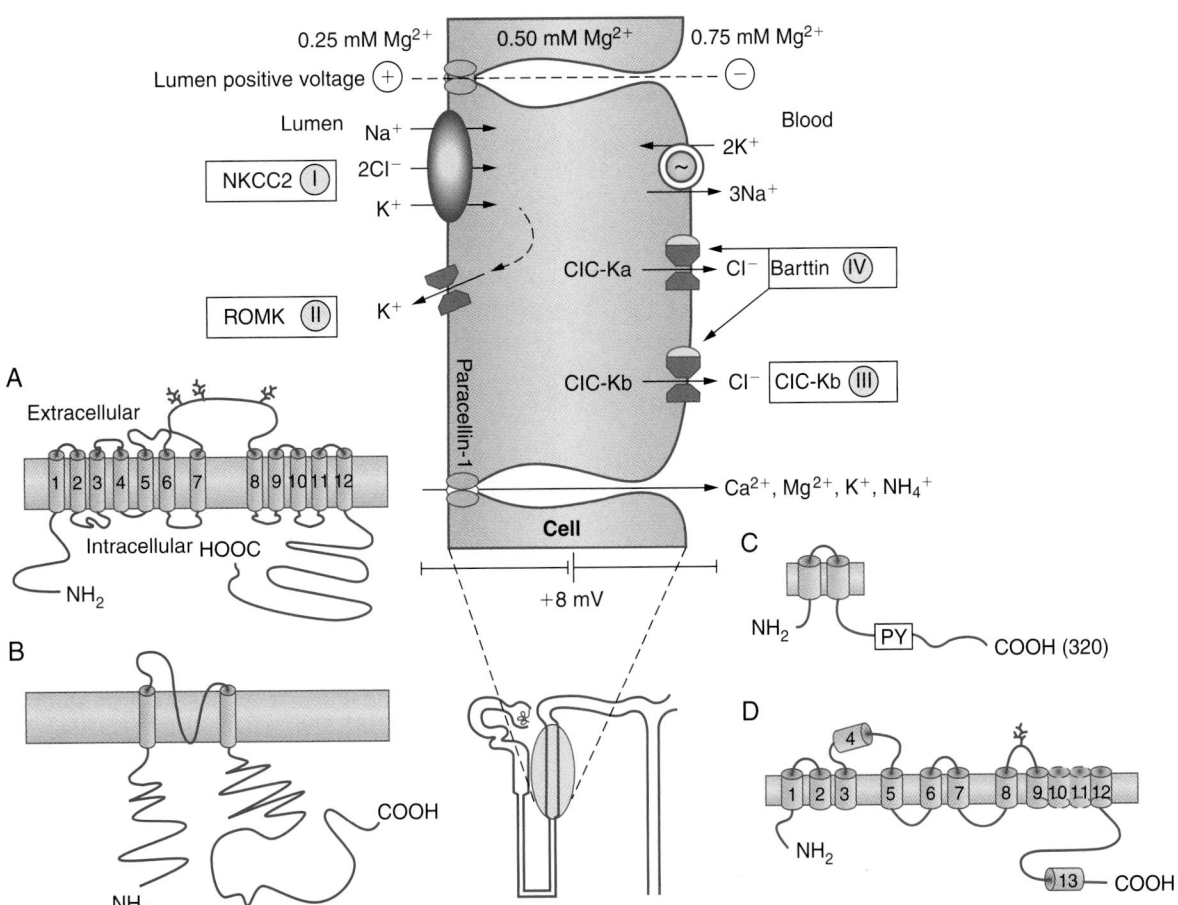

FIGURE 36-11. Bartter syndrome is secondary to loss-of-function mutations in (1) the bumetamide-sensitive $Na^+/K^+/2Cl^-$ cotransporter NKCC2 (type I); (2) the inwardly rectifying renal potassium channel ROMK (type II); (3) the renal chloride channel CLCNKB (type III); and (4) Barttin (type IV). Familial hypomagnesemia with hypercalciuria and nephrocalcinosis is secondary to loss-of-function of paracellin-1. Magnesium reabsorption in the thick ascending loop of Henle is also represented.

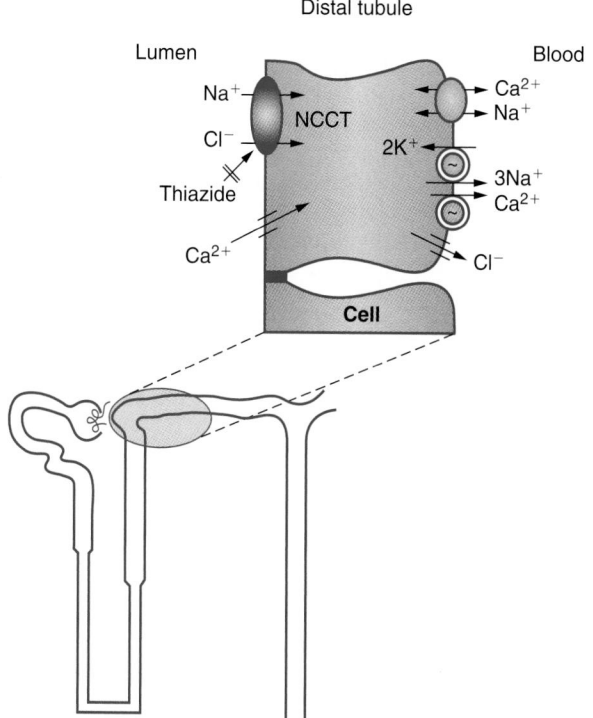

FIGURE 36-12. Gitelman syndrome: loss-of-function mutation of the thiazide-sensitive Na+/Cl− cotransporter.

as an essential activator β-subunit for ClC-Ka and ClC-Kb chloride channels (see Fig. 36-11).

Clinical Presentation

Most cases of Bartter syndrome present antenatally or neonatally. Polyhydramnios and premature labor are a common finding.[298] Polyuria and polydipsia are always present. Postnatal findings include failure to thrive, growth retardation, dehydration, low blood pressure, muscle weakness, seizures, tetany, paresthesias, and joint pain from chondrocalcinosis.[299] In contrast to patients with Gitelman syndrome, those with Bartter syndrome are virtually always hypercalciuric and normomagnesemic. Nephrocalcinosis occurs almost universally in Bartter patients harboring NKCC2 and ROMK mutations, but in only 20% of those harboring ClC-Kb mutations.[295] This could be attributable to lower urine calcium excretion. Patients with ROMK mutations present with hyperkalemia at birth, which converts to hypokalemia within the first weeks of life.[300] Thus, they can be misdiagnosed with pseudohypoaldosteronism type I. They do not need important K+ supplementation, contrary to other Bartter patients. This could be explained by the fact that ROMK, in addition to being required for sodium reabsorption in the thick ascending limb, is also expressed in the collecting duct. The prevailing potassium phenotype can thus shift. Sensorineural deafness is seen in Bartter patients harboring mutations in Barttin, as it is an essential subunit of chloride channels in the inner ear.[301] Barttin mutations are usually associated with a extremely severe phenotype with intrauterine onset, profound renal salt and water wasting, renal failure, sensorineural deafness, and motor retardation.[302]

Treatment

The treatment of Bartter syndrome usually involves potassium supplements, spironolactone, and nonsteroidal anti-inflammatory drugs. Indomethacin has been widely used,[303] as elevated levels of urinary prostaglandin E_2 have provided a rationale. Angiotensin I–converting enzyme inhibitors have been used successfully in conjunction with potassium supplements.[304, 305] Therapy should lead to catch-up growth in infants.[306-308]

Gitelman Syndrome
Pathogenesis

Gitelman syndrome (OMIM 263800) is a milder disorder compared with Bartter syndrome,[309] and is usually diagnosed in adults. It is also inherited as an autosomal recessive trait, and is genetically homogeneous, as it results from inactivating mutations in the *SLC12A3* gene encoding the thiazide-sensitive Na+/Cl− cotransporter, or *NCCT*.[292, 310] This is expected to result in sodium and cloride wasting with secondary hypovolemia and metabolic alkalosis. Activation of the renin-angiotensin-aldosterone system from volume depletion, in addition to increased sodium load to the cortical collecting duct, leads to increased sodium reabsorption by the epithelial sodium channel, counterbalanced by potassium and hydrogen excretion, resulting in hypokalemia and metabolic alkalosis. A mouse model of Gitelman syndrome also shows the human features of the disorder,[311] and confirms that it is a milder phenotype compared with Bartter syndrome.

Clinical Presentation

Unlike Bartter syndrome (Table 36-6), Gitelman syndrome does not present symptomatically in the neonatal period. It is often discovered incidentally. Patients have hypokalemic metabolic alkalosis, but in contrast with Bartter syndrome, they are hypocalciuric and hypomagnesemic, and do not have signs of overt volume depletion.[293] Hypothetically, stimulation of calcium absorption by the distal tubule has been attributed to (1) decreased apical Na+ reabsorption, driving the basolateral Na+/Ca2+ exchanger[312] and apical Ca2+ uptake; and (2) decreased intracellular Cl− concentration, which hyperpolarizes the apical membrane and stimulates Ca2+ uptake[313] via calcium channels.[314] Polyuria and polydipsia are not features of Gitelman syndrome. Arthritis due to chondrocalcinosis in several joints has been described.[315, 316] Urinary prostaglandin E_2 levels are normal,[317] compatible with the poor response to prostanoid synthetase inhibition. The major differential diagnosis of Gitelman syndrome is with diuretic abuse, laxative abuse, and chronic vomiting. A careful history, as well as measurement of urinary chloride and detection of diuretics, should help differentiate between these conditions.

Treatment

The treatment of Gitelman syndrome includes potassium supplementation and spironolactone.[318] Nonsteroidal anti-inflammatory drugs are usually not helpful, as prostaglandin levels are normal.

TABLE 36-6

Clinical Differences between Bartter and Gitelman Syndromes

	BARTTER SYNDROME				GITELMAN SYNDROME
	Type I (NKCC2)	Type II (ROMK)	Type III (CLCNKB)	Type IV (Barttin)	
Polyhydramnios	+	+	+	+	−
Failure to thrive	+	+	+	+	−
Growth retardation	+	+	+	+	−
Polyuria	+	+	+	+	−
Polydipsia	+	+	+	+	−
Muscle cramps/spasm	−	−	−	−	±
Chondrocalcinosis	−	−	−	−	±
Nephrocalcinosis	+	+	−	+	−
Sensorineural deafness	−	−	−	+	−

INHERITED HYPOKALEMIC HYPERTENSIVE DISORDERS

Excess secretion of aldosterone or other mineralocorticoids or abnormal sensitivity to mineralocorticoids may result in hypertension, suppressed plasma renin activity, metabolic alkalosis, and hypokalemia. However, most patients with hypokalemia and hypertension have essential hypertension associated with the use of diuretics or secondary aldosteronism from renal artery stenosis, or primary hyperaldosteronism from adrenal gland hyperplasia or adenoma. Hereditary hypokalemic hypertensive disorders are rare and affect electrolyte handling by the kidney (reviewed in references 319, 320, 321). The molecular basis of several traits associated with hypertension has been elucidated: congenital adrenal hyperplasia, the glucocorticoid-remediable aldosteronism (GRA), the syndrome of apparent mineralocorticoid excess (AME), activating mutations of the mineralocorticoid receptor, and Liddle syndrome. All these conditions are a consequence of abnormal biosynthesis, metabolism, or the action of steroid hormones and are characterized primarily by low or low-normal plasma renin, normal or low serum potassium, and salt-sensitive hypertension, suggesting enhanced mineralocorticoid activity.

Congenital Adrenal Hyperplasia

Inherited abnormalities in steroid biosynthesis cause hypertension in some cases of congenital adrenal hyperplasia. These autosomal recessive disorders arise from deficiencies of key enzymes of the steroid biosynthesis pathway (reviewed in references 322, 323). Hypertension usually accompanies a characteristic phenotype with abnormal sexual differentiation. The decrease in cortisol production causes an increase in adrenocorticotropic hormone (ACTH) secretion and subsequent hyperplasia of the adrenal glands. The phenotypes are determined by deficiencies as well as overproduction of steroids unaffected by the enzymatic defect. Hypertension is observed in only two of the three major subtypes of congenital adrenal hyperplasia (11β-hydroxylase and 17α-hydroxylase deficiencies), as metabolic blockade distal to 21α-hydroxylase allows the formation of 21-hydroxyl groups necessary for mineralocorticoid precursor biosynthesis. Other clinical manifestations are dependent on the effects of the enzymatic defect on androgen biosynthesis with either an increase (11β-hydroxylase) or a decrease (17α-hydroxylase) in

androgen production. In both deficiencies, overproduction of cortisol precursors that are metabolized to mineralocorticoid agonists or that have intrinsic mineralocorticoid activity induces volume and salt-dependent forms of hypertension. The elevated zona fasciculata deoxycorticosterone (DOC) produces mineralocorticoid hypertension with suppressed renin and reduced potassium concentrations. Aldosterone, the most important mineralocorticoid, regulated electrolyte excretion and intravascular volume mainly through its effects on renal distal convoluted tubules and cortical collecting ducts.

11β-Hydroxylase Deficiency

Inactivating mutations in the gene encoding 11β-hydroxylase (*OMIM 202010*)[324] cause the second most common form of congenital adrenal hyperplasia, representing 5% of cases (90% are caused by 21-hydroxylase deficiency). This disease is associated with excess production of DOC, 18-deoxycortisol, and androgens. By virtue of the significant intrinsic mineralocorticoid activity of DOC, subjects harboring mutations in both alleles of the gene exhibit hypokalemic hypertension. Because the androgen pathway is unaffected, prenatal masculinization occurs in females and postnatal virilization occurs in both sexes. The diagnosis of 11β-hydroxylase is made by the detection of increased levels of DOC and 18-deoxycortisol.[325] Treatment consists of exogenous corticoids, which inhibit ACTH secretion. Correction of mild salt wasting from reduced mineralocorticoid production may be necessary.[326]

17α-Hydroxylase Deficiency

17α-hydroxylase deficiency (OMIM 202110) results in reduced conversion of pregnenolone to progesterone and androgens and absent sex hormone production. The absence of sex hormone formation in both the adrenal glands and gonads causes hypogonadism and male pseudohermaphroditism, and is usually detected at adolescence because of failure to undergo puberty. Elevated glucocorticoid-suppressible levels of DOC and corticosterone, as well as their 18-hydroxylated products, are responsible for hypertension, hypokalemia, and renin and aldosterone suppression.[327] The clinical features vary depending on the enzymatic activity affected.[322, 328] In severe 17α-hydroxylase deficiency, 17α-hydroxylase and 17,20-lyase activities are reduced or absent. This results in excess mineralocorticoid activity and hypertension and produces a female phenotype resulting from absent sex steroid production in the adrenals and gonads. Partial 17α-hydroxylase deficiency leads to sexual ambiguity in males, without hypertension. Corticosteroid replacement corrects ACTH levels and hypertension. Females usually require hormonal therapy. Genetic males reared as females also require estrogen replacement. Genetic males reared as males require surgical correction of their external genitalia and androgen replacement therapy.[322]

Liddle Syndrome

Pathogenesis

Liddle syndrome (OMIM 177200) is an autosomal dominant form of hypertension characterized by hypokalemia and low levels of plasma renin and aldosterone, resulting from either premature termination or frameshift mutations in the

COOH-terminal domain of the epithelial sodium channel β- or γ-subunits.[320, 329] The amiloride-sensitive ENaC is a tetramer formed by the assembly of three homologous subunits, α, β, and γ, with the α-subunit being present in two copies[330] (Fig. 36-13). These subunits contain a large extracellular loop, located between two transmembrane α-helices. The NH₂- and COOH-terminal segments are cytoplasmic and contain potential regulatory segments that are able to modulate the activity of the channel. ENaC activity is tightly controlled by several distinct hormonal systems, including corticosteroids and vasopressin. In the kidney and colon, aldosterone is the major sodium-retaining hormone, acting by stimulation of Na⁺ reabsorption through the epithelium. In Liddle syndrome, mutations within the cytoplasmic COOH-terminus of the β- and γ- subunits of ENaC lead to hyperactivity of the channel. These mutations systematically delete or alter a conserved proline-rich amino acid sequence referred to as the PY motif.[329] The identification of specific

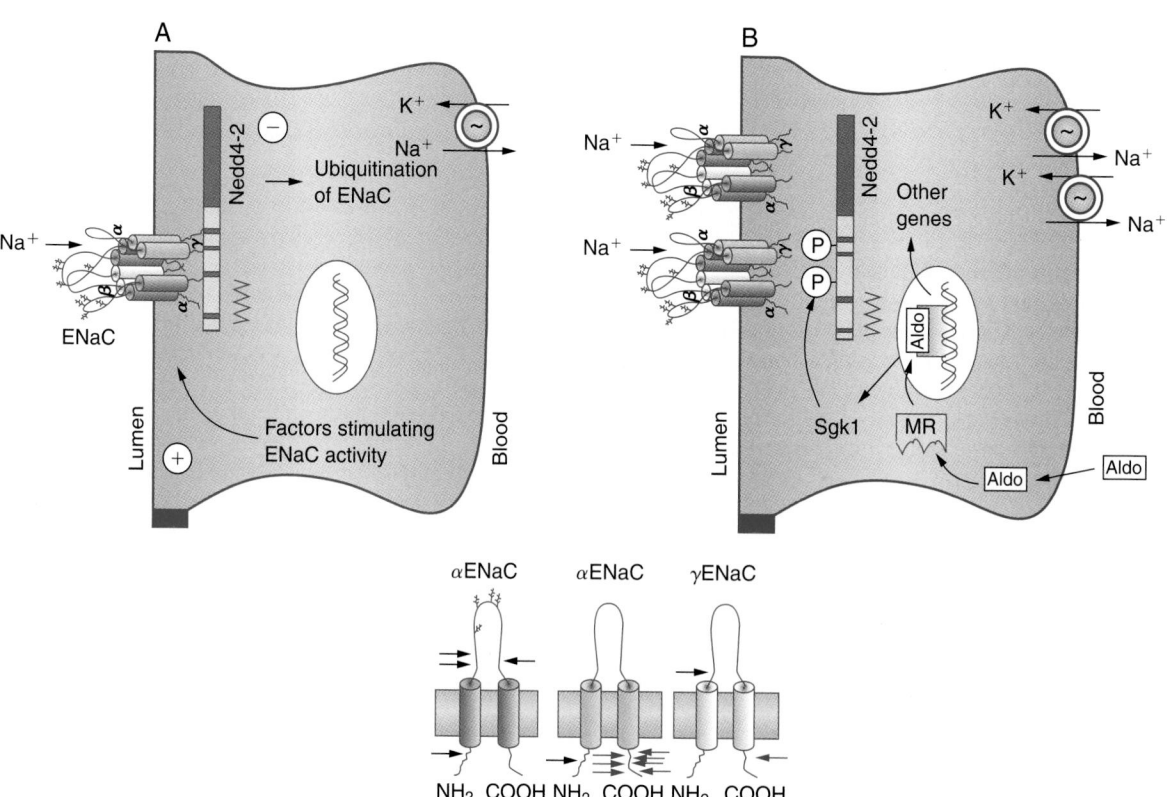

FIGURE 36-13. The epithelial Na⁺ channel (ENaC) is composed of two α-, one β-, and one γ-subunit surrounding the channel pore.[330] Each subunit has two transmembrane domains with short cytoplasmic NH₂ and COOH termini and a large ectocytoplasmic loop. Mutations in subunits of ENaC cause either Liddle syndrome (β- or γ-subunit) or the autosomal recessive form of pseudohypoaldosteronism type 1 (α-, β-, or γ-subunit).[465] The autosomal dominant form of pseudohypoaldosteronism type 1 is secondary to mutations in the mineralocorticoid receptor gene.[365] These ENaC and mineralocorticoid receptor mutations recapitulate the main pathway for Na⁺ reabsorption and potassium secretion across the principal cell of the cortical and medullary collecting duct. Sodium transport in tight epithelia of the distal nephron is mediated by the ENaC and the Na⁺,K⁺-ATPase. The ENaC is located at the apical membrane and constitutes the rate-limiting step for electrogenic sodium transport, whereas the Na⁺,K⁺-ATPase, located at the basolateral membrane, creates the driving form for this process. Note that only the α-subunit is glycosylated. The mechanism of ENaC expression in an aldosterone-sensitive epithelial cell is also represented. **A,** In a resting state, few ENaCs, which facilitate Na⁺ reabsorption in a rate-limiting fashion, are resident in the apical membrane. Factors known to enhance ENaC surface expression and activity are counterbalanced by retrieval of these channels from the membrane through the ubiquitination pathway mediated by Nedd4-2. **B,** Shortly after aldosterone exposure and binding to the mineralocorticoid receptor, transcriptional stimulation of SgK1 leads to phosphorylation of Nedd4-2, which subsequently disrupts ENaC/Nedd4-2 interactions. In this situation, ubiquitination of ENaCs is reduced, thus favoring ENaC residence in the apical membrane and enhanced Na⁺ reabsorption.

Nedd4 (for all subunits) and α-spectrin (for the α-subunit only) binding domains within the cytosolic COOH-terminal region of the ENaC subunits suggests that interactions with cytoskeletal elements control the expression of the ENaC at the apical membrane.[331, 332] Nedd4 and α-spectrin appear to play a role in the assembly, insertion, and retrieval of the ENaC subunits in the plasma membrane.[333] Expression studies have not definitively resolved whether the mutations associated with Liddle syndrome induce constitutive activation of the channel due to an increase in the number of channels[334] or to an increased open probability of individual channels.[335] Recent work has supported the hypothesis that the ENaC is removed from the plasma membrane through endocytosis and that Liddle syndrome mutations lead to the loss of endocytosis of these channels.[336] Mutations affecting the Nedd4 binding domain affect ubiquitination of ENaCs, thus favoring ENaC residence in the apical membrane and enhanced Na[+] reabsorption (reviewed in reference 337).

Clinical Presentation

Constitutive activation of the ENaC, manifested by continuing Na[+] channel activity, causes inappropriate renal Na[+] reabsorption, blunted Na[+] excretion, and low-renin hypertension (see review in reference 338). The features of this syndrome were described by Liddle and colleagues in 1963 in a large pedigree,[339] and were normalized by triamterene but not by spironolactone, a mineralocorticoid receptor antagonist. Affected individuals are at increased risk of cerebrovascular and cardiovascular accidents, but renal failure is notoriously rare. Liddle syndrome can be differentiated from other rare mendelian forms of low-renin hypertension with urinary or plasma hormonal profiles. GRA is associated with increased production of 18-hydroxycortisol and aldosterone metabolites. Apparent mineralocorticoid excess (reviewed in reference 340) is associated with increased urinary cortisol (tetrahydrocortisol) versus cortisone (tetrahydrocortisone) metabolites (Table 36-7).

Treatment

Hypertension is not improved by mineralocorticoid receptor inhibitors but can be corrected by a low-salt diet and ENaC antagonists (amiloride triamterene).

Apparent Mineralocorticoid Excess
Pathogenesis

The syndrome of apparent mineralocorticoid excess (AME; OMIM 207765) is a rare recessive disorder that results in hypokalemic hypertension, with low serum levels of renin and aldosterone (reviewed in references 341, 342). AME is due to a deficiency of 11β-hydroxysteroid dehydrogenase type 2 (11β-HSD2) enzymatic activity. The 11β-HSD2 enzyme is responsible for the conversion of cortisol to the inactive metabolite cortisone and therefore protects the mineralocorticoid receptors from cortisol intoxication. It is high-affinity dehydrogenase that catalyzes the rapid inactivation of glucocorticoids, thus ensuring selective access of aldosterone to otherwise nonselective mineralocorticoid receptors in the distal nephron (reviewed in references 343, 344). In AME, cortisol acts as a potent mineralocorticoid and causes salt retention hypertension and hypokalemia with a suppression of the renin-angiotensin-aldosterone system. Loss-of-function mutations of the 11β-HSD2 gene have been shown to explain the phenotype.[345-347] The milder phenotype, or type 2 variant, also results from abnormal activity of the enzyme.[348] The observation that under certain circumstances cortisol can act as a potent mineralocorticoid also explains the hypertension and hypokalemia in other disorders. For example, in Cushing syndrome, extremely high cortisol levels can overcome the ability of 11β-HSD2 to convert cortisol to cortisone. In addition, inhibition of 11β-HSD2 by licorice (glycyrrhizic acid) explains increased activation of the mineralocorticoid receptor and the subsequent hypertension.[349]

Clinical Presentation

AME is associated with severe juvenile low-renin hypertension, hypokalemic alkalosis, low birth weight, failure to thrive, poor growth, and nephrocalcinosis.[350] The urinary metabolites of cortisol demonstrate an abnormal ratio, with predominance of cortisol metabolites, that is, tetrahydrocortisol plus 5 α-tetrahydrocortisol/tetrahydrocortisone in the range 6.7 to 33, whereas the normal ratio is 1.0.[351] The milder form of AME (type 2), also due to mutations in the 11β-HSD2 gene, has similar clinical features but lacks the typical urinary steroid profile, that is, biochemical analysis reveals a

TABLE 36-7

Urinary Steroid Profiles in Mendelian Forms of Low-Renin Hypertension

	LIDDLE SYNDROME	GLUCOCORTICOID-REMEDIABLE ALDOSTERONISM	APPARENT MINERALOCORTICOID EXCESS
Aldosterone	Decreased	Increased	Decreased
TH-aldo	Decreased	Increased	Decreased
18-Hydroxy-TH-Aldo	Decreased	Increased	Decreased
18-Hydroxycortisol-F	Not detected	Increased	Not deected
Tetrahydrocortisol (TH-F)	Normal	Normal	Increased
Tetrahydrocortisone (TH-E)	Normal	Normal	Decreased
TH-F/TH-E	Normal	Normal	Increased

TH-aldo, tetrahydroxyaldosterone.

Data from Warnock DG: Liddle syndrome: An autosomal dominant form of human hypertension. Kidney Int 53:18-24, 1998.

moderately elevated cortisol-to-cortisone metabolite ratio. In the study of a large Sardinian consanguineous family,[348] affected individuals were 30 years or age of older, and had both mineralocorticoid hypertension and evidence of impaired metabolism of cortisol to cortisone. The heterozygote state was phenotypically normal but associated with subtle defects in cortisol metabolism.

Treatment

The treatment of AME is sodium restriction and either triamterene or amiloride. Spironolactone is not effective. Additional antihypertensive agents can be used as needed (vasodilators, β-blockers), particularly in older patients.

Autosomal Dominant Early-Onset Hypertension with Severe Exacerbation during Pregnancy

Autosomal dominant early-onset hypertension with severe exacerbation during pregnancy (OMIM 605115) is a rare disorder that is associated with activating mutations in the mineralocorticoid receptor.[352] By screening the mineralocorticoid receptor (MR) in 75 patients with early onset of severe hypertension, Geller and colleagues identified a 15-year-old boy with severe hypertension, suppressed plasma renin activity, low aldosterone, and no other underlying cause of hypertension, harboring a heterozygous missense mutation (S810L) in the MR gene.[352] This mutation alters an amino acid that is conserved in all MRs from *Xenopus* to human, but is not found in other nuclear receptors. Twenty-three relatives of the proband were evaluated. Remarkably, 11 had been diagnosed with severe hypertension before age 20, a rare trait in the general population, whereas the remaining 12 had unremarkable blood pressures. Comparison of the clinical features of carriers of the mutant allele with noncarriers revealed a marked increase in blood pressure among carriers even though they were taking antihypertensive medication, as well as suppression of aldosterone secretion. There was a nonsignificant trend toward lower serum potassium. Of note, three deceased family members with early-onset hypertension died of heart failure before age 50. The MR S810L mutation results in constitutive MR activity and altered receptor specificity, with progesterone and other steroids lacking 21-hydroxyl groups, normally MR antagonists, becoming potent agonists. Spironolactone was also a potent agonist of

MR L810, suggesting that this medication is contraindicated in MR L810 carriers.

That progesterone levels normally increase 100-fold in pregnancy, reaching concentrations of 500 nM, suggested that females with MR L810 might develop severe hypertension in pregnancy. Two MR L810 carriers had undergone five pregnancies; all had been complicated by marked exacerbation of hypertension. Aldosterone levels, which normally increase 10-fold in pregnancy, were undetectable.

Glucocorticoid-Remediable Hyperaldosteronism
Pathogenesis

Glucocorticoid-remediable hyperaldosteronism (OMIM 103900), also known as familial hyperaldosteronism type I, aldosteronism sensitive to dexamethasone, glucocorticoid-suppressible hyperaldosteronism, and syndrome of ACTH-dependent hyperaldosteronism, is an autosomal dominant form of hypertension caused by a chimeric gene duplication (Fig. 36-14) arising from unequal crossover between aldosterone synthase and 11β-hydroxylase,[353] two highly similar genes with the same transcriptional orientation lying 45,000 bp apart on chromosome 8. Humans have two isozymes with 11β-hydroxylase activity that are required for cortisol and aldosterone synthesis, respectively. CYP11B1 (11β-hydroxylase) is expressed at high levels and is regulated by ACTH, whereas CYP11B2 (aldosterone synthase) is normally expressed at low levels and is regulated by angiotensin II. In addition to 11β-hydroxylase activity, the latter enzyme has 18-hydroxylase and 18-oxidase activities and thus can synthesize aldosterone from deoxycorticosterone (reviewed in reference 354). Thus, the unequal crossover between the two genes results in the aldosterone synthase gene being under the control of regulatory promoter sequences of the 11β-hydroxylase. The chimeric gene product is expressed at high levels in both the zona glomerulosa and zona fasciculata and is controlled by ACTH. This leads to increased production of 18-hydroxycortisol and aldosterone metabolites.

Clinical Presentation

The phenotype of glucose-remediable aldosteronism (GRA) is highly variable.[355] Affected individuals can have mild hypertension and normal biochemistry, and be clinically

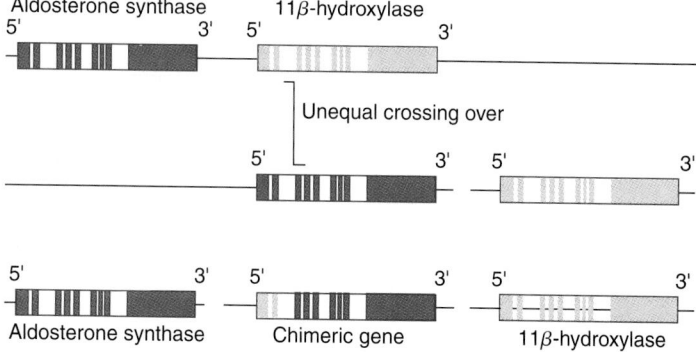

FIGURE 36-14. The chimeric gene duplication causing glucocorticoid-remediable aldosteronism (GRA). Both genes are linked on chromosome 8 and are separated by 45 kb.[466]

indistinguishable from patients with essential hypertension. However, some subjects have early onset of severe hypertension, hypokalemia, and metabolic alkalosis. GRA can be associated with high morbidity and mortality from early onset of hemorrhagic stroke and ruptured intracranial aneurysms.[356] In a study of 376 patients from 27 genetically proven GRA pedigrees, 48% of all GRA pedigrees and 18% of all GRA patients had cerebrovascular complications, which is similar to the frequency of aneurysm in adult polycystic kidney disease.[356] The diagnosis is usually established by measuring 18-hydroxy- or 18-oxocortisol metabolites in the urine or with the dexamethasone suppression test.[357] GRA patients produce high levels of 18-hydroxy- or 18-oxocortisol, steroids that are normally secreted in negligible amounts in normal subjects. In addition, because they secrete aldosterone in response to ACTH, glucocorticoid administration can suppress excessive aldosterone secretion.[358] The dexamethasone suppression test is a variably reliable method for establishing the diagnosis. Subjects without the disease, that is, those with an aldosterone-producing adenoma or with idiopathic hyperaldosteronism, can suppress aldosterone secretion.[359] The diagnosis of GRA can be definitively established demonstrating the chimeric gene by molecular techniques.[353]

Treatment

Simple glucocorticoid replacement is the treatment for GRA. Salt restriction and ENaC inhibition or spironolactone are also effective.

Familial Hyperaldosteronism Type II

Familial hyperaldosteronism type II (FH-II) (OMIM 605635) is characterized by hypersecretion of aldosterone due to adrenocortical hyperplasia, an aldosterone-producing adenoma, or both. In contrast to familial hyperaldosteronism type I, FH-II is not suppressible by dexamethasone. Stowasser and colleagues[357] reported five families with this phenotype with a segregation pattern supporting dominant inheritance. Analysis of an extended kindred has found linkage between FH-II and markers on chromosome 7p22.[360]

INHERITED HYPERKALEMIC HYPOTENSIVE DISORDERS

Pseudohypoaldosteronism Type I
Pathogenesis

Pseudohypoaldosteronism type I (PHA-I) is a rare genetically heterogeneous disorder. There are two subtypes of PHA-I.[361, 362] An autosomal recessive form (OMIM 264350) with severe manifestations that persist into adulthood, and an autosomal dominant form (OMIM 177735) with milder manifestations that remits with age. There are "sporadic" cases as well. The autosomal recessive form is caused by inactivating mutations in any of the three subunits (α, β, γ) of the ENaC.[363, 364] The autosomal dominant form is due to mutations in the MR gene.[365] It is postulated that heterozygous MR mutations result in haploinsufficiency or in dominant negative actions. At least some sporadic cases are caused by

mutations in the MR gene.[365] Homozygous mutations are probably lethal in humans as knockout mice show an important salt-wasting syndrome and die a few days after birth.[366]

Clinical Presentation

The clinical contrast between PHA-I due to ENaC or MR mutations is striking.[362] Autosomal *recessive* PHA-I is manifested neonatally or in childhood and is characterized by renal salt wasting, hypotension, hyperkalemia, metabolic acidosis, and, on occasion, failure to thrive. Other biologic features include hyponatremia, high plasma and urinary aldosterone levels despite hyperkalemia, and elevated plasma renin activity. The differential diagnosis has to be made with aldosterone synthase deficiency, salt-wasting forms of congenital adrenal hyperplasia, and adrenal hypoplasia congenita, each of which causes aldosterone deficiency, and is associated with hyponatremia, hyperkalemia, hypovolemia, elevated plasma renin activity, and sometimes shock and death (reviewed in reference 367). Bartter syndrome from mutations in the ROMK gene can also manifest in the neonatal period with a similar (transient) clinical picture.

Autosomal *dominant* PHA-I manifests with milder manifestations with remission of the syndrome with age. This is consistent with progressively reduced dependence on aldosterone.

Treatment

Treatment consists of salt supplementation, which can greatly improve hyponatremia, hyperkalemia, and growth. Administration of aldosterone, fludrocortisone, and deoxycorticosterone is usually not helpful. Patients with the recessive form usually need lifelong treatment for salt wasting and hyperkalemia, whereas in the dominant form, treatment can usually be withdrawn in adulthood.[320]

INHERITED HYPERKALEMIC HYPERTENSIVE DISORDERS

Pseudohypoaldosteronism Type II
Pathogenesis

Pseudohypoaldosteronism type II (PHA-II; OMIM 145260), also known as familial hyperkalemia and hypertension or Gordon syndrome, is a volume-dependent low-renin form of hypertension characterized by persistent hyperkalemia despite a normal renal GFR.[368, 369] Hypertension is attributable to increased renal salt reabsorption and the hyperkalemia to reduced renal K^+ excretion. Reduced renal H^+ secretion is also commonly seen, resulting in metabolic acidosis.[368] The features of PHA-II are chloride-dependent, because they are corrected when infusion of sodium sulfate or sodium bicarbonate is substituted for sodium chloride.[370, 371] In addition, these abnormalities are ameliorated by thiazide diuretics, which inhibit salt reabsorption in the distal nephron. In the distal convoluted tubule (DCT), salt reabsorption is mediated by the electroneutral Na^+/Cl^- cotransporter. In the cortical collecting duct (CCD), Na^+ is reabsorbed by the ENaC, with this electrogenic step providing the electrical driving force for K^+ and H^+ secretion.

The disease is genetically heterogeneous and three loci have now been mapped to chromosomes 17, 1, and 12.[372, 373] Recently, two genes causing PHA-II were identified on chromosomes 12 and 17.[374] Both genes encode members of the WNK family of serine-threonine kinases that localize to the distal nephron. Disease-causing mutations in *WNK1* are large intronic deletions that increase *WNK1* expression. The mutations in *WNK4* are missense, and cluster in a short, highly conserved segment. WNK4 negatively regulates surface expression of NCCT, thus implicating loss of this regulation in the molecular pathogenesis of the disorder.[375] WNK1 is present throughout the cytoplasm, whereas WNK4 is present exclusively in intercellular junctions in the DCT and in both the cytoplasm and intercellular junctions in the CCD.[374] The action of these kinases may serve to increase transcellular or paracellular Cl^- conductance in the collecting duct, thereby increasing salt reabsorption and intravascular volume, while concomitantly dissipating the electrical gradient and diminishing K^+ and H^+ secretion. Recent data suggest that WNK1 plays a general role in the regulation of epithelial Cl^- flux.[376]

Clinical Presentation

PHA-II is usually diagnosed in adults but is also seen neonatally.[377] The severity of hyperkalemia varies greatly and is influenced by prior intake of diuretics and salt. Causes of spurious elevation of potassium (hemolysis, prolonged first clenching during venipuncture, trauma) should be ruled out before this diagnosis is made. In its most severe form, it is associated with muscle weakness (from hyperkalemia), short stature, and intellectual impairment.[368] Mild hyperchloremia, metabolic acidosis, and suppressed plasma renin activity are findings variably associated with the trait. The plasma renin response to upright posture or to a low-sodium diet is blunted.[378] Aldosterone levels vary from low to high depending on the level of hyperkalemia. Urinary concentrating ability, acid excretion, and proximal tubular function are all normal.

Treatment

Treatment with thiazide diuretics reverses all the biochemical abnormalities. Lower than average doses can be given if overcorrection is seen. Loop diuretics can also be used.

INHERITED DISORDERS OF RENAL MAGNESIUM HANDLING

Magnesium is the second most abundant intracellular cation and plays an important role in protein synthesis, nucleic acid stability, neuromuscular excitability, and oxidative phosphorylation. Under normal conditions, extracellular magnesium concentration is maintained at nearly constant values. Hypomagnesemia results from decreased dietary intake, intestinal malabsorption, or renal loss.

Primary hypomagnesemia is composed of a heterogeneous group of disorders characterized by renal and intestinal Mg^{2+} wasting, often associated with hypercalciuria.[379, 380] The genetic basis and cellular defects of a number of primary hypomagnesemias have been elucidated over the past decade. These include (1) hypomagnesemia with hypercalciuria and nephrocalcinosis, a recessive condition caused by mutations

of the claudin 16 gene (chromosome 3q27); (2) autosomal dominant hypomagnesemia caused by isolated renal magnesium wasting (chromosome 11q23); (3) hypomagnesemia with secondary hypocalcemia, an early-onset, autosomal recessive disease (chromosome 9q12-22.2); (4) autosomal dominant hypoparathyroidism, a variably hypomagnesemic disorder caused by inactivating mutations of the extracellular Ca^{2+}-sensing receptor (chromosome 3q13.3-21); and (5) Gitelman syndrome, a recessive form of hypomagnesemia caused by mutations in the distal tubular NaCl cotransporter gene, *SLC12A3* (chromosome 16q13). These inherited conditions affect different nephron segments and different cell types and lead to variable but increasingly distinguishable phenotypic presentations.

Familial Hypomagnesemia with Hypercalciuria and Nephrocalcinosis

The syndrome of renal hypomagnesemia with hypercalciuria and nephrocalcinosis (OMIM 248250) is a rare autosomal recessive trait characterized by profound Mg^{2+} wasting that results in severe hypomagnesemia that is not corrected by oral or intravenous magnesium supplementation.[381] Renal calcium wasting leads to parenchymal calcification and renal failure. Other clinical findings include polyuria and polydipsia, ocular abnormalities, recurrent urinary tract infections, and recurrent renal colics with stone passage. Bilateral nephrocalcinosis is observed in all cases. Every patient shows hypomagnesemia with inappropriately high urinary Mg^{2+} excretion (Mg^{2+} fractional excretions of 16.2 ± 7.1%).[381] Hypercalciuria is present in every case save those with advanced renal insufficiency. Serum PTH levels are abnormally high. Serum calcium, phosphorus, and potassium and urinary excretion of uric acid and oxalate are normal. Neither chronic oral Mg^{2+} administration nor thiazide diuretics normalize serum Mg^{2+} levels or urinary Ca^{2+} excretion. Renal function worsens in every case, with several patients requiring chronic dialysis. The progression rate of renal insufficiency correlates with the severity of nephrocalcinosis. After kidney graft, tubular handling of Mg^{2+} and Ca^{2+} is normal.

The disorder is caused by mutations in paracellin-1,[382] a protein located in tight junctions of the thick ascending limb of the loop of Henle related to the claudin family of tight junction proteins (see Fig. 36-11).

Familial Hypomagnesemia with Secondary Hypocalcemia

Familial hypomagnesemia with secondary hypocalcemia (OMIM 602014) is an autosomal recessive disease that results in electrolyte abnormalities shortly after birth. Affected individuals show severe hypomagnesemia and hypocalcemia, which lead to seizures and tetany. The disorder has been thought to be caused by a defect in the intestinal absorption of magnesium, rather than by abnormal renal loss of magnesium. Mutations of *TRPM6* cause hypomagnesemia[383, 384] because of abnormal renal magnesium excretion. TRPM6 protein is a new member of the long transient receptor potential channel (TRPM) family. It is similar to *TRPM7*, which encodes a protein with features of a Ca^{2+}- and Mg^{2+}-permeable divalent cation channel. TRPM7 is particular in being both an ion channel and a serine/threonine kinase.[385]

Restoring the concentrations of serum magnesium to normal values by high-dose magnesium supplementation can overcome the apparent defect in magnesium absorption and in serum concentrations of calcium. Lifelong magnesium supplementation is required to overcome the defect in magnesium handling.

Isolated Dominant Hypomagnesemia with Hypocalciuria

This is a rare autosomal dominant disorder (OMIM 154020) caused by a dominant negative mutation of the *FXYD2* gene resulting in a trafficking defect of the γ-subunit of the Na^+,K^+-ATPase at the basolateral membrane of the DCT[386] (Fig. 36-15). Defective activity of the Na^+,K^+- ATPase can lead to either depolarization, reduced intracellular K^+, or increased intracellular Na^+. Experiments with mouse cell lines have yielded evidence for the existence of Mg^{2+} channels in the DCT,[387] and abnormal Na^+,K^+-ATPase activity in the DCT could then lead to reduced Mg^{2+} influx and Mg^{2+} wasting.

Calcium/Magnesium-Sensing Receptor–Associated Disorders

An important regulator of magnesium homeostasis is the Ca^{2+}/Mg^{2+}-sensing receptor CASR.[388] Activating mutations of the *CASR* gene were first described in families affected with autosomal dominant hypocalcemia (ADH). Affected individuals present with hypocalcemia, hypercalciuria, and polyuria, and about 50% of these patients have hypomagnemia.[380]

DIABETES INSIPIDUS

Pathogenesis

The conservation of water by the human kidney is a function of the complex architecture of renal tubules within the renal medulla.[389] The principal cells of the renal collecting tubules are responsive to the neurohypophysial antidiuretic hormone arginine vasopressin (AVP). The major action of AVP is to facilitate urinary concentration by allowing water to be transported passively down an osmotic gradient between the tubular fluid and the surrounding interstitium.

The first step in the antidiuretic action of AVP is its binding to the vasopressin V_2 receptor (AVPR2 in Fig. 36-16) located on the basolateral membrane of collecting duct cells. This step initiates a cascade of events—receptor-linked activation of G protein (G_s), activation of adenylyl cyclase, production of cyclic AMP (cAMP), and stimulation of protein kinase A (PKA)—that leads to the final step in the antidiuretic action of AVP, that is, the exocytic insertion of specific water channels, aquaporin-2 (AQP-2), into the luminal

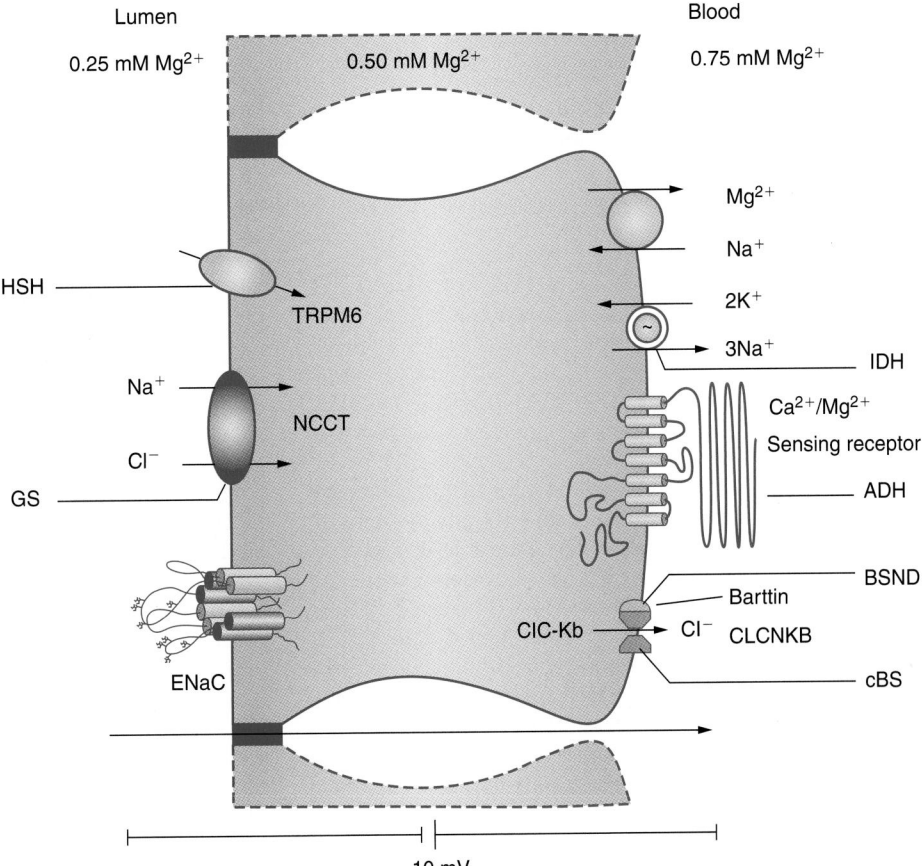

DISTAL CONVOLUTED TUBULE

FIGURE 36-15. Magnesium reabsorption in the distal convoluted tubule. In this segment, magnesium is reabsorbed by an active transcellular pathway involving an apical entry step probably via a magnesium-permeable ion channel and a basolateral exchange mechanism, presumably an Na^+/Mg^{2+} exchanger. The molecular identity of this exchanger is still unknown. HSH, hypomagnesemia with secondary hypocalciuria; GS, Giltelman syndrome; IDH, isolated dominant hypomagnesemia; ADH, autosomal dominant hypoparathyroidism; BSND, antenatal Bartter syndrome with sensorineural deafness; cBS, classic Bartter syndrome. (Modified from Konrad M, Weber S: Recent advances in molecular genetics of hereditary magnesium-losing disorders. J Am Soc Nephrol 14:249-260, 2003.)

OUTER AND INNER MEDULLARY COLLECTING DUCT

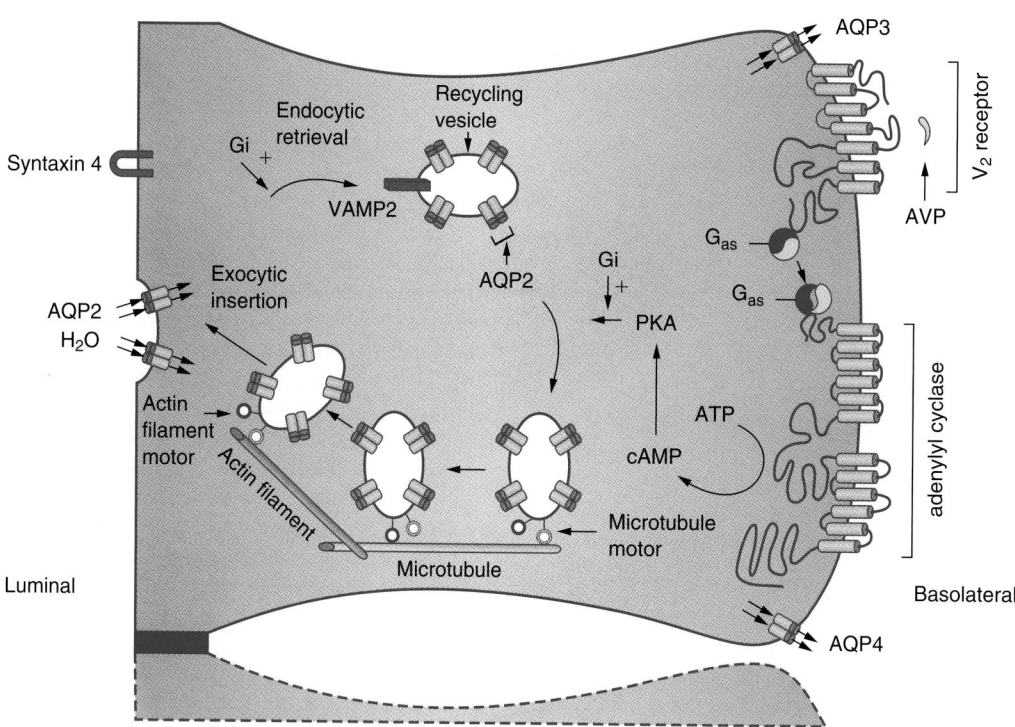

FIGURE 36-16. Schematic representation of the effect of arginine vasopressin (AVP) to increase water permeability in the principal cells of the collecting duct. Please note that Na^+ reabsorption, through the epithelial Na^+ channel (ENaC) is not represented. AVP is bound to the $V_2^{\frac{1}{2}}$ receptor (a G protein–linked receptor) on the basolateral membrane. The basic process of G protein–coupled receptor signaling consists of three steps: (1) a heptahelical receptor that detects a ligand (in this case, AVP) in the extracellular milieu, (2) a G protein that dissociates into α-subunits bound to guanosine triphosphate (GTP) and β- and γ-subunits after interaction with the ligand-bound receptor, and (3) an effector (in this case, adenylyl cyclase) that interacts with dissociated G protein subunits to generate small-molecule second messengers. AVP activates adenylyl cyclase, increasing the intracellular concentration of cyclic adenosine monophosphate (cAMP). The topology of adenylyl cyclase is characterized by two tandem repeats of six hydrophobic transmembrane domains separated by a large cytoplasmic loop and terminates in a large intracellular tail. Generation of cAMP follows receptor-linked activation of the heteromeric G protein (G_s) and interaction of the free $G_{\alpha s}$-chain with the adenylyl cyclase catalyst. Protein kinase A (PKA) is the target of the generated cAMP. Cytoplasmic vesicles carrying the water channel proteins (represented as homotetrameric complexes) are fused to the luminal membrane in response to AVP, thereby increasing the water permeability of this membrane. Microtubules and actin filaments are necessary for vesicle movement toward the membrane. The mechanisms underlying docking and fusion of aquaporin-2 (AQP-2)–bearing vesicles are not known. The detection of the small GTP binding protein Rab3a, synaptobrevin 2, and syntaxin 4 in principal cells suggests that these proteins are involved in AQP-2 trafficking.[467] When AVP is not available, water channels are retrieved by an endocytic process, and water permeability returns to its original low rate. AQP-3 and AQP-4 water channels are expressed on the basolateral membrane.

membrane, thereby increasing the water permeability of that membrane. These water channels are members of a superfamily of integral membrane proteins that facilitate water transport.[390-393] Aquaporin-1 (AQP-1, also known as CHIP, channel-forming integral membrane protein of 28 kDa) was the first protein shown to function as a molecular water channel and is constitutively expressed in mammalian red blood cells, renal proximal tubules, thin descending limbs of the loop of Henle, and other water-permeable epithelia.[394] Murata and colleagues[395] have described an atomic model of AQP-1 at 3.8-Å resolutions, and "real-time" molecular dynamics simulations of water permeation through human AQP-1 have been obtained by de Groot and Grubmüller.[396] The latter have proposed that conserved fingerprint (asparagine-proline-alanine [NPA]) motifs form a selectivity-determining region; a second (aromatic/arginine) region is also proposed to function as a proton filter. These data have thus solved a long-standing physiologic puzzle—how membranes can be freely permeable to water but impermeable to protons. At the subcellular level, AQP-1 is localized in both apical and basolateral plasma membranes that may represent entrance and exit routes for transepithelial water transport. In contrast to AQP-2, limited amounts of AQP-1 are localized in membranes of vesicles or vacuoles. In the basolateral membranes, AQP-1 is localized to both basal and lateral infoldings. AQP-2 is the vasopressin-regulated water channel in renal collecting ducts. It is exclusively present in principal cells of inner medullary collecting duct cells and is diffusely distributed in the cytoplasm in the euhydrated condition, whereas apical staining of AQP-2 is intensified in the dehydrated condition or after vasopressin administration. These observations are thought to represent the exocytic insertion of preformed water channels from intracellular vesicles into the apical plasma membrane (the shuttle hypothesis) (see Fig. 36-16). AQP-3 and AQP-4 are the water channels in basolateral membranes of renal medullary collecting ducts. In addition, vasopressin also increases the water reabsorptive capacity of the kidney by regulating the urea transporter UT-A1 expressed in the innermedullary collecting duct, predominantly in its terminal part.[397, 398]

In nephrogenic diabetes insipidus (NDI), the kidney is unable to concentrate urine despite normal or elevated concentrations of AVP. In congenital NDI, the obvious clinical manifestations of the disease, that is, polyuria and polydipsia, are present at birth and need to be immediately recognized to avoid severe episodes of dehydration. Most (>90%) congenital NDI patients have mutations in the *AVPR2* gene, the Xq28 gene coding for the vasopressin V_2 (antidiuretic) receptor. In fewer than 10% of the families studied, congenital NDI has an autosomal recessive inheritance and mutations have been identified in the AQP-2 gene (*AQP2*) located in chromosome region 12q13, that is, the vasopressin-sensitive water channel. One hundred eighty-three different putative disease-causing mutations in the *AVPR2* gene have now been published in 284 unrelated families with X-linked NDI. When studies in vitro, most *AVPR2* mutations lead to receptors that are trapped intracellularly and are unable to reach the plasma membrane. A minority of the mutant receptors reach the cell surface but are unable to bind AVP or to trigger an intracellular cAMP signal. Similarly, *AQP2* mutant proteins are trapped intracellularly and cannot be expressed at the luminal membrane. This AQP2-trafficking defect is correctable, at least in vitro, by chemical chaperones. Other inherited disorders with mild, moderate, or severe inability to concentrate urine include the Bartter syndrome (MIM 601678),[299] cystinosis, and autosomal dominant hypocalcemia.[35, 380, 399]

Clinical Presentation

LOSS-OF-FUNCTION MUTATIONS OF THE *AVPR2*

X-linked NDI (OMIM 304800) is secondary to *AVPR2* mutations which result in loss-of-function or dysregulation of the V_2 receptor.[400]

Males who have an *AVPR2* mutation have a phenotype characterized by early dehydration episodes, hypernatremia, and hyperthermia as early as the first week of life. Dehydration episodes can be so severe that they lower arterial blood pressure to a degree that is not sufficient to sustain adequate oxygenation to the brain, kidneys, and other organs. Mental and physical retardation and renal failure are the classic "historical" consequences of late diagnosis and lack of treatment. Heterozygous females exhibit variable degrees of polyuria and polydipsia because of skewed X chromosome inactivation.[401, 402]

The "historical" clinical characteristics include hypernatremia, hyperthermia, mental retardation, and repeated episodes of dehydration in early infancy.[403-406] Mental retardation, a consequence of repeated episodes of dehydration, was prevalent in Crawford and Bode's study,[403] in which only 9 of 82 patients (11%) had normal intelligence. Early recognition and treatment of X-linked NDI with an abundant intake of water allows a normal life span with normal physical and mental development.[407] Two characteristics suggestive of X-linked NDI are the familial occurrence and the confinement of mental retardation to male patients. It is then tempting to assume that the family described in 1892 by McIlraith[408] and discussed by Reeves and Andreoli[409] was an X-linked NDI family. Lacombe[410] and Weil[411] described a familial form of diabetes insipidus with an autosomal type of transmission and without any associated mental retardation.

The descendants of the family originally described by Weil were later found to have autosomal dominant NDI (OMIM192340), a now well-characterized entity secondary to mutations in the prepro-arginine-vasopressin-neurophysin II gene (*prepro-AVP-NPII*).[412-415] Patients with autosomal dominant NDI retain some limited capacity to secrete AVP during severe dehydration and the polyuria-polydipsic symptoms usually appear after the first year of life[415] when the infant's demand for water is more likely to be understood by adults.

The early symptomatology of the nephrogenic disorder and its severity in infancy was clearly described by Crawford and Bode.[403] The first manifestations of the disease can be recognized during the first week of life. The infants are irritable, cry almost constantly, and, although eager to suck, will vomit milk soon after ingestion unless prefed with water. The history given by the mothers often includes persistent constipation, erratic unexplained fever, and failure to gain weight. Even though the patients characteristically show no visible evidence of perspiration, increased water loss during fever or in warm weather exaggerates the symptoms. Unless the condition is recognized early, children will experience frequent bouts of hypertonic dehydration, sometimes complicated by convulsions or death; mental retardation is a frequent consequence of these episodes. The intake of large quantities of water, combined with the patient's voluntary restriction of dietary salt and protein intake, lead to hypocaloric dwarfism beginning in infancy. Affected children frequently develop lower urinary tract dilation and obstruction, probably secondary to the large volume of urine produced.[416] Dilation of the lower urinary tract is also seen in primary polydipsic patients and in patients with NDI.[417, 418] Chronic renal insufficiency may occur by the end of the first decade of life and could be the result of episodes of dehydration with thrombosis of the glomerular tufts.[403]

In 1989, we observed that the administration of 1-deamino-8-D-arginine vasopressin (desmopressin acetate, DDAVP), a V_2 receptor agonist, increased plasma cAMP concentrations in normal subjects but had no effect in 14 male patients with X-linked NDI.[419] Intermediate responses were observed in obligate carriers of the disease, possibly corresponding to half of the normal receptor response. Based on these results, we predicted that the defective gene in these patients with X-linked NDI was likely to code for a defective V_2 receptor.[419] Since that time, a number of experimental results have confirmed our hypothesis:(1) The NDI locus was mapped to the distal region of the long arm of the X chromosome, Xq28[420-423]; (2) the V_2 receptor was identified as a candidate gene for NDI[424]; (3) the human V_2 receptor was cloned[425]; and (4) 183 putative disease-causing mutations have now been identified in the V_2 receptor and the list of mutations is expanding (Fig. 36-17).

Generally, X-linked NDI is a rare disease with an estimated prevalence of approximately 8.8 per million male live births in the Province of Quebec (Canada) during the 10-year period 1988 to 1997.[402] In defined regions of North America, however, the prevalence is much higher: we estimated the incidence in Nova Scotia and New Brunswick (Canada) to be 58 per million for the 10-year period 1988 to 1997.[402] It is assumed that the patients in these regions are progeny of common ancestors. An example is the Mormon pedigree, with its members residing in Utah (Utah families); this pedigree was originally described by Cannon.[426]

The "Utah mutation" is a nonsense mutation (L312X) predictive of a receptor that lacks transmembrane domain 7 and the intracellular COOH-terminus.[427] The largest known kindred with X-linked NDI is the Hopewell family, named after the Irish ship *Hopewell*, which arrived in Halifax, Nova Scotia, in 1761.[428] Aboard the ship were members of the Ulster Scot clan, descendants of Scottish Presbyterians who migrated to Ulster in Ireland in the 17th century and left Ireland for the New World in the 18th century. Whereas families arriving with the first emigration wave settled in northern Massachusetts in 1718, the members of the second emigration wave, passengers of the *Hopewell*, settled in Colchester County, Nova Scotia. According to the "Hopewell hypothesis,"[428] most NDI patients in North America are progeny of female carriers of the second emigration wave. This assumption is mainly based on the high prevalence of NDI among descendants of the Ulster Scots residing in Nova Scotia. In two villages with a total of 2500 inhabitants, 30 patients have been diagnosed, and the carrier frequency has been estimated at 6%.[420] Given the numerous mutations found in North American X-linked NDI families,

the Hopewell hypothesis cannot be upheld in its originally proposed form. However, among X-linked NDI patients in North America, the W71X (the Hopewell mutation) mutation is more common than another *AVPR2* mutation. It is a null mutation (W71X[427, 429]) predictive of an extremely truncated receptor consisting of the extracellular NH₂-terminus, the first transmembrane domain, and the NH₂-terminal half of the first intracellular loop. Because the original carrier cannot be identified,[420] it is not clear whether the Hopewell mutation was brought to North America by *Hopewell* passengers or by other Ulster Scot immigrants. One hundred eighty-three different putative disease-causing mutations in the *AVPR2* gene have now been reported in 284 unrelated families with X-linked NDI (see Fig. 36-17). The diversity of *AVPR2* mutations found in many ethnic groups (whites, Japanese, African-Americans, Africans) and the rareness of the disease is consistent with an X-linked recessive disease that in the past was lethal for male patients and was balanced by recurrent mutations. In X-linked NDI, loss of mutant alleles from the population occurs because of the higher mortality of affected males compared with healthy males,

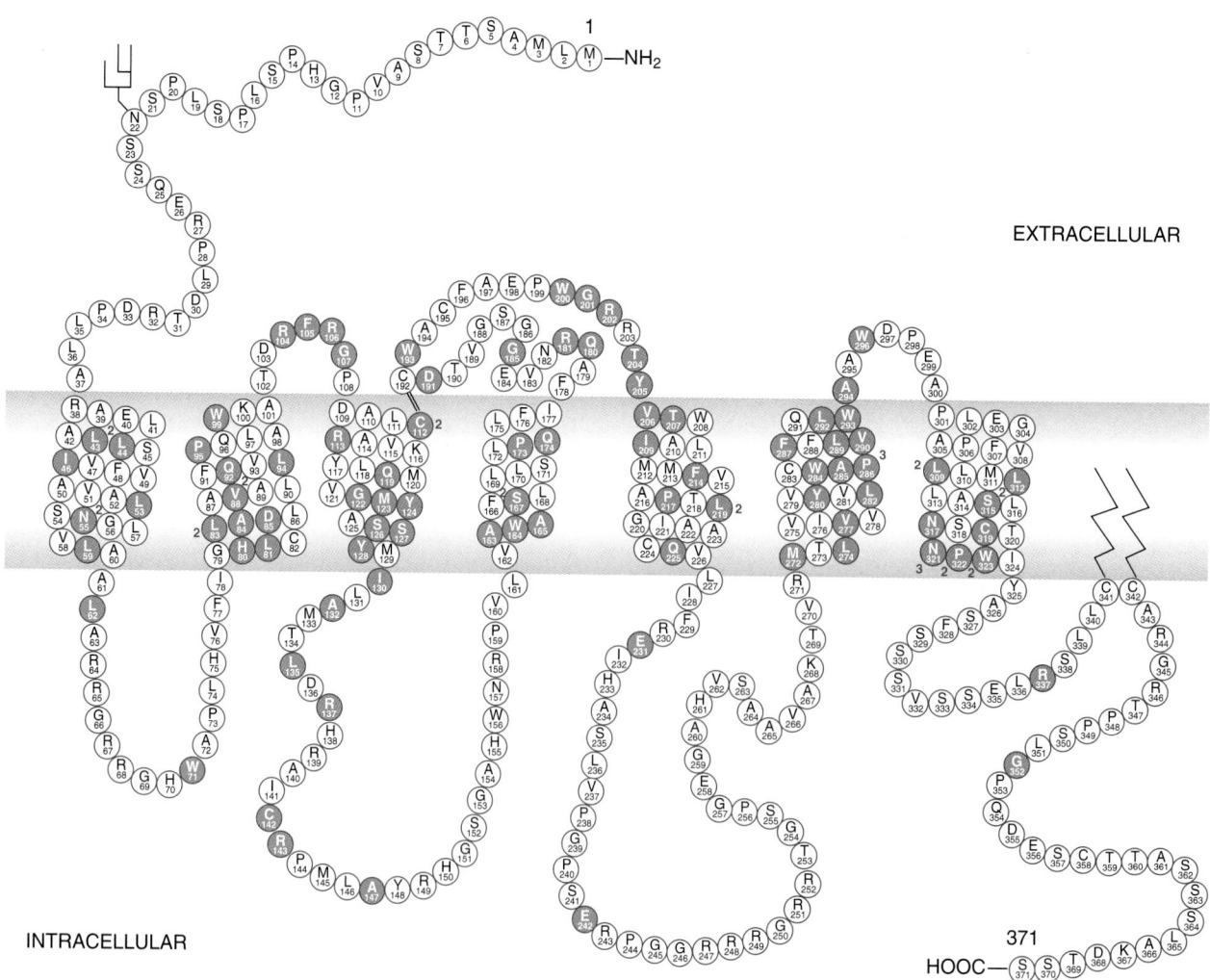

FIGURE 36-17. Schematic representation of the V₂ receptor and identification of 183 putative disease-causing *AVPR2* mutations. Predicted amino acids are given as the one-letter code. Solid symbols indicate missense or nonsense mutations; a number indicates more than one mutation in the same codon. The names of the mutations were assigned according to recommended nomenclature.[468] The extracellular, transmembrane, and cytoplasmic domains are defined according to Mouillac and colleagues.[469] The common names of the mutations are listed by type. Eighty-nine missense, 18 nonsense mutations, 45 frameshift, seven inframe deletions or insertions, four splice-site, as well as 19 large deletions and one complex mutation have been identified.

whereas gain of mutant alleles occurs by mutation. If affected males with a rare X-linked recessive disease do not reproduce and if mutation rates are equal in mothers and fathers, then, at genetic equilibrium, one third of new cases of affected males will be due to new mutations. We and others have described ancestral mutations, de novo mutations, and potential mechanisms of mutagenesis.[402, 430] These data are reminiscent of those obtained from patients with late-onset autosomal dominant retinitis pigmentosa. In one fourth of patients, the disease is caused by mutations in the light receptor rhodopsin. Here too, many different mutations (approximately 100) spread throughout the coding region of the rhodopsin gene have been found.[431]

The basis of loss-of-function or dysregulation on 28 different mutant V_2 receptors (including nonsense, frameshift, deletion, or missense mutations) has been studied using in vitro expression systems. Most of the mutant V_2 receptors tested were not transported to the cell membrane and were thus retained within the intracellular compartment.[432] Schöneberg and co-workers[433, 434] pharmacologically rescued truncated or missense V_2 receptors by coexpression of a polypeptide consisting of the last 130 amino acids of the V_2 receptor. Four of the six truncated receptors (E242X, 804delG, 834delA, and W284X) and the missense mutant Y280C regained considerable functional activity as demonstrated by

an increase in the number of binding sites and stimulation of adenylate cycles activity. These in vitro results are potentially promising avenues for the gene therapy of *AVPR2* mutations if a sufficient number of complemented receptors could be expressed on the cell surface. Our group also demonstrated that misfolded *AVPR2* mutants could be rescued in vitro,[435] but also in vivo,[436] by nonpeptide vasopressin antagonists acting as pharmacologic chaperones. This new therapeutic approach could be applied to the treatment of several hereditary diseases resulting from errors in protein folding and kinesis.

Only three *AVPR2* mutations (D85N, G201D, P322S) have been associated with a mild phenotype.[437, 438] In general, the male infants bearing these mutations are identified later in life and the "classic" episodes of dehydration are less severe. This mild phenotype is also found in expression studies: the mutant proteins are expressed on the plasma membrane of cells transfected with these mutants and demonstrate a stimulation of cAMP for higher concentrations of agonists.[432, 438]

LOSS-OF-FUNCTION MUTATIONS OF *AQP2*

The *AQP2* gene is located in chromosome region 12q13. Males and females affected with congenital NDI have been described who are homozygous for a mutation in the *AQP2* gene or carry two different mutations[437, 439-443] (Fig. 36-18).

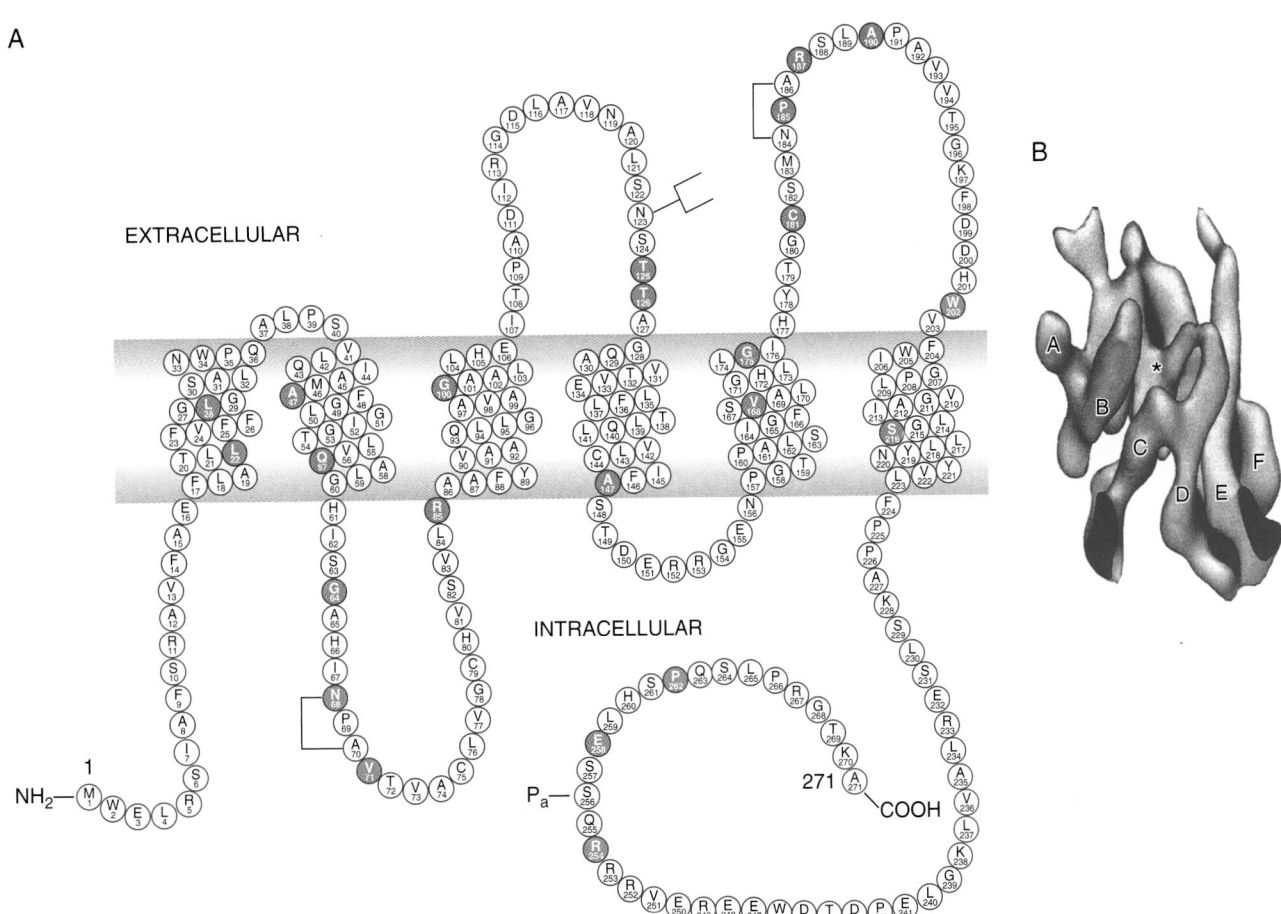

FIGURE 36-18. A representation of aquaporin-2 (AQP2) protein and identification of 32 putative disease-causing *AQP2* mutations. A monomer is represented with six transmembrane helices. The location of the protein kinase A phosphorylation site (Pa) is indicated. The extracellular, transmembrane, and cytoplasmic domains are defined according to Deen and colleagues.[439] Solid symbols indicate the location of the mutations. The common names of the mutations are listed by type. Twenty-two missense, two nonsense, six frameshift, as well as two splice-site mutations, have been identified.

The oocytes of the African clawed frog (*Xenopus laevis*) have provided a most useful test-bed for looking at the functioning of many channel proteins. Oocytes are large cells that are just about to become mature eggs ready for fertilization. They have all the normal translation machinery of living cells and so they will respond to the injection of mRNA by making the protein for which it codes. Functional expression studies showed that *Xenopus* oocytes injected with mutant cRNA had an abnormal coefficient of water permeability, whereas *Xenopus* oocytes injected with both normal and mutant cRNA had a coefficient of water permeability similar to that of normal constructs alone. These findings provide conclusive evidence that NDI can be caused by homozygosity for mutations in the *AQP2* gene. A patient with a partial phenotype has also been described to be a compound heterozygote for the L22V and C181W mutations.[443] Immunolocalization of AQP2-transfected CHO cells showed that the C181W mutant had an endoplasmic reticulum–like intracellular distribution, whereas L22V and wild-type AQP2 showed endosome and plasma membrane staining. The authors suggested that the L22V mutation was key to the patient's unique response to desmopressin. The leucine 22 residue might be necessary for proper conformation or for binding of another protein important for normal targeting and trafficking of the molecule. More recently, we obtained evidence to suggest that both autosomal dominant and autosomal recessive NDI phenotypes could be secondary to novel mutations in the *AQP2* gene.[444-447] Reminiscent of expression studies done with AVPR2 proteins, Mulders, Deen, Tamarappoo, and Verkman and their co-workers also demonstrated that the major cause underlying autosomal recessive NDI is the misrouting of AQP2 mutant proteins.[442,448-452] To determine if the severe AQP2-trafficking defect observed with the naturally occurring mutations T126M, R187C, and A147T is correctable, cells were incubated with the chemical chaperone glycerol for 48 hours. Redistribution of AQP2 from the endoplasmic reticulum to the membrane-endosome fractions was observed by immunofluorescence. This redistribution was correlated to improved water permeability measurements.[449] It will be important to correct this defective AQP2-trafficking in vivo.

POLYURIA, POLYDIPSIA, ELECTROLYTE IMBALANCE, AND DEHYDRATION IN CYSTINOSIS

Polyuria may be as mild as persistent enuresis and as severe as to contribute to death from dehydration and electrolyte abnormalities in infants with cystinosis who have acute grastroenteritis.[35]

POLYURIA IN HEREDITARY HYPOKALIEMIC SALT-LOSING TUBULOPATHIES

Patients with polyhydramnios, hypercalciuria, and hypo- or isothenuria have been found to bear *KCNJ1* (ROMK) and *SLC12A1* (NKCC2) mutaions.[293,299] Patients with polyhydramnios, profound polyuria, hyponatremia, hypochloremia, metabolic alkalosis, and sensorineural deafness were found to bear *BSND* mutations.[297,301,302,453] These studies demonstrate the critical importance of the proteins ROMK, NKCC2, and Barttin to transfer NaCl in the medullary interstitium and

thereby to generate, together with urea, a hypertonic milieu (see Fig. 36-11).

CARRIER DETECTION, PERINATAL TESTING, AND TREATMENT

We encourage physicians who follow families with X-linked and autosomal recessive NDI to recommend mutation analysis before the birth of an infant because early diagnosis and treatment can avert the physical and mental retardation associated with episodes of dehydration. Diagnosis of X-linked NDI was accomplished by mutation testing of cultured amniotic cells (n=5), chorionic villus samples (n=4), or cord blood obtained at birth (n=17) in 23 of our patients. Twelve males were found to bear mutant sequences, seven males were not affected, and four females were not carriers. The affected patients were immediately treated with abundant water intake, a low-sodium diet, and hydrochlorothiazide. They never experienced episodes of dehydration, and their physical and mental development is normal. Gene analysis is also important for the identification of nonobligatory female carriers in families with X-linked NDI. Most females heterozygous for a mutation in the V_2 receptor do not present with clinical symptoms; few are severely affected (see references 402, 454, 455 and Bichet, unpublished observations). Mutational analysis of polyuric patients with cystinosis or hypokalemic salt-losing tubulopathy is also of importance for a definitive molecular diagnosis.

All complications of congenital NDI are prevented by an adequate water intake. Thus, patients should be provided with unrestricted amounts of water from birth to ensure normal development. In addition to a low-sodium diet, the use of diuretics (thiazides) or indomethacin may reduce urinary output. This advantageous effect has to be weighed against the side effects of these drugs (thiazides: electrolyte disturbances; indomethacin: reduction of the GFR and gastrointestinal symptoms). Many affected infants frequently vomit due to an exacerbation of physiologic gastroesophageal reflux. These young patients often improve with the absorption of an H_2 blocker and with metoclopramide (which could induce extrapyramidal symptoms) or with domperidone, which seems to be better tolerated and efficacious.

REFERENCES

1. Bergeron M, Gougoux A, Noël J, et al: The renal Fanconi syndrome. *In* Scriver CR, Beaudet AL, Sly WS, et al (eds): The Metabolic and Molecular Bases of Inherited Disease, 8th ed. New York, McGraw-Hill, 2001, pp 5023-5038.
2. Diamond GL, Zalups RK: Understanding renal toxicity of heavy metals. Toxicol Pathol 26:92-103, 1998.
3. Aronsson S, Engleson G, Jagenburg R, et al: Long-term dietary treatment of tyrosinosis. J Pediatr 72:620-627, 1968.
4. Levin B, Snodgrass GJ, Oberholzer VG, et al: Fructosaemia. Observations on seven cases. Am J Med 45:826-838, 1968.
5. Cusworth DC, Dent CE, Flynn FV: The aminoaciduria in galactosemia. Arch Dis Child 30:150-155, 1957.
6. Adams RG, Harrison JF, Scott P: The development of cadmium-induced proteinuria, impaired renal function, and osteomalacia in alkaline battery workers. Q J Med 38:425-443, 1969.
7. Morris RC Jr: An experimental renal acidification defect in patients with hereditary fructose intolerance. I. Its resemblance to renal tubular acidosis. J Clin Invest 47:1389-1398, 1968.
8. Sanjad SA, Kaddoura RE, Nazer HM, et al: Fanconi's syndrome with hepatorenal glycogenosis associated with phosphorylase *b* kinase deficiency. Am J Dis Child 147:957-959, 1993.

9. McKusick VA: Online Mendelian Inheritance in Man (OMIM). Baltimore, McKusick-Nathans Institute for Genetic Medicine, Johns Hopkins University and National Center for Biotechnology Information, National Library of Medicine, 2000. World Wide Web URL: Available at http://www.ncbi.nlm.nih.gov/omin/.

10. Lloyd S, Pearce S, Fisher S, et al: A common molecular basis for three inherited kidney stone diseases. Nature 379:445-449, 1996.

11. Lloyd SE, Gunther W, Pearce SH, et al, Characterisation of renal chloride channel, *CLCN5*, mutations in hypercalciuric nephrolithiasis (kidney stones) disorders. Hum Mol Genet 6:1233-1239, 1997.

12. Presley JF, Mayor S, McGraw TE, et al: Bafilomycin A1 treatment retards transferrin receptor recycling more than bulk membrane recycling. J Biol Chem, 272:13929-13936, 1997.

13. Jentsch TJ, Stein V, Weinreich F, et al: Molecular structure and physiological function of chloride channels. Physiol Rev 82:503-568, 2002.

14. Steinmeyer K, Schwappach B, Bens M, et al: Cloning and functional expression of rat CLC-5, a chloride channel related to kidney disease. J Biol Chem 270:31172-31177, 1995.

15. Gunther W, Luchow A, Cluzeaud F, et al: ClC-5, the chloride channel mutated in Dent's disease, colocalizes with the proton pump in endocytotically active kidney cells. Proc Natl Acad Sci U S A 95:8075-8080, 1998.

16. Devuyst O, Christie PT, Courtoy PJ, et al: Intra-renal and subcellular distribution of the human chloride channel, CLC-5, reveals a pathophysiological basis for Dent's disease. Hum Mol Genet 8:247-257, 1999.

17. Schwake M, Friedrich T, Jentsch TJ: An internalization signal in ClC-5, an endosomal Cl⁻ channel mutated in Dent's disease. J Biol Chem 276:12049-12054, 2001.

18. Rotin D, Kanelis V, Schild L: Trafficking and cell surface stability of ENaC. Am J Physiol Renal Physiol 281:F391-399, 2001.

19. Piwon N, Gunther W, Schwake M, et al: ClC-5 Cl⁻-channel disruption impairs endocytosis in a mouse model for Dent's disease. Nature 408:369-373, 2000.

20. Hilpert J, Nykjaer A, Jacobsen C, et al: Megalin antagonizes activation of the parathyroid hormone receptor. J Biol Chem 274:5620-5625, 1999.

21. Nykjaer A, Dragun D, Walther D, et al: An endocytic pathway essential for renal uptake and activation of the steroid 25-(OH) vitamin D₃. Cell 96:507-515, 1999.

22. Nykjaer A, Fyfe JC, Kozyraki R, et al: Cubilin dysfunction causes abnormal metabolism of the steroid hormone 25(OH) vitamin D(3). Proc Natl Acad Sci U S A, 98:13895-13900, 2001.

23. Scheinman S: X-linked hypercalciuric nephrolithiasis: Clinical syndromes and chloride channel mutations. Kidney Int 53:3-17, 1998.

24. Wang SS, Devuyst O, Courtoy PJ, et al: Mice lacking renal chloride channel, CLC-5, are a model for Dent's disease, a nephrolithiasis disorder associated with defective receptor-mediated endocytosis. Hum Mol Genet 9:2937-2945, 2000.

25. Wrong O, Norden A, Feest T: Dent's disease; a familial proximal renal tubular syndrome with low-molecular-weight proteinuria, hypercalciuria, nephrocalcinosis, metabolic bone disease, progressive renal failure and a marked male predominance. Q J Med, 87:473-493, 1994.

26. Kelleher CL, Buckalew VM, Frederickson ED, et al: CLCN5 mutation Ser244Leu is associated with X-linked renal failure without X-linked recessive hypophosphatemic rickets [see comments]. Kidney Int 53:31-37, 1998.

27. Bonnardeaux A, Lapointe JY, Bichet DG: Chloride channels and hypercalciuria: An unturned stone. J Clin Invest 99:819-821, 1997.

28. Frymoyer P, Scheinman S, Dunham P, et al: X-linked recessive nephrolithiasis with renal failure. N Engl J Med 325:681-686, 1991.

29. Igarashi T, Hayakawa H, Shiraga H, et al: Hypercalciuria and nephrocalcinosis in patients with idiopathic low-molecular-weight proteinuria in Japan: Is the disease identical to Dent's disease in United Kingdom? Nephron 69:242-247, 1995.

30. Morimoto T, Uchida S, Sakamoto H, et al: Mutations in CLCN5 chloride channel in Japanese patients with low molecular weight proteinuria. J Am soc Nephrol, 9:811-818, 1998.

31. Lloyd SE, Pearce SH, Gunther W, et al: Idiopathic low molecular weight proteinuria associated with hypercalciuric nephrocalcinosis in Japanese children is due to mutations of the renal chloride channel (CLCN5). J Clin Invest 99:967-974, 1997.

32. Hunt DD, Stearns G, Eroning EC, et al: Long term study of a family with the Fanconi syndrome and cystinuria. Surg Forum 16:462-464, 1965.

33. Friedman AL, Trygstad CW, Chesney RW: Autosomal dominant Fanconi syndrome with early renal failure. Am J Med Genet 2:225-232, 1978.

34. Brenton DP, Isenberg DA, Cusworth DC, et al: The adult presenting idiopathic Fanconi syndrome. J Inherit Metab Dis 4:211-215, 1981.

35. Gahl WA, Thoene JG, Schneider JA: Cystinosis. N Engl J Med 347:111-121, 2002.

36. Town M, Jean G, Cherqui S, et al: A novel gene encoding an integral membrane protein is mutated in nephropathic cystinosis. Nat Genet 18:319-324, 1998.

37. Kalatzis V, Cherqui S, Antignac C, et al: Cystinosin, the protein defective in cystinosis, is a H(+)-driven lysosomal cystine transporter. EMBO J 20:5940-5949, 2001.

38. Gahl W, Thoene J, Schneider J: Cystinosis: A disorder of lysosomal membrane transport. *In* Scriver C, Beaudet A, Sly W, et al (eds): The Metabolic and Molecular Bases of Inherited Disease, 8th ed. New York McGraw-Hill, 2001, pp 5085-5108.

39. Attard M, Jean G, Forestier L, et al: Severity of phenotype in cystinosis varies with mutations in the *CTNS* gene: Predicted effect on the model of cystinosin. Hum Mol Genet 8:2507-2514, 1999.

40. Gahl WA, Schneider JA, Thoene JG, et al: Course of nephropathic cystinosis after age 10 years. J Pediatr 109:605-608, 1986.

41. Fivush B, Green OC, Porter CC, et al: Pancreatic endocrine insufficiency in posttransplant cystinosis. Am J Dis Child 141:1087-1089, 1987.

42. Charnas LR, Luciano CA, Dalakas M, et al: Distal vacuolar myopathy in nephropathic cystinosis. Ann Neurol 35:181-188, 1994.

43. Wuhl E, Haffner D, Gretz N, et al: Treatment with recombinant human growth hormone in short children with nephropathic cystinosis: No evidence for increased deterioration rate of renal function. The European Study Group on Growth Hormone Treatment in Short Children with Nephropathic Cystinosis. Pediatr Res 43(4 pt 1):484-488, 1998.

44. Gahl WA, Reed GF, Thoene JG, et al: Cysteamine therapy for children with nephropathic cystinosis. N Engl J Med 316:971-977, 1987.

45. Markello TC, Bernardini IM, Gahl WA: Improved renal function in children with cystinosis treatment with cysteamine. N Engl J Med 328:1157-1162, 1993.

46. Bradbury JA, Danjoux JP, Voller J, et al: A randomised placebo-controlled trial of topical cysteamine therapy in patients with nephropathic cystinosis. Eye 5(pt 6):755-760, 1991.

47. Kashtan CE, McEnery PT, Tejani A, et al: Renal allograft survival according to primary diagnosis: A report of the North American Pediatric Renal Transplant Cooperative Study. Pediatr Nephrol 9:679-684, 1995.

48. Chou JY: The molecular basis of type 1 glycogen storage disease. Curr Mol Med, 1:25-44, 2001.

49. Lei KJ, Shelly LL, Pan CJ, et al: Mutations in the glucose-6-phosphatase gene that cause glycogen storage disease type 1a. Science 262:580-583, 1993.

50. Lei KJ, Pan CJ, Shelly LL, et al: Identification of mutations in the gene for glucose-6-phosphatase, the enzyme deficient in glycogen storage disease type 1a. J Clin Invest, 93:1994-1999, 1994.

51. Shieh JJ, Terzioglu M, Hiraiwa H, et al: The molecular basis of glycogen storage disease type1a: Structure and function analysis of mutations in glucose-6-phosphatase. J Biol Chem 277:5047-5053, 2002.

52. Marcolongo P, Barone V, Priori G, et al: Structure and mutation analysis of the glycogen storage disease type 1b gene. FEBS Lett 436:247-250, 1998.

53. Hiraiwa H, Pan CJ, Lin B, et al: Inactivation of the glucose-6-phosphate transporter causes glycogen storage disease type 1b. J Biol Chem 274:5532-5536, 1999.

54. Lin B, Hiraiwa H, Pan CJ, et al: Type-1c glycogen storage disease is not caused by mutations in the glucose-6-phosphate transporter gene. Hum Genet 105:515-517, 1999.

55. Pears JS, Jung RT, Hopwood D, et al: Glycogen storage disease diagnosed in adults. Q J Med 82:207-222, 1992.

56. Chen YT: Type I glycogen storage disease: Kidney involvement, pathogenesis and its treatment. Pediatr Nephrol 5:71-76, 1991.

57. Chen YT, Van Hove JL: Renal involvement in type I glycogen storage disease. Adv Nephrol Necker Hosp 24:357-365, 1995.

58. Reitsma-Bierens WC, Smit GP, Troelstra JA: Renal function and kidney size in glycogen storage disease type I. Pediatr Nephrol 6:236-238, 1992.

59. Restaino I, Kaplan BS, Stanley C, et al: Nephrolithiasis, hypocitraturia, and a distal renal tubular acidification defect in type 1 glycogen storage disease. J Pediatr 122:392-396, 1993.

60. Matsuo N, Tsuchiya Y, Cho H, et al: Proximal renal tubular acidosis in a child with type 1 glycogen storage disease. Acta Paediatr Scand 75:332-335, 1986.

61. Chen YT, Scheinman JI, Park HK, et al: Amelioration of proximal renal tubular dysfunction in type I glycogen storage disease with dietary therapy. N Engl J Med 323:590-593, 1990.

62. Verani R, Bernstein J: Renal glomerular and tubular abnormalities in glycogen storage disease type I. Arch Pathol Lab Med 112:271-274, 1988.

63. Greene HL, Slonim AE, O'Neill JA Jr, et al: Continuous nocturnal intragastric feeding for management of type 1 glycogen-storage disease. N Engl J Med 294:423-425, 1976.

64. Wolfsdorf JI, Crigler JF Jr: Cornstarch regimens for nocturnal treatment of young adults with type I glycogen storage disease. Am J Clin Nutr 65:1507-1511, 1997.

65. Wolfsdorf JI, Crigler JF Jr: Biochemical evidence for the requirement of continuous glucose therapy in young adults with type 1 glycogen storage disease. J Inherit Metab Dis 17:234-241, 1994.

66. Mitchell GA, Lambert M, Tanguay RM: Hepatorenal tyrosinemia. In Scriver CR, Beaudet AL, Sly WS, et al (eds): The Metabolic and Molecular Bases of Inherited Disease, 8th ed. New York, McGraw-Hill, 2001, pp 1785-1798.

67. Phaneuf D, Lambert M, Laframboise R, et al: Type 1 hereditary tyrosinemia. Evidence for molecular heterogeneity and identification of a causal mutation in a French Canadian patient. J Clin Invest 90:1185-1192, 1992.

68. Heyer E, Tremblay M: Variability of the genetic contribution of Quebec population founders associated to some deleterious genes. Am J Hum Genet 56:970-978, 1995.

69. St-Louis M, Tanguay RM: Mutations in the fumarylacetoacetate hydrolase gene causing hereditary tyrosinemia type I: Overview. Hum Mutat 9:291-299, 1997.

70. Timmers C, Grompe M: Six novel mutations in the fumarylacetoacetate hydrolase gene of patients with hereditary tyrosinemia type I. Hum Mutat 7:367-369, 1996.

71. Ploos van Amstel JK, Bergman AJ, van Beurden EA, et al: Hereditary tyrosinemia type1: Novel missense, nonsense and splice consensus mutations in the human fumarylacetoacetate hydrolase gene; variability of the genotype-phenotype relationship. Hum Genet 97:51-59, 1996.

72. Bergman AJ, van den Berg IE, Brink W, et al: Spectrum of mutations in the fumarylacetoacetate hydrolase gene of tyrosinemia type 1 patients in northwestern Europe and Mediterranean countries. Hum Mutat 12:19-26, 1998.

73. Kubo S, Sun M, Miyahara M, et al: Hepatocyte injury in tyrosinemia type 1 is induced by fumarylacetoacetate and is inhibited by caspase inhibitors. Proc Natl Acad Sci U S A, 95:9552-9557, 1998.

74. Weinberg AG, Mize CE, Worthen HG: The occurrence of hepatoma in the chronic form of hereditary tyrosinemia. J Pediatr 88:434-438, 1976.

75. Jorquera R, Tanguay RM: The mutagenicity of the tyrosine metabolite, fumarylacetoacetate, is enhanced by glutathione depletion. Biochem Biophys Res Commun 232:42-48, 1997.

76. Mitchell G, Larochelle J, Lambert M, et al: Neurologic crises in hereditary tyrosinemia. N Engl J Med 322:432-437, 1990.

77. Spencer PD, Medow MS, Moses LC, et al: Effects of succinylacetone on the uptake of sugars and amino acids by brush border vesicles. Kidney Int 34:671-677, 1988.

78. Roth KS, Carter BE, Higgins ES: Succinylacetone effects on renal tubular phosphate metabolism: A model for experimental renal Fanconi syndrome. Proc Soc Exp Biol Med 196:428-431, 1991.

79. Paradis K, Weber A, Seidman EG, et al: Liver transplantation for hereditary tyrosinemia: The Quebec experience. Am J Hum Genet 47:338-342, 1990.

80. Holme E, Lindstedt S: Diagnosis and management of tyrosinemia type I. Curr Opin Pediatr 7:726-732, 1995.

81. Laine J, Salo MK, Krogerus L, et al: The nephropathy of type I tyrosinemia after liver transplantation. Pediatr Res 37:640-645, 1995.

82. Holton JB, Walter JH, Tyfield LA: Galactosemia. In Scriver CR, Beaudet AL, Sly WS, Valle D, et al (eds): The Metabolic and Molecular Bases of Inherited Disease, 8th ed. New York, McGraw-Hill, 2001, pp, 1553-1587.

83. Chung MA: Galactosemia in infancy: Diagnosis, management, and prognosis. Pediatr Nurs 23:563-569, 1997.

84. Reichardt JK, Woo SL: Molecular basis of galactosemia: Mutations and polymorphisms in the gene encoding human galactose-1-phosphate uridylyltransferase [published erratum appears in Proc Natl Acad Sci U S A 88:7457, 1991]. Proc Natl Acad Sci U S A 88:2633-2637, 1991.

85. Holton JB. Galactosaemia: Pathogenesis and treatment. J Inherit Metab Dis 19:3-7, 1996.

86. Nussbaum RL, Suchy SF: The oculocerebrorenal syndrome of Lowe (Lowe syndrome). In Scriver CR, Beaudet AL, Sly WS, et al (eds): The Metabolic and Molecular Bases of Inherited Disease, 8th ed. New York, McGraw-Hill, 2001, pp 6257-6266.

87. Attree O, Olivos IM, Okabe I, et al: The Lowe's oculocerebrorenal syndrome gene encodes a protein highly homologous to inositol polyphosphate-5-phosphatase. Nature 358:239-242, 1992.

88. Lin T, Orrison BM, Leahey AM, et al: Spectrum of mutations in the OCRL1 gene in the Lowe oculocerebrorenal syndrome. Am J Hum Genet 60:1384-1388, 1997.

89. Zhang X, Jefferson AB, Auethavekiat V, et al: The protein deficient in Lowe syndrome is a phosphatidylinositol-4,5-bisphosphate 5-phosphatase. Proc Natl Acad Sci U S A 92:4853-4856, 1995.

90. Charnas LR, Bernardini I, Rader D, et al: Clinical and laboratory findings in the oculocerebrorenal syndrome of Lowe, with special reference to growth and renal function. N Engl J Med 324:1318-1325, 1991.

91. Culotta VC, Gitlin JD: Disorders of copper transport. In Scriver CR, Beaudet AL, Sly WS, et al (eds): The Metabolic and Molecular Bases of Inherited Disease, 8th ed. New York, McGraw-Hill, 2001, pp 3105-3126.

92. Bull PC, Thomas GR, Rommens JM, et al: The Wilson disease gene is a putative copper transporting P-type. ATPase similar to the Menkes gene [published erratum appears in Nat Genet: 214, 1994.] Nat Genet 5:327-337, 1993.

93. Petrukhin K, Fischer SG, Pirastu M, et al: Mapping, cloning and genetic characterization of the region containing the Wilson disease gene. Nat Genet 5:338-343, 1993.

94. Tanzi RE, Petrukhin K, Chernov I, et al: The Wilson disease gene is a copper transporting ATPase with homology to the Menkes disease gene. Nat Genet 5:344-350, 1993.

95. Yamaguchi Y, Heiny ME, Gitlin JD: Isolation and characterization of a human liver cDNA as a candidate gene for Wilson disease. Biochem Biophys Res Commun 197:271-277, 1993.

96. Lutsenko S, Cooper MJ: Localization of the Wilson's disease protein product to on mitochondria. Proc Natl Acad Sci U S A 95:6004-6009, 1998.

97. Sozeri E, Feist D, Ruder H, et al: Proteinuria and other renal functions in Wilson's disease. Pediatr Nephrol 11:307-311, 1997.

98. Wiebers DO, Wilson DM, McLeod RA, et al: Renal stones in Wilson's disease. Am J Med 67:249-254, 1979.

99. Azizi E, Eshel G, Aladjem M.: Hypercalciuria and nephrolithiasis as a presenting sign in Wilson disease [see comments]. Eur J Pediatr 148:548-549, 1989.

100. Itami N, Akutsu Y, Tochimaru H, et al: Hypercalciuria and nephrolithiasis in Wilson disease [letter; comment]. Eur J Pediatr 149:145, 1989.

101. Hoppe B, Neuhaus T, Superti-Furga A, et al: Hypercalciuria and nephrocalcinosis, a feature of Wilson's disease. Nephron 65:460-462, 1993.

102. Elsas LG, Hayslett JP, Spargo BH, et al: Wilson's disease with reversible renal tubular dysfunction. Correlation with proximal tubular ultrastructure. Ann Intern Med 75:427-433, 1971.

103. Scheinberg IH, Sternlieb I: Wilson's Disease. Philadelphia, WB Saunders, 1984.

104. Walshe JM: Copper chelation in patients with Wilson's disease. A comparison of penicillamine and triethylene tetramine dihydrochloride. Q J Med 42:441-452, 1973.

105. Brewer GJ, Johnson V, Dick RD, et al: Treatment of Wilson disease with ammonium tetrathiomolybdate. II. Initial therapy in 33 neurologically affected patients and follow-up with zinc therapy. Arch Neurol 53:1017-1025, 1996.

106. Bax RT, Hassler A, Luck W, et al: Cerebral manifestation of Wilson's disease successfully treated with liver transplantation. Neurology 51:863-865, 1998.

107. Steinmann B, Gitzelmann R, Van den Berghe G: Disorders of fructose metabolism. In Scriver CR, Beaudet AL, Sly WS, et al (eds): The Metabolic and Molecular Bases of Inherited Disease, 8th ed. New York, McGraw-Hill, 2001, pp 1489-1520.

108. Ali M, Rellos P, Cox TM: Hereditary fructose intolerance. J Med Genet 35:353-365, 1998.

109. James CL, Rellos P, Ali M, et al: Neonatal screening for hereditary fructose intolerance: Frequency of the most common mutant aldolase B allele (A149P) in the British population. J Med Genet 33:837-841, 1996.

110. Lu M, Holliday LS, Zhang L, et al: Interaction between aldolase and vacuolar H⁺- ATPase: Evidence for direct coupling of glycolysis to the ATP-hydrolyzing proton pump. J Biol Chem 276:30407-30413, 2001.

111. Part 8, Amino Acids. *In* Scriver C, Beaudet A, Sly W, et al (eds): The Metabolic and Molecular Bases of Inherited Disease, 8th ed. New York, McGraw Hill, 2001, pp 1667-2105.

112. Wilcken B, Smith A, Brown DA: Urine screening for aminoacidopathies: Is it beneficial? Results of a long-term follow-up of cases detected by screening one millon babies. J Pediatr 97:492-497, 1980.

113. Silbernagl S: The renal handling of amino acids and oligopeptides. Physiol Rev 68:911-1007, 1988.

114. Levy HL, Madigan PM, Shih VE: Massachusetts metabolic disorders screening program. I. Technics and results of urine screening. Pediatrics 49:825-836, 1972.

115. Crawhall JC, Purkiss P, Watts RW, et al: The excretion of amino acids by cystinuric patients and their relatives. Ann Hum Genet 33:149-169, 1969.

116. Turner B, Brown DA: Amino acid excretion in infancy and early childhood. A survey of 200,000 infants. Med J Aust 1:62-65, 1972.

117. Weinberger A, Sperling O, Rabinovitz M, et al: High frequency of cystinuria among Jews of Libyan origin. Hum Hered 24:568-572, 1974.

118. Chillaron J, Roca R, Valencia A, et al: Heteromeric amino acid transporters: Biochemistry, genetics, and physiology. Am J Physiol Renal Physiol 281:F995-F1018, 2001.

119. Dello Strologo LD, Pras E, Pontesilli C, et al: Comparison between *SLC3A1* and *SLC7A9* cystinuria patients and carriers: A need for a new classification. J Am Soc Nephrol 13:2547-2553, 2002.

120. Reig N, Chillaron J, Bartoccioni P, et al: The light subunit of system b(o,+) is fully functional in the absence of the heavy subunit. EMBO J 21:4906-4914, 2002.

121. Pras E, Arber N, Aksentijevich I, et al: Localization of a gene causing cystinuria to chromosome 2p. Nat Genet 6:415-419, 1994.

122. Chillaron J, Estevez R, Samarzija I, et al: An intracellular trafficking defect in type I cystinuria rBAT mutants M467T and M467K. J Biol Chem 272:9543-9549, 1997.

123. Feliubadalo L, Font M, Purroy J, et al: Non-type I cystinuria caused by mutations in *SLC7A9*, encoding a subunit (bo, +AT) of rBAT. International Cystinuria Consortium. Nat Genet 23:52-57, 1999.

124. Wollaston WH: On cystic oxide: A new species of urinary calculus. Trans R Soc London 100:223-230, 1810.

125. Berzelius JJ: Calculus urinaries. Traite Chem 7:424, 1833.

126. Garrod AE: Inborn errors of metabolism. Lancet 2:73, 142, 214, 1908.

127. Wells RG, Hediger MA: Cloning of a rat kidney cDNA that stimulates dibasic and neutral amino acid transport and has sequence similarity to glucosidases. Proc Natl Acad Sci U S A 89:5596-5600, 1992.

128. Bertran J, Magagnin S, Werner A, et al: Stimulation of system y(+)-like amino acid transport by the heavy chain of human 4F2 surface antigen in *Xenopus laevis* oocytes. Proc Natl Acad Sci U S A 89:5606-5610, 1992.

129. Lee WS, Wells RG, Sabbag RV, et al: Cloning and chromosomal localization of a human kidney cDNA involved in cystine, dibasic, and neutral amino acid transport. J Clin Invest 91:1959-1963, 1993.

130. von Udransky L, Baumann E: Über das Vorkommen von Diaminen, sogenannten Ptomainen, bei Cystinurie. Z Physiol Chem 13:562-594, 1889.

131. Asatoor AM, Lacey BW, London DR, et al: Amino acid metabolism in cystinuria. Clin Sci 23:285-304, 1962.

132. Milne MD, Asatoor AM, Edwards KDG, et al: The intestinal absorption defect in cystinuria. Gut 2:323-337, 1961.

133. Thier S, Fox M, Segal S, et al: Cystinuria: In vitro demonstration of an intestinal transport defect. Science 143:482-484, 1964.

134. Magagnin S, Bertran J, Werner A, et al: Poly(A) + RNA from rabbit intestinal mucosa induces b0, + and y⁺ amino acid transport activities in *Xenopus laevis* oocytes. J Biol Chem 267:15384-15390, 1992.

135. Hellier MD, Perrett D, Holdsworth CD: Dipeptide absorption in cystinuria. BMJ J 4:782-783, 1970.

136. Silk DB: Progress report. Peptide absorption in man. Gut 15:494-501, 1974.

137. Whelan DT, Scriver CR: Hyperdibasicaminoaciduria: An inherited disorder of amino acid transport. Pediatr Res 2:525-534, 1968.

138. Brodehl J, Gellissen K, Kowalewski S: Isolated cystinuria (without lysin-, ornithin- and argininuria) in a family with hypocalcemic tetany. Monatsschr Kinderheilkd 115:317-320, 1967.

139. Goodyer P, Saadi I, Ong P, et al: Cystinuria subtype and the risk of nephrolithiasis. Kidney Int 54:56-61, 1998.

140. Stein W: A chromatographic investigation of the amino acid constituents of normal urine. J Biol Chem 201:45, 1953.

141. Crawhall JC, Saunders EP, Thompson CJ: Heterozygotes for cystinuria. Ann Hum Genet 29:257-269, 1966.

142. Perez-Ruiz T, Martinez-Lozano C, Tomas V, et al: Spectrofluorimetric flow injection method for the individual and successive determination of L-cysteine and L-cystine in pharmaceutical and urine samples. Analyst 117:1025-1028, 1992.

143. Birwe H, Hesse A: High-performance liquid chromatographic determination of urinary cysteine and cystine. Clin Chim Acta 199:33-42, 1991.

144. Hambaeus L: Comparative studies of the value of two cyanide-nitroprusside methods in the diagnosis of cystinuria. Scand J Lab Clin Invest 15:657, 1963.

145. Barbey F, Joly D, Rieu P, et al: Medical treatment of cystinuria: Critical reappraisal of long-term results. J Urol 163:1419-1423, 2000.

146. Zinneman HH, Jones JE: Dietary methionine and its influence on cystine excretion in cystinuric patients. Metabolism 15:915-921, 1966.

147. Kolb FO, Earll JM, Harper HA: "Disappearance" of cystinuria in a patient treated with prolonged low methionine diet. Metabolism 16:378-381, 1967.

148. Jaeger P, Portmann L, Saunders A, et al: Anticystinuric effects of glutamine and of dietary sodium restriction. N Engl J Med 315:1120-1123, 1986.

149. Norman RW, Manette WA: Dietary restriction of sodium as a means of reducing urinary cystine. J Urol 143:1193-1195, 1990.

150. Peces R, Sanchez L, Gorostidi M, et al: Effects of variation in sodium intake on cystinuria. Nephron 57:421-423, 1991.

151. Dent CE, Senior B: Studies on the treatment of cystinuria. Br J Urol 27:317, 1955.

152. Crawhall JC, Scowen EF, Watts RWE: Effect of penicillamine on cystinuria. BMJ 1:585-590, 1963.

153. Howard-Lock HE, Lock CJ, Mewa A, et al: D-Penicillamine: Chemistry and clinical use in rheumatic disease. Semin Arthritis Rheum 15:261-281, 1986.

154. Jaffe IA: Adverse effects profile of sulfhydryl compounds in man. Am J Med 80:471-476, 1986.

155. Jaffe IA, Altmann K, Merryman P: The antipyridoxine effect of penicillamine in man. J Clin Invest 43:1869-1873, 1964.

156. Stephens AD: Cystinuria and its treatment: 25 years experience at St. Bartholomew's Hospital. J Inherit Metab Dis 12:197-209, 1989.

157. Combe C, Deforges-Lasseur C, Chehab Z, et al: Cystine lithiasis and its treatment with D-penicillamine. The experience in a nephrology service in a 23-year period. Apropos of 26 patients [in French]. Ann Urol (Paris) 27:79-83, 1993.

158. King JS Jr: Treatment of cystinuria with alpha-mercaptopropionylglycine: A preliminary report with some notes on column chromatography of mercaptans. Proc Soc Exp Biol Med 129:927-932, 1968.

159. Hautmann R, Terhorst B, Stuhlsatz HW, et al: Mercaptopropionylglycine: A progress in cystine stone therapy. J Urol 117:628-630, 1977.

160. Denneberg T, Jeppsson JO, Stenberg P: Alternative treatment of cystinuria with α-mercaptopropionylglycine, Thiola. Proc Eur Dial Transplant Assoc 20:427-433, 1983.

161. Lindell A, Denneberg T, Hellgren E, et al: Clinical course and cystine stone formation during tipronin treatment. Urol Res 23:111-117, 1995.

162. Pak CY, Fuller C, Sakhaee K, et al: Management of cystine nephrolithiasis with α-mercaptopropionylglycine. J Urol 136:1003-1008, 1986.

163. Martin X, Salas M, Labeeuw M, et al: Cystine stones: The impact of new treatment. Br J Urol 68:234-239, 1991.

164. Soble JJ, Streem SB: Contemporary management of cystinuric patients. Tech Urol 4:58-64, 1998.

165. Simell O: Lysinuric protein intolerance and other cationic aminoacidurias. *In* Scriver CR, Beaudet AL, Sly WS, et al (eds): The Metabolic and Molecular Bases of Inherited Disease, 8th ed. New York, McGraw-Hill, 2001, pp 4933-4956.

166. Parto K, Svedstrom E, Majurin ML, et al: Pulmonary manifestations in lysinuric protein intolerance. Chest 104:1176-1182, 1993.

167. Kato T, Mizutani N, Ban M: Hyperammonemia in lysinuric protein intolerance. Pediatrics 73:489-492, 1984.

168. Parto K, Kallajoki M, Aho H, et al: Pulmonary alveolar proteinosis and glomerulonephritis in lysinuric protein intolerance. Case reports and autopsy findings of four pediatric patients. Hum Pathol 25:400-407, 1994.

169. McManus DT, Moore R, Hill CM, et al: Necropsy findings in lysinuric protein intolerance. J Clin Pathol 49:345-347, 1996.

170. Carpenter TO, Levy HL, Holtrop ME, et al: Lysinuric protein intolerance presenting as childhood osteoporosis. Clinical and skeletal response to citrulline therapy. N Engl J Med 312:290-294, 1985.

171. Borsani G, Bassi MT, Sperandeo MP, et al: SLC7A7, encoding a putative permease-related protein, is mutated in patients with lysinuric protein intolerance. Nat Genet 21:297-301, 1999.

172. Torrents D, Mykkanen J, Pineda M, et al: Identification of SLC7A7, encoding y+LAT-1, as the lysinuric protein intolerance gene. Nat Genet 21:293-296, 1999.

173. Mykkanen J, Torrents D, Pineda M, et al: Functional analysis of novel mutations in y(+)LAT-1 amino acid transporter gene causing lysinuric protein intolerance (LPI). Hum Mol Genet 9:431-438, 2000.

174. Palacin M, Estévez P, Bertran J, et al: Molecular biology of mammalian plasma membrane amino acid transporters. Physiol Rev 78:969-1054, 1998.

175. Estevez R, Camps M, Rojas AM, et al: The amino acid transport system y+L/4F2hc is a heteromultimeric complex. FASEB J 12:1319-1329, 1998.

176. Smith DW, Scriver CR, Tenenhouse HS, et al: Lysinuric protein intolerance mutation is expressed in the plasma membrane of cultured skin fibroblasts. Proc Natl Acad Sci U S A 84:7711-7715, 1987.

177. Parenti G, Sebastio G, Strisciuglio P, et al: Lysinuric protein intolerance characterized by bone marrow abnormalities and severe clinical course. J Pediatr 126:246-251, 1995.

178. Yoshida Y, Machigashira K, Suehara M, et al: Immunological abnormality in patients with lysinuric protein intolerance. J Neurol Sci 134:178-182, 1995.

179. Rajantie J, Simell O, Perheentupa J: Oral administration of epsilon N-acetyllysine and homocitrulline in lysinuric protein intolerance. J Pediatr 102:388-390, 1983.

180. Rajantie J, Simell O, Perheentupa J: Oral administration of urea cycle intermediates in lysinuric protein intolerance: Effect on plasma and urinary arginine and ornithine. Metabolism 32:49-51, 1983.

181. Baron DN, Dent CE, Harris H, et al: Hereditary pellagra-like skin rash with temporary cerebellar ataxia. Constant renal amino-aciduria. And other bizarre biochemical features. Lancet 2:421-428, 1956.

182. Levy HL: Hartnup disorder. In Scriver C, Beaudet A, Sly W, et al (eds): The Metabolic and Molecular Bases of Inherited Disease, 8th ed. New York, McGraw-Hill, 2001, pp 4957-4969.

183. Levy HL: Genetic screening. Adv Hum Genet 4:104, 1973.

184. Wilcken B, Yu JS, Brown DA: Natural history of Hartnup disease. Arch Dis Child 52:38-40, 1977.

185. Scriver CR, Mahon B, Levy HL, et al: The Hartnup Phenotype: Mendelian transport disorder, multifactorial disease. Am J Hum Genet 40:401-412, 1987.

186. Leonard JV, Marrs TC, Addison JM, et al: Intestinal absorption of amino acids and peptides in Hartnup disorder. Pediatr Res 10:246-249, 1976.

187. Oakley A, Wallace J: Hartnup disease presenting in an adult. Clin Exp Dermatol 19:407-408, 1994.

188. Chesney R: Iminoglycinuria. In Scriver C, Beaudet A, Valle D, et al (eds): The Metabolic and Molecular Bases of Inherited Disease, 8th ed. New York, McGraw-Hill, 2001, pp 4971-4981.

189. Brodehl J, Gellissen K: Endogenous renal transport of free amino acids in infancy and childhood. Pediatrics 42:395, 1968.

190. Tenenhouse HS, Murer H: Disorders of renal tubular phosphate transport. J Am Soc Nephrol 14:240-247, 2003.

191. Walling MW: Intestinal Ca and phosphate transport: Differential responses to vitamin D3 metabolites. Am J Physiol 233:E488-494, 1977.

192. Birge SJ, Miller R: The role of phosphate in the action of vitamin D on the intestine. J Clin Invest 60:980-988, 1977.

193. Finch JL, Brown AJ, Kubodera N, et al: Differential effects of 1,25-(OH)2D3 and 22-oxacalcitriol on phosphate and calcium metabolism. Kidney Int 43:561-566, 1993.

194. Portale AA, Halloran BP, Morris RC Jr: Physiologic regulation of the serum concentration of 1,25-dihydroxyvitamin D by phosphorus in normal men. J Clin Invest 83:1494-1499, 1989.

195. Portale AA, Halloran BP, Murphy MM, et al: Oral intake of phosphorus can determine the serum concentration of 1,25-dihydroxyvitamin D by determining its production rate in humans. J Clin Invest 77:7-12, 1986.

196. Gmaj P, Murer H: Cellular mechanisms of inorganic phosphate transport in kidney. Physiol Rev 66:36-70, 1986.

197. Murer H, Forster I, Hilfiker H, et al: Cellular/molecular control of renal Na/Pi-cotransport. Kidney Int Suppl 65:S2-10, 1998.

198. Gray RW, Wilz DR, Caldas AE, et al: The importance of phosphate in regulating plasma 1,25-(OH)2 vitamin D levels in humans: Studies in healthy subjects in calcium-stone formers and in patients with primary hyperparathyroidism. J Clin Endocrinol Metab 45:299-306, 1977.

199. Maierhofer WJ, Gray RW, Lemann J Jr: Phosphate deprivation increases serum 1,25-(OH)2 vitamin D concentrations in healthy men. Kidney Int 25:571-575, 1984.

200. Takeyama K, Kitanaka S, Sato T, et al: 25-Hydroxyvitamin D3 1α-hydroxylase and vitamin D synthesis. Science 277:1827-1830, 1997.

201. Carpenter TO, Shiratori T: Renal 25-hydroxyvitamin D-1 α-hydroxylase activity and mitochondrial phosphate transport in Hyp mice. Am J Physiol 259(6 pt 1):E814-821, 1990.

202. Consortium TH: A gene (PEX) with homologies to endopeptidases is mutated in patients with X-linked hypophosphatemic rickets. The HYP Consortium. Nat Genet 11:130-136, 1995.

203. Lipman ML, Panda D, Bennett HPJ, et al: Cloning of human PEX cDNA. Expression, subcellular localization, and endopeptidase activity. J Biol Chem 273:13729-13737, 1998.

204. Guo R, Quarles LD: Cloning and sequencing of human PEX from a bone cDNA library: Evidence for its developmental stage-specific regulation in osteoblasts. J Bone Miner Res 12:1009-1017, 1997.

205. Ruchon AF, Marcinkiewicz M, Siegfried G, et al: Pex mRNA is localized in developing mouse osteoblasts and odontoblasts. J Histochem Cytochem 46:459-468, 1998.

206. Holm IA, Huang X, Kunkel LM: Mutational analysis of the PEX gene in patients with X-linked hypophosphatemic rickets. Am J Hum Genet 60:790-797, 1997.

207. Rowe PS, Oudet CL, Francis F, et al: Distribution of mutations in the PEX gene in families with X-linked hypophosphataemic rickets (HYP). Hum Mol Genet 6:539-549, 1997.

208. Beck L, Soumounou Y, Martel J, et al: Pex/PEX tissue distribution and evidence for a deletion in the 3′ region of the Pex gene in X-linked hypophosphatemic mice. J Clin Invest 99:1200-1209, 1997.

209. Meyer RA, Jr., Meyer MH, Gray RW: Parabiosis suggests a humoral factor is involved in X-linked hypophosphatemia in mice. J Bone Miner Res 4:493-500, 1989.

210. Nesbitt T, Coffman TM, Griffiths R, et al: Crosstransplantation of kidneys in normal and Hyp mice. Evidence that the Hyp mouse phenotype is unrelated to an intrinsic renal defect. J Clin Invest 89:1453-1459, 1992.

211. Boneh A, Tenenhouse HS: Protein kinase C in mouse kidney: Subcellular distribution and endogenous substrates. Biochem Cell Biol 66:262-272, 1988.

212. Boneh A, Tenenhouse HS: Protein kinase C in mouse kidney: Effect of the Hyp mutation and phosphate deprivation. Kidney Int 37:682-688, 1990.

213. Tenenhouse HS, Henry HL: Protein kinase activity and protein kinase inhibitor in mouse kidney: Effect of the X-linked Hyp mutation and vitamin D status. Endocrinology 117:1719-1726, 1985.

214. Boneh A, Mandla S, Tenenhouse HS: Phorbol myristate acetate activates protein kinase C, stimulates the phosphorylation of endogenous proteins and inhibits phosphate transport in mouse renal tubules. Biochim Biophys Acta 1012:308-316, 1989.

215. Henry HL: Influence of a tumor promoting phorbol ester on the metabolism of 25-hydroxyvitamin D3. Biochem Biophys Res Commun 139:495-500, 1986.

216. Tenenhouse H, Econs M: Mendelian hypophosphatemias. In Scriver C, Beaudet A, Sly W, et al: The Metabolic and Molecular Bases of Inherited Disease, 8th ed. New York, McGraw-Hill, 2001, pp 5039-5083.

217. Scriver CR, Reade TM, DeLuca HF, et al: Serum 1,25-dihydroxyvitamin D levels in normal subjects and in patients with hereditary rickets or bone diasease. N Engl J Med 299:976-979, 1978.

218. Lyles KW, Clark AG, Drezner MK: Serum 1,25-dihydroxyvitamin D levels in subjects with X-linked hypophosphatemic rickets and osteomalacia. Calcif Tissue Int 34:125-130, 1982.

219. Orstavik KH, Orstavik RE, Halse J, et al: X chromosome inactivation pattern in female carriers of X linked hypophosphataemic rickets. J Med Genet 33:700-703, 1996.

220. Whyte MP, Schranck FW, Armamento-Villareal R: X-linked hypophosphatemia: A search for gender, race, anticipation, or parent

of origin effects on disease expression in children. J Clin Endocrinol Metab 81:4075-4080, 1996.

221. Berndt M, Ehrich JH, Lazovic D, et al: Clinical course of hypophosphatemic rickets in 23 adults. Clin Nephrol 45:33-41, 1996.

222. Tieder M, Modai D, Samuel R, et al: Hereditary hypophosphatemic rickets with hypercalciuria. N Engl J Med 312:611-617, 1985.

223. Tieder M, Modai D, Shaked U, et al: "Idiopathic" hypercalciuria and hereditary hypophosphatemic rickets. Two phenotypical expressions of a common genetic defect. N Engl J Med 316:125-129, 1987.

224. Kitanaka S, Takeyama K, Murayama A, et al: Inactivating mutations in the 25-hydroxyvitamin D_3 1α-hydroxylase gene in patients with pseudovitamin D–deficiency rickets. N Engl J Med 338:653-661, 1998.

225. Fu GK, Lin D, Zhang MY, et al: Cloning of human 25-hydroxyvitamin D-1α-hydroxylase and mutations causing vitamin D–dependent rickets type 1. Mol Endocrinol 11:1961-1970, 1997.

226. Monkawa T, Yoshida T, Wakino S, et al: Molecular cloning of cDNA and genomic DNA for human 25-hydroxyvitamin D_3 1α-hydroxylase. Biochem Biophys Res Commun 239:527-533, 1997.

227. Fu GK, Portale AA, Miller WL: Complete structure of the human gene for the vitamin D 1α-hydroxylase, P450c1α. DNA Cell Biol 16:1499-1507, 1997.

228. Liberman UA, Marx SJ: Vitamin D and other calciferols. *In* Scriver CR, Beaudet AL, Sly WS, et al: The Metabolic and Molecular Bases of Inherited Disease, 8th ed. New York, McGraw-Hill, 2001, pp 4223-4240.

229. Wiese RJ, Goto H, Prahl JM, et al: Vitamin D–dependency rickets type II. Truncated vitamin D receptor in three kindreds. Mol Cell Endocrinol 90:197-201, 1993.

230. Cockerill FJ, Hawa NS, Yousaf N, et al: Mutations in the vitamin D receptor gene in three kindreds associated with hereditary vitamin D resistant rickets. J Clin Endocrinol Metab 82:3156-3160, 1997.

231. Elsas LJ, Longo N: Glucose transporters. Annu Rev Med 43:377-393, 1992.

232. Barfuss DW, Schafer JA: Differences in active and passive glucose transport along the proximal nephron. Am J Physiol 241:F322-332, 1981.

233. Turner RJ, Moran A: Heterogeneity of sodium-dependent D-glucose transport sites along the proximal tubule: Evidence from vesicle studies. Am J Physiol 242:F406-414, 1982.

234. Wells RG, Pajor AM, Kanai Y, et al: Cloning of a human kidney cDNA with similarity to the sodium-glucose cotransporter. Am J Physiol 263(3 pt 2):F459-465, 1992.

235. Kanai Y, Lee WS, You G, et al: The human kidney low affinity Na$^+$ glucose cotransporter SGLT2. Delineation of the major renal reabsorptive mechanism for D-glucose. J Clin Invest 93:397-404, 1994.

236. You G, Lee WS, Barros EJ, et al: Molecular characteristics of Na(+)-coupled glucose transporters in adult and embryonic rat kidney. J Biol Chem 270:29365-29371, 1995.

237. Turk E, Wright EM: Membrane topology motifs in the SGLT cotransporter family. J Membr Biol 159:1-20, 1997.

238. Loo DD, Zeuthen T, Chandy G, et al: Cotransport of water by the Na$^+$ glucose cotransporter. Proc Natl Acad Sci U S A 93:13367-13370, 1996.

239. Mueckler M: Facilitative glucose transporters. Eur J Biochem 219:713-725, 1994.

240. Dominguez JH, Camp K, Maianu L, et al: Glucose transporters of rat proximal tubule: Differential expression and subcellular distribution. Am J Physiol 262(5 pt 2):F807-812, 1992.

241. Shannon J, Fisher S: The renal tubular reabsorption of glucose in the normal dog. Am J Physiol 122:765-774, 1938.

242. Smith H, Goldring W, Chasis H, et al: The application of saturation methods to the study of glomerular and tubular function in the human kidney. Mt Sinai J Med 10:59-108, 1943.

243. Ruhnau B, Faber OK, Borch-Johnsen K, et al: Renal threshold for glucose in non-insulin-dependent diabetic patients. Diabetes Res Clin Pract 36:27-33, 1997.

244. Brodehl J, Oemar BS, Hoyer PF: Renal glucosuria. Pediatr Nephrol 1:502-508, 1987.

245. Sankarasubbaiyan S, Cooper C, Heilig CW: Identification of a novel form of renal glucosuria with overexcretion of arginine, carnosine, and taurine. Am J Kidney Dis 37:1039-1043, 2001.

246. Marble A: Non-diabetic mellituria. *In* Joslin E, Root H, White P, Marble A (eds): The Treatment of Diabetes Mellitus. Philadelphia, Lea & Febiger, 1959.

247. Wright EM, Martin MG, Turk E: Familial glucose-galactose malabsorption and hereditary renal glycosuria. *In* Scriver CR, Beaudet AL, Sly WS, et al (eds): The Metabolic and Molecular Bases of Inherited Disease, 8th ed. New York, McGraw-Hill, 2001, pp 4891-4908.

248. Oemar BS, Byrd DJ, Brodehl J: Complete absence of tubular glucose reabsorption: A new type of renal glucosuria (type O). Clin Nephrol 27:156-160, 1987.

249. Bagga A, Shankar V, Moudgil A, et al: Type O renal glucosuria. Acta Paediatr Scand 80:116-119, 1991.

250. Hjarne VA: Study of orthoglycaemic glycosuria with particular reference to its heritability. Acta Med Scand 67:422, 1937.

251. De Marchi S, Cecchin E, Basile A, et al: Close genetic linkage between HLA and renal glycosuria. Am J Nephrol 4:280-286, 1984.

252. Elsas LJ, Busse D, Rosenberg LE: Autosomal recessive inheritance of renal glycosuria. Metabolism 20:968-975, 1971.

253. Sakamoto O, Ogawa E, Ohura T, et al: Mutation analysis of the *GLUT2* gene in patients with Fanconi-Bickel syndrome. Pediatr Res 48:586-589, 2000.

254. Santer R, Schneppenheim R, Dombrowski A, et al: Mutations in *GLUT2*, the gene for the liver-type glucose transporter, in patients with Fanconi-Bickel syndrome. Nat Genet 17:324-326, 1997.

255. van den Heuvel LP, Assink K, Willemsen M, et al: Autosomal recessive renal glucosuria attributable to a mutation in the sodium glucose cotransporter (SGLT2). Hum Genet 111:544-547, 2002.

256. Muhlbauer RC, Fleisch H: Abnormal renal glucose handling in X-linked hypophosphataemic mice. Clin Sci (Colch) 80:71-76, 1991.

257. Laplane R, Polonovski C, Etienne M, et al: L'intolérance aux sucres a transfert intestinal actif. Arch Fr Pediatr 19:895, 1962.

258. Lindquist B, Meeuwisse GW: Chronic diarrhea caused by monosaccharide malabsorption. Acta Pediatr 51:674, 1962.

259. Martin MG, Turk E, Lostao MP, et al: Defects in Na$^+$ glucose cotransporter (SGLT1) trafficking and function cause glucose-galactose malabsorption. Nat Genet 12:216-220, 1996.

260. Turk E, Klisak I, Bacallao R, et al: Assignment of the human Na$^+$/glucose cotransporter gene SGLT1 to chromosome 22q13.1. Genomics 17:752-754, 1993.

261. Turk E, Zabel B, Mundlos S, et al: Glucose/galacose malabsorption caused by a defect in the Na$^+$/glucose cotransporter. Nature 350:354-356, 1991.

262. Wright EM, Turk E, Zabel B, et al: Molecular genetics of intestinal glucose transport. J Clin Invest 88:1435-1440, 1991.

263. DuBose T, Alpern R: Renal tubular acidosis. *In* Scriver C, Beaudet A, Sly W, et al (eds): The Metabolic and Molecular Bases of Inherited Disease, 8th ed. New York, McGraw Hill, 2001, 4983-5021.

264. Alper SL: Genetic diseases of acid-base transporters. Annu Rev Physiol 64:899-923, 2002.

265. Boron WF, Fong P, Hediger MA, et al: The electrogenic Na/HCO$_3$ cotransporter. Wien Klin Wochenschr 109:445-456, 1997.

266. Igarashi T, Inatomi J, Sekine T, et al: Mutations in *SLC4A4* cause permanent isolated proximal renal tubular acidosis with ocular abnormalities. Nat Genet 23:264-266, 1999.

267. Usui T, Hara M, Satoh H, et al: Molecular basis of ocular abnormalities associated with proximal renal tubular acidosis. J Clin Invest 108:107-115, 2001.

268. Sly WS, Hewett-Emmett D, Whyte MP, et al: Carbonic anhydrase II deficiency identified as the primary defect in the autosomal recessive syndrome of osteopetrosis with renal tubular acidosis and cerebral calcification. Proc Natl Acad Sci U S A 80:2752-2756, 1983.

269. Sly WS, Whyte MP, Sundaram V, et al: Carbonic anhydrase II deficiency in 12 families with the autosomal recessive syndrome of osteopetrosis with renal tubular acidosis and cerebral calcification. N Engl J Med 313:139-145, 1985.

270. Roth DE, Venta PJ, Tashian RE, et al: Molecular basis of human carbonic anhydrase II deficiency. Proc Natl Acad Sci U S A 89:1804-1808, 1992.

271. Whyte MP: Carbonic anhydrase II deficiency. Clin Orthop 294:52-63, 1993.

272. Hu PY, Ernst AR, Sly WS, et al: Carbonic anhydrase II deficiency: Single-base deletion in exon-7 is the predominant mutation in Caribbean Hispanic patients. Am J Hum Genet 54:602-608, 1994.

273. Bregman H, Brown J, Rogers A, et al: Osteopetrosis with combined proximal and distal renal tubular acidosis. Am J Kidney Dis 2:357-362, 1982.

274. Ismail EA, Abul Saad S, Sabry MA: Nephrocalcinosis and urolithiasis in carbonic anhydrase II deficiency syndrome. Eur J Pediatr 156:957-962, 1997.

275. Lai LW, Chan DM, Erickson RP, et al: Correction of renal tubular acidosis in carbonic anhydrase II–deficient mice with gene therapy. J Clin Invest 101:1320-1325, 1998.

276. Karet FE: Inherited distal renal tubular acidosis. J Am Soc Nephrol 13:2178-2184, 2002.

277. Bruce LJ, Cope DL, Jones GK, et al: Familial distal renal tubular acidosis is associated with mutations in the red cell anion exchange (band 3, *AE1*) gene. J Clin Invest 100:1693-1707, 1997.

278. Jarolim P, Shayakul C, Prabakaran D, et al: Autosomal dominant distal renal tubular acidosis is associated in three families with heterozygosity for the R589H mutation in the AE1 (band 3) Cl$^-$/HCO$_3^-$ exchanger. J Biol Chem 273:6380-6388, 1998.

279. Karet FE, Gainza FJ, Györy AZ, et al: Mutations in the chloride-bicarbonate exchanger gene *AE1* cause autosomal dominant but not autosomal recessive distal renal tubular acidosis. Proc Natl Acad Sci U S A 95:6337-6342, 1998.

280. Devonald MA, Smith AN, Poon JP, et al: Non-polarized targeting of AE1 causes autosomal dominant distal renal tubular acidosis. Nat Genet 33:125-127, 2003.

281. Tanphaichitr VS, Sumboonnanonda A, Ideguchi H, et al: Novel *AE1* mutations in recessive distal renal tubular acidosis loss-of-function is rescued by glycophorin A. J Clin Invest 102:2173-2179, 1998.

282. Karet FE, Finberg KE, Nelson RD, et al: Mutations in the gene encoding B1 subunit of H$^+$-ATPase cause renal tubular acidosis with sensorineural deafness. Nat Genet 21:84-90, 1990.

283. Stover EH, Borthwick KJ, Bavalia C, et al: Novel *ATP6V1B1* and *ATP6V0A4* mutations in autosomal recessive distal renal tubular acidosis with new evidence for hearing loss. J Med Genet 39:796-803, 2002.

284. Smith AN, Skaug J, Choate KA, et al: Mutations in *ATP6N1B*, encoding a new kidney vacuolar proton pump 116-kD subunit, cause recessive distal renal tubular acidosis with preserved hearing. Nat Genet 26:71-75, 2000.

285. Karet FE, Finberg KE, Nayir A, et al: Localization of a gene for autosomal recessive distal renal tubular acidosis with normal hearing (rdRTA2) to 7q33-34. Am J Hum Genet 65:1656-1665, 1999.

286. Bartter FC, Pronove P, Gill JRJ, et al: Hyperplasia of the juxtaglomerular complex with hyperaldosteronism and hypokalemic alkalosis. A new syndrome. Am J Med 33:811-828, 1962.

287. Guay-Woodford LM: Bartter syndrome: Unraveling the pathophysiologic enigma. Am J Med 105:151-161, 1998.

288. Kurtz I: Molecular pathogenesis of Bartter's and Gitelman's syndromes [clinical conference]. Kidney Int 54:1396-1410, 1998.

289. Fanconi A, Schachenmann G, Nussli R, et al: Chronic hypokalaemia with growth retardation, normotensive hyperrenin-hyperaldosteronism ("Bartter's syndrome"), and hypercalciuria. Report of two cases with emphasis on natural history and on catch-up growth during treatment. Helv Paediatr Acta 26:144-163, 1971.

290. McCredie DA, Rotenberg E, Williams AL: Hypercalciuria in potassium-losing nephropathy: A variant of Bartter's syndrome. Aust Paediatr J 10:286-295, 1974.

291. Ohlsson A, Sieck U, Cumming W, et al: A variant of Bartter's syndrome. Bartter's syndrome associated with hydramnios, prematurity, hypercalciuria and nephrocalcinosis. Acta Paediatr Scand 73:868-874, 1984.

292. Simon D, Nelson-Williams C, Johnson Bia M, et al: Gitelman's variant of Bartter's syndrome, inherited hypokalemic alkalosis, is caused by mutations in the thiazide-sensitive Na-Cl cotransporter. Nat Genet 12:24-30, 1996.

293. Bettinelli A, Bianchetti MG, Girardin E, et al: Use of calcium excretion values to distinguish two forms of primary renal tubular hypokalemic alkalosis: Bartter and Gitelman syndromes. J Pediatr 120:38-43, 1992.

294. Simon D, Karet F, Hamdan J, et al: Bartter's syndrome, hypokalemic alkalosis with hypercalciuria, is caused by mutations in the Na-K-Cl cotransporter NKCC2. Nat Genet 13:183-188, 1996.

295. Simon DB, Karet FE, Rodriguez-Soriano J, et al: Genetic heterogeneity of Bartter's syndrome revealed by mutations in the K$^+$ channel, ROMK. Nat Genet 14:152-156, 1996.

296. Simon DB, Bindra RS, Mansfield TA, et al: Mutations in the chloride channel gene, CLCNKB, cause Bartter's syndrome type III. Nat Genet 17:171-178, 1997.

297. Birkenhager R, Otto E, Schurmann MJ, et al: Mutation of BSND causes Bartter syndrome with sensorineural deafness and kidney failure. Nat Genet 29:310-314, 2001.

298. Sieck UV, Ohlsson A: Fetal polyuria and hydramnios associated with Bartter's syndrome. Obstet Gynecol 63(suppl 3):22S-24S, 1984.

299. Peters M, Jeck N, Reinalter S, et al: Clinical presentation of genetically defined patients with hypokalemic salt-losing tubulopathies. Am J Med 112:183-190, 2002.

300. Simon DB, Cruz DN, Hamdan J, et al: A unique phenotype in type II Bartter's syndrome reveals a K$^+$ secretory defect [abstract]. J Am Soc Nephrol 9:111a, 1998.

301. Estevez R, Boettger T, Stein V, et al: Barttin is a Cl$^-$ channel β-subunit crucial for renal Cl$^-$ reabsorption and inner ear K$^+$ secretion. Nature 414:558-561, 2001.

302. Jeck N, Reinalter SC, Henne T, et al: Hypokalemic salt-losing tubulopathy with chronic renal failure and sensorineural deafness. Pediatrics 108:E5, 2001.

303. Verberckmoes R, van Damme BB, Clement J, et al: Bartter's syndrome with hyperplasia of renomedullary cells: Successful treatment with indomethacin. Kidney Int 9:302-307, 1976.

304. Winterborn MH, Hewitt GJ, Mitchell MD: The role of prostaglandins in Bartter's syndrome. Int J Pediatr Nephrol 5:31-38, 1984.

305. Scherling B, Verder H, Nielsen MD, et al: Captopril treatment in Bartter's syndrome. Scand J Urol Nephrol 24:123-125, 1990.

306. Tsunoda S, Tsushima T, Nishioka T, et al: Familial Bartter's syndrome and the effect of indomethacin in one family member. J Urol 127:1000-1005, 1982.

307. Proesmans W, Massa G, Vanderschueren-Lodeweyckx M: Growth from birth to adulthood in a patient with the neonatal form of Bartter syndrome. Pediatr Nephrol 2:205-209, 1988.

308. Mackie FE, Hodson EM, Roy LP, et al: Neonatal Bartter syndrome—use of indomethacin in the newborn period and prevention of growth failure. Pediatr Nephrol 10:756-758, 1996.

309. Gitelman HJ, Graham JB, Welt LG: A new familial disorder characterized by hypokalemia and hypomagnesemia. Trans Assoc Am Physicians 79:221-235, 1966.

310. Lemmink HH, Knoers NV, Karolyi L, et al: Novel mutations in the thiazide-sensitive NaCl cotransporter gene in patients with Gitelman syndrome with predominant localization to the C-terminal domain. Kidney Int 54:720-730, 1998.

311. Schultheis PJ, Lorenz JN, Meneton P, et al: Phenotype resembling Gitelman's syndrome in mice lacking the apical Na$^+$-Cl$^-$ cotransporter of the distal convoluted tubule. J Biol Chem 273:29150-29155, 1998.

312. White KE, Gesek FA, Reilly RF, et al: NCX1 Na/Ca exchanger inhibition by antisense oligonucleotides in mouse distal convoluted tubule cells. Kidney Int 54:897-906, 1998.

313. Gesek FA, Friedman PA: Mechanism of calcium transport stimulated by chlorothiazide in mouse distal convoluted tubule cells. J Clin Invest 90:429-438, 1992.

314. Barry EL, Gesek FA, Yu ASL, et al: Distinct calcium channel isoforms mediate parathyroid hormone and chlorothiazide-stimulated calcium entry in transporting epithelial cells. J Membr Biol 161:55-64, 1998.

315. Bauer FM, Glasson P, Vallotton MB, et al: Bartter's syndrome, chondrocalcinosis and hypomagnesemia [in German]. Schweiz Med Wochenschr 109:1251-1256, 1979.

316. Smilde TJ, Haverman JF, Schipper P, et al: Familial hypokalemia/hypomagnesemia and chondrocalcinosis. J Rheumatol 21:1515-1519, 1994.

317. Luthy C, Bettinelli A, Iselin S, et al: Normal prostaglandinuria E$_2$ in Gitelman's syndrome, the hypocalciuric variant of Bartter's syndrome. Am J Kidney Dis 25:824-828, 1995.

318. Colussi G, Rombola G, De Ferrari ME, et al: Correction of hypokalemia with antialdosterone therapy in Gitelman's syndrome. Am J Nephrol 14:127-135, 1994.

319. Lifton RP: Genetic determinants of human hypertension. Proc Natl Acad Sci U S A 92:8545-8551, 1995.

320. Gharavi A, Lifton RP: The inherited basis of blood pressure variation and hypertension. *In* Scriver C, Beaudet A, Sly W, et al (eds): The Metabolic and Molecular Bases of Inherited Disease, 8th ed. New York, McGraw-Hill, 2001, pp 5399-5417.

321. Lifton RP, Gharavi AG, Geller DS: Molecular mechanisms of human hypertension. Cell 104:545-556, 2001.

322. Donohoue PA, Parker K, Migeon CJ: Congenital adrenal hyperplasia. *In* Scriver CR, Beaudet AL, Sly WS, et al (eds): The Metabolic and Molecular Bases of Inherited Disease, 8th ed. New York, McGraw-Hill, 2001, pp 4077-4115.

323. White PC: Inherited forms of mineralocorticoid hypertension. Hypertension 28:927-936, 1996.

324. Curnow KM, Slutsker L, Vitek J, et al: Mutations in the CYP11B1 gene causing congenital adrenal hyperplasia and hypertension cluster in exons 6,7, and 8. Proc Natl Acad Sci U S A 90:4552-4556, 1993.

325. New MI: Diagnosis and management of congenital adrenal hyperplasia. Annu Rev Med 49:311-328, 1998.

326. Wedell A: An update on the molecular genetics of congenital adrenal hyperplasia: Diagnostic and therapeutic aspects. J Pediatr Endocrinol Metab 11:581-589, 1998.

327. Kater CE, Biglieri EG: Disorders of steroid 17α-hydroxylase deficiency. Endocrinol Metab Clin North Am 23:341-357, 1994.

328. Biglieri EG, Kater CE: 17α-Hydroxylation deficiency. Endocrinol Metab Clin North Am 20:257-268, 1991.

329. Shimkets R, Warnock D, Bositis C, et al: Liddle's syndrome: Heritable human hypertension caused by mutations in the β subunit of the epithelial sodium channel. Cell 79:407-414, 1994.

330. Firsov D, Gautschi I, Merillat AM, et al: The heterotetrameric architecture of the epithelial sodium channel (ENaC). EMBO J 17:344-352, 1998.

331. Rotin D, Bar-Sagi D, O'Brodovich H, et al: An SH3 binding region in the epithelial Na$^+$ channel (alpha rENaC) mediates its localization at the apical membrane. EMBO J 13:4440-4450, 1994.

332. Staub O, Dho S, Henry P, et al: WW domains of Nedd4 bind to the proline-rich PY motifs in the epithelial Na$^+$ channel deleted in Liddle's syndrome. EMBO J 15:2371-2380, 1996.

333. Dinudom A, Harvey KF, Komwatana P, et al: Nedd4 mediates control of an epithelial Na$^+$ channel in salivary duct cells by cytosolic Na$^+$. Proc Natl Acad Sci U S A 95:7169-7173, 1998.

334. Snyder PM, Price MP, McDonald FJ, et al: Mechanism by which Liddle's syndrome mutations increase activity of a human epithelial Na$^+$ channel. Cell 83:969-978, 1995.

335. Firsov D, Schild L, Gautschi I, et al: Cell surface expression of the epithelial Na channel and a mutant causing Liddle syndrome: A quantitative approach. Proc Natl Acad Sci U S A 93:15370-15375, 1996.

336. Shimkets RA, Lifton RP, Canessa CM: The activity of the epithelial sodium channel is regulated by clathrin- mediated endocytosis. J Biol Chem 272:25537-25541, 1997.

337. Farman N, Boulkroun S, Courtois-Coutry N: Sgk: An old enzyme revisited. J Clin Invest 110:1233-1234, 2002.

338. Warnock DG: Liddle syndrome: An autosomal dominant form of human hypertension. Kidney Int 53:18-24, 1998.

339. Liddle G, Bledsoe T, Coppage W: A familial renal disorder simulating primary aldosteronism but with negligible aldosterone secretion. Trans Assoc Am Physicians 76:199-213, 1963.

340. White PC, Mune T, Rogerson FM, et al: Molecular analysis of 11β-hydroxysteroid dehydrogenase and its role in the syndrome of apparent mineralocorticoid excess. Steroids 62:83-88, 1997.

341. Cooper M, Stewart PM: The syndrome of apparent mineralocorticoid excess [editorial]. Q J Med 91:453-455, 1998.

342. White PC: 11β-Hydroxysteroid dehydrogenase and its role in the syndrome of apparent mineralocorticoid excess. Am J Med Sci 322:308-315, 2001.

343. Seckl JR, Chapman KE: Medical and physiological aspects of the 11β-hydroxysteroid dehydrogenase system. Eur J Biochem 249:361-364, 1997.

344. White PC, Mune T, Agarwal AK: 11β-Hydroxysteroid dehydrogenase and the syndrome of apparent mineralocorticoid excess. Endocr Rev 18:135-156, 1997.

345. Mune T, Rogerson FM, Nikkila H, et al: Human hypertension caused by mutations in the kidney isozyme of 11β-hydroxysteroid dehydrogenase. Nat Genet 10:394-399, 1995.

346. Wilson RC, Harbison MD, Krozowski ZS, et al: Several homozygous mutations in the gene for 11β-hydroxysteroid dehydrogenase type 2 in patients with apparent mineralocorticoid excess. J Clin Endocrinol Metab 80:3145-3150, 1995.

347. Stewart PM, Krozowski ZS, Gupta A, et al: Hypertension in the syndrome of apparent mineralocorticoid excess due to mutation of the 11β-hydroxysteroid dehydrogenase type 2 gene. Lancet 347:88-91, 1996.

348. Li A, Tedde R, Krozowski ZS, et al: Molecular basis for hypertension in the "type II variant" of apparent mineralocorticoid excess. Am J Hum Genet 63:370-379, 1998.

349. Stewart PM, Wallace AM, Valentino R, et al: Mineralocorticoid activity of liquorice: 11β-Hydroxysteroid dehydrogenase deficiency comes of age. Lancet 2:821-824, 1987.

350. Wilson RC, Dave-Sharma S, Wei JQ, et al: A genetic defect resulting in mild low-renin hypertension. Proc Natl Acad Sci U S A 95:10200-10205, 1998.

351. Dave-Sharma S, Wilson RC, Harbison MD, et al: Examination of genotype and phenotype relationships in 14 patients with apparent mineralocorticoid excess. J Clin Endocrinol Metab 83:2244-2254, 1998.

352. Geller DS, Farhi A, Pinkerton N, et al: Activating mineralocorticoid receptor mutation in hypertension exacerbated by pregnancy. Science 289:119-123, 2000.

353. Lifton R, Dluhy R, Powers M, et al: A chimaeric 11β-hydroxylase/aldosterone synthase gene causes glucocorticoid-remediable hyperaldosteronism and human hypertension. Nature 355:262-265, 1992.

354. White PC, Curnow KM, Pascoe L: Disorders of steroid 11β-hydroxylase isozymes. Endocr Rev 15:421-438, 1994.

355. Gates LJ, MacConnachie AA, Lifton RP, et al: Variation of phenotype in patients with glucocorticoid remediable aldosteronism. J Med Genet 33:25-28, 1996

356. Litchfield WR, Anderson BF, Weiss RJ, et al: Intracranial aneurysm and hemorrhagic stroke in glucocorticoid-remediable aldosteronism. Hypertension 31(1 pt 2):445-450, 1998.

357. Stowasser M, Huggard PR, Rossetti TR, et al: Biochemical evidence of aldosterone overproduction and abnormal regulation in normotensive individuals with familial hyperaldosteronism type I. J Clin Endocrinol Metab 84:4031-4036, 1999.

358. Litchfield WR, New MI, Coolidge C, et al: Evaluation of the dexamethasone suppression test for the diagnosis of glucocorticoid-remediable aldosteronism. J Clin Endocrinol Metab 82:3570-3573, 1997.

359. Fardella CE, Pinto M, Mosso L, et al: Genetic study of patients with dexamethasone-suppressible aldosteronism without the chimeric CYP11B1/CYP11B2 gene. J Clin Endocrinol Metab 86:4805-4807, 2001.

360. Lafferty AR, Torpy DJ, Stowasser M, et al: A novel genetic locus for low renin hypertension: Familial hyperaldosteronism type II maps to chromosome 7 (7p22). J Med Genet 37:831-835, 2000.

361. Hanukoglu A: Type I pseudohypoaldosteronism includes two clinically and genetically distinct entities with either renal or multiple target organ defects. J Clin Endocrinol Metab 73:936-944, 1991.

362. Bonny O, Rossier BC: Disturbances of Na/K balance: Pseudohypoaldosteronism revisited. J Am Soc Nephrol 13:2399-2414, 2002.

363. Chang SS, Grunder S, Hanukoglu A, et al: Mutations in subunits of the epithelial sodium channel cause salt wasting with hyperkalaemic acidosis, pseudohypoaldosteronism type 1. Nat Genet 12:248-253, 1996.

364. Strautnieks SS, Thompson RJ, Gardiner RM, et al: A novel splice-site mutation in the gamma subunit of the epithelial sodium channel gene in three pseudohypoaldosteronism type 1 families. Nat Genet 13:248-250, 1996.

365. Geller DS, Rodriguez-Soriano J, Vallo Boado A, et al: Mutations in the mineralocorticoid receptor gene cause autosomal dominant pseudohypoaldosteronism type I. Nat Genet 19:279-281, 1998.

366. Berger S, Bleich M, Schmid W, et al: Mineralocorticoid receptor knockout mice: Pathophysiology of Na$^+$ metabolism. Proc Natl Acad Sci U S A 95:9424-9429, 1998.

367. White PC: Abnormalities of aldosterone synthesis and action in children [see comments]. Curr Opin Pediatr 9:424-430, 1997.

368. Gordon R, Klemm S, Tunny T, et al: Gordon's syndrome: A sodium-volume–dependent form of hypertension with a genetic basis. *In* Laragh J, Brenner B (eds): Hypertension: Pathophysiology, Diagnosis, and Management, 2nd ed. New York, Raven Press, 1995, pp 2111-2123.

369. Achard JM, Disse-Nicodeme S, Fiquet-Kempf B, et al: Phenotypic and genetic heterogeneity of familial hyperkalaemic hypertension (Gordon syndrome). Clin Exp Pharmacol Physiol 28:1048-1052, 2001.

370. Schambelan M, Sebastian A, Rector FC Jr: Mineralocorticoid-resistant renal hyperkalemia without salt wasting (type II pseudohypoaldosteronism): Role of increased renal chloride reabsorption. Kidney Int 19:716-727, 1981.

371. Take C, Ikeda K, Kurasawa T, et al: Increased chloride reabsorption as an inherited renal tubular defect in familial type II pseudohypoaldosteronism. N Engl J Med 324:472-476, 1991.

372. Mansfield TA, Simon DB, Farfel Z, et al: Multilocus linkage of familial hyperkalaemia and hypertension, pseudohypoaldosteronism type II, to chromosomes 1q31-42 and 17p11-q21. Nat Genet 16:202-205, 1997.

373. Disse-Nicodeme S, Achard JM, Desitter I, et al: A new locus on chromosome 12p13.3 for pseudohypoaldosteronism type II, an autosomal dominant form of hypertension. Am J Hum Genet 67:302-310, 2000.

374. Wilson FH, Disse-Nicodeme S, Choate KA, et al: Human hypertension caused by mutations in WNK kinases. Science 293:1107-1112, 2001.

375. Wilson FH, Kahle KT, Sabath E, et al: Molecular pathogenesis of inherited hypertension with hyperkalemia. The Na-Cl cotransport is inhibited by wild-type but not mutant WNK4. Proc Natl Acad Sci U S A 100:680-684, 2003.

376. Choate KA, Kahle KT, Wilson FH, et al: WNK1, a kinase mutated in inherited hypertension with hyperkalemia, localizes to diverse Cl⁻-transporting epithelia. Proc natl Acad Sci U S A 100:663-668, 2003.

377. Gereda JE, Bonilla-Felix M, Kalil B, et al: Neonatal presentation of Gordon syndrome. J Pediatr 129:615-617, 1996.

378. Isenring P, Lebel M, Grose JH: Endocrine sodium and volume regulation in familial hyperkalemia with hypertension. Hypertension 19:371-377, 1992.

379. Cole DE, Quamme GA: Inherited disorders of renal magnesium handling. J Am Soc Nephrol 11:1937-1947, 2000.

380. Konrad M, Weber S: Recent advances in molecular genetics of hereditary magnesium-losing disorders. J Am Soc Nephrol 14:249-260, 2003.

381. Praga M, Vara J, Gonzalez-Parra E, et al: Familial hypomagnesemia with hypercalciuria and nephrocalcinosis. Kidney Int 47:1419-1425, 1995.

382. Simon DB, Lu Y, Choate KA, et al: Paracellin-1, a renal tight junction protein required for paracellular Mg²⁺ resorption [see comments]. Science 285:103-106, 1999.

383. Schlingmann KP, Weber S, Peters M, et al: Hypomagnesemia with secondary hypocalcemia is caused by mutations in TRPM6, a new member of the TRPM gene family. Nat Genet 31:166-170, 2002.

384. Walder RY, Landau D, Meyer P, et al: Mutation of TRPM6 causes familial hypomagnesemia with secondary hypocalcemia. Nat Genet 31:171-174, 2002.

385. Nadler MJ, Hermosura MC, Inabe K, et al: LTRPC7 is a Mg²⁺ ATP-regulated divalent cation channel required for cell viability. Nature 411:590-595, 2001.

386. Meij IC, Koenderink JB, van Bokhoven H, et al: Dominant isolated renal magnesium loss is caused by misrouting of the Na(+), K(+)-ATPase γ-subunit. Nat Genet 26:265-266, 2000.

387. Dai LJ, Friedman PA, Quamme GA: Cellular mechanisms of chlorothiazide and cellular potassium depletion on Mg²⁺ uptake in mouse distal convoluted tubule cells. Kidney Int 51:1008-1017, 1997.

388. Brown EM, Gamba G, Riccardi D, et al: Cloning and characterization of an extracellular Ca(2+)-sensing receptor from bovine parathyroid. Nature 366:575-580, 1993.

389. Sands JM: Molecular approaches to urea transporters. J Am Soc Nephrol 13:2795-2806, 2002.

390. Verkman AS, Mitra AK: Structure and function of aquaporin water channels. Am J Physiol Renal Physiol 278:F13-F28, 2000.

391. Borgnia M, Nielsen S, Engel A, et al: Cellular and molecular biology of the aquaporin water channels. Annu Rev Biochem 68:425-458, 1999.

392. Sansom MS, Law RJ: Membrane proteins: Aquaporins—channels without ions. Curr Biol 11:R71-73, 2001.

393. Kozono D, Yasui M, King LS, et al: Aquaporin water channels: Atomic structure molecular dynamics meet clinical medicine. J Clin Invest 109:1395-1399, 2002.

394. Agre P, Preston GM, Smith BL, et al: Aquaporin CHIP: The archetypal molecular water channel. Am J Physiol 34:F463-F476, 1993.

395. Murata K, Mitsuoka K, Hirai T, et al: Structural determinants of water permeation through aquaporin-1. Nature 407:599-605, 2000.

396. de Groot BL, Grubmüller H: Water permeation across biological membranes: Mechanism and dynamics of aquaporin-1 and GlpF. Science 294:2353-2357, 2001.

397. Shayakul C, Steel A, Hediger MA: Molecular cloning and characterization of the vasopressin-regulated urea transporter of rat kidney collecting ducts. J Clin Invest 98:2580-2587, 1996.

398. Yang B, Bankir L, Gillespie A, et al: Urea-selective concentrating defect in transgenic mice lacking urea transporter UT-B. J Biol Chem 277:10633-10637, 2002.

399. Kalatzis V, Antignac C: Cystinosis: From gene to disease. Nephrol Dial Transplant 17:1883-1886, 2002.

400. Oksche A, Rosenthal W: The molecular basis of nephrogenic diabetes insipidus. J Mol Med 76:326-337, 1998.

401. Nomura Y, Onigata K, Nagashima T, et al: Detection of skewed X-inactivation in two female carriers of vasopressin type 2 receptor gene mutation. J Clin Endocrinol Metab 82:3434-3437, 1997.

402. Arthus M-F, Lonergan M, Crumley MJ, et al: Report of 33 novel AVPR2 mutations and analysis of 117 families with X-linked nephrogenic diabetes insipidus. J Am Soc Nephrol 11:1044-1054, 2000.

403. Crawford JD, Bode HH: Disorders of the posterior pituitary in children. In Gardner LI (ed.): Endocrine and Genetic Diseases of Childhood and Adolescence, 2nd ed. Philadelphia, WB Saunders, 1975, pp 126-158.

404. Forssman H: On the mode of hereditary transmission in diabetes insipidus. Nord Med 16:3211-3213, 1942.

405. Waring AG, Kajdi L, Tappan V: Congenital defect of water metabolism. Am J Dis Child 69:323-325, 1945.

406. Williams RM, Henry C: Nephrogenic diabetes insipidus transmitted by females and appearing during infancy in males. Ann Intern Med 27:84-95, 1947.

407. Niaudet P, Dechaux M, Trivin C, et al: Nephrogenic diabetes insipidus: Clinical and pathophysiological aspects. Adv Nephrol Necker Hosp 13:247-260, 1984.

408. McIlraith CH: Notes on some cases of diabetes insipidus with marked family and hereditary tendencies. Lancet 2:767-768, 1892.

409. Reeves WB, Andreoli TE: Nephrogenic diabetes insipidus. In Scriver CR, Beaudet AL, Sly WS, et al (eds): The Metabolic Basis of Inherited Disease, 7th ed. New York, McGraw-Hill, 1995, pp 3045-3071.

410. Lacombe UL: De la polydipsie [thesis No. 99]. Paris: Imprimerie et Fonderie de Rignoux, 1841.

411. Weil A: Ueber die hereditäre Form des Diabetes insipidus. Virchows Arch 95:70-95, 1884.

412. Camerer JW: Eine Ergänzung des Weilschen Diabetes-insipidus-Stammbaumes. Archiv für Rassen und Gesellschaftshygiene Biologie 28:382-385, 1935.

413. Dölle W: Eine weitere Ergänzung des Weilschen Diabetes-insipidus-Stamm. Z Menschliche Vererbungs Konstitutionslehre 30:372-374, 1951.

414. Weil A: Ueber die hereditare form des diabetes insipidus. Dtsch Arch Klin Med 93:180-290, 1908.

415. Rittig R, Robertson GL, Siggaard C, et al: Identification of 13 new mutations in the vasopressin-neurophysin II gene in 17 kindreds with familial autosomal dominant neurohypophyseal diabetes insipidus. Am J Hum Genet 58:107-117, 1996.

416. Streitz JMJ, Streitz JM: Polyuric urinary tract dilatation with renal damage. J Urol 139:784-785, 1988.

417. Boyd SD, Raz S, Ehrlich RM: Diabetes insipidus and nonobstructive dilatation of urinary tract. Urology 16:266-269, 1980.

418. Gautier B, Thieblot P, Steg A: Mégauretère, mégavessie et diabète insipide familial. Semin Hop 57:60-61, 1981.

419. Bichet DG, Razi M, Arthus M-F, et al: Epinephrine and dDAVP administration in patients with congenital nephrogenic diabetes insipidus. Evidence for a pre-cyclic AMP V₂ receptor defective mechanism. Kidney Int 36:859-866, 1989.

420. Bichet DG, Hendy GN, Lonergan M, et al: X-linked nephrogenic diabetes insipidus: From the ship Hopewell to restriction fragment length polymorphism studies. Am J Hum Genet 51:1089-1102, 1992.

421. Kambouris M, Dlouhy SR, Trofatter JA, et al: Localization of the gene for X-linked nephrogenic diabetes insipidus to Xq28. Am J Med Genet 29:239-246, 1988.

422. Knoers N, van der Heyden H, van Oost BA, et al: Three-point linkage analysis using multiple DNA polymorphic markers in families with X-linked nephrogenic diabetes insipidus. Genomics 4:434-437, 1989.

423. van den Ouweland AM, Knoop MT, Knoers VV, et al: Colocalization of the gene for nephrogenic diabetes insipidus (DIR) and the vasopressin type 2 receptor gene (AVPR2) in the Xq28 region. Genomics 13:1350-1352, 1992.

424. Jans DA, van Oost BA, Ropers HH, et al: Derivatives of somatic cell hybrids which carry the human gene locus for nephrogenic diabetes insipidus (NDI) express functional vasopressin renal V₂-type receptors. J Biol Chem. 265:15379-15382, 1990.

425. Birnbaumer M, Seibold A, Gilbert S, et al: Molecular cloning of the receptor for human antidiuretic hormone. Nature 357:333-335, 1992.

426. Cannon JF: Diabetes insipidus clinical and experimental studies with consideration of relationships. Arch Intern Med 96:215-272, 1955.

427. Bichet DG, Arthus M-F, Lonergan M, et al: X-linked nephrogenic diabetes insipidus mutations in North America and the Hopewell hypothesis. J Clin Invest 92:1262-1268, 1993.

428. Bode HH, Crawford JD: Nephrogenic diabetes insipidus in North America: The Hopewell hypothesis. N Engl J Med 280:750-754, 1969.

429. Holtzman EJ, Kolakowski LF, O'Brien D, et al: A null mutation in the vasopressin V$_2$ receptor gene (*AVPR2*) associated with nephrogenic diabetes insipidus in the Hopewell kindred. Hum Mol Genet 2:1201-1204, 1993.

430. Bichet DG, Birnbaumer M, Lonergan M, et al: Nature and recurrence of *AVPR2* mutations in X-linked nephrogenic diabetes insipidus. Am J Hum Genet 55:278-286, 1994.

431. Vaithinathan R, Berson EL, Dryja TP: Further screening of the rhodopsin gene in patients with autosomal dominant retinitis pigmentosa. Genomics 21:461-463, 1994.

432. Ala Y, Morin D, Mouillac B, et al: Functional studies of twelve mutant V$_2$ vasopressin receptors related to nephrogenic diabetes insipidus: Molecular basis of a mild clinical phenotype. J Am Soc Nephrol 9:1861-1872, 1998.

433. Schöneberg T, Yun J, Wenkert D, et al: Functional rescue of mutant V$_2$ vasopressin receptors causing nephrogenic diabetes insipidus by a coexpressed receptor polypeptide. EMBO J 15:1283-1291, 1996.

434. Schöneberg T, Sandig V, Wess J, et al: Reconstitution of mutant V$_2$ vasopressin receptors by adenovirus-mediated gene transfer. J Clin Invest 100:1547-1556, 1997.

435. Morello JP, Salahpour A, Laperrière A, et al: Pharmacological chaperones rescue cell-surface expression and function of misfolded V$_2$ vasopressin receptor mutants. J Clin Invest 105:887-895, 2000.

436. Bichet DG, Bouvier M, Brouard R, et al: Decrease in urine volume and increase in urine osmolality after SR49059 administration in five adult male patients with X-linked nephrogenic diabetes insipidus [abstract]. J Am Soc Nephrol 13:40A, 2002.

437. Vargas-Poussou R, Forestier L, Dautzenberg MD, et al: Mutations in the vasopressin V$_2$ receptor and aquaporin-2 genes in 12 families with congenital nephrogenic diabetes insipidus. J Am Soc Nephrol 8:1855-1862, 1997.

438. Sadeghi H, Robertson GL, Bichet DG, et al: Biochemical basis of partial NDI phenotypes. Mol Endocrinol 11:1806-1813, 1997.

439. Deen PMT, Verdijk MAJ, Knoers NVAM, et al: Requirement of human renal water channel aquaporin-2 for vasopressin-dependent concentration of urine. Science 264:92-95, 1994.

440. van Lieburg AF, Verdijk MAJ, Knoers NVAM, et al: Patients with autosomal nephrogenic diabetes insipidus homozygous for mutations in the aquaporin 2 water-channel gene. Am J Hum Genet 55:648-652, 1994.

441. Hochberg Z, van Lieburg A, Even L, et al: Autosomal recessive nephrogenic diabetes insipidus caused by an aquaporin-2 mutation. J Clin Endocrinol Metab 82:686-689, 1997.

442. Mulders SB, Knoers NVAM, van Lieburg AF, et al: New mutations in the *AQP2* gene in nephrogenic diabetes insipidus resulting in functional but misrouted water channels. J Am Soc Nephrol 8:242-248, 1997.

443. Canfield MC, Tamarappoo BK, Moses AM, et al: Identification and characterization of aquaporin-2 water channel mutations causing nephrogenic diabetes insipidus with partial vasopressin response. Hum Mol Genet 6:1865-1871, 1997.

444. Mulders SM, Bichet DG, Rijss JPL, et al: An aquaporin-2 water channel mutant which causes autosomal dominant nephrogenic diabetes insipidus is retained in the Golgi complex. J Clin Invest 102:57-66, 1998.

445. Kuwahara M, Iwai K, Ooeda T, et al: Three families with autosomal dominant nephrogenic diabetes insipidus caused by aquaporin-2 mutations in the C-terminus. Am J Hum Genet 69:738-748, 2001.

446. Marr N, Bichet DG, Lonergan M, et al: Heteroligomerization of an aquaporin-2 mutant with wild-type aquaporin-2 and their misrouting to late endosomes/lysosomes explains dominant nephrogenic diabetes insipidus. Hum Mol Genet 11:779-789, 2002.

447. Kamsteeg E-J, Bichet DG, Konings IBM, et al: Misrouting of wild-type aquaporin-2 water channels to the basolateral membrane after heterotetramerization with *AQP2* mutant explains dominant nephrogenic diabetes insipidus. Submitted for publication.

448. Deen PMT, Croes H, van Aubel RAMH, et al: Water channels encoded by mutant aquaporin-2 genes in nephrogenic diabetes insipidus are impaired in their cellular routing. J Clin Invest 95:2291-2296, 1995.

449. Tamarappoo BK, Verkman AS: Defective aquaporin-2 trafficking in nephrogenic diabetes insipidus and correction by chemical chaperones. J Clin Invest 101:2257-2267, 1998.

450. Levin MH, Haggie PM, Vetrivel L, et al: Diffusion in the endoplasmic reticulum of an aquaporin-2 mutant causing human nephrogenic diabetes insipidus. J Biol Chem 276:21331-21336, 2001.

451. Marr N, Bichet DG, Hoefs S, et al: Cell-biologic and functional analyses of five new aquaporin-2 missense mutations that cause recessive nephrogenic diabetes insipidus. J Am Soc Nephrol 13:2267-2277, 2002.

452. Lin SH, Bichet DG, Sasaki S, et al: Two novel aquaporin-2 mutations responsible for congenital nephrogenic diabetes insipidus in Chinese families. J Clin Endocrinol Metab 87:2694-2700, 2002.

453. Waldegger S, Jeck N, Barth P, et al: Barttin increases surface expression and changes current properties of ClC-K channels. Pflugers Arch 444:411-418, 2002.

454. Oksche A, Dickson J, Schülein R, et al: Two novel mutations in the vasopressin V$_2$ receptor gene in patients with congenital nephrogenic diabetes insipidus. Biophys Biochem Res Com 205:552-557, 1994.

455. van Lieburg AF, Verdijk MAJ, Schoute F, et al: Clinical phenotype of nephrogenic diabetes insipidus in females heterozygous for a vasopressin type 2 receptor mutation. Hum Genet 96:70-78, 1995.

456. Milavetz JJ, Popovtzer MM: Angiotensin-converting enzyme inhibitors and glycosuria. Arch Intern Med 152:1081-1083, 1992.

457. George AL Jr, Bianchi L, Link EM, et al: From stones to bones: The biology of ClC chloride channels. Curr Biol 11:R620-628, 2001.

458. Chen WM, Deng HW: A general and accurate approach for computing the statistical power of the transmission disequilibrium test for complex disease genes. Genet Epidermiol 21:53-67, 2001

459. Pan C-J, Lei K-J, Chen H, et al: Ontogeny of the murine glucose-6-phosphatase system. Arch Biochem Biophys 358:17-24, 1998.

460. Portale AA, Miller WL: Hereditary rickets revealed. Kidney Int 54:1762-1764, 1998.

461. Wright EM: Genetic disorders of membrane transport. I. Glucose galactose malabsorption. Am J Physiol Gastrointest Liver Physiol 275:G879-G882, 1998.

462. Haycock GB: Isolated defects of tubular function. *In* Davison AM, Cameron JS, Grünfeld J-P, et al (eds): Oxford Textbook of Clinical Nephrology, 2nd ed. New York, Oxford University Press, 1998, pp 1039-1069.

463. Alper SL: The band 3-related AE anion exchanger gene family. Cell Physiol Biochem 4:265-281, 1994.

464. Abrahams JP, Leslie AGW, Lutter R, et al: Structure at 2.8 Å resolution F$_1$-ATPase from bovine heart mitochondria. Nature 370:621-628, 1994.

465. Rossier BC: *Cum Grano Salis*: The epithelial sodium channel and the control of blood pressure. J Am Soc Nephrol 8:980-992, 1997.

466. Lifton RP: Molecular genetics of human blood pressure variation. Science 272:676-680, 1996.

467. Valenti G, Procino G, Liebenhoff U, et al: A heterotrimeric G protein of the G$_i$ family is required for cAMP-triggered trafficking of aquaporin 2 in kidney epithelial cells. J Biol Chem 273:22627-22634, 1998.

468. Antonarakis S, and the Nomenclature Working Group: Recommendations for a nomenclature system for human gene mutations. Nomenclature Working Group. Hum Mutat 11:1-3, 1998.

469. Mouillac B, Chini B, Balestre M-N, et al: The binding site of neuropeptide vasopressin V$_{1a}$ receptor. J Biol Chem 270:25771-25777, 1995.

CHAPTER 37

Cystic Diseases of the Kidney

Jared J. Grantham and Franz Winklhofer

DEVELOPMENT OF RENAL CYSTS

Cysts are common renal abnormalities that, on direct inspection of the kidneys, are usually visible to the naked eye. They are composed of a layer of tubular epithelium enclosing a cavity filled with urine-like liquid or semisolid material. Although they are extremely rare in infants and young children, the prevalence of cysts increases with age. Renal cysts may develop in epithelial structures that begin in any tubular segment between the Bowman capsule and the tip of the renal papilla. The propensity of certain tubular segments to develop cysts appears to depend on the nature of the underlying disorder that provokes cyst formation. A relatively large number of clinical conditions are associated with renal cysts (Table 37-1).

TABLE 37-1

Classification of Renal Cysts

Hereditary polycystic kidney disease
    Autosomal dominant polycystic kidney disease
    Autosomal recessive polycystic kidney disease
Acquired cystic kidney disease (in azotemia and dialysis)
Cystic diseases of the renal medulla
    Medullary cystic disease
        Autosomal recessive
        Autosomal dominant
    Medullary sponge kidney
Simple cysts
Cystic renal dysplasia
Miscellaneous renal cystic disorders
    Hereditary
        Tuberous sclerosis
        von Hippel–Lindau disease
    Nonhereditary
        Solitary multilocular cysts
        Pyelocalyceal cysts
        Renal lymphangiomatosis
        Hilar and perinephric pseudocysts

Because they are the most obvious pathologic features in these disorders, cysts have been a focus of attention. Several facts have emerged from studies of pathology and pathogenesis of cystic disorders in humans and laboratory animals: (1) all cysts, whether acquired or inherited, develop from pre-existing renal tubule segments; (2) after achieving a size of perhaps a few millimeters, most cysts lose their attachments to their parent nephron segment; (3) the cyst-lining epithelium generally shows abnormal cellular differentiation and sustained proliferation; (4) the usually reabsorptive tubular epithelium is transformed into one that is capable of significant volume secretion that involves solute transport and cyclic adenosine monophosphate (cAMP) mechanisms; (5) there must be appropriate remodeling of the extracellular matrix to accommodate the enlarging cysts; and (6) the proliferation, secretion, and matrix remodeling are undoubtedly modulated by endocrine, paracrine, juxtacrine, and autocrine factors that would be important determinants of how fast the cysts grow and how rapidly renal insufficiency develops in cystic disease states.[1, 2]

The fundamental processes that are essential for the development and progressive enlargement of renal cysts include (1) proliferation of epithelial cells in segments of renal tubule, (2) disturbed organization and metabolism of the tubulointerstitial extracellular matrix, and (3) accumulation of fluid within the expanding tubule segment (Fig. 37-1).

Epithelial Proliferation

Renal cysts are benign neoplasms that arise from individual cells or restricted segments of renal tubule.[3-6] In the laboratory, they have been created by transgenetic insertion of activated proto-oncogenes and growth factor genes into rodents, which primarily drives the proliferation of renal cells. It may be supposed, therefore, that almost any process that stimulates coherent renal cell proliferation with the maintenance of epithelial polarity has the potential to generate the cyst phenotype.

Targeted disruption of genes has created cystic changes in renal tubules, but the clinical features of autosomal dominant

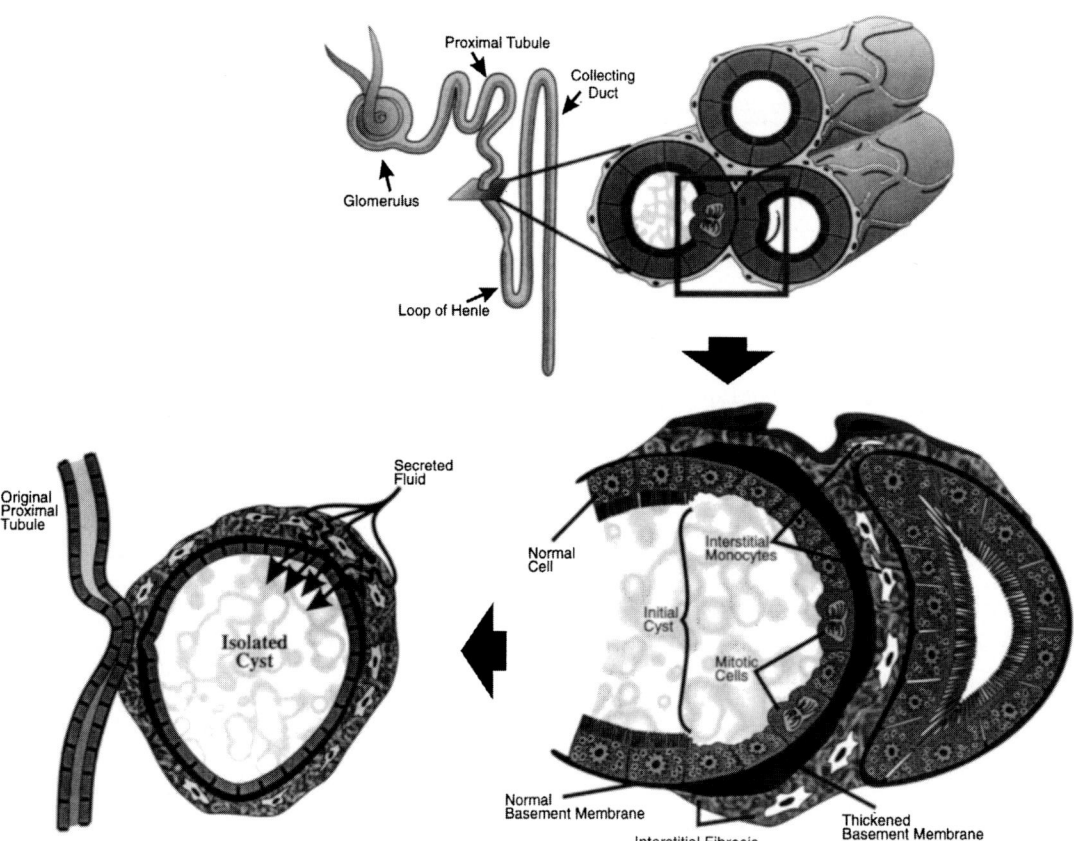

FIGURE 37-1. Evolution of cysts from renal tubules. Abnormal proliferation of tubule epithelium begins in a single cell after a "second hit" process disables the function of the normal allele. Repeated cycles of cell proliferation lead to expansion of the tubule wall into a cyst. The cystic epithelium is associated with thickening of the adjacent tubule basement membrane and with an influx of inflammatory cells into the interstitium. The cystic segment eventually separates from the original tubule, and net epithelial fluid secretion contributes to the accumulation of liquid within the cyst cavity.

disease in humans have not been faithfully reproduced in rodent models.[7, 8] Although the discrete pathways leading to increased proliferation have not been completely mapped, there is a general appreciation that the rate of cell mitogenesis and growth can be modulated by autocrine, paracrine, and juxtacrine factors that activate the classic receptor-tyrosine kinase (RTK), extracellular signal-regulated kinase (ERK), and adenylyl cyclase (cAMP) pathways.[9-11]

Fluid Accumulation

The feature that most readily differentiates renal cysts from solid neoplasms is the relatively large amount of fluid trapped within them. Cysts that develop in otherwise normal, functioning kidney tissue are initially attached to tubule segments that receive a derivative of glomerular filtrate (urine). However, as the cysts enlarge, most of them apparently lose their connections with the original renal tubule and become isolated sacs.[4] In these isolated sacs of liquid, transepithelial secretion of electrolytes and fluid appears to be the only mechanism for accumulation of the liquid within them.[12, 13] Although the fluid within renal cysts contributes the greatest mass in kidneys enlarged by cystic disease and may be the cause of symptoms and signs, it seems unlikely that fluid accumulation is primarily responsible for the development of renal cysts.

The finding of fluid secretion in renal epithelial cysts led to a reinvestigation of fluid secretion mechanisms in otherwise normal renal tubules. Recent evidence indicates that, beyond the loop of Henle, tubule cells have the capacity to secrete solutes and fluid on stimulation with cAMP.[14] This secretory flux operates in competition with the more powerful mechanism by which Na^+ is absorbed through apical epithelial Na^+ channels (ENaC). Under conditions in which Na^+ absorption is diminished, the net secretion of NaCl and fluid can be observed at rates that could have a significant impact on the net economy of body salt and water content. Thus, renal cystic disease has led to a heightened appreciation of an ancient solute and water secretory mechanism that has been largely overlooked in modern studies of renal physiology.[15]

Tubulointerstium-Extracellular Matrix

Abnormalities of the extracellular matrix in and about renal cysts are seen in all cystic disorders.[16-18] In acquired cystic kidney disease, a condition in which a primary renal pathologic disorder such as glomerulonephritis or diabetes mellitus destroys renal parenchyma (see later discussion), renal cysts may arise from residual nephrons embedded in the fibrous residue.[19] This finding raises the possibility that acquired abnormalities in the extracellular matrix may be instrumental in causing renal cysts. The observation that some hereditary renal cystic disorders are associated with aneurysms of arteries, abdominal hernias, and abnormally compliant heart valves is consistent with the view that extracellular matrix abnormalities may have a primary role in the formation of renal cysts. Evidence indicates that, in the early stages of renal cyst development, changes in expression of collagen I and IV,[20] metalloproteinase activators and inhibitors,[21-23] integrins,[24] and β-catenin[25-28] may forecast a vital role for extracellular matrix remodeling in the pathogenesis of renal cysts.

HEREDITARY POLYCYSTIC KIDNEY DISORDERS

Autosomal dominant polycystic kidney disease (ADPKD) and autosomal recessive polycystic kidney disease (ARPKD) are the principal examples of single-gene disorders that cause the polycystic kidney phenotype. ADPKD is caused by genetic mutations in genes on chromosomes 16 (*PKD1*)[29] and 4 (*PKD2*)[30] and possibly one other site. *PKD1* and *PKD2* encode proteins (polycystins) that appear to be members of a group of interactive molecules linked together in a way that transduces signals from the extracellular matrix to processes that govern cellular proliferation, differentiation, and transport within cells (Fig. 37-2).[31-33] Polycystin-1 appears to serve as a

receptor that binds to and activates polycystin-2, leading to the rapid flux of Ca^{2+} through nonspecific cation channels formed by the polycystin-2 proteins.[34, 35] In the process, a G protein-binding site is activated as well. Increased Ca^{2+} flux and G protein activation appear to be principal elements in the determination of normal tubule morphogenesis and growth.[36, 37]

Numerous mutations (deletion, missense, and frameshift) have been identified in the genes encoding polycystins type 1 and type 2, all of which appear to diminish the functions of the proteins. Dozens of different intragenic mutations have been described. Those occurring in the 3′ end of the gene appear to generate a more severe disease phenotype than those in the 5′ end.[38] A germline mutation in one of the PKD genes is necessary to cause the cyst phenotype, but cells heterozygous for either *PKD1* or *PKD2* mutations do not form cysts. A second "hit" or somatic mutation of the allele inherited from the normal parent is required to initiate cyst formation.[39, 40] This accounts for the focal nature of cyst formation. Cysts that do form in fewer than 1% of the tubules reflect the clonal growth of cells lacking a functional polycystin, either the PKD1 or the PKD2 type. Yet knowledge of cystogenesis remains incomplete. In animals in which both copies of the *PKD1* or *PKD2* genes have been altered by mutation, many more cysts develop and create a rapidly progressive form of ADPKD, but in the final analysis the cysts still derive from only a small minority of renal tubule cells. More than likely,

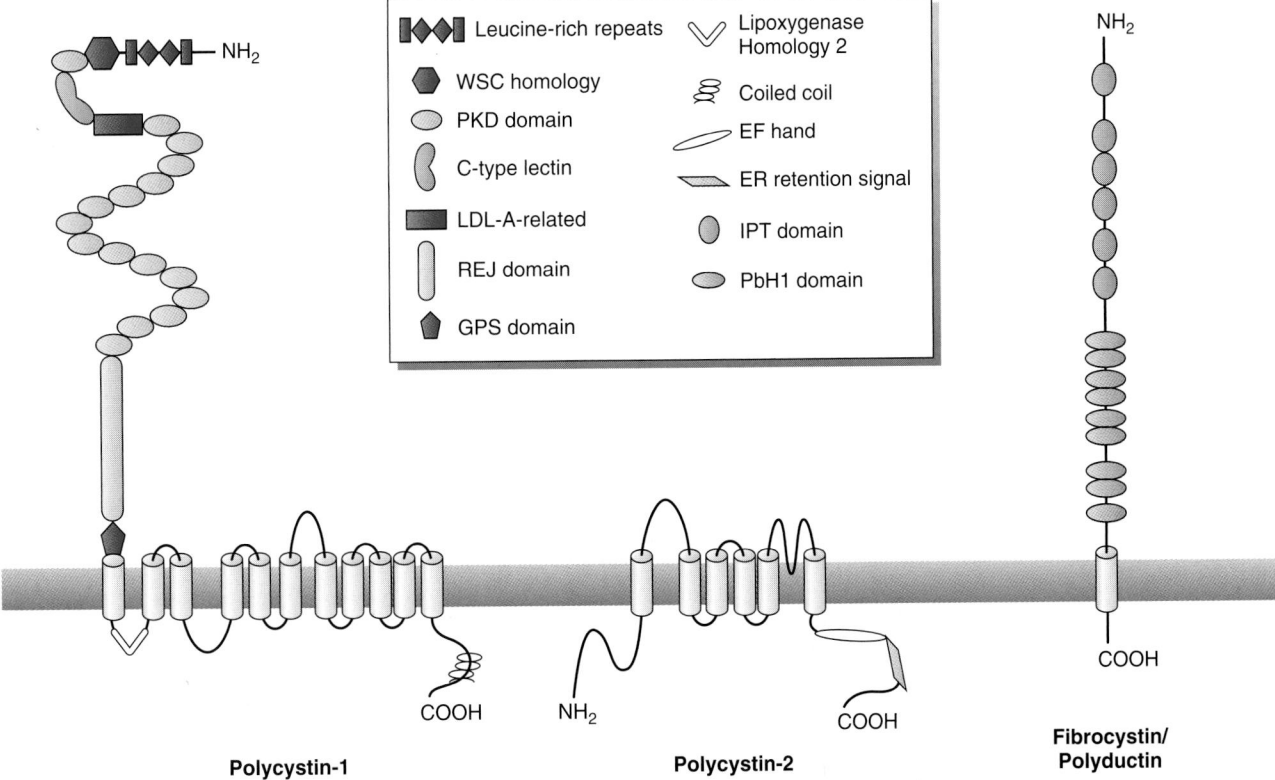

FIGURE 37-2. Structure of polycystin-1, polycystin-2, and fibrocystin/polyductin. Polycystin-1 and -2 are transcribed from DNA coding regions in chromosomes 16 and 4. Polycystin-1 has a long extracellular region, with several segments homologous with domains identified in other proteins that interact with interstitial proteins, and an intracellular tail that interacts with the cytoplasmic terminus of polycystin-2. Polycystin-1 probably is a receptor for an extracellular ligand that signals intracellular processes through interaction with polycystin-2. Fibrocystin/polyductin is transcribed from a DNA coding region in chromosome 6. The protein has a single transmembrane-spanning region, a long extracellular portion, and a relatively short intracellular tail. Fibrocystin/polyductin is found in apical cilia and is thought to mediate mechanosensory and chemosensory processes in renal tubule epithelial cells. PKD, polycystic kidney disease. (From Igarashi P, Somlo S: Genetics and pathogenesis of PKD. J Am Soc Nephrol 13:2384-2398, 2002, with permission.)

environmental or epigenetic factors have important roles in determining the pace of cystogenesis.

The gene for ARPKD (*PKHD1*), located on chromosome 6, encodes a relatively large protein called fibrocystin (polyductin)[38, 41, 42] (see Fig. 37-2). The cellular location of fibrocystin has not been defined, but other proteins that, when mutated, cause recessive PKD phenotypes similar to that seen in ARPKD have been localized to apical cilia of renal epithelial cells.[35] It is proposed that these novel ciliary proteins are involved in the transmission of signals derived from urine flow and chemical composition to mechanisms that determine the size and configuration of specific renal tubular segments.

It is well known that inheritance of a single mutated *PKHD1* gene does not cause renal cysts to form. In this disorder, the inheritance of two mutated alleles, one from each parent, is required for disease expression. Initial studies show, however, that different intragenic mutations occur in the parents more commonly than not. This may account for some of the phenotypic variability that is common in ARPKD.

Autosomal Dominant Polycystic Kidney Disease

ADPKD affects between 1 in every 500 and 1 in every 1000 individuals.[43] It is found on all continents and in all racial and ethnic groups. The most common of the polycystic kidney disorders, ADPKD is inherited as an autosomal dominant trait with complete penetrance. Therefore, each child of an affected parent has a 50% chance of inheriting the abnormal gene. About 40% of patients are unable to give a family history consistent with ADPKD, and this has suggested the possibility of a high spontaneous mutation rate or, alternatively, the possibility that environmental or epidemiologic factors strongly affect the expression of ADPKD. The most common genotype, that involving mutated *PKD1*, affects approximately 85%, that involving *PKD2* affects 15%, and a possible third type affects a very small percentage of known cases. The prevalence in the United States is approximately 600,000. In most respects, PKD1 and PKD2 disease is clinically similar, except that the less common genotype progresses to end-stage renal failure (ESRD) about 10 years later than does PKD1.[44]

ADPKD may not be clinically apparent until the third or fourth decade of life. Uncommonly, some patients are symptomatic before that time, and many patients are unaware of renal cysts until they are discovered by chance in later life. It has been projected that 100% of gene carriers will show evidence of the disease by the age of 80 years, but only about half of patients will progress to renal failure.[45] There is no way to predict in young patients whether or when renal failure will develop, although several risk factors (hypertension, renal hemorrhage, multiple pregnancies, male gender, PKD1 disease genotype) have been identified that are associated with a more rapid course.

Pathology

The kidneys usually are diffusely cystic and, although enlarged, maintain their general reniform shape (Fig. 37-3). In well-developed disease, both kidneys are abnormal, although one of the pair may be considerably larger than the other, and, even within one kidney, the extent of the process may be irregular. In one series, the combined kidney weight was 943 ± 664 g (mean $\pm$ SD) in 19 patients without azotemia, 1143 ± 733 g in 11 patients with mild azotemia, and about 3500 ± 2000 g in 57 patients with moderate azotemia or with renal failure requiring dialysis.[46] The combined volume of normal kidneys is approximately 330 cm^3.

Both the outer and the cut surfaces show numerous, usually spherical, cysts ranging in size from barely visible to several centimeters in diameter. The papillae and pyramids are distinguishable in early cases but difficult or impossible to identify in advanced examples, and the calyces and pelves are often greatly distorted. The cysts are usually distributed fairly evenly throughout both the cortical and medullary parenchyma, but their sizes may be highly diverse. Though it is unusual, striking asymmetry of cyst development may be seen.

Nephron reconstruction and dissection studies have shown the cysts to begin as outpouchings from preexisting renal tubules.[47] With enlargement beyond a few millimeters in diameter, however, it appears that about 75% of cysts become totally detached from their tubule of origin.[4, 48] In the early stages of the disease, the noncystic parenchymal elements appear relatively normal because less than 1% of the total tubules appear to become cystic. About three quarters of the cysts maintain an electrolyte composition of the fluid over

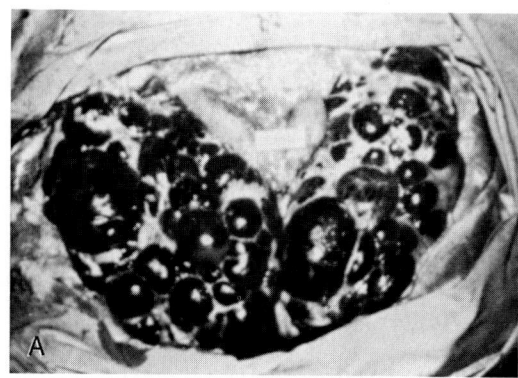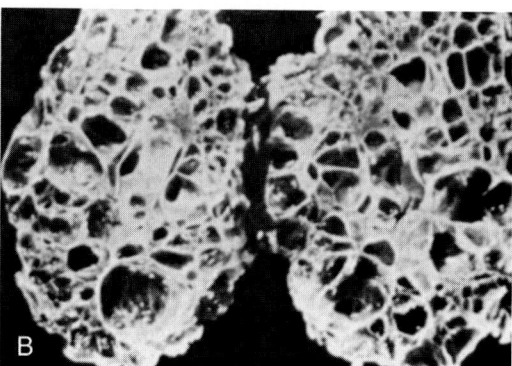

FIGURE 37-3. Autosomal dominant polycystic kidney disease (ADPKD) in situ (**A**) and on cut section (**B**). Note diffuse, bilateral distribution of cysts. (Courtesy of FE Cuppage, Kansas City, KS.)

the years consistent with proximal tubule-like function. The cells in the vast majority of the cysts are not typical of fully differentiated, mature renal tubular epithelium (Fig. 37-4D) and are thought to be undifferentiated or relatively immature. The tubule origin of these nondescript cysts is unknown, although studies in ESRD kidneys indicate that most of them retain histochemical features of distal and collecting tubules.[49] On the other hand, a few cysts exhibit residual morphologic features consistent with glomerular, proximal, or collecting duct origin (see Figs. 37-4A, B, and C, respectively). A minority of the cysts continue to function, as evinced by their capacity to generate transepithelial electrical

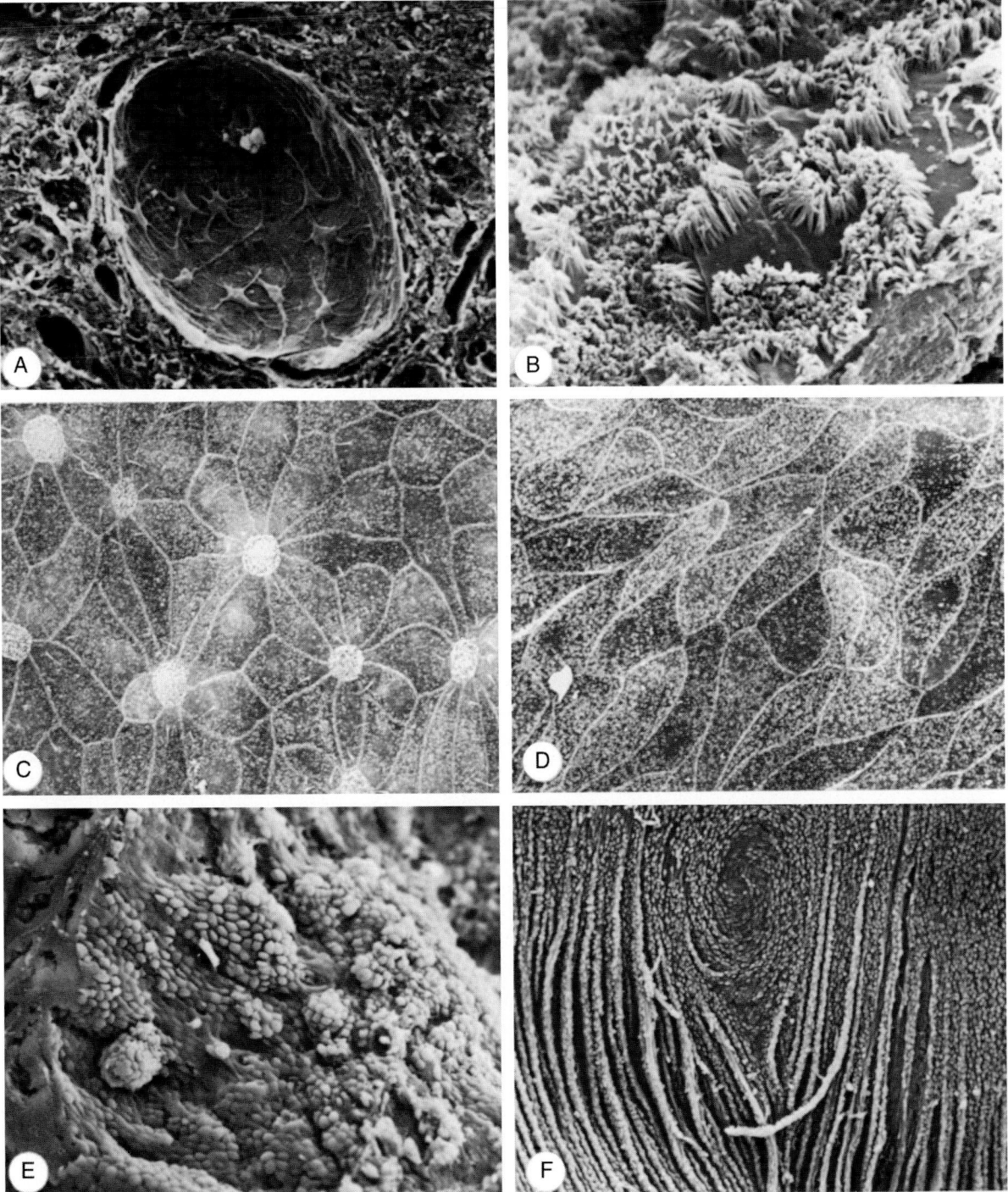

FIGURE 37-4. Scanning electron micrographs of cyst-lining epithelium in autosomal dominant polycystic kidney disease: **A,** typical of glomerular visceral layer (×250); **B,** typical of proximal tubule (×3000); **C,** typical of cortical collecting duct (×1000); **D,** epithelium not typical of any normal tubule segment (×1000); **E,** micropolyps (×250); **F,** cord-like hyperplasia (×80). (From Grantham JJ, Geiser JL, Evan AP: Cyst formation and growth in autosomal dominant polycystic kidney disease. Kidney Int 31:1145-1152, 1987, with permission.)

gradients[50-52] and to secrete NaCl and fluid[53] in vitro. In the final analysis, the electrolyte composition of cyst fluid in advanced ADPKD is determined by the tubule site of origin, the access of the cyst to glomerular filtrate (as opposed to filling exclusively with secreted fluid), the extent of cellular dedifferentiation, and the effects of hormone, paracrine, and autocrine factors on transepithelial electrolyte and fluid transport.[12, 13] The minority cysts (about 25%) with relatively low Na^+ concentrations in relation to plasma and tight apical intercellular junctions probably derive from distal or collecting tubules, whereas the majority cysts (75%) with Na^+ levels approximating that of plasma and relatively leaky apical junctions probably represent the cysts with epithelium that is less well differentiated than that of the low-Na^+ cysts.

The question of function in the cyst wall has been answered in a most direct manner. In a study of carefully dissected individual cysts from adult patients with ADPKD, cyst fluid was found to accumulate at rates of 0.1 to 1.0 mL/day, more than sufficient to account for the in vivo growth rate.[53] Secretion may be dependent on powerful secretagogues (arginine vasopressin [AVP], prostaglandin E_2 [PGE_2], adrenergic agonists, adenosine, and unidentified lipids) that stimulate the cAMP mechanism.[54, 55] Increased levels of intracellular cAMP activate chloride channels in the apical plasma membranes, allowing the secretion of this ion from the extracellular medium into the urine. The cystic fibrosis transmembrane conductance regulator (CFTR), best known for its failure in cystic fibrosis owing to mutation, is an ancient chloride channel that is normally harbored in most tubule epithelial cells. In the isolated cysts where no glomerular filtrate can enter, it appears that the absorptive machinery for Na^+ is down-regulated, and that for Cl^- transport through CFTR is up-regulated, leading to reversal of the net solute flux from absorption to secretion. Net solute and fluid secretion can also be demonstrated in normal renal tubules in vitro by inhibiting the ENaC channel with amiloride, uncovering net secretion after stimulation with cAMP agonists.[14]

About one half of young adults with ADPKD have cysts of the liver, and the prevalence increases with age to as high as 90% in patients whose life is prolonged by renal replacement therapy.[46, 56] These cysts, like renal cysts in ADPKD, are products of "second hit" somatic mechanisms.[57] Cyst number and size correlate positively with female gender and occurrence of pregnancy.[58] The cysts are lined by a single layer of columnar epithelium resembling that of the biliary tract and contain fluid that resembles the composition of serum. They do not communicate with the biliary system. Liver dysfunction and portal hypertension rarely occur, regardless of the size and number of cysts. The liver cysts may continue to grow and to appear de novo after institution of renal replacement therapy. They may become infected and have been the site of origin of cholangiocellular carcinoma.[46] There is a rare association with congenital dilation of intrahepatic bile ducts.[59] There also are a few reported kindreds in which the hepatic change is indistinguishable from that seen in congenital hepatic fibrosis.[60]

Epithelial cysts in organs other than the liver are less common. About 10% of patients have cysts, increased connective tissue, and duct proliferation in the pancreas. Fewer than 5% have cysts in the spleen. About 5% have arachnoid cysts.[61] Cysts of the thyroid, ovary, endometrium, seminal vesicle, and epididymis have been reported but are uncommon.

Pathogenesis of Renal Failure

ESRD develops before the end of the seventh decade of life in approximately 50% of individuals with PKD1 or PKD2 disease.[45] Renal cysts develop in fewer than 1% of renal tubules, so the staggering loss of renal function in patients with ESRD cannot be attributed to cystic segments' simply blocking the excretion of urine by individual renal tubules. Rather, as the cysts progressively expand, they encroach on adjacent parenchyma. In this way, the individual cysts may amplify their effect to compromise function in adjacent noncystic renal tubules and glomeruli. The "pressure" of the expanding cysts, the consequence of cyst epithelial cell proliferation and the secretion of NaCl and fluid into the lumen, may distort the delicate tubulointerstitial network of capillaries, lymphatics, arterioles, and venules, leading to functional disturbances of the surrounding parenchyma. This abnormality in the interstitium is thought to lead to apoptosis in otherwise normal tissue.[62] Hypertrophy of nephrons and glomeruli compensates for the loss of parenchymal mass for several years, but ultimately the amount of noncystic parenchyma decreases so that, at the end stage, only the survivor cysts remain.

Some patients almost seem to be immune to the effects of the cysts to initiate tubulointerstitial fibrogenesis and apoptosis, and these patients maintain life-sustaining renal function for a normal life expectancy. The relatively harmless presence of cysts in these individuals raises the possibility that modifier genes,[63] environmental factors,[64] susceptibility to second hits, or unique features of the genomic mutations[65] may have important roles in the final functional outcome.

Hypertension is thought to develop secondary to the stretching of arteries and arterioles across expanding cysts or to disturbances in the microvasculature, leading to increased secretion of renin and generation of angiotensin II.[66-68] Hypertension accelerates the tubulointerstitial process leading to fibrosis. Patients with hypertension of early onset progress to ESRD faster than those who are normotensive.[44] Despite this evidence, treatment with antiangiotensin drugs has not been shown to be renoprotective.[69] More than likely, this failure is due to the relatively late application of angiotensin-converting enzyme (ACE) inhibitors and angiotensin receptor blockers in the course of the disease.

ADPKD is a striking example of the inadequacy of clinical measurements of glomerular filtration rate (GFR) in predicting the future course of slowly progressive renal diseases. In ADPKD, relatively young patients with normal GFR may have profoundly distorted renal anatomy and extreme renal enlargement, clear evidence that the disease has progressed to a remarkable extent. Yet, the GFR often indicates that the absolute rate of filtration is within normal limits. Commonly overlooked is the fact that GFR is maintained within the normal range in patients with advanced cystic change through compensatory filtration in residual glomerular/tubular units. Despite profound hyperfiltration in residual glomeruli, glomerulosclerotic lesions do not develop in ADPKD.[70] Only after the compensatory mechanisms fail is a fall in GFR seen, and usually this is relatively precipitous, suggesting to clinicians that the "disease" has taken a sudden change for the worse (Fig. 37-5). In fact, the disease has been progressing at a relatively stable rate for many years, reflected by systemic hypertension and the

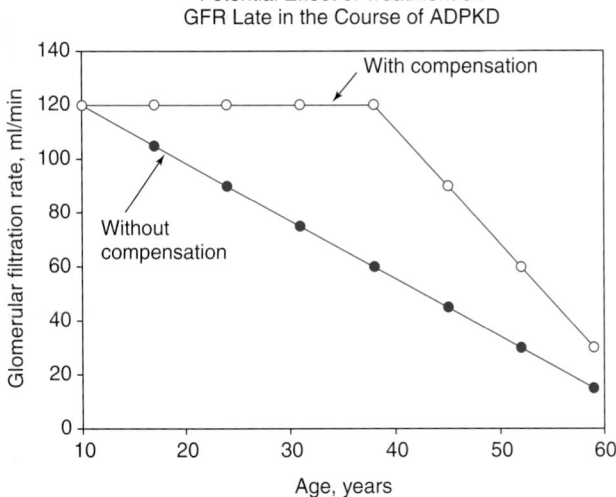

Potential Effect of Treatment on
GFR Late in the Course of ADPKD

FIGURE 37-5. Effects of compensatory maintenance of glomerular filtration rate (GFR) on the pattern of progression in autosomal dominant polycystic kidney disease (ADPKD). It was assumed that, beginning at the age of 10 years, the patient loses each year an amount of parenchyma that normally contributes 2 mL/min of GFR. It was further assumed that each residual normal glomerulus can double the single-nephron GFR by compensatory mechanisms (as evinced in normal individuals by the maintenance of total GFR after uninephrectomy for kidney donation). As seen in the model, total GFR is maintained until parenchymal loss precludes complete compensation; at that point, total GFR begins to fall at a rate that appears more "precipitous" than what had actually occurred. This model illustrates that GFR is a poor indicator of ADPKD progression and that more sensitive markers of parenchymal loss are needed to facilitate earlier monitoring.

excretion of albumin above normal limits.[71] Recent studies suggest that in diseases like ADPKD lacking glomerular lesions, this proteinuria may be a reflection of tubulointerstitial factors.[72]

Tubulointerstitial inflammation, fibrosis, and cysts have been discovered in animals with inherited or acquired renal cystic disease. Various chemicals administered to rodents have been found to cause acute renal injury and cysts.[73] In these models, the renal cystic disease is always accompanied by tubulointerstitial inflammation and fibrosis, and in some cases the changes in the interstitium appear to precede the development of the cysts. Type I and type IV collagen are expressed very early in mice and rats with inherited types of PKD in association with dilatation of renal tubules, which eventually become full-blown cysts.[23, 74, 75] The potential role of leukocytes has been emphasized by studies illustrating that endotoxin can enhance cyst formation in germ-free rats fed nordihydroguaiaretic acid and in association with interstitial infiltrates in the hereditary T cell–mediated autoimmune nephritis of kd/kd mice.[76, 77] Monocytes have been identified in the interstitium of rats with ADPKD in association with the increased expression of monocyte chemotactic protein-1 (MCP-1) and osteopontin in cyst epithelial cells.[78] MCP-1 is found in cyst fluids in high concentrations and is excreted in the urine of patients with ADPKD before there are detectable changes in GFR.[79] Of interest in this regard is the finding that treatment of rats and mice with inherited forms of PKD with methylprednisolone reduced renal size, decreased interstitial inflammation, and improved

renal function.[80] Despite these tantalizing associations, in the final analysis the exact pathogenetic roles of tubulointerstitial inflammation and fibrosis in the initiation of cyst formation and the progressive loss of renal function remain to be elucidated.

At the end stage of the disease, the kidneys are usually several times larger than normal and exhibit innumerable fluid-filled cysts that make up almost all of the total renal mass. In these far-advanced cases, only scant normal-appearing parenchyma may be found in isolated patches. There is abundant fibrous tissue plastered along the surface of the kidneys beneath the capsule, and on the cut surface of transected kidneys cysts may be found encapsulated by fibrous bands. Tubulointerstitial fibrosis and arteriolar sclerosis are cardinal features of the end-stage polycystic kidney.[81] The disappearance of noncystic parenchyma implicates apoptosis as a primary mechanism in progressive renal dysfunction in ADPKD.[62]

Diagnosis

In its fully developed form, ADPKD is not difficult to diagnose. Most polycystic kidneys are enlarged bilaterally and have irregular surfaces that can be felt on careful palpation. Many patients will have noticed increased abdominal girth. An enlarged liver with palpable cysts adds further strength to the diagnosis. On careful questioning, a family history of ADPKD, or consistent with ADPKD, can be obtained in about 60% of newly recognized cases. As described later, many patients report pain that may be associated with gross and microscopic hematuria. Hypertension is common, as are the signs and symptoms of renal infection and lithiasis.

The early stages of ADPKD are not usually reflected in the urinalysis. There may be a defect in maximum concentrating ability, but urinary dilution remains intact.[82] There is no salt wasting, except in the late stages of the disease, and urinary acidification is normal.[83] Massive proteinuria is rare and, if found, should prompt a search for an additional renal disorder. In the middle to late stages of the disease (20 to 40 years of age), mild persistent proteinuria (greater than 200 mg/day) may be found in 20% to 40% of cases. Patients with proteinuria may also excrete doubly refractile lipid bodies (oval fat bodies).[84] The blood erythrocyte count and hematocrit may be increased above normal, possibly because of abnormal erythropoietin production by cysts, and patients with end-stage ADPKD do not have anemia as profound as that occurring in other types of terminal renal disease. In the absence of complications, blood coagulation study results and leukocyte and platelet counts are normal.[85]

Diagnosis can be confirmed by several radiologic tests. In more advanced cases, intravenous urography shows marked deformity of the collecting system with thinning of calyces and infundibula, but this test is no longer used to screen patients at risk for ADPKD. Ultrasonography, the preferred screening method, reveals multiple echo-free areas in both kidneys (Fig. 37-6). Ultrasound studies of children and older adults in conjunction with DNA linkage analyses have led to the development of criteria to minimize false-positive and false-negative results.[45, 86, 87] To ensure a proper diagnosis, patients younger than 30 years of age should have at least two cysts in at least one of the kidneys. Simple cysts are rare in this population. Patients between the ages of 30 and 59 years should have at least two cysts in each kidney, and patients older than 60 years of age should have at least four cysts in each kidney.

We prefer computed tomography (CT) with contrast enhancement in cases in which ultrasonography is equivocal.[88, 89] CT readily distinguishes between solid and liquid renal masses and portrays the diffuse distribution of large and small cysts, a characteristic that is important in differentiating ADPKD from multiple simple cysts (Fig. 37-7A). The contrast-enhancing component of the CT scan can also be valuable in judging the prognosis for renal function (see Fig. 37-7B). Because the contrast material is concentrated in the normal renal tubules, the intensity and relative volume of contrast-enhanced parenchyma are a direct reflection of the amount of relatively unaffected renal parenchyma. CT also reveals small cysts in the liver, a finding that further helps to differentiate ADPKD from acquired cystic disorders.

CT has limitations in young children because of the exposure to ionizing radiation. However, recent upgrades in magnetic resonance imaging (MRI) technology offer a highly useful alternative to CT in unusual cases (Fig. 37-8). In MRI studies, patients are administered an intravenous contrast agent (gadolinium) that has no renal toxicity and few other side effects (see Fig. 37-8A, C). This agent conveys the same information as iodinated compounds do in respect to tubular function and parenchymal volume. Heavy-weighted T2 images permit the detection of cysts only 2 to 3 mm in diameter with great certainty (see Fig. 37-8B, D). In our opinion, heavy-weighted T2 MRI is the most sensitive method currently available for diagnosis of ADPKD in very early stages of the disease.

Radioisotope scanning methods using iodine 131 (^{131}I)-labeled hippurate or technetium 99m (^{99m}Tc) have limited usefulness for diagnosis but are of value in assessing and comparing renal tubule function and glomerular filtration between the two kidneys.

Gene linkage analysis can be used to determine obligate ADPKD gene carriers, but this method has not gained widespread clinical use. In individuals (including fetuses) who are at risk but who have no radiographically defined cysts, genetic linkage analysis may be useful to identify, with an accuracy greater than 99%, those predisposed to develop ADPKD.[90] The test, however, has practical limitations. At least two family members with unequivocal ADPKD must be willing to provide blood samples in order to determine the marker alleles that are critical for ascertaining the status of the individual at risk. Testing should be performed only after the patient has been educated about the risks and benefits of knowing that he or she has ADPKD. Benefits include the knowledge of being free of the ADPKD genotype, genetic counseling, and early intervention in dealing with some of the complications of ADPKD and in selection of genetically unaffected family members in consideration for living related donor renal transplantation.[91] Potential risks include difficulty in gaining employment and insurance.

Recently a mutation analysis based on a high-performance liquid chromatographic (HPLC) method has been introduced as a means of diagnosing ADPKD.[38] The test is

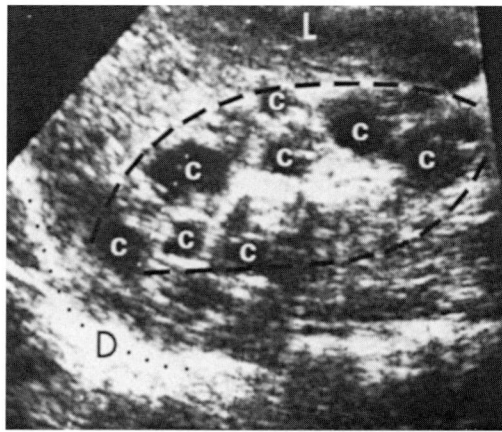

FIGURE 37-6. Autosomal dominant polycystic kidney disease seen in a parasagittal or longitudinal sonogram. This view of the right kidney was obtained with the patient in the right anterior oblique position. The approximate outline of the kidney is shown by the broken line. Some of the larger renal cysts are indicated by C. The liver (L) is at the top of the figure. The right dome of the diaphragm (D) is at the lower left.

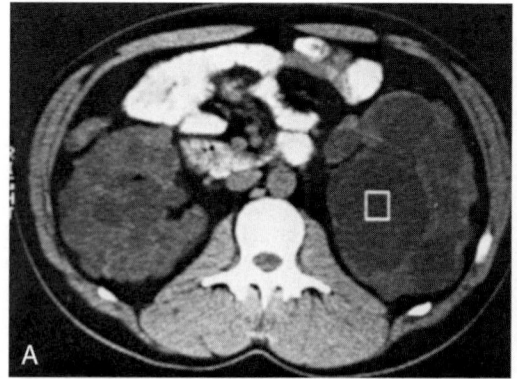
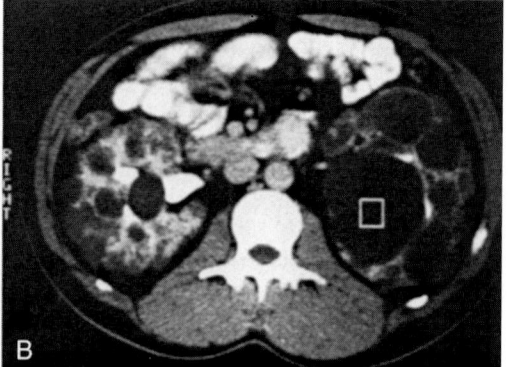

FIGURE 37-7. Computed tomography scans of polycystic kidneys. The patient (male) has autosomal dominant polycystic kidney disease, and the serum creatinine level is within the normal range. An oral contrast agent was given to highlight the intestine. **A,** Computed tomographic scan without contrast. **B,** Computed tomographic scan at the same level as **A** but after intravenous infusion of iodinated radiocontrast material. The cursor *(box)* is used to determine the relative density of cyst fluid, which in this case is equal to that of water. Contrast enhancement highlights functioning parenchyma, which here is concentrated primarily in the right kidney. The renal collecting system also is highlighted by contrast material in both kidneys.

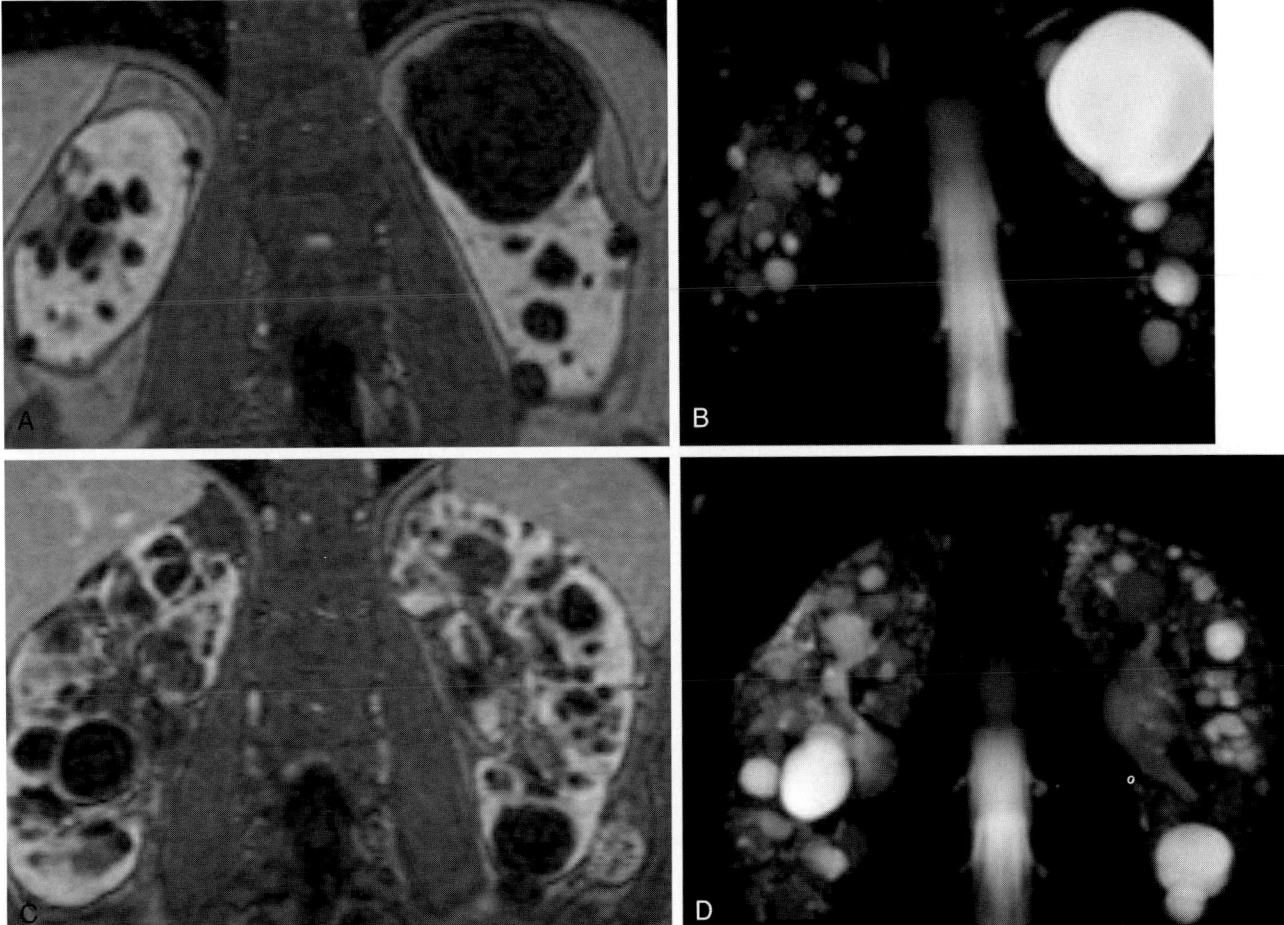

FIGURE 37-8. Magnetic resonance imaging studies of two female patients, with mild and moderately severe disease. In neither subject was the serum creatinine value higher than 1.1 mg/dL. In panels **A** and **C**, gadolinium was infused intravenously a few minutes before the scan was obtained. The residual, normal parenchyma between cysts is highlighted by gadolinium. In panels **B** and **D**, heavy-weighted T2 images are shown at the same kidney level as in **A** and **C**. The cysts are emphasized, illustrating that cysts smaller than 3 mm can be detected.

expensive and, given the fact that the entire universe of mutations in *PKD1* and *PKD2* has not been cataloged, it cannot give definitive information in about 25% of those tested. This test is currently being used as a research tool in several centers, but widespread clinical application has not been enthusiastically endorsed.

The primary and secondary criteria supporting the diagnosis of ADPKD are listed in Table 37-2. Owing to the widespread distribution of the mutated gene products (polycystins), several extrarenal manifestations can be useful in supporting the diagnosis of ADPKD, including cerebral aneurysms, hepatic cysts, cardiac valvular lesions, hernias[92] (abdominal and inguinal), drooping upper eyelids,[93] and seminal vesicle cysts.[94, 95] ADPKD must be differentiated from ARPKD in children and from tuberous sclerosis, multiple simple cysts, multicystic dysplastic kidney, von Hippel-Lindau syndrome, and acquired cystic kidney disease.

Therapy

BASIC FLUID AND ELECTROLYTES

Na$^+$ conservation is usually normal in the early stages of the disease; however, it is important to monitor blood pressure and extracellular volume status (edema) carefully and to

TABLE 37-2

Clinical Criteria for Diagnosis of Autosomal Dominant Polycystic Kidney Disease

Primary criteria
  More than three fluid-filled cysts scattered diffusely throughout renal cortex and medulla of both kidneys
  Definite history of polycystic kidney disease in genetically related family members
Secondary criteria
  Polycystic liver
  Renal insufficiency
  Abdominal hernia
  Cardiac valvular lesions
  Cysts of pancreas
  Aneurysms of cerebral arteries
  Seminal vesicle cysts
  Drooping eyelids

make appropriate adjustments in therapy. Na$^+$ restriction to less than 100 mEq/day may be necessary in those with arterial hypertension. The use of diuretics is problematic. Diuretics (thiazides) may be helpful in the management of hypertension and calcium lithiasis; on the other hand, they have the potential to cause hypokalemia, which has been associated with the development of cysts in individuals with otherwise normal kidneys[96] and may, therefore, increase the growth of cysts in ADPKD. Diuretics alone may not be sufficient to control blood pressure in these patients, and supplementation with antirenin agents seems helpful.[97] Potassium-sparing agents (amiloride, spironolactone) may be useful in preventing hypokalemia.

Patients with early ADPKD may have a diminished ability to concentrate their urine maximally.[82] Nocturia may be the only symptom of this defect, and no specific therapy is indicated. Water intake sufficient to produce 1.5 to 2 L of urine is usually sufficient unless the patient has renal calculi or infection requiring higher urine volume flow rates. The impact of urine flow rate on disease progression should be evaluated prospectively in a well-controlled study that includes patients with normal renal function.

PHYSICAL ACTIVITY AND LIFESTYLE

Most patients with ADPKD require no modification in physical activity or lifestyle in the early stages of the disease. Evidence indicates that recurrent bouts of gross hematuria, usually related to direct trauma, are associated with a faster decline of renal function than otherwise[98, 99]; therefore, avoidance of renal trauma seems prudent. Patients probably should not participate in strenuous athletics in which the abdomen may be traumatized repeatedly.

MANAGEMENT OF PAIN

Pain is the most common symptom in ADPKD.[100] It may be perceived as a unilateral or bilateral vague sense of heaviness or as a dull aching to knifelike and stabbing pain. When chronic, it may be disabling and may lead to analgesic abuse. The cause is often unknown, but medium-sized blood vessels evidently rupture occasionally and cause extravasation of blood either into cysts or perinephric tissues. Perinephric hemorrhage may be associated with intense discomfort and obvious changes in the configuration of the abdomen detected on direct physical examination, but even these hemorrhages can usually be treated with bed rest and analgesics. After counseling, most patients recognize the problem as a transient disorder.

When pain is unrelenting, however, one must consider the possibility of renal infection, stones, or tumors.

Therefore, renal pain that changes in character or that lasts for longer than a few days should be evaluated, especially if it is associated with gross or microscopic hematuria. Pain in association with fever, weight loss, anemia, and a striking change in the configuration of the kidney should raise the suspicion of renal malignancy. The most reliable diagnostic signs of malignancy are the appearance of a solid mass structure by sonography, speckled calcifications in the suspected tumor mass as assessed by conventional radiography or CT, the appearance of material within the cyst with a CT density greater than water, and a typical arteriographic appearance after infusion of radiocontrast material into the renal artery or enhancement of tissue within the cyst after intravenous infusion of contrast medium followed by CT or MRI. Fortunately, this complication is rare.

Pain may also be associated with the enlargement of one or more cysts in a kidney, and some relief may be obtained

by percutaneous aspiration of fluid combined with instillation of a sclerosing agent.[101] Alternatively, surgical techniques may be of value for those who have extremely large kidneys filled with cysts. Surgical aspiration and unroofing of cysts has been reintroduced for the treatment of severe pain.[102, 103] When performed in specialized centers where large numbers of cases are treated, this radical therapy may produce relief that lasts for several years. Percutaneous laparoscopic methods have been developed for cyst unroofing or total nephrectomy with reasonably good outcomes.[104-109]

In some patients who fail surgical treatments, the persistent pain can not be attributed to specific cysts or pathologic processes. These individuals are vulnerable to drug addiction and, in extreme cases, suicide. Pain management in specialized centers can be life-saving if the usual measures fail. Opiates delivered by transcutaneous patches have proved to be highly effective in some patients, as have perinephric injections of local anesthetics, transcutaneous nerve stimulation (TENS), hypnotherapy, and transcendental meditation.

HEMATURIA AND INTRARENAL HEMORRHAGE

Hematuria is usually caused by the rupture of a cyst into the pelvis of the kidney. It appears suddenly and persists as macroscopic or microscopic bleeding for several days. In addition to vascular rupture into cysts, hematuria may be caused by renal stone, infection of cysts, or malignant tumors. On rare occasions, it may not be related to the cysts at all. Glomerulonephritis has been described to occur incidentally with ADPKD, so the urine sediment should be examined carefully for casts at some point in all instances of bleeding. Reduced physical activity or bed rest is usually sufficient to control the bleeding.

Desmopressin acetate (DDAVP) and aprotinin may be of benefit in controlling severe bleeding.[110] Transcatheter arterial infarction has been used to control recurrent hemorrhage in ADPKD and would seem to be of some value in patients with severe renal blood loss for whom dialysis is imminent or extant.[111, 112] It probably should not be used in kidneys with established infection. In patients who have reasonably normal renal function, every effort should be made to preserve that function. Bleeding may occur into cysts located near the renal pelvis and thus may cause obstruction to urine flow. Surgical removal of the clots and the dome of the cyst may permanently restore function in those cases.

RENAL INFECTION

Parenchymal pyogenic bacterial infection is a major problem for patients with ADPKD, particularly for women.[113] Diffuse pyelonephritis is the most common manifestation of parenchymal infection, but one or more cysts may become infected, and, as with any deep-seated abscess, the condition may be difficult to treat. If it is associated with fever, diaphoresis, bacteremia, leukocytosis, bacteriuria, pus casts in the urine, and exquisite tenderness on deep palpation of the kidneys, the diagnosis of diffuse parenchymal infection is ensured, and treatment can be initiated as for individuals without renal cysts. However, the pattern of symptoms and signs is not always so clear, and usually empiric judgments must be made. Cyst infection commonly is unilateral and, unless accompanied by pyelonephritis, may not be associated with bacteriuria or bacteremia. In our experience, localized tenderness over a region of a palpable kidney has been a reliable indicator of an infected cyst or cysts. Infected cysts may also be suspected if the infection fails to respond to conventional parenteral therapy.[114] CT has detected increased cyst wall thickness, and radioactive gallium or indium scans have identified infected foci in polycystic kidneys. Little is known about the invading organisms in most cases of infected cysts. Coliform, staphylococcal, and bacteroides organisms have been isolated from cyst fluid aspirates in some patients. The finding of low oxygen tension (PO_2 less than 40 mm Hg) in some cysts has raised the possibility that anaerobic organisms might grow in such an environment.

It has been suggested that ADPKD may be a member of a growing class of emerging infectious diseases.[115-120] Bacterial endotoxin and fungal β-D-glucans were found in cyst fluids from human kidneys with ADPKD, and tissue samples and serologic tests revealed a variety of fungal antigens in ADPKD but not in healthy kidney tissue. Given the surprising role of *Helicobacter pylori* in duodenal ulcer pathogenesis, the potential impact of indolent infections must be studied carefully in ADPKD.

PKD presents a problem in regard to the choice of antibiotics for treatment. Most of the cysts are permeable to polar antibiotics, such as cephalosporins and aminoglycosides. However, a minority of the cysts are relatively impermeable, and in these cases, lipophilic drugs are the only antibiotics that can penetrate the cysts sufficiently to achieve bacteriocidal levels within the fluid (Fig. 37-9).[121-124] It is suggested, therefore, that parenteral lipid-soluble drugs, such as ciprofloxacin (and newer derivatives), chloramphenicol, erythromycin, tetracyclines, and trimethoprim, may be useful if cephalosporins, penicillin derivatives, and aminoglycosides fail to eradicate the infection.

Once the patient is afebrile and has a normal blood leukocyte count, sterile urine, and no leukocytes in the urine sediment,

we recommend the administration of an oral bacteriocidal antibiotic until there is no renal pain on deep palpation and for an indefinite period thereafter. There are no clear-cut hard and fast rules to guide the duration of therapy. In our experience, these infections frequently relapse after 3 weeks of oral therapy, and in some cases it has been necessary to administer lipophilic antibiotics for longer than 1 year.

Eradication of infection in polycystic kidneys with intrapelvic urinary stones may be difficult or impossible until the stones are removed. Urinary tract infections are more prevalent in female patients,[114] as is true in the non-PKD population, and for prevention we specifically recommend showers rather than tub baths, frequent voiding, good perineal hygiene, and voiding immediately after intercourse. All patients are advised to refuse urinary tract instrumentation procedures unless absolutely necessary. Occasionally, renal infection is so serious and intractable that nephrectomy is necessary. This should be a last resort in patients with good renal function and should be used only after parenteral antibiotics have been administered unsuccessfully.

HYPERTENSION

Arterial hypertension develops in more than half of patients with ADPKD at some time during the course of their disease[67, 68, 98, 125-128] It often antedates measurable changes in renal function by several years. Blood pressure that is disproportionately high in relation to age may be a problem for young individuals with ADPKD.[129, 130] Left ventricular mass may be greater than normal in children, owing to a subtle increase in mean arterial pressure, and is clearly higher in adult ADPKD patients with hypertension. The cause of the hypertension in patients with ADPKD is unknown. Difficulties in ascribing etiology probably stem from the fact that ADPKD is a lifelong condition that affects different elements of renal function and blood pressure regulation at different stages of the disease. The renin-angiotensin-aldosterone system undoubtedly has an important role, but abnormalities in the production of renin and angiotensin do not account for all instances of hypertension.[126, 131, 132] The extracellular fluid volume is clearly expanded in patients well before the onset of renal failure. Nevertheless, they can excrete an intravenous load of NaCl and water faster than normal individuals do,[133] and studies indicate that there is a change in the pressure-natriuresis curve that can be corrected by the administration of an ACE inhibitor.[134] A greater increase in plasma atrial natriuretic peptide in hypertensive ADPKD subjects compared with normotensive subjects is most likely a consequence of the increase in extracellular and plasma fluid volumes. Co-inherited genes that predispose an individual to essential hypertension may also have a complicating impact in patients with ADPKD. Increased activity of the sympathetic nervous system has been implicated in the genesis of hypertension.[135]

It generally is agreed that in ADPKD, as in other renal disorders, hypertension is one of the important risk factors for progression of renal insufficiency as well as a contributor to overall cardiovascular morbidity.[44, 67, 125, 136] Current recommendations for blood pressure targets derive from studies of renal diseases in general. In view of the fact that ADPKD is present at birth and subtle hypertension may extend over decades, physicians should carefully monitor blood pressure and select a target value appropriate for the

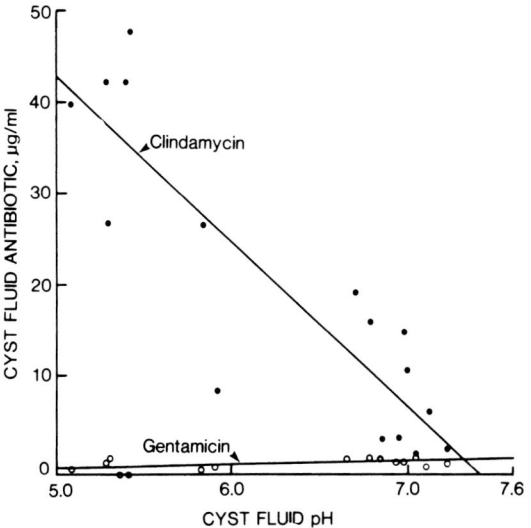

FIGURE 37-9. Antibiotic accumulation in renal cysts of a patient with autosomal dominant polycystic kidney disease. Clindamycin and gentamicin were administered for several days preceding a unilateral nephrectomy to establish proof of principle. Clindamycin (lipophilic) levels in cyst fluids were inversely proportional to cyst fluid pH. By contrast, gentamicin (lipophobic) levels were uniformly low and independent of cyst fluid pH. (From Schwab S, Hinthorn D, Diederich D, et al: pH-Dependent accumulation of clindamycin in a polycystic kidney. Am J Kidney Dis 3:63, 1983.)

age and gender of the patient.[130, 137] Moderate sodium restriction is prudent in most ADPKD patients with hypertension, as are weight control and regular exercise.

ACE inhibitors and angiotensin receptor blockers are effective in the treatment of hypertension in patients with ADPKD.[68, 138] Although interference with the action of angiotensin is highly effective, especially in the early stages of the disease, ACE inhibitors have been associated with severe renal hemorrhage and sudden renal failure in individuals with relatively large kidneys.[139] Any drug that undermines compensatory glomerular filtration in residual nephrons, including angiotensin blockers, β-blockers, α-adrenergic agents, or Ca^{2+} channel blockers, would give an exaggerated decline in clearance and the appearance of a rapid acceleration of the disease. Therefore, prudent use and interpretation of the effects of these powerful agents is of utmost importance.

Ca+ channel blockers are highly effective in ADPKD, and β-adrenergic blockers and α_2-adrenergic agonists may be helpful in refractory cases. In selected cases in which the volume component cannot be controlled by salt restriction, the cautious use of diuretics may be beneficial.

ARTERIAL ANEURYSMS

Cerebral aneurysms, potentially one of the most devastating complications of ADPKD, occur in fewer than 5% of all ADPKD patients. However, in patients with a clear family history of cerebral aneurysm, the risk increases to about 20%.[61, 140, 141] They are noted in both PKD1 and PKD2 disease. The cause of the aneurysms is unknown, although the high expression of polycystin within blood vessels implicates a potential link between these mutated proteins and the structural defect in the blood vessels.[142-144]

Because most patients with ADPKD do not experience this complication, screening is usually reserved for individuals with a family history of aneurysm and those who have symptoms consistent with intracerebral pathology.

Magnetic resonance angiography is the preferred method to screen for aneurysm. Confirmation by conventional angiography further delineates the shape and location of the aneurysm if surgical excision is contemplated. A decision to operate on the aneurysm depends on many factors, including the size, position, and accessibility of the lesion and the experience of the surgeon with similar cases.

The central nervous system vascular lesions may be more diffuse than previously believed. Diffuse arterial dolichoectasias of the anterior and posterior circulation have been reported.[145, 146] This association is important because it may predispose to arterial dissection and stroke. Aggressive management of hypertension is essential to reduce the risk of aneurysmal rupture. An increase in intracranial arachnoid cysts has been observed, but these lesions usually are not problematic.[147]

A number of cardiovascular abnormalities have been found in conjunction with ADPKD. Cardiac valvular lesions[148, 149] and coronary artery and aortic aneurysms[150-153] have been detected in patients with ADPKD, but it is not known whether their prevalence is uniquely increased.

NEPHROLITHIASIS

Calcifications develop in patients with ADPKD within the kidney parenchyma (nephrocalcinosis) and within the urinary collecting system (nephrolithiasis) (Fig. 37-10). The incidence of renal stone formation is approximately 20%.[154] CT is the most sensitive technique for the detection of renal stones and their differentiation from nephrocalcinosis.[155] The stones are most frequently composed of uric acid, or calcium oxalate, or both. Distal acidification defects, abnormal transport of ammonium, low urine pH, and hypocitraturia may be important factors in the pathogenesis of stones.

The treatment of urinary lithiasis is not different from that in patients without ADPKD. Adequate urine flow rate is a central element of therapy. Thiazide diuretics may be used for hypercalciuric states, and potassium citrate has a role when uric acid lithiasis, hypocitraturia, and a distal acidification defect are present in association with renal stones. Uric acid stones can be dissolved despite the anatomic distortion and local stasis of urine caused by cysts impinging on the collecting system. Extracorporeal shock-wave lithotripsy and percutaneous nephrostolithotomy have been used safely for the removal of stones from polycystic kidneys.[156, 157]

LIVER AND GASTROINTESTINAL FINDINGS

The development of hepatic cysts lags far behind that of renal cysts in ADPKD. Liver cysts are rarely found before puberty, but by the age of 50 years, 80% of patients have

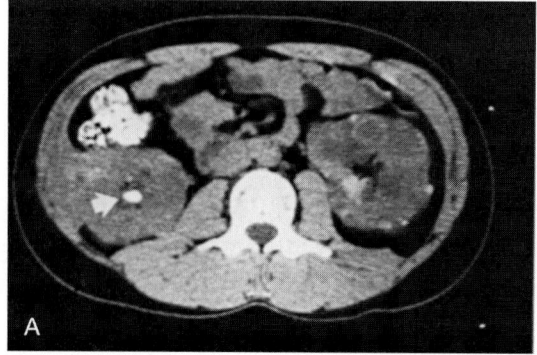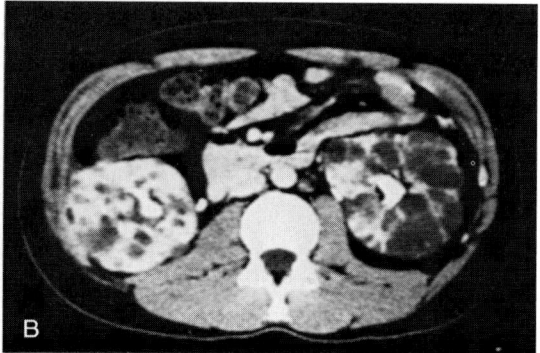

FIGURE 37-10. Computed tomography (CT) scan of polycystic kidneys in a male patient with serum creatinine level within the normal range. **A,** CT scan without contrast shows a radiopaque stone in the pelvis of the right kidney *(arrow)*. **B,** CT scan after intravenous administration of an iodinated radiocontrast agent. The stone now is obscured by contrast medium in the renal pelvis.

radiographically defined liver cysts.[158] Individuals with hepatic cystic disease appear to have worse renal function than those without hepatic cysts. Women generally have greater liver involvement with cysts than men do, and it is not uncommon for the liver cysts to accelerate in size and number after pregnancy. Estrogen replacement may increase the rate of liver cyst growth in postmenopausal women.[159] If symptoms demand the use of estrogenic substances to maintain quality of life, transcutaneous administration of reduced amounts of the agents that are given orally has theoretical advantage, although this has not been formally evaluated. Rarely, hepatic cysts can enlarge enough to cause hepatic venous outflow obstruction and subsequent portal hypertension.[160] The liver may become massively enlarged, even though hepatocellular function remains intact (Fig. 37-11).[161] In cases in which hepatocellular function is impaired, causes other than ADPKD (e.g., hepatitis) should be considered.

Pain, distention, and inanition have been successfully alleviated by partial hepatectomy in extreme cases of liver enlargement.[162] Total hepatectomy is the practice for treating massive hepatomegaly in some centers, but the long-term benefits of this treatment, compared with those of subtotal hepatic resection, have not been determined.[163, 164] Solitary, painful hepatic cysts can be drained percutaneously and fluid reaccumulation aborted by sclerotherapy.

Cysts are occasionally found in the pancreas and spleen. Diverticulosis has been reported in 80% of patients with ADPKD, but one study questioned whether the prevalence of diverticulosis is greater in ADPKD patients than in the population at large.[165] If diverticulitis occurs after transplantation, it can be a serious problem.[166]

PREGNANCY

Women with more than three pregnancies may experience an earlier onset of renal insufficiency than otherwise.[98] Normotensive women with ADPKD usually have uncomplicated pregnancies; however, in those with hypertension beforehand, there is a higher risk for fetal and maternal complications.[167]

END-STAGE DISEASE, DIALYSIS, AND TRANSPLANTATION

ADPKD progresses to the end stage in approximately 45% of affected individuals by 60 years of age.[45] Progression appears to be faster in those who have PKD1 as opposed to PKD2 disease,[44] although considerable variability is observed in the onset of ESRD within families of individuals bearing the same genotype. Consequently, comorbid factors (genetic and nongenetic) probably have strong modifying influences on the progression of the disease. In ADPKD patients with moderate-to-severe renal failure, the glomerular filtration rate appears to decline almost twice as fast as in other types of progressive renal diseases (excluding diabetic nephropathy).[168] However, this relatively rapid decline at the end of the disease process may be misleading because of the long-term compensatory hyperfiltration in residual glomeruli that occurs in slowly (ADPKD) as opposed to more rapidly progressive (diabetic nephropathy) renal diseases (see earlier discussion and Fig. 37-5). Women with ADPKD appear to progress to the end stage at a slower rate than do men.[169]

In retrospective analyses, hypertension has been associated with a more rapid decline in renal function.[44,67] Conversely, a prospective study of ADPKD subjects as a subgroup in the Modification of Diet in Renal Disease Study showed no discernible effect of mildly elevated blood pressure on the rate of decline in GFR, but these patients had progressed to an advanced stage of the disease before the effects of antihypertensive agents were evaluated.[168] A more recent study using historical controls indicated that treatment with antihypertensive agents may protect renal function as well as other cardiovascular side effects.[170] Studies in laboratory animals with hereditary cystic diseases suggest that the early control of hypertension, before severe tubulointerstitial fibrosis supervenes, may preserve renal function.[171, 172] A genetic predisposition to primary hypertension may be associated with an earlier onset of ESRD in ADPKD,[173] although an association of the angiotensin I-converting enzyme gene deletion polymorphism and the early onset of ESRD in ADPKD is controversial.[174, 175]

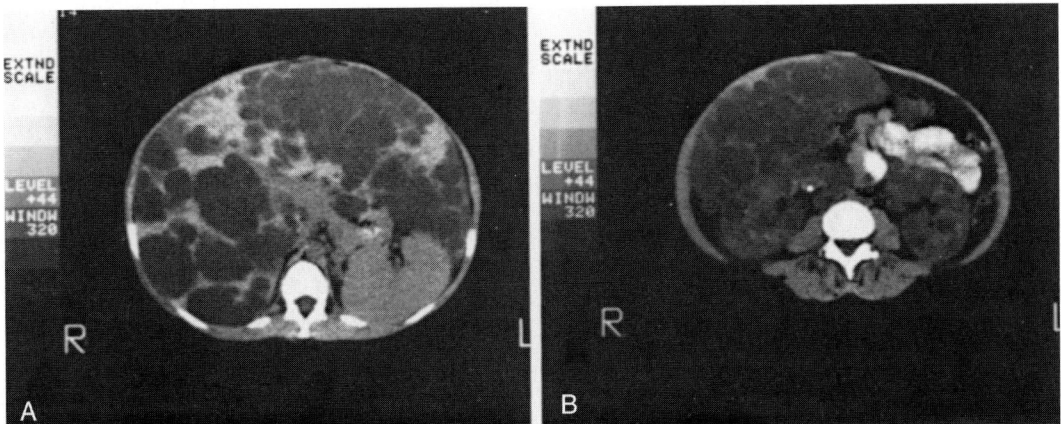

FIGURE 37-11. Computed tomography (CT) scan of polycystic liver and kidneys in female patient with autosomal dominant polycystic kidney disease. The serum creatinine level and liver function test results were within the normal range. An oral contrast agent was given to highlight the intestine, but no intravenous contrast was used. **A,** There is massive enlargement of the liver due to intraparenchymal cysts. **B,** CT scan at a lower level in the abdomen shows cystic kidneys and the lower portion of the cystic liver.

Male gender is a predisposing factor in renal disease progression.[44] Earlier onset of renal failure in both sexes has been related to the PKD1 as opposed to the PKD2 genotype, younger age at diagnosis, larger kidneys, episodes of gross and microscopic hematuria, and moderate-to-severe proteinuria.[1]

Dialysis has been used for more than two decades to treat patients with end-stage ADPKD. Such patients may have higher hematocrit values, without erythropoietin supplementation, than do individuals with other renal diseases. Complications associated with ADPKD subjects undergoing hemodialysis or peritoneal dialysis include rupture of cerebral artery aneurysm, abdominal and inguinal hernias, pyelonephritis, infected renal and hepatic cysts, and massive kidneys and livers requiring resection for symptomatic relief.[176, 177] ADPKD patients do as well or better than others with nondiabetic renal disorders.

Renal transplantation is used routinely to treat patients with end-stage ADPKD. Post-transplantation patient and kidney survival rates appear to be equal if not better than those in other renal disorders. Most ADPKD patients receive the allograft with their native kidneys in place.[178] Native kidneys appear to diminish in size in most patients, but occasionally, persistent enlargement necessitates nephrectomy. Indications for pretransplantation bilateral nephrectomy include severe pain, unrelenting infection, persistent bacteriuria, recurrent severe urinary tract hemorrhage, renal neoplasm, nephrolithiasis, and extreme kidney size with compression of intra-abdominal vessels and viscera leading to symptoms. Other post-transplantation complications associated with ADPKD include cerebral vascular bleeding from aneurysms and peritonitis secondary to ruptured colonic diverticula. Screening for aneurysm was discussed earlier. Colon complications can be diminished if patients are monitored before and after transplantation and segments of bowel with heavy densities of diverticula are resected.[179]

COUNSELING

Guilt and denial are prominent coping patterns in families with ADPKD.[180] Approximately 75% of affected patients indicate knowledge of a family history of ADPKD at the time of diagnosis. In patients with symptoms of ADPKD, a diagnosis should be established after informed consent. We recommend that screening of asymptomatic individuals be considered only for adults (older than 18 years of age). If a patient with the rights of majority in the state in which counseling takes place decides to undergo diagnostic studies to determine the presence or absence of ADPKD, it is reasonable to proceed with physical examination, renal ultrasound examination, urinalysis, and measurement of serum creatinine and urea nitrogen concentrations. Ultrasound screening of those at risk for ADPKD should be performed only after the individual has been apprised of the benefits and the risks of diagnosis. If the ultrasound findings are equivocal or negative in the hands of an experienced radiologist, we recommend heavy-weighted T2 MRI as the best method to rule out cystic disease (see Fig. 37-8).

Benefits that follow testing include the peace of mind that comes from ruling out ADPKD; the opportunity for early management of treatable complications (hypertension, urinary tract infections, impaired renal function, and cerebral aneurysms); and information useful for family planning.

Consequences that weigh against presymptomatic testing include the possibility of medical disqualification for certain careers, medical insurance, and life insurance; loss of the psychological denial defense; and the lack of a specific treatment or cure. In our experience, most asymptomatic individuals at 50% risk for ADPKD do elect not to undergo screening. We advise these individuals to have regular medical examinations that include blood pressure measurements and urinalyses. Those with a family history of cerebral aneurysms probably should be encouraged to undergo screening for renal cysts, with the understanding that a positive diagnosis would be reason to screen also for cerebral aneurysm.

Outstanding material to educate patients and their families about ADPKD can be obtained through the Polycystic Kidney Disease Foundation (www.PKDcure.org).

Prognosis

Once a patient has begun to show a significant decrease in creatinine clearance, the prognosis for the progression of the disease can be judged relatively accurately from the relationship between the reciprocal of the plasma creatinine concentration ($1/P_{Cr}$) and time.[181] Barring intercurrent infections, ureteral obstruction, or other complications, a persistent loss of a fixed amount of creatinine clearance then usually occurs each year and is reflected in a linear decline in $1/P_{Cr}$ versus time. This relationship is valid after the serum creatinine level begins to rise appreciably. In other words, some patients may have normal glomerular filtration rates and plasma creatinine levels for up to 40 years and only then enter into a phase of relatively precipitous decline in $1/P_{Cr}$ as their creatinine clearance rate begins to fall and their serum creatinine concentration rises.

For patients with ADPKD, the probability of being alive and not having ESRD is about 77% at age 50, 57% at age 58, and 52% at age 73 years.[182] How then does one give more specific advice to patients in the age range 20 to 50 years who have ostensibly normal GFR and enlarged, cystic kidneys? We have found that CT and MRI studies with enhancement by radiocontrast and gadolinium, respectively, give the physician grounds for judging the prognosis of life-sustaining renal function over the next decade (see Figs. 37-7, 37-8, 37-10). In a retrospective study using quantitative morphometric analysis of sequential contrast-enhanced CT images, we found that study patients who had less than 43% of renal volume occupied by cysts in the initial scan did not progress to ESRD over the next 8 to 10 years.[183] Conversely, all of those with fractional cyst involvement higher than 43% developed ESRD over this same interval. We found that with careful inspection of CT scans it was possible to estimate the fraction of cyst volume qualitatively to a reasonable degree without resorting to quantitative analysis. To be of greatest value, these findings must be confirmed in a larger study, but until that is done we believe that nephrologists can use CT and MRI scans to reasonably judge prognosis in nonazotemic patients at the extremes of renal cystic change. Those with low degrees of renal volume replacement by cysts can be reassured that they have several years of useful renal function. Those with more extensive changes can be prepared for the dialysis and transplantation treatments that lie ahead.

There is no specific therapy directed at the polycystic disease process that is generally held to be of benefit. In early reports, surgical unroofing of surface cysts (Rovsing's procedure) was reported to increase rather than decrease the progression to renal insufficiency. However, more recent studies suggest that careful cyst aspiration or unroofing relieves pain and hypertension and has no untoward effect on renal function.[102] Laparoscopic approaches have been developed to unroof cysts and relieve symptoms.[104, 106, 108, 184]

Reduction in dietary protein intake has had disappointing results on slowing the progression of renal insufficiency,[168] but this treatment has usually been introduced after the disease has entered the advanced stage. Studies in rodents with polycystic disorders that mimic ADPKD have shown that several exogenous factors can affect the rate at which the disease progresses.[1, 10, 185] Factors that accelerate the rate of functional decline include increased dietary protein, acidosis, low-potassium diet, and the administration of oxidant compounds or testosterone.[64, 96, 186-189] Progression of the disease can be slowed by the administration of a low-protein diet, diets in which soy protein is substituted for ordinary chow protein, alkalinizing salts, lovastatin, probucol, methylprednisolone, and castration.[64, 80, 189, 190] The extent to which these factors that affect disease progression in rodents may be applicable to human ADPKD remains to be determined.

Autosomal Recessive Polycystic Kidney Disease

ARPKD is a rare disorder that occurs once in 6000 to 55,000 live births.[191, 192] It is inherited as an autosomal recessive trait and therefore may occur in siblings but never in the parents. The disease is observed in one fourth of the offspring of parents carrying a mutated recessive gene. Most patients do not have homozygous mutations, and this heterogeneity perhaps accounts for some of the variability in the clinical expression of the disease. The genetic defect has been localized to a large gene in chromosome 6, *PKHD1*, which encodes a protein composed of 4704 amino acids called fibrocystin [41]/polyductin.[193] There is speculation that this protein will be localized to apical cilia of collecting duct cells based on the detection there of other cyst-causing genetic disorders in mice.[194] Perhaps 50% of individuals with ARPKD die from renal insufficiency and pulmonary maldevelopment within hours or days after birth.[195] The remaining patients have a milder form that may not be problematic until later in infancy, childhood, or early adult life.[196, 197] Those who survive the neonatal period have a 50% to 80% chance of surviving at least to age 15 years.[198] A common name used for this disease, infantile polycystic kidney disease, does not accurately describe the nature of the disease, and the bleak prognosis that came to be associated with that term is not always justified.

Pathology

ARPKD affects both the kidneys and the liver in approximately inverse proportions. That is, the disease may be viewed as a spectrum ranging from severe renal damage and mild liver change at one end to mild renal damage and severe liver change at the other. The form with severe renal damage is the more common and is the form that is manifested at or near the time of birth. The form with less severe renal damage and more severe liver damage is less common and usually is manifested in infancy or later.

If ARPKD appears in the perinatal period, it usually is rapidly fatal because of pulmonary hypoplasia, atelectasis, and pulmonary insufficiency, with or without other features of the Potter sequence. The kidneys in such cases are symmetrically and bilaterally enlarged to 10 times normal (Figs. 37-12 and 37-13) and may be the cause of dystocia because of their size. Average combined weight of the kidneys in one series was about 300 g (range, 240 to 563 g), compared with a normal combined weight of about 25 g.[199] The cortical surfaces show innumerable 1- to 2-mm or smaller cysts that, on cut section (see Fig. 37-12), are seen to be continuous with radially oriented, 1- to 8-mm-diameter fusiform or cylindrical channels that occupy the entire kidney. These channels are lined by nondescript cuboidal epithelium and are found

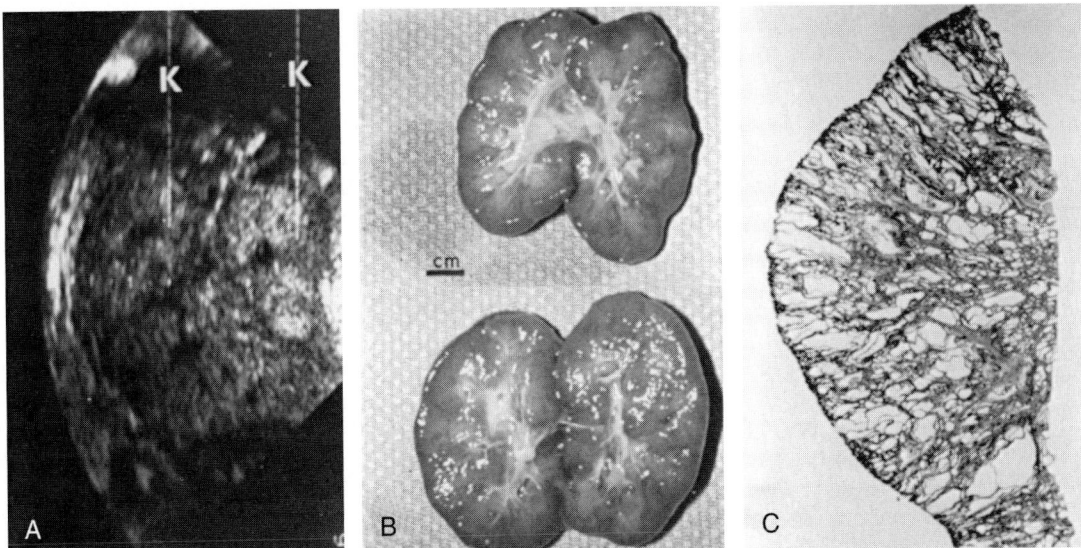

FIGURE 37-12. Autosomal recessive polycystic kidney disease in a 32-week fetus. **A,** Sonogram showing cystic kidneys (K) of fetus in utero. Gross (**B**) and microscopic (**C**) sections show radially oriented cysts of collecting ducts.

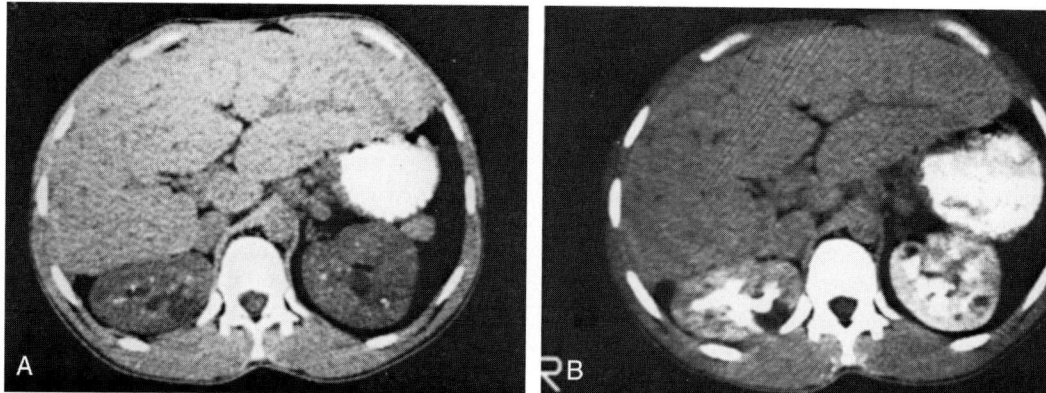

FIGURE 37-13. Computed tomography (CT) scan of autosomal recessive polycystic kidney disease in an 18-year-old male patient with serum creatinine and liver function test results within normal ranges. The patient had clinical evidence of portal hypertension (gastric varices, enlarged spleen). Oral contrast was given to highlight the intestines. **A,** CT scan without contrast enhancement. The liver is enlarged but not cystic. The kidneys are slightly enlarged and contain focal radiodense areas (nephrolithiasis). **B,** CT scan with intravenous iodinated radiocontrast showing cystic areas in both kidneys. The renal calcifications are now obscured by contrast medium in the collecting systems.

by microdissection and by histochemical and specific binding studies[200, 201] to be dilated terminal branches of collecting ducts. A few small, saccular outpouchings from medullary collecting ducts also are found. Perhaps 60% to 90% of all collecting ducts are involved. As the disease progresses, an overall reduction in size may occur. Medullary ductal ectasia continues to be prominent and in kidneys from young adults may be the only obvious abnormality.[202] The picture therefore also resembles, and may be confused with, that in medullary sponge kidney, a completely separate and distinct disease with a far different prognosis (see later discussion). Renal calcifications are common in children with ARPKD.[203] Hypocitraturia and acidification defects resulting from renal insufficiency are the leading factors that contribute to the pathogenesis of calcifications.

The hepatic lesion is diffuse but limited to the portal areas. The parenchyma is unremarkable, and there is no cirrhosis in the usual sense. The central portal bile ducts are absent or reduced in number, and there is hypoplasia of portal veins. Bulbar protrusions from the walls of dilated ducts also occur, and sometimes bridges form. This malformation has been found to occur occasionally as an isolated event (Caroli disease), but most often it is associated with ARPKD.[204]

Diagnosis

The clinical presentation of ARPKD in the newborn is characterized by a history of oligohydramnios and often by a difficult delivery because of the enlarged fetal kidneys. Severely affected infants also may have Potter facies and respiratory distress on the basis of pulmonary hypoplasia and atelectasis. Pneumomediastinum and pneumothorax are common, and pneumonia may develop. Renal function usually is compromised, but death from renal insufficiency is uncommon in the newborn period. Hypertension often develops in the first several months and may be complicated by cardiac hypertrophy, endocardial fibroelastosis, congestive heart failure, and the onset of renal failure. Older children and adolescents may present with symptoms and signs referable to their hepatic fibrosis and portal hypertension,

including gastrointestinal bleeding from varices, portal thrombosis, and hepatosplenomegaly that is possibly complicated by hypersplenism with thrombocytopenia, anemia, and leukopenia. Liver function tests are usually normal. There also may be renal failure and a concentrating defect with secondary effects, including anemia, growth failure, and renal osteodystrophy.

Sonography is the most important diagnostic tool for initial screening purposes as well as for prenatal diagnosis.[205, 206] The typical sonogram (see Fig. 37-12) shows enlarged kidneys with increased echogenicity in the cortex and medulla. It also shows poor definition of the collecting system and rather fuzzy delineation of the kidneys from surrounding tissues. Macrocystic changes may be observed in the kidneys of older patients. CT also has been used with success for diagnostic purposes (see Fig. 37-13), but it is limited to those patients who are able to cooperate during the performance of the test and involves exposure to ionizing radiation,[207] so it is generally unsuitable for very young children. CT can delineate fine details of renal architecture in patients with a doubtful diagnosis. MRI, which does not use ionizing radiation, may be a useful method for the diagnosis of ARPKD. Nonetheless, in children, it still may be difficult to distinguish between ARPKD and ADPKD. The presence of hepatic fibrosis with biliary dysgenesis strongly suggests the diagnosis of ARPKD. Genetic linkage and direct mutational analysis hold promise of more precise diagnosis and characterization of the disease in individual patients.

Therapy

The newborn with large kidneys and Potter sequence who has a history of oligohydramnios probably is in a terminal phase. Those with pulmonary hypoplasia usually succumb to pulmonary insufficiency within the first few days. Nonetheless, until the degree of the pulmonary insufficiency and its cause (pulmonary hypoplasia, pneumothorax, pneumomediastinum, atelectasis, pneumonia, abdominal mass, heart failure) can be assessed fully, artificial ventilation and aggressive resuscitative measures are indicated. Removal of extremely large kidneys has been necessary in a few cases to improve ventilation. Early institution of dialysis has been used successfully.

RENAL INSUFFICIENCY. Patients with less severe ARPKD who survive the newborn period often have near-normal renal function at the time of presentation and thereafter may show stable or even increasing creatinine clearance values during the first 36 months. The enlarged kidneys often appear to decrease in relative size, a phenomenon that appears to be associated with slowly progressive renal insufficiency, anemia, renal osteodystrophy, and hypertension.

The management of chronic renal failure in children with ARPKD should follow the same general guidelines used for any child with established chronic renal insufficiency. That is, children with ARPKD probably should be accepted for dialysis and transplantation on the same terms as other children with ESRD. However, in view of the fact that the associated fibrosing liver disorder may be progressive and untreatable except by liver transplantation, these patients must be classified as high-risk candidates for hemodialysis, peritoneal dialysis, and renal transplantation.

Edema is a common complication and presumably is caused by impaired renal and/or hepatic function. It may be treated by a combination of salt restriction and diuretics but usually requires the more potent loop diuretics, such as furosemide, ethacrynic acid, or bumetanide.

HYPERTENSION. Arterial hypertension has been observed in many patients with ARPKD, either initially or later in the course. It appears to be persistent in most cases but occasionally may diminish or disappear.

Although the proximate cause is not known, most patients respond favorably to salt restriction and the usual antihypertensive drugs (diuretics, vasodilators). There appear to be no unique requirements for specific types of antihypertensive drugs. The much improved prognosis for ARPKD in years has been attributed in large part to the control of hypertension.

HEPATIC INSUFFICIENCY. Hepatocellular function is rarely deranged, and enzyme values are only occasionally mildly elevated. Increased bilirubin or enzyme values suggest the possibility of cholangitis. Signs of portal hypertension usually develop between the ages of 5 and 10 years and must therefore be assessed relatively frequently. Esophageal and gastric varices have been observed frequently in these patients, and gastrointestinal hemorrhage can be life-threatening. Patients with splenomegaly secondary to portal hypertension may have hypersplenism with leukopenia, thrombocytopenia, and anemia. Portacaval and splenorenal shunts have been successful in such children, but the incidence of surgical morbidity has been high. Postoperative renal failure may occur, and hemodialysis must then be available in that period. Splenectomy may be indicated in some cases, but it increases susceptibility to overwhelming bacterial infections and may hinder posttransplantation immunosuppressive medication. If intrahepatic bile duct dilation is prominent (Caroli disease), recurrent cholangitis may be a problem.

URINARY TRACT INFECTION. Like patients with other renal cystic disorders, ARPKD patients are usually susceptible to urinary tract infections and should not be subjected to unnecessary instrumentation. Retrograde ureteral and bladder catheterizations usually can be avoided by use of the new, noninvasive diagnostic techniques. There have been no large series or even anecdotal clinical reports regarding specific treatment of urinary tract infections in these patients,

but a therapeutic approach similar to that discussed in regard to ADPKD seems reasonable.

COUNSELING. Parents who give birth to a child with ARPKD can be advised that, on a statistical basis, each of their children will have a 25% chance of having the disease and a 50% chance of being a carrier of the abnormal gene. Persons with the disease who live long enough to become parents face a low risk of having children with the disease, provided that their spouses are not relatives. Emotional support and education of patient families can be obtained through the Polycystic Kidney Foundation (www.PKDcure.org).

ACQUIRED CYSTIC KIDNEY DISEASE

It was reported in 1977 that some patients maintained on hemodialysis for relatively long periods develop multiple cysts in their remnant kidneys.[208] Since then, many additional cases have been reported and reviewed.[19] The phenomenon is now more popularly called acquired cystic kidney disease (ACKD), and it is known to develop[209] not only in patients undergoing hemodialysis but also, with approximately equal incidence and severity, in patients receiving peritoneal dialysis. It occurs even in those patients, including children, who are chronically azotemic without dialysis. It can affect native kidneys as well as chronically rejected transplanted kidneys, and it has been described in all forms of chronic renal disease. Acquired cysts are found in 7% to 22% of patients with renal failure and serum creatinine values exceeding 3 mg/dL before dialysis, in 44% of patients with less than 3 years of dialysis, and in 75% of patients with more than 3 years of dialysis.[210] In another study, the incidence was 35% in patients with less than 2 years of dialysis, 58% with 2 to 4 years, 75% with 4 to 8 years, and 92% with dialysis for longer than 8 years.[209] The cysts are known to regress in some patients after successful renal transplantation, although cyclosporine has been incriminated as predisposing native kidneys to cyst formation.[211, 212]

A very important additional feature in acquired renal cystic disease has been the occurrence of renal tumors.[212-217] Metastases have been present in 27% of the cases.[218, 219] Carcinoma in dialysis patients is three times more common in the presence than in the absence of acquired renal cysts, and it is six times more common in large cystic kidneys than in small cystic kidneys. Overall, the incidence of renal malignancy in dialysis patients has sometimes been estimated to be 57 to 134 times greater than in the general population.[217]

Pathology

The kidneys usually are equally involved. They may be small, large, or normal in size, even when totally involved by cysts. Most weigh less than 100 g, and about 30% of reported examples weigh less than 50 g. On the other hand, about 25% weigh more than 150 g, and a few exceptional specimens weigh more than 1000 g (Fig. 37-14). In nephrectomy and autopsy specimens, the cysts have varied in number and type from a few subcapsular cysts up to 2 to 3 cm in diameter to numerous smaller cysts that are diffusely distributed. The cysts sometimes are visible on the external surface, may appear to concentrate near the pelvis or corticomedullary junction on cut section, and may be unilocular

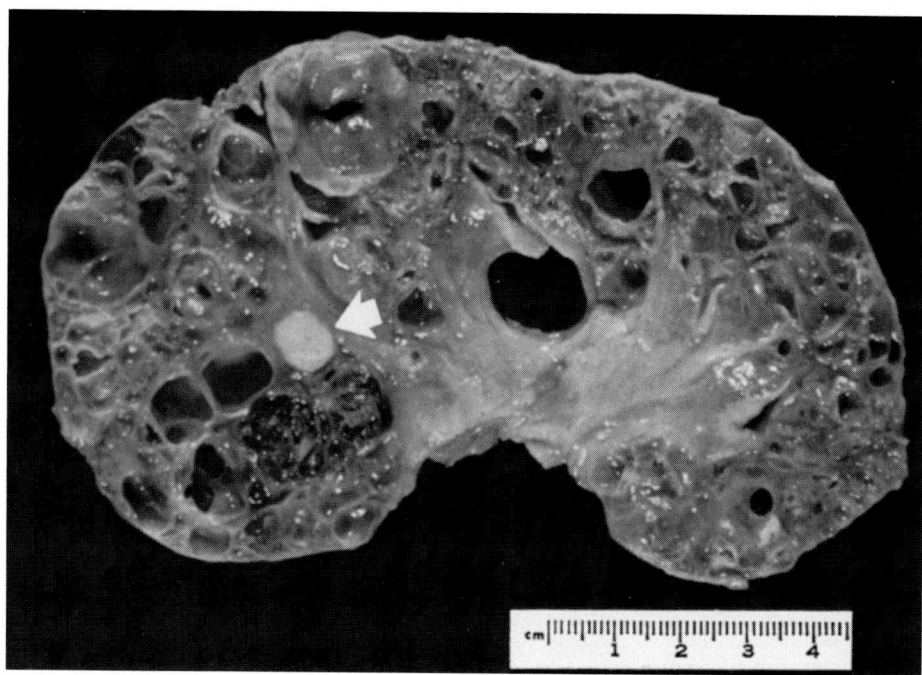

FIGURE 37-14. Acquired cystic disease in 320-g kidney from a patient with a 10-year history of hemodialysis. There were bilateral, multifocal renal cell carcinomas *(arrow)* with multiple systemic metastases.

or multilocular. They may occupy a small portion of the renal mass or, occasionally, such a large portion that the appearance of ADPKD is simulated. Microdissection studies have demonstrated the continuity of the cysts with both proximal and distal tubules and have suggested their origin both in the fusiform dilation of tubule segments and in multiple small tubule diverticula.[220] Because the glomeruli serving the cystic tubule segments often are found to be sclerotic and presumably nonfunctional, the cyst fluid may fill by transepithelial fluid secretion rather than by glomerular filtration.

The cysts most often contain a clear fluid in which the ratio of Na^+ in cyst fluid to the concentration in serum is approximately 1.0, and that for creatinine is considerably greater than 1.0, a composition distinct from that in simple cysts or in the cysts of ADPKD. The cyst fluid occasionally is hemorrhagic, and hemorrhage is sometimes the most prominent feature, with rupture into the pelvis or retroperitoneal area. Microscopically, the original renal tissue is usually very disorganized and contains sclerotic glomeruli, atrophic tubules, and interstitial fibrosis typical of most ESRD, regardless of cause. Hemosiderin-laden macrophages and crystals (usually oxalate) may be prominent in the interstitium. The cyst walls themselves are often not impressive and, regardless of the location, are usually lined only by a flattened cuboidal epithelium.

In a significant fraction of reported cases, the cysts have contained single or, more often, multiple papillary, tubular, or solid neoplasms arising from the cyst lining and consistent with renal cell "adenomas" or adenocarcinomas. The cytology of these tumors is usually not markedly anaplastic, even in cases in which metastases have been documented. The genetic changes underlying the development of most of these tumors are different from those occurring in sporadic clear cell renal cell carcinomas.[219] Whether tumors are more common in the dialyzed patients than in

the uremic, nondialyzed patients also is not clear, and conflicting reports have appeared.[221, 222]

The development of the cysts and tumors seems to be tied to the pronounced epithelial hyperplasia observed microscopically. The hyperplasia, in turn, seems to be a result of the uremic state, even though there appears to be no relation between the occurrence of acquired cysts and the efficacy of dialysis. If ACKD already is present at the time of successful transplantation, that process seems to regress or at least not to increase in severity. Conceivably, the loss of renal mass causes the production of renotropic factors that stimulate hyperplasia. Patients with successful renal allografts usually do not develop cystic disease in their native kidneys, although some reports indicate that renal cancer may develop with a frequency almost equal to that observed in dialysis patients who have not received renal allografts.[223, 224]

Diagnosis

ACKD develops insidiously. Most patients have no symptoms, but when symptoms do occur, gross hematuria, flank pain, renal colic, fever, palpable renal mass, and rising hematocrit are most common. Symptoms associated with renal neoplasm also are uncommon but again include gross hematuria, fever, and back or flank pain, with rising or falling hematocrit, and the complications of metastases. After the rupture of cysts, a large retroperitoneal or perirenal hemorrhage may produce acute pain, hypotension, and shock. Sonography reveals the bilateral cystic process in advanced cases and is useful in the detection of neoplasms, particularly in patients who have chronic renal failure not treated with dialysis and in whom the use of contrast medium might cause a further deterioration in renal function. However, CT, with or without contrast enhancement, is the preferred diagnostic technique and is more capable of distinguishing between kidneys with a few simple cysts and those with multiple acquired cysts (Fig. 37-15). MRI, with or without gadolinium enhancement, may also be useful, particularly for the diagnosis of neoplasms, as an alternative to contrast-enhanced CT in nondialyzed patients and in those cases in which the CT findings are indeterminate.[225] Distinction from ADPKD and from multiple simple cysts usually is suggested by the generally smaller size of the kidneys and of the individual cysts in ACKD, by the usual absence of hepatic cysts, and by the family and patient histories.

Therapy

Bleeding episodes, either intrarenal or perirenal, often may be treated conservatively with bed rest and analgesics. Persistent hemorrhage, however, may require nephrectomy or therapeutic renal embolization and infarction. Because the risk of undetected renal cell carcinoma is high in patients with retroperitoneal hemorrhage, nephrectomy is recommended in those cases in which carcinoma cannot be ruled out. If a few larger cysts are associated with flank pain, percutaneous aspiration (with cytologic examination) is a reasonable temporizing measure. ACKD may regress after successful renal transplantation (see Fig. 37-15B).

Because renal cell carcinoma is an important complication of ACKD, CT screening has been recommended after 3 years of dialysis, followed by screening for neoplasm at 1- or 2-year intervals thereafter. However, because renal cell carcinoma is actually a relatively rare cause of death among dialysis patients, it also has been suggested that a more aggressive renal imaging program and, indeed, even an annual screening program, would be unlikely to reduce the mortality of dialysis patients significantly and therefore would not be justified from a financial standpoint.[226] In the end, the clinical decision must be based on the individual patient, with consideration given both to the known risk factors for carcinoma, including prolonged dialysis, the presence of ACKD, large kidneys, and male sex, and to the patient's age and general fitness.

Renal masses larger than 3 cm detected in ACKD are treated by excision. For tumors smaller than 3 cm, some physicians advise nephrectomy for the acceptable surgical candidate, whereas others recommend annual CT follow-up with resection if the lesions enlarge. Although metastases are statistically less likely to occur from small than from large tumors, small tumor size is not a guarantee against metastasis. Resection even of small neoplasms seems prudent in preparation for transplantation. Even though carcinoma in the setting of ACKD is often multicentric and bilateral, unilateral nephrectomy for tumor does not mandate the removal of an apparently tumor-free contralateral kidney. Instead, frequent monitoring of the contralateral kidney is advised.

CYSTIC DISEASE OF THE RENAL MEDULLA

There are two distinct diseases that primarily involve structures of the renal medulla. Both are associated with variable enlargement of the distal tubules and collecting ducts and with interstitial fibrosis and inflammation of a variable extent. One of them, medullary cystic disease (MCD), progresses to ESRD, and the other, medullary sponge kidney, is a relatively benign condition.

Medullary Cystic Disease

MCD manifests clinically as both autosomal dominant and autosomal recessive conditions. The different genotypes appear grossly similar, but the recessive type, called nephronophthisis (NPH), appears typically in infants and small children, whereas the dominant form may be detected along the entire spectrum of age. The different genotypes share a common and characteristic renal histologic triad of tubular basement membrane disintegration, tubular atrophy with cyst development, and interstitial cell infiltration together with extensive fibrosis. The clinical assessment of individual patients and families is complicated by the fact that autosomal

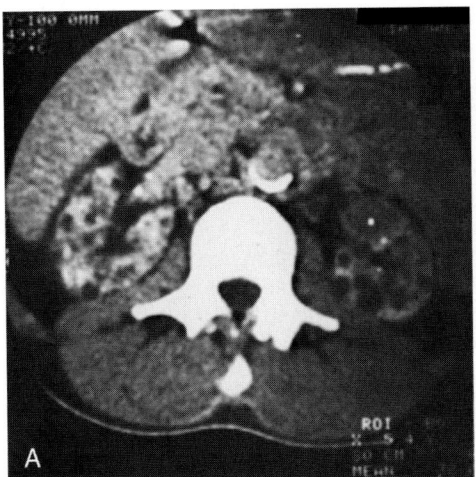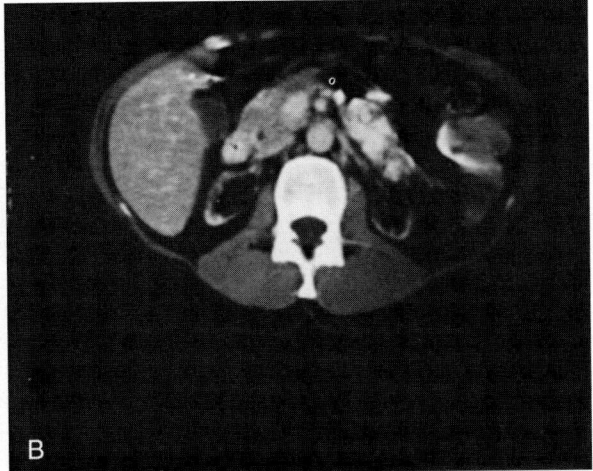

FIGURE 37-15. Acquired renal cystic disease. **A,** Computed tomogram with intravenous contrast. This male patient had renal failure due to diabetic nephropathy and had received hemodialysis for 6 years before this examination. There is bilateral renal enlargement with diffuse cysts in cortex and medulla. A solid tissue tumor *(cursor)* is seen in the anterior part of the left kidney. **B,** Computed tomogram of original kidneys in a patient with a functioning renal allograft. Note the marked atrophy of the renal parenchyma, in contrast to the cystic changes seen in **A.**

dominant (ADMCKD) and the autosomal recessive (NPH) forms exhibit considerable genetic heterogeneity. NPH appears to progress to ESRD at an earlier age than ADMCKD.

ADMCKD has been mapped to chromosomes 1q21 (*ADMCKD1*) and 16p12 (*ADMCKD2*). ADMCKD is characterized by structural renal tubular defects that result in salt wasting and a reduction in urinary concentration. The condition has clinical and morphologic similarities to NPH, which has been localized to three genetic loci: *NPH1* on chromosome 2q12-q13,[227, 228] *NPH2* on chromosome 3q22,[229] and *NPH3* on chromosome 3q21-q22.[230] The gene product of *NPH1* is nephrocystin, a novel protein of unknown function that contains an src-homology 3 domain.[231] NPH seen in association with retinal degeneration, familial retinitis pigmentosa, and pigmentary optic atrophy has been termed *renal-retinal dysplasia*. Associated defects of the skeletal and central nervous system are seen less frequently.

Pathology

The kidneys in these related disorders cannot be distinguished pathologically. They are moderately small with a finely but irregularly granular capsular surface. On cut section, the cortex and medulla are both thinned. The corticomedullary margin is indistinct but is the site of a variable number of spherical, thin-walled cysts that contain fluid resembling normal urine (Fig. 37-16). Similar cysts also may be present in the deeper medulla and papilla.[232, 233] Whereas most kidneys also have a variable number of minute cortical cysts, perhaps 25% have no grossly visible cysts. At the corticomedullary junction, there is a sparse and sometimes nodular chronic inflammatory cell infiltrate. Tubule segments of a single nephron may be encompassed by very dense sclerotic interstitium continuous with peritubular membranes. Microdissections have shown the nephrons to be altered by numerous small diverticula and to be highly variable in size. The cysts are separate objects not directly related to the diverticula and are limited to the distal convoluted and collecting tubule segments. Transmission and scanning electron microscopy show the cysts to be lined by a single layer of epithelium varying from cuboidal or columnar cells that lack microvilli to squamous cells resembling those of the loop of Henle. The tubule basement membranes

frequently are excessively thickened, even fairly early in the course of the disease. Free communication is seen between cysts and nondilated tubules.

Diagnosis

The diagnosis of MCD should be suspected in patients with ESRD in childhood and in azotemic adults with a familial history of renal disease. Genetic linkage analysis may be helpful in arriving at a diagnosis.[231] It is fairly common, at least in the sense that it may account for 1% to 5% of all patients who reach dialysis or transplantation and for 10% to 20% of cases of renal failure in childhood. Clinical presentation usually is in the first or second decade of life but may occur as late as the seventh decade. Excretory urography shows the defect as inhomogeneous streaking confined to the medulla and as resulting from the accumulation of contrast material in the collecting ducts. Sonography, CT, and MRI may be helpful diagnostic procedures, especially for those patients with relatively small medullary cysts that cannot be diagnosed unequivocally with the usual urographic procedures.[234] Open renal biopsy may be the only certain way to make the diagnosis.

Within a family structure, the disease appears to be inherited in a relatively uniform way. For example, patients who manifest renal insufficiency in childhood usually have a form of the disease that is transmitted as an autosomal recessive trait and that presents in a 4- to 10-year-old child with a history of polydipsia, polyuria, pallor, lethargy, and growth retardation. Progression to the end stage of the disease then occurs before the age of 20 years. In the adult form, the clinical presentation is similar with the exceptions that growth retardation and a long history of anemia and other manifestations of ESRD are usually not found and discovery may be delayed until the sixth or seventh decade of life. These adult patients may pass through a period in which they have urinary concentration defects sufficient to cause serious Na^+ wastage, hyponatremia, and extracellular fluid volume contraction. We remember one of these patients well for the fact that he ate approximately 20 g of rock salt and drank 5 to 6 L of fluid each day to maintain blood pressure in an acceptable range. Fractional excretion of Na^+ in the urine, estimated by C_{Na}/C_{inulin}, was approximately 50% in that patient.

It is unusual for patients with MCD to have flank pain, hypertension, hematuria, or renal calculi. This feature stands in contrast to polycystic disease or medullary sponge kidney.

Sodium Wasting

It has been suggested that salt wasting is a cardinal sign of MCD. Although this may be true during certain periods of a patient's life, it is usually a transient condition just preceding the development of ESRD. Presumably, the renal salt wasting occurs secondary to anatomic abnormalities in the distal tubules, collecting ducts, and tubular structures in the medulla, although the cysts themselves may not be directly responsible. It occasionally is associated with hyperreninemia and juxtaglomerular cell hyperplasia, probably secondary to salt depletion. Salt wasting is managed by determining the amount of Na^+ replacement needed to maintain a stable upright position and blood pressure. Some patients require

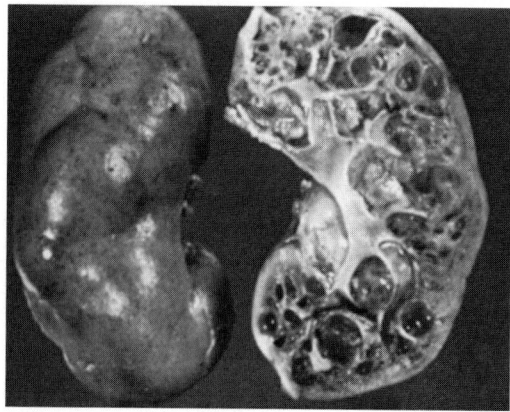

FIGURE 37-16. Outer and cut surface of kidney with severe medullary cystic disease.

vast quantities of NaCl and water to maintain Na$^+$ balance. Should oral intake be interrupted for some reason, intravenous salt and water replacement is mandatory.

On the other hand, as the disease progresses to end stage, it is not uncommon for patients to retain Na$^+$ and to become hypertensive as the number of residual functioning nephrons decreases. At this point, the Na$^+$ and water intake must be reduced to prevent expansion of the extracellular fluid volume.

When acidosis occurs, the diet should be altered to reduce acid residues, and oral sodium bicarbonate should be given in addition to NaCl. The acidosis and hyperkalemia encountered in this disorder are probably caused by a defect in distal tubule handling of Na$^+$, K$^+$, and H$^+$. These disorders are corrected by altering the dietary intake of K$^+$ and H$^+$ and by use of K$^+$-binding ion exchange resins.

Anemia

These patients may have profound anemia that appears earlier than is usual for other diseases leading to renal insufficiency. No specific therapy is known.

Renal Insufficiency

The onset of renal insufficiency in this disorder is usually insidious and is not unique except for the occasional patient with salt wasting. In two patients with MCD, the 1/P$_{Cr}$ relationship was linear over a period of 100 months and indicated that a constant amount of creatinine clearance was being lost per unit time.[235] Clinical infection of the kidney appears to be relatively uncommon in MCD and does not appear to be a major factor in the development of chronic renal failure. Secondary hyperparathyroidism, renal osteodystrophy, and neuropathy may be observed. At the end stage, renal insufficiency can be managed by dialysis or renal transplantation or both.

Counseling

The uncertain pattern of genetic transmission in MCD is a severe obstacle in advising family members of the propensity for genetic transmission and in selecting donors for renal transplantation. If the transplant recipient's renal morphology suggests chronic interstitial nephritis and a living related transplant donor is considered, an extensive search should be made to detect renal disease within the family. Unilateral nephrectomy of the recipient may be necessary to make sure that there are no cysts that might implicate a familial medullary cystic disorder.

The concept of genetic heterogeneity is well established for MCD, and it has been emphasized that the patterns of presentation in children and in adults do not necessarily indicate different disorders. For example, in one study, the parents of 21 patients with childhood onset of MCD also had renal disease in childhood, a situation suggesting autosomal dominant, rather than recessive, inheritance.[236] Therefore, when dealing with MCD, it would seem to be a good rule to consider the disorder to be dominantly inherited until proved otherwise by careful family study. Only when specifically warranted by family study should counseling be directed toward a recessive or a dominant pattern.

Medullary Sponge Kidney

Medullary sponge kidney usually is not recognized until the fourth or fifth decade, when secondary calcareous or infective complications emerge. Progression to renal failure is uncommon. The incidence of this disease is approximately 1 in 5000 in the general population and perhaps 1 in 1000 in patients studied in urology clinics.[237] However, at least a mild degree of the condition may be found in about 20% of patients with nephrolithiasis, the incidence in males being about half that in females.[238] Although most cases appear sporadically, family tendencies have been reported. Curiously, as many as 25% of patients with medullary sponge kidney may have hemihypertrophy of the body, and about 10% of patients with hemihypertrophy also have medullary sponge kidney.[239] Although the affected kidney does not closely resemble a sea sponge, the term *medullary sponge kidney* is common usage. Alternate terms, such as precalyceal canalicular ectasia and cystic dilation of renal collecting ducts, are more accurate but are not widely accepted.

Pathology

The only visible abnormality in this disease is the marked spherical, oval, or irregular enlargement of the medullary and inner papillary portions of collecting ducts. One or several papillae may be affected, and the lesions are bilateral in 70% of cases. Unilateral involvement of only one pyramid is quite uncommon. The dilated ducts communicate proximally with collecting tubules of normal size and often show a relative constriction to approximately normal diameter at the point of their communication with the calyx. Their diameter is often 1 to 3 mm, occasionally 5 mm, and rarely up to 7.5 mm.[237] They may contain clear, jelly-like or dry brown material or, frequently, small calculi. Free calculi are found in about 60% of symptomatic patients. Complications, such as lithiasis with infection and intrarenal obstruction, are common, and secondary changes of the cortex and medulla are seen accordingly. The kidney is otherwise normal in its architecture and development.

Diagnosis

The disease is associated with gross and microscopic hematuria that may be recurrent and with urinary tract infections that often are the first signs of an underlying abnormality. Nephrolithiasis with renal colic, loin pain, and excretion of small stones is also a prominent feature. The disease seldom progresses to ESRD, although reduced glomerular filtration rates have been observed, and perhaps 10% of patients have a relatively poor prognosis because of recurring urolithiasis, bacteriuria, septicemia, and probably pyelonephritis. The most commonly recognized functional abnormalities include defective urinary solute concentrating ability, inability to reduce the urinary pH to a minimum value of 5.5, and systemic acidosis secondary to renal tubular acidosis.[240] Diagnosis is by intravenous urography, which shows radial, linear striations in the papillae or cystic collections of contrast medium in the ectatic collecting ducts (Fig. 37-17). Calcium precipitates also collect in the ectatic collecting duct segments to give, in some patients, a characteristic radiographic pattern

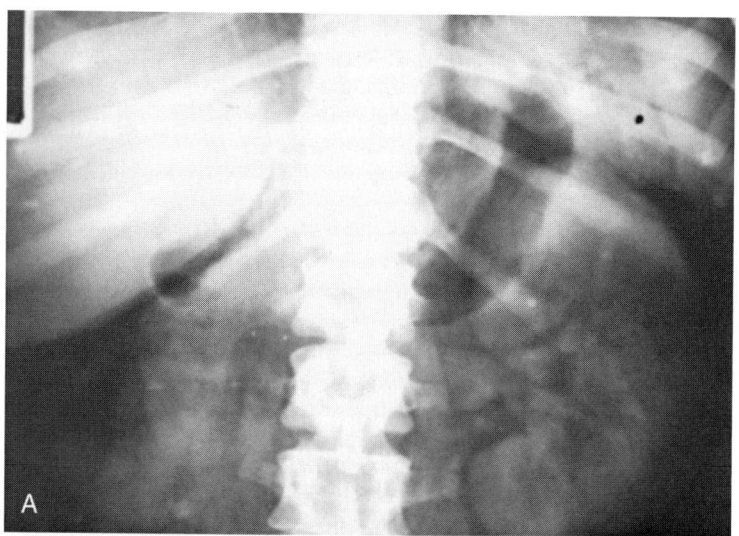

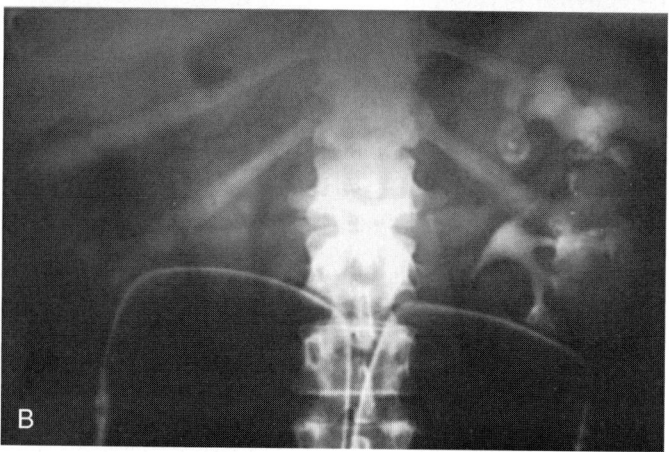

FIGURE 37-17. Medullary sponge kidney. **A,** Plain roentgenogram of a large solitary left kidney containing several calcific densities. **B,** Urogram showing the pronounced tubular ectasia of all papillae that is typical of medullary sponge abnormality. (Courtesy of G. D. Dixon, Kansas City, MO.)

that is obscured by radiocontrast material. Sonography and CT usually are not necessary but may resolve confusion with papillary necrosis or, rarely, even with polycystic disease or transitional cell carcinoma.

Renal Tubule Acidosis

The renal tubule acidosis in this condition has not been characterized beyond recognition that it is of the classic "distal" type. The impact of bicarbonate therapy on the pathogenesis of nephrolithiasis has not been examined critically in patients with complete or incomplete renal tubule acidosis of this type. Because oral administration of alkali increases, rather than decreases, the urinary pH, there might be some risk of promoting calculus formation in patients who have calcium phosphate stones in their ectatic tubules.

Nephrolithiasis

Renal stones consisting of calcium oxalate, calcium phosphate, and other types of calcium salts commonly form in the ectatic collecting ducts in this disease. Nephrolithiasis is therefore a common clinical problem. In studies in which there are strict criteria for the quality of acceptable intravenous urograms, the incidence of medullary sponge kidney

has been about 13% in patients with calcium urolithiasis but only about 2% in otherwise normal patients.[238] Among all calcium stone formers, women have a greater incidence of medullary sponge kidney than do men.[241]

The possible relationship between hyperparathyroidism and medullary sponge kidney has been emphasized, and it has been postulated that renal Ca^{2+} loss causes a reduction in plasma ionized Ca^{2+} concentration that in turn stimulates the secretion of parathyroid hormone. It is thought that this process may ultimately cause the formation of parathyroid adenomas.

In a critical examination of Ca^{2+} excretion in patients with medullary sponge kidney and other stone-forming disorders, absorptive hypercalciuria was the most common abnormality in medullary sponge kidney, occurring in 59% of patients, whereas only 18% had hypercalciuria resulting from renal Ca^{2+} leak.[242] It is generally held that patients with medullary sponge kidneys and renal stones have the same spectrum of metabolic abnormalities as appears in the overall population of stone formers and should be so evaluated and treated. Asymptomatic patients found incidentally to have medullary sponge kidney require no specific therapy but should have yearly routine urinalysis. As a general rule, patients with nephrolithiasis should excrete about 2 L of urine each day to reduce the propensity for calcium salts to precipitate in the collecting ducts and renal pelves. Patients with hypercalciuria may benefit from long-term therapy with thiazide diuretics, but this treatment may elevate plasma Ca^{2+} levels. For patients with calcium urolithiasis and normal urinary Ca^{2+} excretion, oral phosphate therapy may be useful. There are no reports of an increased incidence of hyperuricosuria in patients with medullary sponge kidney, but of course this possibility should be kept in mind in the routine evaluation of such a patient. If hyperuricosuria is observed, a trial of allopurinol may slow the formation of urinary stones.

In some instances, the persistence of renal stone formation in kidneys with medullary sponge disease has been associated with significant morbidity from the pain of urolithiasis and urinary tract infection with persistent bacteriuria.

Renal abscesses are a rare complication that may require prolonged antibiotic therapy or surgical drainage. In some cases, especially those in which the tubule ectasia is unilateral or segmental, a unilateral or partial nephrectomy has resulted in sustained freedom from nephrolithiasis, urolithiasis, and urosepsis. Because medullary sponge kidney is usually a bilateral disorder, however, partial or complete nephrectomy should be undertaken cautiously and only after careful evaluation indicates that sufficient function will remain to sustain life. Patients with medullary sponge kidney appear to be more susceptible to urinary tract infections, and routine preventive measures seem warranted, especially in female patients. Patients who recurrently form and pass stones may benefit from lithotripsy.

Counseling

Most patients discovered incidentally to have medullary sponge kidney can be advised that the disorder is benign and that they can anticipate no serious morbidity or mortality from it. On the other hand, nephrolithiasis can be a difficult problem in symptomatic patients. A clear familial transmission of this disease has not been established. If there is a history of medullary sponge disease in the family, however, detailed investigation is advisable to determine a potential genetic pattern of transmission.

SIMPLE CYSTS

Simple cysts are the most common cystic abnormality encountered in human kidneys. They may be solitary or multiple and are filled with a fluid that is chemically similar to an ultrafiltrate of plasma. They are very rare in children and increase in frequency approximately linearly with age. In autopsy studies and in incidental CT findings of the abdomen, they are found in approximately 50% of patients at 50 years of age. On the other hand, ultrasound may turn up a somewhat lower percentage. Simple cysts do not appear to be associated with any decrease in renal function and, almost by definition, are not hereditary. Early work suggested that simple cysts develop in the renal parenchyma as a consequence of ischemia, but the exact mechanism remains obscure. Some information indicates that simple cysts, like other cystic structures in the cortex and medulla, probably develop from preexisting tubules and perhaps derive from tubule diverticulae.[243, 244] In contrast to cysts in ADPKD, electrolyte gradients typical of proximal and distal

cysts have not been found. The cyst walls also appear to be relatively impermeable to low-molecular-weight solutes and to antibiotics.[245] Nonetheless, the turnover of cyst fluid may be as great as 20 times per day, as measured by ^3H_2O diffusion.[246]

Pathology

Simple cysts may be unilateral or bilateral, and they are usually spherical and unilocular. There may be only one or a few per kidney, but rarely they may be so numerous as to be confused with ADPKD or with acquired PKD. The cysts are often cortical and distort the renal contour, but they may be deep cortical or apparently medullary in origin. They do not communicate with the renal pelvis. Cyst diameters of 0.5 to 1 cm are common, but 3- to 4-cm cysts are not unusual. Rare cysts have been reported to contain many liters of fluid. The cyst fluid is usually urine-like in appearance but may occasionally be blood stained or, rarely, have the consistency of glazier's putty. Hydrostatic pressure within the cysts averages 15 mm Hg but has a wide range (−1 to +42 mm Hg), even among cysts in the same kidney. The walls typically are thin and transparent but may become thickened, fibrotic, opaque, and even calcified as the presumed result of earlier infection. Microscopically, the cysts compress adjacent, otherwise normal tissue and are lined by a single layer of simple, flattened epithelium that may appear to be discontinuous.

Diagnosis

Most simple cysts are found on routine urographic examinations. With increasing use of abdominal sonography, CT, and MRI, they are being recognized more frequently (Fig. 37-18). They are far more common in adults than in children. Patients, particularly children, occasionally present with a palpable abdominal mass, hematuria after abdominal trauma, or mild proteinuria. Simple cysts also have been associated with urethral valves or prostatic hyperplasia, with caliceal obstruction, hematuria, and massive calicovenous reflux, erythrocytosis, and intestinal or biliary obstruction. Hypertension has been attributed to simple cysts in a few cases, and occasionally a patient with an infected cyst may present with flank pain, pyuria, fever, and leukocytosis and, rarely, with perforation with disastrous results. In the vast majority of cases, however, the simple cysts are asymptomatic, and the major problem becomes one of differentiating between simple cyst and malignant mass.

With lesions as common as simple cysts, it is not surprising that the coincidence of simple cyst and tumor in the same kidney is 2% to 4%. Nonetheless, it is very uncommon to find a neoplasm actually arising within a cyst, and with modern diagnostic techniques the risk of failure to recognize cancer in association with a cyst is quite small.[247, 248] Therefore, in asymptomatic patients with a few small and unequivocal simple cysts discovered by urography, CT, or MRI, further evaluation, except perhaps for periodic follow-up by sonography, is probably not indicated in the absence of fever, leukocytosis, hematuria, or renal discomfort. Conversely, if the renal mass discovered on urography is of questionable nature or indeterminate, sonography is probably the next logical step. After that would be CT, using as suggested criteria for benign cyst a homogeneous attenuation value of near-water density, no enhancement with

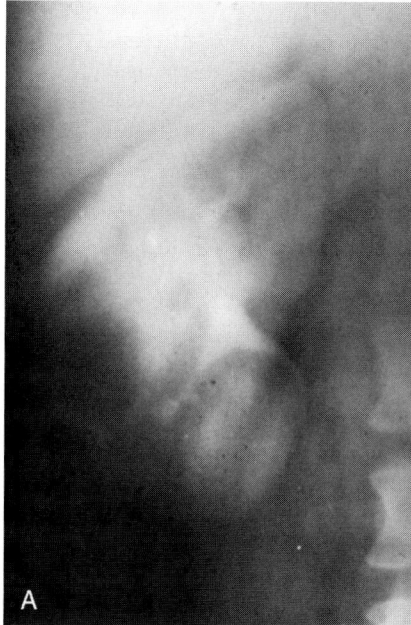
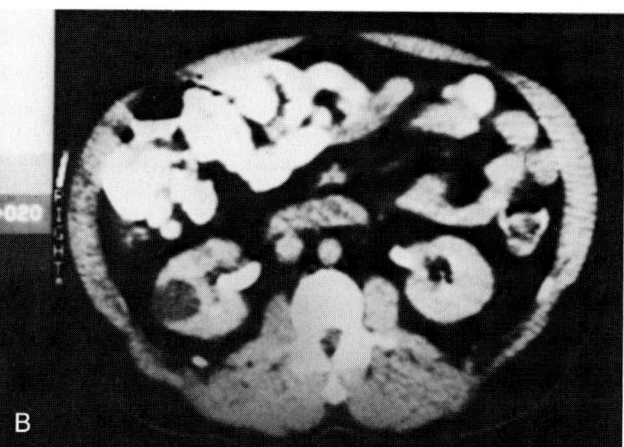

FIGURE 37-18. Simple renal cysts. **A,** Solitary cortical cyst of right kidney seen by intravenous urography. **B,** Solitary cyst of right renal cortex seen by computed tomography with intravenous contrast enhancement. Oral contrast material was given to highlight the intestine.

intravenous contrast material, no measurable thickness of the cyst wall, and a smooth interface with renal parenchyma. If these criteria are not met, the cyst falls into an indeterminate or solid category, and surgical exploration is recommended. MRI with and without gadolinium enhancement may be of some help, as may be the finding of calcification. Two percent of simple cysts and 10% of renal cell carcinomas contain Ca^{2+} deposits, but calcification in simple cysts appears to be peripheral, whereas that in tumors is more central. Nonetheless, it has been said that calcification within a renal mass lesion should be considered to reflect malignancy until proved otherwise.

Percutaneous cyst puncture to confirm a benign cause has been advocated in the past, but more recently was argued to be unnecessary in view of the high probability of correct diagnosis by CT. If cyst puncture is performed, the character of the aspirated fluid is of special importance. Simple cyst fluid is usually straw colored and clear and is free of erythrocytes, leukocytes, and atypical cells. By contrast, fluid aspirated from cystic malignant tumors is usually bloody or dark colored, has a high content of cholesterol and total lipids, and contains malignant cells on cytologic examination.

No rigid criteria have been adopted for the use of CT, sonography, arteriography, MRI, and cyst puncture in the evaluation of patients with questionable renal mass lesions. Clearly, all of these techniques have some value in their own right in selected cases. The quality and availability of the equipment and the expertise of the radiologist also figure prominently in the approach to the renal mass in individual institutions. There is insufficient information determined prospectively to decide whether CT can completely supplant ultrasound and angiographic evaluation of renal mass lesions. Until such studies are performed, it seems reasonable to employ arteriography, ultrasound, CT, and MRI together in the evaluation of questionable cystic lesions of the kidney.

Therapy

The management of symptomatic renal cysts can take several forms. Most intermediate-sized cysts can be aspirated percutaneously, and a sclerosing agent can be instilled into the cavity in an attempt to prevent recurrence. Symptomatic cysts greater than 500 mL in volume are usually drained surgically. Laparoscopic methods are now used routinely.

Hypertension has been attributed to simple cysts in a few patients and sometimes has disappeared after successful aspiration of the cyst fluid or operative removal of the cyst. Renal vein plasma renin activity is usually elevated in such cases, and the mechanism is thought to be compression of adjacent vessels by cysts with selective renal ischemia and increased renin production.

Several examples of infected simple renal cysts have been reported in association with flank pain, pyuria, fever, and leukocytosis. Differentiation from renal abscess may be difficult, but it has been suggested that the clinical triad of acute pyelonephritis, a vascular mass lesion in the kidney, and ipsilateral pleural effusion is more characteristic of abscess. Enterobacteriaceae, staphylococci, and *Proteus* species organisms have been encountered most frequently in infected cysts. An operative approach is usually taken, but percutaneous aspiration and drainage of infected cysts also have been used. Conservative treatment has not been specifically evaluated. If simple cysts cause calyceal obstruction, cyst drainage or enucleation is recommended to relieve the obstruction and the potential for urinary tract infection.

RENAL DYSPLASIA

The term *renal dysplasia* implies that the anlagen of the kidney, the ureteric bud and the metanephric blastema, have both formed embryologically but subsequently have failed to interact and develop in a normal way. In practice, it has come to mean any developmental abnormality resulting from anomalous metanephric differentiation and is applied to any kidney that contains structures that do not recapitulate any stage in the normal renal development. Renal dysplasia therefore includes a spectrum of renal defects with certain features in common. Most dysplastic kidneys are associated either with an abnormally located ureteral orifice or with urinary tract anomalies that are expected to produce unilateral, bilateral, or segmental urinary obstruction.

Many, but not all, are associated with renal cystic changes. In general, the most severely dysplastic kidneys are nonfunctional, have no patent connection to the urinary bladder, and remain asymptomatic if unilateral. Less severely dysplastic kidneys may have near-normal function and manifest with clinical symptoms and signs related only to their size or to their increased susceptibility to infection. Renal dysplasia most often appears sporadically. In a small minority of cases there is a familial tendency.

Pathology

Although most dysplastic kidneys are grossly deformed in a fairly characteristic way, most authors accept only two absolute criteria for dysplasia, and both of those require histologic confirmation (Fig. 37-19).[249] Of greater importance is the finding of primitive ducts encompassed by mantles of variably differentiated mesenchyma and lined by cuboidal to columnar, sometimes ciliated, epithelium unlike that in any normally developing or mature ducts. Somewhat less important because of its variable presence is the finding of metaplastic cartilage. Primitive or fetal glomeruli with cuboidal epithelium, primitive tubules, and ductules surrounded by narrow collars of laminated connective tissue. Cysts of glomerular, tubule, and ductal origin may also be present, but because they might represent either a maldevelopment or a histologically similar degenerative change in previously normal but immature structures, they do not provide absolute evidence of parenchymal maldevelopment.

Cyst formation may accompany any dysplastic defect as an incidental feature. Microdissection studies have shown the cysts to occur most often at the terminal ends of short primitive ducts in the most severely dysplastic kidneys and at the ends or along the course of collecting tubules and terminal duct branches in less severe cases. However, that cysts may or may not be present or, more accurately and with few exceptions, they may range in size and number from small and few to large and numerous.

Because of the varying degrees and distributions of the dysplastic lesions as well as the varying sizes and distributions of incidental cysts, it is apparent that dysplastic kidneys can be large or small, cystic or noncystic, and approximately normal in shape or grossly distorted. The most distorted cystic examples are said to resemble a bunch of grapes (Fig. 37-20).

Diagnosis

The clinical presentation and diagnosis of renal dysplasia is very much determined by the extent of the dysplastic involvement and by the degree of associated urinary obstruction.[250-253] It is convenient, therefore, to consider two major clinicopathologic subsets of renal dysplasia that, for lack of a less confusing and more commonly accepted terminology, we shall call total and subtotal dysplasia. A third, very uncommon, subset of hereditary dysplasia is discussed separately.

TOTAL DYSPLASIA. Kidneys with severe dysplasia involving both the cortex and the medulla (i.e., dysplasia affecting the total kidney) are almost always, if not invariably, associated with ureteral or ureteropelvic absence or atresia. They contain solid areas consistent with rudimentary lobules but otherwise lack normal pyelocalyceal development and lobular organization. A maldevelopment beginning in early gestation therefore appears likely. Small, solid kidneys, termed *aplastic*, and variably enlarged (up to several hundred grams), grossly cystic kidneys, termed *multicystic* (see Fig. 37-20), represent a spectrum ranging from small fibrotic nubbins at one end to large cystic masses at the other. All kidneys in this group are nonfunctional and are not visualized on excretory urograms, although high-dose urography may sometimes result in opacification of cyst walls, and delayed films may demonstrate retention of contrast medium. The ureter is found to be absent or atretic on retrograde pyelography. Cyst walls often calcify in older patients and may be seen as ring-like densities in the region

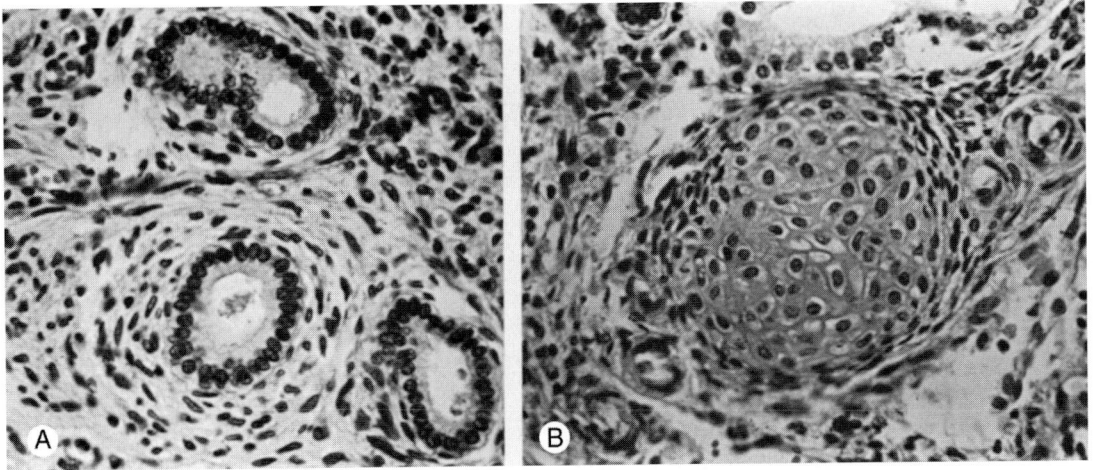

FIGURE 37-19. Renal dysplasia. The diagnostic microscopic features include primitive ducts (**A**) and metaplastic cartilage (**B**).

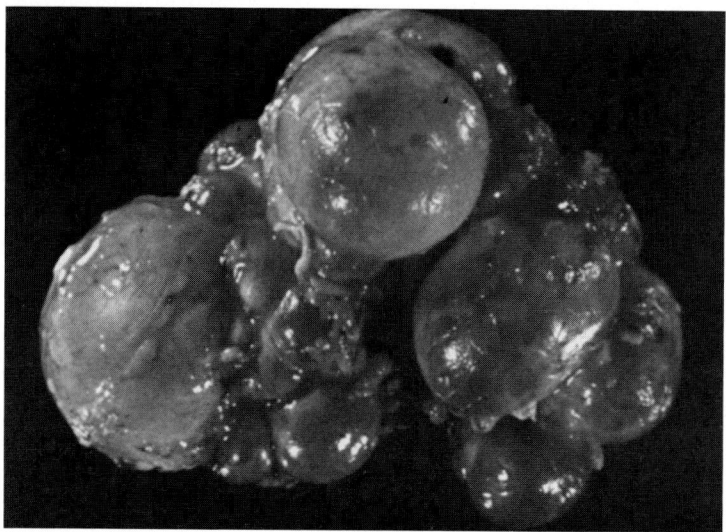

FIGURE 37-20. Severe renal cystic dysplasia (multicystic kidney). The renal architecture is markedly distorted.

of the kidney. The renal artery is usually very small or absent. Sonography and CT also are useful in diagnosis, and sonography has revealed multicystic kidneys in fetuses in utero.

Bilateral total dysplasia is fatal in the newborn period in association with the Potter sequence of oligohydramnios and pulmonary insufficiency. If present as a unilateral isolated abnormality, however, a totally dysplastic kidney usually remains asymptomatic and is discovered incidentally during a renal or abdominal evaluation for unrelated reasons. In contrast to the less severely dysplastic kidneys that do have patent ureters (discussed later), these kidneys are not associated with hypertension or with infection. However, dysplastic kidneys frequently are ectopic, and a pelvic kidney is likely to be dysplastic. There is a high incidence of bilateral defects (80%) and of other major anomalies in multiple organ systems that call attention to a diffuse embryonic defect.

The so-called multicystic variety of total renal dysplasia is about three times more common than the noncystic atrophic, or "hypodysplastic," variety and is the most common type of renal cystic disease diagnosed throughout childhood. It also is the most common cause of abdominal mass in infancy and the most common type of bilateral cystic disease in newborns. The incidence is approximately 0.02 to 0.05 per 100,000 hospital admissions. Bilateral involvement is far less common than unilateral.

SUBTOTAL DYSPLASIA. In contrast to the severely dysplastic kidneys with complete urinary obstruction, kidneys with partly normal development and dysplasia in only a medullary, cortical, or focal distribution are associated with evidence of less severe urinary obstruction in conditions such as ureteral narrowing, megaureter, megacystic megaureter, posterior urethral valves or constriction, ectopic ureter with or without ureterocele, prune-belly syndrome, and developmental neurospinal bladder dysfunction. Segmental dysplasia is most common in the upper pole in association with ectopic ureterocele. In general, urethral or other obstruction severe enough to be apparent shortly after birth is often accompanied by dysplasia of this type, whereas similar obstruction not manifesting until later childhood usually is not.

Kidneys with less than total dysplasia are functional to some extent and do appear on excretory urograms.

Those with patent ureters also appear to be unusually liable to ascending infection. The incidence of contralateral and extraurinary tract anomalies is quite high.

FAMILIAL AND HEREDITARY DYSPLASIA. Early interference with renal organogenesis would explain the occasionally severe dysplasias seen in Meckel and sometimes in Zellweger, Jeune, and oral-facial-digital syndromes. With these exceptions, however, the lesions tend to be mild, perhaps even limited to mildly abnormal glomeruli with cystic capsules (termed *peripheral cortical microcysts*), and usually produce no renal insufficiency.[254, 255]

Therapy

Bilateral totally dysplastic kidneys are rapidly fatal in the newborn period and require only supportive therapy. On the other hand, unilateral totally dysplastic, aplastic, or multicystic kidneys are usually asymptomatic and probably require only occasional follow-up. Neoplasms, both benign and malignant, have been reported in multicystic kidneys but are sufficiently rare that prophylactic nephrectomy is not warranted.

MISCELLANEOUS CYSTIC DISORDERS

Tuberous Sclerosis

In this disease complex, hamartomatous tumors may develop in the skin, brain, retina, bone, liver, heart, lung, and kidney.[256] Renal angiomyolipomas are found in as many as 50% of the patients and must be distinguished from multiple renal cysts, which occur less commonly. The tubular cysts in this disease are lined by a very distinct, perhaps unique epithelium of markedly hypertrophic and hyperplastic cells with prominent eosinophilic cytoplasm bearing some resemblance to that of the proximal tubule. The combination of cystic kidneys and angiomyolipomas has been said to be virtually pathognomonic for tuberous sclerosis.[257] The cysts may be quite large, and renal impairment, although relatively uncommon, may occur before other evidence of the syndrome. Hypertension is a major manifestation of the renal abnormality. There have been several reports of associated renal carcinoma.

Tuberous sclerosis has an incidence of approximately 1:10,000. It is inherited by autosomal dominant transmission, so family history is important in the diagnostic workup. There are two genotypes: *TSC1* is located on chromosome 9q32p34 and encodes a protein called hamartin[258]; *TSC2* is located next to *PKD1* on chromosome 16p13 and encodes a protein called tuberin.[259] Hamartin and tuberin appear to function together in a tumor-suppressor role.[260] Deletion of portions of *PKD1* and *TSC2* leads to an aggressive form of polycystic kidney disease. Sonography, CT, MRI, and arteriography are of value in distinguishing the multiple renal cysts from the more common angiomyolipomas in this disease.

von Hippel–Lindau Syndrome

This syndrome includes cerebellar and retinal hemangioblastomas, pancreatic cysts and carcinoma, and renal cysts and tumors. Numerous irregularly distributed renal cysts up to several centimeters in diameter are found in about 65% of patients. They occasionally are sufficiently numerous to simulate ADPKD. The cyst lining is a flattened, nondescript or cuboidal epithelium that focally may show nodular hyperplasia with apparent progression to clear cell carcinoma. These malignant tumors are often multiple and bilateral. Carcinomas occur in about one fourth of cases, metastasize in about half of those, and cause death in about one third.[261]

This disease is inherited by autosomal dominant transmission, and patients usually present in the third or fourth decade with visual or central nervous system complaints.[262] The gene defect has been localized to the short arm of chromosome 3 and has been linked to an oncogene locus that is possibly involved in spontaneous renal cell carcinoma. Because the chance of cancer existing in a cyst wall or a solid tumor probably is large, family screening and early diagnosis are imperative. MRI and CT are helpful in evaluating the renal lesions, and annual or semiannual examination is recommended for patients at risk, beginning in the second decade. A conservative approach has been advocated for the treatment of the associated renal adenocarcinomas.

Solitary Multilocular Cysts

Also termed benign cystic nephroma or papillary cystadenoma, these rare lesions are neoplasms arising from metanephric blastema. On cut surface, the mass contains numerous individual cysts ranging from a few millimeters to a few centimeters in diameter and filled with clear fluid. Thin and delicate fibrous septa separate the locules and continue into a fibrous capsule that sharply circumscribes the lesion. Microscopically, cysts and dilated tubules are surrounded by a loose mesenchymal stroma that contains clusters of small, poorly developed tubules. No cartilage or other strictly identifiable dysplastic structures are found within the lesion, although smooth muscle and cartilage have been described in the capsule.

Multilocular cysts have very distinctive bimodal age and sex distributions. In one study, 88% of the lesions in males manifested during the first 3 years of life, whereas in females, 37% of the lesions manifested between the ages of 10 months and 15 years and 63% between the ages of 31 and 69 years, predominantly in the fifth and sixth decades. They usually are fairly large (5 to 10 cm in diameter) and often replace one pole. They also are capable of rapid growth and may be found in kidneys observed to be normal only a few years earlier. Even though these lesions are generally considered to be benign, extension beyond the renal capsule may be present.

Furthermore, in 19 of the 200 or so reported cases, the multilocular mass has contained foci of nephroblastoma, sarcoma, or renal cell carcinoma. Three of four patients with sarcoma subsequently died from metastases.[263] Nonetheless, after angiographic and sonographic distinction from other potentially dangerous segmental renal lesions (particularly Wilms tumor and neuroblastoma in children), multilocular cysts require no specific therapy or, at most, partial nephrectomy.

Pyelocalyceal Cysts

Also termed pyelocalyceal diverticula or calyceal or pyelorenal cysts or diverticula, these lesions represent congenital, probably developmental, saccular diverticula from a minor calyx (type I) or from the pelvis or adjacent major calyx (type II). Type I is more common, is usually located in the poles (especially the upper), and tends to be smaller and less often symptomatic than the centrally located type II variety. Both types are usually less than 1 cm in diameter but occasionally may be quite large. The cysts are encompassed by a muscularis, are lined by a usually chronically inflamed transitional epithelium, and usually contain cloudy fluid or frank pus that may be expressed with applied pressure. Transitional cell carcinoma arising in a pyelocalyceal cyst has been reported rarely.

Pyelocalyceal cysts occur sporadically, affect all age groups, and are almost always unilateral. They may be detected in as many as 0.5% of excretory urograms but usually are small and asymptomatic. Symptomatic lesions are more often of larger or medium size; patients present with loin pain and evidence of recurrent pyelonephritis. Calculi are present within the cyst cavity in 10% to 40% of cases but are rarely passed. They may, however, be the cause of outlet obstruction and spontaneous cyst rupture into the perinephric space.

Renal Lymphangiomatosis

Also known as hilar lymphangiectasis, pericalyceal or paracalyceal lymphangiectasis, peripelvic or parapelvic lymphangiectasis, or polycystic disease of the renal sinus, renal lymphangiomatosis consists of cystically dilated renal lymphatic channels. They may be limited to the hilar region adjacent to major blood vessels, or they may extend approximately to the level of the corticomedullary junction. Occasionally, they may also involve the renal capsule and adjacent areas and may simulate polycystic disease. The cysts may be single and unilateral, multiple and unilateral, or multiple and bilateral. The fluid contains albumin, lipid, and cholesterol and therefore does not resemble urine. Renal lymphangiomas are usually asymptomatic and are found incidentally. Sometimes, however, they result in presentation as a mass; as a cause of urinary obstruction, calculus formation, or infection; and perhaps even as a cause of renal ischemia and hypertension. Diagnosis can be made by CT and sonography.[264, 265]

Hilar and Perinephric Pseudocysts

Hilar cysts are unlined, spherical accumulations of clear, fat droplet–containing fluid within compressed fat of the renal sinus. They evidently result from atrophy of fat in debilitated patients. Perinephric pseudocysts are unlined spaces filled with urine extravasated into the perirenal fascia after traumatic or spontaneous rupture of an underlying renal cyst. Some degree of chronic ureteral obstruction is probably also required, and extravasation may continue unless bleeding and clotting intervene. There is a characteristic radiologic and CT appearance. The most serious clinical complication is urinary obstruction requiring surgical intervention. Treatment otherwise is directed to the underlying cause. Nephrectomy may be required in half of the cases.

REFERENCES

1. Grantham J, Cowley BJ, Torres VE: Progression of autosomal dominant polycystic kidney disease (ADPKD) to renal failure. *In* Seldin D, Giebisch G (eds): The Kidney: Physiology and Pathophysiology, Vol 2. Philadelphia, Lippincott Williams & Wilkins, 2000, pp 2513-2536.
2. Grantham JJ: Polycystic kidney disease: From the bedside to the gene and back. Curr Opin Nephrol Hypertens 10:533-542, 2001.
3. Evan AP, Gardner KD Jr, Bernstein J: Polypoid and papillary epithelial hyperplasia: A potential cause of ductal obstruction in adult polycystic disease. Kidney Int 16:743-750, 1979.
4. Grantham JJ, Geiser JL, Evan AP: Cyst formation and growth in autosomal dominant polycystic kidney disease. Kidney Int 31:1145-1152, 1987.
5. Gregoire JR, Torres VE, Holley KE, Farrow GM: Renal epithelial hyperplastic and neoplastic proliferation in autosomal dominant polycystic kidney disease. Am J Kidney Dis 9:27-38, 1987.
6. Nadasdy T, Laszik Z, Lajoie G, et al: Proliferative activity of cyst epithelium in human renal cystic diseases. J Am Soc Nephrol 5:1462-1468, 1995.
7. Lu W, Peissel B, Babakhanlou H, et al: Perinatal lethality with kidney and pancreas defects in mice with a targetted Pkd1 mutation. Nat Genet 17:179-181, 1997.
8. Wu G, D'Agati V, Cai Y, et al: Somatic inactivation of Pkd2 results in polycystic kidney disease. Cell 93:177-188, 1998.
9. Sweeney WE, Chen Y, Nakanishi K, et al: Treatment of polycystic kidney disease with a novel tyrosine kinase inhibitor. Kidney Int 57:33-40, 2000.
10. Grantham JJ: Time to treat polycystic kidney diseases like the neoplastic disorders that they are. Kidney Int 57:339-340, 2000.
11. Qian Q, Harris PC, Torres VE: Treatment prospects for autosomal-dominant polycystic kidney disease. Kidney Int 59:2005-2022, 2001.
12. Sullivan LP, Wallace DP, Grantham JJ: Epithelial transport in polycystic kidney disease. Physiol Rev 78:1165-1191, 1998.
13. Sullivan LP, Wallace DP, Grantham JJ: Chloride and fluid secretion in polycystic kidney disease. J Am Soc Nephrol 9:903-916, 1998.
14. Wallace DP, Rome LA, Sullivan LP, Grantham JJ: cAMP-dependent fluid secretion in rat inner medullary collecting ducts. Am J Physiol Renal Physiol 280:F1019-F1029, 2001.
15. Grantham JJ, Wallace DP: Return of the secretory kidney. Am J Physiol Renal Physiol 282:F1-F9, 2002.
16. Carone FA, Makino H, Kanwar YS: Basement membrane antigens in renal polycystic disease. Am J Pathol 130:466-471, 1988.
17. Wilson PD, Norman JT, Kuo NT, Burrow CR: Abnormalities in extracellular matrix regulation in autosomal dominant polycystic kidney disease. Contrib Nephrol 118:126-134, 1996.
18. Wilson PD, Hreniuk D, Gabow PA: Abnormal extracellular matrix and excessive growth of human adult polycystic kidney disease epithelia. J Cell Physiol 150:360-369, 1992.
19. Grantham JJ: Acquired cystic kidney disease. Kidney Int 40:143-152, 1991.
20. Schafer K, Bader M, Gretz N, et al: Focal overexpression of collagen IV characterizes the initiation of epithelial changes in polycystic kidney disease. Exp Nephrol 2:190-195, 1994.
21. Rankin CA, Suzuki K, Itoh Y, et al: Matrix metalloproteinases and TIMPS in cultured C57BL/6J-cpk kidney tubules. Kidney Int 50:835-844, 1996.
22. Rankin CA, Itoh Y, Tian C, et al: Matrix metalloproteinase-2 in a murine model of infantile-type polycystic kidney disease. J Am Soc Nephrol 10:210-217, 1999.
23. Schaefer L, Han X, Gretz N, et al: Tubular gelatinase A (MMP-2) and its tissue inhibitors in polycystic kidney disease in the Han:SPRD rat. Kidney Int 49:75-81, 1996.
24. Wilson PD, Burrow CR: Cystic diseases of the kidney: Role of adhesion molecules in normal and abnormal tubulogenesis. Exp Nephrol 7:114-124, 1999.
25. Wilson PD: Polycystin: New aspects of structure, function, and regulation. J Am Soc Nephrol 12:834-845, 2001.
26. Geng L, Burrow CR, Li HP, Wilson PD: Modification of the composition of polycystin-1 multiprotein complexes by calcium and tyrosine phosphorylation. Biochim Biophys Acta 1535:21-35, 2000.
27. van Adelsberg J: Polycystin-1 interacts with E-cadherin and the catenins: Clues to the pathogenesis of cyst formation in ADPKD? Nephrol Dial Transplant 15:1-2, 2000.
28. Rodova M, Islam MR, Maser RL, Calvet JP: The polycystic kidney disease-1 promoter is a target of the beta-catenin/T-cell factor pathway. J Biol Chem 277:29577-29583, 2002.
29. Reeders ST, Breuning MH, Davies KE, et al: A highly polymorphic DNA marker linked to adult polycystic kidney disease on chromosome 16. Nature 317:542-544, 1985.
30. Kimberling WJ, Kumar S, Gabow PA, et al: Autosomal dominant polycystic kidney disease: Localization of the second gene to chromosome 4q13-q23. Genomics 18:467-472, 1993.
31. Hughes J, Ward CJ, Peral B, et al: The polycystic kidney disease 1 (PKD1) gene encodes a novel protein with multiple cell recognition domains. Nat Genet 10:151-160, 1995.
32. International Polycystic Kidney Disease Consortium: Polycystic kidney disease: The complete structure of the PKD1 gene and its protein. The International Polycystic Kidney Disease Consortium. Cell 81:289-298, 1995.
33. American PKD1 Consortium: Analysis of the genomic sequence for the autosomal dominant polycystic kidney disease (PKD1) gene predicts the presence of a leucine-rich repeat. Hum Mol Genet 4:575-582, 1995.
34. Somlo S, Ehrlich B: Human disease: Calcium signaling in polycystic kidney disease. Curr Biol 11:R356-R360, 2001.
35. Igarashi P, Somlo S: Genetics and pathogenesis of polycystic kidney disease. J Am Soc Nephrol 13:2384-2398, 2002.
36. Calvet JP, Grantham JJ: The genetics and physiology of polycystic kidney disease. Semin Nephrol 21:107-123, 2001.
37. Delmas P, Nomura H, Li X, et al: Constitutive activation of G-proteins by polycystin-1 is antagonized by polycystin-2. J Biol Chem 277:11276-11283, 2002.
38. Harris PC: Molecular basis of polycystic kidney disease: PKD1, PKD2 and PKHD1. Curr Opin Nephrol Hypertens 11:309-314, 2002.
39. Qian F, Watnick TJ, Onuchic LF, Germino GG: The molecular basis of focal cyst formation in human autosomal dominant polycystic kidney disease type I. Cell 87:979-987, 1996.
40. Brasier JL, Henske EP: Loss of the polycystic kidney disease (PKD1) region of chromosome 16p13 in renal cyst cells supports a loss-of-function model for cyst pathogenesis. J Clin Invest 99:194-199, 1997.
41. Ward CJ, Hogan MC, Rossetti S, et al: The gene mutated in autosomal recessive polycystic kidney disease encodes a large, receptor-like protein. Nat Genet 30:259-269, 2002.
42. Nagasawa Y, Matthiesen S, Onuchic LF, et al: Identification and characterization of Pkhd1, the mouse orthologue of the human ARPKD gene. J Am Soc Nephrol 13:2246-2258, 2002.
43. Gabow P: Definition and natural history of autosomal dominant polycystic kidney disease. *In* Watson ML, Torres VE (eds): Polycystic Kidney Disease. Oxford, Oxford University Press, 1996, pp 333-355.
44. Johnson AM, Gabow PA: Identification of patients with autosomal dominant polycystic kidney disease at highest risk for end-stage renal disease. J Am Soc Nephrol 8:1560-1567, 1997.
45. Parfrey PS, Bear JC, Morgan J, et al: The diagnosis and prognosis of autosomal dominant polycystic kidney disease. N Engl J Med 323:1085-1090, 1990.

46. Levine E, Cook LT, Grantham JJ: Liver cysts in autosomal-dominant polycystic kidney disease: Clinical and computed tomographic study. AJR Am J Roentgenol 145:229-233, 1985.

47. Baert L: Hereditary polycystic kidney disease (adult form): A microdissection study of two cases at an early stage of the disease. Kidney Int 13:519-525, 1978.

48. Evan AP, McAteer JA: Cyst cells and cyst walls. *In* Gardner KD Jr, Bernstein J (eds): The Cystic Kidney. Boston, Kluwer, 1990, pp 21-42.

49. Verani RR, Silva FG: Histogenesis of the renal cysts in adult (autosomal dominant) polycystic kidney disease: A histochemical study. Mod Pathol 1:457-463, 1988.

50. Gardner KD Jr: Composition of fluid in twelve cysts of a polycystic kidney. N Engl J Med 281:985-988, 1969.

51. Cuppage FE, Huseman RA, Chapman A, Grantham JJ: Ultrastructure and function of cysts from human adult polycystic kidneys. Kidney Int 17:372-381, 1980.

52. Gardner KD Jr, Burnside JS, Skipper BJ, et al: On the probability that kidneys are different in autosomal dominant polycystic disease. Kidney Int 42:1199-1206, 1992.

53. Ye M, Grantham JJ: The secretion of fluid by renal cysts from patients with autosomal dominant polycystic kidney disease. N Engl J Med 329:310-313, 1993.

54. Grantham JJ, Ye M, Davidow C, et al: Evidence for a potent lipid secretagogue in the cyst fluids of patients with autosomal dominant polycystic kidney disease. J Am Soc Nephrol 6:1242-1249, 1995.

55. Grantham JJ, Schreiner GF, Rome L, et al: Evidence for inflammatory and secretagogue lipids in cyst fluids from patients with autosomal dominant polycystic kidney disease. Proc Assoc Am Physicians 109:397-408, 1997.

56. Torres VE: Polycystic liver disease. Contrib Nephrol 115:44-52, 1995.

57. Watnick TJ, Torres VE, Gandolph MA, et al: Somatic mutation in individual liver cysts supports a two-hit model of cystogenesis in autosomal dominant polycystic kidney disease. Mol Cell 2:247-251, 1998.

58. Gabow PA, Johnson AM, Kaehny WD, et al: Risk factors for the development of hepatic cysts in autosomal dominant polycystic kidney disease. Hepatology 11:1033-1037, 1990.

59. Terada T, Nakanuma Y: Congenital biliary dilatation in autosomal dominant adult polycystic disease of the liver and kidneys. Arch Pathol Lab Med 112:1113-1116, 1988.

60. Cobben JM, Breuning MH, Schoots C, et al: Congenital hepatic fibrosis in autosomal-dominant polycystic kidney disease. Kidney Int 38:880-885, 1990.

61. Torres VE, Wiebers DO, Forbes GS: Cranial computed tomography and magnetic resonance imaging in autosomal dominant polycystic kidney disease. J Am Soc Nephrol 1:84-90, 1990.

62. Woo D: Apoptosis and loss of renal tissue in polycystic kidney diseases. N Engl J Med 333:18-25, 1995.

63. Woo DD, Nguyen DK, Khatibi N, Olsen P: Genetic identification of two major modifier loci of polycystic kidney disease progression in pcy mice. J Clin Invest 100:1934-1940, 1997.

64. Cowley BD, Jr, Grantham JJ, Muessel MJ, et al: Modification of disease progression in rats with inherited polycystic kidney disease. Am J Kidney Dis 27:865-879, 1996.

65. Harris PC: Autosomal dominant polycystic kidney disease: Clues to pathogenesis. Hum Mol Genet 8:1861-1866, 1999.

66. Gabow PA, Chapman AB, Johnson AM, et al: Renal structure and hypertension in autosomal dominant polycystic kidney disease. Kidney Int 38:1177-1180, 1990.

67. Watson ML: Hypertension in polycystic kidney disease. *In* Watson ML, Torres VE (eds): Polycystic Kidney Disease. Oxford, Oxford University Press, 1996, pp 407-429.

68. Ecder T, Schrier RW: Hypertension in autosomal-dominant polycystic kidney disease: Early occurrence and unique aspects. J Am Soc Nephrol 12:194-200, 2001.

69. Maschio G, Alberti D, Janin G, et al: Effect of the angiotensin-converting-enzyme inhibitor benazepril on the progression of chronic renal insufficiency. The Angiotensin-Converting-Enzyme Inhibition in Progressive Renal Insufficiency Study Group. N Engl J Med 334:939-945, 1996.

70. Zeier M, Fehrenbach P, Geberth S, et al: Renal histology in polycystic kidney disease with incipient and advanced renal failure. Kidney Int 42:1259-1265, 1992.

71. Chapman AB, Johnson AM, Gabow PA, Schrier RW: Overt proteinuria and microalbuminuria in autosomal dominant polycystic kidney disease. J Am Soc Nephrol 5:1349-1354, 1994.

72. Russo LM, Bakris GL, Comper WD: Renal handling of albumin: A critical review of basic concepts and perspective. Am J Kidney Dis 39:899-919, 2002.

73. Gattone VH, Grantham JJ: Understanding human cystic disease through experimental models. Semin Nephrol 11:617-631, 1991.

74. Schaefer L, Han X, Gretz N, Schaefer RM: Alterations of cathepsins B, H and L in proximal tubules from polycystic kidneys of the Han:SPRD rat. Kidney Int 50:424-431, 1996.

75. Schafer K, Gretz N, Bader M, et al: Characterization of the Han:SPRD rat model for hereditary polycystic kidney disease. Kidney Int 46:134-152, 1994.

76. Gardner KD Jr, Evan AP, Reed WP: Accelerated renal cyst development in deconditioned germ-free rats. Kidney Int 29:1116-1123, 1986.

77. Kelly CJ, Neilson EG: The interstitium of the cystic kidney. *In* Gardner KD Jr, Bernstein JB (eds): The Cystic Kidney. Boston, Kluwer, 1996, pp 43-53.

78. Cowley BD Jr, Ricardo SD, Nagao S, Diamond JR: Increased renal expression of monocyte chemoattractant protein-1 and osteopontin in ADPKD in rats. Kidney Int 60:2087-2096, 2001.

79. Zheng D, Cowley BDJ, Wolfe M, et al: Monocyte chemoattractant protein-1 (MCP-1) in urine and cyst fluid of patients with autosomal dominant polycystic kidney disease (ADPKD). J Am Soc Nephrol 13:507A, 2002.

80. Gattone VH 2nd, Cowley BD Jr, Barash BD, et al: Methylprednisolone retards the progression of inherited polycystic kidney disease in rodents. Am J Kidney Dis 25:302-313, 1995.

81. Ritz E, Zeier M, Waldherr R: Progression to renal insufficiency. *In* Watson ML, Torres VE (eds): Polycystic Kidney Disease. Oxford, Oxford University Press, 1996, pp 430-449.

82. Gabow PA, Kaehny WD, Johnson AM, et al: The clinical utility of renal concentrating capacity in polycystic kidney disease. Kidney Int 35:675-680, 1989.

83. Preuss H, Geoly K, Johnson M, et al: Tubular function in adult polycystic kidney disease. Nephron 24:198-204, 1979.

84. Duncan KA, Cuppage FE, Grantham JJ: Urinary lipid bodies in polycystic kidney disease. Am J Kidney Dis 5:49-53, 1985.

85. Ravine D, Gibson RN, Walker RG, et al: Evaluation of ultrasonographic diagnostic criteria for autosomal dominant polycystic kidney disease 1. Lancet 343:824-827, 1994.

86. Ravine D, Gibson RN, Donlan J, Sheffield LJ: An ultrasound renal cyst prevalence survey: Specificity data for inherited renal cystic diseases. Am J Kidney Dis 22:803-807, 1993.

87. Gabow PA, Kimberling WJ, Strain JD, et al: Utility of ultrasonography in the diagnosis of autosomal dominant polycystic kidney disease in children. J Am Soc Nephrol 8:105-110, 1997.

88. Levine E, Grantham JJ: The role of computed tomography in the evaluation of adult polycystic kidney disease. Am J Kidney Dis 1:99-105, 1981.

89. Levine E, Grantham JJ: Radiology of cystic kidneys. *In* Gardner KD Jr, Bernstein J (eds): The Cystic Kidney. Boston, Kluwer, 1990, pp 1781-1206.

90. Koptides M, Deltas CC: Autosomal dominant polycystic kidney disease: Molecular genetics and molecular pathogenesis. Hum Genet 107:115-126, 2000.

91. Sujansky E, Kreutzer SB, Johnson AM, et al: Attitudes of at-risk and affected individuals regarding presymptomatic testing for autosomal dominant polycystic kidney disease. Am J Med Genet 35:510-515, 1990.

92. Morris-Stiff G, Coles G, Moore R, et al: Abdominal wall hernia in autosomal dominant polycystic kidney disease. Br J Surg 84:615-617, 1997.

93. Meyrier A, Simon P: Drooping upper eyelids and polycystic kidney disease. J Am Soc Nephrol 5:1266-1270, 1994.

94. Hihara T, Ohnishi H, Muraishi O, et al: MR imaging of seminal vesicle cysts associated with adult polycystic kidney disease. Radiat Med 11:24-26, 1993.

95. Belet U, Danaci M, Sarikaya S, et al: Prevalence of epididymal, seminal vesicle, prostate, and testicular cysts in autosomal dominant polycystic kidney disease. Urology 60:138-141, 2002.

96. Torres VE, Young WF Jr, Offord KP, Hattery RR: Association of hypokalemia, aldosteronism, and renal cysts. N Engl J Med 322:345-351, 1990.

97. Ecder T, Edelstein CL, Fick-Brosnahan GM, et al: Diuretics versus angiotensin-converting enzyme inhibitors in autosomal dominant polycystic kidney disease. Am J Nephrol 21:98-103, 2001.

98. Gabow PA, Johnson AM, Kaehny WD, et al: Factors affecting the progression of renal disease in autosomal-dominant polycystic kidney disease. Kidney Int 41:1311-1319, 1992.

99. Gabow PA, Duley I, Johnson AM: Clinical profiles of gross hematuria in autosomal dominant polycystic kidney disease. Am J Kidney Dis 20:140-143, 1992.

100. Bajwa ZH, Gupta S, Warfield CA, Steinman TI: Pain management in polycystic kidney disease. Kidney Int 60:1631-1644, 2001.

101. Uemasu J, Fujiwara M, Munemura C, et al: Effects of topical instillation of minocycline hydrochloride on cyst size and renal function in polycystic kidney disease. Clin Nephrol 39:140-144, 1993.

102. Elzinga LW, Barry JM, Torres VE, et al: Cyst decompression surgery for autosomal dominant polycystic kidney disease [see comments]. J Am Soc Nephrol 2:1219-1226, 1992.

103. Fleming TW, Barry JM: Bilateral open transperitoneal cyst reduction surgery for autosomal dominant polycystic kidney disease. J Urol 159:44-47, 1998.

104. Elashry OM, Nakada SY, Wolf JS Jr, et al: Laparoscopy for adult polycystic kidney disease: A promising alternative. Am J Kidney Dis 27:224-233, 1996.

105. Brown JA, Torres VE, King BF, Segura JW: Laparoscopic marsupialization of symptomatic polycystic kidney disease. J Urol 156:22-27, 1996.

106. Dunn MD, Portis AJ, Naughton C, et al: Laparoscopic cyst marsupialization in patients with autosomal dominant polycystic kidney disease. J Urol 165:1888-1892, 2001.

107. Seshadri PA, Poulin EC, Pace D, et al: Transperitoneal laparoscopic nephrectomy for giant polycystic kidneys: A case control study. Urology 58:23-27, 2001.

108. Rehman J, Landman J, Andreoni C, et al: Laparoscopic bilateral hand assisted nephrectomy for autosomal dominant polycystic kidney disease: Initial experience. J Urol 166:42-47, 2001.

109. Lifson BJ, Teichman JM, Hulbert JC: Role and long-term results of laparoscopic decortication in solitary cystic and autosomal dominant polycystic kidney disease. J Urol 159:702-705; discussion 705-706, 1998.

110. Zwettler U, Zeier M, Andrassy K, et al: Treatment of gross hematuria in autosomal dominant polycystic kidney disease with aprotinin and desmopressin acetate. Nephron 60:374, 1992.

111. Harley JD, Shen FH, Carter SJ: Transcatheter infarction of a polycystic kidney for control of recurrent hemorrhage. AJR Am J Roentgenol 134:818-820, 1980.

112. Ubara Y, Tagami T, Sawa N, et al: Renal contraction therapy for enlarged polycystic kidneys by transcatheter arterial embolization in hemodialysis patients. Am J Kidney Dis 39:571-579, 2002.

113. Schwab SJ, Bander SJ, Klahr S: Renal infection in autosomal dominant polycystic kidney disease. Am J Med 82:714-718, 1987.

114. Grunfeld JP, Bennett WM: Clinical aspects of autosomal dominant polycystic kidney disease. Curr Opin Nephrol Hypertens 4:114-120, 1995.

115. Miller-Hjelle MA, Hjelle JT, Jones M, et al: Polycystic kidney disease: An unrecognized emerging infectious disease? Emerg Infect Dis 3:113-127, 1997.

116. Hjelle JT, Waters DC, Golinska BT, et al: Autosomal recessive polycystic kidney disease: Characterization of human peritoneal and cystic kidney cells in vitro. Am J Kidney Dis 15:123-136, 1990.

117. Miller MA, Prior RB, Horvath FJ, Hjelle JT: Detection of endotoxiuria in polycystic kidney disease patients by the use of the limulus amebocyte lysate assay. Am J Kidney Dis 15:117-122, 1990.

118. Hjelle JT, Miller-Hjelle MA, Poxton IR, et al: Endotoxin and nanobacteria in polycystic kidney disease. Kidney Int 57:2360-2374, 2000.

119. Kajander EO, Ciftcioglu N, Miller-Hjelle MA, Hjelle JT: Nanobacteria: Controversial pathogens in nephrolithiasis and polycystic kidney disease. Curr Opin Nephrol Hypertens 10:445-452, 2001.

120. Ciftcioglu N, Miller-Hjelle MA, Hjelle JT, Kajander EO: Inhibition of nanobacteria by antimicrobial drugs as measured by a modified microdilution method. Antimicrob Agents Chemother 46:2077-2086, 2002.

121. Muther RS, Bennett WM: Cyst fluid antibiotic concentrations in polycystic kidney disease: Differences between proximal and distal cysts. Kidney Int 20:519-522, 1981.

122. Schwab S, Hinthorn D, Diederich D, et al: PH-dependent accumulation of clindamycin in a polycystic kidney. Am J Kidney Dis 3:63-66, 1983.

123. Elzinga LW, Golper TA, Rashad AL, et al: Trimethoprim-sulfamethoxazole in cyst fluid from autosomal dominant polycystic kidneys. Kidney Int 32:884-888, 1987.

124. Elzinga LW, Golper TA, Rashad AL, et al: Ciprofloxacin activity in cyst fluid from polycystic kidneys. Antimicrob Agents Chemother 32:844-847, 1988.

125. Iglesias CG, Torres VE, Offord KP, et al: Epidemiology of adult polycystic kidney disease, Olmsted County, Minnesota: 1935–1980. Am J Kidney Dis 2:630-639, 1983.

126. Chapman AB, Johnson A, Gabow PA, Schrier RW: The renin-angiotensin-aldosterone system and autosomal dominant polycystic kidney disease [see comments]. N Engl J Med 323:1091-1096, 1990.

127. Chapman AB, Gabow PA: Hypertension in autosomal dominant polycystic kidney disease. Kidney Int Suppl 61:S71-S73, 1997.

128. Ecder T, Edelstein CL, Fick-Brosnahan GM, et al: Progress in blood pressure control in autosomal dominant polycystic kidney disease. Am J Kidney Dis 36:266-271, 2000.

129. Sedman A, Bell P, Manco-Johnson M, et al: Autosomal dominant polycystic kidney disease in childhood: A longitudinal study. Kidney Int 31:1000-1005, 1987.

130. Zeier M, Geberth S, Schmidt KG, et al: Elevated blood pressure profile and left ventricular mass in children and young adults with autosomal dominant polycystic kidney disease. J Am Soc Nephrol 3:1451-1457, 1993.

131. Bell PE, Hossack KF, Gabow PA, et al: Hypertension in autosomal dominant polycystic kidney disease. Kidney Int 34:683-690, 1988.

132. Brkljacic B, Sabljar-Matovinovic M, Putarek K, et al: Renal vascular resistance in autosomal dominant polycystic kidney disease: Evaluation with color Doppler ultrasound. Acta Radiol 38:840-846, 1997.

133. Torres VE, Wilson DM, Offord KP, et al: Natriuretic response to volume expansion in polycystic kidney disease. Mayo Clin Proc 64:509-515, 1989.

134. Torres VE, Wilson DM, Burnett JC Jr, et al: Effect of inhibition of converting enzyme on renal hemodynamics and sodium management in polycystic kidney disease. Mayo Clin Proc 66:1010-1017, 1991.

135. Klein IH, Ligtenberg G, Oey PL, et al: Sympathetic activity is increased in polycystic kidney disease and is associated with hypertension. J Am Soc Nephrol 12:2427-2433, 2001.

136. Neumann J, Ligtenberg G, Klein IH, Blankestijn PJ: Pathogenesis and treatment of hypertension in polycystic kidney disease. Curr Opin Nephrol Hypertens 11:517-521, 2002.

137. Li Kam Wa TC, Macnicol AM, Watson ML: Ambulatory blood pressure in hypertensive patients with autosomal dominant polycystic kidney disease. Nephrol Dial Transplant 12:2075-2080, 1997.

138. Watson ML, Macnicol AM, Allan PL, Wright AF: Effects of angiotensin converting enzyme inhibition in adult polycystic kidney disease. Kidney Int 41:206-210, 1992.

139. Chapman AB, Gabow PA, Schrier RW: Reversible renal failure associated with angiotensin-converting enzyme inhibitors in polycystic kidney disease [see comments]. Ann Intern Med 115:769-773, 1991.

140. Chapman AB, Rubinstein D, Hughes R, et al: Intracranial aneurysms in autosomal dominant polycystic kidney disease [see comments]. N Engl J Med 327:916-920, 1992.

141. Nakajima F, Shibahara N, Arai M, et al: Intracranial aneurysms and autosomal dominant polycystic kidney disease: followup study by magnetic resonance angiography. J Urol 164:311-313, 2000.

142. Watnick T, Phakdeekitcharoen B, Johnson A, et al: Mutation detection of PKD1 identifies a novel mutation common to three families with aneurysms and/or very-early-onset disease. Am J Hum Genet 65:1561-1571, 1999.

143. Torres VE, Cai Y, Chen X, et al: Vascular expression of polycystin-2. J Am Soc Nephrol 12:1-9, 2001.

144. Griffin MD, Torres VE, Grande JP, Kumar R: Vascular expression of polycystin. J Am Soc Nephrol 8:616-626, 1997.

145. Schievink WI, Torres VE, Piepgras DG, Wiebers DO: Saccular intracranial aneurysms in autosomal dominant polycystic kidney disease. J Am Soc Nephrol 3:88-95, 1992.

146. Schievink WI, Torres VE, Wiebers DO, Huston J 3rd: Intracranial arterial dolichoectasia in autosomal dominant polycystic kidney disease. J Am Soc Nephrol 8:1298-1303, 1997.

147. Schievink WI, Huston J 3rd, Torres VE, Marsh WR: Intracranial cysts in autosomal dominant polycystic kidney disease. J Neurosurg 83:1004-1007, 1995.

148. Leier CV, Baker PB, Kilman JW, Wooley CF: Cardiovascular abnormalities associated with adult polycystic kidney disease. Ann Intern Med 100:683-688, 1984.

149. Hossack KF, Leddy CL, Johnson AM, et al: Echocardiographic findings in autosomal dominant polycystic kidney disease. N Engl J Med 319:907-912, 1988.

150. Chapman JR, Hilson AJ: Polycystic kidneys and abdominal aortic aneurysms. Lancet 1:646-647, 1980.

151. Montoliu J, Torras A, Revert L: Polycystic kidneys and abdominal aortic aneurysms. Lancet 1:1133-1134, 1980.

152. Torra R, Nicolau C, Badenas C, et al: Abdominal aortic aneurysms and autosomal dominant polycystic kidney disease. J Am Soc Nephrol 7:2483-2486, 1996.

153. Hadimeri H, Lamm C, Nyberg G: Coronary aneurysms in patients with autosomal dominant polycystic kidney disease. J Am Soc Nephrol 9:837-841, 1998.

154. Torres VE, Erickson SB, Smith LH, et al: The association of nephrolithiasis and autosomal dominant polycystic kidney disease. Am J Kidney Dis 11:318-325, 1988.

155. Torres VE, Wilson DM, Hattery RR, Segura JW: Renal stone disease in autosomal dominant polycystic kidney disease. Am J Kidney Dis 22:513-519, 1993.

156. Delakas D, Daskalopoulos G, Cranidis A: Extracorporeal shock-wave lithotripsy for urinary calculi in autosomal dominant polycystic kidney disease. J Endourol 11:167-170, 1997.

157. Ng CS, Yost A, Streem SB: Nephrolithiasis associated with autosomal dominant polycystic kidney disease: Contemporary urological management. J Urol 163:726-729, 2000.

158. Everson GT: Hepatic cysts in autosomal dominant polycystic kidney disease. Am J Kidney Dis 22:520-525, 1993.

159. Sherstha R, McKinley C, Russ P, et al: Postmenopausal estrogen therapy selectively stimulates hepatic enlargement in women with autosomal dominant polycystic kidney disease. Hepatology 26:1282-1286, 1997.

160. Torres VE, Rastogi S, King BF, et al: Hepatic venous outflow obstruction in autosomal dominant polycystic kidney disease. J Am Soc Nephrol 5:1186-1192, 1994.

161. Everson GT, Scherzinger A, Berger-Leff N, et al: Polycystic liver disease: Quantitation of parenchymal and cyst volumes from computed tomography images and clinical correlates of hepatic cysts. Hepatology 8:1627-1634, 1988.

162. Que F, Nagorney DM, Gross JB Jr, Torres VE: Liver resection and cyst fenestration in the treatment of severe polycystic liver disease. Gastroenterology 108:487-494, 1995.

163. Chen MF: Surgery for adult polycystic liver disease. J Gastroenterol Hepatol 15:1239-1242, 2000.

164. Pirenne J, Aerts R, Yoong K, et al: Liver transplantation for polycystic liver disease. Liver Transpl 7:238-245, 2001.

165. Dominguez Fernandez E, Albrecht KH, et al: Prevalence of diverticulosis and incidence of bowel perforation after kidney transplantation in patients with polycystic kidney disease. Transpl Int 11:28-31, 1998.

166. Lederman ED, McCoy G, Conti DJ, Lee EC: Diverticulitis and polycystic kidney disease. Am Surg 66:200-203, 2000.

167. Chapman AB, Johnson AM, Gabow PA: Pregnancy outcome and its relationship to progression of renal failure in autosomal dominant polycystic kidney disease. J Am Soc Nephrol 5:1178-1185, 1994.

168. Klahr S, Breyer JA, Beck GJ, et al: Dietary protein restriction, blood pressure control, and the progression of polycystic kidney disease. Modification of Diet in Renal Disease Study Group. [Published erratum appears in J Am Soc Nephrol 6:1318, 1995.] J Am Soc Nephrol 5:2037-2047, 1995.

169. Gretz N, Zeier M, Geberth S, et al: Is gender a determinant for evolution of renal failure? A study in autosomal dominant polycystic kidney disease. Am J Kidney Dis 14:178-183, 1989.

170. Ecder T, Chapman AB, Brosnahan GM, et al: Effect of antihypertensive therapy on renal function and urinary albumin excretion in hypertensive patients with autosomal dominant polycystic kidney disease. Am J Kidney Dis 35:427-432, 2000.

171. Keith DS, Torres VE, Johnson CM, Holley KE: Effect of sodium chloride, enalapril, and losartan on the development of polycystic kidney disease in Han:SPRD rats. Am J Kidney Dis 24:491-498, 1994.

172. Ogborn MR, Sareen S, Pinette G: Cilazapril delays progression of hypertension and uremia in rat polycystic kidney disease. Am J Kidney Dis 26:942-946, 1995.

173. Geberth S, Stier E, Zeier M, et al: More adverse renal prognosis of autosomal dominant polycystic kidney disease in families with primary hypertension. J Am Soc Nephrol 6:1643-1648, 1995.

174. Baboolal K, Ravine D, Daniels J, et al: Association of the angiotensin I converting enzyme gene deletion polymorphism with early onset of ESRF in PKD1 adult polycystic kidney disease. Kidney Int 52:607-613, 1997.

175. Uemasu J, Nakaoka A, Kawasaki H, et al: Association between angiotensin converting enzyme gene polymorphism and clinical features in autosomal dominant polycystic kidney disease. Life Sci 60:2139-2144, 1997.

176. Christophe JL, van Ypersele de Strihou C, Pirson Y: Complications of autosomal dominant polycystic kidney disease in 50 haemodialysed patients: A case-control study. The U.C.L. Collaborative Group. Nephrol Dial Transplant 11:1271-1276, 1996.

177. Pirson Y, Christophe JL, Goffin E: Outcome of renal replacement therapy in autosomal dominant polycystic kidney disease. Nephrol Dial Transplant 11:24-28, 1996.

178. Knispel HH, Klan R, Offermann G, Miller K: Transplantation in autosomal dominant polycystic kidney disease without nephrectomy. Urol Int 56:75-78, 1996.

179. Andreoni KA, Pelletier RP, Elkhammas EA, et al: Increased incidence of gastrointestinal surgical complications in renal transplant recipients with polycystic kidney disease. Transplantation 67:262-266, 1999.

180. Manjoney DM, McKegney FP: Individual and family coping with polycystic kidney disease: The harvest of denial. Int J Psychiatry Med 9:19-31, 1978.

181. Grantham JJ: Polycystic kidney disease: A predominance of giant nephrons. Am J Physiol 244:F3-F10, 1983.

182. Bear JC, McManamon P, Morgan J, et al: Age at clinical onset and at ultrasonographic detection of adult polycystic kidney disease: Data for genetic counselling. Am J Med Genet 18:45-53, 1984.

183. Sise C, Kusaka M, Wetzel LH, et al: Volumetric determination of progression in autosomal dominant polycystic kidney disease by computed tomography. Kidney Int 58:2492-2501, 2000.

184. Dunn MD, Portis AJ, Elbahnasy AM, et al: Laparoscopic nephrectomy in patients with end-stage renal disease and autosomal dominant polycystic kidney disease. Am J Kidney Dis 35:720-725, 2000.

185. Torres VE: New insights into polycystic kidney disease and its treatment. Curr Opin Nephrol Hypertens 7:159-169, 1998.

186. Torres VE, Berndt TJ, Okamura M, et al: Mechanisms affecting the development of renal cystic disease induced by diphenylthiazole. Kidney Int 33:1130-1139, 1988.

187. Torres VE, Bengal RJ, Litwiller RD, Wilson DM: Aggravation of polycystic kidney disease in Han:SPRD rats by buthionine sulfoximine. J Am Soc Nephrol 8:1283-1291, 1997.

188. Torres VE, Cowley BD Jr, Branden MG, et al: Long-term ammonium chloride or sodium bicarbonate treatment in two models of polycystic kidney disease. Exp Nephrol 9:171-180, 2001.

189. Cowley BD Jr, Rupp JC, Muessel MJ, Gattone VH 2nd: Gender and the effect of gonadal hormones on the progression of inherited polycystic kidney disease in rats. Am J Kidney Dis 29:265-272, 1997.

190. Gile RD, Cowley BD Jr, Gattone VH 2nd, et al: Effect of lovastatin on the development of polycystic kidney disease in the Han:SPRD rat. Am J Kidney Dis 26:501-507, 1995.

191. Blyth H, Ockenden BG: Polycystic disease of kidney and liver presenting in childhood. J Med Genet 8:257-284, 1971.

192. Zerres K, Rudnik-Schoneborn S, Steinkamm C, Mucher G: Autosomal recessive polycystic kidney disease. Nephrol Dial Transplant 11:29-33, 1996.

193. Onuchic LF, Furu L, Nagasawa Y, et al: PKHD1, the polycystic kidney and hepatic disease 1 gene, encodes a novel large protein containing multiple immunoglobulin-like plexin-transcription-factor domains and parallel beta-helix 1 repeats. Am J Hum Genet 70:1305-1317, 2002.

194. Yoder BK, Hou X, Guay-Woodford LM: The polycystic kidney disease proteins, polycystin-1, polycystin-2, polaris, and cystin, are co-localized in renal cilia. J Am Soc Nephrol 13:2508-2516, 2002.

195. Cole BR, Conley SB, Stapleton FB: Polycystic kidney disease in the first year of life. J Pediatr 111:693-699, 1987.

196. Zerres K, Rudnik-Schoneborn S, Deget F, et al: Autosomal recessive polycystic kidney disease in 115 children: Clinical presentation, course and influence of gender. Arbeitsgemeinschaft fur Padiatrische, Nephrologie. Acta Paediatr 85:437-445, 1996.

197. Roy S, Dillon MJ, Trompeter RS, Barratt TM: Autosomal recessive polycystic kidney disease: Long-term outcome of neonatal survivors. Pediatr Nephrol 11:302-306, 1997.

198. Gagnadoux MF, Habib R, Levy M, et al: Cystic renal diseases in children. Adv Nephrol Necker Hosp 18:33-57, 1989.

199. Potter EL: Normal and Abnormal Development of the Kidney. Chicago, Year Book Medical Publishers, 1972.

200. Verani R, Walker P, Silva FG: Renal cystic disease of infancy: results of histochemical studies. A report of the Southwest Pediatric Nephrology Study Group. Pediatr Nephrol 3:37-42, 1989.

201. Faraggiana T, Bernstein J, Strauss L, Churg J: Use of lectins in the study of histogenesis of renal cysts. Lab Invest 53:575-579, 1985.

202. Six R, Oliphant M, Grossman H: A spectrum of renal tubular ectasia and hepatic fibrosis. Radiology 117:117-122, 1975.

203. Lucaya J, Enriquez G, Nieto J, et al: Renal calcifications in patients with autosomal recessive polycystic kidney disease: prevalence and cause. AJR Am J Roentgenol 160:359-362, 1993.

204. Nakanuma Y, Terada T, Ohta G, et al: Caroli's disease in congenital hepatic fibrosis and infantile polycystic disease. Liver 2:346-354, 1982.

205. Reuss A, Wladimiroff JW, Stewart PA, Niermeijer MF: Prenatal diagnosis by ultrasound in pregnancies at risk for autosomal recessive polycystic kidney disease. Ultrasound Med Biol 16:355-359, 1990.

206. Zerres K, Mucher G, Becker J, et al: Prenatal diagnosis of autosomal recessive polycystic kidney disease (ARPKD): Molecular genetics, clinical experience, and fetal morphology. Am J Med Genet 76:137-144, 1998.

207. Berger PE, Munschauer RW, Kuhn JP: Computed tomography and ultrasound of renal and perirenal diseases in infants and children: Relationship to excretory urography in renal cystic disease, trauma and neoplasm. Pediatr Radiol 9:91-99, 1980.

208. Dunnill MS, Millard PR, Oliver D: Acquired cystic disease of the kidneys: A hazard of long-term intermittent maintenance haemodialysis. J Clin Pathol 30:868-877, 1977.

209. Mickisch O, Bommer J, Bachmann S, et al: Multicystic transformation of kidneys in chronic renal failure. Nephron 38:93-99, 1984.

210. Ishikawa I: Acquired cystic disease: Mechanisms and manifestations. Semin Nephrol 11:671-684, 1991.

211. Lien YH, Hunt KR, Siskind MS, Zukoski C: Association of cyclosporin A with acquired cystic kidney disease of the native kidneys in renal transplant recipients. Kidney Int 44:613-616, 1993.

212. Levine E, Slusher SL, Grantham JJ, Wetzel LH: Natural history of acquired renal cystic disease in dialysis patients: A prospective longitudinal CT study. AJR Am J Roentgenol 156:501-506, 1991.

213. Levine E, Grantham JJ, Slusher SL, et al: CT of acquired cystic kidney disease and renal tumors in long-term dialysis patients. AJR Am J Roentgenol 142:125-131, 1984.

214. Grantham JJ, Levine E: Acquired cystic disease: Replacing one kidney disease with another. Kidney Int 28:99-105, 1985.

215. Ishikawa I, Kovacs G: High incidence of papillary renal cell tumours in patients on chronic haemodialysis. Histopathology 22:135-139, 1993.

216. Ishikawa I, Saito Y, Onouchi Z, et al: Development of acquired cystic disease and adenocarcinoma of the kidney in glomerulonephritic chronic hemodialysis patients. Clin Nephrol 14:1-6, 1980.

217. Ishikawa I, Saito Y, Shikura N, et al: Ten-year prospective study on the development of renal cell carcinoma in dialysis patients. Am J Kidney Dis 16:452-458, 1990.

218. Hughson MD, Buchwald D, Fox M: Renal neoplasia and acquired cystic kidney disease in patients receiving long-term dialysis. Arch Pathol Lab Med 110:592-601, 1986.

219. Hughson MD, Hennigar GR, McManus JF: Atypical cysts, acquired renal cystic disease, and renal cell tumors in end stage dialysis kidneys. Lab Invest 42:475-480, 1980.

220. Vandeursen H, Van Damme B, Baert J, Baert L: Acquired cystic disease of the kidney analyzed by microdissection. J Urol 146:1168-1172, 1991.

221. Krempien B, Ritz E: Acquired cystic transformation of the kidneys of haemodialysed patients. Virchows Arch A Pathol Anat Histol 386:189-200, 1980.

222. Miach PJ, Dawborn JK, Xipell J: Neoplasia in patients with chronic renal failure on long-term dialysis. Clin Nephrol 5:101-104, 1976.

223. Doublet JD, Peraldi MN, Gattegno B, et al: Renal cell carcinoma of native kidneys: Prospective study of 129 renal transplant patients. J Urol 158:42-44, 1997.

224. Kliem V, Kolditz M, Behrend M, et al: Risk of renal cell carcinoma after kidney transplantation. Clin Transplant 11:255-258, 1997.

225. Levine E: Renal cell carcinoma in uremic acquired renal cystic disease: Incidence, detection, and management. Urol Radiol 13:203-210, 1992.

226. Sarasin FP, Wong JB, Levey AS, Meyer KB: Screening for acquired cystic kidney disease: A decision analytic perspective. Kidney Int 48:207-219, 1995.

227. Konrad M, Saunier S, Heidet L, et al: Large homozygous deletions of the 2q13 region are a major cause of juvenile nephronophthisis. Hum Mol Genet 5:367-371, 1996.

228. Medhioub M, Cherif D, Benessy F, et al: Refined mapping of a gene (NPH1) causing familial juvenile nephronophthisis and evidence for genetic heterogeneity. Genomics 22:296-301, 1994.

229. Omran H, Fernandez C, Jung M, et al: Identification of a new gene locus for adolescent nephronophthisis, on chromosome 3q22 in a large Venezuelan pedigree. Am J Hum Genet 66:118-127, 2000.

230. Omran H, Haffner K, Burth S, et al: Evidence for further genetic heterogeneity in nephronophthisis. Nephrol Dial Transplant 16:755-758, 2001.

231. Hildebrandt F, Otto E: Molecular genetics of nephronophthisis and medullary cystic kidney disease. J Am Soc Nephrol 11:1753-1761, 2000.

232. Zollinger HU, Mihatsch MJ, Edefonti A, et al: Nephronophthisis (medullary cystic disease of the kidney): A study using electron microscopy, immunofluorescence, and a review of the morphological findings. Helv Paediatr Acta 35:509-530, 1980.

233. Pascal RR: Medullary cystic disease of the kidney: Study of a case with scanning and transmission electron microscopy and light microscopy. Am J Clin Pathol 59:659-665, 1973.

234. Elzouki AY, al-Suhaibani H, Mirza K, al-Sowailem AM: Thin-section computed tomography scans detect medullary cysts in patients believed to have juvenile nephronophthisis. Am J Kidney Dis 27:216-219, 1996.

235. Mitch WE, Walser M, Buffington GA, Lemann J Jr: A simple method of estimating progression of chronic renal failure. Lancet 2:1326-1328, 1976.

236. Steele BT, Lirenman DS, Beattie CW: Nephronophthisis. Am J Med 68:531-538, 1980.

237. Kutper BT: Medullary sponge kidney. In Gardner KD Jr (ed): Cystic Diseases of the Kidney. New York, John Wiley and Sons, 1976, pp 151-171.

238. Yendt ER: Medullary sponge kidney. In Gardner KD Jr, Bernstein J (eds): The Cystic Kidney. Boston, Kluwer, 1990, pp 379-391.

239. Indridason OS, Thomas L, Berkoben M: Medullary sponge kidney associated with congenital hemihypertrophy. J Am Soc Nephrol 7:1123-1130, 1996.

240. Osther PJ, Mathiasen H, Hansen AB, Nissen HM: Urinary acidification and urinary excretion of calcium and citrate in women with bilateral medullary sponge kidney. Urol Int 52:126-130, 1994.

241. Parks JH, Coe FL, Strauss AL: Calcium nephrolithiasis and medullary sponge kidney in women. N Engl J Med 306:1088-1091, 1982.

242. O'Neill M, Breslau NA, Pak CY: Metabolic evaluation of nephrolithiasis in patients with medullary sponge kidney. JAMA 245:1233-1236, 1981.

243. Baert L, Steg A: On the pathogenesis of simple renal cysts in the adult: A microdissection study. Urol Res 5:103-108, 1977.

244. Baert L, Steg A: Is the diverticulum of the distal and collecting tubules a preliminary stage of the simple cyst in the adult? J Urol 118:707-710, 1977.

245. Muther RS, Bennett WM: Concentration of antibiotics in simple renal cysts. J Urol 124:596, 1980.

246. Jacobsson L, Lindqvist B, Michaelson G, Bjerle P: Fluid turnover in renal cysts. Acta Med Scand 202:327-329, 1977.

247. Lang EK: Renal cyst puncture studies. Urol Clin North Am 14:91-102, 1987.

248. Steg A: Renal cysts in adults: III. Clinical aspect and diagnostical approach, based on the analysis of 1,342 cases. Eur Urol 2:209-212, 1976.

249. Piel C: Congenital multicystic kidney. In Gardner KD Jr, Bernstein J (eds): The Cystic Kidney. Boston, Kluwer, 1990, pp 393-411.

250. Bernstein J, Brough AJ, McAdams AJ: The renal lesion in syndromes of multiple congenital malformations: Cerebrohepatorenal syndrome; Jeune asphyxiating thoracic dystrophy; tuberous

sclerosis; Meckel syndrome. Birth Defects Orig Artic Ser 10:35-43, 1974.

251. Bernstein J: The multicystic kidney and hereditary renal adysplasia. Am J Kidney Dis 18:495-496, 1991.

252. Bernstein J: A classification of renal cysts. Perspect Nephrol Hypertens 4:7-30, 1976.

253. Bernstein J: The classification of renal cysts. Nephron 11:91-100, 1973.

254. Bernstein J: Morphology of inherited renal developmental abnormalities. Birth Defects Orig Artic Ser 6:9-11, 1970.

255. Bernstein J: Is unilateral multicystic renal dysplasia sometimes heritable, and what is the risk of recurrence? Pediatr Nephrol 4: 662, 1990.

256. Torres VE: Tuberous sclerosis complex. *In* Watson ML, Torres VE (eds): Polycystic Kidney Disease. Oxford, Oxford University Press, 1996, pp 282-308.

257. Bernstein J: Renal cystic disease in the tuberous sclerosis complex. Pediatr Nephrol 7:490-495, 1993.

258. van Slegtenhorst M, de Hoogt R, Hermans C, et al: Identification of the tuberous sclerosis gene TSC1 on chromosome 9q34. Science 277:805-808, 1997.

259. Identification and characterization of the tuberous sclerosis gene on chromosome 16. The European Chromosome 16 Tuberous Sclerosis Consortium. Cell 75:1305-1315, 1993.

260. Tee AR, Fingar DC, Manning BD, et al: Tuberous sclerosis complex-1 and -2 gene products function together to inhibit mammalian target of rapamycin (mTOR)-mediated downstream signaling. Proc Natl Acad Sci U S A 23:23, 2002.

261. Richards RD, Mebust WK, Schimke RN: A prospective study on von Hippel-Lindau disease. J Urol 110:27-30, 1973.

262. Michels V: Von Hippel-Lindau disease. *In* Watson ML, Torres VE (eds): Polycystic Kidney Disease. Oxford, Oxford University Press, 1996, pp 309-330.

263. Madewell JE, Goldman SM, Davis CJ Jr, et al: Multilocular cystic nephroma: A radiographic-pathologic correlation of 58 patients. Radiology 146:309-321, 1983.

264. Murray KK, McLellan GL: Renal peripelvic lymphangiectasia: Appearance at CT. Radiology 180:455-456, 1991.

265. Meredith WT, Levine E, Ahlstrom NG, Grantham JJ: Exacerbation of familial renal lymphangiomatosis during pregnancy. AJR Am J Roentgenol 151:965-966, 1988.

CHAPTER 38

Diabetic Nephropathy

Hans-Henrik Parving, Michael Mauer, and Eberhard Ritz

Although proteinuria had been demonstrated in diabetic patients since the 18th century[1] it was Bright who in 1836 postulated that albuminuria could reflect a serious renal disease specific to diabetes.[2] One hundred years later, Kimmelstiel and Wilson[3] described the nodular glomerular intercapillary lesions in long-standing type 2 diabetic patients suffering from the clinical syndrome of heavy proteinuria and renal failure accompanied by arterial hypertension. Persistent albuminuria (>300 mg/24 hours or 200 μg/minute) is the hallmark of diabetic nephropathy which can be diagnosed clinically if the following additional criteria are fulfilled: presence of diabetic retinopathy and the absence of clinical or laboratory evidence of other kidney or renal tract disease.[4, 5] This clinical definition of diabetic nephropathy is valid in both type 1 diabetes and type 2 diabetes.[4, 6]

During the last decade several longitudinal studies have shown that raised urinary albumin excretion (based on a single measurement) below the level of clinical albuminuria (obtained with Albustix), so-called microalbuminuria, strongly predicts the development of diabetic nephropathy in both type 1[7-10] and type 2 diabetes.[11-13] *Microalbuminuria* is defined as urinary albumin excretion greater than 30 mg/24 hours (20 μg/minute), and less than or equal to 300 mg/24 hours (200 μg/minute) irrespective of how the urine is collected.[14]

Nephropathy is a major cause of illness and death in diabetes. Indeed, the excess mortality in diabetes occurs mainly in proteinuric diabetic patients and results not only from end-stage renal disease (ESRD) but also from cardiovascular disease (CVD), the latter particularly in type 2 diabetic patients.[15-32] Diabetic nephropathy is the single most common cause of ESRD in Europe, Japan, and the United States, with diabetic patients accounting for 25% to 45% of all patients enrolled in ESRD programs.

PATHOLOGY OF THE KIDNEY IN DIABETES

This section outlines renal pathology in type 1 diabetes, followed by a comparison of the similarities and differences in renal pathology in type 2 diabetes. Taken together, diabetic nephropathology in type 1 diabetic patients is unique to this disease (Table 38-1).[33-35] Thickening of the glomerular basement membrane (GBM) is the first change that can be quantitated (Fig. 38-1A and C).[36] Thickening of tubular basement membranes (TBMs) parallels this GBM thickening (Fig. 38-2).[37, 38] Afferent and efferent glomerular arteriolar hyalinosis can also be detected within 3 to 5 years after onset of diabetes or following transplantation of a normal kidney into the diabetic patient.[39] This can eventuate in the total replacement of the smooth muscle cells of these small vessels by waxy, homogeneous, translucent-appearing periodic acid–Shiff (PAS)–positive material (Fig. 38-3A and B) consisting of immunoglobulins, complement, fibrinogen, albumin, and other plasma proteins.[40, 41] Arteriolar hyalinosis, glomerular capillary subendothelial hyaline (hyaline caps), and capsular drops along the parietal surface of the Bowman capsule (Fig. 38-3C) make up the so-called exudative lesions of diabetic nephropathy. These lesions may be capable of triggering inflammatory cascades in that they can fix heterologous complement.[42]

Increases in the fraction of the glomerulus occupied by the mesangium [Vv(Mes/glom)] can be documented only after 4 to 5 years of type 1 diabetes,[36] probably because there is more glomerulus-to-glomerulus variability in this parameter among normal individuals[43] and because its measurement is less precise than that of GBM width. Alternatively, this may be because the relationship of mesangial expansion to diabetes duration is nonlinear, with slow development earlier and

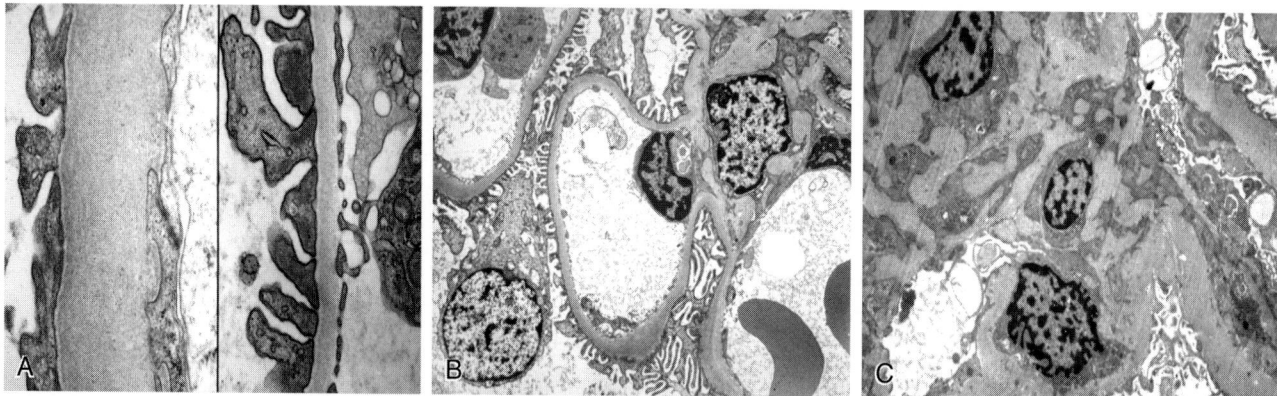

FIGURE 38-1. Electron microscopic photomicrographs: **A,** Normal glomerular basement membrane (GBM) on the left compared to thickened GBM from a proteinuric type 1 diabetic patient on the right. **B,** Normal glomerular capillary loops and mesangial zone. **C,** Thickened glomerular basement membrane (GBM), mesangial expansion (predominantly with mesangial matrix), and capillary luminal narrowing in a proteinuric type 1 diabetic patient.

TABLE 38-1

Pathology of Diabetic Nephropathy in Patients with Type 1 Diabetes and Proteinuria

ALWAYS PRESENT	OFTEN OR USUALLY PRESENT	SOMETIMES PRESENT
Glomerular basement membrane thickening[a]	Kimmelstiel-Wilson nodules (nodular glomerulosclerosis)[a]; global glomerular sclerosis; focal-segmental glomerulosclerosis atubular glomeruli	Hyaline "exudative" leisons (subendothelial)[b]
Tubular basement membrane thickening[a]		Capsular drops[b]
Mesangial expansion with predominance of increased mesangial matrix (diffuse glomerulosclerosis)[a]	Foci of tubular atrophy	Atherosclerosis
Interstitial expansion with predominance of increased extracellular matrix material		Glomerular microaneurysms
Increased glomerular basement membrane, tubular basement membrane, and Bowman capsule staining for albumin and IgG[a]	Afferent and efferent arteriolar hyalinosis[a]	

[a]In combination, diagnostic of diabetic nephropathy.
[b]Highly characteristic of diabetic nephropathy.

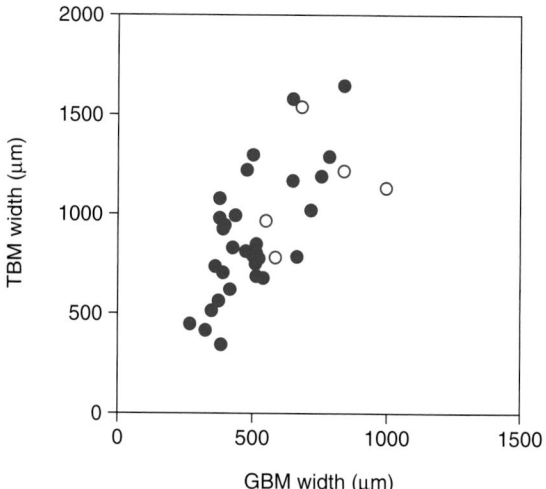

FIGURE 38-2. Relationship of proximal tubular basement membrane (TBM) width and glomerular basement membrane (GBM) width in 35 type 1 diabetic patients, 25 of whom were normoalbuminuric. The hypertensive patients are represented by the open circles. $r = .64$, $P < .001$. (From Brito PL, Fioretto P, Drummond K, et al: Proximal tubular basement membrane width in insulin-dependent diabetes mellitus. Kidney Int 53:754-761, 1998.)

more rapid development later in the disease. This mesangial expansion is primarily due to absolute and relative increases in the mesangial matrix, with lesser contribution from fractional increases in mesangial cell volume (Fig. 38-1C and 38-4).[44] The first change in the volume fraction of cortex which is interstitium [Vv(Int/cortex)] is a decrease in this parameter,[45] perhaps due to the expansion of the tubular compartment of the cortex. In contrast to the mesangium, initial interstitial expansion is primarily due to an increase in the cellular component of this renal compartment.[46] Increase in interstitial extracellular matrix (ECM) fibrillar collagen is a relatively late finding in this disease, measurable only in patients with an already established decline in glomerular filtration rate (GFR).[46]

These various lesions of diabetic nephropathy can progress at varying rates within and between type 1 diabetic patients,[47, 48] and, as discussed below, this is even more the case in type 2 diabetes. For example, GBM width and Vv(Mes/glom) are not highly correlated with one another; some patients have relatively marked GBM thickening without much mesangial expansion and others the converse (Fig. 38-5).[33, 47] Ultimately,[33, 47, 48] marked renal extracellular basement membrane accumulation resulting in extreme mesangial expansion occurs in the vast majority of type 1 diabetic

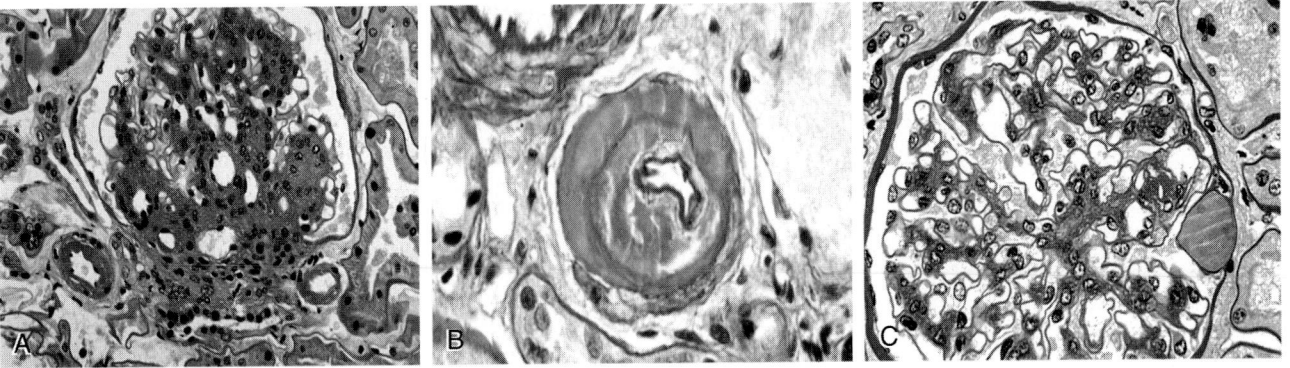

FIGURE 38-3. Light microscopic photomicrographs: **A,** Afferent and efferent arteriolar hyalinosis in a glomerulus from a type 1 diabetic patient. The glomerulus shows diffuse and nodular mesangial expansion (PAS stain). **B,** A glomerular arteriole showing almost completed replacement of the smooth muscle wall by hyaline material and luminal narrowing (PAS stain). **C,** A glomerulus with minimal mesangial expansion and a capsular drop at 3 o'clock (PAS stain).

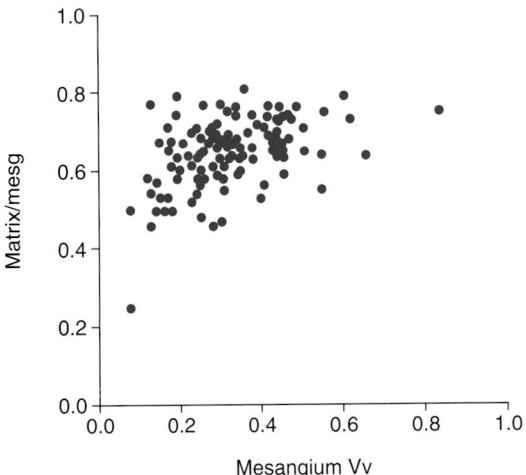

FIGURE 38-4. Mesangial matrix expressed as a fraction of the total mesangium (matrix/mesg) plotted against mesangial fractional volume (mesangium Vv) in long-standing type 1 diabetic patients. The normal value for matrix/mesg is approximately 0.5. Note that most diabetic patients have elevated values for matrix/mesg whether or not there is an increase in mesangium Vv (i.e., values > 0.24). (From Steffes MW, Bilous RW, Sutherland DER, Mauer, SM: Cell and matrix components of the glomerular mesangium in type 1 diabetes. Diabetes 41:679-684, 1992).

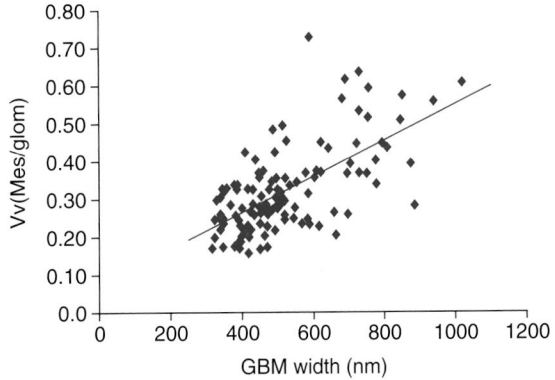

FIGURE 38-5. Relationship between glomerular basement membrane (GBM) width and mesangial fractional volume [Vv(mes/glom)] in 125 long-standing type 1 diabetic patients, 88 of whom were normoalbuminuric, 17 microalbuminuric, and 18 proteinuric. $r = .58$, $P < .001$.

patients who develop overt diabetic nephropathy manifesting as proteinuria, hypertension, and declining GRF (see below).

The diffuse and generalized process of mesangial expansion has been termed *diffuse diabetic glomerulosclerosis* (Fig. 38-6A-C). *Nodular glomerulosclerosis* (Kimmelstiel-Wilson nodular disease) represents areas of marked mesangial expansion appearing as large round fibrillar mesangial zones, with palisading of mesangial nuclei around the periphery of the nodule and extreme compression of the associated glomerular capillaries (Fig. 38-7C). This is typically a focal and segmental change which likely results from glomerular capillary wall detachment from a mesangial anchoring point with consequent microaneurysm formation (Fig. 38-7A)[49] and subsequent filling of the resultant space with mesangial matrix material (Fig. 38-7B). Approximately 50% of proteinuric type 1 diabetic patients have at least a few glomeruli with nodular lesions. Typically, this occurs in patients with

moderate to severe diffuse diabetic glomerulosclerosis but there are some patients with occasional nodular lesions who have little or no diffuse mesangial expansion, suggesting that these two forms of diabetic mesangial expansion may, at least in part, have a different pathogenesis.

As mentioned above, most (about two thirds) of the mesangial expansion in diabetes is due to increased mesangial matrix and one third is due to mesangial cell expansion. The mesangial matrix fraction of mesangial volume is increased in diabetic patients, often even in those in whom Vv(Mes/glom) is still within the normal range (see Fig. 38-4).[44] The relative contribution of cell number versus cell size to the expansion of the cellular component of the mesangium is currently unknown.

Diabetic nephropathology is primarily the consequence of ECM accumulation, which must result from an imbalance in renal ECM dynamics whereby over many years the rate of ECM production exceeds the rate of removal. The accumulation of mesangial, GBM, TBM, and ECM materials probably represents the accumulation of intrinsic ECM components of these structures, including types IV and VI collagen, laminin, and fibronectin,[50] as well as additional intrinsic components not yet identified. However, not all renal ECM components change in parallel in diabetic nephropathy. Thus, alpha 3 and alpha 4 chains of type IV collagen increase

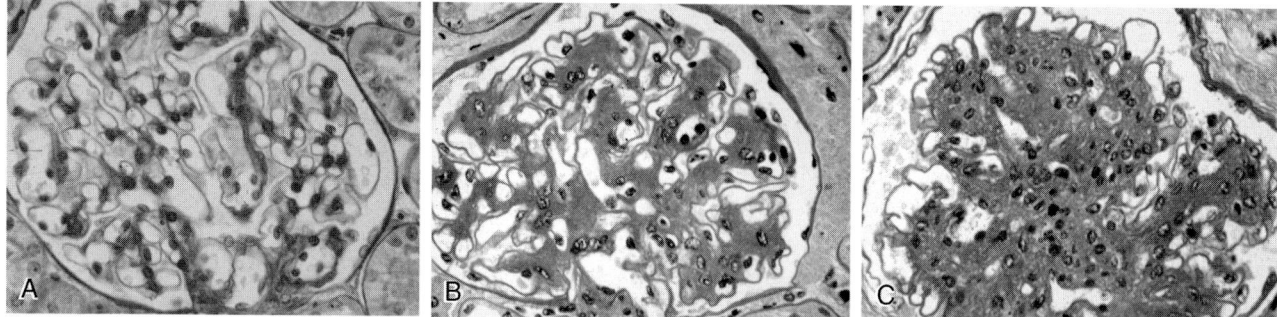

FIGURE 38-6. Light microscopic photomicrographs (PAS stain): **A,** A normal glomerulus. **B,** A glomerulus from a normoalbuminuric type 1 diabetic patient with glomerular basement membrane (GBM) thickening and moderate mesangial expansion, **C,** A glomerulus from a type 1 diabetic patient with overt diabetic nephropathy and severe diffuse mesangial expansion.

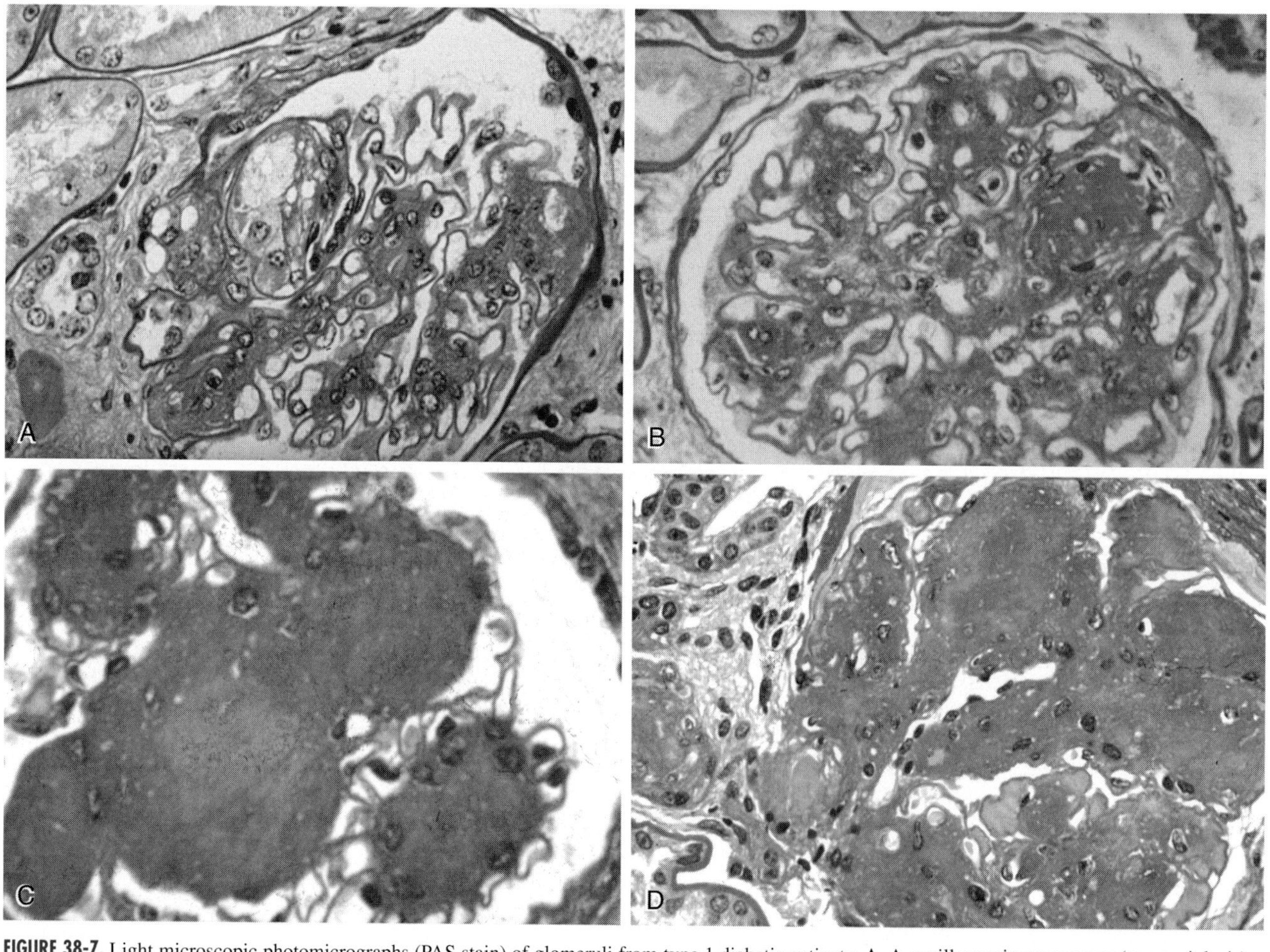

FIGURE 38-7. Light microscopic photomicrographs (PAS stain) of glomeruli from type 1 diabetic patients: **A,** A capillary microaneurysm (mesangiolysis) at 11 o'clock. **B,** Nodule formation within a capillary microaneurysm. **C,** Nodular glomerulosclerosis (Kimmelstiel-Wilson nodules). **D,** End-stage diabetic glomerular changes with nearly complete capillary closed.

in density in the GBM of patients with diabetic renal lesions, whereas alpha 1 and alpha 2 chains decrease in the density of their distribution in the mesangium and in the subendothelial space.[51, 52] The glomerular expression of "scar" collagen is very late in the evolution of diabetic glomerulopathy, occurring primarily in association with global glomerular sclerosis.[50, 51] The understanding of which ECM components are accumulating in the mesangium, GBM, and TBM in diabetes is far from complete.[52, 53] Thus, quantitative electron microscopic immunohistochemical studies of mesangial types IV[52] and VI collagen[53] (the dominant mesangial ECM molecules) have shown reduced density per mesangial matrix area or volume in patients with advanced mesangial expansion, although the absolute amount of these ECM components per glomerulus is increased due to the massive increase in mesangial matrix. Consequently, the nature of ECM accumulation in diabetes remains to be fully elucidated.

As the disease progresses toward renal insufficiency, more glomeruli become totally sclerosed or have closure of glomerular capillary lumens in incompletely scarred glomeruli due to massive mesangial expansion (Fig. 38-7D). However, an increased fraction of glomeruli may become globally sclerosed in type 1 diabetic patients without other glomeruli showing marked mesangial changes.[54] Hørlyck and colleagues[55] found that the distribution pattern of scarred glomeruli in diabetic patients was often not random but, more often than by chance, oriented in the plane vertical to the capsule of the kidney. This suggested that glomerular scarring in diabetes could result, at least in part, from obstruction of medium-sized renal arteries.[55] In fact, patients with increased numbers of globally sclerosed glomeruli have more severe arteriolar hyalinosis lesions.[54] In general, global glomerular sclerosis and mesangial expansion are correlated in type 1 diabetic patients,[54, 56] but this may be less often the case in type 2 diabetes (see later).

Finally, careful examination of light microscopic serial sections from proteinuric type 1 diabetic patients has revealed a high incidence of atubular glomeruli, that is, nonsclerosed glomeruli without attachment to a proximal tubule (B. Najafian, M. Mauer, unpublished data). This phenomenon, described in animal models[57] and human diseases, including pyelonephritis[58] and renal artery stenosis,[59] could be important in the evolution of diabetic nephropathy.

When patients with diabetes of at least 10 years' duration with no other selection criteria are studied by research renal biopsies, there are significant but only imprecise relationships between renal pathology and diabetic duration.[47] This is consistent with the marked variability in susceptibility to diabetic nephropathy, with some patients in renal failure after 15 years of diabetes and others without complications despite having type 1 diabetes for many decades.

Immunohistochemistry

Renal extracellular membranes, including GBM, TBM, and the Bowman capsule, demonstrate increased intensity of immunofluorescent linear staining for plasma proteins, especially albumin and immunoglobulin G (IgG).[41] These changes are seen in all type 1 diabetic patients, whether significant lesions of diabetic nephropathy are developing or not[41] and have been documented in normal kidneys transplanted into type 1 diabetic patients.[41] Although these proteins localize to these membranes, in part due to their negative charge characteristics,[60] additional stronger binding processes must be operative because elution of these proteins requires markedly acid conditions or collagenase treatment.[61] As these abnormalities appear to be unrelated to disease risk, their only clinical importance is that they not be confused with other entities, such as anti-GBM antibody disorders.

Structural-Functional Relationships in Diabetic Nephropathy

Mesangial expansion is the major lesion of diabetic nephropathy leading to renal dysfunction in type 1 diabetes patients.[47] Mesangial expansion out of proportion to increases in

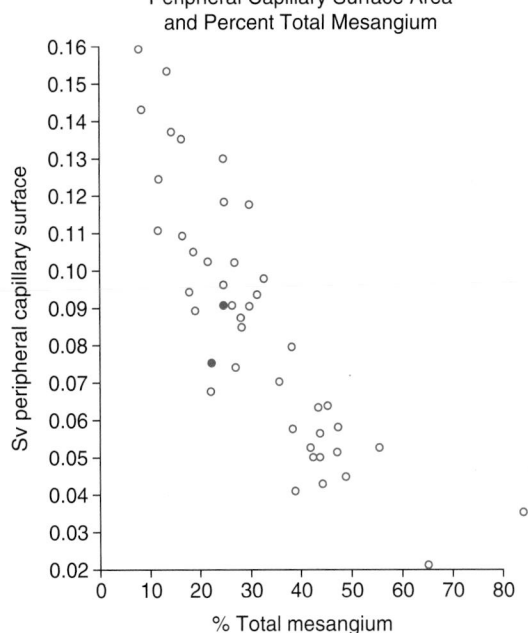

FIGURE 38-8. Relationship of mesangial fractional volume (% total mesangium) and filtration surface density [Sv(peripheral capillary/surface)] in type 1 diabetes patients.

glomerular volume [i.e., increased Vv(Mes/glom)] is correlated precisely with a decrease in peripheral GBM filtration surface density [Sv(PGBM/glom)] (Fig. 38-8)[47] and filtration surface per glomerulus (S/G) is highly correlated with GFR in type 1 diabetes.[62] Vv(Mes/glom) is closely related to the urinary albumin excretion rate (AER)[47,48] (Fig. 38-9A) and is a strong concomitant of hypertension.[47, 56] Thus, all of the clinical manifestations of diabetic nephropathy are related to mesangial expansion and the consequent restriction of the filtration surface. Although GBM width is also directly correlated with blood pressure and AER (Fig. 38-10A) and inversely correlated with GFR, the relationships are weaker than those seen with Vv(Mes/glom).[47, 48] However, Vv(Mes/glom) and GBM width, together, explain a remarkable 59% of the variability in AER in type 1 diabetic patients, with the AER ranging from normoabuminuria to proteinuria.[48]

Glomerular epithelial (podocyte) cell structure[63-65] and number[65] are also related to glomerular permeability alterations in diabetes, although it is currently difficult to sort out cause from effect in these relationships. Thus, foot process width increases and filtration slit-length density decreases as AER increases in type 1 diabetic patients.[63-65] Decreased podocyte number has been described in proteinuric type 2 Pima Indian patients although the number of other cells (mesangial and endothelial cells) were increased in these patients.[65] Also, heparan sulfate proteoglycans, presumably an epithelial cell product important in glomerular charge–based permselectivity, is decreased in density in the lamina rara externa in proportion to the increase in AER in type 1 diabetic patients.[66] Whether the addition of epithelial cell structural variables would reduce the residual unexplained variability in AER or GFR in diabetic nephropathy has not been tested. If true, this would support the idea that

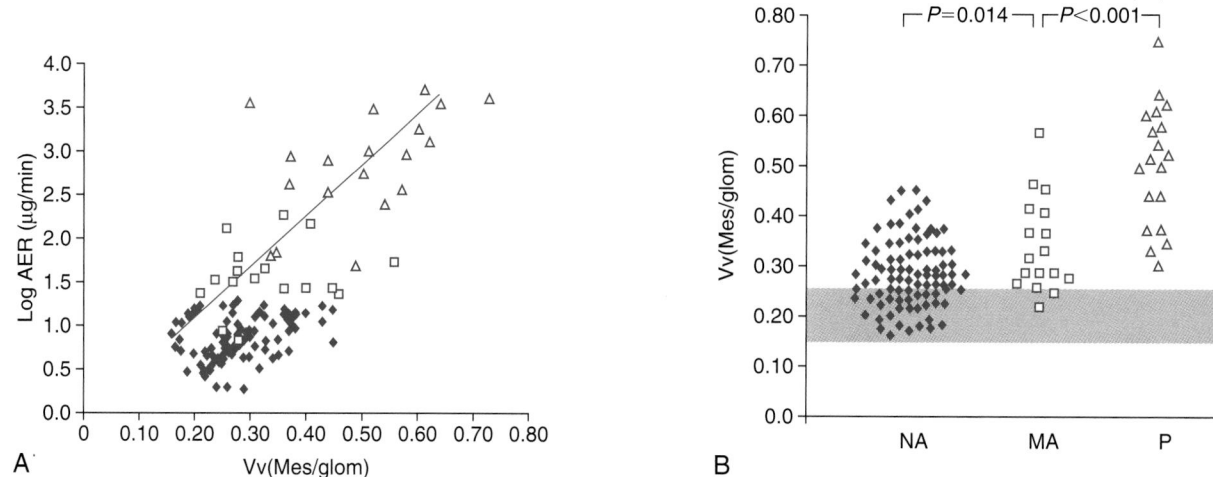

FIGURE 38-9. A, Correlation between mesangial fractional volume [Vv(Mes/glom)] and albumin excretion rate (AER) in 124 patients with type 1 diabetes. ♦, normoalbuminuric patients; □, microalbuminuric patients; Δ, proteinuric patients. r = .75, P < .001. **B,** Vv(Mes/glom) in 88 normoalbuminuric (NA), 17 microalbuminuric (MA), and 19 proteinuric (P) patients with type 1 diabetes. The hatched area represents the mean ± 2 SD in a group of 76 age-matched normal control subjects. All groups are different from control subjects. (From Caramori ML, Kim Y, Huang C, et al: Cellular basis of diabetic nephropathy: 1. Study design and renal structural-functional relationships in patients with long-standing type 1 diabetes. Diabetes 51:506-513, 2002.)

podocyte alterations contribute to proteinuria and renal insufficiency.

The total peripheral capillary filtration surface is highly correlated with GFR across the spectrum from hyperfiltration to renal insufficiency,[62, 67, 68] and hyperfiltration in type 1 diabetes is associated with increased filtration surface.[62, 67, 68] Nonetheless, as already noted, diabetic glomerulopathy structural parameters explain only a minority of GFR variability in type 1 diabetic patients.[48] Percent global sclerosis[54] and interstitial expansion[35] are also correlated with the clinical manifestations of diabetic nephropathy and are, to some extent, independent predictors of renal dysfunction and

hypertension in type 1 diabetes. In fact, some have argued that renal dysfunction in diabetes is primarily consequent to interstitial rather than glomerular lesions.[69-71] However, the finding that the interstitium is more closely related to renal dysfunction in diabetes than glomerular changes is seen in studies where most, if not all, patients have elevated serum creatinine values and where the interstitium is carefully measured but the glomerular structure is subjectively estimated.[69-71] It thus appears that during most of the natural history of diabetic nephropathy, glomerular parameters appear to be more important determinants of renal dysfunction, whereas interstitial changes may be a stronger determinant of the rate of

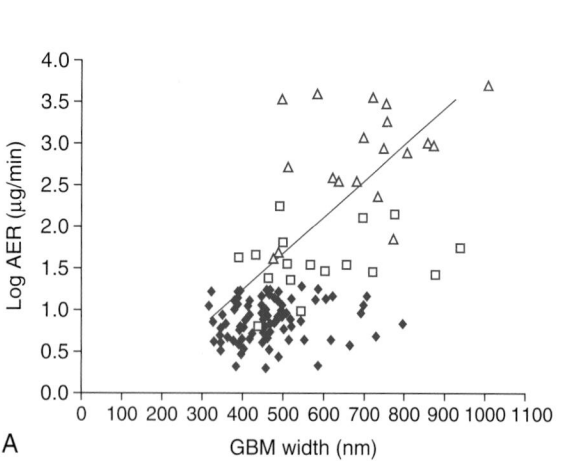

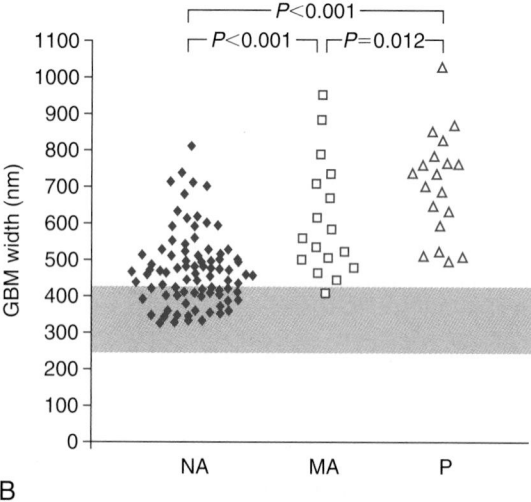

FIGURE 38-10. A, Correlation between glomerular basement membrane (GBM) width and albumin excretion rate (AER) in 124 patients with type 1 diabetes. ♦, normoalbuminuric patients; □, microalbuminuric patients; Δ, proteinuric patients. r =.62, P < .001. **B,** GBM width in 88 normoalbuminuric (NA), 17 microalbuminuric (MA), and 19 proteinuric (P) patients with type 1 diabetes. The hatched area represents the mean ± 2 SD in a group of 76 age-matched normal control subjects. All groups are different from control subjects. (From Caramori ML, Kim Y, Huang C, et al: Cellular basis of diabetic nephropathy:1. Study design and renal structural-functional relationships in patients with long-standing type 1 diabetes. Diabetes 51:506-513, 2002.)

progression from moderate renal insufficiency (serum creatinine >200 mg/dL) to terminal uremia.[72] Further, as mentioned above, in the first decade of diabetes, Vv(Int/cortex) is decreased[45] whereas Vv(Mes/glom) and GBM width are already increased. Moreover, early interstitial expansion in type 1 diabetes is mainly due to expansion of the cellular component of this compartment and increased interstitial fibrillar collagen is seen in patients whose GFR is already reduced.[46] These and other findings suggest that the interstitial and glomerular changes of diabetes have somewhat different pathogenetic mechanisms and that advancing interstitial fibrosis generally follows the glomerular processes in type 1 diabetes.

Microalbuminuria and Renal Structure

As discussed elsewhere in this chapter, persistent microalbuminuria is a strong predictor of the development of clinical nephropathy, whereas the absence of microalbuminuria in long-standing type 1 diabetic patients indicates a relatively lower likelihood of overt nephropathy. Proteinuria in type 1 diabetes of 10 or more years' duration is typically associated with advanced diabetic glomerular pathology in type 1 diabetes patients.[47, 48] One might reason that microalbuminuria is therefore associated with underlying renal structural changes that are predictive of the ultimate progression of this pathology. However, the relationship of renal structural changes to these low levels of albuminuria (i.e., normal or microalbuminuria) are complex and incompletely understood. Normoalbuminuric patients with long-standing type 1 diabetes (mean of ≈20 years), as a group, have increased GBM width and Vv(Mes/glom).[48, 73] The structural parameters within this group vary from within the normal range to rather advanced abnormalities which overlap with patients with microalbuminuria and proteinuria (Fig. 38-9B and 38-10B).[48,73] Patients with microalbuminuria AER (20–200 µg/minute) have even greater GBM and mesangial expansion, with almost no values in the normal range, but overlap with normoalbuminuric and proteinuric patients (see Figs. 38-9B and 38-10B).[48, 73] The incidence of hypertension and reduced GFR is greater in patients with microalbuminuria.[48, 73] Thus, microalbuminuria appears to be a marker of more advanced lesions as well as other functional disturbances.[48, 73] Although available data from longitudinal biopsy studies are sparse, preliminary studies suggest that greater GBM width in baseline biopsies of normoalbuminuric patients is predictive of later clinical progression. More extensive studies in normoalbuminuric and similar studies in microalbuminuric patients are needed. Finally some normoalbuminuric long-standing type 1 diabetic patients, particularly females with retinopathy or hypertension, have reduced GFR, and this is associated with worse diabetic glomerulopathy lesions (M.L. Caramori, M. Mauer, unpublished data). Thus, increased AER is not always the initial clinical indicator of diabetic nephropathy, and GFR measurements may be indicated, especially in normoalbuminuric female patients with the above characteristics.

Risk Factors for Nephropathy May Be Intrinsic to the Kidney

Nondiabetic members of identical twin pairs discordant for type 1 diabetes have glomerular structure [GBM width and Vv(Mes/glom)] within the normal range.[37] In every pair studied, the diabetic twin had higher values for GBM and TBM width and Vv(Mes/glom) than the nondiabetic twin. Several diabetic twins had values for GBM width and Vv(Mes/glom) that were within the range of normal and had "lesions" only in comparison with their nondiabetic twin,[37] whereas others had severe lesions and overt diabetic nephropathy. Thus, given sufficient duration, probably all type 1 diabetic patients have structural changes that are similar in their direction but vary markedly between individuals in the rate at which these lesions develop.

The GBM width, Vv(Mes/glom), or Vv(MM/glom) of the nondiabetic twins did not predict the rate of development of diabetic glomerulopathy lesions in the diabetic twins, indicating that genetic determinants of variability in these parameters within the normal range before the onset of diabetes do not represent risk factors for diabetic nephropathy (unpublished analyses). There is a growing body of information, discussed elsewhere in this chapter, which supports the view that, in addition to glycemia as a risk factor, genetic variables confer susceptibility or resistance to diabetic nephropathy. [An extension of this concept is the hypothesis that these genetic propensities are expressed in the renal tissues' responses to the diabetic state.] This is supported by the marked variability in the rate of development of kidney lesions of diabetic nephropathy in transplanted kidneys, despite the fact that the recipients all had ESRD secondary to diabetic nephropathy.[74] This variability is only partially explained by differences in glycemic control in the post-transplant period and argues for genetically determined tissue responses as important in this recurrence process.[74] Preliminary data indicating that the in vitro behavior of skin fibroblasts of kidney transplant donors is predictive of the rate of development of GBM thickening in type 1 diabetic kidney transplant recipients further corroborate this concept (J. Walker, L. Ng, G. Viberti, M, Mauer, unpublished data).

Glomerular volume and number could be structural determinants of nephropathy risk. Mean glomerular volumes were higher in patients developing diabetic nephropathy after 25 years of type 1 diabetes compared to a group that developed nephropathy after only 15 years.[75] These studies suggest that as mesangial expansion develops, glomerular volume increases, and the studies of Østerby and colleagues.[67] support this view. These studies further suggest that those patients unable to respond to mesangial expansion with glomerular enlargement will more quickly develop overt nephropathy than those whose glomeruli enlarge, with compensatory preservation of glomerular filtration surface. The number of glomeruli per kidney can vary markedly among normal individuals and diabetic patients[76, 77] and it has been suggested that fewer glomeruli per kidney could be a risk factor for diabetic nephropathy.[78] Diabetic patients with advanced renal failure have reduced numbers of glomeruli but this likely results from resorption of sclerotic glomeruli.[77] In this same study,[77] there was a small subgroup of type 1 diabetic patients with proteinuria whose glomerular number was not different from that of patients without proteinuria. If reduced glomerular number were a risk factor, proteinuric patients without advanced renal failure would be predicted to have fewer glomeruli, but this was not the case.[77] Finally, the severity of diabetic glomerulopathy lesions in type 1 diabetic renal transplant recipients (one-kidney patients) is virtually identical to that seen in biopsies of native kidneys of type 1 diabetic patients (two-kidney patients) matched for diabetes duration with the length of exposure of the allograft to the diabetic state (reference 74 and S. Chang, M. Mauer, unpublished data). These findings argue against reduced glomerular number as a risk factor for the genesis of diabetic nephropathology. However, it is reasonable to suppose that reduced glomerular number would be associated with more rapid progression to ESRD once advanced lesions and overt diabetic nephropathy had developed.

A Comparsion of Nephropathy in Type 1 and Type 2 Diabetes

Renal pathology and structural-functional relationships have been less well studied in type 2 diabetic patients, despite the fact that 80% or more of diabetic ESRD patients have type 2 diabetes. Proteinuric white Danish type 2 diabetic patients were reported to have structural changes similar to proteinuric type 1 diabetic patients and the severity of these changes was strongly correlated with the subsequent rate of decline of GFR.[79] However, this report also described greater heterogeneity in glomerular structure in these type 2 patients than the authors had seen in type 1 patients, with some type 2 proteinuric patients having little or no diabetic glomerulopathy.[79] A study of 52 microalbuminuric and proteinuric northern Italian type 2 diabetic patients defined three general groups of abnormalities.[80] About one third of the patients had changes of diabetic nephropathy similar to those typically seen in type 1 diabetes, including glomerular hypertrophy, mesangial expansion, and arteriolar hyalinosis. One third had a marked increase in the percentage of globally sclerosed glomeruli associated with severe tubulointerstitial lesions, whereas nonsclerosed glomeruli showed only mild diabetic changes. In the third group there were typical changes of diabetic glomerulopathy and superimposed changes of proliferative glomerulonephritis, membranous nephropathy and so on.[80] In another Danish study, three fourths of proteinuric type 2 diabetic patients had diabetic nephropathology[6] but one fourth had a variety of nondiabetic glomerulopathies, including "minimal lesions", glomerulonephritis, mixed diabetic and glomerulonephritis changes, or chronic glomerulonephritis. All patients with proteinuria and diabetic retinopathy had diabetic nephropathy; only 40% of patients without retinopathy had diabetic nephropathy. A British study found similar results.[81] It is very likely that these high incidences of diagnosis other than or in addition to diabetic nephropathy represent a selection bias, as many patients in these studies had clinical indications for kidney biopsies, often because of atypical clinical courses or findings. In fact, the likelihood of finding nondiabetic renal disease among type 2 diabetic patients is highly influenced by a center's clinical indications for renal biopsy in type 2 diabetic patients (T. Bertani, personal communication, 2002).

Structural-Functional Relationships in Type 2 Diabetic Nephropathy

Renal structural-functional relationships in Japanese type 2 diabetic patients were initially reported to be similar to those in type 1 patients.[82] However, a more recent study has indicated greater heterogeneity in Japanese type 2 diabetic patients, with some microalbuminuric and proteinuric patients having normal glomerular structural parameters.[83] Østerby and co-workers found less advanced glomerular changes in type 2 versus type 1 diabetic patients with similar AERs.[79] However, the type 1 patients had lower GFR levels than type 2 patients with similar AERs.[79] These findings could reflect much larger glomerular volumes in the type 2 patients, with associated preservation of filtration surface. In fact, GFR and filtration surface per glomerulus were correlated in these patients.[79] However, the explanation for the proteinuria in these type 2 patients was, at least in part, unexplained. Vv(Mes/glom) increased progressively from early to long-term diabetes, with clinical findings ranging from normoalbuminuria, to microalbuminuria, to clinical nephropathy[65] in type 2 diabetic Pima Indian patients. Global glomerular sclerosis was correlated inversely with GFR in these Pima Indian patients.[65] These authors also suggested, as noted earlier, glomerular podocyte loss was related to proteinuria in these patients, although this was not seen in microalbuminuric patients, and thus would more likely be a progression factor rather than a factor in the genesis of diabetic glomerulopathy. In fact, reduced podocyte number predicted the rate of increase in AER over 4 years in these patients and was a somewhat stronger predictor than Vv(Mes/glom). Moreover, studies in white type 2 diabetic patients showed that reduced podocyte numeric density (number/glomerular volume) was already present in microalbuminuric patients and was correlated with AER, although the number of podocytes per glomerulus was not significantly changed compared to normoalbuminuric patients (M. Della-Vestra, P. Fioretto, personal communication, 2002). Further studies along these lines could be of great interest and would help to explain why some type 2 diabetic patients have microalbuminuria or proteinuria with GBM width and Vv(Mes/glom) still in the normal range.

The less precise correlation between glomerular structure and renal function in type 2 versus type 1 diabetic patients may also be related to the more complex patterns of renal injury seen in type 2 diabetic patients.[84] Three categories of renal structure were described in research biopsies in white northern Italian microalbuminuric type 2 diabetic patients.[84] In category I (CI, ≈30%) renal structure by light microscopy was normal or near normal. In category II (CII, ≈30%) patients had typical diabetic nephropathology as usually seen in type 1 diabetes, with roughly balanced severity of glomerular, tubulointerstitial, and arteriolar changes. Category III (CIII, ≈40%) patients had atypical structural patterns. These patients had absent or only mild glomerular diabetic changes with disproportionately severe tubulointerstitial injury, glomerular arteriolar hyalinosis, or global glomerular sclerosis. CIII patients also had higher body mass index and less proliferative retinopathy than CII patients. Thus, the CII patients in this study may be similar to the type 2 diabetic patients with retinopathy in the Danish studies mentioned earlier.[6] This might reflect the heterogeneous nature of type 2 diabetes per se or different responses of the kidney to diabetes at different ages.

These findings are relevant to prognosis, in that the patients with more typical electron microscopic morphometric diabetic glomerulopathy findings were far more likely to have progressive loss of GFR over the next 4 years of follow-up.[85]

This was confirmed in a study of proteinuric Danish type 2 diabetic patients where those with light microscopic changes of diabetic glomerulopathy had much more rapid decline in GFR over a median of 7.7 years of follow-up.[86]

In summary, it appears that renal structural changes in type 2 diabetes are relatively heterogeneous and diabetic glomerulopathy lesions are less severe than in type 1 patients with similar renal dysfunction. Approximately 40% of the patients show atypical renal injury patterns and these patterns are associated with higher body mass index and less diabetic retinopathy. Further cross-sectional and longitudinal studies in type 2 diabetic patients are required before these complexities can be better understood.

It is possible that the atypical manifestations of renal injury in type 2 diabetes could be related to the pathogenesis of type 2 diabetes per se. Thus, obesity, hypertension, increased plasma triglyceride levels, decreased high-density lipoprotein cholesterol concentrations, and accelerated atherosclerosis accompany hyperglycemia in many type 2 diabetic patients in what Reaven termed *syndrome X*.[87] Renal dysfunction in syndrome X, which could clinically simulate nephropathy in type 2 diabetes, could then be the consequence of hypertensive nephrosclerosis, hyperlipidemic renal vascular atherosclerosis, renal hypoperfusion due to congestive heart failure, or the synergistic effects of these multiple factors. The increased risk of clinical renal disease in certain subgroups, such as African Americans, could represent the differential renal consequence of one or more of these pathogenetic influences, for example, the differences in the renal structural consequences of hypertension in African American and white patients.[88]

Other Renal Disorders in Diabetic Patients

It has been reported that renal disorders such as nil lesion nephrotic syndrome[89] and membranous nephropathy[90] occur with greater frequency in the type 1 patient population than among nondiabetics. In fact, fewer than 1% of type 1 patients with 10 or more years of diabetes and fewer than 4% of those with proteinuria and long diabetes duration will have conditions other than, or in addition to, diabetic nephropathy (personal observations). As already discussed, proteinuric type 2 diabetic patients without retinopathy may have a high incidence of atypical renal biopsies or other diseases. Proteinuria in type 1 diabetic patients with less than 10 years of diabetes duration or type 2 diabetic patients without retinopathy should be thoroughly evaluated for other renal diseases and renal biopsy for diagnosis and prognosis should be strongly considered.

Diabetic Nephropathy Lesions Are Reversible

Rats with long-term diabetes induced by islet cell toxins develop mesangial expansion which, by semiquantitative light microscopic studies, reverses within 2 months after transplantation of a kidney with these lesions into normal rats.[56] Similarly, mesangial expansion after 7 months of diabetes reverses within 2 months after normoglycemia is induced by islet transplantation.[91] Electron microscopic morphometric studies show that mesangial expansion in diabetic rats is due equally to expansion of the matrix and cellular components, and both normalize after islet transplantation.[92] However,

increased GBM width in these rats did not improve over this time.[93] It was thus surprising that no improvement in diabetic nephropathy lesions was found at 5 years after establishment of normoglycemia following successful pancreatic transplantation[94] in type 1 patients with diabetes duration of approximately 20 years. However, after 10 years of normoglycemia these same patients had marked reversal of diabetic glomerulopathy lesions. Thus GBM and TBM width were reduced at 10 years compared to the baseline and 5-year values, with several patients having measures at 10 years that had returned to the normal range (Fig. 38-11A and B).[95] Similar results were obtained with Vv(Mes/glom), primarily in association with a marked decrease in mesangial matrix fractional volume (Fig. 38-11C and D). Remarkable glomerular architectural remodeling was seen by light microscopy, including the complete disappearance of Kimmelstiel-Wilson nodular lesions (Fig. 38-12).[95] The reason for the long delay in this reversal process is not understood. Regardless of the mechanism, it seems logical that relevant renal cells must be able to recognize their abnormal ECM environment and must be able to initiate and sustain an opposite ECM imbalance where the rate of ECM removal exceeds that of ECM production. This is clearly not the normal situation because, throughout adult life, GBM width and Vv(Mes/glom) remain quite constant consistent with balanced ECM production and removal.[43]

EPIDEMIOLOGY OF MICROALBUMINURIA AND DIABETIC NEPHROPATHY

Prevalence and Incidence

Table 38-2 displays the prevalence, incidence, and cumulative incidence of abnormally elevated urinary albumin excretion in type 1 and type 2 diabetes. The overall prevalence of micro- and macroalbuminuria is around 30% to 35% in both types of diabetes. However, the range in prevalence of diabetic nephropathy is much wider in type 2 diabetic patients. This is mainly explained by ethnic differences. The highest prevalence is found in Native Americans followed by black Americans, Mexican Americans, Asian Indians, and European white patients.[96, 97] It should be stressed that good agreement has been documented between the clinic- and population-based studies. The cumulative incidence of persistent proteinuria in type 1 diabetic patients diagnosed before 1942 was about 40% to 50% after 25 to 30 years' duration, but it has declined to 25% to 30% in type 1 diabetic patients diagnosed after 1953.[19, 23, 24, 98, 99] This so-called calendar effect has unfortunately not been seen in European white type 2 diabetic patients.[27] The reason for the declining cumulative incidence of proteinuria in type 1 diabetic patients is unknown, but improved diabetes care and control have been suggested,[100] in addition to a general decline in nondiabetic glomerulopathies.

Diabetic nephropathy rarely develops before 10 years' duration of type 1 diabetes, whereas approximately 3% of newly diagnosed type 2 diabetic patients have overt nephropathy.[101] The incidence peak (3% per year) is usually found between 10 and 20 years of diabetes, after which a progressive decline in incidence takes place.[18, 22] Thus, the risk of developing diabetic nephropathy for a normoalbuminuric patient with a diabetes duration of greater than 30 years is very

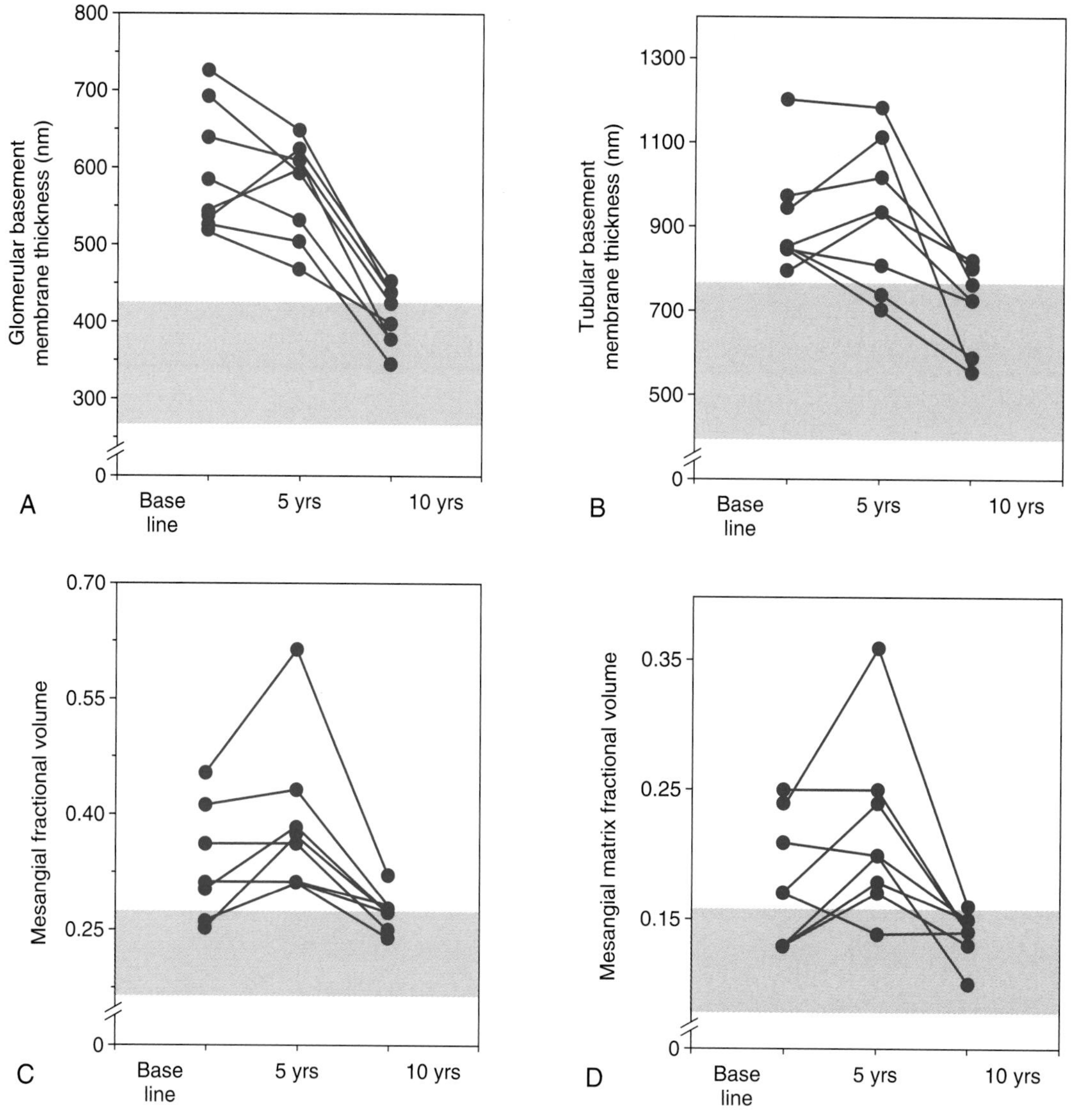

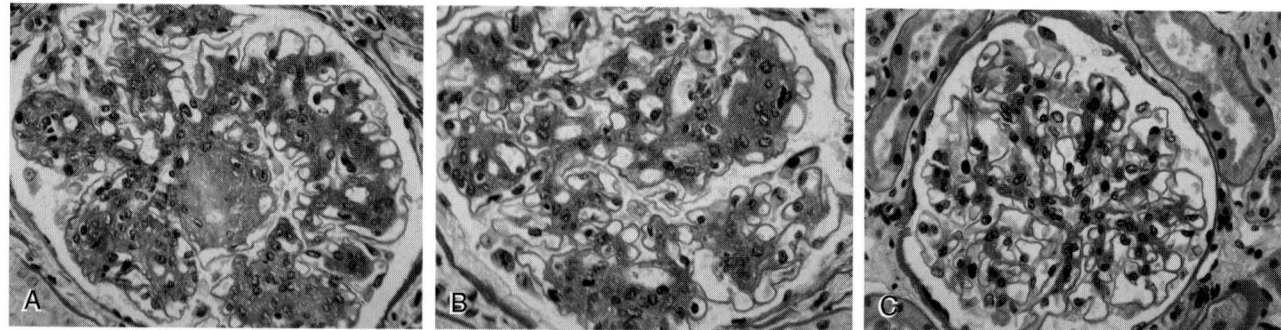

FIGURE 38-11. Thickness of the glomerular basement membrane (GBM). (**A**) thickness of the tubular basement membrane (TBM), (**B**) mesangial fractional volume (**C**), and mesangial-matrix fractional volume (**D**) at baseline, and 5 and 10 years after pancreas transplantation. The shaded area represents the normal ranges obtained in the 66 age-and sex-matched normal controls (mean ± 2 SD). Data for individual patients are connected by lines. (From Fioretto P, Steffes MW, Sutherland DER, et al: Reversal of lesions of diabetic nephropathy after pancreas transplantation. N Engl J Med 339:69-75, 1998.)

FIGURE 38-12. Light microscopic photomicrographs (PAS stain) of renal biopsy specimens obtained before and after pancreas transplantation from a 33-year-old woman with type 1 diabetes of 17 years' duration at the time of transplantation. **A,** Typical glomerulus from the baseline biopsy specimen, which is characterized by diffuse and nodular (Kimmelstiel-Wilson) diabetic glomerulopathy. **B,** Typical glomerulus 5 years after transplantation with persistence of the diffuse and nodular lesions. **C,** Typical glomerulus 10 years after transplantation, with marked resolution of diffuse and nodular mesangial lesions and more open glomerular capillary lumens. (From Fioretto P, Steffes MW, Sutherland DER, et al: Reversal of lesions of diabetic neuropathy after pancreas transplantation. N Engl J Med 339:69-75, 1998.)

TABLE 38-2

Prevalence, Incidence, and Cumulative Incidence of Microalbuminuria and Nephropathy in Diabetes (Median and Range Indicated)

	CLINIC-BASED		POPULATION-BASED
	Type 1	Type 2	Type 2
Prevalence (%) of:			
Microalbuminuria[101, 103, 182, 572-578]	13 (9-20)	25 (13-27)	20 (17-21)
Macroalbuminuria[101, 572, 574, 576, 577, 579-591]	15 (8-22)	14 (5-48)	16 (9-46)
Incidence of macroalbuminuria (%/yr)[18, 24, 25, 27, 592]	1.2 (0-3)	1.5 (1-2)	–
Cumulative incidence of macroalbuminuria (%/25 yr)[18, 24, 25, 27, 592]	31 (28-34)	28 (25-31)	–

TABLE 38-3

Predictive Value of Microalbuminuria for the Development of Diabetic Nephropathy

STUDY	NO. OF PATIENTS	OBSERVATION PERIOD (yr)	CUTOFF URINARY ALBUMIN EXCRETION RATE (μg/minute)	PATIENTS DEVELOPING NEPHROPATHY (%)
Parving et al.[7]	23 IDDM	6	>28	75
			<28	13
Viberti et al.[8]	63 IDDM	14	>30	87
			<30	4
Mogensen & Christensen[9]	43 IDDM	10	>15	86
			<15	0
Mathiesen et al.[10]	71 IDDM	6	>70	100
			<70	5
Mogensen[11]	180 NIDDM	9	>30*	22
			<30*	5
Nelson et al.[12]	439 NIDDM	4	>30†	34
			<30†	4
Ravid et al.[13]	49 NIDDM	5	>20	42
			<20	–

*Albumin μg/mL.

†Albumin creatinine ratio.

low. This changing pattern of risk indicates that the magnitude of exposure to diabetes is not sufficient to explain the development of diabetic nephropathy, and suggests that only a subset of patients are susceptible to kidney complications.

Microalbuminuria Predicts Nephropathy

The type 1 diabetic subpopulation at risk may now be identified fairly accurately by the detection of microalbuminuria.[7-10] Several longitudinal studies have shown that microalbuminuria strongly (predictive power of 80%) predicts the development of diabetic nephropathy in type 1 diabetic patients (Table 38-3).

Type 1 diabetic patients with microalbuminuria have a median risk ratio of 21 for developing diabetic nephropathy, whereas the risk ratio for developing diabetic nephropathy ranges from 4.4 to 21 (median 8.5) in microalbuminuric type 2 diabetic patients.[102] In addition to microalbuminuria, several other risk factors or markers for development of diabetic nephropathy have been documented or suggested as discussed in detail later (Table 38-4).

TABLE 38-4

Risk Factors and Markers for Development of Nephropathy in Type 1 and Type 2 Diabetic Patients

RISK FACTORS/MARKERS	TYPE 1	TYPE 2
Normoalbuminuria (above median)[172, 173, 593]	+	+
Microalbuminuria[7-13, 594]	+	+
Sex[4, 18, 22, 101, 595]	M>F	M>F
Familial clustering[596-600]	+	+
Predisposition to arterial hypertension[214-217, 219, 601]	±	+
Increased sodium/lithium countertransport[215, 216, 601-608]	±	–
Ethnic conditions[96, 97]	+	+
Onset of IDDM before age 20 yr[22, 24, 109]	+	?
Glycemic control[585, 594, 609-611]	+	±
Hyperfiltration[166-171, 230]	±	±
Prorenin[612-617]	+	?
Smoking[168, 618-622]	+	?
Cholesterol[172, 173, 623]	+	+
Presence of retinopathy[79, 172, 173, 229, 624]	+	+

+, Present; –, not present; ±, may be present or absent; ?, no relevant information.

Prognosis in Microalbuminuria

A recent meta-analysis has demonstrated that microalbuminuria is a strong predictor of total and cardiovascular mortality and cardiovascular morbidity in diabetic patients[103] (Table 38-5). Accordingly, microalbuminuria predicts coronary and peripheral vascular disease and death from CVD in the general nondiabetic population.[104-106] The mechanisms linking microalbuminuria and death from CVD are poorly understood. Microalbuminuria has been proposed as a marker of widespread endothelial dysfunction which might predispose to enhanced penetrations in the arterial wall of atherogenic lipoprotein particles[107]; as a marker of established cardiovascular disease[108]; and microalbuminuria is associated with an excess of well-known and potential cardiovascular risk factors.[108] Raised blood pressure,[10, 109-111] dyslipoproteinemia,[112-116] increased platelet aggregability,[113] endothelial dysfunction,[117-122] insulin resistance, and hyperinsulinemia[123, 124] have been demonstrated in microalbuminuria diabetic patients. Autonomic neuropathy, which is also associated with microalbuminuria, predicts death (often sudden) from CVD in diabetic patients,[125] whereas the prevalence of coronary heart disease based on Minnesota coded electrocardiograms (ECGs) is not increased in microalbuminuric non-insulin-dependent diabetes mellitus (NIDDM) patients.[101] Recent echocardiographic studies have revealed impaired diastolic function and cardiac hypertrophy in microalbuminuric insulin-dependent (IDDM) and NIDDM patients.[126-129] Left ventricular hypertrophy predisposes the individual to ischemic heart disease, ventricular arrhythmia, sudden death, and heart failure.[130]

Prognosis in Diabetic Nephropathy

In a cohort of 1030 type 1 diabetic patients diagnosed between 1933 and 1952, patients not developing proteinuria had a low and constant relative mortality, whereas patients with proteinuria had on average a 40 times higher relative mortality.[21, 22] Type 1 diabetic patients with proteinuria showed the characteristic bell-shaped relationship between diabetes duration and age and relative mortality of 110 in females and 80 in males in the age interval of 34 to 38 years. Several other studies have confirmed the poor prognosis in type 1 diabetic patients suffering from diabetic nephropathy, as reviewed by Borch-Johnsen.[22] In three early studies which described the natural course of diabetic nephropathy in type 1 diabetic patients,[18, 24, 131] the cumulative death rate 10 years after onset of nephropathy ranged from 50% to 77%. The 50% figure is a minimum value as Krolewski and co-workers[24] included only death due to ESRD. Two studies have shown a decreasing relative mortality with increasing calendar year of diagnosis, the major decrease occurring between 1941 and 1955.[19, 24]

The overall decrease in relative mortality from 1933 to 1972 was 40% and is partly explained by the decrease in the cumulative incidence of proteinuria. Unfortunately, this calendar effect is not seen in proteinuric type 2 diabetic patients, and subsequently no improved prognosis has been reported.[27] However, the prognostic importance of proteinuria in type 2 patients is considerably less than in type 1 diabetes. Proteinuria confers a 3.5 times higher risk of death, and the concomitant presence of arterial hypertension increases this relative risk to 7 in Pima Indians with type 2 diabetes.[26] European type 2 diabetic patients with proteinuria have a fourfold excess of premature death compared to patients without proteinuria.[132] The cumulative death rate 10 years after onset of abnormally elevated urinary albumin excretion in European type 2 diabetic patients was 70% compared to 45% in normoalbuminuric type 2 diabetic patients.[133, 134]

ESRD is the major cause of death, accounting for 59% to 66% of deaths in type 1 diabetic patients suffering from nephropathy.[17, 18, 22] The cumulative incidence of ESRD 10 years after onset of proteinuria in proteinuric type 1 diabetic patients is 50%,[24] compared to 3% to 11% in proteinuric

TABLE 38-5

Microalbuminuria as Predictor of Mortality in Diabetes Mellitus

STUDY	NO. OF PATIENTS	OBSERVATION PERIOD (yr)	CUTOFF URINARY ALBUMIN EXCRETION RATE (μg/minute)	MORTALITY (%)
*Mogensen[11]	204 NIDDM	9	>30[†]	78
			<30[†]	49
*Jarret et al.[625]	44 NIDDM	14	>10	91
			<10	22
Mattock et al.[626]	141 NIDDM	3.4	>20	28
			<20	4
MacLeod et al.[627]	400 NIDDM	8	>11	52
			<11	30
Atkinson et al.[628]	216 NIDDM	8	>35[†]	47
			<35[†]	21
Gall et al.[629]	328 NIDDM	5	>20	20
			<20	8
Stiegler et al.[630]	290 NIDDM	3	>20[†]	10
			<20[†]	5
Rossing et al.[32]	774 IDDM	10	>20	25
			<20	15

*Retrospective studies.
†Albumin per milliliter.

European type 2 diabetic patients[135] and 65% in proteinuric Pima Indians with type 2 diabetes.[136] However, renal insufficiency was defined as a serum creatinine greater than or equal to 2.0 mg/dL in the Pima Indian study. Of the excess mortality associated with type 2 diabetes in this population, 97% was found in patients with proteinuria, 16% of deaths were ascribed to ESRD, and 22% were due to CVD.[26] CVD is also a major cause of death (15%-25%) in type 1 diabetic patients with nephropathy, despite the relatively low age at death[18, 22] Borch-Johnsen and Kreiner[20] studied a cohort of 2890 type 1 diabetic patients and demonstrated that the relative mortality from CVD was 37 times higher in proteinuric type 1 diabetic patients compared to the general population. Abnormalities in well-established cardiovascular risk factors alone cannot account for this finding. In recent years several studies have shown abnormally raised levels of serum apolipoprotein (a) to be a strong independent risk factor for premature ischemic heart disease in nondiabetic subjects.[137] However, studies in type 1 and type 2 diabetic patients suffering from diabetic nephropathy have yielded conflicting results.[114-116, 138] Most studies have demonstrated that a familial predisposition to CVD is present in type 1 diabetic patients with diabetic nephropathy.[139-142] Increased left ventricular hypertrophy, an established CVD risk factor, and a decrease in diastolic function occur early in the course of diabetic nephropathy.[143] Left ventricular hypertrophy is a well-established risk factor for CVD. Increased plasma homocysteine concentration is also a CVD risk factor and predicts mortality in type 2 diabetic patients with albuminuria.[144] Recently, we demonstrated that increased urinary albumin excretion, endothelial dysfunction, and chronic inflammation are interrelated processes that develop in parallel, progress with time, and are strongly and independently associated with risk of death in type 2 diabetes.[145]

CLINICAL COURSE AND PATHOPHYSIOLOGY

A preclinical phase consisting of a normo-and a microalbuminuria stage and a clinical phase characterized by albuminuria are well documented in both type 1 and type 2 diabetic patients.

Normoalbuminuria

In 1934, Cambier suggested that GFR is increased in some patients suffering from diabetes mellitus.[146] Numerous studies have confirmed and extended this observation in type 1 diabetic patients.[147-154] Approximately one third of type 1 diabetic patients will have a GFR above the upper normal range of age-matched healthy nondiabetic subjects. The degree of hyperfiltration is less in type 2 diabetic patients[155, 156] and reported lacking in some studies.[157] The GFR elevation is particularly pronounced in newly diagnosed diabetic patients and during other intervals with poor metabolic control. Intensified insulin treatment and near-normal blood glucose control reduce GFR toward normal levels after a period of days to weeks in both type 1 and type 2 diabetic patients.[147, 151, 153, 155, 158, 159] Additional metabolites, vasoactive hormones, and increased kidney and glomerular size have been suggested as mediators of hyperfiltration in diabetes, as reviewed by Christiansen[147] (Table 38-6).

TABLE 38-6

Mediators of Hyperfiltration in Diabetes

Glucose[147, 151, 631, 632]
Ketone bodies[633]
Insulin[634]
Growth harmone[635, 636]
Glucagon[637]
High protien intake[638]
Prostaglandins[251, 639, 640]
Atrial natriuretic peptide[641-643]
Nitric oxide[644]
Glomerulopressin[645]
Sodium/lithium countertransport[605]
Kidney and glomerular enlargement[147, 152, 153, 161, 162, 207, 308, 309, 646]

Four factors regulate GFR.[160] First, the glomerular plasma flow influences the mean ultrafiltration pressure and thereby the GFR. Enhanced renal plasma flow (RPF) has been demonstrated in type 1 and type 2 diabetic patients with elevated GFR.[147, 151, 155, 159] A second factor is the systemic oncotic pressure, which is reported to be normal as calculated from plasma protein concentrations.[147, 151] The third determinant of GFR is the glomerular transcapillary hydraulic pressure difference, which cannot be measured in humans. However, the demonstrated increase in filtration fraction is compatible with the enhanced transglomerular hydraulic pressure difference.[147, 151] The last determinant of GFR is the glomerular ultrafiltration coefficient, K_f which is determined by the product of the hydraulic conductance of the glomerular capillary and the glomerular capillary surface area available for filtration. The total glomerular capillary surface area is clearly increased already at the onset of human diabetes.[161, 162]

Studies in insulin-treated experimental diabetic rats have revealed hyperfiltration, hyperperfusion, enhanced glomerular capillary hydraulic pressure, reduced proximal tubular pressure, unchanged systemic oncotic pressure, and unchanged or slightly elevated K_f.[163, 164] Several studies suggest that insulin-like growth factor-I plays a major role in the initiation of renal and glomerular growth in diabetic animals, as reviewed by Flyvbjerg.[165]

Longitudinal studies suggest that hyperfiltration is a risk factor for subsequent increase in urinary albumin excretion and development of diabetic nephropathy in type 1 diabetic patients,[166-168] but conflicting results have also been reported.[169, 170] The prognostic significance of hyperfiltration in type 2 diabetic patients is still debated.[171] Six prospective cohort studies investigating normoalbuminuric type 1 and type 2 diabetic patients for 4 to 10 years revealed that minimal elevation of urinary albumin excretion, poor glycemic control, hyperfiltration, elevated arterial blood pressure, retinopathy, and smoking contribute to the development of persistent microalbuminuria and overt diabetic nephropathy.[168, 172-176] Because several of those risk factors are modifiable, intervention is feasible, as discussed later.

Microalbuminuria

In 1969, Keen and colleagues[177] demonstrated elevated urinary albumin excretion in newly diagnosed type 2 diabetes. The same phenomenon was also documented in newly diagnosed or short-term type 1 diabetic patients in poor glycemic control.[178] This abnormal but subclinical albumin excretion rate has been termed *microalbuminuria* and it can be normalized by improved glycemic control. In addition to hyperglycemia, many other factors can induce microalbuminuria in diabetic patients such as hypertension, massive obesity, heavy exercise, various acute or chronic illnesses, and cardiac failure.[179, 180] Furthermore, the day-to-day variation in the urinary AER is high, 30% to 50%,[181] and consequently more than one urine sample is needed to determine whether an individual patient has persistent microalbuminuria. Urinary albumin excretion within the microalbuminuric range (30-300 mg/24 hours) in at least two out of three consecutive nonketotic sterile urine samples is the generally accepted definition of persistent microalbuminuria. Persistent microalbuminuria has not been detected in type 1 diabetic children younger than age 12 years[182] and is exceptional in the first 5 years of diabetes.[183] The annual rate of rise of urinary albumin excretion is about 20% in both type 2[13] and type 1 diabetic patients with persistent microalbuminuria.[184]

The excretion of albumin in the urine is determined by the amount filtered across the glomerular capillary barrier and the amount reabsorbed by the tubular cells. A normal urinary beta$_2$-microglobulin excretion rate in microalbuminuria suggests that albumin derives from enhanced glomerular leakage rather than from reduced tubular reabsorption of protein. The transglomerular passage of macromolecules is governed by the size- and charge-selective properties of the glomerular capillary membrane and the hemodynamic forces operating across the capillary wall.[185] Alterations in glomerular pressure and flow influence both the diffusive and the convecting driving forces for transglomerular passage of proteins.[186] Studies using renal clearance of endogenous plasma proteins or dextrans have not detected a simple size-selective defect.[151, 178, 187-191] Determination of the IgG/IgG$_4$ ratio suggests that loss of glomerular charge-selectivity procedes or accompanies the formation of new glomerular macromolecular pathways in the development of diabetic nephropathy.[189] Reduction in the negatively charged moieties of the glomerular capillary wall, particularly sialic acid and heparan sulfhate, have been suggested,[108, 192] but not confirmed.[66, 193] Long-term diabetes in spontaneously hypertensive rats is associated with a reduction in both gene and protein expression of nephrin within the kidney.[194] Changes in podocyte number and morphology have been implicated in the pathogenesis of proteinuria and progression of diabetic kidney disease.[65, 195-197] Filtration fraction is presumed to reflect the glomerular hydraulic pressure, and microalbuminuric type 1 diabetic patients have elevated filtration both at rest and during exercise compared to normal controls.[198] A close correlation between filtration fraction and urinary albumin excretion has been demonstrated as well. The demonstration that microalbuminuria diminishes promptly with acute reduction in arterial blood pressure argues for reversible hemodynamic factors playing an important role in the pathogenesis of microalbuminuria.[199] Imanishi and colleagues have demonstrated that glomerular hypertension is present in type 2 diabetic patients with early nephropathy and is closely correlated with increased urinary albumin excretion. In addition, it should be mentioned that increased pressure has been demonstrated in the nail fold capillaries of microalbuminuric type 1 diabetic patients.[201]

GFR measured with the single injection[51]Cr-EDTA (ethylenediaminetetracetic acid) plasma clearance method or the renal clearance of inulin is normal or slightly elevated in type 1 diabetic patients with microalbuminuria.[202-204] Prospective studies have demonstrated that GFR remains stable at normal or supranormal levels for at least 5 years if clinical nephropathy does not develop.[205] Nephromegaly is still present and even more pronounced in microalbuminuric compared to normoalbuminuric type 1 diabetic patients.[206, 207]

Changes in tubular function take place early in diabetes and are related to the degree of glycemic control. The proximal tubular reabsorption of fluid, sodium, and glucose is enhanced.[208] This process could diminish distal sodium delivery and thereby stimulate a tubuloglomerular feedback–mediated enhancement of GFR.[209-211] A direct effect of insulin increasing distal sodium reabsorption has also been demonstrated.[208, 212] The consequences of these alterations in tubular transport for overall kidney function are unknown.

Several studies have demonstrated blood pressure elevation in children and adults with type 1 diabetes and microalbuminuria.[10, 109, 111, 182] The prevalence of arterial hypertension (Joint National Committee [JNC-V] criteria ≥ 140/90 mm Hg) in adult type 1 diabetic patients increases with albuminuria, being 42%, 52%, and 79% in subjects with normo-, micro-, and macroalbuminuria, respectively.[109, 213] The prevalence of hypertension in type 2 diabetes (mean age 60 years) was higher. 71%, 90% and 93% in the normo-, micro-, and macroalbuminuria groups, respectively.[101, 213] A genetic predisposition to hypertension in type 1 diabetic patients developing diabetic nephropathy has been suggested[214] but other studies did not confirm the concept.[215-218] Recently we have confirmed the original finding by applying 24-hour blood pressure measuring in a large group of parents to type 1 diabetic patients with and without diabetic nephropathy.[219] In addition, the cumulative incidence of hypertension was higher among parents of proteinuric patients, with a shift toward younger age at onset of hypertension in this group. However, the difference in prevalence of parental hypertension was not evident using office blood pressure measurements. Several studies have reported that sodium and water retention play a dominant role in the initiation and maintenance of systemic hypertension in microalbuminuria and diabetic nephropathy, whereas the contribution of the renin-angiotensin-aldosterone system is smaller.[203, 220-222]

Diabetic Nephropathy

Diabetic nephropathy is a clinical syndrome characterized by persistent albuminuria (>300 mg/24 hours), a relentless decline in GFR, and raised arterial blood pressure.[4, 223] While albuminuria is the first sign, peripheral edema is the first symptom of diabetic nephropathy.[224] Fluid retention is frequently observed early in the course of this kidney disease, that is, at a stage with well-preserved renal function and only slight reduction in serum albumin.[224] A recent study suggests that capillary hypertension, increased capillary surface area, and reduced capillary reflection coefficient for plasma proteins contribute to the edema formation, whereas the washout of subcutaneous interstitial protein tends to prevent the progressive edema formation in diabetic nephropathy.[225, 226]

Most studies dealing with the natural history of diabetic nephropathy have demonstrated a relentless, often linear but highly variable rate of decline in GFR ranging from 2 to 20 mL/minute/year, with a mean of 12 mL/minute/year.[223, 227, 228] Type 2 diabetic patients suffering from nephropathy display the same degree of loss in filtration power and in variability of GFR.[229, 230] Morphologic studies in both type 1 and type 2 diabetic patients have demonstrated a close inverse correlation between the degree of glomerular and tubulointerstitial lesions on the one side and the GFR level on the other side, as discussed in detail previously. Myers and co-workers[231-236] have demonstrated a reduction in the number of restrictive pores leading to loss of ultrafiltration capacity (K_f) and impairment of glomerular barrier size-selectivity leading to progressive albuminuria and IgGuria in diabetic nephropathy. Furthermore, the extent to which ultrafiltration capacity is impaired appears to be related to the magnitude of the defect in the barrier size-selectivity. A defect in the glomerular barrier size-selectivity has also been demonstrated in type 2 diabetic patients with diabetic nephropathy.[237] The reduction in RPF is proportional to the reduction in GFR (filtration fraction unchanged), and the impact on GFR is partially offset by the diminished systemic colloid osmotic pressure.

Several putative promoters of progression in kidney function have been studied in type 1 diabetes[227, 238-244] and type 2 diabetes[229] patients with nephropathy. A close correlation between blood pressure and the rate of decline in GFR has been documented in type 1 and type 2 diabetic patients.[72, 242, 244-247] This suggests that systemic blood pressure accelerates the progression of diabetic nephropathy. Previously, the adverse impact of systemic hypertension on renal function and structure was thought to be mediated through vasoconstriction and arteriolar nephrosclerosis.[248] However, evidence from rat models shows that systemic hypertension is transmitted to the single glomerulus in such a way as to lead to hyperfusion and increased capillary pressure.[249, 250] Intraglomerular hypertension has also been documented directly in streptozotocin-induced diabetic rats[249, 251] and estimated to prevail in human diabetes, particularly that complicated by kidney disease.[200] Impaired or abolished renal autoregulation of GFR and RPF as demonstrated in type 1 and type 2 diabetic patients with nephropathy contribute to increase vulnerability to hypertension or ischemic injuries of glomerular capillaries.[252, 253] Defective autoregulation of GFR has been demonstrated in streptozotocin-induced diabetic rats during hyperglycemia,[254] but studies in humans with type 2 diabetes revealed no impact of glycemic control on GFR autoregulation.[255] Originally, Remuzzi and Bertani[256] suggested that proteinuria itself may contribute to renal damage. In 1972 Watkins and co-workers[238] demonstrated that type 1 diabetic patients with diabetic nephropathy and nephrotic-range proteinuria (>3 g/24 hours) had the worst prognosis. Several observational studies and treatment trials have confirmed and extended these findings to also include subnephrotic-range proteinuria.[26, 72, 240, 245, 257]

For many years it was believed that once albuminuria had become persistent, then glycemic control had lost its beneficial impact on kidney function and structure, and consequently the concept of "point of no return" was advocated by many investigators, as reviewed by Parving.[258] This misconception was based on studies with few patients, applying inappropriate methods for monitoring kidney function (serum creatinine) and glycemic control (random blood glucose). Several more recent studies dealing with large numbers of type 1 diabetic patients have documented the important impact of glycemic control on progression of diabetic nephropathy.[245, 247, 257, 259-263] In contrast, most of the studies dealing with proteinuric type 2 diabetic patients have failed to demonstrate any significant impact,[226, 229, 264] with one exception.[265] Nearly all studies in type 1 and type 2 diabetic patients have demonstrated a correlation between serum cholesterol concentration and progression of diabetic nephropathy, at least in univariate analysis,[226, 229, 242, 244-247] and some have failed to demonstrate cholesterol as an independent risk factor in multiple regression analysis.

Dietary protein restriction retards the progression of renal disease in virtually every experimental animal model tested.[248] Surprisingly, all major observational studies in type 1 and type 2 diabetic patients with diabetic nephropathy have failed to demonstrate an impact of dietary protein intake on the rate of decline in GFR.[226, 229, 230, 245-247, 259-261, 267] Some but not all studies suggest that smoking may act as a progression promoter in both type 1 and type 2 diabetic patients with proteinuria,[268, 269] but, larger, long-term studies have not been able to confirm that.[270]

The insertion (I)/deletion (D) polymorphism of the gene for angiotensin-converting enzyme, the ACE gene (ACE/ID), is strongly associated with the level of circulating ACE and increased risk of coronary heart disease (CHD) in nondiabetic and diabetic patients.[271, 272] The plasma ACE level in DD subjects is about twice that of II subjects, with ID subjects having intermediate levels.[273] Yoshida and colleagues[274] followed 168 proteinuric type 2 diabetic patients over 10 years. Analysis of the clinical course of the three ACE genotypes revealed that the majority (95%) of patients with the DD genotype progressed to ESRD within 10 years. Moreover, the DD genotype appeared to increase mortality once dialysis was initiated. Two recent studies have confirmed that the D allele had a deleterious effect on kidney function.[275, 276] Finally, more severe diabetic glomerulopathy lesions have been documented both during development and progression of renal disease in type 2 diabetic patients with the D allele.[277] Furthermore, microalbuminuric type 1 patients carrying the D allele have an increased progression of diabetic glomerulopathy, a finding based on renal biopsies taken at baseline and after 26 to 48 months of follow-up.[278]

We showed an accelerated initial and sustained loss of GFR during ACE inhibitor treatment of albuminuric type 1 patients homozygous for the DD polymorphism of the ACE gene.[279] The DD genotype independently influenced the sustained rate of decline in GFR or, in other words, acted as a progression promoter. Four other studies have demonstrated that the D allele is a risk factor for an accelerated course of diabetic nephropathy in patients with type 1 diabetes,[261, 280-282] although in one of the studies the tendency toward a more rapid decline in renal function in the DD genotype was not significant.[280] The potential contribution from other relevant candidate genes remains to be evaluated.

Pregnancy in women with diabetic nephropathy is accompanied by an increase in complications such as hypertension and proteinuria and by increases in prematurity and fetal loss. The impact of pregnancy on the long-term course of renal function in women with diabetic nephropathy has not been clarified until recently. Our study suggests that pregnancy has no adverse long-term impact on kidney function and survival in type 1 diabetic patients with well-preserved kidney function (serum creatinine at start of pregnancy <100 μmol/L) suffering from diabetic nephropathy.[283]

Nondiabetic glomerulopathy is very rare in proteinuric type 1 diabetic patients, whereas this condition is common in proteinuric type 2 diabetic patients without retinopathy.[284] A prevalence of biopsies with normal glomerular structure or nondiabetic kidney diseases of approximately 30% was demonstrated. Furthermore, a more rapid decline in GFR and a progressive rise in albuminuria in type 2 diabetic patients with diabetic glomerulopathy compared to type 2 without has been demonstrated.[86, 285]

Systemic blood pressure elevation to a hypertensive level is an early and frequent phenomenon in diabetic nephropathy.[101, 109, 223, 286, 287] Furthermore, nocturnal blood pressure elevation ("non-dippers") occurs more frequently in type 1 and type 2 diabetic patients with nephropathy.[288, 289] An exaggerated blood pressure response to exercise has also been reported in long-standing IDDM patients with microangiopathy.[290] Finally, the increase in glomerular pressure consequent to nephron reduction may be accentuated by concomitant diabetes, as suggested in animal studies.[291]

Extrarenal Complications in Diabetic Nephropathy

Diabetic retinopathy is present in virtually all type 1 diabetic patients with nephropathy,[109] whereas only 50% to 60% of proteinuric NIDDM patients suffer from retinopathy.[101, 292] Absence of retinopathy should require further investigation for nondiabetic glomerulopathies.[5, 6, 293] Blindness due to severe proliferative retinopathy or maculopathy is approximately five times greater in type 1 and type 2 diabetic patients with nephropathy compared to normoalbuminuric patients.[101, 109] Macroangiopathy, for example, stroke, carotid artery stenosis, CHD, and peripheral vascular disease are two to five times more common in nephropathic patients.[101, 292, 294-296]

Peripheral neuropathy is present in almost all patients with advanced nephropathy. Foot ulcers with sepsis leading to amputation occur frequently (>25%), probably due to a combination of neural and arterial disease.[297] Autonomic neuropathy may be asymptomatic and simply manifest as abnormal cardiovascuar reflexes, or it may result in debilitating symptoms. Nearly all patients suffering from nephropathy have grossly abnormal autonomic function tests. Grenfell and Watkins[297] reported that over half of the patients with advanced nephropathy had symptoms of autonomic neuropathy: gustatory sweating, impotence, postural hypotension, and diarrhea. Diabetic cystopathy is also a frequent (>30%) problem in these patients.[298]

TREATMENT

The major therapeutic interventions which have been investigated include near-normal blood glucose control, antihypertensive treatment, lipid lowering, and restriction of dietary proteins. The impact of these three treatment modalities on progression from normo- to microalbuminuria (primary prevention), from microalbuminuria to diabetic nephropathy (secondary prevention), and from diabetic nephropathy to ESRD will be described and discussed.

Glycemic Control
Primary Prevention

Strict metabolic control achieved by insulin treatment or islet cell transplantation normalizes hyperfiltration, hyperperfusion, and glomerular capillary hypertension and reduces the rate of rise in urinary albumin excretion in experimental diabetic animals.[92, 299-307] The treatment also mitigates the development of diabetic glomerulopathy, but the glomerular enlargement remains unaffected.[91, 300, 301] Risk factors for progression from normoalbuminuria to micro- and macroalbuminuria have been identified (see Table 38-4). Short-term near-normal blood glucose control in normoalbuminuric type 1 diabetic patients reduces GFR, RPF, and the urinary AER, which in some,[178, 308-310] but not all,[147] investigations were accompanied by a reduction in the enlarged kidney. Increased kidney size is associated with an exaggerated renal response to amino acid infusion and studies suggest that both abnormalities can be corrected by 3 weeks of intensive insulin treatment.[311] A meta-analysis of long-term (8-60 months) intensive blood glucose control has documented a beneficial effect on the progression from normo- to microalbuminuria in type 1 diabetic patients.[312] The odds ratio for progression from normo- to microalbuminuria ranged from 0.22 to 0.40 in the intensive treatment groups.[313-318] A worsening of diabetic retinopathy was observed during the initial months of intensive therapy but in the longer term the rate of deterioration was slower than it was in the conventionally treated type 1 diabetic patients.[319] Side effects are a major concern with intensive therapy and the frequency of severe hypoglycemia and diabetic ketoacidosis was greater in several studies.[312] In the Diabetes Control and Complications trial (DCCT)[320] intensive therapy reduced the occurrence of microalbuminuria by 39% (95% confidence interval [CI], 21%-52%), and that of albuminuria by 54% (95% CI, 19% to 74%), when analyzing the two cohorts combined. Despite this, however, 16% in the primary prevention and 26% in the secondary prevention cohort developed microalbuminuria during the 9 years of intensive treatment. This clearly documents the need for additional treatment modalities to avoid or reduce the burden of diabetic nephropathy.

A much smaller study with a design similar to the DCCT in Japanese type 2 diabetic patients also showed a beneficial effect on progression of normoalbuminuria to micro- and macroalbuminuria.[321] This study has been confirmed and extended by the U.K. Prospective Diabetes Study (UKPDS) data documenting a progressive beneficial effect of intensive metabolic control on the development of microalbuminuria and overt proteinuria.[322]

Secondary Prevention

Several modifiable risk factors (level of urinary albumin excretion, hemoglobin A_{1c} (HbA_{1c}), smoking, blood pressure, and serum cholesterol concentration) for progression from microalbuminuria to overt diabetic nephropathy have been identified in clinical trials of type 1 and type 2 diabetic patients.[13, 323-326]

TABLE 38-7

Randomized Studies Comparing the Renal Effects of Intensive (I) Blood Glucose Control vs Conventional (C) Treatment in Type 1 Diabetic Patients with Microalbuminuria

STUDY	FOLLOW-UP (YR)	BASELINE NO. WITH MICROALBUMINURIA	END OF STUDY NORMOALBUMINURIA	MICROALBUMINURIA	NEPHROPATHY	CHANGE IN URINARY ALBUMIN EXCRETION RATE (%/YR)	
DCCT[320]							
I		38	23	11	4	2.5	
	6.5						P < .09
C		35	18	11	6	11	
Stockholm study[647]							
I		8	2	4	2	−2.6	
	7.5						P = .04
C		13	4	5	4	11.8	
Microalbuminuria Collaborative Study Group UK[648]							
I		36	12	17	6		
	5						P = .31
C		34	12	16	6		
Steno study[649]							
I		18	3	15	0	−9	
	2						P < .05
C		18	5	8	5	7	
Oslo study[650]							
I		9	4	4	1	10.8	
	2						NS
C		9	1	7	1	5.8	
All studies							
I		109*	44	51	13		
C		109*	40	47	22		

Chi-square test, P = .26 for distribution between the three groups, and P = .15 for progression to nephropathy.
DCCT, Diabetes Control and Complications Trial Research Group.

The renal impact of intensive diabetic treatment versus conventional diabetic treatment on progression or regression of microalbuminuria in type 1 diabetic patients has shown conflicting outcomes (Table 38-7). These disappointing results might partly be due to the relatively short length of the follow-up period, as the UKPDS study with 15 years of follow-up documented a progressive beneficial effect with time on the development of proteinuria and a twofold increase in plasma creatinine.[322] Furthermore, pancreatic transplantation can reverse glomerulopathy in patients with type 1 diabetes and normo- (n = 3) or microalbuminria (n = 4), but reversal requires more than 5 years of normoglycemia.[95] Recently, we demonstrated that intensified multifactorial intervention (pharmacologic therapy targeting hyperglycemia, hypertension, dyslipidemia, and microalbuminuria) in patients with type 2 diabetes and microalbuminuria substantially slows progression to nephropathy, retinopathy, and autonomic neuropathy.[327]

Nephropathy

The impact of improved metabolic control on progression of kidney function in IDDM patients with nephropathy has been disappointing.[328, 329] The rate of decline in GFR and the rises in proteinuria and systemic blood pressure were not affected by improved glycemic control. However, it should be stressed that none of the trials were randomized and the number of patients investigated was small. In contrast, most major prospective observational studies have indicated an important role for glycemic control in the progression of diabetic nephropathy, as discussed earlier.[245, 247, 257-261]

Blood Pressure Control
Primary Prevention

Originally, Zatz and co-workers[330] showed that prevention of glomerular capillary hypertension in normotensive insulin-treated streptozotocin-induced diabetic rats effectively protects against the subsequent development of proteinuria and focal and segmental glomerular structural lesions. Jackson and colleagues[239] confirmed the beneficial effect of ACE inhibitors in uninephrectomized rats made diabetic by streptozotocin. Anderson and co-workers[331, 332] have demonstrated that anti-hypertensive therapy slows the development of diabetic glomerulopathy but the ACE inhibitors afford superior long-term protection compared to triple therapy with reserpine, hydralazine, and hydrochlorothiazide or a calcium channel blocker (nifedipine). Recent observations are consistent with the concept that glomerular hypertension is a major factor in the pathogenesis of experimental diabetic glomerulopathy, and indicate that lowering of systemic blood pressure without concomitant reduction of glomerular capillary pressure may be insufficient to prevent glomerular injury.[331-333] Lowering of systemic blood pressure by ACE inhibitors or conventional antihypertensive treatment affords significant renoprotection in spontaneously hypertensive streptozotocin-induced diabetic rats.[334] No specific benefit of ACE inhibitors was observed in this hypertensive model in contrast to the normotensive models mentioned earlier. Three randomized placebo-controlled trials in normotensive type 1 and type 2 diabetic patients with normal AERs have suggested a beneficial effect on the development of microalbuminuria.[335-337] In contrast to these three studies, which were carried out as placebo-controlled trials, the literature contains three new studies comparing the effect of ACE inhibitors versus a long-acting dihydropyridine calcium antagonist[338, 339] or β-blockade[340] in hypertensive type 2 diabetic patients with normoalbuminuria. All three studies reported a similar beneficial renoprotective effect of blood pressure reduction with and without ACE inhibition. Furthermore, the UKPDS study reported that by 6 years a smaller proportion of patients in the group under tight blood pressure control had developed microalbuminuria and had a 29% reduction in risk ($P <.009$), with a nonsignificant 39% reduction in the risk of proteinuria ($P = .061$).[340] Beneficial effects of aggressive blood pressure control in normotensive (<160/90 mm Hg) type 2 diabetic patients on albuminuria, retinopathy, and incidence of stroke have recently been demonstrated.[341] The results were the same whether enalapril or nisoldipine were used as the initial blood pressure–lowering drug. Originally, the EUCLID study group[342] demonstrated a significant beneficial effect of ACE inhibitors on progression of diabetic retinopathy and development of proliferative retinopathy in type 1 diabetic patients.

Secondary Prevention

A meta-analysis of 12 trials in 698 type 1 diabetic patients with microalbuminuria who were followed for at least 1 year has revealed that ACE inhibitors reduced the risk of progression to macroalbuminuria compared to that of the placebo group (odds ratio 0.38 [95% CI, 0.25-0.57]).[343] Regression to normoalbuminuria was three times greater than in the patients receiving placebo. At 2 years, the urinary AER was 50% lower in patients taking ACE inhibitors than in those receiving placebo. Furthermore, we showed that the beneficial effect of ACE inhibitors on preventing progression from microalbuminuria to overt nephropathy is long-lasting (8 years) and, more important, it is associated with preservation of normal GFR.[344] Recent data from a double-blind randomized study lasting 3 years show that long-acting dihydropyridine calcium antagonists are as effective as ACE inhibitors in delaying the occurrence of macroalbuminuria in normotensive patients with type 1 diabetes with persistent microalbuminuria.[345] Finally, agents blocking the effect of renal artery stenosis (RAS) have a beneficial impact on glomerular structural changes in type 1 and type 2 diabetic patients with early diabetic glomerulopathy.[346-348]

In 1993, Borch-Johnsen and colleagues[184] analyzed the cost-benefit ratio of screening for, and antihypertensive treatment of, early renal disease indicated by microalbuminuria in type 1 diabetic patients. The authors concluded that screening and intervention programs are likely to be lifesaving and lead to considerable economic savings.

The impact of ACE inhibitors in microalbuminuric type 2 diabetic patients has also been evaluated. A randomized study[349] of diabetic patients with microalbuminuria treated with perindopril or nifedipine for 12 months was conducted. Both treatments significantly reduced mean arterial blood pressure and the urinary AER. Unfortunately, the study dealt with a heterogeneous group of hypertensive or normotensive type 1 or type 2 diabetic patients. Ravid and associates[13] conducted a double-blind randomized study in 94 normotensive microalbuminuria NIDDM patients receiving enalapril or placebo for 5 years. Kidney function remained stable and only 12% of the patients in the actively treated group developed diabetic nephropathy, whereas kidney function declined by 13%, and 42% of the patients receiving placebo developed nephropathy. These data have been confirmed.[325, 326, 341, 350]

Antihypertensive treatment has a renoprotective effect in hypertensive patients with type 2 diabetes and microalbuminuria.[327, 337-340, 351-356] There has been conflicting evidence regarding the existence of a specific renoprotective effect—that is, a beneficial effect on kidney function beyond the hypotensive effect—of agents that block the renin-angiotensin system in patients with type 2 diabetes and microalbuminuria.[327, 337-340, 351-356] The inconclusive nature of the previous evidence may have been due in part to the small size of the patient groups studied and the short duration of antihypertensive treatment in most previous trials. An exception is the long-lasting UKPDS, which suggested the equivalence of a β-blocker and an angiotensin I–converting enzyme inhibitor.[340] Therefore, we evaluated the renoprotective effect of an angiotensin II receptor antagonist, irbesartan in hypertensive patients with type 2 diabetes and microalbuminuria—the IRMA 2 trial.[357]

A total of 590 hypertensive patients with type 2 diabetes and microalbuminuria were enrolled in this multinational, randomized double-blind, placebo-controlled study of irbesartan at a dose of either 150 or 300 mg/day and followed for 2 years. The primary outcome was the time to onset of diabetic nephropathy, defined by persistent albuminuria in overnight specimens, with a urinary AER that was greater than 200 μg/minute and at least 30% higher than the baseline level. The baseline characteristics in the three groups were similar. Ten of the 194 patients in the 300-mg group (5.2%) and 19 of the 195 patients in the 150-mg group (9.7%) reached the primary end point, as compared with 30 of the

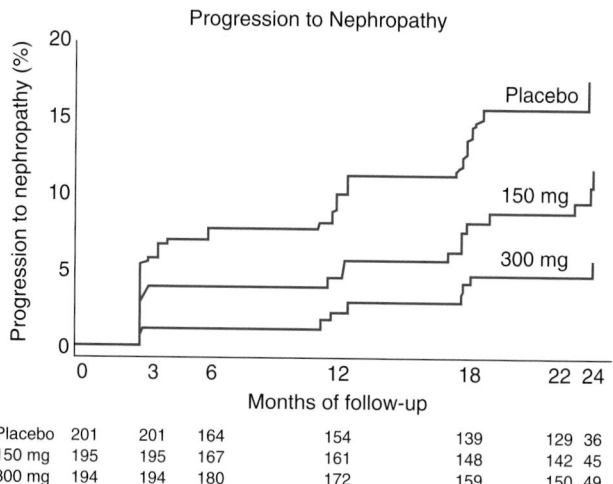

Months of follow-up					
	0	3	6	12	18	22 24

Placebo   201   201   164   154   139   129 36
150 mg   195   195   167   161   148   142 45
300 mg   194   194   180   172   159   150 49

FIGURE 38-13. Probability of progression to diabetic nephropathy during treatment with irbesartan 150 mg/day, 300 mg/day, or placebo in hypertensive type 2 diabetic patients with persistent microalbuminuria. The difference between placebo and irbesartan 150 mg/day was not significant ($P = .80$ by long-rank test) but significant when compared to irbesartan 300 mg/day ($P < .001$ by log-rank test).

201 patients on placebo (14.9%) (hazard ratio 0.30 [95% CI, 0.14-0.61; $P < .001$] and 0.61 [95% CI, 0.34-1.08; $P = .08$] for the two irbesartan groups, respectively). (Fig 38-13). The average blood pressure during the course of the study was 144/83 mm Hg in the placebo group, 143/83 mm Hg in the 150-mg group and 141/83 mm Hg in the 300-mg group ($P = .004$ for the comparison of systolic blood pressure between the placebo group and the combined irbesartan groups). Serious adverse events were less frequent among the patients treated with irbesartan ($P = .02$). The IRMA 2 study demonstrated that irbesartan is renoprotective independent of its blood pressure–lowering effect in patients with type 2 diabetes and microalbuminuria.

In 1995 a consensus report on the detection, prevention, and treatment of diabetic nephropathy with special reference to microalbuminuria was published.[358] Improved blood glucose control (HbA$_{1c}$ < 7.5%-8%) and treatment with ACE inhibitors was recommended. Based on the trials with angiotensin II receptor blockers (ARBs), the American Diabetes Association now recommends: "In hypertensive Type 2 diabetic patients with microalbuminuria or clinical albuminuria, ARBs are the initial agents of choice."[359]

Nephropathy

From a clinical point of view the ability to predict the long-term effect on kidney function of a recently initiated treatment modality, for example, antihypertensive therapy, would be of great value as this could allow for early identification of patients in need of an intensive or alternative therapeutic regimen. In two prospective studies dealing with conventional antihypertensive treatment and ACE inhibitors, we found that the initial reduction in albuminuria (surrogate end point) predicted a beneficial long-term treatment effect on rate of decline in GFR in diabetic nephropathy (principal end point).[360, 361] These findings have been confirmed and extended.[247, 362] Furthermore, similar findings have been demonstrated in nondiabetic nephropathies.[363, 364]

The antiproteinuric effect of ACE inhibitors in patients with diabetic nephropathy varies considerably. Individual differences in the renin-angiotensin system may influence this variation. Therefore, we tested the potential role of an insertion (I)/deletion (D) polymorphism of the ACE gene on this early antiproteinuric responsiveness in an observational follow-up study of young hypertensive type 1 diabetic patients with diabetic nephropathy.[365] Our data showed that type 1 diabetic patients with the II genotype are particularly susceptible to commonly advocated renoprotective treatment. In 1987, the EUCLID Study Group[366] demonstrated that the urinary AER during lisinopril treatment was 57% lower in the II group, 19% lower in the ID group, and 19% higher in the DD group as compared to placebo. Furthermore, the polymorphism of the ACE gene predicts the therapeutic efficacy of ACEI inhibitors against progression of nephropathy in type 2 diabetic patients.[367] All previous studies in diabetic and nondiabetic nephropathies have demonstrated that the deletion polymorphism of the ACE gene, particularly the DD genotype, is a risk factor for an accelerated loss of kidney funciton.[275, 276, 279-282, 368-372] Furthermore, the ACE deletion polymorphism reduces the long-term beneficial effect of ACE inhibitors on progression of diabetic and nondiabetic kidney disease.[279, 370] These findings suggest that

the DD genotype patient should be offered more aggressive ACE inhibitors or treatment with the new ARBs or dual blockade of the RAS.

In an attempt to overcome this interaction we evaluated the short- and long-term renoprotective effect in diabetic nephropathy of losartan in type 1 diabetic patients homozygous for either the I or the D allele.[373, 374] Our data suggest that ARBs offer similar short- and long-term renoprotective and blood pressure–lowering effects in albuminuric hypertensive type 1 diabetic patients with the ACE II and DD genotypes. Head-to-head comparisons of ACE inhibitors versus ARBs suggest similar ability to reduce albuminuria and blood pressure in diabetic patients with elevated urinary albumin excretion.[375-377] These results indicate that the reduction in albuminuria and blood pressure induced by ACE inhibition is primarily caused by interference with the RAS. Because reduction of proteinuria is a prerequisite of successful long-term renoprotection, we investigated whether individual patient factors are determinants of antiproteinuric efficacy.[378] The study suggests that patients responding favorably to one class of antiproteinuric drugs also respond favorably to other classes of available drugs. Furthermore, in dose escalation studies of different ARBs we have demonstrated that the optimal renoprotective dose of losartan is 100 mg/day and 16 mg/day for candesartan.[379, 380] Unfortunately, we do not know the optimal renoprotective dose of the various ACE inhibitors. However, recent short-term studies suggest that dual blockade of the RAS may offer additional renal and cardiovascular protection in diabetic patients with elevated AERs.[381-384] Recently, Nakao and colleagues[385] performed a long-term (4 years) double-blind randomized trial in 263 nondiabetic renal disease patients in Japan. Patients were randomly assigned an ARB (losartan 100 mg/day), an ACE inhibitor (trandolapril 3 mg/day), or a combination of both drugs at equivalent doses. By the end of follow-up, 22.5% of the losartan-treated patients, 23.3% of the trandolapril-treated patients, and 11.4% in the combination group had reached the combined end point of doubling of the baseline serum creatinine concentration or ESRD (log-rank test $P = .02$). In accordance, animal studies suggest that low-dose dual blockade of RAS achieves more important reduction in kidney tissue angiotensin II activity compared to high doses of captopril or losartan.[386] Finally, it should be mentioned that ARBs reduce blood pressure without adversely altering the ability to autoregulate GFR in diabetic patients.[387]

Initiation of antihypertensive treatment usually induces an initial drop in GFR that is three to five times higher per unit of time than during the sustained treatment period.[388] This phenomenon occurs with conventional antihypertensive treatment with β-blockers or diuretics and when ACE inhibitors are used. Whether this initial phenomenon is reversible (hemodynamic) or irreversible (structural damage) after prolonged antihypertensive treatment has recently been investigated. In type 1 patients suffering from diabetic nephropathy, our results render some support to the hypothesis that the faster initial decline in GFR is due to a functional (hemodynamic) effect of antihypertensive treatment which does not become attenuated over time, whereas the subsequent slower decline reflects the beneficial effect on progression of nephropathy.[388] A similar effect has been demonstrated in nondiabetic glomerulopathies.[389] In contrast, our results suggest that the faster initial decline in GFR after initiating antihypertensive therapy in hypertensive type 2 patients with diabetic nephropathy is due an irreversible effect.[390]

In 1982, Mogensen described a beneficial effect of long-term antihypertensive treatment in five hypertensive men with type 1 diabetes and nephropathy.[391] Our prospective study, initiated in 1976, has demonstrated that early and aggressive antihypertensive treatment reduces albuminuria and the rate of decline in GFR in young men and women with type 1 diabetes and nephropathy.[392-394] Figure 38-14 illustrates the mean value for arterial blood pressure, GFR, and albuminuria in nine patients receiving long-term (>9 years) treatment with metoprolol, furosemide, and hydralazine.[394] Note that the data are consistent with a time-dependent renoprotective effect of antihypertensive treatment that in the long term might lead to regression of the disease (ΔGFR $\leq$ 1 mL/minute/year), at least in some patients. The same progressive benefit—ΔGFR with time—has been demonstrated in nondiabetic renal diseases.[395] Regression of kidney disease (ΔGFR $\leq$ 1 mL/minute/year) has been documeted in a sizable fraction (22%) of type 1 patients receiving aggressive antihypertensive therapy for diabetic nephropathy.[396] Remission of proteinuria for at least 1 year (proteinuria $\leq$ 1 g/24hours) has been described in patients with type 1 diabetes participating in the captopril collaborative study.[397] Eight of 108 patients experienced remission during long-term follow-up.[397] We recently confirmed and extended these findings in a long-term prospective observational study of 321 patients with type 1 diabetes and nephropathy.[398] The remission group, not surprisingly, is characterized by slow progression of diabetic nephropathy and an improved cardiovascular risk profile.

At the end of the 1980s, reports appeared that described a beneficial effect of ACE inhibitors on albuminuria and rate of decline in GFR.[399-402] In 1992, Björck and co-workers suggested that ACE inhibitors in diabetic nephropathy confer renoprotection, for example, a beneficial effect on renal function and structure above and beyond that expected from the blood pressure–lowering effect alone.[403] Their investigation was a prospective, open, randomized study lasting for 2.2 years in patients with type 1 diabetes. In 1993 Lewis and colleagues in the Collaborative Study Group demonstrated a significant risk reduction from doubling of serum creatinine concentrations in patients with type 1 diabetes and nephropathy who received captopril (48%; 95% CI, 16%-69%).[404] In comparison, the placebo-treated patients received conventional antihypertensive treatment, excluding calcium channel blockers. We recently reported that long-term treatment (4 years) with an ACE inhibitor or a long-acting dihydropyridine calcium antagonist has similar beneficial effects on progression of diabetic nephropathy in hypertensive patients with type 1 diabetes.[405]

Thus, interruption of the RAS slows the progression of renal disease in patients with type 1 diabetes but similar data

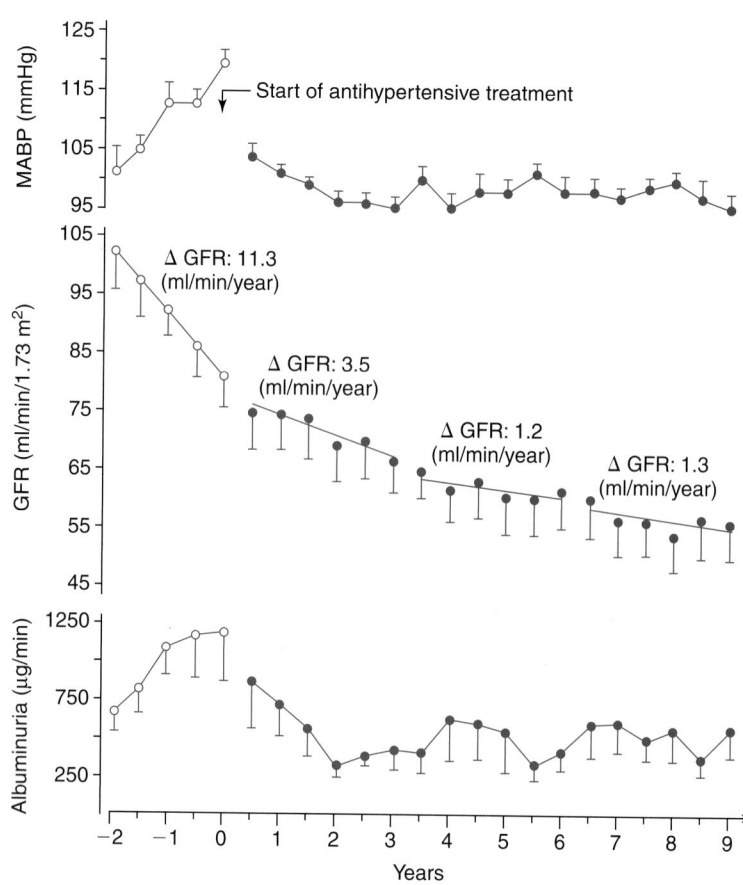

The Effect of Antihypertensive Treatment Upon Kidney Function in 9 IDDM Patients with Diabetic Nephropathy

FIGURE 38-14. Average course of mean arterial blood pressure, GFR, and albumin before (○) and during (●) long-term effective antihypertensive treatment of nine type I patients suffering from diabetic nephropathy. (From Parving H-H, Rossing P, Hommel E, Smidt UM:Angiotensin converting enzyme inhibition in diabetic nephropathy: Ten years experience, Am J Kidney Dis 26:99-107, 1998, with permission.

are not available for patients with type 2 diabetes.[339, 406-409] Against this background, two large multinational, double-blind, randomized placebo-controlled trials with ARBs were carried out in comparable populations of hypertensive patients with type 2 diabetes, proteinuria, and elevated serum creatinine levels.[410, 411] In both trials, the primary outcome was the composite of a doubling of the baseline serum creatinine concentration, ESRD, or death. A comparison of the benefits obtained in the RENAAL (*r*eduction of *e*nd points in *N*IDDM with the *a*ngiotensin II *a*ntagonist *l*osartan) study versus the IDNT (Irbesartan Diabetic Nephropathy Trial) is shown in Table 38-8. Side effects were low and fewer than 2% of the patients had to stop ARBs because of severe hyperkalemia. The number of sudden deaths in the different groups was similar. The two landmark studies led to the following conclusion. Losartan and Irbesartan conferred significant renal benefits in patients with Type 2 diabetes and nephropathy. This protection is independent of the reduction in blood pressure it causes. The ARBs are generally safe and well tolerated. A recent meta-analysis of IRMA 2[357] and the two earlier mentioned ARB trials[410, 411] revealed a significant risk reduction (15%) of cardiovascular events as compared with those in the control groups.[412] As mentioned earlier, based on the three outcome trials with ARBs, the American Diabetes Association recommends ARBs as the initial agents of choice in the treatment of type 2 diabetic patients with microalbuminuria or clinical albuminuria.[359]

Parving and co-workers[413, 414] have assessed the effect of long-term antihypertensive therapy on prognosis in diabetic nephropathy. All type 1 diabetic patients who developed diabetic nephropathy between 1974 and 1978 were enrolled at Steno Diabetes Center (Gentofte, Denmark). Forty-five patients were followed until death or for at least 16 years. The medium follow-up was 16 (4-21) years. Mean blood pressure at the start of antihypertensive treatment was 148/95 ± 15/15 mm Hg. Systolic blood pressure remained unchanged, whereas diastolic blood pressure decreased significantly (0.9 mm Hg/per year) during antihypertensive treatment. The cumulative death rate was 18% (95% CI, 8%-32%) 10 years after onset of proteinuria, in contrast to previous reports of 50% to 77% 10 years after onset of nephropathy.[413] The median survival time in our study exceeded 16 years. Furthermore, serum creatinine was 116 (74-311) µmol/L in the surviving 23 patients. Uremia was the main cause of death (64%) in the study of Parving and co-workers, as in

the three previous studies dealing with the natural course of diabetic nephropathy[18, 29, 414] (Fig. 38-15). Mathiesen and colleagues[415] showed that the survival of type 1 diabetic patients with nephropathy improved substantially because early effective antihypertensive treatment had become routine treatment in their clinic. We confirmed and extended these results in another long-term observational follow-up study by showing that the median survival time was 13.9 years (95% CI, 11.8-17.2 years) in 263 type 1 patients suffering from diabetic nephropathy.[32] The study also revealed that death due to ESRD (dying with serum creatinine concentration > 500 µmol/L) was reduced to 35%.

The first information on progression based on a randomized, double-blind placebo-controlled antihypertensive treatment trial was presented by the collaborative study group on the effect of ACE inhibition with captopril in diabetic nephropathy.[404] This study, lasting on average 2.7 years, demonstrated a risk reduction of 61% (95% CI, 26-80%; *P* = .002) in the subgroup of 102 patients with baseline serum creatinine concentration greater than 133 µmol/L and 46% (*P* = .14) in the 307 patients with serum creatinine

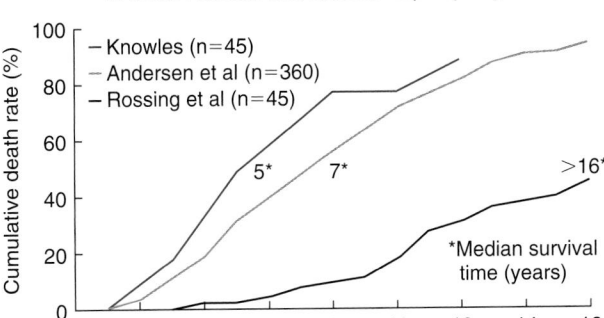

FIGURE 38-15. Cumulative death rate during the natural history of diabetic nephropathy in type I patients (N = 45, Knowles[131]; N = 360, Andersen et al.[18], N = 45, Rossing et al.[18, 29, 414]) compared with patients who had effective antihypertensive treatment (N = 45, Parving et al.)[414] (From Parving H-H, Jacobsen P, Rossing K, et al: Benefits of long-term antihypertensive treatment on prognosis in diabetic nephropathy. Kidney Int 49:1778-1782, 1996, with permission.)

TABLE 38-8

RENAAL and IDNT Results: Comparison of Primary Composite End Point and Components

COMPOSITE END POINT	RISK REDUCTION (% (95% CI))			
	Losartan vs. Placebo (80)	Irbesartan vs. Placebo (81)	Irbesartan vs. Amlodipine (81)	Amlodipine vs. Placebo (81)
DsCr, ESRD, death	16 (2, 28)	20 (3, 34)	23 (7, 37)	−4 (14, −25)
DsCr	25 (8, 39)	33 (13, 48)	37 (19, 52)	−6 (16, −35)
ESRD	28 (11, 42)	23 (−3, 43)	23 (−3, 43)	0 (−32, 24)
Death	−2 (−27, 19)	8 (−31, 23)	−4 (23, −40)	12 (−19, 34)
ESRD or death	20 (5, 32)	—	—	—

CI, confidence interval; DsCr, doubling of serum creatinine; ESRD, end-stage renal disease; IDNT, Irbesartan Diabetic Nephropathy Trial; RENAAL, reduction of end points in NIDDM with the angiotensin II, antagonist losartan study.

concentrations at baseline below 133 µmol/L, for the occurrence of death or progression to dialysis or transplantation in type 1 diabetic patients treated with captopril versus placebo. An economic analysis of the use of captopril in diabetic nephropathy revealed that ACE inhibitors provide significant savings in the health care costs.[416]

In conclusion, the prognosis of type 1 diabetic patients suffering from diabetic nephropathy has improved during the past decade, largely because of effective antihypertensive treatment with conventional drugs (β-blockers, diuretics) and ACE inhibitors. Unfortunately, scanty information on this important issue is available in NIDDM patients with diabetic nephropathy.

Lipid Lowering

In 1982, Moorhead and colleagues[417] hypothesized that hyperlipidemia promotes progression of chronic renal disease after the initiating event has damaged the glomerular capillary wall, thereby allowing increased passage of lipids and lipoproteins into the mesangium. Our recent study of 301 type 1 diabetic patients followed for 7 years indicates that elevated serum cholesterol acts as an independent promoter of progression.[18] By contrast, the renoprotective effect of 3-hydroxy-3 methyl-glutaryl–coenzyme A (HMG-CoA) reductase inhibitors in patients with type 1 or type 2 diabetes with micro- or macroalbuminuria appears to be highly variable, as reviewed by Moorhead's group.[417] However, all nine studies are of short duration, dealing with a small number of patients and only evaluating the surrogate end point: urinary albumin excretion. Large long-term, double-blind, randomized trials with hard end points, for example, doubling of serum creatinine, progression to ESRD, are urgently needed.

Dietary Protein Restriction

Dietary protein restriction, which limits glomerular capillary pressures and flows in rats, was utilized by Zatz and co-workers[418, 419] to further clarify the role of hemodynamic factors in the pathogenesis of experimental diabetic glomerulopathy. After 14 months of streptozotocin-induced diabetes, protein-restricted rats exhibited virtually no albuminuria or glomerular structural lesions and glomerular capillary pressure was normalized. Short-term studies in normoalbuminuric, microalbuminuric, and macroalbuminuric type 1 diabetic patients have shown that a low-protein diet (0.6-0.8 g/kg/day) reduces urinary albumin excretion and hyperfiltration, independent of changes in glucose control and blood pressure.[420-422] Longer-term trials in type 1 patients with diabetic nephropathy suggest that protein restriction reduces the progression of kidney function,[423, 424] but the interpretation has been challenged.[425, 426] Pedrini and colleagues[427] performed a meta-analysis based on three of these studies,[421, 423, 424] and two additional short-term studies lasting less than 1.5 years.[428, 429] They concluded that dietary protein restriction effectively slows the progression of diabetic renal disease, but the conclusion has been disputed.[430, 431] Most recently, we reported a 4-year prospective, controlled trial with concealed randomization comparing the effects of a low-protein diet with a usual-protein diet in 82 type 1 diabetic patients with progressive diabetic nephropathy.[432] ESRD or death occurred in 27% of patients on the usual-protein diet compared with 10% on the low-protein diet (log-rank test $P = .04$). The relative risk of ESRD or death was 0.23 (0.07-0.72) for patients assigned to a low-protein diet, after an adjustment at baseline for the presence of CVD.

END-STAGE RENAL DISEASE IN DIABETIC PATIENTS

Epidemiology

Diabetic nephropathy has become the leading cause of ESRD in most Western countries.[433] According to the U.S. Renal Data System, in 1999 diabetic nephropathy was the primary diagnosis in 42.8% (38,160 out of 89,252) of ESRD patients,[434] an increase of 238% since 1990. In 2000 the actual proportion of diabetics varied considerably among countries, for example, it was 14.6% in the Netherlands, 22% in Australia, 25% in Sweden, and 36.1% in Germany, but was consistently on the rise in all countries. Registry figures tend to underestimate the renal burden of diabetes; we found that diabetes was present in no less than 48.9% of patients admitted for renal replacement therapy in Heidelberg.[435] Clinical features of classic Kimmelstiel-Wilson disease were found only in 60%, however. Atypical presentation consistent with ischemic nephropathy accounted for 13%, and known primary renal disease (e.g., polycystic disease, analgesic nephropathy, glomerulonephritis) with superimposed diabetes accounted for 27% of the cases. Survival of the diabetic on hemodialysis is smaller[436] whether or not diabetic or primary nondiabetic renal disease accounts for end-stage renal failure. In the Heidelberg series diabetes had not been diagnosed at the time of admission in 11% of these patients, presumably because the patients had lost weight secondary to anorexia, thus self-correcting hyperglycemia. The great majority, that is, 94%, suffered from type 2 diabetes and in all countries it is primarily patients with type 2 diabetes whose number is consistently on the rise.[433]

The diabetic patient with ESRD has several options for renal replacement therapy:

1. Transplantation (kidney only, simultaneous pancreas plus kidney, pancreas after kidney)
2. Hemodialysis (HD)
3. Continuous ambulatory peritoneal dialysis (CAPD).

There is consensus that today medical rehabilitation and survival are best after transplantation, particularly after transplantation of pancreas plus kidney. The results of CAPD and HD are inferior to transplantation but comparable between CAPD and HD.

Management of the Patient with Advanced Renal Failure

The diabetic patient with advanced renal failure has usually a much higher burden of *microvascular* and *macrovascular* complications (Table 38-9) than the diabetic patient without or with the early stages of diabetic nephropathy. The morbidity of these diabetic patients with advanced renal failure is usually more severe than that of the average patient seen in the diabetes outpatient clinic. The diabetic patient with advanced renal impairment, even if he or she is asymptomatic, must

TABLE 38-9

Major Microvascular and Macrovascular Complications in Patients with Diabetic Nephropathy

Microvascular complications
  Retinopathy
  Polyneuropathy, including autonomic neuropathy (gastroparesis,
    diarrhea/obstipation, detrusor paresis, painless myocardial ischemia,
    erectile dysfunction, supine hypertension/orthostatic hypotension)
Macrovascular complications
  Coronary heart disease, left ventricular hypertrophy, congestive
    heart failure
  Cerebrovascular complications (stroke)
  Peripheral artery occlusive disease
Mixed complications
  Diabetic foot (neuropathic, vascular)

TABLE 38-10

Frequent Therapeutic Challenges in the Diabetic Patient with Renal Failure

Hypertension (blood pressure amplitude, circadian rhythm)
Hypervolemia
Glycemic control (insulin half-life, accumulation of oral hypoglycemic
  agents)
Malnutrition
Bacterial Infections (diabetic foot)
Timely creation of vascular access

therefore be monitored at regular intervals for timely detection of these complications (opthalmologic examination at half-yearly intervals, cardiac and angiologic status yearly, foot inspection at each visit).

The physician in charge of a diabetic patient with impaired renal function has to face a spectrum of therapeutic challenges, which are listed in Table 38-10. The most vexing clinical problems are related to CHD and autonomic polyneuropathy.

Hypertension

At any given level of GFR, blood pressure tends to be higher in diabetic compared to nondiabetic patients with renal failure. Because of their beneficial effect on cardiovascular complications[437] and progression,[357, 404, 410, 411, 38] ACE inhibitors or ARBs are obligatory unless there are contraindications, for example, an acute increase in serum creatinine (RAS, hypovolemia, congestive heart failure) or hyperkalemia resistant to corrective maneuvers, such as loop diuretics, dietary potassium restriction, or correction of metabolic acidosis. Because of their marked propensity to retain salt, patients with diabetic nephropathy have a marked tendency to develop hypervolemia and edema.[438] Therefore, dietary salt restriction and the use of loop diuretics are usually indicated. At least in monotherapy thiazides are not sufficient once GFR is below 30 to 50 mL/minute. When the creatinine concentration is elevated, multidrug therapy is usually necessary to normalize blood pressure with, on average, three to five antihypertensive agents. In these patients hypertension is also characterized by a high blood pressure amplitude (as a result of increased aortic stiffness) and by an attenuated nighttime decrease in blood pressure which in itself is a potent risk predictor.[439]

Glucose Control

On the one hand, renal failure causes, among other problems, insulin resistance by accumulation of a (hypothetical) circulating factor interfering with the action of insulin. As a result, there is a tendency to develop impaired glucose tolerance and hyperglycemia. Insulin resistance is improved after the start of dialysis.

On the other hand, the half-life of insulin is prolonged, causing a tendency to develop hypoglycemic episodes. This risk is further compounded by anorexia and by accumulation of most sulfonylurea compounds (with the exception of gliquidone or glimepiride). Glinides and glitazones do not accumulate, but long-term safety data in renal failure are not available.

It follows that glycemia as the result of these opposing influences is difficult to predict and thus close monitoring of glycemia is advisable. There is an increasing trend to use short-acting insulins more liberally in these patients, particularly during intercurrent illness (infections, surgery), and insulin treatment is also useful to combat catabolism and malnutrition.

Malnutrition

Patients are often severely catabolic and are predisposed to develop malnutrition, particularly during periods of intercurrent illness and fasting, but also from ill-advised recommendation of protein-restricted diets, particularly when these anorectic patients concomitantly reduce energy intake. Malnutrition is a potent independent predictor of mortality[440] and its presence justifies an early start of renal replacement treatment. Anorectic obese patients with type 2 diabetes and advanced renal failure often undergo massive weight loss leading to normalization of fasting and even postloading glycemia. The diagnosis of Kimmelstiel-Wilson disease then requires documentation of retinopathy or renal biopsy. Wasting with low muscle mass is an important cause why physicians misjudge the severity of renal failure, because at any given level of GFR, serum creatinine concentrations are then spuriously low. This contributes to dosing errors of drugs which accumulate in renal failure and may also contribute to the belated start of renal replacement therapy. It is advisable to measure or estimate (Cockroft-Gault formula) creatinine clearance in cases of doubt.

Acute and "Acute-on-Chronic" Renal Failure

Multimorbid diabetic patients with nephropathy are particularly prone to develop acute renal failure (ARF), very often when serum creatinine is already elevated ("acute on chronic"). In the Heidelberg program, 27% of patients with ARF had diabetes.[435] The most common causes were emergency cardiologic interventions involving administration of radiocontrast, septicemia, low cardiac output, and shock. The high susceptibility of the kidney to ischemic injury, at least in experimental diabetes, may be a contributory factor.[441] Not infrequently, ARF necessitates HD culminating in irreversible chronic renal failure. This mode of presentation as irreversible ARF has a particularly poor prognosis.[442] Prevention of radiocontrast-induced ARF necessitates adequate hydration of the patient with saline as well as temporary interruption of diuretics and possibly ACE inhibitor treatment.[443]

Vascular Access

Timely creation of vascular access is of overriding importance. It should be considered when the GFR is approximately 20 to 25 mL/minute. Although venous runoff problems are not unusual (venous occlusion from infections or infusions and hypoplastic veins, particularly in elderly female diabetics), inadequate arterial inflow is increasingly recognized as the major cause of fistula malfunction. If distal arteries are severely sclerotic, anastomosis at a more proximal level may be necessary. Use of native vessels is clearly the first choice[444] and results of grafts are definitely inferior. It is often necessary to create an upper arm native arteriovenous fistula[444-446] or use more sophisticated approaches.[447] Arteriosclerosis of arm arteries not only jeopardizes fistula flow but also predisposes to the steal phenomenon with ensuing finger gangrene.[448]

Initiation of Renal Replacement Therapy

Many nephrologists would agree that renal replacement therapy should be started earlier than in nondiabetic patients and at a GFR of approximately 15 mL/minute. An even earlier start may be justified when hypervolemia and blood pressure become uncontrollable, when the patient is anorectic and cachectic, and when the patient vomits the combined results of uremia and gastroparesis.

Hemodialysis

In recent years survival of diabetic patients on HD has tended to improve. Several years ago the 5-year survival in type 2 diabetic patients on HD did not exceed 10% in Germany,[449] but it has recently risen to approximately 30% and astonishingly good survival rates, for example, 50% at 5 years in dialysed diabetic patients, have been reported from East Asia. To a large extent these differences between countries may reflect the frequency of cardiovascular death in the background populations.

Intradialytic and Interdialytic Blood Pressure

Diabetic patients receiving dialysis tend to be more hypertensive than dialyzed nondiabetic patients. In diabetic patients blood pressure is exquisitely volume-dependent. The problem is compounded by the fact that patients are predisposed to intradialytic hypotension, so that it is difficult to reach the target "dry weight" by ultrafiltration. Nevertheless, reduced dietary salt intake and ultrafiltration may permit control of hypertension without medication, but many patients need antihypertensive drugs. The main causes of intradialytic hypotension are, on the one hand, disturbed counterregulation (autonomous polyneuropathy) and, on the other hand, disturbed left ventricular compliance so that cardiac output decreases abruptly when left ventricular filling pressure diminishes during ultrafiltration.[450] One or more of the following approaches are useful to avoid intradialytic hypotension: long dialysis sessions, omission of antihypertensive agents immediately before dialysis sessions, controlled ultrafiltration, and correction of anemia by erythropoietin therapy. If nothing works, however, alternative treatment modalities, such as hemofiltration and CAPD, should be considered. Intradialytic hypotension increases

the risk of cardiac death by a factor of three.[436] Intradialytic hypotension also predisposes to myocardial ischemia, arrhythmia, deterioration of maculopathy, and (particularly in the elderly) nonthrombotic mesenteric infarction.

Pulse pressure and impaired elasticity of central arteries are major predictors of death and of cardiovascular events in nonuraemic patients. They are also significant predictors of death in nondiabetic patients, but, for uncertain reasons, not in diabetic patients on HD.[451]

Cardiovascular Problems

Why is survival of diabetic patients on HD (and CAPD) inferior compared to nondiabetic patients? According to a Canadian study,[452] 31% of diabetic patients on HD died from cardiovascular causes. Compared to 14% in nondiabetic controls, cardiovascular mortality accounted for 59% of overall deaths in diabetic patients.

Stack and Bloembergen[453] examined the prevalence of CHD in a national random sample of patients entering renal replacement programs and noted that the prevalence of CHD was significantly higher in diabetic compared to nondiabetic patients, the difference between the two groups even exceeding that observed between in sexes (Fig. 38-16).

Diabetic patients are at a greater risk of acquiring CHD in the predialytic phase. The odds ratio to develop new CVD was 5.35 for diabetic patients with established kidney disease who were not yet on dialysis.[454] This explains the high prevalence of cardiovascular complications when diabetic patients enter dialysis programs. The rate of onset of ischemic heart disease was strikingly and significantly higher in diabetic compared to nondiabetic patients on HD.[452-455]

The diabetic patient is also at higher risk when coronary complications supervene. When myocardial infarction develops, short-term and long-term survival are very poor in all HD patients, but poorest in the diabetic patient on HD: 62.3% versus 55.4% in the nondiabetic patient after 1 year and 93.3% versus 86.9% after 5 years.[456] Diabetic patients are also more prone to develop cardiac arrest during dialysis

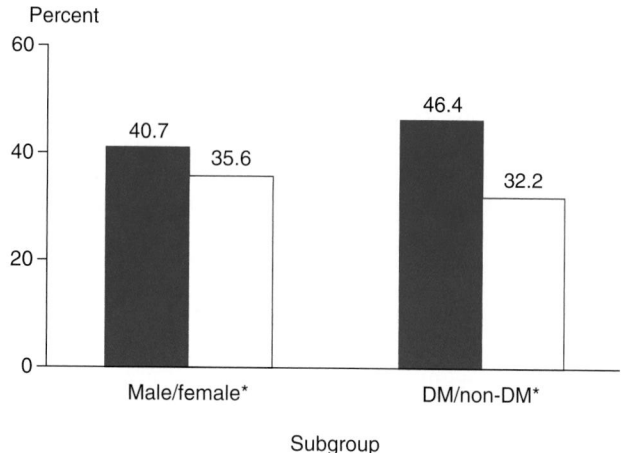

FIGURE 38-16. Prevalence of coronary artery disease (CAD) according to sex and the presence of diabetes mellitus (DM). *$P < .001$ for each pair. (Data from Foley RN, Culleton BF, Parfrey PS, et al: Cardiac disease in diabetic end-stage renal disease. Diabetologia 40:1307-1312, 1997.)

sessions[457] and to sudden death in the dialysis interval. These complications are presumably not fully explained by the severity of stenosing coronary lesions. It is true that in dialyzed diabetic patients coronary calcification is more pronounced[458] and that complex triple-vessel lesions are more frequent. In agreement with our experience, Varghese and colleagues[459] found triple-vessel lesions in 27% of diabetic compared to 12% of nondiabetic patients. Nevertheless, the impact of ischemic heart disease is presumably amplified by frequently coexisting cardiac abnormalities such as congestive heart failure, left ventricular hypertrophy, and disturbed sympathetic innervation,[460, 461] as well as microvessel disease with diminished coronary reserve and deranged cardiomyocyte metabolism.[462] Such functional abnormalities, particularly insufficient NO-dependent vasodilator reserve and deranged sympathetic innervation, have been documented even in the earliest stages of diabetes.[463] They are also present in dialyzed diabetic patients.[460]

Therapeutic challenges are prevention in the asymptomatic and intervention in the symptomatic patient. With respect to prevention, unfortunately, little evidence-based information is available. Observational studies suggest that good glycemic control before[464] or during dialysis[465] reduces overall and cardiovascular mortality. It is also sensible to reduce afterload (blood pressure control) and preload (hypervolemia). The value of lipid lowering by statins has not been proved but is currently being investigated in type 2 diabetic patients on HD.[466] Diabetic patients with renal failure are characterized by premature and more pronounced anemia so that timely and effective treatment with recombinant human erythropoietin (rhEPO) is advisable.[467] If one can extrapolate the results of the Heart Outcomes Prevention Evaluation (HOPE) study[437] and the Losartan Intervention for Endpoint Reduction in Hypertension (LIFE) study[468] to ESRD, pharmacologic blockade of the renin-angiotensin system using ACE inhibitors or ARBs is also well advised. In view of the importance of disturbed sympathetic innervation,[463] it is surprising that β-blockers are only sparing when administered to dialyzed diabetic patients,[469] although better survival on β-blockers has been shown in observational studies[470] and improvement of heart function in dialyzed patients with carvedilol has been documented in a controlled interventional study.[471]

In the patient with symptomatic CHD, active intervention, for example, percutaneous transluminal coronary angioplasty (PTCA) or CABG (coronary artery bypass graft) was shown to be superior to medical treatment alone.[472] In a small series after 8.4 months of follow-up, 15% of the surgically managed patients had a cardiovascular end point compared with 77% in the medically managed group. Because patients often fail to complain of pain, and because screening tests such as exercise ECG and thallium scintigraphy are notoriously poor predictors, one should resort directly to coronary angiography if there is any suspicion of CHD.

No dogmatic statements concerning type of intervention are possible in the absence of evidence from controlled studies. Retrospective interventional studies[473-475] have consistently shown more adverse outcomes in diabetic compared to nondiabetic patients treated either with CABG or PTCA. After PTCA the coronary reocclusion rate is devastating: 70% at 1 year, even in nondiabetic HD patients. Small series suggest markedly better outcomes after PTCA plus stenting compared to PTCA alone,[476] but the frequency of diffuse

three-vessel disease with heavy calcification in dialysed diabetic patients remains a major problem.[477] A recent retrospective analysis of dialysed diabetics suggested that CABG using internal mammary grafts (but not CABG using venous grafts) yielded superior outcome compared to PTCA with or without stenting.[475] In view of the fact that renal failure per se aggravates insulin resistance, the results of the Diabetes Mellitus, Insulin Glucose Infusion in Acute Myocardial Infarction (DIGAMI) study,[478] which show that strict normalization of blood glucose by insulin and glucose infusion dramatically reduces early and late mortality in diabetic patients with myocardial infarction, are relevant.

Metabolic Control

Dialysis partially reverses insulin resistance so that insulin requirements often become less than before dialysis. Even patients with type 1 diabetes may occasionally lose their need for insulin, at least transiently, upon institution of HD. In other patients, however, insulin requirements increase, presumably because anorexia is reversed so that appetite and food consumption increase. It is most convenient to use dialysates that contain glucose, usually about 200 mg/mL. This allows insulin to be administered at the usual times of day, reduces the risk of hyperglycemic or hypoglycemic episodes,[406] and causes fewer hypotensive episodes.[479]

Adequate control of glycemia is important because hyperglycemia causes thirst, high fluid intake, and hypovolemia, as well as an osmotic shift of water and K^+ from the intracellular to the extracellular space. This leads to circulatory congestion and hyperkalemia. Diabetics with poor glucose control are also more susceptible to infection. Finally, in dialyzed diabetic patients, hyperglycemia definitely increases the risk of death, mainly from CVD.[465]

Assessment of glycemic control using HbA_{1c} is confounded by carbamylation of hemoglobin, by altered red blood cell survival, and by assay interference from uremia.[480] HbA_{1c} values above 7.5% cause modest overestimation of hyperglycemia in diabetic patients with ESRD.

Diminished insulin-mediated glucose uptake as evidence of insulin resistance has been noted in the hearts of uremic animals[481] and this has been related to reduced ischemia tolerance of the heart.[462] In view of the dramatic results of insulin and glucose administration after myocardial infarction[478] and the benefit from intensive insulin therapy in critically ill patients, particularly those with ARF,[482] insulin should presumably be administered more generously and this might also be beneficial in the control of malnutrition and anemia management.[483]

Malnutrition

Because of anorexia and prolonged habituation to dietary restriction, the dietary intake of diabetic patients on HD often falls short of adequate energy (30-35 kcal/kg/day) and protein (1.3 g/kg/day) intake. By x-ray absorptiometry Okuno and co-workers documented a decrease in body fat mass in diabetic compared to nondiabetic patients.[484] This is particularly undesirable because malnutrition is a potent predictor of death. It is of concern that malnutrition and microinflammation tend to be more common in diabetic patients.[485] Surprisingly, conventional indicators of malnutrition are not predictive of survival in diabetic patients, however.[486]

Miscellaneous

In the past *visual prognosis* in dialyzed diabetics was extremely poor. Despite the use of heparin, de novo amaurosis on HD has become very unusual.

On average, *hyperparathyroidism* tends to be much less pronounced in diabetic compared to nondiabetic patients on HD.[487]

There are several reports that for unknown reasons *EPO requirements* are less in dialyzed patients.[488, 489] The reasons for this are currently under investigation. *Dyslipidemia*, that is, the total cholesterol value and the low-density–high-density lipoprotein cholesterol ratio, predict cardiac death in dialyzed diabetic, but not in nondiabetic, patients.[490] Cholesterol concentrations are often within the "normal" range, but lipoprotein subfractions are clearly abnormal.[491] Whether statins will reduce cardiovascular end points is currently under investigation.[466]

Amputation

At entry into dialysis 16% of diabetic patients have undergone amputation, most above-the-ankle amputation.[492] The distinction between, and the separate treatment of, neuropathic and vascular foot lesions are crucial to improving the outcome of diabetic foot lesions.[492]

Peritoneal Dialysis

According to the U.S. Renal Data System,[434] 7.1% of all patients with diabetes receiving renal replacement therapy are treated with peritoneal dialysis (PD), 75.4% receive maintenance HD, and 17.5% undergo transplantation. The proportion of diabetic patients treated by peritoneal dialysis varies greatly among countries, illustrating that selection of treatment modalities is also strongly influenced by logistics and reimbursement policies and not only by medical considerations. There are very good a priori reasons to offer initially CAPD treatment to diabetic patients. In diabetic patients with ESRD, forearm vessels are often sclerosed, so that it is not possible to create a fistula. The alternative of hemodialysis via intravenous catheters (instead of arteriovenous fistulas or grafts) is not sufficient in the long run, because blood flow is low and the risk of infection is high. Long-term dialysis via catheter was identified as one major predictor of poor patient survival on HD.[493]

There are additional reasons for offering PD as the initial mode of renal replacement therapy to the diabetic patient. According to Heaf and co-workers, during the first 2 years survival is better for patients treated with PD compared to HD and this was also true for diabetic patients,[494] except the very elderly.[495]

A survival advantage is no longer demonstrable beyond the second year (presumably because by then residual renal function has decayed). Moreover, PD provides slow and sustained ultrafiltration without rapid fluctuations of fluid volumes and electrolyte concentrations, features which are advantageous for blood pressure control and prevention of heart failure.

An interesting concept has been proposed by Van Biesen and colleagues.[496] Patients who started on PD and who were then transferred to HD when residual renal function had decayed had better long-term survival than patients who started on HD and remained on HD throughout. As a potential explanation it has been proposed that an early start on CAPD prevents organ damage accumulating in the late stages of uremia. Survival of patients who had remained on CAPD for more than 48 months was inferior compared to patients on HD, presumably because CAPD is no longer sufficiently effective when residual renal function has gone, at least in heavier patients. It is also relevant that CAPD treatment presents no surgical contraindications to renal transplantation.

In the past an idea had been advanced which seems a priori attractive—to administer insulin by injection into the CAPD fluid with the goal of providing insulin via the "physiologic" portal route. Unfortunately, there are practical problems: uncertaincy of dosage because insulin binds to the surface of dialysis bags and tubing[497] and may be degraded by insulinases in the peritoneum.[498] Moreover, absorption from the peritoneal cavity shows large interindividual variation. There is no firm evidence that the procedure permits better control of glycemia or dyslipidemia.[499] As a result, most nephrologists no longer use this approach.

Although protein is lost across the peritoneal membrane, the main nutritional problem is gain of glucose and calories because high glucose concentrations in the dialysate are necessary for osmotic removal of excess body fluid. This leads to weight gain and obesity. Daily glucose absorption is 100 to 150 g, because a CAPD patient is exposed to 3 to 7 tons of fluid containing 50 to 175 kg of glucose per year. The use of glucose-containing fluids has another interesting disadvantage. Heat sterilization of glucose under acid conditions creates highly reactive glucose degradation products such as methylglyoxal, glyoxal, formaldehyde, 3-deoxyglucosone, and 3,4-dideoxyglucosone-3-ene.[500] GDPs are cytotoxic and lead also to the formation of advanced glycation end products. Even in nondiabetic patients on CAPD, deposits of advanced glycation end products are found in the peritoneal membrane accompanied by fibrogenesis and neoangiogenesis. This observation led to the snappy but misleading term "local diabetes mellitus".[501] Heat sterilization of two-compartment bags circumvents the generation of toxic glucose degradation products. In prospective studies, CAPD fluid thus sterilized was much less toxic than conventional CAPD fluid despite high glucose concentration.[502]

Transplantation
Kidney Transplantation

There is consensus that medical rehabilitation of the diabetic patient with uremia is best after transplantation.[503] Although survival of the diabetic patient with a kidney graft is worse compared with a grafted nondiabetic patient, the gain in life expectancy of the diabetic patient with a graft, compared with the dialyzed diabetic patient on the waiting list, is proportionally much greater than in the nondiabetic patient, because survival of the diabetic patient is so much poorer on dialysis. The higher mortality of the diabetic with a kidney graft is mainly explained as the consequence of preexisting vascular disease,[504] left ventricular hypertrophy, and post-transplant hypertension. Wolfe and colleagues[503] calculated an adjusted relative risk of death in transplant recipients, compared with patients on the waiting list, of 0.27 for diabetic patients versus 0.39 in patients with glomerulonephritis. Obviously, the perioperative risk is higher in diabetic than in nondiabetic patients, but nevertheless in diabetic patients the predicted survival on the waiting list was 8 years and after transplantation, 19 years. The majority of diabetic patients receiving a transplant are currently (C peptide–negative) type 1, although in carefully selected type 2 diabetic patients who had received kidney grafts, graft and patient survival are impressive.[505] Diabetic patients must be subjected to rigorous pretransplantation evaluation which in most centers includes routine coronary angiography.[506] As an alternative Manske has devised an algorithm to identify the diabetic patient who should receive screening tests before transplantation.[507] Patients should also be examined by Doppler sonography of pelvic arteries and, if necessary, angiography, to avoid placement of a renal allograft into an iliac artery with compromised arterial flow at risk of ischemia of the extremity and amputation.

Kidney-Plus-Pancreas Transplantation

Despite great excitement over the seminal double transplantation performed by Lillehei[508] in Minneapolis, the results of the alternative procedure, simultaneous pancreas and kidney transplantation (SPK), remained disappointing for a long time. The breakthrough came with the introduction of calcineurin inhibitors and low-steroid protocols. In an impressivly large single-center experience comprising 335 patients, Becker and co-workers[509] recently showed that survival of patients with SPK approached that of patients transplanted for nondiabetic renal disease and was clearly superior to diabetic recipients of living donor kidney grafts and particularly of cadaver kidney grafts (Fig. 38-17). The Kaplan-Meier estimate of patient survival in 215 SPK versus 111 live donor kidney graft recipients after 10 years was 82% versus 71%. The annual mortality rate was 1.5% for SPK recipients, 3.65% for living donor kidney graft recipients,

and 6.27% for cadaver donor kidney graft recipients. Reversibility of established microvascular complications after SPK is minor at best with the important exception of autonomic polyneuropathy,[510] particularly improved cardiorespiratory reflexes potentially contributing to increased survival,[511] and some improvement in nerve conduction.[512] Further benefits include improved gastric and bladder function,[513] as well as superior quality of life, better metabolic control,[514] and improved survival,[509] so that today SPK should be the preferred treatment for the type 1 diabetic who meets the selection criteria. As of the end of 2001, more than 17,000 pancreas transplants had been performed,[515] the majority (70%) in the United States. Graft survival at 1 year is 83%. There is an increasing tendency for early or even preemptive SPK. Because graft outcome is progressively more adverse with increasing time spent on HD,[516] the latter is sensible. In the United States diabetics younger than 55 years of age are usually considered for SPK at a GFR of less than 40 mL/minute, whereas criteria in Europe are more conservative, requiring a GFR of less than 20 mL/minute.[514] Exclusion criteria are, among others, active smoking, morbid obesity, (uncorrected) CVD, and so on. The indications for pancreas transplantation in nonuremic patients have not been established.

Pancreas-After-Kidney Transplantation

An alternative strategy must be considered in the diabetic patient who has a live kidney donor: to first transplant the living donor kidney, and subsequently, once stable renal function is achieved (GFR > 50mL/minute), to transplant a cadaver donor pancreas. The outcomes are satisfactory.[517]

Transplantation of pancreas segments obtained from living donors is still an experimental procedure.[518]

Procedure and Management

Today the preferred SPK technique is enteric drainage. Bladder drainage has been increasingly abandoned because of irritation of mucosa, development of strictures, bicarbonate wasting with metabolic acidosis, recurrent urinary tract infections (UTIs), and reflux pancreatitis. Elimination or exocrine duct injection is no longer performed.

Oral glucose tolerance normalizes unless the graft is damaged by ischemia or subclinical rejection related to HLA-DR mismatch.[519] Most investigators find either normalization of insulin sensitivity[520] or some impairment of insulin-stimulated nonoxidated glucose metabolism[521] with hepatic insulin resistance,[522] possibly related to insulin delivery into the systemic circulation (as opposed to physiologic delivery into the portal circulation).[523] Impressive normalization of lipoprotein lipase activity and of the lipid spectrum pointing to reduced atherogenic risk[524, 525] have also been reported. Finally, insulin-mediated protein turnover is normalized.[526]

An interesting issue is whether graft rejection affects kidney and pancreatic grafts in parallel. Although this is mostly so (permitting use of renal function as a surrogate marker of rejection in the pancreas), it is by no means obligatory, although episodes of isolated rejections of the pancreas are rare so that monitoring the kidney graft is the usual procedure. The pancreatic graft can be monitored by duplex sonography, if necessary. Pancreas graft biopsy is used to distinguish graft

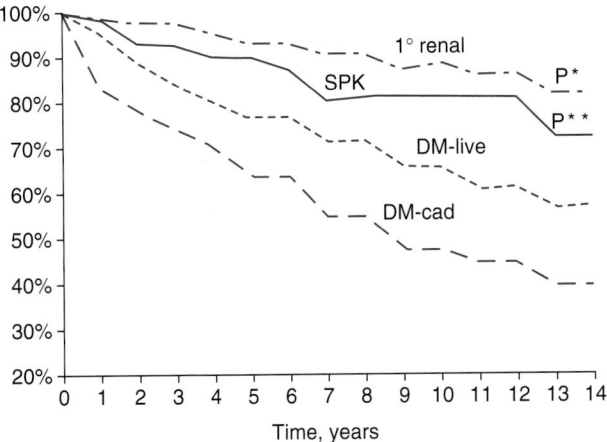

FIGURE 38-17. Kaplan-Meier estimates of simultaneous pancreas-kidney (SPK), diabetic cadaveric (DM-cad), live-donor (DM-live), and primary renal disease cohort (1° renal) transplant patient survival. *P = .0029 1° vs. all others; **P = .004 SPK vs. DM-cad, DM-live. (Data from Kelly WD, Lillehei RC, Merkel FK, et al: Allotransplantation of the pancreas and duodenum along with the kidney in diabetic nephropathy. Surgery 61:827-837, 1967.)

pancreatitis from immune injury to the graft. Pancreas grafts are usually lost because of alloimmunity reactions, but in rare cases graft loss resulting from destruction by autoimmume mechanisms has been described.[527] Recurrence of autoimmune inflammation with selective loss of insulin-producing beta cells (while sparing glucagon, somatostatin, and pancreatic polypeptide–secreting cells) and lymphocytic infiltration had been noted in the pioneering era when segmental pancreatic grafts were performed in monozygotic twins and when insulitis often recurred in the recipient.[528] In our day this has become rare, presumably because immunosuppression keeps autoimmunity under control. Rejection of the pancreas responds poorly to steroid treatment. Its treatment should always include T cell antibodies.

Poorly understood late problems after SPK include carpal tunnel syndrome[529] and bone fractures.[530]

At present, an immunosuppression protocol based on tacrolimus and mycophenolate mofetil (MMF) is used as the standard in most centers around the world.[531] In 72% of patients treated with this combination it is possible to withdraw steroids within the first year after SPK.[532] One-year rejection rates of 20% are reported for SPK patients remaining on tacrolimus–mycophenolate mofetil immunosuppression.[533] The role of sirolimus is currently under investigation.

Islet Cell Transplantation

Although advanced procedures such as transplantation of stem cells or precursor cells, transplantation of encapsulated islet cells, islet xenotransplants, and insulin gene therapy are still beyond the horizon, islet cell transplantation has so far yielded some interesting, but not yet definitive, results. As of 2002 worldwide, 439 patients had received islet cell transplants, mainly in eight major centers. Patient survival was 79%, and 14% of patients were off insulin, but measurable C peptide values greater than 0.5 ng/mL as evidence of residual islet function were noted in 45% of patients. Minor intraportal insulin secretion may be relevant because it may normalize hepatic glucose production.[534] This area got a major boost with the observations of Shapiro and co-workers[535] who reported on successful islet transplantation achieving insulin independence in seven consecutive patients using a steroid-free immunosuppression regimen consisting of sirolimus, tacrolimus, and taclizumab. The generalizability of the results is currently being evaluated by a multicenter study.

Diabetes in Nondiabetic Kidney Graft Recipients

A new aspect is the recent recognition that de novo appearance of type 2 diabetes is a frequent occurrence after renal transplantation in nondiabetic patients which is seen in up to 20% of patients.[536] This is presumably the combined result of the diabetogenic action of calcineurin inhibitors, particularly tacrolimus, and the unmasking of diabetes in individuals genetically predisposed to diabetes mellitus. It is interesting that de novo type 2 diabetes was particularly associated with hepatitis C infection in several series.[537]

It is also of note that recently—in contrast with past teaching—transplantation of the kidneys of diabetic cadaver donors has been adopted and proposed as a measure to expand the donor pool.[538]

BLADDER DYSFUNCTION

Bladder dysfunction as a sequela of autonomous diabetic polyneuropathy is frequent in diabetic patients, leading to straining, hesitancy, and the sensation of incomplete emptying of the bladder, but disabling symptoms are rare (with the exception of the frail elderly).

Because of its association with autonomous polyneuropathy, it is not surprising that bladder dysfunction is frequently associated with postural hypotension, gastroparesis, constipation, and nocturnal diarrhea.

In classic cases, cystometry shows increased bladder volume at first desire to void and increased maximal bladder capacity associated with decreased detrusor contractility.[539] These abnormalities appear very early.[540] Bladder dysfunction is of interest in two respects. First, it has often been stated that cystopathy is related to progression when an element of obstructive uropathy is superimposed on diabetic nephropathy. Torffvit and associates,[541] however, failed to note any relation to progression. Second, and possibly more important, cystopathy with residual volume after voiding renders eradication of UTI difficult.

Some studies showed that diabetic cystopathy is not the most common urodynamic finding in patients with diabetes mellitus and voiding dysfunction.[542] This observation underlines the necessity of careful urodynamic studies. Kaplan and co-workers[542] found bladder outlet obstruction in 36% of male diabetic patients with voiding dysfunction. This observation is in agreement with the finding of Menendez and colleagues,[543] who evaluated the urodynamic changes in IDDM patients with ESRD. Abnormal urodynamic findings were found in 84% of patients: the bladder was hypersensitive in 39% and hyposensitive in 30% of the cases. Acute decompensation may be provoked by anticholinergics. Starer and Libow[544] examined diabetic patients who were incontinent. Cystometry showed involuntary contractions in 61% of patients, normal voluntary contractions in 13%, and subnormal or absent contractions in 26%. This study shows that classic urinary retention secondary to autonomic neuropathy is not the most common cause of urinary incontinence in the diabetic.

URINARY TRACT INFECTION

It is not absolutely certain whether the frequency of bacteriuria is higher in diabetic patients, but there is no doubt that symptomatic UTIs are more severe and more aggressive.

The hypothesis of higher prevalence of UTI in diabetes goes back to the studies of Vejlsgaard,[545] who noted a higher prevalence of bacteriuria, that is, of greater than 10^5 colony-forming units per milliliters urine in female (18.8% vs. 7.9% in control) but not male diabetics. Such UTI was mostly asymptomatic (33%).

A higher prevalence of UTI was also found in pregnant diabetic patients and was related to the presence of retinopathy, presumably as a surrogate marker for autonomous polyneuropathy. This issue has remained controversial, and some prospective studies have failed to resolve it. A higher prevalence in diabetic women was noted by Balasoiu[546] and Zhanel and their associates,[547] but not by Brauner and co-workers.[548]

Virulence factors in *Escherichia coli* isolated from diabetic women with asymptomatic bacteriuria did not differ from those in nondiabetic women.[549] As compared with nondiabetic women, diabetic women with bacteriuria reported significantly more past UTIs. UTIs may also pose problems after renal transplantation.[550]

Symptomatic UTIs tend to run a more aggressive course. [Recent studies show that by multivariate analysis diabetes and poor glycemic control were independent factors associated with upper urinary tract involvement.[551]] UTIs in diabetes also lead to complications, such as prostatic abscess,[552] emphysematous cystitis and pyelonephritis,[552, 553] intrarenal abscess formation, renal carbuncle,[554] and penile necrosis (Fournier disease).[555] One particular complication is renal papillary necrosis,[556] known since the 19th century[557] and rediscovered in the 1930s.[558] In a large autopsy series, Ditscherlein[559] found papillary necrosis in approximately 10% of 400 diabetic patients. This has not been confirmed in our more recent autopsy series.[560] Among hundreds of diabetic patients in our unit, clinical evidence of this complication was found only once. There may be a secular trend of diminishing incidence, possibly related to earlier and more frequent administration of antibiotics. Papillary necrosis should be suspected in diabetic patients with recurrent episodes of UTI, renal colic, hematuria, or obstructive uropathy.

Septicemia and extrarenal bacterial metastases are common and may manifest as endophthalmitis,[561] spondylitis,[562] and iliopsoas abscess formation,[563] particularly after UTI with methicillin-resistant staphylococci.[564]

In community-acquired UTI, the predominant microbe is *E. coli*, but *Klebsiella* is more frequently found in diabetic patients than in control subjects[565]; exotic microbes such as *Pasteurella multocida*[566]; staphylococci, including methicillin-resistant staphylococci[563]; and fungi, particularly *Candida*, may also be found.[567, 568]

The reasons for the potentially higher frequency and the definitely higher severity of UTI in diabetes are not known but may include more favorable conditions for bacterial growth (glucosuria), defective neutrophil function, increased adherence to uroepithelial cells,[569] and impaired bladder evacuation (detrusor paresis).

As to the management of UTI, no clear benefits of antibiotic treatment have been demonstrated for treatment of asymptomatic bacteriuria in diabetic patients.[570] Community-acquired symptomatic lower UTI may be managed with trimethoprim, trimethoprim with sulfamethoxazole, or gyrase inhibitors.[571] For nosocomially acquired UTI, sensitivity tests and sensitivity-directed antibiotic intervention are necessary. Invasive candiduria can be managed with amphotericin by irragation or systemic administration of fungicidal substances.

REFERENCES

1. Rollo J: Cases of Diabetes Mellitus, 2nd ed. London, Dilly, 1798.
2. Bright R: Cases and observations illustrative of renal disease accompanied with the secretion of albuminous urine. Guy Hosp Rep 1:338-400, 1836.
3. Kimmelstiel P, Wilson C: Intercapillary lesions in the glomeruli of the kidney. Am J Pathol 12:83-96, 1936.
4. Deckert T, Parving H-H, Andersen AR, et al: Diabetic nephropathy. A clinical and morphometric study. *In* Eschwege E (ed): Advances in Diabetes Epidemiology. Amsterdam, Elsevier Biomedical Press, 1982, pp 235-243.
5. Grenfell A, Bewick M, Parsons V, et al: Non-insulin-dependent diabetes and renal replacement therapy. Diabet Med 5:172-176, 1988.
6. Parving H-H, Gall M-A, Skøtt P, et al: Prevalence and causes of albuminuria in non-insulin-dependent diabetic patients. Kidney Int 41:758-762, 1992.
7. Parving H-H, Oxenbøll B, Svendsen PA, et al: Early detection of patients at risk of developing diabetic nephropathy. Acta Endocrinol 100:550-555, 1982.
8. Viberti GC, Hill RD, Jarrett RJ, et al: Microalbuminuria as a predictor of clinical nephropathy in insulin-dependent diabetes mellitus. Lancet 1:1430-1432, 1982.
9. Mogensen CE, Christensen CK: Predicting diabetic nephropathy in insulin-dependent patients. N Engl J Med 311:89-93, 1984.
10. Mathiesen ER, Oxenbøll B, Johansen K, et al: Incipient nephropathy in type 1 (insulin-dependent) diabetes. Diabetologia 26:406-410, 1984.
11. Mogensen CE: Microalbuminuria predicts clinical proteinuria and early mortality in maturity onset diabetes. N Engl J Med 310:356-360, 1984.
12. Nelson RG, Knowler WC, Pettitt DJ, et al: Assessing risk of overt nephropathy in diabetic patients from albumin excretion in untimed urine specimens. Arch Intern Med 151:1761-1765, 1991.
13. Ravid M, Savin H, Jutrin I, et al: Long-term stabilizing effect of angiotensin-converting enzyme inhibition on plasma creatinine and on proteinuria in normotensive type II diabetic patients. Ann Intern Med 118:577-581, 1993.
14. Mogensen CE, Chachati A, Christensen CK, et al: Microalbuminuria: An early marker of renal involvement in diabetes. Uremia Invest 9:85-95, 1985.
15. Deckert T, Poulsen JE, Larsen M: Prognosis of diabetics with diabetes onset before the age of thirty-one. I. Survival, causes of death and complications. Diabetologia 14:363-370, 1978.
16. Deckert T, Poulsen JE, Larsen M: The prognosis of insulin-dependent diabetes mellitus and the importance of supervision. Acta Med Scand 624 (suppl):48-53, 1979.
17. Andersen AR, Andersen JK, Christiansen JS, Deckert T: Prognosis for juvenile diabetics with nephropathy and failing renal function. J Cardiovasc Pharmacol 203:131-134, 1978.
18. Andersen AR, Christiansen JS, Andersen JK, et al: T. Diabetic nephropathy in type 1 (insulin-dependent) diabetes: An epidemiological study. Diabetologia 25:496-501,1983.
19. Borch-Johnsen K, Kreiner S, Deckert T: Mortality of type 1 (insulin-dependent) diabetes mellitus in Denmark: A study of relative mortality in 2,930 Danish type 1 diabetic patients diagnosed from 1933 to 1972. Diabetologia 29:767-772, 1986.
20. Borch-Johnsen K, Kreiner S: Proteinuria: Value as predictor of cardiovascular mortality in insulin dependent diabetes mellitus. BMJ 294:1651-1654, 1987.
21. Borch-Johnsen K, Andersen PK, Deckert T: The effect of proteinuria on relative mortality in type 1 (insulin-dependent) diabetes mellitus. Diabetologia 28:590-596, 1985.
22. Borch-Johnsen K: The prognosis of insulin-dependent diabetes mellitus. An epidemiological approach. Dan Med Bull 39:336-349, 1989.
23. Green A, Borch-Johnsen K, Andersen PK, et al: Relative mortality of type 1 (insulin-dependent) diabetes in Denmark:1933-1981. Diabetologia 28:339-342, 1985.
24. Krolewski AS, Warram JH, Christlieb AR, et al: The changing natural history of nephropathy in type 1 diabetes. Am J Med 78:785-794, 1985.
25. Nelson RG, Newman JM, Knowler WC, et al: Incidence of end-stage renal disease in type 2 (non-insulin-dependent) diabetes mellitus in Pima Indians. Diabetologia 31:730-736, 1988.
26. Nelson RG, Pettitt DJ, Carraher MJ, et al: Effect of proteinuria on mortality in NIDDM. Diabetes 37:1499-1504, 1988.
27. Ballard DJ, Humphrey LL, Melton LJ III, et al: Epidemiology of persistent proteinuria in type II diabetes mellitus. Population-based study in Rochester, Minnesota. Diabetes 37:405-412, 1988.
28. Humphrey LL, Ballard DJ, Frohnert PP, et al: Chronic renal failure in non-insulin-dependent diabetes mellitus. A population-based study in Rochester, Minnesota. Ann Intern Med 111:788-796, 1989.
29. Knowles HCJ: Magnitude of the renal failure problem in diabetic patients. Kidney Int Suppl 6:S2-S7, 1974.
30. Breyer JA: Diabetic nephropathy in insulin-dependent patients. Am J Kidney Dis 20:533-547, 1992.
31. Gall M-A, Borch-Johnsen K, Hougaard P, et al: Albuminuria and poor glycemic control predicts mortality in NIDDM. Diabetes 44:1303-1309, 1995.

32. Rossing P, Hougaard P, Barch-Johnsen K, Parving H-H: Predictors of mortality in insulin dependent diabetes: 10 year follow-up study. BMJ 313:779-784, 1996.

33. Mauer SM: Structural-functional correlations of diabetic nephropathy. Kidney Int 45:612-622, 1994.

34. Mauer SM, Steffes MW, Brown DM: The kidney in diabetes. Am J Med 7:603-612, 1981.

35. Lane PH, Steffes MW, Fioretto P, Mauer SM: Renal interstitial expansion in insulin-dependent diabetes mellitus. Kidney Int 43:661-667, 1993.

36. Østerby R: Early phases in the development of diabetic glomerulopathy. A quantitative electron microscopic study. Acta Med Scand 574 (suppl):1-80, 1975.

37. Steffes MW, Sutherland DER, Goetz FC, et al: Studies of kidney and muscle biopsy specimens from identical twins discordant for type I diabetes mellitus. N Engl J Med 312:1282-1287, 1985.

38. Brito PL, Fioretto P, Drummond K, et al: Proximal tubular basement membrane width in insulin-dependent diabetes mellitus. Kidney Int 53:754-761, 1998.

39. Mauer SM, Barbosa J, Vernier RL, et al: Development of diabetic vascular lesions in normal kidneys transplanted into patients with diabetes mellitus. N Engl J Med 295:916-920, 1976.

40. Brown DM, Mauer SM: Diabetes mellitus. In Holliday M, Barratt M, Vernier RL (eds): Pediatric Nephrology. Baltimore: Williams & Wilkins. 1987, pp 513-519.

41. Mauer SM, Miller K, Goetz FC, et al: Immunopathology of renal extracellular membranes in kidneys transplanted into patients with diabetes mellitus. Diabetes 25:709-712, 1976.

42. Burkholder PM: Immunohistopathologic study of localized plasma proteins and fixation of guinea pig complement in renal lesions of diabetic glomerulosclerosis. Diabetes 14:755-770, 1965.

43. Steffes MW, Barbosa J, Basgen JM, et al: Quantitative glomerular morphology of the normal human kidney. Lab Invest 49:82-86, 1983.

44. Steffes MW, Bilous RW, Sutherland DER, Mauer SM: Cell and matrix components of the glomerular mesangium in type 1 diabetes. Diabetes 41:679-684, 1992.

45. Drummond K, Mauer M: The early natural history of nephropathy in type 1 diabetes: II. Early renal structural changes in type 1 diabetes. Diabetes 51:1580-1587, 2002.

46. Katz A, Caramori ML, Sisson-Ross S, et al: An increase in the cell component of the cortical interstitium antedates interstitial fibrosis in type 1 diabetic patients. Kidney Int 61:2058-2066, 2002.

47. Mauer SM, Steffes MW, Ellis EN, et al: Structural-functional relationships in diabetic nephropathy. J Clin invest 74:1143-1155, 1984.

48. Caramori ML, KimY, Huang C, et al: Cellular basis of diabetic nephropathy: 1. Study design and renal structural-functional relationships in patients with long-standing type 1 diabetes. Diabetes 51:506-513, 2002.

49. Saito Y, Kida H, Takeda S, et al: Mesangiolysis in diabetic glomeruli: Its role in the formation of nodular lesions. Kidney Int 34:389-396, 1988.

50. Falk RJ, Scheinman JI, Mauer SM, Michael AF: Polyantigenic expansion of basement membrane constituents in diabetic nephropathy. Diabetes 32(suppl 2):34-39, 1983.

51. Kim Y, Kleppel MM, Butkowski R, et al: Differential expression of basement membrane collagen chains in diabetic nephropathy. Am J Pathol 138:413-420, 1991.

52. Zhu D, Kim Y, Steffes MW, et al: Glomerular distribution of type IV collagen in diabetes by high resolution quantitative immunochemistry. Kidney Int 45:425-433, 1994.

53. Moriya T, Groppoli T J, Kim Y, Mauer M: Quantitative immunoelectron microscopy of type VI collagen in glomeruli in type I diabetic patients. Kidney Int 59:317-323, 2001.

54. Harris RD, Steffes MW, Bilous RW, et al: Global glomerular sclerosis and glomerular arteriolar hyalinosis in insulin dependent diabetes. Kidney Int 40:107-114, 1991.

55. Hørlyck A, Gundersen HJG, Østerby R: The cortical distribution pattern of diabetic glomerulopathy. Diabetologia 29:146-150, 1986.

56. Mauer SM, Sutherland DER, Steffes MW: Relationship of systemic blood pressure to nephropathology in insulin-dependent diabetes mellitus. Kidney Int 41:736-740, 1992.

57. Marcussen N, Ottosen PO, Christensen S: Ultrastructural quantitation of atubular and hypertrophic glomeruli in rats with lithium-induced chronic nephropathy. Virchows Arch 417:513-522, 1990.

58. Marcussen N: Atubular glomeruli and the structural basis for chronic renal failure. Lab Invest 66:265-284,1992.

59. Marcussen N: Atubular glomeruli in renal artery stenosis. Lab invest 65:558-565,1991.

60. Melvin T, Kim Y, Michael AF: Selective binding of IgG4 and other negatively charged plasma proteins in normal and diabetic human kidneys. Am J Pathol 115:443-446, 1984.

61. Michael AF, Brown DM: Increased concentration of albumin in kidney basement membranes in diabetes mellitus. Diabetes 30:843-846, 1981.

62. Ellis EN, Steffes MW, Goetz FC, et al: Glomerular filtration surface in type 1 diabetes mellitus. Kidney Int 29:889-894, 1986.

63. Ellis EN, Steffes MW, Chavers BM, Mauer SM: Observations of glomerular epithelial cell structure in patients with type 1 diabetes mellitus. Kidney Int 32:736-741, 1987.

64. Bjørn SF, Bangstad H-J, Hanssen KF: Glomerular epithelial foot processes and filtration slits in IDDM diabetlic patients. Diabetologia 38:1197-1204, 1995.

65. Pagtalunan ME, Miller PL, Jumping-Eagle S: Podocyte loss and progressive glomerular injury in type II diabetes. J Clin Invest 99:342-348, 1996.

66. Vernier RL, Steffes MW, Sisson-Ross S, Mauer SM: Heparan sulfate proteoglycan in the glomerular basement membrane in type 1 diabetes mellitus. Kidney Int 41:1070-1080, 1992.

67. Østerby R, Gundersen HJG, Nyberg G, Aurell M: Advanced diabetic glomerulopathy. Quantitative structural characterization of non-occluded glomeruli. Diabetes 36:612-619, 1987.

68. Hirose K, Tsuchida H, Østerby R, Gundersen HJG: A strong correlation between glomerular filtration rate and filtration surface in diabetic kidney hyperfunction. Lab Invest 43:434-437, 1980.

69. Thomsen OF, Andersen AR, Christiansen JS, Deckert T: Renal changes in long-term type 1 (insulin-dependent) diabetic patients with and without clinical nephropathy: A light microscopic, morphometric study of autopsy material. Diabetologia 26:361-365, 1984.

70. Bader R, Bader H, Grund KE, et al: A. Structure and function of the kidney in diabetic glomerulosclerosis: Correlations between morphological and functional parameters. Pathol Res Pract 167:204-216, 1980.

71. Bohle A, Wehrmann M, Bogenschutz O, et al: The pathogenesis of chronic renal failure in diabetic nephropathy. Investigation of 488 cases of diabetes glomerulosclerosis. Pathol Res Pract 187:251-259, 1991.

72. Taft JL, Nolan CJ, Yeung SP, et al: Clinical and histological correlations of decline in renal function in diabetic patients with proteinuria. Diabetes 43:1046-1051, 1994.

73. Fioretto P, Steffes MW, Mauer SM: Glomerular structure in nonproteinuric IDDM patients with various levels of albuminuria. Diabetologia 43:1358-1364, 1994.

74. Mauer SM, Goetz FC, McHugh LE, et al: Long-term study of normal kidneys transplanted into patients with type I diabetes. Diabetes 38:516-523, 1989.

75. Bilous RW, Mauer SM, Sutherland DER, Steffes MW: Mean glomerular volume and rate of development of diabetic nephropathy. Diabetes 38:1142-1147, 1989.

76. Nyengaard JR, Bendtsen TF: Glomerular number and size in relation to age, kidney weight, and body surface in normal man. Anat Rec 232:194-201; 1992.

77. Bendtsen TF, Nyengaard JR: The number of glomeruli in type 1 (insulin-dependent) and type 2 (non-insulin-dependent) diabetic patients. Diabetologia 35:844-850, 1992.

78. Brenner BM, Garcia DL, Anderson S: Glomeruli and blood pressure. Less of one, more the other? Am J Hypertens 1:335-347, 1988.

79. Østerby R, Gall M-A, Schmitz A, et al: Glomerular structure and function in proteinuric type 2 (non-insulin-dependent) diabetic patients. Diabetologia 36:1064-1070, 1993.

80. Gambara V, Mecca G, Remuzzi G, Bertani T: Heterogeneous nature of renal lesions in type II diabetes. J Am Soc Nephrol 3:1458-1466, 1993.

81. Lipkin GW, Yeates C, Howie A, et al: More than one third of type 2 diabetics with renal disease do not have diabetic nephropathy: A Prospective study [abstract]. J Am Soc Nephrol 5:379A, 1994.

82. Hayashi H, Karasawa R, Inn H, et al: An electron microscopic study of glomeruli in Japanese patients with non-insulin dependent diabetes mellitus. Kidney Int 41:749-757, 1992.

83. Moriya T, Moriya R, Yajima Y, et al: Urinary albumin as an indicator of diabetic nephropathy lesions in Japenese type 2 diabetic patients. Nephron 91:292-299, 2002.

84. Fioretto P, Mauer SM, Brocco E, et al: Patterns of renal injury in NIDDM patients with microalbuminuria. Diabetologia 39:1569-1576, 1996.

85. Nosadini R, Velussi M, Brocco E, et al: Course of renal function in type 2 diabetic patients with abnormalities of albumin excretion rate. Diabetes 49:476-484, 2000.

86. Christensen PK, Larsen S, Horn T, et al: Renal function and structure in albuminuric type 2 diabetes without retinopathy. Nephrol Dial Transplant 16:2337-2347, 2001.

87. Reaven GM: Syndrome X: 6 years later. J Intern Med Suppl 736:13-22, 1994.

88. Marcantoni C, Ma LJ, Federspiel C, Fogo AB: Hypertensive nephrosclerosis in African Americans versus Caucasians. Kidney Int 62:172-180, 2002.

89. Urizar RE, Schwartz A, Top F Jr, Vernier RL: The nephrotic syndrome in children with diabetes mellitus of recent onset. N Engl J Med; 281:173-181, 1969.

90. Cavallo T, Pinto JA, Rajaraman S: Immune complex disease complicating diabetic glomerulosclerosis. Am J Nephrol 4:347-354, 1984.

91. Mauer SM, Steffes MW, Sutherland DER, et al: Studies of the rate of regression of the glomerular lesions in diabetic rats treated with pancreatic islet transplantation. Diabetes 24:280-285, 1974.

92. Steffes MW, Brown DM, Basgen JM, Mauer SM: Amelioration of mesangial volume and surface alterations following islet transplantation in diabetic rats. Diabetes 29:509-515, 1980.

93. Steffes MW, Brown DM, Basgen JM, et al: Glomerular basement membrane thickness following islet transplantation in the diabetic rat. Lab Invest 41:116-118, 1979.

94. Fioretto P, Mauer SM, Bilous RW, et al: Effects of pancreas transplantation of glomerular structure in insulin-dependent diabetic patients with their own kidneys. Lancet 342:1193-1196, 1993.

95. Fioretto P, Steffes MW, Sutherland DER, et al: Reversal of lesions of diabetic nephropathy after pancreas transplantation. N Engl J Med 339:69-75,1998.

96. Pugh JA: The epidemiology of diabetic nephropathy. Diabetes Metab Rev 5:531-546, 1989.

97. Cowie CC, Port FK, Wolfe RA, et al: Disparities in incidence of diabetic end-stage renal disease according to race and type of diabetes. N Engl J Med 321:1074-1079, 1989.

98. Hirohata T, MacMahon B, Root HF: The natural history of diabetes. 1. Mortality. Diabetes 16:875-881, 1967.

99. Rossing P, Rossing K, Jacobsen P, Parving H-H: Unchanged incidence of diabetic nephropathy in IDDM patients. Diabetes 44:739-743, 1995.

100. Bojestig M, Arnqvist HJ, Hermansson G, et al: Declining incidence of nephropathy in insulin-dependent diabetes mellitus. N Engl J Med 330:15-18, 1994.

101. Gall M-A, Rossing P, Skøtt P, et al: Prevalence of micro-and macroalbuminuria, arterial hypertension, retinopathy and large vessel disease in European type 2 (non-insulin-dependent) diabetic patients. Diabetologia 34:655-661, 1991.

102. Parving HH, Chaturvedi N, Viberti G, Mogensen CE: Does microalbuminuria predict diabetic nephropathy? Diabetes Care 25:406-407, 2002.

103. Dinneen SF, Gerstein HC: The association of microalbuminuria and mortality in non-insulin-dependent diabetes mellitus. Arch Intern Med 157:1413-1418, 1997.

104. Yudkin JS, Forrest RD, Jackson CA: Microalbuminuria as a predictor of vascular disease in non-diabetic subjects. Lancet 2:530-533, 1988.

105. Damsgaard EM, Frøland A, Jørgensen OD, Mogensen CE: Microalbuminuria as predictor of increased mortality in elderly people. BMJ 300:297-300, 1990.

106. Deckert T, Yokoyama H, Mathiesen ER, et al: Cohort study of predictive value of urinary albumin excretion for atherosclerotic vascular disease in patients with insulin dependent diabetes. BMJ 312:871-874, 1996.

107. Deckert T, Feldt-Rasmussen B, Borch-Johnsen K, et al: Albuminuria reflects widespread vascular damage. The Steno hypothesis. Diabetologia 32:219-226, 1989.

108. Winocour PH: Microalbuminuria. BMJ 304:1196-1197, 1992.

109. Parving H-H, Hommel E, Mathiesen ER, et al: Prevalence of microalbuminuria, arterial hypertension, retinopathy and neuropathy in patients with insulin-dependent diabetes. BMJ 296:156-160, 1988.

110. Feldt-Rasmussen B, Borch-Johnsen K, Mathiesen ER: Hypertension as related to diabetic nephropathy. Hypertension 2(suppl):18-20, 1985.

111. Wiseman MJ, Viberti GC, Mackintosh D, et al: Glycaemia, arterial pressure and micro-aluminuria in type 1 (insulin-dependent) diabetes mellitus. Diabetologia 2:401-405, 1984.

112. Jensen T, Stender S, Deckert T: Abnormalities in plasma concentrations of lipoproteins and fibrinogen in type 1 (insulin-dependent) diabetic patients with increased urinary albumin excretion. Diabetologia 31:142-145, 1988.

113. Jones SL, Close CF, Mattock MB, et al: Plasma lipid and coagulation factor concentrations in insulin-dependent diabetics with microalbuminuria. BMJ 298:487-490, 1989.

114. Kapelrud H, Bangstad H-J, Dahl-Jørgensen K, et al: Serum Lp(a) lipoprotein concentrations in insulin dependent diabetic patients with microalbuminuria.BMJ 303:675-678,1991.

115. Gall M-A, Rossing P, Hommel E, et al: Apolipoprotein(a) in insulin-dependent diabetic patients with and without diabetic nephropathy. Scand J Clin Lab Invest 52:513-521, 1992.

116. Nielsen FS, Voldsgaard Al, Gall M-A, et al: Apolipoprotein(a) and cardiovascular disease in type 2 (non-insulin-dependent) diabetic patients with and without diabetic nephropathy. Diabetologia 36:438-444, 1993.

117. Jensen T: Albuminuria—a marker of renal and generalized vascular disease in insulin-dependent diabetes mellitus. Dan Med Bull 38:134-144, 1991.

118. Jensen T, Feldt-Rasmussen B, Bjerre-Knudsen J, Deckert T: Features of endothelial dysfunction in early diabetic nephropathy. Lancet 2:461-463, 1989.

119. Jenson T: Increased plasma level of von Willebrand factor in insulin-dependent diabetic patients with incipient nephropathy. BMJ 298:27-28, 1989.

120. Feldt-Rasmussen B: Increased transcapillary escape rate of albumin in type 1(insulin-dependent) diabetic patients with microalbuminuria. Diabetologia 29:282-286, 1986.

121. Parving H-H, Nielsen FS, Bang LE, et al: Macro-microangiopathy and endothelial dysfunction in NIDDM patients and without diabetic nephropathy. Diabetologia 39:1590-1597, 1996.

122. Schajkwijk CG, Ligtvoet N, Twaalfhoven H, et al: Amadori albumin in type 1 diabetic patients—correlation with markers of endothelial dysfunction, association with diabetic nephropathy, and localization in retinal capillaries. Diabetes 48:2446-2453, 1999.

123. Groop L, Ekstrand A, Forsblom C, et al: Insulin resistance, hypertension and microalbuminuria in patients with type 2 (non-insulin-dependent) diabetes mellitus. Diabetologia 36:642-647, 1993.

124. Yip J, Mattock MB, Morocutti A, et al: Insulin resistance in insulin-dependent diabetic patients with microalbuminuria. Lancet 342:883-887, 1993.

125. Ewing DJ, Campbell IW, Clarke B: The natural history of diabetic autonomic neuropathy. Q J Med 49:95-108, 1980.

126. Thuesen L, Christiansen JS, Mogensen CE, Henningsen P: Echocardiographic-determined left ventricular wall characteristics in insulin-dependent diabetic patients. Acta Med Scand 224:343-348, 1988.

127. Sampson MJ, Chambers JB, Sprigings DC, Drury PL: Abnormal diastolic function in patients with type 1 diabetes and early nephropathy. Br Heart J 64:266-271, 1990.

128. Sampson MJ, Chambers JB, Sprigings DC, Drury PL: Regression of left ventricular hypertrophy with 1 year of antihypertensive treatment in type 1 diabetic patients with early nephropathy. Diabet Med 8:106-110, 1991.

129. Nielsen FS, Ali S, Rossing P, et al: Left ventricular hypertrophy in non-insulin dependent diabetic patients with and without nephropathy. Diabet Med 14:538-546, 1997.

130. Frolich E, Apstein C, Chobanian AV, et al: The heart in hypertension. N Engl J Med 327:998-1008, 1992.

131. Knowles HCJ: Long term juvenile diabetes treated with unmeasured diet. Trans Assoc Am Physicians 84:95-101, 1971.

132. Morrish NJ, Stevens LK, Head J, et al: A prospective study of mortality among middle-aged diabetic patients (the London cohort of the WHO Multinational Study of Vascular Disease in Diabetics). II: Associated risk factors. Diabetologia 33:542-548, 1990.

133. Schmitz A, Vaeth M: Microalbuminuria: A major risk factor in non-insulin-dependent diabetes. A 10-year follow-up study of 503 patients. Diabet Med 5:126-134, 1988.

134. Schmitz A: The kidney in non-insulin-dependent diabetes. Acta Diabetol 29:47-69, 1992.

135. Mogensen CE, Schmitz A, Christensen CK: Comparative renal pathophysiology relevant to IDDM and NIDDM patients. Diabetes Metab Rev 4:453-483, 1988.

136. Kunzelman CL, Nelson RG, Knowler WC, Pettitt DJ: Proteinuria determines prognosis in type 2 (non-insulin-dependent) diabetes [abstract]. Kidney Int 33:197, 1988.

137. Rhoads GG, Dahlen G, Berg K, et al: Lp(a) lipoprotein as a risk factor for myocardial infarction. JAMA 256:2540-2544, 1986.

138. Tarnow L, Rossing P, Nielsen FS, et al: Increased plasma apolipoprotein(a) levels in IDDM patients with diabetic nephropathy. Diabetes Care 19:1382-1387, 1996.

139. Earle K, Walker J, Hill C, Viberti GC: Familial clustering of cardiovascular disease in patients with insulin-dependent diabetes and nephropathy. N Engl J Med 326:673-677, 1992.

140. de Cosmo S, Bacci S, Piras GP, et al: High prevalence of risk factors for cardiovascular disease in parents of IDDM patients with albuminuria. Diabetologia 40:1191-1196, 1997.

141. Nørgaard K, Mathiesen ER, Hommel E, et al: Lack of familial predisposition to cardiovascular disease in type 1 (insulin-dependent) diabetic patients with nephropathy. Diabetologia 34:370-372, 1991.

142. Tarnow L, Rossing P, Nielsen FS, et al: Cardiovascular morbidity and early mortality cluster in parents of type 1 diabetic patients with diabetic nephropathy. Diabetes Care 23:30-33, 2000.

143. Sato A, Tarnow L, Parving H-H: Prevalence of left ventricular hypertrophy in type 1 diabetic patients with diabetic nephropathy. Diabetologia 42:76-80, 1999.

144. Stehouwer CD, Gall MA, Hougaard P, et al: Plasma homocysteine concentration predicts mortality in non-insulin-dependent diabetic patients with and without albuminuria. Kidney Int 55:308-314, 1999.

145. Stehouwer CD, Gall MA, Twisk JW, et al: Increased urinary albumin excretion, endothelial dysfunction, and chronic low-grade inflammation in type 2 diabetes: Progressive, interrelated, and independently associated with risk of death. Diabetes 51:1157-1165, 2002.

146. Cambier P: Application de la théorie de Rehberg à l'étude clinique des affections rénales et du diabète. Ann Med 35:273-299, 1934.

147. Christiansen JS: On the pathogenesis of the increased glomerular filtration rate in short-term insulin-dependent diabetes. Dan Med Bull 31:349-361, 1984.

148. Ditzel J, Schwartz M: Abnormally increased glomerular filtration rate in short-term insulin-treated diabetic subjects. Diabetes 16:264-267, 1967.

149. Mogensen CE: Glomerular filtration rate and renal plasma flow in short-term and long-term juvenile diabetes mellitus. Scand J Clin Lab Invest 28:91-100, 1971.

150. Mogensen CE: Kidney function and glomerular permeability to macromolecules in early juvenile diabetes. Scand J Clin Lab Invest 28:79-90, 1971.

151. Mogensen CE: Kidney Function and Glomerular Permeability to Macromolecules in Juvenile Diabetes [thesis]. Dan Med Bull 19 (suppl 3):1-40, 1972.

152. Christiansen JS, Gammelgaard J, Frandsen M, Parving H-H: Increased kidney size, glomerular filtration rate and renal plasma flow in short-term insulin-dependent diabetics. Diabetologia 20:451-456, 1981.

153. Christiansen JS, Gammelgaard J, Tronier B, et al: Kidney function and size in diabetics before and during initial insulin treatment. Kidney Int 21:683-688, 1982.

154. Stadler G, Schmid R: Severe functional disorders of glomerular capillaries and renal hemodynamics in treated diabetes mellitus during childhood. Ann Paediatr 193:129-138, 1959.

155. Myers BD, Nelson RG, Williams GW, et al: Glomerular function in Pima Indians with noninsulin-dependent diabetes mellitus of recent onset. J Clin Invest 88:524-530, 1991.

156. Vora J, Dolben J, Dean JD, et al: Renal hemodynamics in newly presenting non-insulin dependent diabetes mellitus. Kidney Int 41:829-835, 1992.

157. Schmitz A, Christensen T, Jensen FT: Glomerular filtration rate and kidney volume in normoalbuminuric non-insulin-dependent diabetics—lack of glomerular hyperfiltration and renal hypertrophy in uncomplicated NIDDM. Scand J Clin Lab Invest 49:103-108, 1989.

158. Schmitz A, Hansen HH, Christensen T: Kidney function in newly diagnosed type 2 (non-insulin-dependent) diabetic patients, before and during treatment. Diabetologia 32:434-439, 1989.

159. Vora J, Dolben J, Williams J, et al: Renal haemodynamics in newly presenting non-proteinuric normotensive non-insulin-dependent diabetic patients (NIDDMs): Changes over two years after diagnosis [abstract]. Diabet Med 10 (suppl 1): S25, 1993.

160. Brenner BM, Humes HD: Mechanics of glomerular ultrafiltration. N Engl J Med 297:148-154, 1977.

161. Mogensen CE, Østerby R, Gundersen HJG: Early functional and morphological vascular renal consequences of the diabetic state. Diabetologia 17:71-76, 1979.

162. Østerby R, Gundersen HJG: Glomerular size and structure in diabetes mellitus. I. Early abnormalities. Diabetologia 11:225-229, 1975.

163. Hostetter TH, Troy JL, Brenner BM: Glomerular hemodynamics in experimental diabetics mellitus. Kidney Int 19:410-415, 1981.

164. Michels LD, Davidman M, Keane WF: Determinants of glomerular filtration and plasma flow in experimental diabetic rats. J Lab Clin Med 9:869-885, 1981.

165. Flyvbjerg A: The role of insulin-like growth factor I in initial renal hypertrophy in experimental diabetes. In Flyvbjerg A, Ørskov H, Alberti KGMM (eds): Growth Hormone and Insulin-like Growth Factor I. London John Wiley and sons, 1993, pp 271-306.

166. Mogensen CE: Early glomerular hyperfiltration in insulin-dependent diabetics and late nephropathy. Scand J Clin Lab Invest 46:201-206, 1986.

167. Rudberg S, Persson B, Dahlquist G: Increased glomerular filtration rate as a predictor of diabetic nephropathy—an 8-year prospective study. Kidney Int 41:822-828, 1992.

168. Rossing P, Hougaard P, Parving H-H: Risk factors for development of incipient and overt diabetic nephropathy in type 1 diabetic patients. Diabetes Care 25:859-864, 2002.

169. Jones SL, Wiseman MJ, Viberti GC: Glomerular hyperfiltration as a risk factor for diabetic nephropathy: Five year report of a prospective study. Diabetologia 34:59-60, 1991.

170. Lervang H-H, Jensen S, Bröchner-Mortensen J, Ditzel J: Early glomerular hyperfiltration and the development of late nephropathy in type 1 (insulin-dependent) diabetes mellitus. Diabetologia 31:723-729, 1988.

171. Vedel P, Obel J, Nielsen FS, et al: Glomerular hyperfiltration in microalbuminuria NIDDM patients. Diabetologia 39:1584-1589, 1996.

172. Microalbuminuria Collaborative Study Group UK: Risk factors for development of microalbuminuria in insulin dependent diabetic patients: A cohort study. BMJ 306:1235-1239, 1993.

173. Gall M-A, Hougaard P, Borch-Johnsen K, Parving H-H: Risk factors for development of incipent and overt diabetic nephropathy in patients with non-insulin-dependent diabetes mellitus: Prospective, observational study. BMJ 314:783-788, 1997.

174. Microalbuminuria Collaborative Study Group UK: Predictors of the development of microalbuminuria in patients with type 1 diabetes mellitus: A seven year prospective study. Diabet Med 16:918-925, 1999.

175. Royal College of Physicians of Edinburgh Diabetes Register Group: Near normal urinary albumin concentrations predict progression to diabetic nephropathy in type 1 diabetes. Diabet Med 17:782-791, 2000.

176. Schultz CJ, Neil H, Dalton R, Dunger D: Risk of nephropathy can be detected before the onset of microalbuminuria during the early years after diagnosis of type 1 diabetes. Diabetes Care 23:1811-1815, 2000.

177. Keen H, Chlouverakis C, Fuller JH, Jarrett RJ: The concomitants of raised blood sugar: Studies in newly-detected hyperglycaemics. II. Urinary albumin excretion, blood pressure and their relation to blood sugar levels. Guys Hosp Rep 118:247-254, 1969.

178. Parving H-H, Noer I, Deckert T, et al: The effect of metabolic regulation on microvascular permeability to small and large molecules in short-term juvenile diabetics. Diabetologia 12:161-166, 1976.

179. Mogensen CE, Vestbo E, Poulsen PL, et al: Microalbuminuria and potential confounders. Diabetes Care 18:572-581, 1995.

180. Parving H-H: Microalbuminuria in essential hypertension and diabetes mellitus. J Hypertens 14:S89-S94, 1996.

181. Feldt-Rasmussen B, Mathiesen ER: Variability of urinary albumin excretion in incipient diabetic nephropathy. Diabetes Nephropathy 3:101-103, 1984.

182. Mathiesen ER, Saurbrey N, Hommel E, Parving H-H: Prevalence of microalbuminuria in children with type 1 (insulin-dependent) diabetes mellitus. Diabetologia 29:640-643, 1986.

183. Viberti GC, Walker JD, Pinto J: Diabetic nephropathy. In Alberti KGMM, DeFronzo RA, Keen H, Zimmet P (eds): International Textbook of Diabetes Mellitus. London, John Wiley and Sons, 1992, pp 1267-1328.

184. Borch-Johnsen K, Wenzel H, Viberti GC, Mogensen CE: Is screening and intervention for microalbuminuria worthwhile in patients with insulin dependent diabetes. BMJ 306:1722-1725, 1993.

185. Brenner BM, Hostetter TH, Humes HD: Molecular basis of proteinuria of glomerular origin. N Engl J Med 298:826-833, 1978.

186. Brenner BM, Bohrer MP, Baylis C, Deen WM: Determinants of glomerular permselectivity: Insights derived from observations in vivo. Kidney Int 12:229-237, 1977.

187. Viberti GC, Mackintosh D, Keen H: Determinants of the penetration of proteins through the glomerular barrier in insulin-dependent diabetes mellitus. Diabetes 32:92-95, 1983.

188. Deckert T, Feldt-Rasmussen B, Djurup R, Deckert M: Glomerular size and charge selectivity in insulin-dependent diabetes mellitus. Kidney Int 33:100-106, 1988.

189. Deckert T, Kofoed-Enevoldsen A, Vidal P, et al: Size-and charge selectivity of glomerular filtration in type 1 (insulin-dependent) diabetic patients with and without albuminuria. Diabetologia 36:244-251, 1993.

190. Scandling JD, Myers BD: Glomerular size-selectivity and microalbuminuria in early diabetic glomerular disease. Kidney Int 41:840-846, 1992.

191. Pietravalle P, Morano S, Christina G, et al: Charge selectivity of proteinuria in type 1 diabetes explored by Ig subclass clearance. Diabetes 40:1685-1690, 1991.

192. Shimomura S, Spiro RG: Studies on macromolecular components of human glomerular basement membrane and alterations in diabetes. Decreased levels of heparan sulfate proteoglycan and laminin. Diabetes 36:374-381, 1987.

193. van den Born J, van Kraats AA, Bakker MAH, et al: Reduction of heparan sulphate–associated anionic sites in the glomerular basement of rats with streptozotocin-induced diabetic nephropathy. Diabetologia 38:1169-1175, 1995.

194. Bonnet F, Cooper ME, Kawachi H, et al: Irbesartan normalizes the deficiency in glomerular nephrin expression in a model of diabetes and hypertension. Diabetologia 44:874-877, 2001.

195. Mifsud SA, Allen TJ, Bertram JF, et al: Podocyte foot process broadening in experimental diabetic nephropathy: Amelioration with renin-angiotensin blockade. Diabetologia 44:878:882, 2001.

196. Nakamura T, Ushiyama C, Suzuki S, et al: Urinary excretion of podocytes in patients with diabetic nephropathy. Nephrol Dial Transplant 15:1379-1383, 2000.

197. Steffes MW, Schmidt D, McCrery R, Basgen JM: Glomerular cell number in normal subjects and in type 1 diabetic patients. Kidney Int 59:2104-2113, 2001.

198. Feldt-Rasmussen B: Microalbuminuria and clinical nephropathy in type 1 (insulin-dependent) diabetes mellitus: Pathophysiological mechanisms and intervention studies. Dan Med Bull 36:405-415, 1989.

199. Hommel E, Mathiesen ER, Edsberg B, et al: Acute reduction of arterial blood pressure reduces urinary albumin excretion in type 1 (insulin-dependent) diabetic patients with incipient nephropathy. Diabetologia 29:211-215, 1986.

200. Imanishi M, Yoshioka K, Konishi Y, et al: Glomerular hypertension as one cause of albuminuria in type II diabetic patients. Diabetologia 42:999-1005, 1999.

201. Sandeman DD, Shore AC, Tooke JE: Relation of skin capillary pressure in patients with insulin-dependent diabetes mellitus to complications and metabolic control. N Engl J Med 327:760-764, 1992.

202. Christensen CK: The pre-proteinuric phase of diabetic nephropathy. Dan Med Bull 38:145-159, 1991.

203. Feldt-Rasmussen B, Mathiesen ER, Deckert T, et al: Central role for sodium in the pathogenesis of blood pressure changes independent of angiotensin, aldosterone and catecholamines in type 1 (insulin-dependent) diabetes mellitus. Diabetologia 30:610-617, 1987.

204. Mathiesen ER: Prevention of diabetic nephropathy: Microalbuminuria and perspectives for intervention in insulin-dependent diabetes. Dan Med Bull 40:273-285, 1993.

205. Mathiesen ER, Feldt-Rasmussen B, Hommel E, et al: Stable glomerular filtration rate in normotensive IDDM patients with stable microalbuminuria. Diabetes Care 20:286-289, 1997.

206. Feldt-Rasmussen B, Hegedüs L, Mathiesen ER, Deckert T: Kidney volume in type 1 (insulin-dependent) diabetic patients with normal or increased urinary albumin excretion: Effect of long-term improved metabolic control. Scand J Clin Lab Invest 51:31-36, 1991.

207. Lawson ML, Sochett EB, Chait PG, et al: Effect of puberty on markers of glomerular hypertrophy and hypertension in IDDM. Diabetes 45:51-55, 1996.

208. Skøtt P: Lithium clearance in the evaluation of segmental renal tubular reabsorption of sodium and water in diabetes mellitus. Dan Med Bull 41:23-37, 1993.

209. Ditzel J, Bröchner-Mortensen J, Kawahara R: Dysfunction of tubular phosphate reabsorption related to glomerular filtration and blood glucose control in diabetic children. Diabetologia 23:406-410, 1982.

210. Woods LL, Mizelle HL, Hall JG: Control of renal hemodynamics in hyperglycemia. Am J Physiol 252:F65:F73, 1987.

211. Blantz RC, Peterson OW, Gushwa L, Tucker BJ: Effect of modest hyperglycemia on tubuloglomerular feedback activity. Kidney Int 22(suppl 12):S206-S212, 1982.

212. DeFronzo RA: The effect of insulin on renal sodium metabolism. Diabetologia 21:165-171, 1981.

213. Tarnow L, Rossing P, Gall M-A, et al: Prevalence of arterial hypertension in diabetic patients before and after the JNC-V. Diabetes care 17:1247-1251, 1994.

214. Viberti GC, Keen H, Wiseman MJ: Raised arterial pressure in parents of proteinuric insulin-dependent diabetics. BMJ 295:515-517, 1987.

215. Walker JD, Tariq T, Viberti GC: Sodium-lithium countertransport activity in red cells of patients with insulin-dependent diabetes and nephropathy and their parents. BMJ 301:635-638, 1990.

216. Jensen JS, Mathiesen ER, Nørgaard K, et al: Increased blood pressure and erythrocyte sodium-lithium countertransport activity are not inherited in diabetic nephropathy. Diabetologia 33:619-624, 1990.

217. Molitch ME, Steffes MW, Cleary PA, Nathan DM: Baseline analysis of renal function in diabetes control and complications trial. Kidney Int 43:668-674, 1993.

218. Stephenson J, Eurodiab IDDM Complications Study Group: Blood pressure and urinary albumin excretion in IDDM [abstract]. Diabetes 42 (suppl 1):29A, 1993.

219. Fagerudd JA, Tarnow L, Jacobsen P, et al: Predisposition to essential hypertension and development of diabetic nephropathy in IDDM patients. Diabetes 47:439-444, 1998.

220. Christlieb AR: Renin, angiotensin, and norepinephrine in alloxan diabetes. Diabetes 23:962-970, 1974.

221. Hommel E, Mathiesen ER, Giese J, et al: On the pathogenesis of arterial blood pressure elevation early in the course of diabetic nephropathy. Scand J Clin Lab Invest 49:537-544, 1989.

222. Parving H-H: Arterial hypertension in diabetes mellitus. *In* Alberti KGMM, DeFronzo RA, Keen H, Zimmet P (eds): International Textbook of Diabetes Mellitus. New York, John Wiley & Sons, 1992, pp 1521-1534.

223. Parving H-H, Smidt UM, Friisberg B, et al: A prospective study of glomerular filtration rate and arterial blood pressure in insulin-dependent diabetics with diabetic nephropathy. Diabetologia 20:457-461, 1981.

224. Malins JM: Clinical Diabetes Mellitus. London: Eyre & Spottiswoode, 1968.

225. Hommel E, Mathiesen ER, Aukland K, Parving H-H: Pathophysiological aspects of edema formation in diabetic nephropathy. Kidney Int 38:1187-1192, 1990.

226. Ritz E, Stefanski A: Diabetic nephropathy in type II diabetes. Am J Kidney Dis 27:167-194, 1996.

227. Mogensen CE: Progression of nephropathy in long-term diabetics with proteinuria and effect of initial antihypertensive treatment. Scand J Clin Lab Invest 36:383-388, 1976.

228. Viberti GC, Bilous RW, Mackintosh D, Keen H: Monitoring glomerular function in diabetic nephropathy. Am J Med 74:256-264, 1983.

229. Gall M-A, Nielsen FS, Smidt UM, Parving H-H: The course of kidney function in type 2 (non-insulin-dependent) diabetic patients with diabetic nephropathy. Diabetologia 36:1071-1078, 1993.

230. Nelson RG, Bennett PH, Beck GJ, et al: Development and progression of renal disease in Pima Indians with non-insulin-dependent diabetes mellitus. N Engl J Med 335:1636-1642, 1996.

231. Myers BD, Nelson RG, Williams GW, et al: Glomerular function in Pima Indians with noninsulin-dependent diabetes mellitus of recent onset. J Clin Invest 88:524-530, 1991.

232. Myers BD, Winetz JA, Chui F, Michaels AS: Mechanisms of proteinuria in diabetic nephropathy: A study of glomerular barrier function. Kidney Int 21:633-641, 1982.

233. Tomlanovich S, Deen WM, Jones HW III, et al: Functional nature of glomerular injury in progressive diabetic glomerulopathy. Diabetes 36:556-565, 1987.

234. Friedman S, Jones HW III, Golbetz HV, et al: Mechanisms of proteinuria in diabetic nephropathy II. A study of the size-selective glomerular filtration barrier. Diabetes 32 (suppl 2):40-46, 1983.

235. Carrie BJ, Myers BD: Proteinuria and functional characteristics of the glomerular barrier in diabetic nephropathy. Kidney Int 17:669-676, 1980.

236. Andersen S, Blouch K, Bialek J, et al: Glomerular permselectivity in early stages of overt diabetic nephropathy. Kidney Int 58:2129-2137, 2000.

237. Gall M-A, Rossing P, Kofoed-Enevoldsen A, et al: Glomerular size- and charge selectivity in type 2 (non-insulin-dependent) diabetic patients with diabetic nephropathy. Diabetologia 37:195-201, 1993.

238. Watkins PJ, Blainey JD, Brewer DB, et al: The natural history of diabetic renal disease. A follow-up study of series of renal biopsies. Q J Med 41:437-456, 1972.

239. Jackson B, Debrevi L, Witty M, Johnson CF: Progression of renal disease: Effects of different classes of antihypertensive therapy. J Hypertens 4 (suppl 5):S269-S271, 1986.

240. Rossing P, Hommel E, Smidt UM, Parving H-H: Impact of arterial blood pressure and albuminuria on the progression of diabetic nephropathy in IDDM patients. Diabetes 42:715-719, 1993.

241. Parving H-H: Impact of blood pressure and antihypertensive treatment on incipient and overt nephropathy, retinopathy, and endothelial permeability in diabetes mellitus. Diabetes Care 14:260-269, 1991.

242. Rossing P: Promotion, prediction, and prevention of progression in diabetic nephropathy. Diabet Med 15:900-919, 1998.

243. Jacobsen P, Rossing K, Tarnow L, et al: Progression of diabetic nephropathy in normotensive type 1 diabetic patients. Kidney Int 56:S101-S105, 1999.

244. Hovind P, Rossing P, Tarnow L, et al: Progression of diabetic nephropathy. Kidney Int 59:702-709, 2001.

245. Yokoyama H, Tomonaga O, Hirayama M, et al: Predictors of the progression of diabetic nephropathy and the beneficial effect of angiotensin-converting enzyme inhibitors in NIDDM patients. Diabetologia 40:405-411, 1997.

246. Krolewski AS, Warram JH, Christlieb AR: Hypercholesterolemia—A determinant of renal function loss and deaths in IDDM patients with nephropathy. Kidney Int 45(suppl 45):S125-S131, 1994.

247. Breyer JA, Bain P, Evans JK, et al: Predictors of the progression of renal insufficiency in patients with insulin-dependent diabetes and overt diabetic nephropathy. Kidney Int 50:1651-1658, 1996.

248. Jacobson HR: Chronic renal failure: pathophysiology. Lancet 338:419-423, 1991.

249. Hostetter TH, Rennke HG, Brenner BM: The case for intrarenal hypertension in the initiation and progression of diabetic and other glomerulopathies. Am J Med 72:375-380, 1982.

250. Brenner BM: Hemodynamically mediated glomerular injury and the progressive nature of kidney disease. Kidney Int 23:647-655, 1983.

251. Jensen PK, Steven K, Blaehr H, et al: The effects of indomethacin on glomerular hemodynamics in experimental diabetes. Kidney Int 29:490-495, 1986.

252. Parving H-H, Kastrup J, Smidt UM, et al: Impaired autoregulation of glomerular filtration rate in type 1 (insulin-dependent) diabetic patients with nephropathy. Diabetologia 27:547-552, 1984.

253. Christensen PK, Hansen HP, Parving H-H: Impaired autoregulation of GFR in hypertensive non-insulin dependent diabetic patients. Kidney Int 52:1369-1374, 1997.

254. Hayashi K, Epstein M, Loutzenhiser R, Forster H: Impaired myogenic responsiveness of the afferent arteriole in streptozotocin-induced diabetic rats: Role of eicosanoid derangements. J Am Soc Nephrol 2:1578-1586, 1992.

255. Christensen PK, Lund S, Parving H-H: The impact of glycaemic control on autoregulation of glomerular filtration rate in patients with non-insulin dependent diabetes. Scand J Clin Lab Invest 61:43-50, 2001.

256. Remuzzi G, Bertani T: Is glomerulosclerosis a consequence of altered glomerular permeability to macromolecules? Kidney Int 38:384-394, 1990.

257. Parving H-H, Rossing P, Hommel E, Smidt UM: Angiotensin converting enzyme inhibition in diabetic nephropathy: Ten years experience. Am J Kidney Dis 26:99-107, 1995.

258. Parving H-H: Renoprotection in diabetes: Genetic and non-genetic risk factors and treatment. Diabetologia 41:745-759, 1998.

259. Nyberg G, Blohmé G, Nordén G: Impact of metabolic control in progression of clinical diabetic nephropathy. Diabetologia 30:82-86, 1987.

260. Mulec H, Blohmé G, Grände B, Björck S: Progression of overt diabetic nephropathy (DN): Role of metabolic control [abstract]. J Am Soc Nephrol 6:453, 1995.

261. Alaveras A, Thomas SM, Sagriotis A, Viberti GC: Promoters of progression of diabetic nephropathy: The relative roles of blood glucose and blood pressure control. Nephrol Dial Transplan 12:71-74, 1997.

262. Mulec H, Blohmé G, Grände B, Björck S: The effect of metabolic control on rate of decline in renal function in insulin-dependent diabetes mellitus with overt diabetic nephropathy. Nephrol Dial Transplant 13:651-655, 1998.

263. Bangstad HJ, Osterby R, Rudberg S, et al: Kidney function and glomerulopathy over 8 years in young patients with type I (insulin-dependent) diabetes mellitus and microalbuminuria. Diabetologia 45:253-261, 2002.

264. Biesenbach G, Janko O, Zazgornik J: Similar rate of progression in the predialysis phase in type I and type II diabetes mellitus. Nephrol Dial Transplant 9:1097-1102, 1994.

265. Wu M-S, Yu C-C, Yang C-W, et al: Poor predialysis glycaemic control is a predictor of mortality in type II diabetic patients on maintenance haemodialysis. Nephrol Dial Transplant 12:2105-2110, 1997.

266. Hasslacher C, Stech W, Wahl P, Ritz E: Blood pressure and metabolic control as risk factors for nephropathy in type 1 (insulin-dependent) diabetes. Diabetologia 28:6-11, 1985.

267. Berglund J, Lins L-E, Lins P-E: Metabolic and blood pressure monitoring in diabetic renal failure. Acta Med Scand 218:401-408, 1985.

268. Orth SR, Ritz E, Schrier RW: The renal risk of smoking. Kidney Int 51:1669-1677, 1997.

269. Sawicki PT, Didjurgeit U, Mühlhauser I, et al: Smoking is associated with progression of diabetic nephropathy. Diabetes Care 17:126-131, 1994.

270. Hovind P, Rossing P, Tarnow L, Parving H-H: Smoking and progression of diabetic nephropathy in type 1 diabetes [abstract]. Diabetologia 45:A361, 2002.

271. Cambien F, Poirier O, Lecerf L, et al: Deletion polymorphism in the gene for angiotensin-converting enzyme is a potential risk factor for myocardial infarction. Nature 359(6396):641-644, 1992.

272. Tarnow L, Cambien F, Rossing P, et al: Insertion/deletion polymorphism in the angiotensin-I-converting enzyme gene is associated with coronary heart disease in IDDM patients with diabetic nephropathy. Diabetologia 38:798-803, 1995.

273. Rigat B, Hubert C, Corvol P, Soubrier F: PCR detection of the insertion/deletion polymorphism of the human angiotensin converting enzyme gene (DCP 1) (dipeptidyl-carboxy peptidase 1). Nucleic Acids Res 20:1433-1433, 1992.

274. Yoshida H, Kuriyama S, Atsumi Y, et al: Angiotensin I converting enzyme gene polymorphism in non-insulin dependent diabetes mellitus. Kidney Int 50:657-664, 1996.

275. Schmidt S, Strojek K, Grzeszczak W, et al: Excess of DD homozygotes in haemodialysed patients with type II diabetes. Nephrol Dial Transplant 12:427-429, 1997.

276. Schmidt S, Ritz E: Angiotensin I converting enzyme gene polymorphism and diabetic nephropathy in type II diabetes. Nephrol Dial Transplant 12:37-41, 1997.

277. Solini A, Dalla VM, Saller A, et al: The angiotensin-converting enzyme DD genotype is associated with glomerulopathy lesions in type 2 diabetes. Diabetes 51:251-255, 2002.

278. Rudberg S, Rasmussen LM, Bangstad H-J, Østerby R: Influence of insertion/deletion polymorphism in the ACE-I gene on the progression of diabetic glomerulopathy in type 1 diabetic patients with microalbuminuria. Diabetes Care 23:544-548, 2000.

279. Parving H-H, Jacobsen P, Tarnow L, et al: Effect of deletion polymorphism of angiotensin converting enzyme gene on progression of diabetic nephropathy during inhibition of angiotensin converting enzyme: Observational follow up study. BMJ 313:591-594, 1996.

280. Björck S, Blohmé G, Sylvén C, Mulec H: Deletion insertion polymorphism of the angiotensin converting enzyme gene and progression of diabetic nephropathy. Nephrol Dial Transplant 12(suppl 2):67-70, 1997.

281. Marre M, Jeunemaitre X, Gallois Y, et al: Contribution of genetic polymorphism in the renin-angiotensin system to the development of renal complications in insulin-dependent diabetes. J Clin Invest 99:1585-1595, 1997.

282. Vlemming LJ, van der Pijl JW, Lemkes HHPJ, et al: The DD genotype of the ACE gene polymorphism is associated with progression of diabetic nephropathy to end stage renal failure in IDDM. Clin Nephrol 51:133-140, 1999.

283. Rossing K, Jacobsen P, Hommel E, et al: Pregnancy and progression of diabetic nephropathy. Diabetologia 45:36-41, 2002.

284. Christensen PK, Larsen S, Horn T, et al: The causes of albuminuria in patients with type 2 diabetes without diabetic retinopathy. Kidney Int 58:1719-1731, 2000.

285. Christensen PK, Gall MA, Parving H-H: Course of glomerular filtration rate in albuminuric type 2 diabetic patients with or without diabetic glomerulopathy. Diabetes Care 23(suppl 2):B14-B20, 2000.

286. Parving H-H, Andersen AR, Smidt UM, et al: Diabetic nephropathy and arterial hypertension. Diabetologia 24:10-12, 1983.

287. Drury PL: Diabetes and arterial hypertension. Diabetologia 24:1-9, 1983.

288. Nielsen FS, Rossing P, Bang LE, et al: On the mechanisms of blunted nocturnal decline in arterial blood pressure in NIDDM patients with diabetic nephropathy. Diabetes 44:783-789, 1995.

289. Torffvit O, Agardh C-D: Day and night variation in ambulatory blood pressure in type 1 diabetes mellitus with nephropathy and autonomic neuropathy. J Intern Med 233:131-137, 1993.

290. Karlefors T: Circulatory studies during exercise with particular reference to diabetics. Acta Med Scand 180 (suppl 449):1-87, 1966.

291. Hostetter TH: Pathogenesis of diabetic glomerulopathy: Hemodynamic considerations. Semin Nephrol 10:219-227, 1990.

292. Marshall SM, Alberti KGMM: Comparison of the prevalence and associated features of abnormal albumin excretion in insulin-dependent and non-insulin-dependent diabetes. Q J Med 70:61-71, 1989.

293. Pollare T, Lithell H, Selinus I, Berne C: Sensitivity to insulin during treatment with atenolol and metoprolol: A randomised, double blind study of the effects on carbohydrate and lipoprotein metabolism in hypertensive patients. BMJ 89:1152-1157, 1991.

294. Thomsen ÅC: The Kidney in Diabetes Mellitus. Copenhagen, Munksgaard, 1965.

295. Jensen T, Borch-Johnsen K, Kofoed-Enevoldsen A, Deckert T: Coronary heart disease in young type 1 (insulin-dependent) diabetic patients with and without diabetic nephropathy: Incidence and risk-factors. Diabetologia 30:144-148, 1987.

296. Jarrett RJ: Cardiovascular disease and hypertension in diabetes mellitus. Diabetes Metab Rev 5:547-558, 1989.

297. Grenfell A, Watkins PJ: Clinical diabetic nephropathy: Natural history and complications. Clin Endocrinol Metab 15:783-805, 1986.

298. Frimondt-Møller C: Diabetic cystopathy. Dan Med Bull 25:49-60, 1978.

299. Jensen PK, Christiansen JS, Steven K, Parving H-H: Strict metabolic control and renal function in the streptozotocin diabetic rat. Kidney Int 31:47-51, 1987.

300. Steffes MW, Mauer SM: Diabetic glomerulopathy in man and experimental animal models. Int Rev Exp Pathol 26:147-175, 1984.

301. Steffes MW, Vernier RL, Brown DM, et al: Diabetic glomerulopathy in the uninephrectomized rat resists amelioration following islet transplantation. Diabetologia 23:347-353, 1982.

302. Steffes MW, Brown DM, Mauer SM: The development, enhancement, and reversal of the secondary complications of diabetes mellitus. Hum Pathol 10:293-299, 1979.

303. Rasch R: Prevention of diabetic glomerulopathy in streptozotocin diabetic rats by insulin treatment: Kidney size and glomerular volume. Diabetolgia 16:125-128, 1979.

304. Rasch R: Prevention of diabetic glomerulopathy in streptozotocin diabetic rats by insulin treatment. Glomerular basement membrane thickness. Diabetologia 16:319-324, 1979.

305. Rasch R: Prevention of diabetic glomerulopathy in streptozotocin diabetic rats by insulin treatment. The mesangial regions. Diabetologia 17:243-248, 1979.

306. Rasch R: Prevention of diabetic glomerulopathy by careful insulin treatment, experimental studies of the mesangial regions [abstract]. Diabetologia 15:264, 1978.

307. Hostetter TH, Meyer TW, Rennke HG, Brenner BM: Influence of strict control of diabetes on intrarenal hemodynamics [abstract]. Kidney Int 23:215, 1983.

308. Mogensen CE, Andersen MJF: Increased kidney size and glomerular filtration rate in early juvenile diabetes. Diabetes 22:706-712, 1973.

309. Mogensen CE, Andersen MJF: Increased kidney size and glomerular filtration rate in untreated juvenile diabetes: Normalization by insulin treatment. Diabetologia 11:221-224, 1975.

310. Wiseman MJ, Saunders AJ, Keen H, Viberti GC: Effect of blood glucose control on increased glomerular filtration rate and kidney size in insulin-dependent diabetes. N Engl J Med 312:617-621, 1985.

311. Tuttle KR, Bruton JL, Perusek M, et al: Effect of strict glycemic control on renal hemodynamic response to amino acid infusion. N Engl J Med 324:1626-1632, 1991.

312. Wang PH, Lau J, Chalmers TC: Meta-analysis of effects of intensive blood-glucose control on late complications of type I diabetes. Lancet 341:1306-1309, 1993.

313. The Kroc Collaborative Study Group: Diabetic retinopathy after two years of intensified insulin treatment. JAMA 260:37-41, 1988.

314. Deckert T, Lauritzen T, Parving H-H, Christiansen JS, Steno Study Group: Effect of two years of strict metabolic control on kidney function in long-term insulin-dependent diabetics. Diabetes Nephropathy 2:6-10, 1983.

315. Beck-Nielsen H, Richelsen B, Mogensen CE, et al: Effect of insulin pump treatment for one year on renal function and retinal morphology in patients with IDDM. Diabetes Care 8:585-589, 1985.

316. Christensen CK, Christiansen JS, Schmitz A, et al: Effect of continuous subcutaneous insulin infusion on kidney function and size in IDDM patients: A 2 year controlled study. J Diabetes Complications 1:91-95, 1987.

317. Dahl-Jørgensen K, Hanssen KF, Kierulf P, et al: Reduction of urinary albumin excretion after 4 years of continuous subcutaneous insulin infusion in insulin-dependent diabetes mellitus. Acta Endocrinol 117:19-25, 1988.

318. Reichard P, Berglund B, Britz A, et al: Intensified conventional insulin treatment retards the microvascular complications of insulin-dependent diabetes mellitus (IDDM): The Stockholm Diabetes Intervention Study (SDIS) after 5 years. J Intern Med 230:101-108, 1991.

319. Brinchmann-Hansen O, Dahl-Jørgensen K, Hanssen KF, Sandvik L: The response of diabetic retinopathy to 41 months of multiple insulin injections, insulin pumps, and conventional insulin therapy. Arch Ophthalmol 106:1242-1246, 1998.

320. The Diabetes Control and Complications Trial Research Group: Effect of intensive therapy on the development and progression of diabetic nephropathy in the diabetes control and complications trial. Kidney Int 47:1703-1720, 1995.

321. Ohkubo Y, Kishikawa H, Araki E, et al: Intensive insulin therapy prevents the progression of diabetic microvascular complications in Japanese patients with non-insulin-dependent diabetes mellitus: A randomized prospective 6-year study. Diabetes Res Clin Pract 28:103-117, 1995.

322. UK Prospective Diabetes Study (UKPDS) Group: Intensive blood-glucose control with sulphonylureas or insulin compared with conventional treatment and risk of complications in patients with type 2 diabetes (UKPDS 33). Lancet 352:837-853, 1998.

323. The Microalbuminuria Captopril Study Group: Captopril reduces the risk of nephropathy in IDDM patients with microalbuminuria. Diabetologia 39:587-593, 1996.

324. Ravid M, Lang R, Rachmani R, Lishner M: Long-term renoprotective effect of angiotensin-converting enzyme inhibition in non-insulin-dependent diabetes mellitus. Arch Intern Med 156:286-289, 1996.

325. Sano T, Kawamura T, Matsumae H, et al: Effects of long-term enalapril treatment on persistent microalbuminuria in well-controlled hypertensive and normotensive NIDDM patients. Diabetes Care 7:420-424, 1994.

326. Ahmad J, Siddiqui MA, Ahmad H: Effective postponement of diabetic nephropathy with enalapril in normotensive type 2 diabetic patients with microalbuminuria. Diabetes Care 20:1576-1581, 1997.

327. Gaede P, Vedel P, Parving H-H, Pedersen O: Intensified multifactorial intervention in patients with type 2 diabetes mellitus and microalbuminuria: The Steno type 2 randomised study. Lancet 353:617-622, 1999.

328. Viberti GC, Bilous RW, Mackintosh D, et al: Long term correction of hyperglycaemia and progression of renal failure in insulin dependent diabetes. BMJ 286:598-602, 1983.

329. Tamborlane WV, Puklin JE, Bergman M, et al: Long-term improvement of metabolic control with the insulin pump does not reverse diabetic microangiopathy. Diabetes Care 5 (suppl 1):58-64, 1982.

330. Zatz R, Dunn BR, Meyer TW, et al: Prevention of diabetic glomerulopathy by pharmacological amelioration of glomerular capillary hypertension. J Clin Invest 77:1925-1930, 1986.

331. Anderson S, Rennke HG, Garcia DL, Brenner BM: Short and long term effects of antihypertensive therapy in the diabetic rat. Kidney Int 36:526-536, 1989.

332. Anderson S, Rennke HG, Brenner BM: Nifedipine versus fosinopril in uninephrectomized diabetic rats. Kidney Int 41:891-897, 1992.

333. Flyihara CK, Padilha RM, Zatz R: Glomerular abnormalities in long-term experimental diabetes. Diabetes 41:286-293, 1992.

334. Cooper ME, Allen TJ, O'Brien RC, et al: Nephropathy in model combining genetic hypertension with experimental diabetes. Diabetes 39:1575-1579, 1990.

335. Kasiske BL, Kalil R, Ma JZ, et al: Effect of antihypertensive therapy on the kidney in patients with diabetes: A meta-regression analysis. Ann Intern Med 1993:118:129-138.

336. Ravid M, Brosh D, Levi Z, et al: Use of enalapril to attenuate decline in renal function in normotensive, normoalbuminuric patients with type 2 diabetes mellitus. Ann Intern Med 128:982-988, 1998.

337. Heart Outcomes Prevention Evaluation (HOPE) Study Investigators: Effects of ramipril on cardiovascular and microvascular outcomes in people with diabetes mellitus: Results of the HOPE study and MICRO-HOPE substudy. Lancet 355:253-259, 2000.

338. Tatti P, Pahor M, Byington RP, et al: Outcome results of the fosinopril versus amlodipine cardiovascular events randomized trial (FACET) in patients with hypertension and NIDDM. Diabetes Care 21:597-603, 1998.

339. Estacio RO, Jeffers BW, Gifford N, Schrier RW: Effect of blood pressure control on diabetic microvascular complications in patients with hypertension and type 2 diabetes. Diabetes Care 23(suppl 2):B54-B64, 2000.

340. UK Prospective Diabetes Study (UKPDS) Group: Efficacy of atenolol and captopril in reducing risk of macrovascular and microvascular complications in type 2 diabetes: UKPDS 39. UK Prospective Diabetes Study Group. BMJ 317:713-720, 1998.

341. Schrier RW, Estacio RO, Esler A, Mehler P: Effects of aggressive blood pressure control in normotensive type 2 diabetic patients on albuminuria, retinopathy and strokes. Kidney Int 61:1086-1097, 2002.

342. Chaturvedi N, Sjolie A-K, Stephenson JM, et al: Effect of lisinopril on progression of retinopathy in normotensive people with type 1 diabetes. Lancet 351:28-31, 1998.

343. The ACE Inhibitors in Diabetic Nephropathy Trialist Group: Should all type 1 diabetic microalbuminuric patients receive ACE inhibitors? A meta-regression analysis. Ann Intern Med 134:370-379, 2001.

344. Mathiesen ER, Hommel E, Hansen HP, et al: Randomised controlled trial of long term efficacy of captopril on preservation of kidney funciton in normotensive patients with insulin dependent diabetes and microalbuminuria. BMJ 319:24-25, 1999.

345. Crepaldi G, Carta Q, Deferrari G, et al: Effects of lisinopril and nifedipine on the progression of overt albuminuria in IDDM patients with incipient nephropathy and normal blood pressure. Diabetes Care 21:104-110, 1998.

346. Rudberg S, Osterby R, Bangstad HJ, et al: Effect of angiotensin converting enzyme inhibitor or beta blocker on glomerular structural changes in young microalbuminuric patients with type I (insulin-dependent) diabetes mellitus. Diabetologia 42:589-595, 1999.

347. Osterby R, Bangstad HJ, Rudberg S: Follow-up study of glomerular dimensions and cortical interstitium in microalbuminuric type 1 diabetic patients with or without antihypertensive treatment. Nephrol Dial Transplant 15:1609-1616, 2000.

348. Cordonnier DJ, Pinel N, Barro C, et al: Expansion of cortical interstitium is limited by converting enzyme inhibition in type 2 diabetic patients with glomerulosclerosis. J Am Soc Nephrol 10:1253-1263, 1999.

349. Melbourne Diabetic Nephropathy Study Group: Comparison between perindopril and nifedipine in hypertensive and normotensive diabetic patients with microalbuminuria. BMJ 302:210-216, 1991.

350. Chan JCN, Cockram CS, Nicholls MG, et al: Comparison of enalapril and nifedipine in treating non-insulin dependent diabetics associated with hypertension: one year analysis. BMJ 305:981-985, 1992.

351. Lacourciere Y, Nadeau A, Poirier L, Tancrede G: Captopril or conventional therapy in hypertensive type II diabetics. Three-year analysis. Hypertension 21(6 pt 1):786-794, 1993.

352. Lebovitz HE, Wiegmann TB, Cnaan A, et al: Renal protective effects of enalapril in hypertensive NIDDM: Role of baseline albuminuria. Kidney Int Suppl 45:S150-S155, 1994.

353. Trevisan R, Tiengo A: Effect of low-dose ramipril on microalbuminuria in normotensive or mild hypertensive non-insulin-dependent diabetic patients. North-East Italy Microalbuminuria Study Group. Am J Hypertens 8:876-883, 1995.

354. Agardh C-D, Garcia-Puig J, Charbonnel B, et al: Greater reduction of urinary albumin excretion in hypertensive type II diabetic patients with incipient nephropathy by lisinopril than by nifedipine. J Hum Hypertens 10:185-192, 1996.

355. Chan JC, Ko GT, Leung DH, et al: Long-term effects of angiotensin-converting enzyme inhibition and metabolic control in hypertensive type 2 diabetic patients. Kidney Int 57:590-600, 2000.

356. Viberti G, Wheeldon NM: Microalbuminuria reduction with valsartan in patients with type 2 diabetes mellitus: A blood pressure-independent effect. Circulation 106:672-678, 2002.

357. Parving H-H, Lehnert H, Bröchner-Mortensen J, et al: The effect of irbesartan on the development of diabetic nephropathy in patients with type 2 diabetes. N Engl J Med 345:870-878, 2001.

358. Mogensen CE, Keane WF, Bennett PH, et al: Prevention of diabetic renal disease with special reference to microalbuminuria. Lancet 346:1080-1084, 1995.

359. American Diabetes Association: Diabetic nephropathy. Diabetes Care 25(suppl 1):585-589, 2002.

360. Rossing P, Hommel E, Smidt UM, Parving H-H: Reduction in albuminuria predicts a beneficial effect on diminishing the progression of human diabetic nephropathy during antihypertensive treatment. Diabetologia 37:511-516, 1994.

361. Rossing P, Hommel E, Smidt UM, Parving H-H: Reduction in albuminuria predicts diminished progression in diabetic nephropathy. Kidney Int Suppl 45:S145-S149, 1994.

362. Mulec H, Johnsen SA, Carlström J, Björck S: Initial decrease in proteinuria after institution of ACE inhibitor treatment predicts long term prognosis for kidney function in overt diabetic nephropathy [abstract]. J Am Soc Nephrol 8:116A, 1997.

363. Apperloo AJ, de Zeeuw D, de Jong PE: Short-term antiproteinuric response to antihypertensive treatment predicts long-term GFR decline in patients with non-diabetic renal disease. Kidney Int Suppl 45:S174-S178, 1994.

364. Peterson JC, Adler S, Burkart JM, et al: Blood pressure control, proteinuria, and the progression of renal disease. The modification of diet in renal disease study. Ann Intern Med 123:754-762, 1995.

365. Jacobsen P, Rossing K, Rossing P, et al: Angiotensin converting enzyme gene polymorphism and ACE inhibition in diabetic nephropathy. Kidney Int 53:1002-1006, 1998.

366. The Euclid Study Group: Randomised placebo-controlled trial of lisinopril in normotensive patients with insulin-dependent diabetes and normoalbuminuria or microalbuminuria. Lancet 349:1787-1792, 1997.

367. Tomonaga O, Ujihara N, Yokoyama H, et al: Angiotensin converting enzyme (ACE) gene polymorphism predicts the effect of ACE inhibitor (ACEI) on the progression of nephropathy in Japanese NIDDM patients [abstract]. J Am Soc Nephrol 8:120A, 1997.

368. Thomas SM, Alaveras A, Margiaglione M, et al: Metabolic and genetic predictors of progression of diabetic kidney disease [abstract]. Diabetic Medicine 14:S17, 1997.

369. Jacobsen P, Tarnow L, Hovind P, et al: Genetic variation in the renin-angiotensin system and progression of diabetic nephrology in type 1 diabetic patients [abstract]. J Am Soc Nephrol 13:247A, 2002.

370. Harden PN, Geddes C, Rowe PA, et al: Polymorphisms in angiotensin-converting-enzyme gene and progression of IgA nephropathy. Lancet 345:1540-1542, 1995.

371. van Essen GG, Rensma PL, de Zeeuw D, et al: Association between angiotensin-converting-enzyme gene polymorphism and failure of renoprotective therapy. Lancet 347:94-95, 1996.

372. Fava S, Azzopardi J, Ellard S, Hattersley AT: ACE gene polymorphism as a prognostic indicator in patients with type 2 diabetes and established renal disease. Diabetes Care 24:2115-2120, 2001.

373. Andersen S, Tarnow L, Cambien F, et al: Renoprotective effects of losartan in diabetic nephropathy: Interaction with ACE insertion/deletion genotype? Kidney Int 62:192-198, 2002.

374. Andersen S, Tarnow L, Cambien F, et al: Long-term renoprotective effects of losartan in diabetic nephropathy: Interaction with ACE insertion/deletion genotype? Diabetes Care 26:1501-1506, 2003.

375. Muirhead N, Feagan BF, Mahon J, et al: The effects of valsartan and captopril on reducing microalbuminuria in patients with type 2 diabetes mellitus: A placebo-controlled trial [abstract]. Curr Ther Res 60:650, 2002.

376. Andersen S, Tarnow L, Rossing P, et al: Renoprotective effects of angiotensin II receptor blockade in type 1 diabetic patients with diabetic nephropathy. Kidney Int 57:601-606, 2000.

377. Lacourciere Y, Belanger A, Godin C, et al: Long-term comparison of losartan and enalapril on kidney function in hypertensive type 2 diabetics with early nephropathy. Kidney Int 58:762-769, 2000.

378. Bos H, Andersen S, Rossing P, et al: Role of patient factors in therapy resistance to antiproteinuric intervention in nondiabetic and diabetic nephropathy. Kidney Int (Suppl) 57:S-32-S-37, 2000.

379. Andersen S, Rossing P, Juhl TR, et al: Optimal dose of losartan for renoprotection in diabetic nephropathy. Nephrol Dial Transplant 17:1413-1418, 2002.

380. Rossing K, Christensen PK, Hansen BV, et al: Optimal dose of candesartan for renoprotection in type 2 diabetic patients with nephropathy: A double-blind randomized crossover study. Diabetes Care 26:150-155, 2003.

381. Mogensen CE, Neldam S, Tikkanen I, et al: Randomised controlled trial of dual blockade of renin-angiotensin system in patients with hypertension, microalbuminuria, and non-insulin dependent diabetes: The candesartan and lisinopril microalbuminuria (CALM) study. BMJ 321:1440-1444, 2000.

382. Jacobsen P, Andersen S, Rossing K, et al: Dual blockade of the renin-angiotensin system in type 1 patients with diabetic nephropathy. Nephrol Dial Transplant 17:1019-1024, 2002.

383. Rossing K, Christensen PK, Jensen BR, Parving HH: Dual blockade of the renin-angiotensin system in diabetic nephropathy: A randomized double-blind crossover study. Diabetes Care 25:95-100, 2002.

384. Hilgers KF, Mann JF: ACE inhibitors versus AT(1) receptor antagonists in patients with chronic renal disease. J Am Soc Nephrol 13:1100-1108, 2002.

385. Nakao N, Yoshimura A, Morita H, et al: Combination therapy of angiotensin-II receptor blocker and angiotensin-converting enzyme inhibitor in non-diabetic renal disease: A randomized, controlled trial in Japan (COOPERATE). Lancet 361:117-124, 2003.

386. Komine N, Khang S, Wead LM, et al: Effect of combining an ACE inhibitor and an angiotensin II receptor blocker on plasma and kidney tissue angiotensin II levels. Am J Kidney Dis 39:159-164, 2002.

387. Christensen PK, Lund S, Parving HH: Autoregulated glomerular filtration rate during candesartan treatment in hypertensive type 2 diabetic patients. Kidney Int 60:1435-1442, 2001.

388. Hansen HP, Nielsen FS, Rossing P, et al: Kidney function after withdrawal of long-term antihypertensive treatment in diabetic nephropathy. Kidney Int 52:S49-S53, 1997.

389. Hansen HP, Rossing P, Tarnow L, et al: Increased glomerular filtration rate after withdrawal of long-term antihypertensive treatment in diabetic nephropathy. Kidney Int 47:1726-1731, 1995.

390. Apperloo AJ, de Zeeuw D, de Jong PE: A short-term antihypertensive treatment-induced fall in glomerular filtration rate predicts long-term stability of renal funciton. Kidney Int 51:793-797, 1997.

391. Mogensen CE: Long-term antihypertensive treatment inhibiting progression of diabetic nephropathy. BMJ 285:685-688, 1982.

392. Parving H-H, Andersen AR, Smidt UM, et al: Early aggressive antihypertensive treatment reduces rate of decline in kidney function in diabetic nephropathy. Lancet 1:1175-1179, 1983.

393. Parving H-H, Andersen AR, Smidt UM, et al: Effect of antihypertensive treatment on kidney function in diabetic nephropathy. BMJ 294:1443-1447, 1987.

394. Parving H-H, Smidt UM, Hommel E, et al: Effective antihypertensive treatment postpones renal insufficiency in diabetic nephropathy. Am J Kidney Dis 22:188-195, 1993.

395. Ruggenenti P, Perna A, Gheradi G, et al: Renal function and requirement for dialysis in chronic nephropathy patients on long-term ramipril: REIN follow-up trial. Lancet 352:1252-1256, 1998.

396. Hovind P, Rossing P, Tarnow L, et al: Remission and regression in the nephropathy of type 1 diabetes when blood pressure is controlled aggressively. Kidney Int 60:277-283, 2001.

397. Wilmer WA, Hebert LA, Lewis EJ, et al: Remission of nephrotic syndrome in type 1 diabetes: Long-term follow-up of patients in the captopril study. Am J Kidney Dis 34:308-314, 1999.

398. Hovind P, Rossing P, Tarnow L, et al: Remission of nephrotic-range albuminuria in type 1 diabetic patients. Diabetes Care 24:1972-1977, 2000.

399. Hommel E, Parving H-H, Mathiesen ER, et al: Effect of captopril on kidney function in insulin-dependent diabetic patients with nephropathy. BMJ 293:466-470, 1986.

400. Parving H-H, Hommel E, Smidt UM: Protection of kidney function and decrease in albuminuria by captopril in insulin dependent diabetics with nephropathy. BMJ 297:1086-1091, 1988.

401. Björck S, Nyberg G, Mulec H, et al: Beneficial effect of angiotensin converting enzyme inhibition on renal function in patients with diabetic nephropathy. BMJ 293:471-474, 1986.

402. Björck S, Johnsen SA, Nyberg G, Aurell M: Contrasting effects of enalapril and metoprolol on proteinuria in diabetic nephropathy. BMJ 300:904-907, 1990.

403. Björck S, Mulec H, Johnsen SA, et al: Renal protective effect of enalapril in diabetic nephropathy. BMJ 304:339-343, 1992.

404. Lewis E, Hunsicker L, Bain R, Rhode R: The effect of angiotensin-converting-enzyme inhibition on diabetic nephropathy. N Engl J Med 329:1456-1462, 1993.

405. Tarnow L, Rossing P, Jensen C, et al: Long-term renoprotective effect of nisoldipine and lisinopril in type 1 diabetic patients with diabetic nephropathy. Diabetes Care 23:1725-1730, 2000.

406. Walker WG, Hermann J, Anderson J, et al: Blood pressure (BP) control slows decline of glomerular filtration rate (GFR) in hypertensive NDDM patients [abstract]. J Am Soc Nephrol 3:339, 1992.

407. Lebovitz H, Cnaan A, Wiegmann TB, et al: Enalapril slows the progression of renal disease in non-insulin dependent diabetes mellitus (NIDDM): Results of a 3-yr multicenter, randomized, prospective, double-blinded study [abstract]. J Am Soc Nephrol 3:335, 1992.

408. Nielsen FS, Rossing P, Gall M-A, et al: Long-term effect of lisinopril and atenolol on kidney function in hypertensive non-insulin-dependent diabetic subjects with diabetic nephropathy. Diabetes 46:1182-1188, 1997.

409. Bakris GL, Copley JB, Vicknair N, et al: Calcium channel blockers versus other antihypertensive therapies on progression of NIDDM associated nephropathy. Kidney Int 50:1641-1650, 1996.

410. Brenner BM, Cooper ME, de Zeeuw D, et al: Effects of losartan on renal and cardiovascular outcomes in patients with type 2 diabetes and nephropathy. N Engl J Med 345:861-869, 2001.

411. Lewis EJ, Hunsicker LG, Clarke WR, et al: Renoprotective effect of the angiotensin-receptor antagonist irbesartan in patients with nephropathy due to type 2 diabetes. N Engl J Med 345:851-860, 2001.

412. Pourdjabbar A, Lapointe N, Rouleau JL: Angiotensin receptor blockers: Powerful evidence with cardiovascular outcomes? Can J Cardiol 18(suppl A):7A-14A, 2002.

413. Parving H-H, Hommel E: Prognosis in diabetic nephropathy. BMJ 299:230-233, 1989.

414. Parving H-H, Jacobsen P, Rossing K, et al: Benefits of long-term antihypertensive treatment on prognosis in diabetic nephropathy. Kidney Int 49:1778-1782, 1996.

415. Mathiesen ER, Borch-Johnsen K, Jensen DV, Deckert T: Improved survival in patients with diabetic nephropathy. Diabetologia 32:884-886, 1989.

416. Rodby RA, Firth LM, Lewis E, the Collaborative Study Group: An economic analysis of captopril in the treatment of diabetic nephropathy. Diabetes Care 19:1051-1061, 1996.

417. Moorhead JF, EI-Nahas M, Chan MK, Varghese Z: Lipid nephrotoxicity in chronic progressive glomerular and tubulo-interstitial disease. Lancet 2:1309-1311, 1982.

418. Zatz R, Meyer TW, Rennke HG, Brenner BM: Predominance of hemodynamic rather than metabolic factors in the pathogenesis of diabetic glomerulopathy. Proc Natl Acad Sci U S A 82:5963-5967, 1985.

419. Zatz R, Brenner BM: Pathogenesis of diabetic microangiopathy. The hemodynamic view. Am J Med 80:443-453, 1986.

420. Cohen D, Dodds RA, Viberti GC: Effect of protein restriction in insulin-dependent diabetics at risk of nephropathy. BMJ 294:795-798, 1987.

421. Dullaart PF, Beusekamp BJ, Meijer S, et al: Long-term effects of protein-restricted diet on albuminuria and renal function in IDDM patients without clinical nephropathy and hypertension. Diabetes Care 16, 2:483-492, 1993.

422. Hansen HP, Christensen PK, Tauber-Lassen E, et al: Low-protein diet and kidney function in insulin-dependent diabetic patients with diabetic nephropathy. Kidney Int 55:621-628, 1999.

423. Walker JD, Bending JJ, Dodds RA, et al: Restriction of dietary protein and progression of renal failure in diabetic nephropathy. Lancet 2:1411-1415, 1989.

424. Zeller KR, Whittaker E, Sullivan L, et al: Effect of restricting dietary protein on the progression of renal failure in patients with insulin-dependent diabetes mellitus. N Engl J Med 324:78-84, 1991.

425. Parving H-H: Low-protein diet and progression of renal disease in diabetic nephropathy [letter]. Lancet 335:411, 1990.

426. Parving H-H: Protein restriction and renal failure in diabetes mellitus. N Engl J Med 324:1743-1744, 1991.

427. Pedrini MT, Levey AS, Lau J, et al: The effect of dietary protein restriction on the progression of diabetic and nondiabetic renal diseases: meta-analysis. Ann Intern Med 124:627-632, 1996.

428. Ciavarella A, Di Mizio G, Stefani S, et al: Reduced albuminuria after dietary protein restriction in insulin-dependent diabetic patients with clinical nephropathy. Diabetes Care 10:407-413, 1987.

429. Barsotti G, Ciardella F, Morelli E, et al: Nutritional treatment of renal failure in type 1 diabetic nephropathy. Clin Nephrol 29:280-287, 1988.

430. Parving H-H: Effects of dietary protein on renal disease. Ann Intern Med 126:330-331, 1997.

431. Shah N, Horwitz RI, Cancato J: Effects of dietary protein on renal disease [letter to editor]. Ann Intern Med 126:331, 1997.

432. Hansen HP, Tauber-Lassen E, Jensen BR, Parving HH: Effect of dietary protein restriction on prognosis in patients with diabetic nephropathy. Kidney Int 62:220-228, 2002.

433. Ritz E, Rychlik I, Locatelli F, Halimi S: End-stage renal failure in type 2 diabetes: A medical catastrophe of worldwide dimensions. Am J Kidney Dis 34:795-808, 1999.

434. National Institute of Diabetes and Digestive and Kidney Diseases: United States Renal Data System: USRDS 2001 Annual Data Report. Bethesda, MD, National Institutes of Health, 2001.

435. Schwenger V, Mussig C, Hergesell O, et al: Incidence and clinical characteristics of renal insufficiency in diabetic patients. Dtsch Med Wochenschr 126:1322-1326, 2001.

436. Koch M, Thomas B, Tschöpe W, Ritz E: Survival and predictors of death in dialysed diabetic patients. Diabetologia 36:1113-1117, 1993.

437. The Heart Outcomes Prevention Evaluation Study Investigators: Effects of an angiotensin-converting-enzyme inhibitor, remipril, on cardiovascular events in high-risk patients. N Engl J Med 342:145-153, 2000.

438. Feldstein CA: Salt intake, hypertension and diabetes mellitus. J Hum Hypertens 16(suppl 1):S48-S51, 2002.

439. Sturrock ND, George E, Pound N, et al: Non-dipping circadian blood pressure and renal impairment are associated with increased mortality in diabetes mellitus. Diabet Med 17:360-364, 2000.

440. Flanigan MJ, Frankenfield DL, Prowant BF, et al: Nutritional markers during peritoneal dialysis: Data from the 1998 Peritoneal Dialysis Core Indicators Study. Perit Dial Int 21:345-354, 2001.

441. Melin J, Hellberg O, Larsson E, et al: Protective effect of insulin on ischemic renal injury in diabetes mellitus. Kidney Int 61:1383-1392, 2002.

443. Chantrel F, Enache I, Bouiller M, et al: Abysmal prognosis of patients with type 2 diabetes entering dialysis. Nephrol Dial Transplant 14:129-136, 1999.

443. Mueller C, Buerkle G, Buettner HJ, et al: Prevention of contrast media-associated nephropathy: Randomized comparison of 2 hydration regimens in 1620 patients undergoing coronary angioplasty. Arch Intern Med 162:329-336, 2002.

444. Konner K: Primary vascular access in diabetic patients: An audit. Nephrol Dial Transplant 15:1317-1325, 2000.

445. Dixon BS, Novak L, Fangman J: Hemodialysis vascular access survival: Upper-arm native arteriovenous fistula. Am J Kidney Dis 39:92-101, 2002.

446. Revanur VK, Jardine AG, Hamilton DH, Jindal RM: Outcome for arteriovenous fistula at the elbow for haemodialysis. Clin Transplant 14(4 pt 1):318-322, 2000.

447. Gefen JY, Fox D, Giangola G, et al: The transposed forearm loop arteriovenous fistula: A valuable option for primary hemodialysis access in diabetic patients. Ann Vasc Surg 16:89-94, 2002.

448. Yeager RA, Moneta GL, Edwards JM, et al: Relationship of hemodialysis access to finger gangrene in patients with end-stage renal disease. J Vasc Surg 36:245-249, 2002.

449. Koch M, Kutkuhn B, Grabensee B, Ritz E: Apolipoprotein A, fibrinogen, age, and a history of stroke are predictors of death in dialysed diabetic patients: A prospective study in 412 subjects. Nephrol Dial Transplant 12:2603-2611, 1997.

450. Daugirdas JT: Pathophysiology of dialysis hypotension: An update. Am J Kidney Dis 38(4 suppl 4):S11-S17, 2001.

451. Tozawa M, Iseki K, Iseki C, Takishita S: Pulse pressure and risk of total mortality and cardiovascular events in patients on chronic hemodialysis. Kidney Int 61:717-726, 2002.

452. Foley RN, Culleton BF, Parfrey PS, et al: Cardiac disease in diabetic end-stage renal disease. Diabetologia 40:1307-1312, 1997.

453. Stack AG, Bloembergen WE: Prevalence and clinical correlates of coronary artery disease among new dialysis patients in the United States: A cross-sectional study. J Am Soc Nephrol 12:1516-1523, 2001.

454. Levin A, Djurdjev O, Barrett B, et al: Cardiovascular disease in patients with chronic kidney disease: Getting to the heart of the matter. Am J Kidney Dis 38:1398-1407, 2001.

455. Foley RN, Parfrey PS: Cardiac disease in the diabetic dialysis patient. Nephrol Dial Transplant 13:1112-1113, 1998.

456. Herzog CA, Ma JZ, Collins AJ: Poor long-term survival after acute myocardial infarction among patients on long-term dialysis. N Engl J Med 339:799-805, 1998.

457. Karnik JA, Young BS, Lew NL, et al: Cardiac arrest and sudden death in dialysis units. Kidney Int 60:350-357, 2001.

458. Raggi P, Boulay A, Chasan-Taber S, et al: Cardiac calcification in adult hemodialysis patients. A link between end-stage renal disease and cardiovascular disease? J Am Coll Cardiol 39:695-701, 2002.

459. Varghese K, Cherian G, Abraham MT, et al: Coronary artery disease among diabetic and non-diabetic patients with end stage renal disease. Ren Fail 23:669-677, 2001.

460. Giordano M, Manzella D, Paolisso G, et al: Differences in heart rate variability parameters during the post-dialytic period in type II diabetic and non-diabetic ESRD patients. Nephrol Dial Transplant 16:566-573, 2001.

461. Hathaway DK, Cashion AK, Milstead EJ, et al: Autonomic dysregulation in patients awaiting kidney transplantation. Am J Kidney Dis 32:221-229, 1998.

462. Amann K, Ritz E: Microvascular disease—the Cinderella of uraemic heart disease. Nephrol Dial Transplant 15:1493-1503, 2000.

463. Standl E, Schnell O: A new look at the heart in diabetes mellitus: From ailing to failing. Diabetologia 43:1455-1469, 2000.

464. Wu MS, Yu CC, Yang CW, et al: Poor pre-dialysis glycaemic control is a predictor of mortality in type II diabetic patients on maintenance haemodialysis. Nephrol Dial Transplant 12:2105-2110, 1997.

465. Morioka T, Emoto M, Tabata T, et al: Glycemic control is a predictor of survival for diabetic patients on hemodialysis. Diabetes Care 24:909-913, 2001.

466. Wanner C, Krane V, Ruf G, et al: Rationale and design of a trial improving outcome of type 2 diabetics on hemodialysis. Die Deutsche Diabetes Dialyse Studie Investigators. Kidney Int Suppl 71:S222-S226, 1999.

467. Dikow R, Schwenger V, Schomig M, Ritz E: How should we manage anaemia in patients with diabetes? Nephrol Dial Transplant 17(suppl 1):67-72, 2002.

468. Lindholm LH, Ibsen H, Dahlof B, et al: Cardiovascular morbidity and mortality in patients with diabetes in the Losartan Intervention for Endpoint Reduction in Hypertension Study (LIFE): A randomised trial against atenolol. Lancet 359:1004-1010, 2002.

469. Zuanetti G, Maggioni AP, Keane W, Ritz E: Nephrologists neglect administration of β-blockers to dialysed diabetic patients. Nephrol Dial Transplant 12:2497-2500, 1997.

470. Goodkin DA, Mapes DL, Held PJ: The dialysis outcomes and practice patterns study (DOPPS): How can we improve the care of hemodialysis patients? Semin Dial 14:157-159, 2001.

471. Cice G, Ferrara L, Di Benedetto A, et al: Dilated cardiomyopathy in dialysis patients—beneficial effects of carvedilol: A double-blind, placebo-controlled trial. J Am Coll Cardiol 37:407-411, 2001.

472. Manske CL, Wang Y, Rector T, et al: Coronary revascularization in insulin-dependent diabetic patients with chronic renal failure. Lancet 340:998-1002, 1992.

473. Matzkies FK, Reinecke H, Regetmeier A, et al: Long-term outcome after percutaneous transluminal coronary angioplasty in patients with chronic renal failure with and without diabetic nephropathy. Nephron 89:10-14, 2001.

474. Hosoda Y, Yamamoto T, Takazawa K, et al: Coronary artery bypass grafting in patients on chromic hemodialysis: Surgical outcome in diabetic nephropathy versus nondiabetic nephropathy patients. Ann Thorac Surg 71:543-548, 2001.

475. Herzog CA, Ma JZ, Collins AJ: Comparative survival of dialysis patients in the United States after coronary angioplasty, coronary artery stenting, and coronary artery bypass surgery and impact of diabetes. Circulation 106:2207-2211, 2002.

476. Le Feuvre C, Dambrin G, Helft G, et al: Clinical outcome following coronary angioplasty in dialysis patients: A case-control study in the era of coronary stenting. Heart 85:556-560, 2001.

477. Hatada K, Sugiura T, Nakamura S, et al: Coronary artery diameter and left ventricular function in patients on maintenance hemodialysis treatment: Comparison between diabetic and nondiabetic patients. Nephron 80:269-273, 1998.

478. Malmberg K: Prospective randomised study of intensive insulin treatment on long term survival after acute myocardial infarction in patients with diabetes mellitus. DIGAMI (Diabetes Mellitus, Insulin Glucose Infusion in Acute Myocardial Infarction) Study Group. BMJ 314:1512-1515, 1997.

479. Simic-Ogrizovic S, Backus G, Mayer A, et al: The influence of different glucose concentrations in haemodialysis solutions on metabolism and blood pressure stability in diabetes patients. Int J Artif Organs 24:863-869, 2001.

480. Joy MS, Cefalu WT, Hogan SL, Nachman PH: Long-term glycemic control measurements in diabetic patients receiving hemodialysis. Am J Kidney Dis 39:297-307, 2002.

481. Ritz E, Koch M: Morbidity and mortality due to hypertension in patients with renal failure. Am J Kidney Dis 21(5 suppl 2):113-118, 1993.

482. Van den BG, Wouters P, Weekers F, et al: Intensive insulin therapy in the critically ill patients. N Engl J Med 345:1359-1367, 2001.

483. Pinero-Pilona A, Litonjua P, Devaraj S, et al: Anemia associated with new-onset diabetes: Improvement with blood glucose control. Endocr Pract 8:276-281, 2002.

484. Okuno S, Ishimura E, Kim M, et al: Changes in body fat mass in male hemodialysis patients: A comparison between diabetics and nondiabetics. Am J Kidney Dis 38(4 suppl 1): S208-S211, 2001.

485. Suliman ME, Stenvinkel P, Heimburger O, et al: Plasma sulfur amino acids in relation to cardiovascular disease, nutritional status, and diabetes mellitus in patients with chronic renal failure at start of dialysis therapy. Am J Kidney Dis 40:480-488, 2002.

486. Cano NJ, Roth H, Aparicio M, et al: Malnutrition in hemodialysis diabetic patients: Evaluation and prognostic influence. Kidney Int 62:593-601, 2002.

487. Inaba M, Nagasue K, Okuno S, et al: Impaired secretion of parathyroid hormone, but not refractoriness of osteoblast, is a major mechanism of low bone turnover in hemodialyzed patients with diabetes mellitus. Am J Kidney Dis 39:1261-1269, 2002.

488. Coladonato JA, Frankenfield DL, Reddan DN, et al: Trends in anemia management among US hemodialysis patients. J Am Soc Nephrol 13:1288-1295, 2002.

489. Page DE, Cheung V, Poirier F: Diabetic patients on peritoneal dialysis need less erythropoietin to maintain adequate hemoglobin. Adv Perit Dial 17:130-131, 2001.

490. Tschöpe W, Koch M, Thomas B, Ritz E: Serum lipids predict cardiac death in diabetic patients on maintenance hemodialysis. Results of a prospective study. The German Study Group Diabetes and Uremia. Nephron 64:354-358, 1993.

491. Shoji T, Ishimura E, Inaba M, et al: Atherogenic lipoproteins in end-stage renal disease. Am J Kidney Dis 38(4 suppl 1):S30-S33, 2001.

492. Schomig M, Ritz E, Standl E, Allenberg J: The diabetic foot in the dialyzed patient. J Am Soc Nephrol 11:1153-1159, 2000.

493. Sehgal AR, Leon JB, Siminoff LA, et al: Improving the quality of hemodialysis treatment: A community-based randomized controlled trial to overcome patient-specific barriers. JAMA 287:1961-1967, 2002.

494. Heaf JG, Lokkegaard H, Madsen M: Initial survival advantage of peritoneal dialysis relative to haemodialysis. Nephrol Dial Transplant 17:112-117, 2002.

495. Winkelmayer WC, Glynn RJ, Mittleman MA, et al: Comparing mortality of elderly patients on hemodialysis versus peritoneal dialysis: A propensity score approach. J Am Soc Nephrol 13:2353-2362, 2002.

496. Van Biesen W, Vanholder RC, Veys N, et al: An evaluation of an integrative care approach for end-stage renal disease patients. J Am Soc Nephrol 11:116-125, 2000.

497. Twardowski ZJ, Nolph KD, McGary TJ, et al: Insulin binding to plastic bags: A methodologic study. Am J Hosp Pharm 40:575-579, 1983.

498. Khanna R, Oreopoulos DG: CAPD in patients with diabetes mellitus. *In* Gokal R (ed): Continuos Ambulatory Peritoneal Dialysis. London, Churchill Livingtone, 1986, pp 291-306.

499. Nevalainen PI, Lahtela JT, Mustonen J, Pasternack A: Subcutaneous and intraperitoneal insulin therapy in diabetic patients on CAPD. Perit Dial Int 16:S288-S291, 1996.

500. Linden T, Cohen A, Deppisch R, et al: 3,4-Dideoxyglucosone-3-ene (3,4-DGE): A cytotoxic glucose degradation product in fluids for peritoneal dialysis. Kidney Int 62:697-703, 2002.

501. Wieslander AP: Cytotoxicity of peritoneal dialysis fluid—is it related to glucose breakdown products? Nephrol Dial Transplant 11:958-959, 1996.

502. Rippe B, Simonsen O, Heimburger O, et al: Long-term clinical effects of a peritoneal dialysis fluid with less glucose degradation products. Kidney Int 59:348-357, 2001.

503. Wolfe RA, Ashby VB, Milford EL, et al: Comparison of mortality in all patients on dialysis, patients on dialysis awaiting transplantation, and recipients of a first cadaveric transplant. N Engl J Med 341:1725-1730, 1999.

504. Hypolite IO, Bucci J, Hshieh P, et al: Acute coronary syndromes after renal transplantation in patients with end-stage renal disease resulting from diabetes. Am J Transplant 2:274-281, 2002.

505. Mieghem AV, Fonck C, Coosemans W, et al: Outcome of cadaver kidney transplantation in 23 patients with type 2 diabetes mellitus. Nephrol Dial Transplant 16:1686-1691, 2001.

506. Zeier M, Ritz E: Preparation of the dialysis patient for transplantation. Nephrol Dial Transplant 17:552-556, 2002.

507. Manske CL, Thomas W, Wang Y, Wilson RF: Screening diabetic transplant candidates for coronary artery disease: Identification of a low risk subgroup. Kidney Int 44:617-621, 1993.

508. Kelly WD, Lillehei RC, Merkel FK, et al: Allotransplantation of the pancreass and duodenum along with the kidney in diabetic nephropathy. Surgery 61:827-837, 1967.

509. Becker BN, Brazy PC, Becker YT, et al: Simultaneous pancreas-kidney transplantation reduces excess mortality in type 1 diabetic patients with end-stage renal disease. Kidney Int 57:2129-2135, 2000.

510. Tyden G, Bolinder J, Solders G, et al: Improved survival in patients with insulin-dependent diabetes mellitus and end-stage diabetic nephropathy 10 years after combined pancreas and kidney transplantation. Transplantation 67:645-648, 1999.

511. Navarro X, Kennedy WR, Aeppli D, Sutherland DER: Neuropathy and mortality in diabetes: Influence of pancreas transplantation. Muscle Nerve 19:1009-1016, 1996.

512. Solders G, Tydén G, Tibell A, et al: Improvement in nerve conduction 8 years combined pancreatic and renal transplantation. Transplant Proc 27:3091, 1995.

513. Hathaway DK, Abell T, Cardoso S, et al: Improvement in autonomic and gastric function following pancreas-kidney versus kidney-alone transplantation and the correlation with quality of life. Transplantation 57:816-822, 1994.

514. Kahl A, Bechstein WO, Frei U: Trends and perspectives in pancreas and simultaneous pancreas and kidney transplantation. Curr Opin Urol 11:165-174, 2001.

515. Gruessner AC, Sutherland DE: Analysis of United States (US) and non-US pancreas transplants reported to the United Network for Organ Sharing (UNOS) and the International Pancreas Transplant Registry (IPTR) as of October 2001. Clin Transpl 41-72, 2001.

516. Mange KC, Joffe MM, Feldman HI: Effect of the use or nonuse of long-term dialysis on the subsequent survival of renal transplants from living donors. N Engl J Med 344:726-731, 2001.

517. Hariharan S, Pirsch JD, Lu CY, et al: Pancreas after kidney transplantation. J Am Soc Nephrol 13:1109-1118, 2002.

518. Gruessner RW, Sutherland DE, Drangstveit MB, et al: Pancreas transplants from living donors: Short and long-term outcome. Transplant Proc 33:819-820, 2001.

519. Pfeffer F, Nauck MA, Benz S, et al: Determinants of a normal (versus impaired) oral glucose tolerance after combined pancreas-kidney transplantation in IDDM patients. Diabetologia 39:462-468, 1996.

520. Cottrell DA: Normalization of insulin sensitivity and glucose homeostasis in type I diabetic pancreas transplant recipients: A 48-month cross-sectional study—A clinical research center study. J Clin Endocrinol Metab 81:3513-3519, 1996.

521. Christiansen E, Vestergaard H, Tibell A, et al: Impaired insulin-stimulated nonoxidative glucose metabolism in pancreas-kidney transplant recipients. Dose-response effects of insulin on glucose turnover. Diabetes 45:1267-1275, 1996.

522. Rooney DP, Robertson RP: Hepatic insulin resistance after pancreas transplantation in type I diabetes. Diabetes 45:134-138, 1996.

523. Barrou Z, Seaquist ER, Robertson RP: Pancreas transplantation in diabetic humans normalizes hepatic glucose production during hypoglycemia. Diabetes 43:661-666, 1994.

524. Hughes TA, Gaber AO, Amiri HS, et al: Kidney-pancreas transplantation: The effect of portal versus systemic venous drainage of the pancreas on the lipoprotein composition. Transplantation 60:1406-1412, 1995.

525. Foger B, Konigsrainer A, Palos G, et al: Effects of pancreas transplantation on distribution and composition of plasma lipoproteins. Metabolism 45:856-861, 1996.

526. Luzi L, Battezzati A, Parseghin G, et al: Combined pancreas and kidney transplantation normalizes protein metabolism in insulin-dependent diabetic-uremic patients. J Clin Invest 93:1948-1958, 1994.

527. Tyden G, Reinholt FP, Sundkvist G, Bolinder J: Recurrence of autoimmune diabetes mellitus in recipients of cadaveric pancreatic grafts. N Engl J Med 335:860-863, 1996.

528. Sutherland DER, Gruessner RWG, Brayman KL, Gruessner A: Pancreas transplantation. *In* Porte D, Scherwin RS (eds): Ellenberg and Rifkin's Diabetes Mellitus. Stamford CT, Appelton & Lange, 1997, pp 1255-1279.

529. Mueller-Felber W, Landgraf R, Reimers CD, et al: High incidence of carpal tunnel syndrome in diabetic patients after combined pancreas and kidney transplantation. Acta Diabetol 30:17-20, 1993.

530. Smets YFC, van der Pijl JW, de Fijter JW, et al: Low bone mass and high incidence of fractures after successful simultaneous pancreas-kidney transplantation. Nephrol Dial Transplant 13:1250-1255, 1998.

531. International Pancreas Transplantation Registry [NEWSLETTER]. 12:4-23, 2000.

532. Kahl A, Bechstein WO, Lorenz F, et al: Long-term prednisolone withdrawal after pancreas and kidney transplantation in patients treated with ATG, tacrolimus, and mycophenolate mofetil. Transplant Proc 33:1694-1695, 2001.

533. Kaufman DB, Leventhal JR, Stuart J, et al:. Mycophenolate mofetil and tacrolimus as primary maintenance immunosuppression in simultaneous pancreas-kidney transplantation: Initial experience in 50 consecutive cases. Transplantation 67:586-593, 1999.

534. Luzi L, Perseghin G, Brendel MD, et al: Metabolic effects of restoring partial beta-cell function after islet allotransplantation in type 1 diabetic patients. Diabetes 50:277-282, 2001.

535. Shapiro AM, Lakey JR, Ryan EA, et al: Islet transplantation in seven patients with type 1 diabetes mellitus using a glucocorticoid-free immunosuppressive regimen. N Engl J Med 343:230-238, 2000.

536. Cosio FG, Pesavento TE, Kim S, et al: Patient survival after renal transplantation: IV. Impact of post-transplant diabetes. Kidney Int 62:1440-1446, 2002.

537. Baid S, Tolkoff-Rubin N, Farrell M, et al:. Tacrolimus-associated posttransplant diabetes mellitus in renal transplant recipients: Role of hepatitis C infection. Transplant Proc 34:1771-1773, 2002.

538. Becker YT, Leverson GE, D'Alessandro AM, et al: Diabetic kidneys can safely expand the donor pool. Transplantation 74:141-145, 2000.

539. Ueda T, Yoshimura N, Yoshida O: Diabetic cystopathy: Relationship to autonomic neuropathy detected by sympathetic skin response. J Urol 157:580-584, 1997.

540. Barkai L, Szabo L: Urinary bladder dysfunction in diabetic children with and without subclinical cardiovascular autonomic neuropathy. Eur J Pediatr 152:190-192, 1993.

541. Torffvit O, Agardh C-D, Mathiasson A: A lack of association between cystopathy and progression of diabetic nephropathy in insulin-dependent diabetes mellitus. Scand J Urol Nephrol 31:365-369, 1997.

542. Kaplan SA, Te AE, Blaivas JG: Urodynamic findings in patients with diabetic cystopathy. J Urol 153:342-344, 1995.

543. Menendez V, Cofan F, Talbot-Wright R, et al:. Urodynamic evaluation in simultaneous insulin-dependent diabetes mellitus and end stage renal disease. J Urol 155:2001-2004, 1996.

544. Starer P, Libow L: Cystometric evaluation of bladder dysfunction in elderly diabetic patients. Arch Intern Med 150:810-813, 1990.

545. Vejlsgaard R: Urinary tract infection and diabetes: Diagnosis and treatment. *In* Mogensen CE (ed): The Kidney and Hypertension in Diabetes mellitus. Boston, Kluwer Academic Publisher, 1996, pp 433-437.

546. Balasoiu D, van Kessel KC, van Kats-Renaud HJ, et al: Granulocyte function in women with diabetes and asymptomatic bacteriuria. Diabetes Care 20:392-395, 1997.

547. Zhanel GG, Nicolle LE, Harding GK: Prevalence of asymptomatic bacteriuria and associated host factors in women with diabetes mellitus. The Manitoba Diabetic Urinary Infection Study Group. Clin Infect Dis 21:316-322, 1995.

548. Brauner A, Flodin U, Hylander B, Ostenson CG: Bacteriuria, bacterial virulence and host factors in diabetic patients. Diabet Med 10:550-554, 1993.

549. Geerlings SE, Brouwer EC, Gaastra W, et al:. Virulence factors of *Escherichia coli* isolated from urine of diabetic women with asymptomatic bacteriuria: Correlation with clinical characteristics. Antonie Van Leeuwenhoek 80:119-127, 2001.

550. Tolkoff-Rubin NE, Rubin RH: The infectious disease problems of the diabetic renal transplant recipient. Infect Dis Clin North Am 9:117-130, 1995.

551. Tseng CC, Wu JJ, Liu HL, et al: Roles of host and bacterial virulence factors in the development of upper urinary tract infection caused by *Escherichia coli*. Am J Kidney Dis 39:744-752, 2002.

552. Arki T, Tofuku Y: A case of diabetes mellitus associated with emphysematous cystitis and prostatic abscess. Jpn Diabetes Soc 37:687-693, 1994.

553. Egawa S, Utsunomiya T, Uchida T, et al: Emphysematous pyelonephritis, ureteritis, and cystitis in a diabetic patient. Urol Int 52:176-178, 1994.

554. Patterson JE, Andriole VT: Bacterial urinary tract infections in diabetes. Infect Dis Clin North Am 9:25-51, 1995.

555. Bali I, Abdu AF, Gloster ES, et al:. Penectomy in diabetic patients undergoing maintenance dialysis. Am J Nephrol 15:152-156, 1995.

556. Eknoyan G: Renal papillary necrosis in diabetic patients. *In* Mogensen CE (ed): The Kidney and Hypertension in Diabetes Mellitus. Boston, Martinus Nijhoff Publishing, pp259-268, 1998.

557. Turner FC: Necrosis of the pyramids of one kidney. Trans Pathol Soc London 159:1887-1888, 1939.

558. Günther GW: Die Papillennekrosen der Niere bei Diabetes. Munch Med Wochenschr 84:1695-1699, 1937.

559. Ditscherlein G: Nierenveränderungen bei Diabetikern. Jena, DDR, VEB Gustav Fischer, 1969.

560. Waldherr R, Ilkenhans C, Ritz E: How frequent is glomerulonephritis in diabetes mellitus type II ? Clin Nephrol 37:271-273, 1992.

561. Walmsley RS, David DB, Allan RN, Kirkby GR: Bilateral endogenous *Escherichia coli* endophthalmitis: A devastating complication in an insulin-dependent diabetic. Postgrad Med J 72:361-363, 1996.

562. Ogata M, Sato A, Takahashi Y, et al: A case of pyogenic spondylitis associated with diabetes mellitus. J Tokyo Womens Med Coll 61:645-650, 1991.

563. Nagaoka T, Mizuno Y, Matsushita S, Mihira Sl: An NIDDM patient with recurrence of an iliopsoas abscess on the opposite side. Jpn Diabetes Soc 36:741-746, 1993.

564. Suzuki H, Miyake T: A case of diabetes mellitus associated with iliopsoas abscess caused by MRSA. Jpn Diabetes Soc 38:965-969, 1995.

565. Lye WC, Chan RKT, Lee EJC, Kumarasinghe G: Urinary tract infections in patients with diabetes mellitus. J Infect 24:169-174, 1992.

566. Kobayashi T, Ieiri T, Asada M, et al: A case of *Pasteurella Multocida* urinary tract infection in non-insulin-dependent diabetes mellitus. Jpn Diabetes Soc 40:341-346, 1997.

567. Leibovici L, Samra Z, Konisberger H, et al:. Bacteremia in adult diabetic patients. Diabetes Care 14:89-94, 1991.

568. Jacobs LG, Skidmore EA, Cardoso LA, Ziv F: Bladder irrigation with amphotericin B for treatment of fungal urinary tract infections. Clin Infect Dis 18:313-318, 1994.

569. Hoepelmann IM: Urinary tract infection in patients with diabetes mellitus. Int J Antimicrob Agents 4:113-116, 1994.

570. Gluckman SJ, Dinubile MJ: Controversial issues in the management of urinary tract infections. Curr Opin Infect Dis 5:50-56, 1992.

571. Stapleton A: Urinary tract infections in patients with diabetes. Am J Med 113:80S-84S, 2002.

572. Mogensen CE: A complete screening of urinary albumin concentration in an unselected diabetic out-patient clinic population. Diabetes Nephropathy 2:11-18, 1983.

573. Viberti GC, Mackintosh D, Bilous RW, et al: Proteinuria in diabetes mellitus: Role of spontaneous and experimental variation of glycaemia. Kidney Int 21:714-720, 1982.

574. Fabre J, Balant LP, Dayer PG, et al:. The kidney in maturity onset diabetes mellitus: A clinical study of 510 patients. Kidney Int 21:730-738, 1982.

575. Kunzelman CL, Knowler WC, Pettitt DJ, Bennett PH: Incidence of nephropathy in type 2 diabetes mellitus in the Pima Indians. Kidney Int 35:681-687, 1989.

576. Damsgaard EM, Mogensen CE: Microalbuminuria in elderly hyperglycaemic patients and controls. Diabetic Med 3:430-435, 1986.

577. Bruno G, Cavallo-Perin P, Bargero G, et al: Prevalence and risk factors for micro-and macroalbuminuria in an Italian population-based cohort of NIDDM subjects. Diabetes Care 19:43-47, 1996.

578. Mogensen CE, Poulsen PL: Epidemiology of microalbuminuria in diabetes and in the background population. Curr Opin Nephrol Hypertens 3:248-256, 1996.

579. Keiding NR, Root HF, Marble A: Importance of control of diabetes in prevention of vascular complications. JAMA 150:964-969, 1952.

580. Berglund J, Lins LE, Lins PE: Predictability in diabetic nephropathy. Acta Med Scand 215:263-270, 1984.

581. Rolfe M: Diabetic renal disease in Central Africa. Diabet Med 5:630-633, 1988.

582. Ishihara M, Yukimura Y, Yamada T, et al:. Diabetic complications and their relationships to risk factors in a Japanese population. Diabetes Care 7:533-538, 1984.

583. Haider Z, Obaidullah S, Din F: A prospective follow-up study of patients with newly diagnosed maturity onset diabetes mellitus. J Pakistan Med Assoc 31:35-38, 1981.

584. Paisey RB, Arredondo LN, Villalobos A, et al: Association of differing dietary, metabolic, and clinical risk factors with microvascular complications of diabetes: A prevalence study of 530 Mexican type II diabetic subjects. II. Diabetes Care 7:428-433, 1984.

585. Pirart J: Diabetes mellitus and its degenerative complications: A prospective study of 4,400 patients observed between 1947 and 1973. Diabetes Care 1:168-188, 1978.

586. Rate RG, Knowler WC, Morse HG, et al: Diabetes mellitus in Hopi and Navajo indians. Diabetes 32:894-899, 1983.

587. Haffner SM, Mitchell BD, Pugh JA, et al: Proteinuria in Mexican Americans and non-Hispanic whites with non-insulin-dependent diabetes mellitus. Diabetes Care 12:530-536, 1989.

588. Kamenetzky SA, Bennett PH, Dippe SE, et al: A clinical and histologic study of diabetic nephropathy in the Pima Indians. Diabetes 23:61-68, 1974.

589. Kawate R, Yamakido, M, Nishimoto Y, et al:. Diabetes mellitus and its vascular complications in Japanese migrants on the Island of Hawaii. Diabetes Care 2:161-170, 1979.

590. Klein R, Klein BEK, Moss SE, DeMets DL: Proteinuria in diabetes. Arch Intern Med 148:181-186, 1988.

591. West KM, Erdreich LJ, Stober JA: A detailed study of risk factors for retinopathy and nephropathy in diabetes. Diabetes 28:501-508, 1980.

592. Kofoed-Enevoldsen A, Borch-Johnsen K, Kreiner S, et al:. Declining incidence of persistent proteinuria in type 1 (insulin-dependent) diabetic patients in Denmark. Diabetes 36:205-209, 1987.

593. Mathiesen ER, Rønn B, Jensen T, et al: Relationship between blood pressure and urinary albumin excretion in development of microalbuminuria. Diabetes 39:245-249, 1990.

594. Rudberg S, Dahlquist G: Determinants of progression of microalbuminuria in adolescents with IDDM. Diabetes Care 19:369-371, 1996.

595. Baldwin DS, Neugarten J: Hypertension and renal diseases. Am J Kidney Dis 10:186-191, 1987.

596. Borch-Johnsen K, Nørgaard K, Hommel E, et al: Is diabetic nephropathy an inherited complication ? Kidney Int 41:719-722, 1992.

597. Seaquist ER, Goetz FC, Rich S, Barbosa J: Familial clustering of diabetic kidney disease: Evidence of genetic susceptibility to diabetic nephropathy. N Engl J Med 320:1161-1165, 1989.

598. Pettitt DJ, Saad MF, Bennett PH, et al: Familial predisposition to renal disease in two generations of Pima Indians with type 2 (non-insulin-dependent) diabetes mellitus. Diabetologia 33:438-443, 1990.

599. The Diabetes Control and Complications Trial Research Group: Clustering of long-term complications in families with diabetes in the Diabetes Control and Complications Trial. Diabetes 46:1829-1839, 1997.

600. Faronato PP, Maioli M, Tonolo G, et al: Clustering of albumin excretion rate abnormalities in Caucasian patients with NIDDM. Diabetologia 40:816-823, 1997.

601. Krolewski AS, Canessa H, Warram JH, et al: Predisposition to hypertension and susceptibility to renal disease in insulin-dependent diabetes mellitus. N Engl J Med 318:140-145, 1988.

602. Mangili R, Bending JJ, Scott GS, et al: Increased sodium-lithium counter transport activity in red cells of patients with insulin dependent diabetes and nephropathy. N Engl J Med 318:146-150, 1988.

603. Gall M-A, Rossing P, Jensen JS, et al: Red Cell Na/Li countertransport in non-insulin-dependent diabetics with diabetic nephropathy. Kidney Int 39:135-140, 1991.

604. Elving LD, Wetzels JFM, de Nobel E, Berden JHM: Erythrocyte sodium-lithium countertransport is not different in type 1 (insulin-dependent) diabetic patients with and without diabetic nephropathy. Diabetologia 34:126-128, 1991.

605. Carr S, Mbanya J-C, Thomas T, et al: Increase in glomerular filtration rate in patients with insulin-dependent diabetes and elevated erythrocyte sodium-lithium countertransport. N Engl J Med 322:500-505, 1990.

606. Ng LL, Davies JE, Siczkowski M, et al: Abnormal Na^+/H^+ antiporter phenotype and turnover of immortalized lymphoblasts from type 1 diabetic patients with nephropathy. J Clin Invest 93:2750-2757, 1994.

607. Koren W, Koldanov R, Pronin VS, et al: Enhanced erythrocyte Na^+/H^+ exchange predicts diabetic nephropathy in patients with IDDM. Diabetologia 41:201-205, 1998.

608. Monciotti CG, Semplicini A, Morocutti A, et al: Elevated sodium-lithium countertransport activity in erythrocytes is predictive of the development of microalbuminuria in IDDM. Diabetologia 40:654-661, 1997.

609. Feldt-Rasmussen B, Deckert T: Is metabolic control a determinant of renal disease progression in type I diabetic nephropathy? J Nephrol 2:58-62, 1993.

610. Hanssen KF, Dahl-Jørgensen K, Lauritzen T, et al: Diabetic control and microvascular complications. Diabetologia 29:677-684, 1986.

611. Krolewski M, Eggers PW, Warram JH: Magnitude of end-stage renal disease in IDDM: A 35 year follow-up study. Kidney Int 50:2041-2046, 1996.

612. Luetscher JA, Kramer FB, Wilson DM, et al: Increased plasma inactive renin in diabetes mellitus. A marker of microvascular complications. N Engl J Med 312:1412-1417, 1985.

613. Wilson DM, Luetscher JA: Plasma prorenin activity and complications in children with insulin-dependent diabetes mellitus. N Engl J Med 323:1101-1106, 1990.

614. Danser AHJ, van den Dorpel MA, Deinum J, et al: Renin, prorenin, and immunoreactive renin in vitreous fluid from eyes with and without diabetic retinopathy. J Clin Endocrinol Metab 68:160-167, 1989.

615. Franken AAM, Derkx FHM, Man in't Veld AJ, et al: High plasma prorenin in diabetes mellitus and its correlation with some complications. J Clin Endocrinol Metab 71:1008-1015, 1990.

616. Daneman D, Crompton CH, Balfe JA, et al: Plasma prorenin as an early marker of nephropathy in diabetic (IDDM) adolescents. Kidney Int 46:1154-1159, 1994.

617. Allen TJ, Cooper ME, Gilbert RE, et al: Serum total renin is increased before microalbuminuria in diabetes. Kidney Int 50:902-907, 1996.

618. Christiansen JS: Cigarette smoking and prevalence of microangiopathy in juvenile-onset insulin-dependent diabetes mellitus. Diabetes Care 1:146-149, 1978.

619. Telmer S, Christiansen JS, Andersen AR, et al: Smoking habits and prevalence of clinical diabetic microangiopathy in insulin-dependent diabetics. Acta Med Scand 215:63-68, 1984.

620. Nordén G, Nyberg G: Smoking and diabetic nephropathy. Acta Med Scand 215:257-261, 1984.

621. Mühlhauser I, Sawicki PT, Berger M: Cigarette smoking as a risk factor for macroproteinuria and proliferative retinopathy in type 1 (insulin-dependent) diabetes. Diabetologia 29:500-502, 1986.

622. Chase HP, Garg SK, Marshall G, et al: Cigarette smoking increases the risk of albuminuria among subjects with type 1 diabetes. JAMA 265:614-617, 1991.

623. Ravid M, Neumann L, Lishner M: Plasma lipids and the progression of nephropathy in diabetes mellitus type II: Effect of ACE inhibitors. Kidney Int 47:907-910, 1995.

624. Stephenson J, Fuller JH, Viberti GC, Sjolie A-K, The EURODIAB IDDM Complications Study Group: Blood pressure, retinopathy and urinary albumin excretion in IDDM. Diabetologia 38:599-603, 1995.

625. Jarrett RJ, Viberti GC, Argyropoulos A, et al: Microalbuminuria predicts mortality in non-insulin-dependent diabetes. Diabet Med 1:17-19, 1984.

626. Mattock MB, Morrish NJ, Viberti GC, et al: Prospective study of microalbuminuria as predictor of mortality in NIDDM. Diabetes 41:736-741, 1992.

627. MacLeod JM, Lutale J, Marshall SM: Excess mortality in type 2 diabetic patients with minimal elevation of albumin excretion [abstract]. Diabetologia 35 (suppl 1), A34, 1992.

628. Atkinson AB, Beatty OL, Ritchie CM, et al: Clinic urinary albumin concentration predicts with mortality and progression to nephropathy in NIDDM: Results of an 8 year prospective study [abstract]. Diabet Med 10 (suppl 1), S4, 1993.

629. Gall M-A, Borch-Johnsen K, Nielsen FS, et al: Micro-and macroalbuminuria as predictors of mortality in non-insulin-dependent diabetes [abstract]. Diabetologia 36(suppl 1), A207, 1993.

630. Stiegler H, Standl E, Schulz K, et al: Morbidity, mortality, and albuminuria in type 2 diabetic patients: A three-year prospective study of a random cohort in general practice. Diabet Med 9:646-653, 1992.

631. Mogensen CE: Glomerular filtration rate and renal plasma flow in normal and diabetic man during elevation of blood sugar levels. Scand J Clin Lab Invest 28:177-182, 1971.

632. Christiansen JS, Frandsen M, Parving H-H: Effect of intravenous glucose infusion on renal function in normal man and in insulin-dependent diabetics. Diabetologia 21:368-373, 1981.

633. Trevisan R, Nosadini R, Fioretto P, et al: Ketone bodies increase glomerular filtration rate in normal man and in patients with type 1 (insulin-dependent) diabetes mellitus. Diabetologia 30:214-221, 1987.

634. Christiansen JS, Frandsen M, Parving H-H: The effect of intravenous insulin infusion on kidney function in insulin-dependent diabetes mellitus. Diabetologia 20:199-204, 1981.

635. Christiansen JS, Gammelgaard J, Ørskov H, et al: Kidney function and size in normal subjects before and during growth hormone administration for one week. Eur J Clin Invest 11:487-490, 1981.

636. Christiansen JS, Gammelgaard J, Frandsen M, et al: Kidney function and size in type 1 diabetic patients before and during growth hormone administration for one week. Diabetologia 22:333-337, 1982.

637. Parving H-H, Christiansen JS, Noer I, et al: The effect of glucagon infusion on kidney function in short-term insullin-dependent juvenile diabetes. Diabetologia 19:350-354, 1980.

638. Kupin WL, Cortes P, Dumler F, et al: Effect on renal function of change from high to moderate protein intake in type I diabetic patients. Diabetes 36:73-79, 1987.

639. Christiansen JS, Rasmussen JF, Parving H-H: Short-term inhibition of prostaglandin synthesis has no effect on the elevated glomerular filtration rate of early insulin-dependent diabetes. Diabet Med 2:17-20, 1985.

640. Esmajtjes E, Fernandez MR, Halperin I, et al: Renal hemodynamic abnormalities in patients with short-term insulin-dependent diabetes mellitus: Role of renal prostaglandins. J Clin Endocrinol Metab 60:1231-1236, 1985.

641. Ortola FV, Ballermann BJ, Anderson S, et al: Elevated plasma arterial natriuretic peptide levels in diabetic rats. Potential mediators of hyperfiltration. J Clin Invest 80:670-674, 1987.

642. Sawicki PT, Heineman L, Rave K, et al: Artrial natriuretic factor in various stages of diabetic nephropathy. J Diabetes Complications 2:207-209, 1988.

643. Jones SL, Perico N, Benigni A, et al: Glomerular filtration rate, extracellular fluid volume and atrial natriuretic factor in insulin-dependent diabetics. Kidney Int 33:268, 1988.

644. Tilton RG, Chang K, Hasan KS, et al: Prevention of diabetic vascular dysfunction by guanidines. Diabetes 42:221-232, 1993.

645. del Castillo E, Fuenzalida R, Uranga J: Increased glomerular filtration rate and glomerulopressin activity in diabetic dogs. Horm Metab Res 2:46-53, 1977.

646. Kroustrup JP, Gundersen HJG, Østerby R: Glomerular size and structure in diabetes mellitus. III. Early enlargement of the capillary surface. Diabetologia 13:207-210, 1977.

647. Reichard P, Nilsson BY, Rosenqvist U: The effect of long-term intensified insulin treatment on the development of microvascular complications of diabetes mellitus. N Engl J Med 329:304-309, 1993.

648. Microalbuminuria Collaborative Study Group UK: Intensive therapy and progressive to clinical albuminuria in patients with insulin dependent diabetes mellitus and microalbuminuria. BMJ 311:973-977, 1995.

649. Feldt-Rasmussen B, Mathiesen ER, Deckert T: Effect of two years of strict metabolic control on progression of incipient nephropathy in insulin-dependent diabetes. Lancet 2:1300-1304, 1986.

650. Bangstad H-J, Østerby R, Dahl-Jørgensen K, et al: Improvement of blood glucose control in IDDM patients retards the progression of morphological changes in early diabetic nephropathy. Diabetologia 37:483-490, 1994.

CHAPTER 39

Nephrolithiasis

Fredric L. Coe, Murray J. Favus, and John R. Asplin

Renal stones generally consist of calcium salts, uric acid, cystine, or struvite (the triple salt of magnesium, ammonium, and phosphate). Calcium stones predominate (Table 39-1).[1-7] Calcium stones are composed of calcium oxalate and calcium phosphate crystals. Calcium oxalate crystals are found in mono- and dihydrate forms, which have different lattice structures and microscopic appearances.[8] Calcium phosphate crystals are usually carbonate apatite or hydroxyapatite, and occasionally brushite (calcium hydrogen phosphate), whitlockite (calcium orthophosphate), and octocalcium phosphate.[5] Pure calcium oxalate stones are more frequent than pure calcium phosphate stones (see Table 39-1). Calcium phosphate crystals are often found mixed with calcium oxalate crystals but the amount of calcium oxalate in mixed stones generally exceeds that of calcium phosphate. The prevalence of calcium phosphate in calcium stones varies significantly from study to study. Some of this difference may be due to the techniques used to analyze stones. Because calcium phosphate salts are usually the minor component in mixed stones, studies that use multiple techniques and analyze the core of the stone separately report higher rates of calcium phosphate in stones.[9, 10] The data in Table 39-1 are based on findings in industrialized areas and relatively affluent cultures. In the past, lower urinary tract stones, mainly arising in the bladder, were far more frequent than upper tract stones[11, 12]; these were usually composed of ammonium acid urate and calcium oxalate and were more common in children than in adults. In less developed countries, such bladder stones are still the major form of urinary stone disease.[13] Our interest here, biased as it is by our own situation, focuses only on the stone types listed in Table 39-1. The incidence rate of upper tract stones has not been well defined in general, but by the end of 1974 rates for one well-defined population were 36 cases per 100,000 per year for women, and for men, 123.6 per 100,000 per year, an increase from 78.5 per 100,000 per year in 1950.[14] The prevalence of kidney stones in the United States varies depending on race, sex, and geographic location.[15] The prevalence in men varies from 4% to 9%, and in women it ranges from 1.7% to 4.1%. Whites are at highest risk for stones, African Americans at lowest risk.

Because calcium, uric acid, cystine, and struvite stones differ from one another in pathogenesis and treatment, each stone type is described separately. However, the clinical manifestations of the stones themselves, that is, the ways in which they disturb the urinary tract, are not closely related to their particular composition.

CALCIUM STONES

Calcium oxalate and calcium phosphate stones make up the principal divisions of nephrolithiasis. Because they are so common, much is known about their natural history. Of the many causes of calcium stones, most are remediable.

Natural History

The patient, usually young, who has formed a single stone tends to view with skepticism a lifetime of preventive efforts and invariably inquires about the likelihood of recurrence. The recurrent stone former usually wonders whether the stone disease will tend to wane with age or become worse.

Recurrence after a Single Stone

Many investigators have reported long-term prospective surveys of recurrence in patients who presented after forming their first stone.[16-19] Recurrence was the rule and was maximal at 2 to 3 years. Thereafter, cumulative recurrence was less dramatic, but 40% to 50% had recurred by 5 years and over 50% to 60% by 10 years. Two of the studies reported follow-up of 20 to 30 years with recurrence rates of 75%.[16, 17] Although it has been said that recurrence is the exception and that a young patient who has formed a single stone is unlikely to form another,[20] these long-term studies suggest otherwise: that recurrence is the rule, usually within 5 to 10 years. Unfortunately, patients who will have stone recurrence cannot be distinguished by laboratory evaluation from those who will not.[18, 21, 22]

TABLE 39-1

Types of Renal Stones Formed and Frequency of Occurrence*

	CALCIUM OXALATE AND CALCIUM PHOSPHATE	CALCIUM OXALATE	CALCIUM PHOSPHATE	URIC ACID	CALCIUM OXALATE AND URIC ACID	CYSTINE	STRUVITE	NUMBER OF STONES
Nordin and Hodgkinson[1]	46.0	14.7	8.0	2.9	—	3.3	25.1	243
Lagergren[2]	44.2	15.1	7.6	1.9	1.7	1.1	28.1	460
Melick and Henneman[3]	30.3	27.1	20.6	12.9	—	2.6	14.8	155
Prien[4]	34.3	32.7	5.3	4.7	1.1	2.9	19.0	1000
Sutor et al.[5]*	35.9	28.5	7.4	1.1	1.4	1.6	24.1	810
Mandel and Mandel[6]	9.9	49.3	8.8	9.8	2.2	0.5	12.4	10163
Koide et al.[7]*	54.6	24.7	6.6	4.4	1.7	1.1	6.4	2724

*Numbers represent the percentage of each stone type in the series.

Course of Untreated Recurrent Nephrolithiasis

It is easy to believe that stones tend to abate with time. We have studied the pattern of stone occurrence in 460 patients before they entered our program and before systematic treatment.[21] For each patient, we estimated new stone occurrences, using old records, radiographs, and patient recollection. When new stones were calculated per patient during each 5-year interval after the first stone, in other words, as recurrent stones per patient per 5 years, the recurrence rate, adjusted for patients at risk, clearly fell. A similar pattern has been observed by Marshall and colleagues[20] in a prospective study.

The idea that stone recurrence decreases with time is identical to stating that the interval between successive stones increases, but this prediction is not true. Of our 460 stone formers, we selected those who had two or more new stone events that were separated by an interval whose duration could be estimated precisely. Among these patients "inter-event" intervals fell with successive stones (Table 39-2). One hundred sixty-eight patients had at least three separate intervals, so that the first and last intervals could be compared. The first interval was larger than the last in 115 of the 168 patients, indicating an accelerating pace of recurrence. In the remainder, the last interval was longer than the first.

Inter-event intervals, unique to individuals, reveal a heterogeneous and complex pattern of recurrence. In a majority of patients, stone disease tends to accelerate; in a minority, it lessens. Thus far, it has been impossible to separate the two groups on the basis of their metabolic disorder, age, sex, or other characteristics.[21] The overall natural history of stone disease appears to be one of chronicity, and the hope of a waning of disease with age is, for most patients, unrealistic.

Inter-event intervals and stone occurrence data conflict; stone frequency seems to fall, even though the interval narrows with successive recurrence. The main reason is that stone counts in populations are a poor way of assessing stone activity. Retrospective studies are biased to the extent that referral to a program tends to occur after a given number of recurrences. More active stone formers are referred a shorter time after the onset of stones. Inactive stone formers contribute long intervals and are the only contributors of stone events in the later years. In a prospective study of recurrence, active stone formers, who have short inter-stone intervals, appear in the

TABLE 39-2

Interevent Intervals* for 256 Calcium Stone Formers

		NUMBER OF STONE EVENTS				
GROUP	NUMBER OF PATIENTS	2	3	4	5	6
All patients	256†	4.48	4.02	2.05	2.05	—
Last interval shorter	115	5.03	3.23	2.08	2.10	1.67
First interval shorter	53	1.70	5.55	2.01	1.79	1.67

*Numbers represent mean intervals, in years, between each event and the preceding event.

†In 168 of the 256 patients, there were at least three separate events; of these, the last interval was shorter than the first in 115 patients. In 88 of these, there were only two separate stone events.

early segments of a recurrence graph, whereas the late segments can reflect only less active patients, who have long intervals and low recurrence rates. In other words, recurrence in a population is misleading when extrapolated to the individual, because it depends on counting stones formed per year by a population whose composition with respect to active and less active stone formers is likely to vary with time.

Special Clinical Problems

Within the large group of patients who form calcium stones there exist small groups of patients who present unusual problems and deserve individual analysis. Women who form stones and become pregnant are often concerned that their disease may have a harmful effect on their pregnancy. Among women with renal stones, complications of pregnancy were not increased above those of the general population except for a slightly higher rate of urinary tract infection.[23] Furthermore, the rate of stone formation during their years of pregnancy was no higher than that observed in the same population during their years in the nonpregnant state. A less detailed retrospective analysis based only on hospital charts confirmed the conclusion that pregnancy and stone disease do not prejudicially affect each other.[24] Women with calcium stones are more likely than men to have medullary sponge kidney.[25]

A small fraction of patients who form calcium stones also form uric acid stones and occasionally form stones composed of both calcium oxalate and uric acid.[26] These patients display an unusually high recurrence rate; the average recurrence rate among 23 such patients was 67.8 stones per 100 patient-years—nearly twice the average rate for calcium stone formers in general. These patients often have a mixture of metabolic disorders involving both calcium and uric acid, and when they do, both disorders must be treated or else stone recurrence will continue.[27]

Another small group of patients, which appears to represent about 11% of calcium stone formers, produces very large numbers of stones. Among 78 such patients, each of whom had formed at least 10 recurrent stones, the average recurrence rate was 172 stones per 100 patient-years. Patients with such frequent recurrences usually display very mild metabolic disorders and may easily be suspected of harboring unusual causes of stones; however, in the one study published so far, the causes of their stones appear to be the same as those usually encountered in calcium stone disease, and their responses to treatment were excellent.[28] The mechanisms responsible for their "accelerated" nephrolithiasis have not been made clear.

Pathogenesis

Saturation

Consider a beaker of water containing crystals of calcium oxalate, well mixed, and at a stable temperature. The crystals have been bathed in the solution for a long time and neither grow nor shrink. The Ca^{2+} and oxalate concentrations in the solution must also be unchanging, because the crystals are of a stable mass. The system is at equilibrium. The product of the free ionized calcium and oxalate concentrations in such a solution is called the equilibrium solubility product. A lower free ion activity product will cause the crystals to dissolve. Such a solution is called undersaturated. A higher free ion activity product will cause the crystals to grow.

Now remove the crystals from the equilibrium system and raise the ion activity product by adding Ca^{2+}, oxalate, or both. The elevated activity product would have caused growth of preformed crystals had they been left in the beaker, but in the absence of solid phase, nothing appears to happen: the solution remains clear, free of crystals. A solution that will cause growth of preformed crystals but not the appearance of new solid phase is called metastable. Raise the activity product sufficiently, however, and new crystals will appear. This point is often called the formation product, or the upper limit of metastability. Above the formation product, a solution is unstable, prone to creating new crystal nuclei. Urine may be undersaturated, metastable, or unstable with respect to calcium oxalate or the stone-forming calcium phosphate crystals.

FACTORS INFLUENCING SATURATION

Renal excretion of Ca^{2+}, oxalate, PO_4^{3-}, and water is a primary determinant of saturation. However, complexation of calcium and oxalate, and urine pH, which influences the relative amounts of mono- and dihydrogen phosphate, alter free ion concentrations drastically and have an importance in regulating saturation at least equal to that of the total concentrations. Ion binding also complicates the measurement of urine saturation; simple concentration measurements give little clue to the actual activity product. Citrate readily complexes Ca^{2+}, reducing the ionized calcium levels[29]; a similar relationship exists for Mg^{2+} and oxalate.[30] For this reason, among others, hypercalciuria, oxaluria, hypocitraturia, unduly alkaline urine, and chronic dehydration all seem to increase the risk of calcium stone formation but are not sufficient to ensure that stones will form.

URINE SATURATION MEASUREMENTS

Pak and colleagues[31] have measured urine saturation by comparing urine chemistries to their equilibrium concentration for a given crystal. They add seed crystals to an aliquot of urine and incubate at 37°C, with stirring, at constant pH, for 2 days. By that time, equilibrium is attained; the crystal mass has become stable. If the activity coefficients for Ca^{2+}, oxalate, and PO_4^{3-}—essentially the fractions of each that are free to react—remain stable throughout the incubation, the ratio of the concentration product at the start to the product after incubation, at equilibrium, must equal the activity product ratio (APR), even though the concentration products themselves do not equal the activity products. Pak and colleagues have shown that the assumption of stable activity coefficients is valid, so the empirical concentration product ratio (CPR) is a valid estimation of the APR, provided the Ca^{2+} concentration is below 5.0 mM and oxalate below 0.5 mM.[31] The upper limit of metastability can be determined by raising the activity product by adding ligand and noting the APR at which solid phase begins to appear.

Others have developed a simpler approach using computer programs to calculate urine free ion activities for Ca^{2+}, oxalate, and PO_4^{3-} from their concentrations and their known tendencies to form soluble complexes with each other and with other ligands such as citrate and sulfate.[31-33] If a calculated free ion activity product, such as the calcium oxalate ion product, is divided by the corresponding equilibrium solubility product, estimated in the same way, the resulting APR estimates the degree of saturation. A ratio above 1 connotes oversaturation; below 1 is undersaturation. The validity of this approach has been confirmed by two studies which showed a strong correlation between the type of stone a patient forms and the prevailing supersaturations (Fig. 39-1) found in two or three 24-hour urine samples as estimated by the computer program Equil2.[34, 35]

OBSERVED URINE SATURATION

Robertson, Pak, and Weber and their colleagues, using different measurements, have accumulated considerable evidence that urine from stone formers is more supersaturated than normal[36-40] (Table 39-3). Probably because of the differences in methods, absolute values differ for the three investigative groups. However, stone formers, whether hypercalciuric, without detectable metabolic disorder (idiopathic), or hyperparathyroid, had higher average values of urine saturation than did normal subjects, whether saturation was measured with respect to calcium oxalate, brushite, octocalcium phosphate, or hydroxyapatite. In the study by Weber and associates,[40] supersaturation for calcium oxalate was higher among hypercalciuric than among normocalciuric patients. Another important observation common to both experimental approaches is that normal urine, on average, is above the equilibrium solubility product, supersaturated, with respect to calcium oxalate. In the case of the data of Pak and of Weber and co-workers,[39, 40] this is a visible fact: added crystals grow in urine from most normal persons. Urine supersaturation with brushite is more variable, being highly dependent on urine pH and calcium. The use of urine measurements to assess supersaturation may be insufficient to

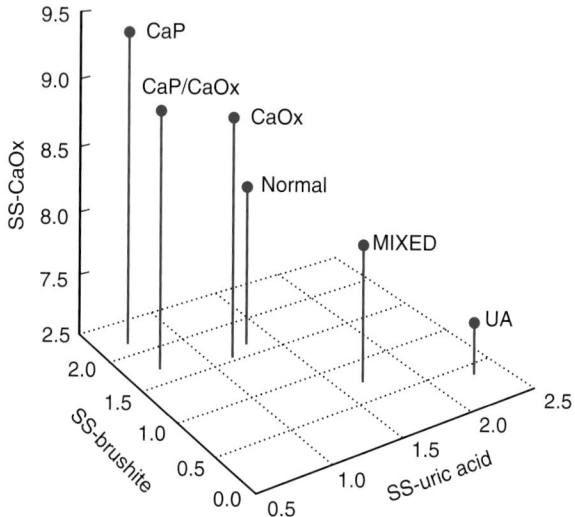

FIGURE 39-1. Relationship of supersaturation (SS) to stone composition in respect to uric acid (UA), brushite, and calcium oxalate (CaOx) in patients with nephrolithiasis. Each spike represents patient groups separated by stone type: pure uric acid stones, mixed calcium oxalate and uric acid stones (MIXED), calcium oxalate stones with no uric acid and less than 20% calcium phosphate, calcium oxalate stones with 20% to 50% calcium phosphate (CaP/CaOx), and stones containing more than 50% calcium phosphate (CaP). Normal, non–stone-forming individuals are included for comparison. (From Asplin J, Parks J, Lingeman J, et al: Supersaturation and stone composition in a network of dispersed treatment sites. J Urol 159:1821-1825, 1998.)

reveal the full crystallization potential that exists in the renal tubule. Hautmann and colleagues[41] have studied Ca^{2+} and oxalate concentrations in tissue from cortex, medulla, and papilla of seven human kidneys. The calcium-oxalate concentration product in the papillae (1×10^{-4} M^2) exceeded that of urine (5×10^{-7} M^2) and those of the medulla and cortex (8×10^{-7} M^2 and 6×10^{-7} M^2, respectively).[41] In addition, high calcium phosphate supersaturation appears to be a frequent event in the tip of the loop of Henle as tubule fluid pH and Ca^{2+} concentration are high due to water extraction in the descending limb.[42]

Limits of Metastability

Urine APR describes whether preexistent crystals, once formed, will grow or shrink while suspended in it; but the APR gives incomplete information about the ability of that urine to produce new crystals. In simple salt solutions the upper limit of metastability for calcium oxalate has been found to occur at an APR of 8.5 by Pak and Holt[39] and 10.0 by Robertson and associates.[32] The small difference in upper limit is mainly methodologic in origin.

Pak and Holt[39] have measured the actual upper limits for calcium oxalate and brushite in human urine samples from normal subjects and from hypercalciuric, normocalciuric, and hyperparathyroid stone formers and have found surprising variability (Fig. 39-2). The APR at the upper limit of metastability (ULM) is higher in normal urine than in a salt solution. The ULM in urine from stone formers is lower than normal, and in primary hyperparathyroidism may be below 8.5, the value observed in simple salt solution. Recently, we have reported studies in which the ULM of calcium oxalate and brushite was measured in urine from calcium stone formers and sex- and age-matched control subjects.[43, 44] We found that the distance between prevailing supersaturation of the urine and the ULM was reduced in stone formers, though the defect was more dramatic for brushite than for calcium oxalate. The closer urine supersaturation is to the ULM, the more likely crystallization and stone formation will occur.

TABLE 39-3

Urine Calcium Oxalate and Calcium Phosphate Activity Product Ratios in Normal Subjects and in Stone Formers

GROUP	NORMAL SUBJECTS	HYPERCALCIURIC STONE FORMERS	NORMOCALCIURIC STONE FORMERS	HYPERPARATHYROIDISM
Calcium oxalate monohydrate				
Robertson*	3 ± 1.2	5.5 ± 1.3	—	—
	10.7 ± 1.3	18.2 ± 1.3		
Pak[†]	1.45 ± 0.70	2.8 ± 1.4	2.2 ± 6.1	2.4 ± 1.1
Weber[‡]	1.97 ± 0.90	3.3 ± 2.2	2.2 ± 1.0	—
Brushite				
Pak[†]	0.35 − 0.26	1.74 ± 0.79	0.9 ± 0.5	1.6 ± 1.1
Marshall[§]	1.15 ± 0.60	1.35 ± 0.70	4 ± 1.4	—
Octocalcium phosphate[‖]	63	79	200	—
Hydroxyapatite[‖]	4.6×10^5	9.1×10^5	2.9×10^8	—

All values are means ± SD.

*From Robertson and co-workers[32, 36, 37] and Marshall and co-workers[38]; values of activity product ratios were calculated from activity products; the equilibrium solubility product (K_{sp}) was taken as 1.7×10^{-9} m^2.

[†]From Pak and Holt[39]; values of activity product ratios were measured by experiments.

[‡]From Weber and co-workers[40]; values of concentration product ratios (see text) were measured by seeding experiments.

[§]From Marshall and co-workers[38]; K_{sp} of brushite was taken as 9.32×10^{-7} m^2; values of activity product ratios were calculated.

[‖]From Marshall and co-workers[38]; K_{sp} of octocalcium phosphate was taken as 2.3×10^{-18} m^2 and of hydroxyapatite as 1.1×10^{-56} m^2.

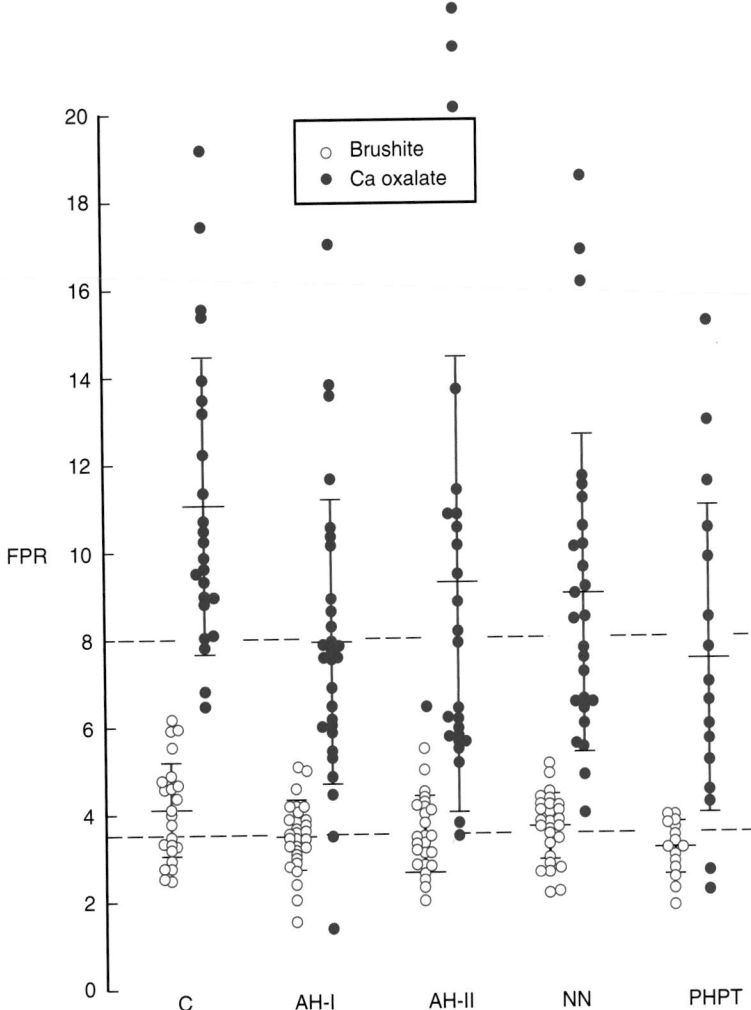

FIGURE 39-2. Urine formation product ratio (FPR) for calcium oxalate and brushite. Each point shows the value for a single urine sample. *Dotted lines* at 8 and 3.6 represent the values of the activity product ratio (APR) at which spontaneous crystallization of calcium oxalate and brushite, respectively, occurs—the so-called formation product ratio. AH-I and AH-II, severe and mild absorptive hypercalciuria respectively; C, control subjects; NN, normocalciuric stone formers; PHPT, primary hyperparathyroidism. Mean values and standard deviations are shown by *horizontal lines*. (From Pak CYC, Holt K: Nucleation and growth of brushite and calcium oxalate in urine of stone formers. Metabolism 25:665, 1976.)

The reduced ULM likely represents a defect of crystallization inhibition in calcium stone formers. Despite their differences, these studies yield similar conclusions. Urine is abnormally saturated in stone formers. Values of APR lie close enough to the ULM, for calcium oxalate and calcium phosphate, that new crystal formation could be expected. Most urine, even from normal persons, is metastable with respect to calcium oxalate, so growth of crystal nuclei into a significant mass is predictable.

Nucleation

Homogeneous nucleation, the spontaneous formation of new crystal nuclei in an oversaturated solution, is uncommon. Usually, particles of dust or debris in solution, irregularities on the surface of the container, or other crystals furnish a surface on which crystal nuclei begin to form at a lower APR than is required for homogeneous nucleation. The very existence of the metastable zone reflects the greater free energy change required to create new nuclei than to enlarge preformed nuclei, so any surface that can serve as a substrate for ions in solution to organize on may act as a heterogeneous nucleus, abridge the costly process of creating a solid phase de novo, and lower the apparent ULM.

The efficiency of heterogeneous nucleation depends on the similarity between the spacing of charged sites on the preformed surface and in the lattice of the crystal that is to grow on that surface. This kind of matching is referred to as epitaxis, and its extent is usually referred to as a good or poor epitaxial relationship.[45] In order to achieve homogeneous nucleation, all potential heterogeneous nuclei must be excluded, an unreasonably difficult task when human urine is under study. So it is probable that the apparent urine formation product ratio (FPR) for any given crystal is conditioned by preformed heterogeneous nuclei and nuclei of other crystals that form as the APR is raised during the experimental determination itself.

A number of urine crystals have good epitaxial matching and behave toward one another as heterogeneous nuclei. Monosodium urate and uric acid are excellent heterogeneous nuclei for calcium oxalate,[46, 47] so uric acid or urate could, by crystallizing, lower the ULM for calcium oxalate. Heterogeneous nucleation may be the mechanism linking hyperuricosuria to calcium oxalate stones,[48-51] a matter discussed later in this chapter. Epitaxial overgrowth of calcium oxalate on a surface of uric acid has been experimentally documented.[52]

Brushite can nucleate calcium oxalate[53] but in vivo it is more likely to transform, above pH 6.9, to hydroxyapatite, which is also an effective nucleating surface for calcium oxalate.[54] Calcium phosphate plaques found in the renal papilla, so-called Randall plaques, may act as nucleating sites for calcium oxalate stones.[55]

The Randall plaque is formed in the interstitium of the papilla but can erode through the papillary epithelium to be exposed to the urine. The plaque provides a preferred nucleating site, lowering the free energy needed for crystallization of calcium oxalate. At the same time the plaque provides an anchoring site allowing the new crystal to be retained in the kidney and have sufficient time to grow to a clinically significant size. The clinical correlates of this phenomenon are the frequent finding of apatite at the core of calcium oxalate stones,[56] and the increased prevalence and severity of Randall plaques in stone formers as compared to non–stone formers.[57]

Crystal Growth and Aggregation

Once present, crystal nuclei will grow if suspended in urine with an APR above 1. Growth and aggregation are critical to stone disease, as microscopic nuclei are too small to cause obstruction or produce symptoms. Crystals are regular lattices, composed of repeating subunits, and they grow by incorporation of calcium and oxalate, or PO_4^{3-}, into new subunits on their surfaces. In metastable solutions, at 37°C, growth rates of calcium oxalate and the stone-forming calcium phosphate crystals are rapid; appreciable changes in macroscopic dimensions occur over hours to days. Growth rate increases with the extent of oversaturation and tends to be most rapid in urines having the highest values of APR.

Small crystals aggregate into larger crystalline masses by electrostatic attraction from the charged surface of the crystals. This process can rapidly increase particle size, producing a crystal that can lodge in the urinary tract. Stone-former urine contains larger crystal aggregates than urine from non–stone formers.[58]

Cell-Crystal Interactions

Finlayson and Reid have proposed that crystals cannot grow or aggregate fast enough to anchor in the urinary tract by obstruction of renal tubules during the normal transit time through the nephron.[59] Crystals must anchor to the renal tubule epithelium or urothelium to grow large enough to be of clinical significance—the fixed particle theory. Although Randall plaques may offer an anchoring or nucleating site, it is also clear that not all stone formers have Randall plaques[57] so an alternative mechanism has been invoked. In vitro studies have shown adherence of calcium oxalate crystals to rat collecting duct epithelial cells,[60] and adherence and subsequent endocytosis of calcium oxalate crystals by monkey kidney epithelial cells.[61] The adherence and uptake of crystals appear to be crystal-specific, greater for calcium oxalate than calcium phosphate.[62, 63] The crystals bind to anionic sites on the cell membrane in a stereospecific fashion.[64] Cells may even act as nucleating sites for crystal formation.[65] Bigelow and associates have shown that phosphatidylserine appears to be a preferred binding site and that enrichment of cell membranes with phosphatidylserine increases calcium oxalate crystal binding by renal epithelial cells in culture.[66] The binding of crystals to the cells can be inhibited by a variety of anionic compounds normally found in urine, which may be part of the normal defense against kidney stones.[67] The importance of the cell-crystal interaction in the pathogenesis of human kidney stone disease is not clear at this time. The cell lines and type of crystal that most closely mimic in vivo events need to be established to link these studies to the disease.

Inhibitors of Growth, Nucleation, and Aggregation

In urine, the upper limit of metastability is higher and crystal growth rates are lower than in a salt solution with the same APR. This fact has provoked chronic interest in the nature of the materials that confer on urine such unusual properties. Both low-molecular-weight compounds and urine macromolecules demonstrate crystallization inhibition.

Pyrophosphate, citrate, and magnesium are the most significant low-molecular-weight crystallization inhibitors. Pyrophosphate increases the formation products of calcium phosphate and calcium oxalate in salt solutions and, by adsorbing to their surfaces, retards the growth of hydroxyapatite[51] and calcium oxalate crystals.[68] Russell and Fleisch[51] have observed average urine pyrophosphate concentrations of 20 to 40 mM in adults, a concentration sufficient to inhibit crystal growth by over 50% in in vitro assays.[68, 69] Bisaz and co-workers[70] found that 77% of hydroxyapatite crystal growth inhibition resided in the low-molecular-weight fraction of a urine ultrafiltrate. Pyrophosphate, citrate, and magnesium were the active low-molecular-weight compounds. Baumann and colleagues[71] showed that pyrophosphate reduced spontaneous calcium oxalate crystallization from a metastable solution. They also found that pyrophosphate inhibited heterogeneous nucleation of calcium oxalate by hydroxyapatite. One study has shown reduced urine pyrophosphate-creatinine ratios in 48% of stone formers, suggesting that low urine pyrophosphate levels may predispose to stone disease.[72] Thus pyrophosphate appears to have significant effects on the nucleation and growth of calcium oxalate and calcium phosphate crystals.

The inhibitory actions of magnesium and citrate are harder to quantitate. Both magnesium and citrate are present in the urine in millimolar concentrations and thus can complex significant amounts of oxalate and calcium, respectively. In many studies it is difficult to sort out the effects of lowering supersaturation by ligand complexation versus true crystallization inhibition. Li and associates,[73] using a continuous crystallizing system, found that magnesium inhibited both nucleation and growth of calcium oxalate, though significant growth inhibition was not seen until the magnesium concentration was 10 mM, above the levels generally found in urine. Robertson and Scurr[74] found little inhibition of calcium oxalate crystallization in the physiologic range of magnesium concentration.

Citrate has been shown to reduce growth, aggregation, and nucleation of calcium oxalate crystals,[74-77] though these studies did not separate complexation of calcium from crystal inhibition. In a carefully performed study of calcium oxalate crystal nucleation, Nicar and co-workers[78] controlled for complexation of calcium by citrate in their assay and were able to show that citrate increased the upper limit of metastability independent of its effects on the calcium oxalate concentration product. However, the effect of calcium complexation was much larger than the direct crystallization inhibition. Tiselius and associates[79] found citrate reduced calcium oxalate aggregation in a saturated crystal system. Such a system would not be affected by calcium complexation by citrate as it had come to chemical equilibrium, suggesting that the aggregation inhibition must be due to direct crystal effects.

Though urinary small molecules do have crystal inhibitory actions, the bulk of the inhibition of calcium oxalate crystallization appears to be in the macromolecular fractions.[69, 79] Ito and Coe[69] observed that strongly acidic peptides, such as poly-L-aspartic or poly-L-glutamic acids, inhibit calcium oxalate crystal growth and that urine appears to contain several glycopeptides that are unusually rich in these two amino acids and that inhibit crystal growth significantly at a low concentration. Since that time a number of macromolecules that inhibit calcium oxalate crystallization have been identified in human urine (Table 39-4). These macromolecules are generally highly anionic, containing large amounts of the acidic amino acids and undergoing extensive post-translational modification with negatively charged side chains. The presumed mode of action of macromolecular inhibitors is through binding of the preferred crystal growth site on a calcium oxalate crystal, thereby slowing crystal growth, or through binding to the crystal and changing surface charge, thus reducing the tendency to aggregate.[80]

Nephrocalcin, a 14-kD glycoprotein, was the first urine protein to be isolated and studied for its crystal inhibitory properties. It contains γ-carboxyglutamic acid (Gla) and has variable amounts of phosphorylation. Nephrocalcin has been shown to inhibit crystal growth,[81] nucleation,[82] and aggregation,[83] as well as inhibiting crystal adhesion to renal epithelial cells.[67] Nephrocalcin from urine of some stone-forming patients[84] is abnormal, lacking Gla and having diminished growth and nucleation inhibition.[82, 84] Unfortunately, nephrocalcin has not been completely purified and sequenced, which has prevented a full exploration of its role in stone disease. Tamm-Horsfall protein is the most abundant urinary protein. It is made in the thick ascending limb of the loop of Henle and can self-aggregate to form urinary casts. Tamm-Horsfall protein strongly inhibits calcium oxalate crystal aggregation[83] but does not alter growth[85] or nucleation.[82] In addition, Tamm-Horsfall protein does not prevent calcium oxalate crystal adherence to cultured renal epithelial cells,[67] but does inhibit endocytosis of crystals by the cells.[62]

Tamm-Horsfall protein from a group of patients with severe accelerated nephrolithiasis does not inhibit aggregation normally,[86] as it appears to be particularly prone to self-aggregation when urine pH is low or calcium is high. Once aggregated into a gel state, the Tamm-Horsfall protein becomes inactive. Schnierle and colleagues[87] reported that Tamm-Horsfall protein from recurrent stone formers has a higher isoelectric point than that of non–stone-forming subjects, though Trewick and Rumsby[88] found no difference in the Tamm-Horsfall protein isoelectric point between patients and controls. Differences in preparation of the protein before analysis may be the reason for the divergent results. Uropontin, the urinary form of osteopontin, is a glycoprotein rich in acidic amino acids. Uropontin is produced in the thin limbs of the loop of Henle and the papillary epithelium.[89] Uropontin inhibits calcium oxalate crystal growth, nucleation, and aggregation in vitro.[90, 91] It is present in human urine at concentrations of 50 to 250 nmol/L, exceeding the range needed for inhibition of calcium oxalate crystallization. Uropontin inhibits adhesion of calcium oxalate to cultured renal epithelial cells,[67] and exposure of cultured renal cells to calcium oxalate crystals increases production of uropontin by the cells, as though the cells were generating a defense against the crystals.[92] Abnormalities of uropontin in stone formers have not been documented at this time.

Three more proteins have recently been described as crystal inhibitors: urinary prothrombin fragment-1, bikunin, and calgranulin. Urinary prothrombin fragment-1, formerly called crystal matrix protein, was initially isolated as the predominant crystal inhibitory protein from calcium oxalate stones.[93, 94] It has been shown by immunohistochemistry to be present in the thick ascending limb of the loop of Henle and in the distal convoluted tubule.[95] It remains unclear how much of the urinary prothrombin-1 fragment derives from filtration versus secretion by the kidney. Prothrombin fragment-1 inhibits aggregation and growth of calcium oxalate crystals.[93] Bikunin, the light chain of inter-α-trypsin inhibitor, has been isolated from urine and shown to inhibit calcium oxalate crystal growth and nucleation.[96, 97] Recently, bikunin and the heavy chains of inter-α-trypsin inhibitor have been isolated from calcium oxalate kidney stones, indicating that multiple fragments of the protein may be involved in preventing stone formation.[98] Marengo and colleagues[99] have shown significant differences in the electrophoretic pattern of inter-α-trypsin inhibitor in Western blots in samples from recurrent stone formers compared to non–stone formers. Whether these differences are the cause or result of stone disease is not known. Calgranulin, an S-100 protein, has been isolated from urine and calcium oxalate kidney stones.[100] It is a potent inhibitor of calcium oxalate growth and aggregation at concentrations found in urine.[101] Calgranulin also has been shown to have inhibitory activity against struvite crystals.[102]

Glycosaminoglycans (GAGs) are polysaccharides formed by the degradation of proteoglycans. Chondroitin sulfate, hyaluronic acid, and heparan sulfate are the most plentiful GAGs found in urine. Heparan sulfate has been shown to have a strong inhibitory activity on calcium oxalate crystal growth and aggregation[103, 104] but little effect on nucleation.[104, 105] GAGs also inhibit the binding of calcium oxalate crystals to renal epithelial cells in culture.[67] Two studies have shown reduced excretion of GAGs in calcium stone formers compared to non–stone-formers.[106, 107]

TABLE 39-4

Urinary Macromolecular Inhibitors of Calcium Oxalate Crystallization

MACROMOLECULE	INHIBITOR ACTIVITY			
	Nucleation	Growth	Aggregation	Cell Adhesion
Nephrocalcin	I	I	I	I
Tamm-Horsfall protein	NI	NI	I	NI
Uropontin	I	I	I	I
Prothrombin-1 fragment	NI	I	I	NT
Bikunin	I	I	I	NT
Calgranulin	NT	I	I	NT
Glycosaminoglycans	?	I	I	I

I, inhibitory activity documented; NI, no inhibitory activity; NT, not tested.

The activity of macromolecular inhibitors is also affected by their environment. Increases in calcium concentration have been shown to alter crystal inhibitory activity, increasing the nucleation inhibition of urine macromolecules but reducing the inhibitory action of chondroitin sulfate.[108] Studies of Tamm-Horsfall protein calcium oxalate aggregation inhibition have shown high urine calcium to reduce inhibition and increase urine citrate to improve inhibition.[109] In order to define the full activity of an inhibitor in vivo, a complete assessment of the interaction of the inhibitor with the urine milieu, as well as interactions between the macromolecules themselves, is required.

An Overview

Oversaturation is the force that drives calcium salts out of solution, into the solid phase. Heterogeneous nuclei may facilitate stone formation by bypassing the thermodynamically costly process of homogeneous nucleation. Inhibitors such as pyrophosphate, citrate, and urinary macromolecules suppress nucleation, increase the supersaturation needed to produce a solid phase, and retard the growth and aggregation of nuclei already formed. In the main established stone-forming conditions, oversaturation, heterogeneous nucleation, and reduced inhibitors all have documented, or at least postulated, roles that vary from one disease to another.[3, 19, 110-112]

Treatment is often successful in reversing stone formation by eliminating those disturbances that enhance the risk of stones or, in some cases, by introducing secondary biochemical changes that compensate for the underlying defect.

Oversaturation occurs in idiopathic hypercalciuria, primary hyperparathyroidism, and hyperoxaluria because of over-excretion, and in hypocitraturia because of increased urine ionized calcium. Hypercalciuria and phosphaturia both occur in renal tubular acidosis (RTA); oversaturation with respect to calcium phosphate salts, which make up most stones in RTA, is also increased by an alkaline urine pH and by low levels of urine citrate, an important Ca^{2+}-binding agent.

Evidence for heterogeneous nucleation in hyperparathyroidism is the finding of urine formation products below those of simple salt solutions. The basis for this finding is not yet clear. Hyperuricosuria may engender urine crystals of uric acid or sodium hydrogen urate, which are efficient heterogeneous nuclei for calcium oxalate.[46, 47, 49] It is not certain whether these crystals are in a gel state.[113]

Robertson and associates[37] reported that there were low levels of urine inhibitors in some hypercalciuric and normocalciuric stone formers and that a urine supersaturation inhibition index distinguished normals from stone formers better than either measurement alone. Another study of urinary inhibitors of calcium oxalate monohydrate crystal growth has shown that the lowest inhibitor levels occur in patients with hypercalciuria but no hyperuricosuria[114] and that samples from normal subjects can be distinguished from those of stone formers no more reliably by a combination of inhibitor and supersaturation measurements than by measurements of inhibition alone. The difference between these studies is probably related to differences in methodology. Our own studies of urine inhibition in stone formers and normal subjects found reduced nucleation inhibition as determined by ULM measurements in both male and female stone formers.[43, 44] We also found calcium oxalate crystal growth inhibition to be

low in stone-forming men but not in stone-forming women. We did not find a defect in crystal aggregation inhibition in stone formers of either sex. Tiselius and colleagues also found a defect in crystal growth inhibition in male stone formers but not in female stone formers.[115] However, the authors also found reduced crystal aggregation. In general, the levels of crystallization inhibitors in the urine of stone formers differ from those in normal subjects, and in consequence of this, their urine samples can be distinguished from samples of normal subjects more reliably when inhibitor content is employed than by the use of supersaturation measurements alone. This fact highlights the presence of low inhibitor levels in stone-forming patients and suggests that inhibitors are important in preventing stones. Which of the many inhibitors thus far identified are the most important in stone disease remains unknown at present.

Table 39-5 shows the frequencies of the main causes of calcium stones. Direct comparisons among the available patient surveys are possible only when the diagnostic criteria and methods for patient selection are similar. The study by Harvey and co-workers[116] included only urine collections and no blood work, so the diagnosis of hyperparathyroidism could not be included. However, this study has the advantage of including patients from throughout the United States, avoiding any geographic or ethnic bias that might be present in a single geographic center. Hypercalciuria was the most common abnormality in all three of the studies presented, with similar degrees of hyperuricosuria and hypocitraturia being reported.[110, 116, 117]

Primary Hyperparathyroidism

All the known manifestations of primary hyperparathyroidism can be accounted for by chronic oversecretion of parathyroid hormone (PTH) and the resultant hypercalcemia (see Chapters 22 and 52). In the past, osteitis fibrosa cystica or renal calculi have been the basis for its detection,[118] although other organ systems may be involved.[119] Today hyperparathyroidism is being discovered mainly as a result of

TABLE 39-5

Occurrence Rates of Established Forms of Calcium Nephrolithiasis

DISORDER	COE[110]	HARVEY ET AL[116]	LEVY ET AL[117]
	(460)*	(3473)†	(1270)
Primary hyperparathyroidism	5.2	X	2.1
Idiopathic hypercalciuria	32.0	35–43	58.8
Hyperuricosuria	26.0	16–19	35.8
Renal tubular acidosis	3.7	X	1.3
Hyperoxaluria	4.6	18–25	8.1
Hypocitraturia	X	22–29	28.0
Idiopathic lithiasis	20.2	X	9.2‡

*Numbers of patients in each survey are shown in parentheses at the top of each column; numbers in the table itself represent the percentage of patients in each survey with specific metabolic disorders. The percentages may exceed 100% in a study because multiple abnormalities can be present in a single patient.

†The occurrence rates are given as a range of percentages that represent the reported rates from four separate regions of the United States.

‡Patients whose only abnormality was low urine volume are included as idiopathic lithiasis.

X, the disorder was not sought.

biochemical screening,[120] and the majority of such patients are asymptomatic. The incidence of primary hyperparathyroidism is now estimated to be about 1 per 1000 adults, based on widespread screening of asymptomatic subjects.[121] Approximately 20% of patients with hyperparathyroidism will develop nephrolithiasis.[120] A single parathyroid adenoma is responsible for hyperparathyroidism in 85% to 95% of patients. Four-gland hyperplasia is found in 5% to 15%, more often in association with familial hyperparathyroidism or as part of the multiple endocrine adenomatosis syndromes.[118, 122] Parathyroid carcinoma is rare, being responsible for fewer than 1% of cases.[118, 122]

Forms of Circulating Parathyroid Hormone

As judged by radioimmunoassay, PTH secretion is under negative feedback control by ionized calcium and, to a lesser extent, magnesium concentration in the serum. Fluctuations in calcium levels result in rapid changes in PTH secretion.[123, 124] Once secreted, the native hormone (Mol wt 9500) is rapidly metabolized,[125] largely into two fragments, in the liver[126, 127] and kidney.[128] It has also been shown that fragments may be secreted from parathyroid glands in vitro.[129] The smaller fragment (Mol wt 3500) is composed of the NH_2-terminal portion of the hormone and possesses biologic activity.[130] The larger fragment contains the middle and COOH-terminal portions of the hormone (Mol wt 5500) and has no biologic activity.[130] The native hormone and the NH_2-terminal fragment undergo rapid clearance from the circulation; the larger middle and COOH-terminal fragment has a half-life 5 to 10 times as long as intact PTH and is excreted by the kidney.[131]

Nature of the Primary Defect

Oversecretion of PTH in primary hyperparathyroidism is due to the increased mass of parathyroid tissue and to an increase in the calcium set-point for PTH release. Most, and perhaps all, parathyroid adenomas are monoclonal in origin.[132] Two genes have been linked to sporadic parathyroid adenomas. In 20% to 40% of parathyroid adenomas there is overexpression of the oncogene cyclin *D1/PRAD1* which leads to parathyroid cell proliferation.[133, 134] In a minority of cases cyclin *D1/PRAD1* activation results from gene rearrangement on chromosome 11, where the cyclin *D1/PRAD1* gene is brought into the region controlling the PTH gene.[135, 136] More commonly, high cyclin D1/PRAD1 levels are secondary to some other defect which increases production of the oncogene. Defects in the *MEN-1* tumor suppressor gene have been found in 10% to 20% of sporadic parathyroid adenomas.[137, 138] Germline mutations in the *MEN-1* gene cause the multiple endocrine neoplasia syndrome type 1. The gene defect in the majority of parathyroid adenomas has not been identified. The calcium-sensing receptor gene was an attractive candidate gene for parathyroid adenomas because the adenomas have an increased set-point for calcium-regulated release of PTH, which is the result of reduced expression of the calcium-sensing receptor in parathyroid adenomas.[139] However, no mutations have been found in the calcium-sensing receptor gene.[140, 141] The reduced expression of calcium-sensing receptor is likely secondary to some other genetic defect, though the reduced calcium sensitivity of the cells may play a key role in promoting cell proliferation.

Calcium Absorption and Balance

Negative Ca^{2+} balance is common (Fig. 39-3).[142-149] Urinary Ca^{2+} losses are offset, though not completely, by a variable increase in gastrointestinal Ca^{2+} absorption as measured by lower fecal Ca^{2+} excretion.[142-149] Fractional Ca^{2+} absorption (percentage of dietary intake absorbed) and the absorptive rate of Ca^{2+} measured by double-isotope techniques or

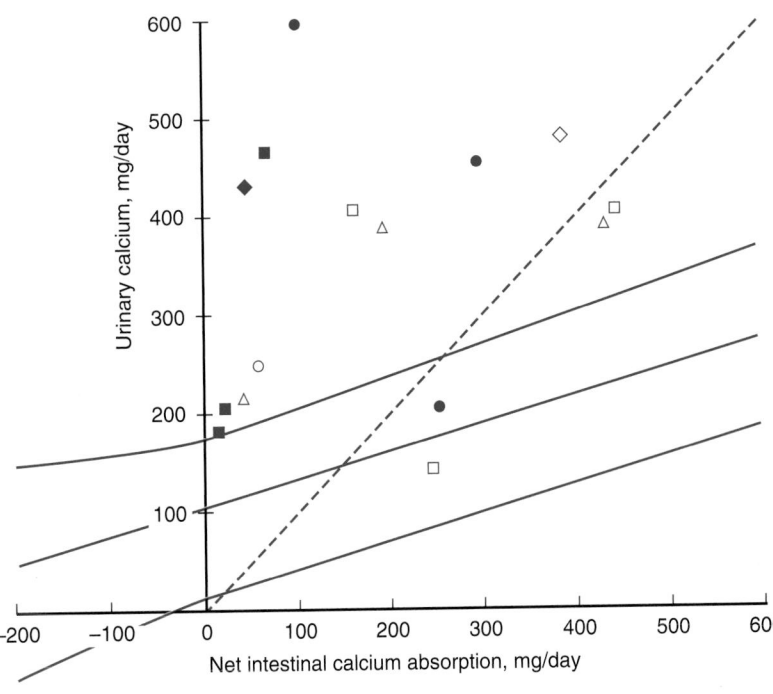

FIGURE 39-3. Relationship of urinary Ca^{2+} excretion to net intestinal Ca^{2+} absorption in patients with primary hyperparathyroidism. Each symbol represents individual patients from different sources: ■, Albright et al.[142]; ●, Aub et al.[143]; ◇, Hodgkinson[144]; □, Lafferty and Pearson[145]; △, Parfitt[147]; ○, Nassim and Higgins[148]; ◆, Bauer et al.[149] *Solid lines* represent the normal mean ±2 SD. Normal data are derived from 6-day balance studies on 195 normal subjects, shown in Figure 39-7. The *dotted line* is the line of identity; points above the line indicate negative Ca^{2+} balance.

TABLE 39-6

Intestinal Calcium Absorption in Patients with Primary Hyperparathyroidism

REFERENCE	METHOD	CALCIUM INTAKE (mg/24 hr)	DOSE ABSORBED (%)*	
			Normal Subjects	Hyperparathyroidism
Birge et al.[150]	$^{47}Ca/^{45}Ca$, PO/IV	800	52.2 ± 13.2 (6)	82.3 ± 15.6 (3)
Pak et al.[151]	Fecal ^{47}Ca	400	50 ± 7 (20)	68 ± 15 (26)
Reeve et al.[152]	$^{47}Ca/^{45}Ca$, PO/IV	850 ± 250	None studied	78.4 ± 16.0 (11)[†]
Kaplan et al.[153]	Fecal ^{47}Ca	400	None studied	68 ± 12 (5)[‡]
				71 ± 12 (12)[†]
Kaplan et al.[154]	Fecal ^{47}Ca	400	48 ± 8 (11)	59 ± 12 (12)[‡]
				64 ± 14 (18)

*Values are mean ± SD; numbers in parentheses represent number of patients studied.
[†]Preoperative.
[‡]After parathyroidectomy.
IV, intravenously; PO, orally.

fecal excretion of an oral dose of ^{47}Ca provide more direct evidence that intestinal absorption is generally increased in hyperparathyroidism (Table 39-6).[150-154] In the few hyperparathyroid patients studied, the contribution of intestinal secretion of Ca^{2+} to fecal Ca^{2+} losses is variable and appears to be unrelated to the level of intestinal Ca^{2+} absorption, Ca^{2+} balance, or serum Ca^{2+} levels.[145, 146] As only 1% of total body Ca^{2+} is extraosseous, the negative Ca^{2+} balance in primary hyperparathyroidism is largely due to loss of bone mineral. Indeed, as fibrosis increases and osteoid accumulates and replaces normal bone, bone mineral content decreases, as measured by quantitative bone histology,[155] retention of ^{47}Ca,[156] and bone densitometry.[157]

Vitamin D is required for intestinal hyperabsorption of Ca^{2+},[158] and PTH is a known stimulator of the production of 1,25-dihydroxyvitamin D_3, the hormonal form of vitamin D known to stimulate Ca^{2+} absorption (see Chapters 22 and 52). Numerous studies[154, 159, 160] have found increased blood levels of 1,25$(OH)_2D_3$ in hyperparathyroid patients, and there is a correlation between 1,25$(OH)_2D_3$ blood levels and the absorption of an oral load of ^{47}Ca. Thus, intestinal Ca^{2+} absorption may be increased in primary hyperparathyroidism because of increased production of 1,25$(OH)_2D_3$. There is conflicting evidence regarding the site of enhanced Ca^{2+} absorption along the intestinal tract. The duodenum normally has the highest rate of Ca^{2+} absorption per unit length, and in one study hyperparathyroid patients absorbed Ca^{2+} maximally in the duodenum.[152] However, in another study, maximal absorption occurred in more distal segments,[150] not in the duodenum.

Dietary calcium contributes to hypercalcemia but is not completely responsible for its maintenance, because hypercalcemia and hypercalciuria persist during fasting.[151] Prolonged dietary calcium restriction[161, 162] lowers serum Ca^{2+} to normal in some, but not all, hyperparathyroid patients. Such calcium restriction will diminish urinary Ca^{2+} excretion uniformly,[147, 161, 162] although efficient tubule reabsorption of Ca^{2+} in some patients serves to maintain the hypercalcemia.[147] Concomitant phosphorus depletion enhances both hypercalcemia and hypercalciuria and may reverse the effects of calcium restriction.[163, 164]

Renal Tubule Calcium Reabsorption

The relative importance of bone mobilization to hypercalcemia appears to be small[147, 165]; intestinal overabsorption and enhanced renal conservation of filtered calcium appear to play the major role. Nordin and Peacock[165] have suggested that the PTH-stimulated increase in distal tubule reabsorption of filtered calcium (see Chapter 22) is quantitatively most important in the maintenance of hypercalcemia in hyperparathyroidism. A further increase in tubule calcium reabsorption occurs during calcium restriction and can maintain hypercalcemia despite a reduced net intestinal absorption of calcium.[147, 166] Enhanced tubule reabsorption of calcium is responsible for normal urinary calcium excretion rates in some hyperparathyroid patients[118, 167] and for the observation that for any given level of serum calcium the urinary calcium excretion is lower in hyperparathyroidism than in other, nonparathyroid types of hypercalcemia (i.e., bone metastasis, sarcoidosis, vitamin D intoxication, multiple myeloma).[165, 167, 168]

Despite the fact that PTH stimulates distal tubule calcium reabsorption, urinary calcium excretion may be greatly elevated in those patients with primary hyperparathyroidism who form renal stones even when hypercalcemia is slight.[169] In a series of 1132 patients with nephrolithiasis, 48 had surgically documented hyperparathyroidism, and 30 of these had extremely mild hypercalcemia, in the range of 10.1 to 11.0 mg/dL (Fig 39-4). Urine calcium excretion exceeded normal in a majority of the patients and was extremely high in a few in whom hypercalcemia was barely evident. Elevated levels of circulating 1,25$(OH)_2D_3$ have been suggested as a cause of the marked hypercalciuria seen in patients such as these,[170] but no differences in serum Ca^{2+}, phosphorus, PTH, 1,25$(OH)_2D_3$, or urinary Ca^{2+} were found between hyperparathyroid stone formers and those without stones.[171] The hypercalciuria is caused by an increase in filtered load of calcium and by reduced Ca^{2+} reabsorption in the thick ascending limb of the loop of Henle. Hypercalcemia activates the calcium-sensing receptor on the basolateral membrane of the ascending loop which suppresses sodium, and subsequently calcium, reabsorption by this segment, resulting in hypercalciuria.[172]

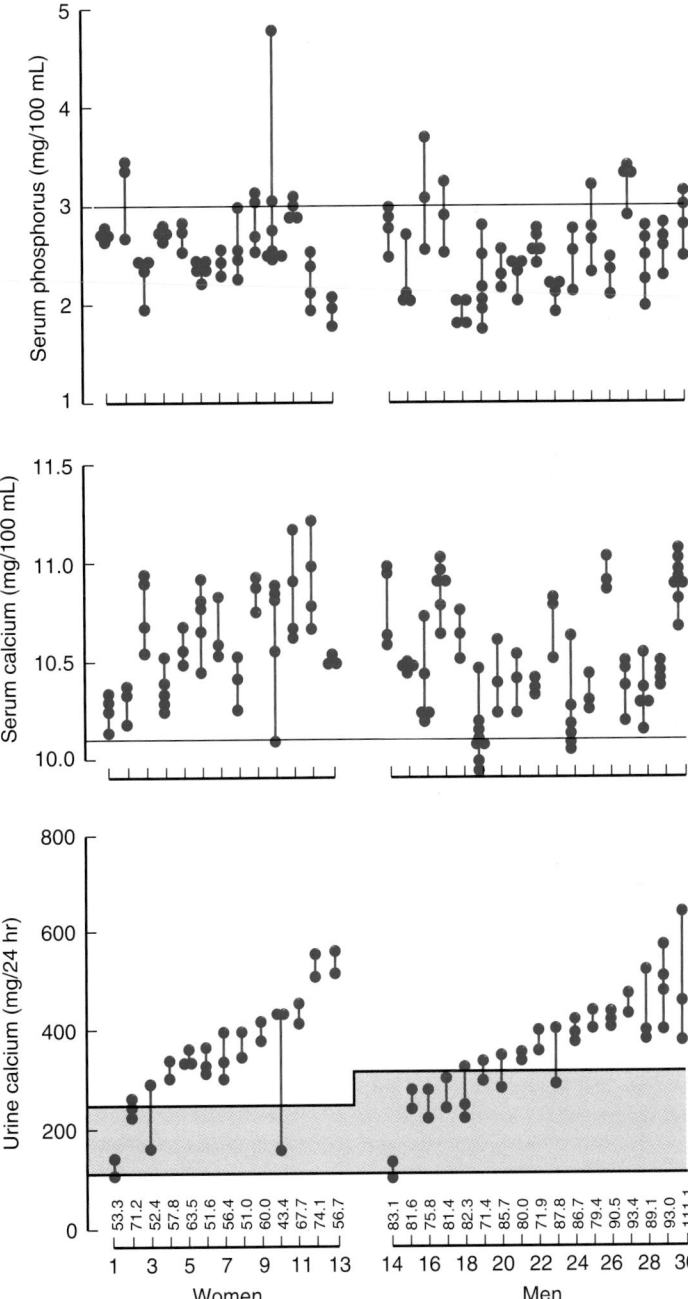

FIGURE 39-4. Selected characteristics of 30 patients with primary hyperparathyroidism, nephrolithiasis, and mild hypercalcemia. The lower limit for serum phosphorus and upper limit for serum Ca^{2+} in the laboratory reporting the study[127] are shown by *solid horizontal lines*; the upper limits for urinary Ca^{2+} excretion are shown in *gray*. Body weight is shown in kilograms for each subject.

Mechanism of Stone Formation

Renal stones in hyperparathyroidism are usually composed of hydroxyapatite, calcium oxalate, or brushite.[173] Mixtures of these crystals may also be found. Stones often recur and become bilateral if the diagnosis is not made early in the course of the disease. Nephrocalcinosis may be the only renal manifestation of hyperparathyroidism. Less commonly, parenchymal calcification may be accompanied by calculi in the renal pelvis and ureters. The presence of nephrocalcinosis should prompt a diagnostic evaluation to exclude hyperparathyroidism, but there are other causes of that syndrome.

The physicochemical composition of urine is favorable to the nucleation and growth of calcium salts.[174] The APRs for calcium oxalate and brushite are elevated in hyperparathyroid urine, mainly because of hypercalciuria.[39] Oxalate excretion is unremarkable; phosphorus excretion may not be elevated despite reduced phosphate reabsorption, because chronic phosphaturia tends to cause a negative phosphorus balance.[144] Nordin[175] has suggested that brushite stone formation may be enhanced by undue urine alkalinity. Although hyperchloremia and lowered blood CO_2 content are observed in some hyperparathyroid patients,[176] urine pH is not abnormally alkaline,[39] and the magnitude of the acidosis is negligible when renal glomerular function is normal,[177] suggesting that altered acid-base metabolism in hyperparathyroidism does not contribute to stone formation. Also unexplained are the low values of FPR for calcium oxalate and brushite (see Fig. 39-2).

Diagnosis

Despite advances in the measurement of immunoreactive PTH (iPTH) and other adjunctive maneuvers, the diagnosis of primary hyperparathyroidism still depends on the demonstration of hypercalcemia and the exclusion of other causes (Table 39-7). In general, multiple serum samples should be studied, and even modest elevations of calcium concentration should be accorded considerable weight, if consistent. The value of serum PTH levels depends on the assay that is used. Historically, radioimmunoassays using midmolecule, COOH-terminal antibodies have been used, with false-negative results in 10% to 20% of patients.[178, 179] Also, radio-immunoassays often failed to show an appropriately suppressed PTH level in hypercalcemia of malignancy.[180] Immunometric assays recognize only the intact PTH molecule by using two antibodies directed against different sites of the PTH molecule.[181] The immunometric assays distinguish hyperparathyroidism and hypercalcemia of malignancy with a high level of reliability,[180, 182] and show elevated PTH levels in 90% of patients with hyperparathyroidism. The sensitivity of the immunometric assay is improved with the use of a nomogram relating PTH to serum calcium levels (Fig. 39-5), as

PTH levels will not be appropriately suppressed in hyperparathyroidism.[180, 182] Urinary excretion of adenosine 3',5' cyclic monophosphate (cAMP) has also been used in the diagnostic evaluation of hyperparathyroid patients. PTH exerts its effects on the kidney through activation of the membrane-associated adenyl cyclase in cortical tubules[183] and therefore increases cAMP in renal tissue and in the urine. The clinical utility of urinary cAMP determinations has been limited by overlap between normal and hyperparathyroid subjects,[184-186] as well as the finding of elevated levels in some cases of familial hypocalciuric hypercalcemia and humoral hypercalcemia of malignancy.[187]

Despite improved iPTH assays, diagnosis of the cause of hypercalcemia may be difficult in certain situations. Perhaps the most interesting of these is familial hypocalciuric hypercalcemia.[188] In this condition, hypercalcemia is associated with normal or subnormal urinary calcium excretion rates. The disorder has been shown to be due to inactivating mutations in the calcium-sensing receptor.[189] Serum iPTH levels and urine cAMP may be normal or slightly elevated, but the hypocalciuria is not dependent on PTH.[190, 191] In one kindred, iPTH levels increased with age, becoming frankly elevated by age 30, making distinction from primary hyperparathyroidism difficult.[192] Patients with this disease do not form renal stones because urinary calcium levels are low. They are best separated from patients with primary

TABLE 39-7

Causes of Hypercalcemia

Excessive parathyroid hormone secretion
  Primary hyperparathyroidism
  After rental transplant
  Lithium therapy
Malignant neoplasm
  Humoral hypercalcemia of malignancy
    Lung: squamous cell carcinoma
    Kidney: hypernephroma
    Other: pancreas, hepatoma, ovary, uterus, bladder, and others
  Bone invasion
    Metastasis from carcinoma: lung, breast, and others
    Multiple myeloma
    Leukemia, lymphoma
Excessive vitamin D activity
  Vitamin D supplementation
  Idiopathic hypercalcemia of infancy
  Lymphoma
  Granulomatous disease
    Sarcoidosis
    Tuberculosis
    Silicosis
    Leprosy
    Plasma cell granuloma
Excessive calcium intake
  Milk-alkali syndrome
Increased bone turnover
  Rapidly progressive osteporosis of childhood
  Thyrotoxicosis
  Paget disease with immobilization
Other causes
  Familial hypocalciuric hypercalcemia
  Adrenal insufficiency
  Thiazide diuretic therapy
  Theophylline therapy
  Recovery phase of acute tubule necrosis
  Generalized periostitis
  Hypothyroidism
  Vitamin A intoxication
  Acquired immunodeficiency syndrome
  Pheochromocytoma

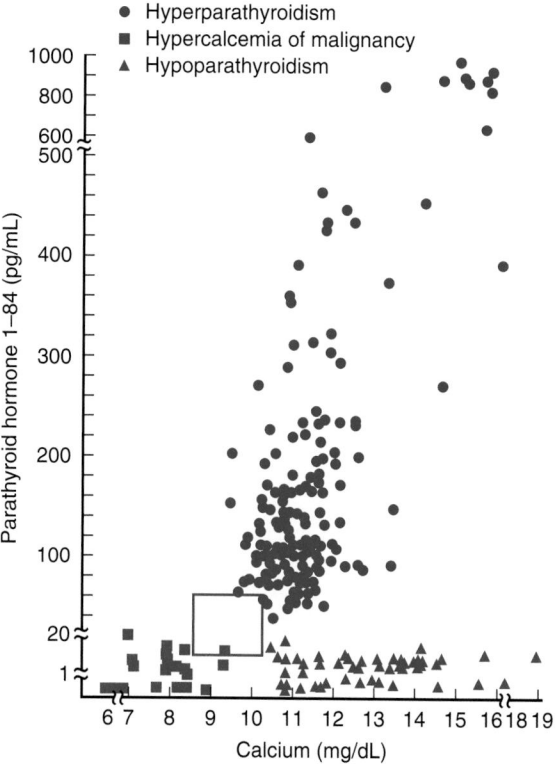

FIGURE 39-5. Results of parathyroid hormone (PTH)-(1-84) immunometric assay in 101 patients with surgically confirmed hyperparathyroidism, 79 patients with hypercalcemia of malignancy, and 23 patients with hypoparathyroidism. The area within the box represents normal serum Ca^{2+} and serum PTH concentrations. (From Nussbaum S, Potts J: Immunoassays for parathyroid hormone 1-84 in the diagnosis of hyperparathyroidism. J Bone Miner Res 6 [suppl 2]:S43-S50, 1991.)

hyperparathyroidism by having a urinary calcium-to-creatinine clearance ratio (Ca^{2+}/creat) of 0.01 or below.[190] Because the disease is inherited as an autosomal dominant trait, screening family members should uncover hypercalcemia in 50% of first-degree relatives. Humoral hypercalcemia of malignancy may be difficult to distinguish from hyperparathyroidism, as both present as hypercalcemia with hypercalciuria. PTH-related peptide has been identified as a mediator of humoral hypercalcemia of malignancy.[193-195] The PTH-related peptide has a high degree of homology with the first 13 amino acids at the biologically active NH_2-terminal end of PTH. The combination of an elevated PTH-related peptide by immunoassay and suppressed intact PTH should clearly separate humoral hypercalcemia of malignancy from hyperparathyroidism.

Treatment

Removal of adenomal or hyperplastic glands is indicated in patients with stone or bone disease and in those with pancreatitis, peptic ulcer, muscle weakness and fatigue, or changes in sensorium, and when serum calcium exceeds 12 mg/100 mL. However, many patients are asymptomatic, discovered by routine screening; for them, the decision for surgery depends on the natural history of their disease. Purnell and associates[179] followed 147 patients with mild asymptomatic hyperparathyroidism for up to 5 years. Twenty percent eventually underwent surgery, but progression of the disease—increasing serum calcium, development of osteitis fibrosa, renal calculus formation—was responsible for only 14% of this 20%. The rest had surgery because of the inconvenience of yearly re-evaluation and anxiety about their uncured disease. Silverberg and co-workers[120] evaluated 121 patients with mild hyperparathyroidism and found stable serum and urine chemistries at up to a decade of follow-up in those patients who did not have surgery. A National Institutes of Health (NIH) consensus conference recommended surgery for asymptomatic patients with markedly elevated serum calcium, low bone mineral density, reduced creatinine clearance, urinary calcium greater than 400 mg/24 hours, age less than 50 years, and for patients with inadequate medical follow-up.[196]

At surgery, it is important to identify and biopsy all four parathyroid glands, as adenomas, although usually single, may be multiple, and four-gland hyperplasia may be difficult to distinguish from a single small adenoma.[118, 179] Preoperative localization of parathyroid glands has improved with the utilization of noninvasive techniques such as high-resolution ultrasound, computed tomography (CT), radionuclide scans, and magnetic resonance imaging (MRI).[197-200] However, it is not clear that these procedures improve outcome in first-time surgery performed by an experienced surgeon.[201] Preoperative localization is essential for patients undergoing re-exploration for recurrent hypercalcemia. If noninvasive techniques are inadequate, selective catheterization of thyroid veins with measurement of PTH levels may localize the parathyroid glands.[202]

In the immediate postoperative period, serum calcium may fall to the hypocalcemic range, and calcium is required if the patient becomes symptomatic. It is important to distinguish the cause of the hypocalcemia. A massive shift of calcium, magnesium, and phosphorus into bone can cause both serum calcium and serum phosphorus levels to be low, and this occurs mainly in patients with osteitis fibrosa cystica, who often display the hungry bone syndrome postoperatively. Magnesium, as well as calcium, may be needed to prevent or treat tetany during the first 48 to 96 hours after surgery. Hypocalcemia with hyperphosphatemia indicates temporary or permanent hypoparathyroidism; calcium supplements and vitamin D may be required on a chronic basis.

Postoperative phosphorus levels greater than 6 mg/dL strongly suggest permanent parathyroid gland damage.[186] Measurement of PTH can distinguish the cause of the hypocalcemia (i.e., low or undetectable in hypoparathyroidism and elevated in the hungry bone syndrome) and chart the subsequent course of recovery.[179]

Medical therapy may be used for patients deemed not to be surgical candidates. Dietary salt restriction reduces urine calcium excretion[203] and may be helpful in preventing stones in patients not having surgery. Estrogen or progestin therapy reduces serum Ca^{2+} levels and may slow bone loss in postmenopausal women with primary hyperparathyroidism.[204-207] Estrogens inhibit the action of PTH on bone but do not alter PTH secretion.[205, 206] However, recent concerns regarding the safety of hormone replacement therapy may limit use of estrogens, especially as some subjects may require high doses of estrogen to reduce serum Ca^{2+}.[208] Bisphosphonates, which inhibit osteoclast function, are effective in controlling hypercalcemia with short-term use.[209] When used chronically, bisphosphonates have been shown to improve bone mineral density during therapy lasting up to 2 years, without adverse effect.[210, 211] Hypercalciuria does not improve, and serum Ca^{2+} remains unchanged. There have been no studies of stone formation during treatment with bisphosphonates. The safety and efficacy of bisphosphonates in primary hyperparathyroidism beyond 2 to 3 years of treatment is not known. Recently, calcimimetic agents have been studied in the treatment of primary hyperparathyroidism. Calcimimetics are small organic molecules that increase the sensitivity of the calcium-sensing receptor to calcium. Calcimimetics have been shown to reduce serum PTH and Ca^{2+} in hyperparathyroidism.[212, 213] Calcimimetics have been used in humans for up to 6 months and appear to be well tolerated. Urine Ca^{2+} excretion remains unchanged during therapy, perhaps due to the activation of the renal calcium-sensing receptor in the loop of Henle. Calcimimetic agents have not yet been approved for clinical use.

EFFECT OF TREATMENT

After successful surgery, serum Ca^{2+} becomes normal and Ca^{2+} balance returns toward normal.[144-146] Gastrointestinal Ca^{2+} absorption decreases[146, 152] and hypercalciuria abates.[118, 144, 169] Cessation of hypercalciuria presumably accounts for the marked decrease in the rate of stone formation compared with that observed in the preoperative period.[169, 214, 215] It also results in a decline in calcium oxalate supersaturation from a CPR of 3.20 ± 0.56 to 1.53 ± 0.21 ($P < .05$) and an increase in the ULM for calcium oxalate from 7.19 ± 1.19 to 12.99 ± 1.69 ($P < .001$).[216] Pratley and colleagues[217] found 28 of their 54 patients well 1 to 10 years after successful parathyroidectomy; however, 8 of the 54 patients had residual renal disease in the form of persistent renal calculi, nephrocalcinosis, urinary tract infection, or increasing blood urea nitrogen (BUN). Britton and associates[218] found 20 of 52 patients well, but the remaining 32 had continued renal and stone disease; 9 developed elevated BUN or creatinine during postoperative follow-up. Parks and colleagues[169] observed recurrent stones in only 1 of 48 patients; this patient remained hypercalciuric despite curative parathyroidectomy. Silverberg and co-workers[120] had 20 patients with kidney stones in their series. The 12 patients who had parathyroidectomy did not have stone recurrence, whereas 6 of the 8 who did not have surgery had recurrence of their stones. Also noted was a marked improvement in bone mineral density in those undergoing surgery, with no change in bone mineral in those not having surgery.

Hypertension may accompany hyperparathyroidism, although the pathogenesis is not known.[118, 186] Britton and associates found that of 20 patients with hyperparathyroidism and hypertension, only 1 became normotensive following parathyroidectomy, and 17 of 33 who were normotensive before surgery developed hypertension in the follow-up period.[218] Patients with osteitis fibrosa appear to suffer more severe renal damage than those presenting with renal calculi alone.[215] However, renal damage in patients with nephrocalcinosis, as opposed to that in patients with calculi alone, was as severe as that in patients with osteitis fibrosa.[219]

Idiopathic Hypercalciuria

Between 30% and 50% of calcium stone formers excrete in their urine more Ca^{2+} than normal people customarily do, above 300 mg/24 hours (men), 250 mg/24 hours (women), or 4 mg/kg body weight/24 hours (either sex), and are therefore labeled hypercalciuric (see Table 39-5). Hypercalciuria is termed "idiopathic" if serum Ca^{2+} is normal and if sarcoidosis, RTA, hyperthyroidism, malignant tumors, rapidly

progressive bone disease, immobilization, Paget disease, Cushing disease (or syndrome), and furosemide administration—the usual causes of normocalcemic hypercalciuria—can be excluded. Virtually all normocalcemic hypercalciuria encountered in patients with nephrolithiasis is idiopathic.[110]

Idiopathic hypercalciuria has been shown clearly to have a genetic origin. In a study of the families of nine patients with idiopathic hypercalciuria and nephrolithiasis, hypercalciuria was documented in 19 of 44 first-degree relatives.[220] The pattern of inheritance in consecutive generations and at a high frequency within generations (Fig. 39-6) is compatible with an inherited trait that has the broad characteristics of autosomal dominant transmission. A similar pattern of inheritance was demonstrated in another large family.[221] However, both studies contain subjects who appear to be exceptions to an autosomal dominant inheritance. Goodman and co-workers[222] have reanalyzed these studies and propose that idiopathic hypercalciuria is a polygenic disorder with regulation by two codominant alleles. Idiopathic hypercalciuria has also been shown to occur in children at the same rate as that observed in adults.[223] Spontaneous hypercalciuria that resembles this condition in humans has been described in the laboratory rat,[224] and rats have been successfully bred for hypercalciuria.[225]

One distinct form of genetic hypercalciuria that has been fully characterized is Dent disease, otherwise known as X-linked recessive nephrolithiasis with renal failure.[226, 227] This syndrome includes defective proximal tubule reabsorption, progressive renal failure, nephrolithiasis, and nephrocalcinosis. Rickets has also been reported in some cases. Carrier females do not develop clinical disease but do excrete increased levels of low-molecular-weight proteins, suggesting there is a mild proximal tubule disorder in the carrier state. The gene responsible for the disease has been

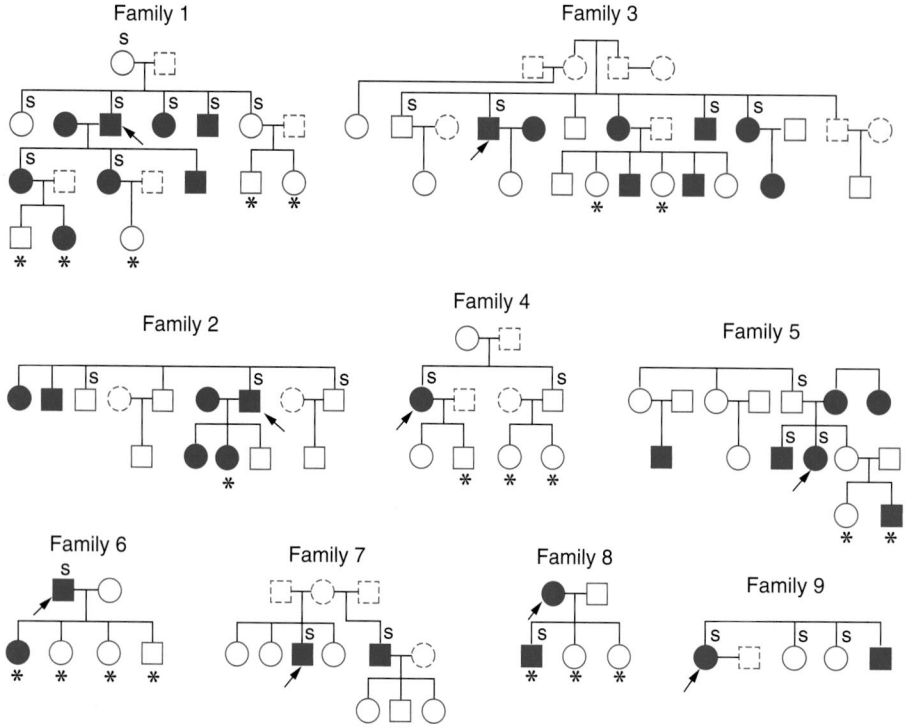

FIGURE 39-6. Family pedigrees of nine probands with idiopathic hypercalciuria. ○ and ■, family members with hypercalciuria; S, stone disease; *, children, defined here as younger than 20 years of age. *Arrows* indicate probands. Interrupted symbols represent relatives who were not studied but who are included to complete the pedigrees. Marginal hypercalciuria was present in four siblings, one each in families 1, 2, 3, and 5; in the mother of proband 4; in two aunts and one niece in family 5; and in one nephew in family 3. Altogether, hypercalciuria occurred in 11 of 24 siblings, 7 of 16 offspring, and 1 of 3 parents of the probands. (From Coe FL, Parks JH, Moore ES: Familial idiopathic hypercalciuria. N Engl J Med 300:337, 1979.)

localized to the short arm of the X chromosome and codes for a voltage-gated chloride channel, CLCN5.[228] A study of stone patients with routine idiopathic hypercalciuria did not reveal any subjects to have mutations in the CLCN5 channel, suggesting it is rarely involved in the pathogenesis of idiopathic hypercalciuria.[229]

Many candidate genes have been studied to determine their role in the pathogenesis of hypercalciuria. Two groups studied the calcium-sensing receptor in families of patients with hypercalciuria and found no association with the disease.[230, 231] Because hypercalciuria may be mediated through high vitamin D activity, the role of 1α-hydroxylase was studied. The investigators found no linkage to calcium excretion or serum calcitriol levels.[232] Vitamin D receptor (VDR) abnormalities could also lead to calcitriol overactivity. Multiple studies have looked for polymorphisms in the VDR gene. Linkage has been reported between stone-forming phenotype or calcium excretion and the VDR gene in some[233-236] but not all studies.[237] Reed and colleagues[238] have mapped a gene defect in idiopathic hypercalciuria to chromosome 1q23.3-q24. The gene apparently encodes a soluble adenylate cyclase.[239] They also report that mutations in the gene not only correlate with hypercalciuria but also with reduction in bone mineral density. Further study is required to determine the prevalence of mutations in this gene in a larger population of patients with idiopathic hypercalciuria.

The pathogenesis of idiopathic hypercalciuria involves excessive intestinal Ca^{2+} absorption and depressed renal tubule Ca^{2+} reabsorption. Excessive urine Ca^{2+} losses are offset by increased intestinal Ca^{2+} absorption, but not always completely; Ca^{2+} balance is negative in over half the patients, suggesting bone loss of Ca^{2+}.

Urine Ca^{2+} is increased without a rise in serum Ca^{2+}, implying that renal tubule Ca^{2+} reabsorption is depressed. Despite many attempts to assign primacy to the bowel, bone, or kidney, the issue is still unresolved.

Intestinal Calcium Absorption

Net Ca^{2+} absorption is the difference between the mucosal absorptive rate and the secretion of Ca^{2+} in biliary, duodenal, and pancreatic fluids. Absorption rates may be measured using oral radiolabeled calcium, but only overall balance studies, in which fecal losses are measured, can quantitate net Ca^{2+} absorption. The mucosal-to-serosal absorptive rate is higher in hypercalciuric than in normal subjects (Table 39-8).[240-246] In 10 studies, normal subjects absorbed an average of 27% to 52% of an oral dose of radioactive calcium, whereas 22% to 80% was absorbed by patients with idiopathic hypercalciuria. If one chooses only the six studies incorporating normal control subjects, the more efficient Ca^{2+} absorption by hypercalciuric subjects is particularly evident. Increased mucosa-to-blood transport of Ca^{2+} but not magnesium has been demonstrated directly by in vivo jejunal perfusion in idiopathic hypercalciuria.[247]

In normal subjects, urine Ca^{2+} excretion rises slowly with net absorption (Fig. 39-7) and Ca^{2+} balance is usually positive when absorption exceeds 200 mg/24 hours. Average net intestinal Ca^{2+} absorption for hypercalciuric patients is higher than in normal subjects, but overlap is extensive (Fig. 39-8).[248-255] At all levels of net absorption, urine Ca^{2+} excretion was higher in hypercalciuric than in normal subjects, so much so that none of the patient data fell within the 95% confidence band derived from studies of normal subjects. For example,

TABLE 39-8

Intestinal Calcium Absorption in Normal Subjects and Patients with Idiopathic Hypercalciuria

			DIETARY CALCIUM ABSORBED (%)*	
REFERENCE	**METHOD**	**CALCIUM INTAKE (mg/24 hr)**	**Normal Subjects**	**Idiopathic Hypercalciuria**
Caniggia et al.[240]	Fecal ^{45}Ca	Free diet†	None studied	22.0 (1)
Birge et al.[150]	^{47}Ca, PO/IV	800	52.2 ± 13.2 (6)	58.5 ± 8.6 (4)
Wills et al.[241]	^{47}Ca, PO/IV	400	49.0 ± 10.0 (4)	76.0 ± 17.0 (5)
Pak et al.[242]	Fecal ^{47}Ca	400	45.6 ± 9.0 (29)	69.7 ± 7.0 (9)
				58.1 ± 13.0 (11)‡
Pak et al.[242]	Fecal ^{47}Ca	400	50.0 ± 7.0 (20)	71.0 ± 7.0 (22)§
				50.0 ± 17.0 (2)‖
Ehrig et al.[243]	^{47}Ca/^{45}Ca, PO/IV	462-952	None studied	47.8 ± 11.0 (22)¶
				37.6 ± 11.0 (22)**
Kaplan et al.[154]	Fecal ^{47}Ca	400	48.0 ± 8.0 (11)	80.0 ± 9.0 (211)§
				73.0 ± 7.0 (3)‖
Shen et al.[244]	^{47}Ca/^{45}Ca, PO/IV	Free diet†	27.0 ± 9.0 (14)	40.0 ± 9.0 (15)
Barilla et al.[245]	Fecal ^{47}Ca	400	None studied	69.5 ± 6.4 (10)§
				70.1 ± 10.4 (8)‖
Zerwekh and Pak[246]	Fecal ^{47}Ca	400	None studied	69.0 ± 7.0 (11)§
				68.0 ± 9.0 (10)§

*Values are mean ± SD; numbers in parentheses represent numbers of patients studied.
†Usual diet but not measured.
‡Eleven patients listed as having normocalcemic primary hyperparathyroidism may be considered hypercalciuric.
§"Absorptive" idiopathic hypercalciuria.
‖"Renal" idiopathic hypercalciuria.
¶Before therapy.
**Three to 16 mo after administration of hydrochlorothiazide was begun.
IV, intravenously; PO, orally.

in the range of 200 to 300 mg of net Ca^{2+} absorption, not 1 of 38 normal subjects excreted as much as 300 mg of Ca^{2+} in their urine, whereas 15 of 16 hypercalciuric patients did (cf. Figs. 39-7 and 39-8). In other words, hypercalciuric patients excreted in their urine an abnormally high percentage of the Ca^{2+} they absorbed from the intestine. Net absorption exceeded 200 mg/24 hours in 55 normal subjects (see Fig. 39-7). Urine Ca^{2+} excretion was less than net absorption, that is, Ca^{2+} balance was positive, in 48. If we allow a generous margin for error (50 mg/24 hours) in the balance data, none of the 55 normal subjects were in negative Ca^{2+} balance. However, among 37 hypercalciuric patients with Ca^{2+} absorption above 200 mg/24 hours, Ca^{2+} excretion exceeded net absorption in 23 patients by more than 50 mg/24 hours (see Fig. 39-8). In other words, negative Ca^{2+} balance was frequent in idiopathic hypercalciuric patients but not in normal subjects.

Renal Tubule Calcium Reabsorption

Two systematic studies have been made of overall fractional Ca^{2+} reabsorption (Table 39-9).[256, 257] In both, the filtered load was calculated from inulin clearance or creatinine clearance and ultrafilterable serum Ca^{2+} concentration, and the fraction of filtered load excreted was calculated for several clearance periods in normal and hypercalciuric subjects. Fractional Ca^{2+} excretion was clearly high in the hypercalciuric subjects. Fractional Ca^{2+} excretion is dependent on sodium excretion in normal and hypercalciuric subjects, increasing as dietary sodium increases.[258, 259] The effects of hydrochlorothiazide and acetazolamide on the tubule handling of Na^+, Mg^{2+}, and Ca^{2+} in patients with fasting hypercalciuria suggest a generalized defect in proximal tubule reabsorption of fluid and electrolytes.[260] Bianchi and colleagues[261] have shown increased activity of Ca^{2+},Mg^{2+}-ATPase in red blood cells from patients with idiopathic hypercalciuria, as well as correlation between the enzyme activity and urine Ca^{2+} excretion in family studies. Ca^{2+},Mg^{2+}-ATPase is also present in the distal tubule and the intestine, suggesting that abnormalities in this enzyme activity may be involved in the pathogenesis of idiopathic hypercalciuria.

Bone Metabolism

There is an increasing body of evidence that the skeleton is involved in the pathogenesis of idiopathic hypercalciuria.

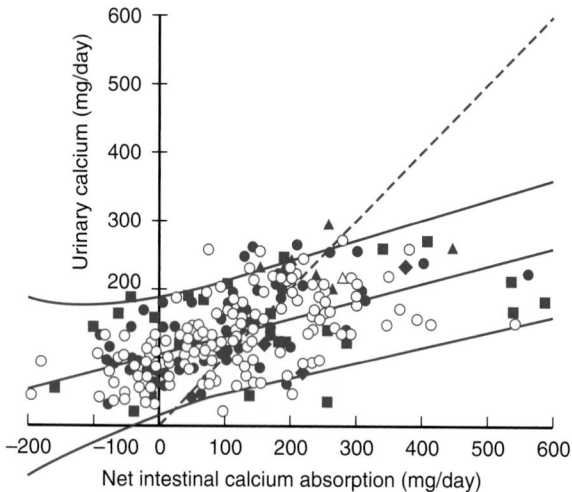

FIGURE 39-7. Urinary Ca^{2+} excretion as a function of net intestinal Ca^{2+} absorption. Data are derived from 6-day balance studies on 195 normal adults. Each symbol represents individual subjects from different sources: ○, Knapp[248]; □, Lafferty and Pearson[145]; ◇, Liberman et al.[249]; △, Edwards and Hodgkinson.[250] *Open symbols* are women and *solid symbols* are men. *Solid lines* represent mean and 2 SD. *Dotted line* is the line of identity; points above the line reflect negative Ca^{2+} balance.

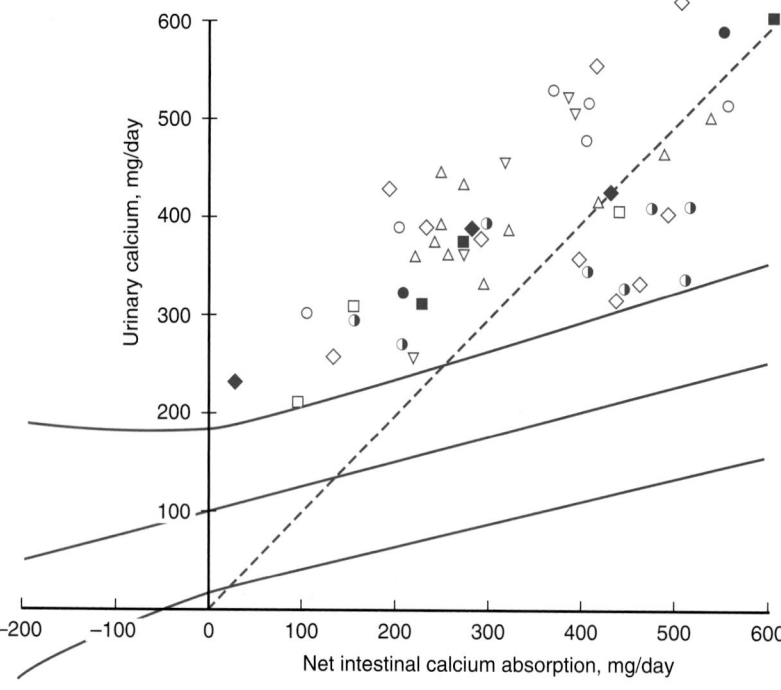

FIGURE 39-8. Urinary Ca^{2+} excretion as a function of net intestinal Ca^{2+} absorption from 6-day balance studies performed on 51 patients with idiopathic hypercalciuria reported as follows: ○, Nassim and Higgins[148]; □, Henneman et al.[251]; ■, Jackson and Dancaster[252]; ◆, Harrison[253]; ●, Dent et al.[254]; ▽, Parfitt et al.[255]; △, Edwards and Hodgkinson[250]; ◇, Liberman et al.[249]; ◖, Lemann (personal communication, 1978). *Solid lines* represent mean and 2 SD derived from balance studies from 195 normal adults, shown in Figure 39-7. *Dotted line* is the line of identity, with positive Ca^{2+} balance below the line.

Certainly, the high rate of negative Ca^{2+} balance in patients with idiopathic hypercalciuria implicates bone involvement, as chronic negative Ca^{2+} balance must involve bone mineral loss. A primary renal Ca^{2+} leak might explain this phenomenon in some patients as a secondary response to the PTH effect. However, negative Ca^{2+} balance is more common than the high-PTH, renal Ca^{2+}-leak subgroup of idiopathic hypercalciuria patients, indicating active involvement of bone in many patients with idiopathic hypercalciuria. Multiple studies have shown that bone mineral density is lower in stone formers than in normal subjects (Table 39-10).[262-265] A variety of methods have been used, all showing at least some subgroup with decreased bone mineral density, even studies that included normocalciuric calcium stone formers.[262, 263] Lawoyin and associates[266] separated the patients into renal leak and absorptive hypercalciuria subgroups and noted low bone mineral density in only those with a renal Ca^{2+} leak. However, Bataille and colleagues[267] found low bone mineral density in idiopathic hypercalciuric patients, including patients with type I absorptive hypercalciuria. Pietschmann and co-workers[268] found reduced vertebral bone mineral density in both absorptive and renal hypercalciuria as compared to normocalciuric stone formers. Radial bone density was the same in all groups. Some of the differences between studies may be due to variations in defining patient subgroups.

Bone turnover has been shown to be increased in idiopathic hypercalciuria. Urinary hydroxyproline is increased in unselected patients with idiopathic hypercalciuria,[269] whereas serum osteocalcin levels were found to be high in patients with renal leak hypercalciuria, but not absorptive hypercalciuria.[270] Bone turnover studies using ^{47}Ca show that idiopathic hypercalciuric patients have increased rates of bone formation and resorption.[249] Bone histology has also been shown to be abnormal.[271, 272] Malluche and co-workers[272] studied 15 patients with absorptive hypercalciuria and found reduced bone matrix apposition and delay of secondary mineralization of osteoid seams. Steinche and colleagues[271] studied 33 idiopathic hypercalciuric patients and found a prolonged mineralization lag time and prolonged formation period, which suggested a mineralization defect, possibly secondary to mild hypophosphatemia.

We have recently published a study linking the stone-forming phenotype to urine Ca^{2+} excretion and bone mineral density.[273] By studying families of hypercalciuric stone formers we were able to include subjects with and without stones and with and without hypercalciuria. In our multivariate analysis we found stone formers had lower amounts of calcium in their diet, yet had the same calcium excretion rate as the non–stone formers. Bone mineral density decreased with increasing urine Ca^{2+} excretion and ammonium excretion in the stone formers, but this association was not found in the non–stone-forming subjects. It appears that stone formers have bones that are primed for demineralization, and

TABLE 39-9

Fraction of Filtered Calcium Excreted in the Urine by Normal and Hypercalciuric Subjects*

REFERENCE	NORMAL SUBJECTS	HYPERCALCIURIC SUBJECTS[†]
Edwards and Hodgkinson[256]	0.94% (7)	2.94% (14) $P < .001$
Peacock and Nordin[257]	1.27% (5)	4.25% (9) $P < .01$

*Number of subjects studied is shown in parentheses next to fractional excretion values.

[†]Urinary Ca^{2+} excretion greater than 300 mg/24 hr (men) or 250 mg/24 hr (women).

TABLE 39-10

Bone Mineral Density and Histology in Patients with Nephrolithiasis

STUDY	METABOLIC DISORDER	NUMBER OF PATIENTS	BONE AREA STUDIED	TECHNIQUE	RESULTS
Lawoyin et al.[266]	RH	44	Distal radius	^{125}Photon absorption	% Normal = 92.5, $P < .001$*
	AH	117			% Normal = 99.8, P NS
Malluche et al.[272]	AH	15	Iliac crest biopsy	Quantitative Histomorphometry	Increased unmineralized osteoid, reduced matrix protein
Barkin et al.[262]	SF	109	Trunk, thighs	Neutron activation	CBI 0.91 ± 0.13, $P < .01$ vs.
	N	115			normal CBI 0.96 ± 0.13
Borghi et al.[264]	DH	20	Vertebral bone	Dual photon absorption	z = −0.3 ± 1.19, P NS[‡]
	DIH	21			z = −1.26 ± 1.18, $P < .02$
Bataille et al.[267]	DH	18	Vertebral bone	Computed tomographic densitometry	% Normal = 91, P NS
	DIH	24			% Normal = 69, $P < .01$
Steinche et al.[271]	IH	33	Iliac crest biopsy	Quantitative Histomorphometry	Increased mineralization lag time, reduced appositional rate
Alhava et al.[263]	MSF	54	Distal radius	γ-Ray attenuation	% Normal = 95.5, $P < .005$
	FSF	21			% Normal = 94.5, $P < .05$
Zanchetta et al.[265]	FRH	23	Vertebral bone	Dual photon absorption	% Normal = 83.8, $P < .0001$
	MRH	15			% Normal = 81.9, $P < .0001$
	FAH	7			% Normal = 83.6, $P < .001$
	MAH	5			% Normal = 94.9, $P < .001$

*% Normal is the bone mineral density in the study population expressed as a percentage of a normal control population.

[†]Results normalized for age and sex using Z scores (value measured minus the mean from age and sex matched normal subjects divided by the standard deviation).

AH, absorptive hypercalciuria; CBI, calcium bone index; DH, dietary hypercalciuria; DIH, dietary independent hypercalciuria; FAH, female absorptive hypercalciuria; FRH, female renal hypercalciuria; FSF, female stone formers; IH, idiopathic hypercalciuria; MAH, male absorptive hypercalciuria; MRH, male renal hypercalciuria; MSF, male stone formers; N, normal; NS, not significant; RH, renal hypercalciuria; SF, unselected stone formers.

dietary factors such as low-calcium and high-acid content provide the driving force.

Models of Hypercalciuria

There are a number of pathophysiologic mechanisms that have been proposed as the etiology of idiopathic hypercalciuria. Kidney, gut, skeleton, PTH, and vitamin D have all been implicated, and certainly no single theory can explain the etiology in every patient, as there are small numbers of patients with clearly defined abnormalities, such as renal phosphate leak or renal Ca^{2+} leak. However, the question of which mechanism is operative in the majority of patients is still a matter of debate.

RENAL VERSUS ABSORPTIVE HYPERCALCIURIA. In general, patients with idiopathic hypercalciuria have been separated into two groups, primary intestinal Ca^{2+} overabsorption or a primary renal tubule Ca^{2+} leak, either of which could produce the findings summarized in Tables 39-8 and 39-9 and in Figures 39-7 and 39-8. Primary intestinal overabsorption would tend to raise postprandial serum Ca^{2+} levels above normal and thereby increase the filtered load of Ca^{2+} (Fig. 39-9, left panel). PTH secretion would be reduced by the hypercalcemia. Since PTH normally stimulates renal tubule Ca^{2+} reabsorption (see Chapter 22), suppression of PTH secretion could reduce Ca^{2+} reabsorption. Hypercalciuria would occur because of decreased reabsorption. A renal leak (see Fig. 39-9, right panel) would cause hypercalciuria. Secondary hyperparathyroidism, from excessive urine Ca^{2+} losses, would stimulate production of $1,25(OH)_2D_3$ and produce intestinal hyperabsorption. Hyperabsorption would elevate postprandial serum Ca^{2+} levels, raise the filtered load, and decrease the magnitude of the secondary hyperparathyroidism. The only way of distinguishing one mechanism from the other is by testing specific predictions, which differ for the two hypothetical models of hypercalciuria. Certain of these predictions are listed in Table 39-11.

Fasting iPTH, urinary Ca^{2+} per gram creatinine or the Ca^{2+}/creat ratio, and cAMP are interrelated and must be considered together. The overabsorption model permits low or normal fasting iPTH (see Fig. 39-9). If repeated bursts of postprandial hypercalcemia were to cause chronic

hypoparathyroidism, fasting iPTH and urine cAMP would be low and the urine Ca^{2+}/creat ratio high (see Table 39-11). If PTH secretion were suppressed only transiently after calcium ingestion, all three fasting measurements would be normal. The absorptive hypothesis predicts a spectrum of fasting values, but it forbids the combination of an elevated fasting urine Ca^{2+}/creat ratio with normal iPTH. The renal model requires an elevated fasting urine Ca^{2+}/creat ratio and a high serum iPTH. Urine cAMP excretion should also be elevated.

High PTH values have been reported in some patients[274, 275] as the renal model demands (see Fig. 39-9, right panel). The question of whether fasting PTH levels are reduced in some patients with idiopathic hypercalciuria is more difficult to answer because assays for PTH vary from one study to another, and many of the assays used had limited ability to detect low levels.[244, 267, 274, 276] Bataille and associates[267]

TABLE 39-11

Predictions of Absorptive and Renal Models of Idiopathic Hypercalciuria

PARAMETER	ABSORPTIVE MODEL	RENAL MODEL
Fasting values		
Serum iPTH	Low or normal	High
Urinary Ca^{2+}	High or normal	High
Urinary cAMP	Low or normal	High
Serum $1,25(OH)_2D_3$	Uncertain	High
Response to thiazide		
Serum iPTH	± Fall	Fall
Urinary Ca^{2+}	Fall	Fall
Ca^{2+} absorption	No fall	Fall
Serum $1,25(OH)_2D_3$	Uncertain	Fall
Response to low-calcium diet		
Serum iPTH	Increase or no change	Increase
Urinary Ca^{2+}	Normal	High
Ca^{2+} balance	Positive or neutral	Negative or neutral
Ca^{2+} excreted ÷ absorbed	Normal	High
Risk of parathyroid adenoma	Normal	High

cAMP, cyclic adenosine monophosphate; iPTH, immunoreactive parathyroid hormone.

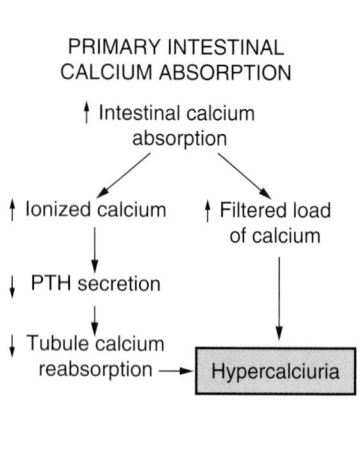

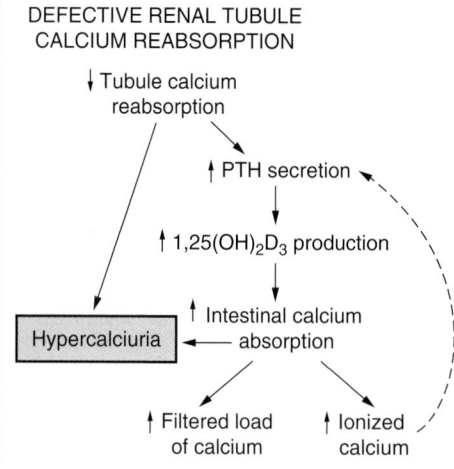

PRIMARY INTESTINAL CALCIUM ABSORPTION

↑ Intestinal calcium absorption

↑ Ionized calcium

↑ Filtered load of calcium

↓ PTH secretion

↓ Tubule calcium reabsorption → Hypercalciuria

DEFECTIVE RENAL TUBULE CALCIUM REABSORPTION

↓ Tubule calcium reabsorption

↑ PTH secretion

↑ $1,25(OH)_2D_3$ production

↑ Intestinal calcium absorption

Hypercalciuria

↑ Filtered load of calcium

↑ Ionized calcium

FIGURE 39-9. Proposed pathogenesis for two alternative models of idiopathic hypercalciuria. *Left*, primary intestinal overabsorption. *Right*, primary defective tubule Ca^{2+} reabsorption. *Dotted line* indicates mechanisms tending to restore PTH secretion toward normal.

studied 42 patients with idiopathic hypercalciuria, using an intact PTH assay. They found only 1 of 16 patients with fasting hypercalciuria with an elevated PTH. The 26 patients with absorptive hypercalciuria had PTH levels that were not different from normals. In most studies of idiopathic hypercalciuric patients, renal leak hypercalciuria is found in the minority of patients. The response of urine Ca^{2+} to a low-calcium diet or cellulose phosphate, a Ca^{2+}-binding ion-exchange resin, has been described by Pak[277, 278] and Bordier[275] and their colleagues. Both groups found a marked fall in absorptive hypercalciuria and, in fact, used this response—along with serum PTH—to classify the patients as absorptive. By hypothesis, urine Ca^{2+} must remain elevated in renal hypercalciuria despite low calcium intake. Bordier[275] and Pak[277, 278] and their colleagues observed this in patients with high PTH, but the data are few.

Pak and associates[279] have developed a simplified outpatient protocol to distinguish between renal and absorptive hypercalciuria. Patients are studied after 7 days of a low-calcium diet (400 mg calcium, 100 mEq NaCl per day). On the last day of the diet, a 24-hour urine sample is collected. At the end of the study diet, urine Ca^{2+} excretion is measured in the fasting state and after a 1-g oral calcium load. Renal hypercalciuria is defined as elevated fasting urine Ca^{2+} (>0.11 mg/100 mL glomerular filtration), and iPTH. Absorptive hypercalciuria type I is defined as normal fasting urine Ca^{2+}, high urinary Ca^{2+} excretion after the oral Ca^{2+} load, hypercalciuria on the calcium-restricted diet, and normal iPTH. Absorptive hypercalciuria type II is the same as type I except for normal urinary Ca^{2+} excretion on the calcium-restricted diet. In a study of

241 consecutive stone-forming patients, Pak and co-workers[279] found 24% had type I absorptive hypercalciuria, 30% had type II, and only 8% had a renal Ca^{2+} leak.

CALCITRIOL EXCESS. When evaluated by the method of Pak and associates, the majority of idiopathic hypercalciuric patients fall into the absorptive group.[278, 279] However, intestinal hyperabsorption does not predict the high incidence of negative Ca^{2+} balance seen in idiopathic hypercalciuric patients. An alternative hypothesis is that of vitamin D excess activity, a situation that would lead to intestinal overabsorption, increased bone resorption, and reduced renal Ca^{2+} reabsorption.

Two studies in normal men have reproduced the clinical characteristics of idiopathic hypercalciuria by the administration of calcitriol. In one report, normal men were studied on a very low-calcium diet (4.2 mmol/day) with and without calcitriol supplementation.[280] Calcitriol supplementation did not result in hypercalcemia. Urine Ca^{2+} and intestinal Ca^{2+} absorption were significantly increased in the men taking calcitriol. Calcium balance was more negative in the men taking calcitriol, indicating bone resorption as the source of Ca^{2+} loss. In a second study,[281] normal men were studied on normal (22 mmol/day) and low-normal (9 mmol/day) calcium diets, on and off calcitriol supplementation. Intestinal Ca^{2+} absorption and urine Ca^{2+} excretion increased during calcitriol therapy but Ca^{2+} balance was unchanged. These two studies are summarized in Figure 39-10. Thus, elevated calcitriol increases urine Ca^{2+} and intestinal Ca^{2+} absorption but only leads to negative Ca^{2+} balance with extreme Ca^{2+} restriction, findings similar to those in most idiopathic

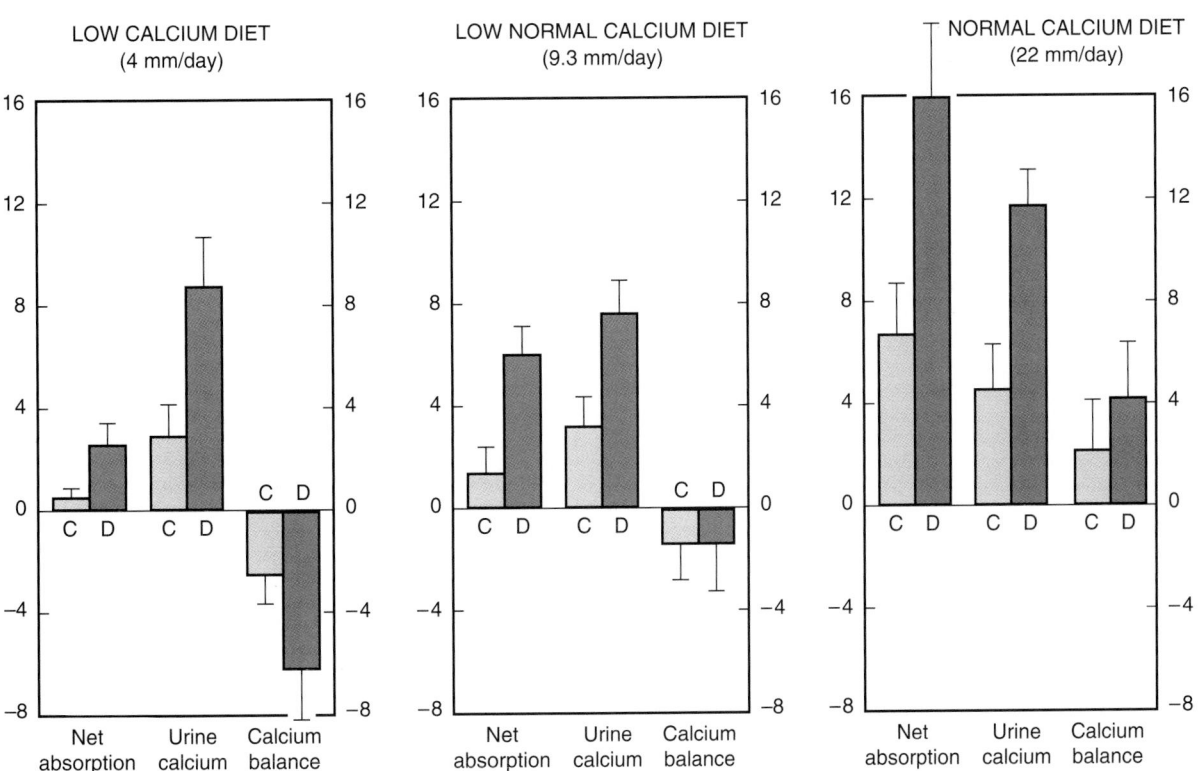

FIGURE 39-10. Intestinal Ca^{2+} absorption, urinary Ca^{2+} excretion, and Ca^{2+} balance in normal men receiving calcitriol (*dark blue bars*) and in control subjects (*gray bars*) at varying levels of calcuim intake. (From Coe FL, Parks JH: Nephrolithiasis: Pathogenesis and Treatment, 2nd ed. Chicago, Year Book Medical Publishers, 1988, p 113. By permission of Mosby–Year Book.)

TABLE 39-12

Serum 1,25(OH)₂D₃ Levels in Normal Subjects and Patients with Idiopathic Hypercalciuria

REFERENCE	SERUM CALCIUM (mg/dL)		SERUM PHOSPHORUS (mg/dL)		SERUM, 1,25(OH)₂D₃ (ng/dL)	
	Normal Subjects	Idiopathic Hypercalciuria Subjects	Normal Subjects	Idiopathic Hypercalciuria Subjects	Normal Subjects	Idiopathic Hypercalciuria Subjects
Shen et al.[244]	10.2 ± 0.2(8)*	10.2 ± 0.5(7)	3.8 ± 0.5	2.6 ± 0.3	3.2 ± 0.4	5.8 ± 2.3
Haussler et al.[283]	—	—	3.8 ± 0.5(18)	2.6 ± 0.4(18)	3.3 ± 0.8	5.2 ± 1.9
Kaplan et al.[154]	9.7 ± 0.5(11)	9.6 ± 0.1(3)†	3.7 ± 0.7	3.6 ± 0.1†	3.4 ± 0.9	6.9 ± 2.3†
	—	9.4 ± 0.3(21)‡		3.7 ± 0.5‡	—	4.5 ± 1.1‡
Gray et al.[160]	9.6 ± 0.3(48)	9.6 ± 0.4(26)	4.0 ± 0.6	3.5 ± 0.6	3.6 ± 1.2	6.2 ± 3.1
Shen et al.[244]	10.0 ± 0.3(15)	9.9 ± 0.3(16)	3.7 ± 0.3	2.9 ± 0.6	3.4 ± 0.7	5.4 ± 1.9
Zerwekh and Pak[246]	—	9.6 ± 0.5(11)‡	—	3.5 ± 0.3‡	—	4.5 ± 1.4‡
		9.7 ± 0.4(10)†		3.5 ± 0.6†		5.2 ± 2.2†
Broadus et al.[284]	9.4 ± 0.2(25)	9.5 ± 0.3(50)	—	—	4.7 ± 1.4	7.7 ± 1.2
Bataille et al.[267]	9.6 ± 0.4(12)	9.5 ± 0.4(24)	3.1 ± 0.3	3.0 ± 0.3	5.0 ± 1.4	6.9 ± 2.4
Coe et al.[285]	9.2 ± 0.6(9)	9.3 ± 0.4(24)	—	—	3.5 ± 0.6	4.1 ± 0.7

*Values are mean ± SD; numbers in parentheses represent numbers of subjects.

†Renal idiopathic hypercalciuria.

‡Absorptive idiopathic hypercalciuria.

hypercalciuric patients. Breslau and associates[282] studied 19 patients with absorptive hypercalciuria, using ketaconazole to suppress calcitriol production. Intestinal Ca^{2+} absorption was measured using ^{47}Ca. Twelve of the 19 subjects reduced Ca^{2+} absorption and urinary Ca^{2+} excretion significantly; the other seven showed no response despite an equal degree of vitamin D suppression as the responders. These findings support the theory that a significant proportion of idiopathic hypercalciuric patients have a disorder of vitamin D regulation as the cause of their disease.

Multiple studies have reported serum 1,25(OH)₂D₃ levels in hypercalciuric and normal subjects (Table 39-12).[244, 283-285] In hypercalciuric patients the 1,25(OH)₂D₃ levels, in general, are above normal. Some studies[154, 246, 286] have separated patients into renal leak and absorptive hypercalciuria groups with higher levels seen in the apparent renal hypercalciuria group. Even in the absence of elevated vitamin D levels, excess calcitriol activity may occur, as has been shown in rats inbred for hypercalciuria. They have high levels of VDR and normal levels of vitamin D, but overabsorb dietary calcium and become hypercalciuric.[287] In a study of patients with absorptive hypercalciuria, peripheral blood monocyte VDR levels were the same as in normal subjects, though 6 of 22 patients clearly had elevated levels.[288] This finding suggests there mey be a subset of hypercalciuric patients with pathophysiology similar to that seen in the rat model. Further work by the same investigators compared restriction length polymorphism of alleles of the VDR gene in normal subjects and patients with absorptive hypercalciuria and found no evidence of the human disease being linked to a common VDR phenotype,[237] nor were mutations in the VDR found. As noted above, some investigators have found some VDR polymorphisms to segregate with the stone-forming phenotype.[233-236]

RENAL PHOSPHATE LEAK. Hypophosphatemia secondary to excess renal phosphate losses stimulates 1,25(OH)₂D₃ production, producing hypercalciuria similar to that of primary 1,25(OH)₂D₃ overproduction. This pattern of abnormalities has been shown in a large kindred from a Bedouin tribe.[289] In a study of 59 members, 9 had the characteristic syndrome of hypophosphatemic rickets, hypercalciuria, and markedly elevated levels of 1,25(OH)₂D₃. Of the remaining 50 asymptomatic members of the tribe, 21 had "idiopathic hypercalciuria," with serum phosphate levels and calcitriol levels between those of normal members of the tribe and the patients with hypophosphatemic rickets. It appears that the magnitude of the hypophosphatemia, through control of 1,25(OH)₂D₃ production, determines which subjects will have isolated hypercalciuria and which will have hypercalciuria and rickets. These findings indicate that a mild renal phosphate leak could produce the syndrome of idiopathic hypercalciuria.

The role of phosphate depletion in idiopathic hypercalciuria in a genral stone-forming population has been studied in a group of stone formers with absorptive hypercalciuria and hypophosphatemia during outpatient evaluation.[290] Serum phosphorus became normal, however, when the patients were studied as inpatients on a controlled diet. Three patients remained hypophosphatemic despite a controlled diet and had elevated levels of serum 1,25(OH)₂D₃; however, after 2 months of phosphate therapy, serum 1,25(OH)₂D₃ was reduced to normal, yet intestinal Ca^{2+} absorption remained elevated. The low phosphorus level observed in the outpatient setting probably reflected a high spontaneous phosphate intake rather than an intrinsic disorder of phosphorus metabolism in all but three patients, and even in these three patients hypophosphatemia could not be linked definitively to the pathogenesis of increased intestinal Ca^{2+} absorption. Though renal phosphate wasting can cause hypercalciuria, it seems to be a relatively uncommon disorder. A recent study of hypercalciuric patients with hypophosphatemia showed that 2 of the 20 subjects studied had a mutation in the gene coding the proximal tubule Na^+/PO_4^{3-} cotransporter which reduced activity of the transporter.[291]

An Attempt at Synthesis

Certainly there is controversy about the studies of the mechanism of idiopathic hypercalciuria. The incidence of any given subtype of hypercalciuria varies from one study to the next.

Some of this may reflect the genetic heterogeneity of the populations studied, but often it is due to the criteria and conditions used to analyze the patients. PTH measurements have been made with a variety of antibodies, but only recently, with the introduction of the intact molecule assay, have low levels been reliably measured. Some of the earlier studies, in which categorization of patients depended on the ability to distinguish low from normal iPTH, may not be accurate. Bataille and co-workers,[267] using an intact PTH assay, found over one third of their hypercalciuric patients unclassifiable by the criteria of Pak and associates[279] as they had high fasting Ca^{2+} with normal PTH levels. Studies of calcitriol supplementation in normal men show that calcitriol excess may cause fasting hypercalciuria,[280] as well as intestinal hyperabsorption, blurring the distinction between renal and absorptive hypercalciuria. In addition, a link has been shown between calcitriol levels and dietary calcium intake in hypercalciuric patients who have high intestinal absorption of Ca^{2+}.[292] However, the calcitriol levels also depend on the length of time on any set calcium intake, making it difficult to compare studies of patients on fixed diets, unless the diets are used for similar lengths of time.

Separation of patients into absorptive and renal leak hypercalciuria groups gave promise of allowing therapy aimed at correcting the underlying pathophysiology. However, the high rate of negative Ca^{2+} balance found in many hypercalciuric patients suggests that simple intestinal overabsorption cannot be the cause in the majority of patients, but rather some form of excess calcitriol activity. The commonly used outpatient evaluations cannot adequately separate these disorders.[279] Prescribing a low-calcium diet for patients with excess calcitriol activity would increase the risk of bone disease.[293] Additional studies are needed to further clarify the role of kidney, intestine, bone, PTH, and calcitriol in the pathogenesis of idiopathic hypercalciuria. Certainly, some marker of calcitriol activity, in addition to calcitriol levels, is needed to clarify the pathogenesis of this disorder.

Treatment

Hypotheses about pathogenesis, particularly the question of primacy, affect the choice of treatment or at least the conviction that a particular treatment is suitable. If primary intestinal overabsorption is saturating the blood with Ca^{2+}, and the kidney is acting as a protective escape port—albeit at the price of an oversaturated urine—a low calcium diet or drugs that reduce Ca^{2+} absorption are appropriate. In contrast, thiazide therapy, but not calcium restriction, is rational for renal hypercalciuria and, presumably, superior to a low-calcium diet, in states of $1,25(OH)_2D_3$ excess. Unfortunately, identifying the pathogenesis of any single patient's hypercalciuria is not easily done, restricting the ability of the practicing physician to carefully tailor therapy.

DIET

A low-calcium diet has long been advocated for the treatment of hypercalciuric stone disease and has been shown to be effective in reducing urine Ca^{2+} excretion.[279] Two large prospective trials showed low dietary calcium intake correlated with a higher risk of new-onset kidney stone disease in both men and women.[294, 295] Though these studies do not

address the treatment of stone formers or provide a mechanism to explain the stone disease, the strong inverse correlation between stone disease and calcium intake calls into question the role of low-calcium diets. One proposed mechanism for this phenomenon is that a low-calcium diet may increase the intestinal absorption of oxalate, reducing the effectiveness of this therapy. No well-controlled studies of dietary calcium restriction have been performed to show the efficacy of stone reduction, though open trials have reported reduction of stone formation of 29% to 47% with dietary manipulation alone.[296, 297] However, the low bone mineral density found in hypercalciuric patients[262, 264, 266, 267] and negative Ca^{2+} balance seen with calcitriol excess[280] makes calcium restriction a potentially dangerous therapy. Idiopathic hypercalciuric patients treated with low-calcium diets have shown bone mineral losses similar to those seen in patients with hyperparathyroidism.[293] Even patients classified as having absorptive hypercalciuria can develop low bone mineral density.[268] Certainly, calcium gluttony should be avoided, but calcium restriction is a therapy which must be used with caution.

Dietary sodium restriction reduces urine Ca^{2+} excretion by reducing GFR and increasing distal Ca^{2+} reabsorption.[258, 259] Salt restriction has been shown to be effective in reducing Ca^{2+} excretion in patients with idiopathic hypercalciuria. In addition, high-salt intake appears to lower urine citrate, another deleterious effect on stone risk.[298] High-protein intake also increases urine Ca^{2+} excretion and causes negative Ca^{2+} balance,[299, 300] so dietary protein restriction would seem to be a prudent recommendation. However, a randomized trial of a low-protein, high-fiber diet in kidney stone formers failed to show a reduction of stone formation.[301]

A recent study by Borghi and colleagues[302] compared the effectiveness of a low-calcium diet to a low-sodium, low-protein, normal-calcium diet. One hundred twenty male hypercalciuric recurrent calcium stone formers were randomized to either a low-calcium (400 mg/day) diet with no sodium or protein restriction or a 1200-mg calcium, low-sodium, low-protein diet. The patients were followed for 5 years. Diet therapy led to a significant reduction in urine Na^+ and urea nitrogen excretion in the patients treated with the low-salt, low-protein diet, showing that the patients were reasonably compliant with the diet. Urine Ca^{2+} excretion fell a similar amount in both diet groups but urine oxalate increased in the low-calcium diet group and decreased in the high-calcium, low-sodium, low-protein diet group (Fig. 39-11). The net effect was that urine calcium oxalate supersaturation fell significantly in the normal-calcium, low-sodium, low-protein diet group. Stone recurrence was significantly lower in the normal-calcium diet group. This study did not directly test the effectiveness of a low-calcium diet in preventing stones as there was no control group without intervention. However, the study did show that urine Ca^{2+} can be reduced by dietary methods other than calcium restriction and produce lower stone rates than a low-calcium diet without the risk of bone demineralization.

As with any type of stone, high-water intake is always the cornerstone of the therapeutic regimen. Increasing urine flow rates lowers urine supersaturation of all stone-forming salts and has been shown to increase the ULM of calcium oxalate.[303] A prospective randomized trial of high-fluid intake has shown greater than a 50% reduction of stone

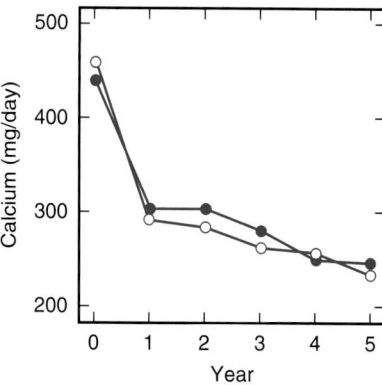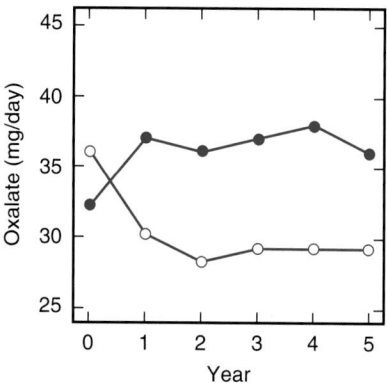

FIGURE 39-11. The effects of a low-calcium diet vs. a normal-calcium, low-sodium, low-protein diet on urine chemistries. In a 5-year randomized prospective study of the effects of dietary intervention on stone formation, patients treated with a normal-calcium, low-sodium, low-protein diet (*open symbols*) had a similar reduction in urine calcium compared with patients given a low-calcium diet (*closed symbols*). However, the subjects on the low-calcium diet had an increase in urine oxalate, whereas those on the normal-calcium, low-sodium, low-protein diet had a decrease in urine calcium. (Data from Borghi L, Schianchi T, Meschi T, et al: Comparison of two diets for the prevention of recurrent stones in idiopathic hypercalciuria. N Engl J Med 346:77-84, 2002.)

recurrence over 5 years.[304] The treated patients reduced their stone risk by increasing 24-hour urine volume to 2.0 to 2.5 L.

CELLULOSE PHOSPHATE

Cellulose phosphate is a Ca^{2+}-binding ion-exchange resin that has been recommended for the treatment of absorptive hypercalciuria. Pak and associates [277] have presented a careful study of 16 patients with severe recurrent calcium phosphate or calcium oxalate stone disease. Although the treatment interval was short, new stones formed during cellulose phosphate treatment were only 7.1% of the number predicted by multiplying the pretreatment recurrence rate, 376 stones per 100 patients per year, by the 41 patient-years of follow-up. It is not certain that equally good results can be obtained in treatment of the more common calcium oxalate stone former. Although cellulose phosphate lowers urine Ca^{2+} markedly, it induces a reciprocal increase in oxalate excretion. In one study, oxalate excretion rose from 30.1 to 60.3 mg/24 hours,[305] and the hyperoxaluria offset the hypocalciuria, so that the mean APR for calcium oxalate fell only 20%, from 2.75 to 2.19. In contrast, the mean APR for calcium phosphate fell dramatically, to less than 1.0 in the 16 patients treated by Pak and associates.[277] Others have confirmed the development of hyperoxaluria in response to cellulose phosphate.[306] One would expect such a drug to prevent calcium phosphate stones, although calcium oxalate stone disease might respond less impressively. The high frequency of negative Ca^{2+} balance in unselected, untreated patients with idiopathic hypercalciuria raises the same concern of bone mineral loss that may complicate low-calcium diets.

THIAZIDE DIURETICS

Thiazide inhibits NaCl but not Ca^{2+} reabsorption in the loop of Henle.[307] Overall, external Na^+ balance becomes normal after a few days of treatment, presumably because delivery of NaCl from more proximal nephron segments falls. Calcium delivery may also fall, leading to decreased urine Ca^{2+} excretion. Thiazide directly stimulates Ca^{2+} reabsorption by the distal convoluted tubule of the rat[308] and may also

have this influence in humans. The studies of the effect of thiazides on intestinal Ca^{2+} transport have shown mixed results, decreasing Ca^{2+} absorption in some patients, but causing no change in others.[148, 243, 245, 246, 309] Two studies from Pak's laboratory[245, 246] showed that hydrochlorothiazide reduced intestinal Ca^{2+} absorption in patients with high-PTH, presumably renal, hypercalciuria, but failed to alter Ca^{2+} absorption in patients with the absorptive form. In contrast, Ehrig and associates[243] showed that Ca^{2+} absorption fell from 59% to 42% in nine hypercalciuric patients with intestinal Ca^{2+} hyperabsorption treated with thiazide. Reduction in urine excretion in the setting of unchanged Ca^{2+} absorption indicates the subject must be in positive Ca^{2+} balance.

Whether thiazide does or does not change intestinal Ca^{2+} absorption, it is likely that thiazide therapy improves Ca^{2+} balance. Coe and associates[309] did formal Ca^{2+} balance studies in seven hypercalciuric patients before and after 6 months of treatment with chlorthalidone. Intestinal Ca^{2+} absorption decreased but Ca^{2+} balance increased because urine Ca^{2+} fell more than intestinal absorption. Studies have indicated that thiazide use in the hypertensive population increases bone mineral[310] and reduces the risk of hip fracture in the elderly.[311] Steiniche and colleagues[312] studied hypercalciuric patients before and 6 months after treatment with hydrochlorothiazide, using histomorphometric analysis of iliac crest biopsies. They found reduced bone turnover during treatment and reduced osteoid thickness, indicating improved mineralization during thiazide therapy.

Thiazide diuretics are the best studied of the treatment interventions for hypercalciuric stone formers. There have been numerous open trials which have suggested the efficacy of thiazides in the treatment of calcium stones. Supersaturation of calcium salts has been shown to fall in response to thiazide therapy as urine Ca^{2+} excretion falls; oxalate excretion is not affected. There have now been seven randomized studies of thiazide-type diuretics in the treatment of recurrent calcium oxalate nephrolithiasis. Although these studies have been reported to show conflicting results, the conflicts are related to the duration of therapy (Table 39-13). The two 1-year trials[313, 314] showed no difference between the

TABLE 39-13

Summary of Seven Randomized Trials of Thiazide Diuretics for Prevention of Calcium Nephrolithiasis

STUDY	DRUG DOSE	NUMBER OF SUBJECTS	YEAR 1			YEAR 2			YEAR 3			P-VALUE AT END OF STUDY
			Drug	Placebo	D/P*	Drug	Placebo	D/P	Drug	Placebo	D/P	
Laerum & Larsen[315]	HCTZ, 25 mg bid	50	18%[†]	30%	0.6	24%	55%	0.43	26%	58%	0.44	$P = .04$
Ettinger et al.[316]	CTD, 25 or 50 mg qd	73	10%	20%	0.5	10%	48%	0.21	20%	50%	0.4	$P < .05$
Mortensen et al.[318]	BFMT, 2.5 mg tid	22	—	—	—	0%	40%	0	—	—	—	$0.05 < P < .1$
Ohkawa et al.[319]	TCM, 4 mg qd	175	—	—	—	8%	14%	0.57	—	—	—	$0.05 < P < .1$
Scholz[313]	HCTZ, 25 mg bid	51	24%	23%	1.04	—	—	—	—	—	—	NS
Brocks[314]	BFMT, 2.5 mg tid	62	15%	17%	0.88	—	—	—	—	—	—	NS
Borghi et al.[317]	Ind 2.5 mg qd	50	15.8%	34%	0.46	15.8%	40%	0.39	15.8%	42.8%	0.37	$P < .02$

*Ratio of drug-treated to placebo-treated subjects with recurrence of stones.

[†]Percent of subjects with recurrence of stones.

BFMT, bendroflumethiazide; bid, twice daily; CTD, chlorthalidone; HCTZ, hydrochlorothiazide; Ind, indapamide; NS, not significant; qd, every day; TCM, trichlormethiazide; tid, three times per day.

placebo and thiazide groups. The three 3-year studies[315-317] showed significant reduction in the number of patients with recurrent stones, but only one of these studies showed significant reductions in stone recurrence rate over the 1-year time period. The other two studies, of intermediate duration,[318, 319] both showed reduction in the number of patients with stone recurrence, though the differences were just short of statistical significance. The study of Ohkawa and co-workers[319] did show a significant reduction in the stone formation rate: 13 stones per 100 patient-years in the thiazide group versus 31 stones per 100 patient-years in the control group. The majority of these trials did not supplement potassium for the patients given thiazide, which would predispose the patients to hypocitraturia and reduce the effectiveness of the drug, nor were drug doses varied to get maximal reduction in urine Ca^{2+}. Thiazides would be expected to be even more effective in clinical practice with appropriate dosing to reach the desired response in urinary Ca^{2+} excretion and with potassium supplementation as needed. These randomized trials are the strongest evidence of effective therapy in the treatment of nephrolithiasis.

Two of the three 3-year randomized trials included hypercalciuric and non-hypercalciuric calcium stone formers and still showed significant reduction in kidney stone formation. The excellent overall therapeutic response suggests that the reduction of urine calcium oxalate saturation is a general approach to Ca^{2+} stone prevention that is useful even in normocalciuric patients, whose calcium oxalate stones must reflect their inability to excrete even normal amounts of calcium and oxalate without forming stones. Laerum and Larsen[315] analyzed hypercalciuric and normocalciuric patients separately, and thiazide was of equal efficacy in both groups. The study by Ohkawa and colleagues[319] included both absorptive and renal hypercalciuric patients and showed similar reductions in the stone formation rate. The effectiveness of thiazide in the other studies, despite its certain use in some absorptive as well as renal hypercalciuric patients, suggests that, as a practical matter, exact pathogenetic distinctions may not be crucial in determining choice of treatment.

Hyperuricosuria

The usual upper limits of daily urine uric acid excretion, 800 mg (men) and 750 mg (women), are exceeded more frequently by calcium stone formers than by normal people (Table 39-14). In hyperuricosuric patients who form calcium stones, stone disease begins at a later average age than usual and is unusually active and severe.[110, 320] Complex mechanisms, not fully understood, link hyperuricosuria to calcium stones. Allopurinol treatment reduces stone formation, so detection of hyperuricosuria is important.

Frequency

Of 460 calcium stone formers in our survey, 26.3% were hyperuricosuric.[110] Hyperuricosuria and idiopathic hypercalciuria coexisted in 11.7% of patients, close to what one might expect based on the independent occurrence rates of these two common disorders. Of our 121 hyperuricosuric patients, 40 men (39%) and 4 women (22%) were hyperuricemic; serum urate values were normal in the rest.

TABLE 39-14

Frequencies of Uric Acid Excretion Rates among Calcium Oxalate Stone Formers and Normal Subjects*

URINARY URATE (mg/24 hr)	MEN N (128)	MEN P (1046)	WOMEN N (77)	WOMEN P (302)
<200	0	0	0	0
200–400	2	1	36	25
400–600	38	17	54	53
600–800	48	50	9	8
800–900	6	14	0	6
900–1000	4	11	—	5
>1000	2	7	—	3

*Numbers represent the percentage of 24-hr urine samples containing the amounts of urate indicated. The total number of urine samples in each group is shown in parentheses.
N, normal subjects; P, stone formers.

TABLE 39-15

Purine and Calorie Intake by Patients and Normal Subjects*

GROUP (n)	PURINE INTAKE (mg/24 hr)	CALORIE INTAKE (cal/24 hr)
Patients (10)	259 ± 29	2109 ± 161
Normal men (5)	155 ± 21	2104 ± 147

*$F = 9.16$, $P < .01$, for patients vs. normal men; values are mean ± SEM.

Other studies have reported hyperuricosuria in 16% to 36% of kidney stone patients.[116, 117] The usual upper limits of normal for uric acid excretion are arbitrary because the distributions of daily uric acid excretion by normal men and women are continuous, not bimodal. However, even if higher limits are used, stone formers still differ from normal (see Table 39-14). The point 2 SD above the normal mean could be used to replace these arbitrary limits, but patients who are most likely to benefit from treatment might not be selected with any greater precision.

Etiology

Coe and co-workers[321] studied purine consumption in hyperuricosuric stone formers and normal subjects. The patients habitually consumed a larger amount of purine than did five well-matched normal subjects whose caloric intake was nearly identical (Table 39-15). The patients preferred to eat more meat, fish, and poultry than did normal subjects and ate a correspondingly smaller amount of breads, grains, and starches.

Hyperuricosuria was not always due entirely to excessive consumption of purine. From a study of normal subjects, it was possible to construct a 95% confidence band relating urine uric acid excretion to purine intake (Fig. 39-12). Three of the 10 patients that we studied excreted more uric acid than did normal subjects eating the same amount of purine. After 7 days of a purine-free diet, these three patients continued to excrete more uric acid than did the normal subjects. Presumably, this surplus uric acid arose from overproduction of uric acid during the course of endogenous purine metabolism.

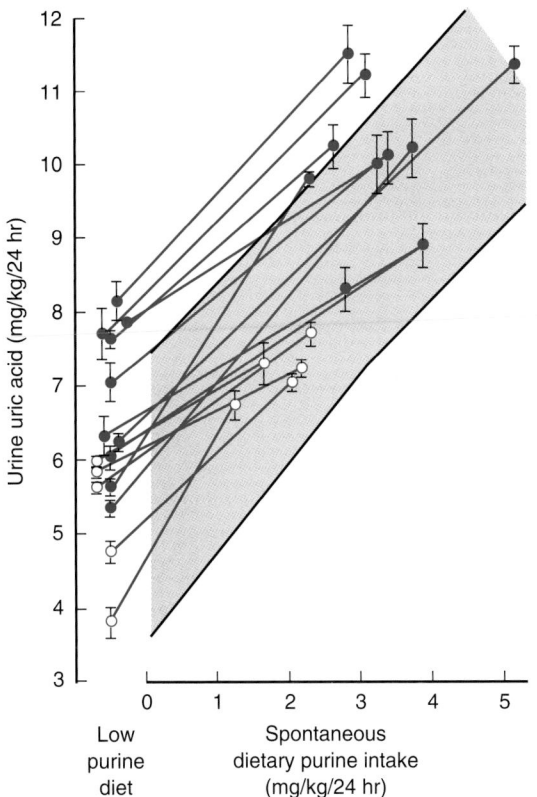

FIGURE 39-12. Relationship between purine intake and uric acid excretion in hyperuricosuric patients compared with that in normal subjects. Uric acid excretion in 3 of the 10 patients (*solid circles*) exceeded the upper limit of the normal range (*shaded area*), indicating an abnormal rate of uric acid excretion. After 7 days of a purine-free diet, these three patients continued to excrete an abnormal amount of uric acid compared with five normal subjects (*open circles*). All values are mean ±1 SEM of three separate determinations. (From Coe FL, Kavalach A: Hypercalciuria and hyperuricosuria in patients with calcium nephrolithiasis. N Engl J Med 291:1344, 1974.)

Mechanism of Stone Formation

The network dimensions of calcium oxalate monohydrate or dihydrate crystals and uric acid crystals match closely enough, within a few percentage points either directly or as integral multiples of one another (Table 39-16), to permit epitaxial growth.[322, 323] Pak and Arnold[46] and we[47] have shown that seed crystals of sodium hydrogen urate or uric acid initiate calcium oxalate precipitation from a metastable solution. Sodium hydrogen urate is effective even though its dimensions[324] do not match those of calcium oxalate very well (see Table 39-16). Although Robertson and colleagues believed otherwise,[325] Pak and co-workers[31] and we[326] have shown that urine is metastably oversaturated with respect to sodium hydrogen urate and uric acid (Table 39-17), so that crystals could form.[326, 327] Crystals of the sodium salt are not found in fresh human urine, but uric acid crystals are common in urine and could be a source of nuclei.

We measured urine supersaturation with respect to monosodium hydrogen urate,[326] using a crystal-seeding technique analogous to that employed for measurement of supersaturation with respect to calcium oxalate. Pak and associates[327] described similar measurements. When urine

TABLE 39-16

Geometric Correspondence between Naturally Occurring Faces of Uric Acid and Calcium Oxalate Crystals

CRYSTALS	FACE	DIMENSIONS (Å)
Uric acid	100	6.21×7.40
Uric acid $\cdot$ 2H$_2$O	100	6.35×7.40
CaOx $\cdot$ H$_2$O*	001	6.28×14.57
CaOx $\cdot$ 2H$_2$O†	101	12.30×7.34
NaH urate $\cdot$ H$_2$O	100	3.567×8.693
	010	9.097×3.567

*Whewellite, or calcium oxalate monohydrate.
†Weddelite, or calcium oxalate dihydrate.

volume and urine pH are controlled experimentally,[327] hyperuricosuria increases urine supersaturation with respect to sodium hydrogen urate. However, when patients with hyperuricosuria consume their own free-choice diet, they produce a urine that has a lower pH than that of normal subjects (see Table 39-17). Because of the low pH, an abnormally high percentage of the total urinary uric acid in these patients is in the form of undissociated uric acid rather than urate. Consequently, supersaturation with respect to monosodium urate is not higher than normal, but urinary undissociated uric acid concentrations are. The solubility of undissociated uric acid in urine is 90 ± 5 mg/L; concentrations in hyperuricosuric patients exceed this solubility limit, whereas concentrations in urine from normal subjects and patients with idiopathic hypercalciuria do not. These findings suggest that undissociated uric acid rather than sodium hydrogen urate would be the favored solid phase in the urine of hyperuricosuric patients. The reason for the low urine pH in patients with hyperuricosuria may be the high intake of meat, fish, and poultry that characterizes their diet.[321]

The clinical role of heterogeneous nucleation is uncertain. Small nuclei of uric acid or urate could lodge in a caliceal niche or in the lumen of a collecting duct and be the center of a calcium oxalate stone. Uric acid itself certainly plugs renal collecting ducts,[328] and urate could do the same. The exposed end of such a plug, bathed perpetually by the flowing urine, is an attractive foundation for a stone. However, proof that heterogeneous nucleation is a link between hyperuricosuria and calcium stones is lacking. Robertson and colleagues[113] have produced another mechanism: adsorption of certain urine crystal growth inhibitors, acid mucopolysaccharides in particular, by urate or uric acid crystals. They suggest that hyperuricosuria may deplete urine of its inhibitors by increasing the mass of uric acid crystals and in this manner predispose to calcium stones. They have found that increasing urine uric acid concentration lowers crystal growth inhibitor activity. However, the mechanism is far from established. Other workers have observed no reduction of urinary crystal growth inhibition in patients with hyperuricosuria.[114, 329] Grover and associates[330] showed that urate promotes crystallization of calcium oxalate independent of the presence of urine macromolecules, and proposed that urate "salts out" calcium oxalate from urine.[329]

TABLE 39-17

Urinary Uric Acid Saturation*

24-HR URINARY VALUES	METABOLIC GROUP				
	Normal (20)	Idiopathic Hypercalciuria (24)	Hyperuricosuria (12)	Both (14)	Neither (17)
Number of samples	24	69	36	42	51
Total uric acid (mg/L)	503 ± 32	421 ± 23	575 ± 28	$616 \pm 27^{\ddagger b}$	462 ± 32
Urine volume (mL)	1268 ± 65	1717 ± 133	1501 ± 79^a	1397 ± 70	1387 ± 90
Urine pH	6.22	5.92	5.62	$5.74^{\dagger b}$	5.67
Undissociated uric acid (mg/L)‡	57 ± 8	84 ± 11	155 ± 21^c	$150 \pm 15^{\dagger d}$	$128 \pm 18^{\dagger b}$
CPR, monosodium hydrogen urate	$2.8 \pm 0.3^\S$	2.2 ± 0.2	2.7 ± 0.2	3.1 ± 0.2	2.2 ± 0.2
[Na$^+$] [urate] (m$^2 \times 10^{-3}$), initial$^\parallel$	37 ± 4	27 ± 3	35 ± 4	$42 \pm 3^\P$	29 ± 3
Sodium concentration (mEq/L)	131 ± 8	118 ± 7	130 ± 7	149 ± 7	132 ± 7

*All values except for the numbers of samples and the numbers of individuals in each metabolic group (in parentheses) are means $\pm$ SEM.

†Differs from control: $^aP < .05$; $^bP < .02$; $^cP < .001$; $^dP < .001$.

‡The mean equilibrium value, determined in 26 urine samples of pH below 5.6 after 48 hr of incubation with crystals of uric acid, was 90 ± 5 (SEM) mg/L. Values were calculated by use of a pK$_a$ of 5.345.

§Based on the study of 16 of the 20 normal subjects who had CPR measurements.

$^\parallel$Before incubation with crystals of sodium hydrogen urate.

¶Men differed from women, $P < .05$.

CPR, concentration product ratio.

Adapted from Coe FL, Strauss AL, Tembe V, Le Dun S: Uric acid saturation in calcium nephrolithiasis. Kidney Int 17:662–668, 1980.

Treatment

Reduction of new stone formation during allopurinol administration is the most compelling evidence for the role of hyperuricosuria in calcium oxalate stone disease. Our treatment studies[48, 110, 331] rely on a comparison of stone production before and during treatment. Allopurinol reduced new stones from the predicted 124.8 (Table 39-18) to 8. Dual treatment with thiazide and allopurinol was equally effective for patients with idiopathic hypercalciuria and hyperuricosuria (see Table 39-18).

Smith[332] has performed a prospective drug trial comparing allopurinol to placebo in the treatment of calcium stone formers with a serum urate level above 6 mg/dL. The rationale for selecting patients was not clear because hyperuricemia by itself has no obvious pertinence to calcium renal stones. Still, there was a dramatic drug effect out to 5 years of follow-up. The definitive study was performed by Ettinger and colleagues[333] in a randomized double-blind trial of allopurinol therapy in hyperuricosuric, normocalciuric calcium oxalate stone formers. There was a significant reduction in calculous events in the group receiving allopurinol, 0.26 stone per patient per year in the placebo group versus 0.12 in the allopurinol group. Actuarial analysis showed the allopurinol-treated patients to have a significantly longer time interval before stone recurrence (Fig. 39-13). The mechanism of allopurinol therapy must be due to decreased urate excretion, as it has been shown that allopurinol, or its metabolite oxypurinol, has no effect on growth or nucleation of calcium oxalate.[334]

It would seem that diet alone, that is, simple reduction of purine intake to a normal level, could be an ideal treatment for the majority of patients, but no published data clearly support or deny this hypothesis. Changing a habit is difficult, especially when the change is quantitative and not the mere omission of a food category. Whether diet modification is a practical and effective treatment remains to be seen.

TABLE 39-18

Effects of Allopurinol on Calcium Stone Formation in Hyperuricosuric Patients*

PARAMETER	HYPERURICOSURIA		HYPERURICOSURIA AND HYPERCALCIURIA	
	P	T	P	T
Number of patients	48		42	
Time (patient-years)	298	186	357	119
Stones formed	200	8	188	6
Stones/patient	4.17	—	4.48	—
Years/patient	6.21	3.90	8.50	2.83
Stones/100 patients/yr	67.1	4.3	52.7	5.0
New stones predicted	—	124.8†	—	62.7†

*Patients with hyperuricosuria were treated with allopurinol; patients with hyperuricosuria and hypercalciuria were treated with allopurinol and thiazide. P and T refer to pretreatment and treatment intervals, respectively.

$^\dagger\chi^2$ for difference between predicted and observed values, 109.3 and 51.3, respectively; $P < .001$ for both.

An alternative therapy was described by Pak and Peterson,[335] who demonstrated reduced stone recurrence rates in hyperuricosuria stone formers treated with potassium citrate. The increased citrate lowers calcium oxalate supersaturation and may inhibit urate-induced crystallization of calcium oxalate.[336]

Renal Tubular Acidosis

Type 1, classic distal RTA, is a cause of nephrocalcinosis and renal stone formation (see Chapter 20). Kidney stones have been seen whether the disease is inherited, secondary to a systemic disease, or occurs sporadically without associated systemic disease. When distal RTA is acquired as a drug- or toxin-induced nephropathy it usually does not cause stones. Proximal RTA (type 2) or any other form of renal

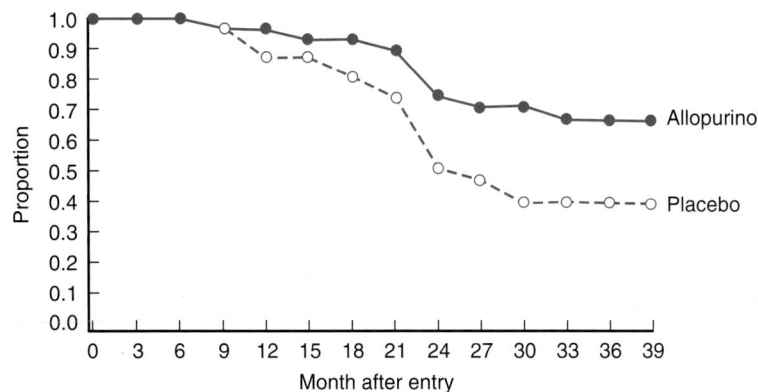

FIGURE 39-13. Life-table plot showing proportion of patients without calculous events during treatment with allopurinol or placebo. (Reprinted with permission from Ethinger B, Tang A, Citron JT, et al: Randomized trial of allopurinol in the prevention of calcium oxalate calculi. N Engl J Med 315:1386-1389, 1986.)

TABLE 39-19

Effect of Distal Renal Tubular Acidosis (Type 1) or Experimental Acid Loading on Calcium Balance

REFERENCE	SUBJECT (AGE AND SEX) AND THERAPY	CALCIUM (mg/24 hr)				
		Intake	Urine	Fecal	Net Absorption	Balance
Albright et al.[339]	13, female	80	163	137	−57	−220
		530	125	460	70	−600
Baines et al.[340]	29, female	457	277	523	−76	−353
Albright et al.[341]	40, female	76	264	39	37	−227
	Alkali therapy	604	475	174	430	−45
Pines and Mudge[342]	28, female	562	215	189	373	158
	Alkali therapy	515	105	376	139	34
	28, female	208	218	175	33	−185
	Alkali therapy	208	144	227	−19	−163
Bauld et al.[343]	29, female	260	120	240	20	−100
	Alkali therapy	260	70	240	20	−50
Greenberg et al.[344]	4, male	743	123	640	103	−20
	Alkali therapy	760	26	406	354	327
Wallach et al.[345]	32, female	458	138	434	24	−114
Weber et al.[346]	Normal subjects*	1204[†]	216	638	388	176
	18 days of acid loading[‡]	1000	580	480	520	−72
Lemann et al.[347]	Normal subjects[§]	1760[‖]	320	1520	240	−80
	12-18 days of acid loading[‡]	1764	1016	1452	312	−704

*Three men and three women.
[†]Mean of six values.
[‡]Acid loading was in the form of NH_4Cl.
[§]Five men.
[‖]Mean of five values.

acidosis associated with renal disease is not usually associated with stones. Stones can occur in the complete form of distal RTA with systemic acidosis or in the incomplete form which expresses deficient renal acidification with acid loading. Stones in RTA result from hypercalciuria, hypocitraturia, and alkaline urine pH. Stones are most often calcium phosphate,[337] though one survey reported a high incidence of calcium oxalate and struvite stones, as well as calcium phosphate.[338]

Hypercalciuria

In contrast to the situation in idiopathic hypercalciuria, intestinal Ca^{2+} absorption is not elevated. It is normal or low (Table 39-19),[339-347] and bone mineral is lost into the urine.

Metabolic acidosis, a result of the renal acidification defect that gives rise to the disease, causes the hypercalciuria. Normal subjects become hypercalciuric if an exogenous acid load, sufficient to produce metabolic acidosis, is administered for at least 7 days.[348] Net intestinal Ca^{2+} absorption does not increase enough to balance urine losses, and Ca^{2+} balance becomes negative.[349] The surplus urine Ca^{2+} arises from bone, as in distal RTA. Alkali therapy at a dose that reverses acidosis reduces urine Ca^{2+} excretion in patients with RTA[350, 351] and improves Ca^{2+} balance in some but not all cases (see Table 39-19); if alkali is discontinued, acidosis and hypercalciuria recur. Intestinal Ca^{2+} absorption is low in these patients, inadequate to compensate for renal Ca^{2+} losses. Preminger and co-workers[352] showed low intestinal Ca^{2+} absorption in a group of patients with incomplete distal RTA which improved with citrate treatment. The changes in Ca^{2+} absorption were independent of vitamin D.

Hypercalciuria is not always secondary to systemic acidosis in RTA. Hypercalciuria may predate RTA, apparently causing renal tubular damage via nephrocalcinosis. This has been shown in some families with hereditary distal RTA, where there is also an autosomal dominant inheritance of hypercalciuria.[353]

Mechanism of Stone Formation

Hypercalciuria and elevated urine phosphorus excretion both tend to raise urine saturation with respect to calcium phosphate, but alkaline urine pH is more important than either one.[354] High pH increases the availability of PO_4^{3-} and HPO_4^{2-}, which are incorporated into octocalcium phosphate and brushite, respectively. Urine citrate excretion is reduced by metabolic acidosis, hypokalemia, and renal insufficiency.[355] The cause of low urine citrate in incomplete RTA is unclear, but it has been suggested that there is a proximal tubule cell intracellular acidosis stimulating citrate utilization.[356] Reduction of the fraction of urine Ca^{2+} bound by citrate raises urine supersaturation of calcium phosphate and calcium oxalate.

Alkali administration is said to reduce stone formation and slow the progress of nephrocalcinosis,[350, 357, 358] but details of the natural history of stones and nephrocalcinosis during treatment are not widely available. Nash and co-workers[350] found stable nephrocalcinosis in four patients. Perhaps the longest cohesive series of treated patients with nephrolithiasis due to hereditary distal RTA is one that describes six patients treated for 7 to 19 years.[337] During 43 patient-years of alkali treatment, only two new stones were formed, one by each of two patients, whereas the pretreatment stone recurrence rate for the group was 96 stones per 100 patient-years. Nephrocalcinosis was present in three of the six patients; it lessened in one and remained unchanged in the other two.[337] A more recent study of nine patients with RTA showed no new stone formation during 3 years of potassium citrate therapy despite a pretreatment stone formation rate of 13 per patient per year.[358] Calcium oxalate supersaturation fell significantly during therapy, but there was not a significant fall in brushite supersaturation, as the increase in citrate and decrease in Ca^{2+} excretion was offset by an increase in urine pH.[358] Renal function tends to stabilize and linear skeletal growth in children tends to resume during alkali therapy.[359]

Hypocitraturia

Hypocitraturia is found in 15% to 60% of stone formers.[360-364] The wide range in the reported prevalence of hypocitraturia reflects differences in the populations studied, as well as differences in the laboratory definition of hypocitraturia. Hypocitraturia may occur as an isolated abnormality or be associated with some other stone-forming risk such as hypercalciuria. Low urine citrates are invariably found in distal RTA (see earlier), chronic diarrheal states, and diuretic-induced hypokalemia, or may be found with no apparent cause, so-called idiopathic hypocitraturia.[29] One of the difficulties in determining the role of citrate in stone disease is that there is no consensus as to what constitutes a

normal citrate level. Some groups report differences in normal subjects related to age and sex[361, 365-367]; others have not found such differences.[364, 368, 369]

Renal Excretion of Citrate

Citrate is freely filtered at the glomerulus, and 65% to 90% is reabsorbed in the proximal tubule.[355] It is a component of the tricarboxylic acid cycle, and the majority of citrate reabsorbed by the kidney is used in oxidative metabolism. Because the tubule does not secrete citrate, the final urinary excretion of citrate is determined by reabsorption in the proximal tubule. The most important regulator of citrate reabsorption is systemic acid-base status. Alkalosis increases and acidosis decreases renal citrate excretion.[355] In acidosis there is increased citrate utilization by the mitochondria resulting in lower intracellular levels of citrate, facilitating citrate reabsorption. Also, lower tubule fluid pH in acidosis converts more $citrate^{-3}$ to $citrate^{-2}$, which is the ionic species that is actively transported.[370] Hypokalemia also reduces urine citrate, presumably by generating an intracellular acidosis in the proximal tubule cell.[371] Hypokalemia may prevent the increase in urine citrate seen with alkalosis.[371]

Mechanism of Stone Formation

Citrate binds Ca^{2+} in the urine, reducing Ca^{2+} activity, resulting in lower supersaturation of calcium salts.[29] Therefore, lowering urine citrate levels is equivalent to increasing urine Ca^{2+} levels in producing supersaturation, the driving force of crystallization. In addition to lowering supersaturation, citrate has direct inhibitory effects on the crystallization of calcium salts. Citrate may also increase the inhibitory activity of urine macromolecules. Hess and co-workers have shown that citrate increases the calcium oxalate aggregation inhibition of Tamm-Horsfall protein in vitro.[109] A prospective study of 33 calcium stone–forming patients showed increased urinary inhibition of calcium oxalate aggregation and increased Tamm-Horsfall protein excretion during therapy with potassium citrate.[372] Thus low urine citrate excretion simultaneously increases urine supersaturation and reduces crystal inhibition, increasing the risk of stone formation.

Treatment

The basis of therapy for hypocitraturia is correction of any underlying disorder that reduces urine citrate, such as acidosis or hypokalemia, or, if the patient has idiopathic hypocitraturia, induction of a mild metabolic alkalosis to increase urine citrate. Any alkali supplement will raise urine citrate levels. However, sodium alkali will increase urine Ca^{2+} excretion, offsetting the benefits of increased urine citrate.[373] Either potassium bicarbonate or potassium citrate may be used. Citrate requires less frequent dosing than bicarbonate as it is metabolized to bicarbonate in the liver.

Citrate is the most frequently used alkali for hypocitraturic patients. There are three randomized trials of citrate therapy in calcium oxalate stone formers. Barcelo and associates[374] did a 3-year double-blind study of potassium citrate in patients with hypocitraturic calcium oxalate stones. The placebo group had no change in the stone formation rate, whereas the potassium citrate–treated group had their stone formation rate decrease from 1.2 to 0.1 stone per patient-year (*P* < .001) (Fig. 39-14). Only 20% of the placebo group remained stone-free during the study as compared to 72% of the treated group. A 3-year double-blind study of potassium magnesium citrate also showed a reduced calcium oxalate stone formation rate with therapy.[375] Of note, the patients in this study had a variety of metabolic abnormalities as the cause of the stones, with only 20% having hypocitraturia. The benefit of citrate therapy was not limited to the patients with hypocitraturia. There has not been a trial directly comparing the efficacy of potassium citrate with potassium magnesium citrate. At this time potassium magnesium citrate has not been approved for clinical use. A third 3-year randomized study using sodium-potassium citrate did not reveal any reduction in stone recurrence in a group of calcium oxalate stone formers.[376] The majority of patients did have hypocitraturia on entry into the study, and the treated group did show an increase in citrate during therapy. The reason for the different outcomes in these studies is not clear; possibly the use of a mixed sodium-potassium salt blunted the antilithogenic response to citrate.[373] In summary, the two positive controlled trials, previous uncontrolled trials showing reduction in stone formation

during citrate therapy,[377, 378] and documentation of reduced urine calcium oxalate supersaturation during citrate therapy support the use of citrate supplements in hypocitraturic calcium stone disease.

Potassium citrate therapy is generally well tolerated, but some patients note significant gastrointestinal side effects, particularly dyspepsia. These side effects may be improved by taking potassium citrate with meals, which will not affect intestinal absorption of the drug.[379] Because alkali will not only increase urine citrate but also raise urine pH, urine calcium phosphate supersaturation may increase. Clinicians should watch for the potential conversion of calcium oxalate stones to calcium phosphate stones if urine pH increases substantially during therapy.

Idiopathic Calcium Lithiasis

Despite a thorough evaluation, a remediable cause of stones will not be found in some patients. Older studies estimated that 20% to 50% of calcium stones were idiopathic, that is, the patients were normocalciuric and free of identifiable metabolic abnormalities.[3, 19, 110, 111] In most of these studies, the metabolic evaluation was not as extensive as it is today. With metabolic evaluation now including the measurement of urine citrate excretion, only 7% to 10% of patients are classified as having idiopathic calcium lithiasis.[117] However, it should be recognized that urinary stone risk factors are continuous variables and the normal limits are somewhat arbitrary.[380] Many patients with idiopathic calcium lithiasis have urine chemistry at the border of the normal limits, which increases urine supersaturation and contributes to stone formation. Identification of the urine chemistries closest to the stone-forming range will allow the clinician to compose a rational therapy for most patients.

Hydration, restriction of dietary protein and sodium, and avoidance of foods that contain excessive oxalate are prudent measures but have not been well studied in patients with recurrent idiopathic calcium lithiasis (Table 39-20). Ettinger[381] and Coe and Parks[382] observed recurrence of stones in more than one half of patients during 2 to 3 years of treatment with diet and hydration. Pharmacologic therapy to further reduce urine supersaturation may be useful if hydration and diet fail to control stone formation.

Orthophosphate

The rationale for using orthophosphate is that urine Ca^{2+} excretion may be reduced by suppressing calcitriol production,[383] and urine excretion of the crystal inhibitor inorganic pyrophosphate increases.[384] Supersaturation with respect to calcium oxalate is reduced.[385] Ettinger and Kolb[386] treated 47 patients who had idiopathic hypercalciuria with potassium acid phosphate (1 g of inorganic phosphorus daily) for up to 4 years (see Table 39-20). The stone formation rate and urine Ca^{2+} excretion did not fall below pretreatment values. The percentage of patients that were stone-free after 2 and 4 years of treatment was greater than that of patients treated by diet and hydration. Subsequently, Ettinger[381] compared acid phosphate, at a dose that provided 1 g of phosphorus daily, to placebo. The drug did not reduce new stone formation, and recurrence rates were above those observed during diet treatment (see Table 39-20). Smith and colleagues[384]

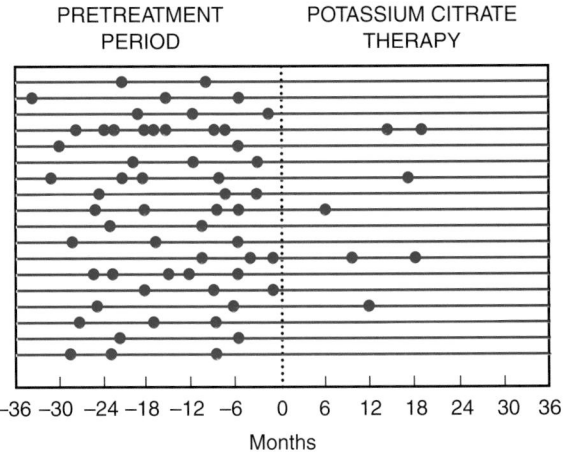

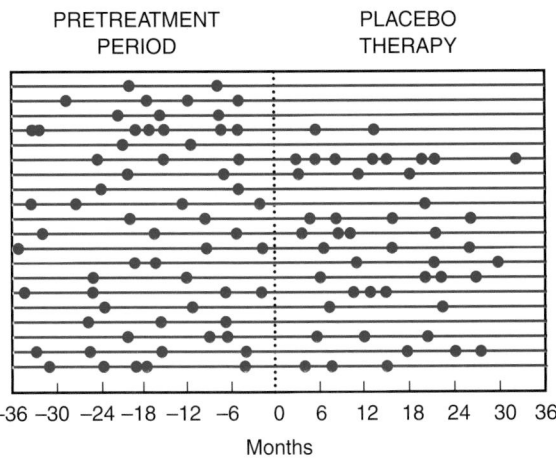

FIGURE 39-14. Effect of potassium citrate therapy (upper panel) vs. placebo (lower panel) on hypocitraturic calcium oxalate stone disease. Each line represents a single patient and each dot represents a new stone formation. (From Barcello P, Wuhl O, Servitge E, et al: Randomized double-blind trial of potassium citrate in idiopathic hypocitraturic calcium nephrolithiasis. J Urol 150:1761-1764, 1993.)

TABLE 39-20

Diet and Hydration and Orthophosphate Therapy for Idiopathic Calcium Stone Disease

TREATMENT	PATIENTS STONE-FREE AT TIME OF FOLLOW-UP*				
	6 Mo	1 Yr	2 Yr	3 Yr	4 Yr
Diet and hydration					
Coe & Parks[320]	79 (34)	71 (34)	43 (28)	47 (15)	46 (13)
Ettinger[381]	85 (26)	77 (26)	66 (15)	46 (13)	—
Orthophosphate					
Ettinger[381]	72 (25)	63 (24)	52 (23)	53 (19)	—
Ettinger and Kolb[386]	89 (47)	—	74 (47)	—	76 (37)
Smith et al.[384]	—	—	—	91 (150)	—
Bernstein and Newton[387]	78 (9)	83 (6)	83 (6)	—	—

*Numbers represent the percentage of patients stone-free on follow-up in each study; numbers of patients at the end of each follow-up interval are shown in parentheses.

treated idiopathic stone formers with twice the dose of orthophosphate daily and achieved better results. In their report, data are presented for the population at an average treatment interval of 3 years (see Table 39-20), but not at the end of each year of the study. Urine Ca^{2+} excretion fell. Bernstein and Newton[387] reported a very small phosphate study involving patients with idiopathic hypercalciuria; their results were comparable to those of Smith (see Table 39-20).

Overall, the effectiveness of orthophosphate is uncertain. Ettinger[381] and Ettinger and Kolb[386] observed no therapeutic effect in their studies, one of which was placebo-controlled. However, the dose they employed was only half as large as that used by Smith and co-workers[384] in their more encouraging study. Furthermore, Ettinger and Ettinger and Kolb used acid phosphate, whereas Smith used neutral phosphate. Lau and associates[388] have shown that acid phosphate administration leads to higher levels of urine Ca^{2+} and lower levels of urine citrate than does neutral phosphate. A reduction in urine supersaturation with respect to calcium oxalate comparable to that achieved with neutral phosphate would not be expected and might be ineffective in preventing calcium renal stones.

Orthophosphate is not always tolerated. The drug is acathartic. Symptoms range from mild abdominal discomfort to persistent diarrhea. With time, intestinal side effects may wane, and paients may adapt. If the drug is begun at half the full dose, symptoms are less prominent, and patient acceptance may be better.

There is also the problem of secondary hyperparathyroidism. Oral phosphate administration to normal subjects and patients with idiopathic hypercalciuria causes a prompt, transient rise in serum PTH and a decline in serum $1,25(OH)_2D_3$.[383, 389] The serum phosphate concentration rises and the Ca^{2+} level falls. During chronic phosphate administration, the serum phosphate level, measured in the postabsorptive state, is normal or low[245, 277, 278] and serum PTH is normal.[386] Each dose of phosphate may, however, provoke transient release of PTH, as in the acute experiment of Reiss and colleagues.[389] A slow-release formulation of neutral phosphate has been studied in a 4-year prospective trial in patients with absorptive hypercalciuria.[390] There was a sustained reduction in urine Ca^{2+} throughout the study. Over 4 years PTH levels increased from 30 pg/mL to 42 pg/mL ($P < .001$) and calcitriol levels fell from 42 to 34 pg/mL ($P < .05$).

There appeared to be no adverse effects from the mild increase in PTH as bone mineral density and urine hydroxyproline were stable and alkaline phosphatase decreased. This slow-release formulation has not been tested for efficacy on stone reduction in a controlled manner and is not yet available for patient care.

Thiazide, Allopurinol, and Citrate

Because our experience with hydration and diet therapy was not encouraging (see Table 39-20), we treated 30 idiopathic stone formers with thiazide and allopurinol in order to lower the calcium oxalate activity product and reduce the availability of heterogeneous nuclei. The results were only mildly encouraging (Fig. 39-15).[382] More patients remained stone-free compared with the 34 patients treated with diet and hydration (see Table 39-20), but the therapeutic response was much less evident than that observed when treating hypercalciuric and hyperuricosuric patients with the same drugs.[110] Either drug may have been sufficient to produce the modest decrease in new stone production, especially thiazide, which by itself appeared to reduce stone recurrence in idiopathic stone formers studied by Yendt.[111] Two of the three 3-year thiazide trials included patients who were not hypercalciuric and yet showed significant reduction in stone formation.[315, 316] Citrate supplementation has also been used in a placebo-controlled trial of unselected calcium stone formers. Stone formation rates improved significantly, suggesting this medication has beneficial effects in patients with and without hypocitraturia.[375]

Hyperoxaluria

Even though oxalate occurs in most kidney stones, hyperoxaluria is found in only 5% to 25% of stone formers.[110, 116, 117] The upper limit of normal for oxalate excretion is usually considered to be 45 mg/day in an adult. When excessive urinary oxalate excretion does occur, it causes stones by raising the saturation of the urine with respect to calcium oxalate.[36, 391] When severe, hyperoxaluria damages the kidneys. Nephrocalcinosis, tubulointerstitial nephritis, functional defects of the renal tubule, azotemia, and frank renal failure all have been reported.

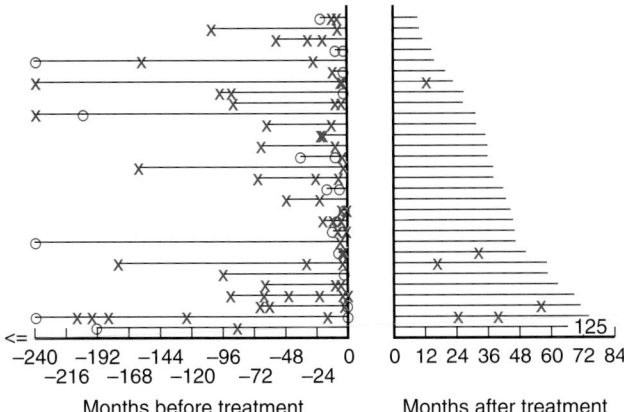

FIGURE 39-15. Course of calcium stone disease in 30 patients with no metabolic disorder before and during combined thiazide and allopurinol administration. Each patient is represented by a *horizontal line*; new stones are represented by *x* and multiple stones by *o*. (From Coe FL: Treated and untreated recurrent calcium nephrolithiasis in patients with idiopathic hypercalciuria, hyperuricosuria or no metabolic disorder. Ann Intern Med 87:404, 1977.)

Oxalate Metabolism

Because humans cannot metabolize oxalate, renal excretion is the major route of oxalate elimination.[392] Oxalate is freely filtered at the glomerulus but in the proximal tubule both secretion and reabsorption have been found.[393] It appears that most normal subjects will have net reabsorption of oxalate, but in settings of severe hyperoxaluria, fractional excretion of over 200% has been documented.[394-396] Urinary oxalate clearance decreases with deterioration of renal function, and serum oxalate levels rise. The retention of oxalate leads to systemic oxalosis as calcium oxalate crystals deposit in the cardiac conduction system, renal parenchyma, joint spaces, blood vessel walls, bone, and elsewhere.

Oxalate is an end product of several metabolic pathways; the amount of oxalate in the urine reflects the sum total of intestinal absorption plus de novo synthesis. Hyperoxaluria may result from increased rates of oxalate production or intestinal hyperabsorption, and these processes serve as a useful basis to classify both hereditary and acquired hyperoxaluric states (Table 39-21). Dietary oxalate intake is estimated to be 50 to 200 mg/day with about 10% being absorbed. Approximately 50% of the oxalate excreted in the urine is absorbed from the diet, and liberal intake of high-oxalate foods can cause frank hyperoxaluria.[397] Intestinal oxalate absorption is not only dependent on the amount of oxalate ingested but also on the bioavailability of the oxalate.[398, 399] If significant amounts of calcium and magnesium are present in the diet, the cations will complex oxalate and reduce its absorption. Diets low in calcium have been shown to increase urine oxalate excretion even when oxalate intake is fixed.[397, 400] Another factor that could influence oxalate absorption is the intestinal flora. Recent studies have shown that oxalate-degrading bacteria are present in the colon of most humans and it has been postulated that loss of these oxalate-degrading bacteria could lead to excess oxalate absorption.[401] Though some retrospective studies have shown lower colonization rates in kidney stone formers than in normal subjects, it is not clear that the loss of

TABLE 39-21

Classification of Hyperoxaluria

Metabolic overproduction of oxalate
    Hereditary (types 1 and 2)
    Pyridoxine deficiency*
    Ethylene glycol ingestion
    Methoxyflurane anesthesia
Gastrointestinal overabsorption of oxalate
    Oxalate overingestion
    Ileal resection
    Celiac sprue
    Pancreatic insufficiency
    Small bowel bypass surgery
    Crohn disease
    Cellulose phosphate ingestion

*Occurs in experimental animals; not of proven clinical significance.

oxalate-degrading bacteria caused hyperoxaluria and kidney stones. Further studies are required to determine the role of these bacteria in the natural history of stone disease.

The two main precursors for endogenous oxalate synthesis are ascorbic acid and glyoxylate. The oxidation of ascorbic acid contributes about 35% of total oxalate production. Oral administration of large doses of ascorbic acid (4 g) increases urinary oxalate in some but not all subjects, suggesting that enzyme activity must be near maximum under usual conditions.[402] The significance of this finding has been questioned because ascorbic acid can be nonenzymatically converted to oxalate in alkaline urine, making analysis of urine oxalate excretion difficult.[403] However, a study in which urine was collected directly from nephrostomy tubes showed increased oxalate excretion when the subjects were given greater than 1000 mg of ascorbic acid.[404] It appears that the ascorbic acid oxidation pathway usually plays little or no role in causing hyperoxaluria, but it may in people taking an excessive ascorbate load.

The oxidation of glyoxylate to oxalate represents the major source of oxalate production in humans.[402] Glyoxylate is mainly produced by the oxidation of glycolate by glycolate oxidase and by oxidative deamination of glycine by D-amino acid oxidase (Fig. 39-16). Glyoxylate can be metabolized to glycine by alanine–glyoxylate aminotransferase (AGT) and to glycolate by D-glycerate dehydrogenase, as this enzyme also possesses hydroxypyruvate reductase and glyoxylate reductase activity.[405] Glyoxylate is also converted to oxalate by either glycolate oxidase or lactate dehydrogenase (LDH), though LDH appears to be the predominant pathway. Conversion of glyoxylate to glycine or glycolate limits the amount of glyoxylate available for oxalate production. Hydroxyproline can be metabolized to glyoxylate and subsequently oxalate. Feeding hydroxyproline to rats increases oxalate excretion and causes calcium oxalate stone formation.[406] Aromatic amino acids can also be converted to oxalate, though the metabolic pathways are not well defined. The contribution of hydroxyproline and aromatic amino acids to daily oxalate production is not known.

Overproduction Hyperoxaluria

Alterations in several of the steps of oxalate synthesis have been implicated in the overproduction hyperoxaluric states.

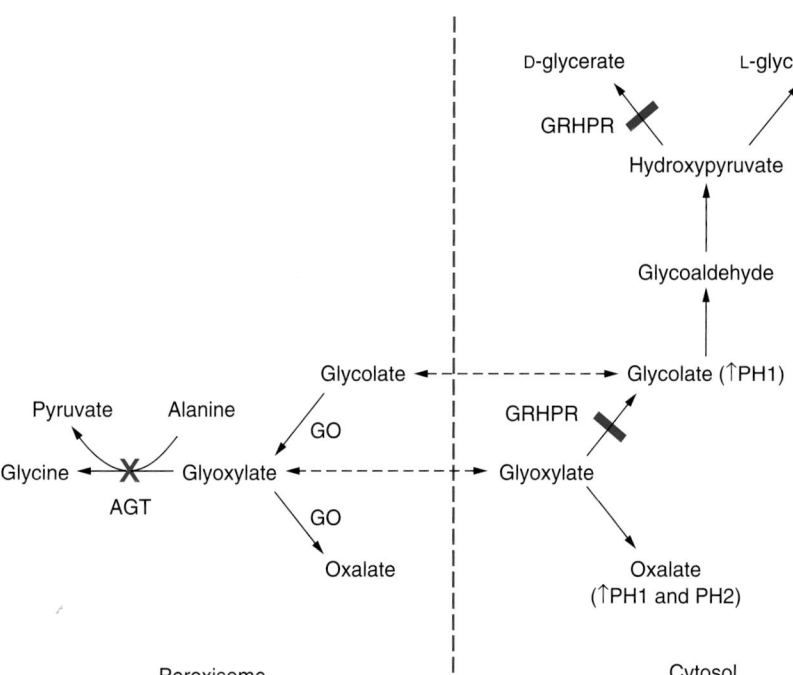

FIGURE 39-16. Oxalate metabolic pathways and metabolic defects in primary hyperoxaluria (PH). The enzyme defect in PH1 is marked by an X. The defects in PH2 are marked by a solid bar. The *dashed arrows* represent bidirectional transport in and out of the peroxisome. AGT, alanine-glyoxylate aminotransferase; GO, glycolate oxidase; GRHPR, glycolate reductase–hydroxypyruvate reductase. (From Asplin JR: Hyperoxaluric calcium nephrolithiasis. Endocrinol Metab Clin North Am 31:927-949, 2002.)

A deficiency in the activity of the peroxisomal enzyme AGT is responsible for primary hyperoxaluria type 1.[407] AGT converts glyoxylate to glycine; a reduction in activity allows more glyoxylate to be converted to oxalate in the cell cytosol and peroxisome. Type 1 primary hyperoxaluria is a heterogeneous disorder with multiple mechanisms for deficient enzyme activity. Forty-five percent of patients completely lack hepatic enzyme activity and have no AGT immunoreactivity on liver biospy, and 20% have immunoreactive AGT in the peroxisome but no detectable enzyme activity.[408] The other 35% have detectable levels of AGT activity, in the range of 3% to 48% of normal, but immunochemical localization shows AGT to be located in the mitochondria rather than the peroxisome.[409] This unusual error of enzyme trafficking places the AGT in an environment where the enzyme functions poorly. Primary hyperoxaluria type 2 is due to a deficiency of a cytosolic enzyme (GRHPR) that functions as a *glyoxylate reductase–hydroxypyruvate reductase*, and glycerate dehydrogenase.[410] The loss of GRHPR activity reduces glyoxylate conversion to glycolate, leading to increased production of oxalate from glyoxylate by LDH in the cytosol. GRHPR deficiency also decreases conversion of hydroxypyruvate to D-glycerate with subsequent overproduction of L-glycerate. Both types of primary hyperoxaluria are inherited as autosomal recessive traits. Another inherited form of hyperoxaluria with hyperglycoluria has been reported in which L-glyceric acid excretion is normal and AGT activity is normal.[411] The metabolic defect in these patients has not been elucidated.

Urinary oxalate excretion in adults is usually 100 to 300 mg/day in both disorders and declines as renal failure ensues. Both disorders may produce recurrent calcium oxalate calculi, progressive renal failure, and oxalosis, beginning as early as childhood. Patients with type 1 disease usually overexcrete glycolate as well as oxalate, but 25% to 30% of patients with primary hyperoxaluria type 1 documented by

liver biopsy will have normal glycolate excretion rates. Those with type 2 disease overexcrete L-glyceric acid and oxalate.[412] Only one case has been reported in which L-glycerate excretion was normal in a patient with primary hyperoxaluria type 2.[413] Though measurements of urinary excretion of glycolate and L-glycerate can aid in diagnosis, a definitive diagnosis of primary hyperoxaluria requires a liver biopsy.[414] Once renal failure has developed, the diagnosis should be suspected from a prior history of stones and evidence of systemic oxalosis.

Treatment of primary hyperoxaluria focuses on reducing oxalate excretion or increasing the solubility of calcium oxalate salts. As with all kidney stone diseases, urine flow should be high, greater than 2.5 L/day in an adult. Because AGT is a pyridoxal phosphate–dependent enzyme, pyridoxine has been used to treat patients with type 1 hyperoxaluria. Pyridoxine in doses of 25 to 1000 mg/day reduces oxalate excretion in 25% to 30% of patients with type 1 hyperoxaluria.[415] Patients who respond to pyridoxine will have some residual AGT activity in liver biopsy samples.[407] In the rat, pyridoxine deficiency is associated with hyperoxaluria by virtue of the reduced transamination of glyoxylate to glycine, making more glyoxylate available for oxidation to oxalate. Pyridoxine deficiency in humans has not been associated with hyperoxaluria and stone formation, but subtle deficiencies in pyridoxine could contribute to some hyperoxaluric conditions. Neutral orthophosphate and magnesium supplements have been used with success,[416, 417] though no controlled trials exist. Milliner and colleagues[418] have reported their long-term outcome in 25 patients with primary hyperoxaluria with a mean follow-up of 12 years. Using the combination of pyridoxine and neutral orthophosphate, they found reduced urine supersaturation and lower rates of crystalluria during therapy. Most important, they found 89% of their patients were free from end-stage renal disease at 10 years of follow-up. Potassium citrate has been shown to reduce calcium oxalate supersaturation and the stone formation rate in children with primary hyperoxaluria,[419] though long-term outcomes are not known.

Acquired overproduction of oxalate follows ingestion of ethylene glycol, which is metabolized via glycolaldehyde to glycolate. The anesthetic methoxyflurane is converted to ethanolamine and then to oxalate. Nephrotoxicities resulting from ethylene glycol and methoxyflurane are discussed in Chapter 34.

Gastrointestinal Overabsorption of Oxalate

Only a small fraction of dietary oxalate is absorbed, but increasing dietary oxalate can lead to significant increases in urine oxalate excretion.[397-399] High-oxalate foods such as spinach, rhubarb, nuts, and chocolate are frequent causes of mild hyperoxaluria, usually in the range of 45 to 80 mg/day. As noted earlier, diets low in calcium can also promote hyperoxaluria by increasing the bioavailability of oxalate.[398, 399] Several gastrointestinal disorders are associated with overabsorption of oxalate and consequent hyperoxaluria.[420-422] Hyperoxaluria with or without calcium oxalate calculi may complicate Crohn disease, celiac sprue, pancreatic insufficiency, and small intestinal bypass surgery for obesity.[423-425] Dietary fat malabsorption with steatorrhea is common to all conditions, and increased luminal free fatty acids may be critical in the development of oxalate overabsorption. There is a positive correlation between fecal fat and hyperoxaluria,[420, 426] whereas patients with jejunocolonic and jejunoileal bypass—procedures that virtually exclude the small intestine—absorb considerable oxalate from the colon. Excessive luminal concentrations of bile salts and long-chain fatty acids enhance oxalate absorption[427] by increasing the permeability of colon epithelium to oxalate.[428] In addition, the free fatty acids bind calcium, which reduces the amount of calcium available to bind oxalate, increasing the amount of oxalate available for absorption. Loss of oxalate-degrading bacteria has been reported in patients with steatorrhea, but the importance of this finding in the overabsorption of oxalate needs to be better defined.[429] Therapy for enteric hyperoxaluria includes control of steatorrhea by dietary restriction of fat, reduced oxalate intake, and the use of cholestyramine, a nonabsorbable anion-exchange resin that binds oxalate in the bowel lumen. Restoration of small bowel continuity should be seriously considered if hyperoxaluria produces clinical manifestations in patients with intestinal bypass. Oral calcium carbonate, 1 to 4 g/day, may be useful in some patients.[430] In general, a low-fat, low-oxalate diet should be used first, followed by oral calcium carbonate or cholestyramine if diet is unsuccessful. Treatment needs to be aggressive as patients can develop renal failure and systemic oxalosis from severe enteric hyperoxaluria.

URIC ACID STONES

Uric acid crystal formation in the urinary tract may manifest itself as crystalluria, stones, or obstruction. In addition, uric acid and its salt, sodium hydrogen urate, may produce intrarenal disease by initiating an inflammatory response to interstitial deposition as a consequence of hyperuricemia. Crystalluria often occurs in uric acid stone formers and is accompanied by dysuria and hematuria. It may occur in the absence of hyperuricemia or hyperuricosuria, and crystals may be present in the urine of normal subjects whenever urine pH is low.

Natural History
Occurrence

Uric acid stones account for 5% to 10% of all renal stones in the United States, but this figure varies in other parts of the globe, with similar figures for Great Britain, a slightly higher incidence in Germany and France, and the highest incidence reported from Israel, where up to 75% of stones are of uric acid composition.[431]

Relationship to Gout

Uric acid stones are more frequent among gouty patients, and stone formation often develops before articular symptoms.[432] The chance of stone formation increases with increasing serum urate levels and urine excretion rates. In one series, 35% of gouty patients with urine uric acid levels of 700 to 1100 mg/24 hours had stones.[433] In a retrospective analysis of patient records, the incidence rate of stones for a patient with newly diagnosed gout was 1 per 114 patients per year.[434]

Pathogenesis

Urine oversaturation with uric acid and subsequent crystal formation are determined largely by urine pH. Uric acid is a weak acid with two dissociable protons having pK_a values of 5.345 and 10.[326] In biologic systems, only the first proton can be dissociated, so when we refer to the salt of uric acid as urate, we mean monohydrogen urate. Urate is more soluble than uric acid, and urate stones are rare, so that urine oversaturation is important only with respect to undissociated uric acid.

Effects of Urine pH

Urine pH changes have a greater impact on uric acid stone formation than does a change in the amount of uric acid excreted. Urine uric acid may increase only two- to threefold, up to 1500 mg/24 hours, whereas a pH change between 5 and 6 will alter the undissociated acid concentration sixfold. Therefore, uric acid stone formation is conditioned more by pH than by daily urine uric acid excretion or urine volume. Normal uric acid excretion by adults is 500 to 800 mg/24 hours in 1.0 to 1.5 L, or 330 to 800 mg/L. So at low urine pH, below 6.2, oversaturation (>96 mg/L of free uric acid)[326] may occur even in normal subjects. The formation of clinically significant crystalluria or stone requires persistent and severe oversaturation due to hyperuricosuria, dehydration, or a markedly acid urine. Fortunately, such conditions are transient in most people.

Factors That Influence Urine pH

The pH of the urine is determined mainly by the quantity of titratable acid excreted and the amount of phosphate available to buffer it. Titratable acid depends on the load of

TABLE 39-22

Etiologic and Pathophysiologic Classification of Uric Acid Stones

	URINE			
ETIOLOGY	pH	NH$_3$	SOURCE OF SURPLUS URINARY URIC ACID	URINE VOLUME
Idiopathic				
Sporadic	Low	Low	NI	N
Familial	Low	Low	NI	N
Associated with hyperuricemia				
Primary gout	Low	Low	Overproduction	N
Lesch-Nyhan syndrome	N	N	Overproduction	N
Glycogen storage disease	N	N	Overproduction	N
Other enzyme defects	N	N	Overproduction	N
Myeloproliferative and other neoplastic disorders	N	N	Overproduction	N
Associated with hyperuricosuria				
Purine gluttony	N	N	Diet	N
Defects in tubule reabsorption	N	N	Reduced intestinal uricolysis	N
Uricosuric drugs	N	N	Reduced intestinal uricolysis	N
Dehydration				
Gastrointestinal diseases	Low	N	NI	Reduced
Losses through the skin	Low	N	NI	Reduced

N, normal; NI, not increased.

protons generated by body metabolism and the rate of NH_4^+ production; NH_4^+ permits the excretion of protons at a high pH, because it is a base. Generally, NH_4^+ constitutes more than one half the total daily acid excretion. Renal acidification and NH_4^+ production are discussed fully in Chapter 11. Uric acid stone formers tend to excrete less NH_4^+, which contributes directly to low urine pH.[432, 435] In addition, gouty patients, and stone formers in particular, have a reduced postprandial alkaline tide (alkaline urine pH).[436] The morning urine pH is generally very low in gouty patients who form uric acid stones.[435] Dehydration, by reducing urine volume, increases urine uric acid concentration and also promotes a fall in urine pH.

Uric Acid Excretion Rate

About two thirds of the daily uric acid load is excreted by the kidneys, and one third is degraded by intestinal uricolysis.[437] Renal handling of uric acid is discussed in Chapter 15. Hyperuricosuric states may derive from defective renal tubule handling of uric acid, which lowers blood uric acid levels and decreases intestinal uricolysis. Diminished uric acid excretion results in hyperuricemia and increased bowel uricolysis.

Either increased dietary purine ingestion or endogenous uric acid overproduction may increase the amount of uric acid that must be excreted daily. Dietary purine is contained mainly in meat, fish, and poultry in the form of nucleoproteins that are degraded by intestinal and pancreatic enzymes. Normally, dietary purine contributes about 50% of urine uric acid. A high purine intake, about 4 mg/kg/day, will cause an elevation of uric acid excretion that is roughly proportional to the amount of surplus purine ingested. Purine nucleosides from dietary sources are split by nucleoside phosphorylase into free purine bases and ribose-1-phosphate. Guanine is deaminated to form xanthine, which, along with hypoxanthine, is subsequently oxidized to uric acid by the enzyme xanthine oxidase. Some patients with gout, probably a minority, overproduce excess uric acid during the course of endogenous purine metabolism and for this reason have hyperuricosuria. Rarely, massive uric acid overproduction from hereditary deficiencies of enzymes that are critical for purine reutilization is a cause of stones. The Lesch-Nyhan syndrome is a well-known example (Table 39-22).

Clinical Classification of Uric Acid Lithiasis

Uric acid stone–forming conditions include a variety of disorders involving disturbances in purine metabolism, renal urate handling, and urine pH. These pathophysiologic mechanisms interact in a complex fashion, and each also serves as a means of classifying this diverse group of disorders (see Table 39-22).

Idiopathic Uric Acid Stones

Both sporadic and familial forms of idiopathic uric acid stones occur. The familial form is inherited as an autosomal dominant trait, and stones are formed at an earlier age than in the sporadic form and are more likely to cause obstruction and subsequent loss of renal function.[438] Men and women are affected equally, and an ethnic predilection (Jews, Italians) has been suggested.[3] A recent study of uric acid stone formers in a small isolated Italian village found two candidate loci for genes associated with uric acid stone formation, one on chromosome 10q21, the other on 20q13.[439] There are no known candidate genes in these regions and further studies are required to determine how these genes might contribute to uric acid stone disease. In the sporadic variety, stone formation or crystalluria usually begins in middle age, with recurrence predictable if the disorder is not treated. Serum and urine uric acid levels are normal in both forms, and the urine pH is invariably low.[440, 441] The mechanism for stone formation is related to the low urine pH. The majority of uric acid stone formers appear to have reduced ammonium excretion as the cause of the low urine pH. Sakhaee and colleagues[441] reported that uric acid stone formers had a higher daily net acid excretion than normal subjects, and the uric acid stone formers excrete a lower percentage of their daily acid load as ammonium. They also found normal subjects had a much greater increase in ammonium excretion than uric acid stone formers after an acute acid load. Kamel and co-workers[442] also found reduced ammonium excretion in 12 of the 14 uric acid stone formers they studied. The other two patients had high ammonium excretion, which, the authors speculated, may be due to an excessive proton load from loss of organic anions in the urine. The etiology of the acid urine in this subgroup requires further investigation.

Gout

Patients with primary gout may also have uric acid stones. The frequency of uric acid stones is directly related to the degree of uricosuria. The disease may be heterogeneous, because uric acid overexcretion persists despite a low-purine diet in some 21% to 28% of gouty subjects. This may be due to overproduction of endogenous purine.[443] In addition, urine pH tends to be low, suggesting a defect in ammonium production. The majority of patients also have a defect in renal urate excretion such that hyperuricemia is required to excrete even normal amounts of uric acid. Uric acid overproduction is incompletely understood; however, certain enzymatic deficiency states involving the purine pathway and resulting in hyperuricemia have been described. These enzyme defects are most clearly expressed when they occur in infants and children with gout and uric acid stones and include the following: deficiency of hypoxanthine-guanine phosphoribosyltransferase (Lesch-Nyhan syndrome), adenine phosphoribosyltransferase deficiency, increased ribose-phosphate pyrophosphokinase, decreased phosphoribosylpyrophosphate (PRPP) substrate utilization, and type 1 glycogen storage disease. It has been estimated that such enzyme defects, albeit in less severe forms, may be involved in the pathogenesis of up to 11% of cases of gout.

Malignant Disease

Myeloproliferative disease and chronic granulocytic leukemia in adults and acute leukemia in childhood are the common neoplastic disorders that cause hyperuricosuria. Massive cell necrosis in response to chemotherapy abruptly increases urine uric acid excretion, which may cause extensive precipitation and urinary tract obstruction. In the absence of chemotherapy, less marked uricosuria may cause uric acid stones.

Gastrointestinal Diseases

Acute diarrheal states and chronic inflammatory bowel disease may increase urine uric acid concentration through excessive water loss and dehydration. Urine pH tends to fall with extracellular volume contraction, increasing the possibility of stone formation.[444] Patients with ileostomy are particularly at risk, and associated small bowel disease (proximal ileum) may contribute to the lowered urine pH through significant bicarbonate loss.[445] Hyperoxaluria may also be present in patients with ileal resection, leading to mixed stones composed of both uric acid and calcium oxalate.[444]

Drug-Induced Stones

Probenecid and aspirin in large doses are both common uricosuric drugs. Hyperuricemic patients respond to these agents with a transient increase in uric acid excretion. Excretion then falls but remains higher than pretreatment levels, owing to reduced intestinal uricolysis.[446] In patients with high dietary purine intake, the efficient excretion of uric acid induced by the drugs may increase the risk of uric acid stone formation or calcium oxalate stone formation.

Treatment
General Measures

The goals of therapy are a regression in the size of preformed stones and the prevention of new ones. These objectives can be achieved only by lowering the urine concentration of protonated uric acid below levels of saturation. The combination of reducing uric acid excretion, increasing urine volume, and increasing urine pH is effective. The available therapeutic tools include fluids, alkali, diet, and allopurinol. Urine volume can be increased to about 2 L/day with minimal inconvenience.

Alkali and Diet

Urine pH should be maintained within the range or 6.0 to 6.5. During the day, this can be achieved by ingestion of alkali, as either bicarbonate or citrate. Citrate may be preferred over bicarbonate as it requires less frequent dosing.[336] With either preparation, 0.5 to 1.5 mEq/kg/day in divided doses is effective. If nocturnal urine pH falls and stone formation persists, a single dose of 250 mg of acetazolamide at bedtime will usually maintain an alkaline urine. Dietary purine may be reduced to avoid periods of transient excessive uric acid excretion.

Allopurinol

Allopurinol is an isomer of hypoxanthine and competes with this purine base as a substrate for xanthine oxidase, thus blocking the oxidation of xanthine or hypoxanthine to uric acid. Also, the drug lowers overall purine synthesis by decreasing the availability of PRPP and by inhibiting the enzyme PRPP amidotransferase.[447] Allopurinol is converted to a biologically active metabolite, oxypurinol, which has a long half-life (18-30 hours) compared with that of the parent compound (60-90 minutes). Oxypurinol is, itself, soluble only to the extent of 350 mg/L. A single case report describes the formation of oxypurinol stones in a woman with regional enteritis and an ileostomy who was treated with a very large dose of allopurinol, 600 mg/day.[448] Allopurinol should be used if stones recur despite fluid and alkali, or if the patient has gout. Allopurinol is also indicated in the dissolution or reduction in size of existing stones and when large, nonobstructing renal pelvic stones are too large to pass. If given prior to chemotherapy for myeloproliferative or lymphoproliferative malignant disease, allopurinol prevents widespread uric acid precipitation. When allopurinol is used for treatment of patients with massive uric acid overproduction, excellent hydration must be maintained. Xanthine kidney stone formation and acute renal failure from intrarenal xanthine crystal deposition have been described in patients with overproduction of uric acid.[449, 450]

CYSTINURIA

Cystinuria is a hereditary disorder of amino acid transport involving the intestinal epithelia and renal tubule cells (see Chapter 36). As a result of abnormal renal tubule transport, large amounts of cystine are excreted in the urine. When overexcretion leads to concentrations higher than the solubility limit, cystine stones tend to form. The prevalence of cystinuria is approximately 1 in 15,000 in the United States.[451] Cystinuria is found in 1% of all patients with nephrolithiasis; in the pediatric age group, 6% to 8% of stone formers will have cystinuria. Renal stones begin to form in the first to fourth decades. Urinary tract obstruction and infection are common. An increased serum creatinine was reported in 17% of subjects in one large series, though estimates of renal insufficiency as measured by renography may be much higher.[452, 453] Calculi tend to occur as staghorn calculi or as multiple and bilateral separate stones and are visible on roentgenograms because of the density of the sulfur in the cystine molecule. Stone recurrence is common; on average, a stone forms every 1 to 4 years.[453] This disease is not to be confused with cystinosis, in which intracellular cystine accumulation leads to widespread tissue damage, including renal failure. In cystinuria, the amino acid accumulates only in the lumen of renal tubules.

Pathogenesis

Amino acids are filtered and normally almost completely reabsorbed by the proximal tubule. Excessive urinary excretion of cystine and the dibasic amino acids in cystinuria occurs with normal or subnormal blood levels, indicating a tubule reabsorption defect in the common transport mechanism for the dibasic amino acids.[454-457] A similar transport defect exists in intestinal epithelial cells. After oral administration of cystine, urinary excretion of cystine does not rise, as it does in normal subjects; urine excretion of orally ingested arginine, lysine, or ornithine is variable and often low.[458, 459] Jejunal perfusion studies have shown defects in arginine as well as cystine absorption,[458] and in vitro studies of specimens of jejunal mucosa obtained by peroral biopsy have confirmed the presence of defects in intestinal transport of these amino acids.

Cystine and dibasic amino acids are reabsorbed in the proximal tubule by a heteromeric transporter located in the apical membrane.[460] The heteromeric transporter is composed of two proteins, a light chain and a heavy chain linked by a single disulfide bond. The light chain of heteromeric amino acid transporters determines the specific amino acids to be reabsorbed; the heavy chain is involved in trafficking of the protein complex to the apical membrane of cells. Recent genetic studies have determined that mutations in the genes encoding the heavy (*SLC3A1*) and the light (*SLC7A9*) chain of the heteromeric transporter cause cystinuria. The *SLC3A1* gene, located on chromosome 2p21, encodes the protein rBAT.[460-462] rBAT is expressed in both the kidney and intestine. The *SLC7A9* gene, located on chromosome 19q13, encodes the light-chain protein b[o, +]AT, which requires association with rBAT to attain proper localization in the cell membrane.[463-465]

Family studies have revealed an autosomal recessive phenotype for cystinuria. However, heterogeneity in the intestinal absorption of cystine in affected patients and in the cystine excretion rate of the parents of probands made it clear that cystinuria was not a homogeneous disease. Before discovery of the genes controlling cystine reabsorption, cystinuria was divided into three subtypes based on the urinary cystine excretion of obligate heterozygotes for the cystine gene. Type I heterozygotes had normal cystine excretion, whereas types II and III had elevated cystine excretion, type II higher than type III.[466] The initial genetic studies found that the type I phenotype was due to mutations in the *SLC3A1* gene, and in vitro studies of the mutated protein showed reduced cystine transport activity.[462, 467, 468] More recent studies have linked both type II and type III cystinuria to the *SLC7A9* gene,[453, 465] which has led to the proposal that the phenotype classification be revised to include only type I and non–type I cystinuria, reflecting the common gene origin. However, detailed studies of phenotype and genotype have shown that some mutations in the *SLC7A9* gene may lead to normal cystine excretion in the heterozygous state, thus mimicking phenotype I.[453] This has led some investigators to propose a genetic classification rather than one based on phenotype. In addition, some patients with cystinuria have not had a mutation found in either of these genes. Patients with unclassified genotype may have mutations in noncoding regions that have not been identified or perhaps a third protein that may be involved in cystine transport. The most likely candidate for a third protein would be an as yet undiscovered light chain that could associate with rBAT. It is likely the classification of cystinuric patients will continue to evolve as the molecular basis of the disease becomes better defined.

Cystine overexcretion raises the urine cystine concentration above the limits of solubility for this most insoluble amino acid. Characteristic hexagonal crystals may be identified in cystinuria, particularly in the first-voided morning urine, which is concentrated and usually acid. The normal adult excretes less than 19 mg of cystine per gram of creatinine in 24 hours,[469] whereas homozygous stone formers usually excrete more than 250 mg/g creatinine; heterozygotes may have normal or moderately increased excretion of cystine.[470] Urinary excretion of the dibasic amino acids arginine, ornithine, and lysine is also increased in homozygous cystinuria and, to a variable extent, in the heterozygous form. However, as the dibasic amino acids are soluble, there is no clinical consequence to their high urine concentrations.

In addition to pure cystine stones, homozygous cystinuric patients are prone to develop calcium oxalate and uric acid stones, as well as cystine stones mixed with other solid phases.[471] This appears to be due to a higher rate of metabolic stone-forming risks than normal. In a study of 27 cystinuric patients, 5 (18%) had hypercalciuria, 6 (22%) had hyperuricosuria, and 10 (44%) had hypocitraturia.[472] Heterozygous cystinuria may carry an increased risk of forming calcium oxalate stones.[473]

Treatment

Therapy is designed to reduce the excretion and increase the solubility of cystine. Lowering urinary cystine concentration by increasing urine volume reduces the likelihood of precipitation and is the basis for clinical treatment. An intake of 4 L/day or more may be required, as patients may excrete up to 1 g/day of cystine. The solubility limit for cystine averages about 300 mg/L, though there is considerable variability in solubility among urine samples, as can be seen in Figure 39-17, making it difficult to gauge exactly the urine flow an individual patient will require to prevent stones.[474] Solubility tends to increase as the urine pH rises, though the most significant increase does not occur until the urine pH is above 7.0 (see Fig. 39-17).[474-476] Aggressive alkalinization should be used in all patients to prevent stone formation. Methionine is a precursor of cystine, and dietary restriction of methionine has been recommended as treatment.[477] However, the reduction in cystine excretion was only 20% in seven patients fed a high-protein diet (140 g/day) and then switched to a low-proten diet (54 g/day).[478] Because methionine is an essential amino acid, long-term restriction may also lead to sulfur amino acid deficiencies. Martensson and colleagues[479] have found low leukocyte glutathione and taurine levels and low urinary sulfate, taurine, and thiosulfate levels, suggesting a mild intracellular cystine deficiency in homozygous cystinuria. Chronic methionine restriction might cause a clinically significant cystine deficiency.

Cystine excretion is linked to sodium excretion, and low-sodium diets have been shown to reduce cystine excretion by 40%.[480, 481] Because high-sodium intake will promote cystine excretion, potassium salts are preferred for alkali therapy. Glutamine has been reported to reduce cystine excretion,[482] but this effect is only present with high-salt intake and is of little clinical benefit.[483]

Pharmacologic therapy is required when patients have not responded to diet, fluid, and alkali therapy. Drug therapy increases cystine solubility by creating a thiol-cysteine

disulfide, which is more soluble than cystine. These thiol-containing drugs may also reduce cystine excretion in addition to increasing cystine solubility.[483] D-Penicillamine and tiopronin are the most commonly used drugs, but they have significant side effects, including rash, proteinuria, nausea, and fever, often forcing discontinuation of the drug.[484] Tiopronin appears to be better tolerated than D-penicillamine.[484] Acetylcysteine is not recommended for therapy as it increases the excretion of cystine.[479] Captopril, a thiol, has been reported to reduce stone formation in some patients with cystinuria and is well tolerated.[485, 486] However the effectiveness of captopril has been questioned by some investigators.[487]

Treatment of large cystine stones can be difficult. The stones are difficult to fragment by extracorporeal shock wave lithotripsy and percutaneous lithotripsy.[488] Stone fragments remain after these procedures in approximately 15% to 50% of patients.[489-491] The holmium:YAG (yttrium-aluminum-garnet) laser may be better at fragmenting the stones than lithotripsy,[492] but there is no consensus as to the preferred approach to cystine stones. Irrigation of the renal pelvis with alkaline solutions can be used to dissolve the remaining fragments after percutaneous or extracorporeal lithotripsy.[489]

STRUVITE (INFECTION) STONES

Struvite ($MgNH_4PO_4 \cdot 6H_2O$) stones form in the renal pelvis and calices only when the urinary tract is infected by a urea-splitting bacterium, usually *Proteus* species.[493] Struvite stones tend to branch and enlarge, and their growth is rapid. Often, they fill the renal collecting systems and assume a staghorn configuration. They frequently grow back after surgical removal because infected chalky fragments have been left behind.

Kidneys are often damaged by obstruction and infection. Because of the size of these calculi, pyelolithotomy is difficult. Infection stones are most destructive and difficult to control. The actual composition of struvite stones in humans is variable in that carbonate apatite [$Ca_{10}(PO_4)_6 \cdot CO_3$] is usually present along with struvite and may even predominate.[494] However, the presence of struvite always implicates urinary tract infection with urea-splitting organisms, whatever the apatite concentration in the stone.

Urea Splitting

Bacterial urease hydrolyzes urea as follows: $(NH_2)_2\text{--}CO \rightarrow H_2O + 2NH_3 + CO_2$. The ammonia hydrolyzes spontaneously to form NH_4OH, wheras the CO_2 hydrates to form H_2CO_3 and then HCO_3^-. Urine pH increases because ammonia hydrolyzes, just as it would if NH_3 were bubbled through it from a storage tank. At a high pH, HCO_3^- loses its proton to become CO_3^{2-}.

The urine conditions produced by ureolysis are unique. Normally, urine NH_4^+ rises only with an acid load or potassium depletion, conditions of low urine pH, and negligible urine carbonate concentration (see Chapter 11). In RTA type 1, the urine is alkaline and may contain bicarbonate, especially during alkali treatment, but urine NH_4^+ levels, though relatively high for the prevailing pH, are very low in absolute concentration (see Chapter 20). In other conditions of

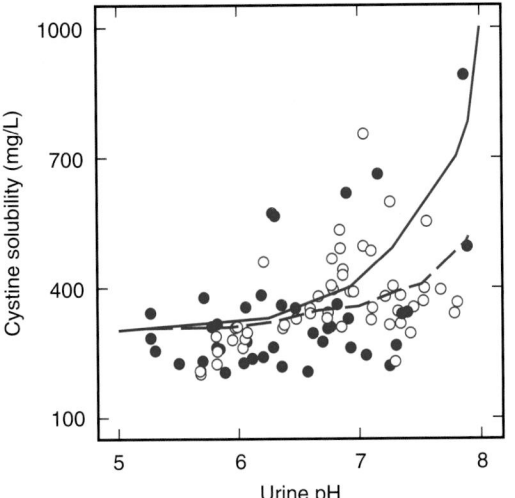

FIGURE 39-17. Effect of pH on cystine solubility in human urine. Cystine solubility (*y* axis) in urine from patients with cystinuria (*open circles*) or from normal subjects or calcium oxalate stone formers (*filled circles*) increased with urine pH (*x* axis). Dent and Senior nomogram[475] (*solid line*) generally overestimated solubility; Marshall and Robertson nomogram[476] (*broken line*) predicts lower solubility than that of Dent and Senior. Both nomograms fail to reflect the large scatter of actual solubility at any given pH. (From Nakagawa Y, Asplin JR, Goldfarb D, et al: Clinical use of cystine supersaturation measurements. J Urol 164: 1481-1485, 2000.)

alkaline urine, such as antacid abuse, urine NH_4^+ is also low. It is only in infection that urease is present in urine, and only urease can elevate NH_4^+, pH, and carbonate concentration at the same time. So it is not surprising that struvite stones arise only from infection and often contain carbonate apatite. All normal urine is undersaturated with respect to struvite,[495, 496] so one could expect dissolution of an infection stone during prolonged antimicrobial treatment if the treatment were successful in eradicating infection. However, normal urine need not be undersaturated with respect to carbonate apatite,[495] only metastable. So whether an infection stone will dissolve depends on its apatite concentration.

Bacteriology

Proteus and *Providencia* species possess urease in over 90% of isolates.[497] Other common urinary pathogens which frequently contain urease include *Klebsiella*, *Pseudomonas*, and enterococci. *Escherichia coli* rarely possesses urease activity.[498] *Ureaplasma urealyticum*, a fastidious bacterium that requires special culture techniques for isolation, has been shown to cause struvite stones.[499] The bacteria produce oversaturation in their own immediate environment, so crystals tend to form around clusters of bacteria. As a result, bacteria permeate every crevice of a struvite-apatite stone. The stone becomes like a harbor; it keeps the bacteria from washing away in the flowing urine. Every fragment of the stone is infected and therefore can enlarge in urine. Bits of a growing stone swept into an uninvolved calyx, or into the bladder, can create a metastatic focus if they adhere to the urothelium. It has been proposed that the high urinary ammonia concentrations interfere with the ability of GAGs to prevent bacterial adhesion to the urothelium, thus increasing the risk of struvite crystals anchoring in the collecting system.[497]

Predisposing Factors

Calcium, uric acid, or cystine stones can become infected, especially as a result of instrumentation of the urinary tract. These patients will tend to have underlying metabolic abnormalities, such as idiopathic hypercalciuria, and maintain relatively well-preserved renal function.[500] Chronic bladder catheterization promotes infection, and *Proteus* or *Pseudomonas* species can predominate despite the use of antimicrobial agents. Patients with spinal cord injury or any other form of neurogenic bladder or in whom ileal diversion of the ureter has been performed are especially prone to forming struvite stones. However, struvite stones also occur without any predisposing cause. They are three times more common in women than in men, presumably because urinary tract infection is much more common in women.[497] Often they grow silently. Radiographic studies performed because of recurrent symptoms of urinary infection, hematuria, or pyuria or because of symptoms not related to the urinary system can disclose a staghorn calculus so large that it fills the renal collecting system and provokes amazement that its symptoms could be so meager.

Treatment

The preferred treatment of a struvite staghorn stone is surgical removal.[501] Untreated staghorn calculi ultimately require nephrectomy in 50% of cases.[502, 503] Open surgical removal had been the procedure of choice and often led to improved renal function if obstruction were present. However, Griffith and colleagues[494] estimated that after 435 such operations, there were recurrences in 118 cases (27%) within 6.3 years, and urinary tract infection persisted after surgery in 129 of 315 cases, or 41%. A more recent study by Silverman and Stamey[504] showed only a 2.2% stone recurrence rate during 7 years of follow-up when open surgery was followed by aggressive lavage of the renal pelvis with hemiacidrin to ensure no stone fragments remained.

Newer procedures have reduced the morbidity of struvite stone removal with reasonably low rates of stone recurrence. Percutaneous nephrolithotomy can completely remove struvite stones in 85% to 90% of kidneys[505, 506] with only a 10% relapse rate in those kidneys rendered stone-free.[507] Extracorporeal shock wave lithotripsy with ureteral stenting has been used as monotherapy for large-volume struvite stones, resulting in stone-free rates of 50% to 75%.[508, 509] The American Urologic Association clinical guidelines recommend a combined approach of percutaneous nephrolithotomy and shock wave lithotripsy as giving the best stone-free rates with the least patient morbidity in patients with struvite staghorn stones.[501] Since the clinical guidelines were published, retrograde ureteroscopy with holmium: YAG laser disruption of stones has become an alternative approach for staghorn stones. Grasso and associates,[510] using a ureteroscopic approach, reported fragmentation of 95% of minor staghorn stones with a 60% stone-free rate at 6 months. No matter which approach is taken, the best long-term results depend on clearing the urinary tract of stone and sterilizing the urine.

Antibiotic treatment and conservative measures may well be preferable to surgery in selected cases. Any metabolic disorder should be treated. Antibiotic use should be based on antibiotic resistance patterns of the infecting organism. Culture of stone material may allow more specific antibiotic therapy directed against the organism producing the stone.[504] Although hope of cure is remote, stone growth can be slowed by reducing the bacterial population. Stamey[511] has reported partial dissolution of stones during chronic antibiotic treatment.

Acetohydroxamic acid (AHA), a compound that inhibits bacterial urease, is another alternative to surgery or an adjunct therapy after surgical reduction of stone mass. Three randomized, double-blind clinical trials have been performed using AHA.[512-514] In all three studies a significant reduction in the rate of stone growth or formation was found. There is a high rate of side effects, which led to significant rates of patient withdrawal from treatment in all three trials. The most common side effects are headache, tremulousness, and anemia. Higher rates of deep venous thrombosis have been reported in patients receiving the active drug in these trials, but the difference has not been statistically significant.

Irrigation of the renal pelvis with acidic solutions can reduce stone burden as both struvite and carbonate apatite dissolve in an acidic environment. Various acid citrate solutions have been used to irrigate the intact unobstructed renal pelvis, although the procedure is potentially very hazardous.[515] Irrigation can lead to renal and ureteral damage and sepsis and must be carried out with great caution. It can be used, however, even in such complex settings as infection stone with ileal conduit urinary diversion.[516] The use of this treatment is usually as an adjunct to open or percutaneous surgery, although it has been used as monotherapy. Oral acidifying agents are not effective in treating struvite stones.

Though many improvements have been made in the medical and surgical approach to struvite stones, a cure may still be difficult to obtain. The correct surgical approach is not always clear, and many patients require multiple procedures. Struvite stones often recur and patients need long-term follow-up and surveillance for urinary tract infections.

REFERENCES

1. Nordin BEC, Hodgkinson A: Urolithiasis, Adv Intern Med 13:155-182, 1967.
2. Lagergren C: Biophysical investigations of urinay calculi. Acta Radiol Scand Suppl 133:1-48, 1956.
3. Melick RA, Henneman PH: Clinical and laboratory studies of 207 consecutive patients in a kidney-stone clinic. N Engl J Med 259:307-314, 1958.
4. Prien EL: Studies in urolithiasis. J Urol 61:821-836, 1949.
5. Sutor DJ, Wooley SE, Illingworth JJ: Some aspects of the adult urinary stone problem in Great Britain and Northern Ireland. Br J Urol 46:275-288, 1974.
6. Mandel NS, Mandel GS: Urinary tract stone disease in the United States veteran population. II. Geographical analysis of variations in composition. J Urol 142:1516-1521, 1989.
7. Koide T, Oka T, Takaha M, et al: Urinary tract stone disease in modern Japan. Eur Urol 12:403-407, 1986.
8. Berenyi M, Frang D, Legrady J: Theoretical and clinical importance of the differentiation between the two types of calcium oxalate hydrate. Int Urol Nephrol 4:34, 1972.
9. Daudon M, Donsimoni R, Hennequin C, et al: Sex and age–related composition of 10167 calculi analyzed by infrared spectroscopy. Urol Res 23:319-326, 1995.
10. Leusmann DB, Blaschke R, Schmandt W: Results of 5035 stone analyses: A contribution to epidemiology of urinary stone disease. Scand J Urol Nephrol 24:205-210, 1990.
11. Ellis H: A History of Bladder Stones. Oxford, Blackwell Scientific Publications, 1969.
12. Sutor DJ, Wooley SE, Illingworth JJ: A geographical and historical survey of the composition of urinary stones. Br J Urol 46:393, 1974.
13. Anderson DA: Historical and geographical differences in the pattern of incidence of urinary stones considered in relation to possible aetiological factors. *In* Hodgkinson A, Nordin BEC (eds): Renal Stone Research Symposium. London, JA Churchill, 1969, p 7.
14. Johnson CM, Wilson DM, O'Fallon WM, et al: Renal stone epidemiology: A 25-year study in Rochester, Minnesota. Kidney Int 16:624-631, 1979.
15. Soucie JM, Thun MJ, Coates RJ, et al: Demographic and geographic variability of kidney stones in the United States. Kidney Int 46:893-899, 1994.
16. Sutherland JW, Parks JH, Coe FL: Recurrence after a single renal stone in a community practice. Miner Electrolyte Metab 11:267-269, 1985.
17. Williams RE: Long-term survey of 538 patients with upper urinary tract stones. Br J Urol 35:416, 1963.
18. Ljunghall S, Danielson BG: A prospective study of renal stone recurrences. Br J Urol 56:122-124, 1984.
19. Blacklock NJ: The pattern of urolithiasis in the Royal Navy. *In* Hodgkinson A, Nordin BEC (eds): Renal Stone Research Symposium. London, JA Churchill, 1969, p 33.
20. Marshall V, White RH, Chaput DE, et al: The natural history of renal and ureteric colic. Br J Urol 47:117, 1975.
21. Coe FL, Keck J, Norton ER: The natural history of calcium urolithiasis. JAMA 238:1519-1523, 1977.
22. Strauss AL, Coe FL, Parks JH: Formation of a single calcium stone of renal origin: Clinical and laboratory characteristics of patients. Arch Intern Med 142:504-507, 1982.
23. Coe FL, Parks JH, Lindheimer MD: Nephrolithiasis during pregnancy. N Engl J Med 298:324-326, 1978.
24. Jones WA, Correa RJ, Ansell JS: Urolithiasis associated with pregnancy. J Urol 122:333, 1979.
25. Parks JH, Coe FL, Strauss AL: Calcium nephrolithiasis and medullary sponge kidney in women. N Engl J Med 306:1088-1091, 1982.
26. Coe FL: Calcium-uric acid nephrolithiasis. Arch Intern Med 138:1090-1093, 1978.
27. Millman S, Strauss AL, Parks JH, et al: Pathogenesis and clinical course of mixed calcium oxalate and uric acid nephrolithiasis. Kidney Int 22:366-370, 1982.
28. Coe FL, Parks JH, Strauss AL: Accelerated calcium nephrolithiasis. JAMA 244:809-810, 1980.
29. Pak CYC: Citrate and renal calculi. Miner Electrolyte Metab 13:257-266, 1987.
30. Hallson PC, Rose GA, Sulaiman S: Magnesium reduces calcium oxalate crystal formation in human whole urine. Clin Sci (Colch) 62:17-19, 1982.
31. Pak CYC, Hayashi Y, Finlayson B, et al: Estimation of the state of supersaturation of brushite and calcium oxalate in urine: A comparison of three methods. J Lab Clin Med 89:891-909, 1977.
32. Robertson WG, Peacock M, Nordin BEC: Activity products in stone-forming and non–stone-forming urine. Clin Sci (Colch) 34:579-594, 1968.
33. Werness PG, Brown CM, Smith LH, et al: Equil2: A basic computer program for the calculation of urinary saturation. J Urol 134:1242-1244, 1985.
34. Asplin J, Parks J, Lingeman J, et al: Supersaturation and stone composition in a network of dispersed treatment sites. J Urol 159:1821-1825, 1998.
35. Parks JH, Coward M, Coe FL: Correspondence between stone composition and urine supersaturation in nephrolithiasis. Kidney Int 51:894-900, 1997.
36. Robertson WG, Peacock M, Nordin BEC: Calcium oxalate crystalluria and urine saturation in recurrent renal stone formers. Clin Sci (Colch) 40:365-374, 1971.
37. Robertson WG, Peacock M, Marshall RW, et al: Saturation-inhibition index as a measure of the risk of calcium oxalate stone formation in the urinary tract. N Engl J Med 294:249-252, 1976.
38. Marshall RW, Cochran M, Robertson WG, et al: The relation between the concentration of calcium salts in the urine and renal stone composition in patients with calcium-containing renal stones. Clin Sci (Colch) 43:433-441, 1972.
39. Pak CYC, Holt K: Nucleation and growth of brushite and calcium oxalate in urine of stone formers. Metabolism 25:665-673, 1976.
40. Weber DV, Coe FL, Parks JH, et al: Urinary saturation measurements in calcium nephrolithiasis. Ann Intern Med 90:180-184, 1979.
41. Hautmann R, Lehmann A, Komor S: Calcium and oxalate concentrations in human renal tissue: The key to the pathogenesis of stone formation. J Urol 123:317-319, 1980.
42. Asplin JR, Mandel NS, Coe FL: Evidence for calcium phosphate supersaturation in the loop of Henle. Am J Physiol 270:F604-F613, 1996.
43. Asplin JR, Parks JH, Chen MS, et al: Reduced crystallization inhibition by urine from men with nephrolithiasis. Kidney Int 56:1505-1516, 1999.
44. Asplin JR, Parks JH, Nakagawa Y, et al: Reduced crystallization inhibition by urine from women with nephrolithiasis. Kidney Int 61:1821-1829, 2002.
45. Nielson AE: Kinetics of Precipitation. New York, Pergamon Press, 1964.
46. Pak CY, Arnold LH: Heterogeneous nucleation of calcium oxalate by seeds of monosodium urate. Proc Soc Exp Biol Med 149:930-932, 1975.
47. Coe FL, Lawton RL, Goldstein RB, et al: Sodium urate accelerates precipitation of calcium oxalate in vitro. Proc Soc Exp Biol Med 149:926-929, 1975.
48. Coe FL, Raisen L: Allopurinol treatment of uric-acid disorders in calcium-stone formers. Lancet 1:129-131, 1973.
49. Coe FL: Hyperuricosuric calcium oxalate nephrolithiasis. Kidney Int 13:418-426, 1978.
50. Fleisch H, Bisaz S: Isolation from urine of pyrophosphate, a calcification inhibitor. Am J Physiol 203:671-675, 1962.
51. Russell RGG, Fleisch H: Inhibitors in urinary stone disease: Role of pyrophosphate in urinary calculi. *In* Cifuentes-Delatte L, Rapado A, Hodgkinson A (eds): Urinary Calculi. Basel, S Karger, 1973, p 307.
52. Deganello S, Coe F: Epitaxy between uric and whewellite: Experimental verification. N Jb Miner Mh 6:270-276, 1983.

53. Meyer JL, Bergert JH, Smith LH: Epitaxial relationships in urolithiasis: The brushite-whewellite system. Clin Sci (Colch) 52:143-148, 1977.

54. Meyer JL, Bergert JH, Smith LH: Epitaxial relationships in urolithiasis: The calcium oxalate monohydrate-hydroxyapatite system. Clin Sci (Colch) 49:369-374, 1975.

55. Randall A: The origin and growth of renal calculi. Ann Surg 105:1009-1027, 1937.

56. Herring LC: Observations on the analysis of ten thousand urinary calculi. J Urol 88:545-555, 1962.

57. Low RK, Stoller ML: Endoscopic mapping of renal papillae for Randall's plaques in patients with urinary stone disease. J Urol 158:2062-2064, 1997.

58. Robertson WG, Peacock M, Nordin BEC: Inhibitors of the growth and aggregation of calcium oxalate crystals in vitro. Clin Chim Acta 43:31-37, 1973.

59. Finlayson B, Reid F: The expectation of free and fixed particles in urinary stone disease. Invest Urol 15:442-448, 1978.

60. Riese RJ, Riese JW, Kleinman JG, et al: Specificity in calcium oxalate adherence to papillary epithelial cells in cultures. Am J Physiol 255:F1025-F1032, 1988.

61. Lieske JC, Walsh-Reitz MW, Toback FG: Calcium oxalate monohydrate crystals are endocytosed by renal epithelial cells and induce proliferation. Am J Physiol 262: F622-F630, 1992.

62. Lieske JC, Toback FG: Regulation of renal epithelial cell endocytosis of calcium oxalate monohydrate crystals. Am J Physiol 264: F800-F807, 1993.

63. Kohjimoto Y, Ebisuno S, Tamura M, et al: Interactions between calcium oxalate monohydrate crystals and Madin-Darby canine kidney cells: Endocytosis and cell proliferation. Urol Res 24: 193-199, 1996.

64. Lieske JC, Toback FG, Deganello S: Face selective adhesion of calcium oxalate dihydrate crystals to renal eptithelial cells. Calcif Tissue Int 58:195-200, 1996.

65. Lieske JC, Toback FG, Deganello S: Direct nucleation of calcium oxalate dihydrate crystals onto the surface of living renal epithelial cells in culture. Kidney Int 54:796-803, 1998.

66. Bigelow MW, Wiessner JH, Kleinman JG, et al: Surface exposure of phosphatidylserine increases calcium oxalate attachment to IMCD cells. Am J Physiol 272:F55-F62, 1997.

67. Lieske JC, Leonard R, Toback FG: Adhesion of calcium oxalate monohydrate crystals to renal epithelial cells is inhibited by specific anions. Am J Physiol 268:F604-F612, 1995.

68. Meyer JL, Smith LH: Growth of calcium oxalate crystals. II. Inhibition by natural urinary crystal growth inhibitors. Invest Urol 13:36-39, 1975.

69. Ito H, Coe FL: Acidic peptide and polyribonucleotide crystal growth inhibitors in human urine. Am J Physiol 233:F455-F463, 1977.

70. Bisaz S, Felix R, Neuman WF, et al: Quantitative determination of inhibitors of calcium phosphate precipitation in whole urine. Miner Electrolyte Metab 1:74-83, 1978.

71. Baumann JM, Ackermann D, Affolter B: The influence of hydroxyapatite and pyrophosphate on the formation product of calcium oxalate at different pHs. Urol Res 17:153-155, 1989.

72. Schwille PO, Rumenapf G, Wolfel G, et al: Urinary pyrophosphate in patients with recurrent urolithiasis and in healthy controls: A reevaluation. J Urol 140:239-245, 1988.

73. Li MK, Blacklock NJ, Garside J: Effects of magnesium on calcium oxalate crystallization. J Urol 133:123-125, 1985.

74. Robertson WG, Scurr DS: Modifiers of calcium oxalate crystallization found in urine. I. Studies with a continuous crystallizer using an artificial urine. J Urol 135:1322-1326, 1986.

75. Rodgers AL, Garside J: The nucleation and growth kinetics of calcium oxalate in the presence of some synthetic urine constituents. Invest Urol 18:484-488, 1981.

76. Hallson PC, Kasidas GP, Samuell CT: The inhibitory activity of some citrate analogues upon calcium crystalluria: Observations using an improved evaporation technique. Urol Int 57:43-47, 1996.

77. Hess B: Simultaneous measurements of calcium oxalate crystal nucleation and aggregation: Impact of various modifiers. Urol Res 23: 231-238, 1995.

78. Nicar MJ, Hill K, Pak CYC: Inhibition by citrate of spontaneous precipitation of calcium oxalate in vitro. J Bone Miner Res 2:215-220, 1987.

79. Tiselius HG, Fornander A, Nilsson M: The effects of citrate and urine on calcium oxalate crystal aggregation. Urol Res 21:363-366, 1993.

80. Hess B, Kok DJ: Nucleation, growth, and aggregation of stone forming crystals. In Coe FL, Favus MJ, Pak CYC, et al (eds): Kidney Stones: Medical and Surgical Management. Philadelphia, Lippincott-Raven, 1996, pp 3-32.

81. Nakagawa Y, Abram V, Kezdy FJ, et al: Purification and characterization of the principal inhibitor of calcium oxalate monohydrate crystal growth in human urine. J Biol Chem 258:12594-12600, 1983.

82. Asplin J, Deganello S, Nakagawa YN, et al: Evidence that nephrocalcin and urine inhibit nucleation of calcium oxalate monohydrate crystals. Am J Physiol 261:F824-F830, 1991.

83. Hess B, Nakagawa Y, Coe FL: Inhibition of calcium oxalate monohydrate crystal aggregation by urine proteins. Am J Physiol 257: F99-106, 1989.

84. Nakagawa Y, Abram V, Parks JH, et al: Urine glycoprotein crystal growth inhibitors. Evidence for a molecular abnormality in calcium oxalate nephrolithiasis. J Clin Invest 76:1455-1462, 1985.

85. Worcester EM, Nakagawa Y, Wabner CL, et al: Crystal adsorption and growth slowing by nephrocalcin, albumin, and Tamm-Horsfall protein. Am J Physiol 255:F1197-F1205, 1988.

86. Hess B, Nakagawa Y, Parks JH, et al: Molecular abnormality of Tamm-Horsfall glycoprotein in calcium oxalate nephrolithiasis. Am J Physiol 260:F569-F578, 1991.

87. Schniele P, Hering F, Seiler H: Isoelectric focusing of Tamm-Horsfall glycoproteins: A simple tool for recognizing recurrent calcium oxalate renal stone formers. Urol Res 24:79-82, 1996.

88. Trewick AL, Rumsby G: Isoelectric focusing of native urinary uromodulin shows no physicochemical differences between stone formers and non–stone formers. Urol Res 27:250-254, 1999.

89. Kleinman JG, Beshensky A, Worcester EM, et al: Expression of osteopontin, a urinary inhibitor of stone mineral crystal growth, in rat kidney. Kidney Int 47:1585-1596, 1995.

90. Shiraga H, Min W, VanDusen WJ, et al: Inhibition of calcium oxalate crystal growth in vitro by uropontin: Another member of the aspartic acid-rich protein superfamily. Proc Natl Acad Sci U S A 89: 426-430, 1992.

91. Asplin JR, Arsenault D, Parks JH, et al: Contribution of human uropontin to inhibition of calcium oxalate crystallization. Kidney Int 53:194-199, 1998.

92. Lieske JC, Hammes MS, Hoyer JR, et al: Renal cell osteopontin production is stimulated by calcium oxalate monohydrate crystals. Kidney Int 51:679-686, 1997.

93. Doyle IR, Marshall VR, Dawson CJ, et al: Calcium oxalate crystal matrix extract: The most potent macromolecular inhibitor of crystal growth and aggregation yet tested in undiluted human urine in vitro. Urol Res 23:53-62, 1995.

94. Stapleton AMF, Ryall RL: Blood coagulation proteins and urolithiasis are linked: Crystal matrix protein is the F1 activation peptide of human prothrombin. Br J Urol 75:712-719, 1995.

95. Stapleton AMF, Seymour AE, Brennan JS, et al: Immunohistochemical distribution and quantification of crystal matrix protein. Kidney Int 44:817-824, 1993.

96. Kobayashi H, Shibata K, Fujie M, et al: Identification of structural domains in inter-alpha-trypsin inhibitor involved in calcium oxalate crystallization. Kidney Int 53:1727-1735, 1998.

97. Atmani F, Khan SR: Characterization of uronic-acid-rich inhibitor of calcium oxalate crystallization isolated from rat urine. Urol Res 23:95-101, 1995.

98. Dawson CJ, Grover PK, Kanellos J, et al: Inter-α-trypsin inhibitor in calcium stones. Clin Sci (Colch) 95:187-193, 1998.

99. Marengo SR, Resnick M, Yang L, et al: Differential expression of urinary inter-alpha-trypsin inhibitor trimers and dimers in normal compared to active calcium oxalate stone forming men. J Urol 159: 1444-1450, 1998.

100. Umekawa T, Kurita T: Calprotectin-like protein is related to soluble organic matrix in calcium oxalate urinary stone. Biochem Mol Biol Int 34:309-313, 1994.

101. Pillay SN, Asplin JR, Coe FL: Evidence that calgranulin is produced by kidney cells and is an inhibitor of calcium oxalate crystallization. Am J Physiol 275:F255-F261, 1998.

102. Asakura H, Selengut JD, Orme- Johnson WH, et al: The effect of purified calprotectin on the nucleation and growth of struvite crystals as assayed by light microscopy. In Pak CYC, Resnick MI, Preminger GM (eds): Urolithiasis 1996. Dallas, Millet the Printer, 1996, pp 199-201.

103. Yamaguchi S, Yoshioka T, Utsunomiya M, et al: Heparan sulfate in the stone matrix and its inhibitory effect on calcium oxalate crystallization. Urol Res 21:187-192, 1993.

104. Suzuki K, Ryall RL: The effect of heparan sulphate on the crystallization of calcium oxalate in undiluted, ultrafiltered human urine. Br J Urol 78:15-21, 1996.

105. Ryall RL, Harnett RM, Hibberd CM, et al: Effects of chondroitin sulphate, human serum albumin and Tamm-Horsfall mucoprotein on calcium oxalate crystallization in undiluted human urine. Urol Res 19:181-188, 1991.

106. Michelacci YM, Glashan RQ, Schor N: Urinary excretion of glycosaminoglycans in normal and stone forming subjects. Kidney Int 36:1022-1028, 1989.

107. Nesse A, Garbossa G, Romero MC, et al: Glycosaminoglycans in urolithiasis. Nephron 62:36-39, 1992.

108. Zerwekh JE, Hwang TI, Poindexter J, et al: Modulation by calcium of the inhibitor activity of naturally occurring urinary inhibitors. Kidney Int 33:1005-1008, 1988.

109. Hess B, Zipperle L, Jaeger P: Citrate and calcium effects on Tamm-Horsfall glycoprotein as a modifier of calcium oxalate crystal aggregation. Am J Physiol 265:F784-F791, 1993.

110. Coe FL: Treated and untreated recurrent calcium nephrolithiasis in patients with idiopathic hypercalciuria, hyperuricosuria, or no metabolic disorder. Ann Intern Med 87:404-410, 1977.

111. Yendt ER: Renal calculi. Can Med Assoc J 102:479, 1970.

112. Hodgkinson A, Pyrah LN: The urinary excretion of calcium and inorganic phosphate in 344 patients with calcium stones of renal origin. Br J Surg 46:10, 1958.

113. Robertson WG, Knowles F, Peacock M: Urinary acid mucopolysaccharide inhibitors of calcium oxalate crystallisation. *In* Fleisch H, Robertson WG, Smith LH, et al (eds): Urolithiasis Research. London, Plenum Press, 1976, pp 331-340.

114. Coe FL, Margolis HC, Deutsch LH, et al: Urinary macromolecular crystal growth inhibitors in calcium urolithiasis. Miner Electrolyte Metab 3:268-275, 1980.

115. Tiselius HG, Bek-Jensen H, Fornander A, et al: Crystallization properties in urine from calcium oxalate stone formers. J Urol 154:940-946, 1995.

116. Harvey JA, Hill KD, Pak CYC: Epidemiology of stone disease in the United States as discerned from a stone risk profile. *In* Walker VR, Sutton RAL, Cameron ECB, et al (eds): Urolithiasis. New York, Plenum Press, 1989, pp 665-667.

117. Levy FL, Adams-Huet B, Pak CYC: Ambulatory evaluation of nephrolithiasis: An update of a 1980 protocol. Am J Med 98:50-59, 1995.

118. Pyrah LN, Hodgkinson A, Anderson CK: Primary hyperparathyroidism. Br J Surg 53:245-316, 1966.

119. Aurbach GD, Mallette LE, Pattern BM, et al: Hyperparathyroidism: Recent studies. Ann Intern Med 79:566, 1973.

120. Silverberg SJ, Shane E, Jacobs TP, et al: A 10-year prospective study of primary hyperparathyroidism with or without parathyroid surgery. N Engl J Med 341:1249-1255, 1999.

121. Boonstra CE, Jackson CE: Hyperparathyroidism detected by routine serum calcium analysis. Ann Intern Med 63:468, 1965.

122. Yendt ER: Disorders of calcium, phosphorus and magnesium metabolism. *In* Maxwell MG, Kleeman CR (eds): Clinical Disorders of Fluid and Electrolyte Metabolism. New York, McGraw-Hill Book Co, 1972, p 401.

123. Sherwood LM, Mayer GP, Care AD, et al: Evaluation by radioimmunoassay of factors controlling the secretion of parathyroid hormone. Nature 209:52, 1966.

124. Sherwood LM, Mayer GP, Romberg CF Jr, et al: Regulation of parathyroid hormone secretion: Proportional control by calcium, lack of effect of phosphate. Endocrinology 83:1043, 1968.

125. Martin IJ, Hruska KA, Freitag JJ, et al: The peripheral metabolism of parathyroid hormone. N Engl J Med 301:1092, 1979.

126. Canterbury JM, Bricker LA, Levey GS, et al: Metabolism of bovine parathyroid hormone. J Clin Invest 55:1245, 1975.

127. D'Amour P, Segre GV, Roth SI, et al: Analysis of parathyroid hormone and its fragments in rat tissues: Chemical identification and microscopical localization. J Clin Invest 63:89, 1979.

128. Catherwood B, Singer FR: Generation of a carboxyl terminal fragment of bovine parathyroid hormone by canine renal plasma membrane. Biochem Biophys Res Commun 57:469-475, 1974.

129. Hanley DA, Takatsuki K, Sultan JM, et al: Direct release of parathyroid hormone fragments from functioning bovine parathyroid glands in vitro. J Clin Invest 62:1247-1254, 1978.

130. Canterbury JM, Levey GS, Reiss E: Activation of renal cortical adenylate cyclase by circulating immunoreactive parathyroid hormone fragments. J Clin Invest 52:524-527, 1973.

131. Segre JV, D'Amour P, Hultman A, et al: Effects of hepatectomy, nephrectomy and nephrectomy/uremia on the metabolism of parathyroid hormone in the rat. J Clin Invest 67:439-448, 1981.

132. Arnold A, Shattuck TM, Mallya SM, et al: Molecular pathogenesis of primary hyperparathyroidism. J Bone Miner Res 17(suppl 2): N30-N36, 2002.

133. Hsi E, Zukerberg LR, Yang WI, et al: Cyclin Dl/PRAD1 expression in parathyroid adenomas: An immunohistochemical study. J Clin Endocrinol Metab 81:1736-1739, 1996.

134. Vasef MA, Brynes RK, Sturm M, et al: Expression of cyclin D1 in parathyroid carcinomas, adenomas, and hyperplasia: A parafin immunohistochemical study. Mod Pathol 12:412-416, 1999.

135. Rosenberg CL, Kim HG, Shows TB, et al: Rearrangement and overexpression of *D11S287E*, a candidate oncogene on chromosome 11q13 in benign parathyroid tumors. Oncogene 6:449-453, 1991.

136. Arnold A, Kim HG, Gaz RD, et al: Molecular cloning and chromosomal mapping of DNA rearranged with the parathyroid hormone gene in a parathyroid adenoma. J Clin Invest 83:2034-2040, 1989.

137. Farnebo F, Teh BT, Kytola S, et al: Alterations of the *MEN1* gene in sporadic parathyroid tumors. J Clin Endocrinol Metab 83:2627-2630, 1998.

138. Heppner C, Kester MB, Agarwal SK, et al: Somatic mutation of the *MEN1* gene in parathyroid tumors. Nat Genet 16:375-377, 1997.

139. Cetani F, Picone A, Cerrai P, et al: Parathyroid expression of calcium-sensing receptor protein and in vivo parathyroid hormone–Ca(2+) set-point in patients with primary hyperparathyroidism. J Clin Endocrinol Metab 85:4789-4794, 2000.

140. Cetani F, Pinchera A, Pardi E, et al: No evidence for mutations in the calcium-sensing receptor gene in sporadic parathyroid adenomas. J Bone Miner Res 14:878-882, 1999.

141. Hosokawa Y, Pollak MR, Brown EM, et al: Mutational analysis of the extracellular Ca sensing receptor gene in human parathyroid tumors. J Clin Endocrinol Metab 80:3107-3110, 1995.

142. Albright F, Bauer W, Claflin D, et al: Studies in parathyroid physiology. III. The effect of phosphate ingestion in clinical hyperparathyroidism. J Clin Invest 11:411, 1932.

143. Aub MC, Tibbets DM, McLean R: The influence of parathyroid hormone, urea, sodium chloride, fat and intestinal activity upon calcium balance. J Nutr 13:635, 1937.

144. Hodgkinson A: Biochemical aspects of primary hyperparathyroidism: Analysis of 50 cases. Clin Sci (Colch) 25:23, 1963.

145. Lafferty FW, Pearson OH: Skeletal, intestinal, and renal calcium dynamics in hyperparathyroidism. J Clin Endocrinol Metab 23:89, 1963.

146. Anderson J, Osborn SC, Tomlinson RWS, et al: Calcium dynamics of the gastrointestinal tract and bone in primary hyperparathyroidism. Q J Med 33:42, 1964.

147. Parfitt AM: Effect of cellulose phosphate and dietary calcium restriction in primary hyperparathyroidism. Clin Sci (Colch) 49:9, 1975.

148. Nassim JR, Higgins BA: Control of idiopathic hypercalciuria. BMJ 1:675-681, 1965.

149. Bauer W, Albright F, Aub JC: A case of osteitis fibrosa cystica (osteomalacia?) with evidence of hyperactivity of the parathyroid bodies. Metabolic study II. J Clin Invest 8:229, 1930.

150. Birge SJ, Peck WA, Berman M, et al: Study of calcium absorption in man: A kinetic analysis and physiologic model. J Clin Invest 48:1705-1713, 1969.

151. Pak CYC, Ohata M, Lawrence EC, et al: The hypercalciurias: Causes, parathyroid functions, and diagnostic criteria. J Clin Invest 54:387-400, 1974.

152. Reeve J, Hesp R, Veall N: Effects of therapy on rate of absorption of calcium from gut in disorders of calcium homeostasis. BMJ 3:310, 1974.

153. Kaplan RA, Snyder WH, Stewart A, et al: Metabolic effects of parathyroidectomy in asymptomatic primary hyperparathyroidism. J Clin Endocrinol Metab 42:415, 1976.

154. Kaplan RA, Haussler MR, Deftos LJ, et al: The role of 1,25-dihydroxyvitamin D in the mediation of intestinal hyperabsorption of calcium in primary hyperparathyroidism and absorptive hypercalciuria. J Clin Invest 59:756-760, 1977.

155. Jowsey J: Bone histology and hyperparathyroidism. Clin Endocrinol Metab 3:267, 1974.

156. Mallette LE, Sode JE, Marx SJ, et al: Total body retention of orally administered ^{47}Ca in primary hyperparathyroidism. J Clin Endocrinol Metab 50:582, 1975.

157. Miller PD, Bilezikian JP: Bone densitometry in asymptomatic primary hyperparathyroidism. J Bone Miner Res 17(suppl 2): N98-N102, 2002.

158. Woodhouse NJY, Doyle FH, Joplin GF: Vitamin-D deficiency and primary hyperparathyroidism. Lancet 2:283, 1971.

159. Brumbaugh PF, Haussler DH, Bressler R, et al: Radioreceptor assay for 1,25-dihydroxyvitamin D_3. Science 183:1089, 1974.

160. Gray RW, Wilz DR, Caldas AE, et al: The importance of phosphate in regulating plasma 1,25 $(OH)_2$ vitamin D levels in humans: Studies in healthy subjects, in calcium stone formers, and in patients with primary hyperparathyroidism. J Clin Endocrinol Metab 45:299-306, 1977.

161. Bauer W, Albright F, Aub JC: Studies of calcium and phosphorus metabolism. II. The calcium excretion of normal individuals on a low-calcium diet; also data on a case of pregnancy. J Clin Invest 7:75, 1929.

162. McGeown MG: Calcium and phosphorus metabolism in the diagnosis of hyperparathyroidism. Urol Int 19:83, 1965.

163. Pronove P, Bell NH, Bartter FC: Production of hypercalciuria by phosphorus deprivation on a low-calcium diet: A new clinical test for hyperparathyroidism. Metabolism 10:364, 1961.

164. Wibell L, Werner I: Serum phosphate and calcium phosphate excretion at different levels of serum calcium. Acta Med Scand 193:16, 1973.

165. Nordin BEC, Peacock M: Role of kidney in regulation of plasma-calcium. Lancet 2:1280, 1969.

166. Transbol I, Hornum I, Hahnemann S, et al: Tubular reabsorption of calcium in the differential diagnosis of hypercalcemia. Acta Med Scand 188:505, 1970.

167. Transbol I, Hahnemann S, Hornum I: The tubular reabsorption of calcium in primary hyperparathyroidism and non-parathyroid hypercalcemia. Acta Med Scand 184:33, 1968.

168. Kleeman CR, Bernstein D, Rockney R, et al: Studies on the renal clearance of diffusible calcium and the role of the parathyroid glands in its regulation. Yale J Biol Med 34:1, 1961.

169. Parks JH, Coe FL, Favus MJ: Hyperparathyroidism in nephrolithiasis. Arch Intern Med 140:1402, 1980.

170. Broadus AE, Horst EL, Lang R, et al: The importance of circulating 1,25-dihydroxyvitamin D in the pathogenesis of hypercalciuria and renal-stone formation in primary hyperparathyroidism. N Engl J Med 302:42, 1980.

171. Pak CYC, Nicar MJ, Peterson R, et al: A lack of unique pathophysiologic background for nephrolithiasis of primary hyperparathyroidism. J Clin Endocrinol Metab 53:536-542, 1981.

172. Riccardi D, Lee W, Lee K, et al: Localization of the extracellular Ca sensing receptor in PTH/PTHrP receptor in rat kidney. Am J Physiol 271:F951-F956, 1996.

173. Hodgkinson A, Marshall RW: Changes in the composition of urinary tract stones. Invest Urol 13:13, 1975.

174. Nicar MJ, Hill K, Pak CY: A simple technique for assessing the propensity for crystallization of calcium oxalate and brushite in urine from the increment in oxalate or calcium necessary to elicit precipitation . Metabolism 32:906-910, 1983.

175. Nordin BEC: Metabolic Bone and Stone Disease. London, Churchill Livingstone, 1973.

176. Muldowney FP, Donohoe JF, Carroll DV, et al: Parathyroid acidosis in uremia. Q J Med 163:32, 1972.

177. Coe FL: Magnitude of metabolic acidosis in primary hyperparathyroidism. Arch Intern Med 134:262-265, 1974.

178. Berson SA, Yalow PS: Parathyroid hormone in plasma in adenomatous hyperparathyroidism, uremia and bronchogenic carcinoma. Science 154:907, 1966.

179. Purnell DC, Scholz DA, Smith LH, et al: Treatment of primary hyperparathyroidism. Am J Med 56:800, 1974.

180. Nussbaum SR, Potts JTJ: Immunoassays for parathyroid hormone 1-84 in the diagnosis of hyperparathyroidism. J Bone Miner Res 6:S43-S50, 1991.

181. Brown RC, Aston JP, Weeks I, et al: Circulating intact parathyroid hormone measured by a two-site immunochemiluminometric assay. J Clin Endocrinol Metab 65:407-414, 1987.

182. Blind E, Schmidt-Gayk H, Scharla S, et al: Two-site assay of intact parathyroid hormone in the investigation of primary hyperparathyroidism and other disorders of calcium metabolism compared with a midregion assay. J Clin Endocrinol Metab 67:353-360, 1988.

183. Melson GL, Chase LR, Aurbach GD: Parathyroid hormone sensitive adenyl cyclase in isolated renal tubules. Endocrinology 86:51, 1970.

184. Kaminsky NI, Broadus AE, Hardman JG, et al: Effects of parathyroid hormone on plasma and urinary adenosine 3',5'-monophosphate in man. J Clin Invest 49:2387, 1970.

185. Neelon FA, Drezner M, Birch BM, et al: Urinary cyclic adenosine monophosphate as an aid in the diagnosis of hyperparathyroidism. Lancet 1:63, 1973.

186. Mallette LE, Bilezikian JP, Heath DA, et al: Primary hyperparathyroidism: Clinical and biochemical features. Medicine (Baltimore) 53:127, 1974.

187. Lafferty FW: Differential diagnosis of hypercalcemia. J Bone Miner Res 6:S51-S59, 1991.

188. Mark SJ, Spiegel AM, Brown EM, et al: Divalent cation metabolism: Familial hypocalciuric hypercalcemia vs typical primary hyperparathyroidism. Am J Med 65:235-242, 1978.

189. Bai M, Janicic N, Trivedi S, et al: Markedly reduced activity of mutant calcium-sensing receptor with an inserted Alu element from a kindred with familial hypocalciuric hypercalcemia and neonatal severe hyperparathyroidism. J Clin Invest 99:1917-1925, 1997.

190. Marx SJ, Stock JL, Attie MF, et al: Familial hypocalciuric hypercalemia: Recognition among patients referred after unsuccessful parathyroid exploration. Ann Intern Med 92:35, 1980.

191. Attie MF, Gill JR, Stock JL, et al: Urinary calcium excretion in familial hypocalciuric hypercalcemia. J Clin Invest 72:667,1983.

192. McMurtry CT, Schranck FW, Walkenhorst DA, et al: Significant developmental elevation in serum parathyroid hormone levels in a large kindred with familial benign (hypocalciuric) hypercalcemia. Am J Med 93:247-258, 1992.

193. Suva LJ, Winslow GA, Wettenhall REH, et al: A parathyroid hormone–related protein implicated in malignant hypercalcemia: Cloning and expression. Science 237:893-896, 1987.

194. Broadus AE, Mangin M, Ikeda K, et al: Humoral hypercalcemia of cancer. N Engl J Med 319:556-563, 1988.

195. Strewler GJ, Stern PH, Jacobs JW, et al: Parathyroid hormone-like protein from human renal carcinoma cells. J Clin Invest 80:1803-1807, 1987.

196. Potts JTJ, Ackerman IP, Barker CF, et al: Diagnosis and management of asymptomatic primary hyperparathyroidism: Consensus development conference statement. Ann Intern Med 144:593-597, 1991.

197. Krubsack AJ, Wilson SD, Lawson TL, et al: Prospective comparison of radionuclide, computed tomographic, sonographic, and magnetic resonance localization of parathyroid tumors. Surgery 106:639-646, 1989.

198. Reading CC, Charboneau JW, James EM, et al: High-resolution parathyroid sonography. AJR Am J Roentgenol 139:539-546, 1982.

199. Auffermann W, Gooding GAW, Okerlund MD, et al: Diagnosis of recurrent hyperparathyroidism: Comparison of MR imaging and other imaging techniques. AJR Am J Roentgenol 150:1027-1033, 1988.

200. Castellani M, Reschini E, Longari V, et al: Role of Tc-99m sestamibi scintigraphy in the diagnosis and surgical decision-making process in primary hyperparathyroid disease. Clin Nucl Med 26:139-144, 2001.

201. Doppman JL, Miller DL: Localization of parathyroid tumors in patients with asymptomatic hyperparathyroidism and no previous surgery. J Bone Miner Res 6:S153-S158, 1991.

202. Eisenberg H, Pallotta J, Sherwood LM: Selective arteriography, venography and venous hormone assay in diagnosis and localization of parathyroid lesions. Am J Med 56:810, 1974.

203. Muldowney FP, Freaney R, Muldowney WP, et al: Hypercalciuria in parathyroid disorders: Effect of dietary sodium control. Am J Kidney Dis 17:323-329, 1991.

204. Marcus R: Estrogens and progestins in the management of primary hyperparathyroidism. J Bone Miner Res 6:S125-S129, 1991.

205. Marcus R, Madvig P, Crim M, et al: Conjugated estrogens in the treatment of postmenopausal women with hyperparathyroidism. Ann Intern Med 100:633-640, 1984.

206. Selby PL, Peacock M: Ethinyl estradiol and norethindrone in the treatment of primary hyperparathyroidism in postmenopausal women. N Engl J Med 314:1418-1509, 1986.

207. Wishart J, Horowitz M, Need A, et al: Treatment of postmenopausal hyperparathyroidism with norethindrone. Arch Intern Med 150: 1951-1953, 1990.

208. Marcus R: The role of estrogens and related compounds in the management of primary hyperparathyroidism. J Bone Miner Res 17 (suppl 2):N146-N149, 2002.

209. Schmidli RS, Wilson I, Espiner EA, et al: Aminopropylidine diphosphonate (APD) in mild primary hyperparathyroidism: Effect on clinical status. Clin Endocrinol 32:293-300, 1990.

210. Rossini M, Gatti D, Isaia G, et al: Effects of oral alendronate in elderly patients with osteoporosis and mild primary hyperparathyroidism. J Bone Miner Res 16:113-119, 2001.

211. Parker CR, Blackwell PJ, Fairbairn KJ, et al: Alendronate in the treatment of primary hyperparathyroid-related osteoporosis: A 2-year study. J Clin Endocrinol Metab 87:4482-4489, 2002.

212. Silverberg SJ, Bone HG, III, Marriott TB, et al: Short-term inhibition of parathyroid hormone secretion by a calcium-receptor agonist in patients with primary hyperparathyroidism. N Engl J Med 337: 1506-1510, 1997.

213. Antoniucci DM, Shoback D: Calcimimetics in the treatment of primary hyperparathyroidism. J Bone Miner Res 17(suppl 2): N141-N145, 2002.

214. McGeown MG: Effect of parathyroidectomy on the incidence of renal calculi. Lancet 1:586, 1961.

215. Edvall CA: Renal function in hyperparathyroidism: A clinical study of 30 cases with special reference to selective renal clearance and renal vein catheterization. Acta Chir Scand Suppl 299:1-55, 1958.

216. Pak CYC: Effect of parathyroidectomy on crystallization of calcium salts in urine of patients with primary hyperparathyroidism. Invest Urol 17:146-148, 1979.

217. Pratley SK, Posen S, Reeve TS: Primary hyperparathyroidism: Experience with 60 patients. Med J Aust 1:42, 1973.

218. Britton DC, Thompson MH, Johnston IDA, et al: Renal function following parathyroid surgery in primary hyperparathyroidism. Lancet 2:74, 1971.

219. Hellstrom J, Ivemark BI: Primary hyperparathyroidism. Acta Chir Scand Suppl 294:1-89, 1962.

220. Coe FL, Parks JH, Moore ES: Familial idiopathic hypercalciuria. N Engl J Med 300:337-340, 1979.

221. Hamed IA, Czerwinski AW, Coats B, et al: Familial absorptive hypercalciuria and renal tubular acidosis. Am J Med 67:385-391, 1979.

222. Goodman HO, Holmes RP, Assimos DG: Genetic factors in calcium oxalate stone disease. J Urol 153:301-307, 1995.

223. Moore ES, Coe FL, McMann BJ, et al: Idiopathic hypercalciuria in children: Prevalence and metabolic characteristics. J Pediatr 92:906-910, 1978.

224. Favus MJ, Coe FL: Evidence for spontaneous hypercalciuria in the rat. Miner Electrolyte Metab 2:150-154, 1979.

225. Bushinsky DA, Favus MJ: Mechanism of hypercalciuria in genetic hypercalciuric rats: Inherited defect in intestinal calcium transport. J Clin Invest 82:1585-1591, 1988.

226. Frymoyer PA, Scheinman SJ, Dunham PB, et al: X-linked recessive nephrolithiasis with renal failure. N Engl J Med 325:681-686, 1991.

227. Scheinman SJ: X-linked hypercalciuric nephrolithiasis: Clinical syndromes and chloride channel mutations. Kidney Int 53:3-17, 1998.

228. Lloyd SE, Pearce SHS, Fisher SE, et al: A common molecular basis for three inherited kidney stone diseases. Nature 379:445-449, 1996.

229. Scheinman SJ, Cox J, Lloyd S, et al: Isolated hypercalciuria with mutation in CLCN5: Relevance to idiopathic hypercalciuria. Kidney Int 57:232-239, 2000.

230. Petrucci M, Scott P, Ouimet D, et al: Evaluation of the calcium-sensing receptor gene in idiopathic hypercalciuria and calcium nephrolithiasis. Kidney Int 58:38-42, 2000.

231. Lerolle N, Coulet F, Lantz B, et al: No evidence for point mutations of the calcium-sensing receptor in familial idiopathic hypercalciuria. Nephrol Dial Transplant 16:2317-2322, 2001.

232. Scott P, Ouimet D, Proulx Y, et al: The 1α-hydroxylase locus is not linked to calcium stone formation or calciuric phenotypes in French-Canadian families. J Am Soc Nephrol 9:425-432, 1998.

233. Ruggiero M, Pacini S, Amato M, et al: Association between vitamin D receptor gene polymorphism and nephrolithiasis. Miner Electrolyte Metab 25:185-190, 1998.

234. Scott P, Ouimet D, Valiquette L, et al: Suggestive evidence for a susceptibility gene near the vitamin D receptor locus in idiopathic calcium stone formation. J Am Soc Nephrol 10:1007-1013, 1999.

235. Chen WC, Chen HY, Lu HF, et al: Association of the vitamin D receptor gene start codon Fok I polymorphism with calcium oxalate stone disease. BJU Int 87:168-171, 2001.

236. Nishijima S, Sugaya K, Naito A, et al: Association of vitamin D receptor gene polymorphism with urolithiasis. J Urol 167:2188-2191, 2002.

237. Zerwekh JE, Hughes MR, Reed BY, et al: Evidence for normal vitamin D receptor messenger ribonucleic acid and genotype in absorptive hypercalciuria. J Clin Endocrinol Metab 80:2960-2965, 1995.

238. Reed BY, Heller HJ, Gitomer WL, et al: Mapping a gene defect in absorptive hypercalciuria to chromosome 1q23.3-q24. J Clin Endocrinol Metab 84:3907-3913, 1999.

239. Reed BY, Gitomer WL, Heller HJ, et al: Identification and characterization of a gene with base substitutions associated with the absorptive hypercalciuria phenotype and low spinal bone density, J Clin Endocrinol Metab 87:1476-1485, 2002.

240. Caniggia A, Gennari C, Cesari L: Intestinal absorption of ⁴⁵Ca in stone-forming patients. BMJ 1:427-429, 1965.

241. Wills MR, Zisman E, Wortsman J, et al: The measurement of intestinal calcium absorption by external radioisotope counting: Application to study of nephrolithiasis. Clin Sci 39:95-106, 1970.

242. Pak CYC, East DA, Sanzenbacher LJ, et al: Gastrointestinal calcium absorption in nephrolithiasis. J Clin Endocrinol Metab 35:261-270, 1972.

243. Ehrig U, Harrison JE, Wilson DR: Effect of long-term thiazide therapy on intestinal calcium absorption in patients with recurrent renal calculi. Metabolism 23:139-149, 1974.

244. Shen FH, Baylink DJ, Nielsen RL, et al: Increased serum 1,25-dihydroxyvitamin D in idiopathic hypercalciuria. J Lab Clin Med 90:955-962, 1977.

245. Barilla DE, Tolentino R, Kaplan RA, et al: Selective effects of thiazide on intestinal absorption of calcium in absorptive and renal hypercalciurias. Metabolism 27:125-131, 1978.

246. Zerwekh JE, Pak CYC: Selective effects of thiazide therapy on serum 1-α,25-dihydryoxyvitamin D and intestinal calcium absorption in renal and absorptive hypercalciurias. Metabolism 29:13-17, 1980.

247. Brannan PG, Morawski S, Pak CYC, et al: Selective jejunal hyperabsorption of calcium in absorptive hypercalciuria. Am J Med 66:425, 1979.

248. Knapp EL: Studies on the urinary excretion of calcium [dissertation]. Ames, Iowa, State University, 1943.

249. Liberman UA, Sperling O, Atsmonia A, et al: Metabolic and calcium kinetic studies in idiopathic hypercalciuria. J Clin Invest 47:2580, 1968.

250. Edwards NA, Hodgkinson A: Metabolic studies in patients with idiopathic hypercalciuria. Clin Sci (Colch) 29:143-157, 1965.

251. Henneman PH, Benedict PH, Forbes AP, et al: Idiopathic hypercalciuria. N Engl J Med 259:802-807, 1958.

252. Jackson WPU, Dancaster C: A consideration of the hypercalciuria in sarcoidosis, idiopathic hypercalciuria, and that produced by vitamin D: A new suggestion regarding calcium metabolism. J Clin Endocrinol Metab 19:658, 1959.

253. Harrison AR: Some results of metabolic investigations in cases of renal stone. Br J Urol 31:398, 1959.

254. Dent CE, Harper CM, Parfitt AM: The effect of cellulose phosphate on calcium metabolism in patients with hypercalciuria. Clin Sci (Colch) 27:417-425, 1964.

255. Parfitt AM, Higgins BA, Nassim JR, et al: Metabolic studies in patients with hypercalciuria. Clin Sci (Colch) 27:463-482, 1964.

256. Edwards NA, Hodgkinson A: Studies of renal function in patients with idiopathic hypercalciuria. Clin Sci (Colch) 29:327, 1965.

257. Peacock M, Nordin BEC: Tubular reabsorption of calcium in normal and hypercalciuric subjects. J Clin Pathol 21:355, 1968.

258. Phillips MJ, Cooke JNC: Relation between urinary calcium and sodium in patients with idiopathic hypercalciuria. Lancet 1:1354-1357, 1967.

259. Kleerman CR, Bohannan J, Bernstein D, et al: Effect of variations in sodium intake on calcium excretion in normal humans. Proc Soc Exp Biol Med 115:29-32, 1964.

260. Sutton RAL, Walker VR: Responses to hydrochlorothiazide and acetazolamide in patients with calcium stones. N Engl J Med 302:709-713, 1980.

261. Bianchi G, Vezzoli G, Cusi D, et al: Abnormal red-cell calcium pump in patients with idiopathic hypercalciuria. N Engl J Med 319:897-901, 1988.

262. Barkin J, Wilson DR, Manuel MA, et al: Bone mineral content in idiopathic calcium nephrolithiasis. Miner Electrolyte Metab 11: 19-24, 1985.

263. Alhava EM, Juuti M, Karjalainen P: Bone mineral density in patients with urolithiasis. Scand J Urol Nephrol 10:154-156, 1976.

264. Borghi L, Meschi T, Guerra A, et al: Vertebral mineral content in diet-dependent and diet-independent hypercalciuria. J Urol 146: 1334-1338, 1991.

265. Zanchetta JR, Rodriguez G, Negri AL, et al: Bone mineral density in patients with hypercalciuric nephrolithiasis. Nephron 73:557-560, 1996.

266. Lawoyin S, Sismilich S, Browne R, et al: Bone mineral content in patients with calcium urolithiasis. Metabolism 28:1250-1254, 1979.

267. Bataille P, Achard JM, Fournier A, et al: Diet, vitamin D and vertebral mineral density in hypercalciuric calcium stone formers. Kidney Int 39:1193-1205, 1991.

268. Pietschmann F, Breslau NA, Pak CY: Reduced vertebral bone density in hypercalciuric nephrolithiasis. J Bone Miner Res 7: 1383-1388, 1992.

269. Sutton RAL, Walker VR: Bone resorption and hypercalciuria in calcium stone formers. Metabolism 35:485-488, 1986.

270. Urivetzky M, Anna PS, Smith AD: Plasma osteocalcin levels in stone disease: A potential aid in the differential diagnosis of calcium nephrolithiasis. J Urol 139:12-14, 1988.

271. Steiniche T, Mosekilde L, Christensen MS, et al: A histomorphometric determination of iliac bone remodeling in patients with recurrent renal stone formation and idiopathic hypercalciuria. APMIS 97: 309-316, 1989.

272. Malluche HH, Tschoepe W, Ritz E, et al: Abnormal bone histology in idiopathic hypercalciuria. J Clin Endocrinol Metab 50:654-658, 1980.

273. Asplin JR, Bauer KA, Kinder JM, et al: Bone mineral density and urine calcium excretion among subjects with and without nephrolithiasis. Kidney Int 63:662-669, 2003.

274. Coe FL, Canterbury JM, Firpo JJ, et al: Evidence for secondary hyperparathyroidism in idiopathic hypercalciuria. J Clin Invest 52:134-142, 1973.

275. Bordier P, Ryckewart A, Gueris J, et al: On the pathogenesis of so-called idiopathic hypercalciuria. Am J Med 63:398, 1977.

276. Burckhardt P, Jaeger P: Secondary hyperparathyroidism in idiopathic renal hypercalciuria: Fact or theory? J Clin Endocrinol Metab 55:550, 1981.

277. Pak CY, Delea CS, Bartter FC: Successful treatment of recurrent nephrolithiasis (calcium stones) with cellulose phosphate. N Engl J Med 290:175-180, 1974.

278. Pak CYC, Kaplan R, Bone H, et al: A simple test for the diagnosis of absorptive, resorptive and renal hypercalciurias. N Engl J Med 292:497, 1975.

279. Pak CYC, Britton F, Peterson R, et al: Ambulatory evaluation of nephrolithiasis: Classification, clinical presentation and diagnostic criteria. Am J Med 69:19-30, 1980.

280. Maierhofer WJ, Gray RW, Cheung HS, et al: Bone resorption stimulated by elevated serum 1,25 (OH) vitamin D concentrations in healthy men. Kidney Int 24:555-560, 1983.

281. Adams ND, Gray RW, Lemann JJ, et al: Effects of calcitriol administration on calcium metabolism in healthy men. Kidney Int 21: 90-97, 1982.

282. Breslau NA, Preminger GM, Adams BV, et al: Use of ketoconazole to probe the pathogenetic importance of 1,25-dihydroxyvitamin D in absorptive hypercalciuria. J Clin Endocrinol Metab 75:1446-1452, 1992.

283. Haussler MR, Baylink DJ, Hughes MR, et al: The assay of 1,25-dihydroxyvitamin D_3: Physiologic and pathologic modulation of circulating hormone levels. Clin Endocrinol Metab 5:15, 1976.

284. Broadus AE, Insoqna KL, Lang R, et al: A consideration of the hormonal basis and phosphate leak hypothesis of absorptive hypercalciuria. J Clin Endocrinol Metab 58:16, 1984.

285. Coe FL, Favus MJ, Crockett T, et al: Effects of low-calcium diet on urine calcium excretion, parathyroid function and serum 1,25(OH)2D₃ levels in patients with idiopathic hypercalciuria and in normal subjects. Am J Med 72:25-32, 1982.

286. Bataille P, Bouillon R, Fournier A, et al: Increased plasma concentrations of total and free 1,25-(OH)2D₃ in calcium stone formers with idiopathic hypercalciuria. Contrib Nephrol 58:137-142, 1987.

287. Li X, Tembe V, Horwitz GM, et al: Increased intestinal vitamin D receptor in genetic hypercalciuric rats. J Clin Invest 91:661-667, 1993.

288. Zerwekh JE, Yu XP, Breslau NA, et al: Vitamin D receptor quantitation in human blood mononuclear cells in health and disease. Mol Cell Endocrinol 96:1-6, 1993.

289. Tieder M, Modai D, Shaked U, et al: "Idiopathic" hypercalciuria and hereditary hypophosphatemic rickets. N Engl J Med 316:125-129, 1987.

290. Barilla DE, Zerwekh JE, Pak CYC: A critical evaluation of the role of phosphate in the pathogenesis of absorptive hypercalciuria. Miner Electrolyte Metab 2: 302, 1979.

291. Prie D, Huart V, Bakouh N, et al: Nephrolithiasis and osteoporosis associated with hypophosphatemia caused by mutations in the type 2a sodium-phosphate cotransporter. N Engl J Med 347: 983-991, 2002.

292. Broadus AE, Insogna KL, Lang R, et al: Evidence for disordered control of 1,25-dihydroxyvitamin D production in absorptive hypercalciuria. N Engl J Med 311:73-80, 1984.

293. Fuss M, Pepersack T, Bergman P, et al: Low calcium diet in idiopathic urolithiasis: A risk factor for osteopenia as great as in primary hyperparathyroidism. Br J Urol 65:560-563, 1990.

294. Curhan GC, Willett WC, Rimm EB, et al: A prospective study of dietary calcium and other nutrients and the risk of symptomatic kidney stones. N Engl J Med 328:833-838, 1993.

295. Curhan GC, Willett WC, Speizer FE, et al: Comparison of dietary calcium with supplemental calcium and other nutrients as factors affecting the risk of kidney stones in women. Ann Intern Med 126:497-504, 1997.

296. Ettinger B: Recurrence of nephrolithiasis: A six-year prospective study. Am J Med 67:245, 1979.

297. Hosking DH, Erickson SB, Van Den Berg CJ, et al: The stone clinic effect in patients with idiopathic calcium urolithiasis. J Urol 130:1115-1118, 1983.

298. Sakhaee K, Harvey JA, Padalino PK, et al: The potential role of salt abuse on the risk for kidney stone formation. J Urol 150:310-312, 1993.

299. Walker RM, Linkswiler HM: Calcium retention in the adult human male as affected by protein intake. J Nutr 102:1297-1302, 1972.

300. Allen LH, Oddoye EA, Margen S: Protein-induced hypercalciuria: A longer term study. Am J Clin Nutr 32:741-749, 1979.

301. Hiatt RA, Ettinger B, Caan B, et al: Randomized controlled trial of a low animal protein, high fiber diet in prevention of recurrent calcium oxalate kidney stones. Am J Epidemiol 144:25-33, 1996.

302. Borghi L, Schianchi T, Meschi T, et al: Comparison of two diets for the prevention of recurrent stones in idiopathic hypercalciuria. N Engl J Med 346:77-84, 2002.

303. Pak CYC, Sakhaee K, Crowther C, et al: Evidence justifying a high fluid intake in treatment of nephrolithiasis. Ann Intern Med 93: 36-39, 1980.

304. Borghi L, Meschi T, Amato F, et al: Urinary volume, water and recurrences in idiopathic calcium nephrolithiasis: A 5-year randomized prospective study. J Urol 155:839-843, 1996.

305. Hayashi Y, Kaplan RA, Pak CYC: Effect of sodium cellulose phosphate therapy on crystallization of calcium oxalate in urine. Metabolism 24:1273-1278, 1975.

306. Backman U, Danielson BG, Johansson G, et al: Treatment of recurrent calcium stone formation with cellulose phosphate. J Urol 123: 9-13, 1980.

307. Edwards BR, Baer PG, Sutton RA, et al: Micropuncture study of diuretic effects on sodium and calcium reabsorption in the dog nephron. J Clin Invest 52:2418-2427, 1973.

308. Costanzo LS, Windhager EE: Calcium and sodium transport by the distal convoluted tubule of the rat. Am J Physiol 235:F492, 1978.

309. Coe FL, Parks JH, Bushinsky DA, et al: Chlorthalidone promotes mineral retention in patients with idiopathic hypercalciuria. Kidney Int 33:1140-1146, 1988.

310. Wasnich RD, Benfante RJ, Yano K, et al: Thiazide effect on the mineral content of bone. N Engl J Med 309:344-347, 1983.

311. LaCroix AZ, Wienpahl J, White LR, et al: Thiazide diuretic agents and the incidence of hip fracture. N Engl J Med 322:286-290, 1990.

312. Steiniche T, Mosekilde L, Christensen MS, et al: Histomorphometric analysis of bone in idiopathic hypercalciuria before and after treatment with thiazide. APMIS 97:302-308, 1989.

313. Scholz D, Schwille PO, Sigel A: Double-blind study with thiazide in recurrent calcium lithiasis. J Urol 128:903-907, 1982.

314. Brocks P, Dahl C, Wolf H: Do thiazides prevent recurrent idiopathic renal calcium stones? Lancet 2:124-125, 1981.

315. Laerum E, Larsen S: Thiazide prophylaxis of urolithiasis: A double-blind study in general practice. Acta Med Scand 215:383-389, 1984.

316. Ettinger B, Citron JT, Livermore B, et al: Chlorthalidone reduces calcium oxalate calculus recurrence but magnesium hydroxide does not. J Urol 139:679-684, 1988.

317. Borghi L, Meschi T, Guerra A, et al: Randomized prospective study of a nonthiazide diuretic, indapamide, in preventing calcium stone recurrences. J Cardiovasc Pharmacol 22(suppl 6):S78-S86, 1993.

318. Mortensen JT, Schultz A, Ostergaard AH: Thiazides in the prophylactic treatment of recurrent idiopathic kidney stones. Int Urol Nephrol 18:265-269, 1986.

319. Ohkawa M, Tokunaga S, Nakashima T, et al: Thiazide treatment for calcium urolithiasis in patients with idiopathic hypercalciuria. Br J Urol 69:571-576, 1992.

320. Coe FL, Parks JH: Nephrolithiasis: Pathogenesis and Treatment, 2nd ed. Chicago, Year Book Medical Publishers, 1988, pp 205-231.

321. Coe FL, Moran E, Kavalach AG: The contribution of dietary purine over-consumption to hyperpuricosuria in calcium oxalate stone formers. J Chronic Dis 29:793-800, 1976.

322. Lonsdale K: Human stones. Science 159:1199, 1968.

323. Lonsdale K: Epitaxy as a growth factor in urinary calculi and gallstones. Nature 217:56-58, 1968.

324. Mandel NS, Mandel GF: Monosodium urate monohydrate, the gout culprit. Am Chem Soc 98:2319, 1976.

325. Robertson WG, Marshall RW, Peacock M, et al: The saturation of urine in recurrent, idiopathic stone formers. *In* Fleisch H, Robertson WG, Smith LH, et al (eds): Urolithiasis Research. London, Plenum Press, 1976, p 335.

326. Coe FL, Strauss AL, Tembe V, et al: Uric acid saturation in calcium nephrolithiasis. Kidney Int 17:662-668, 1980.

327. Pak CYC, Waters O, Arnold L, et al: Mechanism for calcium urolithiasis among patients with hyperuricosuria. J Clin Invest 59:426-431, 1977.

328. Emmerson BT, Graham-Row P: Pathogenesis of the gouty kidney. Kidney Int 8:65, 1975.

329. Grover PK, Ryall RL, Marshall VR: Calcium oxalate crystallization in urine: Role of urate and glycosaminoglycans. Kidney Int 41:149-154, 1992.

330. Grover PK, Ryall RL, Marshall VR: Effect of urate on calcium oxalate crystallization in human urine: Evidence for a promotory role of hyperuricosuria in urolithiasis. Clin Sci (Colch) 79:9-15, 1990.

331. Coe FL, Kavalach AG: Hypercalciuria and hyperuricosuria in patients with calcium nephrolithiasis. N Engl J Med 291:1344-1350, 1974.

332. Smith MJV: Placebo versus allopurinol for renal calculi. J Urol 117:690-692, 1977.

333. Ettinger B, Tang A, Citron JT, et al: Randomized trial of allopurinol in the prevention of calcium oxalate calculi. N Engl J Med 315:1386-1389, 1986.

334. Finlayson B, Burns J, Smith A, et al: Effect of oxipurinol and allopurinol riboside on whewellite crystallization: In vitro and in vivo observations. Invest Urol 17:227-229, 1979.

335. Pak CYC, Peterson R: Successful treatment of hyperuricosuric calcium oxalate nephrolithiasis with potassium citrate. Arch Intern Med 146:863-867, 1986.

336. Pak CYC, Sakhaee K, Fuller C: Successful management of uric acid nephrolithiasis with potassium citrate. Kidney Int 30:422-428, 1986.

337. Coe FL, Parks JH: Stone disease in hereditary distal renal tubular acidosis. Ann Intern Med 93:60-61, 1980.

338. Caruana RJ, Buckalew VM: The syndrome of distal (type 1) renal tubular acidosis: Clinical and laboratory findings in 58 cases. Medicine (Baltimore) 67:84-99, 1988.

339. Albright F, Consolazio WV, Coombs FA, et al: Metabolic studies and therapy in a case of nephrocalcinosis with rickets and dwarfism. Bull Johns Hopkins Hosp 66:7, 1940.

340. Baines GH, Barclay JA, Cooke WT: Nephrocalcinosis associated with hyperchloremia and low plasma bicarbonate. Q J Med 14:113, 1945.

341. Albright F, Burnett CH, Parson W, et al: Osteomalacia and late rickets: The various etiologies met in the United States with emphasis on that resulting from a specific form of renal acidosis, the therapeutic indications for each etiological subgroup, and the relationship between osteomalacia and Milkman's syndrome. Medicine (Baltimore) 25:399, 1946.

342. Pines KL, Mudge GH: Renal tubular acidosis with osteomalacia. Am J Med 11:302, 1951.

343. Bauld WS, MacDonald SA, Hill MC: Effect of renal tubular acidosis on calcium excretion. Br J Urol 30:285, 1958.

344. Greenberg AJ, McNamara H, McCrory WW: Metabolic balance studies in primary renal tubular acidosis: Effects of acidosis on external calcium and phosphorus balances. J Pediatr 69:610, 1966.

345. Wallach S, Baker RK, Nicastri A: Primary renal tubular acidosis and secondary hyperparathyroidism. Am J Med 52:809, 1972.

346. Weber HP, Gray RW, Dominguez JH, et al: The lack of effect of chronic metabolic acidosis on 25-OH-vitamin D metabolism and serum parathyroid hormone in humans. J Clin Endocrinol Metab 43:1047, 1976.

347. Lemann JJ, Litzow JR, Lennon EJ: The effects of chronic acid loads in normal man: Further evidence for the participation of bone mineral in the defence against chronic metabolic acidosis. J Clin Invest 45:1608-1614, 1966.

348. Lemann JJ, Litzow JR, Lennon EJ: Studies of the mechanism by which chronic metabolic acidosis augments urinary calcium excretion in man. J Clin Invest 46:1318-1328, 1967.

349. Lemann JJ, Lennon EJ, Goodman AD, et al: The net balance of acid in subjects given large loads of acid or alkali. J Clin Invest 44:507-517, 1965.

350. Nash MA, Torrado AD, Greifer I, et al: Renal tubular acidosis in infants and children. J Pediatr 80:738, 1972.

351. Coe FL, Firpo JJ: Evidence for mild reversible hyperparathyroidism in distal renal tubular acidosis. Arch Intern Med 135:1485-1489, 1975.

352. Preminger GM, Sakhaee K, Pak CYC: Hypercalciuria and altered intestinal calcium absorption occurring independently of vitamin D in incomplete distal renal tubular acidosis. Metabolism 36:176-179,1987.

353. Buckalew VMJ, Purvis ML, Shulman MG, et al: Hereditary renal tubular acidosis. Medicine (Baltimore) 53:229-254, 1974.

354. Robertson WG, Peacock M, Nordin BEC: Measurement of activity products in urine from stone-formers and normal subjects. *In* Finlayson B, Hench LC, Smith LH (eds): Urolithiasis: Physical Aspects. Washington, DC, National Academy of Science, 1972, p 79.

355. Hamm LL: Renal handling of citrate. Kidney Int 38:728-735, 1990.

356. Donnelly S, Kamel KS, Vasuvattakul S, et al: Might distal renal tubular acidosis be a proximal tubular cell disorder? Am J Kidney Dis 19:272-281, 1992.

357. Wilansky DC, Schneiderman C: Renal tubular acidosis with recurrent nephrolithiasis and nephrocalcinosis. N Engl J Med 257:399, 1957.

358. Preminger GM, Sakhaee K, Skurla C, et al: Prevention of recurrent calcium stone formation with potassium citrate therapy in patients with distal renal tubular acidosis. J Urol 134:20-23, 1985.

359. McSherry E, Morris RCJ: Attainment and maintenance of normal stature with alkali therapy in infants and children with classic renal tubular acidosis. J Clin Invest 61:509, 1978.

360. Rudman D, Kutner MH, Redd SC, et al: Hypocitraturia in calcium nephrolithiasis. J Clin Endocrinol Metab 55:1052-1057, 1982.

361. Minisola S, Rossi W, Pacitti MT, et al: Studies on citrate metabolism in normal subjects and kidney stone patients. Miner Electrolyte Metab 15:303-308, 1989.

362. Menon M, Mahle CJ: Urinary citrate excretion in patients with renal calculi. J Urol 129:1158-1160, 1983.

363. Nicar MJ, Skurla C, Sakhaee K, et al: Low urinary citrate excretion in nephrolithiasis. Urology 21:8-13, 1983.

364. Hosking DH, Wilson JWL, Liedtke RR, et al: Urinary citrate excretion in normal persons and patients with idiopathic calcium urolithiasis. J Lab Clin Med 106:682-689, 1985.

365. Hodgkinson A: Citric acid excretion in normal adults and in patients with renal calculus. Clin Sci (Colch) 23:203-212, 1962.

366. Parks JH, Coe FL: A urinary calcium-citrate index for the evaluation of nephrolithiasis. Kidney Int 30:85-90, 1986.

367. Sarada B, Satyanarayana U: Urinary composition in men and women and the risk of urolithiasis. Clin Biochem 24:487-490, 1991.

368. Nikkila M, Koivula T, Jokela H: Urinary citrate excretion in patients with urolithiasis and normal subjects. Eur Urol 16:382-385, 1989.

369. Marangella M, Bianco O, Grande ML, et al: Patterns of citrate excretion in healthy subjects and patterns with idiopathic stone disease. Contrib Nephrol 58:34-38, 1987.

370. Wright EM: Transport of carboxylic acids by renal membrane vesicles. Annu Rev Physiol 47:127-141, 1985.

371. Evans BM, MacIntyre I, MacPherson CR, et al: Alkalosis in sodium and potassium depletion. Clin Sci (Colch) 16:53-64, 1957.

372. Fuselier HA, Ward DM, Lindberg JS, et al: Urinary Tamm-Horsfall protein increased after potassium citrate therapy in calcium stone formers. Urology 45:942-946, 1995.

373. Lemann JJ, Gray RW, Pleuss JA: Potassium bicarbonate, but not sodium bicarbonate, reduces urinary calcium excretion and improves calcium balance in healthy men. Kidney Int 35:688-695, 1989.

374. Barcelo P, Wuhl O, Servitge E, et al: Randomized double-blind study of potassium citrate in idiopathic hypocitraturic calcium-nephrolithiasis. J Urol 150:1761-1764, 1993.

375. Ettinger B, Pak CY, Citron JT, et al: Potassium-magnesium citrate is an effective prophylaxis against recurrent calcium oxalate nephrolithiasis. J Urol 158:2069-2073, 1997.

376. Hofbauer J, Hobarth K, Szabo N, et al: Alkali citrate prophylaxis in idiopathic recurrent calcium oxalate urolithiasis: A prospective randomized study. Br J Urol 73:362-365, 1994.

377. Pak CY, Fuller C: Idiopathic hypocitraturic calcium-oxalate nephrolithiasis successfully treated with potassium citrate. Ann Intern Med 104:33-37, 1986.

378. Pak CY, Peterson R, Sakhaee K, et al: Correction of hypocitraturia and prevention of stone formation by combined thiazide and potassium citrate therapy in thiazide-unresponsive hypercalciuric nephrolithiasis. Am J Med 79:284-288, 1985.

379. Pak CY, Oh MS, Baker S, et al: Effect of meal on the physiological and physiochemical actions of potassium citrate. J Urol 146:803-805, 1991.

380. Curhan GC, Willett WC, Speizer FE, et al: Twenty-four-hour urine chemistries and the risk of kidney stones among women and men. Kidney Int 59:2290-2298, 2001.

381. Ettinger B: Recurrent nephrolithiasis: Natural history and effect of phosphate therapy. Am J Med 61:200, 1976.

382. Coe FL, Parks JH: Nephrolithiasis: Pathogenesis and Treatment, 2nd ed. Chicago, Year Book Medical Publishers, 1988, pp 1-37.

383. Van Den Berg CJ, Kumar R, Wilson DM, et al: Orthophosphate therapy decreases urinary calcium excretion and serum 1,25-dihydroxyvitamin D concentrations in idiopathic hypercalciuria. J Clin Endocrinol Metab 51:998-1001, 1980.

384. Smith CH, Thomas WC, Arnaud CD: Orthophosphate therapy in calcium renal lithiasis. In Cifuentes-Delatte L, Rapado A, Hodgkinson A (eds): Urinary Calculi. Basel, S Karger, 1973, p 188.

385. Pak CYC, Holt K, Zerwekh J, et al: Effects of orthophosphate therapy on the crystallization of calcium salts in urine. Miner Electrolyte Metab 1:147, 1978.

386. Ettinger B, Kolb FO: Inorganic phosphate treatment of nephrolithiasis. Am J Med 55:32, 1973.

387. Bernstein OS, Newton R: The effect of oral sodium phosphate on the formation of renal calculi and on idiopathic hypercalciuria. Lancet 1:1105, 1966.

388. Lau K, Wolf C, Nussbaum P, et al: Differing effects of acid versus neutral phosphate therapy of hypercalciuria. Kidney Int 16:736, 1979.

389. Reiss E, Canterbury JM, Bercovitz MA, et al: The role of phosphate in the secretion of parathyroid hormone in man. J Clin Invest 49:2146, 1970.

390. Heller HJ, Reza-Albarran AA, Breslau N, et al: Sustained reduction in urinary calcium during long-term treatment with slow release neutral potassium phosphate in absorptive hypercalciuria. J Urol 159:1451-1456, 1998.

391. Hodgkinson A: Relations between oxalic acid, calcium, magnesium and creatinine excretion in normal men and male patients with calcium oxalate kidney stones. Clin Sci Mol Med 46:357-367, 1974.

392. Asplin JR: Hyperoxaluric calcium nephrolithiasis. Endocrinol Metab Clin North Am 31:927-949, 2002.

393. Weinman EJ, Frankfurt SJ, Ince A, et al: Renal tubular transport of organic acids. J Clin Invest 61:801-806, 1978.

394. Williams HE, Johnson GA, Smith LHJ: The renal clearance of oxalate in normal subjects and patients with primary hyperoxaluria. Clin Sci (Colch) 41:213-218, 1971.

395. Kasidas GP, Nemat S, Rose GA: Plasma oxalate and creatinine and oxalate/creatinine clearance ratios in normal subjects and in primary hyperoxaluria. Clin Chim Acta 191:78, 1990.

396. Lindsjo M, Fellstrom B, Danielson BG, et al: Hyperoxaluria or hypercalciuria in nephrolithiasis: The importance of renal tubular functions. Eur J Clin Invest 20:546-554, 1990.

397. Holmes RP, Goodman HO, Assimos DG: Contribution of dietary oxalate to urinary oxalate excretion. Kidney Int 59:270-276, 2001.

398. Brinkley L, McGuire J, Gregory J, et al: Bioavailability of oxalate in foods. Urology 17:534-538. 1981.

399. Brinkley LJ, Gregory J, Pak CYC: A further study of oxalate bioavailability in foods. J Urol 144:94-96, 1990.

400. Marshall RW, Cochran M, Hodgkinson A: Relationships between calcium and oxalic acid intake in the diet and their excretion in the urine of normal and renal-stone forming subjects. Clin Sci (Colch) 43:91-99, 1972.

401. Sidhu H, Schmidt ME, Cornelius JG, et al: Direct correlation between hyperoxaluria/oxalate stone disease and the absence of the gastrointestinal tract-dwelling bacterium *Oxalobacter formigenes*: Possible prevention by gut recolonization or enzyme replacement therapy. J Am Soc Nephrol 10(suppl 14):S334-S340, 1999.

402. Hagler L, Herman RH: Oxalate metabolism. I. Am J Clin Nutr 26:758-765, 1973.

403. Lemann JJ, Hornick LJ, Pleuss JA, et al: Oxalate is overestimated in alkaline urine collected during administration of bicarbonate with no specimen pH adjustment. Clin Chem 35:2107-2110, 1989.

404. Urivetzky M, Kessaris D, Smith AD: Ascorbic acid overdosing: A risk factor for calcium oxalate nephrolithiasis. J Urol 147:1215-1218, 1992.

405. Holmes RP, Assimos DG: Glyoxylate synthesis, and its modulation and influence on oxalate synthesis. J Urol 160:1617-1624, 1998.

406. Bushinsky DA, Asplin JR, Grynpas MD, et al: Calcium oxalate stone formation in genetic hypercalciuric stone-forming rats. Kidney Int 61:975-987, 2002.

407. Danpure CJ: Molecular and clinical heterogeneity in primary hyperoxaluria type I. Am J Kidney Dis 17:366-369, 1991.

408. Cooper PJ, Danpure CJ, Wise PJ, et al: Immunocytochemical localization of human hepatic alanine: Glyoxylate aminotransferase in control subjects and patients with primary hyperoxaluria type 1. J Histochem Cytochem 36:1285-1294, 1988.

409. Danpure CJ, Cooper PJ, Wise PJ, et al: An enzyme trafficking defect in two patients with primary hyperoxaluria type 1: Peroxisomal alanine/glyoxylate aminotransferase rerouted to mitochondria. J Cell Biol 108:1345-1352, 1989.

410. Williams HE, Smith LH: L-Glyceric aciduria: A new genetic variant of primary hyperoxaluria. N Engl J Med 278:233-239, 1968.

411. Van Acker KJ, Eyskens FJ, Espeel MF, et al: Hyperoxaluria with hyperglycoluria not due to alanine:glyoxylate aminotransferase defect: A novel type of primary hyperoxaluria. Kidney Int 50:1747-1752, 1996.

412. Hockaday TDR, Frederick EW, Clayton JE, et al: Studies on primary hyperoxaluria II: Urinary oxalate, glycolate, and glyoxylate measurement by isotope dilution methods. J Lab Clin Med 65:677-687, 1965.

413. Rumsby G, Sharma A, Cregeen DP, et al: Primary hyperoxaluria type 2 without L-glyceriaciduria: Is the disease under-diagnosed? Nephrol Dial Transplant 16:1697-1699, 2001.

414. Danpure CJ, Jennings PR, Watts RWE: Enzymological diagnosis of primary hyperoxaluria type 1 by measurement of hepatic alanine: Glyoxalate aminotransferase activity. Lancet 1:289-291, 1987.

415. Yendt ER, Cohanim M: Response to a physiologic dose of pyridoxine in type I primary hyperoxaluria. N Engl J Med 312:953-957, 1985.

416. Watts RWE, Chalmers RA, Gibbs DA, et al: Studies on some possible biochemical treatments of primary hyperoxaluria. Q J Med 48:259-272, 1979.

417. Smith LHJ, Williams HE: Treatment of primary hyperoxaluria. Mod Treat 4:522-530, 1967.

418. Milliner DS, Eickholt JT, Bergstralh EJ, et al: Results of long-term treatment with orthophosphate and pyridoxine in patients with primary hyperoxaluria. N Engl J Med 331:1553-1558, 1994.

419. Leumann E, Hoppe B, Neuhaus T: Management of primary hyperoxaluria: Efficacy of oral citrate administration. Pediatr Nephrol 7:207-211, 1993.

420. Dobbins JW, Binder HJ: Importance of colon in enteric hyperoxaluria. N Engl J Med 296:298, 1977.

421. Chadwick VS, Elias E, Bell GD, et al: The role of bile acids in the increased intestinal absorption of oxalate after ileal resection. In Matern S, Hackenschmidt J, Bach P, et al (eds): Advances in Bile Acid Research. III. Bile Acid Meeting. Stuttgart, Schattauer Verlag, 1975, p 435.

422. Chadwick VS, Modha K, Dowling RH: Mechanism for hyperoxaluria in patients with ileal dysfunction. N Engl J Med 289:172, 1973.

423. Dowling RH, Rose GA, Sutor DJ: Hyperoxaluria and renal calculi in ileal disease. Lancet 1:1103, 1971.

424. Smith LH, Fromm H, Hoffman AF: Acquired hyperoxaluria, nephrolithiasis and intestinal disease. N Engl J Med 286:137, 1972.

425. Stauffer JQ, Stewart RJ, Bertand G: Acquired hyperoxaluria: Relationship to dietary calcium content and severity of steatorrhea. Gastroenterology 66:783a, 1974.

426. Earnest DL, Johnson G, Williams HE, et al: Hyperoxaluria in patients with ileal resection: An abnormality in dietary oxalate absorption. Gastroenterology 77:1114, 1974.

427. Saunders DR, Sillery J, McDonald GB: Regional differences in oxalate absorption by rat intestine: Evidence for excessive absorption by the colon in steatorrhoea. Gut 16:543-554, 1975.

428. Kathpalia SC, Favus MJ, Coe FL: Evidence for size and charge permselectivity of rat ascending colon: Effects of ricinoleate and bile salts on oxalic acid and neutral sugar transport. J Clin Invest 74: 805-811, 1984.

429. Allison MJ, Cook HM, Milne DB, et al: Oxalate degradation by gastrointestinal bacteria from humans. J Nutr 116:455-460, 1986.

430. Earnest DL, Gaucher S, Admirand WH: Treatment of enteric hyperoxaluria with calcium and aluminum [abstract]. Gastroenterology 70:881A, 1976.

431. Atsmon A, DeVries A, Frank M: Uric Acid Lithiasis. Amsterdam, Elsevier Science Publishing Co, 1963.

432. Yu TF, Gutman AB: Uric acid nephrolithiasis in gout: Predisposing factors. Ann Intern Med 67:1133, 1967.

433. Hall AP, Berry PE, Dawber TR, et al: Epidemiology of gout and hyperuricemia: A long-term population study. Am J Med 42:27, 1967.

434. Fessel WJ: Renal outcomes of gout and hyperuricemia. Am J Med 67:74, 1979.

435. Gutman AB, Yu TF: Urinary ammonium excretion in primary gout. J Clin Invest 44:1474, 1965.

436. Elliot JS, Sharp RF, Lewis L: Urinary pH. J Urol 81:339, 1959.

437. Sorenson LB: The elimination of uric acid in man studied by means of ^{14}C-labelled uric acid. Scand J Clin Lab Invest 12(suppl 54):13, 1960.

438. DeVries A, Frank M, Atsmon A: Inherited uric acid lithiasis. Am J Med 33:880, 1962.

439. Ombra MN, Forabosco P, Casula S, et al: Identification of a new candidate locus for uric acid nephrolithiasis. Am J Hum Genet 68: 1119-1129, 2001.

440. Pak CY, Sakhaee K, Peterson RD, et al: Biochemical profile of idiopathic uric acid nephrolithiasis. Kidney Int 60:757-761, 2001.

441. Sakhaee K, Adams-Huet B, Moe OW, et al: Pathophysiologic basis for normouricosuric uric acid nephrolithiasis. Kidney Int 62: 971-979, 2002.

442. Kamel KS, Cheema-Dhadi S, Halperin ML: Studies on the pathophysiology of the low urine pH in patients with uric acid stones. Kidney Int 61:988-994, 2002.

443. Seegmiller JE, Grayzel AI, Laster L, et al: Uric acid production in gout. J Clin Invest 40:1304, 1961.

444. Bambach CP, Robertson WG, Peacock M, et al: Effect of intestinal surgery on the risk of stone formation. Gut 22:257-263, 1981.

445. Clarke AM, McKenzie RG: Ileostomy and the risk of urinary uric acid stones. Lancet 2:395-397, 1969.

446. Crane C, Lassen UV: The action of probenecid (P-[di-N-propylsulphamylbenzoic acid]) on uric acid excretion and plasma uric acid level in normal human subjects. Acta Pharmacol (Kbh) 11:295, 1955.

447. Fox IH, Wyngaarden JB, Kelley WN: Depletion of erythrocyte phosphoribosylpyrophosphate in man: A newly observed effect of allopurinol. N Engl J Med 283:1177, 1970.

448. Stote RM, Smith LH, Dubb JW, et al: Oxypurinol nephrolithiasis in regional enteritis secondary to allopurinol therapy. Ann Intern Med 92:384-385, 1980.

449. Gomez GA, Stutzman L, Chu TM: Xanthine nephropathy during chemotherapy in deficiency of hypoxanthine-guanine phosphoribosyltransferase. Arch Intern Med 138:1017, 1978.

450. Kranen S, Keough D, Gordon RB, et al: Xanthine-containing calculi during allopurinol therapy. J Urol 133:658-659, 1985.

451. Levy HL, Madigan PM, Shih VE: Massachusetts metabolic disorders screening program. Techniques and results of urine screening. Pediatrics 49:825-835, 1972.

452. Lindell A, Denneberg T, Granerus G: Studies on renal function in patients with cystinuria. Nephron 77:76-85, 1997.

453. Dello SL, Pras E, Pontesilli C, et al: Comparison between SLC3A1 and SLC7A9 cystinuria patients and carriers: A need for a new classification. J Am Soc Nephrol 13:2547-2553, 2002.

454. Dent CE, Senior B, Walshe JM: The pathogenesis of cystinuria. II. Polarographic studies of the metabolism of sulfur-containing amino acids. J Clin Invest 33:1216, 1954.

455. Arrow VK, Westall RG: Amino acid clearance in cystinuria. J Physiol 142:14, 1958.

456. Rosenberg LE, Downing SJ, Segal S: Competitive inhibition of dibasic amino acid transport in rat kidney. J Biol Chem 237:2265, 1962.

457. Fox M, Thier SO, Rosenberg LE, et al: Evidence against a single renal transport defect in cystinuria. N Engl J Med 270:556, 1964.

458. Hellier MD, Holdsworth CD, Perrett D: Dibasic amino acid absorption in man. Gastroenterology 65:613, 1973.

459. Rosenberg LE, Downing S, Durant JL, et al: Cystinuria: Biochemical evidence for three genetically distinct diseases. J Clin Invest 45:365, 1966.

460. Fernandez E, Carrascal M, Rousaud F, et al: rBAT-bo, +AT heterodimer is the main apical reabsorption system for cystine in the kidney. Am J Physiol 283:F540-F548, 2002.

461. Bertran J, Werner A, Chillaron J, et al: Expression cloning of a human renal cDNA that induces high affinity transport of L-cystine shared with dibasic amino acids in Xenopus oocytes. J Biol Chem 268:14842-14849, 1993.

462. Calogne MJ, Volpini V, Bisceglia L, et al: Genetic heterogeneity in cystinuria: The SLC3A1 gene is linked to type I but not to type III cystinuria. Proc Natl Acad Sci U S A 92:9667-9671, 1995.

463. Wartenfield R, Golomb E, Katz G, et al: Molecular analysis of cystinuria in Libyan Jews: Exclusion of the SLC3A1 gene and mapping of a new locus on 19q. Am J Hum Genet 60:624-630, 1997.

464. Bisceglia L, Calogne MJ, Totaro A, et al: Localization, by linkage analysis, of the cystinuria type III gene to chromosome 19q3.1. Am J Hum Genet 60:611-616, 1997.

465. Feliubadalo L, Font M, Purroy J, et al: Non-type I cystinuria caused by mutations in SLC7A9, encoding a subunit of rBAT. Nat Genet 23: 52-57, 1999.

466. Goodyear PR, Clow C, Reade T, et al: Prospective analysis and classification of patients with cystinuria identified in a newborn screening program. J Pediatr 122:568-572, 1993.

467. Gasparini P, Calonge MJ, Bisceglia L, et al: Molecular genetics of cystinuria: Identification of four new mutations and seven polymorphisms, and evidence for genetic heterogeneity. Am J Hum Genet 57:781-788, 1995.

468. Pras E, Raben N, Golomb E, et al: Mutations in the SLC3A1 transporter gene in cystinuria. Am J Hum Genet 56:1297-1303, 1995.

469. Crawhall JC, Purkiss P, Watts RWE, et al: The excretion of amino acids by cystinuric patients and their relatives. Ann Hum Genet 33:149, 1969.

470. Hambraeus L: Comparative studies of the value of two cyanidenitroprusside methods in the diagnosis of cystinuria. Scand J Clin Lab Invest 15:657, 1963.

471. Evans WP, Resnick MI, Boyce WH: Homozygous cystinuria—evaluation of 35 patients. J Urol 127:707-709, 1982.

472. Sakhaee K, Poindexter JR, Pak CYC: The spectrum of metabolic abnormalities in patients with cystine nephrolithiasis. J Urol 141: 819-821, 1989.

473. Resnick MJ, Goodman HO, Boyce WH: Heterozygous cystinuria and calcium oxalate urolithiasis. J Urol 122:52, 1979.

474. Nakagawa Y, Asplin JR, Goldfarb D, et al: Clinical use of cystine supersaturation measurements. J Urol 164:1481-1485, 2000.

475. Dent CE, Senior B: Studies in the treatment of cystinuria. Br J Urol 27:317-331, 1955.

476. Marshall RW, Robertson WG: Nomograms for the estimation of the saturation of urine with calcium oxalate, calcium phosphate, magnesium ammonium phosphate, uric acid, sodium acid urate, ammonium acid urate and cystine. Clin Chim Acta 72:253-260, 1976.

477. Kolb FO, Earle JM, Harper HA: Disappearance of cystinuria in a patient treated with prolonged low methionine diet. Metabolism 16:378, 1967.

478. Rodman JS, Blackburn P, Williams JJ, et al: The effect of dietary protein on cystine excretion in patients with cystinuria. Clin Nephrol 22:273-278, 1984.

479. Martensson J, Denneberg T, Lindell A, et al: Sulfur amino acid metabolism in cystinuria: A biochemical and clinical study of patients. Kidney Int 37:143-149, 1990.

480. Jaeger P, Portman L, Saunders A, et al: Anticystinuric effects of glutamine and of dietary sodium restriction. N Engl J Med 315: 1120-1123, 1986.

481. Norman RW, Manette WA: Dietary restriction of sodium as a means of reducing urinary cystine. J Urol 143:1193-1195, 1990.

482. Miyagi K, Nakada F, Ohshiro S: Effect of glutamine on cystine excretion in a patient with cystinuria. N Engl J Med 301:196, 1979.

483. Lindell A, Denneberg T, Jeppsson JO: Urinary excretion of free cystine and tiopronin-cysteine mixed disulfide during long term tiopronin treatment of cystinuria. Nephron 71:328-342, 1995.

484. Pak CYC, Fuller C, Sakhaee K, et al: Management of cystine nephrolithiasis with α-mercaptopropionylglycine. J Urol 136:1003-1008, 1986.

485. Perazella MA, Buller GK: Successful treatment of cystinuria with captopril. Am J Kidney Dis 21:504-507, 1993.

486. Sloand JA, Lizzo JLJ: Captopril reduces urinary cystine excretion in cystinuria. Arch Intern Med 147:1409-1412, 1987.

487. Michelakakis H, Delis D, Anastasiadou V, et al: Ineffectiveness of captopril in reducing cystine excretion in cystinuric children. J Inherit Metab Dis 16:1042-1043, 1993.

488. Dretler SP: Stone fragility—a new therapeutic distinction. J Urol 139:1124, 1988.

489. Singer A, Das S: Cystinuria: A review of the pathophysiology and management. J Urol 142:669-673, 1989.

490. Martin X, Salas M, Laebeeuw M, et al: Cystine stones: The impact of new treatment. Br J Urol 68:234-239, 1991.

491. Chow GK, Streem SB: Contemporary urological intervention for cystinuric patients: Immediate and long-term impact and implications. J Urol 160:341-345, 1998.

492. Teichman JM, Vassar GJ, Bishoff JT, et al: Holmium:YAG lithotripsy yields smaller fragments than lithoclast, pulsed dye laser or electrohydraulic lithotripsy. J Urol 159:17-23, 1998.

493. Chute R, Suby HI: Prevalence and importance of urea-splitting bacterial infections of the urinary tract in the formation of calculi. J Urol 44:590, 1943.

494. Griffith DP, Gibson JR, Clinton C, et al: Acetohydroxamic acid: Clinical studies of a urease inhibitor in patients with staghorn renal calculi. J Urol 119:9, 1978.

495. Robertson WG, Peacock M: Calcium oxalate crystalluria and inhibitors of crystallization in recurrent renal stone formers. Clin Sci (Colch) 43:499-506, 1972.

496. Elliot JS, Sharp RF, Lewis L: The solubility of struvite in urine. J Urol 80:169, 1959.

497. Griffith DP, Osborne CA: Infection (urease) stones. Miner Electrolyte Metab 13:278-285, 1987.

498. Farmer JJ, Davis BR, Hickman-Brenner FW: Biochemical identification of new species and biogroups of Enterbacteriaceae isolated from clinical specimens. J Clin Microbiol 21:46-76, 1985.

499. Hedelin H, Brorson JE, Grenabo L, et al: *Ureaplasma urealyticum* and upper urinary tract stones. Br J Urol 56:244-249, 1984.

500. Kristensen C, Parks JH, Lindheimer M, et al: Reduced glomerular filtration rate and hypercalciuria in primary struvite nephrolithiasis. Kidney Int 32:749-753, 1987.

501. Segura JW, Preminger GM, Assimos DG, et al: Nephrolithiasis clinical guidelines panel summary report on the management of staghorn calculi. J Urol 151:1648-1651, 1994.

502. Wojewski A, Zajaczkowski T: The treatment of bilateral staghorn calculi of the kidneys. Int Urol Nephrol 5:249, 1974.

503. Singh M, Chapman R, Tressider GC, et al: The fate of the unoperated staghorn calculus. Br J Urol 45:58, 1973.

504. Silverman DE, Stamey TA: Management of infection stones: The Stanford experience. Medicine (Baltimore) 62:44-51, 1983.

505. Kerlan RK, Kahn RK, Laberge JM, et al: Percutaneous removal of renal staghorn calculi. AJR Am J Roentgenol 145:797-801, 1985.

506. Segura JW, Patterson DE, LeRoy AJ, et al: Percutaneous removal of kidney stones: Review of 1000 cases. J Urol 134:1077-1081, 1985.

507. Patterson DE, Segura JW, LeRoy AJ: Long-term follow-up of patients treated by percutaneous ultrasonic lithotripsy for struvite staghorn calculi. J Endourol 1:177, 1987.

508. Michaels EK, Fowler JEJ: Extracorporeal shock wave lithotripsy for struvite renal calculi: Prospective study with extended followup. J Urol 146:728-732, 1991.

509. Miller K, Bachor R, Sauter T, et al: ESWL monotherapy for large stones and staghorn calculi. Urol Int 45:95-98, 1990.

510. Grasso M, Conlin M, Bagley D: Retrograde ureteropyeloscopic treatment of 2 cm or greater upper urinary tract and minor staghorn calculi. J Urol 160:346-351, 1998.

511. Stamey TA: Urinary Infections. Baltimore, Williams & Wilkins, 1972, p 213.

512. Griffith DP, Khonsari F, Skurnick JH, et al: A randomized trial of acetohydroxamic acid for the treatment and prevention of infection-induced urinary stones in spinal cord injury patients. J Urol 140:318-324, 1988.

513. Williams JJ, Rodman JS, Peterson CM: A randomized double blind study of acetohydroxamic acid in struvite nephrolithiasis. N Engl J Med 311:760-764, 1984.

514. Griffith DP, Gleeson MJ, Lee H, et al: Randomized, double-blind trial of Lithostat (acetohydroxamic acid) in the palliative treatment of infection-induced urinary calculi. Eur Urol 20:243-247, 1991.

515. Jacobs SP, Gittes RF: Dissolution of residual renal calculi with hemiacidrin. J Urol 115:2, 1976.

516. Brock WA, Nachtscheim DA, Parsons CL: Hemiacidrin irrigation of renal pelvic calculi in patients with ileal conduit urinary diversion. J Urol 123:345, 1980.

CHAPTER 40

Urinary Tract Obstruction

Mark L. Zeidel and Georgi Pirtskhalaishvili

In a process that is essential for survival, the urinary tract eliminates soluble wastes and toxins from the body. In adults, 1.5 to 2.0 L of urine flows daily from the renal papillae through the ureter, bladder, and urethra in an uninterrupted, unidirectional flow. Any obstruction that interrupts the flow of urine at any point along this path may cause retention of urine and a build-up of pressure, leading to damage to the kidney and interference with its ability to effect excretion of wastes and water and to maintain fluid and electrolyte homeostasis. Because the extent of recovery of renal function in obstructive nephropathy is inversely related to the duration and extent of obstruction, prompt diagnosis and relief of obstruction are the cornerstones of effective management. Fortunately, urinary tract obstruction represents one of the most treatable of kidney diseases.

Several terms with varying definitions have been used to describe urinary tract obstruction.[1, 2] In the following discussion, *hydronephrosis* is defined as a dilation of the renal pelvis and calices proximal to the point of obstruction. *Obstructive uropathy* represents a blockage to urine flow due to a structural or functional derangement anywhere from the tip of the urethra back to the renal pelvis that increases pressure proximal to the site of obstruction. Renal parenchymal damage may or may not occur in the presence of obstructive uropathy. *Obstructive nephropathy* describes functional or pathologic damage to the renal parenchyma resulting from the obstruction anywhere along the urinary tract. It should be noted that hydronephrosis and obstructive uropathy are not interchangeable terms—dilation of the renal pelvis and calices can present without obstruction, and not all cases of urinary obstruction are associated with hydronephrosis.

PREVALENCE AND INCIDENCE

The frequency of urinary tract obstruction varies widely among different patient populations, and depends on age, sex, and concurrent medical conditions. Unfortunately, reports of incidence and prevalence have been based on the studies of selected "populations," such as data from autopsy series and from women with high-risk pregnancies. No data are available for any unselected populations.

In a retrospective review of 59,064 autopsies of persons varying in age from neonate to 80 years, hydronephrosis was noted in 3.1% (2.9% in females and 3.3% in males).[3] In subjects less than 10 years of age, who represented 1.5% of the total autopsies, the principal causes of urinary tract obstruction were neurologic abnormalities or ureteral and urethral strictures. The extent to which these abnormalities were recognized clinically as opposed to being incidental findings is unclear. There was no substantial sex difference until the age of 20 years. Between the ages of 20 and 60, the frequency of urinary obstruction was higher among women than among men, mainly due to the effects of pregnancy and uterine cancer. After age 60, prostatic disease raised the frequency of urinary tract obstruction among men above that among women.

In children under age 15, the frequency of obstruction at autopsy was found to be 2%. Hydronephrosis occurred in 1.5% of the girls and 2.2% of the boys; 80% of the episodes of hydronephrosis were found in subjects under 1 year in age.[4] In more recent autopsy series of 3172 children, 2.5% were found to have urinary tract abnormalities. Hydronephrosis and hydroureter were the most common, constituting 35.9% of all cases.[5] In neither study was it clear what proportion of cases were clinically diagnosed.

Because these autopsy series clearly contained many cases of obstruction that went undetected during life, it appears highly likely that the overall prevalence of urinary tract obstruction is far greater than reports suggest. This conclusion is reinforced by the fact that there are several common but temporary causes of obstruction, such as pregnancy and renal calculi, that contribute to this underestimate.

CLASSIFICATION

Urinary tract obstruction can be classified initially by its duration—acute or chronic.[6] These two categories can be further subdivided according to location (upper or lower urinary tract, supravesical or subvesical, and so on), and further, by whether the obstruction is congenital or acquired. This classification lends itself well to diagnosis and management. Acute obstruction may be associated with sudden onset of the symptoms. Obstruction in the upper urinary tract (ureter or ureteropelvic junction), may present with renal colic. In the lower urinary tract (bladder or urethra), presenting symptoms may include disorders of micturition. Chronic urinary tract obstruction may develop insidiously, presenting with few or only minor symptoms, and with more general manifestations. For example, bladder calculi, recurrent urinary tract infections, and progressive renal insufficiency may all be caused by chronic obstruction. Congenital causes of obstruction arise from developmental abnormalities, whereas acquired lesions develop after birth, either due to disease processes or as a result of medical interventions.

ETIOLOGY

Because congenital and acquired urinary tract obstruction differ to a great degree in cause and clinical course, we will describe them separately.

Congenital Causes of Obstruction

Any level along the urinary tract from the ureteropelvic junction to the tip of urethra can be obstructed because of congenital anomalies, and the obstruction may damage one or both kidneys (Table 40-1). Although some of the lesions are rare, as a group they represent an important cause of urinary tract obstruction, because in younger patients they often lead to severe renal impairment and may result in catastrophic end-stage renal disease.[7]

Obstruction at the ureteropelvic junction is the most common cause of hydronephrosis in fetuses[8] and young children[9] (reported incidence of 5 cases per 100,000 population

TABLE 40-1

Congenital Causes of Urinary Tract Obstruction

Ureteropelvic junction
 Ureteropelvic junction obstruction
Proximal and middle ureter
 Ureteral folds
 Ureteral valves
 Strictures
 Benign fibroepithelial polyps
 Retrocaval ureter
Distal ureter
 Ureterovesical junction obstruction
 Vesicoureteral reflux
 Prune-belly syndrome
 Ureteroceles
Bladder
 Bladder diverticula
 Neurologic conditions (e.g., spina bifida)
Urethra
 Posterior urethral valves
 Urethral diverticula
 Anterior urethral valves
 Urethral atresia
 Labial fusion

per year),[10] and it may affect adults as well.[11, 12] In fact, in one series, more than 50% of patients with congenital ureteropelvic junction obstruction were older than 20 years.[10] Although most cases of ureteropelvic junction obstruction appear to represent sporadic events, familial forms exist, suggesting that in some cases genetic inheritance plays a role.[13] Sixty percent of cases occur on the left side, and two thirds occur in males. In patients detected less than 1 year of age, 20% of cases are bilateral.[14] There is considerable controversy as to whether all cases of obstruction early in life are clinically significant. The widespread use of fetal ultrasound has resulted in detection of many cases that remain asymptomatic and may resolve spontaneously with simple follow-up of the child.[15, 16] Although the majority of cases of ureteropelvic junction obstruction are diagnosed prenatally by ultrasound,[14] the most common clinical presentation in neonates is a flank or abdominal mass.[17] By contrast, adults will generally present with flank pain.[11, 12] Because symptoms of intermittent obstruction may mimic gastrointestinal disease, diagnosis may be delayed. At any age, ureteropelvic junction obstruction may be associated with hypertension, kidney stones, hematuria, or recurrent urinary tract infection.[10-12]

It is thought that ureteropelvic junction obstruction may be caused by an aperistaltic segment of the ureter, which cannot drive urine away from the renal pelvis and down the ureter.[18] Less commonly, the obstruction may be due to an actual stricture of the ureter.[18] Histopathologic studies reveal multiple abnormalities at the ureteropelvic junction. Light microscopic findings may include no abnormality or decreased muscle bulk, infiltration of inflammatory cells, or malorientation of the muscle fibers.[19] Electron microscopy usually demonstrates an abundance of collagen. An association between abnormal angulation at the ureteropelvic junction and the presence of aberrant renal vessels suggest the possibility that the aberrant vessels lead to the functional defect in the ureter,[14, 20] but this remains controversial.[21] For the most part it appears that obstruction does not result from the aberrant vessel but rather from an intrinsic defect of the musculature with the secondary dilated pelvis wrapped around the aberrant vessel. Rarely, fibroepithelial polyps can be the cause of ureteropelvic junction obstruction.[22]

Obstruction can also occur farther down in the proximal or middle ureter. Ureteral folds, which are noncircumferential areas of redundant mucosa, may cause temporary obstruction. They are usually asymptomatic and disappear as the child matures.[23] Ureteral valves, which are transverse folds of redundant ureteral mucosa and smooth muscle, represent uncommon causes of urinary tract obstruction; they may be accompanied by other urinary tract abnormalities.[24, 25] Benign fibroepithelial polyps and congenital strictures[26, 27] of the ureter may also cause obstruction. Abnormal development of the venous system may result in a retrocaval right ureter and its obstruction by the inferior vena cava,[28] producing the classic "fishhook" or "reversed J" sign deformity on an intravenous urogram. This deformity is partial, right-sided, and asymptomatic in early life. It generally goes undetected until the patient reaches adulthood. These patients usually come to clinical attention in their fourth decade, presenting with chronic urinary tract infection and colicky intermittent abdominal pain. Because the lesion is three times more common in males than females, the appearance of urinary tract infection in a male may lead to the diagnosis.

Congenital anomalies of the distal ureter represent another important cause of obstruction. Obstruction at the ureterovesical junction, a functional defect that resembles that seen at the ureteropelvic junction, is the second most common site of congenital ureteral obstruction.[29] These patients may develop striking enlargement of the involved ureter; this is a prominent cause of congenital megaureter.[30, 31] Vesicoureteral reflux results from anatomic abnormalities of the ureterovesical junction and may cause a congenitally enlarged ureter. The reflux may be caused by one or more of several factors, including an abnormally positioned ureteral orifice, a dysmorphic ureter, or bladder outlet obstruction.[32] Megaureter may also occur in prune-belly syndrome, which includes absence of the abdominal musculature, ureteral dilation, and bilateral cryptorchidism.[33, 34] A ureterocele, which is a congenital cystic dilation of the terminal ureter, may also obstruct the ureteral orifice.[35, 36] Ureteroceles may be ectopic, in which case the ureter empties into the bladder at a site other than the lateral angle of the trigone, or they may be orthotopic. Ectopic ureteroceles are often associated with a duplicated collecting system.[35, 37] Orthotopic ureteroceles are less common than ectopic ones; some may be large enough to cause obstruction of both ureters during childhood. They carry a worse prognosis than ureteroceles diagnosed in adults.[38] Large orthotopic ureteroceles may occasionally lead to bladder outlet obstruction as well.[39] Renal duplication with ureteral ectopia may also lead to obstruction and hydronephrosis.[40]

Congenital bladder outlet obstruction may result from mechanical or functional factors. Mechanical factors include bladder diverticula, posterior urethral valves, urethral diverticula, labial fusion, or colonic duplication. Congenital bladder diverticula may obstruct the bladder outlet or one or both ureters,[41] and may even lead to acute renal failure.[42] Posterior urethral valves, seen only in boys at the level of the proximal urethra, are the most common congenital cause of obstruction.[43] Although posterior urethral valves are usually diagnosed during childhood,[44] they may be discovered in adults.[45] Diagnosis is best made by voiding cystourethrography. Perineal ultrasonography also was reported to be very useful, and can visualize the valve itself.[46] In cases of severe obstruction, early surgical intervention may prevent the development of renal failure. Urethral diverticula occur most often in girls and may lead to urethral obstruction.[47] Very rarely, labial fusion may cause urinary obstruction in newborn girls.[48] Colonic duplication, also very rare, may also lead to ureteral obstruction.[49]

Congenital functional disorders result in obstruction because the bladder fails to fill and empty normally. Such disorders are usually due to a neurologic abnormality that most often involves the bladder.[50, 51] Myelodysplasia, typically myelomeningocele with or without hydrocephalus, leads to bladder dysfunction, and is associated with a 10% frequency of hydronephrosis at birth.[50] Because hydronephrosis develops in another 15% of these patients in early childhood,[52] it is important to maintain careful follow-up in this group of patients to prevent later development of renal damage.[50]

Because operative complications may be high,[53, 54] the use of fetal[55, 56] or neonatal[56, 57] surgery for the relief of obstruction remains controversial.[58] Although bilateral obstruction requires intervention, the simple presence of unilateral hydronephrosis does not. Indications for surgery in unilateral hydronephrosis include symptoms of obstruction or impaired function in a presumably salvageable hydronephrotic kidney.

Acquired Causes of Obstruction
Intrinsic Causes

Acquired causes of obstruction may be intrinsic or extrinsic to the urinary tract (Table 40-2). Intrinsic refers to the obstruction resulting from intraluminal or intramural processes; these may be considered according to anatomic location.

Intrinsic intraluminal processes leading to obstruction may be intrarenal or extrarenal. Intrarenal causes arise from formation of crystals or cases within the renal tubules. These include uric acid nephropathy[59]; deposition of crystals of drugs that precipitate in the urine, including sulfonamides,[60] acyclovir,[61] indinavir,[62] and ciprofloxacin[63]; and multiple myeloma.[64] Uric acid nephropathy usually develops as a complication of the use of alkylating agents in the treatment of patients with malignant hematopoietic neoplasms, and the risk of its development relates directly to plasma uric acid concentrations.[59] Uric acid nephropathy may also occur in the setting of disseminated adenomatous carcinoma of the gastrointestinal tract.[65] Sulfonamide crystal deposition, once common, became rare with the introduction of sulfonamides that are more soluble in acid urine than previous ones. However, sulfadiazine, which is used to treat toxoplasmosis in patients with acquired immunodeficiency syndrome (AIDS) because it is relatively lipophilic and penetrates brain, has been associated with intrarenal crystallization and acute renal failure when given in large doses.[60, 66] Ciprofloxacin also may induce crystalluria with stone formation and urinary obstruction.[63] Casts composed of Bence Jones protein obstruct tubules and exert toxic effects on tubular epithelium in patients with multiple myeloma, often leading to the renal failure.[64] As a result of renal damage from Bence Jones protein and other abnormalities frequently seen in patients with multiple myeloma (e.g., amyloidosis and hypercalcemia), renal failure is the second most common cause of death in this patient population.[64] Multiple myeloma may also cause obstructive uropathy due to proteinaceous precipitates in the renal pelvis causing unilateral hydronephrosis.[67]

Several intrinsic intraluminal, extrarenal, or intraureteral processes may also cause obstruction. Nephrolithiasis represents the most common cause of ureteral obstruction in younger men. Twelve percent of the U.S. population form a symptomatic stone at some time in their lives, with a male-to-female predominance of 3:1.[68] Calcium oxalate stones are the most common type; when they cause obstruction, it tends to be acute, unilateral, and intermittent, usually without a long-term impact on renal function. Of course, when a stone obstructs a solitary kidney, the result can be anuric acute renal failure. Less common types of stones, such as struvite (ammonium-magnesium-sulfate) and cysteine stones, are more frequently associated with renal damage because these substances accumulate over time, and often form staghorn calculi. Stones obstruct urine flow at narrowings along the ureter, including the ureteropelvic junction, the pelvic brim (where the ureter arches over the iliac vessels), and the ureterovesical junction.

Other processes that cause ureteral obstruction include papillary necrosis, blood clots, and cystic inflammation. Papillary necrosis[69] may result from sickle cell trait or disease, analgesic abuse, amyloidosis, acute pyelonephritis, or diabetes mellitus. Renal allografts may develop papillary necrosis as well.[70] Acute obstruction may even require surgical intervention.[71]

TABLE 40-2

Acquired Causes of Urinary Tract Obstruction

Intrinsic Processes
Intraluminal
  Intrarenal
    Uric acid nephropathy
    Sulfonamides
    Acyclovir
    Indinavir
    Multiple myeloma
  Intraureteral
    Nephrolithiasis
    Papillary necrosis
    Blood clots
    Fungus balls
Intramural
  Functional
    Diseases
      Diabetes mellitus
      Multiple sclerosis
      Cerebrovascular disease
      Spinal cord injury
      Parkinson disease
    Drugs
      Anticholinergic agents
      Levodopa (α-adrenergic properties)
  Anatomic
    Ureteral strictures
      Schistosomiasis
      Tuberculosis
      Drugs (e.g., nonsteroidal anti-inflammatory agents)
      Ureteral instrumentation
    Urethral strictures
    Benign or malignant tumors of the renal pelvis, ureter, bladder

Extrinsic Processes
Reproductive tract
  Females
    Uterus
      Pregnancy
      Tumor (fibroids, endometrial or cervical cancer)
      Endometriosis
      Uterine prolapse
    Ureteral ligation (surgical)
    Ovary
      Tubo-ovarian abscess
      Tumor
      Cyst
  Male
    Benign prostatic hyperplasia
    Prostate cancer
Malignant neoplasms
  Genitourinary tract
    Tumors of kidney, ureter, bladder, urethra
  Other sites
    Metastatic spread
    Direct extension
Gastrointestinal system
  Crohn disease
  Appendicitis
  Diverticulosis
  Chronic pancreatitis with pseudocyst formation
  Acute pancreatitis
Vascular system
  Arterial aneurysms
    Abdominal aortic aneurysm
    Iliac artery aneurysm
  Venous
    Ovarian vein thrombophlebitis
  Vasculitides
    Systemic lupus erythematosus
    Polyarteritis nodosa
    Wegener granulomatosis
    Schönlein-Henoch purpura
Retroperitoneal processes
  Fibrosis
    Idiopathic
    Drug-induced
    Inflammatory
      Ascending lymphangitis of the lower extremities
      Chronic urinary tract infection
      Tuberculosis
      Sarcoidosis
    Iatrogenic (multiple abdominal surgical procedures)
  Enlarged retroperitoneal nodes
  Tumor invasion
  Tumor mass
  Hemorrhage
  Urinoma
Biologic agents
  Actinomycosis

Blood clots secondary to a benign or malignant lesion of the urinary tract or cystic inflammation of the ureter (ureteritis cystica) can also lead to obstruction and hydronephrosis.[72]

Intrinsic intramural processes that cause obstruction include functional abnormalities resulting in failure of micturition or more rarely of ureteral peristalsis. Functional abnormalities, such as those associated with neurologic dysfunction[73] seen in diabetes mellitus, multiple sclerosis, spinal cord injury, cerebrovascular disease, and Parkinson disease, can be caused by upper motor neuron damage. These can produce involuntary micturition (spastic bladder dysfunction), with the transmissal of increased intravesical pressure retrograde up to the upper urinary tract. Lower spinal tract injury may result in a flaccid, atonic bladder and failure of micturition. This may result in recurrent urinary tract infections.

Various drugs can cause intrinsic intramural obstruction by disrupting the normal function of the smooth muscle of the urinary tract. Anticholinergic agents[74] may decrease bladder contractility, and levodopa[75] may mediate an α-adrenergic increase in bladder outlet resistance. Chronic use of tiaprofenic acid (Surgam) can cause severe cystitis with subsequent ureteral obstruction.[76] When the bladder does not void normally, renal damage may develop as a consequence of recurrent urinary tract infections and back-pressure produced by the accumulation of residual urine.

Acquired anatomic abnormalities of the wall of the urinary tract include ureteral strictures, and benign as well as malignant tumors of the renal pelvis, ureter, bladder, and urethra.[77, 78] Ureteral strictures may occur as a result of radiation therapy for local cancers, such as cervical cancer,[79] or as a result of analgesic abuse.[80] In addition, strictures may develop as a complication of ureteral instrumentation or surgery.

Certain infectious organisms may produce intrinsic obstruction of the urinary tract as well. *Schistosoma haematobium* infects nearly 100 million people worldwide. Though active infection can be treated and obstructive uropathy may resolve, chronic schistosomiasis (bilharziasis) may develop in untreated cases, leading to irreversible ureteral or bladder fibrosis and obstruction.[81] Of other infections, 5% of patients with tuberculosis have genitourinary involvement,[82] predominantly unilateral tuberculous stricture of the ureter.[83] Mycoses such as *Candida albicans* or *Candida tropicalis* infection may also result in obstruction due to intraluminal obstruction (fungus ball) or invasion of the ureteral wall.[84, 85]

Extrinsic Causes

A wide variety of diseases cause acquired extrinsic urinary tract obstruction. Because processes affecting the female reproductive tract such as pregnancy and pelvic neoplasms often cause obstructive uropathy, urinary tract obstruction occurs more often in younger women than in younger men.[2] Noninvasive imaging studies have shown that more than two thirds of women entering their third trimester demonstrate some degree of dilation of the collecting system,[86, 87] most often resulting from mechanical ureteral obstruction.[88] This temporary form of obstruction usually develops as the ureter crosses the pelvic brim, and affects the right ureter more often than the left.[86] The vast majority of these are subclinical and appear to resolve completely soon after delivery.[89] Clinically significant obstructive uropathy almost always presents with flank pain.[90] In these cases, ultrasonography may serve as a useful initial screening test.[17] Magnetic resonance imaging (MRI) can be used if ultrasound (US) data are not conclusive.[91] Of course, the diagnostic evaluation must be tailored to minimize fetal radiation exposure. If the obstruction is significant, a ureteral stent can be placed cystoscopically, and its efficacy monitored with repeated follow-up ultrasonography.[92] The stent can be left in place for the duration of pregnancy, if needed. Although bilateral obstruction during pregnancy can lead to acute renal failure, this is rare.[68, 90] Conditions accompanying pregnancies that may predispose to obstructive uropathy and acute renal failure include multiple fetuses, an incarcerated gravid uterus, polyhydramnios, or a solitary kidney.[93]

Pelvic malignant neoplasms, especially adenocarcinomas of the cervix, represent the second most common cause of extrinsic obstructive uropathy in women.[94] In older women, uterine prolapse may cause obstruction, with hydronephrosis developing in 5% of patients.[95] The prolapse may lead to compression of the ureter by uterine blood vessels. Prolapse has been associated with urinary tract infection, sepsis, pyonephrosis, and renal insufficiency. Genital prolapse due to weakening of the pelvic floor may also result in obstruction.[96, 97] Benign uterine masses or cystic ovary has been reported to cause obstruction, especially as these masses enlarge.[98] Pelvic inflammatory disease, particularly a tubo-ovarian abscess, can also cause obstruction.[99] Pelvic lipomatosis, a disease with an unclear etiology, seen more often in men, is another rare reason for compressive urinary tract obstruction.[100, 101]

Although endometriosis only rarely results in ureteral obstruction,[102-104] it should be pursued as a diagnosis any time a premenopausal woman presents with unilateral obstruction. The onset of obstruction may be insidious, and the process is usually confined to the pelvic portion of the ureter.[105] Ureteral involvement may be intrinsic or extrinsic, with extrinsic compression arising principally from adhesions associated with the endometriosis. Because ureteral involvement often is not suspected, the routine use of excretory urography[106] or computed tomography (CT) is advisable in advanced cases of endometriosis.[107] When surgery is contemplated, it is all the more important to image the ureters, because they cross the anticipated surgical field and may well be near, or attached to, adhesions.[105] It is notable that 52% of inadvertent ligations of the ureter in abdominal and retroperitoneal operations occur in gynecologic procedures.[108]

Above the age of 60 years, obstructive uropathy occurs more commonly in men than in women. Benign prostatic hyperplasia, the most common cause of urinary tract obstruction in men, produces some symptoms of bladder outlet obstruction in 75% of men aged 50 years and older.[109] It appears likely that the proportion of affected older men would be higher if physicians took a detailed history for symptoms. Presenting symptoms of bladder outlet obstruction include urgency, difficulty initiating micturition, dribbling at the end of micturition, incomplete bladder emptying, and nocturia. The diagnosis may be established by history and urodynamic studies. Some claim that imaging studies are useful as well.[110]

Malignant genitourinary tumors occasionally result in urinary tract obstruction. Bladder cancer is the second most common cause (after cervical cancer) of malignant obstruction of the ureter.[2] Prostate cancer may cause obstruction[111] by compression of the bladder neck, invasion of the ureteral orifices, or metastatic involvement of the ureter or pelvic nodes.[112] Although urothelial tumors of the renal pelvis, ureter, and urethra are very rare, they also may lead to urinary obstruction.[113]

Several gastrointestinal processes sometimes cause obstructive uropathy. The inflammation of Crohn disease may extend into the retroperitoneum, leading to obstruction of the ureters,[114, 115] usually on the right side.[116] In addition, gastrointestinal disease with malabsorption may cause oxalosis, leading to nephrolithiasis.[117] Retroperitoneal scarring or abscess formation due to appendicitis in children and young adults[118] or large bowel diverticulitis in older patients[119] may rarely cause obstruction of the right and left ureters, respectively. Fecaloma is another rare cause of bilateral ureteral obstruction.[120] Chronic pancreatitis with pseudocyst formation sometimes causes left ureteral obstruction,[121] and may very rarely cause bilateral obstruction.[122] Right-sided obstruction may be associated with acute pancreatitis.[123]

Vascular abnormalities or diseases may also lead to obstruction. Abdominal aortic aneurysm represents the most common vascular cause of urinary obstruction,[124] due to direct pressure of the aneurysm on the ureter or associated retroperitoneal fibrosis. Aneurysms of the iliac vessels may also cause obstruction.[125] Rarely, the ovarian venous system may cause right ureteral obstruction.[126] In addition, and also rarely, vasculitis caused by systemic lupus erythematosus,[127] polyarteritis nodosa,[128, 129] Wegener granulomatosis[130, 131] and Schönlein-Henoch purpura[132, 133] have been reported to cause obstruction.

Retroperitoneal processes, such as tumor invasion leading to compression and fibrosis, can produce obstruction. The major extrinsic causes of retroperitoneal obstruction, accounting for 70% of all cases, are due to tumors of the cervix, prostate, bladder, colon, ovary, or uterus.[2, 134] When idiopathic, retroperitoneal fibrosis,[135-137] usually involves the middle third of the ureter, and affects men and women equally, predominantly those in the fifth and sixth decades of life. Retroperitoneal fibrosis may also be drug-induced (e.g., methysergide), or it may occur as a consequence of multiple abdominal surgical procedures. It may also be associated with conditions as varied as sarcoidosis, gonorrhea, chronic urinary tract infections, Schönlein-Henoch purpura, biliary tract disease, tuberculosis, and inflammatory processes of the lower extremities with ascending lymphangitis.

Malignant neoplasms can obstruct the urinary tract by metastasis (overall frequency of 1% in one autopsy series),[138] or by direct extension. As noted above, cervical cancer is the most common obstructing malignant neoplasm, followed by bladder cancer.[2, 139, 140] Rare childhood tumors such as pelvic neurofibromas can induce upper urinary tract obstruction in 60% of patients.[141] Wilms tumor obstructs via local compression of the renal pelvis.[142] Miscellaneous inflammatory processes can also result in obstruction. These include granulomatous causes such as sarcoidosis[143] and chronic granulomatous disease of childhood.[144] Amyloid deposits may produce isolated involvement of the ureter. Furthermore, a pelvic mass or inflammatory process associated with actinomycosis may cause external ureteral compression.[145, 146] Retrovesical echinococcal cyst can also impede urine flow.[147] Retroperitoneal malacoplakia can also be a rare cause of urinary obstruction.[148] Hepatitis B–associated polyarteritis nodosa may also result in bilateral hydronephrosis.[149]

Hematologic abnormalities induce obstruction of the urinary tract by a variety of mechanisms. Enlarged retroperitoneal lymph nodes or a tumor mass may compress the ureter.[150] Alternatively, precipitation of cellular breakdown products and paraproteins, as in multiple myeloma, may result in intrinsic obstruction. In patients with clotting abnormalities, blood clots or hematomas may obstruct the urinary tract, as can sloughed papillae in patients with sickle cell disease or analgesic nephropathy. Although leukemic infiltrates rarely cause obstruction in adults, in children they cause obstruction in 5% of patients.[151] Lymphomatous infiltration of the kidney occurs relatively commonly, but obstruction related to ureteral involvement in lymphoma is rarer.[152]

CLINICAL ASPECTS

Patients with urinary tract obstruction may exhibit symptoms referable to the urinary tract. However, even patients with severe obstruction may be asymptomatic, especially when the obstruction develops gradually, or in patients with spinal cord injury.[153] The clinical presentation depends on the rate of onset of the obstruction (acute or chronic), the degree of obstruction (partial or complete), whether the obstruction is unilateral or bilateral, and whether the obstruction is intrinsic or extrinsic. Pain is usually associated with obstruction of sudden onset, as from a kidney stone, blood clot, or sloughed papilla, and appears to result from abrupt stretching of the renal capsule or collecting system. The severity of the pain is thought to correlate with the rate, rather than the degree, of distention. The pain may present as typical renal colic, or, in patients with reflux, the pain may radiate to the flank only during micturition. With ureteropelvic junction obstruction, flank pain may develop when the patient ingests large quantities of fluids or receives diuretics.[154]

Early satiety and weight loss may be another symptom.[155] Ileus or other gastrointestinal symptoms may be associated with the pain, so that it can be difficult to differentiate obstruction for gastrointestinal disease.

Sometimes, symptoms of obstruction include changes in urine output. Urinary tract obstruction is one of the few conditions that can result in anuria; that is, complete obstruction of all nephrons, typically because of bladder outlet obstruction, or obstruction of a solitary kidney at any level. However, obstruction may coexist with no change in urine output. Alternatively, mild episodes of polyuria may alternate with periods of oliguria. Recurrent urinary tract infections may be the only sign of obstruction, particularly in children. As mentioned above, difficulty initiating urination, decreased size or force of the urine stream, postvoiding dribbling, and incomplete emptying are signs of bladder outlet obstruction in patients with prostatic disease.[156] Spastic bladder or irritative symptoms such as dysuria, frequency, and urgency may result from urinary tract infection. The cyclical appearance of obstructive symptoms may also be a sign of endometriosis.[157]

On physical examination, several signs may suggest urinary obstruction. A palpable abdominal mass, especially in neonates, may represent hydronephrosis. A palpable suprapubic mass may represent a distended bladder. On laboratory examination, proteinuria, if present, is generally less than 2 g/day. Microscopic hematuria is a common finding, but gross hematuria may develop occasionally as well.[158] The urine sediment is often unremarkable. Less common manifestations of urinary tract obstruction include deterioration of renal function without apparent cause, hypertension,[159] polycythemia, and abnormal urine acidification and concentration.

DIAGNOSIS

A thorough history and physical examination often lead to detection of urinary tract obstruction, and suggest the reason for it. This focuses the evaluation, so that the minimal amount of time and expense will be incurred in determining the cause of the obstruction.

History and Physical Examination

Important information in the history includes the type and duration of symptoms (voiding difficulties, flank pain, decreased urine output), number of urinary tract infections (especially in children), pattern of fluid intake and urine output, history of stone disease, malignancies, gynecologic diseases, history of recent surgery, AIDS, and drug use.[101]

The physical examination should first focus on an evaluation of the patient's volume status, which will guide fluid therapy. The abdominal examination may reveal hydronephrosis presenting as a flank mass (especially in children), or a distended bladder (as a suprapubic mass). Features of chronic renal failure, such as pallor (anemia), drowsiness (uremia), neuromuscular irritability (metabolic abnormalities), or pericardial friction rub (uremic pericarditis), may also be noted. A thorough pelvic examination in women and a rectal examination for all patients are mandatory. A careful history and a well-directed and complete physical examination often reveal the specific cause of urinary obstruction. Coexistence of obstruction and infection is a urologic emergency and appropriate studies (US, intravenous pyelography, CT) must be performed immediately, so that the obstruction can be relieved promptly.

Laboratory Evaluation

The laboratory evaluation includes urinalysis and examination of the sediment by an experienced observer. Unexplained renal failure with a benign urinary sediment should suggest urinary tract obstruction. Microscopic hematuria without proteinuria may suggest calculus or tumor. Pyuria and bacteriuria may indicate pyelonephritis; bacteriuria alone may suggest stasis. Crystals in a freshly voided specimen should lead to consideration of nephrolithiasis or intrarenal crystal deposition.

Hematologic evaluation should include the hematocrit and mean corpuscular volume (to identify anemia of chronic renal disease), and white blood cell count (to identify possible hematopoietic system neoplasm or infection). Serum electrolytes (Na^+, Cl^-, K^+, and HCO_3^-), blood urea nitrogen concentration, creatinine, Ca^{2+}, phosphorus, Mg^{2+}, uric acid, and albumin levels should be measured. These will help identify disorders of distal nephron function (impaired osmoregulation or acid excretion) and uremia. Urinary chemistries may also suggest distal tubular dysfunction (isosthenuric urine, high urine pH), inability to reabsorb sodium normally (urinary $Na^+ > 20$ mEq/L, fractional excretion of Na^+ [FE_{Na}] > 1%, and osmolality < 350 mOsm). Alternatively, in acute obstruction urinary chemistry values may be consistent with prerenal azotemia (urinary $Na^+ <$ 20 mEq/L, $FE_{Na} <$ 1%, and osmolality > 500 mOsm).[6]

Radiologic Evaluation

The results of the history, physical examination, and initial laboratory studies should guide the radiologic evaluation. Pain, evidence and degree of renal dysfunction, and the presence of infection dictate the speed and nature of the evaluation. A variety of radiologic techniques are available; each has advantages and disadvantages, including the ability to identify the site and cause of the obstruction and to separate functional obstruction from mere dilation of the urinary tract.[160, 161] The risk of radiocontrast in the setting of renal insufficiency, as well as of exposure to radiation in pregnant women, must also be weighed.[17]

Plain Film Imaging of the Abdomen

Abdominal or flank pain in the setting of normal or mildly impaired renal function suggests a renal calculus. In this situation, a plain film of the abdomen (kidney, ureter, and bladder) can provide information on the size and overall contour of the kidneys. In addition, because 90% of calculi are radioopaque, they may be detected along the course of ureter, or in the bladder (Fig. 40-1). Plain films can be performed in pregnant patients with appropriate shielding, if necessary. The plain film may detect radiopaque foreign bodies as well (e.g., stents) (see Fig. 40-1).

Ultrasonography

When obstruction is suspected, ultrasonography is the preferred screening modality[162] because it is highly sensitive

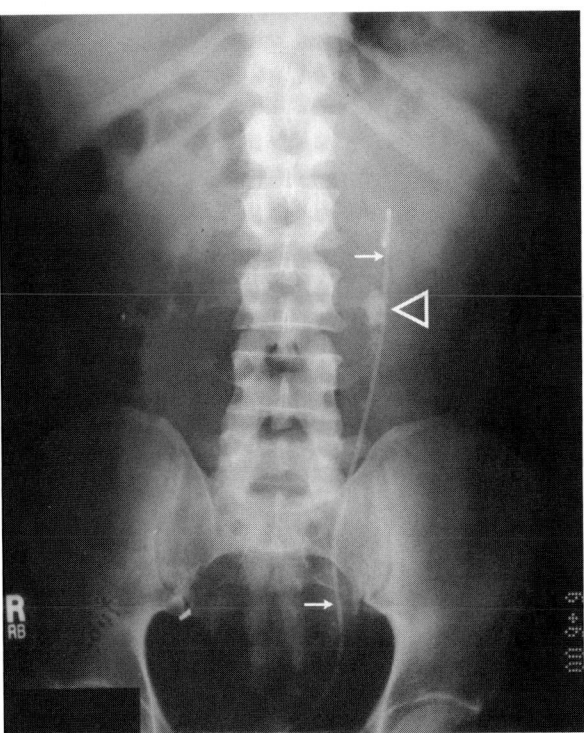

FIGURE 40-1. Plain film of abdomen. Calcifications are seen overlapping left ureter (*arrowhead*). *Small arrows* demonstrate a stent inserted into the kidney to relieve the obstruction.

for hydronephrosis,[163] it is safe and can be repeated frequently, it is low in cost, and lacks ionizing radiation, making it ideal for pregnant patients.[17] Moreover, because no contrast is involved, US is well suited to patients with an elevated or rising serum creatinine level[164, 165] to rule out obstruction as a cause of renal insufficiency, in patients allergic to contrast material, and in pediatric patients. Ultrasonography can determine the size and shape of the kidney, dilation of the pelvis and calices, and may demonstrate thinned cortex in case of severe long-standing hydronephrosis (Fig. 40-2).

Ultrasonography has both high sensitivity and specificity for detecting hydronephrosis, with the rates approaching 90%,[163, 166] even in azotemic patients,[166] when radiocontrast studies are contraindicated. Hydronephrosis will be seen as a dilated collecting system—an anechoic central area surrounded by echogenic parenchyma. The thickness of the renal parenchyma can be measured and may serve as an indirect indicator of the duration of obstruction.

However, in some cases of acute urinary obstruction, US may fail to detect pathology in the first 48 hours,[167] or when hydronephrosis is absent despite obstruction.[168] False-negative results are also possible in cases of dehydration, intrarenal pelvis, staghorn calculi, nephrocalcinosis,[166] retroperitoneal fibrosis,[169] and misinterpretation of caliectasis for cortical cysts.[170] A dilated collecting system without obstruction can be observed in up to 50% of patients with urinary diversion through ileal conduits.[171] Some investigators have developed special obstructive scoring systems (increased echogenicity, parenchymal rims ≤ 5 mm, contralateral hypertrophy, resistive index ratio ≥ 1.10, and so on) to differentiate between obstructing and nonobstructing

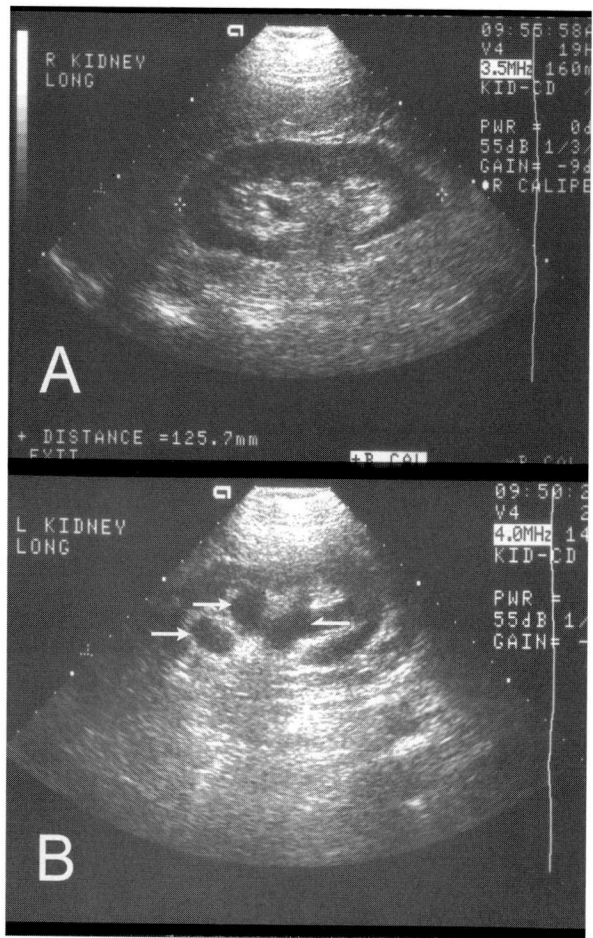

FIGURE 40-2. Renal ultrasound. **A**, Normal kidney. **B**, Hydronephrotic kidney: dilated calices and pelvis (*arrows*).

hydronephrosis on US.[172] False-positive conclusions may be the result of a large extrarenal pelvis, parapelvic cysts,[173] vesicoureteral reflux, or high urine flow rate.[166] In addition, US may only suggest, but not reveal, the presence, or cause of the obstruction.

In conclusion, although US is a useful screening test, it does not depict the functional condition of the kidney, and cannot completely rule out obstruction, especially when prior clinical suspicion is high. Therefore, the diagnosis of obstruction still needs to be considered in patients with worsening renal function, chronic azotemia, or acute changes in renal function or urine output, even in the absence of hydronephrosis on the US.[174]

Antenatal Ultrasonography

Prenatal diagnosis of renal pathology was first described in the 1970s.[175] After that, maternal ultrasonography resulted in a fourfold increase in antenatal detection of congenital urinary tract obstruction.[29] Prenatal hydronephrosis is diagnosed with an incidence of 1 in 100 to 1 in 500 maternal-fetal ultrasonographic studies.[176] Obstructive and nonobstructive processes can both cause dilation of the urinary tract. Obstructive causes include ureteropelvic junction (UPJ)

obstruction (44%), ureterovesical junction obstruction (21%), multicystic dysplastic kidney, ureterocele or ureteral ectopia, duplex kidney (12%), posterior urethral valves (PUVs, 9%), urethral atresia, sacrococcygeal teratoma, and hydrometrocolpos. Nonobstructive causes include vesicoureteral reflux (VUR, 14%), physiologic dilation, prune-belly syndrome, renal cystic disease, and megacalycosis.[177] Increased renal echogenicity and oligohydramnios in the setting of bladder distention are highly predictive (87%) of an obstructive etiology. This finding is important in the prenatal counseling and treatment of boys with bilateral hydronephrosis and marked bladder dilation.[178]

It is generally agreed that persistent postnatal renal abnormalities are present when the anteroposterior diameter of the fetal renal pelvis measures more than 6 mm at less than 20 weeks, more than 8 mm at 20 to 30 weeks, and more than 10 mm at more than 30 weeks of gestation.[179] The long-term morbidity of mild hydronephrosis (pelviectasis without caliceal dilation) is low. Moderate hydronephrosis (dilated pelvis and calices without parenchymal thinning) may be associated with gradual improvement in severity of dilation and drainage, without loss of relative renal function. Cases of severe hydronephrosis (pelvicaliceal dilation with parenchymal thinning) may require surgical intervention for declining renal function, infection, or symptoms. Overall, approximately 5% to 25% of patients with antenatal hydronephrosis will ultimately require surgical intervention.[176, 180] Therefore, long-term follow-up of these patients is required. Almost all patients with antenatal hydronephrosis will have postnatal ultrasonography performed in the first days of life, keeping in mind that most cases of the mild hydronephrosis will be resolved.[181] Functional imaging is required for patients with hydronephrosis. However, in the absence of bilateral hydronephrosis, a solitary kidney, or suspected posterior urethral valve, functional imaging can be deferred until the first 4 to 6 weeks of life.[176] Otherwise, nuclear medicine renal scans should be performed.

All infants with prenatally detected hydronephrosis that is confirmed with postnatal studies should be placed on antibiotic prophylaxis pending the outcome of further evaluation. An infection in the setting of ureteral obstruction can cause significant morbidity in the uroseptic infant, and renal damage is a potential comorbidity. Oral amoxicillin (10 mg/kg/day) is the most commonly used prophylactic antibiotic.[176]

Intravenous Urography

Intravenous urography (IVU; also known as intravenous pyelography, or IVP) is indicated when upper urinary tract obstruction is suggested by history, physical examination, or ultrasonographic findings, in patients with normal renal function, no allergies to contrast material, and not pregnant (Fig. 40-3). Urography may provide both functional and anatomic data, particularly of the ureter, and the location of the obstruction. Until recently it was considered to be the gold standard for imaging in acute renal colic,[182] though recent data have questioned the diagnostic efficacy of IVU.[183] The procedure has drawbacks. The nephrotoxicity of the contrast material may be significant, especially in high-risk patients such as those with diabetes and impaired renal function.[184, 185] Furthermore, kidneys may not be visualized in patients with low glomerular filtration rate (GFR)

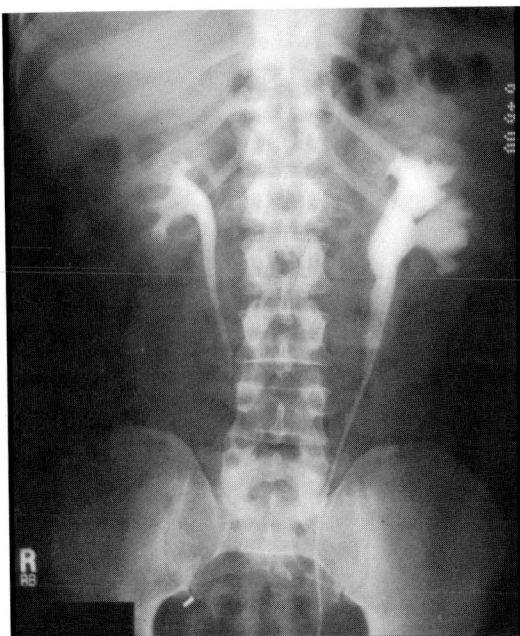

FIGURE 40-3. Intravenous pyelography. Normal right kidney and dilated collecting system on the left. The obstruction was relieved with a stent.

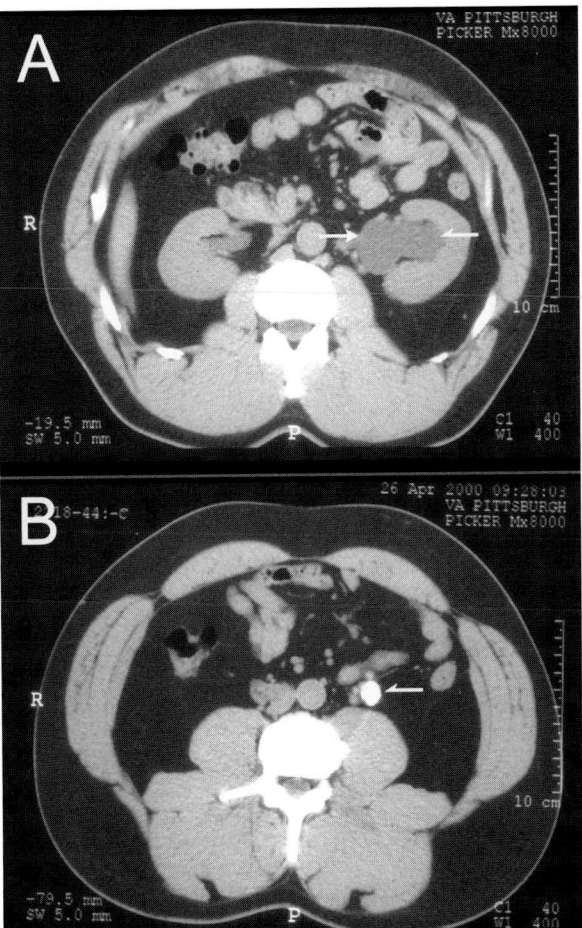

FIGURE 40-4. Computed tomography, noncontrast study. **A,** Left hydronephrosis: dilated renal pelvis (*arrows*), with normal kidney on right. **B,** Reason for obstruction: left midureteral stone (*arrow*).

because of delayed excretion of the contrast agent, or, in cases of severe obstruction, too little contrast material may be excreted on the affected side to allow adequate identification of the site of obstruction. All these concerns have led to replacement of IVU with CT, US, and MRI in many cases. Nevertheless, because it is readily available, well known to most physicians, capable of identifying the site of obstruction in a significant portion of cases (especially in cases of intraluminal noncalculous obstruction), and able to depict the anatomy of the urinary tract, IVU remains a useful and informative diagnostic tool.[186]

Computed Tomography

CT was used earlier, mainly in cases in which US or IVU had failed to identify obstruction.[187] CT has a particular advantage in that it can visualize a dilated collecting system, even without contrast enhancement. It can also be performed much more quickly than IVU, especially when renal impairment or obstruction would delay contrast excretion by the affected kidney in an IVU (Fig. 40-4). Non–contrast-enhanced CT is more effective than IVU in precisely identifying ureteral stones and as effective as IVU in determining the presence or absence of ureteral obstruction.[188, 189] CT can identify even radiolucent stones, because even uric acid stone density is at least 100 HU, which is higher than soft tissue density on CT (usually 10-70 HU). CT is especially good at identifying extrinsic causes of obstruction (e.g., retroperitoneal fibrosis, lymphadenopathy, hematoma). Helical CT is also an accurate and noninvasive method of demonstrating crossing vessels in UPJ obstruction.[190] CT can also detect extraurinary pathology and can establish nonurogenital causes of pain. All of these advantages establish non–contrast-enhanced helical CT as the diagnostic study of

choice for the evaluation of the patient with acute flank pain.[191] CT is very useful in delineating the pelvic organs (bladder, prostate, and so on) as well, and may demonstrate abnormalities such as an obstructed and distended bladder (Fig. 40-5), secondary to an enlarged prostate. US may be the first method of diagnosis in this setting (Fig. 40-6), but CT resolution and depiction of details are usually superior to US.

Isotopic Renography

Isotopic renography, or renal scintigraphy, can diagnose upper urinary tract obstruction while avoiding the risk of radiocontrast agents.[192, 193] Radioisotope is injected intravenously, and its excretion by the kidneys is followed using imaging with a gamma scintillation camera. Although this method gives a functional assessment of the obstructed kidney, anatomic definition is poor. Isotopic renography is typically used to estimate the fractional contribution of each kidney to overall renal function; it may help the urologist to decide whether to repair the obstruction to a kidney or resect it. In addition, the test can be repeated after the relief of obstruction to gauge the extent to which relief of the obstruction has restored renal function.

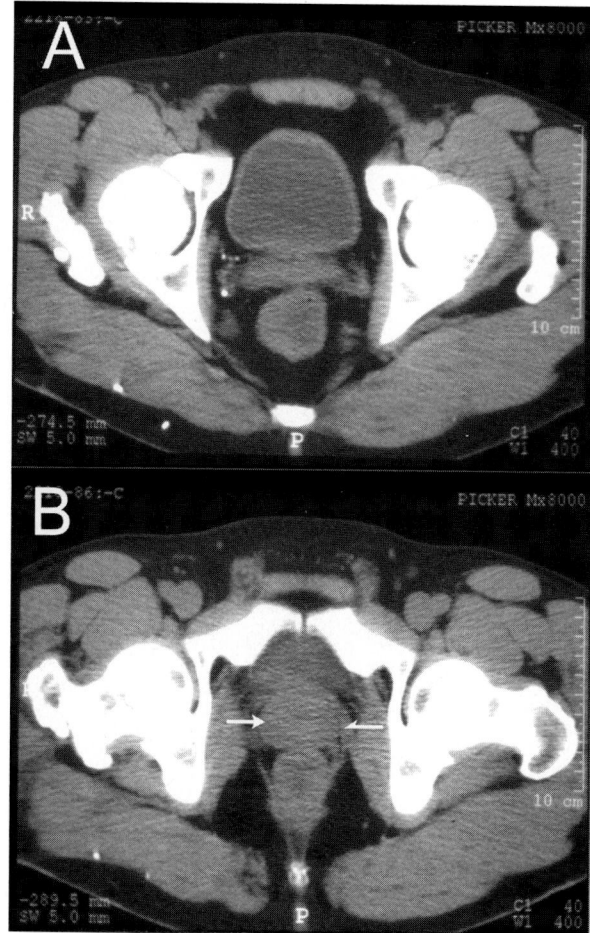

FIGURE 40-5. Computed tomography of the pelvis. **A**, Large postvoiding residual urine in the bladder. **B**, Enlarged prostate (*arrows*), leading to urinary retention.

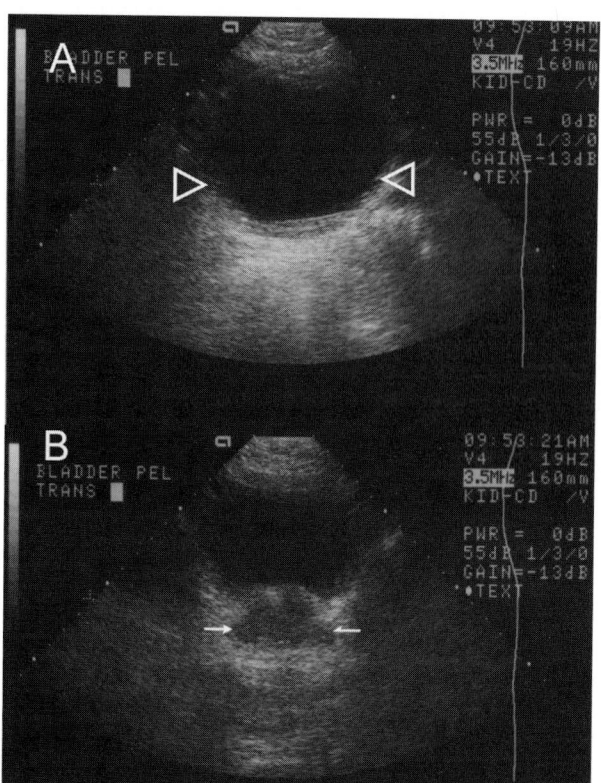

FIGURE 40-6. Pelvic ultrasound. **A**, Distended bladder (*arrowheads*). **B**, Enlarged prostate (*arrows*), causing infravesical urinary obstruction.

Diuretic renography was introduced into clinical practice in 1978,[194] and can be used to distinguish between dilation with obstruction and dilation without obstruction. Following administration of radioisotope, when the isotope appears in the renal pelvis, a loop diuretic such as furosemide is given intravenously. If stasis is causing the dilation, the induced diuresis results in prompt washout of the tracer from the renal pelvis. By contrast, when dilation is caused by obstruction, the washout does not occur.[195] Data can be interpreted visually or by quantitative measurement of the half-life ($t_{1/2}$) for the clearance of the tracer from the collecting system.[196] It is generally accepted that the clearance of the isotope from the collecting system with $t_{1/2}$ less than 15 minutes is normal, and a $t_{1/2}$ of more than 20 minutes usually depicts obstruction. Clearance of the tracer with a $t_{1/2}$ between 15 and 20 minutes is considered equivocal. An absent or blunted response to the diuretic resulting from decreased renal function makes interpretation of the test difficult and limits its usefulness.[197]

Magnetic Resonance Imaging

MRI can be used to explore the urinary tract when obstruction is suspected. Because MRI does not use ionizing radiation and because gadolinium contrast agents are essentially nonnephrotoxic, MRI is especially useful in children, women of childbearing age, and patients with renal insufficiency or renal allografts.[198, 199] It provides improved spatial resolution with avoidance of ionizing radiation and iodinated contrast agents,[200] and it is superior to IVU in detecting obstruction in the presence of severe renal failure. However, MRI today is not clearly superior to other imaging methods,[201] and provides no substantial diagnostic advantages in comparison to combined US and CT. In addition, it cannot demonstrate urinary calculi[200] and it is more expensive than other modalities.[101]

Whitaker Test

The Whitaker test, which involves measurement of pressures and flows, is the only direct clinical test of renal outflow resistance.[202] This approach has been considered to be the gold standard for the evaluation of upper urinary tract dilation.[101] It provides urodynamic evidence of a mechanical obstruction of the upper urinary tract at a given flow rate. The patient is placed in the prone position on the fluoroscopic table, with a catheter in the bladder. A cannula is inserted percutaneously into the renal pelvis, and connected to a pressure transducer. Pressure in the bladder is also monitored. A mixture of saline and contrast material is infused through the renal cannula at a rate of 10 mL/minute, and pressures are monitored. The presence of contrast material allows fluorographic monitoring of the procedure as well, to define the site of the possible obstruction.[203] The urinary tract is considered nonobstructed if renal pelvic pressure is less than 15 cm H_2O, equivocal at a pressure between 15 and 22 cm H_2O, and obstructed if pressure exceeds 22 cm H_2O.[204] With the advent of imaging techniques, and because of its invasiveness, pressure-flow studies are not often used today, and have been replaced to some degree by diuretic renography. However, in cases of extreme upper tract dilation or poor renal function, precluding the adequate diuretic response, the Whitaker test may be considered.

Retrograde and Antegrade Pyelography

When the tests described earlier do not provide adequate anatomic detail, or when obstruction must be promptly relieved (bilateral obstruction, obstruction of solitary kidney, symptomatic infection in the obstructed system), more invasive investigation, with a combination of treatments, may be necessary. Retrograde pyelography is performed by cystoscopically guided cannulation of the ureteral orifice and contrast injection.[205, 206] In cases of complete obstruction, contrast may not reach the kidney, but the procedure will help to define the lower level of the obstruction. Retrograde pyelography can be combined with placement of a ureteral stent to relieve an obstruction, or with possible stone extraction. The risk of introducing infection proximal to the obstruction must be kept in mind, and the obstruction should be relieved immediately after retrograde pyelography. Antegrade pyelography is performed by percutaneous cannulation of the kidney, and injection of the contrast material into the kidney and ureter.[205, 206] This procedure should establish the proximal level of obstruction, and may also serve as a first step in relieving obstruction by means of percutaneous nephrostomy (Figs. 40-7 and 40-8).

PATHOPHYSIOLOGY OF OBSTRUCTIVE NEPHROPATHY

Although acquired obstructive nephropathy in humans is usually partial and prolonged in its time course, most mechanistic studies of renal dysfunction in acquired obstruction use models of acute complete obstruction, usually for 24 hours. In these models, the extent of obstruction is clear and reproducible, and the results are not confounded by changes in renal structure brought on by inflammation or fibrosis. Complete obstruction of short duration strikingly alters renal blood flow, glomerular filtration, and tubular function, while producing minimal anatomic changes in blood vessels, glomeruli, and tubules.[2, 20]

Effects of Obstruction on Glomerular Filtration

Obstruction can profoundly alter many components of glomerular function. The extent of the disturbance depends on the severity and duration of the obstruction, whether it is unilateral or bilateral, and the extent to which the obstruction has been relieved or persists.[2, 20] In defining the effects of obstruction on glomerular filtration, we must review aspects of normal GFR. Whole-kidney GFR depends on the filtration rate of all functioning glomeruli and the proportion of glomeruli actually filtering. Single-nephron GFR (SNGFR) is determined by the blood flow in the glomerulus, the net ultrafiltration pressure across the glomerular capillary, and

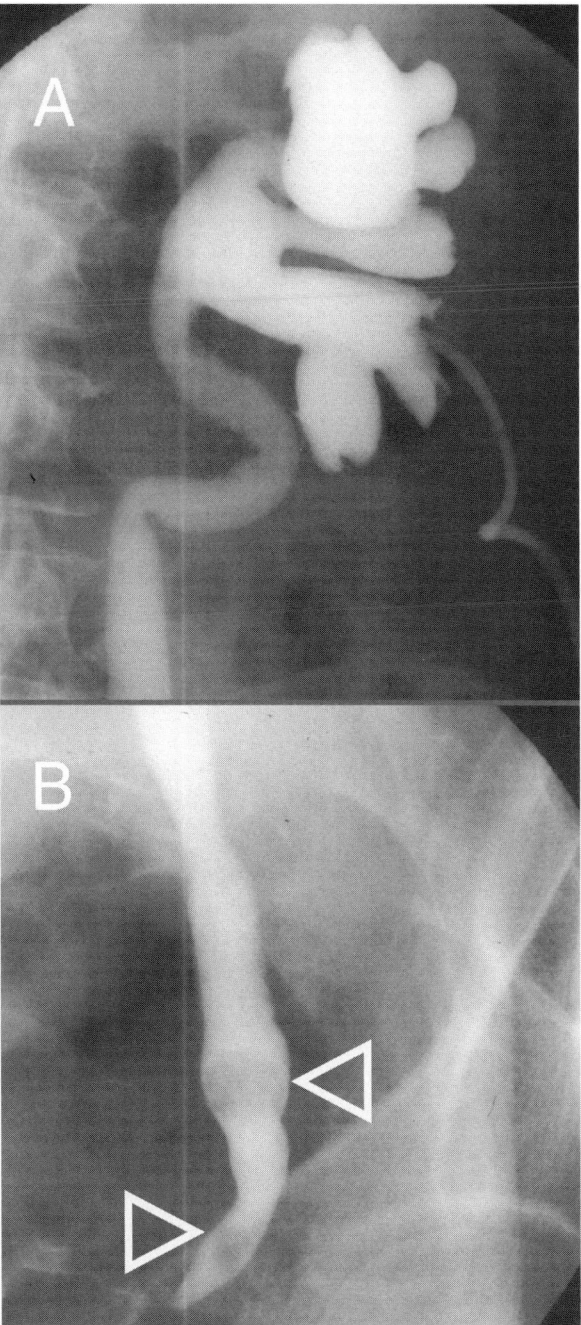

FIGURE 40-7. Antegrade pyelography. **A,** Dilated renal pelvis and calices on left. **B,** Stones (*arrowheads*) as filling defects in the distal ureter (not seen on plain film). Intravenous pyelography was unsuccessful owing to the obstructed and malfunctioning kidney.

the ultrafiltration coefficient (K_f). Glomerular blood flow and the hydraulic pressure in the glomerular capillary (P_{GC}) are determined by the resistances of the afferent (R_A) and efferent (R_E) arterioles. Net ultrafiltration pressure is determined by P_{GC}, the hydraulic pressure of the Bowman space (which equals the proximal tubule hydraulic pressure, P_T), and the differences in oncotic pressure between the glomerular capillary and Bowman space. K_f is determined by the permeability properties of the filtering surface and the surface area available for filtration. Obstruction can alter one or all of the determinants of glomerular filtration.

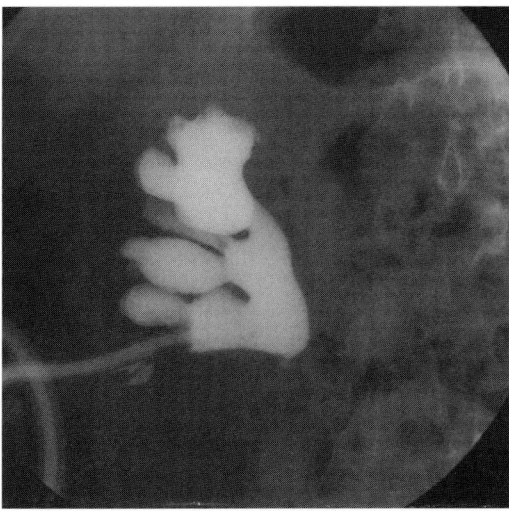

FIGURE 40-8. Antegrade pyelography. No contrast is entering the ureter because of the obstructed and dilated right renal pelvis (the patient has retroperitoneal fibrosis).

The Early, Hyperemic Phase

In the immediate 2 to 3 hours following the onset of unilateral ureteral obstruction, the blockage of antegrade urine flow markedly increased P_T. This increase in pressure in the Bowman space would be expected to halt GFR immediately.[207-209] However, during this early phase of obstruction, the afferent arterioles dilate, decreasing R_A, increasing P_{GC}, and counteracting the increase in P_T.[207, 208] Because this vasodilator or "hyperemic response" occurs in denervated kidneys in situ and in isolated perfused kidneys,[210, 211] it must result from intrarenal mechanisms. In fact, glomeruli of individual nephrons exhibit the same response when antegrade urine flow is blocked by placement of a wax block in the tubule of the nephron.[212]

Many mechanisms have been proposed for this afferent vasodilation, including increases in vasodilator hormones such as prostaglandins, regulation by the macula densa, and a direct myogenic reflex.[31] This hyperemic response is not attenuated by renal nerve stimulation or infusion of catecholamines.[213] Efforts have been made to link this response to changes in interstitial pressure.[210, 214]

Because obstruction reduces urine flow past the macula densa, this structure induces afferent vasodilation, as occurs during tubuloglomerular feedback responses,[212] when reduced distal tubular flow past the macula densa induces falls in R_A and increased P_{GC}, so that SNGFR rises. However, micropuncture studies have shown that the obstruction to flow along the tubule itself is critical to afferent vasodilation. In these studies, flow past the macula densa was blocked, but P_T was maintained at normal levels by an additional puncture of the tubule proximal to the blockage of flow to the macula densa.[208] In such nephrons the increase in P_{GC} observed in obstructed tubules did not occur, indicating that the obstruction itself and not the macula densa stimulates afferent vasodilation.[208]

Because the hyperemic response to obstruction can be blocked by indomethacin, it appears likely that vasodilator prostaglandins are critical to afferent vasodilation.[209, 215, 216] However, in bilateral obstruction, the afferent vasodilation

response is absent or markedly attenuated.[2, 20, 214] There is evidence that renal nerve activity explains the absence of the hyperemic response in bilateral ureteral obstruction. Obstruction of the left kidney has been shown to augment afferent renal nerve activity from the left kidney and efferent nerve activity to the right kidney. The increase in efferent nerve activity to the right kidney was accompanied by reduced blood flow to that kidney. This vasoconstrictor response was ablated by denervation of either the left or right kidney before induction of left ureteral obstruction. These results suggest that, in the setting of bilateral ureteral obstruction, increased afferent renal nerve traffic triggers vasoconstrictive renorenal reflex activity that counteracts the early intrinsic renal vasodilator effects of obstruction.[214]

The Late, Vasoconstrictive Phase

Once obstruction is well established, glomerular filtration ceases. Therefore, efforts to study the regulation of SNGFR later in obstruction have measured determinants of GFR immediately after release of obstruction.[2, 217] Using this approach, investigators have shown that after 3 hours of unilateral obstruction, and through 12 to 24 hours of obstruction, renal blood flow progressively declines.[218-220] Interestingly, after an initial rise in tubular pressures, these also decline, so that by 24 hours renal plasma flow, GFR, and intratubular pressures have all dropped below normal values.[207, 209, 219-222] At this point, examination of regional blood flow in the kidney by injections of silicone rubber reveal large areas of the cortical vascular bed that are not perfused or are underperfused.[2, 209, 219, 220, 223] Depending on the species, the different vascular beds in the outer and juxtamedullary cortex receive differing proportions of the renal blood flow. On this basis, reduced whole-kidney GFR at this stage of obstruction is due, in large part, to nonperfusion of many glomeruli.

At this stage of obstruction, SNGFR is also decreased markedly, because of afferent vasoconstriction, which, in turn, reduces P_{GC}.[221, 224] Importantly, P_{GC} responds in the same manner when the individual nephron is blocked with oil for 24 hours before micropuncture measurements are performed.[225] These results indicate that, like the early hyperemic response, the late vasoconstrictive response to obstruction is due primarily to intrarenal mechanisms. In the setting of bilateral obstruction, renal blood flow is reduced to 30% to 60% below normal.[221, 224, 226] (Table 40-3). Although SNGFR falls to a similar degree in unilateral and bilateral

TABLE 40-3

Glomerular Hemodynamics in Ureteral Obstruction*

STAGE OF OBSTRUCTION	P_T	R_A	P_{GC}	SNGFR
1-2 hr unilateral	↑↑	↓	↑	=
24 hr unilateral	=	↑↑	↓	↓↓
24 hr bilateral	↑↑	=	=	↓↓
After release: 24 hr unilateral	↓	↑↑	↓↓	↓↓
After release: 24 hr bilateral	=	↑↑	↓	↓↓

*See text for discussion and references. P_T, proximal tubule hydraulic pressure; R_A, afferent arteriole resistance; P_{GC}, hydraulic pressure of Bowman space; =, unchanged; ↑, increased; ↑↑, markedly increased; ↓, reduced; ↓↓, markedly reduced.

obstruction, the mechanisms involved are different in the two conditions. In unilateral obstruction, reduced P_{GC} lowers the driving pressure for filtration when set against a nearly normal P_T. However, in bilateral obstruction, P_{GC} remains normal and GFR is reduced by a highly elevated P_T.[221] These results suggest that systemic factors, such as accumulation of extracellular fluid volume and urea, renal nerve activity, and increases in natriuretic substances, modulate the vasoconstrictive effect of obstruction on the affected kidney.[226]

Regulation of the Glomerular Filtration Rate in the Postobstructive Period

The extent of reductions in renal blood flow and GFR after release of obstruction varies with the species studied and the duration of obstruction.[209, 220, 227, 228] After release of 24 hours of unilateral obstruction the GFR remains below 50% of normal in dogs and 25% of normal in rats; renal blood flow remains markedly reduced in both species.[2] After release of bilateral ureteral obstruction, renal blood flow reaches levels higher than that observed following unilateral obstruction, but the GFR remains markedly attenuated. Reduction in whole-kidney GFR results from nonperfusion or underperfusion of many glomeruli, as shown in silicone rubber injections.[209, 219, 220] In nephrons with perfused glomeruli, the fall in P_T that accompanies release of obstruction is matched by a similar drop in P_{GC} so that the driving force for glomerular filtration remains low.[221, 224] The drop in P_{GC} results from intense afferent vasoconstriction at this point following release of both unilateral and bilateral obstruction. In addition, a sharp reduction in K_f also augments the fall in GFR at this point following release of unilateral and bilateral obstruction.[221, 224, 229]

Several mechanisms contribute to afferent vasoconstriction and a reduced K_f. First, release of obstruction strikingly augments the flow of tubular fluid past the macula densa. Although the absolute rate of flow is still far below normal, the macula densa likely senses the dramatic *change* in the rate of flow, and this may lead to vigorous vasoconstriction.[2] In favor of this view, the sensitivity of the tubuloglomerular feedback mechanism is enhanced in unilateral, but not bilateral, obstruction, suggesting that the ability of the mechanism to regulate afferent arteriolar tone is modulated by the extrarenal hormonal milieu.[230]

It is also likely that angiotensin II participates actively in afferent vasoconstriction and reduced K_f following release of ureteral obstruction. Ureteral obstruction promptly increases renal vein renin levels at a time when renal blood flow is normal or elevated,[231-233] but at later time points, renal vein renin levels return to normal.[231-233] In addition, infusion of captopril reduced the declines in renal blood flow and GFR observed in both unilateral and bilateral obstruction.[229, 231, 234, 235] Because inhibition of angiotensin-converting enzyme can also increase kinin activity, these experiments were repeated during infusions of either carboxypeptidase B, which destroys kinins, or aproninin, which blocks kinin generation. Captopril remained equally effective in the presence of either agent, indicating that captopril acted to reduce R_A by blocking generation of angiotensin II. Although K_f was not measured in these studies, it appears likely that increased angiotensin II may also help decrease K_f following release of obstruction.[229]

Several lines of evidence indicate that thromboxane A_2 (TXA_2) may also play a major role in postobstructive vasoconstriction.[231, 236] Early studies in chronically hydronephrotic kidneys showed an increase in TXA_2 (measured by accumulation of its more stable metabolite, TXB_2) accumulation.[236] Administration of thromboxane synthase inhibitors into the renal artery (but not systemically[237]) under conditions shown to reduce renal TXA_2 generation[238] ameliorated the vasoconstrictive effects of release of obstruction; both whole-kidney GFR and renal blood flow were increased.[231, 234, 238, 239] Glomerular micropuncture following relief of obstruction showed that a thromboxane synthase inhibitor reduced R_A and increased K_f.[229] On the basis of these results, it appears that TXA_2 is generated in the kidney following release of obstruction and mediates afferent vasoconstriction and reductions in K_f. However, the source of the TXA_2 is unclear.

In some,[240] but not all[241, 242] cases, glomeruli isolated from obstructed kidneys have shown increased ability to synthesize TXA_2. Although such increases could reduce K_f, the afferent arteriole is upstream of the glomerulus, and unlikely to respond to glomerular thromboxane generation. Further studies have implicated inflammatory cells. During the first 24 hours of obstruction, macrophages and suppressor T cells migrate to the renal cortex and medulla, reaching levels 15-fold higher than basal level.[243] Release of obstruction leads to a gradual decline in these leukocyte populations in the kidney. The appearance of these cells parallels the increase in TXA_2 release and the fall in GFR observed in obstruction.[243] Moreover, renal irradiation in the setting of obstruction reduces leukocyte accumulation and urinary TXB_2 excretion (an index of renal TXA_2 generation), and increases GFR above levels seen with obstruction alone. These results indicate that obstruction stimulates immigration of inflammatory leukocytes which, in turn, generate vasoconstrictors such as TXA_2.[243, 244] These vasoconstrictors appear to contribute to the increased R_A and decreased GFR observed following release of obstruction.

Because irradiation only partially blocked the decrease in GFR, it is likely that renal cells themselves release important mediators. Indeed, glomeruli isolated from obstructed kidneys showed increased eicosanoid synthesis after angiotensin II stimulation.[245] In addition, treatment of obstructed animals with converting enzyme inhibitors enhanced GFR and reduced TXA_2 generation by glomeruli isolated from these animals.[246]

Because vasoconstriction is less severe in animals with bilateral ureteral obstruction, it is likely that extrarenal factors play a major role in modulating the hemodynamic response of the kidney to obstruction and release of obstruction. We have already mentioned the renorenal reflexes stimulated in bilateral obstruction reduce the compensatory vasodilator response normally observed in the early stages of unilateral obstruction. Multiple additional factors, including accumulation of volume and solutes such as urea, atrial natriuretic peptide (ANP) and its congeners, and other natriuretic substances may ameliorate the vasoconstrictive effects of obstruction when both ureters are ligated. Following 24 hours of obstruction, GFR is preserved to some degree if the contralateral kidney is also obstructed or removed.[247] In addition, in animals following release of 24 hours of unilateral obstruction, if the urea, salt, and water content of the urine from the contralateral kidney is reinfused into the animal, a striking increase in GFR over standard unilateral obstruction is observed.[247, 248] On the basis of these and other studies, it appears that urea and other excreted urine solutes have a protective effect, and can ameliorate vasoconstriction following release of ureteral obstruction.[247, 248]

It is also likely that ANP reduces the vasoconstrictive effects of release of obstruction. Animals and humans with bilateral obstruction undergo volume expansion, which stimulates ANP release.[249] Enhanced release and reduced ANP degradation in obstructed kidneys lead to marked increases in circulating levels of ANP.[249] In line with this view, ANP levels have been shown to rise markedly in bilateral, but not unilateral, obstruction.[234, 249] In the basal state, ANP at high levels augments renal blood flow and GFR by direct vasodilation of afferent arterioles, constriction of efferent arterioles, and an increase in K_f.[249] In addition, ANP antagonizes release of renin by the macula densa, lowering levels of angiotensin II. On this basis, it is not surprising that infusions of ANP can enhance GFR in the setting of unilateral or bilateral ureteral obstruction.[234, 250]

Prostaglandin E_2 (PGE_2) and nitric oxide may also reduce vasoconstriction in obstruction. Renal PGE_2 levels increase markedly in obstruction (see later) and in states of extracellular volume expansion, as occurs in bilateral ureteral obstruction. Given the vasodilator effects of PGE_2, it appears likely that increased levels could ameliorate falls in GFR in obstruction. Bilateral obstruction may reduce generation of NO, leading to a net vasoconstrictive effect.[245]

In summary, both intra- and extrarenal factors combine to profoundly decrease GFR during and immediately after release of obstruction. The decrease in GFR is caused by a sharp reduction in the number of perfused glomeruli and by a reduction in the SNGFR of functioning nephrons. Decreased K_f and increased R_A reduce SNGFR. Increases in various vasoconstrictors, such as angiotensin II and TXA_2, as well as other vasoconstrictors, some coming from inflammatory cells, augment these hemodynamic effects. In the setting of bilateral obstruction, retention of urea and other solutes, as well as volume expansion and increases in circulating levels of vasodilators such as ANP, help to offset these vasoconstrictive effects, but only partially.

Recovery of Glomerular Function after Relief of Obstruction

The extent of recovery of glomerular filtration following release of obstruction depends on several factors, including the duration and extent of obstruction, the presence or absence of a functioning contralateral kidney, the presence or absence of associated infection, and the level of preobstruction renal blood flow.[227] In dogs subjected to a 1-week period of complete unilateral ureteral obstruction, GFR fell to 25% of normal on release of the obstruction and recovered gradually to 50% of normal levels 2 years later.[251] In rats, release of unilateral ureteral obstruction of 7 and 14 days' duration left residual GFR at 17% and 9% of control levels, respectively, when the contralateral kidney was left in place, and 31% and 14% when the animals underwent contralateral nephrectomy at the time of release of the obstruction.[222] A similar beneficial effect on the obstructed kidney of contralateral nephrectomy was observed in rats subjected to chronic partial obstruction.[222] As discussed

earlier, this beneficial effect likely results from the accumulation of urea and other solutes and increased levels of ANP when the functioning contralateral kidney is absent.

The partial recovery of total renal GFR following release of obstruction masks a very uneven distribution of blood flow and nephron function. In micropuncture studies, some nephrons never regain filtration function, whereas others reveal striking hyperfiltration.[227] It appeared in some studies that surface nephrons exhibited normal SNGFR, whereas the whole-kidney GFR was reduced to 18% of normal.[252] These results suggest that chronic partial obstruction causes selective damage to juxtamedullary and deep cortical nephrons.[219, 227, 252] Similarly, studies of the long-term outcome of complete 24-hour ureteral obstruction revealed that total renal GFR recovered to normal levels by 14 and 60 days after release of obstruction. However, 15% of the glomeruli were not filtering in recovered kidneys, and other nephrons were hyperfiltering. In this model of complete obstruction, there appeared to be no selective advantage for surface glomeruli over deep cortical and juxtamedullary glomeruli.[227]

Effects of Obstruction on Tubule Function

Obstruction severely impairs the ability of renal tubules to transport Na^+, K^+, and H^+, and reduces their ability to concentrate and dilute the urine (Table 40-4).[2, 253] The resulting inability to reabsorb water and solutes helps cause postobstructive diuresis and natriuresis. As is the case with glomerular filtration, the extent of disruption of tubular transport depends directly on the duration and severity of the obstruction. Pathologically, prolonged obstruction leads to profound tubular atrophy and chronic interstitial inflammatory changes, whereas at early time points following the onset of obstruction, such as at 24 hours, there are only slight structural and ultrastructural changes.[254, 255] These changes include some mitochondrial swelling, modest blunting of basolateral interdigitations in the thick ascending limb and proximal tubule epithelial cells, as well as flattening of the epithelium and some widening of the intercellular spaces in the collecting ducts.[254, 255] The only cell death at early time points is observed at the very tip of the papilla, where focal necrosis may be observed.[254] Because there is so little cell damage, and because of the simplicity of the model, most investigators have examined the effect of 24 hours of complete ureteral obstruction on tubular function. As with glomerular filtration, impairment of tubular transport in obstruction is due both to direct damage to tubular epithelial cells and the action of extratubular hormones, arising both from the kidney and extrarenal sources.

Effects of Obstruction on Tubular Sodium Reabsorption

Following release of unilateral ureteral obstruction of 24 hours' duration, volume excretion from the postobstructed kidney is normal to slightly increased[2, 226, 247, 256] (see Table 40-4). However, as noted earlier, this normal level of volume excretion occurs in the setting of a markedly impaired (20% of normal) GFR. On this basis the fractional excretion of sodium FE_{Na} is markedly elevated in the postobstructed kidney. With bilateral obstruction, salt and water excretion is markedly elevated, up to five to nine times normal.[2, 226, 257, 258] In this setting, GFR is also decreased, so that FE_{Na} may be 20-fold higher than normal.

The micropuncture studies described in Table 40-4 demonstrate that the reabsorption defect following release of obstructive nephropathy is localized similarly in both unilateral and bilateral ureteral obstruction. In superficial nephrons,

TABLE 40-4

Segmental Reabsorption in Superficial and Juxtamedullary Nephrons and in Collecting Ducts in Normal Rats after Release of Bilateral or Unilateral Obstruction

SITE	WATER REMAINING (%)	Na⁺ REMAINING (%)
Normal		
S_1	100	100
S_2	44	44
S_3	26	14
S_4	9.4	5
J_1	100	100
J_2	12	40
CD_1	3.3	2
CD_2	0.4	0.6
After Bilateral Obstruction		
S_1	100	100
S_2	45	45
S_3	40	22
S_4	25	7
J_1	100	100
J_2	42	62
CD_1	8	6
CD_2	16.7	12
After Unilateral Obstruction		
S_1	100	100
S_2	26	26
S_3	21	12
S_4	3.2	1.9
J_1	100	100
J_2	42	52
CD_1	4.2	3.8
CD_2	2.9	2.5

S_{1-4}, values found in superficial nephrons: S_1, Bowman space; S_2, end of proximal convoluted tubule; S_3, earliest portion of distal tubule; S_4, end of distal tubule/beginning of collecting duct. J_{1-2}, values found in juxtamedullary nephrons; J_1, Bowman space; J_2, tip of loop of Henle. CD_1, collecting duct at base of papilla, first accessible portion of inner medullary collecting duct; CD_2, end of collecting duct as it opens into renal pelvis.

proximal tubule reabsorption is normal to enhanced in the S1 and S2 segments. By contrast, in juxtamedullary nephrons, increased proportions of filtered salt and water delivered to the loop of Henle (J_1 and J_2 in Table 40-4) reveal decreased reabsorption. Delivery of salt and water to the first accessible portion of the inner medullary collecting duct, labeled CD_1, was also increased, and net salt and water reabsorption along the inner medullary collecting duct (between CD_1 and CD_2) was diminished in both bilateral and unilateral obstruction. In fact, in bilateral obstruction, there was net addition or secretion of salt and water into the lumen of the inner medullary collecting duct.[257] On the basis of these results, it appears that net salt and water reabsorption was diminished in the medullary thick ascending limb (MTAL), the distal convoluted tubule, and the entire length of the collecting duct, including its cortical, outer medullary, and inner medullary segments.

These studies in whole animals have been confirmed and extended by a series of studies from multiple laboratories using isolated perfused tubule and cell suspension preparations (Table 40-5). Isolated perfused superficial proximal convoluted tubules (SPCTs) taken from animals with unilateral or bilateral obstruction exhibited normal volume reabsorption (J_V).[259] By contrast, J_V in proximal straight tubules, which are derived from juxtamedullary nephrons, was markedly impaired in both forms of obstruction.[259] To determine the rate of MTAL volume reabsorption, the ability of the isolated tubules to reabsorb Cl^- from the lumen was measured (ΔC^-). As shown in Table 40-5, MTAL isolated from unilaterally and bilaterally obstructed animals exhibited similar profound impairment of reabsorptive capacity.[259] This interpretation was confirmed in studies of freshly prepared suspensions of MTAL cells from obstructed kidneys, in which transport-dependent oxygen consumption, which denotes salt reabsorptive capacity, was markedly reduced.[260]

Measurements of collecting duct salt reabsorption relied on determining the rate of removal of isotopic sodium from the lumen of perfused cortical collecting ducts. As shown in Table 40-5, in unilateral obstruction this rate was markedly reduced.[259] In addition, another indicator of transport capacity, the transepithelial voltage, was also reduced in both unilateral and bilateral obstruction.[261] Because the function of the collecting duct is markedly dependent on the mineralocorticoid state of the animal, it is important to note that these decreases in collecting duct reabsorptive capacity occurred in tubules taken from obstructed kidneys, whether or not the animal had been pretreated with mineralocorticoid.[259, 261, 262]

TABLE 40-5

Function of Isolated Perfused Tubules in Obstructive Nephropathy

	J_V SPCT (nL/mm/minute)	J_V PST (nL/mm/minute)	ΔCl^- MTAL (mEq/L)	$^{22}Na^+$ FLUX (pmol/mm/minute)	J_V CCT (+ ADH) (nL/mm/minute)
Control	0.75 ± 0.08	0.25 ± 0.02	-37 ± 3	38.2 ± 4.0	0.90 ± 0.08
Unilateral obstruction	0.73 ± 0.11	0.12 ± 0.03	-9 ± 1	26.2 ± 3.3	0.22 ± 0.04
Bilateral obstruction	0.80 ± 0.08	0.16 ± 0.02	-10 ± 1		0.23 ± 0.04

J_V, volume reabsorption; SPCT, superficial proximal convoluted tubule; PST, proximal straight tubule; ΔCl^-, change in Cl^- concentration; MTAL, medullary thick ascending limb; CCT, cortical collecting tubule; ADH, antidiuretic hormone.
Data from references 259, 260, 262.

Because it is highly branched and difficult to perfuse in vitro, transport in the inner medullary collecting duct has been studied in cell suspensions. In these preparations, transport-dependent oxygen consumption was markedly reduced in cells isolated from animals with bilateral obstruction.[263]

Taken together, the data derived from in vivo micropuncture and in vitro tubule perfusion and cell suspension studies reveal a striking impairment of volume reabsorption in the proximal straight tubule, the MTAL, and the entire collecting duct. As these functional derangements occur in the absence of clear-cut ultrastructural damage, it appears that obstruction induces a selective lesion in the cellular mechanisms of active transport. Because the lesion appears similar in both unilateral and bilateral obstruction,[259, 262] a major component of impaired active transport is likely due to direct tubular cell injury, rather than to the continuous action of natriuretic substances. Of course, the apparent secretion of salt and water in the inner medullary collecting duct of animals following release of bilateral obstruction (see Table 40-4) may be due to the overlay of natriuretic substances on a baseline of impaired tubular salt reabsorption (see later).

Using cell suspensions it is possible to begin to identify the mechanisms by which tubular epithelial cells exhibit impaired salt reabsorption in the setting of obstruction. Active Na^+ transport in tubule epithelia requires an apical entry step (e.g., $Na^+/K^+/2Cl^-$ cotransporter in MTAL or epithelial Na^+ channels [ENaCs] in the collecting duct) coupled to the basolateral Na^+, K^+-ATPase. In addition, the cell must generate sufficient adenosine triphosphate (ATP) to fuel active transport by the ATPase. In suspensions of MTAL cells from obstructed kidneys, furosemide-sensitive oxygen consumption was markedly reduced,[260] indicating reduced activity of the apical $Na^+/K^+/2Cl^-$ cotransporter in these cells. Quantification of the amount of cotransporter protein with isotopic bumetanide binding revealed a marked reduction in the number of membrane binding sites, with no change in affinity of binding, suggesting that obstruction down-regulates the expression of the cotransporter protein on the membrane surface.[260] More recent studies using specific antibodies to the cotransporter have confirmed that obstruction diminishes expression of the cotransporter protein on the apical surface of MTAL cells.[264] To determine whether obstruction down-regulated the activity of the Na^+, K^+-ATPase as well, ouabain-sensitive oxygen consumption was measured, and was also found to be markedly diminished. Measurement of ouabain-sensitive ATPase in the suspensions revealed marked reductions in activity in cells from obstructed kidneys, a finding explained by reduced expression of both α- and β-subunits in the preparations from obstructed kidneys.[260] Examination of messenger RNA (mRNA) levels revealed that the down-regulation of pump subunits in obstruction was due to both transcriptional and post-transcriptional mechanisms.[265]

Results in inner medullary collecting duct cell suspensions closely paralleled those in the MTAL. Suspensions from obstructed animals revealed marked decreases in amiloride-sensitive oxygen consumption and in the rate of entry of isotopic sodium in hyperpolarized cells.[263] These results were in concert with the prior finding of decreased apical membrane conductance in tubules from obstructed, as compared with control animals.[261] These results demonstrated a striking down-regulation of Na^+ channel of ENaC activity.

More recent studies with specific antisera against ENaC subunits have revealed reduced expression of ENaC proteins on the apical membranes of collecting duct cells in obstructed animals.

As occurred in MTAL cells, the rates of ouabain-sensitive oxygen consumption and of ouabain-sensitive ATPase were markedly diminished in inner medullary collecting duct cells from obstructed animals, and the levels of both pump subunits were also reduced in these preparations.[263] Patterns of mRNA expression were also similar to those in MTAL, indicating transcriptional and post-transcriptional down-regulation of pump subunit expression.

With the availability of specific antisera directed against Na^+ transporter proteins, recent studies have extended the results in thick ascending limb and inner medullary collecting duct to the proximal tubule and distal convoluted tubule. In unilateral ureteral obstruction, the overall synthesis and apical localization of the apical Na^+/H^+ exchanger (NHE_3) and the Na^+/PO_4^{3-} exchanger (NaPi-2) were strikingly decreased in the proximal tubule.[264] It appears that these decreases occurred in both the proximal convoluted and proximal straight tubule, even though the micropuncture and tubule perfusion studies cited earlier revealed preserved proximal convoluted tubule salt reabsorption and inhibition of proximal straight tubule reabsorption.[264] The same study demonstrated significant down-regulation of total transporter protein and apical membrane expression of the distal tubule Na^+/Cl^- cotransporter, indicating that obstruction likely reduces convoluted tubule Na^+ reabsorption by mechanisms similar to those observed in the thick ascending limb and collecting duct.[264]

Taken together, these results suggest a generalized down-regulation of transporter activities in tubule epithelial cells subjected to obstruction. Interestingly, metabolic studies have shown that obstruction reduces activities as well of several enzymes of the oxidative and glycolytic pathways, findings that suggest down-regulation of metabolic capacity for energy generation in these cells. It is also notable that these changes in metabolic capacity are reflected in the MTAL in reductions in the extent of basolateral infolding and in the density of mitochondria in tubules of obstructed kidneys.[254] Studies in the MTAL and collecting duct cell suspensions from obstructed kidneys, however, demonstrate decreases in transport-dependent but not transport-independent oxygen consumption, indicating that the rate of ATP generation (oxygen consumption) is not rate-limiting for active transport in these cells.[260, 263] On this basis, it appears more likely that metabolic machinery (as reflected in enzyme activities, basolateral infolding, and mitochondrial density) is down-regulated in response to a decrease in active transport.

The signals involved in down-regulation by obstruction of transporter activity and expression in tubular epithelial cells remain unclear. Possible signals include the halting of urine flow, changes in blood flow to the tubules or in interstitial pressure, and generation of natriuretic substances in the kidney that result in long-term inhibition of transporter function.

Obstruction causes cessation or near cessation of urine flow. With the halting of urine flow, sodium delivery to each tubular segment stops, and apical membrane Na^+ entry slows dramatically because the electrochemical gradients for Na^+ entry between the stationary apical fluid and the cell interior become increasingly unfavorable. The reduction in

Na$^+$ entry might then serve as the signal for down-regulation of transporter activity or expression. In both MTAL and inner medullary collecting duct cells, reduction of Na$^+$ entry by furosemide or amiloride, respectively, promptly reduces ouabain-sensitive oxygen consumption,[260, 266-268] indicating down-regulation of Na$^+$, K$^+$-ATPase. In addition, in mineralocorticoid-clamped animals, chronic inhibition of Na$^+$ entry at the MTAL or cortical collecting duct by administration of furosemide or amiloride, respectively, reduced the levels of ouabain-sensitive ATPase in microdissected tubule segments.[269, 270]

These results suggest that halting urine flow might represent a major signaling mechanism by which obstruction down-regulates Na$^+$ transport.[267] To test this idea, apical Na$^+$ entry was inhibited for 24 hours in a cell line that mimics cortical collecting duct cells, A6 cells, grown on permeable supports. Blockade of apical Na$^+$ entry, achieved either the substitution of another cation for Na$^+$ in the apical solution, or apical application of amiloride, resulted in striking down-regulation of apical Na$^+$ entry for some hours after the blockade was removed.[271] Recent studies have shown that this down-regulation is accompanied by selective reduction in the levels of expression of the β-, but not the α- or γ-subunits of ENaC in the apical membranes of the A6 cells. In addition, total cell synthesis of both pump subunits was down-regulated, although basolateral membrane expression appeared to be normal.[272] These results provide direct evidence that reductions in the rate of Na$^+$ entry, which may occur when urine flow is blocked, can directly down-regulate Na$^+$ transport in renal epithelial cells. The discordant regulation of the different subunits of the ENaC observed in this model may provide some insights into the mechanisms of channel regulation.

In addition to the direct effects of halting urine flow, changes in intrarenal hormones also play a major role in the reduction of salt transport observed with obstruction. It has been shown repeatedly that obstruction markedly accelerates the already-rapid generation of PGE$_2$ in the renal medulla.[236, 238, 241, 273, 274] Studies in isolated perfused tubules and in cell suspensions have shown that PGE$_2$ inhibits Na$^+$ reabsorption rapidly in the MTAL, as well as in the cortical and inner medullary collecting ducts, and that a major component of the inhibition occurs at the Na$^+$, K$^+$-ATPase.[275-280] PGE$_2$ has been shown to reduce trafficking of Na$^+$, K$^+$-ATPase to the plasma membrane,[281] and chronic blockade of cyclooxygenase with indomethacin increases pump activity,[282] indicating that, by several mechanisms, PGE$_2$ can regulate the activity and expression of the sodium pump. On the basis of these results, it is likely that obstruction reduces sodium pump activity in tubular epithelia by increasing renal levels of PGE$_2$.

As discussed earlier, obstruction induces a monocellular infiltrate in the kidney[243]; this infiltrate tends to follow a peritubular distribution.[243] When obstructed kidneys were irradiated, the level of medullary inflammation was diminished, and there was a modest decrease in the fractional excretion of sodium.[244]

In summary, obstruction reduces net reabsorption of salt in several nephron segments, including the proximal straight tubule, the MTAL, and the cortical and inner medullary collecting ducts, by down-regulating the expression and activities of specific transporter proteins. Several signals mediate this down-regulation, including the cessation of urine flow

with its attendant reduction of the rate of Na$^+$ entry across the apical membrane, increased levels of natriuretic substances such as PGE$_2$, and infiltration of the obstructed kidney by mononuclear cells.

When both ureters are obstructed, extrarenal factors markedly enhance the tendency to waste salt that is already present in the obstructed kidney. One mechanism involves the volume expansion that occurs when total renal function is ablated with bilateral obstruction. Volume expansion down-regulates the sympathetic nervous system, reduces circulating levels of aldosterone, and, along with reduced renal clearance, increases levels of ANP. Reduced sympathetic tone and aldosterone, coupled with increased ANP, will markedly stimulate salt excretion. ANP may represent a particularly important mediator of salt wasting in bilateral obstruction. Levels of ANP are markedly elevated in bilateral, but not unilateral, obstruction.[234] ANP enhances salt wasting at several nephron segments. By blocking renin release in the macula densa and angiotensin action in the proximal tubule, ANP reduces proximal tubule salt reabsorption.[234, 249, 250] ANP also reduces aldosterone release, and directly inhibits salt reabsorption in the collecting ducts.[234, 249, 250] In agreement with this mechanism, infusion of ANP into animals in which obstruction has just been released leads to marked increases in salt and water excretion.[234] Moreover, efforts to reduce circulating ANP levels following bilateral obstruction attenuated salt excretion somewhat.[234]

In addition, accumulation of urea and other solutes, some of which are natriuretic, enhance salt wasting by obstructed kidneys. In models of release of 24 hours of unilateral obstruction, removal or obstruction of the contralateral kidney markedly enhances salt wasting by the obstructed kidney.[247] If the contralateral kidney is left in place but amounts of urea, salt, and water equivalent to what the contralateral kidney is excreting are infused into the animal, there is a striking increase in salt excretion in both the obstructed and the contralateral kidney.[247, 248] This effect occurred as well when the fluid was infused into a normal animal.[248] On this basis, bilateral obstruction induces hormonal changes and promotes accumulation of solutes and volume that together enhance natriuresis from the obstructed kidney.

Effects of Obstruction on Urinary Concentration and Dilution

Because the renal tubules in obstructive nephropathy lose the ability to concentrate and dilute the urine, urine osmolality following release of obstruction in humans and experimental animals approaches that of plasma.[2, 20] Dilution of the urine requires that the thick ascending limb reabsorb salt without water and that the collecting duct maintain the dilute urine by not reabsorbing water along its length, despite the presence of a concentrated medullary interstitium.[283, 284] Concentration of the urine requires active salt reabsorption in the thick limb and the action of the countercurrent multiplier to generate a concentrated medullary interstitium, as well as the ability of the collecting duct to insert aquaporin-2 water channels into the apical membrane in response to antidiuretic hormone.[283, 284]

Obstructive nephropathy disrupts several of these mechanisms. As noted above, obstruction markedly attenuates

MTAL salt reabsorption, limiting the kidney's ability to dilute the urine and to generate a high osmolality in the medullary interstitium. Indeed, interstitial osmolality has been shown to be reduced in obstructed kidneys.[2] In addition, collecting ducts isolated from obstructed kidneys reveal normal basal water permeabilities, but a marked diminution in the ability of the tubule to increase water permeability in response to antidiuretic hormone or other stimulants of cyclic adenosine monophosphate (cAMP) accumulation in the cells. As was the case with salt transport, the effects were similar in unilateral and bilateral obstruction.[259, 262] Detailed mechanistic studies have demonstrated that obstruction markedly reduces transcription of mRNA encoding aquaporin-2, as well as synthesis of aquaporin-2 water channels, and that collecting duct cells in obstructed kidneys do not traffic aquaporin-2–containing vesicles effectively to the apical surface in response to vasopressin or increased cAMP.[284-287] Part of this failure in trafficking relates to a diminution of phosphorylation of aquaporin-2 in obstructed kidneys.[288] In addition, unilateral ureteral obstruction markedly decreased synthesis and deployment to the basolateral membrane of aquaporin-3 and -4; when aquaporin-2 is in the apical membrane, these aquaporins mediate the flux of water across the basolateral membrane.[288] Interestingly, expression of aquaporin-2 remains suppressed for 7 days following relief of the obstruction, and the rise in urinary concentration parallels the recovery in aquaporin-2 expression.[284-287, 289] The fact that the tubules did not respond to cAMP indicates that the lesion is at a site beyond the receptor for antidiuretic hormone. Finally, in unilateral obstruction, the contralateral kidney also exhibited reduced ability to concentrate the urine and a diminution of aquaporin-2 expression below the levels observed in sham-operated controls.[287]

On the basis of these results, the defect in urinary dilution in obstruction is likely due to reduced ability of the thick ascending limb to dilute the urine by transporting salt from the lumen of the tubule to its basolateral side. It appears that the collecting duct in obstructed kidneys maintains its low water permeability in the absence of antidiuretic hormone, so that the failure to dilute the urine is not due to collapse of osmotic gradients in the collecting duct. The inability to concentrate the urine results from inability of the thick limb to generate a concentrated interstitium, and inability of the collecting duct to synthesize and to traffic aquaporin-2 water channels in response to antidiuretic hormone.

Effects of Relief of Obstruction on Urinary Acidification

Obstruction dramatically reduces urinary acidification in both experimental animals and humans. In humans, release of obstruction does not lead to bicarbonaturia, suggesting that proximal tubular bicarbonate reclamation is maintained. By contrast, in both experimental animals and patients following release of obstruction, the urine pH does not decrease in response to an acid load, indicating that obstruction impairs the ability of the distal nephron to acidify the urine.[273, 290, 291] This defect likely resides in the collecting duct.[290, 291]

Reduced acidification by the collecting duct could result from defective H^+ (H^+, ATPase or H^+, K^+-ATPase) or HCO_3^- (e.g., Cl^-/HCO_3^- exchange) pathways, backleak of protons down their electrochemical gradient from the lumen into the

interstitium, or, in the cortical collecting duct, the failure to generate a sufficiently lumen-negative transepithelial voltage.[290-292] Several studies have shown that obstruction reduces the activity of apical ENaC in the cortical collecting duct, an effect that would reduce the luminal negativity of this segment, resulting in reduced acidification. Such an effect has been demonstrated in the rat outer medullary collecting duct,[290] but was not seen in the rabbit cortical collecting duct.[291] These results reveal a species difference between rat and rabbit.

In the rat inner medullary collecting duct (studied by micropuncture) and in isolated perfused rat and rabbit outer medullary collecting duct, obstruction causes a large decrease in acidification rates.[290] Because Na^+ transport does not play a major role in acidification in these segments, the defect must be due to direct down-regulation of acid or HCO_3^- transport pathways, or back-leak of protons from lumen to interstitium.[292] At low perfusion rates, outer medullary collecting ducts from obstructed animals generated steep pH gradients,[290] indicating that obstruction does not interfere with the ability of the tubule to block back-flux of protons. However, at high perfusion rates, acidification was markedly lower in tubules from obstructed, as opposed to normal, kidneys,[290] demonstrating that obstruction inhibits activity or expression of H^+ or HCO_3^- transport pathways.

To define the mechanisms by which obstruction reduces acid secretion by the collecting duct, specific antisera directed against the Cl^-/HCO_3^- exchanger and subunits of the H^+, ATPase were used to examine the expression of these transporters in collecting ducts of unilaterally obstructed, contralateral, and control kidney.[292] Two possible mechanisms of reduced acid secretion were explored. One possibility was that the intercalated cells in obstructed kidneys would exhibit a high proportion of "reverse" orientation, with the proton pump in the basolateral membrane, and the Cl^-/HCO_3^- exchanger in the apical membrane. The other possibility was that the orientation of intercalated cells would not change, but there would be reduced expression of the H^+ or HCO_3^- transporter. Immunofluorescence studies showed that the orientation of the intercalated cells was not affected by obstruction. In addition, immunoblots of extracts of renal cortex and medulla of control, unilaterally obstructed or contralateral kidneys showed no change in total expression of H^+, ATPase.[292] Obstruction did attenuate the expression of H^+, ATPase along the apical membranes of intercalated cells. In obstructed kidneys, fewer intercalated cells exhibited an apical labeling pattern and many that did showed discontinuities or gaps in apical membrane labeling.[292] These results suggest that obstruction inhibits trafficking of H^+, ATPase to the apical membranes of intercalated cells. However, this disorder alone cannot account for the entire acidification defect in obstructive nephropathy, because the disturbed trafficking resolves as the obstruction persists, while the acidification defect remains.[292] In addition, the extent of the decrease in labeling appears to be too small to account for the profound defect in acidification.

In addition to defects in collecting duct H^+ transport, reduced generation of ammonia in the proximal tubule may also contribute to reduced acid excretion in kidneys released from obstruction. Cortical slices of obstructed kidneys exhibit reduced ability to generate ammonia from glutamine at several steps along this metabolic pathway, including reductions in glutamine uptake and oxidation, generation of glucose and ammonia, and oxygen consumption.[293, 294]

Effects of Relief of Obstruction of Excretion of Potassium

In parallel with the increase in sodium excretion, potassium excretion increases markedly following release of bilateral obstruction.[295, 296] Micropuncture and microcatheterization studies show that proximal potassium reabsorption is unchanged by obstruction while potassium is more avidly secreted in the collecting duct, likely due to increased distal delivery of sodium and volume following release of obstruction.[257, 295] By contrast, following release of unilateral obstruction, potassium excretion falls roughly in proportion to the reduction in GFR,[297] an effect that may be related to reduced distal delivery of sodium. However, administration of sodium sulfate in this state does not stimulate potassium excretion in obstructed kidneys as it does in controls, suggesting that collecting ducts in unilateral obstructed kidneys have an intrinsic defect in potassium secretion.[298] The kaliuretic effect observed in bilateral obstruction may well be due as well to the influence of elevated levels of ANP, which, at high levels, can stimulate potassium secretion in the distal nephron.

Effects of Relief of Obstruction on Excretion of Phosphate and Divalent Cations

When bilateral ureteral obstruction is relased, phosphate excretion rises in proportion to sodium excretion.[299] Phosphate restriction before the release of the obstruction prevents phosphate accumulation during bilateral obstruction, thereby blocking the increase in phosphate excretion.[299] In addition, phosphate wasting of similar magnitude to that observed following release of bilateral obstruction can be duplicated by phosphate loading of normal animals.[299] By contrast, release of unilateral obstruction results in phosphate retention, likely due to reduced GFR and avid proximal phosphate reabsorption.[300] Calcium excretion may be increased or decreased, depending on whether the obstruction is unilateral or bilateral, and depending on the species studied.[299, 301] Magnesium excretion is markedly increased following release of either bilateral or unilateral obstruction. This magnesium wasting probably occurs because both forms of obstruction markedly attenuate thick ascending limb sodium reabsorption, leading to reduced positive luminal transepithelial voltages and therefore a reduced driving force for lumen-to-basolateral magnesium flux across the paracellular pathway.[301]

Effects of Obstruction on Metabolic Pathways and Gene Expression

Obstruction inhibits oxidative metabolism and promotes anaerobic respiration, leading to decreased ATP levels, and increased levels of adenosine diphosphate (ADP) and AMP.[294, 302, 303] In addition, obstruction alters a wide variety of metabolic enzymes, as well as the expression of many different gene products.[255, 294, 303-305] These changes are summarized in Table 40-6. Many of these changes are difficult to link mechanistically with changes in GFR or tubular transport function observed in obstruction. It is possible,

however, that reduced ability to generate ATP, along with reductions in Na^+, K^+-ATPase expression, contributes to the natriuresis observed following release of obstruction (see earlier discussion).

A great deal of experimental work has focused on the renal effects of longer-term obstruction. A common model is application of unilateral ureteral obstruction for 1 week or more. These studies focus on the mechanisms of long-term renal damage and fibrosis, and have identified a variety of factors that likely mediate damage and determine long-term outcome. In some studies, longer-term obstruction is used as a model for chronic renal damage due to other causes. This body of work is well summarized in a recent review.[306]

Fetal Urinary Obstruction

Fetal urinary obstruction may lead to changes in tissue differentiation. Experiments in animal models reveal that fetal obstruction causes aberrations of morphogenesis, gene expression, cell turnover, and urine composition.[307] The earlier the kidney is obstructed in utero, the greater will be the changes in renal tissue.[308] After birth, obstruction may affect renal growth, especially in neonates and during the first year of life, but the obstruction will not cause tissue dedifferentiation.

Studies demonstrated the up-regulation of the renin-angiotensin system, as well as involvement of other substrates (transforming growth factor-$\beta 1$, endothelin-1, and so on).[309, 310] The exact mechanisms of action of these molecules in the alteration of renal morphogenesis are not fully understood. It is not well known either if obstruction alone is enough to induce renal dysplasia,[311, 312] or if the latter results from secondary obstruction-induced mesenchymal disruption. To know the exact role of obstruction in the

TABLE 40-6

Effects of Urinary Tract Obstruction on Renal Enzymes and Renal Gene Expression

Changes in Energy and Substrate Metabolism
Decreased oxygen consumption
Decreased substrate uptake
Increased anaerobic glycolysis
Decreased ATP/(ADP+AMP)
Decreased ammoniagenesis

Changes in Enzyme Activity
Decreased
  Alkaline phosphatase
  Na^+, K^+-ATPase
  Glucose-6-phosphatase
  Succinate dehydrogenase
  NADH/NADHP dehydrogenase
Increased
  Glucose-6-phosphate dehydrogenase
  Phosphogluconate dehydrogenase

Changes in Gene Expression
Reduction in glomerular $G_{\alpha s}$ and $G_{\alpha q/11}$ proteins
Reduction in pre-proepidermal growth factor and Tamm-Horsfall protein
Transient induction of growth factors FOS and MYC
Striking induction of cellular damage (*TRPM2*) genes

kidney malformation is very important clinically, because it is now possible to relieve obstruction in utero. If urinary obstruction is not the cause of subsequent renal impairment, then some may argue whether it is worthwhile to relieve the obstruction in utero. However, more recent studies suggest that in utero obstruction causes pulmonary hyperplasia and renal impairment directly or indirectly, leading to significant morbidity and mortality.[313] In addition, shunting of obstructed kidneys in animals before the end of nephrogenesis may allow reversal of the arrest of glomerulogenesis seen in this setting,[314] favoring early intervention. Since fetal intervention can be associated with frequent complications and a high rate of fetal wastage, subjects for the intervention should be carefully chosen. Fetal renal biopsy, which demonstrated a 50% to 60% success rate, correlates well with outcome and has few maternal complications.[315] It may be used as one of the methods to determine treatment strategy. Studies demonstrate that antenatal intervention may help fetuses with the most severe forms of obstructive uropathy, otherwise usually associated with a fatal neonatal course.[316] Methods of intervention (especially endoscopic surgery) also need refinement before they can be recommended for broader use.[313]

TREATMENT OF URINARY TRACT OBSTRUCTION AND RECOVERY OF RENAL FUNCTION

Once the presence of obstruction is established, intervention is usually indicated to relieve it. The type of intervention depends on the location of the obstruction, its degree, and its etiology, as well as the presence or absence of concomitant diseases and complications, and the general condition of the patient.[205] The first step usually involves prompt relief of the obstruction, followed by the definitive treatment. Infravesical obstruction (e.g., benign prostatic hyperplasia or urethral stricture) can be easily relieved with placement of a urethral catheter. If the urethra is impassable, suprapubic cystostomy may be necessary. Alternatively, insertion of a nephrostomy tube or ureteral stent may be indicated when supravesical urinary obstruction is present. The urgency of the intervention depends on the degree of renal function, the presence or absence of infection, and the overall risk of the procedure.[317] The presence of the infection in an obstructed urinary tract, or urosepsis, is a urologic emergency that requires prompt relief of the obstruction, in addition to antibiotic treatment. Acute renal failure, associated with bilateral ureteral obstruction or with the obstruction of single functioning kidney, also calls for emergent intervention.

Calculi, the most common form of acute unilateral urinary obstruction, can usually be managed conservatively with analgesics to control the exquisite pain that they cause, and intravenous fluids to increase urine flow. Ninety percent of stones smaller than 5 mm pass spontaneously, but as stones get larger, it becomes progressively less likely that they will pass spontaneously. Surgery or instrumentation is indicated for persistent obstruction, uncontrollable pain, or urinary tract infection. Current possibilities for treatment include cystoscopic placement of ureteral stents, nephrostomy with urine drainage, extracorporeal shock wave lithotripsy (which many require ureteral stent placement if the patient is symptomatic),[318] and ureteroscopy with stone fragmentation (usually with laser lithotripsy). Large renal stones can be fragmented through nephrostomy. These newer approaches have all but eliminated the need for open surgical procedures.[206]

Intramural or extrinsic ureteral obstruction may be relieved by placement of a ureteral stent through the cystoscope.[319] If this cannot be accomplished, or is ineffective (especially in cases of extrinsic ureteral compression by the tumors), then nephrostomy tubes will need to be inserted to effect prompt relief of the obstruction.[320]

For infravesical obstruction due to benign prostatic hyperplasia, surgery can be safely delayed or completely avoided in patients with minimal symptoms, lack of infection, and an anatomically normal upper urinary tract.[321] If needed, transurethral resection of the prostate, laser ablation, or other techniques can be used for definitive treatment. Internal urethrotomy with direct visualization may be effective in the treatment of urethral strictures, as dilation usually has only temporary effect. Suprapubic cystostomy may be necessary in patients with impassable urethral strictures, followed by open urethroplast to restore urinary tract continuity, when possible.

Patients with neurogenic bladder require a variety of approaches, including frequent voiding, often by external compression, medications to stimulate bladder activity or relax the urethral sphincter, and intermittent catheterization using meticulous technique to avoid infection.[322, 323] Long-term indwelling bladder catheters should be avoided because they increase the risk of infection and renal damage. If more conservative measures such as frequent voiding or intermittent catheterization are not effective, ileovesicostomy or other forms of urinary diversion should be considered. Electrical stimulation has also been attempted with varying success.[324]

In many forms of obstruction, initial stabilization of the patient's condition is followed by a decision as to whether to continue observation or to move on to definitive surgery or nephrectomy. The actual course chosen depends on the likelihood that renal function will improve with the relief of obstruction. Factors that affect the decision of whether to operate and what form of surgical intervention to use include the age and general condition of the patient, the appearance and function of the obstructed kidney and the contralateral one, the cause of the obstruction, and the presence of infection.[205] The extent of recovery of renal function depends on the extent and duration of the obstruction.

A detailed discussion of the indications and surgical techniques for intervention to treat urinary tract obstruction is beyond the scope of this chapter, and may be found in other sources.[325, 326]

Estimating Renal Damage and Potential for Recovery

As noted earlier, when deciding whether to bypass or reconstruct drainage of an obstructed kidney rather than excise it, the potential for meaningful recovery of function in the affected kidney represents a critical issue. In many cases, obstruction may be partial, so that it is difficult on the basis of the history alone to predict the outcome. In addition, imaging studies that reveal the anatomy of the obstructed kidney such as ultrasonography or IVU predict the extent of functional recovery poorly, because the extent of anatomic distortion during obstruction correlates poorly with the extent of recovery once the obstruction is relieved.[101] Isotopic renography with a variety of isotopes can be used to examine renal function, as outlined earlier. This approach is a far more reliable indicator of potential renal function when applied well after temporary drainage of the obstructed kidney (e.g., by nephrostomy tubes) has been achieved than if it is performed while the obstruction is still present.[101] Of course, anatomic studies will reveal the remaining size and volume of the kidney, and can provide some idea of the extent to which the tissue remains viable. All of these considerations figure into the clinical judgment as to whether attempts should be made to salvage the kidney.

Recovery of Renal Function after Prolonged Obstruction

In patients, the potential for recovery of renal function depends primarily on the extent and duration of the obstruction, but other factors, such as the presence of other illnesses and the presence or absence of urinary tract infection, play an important role as well. In dogs subjected to 40 days of ureteral ligation, release of the obstruction led to no recovery of renal function. However, recovery of renal function in humans has been documented following release of obstruction of 69 days or longer.[327, 328] Because it is difficult to predict whether renal function will recover when temporary relief of obstruction has been achieved, it makes sense to measure function repeatedly with isotopic renography over time, before deciding on a definitive surgical course. Chronic bilateral obstruction, as seen in benign prostatic hyperplasia, can cause chronic renal failure, especially when the obstruction is of prolonged duration and when it is accompanied by urinary tract infections.[329, 330] Progressive loss of renal function can be slowed or halted by relieving the obstruction and treating the infection.[331]

When obstruction has been relieved and there is poor return of renal function, interstitial fibrosis and inflammation may have supervened. To ensure that there is no other process hampering recovery of renal function, renal biopsy may be indicated. As noted earlier, studies in experimental animals have implicated a variety of factors in chronic renal failure due to prolonged obstruction, including excessive production of renal vasoconstrictors such as renin and angiotensin,[332] growth factors that may enhance fibrosis,[333] and ammoniagenesis, which also affects cell growth.[306, 334] Based on these findings, inhibitors like captopril have been shown to ameliorate to some degree the long-term damage observed following prolonged obstruction.[235, 335]

POSTOBSTRUCTIVE DIURESIS

Release of obstruction can lead to marked natriuresis and diuresis with the wasting of potassium, phosphate, and divalent cations. It is notable that clinically significant postobstructive diuresis usually occurs only in the setting of prior bilateral obstruction, or unilateral obstruction of a solitary functioning kidney. The mechanisms involved have been described in detail earlier and involve the combination of intrinsic damage to tubular salt, solute, and water reabsorption, as well as the effects of volume expansion,

solute (e.g., urea) accumulation, and attendant increases in natriuretic substances such as ANP.[245, 262, 336-340] When the obstruction is unilateral and there is a functioning contralateral kidney, the volume expansion, solute accumulation, and increases in natriuretic substances do not occur, and the contralateral kidney may retain salt and water, resulting in some compensation for the natriuresis and diuresis occurring in the postobstructive kidney. Management of the patient with postobstructive diuresis focuses on avoiding severe volume depletion due to salt wasting, and other electrolyte imbalances, such as hypokalemia, hyponatremia, hypernatremia, and hypomagnesemia.

Postobstructive diuresis is usually self-limited. It usually lasts for several days to a week, but may, in rare cases, persist for months.[331] Acute massive polyuria or prolonged postobstructive diuresis may deplete the patient of Na^+, K^+, Cl^-, HCO_3^-, and water, as well as divalent cations and phosphate. Volume or free water replacement is appropriate only when the salt and water losses result in volume depletion or a disturbance of osmolality. In many cases, excessive volume or fluid replacement prolongs the diuresis and natriuresis. Because the initial urine is isosthenuric, with an initial Na^+ of approximately 80 mEq/L, an appropriate starting fluid for replacement may be 0.45% saline, given at a rate somewhat slower than that of the urine output. During this period, meticulous monitoring of vital signs, volume status, urine output, and serum and urine chemistry and osmolality is imperative. This will determine the need for ongoing replacement of salt, free water, and other electrolytes. With massive diuresis, these measurements will need to be repeated frequently, up to four times daily, with frequent adjustment of replacement fluids, as needed.

REFERENCES

1. Bricker NS, Klahr S: Obstructive nephropathy. *In* Strauss MB, Welt LG (eds): Diseases of the Kidney. Boston, Little, Brown, 1971, pp 997-1037.
2. Yarger WE: Urinary tract obstruction. *In* Brenner BM, Rector FC (ed): The Kidney, 4th ed. Philadelphia, WB Saunders, 1991, pp 1768-1808.
3. Bell ET: Renal Diseases. Philadelphia, Lea & Febiger, 1950.
4. Campbell MF: Urinary obstruction. *In* Campbell MF, Harrison JH (eds): Urology. Philadelphia, WB Saunders, 1970, pp 1772-1793.
5. Tan PH, Chiang GS, Tay AH: Pathology of urinary tract malformations in a paediatric autopsy series. Ann Acad Med Singapore 23: 838-843, 1994.
6. Klahr S, Buerkert J, Morrison A: Urinary tract obstruction. *In* Brenner BM, Rector FCJ (eds): The Kidney, 3rd ed. Philadelphia, WB Saunders, 1986, pp 1443-1490.
7. System URD: USRDS 1993 Annual Data Report. Bethesda, MD, National Institutes of Health, National Institute of Diabetes and Digestive and Kidney Diseases, 1993.
8. Snyder HM 3rd, Lebowitz RL, Colodny AH, et al: Ureteropelvic junction obstruction in children. Urol Clin North Am 7:273-290, 1980.
9. Young DW, Lebowitz RL: Congenital abnormalities of the ureter. Semin Roentgenol 21:172-187, 1986.
10. Graversen HP, Tofte T, Genster HG: Ureter-pelvic stenosis. Int Urol Nephrol 19:245-251, 1987.
11. Lowe FC, Marshall FF: Ureteropelvic junction obstruction in adults. Urology 23:331-335, 1984.
12. Clark WR, Malek RS: Ureteropelvic junction obstruction. I. Observations on the classic type in adults. J Urol 138:276-279, 1987.
13. Buscemi M, Shanske A, Mallet E, et al: Dominantly inherited ureteropelvic junction obstruction. Urology 26:568-571, 1985.
14. Elder JS, Duckett JW: Perinatal urology. *In* Gillenwater JY, Grayhack JT, Howards SS, Duckett JW (eds): Adult and Pediatric Urology. St Louis, Mosby-Year Book, 1991, pp 1711-1810.

15. Rickwood AM, Godiwalla SY: The natural history of pelvi-ureteric junction obstruction in children presenting clinically with the complaint. Br J Urol 80:793-796, 1997.

16. Peters CA: Urinary tract obstruction in children. J Urol 154:1874-1883, 1995.

17. Murthy LN: Urinary tract obstruction during pregnancy: Recent developments in imaging. Br J Urol 80 (suppl 1):1-3, 1997.

18. Novick AC: Surgery of the kidney. In Walsh PC, Retik AB, Vaughan ED, Wein AJ (eds): Campbell's Urology, 8th ed. Philadelphia, WB Saunders, 2002, pp 3570-3644.

19. Hanna MK, Jeffs RD, Sturgess JM, et al: Ureteral structure and ultrastructure. Part II. Congenital ureteropelvic junction obstruction and primary obstructive megaureter. J Urol 116:725-730, 1976.

20. Klahr S, Harris KPG: Obstructive uropathy. In Seldin DW, Giebisch G (eds): The Kidney: Physiology and Pathophysiology, 2nd ed. New York, Raven Press, 1992, pp 3327-3369.

21. Hanna MK: Some observations on congenital ureteropelvic junction obstruction. Urology 12:151-159, 1978.

22. Karaca I, Sencan A, Mir E, et al: Ureteral fibroepithelial polyps in children. Pediatr Surg Int 12:603-604, 1997.

23. Stephens FD: Primary obstructing megaureter. In Stephens FD (ed): Congenital Malformations of the Urinary Tract. New York, Praeger Publishers, 1983, pp 267-281.

24. Wall B, Wachter HE: Congenital ureteral valve: Its role as a primary obstructive lesion: Classification of the literature and report of an authentic case. J Urol 129:1222-1224, 1983.

25. Sant GR, Barbalias GA, Klauber GT: Congenital ureteral valves—an abnormality of ureteral embryogenesis? J Urol 133:427-431, 1985.

26. Ayyat FM, Adams G: Congenital midureteral strictures. Urology 26:170-172, 1985.

27. Macksood MJ, Roth DR, Chang CH, et al: Benign fibroepithelial polyps as a cause of intermittent ureteropelvic junction obstruction in a child: A case report and review of the literature. J Urol 134:951-952, 1985.

28. Eidelman A, Yuval E, Simon D, et al: Retrocaval ureter. Eur Urol 4:279-281, 1978.

29. Brown T, Mandell J, Lebowitz RL: Neonatal hydronephrosis in the era of sonography. AJR Am J Roentgenol 148:959-963, 1987.

30. Tanagho EA: The anatomy and function of ureterovesical junction. Br J Urol 35:151-165, 1963.

31. Woodburne RT: Anatomy of the ureterovesical junction. J Urol 92:431-435, 1964.

32. Lockhart JL, Singer AM, Glenn JF: Congenital megaureter. J Urol 122:310-314, 1979.

33. Welch KJ, Kraney GP: Abdominal musculature deficiency syndrome prune belly. J Urol 111:693-700, 1974.

34. Coplen DE: Prune belly syndrome. In Gillenwater JY, Grayhack JT, Howards SS, Mitchell ME (eds): Adult and Pediatric Urology. Philadelphia, Lippincott Williams & Wilkins, 2002, pp 2209-2225.

35. Fenelon MJ, Alton DJ: Prolapsing ectopic ureteroceles in boys. Radiology 140:373-376, 1981.

36. Kojima Y, Hayashi Y, Maruyama T, et al: 49,XXXXY syndrome with hydronephrosis caused by intravesical ureterocele. Urol Int 63:212-214, 1999.

37. Newman LB, McAlister WH, Kissane J: Segmental renal dysplasia associated with ectopic ureteroceles in childhood. Urology 3:23-26, 1974.

38. Snyder HM, Johnston JH: Orthotopic ureteroceles in children. J Urol 119:543-546, 1978.

39. Sekine H, Kojima S, Mine M, et al: Intravesical ureterocele presenting bladder outlet obstruction in an adult male. Int J Urol 3:74-76, 1996.

40. Lee SS, Sun GH, Yu DS, et al: Giant hydronephrosis of a duplex system associated with ureteral ectopia: A cause of retrograde ejaculation. Arch Androl 45:19-23, 2000.

41. Livne PM, Gonzales ET Jr: Congenital bladder diverticula causing ureteral obstruction. Urology 25:273-276, 1985.

42. Kwan DJ, Lowe FC: Congenital bladder diverticulum: An unusual presentation with abdominal mass, urinary retention, and renal failure in a young adult. Urol Rodiol 14:194-196, 1992.

43. Glassberg KI: Current issues regarding posterior urethral valves. Urol Clin North Am 12:175-185, 1985.

44. Kurth KH, Alleman ER, Schroder FH: Major and minor complications of posterior urethral valves. J Urol 126:517-519, 1981.

45. Martin J, Anderson J, Raz S: Posterior urethral valves in adults: A report of 2 cases. J Urol 118:978-979, 1977.

46. Cohen HL, Susman M, Haller JO, et al: Posterior urethral valve: Transperineal US for imaging and diagnosis in male infants. Radiology 192:261-264, 1994.

47. Freeny PC: Congenital anterior urethral diverticulum in the male. Radialogy 111:173-174, 1974.

48. Norbeck JC, Ritchey MR, Bloom DA: Labial fusion causing upper urinary tract obstruction. Urology 42:209-211, 1993.

49. Novotny MJ, Graves GG, Couillard DR: Ureteral obstruction due to colonic duplication. J Urol 166:216, 2001.

50. Bauer SB: Neurologic dysfunction of the lower urinary tract in children. In Walsh PC, Retik AB, Vaughan ED, Wein AJ (eds): Campbell's Urology, 7th ed. Philadelphia, WB Saunders, 1998, pp 2019-2054.

51. McLorie GA, Perez-Marero R, Csima A, et al: Determinants of hydronephrosis and renal injury in patients with myelomeningocele. J Urol 140(5 pt 2):1289-1292, 1988.

52. Shochat SJ, Perlmutter AD: Myelodysplasia with severe neonatal hydronephrosis: The value of urethral dilatation. J Urol 107:146-148, 1972.

53. Thorup J, Mortensen T, Diemer H, et al: The prognosis of surgically treated congenital hydronephrosis after diagnosis in utero. J Urol 134:914-917, 1985.

54. Wolpert JJ, Woodard JR, Parrott TS: Pyeloplasty in the young infant. J Urol 142(2 pt 2):573-575, 1989.

55. Fine RN: Diagnosis and treatment of fetal urinary tract abnormalities. J Pediatr 121:333-341, 1992.

56. Crombleholme TM, Harrison MR, Longaker MT, et al: Prenatal diagnosis and management of bilateral hydronephrosis. Pediatr Nephrol 2:334-342, 1988.

57. Mandell J, Peters CA, Retik AB: Current concepts in the perinatal diagnosis and management of hydronephrosis. Urol Clin North Am 17:247-262, 1990.

58. Allen TD: The swing of the pendulum. J Urol 148(2 pt 2):534-535, 1992.

59. Conger JD: Acute uric acid nephropathy. Semin Nephrol 1:69-74, 1981.

60. Simon DI, Brosius FC 3rd, Rothstein DM: Sulfadiazine crystalluria revisited. The treatment of Toxoplasma encephalitis in patients with acquired immunodeficiency syndrome. Arch Intern Med 150:2379-2384, 1990.

61. Sawyer MH, Webb DE, Balow JE, et al: Acyclovir-induced renal failure. Clinical course and histology. Am J Med 84:1067-1071, 1988.

62. Deeks SG, Smith M, Holodniy M, et al: HIV-1 protease inhibitors. A review for clinicians. JAMA 277:145-153, 1997.

63. Chopra N, Fine PL, Price B, et al: Bilateral hydronephrosis from ciprofloxacin induced crystalluria and stone formation. J Urol 164:438, 2000.

64. Defronzo RA, Humphrey RL, Wright JR, et al: Acute renal failure in multiple myeloma. Medicine (Baltimore) 54:209-223, 1975.

65. Crittenden DR, Ackerman GL: Hyperuricemic acute renal failure in disseminated carcinoma. Arch Intern Med 137:97-99, 1977.

66. Molina JM, Belenfant X, Doco-Lecompte T, et al: Sulfadiazine-induced crystalluria in AIDS patients with Toxoplasma encephalitis. AIDS 5:587-589, 1991.

67. Waugh DA, Ibels LS: Multiple myeloma presenting as recurrent obstructive uropathy. Aust N Z J Med 10:555-558, 1980.

68. Johnson CM, Wilson DM, O'Fallon WM, et al: Renal stone epidemiology: A 25-year study in Rochester, Minnesota. Kidney Int 16: 624-631, 1979.

69. Eknoyan G, Qunibi WY, Grissom RT, et al: Renal papillary necrosis: An update. Medicine (Baltimore) 61:55-73, 1982.

70. Shapeero LG, Vordermark JS: Papillary necrosis causing hydronephrosis in the renal allograft. Sonographic findings. J Ultrasound Med 8:579-581, 1989.

71. Jameson RM, Heal MR: The surgical management of acute renal papillary necrosis. Br J Surg 60:428-430, 1973.

72. Amos AM, Figlesthaler WM, Cookson MS: Bilateral ureteritis cystica with unilateral ureteropelvic junction obstruction. Tech Urol 5:108-112, 1999.

73. Wein AJ: Neuromuscular dysfunction of the lower urinary tract and its treatment. In Walsh PC, Retik AB, Vaughan ED, Wein AJ (eds): Campbell's Urology, 7th ed. Philadelphia, WB Saunders, 1998, 953-1006.

74. Novicki DE, Willscher MK: Case profile: Anticholinergic-induced hydronephrosis. Urology 13:324-325, 1979.

75. Murdock MI, Olsson CA, Sax DS, et al: Effects of levodopa on the bladder outlet. J Urol 113:803-805, 1975.

76. Crew JP, Donat R, Roskell D, et al: Bilateral ureteric obstruction secondary to the prolonged use of tiaprofenic acid. Br J Clin Pract 51:59-60, 1997.

77. Kanematsu M, Hoshi H, Imaeda T, et al: Renal pelvic and ureteral carcinoma with huge hydronephrosis: US, CT, and MR findings. Radiol Med (Torino) 14:321-323, 1996.

78. Hadas-Halpern I, Farkas A, Patlas M, et al: Sonographic diagnosis of ureteral tumors. J Ultrasound Med 18:639-645, 1999.

79. Graham JB, Abad RS: Ureteral obstruction due to radiation. Am J Obstet Gynecol 99:409-412, 1967.

80. MacGregor GA, Jones NF, Barraclough MA, et al: Ureteric stricture with analgesic nephropathy. BMJ 2:271-272, 1973.

81. Nash TE, Cheever AW, Ottesen EA, et al: Schistosome infections in humans: Perspectives and recent findings. NIH conference. Ann Intern Med 97:740-754, 1982.

82. Christensen WI: Genitourinary tuberculosis: Review of 102 cases. Medicine (Baltimore) 53:377-390, 1974.

83. Murphy DM, Fallon B, Lane V, et al: Tuberculous stricture of ureter. Urology 20:382-384, 1982.

84. Aragona F, Passerini Glazel G, Pavanello L, et al: Upper urinary tract obstruction in children caused by *Candida* fungus balls. Eur Urol 11:188-191, 1985.

85. Scerpella EG, Alhalel R: An unusual cause of acute renal failure: Bilateral ureteral obstruction due to *Candida tropicalis* fungus balls. Clin Infect Dis 18:440-442, 1994.

86. Fayad MM, Youssef AF, Zahran M, et al: The ureterocalyceal system in normal pregnancy. A study using isotope renography and intravenous pyelography. Acta Obstet Gynecol Scand 52:68-76, 1973.

87. Murao F: Ultrasonic evaluation of hydronephrosis during pregnancy and puerperium. Gynecol Obstet Invest 35:94-98, 1993.

88. LaPata RE, McElin TW, Adelson BH: Ureteral obstruction due to compression by the gravid uterus. Am J Obstet Gynecol 106:941-942, 1970.

89. Klein EA: Urologic problems of pregnancy. Obstet Gynecol Surv 39:605-615, 1984.

90. Bennett AH, Adler S: Bilateral ureteral obstruction causing anuria secondary to pregnancy. Urology 20:631-633, 1982.

91. Roy C, Saussine C, LeBras, Y, et al: Assessment of painful ureterohydronephrosis during pregnancy by MR urography. Eur Radiol 6:334-338, 1996.

92. Loughlin KR: Management of acute ureteral obstruction in pregnancy utilizing ultrasound-guided placement of ureteral stents. Urology 43: 412, 1994.

93. D'Elia FL, Brennan RE, Brownstein PK: Acute renal failure secondary to ureteral obstruction by a gravid uterus. J Urol 128:803-804, 1982.

94. Beach EW: Urologic complications of cancer of uterine cervix. J Urol 68:178-189, 1952.

95. Kontogeorgos L, Vassilopoulos P, Tentes A: Bilateral severe hydroureteronephrosis due to uterine prolapse. Br J Urol 57:360-361, 1985.

96. Melser M, Miles BJ, Kastan D, et al: Chronic renal failure secondary to post-hysterectomy vaginal prolapse. 38:361-363, 1991.

97. Gomes CM, Rovner ES, Banner MP, et al: Simultaneous upper and lower urinary tract obstruction associated with severe genital prolapse: Diagnosis and evaluation with magnetic resonance imaging. Int Urogynecol J 12:144-146, 2001.

98. Resnick MI, Kursh ED: Extrinsic obstruction of the ureter. *In* Walsh PC, Retik AB, Vaughan ED, Wein AJ (eds): Campbell's Urology, 7th ed. Philadelphia, WB Saunders, 1998, pp 387-422.

99. Philips JC: Spectrum of radiologic abnormalities due to tubo-ovarian abscess. Radiology 110:307-311, 1974.

100. Carpenter AA: Pelvic lipomatosis: Successful surgical treatment. J Urol 110:397-399, 1973.

101. Gulmi FA, Felsen D, Vaughan ED Jr: Pathophysiology of urinary tract obstruction. *In* Walsh DS, Retik AB, Vaughan ED Jr, Wein AJ (eds): Campbell's Urology, 8th ed. Philadelphia, WB Saunders, 2002, pp 411-462.

102. Sakellariou PG, Protopapas AG, Kyritsis NI, et al: Retroperitoneal endometriosis causing cyclical ureteral obstruction. Eur J Obstet Gynecol Reprod Biol 67:59-62, 1996.

103. Deprest J, Marchal G, Brosens I: Obstructive uropathy secondary to endometriosis. N Engl J Med 337:1174-1175, 1997.

104. Vercellini P, Pisacreta A, Pesole A, et al: Is ureteral endometriosis an asymmetric disease? Br J Obstet Gynaecol 107:559-561, 2000.

105. Klein RS, Cattolica EV: Ureteral endometriosis. Urology 13:477-482, 1979.

106. Kane C, Drouin P: Obstructive uropathy associated with endometriosis. Am J Obstet Gynecol 151:207-211, 1985.

107. Nasu K, Narahara H, Hayata T, et al: Ureteral obstruction caused by endometriosis. Gynecol Obstet Invest 40:215-216, 1995.

108. Dowling RA, Corriere JN Jr, Sandler CM: Iatrogenic ureteral injury. J Urol 135:912-915, 1986.

109. Peters CA, Walsh PC: The effect of nafarelin acetate, a luteinizing-hormone–releasing hormone agonist, on benign prostatic hyperplasia. N Engl J Med 317:599-604, 1987.

110. Alam AM, Sugimura K, Okizuka H, et al: Comparison of MR imaging and urodynamic findings in benign prostatic hyperplasia. Radiol Med 18:123-128, 2000.

111. Mukouyama H, Sugaya K, Ogawa Y, et al: Poorly differentiated sarcoma of the prostate causing obstructive acute renal failure: a case report. Int J Urol 6:615-619, 1999.

112. Marks LS, Gallo DA: Ureteral obstruction in the patient with prostatic carcinoma. Br J Urol 44:411-416, 1972.

113. Batata MA, Whitmore WF, Hilaris BS, et al: Primary carcinoma of the ureter: A prognostic study. Cancer 35:1626-1632, 1975.

114. Present DH, Rabinowitz JG, Banks PA, et al: Obstructive hydronephrosis in regional ileitis. N Engl J Med 280:523-528, 1963.

115. Ben-Ami H, Lavy A, Behar DM, et al: Left hydronephrosis caused by Crohn disease successfully treated conservatively. Am J Med Sci 320:286-287, 2000.

116. Schofield PF, Staff WG, Moore T: Ureteral involvement in regional ileitis (Crohn's disease). J Urol 99:412-416, 1968.

117. Shield DE, Lytton B, Weiss RM, et al: Urologic complications of inflammatory bowel disease. J Urol 115:701-706, 1976.

118. Cook GT: Appendiceal abscess causing urinary obstruction. J Urol 101:212-215, 1969.

119. Bissada NK, Redman JF: Ureteral complications in diverticulitis of the colon. J Urol 112:454-456, 1974.

120. Knobel B, Rosman P, Gewurtz G: Bilateral hydronephrosis due to fecaloma in an elderly woman. J Clin Gastroenterol 30:311-313, 2000.

121. Kiviat MD, Miller EV, Ansell JS: Pseudocysts of the pancreas presenting as renal mass lesions. Br J Urol 43:257-262, 1971.

122. Gibson GE, Tiernan E, Cronin CC, et al: Reversible bilateral ureteric obstruction due to a pancreatic pseudocyst. Gut 34:1267-1278, 1993.

123. Morehouse HT, Thornhill BA, Alterman DD: Right ureteral obstruction associated with pancreatitis. Urol Radiol 7:150-152, 1985.

124. Loughlin K, Kearney G, Helfrich W, et al: Ureteral obstruction secondary to perianeurysmal fibrosis. Urology 24:332-336, 1984.

125. Safran R, Sklenicka R, Kay H: Iliac artery aneurysm: A common cause of ureteral obstruction. J Urol 113:605-609, 1975.

126. Schapira HE, Mitty HA: Right ovarian vein septic thrombophlebitis causing ureteral obstruction. J Urol 112:451-453, 1974.

127. Weisman MH, McDanald EC, Wilson CB: Studies of the pathogenesis of interstitial cystitis, obstructive uropathy, and intestinal malabsorption in a patient with systemic lupus erythematosus. Am J Med 70:875-881, 1981.

128. Melin JP, Lemaire P, Birembaut P, et al: Polyarteritis nodosa with bilateral ureteric involvement. Nephron 32:87-89, 1982.

129. Lie JT: Retroperitoneal polyarteritis nodosa presenting as ureteral obstruction. J Rheumatol 19:1628-1631, 1992.

130. Adelizzi RA, Shockley FK, Pietras JR: Wegener's granulomatosis with ureteric obstruction. J Rheumatol 13:448-451, 1986.

131. Plaisier EM, Mougenot B, Khayat R, et al: Ureteral stenosis in Wegener's granulomatosis. Nephrol Dial Transplant 12:1759-1761, 1997.

132. Kher KK, Sheth KJ, Makker SP: Stenosing ureteritis in Henoch-Schönlein purpura. J Urol 129:1040-1042, 1983.

133. Pfister C, Liard-Zmuda A, Dacher J, et al: Total bilateral ureteral replacement for stenosing ureteritis in Henoch-Schönlein purpura. Eur Urol 38:96-99, 2000.

134. Wagenknecht LV, Hardy JC: Value of various treatments for retroperitoneal fibrosis. Eur Urol 7:193-200, 1981.

135. Keith DS, Larson TS: Idiopathic retroperitoneal fibrosis. J Am Soc Nephrol 3:1748-1752, 1993.

136. Adam U, Mack D, Forstner R, et al: Conservative treatment of acute Ormond's disease. Tech Urol 5:54-56, 1999.

137. Marzano A, Trapani A, Leone N, et al. Treatment of idiopathic retroperitoneal fibrosis using cyclosporin. Ann Rheumat Dis 60: 427-428, 2001.

138. Cohen WM, Freed SZ, Hasson J: Metastatic cancer to the ureter: A review of the literature and case presentations. J Urol 112:188-189, 1974.

139. Goldman SM, Fishman EK, Rosenshein NB, et al: Excretory urography and computed tomography in the initial evaluation of patients with cervical cancer: Are both examinations necessary? AJR Am J Roentgenol 143:991-996, 1984.

140. Jones CR, Woodhouse CR, Hendry WF: Urological problems following treatment of carcinoma of the cervix. Br J Urol 56:609-613, 1984.

141. Blum MD, Bahnson RR, Carter MF: Urologic manifestations of von Recklinghausen neurofibromatosis. Urology 26:209-217, 1985.

142. David HS, Lavengood RW Jr: Bilateral Wilms' tumor. Treatment, management, and review of the literature. Urology 3:71-78, 1974.

143. Schoenfeld RH, Belville WD, Buck AS, et al: Unilateral ureteral obstruction secondary to sarcoidosis. Urology 25:57-59, 1985.

144. Bloomberg SD, Neu HC, Ehrlich RM, et al: Chronic granulomatous disease of childhood with renal involvement. Urology 4:193-197, 1974.

145. Maeda H, Shichiri Y, Kinoshita H, et al: Urinary undiversion for pelvic actinomycosis: A long-term follow up. Int J Urol 6:111-113, 1999.

146. de Feiter PW, Soeters PB: Gastrointestinal actinomycosis: An unusual presentation with obstructive uropathy: Report of a case and review of the literature. Dis Colon Rectum 44:1521-1525, 2001.

147. Emir L, Karabulut A, Balci U, et al: An unusual cause of urinary retention: A primary retrovesical echinococcal cyst. Urology 56:856, 2000.

148. Mark IR, Mansoor A, Derias N, et al: Retroperitoneal malacoplakia: An unusual cause of ureteric obstruction. Br J Urol 76:520-521, 1995.

149. Casserly LF, Reddy SM, Rennke HG, et al: Reversible bilateral hydronephrosis without obstruction in hepatitis B–associated polyarteritis nodosa. Am J Kidney Dis 34:E11, 1999.

150. Talreja D, Opfell RW: Ureteral metastasis in carcinoma of the breast. West J Med 133:252–254, 1980.

151. Gore RM, Shkolnik A: Abdominal manifestations of pediatric leukemias: Sonographic assessment. Radiology 143:207-210, 1982.

152. Richmond J, Sherman RSD: Renal lesions associated with malignant lymphomas. Am J Med 32:184-207, 1962.

153. Vaidyanathan S, Singh G, Soni BM, et al: Silent hydronephrosis/pyonephrosis due to upper urinary tract calculi in spinal cord injury patients. Spinal Cord 38:661-668, 2000.

154. Covington T, Reeser W: Hydronephrosis associated with overhydration. J Urol 63:438-445, 1950.

155. Tebyani N, Candela J, Patel H, et al: Ureteropelvic junction obstruction presenting as early satiety and weight loss. J Endourol 13:445-446, 1999.

156. Chute CG, Panser LA, Girman CJ, et al: The prevalence of prostatism: A population-based survey of urinary symptoms. J Urol 150:85-89, 1993.

157. Akcay A, Altun B, Usalan C, et al: Cyclical acute renal failure due to bilateral ureteral endometriosis. Clin Nephrol 52:179-182, 1999.

158. Shimada K, Katsumi T, Fujita H: Appendiceal granuloma causing bilateral hydronephrosis and macroscopic haematuria. Br J Urol 48:418, 1976.

159. Whiting JC, Stanisic TH, Drach GW: Congenital ureteral valves: Report of 2 patients, including one with a solitary kidney and associated hypertension. J Urol 129:1222-1224, 1983.

160. Koelliker SL, Cronan JJ: Acute urinary tract obstruction. Imaging update. Urol Clin North Am 24:571-582, 1997.

161. Shokeir AA: The diagnosis of upper urinary tract obstruction. Br J Urol 83:893-900, 1999.

162. Coleman BG: Ultrasonography of the upper genitourinary tract. Urol Clin North Am 12:633-644, 1985.

163. Rao KG, Hackler RH, Woodlief RM, et al: Real-time renal sonography in spinal cord injury patients: Prospective comparison with excretory urography. J Urol 135:72-77, 1986.

164. Stuck KJ, White GM, Granke DS, et al: Urinary obstruction in azotemic patients: Detection by sonography. AJR Am J Roentgenol 149:1191-1193, 1987.

165. Gottlieb RH, Weinberg EP, Rubens DJ, et al: Renal sonography: Can it be used more selectively in the setting of an elevated serum creatinine level? Am J Kidney Dis 29:362-367, 1997.

166. Talner LB: Urinary obstruction. In Pollack HM (eds): Clinical Urology: An Atlas and Textbook of Urological Imaging. Philadelphia, WB Saunders, 1990, pp 1535-1628.

167. Papanicolaou N: Urinary tract imaging and intervention: Basic principles. In Walsh PC, Retik AB, Vaughan ED, Wein AJ (eds): Campbell's Urology, 7th ed. Philadelphia, WB Saunders, 1998, pp 170-260.

168. Maillet PJ, Pelle-Francoz D, Laville M, et al: Nondilated obstructive acute renal failure: Diagnostic procedures and therapeutic management. Radiology 160:659-662, 1986.

169. Lalli AF: Retroperitoneal fibrosis and inapparent obstructive uropathy. Radiology 122:339-342, 1977.

170. Amis ES Jr, Cronan JJ, Pfister RC, et al: Ultrasonic inaccuracies in diagnosing renal obstruction. Urology 19:101-105, 1982.

171. Cronan JJ, Amis ES, Scola FH, et al: Renal obstruction in patients with ileal loops: US evaluation. Radiology 158:647-648, 1986.

172. Garcia-Pena BM, Keller MS, Schwartz DS, et al: The ultrasonographic differentiation of obstructive versus nonobstructive hydronephrosis in children: A multivariate scoring system. J Urol 158:560-565, 1997.

173. Cronan JJ, Amis ES Jr, Yoder IC, et al: Peripelvic cysts: An impostor of sonographic hydronephrosis. J Ultrasound Med 1:229-236, 1982.

174. Charasse C, Camus C, Darnault P, et al: Acute nondilated anuric obstructive nephropathy on echography: Difficult diagnosis in the intensive care unit. Intensive Care Med 17:387-391, 1991.

175. Garrett WJ, Grunwald G, Robinson DE: Prenatal diagnosis of fetal polycystic kidney by ultrasound. Aust N Z J Obstet Gynaecol 10: 7-9, 1970.

176. Roth JA, Diamond DA: Prenatal hydronephrosis. Curr Opin Pediatr 13:138-141, 2001.

177. Reddy PP, Mandell J: Prenatal diagnosis. Therapeutic implications. Urol Clin North Am 25:171-180, 1998.

178. Kaefer M, Peters CA, Retik AB, et al: Increased renal echogenicity: A sonographic sign for differentiating between obstructive and nonobstructive etiologies of in utero bladder distension. J Urol 158 (3 pt 2):1026-1029, 1997.

179. Siemens DR, Prouse KA, MacNeily AE, et al: Antenatal hydronephrosis: Thresholds of renal pelvic diameter to predict insignificant postnatal pelviectasis. Tech Urol 4:198-201, 1998.

180. Woodward M, Frank D: Postnatal management of antenatal hydronephrosis. Br J Urol Int 89:149-156, 2002.

181. Feldman DM, DeCambre M, Kong E, et al: Evaluation and follow-up of fetal hydronephrosis. J Ultrasound Med 20:1065-1069, 2001.

182. Mutazindwa T, Husseini T: Imaging in acute renal colic: The intravenous urogram remains the gold standard. Eur J Radiol 23:238-240, 1996.

183. Little MA, Stafford Johnson DB, O'Callaghan JP, et al: The diagnostic yield of intravenous urography. Nephrol Dial Transplant 15:200-204, 2000.

184. Coggins CH, Fang LST: Acute renal failure associated with antibiotics, anesthetic agents and radiographic contrast agents. In Brenner BM, Lazarus JM (eds): Acute Renal Failure. New York, Churchill Livingstone, 1988, pp 295-352.

185. Parfrey PS, Griffiths SM, Barrett BJ, et al: Contrast material–induced renal failure in patients with diabetes mellitus, renal insufficiency, or both. A prospective controlled study. N Engl J Med 320:143-149, 1989.

186. Dalla Palma L: What is left of i.v. urography? Eur Radiol 11: 931-939, 2001.

187. Bosniak MA, Megibow AJ, Ambos MA, et al: Computed tomography of ureteral obstruction. AJR Am J Roentgenol 138:1107-1113, 1982.

188. Smith RC, Rosenfield AT, Choe KA, et al: Acute flank pain: Comparison on non–contrast-enhanced CT and intravenous urography. Radiology 194:789-794, 1995.

189. Boridy IC, Kawashima A, Goldman SM, et al: Acute ureterolithiasis: Nonenhanced helical CT findings of perinephric edema for prediction of degree of ureteral obstruction. Radiology 213:663-667, 1999.

190. Lacey NA, Massouh H: Use of helical CT in assessment of crossing vessels in pelviureteric junction obstruction. Clin Radiol 55:212-216, 2000.

191. Dorio PJ, Pozniak MA, Lee FT Jr, et al: Non–contrast-enhanced helical computed tomography for the evaluation of patients with acute flank pain. Med J 98:30-34, 1999.

192. Testa HJ: Nuclear Medicine. In O'Reilly PH, George NJR, Weiss RM (eds): Diagnostic Techniques in Urology. Philadelphia, WB Saunders, 1990, pp 99-118.

193. English PJ, Testa HJ, Lawson RS, et al: Modified method of diuresis renography for the assessment of equivocal pelviureteric junction obstruction. Br J Urol 59:10-14, 1987.

194. O'Reilly PH, Testa HJ, Lawson RS, et al: Diuresis renography in equivocal urinary tract obstruction. Br J Urol 50:76-80, 1978.

195. O'Reilly PH, Lawson RS, Shields RA, et al: Idiopathic hydronephrosis—the diuresis renogram: A new non-invasive method of assessing equivocal pelviureteral junction obstruction. J Urol 121:153-155, 1979.

196. Conway JJ: "Well-tempered" diuresis renography: Its historical development, physiological and technical pitfalls, and standardized technique protocol. Semin Nucl Med 22:74-84, 1992.

197. Upsdell SM, Leeson SM, Brooman PJ, et al: Diuretic-induced urinary flow rates at varying clearances and their relevance to the performance and interpretation of diuresis renography. Br J Urol 61:14-18, 1988.

198. Dockery WD, Stolpen AH: State-of-the-art magnetic resonance imaging of the kidneys and upper urinary tract. J Endourol 13: 417-423, 1999.

199. Jung P, Brauers A, Nolte-Ernsting CA, et al: Magnetic resonance urography enhanced by gadolinium and diuretics: A comparison with conventional urography in diagnosing the cause of ureteric obstruction. Br J Urol Int 86:960-965, 2000.

200. Rothpearl A, Frager D, Subramanian A, et al: MR urography: Technique and application. Radiology 194:125-130, 1995.

201. Roy C, Saussine C, Guth S, et al: MR urography in the evaluation of urinary tract obstruction. Abdom Imaging 23:27-34, 1998.

202. Wolf JS Jr, Siegel CL, Brink JA, et al: Imaging for ureteropelvic junction obstruction in adults. J Endourol 10:93-104, 1996.

203. Whitaker RH: Perfussion pressure flow studies. In O'Reilly PH, George NJ, Weiss RM (eds): Diagnostic Techniques in Urology. Philadelphia, WB Saunders, 1990, pp 135-141.

204. Whitaker RH, Buxton-Thomas MS: A comparison of pressure flow studies and renography in equivocal upper urinary tract obstruction. J Urol 131:446-449, 1984.

205. Streem SB, Franke JJ, Smith AJ: Management of upper urinary tract obstruction. In Walsh DS, Retik AB, Vaughan ED Jr, Wein AJ, (eds): Campbell's Urology, 8th ed. Philadelphia, WB Saunders, 2002, pp 463-512.

206. Streem SB, Preminger GM. Surgical management of calculous diseases. In Gillenwater JY, Grayhack JT, Howards SS, Mitchell ME (eds): Adult and Pediatric Urology, 4th ed. Philadelphia, Lippincott Williams & Wilkins, 2002, pp 393-448.

207. Dal Canton A, Stanziale R, Corradi A, et al: Effects of acute ureteral obstruction on glomerular hemodynamics in rat kidney. Kidney Int 12:403-411, 1977.

208. Ichikawa I: Evidence for altered glomerular hemodynamics during acute nephron obstruction. Am J Physiol 242:F580-F585, 1982.

209. Gaudio KM, Siegel NJ, Hayslett JP, et al: Renal perfusion and intratubular pressure during ureteral occlusion in the rat. Am J Physiol 238:F205-F209, 1980.

210. Vaughan ED Jr, Shenasky JH 2nd, Gillenwater JY: Mechanism of acute hemodynamic response to ureteral occlusion. Invest Urol 9: 109-118, 1971.

211. Navar LG, Baer PG: Renal autoregulatory and glomerular filtration responses to gradated ureteral obstruction. Nephron 7:301-316, 1970.

212. Wright FS, Briggs JP: Feedback control of glomerular blood flow, pressure, and filtration rate. Physiol Rev 59:958-1006, 1979.

213. Schramm LP, Carlson DE: Inhibition of renal vasoconstriction by elevated ureteral pressure. Am J Physiol 228:1126-1133, 1975.

214. Francisco LL, Hoversten LG, DiBona GF: Renal nerves in the compensatory adaptation to ureteral occlusion. Am J Physiol 238: F229-F234, 1980.

215. Allen JT, Vaughan ED Jr, Gillenwater JY: The effect of indomethacin on renal blood flow and ureteral pressure in unilateral ureteral obstruction in awake dogs. Invest Urol 15:324-327, 1978.

216. Blackshear JL, Wathen RL: Effects of indomethacin on renal blood flow and renin secretory responses to ureteral occlusion in the dog. Miner Electrolyte Metab 1:271-278, 1978.

217. Harris RH, Gill JM: Changes in glomerular filtration rate during complete ureteral obstruction in rats. Kidney Int 19:603-608, 1981.

218. Moody TE, Vaughn ED Jr, Gillenwater JY: Relationship between renal blood flow and ureteral pressure during 18 hours of total unilateral ureteral occlusion. Implications for changing sites of increased renal resistance. Invest Urol 13:246-251, 1975.

219. Harris RH, Yarger WE: Renal function after release of unilateral ureteral obstruction in rats. Am J Physiol 227:806-815, 1974.

220. Yarger WE, Griffith LD: Intrarenal hemodynamics following chronic unilateral ureteral obstruction in the dog. Am J Physiol 227: 816-826, 1974.

221. Dal Canton A, Corradi A, Stanziale R, et al: Glomerular hemodynamics before and after release of 24-hour bilateral ureteral obstruction. Kidney Int 17:491-496, 1980.

222. Provoost AP, Molenaar JC: Renal function during and after a temporary complete unilateral ureter obstruction in rats. Invest Urol 18:242-246, 1981.

223. Jaenike JR: The renal functional defect of postobstructive nephropathy. The effects of bilateral ureteral obstruction in the rat. J Clin Invest 51:2999-3006, 1972.

224. Dal Canton A, Corradi A, Stanziale R, et al: Effects of 24-hour unilateral ureteral obstruction on glomerular hemodynamics in rat kidney. Kidney Int 15:457-462, 1979.

225. Tanner GA: Effects of kidney tubule obstruction on glomerular function in rats. Am J Physiol 237:F379-F385, 1979.

226. Yarger WE, Aynedjian HS, Bank N: A micropuncture study of postobstructive diuresis in the rat. J Clin Invest 51:625-637, 1972.

227. Bander SJ, Buerkert JE, Martin D, et al: Long-term effects of 24-hr unilateral ureteral obstruction on renal function in the rat. Kidney Int 28:614-620, 1985.

228. Ichikawa I, Brenner BM: Local intrarenal vasoconstrictor-vasodilator interactions in mild partial ureteral obstruction. Am J Physiol 236: F131-F140, 1979.

229. Ichikawa I, Purkerson ML, Yates J, et al: Dietary protein intake conditions the degree of renal vasoconstriction in acute renal failure caused by ureteral obstruction. Am J Physiol 249(1 pt 2):F54-F61, 1985.

230. Wahlberg J, Stenberg A, Wilson DR, et al: Tubuloglomerular feedback and interstitial pressure in obstructive nephropathy. Kidney Int 26:294-301, 1984.

231. Yarger WE, Schocken DD, Harris RH: Obstructive nephropathy in the rat: Possible roles for the renin-angiotensin system, prostaglandins, and thromboxanes in postobstructive renal function. J Clin Invest 65:400-412, 1980.

232. Vaughan ED Jr, Sweet RC, Gillenwater JY: Peripheral renin and blood pressure changes following complete unilateral ureteral occlusion. J Urol 104:89-92, 1970.

233. Moody TE, Vaughan ED Jr, Wyker AT, et al: The role of intrarenal angiotensin II in the hemodynamic response to unilateral obstructive uropathy. Invest Urol 14:390-397, 1977.

234. Purkerson ML, Blaine EH, Stokes TJ, et al: Role of atrial peptide in the natriuresis and diuresis that follows relief of obstruction in rat. Am J Physiol 256(4 pt 2):F583-F589, 1989.

235. McDougal WS: Pharmacologic preservation of renal mass and function in obstructive uropathy. J Urol 128:418-421, 1982.

236. Morrison AR, Benabe JE: Prostaglandins in vascular tone in experimental obstructive nephropathy. Kidney Int 19:786-790, 1981.

237. Strand JC, Edwards BS, Anderson ME, et al: Effect of imidazole on renal function in unilateral ureteral-obstructed rat kidneys. Am J Physiol 240:F508-F514, 1981.

238. Klotman PE, Smith SR, Volpp BD, et al: Thromboxane synthetase inhibition improves function of hydronephrotic rat kidneys. Am J Physiol 250(2 pt 2):F282-F287, 1986.

239. Loo MH, Egan D, Vaughan ED Jr, et al: The effect of the thromboxane A$_2$ synthesis inhibitor OKY-046 on renal function in rabbits following release of unilateral ureteral obstruction. J Urol 137: 571-576, 1987.

240. Yanagisawa H, Morrissey J, Morrison AR, et al: Eicosanoid production by isolated glomeruli of rats with unilateral ureteral obstruction. Kidney Int 37:1528-1535, 1990.

241. Folkert VW, Schlondorff D: Altered prostaglandin synthesis by glomeruli from rats with unilateral ureteral ligation. Am J Physiol 241:F289-F299, 1981.

242. Schlondorff D, Folkert VW: Prostaglandin synthesis in glomeruli from rats with unilateral ureteral obstruction. Adv Prostaglandin Thromboxane Leukot Res 7:1177-1179, 1980.

243. Schreiner GF, Harris KP, Purkerson ML, et al: Immunological aspects of acute ureteral obstruction: Immune cell infiltrate in the kidney. Kidney Int 34:487-493, 1988.

244. Harris KP, Schreiner GF, Klahr S: Effects of leukocyte depletion on the function of the postobstructed kidney in the rat. Kidney Int 36:210-215, 1989.

245. Reyes AA, Karl IE, Klahr S: Bilateral ureteral obstruction decreases plasma and tissue L-arginine, the substrate for EDRF synthesis. J Am Soc Nephrol 3:551, 1992.

246. Yanagisawa H, Morrissey J, Morrison AR, et al: Role of ANG II in eicosanoid production by isolated glomeruli from rats with bilateral ureteral obstruction. Am J Physiol 258 (1 pt 2): F85-F93, 1990.

247. Harris RH, Yarger WE: The pathogenesis of post-obstructive diuresis. The role of circulating natriuretic and diuretic factors, including urea. J Clin Invest 56:880-887, 1975.

248. Harris RH, Yarger WE: Urine-reinfusion natriuresis: Evidence for potent natriuretic factors in rat urine. Kidney Int 11:93-105, 1977.

249. Brenner BM, Ballermann BJ, Gunning ME, et al: Diverse biological actions of atrial natriuretic peptide. Physiol Rev 70:665-699, 1990.

250. Purkerson ML, Klahr S: Prior inhibition of vasoconstrictors normalizes GFR in postobstructed kidneys. Kidney Int 35:1305-1314, 1989.

251. Kerr WS: Effect of complete ureteral obstruction for one week on kidney function. J Appl Physiol 6:762-772, 1954.

252. Wilson DR: Micropuncture study of chronic obstructive nephropathy before and after release of obstruction. Kidney Int 2:119-130, 1972.

253. Stone DK, Seldin DW, Kokko JP, et al: Mineralocorticoid modulation of rabbit medullary collecting duct acidification. A sodium-independent effect. J Clin Invest 72:77-83, 1983.

254. Nagle RB, Bulger RE, Cutler RE, et al: Unilateral obstructive nephropathy in the rabbit. I. Early morphologic, physiologic, and histochemical changes. Lab Invest 28:456-467, 1973.

255. McDougal WS, Rhodes RS, Persky L: A histochemical and morphologic study of postobstructive diuresis in the rat. Invest Urol 14: 169-176, 1976.

256. Wilson DR: The influence of volume expansion on renal function after relief of chronic unilateral ureteral obstruction. Kidney Int 5:402-410, 1974.

257. Sonnenberg H, Wilson DR: The role of the medullary collecting ducts in postobstructive diuresis. J Clin Invest 57:1564-1574, 1976.

258. Buerkert J, Martin D, Head M, et al: Deep nephron function after release of acute unilateral ureteral obstruction in the young rat. J Clin Invest 62:1228-1239, 1978.

259. Hanley MJ, Davidson K: Isolated nephron segments from rabbit models of obstructive nephropathy. J Clin Invest 69:165-174, 1982.

260. Hwang SJ, Haas M, Harris HW Jr, et al: Transport defects of rabbit medullary thick ascending limb cells in obstructive nephropathy. J Clin Invest 91:21-28, 1993.

261. Miyata Y, Muto S, Ebata S, et al: Sodium and potassium transport properties of the cortical collecting duct following unilateral ureteral obstruction. J Am Soc Nephrol 3:815, 1992.

262. Campbell HT, Bello-Reuss E, Klahr S: Hydraulic water permeability and transepithelial voltage in the isolated perfused rabbit cortical collecting tubule following acute unilateral ureteral obstruction. J Clin Invest 75:219-225, 1985.

263. Hwang SJ, Harris HW Jr, Otuechere G, et al: Transport defects of rabbit inner medullary collecting duct cells in obstructive nephropathy. Am J Physiol 264(5 pt 2):F808-F815, 1993.

264. Li C, Wang W, Kwon TH, et al: Altered expression of major renal Na transporters in rats with unilateral ureteral obstruction. Am J Physiol Renal Physiol 284:F155-F166, 2003.

265. Hwang S, Hu G, Charness ME, et al: Regulation of Na/K-ATPase expression in obstructive uropathy [abstract]. Clin Res 41:141A, 1993.

266. Zeidel ML, Seifter JL, Lear S, et al: Atrial peptides inhibit oxygen consumption in kidney medullary collecting duct cells. Am J Physiol 251(2 pt 20):F379-F383, 1986.

267. Zeidel ML: Hormonal regulation of inner medullary collecting duct sodium transport. Am J Physiol 265(2 pt 2):F159-F173, 1993.

268. Eveloff J, Bayerdorffer E, Silva P, et al: Sodium-chloride transport in the thick ascending limb of Henle's loop. Oxygen consumption studies in isolated cells. Pflugers Arch 389:263-270, 1981.

269. Grossman EB, Hebert SC: Modulation of Na-K-ATPase activity in the mouse medullary thick ascending limb of Henle. Effects of mineralocorticoids and sodium. J Clin Invest 81:885-892, 1988.

270. Petty KJ, Kokko JP, Marver D: Secondary effect of aldosterone on Na-K-ATPase activity in the rabbit cortical collecting tubule. J Clin Invest 68:1514-1521, 1981.

271. Rokaw MD, Sarac E, Lechman E, et al: Chronic regulation of transepithelial Na$^+$ transport by the rate of apical Na$^+$ entry. Am J Physiol 270(2 pt 1):C600-C607, 1996.

272. Wang J-M, Hui D, Edinger RS, et al: Intrinsic regulation of Na$^+$ transport in A6 cells [abstract]. J Am Soc Nephrol 9:A250, 1998.

273. Okegawa T, Jones PE, DeSchryver K, et al: Metabolic and cellular alterations underlying the exaggerated renal prostaglandin and thromboxane synthesis in ureter obstruction in rabbits. Inflammatory response involving fibroblasts and mononuclear cells. J Clin Invest 71:81-90, 1983.

274. Smith WL, Bell TG, Needleman P: Increased renal tubular synthesis of prostaglandins in the rabbit kidney in response to ureteral obstruction. Prostaglandins 18:269-277, 1979.

275. Lear S, Silva P, Kelley VE, et al: Prostaglandin E$_2$ inhibits oxygen consumption in rabbit medullary thick ascending limb. Am J Physiol 258(5 pt 2): F1372-F1378, 1990.

276. Jabs K, Zeidel ML, Silva P: Prostaglandin E$_2$ inhibits Na$^+$-K$^+$-ATPase activity in the inner medullary collecting duct. Am J Physiol 257(3 pt 2):F424-F430, 1989.

277. Stokes JB, Kokko JP: Inhibition of sodium transport by prostaglandin E$_2$ across the isolated, perfused rabbit collecting tubule. J Clin Invest 59:1099-1104, 1977.

278. Stokes JB: Sodium and potassium transport by the collecting duct. Kidney Int 38:679-686, 1990.

279. Stokes JB: Effect of prostaglandin E$_2$ on chloride transport across the rabbit thick ascending limb of Henle. Selective inhibitions of the medullary portion. J Clin Invest 495-502, 1979.

280. Strange K: Ouabain-induced cell swelling in rabbit cortical collecting tubule: NaCl transport by principal cells. J Membr Biol 107: 249-261, 1989.

281. Marver D, Bernabe J: Inhibition of Na/K-ATPase by PGE$_2$ [abstract]. J Am Soc Nephrol 3:500A, 1992.

282. Cordova HR, Kokko JP, Marver D: Chronic indomethacin increases rabbit cortical collecting tubule Na$^+$-K$^+$-ATPase activity. Am J Physiol 256(4 pt 2):F570-F576, 1989.

283. Zeidel ML, Strange K, Emma F, et al: Mechanisms and regulation of water transport in the kidney. Semin Nephrol 13:155-167, 1993.

284. Harris HW Jr, Strange K, Zeidel ML: Current understanding of the cellular biology and molecular structure of the antidiuretic hormone–stimulated water transport pathway. J Clin Invest 88:1-8, 1991.

285. Zeidel ML: Recent advances in water transport. Semin Nephrol 18:167-177, 1998.

286. Frokiaer J, Marples D, Knepper MA, et al: Bilateral ureteral obstruction downregulates expression of vasopressin-sensitive AQP-2 water channel in rat kidney. Am J Physiol 270(4 pt 2): F657-F668, 1996.

287. Frokiaer J, Christensen BM, Marples D, et al: Downregulation of aquaporin-2 parallels changes in renal water excretion in unilateral ureteral obstruction. Am J Physiol 273(2 pt 2):F213-F223, 1997.

288. Li C, Wang W, Knepper MA, et al: Downregulation of renal aquaporins in response to unilateral ureteral obstruction. Am J Physiol 284:F1066-F1079, 2003.

289. Li C, Wang W, Kwon TH, et al: Downregulation of AQP1, -2, and -3 after ureteral obstruction is associated with a long-term urine-concentrating defect. Am J Physiol Renal Physiol 281:F163-F171, 2001.

290. Ribeiro C, Suki WN: Acidification in the medullary collecting duct following ureteral obstruction. Kidney Int 29:1167-1171, 1986.

291. Laski ME, Kurtzman NA: Site of the acidification defect in the perfused postobstructed collecting tubule. Mine Electrolyte Metab 15:195-200, 1989.

292. Purcell H, Bastani B, Harris KP, et al: Cellular distribution of H(+)-ATPase following acute unilateral ureteral obstruction in rats. Am J Physiol 261(3 pt 2):F365-F376, 1991.

293. Blondin J, Purkerson ML, Rolf D, et al: Renal function and metabolism after relief of unilateral ureteral obstruction. Proc Soc Exp Biol Med 150:71-76, 1975.

294. Klahr S, Schwab SJ, Stokes TJ: Metabolic adaptations of the nephron in renal disease. Kidney Int 29:80-89, 1986.

295. Buerkert J, Head M, Klahr S: Effects of acute bilateral ureteral obstruction on deep nephron and terminal collecting duct function in the young rat. J Clin Invest 59:1055-1065, 1977.

296. McDougal WS, Wright FS: Defect in proximal and distal sodium transport in postobstructive diuresis. Kidney Int 2:304-317, 1972.

297. Buerkert J, Martin D, Head M: Effect of acute ureteral obstruction on terminal collecting duct function in the weanling rat. Am J Physiol 236:F260-F267, 1979.

298. Thirakomen K, Kozlov N, Arruda JA, et al: Renal hydrogen ion secretion after release of unilateral ureteral obstruction. Am J Physiol 231:1233-1239, 1976.

299. Beck N: Phosphaturia after release of bilateral ureteral obstruction in rats. Am J Physiol 237:F14-F19, 1979.

300. Purkerson ML, Rolf DB, Chase LR, et al: Tubular reabsorption of phosphate after release of complete ureteral obstruction in the rat. Kidney Int 5:326-336, 1974.

301. Purkerson ML, Slatopolsky E, Klahr S: Urinary excretion of magnesium, calcium, and phosphate after release of unilateral ureteral obstruction in the rat. Miner Electrolyte Metab 6:182-189, 1981.

302. Stecker JF Jr, Vaughan ED Jr, Gillenwater JY: Alteration in renal metabolism occurring in ureteral obstruction in vivo. Surg Gynecol Obstet 133:846-848, 1971.

303. Nito H, Descoeudres C, Kurokawa K, et al: Effect of unilateral obstruction on renal cell metabolism and function. J Lab Clin Med 91:60-71, 1978.

304. Storch S, Saggi S, Megyesi J, et al: Ureteral obstruction decreases renal prepro-epidermal growth factor and Tamm-Horsfall expression. Kidney Int 42:89-94, 1992.

305. Sawczuk IS, Hoke G, Olsson CA, et al: Gene expression in response to acute unilateral ureteral obstruction. Kidney Int 35:1315-1319, 1989.

306. Klahr S, Morrissey J: Obstructive nephropathy and renal fibrosis. Am J Physiol Renal Physiol 283:F861-F875, 2002.

307. Attar R, Quinn F, Winyard PJ, et al: Short-term urinary flow impairment deregulates PAX2 and PCNA expression and cell survival in fetal sheep kidneys. Am J Pathol 152:1225-1235, 1998.

308. Beck AD: The effect of intra-uterine urinary obstruction upon the development of the fetal kidney. J Urol 105:784-789, 1971.

309. Ayan S, Roth JA, Freeman MR, et al: Partial ureteral obstruction dysregulates the renal renin-angiotensin system in the fetal sheep kidney. Urology 58:301-306, 2001.

310. Klahr S: Urinary tract obstruction. Semin Nephrol 21:133-145, 2001.

311. Berman DJ, Maizels M: The role of urinary obstruction in the genesis of renal dysplasia. A model in the chick embryo. J Urol 128: 1091-1096, 1982.

312. Peters CA, Carr MC, Lais A, et al: The response of the fetal kidney to obstruction. J Urol 148(2 pt 2):503-509, 1992.

313. Agarwal SK, Fisk NM: In utero therapy for lower urinary tract obstruction. Prenat Diagn 21:970-976, 2001.

314. Edouga D, Hugueny B, Gasser B, et al: Recovery after relief of fetal urinary obstruction: Morphological, functional and molecular aspects. Am J Physiol Renal Physiol 281:F26-F37, 2001.

315. Bunduki V, Saldanha LB, Sadek L, et al: Fetal renal biopsies in obstructive uropathy: Feasibility and clinical correlations—preliminary results. Prenat Diagn 18:101-109, 1998.

316. Freedman AL, Johnson MP, Smith CA, et al: Long-term outcome in children after antenatal intervention for obstructive uropathies. Lancet 354:374-377, 1999.

317. Chevalier RL, Klahr S: Therapeutic approaches in obstructive uropathy. Semin Nephrol 18:652-658, 1998.

318. Auge BK, Preminger GM: Ureteral stents and their use in endourology. Curr Opin Urol 12:217-222, 2002.

319. Eiley DM, McDougall EM, Smith AD: Techniques for stenting the normal and obstructed ureter. J Endourol 11:419-429, 1997.

320. Watson G: Problems with double-J stents and nephrostomy tubes. J Endourol 11:413-417, 1997.

321. Lepor H, Lowe FC: Evaluation and nonsurgical management of benign prostatic hyperplasia. *In* Walsh DS, Retik AB, Vaughan ED, Wein AJ (eds): Campbell's Urology, 8th ed. Philadelphia, WB Saunders, 2002, pp 1337-1378.

322. Wyndaele JJ: Intermittent catheterization: Which is the optimal technique? Spinal Cord 40:432-437, 2002.

323. Nijman RJ: Neurogenic and non-neurogenic bladder dysfunction. Curr Opin Urol 11:577-583, 2001.

324. Jezernik S, Craggs M, Grill WM, et al: Electrical stimulation for the treatment of bladder dysfunction: Current status and future possibilities. Neurol Res 24:413-430, 2002.

325. Gillenwater JY, Grayhack JT, Howards SS, et al: Adult and Pediatric Urology, 4th ed. Philadelphia, Lippincott Williams & Wilkins, 2002.

326. Walsh PC, Retik AB, Vaughan ED, et al: Campbell's Urology, 8th ed. Philadelphia, WB Saunders; 2002.

327. Lewis HY, Pierce JM: Return of renal function after relief of complete ureteral obstruction of 69 days' duration. J Urol 88:377-379, 1962.

328. Shapiro SR, Bennett AH: Recovery of renal function after prolonged unilateral ureteral obstruction. J Urol 115:136-140, 1976.

329. Bishop MC: Diuresis and renal functional recovery in chronic retention. Br J Urol 57:1-5, 1985.

330. Sarmina I, Resnick MI: Obstructive uropathy in patients with benign prostatic hyperplasia. J Urol 141:866-869, 1989.

331. Bricker NS, Shwayri EI, Readan JB, et al: An abnormality in renal function resulting from urinary tract obstruction. Am J Med 23: 554-564, 1957.

332. Ibrahim HN, Rosenberg ME, Hostetter TH: Role of the renin-angiotensin-aldosterone system in the progression of renal disease: A critical review. Semin Nephrol 17:431-440, 1997.

333. Egido J: Vasoactive hormones and renal sclerosis. Kidney Int 49: 578-597, 1996.

334. Chobanian MC, Julin CM: Angiotensin II stimulates ammoniagenesis in canine renal proximal tubule segments. Am J Physiol 260 (1 pt 2):F19-F26, 1991.

335. Moridaira K, Morrissey J, Fitzgerald M, et al: ACE inhibition increases expression of the ETB receptor in kidneys of mice with unilateral obstruction. Am J Physiol Renal Physiol 284:F209-F217, 2003.

336. Massry SG, Schainuck LI, Goldsmith C, et al: Studies on the mechanism of diuresis after relief of urinary-tract obstruction. Ann Intern Med 66:149-158, 1967.

337. Muldowney FP, Duffy GJ, Kelly DG, et al: Sodium diuresis after relief of obstructive uropathy. N Engl J Med 274:1294-1298, 1966.

338. Peterson LJ, Yarger WE, Schocken DD, et al: Post-obstructive diuresis: a varied syndrome. J Urol 113:190-194, 1975.

339. Purkerson ML, Klahr S: Protein intake conditions the diuresis seen after relief of bilateral ureteral obstruction in the rat. Proc Soc Exp Biol Med 177:62-68, 1984.

340. Gulmi FA, Mooppan UM, Chou S, et al: Atrial natriuretic peptide in patients with obstructive uropathy. J Urol 142(2 pt 1):268-272, 1989.

CHAPTER 41

Renal Neoplasia

Eric Jonasch, Daniel J. George, and Michael B. Atkins

Malignant neoplasms involving the renal parenchyma and renal pelvis may be primary or secondary in origin. Although metastatic lesions statistically outnumber primary lesions, the former are usually asymptomatic and either are discovered only at postmortem examination or are of little clinical consequence.

Renal cell carcinomas (RCCs) arise within the renal cortex and account for about 80% to 85% of all primary renal neoplasms. Transitional carcinomas arising from the renal pelvis are the next most common and account for 7% to 8% of primary renal neoplasms. Other parenchymal epithelial tumors, such as oncocytomas, collecting duct tumors, and renal sarcomas, are uncommon but are becoming more frequently recognized pathologically. Nephroblastoma (Wilms tumor) is common in children and accounts for 5% to 6% of all primary renal tumors.

This chapter focuses on the epidemiology, pathology, genetics, clinical and radiographic manifestations, staging methods, and surgical and systemic management of RCC. A brief description of the biology and management of the less common tumors is also presented.

RENAL CELL CARCINOMA

Epidemiology

In 2002 it was estimated that renal cell and renal pelvic cancer would develop in 31,800 people in the United States and that 11,600 would die of the disease.[1] RCC is responsible for 2% to 3% of all cancers and 2% of all cancer deaths. Worldwide, the mortality from RCC was estimated to exceed 91,000 in the year 2000.[2]

The incidence varies widely from country to country, with the highest rates found in northern Europe and North America.[2] Although the incidence is reported to be lower in individuals living in African countries,[2] it is equivalent among whites and blacks living in the United States.[3] Historically, RCC was twice as common in men as women, but more recent data suggest that this gap is beginning to narrow.[3] RCC occurs predominantly in the sixth to eighth decade and is uncommon in patients younger than 40 years. A 40-year-old man's lifetime risk of RCC is 1.27%, and the risk of death is 0.51%.[4]

The incidence of RCC steadily increased from 1935 to 1989 in both females (0.7 to 4.2 per 100,000) and males (1.6 to 9.6 per 100,000). More recent data indicate that the incidence may be leveling off and that the number of deaths is actually decreasing.[5] The 5-year survival rate of patients with kidney cancer has improved from 52% for those with cancer diagnosed between 1974 and 1976 to 60% for those with cancer diagnosed between 1986 and 1993.[5] The latter fact is probably a consequence of the increasingly common diagnosis of disease at earlier stages, which is more amenable to surgical cure, than to any improvement in systemic therapy.

Numerous environmental and clinical factors have been implicated in the etiology of RCC, including tobacco use, urbanization, and exposure to cadmium, asbestos, and petroleum byproducts.[6-9] Cigarette smoking doubles the likelihood of RCC and contributes to as many as a third of all cases.[6, 10, 11] Cadmium workers who smoke have been reported to have a particularly high incidence of RCC.[12] The current leveling-off of the incidence of RCC and the increased relative prevalence in women may result from changes in the incidence and demographics of cigarette smokers. Obesity is also a risk factor, particularly in women, in whom there is a linear relationship between increasing body weight and the risk of RCC.[11] Additional clinical factors associated with the development of RCC include hypertension,[11] unopposed estrogen therapy,[13] analgesic abuse,[14, 15] and acquired polycystic disease of the kidney, which develops in patients receiving dialysis for end-stage renal disease.[16] In the latter condition, the risk of development of kidney cancer has been estimated to be 30 times greater than in the general population.[17] In particular, it is estimated that acquired cystic disease develops in 20% to 90% of patients receiving long-term dialysis, depending on the duration of dialysis,[18] and that RCC develops in 3.8% to 4.2% of these patients.[16, 19, 20] Although many of these cancers are clinically insignificant, some can have an aggressive course[21-23]; consequently, careful surveillance of patients with end-stage renal disease, particularly those receiving long-term dialysis, with ultrasonography and computed tomography (CT) has been recommended.

Genetic factors have also been implicated in the etiology of RCC and include tuberous sclerosis,[24] autosomal dominant adult polycystic kidney disease,[25] and von Hippel-Lindau (VHL) disease.[26] Although most RCCs are sporadic, factors suggesting a hereditary cause include first-degree relatives with the disease,[10, 27-29] onset before the age of 40, and bilateral or multifocal disease.[30] Several kindreds with familial clear cell carcinoma have been identified that have consistent abnormalities on the short arm of chromosome 3.[31-34] Other kindred with papillary tumors have been identified with different genetic abnormalities,[35] thus suggesting that these tumors represent distinct disease entities. A more detailed discussion of the molecular biology of RCC is provided in a later section.

VHL disease is transmitted in an autosomal dominant fashion and is characterized by a predisposition to various neoplasms, including RCC (with clear cell histology) and renal cysts, retinal angiomas, spinocerebellar hemangioblastomas, pheochromocytomas, and pancreatic carcinomas and cysts.[26] Renal cysts are frequently multiple and bilateral. RCC develops in about a third of all patients and is a major cause of death in VHL patients. Cloning of the VHL gene in 1993[36] and subsequent functional and structural characterization of the gene product[37-39] have contributed greatly to our understanding of the genetics of this disease and RCC in general.

Pathology and Cytogenetics

RCC was first reported by Konig in 1826. In 1883, Grawitz hypothesized on histologic grounds that RCCs arose from rests of adrenal tissue within the kidney.[3] Although immunohistologic and ultrastructural analyses currently point to the proximal renal tubule as the true cell of origin,[40] the term "hypernephroma" continues to be incorrectly applied to these cancers.

Renal cell tumors occur with equal frequency in the right and left kidney and are distributed equally throughout the kidney.[41] The average diameter is about 7 cm, but tumors have ranged from less than 2 cm to larger than 25 cm in diameter. Previously, renal lesions smaller than 2 to 3 cm in size were considered to be benign adenomas. Such distinction between benign and malignant tumors is no longer made on the basis of size but rather on basic histologic criteria. Even small tumors have been determined to frequently represent renal carcinoma. Therefore, from a practical standpoint, all solid renal masses require resection for accurate histologic diagnosis.

RCCs have historically been classified according to cell type (clear, granular, spindle, or oncocytic) and growth pattern (acinar, papillary, or sarcomatoid).[41] This classification has undergone a transformation to more accurately reflect the morphologic, histochemical, and molecular basis of differing types of adenocarcinomas (Table 41-1).[42-44] Based on these studies, five distinct subtypes have been identified: clear cell, chromophilic (papillary), chromophobic, oncocytic, and collecting duct (Bellini duct) tumors. Each of these tumors has a unique growth pattern, cell of origin, and cytogenetic characteristics. Table 41-1 summarizes this information and more accurately reflects the increased knowledge of the molecular and genetic abnormalities of these lesions.

Clear cell carcinomas make up 75% to 85% of tumors and are characterized by a deletion in one or both copies of chromosome 3p.[45] A higher nuclear grade (Fuhrman classification) or the presence of a sarcomatoid pattern correlates with a poorer prognosis.[46, 47] Chromophilic or papillary carcinomas make up 15% of renal cancers, are often multifocal and bilateral, and are commonly manifested as small tumors.[48] These tumors also appear to arise from the proximal tubule but are both morphologically and genetically distinct from clear cell carcinoma. Chromophilic carcinomas have been

TABLE 41-1

Pathologic Classification of Renal Cell Carcinoma

CARCINOMA TYPE	GROWTH PATTERN	CELL OF ORIGIN	CYTOGENETIC CHARACTERISTICS		INCIDENCE (%)
			Major	Minor	
Clear cell	Acinar or sarcomatoid	Proximal tubule	−3p	+5, +7, +12, −6q, −8p −9, −14q, −Y	75-85
Chromophilic*	Papillary or sarcomatoid	Proximal tubule	+7, +17, −Y	+12, +16 +20, −14	12-14
Chromophobic	Solid, tubular, or sarcomatoid	Intercalated cell of cortical collecting duct	Hypodiploidy	—	4-6
Oncocytic	Typified by tumor nests	Intercalated cell of cortical collecting duct	Undetermined†	—	2-4
Collecting duct	Papillary or sarcomatoid	Medullary collecting duct	Undetermined†	—	1

*These tumors were previously classified as papillary tumors.
†This classification is based on the work of Storkel and van den Berg.[43]

reported to have multiple genetic abnormalities, including monosomy Y, trisomy 7, and trisomy 17,[49] but no abnormalities in 3p.[50] Although these tumors often have a low stage at initial evaluation and are thus thought to have a more favorable prognosis,[48,51] in advanced stages, they can be as aggressive as clear cell lesions.

Chromophobic carcinomas make up about 4% of all RCCs. Histologically, they are composed of sheets of cells that are uniformly darker cells than those of the usual clear cell carcinoma, with a peripheral eosinophilic granularity. These cells lack the abundant lipid and glycogen characteristic of the usual RCC and are believed to arise from the intercalated cells of the renal collecting ducts.[52-54] They have a hypodiploid number of chromosomes, but also no 3p loss.[55-57] Chromophobic carcinomas are usually well circumscribed, and patients with these tumors generally have an excellent prognosis.

Renal oncocytomas are infrequent, but increasingly recognized tumors.[58-60] Oncocytomas are composed of a pure population of oncocytes, large, well-differentiated neoplastic cells with intensely eosinophilic granular cytoplasm. The cytoplasm of these cells is packed with mitochondria, thus leading to their histologic appearance. Immunohistochemical studies suggest that oncocytomas probably also arise from the intercalated cells of the distal collecting tubules.[59] Pathologic differentiation of a typical renal oncocytoma from oncocytic RCC can be difficult. Some series suggest that 3% to 7% of solid renocortical tumors, previously classified as RCCs, are in fact oncocytomas.[58] Grossly, oncocytomas are generally well encapsulated and are only rarely invasive. Larger oncocytomas frequently have a stellate, central fibrous scar, which is often visible on preoperative radiologic studies. Renal oncocytomas almost invariably have a benign clinical behavior and are rarely associated with metastases, even when the primary tumor is very large. Although nephrectomy is usually the treatment of choice for large renal masses, the possibility of an oncocytoma should be considered with incidentally discovered small renal masses or tumors in a solitary kidney, and thought should be given to performing a nephron-sparing partial, rather than a radical nephrectomy.

Collecting duct (Bellini duct) tumors are also very rare but are frequently very aggressive in behavior.[61] This tumor is located in the renal medulla and pelvis and thus is usually characterized by gross hematuria. In contrast to clear cell carcinomas, these tumors produce mucin and react with antibodies to both high- and low-molecular-weight keratins.[62] Sarcomatoid variants have also been noted. Neither oncocytomas nor collecting duct tumors have been associated with a consistent pattern of genetic abnormalities.

Molecular Biology

Individuals who inherit a mutated version of the VHL tumor suppressor gene are predisposed to clear cell RCC, which is the most common form of kidney cancer. Tumor development in this setting is linked to somatic inactivation of the remaining wild-type allele. Moreover, biallelic VHL inactivation as a result of somatic mutations or hypermethylation (or both) is observed in over 50% of sporadic clear cell carcinomas. Restoration of VHL function in VHL (−/−) RCC cell lines suppresses their ability to form tumors in nude mice xenograft assays, in keeping with the notion that VHL is a renal cancer tumor suppressor gene.[63]

VHL-associated tumors are typically hypervascular and occasionally lead to the overproduction of red blood cells (polycythemia)[64] because of the overabundant production of vascular endothelial growth factor (VEGF) and erythropoietin, respectively. Based on the knowledge that these two genes can be induced by hypoxia, several groups went on to show that cells lacking the VHL gene product are unable to suppress the accumulation of hypoxia-inducible genes, including VEGF, under well-oxygenated conditions.[65-67] In short, whereas normal cells produce hypoxia-inducible mRNA only under hypoxic conditions, cells lacking pVHL produce such mRNA constitutively.

The HIF family of transcription factors is at the center of maintaining oxygen homeostasis, and these factors regulate a variety of hypoxia-inducible genes. At present, several dozen HIF target genes have been identified, including those for VEGF, platelet-derived growth factor (PDGF), and erythropoietin. Their protein products play critical roles in the cellular and systemic physiologic responses to hypoxia, including glycolysis, erythropoiesis, angiogenesis, and vascular remodeling.[68] Recently, another HIF target, transforming growth factor-α (TGF-α), has been shown to be a powerful renal epithelial cell mitogen and probably contributes to the development of RCC.[69-71] Overproduction of both TGF-α and its receptor (epidermal growth factor receptor [EGFR]) is common in RCC.

HIF is a heterodimer composed of HIF-α and HIF-β subunits.[68] Whereas the HIF-β subunit is constitutively expressed, HIF-α is normally degraded in the presence of oxygen and accumulates only under hypoxic conditions.[72,73] A 200–amino acid, oxygen-dependent degradation domain described by Huang and colleagues lies within the central region of HIF-1α.[74,75] This region is sufficient to target HIF for degradation by the ubiquitin-proteasome pathway in the presence of oxygen.[75,76] pVHL recognizes an approximately 20–amino acid residue, peptidic determinant corresponding to HIF-1α residues 556 to 575 within the oxygen-dependent degradation domain. Several recent papers have shown that the interaction of pVHL with this peptide is governed by an oxygen-dependent, post-translational modification involving hydroxylation of the HIF-1α proline residue 564 or the HIF-2α proline residue 531.[72, 74-76] Thus, in the presence of oxygen, this residue becomes hydroxylated and HIF is recognized and polyubiquitinated by pVHL. In the absence of oxygen, the modification does not take place and pVHL does not bind to HIF.

A unique subset of RCC consists of papillary renal cell carcinoma (PRC). In hereditary cases, PRC is characterized by the formation of multiple bilateral tumors with trisomy of chromosomes 7 and 17.[77] Recently, the hereditary PRC gene was identified on chromosome 7q31.1-34, and germline missense mutations in the tyrosine kinase domain of the c-*met* proto-oncogene were detected in several hereditary PRC families.[78] In sporadic PRC, mutations of the c-*met* proto-oncogene have been detected in 13% of PRC patients with no family history of kidney cancer.[79] These mutations are oncogenic and create a constitutively active, ligand-independent autophosphorylation of c-Met. These data may underestimate the significance of alterations in c-Met because other mutations, chromosomal duplications (e.g., trisomy 7), and epigenetic events probably increase the frequency of c-MET activation. The ligand for c-Met is hepatocyte growth factor (HGF), also referred to as scatter factor (SF).[80]

HGF-Met signaling has been shown to trigger a variety of cellular responses that vary according to the cellular context. In vivo, HGF/c-Met signaling probably plays a role in growth, invasion, tumor metastasis, angiogenesis, wound healing, and tissue regeneration.[81, 82] A key biologic function has been cell scattering. The process of cell scattering can be divided into three phases, namely, cell spreading, cell-cell dissociation, and cell migration.[83] The HGF–c-Met axis also entails increased cell motility, invasion, and metastasis. c-Met stimulation promotes cell movement, causes epithelial cells to disperse ("scatter") and endothelial cells to migrate, and promotes chemotaxis.

The development of RCC may also involve alterations in genes whose products control cell division, including genes in the *ras* family and the *p53* tumor suppressor gene. Although mutations in the *p53* gene are infrequent in RCCs, the p53 protein is overexpressed in about 50% of all RCCs and may be associated with a more aggressive tumor.[84,85] Such *p53* mutations have been implicated in interleukin-6 (IL-6) overexpression in other tumors,[86] and IL-6 overexpression could contribute to many of the protean clinical manifestations that are often seen with high-grade or advanced renal carcinoma, such as fever, anemia, and liver function test abnormalities (see later). The fact that IL-6 expression has also been implicated in reduced responsiveness to immunotherapy[87] gives this potential connection additional clinical relevance. Nonetheless, the exact significance of these various genetic abnormalities and their true relationship to the pathogenesis and clinical biology of RCC remain to be fully elucidated.

Clinical and Laboratory Features

The clinical manifestation of RCC can be extremely variable. Many tumors are clinically occult for much of their course, thus delaying diagnosis. Indeed, 25% to 30% of individuals have distant metastases, and an additional 25% have locally advanced disease at diagnosis.[44, 88] By contrast, other patients harboring RCC experience a wide array of symptoms or have a variety of laboratory abnormalities, even in the absence of metastatic disease. This propensity of RCC to be manifested as a panoply of diverse and often obscure signs and symptoms has led to its being labeled the "internist's tumor."

In a review of 309 consecutive patients undergoing nephrectomy for RCC, Skinner and co-authors[89] reported in 1971 that hematuria was the most common initial symptom, followed by abdominal mass, pain, and weight loss. Gibbons and associates expanded on these observations a few years later[90] (Table 41-2). With the increased frequency of the incidental diagnosis of RCC[91] (only 7% of cases in 1971), it is likely that the incidence of the specific initial features described by Skinner and colleagues is an overestimate.

The classic triad of flank pain, hematuria, and a palpable abdominal renal mass occurred in only about 9% of Skinner and colleagues' patients,[89, 92] and when it did, the disease had often already metastasized. Hematuria, gross or microscopic, is usually observed only if the tumor has invaded the

TABLE 41-2

Initial Symptoms and Signs in Patients with Renal Cell Carcinoma in Two Series

SYMPTOM OR SIGN	IN 309 PATIENTS* (%)	IN 110 PATIENTS† (%)
Hematuria	59	37
Abdominal or flank mass	45	21
Pain	41	21
Weight loss	28	30
Symptoms from metastases	10	
Classic triad	9	
Acute varicocele	2	

*Data from Skinner and colleagues.[89]

†Data from Gibbons and colleagues.[90]

From Richie JP, Garnick MB: Primary renal ureteral cancer. *In* Rieselbach RE, Garnick MB (eds): Cancer and the Kidney. Philadelphia, Lea & Febiger, 1982, p 662.

collecting system. Gibbons and associates[90] reported the absence of gross or microscopic hematuria in 63% of their patients with proven RCC. An abdominal or flank mass is more commonly palpated in thin adults and those with tumors involving the lower pole of the kidney. The mass is generally firm, homogeneous, and nontender and moves with respiration. Occasionally, hemorrhage into the tumor may cause exquisite pain and tenderness on palpation. Substantial bleeding may lead to clot formation and "clot colic." A sudden onset of scrotal varicocele was reported in up to 11% of patients.[93] Most varicoceles are left sided and typically fail to empty in the recumbent position. These symptoms are usually indicative of obstruction of the gonadal vein at its entry point into the left renal vein by tumor thrombus. This clinical finding should always raise the possibility of an associated neoplasm within the kidney. Often, symptoms or signs related to metastases prompt medical evaluation.[88] Most (75%) patients initially seen with metastatic disease have lung involvement. Other common sites include lymph nodes, bone, and liver. Patients may have pathologic fractures, cough, hemoptysis, dyspnea related to pleural effusions, or palpable nodal masses. Clear cell pathology in the metastatic lesion or the finding of a renal mass on staging CT (or both) usually leads to the proper diagnosis.

A number of patients with RCC experience systemic symptoms or paraneoplastic syndromes.[94] The frequency of these various syndromes in combined series of more than 900 patients is detailed in Table 41-3.

Fever is one of the more common manifestations of RCC and occurs in up to 20% of patients.[95] It is usually intermittent and often accompanied by night sweats, anorexia, weight loss, and fatigue. Secondary amyloidosis is found in 3% to 5% of patients.[94, 96] Anemia has been reported in 29% to 88% of patients with RCC[93, 97-99] and frequently precedes the diagnosis by several months. Although hematuria, hemolysis, or bone marrow replacement by tumor may be contributing factors, the anemia is often out of proportion to these factors. It can be either normocytic or microcytic and is frequently associated with both a low serum iron titer and low iron-binding capacity, typical of the anemia of chronic disease. Hepatic dysfunction in the absence of metastatic disease was noted and labeled "Stauffer syndrome"[100] in

TABLE 41-3

Paraneoplastic Syndromes Associated with Renal Cell Cancer Syndrome

	INCIDENCE (%)
Anemia	20-40
Cachexia, fatigue, weight loss	33
Fever	30
Hypertension	24
Hypercalcemia	10-15
Hepatic dysfunction (Stauffer syndrome)	3-6
Amyloidosis	3-5
Erythrocytosis	3-4
Enteropathy	3
Neuromyopathy	3

From McDougal WS, Garnick MB: Clinical signs and symptoms of kidney cancer. *In* Vogelzang NJ, Scardino PT, Shipley WU, et al (eds): Comprehensive Textbook of Genitourinary Oncology. Baltimore, Williams & Wilkins, 1996.

1961. This syndrome, manifested by abnormal liver function test results (particularly elevated alkaline phosphatase, α_2-globulin, and transaminases) and a prolonged prothrombin time, occurs in up to 7% of patients with RCC.[100, 101] Hepatic dysfunction frequently occurs in association with fever, weight loss, and fatigue. The syndrome probably results from the overproduction of cytokines by the tumor, such as granulocyte-macrophage colony-stimulating factor or possibly IL-6.[102, 103] Even though the laboratory abnormalities and other symptoms often revert to normal after nephrectomy, this syndrome is thought to portend a poor prognosis, with few patients surviving 5 years without recurrence.[104] Plasma fibrinogen is frequently elevated in patients with RCC and may correlate with tumor stage and disease activity.[105] Acquired dysfibrinogenemia has been associated with RCC and can be a sensitive plasma marker for the disease and for tumor progression.[106]

Hormones produced by RCCs include parathyroid-like hormone, gonadotropins, placentolactogen, adrenocorticotropic hormone–like substance, renin, erythropoietin, glucagon, and insulin.[107] Several of these hormones have been associated with specific paraneoplastic phenomena. Erythrocytosis, defined as a hematocrit greater than 55 mL/dL, occurs in almost 4% of patients with RCC. Constitutive erythropoietin production by renal cancer cells has been demonstrated by Da Silva and colleagues.[108] Because VHL gene products have been shown to be involved in the regulation of hypoxia-induced proteins,[109] it is conceivable that the erythrocytosis seen in many patients with VHL and some patients with RCC may be directly related to inactivation of the gene.

Hypercalcemia occurs in up to 15% of all patients with RCC. The presence of hypercalcemia has been recognized as an independent negative prognostic factor in patients with metastatic RCC and is usually associated with lytic bone metastases.[110, 111] Hypercalcemia can occur in the absence of osseous metastases, and ectopic production of parathyroid hormone–related peptide by the primary tumor has been documented in these cases.[112-115] In other patients, elevated prostaglandin levels have been implicated in the development of hypercalcemia, which may respond to indomethacin.[116]

Long-acting bisphosphonates such as pamidronate or zolendronic acid are the treatment of choice in RCC patients with metastatic disease and hypercalcemia. These agents may be especially beneficial in patients with lytic bone metastases, in whom such therapy might also reduce the incidence of pathologic fractures.[117-120]

Radiologic Diagnosis

The more widespread use of ultrasonography and CT for other indications has led to the increased detection of RCC as an incidental finding.[91] Incidental detection of renal carcinoma may account for as much as 40% of all diagnoses in well-served medical communities. As discussed in the subsequent section, the prognosis for patients whose tumors were diagnosed incidentally is more favorable than for those who present with symptoms because the former group consists of patients with smaller tumors that tend to be confined to the kidney.[121]

For patients with symptoms suggestive of RCC, numerous radiologic approaches are available for evaluation of the kidney. With the advent of CT, magnetic resonance imaging (MRI), and sophisticated ultrasonography, many of the more invasive procedures of the past have gone out of practice. Although intravenous pyelography remains useful in the evaluation of hematuria, CT and ultrasonography are the mainstays of evaluation of a suspected renal mass. As seen on CT, the typical RCC is generally larger than 4 cm in diameter, has a heterogeneous density, and enhances with contrast (Fig. 41-1).[122, 123] Ultrasonography, though less sensitive than CT in picking up renal masses,[124] is particularly useful in differentiating between a simple benign cyst and a more complex cyst or a solid tumor (Fig. 41-2). The advent of real-time and gray-scale ultrasonography has improved the ability of sonar techniques to delineate homogeneous (sonolucent) from heterogeneous lesions with internal echoes.[125] Smith and Bennett[126] found that ultrasonography alone had a sensitivity of 97%, a specificity of 97%, and a false-negative rate of only 1% in differentiating a benign cyst from a potentially malignant tumor. As a consequence, renal cysts rarely require biopsy to rule out malignancy. Selective renal arteriography, a mainstay of diagnosis in the past, is now rarely used. The typical RCC usually appears on a renal arteriogram as a well-vascularized lesion that exhibits tumor vessels, venous lakes within the tumor, puddling of contrast medium in vascular spaces, or necrotic areas of the tumor and shunting of contrast medium rapidly into the renal vein (Fig. 41-3). Renal arteriography is generally used only in selected cases in which preoperative mapping of the vasculature is necessary, such as when nephron-sparing surgery is contemplated. MRI with gadolinium contrast is superior to CT for evaluating the inferior vena cava if tumor extension into this vessel is suspected.[127] MRI is also a useful adjunct to ultrasonography in the evaluation of renal masses if radiographic contrast cannot be administered because of allergy or inadequate renal function.

Although most solid renal masses are RCCs, some benign lesions complicate the diagnosis. The most common of these rare tumors are angiomyolipomas (renal hamartomas). Unless very small, angiomyolipomas are readily distinguishable from RCC by the finding of a distinctive fat

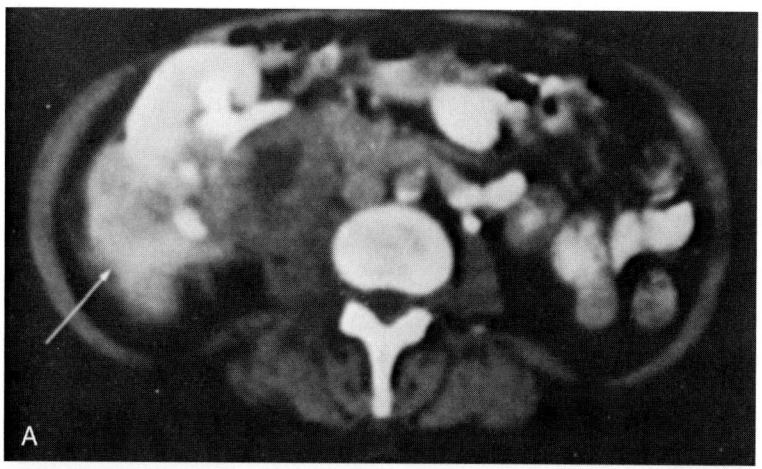

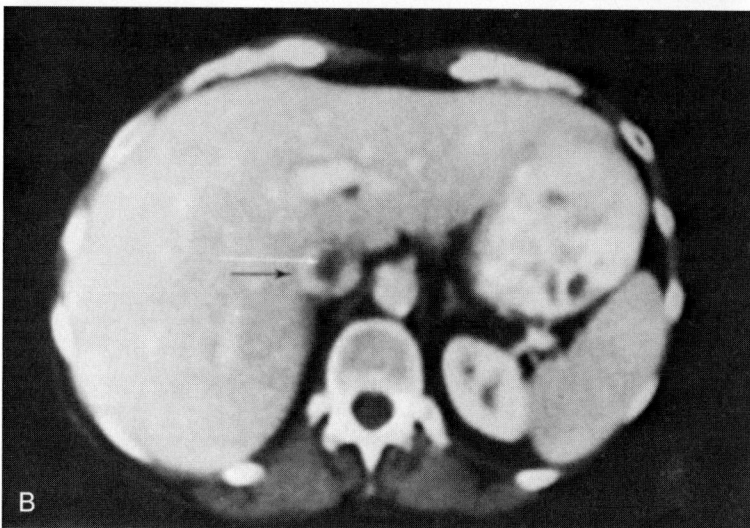

FIGURE 41-1. A, A computed tomographic (CT) scan reveals massive renal cell carcinoma arising from the right kidney *(arrow)* and pushing the kidney anteriorly. Note the distortion of the collecting system. **B,** A CT scan of the same patient demonstrates tumor thrombus *(white arrow)* in the center of the inferior vena cava *(black arrow).* This section was taken at the upper pole of the left kidney and craniad to the right kidney. (From Richie JP, Garnick MB: Primary renal and ureteral cancer. *In* Rieselbach RE, Garnick MB [eds]: Cancer and the Kidney. Philadelphia, Lea & Febiger, 1982, p 662.)

density on CT.[129] However, given that several reports have shown that macroscopic fat can be detected within RCCs, it may no longer be possible to dismiss all fat-containing lesions as benign.[130] As mentioned previously, renal oncocytomas have been described on CT as a central stellate scar within a homogeneous, well-circumscribed solid mass.[58] This finding, however, is nonspecific and does not exclude the diagnosis of clear cell carcinoma.

The role of radionucleotide bone scanning in the initial diagnosis and preoperative staging of RCC is unclear. Although bone scan has high sensitivity for the detection of osteoblastic metastases, RCC usually produces osteolytic lesions that may be missed by bone scan. Atlas and co-workers suggested that the combination of bone pain at initial evaluation and elevated serum alkaline phosphatase levels was comparable to bone scan in evaluating patients with RCC.[131] Others have questioned the sensitivity and usefulness of alkaline phosphatase as a stand-alone test.[132, 133] Koga and associates found bone scan to have a sensitivity of 94% and a specificity of 86%, with low yield in patients with earlier-stage primary tumors. They recommended omitting bone scan in patients with T1 to T3a tumors and no bone pain.[134] Others found that bone scan provided little additional information in patients, even those with a high pretest probability of having metastatic disease.[135, 136]

A number of published studies have evaluated the role of positron emission tomography (PET) in the detection and management of RCC primary and metastatic lesions.[137-144] For detection of primary lesions, Bachor and co-authors reported correct preoperative identification with PET in 20 of 26 pathologically proven RCC primaries; in addition, three benign lesions were inappropriately PET positive.[142] Goldberg and colleagues correctly identified 9 of 10 malignant primaries and 7 of 8 benign cysts before pathologic confirmation.[144] Most recently, of 17 patients with known or suspected primary tumors, Ramdave and co-workers demonstrated pathologically confirmed true-positive findings in 15 cases, true-negative findings in 1, and false-negative findings in 1.[137] Taken together, these reports suggest a fairly high degree of sensitivity and specificity in providing accurate biologic information on renal lesions, and PET can provide data complementary to that obtained with CT and MRI. Nevertheless, because of its expense, lack of general availability, and limited, if any advantages over CT, PET is unlikely to be used as a stand-alone study in the evaluation of a patient with a solid renal mass.

In the restaging and follow-up of RCC, PET provides information that is complementary to conventional imaging and can alter management decisions.[137, 139, 140] Once again, PET scanning has not been prospectively validated as a

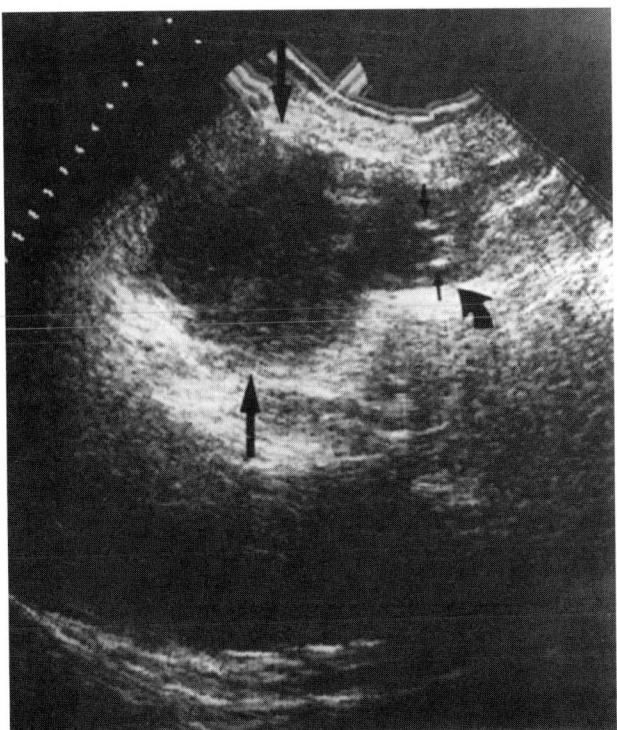

FIGURE 41-2. An ultrasound scan reveals a large, poorly marginated mass *(large arrows)* with internal echoes distorting the upper pole of the kidney (parasagittal posterior view). Note the normal echoes *(small arrows)* from the collecting system in the normal-appearing lower pole *(curved arrow).* (From D'Orsi CJ, Kaplan WD: The radiologic and radionuclide evaluation of the kidney. *In* Rieselbach RE, Garnick MB [eds]: Cancer and the Kidney. Lea & Febiger, Philadelphia, 1982, pp 56-102.)

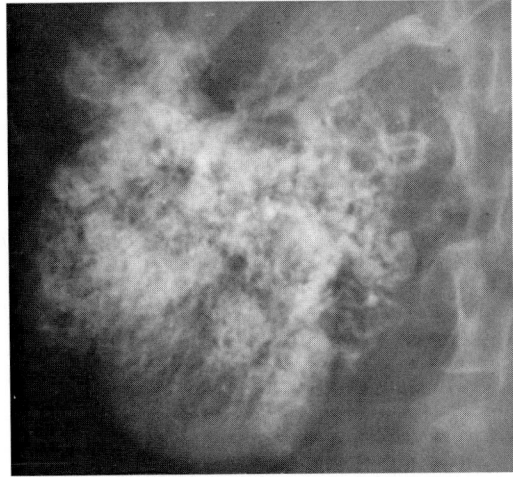

FIGURE 41-3. Selective right renal arteriogram demonstrating typical tumor hypervascularity with puddling in a patient with renal cell carcinoma.

stand-alone study, but it may provide valuable biologic insight on lesions of uncertain significance.

Staging and Prognosis

After the presumptive diagnosis of renal carcinoma has been made, attention must be turned to delineation of the extent of involvement of regional and distant metastatic sites.

TABLE 41-4

Sites and Frequencies of Metastases in Renal Cell Carcinoma

SITE	INCIDENCE (%)
Lung	50-60
Lymph node	30-40
Liver	30-40
Bone	30-40
Adrenal	20
Opposite kidney	10
Brain	5

From McDougal WS, Garnick MB: Clinical signs and symptoms of kidney cancer. *In* Vogelzang NJ, Scardino PT, Shipley WU, et al (eds): Comprehensive Textbook of Genitourinary Oncology. Baltimore, Williams & Wilkins, 1996.

Renal carcinomas can grow locally into very large masses and invade through surrounding fascia into adjacent organs. The most common sites of metastasis are the regional lymphatics, lungs, bone, liver, brain, ipsilateral adrenal gland, and contralateral kidney. The frequency of metastasis to these sites is presented in Table 41-4.[145, 146] Metastases to unusual sites, such as the thyroid gland, pancreas, mucosal surfaces, skin, and soft tissue, are not uncommon in this disease. CT of the abdomen is the principal radiologic tool for defining the local/regional extent of RCC. Although this technique has been recognized to have difficulty in determining the nature of minimally enlarged regional lymph nodes and the cephalad extent of disease within the renal vein, its accuracy in staging RCC is close to 90%.[122] Staging evaluation should also include CT of the chest and a bone scan. Approximately 2% of patients present with bilateral tumors, and 25% to 30% of patients have overt metastases at initial evaluation.[146] If metastatic disease is suspected on the basis of staging studies, pathologic confirmation is usually required before therapy is contemplated. It is often easier and more useful to perform a biopsy on a metastatic site rather than on the primary tumor. CT- or ultrasound-guided percutaneous needle biopsy of a suspected lung, liver, lymph node, adrenal, or sometimes even a skeletal metastasis frequently yields diagnostic material. Mediastinoscopy, bronchoscopy, and thoracoscopy are also frequently useful techniques.

The TNM staging system for RCC (Table 41-5) has largely supplanted the previously used system of Robson. The current staging system as modified in 1998 by the American Joint Committee on Cancer has advantages over the Robson system in that it more clearly separates the various components of locally invasive tumor and quantifies the extent of lymph node and vascular involvement, thereby more explicitly defining the anatomic extent of disease. In addition, the 1998 modification takes into account the finding that even large tumors can have a favorable prognosis if confined to the kidney. Pathologic stage remains the most consistent single prognostic variable that influences survival. Survival based on stage is displayed in Table 41-6.

The more widespread use of ultrasonography and CT for other indications has led to the increased detection of RCC as an incidental finding.[91] The prognosis for patients whose tumors were diagnosed incidentally is more favorable than

TABLE 41-5

TNM Staging for Renal Cell Carcinoma

Primary Tumor (T)

TX	Primary tumor cannot be assessed
T0	No Evidence of primary tumor
T1	Tumor 7 cm or less in greatest dimension, limited to the kidney
T2	Tumor more than 7 cm in greatest dimension, limited to the kidney
T3	Tumor extends into major veins or invades adrenal gland or perinephric tissue, but not beyond Gerota fascia
T3a	Tumor invades adrenal gland or perinephric tissue, but not beyond Gerota fascia
T3b	Tumor grossly extends into renal vein(s) or vena cave below diaphragm
T3c	Tumor grossly extends into vena cava above diaphragm
T4	Tumor invades beyond Gerota fascia

Regional Lymph Nodes (N)*

NX	Regional lymph nodes cannot be assessed
N0	No regional lymph node metastasis
N1	Metastasis in a single regional lymph node
N2	Metastasis in more than one regional lymph node

Distant Metastasis (M)

MX	Distant metastasis cannot be assessed
M0	No distant metastasis
M1	Distant metastasis

*Laterality does not affect the N classification.

TABLE 41-6

Correlation of Stage Grouping with Survival in Patients with Renal Cell Cancer

STAGE GROUPING				5-YEAR SURVIVAL (%)
I	T1	N0	M0	90-95
II	T2	N0	M0	70-85
III	T3a	N0	M0	50-65
	T3b	N0	M0	50-65
	T3c	N0	M0	45-50
	T1	N1	M0	25-30
	T2	N1	M0	25-30
	T3	N1	M0	15-20
IV	T4	Any N	M0	10
	Any T	N2	M0	10
Any T	Any N	Any N	M1	<5

M, distant metastasis; N, nodes; T, tumor.

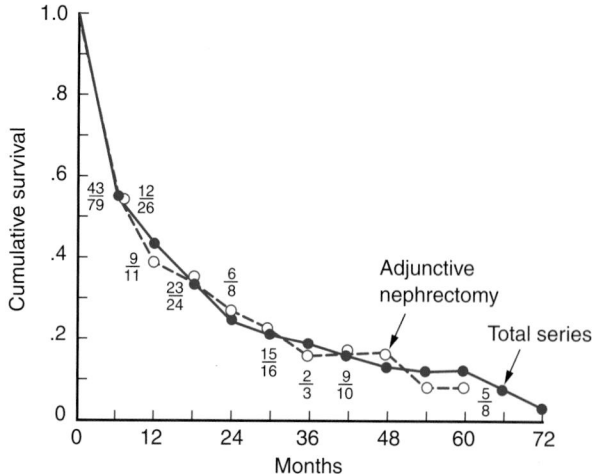

FIGURE 41-4. Survival rates in a series of 86 patients with metastatic renal cell carcinoma treated by various modalities are compared with the survival of patients treated with adjunctive nephrectomy. (From DeKernion JB, Ramming KP, Smith RB: Natural history of metastatic renal cell carcinoma: Computer analysis. J Urol 120:148, 1978.)

for those who present with symptoms because the former group consists of patients with earlier-stage disease. Specifically, patients with incidentally detected renal carcinoma typically have smaller tumors that tend to be confined to the kidney.[121]

Other factors in addition to stage have a bearing on prognosis. For example, oncocytomas rarely metastasize, even when they are large, and therefore have a more favorable prognosis. Although chromophobe and papillary tumors are generally thought to have a better prognosis than clear cell tumors, they appear to be less responsive to systemic therapy; therefore, when metastatic, these tumors may actually have a worse prognosis. Collecting duct cancer is an aggressive disease that tends to occur in younger patients and metastasize early. For clear cell carcinoma, clinical factors

that influence survival include performance status and the presence of paraneoplastic signs or symptoms such as anemia, hypercalcemia, hepatopathy, fever, or weight loss.[147-149] Various microscopic features, such as Fuhrman nuclear grade, sarcomatoid histology, or granular cytoplasm, and biologic features, such as IL-6 or VEGF production, also may be useful in predicting survival.[10, 84-86, 148] UCLA investigators determined the following clinical features at initial evaluation to be independent of stage and associated with poor survival: an Eastern Cooperative Oncology Group (ECOG) performance status of 2 or more, weight loss of more than 10% within the past 6 months, erythrocyte sedimentation rate higher than 50 mm/hr, and hemoglobin less than 10 mg/dL.[150] In addition, Motzer and colleagues recently examined features predictive of survival in 670 patients with stage IV disease enrolled in clinical trials at Memorial Sloan-Kettering Cancer Center. Significant factors predictive of a poor outcome in multivariate analysis included Karnofsky performance status less than 80%, hemoglobin less than 10 mg/dL, serum lactate dehydrogenase greater than 1.5 times the upper limit of normal, corrected serum calcium greater than 10 mg/dL, and lack of previous nephrectomy. A risk model was created with these five factors to assign patients to one of three groups: those with zero risk factors (favorable risk), those with one or two risk factors (intermediate risk), and those with three or more risk factors (poor risk). Median survival for the group as a whole was 10 months, but it ranged from 15 months for patients with favorable risk down to 4 months for those with poor risk (Fig. 41-4). Although survival was also superior in patients who were treated more recently and in those who had received interferon (INF) alfa– or IL-2–based therapy (or both), it was uncertain whether these two observations were causally related. In a subsequent analysis examining 463 patients who had received IFN-based therapy, similar prognostic factors were identified, and the median overall survival was 13 months—ranging from 30 months for patients with favorable risk down to 5 months for those in the poor-risk group.[151]

Surgical Management

Nephrectomy

The mainstay of treatment of primary RCC is surgical excision or nephrectomy. Nephrectomy is the only proven curative modality. Radical nephrectomy, which involves early ligation of the renal artery and renal vein and en bloc excision of the kidney with the surrounding Gerota fascia and ipsilateral adrenal gland, became the procedure of choice in the 1960s.[152] A 5-year survival rate of 66% was reported with this procedure, which compares favorably with the previously reported surgical survival rate of 48% for simple nephrectomy. Various surgical approaches are available for effective performance of this procedure.[152-154] The thoracoabdominal approach described by Chute and associates[154] offers the distinct advantage of palpation of the ipsilateral lung cavity and mediastinum and the opportunity to resect a solitary pulmonary metastasis. Alternative approaches include an extrapleural supracostal incision or an anterior transabdominal incision. Regardless of which approach is used, the principle of early ligation of the vascular pedicle is important to prevent dissemination of tumor at the time of surgery.

With better understanding of tumor biology and changing patterns of initial clinical findings, the value of radical nephrectomy is being reassessed. Involvement of the ipsilateral adrenal gland occurs only 4% of the time, and in most instances, such involvement is associated with direct extension from a large upper pole lesion or the presence of nodal or distant metastases.[155-157] Therefore, adjunctive ipsilateral adrenalectomy rarely contributes significantly to the value of surgery. Furthermore, adjunctive adrenal resection may limit options for effectively treating contralateral adrenal metastases should they arise. As a consequence, adrenalectomy is often reserved for patients with large upper pole lesions or those with solitary ipsilateral adrenal metastases identified on preoperative staging studies. Paul and co-workers demonstrated that tumor size and M stage were the best preoperative predictors of adrenal involvement, and they suggested that adrenalectomy not be performed if the primary tumor was less than 8 cm in size and staging studies were negative.[158]

The benefit of performing regional lymph node dissection in conjunction with radical nephrectomy is controversial. With improved preoperative CT staging, the incidence of unsuspected nodal metastases is low. Furthermore, in patients without clinically evident distant metastases, nodal involvement is found at surgery in only 10% to 20% of patients.[159-161] Although the 5-year survival rate of patients with microscopic nodal involvement (N1M0 disease) can be as high as 50%, less than 25% of patients with N2 or N3 disease and no distant metastases are disease free at 2 years.[162] Although regional lymphadenectomy adds little in terms of operative time or risk, its benefit is largely limited to the prognostic information that it provides. Regional lymph node dissection should be limited to patients being considered for adjuvant treatment protocols (see later).

Nephron-Sparing Surgery

The generally accepted criteria for consideration of nephron-sparing or partial nephrectomy are listed in Table 41-7. Such patients include those with bilateral tumors, tumor in a

TABLE 41-7

Indications for Nephron-Sparing Surgery

Absolute

Bilateral tumors
Tumor in solitary kidney
Tumor in functionally solitary kidney
Patients with compromised renal function
Multiple recurrent tumors (von Hippel-Lindau)

Relative

Localized tumor with progressive disorder that may impair renal function
History of familial renal cell carcinoma
Oncocytoma (preoperative pathologic diagnosis)

Elective

Small (<4-5 cm) polar tumors in patients with normal contralateral kidney

Controversial

Large (>5 cm) tumors in patients with normal contralateral kidney
Centrally located tumors in patients with normal contralateral kidney

solitary kidney, or compromised renal function.[163, 164] The rate of recurrence in the partially resected kidney ranges from 4% to 10% in older series[163-169] and reflects the fact that many patients treated in this manner had large or multifocal tumors. Overall survival was similar to that of patients with comparable-stage disease who underwent radical nephrectomy.[4, 170, 171]

Complications of nephron-sparing surgery include, in decreasing frequency of occurrence, urinary fistulas (7.4%), acute tubular necrosis (6.3%), the need for temporary or permanent dialysis (4.9%), and bleeding (1.9%).[172] Two small studies suggest that a 1- to 2-cm margin is not necessary to ensure local control with smaller tumors and that even a 1-mm margin is sufficient.[173, 174] More extensive prospective data are needed to validate this concept, but it suggests that at least in sporadic RCC, no infiltrative component exists that requires wider excision. A retrospective cost analysis of partial versus radical nephrectomy in 120 cases performed between 1991 and 1997 did not demonstrate any significant difference.

Because of the favorable results seen with nephron-sparing surgery and the increasing number of smaller, incidentally discovered tumors, nephron-sparing surgery has been increasingly used to treat patients with small (<4 cm), polar tumors and a normal contralateral kidney. The primary concern with this approach is that a multicentric tumor would go unrecognized and result in recurrent disease in the salvaged kidney. With highly sensitive preoperative staging, increasing use of three-dimensional reconstruction of CT images, and the use of intraoperative ultrasound, such an occurrence should be relatively rare.[175] Furthermore, patients with multicentric tumors in one kidney are more likely to also have disease in the contralateral kidney, thus supporting a nephron-sparing approach. In patients with small, solitary tumors, the proportion who have local recurrence is 0% to 7%,[172] with a number of series reporting no local recurrence,[164, 166, 171, 176-181] thus further supporting the use of this procedure in appropriately selected patients. Several retrospective series[182, 183-186] and one prospective study[179] compared survival after radical versus nephron-sparing surgery in patients with localized RCC and demonstrated equivalent survival. Nevertheless, most urologists recommend completion nephrectomy in patients documented to have sarcomatoid histology on frozen section or evidence of renal vein invasion.[188] European investigators are conducting a trial in which patients with primary tumors smaller than 5 cm are randomly assigned to undergo either partial or radical nephrectomy. This study should definitively address concerns regarding local recurrence and its impact on overall survival.

The role of partial nephrectomy performed with techniques such as "bench dissection" in patients with larger tumors or centrally located tumors still remains controversial.[189, 190] Partial nephrectomy for this population should be restricted to patients participating in clinical studies.

Laparoscopic Nephrectomy

In 1991, Clayman and co-authors published the first case report of laparoscopic nephrectomy in an 85-year-old woman with RCC.[191] Since then, a number of groups have presented increasingly large series of patients who underwent this procedure.[192-196]

In 1998, a five-institution retrospective review of 157 patients who underwent laparoscopic nephrectomy demonstrated no port site or renal fossa recurrence at a mean follow-up of 19.2 months (range, 1 to 72; 51 patients with 2 or more years' follow-up).[197] Longer follow-up plus comparison to patients undergoing radical nephrectomy was reported in 2002 in a study comparing 64 patients who underwent laparoscopic nephrectomy with 69 treated by open radical nephrectomy.[198] Median follow-up was 54 months for laparoscopic and 69 months for open procedures. Tumors removed via open techniques were on the average larger (6.2 versus 4.3 cm, $P < .001$) than those removed via laparoscopic techniques. Nevertheless, overall survival and disease-free survival were not different between the groups, and this result did not change when stratification of both groups by TNM staging was performed. Meraney and colleagues reported a financial analysis and the operative times of 18 open nephrectomies in comparison to 20 initial and 15 more recent laparoscopic radical nephrectomies.[199] With increased experience, total intraoperative and postoperative costs became less for patients undergoing the less invasive procedure because of the shorter postoperative stay. Although no randomized study has been conducted, the data to date strongly suggest that laparoscopic radical nephrectomy is a viable alternative to an open procedure, with equivalent surgical efficacy and safety and substantially reduced postoperative recovery time.

Most recently, laparoscopic techniques are being applied in the nephron-sparing setting.[200-202] Hemostasis and caliceal repair have been the major theoretical concerns, and thus far, nephron-sparing laparoscopic surgery has been reserved for patients with small, peripheral or exophytic tumors. As surgical experience increases, the use of this approach will probably become more prevalent.

Radiofrequency Ablation

Efforts to develop less invasive techniques have led to the use of radiofrequency ablation (RFA) in patients with small renal tumors, multiple lesions, impaired renal function, solitary kidneys, or significant surgical risks (or any combination of these factors). In 1997, Zlotta and co-workers demonstrated the early ex vivo and in vivo preoperative safety of this procedure in renal lesions.[203] In 1999, McGovern and co-authors published the first case report of a renal lesion completely treated with RFA,[204] followed a year later by a series of eight patients.[205] Radiographic contrast enhancement was used as a surrogate marker of efficacy. Six of nine treated tumors demonstrated freedom from enhancement with a mean 10-month follow-up. Most recently, the same group published a series of 42 tumors in 34 individuals treated with RFA.[206] All 29 exophytic tumors (mean size, 3.2 cm; size range, 1.1 to 5.0 cm) were completely ablated, as were 2 parenchymal tumors. The remaining 11 tumors had a component in the renal sinus. For large (>3.0 cm) tumors, the presence of a tumor component in the renal sinus was a significant negative predictor of technical success; only 5 of these 11 tumors were completely treated versus 11 of 11 tumors without a renal sinus component. Series from other centers[207, 208] have demonstrated similar efficacy and no instance of tumor dissemination or progression. However, Rendon and colleagues reported on 10 patients treated with RFA before surgical removal of small (mean diameter, 2.4 cm) renal lesions[209]: 4 in the perioperative period and 6 at 1 week before surgery. Though safe, pathologic analysis of tumor viability demonstrated between 90% and 100% tumor destruction, with small foci of viable tumor present in several cases. The clinical relevance of these small foci is unclear but demonstrates that careful patient selection and postprocedure follow-up, as well as possible improvement in technology, are all needed for RFA of renal tumors.[206]

Surveillance

Surveillance has also been considered for patients with multiple or bilateral tumors, such as those seen in patients with VHL. Some have advocated waiting until the largest lesion is greater than 3 cm before performing partial nephrectomy.[176] In the past, others have suggested bilateral nephrectomies with transplantation for this population.[171] As improvements occur in nephron-sparing surgery and minimally invasive ablation, surveillance will probably become less common and more drastic approaches such as transplantation less necessary.

Vena Caval Involvement

Inferior vena caval involvement with tumor thrombus is found in about 5% of patients undergoing radical nephrectomy.[210] It occurs more frequently with right-sided tumors and is commonly associated with metastases. Venal caval obstruction may produce various clinical manifestations, including abdominal distention with ascites, hepatic dysfunction—possibly related to Budd-Chiari syndrome, nephrotic syndrome, caput medusa, varicocele, malabsorption, and pulmonary emboli.[210] The anatomic location of the tumor thrombus is important prognostically. Although survival rates in patients with subdiaphragmatic lesions approach 50%, patients with supradiaphragmatic thrombi do considerably less well.[211, 212] A team of specialists is usually required for the surgical management of these patients, particularly if tumor thrombectomy of an intracardiac tumor is contemplated. Even in experienced centers, operative mortality may be as high as 5% to 10%.[213, 214] A minimally invasive technique for extracting supradiaphragmatic thrombus was described by Fitzgerald and colleagues[215]; if generally applicable, this technique may significantly reduce the perioperative morbidity and mortality associated with this type of surgery and shorten the recovery time. Five-year survival in patients with coexisting nodal or systemic metastases is extremely low,[210] and consequently, thrombectomy in this situation should be considered only in the context of a potentially active systemic therapeutic trial, if at all.

Angioinfarction

Angioinfarction is performed with or without nephrectomy for the treatment of patients with metastatic or locally advanced RCC.[216] This approach has been used to reduce vascularity and the consequent risk of hemorrhage during nephrectomy in patients with large, marginally resectable primaries and to control symptoms such as bleeding or pain in patients with unresectable tumors or distant metastases.[217] Several techniques have been developed for embolizing the renal artery, including gelatin sponge pads (Gelfoam), alcohol, and Silastic spheres.[88] Most patients experience pain, fever, and nausea after the procedure that may last several days. Although some investigators have reported regression of distant metastases after sequential angioinfarction and nephrectomy, a survival benefit has not been documented relative to patients undergoing nephrectomy alone.[218, 219]

Debulking Nephrectomy

Patients with RCC who present with metastatic disease have typically been thought to have a poor prognosis, with no 5-year survivors reported in some series.[220] Regression of distant metastases after removal of the primary tumor is an infrequent event that occurred in only 4 of 474 patients (0.8%) in a 1977 database compiled from nine series of patients who underwent debulking nephrectomy.[221] Contemporaneous data on patients undergoing debulking nephrectomy did not show a survival advantage relative to the whole group of patients presenting with metastatic disease.[222]

Responses to immunotherapy are uncommon in patients with primary tumors in place,[223-226] possibly because of the immunosuppressive effects of the primary tumor. Consequently, many groups have advocated that patients presenting with metastatic disease undergo debulking nephrectomy before immunotherapy commences. Two randomized studies have demonstrated a significant survival advantage in patients with metastatic disease who underwent nephrectomy before embarking on a course of IFN therapy.[227, 228] Important caveats to these papers are that nephrectomy did not improve the response to immunotherapy per se and the margin of survival improvement was substantial only in patients with a performance status of 0 or 1. UCLA investigators reported a median survival of 16.7 months and a 19.6% 5-year survival rate in patients treated with IL-2–containing therapy after debulking nephrectomy.[229] In addition, the Cytokine Working Group reported a 21% to 24% response rate in patients who received either low-dose IL-2 and IFN or high-dose IL-2 after recent

nephrectomy.[230] These two analyses suggest that IL-2–based therapy should be considered after nephrectomy in patients with metastatic renal cancer.

Several other reports have indicated that anywhere from 13% to 77% of patients treated in this manner never make it to immunotherapy because of complications of treatment or rapid, symptomatic disease progression,[231-234] thus further emphasizing the need for patient selection if debulking nephrectomy is to be entertained. In recognition of this shortcoming, Fallick and associates[235] developed strict criteria for determining which patients should be subjected to debulking nephrectomy before receiving systemic IL-2 therapy. The criteria used are displayed in Table 41-8.

Palliative Nephrectomy

Although severe local symptoms such as bleeding and pain, systemic symptoms such as fatigue or fever, and laboratory abnormalities such as hypercalcemia have been frequent justification for nephrectomy in the past, such "palliative nephrectomies" are rarely necessary now.[236] Pain and bleeding can often be controlled with systemic pain medication and angioinfarction, clot colic can be minimized with ureteral stents and hydration, and hypercalcemia, fatigue, fever, and other systemic symptoms can often be controlled with nonsteroidal anti-inflammatory drugs, bisphosphonates, hydration, and appetite stimulants such as medroxyprogesterone.[237]

Resection of Metastatic Disease

Surgical resection of metastatic disease has been actively pursued in certain clinical situations. Patients who present with a solitary metastasis have decreased survival relative to patients in whom a metastasis develops after the primary tumor is removed.[222] Nonetheless, it is common to resect solitary metastases or oligometastases, often in the ipsilateral lung or adrenal gland, in conjunction with nephrectomy, with the occasional patient remaining disease free longterm.[238, 239] On the other hand, 5-year survival rates as high as 50% have been reported for patients undergoing resection of isolated metachronous metastases.[224, 240, 241]

Another situation in which resection of metastases has been considered is after effective systemic therapy. Salvage surgery of residual disease after response to systemic IL-2

TABLE 41-8

Criteria for Nephrectomy before Interleukin-2–based Immunotherapy

Greater than 75% debulking of total tumor burden technically feasible
No central nervous system, bone, or liver metastases
Adequate pulmonary and cardiac function
No active infection or significant comorbid condition
ECOG performance status 0 or 1
Predominantly clear cell history*

*Not required before surgery; however, patients in whom pretreatment biopsies reveal a predominant non–clear histology are excluded.

ECOG, Eastern Cooperative Oncology Group.

Adapted from Fallick ML, McDermott DF, LaRock D, et al: Nephrectomy prior to interleukin-2 therapy for patients with metastatic renal cell carcinoma. J Urol 158:1691-1695, 1997.

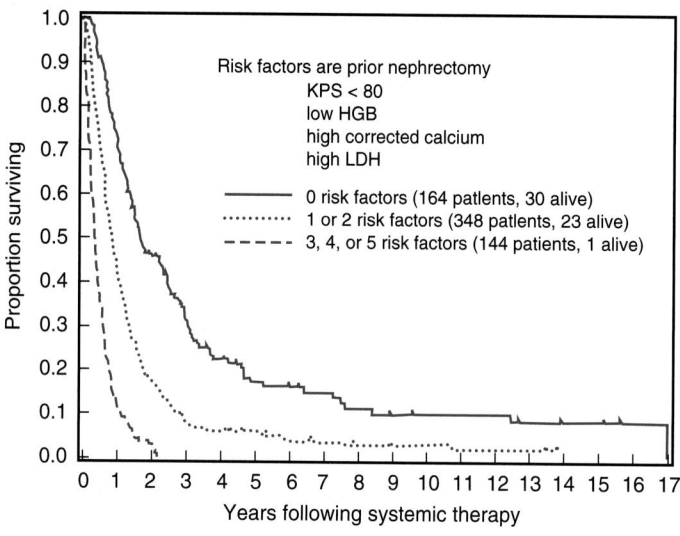

FIGURE 41-5. Prognosis of patients with metastatic renal cell carcinoma. (From Motzer RJ, Mazumdar M, Bacik J, et al: Survival and prognostic stratification of 670 patients with advanced renal cell carcinoma. J Clin Oncol 17:2530-2540, 1999.)

therapy has been effective. Most of the patients who underwent resection while still in response remain disease free long-term.[242-245] Pathologic examination frequently shows an active lymphoidal infiltrate surrounding the residual tumor (Fig. 41-5) or, at times, no evidence of residual tumor.

Radiation Therapy

Adjuvant to Nephrectomy

Studies looking at the possible benefit of adjuvant radiation therapy are few and inconclusive. Only one nonrandomized trial[94] suggested some benefit, whereas two additional studies found no benefit from postoperative irradiation. All these studies used relatively primitive irradiation techniques and schedules that also resulted in a high incidence of complications, including severe liver and other toxicities. A mortality rate of up to 19% was noted.[246] Preoperative radiotherapeutic approaches have produced similarly disappointing results, but trial designs were equally flawed.[247] No well-designed clinical trial of either preoperative or postoperative irradiation in appropriately staged patients with RCC has yet been conducted. In the absence of such data, adjuvant radiation therapy should be considered unproved and be used only in an investigational setting.

Radiation Therapy for Metastatic Disease

The major sites of systemic metastases include the lung, bone, and brain. Radiation treatment of disease in these areas can provide palliation of bone pain, prevention of cord compression or fracture, regression of central nervous system metastases, or control of hemoptysis or airway obstruction. Objective responses occur in about 50% of patients with symptomatic skeletal metastases.[248, 249] Symptomatic improvement is often achieved even in the absence of radiographically documented tumor regression. Radiation therapy is also highly effective in controlling

hemorrhage from bronchial mucosal lesions. Palliation of large renal bed recurrences by external beam irradiation has been unsatisfactory. Some relief of pain has been achieved in about 50% of patients, but it is usually of short duration. In patients with brain metastases, whole-brain radiation therapy alone has not demonstrated significant efficacy.[250] Stereotactic radiosurgery has been reported to be effective in selected patients with small (<3 cm) central nervous system metastases from RCC.[251-253] The presence of more than one brain lesion indicated a higher likelihood for the development of subsequent new brain metastases.[252] Mori and co-authors[251] reported that whole-brain irradiation did not decrease the risk for subsequent new brain tumors, thus suggesting that such treatment may even be omitted in patients who undergo stereotactic radiosurgery. A confirmatory, phase II ECOG trial is now under way.

Systemic Therapy

Although surgical resection of localized disease can be curative, many patients later experience recurrence, and 50% of patients present with either regional or metastatic disease. The prognosis for recurrent or metastatic RCC is poor, with an overall median survival of 12 months.

Patient selection may greatly influence the response rate and survival, and this factor must be kept in mind when evaluating any phase II study. In a multivariate analysis performed in the era before immunotherapy, Elson and associates[254] identified initial ECOG performance status of 0 or 1, a disease-free interval of longer than 1 year, and absence of previous cytotoxic chemotherapy or significant recent weight loss as the strongest predictors of prolonged survival. They divided patients into five prognostic subgroups based on the number of risk factors present. Median survival for these groups ranged from 2.1 to 12.8 months. In other analyses, patients with a single site of metastatic disease and a good performance status appeared to have a more favorable prognosis, with a 29% survival rate at 2 years,[238] and to have a response rate four to five times that of patients with a lower performance status or disease involving multiple sites, particularly the liver or bone, or with intact primaries.[225, 226] Treatment options over the years have included hormonal therapy, chemotherapy, and immunotherapy; however, more recently, attention has been given to more molecularly based targeted therapeutic approaches.

Hormonal Therapy

Numerous trials have explored the role of hormonal therapy in the treatment of patients with metastatic RCC (Table 41-9). These studies were prompted by preclinical studies of estrogen-induced RCC in the Syrian hamster, in which progesterone was shown to be effective in inhibiting both tumor development and tumor growth.[255] Progestins have been the most actively studied clinically as well and have produced response rates ranging from 0% to 20%. Other hormonal agents such as androgens (or antiestrogens) and combinations of hormones and chemotherapy have also produced responses in less than 10% of patients.[256] Subsequent studies using more strictly defined tumor response criteria have consistently produced response rates of only 1% to 2% (see Table 41-9).[257] In reviewing the data on medroxyprogesterone,[258] it was concluded that irrespective of dose or schedule, human RCC is neither hormone dependent nor hormone responsive. Nonetheless, patients with severe anorexia and weight loss may occasionally derive significant symptomatic relief from the administration of medroxyprogesterone, even in the absence of any direct antitumor effect.

Chemotherapy

Many studies of single-agent chemotherapy have been performed, with most agents showing minimal or no activity (Table 41-10).[256] In a review of the chemotherapy literature, Yagoda and co-workers[259] reported a 4% overall response rate in 3635 patients treated with various chemotherapy approaches. Most responses were of poor quality and were rarely associated with a survival advantage, even for the responding patients. The most active drug has been vinblastine, which was reported to produce response rates of approximately 8% to 25%. In a large-scale Scandinavian trial comparing vinblastine with vinblastine plus IFN alfa, however, the vinblastine arm produced tumor responses in only 2.5% of the 81 patients studied.[260] Median time to progression was 2.1 months, and median survival was only 8.8 months for the patients in the vinblastine arm, further

emphasizing the limited antitumor activity of this agent. Response rates with combination chemotherapy regimens are slightly better, but these regimens are also associated with increased toxicity and do not appear to produce a survival benefit relative to single-agent chemotherapy.[256] Hrushesky and colleagues[261] reported a response rate of 20% in 56 patients treated with continuous-infusion floxuridine modified by circadian rhythm; however, other studies have documented this response rate to be closer to 5%.[262] More recently, gemcitabine chemotherapy has been studied in RCC. As a single agent, response rates between 6% and 30% are reported.[263-265] In a recently reported trial, a combination of gemcitabine and 5-fluorouracil (5-FU) demonstrated a response rate of 17% in 41 patients with metastatic RCC.[266] Median progression-free survival in this pretreated group of patients was 28.7 weeks. Efforts are under way in a number of centers to verify these results. In addition, major responses have been reported with cisplatin- and taxane-based therapy in patients with collecting duct tumors.[267] Given that these variant renal cancers respond poorly to IL-2–based therapy (see later), consideration should be given to the first-line use of such cytotoxic chemotherapy regimens in patients with variant (non–clear cell) histology.

Analysis of surface protein expression by kidney cells has revealed a potential mechanism for the profound chemotherapy resistance exhibited by RCCs. The proximal tubule cells of the renal kidney, the purported source of RCCs, have been shown to contain markedly elevated mRNA levels for the multidrug resistance protein (P-glycoprotein/P-170),[268] and the corresponding multidrug resistance gene appears to be overexpressed in most RCCs.[269] Duensing and colleagues[270] correlated P-glycoprotein expression in primary RCCs with a poor overall prognosis, thus suggesting a role for this protein in tumor biology and progression. Other mechanisms of multidrug resistance have also been identified in renal carcinoma cell lines.[271] Efforts to overcome

TABLE 41-10

Single-Agent Activity in Renal Cell Cancer

AGENT	PATIENTS (NO.)	RESPONSE (NO.)	% RANGE	
Vinblastine	296	47	16	(8-25)
5-Fluorouracil	201	10	5	(0-8)
6-Mercaptopurine	73	5	7	(0-17)
Hydroxyurea	140	16	11	(5-20)
Cyclophosphamide	132	12	9	(0-21)
Doxorubicin	65	0	0	
Nitrogen mustard	45	2	4	(4-10)
CCNU	59	4	7	
BCNU	11	0	0	
Streptozocin	15	0	0	
Methyl GAG	54	4	7	(0-16)
Cisplatin	60	0	0	
Chlorambucil	37	6	16	(14-17)
Actinomycin D	37	1	3	(0-11)
Mitomycin C	28	4	14	(11-50)

BCNU, 1,3-*bis*-(2-chloroethyl)-1-nitrosourea (carmustine); CCNU, 1-(2-chloroethyl)-3-cyclohexyl-1-nitrosourea (lomustine); Methyl GAG, Methylglyoxal-*bis*-guanylhydrazone.

Modified from Richie JP, Garnick MB: Primary renal and ureteral cancer. *In* Rieselbach RE, Garnick MB (eds): Cancer and the Kidney. Philadelphia, Lea & Febiger, 1982, p 662.

TABLE 41-9

Hormone Therapy in Advanced Renal Cell Carcinoma*

THERAPY	PATIENTS (NO.)	% RESPONSE (RANGE)
Progestational agents	695	5 (0-17)
Androgenic agents	190	3 (0-14)
Hormonal responses by year of reporting		
1967-1971	228	17
1971-1976	415	2

*Modified from Bodey.[257]

From Richie JP, Garnick MB: Primary renal and ureteral cancer. *In* Rieselbach RE, Garnick MB (eds): Cancer and the Kidney. Philadelphia, Lea & Febiger, 1982, p 662.

these multidrug resistance mechanisms by coadministration of agents that block the multidrug resistance pathway, such as cyclosporine or its derivative PSC 833, have been disappointing,[272, 273] but additional efforts to deal with this problem are ongoing and might yet show some benefit.

Immunotherapy

Immunotherapeutic strategies for RCC have included non-specific stimulators of the immune system, specific antitumor immunotherapy, adoptive immunotherapy, and partially purified or recombinant cytokines. These strategies have been extensively reviewed elsewhere.[274, 275] Many of these approaches have shown some antitumor activity in this disease. Several of these therapies involve laboriously prepared, crude preparations in which the active moieties remain uncertain; consequently, most have been abandoned in favor of the use of purified cytokine-based strategies. Although a number of cytokines have shown antitumor activity in patients with RCC, the most consistent results have been reported with IFN alfa and IL-2. Even though the mechanism of action of these cytokines is incompletely understood, the induction of an antitumor response in mice by IFN alfa and IL-2 has been linked to direct killing of tumor cells by activated T and natural killer cells, as well as to the antiangiogenic effects of these agents.

INTERFERONS

IFN alfa has undergone extensive clinical evaluation for the treatment of metastatic RCC over the past 2 decades. The results of these investigations are thoroughly described in several reviews.[276-278] Despite the use of a variety of preparations, doses, and schedules, most studies have shown antitumor activity, with the overall response rate being approximately 15%. Responses were often delayed in onset, with median time to response being approximately 4 months. Most responses were partial and short lived (median response duration, 6 to 7 months). About 2% of patients have had complete responses, with only an occasional patient having a response persist in excess of 1 year after therapy.[278] Although no clear dose-response relationship exists, daily doses in the 5- to 10-MU range appear to have the highest therapeutic index.[278] The toxicity of IFN includes flulike symptoms such as fever, chills, myalgia, and fatigue, as well as weight loss, altered taste, depression, anemia, leukopenia, and elevated liver function test results. Most side effects, especially the flulike symptoms, tend to diminish with time during chronic therapy.

Recent studies have suggested that the antitumor effects of IFN are quite limited. For example, a phase III trial by the French Immunotherapy Group in which IFN was compared with both IL-2 and IL-2 plus IFN reported a response rate of only 7.5% for the IFN arm and a 1-year event-free survival rate of only 12%.[279] In addition, in a Southwest Oncology Group (SWOG) study comparing IFN alone with debulking nephrectomy followed by IFN, tumor responses were reported in less than 5% of patients receiving either treatment approach. Nonetheless, recent phase III studies have suggested that IFN may have a modest impact on survival in patients with advanced renal cancer. For example, a phase III trial comparing IFN alfa-2a plus vinblastine chemotherapy with vinblastine alone reported a median survival of 67.6 weeks for the IFN plus vinblastine arm versus 37.8 weeks for patients receiving vinblastine alone (P = .0049). In another trial that randomized patients with advanced disease to either IFN or megestrol (Megace), a 28% reduction in the risk of death was noted in the IFN group (P = .017) and a 2.5-month improvement in median survival.

Efforts to improve on the clinical activity of IFN alfa have included combinations with 5-FU, cis-retinoic acid, IFN gamma, thalidomide, and IL-2. For the most part, these strategies have met with limited success, with occasionally promising phase II data[280, 281] failing to be confirmed in phase III trials.

Responses have been reported with IFN gamma as well, although its antitumor activity has, in general, been inferior to that seen with IFN alfa. Phase I and II studies of recombinant human IFN gamma-1b, administered at a variety of doses and schedules, produced an average overall response rate of 11.5%.[282-287] These studies primarily used escalating or maximal tolerated doses of IFN gamma. Of interest, one study by Aulitzky and associates[288] used 100 mg of IFN gamma once weekly, a dose that produced no side effects and optimal up-regulation of neopterin, a biologic marker for macrophage activation, and showed six responses (two complete and four partial) in 20 evaluable patients (response rate, 30%; 95% confidence limits, 12% to 54%). These encouraging results led to a large-scale, randomized, double-blind phase III trial comparing placebo with IFN gamma (60 mg/m^2) administered subcutaneously once weekly. Unfortunately, this Canadian Urologic Oncology Group Trial failed to show any benefit for IFN gamma relative to placebo in either terms of response rate, time to disease progression, or overall survival.[289] In summary, despite some promising early clinical results and the potential identification of surrogate markers of immune activation, single-agent IFN gamma therapy appears to have little or no activity in this disease.

INTERLEUKIN-2 THERAPY

Clinical investigation of IL-2 in RCC began in the mid-1980s. Initial studies were performed with high-dose bolus IL-2 and lymphokine-activated killer (LAK) cells because animal studies had shown a steep dose-response curve for IL-2 and benefit for the addition of LAK cells.[290] Dramatic and durable responses were reported in a small subset of patients.[291] Subsequent clinical studies have shown that high-dose bolus IL-2 possesses antitumor activity that is essentially equivalent to the combination of IL-2 and LAK cells.[292-294]

High-Dose Interleukin-2 Investigations

In 1992, high-dose bolus IL-2 received U.S. Food and Drug Administration (FDA) approval for metastatic RCC based on data from 255 patients treated in seven clinical trials at 21 institutions.[228] In these studies, recombinant IL-2 (Proleukin) (600,000 to 720,000 IU/kg) was administered by 15-minute intravenous infusion every 8 hours on days 1 to 5 and 15 to 19 (maximum, 28 doses). Treatment was repeated at approximately 12-week intervals in responding patients for a maximum of three cycles. Because of considerable toxicity associated with this regimen (hypotension, capillary leak), treatment had to be administered in a setting capable of providing a level of care comparable to that in an intensive care unit, and such treatment was restricted to carefully selected patients with excellent organ function treated at experienced treatment centers.

Data presented to the FDA showed objective responses in 36 of the 255 patients (response rate, 14%).[228] Twelve (5%) complete responses and 24 (9%) partial responses were achieved. At that time, the median duration of response was 23.2 months for all responders (18.8 months for partial responders and no median reached for complete responders). Fourteen of the responding patients (39%) began therapy with tumor burdens greater than 50 cm^2 on pretreatment scans, and 60% of the partial responders had greater than 90% regression of all measurable disease. The quality and durability of these responses were what prompted FDA approval in spite of the relatively low response rate and high level of toxicity.

Follow-up data on these patients have been accumulated through late 1998 (median follow-up, 8 years). The clinical results appear to have steadily improved over time. Seventeen patients (7%) were classified as complete responders and 20 (8%) as partial responders. Survival for the group as a whole was 16.3 months, with 10% to 15% of patients estimated to remain alive 5 to 10 years after treatment with high-dose IL-2. Response duration curves for all responders are displayed in Figure 41-6. The median response duration for all objective responders was 54 months, with a range of 3 to over 131 months. The median response duration for partial responders was 20 months and had still not been reached for complete responders, but it was at least 80 months at the time of that analysis. Eleven patients underwent resection of residual disease, either while still in response or after limited site progression, and 9 remained progression free for a minimum of 65 months. Therefore, a large percentage of responding patients, particularly those remaining free of progression for longer than 2 years or those resected to disease-free status after responding to high-dose IL-2, appear unlikely to progress and may actually be "cured."

Alternative Interleukin-2–Based Regimens

Several investigators have evaluated regimens involving IL-2 administered by alternative routes or in lower doses in an attempt to reduce toxicity. Although encouraging initial response rates have been reported by some investigators, follow-up data and information on response durations have been lacking. Continuous intravenous infusion of IL-2 and LAK cell regimens appeared to produce tumor response rates similar to those seen with high-dose bolus intravenous IL-2.[295-297] Though more convenient to administer, continuous-infusion regimens, on a milligram-per-milligram basis, were actually more toxic than high-dose bolus IL-2. Even with an approximate fivefold reduction in the amount of IL-2 administered per day, the toxicity of continuous-infusion IL-2 was roughly equivalent to that of high-dose bolus IL-2.[296] Furthermore, omitting the LAK cells or reducing the dose of IL-2 further to enable prolonged administration while producing enhanced immune activation appeared to limit antitumor activity.[298, 299]

Sleijfer and colleagues[300] investigated IL-2 administered by daily subcutaneous injection in an outpatient setting. They reported a 22% response rate (two complete and four partial responses) in 27 patients, with the complete responses continuing at 19 and 17 months at the time of publication in 1992. Additional information has not been forthcoming. Yang and associates[301] reported a 15% response rate (7% complete and 8% partial) in 65 patients receiving 10% of the standard high-dose IL-2 regimen (72,000 IU/kg[302] intravenously every 8 hours on days 1 to 5 and 15 to 19). A randomized trial comparing standard high-dose IL-2 with this 10% dose regimen has recently been completed by the National Cancer Institute Surgery Branch. A third arm involving IL-2 administered subcutaneously according to a schedule similar to that described by Sleijfer and co-workers was added later.[303] Although the low-dose intravenous and subcutaneous IL-2 regimens produced significantly less hypotension, thrombocytopenia, malaise, pulmonary toxicity,

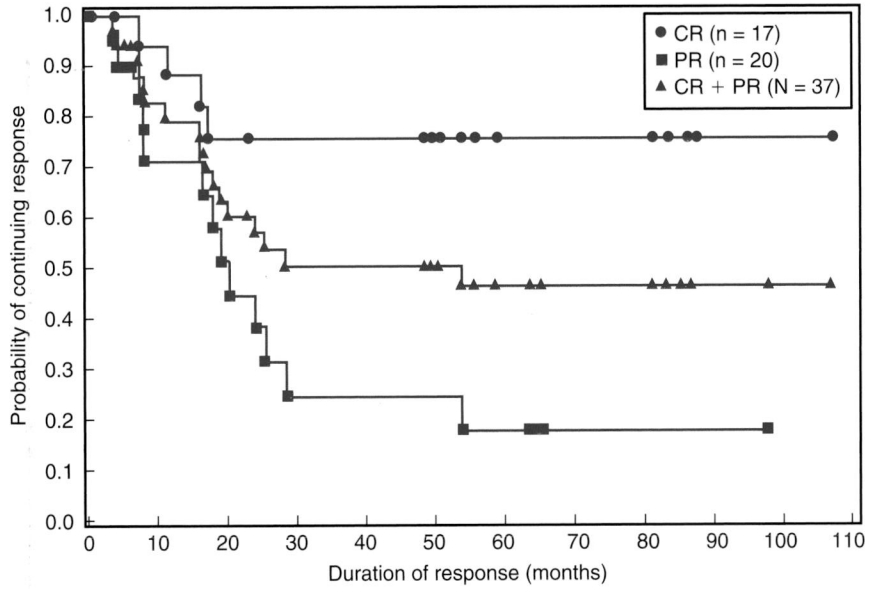

FIGURE 41-6. Response durations for high-dose interleukin-2–based therapy.

and neurotoxicity than standard high-dose IL-2 did, because the side effects of high-dose IL-2 were of short duration, overall quality of life was actually comparable between the treatment arms. Although overall survival was not significantly different between the treatment arms, the response rate was significantly higher for high-dose IL-2 (21% versus 13% and 10% for the two lower-dose IL-2 regimens), and a trend toward improved response duration was noted with high-dose IL-2.[304] These data suggested that high-dose IL-2 remained the optimal treatment for patients who could safely tolerate such intensive therapy.

Toxicity Reduction Strategies

IL-2 is a potent inducer of proinflammatory cytokines such as IL-1, tumor necrosis factor-α (TNF-α), and IFN-γ.[305-307] These substances and others, including nitric oxide,[308] probably play a major role in IL-2 toxicity. Tumor responses, on the other hand, are thought to be mediated through cellular immune mechanisms, which raises the possibility of dissociating the toxicity of IL-2 from its antitumor effect by combining IL-2 with various inhibitors of secondary cytokine function. The addition of dexamethasone was shown to prevent the usual induction of TNF-α by IL-2, and it significantly reduced treatment-related toxicity. However, potential interference with antitumor efficacy limited this approach.[309, 310] The use of more selective inhibitors of secondary cytokine function (e.g., CT1501R, CNI-1493, or soluble TNF-α or IL-1 receptors), despite promise in animal models, has not been able to significantly block IL-2 toxicity clinically.[311-314] Future exploration of this approach will probably require combinations of cytokine antagonists or the use of novel antagonists of secondary cytokines with more pluripotent inhibitory effects.

Interleukin-2 and Interferon Alfa Combinations

Attempts to improve efficacy have included the addition of IFN alfa and then 5-FU to IL-2. In addition to its modest single-agent antitumor activity in patients with RCC, IFN alfa up-regulates expression of HLA class I and tumor-associated antigens, potentially making the tumor cells more immunogenic and possibly more susceptible to IL-2–mediated lysis. Several animal experiments have shown that the combination of IL-2 and type I IFNs enhances effector cell mechanisms and produces antitumor activity superior to that of maximal tolerated doses of the single agents in the same tumor models.[315, 316] Table 41-11 shows the results of several studies involving combinations of IL-2 and IFN alfa. Studies are separated according to the route of IL-2 administration: high-dose intravenous bolus injection, continuous intravenous infusion, subcutaneous injection, or in combination with 5-FU.[226, 317, 318] Although the initial phase I study of high-dose intravenous IL-2 and IFN alfa produced a 31% (11 of 35) response rate in patients with RCC,[317] subsequent high-dose IL-2 and IFN alfa studies achieved response rates that were not clearly better than that of high-dose IL-2 alone.[226, 319-322] Many regimens using combinations of IFN with lower doses of IL-2 administered by different routes, either alone or with 5-FU, were suitable for administration in an outpatient setting. Response rates for these approaches ranged from 22% to 39%.[318, 323-336]

TABLE 41-11

Interleukin-2 and Interferon Alfa Therapy

AUTHOR	IL-2 REGIMEN	N	CR/PR	%
Rosenberg[317]	HD bolus	35	4/7	31
Atkins[226]	HD bolus	28	0/3	11
Sznol[319]	HD bolus	14	1/2	21
Spencer[321]	HD bolus	12	0/1	8
Budd[322]	HD bolus	21	0/2	10
Bergman[339]	HD bolus	36	2/7	25
Figlin[326]	CIV	30	0/9	26
Lipton[324]	CIV	39	6/7	33
Dillman[325]	CIV	3	0/6	7
Morant[340]	CIV	23	5/2	30
Figlin[323]	CIV	22	0/7	32
Besana[327]	CIV	23	1/5	26
Negrier[328]	CIV	140	2/6	19
Atzpodien[329]	SC	34	4/6	29
Palmer[330]	SC	200	7/30	19
Atzpodien[331]	SC	152	9/29	25
Vogelzang[332]	SC	42	1/4	12
Lummen[333]	SC	30	3/4	23
Dutcher[341]	SC	47	2/6	17
Atzpodien[334]	5-FU/IL-2	120	13/34	39
Sella[342]	5-FU/IL-2	19	3/6	47
Hofmockel[336]	5-FU/IL-2	25	3/10	38
Dutcher[343]	5-FU/IL-2	50	1/7	16

CIV, continuous intravenous infusion; CR, complete response; 5-FU, 5-fluorouracil; HD, high dose; IL-2, interleukin-2; PR, partial response; SC, subcutaneous.

Figlin and associates[326] treated patients with low-dose IL-2 administered either by continuous intravenous infusion or by subcutaneous injection on days 1 through 4 together with IFN alfa administered subcutaneously on days 1 and 4.[326] Long-term follow-up data for patients in this trial revealed an overall median duration of response of 23 months and a median duration of survival for responders of 34+ months,[337] although at the time of this report, 10 of 13 responding patients had relapsed and 5 had died. The addition of CD8+-selected tumor-infiltrating lymphocytes culled from pretreatment nephrectomy specimens to this IL-2 and IFN alfa regimen improved the response rate to 34%.[338] However, a large-scale phase III comparison of this approach (omitting the IFN) with IL-2 alone showed no benefit with the addition of CD8+ autologous tumor-infiltrating lymphocytes relative to IL-2 alone.

Atzpodien and colleagues[331] evaluated the combination of IL-2 and IFN alfa both administered subcutaneously at doses suitable for an outpatient setting. Responses were noted in 25% of patients. Subsequently, they developed a regimen that alternated 4 weeks of subcutaneously administered IL-2 and IFN alfa with 4 weeks of combined 5-FU and IFN alfa and reported a response rate of 39% in 120 patients.[334] Response durations and numbers of durable complete responses were not fully reported; however, the median response duration was approximately 12 months for each regimen.

Follow-up trials performed by the Cytokine Working Group failed to confirm the promising results reported by Atzpodien and co-workers.[331] IL-2 and IFN alfa administered subcutaneously with or without weekly 5-FU produced response rates and median survival similar to those observed with high-dose IL-2 alone or high-dose IL-2 and IFN; however, the quality and durability of the responses appeared to be considerably less than those observed with high-dose IL-2.[341] In contrast to the results reported for high-dose IL-2, less than 5% of patients remained disease or progression free at 5 years. However, because these studies were conducted sequentially, selection bias could not be excluded as a cause of these discrepant results.

Investigators in France reported the results of a large-scale, phase III randomized trial comparing intermediate-dose IL-2 administered by continuous intravenous infusion plus subcutaneous IFN alfa with either IL-2 or IFN alfa administered alone.[328] Four hundred twenty-five patients were enrolled. The three treatment groups were well balanced for age and gender, as well as known predictors of response and survival. The response rate and 1-year event-free survival were significantly greater for the combined IL-2 and IFN alfa arm than for either of the single-agent arms, although no significant difference in overall survival was observed among the three groups. Of note, responses were seen in only 6.5% and 7.5% of patients receiving IL-2 or IFN alfa alone, respectively, with only 2.9% and 6.1% of these patients still responding at the week 25 evaluation. Although higher antitumor activity was seen with the combination arm, it was largely due to the very poor activity of the single-agent regimens. How intermediate-dose combinations of IL-2 and IFN alfa compare with high-dose IL-2 alone remained to be established.

The Cytokine Working Group has recently completed a large phase III trial comparing high-dose IL-2 with outpatient, subcutaneously administered IL-2 and IFN alpha. One hundred ninety-three patients were enrolled and 186 were deemed evaluable for response. Patients were stratified according to performance status (ECOG 0 or 1), previous nephrectomy (yes or no), and the presence or absence of hepatic or bone metastases. Tumor responses were seen in 25 of 97 (26%) patients who received high-dose IL-2 versus 10 of 90 (11%) patients who received low-dose IL-2 and IFN ($P = .01$). High-dose IL-2 produced eight complete responses, and nine patients remained progression free at 3 years; with low dose IL-2 and IFN, three patients had complete responses and two patients were progression free at 3 years. Median response durations were similar, but a trend favoring improved survival was noted in patients who received high-dose IL-2, and the trend reached statistical significance in patients with liver or bone metastases. These data once again supported the preferential use of high-dose IL-2 in all patients who have access to such treatment and are deemed able to tolerate the therapy.

Predictors of Response and Survival

Many groups have attempted to determine reliable predictors of response and survival for patients with metastatic RCC who were receiving immunotherapy. Factors that have been variably associated with response are detailed in Table 41-12 and include performance status,[293] the number of organs with metastases (one versus two or more),[328] absence of bone metastases,[226] previous nephrectomy,[225] the degree of treatment-related thrombocytopenia, absence of previous IFN therapy,[344] thyroid dysfunction,[345] rebound lymphocytosis,[346] erythropoietin production,[347] and post-treatment elevations of blood TNF-α and IL-1 levels. Negrier and associates[328] also identified independent predictors of

TABLE 41-12

Factors Associated with Response to Interleukin-2–Based Therapy

FACTOR	AUTHOR
Performance status	Fyfe[293]
Number of metastatic sites	Negrier[328]
Previous nephrectomy	Fisher[225]
Absence of bone metastases	Atkins[226]
Thyroid dysfunction	Atkins[345]
Rebound lymphocytosis	West[346]
Erythropoietin production	Janik[347]
Treatment-related thrombocytopenia	Royal[344]
Low pretreatment IL-6 levels	Blay[87]
No previous IFN therapy	Royal[344]
Post-therapy TNF/IL-1 elevation	Blay[349]

IFN, interferon; IL-6, interleukin-6; TNF, tumor necrosis factor.

rapid disease progression, which was defined as progression within 10 weeks of initiation of therapy. These predictors included more than one metastatic site, disease-free interval of less than 1 year, and the presence of liver metastases or mediastinal nodes, as well as the type of immunotherapy used. Patients with liver metastases, more than one site of disease, and a disease-free interval of less than 1 year had a lower response rate and a median survival of only 6 months, even while receiving combination IL-2 and IFN alfa therapy. Figlin and colleagues[348] identified previous nephrectomy and time from nephrectomy to relaps as important predictors of survival in patients receiving IL-2–based therapy. In their series, patients who received systemic immunotherapy for metastatic disease more than 6 months after nephrectomy had the best median survival and a 3-year survival rate of 46%. Recent data from the Cytokine Working Group phase III trial, mentioned earlier, suggested that disease site factors, such as primary in place or hepatic or bone metastases, may be more predictive of response to low-dose IL-2 and IFN regimens than to high-dose IL-2. Furthermore, this study suggested that the greatest benefit from high-dose IL-2, relative to lower-dose regimens, might be seen in patients with primaries in place or liver and bone metastases (or both). This type of data calls into question the previous studies and suggests that additional predictors of response to IL-2–based therapy are necessary.

Influence of Subtype

Responses most commonly occur in patients with clear cell–type cancer. Occasional responses have been observed in the sarcomatoid and granular variants, but they are usually partial and of shorter duration. Upton and colleagues recently performed a blinded large-scale reanalysis of pathology specimens from patients who received IL-2–based therapy. They determined that response to IL-2 was significantly associated with clear cell histology with alveolar features and the absence of papillary or greater than 50% granular features. Patients with these features in their kidney tumor specimens had a 25% response rate; patients who also had had renal vein involvement had a response rate of over 40%. The results in the kidney tumor specimens were confirmed in a separate analysis of metastatic lesions. In the metastatic setting, responses were limited to patients who had clear cell tumors with the favorable histologic patterns described in the primary tumor specimens. These data strongly suggest that patients with non–clear cell or indeterminate histology or clear cell histology with papillary and greater than 50% granular and no alveolar features should be considered for non-IL-2–based therapy.

Adjuvant Therapy

The ECOG completed a trial comparing adjuvant IFN alfa with observation in patients with high-risk resected RCC. Eligible patients had to be T3b-T3c, T4, and/or N1-N3. Patients were randomly assigned to receive either a year of IFN alfa-n1 (Wellferon) or routine observation. With a minimum follow-up of 36 months and a mean of 68 months overall, no statistically significant difference in disease-free survival was observed between the treatment arms.[350] A smaller study performed by the European Organization for Research in Cancer Therapy (EORTC) also showed no benefit for the adjuvant administration of IFN alfa. Although the results of this study were disappointing, the study was useful in providing information on the natural history of stage III RCC. Specifically, it identified a high-risk group, those with T3c, T4, and/or N2-N3 disease, that had only a 20% to 25% chance of remaining disease free at 2 years.[242] This population was believed to be at sufficient risk of relapse to justify exploration of more aggressive therapy, such as high-dose IL-2, in an effort to prevent or delay relapse. Consequently, the Cytokine Working Group conducted a trial randomly assigning patients who satisfy these high-risk staging criteria to either a single cycle of high-dose IL-2 or observation (with IL-2–based therapy at the time of recurrence). Unfortunately, preliminary review of this trial shows no clear-cut survival benefit for the patients receiving high-dose IL-2 in the adjuvant setting.[351] Thus at the moment, no evidence supports the use of IFN or IL-2 in the adjuvant setting in patients with high-risk renal cancer.

OTHER CYTOKINES

Clinical trials with other cytokines, such as IL-4 and IL-6, have produced only occasional minor responses.[352, 353] A few durable responses have been observed in phase I trials of recombinant human IL-12 (rhIL-12) administered either intravenously[354] or subcutaneously[355]; however, in general, antitumor activity in these studies has been less than predicted by preclinical models. Subsequent clinical investigations have been delayed by the discovery of a peculiar schedule dependency for rhIL-12 whereby a single "test dose" of rhIL-12 has been shown to increase patients' tolerance to subsequent therapy[356] and possibly reduce its antitumor effects. Novel schedules of IL-12[357] and combinations of rhIL-12 with IL-2 have been explored in an effort to sustain the biologic activity of rhIL-12. The results of these clinical trials have been mixed, with considerably more research likely to be required before significant clinical activity for rhIL-12 can be established.

VACCINES

Vaccination with fusions of autologous tumor cells and allogeneic dendritic cells has been shown to induce disease regression in 7 of 17 patients with metastatic renal cancer.[358] Responses were also seen in 3 of 27 patients treated with a vaccine created from tumor lysate–pulsed autologous dendritic cells.[359] Unfortunately, only limited clinical activity was seen with vaccination of fusion cells established from autologous tumor and autologous dendritic cells.[360] Further investigation of this dendritic cell vaccination approach is ongoing, with future efforts likely to include the addition of cytokines such as IL-12 as vaccine adjuvants.

OTHER AGENTS

Given the frequency of biallelic loss of the VHL gene and the associated dysregulation of hypoxia-inducible genes, including the pro-angiogenic growth factors VEGF and PDGF, RCC may be a particularly promising target for antiangiogenic therapy. Among the most promising agents are those that specifically target these growth factors. Phase I studies using bevacizumab, a recombinant humanized anti-VEGF monoclonal antibody, in RCC demonstrated several responses. In a recently reported, randomized phase II study, patients with metastatic RCC who had failed or were not eligible for cytokine therapy were randomized to receive either low-dose bevacizumab (3 mg/kg), high-dose bevacizumab (10 mg/kg), or placebo treatment. The study was discontinued prematurely because of a significant delay in disease progression associated with high-dose bevacizumab in comparison to placebo.[361] Phase III studies of bevacizumab in RCC are planned for the near future. In addition, small molecules that target VEGF and PDGF receptors have shown evidence of clinical response in early phase I studies.[362]

Thalidomide is a putative antiangiogenic agent with initially provocative results in patients with RCC. It has a somewhat unclear mechanism of action but is believed to alter to some extent the expression of angiogenic growth factors in tissues, including VEGF and fibroblast growth factor. Although early anecdotal reports suggested possible objective responses, most reports of even high doses of thalidomide (800+ mg/day) suggest that the agent, at best, results in disease stabilization.[363-366] Toxicity includes somnolence, constipation, fatigue, and with prolonged exposure, peripheral neuropathy.[364] Currently, a large, multicenter, randomized phase III trial is ongoing to determine its clinical efficacy.

CCI-779 is a rapamycin analog that inhibits mammalian target of rapamycin (mTOR) downstream of AKT and results in cell cycle arrest. Atkins and co-authors[367] reported the results of a randomized double-blind phase II trial examining three dose levels of CCI-779 in renal cancer patients who were either refractory to or thought to be poor candidates for cytokine-based therapy.[368] Twenty-nine of the 110 patients enrolled (26%) experienced a partial or minor response. The median time to progression and median survival for all patients were 6 months and 15 months, respectively. The response rate, time to progression, and survival were thought to be encouraging for this population of patients, most of whom had poor prognostic features. No obvious dose effect was evident, with results appearing to be equivalent for doses ranging from 25 to 250 mg. A reanalysis of the trial in which patients were segregated into prognostic groups based on the criteria established by Motzer and colleagues for patients receiving IFN[151] was recently reported.[369] Of note, patients with intermediate and poor prognostic features appeared to benefit most, with a median survival of 19.3 and 8.2 months, respectively, when compared with a median survival of 13.8 and 4.9 months reported in the Motzer database. This study suggests that the population benefiting from CCI-779 may be distinct from the typically good-prognosis patients who benefit from IL-2– or IFN-based therapy (or from both).

Epidermal growth factor (EGF) receptor antagonists, despite the presence of compelling preclinical data, have not yet lived up to their promise. A high rate of EGFR expression on RCC tumors, coupled with loss of VHL resulting in increased expression of TGF-α, supports the presence of an autocrine loop in RCC. Inhibition of this autocrine loop by blocking either the cell surface receptor (EGFR) or the ligand would be expected to result in growth inhibition and clinical response. However, several phase II studies have demonstrated little response to single-agent therapy targeted against EGFR.[370, 371] Nonetheless, the TGF-α–EGFR pathway remains an attractive target, and EGFR blocking agents may have a therapeutic role when given in combination with antagonists to other VHL-regulated growth factors.

Nonmyeloablative Allogeneic Transplantation

Since its inception as a therapy, allogeneic bone marrow transplantation has evolved from a means to achieve chemotherapeutic dose escalation to a form of adoptive immunotherapy.[372] Extensive evidence supports the presence of a graft-versus-malignancy effect in hematologic malignancies,[373, 374] and preclinical data demonstrate the presence of a graft-versus-tumor effect in solid tumors as well.[375-377] In patients with breast cancer, several reports have demonstrated the presence of a graft-versus-tumor effect in the setting of conventional ablative allogeneic transplantation for metastatic disease.[378, 379] Because of the high degree of morbidity and mortality experienced with standard high-dose allogeneic transplantation and evidence supporting the therapeutic importance of the immune-mediated effect of the donor graft, different groups began developing nonmyeloablative allogeneic bone marrow and peripheral blood stem cell transplantation regimens for use in both hematologic and solid tumors.[380-384] The goal of these regimens is to create a conditioning regimen sufficient for proper donor engraftment with the least recipient graft ablation possible.

Preliminary experience with nonmyeloablative allogeneic transplantation in patients with RCC has been reported by a number of centers.[385-388] In all studies, provision existed for post-transplant donor lymphocyte infusion if complete donor chimerism was not achieved. The largest series, reported by Childs and associates,[385] demonstrated a response in 10 of 19 patients after a conditioning regimen of cyclophosphamide and fludarabine. Complete donor chimerism appeared to be a prerequisite for response, as was some degree of graft-versus-host disease. More recently, with the use of thiotepa, cyclophosphamide, and fludarabine conditioning, Bregni and co-authors reported responses in four of seven patients with metastatic RCC after allogeneic nonmyeloablative transplantation.[387] Pedrazzoli and colleagues reported on 17 patients with treatment-refractory solid tumors, 7 of whom had RCC, conditioned with fludarabine and cyclophosphamide.[386] Four

of the patients had a performance status of 2 or poorer, and the remaining three had a performance status of 1. In Pedrazzoli and associates' report, all RCC patients died of progressive disease before day 100. All studies reported substantial hematologic toxicities, as well as graft-versus-host disease. A bad outcome was also consistently associated with poorer pretransplant performance status.

Though promising, nonmyeloablative transplantation requires substantial further development before it can be considered in a larger number of patients. The conditioning regimens need to be rendered less toxic. Post-transplant immunosuppression must be refined to decrease graft failure and graft-versus-host disease and to permit unrelated donor bone marrow to be used. Ideally, as our understanding of the antigens that elicit a graft-versus-RCC response is improved, modification of the donor graft or the donor lymphocyte infusion to enrich for RCC-specific T cell clones may enhance responses. With appropriate tumor antigens in hand, it will also be possible to combine transplantation with vaccination.

RENAL PELVIC TUMORS

The cellular lining of the urinary collecting system originates in the proximal part of the renal pelvis, traverses the ureter and urinary bladder, and terminates in the distal end of the urethra; it is composed of transitional epithelium or urothelium. This entire surface may be affected by carcinogenic influences, which may help explain the multiplicity in time and place of "urothelial" tumors, a term some have called "polychronotropism." Renal pelvic tumors account for approximately 10% of all primary renal cancers.

Tumors of the upper tract are twice as common in men, usually occur in patients older than 65 years, and are generally unilateral. The disease is more common in the Balkan region (Bulgaria, Greece, Romania, Yugoslavia) and is often bilateral. Similar to urothelial tumors of the urinary bladder, exposure to cigarettes, certain chemicals, plastics, coal, tar, and asphalt may increase the incidence of the disease. Long-term exposure to the analgesic phenacetin, usually ingested over years by women for headache relief, has been associated with the development of renal pelvic tumors.

Although most tumors of the upper tract are transitional cell carcinomas (over 90% of lesions), squamous carcinomas also occur, usually in the setting of chronic infection with kidney stones. Adenocarcinomas and other miscellaneous subtypes are rare.

Initial Features and Diagnostic Evaluation

The most common initial feature is gross hematuria, which occurs in 75% of patients, followed by flank pain in 30%. Evaluation may reveal either a nonfunctioning kidney and nonvisualization of the collecting system or, more commonly, a filling defect of the caliceal system, or renal pelvis, on intravenous pyelography. Exfoliative cytology is commonly positive, as it is in bladder cancers. Positive cytology in the presence of a filling defect of the renal pelvis or ureter confirms the diagnosis. Retrograde pyelography with brush biopsy of suspicious lesions may also yield the diagnosis of cancer. If the diagnosis is still uncertain after pyelography, including a retrograde evaluation, ureteroscopy may be performed to further evaluate the filling defect or obstruction.

Staging and Grading

Transitional cell carcinomas are graded on a scale of I, representing a well-differentiated lesion, to grade IV, or anaplastic and undifferentiated lesions. In a staging system similar to that used for urinary bladder cancer, stage 0 is limited to the mucosa; stage A, invasion into the lamina propria without muscularis invasion; stage B, invasion into the muscularis; stage C, invasion into the serosa; and stage D, metastatic disease. Lymphatic metastases usually indicate that more widespread metastatic disease is or will be present.

Management

For low-grade, low-stage transitional cancers, the general approach to treatment is conservative and consists of local excision and preservation of the kidney parenchyma. Five-year survival rates are usually in excess of 60%. For high-stage and high-grade lesions that have infiltrated into the renal parenchyma, the surgical treatment of choice is nephroureterectomy and removal of a cuff of bladder that encompasses the ipsilateral ureteral orifice. This approach is generally required because of the high likelihood of local recurrence in the bladder at the ureterovesical junction. In patients with regionally advanced or metastatic renal pelvic tumors, systemic chemotherapy, identical to that administered for bladder cancer, is often used. Standard first-line regimens for patients with locally advanced or metastatic transitional cell carcinoma include methotrexate, vinblastine, Adriamycin (doxorubicin), and cisplatin (MVAC); gemcitabine and cisplatin; or paclitaxel and cisplatin. Initial response rates may vary depending on prognostic factors, but long-term survival is poor.

OTHER KIDNEY TUMORS

Renal Sarcomas

Renal sarcomas account for approximately 1% to 2% of primary renal cancers. Fibrosarcomas are the most common and have a poor prognosis as a result of late diagnosis and the presence of locally advanced involvement into the renal vein or metastatic disease at initial evaluation. Five-year survival rates are less than 20%. Other, rarer sarcoma variants may occur and include leiomyosarcoma, rhabdomyosarcoma, osteogenic sarcoma, and liposarcoma.

Wilms Tumor

In children, Wilms tumor (nephroblastoma) is the most common cancer of the kidney and accounts for approximately 400 new cases per year in the United States. The success in managing the disease in the 1990s was achieved by the coordinated efforts of a multidisciplinary team of oncologists, radiation therapists, and surgeons. The disease tends to occur more frequently in African American children. A variety of etiologic factors have been suggested

to increase the risk for Wilms tumor, but a definitive link has not been established with any of these factors.

Genetics

Several well-described genetic abnormalities are associated with Wilms tumor. Patients with Wilms tumor may also manifest other abnormalities, including aniridia, WAGR syndrome (Wilms tumor, aniridia, other genitourinary abnormalities, and mental retardation), Denys-Drash syndrome (Wilms tumor, glomerulitis, pseudohermaphroditism), hemihypertrophy, trisomy 21, other rare physical abnormalities of macroglossia, and developmental sexual disorders.

Abnormalities in *WT1* (chromosome 11p13) and *WT2* (11p15) and mutations at 16q have all been implicated in the molecular genetics of Wilms tumor. Loss of heterozygosity in *WT1* and 16q occur in 20% of patients; inactivation of *WT2* has also been described. Other genetic abnormalities have suggested the presence of additional abnormal chromosomal locations. Patients with trisomy 21[389] and XX/XY mosaicisms have been reported to have an increased incidence of Wilms tumor.

Pathology and Staging

Microscopically, Wilms tumors consist of blastemic, epithelial, and stromal cells, often arranged in patterns that resemble tubule or glomeruloid features. The multipotential aspects of Wilms tumors may be characterized by the presence of teratomatous or teratoid features, including components of mesenchymal structures such as muscle, cartilage, and lipoid tissue. In contrast to these differentiated structures, undifferentiated or sarcomatoid lesions can also occur and are associated with a worse prognosis. The presence of nephrogenic rests in the setting of Wilms tumors is common; they are thought to be precursor lesions. According to Wilimas and associates,[390] these rests are "defined as a focus of persistent nephrogenic cells, some of which can be induced to form a Wilms tumor."

The most common staging system divides Wilms tumor into five categories:

Stage 1: Tumor limited to the kidney and completely excised
Stage 2: Tumor beyond the kidney but completely resected
Stage 3: Residual tumor in the local regional area (e.g., peritoneal implants, lymph nodal involvement)
Stage 4: Hematogenous involvement to metastatic sites
Stage 5: Bilateral involvement at initial evaluation

Initial Features

An abdominal mass, with or without abdominal pain, is the most common finding and occurs in 80% and 40% of cases, respectively. Other physical abnormalities, including aniridia, genitourinary abnormalities, and hemihypertrophy, may occasionally be detected. Hematuria, anemia, hypertension, or acute severe abdominal pain may also be present. An abdominal ultrasound is an important diagnostic test to further evaluate the mass and its anatomic extension, which may include inferior or superior extension into the vena cava. Intravenous pyelography and CT are also warranted. Metastatic evaluation of liver, chest, and bone complement the evaluation. The diagnosis is usually established by surgery. If the diagnostic tests and clinical features suggest the presence of a Wilms tumor, preoperative needle biopsy should be avoided because of the attendant risk of tumor spillage.

Multimodality Management

High cure rates have been achieved with the concerted effort of multimodality teams performing surgery, radiation therapy, and chemotherapy. Surgical removal of the affected kidney, along with examination of the regional lymph nodes, evaluation of the contralateral kidney, and detailed abdominal exploration, is the goal. Removal of all gross tumor should be attempted, and such removal justifies the radical resection that is often called for. Aside from patients with early-stage lesions of favorable histology, most patients receive radiation therapy as an adjunct to surgical removal. Specific recommendations regarding the exact portals used are determined by the operative findings, the histologic subtype, and the presence of evidence of tumor spillage during the resection.

Chemotherapy is an important component of therapy in Wilms tumors. In addition to being used after surgery in conjunction with radiation therapy, neoadjuvant chemotherapy can diminish the size of the primary tumor and induce regression of metastatic lesions. Agents that have activity against Wilms tumor are vincristine, dactinomycin, doxorubicin, etoposide, ifosfamide, and cisplatin, with the first two agents being the most active. Before the extensive use of chemotherapy, the survival rate for patients with stage 2 or 3 tumors was less than 45%. Now, cure rates approaching 80% to 90% are routinely achieved; survival rates of 92% to 97% can be obtained in earlier stages of disease. For patients who experience relapse or for those with poor prognostic features, bone marrow transplantation has been offered with good results.

As these excellent results continue to accumulate, treatment programs aimed at lessening treatment duration and minimizing long-term consequences, such as induction of second tumors, continue to be evaluated. Such programs include the more selective use of radiation therapy and a decrease in the duration of chemotherapy.

REFERENCES

1. Jemal A, Thomas A, Murray T, Thun M: Cancer statistics, 2002. CA Cancer J Clin 52:23-47, 2002.
2. Ferlay J, Bray F, Pisani P, et al: GLOBOCAN 2000: Cancer Incidence, Mortality and Prevalence Worldwide, Version 1.0. 2000, IARCPress, 2001.
3. Grawitz P: Die sogennanten Lipoma der Niere. Virchows Arch Pathol Anat 93:39, 1883.
4. Motzer RJ, Bander NH, Nanus DM: Renal-cell carcinoma. N Engl J Med 335:865-875, 1996.
5. Landis SH, Murray T, Bolden S, Wingo PA: Cancer statistics, 1998. CA Cancer J Clin 48:6-29, 1998.
6. La Vecchia C, Negri E, D'Avanzo B, Franceschi S: Smoking and renal cell carcinoma. Cancer Res 50:5231-5233, 1990.
7. Mandel JS, McLaughlin JK, Schlehofer B, et al: International renal-cell cancer study. IV. Occupation. Int J Cancer 61:601-605, 1995.
8. Maclure M: Asbestos and renal adenocarcinoma: A case-control study. Environ Res 42:353-361, 1987.
9. McLaughlin JK, Blot WJ, Mehl ES, et al: Petroleum-related employment and renal cell cancer. J Occup Med 27:672-674, 1985.
10. McLaughlin JK, Mandel JS, Blot WJ, et al: A population-based case-control study of renal cell carcinoma. J Natl Cancer Inst 72:275-284, 1984.
11. Yu MC, Mack TM, Hanisch R, et al: Cigarette smoking, obesity, diuretic use, and coffee consumption as risk factors for renal cell carcinoma. J Natl Cancer Inst 77:351-356, 1986.
12. Kolonel LN: Association of cadmium with renal cancer. Cancer 37:1782-1787, 1976.
13. Lindblad P, Mellemgaard A, Schlehofer B, et al: International renal-cell cancer study. V. Reproductive factors, gynecologic operations and exogenous hormones. Int J Cancer 61:192-198, 1995.
14. Lornoy W, Becaus S, de Vleechouwer M, et al: Renal cell carcinoma, a new complication of analgesic nephropathy. Lancet 1:1271-2127, 1986.
15. McCredie M, Pommer W, McLaughlin JK, et al: International renal-cell cancer study. II. Analgesics. Int J Cancer 60:345-349, 1995.
16. Denton MD, Magee CC, Ovuworie C, et al: Prevalence of renal cell carcinoma in patients with ESRD pre-transplantation: A pathologic analysis. Kidney Int 61:2201-2209, 2002.
17. Brennan JF, Stilmant MM, Babayan RK, Siroky MB: Acquired renal cystic disease: Implications for the urologist. Br J Urol 67:342-348, 1991.
18. Matson MA, Cohen EP: Acquired cystic kidney disease: Occurrence, prevalence, and renal cancers. Medicine (Baltimore) 69:217-226, 1990.
19. Doublet JD, Peraldi MN, Gattegno B, et al: Renal cell carcinoma of native kidneys: Prospective study of 129 renal transplant patients. J Urol 158:42-44, 1997.
20. Gulanikar AC, Daily PP, Kilambi NK, et al: Prospective pretransplant ultrasound screening in 206 patients for acquired renal cysts and renal cell carcinoma. Transplantation 66:1669-1672, 1998.
21. Grantham JJ, Levine E: Acquired cystic disease: Replacing one kidney disease with another. Kidney Int 28:99-105, 1985.
22. Hughson MD, Buchwald D, Fox M: Renal neoplasia and acquired cystic kidney disease in patients receiving long-term dialysis. Arch Pathol Lab Med 110:592-601, 1986.
23. MacDougall ML, Welling LW, Wiegmann TB: Renal adenocarcinoma and acquired cystic disease in chronic hemodialysis patients. Am J Kidney Dis 9:166-1671, 1987.
24. Washecka R, Hanna M: Malignant renal tumors in tuberous sclerosis. Urology 37:340-343, 1991.
25. Posso M, Safadi D, Van Dyk OJ: Unilateral polycystic or multicystic kidney associated with focal mural renal cell carcinoma: Presentation of a case. J Urol 109:559-563, 1973.
26. Lamiell JM, Salazar FG, Hsia YE: von Hippel-Lindau disease affecting 43 members of a single kindred. Medicine (Baltimore) 68:1-29, 1989.
27. Gago-Dominguez M, Yuan JM, Castelao JE, et al: Family history and risk of renal cell carcinoma. Cancer Epidemiol Biomarkers Prev 10:1001-1004, 2001.
28. Schlehofer B, Pommer W, Mellemgaard A, et al: International renal-cell-cancer study. VI. The role of medical and family history. Int J Cancer 66:723-726, 1996.
29. Mellemgaard A, Engholm G, McLaughlin JK, Olsen JH: Occupational risk factors for renal-cell carcinoma in Denmark. Scand J Work Environ Health 20:160-165, 1994.
30. Gnarra JR, Glenn GM, Latif F, et al: Molecular genetic studies of sporadic and familial renal cell carcinoma. Urol Clin North Am 20:207-216, 1993.
31. Cohen AJ, Li FP, Berg S, et al: Hereditary renal-cell carcinoma associated with a chromosomal translocation. N Engl J Med 301:592-595, 1979.
32. Pathak S, Strong LC, Ferrell RE, Trindade A: Familial renal cell carcinoma with a 3;11 chromosome translocation limited to tumor cells. Science 217:939-941, 1982.
33. Carroll PR, Murty VV, Reuter V, et al: Abnormalities at chromosome region 3p12-14 characterize clear cell renal carcinoma. Cancer Genet Cytogenet 26:253-259, 1987.
34. Zbar B, Brauch H, Talmadge C, Linehan M: Loss of alleles of loci on the short arm of chromosome 3 in renal cell carcinoma. Nature 327:721-724, 1987.
35. Zbar B, Tory K, Merino M, et al: Hereditary papillary renal cell carcinoma. J Urol 151:561-566, 1994.
36. Latif F, Tory K, Gnarra J, et al: Identification of the von Hippel-Lindau disease tumor suppressor gene. Science 260:1317-1320, 1993.

37. Iliopoulos O, Kibel A, Gray S, Kaelin WG Jr: Tumour suppression by the human von Hippel-Lindau gene product. Nat Med 1:822-826, 1995.

38. Stebbins CE, Kaelin WG Jr, Pavletich NP: Structure of the VHL-ElonginC-ElonginB complex: Implications for VHL tumor suppressor function. Science 284:455-461, 1999.

39. Kondo K, Kaelin WG Jr: The von Hippel-Lindau tumor suppressor gene. Exp Cell Res 264:117-125, 2001.

40. Tannenbaum M: Ultrastructural pathology of human renal cell tumors. Pathol Annu 6:249-277, 1971.

41. Richie J, Skinner D: Renal neoplasia. In Brenner B, Rector F (eds): The Kidney. Philadelphia, WB Saunders, 1981, p 2109.

42. Thoenes W, Storkel S, Rumpelt HJ: Histopathology and classification of renal cell tumors (adenomas, oncocytomas and carcinomas). The basic cytological and histopathological elements and their use for diagnostics. Pathol Res Pract 181:125-143, 1986.

43. Storkel S, van den Berg E: Morphological classification of renal cancer. World J Urol 13:153-158, 1995.

44. Garnick M: Primary neoplasms of the kidney. In Brady H, Wilcox C (eds): Therapy in Nephrology and Hypertension: A Companion to Brenner and Rector's The Kidney. Philadelphia, WB Saunders, 1999, pp 337-340.

45. Presti JC Jr, Rao PH, Chen Q, et al: Histopathological, cytogenetic, and molecular characterization of renal cortical tumors. Cancer Res 51:1544-1552, 1991.

46. Weiss LM, Gelb AB, Medeiros LJ: Adult renal epithelial neoplasms. Am J Clin Pathol 103:624-635, 1995.

47. Fuhrman SA, Lasky LC, Limas C: Prognostic significance of morphologic parameters in renal cell carcinoma. Am J Surg Pathol 6:655-663, 1982.

48. Mancilla-Jimenez R, Stanley RJ, Blath RA: Papillary renal cell carcinoma: A clinical, radiologic, and pathologic study of 34 cases. Cancer 38:2469-2480, 1976.

49. Kovacs G, Wilkens L, Papp T, de Riese W: Differentiation between papillary and nonpapillary renal cell carcinomas by DNA analysis. J Natl Cancer Inst 81:527-730, 1989.

50. Kovacs G, Fuzesi L, Emanual A, Kung HF: Cytogenetics of papillary renal cell tumors. Genes Chromosomes Cancer 3:249-255, 1991.

51. Sene AP, Hunt L, McMahon RF, Carroll RN: Renal carcinoma in patients undergoing nephrectomy: Analysis of survival and prognostic factors. Br J Urol 70:125-134, 1992.

52. Thoenes W, Storkel S, Rumpelt HJ, et al: Chromophobe cell renal carcinoma and its variants—a report on 32 cases. J Pathol 155:277-287, 1988.

53. Storkel S, Steart PV, Drenckhahn D, Thoenes W: The human chromophobe cell renal carcinoma: Its probable relation to intercalated cells of the collecting duct. Virchows Arch B Cell Pathol Incl Mol Pathol 56:237-245, 1989.

54. Ortmann M, Vierbuchen M, Fischer R: Sialylated glycoconjugates in chromophobe cell renal carcinoma compared with other renal cell tumors. Indication of its development from the collecting duct epithelium. Virchows Arch 61:123-132, 1991.

55. Akhtar M, Kardar H, Linjawi T, et al: Chromophobe cell carcinoma of the kidney. A clinicopathologic study of 21 cases. Am J Surg Pathol 19:1245-1256, 1995.

56. Speicher MR, Schoell B, du Manoir S, et al: Specific loss of chromosomes 1, 2, 6, 10, 13, 17, and 21 in chromophobe renal cell carcinomas revealed by comparative genomic hybridization. Am J Pathol 145:356-364, 1994.

57. Kovacs A, Kovacs G: Low chromosome number in chromophobe renal cell carcinomas. Genes Chromosomes Cancer 4:267-268, 1992.

58. Lieber MM: Renal oncocytoma: Prognosis and treatment. Eur Urol 18(suppl 2):17-21, 1990.

59. Zerban H, Nogueira E, Riedasch G, Bannasch P: Renal oncocytoma: Origin from the collecting duct. Virchows Arch B Cell Pathol Incl Mol Pathol 52:375-387, 1987.

60. Morra MN, Das S: Renal oncocytoma: A review of histogenesis, histopathology, diagnosis and treatment. J Urol 150:295-302, 1993.

61. Kennedy SM, Merino MJ, Lineham WM, et al: Collecting duct carcinoma of the kidney. Hum Pathol 21:449-456, 1990.

62. Rumpelt HJ, Storkel S, Moll R, et al: Bellini duct carcinoma: Further evidence for this rare variant of renal cell carcinoma. Histopathology 18:115-122, 1991.

63. Pause A, Lee S, Worrell RA, et al: The von Hippel-Lindau tumor-suppressor gene product forms a stable complex with human CUL-2, a member of the Cdc53 family of proteins. Proc Natl Acad Sci U S A 94:2156-2161, 1997.

64. Ohh M, Park CW, Ivan M, et al: Ubiquitination of hypoxia-inducible factor requires direct binding to the beta-domain of the von Hippel-Lindau protein. Nat Cell Biol 2:423-427, 2000.

65. Kamura T, Sato S, Iwai K, et al: Activation of HIF1α ubiquitination by a reconstituted von Hippel-Lindau (VHL) tumor suppressor complex. Proc Natl Acad Sci U S A 97:10430-10435, 2000.

66. Tanimoto K, Makino Y, Pereira T, Poellinger L: Mechanism of regulation of the hypoxia-inducible factor-1 alpha by the von Hippel-Lindau tumor suppressor protein. EMBO J 19:4298-4309, 2000.

67. Cockman ME, Masson N, Mole DR, et al: Hypoxia inducible factor-alpha binding and ubiquitylation by the von Hippel-Lindau tumor suppressor protein. J Biol Chem 275:25733-25741, 2000.

68. Semenza GL: HIF-1 and human disease: One highly involved factor. Genes Dev 14:1983-1991, 2000.

69. Sargent ER, Gomella LG, Belldegrun A, et al: Epidermal growth factor receptor gene expression in normal human kidney and renal cell carcinoma. J Urol 142:1364-1368, 1989.

70. Knebelmann B, Ananth S, Cohen HT, Sukhatme VP: Transforming growth factor alpha is a target for the von Hippel-Lindau tumor suppressor. Cancer Res 58:226-231, 1998.

71. de Paulsen N, Brychzy A, Fournier MC, et al: Role of transforming growth factor-alpha in von Hippel-Lindau (VHL)(-/-) clear cell renal carcinoma cell proliferation: A possible mechanism coupling VHL tumor suppressor inactivation and tumorigenesis. Proc Natl Acad Sci U S A 98:1387-1392, 2001.

72. Masson N, William C, Maxwell PH, et al: Independent function of two destruction domains in hypoxia-inducible factor-alpha chains activated by prolyl hydroxylation. EMBO J 20:5197-5206, 2001.

73. Lonergan KM, Iliopoulos D, Ohh M, et al: Regulation of hypoxia-inducible mRNAs by the von Hippel-Lindau tumor suppressor protein requires binding to complexes containing elongins B/C and Cul2. Mol Cell Biol 18:732-741, 1998.

74. Jaakkola P, Mole DR, Tian YM, et al: Targeting of HIF-alpha to the von Hippel-Lindau ubiquitylation complex by O$_2$-regulated prolyl hydroxylation. Science 292:468-472, 2001.

75. Yu F, White SB, Zhao Q, Lee FS: HIF-1α binding to VHL is regulated by stimulus-sensitive proline hydroxylation. Proc Natl Acad Sci U S A 98:9630-9635, 2001.

76. Bruick RK, McKnight SL: A conserved family of prolyl-4-hydroxylases that modify HIF. Science 294:1337-1340, 2001.

77. Bentz M, Bergerheim US, Li C, et al: Chromosome imbalances in papillary renal cell carcinoma and first cytogenetic data of familial cases analyzed by comparative genomic hybridization. Cytogenet Cell Genet 75:17-21, 1996.

78. Schmidt L, Duh FM, Chen F, et al: Germline and somatic mutations in the tyrosine kinase domain of the MET proto-oncogene in papillary renal carcinomas. Nat Genet 16:68-73, 1997.

79. Schmidt L, Junker K, Nakaigawa N, et al: Novel mutations of the MET proto-oncogene in papillary renal carcinomas. Oncogene 18:2343-2350, 1999.

80. Comoglio PM, Tamagnone L, Boccaccio C: Plasminogen-related growth factor and semaphorin receptors: A gene superfamily controlling invasive growth. Exp Cell Res 253:88-99, 1999.

81. Stella MC, Comoglio PM: HGF: A multifunctional growth factor controlling cell scattering. Int J Biochem Cell Biol 31:1357-1362, 1999.

82. van der Voort R, Taher TE, Derksen PW, et al: The hepatocyte growth factor/Met pathway in development, tumorigenesis, and B-cell differentiation. Adv Cancer Res 79:39-90, 2000.

83. Warburton D, Schwartz M, Tefft D, et al: The molecular basis of lung morphogenesis. Mech Dev 92:55-81, 2000.

84. Uhlman DL, Nguyen PL, Manivel JC, et al: Association of immunohistochemical staining for p53 with metastatic progression and poor survival in patients with renal cell carcinoma. J Natl Cancer Inst 86:1470-1475, 1994.

85. Oda H, Nakatsuru Y, Ishikawa T: Mutations of the p53 gene and p53 protein overexpression are associated with sarcomatoid transformation in renal cell carcinomas. Cancer Res 55:658-662, 1995.

86. Santhanan U, Ray A, Sehgal PB: Repression of the interleukin 6 gene promoter by p53 and the retinoblastoma susceptibility gene product. Proc Natl Acad Sci U S A 88:7605-7609, 1991.

87. Blay JY, Negrier S, Combaret B, et al: Interleukin-6 and metastatic clear renal cell carcinoma: A prognosis factor for response and survival after IL-2 therapy. Abstract presented at the 38th Annual Meeting of the American Society for Clinical Oncology, San Diego, CA, 1992, p 217.

88. Linehan W, Shipley W, Parkinson D: Cancer of the kidney and ureter. *In* DeVita VJ, Hellman S, Rosenberg S (eds): Cancer: Principles and Practices of Oncology. Philadelphia, Lippincott-Raven, 1993, pp 1023-1051.

89. Skinner DG, Colvin RB, Vermillion CD, et al: Diagnosis and management of renal cell carcinoma. A clinical and pathologic study of 309 cases. Cancer 28:1165-1177, 1971.

90. Gibbons RP, Monte JE, Correa RJ Jr, Mason JT: Manifestations of renal cell carcinoma. Urology 8:201-206, 1976.

91. Konnak JW, Grossma HB: Renal cell carcinoma as an incidental finding. J Urol 134:1094-1096, 1985.

92. DeKernion J: Real numbers. *In* Walsh P, Gittes R, Perlmutter A (eds): Campbell's Urology. Philadelphia, WB Saunders, 1986, pp 1294-1342.

93. Pinals R, Krane S: Medical aspects of renal cell carcinoma. Postgrad Med J 38:507-529, 1962.

94. Chisholm GD, Roy RR: The systemic effects of malignant renal tumours. Br J Urol 43:687-700, 1971.

95. Cranston WI, Luff RH, Owen D, Rawlins MD: Studies on the pathogenesis of fever in renal carcinoma. Clin Sci Mol Med 45:459-467, 1973.

96. Spencer D: Secondary amyloidosis in relation to carcinoma of the kidney. Postgrad Med J 47:820-822, 1971.

97. Samaan N: Paraneoplastic studies associated with renal cell carcinoma: A pilot study. J Clin Oncol 6:862, 1987.

98. Cherukuri SV, Johenning PW, Ram MD: Systemic effects of hypernephroma. Urology 10:93-97, 1977.

99. Sufrin G, Mirand EA, Moore RH, et al: Hormones in renal cancer. J Urol 117:433-438, 1977.

100. Walsh PN, Kissane JM: Nonmetastatic hypernephroma with reversible hepatic dysfunction. Arch Intern Med 122:214-222, 1968.

101. Utz DC, Warren MM, Gregg JA, et al: Reversible hepatic dysfunction associated with hypernephroma. Mayo Clin Proc 45:161-169, 1970.

102. Chang SY, Yu DS, Sherwood ER, et al: Inhibitory effects of suramin on a human renal cell carcinoma line, causing nephrogenic hepatic dysfunction. J Urol 147:1147-1150, 1992.

103. Stadler WM, Richards JM, Vogelzang NJ: Serum interleukin-6 levels in metastatic renal cell cancer: Correlation with survival but not an independent prognostic indicator. J Natl Cancer Inst 84:1835-1836, 1992.

104. Boxer RJ, Waisman J, Lieber MM, et al: Renal carcinoma: Computer analysis of 96 patients treated by nephrectomy. J Urol 122:598-601, 1979.

105. Sufrin G, Mink I, Fitzpatrick J, et al: Coagulation factors in renal adenocarcinoma. J Urol 119:727-730, 1978.

106. Dawson NA, Barr CF, Alving BM: Acquired dysfibrinogenemia. Paraneoplastic syndrome in renal cell carcinoma. Am J Med 78:682-686, 1985.

107. Gotoh A, Kitazawa S, Mizuno Y, et al: Common expression of parathyroid hormone–related protein and no correlation of calcium level in renal cell carcinomas. Cancer 71:2803-2806, 1993.

108. Da Silva JL, Lacombe C, Bruneval P, et al: Tumor cells are the site of erythropoietin synthesis in human renal cancers associated with polycythemia. Blood 75:577-582, 1990.

109. Iliopoulos O, Levy AP, Jiang C, et al: Negative regulation of hypoxia-inducible genes by the von Hippel-Lindau protein. Proc Natl Acad Sci U S A 93:10595-10599, 1996.

110. Gelb AB: Renal cell carcinoma: Current prognostic factors. Union Internationale Contre le Cancer (UICC) and the American Joint Committee on Cancer (AJCC). Cancer 80:981-986, 1997.

111. Motzer RJ, Mazumdar M, Bacik J, et al: Survival and prognostic stratification of 670 patients with advanced renal cell carcinoma. J Clin Oncol 17:2530-2540, 1999.

112. O'Grady AS, Morse LJ, Lee JB: Parathyroid hormone–secreting renal carcinoma associated with hypercalcemia and metabolic alkalosis. Ann Intern Med 63:858-868, 1965.

113. Lytton B, Rosof B, Evans J: Parathyroid hormone like activity in renal cell carcinoma producing hypercalcemia. J Urol 93:127, 1965.

114. Goldberg M, Tashjian AH, Order S: Renal adenocarcinoma containing a parathyroid hormone–like substance and associated with marked hypercalcemia. Am J Med 36:805, 1964.

115. Buckle RM, McMillan M, Mallinson C: Ectopic secretion of parathyroid hormone by a renal adenocarcinoma in a patient with hypercalcaemia. BMJ 4:724-6, 1970.

116. Brereton HD, Halushka PV, Alexander RW, et al: Indomethacin-responsive hypercalcemia in a patient with renal-cell adenocarcinoma. N Engl J Med 291:83-85, 1974.

117. Hortobagyi GN, Theriault RL, Porter L, et al: Efficacy of pamidronate in reducing skeletal complications in patients with breast cancer and lytic bone metastases. Protocol 19 Aredia Breast Cancer Study Group. N Engl J Med 335:1785-1791, 1996.

118. Kise H, Kobayashi K, Arima K, et al: [Effect of pamidronate and interferon-alpha on bone and lung metastases and hypercalcemia in a patient with renal cell carcinoma.] Hinyokika Kiyo 42:879-881, 1996.

119. Berenson JR, Rosen RS, Howell A, et al: Zoledronic acid reduces skeletal-related events in patients with osteolytic metastases. Cancer 91:1191-1200, 2001.

120. Major P, Lortholary A, Hon J, et al: Zoledronic acid is superior to pamidronate in the treatment of hypercalcemia of malignancy: A pooled analysis of two randomized, controlled clinical trials. J Clin Oncol 19:558-567, 2001.

121. Tsukamoto T, Kumamoto Y, Yamazaki K, et al: Clinical analysis of incidentally found renal cell carcinomas. Eur Urol 19:109-113, 1991.

122. Johnson CD, Dunnick NR, Cohan RH Illescas FF: Renal adenocarcinoma: CT staging of 100 tumors. AJR Am J Roentgenol 148:59-63, 1987.

123. Jaschke W, van Kaick G, Peters S, Palmtag H: Accuracy of computed tomography in staging of kidney tumors. Acta Radiol Diagn 23:593-598, 1982.

124. Amendola MA, Bree RL, Pollack HM, et al: Small renal cell carcinomas: Resolving a diagnostic dilemma. Radiology 166:637-641, 1988.

125. Schreck WR, Holmes JH: Ultrasound as a diagnostic aid for renal neoplasms and cysts. J Urol 103:281-285, 1970.

126. Smith EH, Bennett AH: The usefulness of ultrasound in the evaluation of renal masses in adults. J Urol 113:525-529, 1975.

127. Semelka RC, Shoenut JP, Magro CM, et al: Renal cancer staging: Comparison of contrast-enhanced CT and gadolinium-enhanced fat-suppressed spin-echo and gradient-echo MR imaging. J Magn Reson Imaging 3:597-602, 1993.

128. Andersen CL, Hostetter G, Grigoryan A, et al: Improved procedure for fluorescence in situ hybridization on tissue microarrays. Cytometry 45:83-86, 2001.

129. Daponte D, Zungri E, Algaba F, sole-Balcells F: [Isolated renal angiomyolipoma. Study of 10 cases.] J Urol (Paris) 89:267-271, 1983.

130. Yamashita Y, Ueno S, Makita O, et al: Hyperechoic renal tumors: Anechoic rim and intratumoral cysts in US differentiation of renal cell carcinoma from angiomyolipoma. Radiology 188:179-182, 1993.

131. Atlas I, Kwan D, Stone N: Value of serum alkaline phosphatase and radionuclide bone scans in patients with renal cell carcinoma. Urology 38:220-222, 1991.

132. Kriteman L, Sanders WH: Normal alkaline phosphatase levels in patients with bone metastases due to renal cell carcinoma. Urology 51:397-399, 1998.

133. Seaman E, Goluboff ET, Ross S, Sawczuk IS: Association of radionuclide bone scan and serum alkaline phosphatase in patients with metastatic renal cell carcinoma. Urology 48:692-695, 1996.

134. Koga S, Tsuda S, Nishikido M, et al: The diagnostic value of bone scan in patients with renal cell carcinoma. J Urol 166:2126-2128, 2001.

135. Henriksson C, Haraldsson G, Aldenborg F, et al: Skeletal metastases in 102 patients evaluated before surgery for renal cell carcinoma. Scand J Urol Nephrol 26:363-366, 1992.

136. Staudenherz A, Steiner B, Puig S, et al: Is there a diagnostic role for bone scanning of patients with a high pretest probability for metastatic renal cell carcinoma? Cancer 85:153-155, 1999.

137. Ramdave S, Thomas GW, Berlangieri SU, et al: Clinical role of F-18 fluorodeoxyglucose positron emission tomography for detection and management of renal cell carcinoma. J Urol 166:825-830, 2001.

138. Brouwers AH, Dorr U, Lang O, et al: 131 I-cG250 monoclonal antibody immunoscintigraphy versus (18 F)FDG-PET imaging in patients with metastatic renal cell carcinoma: A comparative study. Nucl Med Commun 23:229-236, 2002.

139. Safaei A, Figlin R, Hoh CK, et al: The usefulness of F-18 deoxyglucose whole-body positron emission tomography (PET) for re-staging of renal cell cancer. Clin Nephrol 57:56-62, 2002.

140. Seto E, Segall GM, Terris MK: Positron emission tomography detection of osseous metastases of renal cell carcinoma not identified on bone scan. Urology 55:286, 2000.

141. Hoh CK, Seltzer MA, Franklin J, et al: Positron emission tomography in urological oncology. J Urol 159:347-356, 1998.

142. Bachor R, Kotzerke J, Gottfried HW, et al: [Positron emission tomography in diagnosis of renal cell carcinoma.] Urologe A 35:146-150, 1996.

143. Bachor R, Kocher F, Groppengiesser F, et al: [Positron emission tomography. Introduction of a new procedure in diagnosis of urologic tumors and initial clinical results.] Urologe A 34:138-142, 1995.

144. Goldberg MA, Mayo-Smith WW, Papanicolaou N, et al: FDG PET characterization of renal masses: Preliminary experience. Clin Radiol 52:510-515, 1997.

145. McDougal WS, Garnick MB: Clinical signs and symptoms of kidney cancer. *In* Vogelzang SP, Shipley NJ, WU, et al (eds): Comprehensive Textbook of Genitourinary Oncology. Baltimore, Williams & Wilkins, 1996, pp 154-159.

146. Ritchie AW, Chisholm GD: The natural history of renal carcinoma. Semin Oncol 10:390-400, 1983.

147. Fahn HJ, Lee YH, Chen MT, et al: The incidence and prognostic significance of humoral hypercalcemia in renal cell carcinoma. J Urol 145:248-250, 1991.

148. Ljungberg B, Joanssen H, Stenling R: Prognostic factors in renal cell carcinoma. Int Urol Nephrol 20:115-121, 1988.

149. Grignon DJ, Ayala AG, el-Naggar A, et al: Renal cell carcinoma. A clinicopathologic and DNA flow cytometric analysis of 103 cases. Cancer 64:2133-2140, 1989.

150. Tsui KH, Shvarts O, Smith RB, et al: Prognostic indicators for renal cell carcinoma: A multivariate analysis of 643 patients using the revised 1997 TNM staging criteria. J Urol 163:1090-1095, quiz 1295, 2000.

151. Motzer RJ, Bacik J, Murphy BA, et al: Interferon-alfa as a comparative treatment for clinical trials of new therapies against advanced renal cell carcinoma. J Clin Oncol 20:289-296, 2002.

152. Robson C: Radial nephrectomy for renal cell carcinoma. J Urol 89:37, 1963.

153. Waters WB, Richie JP: Aggressive surgical approach to renal cell carcinoma: Review of 130 cases. J Urol 122:306-309, 1979.

154. Chute R, Soutter L, Kerr W: The value of the thoracoabdominal incision in removal of the kidney tumors. N Engl J Med 241:951, 1949.

155. Sagalowsky AI, Kadesky KT, Ewalt DM, Kennedy TJ: Factors influencing adrenal metastasis in renal cell carcinoma. J Urol 151:1181-1184, 1994.

156. Shalev M, Cipolla B, Guille F, et al: Is ipsilateral adrenalectomy a necessary component of radical nephrectomy? J Urol 153:1415-1417, 1995.

157. Gill IS, McClennan BL, Kerbl K, et al: Adrenal involvement from renal cell carcinoma: Predictive value of computerized tomography. J Urol 152:1082-1085, 1994.

158. Paul R, Mordhorst J, Leyh H, Hartung R: Incidence and outcome of patients with adrenal metastases of renal cell cancer. Urology 57:878-882, 2001.

159. Herrlinger A, Schrott KM, Schott G, Sigel A: What are the benefits of extended dissection of the regional renal lymph nodes in the therapy of renal cell carcinoma. J Urol 146:1224-1227, 1991.

160. Giuliani L, Giberti C, Martorana G, Rovida S: Radical extensive surgery for renal cell carcinoma: Long-term results and prognostic factors. J Urol 143:468-473, discussion 473-474, 1990.

161. Phillips E, Messing EM: Role of lymphadenectomy in the treatment of renal cell carcinoma. Urology 41:9-15, 1993.

162. Fleischmann J, Lyskewycz M, Flanigan RC: Staging subcategories and prognosis. Abstract presented at the American Urological Association Annual Meeting, New Orleans, 1997.

163. Moll V, Becht E, Ziegler M: Kidney preserving surgery in renal cell tumors: Indications, techniques and results in 152 patients. J Urol 150:319-323, 1993.

164. Thrasher JB, Robertson JE, Paulson DF: Expanding indications for conservative renal surgery in renal cell carcinoma. Urology 43:160-168, 1994.

165. Licht MR, Novick AC, Goormastic M: Nephron sparing surgery in incidental versus suspected renal cell carcinoma. J Urol 152:39-42, 1994.

166. Morgan WR, Zincke H: Progression and survival after renal-conserving surgery for renal cell carcinoma: Experience in 104 patients and extended followup. J Urol 144:852-857, discussion 857-858, 1990.

167. Marberger M, Pugh RC, Auvert J, et al: Conservation surgery of renal carcinoma: The EIRSS experience. Br J Urol 53:528-532, 1981.

168. Novick AC, Streem S, Montie JE, et al: Conservative surgery for renal cell carcinoma: A single-center experience with 100 patients. J Urol 141:835-839, 1989.

169. Steinbach F, Stockle M, Muller SC, et al: Conservative surgery of renal cell tumors in 140 patients: 21 years of experience. J Urol 148:24-29, discussion 29-30, 1992.

170. Steinbach F, Stockle M, Hohenfellner R: Current controversies in nephron-sparing surgery for renal-cell carcinoma. World J Urol 13:163-165, 1995.

171. Provet J, Tessler A, Brown J, et al: Partial nephrectomy for renal cell carcinoma: Indications, results and implications. J Urol 145:472-476, 1991.

172. Uzzo RG, Novick AC: Nephron sparing surgery for renal tumors: Indications, techniques and outcomes. J Urol 166:6-18, 2001.

173. Sutherland SE, Resnick MI, Maclennan GT, Goldman HB: Does the size of the surgical margin in partial nephrectomy for renal cell cancer really matter? J Urol 167:61-64, 2002.

174. Piper NY, Bischoff JT, Magee C, et al: Is a 1-cm margin necessary during nephron-sparing surgery for renal cell carcinoma? Urology 58:849-852, 2001.

175. Whang M, O'Toole K, Bixon R, et al: The incidence of multifocal renal cell carcinoma in patients who are candidates for partial nephrectomy. J Urol 154:968-970, discussion 970-971, 1995.

176. Bazeed MA, Scharfe T, Becht E, et al: Conservative surgery of renal cell carcinoma. Eur Urol 12:238-243, 1986.

177. Carini M, Selli C, Barbanti G, et al: Conservative surgical treatment of renal cell carcinoma: Clinical experience and reappraisal indications. J Urol 140:725-731, 1988.

178. Selli C, Lapini A, Carini M: Conservative surgery of kidney tumors. Prog Clin Biol Res 370:9-17, 1991.

179. D'Armiento M, Damiano R, Feleppa B, et al: Elective conservative surgery for renal carcinoma versus radical nephrectomy: A prospective study. Br J Urol 79:15-9, 1997.

180. van Poppel H, Bamelis B, Oyen R, Baert L: Partial nephrectomy for renal cell carcinoma can achieve long-term tumor control. J Urol 160:674-678, 1998.

181. Hafez KS, Fergany AF, Novick AC: Nephron sparing surgery for localized renal cell carcinoma: Impact of tumor size on patient survival, tumor recurrence and TNM staging. J Urol 162:1930-1933, 1999.

182. Lee CT, Katz J, Shi W, et al: Surgical management of renal tumors 4 cm. or less in a contemporary cohort. J Urol 163:730-736, 2000.

183. Belldegrun A, Tsui KH, deKernion JB, Smith RB: Efficacy of nephron-sparing surgery for renal cell carcinoma: Analysis based on the new 1997 tumor-node-metastasis staging system. J Clin Oncol 17:2868-2875, 1999.

184. Barbalias GA, Liatsikos EN, Tsintavis A, Nikiforidis G: Adenocarcinoma of the kidney: Nephron-sparing surgical approach vs. radical nephrectomy. J Surg Oncol 72:156-161, 1999.

185. Indudhara R, Bueschen AJ, Urban DA, et al: Nephron-sparing surgery compared with radical nephrectomy for renal tumors: Current indications and results. South Med J 90:982-985, 1997.

186. Lerner SE, Hawkins CA, Blute ML, et al: Disease outcome in patients with low stage renal cell carcinoma treated with nephron sparing or radical surgery. J Urol 155:1868-1873, 1996.

187. Butler BP, Novick AC, Miller DP, et al: Management of small unilateral renal cell carcinomas: Radical versus nephron-sparing surgery. Urology 45:34-40, discussion 40-41, 1995.

188. Novick AC: Partial nephrectomy for renal cell carcinoma. Urology 46:149-152, 1995.

189. Semb C: Partial resection of the kidney: Operative technique. Acta Chir Scand 109:360, 1955.

190. Izes JK, Libertino JA: Partial nephrectomy. *In* Libertino JA (ed): Reconstructive Urologic Surgery. St. Louis, Mosby, 1993, pp 37-46.

191. Clayman RV, Kavoussi LR, Soper NJ, et al: Laparoscopic nephrectomy: Initial case report. J Urol 146:278-282, 1991.

192. Rassweiler JJ, Henkel TO, Potempa DM, et al: The technique of transperitoneal laparoscopic nephrectomy, adrenalectomy and nephroureterectomy. Eur Urol 23:425-430, 1993.

193. Ono Y, Sahashi M, Yamada S, Ohshima S: Laparoscopic nephrectomy without morcellation for renal cell carcinoma: Report of initial 2 cases. J Urol 150:1222-1224, 1993.

194. McDougall E, Clayman RV, Elashry OM: Laparoscopic radical nephrectomy for renal tumor: The Washington University experience. J Urol 155:1180-1185, 1996.

195. Ono Y, Katoh N, Kinukawa T, et al: Laparoscopic radical nephrectomy: The Nagoya experience. J Urol 158:719-723, 1997.

196. Rassweiler J, Fornara P, Weber M, et al: Laparoscopic nephrectomy: The experience of the laparoscopy working group of the German Urologic Association. J Urol 160:18-21, 1998.

197. Cadeddu JA, Ono Y, Clayman RV, et al: Laparoscopic nephrectomy for renal cell cancer: Evaluation of efficacy and safety: A multicenter experience. Urology 52:773-777, 1998.

198. Portis AJ, Yan Y, Landman J, et al: Long-term followup after laparoscopic radical nephrectomy. J Urol 167:1257-1262, 2002.

199. Meraney AM, Gill IS: Financial analysis of open versus laparoscopic radical nephrectomy and nephroureterectomy. J Urol 167: 1757-1762, 2002.

200. Jeschke K, Peschel R, Wakonig J, et al: Laparoscopic nephron-sparing surgery for renal tumors. Urology 58:688-692, 2001.

201. Gettman MT, Bischoff JT, Su LM, et al: Hemostatic laparoscopic partial nephrectomy: Initial experience with the radiofrequency coagulation–assisted technique. Urology 58:8-11, 2001.

202. Gill IS, Desai MM, Kaouk JH, et al: Laparoscopic partial nephrectomy for renal tumor: Duplicating open surgical techniques. J Urol 167:469-467, discussion 475-476, 2002.

203. Zlotta AR, Wildschutz T, Raviv G, et al: Radiofrequency interstitial tumor ablation (RITA) is a possible new modality for treatment of renal cancer: Ex vivo and in vivo experience. J Endourol 11: 251-258, 1997.

204. McGovern FJ, Wood BJ, Goldberg SN, Mueller PR: Radio frequency ablation of renal cell carcinoma via image guided needle electrodes. J Urol 161:599-600, 1999.

205. Gervais DA, McGovern FJ, Wood BJ, et al: Radio-frequency ablation of renal cell carcinoma: Early clinical experience. Radiology 217:665-672, 2000.

206. Gervais DA, McGovern FJ, Arellano RS, et al: Renal cell carcinoma: Clinical experience and technical success with radio-frequency ablation of 42 tumors. Radiology 226:417-424, 2003.

207. Pavlovich CP, Walther MM, Choyke PL, et al: Percutaneous radio frequency ablation of small renal tumors: Initial results. J Urol 167:10-15, 2002.

208. de Baere T, Kuoch V, Smayra T, et al: Radio frequency ablation of renal cell carcinoma: Preliminary clinical experience. J Urol 167:1961-1964, 2002.

209. Rendon RA, Kachura JR, Sweet JM, et al: The uncertainty of radio frequency treatment of renal cell carcinoma: Findings at immediate and delayed nephrectomy. J Urol 167:1587-1592, 2002.

210. Libertino J, Swierzewski D, Swierzewski M: Renal cell carcinoma with extension into the vena cava. In Libertino J (ed): Reconstructive Urologic Surgery. St. Louis, Mosby, 1998, pp 47-54.

211. Cherrie RJ, Goldman DG, Lindner A, deKernion JB: Prognostic implications of vena caval extension of renal cell carcinoma. J Urol 128:910-912, 1982.

212. Hatcher PA, Anderson EE, Paulson DF, et al: Surgical management and prognosis of renal cell carcinoma invading the vena cava. J Urol 145:20-23, discussion 23-24, 1991.

213. Marshall FF, Dietrick DD, Baumgartner WA, Reitz BA: Surgical management of renal cell carcinoma with intracaval neoplastic extension above the hepatic veins. J Urol 139:1166-1172, 1988.

214. Novick AC: Current surgical approaches, nephron-sparing surgery, and the role of surgery in the integrated immunologic approach to renal-cell carcinoma. Semin Oncol 22:29-33, 1995.

215. Fitzgerald JM, Tripathy U, Svensson LG, Libertino JA: Radical nephrectomy with vena caval thrombectomy using a minimal access approach for cardiopulmonary bypass. J Urol 159:1292-1293, 1998.

216. deKernion JB: Treatment of advanced renal cell carcinoma—traditional methods and innovative approaches. J Urol 130:2-7, 1983.

217. Swanson DA, Wallace S, Johnson DE: The role of embolization and nephrectomy in the treatment of metastatic renal carcinoma. Urol Clin North Am 7:719-730, 1980.

218. Flanigan RC: The failure of infarction and/or nephrectomy in stage IV renal cell cancer to influence survival or metastatic regression. Urol Clin North Am 14:757-762, 1987.

219. Swanson DA, Johnson DE, von Eschenbach AC, et al: Angioinfarction plus nephrectomy for metastatic renal cell carcinoma—an update. J Urol 130:449-452, 1983.

220. Middleton RG: Surgery for metastatic renal cell carcinoma. J Urol 97:973-977, 1967.

221. Montie JE, Stewart BH, Straffon RA, et al: The role of adjunctive nephrectomy in patients with metastatic renal cell carcinoma. J Urol 117:272-275, 1977.

222. deKernion JB, Ramming KP, Smith RB: The natural history of metastatic renal cell carcinoma: A computer analysis. J Urol 120:148-152, 1978.

223. Belldegrun A, Koo AS, Bochner B, et al: Immunotherapy for advanced renal cell cancer: The role of radical nephrectomy. Eur Urol 18(suppl 2):42-45, 1990.

224. Belldegrun A, Abi-Aad AS, Figlin RA, deKernion JB: Renal cell carcinoma: Basic biology and current approaches to therapy. Semin Oncol 18(5 suppl 7):96-101, 1991.

225. Fisher RI, Coltman CA Jr, Doroshow JH, et al: Metastatic renal cancer treated with interleukin-2 and lymphokine-activated killer cells. A phase II clinical trial. Ann Intern Med 108:518-523, 1988.

226. Atkins MB, Sparano J, Fisher RI, et al: Randomized phase II trial of high-dose interleukin-2 either alone or in combination with interferon alfa-2b in advanced renal cell carcinoma. J Clin Oncol 11:661-670, 1993.

227. Mickisch GH, Garin A, van Poppel H, et al: Radical nephrectomy plus interferon-alfa–based immunotherapy compared with interferon alfa alone in metastatic renal-cell carcinoma: A randomised trial. Lancet 358:966-970, 2001.

228. Flanigan RC, Salmon SE, Blumenstein BA, et al: Nephrectomy followed by interferon alfa-2b compared with interferon alfa-2b alone for metastatic renal-cell cancer. N Engl J Med 345:1655-1659, 2001.

229. Pantuck AJ, Belldegrun AS, Figlin RA: Nephrectomy and interleukin-2 for metastatic renal-cell carcinoma. N Engl J Med 345:1711-1712, 2001.

230. McDermott D, Flaherty L, Clark J, et al: A randomized phase II trial of high-dose interleukin-2(HD IL2) versus subcutaneous (SC) Il2/interferon (IFN) in patients with metastatic renal cell carcinoma (RCC). Paper presented at the 37th Annual Meeting of the American Society of Clinical Oncology, San Francisco, 2001.

231. Rackley R, Novick A, Klein E, et al: The impact of adjuvant nephrectomy on multimodality treatment of metastatic renal cell carcinoma. J Urol 152:1399-1403, 1994.

232. Taneja SS, Rierce W, Figlin R, Belldegrun A: Immunotherapy for renal cell carcinoma: The era of interleukin-2–based treatment. Urology 45:911-924, 1995.

233. Walther MM, Yang JC, Pass HI, et al: Cytoreductive surgery before high dose interleukin-2 based therapy in patients with metastatic renal cell carcinoma. J Urol 158:1675-1678, 1997.

234. Bennett RT, Lerner SE, Taub HC, et al: Cytoreductive surgery for stage IV renal cell carcinoma. J Urol 154:32-34, 1995.

235. Fallick ML, McDermott DF, LaRock D, et al: Nephrectomy before interleukin-2 therapy for patients with metastatic renal cell carcinoma. J Urol 158:1691-1695, 1997.

236. Kaufman JJ: Cancer of the urogenital tract: Kidney. Reasons for nephrectomy: Palliative and curative. JAMA 204:607-608, 1968.

237. De Conno F, Martini C, Zecca E, et al: Megestrol acetate for anorexia in patients with far-advanced cancer: A double-blind controlled clinical trial. Eur J Cancer 34:1705-1709, 1998.

238. Kavolius JP, Mastorakos DP, Pavlovich C, et al: Resection of metastatic renal cell carcinoma. J Clin Oncol 16:2261-2266, 1998.

239. Dineen MK, Pastore RD, Emrich LJ, Huben RP: Results of surgical treatment of renal cell carcinoma with solitary metastasis. J Urol 140:277-279, 1988.

240. O'Dea MJ, Zincke H, Utz DC, Bernatz PE: The treatment of renal cell carcinoma with solitary metastasis. J Urol 120:540-542, 1978.

241. Tolia BM, Whitmore WF Jr: Solitary metastasis from renal cell carcinoma. J Urol 114:836-838, 1975.

242. Fleischmann JD, Kim B: Interleukin-2 immunotherapy followed by resection of residual renal cell carcinoma. J Urol 145:938-941, 1991.

243. Sherry RM, Pass HI, Rosenberg SA, Yang JC: Surgical resection of metastatic renal cell carcinoma and melanoma after response to interleukin-2–based immunotherapy. Cancer 69:1850-1855, 1992.

244. Atkins MB, Dutcher JP: Renal-cell carcinoma. N Engl J Med 336:809, discussion 810-811, 1997.

245. Rafla S: Renal cell carcinoma. Natural history and results of treatment. Cancer 25:26-40, 1970.

246. Finney R: The value of radiotherapy in the treatment of hypernephroma—a clinical trial. Br J Urol 45:258-269, 1973.

247. Kjaer M, Frederiksen PL, Engelholm SA: Postoperative radiotherapy in stage II and III renal adenocarcinoma. A randomized trial

by the Copenhagen Renal Cancer Study Group. Int J Radiat Oncol Biol Phys 13:665-672, 1987.

248. Fossa SD, Kjolseth I, Lund G: Radiotherapy of metastases from renal cancer. Eur Urol 8:340-342, 1982.

249. Halperin EC, Harisiadis L: The role of radiation therapy in the management of metastatic renal cell carcinoma. Cancer 51:614-617, 1983.

250. Wronski M, Maor MH, Davis BJ, et al: External radiation of brain metastases from renal carcinoma: A retrospective study of 119 patients from the M D Anderson Cancer Center. Int J Radiat Oncol Biol Phys 37:753-759, 1997.

251. Mori Y, Kondziolka D, Flickinger JC, et al: Stereotactic radiosurgery for brain metastasis from renal cell carcinoma. Cancer 83:344-353, 1998.

252. Goyal LK, Suh JH, Reddy CA, Barnett GH: The role of whole brain radiotherapy and stereotactic radiosurgery on brain metastases from renal cell carcinoma. Int J Radiat Oncol Biol Phys 47:1007-1012, 2000.

253. Ikushima H, Tokuuye K, Sumi M, et al: Fractionated stereotactic radiotherapy of brain metastases from renal cell carcinoma. Int J Radiat Oncol Biol Phys 48:1389-1393, 2000.

254. Elson PJ, Witte RS, Trump DL: Prognostic factors for survival in patients with recurrent or metastatic renal cell carcinoma. Cancer Res 48:7310-7313, 1988.

255. Kirkman N, Bacon RL: Estrogen-induced tumors of the kidney: Incidence of renal cancer in intact and gonadectomized male golden hamsters treated with diethylstilbestrol. J Natl Cancer Inst 13: 745-755, 1952.

256. Harris DT: Hormonal therapy and chemotherapy of renal-cell carcinoma. Semin Oncol 10:422-430, 1983.

257. Bodey C: Current status of chemotherapy in metastatic renal cell carcinoma. *In* Johnson D, Samuels M (eds): Cancer of the Genitourinary Tract. New York, Raven Press, 1979, p 67.

258. Kjaer M: The role of medroxyprogesterone acetate (MPA) in the treatment of renal adenocarcinoma. Cancer Treat Rev 15:195-209, 1988.

259. Yagoda A, Petrylak D, Thompson S: Cytotoxic chemotherapy for advanced renal cell carcinoma. Urol Clin North Am 20:303-321, 1993.

260. Pyrhonen S, Salminen E, Lehtonen T, et al: Recombinant interferon alfa-2a with vinblastine vs. vinblastine alone in advanced renal cell carcinoma. A phase II study. Paper presented at the 32nd Annual Meeting of the American Society for Clinical Oncology, Philadelphia, 1996, p 244.

261. Hrushesky WJ, von Roemeling R, Lanning RM, Rabatin JT: Circadian-shaped infusions of floxuridine for progressive metastatic renal cell carcinoma. J Clin Oncol 8:1504-1513, 1990.

262. Dexeus FH, Logothetis CJ, Sella A, et al: Circadian infusion of floxuridine in patients with metastatic renal cell carcinoma. J Urol 146:709-713, 1991.

263. Mertens WC, Eisenhauer EA, Moore M, et al: Gemcitabine in advanced renal cell carcinoma. A phase II study of the National Cancer Institute of Canada Clinical Trials Group. Ann Oncol 4: 331-332, 1993.

264. De Mulder PH, Weissbach L, Jakse G, et al: Gemcitabine: A phase II study in patients with advanced renal cancer. Cancer Chemother Pharmacol 37:491-495, 1996.

265. Casali M, Marcellini M, Casali A, et al: Gemcitabine in pre-treated advanced renal carcinoma: A feasibility study. J Exp Clin Cancer Res 20:195-198, 2001.

266. Rini BI, Vogelzang NJ, Dumas MC, et al: Phase II trial of weekly intravenous gemcitabine with continuous infusion fluorouracil in patients with metastatic renal cell cancer. J Clin Oncol 18: 2419-2426, 2000.

267. Gollob JA, Upton MA, DeWolf WC, Atkins MB: Long-term remission in a patient with metastatic collecting duct carcinoma treated with taxol/carboplatin and surgery. Urology 58:1058, 2001.

268. Fojo AT, Ueda K, Slamon DJ, et al: Expression of a multidrug-resistance gene in human tumors and tissues. Proc Natl Acad Sci U S A 84:265-269, 1987.

269. Fojo AT, Shen DW, Mickley LA, et al: Intrinsic drug resistance in human kidney cancer is associated with expression of a human multidrug-resistance gene. J Clin Oncol 5:1922-1927, 1987.

270. Duensing S, Dallmann I, Grosse J, et al: Immunocytochemical detection of P-glycoprotein: Initial expression correlates with survival in renal cell carcinoma patients. Oncology 51:309-313, 1994.

271. Mickisch GH, Roehrich K, Koessig J, et al: Mechanisms and modulation of multidrug resistance in primary human renal cell carcinoma. J Urol 144:755-759, 1990.

272. Warner E, Tobe S, Pei Y, et al: Phase I trial of vinblastine (VBL) with oral cyclosporin A (CSA) as a multidrug resistance modifier in RCC. Paper presented at the 11th Annual Meeting of the American Society for Clinical Oncology, San Diego, CA, 1992, p 204.

273. Lemon S, Meadows B, Fojo A, et al: A phase I study of infusional vinblastine with p-glycoprotein antagonist PSC 833 in patients with metastatic cancer. Paper presented at the 31st Annual Meeting of the American Society for Clinical Oncology, Los Angeles, 1995, p 479.

274. Quesada JR: Biologic response modifiers in the therapy of metastatic renal cell carcinoma. Semin Oncol 15:396-407, 1988.

275. Muss HB: The role of biological response modifiers in metastatic renal cell carcinoma. Semin Oncol 15(5 suppl 5):30-34, 1988.

276. Neidhart JA: Interferon therapy for the treatment of renal cancer. Cancer 57(8 suppl):1696-1699, 1986.

277. Muss HB: Interferon therapy for renal cell carcinoma. Semin Oncol 14(2 suppl 2):36-42, 1987.

278. Muss HB, Costanzi JJ, Leavitt R, et al: Recombinant alfa interferon in renal cell carcinoma: A randomized trial of two routes of administration. J Clin Oncol 5:286-291, 1987.

279. Negrier S, Caty A, Lesimple T, et al: Treatment of patients with metastatic renal carcinoma with a combination of subcutaneous interleukin-2 and interferon alfa with or without fluorouracil. Groupe Francais d'Immunotherapie, Federation Nationale des Centres de Lutte Contre le Cancer. J Clin Oncol 18:4009-4015, 2000.

280. Neidhart JA, Anderson SA, Harris JE, et al: Vinblastine fails to improve response of renal cancer to interferon alfa-n1: High response rate in patients with pulmonary metastases. J Clin Oncol 9:832-836, 1991.

281. Motzer RJ, Schwartz L, Law TM, et al: Interferon alfa-2a and 13-*cis*-retinoic acid in renal cell carcinoma: Antitumor activity in a phase II trial and interactions in vitro. J Clin Oncol 13:1950-1957, 1995.

282. Garnick MB, Reich SD, Maxwell B, et al: Phase I/II study of recombinant interferon gamma in advanced renal cell carcinoma. J Urol 139:251-255, 1988.

283. Quesada JR, Kurzrock R, Sherwin SA, Gutterman SU: Phase II studies of recombinant human interferon gamma in metastatic renal cell carcinoma. J Biol Response Mod 6:20-27, 1987.

284. Otto U, Conrad S, Schneider AW, Kosterhalfen H: Recombinant interferon gamma in the treatment of metastatic renal cell carcinoma. Results of a phase II trial. Arzneimittelforschung 38:1658-1660, 1988.

285. Phase II study of recombinant human interferon gamma (S-6810) on renal cell carcinoma. Summary of two collaborative studies. Recombinant Human Interferon Gamma (S-6810) Research Group on Renal Cell Carcinoma. Cancer 60:929-933, 1987.

286. Wagstaff J, Smith D, Nelmes P, et al: A phase I study of recombinant interferon gamma administered by s.c. injection three times per week in patients with solid tumours. Cancer Immunol Immunother 25:54-58, 1987.

287. Rinehart JJ, Malspeis L, Young D, Neidhart JA: Phase I/II trial of human recombinant interferon gamma in renal cell carcinoma. J Biol Response Mod 5:300-308, 1986.

288. Aulitzky W, Gastl G, Aulitzky WE, et al: Successful treatment of metastatic renal cell carcinoma with a biologically active dose of recombinant interferon-gamma. J Clin Oncol 7:1875-1884, 1989.

289. Gleave ME, Elhiali M, Fradet Y, et al: Interferon gamma-1b compared with placebo in metastatic renal-cell carcinoma. Canadian Urologic Oncology Group. N Engl J Med 338:1265-1271, 1998.

290. Mazumder A, Rosenberg SA: Successful immunotherapy of natural killer–resistant established pulmonary melanoma metastases by the intravenous adoptive transfer of syngeneic lymphocytes activated in vitro by interleukin 2. J Exp Med 159:495-507, 1984.

291. Rosenberg SA, Lotze MT, Muul LM, et al: A progress report on the treatment of 157 patients with advanced cancer using lymphokine-activated killer cells and interleukin-2 or high-dose interleukin-2 alone. N Engl J Med 316:889-897, 1987.

292. Sunderland MC, Weiss GR: High dose IL-2 treatment of renal cell carcinoma. *In* Atkins MB, Mier JW (eds): Therapeutic Applications of Interleukin-2. New York, Marcel Dekker, 1993, pp 119-142.

293. Fyfe G, Fisher RI, Rosenberg SA, et al: Results of treatment of 255 patients with metastatic renal cell carcinoma who received high-dose recombinant interleukin-2 therapy. J Clin Oncol 13:688-696, 1995.

294. Rosenberg SA, Lotze MT, Yang JC, et al: Prospective randomized trial of high-dose interleukin-2 alone or in conjunction with lymphokine-activated killer cells for the treatment of patients with advanced cancer. J Natl Cancer Inst 85:622-632, 1993.

295. Dillman RO, Oldhan RK, Tauer KW, et al: Continuous interleukin-2 and lymphokine-activated killer cells for advanced cancer: A National Biotherapy Study Group trial. J Clin Oncol 9:1233-1240, 1991.

296. Weiss GR, Margolin KA, Aronson FR, et al: A randomized phase II trial of continuous infusion interleukin-2 or bolus injection interleukin-2 plus lymphokine-activated killer cells for advanced renal cell carcinoma. J Clin Oncol 10:275-281, 1992.

297. Fisher RI, Rosenberg SA, Sznol M, et al: High-dose aldesleukin in renal cell carcinoma: Long-term survival update. Cancer J Sci Am 3(suppl 1):70-72, 1997.

298. Sosman JA, Kohler PC, Hank J, et al: Repetitive weekly cycles of recombinant human interleukin-2: Responses of renal carcinoma with acceptable toxicity. J Natl Cancer Inst 80:60-63, 1988.

299. Caligiuri MA, Murray C, Robertson MJ, et al: Selective modulation of human natural killer cells in vivo after prolonged infusion of low-dose recombinant interleukin-2. J Clin Invest 91:123-132, 1993.

300. Sleijfer DT, Janssen RA, Buter J, et al: Phase II study of subcutaneous interleukin-2 in unselected patients with advanced renal cell cancer on an outpatient basis. J Clin Oncol 10:1119-1123, 1992.

301. Yang JC, Topalian SL, Parkinson D, et al: Randomized comparison of high-dose and low-dose intravenous interleukin-2 for the therapy of metastatic renal cell carcinoma: An interim report. J Clin Oncol 12:1572-1576, 1994.

302. Atkins MB, Lotze MT, Dutcher JP, et al: High-dose recombinant interleukin 2 therapy for patients with metastatic melanoma: Analysis of 270 patients treated between 1985 and 1993. J Clin Oncol 17:2105, 1999.

303. Yang JC, Rosenberg SA: An ongoing prospective randomized comparison of interleukin-2 regimens for the treatment of metastatic renal cell cancer. Cancer J Sci Am 3(suppl 1):79-84, 1997.

304. Yang JC, Rosenberg SA: A 3-arm randomized comparison of high and low dose intravenous and subcutaneous interleukin-2 in the treatment of metastatic renal cancer. J Immunother 25(suppl):33, 2002.

305. Numerof RP, Aronson FR, Mier JW: IL-2 stimulates the production of IL-1 alpha and IL-1 beta by human peripheral blood mononuclear cells. J Immunol 141:4250-4257, 1988.

306. Mier JW, Vachino G, van der Meer JW, et al: Induction of circulating tumor necrosis factor (TNF alpha) as the mechanism for the febrile response to interleukin-2 (IL-2) in cancer patients. J Clin Immunol 8:426-436, 1988.

307. Lotze MT, Matory YL, Ettinghausen SE, et al: In vivo administration of purified human interleukin 2. II. Half life, immunologic effects, and expansion of peripheral lymphoid cells in vivo with recombinant IL 2. J Immunol 135:2865-2875, 1985.

308. Hibbs JB Jr, Westenfelder C, Taintor R, et al: Evidence for cytokine-inducible nitric oxide synthesis from L-arginine in patients receiving interleukin-2 therapy. J Clin Invest 89:867-877, 1992.

309. Mier JW, Vachino G, Kempner MS, et al: Inhibition of interleukin-2–induced tumor necrosis factor release by dexamethasone: Prevention of an acquired neutrophil chemotaxis defect and differential suppression of interleukin-2–associated side effects. Blood 76:1933-1940, 1990.

310. Vetto JT, Papa MZ, Lotze MT, et al: Reduction of toxicity of interleukin-2 and lymphokine-activated killer cells in humans by the administration of corticosteroids. J Clin Oncol 5:496-503, 1987.

311. Trehu EG, Mier JW, Shapiro L, et al: A phase I trial of interleukin-2 in combination with the soluble tumor necrosis factor receptor p75 IgG chimera (TNFR:Fc). J Clin Oncol 15:1052-1062, 1966.

312. Du Bois JS, Trehu EG, Mier JW, et al: Randomized placebo-controlled clinical trial of high-dose interleukin-2 in combination with a soluble p75 tumor necrosis factor receptor immunoglobulin G chimera in patients with advanced melanoma and renal cell carcinoma. J Clin Oncol 15:1052-1062, 1997.

313. Margolin K, Atkins M, Sparano J, et al: Prospective randomized trial of lisofylline for the prevention of toxicities of high-dose interleukin 2 therapy in advanced renal cancer and malignant melanoma. Clin Cancer Res 3:565-572, 1997.

314. McDermott D, Trehn E, DuBois J, et al: Phase I clinical trial of the soluable IL-1 receptor either alone or in combination with high-dose IL-2 in patients with advanced malignancies. Clin Cancer Res 5:1203-1213, 1966.

315. Cameron RB, McIntosh JK, Rosenberg SA: Synergistic antitumor effects of combination immunotherapy with recombinant interleukin-2 and a recombinant hybrid alpha-interferon in the treatment of established murine hepatic metastases. Cancer Res 48:5810-5817, 1988.

316. Iigo M, Sakurai M, Tamura T, et al: In vivo antitumor activity of multiple injections of recombinant interleukin-2 alone and in combination with three different types of recombinant interferon, on various syngeneric murine tumors. Cancer Res 48:260-264, 1988.

317. Rosenberg SA, Lotze MT, Yang JC, et al: Combination therapy with interleukin-2 and alpha-interferon for the treatment of patients with advanced cancer. J Clin Oncol 7:1863-1874, 1989.

318. Dutcher JP, Atkins M, Fisher R, et al: Interleukin-2–based therapy for metastatic renal cell cancer: The cytokine working group experience, 1989-1997 Cancer J Sci Am 3(suppl 1):73-78, 1997.

319. Sznol M, MMier JW, Sparano J, et al: A phase I study of high-dose interleukin-2 in combination with interferon-alfa 2B. J Biol Response Mod 9:529-537, 1990.

320. Bergmann L, Frenchel K, Weidmann E, et al: Daily alternating administration of high-dose alfa-2b-interferon and interleukin-2 bolus infusion in metastatic renal cell carcinoma. Cancer 72:1733-1742, 1993.

321. Spencer WF, Linehan WM, Walther HM, et al, Immunotherapy with interleukin-2 and alpha-interferon in patients with metastic renal cell cancer with in situ primary cancer. A pilot study. J Urol 147:24-30, 1992.

322. Budd GT, Murthy S, Finke J, et al: Phase I trial of high-dose bolus interleukin-2 and interferon alfa-2a in patients with metastatic malignancy. J Clin Oncol 10:804-809, 1992.

323. Figlin R, et al: Low dose continuous infusion recombinant human interleukin-2 (rII-2) and Roferon-A: An active outpatient regimen for metastatic RCC. Paper presented at the 20th Annual Meeting of the American Society for Clinical Oncology, Washington, DC, 1990.

324. Lipton A, Harvey H, Givant E, et al: Interleukin-2 and interferon-α-2a outpatient therapy for metastatic RCC. J Immunother 13:122-129, 1993.

325. Dillman RO, Church C, Oldham RK, et al: Inpatient continuous-infusion interleukin-2 in 788 patients with cancer. The National Biotherapy Study Group experience. Cancer 71:2358-2370, 1993.

326. Figlin RA, Belldegrun A, Moldawer N, et al: Concomitant admistration of recombinant human interleukin-2 and recombinant interferon alfa-2A: An active outpatient regimen in metastatic renal cell carcinoma. J Clin Oncol 10:414-421, 1992.

327. Besana C, Borri A, Bucci E, et al: Treatment of advanced renal cell cancer with sequential intravenous recombinant interleukin-2 and subcutaneous α-interferon. Eur J Cancer 9:1292-1298, 1994.

328. Negrier S, Escudier B, Lasset C, et al: Recombinant human interleukin-2, recombinant human interferon alfa-2a, or both in metastatic renal-cell carcinoma. Groupe Francais d'Immunotherapie. N Engl J Med 338:1272-1278, 1998.

329. Atzpodien J, Poliwoda H, Kirchner H, et al: Alfa-interferon and interleukin-2 in RCC: Studies in nonhospitalized patients. Semin Oncol 18(suppl 7):108-112, 1991.

330. Palmer PA, Atzpodien J, Philip T, et al: A Comparsion of 2 modes of administration of recombinant interleukin-2: Continous intravennous infusion alone versus subcutaneous administration plus interferon alfa in patients with advanced RCC. Cancer Biother 8:123-136, 1993.

331. Atzpodien J, Lopez Hanninen E, Kirchner, et al: Multi-institutional home therapy trial of recombinant human interleukin-2 and interferon alfa-2 in progressive metastatic renal cell carcinoma. J Clin Oncol 13:497-501, 1995.

332. Vogelzang N, Lipton A, Figlin RA: Subcutaneous interleukin-2 plus interferon alfa-2a in metastatic renal cancer: An outpatient multi-center trail. J Clin Oncol 11:1809-1816, 1993.

333. Lummen G, Goepel M, Mullhoffs S, et al: Phase II study of interferon gamma versus interleukin-2 and interferon a2b in metastatic RCC. J Urol 155:455-458, 1996.

334. Atzpodien J, Kirchner H, Hanninen EL, et al: Interleukin-2 in combination with interferon-alpha and 5-fluorouracil for metastatic renal cell cancer. Eur J Cancer 29A(suppl 5):6-8, 1993.

335. Sella A, Kilbourn RG, Gray I, et al: Phase I study of interleukin-2 combined with interferon-alpha and 5-fluorouracil in patients with metastatic renal cell cancer. Cancer Biother 9:103-111, 1994.

336. Hofmockel G, Langer W, Theiss M, et al: Immunochemotherapy for metastatic renal cell carcinoma using a regimen of interleukin-2, interferon-alpha and 5-fluorouracil. J Urol 156:18-21, 1996.

337. Gitlitz B, Pierce W, Moldawer N: Long term follow-up and patterns of relapse in metastatic renal cell carcinoma using an outpatient regimen of low dose interleukin-2 (IL-2) and interferon alfa (IFN): The UCLA Kidney Cancer Program. Paper presented at the 30th Annual Meeting of the American Society for Clinical Oncology, Dallas, 1994.

338. Figlin RA, Pierce WC, Kaboo R, et al: Treatment of metastatic renal cell carcinoma with nephrectomy, interleukin-2 and cytokine-primed or CD8(+) selected tumor infiltrating lymphocytes from primary tumor. J Urol 158:740-745, 1997.

339. Bergman L, Frenchel K, Weidmann E, et al: Daily alternating administration of high-dose alfa-2b-interferon and interleukin-2 bolus infusion in metastatic renal cell cancer. Cancer 72:1733-1742, 1993.

340. Morant R, Richter J, Aapro M, et al: Treatment of patients with metastatic renal cell carcinoma with subcutaneous recombinant interferon-alfa 2b and continuous infusion of recombinant interleukin-2: A phase II study. Onkologie 17:254-260, 1994.

341. Dutcher JP, Fisher RI, Weiss G, et al: Outpatient subcutaneous interleukin-2 and interferon-alpha for metastatic renal cell cancer: Five-year follow-up of the Cytokine Working Group Study. Cancer J Sci Am 3:157-162, 1997.

342. Sella A, Zukiwiski A, Robinson E, et al: Interleukin-2 (IL-2) with interferon A (IFN-a) and 5-fluoruracil (5-FU) in patients (pts) with metatatic renal cell carcinoma (RCC). Paper presented at the 30th Annual Meeting of the American Society for Clinical Oncology, Dallas, 1994.

343. Dutcher JP, Atkins M, Fisher R, et al: Interleukin-2–based therapy for metastatic renal cell cancer: The Cytokine Working Group experience, 1989-1997. Cancer J Sci Am 3(suppl 1):73-78, 1997.

344. Royal RE, Steinberg SM, Krouse RS, et al: Correlates of response to IL-2 therapy in patients treated for metastatic renal cancer and melanoma. Cancer J Sci Am 2:91, 1996.

345. Atkins MB, Meir JW, Parkinson DR, et al: Hypothyroidism after treatment with interleukin-2 and lymphokine-activated killer cells. N Engl J Med 318:1557-1563, 1988.

346. West WH, Tauer KW, Yannelli JR, et al: Constant-infusion recombinant interleukin-2 in adoptive immunotherapy of advanced cancer. N Engl J Med 316:898-905, 1987.

347. Janik JE, Sznol M, Urba WJ, et al: Erythropoietin production. A potential marker for interleukin-2/interferon-responsive tumors. Cancer 72:2656-2659, 1993.

348. Figlin R, Gitlitz B, Franklin J, et al: Interleukin-2–based immunotherapy for the treatment of metastatic renal cell carcinoma: An analysis of 203 consecutively treated patients. Cancer J Sci Am 3(suppl):92-97, 1997.

349. Blay J, Combaret V, Negrier S: IL-1 and TNF concentrations as predictive factors of clinical response to IL-2 in patients with renal cell carcinoma. Abstract presented at the 27th Annual Meeting of the American Society for Clinical Oncology, Houston, 1991, p 257.

350. Trump DL, Elson P, Propert K, et al: Randomized controlled trial of adjuvant therapy with lymphoblastoid interferon. Paper presented at the 32nd Annual Meeting of the American Society for Clinical Oncology, Philadelphia, 1996, p 253.

351. Clark JI, Atkins MB, Urba WJ, et al: Adjuvant high-dose bolus interluekin-2 in patients with high-risk renal cell carcinoma—a Cytokine Working Group phase III trial. Paper presented at the 39th Annual Meeting of the American Society for Clinical Oncology, Chicago, 2003.

352. Margolin K, Aronson FR, Sznol M, et al: Phase II studies of recombinant human interleukin-4 in advanced renal cancer and malignant melanoma. J Immunother Emphasis Tumor Immunol 15:147-153, 1994.

353. Weiss GR, Margolin KA, Sznol M, et al: A phase II study of the continuous intravenous infusion of interleukin-6 for metastatic renal cell carcinoma. J Immunother Emphasis Tumor Immunol 18:52-56, 1995.

354. Atkins MB, Robertson MJ, Gordon M, et al: Phase I evaluation of intravenous recombinant human interleukin 12 in patients with advanced malignancies. Clin Cancer Res 3:409-417, 1997.

355. Motzer RJ, Rakhit A, Schwartz LH, et al: Phase I trial of subcutaneous recombinant human interleukin-12 in patients with advanced renal cell carcinoma. Clin Cancer Res 4:1183-1191, 1998.

356. Leonard JP, Sherman ML, Fisher GL, et al: Effects of single-dose interleukin-12 exposure on interleukin-12–associated toxicity and interferon-gamma production. Blood 90:2541-2548, 1997.

357. Gollob JA, Mier JW, Veenstra K, et al: Phase I trial of twice-weekly intravenous interleukin 12 in patients with metastatic renal cell cancer or malignant melanoma: Ability to maintain IFN-gamma induction is associated with clinical response. Clin Cancer Res 6:1678-1692, 2000.

358. Kugler A, Stuhler G, Walden P, et al: Regression of human metastatic renal cell carcinoma after vaccination with tumor cell-dendritic cell hybrids [see comments]. Nat Med 6:332-336, 2000.

359. Holtl L, Zelle-Rieser C, Gander H, et al: Immunotherapy of metastatic renal cell carcinoma with tumor lysate–pulsed autologous dendritic cells. Clin Cancer Res 8:3369-3376, 2002.

360. Avigan D: Dendritic cells: Development, function and potential use for cancer immunotherapy. Blood Rev 13:51-64, 1999.

361. Yang JC, Rosenberg SA: A randomized double-blind placebo-controlled trial of bevacizumab (anti-VEGF antibody) demonstrating a prolongation in time to progression in patients with metastatic renal cancer. Paper presented at the 38th Annual Meeting of the American Society for Clinical Oncology, Orlando, FL, 2002, p 15.

362. George D, Jonasch E, Hart L, et al: Dose-escalating and pharmacokinetic (PK) study of the VEGF-receptor inhibitor PTK787/ZK 222584 (PTK/ZK) in patients with advanced renal cell or prostate carcinomas. Paper presented at a Meeting of the American Society for Cancer Research, National Cancer Institute, and European Organization for Research in Cancer Therapy, 2001.

363. Minor DR, Monroe D, Damico LA, et al: A phase II study of thalidomide in advanced metastatic renal cell carcinoma. Invest New Drugs 20:389-393, 2002.

364. Daliani DD, Papandreou CN, Thall PF, et al: A pilot study of thalidomide in patients with progressive metastatic renal cell carcinoma. Cancer 95:758-765, 2002.

365. Escudier B, Lassau N, Couanet D, et al: Phase II trial of thalidomide in renal-cell carcinoma. Ann Oncol 13:1029-1035, 2002.

366. Motzer RJ, Berg W, Ginsberg M, et al: Phase II trial of thalidomide for patients with advanced renal cell carcinoma. J Clin Oncol 20:302-306, 2002.

367. Atkins MB, Hidalgo M, Stadler WM, et al: A randomized double-blind phase 2 study of intravenous CCI-779 administered weekly to patients with advanced renal cell carcinoma. Paper presented at the 38th Annual Meeting of the American Society for Clinical Oncology, Orlando, FL, 2002.

368. Atkins MB, Hidalgo M, Stadler WM, et al: A randomized double-blind phase II study of intravenous CCI-779 administered weekly to patients with advanced renal cell carcinoma (RCCA). Paper presented at the 38th Annual Meeting of the American Society for Clinical Oncology, Orlando, FL, 2002.

369. Hidalgo M, Atkins M, Stadler M, et al: A randomized double-blind phase 2 study of intravenous (IV) CCI-779 administered weekly to patients with advanced renal cell carcinoma (RCC): Prognostic factor analysis. Paper presented at the 39th Annual Meeting of the American Society for Clinical Oncology, Chicago, 2003.

370. Druker BJ, Schwartz L, Marion S, Motzer R: Phase II trial of ZD 1839 (Iressa), and EGF receptor inhibitor, in patients with renal cell carcinoma. Paper presented at the 38th Annual Meeting of the American Society for Clinical Oncology, Orlando, FL, 2002.

371. Wang P, Fredin P, Davis CG, Yang XD: Therapeutic potential of ABX-EGF, a fully human anti-EGF receptor monoclonal antibody, for the treatment of renal cell carcinoma. Paper presented at the 38th Annual Meeting of the American Society for Clinical Oncology, Orlando, FL, 2002.

372. Gale RP, Champlin RE: How does bone-marrow transplantation cure leukaemia? Lancet 2:28-30, 1984.

373. Weiden PL, Sullivan KM, Flournoy N, et al: Antileukemic effect of chronic graft-versus-host disease: Contribution to improved survival after allogeneic marrow transplantation. N Engl J Med 304:1529-1533, 1981.

374. Weiden PL, Flournoy M, Thomas ED, et al: Antileukemic effect of graft-versus-host disease in human recipients of allogeneic-marrow grafts. N Engl J Med 300:1068-1073, 1979.

375. Moscovitch M, Slavin S: Anti-tumor effects of allogeneic bone marrow transplantation in (NZB $\times$ NZW)F_1 hybrids with spontaneous lymphosarcoma. J Immunol 132:997-1000, 1984.

376. Morecki S, Moshel Y, Gelfend Y, et al: Induction of graft vs. tumor effect in a murine model of mammary adenocarcinoma. Int J Cancer 71:59-63, 1997.

377. Morecki S, Yacovlev E, Diab A, Slavin S: Allogeneic cell therapy for a murine mammary carcinoma. Cancer Res 58:3891-3895, 1998.

378. Ueno NT, Rondon G, Mirza NQ, et al: Allogeneic peripheral-blood progenitor-cell transplantation for poor-risk patients with metastatic breast cancer. J Clin Oncol 16:986-993, 1998.

379. Eibl B, Schwaighofer H, Nachbaur D, et al: Evidence for a graft-versus-tumor effect in a patient treated with marrow ablative chemotherapy and allogeneic bone marrow transplantation for breast cancer. Blood 88:1501-1508, 1996.

380. Childs R, Clave E, Contentin E, et al: Engraftment kinetics after non-myeloablative allogeneic peripheral blood stem cell transplantation: Full donor T-cell chimerism precedes alloimmune responses. Blood 94:3234-3241, 1999.

381. Sykes M, Preffer F, McAfee S, et al: Mixed lymphohaemopoietic chimerism and graft-versus-lymphoma effects after nonmyeloablative therapy and HLA-mismatched bone-marrow transplantation [see comments]. Lancet 353:1755-1759, 1999.

382. Khouri IF, Keating M, Korbling M, et al: Transplant-lite: Induction of graft-versus-malignancy using fludarabine-based nonablative chemotherapy and allogeneic blood progenitor-cell transplantation as treatment for lymphoid malignancies [see comments]. J Clin Oncol 16:2817-2824, 1998.

383. Spitzer TR, McAfee S, Sackstein R, et al: Intentional induction of mixed chimerism and achievement of antitumor responses after non-myeloablative conditioning therapy and HLA-matched donor bone marrow transplantation for refractory hematologic malignancies. Biol Blood Marrow Transplant 6:309-320, 2000.

384. Slavin S, Nager A, Naparstek E, et al: Nonmyeloablative stem cell transplantation and cell therapy as an alternative to conventional bone marrow transplantation with lethal cytoreduction for the treatment of malignant and nonmalignant hematologic diseases. Blood 91:756-763, 1998.

385. Childs R, Chernoff A, Contentin N, et al: Regression of metastatic renal-cell carcinoma after nonmyeloablative allogeneic peripheral-blood stem-cell transplantation. N Engl J Med 343: 750-758, 2000.

386. Pedrazzoli P, Da Prada GA, Georgiani G, et al: Allogeneic blood stem cell transplantation after a reduced-intensity, preparative regimen: A pilot study in patients with refractory malignancies. Cancer 94:2409-2415, 2002.

387. Bregni M, Dodero A, Peccatori J, et al: Nonmyeloablative conditioning followed by hematopoietic cell allografting and donor lymphocyte infusions for patients with metastatic renal and breast cancer. Blood 99:4234-4236, 2002.

388. Rini BI, Zimmerman TM, Gajewski TF, et al: Allogeneic peripheral blood stem cell transplantation for metastatic renal cell carcinoma. J Urol 165:1208-1209, 2001.

389. Wolk A, Gridley G, Niwa S, et al: International renal cell cancer study. VII. Role of diet. Int J Cancer 65:67-73, 1996.

390. Wilimas JA, Magill L, Parham DM, et al: Is renal salvage feasible in unilateral Wilms' tumor? Proposed computed tomographic criteria and their relation to surgicopathologic findings. Am J Pediatr Hematol Oncol 12:164-167, 1990.

SECTION IV

Pathophysiology of Renal Disease

CHAPTER 42

Renal and Systemic Manifestations of Glomerular Disease

Sharon Anderson, Radko Komers, and Barry M. Brenner

PROTEINURIA

Proteinuria characterizes most forms of glomerular injury and causes or contributes to all of the complications of the nephrotic syndrome. This section reviews the physiology and pathophysiology of glomerular permselectivity in clinical and experimental glomerular diseases. Extensive discussion of the mechanisms of proteinuria may also be found in several reviews.[1-7]

Physiologic Basis of Permselectivity

The glomerular capillary wall (GCW) is extremely permeable to water and small solutes, yet imposes a formidable barrier to the passage of plasma proteins. This permselectivity has been evaluated by characterizing the extent to which the GCW discriminates among molecules of different size, charge, and configuration. Classically, measurement of the Bowman space–to–plasma concentration ratio (the "sieving coefficient," θ) for various proteins in the rat has been determined by direct sampling via micropuncture techniques.[1] These studies indicate that small substances appear in the glomerular filtrate in concentrations similar to those in plasma whereas serum albumin is filtered to a much lesser extent (<0.1% that of inulin).

The most extensively used method to quantify glomerular capillary permselectivity involves measurement of the fractional clearance of test macromolecules. For a particular test solute *(m)*, fractional clearance is defined as the urinary clearance of *m* divided by the glomerular filtration rate (GFR). With the clearance of inulin used to measure GFR, fractional clearance of *m* is calculated from the urine and plasma concentrations of inulin *(I)* and *m* as follows:

$$\text{Fractional clearance of m} = \frac{C_{mu}C_{Ia}}{C_{ma}C_{Iu}}$$

where *C* refers to solute concentration and the second subscript denotes urine *(u)* or afferent arteriolar (systemic) plasma *(a)*. If, like inulin, the test macromolecule is not reabsorbed or secreted, its fractional clearance will exactly equal its Bowman space–to–plasma concentration ratio, θ.[5]

Proteins are not ideal test markers for such studies because of variations in size, charge, and shape, as well as tubule reabsorption of filtered protein. These difficulties may be circumvented with the use of a variety of exogenous nonprotein polymers, including dextran, dextran sulfate, diethylaminoethyl (DEAE) dextran, polyvinylpyrrolidone, Ficoll, and polyethylene glycol.[1] Much of the available permselectivity data relate to the use of dextran. However, as discussed later, Ficoll has been evaluated and appears to be superior.[6, 8]

Permselectivity Based on Molecular Size

The use of neutral dextran to analyze glomerular size selectivity is illustrated in the middle curve of Figure 42-1.[9-11] Measurement of the molecular radii of discrete dextran fractions is based on their elution from gel chromatographic columns calibrated with several proteins of known Stokes-Einstein radius.[5] A value of 1.0 on the ordinate denotes a dextran clearance equal to that of inulin (e.g., no measurable resistance to the filtration of dextran). Measurable restriction to filtration of neutral dextran does not occur until the effective radius exceeds about 20 Å.

As dextran size increases, fractional dextran clearance (θ_D) decreases progressively and approaches zero at dextran radii of at least 40 Å.

Theoretical Interpretation of Size Selectivity

ISOPOROUS MODELS. The most useful theoretical descriptions of macromolecular transport across the GCW are based on the concept of hindered movement of solutes through water-filled pores.[12] By using such theoretical analysis, dextran filtration data such as those in Figure 42-1 are accurately predicted by models that envision transport as taking place through numerous, identical cylindrical pores with a radius of approximately 55 Å. Solutes are regarded as solid spheres whose movement through pores occurs by diffusion and convection. Fluxes are hindered both by a partitioning phenomenon in which the macromolecule is partially excluded by virtue of its shape, size, or charge and by a hydrodynamic effect related to the nearby presence of the pore wall.[6, 13] For uncharged spherical molecules, interactions between solute and membrane depend on a single parameter, λ, the ratio of solute molecule radius to pore radius. Solute flux declines toward zero as solute size approaches that of the pore, whereas no hindrance is attributable to the pore if the pore is relatively large.

With these concepts in mind, the flux (J_T) of an uncharged solute *(T)* across the GCW may be expressed in terms of the following: C_T, the concentration of *T* in glomerular capillary plasma; J_v, the local glomerular transcapillary volume flux; D_T, the diffusivity of *T* in bulk solution; *f*, the fraction of the capillary surface area occupied by pores; *l*, the length of the pores; and hindrance factors that are each unique functions

of *l*. For relatively high fluid flow rates through the pore and for large solutes that diffuse poorly, solute movement is primarily via convection. For lower fluid flow rates or small solutes that diffuse rapidly, or for both, solute movement is governed primarily by diffusion.

The rate of filtration of solute T is dependent on two independent glomerular membrane properties: K_f, the glomerular capillary ultrafiltration coefficient, and r_p, the apparent glomerular pore radius. This term may be evaluated by fitting experimentally observed values of θ into the model. A more complete discussion of the theories of partitioning and hindered particle motion may be found in several reviews.[1, 6, 14, 15]

Application of this theoretical model to the data in Figure 42-1 results in calculated values of r_p that are relatively independent of molecular size, with an average of about 47 Å. Presumably, all molecules "see" the same pores, so the finding that the "best-fit" value of r_p is independent of molecular size confirms that the theory successfully correlates most of the available data. Values of θ calculated with the use of the theory for neutral dextran are shown by the middle solid curve in Figure 42-1. In this case, a pore radius of 47 Å provides an excellent fit to the data presented, except for molecular radii smaller than 24 Å, for which the isoporous theory appears to underestimate dextran transport.

An additional parameter that may be derived from values of K_f and r_p is the ratio of total pore area to pore length, *fS/l*, where *f* is the fraction of the capillary surface area *(S)* occupied by pores and *l* represents pore length. For pores of a given radius and length, this parameter is a measure of "pore density," the apparent number of pores per unit area of the GCW. Assuming that *l* is roughly the thickness of the glomerular basement membrane (GBM), the dextran data yield an estimate of f to be about 0.1,[16] thus suggesting that some 10% of the glomerular capillary surface area is perforated by pores.

HETEROPOROUS MODELS. Theoretical calculations indicate that the normal GCW behaves much as an isoporous filter with a pore radius of about 50 to 55 Å.[10, 17] This approach has proved most useful in interpreting data for dextrans with effective molecular radii of about 20 to 45 Å. However, in some human diseases, experimental data were found to be incompatible with the isoporous theory. In these proteinuric patients, θ_D was enhanced for the largest dextrans (>45 Å), but it was often decreased for the smallest dextrans when compared with normal subjects (Fig. 42-2).[18] These findings suggested that the selective increase in filtration of large dextrans could be explained by the emergence of a second population of pores, fewer in number but with larger radii, and thus suggested the need for a heteroporous description of functional GCW characteristics. Accordingly, Deen and colleagues[18] formulated a heteroporous model of glomerular size selectivity designed to account for the experimental observations.

The rationale for this model can be appreciated from a consideration of fractional IgG clearances obtained from subjects with extensive proteinuria.[18] The large size of IgG ($r = 55$ Å) makes it likely that its passage into the Bowman space is most directly related to the extent of the size-selective defect. As shown in a study of 70 nephrotic patients, considerable variability in IgG excretion was found, with fractional IgG clearances spanning three orders of magnitude, which were used to arbitrarily define three grades of

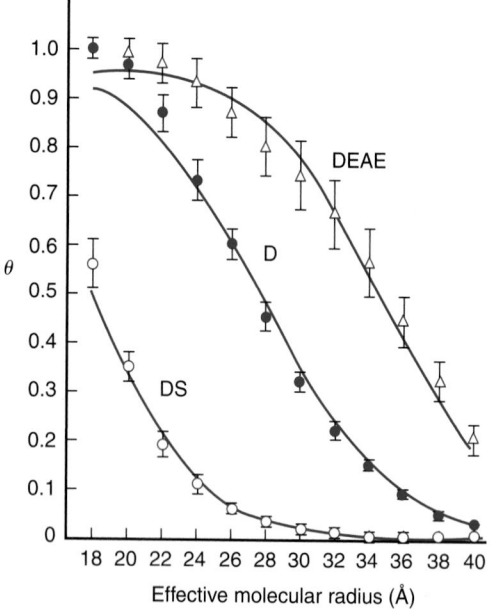

FIGURE 42-1. Filtrate-to-plasma concentration ratio (θ) as a function of molecular size for tritiated dextran sulfate (DS), neutral dextran (D), and diethylaminoethyl dextran (DEAE). Data points are means ± SE measured in the normal Munich-Wistar rat.[9, 10] All three *solid curves* were calculated theoretically by using the membrane parameters: $K_f = 4.8$ nL/ (min · mm Hg), $r_p = 47$ Å, and $C_m = 165$ mEq/L. (From Deen WM, Satvat B, Jamieson JM: Theoretical model for glomerular filtration of charged solutes. Am J Physiol 238:F126, 1980.)

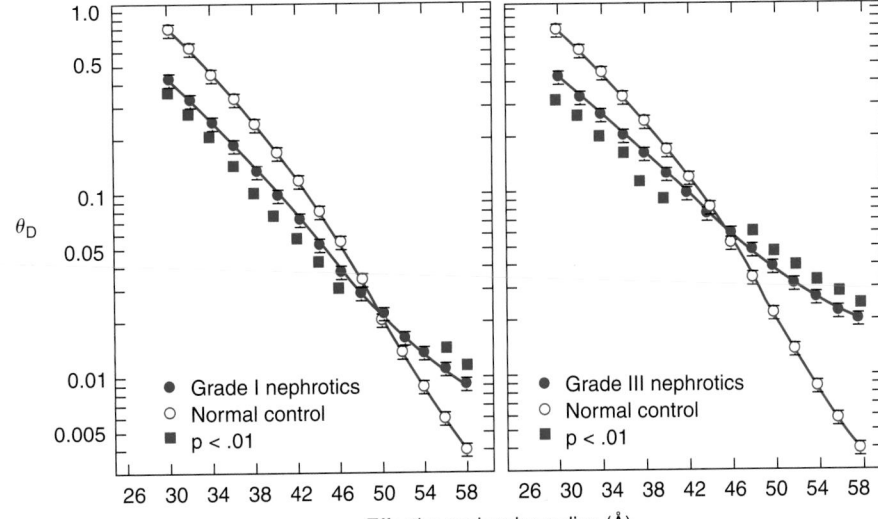

FIGURE 42-2. Fractional dextran clearances (θ_D) plotted as a function of molecular radius. Grade I *(left)* and grade III *(right)* nephrotic patients are compared with normal controls. Values are means ± SE. (From Deen WM, Bridges CR, Brenner BM, Myers BD: Heteroporous model of glomerular size selectivity: Application to normal and nephrotic humans. Am J Physiol 249:F374, 1985.)

increasing barrier injury.[17] Minimal IgG leakage (grade I) was associated with a low selectivity index (C_{IgG}/C_{alb}), an indication that the GCW was highly permeable to albumin but still relatively impermeable to IgG. At the opposite extreme (grade III), high rates of IgG leakage were associated with a high selectivity index, an indication that the GCW did not discriminate between the smaller albumin and the larger IgG molecule. As is shown in Figure 42-2,[18] similarities in sieving curves were noted in all grades of injury, with depressed values of θ_D for smaller and relatively impermeant dextrans and enhanced values of θ_D for larger macromolecules. However, the curves differed at the point at which the dextran sieving curve intersected that of normal subjects: it occurred earlier with increasing IgG leakage (at $r = 54$ Å in grade I and at $r = 46$ Å in grade III). In addition, the large-radius end of the sieving curve deviated more prominently from normal with increasing injury.

These data are inconsistent with the concept of the GCW as an isoporous filter in that no single population of pores of identical size could simultaneously account for restricted transport of smaller dextrans and enhanced transport of larger dextrans. Rather, the data more closely fit a model of solute transport through a heteroporous membrane with a subpopulation of large pores. This model assumes that most of the GCW is perforated by cylindrical pores of radius r_o and that a smaller portion of the GCW is permeated by large, nondiscriminatory "shunt" pathways that do not exhibit size selectivity. The portion of the GCW permeated by shunt pores is denoted ω_o, a parameter that quantitates the magnitude of the size selectivity defect. The fractional area of the membrane occupied by this shunt pathway, though small, increases with each successive grade of barrier injury. This subpopulation of large pores is presumed to allow passage of IgG and probably most of the filtered albumin. Therefore, nonselective heavy proteinuria appears to result from loss of barrier size selectivity, which renders the glomerular membrane more porous to large plasma proteins.[18]

LOGNORMAL MODELS. In some cases, the isoporous plus shunt model has not accurately fit the data, and better results are obtained with a model that assumes a lognormal distribution of pore radii.[8, 19] This distribution is characterized

by u, the mean pore radius, and s, the spread of the distribution.[19] The model has been further refined by calculation of the theoretical fraction of filtrate volume passing through the largest pores. Remuzzi and associates[19] used this model to define an index of the size of the largest pores in the GCW. By definition, 5% of the glomerular filtrate passes through pores with radii greater than $r^*(5\%)$, and 1% passes through pores with radii greater than $r^*(1\%)$.

Although most of the permselectivity data have been obtained with the use of dextran as a marker, a consistent problem has been the finding that θ for normal subjects tends to be large, given the absence of proteinuria. Thus, dextran appears to overestimate the true θ. Oliver and co-authors[8] proposed that Ficoll, which behaves more like an ideal spherical molecule than dextran does, is a better probe of glomerular pore size; the use of Ficoll is now being extended to studies in rats, humans, and in vitro models.[20-22] In normal rats, θ for dextran significantly exceeds that for Ficoll at all molecular sizes, being nearly 10 times that of Ficoll for an r_s greater than 30 Å, and values of θ for Ficoll approximate previously reported values for uncharged glomerular proteins. For Ficoll, a lognormal plus shunt pathway model was found to be the most effective (Fig. 42-3).[8]

Permselectivity Based on Molecular Charge

The charge-selective characteristics of the GCW have traditionally been evaluated with negatively charged markers such as dextran sulfate (DS). In a normal kidney, fractional DS clearance (θ_{DS}) is lower than that for neutral dextran at any given molecular radius (see Fig. 42-1).[5, 11] Conversely, positively charged molecules pass through more freely (see Fig. 42-1).[10] The importance of molecular charge is further demonstrated in proteinuric diseases. In a model of nephrotoxic serum nephritis, Chang and co-workers noted that θ_D for neutral dextran was less than that seen in normal rats (Fig. 42-4),[5, 10, 23-26] and thus these molecules could not account for the observed proteinuria; if albumin behaved like neutral dextran, albumin excretion should decrease rather than increase. Similarly, fractional clearances of cationic DEAE dextran were reduced and therefore could

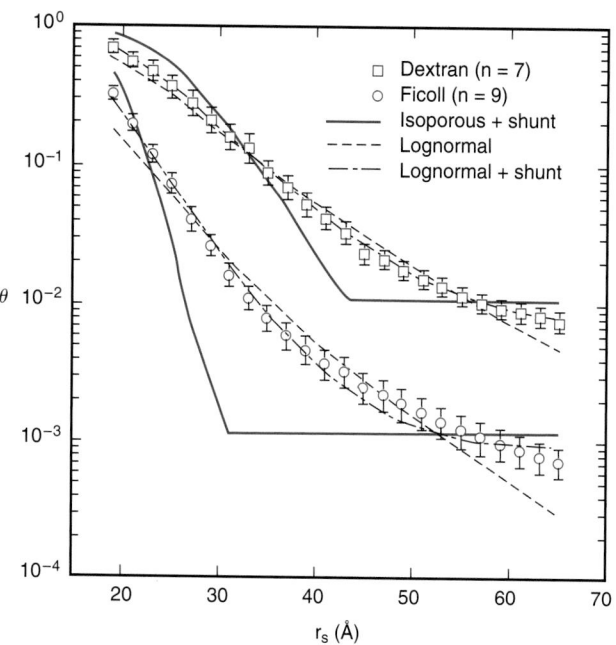

FIGURE 42-3. Sieving coefficient (θ) of dextran and Ficoll as a function of molecular radius (r_s) in normal rats. Experimental values are means ± SE; *curves* represent the best fits to the data obtained with the three types of pore size distribution. (From Oliver JD III, Anderson S, Troy JL, et al: Determination of glomerular size-selectivity in the normal rat with Ficoll. J Am Soc Nephrol 3:214, 1992.)

not explain the proteinuria. However, for any molecular size, θ_{DS} in rats with nephrotoxic serum nephritis was substantially greater than that observed in normal animals.[26] These observations suggested that the albuminuria in this disorder was a specific consequence of the reduction in fixed negative charge of the diseased GCW.

It should be noted that in recent years, the concept of DS as an appropriate marker to assess charge selectivity has been challenged by observations that it is not as inert a tracer as once believed and that earlier studies probably overestimated the effects of charge.[6] For example, Guasch and colleagues[27] found that DS binds with plasma proteins. Furthermore, cellular uptake and intracellular desulfation of DS may affect the interpretation of fractional clearance

data.[28] A detailed discussion of controversies in this field may be found in a recent review.[6] Though not believed to invalidate the concept of charge selectivity, these observations indicate a need for further study in this area.

Permselectivity Based on Molecular Configuration

To compare sieving of molecules with different conformations (i.e., a linear coil for dextran versus lobular proteins), the effects of molecular shape or configuration must be taken into account. Bohrer and associates[29] compared the fractional clearance of neutral dextran with that of Ficoll, an uncharged cross-linked copolymer of sucrose and epichlorohydrin. At any given effective radius, the flexible coil dextran was filtered more readily than Ficoll, a nearly rigid sphere; the superior accuracy of Ficoll was subsequently confirmed, as described earlier.[8] These studies suggest that protein configuration also plays a role in filtration, although size and charge appear to be more important.[1]

ANATOMIC AND FUNCTIONAL BARRIER TO FILTRATION OF MACROMOLECULES. The classic view of the anatomic barrier to the filtration of protein, as well as the changes that result in pathologic proteinuria, has been extensively reviewed[2] and will be briefly summarized here. As detailed later, the past few years have seen a major advance in our insight into this process through the discovery of nephrin and associated studies of the molecular nature of the slit diaphragm.

Early studies concluded that the GBM was the component of the GCW that restricted the passage of macromolecules.[30] Subsequent studies were consistent with this "single-barrier" hypothesis[2] until examination of the behavior of peroxidative tracers suggested that the slit diaphragm was an effective barrier to filtration.[31, 32] Later studies led to the "double-barrier" hypothesis: that the GBM restricts the passage of larger macromolecules whereas slit diaphragms regulate the passage of smaller ones.[33] However, this hypothesis failed to explain the findings that some relatively large tracers were restricted just beneath the slit diaphragm and some were completely restricted at the level of the inner layers of the GBM, so the potential contribution of charge needed to be addressed. Rennke and colleagues[34] used several ferritin fractions of similar size with varying isoelectric

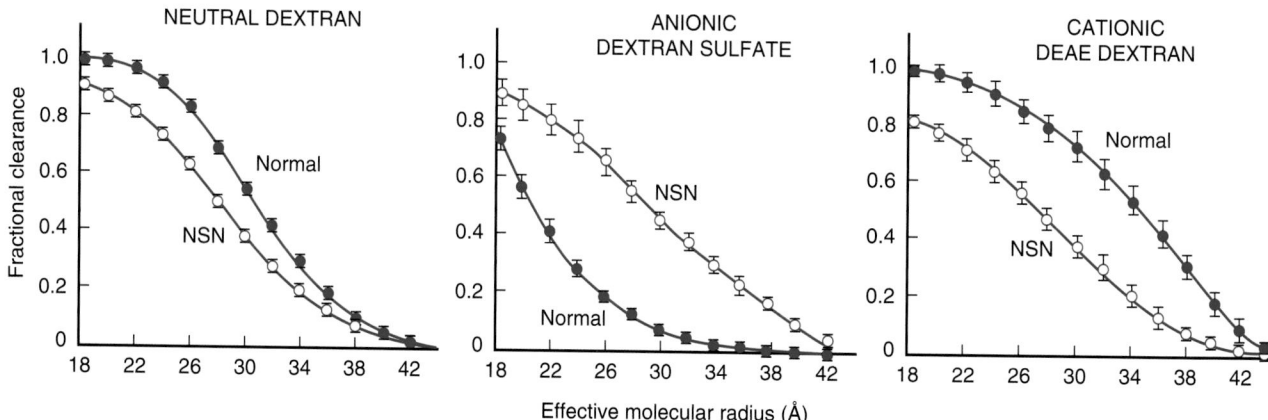

FIGURE 42-4. Fractional clearance of neutral dextran *(left)*, anionic dextran sulfate *(middle)*, and cationic diethylaminoethyl (DEAE) dextran *(right)* plotted as a function of effective molecular radii for normal rats and those with nephrotoxic serum nephritis (NSN). (From Brenner BM, Hostetter TH, Humes HD: Molecular basis of proteinuria of glomerular origin. N Engl J Med 298:926, 1978.)

points (pIs). A stepwise increase in the pI of ferritin resulted in a proportionate increase in its permeation into the GBM, with the more negatively charged particles penetrating furthest. Thus, these studies pointed to the existence of an intrinsic electrical charge in the GBM that was imparted by fixed anionic sites.[34]

These anionic sites have been localized to the surfaces of endothelial and epithelial cells, as well as the GBM interposed between these cells.[2, 35, 36] The glomerular epithelial cell and its foot processes are covered with a surface coat of acidic glycoproteins (sialoproteins or glomerular polyanion) that are highly negatively charged. Stainable polyanion has been identified to be podocalyxin, a sialoprotein that carries most of the glomerular sialic acid.[37] The epithelial slit diaphragm also consists, in part, of glycosialoproteins,[38] as does the endothelial cell coat.

The biochemical composition of the GBM has been extensively studied.[2, 39] The GBM consists of two classes of glycopeptides, a nonpolar collagen-like component and another more polar noncollagen fraction of asparagine-linked polysaccharide units. Glomerular epithelial cells are capable of synthesizing all major GBM components. Integral components of the GBM include type IV collagen, laminin, entactin/nidogen, and various proteoglycans, including chondroitin sulfate proteoglycan and heparan sulfate proteoglycan (HS-PG). Of the latter, HS-PG has been shown to be particularly important in imparting charge selectivity to the GBM.[2, 40] HS-PG is distributed throughout the GBM, but concentrated in the lamina rara interna and externa.[41] Normally, polyanions (particular HS-PG) act as "anticlogging" agents to prevent the adsorption of plasma protein so that ultrafiltration may proceed.[42, 43] Many studies have indicated the importance of anionic sites and HS-PG specifically in the defense against proteinuria.[44, 45] However, as discussed in the next section, newer evidence points away from a predominant role of the GBM in filtration barrier function.

Newer Concepts in Glomerular Permeability

Tracer studies as described earlier cannot differentiate the effects of hemodynamic and hormonal influences from the properties intrinsic to glomerular filtration. Innovative models have been developed to assess glomerular permeability in vitro. Daniels and co-workers[22, 46-48] examined the diffusion of fluorescent macromolecules across individual glomerular capillaries in intact glomeruli by confocal microscopy. With this method, the relative contribution of glomerular cells may be assessed by comparing intact with acellular glomeruli from which cells have been removed and leaving the GBM with some residual mesangial matrix. Studies in this system showed that θ_D in intact glomeruli is much less than that for the GBM alone; most of the size and charge selectivity of the GCW resides in the cells rather than in the GBM. In vivo studies have provided further confirmation of the importance of podocytes[49] and slit diaphragms[6, 50] in the restrictive properties of the GCW.

Traditional observations of changes in the structure of glomerular epithelial cells in various clinical proteinuric diseases prompted speculation that defects in that region might be responsible for increased GCW permeability.[51] More recently, alterations in several epithelial cell proteins, including megalin,[52] glomerular epithelial protein-1

(GLEPP-1),[53] the Wilms tumor gene protein (WT-1),[54] and nephrin,[55] have been associated with nephrotic syndromes. Nephrin, which localizes to the slit diaphragm of visceral epithelial cells, is mutated in a severe form of congenital nephrotic syndrome *(NPHS1)*.[55] Newer candidates genes identified as potentially being associated with nephrotic syndromes now include *Mpv 17*,[56] *NPHS2*,[57] and *NEPH1*.[58]

Influence of Hemodynamic Factors on Filtration of Macromolecules: General Considerations

Hemodynamic factors influence the filtration of macromolecules. Often, θ varies inversely with the single-nephron GFR (SNGFR).[1, 11, 59] Thus, filtration of macromolecules is influenced not only by the intrinsic membrane properties of the GCW but also by other determinants of SNGFR: Q_A, the glomerular capillary plasma flow rate; ΔP, the glomerular transcapillary hydraulic pressure difference; and C_A, the afferent arteriolar plasma protein concentration. The absolute single-nephron clearance of a macromolecule is given by the product $\theta \times$ SNGFR.[11, 15] Absolute clearance usually increases as Q_A is elevated, but less than in proportion to SNGFR; hence, θ decreases. The effect of Q_A is explained by considering that at a high flow rate, a given amount of filtrate produces a smaller increase in the plasma concentration of the test solute, thus making the increased filtration of neutral molecules less than that of water and thereby decreasing θ. Absolute macromolecular clearance rates also increase as ΔP rises. For neutral and anionic macromolecules, this increase is less than the increase in SNGFR, and as a result, θ decreases. For highly anionic molecules, this trend reverses at sufficiently high ΔP, and θ may increase. The opposite behavior is observed for positively charged macromolecules, with θ increasing with rising ΔP. The theoretical effects of C_A on θ are similar to those for inverse changes in ΔP because C_A and ΔP exert opposing effects on SNGFR. The actual effects of changes in C_A are likely to be more complicated because of parallel changes in K_f.[60] Hemodynamic factors may also influence rates of volume flux through the shunt pathway (see later).

Evaluation of the Filtration Barrier in Glomerular Disease
Animal Models of Glomerular Disease

Tracer macromolecules have been used in a number of experimental proteinuric models to characterize the glomerular permeability defects that result in proteinuria, as well as the response to therapeutic interventions. Not surprisingly, all such models exhibit impaired glomerular size selectivity with the passage of large molecules through the glomerular barrier. This defect has been noted in diverse animal models, including renal ablation,[61-63] diabetes,[20] and many others.[64] In some models, a charge-selective defect has also been seen. For example, a reduction in renal mass leads to hypertension and proteinuria, with elevated SNGFR, Q_A, and ΔP and reduced K_f. In this model, the proteinuria is due to defects in both size and charge selectivity,[61-63] with resultant increased flux through the shunt pathway. Peak pore size *(u)* is decreased whereas the width of the pore size distribution *(s)* is increased; both $r^*(5\%)$ and $r^*(1\%)$ increase

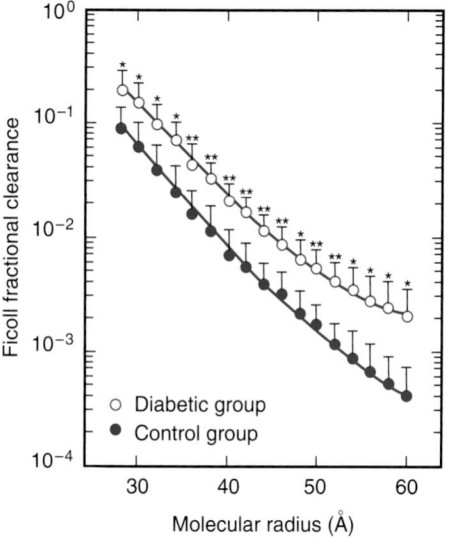
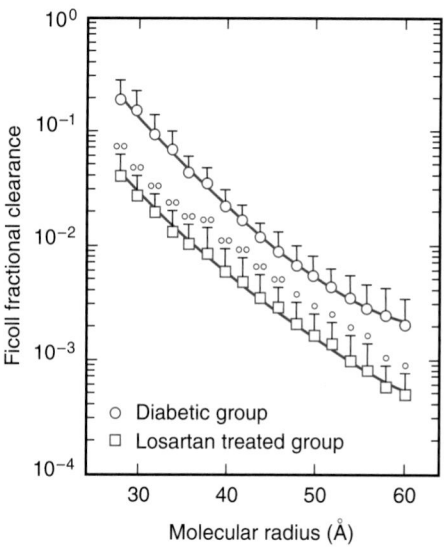

FIGURE 42-5. Fractional clearance of Ficoll as a function of molecular radius (Å) in diabetic and nondiabetic control rats *(left)* and in diabetic rats treated with losartan *(right)*. Values are means ± SE. *$P < .05$; **$P < .01$ versus controls; °$P < .05$; °°$P < .01$ versus the diabetic group. (From Remuzzi A, Perico N, Amuchastegui CS, et al: Short- and long-term effect of angiotensin II receptor blockade in rats with experimental diabetes. J Am Soc Nephrol 4:40, 1993.)

as well.[63] Another prominent example is diabetic nephropathy, a model with similar hemodynamic changes (see Chapter 38). Studies using Ficoll in diabetic rats found impaired size selectivity at all molecular radii tested (Fig. 42-5); in addition, the pore size distribution was shifted toward larger radii, as reflected by increases in *u*, w_o, and $r*(1\%)$.[20]

Another model is produced by injecting puromycin aminonucleoside into rats, which induces massive proteinuria and predominant epithelial cell injury. Ultrastructural studies indicate focal permeability to tracer macromolecules, particularly in areas of epithelial detachment from the GBM,[33, 65] along with altered distribution of anionic sites and sulfation of heparan sulfate.[44] In a puromycin aminonucleoside regimen that results in diminution of K_f with relative preservation of ΔP, Q_A, and K_f, θ_D for neutral dextrans 38 Å and smaller is decreased, whereas θ_{DS} is enhanced. Because glomerular hemodynamics is normal in this model, these data suggest a functional loss of the electrostatic barrier.[66] The θ_D of neutral dextrans larger than 38 Å is also increased, thus suggesting that a size-selective defect likewise contributes to proteinuria in this model.[67] Injection of neutral dextran into rats with doxorubicin (Adriamycin) nephrosis results in increased clearance of molecules larger than 40 Å.[19, 68] The lognormal model indicates increases in *u* and *s,* as well as in $r*(1\%)$ and $r*(5\%)$.[19] The role of a charge-selective defect is controversial.[19, 68] Studies in other models have been reviewed recently.[64]

Effects of Hemodynamic Changes on Glomerular Permselectivity

The influence of hemodynamic changes on glomerular permselectivity has also been widely studied. Acute hypertension induced by angiotensin II (AII) enhances protein filtration,[9] and AII also plays a role in the model of partial renal vein constriction.[69] This maneuver led to a marked decrease in Q_A with a lesser decrease in SNGFR, an increase in ΔP, and an increase in θ_D for dextrans larger than 44 Å. The AII receptor antagonist saralasin normalized glomerular hemodynamics. Fractional clearance of dextrans larger than 46 Å fell toward normal, whereas clearance of dextrans smaller than 40 Å was unaffected. The radius of the small selective pores and the index for fractional volume flux through these pores were relatively unaffected. However, renal vein constriction induced a 10-fold increase in the fraction of filtrate passing through larger, nonselective pores. About half the increase was reversed with saralasin. Thus, these data suggested that AII enhances proteinuria by inducing reversible changes in the sieving properties of the GCW, specifically by increasing flow through the shunt pathway, and that these changes might relate to perturbations in ΔP.[69] The action of AII is somewhat variable, however. Clinical studies have failed to find such an effect of AII in nephrotic subjects, whereas AII did increase fractional neutral dextran clearance in normal subjects; however, the effect could be attributed solely to hemodynamic factors.[70]

Human Glomerular Disease

PROTEIN CLEARANCE AND SELECTIVITY INDEX. Nephrotic-range proteinuria is associated with the passage of large plasma proteins into urine. The permselective characteristics of such glomeruli have been determined by measurement of the urinary clearance of proteins of graded size.[71] The smallest proteins, usually albumin (36 Å) or transferrin (38 Å), have been used as reference markers. When the clearance ratio of larger test proteins to that of the reference protein is plotted as a function of molecular weight, an inverse relationship is seen, which suggests that the diseased glomerulus continues to discriminate among proteins of increasing size but that the pore size distribution is shifted to pores of larger size. Thus, two categories of clinical proteinuria have been designated "selective" and "nonselective." Selective proteinuria is characterized by a relatively sharp molecular size cutoff; the proteinuria consists primarily of relatively small albumin molecules. Nonselective proteinuria contains a large proportion of larger plasma proteins, particularly IgG. When the selectivity index (the clearance ratio of a large protein such as IgG to that of a smaller protein such as albumin) is less than 0.2, the proteinuria is considered to be selective, whereas values greater than 0.2 indicate nonselective proteinuria.

This method, though relatively simple, has some theoretical limitations. The test proteins used have different pIs in physiologic solution, and the technique is unable to take into account changes in glomerular charge selectivity. Similarly, the technique cannot account for changes in tubular reabsorption of proteins, the protein catabolic capacity, or a potential selective increase in the glomerular filtration of one or more proteins. In view of these limitations, dextran (and, more recently, Ficoll) clearance techniques have been used to characterize clinical alterations in glomerular permselectivity.

STUDIES OF GLOMERULAR BARRIER FUNCTION IN CLINICAL GLOMERULAR DISEASE. The defective permselectivity in various forms of clinical proliferative glomerulonephritis was examined by determining the fractional clearance of dextran and IgG.[72] The θ_D values of smaller dextrans were similar regardless of the magnitude of IgG excretion, whereas those of larger dextrans were elevated in patients excreting larger amounts of IgG. These data could be best explained by the existence of a second population of larger pores (i.e., the shunt pathway). This model predicted that the passage of macromolecules such as IgG may be totally unrestricted in the damaged segment, and in fact, the filtered load of IgG was sufficiently large to account for the urinary IgG content. Thus, it was conceivable that IgG passage was entirely through the larger pores whereas passage of the smaller albumin molecule was more likely due to a charge-selective defect in the small-pore component of the GCW. The estimated radius of small pores was similar in the two groups, but the radius of larger pores was increased in patients with greater urinary loss of IgG.[72] These data suggested that when glomerulonephritis is associated with selective proteinuria, the major abnormality is in the charge-selective barrier to smaller proteins, whereas in glomerulonephritis associated with nonselective proteinuria and massive IgG loss, the GCW exhibits a subpopulation of enlarged pores that are highly permeable to proteins of large size and variable charge.

Subsequent studies have found that in many human glomerular diseases, the permselectivity defect consists of a combination of impaired size and charge selectivity and increased volume through the shunt pathway. To cite just a few of many examples, this pattern has been suggested in patients with minimal change disease,[17, 27, 73] membranous nephropathy,[21, 74-76] and diabetic nephropathy.[77-79] In diabetes, the dextran clearance profile changes in the evolutionary stages of diabetic nephropathy.[79-87] In patients with microalbuminuria (<300 mg/day), studies using IgG[80] and neutral dextrans[81] confirm the presence of a size-selective defect. Filtration of dextrans smaller than 48 Å is increased and that of larger dextrans is enhanced with increased filtrate volume through the shunt pathway.[81] Studies in subjects with overt nephropathy indicate qualitatively similar changes, though enhanced in magnitude.[80, 81] The data are also most consistent with the presence of a concomitant charge-selective defect. Indeed, the charge defect may even precede the size defect.[82] In diabetic patients, glycosylation of proteins may contribute to the problem inasmuch as glycosylated proteins, including albumin, appear in urine more readily than nonglycosylated forms do[83] and nonenzymatic glycation of albumin increases its permeability through the GBM in vitro.[84] In addition, it is possible that shape changes

contribute to diabetic proteinuria and that the density of sites that attract polyanions may be increased in diabetic patients.[85] The present data suggest that the primary abnormality in diabetes is a size-selective defect, but that charge and perhaps shape selectivity defects also contribute.[77, 81]

Interventions and Modulation of Permselectivity

Many pathophysiologic and therapeutic interventions that are known to influence proteinuria have been explored by using the aforementioned techniques. Most of the studies have assessed size, but not charge permselectivity. Interventions such as plasma volume (PV) expansion,[5, 86] dietary protein restriction,[19, 61, 87] and others[64] restore normal glomerular size selectivity. Of note, although some antihypertensive regimens tend to reverse size-selective defects, others do not. Moreover, interventions that successfully restore size selectivity do not do so in a uniform manner. Although many interventions reduce permeability only for larger dextrans, drugs that block AII formation (angiotensin-converting enzyme [ACE] inhibitors and the AII receptor antagonist losartan) appear in some cases to reduce the clearance of neutral dextrans of all sizes[20, 88, 89] (as shown in Fig. 42-5).[20] In other cases, however, the same interventions were found to reduce the clearance of only the largest macromolecules.[63,90] The ability of ACE inhibition to improve size selectivity has been shown in type 1 diabetic patients,[91, 92] but it may be less consistent in type 2 diabetes.[93]

Clinical Consequences of Proteinuria

Loss of albumin and other proteins into urine is the hallmark of nephrotic syndrome and a proximate or contributing cause to virtually all the systemic complications of this disorder. As depicted in Figure 42-6[94] and detailed later, increased filtration of plasma proteins contributes to hypoalbuminemia and its complications, to hyperlipidemia, to alterations in coagulation factors, and to alterations in cellular immunity, hormonal status, and mineral and electrolyte metabolism (for reviews, see references 94 to 98).

HYPOALBUMINEMIA

Pathogenesis of Hypoalbuminemia

The hypoalbuminemia of nephrotic syndrome results from multiple abnormalities in albumin homeostasis and is only partially explained by urinary albumin loss.[3, 94-99] Normal albumin metabolism is schematized in the upper panel of Figure 42-7.[98] The liver normally synthesizes 12 to 14 g/day of albumin, 90% of which is catabolized in extrarenal sites, primarily the vascular endothelium.[100, 101] About 10% of the albumin synthesized daily is catabolized in the kidney, mainly by proximal tubule reabsorption of filtered albumin.[102] About 150 g of albumin (or 30% to 50% of the total exchangeable pool) is located intravascularly, with the remainder in interstitial fluid, mostly skin and muscle.[103] The fractional catabolic rate, or the percentage of the plasma pool that is catabolized daily, is about 6% to 10%.[100, 104, 105] Thus, nephrotic hypoalbuminemia could result from some combination of urinary loss, decreased or insufficiently

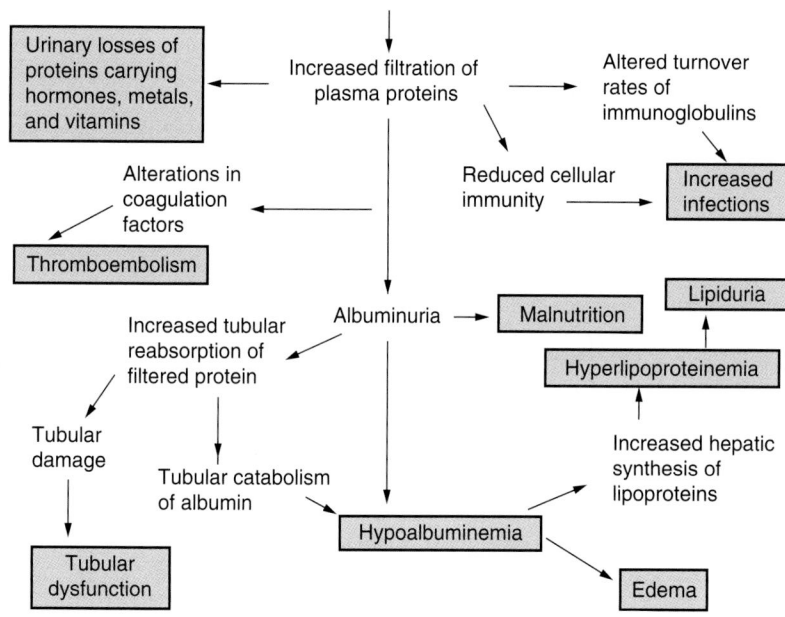

FIGURE 42-6. Pathophysiology of nephrotic syndrome. All abnormalities originate from increased glomerular permeability to plasma proteins; hypoalbuminemia initiates the major manifestations. (From Bernard DB: Extrarenal complications of the nephrotic syndrome. Kidney Int 33:1184, 1988.)

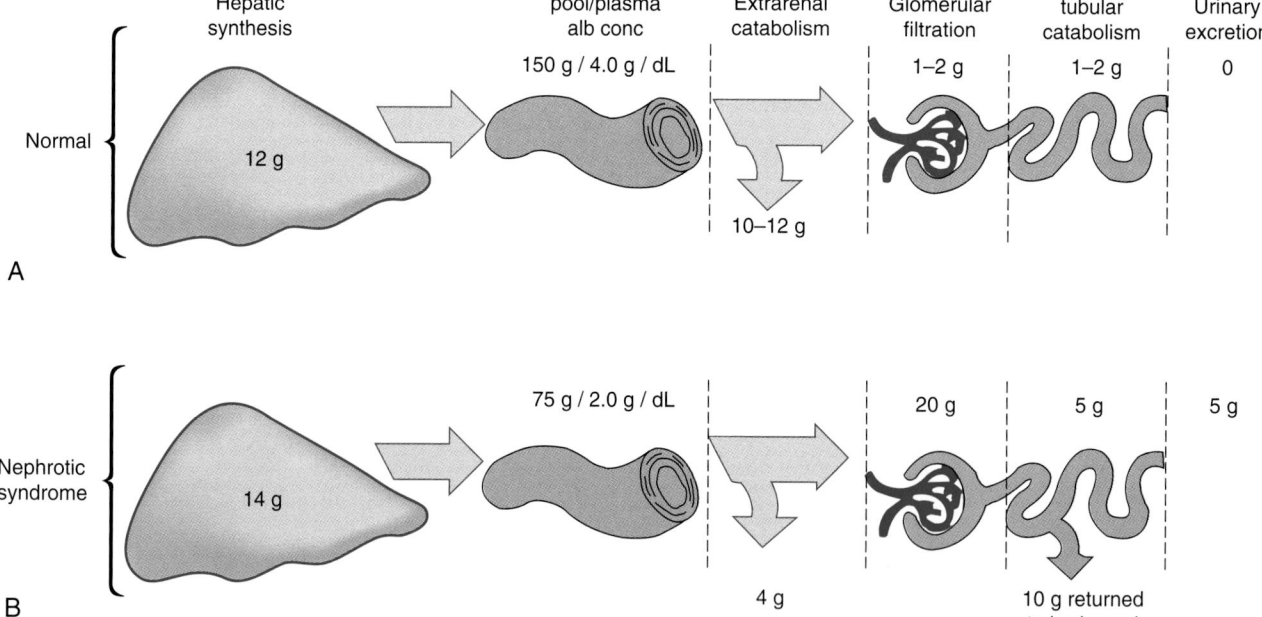

FIGURE 42-7. Daily albumin turnover in normal individuals (**A**) and in patients with nephrotic syndrome (**B**). (Reproduced from Bernard DB: Metabolic complications in nephrotic syndrome: Pathophysiology and complications. *In* Brenner BM, Stein JH [eds]: The Nephrotic Syndrome, Vol 9. New York, Churchill Livingstone,1982.)

increased hepatic albumin synthesis, increased albumin catabolism, or altered albumin distribution.[3, 99]

EXTRACORPOREAL LOSSES. The magnitude of hypoalbuminemia tends to increase with increasing proteinuria, but significant hypoalbuminemia can occur in the presence of urinary loss of only a few grams of albumin per day. Urinary losses alone should not necessarily lead to hypoalbuminemia because the liver can easily augment albumin synthesis and thus compensate for such losses.[101] Evidence

for enhanced intestinal albumin loss, or increased albumin catabolism, in the nephrotic syndrome is inconsistent and not compelling.[99] As discussed later, renal albumin catabolism is increased, thereby contributing to the greater tendency to hypoalbuminemia.

HEPATIC ALBUMIN SYNTHESIS. Hepatic albumin synthesis is not impaired and, in fact, may be increased by as much as 300% in the nephrotic syndrome.[106-108] In nephrotic rats, hepatic release of albumin is enhanced,[109] and the relative synthetic rate of albumin is markedly increased, with a comparable increase in albumin mRNA. The relative amounts of several other mRNA molecules, including those encoding for β-fibrinogen, haptoglobin, and metallothionein II, are increased, whereas the amount of mRNA encoding for α_1-acid glycoprotein is decreased.[109, 110] Oncotic pressure may play a role in albumin synthesis in as much as albumin gene expression varies inversely with oncotic pressure in experimental models.[111] That a transcriptional process is mainly responsible is suggested by findings that both steady-state levels and transcription rates of albumin mRNA are increased in the livers of nephrotic rats.[112, 113] However, the increase in hepatic albumin synthesis is not maximal and is inadequate for the degree of hypoalbuminemia; thus, the albumin synthetic response rate is relatively impaired.

ALBUMIN CATABOLISM. In some hypoalbuminemic states, albumin catabolic rates are reduced.[114] In contrast, the possibility that hypoalbuminemia might be exacerbated by a maladaptive increase in albumin catabolism was suggested by Katz and co-authors,[115, 116] who speculated that the increased urinary albumin load might up-regulate tubular albumin catabolism. In that case, most filtered albumin would be catabolized, and thus urinary albumin would represent only a small fraction of the filtered load. In confirmation of this notion, tubule albumin reabsorptive rates increase in rats with nephrotoxic serum nephritis, though variably.[117] Nephrotic rats have protein reabsorption droplets containing both albumin and globulin in the proximal and distal tubule cells,[118] and tubular lysosomal activity increases with an increased urinary protein load.[119] Additional support for the concept comes from evidence of a dual transport system for albumin uptake in the isolated perfused rabbit proximal tubule. This model exhibits both a low-capacity system that becomes saturated once the protein load exceeds physiologic levels and a high-capacity, low-affinity system that permits tubule albumin reabsorptive rates to rise as the filtered load increases.[120] Thus, an increase in the fractional catabolic rate may occur in the nephrotic syndrome.

Micropuncture studies indicate that albumin reabsorption may, in fact, be saturated at near-physiologic levels, so most of the urinary albumin is excreted rather than catabolized,[117, 121, 122] and the albuminuria does not markedly underestimate overall albumin loss. Regardless of whether fractional catabolism is normal or increased, total body albumin stores are markedly decreased in the nephrotic syndrome. The net result is that absolute catabolic rates are normal or decreased.[106, 115, 123, 124] As discussed later, nutritional considerations affect this process. In nephrotic rats, absolute catabolic rates are decreased in rats fed adequate dietary protein but increased in rats receiving a low-protein diet.[123] Although decreased catabolism may serve to preserve total albumin stores in the face of massive albuminuria, it is obviously insufficient to maintain albumin homeostasis.

ALBUMIN DISTRIBUTION. In nephrotic syndrome, the extravascular albumin pool is even more depleted than the intravascular pool,[125, 126] the mechanisms of which are discussed later. However, although mobilization of extravascular albumin represents an early response to acute albumin loss, this compensatory mechanism is clearly inadequate in the setting of continuing albumin loss, as in nephrotic syndrome.

Regulation of Albumin Metabolism in Nephrotic Syndrome

Several factors contribute to regulation of albumin metabolism and probably contribute to dysregulation in nephrotic syndrome.[99, 124] The most widely studied factors regulating albumin synthesis are serum oncotic pressure and nutritional status (particularly dietary protein intake).

Whereas albumin synthesis in an isolated perfused liver preparation is inversely proportional to the oncotic pressure of the bathing solution,[127] albumin synthetic rates do not correspond to either serum albumin concentration or oncotic pressure in nephrotic patients.[107, 115] It has been postulated that the hepatic albumin synthetic rate is more directly determined by changes in the hepatic extravascular interstitial albumin pool than by plasma characteristics and that this hepatic pool is not depleted in nephrotic syndrome and thus albumin synthesis is not stimulated.[127, 128] More recently, it has been suggested that some serum factor or factors in hypo-oncotic states may stimulate albumin synthesis. In support of this hypothesis, incubation of rat hepatocytes with serum from nephrotic rats led to increased albumin and transferrin synthesis, even when oncotic pressure in the medium was normalized.[129]

Dietary factors also play a role. Kaysen and associates[113] found that albumin synthesis and serum albumin were not correlated in nephrotic rats fed a low-protein diet but that in the presence of high protein intake, albumin synthetic rates varied inversely with serum albumin. Increasing dietary protein intake in nephrotic rats results in increased hepatic albumin mRNA content, as well as increased transcription, whereas decreased dietary protein intake limits hepatic albumin synthesis.[113, 130] Hepatic albumin synthesis may also respond to changes in dietary fat intake,[131] as well as to the relative proportion of protein to nonprotein calories.

These observations suggest that in nephrotic syndrome, the optimal diet would include adequate caloric intake with a moderate- to high-protein diet. However, increasing dietary protein intake does not increase serum albumin or body albumin pools in nephrotic animals[123, 132] or patients.[123] As depicted in Figure 42-8,[123] feeding a high-protein diet markedly stimulates hepatic albumin synthesis in nephrotic rats.[123, 130] This beneficial effect does not correct hypoalbuminemia, however, because dietary protein supplementation also increases urinary protein loss. This unfortunate consequence of a high-protein diet also occurs in nephrotic patients; those eating a high-protein diet exhibit higher albumin synthetic rates, but also increased albuminuria, which results in no change in serum albumin levels.[123]

Factors contributing to enhanced proteinuria in the setting of a high-protein diet may include increased renal blood flow and GFR, with enhanced fractional renal clearance of albumin,[133] and stimulation of the renin-angiotensin system.[134] The exact dietary component of protein that stimulates albumin synthesis is unknown but does not appear to be either arginine[135] or branched-chain amino acids.[136] However, the net result is that despite the enhanced albumin synthesis, increased urinary losses predominate, so the serum albumin concentration and body albumin pools are further reduced.[132] Experimentally, blockade of the renin-angiotensin system in the setting of a high-protein diet

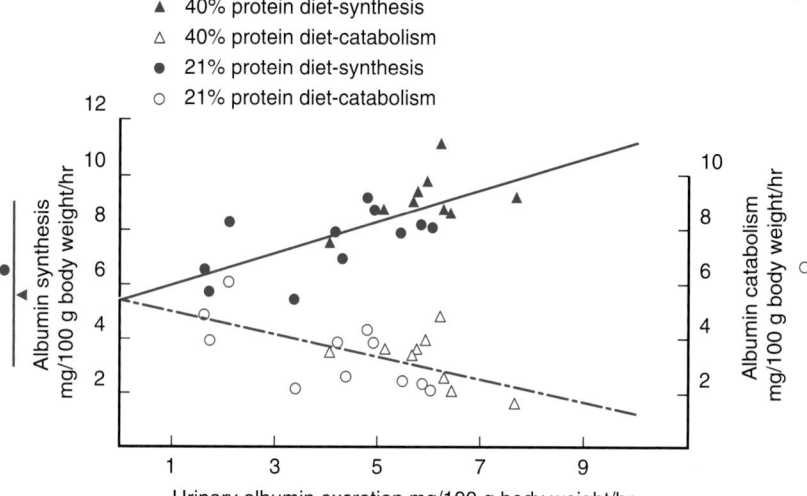

FIGURE 42-8. Relationship between albumin synthesis, catabolism, and albuminuria in nephrotic rats fed 21% or 40% protein diets. (From Kaysen GA, Kirkpatrick WG, Couser WG: Albumin homeostasis in the nephrotic rat: Nutritional considerations. Am J Physiol 247:F192, 1984.)

allows increased hepatic synthesis but limits proteinuria, thereby allowing some amelioration of the hypoalbuminemia.[130, 132] In nephrotic patients, both dietary protein restriction and ACE inhibition reduce proteinuria; however, protein restriction also reduces hepatic albumin synthesis, whereas albumin synthetic rates are maintained with ACE inhibition.[137]

Hormones such as insulin,[138] thyroid hormone,[139] growth hormone,[140] and glucocorticoids[141] are all needed for albumin synthesis, but their relevance to nephrotic hypoalbuminemia is not well understood. Albumin synthesis is suppressed in the presence of inflammation,[142] and it is possible that elevated levels of lymphokines such as tumor necrosis factor[143] interfere with albumin synthesis in nephrotic syndrome.

In summary, nephrotic hypoalbuminemia is characterized by large urinary albumin losses and a marked reduction in the total exchangeable albumin pool. Mechanisms tending to counteract these forces are mobilization of extravascular pools, increases in albumin synthesis, and decreased albumin catabolism. However, these compensatory mechanisms are insufficient to correct the hypoalbuminemia. Comparisons between normal and nephrotic albumin homeostasis are schematized in the bottom panel of Figure 42-7.[98] Normally, hepatic synthesis equals the amount catabolized, with a yield of 1 to 2 g, which undergoes glomerular filtration and proximal tubular catabolism. In the nephrotic state, hepatic synthesis may be slightly increased, but the plasma albumin pool is smaller because catabolism is proportionally enhanced. Larger amounts are presented to the glomerulus, thereby resulting in both increased urinary loss and enhanced tubule catabolism.

Consequences of Hypoalbuminemia

Hypoalbuminemia causes or exacerbates numerous complications of the nephrotic syndrome, including abnormalities in blood volume and composition, edema formation, impaired renal function, increased platelet aggregability, enhanced potential for drug toxicity, and hyperlipidemia.

Edema Formation and Blood Volume Homeostasis

Nephrotic edema does not result solely from hypoalbuminemia. Transcapillary fluid flux (J_v) across a membrane is defined by the Starling relationship: $J_v = L_p(\Delta P - \Delta \Pi)$, where ΔP and $\Delta \Pi$ are the transmembrane hydrostatic and oncotic gradients, respectively; L_p is the hydraulic conductivity of the membrane; and s is the reflection coefficient for plasma proteins, mainly albumin.[144-146] The balance of Starling forces at the arteriolar end of the capillary ($\Delta P > \Delta \Pi$) favors net filtration of fluid into the interstitium.[144] However, ongoing fluid transudation (edema accumulation) is normally limited by at least three protective mechanisms. First, the lymphatics expand and proliferate so that increased lymphatic flow provides protection. Second, transudation of protein-free filtration into the interstitium reduces interstitial oncotic pressure (Π_{IF}), thus decreasing ΔP and slowing ultrafiltration. Third, fluid flux tends to increase interstitial hydrostatic pressure (Π_{IF}), thereby reducing ΔP and further slowing filtration.[147]

Furthermore, the compliance characteristics of the interstitium resist fluid accumulation.[148, 149] Compartmentalization within the interstitial space prevents rapid local translocation of fluid in subcutaneous and subserosal tissue. Thus, the appearance of edema in glomerulonephritis implies substantial disruption of the normal defenses against edema formation.[145] Generalized edema therefore implies substantial and ongoing renal Na+ retention, further supporting the concept that intrarenal mechanisms prevail in the pathogenesis of the Na+ retention associated with glomerular disease (see later).[150-152]

RELATIONSHIP OF EDEMA FORMATION TO REDUCED PLASMA ONCOTIC PRESSURE. According to the traditional view of nephrotic edema formation, hypoalbuminemia lowers the colloid oncotic pressure of blood, thereby favoring movement of water from the vascular to the interstitial space. However, continued edema formation would require disruption of normal defenses against edema, and evidence for such derangement is not clearly found. For example, in nephrotic patients, hypoalbuminemia is accompanied by a fall in Π_{IF} sufficient to substantially retard interstitial fluid accumulation.[153] Values of Π_{IF} in nephrotic animals and patients also fall virtually in parallel with the decrease in plasma colloid osmotic pressure and serum albumin levels, thus maintaining net transcapillary ΔP in the normal range.[154-156] Patients studied during relapse and remission show almost equivalent changes in interstitial and plasma colloid osmotic pressure.[156] The reduction in Π_{IF} results in part from acceleration of lymphatic flow, which in turn returns interstitial protein to the intravascular space.[156-158] It has been suggested that this "wash-down" phenomenon is triggered by a slight increase in interstitial volume and hydraulic pressure induced by the initial loss of fluid into the interstitium. Body albumin pools are thus redistributed so that a greater fraction is located in the intravascular space; the interstitial albumin concentration may be as low as 5% of that in plasma in nephrotic patients.[125] These events thus serve to maintain blood volume and defend against edema formation.[3, 98]

Accordingly, it appears that substantial disruption of the renal mechanisms responsible for extracellular fluid homeostasis, rather than the level of hypoalbuminemia per se, is the primary determinant of the severity of edema formation. In assessing the relative contribution of hypoalbuminemia to edema formation, it is necessary to take into consideration the prevailing intravascular volume as well.

RELATIONSHIP OF EDEMA FORMATION TO THE PREVAILING INTRAVASCULAR VOLUME. One postulated scenario linking hypoalbuminemia to edema formation relates to "underfill mechanisms," as depicted in Figure 42-9.[152, 159-163] According to this scenario, reductions

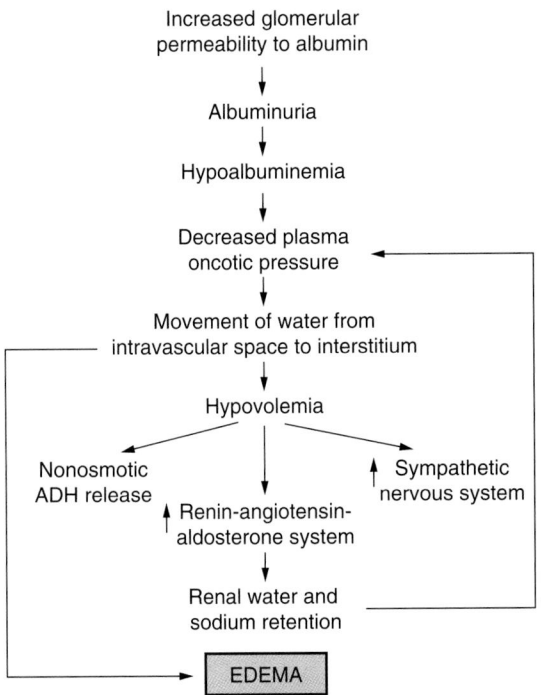

FIGURE 42-9. The "underfill" mechanism of edema formation. Hypovolemia (resulting from hypoalbuminemia and decreased plasma oncotic pressure) is viewed as the key event promoting Na⁺ and water retention by the kidney. (From Perico N, Remuzzi G: Edema of the nephrotic syndrome: The role of the atrial peptide system. Am J Kidney Dis 22:355, 1993.)

in serum albumin, and therefore plasma oncotic pressure, lead to edema formation, but also to hypovolemia. The reduced PV then triggers compensatory mechanisms (e.g., nonosmotic vasopressin release, the renin-angiotensin-aldosterone system, and the sympathetic nervous system) that stimulate renal Na⁺ and water retention. The latter serve to restore intravascular volume but also exacerbate hypoalbuminemia, so edema formation continues. However, some experimental observations are at odds with this hypothesis.[95, 145, 159, 161] First, the clinical syndrome of congenital analbuminemia is not necessarily associated with edema,[164] nor is the transcapillary $\Delta\Pi$ abnormal in analbuminemic rats.[165] Second, the presence of hypovolemia is questionable. The evidence against hypovolemia as the proximate cause of Na⁺ retention is threefold: an inability to document hypovolemia by direct measurements, an inability to consistently find changes in hormonal modulators compatible with hypovolemia, and failure of predicted changes to occur after remission or diuretic therapy. In nephrotic patients, PV and blood volume are not usually reduced; in fact, they are generally normal or even expanded.[166-175]

Many of the available studies actually note a range of PV in patients studied. Moreover, methodologic differences and limitations in blood and PV measurements may interfere with the interpretation of these studies.[152, 162, 168] Nonetheless, it should be possible to indirectly estimate blood volume by measurement of vasoactive hormones that change in response to altered intravascular volume. Thus, reduced intravascular volume should be reflected by elevated values for hematocrit and plasma renin activity (PRA), aldosterone, arginine vasopressin (AVP), and norepinephrine concentrations and reduced values for atrial natriuretic peptide (ANP). Such functional evidence of hypovolemia is not consistently found in nephrotic syndrome.[98, 152, 159, 161, 168] PRA and aldosterone levels tend to be reduced and are not always well correlated with changes in blood volume.[166, 167, 169, 171] Similarly, plasma levels of norepinephrine, AVP, and ANP tend to be normal (or inconsistently changed).[168, 170, 176, 177] Moreover, PV expansion by infusion of hyperoncotic plasma[178] or salt-poor albumin[179] and head-out water immersion[180, 181] does not regularly result in diuresis or natriuresis. However, despite the lack of a uniform response, some studies find evidence consistent with hypovolemia and a natriuretic response to these maneuvers.[152, 162, 178, 182]

Evidence from patients undergoing remission from nephrotic syndrome is likewise unclear. In responsive patients, steroid therapy leads to diuresis and natriuresis before any change in serum albumin. PRA and aldosterone levels are initially high and fall during natriuresis. After resolution of the edema, PRA and aldosterone again rise to high levels, whereas plasma albumin and blood volume remain low; however, Na⁺ retention does not occur, and Na⁺ balance is maintained.[169] Thus, the absence of Na⁺ retention in the setting of evidence of hypovolemia and hypoalbuminemia during remission points to an intrarenal defect as the probable cause of edema during the nephrotic syndrome. Resolution of this intrarenal defect is characterized by an increase in the filtration fraction, again suggesting that natriuresis results from renal repair rather than changes in blood volume.[183]

Taken together, these observations suggest a wide spectrum in prevailing PVs. Indeed, one study found a suggestion of two populations of patients. Those with steroid-responsive minimal change disease tended to have volume contraction and high PRA values, whereas patients with more advanced steroid-resistant disease exhibited PV expansion and suppression of the renin axis.[166] In head-out water immersion studies, the natriuretic response was correlated with the pre-immersion state of Na+ balance.[181] Further evidence comes from studies of nephrotic rats in the presence or absence of PV expansion induced by a reduction in renal mass.[184] Rats with chronic renal failure exhibited PV expansion that progressed when they became nephrotic; edema formation did not occur in the presence of chronic renal failure or nephrotic syndrome alone, only when nephrotic rats were PV expanded.[184] These data have important therapeutic implications. The evidence suggests that edema is not necessary for maintenance of blood volume and, as a corollary, that vigorous treatment of edema with diuretics does not cause failure to maintain blood volume.[170, 185]

ROLE OF INTRARENAL MECHANISMS. No single mechanism accounts for edema formation in all nephrotic patients. However, changes in blood volume are not solely sufficient to explain the avid Na+ retention that occurs clinically. Most of the available evidence implicates a primary intrarenal defect in this disorder. This hypothesis, termed the "overfill theory," is schematized in Figure 42-10.[152] According to this hypothesis, a primary increase in renal Na+ retention leads to extracellular fluid volume expansion, altered Starling forces, and edema formation. Evidence in support of this mechanism comes from observations that Na+ retention occurs only in the ipsilateral kidney of dogs[186] and rats[150, 187] with unilateral glomerulonephritis. Micropuncture and other studies have localized the primary Na+ handling abnormality to the distal nephron.[150] Moreover, the reduction in GFR that is often present would further limit urinary Na+ excretion and thus contribute to renal sodium retention.

The mechanism by which Na+ handling is altered in the distal tubule is beginning to be understood. Considerable attention has focused on the role of ANP. Clinical[188, 189] and experimental[190, 191] studies have documented renal ANP resistance (i.e., blunted or absent natriuretic responses to

ANP) in nephrotic syndrome. ANP resistance is confined to the ipsilateral kidney in unilateral glomerulonephritis,[191] thus suggesting a role for this hormone in primary renal Na+ retention. Although the mechanisms of ANP resistance are still being unraveled, some evidence relates this abnormality to heightened efferent sympathetic nervous activity.[192] At the level of the tubule cell, evidence suggests that the problem is accelerated breakdown of normally produced cyclic guanosine monophosphate.[193-195]

Recently, insight has been gained into the molecular mechanisms of renal sodium avidity. The hydrolytic and transport activities of sodium-potassium-adenosinetriphosphatase (Na+,K+-ATPase) are increased in the cortical collecting duct in nephrotic rats.[196] The proportional increases in Na+,K+-ATPase activity, cell surface expression, and total cellular content are associated with increased amounts of α- and β-subunit mRNA.[196] In principal cells from nephrotic rats, ENaC activity is increased in the absence of transcriptional induction of the mRNA encoding any of the ENaC subunits.[197] Therefore, Na+ retention in the cortical collecting duct appears to be due, at least in part, to coordinated overactivity of the Na+,K+-ATPase and ENaC sodium transporters.[196] Finally, a role for the proximal tubule has been invoked with the observation that Na+ retention may also be associated with a shift of the cortical Na+/H+ exchanger NHE3 from an inactive to an active pool.[198]

Though less well studied, the mechanisms underlying abnormalities in water handling in experimental nephrotic syndrome have begun to be determined by recent molecular studies. These studies have noted reduced renal medullary water channel expression,[199] impaired aquaporin and urea transporter expression,[200] and decreased abundance of thick ascending limb Na+ transporters.[201]

Alterations in Renal Function

The Starling equation would predict that hypoalbuminemia and thus lower plasma colloid oncotic pressure would reduce the forces opposing ultrafiltration, thereby increasing glomerular filtration. However, clinical[202] and experimental[203, 204] studies indicate that such is not the case and that values of GFR are in fact reduced in conditions of reduced plasma protein levels. To examine the influence of plasma protein concentration on the determinants of glomerular filtration, Baylis and co-workers[60] acutely changed the plasma protein concentration in normal rats. When the protein concentration was reduced, observed values for SNGFR were lower than predicted values; this failure of SNGFR to rise resulted from a concomitant reduction in K_f, the glomerular capillary ultrafiltration coefficient.[60]

Reduced values of SNGFR, primarily caused by a reduction in K_f, have subsequently been observed in some,[204] but not all[205] experimental models of nephrotic syndrome; these differences in SNGFR derive, in part, from the presence or absence of compensatory elevations in the glomerular capillary hydraulic pressure ΔP. Studies in a unique strain of rats with no circulating albumin, the Nagase analbuminemic rat, have yielded further insight into the role of serum albumin in the regulation of GFR. Plasma oncotic pressure is modestly reduced in this strain, but a comparable reduction in Π_{IF} yields a fairly normal transcapillary $\Delta\Pi$ and normal extracellular fluid volume. GFR and renal plasma flow

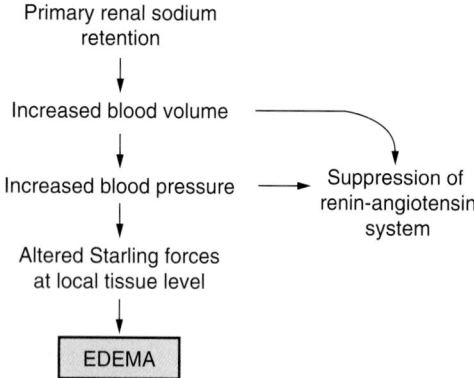

FIGURE 42-10. The "overfill" mechanism of edema formation. The abnormal renal Na+ retention is viewed as the primary event that through the increased plasma volume leads to alteration of the Starling forces at the local tissue level. (From Perico N, Remuzzi G: Edema of the nephrotic syndrome: The role of the atrial peptide system. Am J Kidney Dis 22:355, 1993.)

values are comparable to those in normal rats; the constancy of the GFR relates in part to the elevation in K_f values because glomerular capillary pressure is somewhat reduced.[206] These observations suggest that serum albumin per se may not have a direct effect on K_f or that other factors may mitigate the effects of hypoalbuminemia on K_f in the chronic setting.

Innovative methods for estimating values of SNGFR and its determinants in humans have also suggested that a reduction in K_f commonly accompanies clinical glomerulonephritis as well. For example, this pattern has been observed in patients with progressive lupus nephritis,[207] sickle cell anemia,[208] minimal change disease,[209] and membranous nephropathy.[210]

It should be noted that calculations of plasma oncotic pressure are generally performed by using the equation of Landis and Pappenheimer, in which the albumin-globulin ratio slightly exceeds unity.[1] In the presence of severe hypoalbuminemia, this equation tends to overestimate values for colloid osmotic pressure and, therefore, to underestimate values for the ultrafiltration pressure used to calculate K_f. Accordingly, Miller and Meyer[211] derived the equations required for modifying the Landis-Pappenheimer relationship in this setting. Subsequently, studies have confirmed that in nephrotic patients, Π should be directly determined by membrane osmometry rather than calculated from the protein concentration.[212]

Alterations in Drug Pharmacokinetics

Renal failure induces changes in all aspects of drug handling, including changes in bioavailability, the volume of distribution, renal drug metabolism, and renal excretion of drug or its metabolites, or both.[213] Principles and guidelines for modification of drug dosage in renal insufficiency are readily available[214, 215] and are detailed in Chapter 66. The nephrotic syndrome poses special problems in drug handling and enhanced potential for both drug resistance and drug toxicity.

Hypoalbuminemia limits sites available for protein binding, thus increasing the amount of circulating free drug and potentially increasing first-pass hepatic drug removal. In addition, binding of organic acids and bases is altered in hypoalbuminemic states; the effect on organic acids is the more prominent.[216] In nephrotic patients, reduced protein binding results both from hypoalbuminemia and from a decrease in albumin's affinity for drugs. Accordingly, the unbound fraction of acidic drugs, including salicylate and phenytoin, may be markedly increased.[215] The clinical consequences of altered protein binding may be difficult to predict: decreased binding allows for a higher concentration of free drug, but this effect may be counteracted by a larger volume of distribution or faster metabolism of the drug (or both). Furthermore, protein binding may enhance tubule drug secretion; the lesser protein binding in nephrotic syndrome may result in delayed renal excretion of some drugs.[213] Thus, in nephrotic patients, phenytoin is less protein bound, but the available free drug is more rapidly metabolized in the liver, so plasma levels are not elevated and the dosage need not be adjusted. In contrast, other protein-bound drugs, including prednisone and benzodiazepines, achieve significantly higher drug levels in nephrotic patients, with an enhanced risk of toxicity.[215] Edema and ascites may increase the apparent volume of distribution of drugs that are highly water soluble or protein bound, thereby resulting in inadequate plasma levels; this effect is particularly prominent with aminoglycoside antibiotics.[213]

The actions of diuretics are substantially altered in renal insufficiency and nephrotic syndrome, thereby contributing to the observed resistance to these drugs in this state.[217-222] The unbound fraction of furosemide increases markedly in severely hypoalbuminemic patients.[223] Nephrotic patients with a normal GFR deliver normal amounts of loop diuretics into the urine, but drug delivery is decreased in the setting of renal insufficiency.[224] When proteinuria is also present, a substantial amount of furosemide may bind to urinary proteins, thereby reducing the amount of active, unbound drug in urine.[225, 226] Tubule albumin blunts the inhibitory effects of furosemide on fractional loop Cl^- reabsorption,[227] whereas agents that block albumin-furosemide binding in the proximal tubule, such as warfarin and sulfisoxazole, partially restore diuretic responsiveness in experimental animals.[228] However, a careful study found that sulfisoxazole was ineffective in nephrotic patients.[229] Nephrotic patients exhibit abnormal pharmacodynamic responses to furosemide in addition to the binding effects,[224] so the renal response to the drug is diminished even when adequate amounts of unbound, active drug reach the site of action. Furthermore, animal studies indicate that furosemide is less potent in inhibiting Cl^- reabsorption in the loop in nephrotic rats.[230] Thus, both the pharmacodynamics and pharmacokinetics of loop diuretics are altered in nephrotic syndrome. Single intravenous doses of 80 to 120 mg may be required to attain therapeutic levels of furosemide in urine, but doses above this range are unlikely to achieve any added therapeutic response.[218, 221]

That hypoalbuminemia and altered protein binding are important factors in the resistance to diuretics is further supported by studies in a strain of analbuminemic rats.[231] When compared with normal rats, these rats exhibited resistance to furosemide, with more rapid plasma disappearance of the drug and a larger total plasma clearance and volume of distribution. Injection of furosemide bound to albumin resulted in natriuresis, with normalization of the plasma disappearance rate and increased urinary excretion of furosemide. Thus, binding to plasma albumin appeared to be necessary for efficient delivery of drug into urine. These investigators then examined hypoalbuminemic patients with furosemide resistance and found that injecting furosemide as an admixture with equimolar albumin produced a diuresis whereas giving either alone was without effect. Whether natriuresis occurred in these patients was not specifically mentioned. Since that time, a preliminary report confirmed a natriuretic response to salt-free albumin mixed with bumetanide,[232] but more recent studies in hypoalbuminemic cirrhotic patients found no benefit to combining albumin with furosemide.[233, 234] Because administration of large amounts of albumin alone is both ineffective and expensive, this therapeutic combination will require clear validation before its routine use can be recommended.

Therapy for glomerular disease or nephrotic syndrome may also be associated with drug interactions.[215] For example, corticosteroids may inhibit hepatic microsomal enzymes, thereby altering the metabolism of other drugs. Cyclophosphamide is not associated with significant drug interactions, but clinically important drug interactions may be seen with other immunosuppressive drugs, including cyclosporine and azathioprine, as well as with diuretics and antihypertensive agents.[215]

Alterations in Platelet Function

Hypoalbuminemia may contribute to abnormal platelet function in nephrotic patients because conversion of arachidonic acid to metabolites that aggregate platelets is regulated by albumin.[235] In the presence of hypoalbuminemia, arachidonic acid may be metabolized to platelet-aggregating substances such as endoperoxides and thromboxane A_2.[236] In support of this notion, the degree of platelet dysfunction tends to correlate with the severity of hypoalbuminemia and proteinuria.[237] Platelets from nephrotic patients are refractory to adenylate cyclase stimulation by prostaglandin E_1, further enhancing the tendency toward increased platelet aggregation.[238] However, a firm correlation between the plasma albumin concentration and platelet aggregability is not well established clinically.[239, 240]

HYPERLIPIDEMIA

Hyperlipidemia is a frequent complication of nephrotic syndrome. Marked dysregulation of lipid metabolism occurs, with both quantitative and qualitative abnormalities in plasma lipids and lipoproteins. The precise pathogenesis, clinical consequences, and optimal treatment of nephrotic hyperlipidemia are still being investigated. However, recent studies have identified a number of new mechanisms responsible for derangements of lipid metabolism in nephrotic syndrome. There is also increasing evidence of a broadening range of therapeutic options for these disorders. Although hyperlipidemia is associated with chronic renal diseases of every etiology,[241, 242] it is most striking in nephrotic syndrome, where such changes occur even when the GFR remains normal.

Lipid Abnormalities in Nephrotic Syndrome

The nephrotic syndrome is characterized by abnormalities in virtually every aspect of lipid and lipoprotein metabolism, as depicted in Figure 42-11.[243-246] Increased levels of the apolipoprotein B (apo B)-containing lipoproteins, very low density (VLDL), intermediate-density (IDL), and low-density (LDL) lipoproteins result in hypercholesterolemia, sometimes with hypertriglyceridemia. Cholesterol and phospholipid levels rise early in the course of the disease, whereas triglyceride (TG) elevations are more commonly found with more severe disease. Total HDL levels are usually normal, but in severely proteinuric patients, HDL may be lost in the urine, with resultant reduced levels.[243-249] Subtype analysis demonstrates an abnormal distribution with significant reductions in the protective subtype HDL2.[245, 248, 249] Plasma concentrations of lipoprotein (a) [Lp(a)] are also elevated in nephrotic syndrome.[245, 246, 250-253] In addition, nephrotic patients show qualitative abnormalities in lipoprotein composition. The cholesterol-TG ratio is

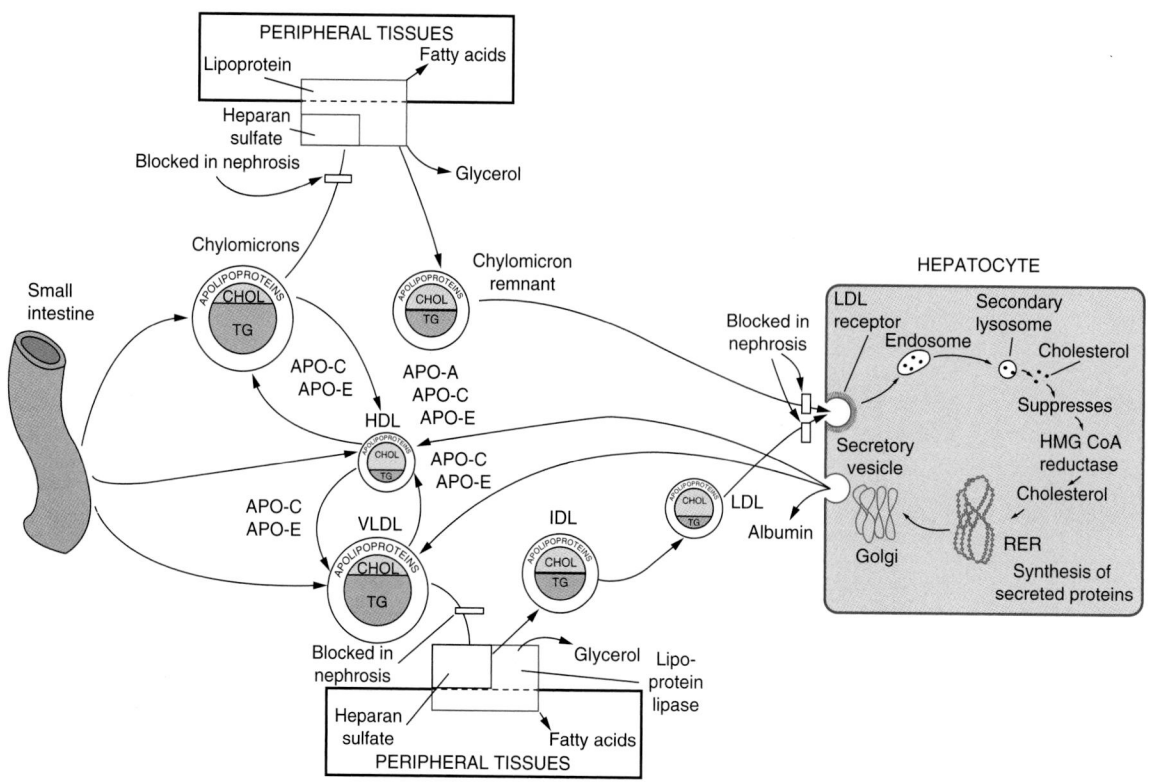

FIGURE 42-11. Normal pathways of lipoprotein metabolism and potential derangements occurring in the nephrotic syndrome. (From Kaysen GA: Hyperlipidemia in the nephrotic syndrome. Am J Kidney Dis 12:548, 1988.)

elevated in all classes of lipoproteins, which also tend to be enriched with cholesterol ester.[245] The highly atherogenic small LDL-III fraction is elevated as well.[254] The apolipoprotein content is also abnormal, with reduced apo C and E despite elevations in apo B, C-II, and E and an increased ratio of apo C-III to apo C-II.[247, 255, 256] Taken together, these abnormalities result in an increased atherogenic profile.[247, 256-258]

Pathogenesis of Nephrotic Hyperlipidemia

Nephrotic hyperlipidemia results from both overproduction and impaired catabolism or composition of serum lipids and lipoproteins. One of the major issues under investigation is whether the lipid abnormalities in nephrotic syndrome arise as a consequence of hypoalbuminemia or proteinuria. Early clinical studies demonstrated links between hypoalbuminemia per se and dysregulation of lipid metabolism in nephrotic syndrome. In general, the severity of hyperlipidemia tends to correlate with the severity of hypoalbuminemia. In addition, remission of nephrotic syndrome is usually associated with a decrease in serum cholesterol as the albumin level rises, whereas albumin infusion acutely raises serum albumin and lowers serum cholesterol levels.[98, 248, 259, 260] Because hepatic synthetic rates of albumin and lipoproteins react to similar stimuli and follow the same synthetic pathways, it has been hypothesized that increased lipoprotein synthesis was simply a side effect of increased albumin synthesis. However, although albumin synthesis is increased, no clear correlation has been found between hyperlipidemia and the rate of albumin synthesis in nephrotic patients. Kaysen and colleagues[261] showed that serum cholesterol levels in nephrotic patients were dependent only on the renal clearance of albumin and were totally independent of albumin synthetic rates but that serum TG levels showed some dependence on albumin synthesis. Similarly, serum lipid levels in nephrotic rats correlated with proteinuria and not with albumin synthetic rates.[262] An alternative stimulus may be the reduction in plasma oncotic pressure. Infusion of either albumin or dextran into nephrotic patients and animals reduces serum lipid levels, thus suggesting that low plasma oncotic pressure may stimulate hepatic lipoprotein synthesis.[260, 263, 264]

Intensive research in this area has identified numerous pathogenetic mechanisms responsible for these complex alterations in lipid metabolism. It is now apparent that reductions in plasma albumin levels or oncotic pressure, as well as the direct consequences of proteinuria, contribute to lipid alterations in nephrotic syndrome. As discussed later, these major factors operate on various levels of the lipid metabolic pathways. Metabolism of lipoproteins is closely linked. For purposes of this review, defects in the metabolism of individual fractions will be discussed separately. However, the reader should be aware that one mechanism may alter the levels and composition of multiple lipoproteins.

Alterations in Low-Density Lipoprotein Metabolism

Increased synthesis seems to be the principal mechanism responsible for the higher levels of LDL in nephrotic syndrome. It has been proposed that some nephrotic patients have increased absolute LDL apo B-100 synthetic rates, greater than VLDL apo B-100 and independent of VLDL synthesis, thus suggesting an alternative secretory pathway for LDL that bypasses VLDL delipidation. Previous studies of LDL metabolism have produced conflicting results, many of which could result from methodologic differences.[265, 266] Recent studies have avoided some of the problems involving measurement of apo B-100 synthesis by using endogenous labeling of lipoproteins with valine labeled with stable isotopes. Importantly, increased LDL apo B synthesis did not correlate with the synthetic rate of albumin.[265]

Plasma levels and the activity of cholesterol ester transfer protein (CETP) are enhanced in nephrotic syndrome.[267] This protein mediates the transfer of esterified cholesterol from HDL to VLDL remnants to yield LDL. In addition to the defects discussed earlier, acquired defects in LDL clearance have also been described. Some studies have demonstrated reduced receptor-mediated LDL clearance with associated increases in LDL catabolism via alternative pathways.[268, 269] Increases in hepatic cholesterol concentrations could contribute to hyperlipidemia both by increasing VLDL production and by down-regulating expression of LDL receptors.[245] Others have suggested that LDL kinetics and pathogenetic mechanisms differ markedly in patients with hypercholesterolemia alone versus those with concurrent hypertriglyceridemia, with overproduction of LDL found only in patients with combined hyperlipidemia.[270]

Alterations in Very Low Density Lipoprotein Metabolism

The increased VLDL levels in nephrotic syndrome occur predominantly as a result of impaired VLDL clearance. Early studies demonstrated defective chylomicron clearance in nephrotic rats.[262] This phenomenon correlated with proteinuria rather than hypoalbuminemia because the serum half-life of chylomicrons remained normal in analbuminemic rats whereas it was markedly impaired in hypoalbuminemic nephrotic animals. In addition, plasma TG levels are higher in nephrotic than in analbuminemic rats despite similar increases in hepatic TG production.[271] Defective VLDL clearance has also been documented in nephrotic patients.[265]

As a major determinant of chylomicron and VLDL clearance, the functional integrity of lipoprotein lipase (LPL) has been a logical focus for study in this area. Reduced LPL activity in nephrotic patients was proposed by Garber and associates.[272] Earlier reports suggested that decreased LPL activity may relate to the increased levels of circulating free fatty acids that result from hypoalbuminemia and the lowered protein-binding capacity of plasma. The increased free fatty acid level contributes by providing the lipid substrate for increased hepatic lipoprotein synthesis and by leading to decreased activity of LPL.[273, 274]

LPL is attached to the endothelium by ionic bonding to a negatively charged matrix of glycosaminoglycans such as heparan sulfate.[3, 273] This endothelium-bound LPL is an active, metabolically important pool, and earlier studies demonstrated that it is reduced in nephrotic rats[262, 275] and patients.[276] Urinary excretion is markedly increased in nephrotic patients,[274] and circulating levels of heparan sulfate are reduced in nephrotic plasma and contribute to the decrease in LPL activity.[3] In support of this concept, studies in nephrotic rats show that the markedly delayed plasma disappearance of radiolabeled chylomicrons may be completely normalized by injection of minute amounts of purified urinary heparan sulfate.[3, 277] The heparan sulfate deficiency may also result from deficient hepatic synthesis of glycosaminoglycans. Nephrotic syndrome is characterized by excessive urinary losses of orosomucoid, a plasma glycoprotein synthesized by the liver. Urinary losses may lead to an increase in hepatic synthesis with a resultant excessive drain of key sugar intermediates from liver parenchymal cells, thus limiting the substrates available for heparan sulfate synthesis.[3] Because the endothelial pool of LPL in Nagase analbuminuric rats is reduced to the same extent as in nephrotic rats but TG levels are much higher in the latter model, it has been hypothesized that in addition to defects in endothelial LPL, other important determinants of VLDL levels are present in nephrotic syndrome.

Indeed, more recent studies have revealed abnormalities in other determinants of VLDL clearance. In two different models of nephrotic syndrome, Liang and Vaziri[278, 279] demonstrated that elevated serum TG levels are in part attributable to reduced VLDL receptor and LPL expression. Reductions in VLDL receptor protein and mRNA were inversely related to plasma VLDL and TG concentrations. The same group implicated secondary hyperparathyroidism in the reduced LPL and hepatic lipase activity of proteinuric rats with progressive renal failure and suggested that because of depletion of hepatic LPL in nephrotic rats, there is no liver compensation for the LPL defect.[280] Furthermore, defective receptor-mediated clearance and a metabolic defect in recognition and removal by the liver may underlie the elevated remnant particles in nephrotic syndrome.[3, 281] The signal for recognition of VLDL remnants by a liver "receptor site" may be LPL, an associated cofactor such as heparan sulfate, or certain apolipoproteins, and it has been hypothesized that the observed deficiencies in LPL or heparan sulfate (or both) may be responsible for failure of recognition and, hence, defective removal of these particles.[3]

VLDL isolated from nephrotic rats hydrolyzes at a different rate in in vitro systems than it does in control animals.[282] Shearer and colleagues[283] perfused hearts from normal, analbuminemic, and nephrotic rats with chylomicrons and found identical clearance of these particles in analbuminemic and nephrotic rats. These observations clearly suggest that altered structure or composition of TG-rich lipoproteins must play a role in altered VLDL clearance. In both studies, the defects in lipolysis in nephrotic rats were corrected by HDL, thus suggesting that a component within HDL played a role in the pathophysiology of these alterations. To facilitate VLDL receptor-mediated and LPL-mediated clearance, HDL supplies VLDL with most of the apo E and apo C. Alterations in these molecules in nephrotic syndrome have been described; apo E is reduced in the HDL of nephrotic rats and in the VLDL of nephrotic patients.[256] Apo C has been found to be markedly reduced per unit of VLDL in nephrotic patients[255, 256] despite normal or even increased plasma levels. Reductions in VLDL apo C and apo E correlate with particle size.[256] Thus, in addition to reduced LPL activity, VLDL clearance in nephrotic syndrome is delayed because of altered composition.

VLDL synthesis has been also evaluated. Earlier reports suggested increased VLDL synthesis related at least in part to reductions in plasma albumin or oncotic pressure.[261, 262, 271] Furthermore, apo B synthesis may be increased in some nephrotic patients.[265, 284] Experimental support for increased VLDL synthesis comes from the observation that levels of apo B mRNA are reduced in cultured hepatocytes when albumin or dextran is added to the medium and increased in the presence of hypo-oncotic medium.[111, 285, 286] However, more recent data indicate normal or even decreased VLDL secretion and no correlation with albumin synthesis in experimental and clinical nephrotic syndrome.[265, 283]

Alterations in High-Density Lipoprotein

Nephrotic syndrome is associated with specific abnormalities in enzymatic functions required for effective function of HDL. Diminished activity of the enzyme lecithin-cholesterol acyltransferase (LCAT) appears to contribute to the lipoprotein abnormalities in nephrotic syndrome.[287-289] LCAT is involved in catalyzing the esterification of cholesterol and its incorporation into HDL particles, as well as the conversion of HDL3 to HDL2. Low LCAT levels would impair this HDL maturation, in turn reducing the transfer of apo C-II to VLDL and thus inhibiting the catabolism of TG-rich lipoproteins.[245] Nephrotic patients have a distribution in HDL isoforms that corresponds to the LCAT defect—the higher-molecular-weight HDL2 is reduced and replaced by an increase in the lower-molecular-weight HDL3. Recent observations have demonstrated that the LCAT deficiency in nephrotic rats is due to urinary losses.[289] In contrast to nephrotic rats, Nagase analbuminemic rats do not demonstrate substantial LCAT alterations. However, earlier studies suggested that hypoalbuminemia could also play a role by increasing levels of free (unbound) lysolecithin, an inhibitor of LCAT.[3, 290]

Increased hepatic production and elevated plasma CETP levels may contribute to HDL abnormalities in nephrotic patients.[267] As a mediator of transfer of esterified cholesterol from HDL to VLDL, elevated levels might contribute to cholesterol enrichment of TG-rich lipoproteins, as well as the observed reductions in HDL2.[267, 288, 291] Braschi and coworkers[267] demonstrated that the enhanced CETP activity in nephrotic patients could be attributed to marked increases in the proportion of lipoprotein-bound nonesterified fatty acids that are responsible for increases in the negative charge of nephrotic lipoproteins.

Elevated HDL in nephrotic rats is associated with apo A-I enrichment of HDL particles.[292, 293] This abnormality has been linked to hypoalbuminemia and reduced oncotic pressure, and the accumulation of apo A-I–rich HDL is due to increased hepatic synthesis and reduced catabolism of HDL and apo A-I.[292, 293] Importantly, the relevance of these observations for human studies is unknown. Unlike experimental models, fractional apo A-I in nephrotic patients is increased because of the increase in CETP that is absent in rats. CETP mediates conversion of the larger HDL2 to the smaller HDL3, which has less affinity for apo A-I, and thus indirectly facilitates clearance of apo A-I.[294] Finally, the altered plasma HDL levels and composition in nephrotic rats are at least partly attributable to reduced protein expression of SR-B1.[295] This molecule has been identified as an HDL receptor responsible for the clearance of these particles.

Lipoprotein (a)

Persuasive evidence indicates that Lp(a) is increased in nephrotic patients.[245, 246, 251-253] In view of the atherogenic potential of Lp(a), these findings are important. The principal mechanism leading to elevations in Lp(a) in nephrotic patients seems to be increased synthesis alone.[251, 253] Lp(a) is related to apo B synthesis in nephrotic humans.[252, 253] As demonstrated by Noto and colleagues,[252] Lp(a) levels in nephrotic children inversely correlate with apo(a) isoform size and plasma albumin levels, but not with the proteinuria–creatinine clearance ratio.

Cholesterol Synthesis

Cholesterol content is increased in most of the nephrotic lipoproteins. These abnormalities could be explained by some of the abnormalities in lipoprotein function and composition discussed earlier. In addition, some evidence indicates enhanced hepatic cholesterol synthesis in experimental nephrotic syndrome. One factor that might contribute to increased cholesterogenesis is greater availability of the cholesterol precursor mevalonic acid. Circulating mevalonate is metabolized in the kidney, and both renal excretion and renal metabolism of this substance are impaired in the nephrotic state.[296] Several studies have demonstrated enzymatic defects in the liver of nephrotic rats that can collectively enhance hepatic cholesterol synthesis. These studies have shown increased hepatic activity of hydroxymethylglutaryl–coenzyme A (HMG-CoA) reductase, the rate-limiting enzyme in cholesterol biosynthesis, in nephrotic rats.[245, 296, 297] In contrast, hepatic expression of cholesterol 7α-hydroxylase, the rate-limiting enzyme responsible for conversion of cholesterol to bile acids, is reduced in nephrotic rats.[298] Most recently, marked up-regulation of hepatic acetyl coenzyme A: cholesterol acyltransferase (ACAT) has been described in nephrotic rats.[289] This multifunctional enzyme is involved in the catalysis of intracellular cholesterol esterification and is responsible for lowering intracellular free cholesterol. By lowering hepatic free cholesterol, ACAT up-regulation may be responsible for the aforementioned defects in HMG-CoA reductase and 7α-hydroxylase activity and the enhanced cholesterol synthesis. Furthermore, enhanced ACAT activity leads to intracellular accumulation of cholesterol ester. Increases in hepatic cholesterol concentrations could contribute to hyperlipidemia both by increasing VLDL production and by down-regulating the expression of LDL receptors.[245] In the vascular system, this phenomenon leads to foam cell formation and atherosclerosis.[299, 300] It should be noted that increases in expression or activity of hepatic HMG-CoA reductase in animals with nephrotic syndrome are not uniform findings. Thabet and co-workers[301] did not find persistently increased mRNA liver expression of this enzyme, thus suggesting that an increase in cholesterol biosynthetic capacity is not necessary for maintenance of nephrotic hypercholesterolemia.

Results of studies in humans are contradictory. Turnover studies using radiolabeled glycerol and mevalonate have suggested increases in cholesterol synthesis.[245] In contrast, the serum lathosterol-to-cholesterol ratio, an index of cholesterol synthesis, is not elevated and does not change in response to antiproteinuric treatment.[302] Whether increased cholesterogenesis actually occurs in human nephrotic syndrome therefore remains unclear.

Clinical Consequences of Nephrotic Hyperlipidemia

Many of the lipid abnormalities in nephrotic syndrome are significant risk factors for atherosclerotic cardiovascular (CV) disease in the general population, including increases in total cholesterol, LDL- and VLDL-cholesterol, apo B, and Lp(a) and reductions in HDL2 cholesterol. Furthermore, additional risk factors, such as hypertension, endothelial dysfunction, and hypercoagulability, may also contribute to the risk of atherosclerotic CV disease. A small study found elevated plasma homocysteine levels in nephrotic patients as well.[303] Nonetheless, evidence that CV risk is indeed increased in these patients remains controversial, and prospective long-term data are not available. Studies that have tried to define CV risk in nephrotic patients have been flawed by inclusion of patients with minimal change disease, which typically remits; diabetes, which is inherently atherogenic; or failure to control for the presence of other risk factors. Early studies, which included relatively young patients, contained small numbers, and were retrospective in design, have not uniformly found an increased risk of CV events.[304-306] However, in a retrospective analysis of 142 nephrotic patients without diabetes, Ordonez and colleagues[307] found that after correction for hypertension and smoking, the relative risk of myocardial infarction was increased 5.5-fold and that of coronary death was increased 2.8-fold in comparison to non-nephrotic controls. In addition, Falaschi and co-workers[308] evaluated the carotid intima-media wall thickness (IMT) in young patients with lupus as a marker of early atherosclerosis and CV risk. Patients with nephrotic-range proteinuria had a significantly higher IMT than did those without. The IMT did not correlate with the lupus activity score or other possible risk factors except for proteinuria, thus suggesting a higher risk of early atherosclerosis even in this young age group.[308]

Recent studies have focused on alterations in endothelial function associated with nephrotic syndrome. These complex changes with multifactorial etiology may be a common denominator of the clinical consequences of nephrotic syndrome, such as atherosclerosis, hypertension, and hypercoagulability. Nephrotic patients may exhibit impaired endothelium-dependent relaxation[309, 310] and decreased total plasma antioxidant potential.[311] Hyperlipidemia itself is also a risk factor for impaired endothelial function. Altered lysophosphatidylcholine metabolism, linked to both hyperlipidemia and hypoalbuminemia, is another factor responsible for the endothelial dysfunction in nephrotic syndrome.[312]

Hyperlipidemia probably contributes to other adverse consequences of nephrotic syndrome. The increased platelet aggregation tends to correlate with the magnitude of hyperlipidemia.[236] Hyperlipidemia may also contribute to the increased susceptibility of nephrotic patients to infection inasmuch as serum from nephrotic patients inhibits lymphocyte proliferation in response to specific and nonspecific antigen stimulation.[313] In addition to increasing the risk for CV disease, Lp(a), which may act to inhibit plasminogen, could contribute to hypercoagulability. Finally, the role of hyperlipidemia as a risk factor for progression of glomerular injury is discussed in detail in Chapter 43.

Therapy for Nephrotic Hyperlipidemia

In view of the magnitude of the CV risk in this population, further studies are needed to establish the need for aggressive hypolipidemic therapy.[257] In general, attempts to modify the lipoprotein profile may be worthwhile in patients with unremitting nephrotic syndrome, particularly if other CV risk factors are present. The principles of therapy are similar to those in other populations and include alterations in diet, the use of pharmacologic agents, and attention to other CV risk factors. Although few studies have systematically looked at the impact of standard dietary therapy in proteinuric patients, a moderate reduction in dietary cholesterol intake appears to be relatively ineffective.[314] Studies of vegetarian soy diets that are low in protein and rich in monounsaturated and polyunsaturated fatty acids have demonstrated improvements in serum cholesterol, LDL, and apo B in patients with proteinuria.[315] Supplementation of this diet with fish oil was not of additional benefit,[316] although it may provide some beneficial effect on TG levels.[245, 315]

More promising are pharmacologic approaches, particularly the statins. Fibric acid derivatives have a more prominent effect on TG metabolism than on cholesterol. Early studies with clofibrate found a frequent complication of muscle toxicity.[317] In one study of 11 patients treated with gemfibrozil, TG levels fell and HDL levels rose, with little change in total cholesterol or LDL-cholesterol levels.[318] Controlled prospective studies have indicated that colestipol and probucol may also have modest hypolipidemic effects.[319, 320]

The preferred agents in nephrotic patients are HMG-CoA reductase inhibitors, which induce the greatest and most consistent hypolipidemic effect.[246, 320] Lovastatin, simvastatin, and pravastatin are all beneficial and well tolerated and result in reductions in total cholesterol, LDL, apo B-100, and TG and increases in HDL.[321-328] Lp(a) levels may also be reduced by statins.[329, 330] However, the literature regarding Lp(a) is inconsistent. In the largest reported study, Olbricht and co-authors[328] conducted a prospective, randomized, placebo-controlled trial of 102 patients with glomerulonephritis and at least 3 g of proteinuria per day. With simvastatin, mean changes from baseline in total cholesterol, LDL-cholesterol, HDL-cholesterol, and serum TG were −39%, −47%, +1%, and −30%; serum Lp(a) was not affected. The final outcomes of the study have not yet been reported. Another recent study demonstrated a possible benefit of combinations of statins with fibrates.[331] Other than lipid lowering, the beneficial effects of statins may include a reduction in platelet aggregation and procoagulant factors, inhibition of mesangial cell proliferation and matrix accumulation, and anti-inflammatory effects.[246]

In addition to standard hypolipidemic therapies, interventions that reduce proteinuria may also indirectly improve serum lipid profiles. Several studies of ACE inhibitor therapy have demonstrated improvement in lipid profiles, including reductions in Lp(a).[332-335] Similar changes occur after the administration of losartan, an AII receptor antagonist.[336] Finally, several reports have indicated beneficial effects of lipoprotein apheresis on severely hyperlipidemic nephrotic patients,[337-339] although evidence of long-term outcomes from this intervention are currently lacking.[340]

HYPERTENSION

Hypertension frequently accompanies glomerular diseases with a nephritic pattern and may accompany nephrotic diseases as well. Although exceptions exist, hypertension in the absence of renal insufficiency is more likely to be present in primary glomerular diseases than in diseases of tubulointerstitial origin. The relationship between hypertension and glomerular disease has been the subject of several reviews[341-343] and is discussed in detail in Chapter 47.

Multiple factors are likely to play a role in the pathogenesis of hypertension associated with glomerular disease.[344] In patients with severe renal functional impairment and with an acute nephritic syndrome and extracellular volume expansion, hypertension is generally volume dependent and is responsive to interventions that ameliorate the volume overload.[151, 345] In addition, elevated peripheral vascular resistance may contribute to hypertension, even in the presence of volume expansion. Although absolute values of plasma renin and AII in such patients may be normal, they are also inappropriately high for the degree of PV expansion, thus suggesting resetting of the Na^+-volume-renin feedback mechanism.[344, 345] In nephrotic syndrome, hypertensive patients also appear to fall in the group with PV expansion,[166, 167] with blood pressures falling after remission or diuretic therapy.[346] Though not well studied, urinary loss of an antihypertensive substance is a possibility. For example, nitric oxide circulates bound to albumin.[347]

HEMATOLOGIC ABNORMALITIES
(See also Chapter 49)

Hypercoagulable State and Renal Vein Thrombosis

The nephrotic syndrome is frequently complicated by an enhanced tendency for intravascular coagulation, with a consequent risk of thromboembolic complications. The most common manifestation is the development of renal vein thrombosis, which is most frequently associated with membranous glomerulonephritis. Prospective studies of the incidence of renal vein thrombosis in patients with membranous nephropathy indicated an average incidence of about 35%, with individual studies finding a range of 5% to 62%.[236, 348, 349] The incidence is much lower in other forms of glomerulonephritis, for unknown reasons.

Thrombosis is not limited to the renal venous circulation, although this site predominates. The incidence of thrombotic complications at other sites ranges from 8% to 44%, with an average of about 20%.[348-350] Of such complications, pulmonary embolism is the most frequent and serious. In a study of 204 children and 116 adults with nephrotic syndrome, children exhibited a lower incidence of events than adults did.[351] However, the complications tended to be more severe in children, almost half of whom exhibited arterial

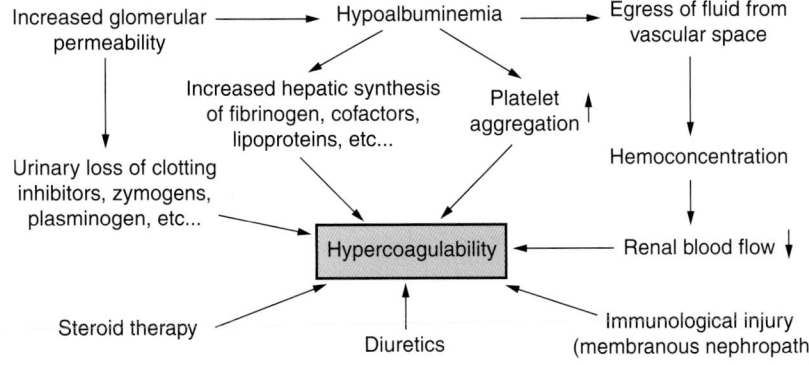

FIGURE 42-12. Schematic representation of pathogenetic factors leading to hypercoagulability, thromboembolic phenomena, and renal vein thrombosis in nephrotic syndrome. (From Llach F: Hypercoagulability, renal vein thrombosis, and other thrombotic complications of nephrotic syndrome. Kidney Int 28:429, 1985.)

thrombosis.[351] As mentioned earlier, the relative risk of coronary thrombotic events is increased in these patients,[307] and hypercoagulability could well contribute to this finding.

Pathogenesis of Hypercoagulability

The numerous abnormalities in the coagulation and hemostasis systems that accompany nephrotic syndrome have been extensively reviewed[94, 95, 236, 348, 352] and will be briefly summarized here. These abnormalities include alterations in the levels and activity of factors in the intrinsic and extrinsic coagulation cascades, levels of antithrombotic and fibrinolytic components of plasma, platelet counts and platelet function, blood viscosity, and other factors. A pathogenetic mechanism for these abnormalities is depicted in Figure 42-12,[236] and reported abnormalities are summarized in Table 42-1. As reviewed by Llach,[236] abnormalities of coagulation in the nephrotic syndrome may relate to each of the five major functional classes of coagulation components: (1) zymogens (factors II, V, VII, IX, X, XI, and XII), which are activated to enzymes, and cofactors (factors V and VIII), which accelerate the conversion of zymogens; (2) fibrinogen; (3) the fibrinolytic system; (4) clotting inhibitors; and (5) components of platelet reaction and thrombogenesis.

TABLE 42-1

Coagulation Abnormalities in Nephrotic Syndrome

Alterations in zymogens and cofactors
    Deficiency in factors IX, XI, XII
    Increased levels of factor II and combined factors VII and X
    Increased levels of factors V and VIII
Increased plasma fibrinogen levels
Alterations in the fibrinolytic system
    Deficiency of plasma plasminogen
    Low antiplasmin activity (α_1-antitrypsin)
    Increased antiplasmin activity (α_2-macroglobulin fraction)
    Increased α_1-antiplasmin
Alterations in coagulation inhibitors
    Deficiency of antithrombin III
    Deficiency of protein S
    Deficiency of protein C (possible)
Alterations in platelet function
    Enhanced platelet aggregability
    Increased levels of β-thromboglobulin

Data modified from Llach F: Hypercoagulability, renal vein thrombosis, and other thrombotic complications of nephrotic syndrome. Kidney Int 28:429, 1985.

Alterations in Zymogens and Cofactors

Most studies have noted deficiencies in levels of factors IX, XI, and XII,[352-357] which are likely to relate to urinary loss of these low-molecular-weight proteins. Deficient factor XII levels are particularly important because this factor regulates coagulation activity, as well as the fibrinolytic and kinin-kallikrein pathways.[358] Increases in the level of factor II and combined factors VII and X have also been noted.[359] These zymogen abnormalities usually normalize with clinical remission of nephrotic syndrome.[353] The nephrotic syndrome is also characterized by increased levels of the cofactors V and VIII, which may correlate inversely with the level of serum albumin.[359-361] The serum elevations appear to result from increased hepatic synthesis, perhaps in response to the decreased oncotic pressure or hypoalbuminemia (or both). These abnormalities in zymogens and cofactors have not been clearly associated with thrombotic complications.[236]

Alterations in Fibrinogen Levels and the Fibrinolytic System

The nephrotic syndrome is associated with elevated plasma fibrinogen levels,[351, 359-361] which most probably result from increased hepatic synthesis and normal catabolic rates.[362] Fibrinogen levels correlate directly with urinary protein and serum cholesterol levels and inversely with serum albumin levels.[359-361] Fibrinogen is an important determinant of plasma viscosity, and the increased levels may be of pathogenetic importance in the hypercoagulability of nephrotic syndrome. Indeed, by inducing fibrin deposition, hyperfibrinogenemia may be a major factor determining thrombotic risk.[363]

The data on fibrinolytic abnormalities, which are associated with thrombosis in other conditions, are conflicting in nephrotic syndrome. Several studies have found deficiencies in plasma levels of plasminogen, with the decrease correlating with the magnitude of hypoalbuminemia and proteinuria.[364-366] Other reported abnormalities include low antiplasmin activity (α_1-antitrypsin)[360] and increased antiplasmin activity (α_2-macroglobulin fraction, which is the primary plasmin inhibitor and may be the most reliable marker of renal vein thrombosis).[367]

Alterations in Coagulation Inhibitors

Nephrotic patients exhibit increased urinary losses and decreased plasma levels of the protease inhibitor antithrombin

III (ATIII), the most important inhibitor of coagulation and thrombin.[351, 368] Deficient serum levels of ATIII are sometimes,[367] though not always[369] correlated with thromboembolic phenomena in nephrotic patients. ATIII deficiency, a defect that is reversible with steroid therapy,[370] occurs commonly, but not universally in nephrotic syndrome.[236]

Abnormalities in other coagulation inhibitors, including protein C and protein S, may also occur in nephrotic syndrome; congenital deficiencies of each of these proteins are associated with recurrent venous thrombosis.[371, 372] Both these proteins are found in the urine of nephrotic patients.[373, 374] Levels of total protein S and protein C antigens are elevated, but the activity of protein S is reduced because of a significant reduction in free (active) protein S levels, a consequence of elevated urinary losses.[374] Protein C anticoagulant activity is elevated, although a marked reduction in specific activity has been noted. Nephrotic patients may exhibit elevations in serum thrombin activatable fibrinolysis inhibitor (TAFI), as well as a deficiency in protein Z, two additional factors that may predispose to thrombosis.[375] A reduction in tissue factor pathway inhibitor (TFPI) has been postulated, but one study found that proteinuria was in fact associated with increased TFPI levels, so the thrombotic tendencies cannot be ascribed to TFPI deficiency.[376]

Alterations in Platelet Function

Platelet counts in nephrotic patients tend to be normal or elevated.[359, 360] Platelet aggregability may be increased[240, 369, 377]; the potential contributions of hyperlipidemia and hypoalbuminemia to this abnormality are discussed earlier. Nephrotic patients may also exhibit elevations in β-thromboglobulin, a specific protein released by platelets on aggregation.[378, 379]

In summary, numerous coagulation abnormalities are found in nephrotic syndrome. In addition to the factors described earlier, nephrotic syndrome may be characterized by increased blood viscosity[379, 380] as a result of both hyperlipidemia and increased fibrinogen. Steroid therapy may also exacerbate hypercoagulability in nephrotic patients.[381]

The specific role of each of these abnormalities in the pathogenesis of thromboembolic complications remains incompletely defined.[236] An increased tendency toward thrombotic events has been correlated with increased α_2-antiplasmin levels,[367] and the presence of factor XII and prekallikrein in subepithelial deposits has been noted in patients with membranous glomerulonephritis.[382] However, a prospective study of nephrotic adults monitored for an average of 21 months found significant increases in factor I, factor VIIIc, factor VIIIr:Ag, α_1-antitrypsin, and α_2-macroglobulin, as well as platelet hyperaggregability, in the group as a whole, but no correlation between these abnormalities and thromboembolic events. Low levels of ATIII and severe hypoalbuminemia were of no predictive value for thromboembolic events.[369] Of five patients with three potential risk factors (severe hypoalbuminemia, low ATIII levels, and platelet hyperaggregability), none had thromboembolic complications during the course of the study. Thus, although the nephrotic syndrome features prominent hematologic abnormalities and a tendency toward thromboembolic complications, the relationship between these problems remains to be completely defined.

HORMONAL AND OTHER SYSTEMIC MANIFESTATIONS

Other systemic manifestations of glomerular disease, which are covered in detail elsewhere in this volume, include enhanced susceptibility to infection,[96, 98, 383] possibly as a result of urinary loss of components of the alternative complement pathway, including factor B, and loss of IgG.[383] IgG synthesis may also be impaired.[384, 385] Deficiencies of trace metals such as copper, zinc, and iron may occur.[386-389] Urinary losses of thyroxine-binding globulin, triiodothyronine, and thyroxine have been noted, although patients remain clinically euthyroid.[390, 391] Urinary levels of corticosteroid-binding globulin[392] and insulin-like growth factor type I[393] are elevated, although the clinical consequences are unclear. Abnormalities in Ca^{2+} and vitamin D metabolism, such as hypocalcemia, hypocalciuria, and low serum levels of vitamin D, also characterize the nephrotic syndrome.[98, 394] It is not clear that clinically significant hypovitaminosis D occurs in the majority of nephrotic patients,[95] but a recent study found an increased incidence of isolated osteomalacia and bone resorption in association with defective mineralization in patients with sustained nephrotic syndrome.[395] Urinary levels of erythropoietin are increased, and plasma levels fail to rise despite anemia[396]; erythropoietin deficiency can occur and cause anemia even in the setting of normal kidney function.[397] Transferrin synthesis is increased, but not sufficiently to replace urinary losses.[398] Finally, extrarenal protein loss in the presence of inadequate protein intake may be associated with negative nitrogen balance and protein malnutrition.[99]

REFERENCES

1. Maddox DA, Deen WM, Brenner BM: Glomerular filtration. *In* Windhager EE (ed): Handbook of Physiology. Section 8, Renal Physiology. New York, Oxford University Press, 1992, pp 545-638.
2. Kanwar YS, Liu ZZ, Kashihara N, et al: Current status of the structural and functional basis of glomerular filtration and proteinuria. Semin Nephrol 4:390-413, 1991.
3. Kaysen GA, Myers BD, Couser WG, et al: Mechanisms and consequences of proteinuria. Lab Invest 54:479-498, 1986.
4. Timpl R: Recent advances in the biochemistry of glomerular basement membrane. Kidney Int 30:293-298, 1986.
5. Chang RL, Ueki IF, Troy JL, et al: Permselectivity of the glomerular capillary wall to macromolecules. II. Experimental studies in rats using neutral dextran. Biophys J 15:887-906, 1975.
6. Deen WM, Lazzara MJ, Myers BD: Structural determinants of glomerular permeability. Am J Physiol 281:F579-F596, 2001.
7. Raats CJL, van den Born J, Berden JHM: Glomerular heparan sulfate alterations: Mechanisms and relevance for proteinuria. Kidney Int 57:385-400, 2000.
8. Oliver JD III, Anderson S, Troy JL, et al: Determination of glomerular size-selectivity in the normal rat with Ficoll. J Am Soc Nephrol 3:214-228, 1992.
9. Bohrer MP, Deen WM, Robertson CR, et al: Mechanism of angiotensin II–induced proteinuria in the rat. Am J Physiol 233: F13-F21, 1977.
10. Bohrer MP, Baylis C, Humes HD, et al: Permselectivity of the glomerular capillary wall. Facilitated filtration of circulating polycations. J Clin Invest 61:72-78, 1978.
11. Deen WM, Satvat B, Jamieson JM: Theoretical model for glomerular filtration of charged solutes. Am J Physiol 238:F126-F139, 1980.
12. Pappenheimer JR: Passage of molecules through capillary walls. Physiol Rev 33:387-423, 1953.

13. Anderson JL, Quinn JA: Restricted transport in small pores: A model for steric exclusion and hindered particle motion. Biophys J 14: 130-150, 1974.

14. Brenner BM, Baylis C, Deen WM: Transport of molecules across renal glomerular capillaries. Physiol Rev 56:502-534, 1976.

15. Deen WM, Bridges CR, Brenner BM: Biophysical basis of glomerular permselectivity. J Membr Biol 71:1-10, 1983.

16. Deen WM, Bohrer MP, Brenner BM: Macromolecule transport across glomerular capillaries: Application of pore theory. Kidney Int 16: 353-365, 1979.

17. Winetz JA, Robertson CR, Golbetz HV, et al: The nature of the glomerular injury in minimal change and focal sclerosing glomerulopathies. Am J Kidney Dis 1:91-98, 1981.

18. Deen WM, Bridges CR, Brenner BM, et al: Heteroporous model of glomerular size selectivity: Application to normal and nephrotic humans. Am J Physiol 249:F374-F389, 1985.

19. Remuzzi A, Battaglia C, Rossa L, et al: Glomerular size selectivity in nephrotic rats exposed to diets with different protein contents. Am J Physiol 253:F318-F327, 1987.

20. Remuzzi A, Perico N, Amuchastegui CS, et al: Short- and long-term effect of angiotensin II receptor blockade in rats with experimental diabetes. J Am Soc Nephrol 4:40-49, 1993.

21. Blouch K, Deen WM, Fauvel J-P, et al: Molecular configuration and glomerular size selectivity in healthy and nephrotic humans. Am J Physiol 273:F430-F437, 1997.

22. Bolton GR, Deen WM, Daniels BS: Assessment of the charge selectivity of glomerular basement membrane using Ficoll sulfate. Am J Physiol 274:F889-F896, 1998.

23. Chang RL, Deen WM, Robertson CR, et al: Permselectivity of the glomerular capillary wall. III. Restricted transport of polyanions. Kidney Int 8:212-218, 1975.

24. Brenner BM, Hostetter TH, Humes DH: Molecular basis of proteinuria of glomerular origin. N Engl J Med 298:826-833, 1978.

25. Chang RLS, Deen WM, Robertson CR, et al: Permselectivity of the glomerular capillary wall: Studies of experimental glomerulonephritis in the rat using neutral dextran. J Clin Invest 57:1272-1280, 1976.

26. Bennett CM, Glassock RJ, Chang RLS, et al: Permselectivity of the glomerular capillary wall: Studies of experimental glomerulonephritis in the rat using dextran sulfate. J Clin Invest 57:1287-1294, 1976.

27. Guasch A, Deen WM, Myers BD: Charge selectivity of the glomerular filtration barrier in healthy and nephrotic humans. J Clin Invest 92:2274-2282, 1993.

28. Vyas SV, Parker JA, Comper WD: Uptake of dextran sulphate by glomerular intracellular vesicles during kidney ultrafiltration. Kidney Int 47:945-950, 1995.

29. Bohrer MP, Deen WM, Robertson CR, et al: Influence of molecular configuration on the passage of macromolecules across the glomerular capillary wall. J Gen Physiol 74:583-593, 1979.

30. Farquhar MG, Wissig SL, Palade GE: Glomerular permeability. I. Ferritin transfer across the normal glomerular capillary wall. J Exp Med 113:47-91, 1961.

31. Graham RC, Karnovsky MJ: Glomerular permeability: Ultrastructural cytochemical studies using peroxidases as protein tracers. J Exp Med 124:1123-1134, 1966.

32. Graham RC, Kellermeyer RW: Bovine lactoperoxidase as a cytochemical protein tracer for electron microscopy. J Histochem Cytochem 16:275-278, 1968.

33. Venkatachalam MA, Cotran RS, Karnovsky MJ: An ultrastructural study of glomerular permeability in aminonucleoside nephrosis using catalase as a tracer protein. J Exp Med 132:1168-1180, 1970.

34. Rennke HG, Cotran RS, Venkatachalam MA: Role of molecular charge in glomerular permeability: Tracer studies with cationized ferritins. J Cell Biol 67:638-646, 1975.

35. Venkatachalam MA, Rennke HG: The structural and molecular basis of glomerular filtration. Circ Res 43:337-347, 1978.

36. Caulfield JP, Farquhar MG: Distribution of anionic sites in glomerular basement membranes: Their possible role in filtration and attachment. Proc Natl Acad Sci U S A 73:1646-1651, 1976.

37. Kerjaschki D, Sharkey DJ, Farquhar MG: Identification and characterization of podocalyxin—the major sialoprotein of the renal glomerular epithelial cell. J Cell Biol 98:1591-1596, 1984.

38. Dekan G, Gabel CA, Farquhar MG: Sulfate contributes to the negative charge of podocalyxin—the major sialoglycoprotein of the filtration slits. Proc Natl Acad Sci U S A 88:5398-5402, 1991.

39. Miner JH: Renal basement membrane components. Kidney Int 56:2016-2024, 1999.

40. Kanwar YS, Farquhar MG: Presence of heparan sulfate in the glomerular basement membrane. Proc Natl Acad Sci U S A 76:1303-1307, 1979.

41. Kanwar YS, Veis A, Kimura JH, et al: Characterization of heparan sulfate proteoglycan of glomerular basement membranes. Proc Natl Acad Sci U S A 81:762-766, 1984.

42. Kanwar YS, Rosenzweig LJ: Clogging of the glomerular basement membrane. J Cell Biol 93:489-494, 1982.

43. Kanwar YS, Rosenzweig LJ: Altered glomerular permeability as a result of focal detachment of visceral epithelium. Kidney Int 21:565-574, 1982.

44. Kanwar YS, Jakubowski ML: Unaltered anionic sites of glomerular basement membrane in aminonucleoside nephrosis. Kidney Int 25:613-618, 1984.

45. Groggel GC, Stevenson J, Hovingh P, et al: Changes in heparan sulfate correlate with increased glomerular permeability. Kidney Int 33:517-523, 1988.

46. Daniels BS, Hauser EB, Deen WM, et al: Glomerular basement membrane: In vitro studies of water and protein permeability. Am J Physiol 262:F919-F926, 1992.

47. Daniels BS, Deen WM, Mayer G, et al: Glomerular permeability barrier in the rat: Functional assessment by in vitro methods. J Clin Invest 92:929-936, 1993.

48. Daniels BS: Increased albumin permeability in vitro following alterations of glomerular charge is mediated by the cells of the filtration barrier. J Lab Clin Med 124:224-230, 1994.

49. Laurens W, Battaglia C, Foglieni C, et al: Direct podocyte damage in the single nephron leads to albuminuria in vivo. Kidney Int 47:1078-1086, 1995.

50. Blantz RC, Gabbai FB, Peterson O, et al: Water and protein permeability is regulated by the glomerular epithelial slit diaphragm. J Am Soc Nephrol 4:1957-1964, 1994.

51. Fogo A. Nephrotic syndrome: Molecular and genetic basis. Nephron 85:8-12, 2000.

52. Farquhar MG, Saito A, Kerjaschki D, Orlando RA: The Heyman nephritis antigenic complex: Megalin (gp330) and RAP. J Am Soc Nephrol 6:35-47, 1995.

53. Sharif K, Goyal M, Kershaw D, et al: Podocyte phenotypes as defined by expression and distribution of GLEPP1 in the developing glomerulus and in nephritic glomeruli from MCD, CNF, and FSGS. A dedifferentiation hypothesis for the nephritic syndrome. Exp Nephrol 6:234-244, 1998.

54. Barison L, Kriz W, Mundel P, D'Agati V: The dysregulated podocyte phenotype: A novel concept in the pathogenesis of collapsing idiopathic focal segmental glomerulosclerosis and HIV-associated nephropathy. J Am Soc Nephrol 10:51-60, 1999.

55. Kestilä M, Lenkkeri U, Männikko M, et al: Positionally cloned gene for a novel glomerular protein—nephrin—is mutated in congenital nephrotic syndrome. Mol Cell 1:575-582, 1998.

56. Weiher H, Noda T, Gray DA, et al: Transgenic mouse model of kidney disease: Insertional inactivation of ubiquitously expressed gene leads to nephrotic syndrome. Cell 62:425-545, 1990.

57. Boute N, Gribouval O, Roselli S, et al: NPHS2, encoding the glomerular protein podocin, is mutated in autosomal recessive steroid-resistant nephrotic syndrome. Nat Genet 24:349-354, 2000.

58. Sellin L, Huber TB, Gerke P, et al: NEPH1 defines a novel family of podocin interacting proteins. FASEB J 17:115-117, 2003.

59. Chang RLS, Robertson CR, Deen WM, et al: Permselectivity of the glomerular capillary wall to macromolecules: I. Theoretical considerations. Biophys J 15:861-866, 1975.

60. Baylis C, Ichikawa I, Willis WT, et al: Dynamics of glomerular ultrafiltration. IX. Effects of plasma protein concentration. Am J Physiol 232:F58-F64, 1977.

61. Olson JL, Hostetter TH, Rennke HG, et al: Altered glomerular permselectivity and progressive sclerosis following extreme ablation of renal mass. Kidney Int 22:112-126, 1982.

62. Yoshioka T, Shiraga H, Yoshida Y, et al: "Intact nephrons" as the primary origin of proteinuria in chronic renal disease: Study in the rat model of subtotal nephrectomy. J Clin Invest 82:1614-1623, 1988.

63. Mayer G, Lafayette RA, Oliver J, et al: Effects of angiotensin II receptor blockade on remnant glomerular permselectivity. Kidney Int 43:346-353, 1993.

64. Anderson S, Tank JE, Brenner BM: Renal and systemic manifestations of glomerular disease. *In* Brenner BM (ed): The Kidney, 6th ed. Philadelphia, WB Saunders, 2000, pp 1871-1900.

65. Ryan GB, Karnovsky MJ: An ultrastructural study of the mechanisms of proteinuria in aminonucleoside nephrosis. Kidney Int 8:219-232, 1975.

66. Bohrer MP, Baylis C, Robertson CR, et al: Mechanism of the puromycin-induced defects in the transglomerular passage of water and macromolecules. J Clin Invest 60:152-161, 1977.

67. Olson JL, Rennke HG, Venkatachalam MA: Alterations in the charge and size selectivity barrier of the glomerular filter in aminonucleoside nephrosis in rats. Lab Invest 44:271-279, 1981.

68. Weening JJ, Rennke HG: Glomerular permeability and polyanion in Adriamycin nephrosis in the rat. Kidney Int 24:152-159, 1983.

69. Yoshioka T, Mitarai T, Kon VE, et al: Role for angiotensin II in a overt functional proteinuria. Kidney Int 30:538-545, 1986.

70. Loon N, Shemesh O, Morelli E, et al: Effect of angiotensin II infusion on the human glomerular filtration barrier. Am J Physiol 257: F608-F614, 1989.

71. Joachim GR, Cameron JS, Schwartz M, et al: Selectivity of protein excretion in patients with the nephrotic syndrome. J Clin Invest 43:2332-2340, 1964.

72. Myers BD, Okarma TB, Friedman S, et al: Mechanisms of proteinuria in human glomerulonephritis. J Clin Invest 70:732-743, 1982.

73. Carrie BJ, Salyers WR, Myers BD: Minimal change nephropathy: An electrochemical disorder of the glomerular membrane. Am J Med 70:262-268, 1981.

74. Shemesh O, Ross JC, Deen WM, et al: Nature of the glomerular capillary injury in human membranous glomerulopathy. J Clin Invest 77:868-877, 1986.

75. Guasch A, Sibley RK, Huie P, et al: Extent and course of glomerular injury in human membranous glomerulopathy. Am J Physiol 263:F1034-F1043, 1992.

76. Hladunewich MA, Lemley KV, Blouch KL, Myers BD: Determinants of GFR depression in early membranous nephropathy. Am J Physiol Renal Physiol 284:F1014-F1022, 2003.

77. Meyer TW: Mechanisms of proteinuria in diabetic renal disease. Semin Nephrol 10:194-202, 1990.

78. Lemley KV, Blouch K, Abdulla I, et al: Glomerular permselectivity at the onset of nephropathy in type 2 diabetes mellitus. J Am Soc Nephrol 11:2095-2105, 2000.

79. Andersen S, Blouch K, Bialek J, et al: Glomerular permselectivity in early stages of overt diabetic nephropathy. Kidney Int 58:2129-2137, 2000.

80. Viberti GC, Mackintosh D, Keen H: Determinants of the penetration of proteins through the glomerular barrier in insulin-dependent diabetes mellitus. Diabetes 32(suppl 2):92-95, 1983.

81. Scandling JD, Myers BD: Glomerular size-selectivity and microalbuminuria in early diabetic glomerular disease. Kidney Int 41:840-846, 1992.

82. Deckert T, Kofoed-Enevoldsen A, Vidal P, et al: Size- and charge-selectivity of glomerular filtration in type I (insulin-dependent) diabetic patients with and without albuminuria. Diabetologia 36: 244-251, 1993.

83. Ghiggeri GM, Candiano G, Delfino G, et al: Electrical charge of serum and urinary albumin in normal and diabetic humans. Kidney Int 28:168-177, 1985.

84. Daniels BS, Hauser EB: Glycation of albumin, not glomerular basement membrane, alters permeability in an in vitro model. Diabetes 41:1415-1421, 1992.

85. Melvin T, Kim Y, Michael AF: Selective binding of IgG4 and other negatively charged plasma proteins in normal and diabetic human kidneys. Am J Pathol 115:443-446, 1984.

86. Shemesh O, Deen WM, Brenner BM, et al: Effect of colloid volume expansion on glomerular barrier size-selectivity in humans. Kidney Int 29:916-923, 1986.

87. Rosenberg ME, Swanson JE, Thomas BL, et al: Glomerular and hormonal responses to dietary protein intake in human renal disease. Am J Physiol 253:F1083-F1090, 1987.

88. Remuzzi A, Puntoriere S, Battaglia C, et al: Angiotensin converting enzyme inhibition ameliorates glomerular filtration of macromolecules and water and lessens glomerular injury in the rat. J Clin Invest 85:541-549, 1990.

89. Rosenberg ME, Hostetter TH: Comparative effects of antihypertensives on proteinuria: Angiotensin-converting enzyme versus α1-antagonist. Am J Kidney Dis 18:472-F482, 1991.

90. Remuzzi A, Perticucci E, Ruggenenti P, et al: Angiotensin converting enzyme inhibition improves glomerular size-selectivity in IgA nephropathy. Kidney Int 39:1267-1273, 1991.

91. Morelli E, Loon N, Meyer T, et al: Effects of converting-enzyme inhibition on barrier function in diabetic glomerulopathy. Diabetes 39:76-82, 1990.

92. Remuzzi A, Ruggenenti P, Mosconi L, et al: Effect of low-dose enalapril on glomerular size-selectivity in human diabetic nephropathy. J Nephrol 6:36-43, 1993.

93. Ruggenenti P, Mosconi L, Sangalli F, et al: Glomerular size-selective dysfunction in NIDDM is not ameliorated by ACE inhibition or calcium channel blockade. Kidney Int 55:984-994, 1999.

94. Bernard DB: Extrarenal complications of the nephrotic syndrome. Kidney Int 33:1184-1202, 1988.

95. Harris RC, Ismail N: Extrarenal complications of the nephrotic syndrome. Am J Kidney Dis 23:477-497, 1994.

96. Abrass CK: Clinical spectrum and complications of the nephrotic syndrome. J Invest Med 45:143-153, 1997.

97. Orth SR, Ritz E: The nephrotic syndrome. N Engl J Med 338: 1202-1211, 1998.

98. Bernard DB: Metabolic complications in nephrotic syndrome: Pathophysiology and complications. *In* Brenner BM, Stein JH (eds): The Nephrotic Syndrome. New York, Churchill Livingstone, 1982, pp 85-120.

99. Kaysen GA: Albumin metabolism in the nephrotic syndrome: The effect of dietary protein intake. Am J Kidney Dis 12:461-480, 1988.

100. Rothschild MA, Oratz M, Schreiber SS: Albumin synthesis. N Engl J Med 286:748-757, 1972.

101. Kaysen GA, Schoenfeld PY: Albumin homeostasis in patients undergoing continuous ambulatory peritoneal dialysis. Kidney Int 25: 107-114, 1984.

102. Sellers AL, Katz J, Bonorris G, et al: Determination of extravascular albumin in the rat. J Lab Clin Med 68:177-185, 1966.

103. Katz J, Bonorris G, Okuyama S, et al: Albumin synthesis in perfused liver of normal and nephrotic rats. Am J Physiol 212:1255-1260, 1967.

104. Katz J, Rosenfeld S, Sellers AL: Role of the kidney in plasma albumin catabolism. Am J Physiol 198:814-818, 1960.

105. Yedgar S, Carew TW, Pittman RC, et al: Tissue sites of catabolism of albumin in rabbits. Am J Physiol 244:E101-E107, 1983.

106. Gitlin D, Janeway CA, Farr LE: Studies on the metabolism of plasma proteins in the nephrotic syndrome. I. Albumin, gamma-globulin, and iron-binding globulin. J Clin Invest 35:44-56, 1956.

107. Kaysen GA, Gambertoglio J, Jimenez I, et al: Effect of dietary protein intake on albumin homeostasis in nephrotic patients. Kidney Int 29:572-577, 1986.

108. Ballmer PE, Weber BK, Roy-Chaudhury P, et al: Elevation of albumin synthesis rates in nephrotic patients measured with [1-13C]leucine. Kidney Int 41:132-138, 1992.

109. Yamauchi A, Yamamoto S, Fukuhara Y, et al: Oncotic pressure regulates the levels of albumin mRNA and apolipoprotein B mRNA in cultured rat hepatoma cells (H411E). Abstract. Kidney Int 35:441, 1989.

110. Sun X, Martin V, Weiss RH, et al: Selective transcriptional augmentation of hepatic gene expression in the rat with Heymann nephritis. Am J Physiol 264:F441-F447, 1993.

111. Pietrangelo A, Panduro A, Chowdhury JR, et al: Albumin gene expression is down-regulated by albumin or macromolecule infusion in the rat. J Clin Invest 89:1755-1760, 1992.

112. Yamauchi A, Imai E, Noguchi T, et al: Albumin gene transcription is enhanced in liver of nephrotic rats. Am J Physiol 254:E676-E679, 1988.

113. Kaysen GA, Jones H Jr, Martin V, et al: A low protein diet restricts albumin synthesis in nephrotic rats. J Clin Invest 81:1623-1629, 1989.

114. Hoffenberg R, Gordon AH, Black EG, Louis LN: Plasma protein catabolism by the perfused rat liver: The effect of alteration of albumin concentration and dietary protein depletion. Biochem J 118:401-404, 1970.

115. Katz J, Sellers AL, Bonorris G: Effect of nephrectomy on plasma albumin catabolism in experimental nephrosis. J Lab Clin Med 63:680-686, 1964.

116. Katz J, Bonorris G, Sellers AL: Albumin metabolism in aminonucleoside nephrotic rats. J Lab Clin Med 62:910-934, 1963.

117. Galaske RG, Baldamus CA, Stolte H: Plasma protein handling in the rat kidney: Micropuncture experiments in the acute heterologous phase of anti-GBM-nephritis. Pflugers Arch 375:269-277, 1978.

118. Exaire E, Pollak VE, Pesce AJ, et al: Albumin and gamma-globulin in the nephron of the normal rat and following the injection of aminonucleoside. Nephron 9:42-54, 1972.

119. Olbricht CJ, Cannon JK, Tisher CC: Cathepsin B and L in nephron segments of rats with puromycin aminonucleoside nephrosis. Kidney Int 32:354-361, 1987.

120. Park CH, Maack T: Albumin absorption and catabolism by isolated perfused proximal convoluted tubules of the rabbit. J Clin Invest 73:767-778, 1984.

121. Eisenbach GM, van Liew JB, Boylan JW: Effect of angiotensin on the filtration of protein in the rat kidney: A micropuncture study. Kidney Int 8:80-87, 1975.

122. Landwehr DM, Carvallo JS, Oken DE: Micropuncture studies of the filtration and absorption of albumin by nephrotic rats. Kidney Int 11:9-17, 1977.

123. Kaysen GA, Kirkpatrick WG, Couser WG: Albumin homeostasis in the nephrotic rat: Nutritional considerations. Am J Physiol 247:F192-F202, 1984.

124. Kaysen GA, Al Bander H: Metabolism of albumin and immunoglobulins in the nephrotic syndrome. Am J Nephrol 10(suppl 1):36-42, 1990.

125. Jensen H, Rossing N, Anderson SB, et al: Albumin metabolism in the nephrotic syndrome in adults. Clin Sci 33:445-457, 1967.

126. Sellers AL, Katz J, Bonorris G: Albumin distribution in the nephrotic rat. J Lab Clin Med 71:511-516, 1968.

127. Oritz M: Oncotic pressure and albumin synthesis. In Bianchi R, Mariani AS, McFarlane AS (eds): Plasma Protein Turnover. Baltimore, University Park, 1976, pp 223-237.

128. Rothschild MA, Oratz M, Evans CD, et al: Role of hepatic interstitial albumin in regulating albumin synthesis. Am J Physiol 210:57-62, 1966.

129. Sun X, Kaysen GA: Albumin and transferrin synthesis are increased in H4 cells by serum from analbuminemic or nephrotic rats. Kidney Int 45:1381-1387, 1994.

130. Kaysen GA, Jones H Jr, Hutchison FN: High protein diets stimulate albumin synthesis at the site of albumin mRNA transcription. Kidney Int 36(suppl 27):168-172, 1989.

131. Castro CE, Sevall JS: Hepatic level of rat albumin messenger RNA is influenced by factors other than dietary protein. J Nutr 115:491-495, 1985.

132. Hutchison FN, Schambelan M, Kaysen GA: Modulation of albuminuria by dietary protein and converting enzyme inhibition. Am J Physiol 253:F719-F725, 1987.

133. Kaysen GA, Rosenthal C, Hutchison FN: GFR increases before renal mass or ODC activity increase in rats fed high protein diets. Kidney Int 36:441-446, 1989.

134. Paller MS, Hostetter TH: Dietary protein increases plasma renin and reduces pressor activity to angiotensin II. Am J Physiol 251:F34-F39, 1986.

135. Kaysen GA, Martin VI, Jones H Jr: Arginine augments neither albuminuria nor albumin synthesis caused by high-protein diets in nephrosis. Am J Physiol 263:F907-F914, 1992.

136. Kaysen GA, Al-Bander H, Martin VI, et al: Branch chain amino acids augment neither albuminuria nor albumin synthesis in nephrotic rats. Am J Physiol 260:F177-F184, 1991.

137. Don B, Kaysen GA, Hutchison F, et al: The effect of angiotensin converting enzyme inhibition and protein restriction in the treatment of proteinuria. Am J Kidney Dis 17:10-17, 1991.

138. Peavey DE, Taylor JM, Jefferson LS: Correlation of albumin production rates and albumin mRNA levels in livers of normal, diabetic and insulin-treated diabetic rats. Proc Natl Acad Sci U S A 75:5879-5883, 1978.

139. Siddiqui UA, Goldflam T, Goodridge AG: Nutritional and hormonal regulation of the translatable levels of malic enzyme and albumin mRNAs in avian liver cells in vivo and in culture. J Biol Chem 256:4544-4550, 1981.

140. Kernoff LM, Pimstone BL, Solomon J, et al: The effect of hypophysectomy and growth hormone replacement on albumin synthesis and catabolism in the rat. Biochem J 124:529-535, 1971.

141. Moshage HJ, Haard HJW, Princen HMG, et al: The influence of glucocorticoid on albumin synthesis and its messenger RNA in rat in vivo and in hepatocyte suspension culture. Biochim Biophys Acta 824:27-33, 1985.

142. Moshage HJ, Janssen JAM, Franssen JH, et al: Study of the molecular mechanism of decreased liver synthesis of albumin in inflammation. J Clin Invest 79:1635-1641, 1987.

143. Suranyi MG, Guasch A, Hall BM, et al: Elevated levels of tumor necrosis factor in the nephrotic syndrome in humans. Am J Kidney Dis 21:251-259, 1993.

144. Intaglietta M, Zweifach BW: Microcirculatory basis of fluid exchange. Adv Biol Med Phys 15:111-159, 1974.

145. Vande Walle JGJ, Donckerwolcke RA: Pathogenesis of edema formation in the nephrotic syndrome. Pediatr Nephrol 16:283-293, 2001.

146. Deschênes G, Feraille E, Doucet A: Mechanisms of oedema in nephrotic syndrome: Old theories and new ideas. Nephrol Dial Transplant 18:454-456, 2003.

147. Bradley SE: The pathophysiology of hypoproteinemic edema. Contrib Nephrol 21:75-80, 1980.

148. Aukland K, Nicolaysen G: Interstitial fluid volume: Local regulatory mechanisms. Physiol Rev 61:556-643, 1981.

149. Brace RA, Guyton A: Effect of hindlimb isolation procedure on isogravimetric capillary pressure and transcapillary fluid dynamics in dogs. Circ Res 38:192-196, 1976.

150. Ichikawa I, Rennke HG, Hoyer JR, et al: Role for intrarenal mechanisms in the impaired salt excretion of experimental nephrotic syndrome. J Clin Invest 71:91-103, 1983.

151. Glassock RJ: Sodium homeostasis in acute glomerulonephritis and the nephrotic syndrome. Contrib Nephrol 23:181-203, 1980.

152. Schrier RW: Pathogenesis of sodium and water retention in high-output and low-output cardiac failure, nephrotic syndrome, cirrhosis, and pregnancy. N Engl J Med 319:1065-1076, 1988.

153. Noddeland H, Riisnes SM, Fadnes HO: Interstitial fluid colloid osmotic and hydrostatic pressures in subcutaneous tissue of patients with nephrotic syndrome. Scand J Clin Lab Invest 42:139-146, 1982.

154. Reed RK: Interstitial fluid volume, colloid osmotic and hydrostatic pressure in rat skeletal muscle: Effect of hypoproteinemia. Acta Physiol Scand 112:141-147, 1981.

155. Golden MHN, Golden BE, Jackson AA: Albumin and nutritional oedema. Lancet 1:114-116, 1980.

156. Koomans HA, Kortlandt W, Geers AB, et al: Lowered protein content of tissue fluid in patients with the nephrotic syndrome: Observations during disease and recovery. Nephron 40:391-395, 1985.

157. Fadnes HO, Pape JF, Sundsfjord JA: A study on oedema mechanism in nephrotic syndrome. Scand J Clin Lab Invest 46:533-538, 1986.

158. Fadnes HO, Reed RK, Aukland K: Mechanisms regulating interstitial fluid volume. Lymphology 11:165-257, 1978.

159. Perico N, Remuzzi G: Edema of the nephrotic syndrome: The role of the atrial peptide system. Am J Kidney Dis 22:355-366, 1993.

160. Brown E, Hopper J Jr, Wennesland R: Blood volume and its regulation. Annu Rev Physiol 19:231-254, 1957.

161. Humphreys MH: Mechanisms and management of nephrotic edema. Kidney Int 45:266-281, 1994.

162. Schrier RW, Fassett RG: A critique of the overfill hypothesis of sodium and water retention in the nephrotic syndrome. Kidney Int 53:1111-1117, 1998.

163. Andreoli TE: Edematous states: An overview. Kidney Int 51(suppl 58):2-10, 1997.

164. Benhold H, Klaus D, Scheurlen PG: Volume regulation and renal function in analbuminemia. Lancet 2:1169-1170, 1960.

165. Joles JA, Willekes-Koolschijn N, Braam B, et al: Colloid osmotic pressure in young analbuminemic rats. Am J Physiol 257:F23-F28, 1989.

166. Meltzer JL, Keim HJ, Laragh JH, et al: Nephrotic syndrome: Vasoconstriction and hypervolemic types indicated by renin-sodium profiling. Ann Intern Med 91:688-696, 1979.

167. Dorhout Mees EJ, Roos JC, Boer P, et al: Observations on edema formation in the nephrotic syndrome in adults with minimal lesions. Am J Med 67:378-384, 1979.

168. Dorhout Mees EJ, Geers AB, Koomans HA: Blood volume and sodium retention in the nephrotic syndrome: A controversial pathophysiological concept. Nephron 36:201-211, 1984.

169. Brown EA, Markandu N, Sagnella GA, et al: Sodium retention in nephrotic syndrome is due to an intrarenal defect: Evidence from steroid-induced remission. Nephron 39:290-295, 1985.

170. Koomans HA, Geers AB, Dourhout Mees EJ, et al: Lowered tissue-fluid oncotic pressure protects the blood volume in the nephrotic syndrome. Nephron 42:317-322, 1986.

171. Shapiro MD, Nicholls KM, Groves BM, et al: Role of glomerular filtration rate in the impaired sodium and water excretion of patients with the nephrotic syndrome. Am J Kidney Dis 8:81-87, 1986.

172. Vande Walle J, Donckerwolcke R, Boer P, et al: Blood volume, colloid osmotic pressure and F-cell ratio in children with the nephrotic syndrome. Kidney Int 49:1471-1477, 1996.

173. Geers AB, Koomans H, Boer P, et al: Plasma and blood volumes in patients with the nephrotic syndrome. Nephron 38:170-173, 1984.

174. Donckerwolcke RA, Vande Walle JG: Pathogenesis of edema formation in the nephrotic syndrome. Kidney Int 51(suppl 58): 72-74, 1997.

175. Joles J, Rabelink T, Braam B, et al: Plasma and blood volumes in patients with the nephrotic syndrome. Nephron 38:170-173, 1984.

176. Tulassay T, Rascher W, Lange RE, et al: Atrial natriuretic peptide and other vasoactive hormones in nephrotic syndrome. Kidney Int 31:1391-1395, 1987.

177. Usberti M, Federico S, Meccariello S, et al: Role of plasma vasopressin in the impairment of water excretion in nephrotic syndrome. Kidney Int 25:422-429, 1984.

178. Koomans HA, Geers AB, van der Meiracker AH, et al: Effects of plasma volume expansion on renal salt handling in patients with the nephrotic syndrome. Am J Nephrol 4:227-234, 1984.

179. Brown EA, Markandu ND, Sagnella GA, et al: Evidence that some mechanism other than the renin system causes sodium retention in nephrotic syndrome. Lancet 2:1237-1240, 1982.

180. Berlyne GM, Sutton J, Brown C, et al: Renal salt and water handling in water immersion in the nephrotic syndrome. Clin Sci 61:605-610, 1981.

181. Krishna GG, Danovitch GM: Effects of water immersion on renal function in the nephrotic syndrome. Kidney Int 21:395-401, 1982.

182. Rascher W, Tulassay T, Seyberth HW, et al: Diuretic and hormonal responses to head-out water immersion in nephrotic syndrome. J Pediatr 109:609-614, 1986.

183. Koomans HA, Boer WH, Dorhout Mees EJ: Renal function during recovery from minimal lesions nephrotic syndrome. Nephron 47:173-178, 1987.

184. Kaysen GA, Pukert TT, Menke DJ, et al: Plasma volume expansion is necessary for edema formation in the rat with Heymann nephritis. Am J Physiol 248:F247-F253, 1985.

185. Fauchald P, Noddeland H, Norseth J: An evaluation of ultrafiltration as treatment of diuretic-resistant oedema in nephrotic syndrome. Acta Med Scand 217:127-131, 1985.

186. Wagnild JP, Gutmann FD: Functional adaptation of nephrons in dogs with acute progressing to chronic experimental glomerulonephritis. J Clin Invest 57:1575-1589, 1976.

187. Chandra M, Hoyer JR, Lewy JE: Renal function in rats with unilateral proteinuria produced by renal perfusion with aminonucleoside. Pediatr Res 15:340-344, 1976.

188. Peterson C, Madsen B, Perlmann A, et al: Atrial natriuretic peptide and the renal response to hypervolemia in nephrotic humans. Kidney Int 34:825-831, 1988.

189. Shapiro MD, Hasbargen J, Hensen J, et al: Role of aldosterone in the sodium retention of patients with nephrotic syndrome. Am J Nephrol 10:44-48, 1990.

190. Perico N, Delaini F, Lupini C, et al: Renal response to atrial peptides is reduced in experimental nephrosis. Am J Physiol 252:F654-F660, 1987.

191. Perico N, Delaini F, Lupini C, et al: Blunted excretory response to atrial natriuretic peptide in experimental nephrosis. Kidney Int 36:57-64, 1989.

192. DiBona GF, Herman PJ, Sawin LL: Neural control of renal function in edema-forming states. Am J Physiol 254:R1017-R1024, 1988.

193. Valentin J-P, Qiu CQ, Muldowney WP, et al: Cellular basis for blunted volume expansion natriuresis in experimental nephrotic syndrome. J Clin Invest 90:1302-1312, 1992.

194. Valentin J-P, Ying W-Z, Sechi LA, et al: Phosphodiesterase inhibitors correct resistance to natriuretic peptides in rats with Heymann nephritis. J Am Soc Nephrol 7:582-593, 1996.

195. Valentin J-P, Ying W-Z, Couser WG, et al: Extrarenal resistance to atrial natriuretic peptide in rats with experimental nephrotic syndrome. Am J Physiol 274:F556-F563, 1998.

196. Deschênes G, Gonin S, Zolty E, et al: Increased synthesis and AVP unresponsiveness of Na,K-ATPase in collecting duct from nephrotic rats. J Am Soc Nephrol 12:2241-2252, 2001.

197. Lourdel S, Zecevic M, Marc Paulais M, et al: ENaC activation in experimental nephrotic syndrome. Abstract. J Am Soc Nephrol 12:138, 2001.

198. Besse-Eschmann V, Klisic J, Nief V, et al: Regulation of the proximal tubular sodium/proton exchanger NHE3 in rats with puromycin

199. aminonucleoside (PAN)-induced nephrotic syndrome. J Am Soc Nephrol 13:2199-2206, 2002.

199. Apostol E, Ecelbarger CA, Terris T, et al: Reduced renal medullary water channel expression in puromycin aminonucleoside–induced nephrotic syndrome. J Am Soc Nephrol 8:15-24, 1997.

200. Fernández-Llama P, Andrews P, Nielsen S, et al: Impaired aquaporin and urea transporter expression in rats with Adriamycin-induced nephrotic syndrome. Kidney Int 53:1244-1253, 1998.

201. Fernández-Llama P, Andrews P, Ecelbarger CA, et al: Concentrating defect in experimental nephrotic syndrome: Altered expression of aquaporins and thick ascending limb Na+ transporters. Kidney Int 54:170-179, 1998.

202. Klahr S, Alleyne GAO: Effects of chronic protein-calorie malnutrition on the kidney. Kidney Int 3:129-141, 1973.

203. Vereerstraeten P, Toussaint C: Effects of plasmapheresis on renal hemodynamics and sodium in dogs. Pflugers Arch 306:92-102, 1969.

204. Anderson S, Diamond JR, Karnovsky MJ, et al: Mechanisms underlying transition from acute glomerular injury to late glomerular sclerosis in a rat model of nephrotic syndrome. J Clin Invest 82:1757-1768, 1988.

205. Meyer TW, Rennke HG: Increased single-nephron protein excretion after renal ablation in nephrotic rats. Am J Physiol 255: F1243-F1248, 1988.

206. Sanfelice NFT, Fujihara CK, Marcondes M, et al: Glomerular hemodynamics and fluid compartments in the analbuminemic rat. Abstract. Kidney Int 35:473, 1989.

207. Buckheit JB, Olshen RA, Blouch K, et al: Modeling of progressive glomerular injury in humans with lupus nephritis. Am J Physiol 273:F158-F169, 1997.

208. Guasch A, Cua M, Mitch WE: Early detection and the course of glomerular injury in patients with sickle cell anemia. Kidney Int 49:786-791, 1996.

209. Guasch A, Myers BD: Determinants of glomerular hypofiltration in nephrotic patients with minimal change nephropathy. J Am Soc Nephrol 4:1571-1581, 1998.

210. Squarer A, Lemley KV, Ambalavanan S, et al: Mechanisms of progressive glomerular injury in membranous nephropathy. J Am Soc Nephrol 9:1389-1398, 1998.

211. Miller PL, Meyer TW: Plasma protein concentration and colloid osmotic pressure in nephrotic rats. Kidney Int 34:220-223, 1988.

212. Canaan-Kühl, Venkatraman ES, Ernst SIB, et al: Relationships among protein and albumin concentrations and oncotic pressure in nephrotic plasma. Am J Physiol 264:F1052-F1059, 1993.

213. Aronoff GR, Abel SR: Principles of administering drugs to patients with renal failure. In Bennett WM, McCarron DA, Brenner BM, Stein JH (eds): Pharmacotherapy of Renal Disease and Hypertension. New York, Churchill Livingstone, 1987, pp 1-20.

214. Aronoff GR, Berns JS, Brier ME, et al: Drug Prescribing in Renal Failure. Philadelphia, American College of Physicians, 1999.

215. Morrison G, Audet PR, Singer I: Clinically important drug interactions for the nephrologist. In Bennett WM, McCarron DA, Brenner BM, Stein JH (eds): Pharmacotherapy of Renal Disease and Hypertension. New York, Churchill Livingstone, 1987, pp 49-98.

216. Reidenberg MN: The biotransformation of drugs in renal failure. Am J Med 62:482-489, 1977.

217. Brater DC: Resistance to diuretics: Emphasis on a pharmacological perspective. Drugs 22:477-494, 1981.

218. Brater DC, Voelker JR: Use of diuretics in patients with renal disease. In Bennett WM, McCarron DA, Brenner BM, Stein JH (eds): Pharmacotherapy of Renal Disease and Hypertension. New York, Churchill Livingstone, 1987, pp 115-148.

219. Ellison DH: The physiological basis of diuretic synergism: Its role in treating diuretic resistance. Ann Intern Med 114:886-894, 1991.

220. Kirchner KA: Mechanisms of diuretic resistance in nephrotic syndrome. In Puschett JB, Greenberg A (eds): Diuretics IV: Chemistry, Pharmacology and Clinical Applications. Amsterdam, Elsevier Science, 1993, pp 435-460.

221. Brater DC: Diuretic therapy. N Engl J Med 339:387-395, 1998.

222. Wilson CS: New insights into diuretic use in patients with chronic renal disease. J Am Soc Nephrol 13:798-805, 2002.

223. Andreasen F: Determination of furosemide in blood plasma and its binding to proteins in normal plasma and in plasma from patients with acute renal failure. Acta Pharmacol Toxicol 32:417-423, 1973.

224. Keller E, Hoppe-Seyler G, Schollmeyer P: Disposition and diuretic effect of furosemide in the nephrotic syndrome. Clin Pharmacol Ther 32:442-449, 1982.

225. Smith DE, Hyneck ML, Berardi RR, et al: Urinary protein binding, kinetics and dynamics of furosemide in nephrotic patients. J Pharm Sci 74:603-608, 1985.

226. Voelker JR, Jameson DM, Brater DC: In vitro evidence that urine composition affects the fraction of active furosemide in the nephrotic syndrome. J Pharmacol Exp Ther 250:772-778, 1989.

227. Kirchner KA, Voelker JR, Brater DC: Intratubular albumin blunts the response to furosemide: A mechanism for diuretic resistance in nephrotic syndrome. J Pharmacol Exp Ther 252:1097-1101, 1990.

228. Kirchner KA, Voelker JR, Brater DC: Binding inhibitors restore furosemide potency in tubule fluid containing albumin. Kidney Int 40:418-424, 1991.

229. Agarwal A, Gorski JC, Sundblad K, Brater DC: Urinary protein binding dose not affect response to furosemide in patients with nephrotic syndrome. J Am Soc Nephrol 11:1100-1105, 2000.

230. Kirchner KA, Voelker JR, Brater DC: Tubular resistance to furosemide contributes to the attenuated diuretic response in nephrotic rats. J Am Soc Nephrol 2:1201-1207, 1992.

231. Inoue M, Okajima K, Itoh K, et al: Mechanism of furosemide resistance in analbuminemic rats and hypoalbuminemic patients. Kidney Int 32:198-202, 1987.

232. Fernandez J, Roth D, Bourgoignie J: Treatment of refractory edema in hypoalbuminemic patients with bumetanide and albumin. Abstract. Am J Kidney Dis 20:4, 1992.

233. Chalasani N, Gorski JC, Horlander JC Sr, et al: Effects of albumin/furosemide mixtures on responses to furosemide in hypoalbuminemic patients. J Am Soc Nephrol 12:1010-1016, 2001.

234. Fliser D, Zurbruggen I, Mutschler E, et al: Coadministration of albumin and furosemide in patients with the nephrotic syndrome. Kidney Int 55:629-634, 1999.

235. Yoshida A, Aoki N: Release of arachidonic acid from human platelets: A key role for the potentiation of platelet aggregability in normal subjects as well as in those with the nephrotic syndrome. Blood 52:969-978, 1978.

236. Llach F: Hypercoagulability, renal vein thrombosis, and other thrombotic complications of nephrotic syndrome. Kidney Int 28:429-439, 1985.

237. Bang N, Tygstad C, Schroeder J, et al: Enhanced platelet function in glomerular renal disease. J Lab Clin Med 81:651-660, 1973.

238. Remuzzi G, Mecca G, Marchest D, et al: Platelet hyperaggregability and the nephrotic syndrome. Thromb Res 16:345-354, 1979.

239. Bennett A, Cameron JS: Platelet hyperaggregability in the nephrotic syndrome which is not dependent on arachidonic acid metabolism or on plasma albumin concentration. Clin Nephrol 27:182-188, 1987.

240. Rabelink TJ, Zwanginga JJ, Koomans HA, et al: Thrombosis and hemostasis in renal disease. Kidney 46:287-296, 1994.

241. Appel G: Lipid abnormalities in renal disease. Kidney Int 39:169-183, 1991.

242. Attman P-O, Samuelsson O, Alaupovic P: Lipoprotein metabolism and renal failure. Am J Kidney 21:573-592, 1993.

243. Kaysen GA: Hyperlipidemia of the nephrotic syndrome. Am J Kidney Dis 39(suppl 31):8-15, 1991.

244. Massy ZA, Kasiske BL: Hyperlipidemia and its management in renal disease. Curr Opin Nephrol Hypertens 5:141-146, 1996.

245. Wheeler DC, Bernard DB: Lipid abnormalities in the nephrotic syndrome: Causes, consequences and treatment. Am J Kidney Dis 23:331-346, 1994.

246. Wheeler DC: Lipid abnormalities in the nephrotic syndrome: The therapeutic role of statins. J Nephrol 14(suppl 4):70-75, 2001.

247. Joven J, Villabona C, Vilella E, et al: Abnormalities of lipoprotein metabolism in patients with the nephrotic syndrome. N Engl J Med 323:579-584, 1990.

248. Muls E, Rosseneu M, Daneels R, et al: Lipoprotein distribution and composition in the human nephrotic syndrome. Atherosclerosis 54:225-237, 1985.

249. Short CD, Durrington PN, Mallick NP, et al: Serum and urinary high density lipoproteins in glomerular disease with proteinuria. Kidney Int 29:1224-1228, 1986.

250. Wanner C, Rader D, Bartens W, et al: Elevated plasma lipoprotein(a) in patients with the nephrotic syndrome. Ann Intern Med 119:263-269, 1993.

251. de Sain-van der Velden MG, Reijngoud DJ, Kaysen GA, et al: Evidence for increased synthesis of lipoprotein(a) in the nephrotic syndrome. J Am Soc Nephrol 9:1474-1481, 1998.

252. Noto D, Barbagallo CM, Cascio AL, et al: Lipoprotein(a) levels in relation to albumin concentration in childhood nephrotic syndrome. Kidney Int 55:2433-2439, 1999.

253. Stenvinkel P, Berglund L, Ericsson S, et al: Low-density lipoprotein metabolism and its association to plasma lipoprotein(a) in the nephrotic syndrome. Eur J Clin Invest 27:169-177, 1997.

254. Deighan CJ, Caslake MJ, McConnell M, et al: The atherogenic lipoprotein phenotype: Small dense LDL and lipoprotein remnants in nephrotic range proteinuria. Atherosclerosis 157:211-220, 2001.

255. Kashyap ML, Srivastava LS, Hynd BA, et al: Apolipoprotein CII and lipoprotein lipase in human nephrotic syndrome. Atherosclerosis 35:29-40, 1980.

256. Deighan CJ, Caslake MJ, McConnell M, et al: Patients with nephrotic-range proteinuria have apolipoprotein C and E deficient VLDL1. Kidney Int 58:1238-1246, 2000.

257. Keane WF, St Peter JV, Kasiske BL: Is the aggressive management of hyperlipidemia in nephrotic syndrome mandatory? Kidney Int 42(suppl 38):134-141, 1992.

258. Radhakrishnan J, Appel AS, Valeri A, et al: The nephrotic syndrome, lipids, and risk factors for cardiovascular disease. Am J Kidney Dis 22:135-142, 1993.

259. Appel GB, Blum CB, Chien S, et al: The hyperlipidemia of the nephrotic syndrome: Relation to plasma albumin concentration, oncotic pressure, and viscosity. N Engl J Med 312:1544-1548, 1985.

260. Baxter JH, Goodman HC, Allen JC: Effects of albumin infusion on serum lipids and lipoproteins in nephrosis. J Clin Invest 40:490-498, 1961.

261. Kaysen GA, Gambertoglio J, Felts J, et al: Albumin synthesis, albuminuria, and hyperlipemia in nephrotic patients. Kidney Int 31:1368-1376, 1987.

262. Davies RW, Staprans I, Hutchison FN, et al: Proteinuria, not altered albumin metabolism, affects hyperlipidemia in the nephrotic rat. J Clin Invest 86:600-605, 1990.

263. Allen JC, Baxter JH, Goodman HC: Effects of dextran, polyvinylpyrrolidone and gamma globulin on the hyperlipidemia of experimental nephrosis. J Clin Invest 40:499-508, 1961.

264. Heymann W, Nash G, Gilkey C, et al: Studies on the causal role of hypoalbuminemia in experimental nephrotic hyperlipemia. J Clin Invest 37:808-819, 1958.

265. de Sain-van der Velden MG, Kaysen GA, Barrett HA, et al: Increased VLDL in nephrotic patients results from a decreased catabolism while increased LDL results from increased synthesis. Kidney Int 53:994-1001, 1998.

266. Kaysen GA, de Sain-van der Velden MG: New insights into lipid metabolism in the nephrotic syndrome. Kidney Int Suppl 71:18-21, 1999.

267. Braschi S, Masson D, Rostoker G, et al: Role of lipoprotein-bound NEFAs in enhancing the specific activity of plasma CETP in the nephrotic syndrome. Arterioscler Thromb Vasc Biol 17:2559-2567, 1997.

268. Warwick GL, Packard CJ, Demant T, et al: Metabolism of apolipoprotein B–containing lipoproteins in subjects with nephrotic-range proteinuria. Kidney Int 40:129-138, 1991.

269. Warwick GL, Caslake MH, Boulton-Jones M, et al: Low-density lipoprotein metabolism in the nephrotic syndrome. Metabolism 39:187-192, 1990.

270. Vega GL, Toto RD, Grundy SM: Metabolism of low-density lipoproteins in nephrotic dyslipidemia: Comparison of hypercholesterolemia alone and combined hyperlipidemia. Kidney Int 47:579-586, 1995.

271. Joles JA, Bijleveld C, van Tol A, et al: Plasma triglyceride levels are higher in nephrotic than in analbuminemic rats despite a similar increase in hepatic triglyceride secretion. Kidney Int 47:566-572, 1994.

272. Garber DW, Gottlieb BA, Marsh JB, et al: Catabolism of very low density lipoproteins in experimental nephrosis. J Clin Invest 74:1375-1383, 1984.

273. Olivecrona T, Bengtsson G, Markland SE, et al: Heparin–lipoprotein lipase interactions. Fed Proc 36:60-65, 1977.

274. Staprans I, Garon SJ, Hooper J, et al: Characterization of glycosaminoglycans in urine from patients with nephrotic syndrome and control subjects, and their effects on lipoprotein lipase. Biochim Biophys Acta 678:414-422, 1981.

275. Kaysen GA, Pan XM, Couser WG, et al: Defective lipolysis persists in hearts of rats with Heymann nephritis in the absence of nephrotic plasma. Am J Kidney Dis 22:128-134, 1993.

276. Yamada M, Matsuda I: Lipoprotein lipase in clinical and experimental nephrosis. Clin Chim Acta 30:787-794, 1970.

277. Staprans I, Felts JM, Couser WG: Glycosaminoglycans and chylomicron metabolism in control and nephrotic rats. Metabolism 36:496-501, 1987.

278. Liang K, Vaziri ND: Gene expression of lipoprotein lipase in experimental nephrosis. J Lab Clin Med 130:387-394, 1997.

279. Liang KH, Vaziri ND: Acquired VLDL receptor deficiency in experimental nephrosis. Kidney Int 51:1761-1765, 1997.

280. Vaziri ND, Wang XQ, Liang K: Secondary hyperparathyroidism downregulates lipoprotein lipase expression in chronic renal failure. Am J Physiol 273:F925-930, 1997.

281. Liang K, Vaziri ND: Down-regulation of hepatic lipase expression in experimental nephrotic syndrome. Kidney Int 51:1933-1937, 1997.

282. Furukawa S, Hirano T, Mamo JC, et al: Catabolic defect of triglyceride is associated with abnormal very-low-density lipoprotein in experimental nephrosis. Metab Clin Exp 39:101-107, 1990.

283. Shearer GC, Stevenson FT, Atkinson DN, et al: Hypoalbuminemia and proteinuria contribute separately to reduced lipoprotein catabolism in the nephrotic syndrome. Kidney Int 59:179-189, 2001.

284. Demant T, Mathes C, Gutlich K, et al: A simultaneous study of the metabolism of apolipoprotein B and albumin in nephrotic patients. Kidney Int 54:2064-2080, 1998.

285. Pullinger CR, North JD, Teng BB, et al: The apolipoprotein B gene is constitutively expressed in HebG2 cells: Regulation of secretion by oleic acid, albumin, and insulin, and measurement of the mRNA half-life. J Lipid Res 30:1065-1077, 1989.

286. Yamaguchi A, Fukuhara Y, Yamamoto S, et al: Oncotic pressure regulates gene transcription of albumin and apolipoprotein B in cultured rat hepatoma cells. Am J Physiol 263:C397-C404, 1992.

287. Moorhead JF, El Nahas AM, Harry D, et al: Focal glomerulosclerosis and nephrotic syndrome with partial lecithin:cholesterol acetyltransferase deficiency and discoidal high density lipoprotein in plasma and urine. Lancet 1:936-938, 1983.

288. Dullaart RPG, Gamsevoort RT, Dollescjeo BD, et al: Role of elevated LCAT and CETP activities in abnormal lipoproteins from proteinuric patients. Kidney Int 44:91-97, 1993.

289. Vaziri ND, Liang K, Parks JS: Acquired lecithin-cholesterol acyltransferase deficiency in nephrotic syndrome. Am J Physiol 280:F823-F828, 2001.

290. Cohen L, Cramp DG, Lewis AD, et al: The mechanism of hyperlipidaemia in nephrotic syndrome: Role of low albumin and the LCAT reaction. Abstract. Clin Chim Acta 104:393, 1980.

291. Moulin P, Appel GB, Ginsberg HN, et al: Increased concentration of plasma cholesteryl transfer protein in nephrotic syndrome: Role in dyslipidemia. J Lipid Res 33:1817-1822, 1992.

292. Sun X, Jones H Jr, Joles JA, et al: Apolipoprotein gene expression in analbuminemic rats and in rats with Heymann nephritis. Am J Physiol 262:F755-F761, 1992.

293. Kaysen GA, Hoye E, Jones H Jr: Apolipoprotein AI levels are increased in part as a consequence of reduced catabolism in nephrotic rats. Am J Physiol 268:F532-F540, 1995.

294. Tall AR: Plasma high density lipoproteins. Metabolism and relationship to atherogenesis. J Clin Invest 86:379-384, 1990.

295. Liang K, Vaziri ND: Down-regulation of hepatic high-density lipoprotein receptor, SR-B1, in nephrotic syndrome. Kidney Int 56:621-626, 1999.

296. Golper TA, Feingold KR, Fulford MH, et al: The role of circulating mevalonate in nephrotic hypercholesterolemia in the rat. J Lipid Res 27:1044-1051, 1986.

297. Vaziri ND, Liang KH: Hepatic HMG-CoA reductase gene expression during the course of puromycin-induced nephrosis. Kidney Int 48:1979-1985, 1995.

298. Liang KH, Oveisi F, Vaziri ND: Gene expression of hepatic cholesterol 7 alpha-hydroxylase in the course of puromycin-induced nephrosis. Kidney Int 49:855-860, 1996.

299. Bocan TM, Krause BR, Rosebury WS, et al: The ACAT inhibitor avasimibe reduces macrophages and matrix metalloproteinase expression in atherosclerotic lesions of hypercholesterolemic rabbits. Arterioscler Thromb Vasc Biol 20:70-79, 2000.

300. Bocan TM, Krause BR, Rosebury WS, et al: The combined effect of inhibiting both ACAT and HMG-CoA reductase may directly induce atherosclerotic lesion regression. Atherosclerosis 157:97-105, 2001.

301. Thabet MA, Challa A, Chan JCM, et al: Studies of alteration of hepatic cholesterol metabolism in puromycin-induced nephrotic syndrome in rats. Kidney Int 44:789-794, 1993.

302. Dullaart RPG, Gansevoort RT, Sluiter WJ, et al: The serum lathosterol to cholesterol ratio, an index of cholesterol synthesis, is not elevated in patients with glomerular proteinuria and is not associated with improvement in hyperlipidemia in response to antiproteinuric treatment. Metabolism 45:723-730, 1996.

303. Joven J, Arcelus R, Camps J, et al: Determinants of plasma homocyst(e)ine in patients with nephrotic syndrome. J Mol Med 78:147-154, 2000.

304. Berlyne GM, Mallick NP: Ischaemic heart disease as a complication of nephrotic syndrome. Lancet 2:399-440, 1969.

305. Wass VJ, Jarrett RJ, Chilvers C, et al: Does the nephrotic syndrome increase the risk of cardiovascular disease? Lancet 2:664-667, 1979.

306. Wass V, Cameron JS: Cardiovascular disease and the nephrotic syndrome: The other side of the coin. Nephron 27:58-61, 1981.

307. Ordonez JD, Hiatt R, Killebrew EJ, et al: The increased risk of coronary heart disease associated with nephrotic syndrome. Kidney Int 44:638-642, 1993.

308. Falaschi F, Ravelli A, Martignoni A, et al: Nephrotic-range proteinuria, the major risk factor for early atherosclerosis in juvenile-onset systemic lupus erythematosus. Arthritis Rheum 43:1405-1409, 2000.

309. Stroes ESG, Joles JA, Chang P, et al: Impaired endothelial function in patients with nephrotic range proteinuria. Kidney Int 48:544-550, 1995.

310. Watts GF, Herrmann S, Dogra GK, et al: Vascular function of the peripheral circulation in patients with nephrosis. Kidney Int 60:182-189, 2001.

311. Dogra G, Ward N, Croft KD, et al: Oxidant stress in nephrotic syndrome: Comparison of F(2)-isoprostanes and plasma antioxidant potential. Nephrol Dial Transplant 16:1626-1630, 2001.

312. Vuong TD, de Kimpe S, de Roos R, et al: Albumin restores lysophosphatidylcholine-induced inhibition of vasodilation in rat aorta. Kidney Int 60:1088-1096, 2001.

313. Lenorsky C, Jordan SC, Ladisch S: Plasma inhibition of lymphocyte proliferation in nephrotic syndrome: Correlation with hyperlipidemia. J Clin Immunol 2:276-281, 1982.

314. D'Amico G, Gentile MG: Influence of diet on lipid abnormalities in human renal disease. Am J Kidney Dis 22:151-157, 1993.

315. Gentile MG, Fellin G, Cofano F, et al: Treatment of proteinuric patients with vegetarian soy diet and fish oil. Clin Nephrol 40: 315-320, 1993.

316. Hall AV, Parbtani A, Clark WF, et al: Omega-3 fatty acid supplementation in primary nephrotic syndrome: Effects on plasma lipids and coagulopathy. J Am Soc Nephrol 3:1321-1329, 1992.

317. Langer T, Levy RI: Acute muscular syndrome associated with administration of clofibrate. N Engl J Med 279:856-858, 1968.

318. Groggel GC, Cheung AK, Ellis-Benigni K, et al: Treatment of the nephrotic hyperlipoproteinemia with gemfibrozil. Kidney Int 36:266-271, 1989.

319. Valeri A, Gelfand J, Blum C, et al: Treatment of the hyperlipidemia of the nephrotic syndrome: A controlled trial. Am J Kidney Dis 8:388-396, 1986.

320. Massy ZA, Ma JZ, Louis TA, et al: Lipid-lowering therapy in patients with renal disease. Kidney Int 48:188-198, 1995.

321. Golper TA, Illingworth DR, Morris CD, et al: Lovastatin in the therapy of multifactorial hyperlipidemia associated with proteinuria. Am J Kidney Dis 13:312-320, 1989.

322. Vega GL, Grundy SM: Lovastatin therapy in nephrotic hyperlipidemia: Effects on lipoprotein metabolism. Kidney Int 33:1160-1165, 1988.

323. Rabelink AJ, Hene RJ, Erkelens DW, et al: Effects of simvastatin and cholestyramine on lipoprotein profile in hyperlipidaemia of nephrotic syndrome. Lancet 2:1335-1338, 1988.

324. Thomas ME, Harris KPG, Ramaswamy C, et al: Simvastatin therapy for hypercholesterolemic patients with nephrotic syndrome or significant proteinuria. Kidney Int 44:1124-1129, 1993.

325. Kasiske BL, Velosa JA, Halstenson CE, et al: The effects of lovastatin in hyperlipidemic patients with the nephrotic syndrome. Am J Kidney Dis 15:8-15, 1990.

326. Spitalewitz S, Porush JG, Cattran D, et al: Treatment of hyperlipidemia in the nephrotic syndrome: The effects of pravastatin therapy. Am J Kidney Dis 22:143-150, 1993.

327. Warwick GL, Packard CJ, Murray L, et al: Effect of simvastatin on plasma lipid and lipoprotein concentrations and low-density lipoprotein metabolism in the nephrotic syndrome. Clin Sci 82:701-708, 1992.

328. Olbricht CJ, Wanner C, Thiery J, et al: Simvastatin in nephrotic syndrome. Kidney Int 56(suppl 71):113-116, 1999.

329. Brown CD, Azrolan N, Thomas L, et al: Reduction of lipoprotein(a) following treatment with lovastatin in patients with unremitting nephrotic syndrome. Am J Kidney Dis 26:170-177, 1995.

330. Wanner C, Boehler J, Eckardt HG, et al: Effects of simvastatin on lipoprotein(a) and lipoprotein composition in patients with nephrotic syndrome. Clin Nephrol 41:138-143, 1994.

331. Deighan CJ, Caslake MJ, McConnell M, et al: Comparative effects of cerivastatin and fenofibrate on the atherogenic lipoprotein phenotype in proteinuric renal disease. J Am Soc Nephrol 12:341-348, 2001.

332. Keilani T, Schlueter WA, Levin ML, et al: Improvement of lipid abnormalities associated with proteinuria using fosinopril, an angiotensin converting enzyme inhibitor. Ann Intern Med 18:246-254, 1993.

333. Gansevoort RT, Heeg JE, Dikkeschei BD, et al: Symptomatic antiproteinuric treatment decreases serum lipoprotein(a) concentration in patients with glomerular proteinuria. Nephrol Dial Transplant 9:244-250, 1994.

334. Praga M, Hernandez E, Montoyo C, et al: Long-term beneficial effects of angiotensin-converting enzyme inhibition in patients with nephrotic syndrome. Am J Kidney Dis 20:242-248, 1992.

335. Ruggenenti P, Mise N, Pisoni R, et al: Diverse effects of increasing lisinopril doses on lipid abnormalities in chronic nephropathies. Circulation 107:586-592, 2003.

336. de Zeeuw D, Gansevoort RT, Dullaart RPF, et al: Angiotensin II antagonism improves the lipoprotein profile in patients with nephrotic syndrome. J Hypertens 13(suppl):53-58, 1995.

337. Brunton C, Varghese Z, Moorhead JF: Lipopheresis in the nephrotic syndrome. Kidney Int 56(suppl 71):6-9, 1999.

338. Muso E, Mune M, Fujii Y, et al: Low density apheresis therapy for steroid-resistant nephrotic syndrome. Kidney Int 56(suppl 71):122-125, 1999.

339. Stenvinkel P, Alvestrand A, Angelin B, et al: LDL-apheresis in patients with nephrotic syndrome: Effects on serum albumin and urinary albumin excretion. Eur J Clin Invest 30:866-870, 2000.

340. Thompson GR: LDL apheresis. Atherosclerosis 167:1-13, 2003.

341. Kincaid-Smith P, Whitworth JA: Pathogenesis of hypertension in chronic renal disease. Semin Nephrol 8:155-162, 1988.

342. Cameron JS: Hypertension in glomerulonephritis. Contrib Nephrol 54:103-112, 1987.

343. Baldwin DS, Neugarten J: Hypertension and renal diseases. Am J Kidney Dis 10:186-191, 1987.

344. Herrera Acosta J: Hypertension in chronic renal disease. Kidney Int 22:702-712, 1982.

345. Powell HR, Rotenberg E, Williams AL, et al: Plasma renin activity in acute poststreptococcal glomerulonephritis and the hemolytic-uraemic syndrome. Arch Dis Child 49:802-807, 1974.

346. Küster S, Mehls O, Seidel C, et al: Blood pressure in minimal change and other types of nephrotic syndrome. Am J Nephrol 10(suppl 1):76-80, 1990.

347. Stamler JS, Jaraki O, Osborne J, et al: Nitric oxide circulates in mammalian plasma primarily as an S-nitroso adduct of serum albumin. Proc Natl Acad Sci U S A 89:7674-7677, 1992.

348. Llach F: Hypercoagulability, renal vein thrombosis, and other thromboembolic complications. *In* Brenner BM, Stein JH (eds): The Nephrotic Syndrome. New York, Churchill Livingstone, 1982, pp 121-144.

349. Hoyer PF, Gonda S, Barthels M, et al: Thromboembolic complications in children with nephrotic syndrome. Acta Paediatr Scand 75:804-810, 1986.

350. Sullivan MJ III, Hough DR, Agodoa LCY: Peripheral arterial thrombosis due to the nephrotic syndrome: The clinical spectrum. South Med J 76:1011-1016, 1983.

351. Mehls O, Andrassy K, Koderisch J, et al: Hemostasis and thromboembolism in children with nephrotic syndrome: Differences from adults. J Pediatr 110:862-867, 1987.

352. Cameron JS: Coagulation and thromboembolic complications in the nephrotic syndrome. Adv Nephrol 13:75-114, 1984.

353. Handley DA, Lawrence JR: Factor IX deficiency in the nephrotic syndrome. Lancet 1:1079-1081, 1967.

354. Natelson EA, Lynch EC, Hetting RA, et al: Acquired factor IX deficiency in the nephrotic syndrome. Ann Intern Med 73:373-378, 1970.

355. Green D, Arruda H, Honig G, et al: Urinary loss of clotting factor due to hereditary membranous nephropathy. Am J Clin Pathol 65:376-383, 1976.

356. Honig GR, Lindley A: Deficiency of Hageman factor (factor XII) in patients with nephrotic syndrome. J Pediatr 78:633-637, 1971.

357. Saito H, Goodnough LT, Makker SP, et al: Urinary excretion of Hageman factor (factor XII) and the presence of nonfunctional Hageman factor in the nephrotic syndrome. Am J Med 70:531-534, 1981.

358. Vaziri ND, Ngo J-CT, Ibsen KH, et al: Deficiency and urinary loss of factor XII in adult nephrotic syndrome. Nephron 32:342-346, 1982.

359. Kendall AG, Lohmann RE, Dossetor JB: Nephrotic syndrome: A hypercoagulable state. Arch Intern Med 127:1021-1027, 1971.

360. Kanfer A, Kleinknecht D, Broyer M, et al: Coagulation studies in 45 cases of nephrotic syndrome without uremia. Thromb Diathes Haemorrh 24:562-571, 1970.

361. Thompson C, Forbes CD, Prentice CRM, et al: Changes in blood coagulation and fibrinolysis in the nephrotic syndrome. Q J Med 43:399-407, 1974.

362. Takeda Y, Chen A: Fibrinogen metabolism and distribution in patients with the nephrotic syndrome. J Lab Clin Med 70:678-685, 1967.

363. Zwaginga JJ, Koomans HA, Sixma JJ, et al: Thrombus formation and platelet-vessel wall interaction in the nephrotic syndrome under flow conditions. J Clin Invest 93:204-211, 1994.

364. Edward N, Young DP-G, MacLeod M: Fibrinolytic activity in plasma and urine in chronic renal disease. J Clin Pathol 17:365-368, 1964.

365. Wu KK, Koak JC: Urinary plasminogen and chronic glomerulonephritis. Am J Clin Pathol 60:915-919, 1973.

366. Lau SO, Tkachuk JY, Hasegawa DK, et al: Plasminogen and antithrombin III deficiencies in the childhood nephrotic syndrome associated with plasminogenuria and antithrombinuria. J Pediatr 96:390-392, 1980.

367. Du XH, Glas-Greenwalt P, Kant KS, et al: Nephrotic syndrome with renal vein thrombosis: Pathogenetic importance of a plasmin inhibitor (a2-antiplasmin). Clin Nephrol 24:186-191, 1985.

368. Kauffman RH, Veltkamp JJ, Van Tilburg NC, et al: Acquired antithrombin III deficiency and thrombosis in the nephrotic syndrome. Am J Med 65:607-613, 1978.

369. Robert A, Olmer M, Sampol J, et al: Clinical correlation between hypercoagulability and thrombo-embolic phenomena. Kidney Int 31:830-835, 1987.

370. Thaler E, Blazar E, Kopsa H, et al: Acquired anti-thrombin III deficiency in patients with glomerular proteinuria. Haemostasis 7:257-272, 1978.

371. Griffin JH, Evati B, Zimmerman TS, et al: Deficiency of protein C in congenital thrombotic disease. J Clin Invest 68:1370-1373, 1981.

372. Comp PC, Esmon DT: Recurrent venous thromboembolism in patients with a partial deficiency of protein S. N Engl J Med 311:1525-1528, 1984.

373. Mannucci PM, Valsecchi C, Bottaso B, et al: High plasma levels of protein C activity and antigen in the nephrotic syndrome. Thromb Haemost 55:31-33, 1986.

374. Vigano-D'Angelo S, D'Angelo A, Kaufman CE Jr, et al: Protein S deficiency occurs in the nephrotic syndrome. Ann Intern Med 107:42-47, 1987.

375. Malyszko J, Malyszko JS, Mysliwiec M: Markers of endothelial injury and thrombin activatable fibrinolysis inhibitor in nephrotic syndrome. Blood Coagul Fibrinolysis 13:615-621, 2002.

376. Ariens RA, Mioa M, Rivolta E, et al: High levels of tissue factor pathway inhibitor in patients with nephrotic proteinuria. Thromb Haemost 82:1020-1023, 1999.

377. Boneu B, Boissou F, Abbal M, et al: Comparison of progressive antithrombin activity and concentration of three thrombin inhibitors in nephrotic syndrome. Thromb Haemost 46:623-625, 1981.

378. Andrassy K, Depperman D, Walter E, et al: Is beta thromboglobulin a useful indicator of thrombosis nephrotic syndrome? Thromb Haemost 42:486, 1979.

379. McGinley E, Lowe GDO, Boulton-Jones M, et al: Blood viscosity and hemostasis in nephrotic syndrome. Thromb Haemost 49:155-157, 1983.

380. Ozanne P, Francis RB, Meiselman HJ: Red blood cell aggregation in nephrotic syndrome. Kidney Int 23:519-525, 1983.

381. Mukherjee AP, Toh BH, Chan GL, et al: Vascular complications in nephrotic syndrome: Relationship of steroid therapy and accelerated thromboplastin generation. BMJ 4:273-276, 1970.

382. Berger J, Yaneva H: Hageman factor deposition in membranous nephropathy. Transplant Proc 3:472-473, 1982.

383. McLean RH, Forsgren A, Bjorksten B, et al: Decreased serum factor B concentration associated with decreased opsonization of *Escherichia coli* in idiopathic nephrotic syndrome. Pediatr Res 11:910-916, 1977.

384. Heslan JM, Lautie JP, Intrator L, et al: Impaired IgG synthesis in patients with the nephrotic syndrome. Clin Nephrol 18:144-147, 1982.

385. Ogi M, Yokoyama H, Tomosugi N, et al: Risk factors for infection and immunoglobulin replacement therapy in adult nephrotic syndrome. Am J Kidney Dis 24:427-4436, 1994.

386. Stec J, Podracká L, Pavkovceková O, et al: Zinc and copper metabolism in nephrotic syndrome. Nephron 56:186-187, 1990.

387. Pedraza-Chaverrí J, Torres-Rodríguez GA, Cruz C, et al: Copper and zinc metabolism in aminonucleoside-induced nephrotic syndrome. Nephron 66:87-92, 1994.

388. Perrone L, Gialanella G, Giordano V, et al: Impaired zinc metabolic status in children affected by idiopathic nephrotic syndrome. Eur J Pediatr 149:438-440, 1990.

389. Ellis D: Anemia in the course of the nephrotic syndrome secondary to transferrin depletion. J Pediatr 90:953-955, 1977.

390. Afrasiabi MA, Vaziri ND, Gwinup G, et al: Thyroid function studies in the nephrotic syndrome. Ann Intern Med 90:335-338, 1979.

391. Fonseca V, Thomas M, Sweny P: Can urinary thyroid hormone loss cause hypothyroidism? Lancet 338:475-476, 1991.

392. Musa BU, Seal US, Doe RP: Excretion of corticosteroid-binding globulin, thyroxine-binding globulin and total protein in adult males with nephrosis: Effect of sex hormones. J Clin Endocrinol 27:768-774, 1967.

393. Haffner D, Tönshoff B, Blum WF, et al: Insulin-like growth factors (IGFs) and IGF binding proteins, serum acid-labile subunit and growth hormone binding protein in nephrotic children. Kidney Int 52:802-810, 1997.

394. Khamiseh G, Vaziri N, Oveisi F, et al: Vitamin D absorption, plasma concentration and urinary excretion of 25(OH) vitamin D in nephrotic syndrome. Proc Soc Exp Biol Med 196:210-213, 1991.

395. Mittal SK, Dash SC, Tiwari SC, et al: Bone histology in patients with nephrotic syndrome and normal renal function. Kidney Int 55:1912-1919, 1999.

396. Vaziri ND, Kaupke CJ, Barton CH, et al: Plasma concentration and urinary excretion of erythropoietin in adult nephrotic syndrome. Am J Med 92:35-40, 1992.

397. Feinstein S, Becker-Cohen R, Algur N, et al: Erythropoietin deficiency causes anemia in nephrotic children with normal kidney function. Am J Kidney Dis 37:736-742, 2001.

398. Prinsen BHCMT, de Sain-Van der Velden MGM, Kaysen GA, et al. Transferrin synthesis is increased in nephrotic patients insufficiently to replace urinary losses. J Am Soc Nephrol 12:1017-1025, 2001.

CHAPTER 43

Adaptation to Nephron Loss

Maarten W. Taal, Valerie A. Luyckx, and Barry M. Brenner

The kidney's primary function of maintaining constancy of the extracellular fluid (ECF) volume and composition is remarkably well preserved until late in the course of chronic renal disease (CRD). When nephrons are lost through disease or surgical ablation, the least affected or remaining nephrons undergo remarkable adaptive physiologic responses resulting in nephron hypertrophy and hyperfunction that combine to compensate for the acquired loss of renal function. Appropriate kidney function requires close integration of glomerular and tubular functions. Indeed, the preservation of glomerulotubular balance seen until the terminal stages of chronic renal failure (CRF) is fundamental to the *intact nephron hypothesis* of Bricker which essentially states that as CRF advances, kidney function is supported by a diminishing pool of functioning (or hyperfunctioning) nephrons, rather than relatively constant numbers of nephrons, each with diminishing function.[1] This concept has important implications for the mechanisms of disease progression in CRF.

Two decades ago, clinical studies of patients with CRD established that once the glomerular filtration rate (GFR) fell below a critical level, a relentless progression to end-stage renal failure inevitably ensued, even when the initial disease activity had abated. The rate of decline of GFR in a given individual followed a near constant linear relationship with time, enabling remarkably accurate predictions of the date at which end-stage renal failure would be reached and renal replacement therapy required.[2] Among patients with diverse renal diseases, the gradient of the GFR/time relationship was found to be a characteristic of individual patients rather than typical of their specific renal diseases.[2, 3] This observation suggested that CRD advanced by means of a programmed course, irrespective of the primary nephropathy, and that the progressive nature of renal disease could perhaps be attributed to a final "common pathway" of mechanisms.

Within this framework, Brenner and colleagues formulated a unifying hypothesis for renal disease progression based on developments in experimental renal physiology of the same era.[4] The central tenets of the common pathway theory state that CRD progression occurs, in general, through focal nephron loss and that the adaptive responses of surviving nephrons, although initially serving to increase single-nephron GFR (SNGFR) and offset the overall loss in clearance, ultimately prove detrimental to the kidney. Over time, glomerulosclerosis and tubular atrophy further reduce nephron number, fueling a self-perpetuating cycle of nephron destruction and culminating in uremia.

The notion that the loss of functioning renal mass might prove detrimental to the rest of the kidney has been considered for several decades. In the mid-20th century, Thomas Addis[5] noted that kidneys facing increased excretory loads underwent hypertrophy and were prone to develop proteinuria and "cylinduria," which are recognized signs of glomerular injury. Addis envisaged that the kidney did "work" in excreting solute loads and reasoned that renal hypertrophy, whether occurring focally, in humans as the sequel to an episode of acute glomerulonephritis, or globally, as the sequel to experimental reduction of total renal mass in rats, was analogous to increased cardiac work in systemic hypertension, leading to hypertrophy of myocytes. Thus, he suggested that adaptive renal hypertrophy was an undesirable manifestation of overwork. Although the notion that the kidney does "work" in direct proportion to its excretory solute load runs contrary to current understanding of renal physiology, Addis clearly appreciated that nephron responses to increased functional demands could be maladaptive. It was not until the advances in experimental renal physiology in rodents made three decades later, however, that Addis's concept of the importance of workload per nephron could be fully realized.[4]

In this chapter we describe in detail the functional and structural adaptations observed in remaining nephrons after substantial reductions in functioning renal mass and the mechanisms thought to be responsible for them. We then consider how these changes may, in time, prove maladaptive and contribute to the progressive renal injury just described. Given the growing worldwide burden of CRD that causes substantial morbidity and mortality in individuals and threatens to overwhelm health care systems, it could be argued that the further elucidation of the mechanisms of CRD progression resulting in more effective interventions to slow its advance should remain among the highest priorities of nephrologists today.

STRUCTURAL AND FUNCTIONAL ADAPTATION OF THE KIDNEY TO NEPHRON LOSS

Alterations in Glomerular Physiology

Glomerular hemodynamic responses to nephron loss have largely been studied in animals subjected to surgical ablation of renal mass. As early as 1947 it was recognized that unilateral nephrectomy in rats resulted in a rapid increase in function of the remaining kidney, such that the GFR eventually achieved 70% to 85% of the previous two-kidney value.[6] Increased GFR is detectable 3 days after nephrectomy and is maximal 2 to 3 weeks later.[7] Because no new nephrons are formed in mature rodents,[8-13] the rise in GFR in this setting represents the summation of increases in filtration rate in the remaining nephrons.

The detailed study of glomerular hemodynamics was made possible by the identification of a rat strain, Munich-Wistar, that is unique in bearing glomeruli on the kidney surface. This allowed micropuncture of the glomerulus and direct measurement of intraglomerular pressures as well as sampling of blood from afferent and efferent arterioles. These techniques made possible the study of mechanisms underlying compensatory increases in GFR after renal mass ablation. Increases in whole kidney GFR at 2 to 4 weeks after unilateral nephrectomy were reflected in an increase in SNGFR averaging 83%, an effect achieved in large part by an increase in glomerular plasma flow rate (Q_A), which, in turn, resulted from dilation of both afferent and efferent arterioles. Although systemic blood pressure was not elevated, glomerular capillary hydraulic pressure (P_{GC}) and the glomerular transcapillary pressure difference (ΔP) were increased significantly after uninephrectomy, accounting for an estimated 25% of the rise in SNGFR.[14] The glomerular ultrafiltration coefficient, K_f (the product of glomerular hydraulic permeability and surface area available for filtration), was unaltered at this stage but may become elevated later.[15]

With more extensive nephron loss, even greater compensatory increases in SNGFR were observed.[16] In Munich-Wistar rats studied 7 days after unilateral nephrectomy and infarction of five sixths of the contralateral kidney, SNGFR in the remnant was more than double that of two-kidney controls. This increment was again attributable to large increases in Q_A and to a substantial rise in P_{GC}. Efferent and afferent arteriolar resistances were reduced to half or less of control values.[17] Changes in K_f after extensive renal mass ablation appear to be time dependent, with a decrease reported

at 2 weeks after surgery[18] and an increase at 4 weeks.[19] Further studies indicated that glomerular hemodynamic responses to nephron loss seem to be similar between the superficial cortical and juxtamedullary nephrons.[20] The rise in SNGFR associated with renal mass ablation is often referred to as *glomerular hyperfiltration,* and the elevated P_{GC} is termed *glomerular hypertension.* Together these terms encompass the central concepts underlying the hemodynamic adaptations in the remnant kidney.

Glomerular hemodynamic adaptations to nephron loss may show interspecies variation. In dogs, increases in SNGFR observed 4 weeks after three-fourths or seven-eighths nephrectomy were attributable largely to increases in Q_A and K_f. In contrast to the findings in rodents, ΔP was only modestly elevated. After ablation of seven eighths of their renal mass, dogs developed a significant rise in P_{GC} independent of arterial pressure, as a result of relatively greater relaxation of afferent versus efferent arterioles.[21]

In humans, the effects of nephron loss on the physiology of the remnant kidney have been studied mainly in healthy individuals undergoing donor nephrectomy for kidney transplantation. Inulin clearance studies of the earliest kidney donors revealed that the GFR in the donor's remaining kidney had increased to 65% to 70% of the previous two-kidney value by 1 week post nephrectomy.[22, 23] A meta-analysis of data from 48 studies that included 2988 living kidney donors estimated that GFR decreased, on average, by only 17 mL/minute after uninephrectomy.[24] These observations imply that single kidney GFR (and therefore also the average SNGFR) increases by 30% to 40% after uninephrectomy in humans. There is currently no method for estimating SNGFR or P_{GC} in vivo, and more detailed assessments of glomerular hemodynamics in humans have thus not yet been possible.

Mediators of the Glomerular Hemodynamic Responses to Nephron Loss

The factors that are sensed after renal mass ablation and serve as signals to initiate the adjustments in glomerular hemodynamics responsible for the increase in remnant kidney GFR remain ill defined. However, the effector mechanisms have been studied extensively and the hemodynamic changes can be attributed to the net effects of complex interactions of several factors, each having specific, and sometimes opposing, actions on the various determinants of glomerular ultrafiltration. Several vasoactive substances, including angiotensin II (AII), natriuretic peptides (NPs), endothelins (ETs), and prostaglandins (PGs), have been implicated in this process. Moreover, sustained increases in SNGFR also require resetting of the autoregulatory mechanisms that normally govern GFR and renal plasma flow (RPF).

Renin-Angiotensin System

Angiotensin II appears to play a critical role in the development of glomerular capillary hypertension after renal ablation and may also contribute to changes in K_f. Acute infusion of AII in normal rats results in a rise in P_{GC}, owing to a greater increase in efferent than afferent resistance and to reductions in Q_A and K_f.[25-27] Chronic administration of

AII for 8 weeks resulted in systemic hypertension, lowered single kidney GFR and, with the exception of K_f, elicited similar glomerular hemodynamic changes to those observed after acute infusion in both normal and uninephrectomized rats.[15] The importance of the influence of endogenous AII on glomerular hemodynamics in remnant kidneys was revealed by studies with pharmacologic inhibitors of the renin-angiotensin system (RAS). Chronic treatment of five-sixths nephrectomized rats with either angiotensin-converting enzyme inhibitors (ACEIs)[28, 29] or AII (subtype 1) receptor antagonists (AT$_1$RA)[30, 31] results in normalization of P_{GC} through reduction in systemic blood pressure and dilatation of both afferent and efferent arterioles. SNGFR, however, remains elevated owing to an increase in K_f. Furthermore, acute infusion of an ACEI or saralasin, a peptide analog receptor antagonist of AII, was found to normalize P_{GC} in five-sixths nephrectomized rats through efferent arteriolar dilatation, without affecting mean arterial pressure (MAP).[18, 32] It is unclear why these findings could not be confirmed with the AT$_1$RA losartan.[33]

These effects of RAS inhibition imply that there is increased local activity of endogenous AII, yet plasma renin levels are reduced after five-sixths nephrectomy.[28] This suggests differential regulation of the systemic versus intrarenal RAS and that AII is formed locally. Renin mRNA and protein levels are both increased in glomeruli adjacent to the infarction scar in five-sixths nephrectomized rats.[34-36] These findings have led to speculation that ablating renal mass by infarction activates the RAS by creating a margin of ischemic tissue around the organizing infarct, explaining the greater severity of hypertension and glomerulosclerosis obtained than that observed when renal mass is excised surgically.[37] Detailed studies of intrarenal AII levels after five-sixths nephrectomy achieved by infarction have confirmed these findings by showing higher AII levels in the peri-infarct portion of the kidney than the intact portion at all time points.[38] On the other hand, the studies also showed that the rise in intrarenal AII after five-sixths nephrectomy was transient. Although AII levels in the peri-infarct portion were elevated compared with sham-operated controls at 2 weeks after surgery, they were not statistically different at 5 or 7 weeks. In the intact portion of the remnant kidney, AII levels were similar to controls at 2 and 5 weeks and were lower at 7 weeks.[38] Sustained increases in intrarenal AII levels are therefore not required to maintain the hypertension and progressive renal injury characteristic of this model. Nevertheless, subsequent studies have shown that the renoprotective effects of ACEI and AT$_1$RA treatment are associated with a reduction in intrarenal AII levels in both the peri-infarct and intact portions of the remnant kidney.[39] In contrast, treatment with the dihydropyridine calcium antagonist nifedipine did not reduce proteinuria despite lowering blood pressure to the same levels as the RAS antagonists and was associated with an increase in intrarenal AII.[39] Thus, intrarenal AII appears to play a central role in the pathogenesis of hypertension and renal injury in this model even in the absence of sustained increases in AII levels. Further research is required to fully explain these findings. It could be argued that apparently normal intrarenal AII levels are inappropriately high in the context of the hypertension and ECF volume expansion in these animals or that the average intrarenal AII levels measured may have failed to detect important local elevations of AII.

Endothelins

Renal production of ETs is increased after five-sixths nephrectomy, raising the possibility that these potent vasoconstrictor peptides may also contribute to the characteristic adjustments in glomerular hemodynamics described earlier.[40, 41] Acute infusion of ET consistently elicits dose-dependent reductions in RPF and GFR in normal rats and dogs.[42-45] Chronic infusion of ET-3 in normal rats resulted in sustained reductions in RPF and GFR, likely caused by constriction of both afferent and efferent arterioles, with resultant reductions in Q_A and SNGFR.[46] Inconsistencies in the observed effects of ETs on P_{GC} may reflect differences in experimental conditions influencing the relative effects on afferent and efferent arterioles.[47-50] Most studies, however, have reported a reduction in K_f after ET infusion.[47-50]

Natriuretic Peptides

Atrial natriuretic peptide (ANP) and other structurally related natriuretic peptides (NPs) mediate, in large part, the functional adaptations in tubular sodium reabsorption that maintain sodium excretion in five-sixths nephrectomized rats.[51, 52] NPs also contribute to the observed increases in GFR and RPF. Circulating ANP levels are elevated in five-sixth nephrectomized rats,[52, 53] and acute administration of an NP antagonist elicited profound decreases in GFR and RPF in rats on a high salt diet but not in those subjected to sodium restriction.[54] It may be inferred from studies in which pharmacologic doses of exogenous ANP were administered to normal rats that the increased baseline GFR was caused by elevated P_{GC}, which, in turn, resulted from significant afferent arteriolar dilatation.[55] In the previously described experiments some residual elevation in remnant kidney GFR appeared to persist even after the NP system was suppressed by sodium restriction or an NP receptor antagonist. This suggests that factors other than NPs make contributions to the preglomerular vasodilatation associated with glomerular hyperfiltration after renal mass ablation.

Eicosanoids

Renal PGs, another family of potent vasoactive molecules present in abundance in the kidney, may also play a role in mediating glomerular hyperfiltration. Urinary excretion per nephron of both vasodilator and vasoconstrictor PGs is increased in rats and rabbits after renal mass ablation.[56-59] Infusion of PGE$_2$, PGI$_2$, or 6-keto PGE$_1$ into the renal artery elicits significant renal vasodilatation.[60] Whereas acute inhibition of PG synthesis by infusion of indomethacin has no effect on GFR or glomerular hemodynamics in normal rats, after three-fourths or five-sixths nephrectomy, indomethacin lowers both SNGFR and Q_A.[57, 58] The relative effects of PG synthesis inhibitors on afferent and efferent arterioles may vary with time after nephrectomy. Afferent arteriolar constriction was the predominant finding reported at 24 hours after surgery, whereas constriction of both afferent and efferent arterioles was observed at 3 to 4 weeks.[57, 58] Although some contribution of thromboxanes to glomerular hemodynamic adjustments in five-sixths nephrectomized rats is suggested by the increase in GFR noted after acute infusion of a selective thromboxane synthesis inhibitor,[59] the general impression, although not entirely uniform,[61] is one of the combined effects of vasodilator prostaglandins outweighing those of the vasoconstrictors.

Nitric Oxide

Intravenous infusion of nitric oxide synthase (NOS) inhibitors results in systemic and renal vasoconstriction in rats,[62, 63] dogs,[64, 65] and rabbits[66] and a reduction in GFR in rats and dogs. Chronic NOS inhibition in five-sixths nephrectomized rats produced elevations in systemic blood pressure and P_{GC} without affecting GFR.[67] Thus, nitric oxide (NO) appears to exert a tonic effect on the physiologic maintenance of systemic blood pressure and renal perfusion under resting conditions. It is unclear, however, whether NO plays a specific role in the adaptive hemodynamic changes that follow renal mass ablation. MAP, renal vascular resistance, renal blood flow (RBF), and GFR all changed to a similar extent after acute infusion of an NOS inhibitor, irrespective of whether given to normal, uninephrectomized, or five-sixths nephrectomized rats. It therefore appears that NO retains a tonic influence on systemic and renal hemodynamics in the context of renal mass ablation but is not a specific determinant of the adaptive changes in glomerular hemodynamics.[63] This notion is further supported by a recent study in which treatment with an inhibitor of inducible NO synthase had no effect on GFR, RPF, or P_{GC} in five-sixths nephrectomized rats.[67a]

Adjustments in Renal Autoregulatory Mechanisms

After extensive renal mass ablation, there is a marked readjustment of the autoregulatory mechanisms that control RPF and GFR.[68, 69] No studies have addressed directly the contribution of myogenic mechanisms to the changes in renal autoregulation after renal mass ablation but the tubuloglomerular feedback system is reset to permit and sustain the elevations in SNGFR and P_{GC} described earlier.[70, 71] Resetting appears to occur as early as 20 minutes after unilateral nephrectomy,[72] in proportion to the extent of renal ablation; the adjustments observed after uninephrectomy are of lesser magnitudes than those seen after five-sixths nephrectomy.[70]

As is readily appreciated from the previous discussion, the adjustments in glomerular hemodynamics seen after renal mass ablation represent the net effect of several endogenous vasoactive factors. AII, vasoconstrictor PGs, and possibly ETs constrict both afferent and efferent arterioles, whereas NPs and vasodilator PGs dilate the preglomerular vessels.

A net fall in preglomerular vascular resistance may therefore be expected, yet efferent arteriolar resistance may increase. The role of bradykinin, a potent vasodilator that is elevated in the remnant kidney,[38] remains to be defined. Together with transmission of a greater proportion of the raised systemic blood pressure to the glomerular capillary network, these alterations in microvascular resistances result in elevations in Q_A, P_{GC}, ΔP, and SNGFR (Table 43-1).

Renal Hypertrophic Responses to Nephron Loss

The notion that a single kidney enlarges to compensate for the loss of its partner has been entertained since antiquity. Aristotle (384-322 BC) noted the sufficiency of a single kidney to sustain life in animals and that such kidneys were enlarged.[73, 74] In preparation for the first human nephrectomy in 1869 a German surgeon, Gustav Simon, uninephrectomized dogs and noted a 1.5-fold increase in the size of the remaining kidney at 20 days.[73, 74] Compensatory renal hypertrophy has been studied in a variety of species, including rats, mice, guinea pigs, rabbits, cats, dogs, pigs, baboons, and toads.[75] In recent years, the majority of experimental work has been conducted in rodents subjected to uninephrectomy, although hypertrophic responses have also been studied in response to unilateral ureteric obstruction[76-80] or after nephrotoxin administration,[81] presumably reflecting hypertrophy of the least injured nephrons.

Whole-Kidney Hypertrophic Responses

Among the earliest responses to unilateral nephrectomy are biochemical changes that precede cell growth. Increased incorporation of choline, a precursor of cell membrane phospholipid, has been detected as early as 5 minutes[82, 83] and increased choline kinase activity at 2 hours after nephrectomy.[84] Activity of ornithine decarboxylase, the enzyme catalyzing the first step of polyamine synthesis, is elevated at 45 to 120 minutes and polyamine levels peak at 1 to 2 days after nephrectomy.[85-87] Early alterations in mRNA metabolism have also been observed. Although there is no change in the half-life or cytoplasmic distribution of mRNA, a near 25% increase in the fraction of newly synthesized poly(A)-deficient mRNA occurs within 1 hour of uninephrectomy, and total RNA synthesis in the kidney increases by 25% to 100% relative to that in the liver.[88-90] Ribosomal RNA synthesis is increased by 40% to 50% at 6 hours.[91] The rate of protein synthesis is increased at 2 hours and is nearly doubled

TABLE 43-1

Hemodynamic Effects of Vasoactive Molecules Mediating Glomerular Hemodynamic Adaptations after Partial Renal Mass Ablation

	R_A	R_E	P_{GC}	Q_A	K_f	SNGFR	RPF	GFR
Angiotensin II[15, 28-31]	↑	↑↑	↑	↓	↓↔	↓↔	↓	↔
Endothelins[42-50]	↑↔	↑	↑↔	↓	↓↔	↓↔	↓	↓↔
Natriuretic peptides[54, 55]	↓	↑ (?)	↑	↔	↔	↑	↑↔	↑
Prostaglandins[57, 58, 60]	↓	↓	↔	↑	↑	↑	↑	↑
Observed changes after partial renal ablation[16-20]	↓↓	↓	↑	↑	↑↓	↑	−	↓

GFR, Glomerular filtration rate; K_f, glomerular ultrafiltration coefficient; P_{GC}, glomerular capillary hydraulic pressure; Q_A, glomerular plasma flow rate; R_A, afferent arteriolar resistance; R_E, efferent arteriolar resistance; RPF, renal plasma flow; SNGFR, single nephron glomerular filtration rate.

at 3 hours.[92] Data on cyclic nucleotide levels, which are thought to affect cell growth and proliferation, are conflicting. Some studies report elevated levels of cyclic guanosine monophosphate (cGMP) in the remaining kidney as early as 10 minutes after surgery,[93-95] whereas others have found no consistent changes in cyclic adenosine monophosphate (cAMP) or cGMP levels.[96]

Early biochemical changes are followed by a period of rapid growth. DNA synthesis is increased at 24 hours, and increased numbers of mitotic figures are evident at 28 to 36 hours. Both reach a maximum increase of 5- to 10-fold at 40 to 72 hours.[75, 97-100] Kidney weight is increased at 48 to 72 hours and, on average, achieves a 35% gain at 2 to 3 weeks (Fig. 43-1).[75, 101] Because nephron number is fixed shortly after birth in most species, this gain in kidney weight is attributable to increased nephron size. Growth is thought to occur largely through cell hypertrophy, accounting for 80% of the increase in renal mass seen in adult animals and, to a lesser extent, through hyperplasia.[92] Renal mass continues to rise for 1 to 2 months until a 40% to 50% increase is achieved.[75] The degree of compensatory growth is a function of the extent of renal ablation. Uninephrectomy has been shown to provoke an 81% increase of residual renal mass at 4 weeks compared with an increase of 168% after 70% renal ablation. Normal controls gained 31% in kidney weight over the same period.[102] Age diminishes renal hypertrophic responses: after uninephrectomy, greater increases in kidney weight and more extensive hyperplasia was observed in 5-day- versus 55-day-old rats[75, 103] and aging rats exhibited gains in kidney weight of only one third to three fourths of those seen in younger controls.[75, 104-106]

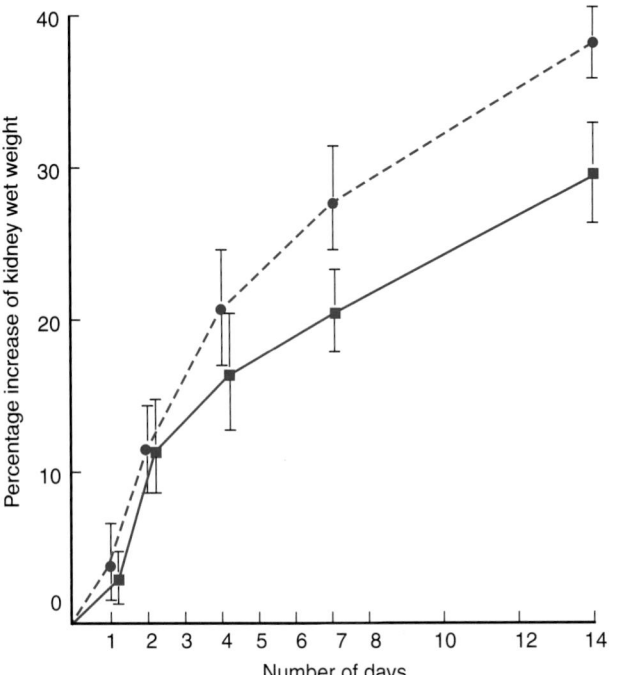

FIGURE 43-1. Rate of compensatory renal growth after unilateral nephrectomy *(circles)* and ureter ligation *(squares)*. (Reproduced with permission from Dicker SE, Shirley DG: Compensatory hypertrophy of the contralateral kidney after unilateral ureteral ligation. J Physiol [Lond] 220:199-210, 1972.)

In humans, radiologic studies estimating gain in renal size after uninephrectomy based on CT or intravenous urograms reported average increases of 3.3% to 9% in renal length,[107-110] 18% to 23% in renal size "index" (product of length and width),[107, 111] or 20% in renal cross-sectional area, as assessed by planimetry.[112] One study, however, was unable to detect any increase in average renal length.[113] Ultrasound estimates report increases of 19% to 100% in kidney volume[114-116] and CT studies show an increase of 30% to 53% in renal cross-sectional area.[117, 118] Interpretation of these data is complicated by the small numbers of subjects, wide variation in the time intervals between nephrectomy and assessment of renal size, and differing indications for nephrectomy.

Glomerular Enlargement

The principal morphometric change observed in glomeruli after uninephrectomy is an increase in volume.[119-123] Glomerular enlargement appears to parallel whole-kidney growth and has been detected as early as 4 days after surgery.[122] The degree of enlargement of superficial and juxtamedullary glomeruli is similar. Proportionally similar increases in number and size of all cell types occur, with preservation of the relative volumes of different glomerular components.[120, 121] There is consensus that glomerular capillaries increase in length and number (i.e., more branching), but most studies show that diameter or cross-sectional surface area of the glomerular capillaries remains constant or increases only minimally.[120, 121, 124, 125] Transplantation of hypertrophied kidneys into uninephrectomized recipients has demonstrated regression of glomerular hypertrophy within 3 weeks, yet the increase in capillary length was maintained.[125]

Glomerular hypertrophy, as evidenced by elevated RNA/DNA and protein/DNA ratios and by increased glomerular volume (V_G) on electron microscopy, has been detected at 2 days after five-sixths nephrectomy.[126] The initial increase in V_G was caused, almost entirely, by increases in visceral epithelial cell volume, whereas, at 14 days, the increase in V_G was largely accounted for by mesangial matrix expansion. Although several studies report glomerular capillary lengthening after five-sixths nephrectomy, few have detected any increase in cross-sectional area or diameter of the glomerular capillaries.[127-130] These observations should, however, be considered in the light of important technical considerations. In vitro perfusion of isolated glomeruli demonstrates that V_G increases as perfusion pressure is raised through physiologic and pathophysiologic ranges. Moreover, glomerular capillary "compliance" in these studies was a function of the baseline V_G and glomeruli obtained from remnant kidneys post five-sixths nephrectomy had a higher compliance than those from control animals.[131] These findings have two important implications. First, although glomerular pressures are only minimally elevated after uninephrectomy, the glomerular capillary hypertension associated with more extensive renal ablation is likely to contribute significantly to the increase in V_G. Second, estimates of V_G in tissues that have not been perfusion fixed at the appropriate blood pressure should be interpreted with caution. Direct comparison of V_G in perfusion-fixed versus immersion-fixed kidney from the same rats yielded estimates of V_G in immersion-fixed samples that were 61% lower than those from perfusion-fixed kidneys.[132]

Mechanisms of Renal Hypertrophy

Despite more than a century of research that has identified a large number of mediators or modulators of renal hypertrophy, the identities of the specific factors that regulate hypertrophy and the stimuli to which these factors respond remain elusive. Renal innervation does not appear to play a role because kidneys transplanted into bilaterally nephrectomized rats exhibit the same degree of hypertrophy after 3 weeks as kidneys remaining after uninephrectomy.[133] The absence of any reduction in renal hypertrophy when rats are treated with an ACEI after uninephrectomy indicates that the RAS also does not play a major role.[134] Several hypotheses have been advanced to account for the observed changes that are associated with renal hypertrophy and are summarized here. Currently, however, none is able to explain satisfactorily all of the reported observations.

Solute Load

The notion that hypertrophy after uninephrectomy is stimulated by the need for the remaining kidney to excrete larger amounts of metabolic waste products, necessitating more excretory "work," was proposed by Sacerdotti in 1896. Subsequently, it became apparent that urea excretion is largely a function of glomerular filtration, whereas the main energy-requiring function of the renal tubules is reabsorption of filtered electrolytes (principally sodium) and water. The hypothesis was therefore modified to view hypertrophy as a response to the increased demand for water and solute reclamation imposed by increased SNGFR (solute load hypothesis).[74, 135] Several lines of evidence support the concepts underlying the "solute load hypothesis." In the remnant kidney, proximal tubule sodium absorption increases in parallel with GFR (glomerulotubular balance)[136] and tubules continue to display enhanced fluid reabsorption in vitro,[137, 138] implying that the adaptive changes are intrinsic to the tubular epithelial cells. In chronic glomerulonephritis, a lesion characterized by marked heterogeneity in SNGFR, there is preservation of the SNGFR-to-proximal fluid reabsorption ratio[139, 140] and a close correlation between glomerular and proximal tubule hypertrophy.[141] Moreover, sustained increases in GFR in the absence of renal mass ablation result in renal hypertrophy in some conditions, including pregnancy (in some but not all studies),[142-145] and diabetes mellitus.[146-148]

On the other hand, experimental maneuvers dissociating renal solute load from hypertrophy appear to contradict the solute load hypothesis. Total diversion of urine from one kidney into the peritoneum by ureteroperitoneostomy is associated with an increase in GFR in the contralateral kidney of similar magnitude to that seen after uninephrectomy but no increase in renal mass or mitotic activity.[149-151] In another example, potassium depletion results in renal hypertrophy without any increase in GFR.[152-154] Moreover, the findings that some of the early biochemical changes associated with hypertrophy precede increases in glomerular filtration or sodium reabsorption argue against a causal association of hypertrophy and increased solute load.[135] It is, however, possible to offer alternative explanations for each of the these observations. The lack of hypertrophy with urinary diversion may be caused by accumulation of a growth inhibitor[74] or reflect the peritonitis and loss of body weight that inevitably accompany the procedure and that have been shown to inhibit hypertrophy after uninephrectomy.[155] Rats receiving intravenous infusion of half of the daily urine output develop increases in GFR and renal weight of similar magnitude to those observed after uninephrectomy, supporting the concept of an association between excretory solute load and hypertrophy.[156] The renal hypertrophic response to potassium depletion is characterized by unique morphologic changes in the medulla and papilla and may be under the control of mediators that are separate to those involved in the response to uninephrectomy.[74, 153] Data on the temporal associations of the initial responses to uninephrectomy are conflicting. Some studies suggest that hypertrophy precedes any increase in GFR[7, 135] whereas others have observed increases in RBF or GFR at time points similar to those for the early biochemical changes.[157, 158] Moreover, the very early biochemical changes described earlier are not necessarily specific for hypertrophy.[74] Despite these conflicting data, there is nevertheless considerable evidence of an association between GFR and proximal tubule hypertrophy that may play a role in stimulating renal growth in the remnant kidney.

Renotropic Factors

Failure of the "solute load hypothesis" to explain all of the experimental data has led others to propose instead that the primary stimulus for renal hypertrophy is a change in renal mass and that renal growth is under the control of specific growth or inhibitory factors. Evidence in support of this theory is derived from three types of experiments.[159] In the first, a stable connection is established between the extracellular space and microcirculation of two animals (parabiosis) and the effects of renal mass ablation in one animal are assessed in the intact kidneys of its partner. In an early experiment in mice, in which parabiosis was established by the creation of a common peritoneal cavity, uninephrectomy in one animal resulted in hypertrophy of the contralateral kidney and, to a lesser extent, of both kidneys of the parabiotic partner. Bilateral nephrectomy in one partner or triple nephrectomy produced incremental degrees of hypertrophy in the remaining kidney(s).[160] Similar experiments in parabiotic rats, however, detected no evidence of hypertrophy (as assessed by tritiated [3H] thymidine uptake) in the intact partners[161] or detected an effect after uninephrectomy but not bilateral nephrectomy.[162] Appreciation that the degree of shared circulation via interconnected capillaries in these experiments was indeterminate[161, 163] prompted others to conduct cross-circulation experiments in pairs of animals with direct, reciprocal arterial to venous connections. Although one early experiment failed to demonstrate any evidence of renal hypertrophy in the intact partner of a uninephrectomized rat,[163] subsequent studies in cross-circulating pairs found significant renal hypertrophy in the partners of bilaterally nephrectomized rats.[164-168] Furthermore, the hypertrophy was rapidly reversed after cessation of cross circulation.[165] In a related experiment, in vitro perfusion of normal kidneys with blood from uninephrectomized dogs resulted in a 75% increase in 3H-adenine uptake as compared with kidneys perfused with blood from normal dogs.[169] On the other hand, bilateral ureteric obstruction did not result in the early increase in the renal RNA/DNA ratio of the parabiotic partner seen after bilateral nephrectomy.[167]

A second strategy has been to inject serum or plasma from uninephrectomized animals into intact subjects and then assess renal hypertrophy by radiolabeled thymidine uptake or mitotic count. Although studies using single small intraperitoneal or subcutaneous doses were negative,[170-172] the administration of repeated, large doses by intraperitoneal or intravenous routes elicited renal hypertrophy in most[173-175] cases.[176]

The data that most consistently support the existence of a renotropic factor are derived from in vitro experiments in which renal tissues are incubated in the presence or absence of plasma or serum from rats subjected to renal mass ablation. Evidence for hypertrophy has generally been assessed by incorporation of radiolabeled thymidine or uridine into DNA or RNA, respectively. Experiments using dry weight and protein content of renal tissue slices as markers of hypertrophy yielded similar findings.[177] In the first experiment of this kind, Ogawa and associates[178] demonstrated increased numbers of mitoses in rat renal outer medulla cells incubated in the presence of serum taken from rats 2 days after uninephrectomy. This effect was organ specific but not species specific. Subsequent studies have not been able to confirm an effect on renal medullary cells, but studies on rat renal cortical slices or fragments have consistently demonstrated increased uptake of radiolabeled nucleotides after incubation with serum from uninephrectomized animals.[179-183] Activity is maximal in serum obtained 10 to 30 hours[180, 181] after nephrectomy and is tissue specific.[179, 181] That a tissue factor produced by kidneys and up-regulated after nephrectomy may be required for the activity of a circulating "renotropin" is suggested by experiments in which kidney extract from rats taken 20 hours after uninephrectomy, in the presence of normal rat serum, was found to stimulate ^{3}H-thymidine incorporation in normal renal cortex. In contrast, addition of the same extract in the absence of the serum tended to depress ^{3}H-thymidine uptake. Furthermore, culture with uninephrectomy kidney extract and uninephrectomy serum resulted in greater uptake of ^{3}H-thymidine than addition of either uninephrectomy kidney extract together with normal serum, or normal kidney extract together with uninephrectomy serum.[181] Synergy may account for the tissue specificity of renotropin, because incubation of liver slices with both uninephrectomy kidney extract and uninephrectomy serum produces an increase in thymidine uptake that is not observed with uninephrectomy serum alone.[184] Serum taken from bilaterally nephrectomized animals lacks renotropic effects, but these can be restored after dialysis of the serum, suggesting the presence of renotropin inhibitory factors that accumulate in the absence of renal function.[179, 181] Similarly, ^{32}P incorporation into phospholipids was stimulated by serum obtained from uninephrectomized rats within 1 hour after surgery.[185] Studies in other species, including hamsters,[186] rabbits,[187, 188] and humans,[188] have reported similar findings. Only one study failed to demonstrate renotropic activity in uninephrectomy serum,[189] possibly because of important methodologic differences.[159] Although the specific identity of renotropin remains elusive, several lines of evidence suggest that it is a small protein. Retention of activity after ultrafiltration, dialysis, and removal of albumin from serum implies that renotropin is a molecule of 12 to 25 kD with no significant binding to albumin.[181, 190]

Harris and colleagues conducted a series of similar experiments to seek renotropic factor activity in urine. Transfer of the factor was demonstrated by increased renal growth after intravenous infusion of half of the daily volume of urine from one rat into another. Fractionation of urine by ultrafiltration showed the renotropic activity to be associated with fractions of molecular weight of 10 kD or greater, thus excluding small solutes such as urea, ammonia, acids, or amino acids as the renotropic factor. Activity was only modestly and transiently decreased after uninephrectomy, implying an extrarenal site of production. Only a small decrease in activity was observed after heating to 100° C.[191]

Several hypotheses have been advanced to reconcile the just-described observed effects and operation of a putative renotropic system. It has variously been proposed that (1) renotropin is a circulating substance normally catabolized or excreted by the kidneys[192]; (2) renal growth is regulated by a specific renotropin-producing tissue that is inhibited by a factor produced by normal kidneys[75]; and (3) renal growth is tonically inhibited by a substance produced by normal kidneys, a decrease in the levels of which induces an enzyme in the renal cortex that cleaves a circulating precursor of renotropin to produce the active molecule.[166, 193-198]

Endocrine Effects

Several of the major endocrine systems influence renal growth but each lacks selective effects on the kidney. There is little evidence that any of these systems represent the specific mediators of compensatory renal hypertrophy. Although early experiments suggested that hypophysectomy inhibits compensatory hypertrophy after uninephrectomy,[199-204] later studies that controlled for the reduction in renal mass that usually accompanies hypopituitarism demonstrated a degree of hypertrophy comparable to that seen in normal rats.[205-207] Nevertheless, specific renotropic activity has been identified in a subfraction of ovine pituitary extract that is not due to growth hormone (GH) or adrenocorticotropic hormone and that is not dependent on testicular steroidogenesis.[208] Further purification revealed that this activity is associated with a lutropin-like substance.[209] Uninephrectomy is accompanied by a transient increase in the pulsatile release of GH, suggesting a role for this hormone in the early phase of hypertrophy. When the increase in GH was prevented by administration of an antagonist to GH-releasing factor, renal hypertrophy at 48 hours after surgery was significantly less than in controls.[210]

Adrenal hormones appear to play little role in renal hypertrophy. Adrenalectomy does not inhibit compensatory growth after uninephrectomy,[200] although one study observed a decrease in mitotic activity.[202] Whereas renal weight relative to body weight is reduced in hypothyroidism[211] and increased by excess thyroid hormone,[212] compensatory hypertrophy still occurs in thyroidectomized rats.[213] Progesterone and estradiol in excess[75, 214] or ovariectomy[212] have little effect on renal weight, but testosterone appears to play a role, as evidenced by a decrease in kidney and body weight after orchidectomy[212, 215] and an increase in kidney weight with excess testosterone.[214] Although orchidectomy does not inhibit hypertrophy after uninephrectomy, exogenous testosterone did increase the amount of hypertrophy observed in some studies.[215-218]

Growth Factors

Of the numerous growth factors and their receptors that have been localized in the kidney, at least three are associated with renal hypertrophy.[219, 220] Renal insulin-like growth factor-1 (IGF-1) levels are elevated at 1 to 5 days after uninephrectomy and start to decline within days.[221-225] Although serum levels of IGF-1 were not different from controls in one study[222] and showed a small decrease compared with baseline in another,[223] Shohat and co-workers found an increase at 10 days that was still present on day 60.[225] Epidermal growth factor (EGF) in the remaining kidney is increased on day 1 in mice[226] and by day 5 in rats.[227] In addition, EGF has been shown to induce IGF-1 mRNA production in collecting duct cells in vitro, suggesting the existence of a local paracrine system.[228] That IGF-1 may be induced independent of GH in the setting of renal hypertrophy is illustrated by preservation of the increase in renal IGF-1 in hypophysectomized[221] and GH-deficient rats.[229] Increased mRNA levels for both hepatocyte growth factor (HGF) and its receptor, c-met, have been demonstrated in the remaining kidney as early as 6 hours after uninephrectomy.[230, 231] In another study the rise in HGF message was found to be nonspecific, occurring in both liver and kidney and also in sham-operated rats, whereas the increase in mRNA for c-met was specific for the outer renal medulla.[232] Despite these associations, the timing of the changes in growth factor levels remains unclear. Whereas some investigators report early increases,[223, 226] several others report changes only at time points when significant hypertrophy is already present, thus failing to provide convincing evidence that they represent the proximal effectors in a renotropic system.[221, 222, 224, 225, 227]

Failure to identify a specific "renotropin" has led some to suggest instead that renal hypertrophy occurs as a result of increased sensitivity of renal cells to prevailing levels of growth-promoting factors. This enhanced sensitivity, it is argued, may result from changes in the intracellular environment brought about by responses to increased glomerular filtration, such as the increase in Na^+/H^+ exchange seen in proximal tubule cells after renal mass reduction.[74] As can readily be appreciated from the previous discussion, many factors have been associated with compensatory renal hypertrophy but a unifying hypothesis that adequately accounts for them all remains elusive. It is likely that multiple pathways are involved. Some factors appear to control normal renal growth and may have a permissive or modulating role compensatory hypertrophy, whereas others act as specific mediators of the dynamic processes that follow a reduction in renal mass.

ADAPTATION OF SPECIFIC TUBULE FUNCTIONS IN RESPONSE TO NEPHRON LOSS

As noted earlier, the bulk of the increase in renal mass after uninephrectomy is caused by hypertrophy of the proximal nephron.[233] The more distal nephron segments also enlarge, but to a lesser extent. In uninephrectomized rats, the proximal convoluted tubule is increased on average by 17% in luminal diameter and 35% in length, yielding a 96% increase in total volume; the distal convoluted tubule is enlarged by 12% in luminal diameter and 17% in length, yielding a 25% increase in total volume.[234] Maintenance of homeostasis for various solutes in the presence of a declining GFR requires highly integrated responses from each tubule segment. Although some solutes including creatinine and urea are chiefly cleared by glomerular filtration and therefore rise gradually in plasma with declining GFR, for others, the tubule solute handling adapts so that plasma levels remain constant, virtually until end-stage renal failure is reached (Fig. 43-2).

Adaptation in Proximal Tubule Solute Handling

In renal ablation models, as with the increase in remnant kidney SNGFR, the extent to which proximal tubule enlarges is inversely proportional to the remnant kidney mass.[235] Proximal tubule enlargement is associated with an increase in proximal reabsorption. In studies of both animals and humans with reduced renal mass, the increase in proximal reabsorption observed was found to be proportional both to the increase in remnant kidney GFR and to the increase in tubular volume.[236, 237] Similarly, in proximal tubules isolated from remnant kidneys, the observed increase in transtubular fluid flux was proportional to the increases in size and protein content of the tubule epithelial cells.[137, 138] Folding of the basolateral membrane of the proximal tubule epithelium was also found to increase, resulting

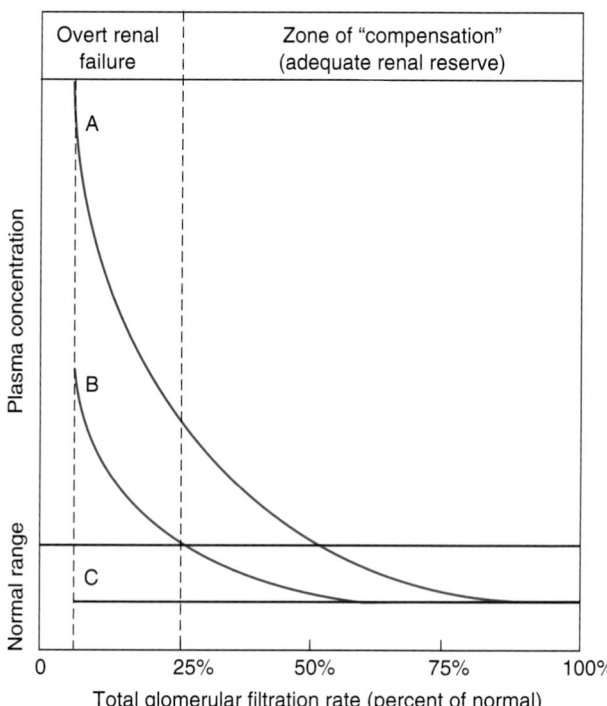

FIGURE 43-2. *Representative patterns of adaptation for different types of solutes in body fluids in chronic renal failure. Pattern A: rise in serum concentration with each permanent reduction in glomerular filtration rate (e.g., creatinine). Pattern B: rise in serum concentration only after GFR falls below a critical value owing to adaptive increases in tubular secretion (e.g., phosphate). Pattern C: serum concentration remains normal through almost entire period of progression of renal failure (e.g., sodium). (Modified from Bricker NS, et al: In Brenner BM, Rector FC [eds]: The Kidney, 2nd ed. Philadelphia, WB Saunders, 1981.)*

in augmentation of the basolateral surface area, in proportion to the increase in cell volume.[238] This increase in surface area was accompanied by an increase in activity of Na+,K+-ATPase, the membrane pump that generates the main driving force for proximal tubule solute transport.[238]

Increases in proximal tubule size and surface area are not, however, the only determinants of increased transport activity in this nephron segment. Fluid reabsorption in isolated proximal tubule segments increases within 24 hours of nephrectomy, that is, when GFR is already increasing but well before significant hypertrophy occurs, implying an intrinsic tubular epithelial cell adaptation to nephron loss.[136] This observation also raises the possibility that the increases in proximal tubular reabsorption occurring in response to nephron loss are driven by the increase in SNGFR and further implies that the increased reabsorptive load could stimulate hypertrophy.[136] Because solute reclamation is an energy-requiring process, it is not surprising that in uninephrectomized rabbits the increase in proximal tubule volume was accompanied by a proportional increase in mitochondrial volume.[239] The observation that the increase in renal mass is outstripped by the rise in GFR in models of progressive nephron loss implies that renal energy consumption per unit of remnant renal mass increases as renal function declines.[234]

The rise in SNGFR that occurs in the remnant kidney presents increased loads of glucose, amino acids, and other solutes that would normally be reabsorbed entirely in the proximal tubule, provided the maximal transport capacity was not exceeded. Maximal proximal tubular reabsorptive capacities for glucose and amino acids have been shown to increase in proportion to tubule mass after partial renal ablation.[240, 241] Some metabolic functions of proximal tubules are also augmented in the remnant kidney, so as to maintain adequate plasma levels of important metabolites including citrulline, arginine, and serine.[242, 243] Other proximal tubule functions, however, are not adjusted in proportion to proximal tubule mass: fractional phosphate reabsorption is decreased whereas ammoniagenesis increases.[240, 244-246] These adaptations are appropriate homeostatic responses that permit continued excretion of daily phosphate and acid loads, respectively, as the number of functioning nephrons declines.

Loop of Henle and Distal Nephron

Although there is little change in cross-sectional area in the thick ascending limb of the loop of Henle,[233] fluid reabsorption in this segment also increases in proportion to SNGFR.[234] In contrast, both the distal tubule and the cortical collecting duct enlarge in response to nephron loss.[233, 234] Unlike the proximal tubule, however, where the increased reabsorptive capacity is chiefly caused by increased tubule dimensions, the increased reabsorptive capacity observed in the distal segments is far greater than would be expected for the corresponding increase in tubule volume, implying a major adaptive increase in active solute transport.[234] Levels of mRNA for the Na+/myoinositol cotransporter (SMIT) and Na+/Cl−/betaine-γ-amino-N-butyric acid transporter (BGT-1) are increased in the cortex and outer medulla of remnant kidneys from five-sixths nephrectomized rats.[247] Likewise, potassium secretion by the distal nephron increases in

compensation for nephron loss, facilitated by an increased basolateral surface area of cortical collecting duct principal cells and an increase in Na+,K+-ATPase activity.[248-250]

Glomerulotubular Balance

Micropuncture studies have confirmed that proximal tubular reabsorption remains proportional to glomerular filtration over a wide range of SNGFR in both glomerular and tubulointerstitial diseases.[251, 252] This glomerulotubular balance is critical to the physiologic integrity of remnant nephron function and, hence, ECF homeostasis. Compensatory increases in SNGFR in surviving nephrons must be accompanied by similar increases in proximal tubular solute and water reabsorption, so as to avoid overwhelming the distal nephron transport capacity and disrupting its regulation of the volume and composition of the final urine. Conversely, reductions in SNGFR in damaged nephrons must be matched by similar reductions in proximal tubular reabsorption so as to maintain adequate solute and water delivery to the distal tubule, again permitting excretion of urine of appropriate volume and composition.

Glomerulotubular balance is maintained as follows: The degree of single nephron hyperfiltration occurring as a consequence of nephron loss determines the passive Starling forces operating in the postglomerular microcirculation, which, in turn, govern net transtubular solute reabsorption.[253] Increases in SNGFR associated with an increased filtration fraction result in elevated postglomerular capillary protein concentrations, which determine nonlinear increases in oncotic pressure, Π_E, the major determinant of peritubular capillary reabsorptive force (P_r). Reductions in SNGFR, in contrast, result in a lowered peritubular oncotic pressure, thereby reducing P_r. Thus, SNGFR and proximal tubular reabsorption remain in direct proportion to one another. Prevention of hyperfiltration by dietary protein restriction has been shown to abrogate the increase in proximal fluid reabsorption in the remnant kidney, underscoring the dependence of proximal tubular function on the level of glomerular filtration.[253] In the remnant kidney of rats subjected to extensive renal mass ablation, absolute fluid reabsorption was found to be markedly increased in proximal portions of both superficial and juxtamedullary nephrons, yet fluid delivery to the more distal segments of the nephron was also somewhat increased.[254] In the setting of nephron loss, sodium reabsorption by the loop of Henle has been shown to remain proportional to sodium delivery to that segment, indicating preservation of tubulotubular balance, a mechanism that maintains appropriate distal solute and water delivery in the presence of progressive nephron loss. Until the adaptive capacities of these mechanisms are finally exhausted, the operation of glomerulotubular balance and tubulotubular balance ensures that the distal tubule mechanisms that determine final urine composition are not overwhelmed by unregulated distal delivery of water and solute.[140] In keeping with these physiologic observations, morphologic studies have shown that within the same kidney, nephrons associated with damaged glomeruli are usually atrophic and presumably hypofunctioning, whereas those associated with healthier glomeruli are usually hypertrophic and hyperfunctioning.[255]

To maintain homeostasis in the presence of continued food and water intake, specific mechanisms that enhance single nephron water and solute excretion must come into play, in addition to the adjustments in SNGFR and tubular reabsorption that occur in response to nephron loss. These mechanisms are not unique to the setting of renal insufficiency, however, and are also engaged when the normal kidney is challenged to excrete extraordinary loads of solute and water. In general, the adaptive physiology of the chronically injured kidney is adequate to preserve homeostasis for many solutes under baseline conditions but the adaptive capacity may easily become overwhelmed by fluctuations in fluid intake and especially by increases in electrolyte and acid loads. Patients with CRF are therefore susceptible to develop volume overload, volume loss, hyperkalemia, and acidosis when the excretory capacity of the kidney is challenged by relatively modest increases in excretory demands.

Sodium Excretion and Extracellular Fluid Volume Regulation

In CRF, the ECF volume is often maintained very close to normal until end stage is reached.[256] This remarkable feat is accomplished by an increase in fractional sodium excretion (FE_{Na}) in inverse proportion to the decline in GFR.[257] Many studies have been carried out in an attempt to identify which nephron segments are responsible for the decrease in sodium reabsorption: micropuncture studies in uninephrectomized rats have shown that tubule fluid transit times, as well as the half-time for reabsorption of a stationary saline droplet in the proximal tubule lumen, were not different from controls[234]; in remnant kidneys of rats receiving high-, normal-, or low-sodium diets, *absolute* sodium reabsorption was found to increase but *fractional* sodium and fluid reabsorption were found to decrease in all groups[258]; micropuncture studies in dogs and rats have failed to detect significant reductions in fractional proximal tubule fluid and sodium reabsorption[259]; distal sodium delivery was found to be markedly increased in the rat remnant kidney[258]; increased solute transport activity has been demonstrated in distal tubule of uninephrectomized rats[234]; and under conditions of hydropenia and salt loading, sodium reabsorption by the medullary collecting duct of the rat remnant kidney was markedly reduced.[260] Taken together, these data suggest that proximal fractional reabsorption remains largely unchanged and that, in the setting of renal insufficiency, adjustments in sodium excretion occur predominantly in the loop and distal nephron segments.[261]

In addition to load-dependent tubular adaptations in sodium handling, sodium excretion is also modulated by hormonal influences. Levels of NPs are elevated in CRF as a result of reduced clearance and in response to alterations in sodium and volume status.[262] In rats with extensive renal mass ablation, plasma ANP levels may be restored toward normal levels by dietary sodium restriction, but, in response to increases in sodium intake, they rise progressively along with sodium excretion.[52] The notion that ANP plays an important role in mediating adaptive changes in sodium excretion in the setting of renal ablation is confirmed by observations that administration of an NP receptor antagonist reduced both FE_{Na} and GFR in five-sixths nephrectomized rats receiving either normal or high-salt diets but did not alter these variables in rats fed low-salt diets.[263] Significantly, NPs not only modulate sodium excretion but may also contribute to the

attendant glomerular hyperfiltration and thereby further exacerbate renal injury (see earlier).

Systemic hypertension has also been proposed by Guyton and associates as a contributor to the increase in FE_{Na} observed with renal insufficiency.[264] Their hypothesis states that a constant sodium intake in the presence of a reduced number of functioning nephrons leads to positive sodium balance as a result of reduced excretory capacity. Positive sodium balance leads to an increase in ECF volume and a rise in systemic blood pressure that, in turn, leads to an increase in FE_{Na} and reestablishes the steady state. In support of this hypothesis, salt intake has been shown to be critical to the development of hypertension in subtotally nephrectomized dogs and uremic patients have been found to exhibit marked sodium retention when treated with vasodilating antihypertensive agents.[265] On the other hand, a lowered salt intake in five-sixths nephrectomized rats does not prevent the development of systemic hypertension,[129] suggesting that sodium excretion and hypertension are not always interdependent in the setting of extensive renal mass ablation. Sodium conservation, on the other hand, is also impaired with renal insufficiency and, in response to an acute reduction in sodium intake, most patients were unable to reduce sodium excretion below 20 to 30 mEq/day.[266] Interestingly, when sodium intake was decreased gradually, salt-wasting patients with CRF were able to maintain sodium balance and reduce their sodium excretion to below 10 mEq/day.[267] The "salt-losing" tendency associated with CRD appears to be dependent on the salt load per nephron and may therefore be reversible with adequate dietary sodium restriction. Other factors modulating FE_{Na} in the setting of renal insufficiency include changes in sympathetic nervous system activity, aldosterone, PGs, and parathyroid hormone levels.[261, 268] Sodium homeostasis and volume regulation are discussed in further detail in Chapters 9, 18, and 19.

Urinary Concentration and Dilution

ECF homeostasis is usually well maintained until renal insufficiency is far advanced, when the ability of the kidney to excrete a volume load becomes significantly reduced.[261] Normal generation of solute-free water is about 12 mL per 100 ml of GFR and is dependent on dilution of tubule fluid in the thick ascending limb, maintenance of low water permeability in the distal nephron segments in the absence of antidiuretic hormone (ADH), and decreased hypertonicity of the medullary interstitium during water diuresis. Although the single nephron capacity to excrete free water per milliliter of GFR is not reduced in patients with advanced renal disease,[269] the absolute reduction in GFR reduces the overall capacity of the kidney to excrete a water load. Patients with CRF therefore cannot adequately dilute their urine and are prone to water intoxication and hyponatremia. Hypothetically, in addition to excretion of the equivalent of 2 L of "isotonic urine" per day (obligatory excretion of 600 mOsm/day), normal kidneys, with a GFR of 150 L/day, can excrete up to 18 L of free water, whereas failing kidneys, with a GFR of 15 L/day, can only excrete about 1.8 L of free water per day. The minimum urinary osmolality achievable by normal kidneys would therefore approach 30 mOsm/L (600 mOsm/20 L), whereas that of diseased kidneys would be 160 mOsm/L (600 mOsm/3.8 L).

Urinary concentration is also impaired in renal insufficiency. Normal urinary concentration requires preservation of the countercurrent mechanism to maintain hypertonicity of the medullary interstitium and normal water transport across the distal nephron segments in response to ADH. Maximal urinary osmolality in normal subjects is about 1200 mOsm/L. As GFR decreases, however, maximal urinary osmolality falls and with a GFR of 15 mL/minute is reduced to about 400 mOsm/L.[270] A normal individual can therefore excrete the obligatory daily 600 mOsm in as little as 0.5 L of urine, whereas the patient with a GFR of 15 mL/minute can excrete the same load in a minimum of 1.5 L. Part of the defect in urinary concentration observed in renal injury may be attributed to the high solute load imposed per surviving nephron. In patients with chronic renal insufficiency, however, the osmotic effect of urea was shown to be inadequate to account fully for the reduction in maximal urine concentration, indicating that factors other than osmotic diuresis contribute to reduction in urinary concentrating ability in these patients.[270] Furthermore, in patients with chronic primary glomerulonephritis, reduction in urine concentrating capacity was found to correlate significantly with the degree of medullary fibrosis on renal biopsy,[271] suggesting that disruption of the medullary architecture, with the consequent loss of medullary hypertonicity, may result in disproportionate impairment of urinary concentrating ability at any given level of GFR. Consistent with this observation, patients with primary tubulointerstitial injury (e.g., analgesic nephropathy and sickle cell disease) have markedly impaired urinary concentrating abilities, even early in the course of their illness.[270, 272, 273] Similarly, in animal experiments, surgical exposure of the renal papilla in intact hydropenic rats was found to lead to reduction in urinary osmolality because of the accompanying alterations in vasa recta flow and ensuing washout of medullary solutes.[274] Interestingly, similar exposure of papillae in rats with remnant kidneys did not affect urinary osmolality, presumably because medullary solute washout had already occurred owing to the adaptive responses to nephron loss. Urinary concentration also depends on water reabsorption in the distal nephron segments of the remnant nephron. Reduction in water reabsorption may be the result of several mechanisms in the failing kidney. Defective cyclic AMP-mediated response to ADH may render the cortical collecting duct resistant to the effects of ADH, resulting in increased water delivery to the papillary collecting duct.[275] Urinary osmolality is inversely proportional to fractional water delivery to the papillary collecting duct in five-sixths nephrectomized rats, despite an increase in absolute water reabsorption per functioning collecting tubule when compared with controls.[274] Patients with renal insufficiency are therefore prone to volume depletion in the presence of water deprivation or impaired thirst mechanisms. More commonly, the inability to concentrate urine becomes manifest as nocturia, which develops as renal function deteriorates. Urinary concentrating and diluting mechanisms are discussed in further detail in Chapter 14.

Potassium Excretion

To maintain potassium homeostasis in the presence of continued dietary intake and a reduced number of functioning nephrons, potassium excretion per nephron must increase.

In both normal and diseased kidneys, almost all of the filtered potassium is reabsorbed in the proximal tubule and loop of Henle. Potassium excretion is therefore determined predominantly by distal secretion,[261, 276] although a reduction in potassium reabsorption by the loop of Henle has been shown to contribute to increased potassium excretion in rats with reduced renal mass.[277] In both normal and partially nephrectomized dogs, urinary potassium excretion was found to correlate directly with serum potassium concentration.[278] Similarly, in intact and uninephrectomized rats, net potassium secretion in the distal convoluted tubule occurred only during potassium infusion, whereas potassium secretion by cortical collecting tubules (CCTs) occurred under all conditions, and was greater after uninephrectomy.[276] Other studies have confirmed that the CCT is an important site of potassium secretion in the remnant kidney.[248, 260] Secretion of potassium by CCTs isolated from remnant kidneys of rabbits fed normal or high-potassium diets was shown to persist in vitro and to be directly related to the dietary potassium content,[248] indicating an intrinsic tubular adaptation to potassium load. This adaptation was absent in CCTs from rabbits in which dietary potassium had been reduced in proportion to the amount of renal mass lost. In addition to variation with dietary potassium load, the increase in potassium secretion by remnant CCTs was also found to correlate with plasma aldosterone levels but not with intracellular potassium concentration or Na^+,K^+-ATPase activity.[248] In contrast, however, others have reported an increase in cortical and outer medullary Na^+,K^+-ATPase activity in homogenates from rat remnant kidneys that was abrogated when potassium intake was reduced in proportion to the reduction in GFR.[250] Finally, the frequent occurrence of hyperkalemia in patients with chronic renal insufficiency after treatment with an aldosterone antagonist or an ACEI suggests that "normal" aldosterone levels are required to maintain adequate potassium excretion in this population.[279, 280] In general, therefore, the increase in potassium secretion by surviving nephrons appears to be predominantly determined by the rise in plasma potassium after potassium ingestion and by intrinsic tubular adaptation to the increased filtered potassium load.[250, 276, 278] In both dogs and patients with chronic renal insufficiency, however, the kaliuretic response to an oral potassium load is attenuated compared with normal subjects despite higher serum potassium levels.[278, 281] The eventual, complete excretion of a potassium load, therefore, occurs at the expense of a prolonged increase in serum potassium. Control of potassium excretion is discussed further in Chapters 10 and 21.

Acid-Base Regulation

Reduction of GFR in patients with CRD is associated with the development of systemic metabolic acidosis, owing to a reduction in serum bicarbonate concentration.[282] Normal acid-base balance requires reabsorption of filtered bicarbonate, excretion of titratable acid, ammonia generation, and acidification of tubular luminal fluid by the distal nephron.[261] In CRD, acidosis develops as a result of varying degrees of impairment in each of these processes.[283]

Reduction in renal ammonia synthesis is the greatest limitation to acid excretion in CRD. Low serum bicarbonate levels result in maintenance of acid urine, which stimulates proximal tubule ammoniagenesis and also protonates ammonia, resulting in its entrapment as ammonium in the tubule lumen. Net ammonia production per hypertrophied proximal tubule has been shown to increase in response to nephron loss.[245, 275] With decreasing GFR, however, this increase becomes inadequate to compensate for further nephron loss, and absolute ammonia excretion falls.[246] In addition, disruption of the tubulomedullary ammonium concentration gradient as a result of structural injury may impair ammonia trapping and therefore reduce ammonium excretion.[246, 284] Bicarbonate reabsorption by the nephron occurs predominantly in association with sodium reclamation in the proximal tubule and is dependent on generation of a proton gradient in the distal nephron. Conflicting data with respect to bicarbonate reabsorption in remnant kidneys may reflect species differences. In dogs with remnant kidneys, bicarbonate reabsorption was shown to be increased at both proximal and distal micropuncture sampling sites compared with intact controls.[285] In contrast, bicarbonate reabsorption per unit GFR has been shown to be reduced in both humans and rats with CRD[261] and some patients with renal insufficiency demonstrate bicarbonate wasting until serum bicarbonate drops below 20 mEq/L.[286] Bicarbonate reabsorption is also reduced in the settings of hyperkalemia, increased ECF, and hyperparathyroidism, all of which may come in to play in patients with chronic renal insufficiency.[287-289] Distal urinary acidification tends to be relatively well preserved in patients with CRD, and urinary pH, although higher than in normal individuals with experimental acidosis, is usually about 5.[282] Urinary excretion of titratable acid is also generally well preserved in the setting of nephron loss, as a consequence of increased fractional phosphate excretion.[240, 246, 261] As renal failure progresses, acid excretion becomes more dependent on excretion of titratable acid. Renal acidification mechanisms are discussed more comprehensively in Chapters 11 and 20.

Calcium and Phosphate

Derangements of calcium and phosphate metabolism occurring with renal insufficiency are not only the result of impaired urinary excretion of these solutes but also of associated abnormalities in vitamin D metabolism and parathyroid hormone (PTH) secretion. With progressive renal dysfunction, 1-hydroxylation of vitamin D by the kidney decreases; calcium absorption from the gut decreases; serum calcium tends to decrease; serum phosphate tends to increase; and PTH secretion increases. In response to increased PTH, calcium is mobilized from bone, renal phosphate excretion is enhanced, and the steady-state becomes reestablished, with secondary hyperparathyroidism as the "trade-off."[290] In CRD, serum phosphate does not increase until GFR falls below 20 mL/minute and phosphate balance is maintained predominantly by an increase in fractional phosphate excretion.[291] With moderate renal insufficiency, therefore, filtered phosphate is not greatly increased and the increase in phosphate excretion must be achieved by a reduction in phosphate reabsorption per nephron.[292] With more severe reductions in GFR, however, phosphate excretion is maintained by an increase in serum phosphate as well as by reduced reabsorption per nephron. Sodium-dependent phosphate transport measured in proximal tubular brush border membrane vesicles prepared from the remnant kidneys of dogs was shown to be decreased

when compared with that in vesicles derived from normal dogs.[240] Interestingly, however, this decrease was abolished if the partially nephrectomized dog had also undergone parathyroidectomy, indicating that PTH plays an important role in proximal tubular adaptation to phosphate excretion. Studies of isolated proximal tubules from euparathyroid uremic rabbits showed a reduction in net phosphate flux per unit of reabsorptive surface area and an increase in sensitivity to PTH.[244] The authors postulated that the number of PTH receptors per tubule must increase in the remnant kidney, concomitant with tubular hypertrophy. The levels of mRNA encoding the sodium coupled phosphate transporter NaP$_i$-2 are reduced by approximately 50% in remnant kidneys from five-sixths nephrectomized rats.[293] In contrast, tubules from hyperparathyroid uremic rabbits demonstrated reduced PTH sensitivity, consistent with down-regulation or persistent occupancy of the PTH receptors. On the other hand, studies in animals with reduced renal mass subjected to parathyroidectomy have shown that fractional excretion of phosphate remains inversely proportional to the reduction in GFR,[294] indicating that phosphate excretion is not entirely dependent on the presence of PTH. Whereas most of the reduction in phosphate reabsorption is achieved in the proximal tubule, there is also some evidence of increased fractional phosphate excretion by the distal tubule in uremic dogs and rats.[295-297] As kidney failure advances, renal 1-hydroxylation of vitamin D decreases and, as a result, calcium absorption from the gut is reduced.[298] In renal failure, fractional intestinal calcium absorption is inversely proportional to blood urea nitrogen.[298] Calcium excretion, on the other hand, varies widely in patients with renal disease, probably owing to differences in diet, heterogeneity of vitamin D production, and predominance of glomerular versus tubulointerstitial injury.[299] In normal individuals, calcium excretion is mediated by suppression of PTH-induced reabsorption in the distal nephron and by suppression of PTH-independent mechanisms in the thick ascending limb. In patients with CRD, fractional calcium excretion remains unchanged until GFR falls below 25 mL/minute, when fractional excretion increases owing to the obligatory solute diuresis.[261] Absolute calcium excretion, however, remains low. Hypocalciuria in patients with chronic renal insufficiency has been shown to be caused, in part, by the attendant hyperparathyroidism.[300] Similar findings were obtained in rats with reduced renal mass, in which parathyroidectomy resulted in increased calcium excretion compared with nonparathyroidectomized controls.[301] Renal calcium clearance has been found to be increased in patients with tubulointerstitial disease and in rats with surgical papillectomy, suggesting that regulation of calcium reabsorption depends on intact medullary structures and that regulation of calcium excretion may be largely modulated by the distal nephron segments.[261, 299, 301] The potential contributions of calcium and phosphate to renal disease progression are discussed later. Calcium and phosphate metabolism is also discussed in greater detail in Chapters 12, 22, and 52.

LONG-TERM ADVERSE CONSEQUENCES OF ADAPTATIONS TO NEPHRON LOSS

The adverse effects of extensive renal mass reduction have been appreciated since 1932, when rats subjected to partial nephrectomy were observed to develop hypertension, albuminuria, remnant kidney hypertrophy, and azotemia.[302] Detailed histopathologic studies performed several decades later revealed that early hypertrophy in rat remnant kidneys after five-sixths nephrectomy was followed by mesangial accumulation of hyaline material that progressively encroached on capillary lumens, obliterating Bowman's space and finally resulting in global sclerosis of the glomerulus.[303] These findings, together with the observation that sclerosed glomeruli are a common finding in human CRD of diverse causes, led the authors to speculate that the pathologic findings described were a consequence of glomerular hyperfiltration resulting from a reduction in nephron number.[303] The five-sixths nephrectomy model has been extensively studied, and considerable progress has been made in elucidating how the physiologic adaptations of remaining nephrons that initially permit greatly augmented function per nephron ultimately produce a complex series of adverse effects that eventuate in progressive renal injury and an inexorable decline in function.

Hemodynamic Factors

As early as 1 week after extensive renal mass ablation, glomerular hyperfiltration and glomerular capillary hypertension were associated with morphologic changes, including visceral epithelial cell cytoplasmic attenuation, protein reabsorption droplets and foot process fusion, mesangial expansion, and focal lifting of endothelial cells from the basement membrane.[17] Evidence that these morphologic changes were a consequence of the glomerular hemodynamic alterations was provided by studies in rats subjected to extensive renal mass ablation and fed a low-protein diet. This intervention prevented the hemodynamic changes, effectively normalizing Q_A, P_{GC}, and SNGFR and also largely attenuated the structural lesions observed in rats on a standard diet.[17] Similar findings were subsequently described in a variety of animal models of CRD, including diabetic nephropathy[148, 304] and deoxycorticosterone (DOCA)-salt hypertension.[305] Together, these observations led Brenner and colleagues to propose that the hemodynamic adaptations after renal mass ablation ultimately prove injurious to glomeruli and initiate processes that eventuate in glomerulosclerosis. The resulting obliteration of further glomeruli would induce hyperfiltration in remaining, less affected glomeruli, thereby establishing a vicious cycle of progressive nephron loss. This vicious cycle therefore constituted a "common pathway" for renal damage that could account for the inexorable progression of CRD, regardless of the cause of the initial renal injury.[4] The hypothesis also explained the finding of both atrophic and hypertrophic nephrons typically encountered in chronically diseased kidneys.[141] Further evidence supportive of the "hyperfiltration hypothesis" was gleaned from the study of experimental diabetic nephropathy in which glomerular hyperfiltration was also found to be a forerunner of glomerular pathology.[17, 304] Maneuvers such as unilateral nephrectomy, which exacerbates hyperfiltration in the remaining kidney, were also found to exacerbate diabetic renal injury.[306] Furthermore, when the kidney was shielded from elevated perfusion pressure and from glomerular capillary hypertension by creating unilateral renal artery stenosis, the ipsilateral kidney was protected against the development of diabetic injury, which progressed unabated

in the contralateral kidney.[307] In addition, when glomerular hyperfiltration was reversed in five-sixths nephrectomized rats by transplantation of an isogeneic kidney, hypertension and proteinuria were ameliorated and glomerular injury was limited.[308] Similarly, augmenting renal mass in Fisher-to-Lewis rats normalized P_{GC} and greatly reduced the development of chronic renal allograft injury.[309, 310] Direct evidence that similar mechanisms may operate in human kidneys is derived from a study of 14 patients with solitary kidneys who had undergone varying degrees of partial nephrectomy of the remaining kidney for malignancy.[311] Before renal-sparing surgery, proteinuria was absent in all patients. Although serum creatinine remained stable after an initial rise of 50% in 12 patients, the 2 patients subjected to the most extensive nephrectomy (75% and 67%, respectively) developed progressive renal failure and required long-term dialysis. Moreover, among the remaining patients, seven developed proteinuria, the levels of which were inversely related to the amount of renal tissue preserved. Renal biopsy specimens in four patients with moderate to severe proteinuria showed focal segmental glomerulosclerosis (FSGS),[311] which later morphometric analysis revealed to involve virtually all glomeruli examined.[312]

The importance of glomerular hemodynamic factors in the development of progressive renal injury was further illustrated by studies that reported dramatic protective effects against the development of glomerulosclerosis after chronic inhibition of the RAS with either an ACEI or AT_1RA in five-sixths nephrectomized rats.[28-31] Micropuncture studies showed that like the low-protein diet, the renoprotective effects of RAS inhibition were associated with near-normalization of the P_{GC}, yet, in contrast to the effects of dietary protein restriction, SNGFR remained elevated.[313] This suggested that glomerular capillary hypertension, rather than hyperfiltration per se, was the key factor in the initiation and progression of glomerular injury. Confirmation of this view came from an experiment in which rats were treated with a combination of reserpine, hydralazine, and hydrochlorothiazide ("triple therapy") to lower arterial pressure to levels similar to those obtained with an ACEI. In contrast to the glomerular hemodynamic effects of the ACEI, however, triple therapy did not alleviate glomerular hypertension or proteinuria and glomerular injury progressed unabated (Fig. 43-3).[29, 30] Interestingly, within the context of pharmacologic inhibition of the RAS, the level to which systemic blood pressure is reduced remains a critical determinant of the extent of the renal protection conferred.[314] The effectiveness of both ACEIs and AT_1RA in lowering glomerular pressure and ameliorating glomerular injury has since been observed in several other animal models of CRD. These include, but are not restricted to, models of diabetic nephropathy,[148, 315, 316] hypertensive renal disease,[317, 318] experimental chronic renal allograft failure (a model that lacks systemic hypertension but exhibits glomerular capillary hypertension),[319-321] age-related glomerulosclerosis,[322, 323] and obesity-related glomerulosclerosis.[324] It is noteworthy that the phase of transition from an acute, nonhypertensive experimental injury induced by puromycin aminonucleoside administration, to a chronic nephropathy characterized by proteinuria and glomerulosclerosis, is also associated with the development of glomerular capillary hypertension.[325] That similar mechanisms are relevant in human CRD

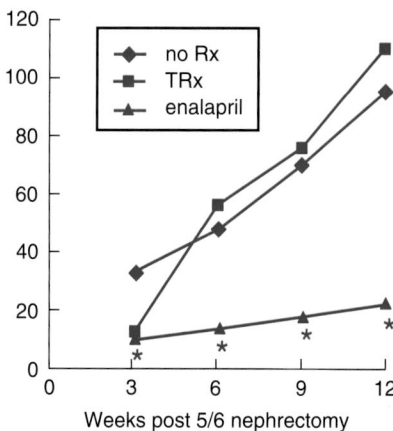

FIGURE 43-3. Proteinuria levels after 5/6 nephrectomy in untreated rats (NX) versus treatment with triple therapy (reserpine, hydralazine and hydrochlorothiazide-TRX) (NX + TRX) or enalapril (NX + CEI). Despite equivalent levels of blood pressure control, enalapril therapy almost completely prevented proteinuria and glomerulosclerosis whereas triple therapy afforded no renoprotection. *P < .05 vs. untreated controls. (Reproduced with permission from Anderson S, Rennke HG, Brenner BM, et al: Therapeutic advantage of converting enzyme inhibitors in arresting progressive renal disease associated with systemic hypertension in the rat. J Clin Invest 77:1993-2000, 1986.)

progression has been strongly suggested by the results of clinical trials showing substantial renoprotective effects with ACEI and AT_1RA treatment.[326-329] The importance of glomerular capillary hypertension has been further illustrated by studies of the effects of omapatrilat, a vasopeptidase inhibitor. Micropuncture studies after five-sixths nephrectomy showed even greater lowering of P_{GC} with omapatrilat than with ACEI treatment, despite equivalent effects on systemic blood pressure. In subsequent chronic studies, omapatrilat produced more effective renoprotection than the ACEI.[330] Thus, among the determinants of glomerular hyperfiltration, glomerular capillary hypertension has been identified as a critical factor in the initiation and progression of glomerular injury. In contrast to the RAS, the role of ETs in mediating glomerular capillary hypertension and experimental renal disease progression is far less well defined. Pharmacologic blockade of ET receptors has been shown to ameliorate disease progression in some studies, but glomerular hemodynamics were not investigated and the mechanisms involved therefore require further elucidation.[331-333]

Mechanisms of Hemodynamically Induced Injury

Mechanical Stress

Several mechanisms have been proposed whereby elevated P_{GC} may result in glomerular cell injury. According to the Law of Laplace (which states that wall tension of a cylinder is equal to the product of its radius and the intraluminal pressure), a rise in P_{GC} produces an increase in capillary wall tension that results in stretching of the glomerular capillary wall, owing to its high mechanical compliance.[131] Experimental evidence suggests that this stretching may have adverse consequences for all three major cell types in the glomerulus. Furthermore, recent advances in the study of cellular responses to mechanical stress raise the possibility that glomerular

hyperperfusion may also promote the development of glomerulosclerosis through more subtle and complex pathways that induce profibrotic phenotypic alterations in glomerular cells.[334]

Endothelial Cells

The vascular endothelium serves multiple complex functions, including acting as a dynamic barrier to leukocytes[335] and plasma proteins, secretion of vasoactive factors (prostacyclin, NO, and ET), conversion of AI to AII,[336] and expression of cell adhesion molecules. It is also the first cellular structure in the kidney that encounters the mechanical forces imparted by glomerular hyperperfusion. After extensive renal mass reduction, endothelial cells are activated or injured, resulting in detachment and exposure of the basement membrane. This, in turn, may induce platelet aggregation, deposition of fibrin, and intracapillary microthrombus formation.[17, 337, 338] In addition to direct cellular injury, exposure of endothelial cells to the shear stress, cyclic stretch, or pulsatile barostress that results from glomerular hyperperfusion may also increase expression of cell surface adhesion molecules, cytokines, and major histocompatibility complex molecules; increase platelet adhesiveness; and alter endothelial barrier functions.[339-341] In vitro, shear stress can stimulate expression of the adhesion molecule, intercellular adhesion molecule (ICAM)-1, on endothelial cell surfaces.[342] Ambient barometric pressure has been shown to enhance expression of ET[343] and basic fibroblast growth factor bFGF[344] by endothelial cells. Cyclic stretch induced endothelial cell proliferation, increased cyclic AMP generation,[345] and enhanced ET release in endothelial cell cultures.[346, 347] These effects may be mediated by Ca^{2+} entry into endothelial cells through mechanosensitive ion channels in the cell surface membrane.[348, 349] Mechanical stress-induced alterations in endothelial synthesis of vasoactive and growth-promoting factors may shift the local balance to favor the vasoconstrictive and growth-promoting effects of factors such as ETs and AII over the growth-inhibitory properties of molecules such as prostacyclin, heparan sulfate, and NO.[350] Transforming growth factor (TGF)-β, another product of activated endothelial cells that is up-regulated in glomerular endothelium in five-sixths nephrectomized rats,[351] may have a dual role, having the potential to act as a growth promoter at low levels and a suppresser at higher levels.[352] The complexity of endothelial responses to mechanical stress is underscored by the finding that the supernatant of cells cultured under sustained shear stress conditions has an antiproliferative effect on cultured mesangial cells.[353] Macrophage chemoattractant protein (MCP)-1, as well as being responsive to its classic cytokine inducers, interleukin (IL)-1, tumor necrosis factor (TNF)-α, interferon (IFN)-γ, and lipopolysaccharide,[354] is also up-regulated in endothelial cells exposed to laminar shear stress[355] and is overexpressed in the arteries of rats with hypertension.[356] Furthermore, endothelial cells may contribute autocrine and paracrine effects through classic cytokine signaling mechanisms. For example, activated endothelial cells may release TNF-α, an autocrine inducer of endothelial adhesion molecule expression,[357-359] and release cytokines and thrombogenic substances. Expression of endothelial cell adhesion molecules could, in turn, lead to indirect amplification of endothelial cell activation through TNF-α or other cytokines (e.g., IL-1) derived from adjacent glomerular cells or monocytes tethered to the endothelium.[360] Biomechanical activation has been described as an "emerging paradigm" in endothelial cell biology[361]; and although the notion of a role for endothelial activation in transducing the adverse effects of glomerular hyperperfusion is intriguing, further studies focusing on glomerular endothelial pathophysiologic responses to mechanical stress are awaited.

Recent studies have shed further light on the potential importance of endothelial cell injury in progressive renal injury. It has been recognized for some time that segmental glomerulosclerosis is associated with focal obliteration of capillary loops[362] and that interstitial fibrosis is associated with loss of peritubular capillaries.[363] Recently it has been shown that this loss of capillaries in the remnant kidney is associated with a decrease in endothelial cell proliferation and reduced constitutive expression of vascular endothelial growth factor (VEGF) by podocytes and renal tubule cells as well as by increased expression of the antiangiogenic factor thrombospondin-1 by the renal interstitium.[364] Because VEGF is an important endothelial cell angiogenic, survival, and trophic factor, these findings suggest that capillary loss may be in part due to failure of recovery from hemodynamically mediated endothelial cell injury. Furthermore, short-term treatment of rats with VEGF ameliorated both glomerular and peritubular capillary loss after five-sixths nephrectomy.[365] This preservation of capillaries was associated with a trend toward less glomerulosclerosis and significantly less interstitial deposition of type III collagen, as well as better preservation of renal function. Long-term studies are required to evaluate further the potential benefit of improving renal angiogenesis in the setting of progressive renal injury.

Mesangial Cells

Subjecting mesangial cells to cyclical stretch or strain in vitro has also been shown to induce proliferation[366] and synthesis of matrix constituents including collagen[367, 368] or to switch mesangial cell phenotype to overexpress extracellular matrix (ECM) constituents and promote fibrogenesis.[369] Transduction of mechanical forces by mesangial cells has been associated with tyrosine phosphorylation[370] and protein kinase C–induced increases in S-6 kinase activity.[371] Mesangial cells cultured at ambient pressures of 50 to 60 mm Hg, that is, levels corresponding to glomerular capillary hypertension, show enhanced synthesis and secretion of ECM when compared with cells grown at "normal" pressures of 40 to 50 mm Hg.[372] Interestingly, when this maneuver was applied to cultured macrophages, the higher pressure was associated with increased secretion of factors that induced mesangial cell proliferation.[372] Cyclic stretch stimulates mesangial cell synthesis of the profibrotic growth factors, TGF-β,[373] and connective tissue growth factor (CTGF)[374] as well as increased expression of TGF-β receptors.[375] Because TGF-β is closely associated with fibrotic states, it has been suggested that TGF-β may represent the link between glomerular capillary hypertension and glomerulosclerosis.[376] Cyclic stretch also activates a cellular RAS in cultured mesangial cells,[377] and AII in turn may also induce TGF-β synthesis.[378] Exposure of mesangial cells to barostress, achieved by culture under increased barometric

pressure, also stimulates expression of cytokines, including platelet-derived growth factor (PDGF)-B[379] and MCP-1.[380]

Podocytes

As mentioned earlier, podocytes display morphologic evidence of injury as early as 1 week after extensive renal mass reduction.[17] Subsequent studies have identified similar evidence of podocyte injury at 6 months after uninephrectomy[381] and after renal ablation in rats with doxorubicin (Adriamycin)-induced nephropathy.[382] Detailed in vitro studies have revealed that podocytes respond to cyclic stretching by undergoing reversible Ca^{2+} influx- and Rho kinase-dependent reorganization of the actin cytoskeleton, a response not seen in fibroblast or epithelial cell lines.[383] This specific mechanosensitivity suggests that podocytes may also respond to mechanical forces resulting from glomerular hypertension, but further studies are required to elucidate the nature and relevance of this response.

Cellular Infiltration in Remnant Kidneys

A cellular infiltrate composed predominantly of macrophages and smaller numbers of lymphocytes accompanies clinical and experimental FSGS.[384-388] The presence of glomerular macrophages has led to the development of secondary focal glomerulosclerosis after extensive renal mass ablation being compared with the pathogenesis of arteriosclerosis.[389] In the latter setting, overexpression of endothelial adhesion molecules[390] is associated with passage of leukocytes across the endothelium, where monocytic infiltrates are believed to contribute to subintimal proliferation by releasing cytokines and growth factors.[391] Similarly, the observed up-regulation of renal endothelial adhesion molecules may facilitate egress of leukocytes from the circulation into the mesangium, where they may participate in further renal injury. The recruited cellular infiltrate may constitute an abundant source of potent pleiotropic cytokine products that, in turn, influence other infiltrating leukocytes, dendritic cells, and kidney cells, stimulating cell proliferation, elaboration of ECM components, increased endothelial adhesiveness, as well as alterations in renal hemodynamics. Evidence is now emerging that these proposed mechanisms, based largely on in vitro observations, are indeed relevant in vivo. In the two-kidney, one-clip model of renovascular hypertension, up-regulated expression of adhesion molecules and TGF-β as well as cell infiltration is observed only in the nonclipped kidney that is exposed to the hypertensive perfusion pressure.[392, 393] In the five-sixths nephrectomy model, coordinated up-regulation of a variety of cell adhesion molecules, cytokines, and growth factors in association with macrophage infiltration has been observed at time points that precede the development of severe glomerulosclerosis.[394-396] Furthermore, prevention of renal injury with ACEI or AT$_1$RA treatment was associated with inhibition of cytokine up-regulation and prevention of renal infiltration by macrophages.[396] Finally, infiltrating monocyte/macrophages have been shown to express increased TGF-β in remnant kidneys.[397]

Several lines of evidence suggest that this cellular infiltrate does contribute to renal injury and is not merely a consequence of it. In one study, multiple linear regression analysis identified glomerular macrophage infiltration in the remnant kidney as a major determinant of mesangial matrix expansion and adhesion formation between Bowman's capsule and glomerular tufts.[398] Furthermore, depletion of leukocytes in rats by irradiation delayed the onset of glomerular injury after renal ablative surgery.[385] Recently, several studies have reported amelioration of the cellular infiltrate and renal injury in the five-sixths nephrectomy model after treatment with the immunosuppressive agent mycophenolate mofetil.[399-402] Together, these data are consistent with the notion that chronic inflammatory processes are activated in the remnant kidney. Interestingly, the anti-inflammatory agent nitroflurbiprofen, which is also a NO donor, has a modest effect to ameliorate remnant kidney injury after five-sixths nephrectomy.[403]

Infiltrating cells, although present in the glomeruli of remnant kidney, are chiefly distributed in the tubulointerstitial regions.[384-386] Their role in the development of the tubulointerstitial fibrosis that accompanies glomerulosclerosis is unclear. It is possible that interstitial infiltrates are recruited as the result of tubulointerstitial cell activation by the downstream effects of cytokines released in the glomeruli. More recently, the proinflammatory phenotype of tubular epithelial cells that take up filtered proteins is thought to account for the expression of cell adhesion and chemoattractant molecules that recruit macrophages and other monocytic cells to tubulointerstitial areas.[404] The potential role for macrophages in the development of tubulointerstitial injury is intriguing, but, at present, the evidence for such a role remains largely associative. The notion that transdifferentiation (dedifferentiation or retrodifferentiation) of renal tubule epithelial cells to a myofibroblast phenotype represents an important step in the development of tubulointerstitial fibrosis[405] has been raised by the finding that renal tubule cells in the remnant kidney of five-sixths nephrectomized rats expressed α-smooth muscle actin, a myofibroblast marker not usually expressed by epithelial cells.[406] The significance of this interesting observation remains to be determined. Interstitial myofibroblasts are thought to contribute to tubulointerstitial fibrosis after five-sixths nephrectomy in association with increased expression of PDGF expression by distal tubule and collecting duct epithelial cells.[407]

The importance of factors acting "downstream" from the hemodynamic changes in the common pathway mechanisms of CRD progression has been demonstrated by studies using a peroxisome proliferator-activated receptor γ (PPARγ) receptor agonist.[408] These compounds have been introduced as antidiabetic agents that improve insulin resistance in type 2 diabetes mellitus. The PPARγ receptor is a member of the nuclear receptor superfamily of transcriptional factors, and in vitro studies suggest that PPARγ receptor agonists may have a wide range of effects, including modulation of adipocyte differentiation, macrophage function, and activation of other transcription factors.[408] Rats treated with a PPARγ receptor agonist after five-sixths nephrectomy evidenced significant attenuation of the proteinuria and glomerulosclerosis observed in untreated rats, despite the failure of treatment to lower blood pressure. This renoprotection was observed in association with marked reductions in glomerular cell proliferation, glomerular macrophage infiltration, and renal expression of plasminogen activator inhibitor (PAI)-1 and TGF-β.[408] The authors speculate that some of these effects may have resulted from the known

actions of PPARγ receptor activation to antagonize the activities of the transcription factors AP-1 and NF-κB. These findings strongly support the hypothesis that downstream cellular and molecular mediators of the effects of glomerular hemodynamic adaptations are critical to progressive renal injury after nephron loss. Treatments that antagonize these mediators may therefore be of benefit in slowing the rate of progression of CRD.

Nonhemodynamic Factors in the Development of Nephron Injury after Extensive Renal Mass Ablation

The weight of evidence in support of the hypothesis that glomerular hemodynamic adaptations are central to progressive renal injury does not exclude the possibility that the kidney may also be affected by a variety of factors not directly attributable to hemodynamic changes. These nonhemodynamic factors have been extensively studied in recent years and may offer new therapeutic targets for future renoprotective interventions.

Transforming Growth Factor-β

TGF-β is increasingly being associated with chronic fibrotic states, including CRD.[409] In vitro, TGF-β elicits overproduction of ECM constituents by mesangial cells and its expression is increased in several experimental models of renal disease, including diabetic nephropathy,[410, 411] anti-Thy-1 glomerulonephritis,[376] doxorubicin-induced nephropathy,[412] and chronic allograft nephropathy,[413] as well as in human glomerulonephritis,[414, 415] HIV nephropathy,[416] diabetic nephropathy,[410] and chronic allograft nephropathy.[417] The role of TGF-β in renal fibrosis is further illustrated by experiments in which transfection of the gene for TGF-β into one renal artery produced ipsilateral renal fibrosis.[418] Moreover, transfection of the gene for decorin, the naturally occurring inhibitor of TGF-β, into skeletal muscle limited the progression of renal injury in anti-Thy-1 glomerulonephritis.[419] In five-sixths nephrectomized rats a twofold to threefold increase in remnant kidney mRNA levels for TGF-β was observed and in situ hybridization revealed elevations in TGF-β mRNA throughout glomeruli, tubules, and interstitium. Treatment with an ACEI or an AT$_1$RA resulted in substantial renal protection and prevented up-regulation of TGF-β.[396, 397] Furthermore, in rats treated with an ACEI or an AT$_1$RA the extent of glomerulosclerosis correlated closely with remnant kidney TGF-β mRNA levels.[314] Recently, another fibrogenic molecule, connective tissue growth factor (CTGF), that has been associated with tissue fibrosis has also been observed to be overexpressed in kidney biopsy specimens from patients with a variety of renal diseases.[420] The specific induction of CTGF expression by exogenous TGF-β in mesangial cells[374, 421] and fibroblasts,[422] together with the finding that blocking antibodies to TGF-β inhibited increased CTGF expression in mesangial cells exposed to high glucose concentrations,[421] suggests that CTGF may serve as a downstream mediator of the profibrotic effects of TGF-β.[423]

Angiotensin II

As discussed earlier, AII plays a central role in the glomerular hemodynamic adaptations observed after renal mass ablation.

Nevertheless, experimental studies have revealed several nonhemodynamic effects of AII that may also be important in CRD progression (Fig. 43-4): In isolated, perfused kidneys, infusion of AII results in loss of glomerular size permselectivity and proteinuria, an effect that has been attributed to both hemodynamic effects of AII resulting in elevations in P_{GC}, and a direct effect of AII on glomerular permselectivity.[424] In vitro AII has been shown to stimulate mesangial cell proliferation and induce expression of TGF-β, resulting in increased synthesis of ECM.[378] In vivo, transfection of rat kidneys with human genes for renin and angiotensinogen resulted in glomerular ECM expansion within 7 days.[425] AII also stimulates production of plasminogen activator inhibitor-1 (PAI-1) by endothelial cells and vascular smooth muscle cells[426-428] and may therefore further increase accumulation of ECM through inhibition of ECM breakdown by matrix metalloproteinases that require conversion to an active form by plasmin. Reports indicate that AII may directly induce the transcription of a variety of cell adhesion molecules and cytokines through activation of the transcription factor NF-κB[429] and may also directly stimulate monocyte activation.[430] Finally, AII may have fibrogenic effects via mineralocorticoids. Aldosterone has been shown to stimulate the laying down of collagen in the myocardium, and myocardial fibrosis may be inhibited by spironolactone.[431, 432] In the remnant kidney model, coadministration of aldosterone with pharmacologic blockers of the RAS was found to negate the renoprotective effects of the latter.[433] It is uncertain, however, if the profibrotic effects of aldosterone can be entirely dissociated from its hemodynamic effects through sodium and extracellular volume homeostasis.

Hepatocyte Growth Factor

Recent investigations have shed light on the role of HGF as a potential antifibrotic factor in CRD. Initial studies focused on the property of HGF to ameliorate tubule cell injury in models of renal ischemia,[434, 435] but studies in models of CRD suggest that HGF may also ameliorate chronic renal injury through its mitogenic, morphogenic, and antiapoptotic actions.[436] As discussed earlier, HGF is up-regulated in the remaining kidney after uninephrectomy and may play a role in compensatory renal hypertrophy.[230] In one study it was confirmed that HGF and its receptor, c-met, are also up-regulated in the remnant kidney after five-sixths nephrectomy.[437] Furthermore, blockade of HGF action with anti-HGF antibodies resulted in a more rapid decline in GFR and more severe renal fibrosis that was associated with increased ECM accumulation and a greater number of myofibroblasts in the interstitium and tubules. Moreover, in vitro studies revealed that HGF decreased ECM accumulation in proximal tubule cell cultures by increasing expression of collagenases such as matrix metalloproteinase-9 (MMP-9) and decreasing the expression of the endogenous inhibitors of MMPs, tissue inhibitors of matrix metalloproteinase-1 (TIMP-1) and TIMP-2.[437] Further experiments have confirmed the renoprotective role of HGF: the renoprotective effects of ACEI and AT₁RA are associated with increased renal expression on HGF mRNA[438]; treatment with anti-HGF antibodies resulted in increased TGF-β levels in a mouse model of chronic glomerulonephritis[439]; HGF treatment ameliorated the progression of chronic allograft nephropathy in a renal transplant model[440]; HGF blocked the TGF-β–induced transdifferentiation of tubule epithelial cells to myofibroblasts[441]; and exogenous HGF administration[441] or HGF overexpression[442] blocked myofibroblast activation and prevented interstitial fibrosis in the unilateral ureteric obstruction model. In contrast, other studies have reported adverse renal effects associated with excess HGF exposure: transgenic mice that overexpressed HGF developed progressive renal disease characterized by tubular hypertrophy, glomerulosclerosis, and cyst formation[443] and HGF administration

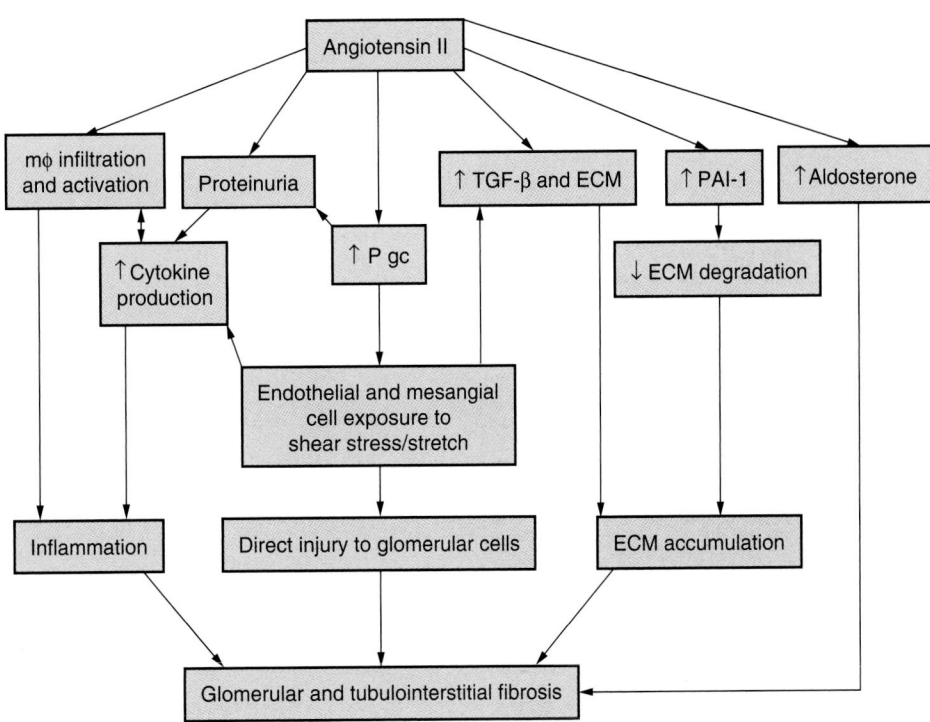

FIGURE 43-4. Scheme depicting the central role of angiotensin II, through hemodynamic and nonhemodynamic effects, in the pathogenesis of progressive renal injury and fibrosis after nephron loss. ECM, extracellular matrix; mφ, macrophage; PAI-1, plasminogen activator inhibitor-1; P_{GC}, glomerular capillary hydraulic pressure; TGF-β, transforming growth factor-β. (Reproduced with permission from Taal MW, Brenner BM: Renoprotective benefits of RAS inhibition: From ACEI to angiotensin II antagonists. Kidney Int 57:1803-1817, 2000.)

resulted in more rapid deterioration of creatinine clearance as well as increased albuminuria in obese db diabetic mice.[444] Available evidence thus suggests that HGF may play a role in ameliorating chronic renal injury but that inappropriate or excessive exposure to HGF may have adverse renal effects.

Hypertrophy

The consistent observation of renal and, in particular, glomerular hypertrophy after renal mass reduction has prompted investigators to propose that processes involved in, or resulting from, hypertrophy may contribute to progressive renal injury in CRD.[445, 446] The well-documented observation that both renal and glomerular hypertrophy precede the development of diabetic nephropathy[147] and the finding of a positive association between glomerular size and early sclerosis in rats subjected to renal mass ablation[447] suggested that hypertrophy may play a direct role in pathogenesis of glomerulosclerosis. This notion was further supported by the observation that PVG/c rats, which show the same increase in whole kidney GFR as Wistar rats after unilateral nephrectomy, do not develop the glomerular hypertrophy or the lesions of FSGS seen in the remaining kidney of Wistar rats at 1 year after nephrectomy.[448] On the other hand, the same study reported greater numbers of nephrons per kidney in PVG/c than Wistar rats, and because glomerular hemodynamics were not studied, these data should be interpreted with caution. Several clinical observations also support an association between glomerular hypertrophy and renal injury. Oligomeganephronia, a rare congenital condition in which nephrons number 25% of normal or less, is characterized by marked hypertrophy of the remaining glomeruli and development of proteinuria and renal failure in adolescence, with FSGS as the typical renal biopsy finding.[449-451] In children with minimal change disease, a glomerulopathy generally associated with spontaneous remission and lack of progression to renal failure, investigators noted an association between glomerular size and the risk of developing FSGS and renal failure.[452]

Two forms of intervention have been employed in an attempt to interrupt the development of glomerular hypertrophy after renal mass reduction and thereby assess its role in renal disease progression. Rats subjected to five-sixths nephrectomy were compared with rats in which two thirds of the left kidney was infarcted and the right ureter drained into the peritoneal cavity (an intervention that apparently results in decreased renal clearance without compensatory renal hypertrophy). Micropuncture studies confirmed similar degrees of elevation of P_{GC} and SNGFR in both models. At 4 weeks, however, the maximal planar area of the glomerulus was significantly less and glomerular injury, as assessed by sclerosis index, significantly reduced in ureteroperitoneostomized rats versus five-sixths nephrectomized controls. Accordingly, the authors concluded that glomerular hypertrophy was more important than glomerular capillary hypertension in the progression of glomerular injury in this model.[453] Dietary sodium restriction has also been utilized to inhibit renal hypertrophy after five-sixths nephrectomy. Although sodium restriction had no effect on glomerular hemodynamics, glomerular volume was significantly reduced in five-sixths nephrectomized rats fed low versus normal

sodium diets. Moreover, urinary protein excretion was lower and glomerulosclerosis was less severe in rats on restricted sodium intake.[129] These findings were extended by another study in which the effect of sodium restriction in preventing glomerular hypertrophy and ameliorating glomerular injury was confirmed but that also found that these benefits were overcome by administration of an androgen that stimulated glomerular hypertrophy despite sodium restriction. Glomerular hemodynamics were similar among the groups.[454]

Glomerular hypertrophy may contribute to glomerulosclerosis through a number of different mechanisms. According to the law of Laplace, the increase in glomerular volume could result in an increase in capillary wall tension only if the capillary wall diameter was also increased. Cyclic stretch would then exert degrees of stress capable of damaging epithelial, mesangial, and endothelial cells, as described earlier. Alternatively, glomerulosclerosis may be viewed as a maladaptive growth response after loss of renal mass and resulting in excessive mesangial proliferation and ECM production.[445] In the past there has tended to be a dichotomy of viewpoints regarding the relative importance of hemodynamic factors or hypertrophy in the pathogenesis of glomerulosclerosis.[445, 446, 455] Proponents of the "hypertrophy hypothesis" have pointed out that in some experiments a disassociation between glomerular hemodynamic changes and glomerulosclerosis has been observed[456-458] and that in one study antihypertensive therapy was renoprotective without lowering P_{GC}.[447] On the other hand, those favoring the "hemodynamic hypothesis" have noted that treatment with $ACEI$[29] or AT_1RA[31] in five-sixths nephrectomized rats resulted in renal protection without preventing glomerular enlargement.[29] Furthermore, in the experiment of Yoshida and co-workers rats subjected to ureteroperitoneostomy developed significantly more glomerulosclerosis than sham-operated controls despite a lack of increase in glomerular size.[453] Moreover, many of the studies purporting to show a positive association between glomerular hypertrophy and sclerosis failed to report glomerular hemodynamic data.[455] Recently, however, positions have emerged that, although continuing to regard raised glomerular capillary pressure as the critical factor in initiating glomerulosclerosis, also acknowledge that glomerular hypertrophy and other pathogenetic mechanisms may act in concert with hemodynamic factors in a complex interplay that eventuates in progressive renal injury (Fig. 43-5).[334, 459]

Altered Glomerular Permselectivity to Plasma Proteins

Abnormal excretion of protein in the urine is the hallmark of experimental and clinical glomerular disease. Whereas immune complex deposition and resulting inflammation account for abnormal permeability of the glomerular filtration barrier to proteins in glomerulonephritis, studies in rats subjected to extensive renal ablation have shown loss of glomerular barrier function to proteins of similar molecular size, yet in the apparent absence of primary immune-mediated renal injury or inflammatory response. Sieving studies using dextrans and other macromolecules in rats 7 or 14 days after five-sixths nephrectomy revealed loss of both size and charge-selectivity of the glomerular filtration barrier. Ultrastructural examination of the remnant kidneys revealed detachment of glomerular endothelial cells and visceral epithelial cells

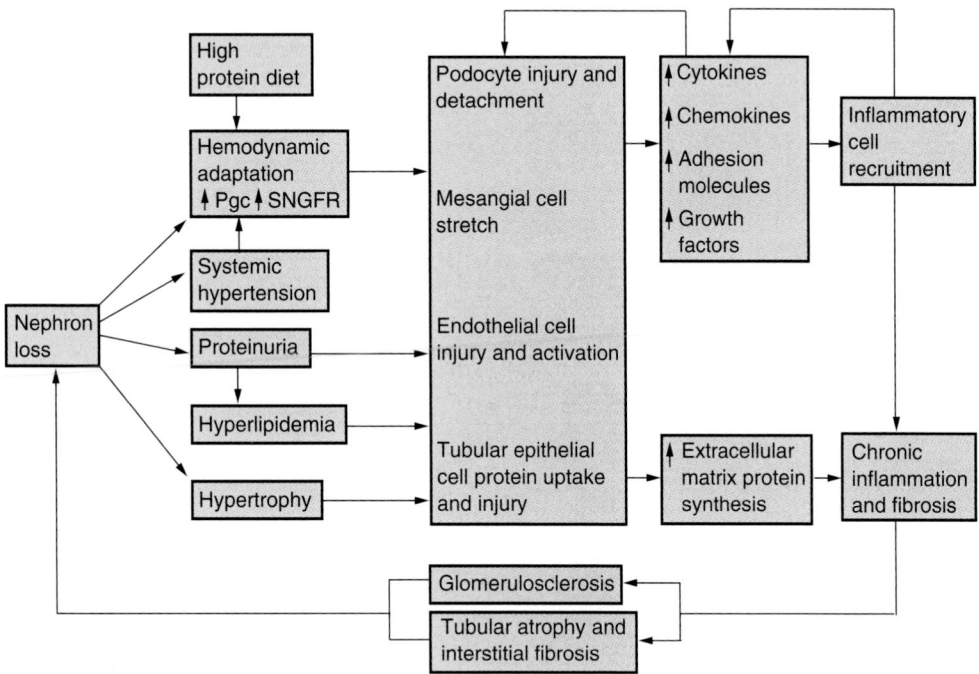

FIGURE 43-5. Scheme hypothesizing the interaction of hemodynamic and nonhemodynamic factors in the "common pathway" of mechanisms contributing to progressive nephron loss in chronic renal disease. P_{GC}, glomerular capillary hydraulic pressure; SNGFR, single-nephron glomerular filtration rate. (Reproduced from Mackenzie HS, et al: *In* Brenner BM [ed]: The Kidney, 6th ed. Philadelphia, WB Saunders, 2000.)

from the glomerular basement membrane. In addition, protein reabsorption droplets and attenuation of cytoplasm resulting in bleb formation was observed in podocytes. The authors concluded that the altered permselectivity may be caused, in part, by separation of endothelial cells from the glomerular basement membrane, allowing access of macromolecules, and, in part, to loss of anionic sites in the lamina rara externa, resulting in both loss of charge-selectivity and detachment of podocytes.[460] A direct role for AII in modulating glomerular capillary permselectivity is suggested by the observation of marked increases in urinary protein excretion during infusion of AII in normal rats.[461, 462] Whereas one group of investigators has attributed this to a direct effect of AII on the cellular components of the glomerular filtration barrier, resulting in opening of interendothelial junctions and epithelial cell disruption,[461] others have shown that the increase in proteinuria may be accounted for almost completely by the associated hemodynamic changes, principally a reduction in Q_A and an increase in filtration fraction.[462] On the other hand, the notion that AII may mediate changes in glomerular permselectivity independent of its effects on glomerular hemodynamics is supported by studies in an isolated perfused rat kidney preparation in which infusion of AII augmented urinary protein excretion and enhanced the clearance of tracer macromolecules independent of any change in filtration fraction.[424]

Proteinuria, long considered simply a marker of glomerular injury, has been implicated in experimental studies as an effector of injury processes involved in renal disease progression, especially those resulting in tubulointerstitial fibrosis. In rats with aminonucleoside-induced nephrotic syndrome the proteinuric phase of the disease was associated with an acute interstitial nephritis, the intensity of which

correlated closely with the severity of the proteinuria.[463, 464] Furthermore, in an overload proteinuria model induced by daily intraperitoneal administration of bovine serum albumin to uninephrectomized rats, proximal tubule cell injury and interstitial infiltration of macrophages and lymphocytes were evident after 1 week.[465] The severity of the proteinuria showed a positive correlation with the intensity of the infiltrate. At 4 weeks, focal areas of chronic interstitial inflammation were noted.[465] A causative association between excessive proteinuria and interstitial inflammation has been suggested by in vitro studies of proximal tubule epithelial cells cultured in media supplemented with high concentrations of albumin, IgG, or transferrin. Cellular uptake of these proteins was observed to increase secretion of ET-1,[466] MCP-1,[467] and RANTES.[468] Electrophoretic mobility shift assay of cell nucleus extracts in the latter study revealed intense activation of the transcription factor NF-κB that was dependent on the concentration of protein in the medium. Furthermore, the liberation of these molecules was noted to be predominantly from the basolateral aspect of the cells. This would be in keeping with secretion into the renal interstitium in vivo, thereby contributing to the development of tubulointerstitial inflammation and fibrosis. It has been proposed that the mechanism for cytokine induction in renal tubule epithelial cells that ingest excessive amounts of protein resembles that operating in virus-infected cells, where accumulation of viral protein in the endoplasmic reticulum activates the transcription factor NF-κB.[404, 469] Alternatively, the increased lysosomal enzyme activity associated with protein ingestion may result in leakage of lysosomal enzymes into the cell cytoplasm causing cell injury that could then provoke reactive inflammation and scarring.[470-473]

The relevance of these findings to the processes occurring in vivo has been borne out by studies in rats. In the protein-overload model, the development of proteinuria at 1 week was associated with significant increases in TGF-β at both protein and mRNA levels, in interstitial as well as proximal tubule cells.[474] Similarly, renal cortical mRNA levels encoding the macrophage chemoattractant osteopontin were increased on day 4 and immunofluorescence localized increased osteopontin staining to cortical tubules at day 7. MCP-1 and osteopontin mRNA and protein levels were elevated at 2 and 3 weeks. Furthermore, a significant effect of proteinuria on molecules involved in ECM protein turnover was observed. Although mRNA levels for various renal matrix proteins were variable, staining for the proteins in the cortical interstitium increased progressively. Levels of mRNA for the protease inhibitors PAI-1 and TIMP-1 were elevated at 2 weeks, at which time significant renal fibrosis was present.[474] In other models of proteinuric renal disease including five-sixths nephrectomy and passive Heymann nephritis, accumulation of albumin and IgG by proximal tubule cells occurred before infiltration of the interstitium by macrophages and major histocompatibility complex-II positive mononuclear cells. The infiltrates localized to areas where proximal tubule cells stained positive for intracellular IgG or where luminal casts were present. Furthermore, proximal tubule cells that stained positive for IgG also showed evidence of increased osteopontin production.[475] Studies in the five-sixths nephrectomy model have suggested that tubulointerstitial injury may play an important role in the decline of GFR, especially in the late stages of progressive renal injury.[476] By examining serial sections of remnant kidneys, the investigators were able to show that in association with a doubling in serum creatinine there was a substantial increase in the proportion of glomeruli no longer connected to glomeruli (atubular glomeruli) or connected to atrophic tubules. The majority of these glomeruli were not globally sclerosed, implying that the tubular injury was responsible for the final loss of function in these glomeruli. The authors speculate that the absorption of excess filtered protein may play an important role in this tubular injury.[476] Earlier findings that renal function is associated more closely with tubulointerstitial injury than glomerulosclerosis in human renal disease suggest that similar mechanisms may operate in human renal disease.[477, 478]

Proteins other than albumin or immunoglobulin may also play a role in the progression of chronic nephropathies. Although normally absent from tubular fluid, complement components C3 and C5b-9 neoantigen were observed along the luminal border of tubule epithelial cells in the protein overload proteinuria model.[465] To examine the role of filtered complement in renal injury, rats with puromycin aminonucleoside nephrosis were subjected to complement depletion with cobra venom factor or inhibition of complement activation by administration of soluble recombinant human complement receptor type 1, before the onset of proteinuria. In control rats, proximal tubular degeneration, interstitial leukocyte infiltrate, and renal impairment (as assessed by inulin and p-aminohippurate [PAH] clearances) occurred at 7 days, together with positive staining for C3 and C5b-9 along the proximal tubule brush border. Both interventions were associated with significantly less tubulointerstitial pathology and greater clearance of PAH but not inulin,

whereas the severity of the proteinuria was unaffected, suggesting that filtered complement plays a significant role in the tubulointerstitial injury associated with proteinuria.[479] High-density (HDL) and low-density (LDL) lipoproteins have been identified in the urine, renal interstitium, and tubule cells in renal biopsy specimens of patients with nephrotic syndrome.[480] In vitro, cultured human proximal tubule epithelial cells take up LDL and HDL.[481] Oxidized LDL may cause tubule cell injury, and exposure of tubule epithelial cells to HDL is associated with increased synthesis of ET-1.[481, 482] A role has also been proposed for compounds bound to filtered proteins such as IGF-1, which has been detected in increased amounts in the proximal tubular fluid of rats with doxorubicin nephrosis. Proximal tubule cells cultured in the presence of proximal tubular fluid from nephrotic rats exhibit enhanced cell proliferation and increased secretion of type I and type IV collagen. Both effects were inhibited by neutralizing IGF-1 receptor antibodies.[483] In experimental models of proteinuric renal disease, filtered proteins have also been found to accumulate in the glomerular mesangium[460, 484, 485] and may therefore contribute to glomerular as well as tubulointerstitial injury. Further support for this notion is derived from a meta-analysis of 57 studies of experimental CRD that found a consistent positive correlation between the severity of proteinuria and the extent of glomerulosclerosis.[486] Lipoproteins, in particular, accumulate in the glomeruli of patients with glomerulonephritis.[487, 488] Furthermore, LDL stimulates mesangial cells to proliferate in vitro[489, 490] and enhances mesangial cell synthesis of the ECM protein fibronectin.[491] LDL exposure is also associated with increased mesangial cell mRNA levels for MCP-1[491] and PDGF.[490] Oxidation of LDL by mesangial cells or macrophages may enhance its toxicity.[489] Thus, accumulation of proteins in the mesangium may stimulate a number of different mechanisms that contribute to glomerulosclerosis.

Although establishing cause-effect relationship between proteinuria and renal injury in humans is difficult, several clinical studies provide strong evidence in support of this notion. A meta-analysis of 17 clinical studies of CRD revealed a positive correlation between the severity of proteinuria and the extent of biopsy-proven glomerulosclerosis.[486] Observations from the Modification of Diet in Renal Disease (MDRD) trial also suggest that proteinuria is an independent determinant of CRD progression: greater levels of baseline proteinuria were strongly associated with more rapid declines in GFR; and reduction of proteinuria, independent of reduction in blood pressure, was associated with lesser rates of decline in GFR. Furthermore, the degree of benefit achieved by lowering blood pressure below usual target levels was highly dependent on the level of baseline proteinuria.[492] Similar findings were obtained in the Ramipril Efficacy In Nephropathy (REIN) trial. Higher baseline proteinuria was associated with more rapid rates of decline in GFR. In patients with pretreatment urinary protein excretion in excess of 3 g/day, treatment with ramipril reduced proteinuria to an extent that correlated inversely with the subsequent rate of decline in GFR. Treatment with other antihypertensives to achieve equivalent levels of blood pressure control did not decrease proteinuria and was associated with a higher rate of decline in GFR and an increased risk of reaching the combined end point of doubling of the baseline serum creatinine or end-stage renal failure.[327] A meta-analysis that included data from 1860 patients with nondiabetic CRD confirmed these findings and showed that during antihypertensive treatment the current level of proteinuria was a powerful predictor of the combined end point of doubling of baseline serum creatinine or onset of end-stage renal disease (ESRD, relative risk 5.56 for each 1.0 g/day of proteinuria).[493] Taken together, the evidence from experimental and clinical studies provides credible support for the hypothesis that excessive filtration of proteins due to impaired glomerular permselectivity directly damages the kidney. Whether or not this is so, the close association between the severity of proteinuria and renal prognosis implies that reduction of proteinuria should be regarded as an important independent therapeutic goal in clinical strategies seeking to slow the rate of progression of CRD.

INSIGHTS FROM MODIFIERS OF CHRONIC RENAL DISEASE PROGRESSION

Dyslipidemia

In 1982, Moorhead and colleagues advanced the hypothesis that abnormalities in lipid metabolism may contribute to the progression of CRD.[494] Glomerular injury, accompanied by an alteration in basement membrane permeability, was envisaged as the initiator of a vicious cycle of hyperlipidemia and progressive glomerular injury. They proposed that urinary losses of albumin and lipoprotein lipase activators result in an increase in circulating LDLs, which in turn bind to the glomerular basement membrane, further impairing its permselectivity; filtered lipoproteins accumulate in the mesangium, stimulating ECM synthesis and mesangial cell proliferation; and filtered LDLs are taken up and metabolized by the tubules, leading to cell injury and interstitial disease. Notably, this hypothesis did not propose hyperlipidemia as an initiating factor in renal injury but rather as a participant in a self-sustaining mechanism of disease progression.

Several lines of experimental evidence confirm the association between dyslipidemia and renal injury. Both intact and uninephrectomized rats with dietary-induced hypercholesterolemia developed more extensive glomerulosclerosis than their normocholesterolemic controls, and the severity of glomerulosclerosis correlated with serum cholesterol levels[495-497]; aging female Nagase analbuminemic rats (NAR) have endogenous hypertriglyceridemia and hypercholesterolemia and develop proteinuria and glomerulosclerosis by 9 and 18 months of age, respectively, whereas male NAR have lower lipid levels and have no glomerulosclerosis by 22 months of age.[498] Interestingly, ovariectomy in female NAR lowers triglyceride levels and reduces their renal injury. In seeming contradiction, however, young and aging male Sprague-Dawley rats developed more extensive glomerulosclerosis than age- and sex-matched NAR despite increased cholesterol levels in the NAR.[499] Triglyceride levels, however, were lower in the NAR, again suggesting an independent role for triglycerides in lipid-mediated renal injury. The association of hypercholesterolemia and renal disease has not been observed consistently across species; for example, Watanabe hyperlipidemic rabbits do not develop renal injury despite elevations in serum lipids.[500] A consistent pattern emerges, however, of an interaction between hyperlipidemia and various models of renal injury. Cholesterol feeding has been shown to exacerbate glomerulosclerosis in uninephrectomized rats, in prediabetic rabbits, in rats with puromycin aminonucleoside nephropathy (PAN), and in the unclipped kidney of rats with two-kidney, one-clip hypertension.[495, 497, 501, 502] When hypertension and dyslipidemia are superimposed, a synergistic effect that dramatically accelerates renal functional deterioration is observed.[503, 504]

In humans, the extent of the role of lipids in initiation and progression of renal disease remains unclear. At autopsy, a highly significant correlation was found between the presence of systemic atherosclerosis and the percentage of sclerotic glomeruli in normal individuals, fostering speculation that the development of glomerulosclerosis may be analogous to that of atherosclerosis.[505] A study designed to identify the clinical correlates of hypertensive ESRD found a strong association between atherosclerosis and hypertensive ESRD among older white patients.[506] The common forms of primary hypercholesterolemia, however, are not associated with an increased incidence of renal disease in the general population.[507, 508] In contrast, primary renal injury has been described in association with inherited disorders of lipoprotein metabolism, such as familial elevations of lipoproteins (a), B-100, and E[509-516] and congenital lecithin-cholesterol acyltransferase (LCAT) deficiency.[517] In the latter condition, renal injury may recur post-transplantation implying a causal role for LCAT deficiency.[503] The pathologic hallmark of lipoprotein-associated renal injury, lipoprotein glomerulopathy (LPG), is the presence of lipid thrombi that stain positive for lipoproteins E and B within dilated glomerular capillaries.[516] Indirect evidence of a role for hyperlipidemia in renal injury is derived from study of patients with morbid obesity and the nephrotic syndrome who have a propensity to develop glomerulosclerosis in association with hyperlipidemia.[518-520] Weight loss ameliorates the severity of proteinuria, and CRD in these patients and is associated with a favorable effect on the serum lipid profile.[521]

Whereas primary lipid-mediated renal injury is relatively rare among patients with CRD, the latter is frequently accompanied by elevations in serum lipids, as a result of urinary loss of albumin and lipoprotein lipase activators, defective clearance of triglycerides, modification of LDL by advanced glycation end products, reduced plasma oncotic pressure, adverse effects of medication, and underlying systemic diseases.[522-524] Among a cohort of adult patients with chronic renal insufficiency, the most frequent lipid abnormalities noted were hypertriglyceridemia and low HDL as well as increased apolipoprotein levels.[525] Furthermore, in a study of 631 routine renal biopsy specimens, lipid deposits were detected in nonsclerotic glomeruli in 8.4% of kidneys and staining for apo B was positive in approximately one fourth of the specimens, suggesting that lipid deposition is not infrequent in diverse renal diseases.[487] Several epidemiologic studies have found a strong association between renal disease progression and dyslipidemia: in the MDRD study, low serum HDL cholesterol was found to be an independent predictor of more rapid rates of decline in GFR[526]; elevated apo B has been found to correlate strongly with functional deterioration in both diabetic and nondiabetic patients with renal disease[512]; hypercholesterolemia was shown to be a predictor of loss of renal function in both type 1 and type 2 diabetics[527-530]; and in nondiabetics, renal disease progression advanced more rapidly in patients with hypercholesterolemia and hypertriglyceridemia, independent of blood pressure control.[531] Not all studies confirm these findings, however: in the Multiple Risk Factor Intervention Trial (MRFIT), dyslipidemias were not associated with a decline in renal function[532]; and in a retrospective analysis of patients with nephrotic syndrome, hypercholesterolemia at diagnosis was not found to be a predictor of renal disease progression.[533] In the latter study, however, both progressors and nonprogressors had markedly elevated serum cholesterol levels that may have confounded the analysis. Interpretation of these data is complicated by the fact that in patients with renal insufficiency dyslipidemias do not occur in isolation and are associated with other factors that also affect renal disease progression, including hypertension, hyperglycemia, and proteinuria. Levels of serum cholesterol and triglycerides have been found to correlate with blood pressure and circulating AII levels in both type 1 and type 2 diabetics with renal disease and to rise with increasing proteinuria in nephrotics.[508, 512, 530, 534-536]

The possible mechanisms whereby hyperlipidemia may contribute to renal injury have not been fully elucidated. Cholesterol feeding has been associated with an increase in mesangial lipid content,[496] glomerular macrophages, and TGF-β as well as fibronectin mRNA levels.[537, 538] Furthermore, reduction of glomerular macrophages by whole-body X-irradiation in the setting of nephrotic syndrome significantly reduced albuminuria without affecting serum lipids, indicating that macrophages play a central role in hyperlipidemic glomerular injury.[538] Mesangial cells express receptors for LDL, and uptake is stimulated by vasoconstrictor and mitogenic peptides such as ET-1 and PDGF.[490] Metabolism of LDL by mesangial cells leads to increased synthesis of fibronectin and MCP-1, which may contribute to mesangial matrix expansion and recruitment of circulating macrophage/monocytes into the glomerulus.[491] Moreover, triglyceride-rich lipoproteins (very low density lipoprotein [VLDL] and intermediate-density lipoprotein [IDL]) induce mesangial cell proliferation and elaboration of IL-6, PDGF, and TGF-β in vitro.[539] Mesangial cells, macrophages, and renal tubule cells all have the capacity to oxidize LDL through formation of reactive oxygen species, a step that may be inhibited by antioxidants and HDL.[481, 513, 540] Oxidized LDL may induce dose-dependent mesangial cell proliferation or mesangial cell death as well as production of TNF-α, eicosanoids, monocyte chemotaxins, and glomerular vasoconstriction. These pathways, together with free radicals generated during LDL oxidation, may each contribute to renal inflammation and injury.[539, 540] Hyperlipidemia is also associated with elevated P_{GC}, raising the possibility of a further pathway to glomerulosclerosis through hemodynamic injury.[496] The elevated P_{GC} appears to be mediated, in part, by an increase in renal vascular resistance that occurs in the context of increased plasma viscosity. In diabetic patients, circulating AII levels have been found to correlate with serum cholesterol[534] and both oxidized LDL and lipoprotein(a) have been shown to stimulate renin production by juxtaglomerular cells in vitro.[513] Moreover, oxidized LDL has been found to reduce nitric oxide synthesis by endothelial cells,[513] raising the possibility that alterations in activity of

the RAS and nitric oxide metabolism could also contribute to the increase in P_{GC} observed with hyperlipidemia.

It would follow that if hyperlipidemia exacerbates renal injury, interventions designed to lower serum lipids should ameliorate disease progression. Treatment with a 3-hydroxyl-3-methylglutaryl coenzyme A (HMG-CoA) reductase inhibitor or clofibric acid in the obese Zucker rat (a strain with endogenous hyperlipidemia and spontaneous glomerulosclerosis) and five-sixths nephrectomized rats (which develop hyperlipidemia secondary to renal insufficiency) resulted in lowering of serum lipid levels, reduction in albuminuria, reduction in mesangial cell DNA synthesis, and attenuation of glomerulosclerosis despite a lack of effect on either systemic blood pressure or P_{GC}.[19, 541, 542] In rats in the nephrotic phase of PAN, HMG-CoA reductase inhibitor treatment resulted in reduction of albuminuria and serum cholesterol, reduction of MCP-1 mRNA expression, and a 77% reduction in glomerular macrophage accumulation.[543] The HMG-CoA reductase inhibitors may therefore exert beneficial effects on renal disease progression, not only by reducing serum lipid levels but also by inhibiting mesangial cell proliferation and mechanisms for the recruitment of macrophages owing to decreased expression of chemotactic factors and cell adhesion molecules.[544] Cholesterol-fed rats with PAN treated with the antioxidants probucol or vitamin E showed significant reductions in proteinuria and glomerulosclerosis compared with untreated controls.[545] Furthermore, plasma VLDL and LDL from the treated animals were less susceptible to in vitro oxidation and less renal lipid peroxidation was evident, implying that lipid peroxidation plays an important role in renal injury associated with hyperlipidemia. In some patients, dietary or pharmacologic lowering of serum lipids has also been associated with a reduction in proteinuria and lower rates of decline in renal function.[546-549] Reduction of proteinuria by either dietary protein restriction or treatment with an ACEI has also been shown to improve serum lipid profiles, an effect that may contribute to subsequent renoprotection.[550, 551] Other studies in patients with CRD, however, have failed to demonstrate significant beneficial effects of lipid-lowering therapy on proteinuria or decline of renal function, despite adequate therapeutic reductions in serum lipids.[546-549, 552, 553] To date there have been no large-scale controlled trials of lipid-lowering therapies in patients with CRD of sufficient size to resolve these issues. Nevertheless, a recent meta-analysis of 12 small studies that included both diabetic and nondiabetic renal disease found that lipid-lowering therapy significantly reduced the rate of decline in GFR (mean reduction of 1.9 mL/minute/year).[554]

Dietary Protein Intake

Increases in dietary protein intake or intravenous protein loading in animals or humans with intact kidneys are associated with increases in renal mass, RBF, and GFR, as well as a decrease in renal vascular resistance.[555-558] The magnitude of the increases in GFR and RBF in response to a protein load is a function of renal reserve. In patients with renal insufficiency, most studies have shown that with a lower baseline GFR the percentage increase in GFR in response to a protein meal is reduced.[556, 557] In contrast, a study comparing the renal response to an oral protein load in patients with moderate and advanced renal failure found a similar percent increase in GFR over baseline in both groups, demonstrating that even with advanced renal disease some renal reserve is still present and that elevated intake of dietary protein may have undesirable effects on glomerular hemodynamics at all levels of renal function.[559]

To understand the mechanisms whereby protein loading acutely augments renal function, various components of protein diets have been examined individually: administration of equivalent quantities of urea, sulfate, acid, and vegetable protein to dogs or humans all failed to reproduce the meat protein–induced rise in GFR.[558, 560, 561] In contrast, feeding or infusion of mixed or individual amino acids (e.g., glycine, L-arginine) was shown to effect increases in GFR of similar magnitude to those seen with meat ingestion.[562, 563] Micropuncture experiments demonstrated that amino acid infusion resulted in increases in Q_A and ΔP, thereby raising SNGFR without affecting the ultrafiltration coefficient.[562] Interestingly, however, perfusion of the isolated kidney with an amino acid mixture resulted in only a modest increase in GFR.[564] Taken together, these observations suggest that amino acids themselves do not have a major direct effect on renal hemodynamics but that their effects are mediated by an intermediate compound generated only in the intact organism. Glucagon, the secretion of which is stimulated by protein feeding, has been proposed as such a mediator. GFR and RBF increase in response to glucagon infusion in dogs.[563] Furthermore, administration of the glucagon antagonist somatostatin consistently blocks amino acid–induced augmentation in renal function both in humans and rats.[562, 565] Large protein meals are also rich in minerals, potassium, phosphate, and acids. Indeed, after feeding a protein meal to dogs, the excretions of sodium, potassium, phosphorus, and urea were found to increase in parallel to the increase in GFR.[560] On the other hand, sodium chloride reabsorption in the proximal tubule and loop of Henle was found to be increased in rats maintained on a high-protein diet.[566, 567] As a result, less sodium and chloride would be delivered to the macula densa, thereby inhibiting tubuloglomerular feedback and adding a further stimulus to renal hyperemia.[567] Because dietary protein does not affect systemic blood pressure,[562, 568] other factors have been suggested to contribute to the renal hemodynamic changes after a protein load. Administration of the NO inhibitor L-NMMA or nonsteroidal anti-inflammatory agents have been shown to blunt the renal hyperemic response to an oral protein load in both rats and humans, invoking a role for NO and prostaglandins.[555, 566] In addition, AII and ET have been proposed as mediators of protein-induced renal injury because low-protein diets have been shown to reduce renal ET-1, ET receptors A and B, and AT_1 receptor mRNA expression in PAN-injected and normal rats.[569, 570]

It has been proposed that the augmented renal function induced by dietary protein may be an evolutionary adaptation of the kidney to the intermittent heavy protein intake of the hunter-gatherer.[4] Renal hyperfunction after a protein load would serve to facilitate excretion of the waste products of protein catabolism and other dietary components thereby achieving homeostasis in the presence of an abrupt increase in consumption in times of nutritional plenty; the subsequent decline of GFR to baseline during the intervals between meals would then favor mechanisms suited to conservation of fluid and electrolytes in times of scarcity. Persistent renal hyperfunction from continuous excessive protein intake, however, leads to renal injury in experimental models. Laboratory animals with intact kidneys that ingest food ad libitum become proteinuric and develop glomerulosclerosis with age.[4, 253, 571] This progression was significantly attenuated by feeding animals on alternate days only.[253] Furthermore, aging rats fed a high-protein diet ad libitum showed marked acceleration and increased severity of renal injury compared with rats receiving a normal protein diet, whereas rats fed a low-protein diet were protected from renal injury.[571] Similarly, in diabetic rats, progression of nephropathy was markedly accelerated in the setting of a high-protein diet and substantially attenuated by a low-protein diet.[304] In this study, kidney weight in high-protein-fed diabetic rats was significantly greater than in diabetic rats receiving normal protein diets, suggesting that protein-induced renal hypertrophy may itself contribute to acceleration of renal functional deterioration. As discussed earlier, the renoprotective effects of dietary protein restriction in experimental animals are associated with virtual normalization of P_{GC} and SNGFR.[17]

Despite unambiguous evidence from experimental studies, confirmation of a beneficial effect of protein restriction in clinical trials has proved elusive. After the publication of several smaller studies that generally suggested a beneficial effect from protein restriction but that suffered from deficiencies in design or patient compliance, a large, multicenter, randomized study, the MDRD study, was conducted to resolve the issue.[572, 585] Patients with moderate CRF (GFR = 25 to 55 mL/minute/1.73m^2) were randomized to "usual" (1.3 g/kg/day) or "low" (0.58 g/kg/day) protein diet (study 1) and 255 patients with severe CRF (GFR = 13 to 24 mL/minute/1.73m^2) to "low" (0.58 g/kg/day) or "very low" (0.28 g/kg/day) protein diet. All causes of CRD were included, but patients with diabetes mellitus requiring insulin therapy were excluded. Patients were also assigned to different levels of blood pressure control. After a mean of 2.2 years of follow-up, the primary analysis revealed no difference in the mean rate of GFR decline in study 1 and only a trend toward a slower rate of decline in the "very low" protein group in study 2. Secondary analyses of the MDRD data, however, revealed that dietary protein restriction probably did achieve beneficial effects. In study 1 "low" protein diet was associated with an initial reduction in GFR that likely resulted from the functional effects of decreased protein intake and not from loss of nephrons. This initial reduction in GFR obscured a later reduction in the rate of GFR decline that was evident after 4 months in the "low" protein group and that may have resulted in more robust evidence of renoprotection had follow-up been continued for a longer period.[573] Further evidence to support a beneficial effect of dietary protein restriction in CRD is derived from a meta-analysis of five randomized, controlled trials (including MDRD study 1). Despite inconclusive findings in several of the individual studies, Pedrini and associates[574] determined that the overall relative risk for renal failure or death was reduced to 0.67 (CI 0.50 to 0.89) with protein restriction, an effect that was not attributable to differences in blood pressure control between the groups. The subject of nutritional therapy in renal disease is discussed in greater detail in Chapter 57.

Calcium and Phosphate Metabolism

A retrospective analysis of 15 patients with nonprogressing CRD (GFRs of 27 to 70 mL/minute, followed for up to 17 years) revealed that the single feature common to all these patients was an enhanced capacity to excrete phosphate when compared with patients with similar GFRs but progressive renal disease.[575] In all of the nonprogressors, serum phosphate and calcium remained within normal limits without use of phosphate binders, calcium supplementation, or vitamin D. This study poses the intriguing question of whether the ability to maintain normal phosphate balance and avoidance of secondary hyperparathyroidism attenuated disease progression in these patients.

Uninephrectomized rats receiving a high-phosphate diet (1%) developed renal calcium and phosphate deposition and tubulointerstitial injury within 5 weeks of nephrectomy.[292] Similar changes were observed in a proportion of intact rats fed a 2% phosphate diet. Phosphate excess, therefore, does appear to have some intrinsic nephrotoxicity that is enhanced in the setting of reduced nephron number. A high-phosphate diet has also been associated with the development of parathyroid hyperplasia and hyperparathyroidism in remnant kidney rats.[576] Moreover, increased circulating parathyroid hormone levels induced by increased phosphate loads may exacerbate renal dysfunction through effects on blood pressure,[577] glucose intolerance, and lipid metabolism.[578, 579] Conversely, in both animals and humans with renal insufficiency, dietary phosphate restriction or treatment with oral phosphate binders has been associated with reductions in proteinuria and glomerulosclerosis and attenuation of disease progression as well as prevention of hyperparathyroidism.[580-583] Dietary phosphate restriction, however, almost inevitably also imposes dietary protein restriction. Given the established beneficial effects of protein restriction on renal disease progression, these data should be interpreted with caution. When phosphate restriction was superimposed on protein restriction in humans, however, renal disease progression was reduced significantly more than with protein restriction alone, implying that phosphate restriction may indeed have an independent beneficial effect.[584]

Calcium-phosphate deposition is a frequent histologic finding in end-stage kidney biopsies, irrespective of the underlying cause of renal failure.[298, 585] Calcium levels in end-stage kidneys have been found to be approximately nine times greater than levels in control kidneys.[585] Histologically, deposits were seen in cortical tubule cells, basement membranes and the interstitium.[585, 586] Furthermore, the severity of renal parenchymal calcification has been found to correlate with the degree of renal dysfunction, implicating calcium-phosphate deposition in disease progression.[580, 582] To determine whether the calcium deposits observed in end-stage kidneys precede or follow renal parenchymal fibrosis, rats with reduced renal mass were maintained on a high phosphate diet, thus ensuring a high calcium-phosphate product. A subgroup was treated with 3-phosphocitrate, an inhibitor of calcium-phosphate deposition.[582] Treatment with 3-phosphocitrate led to a significant reduction in renal injury compared with controls, indicating that calcium-phosphate deposition within the kidney occurs during the evolution of renal injury and exacerbates nephron loss. Calcium deposition in the renal parenchyma is associated with ultrastructural evidence of mitochondrial disorganization and calcium accumulation[586] and may therefore contribute to renal injury through uncoupling of mitochondrial respiration and generation of reactive oxygen species.[587] Mitochondrial calcium deposition was reduced by dietary protein restriction or calcium channel blocker therapy.[586, 587] Other potential roles for cellular calcium in renal disease progression include effects on vascular smooth muscle tone, mesangial cell contractility, cell growth and proliferation, ECM synthesis, and immune cell modulation.[588]

Gender

The age- and sex-adjusted incidence and prevalence of ESRD is greater in men than in women in the United States.[589] Similar trends have been noted elsewhere. A Japanese community-based mass screening program determined that the odds ratio of developing ESRD (if baseline serum creatinine was greater than 1.2 mg/dL for males or 1 mg/dL for females) was almost 50% higher in men than in women.[590] Similarly, in France, studies of factors influencing development of ESRD in patients with moderate and severe renal disease found that disease progression was accelerated in males versus females, especially in those with chronic glomerulonephritis or autosomal dominant polycystic kidney disease (ADPKD). Furthermore, the effect of hypertension as a risk factor for renal disease progression appeared to be greater in males.[591, 592] Many other studies have confirmed these observations for specific renal diseases.[593-601] In general, the prevalence of hypertension and uncontrolled hypertension is higher among men; men tend to consume more protein than women; the prevalence of dyslipidemias is greater in men than premenopausal women. All of these may contribute to the increased severity of renal disease seen in men.[589, 602] These factors do not, however, explain all the observed differences.

Laboratory studies confirm that males also appear to be at greater risk of developing renal disease and of disease progression than females.[603, 604] Age-associated glomerulosclerosis is much more pronounced in male than in female rats, and it is notable that the male propensity for age-related glomerulosclerosis can be prevented by castration.[605] Because gender difference in development of glomerular injury was found to be independent of P_{GC} or glomerular hypertrophy, a role for the sex hormones as modulators of renal injury has been proposed. Ovariectomy, on the other hand, had no effect on the development of glomerular injury seen in nonovariectomized female rats, implying that the presence of androgens, and not the lack of estrogens, promotes renal injury.[605, 606] By contrast, in the hypercholesterolemic Imai rat, the development of spontaneous glomerulosclerosis in males can be significantly reduced by castration or by administration of exogenous estrogens.[607, 608] Interestingly, although administration of testosterone negated the beneficial effect of castration in a dose-dependent manner, despite achieving a fivefold increase in circulating testosterone levels, exogenous testosterone did not overcome the beneficial renoprotective effects conferred on estrogen-treated males. These data again suggest an important role for androgens in the development of renal injury and raise the possibility that estrogens may to some extent counteract the adverse effects of androgens. In an apparently conflicting observation, female Nagase analbuminemic rats develop renal injury of greater severity than afflicts males, a characteristic that is ameliorated by ovariectomy.[498] These rats may be unique, however, in that triglyceride levels, which are higher in females, may have an independent and overriding effect on renal disease propensity. Glomerulosclerosis also develops to a significantly greater extent in male versus female rats subjected to extensive renal ablation.[603] This difference was independent of blood pressure and glomerular hypertrophy, but the degree of glomerulosclerosis and the extent of mesangial expansion each were found to correlate significantly with an increased expression of glomerular procollagen $\alpha 1(IV)$ mRNA in males. Similarly, in aging Munich-Wistar rats, glomerular metalloproteinase activity was found to decrease with age in males but not in females or castrated rats, suggesting that suppression of metalloproteinase activity by androgens could account for the gender difference in disease susceptibility.[609] Finally, estrogens, but not androgens, possess antioxidant activity and have been shown to inhibit mesangial cell LDL oxidation,[610] a property that may contribute to renoprotection.

Arterial Hypertension

Malignant hypertension frequently leads to renal injury, but whether or not less severe forms of hypertension cause "hypertensive nephrosclerosis" remains a subject of debate.[611, 612] The increased risk of developing progressive renal failure with higher levels of blood pressure has been established in several community-based studies[613-615] and is exemplified by findings from the Multiple Risk Factors Intervention Trial (MRFIT).[614] From a population of over 332,000 men screened between 1973 and 1977 for inclusion in the trial, the risk of developing or dying with ESRD over a 15- to 17-year follow-up period was 22-fold higher in patients whose systolic blood pressure at screening averaged 210 mm Hg when compared with those with systolic pressure of less than 120 mm Hg. An important finding was that a close correlation of blood pressure and risk of ESRD was also present at intermediate levels of blood pressure. Renal function was not assessed at screening or during follow-up, however, so it is not possible to establish with any certainty whether higher blood pressure initiated renal disease or accelerated a nephropathy that was already present. Further evidence of the importance of hypertension as a risk factor for ESRD is supplied by the finding that lowering systolic blood pressure by 20 mm Hg reduced the risk of ESRD by two thirds among American veterans.[616]

Although the role of hypertension in initiating renal disease requires further clarification, there is clear evidence that hypertension accelerates the rate of progression of preexisting renal disease, most likely through transmission of raised hydraulic blood pressure to the glomerulus, resulting in exacerbation of glomerular capillary hypertension associated with nephron loss.[4] Among insulin-dependent diabetic patients with diabetic nephropathy, the initiation of antihypertensive therapy resulted in marked reductions in the rates of GFR decline,[617, 618] implying that hypertension, an almost universal consequence of impaired renal function, also contributes to the progression of CRD. Similar observations were subsequently reported among patients with nondiabetic forms of CRD.[619-621] The potential impact of hypertension on the kidney is exemplified by case reports of patients with unilateral renal artery stenosis who manifested diabetic nephropathy or FSGS only in the nonstenotic kidney and not in the stenotic side that was shielded from the hypertension.[622, 623] Uncertainty remains, however, as to what level of blood pressure lowering is required to achieve optimal renoprotection. The MDRD study sought to resolve this issue by directly evaluating whether lower than previously recommended blood pressure targets afforded greater renoprotection than "usual" blood pressure control among patients with predominantly nondiabetic CRD. In addition to the dietary interventions described earlier, patients were randomized to a target MAP of 107 mm Hg or 92 mm Hg. Whereas the primary analysis did not show any overall difference in rate of GFR decline between these groups, patients randomized to the low blood pressure group evidenced an early rapid decrease in GFR, likely owing to associated renal hemodynamic effects, that obscured a later significantly slower rate of GFR decline than that observed in the "usual" blood pressure target group. Furthermore, a higher level of baseline proteinuria was associated with a greater difference in GFR decline between "usual" and low blood pressure groups.[572] Secondary analysis revealed significant correlations between the rate of GFR decline and achieved blood pressure, an effect that was also more marked among those with greater baseline proteinuria.[624] In study 1 (patients with GFR of 25 to 55 mL/minute/1.73m²), rates of GFR decline increased above a MAP of 98 mm Hg among patients with baseline proteinuria of 0.25 to 3.0 g/day and above 92 mm Hg in those with baseline proteinuria greater than 3.0 g/day. In study 2 (patients with GFR of 13 to 24 mL/minute/m²), among patients with baseline proteinuria greater than 1 g/day, higher achieved blood pressure was associated with greater rates of GFR decline at all levels (Fig. 43-6). The authors conclude by recommending a blood pressure goal of less than 125/75 (MAP = 92 mm Hg) for CRD patients with more than 1 g/day of proteinuria and a goal of less than 130/80 (MAP = 98 mm Hg) for those with proteinuria of 0.25 to 1.0 g/day.[624] Because not all the patients in the MDRD study received ACEI, it remains unclear to what extent the level of blood pressure attained remains important in CRD patients receiving ACEI or AT_1RA. However, experimental studies have found systolic blood pressure to be a major determinant of glomerular injury in rats receiving either ACEI or AT_1RA treatment.[314, 625] Moreover, among patients with type 1 diabetes and established nephropathy receiving ACEI, randomization to a low (MAP = 92 mm Hg) versus "usual" (MAP = 100 to 107 mm Hg) target blood pressure was associated with significantly lower levels of proteinuria after 2 years, although there was no significant difference in GFR.[626] A recent finding that intensive blood pressure control was not associated with significantly improved renal function among patients with ADPKD appears to contradict the just discussed findings but, by the authors' own admission, the study may not have had adequate statistical power to detect such a difference.[627]

Nephron Endowment

Severe congenital deficiencies in nephron endowment are associated with progressive glomerular injury in later life, suggesting that congenital nephron deficit results in similar adverse effects as an acquired deficit. Individuals born with

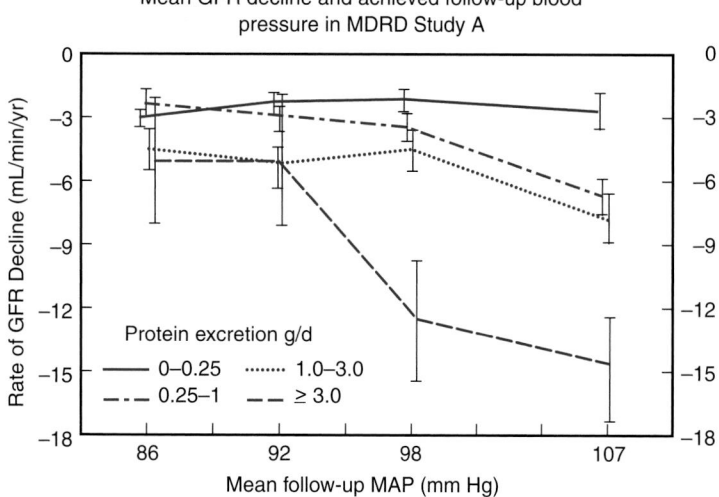

Mean GFR decline and achieved follow-up blood pressure in MDRD Study A

FIGURE 43-6. The interaction of blood pressure reduction and proteinuria at baseline on the rate of decline in glomerular filtration rate (GFR). MAP, mean arterial pressure. (Reproduced with permission from Peterson JC, Adler S, Burkart JM, et al: Blood pressure control, proteinuria, and the progression of renal disease. The Modification of Diet in Renal Disease Study. Ann Intern Med 123:754-62, 1995.)

the rare condition congenital oligomeganephronia have a greatly reduced nephron number and develop glomerulosclerosis and ESRD in adolescence.[451, 628, 629] Similarly, mice with a genetic defect characterized by oligosyndactyly and a congenital shortfall in nephron number of approximately 50% also develop glomerulosclerosis in maturity.[630] Nevertheless, it is possible that the predisposition to develop glomerulosclerosis is conferred by a gene or genes other than those determining nephron number, because the expression of glomerulosclerosis in the oligosyndactyly mouse depends on the genetic background of the strain with which it is outbred.[631]

Recent observations suggest that intermediate deficiencies in nephron number may also be associated with the susceptibility to develop renal disease and systemic hypertension. In experimental models, nephron endowment can be reduced through a variety of interventions, including induction of uterine ischemia,[632] maternal hyperglycemia,[633] treatment of pregnant rats with gentamicin,[634] or maternal dietary protein restriction.[635] Furthermore, reduction of nephron endowment in the latter two models was associated with the development of hypertension and glomerulosclerosis in later life.[634, 636, 637] Further evidence to support a role for nephron endowment in CRD susceptibility is derived from the study of rat strains with different nephron numbers. In male Munich Wistar Fromter (MWF) rats, a 50% reduction in nephron endowment versus control Wistar rats was associated with significant increases in SNGFR and proteinuria.[638] Similarly, spontaneously hypertensive rats have 25% fewer nephrons than their normotensive Wistar Kyoto counterparts[639] and Dahl salt-sensitive rats have 15% fewer nephrons than Dahl salt-resistant rats.[640]

The number of nephrons in human kidneys follows a gaussian distribution and exhibits marked variance among individuals in the "normal" population.[641-643] Although it is traditionally stated that the human kidney contains roughly 1 million nephrons,[641] recent determinations place the average closer to 600,000 nephrons per kidney with a standard deviation greater than 200,000.[642, 643] It appears that this variation may be determined by environmental factors during gestation, as well as by genetics. Low birth weight,

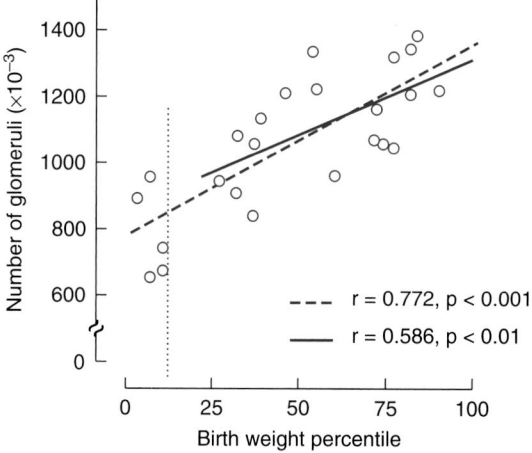

FIGURE 43-7. Graph showing the relationship between birth weight and the number of glomeruli in humans. (Reproduced with permission from Merlet-Benichou C, et al: Fetal nephron mass: Its control and its deficit. *In* Grünfeld J, Bach J, Kreis H [eds]: Advances in Nephrology from the Necker Hospital, Vol 26. St. Louis: Mosby–Year Book, 1997, pp 20-45.)

especially if associated with intrauterine growth retardation, is associated with deficits in nephron number of up to 20%, even in full-term pregnancies.[644, 645] Close correlations have been observed between birth weight and nephron endowment[646, 647, 647a] (Fig. 43-7), and low birth weight may therefore serve as a marker for reduced nephron number. Several clinical studies suggest that variation in nephron endowment may predispose individuals to hypertension and renal disease in later life. A review of 34 studies including over 66,000 subjects concluded that there is an inverse relationship between birth weight and blood pressure in both children and adults.[648] Short stature, a marker of low birth weight, was found among type 1 diabetics to be associated with diabetic nephropathy[649] and low birth weight predicts an increased risk of diabetic nephropathy among Pima Indians.[650] Birth weight may also influence the rate of progression of membranous nephropathy[651] and is associated with increased risk of developing proteinuria in Australian aboriginies.[652]

Moreover, in a recent postmortem study, hypertensive patients were found to have almost 50% fewer glomeruli per kidney than control subjects with normal blood pressure.[652a]

The notion that comparatively subtle variations in nephron number in the "normal" population predisposes to essential hypertension or advances the progression of acquired nephropathies may seem at odds with information amassed from kidney transplant donors and patients uninephrectomized for acquired renal disease. The lack of serious long-term consequences of the single kidney state is often cited to refute the hypothesis that increased excretory burden per nephron has adverse effects. Close inspection of the data does, however, reveal abnormalities that are attributable to the single kidney state. Total GFR in these groups often averages approximately 70% of prenephrectomy values despite the 50% reduction in renal mass, indicating hyperfiltration of the remaining kidney.[653] Although it seems clear that uninephrectomized individuals are not at substantially increased risk of developing progressive renal failure, a meta-analysis of 48 studies that included 2988 uninephrectomized patients revealed small increases in mean systolic and diastolic blood pressures and an increased incidence of proteinuria. Furthermore, the proteinuria increased in magnitude with time in the group, although among those for whom the indication for nephrectomy was organ donation, trauma, obstruction, or calculi, it decreased.[24] These observations have led Brenner and associates to propose that nephron underendowment may represent an important predisposing factor to hypertension and CRD.[654] The glomerular hemodynamic changes associated with mild to moderate congenital nephron deficiencies may not in themselves be sufficient to provoke renal injury but would compound the effects of an acquired renal insult and predispose the individual to progressive renal injury. Thus, CRD is viewed as a "multi-hit" process in which the first "hit" is reduced nephron endowment.[655]

Sympathetic Nervous System

Overactivity of the sympathetic nervous system has been observed in patients with CRD, and several lines of evidence suggest that this may be another factor that contributes to progressive renal injury.[656] The kidneys are richly supplied with afferent sensory and efferent sympathetic innervation and may therefore act as both a source and target of sympathetic activation. That the former is true is suggested by a study that compared postganglionic sympathetic nerve activity (SNA) measured by microelectrodes in the peroneal nerve in normal individuals and hemodialysis patients subdivided into those who retained their native kidneys and those who had undergone bilateral nephrectomy.[657] SNA was 2.5 times higher in non-nephrectomized dialysis patients compared with both normals and nephrectomized patients, in whom SNA was similar. Furthermore, increased SNA was associated with increased vascular tone and mean arterial blood pressure in non-nephrectomized patients. SNA did not vary as a function of age, blood pressure, antihypertensive agents, or body fluid status. The authors speculated that intrarenal accumulation of uremic compounds stimulates renal afferent nerves through chemoreceptors, leading to reflex activation of efferent sympathetic nerves and increased SNA. Other studies, however, have observed increased SNA in the

absence of uremia in patients with renovascular disease[658] or increased norepinephrine secretion in patients with nephrotic syndrome[659] or ADPKD.[660, 661] Furthermore, correction of uremia by renal transplantation does not abrogate the increased SNA.[662] Together, these findings suggest that a variety of forms of renal injury may provoke increased SNA and that uremia is not required for this response.

Evidence from experimental studies indicates that sympathetic overactivity resulting from renal disease may also accelerate renal injury. Ablation of afferent sensory signals from the kidneys by bilateral dorsal rhizotomy in five-sixths nephrectomized rats prevented the expected rise in systemic blood pressure, attenuated the rise in serum creatinine, and reduced the severity of glomerulosclerosis in the remnant kidneys when compared with sham rhizotomized controls.[663] To further investigate whether these benefits were solely attributable to the prevention of hypertension, five-sixths nephrectomized rats were treated with nonhypotensive doses of the sympatholytic drug moxonidine.[664] Despite the lack of effect on blood pressure, moxonidine treatment was associated with lower levels of proteinuria and less severe glomerulosclerosis than in untreated rats. In a similar study, five-sixths nephrectomized rats were treated with the α-blocker phenoxybenzamine, the β-blocker metoprolol, or a combination.[665] As in the previous study, the doses used did not lower blood pressure, but all three treatments significantly lowered albuminuria and almost normalized the reductions in capillary length density (an index of glomerular capillary obliteration) and podocyte number. Metoprolol and combination therapy significantly lowered the glomerulosclerosis index versus untreated controls. Taken together, these results indicate that increased SNA accelerates renal injury independent of its effect on blood pressure and that the adverse effects are not mediated by sympathetic cotransmitters but by catecholamines. Furthermore, sympathetic nerve overactivity has been proposed to contribute to the development of tubulointerstitial injury by reducing peritubular capillary perfusion to the extent that tubular and interstitial ischemia result.[666]

Preliminary evidence suggests that sympathetic overactivity may also be important in the progression of human CRD. Among patients with type 1 diabetes mellitus and proteinuria, evidence of parasympathetic dysfunction (that permits unopposed sympathetic tone) was associated with an increase in serum creatinine over the next 12 months.[667] Furthermore, among 15 normotensive type 1 diabetics, 3 weeks of treatment with moxonidine significantly lowered albumin excretion rates without affecting blood pressure.[668] In another study, chronic treatment with an ACEI, of proven benefit in renoprotection, was associated with a reduction in sympathetic overactivity.[669] In contrast, treatment with amlodipine was associated with increased SNA. Because ACEIs do not readily enter the CNS, it is possible that ACEIs modulate neurotransmitter release in the kidney and reduce afferent signaling. Several questions remain to be answered regarding the role of increased SNA in CRD progression. Although the renoprotective effects of sympatholytic drugs appear to be independent of effects on systemic blood pressure, it is as yet unknown what effect these drugs have on glomerular hemodynamics. Further studies are also required to determine the extent to which chronic inhibition of sympathetic overactivity may be beneficial in a variety of forms of human CRD and whether this benefit is additive to that derived from ACEI treatment.

Ethnicity

African Americans constitute only 12.4% of the total U.S. population but account for 30.8% of the U.S. ESRD population.[670] In the age group from 20 to 44 years, there are 18 African Americans for every white patient with ESRD.[671] The reasons for such obvious discrepancies in prevalence of renal disease among different ethnic groups remain unclear. A retrospective analysis of 340 routine kidney biopsy specimens detected a significantly higher prevalence of FSGS and a significantly lower prevalence of membranous glomerulonephritis and IgA and immunotactoid nephropathies among black versus white patients.[672] Similarly, among pediatric transplant recipients a higher proportion of African American and Hispanic children had FSGS as a primary diagnosis versus whites.[673] The same investigators found that despite similar treatment modalities and similar durations of nephrotic syndrome, black children with FSGS reached ESRD almost twice as frequently as white children.[673] Black children tended to have higher serum levels of creatinine and cholesterol at the disease onset. These data suggest that ethnicity is a determinant of the susceptibility to develop primary glomerular disease.

More significant in terms of patient numbers and morbidity, however, are the racial discrepancies in the incidence of hypertensive and diabetic nephropathies. The incidence of ESRD caused by diabetic nephropathy is fourfold higher among African Americans than among white Americans.[670] It is notable that after controlling for the higher prevalences of diabetes and hypertension as well as age, socioeconomic status, and access to health care, the excess incidence of ESRD caused by diabetes in blacks versus whites was confined to type 2 diabetics.[674] Among type 1 diabetics, blacks were not found to be at higher risk than whites. Indeed, the majority of blacks with diabetic ESRD (77%) have type 2 diabetes whereas the majority of whites with diabetic ESRD (58%) have type 1 diabetes.[675] Among hypertensive patients undergoing treatment, the risk of decline in renal function in black patients was found to be almost twice that of whites.[676] This finding of increased risk persisted after controlling for the effects of diabetes, blood pressure levels, heart failure, and male gender. Similarly, in the MRFIT trial, despite similar levels of blood pressure control in black versus white men, renal function deteriorated more rapidly in the black men.[532] MDRD data also showed the prevalence of hypertension to be higher in blacks versus whites among patients with CRD, despite a higher mean GFR in the black patients.[602] Hypertensive patients were found to have had more rapid progression of renal disease before entry into the study, suggesting that the increased prevalence of hypertension in black versus white patients is likely to be a significant contributor to the accelerated progression of CRD seen in blacks. In a large community-based epidemiologic study, black patients were found to have a 5.6 times higher unadjusted incidence of hypertensive ESRD with respect to the entire study population.[677] This increased incidence was directly related to the prevalence of hypertension, severe hypertension, and diabetes in the study population and inversely related to age at diagnosis of hypertension and socioeconomic status.

After adjustment for these factors the risk of hypertensive ESRD remained 4.5 times greater among blacks compared with whites, providing credible evidence that black patients have an increased susceptibility to renal disease beyond that attributable to their increased prevalence of hypertension and diabetes.

Salt-sensitive hypertension, in particular, is more prevalent in the black population than in the white population.[678] Comparing renal responses to a high sodium intake in salt-sensitive versus salt-resistant patients, RBF was found to decrease in the presence of an increased filtration fraction (implying an increased P_{GC}) in salt-sensitive patients whereas the converse occurred in salt-resistant patients.[611] These observations are consistent with the notion that salt loading injures the glomerulus through glomerular capillary hypertension and that salt-sensitive individuals, and blacks in particular, are at added risk of this form of injury. Several other potential factors contributing to the different prevalence and severity of renal disease among population groups have been analyzed: adjustment for socioeconomic factors reduces, but does not eliminate, the increased odds ratios of African Americans to develop ESRD[670]; and African Americans have lower birth weights than their white counterparts and may therefore have programmed or genetically determined deficits in nephron number, rendering them more susceptible to hypertension and subsequent ESRD.[679, 680] Finally, 40% of African American patients with hypertensive ESRD and 35% with type 2 diabetes–associated ESRD have a first-, second- or third-degree relative with ESRD, implying a strong familial susceptibility to ESRD and therefore a genetic predisposition.[681]

Anemia

Anemia is a frequent consequence of CRD but may also influence its progression. Both acute and chronic anemia are associated with reversible increases in renal vascular resistance and a normal or reduced filtration fraction in animals and humans.[682-684] Conversely, an increase in hematocrit is associated with an increase in filtration fraction.[684-686] The hematocrit-related changes in filtration fraction may be mediated chiefly by passive changes in efferent arteriolar resistance caused by variations in blood viscosity.[684] Consequently, hematocrit may influence renal hemodynamics and thereby affect the rate of progression of CRD.

The effects of anemia on glomerular hemodynamics have been studied in rats subjected to five-sixths nephrectomy, DOCA-salt hypertension, and diabetes.[687-689] Irrespective of the model, anemia was associated with significant amelioration of glomerulosclerosis and consistently associated with reduction in P_{GC}. Reduced P_{GC} arose predominantly through reductions in efferent arteriolar resistance in rats with renal ablation, lowered systolic blood pressure in DOCA-salt rats, and increased afferent arteriolar resistance in diabetic rats. Similarly, in the MWF/Ztm rat, which develops spontaneous glomerulosclerosis with age, anemia induced by dietary iron deficiency was associated with lower blood pressure, reduced urinary protein excretion, and less extensive glomerulosclerosis compared with controls fed a diet of normal iron content.[690] In contrast, however, prevention of anemia by administration of erythropoietin to remnant kidney rats to maintain a normal hematocrit resulted in increased systemic and glomerular blood pressures and markedly increased glomerulosclerosis.[687] On the other hand, recent attention has focused on potential adverse effects of anemia that may promote CRD progression, including induction of hypoxia-inducible factor that in turn binds to the promoter region of several genes that may promote renal scarring, changes in renal sympathetic nerve activity, and increased production of free radicals.[690a] Further studies are required to evaluate the relative importance of the potential beneficial and adverse effects of anemia on the progression of CRD.

Tobacco Smoking

Smoking produces acute sympathetic nervous system activation resulting in tachycardia and an increase in systolic blood pressure of up to 21 mm Hg.[691] Vasoconstriction occurs in several vascular beds, including the kidneys. Among healthy, nonsmoking volunteers, acute exposure to cigarette smoke caused an 11% increase in renovascular resistance accompanied by a 15% reduction in GFR and an 18% decrease in filtration fraction. These effects appear to be mediated, at least in part, by nicotine, because similar responses were observed after chewing nicotine gum.[692] Furthermore, the renal hemodynamic effects of smoking can be blocked by pretreatment with a β-blocker, indicating that β-adrenergic stimulation is also involved.[693] The effects of chronic smoking on the normal kidney are less well defined. Renal plasma flow but not GFR is reduced in chronic smokers, and plasma ET levels are elevated. In one population-based study, chronic smoking was associated with a small increase in creatinine clearance, implying that smoking may cause glomerular hyperfiltration.[694] That these functional abnormalities may result in structural changes to blood vessels is suggested by the observation of abnormal intrarenal vasculature in smokers.[695, 696] Moreover, epidemiologic studies have found smoking to be an important predictor of albuminuria in the general population.[694, 697] In one study, heavy smoking (>20 cigarettes/day) was associated with a relative risk for albuminuria of 1.92.[697] Furthermore, in other epidemiologic studies, smoking has been identified as a significant risk factor for renal dysfunction.[698, 699]

Although more studies are required to elucidate the effects of smoking on healthy kidneys, a growing body of evidence attests to the role of smoking as an important risk factor for disease progression in a variety of forms of CRD. The first published studies focused on diabetic nephropathy. Among type 1 diabetics smoking has been found to be a significant risk factor for the development of microalbuminuria and overt nephropathy.[700-703] Furthermore, smoking was associated with more rapid progression from microalbuminuria to overt nephropathy[704] and with almost double the rate of decline in GFR in nonsmokers.[705] Similar observations have been made among type 2 diabetics.[706-708] Several studies have also reported associations between smoking and accelerated CRD progression among nondiabetic forms of CRD. Among men with ADPKD or IgA nephropathy, a dose-dependent association between smoking and ESRD was observed, with an odds ratio of 5.8 for those with more than 15 pack-years versus less than 5 pack-years.[709] The median time to ESRD was almost halved in smokers versus nonsmokers in patients with lupus nephritis.[710] Among 295 patients with primary glomerulonephritis, those with a serum creatinine value greater than 1.7 mg/dL were significantly more likely to be smokers than those with normal creatinine values.[711] Similarly, among 73 patients with primary renal disease, the rate of decline in GFR was doubled in heavy smokers versus nonsmokers.[712] Finally, smoking was the most powerful predictor of a rise in serum creatinine level among patients with severe essential hypertension.[713]

Mechanisms whereby cigarette smoking may result in renal injury are the subject of ongoing research but are thought to include sympathetic nervous system activation, glomerular capillary hypertension, endothelial cell injury, and direct tubulotoxocity.[714] Among patients with CRD the hemodynamic effects were variable, but smoking was associated with a consistent increase in albumin/creatinine excretion.[692] Analysis of urine from both smokers and nonsmokers has revealed significantly higher excretions of thromboxane- and prostacyclin-derived products in smokers.[715] The authors suggest that increased synthesis of thromboxanes and prostacyclins may have pathologic importance for vascular injury given the biologic effects of these compounds on platelets and smooth muscle cells. An important role for sympathetic nervous system activation was suggested by an experimental study in which sympathetic denervation abrogated renal injury induced by exposure to cigarette smoke condensate.[716] A growing body of evidence thus supports the notion that the kidney is yet another organ that is adversely affected by smoking. Preliminary studies indicate that smoking cessation is therefore another intervention that may contribute to slowing the rate of progression of CRD.[717]

FUTURE DIRECTIONS

The development of pharmacologic inhibitors of the RAS provided powerful and incisive tools to explore renal hemodynamic and other associated adaptations in the setting of progressive renal injury. These physiologic insights paved the way for clinical studies that have now provided clear evidence for the use of ACEI and AT_1RA as the mainstay of renoprotective strategies.[326-329] Nevertheless, these studies have shown at best a halving of the rate of CRD progression. The present era of cell biology and molecular cloning continues to yield new insights into the mechanisms of progressive renal injury that promise to direct researchers to potential new molecular targets for renoprotective interventions. The development of the means to specifically inhibit molecular targets may provide novel forms of therapy for those with CRD and enable physicians to realize the ultimate goal of achieving remission of progressive renal injury in the majority of patients.

REFERENCES

1. Bricker NS: On the meaning of the intact nephron hypothesis. Am J Med 46:1, 1969.
2. Mitch WE, Walser M, Buffington GA, et al: A simple method for estimating progression of chronic renal failure. Lancet 2:1326-1328, 1976.
3. Rutherford WE, Blondin J, Miller JP, et al: Chronic progressive renal disease: Rate of change of serum creatinine. Kidney Int 11:62-70, 1977.
4. Brenner BM, Meyer TW, Hostetter TH: Dietary protein intake and the progressive nature of kidney disease: The role of hemodynamically mediated glomerular injury in the pathogenesis of progressive glomerular sclerosis in aging, renal ablation and intrinsic renal disease. N Engl J Med 307:652-659, 1982.

5. Addis T: Glomerular Nephritis: Diagnosis and Treatment. New York, Macmillan, 1948.

6. Braun-Menendez E, Chiodi H: La funcion renal en la rata blanca despues de la nefrectomia unilateral. Rev Soc Argen Biol 23:21-27, 1947.

7. Katz AI, Epstein FH: Relation of glomerular filtration rate and sodium reabsorption to kidney size in compensatory renal hypertrophy. Yale J Biol Med 40:222-230, 1967.

8. Bonvalet JP, Champion M, Wanstok F, et al: Compensatory hypertrophy in young rats: Increase in the number of nephrons. Kidney Int 1:391-396, 1972.

9. Bonvalet JP: Evidence of induction of new nephrons in immature kidneys undergoing hypertrophy. Yale J Biol Med 51:315-319, 1978.

10. Canter CE, Goss RJ: Induction of extra nephrons in unilaterally nephrectomized immature rats (38525). Proc Soc Exp Biol Med 148:294-296, 1975.

11. Imbert MJ, Berjal G, Moss N, et al: Number of nephrons in hypertrophic kidneys after unilateral nephrectomy in young and adult rats. Pflugers Arch 346:279-290, 1974.

12. Kaufman JM, Hardy R, Hayslett JP: Age-dependent characteristics of compensatory renal growth. Kidney Int 8:21-26, 1975.

13. Larsson L, Aperia A, Wilton P: Effect of normal development on compensatory renal growth. Kidney Int 18:29-35, 1980.

14. Deen WM, Maddox DA, Robertson CR, et al: Dynamics of glomerular ultrafiltration in the rat: VII. Response to reduced renal mass. Am J Physiol 227:556-562, 1974.

15. Miller PL, Rennke HG, Meyer TW: Glomerular hypertrophy accelerates hypertensive glomerular injury in rats. Am J Physiol (Renal Fluid Electrolyte Physiol) 261:F459-F465, 1991.

16. Kaufman JM, Siegel NJ, Hayslett JP: Functional and hemodynamic adaptation to progressive renal ablation. Circ Res 36:286-293, 1975.

17. Hostetter TH, Olson JL, Rennke HG, et al: Hyperfiltration in remnant nephrons: A potentially adverse response to renal ablation. Am J Physiol 241:F85-F93, 1981.

18. Pelayo JC, Quan AH, Shanley PF: Angiotensin II control of the renal microcirculation in rats with reduced renal mass. Am J Physiol (Renal Fluid Electrolyte Physiol) 258:F414-F422, 1990.

19. Kasiske BL, O'Donnel MP, Garvis WJ, et al: Pharmacologic treatment of hyperlipidemia reduces injury in rat 5/6 nephrectomy model of chronic renal failure. Circ Res 62:367-374, 1988.

20. Buerkert J, Martin D, Prasad J, et al: Response of deep nephrons and the terminal collecting duct to a reduction in renal mass. Am J Physiol (Renal Fluid Electrolyte Physiol) 236:F454-F464, 1979.

21. Brown SA, Finco DR, Crowell WA, et al: Single-nephron adaptations to partial renal ablation in the dog. Am J Physiol (Renal Fluid Electrolyte Physiol) 258:F495-503, 1990.

22. Krohn AG, Ogden DA, Holmes JH: Renal function in 29 healthy adults before and after nephrectomy. JAMA 196:322, 1966.

23. Flanigan WJ, Burns RO, Takacs FJ, et al: Serial studies of glomerular filtration rate and renal plasma flow in kidney transplant donors, identical twins, and allograft recipients. Am J Surg 116:788-794, 1968.

24. Kasiske BL, Ma JZ, Louis TA, et al: Long-term effects of reduced renal mass in humans. Kidney Int 48:814-819, 1995.

25. Blantz RC, Konnen KS, Tucker BJ: Angiotensin II effects upon the glomerular microcirculation and ultrafiltration coefficient of the rat. J Clin Invest 57:419-434, 1976.

26. Ichikawa I, Miele JF, Brenner BM: Reversal of renal cortical actions of angiotensin II by verapamil and manganese. Kidney Int 16: 137-147, 1979.

27. Myers B, Deen WM, Brenner BM: Effects of norepinephrine and angiotensin II on the determinants of glomerular ultrafiltration and proximal tubule fluid reabsorption in the rat. Circ Res 37:101-110, 1975.

28. Anderson S, Meyers TW, Rennke HG, et al: Control of glomerular hypertension limits glomerular injury in rats with reduced renal mass. J Clin Invest 76:612-619, 1985.

29. Anderson S, Rennke HG, Brenner BM: Therapeutic advantage of converting enzyme inhibitors in arresting progressive renal disease associated with systemic hypertension in the rat. J Clin Invest 77:1993-2000, 1986.

30. Lafayette RA, Mayer G, Park SK, et al: Angiotensin II receptor blockade limits glomerular injury in rats with reduced renal mass. J Clin Invest 90:766-771, 1992.

31. Mackenzie HS, Troy JL, Rennke HG, et al: TCV116 prevents progressive renal injury in rats with extensive renal mass ablation. J Hypertens 12(suppl 9):S11-S16, 1994.

32. Rosenberg ME, Kren SM, Hostetter TH: Effect of dietary protein on the renin-angiotensin system in subtotally nephrectomized rats. Kidney Int 38:240-248, 1990.

33. Baboolal K, Meyer TW: The effect of acute angiotensin II blockade on renal function in rats with reduced renal mass. Kidney Int 46: 980-985, 1994.

34. Correa-Rotter R, Hostetter TH, Manivel JC, et al: Renin expression in renal ablation. Hypertension 20:483-490, 1992.

35. Pupilli C, Chevalier RL, Carey RM, et al: Distribution and content of renin and renin mRNA in remnant kidney of adult rat. Am J Physiol (Renal Fluid Electrolyte Physiol) 263:F731-F738, 1992.

36. Rosenberg ME, Correa-Rotter R, Inagami T, et al: Glomerular renin synthesis and storage in the remnant kidney in the rat. Kidney Int 40:677-683, 1991.

37. Griffin KA, Picken M, Bidani AK: Method of renal mass reduction is a critical modulator of subsequent hypertension and glomerular injury. J Am Soc Nephrol 4:2023-2031, 1994.

38. Mackie FE, Campbell DJ, Meyer TW: Intrarenal angiotensin and bradykinin peptide levels in the remnant kidney model of renal insufficiency. Kidney Int 59:1458-1465, 2001.

39. Mackie FE, Meyer TW, Campbell DJ: Effects of antihypertensive therapy on intrarenal angiotensin and bradykinin levels in experimental renal insufficiency. Kidney Int 61:555-563, 2002.

40. Benigni A, Perico N, Gaspari F, et al: Increased renal endothelin production in rats with reduced renal mass. Am J Physiol 260:F331-F339, 1991.

41. Orisio S, Benigni A, Bruzzi I, et al: Renal endothelin gene expression is increased in remnant kidney and correlates with disease progression. Kidney Int 43:354-358, 1993.

42. Takabatake T, Ise T, Ohta K, et al: Effects of endothelin on renal hemodynamics and tubuloglomerular feedback. Am J Physiol 263:F103-F108, 1992.

43. Katoh T, Chang H, Uchida S, et al: Direct effects of endothelin in the rat kidney. Am J Physiol 258:F397-F402, 1990.

44. Claria J, Jimenez W, La VG, et al: Effects of endothelin on renal haemodynamics and segmental sodium handling in conscious rats. Acta Physiol Scand 141:305-308, 1991.

45. Munger KA, Takahashi K, Awazu M, et al: Maintenance of endothelin-induced renal arteriolar constriction in rats is cyclooxygenase dependent. Am J Physiol 264:F637-F644, 1993.

46. Martinez F, Deray G, Dubois M, et al: Chronic effects of endothelin-3 on blood pressure and renal haemodynamics in rats. Nephrol Dial Transplant 11:270-274, 1996.

47. Badr KF, Murray JJ, Breyer MD, et al: Mesangial cell, glomerular and renal vascular responses to endothelin in the rat kidney. J Clin Invest 83:336-342, 1989.

48. Kon V, Yoshioka T, Fogo A, et al: Glomerular actions of endothelin in vivo. J Clin Invest 83:1762-1767, 1989.

49. King AJ, Brenner BM, Anderson S: Endothelin: A potent renal and systemic vasoconstrictor peptide. Am J Physiol 256:F1051-F1058, 1989.

50. Munger KA, Takahashi K, Awazu M, et al: Maintenance of endothelin-induced renal arteriolar constriction in rats in cyclooxygenase dependent. Am J Physiol 264:F1091-1097, 1993.

51. Ortola FV, Ballermann BJ, Brenner BM: Endogenous ANP augments fractional excretion of Pi, Ca, and Na in rats with reduced renal mass. Am J Physiol 255:F1091-F1097, 1988.

52. Smith S, Anderson S, Ballerman BJ, et al: Role of atrial natriuretic peptide in adaptation of sodium excretion with reduced renal mass. J Clin Invest 77:1395-1398, 1986.

53. Brandt MA, Fink GD, Chimoskey JE: Plasma atrial natriuretic peptide in conscious rats with reduced renal mass. FASEB J 3:2302-2307, 1989.

54. Zhang PL, Mackenzie HS, Troy JL, et al: Effects of natriuretic peptide receptor inhibition on remnant kidney function in rats. Kidney Int 46:414-420, 1994.

55. Dunn BR, Ichikawa I, Pfeffer JM, et al: Renal and systemic hemodynamic effects of synthetic atrial natriuretic peptide in the anesthetized rat. Circ Res 59:237-246, 1986.

56. Kirschenbaum MA, Serros ER: Effect of prostaglandin inhibition on glomerular filtration rate in normal and uremic rabbits. Prostaglandins 22:245-254, 1981.

57. Nath KA, Chmielewski DH, Hostetter TH: Regulatory role of prostanoids in glomerular microcirculation of remnant nephrons. Am J Physiol 252:F829-F837, 1987.

58. Pelayo JC, Shanley PF: Glomerular and tubular adaptive responses to acute nephron loss in the rat: Effect of prostaglandin synthesis inhibition. J Clin Invest 85:1761-1769, 1990.

59. Stahl RA, Kudelka S, Paravicini M, et al: Prostaglandin and thromboxane formation in glomeruli from rats with reduced renal mass. Nephron 42:252-257, 1986.

60. Jackson EK, Heidemann HT, Branch RA, et al: Low dose intrarenal infusions of PGE2, PGI2, and 6-keto-PGE1 vasodilate the in vivo rat kidney. Circ Res 51:67-72, 1982.

61. Griffin KA, Bidani AK, Picken M, et al: Prostaglandins do not mediate impaired autoregulation or increased renin secretion in remnant rat kidneys. Am J Physiol 263:F1057-F1062, 1992.

62. De Nicola L, Blantz RC, Gabbai FB: Nitric oxide and angiotensin II: Glomerular and tubular interaction in the rat. J Clin Invest 89:1248-1256, 1992.

63. Griffin KA, Bidani AK, Ouyang J, et al: Role of endothelium-derived nitric oxide in hemodynamic adaptations after graded renal mass reduction. Am J Physiol 264:R1254-R1259, 1993.

64. Granger JP, Alberola AM, Salazar FJ, et al: Control of renal hemodynamics during intrarenal and systemic blockade of nitric oxide synthesis in conscious dogs. J Cardiovasc Pharmacol 20(suppl 12):S160-S162, 1992.

65. Yukimura T, Yamashita Y, Miura K, et al: Renal effects of the nitric oxide synthase inhibitor, L-NG-nitroarginine, in dogs. Am J Hypertens 5:484-487, 1992.

66. Denton KM, Anderson WP: Intrarenal haemodynamic and glomerular responses to inhibition of nitric oxide formation in rabbits. J Physiol (Lond) 475:159-167, 1994.

67. Fujihara CK, De NG, Zatz R: Chronic nitric oxide synthase inhibition aggravates glomerular injury in rats with subtotal nephrectomy. J Am Soc Nephrol 5:1498-1507, 1995.

67a. Fujihara CK, Mattar AL, Vieira JM Jr, et al: Evidence for the existence of two distinct functions for the inducible NO synthase in the rat kidney: Effect of aminoguanidine in rats with 5/6 ablation. J Am Soc Nephrol 13:2278-2287, 2002.

68. Bidani AK, Schwartz MM, Lewis EJ: Renal autoregulation and vulnerability to hypertensive injury in remnant kidney. Am J Physiol (Renal Fluid Electrolyte Physiol) 252:F1003-F1010, 1987.

69. Pelayo JC, Westcott JY: Impaired autoregulation of glomerular capillary hydrostatic pressure in the rat remnant nephron. J Clin Invest 88:101-105, 1991.

70. Salmond R, Seney FD: Reset tubuloglomerular feedback permits and sustains glomerular hyperfunction after extensive renal ablation. Am J Physiol (Renal Fluid Electrolyte Physiol) 260:F395-F401, 1991.

71. Braam B, Mitchell KD, Koomans HA, et al: Relevance of the tubuloglomerular feedback mechanism in pathophysiology. Editorial. J Am Soc Nephrol 4:1257-1274, 1993.

72. Müller-Suur R, Norlén B-J, Persson EG: Resetting of tubuloglomerular feedback in rat kidneys after unilateral nephrectomy. Kidney Int 18:48-57, 1980.

73. Peters G: Introduction: History and problems of compensatory adaptation of renal functions and of compensatory hypertrophy of the kidney. Yale J Biol Med 51:235-245, 1978.

74. Fine L: The biology of renal hypertrophy. Kidney Int 29:619-634, 1986.

75. Wesson LG: Compensatory growth and other growth responses of the kidney. Nephron 51:149-184, 1989.

76. Dicker SE, Shirley DG: Compensatory hypertrophy of the contralateral kidney after unilateral ureteral ligation. J Physiol (Lond) 220:199-210, 1972.

77. Mason RC, Ewald BH: Studies on compensatory renal hypertrophy: I. Effect of unilateral ureteral ligation and transection. Proc Soc Exp Biol Med 120:210-214, 1965.

78. Morris GC: Growth of rats' kidneys after unilateral uretero-caval anastomosis. J Physiol (Lond) 258:755-767, 1976.

79. Paulson DF, Fraley EE: Chemical evidence for early but unsustained growth in the obstructed mouse kidney. Am J Physiol 219:872-875, 1970.

80. Paulson DF, Fraley EE: Compensatory renal growth after unilateral ureteral obstruction. Kidney Int 4:22-27, 1973.

81. Kramp RA, MacDowell M, Gottschalk CW, et al: A study by microdissection and micropuncture of the structure and the function of the kidneys and the nephrons of rats with chronic renal damage. Kidney Int 5:147-176, 1974.

82. Lowenstein LM, Toback FG: Metabolic response to renal compensatory growth. Yale J Biol Med 51:395-401, 1978.

83. Toback FG, Smith PD, Lowenstein LM: Phospholipid metabolism in the initiation of renal compensatory growth after acute reduction of renal mass. J Clin Invest 54:91-97, 1974.

84. Bean GH, Lowenstein LM: Choline pathways during normal and stimulated renal growth in rats. J Clin Invest 61:1551-1554, 1978.

85. Austin H, Goldin H, Gaydos D, et al: Polyamine metabolism in compensatory renal growth. Kidney Int 23:581-587, 1983.

86. Brandt JT, Pierce DA, Fausto N: Ornithine decarboxylase activity and polyamine synthesis during kidney hypertrophy. Biochim Biophys Acta 279:184-193, 1972.

87. Desiderio MA, Sessa A, Perin A: Induction of diamine oxidase activity in rat kidney during compensatory hypertrophy. Biochim Biophys Acta 714:243-249, 1982.

88. Halliburton IW, Thomson RY: Early chemical changes in compensatory renal hypertrophy. Biochem J 99:44P-45P, 1966.

89. Ouellette AJ, Malt RA: Noncoordinate regulation of cytoplasmic RNA in compensatory renal hypertrophy. Am J Physiol 237:R360-R365, 1979.

90. Ouellette AJ: Messenger RNA regulation during compensatory renal growth. Kidney Int 23:575-580, 1983.

91. Ouellette AJ, Moonka R, Zelenetz AD, et al: Regulation of ribosome synthesis during compensatory renal hypertrophy in mice. Am J Physiol 253:C506-C513, 1987.

92. Johnson HA, Vera RJ: Compensatory renal enlargement: Hypertrophy versus hyperplasia. Am J Pathol 49:1-13, 1966.

93. Dicker SE: Changes in renal cyclic nucleotides as a trigger to the onset of compensatory renal hypertrophy. Yale J Biol Med 51:381-385, 1978.

94. Schlondorff D, Weber H: Evidence for altered cyclic nucleotide metabolism during compensatory renal hypertrophy and neonatal kidney growth. Yale J Biol Med 51:387-392, 1978.

95. Yusufi AN, Dancona C, Nguyen JL, et al: Early changes of guanylate cyclase and cGMP phosphodiesterase activities in glomeruli and tubules isolated from the remaining kidney after unilateral nephrectomy in the rabbit. Ren Physiol 6:80-86, 1983.

96. Solomon S, Wise PM, Sanborn C, et al: Cyclic nucleotide concentrations in relation to renal growth and hypertrophy. Yale J Biol Med 51:373-379, 1978.

97. Hoang T, Bergeron M: Segmental heterogeneity of enzymatic response during compensatory renal growth. Growth 49:439-449, 1985.

98. Mayfield EJ, Liebelt RA, Bresnick E: Activities of enzymes of deoxyribonucleic acid synthesis after unilateral nephrectomy. Cancer Res 27:1652-1657, 1967.

99. Reiter RJ: Cellular proliferation and deoxyribonucleic acid synthesis in compensating kidneys of mice and the effect of food and water restriction. Lab Invest 14:1636-1643, 1965.

100. Sulkin NM: Cytological studies of the remaining kidney following unilateral nephrectomy in the rat. Anat Rec 105:95-107, 1949.

101. Halliburton IW, Thomson RY: Chemical aspects of compensatory renal hypertrophy. Cancer Res 25:1882-1887, 1965.

102. Kaufman JM, DiMeola HJ, Siegel NJ, et al: Compensatory adaptation of structure and function following progressive renal ablation. Kidney Int 6:10-17, 1974.

103. Celsi G, Jakobsson B, Aperia A: Influence of age on compensatory renal growth in rats. Pediatr Res 20:347-350, 1986.

104. Barrows CH, Roeder LM, Olewine DA: Effect of age on renal compensatory hypertrophy following unilateral nephrectomy in the rat. J Gerontol 17:148-150, 1962.

105. Hayslett JP: Effect of age on compensatory renal growth. Kidney Int 23:599-602, 1983.

106. MacKay EM, MacKay LL, Addis T: The degree of compensatory renal hypertrophy following unilateral nephrectomy. J Exp Med 56:255-265, 1932.

107. Boner G, Sherry J, Rieselbach RE: Hypertrophy of the normal human kidney following contralateral nephrectomy. Nephron 9:364-370, 1972.

108. Donadio JJ, Farmer CD, Hunt JC, et al: Renal function in donors and recipients of renal allotransplantation: Radioisotopic measurements. Ann Intern Med 66:105-115, 1967.

109. Dossetor RS: Renal compensatory hypertrophy in the adult. Br J Radiol 48:993-995, 1975.

110. Tapson JS, Owen JP, Robson RA, et al: Compensatory renal hypertrophy after donor nephrectomy. Clin Radiol 36:307-310, 1985.

111. Ekelund L, Gothlin J: Compensatory renal enlargement in older patients. Am J Roentgenol 127:713-715, 1976.

112. Edgren J, Laasonen L, Kock B, et al: Kidney function and compensatory growth of the kidney in living kidney donors. Scand J Urol Nephrol 10:134-136, 1976.

113. Heideman HD, Rosenbaum HD: A study of renal size after contralateral nephrectomy. Radiology 94:599-601, 1970.

114. Gomez AB, Carrero LV, Diaz GR: Image-directed color Doppler ultrasound evaluation of the single kidney after unilateral nephrectomy in adults. J Clin Ultrasound 25:29-35, 1997.

115. Gudinchet F, Meuli R, Regazzoni B: Compensatory renal growth in children and adults studied by Doppler sonography. J Clin Ultrasound 22:11-15, 1994.

116. Schmitz A, Christensen CK, Christensen T, et al: No microalbuminuria or other adverse effects of long-standing hyperfiltration in humans with one kidney. Am J Kidney Dis 13:131-136, 1989.

117. Prassopoulos P, Gourtsoyiannis N, Cavouras D, et al: CT evaluation of compensatory renal growth in relation to postnephrectomy time. Acta Radiol 33:566-568, 1992.

118. Prassopoulos P, Cavouras D, Gourtsoyiannis N: Pre- and postnephrectomy kidney enlargement in patients with contralateral renal cancer. Eur Urol 24:58-61, 1993.

119. Oliver J: The regulation of renal activity: X. The morphological study. Arch Intern Med 34:258-265, 1924.

120. Olivetti G, Anversa P, Rigamonti W, et al: Morphometry of the renal corpuscle during normal postnatal growth and compensatory hypertrophy: A light microscope study. J Cell Biol 75:573-585, 1977.

121. Olivetti G, Anversa P, Melissari M, et al: Morphometry of the renal corpuscle during postnatal growth and compensatory hypertrophy. Kidney Int 17:438-454, 1980.

122. Seyer-Hansen K, Gundersen HJ, Osterby R: Stereology of the rat kidney during compensatory renal hypertrophy. Acta Pathol Microbiol Immunol Scand 93:9-12, 1985.

123. Shea SM, Raskova J, Morrison AB: A stereologic study of glomerular hypertrophy in the subtotally nephrectomized rat. Am J Pathol 90:201-210, 1978.

124. Nyengaard JR: Number and dimensions of rat glomerular capillaries in normal development and after nephrectomy. Kidney Int 43:1049-1057, 1993.

125. Schwartz MM, Churchill M, Bidani A, et al: Reversible compensatory hypertrophy in rat kidneys: Morphometric characterization. Kidney Int 43:610-614, 1993.

126. Lee GS, Nast CC, Peng SC, et al: Differential response of glomerular epithelial and mesangial cells after subtotal nephrectomy. Kidney Int 53:1389-1398, 1998.

127. Amann K, Irzyniec T, Mall G, et al: The effect of enalapril on glomerular growth and glomerular lesions after subtotal nephrectomy in the rat: A stereological analysis. J Hypertens 11:969-975, 1993.

128. Bidani AK, Mitchell KD, Schwartz MM, et al: Absence of glomerular injury or nephron loss in a normotensive rat remnant kidney model. Kidney Int 38:28-38, 1990.

129. Daniels BS, Hostetter TH: Adverse effects of growth in the glomerular microcirculation. Am J Physiol 258:F1409-F1416, 1990.

130. Schwartz MM, Evans J, Bidani AK: The mesangium in the long-term remnant kidney model. J Lab Clin Med 124:644-651, 1994.

131. Cortes P, Zhao X, Riser BL, et al: Regulation of glomerular volume in normal and partially nephrectomized rats. Am J Physiol 270:F356-F370, 1996.

132. Miller PL, Meyer TW: Effects of tissue preparation on glomerular volume and capillary structure in the rat. Lab Invest 63:862-866, 1990.

133. Churchill M, Churchill PC, Schwartz M, et al: Reversible compensatory hypertrophy in transplanted brown Norway rat kidneys. Kidney Int 40:13-20, 1991.

134. Valentin JP, Sechi LA, Griffin CA, et al: The renin-angiotensin system and compensatory renal hypertrophy in the rat. Am J Hypertens 10:397-402, 1997.

135. Katz AI, Toback FG, Lindheimer MD: The role of renal "work" in compensatory kidney growth. Yale J Biol Med 51:331-337, 1978.

136. Tabei K, Levenson DJ, Brenner BM: Early enhancement of fluid transport in rabbit proximal straight tubules after loss of contralateral renal excretory function. J Clin Invest 72:871-881, 1983.

137. Trizna W, Yanagawa N, Bar-Khayim Y, et al: Functional profile of the isolated uremic nephron. J Clin Invest 68:760-767, 1981.

138. Fine LG, Trizna W, Bourgoignie JJ, et al: Functional profile of the isolated uremic nephron: Role of compensatory hypertrophy in the control of fluid reabsorption by the proximal straight tubule. J Clin Invest 61:1508-1518, 1978.

139. Allison ME, Wilson CB, Gottschalk CW: Pathophysiology of experimental glomerulonephritis in rats. J Clin Invest 53:1402-1423, 1974.

140. Ichikawa I, Hoyer JR, Seiler MW, et al: Mechanism of glomerulotubular balance in the setting of heterogeneous glomerular injury. J Clin Invest 69:185-198, 1982.

141. Oliver J: Architecture of the Kidney in Chronic Bright's Disease. New York, Hoeber, 1939.

142. Baylis C, Rennke HG: Renal hemodynamics and glomerular morphology in repetitively pregnant aging rats. Kidney Int 28:140-145, 1985.

143. Davison JM, Lindheimer MD: Changes in renal haemodynamics and kidney weight during pregnancy in the unanaesthetized rat. J Physiol (Lond) 301:129-136, 1980.

144. Garland HO, Green R, Moriarty RJ: Changes in body weight, kidney weight and proximal tubule length during pregnancy in the rat. Renal Physiol 1:42-47, 1978.

145. Matthews BF: Growth of the maternal kidneys in pregnant mice. Proceedings. J Physiol (Lond) 273:84P, 1977.

146. Mogensen CE, Andersen MJ: Increased kidney size and glomerular filtration rate in untreated juvenile diabetes: Normalization by insulin-treatment. Diabetologia 11:221-224, 1975.

147. Seyer-Hansen K: Renal hypertrophy in streptozotocin-diabetic rats. Clin Sci Mol Med Suppl 51:551-555, 1976.

148. Zatz R, Dunn BR, Meyer TW, et al: Prevention of diabetic glomerulopathy by pharmacological amelioration of glomerular capillary hypertension. J Clin Invest 77:1925-1930, 1986.

149. Bugge-Asperheim B, Kiil F: Examination of growth-mediated changes in hemodynamics and tubular transport of sodium, glucose and hippurate after nephrectomy. Scand J Clin Lab Invest 22:255-265, 1968.

150. Simpson DP: Hyperplasia after unilateral nephrectomy and role of excretory load in its production. Am J Physiol 201:517-522, 1961.

151. Weinman EJ, Renquist K, Stroup R, et al: Increased tubular reabsorption of sodium in compensatory renal growth. Am J Physiol 224:565-571, 1973.

152. Epstein FH, Charney AN, Silva P: Factors influencing the increase in Na-K-ATPase in compensatory renal hypertrophy. Yale J Biol Med 51:365-372, 1978.

153. Toback FG, Ordonez NG, Bortz SL, et al: Zonal changes in renal structure and phospholipid metabolism in potassium-deficient rats. Lab Invest 34:115-124, 1976.

154. Toback FG, Havener LJ, Spargo BH: Stimulation of renal phospholipid formation during potassium depletion. Am J Physiol 233:E212-E218, 1977.

155. Royce PC: Inhibition of renal growth following unilateral nephrectomy in the rat. Proc Soc Exp Biol Med 113:1046-1049, 1963.

156. Harris RH, Best CF: Circulatory retention of urinary factors as a stimulus to renal growth. Kidney Int 12:305-312, 1977.

157. Krohn AG, Peng BB, Antell HI, et al: Compensatory renal hypertrophy: The role of immediate vascular changes in its production. J Urol 103:564-568, 1970.

158. Potter DE, Leumann EP, Sakai T, et al: Early responses of glomerular filtration rate to unilateral nephrectomy. Kidney Int 5:131-136, 1974.

159. Austin HD, Goldin H, Preuss HG: Humoral regulation of renal growth: Evidence for and against the presence of a circulating renotropic factor. Nephron 27:163-170, 1981.

160. Kurnick NB, Lindsay PA: Compensatory renal hypertrophy in parabiotic mice. Lab Invest 19:45-48, 1968.

161. Thompson JW, Lytton B: Compensatory renal hypertrophy in parabiotic rats. J Urol 98:548-551, 1967.

162. Lytton B, Schiff MJ, Bloom N: Compensatory renal growth: Evidence for tissue specific factor of renal origin. J Urol 101:648-652, 1969.

163. Johnson HA, Vera Roman JM: Renal epithelial hyperplasia: Failure to demonstrate a humoral control factor. Cell Tiss Kinet 1:35-41, 1968.

164. Van Vroonhoven TJ, Soler-Montesinos L, Malt RA: Humoral regulation of renal mass. Surgery 72:300-305, 1972.

165. Dijkhuis CM, van UH, Malamud D, et al: Rapid reversal of compensatory renal hypertrophy after withdrawal of the stimulus. Surgery 78:476-480, 1975.

166. Dicker SE, Greenbaum AL: Changes in renal cyclic nucleotide content as a possible trigger to the initiation of compensatory renal hypertrophy in rats. J Physiol 271:505-514, 1977.

167. Obertop H, Malt RA: Lost mass and excretion as stimuli to parabiotic compensatory renal hypertrophy. Am J Physiol 232:F405-F408, 1977.

168. Van Urk H, Malamud D, Soler-Montesinos L, et al: Compensatory hyperplasia with increasing loss of renal mass. Lab Invest 38:674-676, 1978.

169. Shames D, Murphy JJ, Berkowitz H: Evidence for a humoral factor in unilaterally nephrectomized dogs stimulating renal growth in isolated canine kidneys. Surgery 79:573-576, 1976.

170. Connolly JG, Demelker J, Promislow C: Compensatory renal hyperplasia. Can J Surg 12:236-240, 1969.

171. Reiter RJ, McCreight CE: Failure to demonstrate a humoral factor controlling compensatory renal hyperplasia. Anat Rec 148:396-397, 1964.

172. Williams GEG: Studies on the control of compensatory hyperplasia of the kidney in the rat. Lab Invest 11:1295-1302, 1962.

173. Lowenstein LM, Stern A: Serum factor in renal compensatory hyperplasia. Science 142:1479-1480, 1963.

174. Silk MR, Homsy GE, Merz T: Compensatory renal hyperplasia. J Urol 98:36-39, 1967.

175. Vichi FL, Earle DP: Renal hypertrophy factor in serum of nephrectomized rats, with observations on species specificity. Proc Soc Exp Biol Med 135:38-41, 1970.

176. Kurnick NB, Lindsay PA: Mechanism of compensatory renal hypertrophy: Possible role of serum factor. Lab Invest 17:211-216, 1967.

177. Dicker SE, Morris CA: Presence of renotropic factor in plasma of unilaterally nephrectomized rats. J Physiol (Lond) 299:13-27, 1980.

178. Ogawa K, Nowinski WW: Mitosis stimulating factor in serum of unilaterally nephrectomized rats. Proc Soc Exp Biol Med 99:350-353, 1958.

179. Preuss HG, Terryi EF, Keller AI: Renotropic factor(s) in plasma from uninephrectomized rats. Nephron 7:459-470, 1970.

180. Preuss HG, Goldin H: Humoral regulation of compensatory renal growth. Med Clin North Am 59:771-780, 1975.

181. Preuss HG, Goldin H: A renotropic system in rats. J Clin Invest 57:94-101, 1976.

182. Preuss HG, Goldin H: Effects of the rat renotropic system on ^{14}C-uridine incorporation into RNA and RNA precursors. Life Sci 25:497-505, 1979.

183. Castillo O, Robertson D, Goldin H, et al: Autoradiographic studies of the rat renotropic system. Nephron 25:202-206, 1980.

184. Hernandez W, Goldin H, Shivers M, et al: Studies on the tissue specificity of a circulating renotropic factor. Acta Physiol Lat Am 29:117-122, 1979.

185. Kukolja S, Pokrajac N, Banfic H: Plasma from uninephrectomized rats increases ^{32}P incorporation into phospholipids of renal cortical slices. Nephron 43:62-66, 1986.

186. Lyons HJ, Evan AP, McLaren LC, et al: In vitro evidence for a renotrophic factor in renal compensatory hypertrophy. Nephron 13:198-211, 1974.

187. Kanetake H, Yamamoto N: Studies on the mechanism of compensatory renal hypertrophy and hyperplasia in a nephrectomized animal model: I. Evidence for a renotropic growth stimulating factor in uninephrectomized rabbit sera using tissue culture. Invest Urol 18:326-330, 1981.

188. Yamamoto N, Kanetake H, Yamada J: In vitro evidence from tissue cultures to prove existence of rabbit and human renotropic growth factor. Kidney Int 23:624-631, 1983.

189. Cortes P, Levin NW, Martin PR: Ribonucleic acid synthesis in the renal cortex at the initiation of compensatory growth. Biochem J 158:457-470, 1976.

190. Gaydos DS, Goldin H, Jenson B, et al: Partial characterization of a renotropic factor. Ren Physiol 6:139-144, 1983.

191. Harris RH, Hise MK, Best CF: Renotrophic factors in urine. Kidney Int 23:616-623, 1983.

192. Braun-Menéndez E: Evidence for renotrophin as a causal factor in renal hypertension. Circulation 17:696-701, 1958.

193. Dicker SE: Factors influencing compensatory renal hyperplasia. J Physiol (Lond) 214:14P-15P, 1971.

194. Dicker SE, Morris CA: Investigation of a substance of renal origin which inhibits the growth of renal cortex explant in vitro. J Embryol Exp Morphol 31:655-665, 1974.

195. Dicker SE, Morris C: Proceedings: Renal control of kidney growth. J Physiol (Lond) 241:20P-21P, 1974.

196. Dicker SE, Morris CA, Shipolini RA: Proceedings: Inhibition of compensatory renal hypertrophy by the renal cortex. J Physiol (Lond) 258:90P, 1976.

197. Dicker SE, Morris CA, Shipolini R: Regulation of compensatory kidney hypertrophy by its own products. J Physiol (Lond) 269:687-705, 1977.

198. Dicker SE, Morris CA, Pearce FL: Role of a renal arginylesteropeptidase in the production of a renotrophic factor in unilaterally nephrectomized rats. J Physiol (Lond) 315:413-419, 1981.

199. Astarabadi TM, Essex HE: Effect of hypophysectomy on compensatory renal hypertrophy after unilateral nephrectomy. Am J Physiol 173:526-534, 1953.

200. Astarabadi T: The effect of hypophysectomy, adrenalectomy and ACTH administration on compensatory renal hypertrophy in rats. Q J Exp Physiol 48:80-84, 1963.

201. Astarabadi T: The effect of growth and lactogenic hormones on renal compensatory hypertrophy in hypophysectomized rats. Q J Exp Physiol 48:85-92, 1963.

202. Goss RJ, Rankin M: Physiological factors affecting compensatory renal hyperplasia in the rat. J Exp Zool 145:209-216, 1960.

203. McCreight CE, Reiter RJ: Effects of hormones on the renal response to unilateral nephrectomy in hypophysectomized rats. J Exp Zool 166:65-69, 1967.

204. McQueen-Williams M, Thompson KW: The effect of ablation of the hypophysis upon the weight of the kidney of the rat. Yale J Biol Med 12:531-541, 1939.

205. Rolf D, White HL: Endocrine influences on renal compensatory hypertrophy. Endocrinology 53:436-440, 1953.

206. Ross J, Goldman JK: Compensatory renal hypertrophy in hypophysectomized rats. Endocrinology 87:620-624, 1970.

207. Dicker SE, Greenbaum AL, Morris CA: Compensatory renal hypertrophy in hypophysectomized rats. J Physiol (Lond) 273:241-253, 1977.

208. Nicholson WE, Barton RN, Puett D, et al: Evidence for renotropic activity in ovine pituitaries. Endocrinology 105:16-20, 1979.

209. Nomura K, Mizuhira V, Shiihashi M, et al: Renotropic stimulation of DNA synthesis of proximal tubules and endothelial cells in the outer medulla. Nephron 39:255-260, 1985.

210. Haramati A, Lumpkin MD, Mulroney SE: Early increase in pulsatile growth hormone release after unilateral nephrectomy in adult rats. Am J Physiol 266:F628-F632, 1994.

211. Bradley SE, Coelho JB, Sealey JE, et al: Changes in glomerulotubular dimensions, single nephron glomerular filtration rates and the renin-angiotensin system in hypothyroid rats. Life Sci 30:633-639, 1982.

212. Korenchevsky V, Hall K: Correlation between sex hormones, thyroid hormones and desoxycorticosterone as judged by their effects on the weights of organs of gonadectomized rats. Biochem J 35:726-735, 1941.

213. Zeckwer IT: Compensatory growth of the kidney after unilateral nephrectomy in thyroidectomized rats. Am J Physiol 145:531-541, 1945-1946.

214. Ludden JB, Kreuger E, Wright IS: Effect of testosterone propionate, estradiol benzoate and desoxycorticosterone acetate on the kidneys of adult rats. Endocrinology 28:619-623, 1941.

215. Basinger GT, Gittes RF: Effect of testosterone propionate on compensatory renal hypertrophy. Endocrinology 94:599-601, 1974.

216. MacKay EM: Degree of compensatory renal hypertrophy following unilateral nephrectomy: III. Influence of testosterone propionate. Proc Soc Exp Biol Med 45:216-217, 1940.

217. Malt RA, Ohno S, Paddock JK: Compensatory renal hypertrophy in the absence of androgen binding. Endocrinology 96:806-807, 1975.

218. Schlondorff D, Trizna W, De RE, et al: Effect of testosterone on compensatory renal hypertrophy in the rat. Endocrinology 101:1670-1675, 1977.

219. Hammerman MR, O'Shea M, Miller SB: Role of growth factors in regulation of renal growth. Annu Rev Physiol 55:305-321, 1993.

220. Fine LG, Hammerman MR, Abboud HE: Evolving role of growth factors in the renal response to acute and chronic disease. Editorial. J Am Soc Nephrol 2:1163-1170, 1992.

221. Stiles AD, Sosenko IR, D'Ercole AJ, et al: Relation of kidney tissue somatomedin-C/insulin-like growth factor I to postnephrectomy renal growth in the rat. Endocrinology 117:2397-2401, 1985.

222. Fagin JA, Melmed S: Relative increase in insulin-like growth factor I messenger ribonucleic acid levels in compensatory renal hypertrophy. Endocrinology 120:718-724, 1987.

223. Flyvbjerg A, Thorlacius UO, Naeraa R, et al: Kidney tissue somatomedin C and initial renal growth in diabetic and uninephrectomized rats. Diabetologia 31:310-314, 1988.

224. Lajara R, Rotwein P, Bortz JD, et al: Dual regulation of insulin-like growth factor I expression during renal hypertrophy. Am J Physiol 257:F252-F261, 1989.

225. Shohat J, Davidowitz M, Erman A, et al: Serum and renal IGF-I levels after uninephrectomy in the rat. Scand J Clin Lab Invest 57:167-173, 1997.

226. Kanda S, Saha PK, Nomata K, et al: Transient increase in renal epidermal growth factor content after unilateral nephrectomy in the mouse. Acta Endocrinol (Copenh) 124:188-193, 1991.

227. Miller SB, Rogers SA, Estes CE, et al: Increased distal nephron EGF content and altered distribution of peptide in compensatory renal hypertrophy. Am J Physiol 262:F1032-F1038, 1992.

228. Rogers SA, Miller SB, Hammerman MR: Insulin-like growth factor I gene expression in isolated rat renal collecting duct is stimulated by epidermal growth factor. J Clin Invest 87:347-351, 1991.

229. El Nahas AM, Le Carpentier JE, Bassett AH: Compensatory renal growth: Role of growth hormone and insulin-like growth factor-I. Nephrol Dial Transplant 5:123-129, 1990.

230. Ishibashi K, Sasaki S, Sakamoto H, et al: Expressions of receptor gene for hepatocyte growth factor in kidney after unilateral nephrectomy and renal injury. Biochem Biophys Res Commun 187:1454-1459, 1992.

231. Nagaike M, Hirao S, Tajima H, et al: Renotropic functions of hepatocyte growth factor in renal regeneration after unilateral nephrectomy. J Biol Chem 266:22781-22784, 1991.

232. Joannidis M, Spokes K, Nakamura T, et al: Regional expression of hepatocyte growth factor/c-met in experimental renal hypertrophy and hyperplasia. Am J Physiol 267:F231-F236, 1994.

233. Oliver J: The regulation of renal activity: X. The morphologic study. Arch Intern Med 34:258-265, 1924.

234. Hayslett JP, Kashgarian M, Epstein FH: Functional correlates of compensatory renal hypertrophy. J Clin Invest 47:774-782, 1968.

235. Oliver J: New direction in renal morphology: A method, its results and its future. Harvey Lect 40:102-155, 1945.

236. Hayslett JP, Kashgarian M, Epstein FH: Mechanism of change in the excretion of sodium per nephron when renal mass is reduced. J Clin Invest 48:1002, 1969.

237. Pabico RC, McKenna BA, Freeman RB: Renal function before and after unilateral nephrectomy in renal donors. Kidney Int 8:166-175, 1975.

238. Salehmoghaddam S, Bradley T, Mikhail N, et al: Hypertrophy of basolateral Na-K pump activity in the proximal tubule of the remnant kidney. Lab Invest 53:443-452, 1985.

239. Hwang S, Bohman R, Navas P, et al: Hypertrophy of renal mitochondria. J Am Soc Nephrol 1:822-827, 1990.

240. Hruska K, Klahr S, Hammerman MR: Decreased luminal membrane transport of phosphate in chronic renal failure. Am J Physiol 242:F17-F22, 1982.

241. Mitchell AD, Valk WL: Compensatory renal hypertrophy. J Urol 88:11-18, 1992.

242. Wang M, Vyhmeister I, Kopple JD, et al: Effect of protein intake on weight gain and plasma amino acid levels in uremic rats. Am J Physiol 230:1455-1459, 1976.

243. Bouby N, Hassler C, Parvy P, et al: Renal synthesis of arginine in chronic renal failure: In vivo and in vitro studies in rats with 5/6 nephrectomy. Kidney Int 44:676-683, 1993.

244. Yanagawa N, Nissenson RA, Edwards B, et al: Functional profile of the isolated uremic nephron: Intrinsic adaptation of phosphate transport in the rabbit proximal tubule. Kidney Int 23:674-683, 1983.

245. Schoolwerth AC, Sandler RS, Hoffman PM, et al: Effects of nephron reduction and dietary protein content on renal ammoniagenesis in the rat. Kidney Int 7:397-404, 1975.

246. Buerkert J, Martin D, Trigg D, et al: Effect of reduced renal mass on ammonium handling and net acid formation by the superficial and juxtamedullary nephron of the rat: Evidence for reentrapment rather than decreased production of ammonium in the acidosis of uremia. J Clin Invest 71:1661-1675, 1983.

247. Yamauchi A, Sugiura T, Kitamura H, et al: Effects of partial nephrectomy on the expression of osmolyte transporters. Kidney Int 51:1847-1854, 1997.

248. Fine LG, Yanagawa N, Schultze RG, et al: Functional profile of the isolated uremic nephron: Potassium adaptation in the rabbit cortical collecting tubule. J Clin Invest 64:1033-1043, 1979.

249. Zalups RK, Stanton BA, Wade JB, et al: Structural adaptation in initial collecting tubule following reduction in renal mass. Kidney Int 27:636-642, 1985.

250. Schon DA, Silva P, Hayslett JP: Mechanism of potassium excretion in renal insufficiency. Am J Pathol 227:1323-1330, 1974.

251. Allison MEM, Wilson CB, Gottschalk CW: Pathophysiology of experimental glomerulonephritis in rats. J Clin Invest 53:1402-1423, 1974.

252. Kramp RA, MacDowell M, Gottschalk CW, et al: A study by microdissection and micropuncture of the structure and the function of the kidneys and the nephrons of rats with chronic renal damage. Kidney Int 5:147-176, 1974.

253. Brenner BM: Nephron adaptation to renal injury or ablation. Am J Physiol 249:F324-F337, 1985.

254. Pennell JP, Bourgoignie J: Adaptive changes of juxtaglomerular filtration in the remnant kidney. Pflugers Arch 389:131-135, 1981.

255. Marcussen N: Atubular glomeruli and the structural basis for chronic renal failure. Lab Invest 66:265-284, 1992.

256. Mitch WE, Wilcox CS: Disorders of body fluids, sodium and potassium in chronic renal failure. Am J Med 72:536-550, 1982.

257. Slatopolsky E, Elkan IO, Weerts C, et al: Studies on the characteristics of the control system governing sodium excretion in uremic man. J Clin Invest 47:521-530, 1968.

258. Weber H, Lin K-Y, Bricker NS: Effect of sodium intake on single nephron glomerular filtration rate and sodium reabsorption in experimental uremia. Kidney Int 8:14-20, 1975.

259. Bank N, Aynedjian HS: Individual nephron function in experimental bilateral pyelonephritis: I. Glomerular filtration rate and proximal tubular sodium, potassium, and water reabsorption. J Lab Clin Med 68:713-727, 1966.

260. Wilson DR, Sonnenberg H: Medullary collecting duct function in the remnant kidney before and after volume expansion. Kidney Int 15:487-501, 1979.

261. Hayslett JP: Functional adaptation to reduction in renal mass. Physiol Rev 59:137-164, 1979.

262. Woolf AS: Does atrial natriuretic factor contribute to the progression of renal disease? Med Hypoth 31:261-263, 1990.

263. Zhang PL, Mackenzie HS, Troy JL, et al: Effects of natriuretic peptide receptor inhibition on remnant kidney function in rats. Kidney Int 46:418-420, 1993.

264. Guyton AC, Coleman TG, Young DB, et al: Salt balance and long-term blood pressure control. Ann Rev Med 31:15-27, 1980.

265. Dormois JC, Young JL, Nies AS: Minoxidil in severe hypertension: Value when conventional drugs have failed. Am Heart J 90:360-368, 1975.

266. Gonick HC, Maxwell MH, Rubini ME, et al: Functional impairment in chronic renal disease: I. Studies on sodium-conserving ability. Nephron 3:137-152, 1966.

267. Danovitch GM, Bourgoignie JJ, Bricker NS: Reversibility of the "salt-losing" tendency of chronic renal failure. N Engl J Med 296:14-19, 1977.

268. Bricker NS: Sodium homeostasis in chronic renal disease. Kidney Int 21:886-897, 1982.

269. Bricker NS, Dewey RR, Lubowitz H, et al: Observations on the concentrating and diluting mechanisms of the diseased kidney. J Clin Invest 38:516-523, 1959.

270. Mees EJD: Relation between maximal urine concentration, maximal water reabsorption capacity, and mannitol clearance in patients with renal disease. BMJ 1:1159-1160, 1959.

271. Conte G, Dal Canton A, Fuiano G, et al: Mechanism of impaired urinary concentration in chronic primary glomerulonephritis. Kidney Int 27:792-798, 1985.

272. Duback UC, Rosner B, Muller A, et al: Relationship between regular intake of phenacetin-containing analgesics and laboratory evidence of urorenal disease in a working female population of Switzerland. Lancet 1:539-543, 1975.

273. Hatch FE, Culberston JW, Diggs LW: Nature of the renal concentrating defect in sickle cell disease. J Clin Invest 46:336-345, 1967.

274. Pennell JP, Bourgoignie JJ: Water reabsorption by papillary collecting ducts in the remnant kidney. Am J Physiol 242:F657-F663, 1982.

275. Klahr S, Schwab SJ, Stokes TJ: Metabolic adaptations of the nephron in renal disease. Kidney Int 29:80-89, 1986.

276. Bengele HH, Evan A, McNamara ER, et al: Tubular sites of potassium regulation in the normal and uninephrectomized rat. Am J Physiol 234:F146-F153, 1978.

277. Milanes CL, Jamison RL: Effect of acute potassium load on reabsorption in Henle's loop in chronic renal failure in the rat. Kidney Int 27:919-927, 1985.

278. Bourgoignie JJ, Kaplan M, Pincus J, et al: Renal handling of potassium in dogs with chronic renal insufficiency. Kidney Int 20:482-490, 1981.

279. Greenblatt DJ, Koch-Weser J: Adverse reactions to spironolactone. A report from the Boston Collaborative Drug Surveillance Program. JAMA 225:40-43, 1973.

280. Rimmer JM, Horn JF, Gennari FJ: Hyperkalemia as a complication of drug therapy. Arch Intern Med 147:867-869, 1987.

281. Gonick HC, Kleeman CR, Rubini ME, et al: Functional impairment in chronic renal disease: III. Studies of potassium excretion. Am J Med Sci 261:281-261, 1971.

282. Wrong O, Davies HEF: Excretion of acid in renal disease. Q J Med 28:259, 1959.

283. Widmer B, Gerhardt RE, Harrington JT, et al: Serum electrolyte and acid base composition: The influence of graded degrees of chronic renal failure. Arch Intern Med 139:1099-1102, 1979.

284. Finkelstein FO, Hayslett JP: Role of medullary structures in the functional adaptation of renal insufficiency. Kidney Int 6:419-425, 1974.

285. Wong NL, Quamme GA, Dirks JH: Tubular handling of bicarbonate in dogs with experimental renal failure. Kidney Int 25:912-918, 1984.

286. Schwartz WB, Hall PW, Hays RM, et al: On the mechanism of acidosis in chronic renal disease. J Clin Invest 38:39-52, 1959.

287. Muldowney FP, Donohoe JF, Carrol DV, et al: Parathyroid acidosis in uremia. Q J Med 41:321-342, 1972.

288. Purkerson ML, Lubowitz H, White RW, et al: On the influence of extracellular fluid volume expansion on bicarbonate reabsorption in the rat. J Clin Invest 48:1754-1760, 1969.

289. Sastrasinh S, Tanen RL: Effect of plasma potassium on renal NH_3 production. Am J Physiol 244:F383-F391, 1983.

290. Bricker NS: On the pathogenesis of the uremic state: An exposition of the "Trade-off Hypothesis." N Engl J Med 286:1093-1099, 1972.

291. Slatopolsky E, Robson AM, Elkan I, et al: Control of phosphate excretion in uremic man. J Clin Invest 47:1865-1874, 1968.

292. Haut LL, Alfrey AC, Guggenheim S, et al: Renal toxicity of phosphate in rats. Kidney Int 17:722-731, 1980.

293. Brooks DP, Ali SM, Contino LC, et al: Phosphate excretion and phosphate transporter messenger RNA in uremic rats treated with phosphonoformic acid. J Pharmacol Exp Ther 281:1440-1445, 1997.

294. Kraus E, Briefel G, Cheng L, et al: Phosphate excretion in uremic rats: Effects of parathyroidectomy and phosphate restriction. Am J Physiol 248:F175-F182, 1985.

295. Wen S-F, Stoll RW: Renal phosphate adaptation in uraemic dogs with a remnant kidney. Clin Sci 60:273-282, 1981.

296. Campese VM: Neurogenic factors and hypertension in chronic renal failure. J Nephrol 10:184-187, 1997.

297. Bank N, Su WS, Aynedjian H: A micropuncture study of renal phosphate transport in rats with chronic renal failure and secondary hyperparathyroidism. J Clin Invest 61:884-894, 1978.

298. Hsu CH: Are we mismanaging calcium and phosphate metabolism in renal failure? Am J Kidney Dis 29:641-649, 1997.

299. Better OS, Kleeman CR, Gonick HC, et al: Renal handling of calcium, magnesium and inorganic phosphate in chronic renal failure. Isr J Med Sci 3:60-79, 1967.

300. Better OS, Kleeman CR, Maxwell MH, et al: The effect of induced hypercalcemia on renal handling of divalent ions in patients with renal disease. Isr J Med Sci 5:33-42, 1969.

301. Finkelstein FO, Kliger AS: Medullary structures in calcium reabsorption in rats with renal insufficiency. Am J Physiol 233:F197-F200, 1977.

302. Chanutin A, Ferris EB: Experimental renal insufficiency produced by partial nephrectomy. Arch Intern Med 49:767-787, 1932.

303. Shimamura T, Ashton B, Morrison MD: A progressive glomerulosclerosis occurring in partial five-sixths nephrectomized rats. Am J Pathol 79:95-106, 1975.

304. Zatz R, Meyer TW, Rennke HG, et al: Predominance of hemodynamic rather than metabolic factors in the pathogenesis of diabetic glomerulopathy. Proc Natl Acad Sci U S A 82:5963-5967, 1985.

305. Dworkin LD, Hostetter TH, Rennke HG, et al: Hemodynamic basis for glomerular injury in rats with desoxycorticosterone-salt hypertension. J Clin Invest 73:1448-1461, 1984.

306. Steffes MW, Brown DM, Mauer SM: Diabetic glomerulopathy following unilateral nephrectomy in the rat. Diabetes 27:35-41, 1978.

307. Mauer SM, Steffes MW, Azar S, et al: The effects of Goldblatt hypertension on development of the glomerular lesions of diabetes mellitus in the rat. Diabetes 27:738-744, 1978.

308. Ots M, Troy JL, Mackenzie HS, et al: Isograft supplementation slows the progression of chronic experimental renal injury. Abstract. J Am Soc Nephrol 7:1861, 1996.

309. Mackenzie HS, Tullius SG, Heemann UW, et al: Nephron supply is a major determinant of long-term renal allograft outcome in rats. J Clin Invest 94:2148-2152, 1994.

310. Mackenzie HS, Azuma H, Troy JL, et al: Augmenting kidney mass at transplantation abrogates chronic renal allograft injury in rats. Proc Assoc Am Physicians 108:127-133, 1996.

311. Novick AC, Gephardt G, Guz B, et al: Long-term follow-up after partial removal of a solitary kidney. N Engl J Med 325:1058-1062, 1991.

312. Remuzzi A, Mazerska M, Gephardt GN, et al: Three-dimensional analysis of glomerular morphology in patients with subtotal nephrectomy. Kidney Int 48:155-162, 1995.

313. Anderson S, Meyer TW, Rennke HG, et al: Control of glomerular hypertension limits glomerular injury in rats with reduced renal mass. J Clin Invest 76:612-619, 1985.

314. Taal MW, Chertow GM, Rennke HR, et al: Mechanisms underlying renoprotection during renin-angiotensin system blockade. Am J Physiol 280:F343-F355, 2001.

315. Anderson S, Rennke HG, Garcia DL, et al: Short and long term effects of antihypertensive therapy in the diabetic rat. Kidney Int 36:526-536, 1989.

316. Fujihara CK, Padilha RM, Zatz R: Glomerular abnormalities in long-term experimental diabetes: Role of hemodynamic and nonhemodynamic factors and effects of antihypertensive therapy. Diabetes 41:286-293, 1992.

317. Simons JL, Provoost AP, Anderson S, et al: Pathogenesis of glomerular injury in the fawn-hooded rat: Early glomerular capillary hypertension predicts glomerular sclerosis. J Am Soc Nephrol 3:1775-1782, 1993.

318. Ziai F, Ots M, Provoost AP, et al: The angiotensin receptor antagonist, irbesartan, reduces renal injury in experimental chronic renal failure. Kidney Int 50(suppl 57):S-132-S-136, 1996.

319. Mackenzie HS, Ziai F, Nagano H, et al: Candesartan cilexetil reduces chronic renal allograft injury in Fisher→Lewis rats. J Hypertens 15(suppl 6):S21-S25, 1997.

320. Ziai F, Nagano H, Kusaka M, et al: Renal allograft protection with losartan in Fisher→Lewis rats: Hemodynamics, macrophages, and cytokines. Kidney Int 57:2618-2625, 2000.

321. Benediktsson H, Chea R, Davidoff A, et al: Antihypertensive drug treatment in chronic renal allograft rejection in the rat: Effect on structure and function. Transplantation 62:1634-1642, 1996.

322. Remuzzi A, Malanchini B, Battaglia C, et al: Comparison of the effects of angiotensin-converting enzyme inhibition and angiotensin II receptor blockade on the evolution of spontaneous glomerular injury in male MWF/Ztm rats. Exp Nephrol 4:19-25, 1996.

323. Anderson S, Rennke HG, Zatz R: Glomerular adaptations with normal aging and with long-term converting enzyme inhibition in rats. Am J Physiol 267:F35-F43, 1994.

324. Schmitz PG, O'Donnell MP, Kasiske BL, et al: Renal injury in obese Zucker rats: Glomerular hemodynamic alterations and effects of enalapril. Am J Physiol 263:F496-F502, 1992.

325. Anderson S, Diamond JR, Karnovsky MJ, et al: Mechanisms underlying transition from acute glomerular injury to late glomerular sclerosis in a rat model of nephrotic syndrome. J Clin Invest 82:1757-1768, 1988.

326. Lewis EJ, Hunsicker LG, Bain RP, et al: The effect of angiotensin-converting-enzyme inhibition on diabetic nephropathy. N Engl J Med 329:1456-1462, 1993.

327. GISEN (Gruppo Italiano di Studi Epidemiologici in Nefrologia): Randomised placebo-controlled trial of effect of ramipril on decline in glomerular filtration rate and risk of terminal renal failure in proteinuric, non-diabetic nephropathy. Lancet 349:1857-1863, 1997.

328. Lewis EJ, Hunsicker LG, Clarke WR, et al: Renoprotective effect of the angiotensin-receptor antagonist irbesartan in patients with nephropathy due to type 2 diabetes. N Engl J Med 345:851-860, 2001.

329. Brenner BM, Cooper ME, de Zeeuw D, et al: Effects of losartan on renal and cardiovascular outcomes in patients with type 2 diabetes and nephropathy. N Engl J Med 345:861-869, 2001.

330. Taal MW, Nenov VD, Wong W, et al: Vasopeptidase inhibition affords greater renoprotection than angiotensin-converting enzyme inhibition alone. J Am Soc Nephrol 12:2051-2059, 2001.

331. Benigni A, Zola C, Corna D, et al: Blocking both type A and B endothelin receptors in the kidney attenuates renal injury and prolongs survival in rats with remnant kidney. Am J Kidney Dis 27:416-423, 1996.

332. Orth SR, Esslinger JP, Amann K, et al: Nephroprotection of an ET(A)-receptor blocker (LU 135252) in salt-loaded uninephrectomized stroke-prone spontaneously hypertensive rats. Hypertension 31:995-1001, 1998.

333. Amann K, Simonaviciene A, Medwedewa T, et al: Blood pressure—independent additive effects of pharmacologic blockade of the renin-angiotensin and endothelin systems on progression in a low-renin model of renal damage. J Am Soc Nephrol 12:2572-2584, 2001.

334. Hostetter TH: Progression of renal disease and renal hypertrophy. Ann Rev Physiol 57:263-278, 1995.

335. Pober JS, Cotran RS: The role of endothelial cells in inflammation. Transplantation 50:537-544, 1990.

336. Vane JR: The Croonian Lecture, 1993. The endothelium: Maestro of the blood circulation. Philos Trans R Soc Lond B Biol Sci 343:225-246, 1994.

337. Olson JL, de UA, Heptinstall RH: Glomerular hyalinosis and its relation to hyperfiltration. Lab Invest 52:387-398, 1985.

338. Fujihara CK, Limongi DM, Falzone R, et al: Pathogenesis of glomerular sclerosis in subtotally nephrectomized analbuminemic rats. Am J Physiol 261:F256-F264, 1991.

339. Thornhill MH, Wellicome SM, Mahiouz DL, et al: Tumor necrosis factor combines with IL-4 or IFN-g to selectively enhance endothelial cell adhesiveness for T cells. J Immunol 146:592-589, 1991.

340. Pober JS, Cotran RC: Cytokines and endothelial cell biology. Physiol Rev 70:427-451, 1990.

341. Duijvestijn A, Hamann A: Mechanism and regulation of lymphocyte migration. Immunol Today 10:23-28, 1989.

342. Nagel T, Resnick N, Atkinson WJ, et al: Shear stress selectively upregulates intercellular adhesion molecule-1 expression in cultured human vascular endothelial cells. J Clin Invest 94:885-891, 1994.

343. Hishikawa K, Nakaki T, Marumo T, et al: Pressure enhances endothelin-1 release from cultured human endothelial cells. Hypertension 25:449-452, 1995.

344. Acevedo AD, Bowser SS, Gerritsen ME, et al: Morphological and proliferative responses of endothelial cells to hydrostatic pressure: Role of fibroblast growth factor. J Cell Physiol 157:603-614, 1993.

345. Letsou GV, Rosales O, Maitz S, et al: Stimulation of adenylate cyclase activity in cultured endothelial cells subjected to cyclic stretch. J Cardiovasc Surg (Torino) 31:634-639, 1990.

346. Sumpio BE, Widmann MD: Enhanced production of endothelium-derived contracting factor by endothelial cells subjected to pulsatile stretch. Surgery 108:277-281, 1990.

347. Macarthur H, Warner TD, Wood EG, et al: Endothelin-1 release from endothelial cells in culture is elevated both acutely and chronically by short periods of mechanical stretch. Biochem Biophys Res Commun 200:395-400, 1994.

348. Lansman JB, Hallam TJ, Rink TJ: Single stretch-activated ion channels in vascular endothelial cells as mechanotransducers? Nature 325:811-813, 1987.

349. Naruse K, Sokabe M: Involvement of stretch-activated ion channels in Ca^{2+} mobilization to mechanical stretch in endothelial cells. Am J Physiol 264:C1037-C1044, 1993.

350. Vanhoutte PM, Scott BT: The endothelium in health and disease. Tex Heart Inst J 21:62-67, 1994.

351. Lee LK, Meyer TW, Pollock AS, et al: Endothelial cell injury initiates glomerular sclerosis in the rat remnant kidney. J Clin Invest 96:953-964, 1995.

352. ScottBurden T, Vanhoutte PM: Regulation of smooth muscle cell growth by endothelium-derived factors. Tex Heart Inst J 21:91-97, 1994.

353. Morigi M, Zoja C, Figliuzzi M, et al: Supernatant of endothelial cells exposed to laminar flow inhibits mesangial cell proliferation. Am J Physiol 264:C1080-C1083, 1993.

354. Brown Z, Gerritsen ME, Carley WW, et al: Chemokine gene expression and secretion by cytokine-activated human microvascular endothelial cells: Differential regulation of monocyte chemoattractant protein-1 and interleukin-8 in response to interferon-gamma. Am J Pathol 145:913-921, 1994.

355. Shyy JYJ, Lin MC, Han JH, et al: The *cis*-acting phorbol ester 12-O-tetradecanoylp[horbol]-13-acetate-responseive element is involved in shear stress-induced monocyte chemotactic protein-1 expression. Proc Natl Acad Sci U S A 92:8069-8073, 1995.

356. Capers Q IV, Alexander RW, Lou P, et al: Monocyte chemoattractant protein-1 expression in aortic tissues of hypertensive rats. Hypertension 30:1397-1402, 1997.

357. Bebo BJ, Linthicum DS: Expression of mRNA for 55-kDa and 75-kDa tumor necrosis factor (TNF) receptors in mouse cerebrovascular endothelium: Effects of interleukin-1 beta, interferon-gamma and TNF-alpha on cultured cells. J Neuroimmunol 62:161-167, 1995.

358. Whitley MZ, Thanos D, Read MA, et al: A striking similarity in the organization of the E-selectin and beta interferon gene promoters. Mol Cell Biol 14(10):6464-6475, 1994.

359. Savage CO, Brooks CJ, Adu D, et al: Cell adhesion molecule expression within human glomerular and kidney organ culture. J Pathol 181:111-115, 1997.

360. Weyrich AS, McIntyre TM, McEver RP, et al: Monocyte tethering by P-selectin regulates monocyte chemotactic protein-1 and tumor necrosis factor-alpha secretion: Signal integration and NF-kappa B translocation. See comments. J Clin Invest 95:2297-2303, 1995.

361. Gimbrone MA, Nagel T, Topper JN: Biomechanical activation: An emerging paradigm in endothelial adhesion biology. J Clin Invest 99:1809-1813, 1997.

362. Rennke HG, Klein PS: Pathogenesis and significance of nonprimary focal and segmental glomerulosclerosis. Am J Kidney Dis 13:443-456, 1989.

363. Bohle A, Mackensen-Haen S, Wehrmann M: Significance of post-glomerular capillaries in the pathogenesis of chronic renal failure. Kidney Blood Press Res 19:191-195, 1996.

364. Kang DH, Joly AH, Oh SW, et al: Impaired angiogenesis in the remnant kidney model: I. Potential role of vascular endothelial growth factor and thrombospondin-1. J Am Soc Nephrol 12:1434-1447, 2001.

365. Kang DH, Hughes J, Mazzali M, et al: Impaired angiogenesis in the remnant kidney model: II. Vascular endothelial growth factor administration reduces renal fibrosis and stabilizes renal function. J Am Soc Nephrol 12:1448-1457, 2001.

366. Ingram AJ, Ly H, Thai K, et al: Activation of mesangial cell signaling cascades in response to mechanical strain. Kidney Int 55:476-485, 1999.

367. Riser BL, Cortes P, Zhao X, et al: Intraglomerular pressure and mesangial stretching stimulate extracellular matrix formation in the rat. J Clin Invest 90:1932-1943, 1992.

368. Harris RC, Haralson MA, Badr KF: Continuous stretch-relaxation in culture alters rat mesangial cell morphology, growth characteristics, and metabolic activity. See comments. Lab Invest 66:548-554, 1992.

369. Cortes P, Riser BL, Zhao X, et al: Glomerular volume expansion and mesangial cell mechanical strain: Mediators of glomerular pressure injury. Kidney Int 45(Suppl 45):S11-S16, 1994.

370. Hamasaki K, Mimura T, Furuya H, et al: Stretching mesangial cells stimulates tyrosine phosphorylation of focal adhesion kinase pp125FAK. Biochem Biophys Res Commun 212:544-549, 1995.

371. Homma T, Akai Y, Burns KD, et al: Activation of S6 kinase by repeated cycles of stretching and relaxation in rat glomerular mesangial cells: Evidence for involvement of protein kinase C. J Biol Chem 267:23129-23135, 1992.

372. Mattana J, Singhal PC: Applied pressure modulates mesangial cell proliferation and matrix synthesis. Am J Hypertens 8:1112-1120, 1995.

373. Riser BL, Cortes P, Heilig C, et al: Cyclic stretching force selectively up-regulates transforming growth factor-beta isoforms in cultured rat mesangial cells. Am J Pathol 148:1915-1923, 1996.

374. Riser BL, Denichilo M, Cortes P, et al: Regulation of connective tissue growth factor activity in cultured rat mesangial cells and its expression in experimental diabetic glomerulosclerosis. J Am Soc Nephrol 11:25-38, 2000.

375. Riser BL, Ladson-Wofford S, Sharba A, et al: TGF-beta receptor expression and binding in rat mesangial cells: Modulation by glucose and cyclic mechanical strain. Kidney Int 56:428-439, 1999.

376. Ketteler M, Noble NA, Border WA: Transforming growth factor-beta and angiotensin II: The missing link from glomerular hyperfiltration to glomerulosclerosis? Annu Rev Physiol 57:279-295, 1995.

377. Becker BN, Yasuda T, Kondo S, et al: Mechanical stretch/relaxation stimulates a cellular renin-angiotensin system in cultured rat mesangial cells. Exp Nephrol 6:57-66, 1998.

378. Kagami S, Border WA, Miller DE, et al: Angiotensin II stimulates extracellular matrix protein synthesis through induction of transforming growth factor-beta expression in rat glomerular mesangial cells. J Clin Invest 93:2431-2437, 1994.

379. Kato H, Osajima A, Uezono Y, et al: Involvement of PDGF in pressure-induced mesangial cell proliferation through PKC and tyrosine kinase pathways. Am J Physiol 277(1 Pt 2):F105-F112, 1999.

380. Suda T, Osajima A, Tamura M, et al: Pressure-induced expression of monocyte chemoattractant protein-1 through activation of MAP kinase. Kidney Int 60:1705-1715, 2001.

381. Nagata M, Kriz W: Glomerular damage after uninephrectomy in young rats: II. Mechanical stress on podocytes as a pathway to sclerosis. Kidney Int 42:148-160, 1992.

382. Fries JW, Sandstrom DJ, Meyer TW, et al: Glomerular hypertrophy and epithelial cell injury modulate progressive glomerulosclerosis in the rat. Lab Invest 60:205-218, 1989.

383. Endlich N, Kress KR, Reiser J, et al: Podocytes respond to mechanical stress in vitro. J Am Soc Nephrol 12:413-422, 2001.

384. vanGoor H, Fidler V, Weening JJ, et al: Determinants of focal and segmental glomerulosclerosis in the rat after renal ablation: Evidence for involvement of macrophages and lipids. Lab Invest 64:754-765, 1991.

385. vanGoor H, vanderHorst ML, Fidler V, et al: Glomerular macrophage modulation affects mesangial expansion in the rat after renal ablation. Lab Invest 66:564-571, 1992.

386. Saito T, Ootaka T, Sato H, et al: Participation of macrophages in segmental endocapillary proliferation preceding focal glomerular sclerosis. See comments. J Pathol 170:179-185, 1993.

387. Magil AB, Frohlich JJ: Monocytes and macrophages in focal glomerulosclerosis in Zucker rats. Nephron 59:131-138, 1991.

388. Floege J, Alpers CE, Burns MW, et al: Glomerular cells, extracellular matrix accumulation, and the development of glomerulosclerosis in the remnant kidney model. Lab Invest 66:485-497, 1992.

389. Diamond JR, Karnovsky MJ: Focal and segmental glomerulosclerosis: Analogies to atherosclerosis. Kidney Int 33:917-924, 1988.

390. Davies MJ, Gordon JL, Gearing AJ, et al: The expression of the adhesion molecules ICAM-1, VCAM-1, PECAM, and E-selectin in human atherosclerosis. J Pathol 171:223-229, 1993.

391. Ross R: The pathogenesis of atherosclerosis: A perspective for the 1990s. Nature 362:801-809, 1993.

392. Mai M, Geiger H, Hilgers KF, et al: Early interstitial changes in hypertension-induced renal injury. Hypertension 22:754-765, 1993.

393. Wolf G, Schneider A, Wenzel U, et al: Regulation of glomerular TGF-beta expression in the contralateral kidney of two-kidney, one-clip hypertensive rats. J Am Soc Nephrol 9:763-772, 1998.

394. Floege J, Burns MW, Alpers CE, et al: Glomerular cell proliferation and PDGF expression precede glomerulosclerosis in the remnant kidney model. Kidney Int 297-302, 1992.

395. Shultz PJ, DiCorleto PE, Silver BJ, et al: Mesangial cells express PDGF mRNAs and proliferate in response to PDGF. Am J Physiol 255(4 Pt 2):F674-F684, 1988.

396. Taal MW, Zandi-Nejad Z, Weening B, et al: Proinflammatory gene expression and macrophage recruitment in the rat remnant kidney. Kidney Int 58:1664-1676, 2000.

397. Wu LL, Cox A, Roe CJ, et al: Transforming growth factor beta 1 and renal injury following subtotal nephrectomy in the rat: Role of the renin-angiotensin system. Kidney Int 51:1553-1567, 1997.

398. van Goor H, Fidler V, Weening JJ, et al: Determinants of focal and segmental glomerulosclerosis in the rat after renal ablation: Evidence for involvement of macrophages and lipids. Lab Invest 64:754-765, 1991.

399. Fujihara CK, Malheiros D, Zatz R, et al: Mycophenolate mofetil attenuates renal injury in the rat remnant kidney. Kidney Int 54:1510-1519, 1998.

400. Fujihara CK, De Lourdes Noronha I, Malheiros, et al: Combined mycophenolate mofetil and losartan therapy arrests established injury in the remnant kidney. J Am Soc Nephrol 11:283-290, 2000.

401. Remuzzi G, Zoja C, Gagliardini E, et al: Combining an antiproteinuric approach with mycophenolate mofetil fully suppresses progressive nephropathy of experimental animals. J Am Soc Nephrol 10:1542-1549, 1999.

402. Romero F, Rodriguez-Iturbe B, Parra G, et al: Mycophenolate mofetil prevents the progressive renal failure induced by 5/6 renal ablation in rats. Kidney Int 55:945-955, 1999.

403. Fujihara CK, Malheiros DM, Donato JL, et al: Nitroflurbiprofen, a new nonsteroidal anti-inflammatory, ameliorates structural injury in the remnant kidney. Am J Physiol 274:F573-F579, 1998.

404. Remuzzi G, Bertani T: Pathophysiology of progressive nephropathies. N Engl J Med 339:1448-1456, 1998.

405. Strutz F, Muller GA, Neilson EG: Transdifferentiation: A new angle on renal fibrosis. Exp Nephrol 4:267-270, 1996.

406. Ng YY, Huang TP, Yang WC, et al: Tubular epithelial-myofibroblast transdifferentiation in progressive tubulointerstitial fibrosis in 5/6 nephrectomized rats. Kidney Int 54:864-876, 1998.

407. Kliem V, Johnson RJ, Alpers CE, et al: Mechanisms involved in the pathogenesis of tubulointerstitial fibrosis in 5/6-nephrectomized rats. Kidney Int 49:666-678, 1996.

408. Ma LJ, Marcantoni C, Linton MF, et al: Peroxisome proliferator-activated receptor-gamma agonist troglitazone protects against non-diabetic glomerulosclerosis in rats. Kidney Int 59:1899-1910, 2001.

409. Border WA, Noble NA: Fibrosis linked to TGF-beta in yet another disease. J Clin Invest 96:655-656, 1995.

410. Yamamoto T, Nakamura T, Noble NA, et al: Expression of transforming growth factor beta is elevated in human and experimental diabetic nephropathy. Proc Natl Acad Sci U S A 90:1814-1818, 1993.

411. Kato S, Luyckx VA, Ots M, et al: Renin-angiotensin blockade lowers MCP-1 expression in diabetic rats. Kidney Int 56:1037-1048, 1999.

412. Tamaki K, Okuda S, Ando T, et al: TGF-beta 1 in glomerulosclerosis and interstitial fibrosis of Adriamycin nephropathy. Kidney Int 45:525-536, 1994.

413. Hancock WH, Whitley WD, Tullius SG, et al: Cytokines, adhesion molecules, and the pathogenesis of chronic rejection of rat renal allografts. Transplantation 56:643-650, 1993.

414. Niemir ZI, Stein H, Noronha IL, et al: PDGF and TGF-beta contribute to the natural course of human IgA glomerulonephritis. Kidney Int 48:1530-1541, 1995.

415. Yamamoto T, Noble NA, Cohen AH, et al: Expression of transforming growth factor-beta isoforms in human glomerular diseases. Kidney Int 49:461-469, 1996.

416. Yamamoto T, Noble NA, Miller DE, et al: Increased levels of transforming growth factor-beta in HIV-associated nephropathy. Kidney Int 55:579-592, 1999.

417. Shihab FS, Yamamoto T, Nast CC, et al: Transforming growth factor-beta and matrix protein expression in acute and chronic rejection of human renal allografts. J Am Soc Nephrol 6:286-294, 1995.

418. Isaka Y, Fujiwara Y, Ueda N, et al: Glomerulosclerosis induced by in vivo transfection of transforming growth factor-beta or platelet-derived growth factor gene into the rat kidney. J Clin Invest 92:2597-2601, 1993.

419. Isaka Y, Brees DK, Ikegaya K, et al: Gene therapy by skeletal muscle expression of decorin prevents fibrotic disease in rat kidney. Nat Med 2:418-423, 1996.

420. Ito Y, Aten J, Bende RJ, et al: Expression of connective tissue growth factor in human renal fibrosis. Kidney Int 53:853-861, 1998.

421. Murphy M, Godson C, Cannon S, et al: Suppression subtractive hybridization identifies high glucose levels as a stimulus for expression of connective tissue growth factor and other genes in human mesangial cells. J Biol Chem 274:5830-5834, 1999.

422. Igarashi A, Okochi H, Bradham DM, et al: Regulation of connective tissue growth factor gene expression in human skin fibroblasts and during wound repair. Mol Biol Cell 4:637-645, 1993.

423. Clarkson MR, Gupta S, Murphy M, et al: Connective tissue growth factor: A potential stimulus for glomerulosclerosis and tubulointerstitial fibrosis in progressive renal disease. Curr Opin Nephrol Hypertens 8:543-548, 1999.

424. Lapinski R, Perico N, Remuzzi A, et al: Angiotensin II modulates glomerular capillary permselectivity in rat isolated perfused kidney. J Am Soc Nephrol 7:653-660, 1996.

425. Arai M, Wada A, Isaka Y, et al: In vivo transfection of genes for renin and angiotensinogen into the glomerular cells induced phenotypic change of the mesangial cells and glomerular sclerosis. Biochem Biophys Res Commun 206:525-532, 1995.

426. van Leeuwen RT, Kol A, Andreotti F, et al: Angiotensin II increases plasminogen activator inhibitor type 1 and tissue-type plasminogen activator messenger RNA in cultured rat aortic smooth muscle cells. Circulation 90:362-368, 1994.

427. Vaughan DE, Lazos SA, Tong K: Angiotensin II regulates the expression of plasminogen activator inhibitor-1 in cultured endothelial cells: A potential link between the renin-angiotensin system and thrombosis. J Clin Invest 95:995-1001, 1995.

428. Feener EP, Northrup JM, Aiello LP, et al: Angiotensin II induces plasminogen activator inhibitor-1 and -2 expression in vascular endothelial and smooth muscle cells. J Clin Invest 95:1353-1362, 1995.

429. Ruiz-Ortega M, Bustos C, Hernandez-Presa MA, et al: Angiotensin II participates in mononuclear cell recruitment in experimental immune complex nephritis through nuclear factor-kappa B activation and monocyte chemoattractant protein-1 synthesis. J Immunol 161:430-439, 1998.

430. Hahn AW, Jonas U, Buhler FR, et al: Activation of human peripheral monocytes by angiotensin II. FEBS Lett 347:178-180, 1994.

431. Brilla CG, Matsubara LS, Weber KT: Antifibrotic effects of spironolactone in preventing myocardial fibrosis in systemic arterial hypertension. Am J Cardiol 71:12A-16A, 1993.

432. Weber KT, Brilla CG: Pathological hypertrophy and cardiac interstitium: Fibrosis and renin-angiotensin-aldosterone system. Circulation 83:1849-1865, 1991.

433. Greene EL, Kren S, Hostetter TH: Role of aldosterone in the remnant kidney model in the rat. J Clin Invest 98:1063-1068, 1996.

434. Miller SB, Martin DR, Kissane J, et al: Hepatocyte growth factor accelerates recovery from acute ischemic renal injury in rats. Am J Physiol 266(1 Pt 2):F129-F134, 1994.

435. Liu Y, Tolbert EM, Lin L, et al: Up-regulation of hepatocyte growth factor receptor: An amplification and targeting mechanism for hepatocyte growth factor action in acute renal failure. Kidney Int 55:442-453, 1999.

436. Liu Y: Hepatocyte growth factor and the kidney. Curr Opin Nephrol Hypertens 11:23-30, 2002.

437. Liu Y, Rajur K, Tolbert E, et al: Endogenous hepatocyte growth factor ameliorates chronic renal injury by activating matrix degradation pathways. Kidney Int 58:2028-2043, 2000.

438. Matsumoto K, Morishita R, Moriguchi A, et al: Prevention of renal damage by angiotensin II blockade, accompanied by increased renal hepatocyte growth factor in experimental hypertensive rats. Hypertension 34:279-284, 1999.

439. Mizuno S, Matsumoto K, Kurosawa T, et al: Reciprocal balance of hepatocyte growth factor and transforming growth factor-beta 1 in renal fibrosis in mice. Kidney Int 57:937-948, 2000.

440. Azuma H, Takahara S, Matsumoto K, et al: Hepatocyte growth factor prevents the development of chronic allograft nephropathy in rats. J Am Soc Nephrol 12:1280-1292, 2001.

441. Yang J, Liu Y: Blockage of tubular epithelial to myofibroblast transition by hepatocyte growth factor prevents renal interstitial fibrosis. J Am Soc Nephrol 13:96-107, 2002.

442. Yang J, Dai C, Liu Y: Systemic administration of naked plasmid encoding hepatocyte growth factor ameliorates chronic renal fibrosis in mice. Gene Ther 8:1470-1479, 2001.

443. Takayama H, LaRochelle WJ, Sabnis SG, et al: Renal tubular hyperplasia, polycystic disease, and glomerulosclerosis in transgenic mice overexpressing hepatocyte growth factor/scatter factor. Lab Invest 77:131-138, 1997.

444. Laping NJ, Olson BA, Ho T, et al: Hepatocyte growth factor: A regulator of extracellular matrix genes in mouse mesangial cells. Biochem Pharmacol 59:847-853, 2000.

445. Fogo A, Ichikawa I: Evidence for the central role of glomerular growth promoters in the development of sclerosis. Semin Nephrol 9:329-342, 1989.

446. Fogo A, Ichikawa I: Evidence for a pathogenic linkage between glomerular hypertrophy and sclerosis. Am J Kidney Dis 17:666-669, 1991.

447. Yoshida Y, Kawamura T, Ikoma M, et al: Effects of antihypertensive drugs on glomerular morphology. Kidney Int 36:626-635, 1989.

448. Grond J, Beukers JY, Schilthuis MS, et al: Analysis of renal structural and functional features in two rat strains with a different susceptibility to glomerular sclerosis. Lab Invest 54:77-83, 1986.

449. Elfenbein IB, Baluarte HJ, Gruskin AB: Renal hypoplasia with oligomeganephronia. Arch Pathol 97:143-149, 1974.

450. Morita T, Wenzl J, McCoy J, et al: Bilateral renal hypoplasia with oligomeganephronia. Am J Clin Pathol 59:104-112, 1973.

451. McGraw M, Poucell S, Sweet J, et al: The significance of focal segmental glomerulosclerosis in oligomeganephronia. Int J Pediatr Nephrol 5:67-72, 1984.

452. Fogo A, Hawkins EP, Berry PL, et al: Glomerular hypertrophy in minimal change disease predicts subsequent progression to focal glomerular sclerosis. Kidney Int 38:115-123, 1990.

453. Yoshida Y, Fogo A, Ichikawa I: Glomerular hemodynamic changes vs. hypertrophy in experimental glomerular sclerosis. Kidney Int 35:654-660, 1989.

454. Lax DS, Benstein JA, Tolbert E, et al: Effects of salt restriction on renal growth and glomerular injury in rats with remnant kidneys. Kidney Int 41:1527-1534, 1992.

455. Lafferty HM, Brenner BM: Are glomerular hypertension and "hypertrophy" independent risk factors for progression of renal disease? Semin Nephrol 10:294-304, 1990.

456. Bank N, Klose R, Aynedjian HS, et al: Evidence against increased glomerular pressure initiating diabetic nephropathy. Kidney Int 31:898-905, 1987.

457. Fogo A, Yoshida Y, Glick AD, et al: Serial micropuncture analysis of glomerular function in two rat models of glomerular sclerosis. J Clin Invest 82:322-330, 1988.

458. Yoshida Y, Fogo A, Shiraga H, et al: Serial micropuncture analysis of single nephron function in subtotal renal ablation. Kidney Int 33:855-867, 1988.

459. Zatz R: Haemodynamically mediated glomerular injury: The end of a 15-year-old controversy? Curr Opin Nephrol Hypertens 5:468-475, 1996.

460. Olson JL, Hostetter TH, Rennke HG, et al: Altered glomerular permselectivity and progressive sclerosis following extreme ablation of renal mass. Kidney Int 22:112-126, 1982.

461. Eisenbach GM, Van Liew JB, Boylan JW: Effect of angiotensin on the filtration of protein in the rat kidney: A micropuncture study. Kidney Int 8:80-87, 1975.

462. Bohrer MP, Deen WM, Robertson CR, et al: Mechanism of angiotensin II-induced proteinuria in the rat. Am J Physiol 233:F13-F21, 1977.

463. Bertani T, Cutillo F, Zoja C, et al: Tubulo-interstitial lesions mediate renal damage in Adriamycin glomerulopathy. Kidney Int 30:488-496, 1986.

464. Eddy AA, Michael AF: Acute tubulointerstitial nephritis associated with aminonucleoside nephrosis. Kidney Int 33:14-23, 1988.

465. Eddy AA: Interstitial nephritis induced by protein-overload proteinuria. Am J Pathol 135:719-733, 1989.

466. Zoja C, Morigi M, Figliuzzi M, et al: Proximal tubular cell synthesis and secretion of endothelin-1 on challenge with albumin and other proteins. Am J Kidney Dis 26:934-941, 1995.

467. Wang Y, Chen J, Chen L, et al: Induction of monocyte chemoattractant protein-1 in proximal tubule cells by urinary protein. J Am Soc Nephrol 8:1537-1545, 1997.

468. Zoja C, Donadelli R, Colleoni S, et al: Protein overload stimulates RANTES production by proximal tubular cells depending on NF-kappa B activation. Kidney Int 53:1608-1615, 1998.

469. Barnes PJ: Nuclear factor-kB—A pivotal transcription factor in chronic inflammatory diseases. N Engl J Med 336:1066-1071, 1997.

470. Maack T, Mackensie DD, Kinter WB: Intracellular pathways of renal reabsorption of lysozyme. Am J Physiol 221(6):1609-1616, 1971.

471. Olbricht CJ, Cannon JK, Garg LC, et al: Activities of cathepsins B and L in isolated nephron segments from proteinuric and nonproteinuric rats. Am J Physiol 250:F1055-F1062, 1986.

472. Park CH, Maack T: Albumin absorption and catabolism by isolated perfused proximal convoluted tubules of the rabbit. J Clin Invest 73:767-777, 1984.

473. Burton C, Harris KP: The role of proteinuria in the progression of chronic renal failure. Am J Kidney Dis 27:765-775, 1996.

474. Eddy AA, Giachelli CM: Renal expression of genes that promote interstitial inflammation and fibrosis in rats with protein-overload proteinuria. Kidney Int 47:1546-1557, 1995.

475. Abbate M, Zoja C, Corna D, et al: In progressive nephropathies, overload of tubular cells with filtered proteins translates glomerular permeability dysfunction into cellular signals of interstitial inflammation. J Am Soc Nephrol 9:1213-1224, 1998.

476. Gandhi M, Olson JL, Meyer TW: Contribution of tubular injury to loss of remnant kidney function. Kidney Int 54:1157-1165, 1998.

477. Risdon RA, Sloper JC, De Wardener HE: Relationship between renal function and histological changes found in renal-biopsy specimens from patients with persistent glomerular nephritis. Lancet 2:363-366, 1968.

478. Schainuck LI, Striker GE, Cutler RE, et al: Structural-functional correlations in renal disease: II. The correlations. Hum Pathol 1:631-641, 1970.

479. Nomura A, Morita Y, Maruyama S, et al: Role of complement in acute tubulointerstitial injury of rats with aminonucleoside nephrosis. Am J Pathol 151:539-547, 1997.

480. Kashyap ML, Ooi BS, Hynd BA, et al: Sequestration and excretion of high density and low density lipoproteins by the kidney in human nephrotic syndrome. Artery 6:108-121, 1979.

481. Ong ACM, Moorhead JF: Tubular lipidosis: Epiphenomenon or pathogenetic lesion in human renal disease? Kidney Int 45:753-762, 1994.

482. Ong ACM, Jowett TP, Moorhead JF, et al: Human high density lipoproteins stimulate endothelin-1 release by cultured human renal proximal tubular cells. Kidney Int 46:1315-1321, 1994.

483. Hirschberg R: Bioactivity of glomerular ultrafiltrate during heavy proteinuria may contribute to renal tubulo-interstitial lesions: Evidence for a role for insulin-like growth factor I. J Clin Invest 98:116-124, 1996.

484. Purkerson ML, Hoffsten PE, Klahr S: Pathogenesis of the glomerulopathy associated with renal infarction in rats. Kidney Int 9:407-417, 1976.

485. Glasser RJ, Velosa JA, Michael AF: Experimental model of focal sclerosis: I. Relationship to protein excretion in aminonucleoside nephrosis. Lab Invest 36:519-526, 1977.

486. Perna A, Remuzzi G: Abnormal permeability to proteins and glomerular lesions: A meta-analysis of experimental and human studies. Am J Kidney Dis 27:34-41, 1996.

487. Lee HS, Lee JS, Koh HI, et al: Intraglomerular lipid deposition in routine biopsies. Clin Nephrol 36:67-75, 1991.

488. Sato H, Suzuki S, Ueno M, et al: Localization of apolipoprotein(a) and B-100 in various renal diseases. Kidney Int 43:430-435, 1993.

489. Wheeler DC, Persaud JW, Fernando R, et al: Effects of low-density lipoproteins on mesangial cell growth and viability in vitro. Nephrol Dial Transplant 5:185-191, 1990.

490. Grone EF, Abboud HE, Hohne M, et al: Actions of lipoproteins in cultured human mesangial cells: Modulation by mitogenic vasoconstrictors. Am J Physiol 263:F686-F696, 1992.

491. Rovin BH, Tan LC: LDL stimulates mesangial fibronectin production and chemoattractant expression. Kidney Int 43:218-225, 1993.

492. Peterson JC, Adler S, Burkart JM, et al: Blood pressure control, proteinuria, and the progression of renal disease. The Modification of Diet in Renal Disease Study. Ann Intern Med 123:754-762, 1995.

493. Jafar TH, Stark PC, Schmid CH, et al: Proteinuria as a modifiable risk factor for the progression of non-diabetic renal disease. Kidney Int 60:1131-1140, 2001.

494. Moorhead JF, El-Nahas M, Chan MK, et al: Lipid nephrotoxicity in chronic progressive glomerular and tubulo-interstitial disease. Lancet 2:1309-1311, 1982.

495. Peric-Golia L, Peric-Golia M: Aortic and renal lesions in hypercholesterolemic adult, male, virgin Sprague-Dawley rats. Atherosclerosis 46:57-65, 1983.

496. Kasiske B, O'Donnell MP, Schmitz PG, et al: Renal injury of diet-induced hypercholesterolemia in rats. Kidney Int 37:880-891, 1990.

497. Grone HJ, Walli A, Grone E, et al: Induction of glomerulosclerosis by dietary lipids: A functional and morphologic study in the rat. Lab Invest 60:433-446, 1989.

498. Joles JA, van Goor H, van der Horst MLC, et al: High lipid levels in very low density lipoprotein and intermediate density lipoprotein may cause proteinuria and glomerulosclerosis in aging female analbuminemic rats. Lab Invest 73:912-921, 1995.

499. Fujihara CK, Limongi DMZP, De Oliveira HCF, et al: Absence of focal glomerulosclerosis in aging analbuminemic rats. Am J Physiol 262:R947-R954, 1992.

500. Moorhead JF, Brunton C, Fernando RL, et al: Do glomerular atherosclerosis and lipid-mediated tubulo-interstitial disease cause progressive renal failure in man? Blood Purif 14:58-66, 1996.

501. Wellman KF, Volk BW: Renal changes in experimental hypercholesterolemia in normal and in subdiabetic rabbits. Lab Invest 22:36-49, 1970.

502. Rayner HC, Ross-Gilbertson VL, Walls J: The role of lipids in the pathogenesis of glomerulosclerosis in the rat following subtotal nephrectomy. Eur J Clin Invest 20:97-104, 1990.

503. Grone HJ, Walli AK, Grone EF: Arterial hypertension and hyperlipidemia as determinants of glomerulosclerosis. Clin Invest 71:834-839, 1993.

504. Keane WF, Kasiske BL, O'Donnell MP, et al: Hypertension, hyperlipidemia and renal damage. Am J Kidney Dis 21(suppl 2):43-50, 1993.

505. Kasiske B: Relationship between vascular disease and age-associated changes in the human kidney. Kidney Int 31:1153-1159, 1987.

506. Bleyer AJ, Chen R, D'Agostino RB Jr, et al: Clinical correlates of hypertensive end-stage renal disease. Am J Kidney Dis 31:28-34, 1998.

507. Shohat J, Boner G: Role of lipids in the progression of renal disease in chronic renal failure: Evidence from animal studies and pathogenesis. Isr J Med Sci 29:228-239, 1993.

508. Keane WF: Lipids and the kidney. Kidney Int 46:910-920, 1994.

509. Querfeld U, Lang M, Friedrich JB, et al: Lipoprotein(a) serum levels and apolipoprotein(a) phenotypes in children with chronic renal disease. Pediatr Res 34:772-776, 1993.

510. Saito T, Sato H, Kudo K-I: Lipoprotein glomerulopathy: Glomerular lipoprotein thrombi in a patient with hyperlipoproteinemia. Am J Kidney Dis 13:148-153, 1989.

511. Sato H, Suzuki S, Ueno M, et al: Localization of apolipoprotein(a) and B-100 in various renal diseases. Kidney Int 43:430-435, 1993.

512. Samuelsson O, Aurell M, Knight-Gibson C, et al: Apolipoprotein-B-containing lipoproteins and the progression of renal insufficiency. Nephron 63:279-285, 1993.

513. Wanner C, Greiber S, Kramer-Guth A, et al: Lipids and progression of renal disease: Role of modified low density lipoprotein and lipoprotein(a). Kidney Int 52(suppl 63):S-102-S-106, 1997.

514. Oikawa S, Matsunaga A, Saito T, et al: Apolipoprotein E Sendai (arginine-proline): A new variant associated with lipoprotein glomerulopathy. J Am Soc Nephrol 8:820-823, 1997.

515. Ellis D, Orchard TJ, Lombardozzi S, et al: Atypical hyperlipidemia and nephropathy associated with apolipoprotein E homozygosity. J Am Soc Nephrol 6:1170-1177, 1994.

516. Karet FE, Lifton RP: Lipoprotein glomerulopathy: A new role for apolipoprotein E? J Am Soc Nephrol 8:840-852, 1997.

517. Myhre E, Gjone E, Flatmark A, et al: Renal failure in familial lecithin-acyltransferase deficiency. Nephron 18:239-248, 1977.

518. Kasiske BL, Crosson JT: Renal disease in patients with massive obesity. Arch Intern Med 146:1105-1109, 1986.

519. Kasiske B, Napier J: Glomerular sclerosis in patients with massive obesity. Am J Nephrol 5:45-50, 1985.

520. Weisinger JR, Kempson RL, Eldridge FL, et al: The nephrotic syndrome: A complication of massive obesity. Ann Intern Med 81:440-447, 1974.

521. Lamas S, Sanz A, Ruiz A, et al: Weight reduction in massive obesity associated with focal segmental glomerulosclerosis: Another evidence for hyperfiltration? Nephron 56:225-226, 1990.

522. Keane WF, Kasiske BL, O'Donnell MP: Hyperlipidemia and the progression of renal disease. Am J Clin Nutr 47:157-160, 1988.

523. Bucala R, Makita Z, Vega G, et al: Modification of low density lipoprotein by advanced glycation end products contributes to the dyslipidemia of diabetes and renal insufficiency. Proc Natl Acad Sci U S A 91:9441-9445, 1994.

524. Kasiske BL, Ma JZ, Kalil RSN, et al: Effects of antihypertensive therapy on serum lipids. Ann Intern Med 122:133-141, 1995.

525. Monzani G, Bergesio F, Ciuti R, et al: Lipoprotein abnormalities in chronic renal failure and dialysis patients. Blood Purif 14:262-272, 1996.

526. Hunsicker LG, Adler S, Caggiula A, et al: Predictors of progression of renal disease in the Modification of Diet in Renal Disease Study. Kidney Int 51:1908-1919, 1997.

527. Krolewski AS, Warram JH, Christlieb AR: Hypercholesterolemia—a determinant of renal function loss and deaths in IDDM patients with nephropathy. Kidney Int 45(suppl 45):S-125-S-131, 1994.

528. Ravid M, Brosh D, Ravid-Safran D, et al: Main risk factors for nephropathy in type 2 diabetes mellitus are plasma cholesterol levels, mean blood pressure, and hyperglycemia. Arch Intern Med 158:998-1004, 1998.

529. Warram JH, Laffel LM, Ganda OP, et al: Coronary artery disease is the major determinant of excess mortality in patients with insulin-dependent diabetes mellitus and persistent proteinuria. J Am Soc Nephrol 3(4 suppl):S104-S110, 1992.

530. Mulec H, Johnson S-A, Bjorck S: Relation between serum cholesterol and diabetic nephropathy. Lancet 335:1537-1538, 1990.

531. Maschio G, Oldrizzi L, Rugiu C, et al: Serum lipids in patients with chronic renal failure on long-term, protein-restricted diets. Am J Med 87(5N):51N-54N, 1989.

532. Walker WG, Neaton JD, Cutler JA, et al: Renal function change in hypertensive members of the Multiple Risk Factor Intervention Trial. JAMA 268:3085-3091, 1992.

533. Radhakrishnan J, Appel AS, Valeri A, et al: The nephrotic syndrome, lipids, and risk factors for cardiovascular disease. Am J Kidney Dis 22:135-142, 1993.

534. Walker WG: Relation of lipid abnormalities to progression of renal damage in essential hypertension, insulin-dependent and non-insulin-dependent diabetes mellitus. Miner Electrolyte Metab 19:137-143, 1993.

535. Moorhead JF: Lipids and the pathogenesis of kidney disease. Am J Kidney Dis 17:65-70, 1991.

536. Stephenson JM, Kenny S, Stevens LK, et al: Proteinuria and mortality in diabetes: The WHO Multinational Study of Vascular Disease in Diabetes. Diabet Med 12:149-155, 1995.

537. Ding G, Pesek-Diamond I, Diamond JR: Cholesterol, macrophages, and gene expression of TGF-β 1 and fibronectin during nephrosis. Am J Physiol 264:F577-F584, 1993.

538. Diamond JR, Ding G, Frye J, et al: Glomerular macrophages and the mesangial proliferative response in the experimental nephrotic syndrome. Am J Pathol 141:887-894, 1992.

539. Nishida Y, Yorioka N, Oda H, et al: Effect of lipoproteins on cultured human mesangial cells. Am J Kidney Dis 29:919-930, 1997.

540. Wheeler DC, Chana RS, Topley N, et al: Oxidation of low density lipoprotein by mesangial cells may promote glomerular injury. Kidney Int 45:1628-1636, 1994.

541. Kasiske BL, O'Donnell MP, Cleary MP, et al: Treatment of hyperlipidemia reduces glomerular injury in obese Zucker rats. Kidney Int 33:667-672, 1988.

542. O'Donell MP, Kasiske BL, Kim Y, et al: Lovastatin retards the progression of established glomerular disease in obese Zucker rats. Am J Kidney Dis 22:83-89, 1993.

543. Park Y-S, Guijarro C, Kim Y, et al: Lovastatin reduces glomerular macrophage influx and monocyte chemoattractant protein-1 mRNA in nephrotic rats. Am J Kidney Dis 31:190-194, 1998.

544. Keane WF: Lipids and progressive renal failure. Wien Klin Wochenschr 108:420-424, 1996.

545. Lee HS, Jeong JY, Kim BC, et al: Dietary antioxidant inhibits lipoprotein oxidation and renal injury in experimental focal segmental glomerulosclerosis. Kidney Int 51:1151-1159, 1997.

546. Rabelink AJ, Hene RJ, Erkelens DW, et al: Partial remission of nephrotic syndrome in patient on long-term simvastatin. Lancet 335:1045-1046, 1990.

547. Sasaki T, Kurata H, Nomura K, et al: Amelioration of proteinuria with pravastatin in hypercholesterolemic patients with diabetes mellitus. Jpn J Med 29:156-163, 1990.

548. Maschio G, Oldrizzi L, Rugiu C, et al: Effect of dietary manipulation on the lipid abnormalities in patients with chronic renal failure. Kidney Int 39:S-70-S-72, 1991.

549. D'Amico G, Gentile MG: Pharmacological and dietary treatment of lipid abnormalities in nephrotic patients. Kidney Int 39(suppl 31):S-65-S-69, 1991.

550. D'Amico G, Gentile MG, Fellin G, et al: Effect of dietary protein restriction on the progression of renal failure: A prospective randomized trial. Nephrol Dial Transplant 9:1590-1594, 1994.

551. Keilani T, Schlueter WA, Levin ML, et al: Improvement of lipid abnormalities associated with proteinuria using fosinopril, an angiotensin converting enzyme inhibitor. Ann Intern Med 118:246-254, 1993.

552. Spitalewitz S, Porush JG, Cattran D, et al: Treatment of hyperlipidemia in the nephrotic syndrome: The effects of pravastatin therapy. Am J kidney Dis 22:143-150, 1993.

553. Thomas ME, Harris KPG, Ramaswamy C, et al: Simvastatin therapy for hypercholesterolemic patients with nephrotic syndrome or significant proteinuria. Kidney Int 44:1124-1129, 1993.

554. Fried LF, Orchard TJ, Kasiske BL: Effect of lipid reduction on the progression of renal disease: A meta-analysis. Kidney Int 59:260-269, 2001.

555. Krishna GG, Newell G, Miller E, et al: Protein-induced glomerular hyperfiltration: Role of hormonal factors. Kidney Int 33:578-583, 1988.

556. Bosch JP, Lauer A, Glabman S: Short-term protein loading in assessment of patients with renal disease. Am J Med 77:873-879, 1984.

557. Bosch JP, Lew S, Glabman S, et al: Renal hemodynamic changes in humans: Response to protein loading in normal and diseased kidneys. Am J Med 81:809-815, 1986.

558. Wiseman MJ, Hunt R, Goodwin A, et al: Dietary composition and renal function in healthy subjects. Nephron 46:37-42, 1987.

559. Krishna GG, Kapoor SC: Preservation of renal reserve in chronic renal disease. Am J Kidney Dis 17:18-24, 1991.

560. O'Connor WJ, Summerill RA: The excretion of urea by dogs following a meat meal. J Physiol 256:93-102, 1976.

561. O'Connor WJ, Summerill RA: Sulphate excretion by dogs following ingestion of ammonium sulphate or meat. J Physiol 260:597-607, 1976.

562. Meyer TW, Ichikawa I, Zatz R, et al: The renal hemodynamic response to amino acid infusion in the rat. Trans Assoc Am Physicians 96:76-83, 1983.

563. Johannesen J, Lie M, Kiil F: Effect of glycine and glucagon on glomerular filtration and renal metabolic rates. Am J Physiol 233:F61-F66, 1977.

564. Maack T, Johnson V, Tate SS, et al: Effects of amino-acids (AA) on the function of the isolated perfused rat kidney. Abstract. Fed Proc 33:305, 1974.

565. Castellino P, Coda B, DeFronzo RA: The effect of intravenous amino acid infusion on renal hemodynamics in man. Abstract. Kidney Int 27:243, 1985.

566. King A: Nitric oxide and the renal hemodynamic response to proteins. Semin Nephrol 15:405-414, 1995.

567. Seney FD, Persson AEG, Desir GV, et al: Dietary protein: Effect on tubuloglomerular feedback signal and sensing mechanism. Abstract. Kidney Int 27:299, 1985.

568. Anderson S, Brenner BM: Progressive renal disease: A disorder of adaptation. Q J Med 70:185-189, 1989.

569. Nakamura T, Fukui M, Ebihara I, et al: Effects of low-protein diet in glomerular endothelin family gene expression in experimental focal glomerular sclerosis. Clin Sci 88:29-37, 1995.

570. Benabe JE, Wang J, Wilcox JN, et al: Modulation of ANG II receptor and its mRNA in normal rat by low-protein feeding. Am J Physiol 265:F660-F669, 1993.

571. Bertani T, Zoja C, Abbate M, et al: Age-related nephropathy and proteinuria in rats with intact kidneys exposed to diets with different protein content. Lab Invest 60:196-204, 1989.

572. Klahr S, Levey AS, Beck GJ, et al: The effects of dietary protein restriction and blood-pressure control on the progression of chronic renal disease. Modification of Diet in Renal Disease Study Group. N Engl J Med 330:877-884, 1994.

573. Levey AS, Beck GJ, Bosch JP, et al: Short-term effects of protein intake, blood pressure, and antihypertensive therapy on glomerular filtration rate in the Modification of Diet in Renal Disease Study. J Am Soc Nephrol 7:2097-2109, 1996.

574. Pedrini MT, Levey AS, Lau J, et al: The effect of dietary protein restriction on the progression of diabetic and nondiabetic renal diseases: A meta-analysis. Ann Intern Med 124:627-632, 1996.

575. Plante GE: Urinary phosphate excretion determines the progression of renal disease. Kidney Int 36(suppl 27):S-128-S-132, 1989.

576. Denda M, Finch J, Slatopolsky E: Phosphorus accelerates the development of parathyroid hyperplasia and secondary hyperparathyroidism in rats with renal failure. Am J Kidney Dis 28:596-602, 1996.

577. Trachtman H, Chan JCM, Boyle R, et al: The relationship between calcium, phosphorus and sodium intake, race, and blood pressure in children with renal insufficiency: A report of the growth failure in children with renal diseases (GFRD) study. J Am Soc Nephrol 6:126-131, 1995.

578. Bro S, Olgaard K: Effects of excess PTH on nonclassical target organs. Am J Kidney Dis 30:606-620, 1997.

579. Akmal M, Kasim SE, Soliman AR, et al: Excess parathyroid hormone adversely affects lipid metabolism in chronic renal failure. Kidney Int 37:854-858, 1990.

580. Alfrey AC, Zhu J-M: The role of hyperphosphatemia. Am J Kidney Dis 17:53-56, 1991.

581. Delmez JA, Slatopolsky E: Hyperphosphatemia: Its consequences and treatment in patients with chronic renal disease. Am J Kidney Dis 19:303-317, 1992.

582. Lau K: Phosphate excess and progressive renal failure: The precipitation-calcification hypothesis. Kidney Int 36:918-937, 1989.

583. Shimamura T: Prevention of 11-deoxycorticosterone-salt-induced glomerular hypertrophy and glomerulosclerosis by dietary phosphate binder. Am J Pathol 136:549-556, 1990.

584. Barsotti G, Giannoni A, Morelli E, et al: The decline of renal function slowed by very low phosphorus intake in chronic renal patients following a low nitrogen diet. Clin Nephrol 21:54-59, 1984.

585. Ibels LS, Alfrey AC, Huffer WE, et al: Calcification in end-stage kidneys. Am J Med 71:33-37, 1981.

586. Goligorsky MS, Chiamovitz C, Rapoport J, et al: Calcium metabolism in uremic nephrocalcinosis: Preventive effect of verapamil. Kidney Int 27:774-779, 1985.

587. Schrier RW, Shapiro JI, Chan L, et al: Increased nephron oxygen consumption: Potential role in progression of chronic renal disease. Am J Kidney Dis 23:176-182, 1994.

588. Kramer HJ, Meyer-Lehnert H, Mohaupt M: Role of calcium in the progression of renal disease: Experimental evidence. Kidney Int 41(suppl 36):S-2-S-7, 1992.

589. Silbiger SR, Neugarten J: The impact of gender on the progression of chronic renal disease. Am J Kidney Dis 25:515-533, 1995.

590. Iseki K, Ikemiya Y, Fukiyama K: Risk factors of end-stage renal disease and serum creatinine in a community-based mass screening. Kidney Int 51:850-854, 1997.

591. Hannedouche T, Chauveau P, Kalou F, et al: Factors affecting progression in advanced chronic renal failure. Clin Nephrol 39:312-320, 1993.

592. Jungers P, Hannedouche T, Itakura Y, et al: Progression rate to end-stage renal failure in non-diabetic kidney diseases: A multivariate analysis of determinant factors. Nephrol Dial Transplant 10:1353-1360, 1995.

593. Honkanen E, Tornroth T, Gronhagen-Riska C, et al: Long-term survival in idiopathic membranous glomerulonephritis: Can the course be clinically predicted? Clin Nephrol 41:127-134, 1994.

594. Gretz N, Ceccherini I, Kranzlin B, et al: Gender-dependent disease severity in autosomal polycystic kidney disease of rats. Kidney Int 48:496-500, 1995.

595. Wyatt RJ, Kritchevsky SB, Woodford SY, et al: IgA nephropathy: Long-term prognosis for pediatric patients. J Pediatr 127:913-919, 1995.

596. Gabow PA, Johnson AM, Kaehny WD, et al: Factors affecting the progression of renal disease in autosomal-dominant polycystic kidney disease. Kidney Int 41:1311-1319, 1992.

597. Hopper Jr J, Trew P, Biava CG: Membranous nephropathy: Its relative benignity in women. Nephron 29:18-24, 1981.

598. Iseki K, Miyasato F, Oura T, et al: An epidemiologic analysis of end-stage lupus nephritis. Am J Kidney Dis 23:547-554, 1994.

599. Gretz N, Zeier M, Geberth S, et al: Is gender a determinant for evolution of renal failure? A study in autosomal dominant polycystic kidney disease. Am J Kidney Dis 14:178-183, 1989.

600. Murphy BF, Fairley KF, Kincaid-Smith PS: Idiopathic membranous glomerulonephritis: Long-term follow-up in 139 cases. Clin Nephrol 30:175-181, 1988.

601. West KM, Erdreich LJ, Stober JA: A detailed study of risk factors for retinopathy and nephropathy in diabetes. Diabetes 29:501-508, 1980.

602. Buckalew VM Jr, Berg RL, Wang SR, et al: Prevalence of hypertension in 1,795 subjects with chronic renal disease: The modification of diet in renal disease study baseline cohort. Modification of Diet in Renal Disease Study Group. Am J Kidney Dis 28:811-821, 1996.

603. Lombet JR, Adler SG, Anderson PS, et al: Sex vulnerability in the subtotal nephrectomy model of glomerulosclerosis in the rat. J Lab Clin Med 114:66-74, 1989.

604. Kreisberg JI, Karnovsky MJ: Focal glomerulosclerosis in the Fawn-Hooded rat. Am J Pathol 92:637-652, 1978.

605. Baylis C: Age-dependent glomerular damage in the rat: Dissociation between glomerular injury and both glomerular hypertension and hypertrophy: Male gender as a primary risk factor. J Clin Invest 94:1823-1829, 1994.

606. Baylis C, Corman B: The aging kidney: Insights from experimental studies. J Am Soc Nephrol 9:699-709, 1998.

607. Sakemi T, Toyoshima H, Morito F: Testosterone eliminates the attenuating effect of castration on progressive glomerular injury in hypercholesterolemic male Imai rats. Nephron 67:469-476, 1994.

608. Sakemi T, Ohtsuka N, Yoshiyuki T, et al: Testosterone does not eliminate the attenuating effect of estrogen on progressive glomerular injury in estrogen-treated hypercholesterolemic male Imai rats. Kidney Blood Press Res 20:51-56, 1997.

609. Reckelhoff JF, Baylis C: Glomerular metalloproteinase activity in the aging rat kidney: Inverse correlation with injury. J Am Soc Nephrol 3:1835-1838, 1993.

610. Neugarten J, Silbiger SR: Effects of sex hormones on mesangial cells. Am J Kidney Dis 26:147-151, 1995.

611. Campese VM, Karubian F: Salt sensitivity in hypertension: Implications for the kidney. J Am Soc Nephrol 2(2 suppl 1):S53-S61, 1991.

612. Zucchelli P, Zuccala A: The diagnostic dilemma of hypertensive nephrosclerosis: The nephrologist's view. Am J Kidney Dis 21(5 suppl 2):87-91, 1993.

613. Iseki K, Iseki C, Ikemiya Y, et al: Risk of developing end-stage renal disease in a cohort of mass screening. Kidney Int 49:800-805, 1996.

614. Klag MJ, Whelton PK, Randall BL, et al: Blood pressure and end-stage renal disease in men. N Engl J Med 334:13-18, 1996.

615. Perry HM Jr, Miller P, Fornoff JR, et al: Early predictors of 15-year end-stage renal disease in hypertensive patients. Hypertension 25(pt 1):587-594, 1995.

616. Perry HM Jr, Miller JP, Fornoff JR, et al: Early predictors of 15-year end-stage renal disease in hypertensive patients. Hypertension 25(4 pt 1):587-594, 1995.

617. Mogensen CE: Progression of nephropathy in long-term diabetics with proteinuria and effect of initial anti-hypertensive treatment. Scand J Clin Lab Invest 36:383-388, 1976.

618. Parving HH, Andersen AR, Smidt UM, et al: Early aggressive anti-hypertensive treatment reduces rate of decline in kidney function in diabetic nephropathy. Lancet 1:1175-1179, 1983.

619. Bergstrom J, Alvestrand A, Bucht H, et al: Progression of chronic renal failure in man is retarded with more frequent clinical follow-ups and better blood pressure control. Clin Nephrol 25:1-6, 1986.

620. Brazy PC, Fitzwilliam JF: Progressive renal disease: Role of race and antihypertensive medications. Kidney Int 37:1113-1119, 1990.

621. Kes P, Ratkovic-Gusic I: The role of arterial hypertension in progression of renal failure. Kidney Int Suppl 55:S72-S74, 1996.

622. Alkhunaizi AM, Chapman A: Renal artery stenosis and unilateral focal and segmental glomerulosclerosis. Am J Kidney Dis 29:936-941, 1997.

623. Berkman J, Rifkin H: Unilateral nodular diabetic glomerulosclerosis (Kimmelstiel-Wilson): Report of a case. Metabolism 22:715-722, 1973.

624. Peterson JC, Adler S, Burkart JM, et al: Blood pressure control, proteinuria, and the progression of renal disease. Ann Intern Med 123:754-762, 1995.

625. Bidani AK, Griffin KA, Bakris G, et al: Lack of evidence of blood pressure-independent protection by renin-angiotensin system blockade after renal ablation. Kidney Int 57:1651-1661, 2000.

626. Lewis JB, Berl T, Bain RP, et al: Effect of intensive blood pressure control on the course of type 1 diabetic nephropathy. Am J Kidney Dis 34:809-817, 1999.

627. Schrier R, McFann K, Johnson A, et al: Cardiac and renal effects of standard versus rigorous blood pressure control in autosomal-dominant polycystic kidney disease: Results of a seven-year prospective randomized study. J Am Soc Nephrol 13:1733-1739, 2002.

628. Fetterman G, Habib R: Congenital bilateral oligonephronic renal hypoplasia with hypertrophy of nephrons (oligomeganephronia). Am J Clin Pathol 52:199-207, 1969.

629. Carter JE, Lirenman DS: Bilateral renal hypoplasia with oligomeganephronia. Am J Dis Child 120:537-542, 1970.

630. He C, Zalups RK, Henderson DA, et al: Molecular analysis of spontaneous glomerulosclerosis in Os/+ mice, a model with reduced nephron mass. Am J Physiol F266-F273, 1995.

631. He C, Esposito C, Phillips C, et al: Dissociation of glomerular hypertrophy, cell proliferation, and glomerulosclerosis in mouse strains heterozygous for a mutation (Os) which induces a 50% reduction in nephron number. J Clin Invest 97:1242-1249, 1996.

632. Merlet-Bénichou C, Gilbert T, Muffat-Joly M, et al: Intrauterine growth retardation leads to a permanent nephron deficit in the rat. Pediatr Nephrol 8:175-180, 1994.

633. Amri K, Freund N, Vilar J, et al: Adverse effects of hyperglycemia on kidney development in rats: In vivo and in vitro studies. Diabetes 48:2240-2245, 1999.

634. Gilbert T, Lelièvre-Pégorier M, Merlet-Bénichou C: Long-term effects of mild oligonephronia induced in utero by gentamicin in the rat. Pediatr Res 30:450-456, 1991.

635. Mackenzie HS, Luyckx VA, Lawler EV, et al: Reduced glomerular number in the offspring of female rats subjected to dietary protein restriction: A quantitation using unbiased stereological techniques. Abstract. J Am Soc Nephrol 9:616A, 1998.

636. Langley-Evans SC, Welham SJ, Jackson AA: Fetal exposure to a maternal low protein diet impairs nephrogenesis and promotes hypertension in the rat. Life Sci 64:965-974, 1999.

637. Nwagwu MO, Cook A, Langley-Evans SC: Evidence of progressive deterioration of renal function in rats exposed to a maternal low-protein diet in utero. Br J Nutr 83:79-85, 2000.

638. Fassi A, Sangalli F, Maffi R, et al: Progressive glomerular injury in the MWF rat is predicted by inborn nephron deficit. J Am Soc Nephrol 9:1399-1406, 1998.

639. Skov K, Nyengaard JR, Korsgaard N, et al: Number and size of renal glomeruli in spontaneously hypertensive rats. J Hypertens 12:1373-1376, 1994.

640. Azar S, Johnson MA, Hertel B, et al: Single-nephron pressures, flows, and resistances in hypertensive kidneys with nephrosclerosis. Kidney Int 12:28-40, 1977.

641. Moore RA: The total number of glomeruli in the normal human kidney. Anat Rec 48:153-168, 1931.

642. Dunnill M, Halley W: Some observations on the quantitative anatomy of the kidney. J Pathol 110:113-121, 1973.

643. Nyengaard JR, Bendetsen TF: Glomerular number and size in relation to age, kidney weight, and body surface in normal man. Anat Rec 232:194-201, 1992.

644. Hinchliffe SA, Lynch MR, Sargent PH, et al: The effect of intrauterine growth retardation on the development of renal nephrons. Br J Obstet Gynaecol 99:296-301, 1992.

645. Hinchliffe SA, Howard CV, Lynch MR, et al: Renal developmental arrest in sudden infant death syndrome. Pediatr Pathol 13:333-343, 1993.

646. Merlet-Benichou C, Gilbert T, Vilar J, et al: Nephron number: Variability is the rule. Causes and consequences. Lab Invest 79: 515-527, 1999.

647. Manalich R, Reyes L, Herrera M, et al: Relationship between weight at birth and the number and size of renal glomeruli in humans: A histomorphometric study. Kidney Int 58:770-773, 2000.

647a. Hughson M, Farris AB, Douglas-Denton R, et al: Glomerular number and size in autopsied kidneys: The relationship to birth weight. Kidney Int 63:2113-2122, 2003.

648. Law CM, Shiell AW: Is blood pressure inversely related to birth weight? The strength of evidence from a systematic review of the literature. J Hypertens 14:935-941, 1996.

649. Rossing P, Tarnow L, Nielsen FS, et al: Short stature and diabetic nephropathy. BMJ 310:296-297, 1995.

650. Nelson RG, Morgenstern H, Bennett PH: Birth weight and renal disease in Pima Indians with type 2 diabetes mellitus. Am J Epidemiol 148:650-656, 1998.

651. Duncan RC, Bass PS, Garrett PJ, et al: Weight at birth and other factors influencing progression of idiopathic membranous nephropathy. Nephrol Dial Transplant 9:875, 1994.

652. Hoy WE, Rees M, Kile E, et al: A new dimension to the Barker hypothesis: Low birthweight and susceptibility to renal disease. Kidney Int 56:1072-1077, 1999.

652a. Keller G, Zimmer G, Mall G, et al: Nephron number in patients with primary hypertension. N Engl J Med 348:101-108, 2003.

653. Provoost AP, Brenner BM: Long-term follow-up of humans with single kidneys: The need for longitudinal studies to assess true changes in renal function. Curr Opin Nephrol Hypertens 2:521-526, 1993.

654. Brenner BM, Garcia DL, Anderson S: Glomeruli and blood pressure: Less of one, more of the other? Am J Hypertens 1:335-347, 1988.

655. Nenov VD, Taal MW, Sakharova OV, et al: Multi-hit nature of chronic renal disease. Curr Opin Nephrol Hypertens 9:85-97, 2000.

656. Rump LC, Amann K, Orth S, et al: Sympathetic overactivity in renal disease: A window to understand progression and cardiovascular complications of uraemia? Nephrol Dial Transplant 15:1735-1738, 2000.

657. Converse RL Jr, Jacobsen TN, Toto RD, et al: Sympathetic overactivity in patients with chronic renal failure. N Engl J Med 327:1912-1918, 1992.

658. Johansson M, Elam M, Rundqvist B, et al: Increased sympathetic nerve activity in renovascular hypertension. Circulation 99:2537-2542, 1999.

659. Rahman SN, Abraham WT, Van Putten VJ, et al: Increased norepinephrine secretion in patients with the nephrotic syndrome and normal glomerular filtration rates: Evidence for primary sympathetic activation. Am J Nephrol 13:266-270, 1993.

660. Cerasola G, Vecchi M, Mule G, et al: Sympathetic activity and blood pressure pattern in autosomal dominant polycystic kidney disease hypertensives. Am J Nephrol 18:391-398, 1998.

661. Klein IH, Ligtenberg G, Oey PL, et al: Sympathetic activity is increased in polycystic kidney disease and is associated with hypertension. J Am Soc Nephrol 12:2427-2433, 2001.

662. Kosch M, Barenbrock M, Kisters K, et al: Relationship between muscle sympathetic nerve activity and large artery mechanical vessel wall properties in renal transplant patients. J Hypertens 20:501-508, 2002.

663. Campese VM, Kogosov E, Koss M: Renal afferent denervation prevents the progression of renal disease in the renal ablation model of chronic renal failure in the rat. Am J Kidney Dis 26:861-865, 1995.

664. Amann K, Rump LC, Simonaviciene A, et al: Effects of low dose sympathetic inhibition on glomerulosclerosis and albuminuria in subtotally nephrectomized rats. J Am Soc Nephrol 11:1469-1478, 2000.

665. Amann K, Koch A, Hofstetter J, et al: Glomerulosclerosis and progression: Effect of subantihypertensive doses of alpha and beta blockers. Kidney Int 60:1309-1323, 2001.

666. Johnson RJ, Schreiner GF: Hypothesis: The role of acquired tubulointerstitial disease in the pathogenesis of salt-dependent hypertension. Kidney Int 52:1169-1179, 1997.

667. Weinrauch LA, Kennedy FP, Gleason RE, et al: Relationship between autonomic function and progression of renal disease in diabetic proteinuria: Clinical correlations and implications for blood pressure control. Am J Hypertens 11(3 pt 1):302-308, 1998.

668. Strojek K, Grzeszczak W, Gorska J, et al: Lowering of microalbuminuria in diabetic patients by a sympathicoplegic agent: Novel approach to prevent progression of diabetic nephropathy? J Am Soc Nephrol 12:602-605, 2001.

669. Ligtenberg G, Blankestijn PJ, Oey PL, et al: Reduction of sympathetic hyperactivity by enalapril in patients with chronic renal failure. N Engl J Med 340:1321-1328, 1999.

670. Price DA, Owen WF Jr: African-Americans on maintenance dialysis: A review of racial differences in incidence, treatment and survival. Adv Ren Replace Ther 4:3-12, 1997.

671. Striker GE: Kidney disease and hypertension in blacks. Am J Kidney Dis 20:673, 1992.

672. Korbet SM, Genchi RM, Borok RZ, et al: The racial prevalence of glomerular lesion in nephrotic adults. Am J Kidney Dis 27:647-651, 1996.

673. Ingulli E, Tejani A: Racial differences in the incidence and renal outcome of idiopathic focal segmental glomerulosclerosis in children. Pediatr Nephrol 5:393-397, 1991.

674. Brancati FL, Whittle JC, Whelton PK, et al: The excess incidence of diabetic end-stage renal disease among blacks: A population based study of potential explanatory factors. JAMA 268:3079-3084, 1992.

675. Cowie CC, Port FK, Wolfe RA, et al: Disparities in incidence of diabetic end-stage renal disease according to race and type of diabetes. N Engl J Med 321:1074-1079, 1989.

676. Tierney WM, McDonald CJ, Luft FC: Renal disease in hypertensive adults: Effect of race and type II diabetes mellitus. Am J Kidney Dis 13:485-493, 1989.

677. Whittle JC, Whelton PK, Seidler AJ, et al: Does racial variation in risk factors explain black-white differences in the incidence of hypertensive end-stage renal disease? Arch Intern Med 151:1359-1364, 1991.

678. Eisner GM: Hypertension: Racial differences. Am J Kidney Dis 16(4 suppl 1):35-40, 1991.

679. Lopes AAS, Port FK: The low birth weight hypothesis as a plausible explanation for the black/white differences in hypertension, non-insulin-dependent diabetes and end-stage renal disease. Am J Kidney Dis 25:350-356, 1995.

680. David RJ, Collins JW Jr: Differing birth weight among infants of U.S.-born blacks, African-born blacks and U.S.-born whites. N Engl J Med 337:1209-1214, 1997.

681. Freedman BI, Spray BJ, Tuttle AB, et al: The familial risk of end-stage renal disease in African Americans. Am J Kidney Dis 21:387-393, 1993.

682. Aperia AC, Liebow AA, Roberts LE: Renal adaptation to anemia. Circ Res 22:489-500, 1968.

683. Paterson JCS: Effect of chronic anemia on renal function in the dog. Am J Physiol 164:682-685, 1951.

684. Nashat FS, Portal RW: The effects of changes in hematocrit on renal function. J Physiol 193:513-522, 1967.

685. Whitaker W: Some effects of severe chronic anemia on the circulatory system. Q J Med 25:175-183, 1956.

686. Wardener HE, McSwiney RR: Renal hemodynamics in primary polycythemia. Lancet 2:204-205, 1951.

687. Garcia DL, Anderson S, Rennke HG, et al: Anemia lessens and treatment with recombinant human erythropoietin worsens glomerular injury and hypertension in rats with reduced renal mass. Proc Natl Acad Sci U S A 85:6142-6146, 1988.

688. Lafferty HM, King AJ, Troy JL, et al: Normalization of the renal hemodynamic abnormalities of early diabetes in the anemic rat. Abstract. Kidney Int 37:511, 1990.

689. Lafferty HM, Garcia DL, Rennke HG, et al: Anemia ameliorates progressive renal injury in experimental DOCA-Salt hypertension. J Am Soc Nephrol 1:1180-1185, 1991.

690. Puntorieri S, Brugnetti B, Remuzzi G, et al: Renoprotective effect of low iron diet and its consequence on glomerular hemodynamics. Abstract. J Am Soc Nephrol 1:693, 1990.

690a. Deicher R, Hörl WH: Anaemia as a risk factor for the progression of chronic kidney disease. Curr Opin Nephrol Hypertens 12:139-143, 2003.

691. Groppelli A, Giorgi DM, Omboni S, et al: Persistent blood pressure increase induced by heavy smoking. J Hypertens 10:495-499, 1992.

692. Ritz E, Benck U, Franek E, et al: Effects of smoking on renal hemodynamics in healthy volunteers and in patients with glomerular disease. J Am Soc Nephrol 9:1798-1804, 1998.

693. Benck U, Clorius JH, Zuna I, et al: Renal hemodynamic changes during smoking: Effects of adrenoreceptor blockade. Eur J Clin Invest 29:1010-1018, 1999.

694. Halimi JM, Giraudeau B, Vol S, et al: Effects of current smoking and smoking discontinuation on renal function and proteinuria in the general population. Kidney Int 58:1285-1292, 2000.

695. Oberai B, Adams CW, High OB: Myocardial and renal arteriolar thickening in cigarette smokers. Atherosclerosis 52:185-190, 1984.

696. Lhotta K, Rumpelt HJ, Konig P, et al: Cigarette smoking and vascular pathology in renal biopsies. Kidney Int 61:648-654, 2002.

697. Pinto-Sietsma SJ, Mulder J, Janssen WM, et al: Smoking is related to albuminuria and abnormal renal function in nondiabetic persons. Ann Intern Med 133:585-591, 2000.

698. Bleyer AJ, Shemanski LR, Burke GL, et al: Tobacco, hypertension, and vascular disease: Risk factors for renal functional decline in an older population. Kidney Int 57:2072-2079, 2000.

699. Goetz FC, Jacobs DR Jr, Chavers B, et al: Risk factors for kidney damage in the adult population of Wadena, Minnesota: A prospective study. Am J Epidemiol 145:91-102, 1997.

700. Muhlhauser I, Sawicki P, Berger M: Cigarette-smoking as a risk factor for macroproteinuria and proliferative retinopathy in type I (insulin-dependent) diabetes. Diabetologia 29:500-502, 1986.

701. Chase HP, Garg SK, Marshall G, et al: Cigarette smoking increases the risk of albuminuria among subjects with type I diabetes. JAMA 265:614-617, 1991.

702. McKenna K, Thompson C: Microalbuminuria: A marker to increased renal and cardiovascular risk in diabetes mellitus. Scott Med J 42:99-104, 1997.

703. Muhlhauser I, Overmann H, Bender R, et al: Predictors of mortality and end-stage diabetic complications in patients with type 1 diabetes mellitus on intensified insulin therapy. Diabet Med 17:727-734, 2000.

704. Stegmayr B, Lithner F: Tobacco and end stage diabetic nephropathy. BMJ 295:581-582, 1987.

705. Biesenbach G, Janko O, Zazgornik J: Similar rate of progression in the predialysis phase in type I and type II diabetes mellitus. Nephrol Dial Transplant 9:1097-1102, 1994.

706. Mehler PS, Jeffers BW, Biggerstaff SL, et al: Smoking as a risk factor for nephropathy in non-insulin-dependent diabetics. J Gen Intern Med 13:842-845, 1998.

707. Biesenbach G, Grafinger P, Janko O, et al: Influence of cigarette-smoking on the progression of clinical diabetic nephropathy in type 2 diabetic patients. Clin Nephrol 48:146-150, 1997.

708. Pijls LT, de Vries H, Kriegsman DM, et al: Determinants of albuminuria in people with Type 2 diabetes mellitus. Diabetes Res Clin Pract Suppl 52:133-143, 2001.

709. Orth SR, Stockmann A, Conradt C, et al: Smoking as a risk factor for end-stage renal failure in men with primary renal disease. Kidney Int 54:926-931, 1998.

710. Ward MM, Studenski S: Clinical prognostic factors in lupus nephritis: The importance of hypertension and smoking. Arch Intern Med 152:2082-2088, 1992.

711. Stengel B, Couchoud C, Cenee S, et al: Age, blood pressure and smoking effects on chronic renal failure in primary glomerular nephropathies. Kidney Int 57:2519-2526, 2000.

712. Samuelsson O, Attman PO: Is smoking a risk factor for progression of chronic renal failure? Kidney Int 58:2597, 2000.

713. Regalado M, Yang S, Wesson DE: Cigarette smoking is associated with augmented progression of renal insufficiency in severe essential hypertension. Am J Kidney Dis 35:687-694, 2000.

714. Orth SR, Ritz E: The renal risks of smoking: An update. Curr Opin Nephrol Hypertens 11:483-488, 2002.

715. Barrow SE, Ward PS, Sleightholm MA, et al: Cigarette smoking: Profiles of thromboxane- and prostacycline-derived products in human urine. Biochem Biophys Acta 993:121-127, 1989.

716. Odoni G, Ogata H, Viedt C, et al: Cigarette smoking condensate aggravates renal injury in the renal ablation model. Kidney Int 61:2090-2098, 2002.

717. Sawicki PT, Didjurgeit U, Muhlhauser I, et al: Smoking is associated with progression of diabetic nephropathy. Diabetes Care 17:126-131, 1994.

CHAPTER 44

Biology of the Vascular Wall in Hypertension

Bradford C. Berk

The structural changes of the human vascular wall in response to the development of hypertension are well characterized. They include appearance of intimal smooth muscle cells, thickening of the media as a result of increases in smooth muscle cell number or size (or both) as well as matrix deposition, and increased vasa vasorum in the adventitia.[1-5] In the pathogenesis of hypertension, however, the ways in which these structural alterations are related to underlying functional abnormalities and elevated blood pressure remain unclear. Substantial new data suggest that, in the setting of altered hemodynamic forces, genetically determined functional alterations in vessel wall components cause these structural alterations. In turn, the alterations in vessel structure then contribute to increased vascular resistance.

In this chapter, the structural and functional abnormalities of the vessel wall in hypertension are discussed. Figure 44-1 illustrates the conceptual framework for this discussion. In this scheme, a variety of systemic pathogenic stimuli (environmental, genetic, and hormonal) contribute to alterations in vessel structure. The appearance of these alterations is modulated locally by hemodynamic forces, hormones, tissue demand, and nerve activity. These primary changes lead to increased vascular resistance, which, if left uncorrected, contributes to vessel wall growth and remodeling. This creates a vessel whose structure is permanently altered so that vascular resistance increases and thereby raises blood pressure. Simultaneously, there are functional alterations in the cellular components of

the vessel wall (endothelial cells, smooth muscle cells, inflammatory cells, and fibroblasts) that lead to characteristic features of the hypertensive vessel, such as altered reactivity and elasticity. The multiple mechanisms for regulation of these structural and functional changes are apparent in the heterogeneity of responses that have been shown for hypertensive vessels of different sizes (conduit, resistance, microvascular) located in different tissues (e.g., brain, coronary, kidney). Recently, genetic approaches to understand the etiology of hypertension have yielded many new insights and suggest important differences in the causes of hypertension in men versus women, for example.[6, 7]

In this chapter, the structural and functional abnormalities that have been observed in hypertensive vessels are described first, followed by a discussion of the role of specific functional alterations (e.g., increased growth factor production) to cause specific structural changes (e.g., increased smooth muscle cell mass). Finally, the cellular mechanisms that are responsible for these functional alterations are described. In this way, adaptive changes that occur in response to hypertension (e.g., maintenance of cerebral autoregulation) may be analyzed separately from maladaptive changes (e.g., increased atherogenesis). Ultimately, an understanding of the fundamental cellular and molecular abnormalities in hypertension should provide insight into the features of the disease that are genetic and predetermined versus those that are environmental and a consequence of the disease process itself.

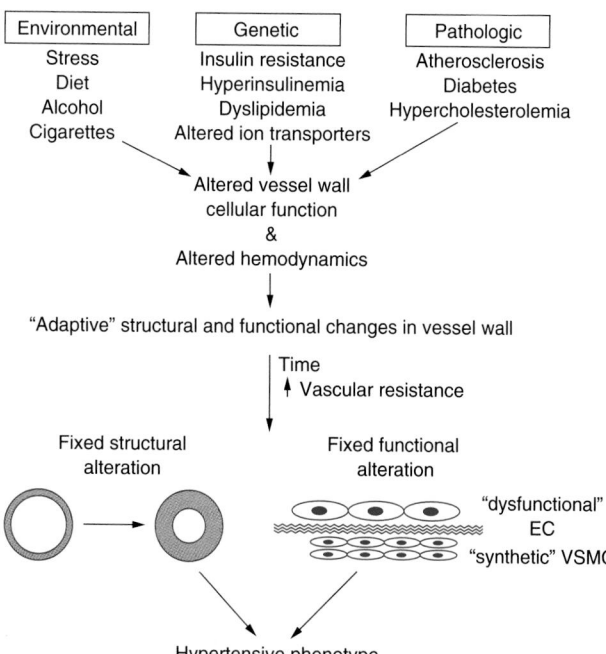

FIGURE 44-1. Model for development of structural and functional alterations characteristic of the hypertensive vessel wall. EC, endothelial cell; VSMC, vascular smooth muscle cell.

VASCULAR MORPHOLOGY AND STRUCTURE IN HYPERTENSION

Morphology

The morphologic changes that occur in vessels during chronic hypertension vary according to vessel size and tissue type.[4, 5, 8, 9] The arterioles are the physical sites for the largest increase in vascular resistance (Fig. 44-2A) and therefore are the most important from a functional point of view. It is clear that the relative proportion of smooth muscle cells to endothelium decreases as vessels become smaller (see Fig. 44-2B), implying less contractile power. However, as the cross-sectional area of the vessel diminishes, the resistance rises to the fourth power. Therefore, a small change in surface area of a small vessel causes a large increase in its resistance. These physical properties explain the fact that arterioles are the most important regulators of blood pressure.

Much of our knowledge of the progression of hypertensive changes in the vessel wall comes from animal models. Among the most important are the rat models of genetic hypertension: the spontaneously hypertensive rat (SHR); its related strain, the stroke-prone SHR; and its normotensive control, the Wistar-Kyoto (WKY) rat. Other common models are the Dahl salt-resistant and salt-sensitive strains and salt-induced hypertensive rats (the one-kidney, one-clip deoxycorticosterone salt rats, which are referred to as one-kidney one-clip hypertensive rats).

The earliest change after onset of hypertension observed in the arterioles of these rat models is a thickening of the media.[10-12] This is the result of at least three processes: matrix deposition, smooth muscle cell hypertrophy (increase in cell size without division), and smooth muscle

cell hyperplasia (increase in cell number). In arterioles and smaller vessels, hyperplasia is more prominent than hypertrophy.[11, 12] In addition, remodeling commonly has been found in these smaller vessels.[2, 3, 8, 13] Remodeling of the vessel occurs when the smooth muscle cells of the media rearrange to create a smaller (or, rarely, larger) lumen without change in number or size (Fig. 44-3). Mulvany and colleagues[14] described several different types of remodeling defined by changes in the size of the vessel (outward for larger and inward for smaller vessels) and by changes in the mass of smooth muscle cells (hypertrophic for increased mass and eutrophic for no change in mass). Next, there may be development of a neointima with appearance of smooth muscle cells inside the internal elastic lamina. Other morphologic features include local areas of endothelial cell denudation and inflammatory cell infiltration. Finally, there may be loss of blood vessels in the tissue, a process termed "rarefaction." It is likely that rarefaction involves programmed cell death or apoptosis that occurs in the absence of inflammation. In human hypertension, less is known regarding the time course of these events, but similar processes are apparent in autopsy specimens and in biopsies of patients with essential hypertension.[4, 5, 8, 13]

In conduit vessels, many of the same events occur, except that smooth muscle cell hypertrophy and endoreduplication are more common. Endoreduplication refers to synthesis of DNA and an increase in chromosome number (e.g., 2N to 4N) without cell division. In most studies, hypertrophy and polyploidy have been documented in the aorta and other large vessels of hypertensive rats to a greater extent than hyperplasia.[11, 12] Owens and Schwartz[11, 12] showed that about 25% of the cells in SHR aorta had undergone S phase with synthesis of DNA, yet had failed to divide. These cells appeared hypertrophied because of their increase in size, but they also had a DNA content that was twice or occasionally four times the normal content. Similar processes have been demonstrated in human hypertensive aorta.

The dominant change in hypertensive conduit vessels, however, is a loss of elasticity. In elderly humans, this is a major cause of systolic hypertension, often referred to as "stiff" arteries. This correlates with vessel morphology in which the elastin and collagen contents increase and the more elastic smooth muscle cells decrease in number because of the death of smooth muscle cells (medial atrophy, necrosis, or apoptosis). An important feature of conduit vessels, not found in smaller vessels, is the vasa vasorum, tiny vessels in the adventitia that supply nutrients and oxygen to the deeper layers of the media. Significant increases in size and number of vasa vasorum occur during chronic hypertension. This process is probably adaptive in the sense that the increased smooth muscle cell mass in the hypertensive vessel requires more oxygen and nutrients.

In the microcirculation, the ratio of endothelial cells to smooth muscle cells is approximately 1:1. Alterations in endothelial cell structure and function therefore have a major impact on hypertensive changes in these vessels. Although chronic hypertension causes little change in the number of smooth muscle cells present in microvessels and no significant increase in the matrix surrounding the smooth muscle cells, there is increased subendothelial matrix. Most importantly, the morphology of the endothelial cell is altered. This morphologic change is associated with

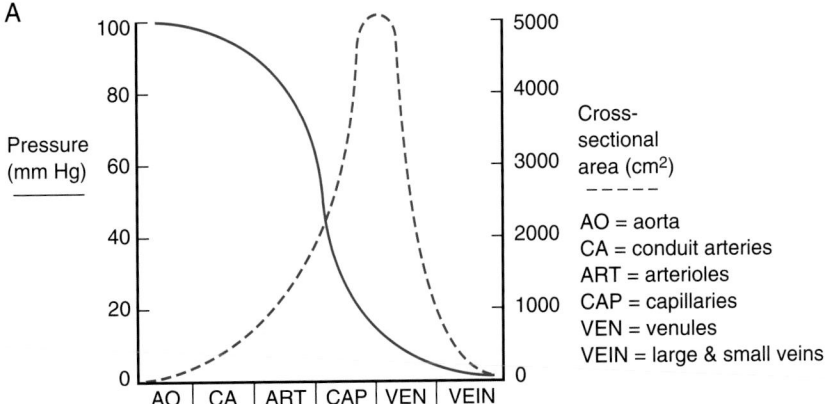

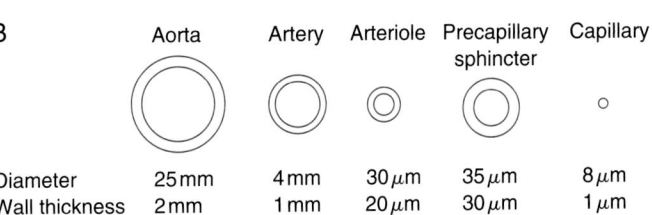

FIGURE 44-2. A, Pressure and cross-sectional area of blood vessels of the normal human systemic circulation. The important features are that the major pressure drop occurs across the arterioles and that the maximal cross-sectional area is represented by the capillaries. (From Berne RM, Levy MN [eds]: Cardiovascular Physiology, 5th ed. St. Louis, Mosby, 1992, p 2.) **B,** Internal diameter and wall thickness of the various blood vessels that constitute the circulatory system. Cross-sections of the vessels are not drawn to scale because of the large range in size from aorta to capillary. (Modified from Burton AC: Relation of structure to function of the tissues of the wall of blood vessels. Physiol Rev 34:619, 1954.)

increased vascular permeability. Electron microscopy shows decreased endothelial cell tight junctions to be the cause.

In summary, morphologic analysis of hypertensive vessels shows alterations in all cellular components as well as matrix. These changes vary depending on vessel size and the duration of hypertension. The hypertensive vessel wall is generally characterized by increased medial thickness or an increased media/lumen ratio of the resistance arterioles. This structural change in the hypertensive vessel causes it to have a mechanical advantage over the normotensive vessel (i.e., greater contractile force). Functionally, this means that there is greater resistance for a given contractile stimulus. Biomechanically, this increase in medial thickness is adaptive because wall stress is normalized as defined by Laplace's law. In the next section, the etiologic interaction

between smooth muscle cell growth and contractile function is examined.

Vascular Structure and Hypertension: Cause or Consequence?

In long-standing essential hypertension, the fundamental abnormality is an increase in peripheral vascular resistance in the setting of normal cardiac output.[15] The increase in resistance occurs even when vessels are fully dilated, indicating that the altered structure of the vessel is the cause, rather than a functional "overactivity."[16] Either or both of two processes may contribute to the structural increase in resistance: (1) increased mass of the vascular wall that causes a narrowing of the lumen[16] (termed inward remodeling by

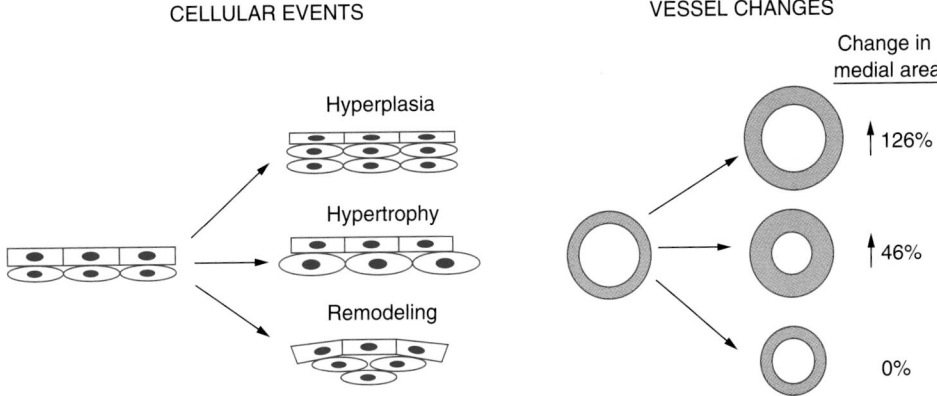

FIGURE 44-3. Model for changes in vessel wall cellular architecture in hypertension. *Left,* Smooth muscle cell hyperplasia, hypertrophy, and remodeling are shown. *Right,* Combinations of smooth muscle cell hypertrophy and remodeling are shown. Progressive increases in media area from bottom to top occur with a small decrease in lumen *(bottom),* a large decrease in lumen *(middle),* and a small increase in lumen *(top).* These changes would be characteristic of an adaptive response to increased pressure by remodeling only, without smooth muscle cell hypertrophy *(bottom);* a maladaptive response to increased pressure with smooth muscle cell hypertrophy, remodeling, or both *(middle);* and an adaptive response to increased pressure and/or flow with smooth muscle cell hypertrophy, remodeling, or both *(top).*

Mulvany[14]), and (2) rarefaction of the vasculature that causes a decrease in the number of parallel circuits.[17] Two questions must be answered to understand whether the structural increase in vessel resistance is a cause or a consequence of hypertension. First, which vessels are responsible? Second, is there a correlation between vascular structure and blood pressure and, if so, what is the nature of this relationship?

The answers to these questions have been provided during the past 10 years by the work of many investigators.[3-5, 11-13, 16, 18, 19] To summarize their important findings:

1. Resistance vessels are the site of the structural changes. These vessels include both the microvasculature (arterioles and precapillary sphincters with lumen diameters smaller than 100 μm) and small arteries (lumen diameters of 100 to 300 μm).
2. There is a strong correlation between vascular structure and blood pressure in a variety of hypertensive models in these resistance vessels.
3. Altered vascular structure is not simply a consequence of increased blood pressure; it is caused by primary functional changes in the cellular components of the vessel wall, mediated by genetic and environmental influences that control cell growth and the neurohormonal milieu.

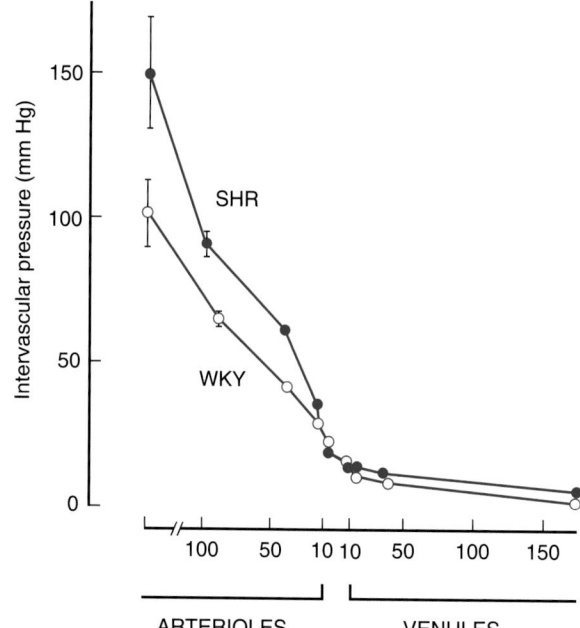

FIGURE 44-4. Pressure profile in the vasculature of the spontaneously hypertensive rat (SHR) and the normotensive Wistar-Kyoto (WKY) rat. The relationship between intravascular pressure and vessel diameter (in micrometers) shows a significantly greater pressure at any diameter in the SHR. (Modified from Mulvany MJ: Vascular structure and smooth muscle contractility in experimental hypertension. J Cardiovasc Pharmacol 6[suppl]:S79, 1987.)

Resistance Vessels: The Primary Site of Structural Change

Analysis of changes in blood pressure across various vascular beds in SHR and renal hypertensive rats demonstrates increased vascular resistance in both the microvasculature and small arteries (100 to 300 μm). Figure 44-4 shows that these vessels are the site where pressure regulation differs in the hypertensive animal compared with the genetically normal animal or normotensive control. These measurements are supported by the morphologic analysis of media thickness and media/lumen ratios, which shows the greatest changes in vessels of this size. In a variety of human hypertensive states, structural changes in these vessels also correlate with blood pressure (e.g., in women with preeclampsia,[20] in patients with uremia,[21] in patients with essential hypertension[8, 22, 23]). Drugs such as angiotensin-converting enzyme inhibitors (ACEI) and angiotensin receptor blockers (ARBs) that are associated with reversal of vessel structure also appear to have their greatest effect on media thickness in these resistance arterioles.[24]

Rarefaction appears to be confined to microvessels in humans and animals.[17, 25] Its importance in the different vascular beds remains to be determined. In particular, because it is difficult to study the microvasculature in humans, the discussion here focuses on changes in small arteries.

Positive Correlation between Vessel Structure and Blood Pressure

In both human patients and hypertensive animals, the fundamental structural abnormality in chronic hypertension is a decrease in the lumen diameter of the resistance vessel. This is explained by an increase in media thickness and media

cross-sectional area. In addition, this change is associated with increased contractile force generation when assayed in vitro. However, when the force generated is expressed in relation to medial mass, there is no inherent difference in the contractile ability of the smooth muscle in the hypertensive vessel compared with that in the normotensive vessel.[23, 26, 27] Therefore, the increased contractile force associated with hypertension is accounted for primarily by the altered structure of the resistance vessels (i.e., improved mechanical advantage relative to normotensive vessels).

A caveat to this last statement is required. As discussed in the following section, many functional alterations in the endothelial cells and smooth muscle cells of hypertensive vessels may modulate the contractile response. This is particularly true for smooth muscle agonists such as α-adrenergic agents, angiotensin II, and vasopressin, whose receptor number and signal transduction coupling to the contractile machinery may be altered. It is also true for endothelial-dependent vasodilation, which is impaired in human and animal models of hypertension. Nonetheless, structural change in resistance vessels is the primary abnormality that characterizes the chronic hypertensive state. It is also clear that underlying genetic and environmental stimuli are responsible for altered endothelial and smooth muscle cell function leading to this structural change (see Fig. 44-1).

The relation between media area and lumen size for SHR and WKY resistance vessels is shown in Figure 44-5. It is clear from the studies by Mulvany and co-workers,[9, 10, 28-30] as assembled in a review,[27] that for lumen sizes between 100 and 300 μm the SHR media area is relatively greater. This is most apparent in vessels larger than 200 μm. As discussed in

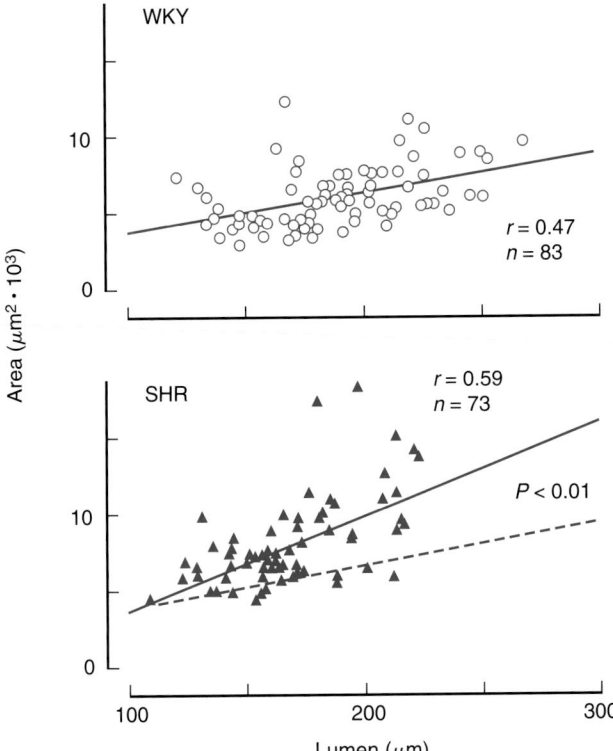

FIGURE 44-5. Relation of cross-sectional area of the media to normalized luminal diameter in mesenteric resistance vessels of 83 WKY rats *(top)* and 73 SHRs *(bottom)*. In the lower panel, the dashed line indicates the regression line for the WKY data redrawn from the top panel. The slopes of the regression lines are different ($P < .01$). (From Mulvany MJ: Vascular structure and smooth muscle contractility in experimental hypertension. J Cardiovasc Pharmacol 6[suppl]:S79, 1987.)

the following section, this alteration in media area is a consequence of vessel remodeling and increased smooth muscle cell size.

There is a strong correlation between media/lumen ratio and the magnitude of blood pressure increase in hypertension.

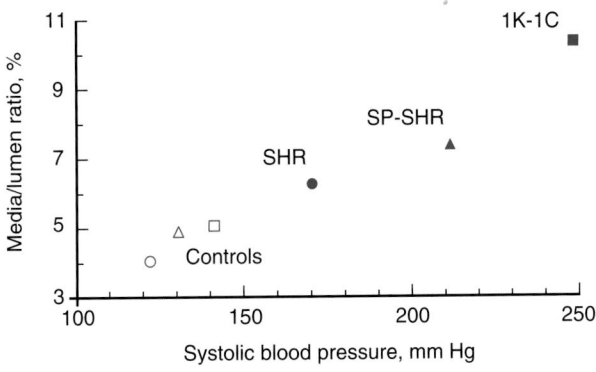

FIGURE 44-6. The media/lumen ratio correlates with the systolic blood pressure in hypertensive rats. Both genetic models of hypertension (spontaneously hypertensive rats [SHR], stroke-prone [SP-SHR]) and induced models (one-kidney one-clip [1K-1C]) show a positive correlation between the blood pressure and the percentage of the media relative to the lumen. (Modified from Mulvany MJ: Vascular structure and smooth muscle contractility in experimental hypertension. J Cardiovasc Pharmacol 6[suppl]:S79, 1987.)

Data from a variety of hypertensive models (SHR, stroke-prone SHR, one-kidney one-clip) show a clear relation between higher blood pressure and greater media/lumen ratio (Fig. 44-6), suggesting cause and effect. Therefore, the elevation of blood pressure in the chronic hypertensive state is caused by a permanent change in vessel structure. Several elegant experiments have indicated that the primary abnormality is in medial growth and/or remodeling and that the increase in blood pressure is secondary rather than primary.[5, 10, 31]

Structural Abnormalities Resulting from Functional Changes in Smooth Muscle Cells Caused by Genetic and Environmental Stimuli

Four lines of evidence support the proposal that abnormalities of the smooth muscle cells in the media (in particular, vessel remodeling and smooth muscle cell growth), rather than blood pressure per se, are the cause of the hypertensive phenotype:

1. Lowering of blood pressure of SHRs with hydralazine fails to normalize the media/lumen ratio in mesenteric arterioles (Fig. 44-7).[28]
2. Treatment of SHRs with inhibitors of the renin-angiotensin system, such as the ACEI captopril,[12, 32] causes much greater reduction in media growth for a given decrease in blood pressure than does treatment with hydralazine or β-blockers (see Fig. 44-7). Similar results were obtained recently in human hypertensive subjects, in whom the ARB losartan was more effective than atenolol at reversing medial hypertrophy.[24] Conversely, subpressor doses of angiotensin II promote smooth muscle cell hypertrophy.[33]
3. Abnormalities in regulation of smooth muscle cell function, such as increased superoxide formation from reduced nicotinamide adenine dinucleotide phosphate (NADPH) oxidase, contribute to hypertension directly and also are a component of angiotensin II–mediated hypertension.[34, 35]
4. The vessel response to hypertension differs in different tissues and vascular beds. For example, control of systolic blood pressure has lowered the incidence of stroke by about 50% but has had less benefit in renal disease associated with hypertension.

The functional abnormalities in the cells that make up the vessel wall and the cellular mechanisms by which medial growth is stimulated are discussed in the following section.

The Smooth Muscle Response: Hypertrophy, Hyperplasia, and Remodeling
Hypertrophy

The most characteristic feature of hypertension is an increase in media mass, known as medial hypertrophy. Medial hypertrophy occurs in most vascular beds during chronic hypertension and may be viewed as adaptive because it returns wall stress to normal. This is accomplished by increasing wall thickness or reducing vessel diameter

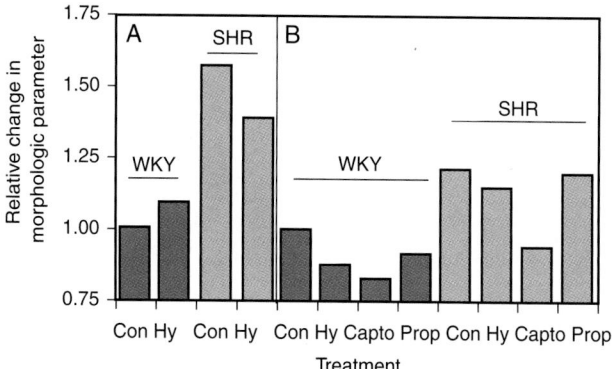

FIGURE 44-7. Captopril, an angiotensin-converting enzyme inhibitor, causes the greatest change in vessel morphology. Spontaneously hypertensive rats (SHR) and normotensive Wistar-Kyoto (WKY) rats were treated between 2 and 5 months of age with hydralazine (Hy, 40 mg/L in drinking water), captopril (Capto, 375 mg/L), and propranolol (Prop, 1.5 mg/L). The changes in media/lumen ratio (**A**) and in media area (**B**) were measured at 5 months. Con, control. (Modified from Owens GK: Influence of blood pressure on development of aortic medial smooth muscle hypertrophy in spontaneously hypertensive rats. Hypertension 9:178, 1987.)

(see Fig. 44-4). Increases in wall thickness result from both increases in smooth muscle cell size (cell hypertrophy) and increases in smooth muscle cell number (cell hyperplasia), as well as deposition of matrix. Decreases in vessel diameter require remodeling, a rearrangement of the vessel wall components. Among the causes of medial hypertrophy, pulse pressure may be more important than mean arterial pressure, as was shown by Heistad and Baumbach.[19, 36] Hypertrophy is a reversible mechanism when it is unaccompanied by endoreduplication. However, after DNA synthesis occurs, the change in cell size is probably irreversible. Therefore, cell hypertrophy caused by protein synthesis is adaptive, whereas hypertrophy associated with DNA synthesis is maladaptive in the sense that the increase in cell size (and the increase in media/lumen ratio) cannot be returned to normal. Because endoreduplication is such a common finding in hypertension and so little is known regarding its mechanisms, this should be an area of future research focus.

As discussed later, several mechanisms have been established for smooth muscle cell hypertrophy, including stimulation by angiotensin II[37, 38] and by transforming growth factor-β (TGF-β).[39] In particular, there is a strong correlation between blood pressure and both the frequency of polyploid smooth muscle cells and the medial smooth muscle content. Conversely, the efficacy of drugs (captopril and hydralazine) in preventing the development of smooth muscle cell polyploidism and medial hypertrophy in the SHR was the same as their efficacy in lowering blood pressure.[12] Of interest, propranolol caused no decrease in smooth muscle hypertrophy despite a decrease in blood pressure of 26 mm Hg (see also Fig. 44-7). These findings suggest that the primary cause of smooth muscle cell polyploidy and hypertrophy associated with endoreduplication is blood pressure itself. However, important secondary roles are suggested by the greater efficacy of ACEIs and ARBs, compared with hydralazine and β-blockers (see later discussion).

Hyperplasia

Hyperplasia also appears to be an important element in human hypertension. This is suggested by the significant increase in smooth muscle cell proliferative rate and the number of cell layers in the media of vessels from animals with chronic hypertension.[40, 41] As described earlier, there is also medial atrophy (due to both necrosis and apoptosis) in conduit vessels associated with loss of smooth muscle cells. If cell death preceded smooth muscle cell growth, hyperplasia could be viewed as an adaptive change. However, the reverse appears to be true: smooth muscle cell proliferation precedes medial necrosis.

Hyperplasia is a slow process in chronic human hypertension. Normal rat aortic smooth muscle cell growth is 0.01% per day.[42] In hypertensive models, this increases to a maximum of 1% per day. Simple calculations indicate that if this rate persisted, an arteriole 30 μm in diameter would occlude in 40 days, based on a medial thickness of 20 μm and cell diameter of 5 μm. This implies that only a certain percentage of cells may be able to replicate (smooth muscle cell heterogeneity) or that there must be only brief periods of proliferation (e.g., environmental stimuli) followed by inhibition of cell growth. Both processes appear to occur and contribute to the proliferation of smooth muscle cells in hypertension. Alternatively, there may be programmed cell death of some proliferating cells, a process termed apoptosis. It has recently been shown that there is increased apoptosis of smooth muscle cells in atherosclerosis, suggesting that when cells enter the cell cycle to proliferate they are also more prone to undergo cell death.[43]

Although smooth muscle cells in the vessel wall appear morphologically similar, it is likely that they are functionally heterogeneous. Several mechanisms could explain this. First, there may be embryonic cells ("progenitors") left from development, similar to those isolated from fetal animals.[44] For example, Schwartz and colleagues[44, 45] showed that proliferating smooth muscle cells isolated from the aorta express unique cytochrome P-450 enzymes that are typical of embryonic smooth muscle cells. Alternatively there may be circulating stem cells that can differentiate into smooth muscle cells.[46]

Second, there may be two types of smooth muscle cells: one that can undergo a dedifferentiation process recapitulating development and hence proliferation and another that is terminally differentiated and therefore able to migrate but not to proliferate. These two types could be genetically determined or could be a consequence of environmental modification. For example, inflammatory cells or oxidized low-density lipoproteins (LDL) may stimulate expression of growth factor receptors in smooth muscle cells, which could then respond to release of growth factors by proliferating. Because smooth muscle cells are sources of many autocrine growth factors, they may be constantly exposed to potential mitogens.

Third, there may be heterogeneity within the vessel wall that modifies the local environment. To take three examples: (1) Variations in hemodynamic forces may cause local gradients in nutrients (e.g., increased residence time of oxidized lipids) or local metabolic requirements (e.g., increased energy metabolism, altered cytoskeleton arrangements).[47-49] Hemodynamic forces are sensed by the vessel, because atherosclerosis develops in regions of low shear stress. Data show that endothelial cell production and release of growth factors are regulated by shear stress.[48-50] (2) Variation in matrix composition may be important, as illustrated by the fact that fibronectin is thought to be growth promoting and laminin growth inhibiting.[51-53] (3) Variations in uptake of circulating cells (e.g., leukocytes) or materials (e.g., LDL) may create different local environments.

In summary, multiple mechanisms may account for the appearance of smooth muscle cell hyperplasia compared with hypertrophy in the various vascular beds.

Remodeling

Remodeling is a complex process that involves changes in all vessel wall components, although smooth muscle cell growth, migration, and matrix changes appear most prominent.[14] It occurs primarily in resistance vessels in hypertension. The process appears to be fundamentally dependent on the presence of an intact endothelium. This has been shown best in growing vessels. In young rats, if one carotid is ligated to decrease flow (but pressure is maintained constant via collateral circulation), the ligated vessel fails to grow, and after 10 weeks it has a diameter only 50% of that of the control carotid.[54, 55] If the endothelium is removed, the normal vessel also fails to grow, establishing the endothelium as critical to vessel growth. In a similar manner, if flow is increased by a graft anastomosis, the subsequent downstream increase in vessel size is dependent on an intact endothelium.[56] Studies have shown that about 70% of the remodeling is a result of nitric oxide production by the endothelium, as determined by inhibiting production of nitric oxide with inhibitors of endothelial nitric oxide synthase (eNOS).[57] Therefore, remodeling in response to flow appears to be an endothelium-dependent process.

Remodeling appears to be important in the changes in arteriolar structure that occur in humans with essential hypertension. In small arteries (200 μm in diameter) obtained from gluteal biopsies of skin and subcutaneous fat of patients with essential hypertension, there was a significant decrease in lumen diameter (17%) and a significant increase in media/lumen ratio (31%) compared with arteries of normotensive subjects.[31] Most important, there was no significant change (10% decrease) in media volume per segment length (media cross-sectional area). This suggests that the dominant change in vessel structure was a rearrangement or remodeling of the lumen without increase in the media mass. It should be noted that a small increase in smooth muscle cell volume (16%) and decrease in smooth muscle cell number (26%) occurred in the hypertensive vessels, values that were not statistically significant.[31] These results suggest a minor role for smooth muscle cell hypertrophy in human essential hypertension and a predominant role for remodeling. Similar results were shown by Short[22] and by Schiffrin and colleagues[24] in chronic human hypertension.

Functional Consequences of Vessel Wall Hypertrophy, Hyperplasia, and Remodeling

Increases in vessel wall thickness caused by hypertrophy, hyperplasia, and remodeling are adaptive responses to hypertension in that they decrease wall stress. Increases in blood pressure increase wall stress, which increases smooth muscle cell work and oxygen consumption. In large vessels, this may drive the oxygen tension to zero, causing tissue hypoxia and smooth muscle cell dysfunction or death.[58-60] As discussed previously, increases in wall thickness and reductions in vessel diameter both act to return wall stress to normal (see Fig. 44-4). Furthermore, if increases in pressure during hypertension were transmitted unabated to arterioles and capillaries, the microcirculation would be damaged. This is especially critical in the cerebral circulation, where increased vascular permeability would rapidly lead to cerebral edema. Therefore, medial hypertrophy may be viewed as adaptive.

Both vascular hypertrophy and remodeling increase the media/lumen ratio. This increases the apparent responsiveness to vasoconstrictor stimuli in that the same increase in smooth muscle cell tone causes a much larger increase in resistance (because the proportionate decrease in lumen diameter is much greater). In larger vessels, there is no significant effect on minimal resistance because the diameter is so large. However, in smaller vessels, the passive properties of the vessel are changed and resting resistance may be substantially increased. It is in this setting that the adaptive compensatory increase in vessel wall thickness (relative to lumen) becomes maladaptive and contributes to hypertension.

FUNCTIONAL ABNORMALITIES IN HYPERTENSION: LINK TO STRUCTURAL ALTERATIONS

The functional abnormalities that have been observed in hypertension are of two types: those related to the passive properties of the vessel and those related to the dynamic properties. Passive properties include the features related to composition of the vessel. Dynamic or active properties refer to the characteristics determined by cellular mechanisms that require energy and change on a moment-to-moment basis.

Alterations in the Passive Properties of Hypertensive Vessels

The most characteristic feature of the passive properties in hypertension is a decrease in compliance or elasticity. It should be noted that the contribution of arterial compliance is dependent on the blood pressure. For example, at high levels of pressure, vessels have active tone and arterial compliance may make little contribution to vascular resistance. At low levels of pressure, vessels have little active tone, so arterial compliance is likely to contribute more to vascular resistance. Such shifts were shown in cerebral vessels of hypertensive rats by Heistad and Baumbach.[19] More recently, it has become clear that arterial stiffness is a major risk factor for vascular disease and contributes to isolated systolic hypertension and increased pulse pressure, especially as observed in elderly hypertensives.[61] The increase in pulse pressure may have specific effects, because pulse pressure due to pulsatile flow induces smooth muscle cell migration via urokinase and matrix metalloprotease (MMP)–dependent mechanisms.[62]

Alterations in the Active Properties of Hypertensive Vessels: Overview

The changes in hypertensive vessels in response to agonists that stimulate relaxation or contraction can be divided into processes associated with impaired vessel relaxation and those associated with augmented vessel contraction. Impaired relaxation has been attributed primarily to dysfunctional endothelium, and augmented contraction has been attributed to enhanced smooth muscle cell vasoreactivity. As discussed later, the endothelium secretes a variety of vasodilators and vasoconstrictors. Decreased relaxation could be caused by impaired production of vasodilating substances or by increased production of vasoconstricting substances, or both. Increased smooth muscle cell responsiveness may result from alterations in the ability of these vasodilating substances to exert their effects or from changes in the ability of smooth muscle cells to respond to the vasodilators. Conversely, there may be increased responsiveness to vaso-constrictors because of increased numbers of receptors or an augmented contractile machinery. All of these disturbances have been observed in different models of hypertension, with different mechanisms being prevalent in different vascular beds and in vessels of different size.

Examples of Altered Active Vessel Properties
Endothelium-Dependent Alterations

There is strong evidence for multiple alterations in endothelial function in hypertension, with increased production of constricting factors and decreased production of relaxing factors.

ENDOTHELIUM-DERIVED RELAXING FACTOR. Perhaps the most important endothelium-derived regulator of vascular tone is endothelium-derived relaxing factor (EDRF). The best known EDRF is nitric oxide (NO). Two abnormalities of endothelial function related to NO were described by Dohi and colleagues[63]: reduced basal release of NO and impaired endothelium-dependent relaxation in response to acetylcholine. The defects in endothelial function in rat hypertensive models are complex, as shown by the fact that impairment of endothelium-dependent relaxation occurs only with certain agonists. For example, in the SHR aorta, the response to acetylcholine is markedly reduced, whereas the response to thrombin is normal and that to histamine is slightly enhanced.[64] In mesenteric resistance arteries of the SHR, the relaxation in response to acetylcholine is impaired, although relaxation in response to endothelium-independent vasodilators such as the NO-donating 3-morpholinosydnoneimine (SIN-1) are normal, suggesting reduced formation of endothelium-derived NO.[63, 65, 66] A likely mechanism is the presence of a more oxidizing environment (increased O_2^-) in the luminal surface that more rapidly degrades NO by formation of peroxyni-trite ($ONOO^-$)[67-69] or a physical barrier in the luminal subendothelial space. Support for the hypothesis of increased reactive oxygen species comes from studies of angiotensin II–induced hypertension, in which increased NADPH oxidase and superoxide production have been demonstrated.[35, 70] Similar findings were observed in patients with essential hypertension, who had impaired

vasorelaxation to endogenous mediators such as bradykinin and increased blood flow.[71, 72]

ENDOTHELIUM-DERIVED VASOCONSTRICTORS. The endothelium may also be a source of vasoconstrictors termed "endothelium-derived constricting factors." For example, in the SHR aorta, high concentrations of acetyl-choline (more than 10^{-6} M) cause an endothelium-dependent contraction that is prevented by phospholipase A_2 inhibitors (e.g., quinacrine) or by cyclooxygenase inhibitors (e.g., indomethacin, meclofenamate).[64] The composition of these factors is unknown. Likely candidates include cyclooxyge-nase products of arachidonic acid and other *cis*-unsaturated fatty acids such as hydroxyeicosatetraenoic acid (HETE) and epoxyeicosatrienoic acid (EET).[73, 74]

Changes in Smooth Muscle Cell–Mediated Tone

The changes in contractile tone of smooth muscle cells in vessels exposed to chronic hypertension present a paradox. On the one hand, some of these cells undergo phenotypic modulation to a "synthetic" as opposed to a "contractile" phenotype, with loss of α_1-actin and smooth muscle myosin.[13, 75] These synthetic growing cells would be expected to be less contractile than normal cells. On the other hand, there is increased tone in hypertension, in part explained by the mechanical advantage of an increased media-to-lumen ratio. However, it is well established that there is increased sensitivity to vasopressors as well. This could be secondary to enhanced calcium sensitivity of the contractile apparatus, calcium-independent mechanisms that regulate tone,[29] depressed endothelium-dependent vasodilation,[76] increased receptor affinity for norepineph-rine,[77] altered coupling of the receptor to downstream effector pathways such as that observed for G proteins,[78, 79] and decreased cyclic nucleotides (cyclic adenosine and guanosine monophosphates) due to increased activity of phosphodiesterases. In summary, it appears that both receptor-coupled and receptor-independent mechanisms are augmented in several hypertensive models.

Changes in Nervous System–Mediated Tone

Several features of the sympathetic nervous system suggest that it contributes to the medial hypertrophy of hyperten-sion. First, norepinephrine and epinephrine are both vaso-constrictors. Vasoconstrictors are generally growth factors for smooth muscle cells,[80] as discussed later. Second, a number of studies have shown that sympathectomy markedly diminishes medial hypertrophy in the SHR model. Lee and colleagues[41] demonstrated that neonatal sympathec-tomy (anti-nerve growth factor antibody and sympa-thectomy) prevented development of SHR hypertension. In these rats, the arteries showed hypertrophy but no evidence of hyperplasia. In another study, infusion of epinephrine increased polyploidy of vascular smooth muscle cells (VSMCs) in the absence of an increase in blood pressure.[81] In addition, propranolol was shown in the deoxycorticos-terone acetate salt hypertensive rat model to prevent the development of polyploidy even when it failed to lower blood pressure.[82] Finally, during development of vessels, sympathectomy inhibits the increase in DNA mass of the vessel, suggesting an important role for the sympathetic nervous system in the formation of blood vessels.[83] Therefore, it appears that sympathectomy and other inhibitors of the sympathetic nervous system inhibit smooth muscle cell growth in hypertensive vessels.

Functional vessel abnormalities in hypertension exist alongside structural abnormalities that are in part adaptive. The next issue to be addressed regards the fundamental pathogenetic mechanisms that underlie these processes. Specifically, what unifying pathogenetic processes could cause both increased media/lumen ratios and altered vascular responsiveness, two features seen almost universally in hypertensive vessels?

THE ENDOTHELIUM IN HYPERTENSION

Endothelium-Derived Vasoactive Mediators

The endothelium has become a focus for research in hypertension because of expanding knowledge regarding its importance as a source of vasoactive mediators and its dysfunction during chronic hypertension. The best-characterized alteration in hypertension is diminished endothelium-dependent relaxation in response to acetylcholine. This has been demonstrated both in mesenteric resistance arteries of hypertensive rats and in the forearm circulation of hypertensive patients.[64, 71, 84] In a study by Panza and colleagues,[71] increased forearm blood flow during intrabrachial infusion of acetylcholine was markedly diminished in hypertensive subjects compared with normotensive individuals, although dilation in response to nitroprusside (a direct smooth muscle cell vasodilator) was unchanged.

This dysfunction is related to a decrease in the effective concentration of EDRF. Furchgott and Zawadzki[85] were the first to establish that the endothelium is the source of an acetylcholine-stimulated vasorelaxing factor, by demonstrating that acetylcholine is a vasodilator in the presence of intact endothelium and a vasoconstrictor in the absence of endothelium. A major advance was made by Moncada's group,[86, 87] who showed that NO could be produced from L-arginine in endothelium. NO is produced in endothelial cells by the eNOS (Fig. 44-8), which is a Ca^{2+}- and calmodulin-dependent enzyme of the flavin-biopterin class. This enzyme is dynamically regulated and can increase production of NO by more than 20-fold within seconds. Stimuli that have been shown to increase NO synthesis include fluid shear stress (increased flow) and a variety of vasomediators, including bradykinin, histamine, norepinephrine, substance P, serotonin, thrombin, and vasopressin. All of these factors probably work by increasing intracellular Ca^{2+} levels and activating the enzyme. There does not seem to be any control of NO release, because NO rapidly diffuses out of the cell. However, before it reaches target cells, it may be inactivated by factors such as reactive oxygen species (O_2^- and OH^-) and iron-containing compounds (e.g., hemoglobin).

As already discussed, NO stimulates soluble guanylate cyclase, which increases cyclic guanosine monophosphate (cGMP). In smooth muscle cells increased cGMP causes relaxation, and in platelets it inhibits adhesion and aggregation.[88] Elevation of cGMP also appears to be growth inhibitory for smooth muscle cells.[89] Therefore, decreased NO production would lead to decreased cGMP in smooth

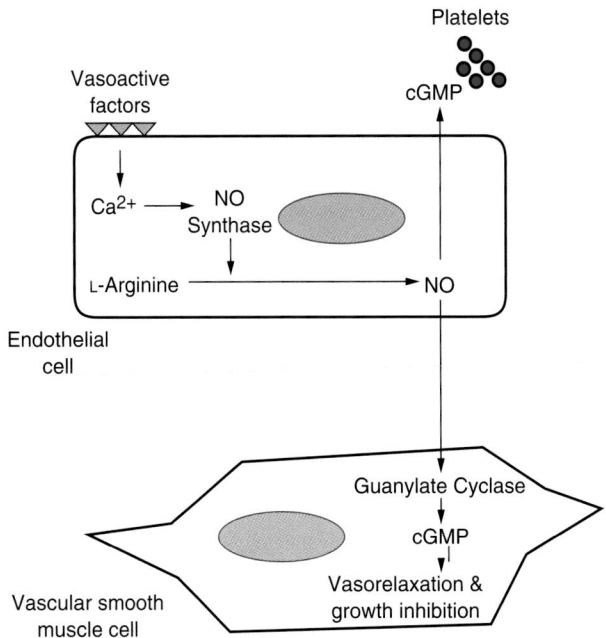

FIGURE 44-8. Nitric oxide (NO) is an important regulator of vessel wall function. In response to a variety of vasoactive factors, including increased fluid shear stress, endothelial cells activate NO synthase, which generates NO from L-arginine. NO diffuses rapidly from the cell and activates guanylate cyclase in target cells. In platelets, this inhibits aggregation; in smooth muscle, it causes vasorelaxation and growth inhibition. cGMP, cyclic guanosine monophosphate.

muscle cells, removing a growth-inhibiting and vasodilating mechanism. Alternatively, induction of cGMP phosphodiesterases by nitrate tolerance and angiotensin II would have a similar effect on growth and tone.[90, 91] This might contribute to increased smooth muscle cell growth in conditions of impaired NO production such as hypercholesterolemia, oxidative stress, and homocystinuria. The critical role of eNOS in these processes has been strengthened by studies using transgenic mice in which eNOS was deleted by homologous recombination. These mice are hypertensive, and after arterial injury they display enhanced VSMC growth and neointima formation.[92, 93]

Abnormalities in Nitric Oxide Action (Function) in Hypertension

Abnormalities in NO function that may contribute to hypertension are related to reduced release of NO and impaired VSMC relaxation in response to NO. Three mechanisms appear most likely to explain the apparent decrease in NO responsiveness:

1. Increased destruction: NO is readily destroyed by several reactive oxygen species as well as by advanced glycosylation end products.[94] Substantial evidence has accumulated that there are increased reactive oxygen species in atherosclerosis and hypertension.[58, 59] In fact, administration of superoxide dismutase (an enzyme that destroys the superoxide radical) decreased blood pressure in the SHR.[69]

2. Decreased production: NO production by NO synthase requires arginine, which appears to be present in excess within the cell. However, it is possible that alterations in activation of NO synthase may limit NO production in response to physiologic stimuli such as increased flow.
3. Impaired endothelial responsiveness to physiologic stimuli: Flow-dependent responses may be altered by changes in coupling of biomechanical forces in response to increases in calcium or other posttranslational mechanisms that regulate eNOS function.[95]

Our knowledge regarding changes that cause impaired smooth muscle cell responsiveness to NO is limited. As illustrated in Figure 44-8, NO exerts its vasodilating effects by increasing cGMP, which activates cGMP-dependent kinase, inhibiting myosin phosphorylation. It appears that this series of intracellular events may be altered in smooth muscle cells exposed to chronic hypertension, as shown by the decreased relaxation in the aorta and carotid of SHRs on administration of a variety of compounds (e.g., nitroprusside, SIN-1) that donate NO and thereby stimulate cGMP.[96]

Myosin light chain kinase is regulated by myosin phosphatase, which is itself regulated by kinases that are effectors for the small G protein, Rho. These kinases, termed Rho kinases, appear to play an important role in blood pressure regulation, as shown by the findings that specific inhibitors of Rho kinase lower blood pressure in hypertensive models.[97]

In summary, the decrease in endothelium-dependent relaxation is one of the fundamental abnormalities in the vessel wall in chronic hypertension.

Several Endothelium-Dependent Functions Are Abnormal in Hypertension

Several other aspects of endothelial dysfunction contribute to the altered function of the vessel wall:

1. There is disruption of the permeability barrier of the endothelium, allowing transudation of lipids and serum proteins. In particular, oxidized lipids may contribute in several ways to abnormal smooth muscle cell growth and endothelial cell dysfunction. For example, LDL induces expression of chemotactic proteins (e.g., monocyte chemotactic peptide-1) that may stimulate transmigration of monocytes and promote residence in the subendothelial space.[98] Subsequent macrophage activation and generation of inflammatory cytokines and reactive oxygen species may cause a more oxidizing vessel environment. This environment would shorten the half-life of NO.
2. There is increased adhesion of circulating blood elements. In particular, there may be expression of leukocyte adhesion molecules such as vascular cell adhesion molecule and endothelial leukocyte adhesion molecule-1 by the endothelium. These inflammatory cells may release a variety of smooth muscle cell growth factors and vasoconstrictors that alter vasoreactivity and promote VSMC growth.
3. The endothelium may release increased amounts of constricting factors that are not normally present.[99]

Two important endothelium-derived constricting factors are endothelin (ET) and cyclooxygenase-dependent contracting factors. ET-1 is a 21-amino-acid peptide that is produced in endothelial cells by many stimuli, including thrombin, TGF-β, and norepinephrine. ET-1 is extremely potent on a molar basis and appears to play an important role in local regulation of vessel tone. Responses to ET are regulated by processing of a 212-amino-acid precursor molecule, secretion of mature ET-1, and receptor expression by smooth muscle cells.[100] Of interest, in many vessels NO and nitrovasodilators are able to inhibit the release of ET, suggesting a self-regulating mechanism.[101]

4. Production of other vasodilating substances, such as prostacyclin and endothelium-derived hyperpolarizing factor, may be decreased. The production of prostacyclin is stimulated in endothelium by fluid shear stress and by many of the same agonists that release NO. However, inhibition of prostacyclin formation shows that it is normally much less important than NO in mediating vasorelaxation.[102] The nature of endothelium-derived hyperpolarizing factor remains unclear, but in certain vessels an endothelium-dependent hyperpolarization of smooth muscle cells has been demonstrated that is mediated by a diffusible substance.[103]

In summary, alterations in EDRFs (especially NO) appear to be critical to the altered function of the hypertensive vessels. Other vasoactive substances derived from the endothelium, including constrictors such as ET-1, cyclooxygenase-derived fatty acids, and platelet-derived growth factor (PDGF), may also be abnormal.[99] However, the evidence that these factors are important in altering resistance vessel function is limited at the present time. Future work should establish the importance of EDRF (and the mechanisms for its dysfunction) in human patients with essential hypertension.

SMOOTH MUSCLE IN HYPERTENSION

Smooth muscle cells have been the focus of research related to the response of vessel walls to hypertension for many years. The morphologic changes in the smooth muscle cells described in the following section indicate their ability to respond to the hemodynamic environment. Despite a clear description of the morphologic modifications associated with hypertension, the biochemical changes responsible for the altered phenotype remain largely unknown. That these morphologic changes are biochemical in nature was suggested by the use of the terms contractile phenotype and synthetic phenotype.[75] As outlined in Table 44-1, contractile cells are spindle-shaped, are located in the media, contract in response to agonists, and express high levels of contractile proteins such as α-actin and smooth muscle cell–specific myosin. Most importantly, these cells do not proliferate initially when placed in tissue culture. In contrast, synthetic phenotype smooth muscle cells are round, may be present in the intima, do not contract, and do not express α-actin or smooth muscle cell–specific myosin. These cells are characterized by large amounts of rough endoplasmic reticulum and secretion of matrix proteins. Most importantly, they

TABLE 44-1

Synthetic and Contractile Smooth Muscle Cells

PROPERTY	CONTRACTILE	SYNTHETIC
Shape	Spindle	Round
Location	Media	Media and intima
Contractility	Yes	Probably not
Proteins	α_1-actin	α_1- and γ-actin
Growth factors	No response to PDGF	Proliferate in response to PDGF
	Do not secrete PDGF	Secrete PDGF

PDGF, platelet derived growth factor.

proliferate when placed in culture. In fact, on being placed in culture, contractile smooth muscle cells undergo a process of phenotypic modulation in which they take on the appearance of synthetic cells and begin to proliferate in response to mitogens. In the following sections, the smooth muscle cell growth response and the biochemical mechanisms unique to hypertension are discussed (see the recent review by Berk[104] for further details).

Smooth Muscle Cells: Phenotypic Plasticity

One of the distinguishing features of smooth muscle cells is the plasticity of their growth responses. As shown in Figure 44-3, smooth muscle cells can respond in three ways to alterations in hemodynamic stress: hyperplasia, hypertrophy, and remodeling. In chronic hypertension, all three responses may be observed in different-sized vessels or even within the same vessel. Although smooth muscle cell plasticity offers an advantage in terms of its adaptability, in hypertensive humans this process may be pathologic. In particular, although hypertrophy and remodeling appear to be reversible, hyperplasia is not. An additional response is endoreduplication, in which DNA synthesis occurs without cell division. This results in a hypertrophic phenotype with excess DNA. At this time, the mechanisms controlling hyperplasia have been best studied, so they are the focus of the discussion that follows. Knowledge of hypertrophy is limited,[105] and information regarding mechanisms for remodeling and endoreduplication is scant.[2, 3, 31]

Smooth Muscle Cell Growth Factors in Hypertension

Growth factors have been isolated and characterized by their ability to stimulate growth of cultured cells. This research approach has caused us to think of growth factors as circulating factors that are released by platelets during injury (e.g., PDGF) or generated from circulating prohormones (e.g., angiotensin I to angiotensin II, prothrombin to thrombin). However, this concept may be the exception rather than the rule. In fact, temporal and spatial expression of growth factors and their receptors is dynamically regulated locally within the vessel wall. New techniques such as in situ hybridization and gene transfer, as well as the availability of antibodies to specific vascular growth factors, have helped define the growth factors that are important in vessel growth. Because several excellent reviews detail the range of growth factors that may stimulate smooth muscle cell growth in the

hypertensive vessel wall,[104, 106-109] the following discussion focuses on specific examples of mechanisms that are probably important in human essential hypertension. Table 44-2 provides a summary for those interested in greater detail.

Vasoconstrictors as Growth Factors

Agonists that act as vasoconstrictors frequently stimulate smooth muscle cell growth; conversely, many growth factors have vasoconstrictor activity. This paradigm has been proved many times over.[37, 63, 80, 110-115] For example, PDGF is a vasoconstrictor,[80] and angiotensin II is a potent smooth muscle cell growth factor.[37, 110] Shared initial signal transduction events activated by vasoconstrictors and growth factors probably account for activation of the growth response. Examples of shared signaling events include activation of phospholipase C, mobilization of intracellular Ca^{2+}, activation of protein kinase C, stimulation of Na^+/H^+ exchange, and stimulation of c-fos messenger RNA (mRNA) expression.[116, 117] As discussed earlier, changes in myosin phosphorylation mediated by activation of Rho kinases and inhibition of myosin phosphatase may represent another shared mechanism for growth factors and vasoconstrictors. These shared initial events are modified by later downstream regulatory mechanisms that determine the nature of the growth response: hypertrophy, hyperplasia, or remodeling.

G Protein Receptor–Coupled Agonists

ANGIOTENSIN II. The importance of angiotensin II in the smooth muscle cell growth response in hypertension was suggested initially by the findings that ACEIs have special beneficial effects on vessel wall function in the SHR,[32] that angiotensin II induces smooth muscle cell growth at subpressor concentrations,[33, 118] and that ACEIs block neointimal proliferation after balloon injury of the rat carotid.[119] More recent molecular evidence has provided stronger support for a role of angiotensin II. First, overexpression of renin in the transgenic rat[120] results in animals with significant hypertension. Conversely, deletion of the angiotensinogen gene[121] or the angiotensin type 1 receptor (AT1R) gene[122] by homologous recombination results in mice with relative hypotension. Second, a likely mechanism for angiotensin II effects is an increase in vascular production of superoxide anion related to alterations in smooth muscle cell enzymes such as NADPH oxidase that produce superoxide.[34, 35, 123] Finally, there is increasing evidence that other angiotensin peptides, specifically angIV (angiotensin 3-8) and angIII (angiotensin 1-7) play an important role in vascular tone in specific vascular beds.[124]

Two caveats to the interpretation of these data should be made. (1) ACEIs also block kinin metabolism and therefore increase the concentration of kinins.[107, 125] The presence of a local vessel wall kinin system is suggested by the findings that both arteries and veins contain a kallikrein-like enzyme and that cultured VSMCs express mRNA for glandular kallikrein.[126] In addition, cultured VSMCs have been shown to release both glandular kallikrein and kininogen.[127] These kinins (e.g., bradykinin) may be important smooth muscle cell growth inhibitors. For example, after rat carotid injury, the inhibition of VSMC growth observed with ACEIs is significantly reduced by coadministration of Hoe 140, an

TABLE 44-2

Smooth Muscle Cell Growth Factors in Essential Hypertension

GROWTH FACTOR	CELL SOURCE	REGULATED BY	COMMENTS
Angiotensin II	SMC	ACE Angiotensinogen Renin	ACE Inhibition, ↓ SHR media ↑ TGF-β, ↑ PDGF A ↑ PDGF β-receptor
Endothelin	EC	TGF-β, Thrombin, angiotensin, arginine vasopressin, shear stress, PDGF AA	↑ SMC growth
Vasopressin	Nerves	Autonomic activity	↑ SMC growth
Epidermal growth factor	Platelets Salivary gland	Unknown, ? testosterone	Synergistic with thrombospondin
Fibroblast growth factor	EC SMC	Unknown	Extracellular matrix Binds to heparans Angiogenic Multiple receptors ↑ Insulin-like growth factor
Thrombin	Liver	EC prothrombotic state	↑ PDGF A, ↑ SMC growth
Insulin-like growth factor (IGF)	SMC	Angiotensin II ↑ Stimulated by PDGF and epidermal growth factor	Regulated by insulin-like growth factor binding proteins Synergistic with PDGF
Platelet derived growth factor (PDGF)	EC SMC	Shear Stress Angiotensin II	↑ Thrombospondin synthesis Receptor-specific interactions for AA, AB, BB forms ↑ IGF
Transforming growth factor (TGF-β)	SMC Platelets	Angiotensin II	↑ and ↓ SMC proliferation Multiple receptors Regulated by binding protein Must be activated by proteases Down-regulates PDGF receptor α-subunits
Norepinephrine and catecholamines	Nerves	Central nervous system	Chemical Sympathectomy ↓ SHR media
Serotonin	Platelets Nerves	EC prothrombotic state	Stimulates endothelial cells to release EDRF ↑ SMC growth directly

ACE, angiotensin-converting enzyme; EC, endothelial cell; EDRF, endothelium-derived relaxing factors; SHR, spontaneously hypertensive rat; SMC, smooth muscle cell.

antagonist for the bradykinin B_2 receptor.[125] These findings suggest that increases in bradykinin as well as decreases in angiotensin II are important in the growth-inhibiting effects of ACEIs. (2) Some of the effect of angiotensin II may be due to facilitated release of norepinephrine from nerve terminals, because α_1-adrenergic blockade also decreases angiotensin II–induced DNA synthesis after injury.[128]

It has become clear that the entire renin-angiotensin system is present within the vessel wall and can act as an autocrine growth mechanism for smooth muscle cells[129, 130]; further, their activity is dynamically regulated. For example, angiotensinogen mRNA is present in the endothelium, medial smooth muscle, and periadventitial fat of normal rat arteries,[131] suggesting that several cell types in the vessel can synthesize angiotensinogen.[130] After balloon injury, the ratio of medial to adventitial angiotensinogen mRNA increases, implying increased production of this angiotensin II precursor in the media. Renin is also present in the vascular wall and cleaves angiotensinogen to angiotensin I. ACE then generates the vasoconstrictor and growth factor angiotensin II. Furthermore, ACE is highly regulated,[132] and increased expression of ACE by endothelial and smooth muscle cells may increase the amounts of angiotensin II present locally in the vessel wall.

It has been suggested that angiotensin II exerts its trophic effects in part through stimulation of PDGF A-chain mRNA and protein production.[59, 133] This has been supported most strongly by experiments in which transfection into VSMCs of antisense PDGF A-chain oligonucleotides inhibited angiotensin II–stimulated protein synthesis by more than 50%.[134, 135] As discussed next, angiotensin II also induces TGF-β mRNA in smooth muscle cells. Gibbons and colleagues[134, 135] observed that, in the presence of a neutralizing antibody to TGF-β, angiotensin II stimulated DNA synthesis and cell division of smooth muscle cells from normotensive rats. Based on this finding, they hypothesized that angiotensin II is a bifunctional growth factor. Angiotensin II stimulated hyperplasia when PDGF A-chain activity was the dominant growth factor expressed, but it stimulated cell hypertrophy when TGF-β activity was dominant.[109, 134, 135] Buhler's group[136] obtained similar findings regarding PDGF A-chain and TGF-β induction by angiotensin II in cultured aortic smooth muscle cells from the SHR. However, other investigators[39] found that angiotensin II induction of TGF-β was associated with enhanced PDGF-stimulated mitogenesis. Although most investigators agree that PDGF A-chain is a weak mitogen for cultured smooth muscle cells by itself, it appears to be critical to the hypertrophic response stimulated by angiotensin II in normotensive smooth muscle cells.[137] The increase in cell volume after exposure to angiotensin II follows a time course similar to that for induction of PDGF A-chain expression, and antibodies against the

PDGF A-chain prevent hypertrophy. Changes in cell redox state mediated by NADPH oxidase have been shown to play an important role in angiotensin II–stimulated hypertrophy; antisense to p22 phox prevented the increase in protein synthesis.[138, 139] These studies indicate that smooth muscle cell growth in hypertension that is mediated by angiotensin II actually involves complex regulation of multiple hormones and their receptors.

CATECHOLAMINES. Classic vasoconstrictors such as catecholamines are potent smooth muscle cell mitogens in certain settings.[112-114] In vitro, it has been shown that norepinephrine stimulates both endoreduplication[114] and hyperplasia.[112] In carotid injury models, Majesky and colleagues[140] showed that α_1-adrenergic stimulation caused PDGF A-chain expression. The importance of this finding was emphasized by the discovery that α_1-adrenergic receptor blockade with prazosin inhibited balloon injury–induced smooth muscle cell proliferation.[128] It appears that norepinephrine may be part of an autocrine growth loop, because α_1-stimulation induced both PDGF A-chain expression[140] and PDGF receptor expression.[141]

ENDOTHELIN. ET-1, the most potent vasoconstrictor yet identified, is a growth factor derived from endothelial cells. It stimulates several proto-oncogenes as well as cell cycle progression.[142] ET-1 is induced by several other smooth muscle cell growth factors, including angiotensin II, vasopressin, and PDGF. However, when administered in serum-free conditions, ET-1 is a weak mitogen, suggesting that its importance is as a comitogen with other growth factors present in the vessel wall.[143, 144] Accumulating data with ET-1 receptor–specific antagonists suggest a potentially important role for ET-1 in pulmonary VSMC proliferation and pulmonary hypertension.[145]

VASOPRESSIN. Both hypertrophy[111] and hyperplasia[115, 146] have been reported in response to vasopressin. These disparate results may have an explanation similar to that for angiotensin II: both positive and negative growth events are stimulated by vasopressin. For example, vasopressin stimulates many of the same early growth events as do classic growth factors, including ET-1. However, it also increases production of prostaglandin E_2 and prostacyclin,[147, 148] which are known to inhibit VSMC growth.[149, 150]

Tyrosine Kinase Receptor–Coupled Agonists

A focus of research has been peptide growth factors synthesized locally in the vessel in an autocrine or paracrine fashion. The role of these growth factors in hypertension has been extensively reviewed.[104, 106, 109, 130, 133, 134, 151] Tables 44-2 and 44-3 summarize the growth factors known to be involved in smooth muscle cell growth. In the following discussion, we address specifically the issue of autocrine or paracrine growth mechanisms, focusing on both positive and negative growth regulatory mechanisms.

PLATELET-DERIVED GROWTH FACTOR. PDGF has been the center of focus because it is made by many cells present in the vessel wall. Endothelial cells and macrophages produce both PDGF A and B chains, whereas adult smooth muscle cells and fibroblasts produce only PDGF A-chain.[152] In the hypertensive vessel, it appears that the dominant PDGF isoform expressed is the PDGF AA homodimer. This isoform can bind only to the PDGF α-α receptor.[153]

TABLE 44-3

Growth Inhibitors in the Vessel Wall

GROWTH INHIBITOR	CELL SOURCE	EFFECT
Heparinoids	EC	Regulates FGF availablity
	SMC	Inhibits SMC Growth
Nitric oxide	EC	↑Cyclic GMP, inhibits SMC
	SMC	↓Platelet aggregation
Prostacyclin	EC	↑cAMP, inhibits SMC
Atrial natriuretic	SMC	↑cGMP, inhibits SMC
peptide	Atria	
	EC	
Kinins	Kininogen	↓SMC growth

cAMP, cyclic adenosine monophospate; cGMP, cyclic guanosine monophosphate; EC, endothelial cell; FGF, fibroblast growth factor; SMC, smooth muscle cell.

However, the dominant PDGF receptor type appears to be the PDGF β-β receptor, which does not bind PDGF AA homodimers.[154, 155] Thus, there is a mismatch between hormone and receptor. This suggests that the source of PDGF for smooth muscle cell growth is likely to be either platelets (which contain all three PDGF isoforms) or macrophages (which have been shown to express PDGF BB). Alternatively, PDGF A-chain may not be that important in smooth muscle cell growth in hypertension. It is unclear what role the PDGF α-α receptor may play.

FIBROBLAST GROWTH FACTOR. The importance of fibroblast growth factor (FGF) as an autocrine or paracrine mediator of smooth muscle cell growth in hypertensive vessels is supported by its diverse actions on other smooth muscle cell growth factors (see Table 44-2). For example, FGF stimulates PDGF A-chain expression,[156] and it induces ACE expression in endothelial cells[157] and in VSMC.[158] PDGF-stimulated smooth muscle cell migration is inhibited by anti-FGF antibody.[159]

INSULIN-LIKE GROWTH FACTOR. The insulin-like growth factors (IGF-1 and IGF-2) are a family of growth factors whose importance in hypertension is increasingly evident. IGF-1 has been the best studied in the vasculature and is thought to be regulated by endocrine, autocrine, and paracrine mechanisms.[160] Work by Delafontaine and colleagues[161] has established that IGF-1 is increased in hypertension. These investigators observed a specific increase in IGF-1 mRNA in the aorta after infrarenal aortic coarctation. Because the cellular actions of IGF-1 are also determined by its protein binding and receptor expression, the precise effect of this increase remains to be determined. However, these investigators have further demonstrated that IGF-1 mRNA is induced by angiotensin II, suggesting that IGF-1 participates in the angiotensin II growth pathway.[162] IGF-1 is also likely to play an important role in vascular remodeling, because it has been shown to stimulate expression of extracellular matrix components such as collagens I and II and elastin.[163] Of great interest is the apparent relationship, in some patients with essential hypertension, among insulin resistance, hyperinsulinemia, and the development of hypertension, which is widely termed the metabolic syndrome.[94] Whether insulin acts as a growth factor by stimulation of its own receptors or by relatively weak interactions with IGF-1 receptors remains to be determined.

Other Smooth Muscle Cell Growth Regulators

TRANSFORMING GROWTH FACTOR-β. The variety of smooth muscle cell responses to TGF-β is daunting. TGF-β receptors are a family of transmembrane proteins that activate serine-threonine kinases.[164] By virtue of stimulating the transcriptional activity of the SMAD proteins, TGF-β modulates function of cells that express the TGF-β receptor.[165] It appears clear that TGF-β expression is increased in hypertension. Aortic smooth muscle cells from SHRs have higher levels than those from WKY control rats,[166] and both the SHRs and one-kidney one-clip hypertensive rats have increased TGF-β expression.[155, 167] In addition, infusion of TGF-β into animals after carotid injury promoted neointimal proliferation, suggesting a mitogenic effect.[168] However, the significance of increased mRNA expression is unclear. TGF-β is secreted in a latent form and then must be proteolyzed to be active. In addition, there is extensive binding of TGF-β to extracellular matrix proteins such as decorin.[169] Therefore, further work is required to demonstrate that there is increased functional TGF-β in hypertensive vessels.

In vitro experiments suggest that TGF-β can be both growth-promoting and growth-inhibiting for smooth muscle cells. At low concentrations (less than 0.1 ng/mL), TGF-β is growth-promoting, which is thought to be due to increased expression of PDGF A-chain and the PDGF α-receptor,[170-172] as well as thrombospondin.[172, 173] At higher concentrations, TGF-β is growth-inhibiting, which may be due to decreased PDGF A-chain and PDGF α-receptor expression.[170, 171] Other investigators have found that TGF-β induces a delayed increase in DNA synthesis associated primarily with cell hypertrophy.[174] The complexity of TGF-β growth

effects is compounded when combinations of growth factors are examined (e.g., PDGF and TGF-β or angiotensin II and TGF-β). For example, smooth muscle cells from SHRs show different growth responses to angiotensin II than those of WKY animals.[39, 175] In SHR smooth muscle cells, angiotensin II is mitogenic, and this correlates with relatively diminished TGF-β expression[175] compared with WKY cells, in which angiotensin II is primarily hypertrophic. As already discussed, TGF-β neutralizing antibody inhibited angiotensin II-induced increases in DNA synthesis.[39, 134, 151] However, exogenous TGF-β, at concentrations similar to those induced by angiotensin II, failed to elicit a mitogenic response in the SHR.[39]

Several new findings may explain these contradictory results. As discussed in detail later, it is now clear that TGF-β is a family of growth factors with several receptors.[176, 177] In particular, because TGF-β is synthesized and secreted in a latent form, storage of this latent molecule by matrix-bound receptors such as decorin[169] and activation of the latent molecule by proteases such as plasmin are critical regulatory steps. In addition, the system that activates TGF-β is highly regulated: TGF-β itself stimulates production of the protease inhibitor plasminogen activator inhibitor-1.[178] Thus, as shown in Figure 44-9, post-translational regulation of TGF-β (activation, storage, and presentation) contributes significantly to its physiologic effects in the vessel wall. Because of the complexity of TGF-β actions, its role in the blood vessel in hypertension requires further investigation.[133, 168, 173, 178, 179]

ATRIAL NATRIURETIC PEPTIDES. The family of atrial natriuretic peptides have been increasingly recognized as important regulators of smooth muscle cell growth in hypertension. There are at least three peptides and their cognate

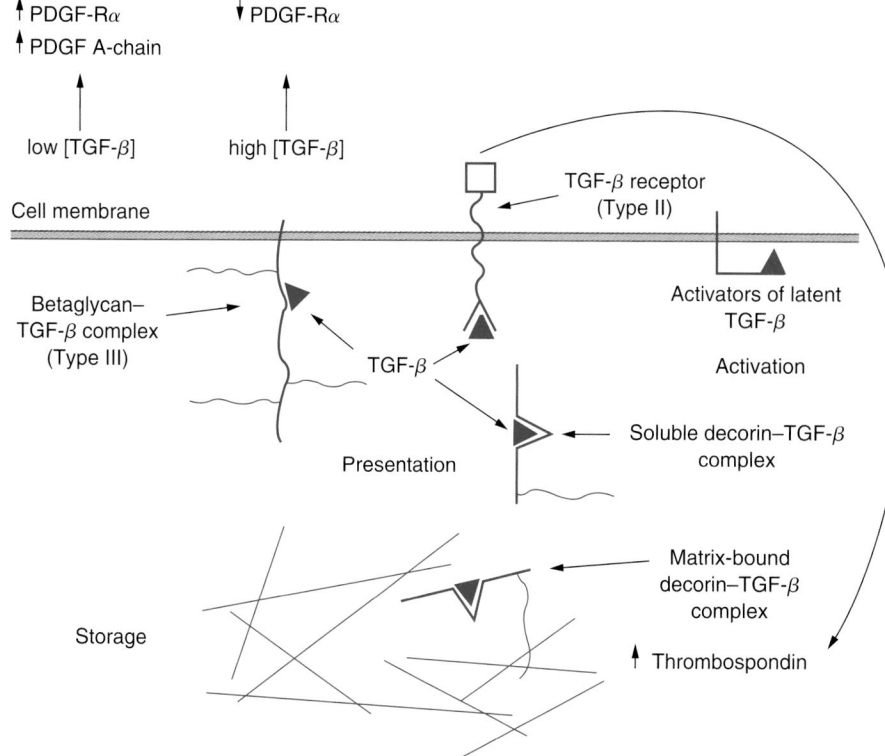

FIGURE 44-9. Interactions of transforming growth factor-β (TGF-β) with extracellular matrix and activator proteases. TGF-β binds to low-affinity sites, including β-glycan and decorin, that determine availability for signal-transducing membrane–associated receptors. TGF-β binding is associated with both positive growth stimulation (platelet-derived growth factor [PDGF] A-chain, PDGF α-receptor, and thrombospondin synthesis) and negative growth effects, particularly at high concentrations (decreased PDGF α-receptor expression and inhibition of activation by plasminogen activator inhibitor-1). (Modified from Ruoslahti E, Yamaguchi Y: Proteoglycans as modulators of growth factor activities. Cell 64:867, 1991. Copyright by Cell Press.)

receptors: A type or ANP, which is produced by atrial myocardium; B type or BNP, which is produced mainly by the myocardium and also is found in brain; and C type or CNP, which is produced by endothelial cells.[180] The three atrial natriuretic peptide receptors that have been described are the A receptor, which binds ANP and BNP and contains intrinsic guanylate cyclase activity; the B receptor, which is structurally related to the A receptor but is activated by CNP; and the C or "clearance" receptor, which has no intrinsic cyclase activity and appears to be involved in clearance of circulating forms of natriuretic peptides.[180-182] The importance of the natriuretic peptide A receptor in the regulation of blood pressure is strongly supported by findings that mice lacking a functional *Npr1* gene coding for the A receptor have elevated blood pressures and hearts exhibiting marked hypertrophy, with interstitial fibrosis resembling that seen in human hypertensive heart disease.[183]

ANP is a vasodilator and inhibits growth of cultured smooth muscle cells.[181, 182] In addition, ANP prevents the hypertrophy of cultured smooth muscle cells stimulated by angiotensin II and TGF-β.[135] Because ANP activates guanylate cyclase, cGMP levels rise. As discussed earlier for NO, elevations in cGMP appear to be growth inhibitory, suggesting that ANP exerts its antiproliferative effects by increasing guanylate cyclase activity.[89] When smooth muscle cells are placed in culture, they rapidly lose guanylate cyclase activity, which may be one form of loss of growth inhibition. Because the intact vessel expresses ANP mRNA,[184] it is possible that the family of atrial natriuretic peptides may be a local autocrine growth-regulating system analogous to the renin-angiotensin system. The potential importance of this system in hypertension is suggested by the demonstration that long-term infusion of low concentrations of ANP in the SHR (insufficient to lower blood pressure) decreased carotid artery media thickness and also inhibited smooth muscle cell hypertrophy (endoreduplication) as measured by nuclear size.[185]

Although CNP has been less studied, it appears to be critical for the ANP autocrine growth loop, because it is highly regulated in endothelial cells. The normally low level of endothelial cell CNP expression is dramatically increased by TGF-β.[186] Receptors for CNP have been demonstrated in both cultured smooth muscle cells[181] and aorta.[187] Activation by CNP increases cGMP, suggesting a hormonally activated receptor that is functionally coupled. In vitro growth inhibition studies show that CNP may be more potent than ANP at inhibiting smooth muscle cell proliferation.[188] Studies with neutral endopeptidase inhibitors that increase circulating atrial natriuretic peptides and lower blood pressure further support the importance of these hormones in blood pressure regulation, although vasodilation may not be common to all vascular beds.[189-191] In summary, this peptide family is emerging as another autocrine or paracrine growth regulatory system for smooth muscle cells that may have special importance in hypertension.

CALCITONIN GENE-RELATED PEPTIDE FAMILY. Calcitonin gene-related peptides (CGRPs), together with calcitonin, amylin, and adrenomedullin, are members of a supergene family. CGRPs are peptides (the parent molecule is CGRP1-37) that act as vasodilators and act by binding to CGRP receptors, two of which have been cloned (CGRP1 and CGRP2).[192] Adrenomedullin is a 52-amino-acid

vasorelaxant peptide that was originally isolated from human pheochromocytoma.[193] Adrenomedullin has 24% amino acid homology with CGRP and is synthesized and secreted by both endothelial cells and smooth muscle cells.[194, 195] In addition to their actions as vasorelaxants, the CGRP family prevent apoptosis in endothelial cells.[196] Adrenomedullin probably inhibits proliferation of VSMC by increasing cyclic adenosine monophosphate.[197, 198] A current working model for these peptides is that CGRP[8-37] a truncated version of CGRP, acts as an adrenomedullin receptor antagonist, because both peptides bind to the adrenomedullin and CGRP1 receptors.[192, 198-200] This model suggests that the relative balance among CGRP peptides, adrenomedullin, and the nature of receptor expression determines the effect of CGRP family members on vascular structure.

EXTRACELLULAR MATRIX, WITH EMPHASIS ON TISSUE REMODELING

The extracellular matrix is a critical regulator of vessel wall function. As already described, changes in conduit vessel elasticity are a hallmark of the chronic hypertensive state. However, the importance of the extracellular matrix has become more evident with the new knowledge that its structure and interactions with growth factors are regulated by many factors. Two concepts are widespread regarding the role of extracellular matrix in hypertension. First, dynamic alterations in vessel structure, such as those that occur with remodeling, are mediated by direct interactions between extracellular matrix and cellular components. Second, changes in extracellular matrix composition indirectly modulate cell function by their effects on growth factor binding and activity and by altering the phenotypic expression of smooth muscle cells, thereby regulating cell responsiveness to growth factors.

Extracellular Matrix Composition and Changes with Hypertension

The extracellular matrix is a complex protein-carbohydrate network consisting of collagens, elastins, proteoglycans, and glycopeptides.[201] Among the proteins that appear to be most highly regulated during vessel growth and remodeling are collagen, elastin, laminin, thrombospondin, fibronectin, and tenascin. During development of hypertension, there are significant increases in both elastin and fibronectin.[52, 53] The interactions between these molecules are regulated by a variety of enzymes, produced by both smooth muscle cells and endothelial cells, that alter the structure of the extracellular matrix. For example, collagenases (primarily matrix MMP-9 and MMP-2) are highly regulated in smooth muscle cells. Expression of proteases such as urokinase and tissue plasminogen activator is stimulated during smooth muscle cell mitogenesis and their induction is also blocked by heparin.[202-204] Conversely, TGF-β stimulates production of the protease inhibitor, plasminogen activator inhibitor-1.[178] This would act as a negative feedback mechanism for production of active TGF-β, by inhibiting the proteases required for activation of latent TGF-β.[133, 178] The relative composition of the extracellular matrix is likely to be important as well. For example, fibronectin promotes the phenotypic modulation of smooth muscle cells to a synthetic proliferative phenotype when cells are placed in culture.[205] In contrast, laminin maintains smooth muscle cells in a contractile form for a prolonged period.[205]

Recent advances in understanding the regulation and specific roles of MMPs has provided insight into the mechanisms responsible for the ordered dissolution of matrix and its reassembly during vessel remodeling. Several papers have discussed the proteases in great detail, so the discussion here focuses only on their role in vessel remodeling.[13, 62, 203] First, the basal levels of the MMPs are themselves regulated by matrix. Second, specific signals are transduced from matrix to cell via matrix receptors termed integrins, which are concentrated in regions of close interaction with the matrix termed focal adhesions or focal contacts. Cooperative signaling by specific integrins expressed in VSMC (e.g., $\alpha 5\beta 1$-integrin, $\alpha 4\beta 1$-integrin) plays an important role in regulating expression of extracellular matrix–remodeling genes such as the MMPs in response to fibronectin and other matrix proteins. Third, there is temporal and spatial regulation of integrin expression that determines the ability to respond to matrix. For example, in animal models of hypertension there are rapid increases in expression of fibronectin[53] and osteopontin.[206] These studies demonstrate the regulated and highly modular way in which information in the extracellular matrix is detected and processed by cell surface receptors.

Extracellular Matrix and Growth Factors

Although many growth factors may have interactions with the extracellular matrix, TGF-β and FGF have the most clearly defined regulatory mechanisms. TGF-β binds to two matrix proteoglycans: β–glycan (type III TGF-β receptor) and decorin.[169] Competition for TGF-β among these receptors may regulate its activity. Because decorin neutralizes TGF-β and its synthesis is stimulated by TGF-β, it may function as a negative regulatory component.

As with TGF-β, binding of FGF to heparan sulfate proteoglycans has been established for several years (Fig. 44-10).[207] This interaction has been thought to serve as both a reservoir of FGF and a proteolytic protective mechanism. It has become clear that heparan sulfate proteoglycans are required for binding of basic FGF to cells, even in the presence of the FGF receptor.[208] Presentation of basic FGF by heparan sulfate may involve its oligomerization or conformational changes. Finally, the membrane heparan sulfate proteoglycan that appears to maintain FGF in an inactive form may be cleaved by glycosylphosphatidylinositol phospholipase C to yield a free heparan sulfate–basic FGF complex.[209] This complex appears to be a powerful mediator of FGF signal transduction.

In summary, the extracellular matrix is a critical regulator of vessel growth and structure by virtue of its own dynamic regulation and because it modulates the activities of both growth-promoting and growth-inhibiting factors.

INCREASED GROWTH FACTOR RESPONSIVENESS: SIGNAL TRANSDUCTION AND ION TRANSPORT

Signal Transduction

The foregoing discussion suggests that the hypertensive vessel exists in a state of increased growth responsiveness which, over time, results in an increased number and/or size of VSMCs. In addition, these cells appear to have both increased and decreased contractile responses to a variety of

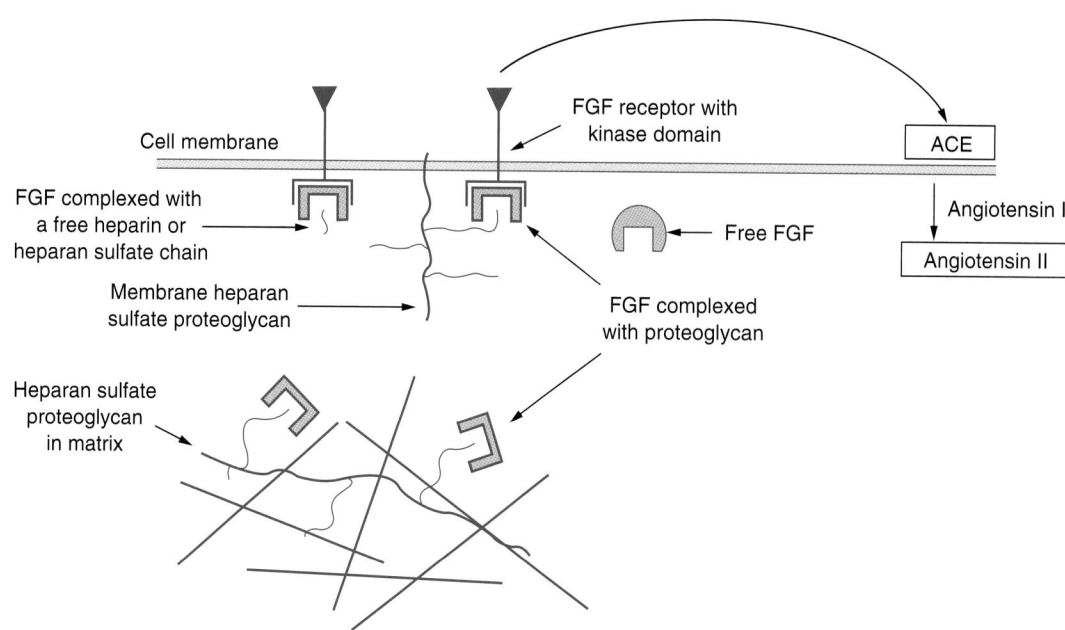

FIGURE 44-10. Interactions of fibroblast growth factor (FGF) with extracellular matrix and activation by heparan sulfates. FGF is shown in a complex with proteoglycans in an inactive form. Free heparin or heparan sulfate (generated from either matrix or cell membrane) presents FGF in a different conformation that is recognized by the cell-associated FGF receptor. Interactions with other growth factors include induction of angiotensin-converting enzyme (ACE). (Modified from Ruoslahti E, Yamaguchi Y: Proteoglycans as modulators of growth factor activities. Cell 64:867, 1991. Copyright by Cell Press.)

factors (measured by the median effective concentrations [EC_{50}] for a given contractile force). This is puzzling when one considers that if some of these cells have undergone phenotypic modulation they may have relatively less contractile machinery. In addition, it appears that the alterations in sensitivity to contractile agonists (e.g., norepinephrine) include both increases and decreases. This has led to the general hypothesis that alterations in the coupling of vasoactive molecules to intracellular events may be a fundamental genetic abnormality of hypertension. Numerous examples of such alterations exist at all steps of signal transduction, from hormone-receptor binding to stimulation of gene expression. For the discussion that follows, we will classify these alterations into three categories: changes in hormone-receptor coupling, alterations in downstream effector pathways, and changes in contractile machinery.

Increased contractile responsiveness may be secondary to up-regulation of receptor number, as has been observed with the epidermal growth factor[143] and with angiotensin II receptors.[38] Altered agonist affinity, as has been described for norepinephrine,[77] may be a consequence of expression of a different receptor subtype or modulation of receptor affinity by intracellular receptor modulators such as guanosine triphosphate (GTP)–binding proteins (G proteins). Recent data show increased expression of a polymorphism (C825T, termed the T allele) in the gene encoding the β3-subunit of G proteins (GNB3) in patients with essential hypertension.[210] The T allele is associated with the occurrence of a splice variant, GNB3-s (encoding G β3-s), in which nucleotides 498 through 620 of exon 9 are deleted. This in-frame deletion causes the loss of 41 amino acids and one WD repeat domain of the G β-subunit and most likely results in altered signal transduction.

There are many alterations in downstream effectors that have been demonstrated in SHR-derived cells compared with WKY-derived cells. For example, phospholipase C–mediated phosphoinositide turnover is stimulated by significantly lower concentrations of thrombin and angiotensin II in the SHR.[211] This would have consequences for downstream events mediated by the two second messengers generated by phospholipase C: inositol trisphosphate, which mobilizes intracellular Ca^{2+}, and diacylglycerol, which stimulates protein kinase C. In fact, increased protein kinase C activity[212, 213] and increased intracellular Ca^{2+},[214, 215] have been demonstrated in VSMC from the SHR. Alterations in growth factor–activated protein kinase cascades have also been found in SHR compared with WKY VSMC, indicating that multiple alterations in signal transduction pathways may contribute to the development of hypertension and altered VSMC growth.[78, 216, 217] An important family of kinases that seems likely to mediate these effects are the mitogen-activated protein kinases (MAP kinases). These kinases integrate signals from both tyrosine kinase and G protein-coupled receptors and mediate a variety of cell responses. Alterations in function of MAP kinases in SHR and WKY VSMC have been demonstrated by several investigators and include increases in the extent of activation and differences in regulation by intracellular mediators such as calcium.[216] The fact that these abnormalities persist in culture suggests that there may be a genetic abnormality in the regulation of these enzymes. Therefore, changes in hormone-receptor coupling, including those mediated by G proteins and downstream effectors such as phospholipases and protein kinases, provide many opportunities for alterations that may contribute to hypertension.

Ion Transport

Many investigators have suggested that a generalized abnormality in membrane function, especially ion transport, may explain the abnormal contractility and growth of SHR VSMCs.[217, 218] Increases in cellular Ca^{2+} fluxes, intracellular Na^{+} concentration, and agonist-induced Ca^{2+} mobilization have been shown in the SHR. In addition, Na^{+} uptake and the activity of Na^{+}-regulating ion transporters such as the sodium-potassium adenosine triphosphatase pump (Na^{+}, K^{+}-ATPase)[219, 220] and the Na^{+}/H^{+} exchanger[38, 143, 221] have been demonstrated in the SHR. As discussed next, the most consistent abnormality in both human essential hypertension and animal models of hypertension has been enhanced Na^{+}/H^{+} exchange.

The growth-activated Na^{+}/H^{+} exchanger (NHE1) is a member of a multigene family whose activity is increased in tissues of hypertensive humans and animals.[222] The exchanger extrudes one H^{+} in exchange for one Na^{+} when decreases in intracellular pH occur. In addition, it is an important regulator of cell volume: when cell shrinkage occurs, Na^{+}/H^{+} exchange is activated and restores cell volume by increasing intracellular Na^{+} (via obligate water entry[223-225]). Rapid increases in Na^{+}/H^{+} exchange activity occur on exposure to growth factors and vasoconstrictors.[85, 186] Activation of protein kinase C and the p44/p42 MAP kinases (extracellular signal-regulated kinases [ERK1/2]) as well as elevation of intracellular Ca^{2+}, have been reported to mediate the stimulatory effects of Na^{+}/H^{+} exchange.[116, 226-228] This stimulation is characterized by a change in affinity for intracellular H^{+} and extracellular Na^{+}.[116, 227]

Evidence indicates that the Na^{+}/H^{+} exchanger participates in signal transduction pathways by which vasoactive agents regulate smooth muscle cell proliferation.[38, 221, 227, 229] The effect of increased Na^{+}/H^{+} exchange on growth would likely be an enhanced sensitivity to mitogens.[38] Because of the activation of the Na^{+}/H^{+} exchanger by both hyperplastic and hypertrophic agents, it has been proposed that abnormal function of this protein may be involved in the pathophysiology of hypertension.[217, 227]

Evidence for dysfunction of the Na^{+}/H^{+} exchanger in hypertension is provided by observations that its activity is increased in neutrophils, lymphocytes, and platelets from SHRs and in platelets and lymphocytes from hypertensive patients.[217, 227, 230] Data from several laboratories[38, 143] indicate that both cultured smooth muscle cells and intact mesenteric arteries from SHR animals[221] have a greater capacity for Na^{+}/H^{+} exchange and altered kinetic characteristics, compared with those from WKY rats. As discussed later, these findings correlate with increased exchanger phosphorylation in SHRs, without change in protein expression or amino acid sequence.[231, 232] The report that immortalized lymphoblasts from patients with a family history of essential hypertension had greater Na^{+}/H^{+} exchange than lymphoblasts from normotensive patients further suggests that this is a genetic property of hypertension. Yet, analysis by restriction fragment length polymorphisms[233] and complementary DNA sequencing[234] has failed to demonstrate the Na⁺/H⁺ exchanger gene itself is a candidate gene for hypertension. There is no evidence for NHE1 mutations or altered NHE1 expression in several hypertensive populations. Studies with the SHR have demonstrated increased activity of the Na⁺/H⁺ exchanger[38, 221] but no change in regulation at the mRNA[235] or protein level.[231, 232] This suggests that the abnormality in Na⁺/H⁺ exchange is a consequence of a posttranslational mechanism. It has become clear that the Na⁺/H⁺ exchanger is regulated by several posttranslational mechanisms that may alter its activity. These include phosphorylation, glycosylation, binding of calmodulin, and binding of accessory proteins that may mediate interactions with the cytoskeleton and integrins.[236-240] The most likely mechanism for increased Na⁺/H⁺ exchange activity in the SHR is related to increased phosphorylation.[231, 232] Our laboratory identified p90RSK as one kinase that phosphorylates NHE1 and increases its activity.[241] Other laboratories have suggested important roles for the Nck-interacting kinase[238] and for ERK1/2.[242]

UNIFYING HYPOTHESIS

To account for the hypertensive phenotype, several mechanisms related to abnormalities in signal transduction and ion transport have been proposed as etiologic. For example, in the SHR, many new insights into the regulation of the kinases and phosphatases responsible for activating and inactivating these proteins suggest that a common regulatory factor or "integrator" may account for multiple changes in hypertensive cells. Unifying hypotheses for this integrator have been based on alterations in ion transport (regulation of intracellular Na⁺ and Ca²⁺) or on alterations in signal transduction mechanisms (G proteins, kinases, and phosphatases).[38, 218, 243, 244] As evidence mounts that many ion transporters are regulated by G protein–coupled receptor–mediated activation of protein kinases,[236, 245, 246] these two hypotheses have come together. In particular, genes for many of the ion transporters have been cloned and sequenced. Comparison of normotensive and hypertensive strains of rats has uniformly failed to identify significant differences in the coding sequences of these transport molecules.[230, 247] It should be noted that changes in the epithelial sodium channel have been described, and mutations (or deletions) that lead to increased sodium reabsorption are associated with significant hypertension.[248] For the Na⁺/H⁺ exchanger, it appears likely that proteins that mediate receptor signal transduction as well as the downstream enzymes that regulate transporter activity, rather than the transporters themselves, contribute to hypertension. Specifically (Fig. 44-11), it is proposed that intracellular signal mediators that are integrators of extracellular stimuli are enhanced in hypertensive VSMC, and that these mediators in turn affect common regulatory events such as ion fluxes and cell cycle genes that cause both increased tone and growth.[78, 79, 212, 213]

By using the Na⁺/H⁺ exchanger as an example, an alteration in phosphorylation of the exchanger would be a likely mechanism, because it would explain both increased smooth muscle cell growth and function. Several growth factors stimulate phosphorylation of the Na⁺/H⁺ exchanger.[246] It is now known that these growth factors activate a cascade of intracellular kinases that include Raf kinase, the MAP kinase kinase

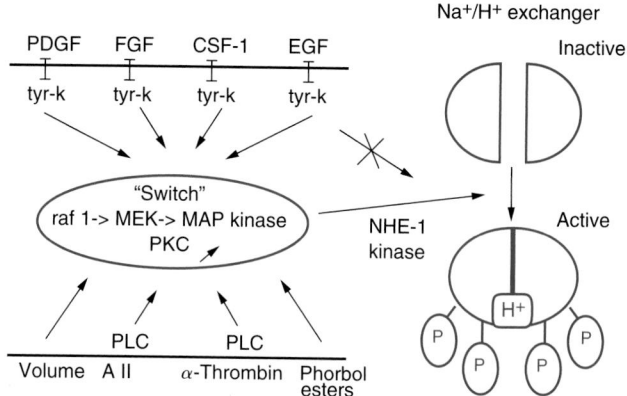

FIGURE 44-11. Model for activation of the Na⁺/H⁺ exchanger by receptor-coupled kinase cascade. Multiple stimuli, including both tyrosine kinases (tyr-k) coupled to growth factor receptors and vasoactive mediators (volume, angiotensin II [AII], α-thrombin, and phorbol esters), activate the mitogen-activated protein kinase (MAP kinase). The MAP kinase then stimulates downstream effector kinases (e.g., the Na⁺/H⁺ exchanger [NHE1] kinase), which in turn activate intracellular ion transporters such as the exchanger.

(or MEK-1, MAP and ERK kinase), and ERK1/2.[249, 250] Inhibition of these kinases by overexpression of a dominant negative mutant of ERK1/2[251] or by treatment with an inhibitor of MEK-1,[252] inhibits growth factor–stimulated mitogenesis and Na⁺/H⁺ exchange activity. Conversely, an increase in the activity of one of these kinases would increase activity of many growth factors, because it acts as a convergence or integration point for multiple stimuli. The increase in kinase activity could arise by several mechanisms: a primary abnormality in its structure that causes increased activity, an abnormality in its regulation that causes it to be overexpressed (increased synthesis or decreased degradation), or a change in the enzymes that regulate its activity (e.g., a phosphatase that inactivates the kinase or a kinase that activates it).

Our laboratory recently identified p90RSK as one candidate NHE1 kinase.[241] Because p90RSK is a downstream substrate for ERK1/2, alteration in p90RSK activity is consistent with previous studies involving ERK1/2 inhibitors. More recently, we showed that p38 acts as a negative regulator of NHE1 by inhibiting ERK1/2 activity.[253] Future work in this rapidly developing field should yield many candidate kinases, such as Nck-interacting kinase[238] and ERK1/2,[242] that mediate these effects. Based on these findings, it appears reasonable that alterations in the function of these intracellular enzymes may cause the multiple abnormalities in VSMC ion transport and growth that are the hallmarks of hypertension at the cellular level.

SUMMARY

The hypertensive vessel wall is typified by abnormalities in structure and function. These alterations include increased smooth muscle cell mass relative to lumen size with an increase in vascular resistance mediated at the level of the resistance arterioles. These alterations appear to be due to a primary abnormality in VSMC growth regulation that is caused by genetic, environmental, and hemodynamic factors. Genetic analysis suggests that at least five or six genes are responsible for essential hypertension.[7, 254] The establishment of transgenic mice and rats[120] that express candidate gene abnormalities should enable the role of these genes to be studied in a tissue-specific manner. Ultimately, delineation of the specific events that alter vascular cell-specific function to a hypertensive phenotype will permit therapy that is more effective in preventing chronic end-organ damage.

REFERENCES

1. Chobanian AV: Corcoran lecture: Adaptive and maladaptive responses of the arterial wall to hypertension. Hypertension 15:666-674, 1990.
2. Mulvany MJ, Aalkjaer C: Structure and function of small arteries. Physiol Rev 70:921-961, 1990.
3. Mulvany MJ: Abnormalities of resistance vessel structure in essential hypertension. Clin Exp Pharmacol Physiol 18:13-20, 1991.
4. Heagerty AM: Changes in vascular morphology in essential hypertension. J Hum Hypertens 1:3-8, 1991.
5. Heagerty AM, Aalkjaer C, Bund SJ, et al: Small artery structure in hypertension: Dual processes of remodeling and growth. Hypertension 21:391-397, 1993.
6. Stoll M, Cowley AW Jr, Tonellato PJ, et al: A genomic-systems biology map for cardiovascular function. Science 294:1723-1726, 2001.
7. Cowley AJ, Stoll M, Greene AS, et al: Genetically defined risk of salt sensitivity in an intercross of brown Norway and Dahl S rats. Physiol Genomics 2:107-115, 2000.
8. Korsgaard N, Mulvany MJ: Cellular hyertrophy in mesenteric resistance vessels from renal hypertensive rats. Hypertension 12:162-167, 1988.
9. Mulvany MJ, Baadrup U, Gundersen HJG: Evidence for hyperplasia in mesenteric resistance vessels of spontaneously hypertensive rats using a three-dimensional dissector. Circ Res 57:794-800, 1985.
10. Mulvany MJ, Hansen PK, Aalkjaer C: Direct evidence that the greater contractility of resistance vessels in spontaneously hypertensive rats is associated with a narrower lumen, a thicker media and a greater number of smooth muscle cell layers. Circ Res 43:854-864, 1978.
11. Owens G, Schwartz S: Alterations in vascular smooth muscle mass in the spontaneously hypertensive rat: Role of cellular hypertrophy, hyperploidy and hyperplasia. Circ Res 51:280-289, 1982.
12. Owens GK: Influence of blood pressure on development of aortic medial smooth muscle hypertrophy in spontaneously hypertensive rats. Hypertension 9:178-187, 1987.
13. Schwartz SM, Majesky MW, Dilley RJ: Vascular remodeling in hypertension and atherosclerosis. *In* Laragh J, Brenner BM (eds): Hypertension: Pathophysiology, Diagnosis and Management. New York, Raven Press, 1990, pp 521-539.
14. Mulvany MJ, Baumbach GL, Aalkjaer C, et al: Vascular remodeling. Hypertension 28:505-506, 1996.
15. Lund-Johansen P: Haemodynamics in essential hypertension: State of the art review. Clin Sci 59:343S-354S, 1980.
16. Folkow B, Grimby G, Thulesius O: Adaptive structural changes of the vascular walls in hypertension and their relation to the control of peripheral resistance. Acta Physiol Scand 44:255-272, 1958.
17. Harper RN, Moore MA, Marr MC, et al: Arteriolar rarefaction in the conjuctiva of human essential hypertensives. Microvasc Res 16:369-372, 1978.
18. Harrison DG, Treasure CB, Mugge A, et al: Hypertension and the coronary circulation: With special attention to endothelial regulation. Am J Hypertens 4:454S-459S, 1991.
19. Heistad DD, Baumbach GL: Cerebral vascular changes during chronic hypertension: Good guys and bad guys. J Hypertens Suppl 10:S71-S75, 1992.
20. Aalkjaer C, Danielsen H, Johannesen P, et al: Abnormal vascular function and morphology in pre-eclampsia: A study of isolated resistance vessels. Clin Sci 69:477-482, 1985.
21. Aalkjaer C, Pedersen EB, Danielsen H, et al: Morphological and functional characteristics of isolated resistance vessels in advanced uraemia. Clin Sci 71:657-663, 1976.
22. Short D: Morphology of the intestinal arterioles in chronic human hypertension. Br Heart J 28:184-192, 1966.
23. Aalkjaer C, Heagerty AM, Petersen KK, et al: Evidence for increased media thickness, increased neuronal amine uptake, and depressed excitation-contraction coupling in isolated resistance vessels from essential hypertensives. Circ Res 61:181-186, 1987.
24. Schiffrin EL, Park JB, Intengan HD, et al: Correction of arterial structure and endothelial dysfunction in human essential hypertension by the angiotensin receptor antagonist losartan. Circulation 101:1653-1659, 2000.
25. Bohlen HG, Gore RW, Hutchins PM: Comparison of microvascular pressures in normal and spontaneously hypertensive rats. Microvasc Res 13:125-130, 1977.
26. Schiffrin EL, Deng LY, Larochelle P: Blunted effects of endothelin upon small subcutaneous resistance arteries of mild essential hypertensive patients. J Hypertension 10:437-444, 1992.
27. Mulvany MJ: Vascular structure and smooth muscle contractility in experimental hypertension. J Cardiovasc Pharmacol 10(suppl 6):S79-S85, 1987.
28. Jespersen LT, Nyborg NCB, Pedersen OL, et al: Cardiac mass and peripheral vascular structure in hydralazine-treated spontaneously hypertensive rats. Hypertension 7:734-741, 1985.
29. Mulvany MJ, Nyborg N: An increased calcium sensitivity of mesenteric resistance vessels in young and adult spontaneously hypertensive rats. Br J Pharmacol 71:585-596, 1980.
30. Mulvany MJ, Nilsson H, Nyborg N, et al: Are isolated femoral resistance vessels or tail arteries good models for the hindquarter vasculature of spontaneously hypertensive rats? Acta Physiol Scand 116:275-283, 1982.
31. Korsgaard N, Aalkjaer C, Heagerty AM, et al: Histology of subcutaneous small arteries from patients with essential hypertension. Hypertension 22:523-526, 1993.
32. Owens GK: Differential effects of antihypertensive drug therapy on vascular smooth muscle cell hypertrophy, hyperploidy and hyperplasia in the spontaneously hypertensive rat. Circ Res 56:525-536, 1985.
33. Griffin SA, Brown WC, MacPherson F, et al: Angiotensin II causes vascular hypertrophy in part by a non-pressor mechanism. Hypertension 17:626-635, 1991.
34. Griendling KK, Minieri CA, Ollerenshaw JD, et al: Angiotensin II stimulates NADH and NADPH oxidase activation in cultured vascular smooth muscle cells. Circ Res 74:1141-1148, 1994.
35. Rajagopalan S, Kurz S, Munzel T, et al: Angiotensin II-mediated hypertension in the rat increases vascular superoxide production via membrane NADH/NADPH oxidase activation: Contribution to alterations of vasomotor tone. J Clin Invest 97:1916-1923, 1996.
36. Christensen KL: Reducing pulse pressure in hypertension may normalize small artery structure. Hypertension 18:722-727, 1991.
37. Geisterfer AAT, Peach MJ, Owens GK: Angiotensin II induces hypertrophy, not hyperplasia, of cultured rat aortic smooth muscle cells. Circ Res 62:749-756, 1988.
38. Berk BC, Vallega G, Muslin AJ, et al: Spontaneously hypertensive rat vascular smooth muscle cells in culture exhibit increased growth and Na+/H+ exchange. J Clin Invest 83:822-829, 1989.
39. Stouffer GA, Owens GK: Angiotensin II-induced mitogenesis of spontaneously hypertensive rat-derived cultured smooth muscle cells is dependent on autocrine production of transforming growth factor-beta. Circ Res 70:820-828, 1992.
40. Halpern W, Warshaw DM, Mulvany MJ: Mechanical and morphological properties of arterial resistance vessels in young and old spontaneously hypertensive rats. Circ Res 45:250-259, 1979.
41. Lee RMKW, Triggle CR, Cheung DWT, et al: Structural and functional consequence of neonatal sympathectomy on the blood vessels of spontaneously hypertensive rats. Hypertension 10:328-338, 1987.
42. Thomas WA, Lee KT, Kim DN: Cell population kinetics in atherogenesis: Cell births and losses in intimal cell mass-derived lesions in the abdominal aorta of swine. Ann N Y Acad Sci 454:305-315, 1985.
43. Bennett MR, Evan GI, Schwartz SM: Apoptosis of human vascular smooth muscle cells derived from normal vessels and coronary atherosclerotic plaques. J Clin Invest 95:2266-2274, 1995.
44. Schwartz SM, Reidy MR, Clowes A: Kinetics of atherosclerosis: A stem cell model. Ann N Y Acad Sci 454:292-304, 1985.
45. Majesky MW, Giachelli CM, Reidy MA, et al: Rat carotid neointimal smooth muscle cells reexpress a developmentally regulated mRNA phenotype during repair of arterial injury. Circ Res 71:759-768, 1992.
46. Dimmeler S, Aicher A, Vasa M, et al: HMG-CoA reductase inhibitors (statins) increase endothelial progenitor cells via the PI 3-kinase/Akt pathway. J Clin Invest 108:391-397, 2001.

47. Ku DN, Giddens DP: Pulsatile flow in a model carotid bifurcation. Arteriosclerosis 3:31-39, 1983.
48. Davies PF: Endothelial cells, hemodynamic forces, and the localization of atherosclerosis. In Ryan US (ed): Endothelial Cells. Boca Raton, FL: CRC Press, 1988, pp 123-139.
49. Davies PF, Zilberberg J, Helmke BP: Spatial microstimuli in endothelial mechanosignaling. Circ Res 92:359-370, 2003.
50. Mitsumata M, Fishel RS, Nerem RN, et al: Fluid shear stress stimulates platelet-derived growth factor expression in endothelial cells. Am J Physiol 265:H3-H8, 1993.
51. Howard PS, Myers JC, Gorfien SF, et al: Progressive modulation of endothelial phenotype during in vitro blood vessel formation. Dev Biol 146:325-338, 1991.
52. Saouaf R, Takasaki I, Eastman E, et al: Fibronectin biosynthesis in the rat aorta in vitro: Changes due to experimental hypertension. J Clin Invest 88:1182-1189, 1991.
53. Takasaki I, Chobanian AV, Sarzani P, et al: Effects of hypertension on fibronectin expression in the rat aorta. J Biol Chem 265:21935-21939, 1990.
54. Langille BL, O'Donnell F: Reductions in arterial diameter produced by chronic decreases in blood flow are endothelium-dependent. Science 231:405-407, 1986.
55. Langille BL, Brownlee RD, Adamson SL: Perinatal aortic growth in lambs: Relation to blood flow changes at birth. Am J Physiol 259:H1247-H1253, 1990.
56. Kohler TR, Kirkman TR, Kraiss LW, et al: Increased blood flow inhibits neointimal hyperplasia in endothelialized vascular grafts. Circ Res 69:1557-1565, 1991.
57. Tronc F, Wassef M, Esposito B, et al: Role of NO in flow-induced remodeling of the rabbit common carotid artery. Arterioscler Thromb Vasc Biol 16:1256-1262, 1996.
58. Crawford DW, Blankenhorn DH: Arterial wall oxygenation, oxyradicals, and atherosclerosis. Atherosclerosis 89:97-108, 1991.
59. Halliwell B: Free radicals, reactive oxygen species and human disease: A critical evaluation with special reference to atherosclerosis. Br J Exp Pathol 70:737-757, 1989.
60. Crawford DW, Back LH, Cole MA, et al: In vivo oxygen transport in the normal rabbit femoral arterial wall. J Clin Invest 65:1498, 1980.
61. Chambless LE, Folsom AR, Davis V, et al: Risk factors for progression of common carotid atherosclerosis: The Atherosclerosis Risk in Communities Study, 1987-1998. Am J Epidemiol 155:38-47, 2002.
62. Redmond EM, Cahill PA, Hirsch M, et al: Effect of pulse pressure on vascular smooth muscle cell migration: The role of urokinase and matrix metalloproteinase. Thromb Haemost 81:293-300, 1999.
63. Dohi Y, Thiel MA, Buhler FR, et al: Activation of endothelial L-arginine pathway in resistance arteries: Effect of age and hypertension. Hypertension 15:170-179, 1990.
64. Luscher TF, Vanhoutte PM: Endothelium-dependent contractions to acetylcholine in the aorta of the spontaneously hypertensive rat. Hypertension 8:344-348, 1986.
65. Dohi Y, Lüscher TF: Endothelin in hypertensive resistance arteries: Intraluminal and extraluminal dysfunction. Hypertension 18:543-549, 1991.
66. Diederich D, Yang Z, Buhler FR, et al: Impaired endothelium-dependent relaxations in hypertensive resistance arteries involve the cyclooxygenase pathway. Am J Physiol 258:H445-H451, 1990.
67. Hunter GC, Dubick MA, Keen CL, et al: Effects of hypertension on aortic antioxidant status in human abdominal aneurysmal and occlusive disease. Proc Soc Exp Biol Med 196:273-279, 1991.
68. Cuccurullo F, Porreca E, Lapenna D, et al: Aortic glutathione-related antioxidant defenses in rabbits subjected to suprarenal aortic coarctation hypertension. J Mol Cell Card 23:727-734, 1991.
69. Nakazono K, Watanabe N, Matsuno K, et al: Does superoxide underlie the pathogenesis of hypertension? Proc Natl Acad Sci U S A 88:10045-10048, 1991.
70. Laursen JB, Rajagopalan S, Galis Z, et al: Role of superoxide in angiotensin II-induced but not catecholamine-induced hypertension. Circulation 95:588-593, 1997.
71. Panza JA, Quyyumi AA, Brush JE, et al: Abnormal endothelium-dependent vascular relaxation in patients with essential hypertension. N Engl J Med 323:22-27, 1990.
72. Harrison DG: Endothelial function and oxidant stress. Clin Cardiol 20(11 Suppl 2):II-11-II-17, 1997.
73. Pratt PF, Falck JR, Reddy KM, et al: 20-HETE relaxes bovine coronary arteries through the release of prostacyclin. Hypertension 31:237-241, 1998.
74. Li PL, Campbell WB: Epoxyeicosatrienoic acids activate K+ channels in coronary smooth muscle through a guanine nucleotide binding protein. Circ Res 80:877-884, 1997.
75. Campbell-Chamley JH, Campbell GR: What controls smooth muscle phenotype. Atherosclerosis 40:347-357, 1981.
76. Falloon BJ, Bund SJ, Tulip JR, et al: In vitro perfusion studies of resistance artery function in genetic hypertension. Hypertension 22:486-495, 1993.
77. Nyborg NCB, Bevan JA: Increased alpha-adrenergic receptor affinity in resistance vessels from hypertensive rats. Hypertension 11:635-638, 1988.
78. Siffert W, Dusing R: Sodium-proton exchange and primary hypertension: An update. Hypertension 26:649-655, 1995.
79. Siffert W, Rosskopf D, Moritz A, et al: Enhanced G protein activation in immortalized lymphoblasts from patients with essential hypertension. J Clin Invest 96:759-766, 1995.
80. Berk BC, Alexander RW, Brock TA, et al: Vasoconstriction: A new activity for platelet-derived growth factor. Science 232:87-90, 1986.
81. Yamori Y, Mano M, Nara Y, et al. Catecholamine-induced polyploidization in aortic smooth muscle cells of hypertensive rats. Circulation 75:I92-I95, 1987.
82. Leitschuh M, Chobanian AV: Inhibition of nuclear polyploidy by propranolol in aortic smooth muscle cells of hypertensive rats. Hypertension 9(Suppl III):III-106-III-109, 1987.
83. Bevan RD, Tsuru H: Functional and structural changes in the rabbit ear artery after sympathetic denervation. Circ Res 49:478-485, 1981.
84. Linder L, Kiowski W, Buhler FR, et al: Indirect evidence for the release of endothelium-derived relaxing factor in human forearm in vivo: Blunted response in essential hypertension. Circulation 81:1762-1767, 1990.
85. Furchgott RF, Zawadzki JV: The obligatory role of endothelial cells in the relaxation of arterial smooth muscle by acetylcholine. Nature 288:373-386, 1980.
86. Palmer RMJ, Ashton DS, Moncada S: Vascular endothelial cells synthesize NO from L-arginine. Nature 333:664-666, 1988.
87. Palmer RMJ, Ferrige AG, Moncada S: Nitric oxide accounts for the biological activity of endothelium-derived relaxing factor. Nature 327:524-526, 1987.
88. Radomsky MW, Palmer RMJ, Moncada S: The anti-aggregatory properties of vascular endothelium: Interactions between prostacyclin and nitric oxide. Br J Pharmacol 92:639-646, 1987.
89. Garg UC, Hassid A: Nitric oxide-generating vasodilators and 8-bromo-cyclic guanosine monophosphate inhibit mitogenesis and proliferation of cultured rat vascular smooth muscle cells. J Clin Invest 83:1774-1777, 1989.
90. Frame MD, Fox RJ, Kim D, et al: Diminished arteriolar responses in nitrate tolerance involve ROS and angiotensin II. Am J Physiol Heart Circ Physiol 282:H2377-H2385, 2002.
91. Kim D, Rybalkin SD, Pi X, et al: Upregulation of phosphodiesterase 1A1 expression is associated with the development of nitrate tolerance. Circulation 104:2338-2343, 2001.
92. Shesely EG, Maeda N, Kim HS, et al: Elevated blood pressures in mice lacking endothelial nitric oxide synthase. Proc Natl Acad Sci U S A 93:13176-13181, 1996.
93. Rudic RD, Shesely EG, Maeda N, et al: Direct evidence for the importance of endothelium-derived nitric oxide in vascular remodeling. J Clin Invest 101:731-736, 1998.
94. Sowers JR: Insulin resistance, hyperinsulinemia, dyslipidemia, hypertension, and accelerated atherosclerosis. J Clin Pharmacol 32:529-535, 1992.
95. Michel T, Feron O: Nitric oxide synthases: Which, where, how, and why? J Clin Invest 100:2146-2151, 1997.
96. Luscher TF, Vanhoutte PM, Raij L: Antihypertensive treatment normalizes decreased endothelium-dependent relaxations in rats with salt-induced hypertension. Hypertension 9:III193-III197, 1987.
97. Uehata M, Ishizaki T, Satoh H, et al: Calcium sensitization of smooth muscle mediated by a Rho-associated protein kinase in hypertension. Nature 389:990-994, 1997.
98. Navab M, Imes SS, Hama SY, et al: Monocyte transmigration induced by modification of low density lipoprotein in cocultures of human aortic wall cells is due to induction of monocyte chemotactic protein 1 synthesis and is abolished by high density lipoprotein. J Clin Invest 88:2039-2046, 1991.
99. Luscher TF, Boulanger CM, Dohi Y, et al: Endothelium-derived contracting factors. Hypertension 19:117-130, 1992.

100. Fabbrini MS, Vitale A, Patrano C, et al: Heterologous *in vivo* processing of human preproendothelin 1 into bioactive peptides. Proc Natl Acad Sci U S A 88:8939-8943, 1991.

101. Boulanger C, Lüscher TF: Release of endothelin from the porcine aorta: Inhibition by endothelium-derived nitric oxide. J Clin Invest 85:587-590, 1990.

102. Yang Z, Stulz P, von Segesser L, et al: Different activation of the endothelial L-arginine and cyclooxygenase pathway in the human internal mammary artery and saphenous vein. Circ Res 68:52-60, 1991.

103. Feletou M, Vanhoutte PM: Endothelium-dependent hyperpolarization of canine coronary smooth muscle. Br J Pharmacol 93:352-357, 1988.

104. Berk BC: Vascular smooth muscle growth: Autocrine growth mechanisms. Physiol Rev 81:999-1030, 2001.

105. Owens GK: Control of hypertrophic versus hyperplastic growth of vascular smooth muscle cells. Am J Physiol 257:H1755-H1765, 1989.

106. Scott-Burden T, Hahn AW, Buhler FR, et al: Vasoactive peptides and growth factors in the pathophysiology of hypertension. J Cardiovasc Pharmacol 20(suppl 1):S55-S64, 1992.

107. Carretero OA, Scicli AG: Local hormonal factors (intracrine, autocrine, and paracrine) in hypertension. Hypertension 18:I58-I69, 1991.

108. De Mey JG, Schiffers PM: Effects of the endothelium on growth responses in arteries. J Cardiovasc Pharmacol 21(suppl 1):S22-S25, 1993.

109. Dzau VJ, Gibbons GH: Endothelium and growth factors in vascular remodeling of hypertension. Hypertension 18:115-121, 1991.

110. Berk BC, Vekshtein V, Gordon HM, et al: Angiotensin II-stimulated protein synthesis in cultured vascular smooth muscle cells. Hypertension 13:305-314, 1989.

111. Geisterfer AAT, Owens GK: Arginine vasopressin-induced hypertrophy of cultured rat aortic smooth muscle cells. Hypertension 14:413-420, 1989.

112. Blaes N, Boissel JP: Growth stimulating effect of catecholamines on rat aortic smooth muscle cells in culture. J Cell Physiol 116:167-172, 1983.

113. Nakaki T, Nakayama M, Yamamoto S, et al: Alpha1-adrenergic stimulation and beta2-adrenergic inhibition of DNA synthesis in vascular smooth muscle cells. Mol Pharmacol 37:30-36, 1990.

114. Printseva OY, Tjurmin AV, Rudchenko SA, et al: Noradrenaline induces the polyploidization of smooth muscle cells: The synergism of second messengers. Exp Cell Res 184:342-350, 1989.

115. Hamada M, Nishio I, Baba A, et al: Enhanced DNA synthesis of cultured vascular smooth muscle cells from spontaneously hypertensive rats: Difference of response to growth factor, intracellular free calcium concentration and DNA synthesizing cell cycle. Atherosclerosis 81:191-198, 1990.

116. Berk BC, Aronow MS, Brock TA, et al: Angiotensin II-stimulated Na+/H+ exchange in cultured vascular smooth muscle cells: Evidence for protein kinase C-dependent and -independent pathways. J Biol Chem 262:5057-5064, 1987.

117. Taubman MB, Berk BC, Izumo S, et al: Angiotensin II induces c-fos mRNA in aortic smooth muscle: Role of Ca^{2+} mobilization and protein kinase C activation. J Biol Chem 264:526-530, 1989.

118. Daemen MJAP, Lombardi DM, Bosman FT, et al: Angiotensin II induces smooth muscle cell proliferation in the normal and injured rat arterial wall. Circ Res 68:450-456, 1991.

119. Powell JS, Clozel JP, Muller RK, et al: Inhibitors of angiotensin-converting enzyme prevent myointimal proliferation after vascular injury. Science 245:186-188, 1989.

120. Mullins JJ, Peters J, Ganten D: Fulminant hypertension in transgenic rats harbouring the mouse Ren-2 gene. Nature 344:541-544, 1990.

121. Tanimoto K, Sugiyama F, Goto Y, et al: Angiotensinogen-deficient mice with hypotension. J Biol Chem 269:31334-31337, 1994.

122. Ito M, Oliverio MI, Mannon PJ, et al: Regulation of blood pressure by the type 1A angiotensin II receptor gene. Proc Natl Acad Sci U S A 92:3521-3525, 1995.

123. Ushio-Fukai M, Zafari AM, Fukui T, et al: p22phox is a critical component of the superoxide-generating NADH/NADPH oxidase system and regulates angiotensin II-induced hypertrophy in vascular smooth muscle cells. J Biol Chem 271:23317-23321, 1996.

124. Benter IF, Diz DI, Ferrario CM: Cardiovascular actions of angiotensin (1-7). Peptides 14:679-684, 1993.

125. Farhy RD, Carretero OA, Ho K-L, et al: Role of kinins and nitric oxide in the effects of angiotensin converting enzyme inhibitors on neointima formation. Circ Res 72:1202-1210, 1993.

126. Saed GM, Carretero OA, MacDonald RJ, et al: Kallikrein messenger RNA in rat arteries and veins. Circ Res 67:510-516, 1990.

127. Oza NB, Schwartz JH, Goud HD, et al: Rat aortic smooth muscle cells in culture express kallikrein, kininogen, and bradykininase activity. J Clin Invest 85:597-600, 1990.

128. van Kleef EM, Smits JFM, De Mey JGR, et al: Alpha1-adrenergic blockade reduces the angiotensin II-induced vascular smooth muscle cell DNA synthesis in the rat thoracic aorta and carotid artery. Circ Res 70:1122-1127, 1992.

129. Dzau VJ: Circulating versus local renin-angiotensin system in cardiovascular homeostasis. Circulation 77(suppl I):4-13, 1988.

130. Dzau VJ, Gibbons GH, Pratt RE: Molecular mechanisms of vascular renin-angiotensin system in neointimal hyperplasia. Hypertension 18(suppl II):II-100–II-5, 1991.

131. Naftilan AJ, Zuo WM, Inglefinger J, et al: Localization and differential regulation of angiotensinogen mRNA expression in the vessel wall. J Clin Invest 87:1300-1311, 1991.

132. Dasarathy Y, Fanburg BL: Involvement of second messenger systems in stimulation of angiotensin converting enzyme of bovine endothelial cells. J Cell Physiol 148:327-335, 1991.

133. Berk BC, Corson MA: Autocrine and paracrine growth mechanisms in vascular smooth muscle. Curr Opin Cardiol 7:739-744, 1992.

134. Koibuchi Y, Lee WS, Gibbons GH, et al: Role of transforming growth factor-beta 1 in the cellular growth response to angiotensin II. Hypertension 21:1046-1050, 1993.

135. Itoh H, Pratt IH, Dzau VJ: Atrial natriuretic polypeptide inhbits hypertrophy of vascular smooth muscle cells. J Clin Invest 86:1690-1697, 1990.

136. Hahn AW, Resink TJ, Bernhardt J, et al: Stimulation of autocrine platelet-derived growth factor AA-homodimer and transforming growth factor beta in vascular smooth muscle cells. Biochem Biophys Res Commun 178:1451-1458, 1991.

137. Berk BC, Rao GN: Angiotensin II-induced vascular smooth muscle cell hypertrophy: PDGF A-chain mediates the increase in cell size. J Cell Physiol 154:368-380, 1993.

138. Ushio-Fukai M, Alexander RW, Akers M, et al: p38 Mitogen-activated protein kinase is a critical component of the redox-sensitive signaling pathways activated by angiotensin II: Role in vascular smooth muscle cell hypertrophy. J Biol Chem 273:15022-15029, 1998.

139. Griendling KK, Ushio-Fukai M: Redox control of vascular smooth muscle proliferation. J Lab Clin Med 132:9-15, 1998.

140. Majesky MW, Daemen MJAP, Schwartz SM: Alpha 1-adrenergic stimulation of platelet-derived growth factor A-chain gene expression in aorta. J Biol Chem 265:1082-1088, 1990.

141. Bobik A, Grinpukel S, Little PJ, et al: Angiotensin II and noradrenaline increase PDGF BB receptors and potentiate PDGF BB stimulated DNA synthesis in vascular smooth muscle. Biochem Biophys Res Commun 166:580-588, 1990.

142. Bobik A, Grooms A, Millar JA, et al: Growth factor activity of endothelin on vascular smooth muscle. Am J Physiol 258:C409-C415, 1990.

143. Scott-Burden T, Resink TJ, Baur U, et al: Epidermal growth factor responsiveness in smooth muscle cells from hypertensive and normotensive rats. Hypertension 13:295-304, 1989.

144. Scott-Burden T, Resink TJ, Hahn AW, et al: Induction of endothelin secretion by angiotensin II: Effects on growth and synthetic activity of vascular smooth muscle cells. J Cardiovasc Pharmacol 17(suppl 7):S96-S100, 1991.

145. Luscher TF, Wenzel RR: Endothelin and endothelin antagonists: Pharmacology and clinical implications. Agents Actions Suppl 45:237-253, 1995.

146. Murase T, Kozawa O, Miwa M, et al: Regulation of proliferation by vasopressin in aortic smooth msucle cells: Function of protein kinase C. Hypertension 10:1505-1511, 1992.

147. Vallotton MB, Wuthrich RP, Lew PD, Capponi AM: Effects of vasopressin and its analogues on rat aortic smooth muscle and renal medullary tubular cells: Characterization of receptor subtypes. J Cardiovasc Pharmacol 8(suppl 7):S5-S11, 1986.

148. Hassid A, Williams C: Vasoconstrictor-evoked prostaglandin synthesis in cultured vascular smooth muscle cells. Am J Physiol 245:C278-C282, 1983.

149. Loesberg C, van Wijk R, Zandvergen J, et al: Cell cycle-dependent inhibition of human vascular smooth muscle cell proliferation by prostaglandin E1. Exp Cell Res 160:117-125, 1985.

150. Morisaki N, Kanzaki T, Motoyama N, et al: Cell cycle-dependent inhibition of DNA synthesis by prostaglandin E2 in cultured rabbit aortic smooth muscle cells. Atherosclerosis 71:165-171, 1988.

151. Gibbons GH, Pratt RE, Dzau VJ: Vascular smooth muscle cell hypertrophy vs. hyperplasia: Autocrine transforming growth factor-beta 1 expression determines growth response to angiotensin II. J Clin Invest 90:456-461, 1992.

152. Libby P, Warner SJC, Salomon RN, et al: Production of platelet-derived growth factor-like mitogen by smooth-muscle cells from human aorta. N Engl J Med 318:1493-1498, 1988.

153. Seifert RA, Hart CE, Phillips PE, et al: Two different subunits associate to create isoform-specific platelet-derived growth factor receptors. J Biol Chem 264:8771-8778, 1989.

154. Sarzani R, Arnaldi G, Chobanian AV: Hypertension-induced changes of platelet-derived growth factor receptor expression in rat aorta and heart. Hypertension 17:888-895, 1991.

155. Sarzani R, Arnaldi G, Takasaki I, et al: Effects of hypertension and aging on platelet-derived growth factor receptor expression in rat aorta and heart. Hypertension 18(suppl III):III93-III99, 1991.

156. Winkles JA, Gay CG: Regulated expression of PDGF A-chain mRNA in human saphenous vein smooth muscle cells. Biochem Biophys Res Commun 180:519-524, 1991.

157. Okabe T, Yamagata K, Fujisawa M, et al: Induction by fibroblast growth factor of angiotensin converting enzyme in vascular endothelial cells in vitro. Biochem Biophys Res Commun 145:1211-1216, 1987.

158. Fishel RS, Thourani V, Eisenberg SJ, et al: Fibroblast growth factor stimulates angiotensin converting enzyme expression in vascular smooth muscle cells. J Clin Invest 95:377-387, 1995.

159. Sato Y, Hamanaka R, Ono J, et al: The stimulatory effect of PDGF on vascular smooth muscle cell migration is mediated by the induction of endogenous basic FGF. Biochem Biophys Res Commun 174:1260-1266, 1991.

160. Sara VR, Hall K: Insulin-like growth factors and their binding proteins. Physiol Rev 70:591-614, 1990.

161. Fath KA, Alexander RW, Delafontaine P: Abdominal coarctation increases insulin-like growth factor I mRNA levels in rat aorta. Circ Res 72:271-277, 1993.

162. Delafontaine P, Lou H: Angiotensin II regulates insulin like growth factor-1 gene expression in vascular smooth muscle cells. J Biol Chem 268:16866-16870, 1993.

163. Goldstein RH, Polliks CF, Pilch PF, et al: Stimulation of collagen formation by insulin and insulin-like growth factor I in culture of human lung fibroblasts. Endocrinology 124:964-970, 1989.

164. Perrella MA, Jain MK, Lee ME: Role of TGF-beta in vascular development and vascular reactivity. Miner Electrolyte Metab 24:136-143, 1998.

165. Attisano L, Wrana JL: MADs and SMADs in TGF beta signalling. Curr Opin Cell Biol 10:188-194, 1998.

166. Hamet P, Hadrava V, Kruppa V, et al: Transforming growth factor beta 1 expression and effect in aortic smooth muscle cells from spontaneously hypertensive rats. Hypertension 17:896-901, 1991.

167. Sarzani R, Brecher P, Chobanian AV: Growth factor expression in aorta of normotensive and hypertensive rats. J Clin Invest 83:1404-1408, 1989.

168. Majesky MW, Lindner V, Twardzik DR, et al: Production of transforming growth factor beta 1 during repair of arterial injury. J Clin Invest 88:904-910, 1991.

169. Ruoslahti E, Yamaguchi Y: Proteoglycans as modulators of growth factor activities. Cell 64:867-869, 1991.

170. Battegay EJ, Raines EW, Seifert RA, et al: TGF-beta induces bimodal proliferation of connective tissue cells via complex control of an autocrine PDGF loop. Cell 63:515-524, 1990.

171. Gronwald RGK, Seifert RA, Bowen-Pope DF: Differential regulation of expression of two platelet-derived growth factor receptor subunits by transforming growth factor-beta. J Biol Chem 264:8120-8125, 1989.

172. Janat MF, Liau G: Transforming growth factor beta 1 is a powerful modulator of platelet-derived growth factor action in vascular smooth muscle cells. J Cell Physiol 150:232-242, 1992.

173. Majack RA, Majesky MW, Goodman LV: Role of PDGF-A expression in the control of vascular smooth muscle cell growth by transforming growth factor-beta. J Cell Biol 111:239-247, 1990.

174. Owens GK, Geisterfer AA, Yang YW, et al: Transforming growth factor-beta-induced growth inhibition and cellular hypertrophy in cultured vascular smooth muscle cells. J Cell Biol 107:771-780, 1988.

175. Hahn AW, Resink TJ, Scott-Burden T, et al: Stimulation of endothelin mRNA and secretion in rat vascular smooth muscle cells: A novel autocrine function. Cell Regul 1:649-659, 1990.

176. Wang X-F, Lin HY, Ng-Eaton E, et al: Expression cloning and characterization of the TGF-b type III receptor. Cell 67:797-805, 1991.

177. Cheifetz S, Hernandez H, Laiho M, et al: Determinants of cellular responsiveness to the three transforming growth factor-beta isoforms. J Biol Chem 265:20533-20538, 1990.

178. Sato Y, Tsuboi R, Lyons R, et al: Characterization of the activation of latent TGF-beta by co-cultures of endothelial cells and pericytes or smooth muscle cells: A self-regulating system. J Cell Biol 111:757-763, 1990.

179. Chen JK, Hoshi H, McKeehan WL: Transforming growth factor type beta specifically stimulates synthesis of proteoglycan in human adult arterial smooth muscle cells. Proc Natl Acad Sci U S A 84:5287-5291, 1987.

180. Koller KJ, Goeddel DV: Molecular biology of the natriuretic peptides and their receptors. Circulation 86:1081-1088, 1992.

181. Suga S-I, Nakao K, Kishimoto I, et al: Phenotype-related alteration in expression of natriuretic peptide receptor in aortic smooth muscle cells. Circ Res 71:34-39, 1992.

182. Nakao K, Ogawa Y, Suga S-I, et al: Molecular biology and biochemistry of the natriuretic peptide system II: Natriuretic peptide receptors. J Hypertens 10:1111-1114, 1992.

183. Oliver PM, Fox JE, Kim R, et al: Hypertension, cardiac hypertrophy, and sudden death in mice lacking natriuretic peptide receptor A. Proc Natl Acad Sci U S A 94:14730-14735, 1997.

184. Gardner DG, Deschepper CF, Baxter JD: The gene for the atrial natriuretic factor is expressed in the aortic arch. Hypertension 9:103-106, 1987.

185. Mourlon-LeGrand MC, Poitevin P, Benessiano J, et al: Effect of a nonhypotensive long-term infusion of ANP on the mechanical and structural properties of the arterial wall in Wistar-Kyoto and spontaneously hypertensive rats. Arterioscl Thromb 13:640-650, 1993.

186. Suga S-I, Nakao K, Itoh H, et al: Endothelial production of C-type natriuretic peptide and its marked augmentation by transforming growth factor B. J Clin Invest 90:1145-1149, 1992.

187. Komatsu Y, Nakao K, Itoh H, et al: Vascular natriuretic peptide. Lancet 340:622, 1992.

188. Porter JG, Catalano R, McEnroe G, et al: C-type natriuretic peptide inhibits growth factor-independent synthesis in smooth muscle cells. Am J Physiol 263:C1001-C1006, 1992.

189. Ferro CJ, Spratt JC, Haynes WG, et al: Inhibition of neutral endopeptidase causes vasoconstriction of human resistance vessels in vivo. Circulation 97:2323-2330, 1998.

190. Trippodo NC, Robl JA, Asaad MM, et al: Effects of omapatrilat in low, normal, and high renin experimental hypertension. Am J Hypertens 11:363-372, 1998.

191. Chatelain RE, Ghai RD, Trapani AJ, et al: Antihypertensive and natriuretic effects of CGS 30440, a dual inhibitor of angiotensin-converting enzyme and neutral endopeptidase 24.11. J Pharmacol Exp Ther 284:974-982, 1998.

192. Bell D, McDermott BJ: Calcitonin gene-related peptide in the cardiovascular system: Characterization of receptor populations and their (patho)physiological significance. Pharmacol Rev 48:253-288, 1996.

193. Kitamura K, Kangawa K, Kawamoto M, et al: Adrenomedullin: A novel hypotensive peptide isolated from human pheochromocytoma. Biochem Biophys Res Commun 192:553-560, 1993.

194. Sugo S, Minamino N, Kangawa K, et al: Endothelial cells actively synthesize and secrete adrenomedullin. Biochem Biophys Res Commun 201:1160-1166, 1994.

195. Sugo S, Minamino N, Shoji H, et al: Production and secretion of adrenomedullin from vascular smooth muscle cells: Augmented production by tumor necrosis factor-alpha. Biochem Biophys Res Commun 203:719-726, 1994.

196. Kato H, Shichiri M, Marumo F, et al: Adrenomedullin as an autocrine/paracrine apoptosis survival factor for rat endothelial cells. Endocrinology 138:2615-2620, 1997.

197. Kano H, Kohno M, Yasunari K, et al: Adrenomedullin as a novel antiproliferative factor of vascular smooth muscle cells. J Hypertens 14:209-213, 1996.

198. Barker S, Kapas S, Corder R, et al: Adrenomedullin acts via stimulation of cyclic AMP and not via calcium signalling in vascular cells in culture. J Hum Hypertens 10:421-423, 1996.

199. Eguchi S, Hirata Y, Kano H, et al: Specific receptors for adrenomedullin in cultured rat vascular smooth muscle cells. FEBS Lett 340:226-230, 1994.

200. Kapas S, Clark AJ: Identification of an orphan receptor gene as a type 1 calcitonin gene-related peptide receptor. Biochem Biophys Res Commun 217:832-838, 1995.

201. Wagner WD: Proteoglycan structure and function as related to atherosclerosis. Ann N Y Acad Sci 454:52-68, 1985.

202. Au YP, Kenagy RD, Clowes AW: Heparin selectively inhibits the transcription of tissue-type plasminogen activator in primate arterial smooth muscle cells during mitogenesis. J Biol Chem 267:3438-3444, 1992.

203. Clowes AW, Clowes MM, Au YPT, et al: Smooth muscle cells express urokinase during mitogenesis and tissue-type plasminogen activator during migration in injured rat carotid artery. Circ Res 67:61-67, 1990.

204. Clowes AW, Clowes MM, Kirkman TR, et al: Heparin inhibits the expression of tissue-type plasminogen activator by smooth muscle cells in injured rat carotid artery. Circ Res 70:1128-1136, 1992.

205. Hedin U, Bottger BA, Forsberg E, et al: Diverse effects of fibronectin and laminin on the phenotypic properties of cultured arterial smooth muscle cells. J Cell Biol 107:307-319, 1989.

206. Ashizawa N, Graf K, Do YS, et al: Osteopontin is produced by rat cardiac fibroblasts and mediates AII-induced DNA synthesis and collagen gel contraction. J Clin Invest 98:2218-2227, 1996.

207. Burgess WH, Maciag T: The heparin-binding (fibroblast) growth factor family of proteins. Ann Rev Biochem 58:575-606, 1989.

208. Yayon A, Klagsbrun M, Esko JD, et al: Cell surface, heparin-like molecules are required for binding of basic fibroblast growth factor to its high affinity receptor. Cell 64:841-848, 1991.

209. Bashkin P, Neufeld G, Gitay GH, et al: Release of cell surface-associated basic fibroblast growth factor by glycosylphosphatidyl-inositol-specific phospholipase C. J Cell Physiol 151:126-137, 1992.

210. Siffert W, Rosskopf D, Siffert G, et al: Association of a human G-protein beta3 subunit variant with hypertension. Nat Genet 18:45-48, 1998.

211. Koutouzov S, Remmal A, Marche P, et al: Hypersensitivity of phospholipase C in platelets of spontaneously hypertensive rats. Hypertension 10:497-504, 1987.

212. Silver PJ, Lepore RE, Cumiskey WR, et al: Protein kinase C activity and reactivity to phorbol ester in vascular smooth muscle from spontaneously hypertensive rats (SHR) and normotensive Wistar Kyoto rats (WKY). Biochem Biophys Res Comm 154:272-277, 1988.

213. Takaori K, Itoh S, Kanayama Y, et al: Protein kinase C activity in platelets from spontaneously hypertensive rats (SHR) and normotensive Wistar Kyoto rats (WKY). Biochem Biophys Res Comm 141:769-773, 1986.

214. Oshima T, Young EW, Bukoski RD, et al: Abnormal calcium handling by platelets of spontaneously hypertensive rats. Hypertension 15:606-611, 1990.

215. Bhalla RC, Webb RC, Singh D, et al: Calcium fluxes, calcium binding, and adenosine cyclic 3',5'-monophosphate-dependent protein kinase activity in the aorta of spontaneously hypertensive and Kyoto Wistar normotensive rats. Mol Pharmacol 14:468-477, 1978.

216. Lucchesi PA, Bell JM, Willis LS, et al: Ca^{2+}-dependent mitogen-activated protein kinase activation in spontaneously hypertensive rat vascular smooth muscle defines a hypertensive signal transduction phenotype. Circ Res 78:962-970, 1996.

217. Rosskopf D, Dusing R, Siffert W: Membrane sodium-proton exchange and primary hypertension. Hypertension 21:607-617, 1993.

218. Resnick LM, Gupta RK, Lewanczuk RZ, et al: Intracellular ions in salt-sensitive essential hypertension: Possible role of calcium-regulating hormones. Contrib Nephrol 90:88-93, 1991.

219. Tamura H, Hopp L, Kino M, et al: Na+-K+ regulation in cultured vascular smooth muscle cell of the spontaneously hypertensive rat. Am J Physiol 250:C939-C947, 1986.

220. Friedman SM: Evidence for enhanced sodium transport in the tail artery of the spontaneously hypertensive rat. Hypertension 1:572-582, 1979.

221. Foster CD, Hill WAG, Honeyman TW, et al: Characterization of Na+-H+ exchange in segments of rat mesenteric artery. Am J Physiol 262:H1651-H1656, 1992.

222. Orlowski J: Na+/H+ exchangers: Molecular diversity and relevance to heart. Ann N Y Acad Sci 874:346-353, 1999.

223. Brayden JE, Halpern W, Brann LR: Biochemical and mechanical properties of resistance arteries from normotensive and hypertensive rats. Hypertension 5:17-25, 1983.

224. Fridovich I: Hypoxia and oxygen toxicity. Adv Neurol 26:256, 1979.

225. Back LH: Analysis of oxygen transport in the vascular region of arteries. Math Biosci 31:285, 1976.

226. Berk BC, Taubman MB, Cragoe EJ Jr, et al: Thrombin signal transduction mechanisms in rat vascular smooth muscle cells: Calcium and protein kinase C-dependent and -independent pathways. J Biol Chem 265:17334-17340, 1990.

227. Hogue D, Michalak M, Fliegel L: The role of ion antiporters in the maintenance of intracellular pH in rat vascular smooth muscle cells. Mol Cell Biochem 102:125-137, 1991.

228. Little PJ, Weissberg PL, Cragoe EJ Jr, et al: Dependence of Na+/H+ antiport activation in cultured rat aortic smooth muscle on calmodulin, calcium, and ATP: Evidence for the involvement of calmodulin-dependent kinases. J Biol Chem 263:16780-16786, 1988.

229. Mitsuka M, Nagae M, Berk BC: Na$^+$-H$^+$ exchange inhibitors decrease neointimal formation after rat carotid injury. Circ Res 73:269-275, 1993.

230. Rosskopf D, Fromter E, Siffert W: Hypertensive sodium-proton exchanger phenotype persists in immortalized lymphoblasts from essential hypertensive patients: A cell culture model for human hypertension. J Clin Invest 92:2553-2559, 1993.

231. Siczkowski M, Davies JE, Ng LL: Na+-H+ exchanger isoform 1 phosphorylation in normal Wistar-Kyoto and spontaneously hypertensive rats. Circ Res 76:825-831, 1995.

232. Siczkowski M, Davies JE, Ng LL: Activity and density of the Na+/H+ antiporter in normal and transformed human lymphocytes and fibroblasts. Am J Physiol 267:C745-C752, 1994.

233. Lifton RP, Hunt SC, Williams RR, et al: Exclusion of the Na+-H+ antiporter as a candidate gene in human essential hypertension. Hypertension 17:8-14, 1991.

234. Dudley CRK, Taylor DJ, Ng LL, et al: Evidence for abnormal Na/H antiport activity detected by phosphorus nuclear magnetic resonance spectroscopy in exercising skeletal muscle of patients with essential hypertension. Clin Sci 79:491-497, 1990.

235. Lucchesi PA, DeRoux N, Berk BC: Na+-H+ exchanger expression in vascular smooth muscle of spontaneously hypertensive and Wistar-Kyoto rats. Hypertension 24:734-738, 1994.

236. Grinstein S, Rothstein A: Mechanisms of regulation of the Na+/H+ exchanger. J Membr Biol 90:1-12, 1986.

237. Lin X, Barber DL: A calcineurin homologous protein inhibits GTPase-stimulated Na-H exchange. Proc Natl Acad Sci U S A 93:12631-12636, 1996.

238. Yan W, Nehrke K, Choi J, et al: The Nck-interacting kinase (NIK) phosphorylates the Na+-H+ exchanger NHE1 and regulates NHE1 activation by platelet-derived growth factor. J Biol Chem 276:31349-31356, 2001.

239. Denker SP, Huang DC, Orlowski J, et al: Direct binding of the Na–H exchanger NHE1 to ERM proteins regulates the cortical cytoskeleton and cell shape independently of H(+) translocation. Mol Cell 6:1425-1436, 2000.

240. Lehoux S, Abe J, Berk BC: 14-3-3 is a serum stimulated Na+/H+ exchanger binding protein. Circulation 100:I-280-1-1, 1999.

241. Takahashi E, Abe J, Gallis B, et al: p90RSK is a serum-stimulated NHE1 kinase: Regulatory phosphorylation of serine 703 of Na+/H+ exchanger isoform-1. J Biol Chem 274:20206-20214, 1999.

242. Wang H, Silva NL, Lucchesi PA, et al: Phosphorylation and regulation of the Na+/H+ exchanger through mitogen-activated protein kinase. Biochemistry 36:9151-9158, 1997.

243. Berk BC, Elder E, Mitsuka M: Hypertrophy and hyperplasia cause differing effects on vascular smooth muscle cell Na+/H+ exchange and intracellular pH. J Biol Chem 265:19632-19637, 1990.

244. Ashida T, Kuramochi M, Omae T: Increased sodium-calcium exchange in arterial smooth muscle of spontaneously hypertensive rats. Hypertension 13:890-895, 1989.

245. Bianchini L, Woodside M, Sardet C, et al: Okadaic acid, a phosphatase inhibitor, induces activation and phosphorylation of the Na$^+$/H$^+$ antiport. J Biol Chem 266:15406-15413, 1991.

246. Sardet C, Fafournoux P, Pouysségur J: a-Thrombin, epidermal growth factor, and okadaic acid activate the Na$^+$/H$^+$ exchanger, NHE-1, by phosphorylating a set of common sites. J Biol Chem 266:19166-19171, 1991.

247. Simonet L, St-Lezin E, Kurtz TW: Sequence analysis of the alpha 1 Na+,K(+)-ATPase gene in the Dahl salt-sensitive rat. Hypertension 18:689-693, 1991.

248. Schild L, Canessa CM, Shimkets RA, et al: A mutation in the epithelial sodium channel causing Liddle disease increases channel activity in the *Xenopus laevis* oocyte expression system. Proc Natl Acad Sci U S A 92:5699-5703, 1995.

249. Lange-Carter CA, Pleiman CM, Gardner AM, et al: A divergence in the MAP kinase regulatory network defined by MEK kinase and raf. Science 260:315-319, 1993.

250. Boulton TG, Nye SH, Robbins DJ, et al: ERKs: A family of protein-serine/threonine kinases that are activated and tyrosine phosphorylated in response to insulin and NGF. Cell 65:663-675, 1991.

251. Pages G, Lenormand P, L'Allemain G, et al: Mitogen-activated protein kinases p42mapk and p44mapk are required for fibroblast proliferation. Proc Natl Acad Sci U S A 90:8319-8323, 1993.

252. Aharonovitz O, Granot Y: Stimulation of mitogen-activated protein kinase and Na^+/H^+ exchanger in human platelets. J Biol Chem 271:16494-16499, 1996.

253. Kusuhara M, Takahashi E, Peterson TE, et al: p38 kinase is a negative regulator of angiotensin II signal transduction in vascular smooth muscle cells: Effects on Na^+/H^+ exchange and ERK1/2. Circ Res 83:824-831, 1998.

254. Jacob HJ, Pettersson A, Wilson D, et al: Genetic dissection of autoimmune type I diabetes in the BB rat. Nat Genet 2:56-60, 1992.

CHAPTER 45

Essential Hypertension

Jon D. Blumenfeld and John H. Laragh

High blood pressure (BP) is a leading risk factor for heart disease, stroke, and kidney failure.[1] It is estimated that 45 million people in the United States are afflicted with hypertension, so it is not surprising that BP measurement is one of the most common reasons for a visit to the doctor's office.[2, 3] Moreover, antihypertensive medications are among the most commonly written prescriptions. Nevertheless, fewer than 30% of all hypertensive patients in this country have their BP adequately controlled[2] (Table 45-1). Even when BP is lowered by antihypertensive medication, the associated reduction in risk of coronary heart disease (CHD) lags well behind stroke.[4, 5] Guidelines for treating high BP have had a limited impact, as indicated by the recent declines in detection and treatment of hypertension and by the 50% drop in the use of "preferred" antihypertensive agents by practicing physicians.[6, 7]

The issues contributing to these problems are complex, but a key factor is the widely held misconception that hypertension is a single disease that can be treated with a single recipe. In this chapter, we focus on the concept that hypertension is a heterogeneous disorder in which patients can be stratified by pathophysiologic characteristics that have direct bearing on the efficacy of targeted antihypertensive medications, on the detection of potentially curable forms of hypertension, and on the risk of cardiovascular complications.

The phenomenon of hypertension was first characterized at the turn of the past century, when Riva-Rocci developed the prototype of the modern sphygmomanometer and so allowed the routine measurement of BP.[8] Korotkov then perfected the sphygmomanometric technique by describing the sounds heard over the brachial artery as the pressure in the cuff is reduced.[9] In general, the upper limits of normal BP in older persons have been considered to be a systolic value of 140 mm Hg and a diastolic value of 90 mm Hg. These figures may be adjusted downward for younger patients to the point that readings in excess of 120/80 mm Hg may be considered hypertensive.[5] Population studies suggest that BP is a continuous variable, with no absolute dividing line between normal and abnormal values.[10] This situation has resulted in an inevitable continuing debate over borderline readings that focuses on whether people with such pressures are normal and on what, in fact, constitutes normalcy.[11, 12] Moreover, studies using 24-hour monitoring techniques and home BP measurements have revealed that significant fractions of patients who appear hypertensive in the office setting do not have hypertension at other times.[13-15]

Early on, however, life insurance studies indicated that relatively higher BPs that are casually recorded, even those that are within the normal range, are statistically associated with increased mortality from cardiovascular complications.[16-18] The Veterans Administration established through a subsequent trial of therapy (principally with diuretics, which were often combined with other agents) that antihypertensive treatment could provide a significant degree of protection against such complications—notably congestive heart failure (CHF), renal failure, and stroke, but not coronary artery disease.[19, 20] From such demonstrations sprang the concept of a medical obligation to treat all cases of hypertension.

TABLE 45-1

Trends in Awareness, Treatment, and Control of High Blood Pressure in Adults*

	NHANES II (1976-1980)	NHANES III (PHASE 1) (1988-1991)	NHANES III (PHASE 2) (1991-1994)
Awareness	51%	73%	68%
Treatment	31%	55%	53%
Control	10%	29%	27%

*Data are percentages of adults aged 18 to 74 years with systolic blood pressure greater than or equal to 140 mm Hg, diastolic pressure greater than or equal to 90 mm Hg, or taking antihypertensive medication.

NHANES, National Health and Nutrition Examination Survey.

Data from Burt VL, Whelton P, Roccella EJ, et al: Prevalence of hypertension in the U.S. population: Results from the Third National Health and Nutrition Examination Survey, 1988-1991. Hypertension 25:305-314, 1995.

Nonetheless, the risks of death and disability associated with hypertension are increased only in the broad statistical sense; a large majority of patients with clearly elevated BP live lives of normal longevity and health.[21, 22] Not only are the risks variable from one person to another but also great variability has been found among hypertensive patients in their responses to antihypertensive treatments, a phenomenon that also suggests no single cause. Thus, risks are apparently not distributed randomly but are concentrated in subgroups that have been difficult to identify. For these and other reasons, hypertension cannot yet be considered a discrete disease entity but must rather be considered a marker common to the course of perhaps several pathologic developments. Thus, hypertension is a physical sign and a risk factor to be assessed in conjunction with other physiologic and environmental factors.

Variant patterns may be recognized. Hypertension may be purely systolic and accompanied by normal or even lowered diastolic pressure. Systolic hypertension usually occurs in the elderly and may be a manifestation of atherosclerosis, the increased systolic pressure resulting from decreased arterial elasticity.[2, 23] Often in the elderly, diastolic pressure is either normal or low, which suggests less or no arteriolar vasoconstriction and a different pathophysiologic process involving changes in the large vessels rather than in the arterioles.[24] Systolic hypertension may also occur as part of a hyperdynamic cardiovascular state, such as that occurring in hyperthyroidism or in younger people who appear to have increased β-adrenergic activity.

Several imprecise terms have been applied to describe patients with high BP. *Labile hypertension* describes an intermittent form of hypertension, also sometimes referred to as prehypertension, neurocirculatory asthenia, or hyperkinetic heart syndrome. This term lacks definition, for investigators have not yet determined whether such patients go on to sustained hypertension with consequent secondary cardiovascular damage. *Borderline hypertension* defines BP readings close to the upper limits of the normal range or only slightly elevated.

Malignant hypertension, a syndrome defined originally by Volhard and Fahr in 1914, is characterized clinically by severe accelerating hypertension with neuroretinopathy or papilledema and by evidence of renal damage.[25] Clinically, it is almost always associated with massive oversecretion of renin and aldosterone and is strikingly relieved by binephrectomy or antirenin drugs but not by total adrenalectomy.[26] On pathologic examination, it is characterized by fibrinoid and necrotizing arteriolitis. This syndrome can occur de novo, but most often it follows preexisting milder forms of hypertension. Malignant hypertension may occur as a complication of essential hypertension and of virtually every form of secondary hypertension, with the notable exception of coarctation of the aorta, a condition in which the renal circulation is protected from the high pressures that occur proximal to the coarctation.[10] *Accelerated hypertension* is a term often used synonymously with malignant hypertension, but sometimes only to imply a significant increase in the pace or severity of the hypertensive process.

In an attempt to clarify the nomenclature, recent guidelines[5] have designated a classification system for BP for adults as optimal (<120/80 mm Hg), normal (<130/85 mm Hg), or high-normal (systolic 130-139 mm Hg or diastolic 85-89 mm Hg). Hypertension is stratified as (systolic/diastolic) stage 1 (140-159 mm Hg or 90-99 mm Hg), stage 2 (160-179 mm Hg or 100-109 mm Hg), and stage 3 ($\geq$ 180 mm Hg or $\geq$ 110 mm Hg).

Some causes of hypertension can now be identified, and some may even be curable (Table 45-2). By definition, these are designated "secondary hypertension." However, the pathophysiologic mechanism in approximately 90% of the hypertensive population resists precise description. Members of this group are classified as having "primary hypertension" or "essential hypertension," signifying that no cause for their disorder has been found. Thus, essential hypertension is a diagnosis (if indeed a confession of ignorance can be called a diagnosis) reached only after known causes of hypertension have been excluded. The diagnostic exclusion process is of vital importance, however, because cure or effective treatment is available for some of the known causes.

Even when known causes have been excluded, the enormous residue defaulted as essential hypertension suggests etiologic variability, reflected by heterogeneity not only in morbidity and mortality but also in the response, or lack of it, to different classes of drugs.[27, 28] Moreover, much of this considerable variability is not well correlated with the BP level.[21, 22] Converging clinical and pharmaceutical research is providing clues to physiologic mechanisms that might explain this variability. In this chapter, we discuss this evidence and its implications for diagnosis and treatment.

EPIDEMIOLOGY

Prevalence

The Third National Health and Nutrition Examination Survey[2] estimated that 24%, or 43 million, of the adult noninstitutionalized U.S. population are hypertensive, when the criteria included systolic BP greater than or equal to 140 mm Hg, diastolic BP greater than or equal to 90 mm Hg, or current treatment for hypertension with prescription medication (Fig. 45-1). The overall hypertension prevalence increases to 50 million, or 27.6% of the U.S. population if the definition is broadened to include those with an average BP of less than 140/90 mm Hg, but who report a history of

TABLE 45-2

Known Causes of Hypertension

Renal Disorders

Renal Parenchymal

　Acute and chronic glomerulonephritis; pyelonephritis; nephrocalcinosis; neoplasms; glomerulosclerosis; interstitial, hereditary, or radiation nephritis

　Obstructive uropathies and hydronephrosis

　Renin-secreting renal tumors (hemangiopericytoma; Wilms, renal cell, pancreatic, ovarian tumors)

　Congenital defect in renal sodium transport (Liddle syndrome)

　Renal trauma

Renovascular

　Renal arterial lesions, occlusions, stenoses, aneurysms, thromboses

　Renal vasculitis or glomerulitis

　Coarctation of the aorta with renal ischemia

　Aortitis with renal ischemia

Adrenocortical Disorders

Cushing syndrome (cortisol excess)

Primary aldosteronism due to adenoma (Conn syndrome)

Pseudoprimary aldosteronism (bilateral adrenocortical hyperplasia)

Congenital or acquired enzymatic defects with excess Na^+-retaining steroids (11β-hydroxylase deficiency, 11β-hydroxysteroid dehydrogenase deficiency, 17-hydroxylase deficiency)

Adrenal carcinoma

Ectopic corticotropin-secreting tumor

Pheochromocytoma (adrenal medullary or extra-adrenal chromaffin tumors secreting norepinephrine or epinephrine)

Other Endocrine Causes

Hypothyroidism (diastolic hypertension)

Hyperthyroidism (systolic hypertension)

Hypercalcemic states, hyperparathyroidism

Acromegaly

Toxemias of Pregnancy

Neurogenic Factors

Increased intracranial pressure

Familial dysautonomia

Acute porphyria, buffer denervation, poliomyelitis, spinal cord injuries

Psychogenic?

Iatrogenic and Other Causes

Oral contraceptive or estrogen therapy

Mineralocorticoid or glucocorticoid therapies, licorice ingestion (i.e., acquired 11β-hydroxysteroid dehydrogenase deficiency)

Sympathomimetic drugs (decongestants)

Antidepressants

Alcohol abuse

Lead toxicity

Monoamine oxidase inhibitors (interactions with other agents)

Excessive salt appetite?

From Blumenfeld JD, Mann SJ, Laragh JH: Clinical evaluation and differential diagnosis of the individual hypertensive patient. *In* Laragh JH, Brenner BM (eds): Hypertension Pathophysiology, Diagnosis, and Management, 2nd ed. New York, Raven Press, 1995, pp 1897-1911.

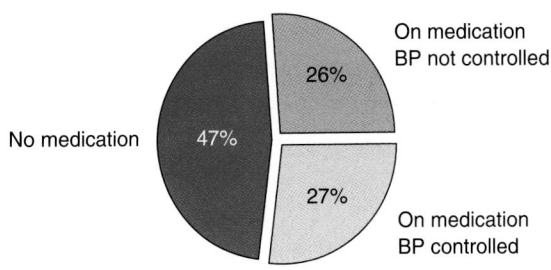

FIGURE 45-1. Treatment and control of hypertension in the United States. Only 53% of hypertensive patients are treated and only 27% have their blood pressure reduced by treatment to a target pressure of 140/90 mm Hg or less. See text. (From National Committee on Prevention, Evaluation, and Treatment of High Blood Pressure: The sixth report of the Joint National Committee on Prevention, Evaluation, and Treatment of High Blood Pressure. Arch Intern Med 157:2413-2446, 1997.)

hypertension and use one or more nonpharmacologic interventions to lower BP.

Systolic pressure increases during adulthood. Although the mean systolic pressure tends to be lower in younger women, after age 60 years it increases at a greater rate and is at least as high as the corresponding values for men (Fig. 45-2). Diastolic pressure increases until age 50 years, when it plateaus and then decreases with advancing age. Consequently, there is an age-related increase in pulse pressure for both men and women.[23, 29] The age-adjusted prevalence of hypertension is 40% higher in the non-Hispanic black population (32.4% vs. 23.3%). These findings may have bearing on the observation that the age-adjusted decline in mortality rates for stroke and CHD during the past 2 decades were less for blacks than for whites. Furthermore, data from the Framingham Heart Study indicate that the residual lifetime risk for developing hypertension stage 1 or higher (≥140/90 mm Hg regardless of treatment) in 55- and 65-year-old participants is 90%.[30] This risk for hypertension in men was 60% higher in the contemporary period (1976-1998) when compared to an earlier period (1952-1976). However, the residual lifetime risk for more severe hypertension (≥160/100 mm Hg) was significantly lower in both sexes during the latter period.

Sodium Intake and Lifestyle Modification

Dietary salt has been implicated because of observations that hypertension and its complications are more common in societies with high sodium chloride intake whereas some primitive tribal societies have low sodium intake and low BPs.[31-35] However, correlation of sodium intake with BP within societies, such as those in the United States, Japan, or New Zealand, has not been possible. This lack of correlation has been most convincingly demonstrated by the Intersalt study, which found no correlation between sodium intake and BP in 48 centers around the world.[31] This observation reflects the variability in BP to dietary sodium restriction among hypertensive patients. Approximately 30% of hypertensive patients will decrease their BP when dietary sodium is markedly reduced, whereas in the majority, pressure is either unchanged or may even increase.[34]

The impact of sodium restriction on hypertensive target organ changes is uncertain. There is evidence that dietary sodium restriction leads to regression of left ventricular hypertrophy (LVH) and reduction of urinary albumin excretion.[36] The National Health and Nutrition Examination Survey (NHANES I) Epidemiologic Follow-up Study, a prospective cohort study, found that among overweight individuals, a 100-mmol or higher sodium intake was associated with a significantly higher risk of stroke and mortality from stroke, CHD, cardiovascular disease, or death from all causes.[35] These findings were independent of baseline systolic BP. However, the associations between sodium intake and risk from these adverse outcomes were *not* found in

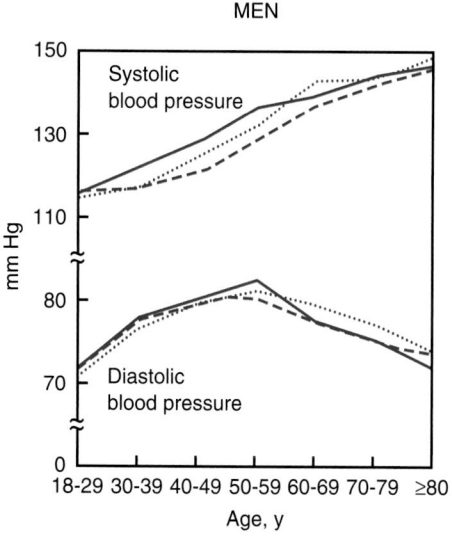

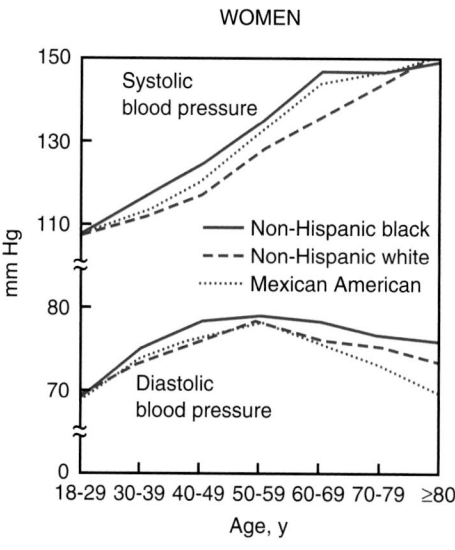

FIGURE 45-2. Systolic and diastolic blood pressure distribution stratified by gender, age, and race. See text. (From Burt VL, Whelton P, Roccella EJ, et al: Prevalence of hypertension in the U.S. population: Results from the Third National Health and Nutrition Examination Survey, 1988-1991. Hypertension 25:305-314, 1995.)

nonobese subjects. The issue is complicated further by two reports that have linked sodium restriction with *higher* rates of myocardial infarction (MI) and of death from cardiovascular and other causes.[35, 37]

The effect of dietary composition on BP was evaluated in the Dietary Approaches to Stop Hypertension (DASH) study.[38] In that study, the effects on BP of either a diet rich in fruits, vegetables, and low-fat dairy products or a control diet were compared. In addition, dietary sodium intake on each diet ranged from high (150 mmol/day), to intermediate (100 mmol/day), to low (50 mmol/day). Compared to the control diet, the DASH diet significantly lowered systolic BP at each level of sodium intake and reduced diastolic BP at high and intermediate levels of sodium intake by (systolic/diastolic) 5.9/2.9 mm Hg (high-sodium diet), 5.0/2.5 mm Hg (intermediate-sodium diet), and 2.2/1.0 mm Hg (low-sodium diet). These statistically significant BP effects were observed in both black and white subjects and were comparable in obese and nonobese subjects.[39] Although this study demonstrated BP reduction by dietary intervention, the application of these findings to the specific treatment of hypertensive patients is limited because the follow-up period was only 30 days.

Body mass index is positively associated with BP. In women, long-term weight gain increases the likelihood of hypertension, whereas long-term weight loss decreases the risk that hypertension will occur.[40] In one study of obese patients, BP remained well controlled in 35% of the group who reduced their weight by 10 pounds, compared with 16% of those in whom weight was unchanged.[41] However, there is wide variability in the individual BP responses to weight reduction and there are no reliable predictors of BP reduction.

Lifestyle modifications, including weight loss, reduced sodium intake, increased physical activity, and limited alcohol consumption, have been established recommendations for the treatment of hypertension, particularly in patients at low risk for cardiovascular complications.[5] Studies of the DASH diet (see above) were so promising that the diet was included in the JNC 6 guidelines as a cornerstone of antihypertensive therapy even though few, relatively small, studies of short duration had been published.

Individually, these nonpharmacologic interventions can modestly reduce BP in some patients. However, when combined, their antihypertensive effect is not additive, and their impact on the progression of hypertensive target organ disease has not been established. In the PREMIER trial, patients with untreated BP, ranging from 120-159/80-95 mm Hg, were randomized to undergo either "established" lifestyle modifications (weight loss ≥15 pounds at 6 months, moderate intensity exercise for 3 hours each week, dietary sodium intake ≤100 mEq, and restricted daily alcohol intake of ≤1 ounce for men and ½ ounce for women) or a combination of these lifestyle modifications and the DASH diet ("established plus DASH"[42]). Intensive contact and counseling was provided to patients in these two study groups. A third group of patients in this study received "advice only" for nonpharmacologic treatment after randomization in one 30-minute session with a registered dietitian. The mean net change in BP (difference between the "established" and the "advice only" group) was 3.7/1.7 mm Hg. The addition of the DASH diet further lowered BP by only 0.6/0.9 mm Hg.

Several factors may account for the disappointing effect of combined lifestyle modification on blood pressure. The authors of this study point to an inadequate "dose" of the DASH diet—mean fruit and vegetable intake was 7.8 servings per day, below the 9.8 servings per day provided in the earlier DASH studies (see above). Another proposed explanation is the so-called subadditivity of interventional effects, referring to the suboptimal adherence to the multiple study interventions. It is also possible that each of these interventions has a common physiologic mechanism of action, and, thus, the dose-response relationship is not linear.[42a] Regardless, the findings of the PREMIER study challenge the recommendation regarding the DASH diet as a central component of combined lifestyle modification for the treatment of hypertension.

Defining the Risk of Hypertensive Complications

Practice guidelines for the treatment of hypertension are traditionally based on the premise that a discrete cut point separates normotension and hypertension. During the past

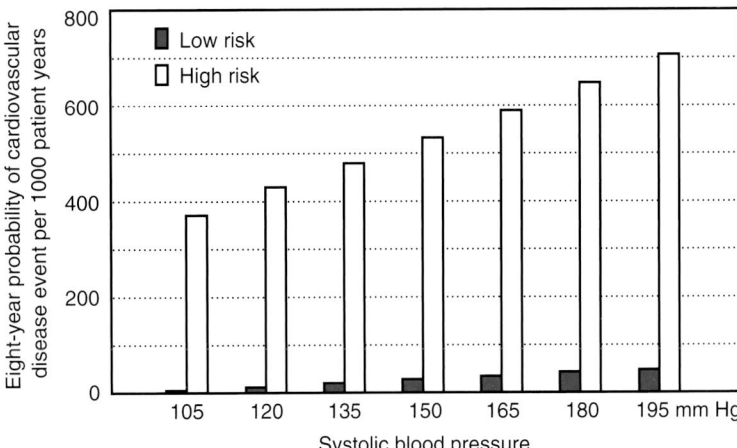

FIGURE 45-3. Absolute and relative risk for a cardiovascular disease event in a high- and low-risk 55-year-old man by systolic blood pressure. See text. (From Alderman MH: Blood pressure management: Individualized treatment based on absolute risk and the potential for benefit. Ann Intern Med 119:329-335, 1993.)

5 decades, antihypertensive treatment strategies have produced improvement in cardiovascular health. However, the impact of these drug treatment strategies is limited because their use in patients is prompted simply because their BP exceeds some arbitrary threshold, even though their risk of stroke and cardiovascular disease is very small. For example, in the Medical Research Council treatment trial of mild hypertension, enrollment of many low-risk patients occurred because mildly elevated BP was required for inclusion (diastolic pressure 90-109 mm Hg). This probably accounted for the finding that only one stroke was prevented for every 850 patients treated for 1 year.[22, 44] This modest benefit comes at a cost because antihypertensive drug treatment per se has risks, particularly electrolyte disturbances and their related complications that occur with first-line agents such as diuretics and β-blockers.[45]

There is, in fact, a continuous, graded, and independent relationship between the height of the BP and the incidence of cardiovascular disease and stroke.[22] However, BP is not the sole determinant of cardiovascular risk. In fact, only some hypertensive individuals will have a heart attack or stroke even at the highest end of the BP range. For example, during 15 years of follow-up in the Framingham study, fewer than one third of patients whose only risk factor was systolic BP exceeding 195 mm Hg had a heart attack or stroke.[22, 46] Conversely, lower BP does not necessarily protect against a cardiovascular event—more than half of all heart attacks and almost half of all strokes occur in persons with normal BP.[22] Thus, there is no threshold BP that distinguishes patients who will have a heart attack or stroke.

To determine the likelihood that treatment will lead to a decrease in risk of CHD or stroke, one must quantify the probability that an event will occur. *Relative risk* describes the increase (or decrease) in the likelihood of an event in one population compared with a reference population—it is a ratio that provides no information about the absolute incidence of events. *Absolute risk* is a term that describes the expected incidence of events and the actual odds for a person to have an event.[22]

By defining absolute risk, one can identify the prognostic differences between patients with identical BPs (Fig. 45-3). For example, the risk of CHD is significantly greater, at every level of BP, for a 55-year-old male smoker with LVH than a 55-year-old male nonsmoker without cardiac enlargement.[1, 22] The relative risk of CHD increases with increasing BP among persons with higher or lower absolute risk. However, the absolute hazard is dramatically different in this example. Persons with lower absolute risk (even those with systolic BP >195 mm Hg), are only one-tenth as likely to have an event as are those of the same age and sex with a systolic BP of 105 mm Hg but at high absolute risk (46 vs. 372/1000 patient-years).[22]

In the Framingham cohort from 1990 to 1995, patients found to have BP greater than or equal to 130/85, 2.4% had high-normal or stage 1 hypertension without other risk factors or other target organ damage, 59.3% were hypertensive with no other cardiovascular risk factors except diabetes mellitus, but who did not have target organ damage, and 38.2% had hypertension with cardiovascular disease.[47] In recognition of this complex interaction among BP, cardiovascular risk, and the presence of genetic, biologic, and behavioral factors that modify it, the BP threshold for antihypertensive treatment has been lowered when other cardiovascular risk factors are present.[5]

Complications of Hypertension
Coronary Heart Disease

Life insurance statistics have established that hypertensive individuals, as a population, have shortened survival and that this vulnerability correlates broadly with increasing levels of arterial BP.[48] The long-term Framingham Heart Study confirmed these findings and demonstrated that high BP is the leading risk factor predisposing to stroke, heart failure, heart attack, and kidney failure.[1] Whether, and how soon, these complications occur in a specific hypertensive patient appears to be strongly determined by the concurrence of other risk factors, such as LVH, glucose intolerance, smoking, hypercholesterolemia, and obesity. Sleep-disordered breathing is also a relatively common factor, although often unrecognized, that is independently associated with hypertension and its cardiovascular complications.[49]

The relative importance of the systolic, diastolic, and, more recently, pulse pressure (defined as the numeric difference between systolic and diastolic pressure) components of

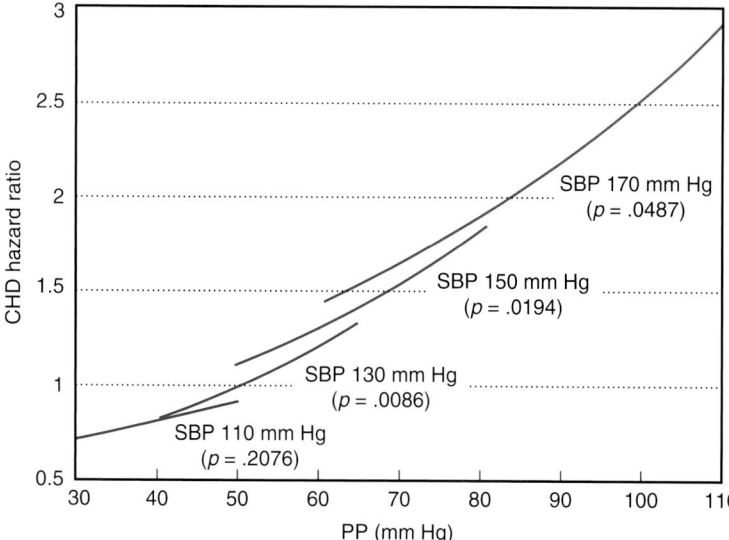

FIGURE 45-4. Joint influences of systolic blood pressure and pulse pressure on coronary heart disease risk in the Framingham Heart Study. Coronary heart disease hazard ratios were set to a reference value of 1.0 for systolic blood pressure (SBP) of 130 mm Hg and pulse pressure (PP) of 50 mm Hg and are plotted for SBP values of 110, 130, 150, and 170 mm Hg, respectively. All estimates were adjusted for age, gender, body mass index, cigarettes smoked daily, and total cholesterol–high-density lipoprotein cholesterol. (From Franklin SS, Khan SA, Wong ND, et al: Is pulse pressure useful in predicting risk for coronary heart disease: The Framingham Heart Study. Circulation 100:354-360, 1999.)

BP as predictors of cardiovascular risk have been analyzed.[29, 50] Below age 50 years, diastolic BP is the strongest predictor. Between age 50 and 59 years, all three BP components are comparable predictors. However, from age 60 years onward, diastolic pressure is negatively related to CHD risk at any given systolic pressure greater than or equal to 120 mm Hg, so that pulse pressure emerged as the best predictor (Fig. 45-4). This finding is especially relevant in the elderly, in whom 65% to 75% of hypertension is of the isolated systolic type.[21] However, the association of CHD risk with pulse pressure is not simply a surrogate for increasing systolic pressure, as there is a much greater increase in risk with increments in pulse pressure without a concurrent rise in systolic pressure than when systolic pressure increases without a corresponding increase in pulse pressure.[29]

There have been reports of excess mortality due to CHD at both low and high levels of diastolic pressure, referred to as a J-curve relationship.[21, 51] Data from the Framingham study suggest that, among patients with an MI but without heart failure, there was a bimodal increase in risk of coronary mortality related to diastolic pressure. By contrast, in healthy people, there was a linear, graded effect of both systolic and diastolic pressures to occurrence of CHD.

LEFT VENTRICULAR HYPERTROPHY. *LVH* is a common manifestation of hypertension that carries with it an ominous prognosis. Electrocardiographic evidence of LVH (ECG-LVH) is present in about 3% to 8% of hypertensive patients.[52] When ECG-LVH is identified, clinical manifestations of CHD occur at a rate that is about threefold higher than in the general population. Moreover, the risks of stroke and heart failure associated with ECG-LVH are actually greater than those following the appearance of ECG changes of MI (ECG-MI).

Echocardiography is a more sensitive measure of left ventricular mass.[52] Thus, about 12% to 30% of relatively unselected hypertensive adult patients will have echocardiographic increases in left ventricular (LV) mass. LV wall thickness and muscle mass are more closely related to 24-hour ambulatory BP measurements than to casual readings. As with ECG-LVH, echocardiographic LVH is a powerful

predictor of morbidity and mortality in hypertensive patients. In a study of patients with initially uncomplicated essential hypertension, LV mass index greater than 125 g/m^2 strongly predicted all-cause mortality and cardiac death.[53] Compared with hypertensive patients with normal LV geometry, those with concentric LVH (increased LV mass and relative wall thickness) had about a 10-fold greater total mortality and about a fivefold higher rate of cardiovascular events. Several mechanisms may contribute to this increased cardiovascular risk, including increased total myocardial oxygen demand of the hypertrophied ventricle and induction of electrophysiologic abnormalities that may predispose to arrhythmias. However, the mechanism(s) that contributes to the relationship between LVH and coronary artery disease has not been elucidated.

Data from the Framingham population illustrates the strong association between BP and LVH.[54] During the period from 1959 to 1989, antihypertensive drug use increased from 2.3% to 24.6% among men and 5.7% to 27.7% among women. As antihypertensive treatment became more prevalent, the age-adjusted prevalence of more severe hypertension (i.e., >160/100 mm Hg) decreased from 18.5% to 9.2% among men and from 28.8% to 7.7% among women. This reduction in BP was accompanied by an age-adjusted decrement in the prevalence of ECG-LVH (men: 4.5%-2.5%; women: 3.6%-1.1%).

PLASMA RENIN ACTIVITY. Several lines of evidence suggest that excess activity of the renin system plays an important role in the pathogenesis of cardiovascular disease: (1) Angiotensin II (AII) infusion causes MI in experimental animal models; (2) drugs that block renin secretion (β-blockers), AII formation (angiotensin-converting enzyme, or ACE, inhibitors), or AII binding (type 1 AII receptor [AT$_1$] blockers) prevent reinfarction and prolong survival in patients with CHD and heart failure; and (3) the risks of MI and stroke in hypertensive patients were greater in those with medium or high plasma renin levels compared to those with low renin levels.[55-59] Alderman and colleagues measured the pretreatment plasma renin activity (PRA) level in more than 1700 patients with mild hypertension and

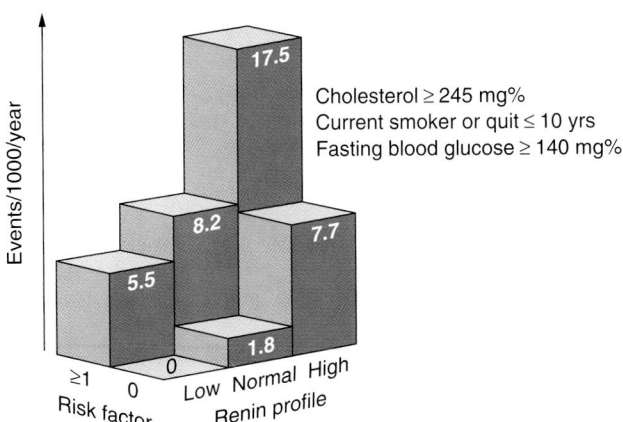

Cholesterol ≥ 245 mg%
Current smoker or quit ≤ 10 yrs
Fasting blood glucose ≥ 140 mg%

FIGURE 45-5. Association between plasma renin activity level and future myocardial infarction in patients with mild hypertension. The incidence of myocardial infarction is related to baseline, pretreatment plasma renin activity among 1717 patients with mild hypertension. Back row represents the 997 patients who had one or more known cardiac risk factors (hypercholesterolemia, diabetes, cigarette use). Front row indicates heart attack rates for patients with no known risk factors. Plasma renin level, before antihypertensive treatment, is a powerful, continuous risk factor that increased the heart attack rate by more than threefold among those who had other risk factors, and by more than sevenfold among those without other risk factors. No heart attacks occurred in 241 patients with low renin levels, suggesting that renin is a continuous variable. These data are further supported by animal studies describing myocardial, cerebral, and renal lesions after injection of renin or angiotensin. (From Alderman HM, Madhaven S, Ooi WL, et al: Association of the renin-sodium profile with the risk of myocardial infarction in patients with hypertension. N Engl J Med 324:1098-1104, 1991.)

then followed them during antihypertensive treatment for approximately 8 years.[60] Despite the comparable level of BP control in the high-, medium-, and low-renin groups, there was a greater incidence of MI in patients with medium or high pretreatment renin levels (Fig. 45-5). This association of cardiovascular risk and a high renin level was especially striking in those without other cardiovascular risk factors— an MI was seven times more likely to occur with a high PRA level than with a normal or low pretreatment PRA level. In fact, when all other cardiovascular risk factors were absent, no MI occurred in patients with low renin levels.[60] Thus, there is a strong independent association between PRA and the incidence of MI in hypertensive patients.

This association between PRA and MI was confirmed and extended in a recent study of both normotensive and hypertensive patients evaluated in an emergency department for suspected MI.[61] The mean PRA level was threefold higher in patients found to have an MI compared to those in whom MI was ruled out. Furthermore, there was a strong association between PRA and MI that was independent of other cardiac risk factors and medication use. Altogether, this evidence suggests a causal role for excess renin system activity in the pathogenesis of MI.

Stroke

Stroke is the most feared and devastating complication of hypertension. Atherothrombotic brain infarction accounts for 60% of stroke and is the most common type in the

hypertensive population. In the Framingham population, the risk of stroke was positively associated with BP, with no critical level below which stroke did not occur.[62] Nevertheless, definite hypertension (≥160/95 mm Hg) was associated with a 2.5-fold higher relative risk of stroke, after adjustment for other known cardiac risk factors. Systolic pressure is more closely associated with atherothrombotic infarction than other factors such as diastolic pressure or pulse pressure.

A study of the population in Rochester, Minnesota, indicates that the incidence of stroke decreased by 46% in the 1970s and by 17% in the 1980s.[62] These decrements were related to the control of hypertension during that period. These findings are consistent with the 42% reduction in stroke that accompanied a 5- to 6-mm fall in diastolic pressure reported in a meta-analysis of placebo-controlled treatment trials of more than 37,000 hypertensive patients.[4] However, the incidence of stroke has increased recently, despite improvement in BP control in the population.[5]

Heart Failure

Heart failure is now one of the leading causes of hospitalization for the Medicare population. Hypertension is the most common condition antedating heart failure, with a two- to threefold higher risk than for normotensive subjects and with a graded increase in risk at higher pressure.[63] Moreover, in the Framingham population, more than 90% of patients with symptomatic heart failure had a history of hypertension.[63] The risk is amplified further when ECG-LVH is present (see earlier discussion). Although MI is a principal cause of systolic dysfunction, fewer than half of hypertensive patients in the Framingham cohort had a history of a prior event. Therefore, diastolic dysfunction may have played an important role in the pathogenesis of heart failure in that hypertensive population.

Chronic Renal Insufficiency

According to the 2000 Annual Data Report of the U.S. Renal Disease Survey, hypertension is the second most common cause of end-stage renal disease (ESRD), accounting for 28% of the patients undergoing dialysis.[64] However, this figure is probably inaccurate because the cause of ESRD is often uncertain. In many cases, hypertension is applied as a diagnosis by default because BP is elevated in the majority of patients when dialysis is initiated. To address this problem, the process of recording the primary cause of ESRD was changed with the new Medical Evidence Form, thereby avoiding many redundant and antiquated diagnoses.

Ischemic nephropathy, which is defined as impairment in glomerular filtration rate (GFR) attributable to hemodynamically significant stenosis of both renal arteries, or to the artery of a solitary kidney, is increasingly recognized as an important cause of ESRD and has been included in this new classification system (see Chapter 46). Prospective and retrospective studies report that as many as 15% of elderly hypertensive patients may have ischemic nephropathy as the cause of ESRD.[65, 66] Previously, ESRD attributed to renal artery stenosis was classified under "hypertension" and ESRD attributed to renal artery occlusion was classified under "other." Neither cholesterol emboli nor atherosclerotic disease were specified in the previous list of detailed renal diagnoses.

Therefore, the true prevalence of ischemic nephropathy in the ESRD population is uncertain at this point.

The relatively low incidence of ESRD is a barrier to assessing a relationship with hypertension and assessing benefits from treatment.[67] Nevertheless, a graded relationship of the incidence of ESRD with both systolic and diastolic BP has been reported in men which is independent of associations between ESRD and other factors such as age, race, income, history of MI, serum cholesterol level, and cigarette use. The estimated risk of ESRD associated with elevated systolic pressure is reportedly greater than that for diastolic pressure.[67] Antihypertension treatment appears to slow the rate of progressive azotemia in nondiabetic patients with preexisting renal disease, although few well-controlled prospective studies have been done.[68a]

Microalbuminuria

Generally defined as urinary albumin excretion between 20 and 200 μg/minute, microalbuminuria is caused by impaired permselectivity of the glomerular capillary that is associated with glomerular hypertension in experimental models of renal injury. In patients with diabetes mellitus, microalbuminuria predicts the onset of frank proteinuria (urine protein >150 mg/day), progressive renal failure, and cardiovascular disease. These complications can be attenuated by effective treatment of hypertension, particularly with a regimen that includes an ACE inhibitor or AT_1 antagonist.[69-71] The increased risk of cardiovascular and peripheral vascular disease associated with microalbuminuria also applies to nondiabetic patients.[72]

There also appears to be a link between hypertensive heart disease and changes in the glomerular hemodynamic profile in essential hypertension. Patients with essential hypertension and LVH reportedly have higher GFR and filtration fraction than those without ventricular hypertrophy.[73] Although albumin excretion was not measured in that study, these findings suggest that glomerular hyperfiltration in patients with hypertension is related to cardiac remodeling and, perhaps, more generalized vascular adaptation.

In a large prospective study of patients with stage II or III hypertension, ECG-LVH, and plasma creatinine less than 1.9 mg/dL, microalbuminuria was found in 23% and macroalbuminuria in 4% of patients.[74] Microalbuminuria was present in 29% of patients with ECG-LVH. It was less prevalent in white patients (22%) than African-American (35%), Asian (36%), or Hispanic patients (37%). Excess albumin excretion was significantly more prevalent in diabetic than in nondiabetic patients. After adjusting for confounding variables, diabetic patients had a 2.4-fold higher prevalence of microalbuminuria and a 5.3-fold higher prevalence of macroalbuminuria.

Effective reduction in BP with antihypertensive medication can decrease the urinary excretion of albumin (see Chapters 43 and 56).[75, 76] Although there is evidence that ACE inhibitors may be more effective in accomplishing this goal, this effect has been reported with several different classes of antihypertensive agents. It has not been established whether the treatment-related reduction in albumin excretion per se is associated with a decline in cardiovascular risk in patients with essential hypertension, or whether this change simply reflects the decline in BP.

Awareness and Treatment

During the period 1976 to 1991, the levels of awareness, treatment, and control of hypertension increased (see Table 45-1). However, from 1991 to 1994 these levels have all decreased despite an ongoing campaign by the National High Blood Pressure Education Program. In general, women are more aware of their hypertension and are more likely than men to have their high BP treated and controlled. Nevertheless, it is estimated that only about half of all hypertensive persons are treated with medication and fewer than half of these have their BP reduced to 140/90 mm Hg or less.[2] Consequently, fewer than 30% of all hypertensive persons in the United States have their hypertension adequately controlled. Comparable, or even lower, response rates have been reported in European studies.[77] These findings coincide with the recent rise in the age-adjusted rate of stroke and the leveling of the previous rate of decline in CHD.[5]

Patient noncompliance with medical therapy accounts, at least partly, for the failure to control high BP. It has been estimated that 50% of hypertensive patients fail to keep follow-up appointments and only 60% follow their prescribed medication regimens.[78] These problems are even more prevalent among the inner-city poor populations in which the 1-year compliance rate for hypertensive patients was 6.2% in the California Medicaid program. The potential causes of noncompliance include lack of awareness, the asymptomatic nature of the disease, and the complexity, cost, and adverse effects of antihypertensive medication.

The failure to control BP is not solely a problem of patient noncompliance or lack of access to medical care. In a recent analysis of practice patterns at the Veterans Affairs hospitals, more than 45% of patients were reported to have BP greater than or equal to 160/95 mm Hg and fewer than 25% with BP less than 140/90 mm Hg.[79] Physicians frequently failed to increase the dose of medications or try new treatments in those with poorly controlled BP, even though patients were monitored relatively frequently.

Natural History of Untreated Essential Hypertension

In the 1950s, Perera observed 500 untreated patients, 150 from before the onset of their hypertension until their death, and another 350 from the uncomplicated phase until their death.[80] The mean survival of these patients after discovery of their hypertension was 20 years. The height of the casually obtained BP had little prognostic value. Some patients with readings above 200 mm Hg systolic survived untreated for more than 35 years. The disease process included an uncomplicated phase lasting about 15 years followed by a phase in which organ complications, largely arteriosclerotic and atherosclerotic, became apparent. Of these complications, 74% were cardiac, 42% were renal, and 32% were retinal. More than half the subjects died of heart disease (principally CHF), 10% to 15% died of cerebral accidents, and about 10% died of renal failure. Malignant hypertension occurred in fewer than 5% of these patients.

Benefits and Limitations of Treatment

The Veterans Administration Cooperative trial of the 1960s was the first major American effort to evaluate the impact of antihypertensive therapy in a group of patients with essential hypertension.[19, 20] Compliant veterans were randomly assigned to placebo or medication, and treatment was rapidly found to result in great improvement of cardiovascular morbidity and mortality in patients with diastolic BPs of 115 to 129 mm Hg. A statistically favorable outcome was shown after 3.3 years of follow-up in patients of the treated group whose diastolic BP was between 105 and 115 mm Hg. The benefit was manifested by a reduced frequency of strokes, CHF, and dissection of the aorta but not of ischemic cardiac events. The benefits of treating patients with moderate to severe hypertension were thus clearly shown.

No benefit was achieved, however, among the patients with diastolic BP below 105 mm Hg. Furthermore, a particularly relevant finding was that the major benefit in the group with diastolic BPs between 105 and 115 mm Hg was realized by those patients who had displayed evidence of preexisting cardiovascular disease on entering the study or who were 50 years of age or older. Among patients who had no preexisting end-organ disease or who were younger than 50 years, no difference in benefit was found between the treated and untreated groups.

One of the first attempts to address some of the issues left unresolved by the original Veterans Administration study was undertaken by the U.S. Public Health Service Hospital Study Group.[81] Although the study was inconclusive—largely because it involved a small sample of 389 subjects whose diastolic pressures were below 104 mm Hg and who had shown no evidence of target organ disease—no differences in mortality were found between the two groups. Increased BP levels, however, and the beginning of LVH were evident in the untreated control subjects. The study's chief value was its demonstration that BP levels in a general population could be controlled.

The benefits of treatment were studied in the early 1970s by the National Institutes of Health in a far broader population (approximately 11,000 subjects screened from 158,000 people in 14 communities), which included women and a higher proportion of asymptomatic patients.[82] This study was the so-called Hypertension Detection and Follow-up Program. Patients were randomly allocated to "stepped-care" intervention or to "referred care." The stepped-care group received drug treatment without cost, whereas patients in the referred group were simply referred to their own physicians. Diastolic BP was substantially reduced in both groups but to a significantly greater degree, with a difference of 5 mm Hg, in the stepped-care group. Because the study did not control for such factors as compliance (in the first group, compliance was encouraged by gratis treatment), distinguishing the benefits of the nature and quality of medical care from the benefits of specific pharmacologic therapy is difficult. The fact that the stepped-care group had a 17% reduction in mortality from all causes (e.g., a significant reduction in cancer mortality was found) supports the notion that aspects of care other than antihypertensive treatment, such as consistent, enthusiastic, and cost-defrayed general care, may have contributed to the observed outcome.

One must also recognize that death rates in both groups were extremely small and that the incremental gain realized by intervention was limited. One reason for these results may have been that most subjects had only mild (90-104 mm Hg diastolic) hypertension. Five-year survivorship in the referred-care group was slightly less than 93%, whereas that in the stepped-care group was slightly more than 94%. Thus, 1000 people would need to be treated continuously for 5 years to derive a similar benefit in 8 patients.

Based on the reduction in mortality achieved by antihypertensive treatment in patients with malignant hypertension and in nonmalignant but severe diastolic hypertension, several randomized controlled treatment trials were performed during the past 4 decades to assess the efficacy of treatment in patients with more modestly elevated BP (Table 45-3). Until the late 1980s, entry criteria included diastolic rather than systolic BP, reflecting the perceptions of cardiovascular risk at that time. Diuretics and β-blockers were the primary drugs tested and most studies done before the mid-1980s used high doses of diuretics.[83] Moreover, patients enrolled in those studies were younger, approximately 50 to 60 years old. In a meta-analysis of 18 antihypertensive treatment trials, including over 48,000 patients with follow-up averaging 5 years, Psaty and colleagues analyzed separately the controlled trials that involved high-dose diuretics (≥ 50 mg hydrochlorothiazide) from those in which lower doses were used.[84] Whereas stroke protection occurred regardless of the drug doses used, the risk of CHD was not decreased by high doses of diuretics and β-blockers.

The clinical impact of diuretic-induced hypokalemia on CHD and stroke risk was highlighted in a recent analysis of data from the Systolic Hypertension in the Elderly Program (SHEP). After 1 year of treatment with a low-dose diuretic, patients randomized to active treatment were more likely to be hypokalemic (serum potassium <3.5 mEq/L) than those randomized to placebo (7.2% vs. 1.0%; $P < .01$). After adjustment for known risk factors, those who received active treatment and who experienced hypokalemia had a similar risk of cardiovascular events, coronary events, and stroke as those randomized to placebo. By contrast, for those in the active treatment group who had normal serum potassium levels, the risk of these events was 51%, 55%, and 72% lower, respectively, among those who had normal serum potassium levels compared with those who experienced hypokalemia. Although renin-angiotensin-aldosterone system activity was not measured in this study, diuretic stimulation of aldosterone often occurs during diuretic therapy [85] and may have contributed to the pathophysiology of this adverse outcome (see later).

In the ALLHAT study, 33,000 relatively high-risk patients with hypertension were treated over a 5-year period with either chlorthalidone (a thiazide-type diuretic), amlodipine (a dihydropyridine calcium channel blocker), or lisinopril (an ACE inhibitor) to achieve a goal BP below 140/90 mm Hg.[43] There was no difference in the primary end point of fatal or nonfatal CHD. However, there were differences in some of the secondary end points. Patients on diuretics were less likely to develop heart failure, cardiovascular disease, or stroke than those treated with the ACE inhibitor. There were small but statistically significant differences in BPs achieved among the three drugs tested. Black subjects and the elderly had a greater decrease in BP when treated with the diuretic than with the ACE inhibitor.

There were several important limitations in the design of ALLHAT that probably influenced the outcomes and interpretation of this study. To achieve the target BP, 60% of patients required combination treatment with at least two

TABLE 45-3

Randomized Placebo-Controlled Trials of Antihypertensive Drug Treatment

TRIAL	NO. OF PATIENTS	ENTRY BP (MM HG)	MEAN AGE (YR)	DURATION (YR)	PRIMARY DRUGS
VA Coop (1967)	143	186/121	51	1.5	D-high
VA Coop (1970)	380	163/104	51	3.3	D-high
Carter[268]	97	>160/110	60-79	4.0	D-high
Barraclough, et al.[269]	116	—/109	56	2.0	D-high
Hypertension-Stroke Coop[270]	452	167/100	59	3.0	D-high
USPHS[271]	389	148/99	44	7.0	D-high
VA-NHLBI[272]	1012	—/93	38	1.5	D-high
HDFP[82]	10,940	170/101	51	5.0	D-high
Oslo[273]	785	155/97	45	5.5	D-high
Australian[274]	3427	165/101	50	4.0	D-high
Kuramoto, et al.[275]	91	168/86	76	4.0	D-high
MRC-I[44]	17,354	161/98	52	5.0	β-B/D-high
EWPHBP[276]	840	182/101	72	4.7	D-low
Coope & Warrender[277]	884	197/100	60	4.4	β-B
SHEP-P[278]	551	172/75	72	2.8	D-low
SHEP Coop[114]	4736	170/77	72	4.5	D-low
STOP-H[279]	1627	195/102	76	2.0	β-B
MRC-II[280]	4396	185/91	70	5.8	β-B/D-low
Syst-Eur[115]	4695	174/86	70	2.0	Nitrendipine
LIFE[89]	9193	174/98	67	4.8	Losartan

β-B, beta-blocker; BP, blood pressure; D-high, diuretic dose ≥50 mg hydrochlorothiazide; D-low, diuretic dose <50 mg hydrochlorothiazide; EWPHBP, European Working Party on High Blood Pressure in the Elderly; HDFP, Hypertension Detection and Follow-up Program; LIFE, Losartan Intervention for Endpoint Reduction in Hypertension Study; MRC, Medical Research Council; NHLBI, National Heart, Lung, and Blood Institute; SHEP, Systolic Hypertension in the Elderly Program; SHEP-P, SHEP pilot study; STOP-H, Swedish Trial in Old Patients; USPHS, U.S. Public Health Service; VA, Veterans Administration.

Adapted from Kaplan N: Kaplan's Clinical Hypertension, 8th ed. Philadelphia, Lippincott Williams & Wilkins, 2002.

antihypertensive drugs at the 5-year follow-up visit. According to the study design, patients who did not reach the goal BP on the diuretic monotherapy could receive a β-blocker. This is a logical choice because it suppresses the activity of the renin system, a mechanism of hypertension that is not blocked but can be stimulated by diuretic therapy (see below). By contrast, patients in the ACE inhibitor treatment group who did not reach the target BP were not allowed by protocol to receive a diuretic or a calcium channel blocker as a second- or third-step agent that would complement its pharmacologic actions (see below). Instead, they were limited to a β-blocker, reserpine, clonidine, and hydralazine as additional therapy. The unfortunate decision to use second-step agents in the ACE inhibitor group that also suppress the renin system or are generally less effective antihypertensive agents, particularly in the elderly and black populations, most likely contributed to the higher BP and greater prevalence of secondary end points. The most striking of these is the 40% greater event rate in black patients randomized to lisinopril.[43a]

Before randomization in ALLHAT, all antihypertensive medications were discontinued before the study drug was begun. The prerandomization drug regimens were not recorded. Thus, the effect of changing drug classes after randomization on the incidence of secondary end points (i.e., heart failure, stroke) could not be evaluated.

The results of ALLHAT are in contrast with the findings of the Second Australian National Blood Pressure Study Group.[43b] In that study, hypertensive patients were randomized to either thiazide-type diuretic or ACE inhibitor treatment. Approximately two-thirds of each group were receiving monotherapy after a 5-year follow-up and the BPs in the two groups were comparable throughout the study. In contrast

with the ALLHAT results, there was a significantly lower rate (−11%) of the primary end point (cardiovascular events or death from any cause) in the ACE inhibitor group, although the incidence of heart failure was similar in both treatment groups of the Australian study. Moreover, unlike in the ALLHAT study, similar second-step drugs were used in both treatment groups, including calcium channel blockers, β-blockers, diuretics, and ACE inhibitors. The methodologic differences in these two studies are substantial. Whether this accounts for their contrasting cardiovascular disease outcomes remains to be defined.

Since 1985, several large randomized placebo-controlled treatment trials have been preformed in elderly patients with isolated systolic hypertension. A meta-analysis of more than 15,000 patients found that antihypertensive treatment (mean BP 10.4/4.1 mm Hg), predominantly with diuretics and β-blockers, significantly reduced all-cause (13%) and cardiovascular (18%) mortality during a 3.8-year follow-up.[86] Furthermore, there were significant reductions in cardiovascular morbidity (23%) and stroke (28%) when compared with placebo. These benefits were greater in male patients with higher baseline risk status, such as prior cardiovascular complications. Accordingly, to prevent one cardiovascular event, treatment for 5 years would be required in the following: 18 men versus 38 women; 19 patients aged 79 years versus 39 patients aged 60 to 69 years; and 16 patients with prior cardiovascular complications versus 37 patients without.

Left Ventricular Hypertrophy

Regression of echocardiographic LVH has been reported during treatment with several classes of antihypertensive medications. In a randomized controlled trial, ACE inhibitor treatment with ramipril decreased LV mass to a greater extent than hydrochlorothiazide, even though 24-hour ambulatory BP was reduced to a lower level during diuretic treatment.[87] In that study, plasma AII levels fell to undetectable levels during ramipril treatment, but increased with hydrochlorothiazide. The dissociation of BP reduction from this marker of hypertensive heart disease (i.e., LV mass) during diuretic therapy may represent a pathophysiologic mechanism for the well-recognized limited reduction in cardiovascular risk during diuretic treatment.[4] This finding strongly suggests that, in addition to the absolute level of BP, AII is also a determinant of LV geometry.[87] These results support the finding of an earlier meta-analysis, that specific drug class was an important determinant of the extent of LV regression (ACE inhibitor >β-blockers = calcium channel blockers = diuretics).[73] Moreover, results of the Heart Outcomes Prevention Evaluation (HOPE) study, in which high-risk patients were randomized to treatment with ramipril or placebo, showed that ramipril decreases the development of ECG-LVH and causes its regression. These changes are independent of BP and are associated with reduced risk of death, MI, and CHF.[88]

These findings suggest that AII is important in the pathogenesis of LVH and related cardiovascular complications. This hypothesis was tested in the Losartan Intervention for Endpoint Reduction (LIFE) study, a randomized controlled trial comparing the effects of losartan and atenolol on cardiovascular morbidity and death in hypertensive patients with ECG-LVH.[89] Losartan treatment was associated with a significant (13%) reduction in the primary composite end point (death, MI, or stroke), attributable to a 25% relative risk reduction for stroke. This was the first study to demonstrate an incremental benefit of a drug above the established benefits of β-blockade. These findings are consistent with results of the HOPE trial, which found that an ACE inhibitor also protects against stroke, beyond reducing BP, in high-risk patients.[56] Moreover, sustained BP reduction in hypertensive patients causes continued decrease in echocardiographic LV mass and prevalence of anatomic LVH for at least 2 years despite only small BP decreases after the first year of treatment with either a β-blocker of AII receptor blocker. These data document cardiac benefit of sustained BP control and suggest that maximum LVH regression with effective antihypertensive treatment requires at least 2 years' duration.[90]

Congestive Heart Failure

Median survival after the diagnosis of CHF in the Framingham cohort was 1.4 years in men and 2.5 years in women.[63] Reports from controlled treatment trials indicate that survival is prolonged by drugs that interrupt renin system activity, including ACE inhibitors and type 1 AII receptor blockers.[59, 91, 92] Moreover, patients with the highest pretreatment levels of AII are most likely to derive benefits in ventricular function, functional class, and prolonged survival during treatment with an ACE inhibitor.[93]

The Antihypertensive and Lipid-Lowering Treatment to Prevent Heart Attack Trial (ALLHAT), a randomized, double-blind, active-controlled clinical trial, reported that hypertensive patients with at least one other cardiovascular risk factor, when treated with doxazosin (an α₁-adrenergic receptor blocker), were twice as likely to develop heart failure (8.13% vs. 4.45%) than patients treated with chlorthalidone.[94]

There was no difference in the primary outcome, fatal or nonfatal MI. Several factors make it difficult to judge whether the CHF rate in the doxazosin group was different from expected in an untreated, comparable group of hypertensive patients, including (1) absence of a placebo control group, (2) greater adherence to drug treatment in the chlorthalidone group, and (3) slightly higher mean systolic pressure (2-3 mm Hg) in the doxazosin group (see above).

Previous studies lend support to the view that α₁-adrenergic receptor blockade may not reduce the risk of CHF. In the Treatment of Mild Hypertension Study, LV mass was reduced in the chlorthalidone group, but not in the doxazosin group.[95] In patients with preexisting heart failure, mortality benefit for combination therapy was reported with isosorbide dinitrate and hydralazine, but not for prazosin, an α₁-receptor blocker.[96] Moreover, based upon data from the SHEP trial, a 3-mm Hg systolic BP could account for a 10% to 20% increase in CHF risk, but is unlikely to explain the doubling of this risk that occurred in the ALLHAT.[97]

Ischemic Stroke

BP increases during acute stroke in previously treated hypertensive and even in previously normotensive patients.[98] When left untreated during an ischemic stroke, BP decreases to baseline level within 1 to 4 days. By contrast, during intracerebral hemorrhage, BP tends to increase to a higher level and does not usually decline as predictably as in ischemic stroke.

Although severe hypertension during an ischemic stroke has been reported to auger a poor prognosis, there is no convincing evidence to support the acute pharmacologic reduction in BP in this setting.[99, 100] A study of hypertensive patients who were otherwise healthy found that autoregulation of cerebral blood flow is reset to a higher level.[101] This has led to questionable conclusion that mean arterial pressure during acute ischemic stroke can be safely lowered by 25% with antihypertensive drug treatment during the first 24 hours.[102] To the contrary, cerebral autoregulation is disrupted during acute ischemic stroke and marked decrements in cerebral blood flow can occur with reductions in BP of that magnitude.[100]

Randomized controlled clinical trials indicate that antihypertensive drug treatment during an ischemic stroke does not improve clinical outcome and, in fact, may worsen it.[103] For example, a large (N = 624), randomized placebo-controlled trial of treatment with antihypertensive medication (i.e., labetalol, nitroprusside) and recombinant tissue plasminogen activator (rt-PA) during ischemic stroke evaluated the potentially greater risk of intracerebral hemorrhage in hypertensive stroke patients.[99] The study found that, in hypertensive patients randomized to receive treatment with rt-PA, antihypertensive treatment after randomization was associated with a fourfold greater risk of death and chronic neurologic impairment when compared with rt-TPA patients who did *not* receive antihypertensive medication after randomization. Furthermore, in patients who were randomized not to receive treatment with rt-PA, antihypertensive therapy after randomization provided *no benefit* in neurologic recovery or death rate. The rt-PA group treated with antihypertensive drugs was more likely to have a more abrupt decline in BP than those who were not treated with antihypertensive medication.

The adverse impact of antihypertensive treatment could not be attributed to other patient characteristics (e.g., age, stroke severity, or severity of hypertension), which were similar in the rt-PA and non-rtPA treatment groups. This important controlled trial highlights that during ischemic stroke (1) there is no demonstrable benefit of antihypertensive treatment regardless of whether concurrent rt-PA treatment is employed, and (2) concurrent treatment with rt-PA and antihypertensive medication appears to have a detrimental effect on clinical outcome, including neurologic recovery and survival.[99]

Precipitous declines in BP during treatment with direct vasodilators (e.g., nitroprusside, nifedipine, hydralazine) may have catastrophic consequences. Calcium channel blocker use has been associated with increased risk of intracerebral bleeding during thrombolytic therapy after an acute MI (Thrombolysis in Myocardial Infarction II study). This has new relevance because thrombolytic therapy is now being used more frequently for patients with nonhemorrhagic stroke.[104] Therefore, calcium channel blockers, especially short-acting nifedipine, should not be used.[105]

Because acute antihypertensive treatment holds the potential for harm and is of unproven benefit, it should be avoided and BP should be allowed to decrease spontaneously during the first few days after an ischemic stroke.[62, 100] Antihypertensive treatment is indicated when there is a concurrent medical condition, such as acute aortic dissection or MI. A single target BP is unlikely to apply to all patients and will likely depend upon the severity of the stroke and the extent of the penumbral zone. This pathophysiologic variability will undoubtedly complicate the management of patients with nonhemorrhagic strokes for whom thrombolytic therapy is being considered (see later).

Hemorrhagic Stroke

Hypertension occurs commonly in the early period following intracerebral hemorrhage. It is more severe and, in contrast to the BP elevation during ischemic stroke, is less likely to spontaneously improve during the first few days after presentation.[98, 100, 106]

Nimodipine, a dihydropyridine calcium channel blocker, significantly improves outcome in patients with subarachnoid hemorrhage. However, transient hypotension is a relatively common side effect of nimodipine, particularly when it is administered intravenously.[107, 108] Although the fall in BP usually responds to hydration, approximately 30% of patients also require treatment with vasoconstrictors (e.g., dopamine, phenylephrine, norepinephrine) to reverse its vasodilating effect. These offsetting therapeutic strategies have unpredictable consequences, particularly now that surgery for ruptured aneurysms is done in older patients with concomitant coronary artery disease.[107]

Treatment with a dihydropyridine calcium channel blocker during the early period after intracerebral or subarachnoid hemorrhage has a significant effect on cerebral hemodynamics.[109] Within 30 minutes after a single dose of short-acting nifedipine, mean arterial pressure falls by 20%, mean intracerebral pressure rises by 40%, and, consequently, cerebral perfusion pressure (CPP) falls by 40%. Patients with higher pretreatment intracerebral pressures (i.e., ≥40 mm Hg) have more marked reductions in CPP. This means that nifedipine promotes cerebral edema, reduction in CPP, and, hence, impairs autoregulation of cerebral blood flow.[109] However, the long-term clinical impact of these results cannot be interpreted fully because the neurologic outcomes of these patients were not reported.

The adverse hemodynamic responses of dihydropyridine calcium channel blockers may account for their limited therapeutic efficacy reported in some treatment trials. For example, the Cooperative Aneurysm Study, a large (N = 906), randomized controlled trial in patients with aneursymal subarachnoid hemorrhage, compared high-dose intravenous nicardipine with a control group treated with volume expansion. In that study, hypotension occurred twice as frequently in the nicardipine group (34.5% vs. 17.5%).[110] Overall neurologic outcome and survival were similar in these two groups at 3-month follow-up even though the incidence of symptomatic vasospasm was greater in the control group than in the nicardipine group.

In summary, data from controlled studies of antihypertensive drug therapy on acute stroke are limited but useful when considering treatment options. The evidence indicates that, in ischemic stroke, BP spontaneously falls to prestroke levels within a few days.[98] There is no evidence from clinical trials to support the use of antihypertensive treatment during acute stroke in the absence of other concurrent disorders (e.g., aortic dissection, heart failure; see later). Moreover, data from laboratory and clinical studies strongly suggest that antihypertensive treatment may adversely affect cerebral autoregulation in acute stroke. In particular, dihydropyridine calcium channel blockers and other direct vasodilators promote inconsistent changes in cerebral hemodynamics that might be detrimental. Although the favorable effect of nimodipine in patients with acute subarachnoid hemorrhage has been established, treatment-induced hypotension may limit its efficacy.

J-Shaped Curve and Antihypertensive Drug Treatment in Stroke

A J-shaped relationship was identified between diastolic BP and the incidence of stroke in treated hypertensive patients participating in the Rotterdam study, a prospective population-based cohort study.[111] The adjusted stroke risk increased at diastolic pressure levels below 65 mm Hg when compared with a reference range of 65 to 74 mm Hg. This observation was confirmed after patients with isolated systolic hypertension were excluded from the analysis. By contrast, in patients untreated for hypertension, there was a continuous increase in stroke incidence with increasing systolic and diastolic BP.

Diabetes mellitus is a common current condition in hypertensive patients. Randomized treatment trials have illustrated that BP control reduces cardiovascular risk and slows the rate of progression of renal insufficiency[112, 113] (see Chapter 38). Data from elderly diabetic patients with isolated systolic hypertension enrolled in the Systolic Hypertension in the Elderly Program (SHEP)[114] and the Syst-Eur trial[115] were analyzed separately from nondiabetic patients. The risk of combined cardiovascular end points was reduced significantly in both diabetic and nondiabetic patients, although the risk of stroke and death were not decreased significantly in the diabetic patients in the SHEP trial.

PHYSIOLOGY OF BLOOD PRESSURE HOMEOSTASIS

Before proceeding with a discussion of the pathophysiology of hypertension, it is necessary to briefly review the factors that control BP homeostasis. Blood pressure is defined as

$$BP = CO \times TPR = (HR \times SV) \times TPR$$

where BP = blood pressure; CO = cardiac output; HR = heart rate; SV = stroke volume; TPR = total peripheral resistance.

Body volume varies directly with total body Na content because Na is the predominant extracellular solute that retains water within the extracellular space. One primary function of the kidneys is to regulate Na and water excretion and, consequently, they also provide a dominant role in the long-term control of BP. To achieve this goal, two important renal mechanisms are utilized. One mechanism regulates extracellular fluid volume by coupling increases or decreases in urinary excretion of salt and water, and the related changes in blood volume and cardiac output, to changes in renal perfusion pressure. This phenomenon has been referred to as pressure natriuresis.[116] The second mechanism employs the renin-angiotensin-aldosterone system, which directly controls peripheral vascular resistance and renal reabsorption of Na and water. Accordingly, the renin system normally functions as a long-term regulator of BP homeostasis.[117]

Pressure Natriuresis

Pressure natriuresis is the increase in urinary excretion of Na and water that occurs when arterial pressure increases. As a consequence of this compensatory renal response, BP is maintained within the normal range.[116] For example, when an experimental animal is infused rapidly with approximately 40% of its own blood volume, cardiac output and urine output increase dramatically. However, only a minor increase in BP occurs because peripheral vascular resistance declines. The subsequent increase in urine flow restores blood volume to normal and so BP is reduced and urinary excretion then falls back to the baseline level. This feedback allows the kidney to regulate BP. Accordingly, the kidney functions as a servo-controller of arterial pressure and exhibits an infinite negative feedback gain for the long-term regulation of arterial pressure by adjusting blood volume.[118]

The quantitative characteristics of pressure natriuresis can be illustrated by examining the relationship between mean arterial pressure and the relative intake and output of sodium (Fig. 45-6). The BP and urinary Na values are obtained after the experimental subject has eaten a diet containing a fixed level of sodium for several days so that salt intake and excretion are equal. This situation is referred to as sodium balance. One striking characteristic of the normal salt-loading renal function curve is that BP remains remarkably constant despite the wide range of sodium intake, even in amounts exceeding 15 times normal. This illustrates the capability of the renal-fluid volume mechanism of returning BP back to a normal level regardless of any initial deviation. Using a term applied to negative feedback systems, this characteristic is referred to as "infinite gain." The kidney regulates the excretion of water and electrolytes through the tightly controlled balance of glomerular filtration, tubular reabsorption, and secretion. These processes are governed by biophysical

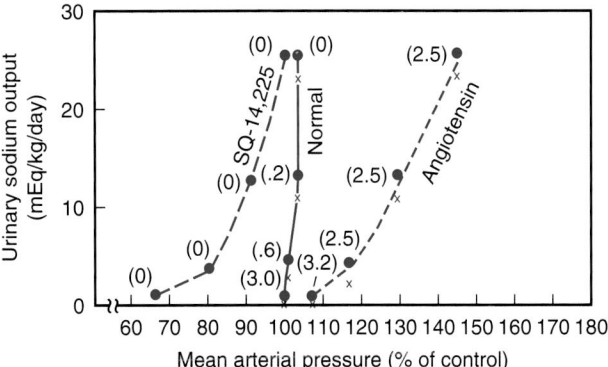

FIGURE 45-6. Pressure-natriuresis relationship. Blood pressure is maintained at a relatively constant level despite 15-fold changes in dietary sodium intake. Renin-angiotensin dependency of blood pressure normally occurs at low sodium intake, whereas sodium-volume dependency of blood pressure occurs during high sodium intake. These are salt-loading renal function curves in three dog models: (1) normal, (2) during angiotensin-converting enzyme inhibitor treatment (SQ-14,225), and (3) during continuous infusion of angiotensin II. The numbers in parentheses represent the calculated levels of circulating angiotensin II, with 1.0 as the normal level. (From Guyton A, Hall J, Coleman T, et al: The dominant role of the kidneys in long-term arterial pressure regulation in normal and hypertensive states. *In* Laragh JH, Brenner BM [eds]: Hypertension: Pathophysiology, Diagnosis, and Management, 2nd ed. New York, Raven Press, 1995, pp 1311-1326.)

characteristics such as transcapillary pressure gradients (see Chapter 8) and by a variety of hormones (see later) and locally acting vasoactive substances (see Chapter 16).

Autoregulation of renal blood flow and GFR prevents increases in renal perfusion pressure from being transmitted to the glomerular or peritubular capillaries (see Chapters 7 and 8). Therefore, the mechanisms promoting pressure natriuresis appear to inhibit tubular reabsorption in the absence of an intrarenal hemodynamic signal. However, blood flow and pressure are not autoregulated in the renal medullary circulation of volume-expanded rats.[119] Vasa recta capillary pressure and renal interstitial hydrostatic pressure (RIHP) increase, whereas pressure in peritubular capillaries in the renal cortex is unchanged. The rise in vasa recta capillary pressure leads to increased RIHP and, consequently, attenuates reabsorption of medullary tubular fluid. Other factors contribute to the pressure-natriuresis phenomenon, including the effect of high medullary pressure and flow to wash out the medullary solute gradient.[118]

In addition to these biophysical factors, it is clear that several endocrine and paracrine factors contribute to the pressure-natriuresis phenomenon and, hence, to the regulation of BP.

Renin-Angiotensin-Aldosterone System

The ability to maintain normal BP at sodium intakes ranging from levels well below normal to those far above normal is a direct effect of the circulating levels of renin AII. The kidneys secrete the enzyme renin from the juxtaglomerular cells in response to a variety of normal or abnormal phenomena that reduce arterial BP, renal perfusion, or sodium chloride load to the macula densa.[117] These include changes in posture or effective circulating fluid volume (i.e., Na depletion, hemorrhage, CHF, nephrotic syndrome, cirrhosis). Baroreceptors in the afferent arterioles, chloride-sensitive receptors in the macula densa and juxtaglomerular apparatus, and efferent renal sympathetic nerve activity all participate in this feedback control. In this way, circulating renin levels are tightly regulated and subject to constant physiologic adjustment.[120-123]

The kidney secretes active renin into the peripheral circulation and thus renin has characteristics of both an enzyme and a hormone.[124] Although prorenin is secreted by the kidney and is also synthesized by extrarenal tissues, there is no evidence that it is converted to active renin in the peripheral circulation. Accordingly, renin of renal origin determines the plasma renin level. This accounts for the observation that, following bilateral nephrectomy, PRA is undetectable.[117] The half-life of renin in the circulation is about 15 to 20 minutes, with its metabolism occurring primarily in the liver. The rate of disappearance from the blood after bilateral nephrectomy suggests a longer half-life, reflecting the accumulation of renin in extravascular fluids. Clearance of renin can also be delayed when hepatic function is impaired.

Under normal circumstances, changes in the biosynthesis and renal secretion of renin are the primary determinants of plasma AII formation. Thus, renin secretion is the rate-limiting step in the regulation of the renin-angiotensin system (Fig. 45-7). Renin cleaves the inactive decapeptide, AI, from angiotensinogen (renin substrate). AI is then converted to the octapeptide AII by ACE, located on the endothelial surface and in the circulation.[124]

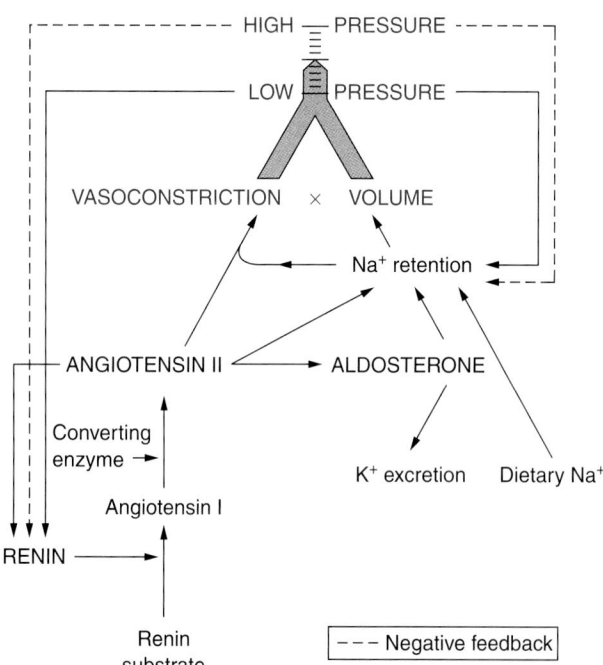

FIGURE 45-7. Regulation of the renin-angiotensin-aldosterone system. Renin, secreted in response to reduced arterial pressure or reduced renal tubule Na$^+$, cleaves angiotensin I from circulating angiotensinogen (renin substrate). Angiotensin-converting enzyme then converts angiotensin I to angiotensin II. Angiotensin II raises pressure by direct arteriolar vasoconstriction, and stimulates adrenal aldosterone secretion; together, aldosterone and angiotensin II cause renal Na$^+$ retention. The resultant fluid accumulation leads to improved flow. These pressure and volume effects in turn lead to suppression of renin release. *Dashed line* indicates negative feedback. (From Laragh JH, Letcher RL, Pickering TG: Renin profiling for modern diagnosis and treatment of hypertension. JAMA 241:151-156, 1979. Copyright 1979, American Medical Association.)

AII is the first effector hormone of the system. It increases BP in several different ways, each of which is mediated by the AT$_1$ receptor. First, it exerts powerful, direct, and immediate vasoconstriction and thus increases peripheral vascular resistance. Second, it promotes Na reabsorption via the Na$^+$/H$^+$ antiporter at the S1 segment of the proximal nephron[125] (see Chapters 9 and 11). Third, and at a slower pace, AII stimulates aldosterone biosynthesis and secretion by the adrenal zona glomerulosa, which, in turn, drives electrogenic reabsorption of Na$^+$ by principal cells in the collecting duct and by mineralocorticoid-responsive tissue in the colon and the sebaceous and salivary glands. The retained Na is responsible for increased extracellular fluid volume that increases BP hydraulically and also may heighten vascular sensitivity to AII and other vasoconstrictors.[124] Together, these multiple effects combine to raise BP and restore fluid volume to the point where the initial signals for renin release (i.e., low BP and renal perfusion pressure) are attenuated or abolished.

In the normotensive individual, when salt intake is increased, circulating renin-AII levels decrease and BP remains within the normal range. Conversely, when sodium intake decreases, renin-AII levels increase without a significant deviation in BP. Thus, BP is kept relatively constant, even when sodium intake is varied from 10 to 1500 mEq/day, because of the reciprocal change in AII levels and body Na content[116] (see Fig. 45-6). By contrast, when the plasma AII concentration is fixed at a relatively high level by a constant infusion of exogenous hormone, then increases in sodium intake result in marked increases in BP (see Fig. 45-6).[116, 126] When the renin system is blocked (e.g., ACE inhibition), then the salt-loading renal function curve is shifted to the left so that BP decreases profoundly at low levels of sodium intake. However, BP remains normal in the absence of AII as long as sodium intake is sufficient.[117]

The concept that long-tem control of arterial BP is determined by the degree of vasoconstriction of the arterial bed located between the aortic valve and the capillaries and by the volume of fluid filling this bed has been referred to as the vasoconstriction-volume hypothesis.[117] Accordingly, it has been well established that renin-mediated vasoconstriction, as reflected by the height of the plasma renin value, is a major factor for sustaining the increased arteriolar tone. In contrast, when plasma renin levels are suppressed in normal subjects who are Na replete, then arteriolar tone is supported by a renin-independent, Na-related support of arteriolar tone.

The dynamic reciprocation between these two forms of vasoconstriction has been demonstrated in several experimental models. For example, the BP response to upright tilt, before and after renin suppression, was examined during high and then low dietary sodium.[116, 117, 127] Normally, plasma renin levels increase significantly during upright posture. However, when renin secretion is blocked by pretreatment with a β-adrenergic receptor blocker (propranolol) during a high-sodium diet, tilting produced no reduction in BP (Fig. 45-8).[127] This indicates that a renin-independent mechanism of vasoconstriction BP was enabled by dietary sodium. When the study was repeated during a low-sodium diet, baseline plasma renin levels were higher and increased further during upright tilt, while BP was maintained. However, when the tilt test was repeated both during a low sodium intake and pretreatment with a β-blocker to suppress renin secretion, all subjects became hypotensive during upright tilt.

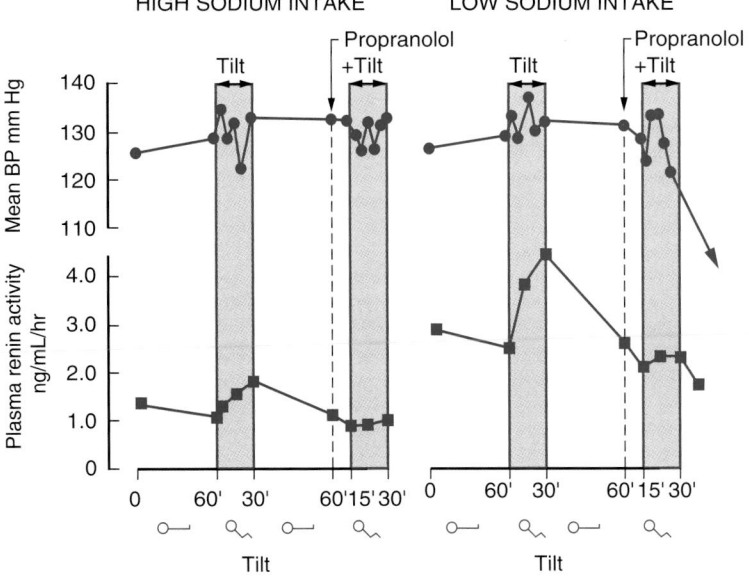

FIGURE 45-8. Interaction of sodium balance and renin system activity on blood pressure (BP). Four patients with uncomplicated hypertension were studied twice—first after ingesting a high-sodium diet (300 mEq/day; left panel) for 5 days and then again after ingesting a low-sodium diet (10 mEq/day; right panel) for 5 days. On the high-sodium diet (*left panel*), BP did not change in response to head-up tilt but the mean renin level increased. However, the defense of BP was independent of the renin level, which was suppressed by intravenous propranolol (0.12 mg/kg) that was administered before the second tilt study. On the low-sodium diet (*right panel*), baseline plasma renin levels were significantly higher than during the high-sodium diet and increased markedly during head-up tilt, although BP was maintained. After propranolol, plasma renin was suppressed and head-up tilt caused severe hypotension. Thus, after removal of both the sodium and renin mechanisms, BP could not be sustained during tilt.[127, 265] (Adapted from Morganti A, Lopez-Ovejero JA, Pickering TG, Laragh JH: Role of the sympathetic nervous system in mediating the renin response to head-up tilt. Their possible synergism in defending blood pressure against postural changes during sodium deprivation. Am J Cardiol 43:600-604, 1979.)

This study illustrates that Na-mediated vasoconstriction does not require participation of the renin system and vice versa. However, when *both* renin-mediated and Na-mediated mechanisms are inactivated, hypotension occurs.

The AII-mediated events described above are a consequence of its interaction with the AT$_1$ receptor, which has been localized to the brain, peripheral blood vessels, adrenal gland, heart, and kidney.[128, 129] Compared with the AT$_1$ receptor, the function of the type 2 AII receptor (AT$_2$) is less well understood. AT$_2$ messenger RNA (mRNA) expression decreases with age, disappearing after the neonatal period, although the receptor has been identified at a reduced level in mature rats.[130] NO synthase inhibition and AT$_2$ receptor blockade both reportedly attenuate the increase in cyclic guanosine monophosphate (cGMP) that is normally provoked by sodium restriction or AII infusion, suggesting that the AT$_2$ receptor may stimulate NO production either directly or through a bradykinin-mediated (B$_2$) mechanism. In support of this concept, mice genetically engineered to be deficient in the AT$_2$ receptor have low renal levels of bradykinin and NO. Those mice are normotensive under basal conditions, but have exaggerated pressor and antinatriuretic responses to AII infusion. These findings raise the possibility of an AT$_2$-bradykinin-NO interaction that may contribute to BP and body volume homeostasis.

Nitric Oxide

There is considerable evidence that NO participates in the regulation of BP, with important influences on BP and renal hemodynamics.[118] In healthy human subjects, inhibition of NO synthase acutely increases BP, peripheral vascular resistance, and fractional excretion of Na.[131] NO is tonically active in the medullary circulation, so that reducing NO production, or vascular responsiveness to it, reportedly enhances the pressure-natriuresis response, followed by reductions in papillary blood flow, renal interstitial hydrostatic pressure, and Na excretion by almost 30%, without corresponding changes in total or cortical renal blood flow

(RBF) or GFR.[118] This mechanism may contribute to the blunted pressure-natriuresis reported in experimental models (see later).

Endothelin

Endothelin (ET) is one of the most potent known vasoconstrictors. Its actions are mediated through two types of receptors, ET$_A$ and ET$_B$, both of which are located on vascular smooth muscle (see Chapter 16). An orally active mixed ET receptor antagonist, bosentan, reduces BP in hypertensive patients to a level that is comparable to enalapril.[132] Bosentan has also been reported to block the effects of an infusion of AII on BP and RBF in rats.[133] This raises the issue of whether a component of these AII actions may be mediated by ET.

Other vasoactive factors, including vasopressin (Chapter 13), prostaglandins (Chapter 17), renal sympathetic nerve activity (Chapter 7), and atrial natriuretic peptide (Chapter 16) also influence the pressure-natriuresis relationship, and hence BP regulation, to varying degrees.[118]

PATHOPHYSIOLOGY OF HYPERTENSION

The central role of the kidneys in BP phenomena was pointed out in 1826, when Richard Bright called attention to a group of patients who had bounding pulse and edema and, at autopsy, demonstrated hardened, contracted kidneys and cardiac hypertrophy.[134] Tigerstedt and Bergman in 1898 identified a humoral substance, which they called renin, in saline extracts of rabbit kidneys.[135] This substance had a powerful capacity to raise BP when injected into another rabbit. Goldblatt's landmark experiment in 1934, in which hypertension similar to the human form was produced hemodynamically by constricting the renal artery of the dog, further documented the kidney's vital role.[136] The organ's importance in physiologic and pathologic BP events was reconfirmed by studies in the 1960s that showed renin and aldosterone to be key elements in a normal servocontrol system that simultaneously regulates electrolyte balance and BP.[26, 137, 138]

Several lines of evidence further support the conclusion that the kidney plays an essential role in the pathogenesis of hypertension.[116, 118] First, in human hypertension and virtually all experimental models of hypertension, the ability to excrete Na is impaired at normal BP. This phenomenon has been demonstrated in renal artery stenosis, aortic coarctation, mineralocorticoid hypertension, surgical reduction of renal mass, glomerulonephritis, long-term infusion of vasoconstrictors,[139] and all genetic rat models of hypertension (see "Impaired Pressure-Natriuresis Relationship"). Second, when renal excretory function is dampened by infusion of Na- and water-retaining hormones (e.g., vasopressin, AII, aldosterone), an increase in renal perfusion pressure is required to restore Na and volume homeostasis (see "Impaired Pressure-Natriuresis Relationship"). Third, all effective antihypertensive drugs shift the pressure-natriuresis relationship back to control levels.[139] Fourth, the BP level in a human or experimental animal renal transplant recipient is directly related to the BP of the kidney donor. For example, to maintain a similar BP level in renal transplant recipients without familial hypertension, a kidney received from a hypertensive donor requires a 10-fold larger increase in the dose of antihypertensive therapy than the transplantation of a kidney from a normotensive donor.[140]

Vascular Remodeling and Pathologic Changes

In essential hypertension, the column of blood in the arterial tree between the aortic valves and the capillaries moves at abnormally high pressure throughout the cardiac cycle of contraction and relaxation. Cardiac output, however, is usually normal or close to normal. Thus, the main determinant of the sustained elevated BP is an increase in peripheral resistance. The increase in vascular resistance, a cardinal characteristic of diastolic hypertension, is commonly related to excessive vasoconstriction of arteriolar smooth muscle, although it can also result, at least in part, from structural changes in these arterioles, from increased blood viscosity, or even perhaps from increased extravascular (interstitial) pressure.[141]

In essential hypertension, physiologic and pathologic renal changes often precede changes identifiable in other organs, but whether they precede or follow the onset of the hypertension itself has not been fully determined. Early hypertensive patients may exhibit no renal structural changes observable by light microscopy.[142-144]

Renal vein catheterization data also indicate that the earliest physiologic lesion of essential hypertension is vascular: the GFR is maintained, whereas total RBF is reduced (increased filtration fraction).[145, 146] This pattern may be explained by diffuse, predominantly efferent, but also afferent vasoconstriction of all nephrons or, alternatively, by selective afferent vasoconstriction with diversion of blood away from some nephrons to maintain near-normal GFR. That renal vasoconstriction can be reversible is shown by the depressor response to pyrogens or to antihypertensive drugs.

This process is unlike that of malignant hypertension, in which gross pathologic change is accompanied by major disruption of renal function.[147] RBF and GFR may be greatly reduced, and the renal vasculature in malignant hypertension, unlike that in essential hypertension, may no longer respond to vasodilators. Indeed, in the more advanced forms of

hypertensive disease, sodium deprivation may be contraindicated, because it may further reduce RBF by provoking renal vasoconstriction. This observation provides a rationale for administering adequate amounts of dietary sodium to azotemic patients who express the so-called uremia par manque du sel.[148]

Under normal circumstances, peripheral resistance is determined predominantly by the precapillary vessels with a lumen diameter of less than 500 μm.[149] In human hypertension and in experimental animal models of hypertension, structural changes in these resistance vessels are commonly observed. In patients with essential hypertension, the characteristic findings include decreased lumen diameter and increased ratio of the diameter of the vascular smooth muscle layer of the vessel (tunica media) to the lumen diameter, referred to as the media-to-lumen ratio.

The Laplace relationship illustrates that these characteristic vascular changes provide an adaptive function by reducing wall tension as follows:

$$T = P \times (r/w)$$

where T = tension per unit of wall layer; P = transmural pressure; r = radius; w = wall thickness.

It is apparent from this relationship that, when the pressure increases, tension (T) remains constant only if the ratio of radius to wall thickness (r/w) decreases proportionately by w thickening or r decreasing or both. When this alteration of vascular structure occurs within the resistance axis, located from the aortic valve up to and including the glomerular capillary membrane, then it contributes to the long-term elevation in BP.[116]

The increase in media-to-lumen ratio of the resistance vessels occurs by the addition of material to either the outer or inner surfaces of the blood vessel wall.[149] This process requires growth (either hyperplasia or hypertrophy) of the cellular components of the blood vessel wall and results in an increase in its cross-sectional area. An alternative process, referred to as vascular remodeling, can result in an increased media-to-lumen ratio through rearrangement of the existing material without an increase in the cross-sectional area of the vessel. For this to occur, a reduction in the external diameter of the blood vessel is required. In human essential hypertension, there is increasing evidence to support the view that vascular remodeling, rather than growth, is the predominant change occurring in resistance vessels.

The hallmark renal vascular lesion in patients with uncomplicated essential hypertension is afferent arteriolar narrowing.[142, 150] This abnormality is characterized by a spectrum of histologic changes, including focal spasm of the otherwise normal afferent arterioles, endothelial edema, vascular smooth muscle hypertrophy, and widening of the internal elastic lamina with deposition of positive acid–Schiff (PAS)–positive material, and degenerative changes and hyalinization with focal luminal narrowing. In addition, juxtaglomerular cells are hyperplastic, signifying increased renin biosynthesis. However, it should be emphasized that these renal vascular changes are focal, with relatively few obsolescent glomeruli being present, thereby supporting the clinical observation that significant nephron loss and overt renal insufficiency are not major contributing factors in the pathogenesis of uncomplicated essential hypertension.

The relevance of this renal lesion to the pathogenesis of essential hypertension is supported by the finding that when the luminal diameter of the distal afferent arteriole is decreased in young spontaneously hypertensive rats (SHRs), hypertension subsequently develops.[151] Moreover, when young SHRs were treated with an ACE inhibitor, the lumen diameter of the afferent arterioles was increased, the media-to-lumen ratio decreased in a dose-dependent manner, and the BP remained low even after the drug was discontinued. By contrast, other agents that had no effect on afferent arteriolar structure did not cause a sustained reduction in BP.[152] These findings support the hypothesis that a subpopulation of nephrons with narrowed afferent arterioles can contribute to the pathogenesis of sustained hypertension.

Thus, the above-described increase in the ratio of preglomerular to postglomerular resistances may cause hypertension by (1) impeding transmission of pressure to the glomerulus, thereby reducing pressure natriuresis and promoting Na retention; (2) enhancing renin-angiotensin-aldosterone secretion by stimulating the macula densa and juxtaglomerular baroreceptor, thereby increasing vasoconstriction and Na reabsorption; and (3) promoting AII-enhanced tubuloglomerular feedback, thereby amplifying the signal whereby distal tubular Na delivery stimulates afferent arteriolar constriction.[116, 151, 153, 154]

Our research indicates that there are two functionally abnormal nephron populations in essential hypertension: (1) a minor subgroup of ischemic hypofiltering nephrons with impaired sodium excretion and with unabated renin secretion that is not turned off by sodium feeding; and (2) a larger subgroup of normal but adapting, hyperfiltering nephrons that excrete the added sodium burden and exhibit chronically suppressed renin secretion with increased GFR and distal sodium supply.[150] The two populations thus resemble the interaction between the two kidneys in the two-kidney, one-clip Goldblatt model of hypertension.

With this nephron heterogeneity, natriuresis by the normal nephrons is blunted by excessive renin-AT production by the neighboring ischemic nephrons. This internephron discord causes excess total body sodium in the face of unsuppressed plasma renin levels—a hallmark hypertensive situation in which total GFR and mean renal renin secretion remain normal. Yet, blockade of this "normal" plasma renin level by ACE inhibitors normalizes sodium balance and BP.[150]

Functional evidence for heterogeneity of nephron function in essential hypertension, comparable to that described in experimental hypertension, derives from data demonstrating the abnormal responses of renin secretion to sodium loading. The natriuretic response to saline infusion in hypertensive patients is more immediate than in normotensive subjects.[155] This response is attenuated when BP is reduced, indicating high arterial pressure is a prerequisite. Furthermore, the magnitude of this natriuresis is inversely related to the baseline PRA, with a consistent reciprocal relationship between the extent of PRA suppression and the fractional excretion of Na during acute infusion of saline. The magnitude of natriuresis was reportedly greatest in patients with primary aldosteronism in whom renin secretion was completely suppressed and PRA levels were the lowest.

Impaired Pressure-Natriuresis Relationship

Disruption of the pressure-natriuresis relationship is a fundamental aspect of human hypertension and of all experimental models of hypertension (see earlier discussion).

The relevance of the renal-fluid volume mechanism and the renin-angiotensin-aldosterone system in the pathogenesis of hypertension can be clearly seen from the results of a series of studies done by Guyton and co-workers.[116, 156, 157] These investigators devised an experimental model in which an electronically controlled hydraulic constrictor was placed around the aorta above the renal arteries in awake animals. With this technique, the renal artery pressure could be maintained at a normal level even though the systemic BP was increased by the simultaneous infusion of vasoactive hormones. When aldosterone was infused at a constant rate for 2 weeks, during which the renal perfusion pressure was maintained at normal baseline levels, Na retention occurred and the systemic pressure rose significantly. By the end of the infusion period, signs of volume overload, including pulmonary edema, were apparent. The rise in systemic pressure was caused initially by Na retention due to the direct renal effects of aldosterone and then was sustained by the impaired pressure natriuresis due to the inability to transmit the elevated pressure to the renal circulation. When the suprarenal constriction was relieved and the renal perfusion pressure allowed to increase to the level of the systemic pressure, a brisk natriuresis and diuresis occurred and systemic pressure decreased. Similar responses were also observed when other vasoactive salt- and water-retaining hormones (e.g., AII, vasopressin) were infused and a rise in renal perfusion pressure was prevented.[116, 157]

Medullary Circulation and Hypertension

Cowley and Roman have elucidated the role of the renal medullary circulation in the normal pressure-natriuresis relationship and in the pathogenesis of hypertension in a variety of experimental animal models.[118] Using laser Doppler flowmetry, these investigators found that, although superficial and deep cortical blood flow are autoregulated when renal perfusion pressure is raised above 100 mm Hg, blood flow to the inner and outer medulla are poorly autoregulated in volume-expanded rats.[118] Accordingly, increases in medullary blood flow and pressure in the vasa recta capillaries result in parallel increases in renal interstitial hydrostatic pressure, loss of the medullary osmotic gradient, and, consequently, increased natriuresis.[118, 158]

The following vasoactive substances contribute to these hemodynamic effects in the renal medulla (see Chapters 7, 16-18).

Nitric Oxide

NO is synthesized by vascular and tubular segments of the renal medulla and contributes importantly to the maintenance of normal renal medullary blood flow. Long-term inhibition of NO production causes sustained hypertension[158] that appears to be related to a shift in the pressure-natriuresis relationship to a higher pressure. Specifically, infusion of inhibitors of nitric oxide synthase into the renal interstitium significantly decreases papillary (but not cortical) blood flow, renal interstitial pressure, and excretion of Na and water.

Angiotensin II

The direct vasodilating effect of NO on the renal medullary circulation appears to have an important role in the defense of BP against elevated levels of circulating vasoconstrictors. AII can shift the pressure-natriuresis relationship to abnormally high levels of arterial pressure. However, there are substantial differences in this response among different species—dogs and humans are highly sensitive, Sprague-Dawley rats are less sensitive, to its renal medullary vasoconstrictor effects.[158] This relative insensitivity of rats to long-term elevations of circulating AII has been attributed to counterregulatory effects of the NO system within the renal medulla. Specifically, neither BP nor blood flow to the renal cortex or medulla was altered in rats infused with AII. By contrast, the same dose of AII, when administered after a threshold dose of an NO synthesis inhibitor (L-NAME) that did not affect RBF or BP, decreased medullary blood flow by 30% and subsequently increased BP by approximately 20 mm Hg.[159] Thus, renal NO production buffers the effects of AII on the renal medullary circulation and, in turn, blunts a related shift in the pressure-natriuresis relationship.[160]

Vasopressin

Vasopressin is a powerful vasoconstrictor that significantly reduces medullary blood flow and blunts natriuresis.[158] However, these effects are not sustained during chronic vasopressin infusion and, consequently, chronic hypertension does not occur. The transient response to vasopressin reflects the divergent effects of the V_1 and V_2 receptors (V_1R and V_2R).[161] Infusion of a selective V_1R agonist reduces medullary blood flow and increases BP. By contrast, V_2R stimulation promotes medullary NO production. When renal medullary NO synthase (NOS) is inhibited by a subpressor dose of N^G-nitro-L-arginine methyl ester, then vasopressin produces a sustained elevation in BP. Endothelial NOS expression is significantly increased in the inner medulla during prolonged vasopressin infusion. Thus, arginine vasopressin (AVP) stimulation of NO production in the renal medulla attenuates the V_1R-mediated vasoconstrictor effects. As with AT, this local counterregulatory response blunts the increase in BP that would otherwise occur during conditions in which vasopressin levels are elevated.[161]

Reactive Oxygen Species

Reactive oxygen species, including the superoxide anion (O_2^-), hydrogen peroxide (H_2O_2), and the hydroxyl radical (OH), have been implicated in the pathogenesis of pathologic processes, including atherogenesis and hypertension.[162] For example, AII stimulates NADH and NADPH activity, which promotes superoxide radical formation and thereby inactivates NO, stimulates monocyte-macrophage migration, and stimulates release of inflammatory cytokines. Furthermore, in a family study of probands with hypertension, H_2O_2 production was heritable and directly related to renin-angiotensin system activity, albeit weakly.[163]

Superoxide dismutase (SOD) constrains the level of reactive oxygen species by producing H_2O_2, a more stable form that is readily converted to water by catalase and glutathione peroxidase. High levels of SOD, achieved either by injection of a recombinant form, by treatment with a liposomal encapsulated product, or with a stable, membrane-permeable SOD mimetic, lowers BP in rat models. Moreover, Makino and co-workers have shown that chronic infusion of an SOD

inhibitor directly into the medullary interstitium significantly reduced medullary blood flow and increased systemic BP.[162] These findings suggest that high levels of superoxide shift the pressure-natriuresis relationship to a higher arterial pressure by impairing medullary blood flow.

Autonomic Nervous System

A popular belief is that hypertension may arise from persistent vasomotor alarm reactions.[164, 165] Hypertensive patients have been reported to respond to such noxious stimuli as mental arithmetic and psychic trauma with increased BP, visceral and skin vasoconstriction, and increased blood flow to muscles. The hemodynamic pattern resembles that occurring after exercise, and investigators believe that it reflects an abnormal conditioned reflex arising in the central nervous system, which suggests that hypertension is an expression of a central nervous system disorder.

In apparent support of this view are animal studies demonstrating severe hypertension with renal damage in a strain of mice subjected to the psychosocial stress of overcrowding.[165] Hypertension has been induced by operant conditioning in primates and dogs, although this type of hypertension is not severe and tends to subside when the stimulus is withdrawn.

Nearly all observers agree that the nervous system may participate importantly in the pathogenesis or maintenance of hypertension. The beneficial effects of tranquilizers, anesthetics, autonomic blocking drugs, and sympathectomy are well recognized. Moreover, the rare tumors of chromaffin tissue (pheochromocytoma), which secrete excessive norepinephrine or epinephrine, constitute a surgically curable cause of hypertension.

With the identification of the buffer nerve system, the catecholamines, the autonomic nervous system, and the subcortical regions of the brain are understood to function in a coordinated way to defend the arterial circulation against acute changes in pressure.[166] Any decrease in arterial BP perceived in the carotid sinus or aortic body results in reduced traffic transmitted by the 9th and 10th cranial nerves to the nucleus tractus solitarius in the medulla. This change causes reduced inhibition of neurogenic activity and a consequent increased sympathetic outflow leading to systemic vasoconstriction and tachycardia. The reverse phenomena (bradycardia and systemic vasodilation) occur with an increase in pressure or flow to baroreceptors in the carotid and aortic regions. The system thus provides instant defense of the circulation and undoubtedly accounts for much of the short-term regulation of BP and tissue perfusion in response to a varity of physiologic stimuli, including posture and exercise.

Can abnormalities in baroreceptor activity chronically affect BP? Dock and associates showed that pithing of the brain could correct Goldblatt hypertension in experimental animals.[167] McCubbin and associates postulated a "resetting" of baroreceptor activity in human hypertension, permitting a new level of BP to become the midpoint for the buffer nerve activity.[168] The human counterpart of buffer nerve hypertension, produced experimentally by denervation of the carotid–aortic body network, has not been convincingly demonstrated, however, and some investigations cast serious doubt on the persistence of buffer nerve hypertension in animals.[169] Such experimental hypertension, rather than resulting in a sustained average increase in mean pressure throughout the day, appears merely to increase upward and downward lability, that is, to produce an *un*buffering. Significantly, neither cardiac hypertrophy nor other target organ vascular disease occurs in these animal models.

Research by Nathan and Reis showed that, in experimental animals, bilateral destruction of the nucleus tractus solitarius can produce acute fulminant hypertension that is sustained in a milder form resembling buffer nerve hypertension.[169] Similar bilateral lesions in dogs have been shown to result in only transient hypertension associated with a sustained increase in peripheral resistance.[170]

Recent studies in a rat model have demonstrated that prolonged infusion with phenylephrine, at a dose sufficient to elevate BP, can cause renal microvascular and tubulointerstitial injury.[171] When the pheynylephrine infusion was withdrawn, BP returned to normal. However, hypertension developed when those animals were fed a high-sodium diet. These findings support the possibility that excess sympathetic nervous system activity may lead to chronic hypertension by inducing renal injury, thereby disrupting the normal pressure-natriuresis relationship.[172] Similar observations have also been reported in animal models, whereby renal injury caused by infusion of other vasoconstrictors (e.g., AII, cyclosporine) has culminated in Na-sensitive hypertension. These observations fit with the general hypothesis that heterogeneity of nephron structure and function plays a key role in the pathogenesis of hypertension.[150]

Thus, the possibility that a central or peripheral disorder of neural behavior may be involved in established human hypertension, although still unproved, remains an extremely attractive subject for future research. The characterization of an interaction of this rapidly acting, centrally controlled system with other, more prolonged pressor mechanisms, such as the renin system, may be fundamental to a complete understanding of BP regulation and the pathogenesis of hypertension.[173]

Nevertheless, despite the attractiveness of these possibilities, numerous biochemical measurements and indirect testing procedures have failed to reveal any convincing evidence that abnormal catecholamine secretion or metabolism, or abnormal nervous system function, participates significantly in the established forms of chronic human hypertension.[174] What does seem clear is that the autonomic nervous system and the subcortical region of the brain coordinate the defense of BP in response to acute stimuli. This defense appears for the most part to be transient, lasting from a few minutes to several hours or until longer-term mechanisms take over. The operation of this system does not seem to be markedly altered in hypertensive patients, except that their diurnal BP patterns may possibly be more labile. Furthermore, investigators have not been able to measure differences in circulating levels of catecholamines or to predict consistently the responses or lack of responses to σ- or β-blocking drugs in individual hypertensive patients.

Several studies suggest that patients with essential hypertension have impaired circulatory homeostasis with abnormal vascular reactivity. When monitored for 24 hours, these patients generally show a resetting of their diurnal BP profile to a higher level, with somewhat wider-than-normal fluctuations in BP.[175] They may also have a wider BP response to various psychic or physical stimuli. They may exhibit abnormal responses (fainting) to venous occlusion of the legs and can exhibit such other vasomotor phenomena as increased flushing, tachycardia, and sweating in response to various stimuli.[176] These phenomena are not necessarily or consistently related to the hypertension itself. They may reflect a relative instability of the individual's circulation compared with that of normotensive people, whose BP level is closer to the midpoint of defensive buffering systems that protect against assaults on the circulation.

Wave Reflection and Systolic Hypertension

Although the left ventricle ejects only a single jet of blood with each contraction, a second waveform can normally be observed in the arterial pressure pulse.[177] This secondary wave is caused by wave reflections that occur at peripheral sites where large-diameter arteries with low resistance branch and narrow into vessels with high resistance. Reflected waves can be identified beyond the high-frequency notch associated with aortic valve closure. These waves have their greatest amplitude at their origin in the peripheral vasculature and have their lowest amplitude in the central thoracic aorta. This behavior accounts for the observation that the systolic and pulse pressures are higher in the peripheral vasculature than in the aorta.

Under normal conditions, wave reflection is coordinated to return to the ascending aorta from the periphery after ventricular ejection has ceased.[177] This is advantageous because the rise in aortic pressure caused by the reflected wave occurs in diastole rather than in systole. As a consequence, diastolic pressure is increased, perfusion pressure to the coronary arteries is augmented, and LV afterload is reduced. However, for the reasons described earlier, this favorable response is associated with amplification of the systolic pressure in the periphery by 20 mm Hg above that in the thoracic aorta and left ventricle.

There is a progressive increase in pulse pressure and pulse wave velocity that occurs with aging.[24, 50] Arterial stiffening occurs because of the decreased elastic fiber content in the vessels. A similar stiffening of the vessels and the concomitant increase in pulse wave velocity can also occur in younger persons with hypertension because wall stress caused by the high pressure is transferred from the elastic fibers to collagen fibers, which are less distensible. When pressure increases, the reflected wave occurs earlier and can move into the systolic part of the wave. When this occurs, systolic pressure is amplified and the diastolic pressure decreases. The magnitude of this increase in systolic pressure can be substantial, averaging over 20 mm Hg in normotensive adults and up to 50 mm Hg in hypertensive patients. This hemodynamic profile is maladaptive because the resulting increase in systolic and LV pressures are associated with increased afterload, augmented myocardial oxygen consumption, LVH, and impaired diastolic and systolic function.

Isolated systolic hypertension, defined as systolic pressure greater than or equal to 140 mm Hg with a diastolic pressure less than or equal to 90 mm Hg, can be attributed to relocation of the reflected wave to systole. This has important clinical implications because the prevalence of isolated systolic hypertension increases after age 60 years and is associated with cardiovascular complications, including stroke and cardiovascular disease.[21, 114, 178]

HUMAN HYPERTENSIVE DISORDERS AS A SPECTRUM OF ABNORMAL PLASMA RENIN AND SODIUM-VOLUME PRODUCTS

An important contribution to the modern understanding of hypertension was the discovery of the involvement of the renin system in high BP states.[117] Clinical studies in normal volunteers demonstrated that prolonged infusion of AII for 10 days or more could produce sustained hypertension with sodium retention.[138] Moreover, this effect could be achieved with diminishingly small doses of AII. Neither the sustained hypertension nor the sodium retention could be produced by norepinephrine infusion. These studies established that AII, which was effective at low concentrations, was unique among known pressor agents in that it could produce and sustain chronic hypertension that was indistinguishable from human essential hypertension. By contrast, norepinephrine infusions do not produce sustained hypertension in normal humans.

This research indicated that the renin system, like other endocrinologic control systems, did not function in isolation but was reactive to other forces, both internal and external, affecting BP and electrolyte balance. Just as a normal level of serum insulin may be defined only in relationship to the concurrent influence of glucose, so a normal level of plasma renin may be defined only in relationship to the concurrent influence of sodium.

This point was demonstrated by the development of a protocol of renin-sodium profiling, in which plasma renin levels were indexed to the current state of sodium intake as determined by a 24-hour sodium excretion analysis.[55, 60, 179, 180] The nomograms obtained from normal subjects (Fig. 45-9; values inside dotted lines) indicate that the plasma renin values are inversely related to sodium intake. At high levels of sodium intake, PRA is suppressed, whereas at low intake PRA is markedly elevated. Despite these wide ranges, BP remains constant. These data indicate that, at low sodium intake, BP is maintained by renin-AII–mediated vasoconstriction, whereas at high sodium intake BP is maintained in the normal range by sodium-volume–mediated vasoconstriction. The dynamic reciprocation of these two forms of vasoconstriction is essential to maintain normal BP homeostasis across a wide range of dietary sodium intakes (see "Physiology of Blood Pressure Homeostasis"). This pattern follows the classic reactive behavior of an endocrinologic control system. With this index of normalcy, the role of the renin system in the various types of hypertension can be examined with the potential for stratifying patients pathophysiologically according to their renin system patterns. This is evident with the observation that,

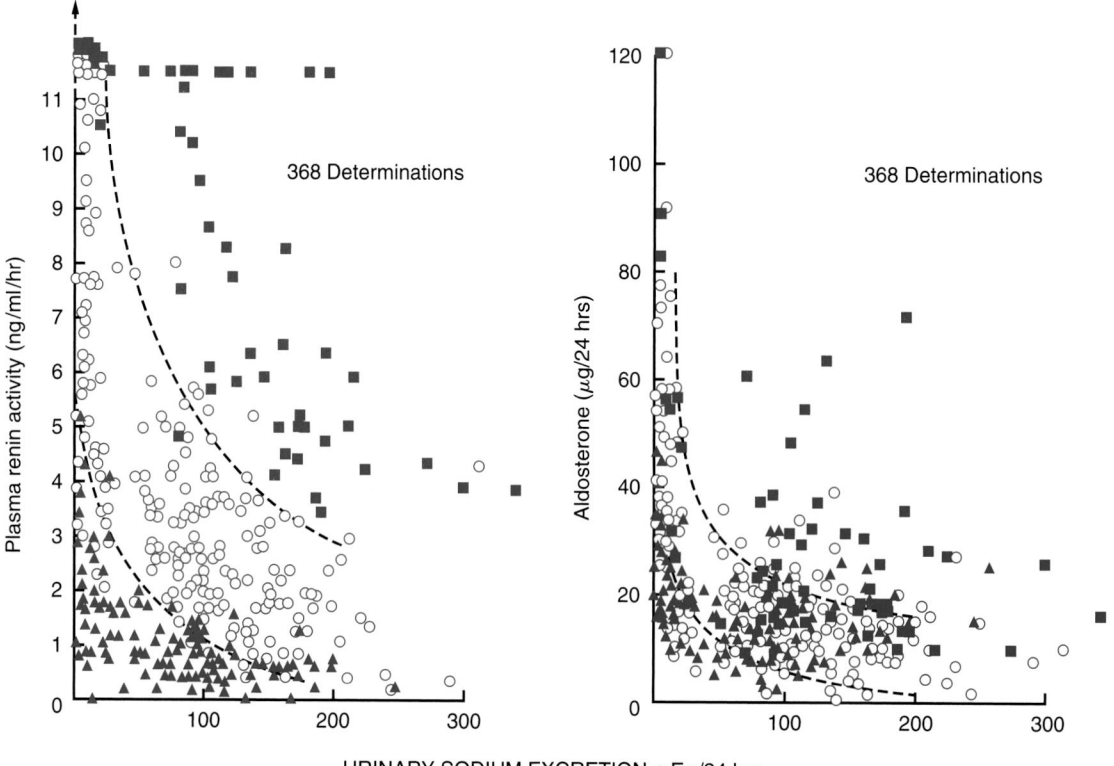

FIGURE 45-9. Relation of the noon ambulatory plasma renin activity (*left*) and the corresponding daily urinary aldosterone excretion (*right*). The *dashed lines* define the normal channel derived from the study of normotensive subjects. A total of 219 patients with untreated essential hypertension were studied, some on several occasions at different levels of sodium intake (closed triangles, low renin; open circles, normal renin; closed squares, high-renin essential hypertension). Three major subgroups are defined by the appropriateness or normalcy of the plasma renin activity to the rate of Na+ excretion, which is used as an index of dietary intake, and of Na+ balance. Additional normal subgroups are defined when aldosterone (*right*) is included in the analysis. Plasma renin activity results are expressed as nanograms of angiotensin I formed per milliliter per hour. Multiply these plasma renin activity values by 0.65 to conform to the National Bureau of Standards angiotensin I reference standard used by the Cardiovascular Center Laboratory at New York Presbyterian Hospital–Weill Medical College, and by Quest Laboratories. (From Brunner HR, Laragh JH, Baer L, et al: Essential hypertension: Renin and aldosterone, heart attack and stroke. N Engl J Med 286:441, 1972.)

although the reciprocal relationship of sodium intake and PRA is similar in hypertensive patients to that of normotensive subjects, renin levels are distributed over a much broader range in hypertensive patients.

The pathophysiologic relevance of this finding is illustrated in Fig. 45-10, in which the most commonly encountered forms of hypertension are stratified according to their renin-sodium profile. The higher renin states (see Fig. 45-10; top four disorders) have the most severe vascular disease, with damage to the heart, brain, and kidneys. Even pheochromocytoma is associated with high renin levels consequent to norepinephrine-induced renal ischemia and direct stimulation of β-adrenergic receptors located on the juxtaglomerular cells.[181] By contrast, the sodium-retaining, high-volume forms of hypertension (see Fig. 45-10; bottom two disorders) have suppressed renin secretion and present with much less vascular disease and better tissue perfusion associated with sodium-volume excess.[55, 60] This is exemplified by low-renin hypertension and primary aldosteronism, both of which are relatively benign long-standing conditions because of better tissue perfusion.[22, 55] The intermediate forms, with mixed renin-sodium excess, develop intermediate degrees of cardiovascular damage. Bilateral renal artery stenosis and aortic coarctation have sodium-volume retention, which only partially suppresses renin secretion. Consequently, these disorders are manifested by pulmonary edema when sodium-volume is in excess.[182]

Renin-Dependent Forms of Hypertension

Malignant Hypertension

The process of malignant hypertension begins with a critical degree of renal microvascular injury due to causes that are not always clear but are generally associated with severe hypertension.[137, 183-185] Renal hypoperfusion triggers a massive release of renin. In its joint vasoconstrictor and Na⁺-retaining effects, systemic pressure increases markedly. The rise in pressure normally suppresses renin production through feedback inhibition (see earlier discussion). However, in malignant hypertension, this regulatory mechanism is impaired and renin secretion continues unabated. A vicious circle results whereby more renin secretion causes more hypertension, causing more renal and systemic arteriolar necrosis, which again causes more renin secretion. In addition, renal sodium excretion is further impaired by the hypersecretion of aldosterone, which is stimulated by high levels of renin and AII. This process is referred to as secondary hyperaldosteronism.

This description of the pathogenesis of malignant hypertension is supported by several observations. Diffuse vasculitis and death result within 1 or 2 days in rats overloaded by simultaneous injections of renin and aldosterone.[186] Moreover, the experience in dialysis patients shows that the BP of patients with malignant hypertension can be lowered to virtually normal values and their arteriolar necrosis improved by bilateral nephrectomy.[187]

An equally convincing demonstration of the causal role of the renin system can be made by its pharmacologic blockade.[188] Drugs that interrupt the renin-angiotensin system (e.g., propranolol and captopril) can normalize and maintain the BP in patients with malignant hypertension, including those in encephalopathic crises.[189-192] In other such patients, the addition of diuretics to antirenin therapy may be required for normalization of BP, illustrating the joint participation of renin and Na⁺ retention.

Renovascular Hypertension

UNILATERAL RENOVASCULAR DISEASE. An experimental analog of human unilateral renovascular disease can be found in the two-kidney Goldblatt model, in which one renal artery of the animal is clipped and the other is left intact.[136, 193] In general, PRA levels are excessively high. The affected kidney, with its decreased renal perfusion pressure beyond a stenotic renal artery, reacts to the situation as if there were systemic hypotension and thus releases renin. The conversion to AII results in vasoconstriction, which raises BP. The elevated systemic BP and increased circulating AII level suppress renin release by the contralateral kidney but not by the ipsilateral kidney, where ischemia and reduced filtration continue beyond the arterial stenosis.

Excess AII promotes inappropriate sodium retention in the contralateral kidney by enhancing proximal tubule sodium reabsorption and also by increasing afferent arteriolar resistance by the tubuloglomerular feedback mechanism.[150, 153] Thus, complete suppression of renin secretion by the contralateral kidney does not counterbalance the uncontrolled release of renin in the affected kidney, because the contralateral kidney is exposed to high circulating AII levels from the ischemic kidney.

The renin system is so clearly involved in unilateral renovascular hypertension that it provides the basis for definitive diagnosis and management. The renin dependency can be demonstrated in animals or in patients by a prompt depressor response to renin system blockade. An acute, marked

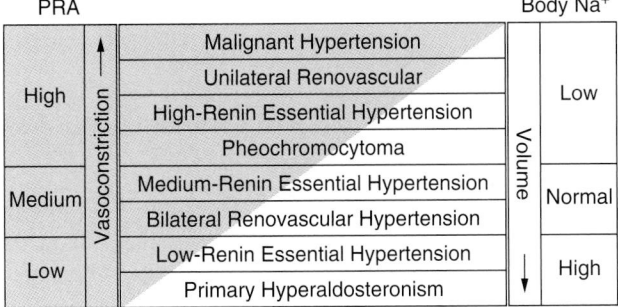

THE LARAGH VASOCONSTRICTION-VOLUME
SPECTRUM OF CLINICAL HYPERTENSION

PRA	Vasoconstriction		Volume	Body Na⁺
High	↑	Malignant Hypertension		Low
		Unilateral Renovascular		
		High-Renin Essential Hypertension		
		Pheochromocytoma		
Medium		Medium-Renin Essential Hypertension		Normal
		Bilateral Renovascular Hypertension		
Low	↓	Low-Renin Essential Hypertension		High
		Primary Hyperaldosteronism		

Normal BP = (PRA) × (Na⁺ ÷ Volume)

FIGURE 45-10. The spectrum of hypertensive disorders stratified according to their renin-sodium relationship. Normal subjects, indicated by the equation at the bottom of the figure, maintain and defend normotension by curtailing renal renin secretion in reaction to a rise in sodium intake or autonomic vasoconstriction, or by proportionally increasing renin secretion in the face of either Na⁺ depletion or hypotension from fluid or blood loss or a neurogenic fall in blood pressure. Hypertensive subjects sustain their higher blood pressures by renal secretion of too much renin for their sodium-volume states, or by renal retention of too much Na⁺ (volume) for their renin level, which often fails to fully turn off as it does in normal subjects. High-renin hypertensive patients are proportionally more vasoconstricted with poorer tissue perfusion and therefore are most susceptible to cardiovascular tissue ischemic damage (see text). BP, blood pressure; PRA, plasma renin activity.

increase in peripheral renin following a single dose of captopril, an ACE inhibitor, is highly suggestive and provides sound reason for pursuing the possibility of curable renovascular hypertension. Renal vein renin sampling after the administration of captopril provides even greater sensitivity, because ACE inhibition produces a pronounced increase in renin release from the ischemic kidney.[194, 195]

Normally, each renal vein renin level is about 25% higher than the renal arterial level, and this determines the normal peripheral level.[196] With renin totally suppressed in the contralateral kidney in unilateral renal disease, the ischemic kidney must produce at least a 50% increment to sustain the peripheral renin level. This response suggests that hypertension is curable and renal function will be maintained after revascularization.

The ability to use these relatively safe, sensitive, and specific diagnostic tests to define curable renovascular hypertension, together with the development of balloon angioplasty as an alternative to surgery, has helped in identifying more cases of curable renovascular disease than was ever suspected.[194] Many patients, now cured by an outpatient procedure, would previously have been labeled as essential hypertension by default and might have been given lifelong antihypertensive drug treatment.

BILATERAL RENOVASCULAR HYPERTENSION. In the patient with bilateral renovascular disease, peripheral renin levels are either "normal" or even slightly reduced.[196] This finding also prevails in the experimental one-kidney Goldblatt model, in which one kidney is clipped and the other removed. When both kidneys are ischemic, the perfusion defect initially stimulates renin production, but at the same time it limits excretion of sodium and water, so BP rises. The result is total-body sodium and volume accumulation to the point where renal perfusion pressure is restored beyond the stenosis. Renin production is thus depressed to normal or even subnormal levels. This restoration of equilibrium in bilateral renovascular disease is accomplished at the cost of volume expansion and systemic hypertension. Because total GFR and nephron number are seriously compromised, the BP elevation is sustained predominantly by sodium retention rather than by AII.[197]

This sodium-volume dependence can be demonstrated in experimental animals with the two forms of renovascular hypertension. Infusion of an AII blocker produces no fall in BP in the one-kidney, one-clip model when dietary salt is not reduced.[198, 199] Similarly, sodium depletion does not produce a fall in BP because the plasma renin level increases sharply, converting sodium-dependent hypertension to renin-dependent hypertension. However, during sodium restriction, anti–renin system drugs lower BP significantly. Thus, in two-kidney, one-clip Goldblatt hypertension and in patients with bilateral renal artery stenosis, elevated BP is maintained by whatever mechanism is available based upon the body sodium content—either renin-AII when body sodium is reduced, or sodium-volume when body Na is replete or in excess. The behavior of the renin system provides an important clue to the underlying mechanism.

Patients with bilateral renovascular disease show a marked decrease of BP and exacerbation of azotemia when treated with an ACE inhibitor, especially when volume-depleted by concurrent diuretic treatment.[200] Furthermore, renal vein renin patterns may be similar to that of unilateral

disease, with lateralization of renin secretion to the predominantly ischemic kidney.[195] Thus, these patients may also have renin-dependent hypertension.

In summary, the pathogenesis of bilateral renovascular hypertension is characterized by the participation of both renin and volume factors. Acute pulmonary edema is much more common in patients with bilateral disease than it is in unilateral disease[182] (see also "Impaired Pressure-Natriuresis Relationship" and Chapter 46). This phenomenon may reflect an inability to handle an acute volume load, as indicated by the natriuresis that occurs after angioplasty.[201]

Sodium-Dependent Forms of Hypertension

The plasma volume factor is largely determined by the body sodium content, as sodium constitutes the major osmotic factor regulating the amount of water in the bloodstream and extracellular space. Available sodium thus determines the fluid pressure of the circulating blood. Plasma protein and red blood cell mass are also key elements in determining circulating whole-blood volume, but these factors appear normal and fixed in most patients with uncomplicated hypertension. Accordingly, sodium contributes crucially to the volume factor that is involved to some extent in all BP phenomena. Thus, when cardiac performance is normal, arteriolar vasoconstriction and the arterial filling volume become the two dynamic final determinants of BP.

The mechanism by which sodium retention exerts its pressor effects is still not completely understood. More than one pathway to the source of low-renin hypertension has become apparent. The first of these indications is that calcium channel blocking drugs lower BP in low-renin patients with essential hypertension.[202] The serum calcium concentration is directly related to PRA, whereas the serum Mg^{2+} concentration is inversely related to PRA.[203] A high-salt diet has also been demonstrated to reduce plasma calcium concentration (most probably because of influx to the cell) to levels similar to those seen in low-renin essential hypertension, and salt restriction has been shown to do the reverse.[204] One may consider the possibility that the influence of dietary sodium on BP may be mediated by changes in the concentration or activity of divalent cations.

The significance of the sodium-calcium relationship takes on additional dimensions considering the central role of cytosolic calcium concentration in vascular smooth muscle contraction.[205] What makes this avenue especially attractive now is the availability of the σ_1-adrenergic blockers doxazosin and terazosin, which selectively block postsynaptic α_1-receptors with specificity unconnected with the widespread side effects associated with the earlier ganglionic blockers.

Significantly, the depressor effects of these agents are particularly selective among low-renin hypertension patients, those also preferred by calcium channel blockers and diuretics.[206] This form of vasoconstriction is related to antecedent sodium-volume retention. Marked orthostatic decreases in BP, as a first-dose response to prazosin, have been inversely correlated with baseline PRA.[207] Furthermore, this σ_1-antagonism stimulated reactive renin secretion when it lowered pressure, again demonstrating reciprocation between renin and nonrenin pressor phenomena. The antihypertensive efficacy of calcium channel blockade is apparently not augmented by sodium depletion and may actually be enhanced by the concurrent liberalization of salt intake.[208]

Sodium may also affect peripheral resistance through its interaction with endothelial-derived vasoactive substances. In rats, dietary sodium loading stimulates the production of NO from the macula densa.[209] Vasodilation of the afferent arteriole counteracts the vasoconstriction generated by the tubuloglomerular feedback response. When NOS is inhibited, mean arterial pressure and renal vascular resistance rise.[131] In this model, greater increases occur during adaptation to a high-sodium intake when compared with a low-sodium intake.[210] These responses appear to be independent of renin system activity. Other mechanisms may also contribute to these effects, including autoregulation-induced changes in arteriolar constriction or changes in the transport or distribution of sodium across cell membranes and between the intravascular and interstitial compartments.

Inherited Forms of Sodium-Sensitive Hypertension

Normal BP homeostasis requires precise regulation of sodium intake and excretion. Accordingly, in a normal day the kidneys reabsorb 99.5% of the 23,000 mEq sodium filtered by the glomerulus. As described above, this process is governed by renal tubular epithelial transport that is regulated in part by the renin-angiotensin-aldosterone system. Disruptions in epithelial transporters or in the hormones that regulate them can lead to clinically significant alterations in BP. Accordingly, mutations in genes that control these processes have been identified in families with rate disorders that cause severe hypertension or hypotension.[211] The pathophysiologic link between Na and BP has been illustrated in cases where gain-of-function and loss-of-function mutations in the same gene regulating sodium reabsorption raise and lower BP, respectively. Increased sodium reabsorption triggers thirst and promotes water reabsorption to maintain the serum sodium concentration at 140 mM, and increases blood volume and BP, whereas impaired sodium reabsorption lowers body volume and pressure.

The following disorders illustrate mechanisms that cause sodium-volume–dependent hypertension.

Adrenocortical Hypertension
Primary Aldosteronism

Primary aldosteronism, or Conn syndrome, is due to autonomous overproduction of aldosterone by a solitary adrenocortical adenoma.[212] The term *pseudoprimary*, or idiopathic, aldosteronism, describes a subgroup characterized instead by diffuse bilateral adrenocortical hyperplasia.[201] Together, these conditions are underdiagnosed and account for at least 1% to 2% of all hypertension. In both disorders, overproduction of aldosterone is sustained, producing a clinical syndrome manifested by sodium and volume retention, low PRA, hypokalemia with excess kaliuresis, and a chloride-unresponsive metabolic alkalosis. "Escape" from the Na$^+$-retaining effects of aldosterone accounts for the enhanced natriuresis of an exogenous sodium load and renal potassium wasting.[213] PRA levels are suppressed because of the sodium-volume expansion, increased renal perfusion pressure, and enhanced sodium chloride delivery to the macula densa.[154, 214]

The magnitude of the hypertension and metabolic abnormalities tends to be more marked when an adenoma is identified as the cause of hyperaldosteronism.[215, 216]

Unilateral adrenalectomy can cure primary aldosteronism when it is caused by a functioning adenoma or, in some cases, by adrenal hyperplasia when aldosterone secretion is comparably autonomous and is confined to one adrenal gland.[215, 216] By contrast, adrenalectomy does not cure hypertension in most patients with idiopathic hyperaldosteronism associated with bilateral hyperplasia. Diagnostic tests that discriminate between primary and pseudoprimary aldosteronism are based on the (1) greater degree of autonomy of aldosterone secretion from renin-angiotensin by the adenoma (i.e., postural stimulation test), (2) elevated plasma levels of 18-hydroxycorticosterone and urinary excretion of novel metabolites of cortisol metabolism (18-hydroxycortisol, 18-oxocortisol) by the adenoma, and (3) lateralization of aldosterone secretion.[217, 218] However, the results of adrenal imaging studies are often inconclusive. Despite the potential for cure, 50% to 60% of patients with an adenoma have persistent hypertension requiring medication after unilateral adrenalectomy. Those most likely to become normotensive are less than 50 years old and have a maximally suppressed PRA before surgery.[215, 219]

Mutations Altering Renal Sodium Channels and Transporters

The discovery by Lifton and co-workers and others of mutations in genes that regulate renal Na have clarified the pathogenesis of several rare forms of low-renin hypertension and provided insights into some of the mechanisms contributing to what remain characterized as low-renin essential hypertension.[211] Mutations that alter sodium reabsorption and BP are summarized below (see Chapter 6).

LIDDLE SYNDROME. Liddle syndrome is characterized by autosomal dominant transmission of early-onset hypertension, hypokalemia with urinary K$^+$ wasting, suppressed PRA, and low aldosterone levels. The responsible gain-of-function mutation has been localized to either the β- or γ-subunit of the epithelial sodium channel (ENaC), which causes a deletion of their cytoplasmic C termini.[220] ENaC with the Liddle mutation, when expressed in cells that lack endogenous Na channels (e.g., *Xenopus* oocytes), generates two to five times more Na$^+$ current. This enhanced Na$^+$ current has been attributed partly to a novel mechanism whereby cell surface expression of ENaC is increased due to inhibition of endocytosis via clathrin-coated pits.[221] Binding of Nedd-4 proteins to the PPXY sequence of ENaC, which normally leads to its ubiquitination and degradation, is impaired by the Liddle mutation.[222] Consequently, sodium reabsorption increases because ENaC clearance from the cell surface is reduced.[223] As with other mendelian forms of hypertension, this mechanism is due to a primary increase in sodium balance.

Mutations in the Mineralocorticoid Receptor

SL810 MUTATION. An autosomal dominant form of hypertension is caused by a mutation in the ligand-binding domain of the mineralocorticoid receptor (MR$_{L810}$).[224] Carriers of this mutation are hypertensive before age 20 years and aldosterone secretion is suppressed. MR$_{L810}$ is constitutively activated in a Cos-7 expression system, with 27% of maximal activity in the absence of aldosterone. Normally, steroids with 17-keto groups (estradiol, testosterone) and those lacking 21-hydroxyl groups (progesterone) are mineralocorticoid receptor antagonists because they bind but do not activate it. However, these steroids are potent activators of the MR_{L810} receptor, with progesterone stimulating mineralocorticoid activity that is indistinguishable from aldosterone. The aberrant nature of MR_{L810} is underscored by the finding that spironolactone, the drug used because of its efficacy as a mineralocorticoid receptor antagonist, instead activates the MR_{L810} receptor.

Progesterone levels normally increase 100-fold during pregnancy, and thus the MR_{L810} mutation may have particular relevance as a cause of gestational hypertension. Geller and colleagues [224] reported two patients with an exacerbation of hypertension, hypokalemia, renal K^+ wasting, and undetectable aldosterone levels. The agonist activity of progesterone has been attributed to the observation that the MR_{L810} mutation alters van der Waals interactions within the ligand-binding domain that eliminate the requirement for a 21-hydroxyl group for receptor activation.[211]

Mutations Affecting Circulating Mineralocorticoid Hormones

APPARENT MINERALOCORTICOID EXCESS. Apparent mineralocorticoid excess type 1 (AME) is characterized by hypertension, low PRA, low urinary aldosterone excretion rate, and increased urinary excretion of metabolites of cortisol rather than cortisone (ratio of free cortisol-cortisone and tetrahydrocortisols-tetrahydrocortisone).[225] Normally, the mineralocorticoid receptor in vitro binds cortisol and aldosterone with equal affinity, whereas cortisone binding is less avid.[226, 227] Although the serum concentration of cortisol is normally 1000-fold greater than aldosterone, cortisol is inactivated by conversion to cortisone at mineralocorticoid-responsive tissues by 11β-hydroxysteroid dehydrogenase (11β-HSD). This allows aldosterone, rather than cortisol, to gain access to the mineralocorticoid receptor. Thus, it is 11β-HSD rather than the mineralocorticoid receptor per se that confers tissue specificity for aldosterone.

AME is caused by reduced conversion of cortisol to cortisone due to impaired activity of the type 1 isoenzyme of 11β-HSD.[228] The serum cortisol is normal and does not aid in the diagnosis. Homozygous inactivating mutations of this enzyme have been identified in patients with AME.[229] Treatment options include (1) blockade of either the mineralocorticoid receptor (e.g., spironolactone) or the renal apical sodium channel (amiloride), or (2) suppression of endogenous cortisol production with dexamethasone, which has a low affinity for the mineralocorticoid receptor.

In other syndromes, such as ectopic corticotropin and excessive ingestion of licorice (which contains glycyrrhizic acid, a competitive inhibitor of 11β-HSD), acquired mineralocorticoid excess occurs because the normal mechanisms of cortisol inactivation are either overwhelmed or attenuated.[230, 231] Cortisol is thus allowed to bind to the type 1 mineralocorticoid receptor with an affinity similar to that of aldosterone. Mineralocorticoid excess syndromes can also be produced by overproduction of deoxycorticosterone and adrenal androgens.[232] In many of these syndromes, sodium-volume

expansion and hypertension suppress renin secretion, and consequently endogenous aldosterone production is markedly decreased. By contrast, in hypertension associated with other forms of Cushing syndrome and chronic oral contraceptive use, the renin-angiotensin-aldosterone system may be inappropriately activated as a consequence of increased production of angiotensinogen or by direct augmentation of vascular reactivity.[233]

GLUCOCORTICOID-REMEDIABLE ALDOSTERONISM. Glucocorticoid-remediable aldosteronism (GRA) is an autosomal dominant disorder characterized by hypertension, suppressed PRA, high levels of C-18 methyloxygenated metabolites of cortisol, normal or elevated levels of aldosterone, and varying degrees of hypokalemia and metabolic alkalosis. The hallmark feature is that exogenous glucocorticoids suppress aldosterone secretion.[211] GRA is caused by a gene duplication resulting from unequal crossing over of the genes that encode the enzymes producing aldosterone and cortisol. The resulting chimeric gene encodes a protein that has aldosterone synthase activity, which activity is expressed in the zona fasiculata under the control of corticotropin, rather than the normal situation whereby aldosterone production in the zona glomerulosa is stimulated by AII. In this situation, cortisol secretion is regulated normally, but aldosterone secretion is excessive. This leads to volume expansion, BP elevation, and suppressed PRA with persistent aldosterone overproduction, the latter driven by corticotropin.

GRA is underdiagnosed because serum K^+ levels are often either mildly decreased or normal. Clinical clues are low PRA family members with onset of hypertension younger than age 20 years.[234-236] Suspected patients and family members can be screened for the chimeric gene. This disorder is associated with a high incidence of early-onset intracranial aneurysm and hemorrhagic stroke, with 48% of all GRA pedigrees and 18% of all GRA patients suffering cerebrovascular complications. This rate is similar to the frequency of aneurysm in polycystic kidney disease.[237] Therefore, all hypertensive family members of a GRA proband should undergo genetic screening and counseling and asymptomatic GRA patients should be screened for an intracranial aneurysm. Treatment includes exogenous glucocorticoids and K^+-sparing diuretics.

Two Forms of Vasoconstriction in Essential Hypertension

The evidence presented thus far illustrates the dynamic reciprocity of two forms of vasoconstriction, mediated by sodium and by renin-angiotensin. These mechanisms are essential to maintain normal BP homeostasis, and when these mechanisms are impaired hypertension occurs. This relationship is clearly evident in the secondary forms of hypertension described earlier, especially malignant hypertension (renin-dependent) and in the disorders of mineralocorticoid excess (sodium-volume–dependent).

The spectral patterns of vasoconstriction demonstrated in the more extreme forms of hypertension described earlier also operate in essential hypertension. When renin profiling is performed and indexed in patients with essential hypertension, about 20% are found to have high renin values and about 30% to have low renin values, with the remaining half distributed between these extremes[238] (see Fig. 45-9).

These findings support the concept that the lower range of renin values mark the presence of sodium-volume–related vasoconstriction and that as one proceeds to the high end of the renin spectrum, the vasoconstriction becomes increasingly renin-mediated. This concept is supported by the observed heterogeneity in BP responses to specifically targeted antihypertensive drugs (Table 45-4). For example, diuretic agents, calcium channel antagonists, and α-adrenergic receptor blockers are especially effective in the low-renin range and become less effective in high-renin patients.[206, 239-241]

TABLE 45-4

Plasma Renin Activity Predicts Blood Pressure Responses to Antihypertensive Drugs

ANTIHYPERTENSIVE DRUG CLASS	PRETREATMENT PRA <0.65	PRETREATMENT PRA ≥0.65
Angiotensin II receptor blocker	+	++++
Angiotensin-converting enzyme inhibitor	+	++++
β-Adrenergic receptor blocker	+	++++
Central α₂-receptor agonist	+	++++
Diuretic	++++	+
Calcium channel blocker	++++	+
α₁-Adrenergic receptor blocker	++++	+

PRA, plasma renin activity.

Adapted from Laragh J: Laragh's lessons in pathophysiology and clinical pearls for treating hypertension. Am J Hypertens 14:491-503, 2001.

+-weakest response to drug, ++++-strongest response to drug.

Drugs that interrupt the renin-angiotensin system (e.g., by ACE inhibitors, AII receptor blockers, or β-blockers; see Table 45-5 and Fig. 45-11; see also later) are most effective in the high-renin forms of hypertension and least effective in the low-renin forms.[189, 242-245] Moreover, the increase in renin-angiotensin-aldosterone system activity that occurs in response to diuretic-induced sodium-volume depletion can blunt the antihypertensive efficacy of diuretics and is an important cause of diuretic resistance (Fig. 45-12). The relevance of this mechanism is supported by the synergistic antihypertensive response that occurs when an anti–renin system drug is added to diuretic treatment in a patient resistant to diuretic monotherapy.[85] The heterogeneity in pathophysiology in essential hypertension can thus be correlated with pharmacologic responsiveness.[28, 117]

EVALUATION AND TREATMENT OF THE INDIVIDUAL PATIENT

General Principles

The evaluation of a new patient with high BP embraces all the principles of good medical practice. It relies on a complete history and physical examination and the routine application of appropriately chosen laboratory tests. A thorough initial evaluation can avoid the prescription of needless or inappropriate drugs for the lifetime commitment that hypertension may often require, and at the start it can reveal

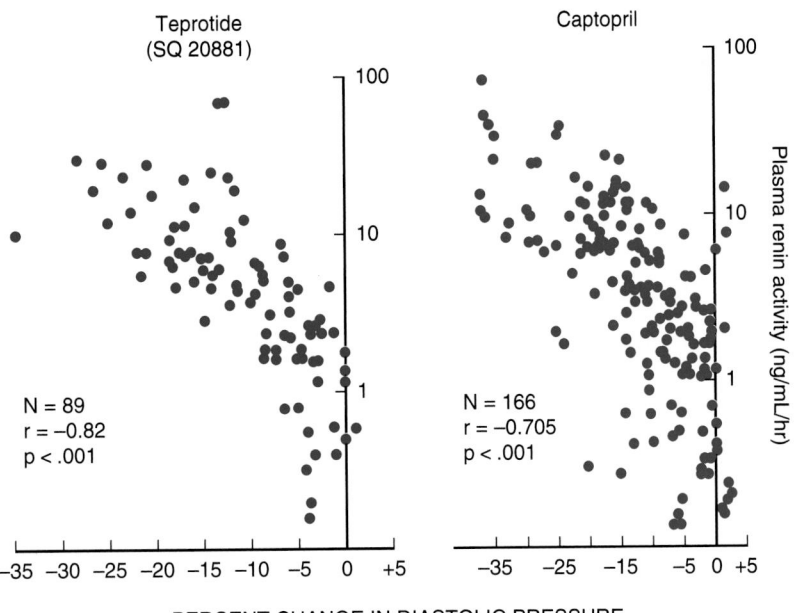

PERCENT CHANGE IN DIASTOLIC PRESSURE

FIGURE 45-11. The acute effects (at 90 minutes) of intravenous- and oral-converting enzyme inhibitors on diastolic blood pressure. With both drugs, the percentage fall in blood pressure is closely related to the pretreatment levels of plasma renin activity in quietly seated, untreated hypertensive patients. The left panel illustrates the effects of the intravenous administration of the nonapeptide isolated from snake venom, teprotide (SQ 20881), to 89 patients; data are replotted from Case, et al.[190] The right panel shows changes in seated diastolic blood pressure in 166 patients 90 minutes after a single oral dose of 25 mg captopril. Notwithstanding the errors in cuff pressure measurements, the data reveal remarkable and extremely similar correlations between the height of the pretreatment plasma renin values and the degree of induced fall in blood pressure. Note that patients with plasma renin values below 1.0 ng/mL/hour usually exhibited no change in pressure. The data in both panels also provide strong indirect evidence that a plasma renin value closely reflects the active role of renin in supporting arterial pressure in hypertensive individuals. Plasma renin activity values are expressed as nanograms of angiotensin I formed per milliliter per hour. Multiply the values in this figure by 0.65 to conform to the National Bureau of Standards angiotensin I reference standard now adopted by our laboratory and commercial laboratories.

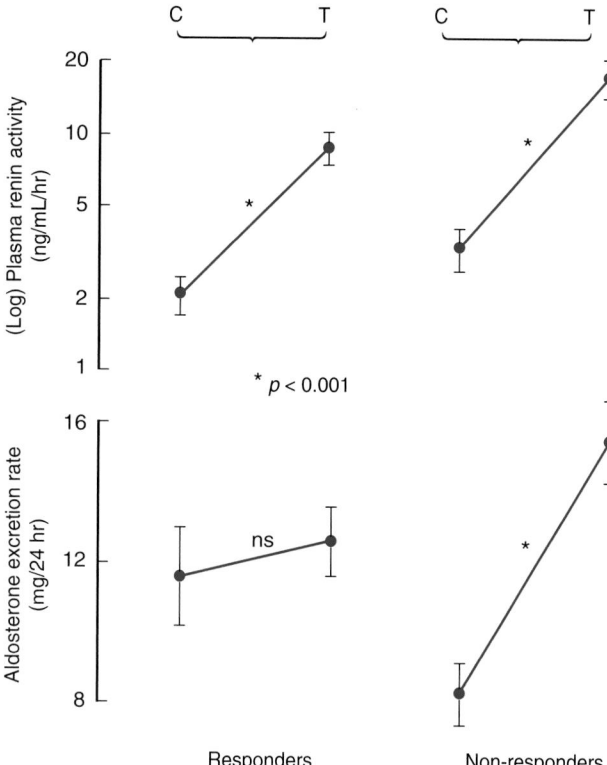

FIGURE 45-12. Relation of blood pressure response and renin system reactivity during antihypertensive treatment with a thiazide-type diuretic. Fifty patients with essential hypertension were treated with chlorthalidone 100 mg/day for 6 weeks and characterized by their blood pressure response (responders = fall in mean pressure ≥10% below pretreatment level; 25 responders, 25 nonresponders). In the responders, the mean pretreatment plasma renin level was lower (2.1 vs. 3.3 ng/mL/hour; $P < .025$) and urine aldosterone was higher (11.6 vs. 8.3 μg/24 hours; $P < .05$) than in nonresponders. During treatment with chlorthalidone, the mean increase in aldosterone was sevenfold higher in the blood pressure nonresponders than in the responders, reflecting the greater rise in plasma renin activity. Changes in body weight, serum K^+, and creatinine were comparable in these groups. These findings suggest that activation of the renin-angiotensin-aldosterone system during diuretic treatment attenuated its antihypertensive efficacy. (From Weber MA, Drayer JI, Rev A, Laragh JH: Disparate patterns of aldosterone response during diuretic treatment of hypertension. Ann Intern Med 87:558-563, 1977.)

surgically curable hypertension or other important medical diseases.

For most hypertensive patients, the pretreatment evaluation is more efficiently accomplished in the office setting. Multiple visits have the advantage of defining the persistence or lability of the hypertensive process. In general, the milder or more labile the hypertension is, the longer the evaluation period will be before commitment to therapy. Except when the hypertension is severe or complications are impending or present, treatment should be withheld throughout the evaluation. For patients already on ineffective therapy, cautious withdrawal of the drugs during the initial evaluation is worthwhile to determine whether the hypertension is persistent or even drug-induced and, in the case of multiple drug therapy, whether all or any of the agents are necessary. Hospitalization is reserved for those patients with severe hypertensive disease, those with impending complications, and those for whom the outpatient data suggest the need for specialized diagnostic procedures.

For some patients receiving relatively simple and well-tolerated therapy, the clinician may decide that the program already in force is adequate and need not be disturbed. However, one should not hesitate to stop medications in those in whom the regimen appears even slightly unsatisfactory or unpalatable. We have observed repeatedly that when hypertension persists in patients receiving multiple drug therapy, the discontinuation of medications gradually and serially usually does not lead to any further rise in BP. Surprisingly often, the BP may actually improve as the medical regimen is simplified. In the Veterans Administration study of severe hypertension (diastolic pressure >110 mm Hg), 15% of those patients in whom all drugs were stopped remained normotensive for the ensuing 18 months of observation.[19] Serial withdrawal of drugs in patients who are poorly controlled with multiple drug therapy puts the physician in the best position for re-evaluating the disease process and setting up new therapeutic strategies.

Goals of the Initial Evaluation

The five major goals of the initial evaluation are to (1) establish whether the hypertension is sustained and might benefit from treatment, (2) define coexisting diseases, (3) characterize other risk factors, (4) identify the presence and extent of target organ damage, and (5) identify or exclude curable causes of the hypertension.

A rational method for selecting drugs for the individual hypertensive patient must be based on an individual pathophysiologic evaluation. The diagnostic workup, aside from the routine complete blood count and urinalysis, includes serum potassium, glucose, blood urea nitrogen, and serum creatinine concentrations; an electrocardiogram (ECG) and baseline echocardiogram for full evaluation of LV mass; and the plasma renin activity level, which is described in the next section.

The first goal of this process is to identify or exclude definable and curable causes of the hypertensive disorder. Doing so may spare many patients a lifetime of needless, costly, and intrusive drug therapy, for often a cure can be accomplished by relatively simple, nonsurgical techniques. Clinical clues that secondary hypertension is present include (1) new onset of hypertension in patients over age 60 years, especially with diastolic BP above 100 mm Hg, (2) BP that is not adequately reduced by multidrug regimen, (3) the presence of diffuse atherosclerotic disease, and (4) hypokalemia while not treated with a diuretic.[246]

The remaining 90% or so of patients, for whom no definable cause for the hypertension can be found but who can be stratified pathophysiologically by the PRA level, are candidates for long-term drug therapy. This statistic assumes, of course, that their hypertension is significant and sustained, is possibly causing target organ damage, and is not responsive to simple nonpharmacologic forms of therapy (weight reduction, exercise, low-salt diet, and alcohol and tobacco withdrawal). For these individuals, the baseline evaluation process informs the selection of the most effective and least counterproductive treatment.

Medical History

Evaluation of the severity and time course of the hypertensive disorder is important to allow planning of the pace of the medical workup and treatment. Normally, the evaluation is accomplished in an unhurried manner during several visits spaced at weekly or biweekly intervals. The initial examination, however, should provide enough information to determine whether the process must be accelerated.

Accordingly, after learning of any current symptoms, one should record the duration of the hypertension, the circumstances of its onset, and the highest known readings. Was the BP elevation merely discovered on routine examination? Has loss of well-being, decline in general vigor, or weight loss occurred? Does the patient have symptoms suggestive of sleep apnea, such as somnolence at work or snoring? Which drugs has the patient tried, and what effect have they produced? Has the patient any agents that may raise BP, such as oral contraceptives, diet pills, antidepressants, cocaine or other illicit drugs, or increased the intake of alcohol?

The neurologic history may disclose headaches. Classically, headaches in hypertensive patients are said to be occipital and pulsatile, most prominent on awakening, and gradually lessening during the day. Possibly, this symptom is no more common in hypertensive patients than in normotensive people. Moreover, studies indicate that when headaches do occur in hypertensive patients, they are not well correlated with the degree of elevation of BP.[247]

Signs and symptoms of autonomic nervous system vasomotor instability seem to be more common among hypertensive patients. These signs include a tendency for flushing, and the patient may report excessive sweating or even a lack of sweating. The symptoms are common side effects of antihypertensive medications, particularly dihydropyridine calcium channel blockers.

Other neurologic symptoms include blurred vision, unsteadiness of gait, depression, insomnia, sluggishness, and in some patients, a decreased libido. Whereas some of these symptoms may be nonspecific, blurred vision may reflect vascular changes in the fundi. More advanced hypertensive disease may also be accompanied by more defined focal sensory or motor neurologic changes, occurring paroxysmally and associated with either transient ischemic attacks or more sustained attacks presaging the onset of hypertensive encephalopathy or stroke. To the extent that these symptoms are related to hypertension, they will improve during successful treatment.

The cardiovascular system may be symptom-free in early or uncomplicated hypertensive disease. Early signs of dysfunction are expressed by palpitations signifying either tachycardia or a forceful heartbeat, by increased fatigability, or by shortness of breath on effort, which probably reflect the increased cardiac work of hypertension or impending heart failure. Young patients with labile pressure or largely systolic hypertension may exhibit tachycardia and signs of an unstable or hyperdynamic circulation. This sort of vasomotor instability can occur in normotensive people. On the other hand, it could at times reflect higher cardiac output and stroke volume, which are described in some patients with early hypertensive disease. Palpitations may also reflect an arrhythmia. Cardiac arrhythmias are more common in hypertensive than in normotensive people, especially in the presence of demonstrable LVH.[248, 249] Because coronary artery disease and MI are more prevalant in hypertensive patients, a history of angina pectoris or documented MI may be elicited. Hypertensive patients with LVH reportedly have a higher mortality rate despite apparent control of BP.

The renal history may reveal antecedent acute glomerulonephritis, proteinuria, hematuria, nocturia, polyuria, or recurrent urinary tract infections. Renal colic or renal trauma should be noted, and the physician should suspect that the hypertension has a renal basis whenever it can be established that the urinary tract symptoms or the proteinuria preceded the hypertension. An abrupt onset of hypertension with rapid progression, especially in young or old patients, should lead the physician to a strong suspicion of renovascular hypertension due to either fibromuscular hyperplasia or an atherosclerotic plaque, respectively. This suspicion is reinforced by retinopathy or by cardiac or renal involvement, all of which are likely to be more prominent in renovascular (renin-dependent) hypertension. Renin-secreting tumors (hemangiopericytoma) of the juxtaglomerular apparatus and Wilms tumor represent rare diseases that are more common in childhood and also may be associated with abrupt and severe hypertension.[250] Polycystic disease is commonly associated with hypertension that is AII-dependent.[251]

Polyuria or nocturia may indicate more severe renal hypertension or a metabolic abnormality such as hypokalemia or hypercalcemia. Inability to concentrate the urine, with polydipsia, polyuria, and nocturia, commonly occurs in patients with primary aldosteronism or malignant hypertension or in chronic renal disorders, including glomerulonephritis, tubulointerstitial nephropathy, or obstructive uropathy. Muscle weakness may accompany hypokalemia or hypercalcemia.

Patients should be asked about their smoking, drinking, exercise, and dietary habits.[5] Obesity can be an important factor in producing or amplifying hypertension.[41] Excessive regular consumption of alcohol can also induce or aggravate hypertension, and in some patients, cessation of the habit may correct the hypertensive process.[252] Tobacco, because it is a known vasoconstrictor, is especially contraindicated in hypertensive subjects, even though no causal relationship between smoking and the development of essential hypertension has been defined.[253] Physical exercise purportedly reduces BP in previously untrained subjects, but more research on this relationship and its claimed benefits is needed.[5] Also, an estimate should be made of the adjustment of the patient to his or her life situation and of any emotional or psychiatric factors that seem relevant. The risk factor analysis is completed by the identification of any target organ damage and of any other coexisting diseases.

Physical Examination
Special Aspects

The general appearance is unrevealing in most patients with hypertension. However, a florid facies—with or without a tendency for rapid color changes, which would suggest vasomotor instability—may signify an underlying metabolic process, perhaps pheochromocytoma, a hyperdynamic circulation, hyperthyroidism, or, alternatively, the anxiety or the vasomotor instability characteristic of some patients with essential hypertension. Chronic alcoholism may also produce some of these signs, and it can also cause hypertension characterized by σ_1-adrenergic activity on withdrawal from alcohol use. A ruddy complexion with a bluish tinge characterizes some patients with essential hypertension and reactive polycythemia (Gaisböck syndrome). High-renin patients with essential hypertension may also present with a dusky appearance associated with vasoconstriction and a higher hematocrit.

Truncal obesity with moon facies, frontal baldness, atrophic extremities with abdominal striae, atrophy of the skin, and spontaneous ecchymoses suggest Cushing syndrome.[254] Multiple neurofibromas or café au lait discoloration of the skin suggests a familial basis for an associated pheochromocytoma. Also, mucosal neuromas may be associated with other components of the syndrome of multiple endocrine neoplasia with hypertension. Renal failure may be expressed by a pale yellowish skin, periorbital and peripheral edema, and uremic breath.

Blood Pressure

In the vast majority of hypertensive patients, elevated BP is the only abnormal finding. Hence, the way in which the BP is measured assumes great importance. The patient should be seated quietly, and a cuff size appropriate to the arm diameter should be chosen. Several readings should be taken, and it is generally recommended that phase 5 of Korotkoff sounds be taken as diastolic pressure. Establishing a diagnosis of hypertension often requires more than one visit, because the pressure tends to fall with repeated measurement. Even after several visits, however, a fairly sizable group of patients show a persistently elevated pressure in the clinic although they are normotensive at other times.[13] This phenomenon, often referred to as "white coat hypertension," can be detected only by including measurements made outside the clinic.[13] These measurements can be obtained by having the patient measure his or her BP at home or by ambulatory monitoring. A knowledge of the patient's BP in these circumstances can be of great value in deciding on the need for treatment and in evaluating its efficacy.

Optic Fundus

Ophthalmoscopic examination of the optic fundi is one of the most valuable clinical tools for assessing target organ damage, the severity and duration of the hypertension, and the urgency for applying treatment. Moreover, patients with retinopathy are more likely to have white matter lesions (WMLs) observed by magnetic resonance imaging than those without retinopathy.[255] The 5-year cumulative incidence of clinical stroke was higher in persons with than without WMLs and in persons with than without retinopathy. Patients with both WMLs and retinopathy had a significantly higher 5-year cumulative incidence of stroke than those without either WMLs or retinopathy (200% vs. 1.4%). Thus, the presence of hypertensive retinopathy has important implications both for acute management and for prognosis.

Heart

In hypertensive disease, the heart is frequently more affected than either the brain or kidneys. Hypertension in adults is a leading cause of cardiac hypertrophy and dilation as well as CHF.

The mechanical effects on the heart of sustained increase of pressure work may be reflected in the physical findings. A forceful apical thrust is common even in early hypertensive disease and may be exaggerated in the so-called hyperdynamic state. In contrast, a sustained, heaving LV pulse indicates significant hypertrophy due to pressure overload. Probably the earliest physical sign of cardiac involvement is the fourth heart sound (S_4), the atrial gallop occasionally heard in normal patients; it is usually audible before cardiac enlargement is detectable, and it is said to reflect a reduced ventricular compliance leading to a more forceful atrial contraction. The fourth heart sound may correlate with the finding of P wave abnormalities on the ECG. The third heart sound, the ventricular gallop, may occur in young subjects with rapid ventricular filling. In older patients, it may be a late manifestation of hypertensive heart disease and reflects the early diastolic compliance abnormality of LV failure.

In severe hypertension, an accentuated aortic second sound may be accompanied by an aortic insufficiency murmur. This soft diastolic murmur may be heard in the second right interspace and along the left sternal border. It suggests dilation of the aortic root and may indicate the need for more urgent therapy. When associated with primary aortic regurgitation disease, hypertension in elderly patients is usually systolic, with a wider pulse pressure. Surgical replacement of the regurgitant aortic valve is usually followed by an increase in diastolic BP. Aortic stenosis in the elderly, usually from calcific valvular disease, is associated with a systolic murmur, a narrow pulse pressure, and a slow carotid upstroke. Diastolic hypertension is rare or mild in this situation.

The syndrome of a hyperkinetic or hyperdynamic circulation may occasionally be encountered in adolescents and young adults with or without hypertension. If present, the hypertension is labile, largely systolic, and accompanied by tachycardia at rest, a forceful apical thrust, and occasional pulsation in the carotid arteries. Whenever this syndrome is encountered, the possibility of metabolic or psychiatric factors should be pursued.

In a younger patient, a harsh systolic murmur over the precordium or midscapular area of the back suggests coarctation of the aorta. This finding should lead the physician to compare the blood pressures in the arms and legs and obtain an echocardiographic examination of the aortic valve, because bicuspid aortic valves commonly occur in association with coarctation of the aorta.

Vascular System

Bruits and thrills, indicative of occlusive disease, are more prevalent in hypertensive patients and may occur throughout the arterial tree. Accordingly, the physician should examine the carotid arteries, abdominal aorta, renal arteries, and femoral arteries. A diastolic component to a bruit or palpable thrill over a peripheral vessel usually suggests a higher-grade stenosis. Systolic bruits without diastolic components tend to be less significant and may have no pathogenic importance when they occur in the abdomen.

A systolic bruit over the carotid artery can be significant. Carotid auscultation should be performed in every patient. The stethoscope is placed over the external carotid in the supraclavicular region as close to the angle of the jaw as possible. Particularly when a precordial bruit is also heard, this approach may help distinguish a transmitted sound from an intrinsic sound.

Bruits can be unilateral or bilateral. They may be audible throughout the cardiac cycle or only during systole. Although bruits are likely to occur with equal frequency in normotensive and hypertensive subjects, they have far graver prognostic significance in the hypertensive person. Although the carotid bruit is a marker for subsequent cardiovascular disease, it does not predict the location of the lesion. Indeed, patients with carotid bruits are more likely to have MI than stroke.

A systolic bruit over the femoral artery suggests atherosclerotic disease but does not necessarily imply occlusion. When pulses in the lower extremities are absent or dampened, coarctation of the aorta should be suspected in a young person, and occlusive aortic femoral disease should be suspected in an older one. The ankle-arm index (AAI = ratio of ankle to arm systolic BP) is a simple, noninvasive, and inexpensive screening test. An AAI value of 0.9 or less has recently been found to be highly predictive of subsequent mortality in several populations, including hemodialysis patients.[256]

Abdomen

The aorta should be palpated carefully in all patients inasmuch as aortic dilation or aneurysm is a highly treatable condition best identified at the initial physical examination. A systolic and diastolic bruit in the upper epigastrium or in one or both upper quadrants of the abdomen suggests renal artery stenosis and should encourage the physician to pursue this diagnosis if other criteria are compatible. A palpable enlargement of one or both kidneys may suggest polycystic renal disease, hydronephrosis, or a renal tumor. Rarely is a pheochromocytoma large enough to be palpable. Purple striae and central obesity are signs of hypercortisolism that should prompt a laboratory evaluation of Cushing syndrome.

Neurologic Examination

Gross neurologic deficits in sensory or motor function, mentation, or mood are not likely to be ignored. More subtle deficits suggesting transient cerebral ischemia or autonomic dysfunction may be overlooked and should be sought clinically, especially when the history is suggestive.

Initial Laboratory Evaluation

The initial laboratory evaluation should include complete blood count and hematocrit together with complete urinalysis; blood urea nitrogen, serum creatinine, serum uric acid, fasting blood glucose, and serum electrolyte measurements; and a lipid profile. If the serum K^+ level is borderline or low (i.e., ≤3.6 mEq/L), the test should be repeated on two or three separate occasions. The serum K^+ concentration serves as a baseline value for the subsequent response to thiazide diuretics and often provides the first laboratory clue to the presence of primary or secondary aldosterone excess. A hemoglobin level is especially relevant in patients with renal disease who are treated with erythropoietin (EPO). Although the hemoglobin level during EPO therapy is generally not closely related to BP, severe hypertension may be more likely to occur when the hemoglobin level rises too rapidly or to excessive levels (see Chapter 58).

With the current widespread use of automated laboratory testing, a variety of other relevant tests may be added at little or no extra cost. Serum Ca^{2+} and circulating thyroid hormone levels may point to parathyroid or thyroid disease, which often exists without clear-cut clinical evidence. Measurement of serum cholesterol, high- and low-density lipoprotein cholesterol, and triglyceride levels are usually offered as part of these automated testing profiles.

When pheochromocytoma is suspected, measurements of catecholamines in plasma or in urine, or in both, and measurement of metanephrines, their urinary metabolites, are essential. The plasma metanephrine level has been reported to be a reliable screening tool because of its high sensitivity and specificity.[257] Cushing syndrome can be screened for by an elevated 24-hour urinary free cortisol level. Urinary aldosterone levels, when combined with measurements of urinary Na^+ and K^+ excretion, are extremely valuable for establishing the diagnosis of primary aldosteronism and other hypertensive situations associated with either low-renin levels or hypokalemia (see earlier discussion). A plasma aldosterone-renin ratio greater than 50 (ng/dL-ng/mL/hour) has been suggested as a simple screening test for this disorder.[215, 258] However, there is some concern that this test may be misleading in patients with low-renin essential hypertension or when it is measured during antihypertensive treatment with agents that affect renin secretion.

Radiography

A chest x-ray examination may be useful as part of every initial workup, particularly in patients older than 50 years. It can reveal a coarctation or aneurysm of the aorta, but is less useful for identifying cardiac hypertrophy. However, other imaging tests (e.g., echocardiography; see below) have largely supplanted its role in the assessment of hypertensive cardiovascular disease.

Electrocardiogram

A routine ECG to identify signs of LVH is highly desirable for all new patients with established high BP. Manifestations of LVH include T wave abnormalities, expressed either by notching or by a biphasic form, particularly in the precordial leads. As LVH progresses, voltage of the R waves increases, and then a characteristic strain pattern involving ST segment depressions and T wave inversion occurs. In addition, approximately 30% of MIs that are evident on ECG are asymptomatic and thus may not be elicited by the history.[1]

Echocardiography

With the advent of echocardiography and its application to the development of highly sensitive methods for examining cardiac structure and function, investigators have been able to study the evolution of cardiac hypertrophy in hypertensive patients with greater precision than before[52] (see "Left Ventricular Hypertrophy"). The possible linkage between cardiac and hormonal heterogeneity in hypertensive diseases may also provide a basis for understanding differences in the effectiveness of various antihypertensive drugs in reversing LVH.

Ambulatory and Home Blood Pressure Monitoring

Ambulatory BP monitoring (ABPM), whereby multiple indirect BP readings are obtained automatically over 1 or more days, is being used to investigate BP patterns in normal individuals and in hypertensive patients. Studies of normotensive subjects show that BP is characterized by a circadian rhythm with peaks during the daytime hours. Blood pressure can also vary with work, activity, emotion, and possibly by race and age.[176, 259, 260]

The cost of ABPM and the reimbursement for this test by third-party payers are important issues. A National Institutes of Health working group report stated that charges for ambulatory BP monitoring by physicians and by scanning services range from $100 to $300, but exceptions have been reported as high as $500.[261] The initial cost of two monitors and related equipment is approximately $12,000 to $15,000. The predominant expense is the long-term cost of antihypertensive medication. If ABPM use successfully identifies patients who have "office" or white coat hypertension, but otherwise have normal BP, and thus may not require medication, then the cost-benefit ratio should be favorable. Medicare and other health insurance providers will cover the cost of ABPM for the diagnosis of white coat hypertension.

Home BP monitoring is used increasingly in the evaluation and treatment of patients with hypertension. Although BP readings are generally higher in the medical office setting, these measurements do not correlate as well as home readings to the presence of abnormal markers for cardiovascular risk (e.g., LVH[14]). Home BP monitors are relatively inexpensive and simple to use. Although they are generally accurate, the patient's technique and the precision and reproducibility of the measurements should be validated during an office visit by the clinician.

Identifying Curable Forms of Hypertension
Renovascular Disease

As pointed out earlier in this chapter, and in Chapter 46, curable and definable forms of hypertension should be identified before long-term drug therapy is contemplated. Rarer causes of chronic hypertension aside, the baseline evaluation has much to offer in detecting the presence or absence of kidney disease, including such surgically curable forms of hypertension as renovascular hypertension, primary aldosteronism, coarctation of the aorta, pheochromocytoma, and Cushing syndrome.

The PRA level, which is either medium or increased in renovascular disease and suppressed in primary aldosteronism, is a valuable primary screen in this endeavor (see earlier discussion). It is no more expensive or complicated than other commonly performed tests (e.g., thyroid and cholesterol), and it is potentially far more relevant, not only because it can enable the absolute diagnosis of curable hypertensive disorders but also because it can be used for physiologic evaluation and treatment planning.

The renin-sodium nomogram, developed by plotting PRA against the 24-hour urinary Na^+ level, provides correction for the fact that renin, as a regulatory hormone, rises normally in response to a low-salt diet and declines in response to a high-salt diet (see Fig. 45-9). As with most laboratory tests, the PRA level is most powerful when its deviations from normal are great. Low or high values lead one to suspect, respectively, adrenocortical or curable renovascular disease. Indeed, the baseline plasma renin and serum K^+ measurements are the essential tools for the exclusion or diagnosis of these types of hypertension. The test originally involved the collection of a 24-hour urine specimen for Na^+ measurement and a venous blood sample for renin measurement that is collected while the patient is seated quietly in the office. However, for expedience, the 24-hour urine collection is not required, unless marked salt depletion is suspected either because of dietary sodium restriction or concurrent illness or medication use.

The matter of excluding curable hypertension has a special meaning and urgency because the possibilities of cure of renovascular disease have multiplied dramatically with the widespread use of screening tests (e.g., captopril test[262]), and the availability of percutaneous transluminal renal angioplasty and renal artery stent placement (see later). At New York–Presbyterian Hospital, balloon dilation has been successfully employed. Approximately two thirds of those patients with normal renal function are able to stop taking drugs completely or have improved BP with antihypertensive medications. If not for today's advanced testing protocols, a large proportion of these patients would be on a lifetime regimen of drugs and would be incorrectly thought to have essential hypertension.

Any untreated hypertensive patient with an ambulatory plasma renin value greater than 1.6 ng/mL/hour is a candidate for further evaluation of unilateral renal artery stenosis. A study of 52 consecutive patients showed no patient with proven unilateral renal disease whose renin level was less than that value.[262] However, renin levels can be lower in azotemic patients with hemodynamically significant bilateral renal artery stenosis because of the impaired Na^+ excretion and volume expansion. This is especially relevant considering the emerging evidence that 15% of the ESRD population may have ischemic nephropathy, due to stenosis of the main renal arteries, as the basis for their progressive azotemia.[65, 66] Proteinuria may occasionally be pronounced in such patients, particularly when one renal artery is totally occluded (see Chapter 46). Therefore, any patient with an abnormal serum creatinine value, regardless of plasma renin values, may also be a candidate for evaluation, especially if there is no other basis for the azotemia.

In patients with plasma renin values greater than 1.6 ng/mL/hour, with a normal serum creatinine concentration, the captopril test is informative in the evaluation of suspected unilateral renovascular hypertension. This test, performed in untreated patients, is based on the remarkable specificity of captopril to inhibit the formation of AII while stimulating a reactive increase in renin secretion from the ischemic kidney. Patients who are Na^+-depleted, because of either a low-salt diet or a diuretic, are ineligible for the test because they start with high renin levels and may show a false-positive increase.[262] To identify such patients, we routinely measure a 24-hour urine sodium and have the patient bring the sample on the day of the captopril test (Table 45-5).

In this test, the patient is seated quietly for 45 minutes and then a blood sample for renin is drawn. A single dose of 25 mg of captopril is then given orally to the quietly seated patient. The patients remains quietly seated and BP is

TABLE 45-5

How to Do a Captopril Test

1. Maintain the patient on normal salt intake; give no diuretics.
2. If possible, withdraw all antihypertensive medications 3 wk before the test.
3. Allow the patient to sit quietly for at least 30 min.
4. Measure blood pressure at 20, 25, and 30 min (average the three readings to obtain baseline reading).
5. Draw a venous blood sample for measurement of baseline renin activity.
6. Administer 25 mg captopril, orally.
7. Measure blood pressure 15, 30, 45, and 60 min after administration of captopril.
8. At 60 min draw a second venous blood sample for measurement of stimulated plasma renin activity.

From Laragh JH: Issues and goals in the selection of first-line drug therapy for hypertension. Hypertension 13(suppl 1):103, 1989.

measured at 10- to 15-minute intervals and a second blood sample for renin is drawn 1 hour after the captopril dose. Captopril is rapidly absorbed, blocking the renin system within 1 hour. Patients with renovascular hypertension react to this blockade with an unusually vigorous rise in renin secretion from the ischemic kidney, whereas those hypertensive patients without renal artery obstruction show little or no plasma renin response.

Table 45-5 lists the procedures for performing the captopril test. *The 60-minute plasma renin response, rather than the BP response, is the discriminator for the diagnosis of renovascular hypertension.* The following criteria are suggestive of the presence of unilateral renal artery stenosis: (1) stimulated PRA 7.8 ng/mL/hour or more by 60 minutes, (2) absolute increase in PRA of 6.5 ng/mL/hour or more, and (3) percent increase in PRA of 150% or more, or 400% or more if the baseline PRA is less than of equal to 1.3 ng/mL/hour.[262] Although a substantial BP decline usually accompanies the marked rise in plasma renin level, this finding is not altogether a reliable indicator of renin dependency or of renovascular hypertension because other transient defenses of the BP level may operate acutely.[262]

A positive captopril test strongly suggests the possibility of renovascular disease. In a series comparing 56 patients with proven renovascular disease with 112 patients with essential hypertension, the captopril test was found to be both highly sensitive and specific for renin-dependent hypertension related to renal artery stenosis. Furthermore, it is perhaps the best screening test for unilateral renovascular disease because it is safe, inexpensive, easy to perform, and avoids the problem of disposal of radiopharmaceutical agents. Although some false-positive results are inevitable, false-negative results are uncommon.

A positive captopril test result does not discriminate between unilateral and bilateral kidney disease, nor does it discriminate between a parenchymal and arteriolar lesion. In patients with a positive captopril test, these questions can be definitively resolved by digital subtraction angiography and by renal vein renin sampling during captopril stimulation. In typical unilateral renovascular disease, renin is secreted from only one kidney; a simple arithmetic analysis of the concentration of renin in each renal vein can be used to identify the renin-secreting kidney and assess its degree of ischemia. At the same time, the peripheral blood level of renin reflects the secretion rate of renin from that kidney.[263]

Primary Aldosteronism

Primary aldosteronism is characterized typically by the following diagnostic triad: (1) serum K^+ level less than 3.5 mEq/L; with urinary K^+ excretion greater than 40 mEq/day; (2) PRA is markedly suppressed—plasma renin levels are typically less than 0.65 ng/mL/hour, but occasionally are as high as 1.0 ng/mL/hour; and (3) elevated 24-hour urinary or plasma aldosterone levels. Because potassium is a major secretagogue of aldosterone, and body potassium is depleted in primary aldosteronism, aldosterone values may not be very high. Therefore, aldosterone levels should be measured after oral potassium supplementation.

If hormonal evidence of primary aldosteronism is found, then physiologic studies to assess the autonomy of aldosterone secretion should be performed. These include measurements of aldosterone during a postural stimulation test and during dietary sodium loading or acute infusion of saline. If these tests are positive, then adrenal vein sampling should be performed to determine whether aldosterone secretion lateralizes. For the following reasons, computed tomography (CT) or other imaging studies should be done *after* measurements of hormone levels confirm the diagnosis of primary aldosteronism: (1) nonfunctioning adenomas are commonly discovered by CT scan, (2) curable forms occur in patients without a distinct adenoma, even when the adrenal glands appear normal, and (3) a dominant adrenal nodule, in a diffusely hyperplastic gland, may appear to be a solitary adenoma.

For those not meeting these criteria, the plasma renin test remains useful as an indicator of (1) the presence and degree of renin-related vasoconstriction for values above 0.65, and (2) the sodium-volume factor for values below 0.65 ng/mL/hour.[238] The PRA is also a determinant of the likelihood or unlikelihood of subsequent cardiac and vascular sequelae. Finally, the PRA simplifies and hastens the drug selection process and the finding of the best single drug or combination for the long term.

Drug Therapy for Essential Hypertension

After performing the initial evaluation, in which the diagnosis of secondary forms of hypertension has been excluded, the clinician is then faced with the treatment of essential hypertension. A relatively small proportion of patients will have a significant response to nonpharmacologic interventions, such as dietary sodium restriction, weight loss, reduction in alcohol intake, and increased exercise.[37, 39, 264] However, pharmacologic treatment will be required in the vast majority of patients with essential hypertension, even in those with initial improvement during nonpharmacologic intervention.

The drug treatment of the hypertensive patient is a complex decision-making process.[265] It is complicated by the fact that there are many pharmacologically distinct drug classes available and that hypertensive patients are not all alike mechanistically so that individual hypertensive patients respond quite differently to the various types of antihypertensive drugs. There are eight major categories of antihypertensive agents: diuretics, specific aldosterone receptor blockers, calcium channel blockers, α-blockers, β-blockers, ACE inhibitors, A_1 receptor blockers, and centrally acting α-agonists (see Chapter 55). The problem of which drug to choose for a particular patient is further complicated by the fact that many different products are available within each class, drugs which are often claimed by their maker to differ importantly from other products in the same class. Such marketing claims can be confusing to physicians and patients. These issues are compounded because the selection of drugs is increasingly limited by contractual agreements between the health insurance and pharmaceutical industries.

The drug selection process is simplified when considering that the basic determinants of BP include sodium-volume and renin-angiotensin vasoconstriction. The plasma renin test, measured in the seated patient, reliably defines the presence and the degree of either the sodium-volume or the renin-vasoconstrictor factor in untreated patients or in those receiving antihypertensive drugs. The renin test is, therefore, central to pathophysiologically based treatment. Thus, hypertensive patients are characterized by the following:

- PRA levels of less than 0.65 ng/mL/hour with predominantly *sodium-volume*–mediated hypertension, or
- PRA levels greater than or equal to 0.65 ng/mL/hour with predominantly plasma *renin-angiotensin*–mediated *vasoconstrictor* hypertension.

The antihypertensive drug classes are divided into two major categories:

1. Drugs that reduce BP because of primary or secondary actions to reduce body sodium and volume content by enhancing renal Na^+ excretion (V drugs).
2. Drugs that lower BP by reducing or blocking the activity of the renin-angiotensin system (R drugs).

A basic principle guiding this approach is that a higher BP per se normally (i.e., in normotensive subjects) suppresses PRA levels so that any hypertensive patient whose PRA is *not* suppressed (≥0.65 ng/mL/hour) has inappropriate amounts of renin in the blood and therefore has a form of hypertension that, at least partly, is renin-dependent. By contrast, hypertensive patients who *do* have suppressed PRA levels (PRA <0.65) have a primarily sodium-volume–dependent hypertension.[265]

Because plasma renin-angiotensin is vasculotoxic for the hypertensive patient, contributing to the pathogenesis of MI, CHF, stroke, and progressive renal failure, drugs that block the renin system (R drugs) should be the initial choice for treatment of those hypertensive patients who do not have suppressed PRA levels. The R drugs include ACE inhibitors, AT receptor blockers, and β-adrenergic receptor blockers.[265]

Those patients with PRA of less than 0.65 ng/mL/hour are treated with an anti–sodium-volume drug (V drug). The V drugs include diuretics, α-adrenergic receptor blockers, and calcium channel blockers.

The Newly Diagnosed or Untreated Hypertensive Patient

The evaluation and treatment process comprises a series of patient visits (Fig. 45-13). At *visit 1* the BP is measured and blood is collected to measure the PRA. At *visit 2* the BP is measured again to confirm that the patient is truly hypertensive and the result of the PRA test is evaluated. If the PRA is greater than or equal to 0.65 ng/mL/hour, the patient is placed into the renin-vasoconstriction–dependent (R) hypertension category. If the PRA is less than 0.65 ng/mL/hour, the patient is placed in the sodium-volume–dependent (V) hypertension category.

RENIN-DEPENDENT HYPERTENSION. A patient in the R category at *visit 2* will be started on a low-dose R drug. At *visit 3* the BP will be measured. If the BP is not controlled, the dose of the R drug will be increased. At *visit 4* if the BP is still not controlled, a V drug will be added to the treatment regimen to reduce the sodium-volume component of the BP. At *visit 5* if the BP is not yet controlled, the V drug dosage will be increased and blood will be drawn to check the PRA level during treatment. At *visit 6*, if the BP is not controlled, the PRA level from visit 5 will determine the change in the treatment regimen. If the PRA level was less than 0.65 ng/mL/hour at visit 5, the R drug will be discontinued at visit 6 and a second V drug added. If the PRA level was between 0.65 and 6.5 ng/mL/hour at visit 5, a second R drug will be added at visit 6 to more effectively block the renin-angiotensin system. If the PRA level was above 6.5 ng/mL/hour, the V drug is discontinued to reduce the reactive rise in renin induced by most V drugs and a second R drug is added.

SODIUM-VOLUME–DEPENDENT HYPERTENSION. A patient in the V category will start on a low-dose V drug. At *visit 3*, about 3 weeks later, the patient will have his or her BP tested again. If the BP is not controlled, the dose of the V drug will be increased. At *visit 4*, if the BP is still not controlled, an R drug will be added to the treatment regimen, based on the rationale that the patient has both a volume and a renin component to the hypertension. At *visit 5*, if the BP is still not controlled, the R drug dosage will be increased and blood will be drawn to check the PRA levels. At *visit 6*, if the BP is still not controlled, the PRA level collected at visit 5 will be used to determine the change in the treatment regimen. If the PRA level remains below 0.65 ng/mL/hour, the R drug will be discontinued and a second V drug added. If the PRA level is between 0.65 and 6.5 ng/mL/hour, a second R drug will be added to block the effects of the reactive rise in plasma renin. If the PRA level is above 6.5 ng/mL/hour, the V drug will be discontinued to eliminate its stimulatory effect on renin secretion and a second R drug will be added.

Patients with Persistent Hypertension despite Drug Treatment

This section provides an approach to antihypertensive drug selection for the patient who presents initially with persistent hypertension despite ongoing drug treatment (Fig. 45-14).

Visit 1 involves measuring the BP and drawing blood to test PRA levels. The appropriate action to take during *visit 2* depends on the current treatment regimen and the PRA level.[265]

PATIENT ON A V DRUG WITH PERSISTENT HYPERTENSION. If the PRA level is below 0.65 ng/mL/hour, the dose of the drug should be increased to a maximum level as long as the PRA remains below 0.65 ng/mL/hour. In such a patient the sodium-volume factor is still operative and contributing to the hypertensive state. As a renin factor is unlikely to be present in any patient with a low renin level, a patient on any V drug who remains hypertensive with a PRA

PROTOCOL I: USING PLASMA RENIN ACTIVITY (PRA) TO GUIDE TREATMENT OF NEW OR UNTREATED HYPERTENSIVE PATIENTS

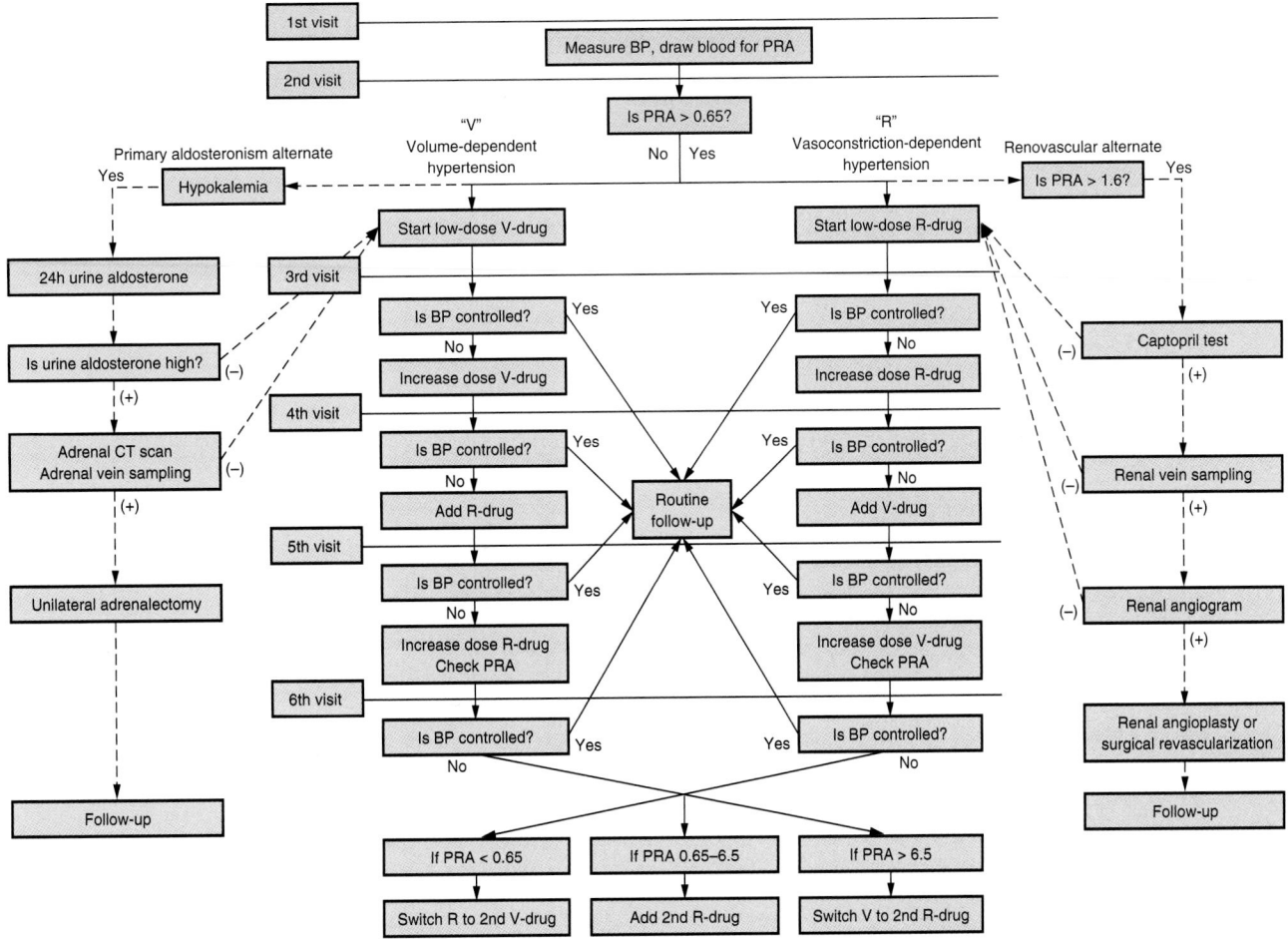

FIGURE 45-13. Diagnosis and treatment of hypertension in the previously untreated patient. The peripheral paths (*gray/dotted lines*) show the alternative decision trees to assess potentially curable forms of hypertension, including renovascular hypertension and primary aldosteronism. See text. (From Laragh J: Laragh's lessons in pathophysiology and clinical pearls for treating hypertension. Lesson XVI: How to choose the correct drug treatment for each hypertensive patient using a plasma renin–based method and the volume-vasoconstriction analysis. Am J Hypertens 14:491-503, 2001.)

level of less than 0.65 ng/mL/hour is unlikely to respond to any R drug. Therefore, if a full dose of a V drug has already been tested, and assuming good compliance, a V drug with a different mechanism of action should then be added (e.g., diuretic added to an α-blocker or calcium channel blocker).

If the PRA level of the V drug–treated patient is between 0.65 and 6.5 ng/mL/hour, an R drug is added to block both volume and vasoconstrictor factors. If the PRA level is above 6.5 ng/mL/hour, the V drug is discontinued and the patient is switched to an R drug to eliminate the confounding renin-stimulatory effect of the V drug.

PATIENT ON AN R DRUG WITH PERSISTENT HYPERTENSION. If the PRA level is below 0.65 ng/mL/hour, then the patient should be changed to a V drug because the low renin level indicates that there is no apparent renin-mediated vasoconstriction. However, if the PRA level is between 0.65 and 6.5 ng/mL/ hour, the dose of the R drug should be maximized. A patient who is unsuccessfully treated with a full dose of any R drug should then have a V drug added as long as PRA is less than 6.5 ng/mL/hour. Finally, if the PRA is above 6.5 ng/mL/hour, a V drug is unlikely to be effective

and a second R drug is added to more effectively block the renin system.

Although the three classes of R drugs all block the renin-angiotensin system, they have different sites of action and may be additive in increasing inhibition of the renin system. Thus, at the recommended maximal therapeutic doses, neither ACE inhibitors nor AT receptor blockers are completely blocking the renin system and a reactive rise in renin secretion may overcome or attenuate the effectiveness of these agents. β-Blockers suppress adrenergically mediated renin release, and can enhance the antihypertensive efficacy of ACE inhibitors and AT receptor blockers.

PATIENT ON MULTIPLE DRUGS WITH PERSISTENT HYPERTENSION. A PRA test on the first visit is extremely helpful for the patient on multiple drugs because it can reveal which mechanism predominates. Thus, PRA values of less than 0.65 ng/mL/hour clearly indicate that sodium-volume excess is present. In this case, the R drug should be stopped and a second V drug added. Conversely, if the PRA is between 0.65 and 6.5 ng/mL/hour, the antirenin limb of treatment needs to be strengthened by the addition of a

PROTOCOL II: USING PLASMA RENIN ACTIVITY (PRA) TO GUIDE TREATMENT OF UNSUCCESSFULLY TREATED PATIENTS
(PATIENT ASSUMED TO BE ON FULL DOSE OF EACH DRUG)

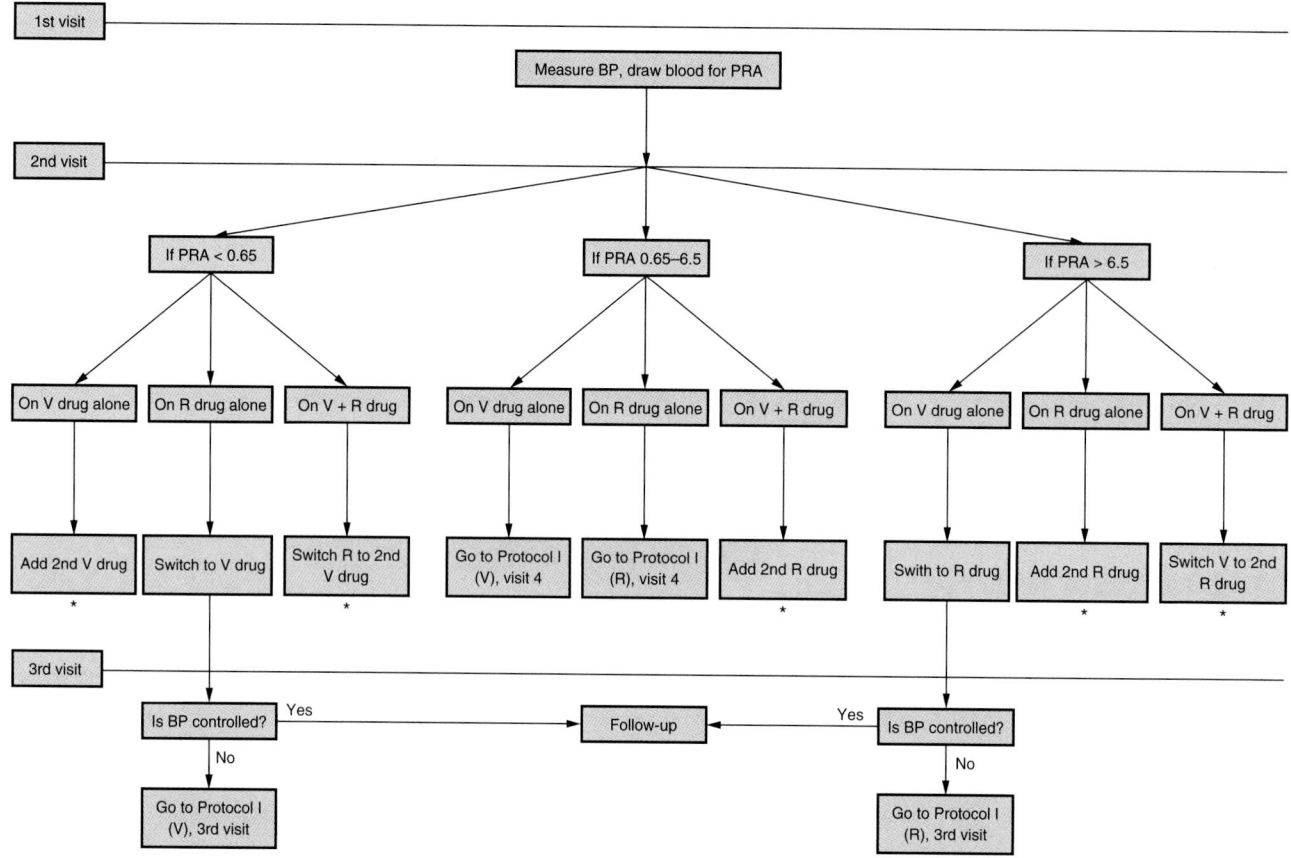

*In exceptionally difficult cases a 3rd V or a 3rd R drug may be necessary, but only if the PRA remains suppressed (<0.65 V) or markedly elevated (>6.5 R)

FIGURE 45-14. Selection of antihypertensive medication in the unsuccessfully treated patients with hypertension. See text. (From Laragh J: Laragh's lessons in pathophysiology and clinical pearls for treating hypertension. Lesson XVI: How to choose the correct drug treatment for each hypertensive patient using a plasma renin–based method and the volume-vasoconstriction analysis. Am J Hypertens 14:491-503, 2001.)

second R drug. Above 6.5 ng/mL/hour, the V drug should be stopped because it may be inducing excessive renin secretion. A second R drug can be added, if necessary.

Our experience using such a protocol at New York–Presbyterian Hospital indicates that about 25% of hypertensive patients will be controlled after the third visit, and that 90% or more will be adequately controlled after the sixth visit. Moreover, in patients referred to us on a multiple drug regimen, we can usually reduce the number of medications.[266]

Other strategies are more widely used for the selection of antihypertensive drug treatment. These approaches vary, but employ an empirical approach that may include in the decision process the patient's age, race, or presence of comorbid conditions (e.g., prostatism) that are unrelated to the pathophysiology of their hypertensive disease and that do not identify a specific marker for vasoconstriction.[5, 267] An interesting alternative approach has been reported in which there is crossover rotation of representatives from each of the main classes of antihypertensive drugs. Although only 39% of patients achieved the target BP (≤140/90 mm Hg) with their first drug, 73% ultimately reached this goal with monotherapy after rotation to another drug class.[28] Moreover, in that crossover study, there were significant correlations between

the BP responses to drugs that block the renin system (ACE inhibitor and β-blocker; $r = .5$; $P < .0001$) and drugs that are active in low-renin hypertension (calcium channel blocker and diuretic; $r = .6$; $P < .01$), but not between the other four pairings of treatments. The marked variability in the efficacy of drug treatment in essential hypertension described in this study, together with the concordance of BP responses found in this study and by the renin-based approach to drug selection (see earlier discussion), highlight the heterogeneity of the pathogenesis and its relevance to the heterogeneity of essential hypertension.

Recapitulation and Summary

Hypertension afflicts 20% or more of the adult population of the world, depending on the arbitrary cutoffs used to define hypertension and normotension. About 90% of hypertension is classified, after exclusion of the known and curable causes (usually kidney or adrenal disorders), as essential hypertension. Historically, adult BP levels of 140/90 mm Hg or above were widely used to define the presence of hypertension. This threshold has recently been lowered with the recognition of other genetic, biologic, and behavioral factors, including age, sex, cigarette use, hypercholesterolemia, diabetes, and, more recently, elevated PRA level.[1, 60]

Clinical trials of diuretic-based stepped-care regimens, in which drugs are added sequentially until the BP is subdued, have established the feasibility and reasonable safety of long-term oral drug regimens. Significant protection has been shown for stroke but, unfortunately, less so for cardiac events (e.g., MI), the latter comprising 80% or so of the added risk burden of being hypertensive. Despite the generally favorable outcomes demonstrated in randomized controlled treatment trials, fewer than half of all patients in the general population have their BP controlled with current drug treatment strategies.[2] Altogether, only about one fourth of all hypertensive patients in the United States, or in other industrialized societies, have their BP controlled.

A serious limitation of the clinical trials to date is that their design and analyses have assumed that all essential hypertension is alike and is a single process amenable to a single-drug treatment recipe. Unfortunately, this is not the case. Essential hypertension is heterogeneous in its hormonal and biochemical patterns and in its prognosis. Thus, clinicians have long known that many patients live a normal life span without cardiac or cerebral sequelae, whereas others, sometimes with lesser elevations in BP, die prematurely of a cardiac event or stroke. Furthermore, practicing physicians are well aware of gross differences in individual responses to the six major drug classes (diuretics, α-blockers, calcium channel antagonists, AII receptor blockers, ACE inhibitors, and β-blockers). Each of these drug types, when randomly selected as monotherapy, will correct hypertension in about 40% to 45% of patients; but for each drug class, *different* subpopulations will respond. Thus, about the same percentage of patients will respond to either diuretic monotherapy or β-blocker monotherapy. However, an individual patient's BP often does not respond to all drugs. When both agents are given concurrently, their effects summate and the combination controls BP in 80% or so of patients. This has prompted the recommendation that initial therapy should include two-drug therapy rather than the goal of achieving for every patient the "best-fit" strategy of using the fewest number of drugs in the lowest amount and frequency. Accordingly, future large-scale clinical trials are not likely to improve our understanding of hypertension and its treatment unless every patient is given a prototype of every drug class and then classified as a nonresponder or responder to each prototype drug studied.

Pressure natriuresis, the increase in urinary excretion of Na^+ and water that occurs when arterial pressure increases, is a predominant mechanism that normally allows the kidney to regulate BP homeostasis. The renin-angiotensin-aldosterone system plays a key role in this feedback control system by its direct effects on peripheral vascular resistance (AII) and volume regulation (AII and aldosterone). Blood pressure elevation occurs when this pressure-natriuresis mechanism is disrupted, for example, by excess activation of the renin system, reduction in renal mass, or impaired regulation of renal blood flow.

Measurement of PRA provides a useful method for understanding the pathophysiology of hypertension in the individual patient. When plasma renin is not suppressed (PRA <0.65 ng/mL/hour), renin-angiotensin is likely to be important in the pathophysiology and thus BP will decrease when treated with drugs that interrupt the renin system (i.e., AT receptor blocker, ACE inhibitor, β-adrenergic receptor blocker). By contrast, when PRA is suppressed (PRA <0.65 ng/mL/hour), then renin-angiotensin is less likely to be a major factor. In the latter case, hypertension is more likely to be sodium-volume–dependent and is more responsive to a diuretic, calcium channel blocker, or α-adrenergic receptor blocker. This strategy is further supported by the observations that, in the hypertensive patient, an elevated PRA level confers increased risk of MI and, when LVH is present, AT receptor blockade decreases the risk of stroke.

In summary, essential hypertension is a heterogeneous disorder that is associated with various hormonal and biochemical abnormalities that have a direct bearing on the individual patient's responsiveness to targeted antihypertensive medications and on the patient's risk of cardiovascular disease, stroke, and renal failure.

REFERENCES

1. Kannel WB, Wilson PWF: Hypertension, other risk factors, and the risk of cardiovascular disease. *In* Laragh JH, Brenner BM (eds): Hypertension: Pathophysiology, Diagnosis and Management, 2nd ed. New York, Raven Press, 1995, pp 99-114.
2. Burt VL, Whelton P, Roccella EJ, et al: Prevalence of hypertension in the U.S. population: Results from the Third National Health and Nutrition Examination Survey, 1988-1991. Hypertension 25:305-314, 1995.
3. Barondess J: The future of generalism. Ann Intern Med 119:153-260, 1993.
4. Collins R, Peto R, MacMahon S, et al: Blood pressure, stroke, and coronary heart disease. Part 2, Short-term reductions in blood pressure: Overview of randomised drug trials in their epidemiological context [see comments]. Lancet 335:827-838, 1990.
5. Joint National Committee on Prevention, Evaluation, and Treatment of High Blood Pressure. The sixth report of the Joint National Committee on Prevention, Detection, Evaluation and Treatment of High Blood Pressure. Arch Intern Med 157:2413-2446, 1997.
6. Siegel D, Lopez J: Trends in antihypertensive drug use in the United States: Do the JNC V recommendations affect prescribing? JAMA 278:1745-1748, 1997.
7. Lenfant C: Reflections on hypertension control rates: A message from the director of the National Heart, Lung, and Blood Institute. Arch Intern Med 162:131-132, 2002.
8. Riva-Rocci S: Un nuovo sfigmomanometro. Gaz Med Torino 47:981, 1896.
9. Korotkov N: A contribution to the problem of methods for the determination of the blood pressure. Izv Imperatorskoi Voen Med Akad 11:365, 1905.
10. Pickering G: High Blood Pressure. London, JA Churchill, 1968.
11. Port S, Demer L, Jennrich R, et al: Systolic blood pressure and mortality. Lancet 355:175-180, 2000.
12. Alderman M: Measures and meaning of blood pressure. Lancet 355:159, 2000.
13. Pickering T: White coat hypertension. Curr Opin Nephrol Hypertens 5:192-198, 1996.
14. Mancia G, Parati G: Ambulatory blood pressure monitoring and organ damage. Hypertension 36:894-900, 2000.
15. Yarows S, Julius S, Pickering T: Home blood pressure monitoring. Arch Intern Med 160:1251-1257, 2000.
16. Blood Pressure Study. New York, Actuarial Society of America and Association of Life Insurance Medical Directors. 1925.
17. Society of Acturaries: Build and Blood Pressure Study. Chicago, Society of Actuaries, 1959.
18. Lew E: Hypertension and longevity. *In* Laragh JH, Brenner BM (eds): Hypertension: Pathophysiology, Diagnosis, and Management. New York, Raven Press, 1990, pp 175-190.
19. Veterans Administration Cooperative Study Group on Antihypertensive Agents: Effects of treatment on morbidity in hypertension. JAMA 202:1028-1034, 1967.

20. Veterans Administration Cooperative Study Group on Antihypertensive Agents: Effects of treatment on morbidity in hypertension. JAMA 213:1143-1152, 1970.

21. Kannel WB: Blood pressure as a cardiovascular risk factor: Prevention and treatment. JAMA 275:1571-1576, 1996.

22. Alderman MH: Blood pressure management: Individualized treatment based on absolute risk and the potential for benefit. Ann Intern Med 119:329-335, 1993.

23. Luc M, Bortel V, Struijker-Boudier H, Safar M: Pulse pressure, arterial stiffness, and drug treatment of hypertension. Hypertension 38:914-921, 2001.

24. O'Rourke M: Mechanical principles in arterial disease. Hypertension 26:2-9, 1995.

25. Volhard E, Fahr T: Die Brightsche Nierenkrankheit Klinik: Pathologie und Altas. Berlin, Springer-Verlag, 1914.

26. Laragh JH, Ulick S, Januszewicz V, et al: Electrolyte metabolism and aldosterone secretion in benign and malignant hypertension. Ann Intern Med 53:259-272, 1960.

27. Materson B, Reda D, Cushman W, et al: Single drug therapy for hypertension in men: A comparison of six antihypertensive agents with placebo. N Engl J Med 328:914-921, 1993.

28. Dickerson JE, Hingorani AD, Ashby MJ, et al: Optimisation of anti-hypertensive treatment by crossover rotation of four major classes. Lancet 353:2008-2013, 1999.

29. Franklin SS, Khan SA, Wong ND, et al: Is pulse pressure useful in predicting risk for coronary heart disease? The Framingham Heart Study. Circulation 100:354-360, 1999.

30. Vasan RS, Beiser A, Seshadri S, et al: Residual lifetime risk for developing hypertension in middle-aged women and men: The Framingham Heart Study. JAMA 287:1003-1010, 2002.

31. Intersalt Cooperative Research Group: Intersalt: An International study of electrolyte excretion and blood pressure. Results for 24 hour urinary sodium and potassium excretion. Intersalt Cooperative Research Group. BMJ 297:319-328, 1988.

32. Laragh JH, Pecker MS: Dietary sodium and essential hypertension: Some myths, hopes, and truths. Ann Intern Med 98(5 pt 2):735-743, 1983.

33. Waldron I, Nowotarski M, Freimer M, et al: Cross-cultural variation in blood pressure: A quantitative analysis of the relationships of blood pressure to cultural characteristics, salt consumption and body weight. Soc Sci Med 16:419-430, 1982.

34. Chrysant SG, Weir MR, Weder AB, et al: There are no racial, age sex, or weight differences in the effect of salt on blood pressure in salt-sensitive hypertensive patients. Arch Intern Med 157:2489-2494, 1997.

35. Alderman MH, Cohen H, Madhavan S: Dietary sodium intake and mortality: The National Health and Nutrition Examiantion Survey (NHANES I). Lancet 351:781-785, 1998.

36. Hinderliter A, Sherwood A, Gullette EC, et al: Reduction of left ventricular hypertrophy after exercise and weight loss in overweight patients with mild hypertension. Arch Intern Med 162:1333-1339, 2002.

37. Alderman MH, Madhavan S, Cohen H, et al: Low urinary sodium is associated with greater risk of myocardial infarction among treated hypertensive men [see comments]. Hypertension 25:1144-1152, 1995.

38. Sacks FM, Svetkey LP, Vollmer WM, et al: Effects on blood pressure of reduced dietary sodium and the Dietary Approaches to Stop Hypertension (DASH) diet. DASH-sodium Collaborative Research Group. N Engl J Med 344:3-10, 2001.

39. Vollmer WM, Sacks FM, Ard J, et al: Effects of diet and sodium intake on blood pressure: Subgroup analysis of the DASH-sodium trial. Ann Intern Med 135:1019-1028, 2001.

40. Huang Z, Willett WC, Manson JE, et al: Body weight, weight change, and risk for hypertension in women. Ann Intern Med 128:81-88, 1998.

41. Whelton PK, Appel LJ, Espeland MA, et al: Sodium reduction and weight loss in the treatment of hypertension in older persons: A randomized controlled trial of nonpharmacologic interventions in the elderly (TONE). TONE Collaborative Research Group. JAMA 279:839-846, 1998.

42. Writing Group of the PREMIER Collaborative Reserch Group: Effects of comprehensive lifestyle modification on blood pressure control: Main results of the PREMIER clinical trial. JAMA 289:2083-2093, 2003.

42a. Pickering TG: Lifestyle modification and blood pressure control: Is the glass half full or half empty? JAMA 289:2131-2132, 2003.

43. ALLHAT Officers and Coordinators for the ALLHAT Collaborative Research Group: Major outcomes in high-risk hypertensive patients randomized to angiotensin-converting enzyme inhibitor or calcium channel blocker vs. diuretic: The Antihypertensive and Lipid-Lowering Treatment to Prevent Heart Attack Trial (ALLHAT). JAMA 288:2981-2997, 2002.

43a. Webber M: Results of the ALLHAT trial: Is the debate about initial antihypertensive drug therapy over? J Clin Hypertens 5:5-8, 2003.

43b. Wing LMH, Reid CM, Ryan P, et al: A comparison of outcomes with angiotensin-converting enzyme inhibitors and diuretics for hypertension in the elderly. N Engl J Med 348:583-592, 2003.

44. Medical Research Council Working Party: MRC trial of treatment of mild hypertension: Principal results. Medical Research Council Working Party. BMJ (Clin Res Ed) 291:97-104, 1985.

45. Siscovick DS, Raghunathan TE, Psaty BM, et al: Diuretic therapy for hypertension and the risk of primary cardiac arrest. N Engl J Med 330:1852-1857, 1994.

46. Madhavan S, Alderman MH: The potential effect of blood pressure reduction on cardiovascular disease. A cautionary note. Arch Intern Med 141:1583-1586, 1981.

47. Lloyd-Jones DM, Evans JC, Larson MG, et al: Cross-classification of JNC VI blood pressure stages and risk groups in the Framingham Heart Study. Arch Intern Med 159:2206-2212, 1999.

48. Lew E: High blood pressure, other risk factors and longevity: The insurance viewpoint. In Laragh JH (ed): Hypertension Manual. New York, Yorke Medical Books, 1974.

49. Young T, Peppard P, Palta M, et al: Population-based study of sleep-disordered breathing as a risk factor for hypertension. Arch Intern Med 157:1746-1752, 1997.

50. Franklin SS: Blood pressure and cardiovascular disease: What remains to be achieved? J Hypertens 19(suppl 3):S3-S8, 2000.

51. Hansson L: The J-shaped curve and how far blood pressure should be lowered. In Laragh JH, Brenner BM, (eds): Hypertension: Pathophysiology, Diagnosis and Management, 2nd ed. New York, Raven Press, 1995, pp 2765-2770.

52. Devereux R, Roman M: Hypertensive cardic hypertrophy: Pathophysiology and clinical characteristics. In Laragh JH, Brenner BM (eds): Hypertension: Pathophysiology, Diagnosis and Management, 2nd ed. New York, Raven Press, 1995, pp 1969-1986.

53. Koren MJ, Devereux RB, Casale PN, et al: Relation of left ventricular mass and geometry to morbidity and mortality in uncomplicated essential hypertension. Ann Intern Med 114:345-352, 1991.

54. Mosterd A, D'Agostina RB, Silbershatz H, et al: Trends in the prevalence of hypertension, antihypertensive therapy, and left ventricular hypertrophy from 1950 to 1989. N Engl J Med 340:1221-1227, 1999.

55. Brunner HR, Laragh JH, Bear L, et al: Essential hypertension: Renin and aldosterone, heart attack and stroke. N Engl J Med 286:441-449, 1972.

56. Yusuf S, Sleight P, Pogue J, et al: Effects of an angiotensin-converting-enzyme inhibitor, ramipril, on cardiovascular events in high-risk patients. The Heart Outcomes Prevention Evaluation Study Investigators. N Engl J Med 342:145-153, 2000.

57. Gavras H, Brown JJ, Lever AF, et al: Acute renal failure, tubular necrosis, and myocardial infarction induced in the rabbit by intravenous angiotensin II. Lancet 2:19-22, 1971.

58. Pfeffer MS, Braunwald E, Moye LA, et al: Effect of captopril on mortality and morbidity in patients with left ventricular dysfunction after myocardial infarction. Results of the Survival and Ventricular Enlargement Trial. N Engl J Med 327:669-677, 1992.

59. Pitt B, Segal R, Martinez FA, Meurers G, et al: Randomized trial of losartan versus captopril in patients over 65 with heart failure (Evaluation of Losartan in the Elderly Study, ELITE). Lancet 349:747-752, 1997.

60. Alderman MH, Madhavan S, Ooi WL, et al: Association of the renin-sodium profile with the risk of myocardial infarction in patients with hypertension [see comments]. N Engl J Med 324:1098-1104, 1991.

61. Blumenfeld JD, Sealey JE, Alderman MH, et al: Plasma renin activity in the emergency department and its independent association with acute myocardial infarction. Am J Hypertens 13:855-863, 2000.

62. Phillips S, Whisnant J: Hypertension and stroke. In Laragh JH, Brenner BM (eds): Hypertension: Pathophysiology, Diagnosis and Management, 2nd ed. New York, Raven Press, 1995, pp 465-478.

63. Levy D, Larson MG, Vasan RS, et al: The progression from hypertension to congestive heart failure. JAMA 275:1557-1562, 1996.

64. USRDS Coordinating Center: United States Renal Data Survey 2000, Annual Data Report. 2000.

65. Mailloux LU, Napolitano B Bellucci, AG: Renal vascular disease causing end-stage renal disease, incidence, clinical correlates and outcomes: A 20-year clinical experience. Am J Kidney Dis 24:662-669, 1994.

66. Scoble JE, Maher ER, Hamilton G, et al: Atherosclerotic renovascular disease causing renal impairment—a case for treatment. Clin Nephrol 31:119-122, 1989.

67. Klag MJ, Whelton PK, Randall BL, et al: Blood pressure and end-stage renal disease in men. N Engl J Med 334:13-18, 1996.

68. Maschio G, Alberti D, Janin G, et al: Effect of the angiotensin-converting-enzyme inhibitor benazepril on the progression of chronic renal insufficiency. The Angiotensin-Converting-Enzyme Inhibition in Progressive Renal Insufficiency Study Group. N Engl J Med 334:939-945, 1996.

69. Lewis EJ, Hunsicker LG, Bain RP, Rohde RD: The effect of angiotensin-converting-enzyme inhibition on diabetic nephropathy. The Collaborative Study Group. N Engl J Med 329:1456-1462, 1993.

70. Brenner BM, Cooper ME, de Zeeuw D, et al: Effects of losartan on renal and cardiovascular outcomes in patients with type 2 diabetes and nephropathy. N Engl J Med 345:861-869, 2001.

71. Lewis EJ, Hunsicker LG, Clarke WR, et al: Renoprotective effect of the angiotensin-receptor antagonist irbesartan in patients with nephropathy due to type 2 diabetes. N Engl J Med 345:851-860, 2001.

72. Yudkin JS, Forrest RD, Jackson CA: Microalbuminuria as predictor of vascular disease in non-diabetic subjects. Islington Diabetes Survey. Lancet 2:530-533, 1988.

73. Schmieder RE, Martus P, Klingbeil A: Reversal of left ventricular hypertrophy in essential hypertension. A meta-analysis of randomized double-blind studies. JAMA 275:1507-1513, 1996.

74. Wachtell K, Olsen MH, Dahlof B, et al: Microalbuminuria in hypertensive patients with electrocardiographic left ventricular hypertrophy: The LIFE study. J Hypertens 20:405-412, 2002.

75. Crippa G: Microalbuminuria in essential hypertension. J Hum Hypertens 16(suppl 1):S74-S77, 2002.

76. Erley CM, Haefele U, Heyne N, et al: Microalbuminuria in essential hypertension. Reduction by different antihypertensive drugs. Hypertension 21(6 pt 1): 810-815, 1993.

77. Mancia G, Sega R, Milesi C, et al: Blood-pressure control in the hypertensive population. Lancet 349:454-457, 1997.

78. Rizzo J: Economics of patient non-compliance—looking at the real world. Cardiol Rev 13:21-26, 1996.

79. Berlowitz DR, Ash AS, Hickey EC, et al: Inadequate management of blood pressure in a hypertensive population. N Engl J Med 339:1957-1963, 1998.

80. Perera G: Hypertensive vascular disease. J Chronic Dis 1:33, 1955.

81. Smith WM: Treatment of mild hypertension: Results of a ten-year intervention trial. Circ Res 40(5 suppl 1): I98-I105, 1977.

82. Hypertension Detection and Follow-up Program Cooperative Group: I. Reduction of mortality in persons with high blood pressure, including hypertension. II Mortality by race, sex, and age. JAMA 242:2562, 1979.

83. Kaplan N: Kaplan's Clinical Hypertension, 8th ed. Philadelphia, Lippincott Williams & Wilkins, 2002.

84. Psaty BM, Smith NL, Siscovick DS, et al: Health outcomes associated with antihypertensive therapies used as first-line agents. A systematic review and meta-analysis. JAMA 277:739-745, 1997.

85. Weber MA, Drayer JI, Rev A, Laragh JH: Disparate patterns of aldosterone response during diuretic treatment of hypertension. Ann Intern Med 87:558-563, 1977.

86. Staessen JA, Gasowski J, Wang JG, et al: Risks of untreated and treated isolated systolic hypertension in the elderly: Meta-analysis of outcome trials. Lancet 355:865-872, 2000.

87. Roman MJ, Alderman MH, Pickering TG, et al: Differential effects of angiotensin converting enzyme inhibition and diuretic therapy on reductions in ambulatory blood pressure, left ventricular mass, and vascular hypertrophy. Am J Hypertens 11(4 pt 1):387-396, 1998.

88. Mathew J, Sleight P, Lonn E, et al: Reduction of cardiovascular risk by regression of electrocardiographic markers of left ventricular hypertrophy by the angiotensin converting enzyme inhibitor ramipril. Circulation 104:1615-1621, 2001.

89. Dahlof B, Devereux RB, Kjeldsen SE, et al: Cardiovascular morbidity and mortality in the Losartan Intervention for Endponit Reduction in Hypertension Study (LIFE): A randomised trial against atenolol. Lancet 359:995-1003, 2002.

90. Devereux RB, Palmieri V, Liu JE, et al: Progressive hypertrophy regression with sustained pressure reduction in hypertension: The Losartan Intervention for Endpoint Reduction Study. J Hypertens 20:1445-1450, 2002.

91. Garg R, Yusuf S: Overview of randomized trials of angiotensin-converting enzyme inhibitors on mortality and morbidity in patients with heart failure. JAMA 273:1450-1456, 1995.

92. Cohn JN, Tognoni G: A randomized trial of the angiotensin-receptor blocker valsartan in chronic heart failure. N Engl J Med 345: 1667-1675, 2001.

93. Swedberg K, Eneroth P, Kjekshus J, Wilhelmsen L: Hormones regulating cardiovascular function in patients with severe congestive heart failure and their relation to mortality. Circulation 82:1730-1736, 1990.

94. ALLHAT: Major cardiovascular events in hypertensive patients randomized to doxazosin vs chlorthalidone: The Antihypertensive and Lipid-Lowering Treatment to Prevent Heart Attack Trial (ALLHAT). ALLHAT Collaborative Research Group. JAMA 283:1967-1975, 2000.

95. Liebson P, Grandits G, Dianzumba S, et al: Comparison of five antihypertensive monotherapies and placebo for change in left ventricular mass in patients receiving nutritional-hygienic therapy in the Treatment of Mild Hypertension Study (TOMHS). Circulation 91:698-706, 1995.

96. Cohn J, Archibald D, Zieche S, et al: Effect of vasodilartor therapy on mortality in congestive heart failure: Results of a Veterans Administration Cooperative Study. N Engl J Med 314:1547-1552, 1986.

97. Kostis J, Davis B, Cutler J, et al: Prevention of heart failure by antihypertensive drug treatment in older persons with isolated systolic hypertension. JAMA 278:212-216, 1997.

98. Wallace J, Levy LL: Blood pressure after stroke. JAMA 246: 2177-2180, 1981.

99. Brott N, Lu M, Kothari R, et al: Hypertension and its treatment in the NINDS rt-PA stroke trial. Stroke 29:1504-1509, 1998.

100. Powers W: Acute hypertension after stroke: The scientific basis for treatment decisions. Neurology 43:461-467, 1993.

101. Strandgaard S: Autoregulation of cerebral blood flow in hypertensive patients. The modifying influence of prolonged antihypertensive treatment on the tolerance to acute, drug-induced hypotension. Circulation 53:720-727, 1976.

102. Calhoun D, Oparil S: Treatment of hypertensive crisis. N Engl J Med 323:1177-1183, 1990.

103. Blumenfeld JD, Laragh JH: Management of hypertensive crises: The scientific basis for treatment decisions. Am J Hypertens 14 (11 pt 1):1154-1167, 2001.

104. Fisher M, Bogousslavsky J: Further evolution toward effective therapy for acute ischemic stroke. JAMA 279:1298-1303, 1998.

105. Grossman E, Messerli FH, Grodzicki T, Kowey P: Should a moratorium be placed on sublingual niedipine capsules given for hypertenive emergencies and pseudoemergencies? [see comments]. JAMA 276:1328-1331, 1996.

106. Feigin V, Rinkel G, Algra A, et al: Calcium antagonists in patients with aneursymal subarachnoid hemorrhage: A systematic review. Neurology 50:876-883, 1998.

107. Radhakrishnan C, Menon D: Haemodynamic effects of intravenous nimodipine following aneurysmal subarachnois hemorrhage: Implications for monitoring. Anaesthesia 52:489-491, 1997.

108. Porchet F, Chiolero R, de Tribolet N: Hypertensive effect of nimodipine during treatment for aneurysmal subarachnoid hemorrhage. Acta Neurochir (Wien) 137:62-69, 1995.

109. Hayashi M, Kobayashi H, Kawano H, et al: Treatment of systemic hypertension and intracranial hypertension in cases of brain hemorrhage. Stroke 19:314-321, 1988.

110. Haley EJ, Kassell N, Torner J: A randomized controlled trial of high-dose intravenous nicardipine in aneurysmal subarachnoid hemorrhage: A report of the Cooperative Aneurysm Study. J Neurosurg 78: 537-547, 1993.

111. Voko V, Bots M, Hofman A, et al: J-shaped relation between blood pressure and stroke in treated hypertension. Hypertension 34:1181-1185, 1999.

112. Hansson L, Zanchetti A, Carruthers SG, et al: Effects of intensive blood-pressure lowering and low-dose aspirin in patients with hypertension: Principal results of the Hypertension Optimal Treatment (HOT) randomised trial. HOT Study Group. Lancet 351:1755-1762, 1998.

113. Adler AI, Stratton IM, Neil HA, et al: Association of systolic blood pressure with macrovascular and microvascular complications of type 2 diabetes (UKPDS 36): Prospective observational study. BMJ 321:412-419, 2000.

114. SHEP Cooperative Research Group: Prevention of stroke by antihypertensive drug treatment in older persons with isolated systolic hypertension. Final results of the Systolic Hypertension in the Elderly Program (SHEP). SHEP Cooperative Research Group. JAMA 265:3255-3264, 1991.

115. Staessen JA, Fagard R, Thijs L, et al: Randomized double-blind comparison of placebo and active treatment for older patients with isolated systolic hypertension. The Systolic Hypertension in Europe (Syst-Eur) Trial Investigators. Lancet 350:757-764, 1997.

116. Guyton A, Hall J, Coleman T, et al: The dominant role of the kidneys in long-term arterial pressure regulation in normal and hypertensive states. *In* Laragh JH, Brenner BM (eds): Hypertension: Pathophysiology, Diagnosis, and Management, 2nd ed. New York, Raven Press, 1995, pp 1311-1326.

117. Laragh JH, Sealey JE: Renin-angiotensin-aldosterone system and the renal regulation of sodium, potassium, and blood pressure homeostasis. *In* Windhager EE (ed): Handbook of Physiology. Renal Physiology. New York, Oxford University Press, 1992, pp 1409-1541.

118. Cowley AW Jr, Roman RJ: The role of the kidney in hypertension. JAMA 275:1581-1589, 1996.

119. Roman RJ, Cowley AW Jr, Garcia-Estan J, Lombard JH: Pressure-diuresis in volume-expanded rats. Cortical and medullary hemodynamics. Hypertension 12:168-176, 1988.

120. Thames MD, DiBona GF: Renal nerves modulate the secretion of renin mediated by nonneural mechanisms. Circ Res 44:645-652, 1979.

121. Osborn JL, Thames MD, DiBona GF: Renal nerves modulate renin secretion during autoregulation. Proc Soc Exp Biol Med 169:432-437, 1982.

122. Osborn J, DiBona G, Thames M: Beta-1 receptor mediation of renin secretion elicited by low-frequency renal nerve stimulation. J Pharmacol Exp Ther 216:265-269, 1981.

123. DiBona GF: Peripheral and central interactions between the renin-angiotensin system and the renal sympathetic nerves in control of renal function. Ann N Y Acad Sci 940:395-406, 2001.

124. Sealey JE, Laragh JH: The renin-angiotensin-aldosterone system for the normal regulation of blood pressure and sodium and potassium homeostatsis. *In* Laragh JH, Brenner BM (eds): Hypertension: Pathophysiology, Diagnosis, and Management, 2nd ed. New York, Raven Press, 1995, pp 1763-1797.

125. Cogan MG: Angiotensin II: A powerful controller of sodium transport in the early proximal tubule. Hypertension 15:451-458, 1990.

126. Ghose RP, Hall PM, Bravo EL: Medical management of aldosterone-producing adenomas. Ann Intern Med 131:105-108, 1999.

127. Morganti A, Lopez-Ovejero JA, Pickering TG, Laragh JH: Role of the sympathetic nervous system in mediating the renin response to head-up tilt. Their possible synergism in defending blood pressure against postural changes during sodium deprivation. Am J Cardiol 43:600-604, 1979.

128. Goodfriend TL, Elliott ME, Catt KJ: Angiotensin receptors and their antagonists. N Engl J Med 334:1649-1654, 1996.

129. Moore AF, Heiderstadt NT, Huang E, et al: Selective inhibition of the renal angiotensin type 2 receptor increases blood pressure in conscious rats. Hypertension 37:1285-1291, 2001.

130. Carey RM, Wang ZQ, Siragy HM: Role of the angiotensin type 2 receptor in the regulation of blood pressure and renal function. Hypertension 35(1 pt 2):155-163, 2000.

131. Haynes WG, Noon JP, Walker BR, Webb DJ: Inhibition of nitric oxide synthesis increases blood pressure in healthy humans. J Hypertens 11:1375-1380, 1993.

132. Krum H, Viskoper RJ, Lacourciere Y, et al: The effect of an endothelin-receptor antagonist, bosentan, on blood pressure in patients with essential hypertension. Bosentan Hypertension Investigators. N Engl J Med 338:784-790, 1998.

133. Herizi A, Jover B, Bouriquet N, Mimran A: Prevention of the cardiovascular and renal effects of angiotensin II by endothelin blockade. Hypertension 31:10-14, 1998.

134. Bright R: Reports of Medical Cases. Selected with a View of Illustrating the Symptoms and Cure of Diseases by a Reference to Morbid Anatomy. London, Longman, Rees, 1827.

135. Tigerstedt R, Bergman P: Niere und Kreislauf, Scand Arch Physiol 8:223, 1898.

136. Goldblatt H, Lynch R, Hanzai R: Studies on experimental hypertension: Production of persistent elevation of systolic blood pressure by means of renal ischemia. J Exp Med 59:347, 1934.

137. Laragh J, Angers M, Kelley W, Lieberman S: Hypotensive agents and pressor substances: The effect of norepinephrine, angiotensin II, and others on the secretory rate of aldosterone in man. JAMA 174:234, 1960.

138. Ames R, Borkowski A, Sicinski A, Laragh J: Prolonged infusions of angiotensin II and norepinephrine and blood pressure, electrolyte balance, aldosterone, and cortisol secretion in normal man and in cirrhosis with ascites. J Clin Invest 44:1171, 1965.

139. Cowley AW Jr, Guyton AC: Baroreceptor reflex effects on transient and steady-state hemodynamics of salt-loading hypertension in dogs. Circ Res 36:536-546, 1975.

140. Guidi E, Menghetti D, Milani S, et al: Hypertension may be transplanted with the kidney in humans: A long-term historical prospective follow-up of recipients grafted with kidneys coming form donors with or without hypertension in their families. J Am Soc Nephrol 7:1131-1138, 1996.

141. Chabanel A, Chien S: Blood viscosity as a factor in human hypertension. *In* Laragh JH, Brenner BM (eds): Hypertension: Pathophysiology, Diagnosis, and Management, 2nd ed. New York, Raven Press, 1995, pp 365-376.

142. Sommers S, Relman A, Smithwick R: Histologic studies of kidney biopsy specimens from patients with hypertension. Am J Pathol 34:685, 1958.

143. Sommers S, McLaughlin R, McAuley R: Pathology of diastolic hypertension as a generalized vascular disease. J Cardiol 9:653, 1962.

144. Sommers S: Hypertension and kidney disease. Prog Cardiovasc Dis 8:210, 1965.

145. Bradley S: Physiology of essential hypertension. Am J Med 4:398, 1948.

146. Hollenberg NK, Adams DF, Solomon H, et al: Renal vascular tone in essential and secondary hypertension: Hemodymanic and angiographic responses to vasdilators. Medicine (Baltimore) 54:29-44, 1975.

147. Bradley S, Bradley G, Tyson C: Renal function in renal diseases. Am J Med 9:766, 1950.

148. Nickel J, Lawrence P, Leifer E, Bradley S: Renal function, electrolyte excretion and body fluids in patients with chronic renal insufficiency before and after sodium depletion. J Clin Invest 32:68, 1953.

149. Mulvaney M: Structural changes in the resistance vessels in human hypertension. *In* Laragh JH, Brenner BM (eds): Hypertension: Pathophysiology, Diagnosis, and Management, 2nd ed. New York, Raven Press, 1995, pp 503-513.

150. Sealey JE, Blumenfeld JD, Bell GM, et al: On the renal basis for essential hypertension: Nephron heterogeneity with discordant renin secretion and sodium excretion causing a hypertensive vasoconstriction-volume relationship. J Hypertens 6:763-777, 1988.

151. Nerrelund H, Choristensen KL, Samani NJ, et al: Early narrowed afferent arteriole is a contributor to the development of hypertension. Hypertension 24:301-308, 1994.

152. Mulvany MJ: Effects of angiotension converting enzyme inhibition on vascular remodelling of resistance vessels in hypertensive patients. J Hypertens Suppl 14:S21-S24, 1996.

153. Mitchell KD, Navar LG: Enhanced tubuloglomerular feedback during peritubular infusions of angiotensins I and II. Am J Physiol 255(3 pt 2):F383-F390, 1988.

154. Skott O, Briggs JP: Direct demonstration of macula densa–mediated renin secretion. Science 237:1618-1620, 1987.

155. Luft F, Grim C, Willis L, et al: Natriuretic response to saline infusion in normotensive and hypertensive man: The role of renin suppression in exaggerated natriuresis. Circulation 55:779-784, 1977.

156. Olsen ME, Hall JE, Montani JP, et al: Mechanisms of angiotensin II natriuresis and antinatriuresis. Am J Physiol 249(2 pt 2):F299-F307, 1985.

157. Olsen ME, Hall JE, Montaini JP, Guyton AC: Angiotensin II natriuresis and anti-natriuresis: Role of renal artery pressure in anaesthetized dogs. J Hypertens Suppl 2:S347-S350, 1984.

158. Cowley AW Jr, Mattson DL, Lu S, Roman RJ: The renal medulla and hypertension. Hypertension 25(4 pt 2):663-673, 1995.

159. Szentivanyi M Jr, Maeda CY, Cowley AW Jr: Local renal medullary L-NAME infusion enhances the effect of long-term angiotensin II treatment. Hypertension 33(1pt 2):440-445, 1999.

160. Madrid MI, Garcia-Salom M, Tornel J, et al: Interactions between nitric oxide and angiotensin II on renal cortical and papillary blood flow. Hypertension 30:1175-1182, 1997.

161. Szentivanyi M Jr, Park F, Maeda CY, Cowley AW Jr: Nitric oxide in the renal medulla protects from vasopressin-induced hypertension. Hypertension 35:740-745, 2000.

162. Makino A, Skelton MM, Zou AP, et al: Increased renal medullary oxidative stress produces hypertension. Hypertension 39(2 pt 2): 667-672, 2002.

163. Lacy F, Kailasam MT, O'Connor DT, et al: Plasma hydrogen peroxide production in human essential hypertension: Role of heredity, gender, and ethnicity. Hypertension 36:878-884, 2000.

164. Folkow B: Psychosocial and central nervous influences in primary hypertension. Circulation 76(1 pt 2):I10-I19, 1987.

165. Henry JP, Liu J, Meehan W: Psychosocial stress and experimental hypertension. *In* Laragh JH, Brenner BM (eds): Hypertension: Pathophysiology, Diagnosis, and Management, 2nd ed. New York, Raven Press, 1995, pp 905-922.

166. Heymans C, Neil E: Reflexogenic Areas of the Cardiovascular System. Boston, Little, Brown and Co, 1958.

167. Dock W, Shidler E, Moy B: The vasomotor center essential in maintaining renal hypertension. Am Heart J 23:513, 1942.

168. McCubbin J, Green J, Page IH: Baroreceptor function in chronic renal hypertension. Circ Res 4:205, 1956.

169. Nathan M, Reis D: Chronic labile hypertension produced by lesions of the nucleus tractus solitarius in the cat. Circ Res 40:72, 1977.

170. Carey RM, Dacey RG, Jane JA, et al: Production of sustained hypertension by lesions in the nucleus tractus solitarii of the American foxhound. Hypertension 1:246-254, 1979.

171. Johnson RJ, Gordon KL, Suga S, et al: Renal injury and salt-sensitive hypertension after exposure to catecholamines. Hypertension 34:151-159, 1999.

172. Johnson RJ, Herrera-Acosta J, Schreiner GF, Rodriguez-Iturbe B: Subtle acquired renal injury as a mechanism of salt-sensitive hypertension. N Engl J Med 346:913-923, 2002.

173. Oparil S, Chen Y-F, Berecek K: The role of the central nervous system in hypertension. *In* Laragh JH, Brenner BM (eds): Hypertension: Pathophysiology, Diagnosis, and Treatment, 2nd ed. New York, Raven Press, 1995, pp 713-740.

174. Kopin I (ed): The Sympathetic Nervous System and Hypertension. New York, Springer-Verlag, 1981.

175. Pickering TG, Harshfield GA, Kleinert HD, et al: Blood pressure during normal daily activities, sleep, and exercise. Comparison of values in normal and hypertensive subjects. JAMA 247:992-996, 1982.

176. Julius S: Hemodynamic, pharmacologic and epidemiologic evidence for behavioral factors in human hypertension. *In* Julius S, Bassett, DR (eds): Behavioral Factors in Hypertension. Amsterdam, Elsevier, 1987.

177. O'Rourke MF, Kelly RP: Wave reflection in the systemic circulation and its implications in ventricular function. J Hypertens 11:327-337, 1993.

178. Kannel WB: Hypertension and the risk of cardiovascular disease. *In* Laragh JH, Brenner BM (eds): Hypertension: Pathophysiology, Diagnosis, and Management. New York, Raven Press, 1995.

179. Ledingham JG, Bull MB, Laragh JH: The meaning of aldosteronism in hypertensive disease. Circ Res 21(suppl 2):177, 1967.

180. Laragh J, Sealey JE, Sommers S: Patterns of adrenal secretion and urinary excretion of aldosterone and plasma renin activity in normal and hypertensive subjects. Circ Res 18(suppl 1):158, 1966.

181. Plouin PF, Chatellier G, Rougeot MA, et al: Plasma renin activity in phaeochromocytoma: Effects of beta-blockade and converting enzyme inhibition. J Hypertens 6:579-585, 1988.

182. Pickering TG, Herman L, Devereux RB, et al: Recurrent pulmonary oedema in hypertension due to bilateral renal artery stenosis: Treatment by angioplasty or surgical revascularisation. Lancet 2:551-552, 1988.

183. Laragh J: The role of aldosterone in man: Evidence for regulation of electrolyte balance and arterial pressure by a renal-adrenal system

184. Laragh J, Ulick S, Januszewicz V: Aldosterone secretion and primary and malignant hypertension. J Clin Invest 39:1091, 1960.

185. Vaughan C, Dealnty N: Hypertensive emergencies. Lancet 356: 411-417, 2000.

186. Masson G, Kashii C, Matsunaga M, Page I: Hypertensive vascular disease induced by heterologous renin. Circ Res 18:219, 1966.

187. Laragh JH, Baer L, Brunner HR, et al: Renin, angiotensin and aldosterone system in pathogenesis and management of hypertensive vascular disease. Am J Med 52:633–652, 1972.

188. Laragh J: The meaning of plasma renin measurements: Renin and sodium volume-medicated (low renin) forms of vasoconstriction in experimental and human hypertension and in the oedematous states of nephrosis and heart failure. J Hypertens 2(suppl 1):141, 1984.

189. Buhler FR, Laragh JH, Baer L, et al: Propranolol inhibition of renin secretion. A specific approach to diagnosis and treatment of renin-dependent hypertensive disease. N Engl J Med 287:1209-1214, 1972.

190. Case DB, Atlas SA, Laragh JH, et al: Clinical experience with blockade of the renin-angiotensin-aldosterone system by an oral converting-enzyme inhibitor (SQ 14,225, captopril) in hypertensive patients. Prog Cardiovasc Dis 21:195-206, 1978.

191. Laragh JH, Case DB, Atlas SA, Sealey JE: Captopril compared with other antirenin system agents in hypertensive patients: Its triphasic effects on blood pressure and its use to identify and treat the renin factor. Hypertension 2:586-593, 1980.

192. Lopez-Ovejero JA, Saal SD, D'Angelo WA, et al: Reversal of vascular and renal crises of scleroderma by oral angiotensin-converting-enzyme blockade. N Engl J Med 300:1417-1419, 1979.

193. Laragh JH: The classification and treatment of essential hypertension using the renin-sodium index for vasoconstriction-volume analysis. Bull Johns Hopkins Hosp 137:184-194, 1975.

194. Pickering TG, Sos TA, Vaughan ED Jr, et al: Predictive value and changes of renin secretion in hypertensive patients with unilateral renovascular disease undergoing successful renal angioplasty. Am J Med 76:398-404, 1984.

195. Pickering TG, Sos TA, James GD, et al: Comparison of renal vein renin activity in hypertensive patients with stenosis of one or both renal arteries. J Hypertens Suppl 33:S291-S293, 1985.

196. Sealey JE, Buhler FR, Laragh JH, Vaughan ED Jr: The physiology of renin secretion in essential hypertension. Estimation of renin secretion rate and renal plasma flow from peripheral and renal vein renin levels. Am J Med 55:391-401, 1973.

197. Tobian L, Coffee K, McCrea P: Contrasting exchangeable sodium in rats with different types of Goldblatt hypertension. Am J Physiol 217:458-460, 1969.

198. Brunner HR, Kirshman JD, Sealey JE, Laragh JH: Hypertension of renal origin: Evidence for two different mechanisms. Science 174:1344-1346, 1971.

199. Gavras H, Brunner HB, Vaughan ED, Laragh JH: Angiotension-sodium interaction in blood pressure maintenance of renal hypertensive and normotensive rats. Science 180:1369-1371, 1973.

200. Hricik DE, Browning PJ, Kapelman R, et al: Captopril-induced functional renal insufficiency in patients with bilateral renal-artery stenoses or renal-artery stenosis in a solitary kidney. N Engl J Med 308:373, 1983.

201. Baer L, Sommers SC, Krakoff LR, et al: Pseudo-primary aldosteronism. An entity distinct from true primary aldosteronism. Circ Res 271(1 suppl 1): 203-220, 1970.

202. Erne P, Bolli P, Bertel O, et al: Factors influencing the hypotensive effects of calcium antagonists. Hypertension 5(4 pt 2):II97-II102, 1983.

203. Resnick LM, Laragh JH, Sealey JE, Alderman MH: Divalent cations in essential hypertension. Relations between serum ionized calcium, magnesium, and plasma renin activity. N Engl J Med 309:888-891, 1983.

204. Resnick LM, Nicholson JP, Laragh JH: Alterations in calcium metabolism mediate dietary salt sensitivity in essential hypertension. Trans Assoc Am Physicians 98:313-321, 1985.

205. van Zweiten P, van Meel J, Timmermans P: Pharmacology of calcium entry blockers' interaction with vascular alpha-adrenoceptors. Hypertension 5(suppl 2):8, 1983.

206. Bolli P, Awann F, Buhler FR: Acute hypotensive response to post-synaptic alpha-blockade with prazosin in low and normal

renin hypertension. J Cardiovasc Pharmacol 2(suppl 3):S399-S405, 1980.

207. Nicholson JP, Resnick LM, Pickering TG, et al: Relationship of blood pressure response and the renin-angiotensin system to first-dose prazosin. Am J Med 78:241-244, 1985.

208. Nicholson JP, Resnick LM, Laragh JH: The antihypertensive effect of verapamil at extremes of dietary sodium intake. Ann Intern Med 107:329-334, 1987.

209. Wilcox CS, Welch WJ, Murad F, et al: Nitric oxide synthase in macula densa regulates glomerular capillary pressure. Proc Natl Acad Sci U S A 89:11993-11997, 1992.

210. Tolins JP, Shultz PJ: Endogenous nitric oxide synthesis determines sensitivity to the pressor effect of salt. Kidney Int 46:230-236, 1994.

211. Lifton RP, Gharavi AG, Geller DS: Molecular mechanisms of human hypertension. Cell 104:545-556, 2001.

212. Conn J, Knopf R, Nesbit R: Clinical characteristics of primary aldosteronism from an analysis of 145 cases. Am J Surg 107:157, 1964.

213. Biglieri E, Forsham P: Studies on the expanded extracellular fluid and the responses to various stimuli in primary aldosteronism. Am J Med 34:564, 1961.

214. Conn J: Plasma renin activity in primary aldosteronism. JAMA 190:222, 1964.

215. Blumenfeld JD, Sealey JE, Schlussel Y, et al: Diagnosis and treatment of primary hyperaldosteronism [see comments]. Ann Intern Med 121:877-885, 1994.

216. Fontes R, Kater C, Biglieri E, Irony I: Reassessment of the predictive value of the postural stimulation test in primary aldosteronsim. Am J Hypertens 4:786-791, 1991.

217. Biglieri E, Lopez J: Clinical and laboratory diagnosis of adenocortical hypertension. Cardiovasc Med 1:335, 1976.

218. Ulick S, Blumenfeld J, Atlas S, et al: The unique steroidogenesis of the aldosteronoma in the differential diagnosis of primary aldosteronism. J Clin Endocrinol Metab 76:873-878, 1992.

219. Streeten DH, Anderson GH Jr, Wagner S: Effect of age on response of secondary hypertension to specific treatment. Am J Hypertens 3(5 pt 1):360-365, 1990.

220. Shimkets RA, Warnock DG, Bositis CM, et al: Liddle's syndrome: Heritable human hypertension caused by mutations in the beta subunit of the epithelial sodium channel. Cell 79:407-414, 1994.

221. Snyder PM: The epithelial Na$^+$ channel: Cell surface insertion and retrieval in Na$^+$ homeostasis and hypertension. Endocr Rev 23:258-275, 2002.

222. Snyder PM, Olson DR, Thomas BC: Serum and glucocorticoid-regulated kinase modulates Nedd4-2-mediated inhibition of the epithelial Na$^+$ channel. J Biol Chem 277:5-8, 2002.

223. Shimkets RA, Lifton RP, Canessa CM: The activity of the epithelial sodium channel is regulated by clathrin-mediated endocytosis. J Biol Chem 272:25537-25541, 1997.

224. Geller DS, Farhi A, Pinkerton N, et al: Activating mineralocorticoid receptor mutation in hypertension exacerbated by pregnancy. Science 289:119-123, 2000.

225. Stewart PM: Mineralocorticoid hypertension. Lancet 353:1341-1347, 1999.

226. Funder JW: Apparent mineralocorticoid excess. Endocrinol Metab Clin North Am 24:613-621, 1995.

227. Arriza JL, Weinberger C, Cerelli G, et al: Cloning of human mineralocorticoid receptor complementary DNA: Structural and functional kinship with the glucocorticoid receptor. Science 237:268-275, 1987.

228. Ulick S, Levine LS, Gunczler P, et al: A syndrome of apparent mineralocorticoid excess associated with defects in the peripheral metabolism of cortisol. J Clin Endocrinol Metab 49:757-764, 1979.

229. Dave-Sharma S, Wilson RC, Harbison MD, et al: Examination of genotype and phenotype relationships in 14 patients with apparent mineralocorticoid excess. J Clin Endocrinol Metab 83:2244-2254, 1998.

230. Farese RV Jr, Biglieri EG, Shackleton CH, et al: Licorice-induced hypermineralocorticoidism. N Engl J Med 325:1223-1227, 1991.

231. Ulick S, Wang JZ, Blumenfeld JD, Pickering TG: Cortisol inactivation overload: a mechanism of mineralocorticoid hypertension in the ectopic adrenocorticotropin syndrome [see comments]. J Clin Endocrinol Metab 74:963-967, 1992.

232. Biglieri EG, Stockigt JR, Schambelan M: Adrenal mineralocorticoids causing hypertension. Am J Med 52:623-632, 1972.

233. Krakoff L: Measurement by radioimmunoassay of angiotensin I concentration in syndromes associated with steroid excess. J Clin Endocrinol Metab 37:110, 1973.

234. Rich GM, Ulick S, Cook S, et al: Glucocorticoid-remediable aldosteronism in a large kindred: Clinical spectrum and diagnosis using a characteristic biochemical phenotype. Ann Intern Med 116:813-820, 1992.

235. Dluhy RG, Lifton RP: Glucocorticoid-remediable aldosteronism (GRA): Diagnosis, variability of phenotype and regulation of potassium homeostasis. Steroids 60:48-51, 1995.

236. Lifton RP, Dluhy RG, Powers M, et al: Hereditary hypertension caused by chimaeric gene duplications and ectopic expression of aldosterone synthase. Nat Genet 2:66-74, 1992.

237. Litchfield WR, Anderson BF, Weiss RJ, et al: Intracranial aneurysm and hemorrhagic stroke in glucocorticoid-remediable aldosteronism. Hypertension 31(1 pt 2):445-450, 1998.

238. Laragh JH: Renin system understanding for analysis and treatment of hypertensive patients: A means to quantify the vasoconstrictor elements, diagnose curable renal and adrenal causes, assess risk of cadiovascular morbidity, and find the best fit drug regimen. *In* Laragh JH, Brenner BM (eds): Hypertension: Pathophysiology, Diagnosis, and Management, 2nd ed. New York, Raven Press, pp 1813-1836.

239. Laragh JH: The renin system in high blood pressure, from disbelief to reality: Converting-enzyme blockade for analysis and treatment. Prog Cardiovasc Dis 21:159-166, 1978.

240. Resnick LM, Nicholson JP, Laragh JH: Calcium, the renin-aldosterone system, and the hypotensive response to nifedipine. Hypertension 10:254-298, 1987.

241. Vaughan ED Jr, Laragh JH, Gavras I, et al: Volume factor in low and normal renin essential hypertension. Treatment with either spironolactone or chlorthalidone. Am J Cardiol 32:523-532, 1973.

242. Case DB, Wallace JM, Keim HJ, et al: Estimating renin participation in hypertension: Superiority of converting enzyme inhibitor over saralasin. Am J Med 61:790-796, 1976.

243. Case DB, Atlas SA, Laragh JH, et al: Use of first-dose response or plasma renin activity to predict the long-term effect of captopril: Identification of triphasic pattern of blood pressure response. J Cardiovasc Pharmacol 2:339-346, 1980.

244. Gavras H, Brunner HR, Laragh JH, et al: An angiotensin-converting enzyme inhibitor to identify and treat vasoconstrictor and volume factors in hypertensive patients. N Engl J Med 291:817-821, 1974.

245. Case DB, Wallace JM, Keim HJ, et al: Possible role of renin in hypertension as suggested by renin-sodium profiling and inhibition of converting enzyme. N Engl J Med 296:641-646, 1977.

246. Anderson G, Blakeman N, Streeten D: Prediction of renovascular hypertension. Am J Hypertens 1:301-304, 1988.

247. Bulpitt CJ, Dollery CT, Carne S: Change in symptoms of hypertensive patients after referral to hospital clinic. Br Heart J 38:121-128, 1976.

248. Messerli FH, Ventura HO, Elizardi DJ, et al: Hypertension and sudden death. Increased ventricular ectopic activity in left ventricular hypertrophy. Am J Med 77:18-22, 1984.

249. McLenachan JM, Henderson E, Morris KI, Dargie HJ: Ventricular arrhythmias in patients with hypertensive left ventricular hypertrophy. N Engl J Med 317:787-792, 1987.

250. Corvol P, Pinet E, Plouin P: Primary reninism. *In* Laragh JH, Brenner BM (eds): Hypertension: Pathophysiology, Diagnosis, and Management, 2nd ed. New York, Raven Press, 1995, pp 2069-2080.

251. Chapman A, Johnson A, Gabow P, Schrier R: The renin-angiotensin-aldosterone system and autosomal dominant polycystic kidney disease. N Engl J Med 323:1091-1096, 1990.

252. Shaper AG, Wannamethee G, Whincup P: Alcohol and blood pressure in middle-aged British men. J Hum Hypertens 2:71-78, 1988.

253. Groppelli A, Giorgi DM, Omboni S, et al: Persistent blood pressure increase induced by heavy smoking. J Hypertens 10:495-499, 1992.

254. Vaughan EJ, Blumenfeld J: The adrenals. *In* Walsh P, Retik A, Vaughan EJ (eds): Campbell's Urology, 7th ed. Philadelphia, WB Saunders, 1998, pp 2915-2972.

255. Wong TY, Klein R, Sharrett AR, et al: Cerebral white matter lesions, retinopathy, and incident clinical stroke. JAMA 288:67-74, 2002.

256. Fishbane S, Youn S, Flaster E, et al: Ankle-arm blood pressure index as a predictor of mortality in hemodialysis patients. Am J Kidney Dis 27:668-672, 1996.

257. Lenders JW, Pacak K, Walther MM, et al: Biochemical diagnosis of pheochromocytoma: Which test is best? JAMA 287:1427-1434, 2002.

258. Hamlet SM, Tunny TJ, Woodland E, Gordon RD: Is aldosterone/renin ratio useful to screen a hypertensive population for primary aldosteronism? Clin Exp Plarmacol Physiol 12:249-252, 1985.

259. James GD, Sealey JE, Muller F, et al: Renin relationship to sex, race and age in a normotensive population. J Hypertens Suppl 4:S387-S389, 1986.

260. James GD, Cates EM, Pickering TG, Laragh JH: Parity and perceived job stress elevate blood pressure in young normotensive working women. Am J Hypertens 2:637-639, 1989.

261. White WB, Grin JM, McCabe EJ: Clinical usefulness of ambulatory blood pressure monitoring. Am J Hypertens 6(6 pt 2):225S-228S, 1993.

262. Muller FB, Sealey JE, Case DB, et al: The captopril test for identifying renovascular disease in hypertensive patients. Am J Med 80:633-644, 1986.

263. Vaughan ED Jr, Buhler FR, Laragh JH, et al: Renovascular hypertension: renin measurements to indicate hypersecretion and contralateral suppression, estimate renal plasma flow, an score for surgical curability. Am J Med 55:402-414, 1973.

264. Freis ED: Improving treatment effectiveness in hypertension. Arch Intern Med 159:2517-2521, 1999.

265. Laragh J: Laragh's lessons in pathophysiology and clinical pearls for treating hypertension. Lesson XVI: How to choose the correct drug treatment for each hypertensive patient using a plasma renin–based method and the volume-vasoconstriction analysis. Am J Hypertens 14:491-503, 2001.

266. Blumenfeld JD, Laragh JH: Renin system analysis: A rational method for the diagnosis and treatment of the individual patient with hypertension. Am J Hypertens 11:894-896, 1998.

267. Preston RA, Materson BJ, Reda DJ, et al: Age-race subgroup compared with renin profile as predictors of blood pressure response to antihypertensive therapy. Department of Veternas Affairs Cooperative Study Group on Antihypertensive Agents. JAMA 280:1168-1172, 1998.

268. Carter A: Hypotensive therapy in stroke survivors. Lancet 1:485-489, 1970.

269. Barraclough M, Joy M, MacGregor G, et al: Control of moderately raised blood pressure. BMJ 3:434-436, 1973.

270. Hypertension-Stroke Cooperative Study Group: Effect of antihypertensive treatment on stroke recurrence. Hypertension-Stroke Cooperative Study Group. JAMA 229:409-418, 1974.

271. Smith W: Treatment of mild hypertension. Hypertension 25(suppl 1):I98-I105, 1977.

272. Perry H, Goldman A, Lavin M, et al: Evaluation of drug treatment in mild hypertension. Ann N Y Acad Sci 304:267-288, 1978.

273. Hegeland A: Treatment of mild hypertension. Am J Med 69:725-732, 1980.

274. Management Committee of the Australian National Blood Pressure Study: The Australian therapeutic trial in mild hypertension. Report by the Management Committee. Lancet 1:1261-1267, 1980.

275. Kuramoto K, Matsushita S, Kuwajima I, Murakami M: Prospective study on the treatment of mild hypertension in the aged. Jpn Heart J 22:75-85, 1981.

276. Amery A, Birkenhager W, Brixko P, et al: Mortality and morbidity results from the European Working Party on High Blood Pressure in the Elderly trial. Lancet 1:1349-1354, 1985.

277. Coope JR, Warrender TS: Randomised trial of treatment of hypertension in elderly patients in primary care. BMJ (Clin Res Ed) 294:179, 1987.

278. Perry HM Jr, Smith WM, McDonald RH, et al: Morbidity and mortality in the Systolic Hypertension in the Elderly Program (SHEP) pilot study. Stroke 20:4-13, 1989.

279. Dahlof B, Lindholm LH, Hansson L, et al: Morbidity and mortality in the Swedish Trial in Old Patients with Hypertension (STOP-Hypertension). Lancet 338:1281-1285, 1991.

280. Medical Research Council Working Party: Medical Research Council trial of treatment of hypertension in older adults: Principal results. MRC Working Party. BMJ 304:405-412, 1992.

Renovascular Hypertension and Ischemic Nephropathy

Stephen C. Textor

Few clinical problems present more complex challenges to nephrologists than managing renovascular hypertension and ischemic nephropathy. When successful, renal revascularization in these disorders can both reverse hypertension and salvage renal function to a remarkable degree. Selecting patients for whom these benefits apply without excessive risks is rarely simple, however. Broad changes in population demographics, imaging technology, and medical therapy related to the renin-angiotensin system, combined with rapidly evolving techniques of renal revascularization, make this a dynamic clinical field.

Renovascular disease presents an interface between many medical disciplines and subspecialties, including internal medicine, cardiovascular disease, interventional radiology, and vascular surgery. It should be recognized that management of renovascular disease remains controversial. Subspecialty groups tend to deal with widely different patient subgroups and clinical issues that shape different points of view. Cardiologists, for example, more commonly encounter patients with widespread coronary and vascular disease at risk for "flash" pulmonary edema than internists who may deal with established hypertensive patients with progressive hypertension and a rise in serum creatinine (Fig. 46-1A and 46-1B). Both of these may represent clinical manifestations of renovascular disease but present different comorbid risk and management issues. It will come as no surprise that perceptions related to renovascular hypertension and ischemic nephropathy sometimes differ among informed clinicians, even when interpreting the same published data.

Nephrologists play a major role in caring for patients with these disorders. Ultimately, renovascular disease threatens blood flow to the kidney. The consequences of impaired blood flow not only affect blood pressure and cardiovascular risk but also threaten the viability of the kidney. It can lead to irreversible loss of kidney function, sometimes designated "ischemic nephropathy" or "azotemic renovascular disease."[1] It must be recognized, however, that renal revascularization is a two-edged sword. The benefits of renal artery interventional procedures include the potential to improve systemic arterial blood pressures and to preserve or salvage renal function. Unfortunately, the risks of renal intervention are well known to nephrologists. The procedures themselves may threaten the viability of the affected kidney through vascular thrombosis, dissection, restenosis, or atheroemboli. The consequences of these events sometimes precipitate the need for renal replacement therapy, including dialysis or transplantation. It is therefore important that nephrologists have a solid foundation related to the risks and benefits of reduced renal perfusion and the implications of both medical management and restoration of renal perfusion pressure.

This chapter undertakes to summarize our current knowledge related to the mechanisms underlying renovascular hypertension and ischemic nephropathy. It addresses the changing demographics and comorbid risk of patients with renovascular disease, the spectrum of clinical manifestations encountered, the implications of disease progression, and the risks and benefits of both medical management and renal revascularization.

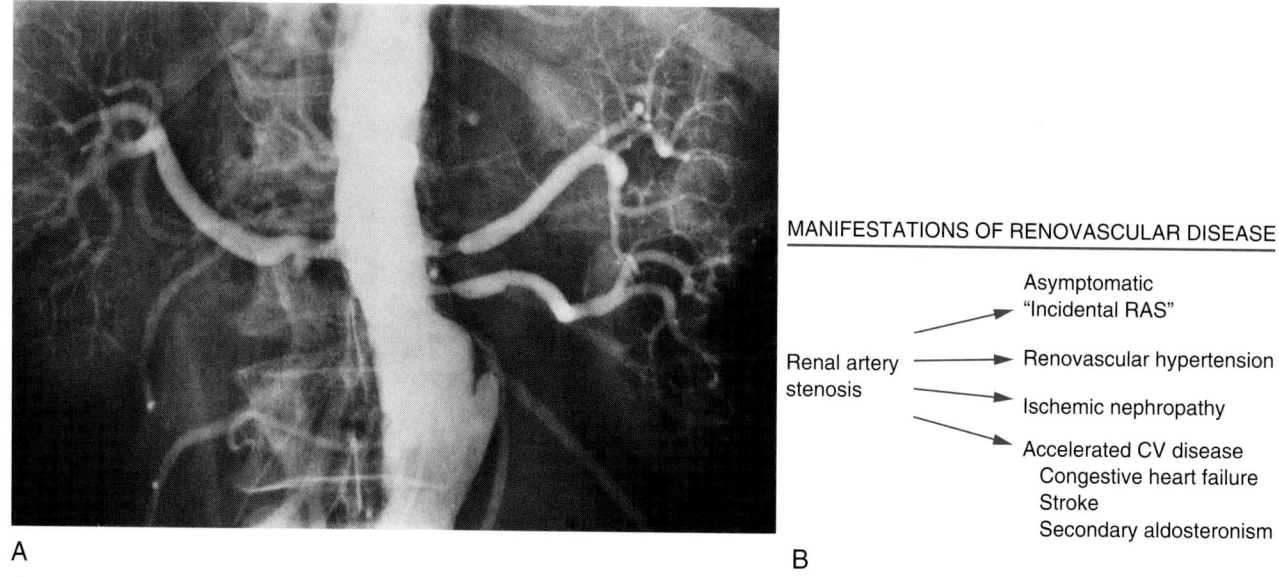

A   B

FIGURE 46-1. A, An aortogram demonstrating renal artery stenosis (RAS) in multiple arteries in a 78-year-old man with hypertension. This image was obtained during lower extremity angiography for symptomatic claudication. Renovascular disease commonly develops in the setting of atherosclerotic disease elsewhere. Identification of an aortic aneurysm is an additional incidental finding. Understanding the role of renal artery disease in a specific patient regarding blood pressure control and kidney function is central to deciding when to consider renal revascularization. In this case, hypertension was easily treated with a single agent and serum creatinine remained stable at 1.3 mg/dL for more than 6 years. **B,** The spectrum of clinical manifestations of renovascular disease ranges from minimal hemodynamic effects to major acceleration of cardiovascular (CV) risk and renal injury. The primary challenge to clinicians is to recognize the specific role renovascular disease plays in each patient.

HISTORICAL PERSPECTIVE

Many of the earliest observations regarding blood pressure regulation are focused upon the role of the kidney. In 1898, Tigerstedt and Bergman established that extracts of the kidney had pressor effects in the whole animal and these authors are credited with the identification of "renin."[2] The sequence of studies leading to the identification of each element in the renin-angiotensin system represents a remarkable series of research ventures spanning a half-century and investigators in many countries. It has been reviewed recently.[3] In 1934, Goldblatt and co-workers provided seminal experiments with the development of an animal model in which reduced renal perfusion regularly produced hypertension.[4] Numerous investigators thereafter addressed the peptide nature of angiotensin, the role of "renin-substrate" or angiotensinogen, the role of nephrectomy in sensitizing the animal to the pressor effects of angiotensin, and the sequential "phases" of hypertension.[5] Activation of the renin-angiotensin system was identified as central in renovascular hypertension.[6, 7] Hence, the renin-angiotensin system owes its discovery and nomenclature primarily to early studies related to regulation of blood pressure by the kidney. Only recently have the many additional actions of angiotensin become evident regarding vascular remodeling, modulation of inflammatory pathways, and interaction with fibrogenic mechanisms.[8-10]

Understanding that reduced renal blood flow produced sustained elevations in arterial pressure led to broad study of the mechanisms of hypertension. Experimental hypertension of the two-kidney, one-kidney renal clip (two-kidney and one-kidney Goldblatt models) represented some of the most extensively studied models of blood pressure and cardiovascular

regulation, as has been emphasized.[7] Translation of these studies to clinical medicine followed soon thereafter. Some forms of hypertension were recognized as "malignant" in character during the late 1930s and 1940s. Few antihypertensive agents were known until the 1950s and intervention consisted mainly of lumbar sympathectomy or extremely low-sodium intake diets, or a combination of both. Recognition that some forms of severe hypertension were secondary to occlusive vascular disease in the kidney led surgeons to undertake unilateral nephrectomy for small kidneys in 1937.[11-13] The fact that some of these were indeed "pressor" kidneys and blood pressure fell to normal levels provided "proof of concept" and led to the more widespread use of nephrectomy. Unfortunately, "cure" of hypertension after nephrectomy was rare, and Homer Smith reviewed the poor results overall in a 1956 paper critical of this practice.[13]

The 1960s marked the introduction of practical methods of vascular surgery which could be applied to restoration of renal blood flow.[14] These carried substantial morbidity, but offered an opportunity to restore the renal circulation and potentially to reverse renovascular hypertension. One result of this development was a series of studies to characterize the functional role of each vascular lesion in producing hypertension, thereby allowing prediction of the outcomes of vascular surgery.[12, 15] A large cooperative study of renovascular hypertension included major vascular centers and reported on the results of more than 500 surgical procedures. These results provided limited support for vascular repair, but highlighted relatively high associated morbidity and mortality, particularly in patients with atherosclerotic disease.[16]

The 1980s and 1990s were characterized by both improved medications and the introduction of endovascular procedures, including percutaneous angioplasty and stents. These both broadened the options for treating patients with vascular disease and raised new issues regarding the timing and overall goals of intervention. Recent developments highlight the need for intensive cardiovascular risk factor reduction and more stringent standards of blood pressure control. Medications have improved dramatically, both as regards efficacy and tolerability. As is emphasized below, broad application of angiotensin-converting enzyme (ACE) inhibitors and angiotensin receptor antagonists for reasons other than hypertension alone has changed the clinical presentation of disorders associated with renal artery stenosis (RAS). Uncontrollable hypertension is now less commonly the reason to intervene in renovascular disease than before. Often the main objective is the long-term preservation of renal function. In recent years, endovascular techniques of angioplasty and stent placement have opened the possibility of renal revascularization with relatively low morbidity in many patients previously considered unacceptable surgical candidates. How and when to apply these tools most effectively in the management of individual patients remain the central challenges to clinicians.

PATHOPHYSIOLOGY

Renal Artery Stenosis versus Renovascular Hypertension

As with most vascular lesions, the presence of a vascular abnormality alone does not translate directly into functional importance. Some degree of RAS can be identified in 20% to 45% of patients undergoing vascular imaging for other reasons, such as coronary angiography or lower extremity peripheral vascular disease.[17] Most of these "incidental" stenoses are of little or no hemodynamic significance. The term "renovascular hypertension" refers to a rise in arterial pressure induced by reduced renal perfusion. A variety of lesions can lead to the syndrome of renovascular hypertension, some of which are listed in Table 46-1. Strictly speaking, the diagnosis of renovascular hypertension is established only in retrospect after successful reversal of hypertension with revascularization.

Studies of vascular obstruction using latex rubber casts indicate that between 70% and 80% of lumen obstruction must occur before measurable changes in blood flow or pressure across the lesion can be detected.[18] When advanced stenosis is present, the fall in pressure and flow develops steeply, as illustrated in Figure 46-2A and B. When lesions have reached a degree of hemodynamic significance, they are deemed to have reached "critical" stenosis.[19]

When renal artery lesions reach critical dimensions, a series of events leads to a rise in systemic arterial pressure and restoration of renal perfusion, as illustrated in Figure 46-3. Hence, one can view the development of rising pressures in this context as an integrated renal response to maintain renal perfusion. It is important to distinguish between experimental models of "clip" stenosis, at which time a sudden change in renal perfusion is induced, and the more common clinical situation of gradually progressive lumen obstruction. In the latter instance, hemodynamic characteristics change slowly and are likely to produce hypertension over a prolonged time interval. The rise in systemic pressure

TABLE 46-1

Examples of Vascular Lesions Producing Renal Hypoperfusion and the Syndrome of Renovascular Hypertension

Unilateral Disease (Analogous to One-Clip, Two-Kidney Hypertension)
Unilateral atherosclerotic renal artery stenosis
Unilateral fibromuscular dysplasia[97]
   Medial fibroplasia
   Perimedial fibroplasia
   Intimal fibroplasia
   Medial hyperplasia
Renal artery aneurysm
Arterial embolus
Arteriovenous fistula (congenital/traumatic)
Segmental arterial occlusion (post-traumatic)
Extrinsic compression of renal artery, e.g., pheochromocytoma
Renal compression, e.g., metastatic tumor

Bilateral Disease or Solitary Functioning Kidney (Analogous to One-Clip, One-Kidney Model)
Stenosis to a solitary functioning kidney
Bilateral renal arterial stenosis
Aortic coarctation
Systemic vasculitis (e.g., Takayasu arteritis, polyarteritis)
Atheroembolic disease

Modified from Textor SC: Pathophysiology of renovascular hypertension. Urol Clin North Am 11:373-381, 1984; and Pohl MA: Renal artery stenosis, renal vascular hypertension and ischemic nephropathy. *In* Schrier RW, Gottschalk CW (eds): Diseases of the Kidney. Boston, Little, Brown, 1997, pp 1367-1423.

restores normal renal perfusion, often with normal-size kidneys and no discernible hemodynamic compromise. If the renal artery lesion progresses further (or is experimentally advanced), the cycle of reduced perfusion and rising arterial pressures recurs until malignant phase hypertension develops.[20] Recent experimental swine models emphasize gradually progressing vascular lesions that mimic human renovascular disease.[21]

A corollary to "critical" arterial stenosis is that reduction of elevated systemic pressures to normal in renovascular hypertension threatens to reduce renal pressures beyond the stenotic lesion. Poststenotic pressures may fall below levels that maintain blood flow. Such underperfusion of the kidney activates counterregulatory pathways and leads to a sequence of events directed toward restoring kidney perfusion. Foremost among these pathways is the release of renin with activation of the renin-angiotensin system.

The Role of the Renin-Angiotensin System in One-Kidney and Two-Kidney Renovascular Hypertension

Reduction in renal perfusion pressures activates the release of renin from juxtaglomerular cells within the affected kidneys.[22, 23] Experimental studies indicate that two-kidney, one-clip models of hypertension can be delayed indefinitely so long as agents that block this system are administered, as illustrated in Figure 46-4.[6, 24]

Demonstration of the role of the renin-angiotensin axis in renovascular hypertension depends in part upon whether or not a contralateral, nonstenotic kidney is present. Classically, human renovascular hypertension is considered analogous to

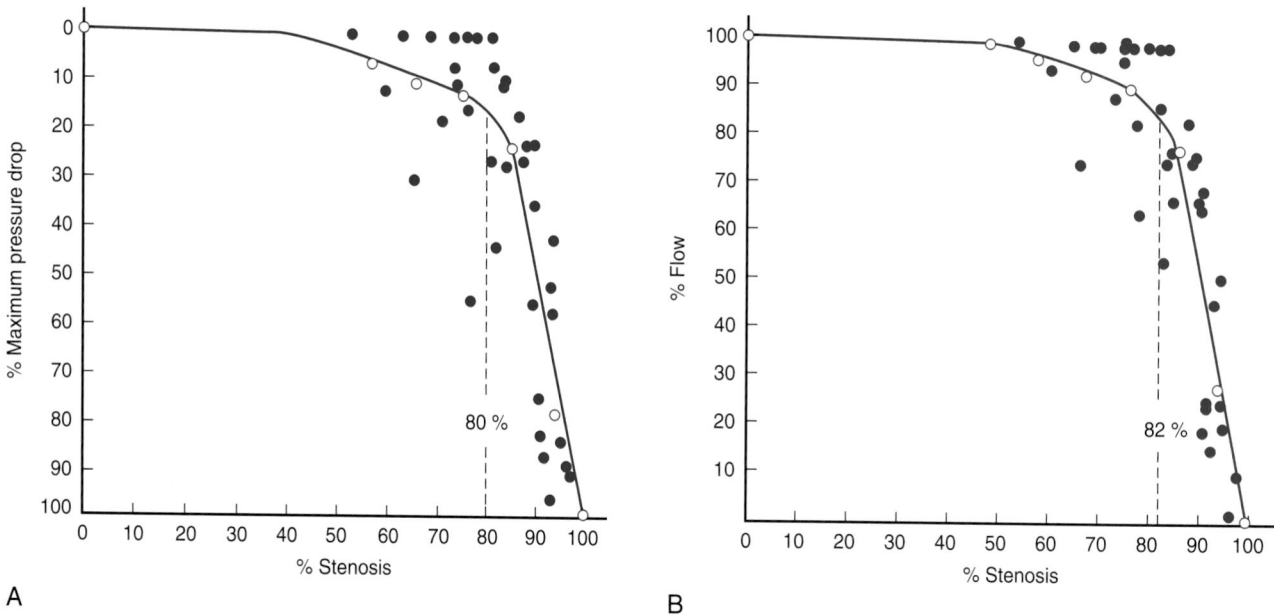

FIGURE 46-2. Measured fall in arterial pressure (**A**) and blood flow (**B**) across stenotic vascular lesions induced in experimental animals. The degree of stenosis was quantitated using latex casts after completion of the experiment. These data indicate that "critical" lesions require 70%-80% luminal obstruction before hemodynamic effects can be detected. (From May AG, Van de Berg L, DeWeese JA, et al: Critical arterial stenosis. Surgery 54:250-259, 1963.)

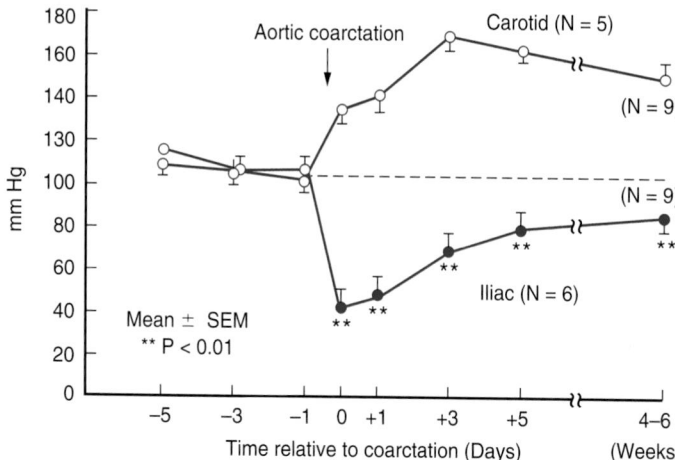

FIGURE 46-3. Systemic arterial pressure (carotid) and poststenotic renal perfusion pressures (iliac) in an aortic coarctation model with the clip placed between the right and left renal arteries. These measurements in conscious animals during development of renovascular hypertension illustrate that renal perfusion pressure is maintained at near-normal levels at the expense of systemic hypertension due to the gradient induced by the stenotic lesion. (From Textor SC, Smith-Powell L: Poststenotic arterial pressure, renal haemodynamics, and sodium excretion during graded pressure reduction in conscious rats with one- and two-kidney coarctation hypertension. J Hypertens 6:311-319, 1988.)

two-kidney, one-clip experimental (Goldblatt) hypertension. The contralateral, nonstenotic kidney is subjected to elevated systemic perfusion pressures. The effect of rising perfusion on pressure is to force natriuresis from the nonstenotic kidney and to suppress renin release.[25-27] Hence, the nonstenotic kidney tends to prevent the rise in systemic pressures, thereby perpetuating reduced perfusion to the stenotic side and fostering continued renin release from the stenotic kidney. Blood pressure in these models is usually demonstrably angiotensin-dependent and associated with elevated circulating levels of plasma renin activity,[28] as illustrated in Figure 46-5. It is important to recognize that the two-kidney, one-clip model of renovascular hypertension forms the basis for many of the early functional studies of surgically curable hypertension in which side-to-side function was compared regarding glomerular filtration, sodium excretion, and so on.[29]

This paradigm is also the basis for comparing kidneys side to side using radionuclide studies, such as captopril renograms and renal vein renin determinations. Unilateral renal ischemia represents a classic model for the study of angiotensin-dependent hypertension and target organ injury.[30-32]

When no such contralateral kidney is present, mechanisms sustaining hypertension differ. This model corresponds to the one-kidney, one-clip (one-kidney Goldblatt) hypertensive animal. Although renin release occurs initially, elevated systemic pressures develop with sodium and volume retention, as there is no sodium excretion by the contralateral kidney. Rising pressures eventually restore renin levels to normal. Hypertension in this model is not demonstrably dependent upon angiotensin II (AII) unless prior sodium depletion is achieved.[33-35] Clinical examples of this situation are those of bilateral RAS or stenosis to a solitary functioning kidney

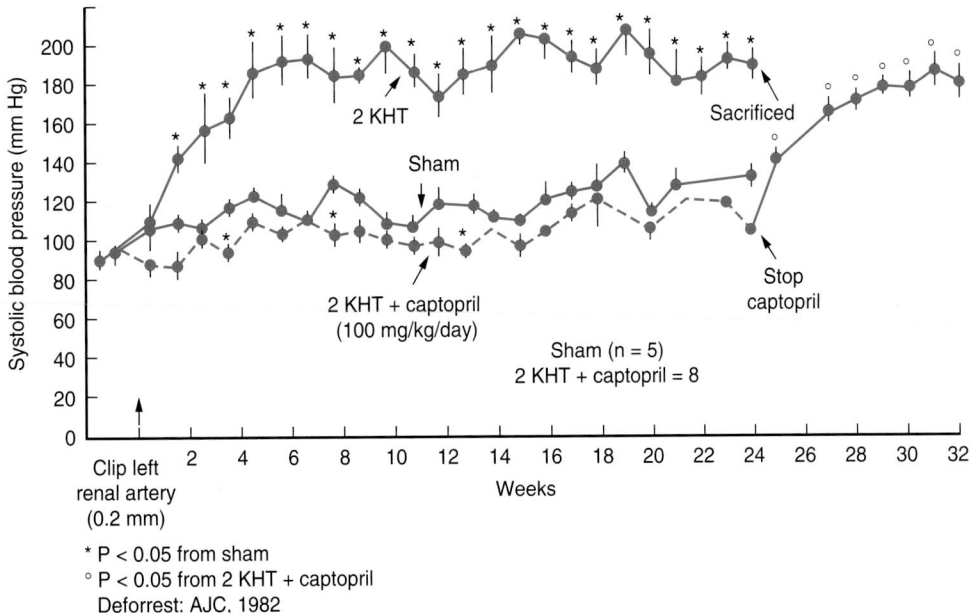

FIGURE 46-4. Blood pressures before and after placement of a renal artery clip in experimental two-kidney, one-clip renovascular hypertension. Administration of an angiotensin-converting enzyme inhibitor (captopril) prevented the development of hypertension so long as it was continued. These data demonstrate the pivotal role of activation of the renin-angiotensin system at the onset of renovascular hypertension. (From DeForrest JM, Knappenberger RC, Antonaccio MJ, et al: Angiotensin II is a necessary component for the development of hypertension in the two-kidney, one-clip rat. Am J Cardiol 49:1515-1517, 1982.)

in which the entire renal mass is affected. In such cases diagnostic comparison of side-to-side renin release is not possible or has little meaning.

Mechanisms Leading to Sustained Renovascular Hypertension

For more than a century, the kidney has been recognized as a source of pressor materials. Identification of components of the renin-angiotensin system has provided a crucial link to understanding these systems. Circulating renin is derived primarily from the kidney in response to a reduction of renal perfusion pressure detected by loss of afferent arteriolar stretch.[36, 37] Renin itself has a biologic activity directed mainly to the enzymatic release of angiotensin I (AI) from its circulating substrate, angiotensinogen, in plasma and possibly other sites. Two further peptides are cleaved from AI through the action of ACE to produce AII. Generation of AII in plasma occurs mainly during passage through the lung. Hence, the signal of reduced kidney pressures is amplified and transmitted to a major vasopressor system which acts throughout the body, accounting for one major mechanism by which renovascular hypertension develops.

The importance of the renin-angiotensin system in renovascular hypertension cannot be overemphasized. As noted above, two-kidney, one-clip renovascular hypertension can be prevented so long as this system is blocked by inhibition of the ACE.[6] The actions of AII are multifold and widespread, as illustrated in Figure 46-6. Activation of this system represents amplification of a local signal within the kidney to activate systemic pressor mechanisms, mediated by increased vascular resistance, sodium retention, and aldosterone stimulation.

Further studies indicate that complex interactions between AII and tissue and cellular systems occur, leading to vascular remodeling, left ventricular hypertrophy, and activation of fibrogenic mechanisms.

Hypertension and peripheral vasoconstriction reflect complex interactions between angiotensin and other vasoactive systems. Renovascular disease leads to disturbances in sympathetic nerve traffic, which may differ between one-kidney and two-kidney models.[38-40] A major transition occurs with recruitment of altered oxidative stress within the systemic vasculature, leading to increased oxygen free radicals.[37, 41] Vascular injury itself produces disturbances in endothelium-derived mechanisms, such as endothelin (ET) production and vasodilator systems, such as prostacyclin.[38, 42-45] That endothelium-derived systems and increased oxidative stress participate in human renovascular disease has been supported by recent clinical studies in patients with both atherosclerotic and fibromuscular RAS.[46] These studies indicate that oxidative stress can be reversed both by infusion of antioxidants and by successful revascularization which can restore vasomotor tone toward normal.

Phases of Development

Experimental models of renovascular hypertension indicate that mechanisms sustaining hypertension change over time (Fig. 46-7). An early phase is characterized by elevated circulating indices of renin activity and hypertension, both of which return to normal after removing the vascular lesion. A second phase has been described with a return of circulating renin activity to normal or low levels, during which hypertension persists and blood pressure can still respond to clip removal. A third phase has been proposed, during

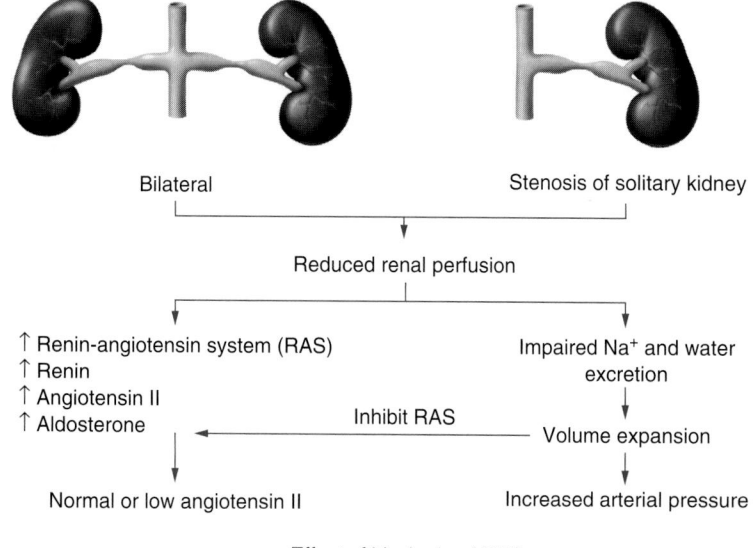

UNILATERAL RENAL ARTERY STENOSIS

Reduced renal perfusion

Increased renal perfusion

↑ Renin-angiotensin system (RAS)
↑ Renin
↑ Angiotensin II
↑ Aldosterone

Suppressed RAS

Increased Na⁺ excretion
(pressure natriuresis)

Angiotensin II–dependent hypertension

Effect of blockade of RAS
Reduced arterial pressure
Enhanced lateralization of diagnostic tests
Glomerular filtration rate (GFR) in stenotic kidney may fall

Diagnostic tests
Plasma renin activity elevated
Lateralized features, e.g., renin levels in renal veins, captopril-enhanced renography

A

BILATERAL RENAL ARTERY STENOSIS

Bilateral

Stenosis of solitary kidney

Reduced renal perfusion

↑ Renin-angiotensin system (RAS)
↑ Renin
↑ Angiotensin II
↑ Aldosterone

Impaired Na⁺ and water
excretion

Inhibit RAS

Volume expansion

Normal or low angiotensin II

Increased arterial pressure

Effect of blockade of RAS
Reduced arterial pressure only after volume depletion
May lower GFR

Diagnostic tests
Plasma renin activity normal or low
Lateralized features: none

B

FIGURE 46-5. A and **B,** Schematic view of two-kidney and one-kidney renovascular hypertension. These models differ by the presence of a contralateral kidney exposed to elevated perfusion pressures in two-kidney hypertension. The nonstenotic kidney tends to allow pressure natriuresis to ensue and produces ongoing stimulation of renin release from the stenotic kidney. The one-kidney model eventually produces sodium retention and a fall in renin with minimal evidence of angiotensin dependency unless sodium depletion is achieved. (From Textor SC: Renovascular hypertension. *In* Johnson RJ, Feehally J [eds]: Comprehensive Clinical Nephrology. London, Mosby, 2000, pp 41.1-41.12.)

which removal of the clip no longer leads to reduction in arterial pressure. These observations have been interpreted to underscore the transition between differing mechanisms of vascular control, some of which no longer depend upon reduced renal perfusion. Some data have been presented to argue that microvascular injury to the contralateral kidney sustains hypertension in this phase.[47] Recent studies in a swine model indicate that the fall in renin activity follows a transition to mechanisms related to oxidative stress with persistent elevation of oxidative metabolites such as isoprostanes.[41] Whether these phases apply directly to human renovascular disease is not known.

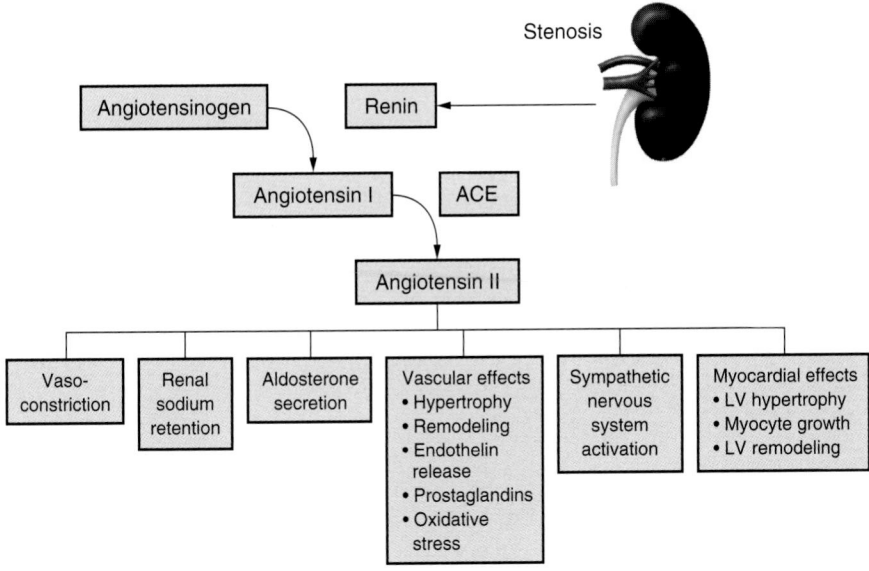

FIGURE 46-6. Schematic view of activation of the renin-angiotensin system beyond a renal artery stenotic lesion. Generation of circulating and local angiotensin II leads to widespread effects, including sodium retention, efferent arteriolar vasoconstriction, and elevated systemic vascular resistance. Studies in recent years implicate angiotensin II in many other pathways of vascular and cardiac smooth muscle remodeling, activation of inflammatory and fibrogenic cytokines, coagulation factors, and induction of other vasoactive systems. ACE, angiotensin-converting enzyme, LV, left ventricular.

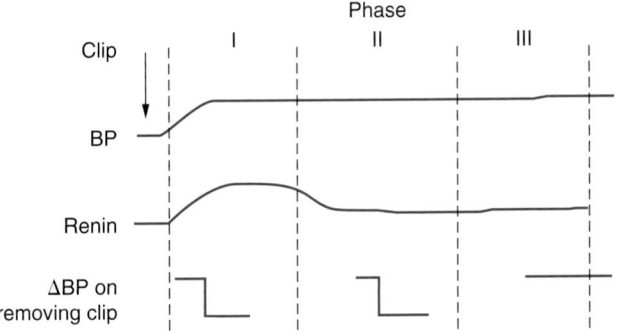

FIGURE 46-7. Depiction of phases observed in experimental renovascular hypertension. Initially high levels of renin activity fall during later phases, despite the fact that removal of the renal artery clip corrects hypertension. These observations support the concept of recruitment of additional vaso-pressor mechanisms after the initial activation of the renin-angiotensin system (see text). Whether human renovascular hypertension follows these patterns precisely is not well known. BP, blood pressure. (From Brown JJ, Davis DL, Morten JJ, et al: Mechanism of renal hypertension. Lancet 1:1219-1221, 1976.)

Mechanisms of Ischemic Nephropathy

Reduced renal perfusion beyond critical stenosis ultimately leads to loss of viable kidney function, as illustrated in Figure 46-8. Patients with stenosis affecting the entire renal mass can develop reduced blood flow and glomerular filtration when poststenotic pressures fall below the range of autoregulation. This process is reversible if pressure is restored or the vascular lesion is removed. If allowed to progress, recurrent reduction in kidney blood flow can produce irreversible fibrosis, as illustrated schematically in Figure 46-9A. The mechanisms by which this occurs may differ from those that govern the development of hypertension. The term "ischemic" nephropathy may itself be a misnomer, as we have discussed previously.[48] Unlike brain or cardiac tissue, the kidney is vastly oversupplied with oxygenated blood, consistent with its function as a filtering organ. Measurements of both renal vein oxygen saturation and erythropoietin in

patients with high-grade renovascular lesions indicate that whole-organ "ischemia" is not present.[49, 50] There may be local areas of deranged oxygen delivery within the kidney.[48, 51]

Reduction of blood flow to the kidney activates numerous pathways of vascular and tissue injury, including increased AII, ET release, and oxidative stress, as noted earlier. Under the right conditions, these factors trigger inflammatory cytokines and fibrogenic mechanisms leading to tissues fibrosis.

Adaptive Mechanisms to Reduced Renal Perfusion

The kidney maintains autoregulation of blood flow in the face of reduced arterial diameters of up to 75%. Under basal conditions, renal blood flow is among the highest of all organs, reflecting its filtration function. Less than 10% of delivered oxygen is sufficient to maintain renal metabolic needs. Under conditions of impaired renal perfusion, oxygen delivery is sometimes maintained by development of collateral vessels,[52] associated with intrarenal redistribution of blood flow. The kidney medulla functions at levels closer to hypoxia than does the cortex, which is efficiently autoregulated.[53] The outer medulla, for example, is continuously at the verge of anoxia and is sensitive to acute changes in perfusion, which produces tubular necrosis. During chronic reduction of blood flow, the medulla is protected somewhat by adaptive maintenance of tissue perfusion at the expense of cortical blood flow, which parallels whole-kidney renal blood flow.[53, 54] Hence, gradual reduction of renal perfusion pressures allows recruitment of protective mechanisms which remain incompletely understood, leading to different functional and morphologic changes from those observed after acute ischemic injury.[55]

A fall in renal blood flow is accompanied by decreased oxygen consumption, in part due to reduced metabolic demands of filtration and tubular solute reabsorption.[50] Eventually, structural atrophy of the renal tubules occurs, partly due to necrosis and apoptosis (Fig. 46-9B). The latter is an active, programmed form of cellular death which appears to be closely regulated and differs from tissue necrosis.[56] Tubular atrophy is potentially reversible and the kidney

BLOOD PRESSURE, RENAL PLASMA FLOW, AND GFR IN PATIENTS WITH BILATERAL RAS
DURING NITROPRUSSIDE INFUSION BEFORE AND AFTER REVASCULARIZATION

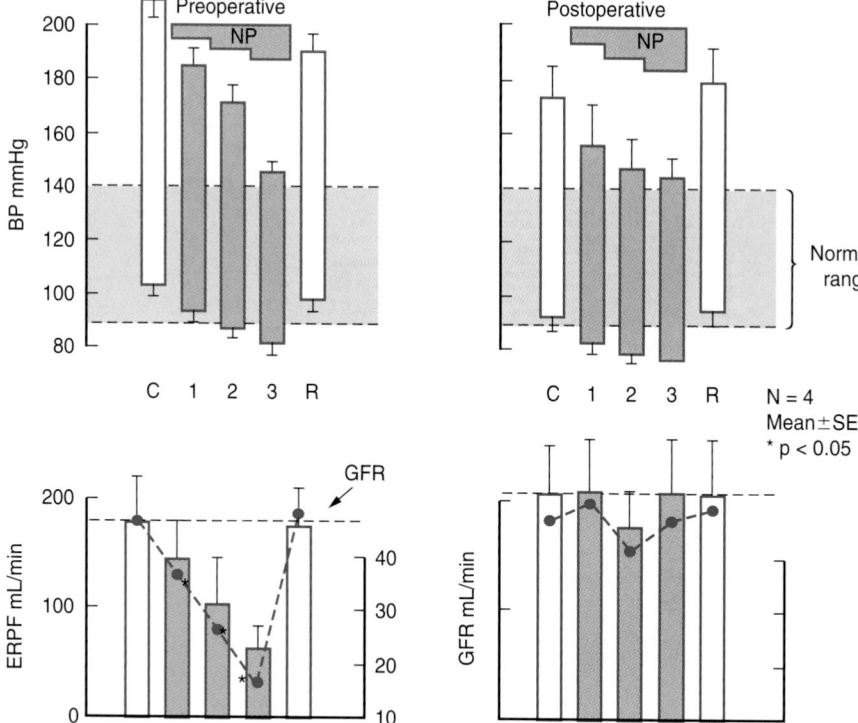

FIGURE 46-8. Renal blood flow and glomerular filtration in patients with critical bilateral renal artery stenosis (RAS) during pressure reduction with sodium nitroprusside. Reduction to normal blood pressures (BPs) produced a reversible fall in both blood flow and glomerular filtration rate (GFR). Studies in the same patients (*right set*) after unilateral surgical revascularization indicate that the sensitivity of blood flow and GFR to pressure reduction can be reversed. ERPF, effective renal plasma flow rate. (From Textor SC, Novick A, Tarazi RC, et al: Critical perfusion pressure for renal function in patients with bilateral atherosclerotic renal vascular disease. Ann Intern Med 102: 309-314, 1985.)

maintains the capacity for tubular cell regeneration under many conditions,[57] features which support the concept that underperfused kidney tissue can achieve a "hibernating" state capable of restoring function if blood flow is restored.[58] Eventually, pathologic examination demonstrates reduced glomerular volume, loss of tubular structures near underperfused glomeruli, and areas of local inflammatory reaction, as illustrated in (Fig. 46-10A and B; see also Color Plate I).

Mechanisms of Tissue Injury in Azotemic Renovascular Disease

The role of AII during renal hypoperfusion is complex. Generation of AII acts to raise perfusion pressure and to protect glomerular filtration by efferent arteriolar constriction, as noted above. AII induces cellular hypertrophy and hyperplasia in several cell types, in addition to stimulating local hormone production and ion transport directly. Experimental infusion of AII leads to parenchymal renal injury with focal and segmental glomerulosclerosis.[59] ACE inhibition and AII receptor blockade in several experimental models diminish renal cell proliferation and suppress infiltration of mononuclear cells which trigger expression of extracellular matrix proteins leading to progressive nephrosclerosis.[60, 61] Recent studies implicate AII in vascular smooth muscle cell growth, platelet aggregation, generation of superoxide radicals, activation of adhesion molecules and macrophages, induction of gene transcription for proto-oncogenes, and oxidation of low-density lipoproteins.[62] These observations underscore tha dual roles of AII, both for adaptation and maintenance of

kidney function and for modulating many steps in the pathologic cascade underlying progressive renal injury.

The vascular endothelium is a source of multiple vasoactive factors, the most widely recognized of which are nitric oxide (NO) and ET.[63] Endothelial *nitric oxide* is synthesized from L-arginine by a family of NO synthases and participates in the regulation of kidney function by counteracting the vasoconstrictor effects of AII.[64] In addition to its effects on blood flow and tubular reabsorption of sodium, NO inhibits growth of vascular smooth muscle cells, mesangial cell hypertrophy and hyperplasia, and synthesis of extracellular matrix.[65] These occur in part by down-regulating expression of ACE[66] and AII genes. Loss of the balance between AII and NO represents a disturbance of tissue homeostasis and may accelerate tissue damage.

A reduction in renal perfusion leads to diminished "shear stress" distal to the stenosis (see Figure 46-9B). This condition reduces production of NO and accelerates release of renin and generation of AII in the stenotic kidney. Hence, the effects of NO are diminished in the poststenotic kidney, allowing predominance of intrarenal vasoconstrictors, including AII and vasoconstrictor prostaglandins such as thromboxane.[67] The decrease in NO allows removal of its antithrombotic effects and inhibition of growth-related responses to tissue injury.

The *endothelin* peptides are a family of potent and long-lasting vasoconstrictor peptides produced and released from endothelial cells. ET itself is released from renal epithelial cells after simulation with a variety of substances such as thrombin and local cytokines, including transforming growth factor-β (TGF-β), interleukin-1 (IL-1), and tumor necrosis

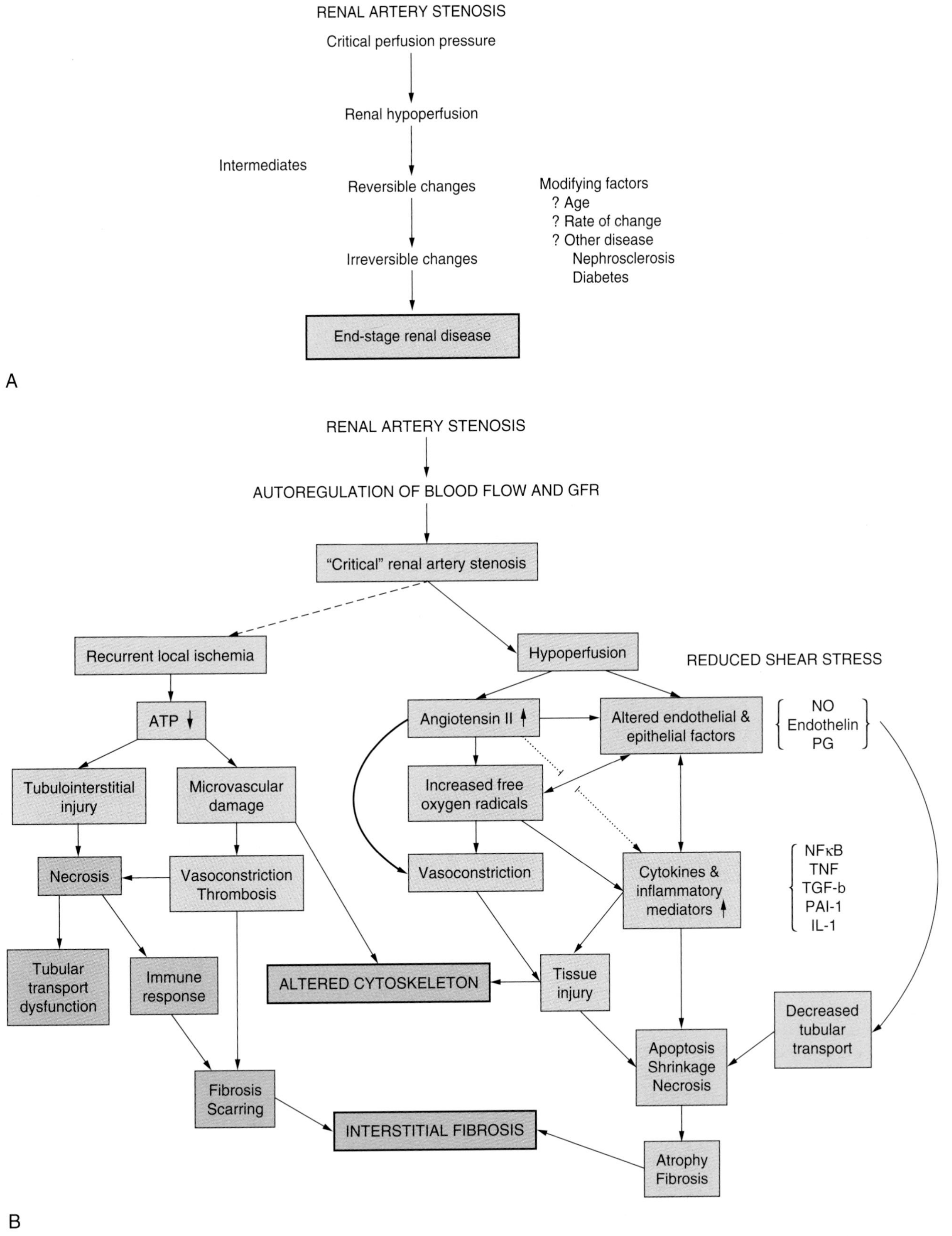

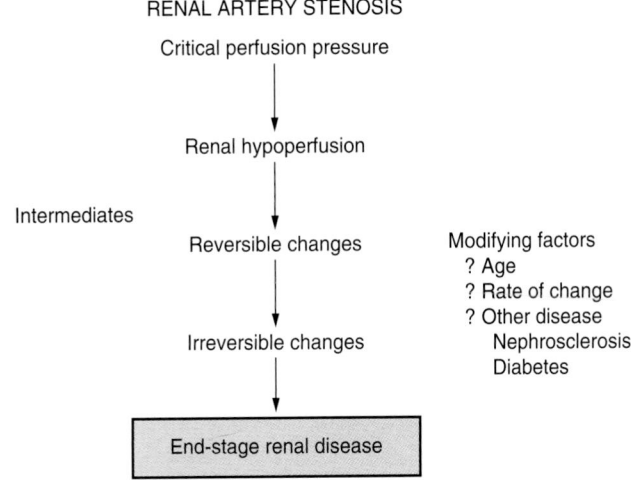

A

B

FIGURE 46-9. A, Schematic depiction of the paradigm underlying the observation that critical reductions in renal perfusion lead at first to reversible decrements in renal function. Ultimately, changes in the kidney parenchyma lose the capacity of reversal and produced end-stage renal failure. **B,** Proposed pathways implicated in ischemic nephropathy. These pathways entail recurrent local ischemia with microvascular injury and reduced perfusion producing activation of endothelial mechanisms of injury and inflammation. Eventually apoptosis and increased oxidative stress activate fibrogenic mechanisms, some of which may be modulated by the renin-angiotensin system and other factors, such as lipid peroxidation. ATP, adenosine triphosphate; GFR, glomerular filtration rate; IL-1, interleukin-1; NFκB, nuclear factor κB; PAI-1, plasminogen activator inhibitor-1; NO, nitric oxide; PG, prostaglandin; TGF-β, transforming growth factor-β; TNF, tumor necrosis factor. (From Lerman L, Textor SC: Pathophysiology of ischemic nephropathy. Urol Clin North Am 28:793-803, 2001.)

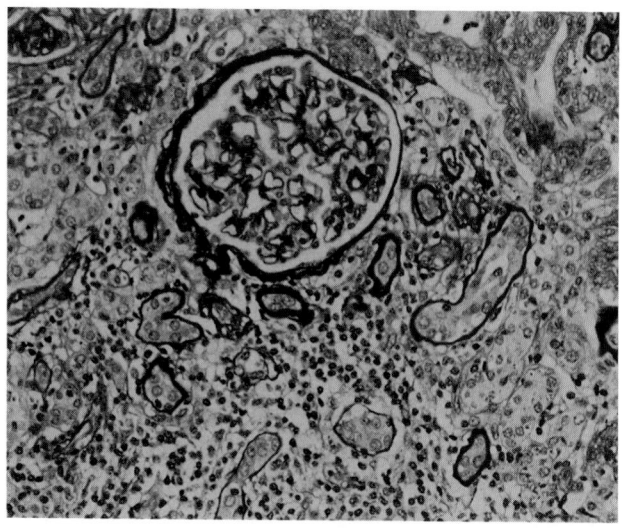

A

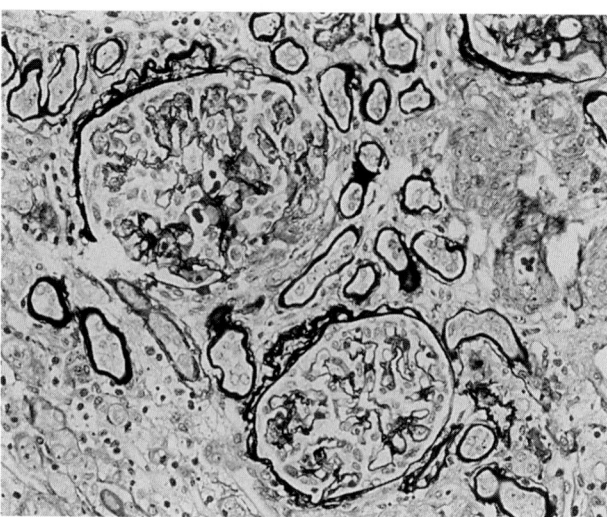

B

FIGURE 46-10. A and **B,** Photomicrographs obtained from a kidney beyond an occlusive renal artery lesion. The glomerular volume is small, with tubular atrophy and interstitial fibrosis with patchy areas of inflammatory cellular infiltrate. (From Textor SC, Wilcox CS: Renal artery stenosis: A common, treatable cause of renal failure? Annu Rev Med 52:421-442, 2001.) See also Color Plate I.

factor (TNF), among others. It must be emphasized that renal ischemia is a potent stimulus for expression of the ET-1 gene in the kidney, which persists for days after resolution of the ischemic injury.[68] Sustained vascular effects of ET may participate in the hypoperfusion, which lasts long beyond the vascular insult to postischemic kidneys.[69]

The kidney is a rich site for production of *prostaglandins* (PGs), which are cyclooxygenase derivatives of arachidonic acid. These materials are produced in arteries, arterioles, and glomeruli in the cortex, where they have important actions to maintain renal blood flow and filtration, particularly under conditions of elevated AII.[70] Enhanced synthesis of prostacyclin (PGI_2) and prostaglandin E_2 (PGE_2) occurs during tissue hypoperfusion and ischemia, which may protect against some forms of hypoxic injury.[71] Conversely, thromboxane A_2 (TXA_2) is a vasoconstrictor prostaglandin

that lowers the glomerular filtration rate (GFR) by reducing renal plasma flow and it can accelerate structural renal damage. It is stimulated by AII production and by production of reactive oxygen species, and may in turn modify hemodynamic actions of AII. TXA_2 modulates ET in actions on vascular permeability[72] which may contribute to interstitial matrix composition and target organ damage. Blockade of TXA_2 receptors thereby can reduce the severity of experimental tissue injury, including acute ischemic damage.[73]

Oxidative stress is a term reflecting an imbalance between tissue oxygen radical–generating systems and radical scavenging systems leading to a shift toward "pro-oxidant" species. This involves the increased presence and toxicity of reactive oxygen species, which in turn can promote the formation of vasoactive mediators, including ET-1, leukotrienes, and $PGF_{2\alpha}$ isoprostanes, which are products of lipid peroxidation. As noted above, these mediators affect renal function and hemodynamics, both by inducing renal vasoconstriction and by changing glomerular capillary ultrafiltration characteristics.[74]

Reactive oxygen species can magnify ischemic renal injury by causing lipid peroxidation of cell and organelle membranes. These disrupt the structural integrity and capacity for cell transport and energy production, particularly within the proximal tubule.[75] Other cytokine pathways, including activation of nuclear factor-κB and growth factors, may play a role.[76]

The role of *transforming growth factor-β* merits emphasis. It belongs to a family of polypeptides which regulate normal cell growth, development, and tissue remodeling after injury.[77] This cytokine is an important fibrogenic factor, which modifies extracellular matrix synthesis by both glomerular and extraglomerular mesenchymal cells. These factors modify both tissue healing and progression to advanced renal failure. TGF-β is essential for tissue repair after many forms of injury, including ischemic injury, during which it participates in restoration of extracellular matrix in proximal tubular basement membranes.[78] However, activation of the angiotensin type 1 (AT_1) receptor stimulates generation of TGF-β which plays a major role in tissue fibrosis[79] through increases in type IV collagen deposition. TGF-β acts synergistically with ET and has interactions with platelet-derived growth factor (PDGF), IL-1, and basic fibroblast growth factor in progressive interstitial fibrosis.[80] Some investigators have proposed that many forms of renal scarring represent an overabundance of TGF-β activity due to failure to suppress its activity after repair of an original injury.[9] Activation of TGF-β develops in experimental models of RAS and is magnified by hypercholesterolemia.[81]

Although whole-kidney oxygen saturation and delivery remain preserved in the poststenotic kidney, it is inescapable that local areas within the kidney likely are exposed to at least *intermittent, recurrent ischemia.* The potential for repetitive acute renal injury to induce long-term irreversible fibrosis is evident from studies of acute heme protein exposure.[82] The hallmark of acute ischemic injury is a rapid decline in cellular adenosine triphosphae (ATP), which in turn allows accumulation of intracellular calcium, activation of phospholipases, and generation of oxygen free radicals.

Tissue ischemia appears to be a common denominator in many forms of tubulointerstitial injury, which is the major prognostic factor in most renal diseases.[51] Such injury is associated commonly with interstitial inflammatory reactions and activation of fibroblasts and heat shock proteins.[83] Injury to the tubular epithelium alters the antigenic profile of these cells, initiating a cell-mediated immune response, sometimes associated with B lymphocyte, T lymphocyte, and macrophage infiltrates.[84] As noted above, sustained tubulointerstitial injury leads to increased TGF-β, enhanced expression of plasminogen activator inhibitor-1 (PAI-1), tissue inhibitor of metalloprotease-1 (TIMP-1), α_1(IV)-collagen, and fibronectin-EIIA, and thus to increased synthesis of extracellular matrix.

Many of the mechanisms mentioned above interact with one another. Taken together, the kidney is subject to a wide variety of vasoactive and inflammatory mediators, which can be disrupted by loss of blood flow and perfusion pressure. These disturbances appear to activate a variety of fibrogenic and local destructive mechanisms, which lead to irreversible parenchymal damage within the kidney.

Consequences of Restoring Renal Blood Flow

As illustrated in Figure 46-9A, restoring renal perfusion can allow recovery of renal function to the extent that these changes remain reversible. At some point, both inflammatory and fibrogenic mechanisms appear to no longer respond with recovery of renal function.

Renal Reperfusion Injury

The course of recovery after restoration of blood supply to an underperfused kidney depends upon the extent and duration of the perfusion injury, in addition to the adequacy of reperfusion.[85] Paradoxically, some tissues subjected to ischemic injury undergo morphologic and functional changes which worsen during the reperfusion phase.[86] This is thought to reflect vascular endothelial injury and activated leukocytes, which may be "primed" to obstruct distal capillaries after restoring perfusion pressure, contributing to a so-called no-reflow phenomenon. Under experimental conditions, reperfusion injury appears to require major degrees of pro-oxidant stress with excess $PGF_{2\alpha}$ isoprostanes and free oxygen radicals, particularly with a deficit of NO.[87] Hence, antioxidants and reactive oxygen metabolite scavengers improve outcomes following experimental reperfusion.[88] Within the kidney, ischemia-reperfusion models are most pronounced in the proximal tubules, with local necrosis and tubular obstruction, as observed in acute tubular necrosis (ATN).

AII may participate in some of these changes as activation of AT_1 receptors impairs glomerular filtration in postischemic kidney.[89] Local imbalance of NO production is particularly prominent within the kidney; it has a dual action with the potential drawback of accelerating reoxygenation injury and initiating lipid peroxidation.[90] However, systemic treatment with NO donors improves renal function and blunts local inflammation before reperfusion in some conditions.[87]

EPIDEMIOLOGY OF RENAL ARTERY STENOSIS

The syndrome of renovascular hypertension can be produced by a wide variety of lesions affecting renal blood flow.

Some of these are listed in Table 46-1. The majority of stenotic lesions consist of "fibromuscular diseases" or atherosclerotic RAS. Of patients with hypertension, previous studies have produced a wide range of estimates as to the prevalence of renovascular hypertension. This range depends heavily upon differences between patient groups studied. In unselected mild to moderate hypertensive populations, the frequency appears to be between 0.6% and 3.0%,[91, 92] whereas in a referral clinic of "elderly" patients, the prevalence may exceed 30%.[93, 94] As noted later, the prevalence of anatomic RAS far exceeds that of renovascular hypertension.

Fibromuscular Disease

Fibromuscular disease (FMD) commonly refers to one of several conditions affecting the intima or fibrous layers of the vessel wall. In some cases multiple layers of the vessel wall may be affected.[95] Reports from arteriograms obtained in "normal" renal organ donors indicate that 3% to 5% of the population may have one of these lesions, many of which are present at an early age and do not affect either renal blood flow or arterial pressure.[96] Such lesions can lead to renovascular hypertension, sometimes associated with dissection or progression. Smoking is a risk factor for disease progression. Medial fibroplasia is the most common subtype, often associated with a "string-of-beads" appearance,[97] as illustrated in Figure 46-11A. Such lesions consist primarily of intravascular "webs," each of which may have only moderate hemodynamic effect. The combination of multiple webs in series, however, can impede blood flow characteristics and activate responses within the kidney to reduced perfusion. FMD lesions have a modest association with dysplastic lesions in other vascular beds, most commonly the carotid artery.[98, 99] The large preponderance of hypertensive cases coming to vascular intervention occur in women, with a bias toward the right renal artery.[96, 100] FMD lesions are classically located away from the origin of the renal artery, often in the midportion of the vessel or at the first arterial bifurcation. Some of these expand to develop small vascular aneurysms. Although less common, other dysplastic lesions, particularly intimal hyperplasia, can progress and lead to renal ischemia and atrophy.[101] Although these are considered commonly a disorder of younger women, they can present at older ages, sometimes combined with atherosclerotic lesions, which magnify the hemodynamic effects. Whereas previous estimates derived from hypertension referral clinics suggested that 25% of patients with renovascular hypertension may have FMD,[102] more recent studies suggest that current rates may be closer to 16%.[103]

Atherosclerosis

Atherosclerosis affecting the renal arteries is the most common renovascular lesion, constituting 75% to 84% of interventional series in recent years. Atherosclerotic renal artery stenosis (ARAS) can be identified commonly with vascular disease affecting other vascular beds.[104] Recent studies in patients undergoing coronary angiography indicate that 19% to 20% have ARAS with greater than 50% narrowing of the renal artery lumen.[17, 105-107] Aortograms obtained in patients with peripheral vascular disease indicate that 30% to 50% of such patients have renal artery lesions of some degree.[108, 109]

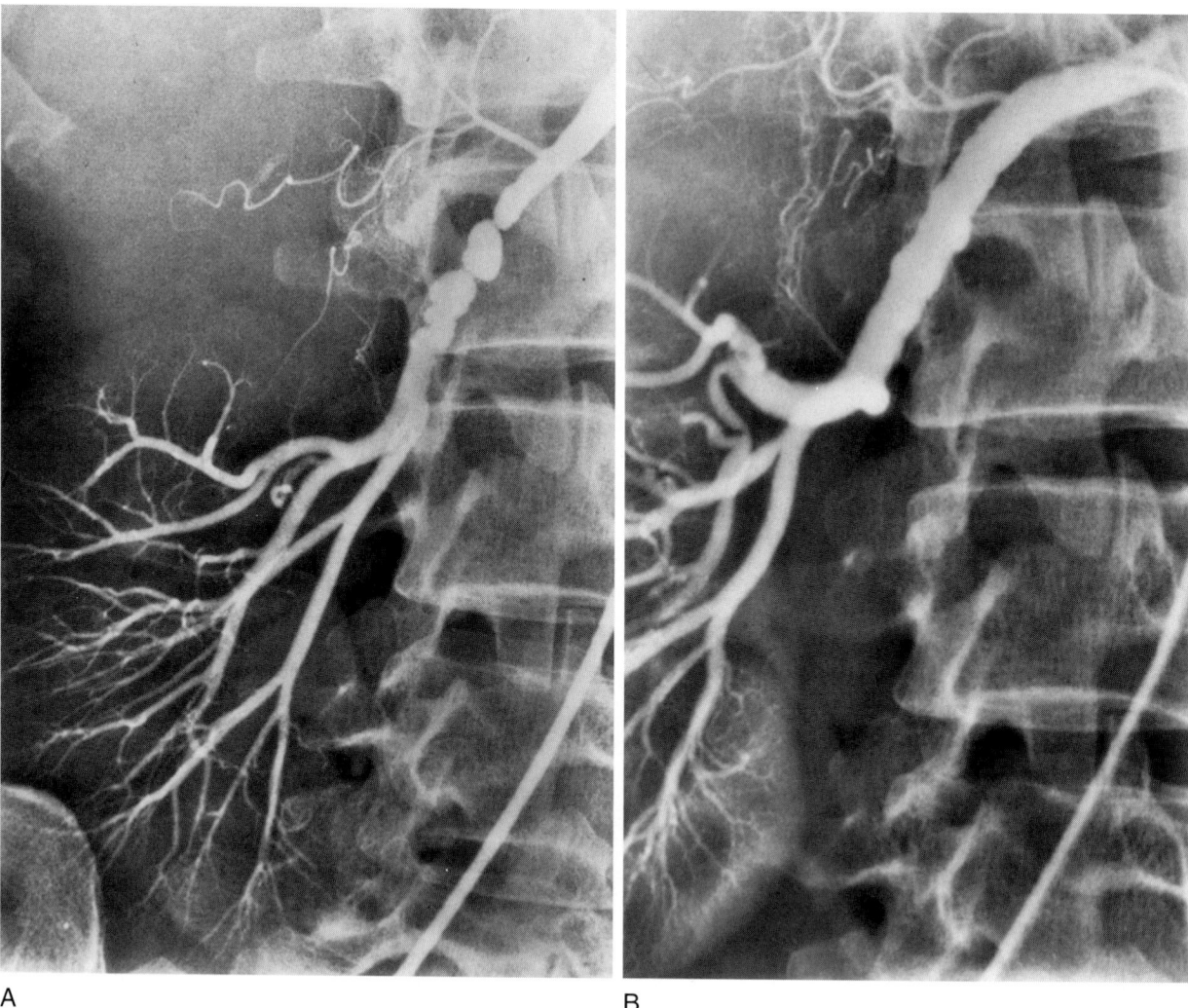

A   B

FIGURE 46-11. **A** and **B**, Angiographic appearance of medial fibroplasia with serial intravascular webs with small aneurysmal dilations between them. These lesions appear in the midportion of the vessel, have strong predilection for the right renal artery, and are most commonly found in women. As shown in **B**, these lesions can often be improved substantially by effective balloon angioplasty.

Table 46-2 summarizes several reports related to the coexistence of atherosclerotic lesions in various vascular territories. The prevalence of such lesions increases with age and with the presence of atherosclerotic risk factors such as elevated cholesterol, smoking, and hypertension.[110] Recent studies indicate that the probability of identifying high-grade RAS in hypertensive patients with azotemia rises from 3.2% in the sixth decade to above 25% in the eighth decade.[111] These figures confirm previous postmortem observations indicating that many patients dying of cardiovascular disease have renal artery lesions at autopsy.[112] The above data underscore the fact that many renal artery lesions remain undetected on clinical grounds (see later).

The location of atherosclerotic disease is most often at the origin of the artery (Fig. 46-12A), although it can be observed anywhere. Many such lesions represent a direct extension of an aortic plaque into the renal arterial segment. It should be emphasized that ARAS is strongly associated with preexisting hypertension, cardiovascular lipid risk, diabetes, smoking, and abnormal renal function.[17, 113]

TABLE 46-2

Prevalence Rates of Atherosclerotic Renal Artery Stenosis in Patients with Vascular Disease Affecting Other Regional Beds Identified by Angiography

STUDY	NO. WITH CAD	RENAL ARTERY STENOSIS (>50%)
Vetrovec et al.[107]	76	22 (29%)
Harding et al.[105]	817	164 (20%)
Rihal et al.[106]	297	57 (19.2%)
	NO. WITH PVD	
Choudhri et al.[109]	100	42 (42%)
Wilms et al.[316]	100	22 (22%)
Olin et al.[110]	318	122 (38%)
Salmon	374	52 (14%)
Swartbol et al.[108]	450	104 (23%)

CAD, coronary artery disease; PVD, peripheral vascular disease.

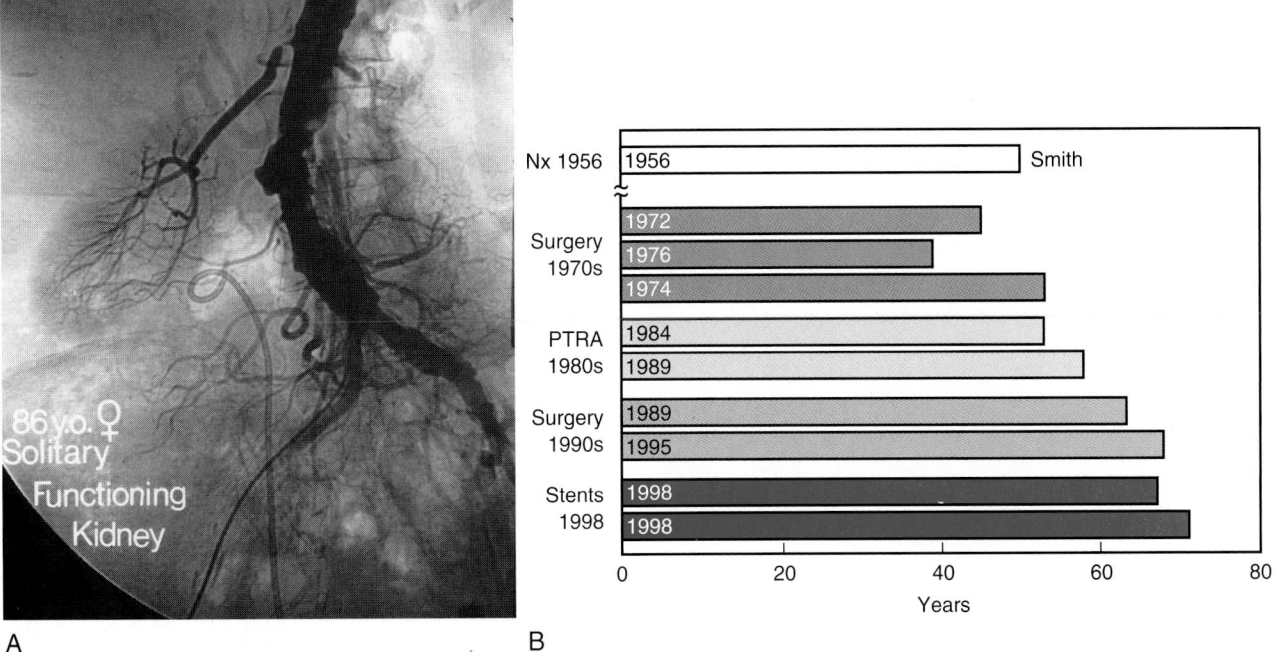

FIGURE 46-12. A, Atherosclerotic disease affecting the abdominal aorta first presenting in an 86-year-old woman. The left renal artery is totally occluded and the right kidney has a tight lesion located at the origin. The aorta has extensive atherosclerotic disease and areas of aneurysmal dilation. This patient presented during acceleration of previously treated hypertension with a cerebral hemorrhage. **B,** Mean age levels from selected interventional series for renovascular disease from the 1950s through the 1990s. This age has increased from age 50 years in the early surgical literature to older than 70 years in recent series with stent-supported angioplasty. Accordingly, management of such patients must factor in comorbid disease risk and the determination of risk-benefit considerations differently in older patients.

CLINICAL FEATURES OF RENOVASCULAR HYPERTENSION

This section examines the demographic and clinical presentation of RAS, primarily as caused by atherosclerotic disease. It emphasizes the role of changing population demographics within the United States, newer antihypertensive agents, and the expanding use of agents which block the renin-angiotensin system for indications other than hypertension. These factors are changing fundamentally the populations at risk for being adversely affected by renal arterial disease and its clinical manifestations. "Uncontrollable" hypertension now is less commonly the main reason for considering renal revascularization. Rather, the hazards of underperfusion to kidney tissue leading to irreversible renal failure have led many to consider revascularization for "preservation" of renal function. Most importantly, it must be emphasized that long-term clinical outcomes in such patients commonly are determined by other disease entities (termed "competing risk") which may have important implications for decisions concerning invasive therapy.[114] The importance of timing of therapy and the evolution of vascular disease over time cannot be overstated.

Fibromuscular Disease versus Atherosclerosis

As noted earlier, renovascular hypertension may develop as a result of many lesions (see Table 46-1). The two most common are the FMDs and atherosclerosis. It must be emphasized that FMDs of the renal artery differ from atherosclerotic diseases in many respects. FMD represents several types of intimal or medial disorders of the vessel wall, commonly affecting midportions of the renal artery in younger persons. These lesions rarely lead to major renal functional loss, although some progression may be seen, particularly in smokers. These lesions appear most often as hypertension of early onset (<30 years of age) and unusual severity. Occasionally, they present as one cause of hypertension during pregnancy. Many lesions respond well to percutaneous angioplasty[115] (see Fig. 46-9B). By contrast, atherosclerotic lesions more commonly arise near the origin of the renal artery and are related to a systemic disorder predisposing to atherosclerosis elsewhere.

As a result, one of the major current controversies in cardiovascular disease is how to identify and monitor clinically significant RAS. This controversy is compounded by changes produced by (1) evolving medical therapy and (2) changing population characteristics.

The Role of Changing Antihypertensive Therapy

Prior to the 1980s, the literature of renovascular disease concerned primarily identification of functionally important lesions in patients with severe hypertension. Drug therapy was limited in scope and often produced poorly tolerated side effects. Most importantly, the range of available drugs failed to include agents capable of interrupting the renin-angiotensin system. As a result, patients commonly appeared with accelerated or malignant hypertension, a large fraction of which was related to RAS. Among 123 patients whose average age was 44 years presenting with accelerated hypertension, more than 30% of whites were identified as having renovascular hypertension.[116] Some patients were reported during this period for whom "urgent" bilateral nephrectomy was undertaken as a lifesaving measure for "untreatable" hypertension.[117] Hence, the evaluation of RAS centered upon identifying those patients whose blood pressures could be improved, perhaps "cured," by renal revascularization.[15, 118]

Since the early 1980s, several new classes of antihypertensive agents have become available and widely used. These include calcium channel blockers and, most important, drugs which functionally block the renin-angiotensin system, such as ACE inhibitors and angiotensin receptor blockers (ARBs). The impact of these agents cannot be overstated. Reviews of medical therapy for renovascular hypertension indicate that regimens using these agents increased the likelihood of achieving good blood pressure control from 46% to more than 90%.[119-121] The concept of emergency bilateral nephrectomy for control of hypertension has almost disappeared. Most important, it is likely that many, if not most, patients with renovascular disease and hypertension now go undetected because blood pressure and renal function are well controlled and stable.[106] This may be happening even more frequently than before with the expansion of use of ACE inhibitors for other reasons, including congestive cardiac failure, proteinuric renal disease, and other constellations of cardiovascular risk factors, particularly since the publication of the Heart Outcomes Prevention Evaluation, (HOPE) trial.[122, 123] Treatment with ACE inhibitors improves survival related to cardiovascular events in patients with renovascular disease, as it does in other conditions.[124] Whether the use of ACE inhibitors or ARBs or both delays the onset of renovascular hypertension in humans, as it does in experimental animals, cannot be established with present data.

Changing Population Demographics

The last several decades have been characterized by longer life spans in many Western countries. This is likely the result of several factors, including major declines in mortality related to stroke and cardiovascular disease. The population group above age 65 years is now the most rapidly growing segment in the United States.[125] One consequence of lower mortality from coronary and cerebrovascular events is the delayed appearance of vascular disease affecting other beds, such as the aorta and kidneys.[126] As a result, clinical manifestations of RAS are appearing in older people, often combined with other comorbid diseases.[127] These features change the clinical presentation (see later) in many respects and may affect the risk-benefit considerations inherent in deciding whether to consider renal revascularization. Series with renal artery intervention now routinely include average age values between 68 and 71 years old, whereas a decade ago the mean age was between 61 and 63 years.[128, 129] These mean values are more than 15 years older than those of the 1960s and 1970s[14, 130] (see Fig. 46-12A and B). As might be expected, the prevalence of advanced coronary disease, congestive heart failure, previous stroke or transient ischemic attack, and aortic disease, as well as impaired renal function, is rising in patients with atherosclerotic renal artery disease.[131]

Clinical Presentation of Renal Artery Stenosis

Manifestations of renal artery disease vary widely across a spectrum illustrated in Figure 46-1 and Table 46-3. As noted earlier this spectrum may range from a purely *incidental finding noted during angiography* for other indications to advancing renal failure leading to the need for dialytic support. As described earlier, multiple mechanisms raise systemic arterial pressure and tend to restore renal perfusion pressures to levels close to baseline.[5, 20, 55, 132] Clinical features of patients with essential hypertension compared with those in patients subjected to revascularization for renovascular hypertension in the cooperative study in the 1960s are summarized in Table 46-3. Many features, including duration of hypertension, age of onset, fundoscopic findings, hypokalemia, and so on, were more common in those with renovascular hypertension, but had limited discriminating or predictive value.[133]

If renal artery lesions progress to critical stenosis, they can produce a *rapidly developing form of hypertension,* which may be severe and associated with polydipsia, hyponatremia, and central nervous system findings.[134, 135] Such cases are most often seen with acute renovascular events, such as sudden occlusion of a renal artery or branch vessel.

More commonly, RAS presents as a progressive *worsening of preexisting hypertension,* often with a modest rise in serum creatinine. Since the prevalence of both hypertension and atherosclerosis rises with age, this disorder must be considered, particularly in older patients with progression of blood

TABLE 46-3

Clinical Features of Patients with Renovascular Hypertension[*]

CLINICAL FEATURE	ESSENTIAL HYPERTENSION (%)	RENOVASCULAR HYPERTENSION (%)
Duration <1 yr	12	24
Age of onset >50 yr	9	15
Family history of hypertension	71	46
Grade 3 or 4 fundi	7	15
Abdominal bruit	9	46
Blood urea nitrogen >20 mg/dL	8	16
Potassium <3.4 mEq/L	8	16
Urinary casts	9	20
Proteinuria	32	46

Syndromes Associated with Renovascular Hypertension[†]

1. Early- or late-onset hypertension (<30 yr/>50 yr)
2. Acceleration of treated essential hypertension
3. Deterioration of renal function in treated essential hypertension
4. Acute renal failure during treatment of hypertension
5. "Flash" pulmonary edema
6. Progressive renal failure

[*]Clinical features that differed (*P* < .05) between closely matched groups of 131 patients with essential and renovascular hypertension are from Simon N, Franklin SS, Bleifer KH, Maxwell MH: Clinical characteristics of renovascular hypertension. JAMA 220:1209-1218, 1972. These observations underscore the potential severity of hypertension in candidates for surgery, but none of these features allows clinical discrimination with confidence (see text).

[†]The "syndromes" should alert the clinician to the possible contribution of renovascular disease in a given patient. The bottom three are most common in patients with bilateral disease, many of whom are treated as "essential hypertension" until these characteristics appear (see text). (From Textor SC: Renovascular hypertension. Endocrinol Metab Clin North Am 23:235-253, 1994.)

pressure elevation. As patients continue to age, some of the most striking examples of renovascular hypertension are those in whom previously well-controlled hypertension has deteriorated to an accelerated rise in systolic blood pressure and target injury, such as stroke. Studies from hypertension referral centers in the Netherlands are instructive in this regard. Of 477 patients undergoing detailed evaluation for RAS because of "treatment resistance," 107 (22.4%) were identified with renovascular disease (>50% stenosis by angiography). Clinical features predictive of RAS included older age, recent progression, other vascular disease (e.g., claudication), an abdominal bruit, and elevated serum creatinine. The authors derived a multivariate regression equation of predictive features for the presence of angiographic RAS. They presented a clinical scoring system to determine the pretest probability of identifying renal artery disease (Fig. 46-13).[103] The strongest predictors include age and serum creatinine. Of note is the fact that clinical features alone could provide pretest predictive value nearly as accurate as radionuclide scans.[103]

Declining renal function during antihypertensive therapy is a common manifestation of progressive renal arterial disease. It is recognized that beyond levels of critical stenosis, blood flow and perfusion pressures to the kidney fall.[136] This can be magnified by a reduction in systemic arterial pressure by any antihypertensive regimen.[137] This phenomenon has become particularly common since the introduction of ACE inhibitors, and more recently with ARBs. A sudden rise in serum creatinine soon after starting these agents may occur due to a loss of transcapillary filtration pressure produced by removing the efferent arteriolar vasoconstrictive effects of AII.[138, 139] This particular "functional" loss of GFR is reversible if detected promptly and should lead the clinician to exclude large vessel vascular disease when it occurs. As may be expected, detectable changes in serum creatinine develop mainly when the entire renal mass is affected, such as with bilateral RAS or stenosis to a solitary functioning kidney.

Other syndromes heralding occult RAS are becoming more commonly recognized. Among the most important are rapidly developing episodes of circulatory congestion (so-called *flash pulmonary edema*).[140, 141] This usually arises in patients with hypertension and with left ventricular systolic function that may be well preserved. Underlying arterial compromise may favor volume retention and resistance to diuretics in such cases. A rapid rise in arterial pressure impairs cardiac function due to rapidly developing diastolic dysfunction. Such episodes tend to be rapid both in onset and in resolution.[142, 143] A similar sequence of events may produce symptoms of crescendo angina from otherwise stable coronary disease.[144] When the role of RAS is identified, renal revascularization can prevent its recurrence.[145, 146]

Another clinical presentation of RAS is *advanced renal failure*, occasionally at end stage requiring renal replacement therapy. This manifestation has received much attention during the past decade, particularly because it raises the

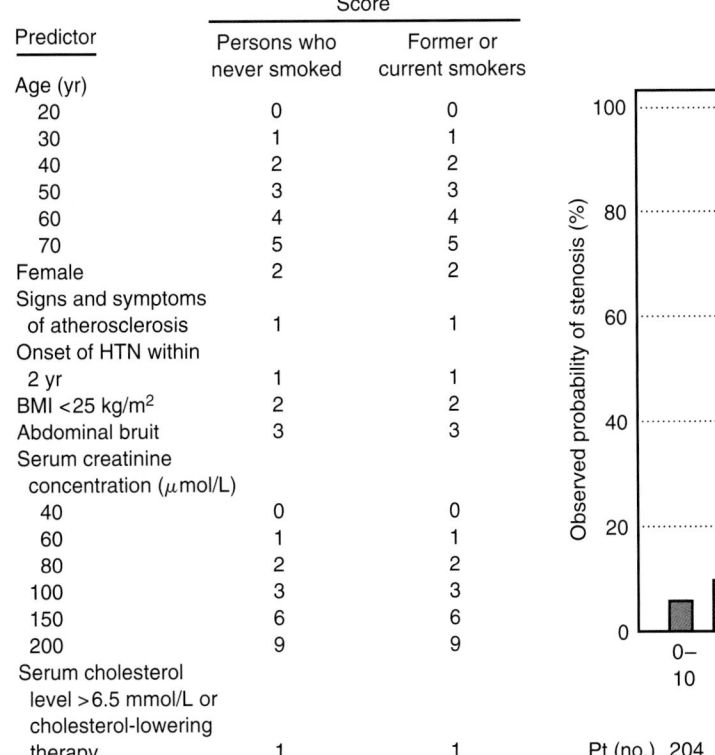
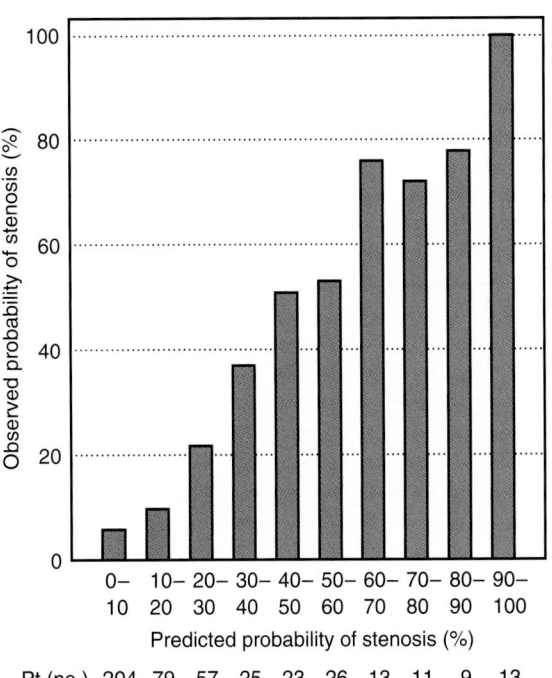

FIGURE 46-13. Probability of identifying renal artery stenosis based upon clinical features. These data were obtained from 477 patients in referral centers for treatment-resistant hypertension in the Netherlands. The overall prevalence was 22.4%, illustrating that even in "enriched" patient populations, renovascular disease is not the most common cause of resistant hypertension. Clinical features allowed selection of patients for testing with relatively high "pretest probability" of disease, which affects the validity of testing schemes. (From Krijnen P, van Jaarsveld BC, Steyerberg EW, et al: A clinical prediction rule for renal artery stenosis. Ann Intern Med 129:705-711, 1998.)

possibility of an undetected, potentially reversible, form of chronic renal failure. As discussed earlier, this is designated by some as "ischemic nephropathy" or "azotemic renovascular disease"[147, 148] and is defined as loss of renal function beyond an arterial stenosis due to impaired renal blood flow.[149] Studies in patients with bilateral RAS indicate that reduction of systemic pressures to normal levels using sodium nitroprusside can abruptly reduce both renal plasma flow and the GFR, indicating that the poststenotic pressures are at critical levels beyond autoregulation (see Fig. 46-8).[136] Some estimates indicate that between 12% and 14% of patients reaching end-stage renal disease (ESRD) with no other identifiable primary renal disease may have occult, bilateral RAS.[127, 150] Patients with vascular lesions affecting the entire renal mass primarily are at risk for losing kidney function on this basis. The role of vascular impairment in producing renal dysfunction is established most firmly when renal revascularization leads to restoration of renal function.[151] Unfortunately, this does not occur commonly, as we have reviewed.[1] Patients with advanced renal dysfunction have high comorbid disease risks associated with cardiovascular disease and commonly have interstitial renal injury on biopsy.[152, 153] Radionuclide studies in patients with atherosclerotic disease commonly identify reduced function unrelated to the presence of stenosis.[154] Those with declining renal function have a poor survival rate regardless of intervention, the strongest predictor of which is a low baseline GFR.[142, 155, 156] Recent attempts to quantitate the prevalence of "ischemic nephropathy" as a cause of ESRD in the United States produce figures rising from 1.4% of new cases in 1991 to 2.1% in 1997. Multivariate analysis indicated that male sex and advancing age correlated positively with this disorder, whereas African ancestry and Asian or Native American background correlated negatively.[157]

The likely benefit of revascularization regarding salvage, or at least stabilization, of renal function is greatest at low levels of azotemia, so this diagnosis is best considered early in its course. Remarkably, RAS can be associated with *proteinuria*, occasionally to nephrotic levels.[158-160] Such proteinuria can diminish or resolve entirely following renal revascularization,[161] leading to the speculation that intrarenal hemodynamic changes or stimulation of local hormonal or cytokine activity alter glomerular membrane permeability in a reversible fashion. Although other glomerular diseases can develop in patients with renal artery disease, including diabetic nephropathy and focal sclerosing glomerulonephritis (FSGN),[162] the presence of proteinuria alone does not establish a second disorder.

Clinical manifestations and prognosis differ when renovascular disease affects one of two kidneys or affects the entire functioning renal mass. Although blood pressure levels may be similar, response to renal revascularization leads to a greater fall in bilateral disease.[163] Most patients with episodic pulmonary edema have bilateral disease or a solitary kidney. Long-term mortality during follow-up is higher when bilateral disease is present, regardless of whether renal revascularization is undertaken.[164] The latter authors argue that the extent and severity of renovascular disease reflects the overall atherosclerotic burden of the individual. Our observations in patients with incidental RAS (>75%) managed without revascularization reemphasize the reduced survival with bilateral disease, despite reasonable blood pressure control, as illustrated in Figure 46-14. The causes of death were mainly related to cardiovascular disease, including stroke and congestive heart failure.

Progressive Vascular Occlusion

Atherosclerosis is a progressive disorder. The clinical manifestations of RAS depend upon the severity and extent of the vascular occlusion. The most ominous of these manifestations, for example, renal failure or pulmonary edema, are related to bilateral disease or stenosis to a solitary functioning kidney and pose the greatest hazard when total arterial occlusion develops. Hence, the impetus to intervene in RAS depends in many cases upon predicting, or establishing, the "natural history" of vascular stenosis within an individual. Retrospective studies of serial angiograms obtained in the 1970s and early 1980s indicated that atherosclerotic lesions progressed to more severe levels in 44% to 63% of patients followed from 2 to 5 years.[104, 165-167] Up to 16% of renal arteries developed total occlusion. More recent prospective studies, either in patients undergoing cardiac catheterization or serial Doppler ultrasound measurements, suggest that current rates of progression may be lower. Zierler and colleagues reported a 20% overall rate of disease progression, with 7% advancing to total occlusion over 3 years.[168] A later report from the same group using different Doppler velocity criteria

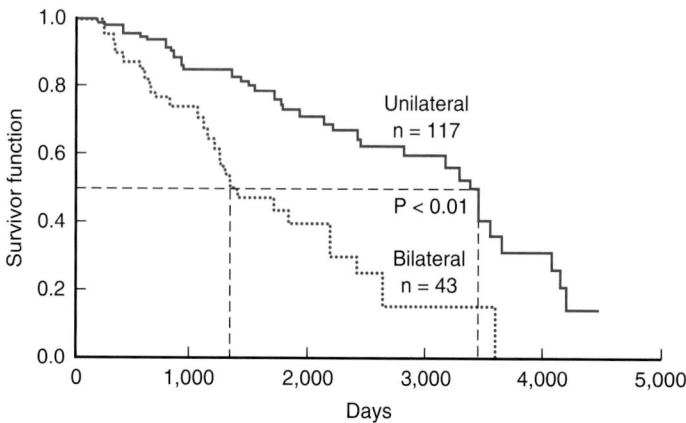

FIGURE 46-14. Kaplan-Meier survival curve of 160 patients managed without renal revascularization. Those with bilateral disease had lower survival, primarily from cardiovascular events. The mean age of patients dying was 79 years. (Data from references 176 and 251.)

suggested higher rates of progressive stenosis. Overall progression was detectable in 31%, but primarily those with the most severe baseline stenosis (>60%) and severe hypertension were more likely to progress (49%) (Fig. 46-15). The occurrence of total occlusion was rare (9/295 or 3%).[169] Data from medical treatment trials suggest that progressive occlusion can develop silently in up to 16% of treated patients.[170]

Importantly, clinical events such as detectable changes in renal fucntion or accelerating hypertension bear only a limited relationship to vascular progression. The occurrence of renal "atrophy" (loss in renal size of 1 cm or more by ultrasound) developed in 20.8% of the most severe lesions in the prospective series.[171] Most series of medically treated patients indicate that despite evident progression of vascular disease, changes in kidney function are modest. Results reported during medical follow-up of 41 patients managed medically, before the introduction of ACE inhibitors, for an average of 36 months identified a loss of renal length in 35%, while a significant rise in serum creatinine developed in 8 of 41 (19.5%) patients.[172] The results of 160 patients with high-grade (>70%) stenosis identified incidentally and managed without revascularization are summarized in Table 46-4. These patients were followed for many years and are divided into cohorts spanning the introduction of ACE inhibitors into clinical practice. Blood pressure control improved during these intervals. Medical management was associated with increased requirements for antihypertensive agents. The number developing clinical progression with refractory hypertension or progressive renal insufficiency fell from 21% in 1980-1984 to less than 10% in the most recent cohort. This conclusion is consistent with recent long-term studies from Europe in which incidental renal artery lesions were not associated with ESRD after more than 9 years of follow-up.[173] These data support the observation that renal artery lesions can remain stable in some patients over many years without adverse clinical effects or evident progression.[174-176] Whether the apparent lower rates of vascular disease progression in recent studies indicate a true change or differences

in study methodology is not yet certain. However, it may be argued that overall rates of atherosclerotic disease progression likely will change with the more widespread use of "statin"-class drugs, aspirin, diminishing tobacco use, and more intense antihypertensive therapy. Hence, progressive vascular occlusion is an important clinical risk but does not occur in all patients.

The Role of Concurrent Diseases

Atherosclerotic RAS rarely occurs as an isolated entity. It is a manifestation of atherosclerotic disease, which ordinarily affects multiple other sites. Follow-up studies related to survival of "incidentally" identified renal arterial disease suggest that the presence of RAS independently predicts mortality, particularly in the presence of elevated serum creatinine.[177] It bears emphasis that the mortality risk of a serum creatinine level above 1.4 mg/dL (but <2.3 mg/dL) for any reason is higher than the risk with normal creatinine levels.[123] The major causes of death are cardiovascular events, including congestive cardiac failure, stroke, and myocardial infarction. It is essential to consider the role of these "competing risks" in planning management of patients with all forms of vascular disease, especially the elderly.[114] These disorders often dominate the clinical outcomes of patients with renal arterial disease, independent of the level of renal function. As one result, it has been difficult to establish improved survival in prospective trials of patients treated with either medical therapy or renal revascularization. While many patients experience more easily controlled blood pressure and some recover renal function, current methods of revascularization are not free of risks. Even after successful renovascular procedures, other comorbid events may obscure long-term benefit, leading some to challenge the cost-effectiveness of renal revascularization.[178, 179] Conversely, others argue that RAS accelerates the cardiovascular risk by increasing arterial pressures, predisposing to both congestive heart failure and renal dysfunction. Hence, they argue

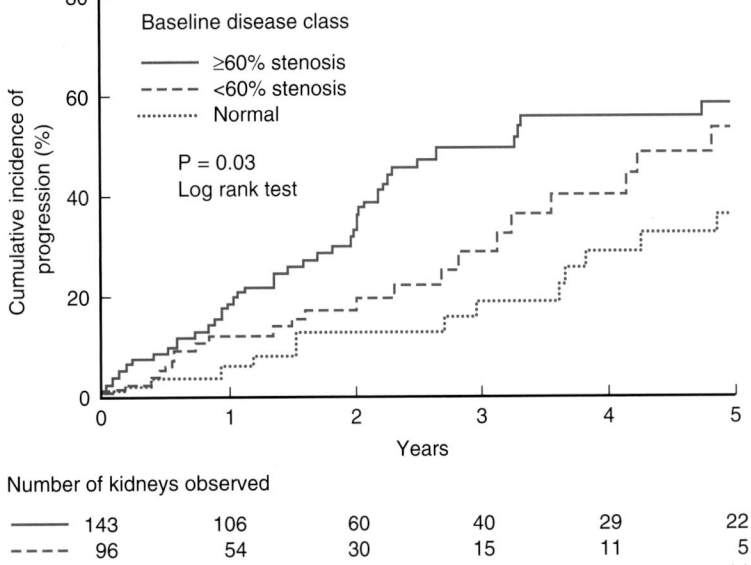

FIGURE 46-15. Cumulative rates of disease progression in atherosclerotic renal artery stenosis, as measured by renal artery Doppler ultrasound. During a follow-up period of 5 years, overall progression was 31%, but those with the most severe baseline lesions progressed in nearly 50% of cases. The progression of vascular disease was not closely related to change in serum creatinine or renal atrophy (see text).

Number of kidneys observed

143	106	60	40	29	22
96	54	30	15	11	5
56	45	36	29	21	14

TABLE 46-4

Incidental Renal Artery Stenosis: Medical Management 1980-1993*

	1980-1984	1985-1989	1990-1994
No.	34	57	69
Age	69.3	70.3	71.5
Mean follow-up (mo)	58	54	35
Blood pressure (mm Hg)			
Initial	172/91	163/88	155/81‡
Last follow-up	163/83†	160/84	154/79
Creatinine (mg/dL)			
Initial	1.6	1.6	1.4
Last follow-up	2.0†	2.1*	2.0*
Renal failure§ (%)	2.9	5.3	7.2
Antihypertensive drugs at follow-up	2.5	2.0	2.1
Angiotensin-converting enzyme inhibitors (%) (initial)		21	41‡,ǁ
Subsequent revascularization (%)	20.6	14	5.7(a)

*These cohorts bridged the period of introduction of angiotensin-converting enzyme inhibitors in treatment of hypertension, during which use rose from 0% to 40.6% of patients. Blood pressures achieved improved during this interval and the number of patients referred for revascularization due to refractory hypertension or progressive renal insufficiency fell from 20.6% to less than 10% over several years of follow-up. Such observations underscore the fact that some patients can be managed medically without adverse effects for many years.

†$P < .01$ at last follow-up vs. initial follow-up.

‡$P < .05$ vs. 1980-1984.

§Creatinine rise ≥50%.

ǁ$P < .05$ vs. 1985-1989.

Data from Chabova V, Schirger A, Stanson AW, et al: Outcomes of atherosclerotic renal artery stenosis managed without revascularization. Mayo Clin Proc 75:437-444, 2000; and Chabova V, Schirger A, Stanson A, Textor SC: Management of renal artery stenosis without revascularization since the introduction of ACE inhibitors [abstract]. J Am Soc Nephrol 10:362A, 1999.

that restoration of renal perfusion should be considered at an early stage.[180] There is a need for a larger prospective evaluation of this proposition in a group of patients stratified by comorbid risk to answer the issues at hand.

DIAGNOSTIC TESTING FOR RENOVASCULAR HYPERTENSION AND ISCHEMIC NEPHROPATHY

Goals of Evaluation

The literature related to the diagnostic evaluation of renovascular hypertension is complex and inconsistent. Some of the confusion likely reflects the widely different patient groups being considered for evaluation and the divergent goals for intervention. It behooves the clinician to identify carefully the objectives when embarking upon a path of sometimes ambiguous and expensive studies (Table 46-5). As with all tests, the reliability and value of diagnostic studies depend heavily on the pretest probability of disease.[181-183] Furthermore, it is essential to consider from the outset exactly what is to be achieved. Is the major goal to exclude high-grade renal artery disease? Is it to exclude bilateral (as opposed to unilateral) disease? Is it to identify stenosis and estimate the potential for clinical benefit from renal revascularization? Is it to evaluate the role of renovascular disease in explaining deteriorating renal function? The specific approach to diagnosis will differ depending upon which of these is the predominant clinical issue.

Noninvasive diagnostic tests for renovascular hypertension and ischemic nephropathy remain imperfect. For the purposes of this discussion, diagnostic tests fall into three general categories (Table 46-6): (1) physiologic and functional studies to evaluate the role of stenotic lesions particularly related to activation of the renin-angiotensin system, (2) perfusion and imaging studies to identify the presence and degree of vascular stenosis, and (3) studies to predict the likelihood of benefit from invasive maneuvers, including renal revascularization.

Physiologic and Functional Studies of the Renin-Angiotensin System

For more than 30 years, efforts have been made to establish the level of activation of the renin-angiotensin system as a marker for underlying renovascular hypertension.[184] Peripheral plasma renin activity conducted under standardized conditions of sodium intake (renin-sodium profiling) and the response of renin to administration of an ACE inhibitor such as captopril have been proposed.[185] While these studies are promising when examined in patients with known renovascular hypertension, they have lower performance as diagnostic tests when applied to wider populations, as we and others have reviewed.[186, 187] In a series of 31 patients studied prior to percutaneous transluminal renal angioplasty (PTRA), combined mathematical models to predict the clinical results indicate a sensitivity of 36% and accuracy of 43%, too low to be used as a major determinant in decision making.[186] Plasma renin activity is sensitive to changes in sodium intake, volume status, renal function, and many medications. The predictive value of such maneuvers is heavily dependent upon the a priori probability of renovascular hypertension.[188] In practice, the major utility of these studies depends upon

TABLE 46-5

Goals of Diagnostic Evaluation and Therapeutic Intervention in Renovascular Hypertension and Ischemic Nephropathy

Goals of Diagnostic Evaluation

Establish presence of renal artery stenosis: location and type of lesion
Establish whether unilateral or bilateral stenosis (or stenosis to a solitary kidney) is present
Establish presence and function of stenotic and nonstenotic kidneys
Establish hemodynamic severity of renal arterial disease
Plan vascular intervention: degree and location of atherosclerotic disease

Goals of Therapy

I. Improved Blood Pressure Control:
   Prevent morbidity and mortality of high blood pressure
   Improve blood pressure control and reduce medication requirement
II. Preservation of Renal Function
   Reduce risk of renal-adverse perfusion from use of antihypertensive agents
   Reduce episodes of circulatory congestion ("flash" pulmonary edema)
   Reduce risk of progressive vascular occlusion causing loss of renal function: "preservation of renal function"
   Salvage renal function; i.e., recover glomerular filtration rate

their negative predictive value, that is, the certainty with which one can exclude significant renovascular disease if the test is negative. Since the negative predictive value rarely exceeds 60% to 70%, these tests offer limited value in clinical decision making.

Measurement of renal vein levels has been widely applied in planning surgical revascularization. These measurements are obtained by sampling renal vein and inferior vena cava blood individually. The level of the vena cava is taken as comparable to the arterial levels in each kidney and allows estimation of the contribution of each kidney to total circulating levels of plasma renin activity.[189] Lateralization is defined usually as a ratio exceeding 1.5 between the renin activity of the stenotic kidney and the nonstenotic kidney.[190] Some authors propose detailed examination not only of the relative ratio between kidneys but the degree of suppression of renin release from the nonstenotic or contralateral kidney.[189] In general, the greater the degree of lateralization, the more probable that clinical blood pressure benefit will accrue from surgical or other revascularization. Results from many studies support the observation that large differences between kidneys identify high-grade RAS.[92, 190, 191] As with many tests of hormonal activation, study conditions are crucial. A number of measures to enhance renin release and magnify differences between kidneys have been proposed, including sodium depletion with diuretic administration, hydralazine, tilt-table stimulation, or captopril.[188] Strong and colleagues demonstrated that nonlateralization can be changed to lateralizing measurements by administration of diuretics between sequential studies.[192] A review of more than 50 studies of renal vein renin measurements indicated that when lateralization could be demonstrated, clinical benefit regarding blood pressure control could be expected in more than 90% of patients.[190] Failure to demonstrate lateralization, however, still was associated with significant benefit in more than 50% of patients.[188] More recent series reached similar conclusions, indicating that the overall sensitivity of renal vein

renin measurements was no better than 65% and that the positive predictive value was 18.5%.[193] For many reasons, renal vein assays are performed less often than before. A major factor is that the goals of renal revascularization have shifted substantially and are often directed toward preservation of renal function, rather than blood pressure control per se. In patients in whom it is important to establish the degree of pressor effect of a specific kidney or site, such as before considering nephrectomy of a pressor kidney, measurement of renal vein renins can provide strong supportive evidence.

Studies of Individual Renal Function

Serum creatinine, iothalamate clearance, and other estimates of the GFR are measures of total renal excretory function and do not address changes within each kidney. They may be influenced by numerous factors, including body mass, protein intake, and age. A large body of literature addresses the potential for individual split renal function studies to establish the functional importance of each kidney in renovascular disease.

Split renal function studies utilize separate ureteral catheters to allow individual urine collection for measurement of separate GFR, renal blood flow, sodium excretion, concentrating ability, and the response to blockade of AII.[29, 194, 195] These studies demonstrate that the hemodynamic effects of renal artery lesions translate directly into functional changes, such as avid sodium retention, before major changes in blood flow occur. They emphasize that autoregulation of blood flow and GFR can occur over a wide range of pressures in humans and may be affected in both stenotic and contralateral kidneys by the effects of AII.[195, 196] These studies require urinary tract instrumentation and provide only indirect information regarding the probability of benefit from revascularization. They are now rarely performed.

Separate renal functional measurements now can be obtained less invasively with radionuclide techniques. These methods use a variety of radioisotopes (e.g., technetium Tc 99m mertiatide or technetium Tc 99m pentetate) to estimate fractional blood flow and filtration to each kidney. Administration of captopril beforehand magnifies differences between kidneys, primarily by delaying excretion of the filtered isotope due to removal of the efferent arteriolar effects of ACE inhibition. Some authors rely upon such measurements to follow progressive renal artery disease and its effect on unilateral kidney function as a guide to consider revascularization.[187, 197] Some authors indicate that serial measurement of individual renal function by radionuclide studies allows more precise identification of progressive ischemic injury to the affected kidney in unilateral renal artery disease than can be determined from the overall GFR.[187, 198]

Noninvasive Imaging and Assessment of the Renal Vasculature

Advances in Doppler ultrasound, radionuclide imaging, magnetic resonance arteriography (MRA), and computed tomographic (CT) angiography continue to introduce major changes in the field of renovascular imaging. The details of these methods are beyond the scope of this discussion.

TABLE 46-6

Noninvasive Assessment of Renal Artery Stenosis

STUDY	RATIONALE	STRENGTHS	LIMITATIONS
Physiologic studies to assess the renin-angiotensin system			
Measurement of peripheral plasma renin activity	Reflects the adequacy of sodium excretion	Measures level of activation of renin-angiotensin system	Low predictive accuracy for renovascular hypertension; results influenced by medications and many other conditions
Measurement of captopril-stimulated renin activity	Produces a fall in pressure distal to the stenosis	Enhances release of renin from stenotic kidney	Low predictive accuracy for renovascular hypertension; results influenced by many other conditions
Measurement of renal vein renin activity	Compares renin release from the two kidneys	Lateralization predictive of improvement in blood pressure with revascularization	Nonlateralization not predictive of failure of blood pressure to improve with revascularization; results influenced by medications and many other conditions
Functional studies to assess overall renal function			
Measurement of serum creatinine	Measures overall renal function	Readily available; inexpensive	Not sensitive to early changes in renal mass or single-kidney function
Urinalysis	Assesses urinary sediment and proteinuria	Readily available; inexpensive	Results are nonspecific and influenced by many other diseases
Nuclear imaging with [^{125}I] iothalamate or chromium ^{Cr}51-labeled pentetate to determine glomerular filtration rate (GFR)	Measures overall GFR	Useful for estimating GFR in patients with normal and abnormal renal function	Expensive; not widely available
Perfusion studies to assess differential renal blood flow			
Captopril renography with technetium Tc 99m mertiatide	Captopril-mediated fall in filtration pressure amplifies differences in renal perfusion	Normal study excludes renovascular hypertension	Multiple limitations in patients with advanced atherosclerosis or creatinine >2.0 mg/dL (177 μmol/L)
Nuclear imaging with technetium Tc 99m mertiatide or technetium Tc 99m pentetate to estimate fractional flow to each kidney	Estimates fractional flow to each kidney	Allows calculation of single-kidney GFR	Results may be influenced by presence of obstructive uropathy
Vascular studies to evaluate renal arteries			
Duplex ultrasonography	Shows renal arteries and measures flow velocity as a means of assessing severity of stenosis	Inexpensive; widely available	Heavily dependent on operator's experience; less useful than invasive angiography for diagnosis of fibromuscular dysplasia and abnormalities in accessory renal arteries
Magnetic resonance angiography	Shows renal arteries and perirenal aorta	Not nephrotoxic; useful in patients with renal failure; provides excellent images	Expensive; less useful than invasive modalities
Computed tomographic angiography	Shows renal arteries and perirenal aorta	Provides excellent images; stents do not cause artifacts	Not widely available; the large volume of contrast medium required is potentially nephrotoxic

Modified from Safian RD, Textor SC: Medical progress: Renal artery stenosis. N Engl J Med 344:431-442, 2001, with permission.

They are addressed more fully elsewhere. What follows is a discussion of some of the specific merits and limitations of each modality as they apply to use in renovascular hypertension and ischemic nephropathy.[183]

Current practice favors limiting invasive arteriography to the occasion of endovascular intervention, for example, placement of stents or angioplasty. Although angiography remains for many the "gold standard" for evaluation of the renal vasculature, its invasive nature, potential hazards, and cost make it most suitable for those in whom intervention is planned, often during the same procedure. As a result, most clinicians favor preliminary noninvasive studies beforehand.

Captopril Renography

Imaging the kidneys before and after administration of an ACE inhibitor (e.g., captopril) provides a functional assessment of the change in blood flow and GFR to the kidney, related to both changes in arterial pressure and removal of the efferent arteriolar effects of AII. The most commonly used radiopharmaceuticals are technetium Tc 99m pentetate and technetium Tcl 99m mertiatide. The latter has clearance characteristics similar to hippuran and is often taken as reflecting renal plasma flow. Both can be used, although specific interpretive criteria differ.[198] Both provide information regarding size and filtration of both kidneys and the change in these characteristics after ACE inhibition allows inferences regarding the dependence of glomerular filtration upon AII. Several studies in patient groups with prevalence rates between 35% and 64% suggest that sensitivity and specificity range between 65% and 96% and 62% and 100% respectively.[198] With high specificity, captopril renography can be applied to populations at low pretest probability with an expectation that a normal study will exclude significant renovascular hypertension in more than 96% of cases.[199] Some series report 100% accurate negative predictive values.[200]

These studies are less sensitive and specific for renovascular disease in the presence of renal insufficiency (usually defined as creatinine >2.0 mg/dL).[201] These performance characteristics deteriorate in patients who cannot be prepared carefully, that is, by withdrawal of diuretics and ACE inhibitors for 4 to 14 days before the study.[198] It should be emphasized that renography provides functional information but no direct anatomic information, that is, the location of renal arterial disease, the number of renal arteries, or associated aortic or ostial disease (Fig. 46-16A and B). Some authors believe that renographic screening of patients using this technique is among the most cost-effective methods of identifying candidates for further diagnostic studies and is superior to functional studies of the renin-angiotensin system.[202] The prospective studies of renovascular disease from the Netherlands did observe changes in the renogram during follow-up, but did not find captopril renography predictive of angiographic findings or outcomes.[170]

Under carefully controlled conditions some authors argue that changes in renographic appearance correlate with the changes in blood pressure to be expected after revascularization.[184, 203] Changes in split renal function indicate that stenotic kidneys regain GFR after revascularization, sometimes with a decrement in the contralateral GFR, thereby leaving overall kidney function unchanged.[204, 205]

Doppler Ultrasound of the Renal Arteries

Duplex interrogation of the renal arteries provides measurements of localized velocities of blood flow. In many institutions, this provides an inexpensive means for measuring vascular occlusive disease at sequential time points, to establish both the diagnosis of RAS and its progression.[169] After renal revascularization, Doppler studies are commonly used to monitor restenosis and target vessel patency[206, 207] (Fig. 46-17A and B). Its main drawbacks relate to the difficulties of obtaining adequate studies in obese patients. The utility and reliability of Doppler ultrasound depend partly

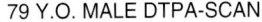
79 Y.O. MALE DTPA-SCAN

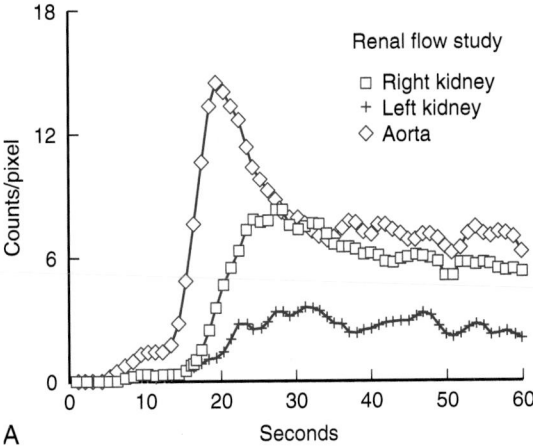
A

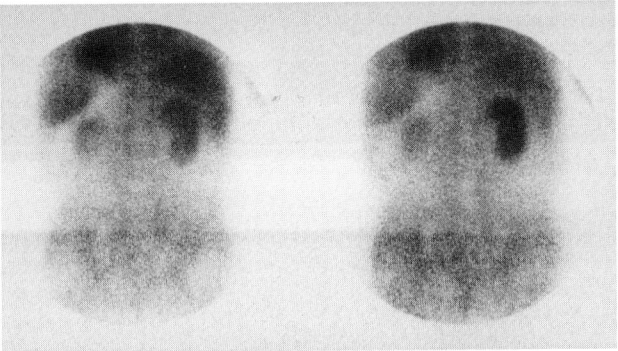
B   79 Y.O. Male
HIPPURAN SCAN

FIGURE 46-16. **A** and **B,** Isotope renography in a patient with unilateral renal artery stenosis. A technetium Tc99m pentetate scan demonstrates delayed circulation and excretion of isotope on the left. A hippuran scan (now replaced with technetium Tc99m metiatide) provided a renogram demonstrating a small kidney with impaired renal function on the affected side.

upon the operator and the time allotted for optimal studies. These factors vary considerably among institutions.

The primary criteria for renal artery studies are a peak systolic velocity above 180 cm/second or a relative velocity above 3.5 as compared to the adjacent aortic flow.[208] Using these criteria, sensitivity and specificity, with angiographic estimates of lesions exceeding 60%, can surpass 90% and 96% respectively,[209, 210] although not universally.[211] When main vessel velocities cannot be determined reliably, segmental waveforms within the arcuate vessels in the renal hilum can be examined. Damping of these waveforms, labeled as "parvus" and "tardus," have been proposed as indirect signs of upstream vascular occlusive phenomena.[212] Recent studies challenge the use of angiographic estimates of stenosis as representing a gold standard altogether.[213] These authors argue that Doppler velocities correlate highly (r = .97) with a truer estimate of vascular occlusion, specifically stenosis determined by intravascular ultrasound.

In our own experience, Doppler study of the renal arteries is highly reliable when adequate imaging of the renal arteries can be obtained. Positive Doppler velocities in an artery clearly identified as the renal artery are rarely later proved

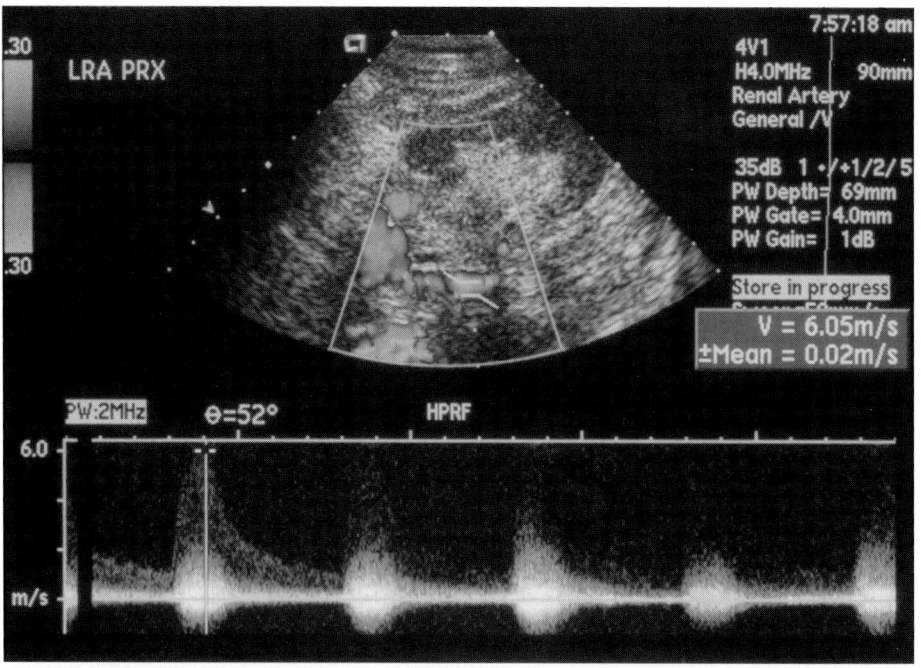

A

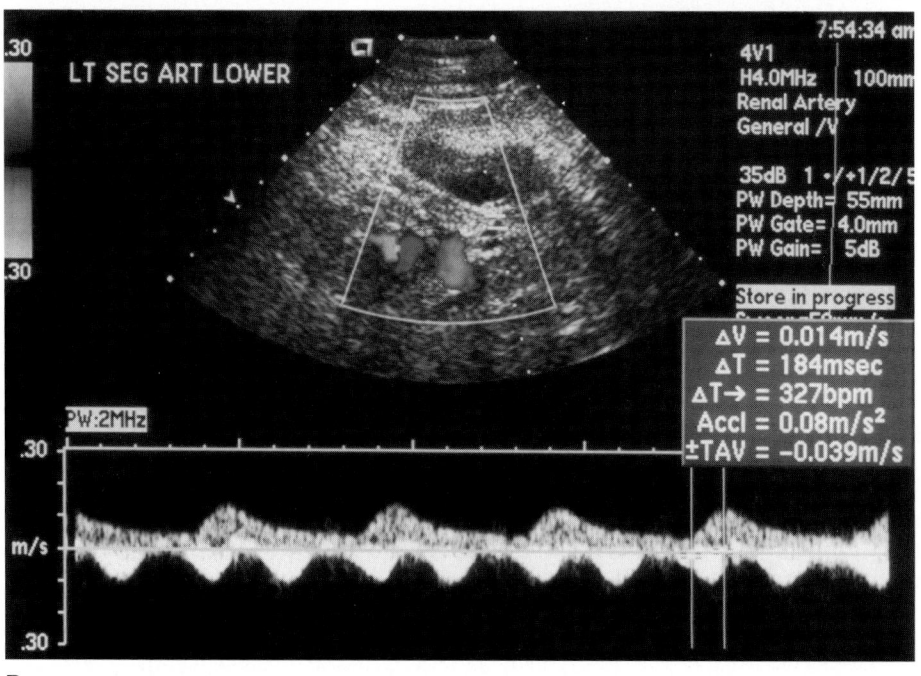

B

FIGURE 46-17. A, Velocity measurements in a patient with high-grade renal artery stenosis affecting the main left renal artery. Proximal segments demonstrate velocities of 605 cm/second, far above the normal upper limit of 180 cm/second. **B,** Segmental branch ultrasound in the distal arteries demonstrates "parvus" and "tardus" dampening of the signal typical of poststenotic waveforms. The utility of these measurements depends upon the ability to obtain reliable identification of vessel segments and the skills of the operator.

to be negative. False-negative studies are more common. In subjects with accessible vessels, Doppler ultrasound provides the most practical means of following vessel characteristics sequentially over time. Drawbacks of renal artery Doppler studies include failure to identify accessory vessels.

Recent studies emphasize the potential for Doppler ultrasound to characterize the small vessel flow characteristics within the kidney. The resistive index provides an estimate of the relative flow velocities in diastole and systole. In a study of 138 patients with RAS, a resistive index above 80 provided an excellent tool for identification of parenchymal renal disease patients who did not respond to renal

revascularization[214] (Fig. 46-18). A sizable portion of this group eventually progressed to renal failure. A resistive index less than 80 was associated with more than 90% favorable blood pressure response and stable or improved renal function. The authors emphasize that accurate predictive power depended upon using the highest resistive index observed, even when present in the nonstenotic kidney.

Magnetic Resonance Angiography

Gadolinium-enhanced MRA of the abdominal and renal vasculature is becoming a mainstay of evaluating renovascular disease in many institutions.[215, 216] This technique is suitable

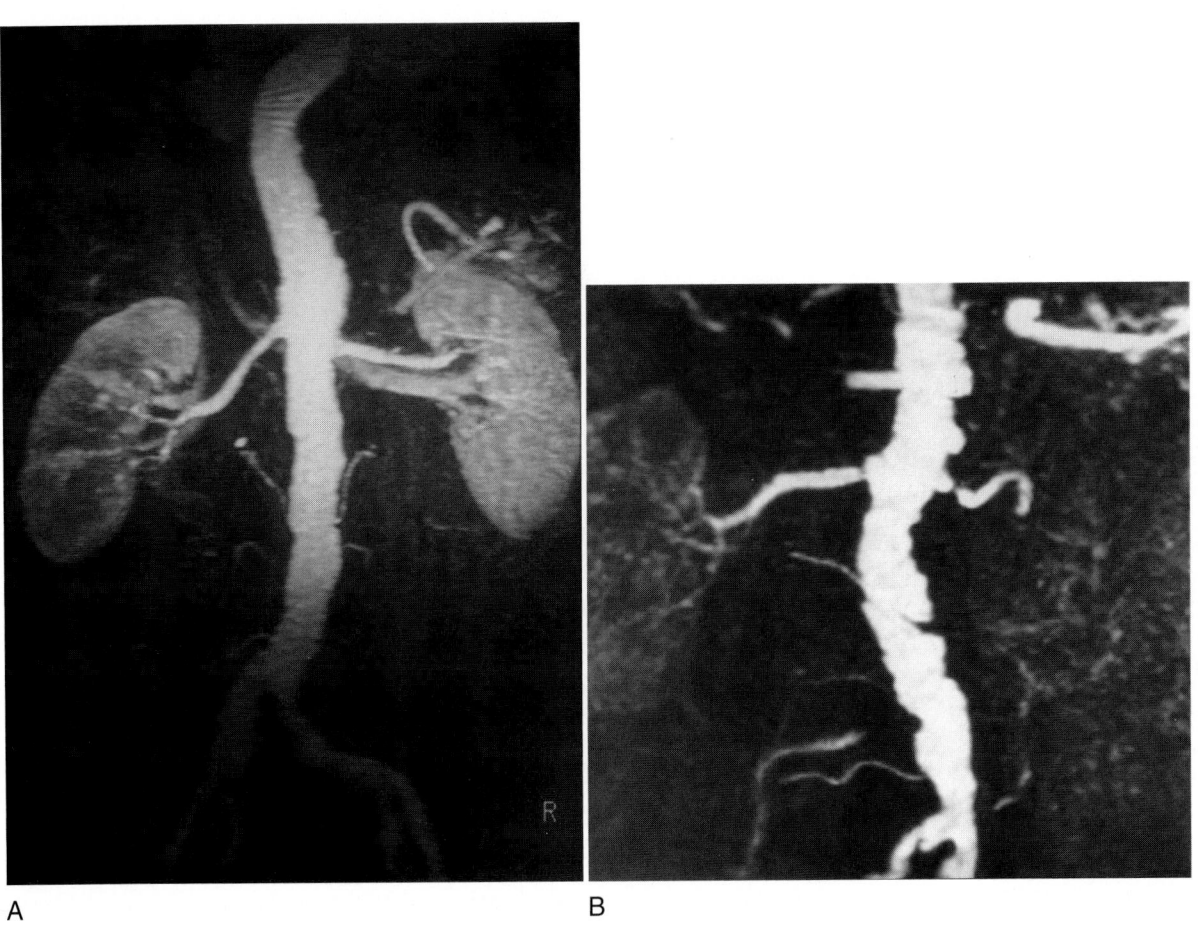

FIGURE 46-18. Mean arterial pressure and number of antihypertensive agents used after renal revascularization in 138 patients with renal artery stenosis. These patients were divided into groups with resistive index of 80 or greater and those less than 80 in the most severely affected kidney. The authors indicate that high resistive index reflects intrinsic parenchymal and small vessel disease in the kidney which does not improve after revascularization. Those with lower indices had both lower blood pressures during follow-up and lower antihypertensive medication requirements. (From Radermacher J, Chavan A, Bleck J, et al: Use of Doppler ultrasonography to predict the outcome of therapy for renal-artery stenosis. N Engl J Med 344:410-417, 2001.)

FIGURE 46-19. A, Gadolinium-enhanced magnetic resonance (MR) angiography demonstrating mild atheromatous disease of the aorta and well-preserved nephrogram bilaterally. The renal arteries have only minimal changes and a venous phase is easily seen showing the renal vein on the left. **B,** MR angiogram in an 82-year-old man with recent hypertension and stroke. The aorta has extensive atheromatous change and both renal arteries have significant vascular lesions. No nephrogram is apparent on the left in this view. The right renal artery also has a substantial signal void near the origin and an accessory renal artery on the right has a near total occlusion in the midportion.

for patients with impaired renal function, as it offers the advantage of nonnephrotoxic imaging agents. No radiation is used. Comparative studies indicate that sensitivity ranges from 83% to 100% and specificity from 92% to 97% in RAS.[217, 218] The nephrogram obtained from gadolinium filtration provides an estimate of relative function and filtration, as well as parenchymal volume.[219]

Examples of MRA are shown in Figure 46-19A and B. Drawbacks include the expense and the tendency to overestimate the severity of lesions, which in fact are shown as a signal void.[216] The limits of resolution with current instrumentation make detection of small accessory vessels limited, and quantitating fibromuscular lesions is difficult with the current technology. Both of these are improving with newer generations of scanners. Signal degradation in the presence of metallic stents render MRA unsuitable for follow-up studies after endovascular procedures in which stents are used.

Computed Tomographic Angiography

CT angiography using "helical" or multiple head scanners and intravenous contrast can provide excellent images of both kidneys and the vascular tree. Resolution and reconstruction techniques render this modality capable of identifying smaller vessels, vascular lesions, and parenchymal characteristics, including stones.[220] When used for detection of RAS, CT angiography agrees well with conventional arteriography (correlation 95%) and sensitivity may reach 98% and specificity 94%.[220, 221] Although this technique offers a noninvasive examination of the vascular tree suitable for kidney donors (as illustrated in Fig. 46-20), for example, it has the drawback of considerable contrast requirement. As a result, it is less ideally suited for evaluation of renovascular hypertension or ischemic nephropathy in patients with impaired renal function.

MANAGEMENT OF RENAL ARTERY STENOSIS AND ISCHEMIC NEPHROPATHY

Considering the array of potential interventions that bear upon renovascular disease and the complexity of these patients, clinicians should formulate a clear set of therapeutic goals. Because each mode of treatment—ranging from medical therapy alone to surgical revascularization—carries with it both benefits and risks, the clinician's task is to weigh the role of each within the context of the individual patient's comorbid disease risk. Rarely is it obvious how best to proceed. In most cases, management of the patient with renovascular disease represents a balance between the pharmacologic management of blood pressure and cardiovascular risk and the optimal timing of renal revascularization. The objective of this section is to provide a framework by which to plan a balanced approach to the patient with unilateral or bilateral RAS. It should be emphasized that consideration of renal artery disease takes place in the broad context of managing other cardiovascular risk factors, including withdrawal of tobacco use, reduction of cholesterol levels, and treatment of diabetes and obesity.

The overall goals of therapy are summarized in Table 46-5. Foremost among these is the goal as stated by the Joint National Committee (JNC) of the National High Blood Pressure Education Program (NHBPEP): "The goal of treating patients with hypertension is to prevent morbidity and mortality associated with high blood pressure..."[222] This task may include the effort to simplify or potentially to eliminate long-term antihypertensive drug therapy. A further goal is to preserve kidney function and to prevent loss of kidney function related to impaired renal blood flow. In some instances, renal revascularization is undertaken to allow improved management of salt and water balance in the process of managing patients with congestive cardiac failure.[139]

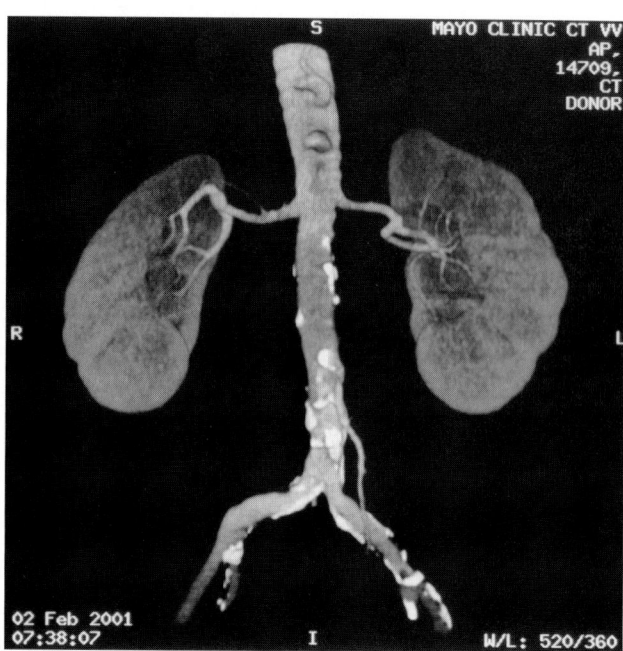

FIGURE 46-20. Computed tomography angiogram using conventional iodinated contrast with three-dimensional reconstruction in an older potential kidney donor. The contrast provides an excellent view of the vascular tree, often demonstrating accessory and polar arteries. Calcified areas of plaque are evident external to the actual blood compartment and are shown as white areas. These images are now standard for kidney donors and provide excellent images. They have the disadvantage for patients with impaired renal function of requiring iodinated contrast.

This may allow safer use of diuretic agents and the ACE inhibitor and ARB classes of medication in patients with critical renal artery lesions to the entire renal mass. Because prospective, randomized trial information is limited in renovascular disease, each patient must be considered individually. What cannot be taken for granted currently is the premise that renal revascularization prolongs life or prevents ESRD.[1] As noted earlier, the burden of atherosclerotic disease associated with RAS is often widespread and the causes of death include a broad array of cardiovascular events. Both endovascular and surgical intervention in the aorta and renal vasculature carry substantial risk that may accelerate morbidity and loss of renal function. As a result, these measures must be considered within the entire context of patient management over time.

Unilateral versus Bilateral Renal Artery Stenosis

Consideration of unilateral versus bilateral RAS differs in some respects. "Bilateral" in this context refers to the circumstances when the entire functional renal mass is affected by vascular occlusion. This may be caused either by bilateral stenoses or stenosis to a solitary functioning kidney. Not only are the putative mechanisms related to blood pressure and volume control different in the presence of a nonstenosed, functioning contralateral kidney with unilateral disease (as outlined earlier under "Pathophysiology") but the potential hazards of intervention and medical therapy differ. Patient survival is reduced in patients with bilateral disease or stenosis to a solitary functioning kidney. Progressive arterial

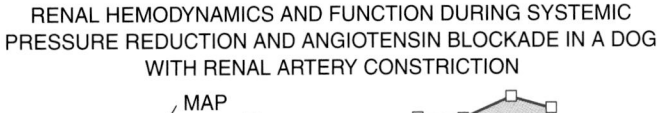

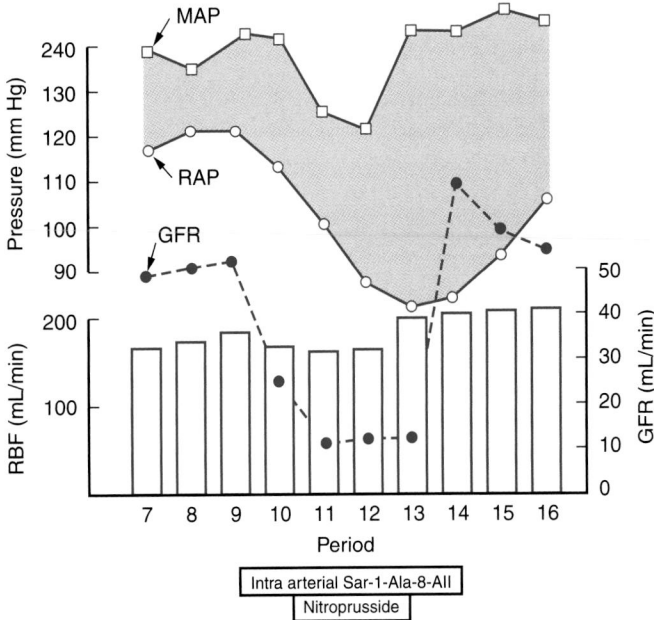

FIGURE 46-21. **A,** Glomerular filtration rate (GFR) falls beyond a renal artery stenotic lesion during blockade of angiotensin II (with intrarenal infusion of Sar-1-ala-8-angiotensin II) and pressure reduction with nitroprusside. The fall in GFR occurs despite preserved renal blood flow (RBF, measured by electromagnetic flow probe). These observations illustrate the role of angiotensin II in maintaining GFR in the poststenotic kidney at low perfusion pressures. **B,** Summary of the effects of angiotensin-converting enzyme (ACE) inhibition on RBF, GFR, and filtration fraction (FF) in normal, moderate, and severe levels of renal artery stenosis. As compared with other antihypertensive agents, ACE inhibitors (and angiotensin receptor blockers) lead to a detectable fall in GFR and FF owing to removal of the efferent arteriolar effects of angiotensin II. When stenosis is sufficiently severe that pressure reduction compromises RBF, the potential for complete occlusion is present, which occurs after pressure reduction with other antihypertensive agents also. (From Textor SC: Renal failure related to ACE inhibitors. Semin Nephrol 17:67-76, 1997.)

disease in this group also poses the most immediate hazard of declining renal function. As noted, patient survival depends upon the extent of vascular involvement[164] regardless of whether renal revascularization is undertaken.

Management of Unilateral Renal Artery Stenosis

Most patients with atherosclerotic renal artery disease have preexisting hypertension. As a result, they are exposed to antihypertensive therapy before identification of the lesion and may be well controlled with only moderate medication use.[106] As noted earlier, such patients commonly come to clinical attention when recognizable clinical progression occurs. Occasionally, clinical decision making is influenced strongly by concerns about the hazards of medical therapy and failure to achieve restored blood flow soon enough. Examination of the results of medical therapy alone is important before evaluating the role of vascular reconstruction or dilation.

Since the introduction of agents that block the renin-angiotensin system, most patients (86%-92%) with unilateral renal artery disease can achieve blood pressure levels of less than 140/90 mm Hg with medical regimens based upon these agents.[120, 121, 223] It must be understood that widespread application of these agents to patients with many forms of cardiovascular disease ensures that subcritical cases of renovascular disease are treated without being identified.

Does the risk of treating unidentified RAS with antihypertensive drug therapy pose a hazard to the patient? This issue is at the crux of clinical debates regarding management of patients with renovascular hypertension. Early studies with experimental "clip" hypertension emphasized renal fibrosis and scarring that occurred in the stenotic kidney in animals treated with ACE inhibitors.[224] Several studies suggest that experimental hypertension may be more prone to pressure reduction and poststenotic renal injury in ACE inhibitor–treated groups as compared to either vasodilators, such as hydralazine or minoxidil, or calcium channel blockers, such as nifedipine.[225, 226] It is well recognized that removal of the efferent arteriolar effects of AII pose the possibility of loss of glomerular filtration in a kidney with reduced renal perfusion (Fig. 46-21A and B).[227] Experimental studies in two-kidney, one-clip rats indicate that the loss of kidney function is sometimes irreversible, although survival is improved in ACE inhibitor–treated animals as compared to minoxidil treatment.[225] The unique role of ACE inhibitors and ARBs must be understood in this regard. Any drug capable of reducing systemic arterial pressure has the potential to lower renal pressures beyond a critical stenosis.[137, 228] As a result, successful antihypertensive therapy in renovascular disease has the theoretical result of reducing blood flow to the poststenotic kidney sufficient to induce vascular occlusion. The unique feature of agents that block the renin-angiotensin system is the reduction of efferent arteriolar resistance sufficient to lower transcapillary filtration pressures, despite preserved blood flow to the glomerulus (see Fig. 46-21B).[227] This property is central to the benefits of this class of agent in "hyperfiltration" states thought to accelerate renal damage in other settings.[229-232] Hence, the fall in glomerular filtration beyond a stenotic lesion can be observed despite relatively preserved plasma flows. The fall in GFR heralds an approaching degree of critical vascular compromise before blood flow itself is reduced.[233] Studies in renovascular hypertensive animals confirm that despite a reduction in filtration, renal structural integrity can be preserved and recovered[234] after removal of the clip or removal of the ACE inhibitor. Hence, it is unlikely that ACE inhibitors or ARBs themselves pose a unique hazard, beyond that attributable to the reduction in renal blood flow.

It is important to recognize that the contralateral kidney usually supports total glomerular filtration despite reduced filtration in the stenotic kidney. Changes in overall GFR may be undetectable. This may be interpreted in several ways. Some authors argue in favor of using split renal function measurements, such as radionuclide renal scans, to detect loss of individual kidney function as a means of timing revascularization.[187] Depending upon the circumstances, loss of one kidney may be an acceptable price to pay if one can assure the patient that the remaining kidney has adequate function and blood supply, as illustrated in Figure 46-22A-C. The fall in GFR from a loss of one kidney represents a loss of GFR similar to that of donating a kidney for renal transplantation or of nephrectomy for malignancy. In such instances, the long-term hazard to the remaining kidney is small, although not negligible.[235-237] As the age and comorbid disease burden of the population at risk rises, the loss of one kidney may pose no great hazard if overall glomerular filtration is adequate. The experience of ACE inhibition in trials of congestive cardiac failure is reassuring in this regard. Thousands of patients with marginal arterial pressures and clinical heart failure have been treated over many years with a variety of ACE inhibitors, and, more recently, with ARBs. These patients are at high risk for undetected renal artery lesions as part of the atherosclerotic burden associated with coronary disease. Although a minor change in creatinine is observed in 8% to 10% of these patients, a rise sufficient to lead to withdrawal of these agents under trial monitoring conditions occurs in only 1% to 2%.[233] Data from patients with high cardiovascular disease risk treated with ramipril included patients with creatinine levels up to 2.3 mg/dL. Those with creatinine levels between 1.4 and 2.3 mg/dL were at higher risk for cardiovascular mortality and had a major survival benefit from ACE inhibition. Close follow-up of kidney function indicated that withdrawal of ACE inhibition due to deterioration of renal function was less than 5% and no greater than placebo.[123]

Medical Therapy versus PTRA

It follows from the foregoing that many patients with unilateral RAS are managed without restoration of blood flow for a long period, sometimes indefinitely. The judgment on endovascular intervention in a specific case revolves about the anticipated outcome, as summarized later. There are a few prospective, randomized trials comparing medical therapy with PTRA upon which to draw. Familiarity with the available trials and their limitations is important for nephrologists. The major features of these trials are summarized in Table 46-7.

Three small trials addressed the relative value of endovascular repair, specifically PTRA as compared to medical therapy in atherosclerotic RAS. To the credit of these investigators, care was taken to standardize blood pressure measurements before and after endovascular repair and to select antihypertensive regimens carefully. All of these trials have limitations, but they are instructive. Webster and co-workers[163] randomized 55 patients with atherosclerotic RAS to either medical therapy or PTRA. Follow-up blood pressures were obtained using a random-zero sphygmomanometer after a run-in period. The run-in period produced considerable reduction in blood pressures in all patients. Those with unilateral disease had no significant difference between medical therapy and PTRA after 6 months. There was greater blood pressure benefit after PTRA in those with bilateral RAS. The authors indicated they were "unable to demonstrate any benefit in respect of renal function or event free survival" during follow-up presented for 40 months.[163] Plouin and colleagues[238] randomized 49 patients with unilateral atherosclerotic RAS of greater than 75% or greater than 60% with lateralizing functional studies. Blood pressure measurements were based upon overnight ambulatory blood pressure monitoring (ABPM), which is thought to yield more reproducible trial data and to be relatively free of placebo or office effects.[239-241] Seven of 26 patients (27%) assigned to medical therapy eventually crossed over to the PTRA group for refractory hypertension. There were six procedural complications in the PTRA group, including branch dissection and segmental infarction. Final blood pressures were not different between groups, but slightly fewer medications were required in the PTRA group. Taken together, the trial of Plouin and colleagues suggested that PTRA produced more complications in the near term, was useful in some medical treatment failures, and required slightly fewer medications after 6 months. The study excluded agents which blocked the renin-angiotensin system (such as ACE inhibitors).[238] The largest randomized, prospective trial included 106 patients enrolled in the DRASTIC (Dutch Renal Artery Stenosis Intervention Cooperative) study.[170] These patients were selected for "resistance" to therapy, including two drugs, and were required to have serum creatinine values below 2.3 mg/dL. Blood pressures were evaluated using automated oscillometric devices at 3 and 12 months after entry. Patients were evaluated on an "intention to treat" basis. Blood pressures did not differ between groups overall at either 3 or 12 months, although the PTRA group was taking fewer medications (2.1 ± 1.3 vs. 3.2 ± 1.5 defined daily doses, $P < .001$). The authors concluded that in the treatment of hypertension and RAS, "angioplasty has little advantage over antihypertensive drug therapy."[170] It cannot be overlooked, however, that 22 of 50 (44%) patients assigned to medical therapy were considered treatment failures and referred for

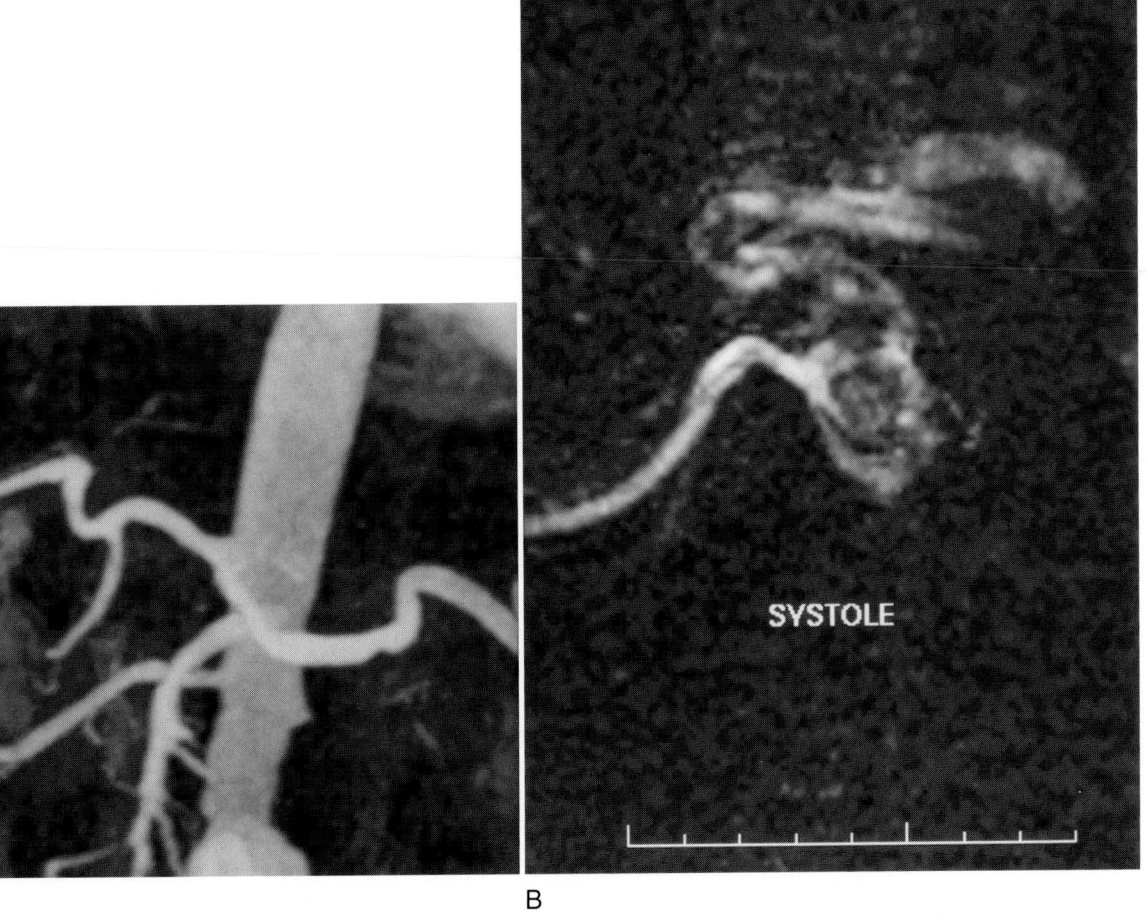

A   B

RECIPROCAL CREATININE IN RENAL ARTERY STENOSIS

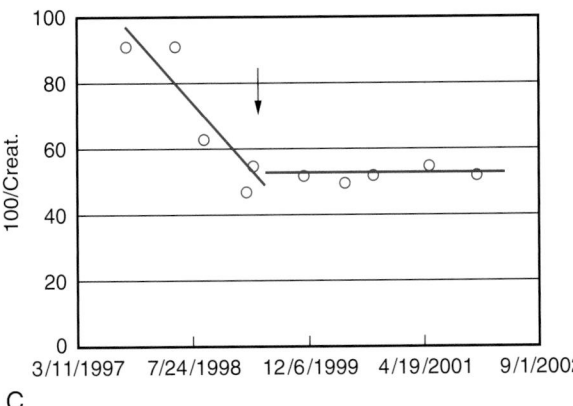

C

FIGURE 46-22. A and **B,** Magnetic resonance angiogram of a 79-year-old man with prostate cancer and worsening hypertension and proteinuria. The aortogram indicates virtually complete occlusion developing to the left kidney, which is confirmed by absense of any systolic flow (**B**). The patency and flow to the right kidney is normal. Addition of an angiotensin receptor blocker (ARB) to his diuretic regimen allowed stable blood pressure and resolution of proteinuria (see text). **C,** As illustrated by the plot of reciprocal creatinine values, this patient's renal function stabilized beyond the time point indicated by the *arrow.* This reflected the time of complete loss of function of the left kidney. Residual function in the solitary, normally perfused kidney has been stable for years. This patient has had no further difficulty for 3 years. In this case, stable renal function and blood pressure were obtained with medical therapy. The decision as to whether renal revascularization should be undertaken depends in part upon other factors, including age and comorbid disease conditions.[242]

PTRA after 3 months. There were several instances of total arterial occlusion in the medical group, compared to none in the angioplasty group. Many clinicians interpret these data to support an important role for PTRA in the management of patients with refractory hypertension and RAS. Regardless of interpretation, these trials offer important insights into current management options. The benefits of endovascular procedures, even in the short term, are moderate compared to

effective antihypertensive therapy. Patients failing to respond to medical therapy often improve after revascularization.[242]

These modest benefits emphasize differences between the current era and the situation a few decades ago. Reports from the 1970s underscore the fact that some patients experienced recurrent episodes of malignant phase hypertension with encephalopathy, fluid retention, and progressive renal insufficiency.[117, 243, 244] Despite medical therapy, some of these

TABLE 46-7

Prospective, Randomized Trials of Medical versus Interventional Therapy for Atherosclerotic Renal Artery Stenosis[*]

AUTHOR/NO. OF PATIENTS	INCLUSION/BP MEASUREMENT	BP OUTCOME (mm Hg)	RENAL OUTCOME	AUTHORS COMMENTS
Webster et al. (1998)[163] N = 55 (unilateral = 27) N = 135 eligible RAS >50%	DBP ≥95 mm Hg, resistant 2 drugs Exclusion: CVA, MI within 3 mo; creatinine (>500 μmol/L) BP: Random-zero device; no ACEI allowed	Unilateral PTRA: 173/95 Med Rx: 161/88 Bilateral PTRA: 152/83 Med Rx: 171/91, P <.01	Creatinine (μmol/L) Bilateral: PTRA: 188 Med Rx: 157 Unilateral: PTRA: 144 Med Rx: 168	"…unable to demonstrate any benefit in respect of renal function or event free survival" (F/U 40 mo)
Plouin et al. (1998)[238] N = 49 (unilateral ASO) RAS >75% or >60%, lateralizing study	Age <75 yr; normal contralateral kidney Exclusion: MHTN CVA, CHF, MI within 6 mo BP: Automated sphygmomanometer, ABPM at 6 mo	PTRA: 140/81 Med Rx: 141/84 No. drugs (DDD): PTRA: 1.0 Med Rx: 1.78, P <.01 Crossover to PTRA: 7/26 (27%)	Creatinine clearance (mL/min): (6 mo) PTRA: 77 Med Rx: 74 Renal artery occlusion PTRA: 0 Med Rx: 0	"BP levels and the proportion of patients given antihypertensive treatment were similar one year after randomization in the control and angioplasty groups, confirming that the BP-lowering effect of angioplasty in the short and medium terms is limited in atherosclerotic RAS."
van Jaarsveld et al. (2000)[170] N = 106 (ASO) RAS >50%	Resistant: 2 drugs; DBP >95 mm Hg or creatinine rise with ACEI Exclusion: creatinine ≥2.3 mg/dL; solitary kidney/total occlusion, kidney <8 cm BP automated oscillometric	BP outcome at 3 mo: PTRA: 169/89 Med Rx: 163/88 At 12 mo: PTRA: 152/84 Med Rx:162/88 No. drugs: 1.9 vs. 2.4; P <.01	Creatinine clearance (mL/min) (3 mo): PTRA: 70 Med Rx: 59 (P = .03) Abnormal renograms PTRA: 36% Med Rx: 70% (P = .002) Renal artery occlusion PTRA 0 Med Rx 8	"In the treatment of patients with hypertension and renal artery stenosis, angioplasty has little advantage over antihypertensive drug therapy"

[*]Summary of three prospective randomized trials comparing medical therapy for renovascular hypertension to percutaneous transluminal renal angioplasty (PTRA). These studies were small and contained selected patient populations. However, they sought to standardize blood pressure outcome measurement and to randomize patients prospectively. Each was different, but all found fewer major benefits accrued in PTRA groups than reported by observational studies alone. Crossover rates from medical to angioplasty arms were significant, however, and emphasize the importance of restoring blood supply in selected patients, particularly those with bilateral disease.[163,170,238]

ABPM, ambulatory blood pressure monitoring; ACEI, angiotensin-converting enzyme inhibitor; ASO, atherosclerosis; BP, blood pressure; CHF, congestive heart failure; CVA, cerebrovascular accident; DBP, diastolic blood pressure; DDD, defined daily doses; F/U, follow-up; MHTN, malignant hypertension; MI, myocardial infarction; RAS, renal artery stenosis.

cases required "urgent bilateral nephrectomy" as a lifesaving measure.[117] The mean age in several of these small series was less than 50 years. In the years since then, malignant hypertension has become less prevalent in most Western countries, although not universally.[245, 246] The introduction of ACE inhibitors and calcium channel blocking drugs in the 1980s has been associated temporally with reduced occurrence of severe hypertension and improved medical management of patients with high-renin states, including renovascular hypertension. More effective medical management, including treatment of patients with renovascular disease, largely has eliminated "urgent" nephrectomy for blood pressure control.

Progressive Renal Artery Stenosis in Medically Treated Patients

As noted, the potential for progressive vascular occlusion is central to management of patients with renovascular disease. It may be argued that failure to revascularize the kidneys exposes the patient to the hazard of undetected, progressive occlusion, potentially leading to total occlusion or irreversible loss of renal function. A firm understanding of the data regarding progressive atherosclerotic disease of the kidney is essential to optimal application of both endovascular and surgical revascularization.

Atherosclerosis is a variably progressive disorder. Proper management of disorders of the carotid, coronary, aortic, and peripheral vasculature recognizes the potential for progression, which occurs at widely different rates among individuals. Medical therapy of vascular disorders should incorporate measures aimed at intensive reduction of risk factors, of which smoking cessation, blood pressure control, and correction of dyslipidemias are paramount.[247-249] Treatment of these risk factors reduces mortality rates related to cardiovascular disease.[222, 250]

How does progressive renal artery occlusive disease affect management of renovascular hypertension? Evident anatomic progression does not reliably predict functional changes in terms of deteriorating blood pressure control or renal function. In the Doppler ultrasound studies from Seattle, a decrement in measured renal size of 1 cm (renal atrophy) developed in 5.5% of those with initially normal vessels and 20.8% of those with baseline stenosis greater than 60% during a follow-up interval of 33 months.[171] Changes in serum creatinine were infrequent but did occur in a subset of patients, particularly those with bilateral RAS. These findings are in general agreement with early studies during medical therapy of renovascular hypertension in which 35% had a detectable fall in measured renal length, but in which 8 of 41 (19%) had a significant rise in creatinine during a follow-up of 33 months.[172] Follow-up of the medical treatment arms during relatively short-term studies fails to show major changes in kidney function, although occasional loss of renal perfusion by radionuclide scan is observed.[170]

How often does management of RAS without revascularization lead to clinical deterioration, either in terms of progression to refractory hypertension or to progressive renal insufficiency? Follow-up of patients with incidentally identified RAS is helpful in this regard. Review of peripheral aortograms identified 69 patients with high-grade RAS (>70%) followed without revascularization for more than 6 months.

Long-term follow-up identified generally satisfactory blood pressure control (by the standards of 1990), although the requirement for further antihypertensive therapy progressed during an average of 36 months of follow-up.[176] Four patients eventually underwent renal revascularization for refractory hypertension or renal dysfunction. Five developed ESRD, of which only one was thought related to RAS directly. Overall, serum creatinine rose from 1.4 mg/dL to 2.0 mg/dL. These data indicated that many such patients could be managed without revascularization for many years and that clinical progression leading to urgent revascularization developed in between 10% and 14% of such patients. Expansion of this data set to 160 patients allowed comparison of different antihypertensive regimens. The rates of progression did not appear to be related to the introduction of ACE inhibitors, although the level of blood pressure control improved in recent years (see Table 46-4).[251] These observations are supported by a recent report of 126 patients with "incidental" RAS compared to 397 patients matched for age. Measured serum creatinine was higher and the calculated (Cockcroft-Gault) GFR was lower in patients with RAS followed for 8 to 10 years. However, none of the patients identified progressed to ESRD. These observations are entirely consistent with the preliminary results of prospective trials of medical versus surgical intervention started in the 1980s.[252] Taken together, these studies indicate that rates of progression of renovascular disease are moderate and occur at widely varying rates. Often, such patients can be managed well without revascularization for many years. The clinical issue in a specific patient frequently hinges on whether the risks of revascularization are truly less than the risks of progression.

While these reports are informative, they leave many questions unanswered. How often does suboptimal blood pressure control in renovascular hypertension accelerate cardiovascular morbidity and mortality? Does one lose the opportunity to reverse hypertension effectively by delaying renal revascularization? The answers to these questions depend upon further prospective studies. It is equally clear that for many patients with progressive disease, optimal long-term stability of kidney function and blood pressure control can be achieved by successful surgical or endovascular restoration of the renal blood supply.

Surgical Treatment of Renovascular Hypertension and Ischemic Nephropathy

Early experience with vascular disease of the kidney was based entirely upon surgical intervention, either nephrectomy or vascular reconstruction, with the objective of "surgical curability."[253] For that reason, many of the original data regarding split renal function measurement were geared toward identifying "functionally" significant lesions as a guide by which patients should be selected for a major surgical procedure. Surgical intervention is less commonly performed in the current era, in part because the age and comorbid risk of patients with atherosclerotic disease commonly favor endovascular procedures when feasible.

Methods of surgical intervention have changed over the decades. A review in 1982 emphasized the role of "ablative" techniques, including partial nephrectomy.[253] Use of ablative operative means was guided by the difficulty of controlling blood pressure during that era. They have become less common since the expansion of tolerable medication regimens, as noted earlier. The recent introduction of laparoscopic techniques, including hand-assisted nephrectomy, may return attention to nephrectomy as a means to reduce medication requirements with low morbidity in high-risk patients.

Surgical series from the 1960s and early 1970s indicated that "cure" of hypertension was achieved in only 30% to 40% of patients, despite attempts at preselection. Survival of groups chosen for surgery appeared to be better than those chosen for medical management.[15, 129] This likely reflected the heavy disease burden and preoperative risks identified in those for whom surgery was not considered.[165, 254] The cooperative studies of renovascular disease in the 1960s and 1970s examined many of the clinical characteristics of renovascular hypertension. These studies identified some of the limitations and hazards of surgical intervention and reported mortality rates of 6.8%, even in excellent institutions.[16, 130] The mean age in these series was 50.5 years. Definitions of operative mortality included events as late as 375 days after the procedure and may overestimate the hazard. Had the authors considered only deaths within the first week, for example, the immediate perioperative mortality would be 1.7%.

Subsequent development of improved techniques for patient selection, including screening for coronary and carotid disease, for renal artery bypass and endarterectomy, and for combined aortic and renal artery repair represent significant elements in the history of major vascular surgery.[12, 253] Several of the options developed for renal artery reconstruction are listed in Table 46-8. The majority of these methods now focus on reconstruction of the vascular supply for preservation of nephron mass. Transaortic endarterectomy can effectively restore circulation to both kidneys. It requires aortic cross-clamping and is often undertaken as part of a combined procedure with aortic replacement.[131, 255] Identification and treatment of carotid and coronary disease led to reductions in surgical morbidity and mortality.[256] By addressing associated cardiovascular risk before surgery, early surgical mortality falls below 2% in patients without other major disease.

TABLE 46-8

Surgical Procedures Applied to Reconstruction of the Renal Artery and to Reversal of Renovascular Hypertension

Ablative surgery: removal of a "pressor" kidney
  Nephrectomy: direct or laparoscopic
  Partial nephrectomy
Renal artery reconstruction (requires aortic approach)
  Renal endarterectomy
  Transaortic endarterectomy
  Resection and reanastomosis: suitable for focal lesions
  Aortorenal bypass graft
Extra-anatomic procedures (may avoid direct manipulation of the aorta);
    require adequate alternate circulation without stenosis at celiac origin)
  Splenorenal bypass graft
  Hepatorenal bypass graft
  Gastroduodenal, superior mesenteric, iliac-to-renal bypass grafts
Autotransplantation with ex vivo reconstruction

Modified from Libertino JA, Zinman L: Surgery for renovascular hypertension. *In* Breslin DL, Swinton NW, Libertino JA, Zinman L (eds): Renovascular Hypertension. Baltimore, Williams & Wilkins, 1982, pp 166-212.

Surgical reconstruction of the renal blood supply usually requires access to the aorta. A variety of alternative surgical procedures have been designed to avoid manipulation of the badly diseased aorta, including those for which previous surgical procedures make access difficult. These include "extra-anatomic" repair of the renal artery using hepatorenal or splenorenal conduits which lower the requirement of manipulation of a badly diseased aorta.[257] It should be emphasized that success with extrarenal conduits depends upon the integrity of the alternative blood supply. Hence, careful preoperative assessment of stenotic orifices of the celiac axis is undertaken before using either the hepatic or splenic arteries.[258] The results of these procedures have been good, both in the short term and during long-term follow-up studies.[259] Analysis of 222 patients treated more than 10 years earlier indicates that these procedures were performed with 2.2% mortality and low rates of restenosis (7.3%) and good long-term survival. The predictors of late mortality were age above 60 years, coronary disease, and previous vascular surgery.

The durability of surgical vascular reconstruction is well established.[260] Follow-up studies after 5 and 10 years for all forms of renal artery bypass procedures indicate excellent long-term patency (>90%) both for renal artery procedures alone and when combined with aortic reconstruction.[261] Results of surgery have been good despite increasing age in the reported series (see Fig. 46-10B). Patient selection has been important in all of these reports. While long-term outcome data are established for surgery, little information is available for endovascular stent procedures, which appear more prone to restenosis and technical failure. This proven record of surgical reconstruction leads some clinicians to favor this approach for younger patients with longer life expectancy.

Few studies have compared endovascular intervention (PTRA without stents) and surgical repair. A single study of nonostial, unilateral atherosclerotic disease in which patients were randomly assigned to surgery or PTRA indicate that while surgical success rates were higher and PTRA was needed on a repeat basis in several cases, the 2-year patency rates were 90% for PTRA and 97% for surgery. The authors favored using PTRA as the initial choice of therapy with a requirement for close follow-up.[262, 263]

In my institution, surgical reconstruction of the renal arteries is most often undertaken as part of aortic surgery. Those with impaired renal function (creatinine ≥2.0 mg/dL) underwent simultaneous aortic and renal procedures in 75% of cases.[131] Recent experience indicates that combining renal revascularization with aortic repair does not increase the risk of the aortic operation substantially.[264] As with endovascular techniques, the results regarding changes in renal function include improvement in 22% to 26%, no change (some consider "stabilization") in 46% to 52%, and progressive deterioration in 18% to 22%.[265-270] These data are illustrated in Figure 46-23. Using intraoperative color flow Doppler ultrasound allows immediate correction of suboptimal results and improved long-term patency.[271] Results from several surgical series are summarized in Table 46-9. Using current techniques, the operative risk is less than 4% in good-risk candidates.[265, 272] Risk factors include advanced age, elevated creatinine (>2.7-3.0 mg/dL) and associated aortic or other vascular disease.[264] The combined risk when multiple comorbid risk factors are present may rise to 15%.[131] In some cases,

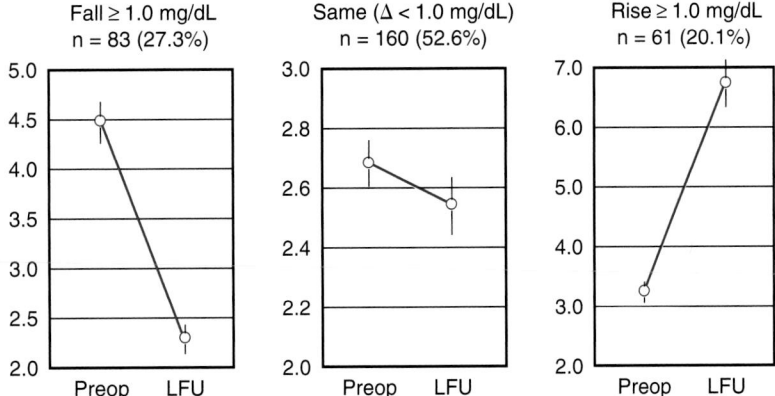

CREATININE IN AZOTEMIC PATIENTS WITH RAS

FIGURE 46-23. Outcomes of renal revascularization in 304 azotemic patients (creatinine > 2.0 mg/dL) with renal artery stenosis (RAS) after renal revascularization. On average, mean serum creatinine did not fall over a follow-up period beyond 36 months. Group mean values obscure major differences in clinical outcomes as shown here. Some patients experience major clinical benefit (defined as a fall in serum creatinine of >1.0 mg/dL) with significant improvement in creatinine levels and durable recovery from renal failure (*left panel*). The largest group has minor change (<1.0 mg/dL), which might be considered "stabilization" of renal function. The degree of benefit in these patients depends upon whether renal function is deteriorating. The data for the group in the *right panel* show the failure to observe consistent overall improvements, because 18% to 22% of patients develop worsening renal function. The exact cause of this deterioration is not clear, although atheroembolic disease is responsible for a portion. This potential hazard of revascularization must be considered when offering these procedures. LFU, latest follow-up. (From Textor SC, Wilcox CS: Renal artery stenosis: A common, treatable cause of renal failure? Annu Rev Med 52:421-442, 2001.)

TABLE 46-9

Surgical Treatment of Renovascular Hypertension and Ischemic Nephropathy

	Renovascular Hypertension[a]		
	"CURED"	**"IMPROVED"**	**NO EFFECT**
Fibromuscular disease 7 series N = 575	Mean[*]: 59% (range 43%-76%)	Mean: 29% (range 14%-39%)	Mean: 12% (range 1.3%-33%)
Atherosclerotic disease 7 series N = 631	Mean[*]: 34% (range 15%-58%)	Mean: 80% (range 21%-75%)	Mean: 16% (range 5%-38%)
	Ischemic Nephropathy[b]		
	"IMPROVED"	**"NO CHANGE"**	**WORSE**
Atherosclerotic disease 7 series after 1990 N = 805	Mean[*]: 41% (range 27%-63%)	Mean: 37% (range 19%-54%)	Mean: 22% (range 4%-42%)

[*]Mean here represents the weighted mean after factoring the number of patients reported in each series.
[a]Modified from Stanley JC: Surgical treatment of renovascular hypertension. Am J Surg 174:102–110, 1997.
[b]Data from references 1, 12, 131, 265, 269, 270, 272, 307, 318.

nephrectomy of a totally infarcted kidney provides major improvement in blood pressure control at low operative risk. The introduction of laparoscopic surgical techniques makes nephrectomy technically feasible in some patients for whom vascular reconstruction is not an option. These series reflect widely variable methods of determining blood pressure benefit as discussed later.

Studies in patients with bilateral renal artery lesions or vascular occlusion to the entire renal mass indicate that restoration of blood flow can lead to preservation of renal function in some cases.[151, 273, 274] Most often, this has been undertaken when a clue to preserved blood supply, sometimes from capsular vessels, is evident by renography. Occasionally, revascularization can lead to functional recovery sufficient to eliminate the need for dialysis.[151]

Endovascular Renal Procedures

The ability to restore renal perfusion in high-risk patients with renovascular hypertension and ischemic nephropathy using endovascular methods represents a major advance in this disorder.[275] Restoration of blood flow to the kidney beyond a stenotic lesion provides the obvious means to improve renovascular hypertension and halt the progression of vascular occlusive injury. The past 2 decades have been characterized by a major shift from surgical reconstruction toward preferential application of endovascular procedures. This shift has enlarged the physician pool engaged in making decisions about renovascular hypertension.

Revascularizing the kidney has both benefits and risks, however. With older patients developing RAS in the context of preexisting hypertension in the present era, the likelihood of cure is small, particularly in atherosclerotic disease. The morbidity of surgical procedures can be substantial, so the ability to convert a diagnostic angiogram into a therapeutic procedure at the same setting is attractive. The true risks and benefits of these procedures are sometimes difficult to ascertain from the published literature. They may vary among institutions depending upon the technical expertise available. As noted later, methods of reporting results regarding clinical outcomes are inconsistent. Although complications are not common, they can be catastrophic,[276] a feature familiar to nephrologists responsible for managing renal failure when it occurs, often related to atheroembolic disease. Wide variability in experience with endovascular procedures is reflected by the observation that their use, including both renal and lower extremity vascular stents, varies more than 14-fold among regions in the United States.[277] The probability of renal angioplasty within 30 days of cardiac catheterization is fourfold higher when cardiologists perform the procedure than when interventional radiologists are responsible. Knowing when to pursue renal revascularization is central to the dilemma of managing renovascular disease. The following section undertakes to summarize the available information for nephrologists active in this field.

The introduction of endovascular stents has accelerated this trend, in part because of the improved technical patency possible with ostial atherosclerotic lesions compared to angioplasty alone. It should be emphasized that much of the shift to endovascular procedures relates to their applicability in elderly patients and the widespread availability of interventional radiology. Whether endovascular repair is comparable to surgical intervention during long-term follow-up is not yet known, at least since the advent of stents.

Interpretation of Observational Studies Related to Endovascular Procedures

Literature reports related to renal revascularization are made more difficult by the fact that these procedures have not been subjected to rigorous evaluation in the form of large, prospective, randomized clinical trials. The few trials performed in recent years have been summarized earlier. The primary body of literature is founded on observational reports of outcomes based upon measurements before and after intervention in patients often selected by means not clearly defined. These reports vary widely, as others have noted.[278, 279] Commonly, they are limited by imprecise definitions of blood pressure measurement and goal levels, widely varied antihypertensive medication administration, time intervals for follow-up, definitions of procedural success, and complications. As a result, the enthusiasm for results of angioplasty, for example, varies according to the series selected.[278] Remarkably, the reported frequency of clinical success, including "cure," falls during later reports of most of these procedures, including both surgery and PTRA.[280, 281] Application of formal blood pressure measurement protocols, including ambulatory monitoring, routinely demonstrates less effect from renal revascularization than those reported from observational studies.[163, 170, 238] Furthermore, use of standardized antihypertensive drug regimens, for example, during a formal "run-in" period, can provide improvements in blood pressure at least equal to revascularization.[163, 282] The same caveats apply when evaluating renal functional outcomes for ischemic nephropathy, although serum creatinine levels and progression to ESRD are more discrete end points than blood pressure levels. Several of the larger trials utilizing PTRA and stents are summarized in Table 46-10.

Angioplasty for Fibromuscular Disease

Most lesions of medical fibroplasia are located at a distance away from the renal artery ostium. Many of these have multiple webs within the vessel, which can be successfully traversed and opened by balloon angioplasty.[283] Experience in the 1980s indicated more than 94% technical success rates.[284] Some of these lesions (approximately 10%) develop restenosis

TABLE 46-10

Outcomes of Renal Artery Stent Placement

	Hypertension		
	"CURED"	**"IMPROVED"**	**NO CHANGE**
14 series N = 678 98% technical success	Weighted mean: 17% Range: 3%-68%	Weighted mean: 47% Range: 5%-61%	Weighted mean: 36% Range: 0%-61%
	Effect on Renal Function in Azotemic Patients		
	"IMPROVED"	**"STABILIZED"**	**WORSE**

14 series reporting
  "impaired renal
  function" N = 496
	Weighted mean: 30%
	Range: 10%-41%
		Weighted mean: 42%
		Range: 32%-71%
			Weighted mean: 29%
			Range: 19%-34%

Modified and summarized from references 207, 287, 288, 290, 302, 319-322.

for which repeat procedures have been used. Clinical benefit regarding blood pressure control has been reported in observational outcome studies in 65% to 75% of patients, although the rates of "cure" are less secure.[100] Cure of hypertension, defined as sustained blood pressure levels less than 140/90 mm Hg with no antihypertensive medications, may be obtained between 35% and 50% of the time. Predictors of cure (normal arterial pressures without medication at 6 months and beyond after PTRA) include lower systolic blood pressures, younger age, and shorter duration of hypertension.[285] Stents are used rarely.

A large majority of patients with FMD are female. The age of detecting hypertension is usually younger than in the series with atherosclerotic disease.[100, 286] In general, such patients have relatively less aortic disease and are at less risk for the major complications of angioplasty. Because the risk for major procedural complications is low, most clinicians favor early intervention for patients with FMD with the hope of reduced antihypertensive medication requirements after successful PTRA.

Angioplasty and Stent Placement for Atherosclerotic Renal Artery Stenosis

Few advances in renovascular disease have been associated with the level of controversy as great as that over the use of endovascular stent placement for atherosclerotic renovascular disease. After the introduction of angioplasty (PTRA) it was soon evident that ostial lesions commonly failed to respond, in part because of extensive recoil of the plaque which extended into the main portion of the aorta.[287, 288] These lesions develop restenosis rapidly, even after early success.[289] Endovascular stents were introduced for ostial lesions in the late 1980s and early 1990s.[290] These agents have been widely accepted by interventional radiologists and cardiologists, despite the fact that none has yet been approved by the Food and Drug Administration (FDA) for use in the renal arteries.

The technical advantage of stents is indisputable. An example of successful renal artery stent placement is shown in Figure 46-24. A prospective comparison between angioplasty alone versus angioplasty with stents indicates that intermediate (6-12 months) vessel patency was 29% and 75% respectively. Restenosis fell from 48% to 14% in patients with stents.[287] As technical success continues to improve, many reports suggest nearly 100% technical success in early vessel patency, although rates of restenosis continue to reach 14% to 25%.[288, 291-295]

The demographic features of patients undergoing renal revascularization have been changing during the last decades.[131] The mean age of patients undergoing either surgery or angioplasty (with or without stents) has climbed from 55 years to more than 75 years, as illustrated in Figure 46-10B. It is likely that many patients are now offered endovascular procedures who otherwise would not be considered candidates for major surgical procedures, such as aortic or renal reconstruction.

What are the outcomes of patients undergoing placement of renal artery stents? These are commonly considered in terms of (1) *blood pressure control* and (2) preservation or salvage of *renal function* in ischemic nephropathy. Results from observational cohort blood pressure studies after stent placement face the same limitations observed with angioplasty alone. Results during follow-up from 1 to 4 years are summarized for representative series in Table 46-10. These have been reviewed elsewhere.[293, 296] Typical falls in blood pressure levels are in the range of 25 to 30 mm Hg systolic, the best predictor of which was the initial systolic blood pressure.[297] Some authors report 42% "improvement" in blood pressure with fewer medications needed, although cures were rare and renal function was unchanged.[292] Careful attention to the degree of residual patency led to more than 91% patency at 1 year and 79% at 5 years in 210 patients with stents.[207] Blood pressures were "cured" or "improved" in more than 80%. In some cases, angina and recurrent congestive cardiac failure subsided.[298, 299] As noted under the trials summarized earlier, prospective randomized controlled trials have been less impressive regarding the benefits of angioplasty. When standardized pressure measurement is applied to both medically treated control groups and interventional groups, the differences in blood pressure are more in the range of 5 to 10 mm Hg. The ambiguity of blood pressure responses in these studies has produced widely different recommendations. These range from "we are left with whether renal angioplasty should be considered at all"[300] to a general conviction expressed within the interventional cardiology community that "open renal arteries are better than closed renal arteries" and that nearly all renal artery lesions should be opened (and probably with placement of stents).[180]

It must be emphasized that these trials face the problem of patient selection, which likely understates the benefit of revascularization. Most trials excluded accelerated hypertension, advancing renal dysfunction, or recent congestive cardiac failure, in which cases successful revascularization can offer major benefit. Importantly, the crossover rate from medical therapy ranged from 26% to 44% in the prospective trials,[170, 241] indicating that medical therapy alone simply does not succeed in a subset of patients with renovascular hypertension.

Several comparisons have been made between stents and angioplasty (PTRA) alone.[294] Remarkably, the differences in clinical outcomes have been relatively small, both as regards changes in blood pressure and in kidney function, despite demonstrably improved vessel patency in patients with stents.[294] A prospective, randomized trial comparing stents with angioplasty for ostial lesions demonstrated nearly identical clinical results regarding both blood pressure and kidney function.[287] These observations tend to emphasize the lack of correlation between target vessel patency alone and the clinical results of renal revascularization.

What are the results regarding *recovery of renal function* with endovascular revascularization? Table 46-10 summarizes some of the recent series. In general, changes in renal function for atherosclerotic RAS, as reflected by serum creatinine levels, have been small.[1] Remarkably, the changes in renal function in azotemic patients after surgical reconstruction are similar.[131, 301] As some have observed, overall group changes in kidney function can be misleading.[175] Careful evaluation of the literature indicates that three distinctly different clinical outcomes are routinely observed. In some instances (approximately 27%), revascularization results in distinct improvement in kidney function. For this group, serum creatinine may fall from a mean value of 4.5 mg/dL to an average of 2.2 mg/dL.[1] There can be no doubt that such

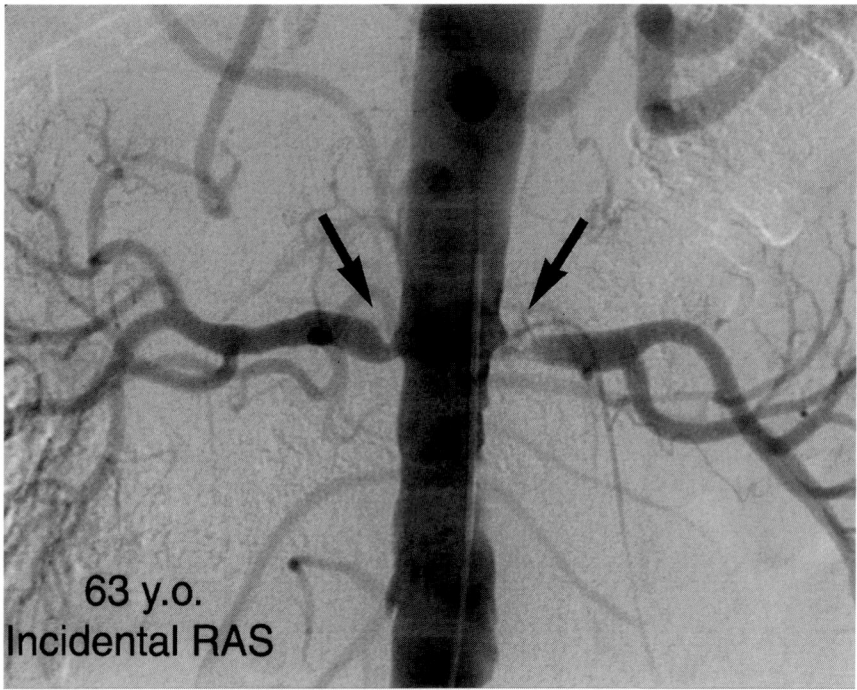

63 y.o.
Incidental RAS

A

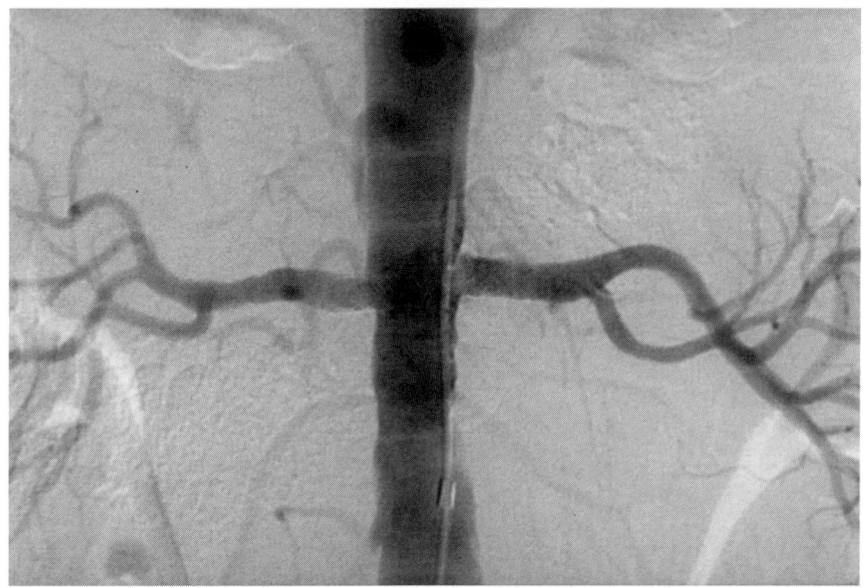

B

FIGURE 46-24. A, Renal aortogram illustrating high-grade, bilateral renal arterial lesions in a 63-year-old man who developed accelerated hypertension a few months earlier. **B,** Aortogram after placement of endovascular stents, illustrating excellent vessel patency and early technical success. This was followed by resolution of the hypertension. (From Textor SC: Progressive hypertension in a patient with "incidental" renal artery stenosis. Hypertension 40:595-600, 2002.)

patients benefit from the procedure and can avoid the major morbidity (and probably mortality) associated with advanced renal failure. The bulk of patients, however, have no measurable change in renal function (approximately 52%). Whether such patients benefit much depends upon the true clinical likelihood of progressive renal injury if the stenotic lesion had been managed without revascularization, as discussed earlier. Those without the risk of progression likely gain little. The most significant concern, however, is the group of patients whose renal function deteriorates further after a revascularization procedure. In most reports, this ranges from 19% to 25%.[1, 302] In some instances, this represents atheroembolic disease, or a variety of complications, including vessel

dissection with thrombosis.[303] Hence, nearly 20% of patients face a relatively rapid progression of renal insufficiency and the potential for requiring renal replacement therapy, including dialysis or renal transplantation.[293, 301, 304] Possible mechanisms of deterioration include atheroembolic injury, which may be nearly universal after any vascular intervention,[305] and acceleration of oxidative stress producing interstitial fibrosis.[61] Whether improving techniques, including the application of distal "protection" devices for endovascular catheters, will reduce these complications is not yet known.

Several studies suggest that progression of renal failure attributed to ischemic nephropathy may be reduced by endovascular procedures.[302, 306] Harden and co-workers

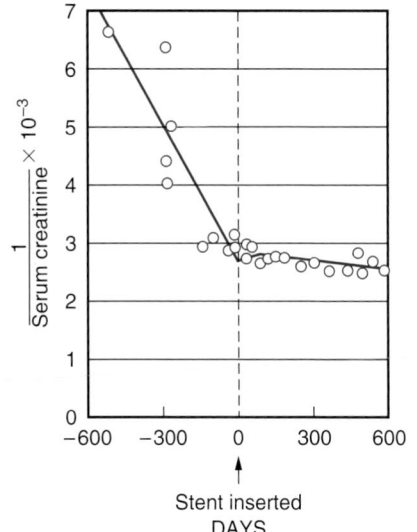 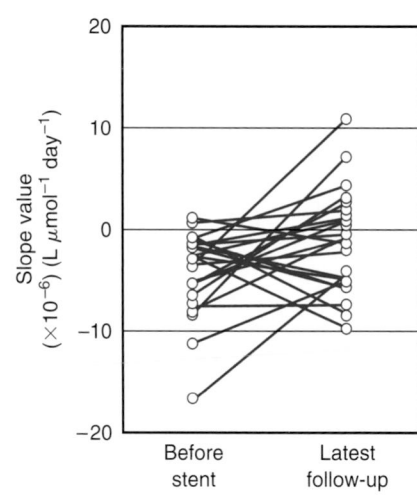

FIGURE 46-25. Reciprocal creatinine plots and calculated slope of declining renal function in 23 of 32 patients followed before and after placement of renal artery stents. These data are presented as reflecting "stabilization" of renal function, although it might be observed that similar plots might be obtained with renal artery occlusion as illustrated in Figure 46-22. Nonetheless, that some patients actually improved has been observed in series with bilateral renal artery stenoses or stenosis to a solitary kidney.[306] (From Harden PN, Macleod MJ, Rodger RS, et al: Effect of renal-artery stenting on progression of renovascular renal failure. Lancet 349:1133-1136, 1997.)

presented reciprocal creatinine plots in 23 of 32 patients suggesting that the slope of loss of the GFR could be favorably changed after placement of renal artery stents, as illustrated in Figure 46-25.[302] It should be emphasized that 69% "improved or stabilized," indicating that 31% did not, as with other series. Caution must be applied regarding the use of reciprocal creatinine plots in this disorder, however. It will be recognized that vascular disease is not a uniform disorder affecting both kidneys nor is it likely to follow a regular and progressive course, in contrast, for example, to diabetic nephropathy. As a result, a gradual loss of renal function with subsequent stabilization might be obtained with unilateral disease leading to total occlusion, as illustrated in Figure 46-22C. Perhaps the most convincing group data in this regard derived from serial renal functional measurement in 33 patients with high-grade (>70%) stenosis to the entire affected renal mass (bilateral disease or stenosis to a solitary functioning kidney) with creatinine levels between 1.5 and 4.0 mg/dL. Follow-up over a mean of 20 months indicate that the slope of GFR loss converted from negative (−0.0079 dL/mg/month) to positive (0.0043 dL/mg/month).[306] These studies agree with other observations that long-term survival is reduced in bilateral disease and that the potential for renal dysfunction and accelerated cardiovascular disease risk is highest in such patients (see earlier discussion).

Predictors of Likely Benefit Regarding Renal Revascularization

Identification of patients most likely to obtain improved blood pressure or renal function after renal revascularization remains an elusive task. As noted, functional tests of renin release, such as measurement of renal vein renin levels, have not performed universally well. Many of these studies are most useful when positive, for example, the likelihood of benefit improves with more evident lateralization, but have relatively poor negative predictive value, that is, when such studies are negative, outcomes of vessel repair may still

be beneficial. As a clinical matter, recent progression of hypertension remains among the most consistent predictors of improved blood pressure after intervention.

Predicting favorable renal functional outcomes is also difficult. Several series indicate that either surgical or endovascular procedures are least likely to benefit those with advanced renal insufficiency, usually characterized by serum creatinine levels above 3.0 mg/dL.[131, 265, 266, 307] Small kidneys, as identified by length less than 8 cm, are less likely to recover function, particularly when little function can be identified on radionuclide renography.[308] Reports of renal resistance index measured by Doppler ultrasound in 5950 patients indicate that identification of lower resistance was a favorable marker for improvement in both GFR and blood pressure, whereas an elevated resistance index was an independent marker for poor outcomes[214] (see Fig. 46-16). None of these is absolute. A recent deterioration of kidney function portends more likely improvement with reconstruction.

Complications of Angioplasty and Stents

Atherosclerotic plaques are commonly composed of multiple layers with calcified, fibrotic, and inflammatory components. Physical expansion of such lesions applies considerable force to the wall and may lead to cracking and release of small particulate debris into the bloodstream. Effective balloon angioplasty and placement of stents requires learning optimal techniques for limiting the damage to blood vessels during the procedure. As a result, optimal results depend upon achieving a level of competence after traversing a learning curve. Reported results vary considerably among centers and are improving with increasing experience.[309] A review of 10 published series with 416 vessels with stents indicates that significant complications arise in 13% of cases, not including those that lead to the need for dialysis. These include several of the events listed in Table 46-11, including hematomas and retroperitoneal bleeding requiring transfusion. Renal function deteriorated in these series on average 26% of the time and 50% (7/14) subjects with

TABLE 46-11

Complications after Percutaneous Transluminal Renal Angioplasty and Renal Artery Stent Placement

Minor (most frequently reported)
  Groin hematoma
  Puncture site trauma
Major (reported in 71/799 treated arteries [9%][294])
  Hemorrhage requiring transfusion
  Femoral artery pseudoaneurysm needing repair
  Brachial artery traumatic injury needing repair
  Renal artery perforation leading to surgical intervention
  Stent thrombosis: surgical or antithrombotic intervention
  Distal renal artery embolus
  Iliac artery dissection
  Segmental renal infarction
  Cholesterol embolism: renal
  Peripheral atheroemboli
  Aortic dissection[303]
Restenosis: 16% (range: 0%-39%)
Deterioration of renal function: 26% (range: 0%-45%)
Mortality attributed to procedure: 0.5%
Procedure-related complications: 51/379 patients in 10 series: 13.5%[293]

Data from references 293, 294, 303.

preprocedure creatinine levels above 400 mmol (4.5 mg/dL) progressed to advanced renal failure requiring dialysis.[293] Most complications are minor, including local hematomas and false aneurysms at the insertion site. Occasional severe complications develop, including aortic dissection,[303] stent migration, and vessel occlusion with thrombosis.[275] Local renal dissections can be managed by judicious application of additional stents. The mortality related directly to this procedure is small, but has been reported as a complication in 0.5% of patients.[293] Restenosis remains a significant clinical limitation. Reported rates vary widely between 13% and 30%, most often within the first 6 to 12 months.[128, 293, 294, 310] Most recent series report 13% to 16% restenoses, sometimes leading to repeat procedures. Whether this will be changed by future use of sirolimus-coated stents, as it has for coronary restenosis, is not yet known.[311]

SUMMARY

Renovascular disease is common, particularly in older people with atherosclerotic disease elsewhere. It can produce a wide array of clinical effects, ranging from asymptomatic "incidental" disease to accelerated hypertension and progressive renal failure. With improved imaging and older patients, significant renal artery disease is detected more often than ever before. Management of cardiovascular risk and hypertension is the primary objective of medical management. It is incumbent upon clinicians to evaluate both the role of renal artery disease in the individual patient and the potential risk-benefit ratio for timing renal revascularization. For most patients, the realistic goals of renal revascularization are to reduce medication requirements and to stabilize renal function over time. Patients with bilateral disease or stenosis to a solitary functioning kidney may achieve a lower risk of circulatory congestion (flash pulmonary edema or its equivalent) and a lower risk for advancing renal failure.

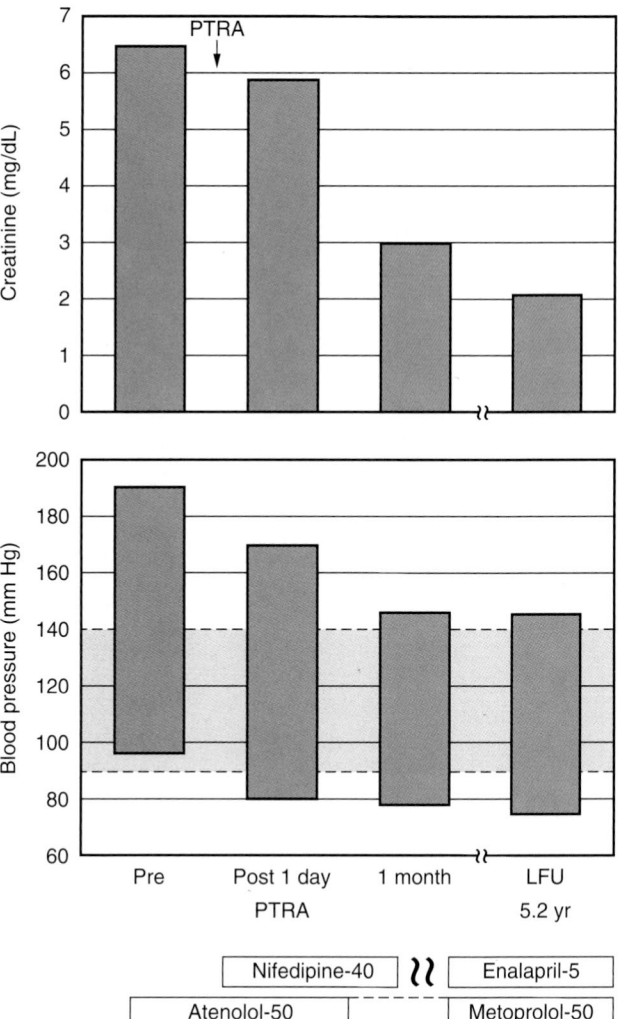

FIGURE 46-26. Serum creatinine and blood pressure levels before and after percutaneous renal artery angioplasty (PTRA) in a patient with bilateral, high-grade renal artery stenoses and recently developing renal failure. Restoration of blood supply to the kidneys led to a fall in creatinine from above 6 mg/dL to 2.1 mg/dL. Improvement in blood pressure control was achieved with administration of an angiotensin-converting enzyme (ACE) inhibitor, which had not been tolerated previously. Such cases illustrate the potential benefits of recognizing and acting to restore kidney function when possible in patients developing ischemic nephropathy. LFU, latest follow-up. (From Textor SC, Wilcox CS: Ischemic nephropathy/azotemic renal vascular disease. Semin Nephrol 20:489-502, 2000.)

As illustrated in Figure 46-26, successful renal revascularization can dramatically restore kidney function and improve long-term blood pressure control in selected patients. It is essential to appreciate the risks inherent in either surgical or endovascular manipulation of the diseased aorta. These include the hazard of atheroembolic complications and potential deterioration of renal function related to the procedure itself (estimated at 20%). Hence, the decision to undertake these procedures should include consideration of whether the potential gain warrants such risks. In many cases, improved blood pressure and recovery of renal function represent complete risk justification. Long-term management of patients with renovascular disease requires a commitment to intensive medical management aimed at reducing atherosclerotic risk.

MANAGEMENT OF RENOVASCULAR HYPERTENSION AND ISCHEMIC NEPHROPATHY

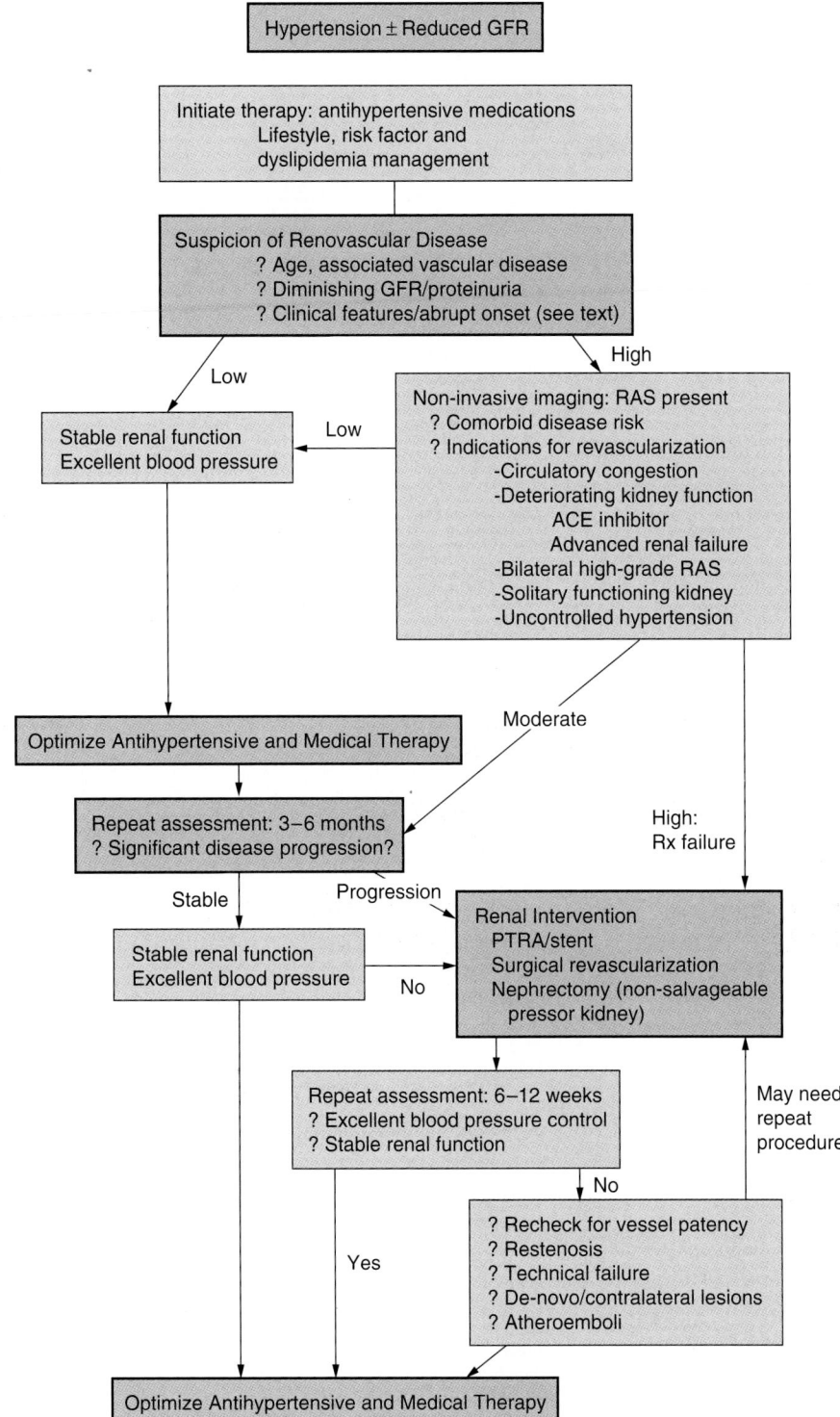

FIGURE 46-27. Algorithm summarizing a general management scheme for patients with renovascular hypertension or ischemic nephropathy, or both. Optimizing antihypertensive and medical therapy of comorbid disease, particularly hyperlipidemia, is paramount to reducing cardiovascular morbidity and mortality in atherosclerotic disease. Decisions regarding timing of renal revascularization procedures depend both upon the clinical manifestations (see text) and whether blood pressures and kidney function remain stable. ACE, angiostensin-converting enzyme; GFR, glomerular filtration rate; PTRA, percutaneous transluminal renal angioplasty; RAS, renal artery stenosis.

One algorithm by which one can pursue this objective is illustrated in Figure 46-27. Application of surgical or endovascular revascularization is one important means of achieving reduced risk and protecting the kidney, but requires frequent reassessment. Follow-up of both blood pressure and renal function is important, particularly because of the potential for restenosis or recurrent disease. Selection of the balance and timing of medical management and revascularization depends largely upon the comorbid disease risks for each patient.

REFERENCES

1. Textor SC, Wilcox CS: Renal artery stenosis: A common, treatable cause of renal failure? Annu Rev Med 52:421-442, 2001.
2. Tigerstedt R, Bergman PG: Niere und Kreislauf. Scand Arch Physiol 8:223-271, 1898.
3. Basso N, Terragno NA: History about the discovery of the renin-angiotensin system. Hypertension 38:1246-1249, 2001.
4. Goldblatt H, Lynch J, Hanzal RE, Summerville WW: Studies on experimental hypertension I: The production of persistent elevation of systolic blood pressure by means of renal ischemia. J Exp Med 59:347-379, 1934.
5. Ferrario CM, McCubbin JW: Renal blood flow and perfusion pressure before and after development of renal hypertension. Am J Physiol 224:102-109, 1973.
6. DeForrest JM, Knappenberger RC, Antonaccio MJ, et al: Angiotensin II is a necessary component for the development of hypertension in the two-kidney, one clip rat. AM J Cardiol 49:1515-1517, 1982.
7. Martinez-Maldonado M: Pathophysiology of renovascular hypertension. Hypertension 17:707-719, 1991.
8. Meyrier A, Hill GW, Simon P: Ischemic renal diseases: New insights into old entities. Kidney Int 54:2-13, 1998.
9. Border WA, Noble NA: Interactions of transforming growth factor-β and angiotensin II in renal fibrosis. Hypertension 31(pt 2):181-188, 1998.
10. Gavras I, Gavras H: Angiotensin II as a cardiovascular risk factor. J Hum Hypertens 16(suppl 2):S2-S6, 2002.
11. Leadbetter WF, Burkland CE: Hypertension in unilateral renal disease. J Urol 39:611-626, 1938.
12. Stanley JC: Surgical treatment of renovascular hypertension. Am J Surg 174:102-110, 1997.
13. Smith HW: Unilateral nephrectomy in hypertensive diseases. J Urol 76:685-701, 1956.
14. Morris GC, DeBakey NE, Cooley DA: Surgical treatment of renal failure of renovascular origin. JAMA 182:609-612, 1962.
15. Hunt JC, Sheps SG, Harrison EG, et al: Renal and renovascular hypertension : A reasoned approach to diagnosis and management. Arch Intern Med 133:988-999, 1974.
16. Franklin SS, Young JD, Maxwell MH, et al: Operative morbidity and mortality in renovascular disease. JAMA 231:1148-1153, 1975.
17. Conlon PJ, O'Riordan E, Kalra PA: Epidemiology and clinical manifestations of atherosclerotic renal artery stenosis. Am J Kidney Dis 35:573-587, 2000.
18. May AG, DeWeese JA, Rob CG: Hemodynamic effects of arterial stenosis. Surgery 53:513-524, 1963.
19. May AG, van Berg L, DeWeese JA, et al: Critical arterial stenosis. Surgery 54:250-259, 1963.
20. Dzau VJ, Siwek LG, Rosen S, et al: Sequential renal hemodynamics in experimental benign and malignant hypertension. Hypertension 3:63-68, 1981.
21. Lerman LO, Schwartz RS, Grande JP, et al: Noninvasive evaluation of a novel swine model of renal artery stenosis. J Am Soc Nephrol 10:1455-1465, 1999.
22. Hollenberg NK: Medical therapy of renovascular hypertension: Efficacy and safety of captopril in 269 patients. Cardiovasc Rev Rep 4:852-876, 1983.
23. Davis JO, Freeman RH: Mechanisms regulating renin release. Physiol Rev 56:1-56, 1976.
24. Freeman RH, Davis JO, Watkins BE, et al: Effects of continuous converting enzyme blockade on renovascular hypertension in the rat. Am J Physiol 236:F21-F24, 1979.
25. Vaughan ED Jr, Buhler FR, Laragh JH, et al: Renovascular hypertension: Renin measurements to indicate hypersecretion and contralateral suppression, estimate renal plasma flow and score for surgery. Am J Med 55:402-414, 1973.
26. Brunner H, Desaulles PA, Regoli D, Gross F: Renin content and excretory function of the kidney in rats with experimental hypertension. Am J Physiol 202:795-799, 1962.
27. Mackenzie HS, Morrill AL, Ploth DW: Pressure dependence of exaggerated natriuresis in two-kidney, one clip Goldblatt hypertensive rats. Kidney Int 27:731-738, 1985.
28. Brunner HR, Kirshmann JD, Sealey JE, Laragh JH: Hypertension of renal origin: Evidence for two different mechanisms. Science 174:1344-1346, 1971.
29. Howard JE, Berthrong N, Gould D, Yendt ER: Hypertension resulting from unilateral renovascular disease and its relief by nephrectomy. Bull Johns Hopkins Hosp 94:51-74, 1954.
30. Floyer MA: Role of the kidney in experimental hypertension. Br Med Bull 13:29-32, 1957.
31. Doyle AE, Duffy SG: Sodium balance and plasma renin activity during the development of two-kidney Goldblatt hypertension in rats. Clin Exp Pharmacol Physiol 7:293-304, 1980.
32. de Simone G, Devereux RB, Volpe M, et al: Relation of left ventricular hypertrophy, afterload, and contractility to left ventricular performance in Goldblatt hypertension. Am J Hypertens 5:292-301, 1992.
33. Brunner HR, Gavras H, Laragh JH: Specific inhibition of the renin-angiotensin system: A key to understanding blood pressure regulation. Prog Cardiovasc Dis 17:87-98, 1974.
34. Gavras H, Brunner HR, Vaughan ED, Laragh JH: Angiotensin-sodium interaction in blood pressure maintenance of renal hypertensive and normotensive rats. Science 180:1369-1370, 1973.
35. Gavras H, Brunner HR, Thurston H, Laragh JH: Reciprocation of renin dependency with sodium-volume dependency in renal hypertension. Science 188:1316-1317, 1975.
36. Cowley AW, Roman RJ: The role of the kidney in hypertension. JAMA 275:1581-1589, 1996.
37. Romero JC, Feldstein AE, Rodriguez-Porcel MG, Cases-Amenos A: New insights into the pathophysiology of renovascular hypertension. Mayo Clin Proc 72:251-260, 1997.
38. Faria FA, Salgado MC: Facilitation noradrenergic transmission by angiotensin in hypertensive rats. Hypertension 19(suppl 2):II30-II35, 1992.
39. Miyajima E, Yamada Y, Yoshida Y, et al: Muscle sympathetic nerve activity in renovascular hypertension and primary aldosteronism. Hypertension 17:1057-1062, 1991.
40. Ploth DW, Roy RN, Huang WC, Navar LG: Impaired renal blood flow and cortical pressure autoregulation in contralateral kidneys of Goldblatt hypertensive rats. Hypertension 3:67-74, 1981.
41. Lerman LO, Nath KA, Rodriguez-Porcel M, et al: Increased oxidative stress in experimental renovascular hypertension. Hypertension 37:541-546, 2001.
42. Ruiz-Ortega M, Gomez-Garre D, et al: Involvement of angiotensin II and endothelin in matrix protein production and renal sclerosis. J Hypertens Suppl 12:S51-S58, 1994.
43. Romero JC, Reckelhoff JF: Role of angiotensin and oxidative stress in essential hypertension. Hypertension 43(pt 2):943-949, 1999.
44. Herizi A, Jover B, Bouriquet N, Mimran A: Prevention of the cardiovascular and renal effects of angiotensin II by endothelin blockade. Hypertension 31(pt 1):10-14, 1998.
45. DiBona G: Central sympathoexcitatory actions of angiotensin II: Role of type 1 angiotensin II receptors. J Am Soc Nephrol 10:S90-S94, 1999.
46. Higashi Y, Sasaki S, Nakagawa K, et al: Endothelial function and oxidative stress in renovascular hypertension. N Engl J Med 346:1954-1962, 2002.
47. Brown JJ, Davies DL, Morton JJ, et al: Mechanism of renal hypertension. Lancet 1:1219-1221, 1976.
48. Lerman L, Textor SC: Pathophysiology of ischemic nephropathy. Urol Clin North Am 28:793-803, 2001.
49. Jensen G, Bjorck S, Nielsen OJ, et al: Diagnostic use of renal vein erythropoietin measurements in patients with renal artery stenosis. Nephrol Dial Transplant 7:400-405, 1992.
50. Nielsen K, Rehling M, Henriksen JH: Renal vein oxygen saturation in renal artery stenosis. Clin Physiol 12:179-184, 1992.
51. Moran K, Mulhall J, Kelly D, et al: Morphological changes and alterations in regional intrarenal blood flow induced by graded renal ischemia. J Urol 148:463-466, 1992.
52. Yune HY, Klatte EC: Collateral circulation to an ischemic kidney. Radiology 119:539-546, 1976.
53. Lerman LO, Bentley MD, Fiksen-Olsen MJ, et al: Pressure dependency of canine intrarenal blood flow within the range of autoregulation. Am J Physiol 268:F404-F409, 1995.
54. Lerman LO, Taler SJ, Textor SC, et al: Computed tomography–derived intrarenal blood flow in renovascular and essential hypertension. Kidney Int 49:846-854, 1996.
55. Textor SC, Smith-Powell L: Post-stenotic arterial pressure, renal haemodynamics and sodium excretion during graded pressure reduction in conscious rats with one- and two-kidney coarctation hypertension. J Hypertens 6:311-319, 1988.

56. Best PJ, Hasdai D, Sangiorgi G, et al: Apoptosis: Basic concepts and implications in coronary artery disease. Arterioscler Thromb Vasc Biol 19:14-22, 1999.

57. Gobe GC, Axelsen RA, Searle JW: Cellular events in experimental unilateral ischemic renal atrophy and in regeneration after contralateral nephrectomy. Lab Invest 63:770-779, 1990.

58. Abdi A, Johns EJ: Importance of the renin-angiotensin system in the generation of kidney failure in renovascular hypertension. J Hypertens 14:1131-1137, 1996.

59. Zou LX, Imig JD, von Thun AM, et al: Receptor-mediated intrarenal angiotensin II augmentation in angiotensin II–infused rats. Hypertension 28:669-677, 1996.

60. Geiger H, Fierlbeck W, Mai B, et al: Effects of early and late antihypertensive treatment on extracellular matrix proteins and mononuclear cells in uninephrectomized SHR. Kidney Int 51:750-761, 1997.

61. Klahr S, Morrissey J: The role of vasoactive compounds, growth factors and cytokines in the progression of renal disease. Kidney Int 57:S7-S14, 2000.

62. Matsusaka T, Hymes J, Ichikawa I: Angiotensin in progressive renal diseases: Theory and practice. J Am Soc Nephrol 7:2025-2043, 1996.

63. Nava E, Luscher TF: Endothelium-derived vasoactive factors in hypertension: Nitric oxide and endothelin. J Hypertens 13:S39-S48, 1995.

64. Aki Y, Tomohiro A, Nishiyama A, et al: The role of basally synthesized nitric oxide in modulating the renal vasoconstrictor action of angiotensin II. Hypertens Res 20:251-256, 1997.

65. Bachmann S, Mundel P: Nitric oxide in the kidney: Synthesis, localization and function. Am J Kidney Dis 24:112-129, 1994.

66. Raij L: Nitric oxide in hypertension: Relationship with renal injury and left ventricular hypertrophy. Hypertension 31:189-193, 1998.

67. Sigmon DH, Beierwaltes WH: Renal nitric oxide and angiotensin II interaction in renovascular hypertrophy. Hypertension 22:237-242, 1993.

68. Ritthaler T, Gopfert T, Firth JD, et al: Influence of hypoxia on hepatic and renal endothelin gene expression. Pflugers Arch 431:587-593, 1996.

69. Firth JD, Ratcliffe PJ: Organ distribution of the three rat endothelin messenger RNAs and the effects of ischemia on renal gene expression. J Clin Invest 90:1023-1031, 1992.

70. Schlondorff D: Renal prostaglandin synthesis: Sites of production and specific actions of prostaglandins. Am J Med 81:1-11, 1986.

71. Chaudhari A, Kirschenbaum MA: Alterations in rabbit renal microvascular prostanoid synthesis in acute renal failure. Am J Physiol 254:F684-F688, 1988.

72. Sirois MG, Filep JG, Rousseau A, et al: Endothelin-1 enhances vascular permeability in conscious rats: Role of thromboxane A2. Eur J Pharmacol 214:119-125, 1992.

73. Himmelstein SI, Klotman PE: The role of thromboxane in two-kidney, one-clip Goldblatt hypertension in rats. Am J Physiol 257:F190-F196, 1989.

74. Bomzon A, Holt S, Moore K: Bile acids, oxidative stress and renal function in biliary obstruction. Semin Nephrol 17:549-562, 1997.

75. Baud L, Ardaillou R: Involvement of reactive oxygen species in kidney damage. Br Med Bull 49:621-629, 1993.

76. Remuzzi G, Bertani T: Pathophysiology of progressive nephropathies. N Engl J Med 339:1448-1456, 1998.

77. Grande JP: Role of transforming growth factor-β in tissue injury and repair. Proc Soc Exp Biol Med 214:27-40, 1997.

78. Basile DP, Martin DR, Hammerman MR: Extracellular matrix–related genes in kidney after ischemic injury: Potential role for TGF β in repair. Am J Physiol 275:F894-F903, 1998.

79. Wolf G, Mueller E, Stahl RA, Ziyadeh FN: Angiotensin II–induced hypertrophy of cultured murine proximal tubular cells is mediated by endogenous transforming growth factor-β. J Clin Invest 92:1366-1372, 1993.

80. Eddy AA: Molecular insights into renal interstitial fibrosis. J Am Soc Nephrol 7:2495-2508, 1996.

81. Chade AR, Rodriguez-Porcel M, Grande JP, et al: Distinct renal injury in early atherosclerosis and renovascular disease. Circulation 106:1165-1171, 2002.

82. Nath KA, Croatt AJ, Haggard JJ, Grande JP: Renal response to repetitive exposure to heme proteins: Chronic injury induced by an acute insult. Kidney Int 57:2423-2433, 2000.

83. Thomas SE, Anderson S, Gordon KL, et al: Tubulointerstitial disease in aging: Evidence for underlying peritubular capillary damage, a potential role for renal ischemia. J Am Soc Nephrol 9:231-242, 1998.

84. Truong LD, Farhood A, Tasby J, Gillum D: Experimental chronic renal ischemia: Morphologic and immunologic studies. Kidney Int 41:1676-1689, 1992.

85. Molitoris BA, Marrs J: The role of cell adhesion molecules in ischemic acute renal failure. Am J Med 106:583-592, 1999.

86. Weight SC, Bell PRF, Nicholson ML: Renal ischaemia-reperfusion injury. Br J Surg 83:162-170, 1996.

87. Garcia-Criado FJ, Eleno N, Santos-Benito F, et al: Protective effect of exogenous nitric oxide on the renal function and inflammatory response in a model of ischemia-reperfusion. Transplantation 66:982-990, 1998.

88. Dauber IM, Lesnefsky EJ, Van Benthuysen KM, et al: Reactive oxygen metabolite scavengers decrease functional coronary microvascular injury due to ischemia-reperfusion. Am J Physiol 260:H42-H49, 1991.

89. Kontogiannis J, Burns KD: Role of AT1 angiotensin II receptors in renal ischemic injury. Am J Physiol 274:F79-F90, 1998.

90. Yu L, Gengaro PE, Niederberger M, et al: Nitric oxide: A mediator in rat tubular hypoxia/reoxygenation injury. Proc Natl Acad Sci U S A 91:1691-1695, 1994.

91. Lewin A, Blaufox MD, Castle H, et al: Apparent prevalence of curable hypertension in the Hypertension Detection and Follow-up Program. Arch Intern Med 145:424-427, 1985.

92. Working Group on Renovascular Hypertension: Detection, evaluation and treatment of renovascular hypertension: Final report. Arch Intern Med 147:820-829, 1987.

93. Svetkey LP, Kadir S, Dunnick NR, et al: Similar prevalence of renovascular hypertension in selected blacks and whites. Hypertension 17:678-683, 1991.

94. Anderson GH, Blakemen N, Streeten DH: The effect of age on prevalence of secondary forms of hypertension in 4429 consecutively referred patients. J Hypertens 12:609-615, 1994.

95. Alimi Y, Mercier C, Bellissier JF, et al: Fibromuscular disease of the renal artery: A new histopathologic classification. Ann Vasc Surg 6:220-224, 1992.

96. Cragg AH, Smith TP, Thompson BH, et al: Incidental fibromuscular dysplasia in potential renal donors: Long-term clinical follow-up. Radiology 172:145-147, 1989.

97. Harrison EG, McCormack LJ: Pathologic classification of renal arterial disease in renovascular hypertension. Mayo Clin Proc 46:161-167, 1971.

98. Morishita R: Possible role of the vascular renin-angiotensin system in hypertension and vascular hypertrophy. Hypertension 19(suppl 2):II-62-II-67, 1992.

99. Rossi G, Rossi A, Zanin L, et al: Excess prevalence of extracranial carotid artery lesions in renovascular hypertension. Am J Hypertens 5:8-15, 1992.

100. Bonelli FS, McKusick MA, Textor SC, et al: Renal artery angioplasty: Technical results and clinical outcome in 320 patients. Mayo Clin Proc 70:1041-1052, 1995.

101. Meaney TF, Dustan HP, McCormack LJ: Natural history of renal arterial disease. Radiology 91:881-887, 1968.

102. Berglund G: Secondary hypertension in the community. *In* Birkenhager WH, Reid JL (eds): Handbook of Hypertension. Amsterdam, Elsevier, 1985, pp 249-254.

103. Krijnen P, Van Jaarsveld BC, Steyerberg EW, et al: A clinical prediction rule for renal artery stenosis. Ann Intern Med 129:705-711, 1998.

104. Hansen KJ: Prevalence of ischemic nephropathy in the atherosclerotic population. Am J Kidney Dis 24:615-621, 1994.

105. Harding MB, Smith LR, Himmelstein SI, et al: Renal artery stenosis: Prevalence and associated risk factors in patients undergoing routine cardiac catheterization. J Am Soc Nephrol 2:1608-1616, 1992.

106. Rihal CS, Textor SC, Breen JF, et al: Incidental renal artery stenosis among a prospective cohort of hypertensive patients undergoing coronary angiography. Mayo Clin Proc 77:309-316, 2002.

107. Vetrovec GW, Landwehr DM, Edwards VL: Incidence of renal artery stenosis in hypertensive patients undergoing coronary angiography. J Intervent Cardiol 2:69-76, 1989.

108. Swartbol P, Thorvinger BOT, Parsson H, Norgren L: Renal artery stenosis in patients with peripheral vascular disease and its correlation to hypertension: A retrospective study. Int Angiol 11:195-199, 1992.

109. Choudhri AH, Cleland JGF, Rowlands PC, et al: Unsuspected renal artery stenosis in peripheral vascular disease. BMJ 301:1197-1198, 1990.

110. Olin JW, Melia M, Young JR, et al: Prevalence of atherosclerotic RAS in patients with atherosclerosis elsewhere. Am J Med 88: 46N-51N, 1990.

111. Coen G, Manni M, Giannoni MF, et al: Ischemic nephropathy in an elderly nephrologic and hypertensive population. Am J Nephrol 18:221-227, 1998.

112. Holley KE, Hunt JC, Brown AL Jr, et al: Renal artery stenosis. A clinical-pathological study in normotensive and hypertensive patients. Am J Med 37:124-132, 1964.

113. Scoble JE: The epidemiology and clinical manifestations of atherosclerotic renal disease. *In* Novick AC, Scoble J, Hamilton G (eds): Renal Vascular Disease. London: WB Saunders, 1996, pp 303-314.

114. Welch HG, Albertsen PC, Nease RF, et al: Estimating treatment benefits for the elderly: The effect of competing risks. Ann Intern Med 124:577-584, 1996.

115. Tegtmeyer CJ, Elson J, Glass TA, et al: Percutaneous transluminal angioplasty: The treatment of choice for renovascular hypertension due to fibromuscular dysplasia. Radiology 143:631-637, 1982.

116. Davis BA, Crook JE, Vestal RE, Oates JA: Prevalence of renovascular hypertension in patients with grade III or IV hypertensive retinopathy. N Engl J Med 301:1273-1276, 1979.

117. Lazarus JM, Hampers CL, Bennett AH, et al: Urgent bilateral nephrectomy for severe hypertension. Ann Intern Med 76:733-739, 1972.

118. Swinton NW, Breslin DJ, Libertino JA, Zinman L: Renovascular hypertension: Therapeutic decisions and results. *In* Breslin DJ, Swinton NW, Libertino JA, Zinman L (eds): Renovascular Hypertension. Baltimore, Williams & Wilkins, 1982, pp 213-221.

119. Hollenberg NK: Medical therapy for renovascular hypertension: A review. Am J Hypertens 1:338s-343s, 1988.

120. Textor SC: ACE inhibitors in renovascular hypertension. Cardiovasc Drugs Ther 4:229-235, 1990.

121. Franklin SS, Smith RD: Comparison of effects of enalapril plus hydrochlorothiazide versus standard triple therapy on renal function in renovascular hypertension. Am J Med 79(suppl 3c):14-23, 1985.

122. Heart Outcomes Prevention Evaluation Study Investigators: Effects of an angiotensin-converting enzyme inhibitor, ramipril, on cardiovascular events in high risk patients. N Engl J Med 342:145-153, 2000.

123. Mann JFE, Gerstein HC, Pogue J, et al, and the HOPE Investigators: Renal insufficiency as a predictor of cardiovascular outcomes and the impact of ramipril: The HOPE randomized trial. Ann Intern Med 134:629-636, 2001.

124. Losito A, Gaburri M, Errico R, et al: Survival of patients with renovascular disease and ACE inhibition. Clin Nephrol 52:339-343, 1999.

125. Schneider E, Guralnik J: The aging of America: Impact on health care costs. JAMA 263:2335-2340, 1990.

126. Winker MA: The emerging epidemic of atherosclerosis. JAMA 281:84-85, 1999.

127. Greco BA, Breyer JA: The natural history of renal artery stenosis: Who should be evaluated for suspected ischemic nephropathy? Semin Nephrol 16:2-11, 1996.

128. Tuttle KF, Chouinard RF, Webber JT, et al: Treatment of atherosclerotic ostial renal artery stenosis with the intravascular stent. Am J Kidney Dis 32:611-622, 1998.

129. Graham RM, Sebel EF, Stokes GS: Surgical intervention in severe and complicated renal hypertension: Report of the Sydney Renal Hypertension Group (1969-1975). Clin Sci Mol Med 51:231s-233s, 1976.

130. Foster JH, Maxwell MH, Franklin SS, et al: Renovascular occlusive disease:Results of operative treatment. JAMA 2231:1043-1048, 1975.

131. Hallett JW, Textor SC, Kos PB, et al: Advanced renovascular hypertension and renal insufficiency: Trends in medical comorbidity and surgical approach from 1970 to 1993. J Vasc Surg 21:750-759, 1995.

132. Dustan HP, Humphries AW, de Wolfe VG, Page IH: Normal arterial pressure in patients with renal arterial stenoses. JAMA 187:1028-1029, 1964.

133. Simon N, Franklin SS, Bleifer KH, Maxwell MH: Clinical characteristics of renovascular hypertension. JAMA 220:1209-1218, 1972.

134. Kaneko K, Shimazaki S, Ino T, et al: Severe hyponatremia in a patient with renovascular hypertension: Case report. Nephron 68:252-255, 1994.

135. Padfield PL, Brown JJ, Lever AF, et al: Changes of vasopressin in hypertension: Cause or effect? Lancet 1:1255-1257, 1976.

136. Textor SC, Novick A, Tarazi RC, et al: Critical perfusion pressure for renal function in patients with bilateral atherosclerotic renal vascular disease. Ann Intern Med 102:309-314, 1985.

137. Textor SC, Novick AC, Steinmuller DR, Streem SB: Renal failure limiting antihypertensive therapy as an indication for renal revascularization. Arch Intern Med 143:2208-2211, 1983.

138. Hricik DE, Browning PJ, Kopelman R, et al: Captopril-induced functional renal insufficiency in patients with bilateral renal-artery stenosis or renal-artery stenosis in a solitary kidney. N Eng1 J Med 308:377-381, 1983.

139. Holm EA, Randlov A, Strandgaard S: Brief report: Acute renal failure after losartan treatment in a patient with bilateral renal artery stenosis. Blood Press 5:360-362,1996.

140. Diamond JR: Flash pulmonary edema and the diagnostic suspicion of occult renal artery stenosis. Am J Kidney Dis 221:328-330, 1993.

141. Missouris CG, Belli AM, MacGregor GA: "Apparent" heart failure: A syndrome caused by renal artery stenoses. Heart 83:152-155, 2000.

142. Johansson M, Herlitz H, Jensen G, et al: Increased cardiovascular mortality in hypertensive patients with renal artery stenosis. Relation to sympathetic activation, renal function and treatment regimens. J Hypertens 17:1743-1750, 1999.

143. Pickering TG, Herman L, Devereux RB, et al: Recurrent pulmonary oedema in hypertension due to bilateral renal artery stenosis: Treatment by angioplasty or surgical revascularisation. Lancet 2:551-552, 1988.

144. Tami LF, McElderry MW, Al-Adli NM, et al: Renal artery stenosis presenting as crescendo angina pectoris. Cathet Cardiovasc Diagn 35:252-256, 1995.

145. Messina LM, Zelenock GB, Yao KA, Stanley JC: Renal revascularization for recurrent pulmonary edema in patients with poorly controlled hypertension and renal insufficiency: A distinct subgroup of patients with arteriosclerotic renal artery occlusive disease. J Vasc Surg 15:73-82, 1992.

146. Stack R: Procedural indications and variables that affect acute outcome. J Invasive Cardiol 10:103-104, 1998.

147. Scoble JE, Maher ER, Hamilton G, et al: Atherosclerotic renovascular disease causing renal impairment—a case for treatment. Clin Nephrol 31:119-122, 1989.

148. Jacobson HR: Ischemic renal disease: An overlooked clinical entity. Kidney Int 34:729-743, 1988.

149. Textor SC, Smith-Powell L: Pathophysiology of renal failure in ischemic renal disease. *In* Novick AC, Scoble J, Hamilton G (eds): Renal Vascular Disease. London, WB Saunders Co, 1996, pp 289-302.

150. Connolly JO, Higgins RM, Walters HL, et al: Presentation, clinical features and outcome in different patterns of atherosclerotic renovascular disease. Q J Med 87:413-421, 1994.

151. Kaylor WM, Novick AC, Ziegelbaum M, Vidt DG: Reversal of end stage renal failure with surgical revascularization in patients with atherosclerotic renal artery occlusion. J Urol 141:486-488, 1989.

152. Cheung CM, Wright JR, Shurrab AE, et al: Epidemiology of renal dysfunction and patient outcome in atherosclerotic renal artery occlusion. J Am Soc Nephrol 13:149-157, 2002.

153. Wright JR, Duggal A, Thomas R, et al: Clinicopathological correlation in biopsy-proven atherosclerotic nephropathy: Implications for renal functional outcome in atherosclerotic renovascular disease. Nephrol Dial Transplant 16:765-770, 2001.

154. Farmer CKT, Cook GJR, Balke GM, et al: Individual kidney function in atherosclerotic nephropathy is not related to the presence of renal artery stenosis. Nephrol Dial Transplant 14:2880-2884, 1999.

155. Wright JR, Shurrab AE, Cheung C, et al: A prospective study of the determinants of renal functional outcome and mortality in atherosclerotic renovascular disease. Am J Kidney Dis 39:1153-1161, 2002.

156. Mailloux LU, Napolitano B, Bellucci AG, et al: Renal vascular disease causing end-stage renal disease: Incidence, clinical correlates, and outcomes: A 20-year clinical experience. Am J Kidney Dis 24:622-629, 1994.

157. Fatica RA, Port FK, Young EW: Incidence trends and mortality in end-stage renal disease attributed to renovascular disease in the United States. Am J Kidney Dis 37:1184-1190, 2001.

158. Chen R, Novick AC, Pohl M: Reversible renin mediated massive proteinuria successfully treated by nephrectomy. J Urol 153:133-134, 1995.

159. Docci D, Moscatelli G, Capponcini C, et al: Nephrotic-range proteinuria in a patient with high renin hypertension: Effect of treatment with an ACE-inhibitor. Am J Nephrol 12:387-389, 1992.

160. Ie EH, Karschner JK, Shapiro AP: Reversible nephrotic syndrome due to high renin state in renovascular hypertension. Neth J Med 46:136-141, 1995.

161. Ben-Chitrit S, Korzets Z, Podjarny E, Bernheim J: Reversal of the nephrotic syndrome due to renovascular hypertension by successful percutaneous angioplasty and stenting. Nephrol Dial Transplant 10:1460-1461, 1995.

162. Alkhunaizi AM, Chapman A: Renal artery stenosis and unilateral focal and segmental glomerulosclerosis. Am J Kidney Dis 29:936-941, 1997.

163. Webster J, Marshall F, Abdalla M, et al: Randomised comparison of percutaneous angioplasty vs continued medical therapy for hypertensive patients with atheromatous renal artery stenosis. J Hum Hypertens 12:329-335, 1998.

164. Conlon PJ, Little MA, Pieper K, Mark DB: Severity of renal vascular disease predicts mortality in patients undergoing coronary angiography. Kidney Int 60:1490-1497, 2001.

165. Wollenweber J, Sheps SG, Davis DG: Clinical course of atherosclerotic renovascular disease. Am J Cardiol 21:60-71, 1968.

166. Schreiber MJ, Pohl MA, Novick AC: The natural history of atherosclerotic and fibrous renal artery disease. Urol Clin North Am 11:383-392, 1984.

167. Tollefson DFJ, Ernst CB: Natural history of atherosclerotic renal arterial disease associated with aortic disease. J Vasc Surg 14:327-331, 1991.

168. Zierler RE, Bergelin RO, Davidson RC, et al: A prospective study of disease progression in patients with atherosclerotic renal artery stenosis. Am J Hypertens 9:1055-1061, 1996.

169. Caps MT, Perissinotto C, Zierler RE, et al: Prospective study of atherosclerotic disease progression in the renal artery. Circulation 98:2866-2872, 1998.

170. van Jaarsveld BC, Krijnen P, Pieterman H, et al. for the Dutch Renal Artery Stenosis Intervention Cooperative Study Group: The effect of balloon angioplasty on hypertension in atherosclerotic renal-artery stenosis. N Engl J Med 342:1007-1014, 2000.

171. Caps MT, Zierler RE, Polissar NL, et al: Risk of atrophy in kidneys with atherosclerotic renal artery stenosis. Kidney Int 53:735-742, 1998.

172. Dean RH, Kieffer RW, Smith BM: Renovascular hypertension: Anatomic and renal functional changes during therapy. Arch Surg 116:1408-1415, 1981.

173. Leertouwer TC, Pattynama PMT, van den Berg-Huysmans A: Incidental renal artery stenosis in peripheral vascular disease: A case for treatment? Kidney Int 59:1480-1483, 2001.

174. Iglesias JI, Hamburger RJ, Feldman L, Kaufman JS: The natural history of incidental renal artery stenosis in patients with aortoiliac vascular disease. Am J Med 109:642-647, 2000.

175. Textor SC: Revascularization in atherosclerotic renal artery disease. Kidney Int 53:799-811, 1998.

176. Chabova V, Schirger A, Stanson AW, et al: Outcomes of atherosclerotic renal artery stenosis managed without revascularization. Mayo Clin Proc 75:437-444, 2000.

177. Conlon PJ, Athirakul K, Kovalik E, et al: Survival in renal vascular disease. J Am Soc Nephrol 9:252-256, 1998.

178. Rimmer JM, Plante DA, Madias NE: Therapeutic decision making in renal vascular hypertension. *In* Novick AC, Scoble J, Hamilton G (eds): Renal Vascular Disease. London, WB Saunders, 1996, pp 245-266.

179. Butterly DW, Schwab SJ: Renal artery stenosis: The case for conservative management. Mayo Clin Proc 75:435-436, 2000.

180. White CJ: Open renal arteries are better than closed renal arteries. Cathet Cardiovasc Diagn 45:9-10, 1998.

181. Mann SJ, Pickering TG: Detection of renovascular hypertension: State of the art: 1992. Ann Intern Med 117:845-853, 1992.

182. Wilcox CS: Use of angiotensin converting enzyme inhibitors for diagnosing renovascular hypertension. Kidney Int 44:1379-1390, 1993.

183. Boudewijn G, Vasbinder C, Nelemans PJ, et al: Diagnostic tests for renal artery stenosis in patients suspected of having renovascular hypertension: A meta-analysis. Ann Intern Med 135:401-411, 2001.

184. Wilcox CS, Williams CM, Smith TB, et al: Diagnostic uses of angiotensin-converting enzyme inhibitors in renovascular hypertension. Am J Hypertens 1:334s-349s, 1998.

185. Mueller FB, Sealey JE, Case DB, et al: The captopril test for identifying renovascular disease in hypertensive patients. Am J Med 80:633-644, 1986.

186. Postma CT, van Oijen AH, Barentsz JO, et al: The value of tests predicting renovascular hypertension in patients with renal artery stenosis treated by angioplasty. Arch Intern Med 151:1531-1535, 1991.

187. Safian RD, Textor SC: Medical progress: Renal artery stenosis. N Engl J Med 344:431-442, 2001.

188. Rudnick MR, Maxwell MH: Limitations of renin assays. *In* Narins RG (ed): Controversies in Nephrology and Hypertension. New York, Churchill Livingstone, 1984, pp 123-160.

189. Vaughan ED: Renovascular hypertension. Kidney Int 27:811-827, 1985.

190. Grim CE, Weinberger MH: Diagnosis of renovascular hypertension: The case for renin assays. *In* Narins RG (ed): Controversies in Nephrology and Hypertension. New York, Churchill Livingstone, 1984, pp 190-122.

191. Simon G, Coleman CC: Captopril-stimulated renal vein renin measurements in the diagnosis of atherosclerotic renovascular hypertension. Am J Hypertens 7:1-6, 1994.

192. Strong CG, Hunt JC, Sheps SG, et al: Renal venous renin activity: Enhancement of sensitivity of lateralization by sodium depletion. Am J Cardiol 27:602-611, 1971.

193. Roubidoux MA, Dunnick NR, Klotman PE, et al: Renal vein renins: Inability to predict response to revascularisation in patients with hypertension. Radiology 178:819-822, 1991.

194. Stamey TA, Nudelman JJ, Good PH, et al: Functional characteristics of renovascular hypertension. Medicine (Baltimore) 40:347-394, 1961.

195. Textor SC, Novick A, Mujais SK, et al: Responses of the stenosed and contralateral kidneys to (Sar-1, Thr-8) AII in human renovascular hypertension. Hypertension 5:796-804, 1983.

196. Textor SC, Tarazi RC, Novick AC, et al: Regulation of renal hemodynamics and glomerular filtration in patients with renovascular hypertension during converting enzyme inhibition with captopril. Am J Med 76:29-37, 1984.

197. Davidson RA, Wilcox CS: Newer tests for the diagnosis of renovascular disease. JAMA 268:3353-3357, 1992.

198. Taylor A: Functional testing: ACEI renography. Semin Nephrol 20:437-444, 2000.

199. Mann JFE: The diagnosis of renovascular hypertension: State of the art 1995. Nephrol Dial Transplant 10:1285-1286, 1995.

200. Canzanello VJ, Textor SC: Noninvasive diagnosis of renovascular disease. Mayo Clin Proc 69:1172-1181, 1994.

201. Fernandez P, Morel R, Jeandot R, et al: Value of captopril renal scintigraphy in hypertensive patients with renal failure. J Nucl Med 40:412-417, 1999.

202. Elliot WJ, Martin WB, Murphy MB: Comparison of two non-invasive screening tests for renovascular hypertension. Arch Intern Med 153:755-764, 1993.

203. Nally JV, Chen C, Fine E, et al: Diagnostic criteria of renovascular hypertension with captopril renography: A consensus statement. Am J Hypertens 4(12 pt 2):749s-752s, 1991.

204. La Batide-Alanore A, Azizi M, Froissart M, et al: Split renal function outcome after renal angioplasty in patients with unilateral renal artery stenosis. J Am Soc Nephrol 12:1235-1241, 2001.

205. Meholic AJ, Saddler MC, Hallin GW, et al: The captopril renogram in percutaneous transluminal angioplasty of the renal arteries. Am J Physiol Imaging 7:36-41, 1992.

206. Bakker J, Beutler JJ, Elgersma OE, et al: Duplex ultrasonography in assessing restenosis of renal artery stents. Cardiovasc Intervent Radiol 22:468-474, 1999.

207. Henry M, Amor M, Henry I, et al: Stents in the treatment of renal artery stenosis: Long-term follow-up. J Endovasc Surg 6:42-51, 1999.

208. Edwards JM, Zaccardi JM, Strandness DE: A preliminary study of the role of duplex scanning in defining the adequacy of treatment of patients with renal artery fibromuscular dysplasia. J Vasc Surg 15:604-609, 1992.

209. Olin JW, Piedmonte MR, Young JR, et al: The utility of duplex ultrasound scanning of the renal arteries for diagnosing significant renal artery stenosis. Ann Intern Med 122:833-838, 1995.

210. Spies KP, Fobbe F, El-Bedewi M, et al: Color-coded duplex sonography for noninvasive diagnosis and grading of renal artery stenosis. Am J Hypertens 8:1222-1231, 1995.

211. Postma CT, van Aalen J, de Boo T, et al: Doppler ultrasound scanning in the detection of renal artery stenosis in hypertensive patients. Br J Radiol 65:857-860, 1992.

212. Stavros AT, Parker SH, Yakes WF, et al: Segmental stenosis of the renal artery: Pattern recognition of tardus and parvus abnormalities with duplex sonography. Radiology 184:487-492, 1992.

213. Radermacher J, Weinkove R, Haller H: Techniques for predicting favorable response to renal angioplasty in patients with renovascular disease. Curr Opin Nephrol Hyper 10:799-805, 2002.

214. Radermacher J, Chavan A, Bleck J, et al: Use of Doppler ultrasonography to predict the outcome of therapy for renal-artery stenosis. N Engl J Med 344:410-417, 2001.

215. Spinosa DJ, Hagspiel KD, Angle JF, et al: Gadolinium-based contrast agents in angiography and interventional radiology: Uses and techniques. J Vasc Intervent Radiol 11:985-990, 2000.

216. King BF: Diagnostic imaging evaluation of renovascular hypertension. Abdom Imaging 20:395-405, 1995.

217. Grist TM: Magnetic resonance angiography of renal artery stenosis. Am J Kidney Dis 24:700-712, 1994.

218. Postma CT, Joosten FB, Rosenbusch G, Thien T: Magnetic resonance angiography has a high reliability in the detection of renal artery stenosis. Am J Hypertens 10:957-963, 1997.

219. Ros PR, Gauger J, Stoupis C, et al: Diagnosis of renal artery stenosis: Feasibility of combining MR angiography, MR renography and gadopentetate-based measurements of glomerular filtration rate. Am J Radiol 165:1447-1451, 1995.

220. Olbricht CJ, Paul K, Prokop M, et al: Minimally invasive diagnosis of renal artery stenosis by spiral computed tomography angiography. Kidney Int 48:1332-1337, 1995.

221. Elkohen M, Beregi JP, Deklunder G, et al: Evaluation of the spiral computed tomography alone and combined with color doppler ultrasonography in the detection of renal artery stenosis: A prospective study of 114 renal arteries. Arch Mal Coeur Vaiss 88:1159-1164, 1995.

222. Sheps SG, Black HR, Cohen JD, et al: The sixth report of the joint national committee on prevention, detection, evaluation, and treatment of high blood pressure. Arch Int Med 157:2413-2446, 1997.

223. Hollenberg NK: Treatment of hypertension: The place of angiotensin-converting enzyme inhibitors in the nineties. J Cardiovasc Pharmacol 20(suppl):S29-S33, 1992.

224. Michel JB, Dussaule JC, Choudat L, et al: Renal damage induced in the clipped kidney of one-clip, two-kidney hypertensive rats during normalization of blood pressure by converting enzyme inhibition. Kidney Int Suppl 31:S168-S172, 1987.

225. Jackson B, Franze L, Sumithran E, Johnston CI: Pharmacologic nephrectomy with chronic angiotensin converting enzyme inhibitor treatment in renovascular hypertension in the rat. J Lab Clin Med 115:21-27, 1990.

226. Mimran A: Renal effects of antihypertensive agents in parenchymal renal disease and renovascular hypertension. J Cardiovasc Pharmacol 19(suppl 6):S45-S50, 1992.

227. Hall JE, Guyton AC, Jackson TE, et al: Control of glomerular filtration rate by renin-angiotensin system. Am J Physiol 233:F366-F372, 1977.

228. Veniant M, Heudes D, Clozel JP, et al: Calcium blockade versus ACE inhibition in clipped and unclipped kidneys of 2K-1C rats. Kidney Int 46:421-429, 1994.

229. Mackenzie HS, Brenner BM: Prevention of progressive renal failure. In Brady H, Wilcox C (eds): Therapy in Nephrology and Hypertension. Philadelphia, WB Saunders, 1999, pp 463-473.

230. Neuringer JR, Brenner BM: Hemodynamic theory of progressive renal disease: A 10-year update in brief review. Am J Kidney Dis 22:98-104, 1993.

231. Ots M, Mackenzie HS, Troy JL, et al: Effects of combination therapy with enalapril and losartan on the rate of progression of renal injury in rats with 5/6 renal mass ablation. J Am Soc Nephrol 9:224-230, 1986.

232. Zatz R, Dunn RB, Meyer TW, et al: Prevention of diabetic glomerulopathy by pharmacological amelioration of glomerular capillary hypertension. J Clin Invest 77:1925-1930, 1986.

233. Textor SC: Renal failure related to ACE inhibitors. Semin Nephrol 17:67-76, 1997.

234. Grone HJ, Warnecke E, Olbricht CJ: Characteristics of renal tubular atrophy in experimental renovascular hypertension: A model of kidney hibernation. Nephron 72:243-252, 1996.

235. Kavoussi LR: Laparoscopic donor nephrectomy. Kidney Int 57:2175-2186, 2000.

236. Kasiske BL, Ma JZ, Louis TA, Swan SK: Long-term effects of reduced renal mass in humans. Kidney Int 48:814-819, 1995.

237. Lau WKO, Blute ML, Weaver AL, et al: Matched comparison of radical nephrectomy vs. nephron-sparing surgery in patients with unilateral renal cell carcinoma and a normal contralateral kidney. Mayo Clin Proc 75:1236-1242, 2000.

238. Plouin PF, Chatellier G, Darne B, Raynaud A: Blood pressure outcome of angioplasty in atherosclerotic renal artery stenosis: A randomized trial. Hypertension 31:822-829, 1998.

239. Fagard RH, Staessen JA, Thijs L, et al: Response to antihypertensive therapy in older patients with sustained and nonsustained systolic hypertension. Circulation 102:1139-1144, 2000.

240. Krakoff LR: Ambulatory blood pressure monitoring can improve cost-effective management of hypertension. Am J Hypertens 6:220S-224S, 1993.

241. Verdecchia P, Porcellati C, Schillaci G, et al: Ambulatory blood pressure: An independent predictor of prognosis in essential hypertension. Hypertension 24:793-801, 1994.

242. Semple PF, Dominczak AF: Detection and treatment of renovascular disease: 40 years on. J Hypertens 12:729-734, 1994.

243. Harington M, Kincaid-Smith P, McMichael J: Results of treatment in malignant hypertension: A seven year experience in 94 cases. BMJ 2:969-980, 1959.

244. Mahony JF, Storey BG, Gibson GR, et al: Bilateral nephrectomy for malignant hypertension. Lancet 1:1036-1038, 1972.

245. Lip GYH, Beevers M, Beevers G: The failure of malignant hypertension to decline: A survey of 24 years experience in a multiracial population in England. J Hypertens 12:1297-1305, 1994.

246. Kitiyakara C, Guzman NJ: Malignant hypertension and hypertensive emergencies. J Am Soc Nephrol 9:133-142, 1998.

247. Wilson PWF, Hoeg JM, D'Agostino RB, et al: Cumulative effects of high cholesterol levels, high blood pressure, and cigarette smoking on carotid stenosis. N Engl J Med 337:516-522, 1997.

248. Pitt B, Waters D, Brown WV, et al: Aggressive lipid-lowering therapy compared with angioplasty in stable coronary artery disease. N Engl J Med 341:70-76, 1999.

249. Howard G, Wagenknecht LE, Burke GL, et al: Cigarette smoking and progression of atherosclerosis: The Atherosclerosis Risk in Communities (ARIC) Study. JAMA 279:119-124, 1998.

250. White HD, Simes RJ, Anderson NE, et al: Pravastatin therapy and the risk of stroke. N Engl J Med 343:317-326, 2000.

251. Chabova V, Schirger A, Stanson A, Textor SC: Management of renal artery stenosis without revascularization since the introduction of ACE inhibitors [abstract]. J Am Soc Nephrol 10:362A, 1999.

252. Uzzo RG, Novick AC, Goormastic M, et al: Medical versus surgical management of atherosclerotic renal artery stenosis. Transplantation Proc 34:723-725, 2002.

253. Libertino JA, Zinman L: Surgery for renovascular hypertension. In Breslin DL, Swinton NW, Libertino JA, Zinman L (eds): Renovascular Hypertension. Baltimore, Williams & Wilkins, 1982, pp 166-212.

254. Strong CG, Hunt JC: Renovascular hypertension. In Office of Director NHLBI (ed): First Joint US-USSR Symposium on Hypertension (NIH Publication No. 79-1272, 317-344). Washington, DC, U.S Department of Health, Education and Welfare, 1979.

255. Dougherty MJ, Hallett JW, Naessens J, et al: Renal endarterectomy vs. bypass for combined aortic and renal reconstruction: Is there a difference in clinical outcome? Ann Vasc Surg 9:87-94, 1995.

256. Novick AC, Straffon RA, Stewart BH, et al: Diminished operative morbidity and mortality following revascularization for atherosclerotic renovascular disease. JAMA 246:749-753, 1981.

257. Novick AC, Ziegelbaum M, Vidt DG, et al: Trends in surgical revascularization for renal artery disease: Ten years' experience. J Urol 257:498-501, 1987.

258. Novick AC: Management of renovascular disease: A surgical perspective. Circulation 83(suppl):I:I-167-I-171, 1991.

259. Steinbach F, Novick AC, Campbell S, Dykstra D: Long-term survival after surgical revascularization for atherosclerotic renal artery disease. J Urol 158:38-41, 1997.

260. Cambria RP, Brewster DC, L'Italien GJ, et al: The durability of different reconstructive techniques for atherosclerotic renal artery disease. J Vasc Surg 20:76-87, 1994.

261. Paty PS, Darling RC III, Lee D, et al: Is prosthetic renal artery reconstruction a durable procedure? An analysis of 489 bypass grafts. J Vasc Surg 34:127-132, 2001.

262. Weibull H, Bergqvist D, Bergentz SE, et al: Percutaneous transluminal renal angioplasty versus surgical reconstruction of atherosclerotic renal artery stenosis: A prospective randomized study. J Vasc Surg 18:841-850, 1993.

263. Weibull H, Bergqvist D, Jonsson K, et al: Long-term results after percutaneous transluminal angioplasty of atherosclerotic renal artery stenosis—the importance of intensive follow-up. Eur J Vasc Surg 5:291-301, 1991.

264. Cambria RP, Brewster DC, L'Italien G, et al: Simultaneous aortic and renal artery reconstruction: Evolution of an eighteen-year experience. J Vasc Surg 21:916-924, 1995.

265. Chaikof EL, Smith RB, Salam AA, et al: Ischemic nephropathy and concomitant aortic disease: A ten-year experience. J Vasc Surg 19:135-146, 1994.

266. Cambria RP, Brewster DC, L'Italien GJ, et al: Renal artery reconstruction for the preservation of renal function. J Vasc Surg 24:371-382, 1996.

267. Alcazar JM, Rodicio JL: Ischemic nephropathy: Clinical characteristics and treatment. Am J Kidney Dis 36:883-893, 2000.

268. Clair DB, Belkin M, Whittemore AD, et al: Safety and efficacy of transaortic renal endarterectomy as an adjunct to aortic surgery. J Vasc Surg 21:926-933, 1995.

269. Hansen KJ, Starr SM, Sands RE, et al: Contemporary surgical management of renovascular disease. J Vasc Surg 16:319-330, 1992.

270. Lamawansa MD, Bell R, House AK: Short-term and long-term outcome following renovascular reconstruction. Cardiovasc Surg 3:50-55, 1995.

271. Dougherty MJ, Hallett JW, Naessens JM, et al: Optimizing technical success of renal revascularization: The impact of intraoperative color-flow duplex ultrasonography. J Vasc Surg 17:849-857, 1993.

272. Libertino JA, Bosco PJ, Ying CY, et al: Renal revascularization to preserve and restore renal function. J Urol 147:1485-1487, 1992.

273. Hansen KJ, Thomason RB, Craven TE, et al: Surgical management of dialysis-dependent ischemic nephropathy. J Vasc Surg 21:197-209, 1995.

274. Ying CY, Tifft CP, Gavras H, Chobanian AV: Renal revascularization in the azotemic hypertensive patient resistant to therapy. N Engl J Med 311:1070-1075, 1984.

275. Textor SC, McKusick MA: Renal artery stenosis. Curr Treatment Options Cardiovasc Med 3:187-194, 2001.

276. Thadhani RI, Camargo CA, Xavier RJ, et al: Atheroembolic renal failure after invasive procedures: Natural history based on 52 histologically proven cases. Medicine (Baltimore) 74:350-358, 1995.

277. Axelrod DA, Fendrick AM, Birkmeyer JD, et al: Cardiologists performing peripheral angioplasties: Impact on utilization. Effective Clin Prac 4:191-198, 2001.

278. Ramsay LE, Waller PC: Blood pressure response to percutaneous transluminal angioplasty for renovascular hypertension: An overview of published series. BMJ 300:569-572, 1990.

279. Englund R, Brown MA: Renal angioplasty for renovascular disease: A reappraisal. J Cardiovasc Surg 32:76-80, 1991.

280. Aurell M, Jensen G: Treatment of renovascular hypertension. Nephron 75:373-383, 1997.

281. Textor SC: Renovascular hypertension. *In* Johnson RJ, Feehally J (eds): Comprehensive Clinical Nephrology. London, Mosby, 2000, pp 41.1-41.12.

282. Taler SJ, Textor SC, Augustine JE: Resistant hypertension: Comparing hemodynamic management to specialist care. Hypertension 39:982-988, 2002.

283. Tegtmeyer CJ, Kellum CD, Ayers C: Percutaneous transluminal angioplasty of the renal artery: Results and long-term follow-up. Radiology 153:77-84, 1984.

284. Tegtmeyer CJ, Selby JB, Hartwell GD, et al: Results and complications of angioplasty in fibromuscular disease. Circulation 83(suppl):I155-I161, 1991.

285. Davidson RA, Barri Y, Wilcox CS: Predictors of cure of hypertension fibromuscular renovascular disease. Am J Kidney Dis 28:334-338, 1996.

286. Dustan HP: Renal arterial disease and hypertension. Med Clin North Am 81:1199-1212, 1997.

287. van de Ven PJ, Kaatee R, Beutler JJ, et al: Arterial stenting and balloon angioplasty in ostial atherosclerotic renovascular disease: A randomized trial. Lancet 353:282-286, 1999.

288. White CJ, Ramee SR, Collins TJ, et al: Renal artery stent placement: Utility in lesions difficult to treat with balloon angioplasty. J Am Coll Cardiol 30:1445-1450, 1997.

289. Tullis MJ, Zierler RE, Glickerman DJ, et al: Results of percutaneous transluminal angioplasty for atherosclerotic renal artery stenosis: A follow-up study with duplex ultrasonography. J Vasc Surg 25:46-54, 1997.

290. Blum U, Krumme B, Fluegel P, et al: Treatment of ostial renal-artery stenoses with vascular endoprostheses after unsuccessful balloon angioplasty. N Engl J Med 336:459-465, 1997.

291. Dorros G, Jaff M, Jain A, et al: Follow-up of primary Palmaz-Schatz stent placement for atherosclerotic renal artery stenosis. Am J Cardiol 75:1051-1055, 1995.

292. Dorros G, Jaff M, Mathiak L, et al: Four-year follow-up of Palmaz-Schatz stent revascularization as treatment for atherosclerotic renal artery stenosis. Circulation 98:642-647, 1998.

293. Isles CG, Robertson S, Hill D: Management of renovascular disease: A review of renal artery stenting in ten studies. Q J Med 92:159-167, 1999.

294. Leertouwer TC, Gussenhoven EJ, Bosch JP, et al: Stent placement for renal arterial stenosis: Where do we stand? A meta-analysis. Radiology 21:78-85, 2000.

295. Textor SC, McKusick M: Can renal artery stenting preserve renal function? An analysis of present data and issues for future investigation. *In* Jaff MR (ed): Endovascular Therapy for Atherosclerotic Renal Artery Stenosis: Present and Future. Armonk, NY, Futura Publishing Co, 2001, pp 121-132.

296. Bloch MJ, Pickering T: Renal vascular disease: Medical management, angioplasty and stenting. Semin Nephrol 20:474-488, 2000.

297. Burket MW, Cooper CJ, Kennedy DJ, et al: Renal artery angioplasty and stent placement: Predictors of a favorable outcome. Am Heart J 139:64-71, 2000.

298. Khosla S, White CJ, Collins TJ, et al: Effects of renal artery stent implantation in patients with renovascular hypertension presenting with unstable angina or congestive heart failure. J Am Coll Cardiol 80:363-366, 1997.

299. Bloch MJ, Trost DW, Pickering TG, et al: Prevention of recurrent pulmonary edema in patients with bilateral renovascular disease through renal artery stent placement. Am J Hypertens 12:1-7, 1999.

300. Ritz E, Mann JFE: Renal angioplasty for lowering blood pressure. N Engl J Med 342:1042-1043, 2000.

301. Hansen KJ, Cherr GS, Craven TE, et al: Management of ischemic nephropathy: Dialysis-free survival after surgical repair. J Vasc Surg 32:472-482, 2000.

302. Harden PN, Macleod MJ, Rodger RS, et al: Effect of renal-artery stenting on progression of renovascular renal failure. Lancet 349:1133-1136, 1997.

303. Bloch MJ, Trost DW, Sos TA: Type B aortic dissection complicating renal artery angioplasty and stent placement. J Vasc Intervent Radiol 12:517-520, 2001.

304. Dejani H, Eisen TD, Finkelstein FO: Revascularization of renal artery stenosis in patients with renal insufficiency. Am J Kidney Dis 36:752-758, 2000.

305. Topol EJ, Yadav JS: Recognition of the importance of embolization in atherosclerotic vascular disease. Circulation 101:570-580, 2000.

306. Watson PS, Hadjipetrou P, Cox SV, et al: Effect of renal artery stenting on renal function and size in patients with atherosclerotic renovascular disease. Circulation 102:1671-1677, 2001.

307. Mercier C, Piquet P, Alimi Y, et al: Occlusive disease of the renal arteries and chronic renal failure: The limits of reconstructive surgery. Ann Vasc Surg 2:166-170, 1990.

308. Lamawansa MD, Bell R, Kumar A, House AK: Radiological predictors of response to renovascular reconstructive surgery. Ann R Coll Surg Engl 77:337-341, 1995.

309. Beek FJ, Kaatee R, Beutler JJ, et al: Complications during renal artery stent placement for atherosclerotic ostial stenosis. Cardiovasc Intervent Radiol 20:184-190, 1997.

310. Taylor A, Sheppard D, Macleod MJ, et al: Renal artery stent placement in renal artery stenosis: Technical and early clinical results. Clin Radiol 52:451-457, 1997.

311. Morice MC, Serruys PW, Sousa JE, et al, for RAVEL Study Group: A randomized comparison of a sirolimus-eluting stent with a standard stent for coronary revascularization. N Engl J Med 346:1773-1780, 2002.

312. Textor SC, Wilcox CS: Ischemic nephropathy azotemic renovascular disease. Semin Nephrol 20:489-502, 2000.

313. Textor SC: Pathophysiology of renovascular hypertension. Urol Clin North Am 11:373-381, 1984.

314. Pohl MA: Renal artery stenosis, renal vascular hypertension and ischemic nephropathy. In Schrier RW, Gottschalk CW (eds): Diseases of the Kidney. Boston, Little, Brown, 1997, pp 1367-1423.

315. Novick AC: Atherosclerotic ischemic nephropathy. Urol Clin North Am 21:195-200, 1994.

316. Wilms G, Marchal G, Penne P, et al: The angiographic incidence of renal artery stenosis in the arteriosclerotic population. Eur J Radiol 10:195-197, 1990.

317. Textor SC: Renovascular hypertension. Endocrinol Metab Clin North Am 23:235-253, 1994.

318. Bredenberg CE, Sampson LN, Ray FS, et al: Changing patterns in surgery for chronic renal artery occlusive diseases. J Vasc Surg 15:1018-1024, 1992.

319. Kuhn FP, Kutkuhn B, Torsello G, Modder U: Renal artery stenosis: Preliminary results of treatment with the Strecker stent. Radiology 180:367-372, 1991.

320. Iannone LA, Underwood PL, Nath A, et al: Effect of primary balloon expandable renal artery stents on long-term patency, renal function, and blood pressure in hypertensive and renal insufficient patients with renal artery stenosis. Cathet Cardiovasc Diagn 37:243-250, 1996.

321. Xue F, Bettman MA, Langdon DR, Wivell WA: Outcome and cost comparison of percutaneous transluminal renal angioplasty, renal arterial stent placement, and renal arterial bypass grafting. Radiology 212:378-384, 1999.

322. Rundback JH, Gray RJ, Rozenblit G, et al: Renal artery stent placement for the management of ischemic nephropathy. J Vasc Intervent Radiol 9:413-420, 1998.

CHAPTER 47

Hypertension and Renal Disease

Joseph L. Izzo, Jr., and Vito M. Campese

AGING, HYPERTENSION, AND RENAL DISEASE: THE VICIOUS CYCLE

In industrialized societies, there is an extremely close relationship among advancing age, chronic hypertension, and progressive impairment of renal function. Indeed, it is unclear whether these elements can be fully separated on a pathophysiologic basis. Hypertension and its partner disorder, diabetes, are the principal reasons for the initiation of renal replacement therapy with dialysis or transplantation. Hypertension remains extremely common in end-stage renal disease (ESRD), occurring in at least 80% of dialysis patients, and chronic kidney disease is the most common cause of secondary hypertension. Together, hypertension and renal disease increase the risk for cardiovascular disease (CVD). Even a modest degree of renal impairment (e.g., a 30% decline in glomerular filtration rate [GFR] or microalbuminuria) dramatically increases the risk for CVD. The fact that only a small minority of people with hypertension develop ESRD is probably best explained by the time interval necessary for renal failure to develop; most hypertensives die of CVD before ESRD occurs.

The Nonlinear Disease Model of Hypertension and Renal Deterioration

The model that underlies this discussion (Fig. 47-1) is based on the premise that the pathogenesis of hypertension and renal disease is not well represented by a linear disease sequence. Rather, the progression of these interrelated disorders involves an interacting series of dysregulatory relationships among several basic physiologic mechanisms, the ultimate product of which is a "vicious cycle" or downward spiral in which worsening hypertension and nephron loss mutually reinforce each other's contribution to "accelerated aging," with premature death from cardiovascular or renal disease. The interactions among the core pathogenetic mechanisms are both initiating and sustaining forces in hypertension and renal disease.

In this model, it is not necessary for any individual component to fall into what would traditionally be considered an

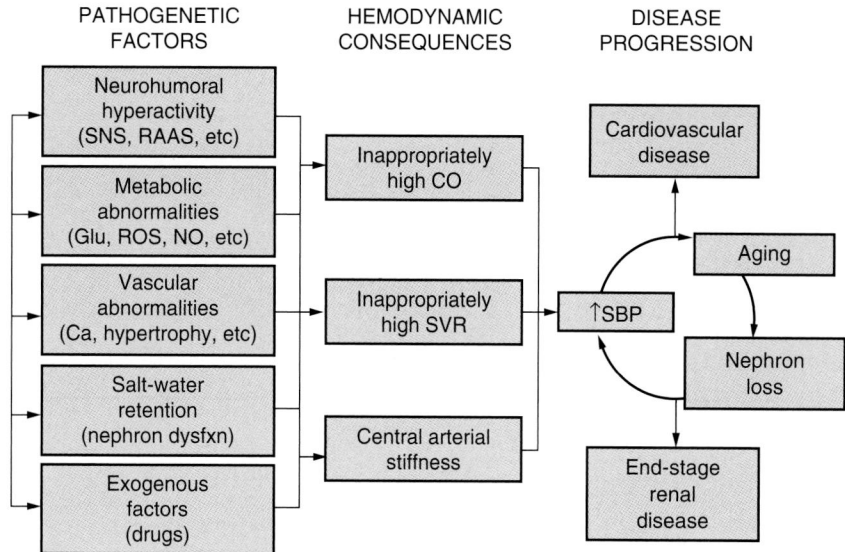

FIGURE 47-1. Hypertension and renal disease. Hypertension and age-related loss of renal function are intimately interrelated and pathogenetically almost inseparable. A series of interactions among several basic pathogenetic factors is responsible for initiation and maintenance of a series of systemic hemodynamic abnormalities that in turn promote acceleration of age-related nephron loss and premature cardiovascular and renal disease. Ca, abnormal cellular calcium flux; CO, cardiac output; dysfxn, dysfunction; Glu, abnormal glucose homeostasis; NO, nitric oxide; RAAS, renin-angiotensin-aldosterone system; ROS, reactive oxygen species; SBP, systolic blood pressure; SNS, sympathetic nervous system; SVR, systemic vascular resistance.

abnormal range of activity to participate in the process; the relative contribution of a given pathogenetic factor can be evaluated only in relation to the relative contribution of the other interactions that are present. In rare situations, such as pheochromocytoma, one overriding mechanism can be identified, but in the vast majority of people no single component predominates. It is also assumed that all factors need not be present simultaneously for the full phenotype to be expressed.

Another closely related concept is dynamic heterogeneity of the interacting factors, many of which counterregulate each other. Because of this feature, high blood pressure (BP) tends to persist over a wide range of physiologic variation, such as that seen with postural change or altered hydration status. The persistence of the contributions of the individual pathogenetic factors also remains important. Such sustaining influences can be demonstrated by the effects of certain drugs (e.g., angiotensin-converting enzyme [ACE] inhibitors) to lower BP while retarding or partially reversing pathologic vascular changes at advanced stages of the process. Also, the proportional contributions of the core pathogenetic factors may vary at different stages of the disorders.

Defining and Applying the Model

In principle, this disease model is not new. More than 50 years ago, Irvine Page constructed his "mosaic model" of hypertension based on these same theoretical principles. What is new today is the immense amount of data from clinical and laboratory studies and a clearer focus on how the ongoing interactions of the major components lead inexorably to abnormal systemic hemodynamics and age-dependent renal disease and CVD.

Five main groups of core pathogenetic factors are discussed here: (1) neurohumoral factors (principally the sympathetic nervous system [SNS]), (2) metabolic factors (the metabolic syndrome and reactive oxygen and nitrogen species), (3) vascular factors (e.g., calcium-mediated vasoconstriction, structural changes), (4) disordered renal salt and water excretion, and (5) exogenous factors (mainly drugs). Accordingly, this chapter is organized from the

perspective of the disease outcomes, looking backward to the hemodynamic and pathogenetic causes of the process. The final section includes suggestions on how to apply the principles developed in the model to clinical practice.

CLINICAL STUDIES

If the argument is true that the fundamental disease characteristics of hypertension are similar across the entire spectrum of renal disease, then it follows logically that the consequences of hypertension should also be similar in those with and without overt renal disease. Observational studies and clinical trial data indicate that this statement is indeed true.

Age and Systolic Hypertension

Age strongly affects the relationship between systolic blood pressure (SBP) and diastolic blood pressure (DBP), both within and between individuals. From age 20 to 50 years, SBP and DBP increase with age in a parallel manner.[1] After 50 years of age, in both men and women and in all demographic groups (whites, blacks, Hispanic Americans) studied in the Third National Health and Nutrition Examination Survey (NHANES III), DBP decreased while SBP continued to rise.[1] This pattern accounts for the increase in pulse pressure (PP = SBP − DBP) that is driven by the age-related increase in stiffness of the aorta and central arteries.[2]

Some investigators have suggested that PP is slightly more important than SBP as a risk factor for coronary events in the general population[3-5] or in persons with ESRD.[6] However, closer scrutiny reveals that the more robust association between PP and coronary events occurs only if the study population includes people older than 60 years of age, as found in studies such as the European Working Party Study on Hypertension in the Elderly, HEP, the Medical Research Council Studies, the Systolic Hypertension in the Elderly Program (SHEP), the Systolic Hypertension in Europe (Syst-EUR) study, and the Systolic Hypertension Treatment in Old People Study.[7] When populations are used that include younger subjects, the superiority of PP over SBP or DBP disappears. In the Prospective Trialists meta-regression follow-up study in 1 million individuals monitored for a mean of 12.7 years, the respective predictive powers of the individual BP components for future ischemic heart disease were as follows: mean BP, 97%; SBP, 93%; DBP, 78%; and PP, 43%.[8] The National Heart, Lung, and Blood Institute has recommended that it is clinically more prudent to base diagnostic and therapeutic recommendations for hypertension on SBP rather than on DBP or PP.[9]

Systolic Hypertension and Cardiovascular Disease Risk

In the general population, both SBP and DBP are continuously related to morbidity and mortality from CVD. Until very recently, standard teaching has held that elevated DBP and inappropriate peripheral vasoconstriction are the central features of the syndrome of chronic hypertension.[9] Today it is almost universally accepted that elevated SBP is the more robust predictor of poor cardiovascular[10, 11] and renal[12] outcomes, and SBP has finally become the principal end point for the classification and treatment of hypertension.[9]

DBP cannot be completely disregarded, however, because it remains a useful predictor of risk in those younger than 50 years of age,[5] especially in African-American men, who are at increased risk for ESRD. The continuous nature of the relationship between SBP and CVD risk has been well established in longitudinal studies, including the Framingham Heart Study and the Multiple Risk Factor Intervention Trial (MRFIT).[10, 11] In the Prospective Trialists database for men or women age 40 to 70 years, each 20 mm Hg increase in SBP (or each 10 mm Hg increase in DBP) doubled the risk of CVD at any level of SBP from 115 to 175 mm Hg (or DBP from 75 to 115 mm Hg).[8] Furthermore, randomized clinical trials have shown unequivocally that lowering SBP lowers cardiovascular morbidity and mortality—by 32% overall for diuretic-based therapy in the SHEP study,[13] and by 31% overall for calcium antagonist–based therapy in the Syst-EUR trial.[14]

Aging, Hypertension, and Loss of Renal Function

The incidence of renal failure is related to age and SBP. In the MRFIT study, after 16 years of follow-up in more than 300,000 men, increased SBP was more robust than DBP as a predictor of ESRD,[12] which was twice as prevalent in African Americans as in whites.[15] SBP and PP are also related to proteinuria, an important marker of chronic kidney disease. In the GUBBIO study, PP and isolated systolic hypertension were significantly related to urinary albumin excretion and prevalence of microalbuminuria in the population. When gender and other variables were controlled, a 15 mm Hg higher PP increased the relative risk of microalbuminuria to 1.7 (95% confidence interval [CI], 1.3 to 2.2) overall and to 5.0 for isolated systolic hypertension (95% CI, 3.2 to 7.8).[16]

With advancing age in industrialized societies, there is a steady decrease in GFR that is accelerated by the presence of hypertension.[12] A meta-regression analysis of recent treatment trials in middle-aged people at risk for progressive kidney disease (largely due to diabetes or hypertension) found that the rate of decline in GFR was inversely related to the baseline SBP[17]; with a baseline SBP of 130 to 140 mm Hg,

the rate of decline in GFR was about 2 mL/min per year, but it was twofold to threefold higher when the baseline SBP was between 150 and 160 mm Hg. In this model (assuming a first-order decay function), it would take a person with an SBP of 130 to 140 mm Hg about 35 to 40 years to experience a doubling of serum creatinine concentration (SCr), whereas someone with an untreated SBP of 150 to 160 mm Hg would reach that point in 12 to 15 years. For an initial SCr of 1.5 mg/dL, a person with an SBP of 150 to 160 mm Hg would require renal replacement therapy within 25 to 30 years. Although death from CVD often supervenes before chronic kidney disease becomes primary, current trends toward increased longevity and improved CVD prevalence and outcome rates suggest a continuing increase in the number of elderly people who develop hypertension-related chronic kidney disease.

Cardiovascular Disease Risk and Renal Failure

Renal failure is a major risk factor for premature CVD and death. In the Heart and Estrogen-Progestin Replacement Study (HERS), women with mild or moderate renal insufficiency (SCr, 1.2 to 1.4 mg/dL or >1.4 mg/dL, respectively) commonly were older, were black, and had a prior history of hypertension, diabetes, or dyslipidemia. They also had increased relative risks for a subsequent cardiovascular event—1.24 (95% CI, 1.0 to 1.5) and 1.57 (95% CI, 1.2 to 2.1), respectively—after adjustment for other risk factors and comorbid conditions. Therefore, renal insufficiency is an independent risk factor for cardiovascular events in postmenopausal women with known coronary artery disease.[18]

Elevations in SCr are independent predictors of poor outcomes in acute coronary syndromes, as reported in a meta-analysis of four large thrombolysis trials involving almost 38,000 patients.[19] In this analysis, if the estimated creatinine clearance was less than 70 mL/min, there was a 21% increase in mortality in the group with ST-segment elevation and a 19% increase for those without ST-segment elevation.[19] Reduced GFR or an estimated creatinine clearance of less than 60 mL/min is a risk factor for heart failure.[20] In the Study of Left Ventricular Dysfunction (SOLVD) Prevention Trial and the SOLVD Treatment Trial, moderate renal impairment was associated with a 41% increased risk in all-cause mortality ($P = .001$), explained largely by heart failure, death, or hospitalization.[20]

Albuminuria also functions as a major cardiovascular risk factor, at least in diabetes.[21, 22] In the Losartan Intervention for Endpoint Reduction (LIFE) study of high-risk hypertension, left ventricular (LV) hypertrophy, abnormal LV geometry, and high LV mass were associated with high albumin excretion rates independent of age, SBP, diabetes, or race.[23] Hypertension is strongly associated with increasing microalbuminuria and decreasing renal function in diabetic Pima Indians.[22] In diabetics overall, it is the presence of hypertension rather than the degree of albuminuria that is most closely associated with glomerular basement membrane thickening and increased mesangial volume on renal biopsy.[24] Inflammatory markers such as C-reactive protein and fibrinogen were found to be elevated in microalbuminuric versus normoalbuminuric subjects, but these associations were relatively weak ($r < .2$).[25] In the same study, a logistic regression model demonstrated that fibrinogen was weakly but independently associated with microalbuminuria, along with hypertension, female gender, waist circumference, and fasting blood glucose concentration.

In patients with ESRD, hypertension remains strongly associated with increased deaths from CVD,[26] and it is the single most important predictor of coronary artery disease in these patients, even more so than cigarette smoking or hypertriglyceridemia. In a cohort study of 432 ESRD patients (261 receiving hemodialysis and 171 peritoneal dialysis) monitored prospectively for an average 3.5 years, each 10 mm Hg rise in mean arterial blood pressure (MAP) increased the relative risk of echocardiographic LV hypertrophy by 48%, de novo heart failure by 44%, and de novo ischemic heart disease by 39%, even after adjusting for age and preexisting diabetes, ischemic heart disease, hemoglobin, and serum albumin.[26] There was a twofold increase in the risk of death from CVD among patients with a predialysis MAP of 98 mm Hg (equivalent to BP 130/80 mm Hg), compared with those whose predialysis MAP was less than 98 mm Hg.[27] Controlled studies are not available on the benefits of antihypertensive therapy for patients receiving hemodialysis or peritoneal dialysis. However, maintaining a controlled BP is considered to be of great importance for long-term survival.[28, 29]

Hypotension as a Risk Factor

Although it is increasingly recognized that maintenance of optimal BP (120/80 mm Hg or below) is desirable, acute hypotension is also potentially dangerous. In individuals with hypotensive episodes, it is common to find increased lability of BP, with extremely high values present as well. This pattern of exaggerated BP variability exposes the individual to risks from both hypertension and hypotension. Postural hypotension (usually defined as a drop of 20 mm Hg SBP or 10 mm Hg DBP on standing) is associated with cerebrovascular disease and with premature death.[30-35]

In ESRD patients, the curve for the relationship between BP and CVD risk is J-shaped or U-shaped.[26, 36, 37] Low MAP is independently associated with increased mortality (by 36% per 10 mm Hg fall, $P < .01$).[26] Port and colleagues[36] examined the U.S. Renal Data System database and found an 86% increase in mortality over a follow-up period of 2 to 3 years among patients with low (<110 mm Hg) predialysis SBP.[36] There are obvious pathophysiologic reasons why low BP may be associated with adverse outcomes in patients with ESRD, the most prominent of which is that exposure to hypertension for several years causes these patients to develop cardiac failure, which lowers BP (so-called reverse causality). Some studies have indicated that short-term survival is actually higher in dialysis patients with hypertension than in those with normal BP values.[37] These studies should be interpreted cautiously, because they not only are small but have very short follow-up periods.

The Metabolic Syndrome and Risk Factor Interactions

Certain traits, including obesity, hypertension, impaired glucose tolerance, and dyslipidemia, occur together more often than would be predicted by chance.[38] This cluster, originally termed the *insulin resistance syndrome*[39, 40] is now known as the *metabolic syndrome* and has been defined in the Adult Treatment Panel (ATP) III guideline as the presence of three

or more of the following: increased waist circumference (>40 inches in men or >35 inches in women), increased BP (>130/85 mm Hg), increased fasting glucose concentration (>110 mg/dL), increased triglycerides (>150 mg/dL), and low concentration of high-density lipoprotein (HDL) cholesterol (<50 mg/dL in women or <40 mg/dL in men). Recent analysis of NHANES III revealed unadjusted and age-adjusted prevalence rates of the metabolic syndrome of 21.8% and 23.7%, respectively, with no gender difference. Age is a major factor, with prevalence ranging from 6.7% among those 20 to 29 years of age to about 43% for those age 70 years or older. Ethnic origins are also important, and the condition is more prevalent among African Americans and Mexican Americans than in other groups.[41]

The long-term impact of the metabolic syndrome is a progressive increase in overall CVD and renal disease risk proportional to the number of components present, as originally documented by the Framingham Heart Study.[10, 42] The nature of the interaction of Framingham risk factors is mostly additive, and subsequent studies extend this principle to renal disease. In the Atherosclerosis Risk in Communities (ARIC) study, the incidence of a significant (>0.4 mg/dL) rise in SCr was 5.1 per 1000 person-years over 2.9 years[43]; individuals with higher triglycerides and lower HDL levels had increased risk for a significant rise in SCr, even after adjustment for race, gender, baseline age, diabetes, SCr, SBP, and antihypertensive medications (all P trends < .02). In the Nord-Trondelag Health Study (HUNT), increases in any BP component (PP, SBP, or DBP) were correlated with microalbuminuria in men and women. However, advanced age, elevated cholesterol, or elevated glucose concentration was also associated with microalbuminuria and a high total risk of CVD. After excluding individuals with Coronary heart disease and untreated hypertension, only age was associated with microalbuminuria in men.[43]

The value of simultaneous management of multiple risk factors was demonstrated in a small study of 160 diabetics by Gaede and coworkers,[44] who randomly assigned patients to standard or intensive care (lifestyle modification, aspirin, and intensive drug management of hyperglycemia, hypertension, dyslipidemia, and microalbuminuria). Those receiving intensive treatment had a significantly lower relative risk of CVD (0.47; 95% CI, 0.24 to 0.73), nephropathy (0.39; 95% CI, 0.17 to 0.87), retinopathy (0.42; 95% CI, 0.21 to 0.86), and autonomic neuropathy (0.37; 95% CI, 0.18 to 0.79), proving the value of multiple risk factor modification. Translated into practical terms, the greater the global CVD risk, the more beneficial is treatment of hypertension and the fewer the number of individuals needed to be treated to prevent a CVD event. The high prevalence of hyperglycemia and dyslipidemia in ESRD patients necessitates extremely aggressive management of these risk factors along with hypertension in this population.

Ambulatory Blood Pressure Monitoring

It has become apparent that assessment of hypertension and its consequences is more reliably and fully accomplished by ambulatory BP monitoring (ABPM) techniques than by casual office readings. The role of ABPM in applied research, diagnosis, and management of hypertension continues to grow.[45, 46]

BLOOD PRESSURE VARIABILITY. The major justification for ABPM is to better assess the patterns and impact of the wide variation in BP that occurs throughout the day. As an overall assessment tool, ABPM is more valuable than clinic readings because ABPM gives a better representation of BP responses to many different situations. The overall waking or sleeping BP is also more representative of an individual's average BP. On an arithmetic basis alone, the more readings that are available, the greater the confidence in the overall mean.[46-48] ABPM is particularly useful in assessing the "white coat syndrome" and in judging responses to antihypertensive medications. The white coat syndrome is present in 10% to 20% of the population, depending on the definition used.[49, 50] The overall prognostic significance of the phenomenon is still debated, but it is clear that the pattern of target organ damage in white-coat hypertensives is substantially less than that observed in individuals with sustained hypertension.[47, 51]

In ESRD patients, ABPM is useful to assess the wide variation in BP caused by dialysis treatments and interdialytic salt and water retention.[52-54] This variability obscures the overall relationship between BP and clinical end points. The average of predialysis and postdialysis BP readings may be a reasonable predictor of mean interdialysis BP, but no method has demonstrated complete reliability.[55] Several investigators have suggested that ABPM or self-measured home BPs may be better markers of interdialytic BP load than BPs obtained at dialysis centers.[54,55]

DIURNAL RHYTHMS. Another important phenomenon described by ABPM is the diurnal rhythm of BP. Normally, SBP and DBP tend to be highest during the morning, followed by a gradual decrease during the course of the day, and an abrupt fall-off during sleep.[56, 57] The circadian rhythm of BP follows the circadian rhythm of blood volume and neurohumoral activation. Specific physiologic BP-related variables that peak in the morning hours include blood volume, plasma norepinephrine, plasma renin activity, cortisol secretion, cardiac output, and α-receptor–dependent vasomotor tone.[58-61] Superimposed on this circadian pattern are the cardiovascular responses to episodic stimuli, which are usually stronger signals than the diurnal rhythm.[62-64] To demonstrate a diurnal pattern, the individual must be isolated from the environment and kept in a supine position. Merely assuming the upright posture causes marked SNS stimulation. The greater role of extrinsic stimulation compared with intrinsic diurnal rhythm is easily demonstrated in rotating shift workers, whose BPs follow their activity levels.[65, 66] Approximately 10% to 25% of patients with essential hypertension fail to manifest normal nocturnal dipping of BP (defined as a nighttime BP fall of more than 10%); these patients are called "nondippers,"[67] and those with a normal circadian rhythm are called "dippers." Correlations between urinary albumin excretion, 24-hour DBP, and nighttime DBP are present in nondippers.[68]

Patients with advanced renal disease[69] and up to 80% of those on maintenance hemodialysis[54, 70, 71] fail to exhibit nocturnal BP dipping. At times, nocturnal BP can be greater than daytime BP in these individuals. Because BP is usually measured during the day, failure to obtain nocturnal readings may lead to the erroneous impression of good BP control.[47] Using ABPM, Agarwal[55] observed that in hemodialysis patients the BP decreased after dialysis and remained low during the first night. By the next morning BP reached predialysis levels, and during the second night it failed to decrease. Mechanisms of abnormal circadian BP control in

renal disease patients may include autonomic dysfunction,[72] reduced physical activity,[73] sleep-disordered breathing,[74, 75] and volume overload.[76] Because the nondipping pattern is also prevalent among salt-sensitive patients with essential hypertension,[77] and because this disturbance regresses with salt restriction[78] or diuretic therapy,[79] volume expansion would seem to be the primary etiologic factor. However, the explanation is probably more complicated, because interdialytic weight gain does not consistently correlate with the phenomenon of nondipping.[80] Furthermore, daily hemodialysis does not normalize nocturnal dipping in all patients, despite more consistent extracellular fluid volume (ECV) and better BP control.[81]

TARGET ORGAN DAMAGE. A large body of evidence from subjects with essential hypertension has shown that ABPM values correlate more closely than office BPs with overall morbidity and with the incidence and timing of cardiovascular complications.[47, 68, 82-86] This is not surprising given the variation in BP that occurs naturally during the day and the greater reliability of a mean ABPM reading compared to a single office reading.[46-48] Verdecchia and co-workers[87] reported an inverse correlation between LV mass index and degree of nocturnal BP reduction. There is also a significant correlation between nighttime SBP or DBP and urinary albumin excretion, and also between 24-hour SBP and albumin excretion in hypertensive patients.[68, 88] Among hemodialysis patients, the absence of normal dipping also predicts adverse cardiovascular events. In other studies, nocturnal BP measurements predicted cardiovascular outcomes only in patients with reproducible BP profiles[89]; because so many dialysis patients have very wide BP variability, the relevance of day/night BP differences is less clear in this population. Some data suggest that predialysis SBP correlates best with cardiac hypertrophy,[90] whereas other reports suggest that postdialysis BP is closer to interdialytic BP as assessed by ABPM.[54]

SYSTEMIC HEMODYNAMICS

Systemic Hemodynamics and the Electrical Model

The traditional view of systemic hemodynamics was derived from a steady-state electrical analog model of the circulation:

Voltage = Current × Impedance

MAP = Cardiac output × Systemic vascular resistance

The electrical model has been extended to clinical practice by assuming that DBP is a reasonable surrogate for mean BP. Virtually all teaching of cardiovascular and renal hemodynamics is based on this approach and the related assumption that chronic hypertension is simply a manifestation of increased systemic vascular resistance (SVR). Although this model is still useful as a teaching aid, it does not explain other critical features of pulsatile flow, dynamic stress responses,[91, 92] or systolic hypertension,[93] and it has also indirectly promoted the use of vasodilator antihypertensive monotherapies that do not provide optimal protection of the cardiovascular system or the kidney.

The notion that people with established hypertension demonstrate a chronic increase in SVR is a gross oversimplification of the problem. First, SVR is measured only under supine resting conditions. Second, the physiologic variation in

SVR is extremely wide within and between individuals, with extremely broad overlap between normal and hypertensive individuals in most studies.[94-96] Postural adaptation is a good example of how hemodynamics can vary in an individual. In the upright position, where venous return is limited by gravitational pooling of blood in the venous system, cardiac output is about 20% to 25% less than in the supine position, yet central BPs remain reasonably constant. In the upright position, the differences in SVR between normal and hypertensive people disappear, and hypertensives maintain a supranormal upright cardiac output (J. L. Izzo, Jr., personal observations). During other stimulated conditions such as dynamic exercise, hypertensives exhibit a slightly supranormal increase in cardiac output with reduced exercise-induced systemic vasodilation.[97] Therefore, over the dynamic range of conditions experienced daily, hypertension exhibits features of both inappropriately high cardiac output and inappropriately high SVR.[98-100] The fact that hemodynamic differences between normotensives and hypertensives are both instantaneous and chronic provides a clue that the SNS participates in the pathogenesis of hypertension, at least in a permissive fashion; no other system in the body is capable of such rapid and dynamic responses.[100]

Systemic hemodynamics in renal failure can be more complex than in essential hypertension, but the natural history of hemodynamic trends tends to be the same as that seen in essential hypertension.[101] Cardiac output tends to remain relatively high as renal disease progresses, because impaired renal salt and water excretion increases blood volume and also because progressive anemia increases stroke volume and heart rate. Chronically, persistence of the BP elevation still depends on both increased cardiac output and SVR. In individuals with ESRD, high-volume proximal fistulas can place an additional demand on cardiac output.

Importance of Systolic Blood Pressure and Pulsatile Flow

The realization that arterial stiffness and SBP are major concerns in hypertension is a relatively recent development,[9, 102] and the full implications of SBP and concepts of pulsatile load[103] have yet to be fully appreciated, from either a physiologic or a clinical perspective. Exploration of this area is likely to yield important new insights and therapies.

CENTRAL ARTERIAL STIFFNESS AND PULSATILE LOAD. From a cardiac perspective, the pulsatile load on the heart is dependent on the integral of the systolic pressure wave at the aortic root. The major components of that integral are as follows:

Pulsatile load ∝ Cardiac output · Cardiac afterload

where

Cardiac output ∝ Heart rate · Contractility

and

Cardiac afterload ∝ Impedance (early and late) · SVR

This view brings several additional features into play, including the major role played by proximal aortic stiffness, which increases impedance during the early part of systole, and the lesser contribution of reflected pressure waves, which augment central systolic pressure during late systole.[93]

AGING, ARTERIAL STIFFNESS, AND WIDE PULSE PRESSURE. Aging is associated with increased SBP, but the pathogenesis of this phenomenon is still incompletely understood. Systolic hypertension is much more prominent in industrialized societies than in less developed ones, and results principally from increased aortic and central arterial stiffness, although distal vasoconstriction also contributes.[104-106] The clinical hallmark of systolic hypertension is a pattern of wide pulse pressure (PP = SBP − DBP) that includes elevated SBP with or without elevated DBP or MAP.

To understand how wide PP occurs, it is necessary to review the role of the central arteries. Normally (i.e., in young people without hypertension), the elastic recoil function of the proximal aorta serves to dampen the impact of pulsatile flow (i.e., it narrows the PP) by retaining a fraction of each cardiac stroke volume during systole and then delivering this retained volume to the distal circulation during diastole.[107] When central arteries stiffen with aging and hypertension, the full stroke volume is delivered through the resistance arterioles during systole, because there is no elastic recoil (i.e., reservoir or "compliance" function) of the aorta. As a result, the amplitude of the pulse wave (the PP) increases or widens, and the systolic peak itself becomes sharper,[108] independent of any changes in cardiac output or systemic resistance. PP has also been reported to be elevated in patients with ESRD,[109] but the etiology of this finding is complex, because ESRD patients not only have stiffer arteries but in many cases demonstrate increased cardiac stroke volume due to anemia, erythropoietin, or other causes.

On a cellular basis, central arterial stiffening is the result of the breakdown of elastin fibers in the face of continued collagen deposition and vascular smooth muscle hypertrophy.[110] The independence of aortic stiffness from vascular resistance in generating systolic hypertension is demonstrated by observations that thiazolium derivatives, which disrupt collagen cross-links formed by advanced glycosylation end products, reduce arterial stiffness and SBP despite the absence of distal vasodilatory effects.[111] In patients with renal failure, there is increased pulse wave velocity, an indicator of increased arterial stiffness.[112, 113] A potential role of angiotensin II (Ang II) in aortic stiffness has been proposed but not proven. Ceiler and colleagues[114, 115] infused Ang II into rats chronically, induced aortic hypertrophy, and found that the Ang II-induced increases in aortic wall mass or smooth muscle tone did not modify the relationship between overall resistance and pressure or between pulsatile compliance and pressure. In essential hypertension, Mitchell and colleagues[116] found that much greater improvements in aortic stiffness (characteristic aortic impedance) could be obtained by combining neutral endopeptidase inhibition (which increases atriopeptins and further augments bradykinin) with ACE inhibition.

PULSATILITY AND THE PERIPHERAL CIRCULATION. Much less well understood is the impact of pulse wave propagation factors on the peripheral circulation, particularly the brain and kidney. A fundamental characteristic of pressure waves is that they are amplified as they travel downstream.[117] Despite the fact that MAP remains constant throughout the arterial tree, PP widens progressively in distal arteries as local SBP increases and DBP decreases. Therefore, the morphology of a distal pulse wave is intrinsically different (basically taller and narrower) than the corresponding wave at the aortic root. One of the basic principles explaining this phenomenon is that for any impedance mismatch (disturbance in the pressure-flow relationship) that occurs in peripheral arteries (due to tapering, branching, stenosis, constriction, or turbulence), part of the pressure wave is reflected backward toward the heart. At the same time, the amplitude of the forward-traveling wave is augmented. Pulse wave morphology is further modified by distal vasoconstriction and additional wave reflections, such that α_1-receptor–mediated vasoconstriction further "sharpens" the peak SBP.[108]

Changes in pulse wave morphology can have major impact on microcirculatory function, including GFR, which is highly pressure dependent. Because GFR is related to the integral of the capillary pulse wave, alterations in the morphology of that wave could have substantial influence on salt and water excretion. Renal pulsatility itself may be a critical function, because kidneys with poor GFR also are poorly pulsatile (as occurs chronically with progressive renal failure and in non-filtering allografts with hyperacute renal shutdown). In fact, a classic model of hypertension, the perinephric scarring model (Page kidney) is characterized by severe hypertension associated with abnormal pulse wave transmission due to renal compression.[118, 119] It is also likely that these pulsatile signals yield information transmitted to the brain via renal afferent nerves, as discussed in the next section.

Pressure-Volume Homeostasis

The dynamic range of counterregulation of flow and resistance must be considered in any discussion of BP regulation. The pressure–flow dysregulation that characterizes chronic hypertension can be characterized as dysregulation of the vasoconstriction–volume axis. Cardiac output is highly dependent on ventricular distention during diastole (preload); ventricular preload is in turn dependent on SNS-mediated peripheral venoconstriction and venous volume. Ventricular performance is diminished by factors that increase impedance to ventricular emptying, mainly SBP and central arterial stiffness. BP itself is only a loosely regulated physiologic variable that is most commonly influenced by the activity of the SNS. Under resting conditions, flow (cardiac output) and impedance (SVR) counterregulate each other, so that BP remains relatively constant. Teleologically, it is probable that SNS-mediated central vasoregulation conferred adaptive advantages by allowing effective adjustments to upright posture but also aided in times of significant hemorrhage or dehydration. It is therefore important to identify whether baroreflex feedback mechanisms that modulate SNS activity continue to function appropriately in hypertension and renal failure or whether they permit excessive BP variability[120] or inappropriately elevated SNS activity.[121-127]

BAROREFLEX CONTROL MECHANISMS. There are two main inhibitory baroreflex sensor systems that control SNS outflow: one responds to changes in arterial pressure (aorto-carotid baroreflexes), the other to changes in cardiac filling (cardiopulmonary baroreflexes). In response to a sudden fall in arterial pressure, the carotid sinus is "unloaded" and afferent signals are sent to the nucleus tractus solitarius (NTS) that disinhibit the SNS, resulting in increased heart rate, enhanced myocardial contractility, and constriction of vascular smooth muscle.[121] The arterial baroreflex system inhibits the SNS during acute rises in SBP via mechanical deformation of the

carotid sinus and ionic signals generated by the carotid sinus endothelium.[128, 129]

Operating in parallel with the arterial system are the low-pressure stretch receptors in the heart and great veins (cardiopulmonary baroreflexes) that sense changes in central blood volume.[121] Decreases in central blood volume (or cardiac preload) lead to SNS activation, whereas salt-loading or ECV expansion suppresses SNS activity.[130, 131] The cardiopulmonary baroreflex system often overrides the aorto-carotid system in controlling SNS and renin-angiotensin activity, especially during postural adaptation or other conditions that affect central blood volume.[132-136] The cardiopulmonary baroreflex system, therefore, is designed to allow counterregulation of blood volume and BP by adjusting the degree of distal arterial and venous constriction to meet the need for appropriate cardiac filling (preload) via centralization of blood volume.

Therefore, during postural adaptation, dehydration, or hemorrhage, cardiac filling pressure is protected by cardiopulmonary baroreflex–mediated SNS activation, which causes systemic and renal vasoconstriction and antinatriuresis. In contrast, with central volume overload, cardiopulmonary baroreflex loading leads to withdrawal of efferent sympathetic tone, causing renal vasodilation, enhanced natriuresis, and dilation of systemic arteries and veins. These effects are independent of aortocarotid baroreflex function.[134]

In humans, cardiopulmonary baroreflexes can be stimulated selectively by lower-body negative pressure, which reduces central blood volume and triggers increased muscle and renal SNS activity, renal and splanchnic vascular resistance, and plasma renin activity.[136-138] When postural adaptation is studied, plasma norepinephrine correlates strongly with reduced cardiac stroke volume in both supine and upright postures.[133]

VASOPRESSIN. When central blood volume or cardiac preload changes, alterations in cardiac mechanoreceptor stretch stimulate afferent cardiopulmonary baroreflex nerves that project fibers to the paraventricular brain region, especially the supraoptic nucleus, which controls the secretion of vasopressin from the posterior pituitary gland. During conditions of reduced venous return or central blood volume, vasopressin release is stimulated in parallel with SNS activation. It is a popular misconception that vasopressin is uniformly a vasoconstrictor hormone; it typically causes vasopressin 1 receptor (V_1R)–mediated constriction in the cerebral, coronary, renal, splanchnic, and cutaneous beds, but it also consistently vasodilates skeletal muscle beds via its actions on V_2Rs.[139]

Vasopressin tends to cause a biphasic pattern of BP change, with elevation (lasting for minutes) followed by subsequent decreases, sometimes to very low levels. Overall, the action of vasopressin may be to redistribute blood flow to muscle beds in times of acute stress, presumably to optimize the defense mechanism to physical threat. Plasma vasopressin is often elevated in essential hypertension[140] and in heart failure,[141] and its hypotensive effects are enhanced in older people with postural hypotension.[142] Vasopressin causes baroreflex blunting in hypertensive animals[143] and in humans with heart failure,[144, 145] facilitating chronic SNS activation. A role for vasopressin in renal failure has not been clearly established, but V_2R stimulation may hasten the progression of renal disease in Brattleboro rats after 5/6 nephrectomy.[146]

NATRIURETIC PEPTIDES. The natriuretic peptide system functions as another buffer to SNS activation during volume depletion.[147] At least three natriuretic peptides are secreted by cardiovascular and neural tissue and are now termed ANP, BNP, and CNP. ANP is secreted principally by cardiac tissue, BNP by the heart and brain, and CNP by the endothelium. The secretion of natriuretic peptides by the heart is highly sensitive to mechanoreceptor stretch and cardiac distention. In times of reduced cardiac filling, natriuretic peptide release is suppressed (while the SNS is stimulated), and in times of increased cardiac filling, natriuretic peptide is released (while the SNS is suppressed). Although natriuretic peptides are powerful suppressants of the SNS and of the activity of the renin-angiotensin-aldosterone system (RAAS), they are also powerful direct vasodilators, and they act directly on renal tubules to promote salt and water excretion. Thus the natriuretic peptide system opposes the SNS.

Plasma levels of natriuretic peptides, particularly ANP and pro-ANP, are usually increased in patients with hypertension, signaling their relative inability to overcome volume retention and higher BP.[148] In patients with ESRD predialysis plasma levels of ANP and pro-ANP are substantially greater than in control subjects, and the ability of cardiac stretch to stimulate natriuretic peptide release is maintained.[149-152] On the other hand, no correlation has been found between predialysis levels of ANP and interdialytic weight gain or between ANP and volume removal with hemodialysis. Therefore, plasma ANP does not appear to be a useful marker of volume status in hemodialysis patients. Cardiac natriuretic peptides are related to LV mass and function in dialysis patients and predict cardiovascular mortality.[153]

INTERACTING PATHOGENETIC FACTORS

It is a central theme of this chapter that the same mechanisms that lead to essential hypertension continue to raise BP throughout the progression of renal disease, including ESRD. The most consistent contributions to elevated BP can be attributed to inappropriate SNS activity, metabolic abnormalities, functional and structural vascular changes, and altered ECV homeostasis. Other drug-related causes also exist. Each of these factors interacts with the others, but during different phases of renal deterioration each may contribute in different proportions.[106]

NEUROHUMORAL FACTORS

Central Nervous System Control Centers and Experimental Hypertension

Elegant studies in the laboratories of Reis and others have identified the functional role of several central nervous system (CNS) nuclei in acute and chronic regulation of BP and SNS activity. Reflex and behavioral BP control is integrated in the rostral ventrolateral (RVL) nucleus of the medulla oblongata, which is sometimes called the vasomotor control center.[154, 155] Cell bodies of efferent SNS cardiovascular stimulatory neurons lie in the C_1 subregion, which also receives and sends neural projections to and from many other CNS centers. There are at least some collateral

synapses of C_1 axons on noradrenergic cell bodies in the spinal cord that offer the opportunity for regional modulation of SNS responses.[156] The most relevant of these regional modulating influences is probably the renorenal reflex, which modifies contralateral renal hemodynamics in response to changes in ipsilateral flow and function.[156]

RVL output is modulated by the overlying NTS, which receives afferent fibers from pressure-sensitive mechanoreceptors in the carotid sinus and aortic arch (aortocarotid baroreflexes) and from cardiopulmonary stretch receptors that sense central volume[157-159] (see earlier discussion). Signals from the NTS inhibit RVL-sympathetic outflow and tend to buffer acute BP changes, as demonstrated by experiments in which ablation of the NTS in rats causes increased SNS outflow, severe BP lability,[160, 161] or severe chronic hypertension,[162, 163] which could be abolished by simultaneous ablation of the RVL.[163] The NTS integrates a variety of signals from stimulatory and inhibitory centers in the brainstem, basal ganglia, and cortex,[157-159] including excitatory input from peripheral chemoreceptor afferent neurons in the kidneys and skeletal muscle that act to increase RVL-sympathetic outflow.[164]

Several periventricular nuclei modulate RVL outflow, including those in the region of the anterolateral third ventricle (AV3V region).[158, 163, 165-168] Of particular importance is an area in the floor of the fourth ventricle, the area postrema, which immediately overlies the NTS. The area postrema does not have a blood–brain barrier,[158, 163, 167, 168] and it is highly sensitive to circulating Ang II, which inhibits the inhibitory effects of the NTS, thus increasing RVL activation and SNS outflow. Stimulation of the area postrema by Ang II is thought to be a major sustaining mechanism in genetic and steroid-induced hypertension.[161, 163, 167, 169]

Abnormalities in hypothalamic function may contribute to essential and renal hypertension. The median preoptic nucleus of the hypothalamus serves to integrate water balance and thirst-sensing mechanisms with cardiovascular signals and may mediate organ-specific responses such as skeletal muscle vasodilation.[170, 171] In addition to acute changes in BP, the hypothalamus may affect long-term BP as well. Ablation of the posterior hypothalamus reduces BP in steroid-induced, genetic, and renal hypertension.[170] Lesions of the anterior hypothalamus dramatically increase BP via massive adrenomedullary stimulation in normotensive rats,[172] whereas electrical stimulation of this region increases sympathetic outflow.[173] Ablation of the paraventricular nucleus prevents the development of hypertension in the spontaneously hypertensive rat.[174]

Sympathetic Nervous System Hyperactivity and Hypertension in Humans

A critical feature common to all forms of chronic hypertension and renal disease is inappropriately elevated SNS activation, which remains present at all stages of both conditions. The popular view, that the SNS is an early trigger to hypertension whose influence on BP wanes over time, is not fully consistent with available data. There is little argument that there is increased SNS activity in early hypertension.[175-177] Goldstein[176] concluded that the majority of studies demonstrated elevated plasma norepinephrine values only in young, borderline hypertensives. In the Tecumseh,

Michigan, study, 37% of hypertensives designated border-line were found to be overweight, with a tendency toward insulin resistance, elevated plasma norepinephrine, fast heart rate, increased cardiac index, and increased forearm blood flow.[177]

There are ample data showing that inappropriate SNS activity remains a major feature in the progression and maintenance of chronic hypertension as well. Increased or inappropriately high SNS activity has been consistently demonstrated by venous plasma norepinephrine values in chronic hypertension. A prospective, 10-year follow-up study in initially normotensive Japanese subjects found higher initial plasma norepinephrine values in those whose BPs subsequently increased than in those who remained normotensive.[178-180] Perhaps most importantly in these studies, the increment in plasma norepinephrine observed during the follow-up period was more closely related to the BP increase observed over the course of the study, consistent with an ongoing role of the SNS in the pathogenesis of chronic hypertension. There is also convincing evidence that the SNS plays a sustaining as well as an initiating role in hypertension at all ages. Messerli[96] and Izzo[181] and their colleagues found significant correlations among advancing age, increased plasma norepinephrine, and BP or elevated vascular resistance in established hypertensives. In the Normative Aging Study, one of the strongest residual relationships among the various parameters tested as determinants of BP was the age-independent relationship between urinary norepinephrine excretion and BP.[182] Increased muscle SNS traffic has also been demonstrated in established hypertension.[183]

Increased Sympathetic Nervous System Activity in Renal Failure

Increased SNS activity is one of the most consistent features of hypertension in uremic animals and humans. In 5/6 nephrectomized (chronic renal failure [CRF]) rats, the turnover rate[184] and the secretion of norepinephrine[185] from the posterior hypothalamus were greater than in control rats. Bilateral dorsal rhizotomy at the level T10 to L3 prevented the increase in BP, the increase in norepinephrine turnover in the posterior hypothalamus, and the progression of renal disease in CRF rats.[186] Therefore, it seems that increased renal sensory impulses transmitted to the CNS activate critical regions in the CNS and are also involved in the control of SNS outflow. Reduced concentrations of SNS inhibitors such as central dopine[187] and β-endorphin and β-lipotropin[188] have been found, and disorders of parasympathetic nervous control have also been identified in renal patients.[189]

In humans with renal failure, there is even more marked hyperactivity of the SNS than in chronic hypertension, as measured by a variety of indices of SNS function, including concentrations of catecholamine degradative enzymes,[190] synthetic enzymes,[191] and plasma catecholamines.[192-199] Plasma norepinephrine levels do not always correlate with moment-to-moment changes in BP[193] but are very consistent over time; they are not simply reflections of reduced clearance, but rather signify marked elevations in norepinephrine turnover.[200] Major increases in muscle SNS traffic in uremic subjects confirm these other findings.[201] In addition, central sympatholytic drugs such as clonidine are extremely effective in uremic hypertension, causing proportional falls in

plasma norepinephrine and BP.[193, 202] Klein and associates[198] observed increased muscle SNS activity in hypertensive patients with polycystic kidney disease regardless of kidney function. Ligtenberg and coworkers[199] reported that increased muscle sympathetic nerve discharge in patients with chronic renal failure was reduced by ACE inhibition, suggesting that abnormal SNS outflow in renal failure is Ang II dependent.

Baroreflex Abnormalities

Arterial baroreceptors exert an important permissive influence in chronic hypertension because of their intrinsic inability to respond to chronic changes in BP, a phenomenon known as baroreflex resetting.[121-127] Reset baroreceptors are still able to respond to acute changes in pressure, but they are not capable of returning BP to normal, so the SNS is never completely suppressed by elevated BP. Although there remains an inverse correlation between resting plasma norepinephrine and arterial baroreflex sensitivity in chronic hypertension,[122] "normal" levels of SNS outflow are still inappropriately elevated. Chronic arterial baroreflex blunting has been linked with aging[124, 125, 203] and with increased Ang II effect.[204, 205] Baroreflex blunting has also been described in animals and patients with renal failure[206-208]; the pathophysiology of the abnormality is unknown but was attributed by one group to abnormal central opioid metabolism.[209] Baroreflex sensitivity is impaired by Ang II or by excess activity of reactive oxygen species (ROS) and improved by increased nitric oxide (NO) activity.[210]

Altered sensitivity of cardiopulmonary baroreflexes may facilitate chronic increases in SNS activity and BP by allowing exaggerated reactivity of the SNS during volume depletion or through impaired suppression of SNS outflow during volume loading. Anderson and colleagues[183] found that borderline hypertensives exhibit augmented muscle SNS activation during salt-loading, compared with normotensives. Hajduczok[124] demonstrated that impaired cardiopulmonary baroreflexes contribute to the age-related increase in SNS activity. In volume loading experiments in dogs with renal failure and hypertension, blunting of both cardiopulmonary and aortocarotid baroreflexes was found.[134] Endogenous membrane pump inhibitors such as ouabain[211, 212] and hormones such as Ang II[213] may modulate cardiopulmonary baroreflex resetting and influence the ability of the cardiopulmonary baroreflex to be suppressed by volume loading.[212]

Renal Nerves

The kidney is highly innervated, and its functional responses are greatly influenced by both sensory and motor nerves.

AFFERENT NERVES. There is a large sensory input from the kidney to the brain that conveys information to the CNS about renal perfusion and metabolism from renal mechanoreceptors and chemoreceptors.[214-216] The two main functional types of renal sensory receptors and afferent nerves are renal baroreceptors, which increase their firing in response to changes in intrarenal pressure or volume, and renal chemoreceptors, which are stimulated by ischemic metabolites or uremic toxins.[217] In rats, chemoceptive sensors are further classified as either R_1 or R_2 based on their resting levels of activity and the types of stimuli that elicit a response. Activation of these chemosensitive receptors stimulates renal afferent nerves that establish connections with integrative nuclei in the CNS.[214] In experimental animals, stimulation of renal afferent nerves by ischemic metabolites such as adenosine or by uremic toxins such as urea evoked reflex increases in SNS activity and BP.[216] Development of renovascular hypertension can be prevented by chemical sympathectomy[218] or thoracolumbar dorsal rhizotomy, which selectively ablates afferent renal nerves.[219] However, once renovascular hypertension is fully established, thoracolumbar dorsal rhizotomy cannot cure it.[220]

EFFERENT NERVES. Efferent renal nerves are extremely important in controlling renal hemodynamics, especially in the integrated neurohumoral responses caused by alterations in physiologic stress states. Volume homeostasis is also very much dependent on renal nerves, as discussed later. Renal nerve stimulation causes renal vasoconstriction[221, 222] and also regulates renin release.[223-225] Juxtaglomerular cells release renin primarily via activation of membrane β_1-adrenoceptors,[226] but α_1-adrenoceptors also stimulate renin release,[221, 222] probably by altering tubular sodium content or macula densa function.[223] Given these interrelationships between the SNS and the RAAS, a permissive role of the SNS in renovascular hypertension could be anticipated. Renal denervation in two-kidney or one-kidney renovascular hypertension lowers BP[227-229] and in the one-kidney model it reduces abnormal hypothalamic norepinephrine metabolism and SNS overactivity.[227, 228] Although excessive renal sympathetic nerve activity tends to raise BP chronically by increasing vascular resistance and promoting salt and water retention, renal sympathetic nerves may also have organ-protective effects. Precapillary arteriolar constriction may serve to protect the kidney from surges in SBP and the attendant barotrauma, thus limiting the increases in glomerular capillary hypertension and slowing the progression of glomerulosclerosis.[230] However, some evidence suggests increased efferent nerve traffic may accelerate progression of renal failure. Dorsal rhizotomy[186] and administration of moxonidine in a dose that failed to lower systolic BP was associated with less glomerulosclerosis.[231]

Renin-Angiotensin-Aldosterone System

Several factors support a role for the RAAS in the pathogenesis of hypertension in patients with chronic renal failure. First, these patients have excessive renin secretion in relation to their ECV status.[232] Second, a direct relationship between plasma renin activity and BP has been found in dialysis patients.[233] Third, aldosterone was shown to contribute to hypertension and renal injury in the remnant kidney model in the rat.[234] Fourth, bilateral nephrectomy was used in prior decades to combat severe hypertension in patients with renal transplantation[235] or ESRD,[236] although it could act through mechanisms other than RAAS suppression, including interruption of afferent renal chemoreflex fibers that may activate the central SNS. Finally, so-called paradoxical or dialysis-refractory hypertension often responds to ACE inhibitors or angiotensin antagonists.

Inappropriately high RAAS activity in renal failure may have a neurogenic origin, but it has also been postulated that intrinsic heterogeneity of nephron function leads to marked overproduction of renin in some nephrons and underproduction in others. In this model, the geometric sum of renin production across the entire kidney is increased.[237] Ang II

exerts other pressor effects, including direct vasoconstriction via stimulation of AT_1 receptors, increased thirst, secretion of aldosterone from the adrenal cortex,[238] and secretion of vasopressin (antidiuretic hormone) from the posterior pituitary.[239] Ang II acts together with catecholamines to promote structural changes such as hypertrophy of cardiac[240] and vascular smooth muscle.[241]

Changing Interactions of the Sympathetic Nervous System and the RAAS

As the two principal acute BP defense mechanisms, the SNS and the RAAS have a unique set of mutually reinforcing actions that affect BP acutely and chronically. As already discussed, renal nerve activation via β_1- and α_1-receptors mediates the release of renin from the juxtaglomerular apparatus, which causes a subsequent increase in circulating Ang II. In turn, Ang II has several stimulatory effects on the SNS that act to sustain or enhance further SNS outflow. First, circulating Ang II stimulates the area postrema, which enhances sympathetic outflow.[161, 163, 167, 169] Second, Ang II acts on stimulatory presynaptic receptors in CNS and peripheral synapses to enhance the amount of norepinephrine (or epinephrine) released during each nerve impulse,[242, 243] similar to the stimulatory function of presynaptic β-receptors. Third, Ang II facilitates norepinephrine-induced vasoconstriction by causing inositide-dependent potentiation of calcium influx.[243, 244] Fourth, Ang II blunts baroreflex suppression of SNS outflow, although there is some controversy in this regard.[205, 211, 213, 245, 246] Ouabain mediates increased RVL-sympathetic outflow and exaggerated BP increases during sodium loading in rats, but this effect is also dependent on CNS AT_1 receptors.[211, 212] CNS ouabain and Ang II also work through a similar final common pathway to resensitize cardiopulmonary baroreflexes and reduce SNS overactivity in rats with heart failure.[247]

In essential hypertension, the relationship between the SNS and the RAAS is complex. This positive interconnection was extensively explored by Esler and colleagues, who in general found mutually reinforcing correlations between the two systems, including higher heart rate and cardiac index among the high-renin hypertensives.[248-250] The degree of BP lowering after β-blockade was also greater in high-renin hypertensives, suggesting that these individuals had so-called neurogenic hypertension.[251] Later studies demonstrated a direct correlation between plasma renin activity and plasma norepinephrine in younger hypertensives.[252] In addition, Schmieder and associates[253] found that mental stress causes supranormal increases in GFR and plasma Ang II in hypertensives compared with normotensives.

Yet the mutually reinforcing relationship between the SNS and the RAAS does not appear to persist as the disorder progresses. At the outset, the baroreflexes blunt the reinforcing effects of the SNS and the RAAS, but baroreflex resetting occurs in chronic hypertension and reduces the overall suppression of the SNS-RAAS axis. Goldsmith and colleagues found that Ang II reduced the forearm vascular response to arterial pressure change in hypertensives[254] and that Ang II reduced the rate of norepinephrine release in patients with heart failure.[255] Pressor sensitivity to Ang II was reduced in conscious uremic dogs[256] and also in uremic patients.[257, 258] The latter finding is consistent with anecdotal clinical experience suggesting that RAAS-blocking drugs are relatively ineffective in patients with ESRD.

A cellular explanation for these findings appears to be related to the importance of the activation state of the SNS and the ambient intracellular calcium concentrations. Fernandez and associates[244] demonstrated that stimulation of AT_1 receptors by Ang II activates cultured sympathetic neurons to release norepinephrine only if basal cytosolic calcium is low; Ang II actually inhibits sympathetic neurons if cytosolic calcium is high.[244] The mechanisms by which the effects of Ang II are switched appear to relate to the ability of Ang II to stimulate calcium extrusion via sodium-calcium exchange in parallel with its ability to enhance calcium influx via AT_1 receptors,[244] similar to its effects in vascular smooth muscle cells.[259, 260] Given the marked SNS activation in uremia and altered vascular status, pressor insensitivity to Ang II may be a systemic manifestation of the events seen in individual neurons and vascular smooth muscle cells. This cellular switching mechanism for Ang II also explains the well-known property of the hormone to desensitize the system to its own actions, which results in a rapid tachyphylaxis to its pressor effects.

Adrenomedullin and Calcitonin Gene–Related Peptide

Other circulating substances modify vascular function. Adrenomedullin was infused systemically and was found to decrease BP in healthy subjects.[261] Similarly, calcitonin gene–related peptide (CGRP) was infused into patients with moderate renal insufficiency and was found to lower BP and increase GFR, but it also increased intraglomerular pressure and Ang II formation.[262] In patients on maintenance hemodialysis, plasma adrenomedullin levels were elevated, even after fluid removal by ultrafiltration,[263] and it was speculated that increased levels of adrenomedullin may partially mitigate the rise in BP observed in hemodialysis patients. Increased plasma neuropeptide Y in response to fluid overload may also participate in hypertension in ESRD.[264]

METABOLIC FACTORS

One of the major breakthroughs in the last several years has been the articulation of the relationship between insulin resistance and hypertension. Another series of breakthroughs has been elucidation of the roles of reactive oxygen and nitrogen species in physiology and disease pathogenesis. All cell types respond to the generation of these highly labile substances in complex multilevel interactions whose individual significance is still a matter of considerable debate. Whether these reactions are generalized or tissue specific remains to be elucidated for most conditions.

The Metabolic Syndrome

The central feature of the metabolic syndrome is obesity, which is strongly and positively correlated with hypertension at all ages, regardless of gender or race.[265-267] There is a strong, three-way association between increased SNS activity, obesity, and insulin resistance.[268-272] In the Tecumseh study, an association among obesity, insulin resistance, and SNS hyperactivity was noted[177]; therefore, increased SNS activity is an underrecognized feature of the metabolic syndrome. Pathophysiologically, it is well accepted that hyperinsulinemia increases SNS activity in animals and humans.[268, 272]

The hypothesis that increased SNS activity causes insulin resistance[273] is consistent with studies showing that when the SNS is activated by lower-body negative pressure, forearm insulin resistance is induced.[274] Another observation consistent with this pattern is that the central sympatholytic drug clonidine lowers SNS output and plasma catecholamines and increases insulin sensitivity in obese dogs.[275] Therefore, a metabolic vicious cycle of obesity, increased SNS activity, and hyperinsulinemia occurs that may be a major sustaining force in hypertension.

Increased RAAS activity may play a role in insulin resistance as well. Ogihara and colleagues[276] found that treatment with tempol in the angiotensin infusion model of hypertension normalized several indices of insulin resistance, including decreased glucose infusion rate in the hyperinsulinemic euglycemic clamp, decreased insulin-induced glucose uptake into isolated skeletal muscle, and enhanced insulin-induced phosphatidylinositol 3 (PI3) kinase activation. Insulin resistance may also somehow stimulate angiotensin production, because the insulin sensitizer troglitazone has been found to suppress Ang II along with insulin signaling in vascular smooth muscle cells.[277] Therefore, similar to the pattern observed for insulin resistance and SNS activity, bidirectional reinforcement may also exist for Ang II and insulin resistance.

Insulin resistance is related in complex ways to renal disease and renal disease progression. Insulin resistance and concomitant hyperinsulinemia have been reported to occur in individuals with polycystic kidney disease or immunoglobulin A nephropathy even with a GFR within the normal range.[278] Abdominal obesity still plays an important role in insulin resistance in dialysis subjects, but the presence of renal failure itself was found to result in insulin resistance in the leaner subjects and in dyslipidemia in all subjects undergoing hemodialysis, compared with control subjects with similar weight.[279]

Insulin resistance remains exercise-sensitive in people with renal impairment or ESRD, and the persistent negative correlation of insulin and maximal aerobic work capacity suggests that these patients might benefit from physical training programs.[280] Uremia is a rapidly reversible cause of insulin resistance. Kobayashi and co-workers[281] performed hyperinsulinemic euglycemic glucose clamp experiments and found that the glucose disposal rate, which was about one-third lower in subjects with ESRD than in normal subjects, could be almost normalized by peritoneal dialysis or hemodialysis. Multiple logistic regression analyses showed that dialysis-induced changes in blood urea nitrogen, hematocrit, and plasma bicarbonate correlated with the change in insulin resistance, further suggesting the presence of a low-molecular-weight substance that functions as an insulin desensitizer in uremia. Glomerular structural damage may be partly related to insulin resistance, because in spontaneously hypertensive rats with 5/6 nephrectomy administered ACE inhibitor, insulin sensitizer (troglitazone), or a combination of the two drugs, similar glomerulosclerosis scores were achieved despite much greater BP lowering by the ACE inhibitor.[282]

Reactive Oxygen Species

Superoxide and other oxygen radicals (ROS) derived from the oxidative metabolism of L-arginine influence cell signaling and gene expression and in some tissues stimulate structural changes such as proliferation, hypertrophy, or remodeling. For example, ROS production within the CNS tends to stimulate neural excitation, and in vascular tissue it tends to cause contraction. Superoxide radicals act directly or through other metabolites such as hydrogen peroxide, which modulates changes in cytosolic calcium concentration.[283] ROS availability is strongly influenced by endogenous enzymatic (e.g., superoxide dismutase) and nonenzymatic (e.g., heme) mechanisms that quench ROS. Ang II stimulates ROS production, and it has been suggested that several of the deleterious effects of this hormone are ROS mediated. ROS production in endothelial cells is strongly influenced by glucocorticoid production.[284]

In experimental hypertension, increased ROS is commonly found. In angiotensin-dependent hypertension, Ortiz and colleagues[285] found that the antioxidants tempol and vitamin E reduced plasma levels of endothelin and oxidative metabolites (thiobarbituric acid–reactive substances, or TBARSs) and prevented the development of sustained BP increases.[285] Other data suggest that ROS production is increased in several experimental animal models of hypertension, including genetic,[286] renovascular,[287, 288] steroid-induced,[289] salt-sensitive,[290] lead-induced,[291] and uremic hypertension.[292] In glucose-fed rats, positive correlations were found among aortic superoxide production, BP, insulin resistance, and superoxide production, along with decreased activity of plasma glutathione peroxidase that could be prevented by lipoic acid treatment.[293]

Whether ROS overproduction leads directly to the initiation or maintenance of hypertension in humans is not clear. In a cross-sectional study, serum vitamins A and E were positively correlated with SBP, whereas α-carotene and β-carotene were inversely correlated with SBP.[294] Therapy with ascorbic acid had little effect on BP in larger studies,[295, 296] although one small study suggested a positive antihypertensive effect.[297] Ascorbic acid had little effect by itself on endothelium-dependent forearm vasoreactivity,[298] but vitamin E may augment statin-related improvement in flow-mediated vasodilation.[299] The failure of antioxidants to positively influence BP and vasomotor tone may simply reflect the difficulty of delivering the proper proportions of scavengers to critical tissue sites. Alternatively, ROS may be important not in directly raising BP but rather in more long-term processes related to tissue damage. There is growing information about abnormal ROS activity in advanced renal disease, especially with respect to ROS-NO interactions.

Nitric Oxide Metabolism

Production of reactive nitrogen species, most notably the ubiquitous vasodilator-neuromodulator NO, is important in excitable tissue because of the far-reaching modulatory effects of these labile intermediaries. The relevance of NO effects to cardiovascular physiology has been demonstrated by many studies in various laboratories. Furchgott and Zawadski[300] first showed that acetylcholine-induced arterial relaxation depended on an intact endothelium which produced a diffusible and transferable substance that relaxed smooth muscle cells. This substance, initially called endothelium-derived relaxing factor (EDRF), was subsequently identified as NO by two different groups.[301, 302] The formation of NO from L-arginine by nitric oxide synthase (NOS) enzymes in vascular endothelial cells is now widely

recognized, and three main isoforms of NOS have been identified. Constitutive NOS (eNOS), is dependent on cytosolic Ca^{2+} and calmodulin. It releases NO for short periods in response to receptor activation or alterations in shear stress, providing a signal transduction mechanism that modulates several physiologic responses, including local vasodilation. Inducible NOS (iNOS) is independent of cytosolic Ca^{2+} and requires the cofactor tetrahydrobiopterin. iNOS is activated by cytokines in various cell types, including macrophages, granulocytes, and endothelial cells, and can be inhibited by glucocorticoids. The third major isoform, nNOS, is found in the neural tissue; it appears to modulate the activity of the SNS.

There is intense investigation of the potential role of NO in hypertension. Regulation of CNS NOS activity may be important in renal parenchymal hypertension. In 5/6 nephrectomized (CRF) rats, norepinephrine turnover rate, NOS mRNA gene expression, and NO_2/NO_3 content have been found to be increased in the posterior hypothalamic nuclei, locus caeruleus, paraventricular nuclei, and rostral ventral medulla.[303] N^wL-nitro-nitro-L-arginine-methyl-ester (L-NAME), an NOS inhibitor, increased BP and norepinephrine turnover rate in several brain nuclei of both control and CRF rats, and a significant relationship was found between the increase in NOS mRNA caused by renal failure and the corresponding increase in norepinephrine turnover rate caused by L-NAME.[303] In a phenol-renal injury model of hypertension, tempol, a superoxide dismutase analog, increased interleukin-1β and nNOS in the posterior hypothalamic and paraventricular nuclei when injected in the lateral ventricle, associated with reduced norepinephrine turnover in the hypothalamus and a reduction in BP. The increases in CNS norepinephrine turnover and BP in the phenol renal injury model are also angiotensin dependent, because they can be blocked by the AT_1 receptor blocker losartan.[304] NO may serve to tonically inhibit SNS activity under normal conditions, but when there is renal failure or excessive RAAS stimulation, increased NO release is insufficient to overcome the chronic SNS overactivity that occurs.

Deficient NO production may also underlie certain aspects of renal failure, vascular disease, and glomerulosclerosis. In 5/6 nephrectomized rats, Vaziri and co-workers[305] observed down-regulation of eNOS and iNOS and suggested that this may contribute to the elevation of BP in these animals. Chronic inhibition of NO synthesis by L-NAME has been developed as a new model of arterial hypertension, and administration of nitro-L-arginine to rats causes systemic hypertension, marked renal vasoconstriction, renal hypoperfusion, reduced GFR, increased filtration fraction, increased plasma renin activity, and increased circulating Ang II.[306, 307] Renal histologic examination in rats subjected to chronic NOS inhibition revealed widespread arteriolar narrowing, focal arteriolar obliteration, and segmental fibrinoid necrosis of the glomeruli, findings that mimic the focal glomerulosclerosis (FGS) observed in conditions in which glomerular capillary pressure is elevated.[308] It is also possible that the increase in GFR seen after a large protein load is an example of recruitment of GFR reserve via NO-dependent mechanisms.

Endogenous NOS inhibitors may influence BP in hypertension and renal disease. Vallance and associates[309] demonstrated in vitro and in vivo that NO synthesis can be inhibited by an endogenous compound, N^GN^G-dimethylarginine (also called asymmetrical dimethylarginine, or ADMA).[309] ADMA levels are increased in Dahl rats[310] and in patients with salt-sensitive hypertension,[311] suggesting that this compound may play a role in this disease, perhaps by reducing the ability of the SNS to be inhibited by volume expansion. There is also speculation that ADMA may be involved in endothelial dysfunction and atherosclerosis.[312] There is a significantly higher plasma level of ADMA and a significantly lower plasma arginine-to-dimethylarginine ratio in ESRD patients, raising the intriguing possibility that hypertension in these patients might be due to inhibition of NO synthesis by endogenous ADMA.[309] It is further possible that reduced plasma ADMA during hemodialysis contributes to the post-dialysis improvement in systemic BP.[313]

Interactions between Reactive Oxygen Species and Nitric Oxide

Interactions between ROS and NO are complex and yield a spectrum of effects that are potentially important in the pathobiology of hypertension and renal disease. ROS appear to have effects on CNS nuclei responsible for SNS control and in some cases may blunt the antisympathetic effects of NO. In some studies, NO appears to be more involved with the maintenance of hypertension in uremia than with its initiation.[314] Sakuma and colleagues[315] showed that N^G-methyl-L-arginine (an NOS inhibitor) increased renal SNS activity and caused systemic hypertension in normal rats, which was ameliorated by spinal cord transection, implying that NO may play a role in the central regulation of sympathetic tone.[315] In the deoxycorticosterone acetate (DOCA)–salt rat model of hypertension, the ROS scavenger tempol suppressed the increased SNS activity independent of NO synthesis, suggesting an independent effect of ROS on SNS activity.[316]

Vasoconstriction can also be induced by quenching NO-mediated vasodilation or through increased production of hydrogen peroxide and peroxynitrite.[317] NO actively reacts with superoxide (O_2^-) and other ROS to produce peroxynitrite ($ONOO^-$), a highly cytotoxic reactive nitrogen species. Peroxynitrite reacts with other proteins, such as tyrosine to produce nitrotyrosine, which can be detected in plasma and tissues. Peroxinitrite is thought to induce oxidative damage to DNA, lipids, and proteins in vascular cells, all of which contribute to cellular damage.[317, 318] Nitrotyrosine is the footprint of the NO-ROS interaction and is used as an indicator of NO oxidation by ROS.[319, 320] Antioxidant therapy partially ameliorates hypertension in uremic rats, presumably by improved vascular tissue NO production and lowered tissue nitrotyrosine.[292] Depletion of glutathione (an endogenous scavenger of ROS) by the glutathione synthase inhibitor buthionine sulfoximine caused a marked elevation of nitrotyrosine (a marker of peroxynitrite) and a marked elevation of BP in rats.[321] Vaziri and colleagues[322] showed that ROS increases in uremic rats are accompanied by increases in NO and that together they produce cytotoxic reactive nitrogen species capable of nitrating proteins and damaging other molecules.

ROS and NO have additional interactions with the SNS-RAAS axis. Ang II is believed to be a major regulator of ROS production in vascular smooth muscle cells, through regulation of the activity of nicotinamide adenine dinucleotide phosphate (NADPH) oxidases.[323, 324] It has also been

speculated that many of the actions of ACE inhibitors and Ang II receptor blockers (ARBs) are mediated at least in part by a reduction of oxidative stress within the vessel wall.[325] Some of the processes affected in vascular smooth muscle cell and fibroblast function and structure involve altered gene expression[326] that in turn modifies function of critical NADPH oxidases, increases adhesion molecule expression, activates matrix metalloproteinases, and induces growth and migration of vascular smooth muscle cells.[327, 328] In turn, NO appears to be able to modulate the action of Ang II and the expression of AT_1 receptors in various sites.[329] Central infusion of Ang II has been shown to decrease nNOS gene expression in the brainstem.[330] The interconnection of the SNS and the RAAS is only partly dependent on NO, however, because blockade of NOS increases SNS activity in conscious animals only after plasma Ang II concentrations increase.[331]

Parathyroid Hormone and Vitamin D

Relationships between calcium metabolic hormones and renin activity have been proposed as mechanisms to explain calcium-induced vasoconstriction and salt sensitivity in essential hypertension.[332] In this model, high-renin forms of hypertension are not vitamin D sensitive. From a hemodynamic standpoint, hypercalcemia appears to cause a selective increase in SVR (cardiac output usually remains unchanged), suggesting increased vascular sensitivity.[333] Insulin resistance has been normalized in uremic animals and in humans with vitamin D treatment (1,25-dihydroxycholecalciferol), with variable effects on parathyroid hormone (PTH) levels.[334]

In rats with CRF, hypercalcemia-induced BP increases are greater than in normal rats.[335] This vascular hyperresponsiveness is reversed by parathyroidectomy, suggesting that the presence of PTH plays an important role in the hypertensive action of hypercalcemia. Hypertension results from secondary hyperparathyroidism, at least in some patients with ESRD. Raine and co-workers[336] studied 36 patients with chronic renal failure and found higher platelet intracellular calcium concentrations ($[Ca^{2+}]i$) in patients with increased serum PTH than in patients with normal serum PTH, with significant correlations between serum PTH, platelet $[Ca^{2+}]i$, and mean AP. Nifedipine therapy was associated with lower platelet $[Ca^{2+}]i$ in ESRD patients with high serum PTH, whereas vitamin D therapy decreased serum PTH, platelet $(Ca^{2+})i$, and mean BP. Treatment of secondary hyperparathyroidism with oral calcium reduces BP in some hemodialysis patients.[337] On the other hand, hypertension in ESRD cannot be due solely to hyperparathyroidism, because parathyroidectomy does not usually normalize BP.[338] Furthermore, dialysis patients occasionally develop hypercalcemia as a result of a variety of causes (exogenous vitamin D, oral calcium supplementation, granulomatous diseases, multiple myeloma, or severe secondary hyperparathyroidism), but corresponding changes in BP are not usually seen.

VASCULAR FACTORS

Functional and pathologic changes in the peripheral vasculature interact with the complex neurohumoral and metabolic alterations to further sustain the vicious cycle of hypertension and renal disease.

Intracellular Calcium and Sodium

In many respects, cytosolic calcium concentration is the final common pathway for vasoconstriction, cardiac contraction, and sympathetic neuronal activity. Excitable cells such as neurons, cardiomyocytes, and vascular smooth muscle cells are essentially "driven" by their cytosolic free calcium concentrations, which are influenced by many extracellular and intracellular signals. Pressor hormones such as norepinephrine activate signal transduction mechanisms that lead to bursts in cytosolic calcium, which in turn drive a series of phosphorylations that lead to actinomyosin contraction or hormone secretion. The potency of calcium as a second messenger is demonstrated by the observation that these cells maintain a 10,000-fold gradient between extracellular and intracellular calcium concentrations. A linear relationship between platelet or lymphocyte $[Ca^{2+}]i$ and BP has been demonstrated in patients with essential hypertension[339] and ESRD.[340]

The major intracellular mechanisms affecting $[Ca^{2+}]i$ are (1) calcium influx through voltage-dependent membrane ion channels, particularly the L-type calcium channel; (2) receptor-operated membrane calcium channels that allow calcium to enter the cell under the influence of hormones such as norepinephrine or Ang II; (3) membrane sodium/calcium exchange, which usually allows passive gradient-driven exchange of extracellular sodium for intracellular calcium; (4) activity of membrane calcium adenosine triphosphatase (ATPase), an energy-dependent process that extrudes calcium into the extracellular space; and (5) specialized proteins that allow passage into the endoplasmic reticulum or the mitochondria. Currently no specific defects in any of these mechanisms have been demonstrated in hypertension or uremia, but several are possible. No direct calcium leak has been found, but the role of cytosolic calcium and calcium flux continues to be a focus of speculation regarding the pathogenesis of hypertension and renal disease.

Many attempts have been made to identify a substance that influences sodium and calcium flux and the consequent increased sensitivity to endogenous pressor factors in hypertension and uremia.[341] One candidate has been an endogenous ouabain-like substance that inhibits the vascular smooth muscle sodium-potassium pump (Na+,K+-ATPase).[342] As a consequence of Na+,K+-ATPase inhibition, intracellular sodium increases. Coupled with this effect, cytosolic calcium also increases owing to reduced membrane sodium/calcium exchange (the Blaustein hypothesis).[343, 344] The net result of this process is thought to be basal vasoconstriction and enhanced vascular responsiveness to pressor agents. It has also been postulated that the increase in intracellular sodium may cause swelling of arteriolar walls, narrowing of the lumen of arterioles, and increased peripheral vascular resistance.[345] Boero and colleagues[346] noted lower erythrocyte Na+,K+-ATPase activity in 38 uremic dialyzed patients than in hypertensive or normotensive subjects, with an inverse correlation between Na+,K+-ATPase activity and peripheral vascular resistance in the hypertensives.[346] Increased secretion of a ouabain-like factor in response to volume expansion occurs in volume-overloaded or hypertensive states, at least in whites,[347] but a direct relationship of this phenomenon to hypertension has not been established. Other unproven speculation holds that increased intracellular sodium could be the result of a membrane sodium leak, which would have the same net effect on $[Ca^{2+}]i$ as that of Na+,K+-ATPase inhibition.

α-Adrenergic Hyperresponsiveness

The importance of peripheral vascular α-adrenergic tone in the maintenance of hypertension was demonstrated by Egan and co-workers,[98] who found increased basal forearm vascular resistance in established hypertensives that could be normalized by α-blockade. Philipp[348] and Kiowski[349] and their colleagues examined the relative contributions of increased plasma norepinephrine and increased α-adrenergic vascular responsiveness in established hypertension. After stratification for BP, a series of hyperbolic relationships between plasma norepinephrine concentration and α-adrenergic responsiveness were found. Patients with high plasma norepinephrine had low α-adrenergic responsiveness, and vice versa.[348] Racial differences in α-adrenergic responsiveness have been described as well. Blacks have greater BP increases during cold and mental stress, and a recent study of black children revealed lower urinary catecholamines despite higher BPs than in their white counterparts.[350] Egan's laboratory has reported that α-adrenergic hyperresponsiveness is linked to increased endothelial fatty acid uptake[351] and perhaps to endothelial dysfunction.

Endothelial Dysfunction

Many investigators have speculated that endothelial dysfunction may play a role in hypertension and in vascular and renal damage, including glomerular membrane breakdown.[352] As the functional interface between the circulating blood and vascular smooth muscle cells, endothelial cells have several key vasomotor modulatory functions.[353, 354] Normal endothelial cells serve as a first barrier to circulating antigens and actively participate in the defense reactions; they play a cardinal role in both preventing and promoting clot formation through their interactions with platelets, the fibrinolytic system, and the clotting cascade; they clear from the blood substances such as norepinephrine and serotonin; they activate peptides such as angiotensin and inactivate others such as bradykinin; they retard thickening and fibrosis of blood vessels through antimitogenic effects; and they play a role in regulating regional blood flow and vascular resistance by transducing signals derived from membrane shear forces. Endothelial cells cause vasodilatation in response to increased flow, shear stress, or certain agonists, a process that is transduced by the release of several mediators, including EDRF (which has been characterized as NO), prostaglandin I_2 (PGI₂), and endothelium-derived hyperpolarizing factor (EDHF). The endothelium may also affect systemic hemodynamics by secreting substances such as endothelin and natriuretic peptides. One common model of vascular tone uses the concept of endothelial dysfunction as a central feature, with excess vasoconstriction occurring when there is an imbalance between an overproduction of ROS and that of other vasoconstrictors or a corresponding underproduction in endogenous vasodilators such as NO.[354]

Whether vascular NO deficiency contributes directly to human hypertension is unclear. Those who argue in favor of a role for the endothelium[354] believe that some degree of tonic endothelial dilatory input is necessary to counteract the intrinsic degree of vasoconstrictor tone that is believed to be present. There have been many types of experiments in essential hypertension that demonstrate reduced endothelial function, as measured by reduced peripheral vasodilation in response to acetylcholine[355] or reduced flow-mediated dilation after forearm ischemia.[356] The degree of endothelial abnormality attributed to essential hypertension is probably an overestimate in these studies, because the investigators did not control for hypercholesterolemia, glucose intolerance, or other factors commonly found in hypertensive patients that directly cause endothelial dysfunction.[357, 358] Furthermore, exogenous nitrates are ineffective chronic antihypertensive drugs. Although they can lower BP acutely in hypertensive crises, there is a minimal long-term effect on SVR or BP.

Endothelial dysfunction induced by dyslipidemia may contribute to renal dysfunction and increased vascular reactivity. When challenged with acetylcholine, the renal vasculature of normal swine dilates, whereas that of hypercholesterolemic animals does not.[359, 360] Chronic antioxidant therapy in these animals appears to normalize the intrarenal vascular hyperreactivity associated with hypercholesterolemia,[361] suggesting a role of ROS in the process.

Endothelins

In 1988, Yanagisawa and colleagues[362] identified a potent 21-amino-acid peptide (endothelin) derived from endothelial cells. Since that time, three endothelin genes have been cloned and three distinct isopeptides have been found that are expressed differently in different tissues: ET1, ET2, and ET3.[363, 364] ET1 is expressed in vascular endothelial cells and in brain, kidney, lung, and other tissues. ET2 and ET3 are expressed in brain, kidney, adrenal glands, and intestine. All ETs are synthesized from a large precursor molecule, pre-proendothelin (pre-pro-ET). Pre-pro-ET1, a 203-amino-acid peptide, is the progenitor of pro-ET (big endothelin), a peptide containing 92 amino acids. ET1 is formed from big endothelin by the action of endothelin-converting enzyme (ECE).

ET2 is the most potent vasoconstrictor, followed by ET1 and ET3. Subpressor doses of ET1 potentiate the vasoconstrictor effects of hormones such as norepinephrine. Calcium antagonists inhibit the pressor and potentiating effects of ET1. In addition to its contractile actions on vascular smooth muscle, ET1 has mitogenic action on vascular smooth muscle cells, mesangial cells, and fibroblasts. It potently contracts nonvascular smooth muscle (bronchial, uterine, intestinal, and urinary bladder), and it has prominent cardiac effects (positive isotropy, chronotropy, and stimulation of ANP release). ET release from endothelial cells is stimulated by cytokines, thrombin, and vasoactive hormones such as epinephrine, Ang II, and vasopressin and is inhibited by local heparans.[365, 366] In addition, physical stimuli such as shear stress can enhance ET production. ET1 plays also an important role as a local vasoactive peptide in the regulation of renal hemodynamic and excretory function.[364] Specific receptors for ET1 exist, and two distinct complementary DNAs of ET receptors have been identified. One—ET_A—is definitely expressed in vascular smooth muscle cells, and the other—ET_B—is also probably present on endothelial cells and may trigger the release of prostacyclin and NO.[367]

The situation with ET receptors is therefore similar to what has been found for Ang II receptors, one (AT_1) being intrinsically associated with vasoconstriction and the other (AT_2) being vasodilatory. Also as with angiotensin receptors, the vasodilatory receptor is less often expressed and therefore may be functionally less important. The order of affinity for the ET_A receptor is ET1 > ET2 > ET3, with ET-1 affinity about 100 times greater than that of ET3. ET_B receptors have equal affinity for all three isoforms.

In rats, endothelin causes a sustained BP elevation.[368] Patients with increased vascular reactivity[369] tend to have high levels of endothelin; increased plasma ET1 levels have been shown in patients with essential hypertension by some investigators[370] but not by others.[371] As with norepinephrine in pheochromocytoma, very high levels of ET1 can cause hypertension by itself, as was shown in two patients with hemangioendothelioma, a rare malignant vascular neoplasm,[372] in whom plasma ET levels were 10- to 15-fold greater than those of patients with essential hypertension. Surgical removal of the tumor resolved the hypertension, but when the tumor recurred in one patient and plasma ET levels increased, hypertension reappeared. A potential role of ET in chronic hypertension is implied by the observation that phosphamidon, a metalloprotease ECE inhibitor, reduces BP in conscious spontaneously hypertensive rats.[373] Endothelin receptor blockers have been tested in human hypertension with mixed effects. Bosentan, a combined ET_A-ET_B blocker, lowers BP in essential hypertension.[374] Schiffrin[375] suggested that the relatively heterogeneous response to nonspecific endothelin receptor blockers can be subdivided as follows: patients with classic high-renin forms of hypertension are poor responders, whereas those with low-renin forms are good responders. Such a distinction, if true, has useful scientific and therapeutic implications.

High ET1 levels are seen in patients with chronic renal failure.[376-378] Suzuki and colleagues[378] also found increased ET3 levels in hemodialysis patients. Miyauchi's group[379] found increased ET1 and ET3 levels in hemodialyzed patients, as well as a positive correlation between ET1 levels and BP. Lebel and associates[380] observed higher ET1 concentrations and mean BPs in patients undergoing hemodialysis, compared with continuous ambulatory peritoneal dialysis, and suggested a link to erythropoietin therapy.[380] Other investigators have suggested that increased ET levels may be influenced by the extracorporeal circuit during hemodialysis.[381]

Prostaglandins

Prostaglandins are complex lipids that are synthesized from arachidonic acid, an unsaturated fatty acid derived from triglycerides subsequently metabolized by lipases, endoperoxidases, and cyclooxygenases to form biologically active metabolites. There are constrictor and dilator prostaglandins, all of which are highly unstable. Moncada and colleagues[382] first demonstrated that the endothelium is the major source of the potent vasodilator prostacyclin (PGI_2), whose synthesis is stimulated by bradykinin through its actions on B_2 receptors.[382] PGI_2 increases levels of cyclic adenosine monophosphate (cAMP) in vascular smooth muscle cells, leading to vasodilatation. It also inhibits platelet adhesion and has thrombolytic and cytoprotective actions. PGI_2 and NO potentiate each other's vascular and platelet antiaggregating effects, even at subthreshold concentrations.[383, 384] Endoperoxides in platelets lead to the generation of thromboxane A_2, which is a potent vasoconstrictor that opposes the vascular actions of PGI_2. A relative deficiency of vasodilator prostaglandin in hypertension and renal disease is being reconsidered in light of observations that potent new nonsteroidal anti-inflammatory drugs (NSAIDs) such as cyclooxygenase-1 inhibitors tend to increase BP[385] or blunt the effects of many different classes of antihypertensive drugs, including ACE inhibitors, ARBs, diuretics, and β-blockers.

Other Vasoactive Substances

Endothelium-derived contracting factors (EDCFs) include PGH_2[386] and epidermal growth factor (EGF), which is a vasoconstrictor and mitogen for smooth muscle cells in vitro.[387] Glomerular mesangial cells express EGF receptors, thus making it possible for EGF to regulate GFR.[387] Other endothelium-derived vasodilators are also present. Feketou and Vanhoutte[388] discovered an endothelium-dependent hyperpolarization factor (EDHF) in the canine femoral artery. EDHF opens vascular smooth muscle calcium-activated potassium (K_{Ca}) channels, allowing potassium efflux, hyperpolarization, and relaxation. Depolarization of smooth muscle cells with high extracellular potassium or inhibitors of K_{Ca} channels blocks this action of EDHF and promotes vasoconstriction. The activity of EDHF is attenuated by ouabain, an Na^+,K^+-ATPase inhibitor, but not by inhibitors of cyclooxygenase or NOS.[388] The chemical identity of EDHF remains controversial. There is some evidence that it is hydrogen peroxide, but others believe that it is potassium itself. In diabetes and hypertension, impairment of EDHF is believed to contribute to endothelial dysfunction.[389]

Arteriolar Hypertrophy and Vascular Damage

Chronic structural changes in large and small blood vessels are themselves important determinants of systemic circulatory adaptations to aging and hypertension. In addition to the age-related stiffening of central arteries, vasculopathic changes in resistance arterioles contribute to the maintenance of chronic hypertension and to renal deterioration. Folkow[390, 391] emphasized the importance of vascular smooth muscle hypertrophy in regulating the vascular responses to SNS-induced systemic vasoconstriction. In this analysis, a thickening of the arteriolar wall, characterized by an increase in the wall-to-lumen ratio, causes a given degree of SNS stimulation, resulting in a disproportional decrease in lumen diameter and a geometric increase in SVR as the thickened arteriolar wall encroaches on the arteriolar lumen.

Ang II,[392] endothelins,[393, 394] and other growth-promoting vasoconstrictors cause vascular smooth muscle hypertrophy in parallel with vasoconstriction, and many of the signal transduction pathways for these events are now reasonably well characterized.[395] In rats, the prohypertrophic effect of Ang II is largely pressure dependent.[392] In humans, the relationship of arteriolar hypertrophy to systemic hemodynamics is complex. At the macrovascular level, Ang II seems to have little effect on pulsatile dynamics, as previously discussed.[115] At the microcirculatory level, Thybo and associates[396] found that despite equal BP reduction at 1 year with β-blocker or ACE inhibitor, the wall-to-lumen ratio of subcutaneous arteries could be reduced by ACE inhibition but not by β-blockade.[396] Overall, the functional significance of the effects of Ang II on vascular smooth muscle hypertrophy remains unclear.

Renal Microvascular Structural Changes: Nephrosclerosis and Glomerulosclerosis

Hypertension and aging cause similar hypertrophic changes in the walls of large arteries and in the small blood vessels of the kidney. Hypertension and the associated renal vasculopathy is associated with a more rapid decline in renal perfusion than is seen in age-adjusted normotensives. The relationship (i.e., vicious cycle) between renal vascular changes, impaired salt excretion, and hypertension was the subject of an excellent review by Johnson and colleagues.[397] As hypertension progresses, renal hypoperfusion is manifested by progressive decreases in total renal blood flow, initially with preservation of GFR.[398] This phase is consistent with early *nephrosclerosis* (defined here as hypertrophy and initial medial fibrosis of preglomerular arterioles) and includes decreased filtration fraction, impairment of pressure-induced natriuresis, and the beginnings of salt sensitivity. As nephrosclerosis progresses, it is easy to conceptualize that it creates a pressure gradient between the systemic circulation and the renal circulation that may also be part of the vicious cycle of renal impairment and chronic hypertension. As hypertension becomes more fixed and BP continues to increase, progressive decreases in renal blood flow are matched by parallel decreases in GFR. At about this point, albuminuria becomes more prominent, and measurable abnormalities of salt and water excretion occur that are indicative of clinically significant *glomerulosclerosis* (defined here as progressive loss of glomerular capillary surface area with glomerular and peritubular fibrosis). The sine qua non of glomerulosclerosis is increased glomerular capillary pressure, with subsequent patchy dropout of tufts of glomerular capillaries, along with mesangial cell hypertrophy and increased glomerular basement membrane permeability to albumin and other proteins and progressive albuminuria.

Nephrosclerosis and glomerulosclerosis are highly interactive; both are highly pressure dependent, increase with age, and are associated with diminished salt excretion and with salt sensitivity.[399-401] The process may be further fostered by heterogeneity of effect across the population of nephrons, with progressive ischemia in certain nephrons and relative sparing of others, which leads to marked overproduction of renin by some nephrons. Despite probable suppression of renin release in other nephrons, the overall effect is inappropriate renin release for a given level of systemic BP. Progressive nephron dropout further accelerates this process in its own vicious cycle.

The role of preglomerular arteries in disease progression is demonstrated by experiments in which the infusion of catecholamines in animal models induces anatomic change and increased sensitivity of BP to salt-loading.[402] Ang II itself causes microvascular lesions when infused chronically into the rat.[403] In addition, it appears that transforming growth factor-β and other cytokines add to the mix by promoting glomerular fibrosis and increasing glomerular permeability to albumin.[404] It may be that the nephrons most affected by nephrosclerosis are somewhat protected from FGS because of the gradient caused by the preglomerular constriction. In contrast, the "unprotected" glomeruli suffer disproportionately from FGS; glomerular capillary dropout within these units accelerates glomerular ischemia and nephron dropout, favoring hyperperfusion of the remaining nephrons. Hyperperfusion, nephrosclerosis, FGS, excessive renin release, and other factors then interact to accelerate the onset of ESRD. The intrinsic heterogeneity of changes across different nephrons is readily apparent on renal biopsy and by itself may be an important part of the pathogenesis of progressive nephron dropout, because of the extremes of dysfunction caused in salt excretion, renin release, and other parameters.

IMPAIRED SALT AND WATER EXCRETION

Pressure-Natriuresis Relationships: The Classic View

In the normal kidney, increased renal perfusion pressure is accompanied by increased salt and water excretion via increased glomerular capillary pressure. Dehydration is then prevented by reflex renal vasoconstriction and intrarenal mechanisms that limit fluid losses as BP returns to normal. As renal disease progresses, salt and water retention becomes more prominent despite systemic BP increases via a phenomenon known as resetting of the pressure-natriuresis curve. According to the Guyton hypothesis,[405-407] chronic hypertension is not possible without a component of chronic volume expansion that is inappropriate for the level of BP. In this model, sodium excess leads initially to volume expansion and increased cardiac output, followed eventually by an increase in total peripheral vascular resistance mediated by altered vascular autoregulation.[405] Closer inspection, however, reveals that this simplified model does not by itself explain all the features of essential hypertension or hypertension with renal disease.

Blood Volume in Hypertension

There are no consistent relationships between blood volume and BP in hypertension. This is not truly surprising given the ability of the cardiovascular system to counterregulate volume and vasoconstriction, as already discussed. Because most of the blood volume resides in the capillaries and venous system, inappropriately high cardiac output can occur when there is sufficient venous volume and venoconstriction to increase cardiac preload and cardiac output. The blood volume is normal in the most individuals with essential hypertension, but as SVR increases with age and hypertension becomes more severe, a strong inverse correlation emerges between blood volume and SVR.[408-410] Relative blood volume expansion occurs in obesity[411] and in the later stages of renal failure,[412] but in the main, chronic systolic hypertension also requires inappropriately high vascular resistance and central arterial stiffness.

Antinatriuretic Effects of Renal Nerve Activation

SNS activity and renal nerves are extremely important in the dynamic regulation of salt and water excretion and in ECV homeostasis. Excess salt and water retention during times of psychological or physiologic stress is likely to be important in contributing to inappropriately high cardiac output. Delayed natriuresis in this model is also important in sustaining the

transient increase in ECV and cardiac output for an abnormally long period. Therefore, if the frequency of significant stressors is sufficiently high, relative volume retention can be sustained. This pattern is probably further exacerbated by the blunting of cardiopulmonary baroreflex suppression of renal sympathetic nerve activity, which has been clearly demonstrated in dogs with renal parenchymal hypertension.[132] SNS activation also causes modifiable activation of the RAAS during mental stress,[413] an additional feature promoting impaired salt and water excretion.

Environmental stress plays an important role in salt and water excretion in animal and human experiments. DiBona and colleagues[414-418] performed a variety of experiments in various animal models to demonstrate how efferent renal nerves transduce stress responses, reduce sodium excretion, and increase BP. In spontaneously hypertensive rats, repeated air jet stress was used to stimulate the SNS. The result was exaggerated renal vasoconstriction and salt and water retention, with increased BP.[419] Later experiments identified the importance of α_2-receptors in CNS control centers in mediating this pattern.[415] In humans, Hollenberg and associates[420] directly measured changes in renal blood flow during mental stress in normotensives with no parental history of hypertension, normotensives with parental history of hypertension, and borderline hypertensives. Renal vasoconstriction was observed during mental stress in borderline hypertensives and to a lesser degree in normotensives with parental history of hypertension. In contrast, normotensives without parental hypertension demonstrated renal vasodilation during mental stress.

The physiologic importance of efferent renal nerves in sodium homeostasis is further demonstrated by observations in animals and humans that a salt-wasting state follows renal denervation[421, 422] or chemical sympathectomy.[423] Renal salt-wasting is a major reason why individuals with autonomic insufficiency have abnormally low blood volume and orthostatic hypotension.[421]

Metabolic Factors and Salt Sensitivity

Salt sensitivity is also associated with the metabolic syndrome and with nondipping status on ABPM.[424] Much attention has focused on the role of insulin in controlling natriuresis, in part through its actions on Na^+,K^+-ATPase and potassium,[425-427] and in part through stimulation of tyrosine kinases, PI3 kinases, and protein kinase C.[428] Yet insulin is a systemic vasodilator that by itself does not cause hypertension during chronic infusions in dogs,[429] lowers BP in humans,[430] and requires concomitant renin-angiotensin activation to cause hypertension in rats.[431] The antinatriuretic effects of insulin infusion in humans are preserved over a wide range of conditions, including insulin resistance status,[432] insulin-dependent and non–insulin-dependent diabetes,[430] salt sensitivity status[433] and hypertension status.[432] Therefore, although insulin may blunt natriuresis, differences in insulin-mediated natriuresis do not explain by themselves the blunting of natriuresis in hypertension and related syndromes. Nevertheless, interactions among dietary salt intake,[434] obesity,[435] RAAS activity,[436, 437] altered endoperoxide and prostaglandin production,[438] and insulin-mediated antinatriuresis are still possible, as are associations with increased SNS activity or altered endothelial function.

Romero and associates systematically investigated the effects of intrarenal NO on natriuresis and BP in animal models. In the rat, NOS blockade is associated with antinatriuresis and hypertension,[439] a finding not affected by inhibition of prostaglandin synthesis.[440] Studies in the dog revealed that natriuresis induced by volume-loading could be blunted by NO synthesis blockade, which was responsible for shifting the pressure–natriuresis curve to require higher BP to maintain natriuresis.[441] Administration of the NO precursor L-arginine limits salt sensitivity in the Dahl rat.[442] Therefore, it is attractive to speculate that reduced renal NOS activity is a cause of impaired natriuresis and renal microcirculatory injury.[443] At the very least, normal endothelial function permits more effective perfusion of the microcirculation and probably provides local modulation.

Extracellular Fluid Volume Status and Blood Pressure in End-Stage Renal Disease

Several studies have shown that short daily hemodialysis treatments can effectively reduce BP, number of antihypertensive medications, and LV mass index.[444-446] Data collected from the Dialysis Morbidity and Mortality Study by the U. S. Renal Data System show that interdialytic weight gain and noncompliance with the dialysis regimen are independent predictors of a higher BP.[447] Normalization of the patient's volume status appears also to correct the nondipping pattern in the circadian BP rhythm that occurs with ECV expansion.[448] Most studies in hemodialysis patients, however, have failed to demonstrate a consistent relationship between postdialytic weight, weight gain between dialysis treatments (i.e., ECV expansion), and BP. In patients with persistently elevated BP despite intense ultrafiltration, sodium and volume excess may play only a secondary role, because exchangeable sodium and ECV are not correlated with BP in these patients.[449-451] The time frame of the dialytic fluid removal may also play a role, because when excessive body fluids were removed with slow dialysis (8 hours × 3 times weekly) and a consistent "dry weight" is achieved, BP 3 months after the initiation of dialysis was controlled in more than 90% of ESRD patients,[452] and this effect was associated with a dramatic reduction in the number of patients requiring antihypertensive drugs (from 89% to about 5%).[452] Reduced ECV alone does not explain the presence of hypertension, because a stable dry weight was achieved in the first month of dialysis treatment, yet BP continued to decrease for another 8 months despite the withdrawal of antihypertensive medications.

In another study, Katzarski and colleagues[453] compared practices in two centers that employed either long (8 hours) or short (3 to 5 hours) hemodialysis with respect to fluid status (bioimpedance, ultrasonographic diameter of the inferior vena cava, and on-line monitoring of changes in blood volume) and BP control. Hypertensive patients had significantly higher volume parameters than those in normotensive patients, and they demonstrated a greater fall in blood volume and BP during dialysis in the short-dialysis group. On the whole, although normotension in dialysis patients can be achieved independently of the duration and dose of dialysis, it may be true that the interdialytic variability of BP is reduced by the longer treatment protocol. It may also be true that judicious use of antihypertensive drugs further

reduces interdialytic BP variability, but this hypothesis has not been adequately tested.

EXOGENOUS FACTORS

Nonsteroidal Anti-inflammatory Drugs

It is now clear that drugs that inhibit prostaglandin synthesis can raise BP, at least in some people. Dedier and associates[385] assessed analgesic use and BP by questionnaire in 51,630 women age 44 to 69 years, who were initially without hypertension or renal disease. Over 8 years (381,078 person-years of follow-up), 10,579 new cases of hypertension were reported. After adjusting for potential confounders, women who used aspirin or acetaminophen on at least 1 day per month or NSAIDs on 5 or more days per month had a higher incidence of hypertension. The risk of developing hypertension in the highest frequency of use category (>22 days per month) compared with no use were as follows: aspirin, 1.21 (95% CI, 1.13 to 1.30); acetaminophen, 1.20 (1.08 to 1.33); and NSAIDs, 1.35 (1.25 to 1.46). For each analgesic type, there was a significant trend toward an increased risk of hypertension with increasing frequency of use ($P < .001$).[385] NSAIDs have also been implicated in the pathogenesis of interstitial renal disease, especially in elderly people.[454, 455] The nonuniformity of effect of NSAIDs on BP is evident from other studies. Alam and colleagues[456] used ABPM to study the interaction of dietary sodium (90 versus 240 mEq/day) and indomethacin in people older than 60 years of age. High-salt diet increased mean SBP by 5.8 mm Hg and DBP by 3.4 mm Hg ($P = .002$), whereas indomethacin increased mean SBP by 2.7 mm Hg ($P = .015$) and had no effect on DBP. High-salt and indomethacin effects were additive; in the hypertensive subgroup, high-salt diet and indomethacin elevated SBP by 10 mm Hg ($P = .0001$) and DBP by 5.3 mm Hg ($P = .006$), with no significant effects in the normotensive group.[456]

Erythropoietin

To maintain an adequate oxygen supply to peripheral tissues, anemia requires a hyperdynamic circulatory state that is characterized by an increase in cardiac output and a decrease in SVR. Clinical and experimental studies have confirmed that increases in hematocrit are accompanied by renal and systemic hemodynamic changes.[457, 458] Polycythemia and associated increased blood viscosity normally lower SVR, because the microvessels dilate in response to better tissue delivery of oxygen.[459] LV mass and end-diastolic diameter also increase in response to the hyperdynamic state. In patients with essential hypertension, elevated hematocrit leads to parallel changes in blood viscosity and SVR.[460] In humans as well as animals, anemia is associated with a proportionately greater increase in renal plasma flow than in GFR, so that filtration fraction tends to decrease. Micropuncture studies in the rat have shown that an acute decrease in hematocrit from 51% to 20% results in an acute increase in glomerular capillary plasma flow, a less steep rise in single-nephron GFR, and a subsequent fall in filtration fraction. Both afferent and efferent arteriolar resistances decrease, resulting in a fall in glomerular capillary pressure.[461] In addition to the direct effects on glomerular hemodynamics, the accompanying increase in blood viscosity also modulates glomerular permselectivity to macromolecules and hence may increase proteinuria.[462] A natural experiment of the effect of chronic polycythemia on progressive renal disease is the massive glomerular enlargement, proteinuria, and progressive glomerulosclerosis observed in cyanotic patients with heart disease, polycythemia, and hyperviscosity.[463]

Recombinant human erythropoietin (rhEPO) has substantially improved the management of anemia and the quality of life in patients with chronic renal failure.[464] However, it can worsen hypertension and increase the requirement for antihypertensive drugs. In rats as in humans, renal insufficiency is a prerequisite for the development of hypertension during rhEPO therapy.[465, 466] Of interest, this adverse effect on BP has not been noted in patients receiving rhEPO for other reasons, suggesting that renal disease may confer a particular susceptibility to the hypertensive action of rhEPO.[466] Patients at greater risk for development of hypertension during rhEPO therapy are those with severe anemia (especially if it is corrected too rapidly) or preexisting hypertension, and perhaps those with their native kidneys. A multicenter study of rhEPO in dialysis patients revealed that a DBP increase of more than 10 mm Hg or an increase in antihypertensive drug use occurred in 88 (35%) of 251 previously hypertensive patients and in 31 (44%) of 71 normotensive patients, of whom 32% required antihypertensive therapy.[467] The rise in BP during rhEPO administration usually occurs within 2 to 16 weeks, although some patients experience a pressor effect several months after the initiation of therapy.

Patients who become hypertensive during rhEPO therapy either have an exaggerated rise in SVR in response to the increase in hematocrit or have a cardiac output that does not decrease to the same extent as that seen in patients who remain normotensive. Of note, the increases in blood viscosity and SVR that are seen during rhEPO therapy do not correlate with BP changes.[468] Therefore, other mechanisms must contribute if BP is elevated. Enhanced pressor responsiveness to norepinephrine or Ang II has been reported.[469, 470] A direct vasoconstrictor action on smooth muscle cells has not been consistently found.[471, 472] A direct stimulatory effects of rhEPO on renal renin mRNA was found in rats despite no change in plasma renin activity and a BP response to ACE inhibition.[473] An increase in platelet cytosolic free calcium was shown in volunteers who received rhEPO,[474] whereas investigators found no correlation between BP and platelet calcium in hemodialyzed patients treated with rhEPO.[475] Administration of rhEPO to normal and uremic rats caused rises in blood and platelet serotonin that were blunted by ketanserin, an antagonist of serotonin 5-HT$_2$ receptors,[476] suggesting a potential role of serotonin in the process. Others have shown that hemodialysis patients on rhEPO therapy manifest increased ET1 levels.[477] There is no evidence that decreased NO activity is responsible for rhEPO-associated hypertension; in fact, NO production is stimulated by administration of rhEPO.[478]

Transplantation and Calcineurin Inhibitors

Cyclosporine A (CyA) and tacrolimus are orally active immunosuppressive agents of the calcineurin inhibitor class that are used in the management of a variety of immunologic diseases and in prevention of allograft rejection in organ transplantation. Hypertension is more common with CyA, which causes vascular hyalinization and hypertension in a dose-related manner. Hemodynamically, there is a chronic increase in peripheral vascular resistance that has been attributed to a direct effect on vascular smooth muscle. CyA also decreases renal blood flow, an effect that is not reversed by ACE inhibition. In vivo, calcineurin inhibitor–induced renal vasoconstriction probably depends to a large degree on activation of the SNS, because renal denervation and α-blocking agents prevent the drug-induced decrease in renal blood flow. Direct measurements in rats and humans have shown that CyA increases the activity of renal afferent and efferent sympathetic nerves and decreases fractional excretion of sodium.[479-482] CyA interactions with the RAAS are complex; acute administration of CyA increases plasma renin activity acutely, but during chronic treatment plasma renin activity levels return to normal or subnormal levels; CyA may also blunt the vascular toxicity of Ang II under certain conditions.[483] CyA increases the production of thromboxane A$_2$ and inhibits the production of PGE$_2$; inhibitors of thromboxane lessen the renal hemodynamic abnormalities caused by CyA. CyA increases the concentration of serotonin in the blood and platelets.[476] CyA can cause magnesium deficiency,[484] but hypokalemia is not usually found.

CLINICAL IMPACT

The foregoing discussion has reviewed in depth the large number of interacting factors that may contribute to the accelerated, age-related downward spiral of increased BP and decreased renal function. Although this process is relatively slow, it ultimately eventuates in CVD and renal deterioration. The most important part of this downward cycle is most certainly the direct effect of hypertension on loss of renal function and the simultaneous ability of renal dysfunction to raise BP. The speed with which the downward spiral proceeds is related to the individual pathogenetic factors and interactions with other cardiovascular risk factors such as dyslipidemia, cigarette smoking, and glucose intolerance. Therefore, disease prevention via fastidious lifestyle modification is the most important overall public health strategy.

The ultimate goal of antihypertensive drug therapy is to reduce cardiovascular morbidity and mortality. Once disease develops, the natural history can be favorably affected by drug therapy in a pattern consistent with the model presented. Of the specific contributions of the five major groups of interacting pathogenetic factors, inappropriate activity of the SNS, increased intracellular calcium concentrations, arteriolar hypertrophy, and inappropriate ECV control are probably most important in sustaining the hypertension. The RAAS may play an important role in renal microcirculatory disease, especially during the early and middle phases of the degenerative process. These features are especially important because drug therapy can blunt their impact and in some cases reverse the overall disease process.

Hypertension without Renal Disease

In the general population, hypertension is diagnosed when BP reaches 140/90 mm Hg.[485] For people with uncomplicated hypertension, renal and cardiovascular outcomes are best prevented by aggressive antihypertensive drug therapy in the form of combination therapy. Thiazide-type diuretics are best used in combination with ACE inhibitors, β-blockers, or ARBs. Calcium antagonists and aldosterone blockers are reasonable alternatives. Management needs in coexisting cardiovascular conditions must be pursued in parallel with antihypertensive drug choices.[485]

Hypertension with Diabetic and Nondiabetic Renal Disease

Treatment of hypertension to retard the rate of renal deterioration is now firmly established as a core principle of management. The threshold BP of 130/80 mm Hg is recommended for antihypertensive drug treatment in hypertensive people with diabetes or renal impairment, defined by either reduced GFR (<60 mL/min, or SCr >1.5 mg/dL in men or >1.3 mg/dL in women) or albuminuria (urinary albumin excretion >300 mg/day or albumin concentration >200 mg/g creatinine).[485] Current guidelines are based largely on data from the Modification in Diet in Renal Disease (MDRD) study.[485-487]

The importance of the RAAS in progressive renal disease is underscored by the positive results from clinical trials in which ACE inhibitors[488, 489] and ARBs[490-492] have proved to be effective when combined with diuretics to reduce the rate of deterioration in SCr or progression of albuminuria. Special attention should be paid to adequate dosing of these agents, as in the irbesartan in patients with type 2 diabetes and microalbuminuria (IRMA2) study, where the higher dose of irbesartan (300 versus 150 mg/day) was clearly superior in protecting the kidney. Calcium antagonists remain effective in reducing BP in renal impairment, suggesting that intracellular calcium is an important determinant of inappropriate vasoconstriction in these patients. Calcium antagonist use in renal disease has been questioned, at least in African Americans with nondiabetic renal disease and proteinuria,[493] but these agents are often necessary to achieve goal BP (<130/80–85 mm Hg). In keeping with the idea that inappropriate ECV plays an increasing role in the hypertension of renal failure, choice of diuretic type becomes increasingly important. Thiazide diuretics are progressively less effective when the GFR falls below 50% of normal (SCr about 2 mg/dL), after which loop diuretics are preferred. BP control often becomes substantially more difficult as GFR declines, and four- or five-drug regimens (including increasing doses of loop diuretics), adrenergic inhibitors, vasodilators, and anti-RAAS drugs are needed.

Hypertension in End-Stage Renal Disease

An ideal goal BP has not been established in ESRD. The Health Care Financing Administration's guidelines suggest that a BP lower than 150/90 mm Hg is a reasonable goal for most patients undergoing hemodialysis.[494] However, this recommendation is not based on clinical evidence. At the other end of the spectrum, the Working Group on Chronic Renal Failure and Renovascular Hypertension recommended a goal BP of less than 130/85 mm Hg.[495] In the only prospective study so far performed in the dialysis population, a BP of 140/90 mm Hg was associated with reduced occurrence of LV hypertrophy and death.[496] These varying recommendations reflect the existing confusion in the literature as to what level of BP predicts better outcome in this patient population.

DIALYSIS. As renal mass declines further, dialysis therapy replaces diuretics for control of ECV, although wide interdialytic fluctuations in BP complicate therapy. In most dialysis patients, BP rises during the interdialytic period in proportion to the amount of sodium and water ingested. To achieve dry weight, there should be a progressive reduction in each postdialysis weight over 4 to 8 weeks, to a point at which BP is reduced during each treatment to acceptable values (SBP <140 mm Hg if possible) but not to levels at which the patient experiences symptoms of excessive sodium depletion (e.g., fatigue, cramps, nausea). When dry weight is achieved and maintained, postdialysis BP becomes normal in most patients and antihypertensive drugs can be reduced. During the initiation of dialysis treatment in patients with SBP greater than 140–159 mm Hg and DBP greater than 90–99 mm Hg who have no major cardiovascular complications, antihypertensive medications are sometimes withheld until dry weight is achieved. If BP remains lower than 150/95 mm Hg between dialyses in lower-risk patients, consideration can be given to controlling BP by dialysis alone, especially in patients who experience intradialytic hypotensive episodes.

A comment on the use of vigorous dialysis instead of drug therapy is warranted. In addition to reducing quality of life through symptoms (e.g., weakness, malaise, nausea, fatigue), overzealous ultrafiltration may cause a more serious group of untoward consequences, including hypotension, compromise of residual renal function, cerebral or coronary ischemic events, and paradoxical hypertension. In contrast, more vigorous ultrafiltration may be necessary in patients with LV failure, acute pulmonary edema, pericardial effusion, or dissecting aneurysm of the aorta. All of these are complex problems that are dependent on the (somewhat arbitrary) assignment of a particular dry weight and the associated choice of vasoactive drugs. Because of the potential adverse consequences, the attending physician and staff must pay close attention to the balance between the dry weight assigned by the nursing staff and the cardiovascular drugs needed to optimize the risk profile. In some cases, a small degree of liberalization of dry weight and a concomitant increase in antihypertensive drugs will improve quality of life.

DRUG THERAPY. If BP remains greater than 160/100 mm Hg, antihypertensive drug therapy is definitely necessary, usually with combinations of two or more drugs. For patients who are already taking antihypertensive medications at the beginning of dialysis, the same drugs should be continued and the dose should be tapered as BP decreases with ultrafiltration. Intensive BP therapy is more effective in some patients than in others, however, and many individuals with galloping chronic renal disease progress rapidly to dialysis despite the ongoing effort to maintain good BP control. Severe hypertension (>180/110 mm Hg) or clinically significant target organ damage (e.g., ischemic heart symptoms, heart failure, cerebrovascular disease, retinopathy, aneurysms) should prompt even more vigorous drug therapy with multidrug regimens.

At some point during the progression to ESRD, vascular and neural sensitivity to Ang II diminishes, as discussed earlier. Therefore, ACE inhibitors and ARBs become less effective in most dialysis patients. The ongoing role of the SNS is evidenced by the continuing utility of clonidine and labetalol to control BP in these patients. In those with more severe hypertension, the role of cellular calcium in perpetuating ongoing vasoconstriction is consistent with the utility of calcium antagonists to lower BP, especially in combination with sympatholytic drugs. If no evident cause for resistant hypertension is found, continuous ambulatory peritoneal dialysis should be consider, because it is generally more effective than hemodialysis for BP control. Given the effectiveness of appropriate dialytic therapy and the power of antihypertensive drug combinations, it is rarely (if ever) necessary to consider renal ablation with surgical or embolic nephrectomy. Loop diuretics have a role in limiting interdialytic weight gain in those few dialysis patients with residual renal function.

PARADOXICAL HYPERTENSION DURING HEMODIALYSIS. Hypertension induced by hemodialysis is a topic that has received little attention.[497] It occurs in a small number of patients, and its causes have not been well delineated. In a few cases, increases in BP late in dialysis may represent dialytic removal of certain water-soluble antihypertensive drugs, including certain ACE inhibitors, minoxidil, and some β-blockers. A more common cause is probably excessive reflex activation of the SNS and the RAAS caused by rapid or exaggerated reduction in venous return and cardiac preload, which activates the cardiopulmonary baroreflexes, which in turn cause central sympathetic stimulation.[498-502] In ESRD patients with native kidneys still present, a favorable response to anti-RAAS drugs is occasionally seen.

Volume overload and cardiac distention may play a role as well. In a study of seven patients with this characteristic, all were found to have marked cardiac dilation; a period of intensified ultrafiltration reduced BP and cardiac size and eliminated the paradoxical elevation of BP during dialysis.[497]

REFERENCES

1. Burt VL, et al: Prevalence of hypertension in the US adult population: Results from the Third National Health and Nutrition Examination Survey, 1988–1991. Hypertension 25:305-313, 1995.
2. O'Rourke M: Arterial stiffness, systolic blood pressure, and logical treatment of arterial hypertension. Hypertension 15:339-347, 1990.
3. Madhaven S, et al: Relation of pulse pressure and blood pressure reduction to the incidence of myocardial infarction. Hypertension 23:395-401, 1994.
4. Franklin SS, Gustin WT, Wong ND: Hemodynamic patterns of age-related changes in blood pressure. Circulation 96:308-315, 1997.
5. Franklin SS, et al: Is pulse pressure more important than systolic blood pressure in predicting coronary heart disease events. Circulation 100:354-360, 1999.
6. Amar J, et al: Nocturnal blood pressure and 24-hour pulse pressure are potent indicators of mortality in hemodialysis patients. Kidney Int 57:2485-2491, 2000.
7. Gasowski J, et al: Pulsatile blood pressure component as predictor of mortality in hypertension: A meta-analysis of clinical trial control. J Hypertens 20:145-151, 2002.
8. Lewington S, et al: Age-specific relevance of usual blood pressure to vascular mortality: A meta-analysis of individual data for one million adults in 61 prospective studies. Lancet 360:1903-1913, 2002.
9. Izzo JL Jr, Levy D, Black HR: Clinical Advisory Statement: Importance of systolic blood pressure in older Americans. Hypertension 35:1021-1024, 2000.
10. Kannel WB, Gordon T, Schwartz MJ: Systolic versus diastolic blood pressure and risk of coronary heart disease. Am J Cardiol 27:335-345, 1971.
11. Neaton JD, Wentworth D: Serum cholesterol, blood pressure, cigarette smoking, and death from coronary heart disease: Overall findings and differences by age for 316,099 white men. Multiple Risk Factor Intervention Trial Research Group. Arch Intern Med 152:56-64, 1992.
12. Klag MJ, et al: Blood pressure and end-stage renal disease in men. N Engl J Med 334:13-18, 1996.
13. Prevention of stroke by antihypertensive drug treatment in older patients with isolated systolic hypertension: Final results of the Systolic Hypertension in the Elderly Program (SHEP). SHEP Cooperative Research Group. JAMA 265:3255-3264, 1991.
14. Staessen JA, et al: Randomised double-blind comparison of placebo and active treatment for older patients with isolated systolic hypertension. The Systolic Hypertension in Europe (Syst-Eur) Trial Investigators. Lancet 350:757-764, 1997.
15. Klag MJ, et al: End-stage renal disease in African American and white men. JAMA 277:1293-1298, 1997.
16. Cirillo M, et al: Pulse pressure and isolated systolic hypertension: Association with microalbuminuria. The GUBBIO Study Collaborative Research. Kidney Int 58:1211-1218, 2000.
17. Kaperonis N, Bakris GL: Blood pressure, antihypertensive therapy, and risk for renal injury in African Americans. Curr Opin Nephrol Hypertens 12:79-84, 2003.
18. Shlipak MG, et al: Renal insufficiency and cardiovascular events in postmenopausal women with coronary heart disease. J Am Coll Cardiol 38:705-711, 2001.
19. Al Suwaidi J, et al: Prognostic implications of abnormalities in renal function in patients with acute coronary syndromes. Circulation 106:974-980, 2002.
20. Dries DL, et al: The prognostic implications of renal insufficiency in asymptomatic and symptomatic patients with left ventricular systolic dysfunction. J Am Coll Cardiol 35:681-689, 2000.
21. Mogensen CE: Microalbuminuria predicts clinical proteinuria and early mortality in maturity-onset diabetes. N Engl J Med 310:356-360, 1984.
22. Nelson RG, et al: Development and progression of renal disease in Pima Indians with non-insulin-dependent diabetes mellitus. Diabetic Renal Disease Study Group. [See comment.] N Engl J Med 335:1636-1642, 1996.
23. Wachtell K, et al: Urine albumin/creatinine ratio and echocardiographic left ventricular structure and function in hypertensive patients with electrocardiographic left ventricular hypertrophy: The LIFE study. Losartan Intervention for Endpoint Reduction. Am Heart J 143:319-326, 2002.
24. Chavers BM, et al: Glomerular lesions and urinary albumin excretion in type I diabetes without overt proteinuria. [See comment.] N Engl J Med 320:966-970, 1989.
25. Festa A, et al: Inflammation and microalbuminuria in nondiabetic and type 2 diabetic subjects: The Insulin Resistance Atherosclerosis Study. Kidney Int 58:1703-1710, 2000.
26. Foley RN, et al: Impact of hypertension on cardiomyopathy, morbidity and mortality in end-stage renal disease. Kidney Int 49:1379-1385, 1996.
27. Charra B: Control of blood pressure in long slow hemodialysis. Blood Purif 12:252-258, 1994.
28. Klooker P, Bommer J, Ritz E: Treatment of hypertension in dialysis patients. Blood Purif 3:15-26, 1985.
29. Foley R, Parfrey P: Cardiovascular disease and mortality in ESRD. J Nephrol 11:239-245, 1998.
30. Masaki KH, et al: Orthostatic hypotension predicts mortality in elderly men: The Honolulu Heart Program. Circulation 98:2290-2295, 1998.
31. Dobkin BH: Orthostatic hypotension as a risk factor for symptomatic occlusive cerebrovascular disease. Neurology 39:30-34, 1989.
32. Raiha I, et al: Prevalence, predisposing factors, and prognostic importance of postural hypotension. Arch Intern Med 155:930-935, 1995.
33. Luukinen H, et al: Prognosis of diastolic and systolic orthostatic hypotension in older persons. Arch Intern Med 159:273-280, 1999.
34. Rutan GH, et al: Orthostatic hypotension in older adults: The Cardiovascular Health Study. CHS Collaborative Research Group. Hypertension 19:508-519, 1992.
35. Wu JS, et al: Postural hypotension and postural dizziness in patients with non-insulin-dependent diabetes. Arch Intern Med 159:1350-1356, 1999.
36. Port FK, et al: Predialysis blood pressure and mortality risk in a national sample of maintenance hemodialysis patients. Am J Kidney Dis 33:507-517, 1999.
37. Salem MM: Hypertension in the haemodialysis population: Any relationship to 2-years survival? Nephrol Dial Transplant 14:125-128, 1999.
38. Ferrannini E, DeFronzo RA: The association of hypertension, diabetes, and obesity: A review. J Nephrol 1:3-15, 1989.

39. Reaven GM: Role of insulin resistance in human disease. Diabetes 37:1595-1607, 1988.

40. DeFronzo RA, Ferrannini E: Insulin resistance: A multifaceted syndrome responsible for NIDDM, obesity, hypertension, dyslipidemia, and atherosclerotic cardiovascular disease. Diabetes Care 14:173-194, 1991.

41. Ford ES, Giles WH, Dietz WH: Prevalence of the metabolic syndrome among US adults: Findings from the third National Health and Nutrition Examination Survey. JAMA 287:356-359, 2002.

42. Kannel WB: Role of blood pressue in cardiovascular morbidity and mortality. Prog Cardiovasc Dis 17:5-24, 1974.

43. Romundstad S, et al: Microalbuminuria, cardiovascular disease and risk factors in a nondiabetic/nonhypertensive population: The Nord-Trondelag Health Study (HUNT, 1995–97), Norway. J Intern Med 252:164-172, 2002.

44. Gaede P, et al: Multifactorial intervention and cardiovascular disease in patients with type 2 diabetes. [See comment.] N Engl J Med 348:383-393, 2003.

45. Zachariah PK, Sheps SG, Smith RL: Clinical use of home and ambulatory blood pressure monitoring. Mayo Clin Proc 64:1436-1446, 1989.

46. Pickering TG, et al: American Society of Hypertension Expert Panel: Conclusions and recommendations on the clinical use of home(self) and ambulatory blood pressure monitoring. Am J Hypertens 9:1-11, 1996.

47. Sokolow M, et al: Relationship between level of blood pressure measured casually and by portable recorders and severity of complications in essential hypertension. Circulation 34:279-298, 1996.

48. Parati G, et al: Limitations of the difference between clinic and day-time blood pressure as a surrogate measure of the "white-coat" effect. Syst-Eur investigators. J Hypertens 16:23-29, 1998.

49. Pickering TG, et al: How common is white coat hypertension? JAMA 259:225-228, 1988.

50. Julius S, et al: "White coat" versus "sustained" borderline hypertensions in Tecumseh, Michigan. Hypertension 16:617-623, 1990.

51. Mancia G, Parati G: Clinical significance of "white coat" hypertension. Editorial comment. Hypertension 16:624-626, 1990.

52. Kooman JP, et al: Blood pressure during the interdialytic period in hemodialysis patients: Estimation of representative blood pressure values. Nephrol Dial Transplant 7:917-923, 1992.

53. Coomer RW, et al: Ambulatory blood pressure monitoring in dialysis patients and estimation of mean interdialytic blood pressure. Am J Kidney Dis 29:678-684, 1997.

54. Peixoto AJ, White WB: Ambulatory blood pressure monitoring in chronic renal disease: Technical aspects and clinical relevance. Curr Opin Nephrol Hypertens 11:507-516, 2002.

55. Agarwal R: Role of home blood pressure monitoring in hemodialysis patients. Am J Kidney Dis 33:682-687, 1999.

56. Millar-Craig MW, Bishop CN, Raftery EB: Circadian variation of blood pressure. Lancet 1:795-797, 1978.

57. Drayer JIM, et al: Circadian blood pressure patterns in ambulatory hypertensive patients. Am J Med 73:493-499, 1982.

58. Muller JE, et al: Circadian variation in the frequency of onset of acute myocardial infarction. N Engl J Med 313:1315-1322, 1985.

59. Tuck ML, Stern N, Sowers JR: Enhanced 24-hour norepinephrine and renin secretion in young patients with essential hypertension: Relation with the circadian pattern of arterial blood pressure. Am J Cardiol 55:112-115, 1985.

60. Panza JA, Epstein SE, Quyyumi AA: Circadian variation in vascular tone and its relation to alpha-sympathetic vasoconstrictor activity. N Engl J Med 325:986-1039, 1991.

61. Minors DS, Waterhouse JM: Circadian Rhythms and the Human. Bristol: Wright, 1990.

62. Pickering TG, et al: Behavioral determinants of 24-hour blood pressure patterns in borderline hypertension. J Cardiovasc Pharmacol 8:89-92, 1986.

63. Cugini P, et al: Postural effects on the circadian rhythm of blood pressure and heart rate in young and elderly subjects. Prog Clin Biol Res 227B:97-105, 1987.

64. Sundberg S, Kohvakka A, Gordin A: Rapid reversal of circadian blood pressure rhythm in shift workers. J Hypertens 6:394-396, 1988.

65. Chau NP, et al: Twenty-four-hour ambulatory blood pressure in shift workers. Circulation 80:341-347, 1989.

66. Baumgart P, et al: Twenty-four-hour blood pressure is not dependent on endogenous circadian rhythm. J Hypertens 7:331-334, 1989.

67. O'Brien E, Sheridan J, O'Malley K: Dippers and non dippers. Lancet 2:397, 1988.

68. Bianchi S, et al: Diurnal variation of blood pressure and microalbuminuria in essential hypertension. Am J Hypertens 7:23-29, 1994.

69. Farmer CK, et al: An investigation of the effect of advancing uraemia, renal replacement therapy and renal transplantation on blood pressure diurnal variability. Nephrol Dial Transplant 12:2301-2307, 1997.

70. Baumgart P, et al: Blood pressure elevation in the night in chronic renal failure, hemodialysis and renal transplantation. Nephron 57:293-298, 1991.

71. Ritz E, et al: Ambulatory blood pressure monitoring: fancy gadgetry or clinically useful exercise? Nephrol Dial Transplant 16:1550-1554, 2001.

72. Perin PC, Maule S, Quadri R: Sympathetic nervous system, diabetes, and hypertension. Clin Exp Hypertens 23:45-55, 2001.

73. O'Shea JC, Murphy MB: Nocturnal blood pressure dipping: A consequence of diurnal physical activity blipping? Am J Hypertens 13:601-606, 2000.

74. Hanly PJ, Pierratos A: Improvement of sleep apnea in patients with chronic renal failure who undergo nocturnal hemodialysis. N Engl J Med 344:102-107, 2001.

75. Zoccali C, et al: Nocturnal hypoxemia, night-day arterial pressure changes and left ventricular geometry in dialysis patients. Kidney Int 53:1078-1084, 1998.

76. Sorof JM, Brewer ED, Portman RJ: Ambulatory blood pressure monitoring and intrerdialytic weight gain in children receiving chronic hemodialysis. Am J Kidney Dis 33:667-674, 1999.

77. Uzu T, et al: Sodium restriction shifts circadian rhythm of blood pressure from nondipper to dipper in essential hypertension. Circulation 96:1859-1862, 1997.

78. Higashi Y, et al: Nocturnal decline in blood pressure is attenuated by NaCl loading in salt-sensitive patients with essential hypertension: Noninvasive 24-hour ambulatory blood pressure monitoring. Hypertension 30:163-167, 1997.

79. Uzu T, Kimura G: Diuretics shift circadian rhythm of blood pressure from nondipper to dipper in essential hypertension. Circulation 100:1635-1638, 1999.

80. Toth L, et al: Diurnal blood pressure variations in incipient and end-stage diabetic renal disease. Diabetes Res Clin Pract 49:1-6, 2000.

81. McGregor DO, et al: Ambulatory blood pressure monitoring in patients receiving long, slow home haemodialysis. Nephrol Dial Transplant 14:2676-2679, 1999.

82. Perloff D, Sokolow M, Cowan R: The prognostic value of ambulatory blood pressures. JAMA 249:2792-2798, 1983.

83. Devereux RB, et al: Left ventricular hypertrophy in patients with hypertension: Importance of blood pressure response to regularly recurring stress. Circulation 3:470-476, 1983.

84. White WB, et al: Average daily blood pressure, not office blood pressure, determines cardiac function in patients with hypertension. JAMA 261:873-877, 1989.

85. Parati G, et al: Relationship of 24-hour blood pressure mean and variability to severity of target-organ damage in hypertension. J Hypertens 5:93-98, 1987.

86. Sluniade K, et al: Silent cerebrovascular disease in the elderly: Correlation with ambulatory pressure. Hypertension 16:692-699, 1990.

87. Verdecchia P, et al: Circadian blood pressure changes and left ventricular hypertrophy in essential hypertension. Circulation 81:528-536, 1990.

88. Cerasola G, et al: Micro-albuminuria as a predictor of cardiovascular damage in essential hypertension. J Hypertens 7:S332-S333, 1989.

89. Omboni S, et al: Reproducibility and clinical value of nocturnal hypotension: Prospective evidence from the SAMPLE study. Study on Ambulatory Monitoring of Pressure and Lisinopril Evaluation. J Hypertens 16:733-738, 1998.

90. Conlon PJ, et al: Predialysis systolic blood pressure correlates strongly with mean 24-hour systolic blood pressure and left ventricular mass in stable hemodialysis patients. J Am Soc Nephrol 7:2658-2663, 1996.

91. Schulte W, Neus H: Hemodynamics during emotional stress in borderline and mild hypertension. Eur Heart J 4:803-809, 1983.

92. Montain SJ, et al: Altered hemodynamics during exercise in older essential hypertensive subjects. Hypertension 12:479-484, 1988.

93. Mitchell GF, Pfeffer MA: Pulsatile hemodynamics in hypertension. Curr Opin Cardiol 14:361-369, 1999.

94. Julius S, Conway J: Hemodynamic studies in patients with borderline blood pressure elevation. Circulation 38:282-288, 1968.

95. Safar ME, et al: Hemodynamic study of 85 patients with borderline hypertension. Am J Cardiol 31:315-319, 1973.

96. Messerli FH, et al: Borderline hypertension: relationship between age, hemodynamics and circulating catecholamines. Circulation 64:760-764, 1981.

97. Wilson MF, et al: Exaggerated pressure response to exercise in men at risk for systemic hypertension. Am J Cardiol 66:731-736, 1990.

98. Egan B, et al: Mechanism of increased alpha adrenergic vasoconstriction in human essential hypertension. J Clin Invest 80:812-817, 1987.

99. Egan B, Schmouder R: The importance of hemodynamic considerations in essential hypertension. Am Heart J 116:594-599, 1988.

100. Izzo JL Jr: Sympathoadrenal activity, catecholamines, and the pathogenesis of vasculopathic hypertensive target-organ damage. Am J Hypertens 2:305S-312S, 1989.

101. Brod J, et al: Development of hypertension in renal disease. Clin Sci 64:141-152, 1983.

102. Black H, et al: The first report of the Systolic and Pulse Pressure (SYPP) Working Group. J Hypertens 17:S1-S12, 1999.

103. Franklin SS: The concept of vascular overload. Cardiology Clin 13:501-507, 1995.

104. Avolio A, et al: Effects of aging on arterial distensibility in populations with high and low prevalence of hypertension: Comparison between urban and rural communities in China. Circulation 71:202-210, 1987.

105. Avolio A: Genetic and environmental factors in the function and structure of the arterial wall. Hypertension 26:23-37, 1995.

106. O'Rourke MF, Kelly RP: Wave reflection in the systemic circulation and its implications in ventricular function. J Hypertens 11:327-337, 1993.

107. Izzo JL Jr: Hypertension in the elderly: A pathophysiologic approach to therapy. J Am Geriatr Soc 30:352-359, 1982.

108. Chadwick RS, Goldstein DS, Keiser HR: Pulse-wave model of brachial arterial pressure modulation in aging and hypertension. Am J Physiol 251:H1-H11, 1986.

109. Tozawa M, et al: Pulse pressure and risk of total mortality and cardiovascular events in patients on chronic hemodialysis. Kidney Int 61:717-726, 2002.

110. Avolio A, Jones D, Tafazzoli-Shadpour M: Quantification of alterations in structure and function of elastin in the arterial media. Hypertension 32:170-175, 1998.

111. Kass DA, et al: Improved arterial compliance by a novel advanced glycation end-product crosslink breaker. Circulation 104:1464-1470, 2001.

112. London GM, et al: Aortic and large artery compliance in end-stage renal failure. Kidney Int, 37:137-142, 1990.

113. Asmar R, et al: Pulse pressure and aortic pulse wave are markers of cardiovascular risk in hypertensive populations. Am J Hypertens 14:91-97, 2001.

114. Brouwers-Ceiler DL, et al: The influence of angiotensin II-induced increase in aortic wall mass on compliance in rats in vivo. Cardiovasc Res 33:478-484, 1997.

115. Ceiler DL, et al: Pressure but not angiotensin II-induced increases in wall mass or tone influences static and dynamic aortic mechanics. J Hypertens 17:1109-1116, 1999.

116. Mitchell GF, et al: Omapatrilat reduces pulse pressure and proximal aortic stiffness in patients with systolic hypertension: Results of the conduit hemodynamics of omapatrilat international research study. Circulation 105:2955-2961, 2002.

117. O'Rourke MF, Yaginuma T: Wave reflections and the arterial pulse. Arch Intern Med 144:366-371, 1984.

118. Takata M, Denton KM, Anderson WP: Renal and systemic vascular conductances in renal wrap hypertension in rabbits. J Hypertens 6:719-722, 1988.

119. Denton KM, Anderson WP, Korner PI: Renal blood flow and glomerular filtration rate in renal wrap hypertension in rabbits. J Hypertens 1:351-355, 1983.

120. Mancia G, et al: Arterial baroreflexes and blood pressure and heart rate variabilities in humans. Hypertension 8:147-153, 1986.

121. Izzo JLJ, Taylor AA: The sympathetic nervous system and baroreflexes in hypertension and hypotension. Curr Hypertens Rep 1:254-263, 1999.

122. Goldstein DS: Arterial baroreflex sensitivity, plasma catecholamines, and pressor responsiveness in essential hypertension. Circulation 68:234-240, 1983.

123. Matsukawa T, et al: Reduced baroreflex changes in muscle sympathetic nerve activity during blood pressure elevation in essential hypertension. J Hypertens 9:537-542, 1991.

124. Hajduczok C, Chapleau MW, Abboud FM: Increase in sympathetic activity with age: II. Role of impairment of cardiopulmonary baroreflexes. Am J Physiol 260:H1121-H1127, 1991.

125. Hajduczok G, et al: Increase in sympathetic activity with age: I. Role of impairment of arterial baroreflexes. Am J Physiol 260:H1113-H1120, 1991.

126. Hajduczok G, Chapleau MW, Abboud FM: Rapid adaptation of central pathways explains the suppressed baroreflex with aging. Neurobiol Aging 12:601-604, 1991.

127. Ebert TJ, et al: Effects of aging on baroreflex regulation of sympathetic activity in humans. Am J Physiol 263:H798-H803, 1992.

128. Chapleau MW, Hajduczok G, Abboud FM: Pulsatile activation of baroreceptors causes central facilitation of baroreflex. Am J Physiol 256:H1735-H1741, 1989.

129. Hajduczok G, et al: Gadolinium inhibits mechanoelectrical transduction in rabbit carotid baroreceptors: Implication of stretch-activated channels. J Clin Invest 94:2392-2396, 1994.

130. Luft FC, et al: Plasma and urinary norepinephrine at extremes of sodium intake in normal man. Hypertension 1:261-266, 1979.

131. Romoff MS, et al: Effect of sodium intake on plasma catecholamines in normal subjects. J Clin Endocrinol Metab 48:26-31, 1979.

132. Thames MD, Johnson LN: Impaired cardiopulmonary baroreflex control of renal nerves in renal hypertension. Circ Res 57:741-747, 1985.

133. Izzo JL Jr, Sander E, Larrabee PS: Effect of postural stimulation on systemic hemodynamics and sympathetic nervous activity in systemic hypertension. Am J Cardiol 65:339-342, 1990.

134. Guo GB, Thames MD: Abnormal baroreflex control in renal hypertension is due to abnormal baroreceptors. Am J Physiol 245:420-428, 1983.

135. Simon AC, et al: Baroreflex sensitivity and cardiopulmonary blood volume in normotensive and hypertensive patients. Br Heart J 39:799-805, 1977.

136. Tidgren B, et al: Renal responses to lower body negative pressure in humans. Am J Physiol 259:F573-F579, 1990.

137. Joyner MJ, Shepherd JT, Seals DR: Sustained increases in sympathetic outflow during prolonged lower body negative pressure in humans. J Appl Physiol 68:1004-1009, 1990.

138. Schmedtje JF Jr, et al: Correlation of plasma norepinephrine and plasma atrial natriuretic factor during lower body negative pressure. Aviat Space Environ Med 61:555-558, 1990.

139. Hirsch AT, et al: Vasopressin-mediated forearm vasodilation in normal humans: Evidence for a vascular vasopressin V2 receptor. J Clin Invest 84:418-426, 1989.

140. Davies R, et al: Plasma vasopressin and blood pressure: Studies in normal subjects and in benign essential hypertension at rest and after postural challenge. Br Heart J 49:528-531, 1983.

141. Goldsmith SR, Francis GS, Cowley AW: Arginine vasopressin and the renal response to water loading in congestive heart failure. Am J Cardiol 58:295-299, 1986.

142. DePaula RB, et al: Contribution of vasopressin to orthostatic blood pressure maintenance in essential hypertension. Am J Hypertens 6:794-798, 1993.

143. Cowley AW, Monos E, Guyton AC: Interaction of vasopressin and the baroreceptor reflex system in the regulation of arterial pressure in the dog. Circ Res 34:505-514, 1974.

144. Hirsch AT, et al: Regional vascular responses to prolonged lower body negative pressure in normal subjects. Am J Physiol 257:H219-H225, 1989.

145. Hirsch AT, Dzau VJ, Creager MA: Baroreceptor function in congestive heart failure: effect on neurohumoral activation and regional vascular resistance. Circulation 75(suppl IV):IV36-IV48, 1987.

146. Bouby N, Hassler C, Bankir L: Contribution of vasopressin to progression of chronic renal failure: Study in Brattleboro rats. Life Sci 65:991-1004, 1999.

147. Levin E, Gardner DG, Samson WK: Natriuretic peptides. N Engl J Med 339:321-328, 1998.

148. Sagnella GA, et al: Raised circulating levels of atrial natriuretic peptides in essential hypertension. Lancet 1:179-181, 1986.

149. Zoccali C, et al: The influence of autonomic failure on plasma ANF concentration in uremic patients on chronic hemodialysis. Clin Nephrol 37:198-203, 1992.

150. Tikkanen I, et al: Plasma level of atrial natriuretic peptide as an indicator of increased cardiac load in uremic patients. Clin Nephrol 34:167-172, 1990.

151. Cannella G, et al: Plasma concentrations of atrial natriuretic peptide in relation to body fluid status in chronic uraemia. Nephrol Dialysis Transplant 2:158-160, 1987.

152. Winters CJ, Vesely DL: Change in plasma immunoreactive N-terminus, C-terminus, and 4,000-dalton midportion of atrial natriuretic factor prohormone with hemodialysis. Nephron 58:17-22, 1991.

153. Zoccali C, et al: Cardiac natriuretic peptides are related to left ventricular mass and function and predict mortality in dialysis patients. J Am Soc Nephrol 12:1508-1515, 2001.

154. Ross CA, et al: Tonic vasomotor control by the rostral ventrolateral medulla: Effect of electrical or chemical stimulation of the area containing C1 adrenaline neurons on arterial pressure, heart rate and plasma catecholamines and vasopressin. J Neurosci 4:474-494, 1984.

155. Reis DJ, Ruggiero DA, Morrison SF: The C1 area of the rostal ventrolateral medulla oblongata. Am J Hypertens 2:363S-374S, 1989.

156. DiBona GF, Rios LL: Renal nerves in compensatory renal response to contralateral renal denervation. Am J Physiol 238:F26-F30, 1980.

157. Fink GD, et al: Central site for pressor action of blood-borne angiotensin in rat. Am J Physiol 239:R358-4361, 1980.

158. Shapiro RE, Miselis RR: The central neural connections of the area postrema of the rat. J Comp Neurol 234:344-364, 1985.

159. Huang ZG, et al: Roles of periaqueductal gray and nucleus tractus solitarius in cardiorespiratory function in the rat brainstem. Respir Physiol 120:185-195, 2000.

160. Nathan MA, Reis DJ: Chronic labile hypertension produced by lesions of the nucleus tractus solitarri in the cat. Circ Res 40:72-80, 1977.

161. Bruner CA, et al: Area postrema ablation and vascular reactivity in deoxycorticosterone-salt-treated rats. Hypertension 11:668-673, 1988.

162. Catelli JM, Sved AF: Lesions of the AV3V region attenuate sympathetic activation but not the hypertension elicited by destruction of the nucleus tractus solitarius. Brain Res 439:330-336, 1988.

163. Mangiapane ML, et al: Lesion of the area postrema region attenuates hypertension in spontaneously hypertensive rats. Circ Res 64:129-135, 1989.

164. Abboud FM: The sympathetic system in hypertension. Hypertension 4(suppl II):II208-II225, 1982.

165. Knuepfer MM, Johnson AK, Brody MJ: Identification of brain stem projections mediating hemodynamic responses to stimulation of the anteroventral third ventricle (AV3V) region. Brain Res 294:305-314, 1984.

166. Brody MJ, et al: The role of the anteroventral third ventricle (AV3V) region in experimental hypertension. Circ Res 43(suppl I):I2-I13, 1978.

167. Fink GD, Bruner CA, Mangiapane ML: Area postrema is critical for angiotensin-induced hypertension in rats. Hypertension 9:355-361, 1987.

168. Undesser KP, et al: Interactions of vasopressin with the area postrema in arterial baroreflex function in conscious rabbits. Circ Res 56:410-417, 1985.

169. Mangiapane ML, Brody MJ: Vasoconstrictor and vasodilator sites within anteroventral third ventricle region. Am J Physiol 253:827-831, 1987.

170. Bunag RD, Eferakeya AD: Immediate hypotensive after effects of posterior hypothalamic lesions in awake rats with spontaneous, renal, or DOCA hypertension. Cardiovasc Res 10:663-671, 1976.

171. Folkow B, Johansson B, Oberg B: A hypothalamic structure with marked inhibitory effect on tonic sympathetic activity. Acta Physiol Scand 47:262-270, 1959.

172. Nathan MA, Reis DJ: Fulminating arterial hypertension with pulmonary edema from release of adrenomedullary catecholamines after lesions of the anterior hypothalamus in the rat. Circ Res 37:226-235, 1975.

173. Takeda K, Bunag RD: Sympathetic hyperactivity during hypothalamic stimulation in spontaneously hypertensive rats. J Clin Invest 62:642-648, 1978.

174. Takeda K, et al: Sympathetic inhibition and attenuation of spontaneous hypertension by PVN lesions in rats. Brain Res 543:296-300, 1991.

175. Miura Y, et al: Plasma noradrenaline concentrations and haemodynamics in the early stage of essential hypertension. Clin Sci Mol Med 55:69S-71S, 1978.

176. Goldstein DS: Plasma norepinephrine in essential hypertension: A study of studies. Hypertension 3:48-52, 1981.

177. Julius S, et al: Hyperkinetic borderline hypertension in Tecumseh, Michigan. J Hypertens 9:77-84, 1991.

178. Masuo K, et al: Differences in insulin and sympathetic responses to glucose ingestion due to family history of hypertension. Am J Hypertens 9:739-745, 1996.

179. Masuo K, et al: Sympathetic nerve hyperactivity precedes hyperinsulinemia and blood pressure elevation in young, nonobese Japanese population. Am J Hypertens 10:77-83, 1997.

180. Masuo K, et al: Familial hypertension, insulin, sympathetic activity, and blood pressure elevation. Hypertension 32:96-100, 1998.

181. Izzo JL Jr, et al: Plasma norepinephrine and age as determinants of systemic hemodynamics in men with established essential hypertension. Hypertension 9:415-419, 1987.

182. Ward KD, et al: Influence of insulin, sympathetic nervous system activity, and obesity on blood pressure: The Normative Aging Study. J Hypertens 14:301-308, 1996.

183. Anderson EA, et al: Elevated sympathetic nerve activity in borderline hypertensive humans: Evidence from direct intraneural recordings. Hypertension 14:177-183, 1989.

184. Bigazzi R, Kogosov E, Campese VM: Altered norepinephrine turnover in the brain of rats with chronic renal failure. J Am Soc Nephrol 4:1901-1907, 1994.

185. Ye S, Ozgur B, Campese VM: Renal afferent impulses, the posterior hypothalamus, and hypertension in rats with chronic renal failure. Kidney Int 51:722-727, 1997.

186. Campese VM, Kogosov E, Koss M: Renal afferent denervation prevents the progression of renal disease in the renal ablation model of chronic renal failure in the rat. Am J Kidney Dis 26:861-865, 1995.

187. Kuchel OG, Shigetomi S: Dopaminergic abnormalities in hypertension associated with moderate renal insufficiency. Hypertension 23(suppl I):I240-I245, 1994.

188. Elias AN, Vasiri ND: Plasma catecholamines in chronic renal disease. Int J Artif Org 8:243-244, 1985.

189. Zucchelli P, et al: Influence of ultrafiltration on plasma renin activity and adrenergic system. Nephron 21:317-324, 1978.

190. Atuk NO, et al: Red blood cell catechol-o-methyl transferase, plasma catecholamines and renin in renal failure. Trans Am Soc Artif Intern Organs 22:195-200, 1976.

191. Lake CR, et al: Plasma levels of norepinephrine and dopamine-beta-hydroxylase in CRF patients treated with dialysis. Cardiovasc Med 1:1099-1111, 1979.

192. Henrich WM, et al: Competitive effects of hypokalemia and depletion on plasma renin activity, aldosterone and catecholamine concentrations in hemodialysis patients. Kidney Int 12:279-284, 1977.

193. Campese VM, et al: Mechanisms of autonomic nervous system dysfunction in uremia. Kidney Int 20:246-253, 1981.

194. Izzo JL Jr, et al: Sympathetic nervous system hyperactivity in maintenance hemodialysis patients. Trans Am Soc Artif Organs 28:604-607, 1982.

195. Ishii M, Ikeda T, Takagi M: Elevated plasma catecholamines in hypertensives with primary glomerular diseases. Hypertension 5:545-551, 1983.

196. Cuche JL, et al: Plasma free, sulfo- and glucuro-conjugated catecholamines in uremic patients. Kidney Int 30:566-572, 1986.

197. Grekas D, et al: Effects of sympathetic and plasma renin activity on hemodialysis hypertension. Clin Nephrol 55:115-120, 2001.

198. Klein IH, et al: Sympathetic activity is increased in polycystic kidney disease and is associated with hypertension. J Am Soc Nephrol 12:2427-2433, 2001.

199. Ligtenberg G, et al: Reduction of sympathetic hyperactivity by enalapril in patients with chronic renal failure. N Engl J Med 340:1321-1328, 1999.

200. Izzo JL Jr, Sterns RH: Abnormal norepinephrine release in uremia. Kidney Int 24(suppl 16):S221-S223, 1983.

201. Converse RL Jr, et al: Sympathetic overactivity in patients with chronic renal failure. N Engl J Med 327:1912-1918, 1992.

202. Izzo JL Jr, et al: Increased plasma norepinephrine and sympathetic nervous activity in essential hypertensive and uremic humans: Effects of clonidine. J Cardiovasc Pharmacol 10(suppl 12):S225-S229, 1987.

203. Randall OS, et al: Relationship of age and blood pressure to baroreflex sensitivity and arterial compliance in man. Clin Sci Mol Med 51:357s-360s, 1976.

204. Ismay JJA, Lumbers ER, Stevens AD: The action of angiotensin II on the baroreflex response of the conscious ewe and the conscious fetus. J Physiol 288:467-479, 1979.

205. Guo GB, Abboud FM: Angiotensin II often rates baroreflex control of heart rate and sympathetic activity. Am J Physiol 246:H80-H89, 1984.

206. Pickering TG, Gribbin B, Oliver DO: Baroreflex sensitivity in patients on long-term hemodialysis. Clin Sci 43:645-647, 1972.

207. Watson AJ, Di Pette D: Baroreflex sensitivity and pressor responses in a rat model of uraemia. Clin Sci 69:637-640, 1985.

208. Rogerson ME, et al: The effect of recombinant human erythropoietin on cardiovascular responses to postural stress in dialysis patients. Clin Autonom Res 3:271-274, 1993.

209. Zoccali C, et al: The role of endogenous opioids in the baroreflex dysfunction of dialysis patients. Proc Eur Dial Transplant Assoc Eur Ren Assoc 21:190-194, 1985.

210. Wong LF, et al: Genetic and pharmacological dissection of pathways involved in the angiotensin II-mediated depression of baroreflex function. FASEB J 16:1595-1601, 2002.

211. Huang BS, Veerasingham SJ, Leenen FH: Brain "ouabain," ANG II, and sympathoexcitation by chronic central sodium loading in rats. Am J Physiol 274:H1269-H1276, 1998.

212. Budzikowski AS, Huang BS, Leenen FH: Brain "ouabain," a neurosteroid, mediates sympathetic hyperactivity in salt-sensitive hypertension. Clin Exp Hypertens 20:119-140, 1998.

213. Murakami H, Liu JL, Zucker IH: Angiotensin II blockade enhances baroreflex control of sympathetic outflow in heart failure. Hypertension 29:564-569, 1997.

214. Faber JE, Brody MJ: Afferent renal nerve-dependent hypertension following acute renal artery stenosis in the conscious rat. Circ Res 57:676-688, 1985.

215. Calaresu FR, Ciriello J: Renal afferent nerves affect discharge rate of medullary and hypothalamic single units in the cat. J Auton Nerv System 3:311-320, 1981.

216. Katholi RE, et al: Intrarenal adenosine produces hypertension by activating the sympathetic nervous system via the renal nerves. J Hypertension 2:349-359, 1984.

217. Recordati G, et al: Renal chemoreceptors. J Auton Nerv Syst 3:237-251, 1981.

218. Dargie HL, Franklin SS, Reid JL: The sympathetic nervous system in renovascular hypertension in the rat. Br J Pharmacol 56:365-374, 1976.

219. Wyss JM, Aboukarsh N, Oparil S: Sensory denervation of the kidney attenuates renovascular hypertension in the rat. Am J Physiol 250: H82-H86, 1986.

220. Wyss JM, Aboukarsh N, Oparil S: Selective lesion of the renal afferents transiently lowers blood pressure in established 1 kidney, 1 clip Goldblatt hypertension. Circulation 70:429-435, 1984.

221. Blair ML, Chen Y-H, Hisa H: Elevation of plasma renin activity by alpha-adrenoceptor agonists in conscious dogs. Am J Physiol 251: E695-E702, 1986.

222. Blair ML: Stimulation of renin secretion by alpha-adrenoceptor agonists. Am J Physiol 244:E37-E44, 1983.

223. Osborn JL, Thames MD, DiBona GF: Role of macula densa in renal nerve modulation of renin secretion. Am J Physiol 242:367-371, 1982.

224. Osborn JL, Roman RJ, Ewens JD: Renal nerves and the development of Dahl salt-sensitive hypertension. Hypertension 11:523-528, 1988.

225. Osborn JL, et al: Long-term increases in renal sympathetic nerve activity and hypertension. Review. Clin Exp Pharmacol Physiol 24:72-76, 1997.

226. Johnson JA, et al: Evidence for an intrarenal beta receptor in control of renin release. Am J Physiol 230:410-418, 1976.

227. Winternitz SR, Katholi RE, Oparil S: Decrease in hypothalamic norepinephrine content following renal denervation in the one-kidney one-clip Goldblatt hypertensive rat. Hypertension 4:369-373, 1982.

228. Katholi RE, Winternitz SR, Oparil S: Role of the renal nerves in the pathogenesis of one-kidney renal hypertension in the rat. Hypertension 3:404-409, 1981.

229. Katholi RE, et al: Importance of the renal nerves in established two-kidney, one clip Goldblatt hypertension in the rat. Hypertension 4:166-174, 1982.

230. Beroniade VC, Lefebvre R, Falardeau P: Unilateral nodular diabetic glomerulosclerosis: Recurrence of an experiment of nature. Am J Nephrol 7:55-59, 1987.

231. Ahann K, Rump LC, Simonaviciene A, et al: Effects of low dose sympathetic inhibition on glomerulosclerosis and albuminuria in subtotally nephrectomized rats. J Am Soc Nephrol 11:1469-1478, 2000.

232. Lazarus JM, Hampers CL, Merrill JP: Hypertension in chronic renal failure: Treatment with hemodialysis and nephrectomy. Arch Intern Med 133:1059-1065, 1974.

233. Weidman P, et al: Plasma renin activity and blood pressure in terminal renal failure. N Engl J Med 285:757-762, 1971.

234. Greene EL, Kren S, Hostetter TH: Role of aldosterone in the remnant kidney model in the rat. J Clin Invest 98:1063-1068, 1996.

235. Curtis JJ, et al: Benefits of removal of native kidneys in hypertension after renal transplantation. Lancet 2:739-742, 1985.

236. Donohue JP, et al: Bilateral nephrectomy: Its role in management of the malignant hypertension of end-stage renal disease. J Urol 106: 488-491, 1971.

237. Laragh JH: Lewis K. Dahl Memorial Lecture. The renin system and four lines of hypertension research: Nephron heterogeneity, the calcium connection, the prorenin vasodilator limb, and plasma renin and heart attack. Hypertension 20:267-279, 1992.

238. Davis JO, Freeman RH: Historical perspectives on the renin-angiotensin-aldosterone system and angiotensin blockade. Am J Cardiol 49:1385-1389, 1982.

239. Gavras I, Mulinari R, Gavras H: Renin-angiotensin and vasopressin in the development of salt-induced hypertension. J Hypertens 6: 999-1002, 1988.

240. Waeber B, Brunner HR: Cardiovascular hypertrophy: Role of angiotensin II and bradykinin. J Cardiovasc Pharmacol 27(suppl 2): S36-S40, 1996.

241. Griffin SA, et al: Angiotensin II causes vascular hypertrophy in part by a non- pressor mechanism. Hypertension 17:626-635, 1991.

242. Zimmerman BG: Adrenergic facilitation by angiotensin: does it serve a physiological function? Clin Sci 60:343-348, 1981.

243. Zimlichman R, et al: Angiotensin II increases cytosolic calcium and stimulates catecholamine release in cultured bovine adrenomedullary cells. Cell Calcium 8:315-325, 1987.

244. Fernandez SF, et al: Modulation of angiotensin II responses in sympathetic neurons by cytosolic calcium. Hypertension 41:56-63, 2003.

245. Lee WB, Lumbers ER: Angiotensin and the cardiac baroreflex response to phenylephrine. Clin Exp Pharmacol Physiol 8:109-117, 1981.

246. Ibsen H, et al: Reflex-hemodynamic adjustments and baroreflex sensitivity during converting enzyme inhibition with MK-421 in normal humans. Hypertension 5:I184-I191, 1983.

247. Huang BS, Yuan B, Leenen FH: Chronic blockade of brain "ouabain" prevents sympathetic hyper-reactivity and impairment of acute baroreflex resetting in rats with congestive heart failure. Can J Physiol Pharmacol 78:45-53, 2000.

248. Esler MD, Nestel PJ: High catecholamine essential hypertension: Clinical and physiological characteristics. Aust N Z J Med 3: 117-123, 1973.

249. Esler MD, Nestel PJ: Renin and sympathetic nervous system responsiveness to adrenergic stimuli in essential hypertension. Am J Cardiol 32:643-649, 1973.

250. Esler MD, Nestel PJ: Essential hypertension with symptoms of hyperkinetic circulation. Med J Aust 2:253-257, 1973.

251. Esler MD: Effect of practolol on blood pressure and renin release in man. Clin Pharmacol Ther 15:484-489, 1974.

252. Esler M, et al: Mild high-renin essential hypertension: Neurogenic human hypertension? N Engl J Med 296:405-411, 1977.

253. Schmieder RE, et al: Glomerular hyperfiltration during sympathetic nervous system activation in early essential hypertension. J Am Soc Nephrol 8:893-900, 1997.

254. Goldsmith SR, Hasking GJ: Angiotensin II inhibits the forearm vascular response to increased arterial pressure in humans. J Am Coll Cardiol 25:246-250, 1995.

255. Goldsmith SR, Hasking GJ, Miller E: Angiotensin II and sympathetic activity in patients with congestive heart failure. J Am Coll Cardiol 21:1107-1113, 1993.

256. Fujii AM, Vatner SF: Direct versus indirect pressor and vasoconstrictor actions of angiotensin in conscious dogs. Hypertension 7:253-261, 1985.

257. Sorensen SS, et al: Hypotension in end-stage renal disease: Effect of postural change, exercise and angiotensin II infusion on blood pressure and plasma concentrations of angiotensin II, aldosterone and arginine vasopressin in hypotensive patients with chronic renal failure treated by dialysis. Clin Nephrol 26:288-296, 1986.

258. Jespersen B, et al: Reduced angiotensin II induced vascular reactivity in chronic renal failure. Scand J Clin Lab Invest 48:705-713, 1988.

259. Monteith GR, et al: Plasma membrane calcium pump-mediated calcium efflux and bulk cytosolic free calcium in cultured aortic smooth muscle cells from spontaneously hypertensive and Wistar-Kyoto normotensive rats. J Hypertens 14:435-442, 1996.

260. Haller H, et al: Intracellular actions of angiotensin II on vascular smooth muscle cells. J Am Soc Nephrol 10(suppl 11):S75-S83, 1999.

261. Lainchbury JG, et al: Adrenomedullin: A hypotensive hormone in man. Clin Sci 92:467-472, 1997.

262. Palla R, et al: Acute effects of calcitonin gene related peptide on renal haemodynamics and renin and angiotensin II secretion in patients with renal disease. Int J Tissue React 17:43-49, 1995.

263. Mallamaci F, et al: Plasma adrenomedullin during acute changes in intravascular volume in hemodialysis patients. Kidney Int 54:1697-1703, 1998.

264. Odar-Cederlof I, et al: Is neuropeptide Y a contributor to volume induced hypertension? Am J Kidney Dis 31:803-808, 1998.

265. Court JM, et al: Hypertension in childhood obesity. Aust Paediatr J 10:296-300, 1974.

266. Kannel WB, et al: The relation of adiposity to blood pressure and development of hypertension: The Framingham study. Ann Intern Med 67:48-49, 1976.

267. Stamler R, et al: Weight and blood pressure findings in hypertension screening of 1 million Americans. JAMA 240:1607-1610, 1978.

268. Rowe JW, et al: Effect of insulin and glucose infusions on sympathetic nervous system activity in normal man. Diabetes 30:219-225, 1981.

269. Sowers JR, et al: Role of the sympathetic nervous system in blood pressure maintenance in obesity. J Clin Endocrinol Metab 54: 1181-1186, 1982.

270. Daly PA, Landsberg L: Hypertension in obesity and NIDDM: Role of insulin and sympathetic nervous system. Diabetes Care 14:240-248, 1991.

271. Facchini FS, Stoohs RA, Reaven GM: Enhanced sympathetic nervous system activity. The linchpin between insulin resistance, hyperinsulinemia, and heart rate. Am J Hypertens 9:1013-1017, 1996.

272. Reaven GM, Lithell H, Landsberg L: Hypertension and associated metabolic abnormalities: The role of insulin resistance and the sympathoadrenal system. N Engl J Med , 334:374-381, 1996.

273. Izzo JL Jr, Swislocki ALM: Symposium on Insulin and Cardiovascular Disease: Workshop III. Insulin resistance: Is it truly the link? Am J Med 90(suppl 2A):26S-31S, 1991.

274. Jamerson K, et al: Vasoconstriction with norepinephrine causes less forearm insulin resistance than a sympathetic reflex vasoconstriction. Hypertension 23:1006-1011, 1994.

275. Rocchini AP, et al: Clonidine prevents insulin resistance and hypertension in obese dogs. Hypertension 32:592, 1998.

276. Ogihara T, et al: Angiotensin II-induced insulin resistance is associated with enhanced insulin signaling. Hypertension 40:872-879, 2002.

277. Fukuda N, et al: Troglitazone inhibits growth and improves insulin signaling by suppression of angiotensin II action in vascular smooth muscle cells from spontaneously hypertensive rats. Atherosclerosis 163:229-239, 2002.

278. Fliser D, et al: Insulin resistance and hyperinsulinemia are already present in patients with incipient renal disease. Kidney Int 53: 1343-1347, 1998.

279. Lee P, et al: The role of abdominal adiposity and insulin resistance in dyslipidemia of chronic renal failure. Am J Kidney Dis 29:54-65, 1997.

280. Eidemak I, et al: Insulin resistance and hyperinsulinaemia in mild to moderate progressive chronic renal failure and its association with aerobic work capacity. Diabetologia 38:565-572, 1995.

281. Kobayashi S, et al: Impact of dialysis therapy on insulin resistance in end-stage renal disease: Comparison of haemodialysis and continuous ambulatory peritoneal dialysis. Nephrol Dialysis Transplant 15:65-70, 2000.

282. Yoshida K, et al: Effects of troglitazone and temocapril in spontaneously hypertensive rats with chronic renal failure. J Hypertens 19:503-510, 2001.

283. Hu Q, et al: Hydrogen peroxide induces intracellular calcium oxillations in human aortic endothelial cells. Circulation 97:268-275, 1998.

284. Suzuki H, et al: In vivo evidence for microvascular oxidative stress in spontaneously hypertensive rats: Hydroethidine microfluorography. Hypertension 25:1083-1089, 1995.

285. Ortiz MC, et al: Antioxidants block angiotensin II-induced increases in blood pressure and endothelin. Hypertension 38:655-659, 2001.

286. Kerr S, et al: Superoxide anion production is increased in a model of genetic hypertension: Role of the endothelium. Hypertension 33: 1353-1358, 1999.

287. Lerman LO, et al: Increased oxidative stress in experimental renovascular hypertension. Hypertension 27:541-546, 2001.

288. Dobrian AD, Schriver SD, Prewitt RL: Role of angiotensin II and free radicals in blood pressure regulation in a rat model of renal hypertension. Hypertension 38:361-366, 2001.

289. Somers MJ, et al: Vascular superoxide production and vasomotor function in hypertension induced by deoxycorticosterone acetate-salt. Circulation 101:1722-1728, 2000.

290. Swei A, et al: A mechanism of oxygen free radicals production in the Dahl hypertensive rat. Microcirculation 6:179-187, 1999.

291. Vaziri ND, Liang K, Ding Y: Increased nitric oxide inactivation by reactive oxygen species in lead-induced hypertension. Kidney Int 56:1492-1498, 1999.

292. Vaziri ND, Oveisi F, Ding Y: Role of increased oxygen free radical activity in the pathogenesis of uremic hypertension. Kidney Int 53:1748-1754, 1998.

293. El Midaoui A, de Champlain J: Prevention of hypertension, insulin resistance, and oxidative stress by alpha-lipoic acid. Hypertension 39:303-307, 2002.

294. Chen J, et al: Serum antioxidant vitamins and blood pressure in the United States population. Hypertension 40:810-816, 2002.

295. Kim MK, et al: Lack of long-term effect of vitamin C supplementation on blood pressure. Hypertension 40:797-803, 2002.

296. Kostis JB, Wilson AC, Lacy CR: Hypertension and ascorbic acid. Lancet 355:1272, 2000.

297. Hajjar IM, et al: A randomized, double-blind, controlled trial of vitamin C in the management of hypertension and lipids. Am J Ther 9:289-293, 2002.

298. Duffy SJ, et al: Effect of ascorbic acid treatment on conduit vessel endothelial dysfunction in patients with hypertension. Am J Physiol Heart Circ Physiol 280:H528-H534, 2001.

299. Neunteufl T, et al: Additional benefit of vitamin E supplementation to simvastatin therapy on vasoreactivity of the brachial artery of hypercholesterolemic men. J Am Coll Cardiol 32:711-716, 1998.

300. Furchgott RF, Zawadski JV: The obligatory role of endothelial cells in the relaxation of arterial smooth muscle by acetylcholine. Nature 288:373-376, 1980.

301. Palmer RM, Ferrige AG, Moncada S: Nitric oxide release accounts for biological activity of endothelium derived relaxing factor. Nature 327:524-526, 1987.

302. Ignarro LJ, et al: Endothelium-derived relaxing factor produced and released from artery and vein is nitric oxide. Proc Natl Acad Sci U S A 84:9265-9269, 1987.

303. Ye S, Nosrati S, Campese VM: Nitric oxide (NO) modulates the neurogenic control of blood pressure in rats with chronic renal failure. J Clin Invest 99:540-548, 1997.

304. Ye S, et al: Losartan reduces central and peripheral sympathetic nerve activity in a rat model of neurogenic hypertension. Hypertension 39:1101-1116, 2002.

305. Vaziri ND, et al: Downregulation of nitric oxide synthase in chronic kidney insufficiency: Role of excess PTH. Am J Physiol Renal Physiol 274:F642-F649, 1998.

306. Hu LR, Manning RJ, Brands MW: Long-term cardiovascular role of nitric oxide in conscious rats. Hypertension 23:185-194, 1994.

307. Johnson RA, Freeman RH: Sustained hypertension in the rat induced by chronic blockade of nitric oxide production. Am J Hypertens 5: 919-922, 1992.

308. Baylis C, Mitruka B, Deng A: Chronic blockade of nitric oxide synthesis in the rat produces systemic hypertension and glomerular damage. J Clin Invest 90:278-281, 1992.

309. Vallance P, et al: Accumulation of an endogenous inhibitor of nitric oxide synthesis in chronic renal failure. Lancet 339:572-575, 1992.

310. Matsuoka H, et al: Asymmetrical imethylarginine, an endogenous nitric oxide synthase inhibitor, in experimental hypertension. Hypertension 29:242-247, 1997.

311. Fujiwara N, et al: Study on the relationship between plasma nitrite and nitrate level and salt sensitivity in human hypertension: Modulation of nitric oxide synthesis by salt intake. Circulation 101:856-861, 2000.

312. Cooke JP: Does ADMA cause endothelial dysfunction? Arterioscler Thromb Vasc Biol 20:2032-2037, 2000.

313. Kielstein JT, et al: Asymmetric dimethylarginine plasma concentrations differ in patients with end-stage renal disease: Relationship to treatment method and atherosclerotic disease. J Am Soc Nephrol 10:594-600, 1999.

314. Sander M, Hansen J, Victor RG: The sympathetic nervous system is involved in the maintenance but not initiation of the hypertension induced by N(omega)-nitro-L-arginine methyl ester. Hypertension 30:64-70, 1997.

315. Sakuma I, et al: N^G-methyl-L-arginine, an inhibitor of L-arginine-derived nitric oxide synthesis, stimulates renal sympathetic nerve activity. Circ Res 70:607-611, 1992.

316. Xu H, Fink GD, Galligan JJ: Nitric oxide-independent effects of tempol on sympathetic nerve activity and blood pressure in DOCA-salt rats. Am J Physiol Heart Circ Physiol 283:H885-H892, 2002.

317. Ballinger SW, et al: Hydrogen peroxide-and peroxynitrite-induced mitochondrial DNA damage and dysfunction in vascular endothelial and smooth muscle cells. Circ Res 86:960-966, 2000.

318. Mihm MJ, Jing L, Bauer JA: Nitrotyrosine causes selective vascular endothelial dysfunction and DNA damage. J Cardiovasc Pharmacol 36:182-187, 2000.

319. Eiserich JP, et al: Formation of nitric oxide-derived inflammatory oxidants by myeloperoxidase in neutrophils. Nature 391:393-397, 1998.

320. Eiserich JP, et al: Nitric oxide rapidly scavenges tyrosine and tryptophan radicals. Biochem J 310:745-749, 1995.

321. Vaziri ND, et al: Induction of oxidative stress by glutathione depletion causes hypertension in normal rats. Hypertension 36:142-146, 2000.

322. Vaziri ND, et al: Enhanced nitric oxide inactivation and protein nitration by reactive oxygen species in renal insufficiency. Hypertension 39:135-141, 2002.

323. Griendling KK, et al: Angiotensin II stimulates NADH and NADPH oxidase activity in cultured vascular smooth muscle cells. Circ Res 74:1141-1148, 1994.

324. Cai H, et al: NAD(P)H oxidase-derived hydrogen peroxide mediates endothelial nitric oxide production in response to angiotensin II. J Biol Chem 277:48311-48317, 2002.

325. Hornig B, et al: Comparative effect of ace inhibition and angiotensin II type 1 receptor antagonism on bioavailability of nitric oxide in patients with coronary artery disease: Role of superoxide dismutase. Circulation 103:799-805, 2001.

326. Rao GN, Berk BC: Active oxygen species stimulate vascular smooth muscle cell growth and proto-oncogene expression. Circ Res 70:593-599, 1992.

327. Rajagopalan S, et al: Reactive oxygen species produced by macrophage-derived foam cells regulate the activity of vascular matrix metalloproteinases in vitro. J Clin Invest 98:2572-2579, 1996.

328. Ushio-Fukai M, et al: P22phox is a critical component of the superoxide generating NADH·NADHP oxidase system and regulates angiotensin II-induced hypertrophy in vascular smooth muscle cells. J Biol Chem 271:23217-23321, 1996.

329. Ichiki T, et al: Downregulation of angiotensin II type 1 receptor gene transcription by nitric oxide. Hypertension 31:342-348, 1998.

330. Calapai G, et al: Effects of water deprivation and angiotensin II intracerebroventricular administration on brain nitric oxide synthase activity. Eur J Pharmacol 360:147-154, 1998.

331. Liu J-L, Murakami H, Zucker IH: Angiotensin II-nitric oxide interaction on sympathetic outflow in conscious rabbits. Circ Res 82:496-502, 1998.

332. Resnick LM: Calcium metabolism in hypertension and allied metabolic disorders. Diabetes Care 14:505-520, 1991.

333. Marone C, Beretta-Piccoli C, Weidmann P: Acute hypercalcemic hypertension in man: Role of hemodynamics, catecholamines and renin. Kidney Int 20:92-96, 1980.

334. Mak RH, Wong JH: The vitamin D/parathyroid hormone axis in the pathogenesis of hypertension and insulin resistance in uremia. Miner Electrolyte Metab 18:156-159, 1992.

335. Iseki K, Massry SG, Campese VM: Effects of hypercalcemia and PTH on blood pressure in normal and renal failure rats. Am J Physiol 250:F924-F929, 1986.

336. Raine AEG, et al: Hyperparathyroidism, platelet intracellular free calcium and hypertension in chronic renal failure. Kidney Int 43:700-705, 1993.

337. Petersen LJ, Rudnicki M, Hjsted J: Long-term oral calcium supplementation reduces diastolic blood pressure in end-stage renal disease: A randomized, double-blind, placebo controlled study. Int J Artif Org 17:37-40, 1994.

338. Ifudu O, et al: Parathyroidism does not correct hypertension in patients on maintenance hemodialysis. Am J Nephrol 18:28-34, 1998.

339. Erne P, et al: Correlation of platelet calcium with blood pressure. N Engl J Med 310:1084-1088, 1984.

340. Schiffl H: Correlation of blood pressure in end-stage renal disease with platelet cytosolic free-calcium concentration. Klin Wochenschr 68:718-722, 1990.

341. Zimlichman RR, et al: Vascular hypersensitivity to noradrenaline: A possible mechanism of hypertension in rats with chronic uremia. Clin Sci 67:161-166, 1984.

342. De Wardener HE, MacGregor GA: Dahl's hypothesis that a saluretic substance may be responsible for a sustained rise in arterial pressure: Its possible role in essential hypertension. Kidney Int 18:1-9, 1980.

343. Hamlyn JM, et al: A circulating inhibitor of $(Na^+ + K^+)$ATPase associated with essential hypertension. Nature 300:650-652, 1982.

344. Blaustein MP, et al: Sodium/calcium exchange in vascular smooth muscle: A link between sodium metabolism and hypertension. Ann N Y Acad Sci 488:199-216, 1986.

345. Tobian LJ, Binion JT: Tissue cations and water in arterial hypertension. Circulation 5:754-758, 1952.

346. Boero R, Guarena C, Berto IM: Pathogenesis of arterial hypertension in chronic uremia: The role of reduced Na^+K^+-ATPase activity. J Hypertens 6(suppl 14):S363-S365, 1988.

347. Hamlyn JM, Hamilton BP, Manunta P: Endogenous ouabain, sodium balance and blood pressure: A review and a hypothesis. J Hypertens 14:151-167, 1996.

348. Philipp T, Distler A, Cordes U: Sympathetic nervous system and blood pressure control in essential hypertension. Lancet 2:959-963, 1978.

349. Kiowski W, van Brummelen P, Buhler FR: Plasma noradrenaline correlates with alpha-adrenoceptor-mediated vasoconstriction and blood pressure in patients with essential hypertension. Clin Sci 57:177S-180S, 1979.

350. Pratt JH: The interaction of norepinephrine excretion with blood pressure and race in children. J Hypertens 10:93-96, 1992.

351. Stepniakowski KT, et al: Fatty acids, not insulin, modulate alpha1-adrenergic reactivity in dorsal hand veins. Hypertension 30:1150-1155, 1997.

352. McGuire PG, et al: Increased deposition of basement membrane macromolecules in specific vessels of the spontaneously hypertensive rat. Am J Pathol 135:291-299, 1989.

353. Vanhoutte PM, et al: Modulation of vascular smooth muscle contraction by the endothelium. Ann Rev Physiol 48:307-320, 1986.

354. Luscher TF: Imbalance of endothelium-derived relaxing and contracting factors: A new concept in hypertension. Am J Hypertens 3:317-330, 1990.

355. Panza JA, et al: Abnormal endothelium-dependent vascular relaxation in patients with essential hypertension. N Engl J Med 323:22-27, 1990.

356. Li J, et al: Non-invasive detection of endothelial dysfunction in patients with essential hypertension. Int J Cardiol 61:165-169, 1997.

357. Sung BH, et al: Insulin-mediated venodilation is impaired in patients with high cholesterol. Hypertension 31:1266-1271, 1998.

358. Sung BH, et al: Vasodilatory effects of troglitazone improve blood pressure at rest and during mental stress in type 2 diabetes mellitus. Hypertension 34:83-88, 1999.

359. Rodriguez-Porcel M, et al: Combination of hypercholesterolemia and hypertension augments renal function abnormalities. Hypertension 37:774-780, 2001.

360. Stulak JM, et al: Impaired renal vascular endothelial function in vitro in experimental hypercholesterolemia. Atherosclerosis 154:195-201, 2001.

361. Stulak J, et al: Renal vascular function in hypercholesterolemia is preserved by chronic antioxidant supplementation. J Am Soc Nephrol 12:1882-1891, 2001.

362. Yanagisawa M, et al: A novel potent vasoconstrictor peptide produced by vascular endothelial cells. Nature 332:411-415, 1988.

363. Luscher TF, et al: Molecular and cellular biology of endothelin and its receptors. J Hypertens 11:7-11, 1993.

364. Clavell AL, Burnett JCJ: Physiologic and pathophysiologic roles of endothelin in the kidney. Curr Opinion Nephrol Hypertens 3:66-72, 1994.

365. Yokokawa K, et al: Heparin suppresses endothelin-1 action and production in spontaneously hypertensive rats. Am J Physiol 263:R1035-R0141, 1992.

366. Yokokawa K, et al: Heparin regulates endothelin production through endothelium-derived nitric oxide in human endothelial cells. J Clin Invest 92:2080-2085, 1993.

367. Schiffrin EL: Endothelin and endothelin antagonists in hypertension. J Hypertens 16:1891-1895, 1998.

368. Kohno M, et al: Prolonged blood pressure elevation after endothelin administration in bilaterally nephrectomized rats. Metabolism 38:712-713, 1989.

369. Predel HG, Meyer-Lehuert H: Plasma concentrations of endothelin in patients with abnormal vascular reactivity: Effects of ergometric exercise of acute saline loading. Life Sci 47:1837-1843, 1990.

370. Saito Y, et al: Increased plasma endothelin level in patients with essential hypertension. N Engl J Med 322:205, 1990.

371. Schiffrin EL, Thibault G: Plasma endothelin in human essetial hypertension. Am J Hypertens 4:303-308, 1991.

372. Yokokawa K, et al: Hypertension associated with endothelin-secreting malignant hemangioendothelioma. Ann Intern Med 114:213-215, 1991.

373. McMahon EG, Palomo MA, Moore WM: Phosphoramidon blocks the pressor activity of big endothelin (1-39) and lowers blood pressure in spontaneously hypertensive rats. J Cardiovasc Pharmacol 17(suppl 7):529-533, 1991.

374. Krum H, et al: The effect of an endothelin-receptor antagonist, bosentan, on blood pressure in patients with essential hypertension: Bosentan Hypertension Investigators. N Engl J Med 338:784-790, 1998.

375. Schiffrin EL: Role of endothelin-1 in hypertension and vascular disease. Am J Hypertens 14:83S-89S, 2001.

376. Koyama H, et al: Plasma endothelin levels in patients with uremia. Lancet 1:991-992, 1989.

377. Shichiri M, et al: Plasma endothelin levels in hypertension and chronic renal failure. Hypertension 15:493-496, 1990.

378. Suzuki N, et al: Endothelin-3 concentrations in human plasma: The increased concentrations in patients undergoing hemodialysis. Biochem Biophys Res Commun 169:809-815, 1990.

379. Miyauchi T, et al: Plasma concentrations of endothelin-1 and endothelin-3 are altered differently in various pathophysiological conditions in humans. J Cardiovasc Pharmacol 17(suppl 7):S394-S397, 1991.

380. Lebel M, et al: Plasma endothelin levels and blood pressure in hemodialysis and in CAPD patients: Effect of subcutaneous erythropoietin replacement therapy. Clin Exp Hypertens 16:565-575, 1994.

381. Warrens AN, et al: Endothelin in renal failure. Nephrol Dial Transplant 5:418-422, 1990.

382. Moncada S, et al: Differential formation of prostacyclin (PGX or PGI2) by layers of the arterial wall: An explanation for the anti-thrombotic properties of vascular endothelium. Thromb Res 11:323-344, 1977.

383. Radomski MW, Palmer RMJ, Moncada S: The anti-aggregating properties of vascular endothelium interaction between nitric oxide and prostacyclin. Br J Pharmacol 92:639-646, 1987.

384. Shimokawa H, et al: Prostacyclin releases EDRF and potentiates its action in the coronary arteries of the pig. Br J Pharmacol 95:1197-1203, 1988.

385. Dedier J, et al: Nonnarcotic analgesic use and the risk of hypertension in US women. Hypertension 40:604-608, 2002.

386. Kato T, et al: Prostaglandin H2 may be the EDCF released by acetylcholine in the aorta of the rat. Hypertension 15:475-481, 1990.

387. Harris RC, et al: Mediation of renal vascular effects of epidermal growth factor by arachidonate metabolites. FASEB J 4:1654-1660, 1990.

388. Feketou M, Vanhoutte PM: Endothelium-dependent hyperpolarization of canine coronary smooth muscle. Br J Pharmacol 93:515-524, 1988.

389. Campbell WB, Gauthier KM: What is new in endothelium-derived hyperpolarizing factors. Curr Opin Nephrol Hypertens 11:177-183, 2002.

390. Folkow B: Cardiovascular structural adaptation: Its role in the initiation and maintenance of primary hypertension. Clin Sci Mol Med 55:3S-22S, 1978.

391. Folkow B: "Structural factor" in primary and secondary hypertension. Hypertension 16:89-101, 1990.

392. Parker SB, Wade SS, Prewitt RL: Pressure mediates angiotensin II-induced arterial hypertrophy and PDGF-A expression. Hypertension 32:452-485, 1998.

393. Cottone S, et al: Influence of vascular load on plasma endothelin-1, cytokines and catecholamine levels in essential hypertensives. Blood Press 7:144-148, 1998.

394. Barton M, et al: ET(A) receptor blockade prevents increased tissue endothelin-1, vascular hypertrophy, and endothelial dysfunction in salt-sensitive hypertension. Hypertension 81:499-504, 1998.

395. Zafari AM, et al: Role of NADH/NADPH oxidase-derived H_2O_2 in angiotensin II-induced vascular hypertrophy. Hypertension 32:488-495, 1998.

396. Thybo NK, et al: Effect of antihypertensive treatment on small arteries of patients with previously untreated essential hypertension. Hypertension 25:474-481, 1995.

397. Johnson RJ, et al: Subtle acquired renal injury as a mechanism of salt-sensitive hypertension. N Engl J Med 346:913-923, 2002.

398. Pessina AC, Casiglia E, Dal Palu C: Aging, hypertension, and renal damage: Generalities and results of the Cardiovascular Study in the Elderly. Am J Kidney Dis 21(5 suppl 2):10-14, 1993.

399. Johnson RJ, et al: Tubulointerstitial injury and loss of nitric oxide synthases parallel the development of hypertension in the Dahl-SS rat. J Hypertens18:1497-1505, 2000.

400. Johnson RJ, et al: Renal injury and salt-sensitive hypertension after exposure to catecholamines. Hypertension 34:151-159, 1999.

401. Thomas SE, et al: Tubulointerstitial disease in aging: Evidence for underlying peritubular capillary damage, a potential role for renal ischemia. J Am Soc Nephrol 9:231-242, 1998.

402. Johnson RJ, et al: Renal injury and salt-sensitive hypertension after exposure to catecholamines. Hypertension 34:134-138, 1999.

403. Johnson RJ, et al: Renal injury from angiotensin II-mediated hypertension. Hypertension 19:464-474, 1992.

404. Gaedeke J, et al: Angiotensin II, TGF-beta and renal fibrosis. Contrib Nephrol 135:153-160, 2001.

405. Coleman TG, et al: Regulation of arterial pressure in the anephric state. Circulation 42:509-514, 1970.

406. Coleman TG, Guyton AC: Hypertension caused by salt loading in the dog: III. Onset transients of cardiac output and other variables. Circ Res 25:153-160, 1969.

407. Hall JE, et al: Long-term regulation of arterial pressure, glomerular filtration and renal sodium reabsorption by angiotensin II in dogs. Clin Sci, 59:87S-90S, 1980.

408. Messerli FH, et al: Essential hypertension in black and white subjects: Hemodynamic findings and fluid volume state. Am J Med 67:27-31, 1979.

409. Messerli FH, et al: Essential hypertension in the elderly: Haemodynamics, intravascular volume, plasma renin activity, and circulating catecholamine levels. Lancet 2:983-986, 1983.

410. Messerli FH: The heterogeneity of essential hypertension: Hemodynamic aspects. Am Heart J 116:590-593, 1988.

411. Messerli FH, et al: Obesity and essential hypertension: Hemodynamics, intravascular volume, sodium excretion, and plasma renin activity. Arch Intern Med 141:81-85, 1981.

412. Ritz E, Koomans HA: New insights into mechanisms of blood pressure regulation in patients with uraemia. Nephrol Dial Transplant 11(suppl 2):52-59, 1996.

413. Allen K, Shykoff BE, Izzo JL Jr: Pet ownership, but not ACE inhibitor therapy, blunts home blood pressure responses to mental stress. Hypertension 38:815-820, 2001.

414. DiBona GF: Role of the renal nerves in hypertension. Semin Nephrol 11:503-511, 1991.

415. Kapusta DR, et al: Selective central alpha-2 adrenoceptor control of regional haemodynamic responses to air jet stress in conscious spontaneously hypertensive rats. J Hypertens 7:189-194, 1989.

416. DiBona GF: Stress and sodium intake in neural control of renal function in hypertension. Hypertension 17(4 suppl):III3-III6, 1991.

417. DiBona GF, Sawin LL: Role of renal nerves in sodium retention of cirrhosis and congestive heart failure. Am J Physiol 260:R298-R305, 1991.

418. DiBona GF, Jones SY: Acute environmental stress overrides cardiac volume receptor reflex in borderline hypertensive rats. J Hypertens 13:63-68, 1995.

419. DiBona GF, Jones SY, Sawin LL: Reflex effects on renal nerve activity characteristics in spontaneously hypertensive rats. Hypertension 30:1089-1096, 1997.

420. Hollenberg NK, Williams GH, Adams DF: Essential hypertension: Abnormal renal vascular and endocrine responses to a mild psychological stimulus. Hypertension 3:11-17, 1981.

421. Wagner HNJ: The influence of autonomic vasoregulatory reflexes on the rate of sodium and water excretion in man. J Clin Invest 36:1319-1327, 1957.

422. Kamm DE, Levinsky NG: The mechanism of denervation natriuresis. J Clin Invest 44:93, 1965.

423. Gill JRJ, Bartter FC: Adrenergic nervous system in sodium metabolism: II. Effects of guanethidine on the renal response to sodium deprivation in normal man. N Engl J Med 275:1466-1471, 1966.

424. Suzuki M, et al: Association of insulin resistance with salt sensitivity and nocturnal fall of blood pressure. Hypertension 35:864-868, 2000.

425. Levinson PD, Iosiphidis AH, Gann DS: Hormone and catecholamine responses accompanying the antinatriuresis of glucose ingestion. Am J Hypertens 2:178-181, 1989.

426. Friedberg CE, et al: Sodium retention by insulin may depend on decreased plasma potassium. Metab Clin Exp 40:201-204, 1991.

427. Feraille E, et al: Sites of antinatriuretic action of insulin along rat nephron. Am J Physiol 263:F175-F179, 1992.

428. Ito O, et al: Tyrosine kinase, phosphatidylinositol 3-kinase, and protein kinase C regulate insulin-stimulated NaCl absorption in the thick ascending limb. Kidney Int 51:1037-1041, 1997.

429. Hall JE, et al: Chronic intrarenal hyperinsulinemia does not cause hypertension. Am J Physiol 260:F663-F669, 1991.

430. Gans RO, et al: Acute hyperinsulinemia induces sodium retention and a blood pressure decline in diabetes mellitus. Hypertension 20:199-209, 1992.

431. Brands MW, et al: Insulin-induced hypertension in rats depends on an intact renin-angiotensin system. Hypertension 29:1014-1019, 1997.

432. Shimamoto K, et al: Insulin sensitivity and the effects of insulin on renal sodium handling and pressor systems in essential hypertensive patients. Hypertension 23(1 suppl):I29-I33, 1994.

433. ter Maaten JC, et al: Renal sodium handling and haemodynamics are equally affected by hyperinsulinaemia in salt-sensitive and salt-resistant hypertensives. J Hypertens 19:1633-1641, 2001.

434. Trevisan R, et al: Enhanced responsiveness of blood pressure to sodium intake and to angiotensin II is associated with insulin resistance in IDDM patients. Diabetes 48:1347-1353, 1998.

435. Rocchini AP: Obesity hypertension, salt sensitivity and insulin resistance. Nutr Metab Cardiovasc Dis 10:287-294, 2000.

436. Grant FD, et al: Low-renin hypertension, altered sodium homeostasis, and an alpha-adducin polymorphism. Hypertension 39:191-196, 2002.

437. Raji A, et al: Insulin resistance in hypertensives: Effect of salt sensitivity, renin status and salt intake. J Hypertens 19:99-105, 2001.

438. Laffer CL, et al: Differential regulation of natriuresis by 20-hydroxyeicosatetraenoic acid in human salt-sensitive versus salt-resistant hypertension. Circulation 107:574-578, 2003.

439. Salazar FJ, et al: Salt-induced increase in arterial pressure during nitric oxide synthesis inhibition. Hypertension 22:49-55, 1993.

440. Garcia-Estan J, et al: Chronic effects of nitric oxide and prostaglandin inhibition on pressure diuresis and natriuresis in rats. Kidney Int Suppl 55:S141-S143, 1996.

441. Villa E, Garcia-Robles R, Romero JC: Effects of hyperinsulinemia on the regulation of regional blood flow and blood pressure in anesthetized dogs: Hemodynamic role of nitric oxide. Am J Hypertens 11:1232-1238, 1998.

442. Chen PY, Sanders PW: L-Arginine abrogates salt-sensitive hypertension in Dahl/Rapp rats. J Clin Invest 88:1559-1567, 1991.

443. Raij L: Nitric oxide, salt sensitivity, and cardiorenal injury in hypertension. Semin Nephrol 19:296-303, 1999.

444. Fagugli RM, et al: Short daily hemodialysis: Blood pressure control and left ventricular mass reduction in hypertensive hemodialysis patients. Am J Kidney Dis 38:371-376, 2001.

445. Kooistra MP, et al: Daily home hemodiaysis in the Netherlands: Effects on metabolic control, haemodynamics, and quality of life. Nephrol Dial Transplant 13:2853-2860, 1998.

446. Taeger J, et al: Daily versus standard hemodialysis: One year experience. Artif Organs 22:558-563, 1998.

447. Rahman M, et al: Interdialytic weight gain, compliance with dialysis regimen, and age are independent predictors of blood pressure in hemodialysis patients. Am J Kidney Dis 35:257-265, 2000.

448. Zucchelli P, Santoro A: Dry weight in hemodialysis: Volemic control. Semin Nephrol 21:286-290, 2001.

449. Schalekamp MADH, et al: Interrelationships between blood pressure, renin, renin substrate and blood volume in terminal renal failure. Clin Sci Mol Med 45:417-428, 1973.

450. Schultze G, Prefke S, Malzahn M: Blood pressure in terminal renal failure: Fluid spaces and renin-angiotensin system. Nephron 25:15-24, 1980.

451. Horl MP, Horl WH: Hemodialysis-associated hypertension: Pathophysiology and therapy. Am J Kidney Dis 39:227-244, 2002.

452. Chazot C, et al: Interdialysis blood pressure control by long haemodialysis sessions. Nephrol Dial Transplant 10:831-837, 1995.

453. Katzarski KS, et al: Fluid state and blood pressure control in patients treated with long and short haemodialysis. Nephrol Dial Transplant 14:369-376, 1999.

454. Griffin MR, Yared A, Ray WA: Nonsteroidal antiinflammatory drugs and acute renal failure in elderly persons. Am J Epidemiol 151:488-496, 2000.

455. Ailabouni W, Eknoyan G: Nonsteroidal anti-inflammatory drugs and acute renal failure in the elderly: A risk-benefit assessment. Drugs Aging 9:341-351, 1996.

456. Alam S, Purdie DM, Johnson AG: Evaluation of the potential interaction between NaCl and prostaglandin inhibition in elderly individuals with isolated systolic hypertension. J Hypertens 17:1195-1202, 1999.

457. Raine AEG: Hypertension, blood viscosity, and cardiovascular morbidity in renal failure: Implications of erythropoietin therapy. Lancet 1:97-100, 1988.

458. Garcia DL, et al: Anemia lessens and its prevention worsens glomerular injury and hypertension in rats with reduced renal mass. Proc Natl Acad Sci U S A 85:6142-6146, 1988.

459. Coleman TG: Hemodynamics of uremic anemia. Circulation 45:510-511, 1972.

460. Letcher RL, et al: Direct relationship between blood pressure and blood viscosity in normal and hypertensive subjects: Role of fibrinogen and concentration. Am J Med 70:1195-1202, 1981.

461. Myers BD, et al: Dynamics of glomerular ultrafiltration in the rat: VIII. Effects of hematocrit. Circ Res 36:425-435, 1975.

462. Simpson LO: Blood viscosity induced proteinuria. Nephron 36:280-281, 1984.

463. Spear GS: The glomerulus in cyanotic congenital heart disease and primary pulmonary hypertension: A review. Nephron 1:238-248, 1964.

464. Eschbach JW, et al: Treatment of anemia of progressive renal failure wuth recombinant human erythropoietin. N Engl J Med 321:158-163, 1989.

465. Poux JM, et al: Uraemia is necessary for erythropoietin-induced hypertension in rats. Clin Exp Pharmacol Physiol 22:769-771, 1995.

466. Adamson JW, Eschbach JW: Treatment of anemia of chronic renal failure with recombinant human erythropoietin. Annu Rev Med 41:349-360, 1990.

467. Eschbach JW, et al: Recombinant human erythropoietin in anemic patients with end-stage renal disease: Results of a Phase III multicenter clinical trial. Ann Intern Med 111:992-1000, 1989.

468. Steffen HM, et al: Peripheral hemodynamics, blood viscosity, and the renin-angiotensin system in hemodialysis patients under therapy with recombinant human erythropoietin. Contrib Nephrol 76:292-298, 1989.

469. Vaziri ND: Mechanism of erythropoietin-induced hypertension. Am J Kidney Dis 33:821-828, 1999.

470. Yamakado M, et al: Mechanisms of hypertension induced by erythropoietin in patients on hemodialysis. Clin Invest Med 14:623-629, 1991.

471. Hand MF, et al: Erythropoietin enhances vascular responsiveness to norepinephrine in renal failure. Kidney Int 48:806-813, 1995.

472. Vaziri ND, et al: In vivo and in vitro pressor effects of erythropoietin in rats. Am J Physiol 269:F838-F845, 1995.

473. Eggena P, et al: Influence of recombinant human erythtropoietin on blood pressure and tissue renin-angiotensin systems. Am J Physiol 261:E642-E646, 1991.

474. van Geet C, et al: Recombinant human erythropoietin increases blood pressure, platelet aggregability and platelet free calcium mobilization in uremic children: A possible link? Thromb Haemost 64:7-10, 1990.

475. Neusser M, Tepel M, Zidek W: Erythropoietin increases cytosolic free calcium concentration in vascular smooth muscle cells. Cardiovasc Res 27:1233-1236, 1993.

476. Mysliwiec J, et al: The effect of tacrolimus (FK506) and cyclosporin A (Cya) on peripheral serotonergic mechanisms in uremic rats. Thromb Res 83:175-181, 1996.

477. Carlini R, Obialo CI, Rothstein M: Intravenous erythropoietin administration increases plasma endothelin and blood pressure in hemodialysis. Am J Hypertens 6:103-107, 1993.

478. del Castillo D, et al: The pressor effect of recombinant human erythropoietin is not due to decreased activity of the endogenous nitric oxide system. Nephrol Dial Transplant 10:505-508, 1995.

479. Morgan BJ, et al: Cyclosporine causes sympathetically mediated elevations in arterial pressure in rats. Hypertension 18:458-466, 1991.

480. Zhang W, et al: Cyclosporine A-induced hypertension involves synapse in renal sensory nerve endings. Proc Natl Acad Sci U S A 97:9765-9770, 2000.

481. Moss NG, Powell SL, Falk RJ: Intravenous cyclosporine activates afferent and efferent renal nerves and causes sodium retention in innervated kidneys in rats. Proc Natl Acad Sci U S A 82:8222-8226, 1985.

482. Zhang W, Victor RG: Calcineurin inhibitors cause renal afferent activation in rats: A novel mechanism of cyclosporine-induced hypertension. Hypertension 13:999-1004, 2000.

483. Lassila M: Interaction of cyclosporine A and the renin-angiotensin system: New perspectives. Curr Drug Metab 3:61-71, 2002.

484. Vannini SD, et al: Permanently reduced plasma ionized magnesium among renal transplant recipients on cyclosporine. Transplant Int 12:244-249, 1999.

485. Chobanian AV, et al: Seventh report of the Joint National Committee on Prevention, Detection, Evaluation, and Treatment of High Blood Pressure: The JNC VII Report. JAMA 289:2560-2572, 2003.

486. Klahr S, et al: The effects of dietary protein restriction and blood-pressure control on the progression of chronic renal disease: Modification of Diet in Renal Disease Study Group. N Engl J Med 330:877-884, 1994.

487. Bakris GL, et al: Preserving renal function in adults with hypertension and diabetes: A consensus approach. National Kidney Foundation Hypertension and Diabetes Executive Committees Working Group. Am J Kidney Dis 36:646-661, 2000.

488. Lewis EJ, et al: The effect of angiotensin-converting-enzyme inhibition on diabetic nephropathy. N Engl J Med 329:1456-1462, 1993.

489. Gisen G: Randomised placebo-controlled trial of effect of ramipril on decline in glomerular filtration rate and risk of terminal renal failure in proteinuric, non-diabetic nephropathy: The REIN Trial. Lancet 349:1857-1863, 1997.

490. Brenner BM, et al: Effects of losartan on renal and cardiovascular outcomes in patients with type 2 diabetes and nephropathy. N Engl J Med 345:861-869, 2001.

491. Lewis EJ, et al: Renoprotective effect of the angiotensin-receptor antagonist irbesartan in patients with nephropathy due to type 2 diabetes. N Engl J Med 345:851-860, 2001.

492. Parving HH, et al: Irbesartan in Patients with Type 2 Diabetes and Microalbuminuria Study Group: The effect of irbesartan on the development of diabetic nephropathy in patients with type 2 diabetes. N Engl J Med 345:870-878, 2001.

493. Wright JT Jr, et al: Effect of blood pressure lowering and antihypertensive drug class on progression of hypertensive kidney disease: Results from the AASK trial [Comment]. JAMA 288:2421-2431, 2002.

494. Health Care Financing Administration: Highlights from the 1996 Core Indicators Project for hemodialysis patients. Dial Transplant 26:188-191, 1997.

495. 1995 Update of the working group reports on chronic renal failure and renovascular hypertension. National High Blood Pressure Education Program Working Group. Arch Intern Med 156:2938-1947, 1996.

496. Foley RN, et al: Impact of hypertension on cardiomyopathy, morbidity and mortality in end-stage renal disease. Kidney Int 49:1379-1385, 1996.

497. Cirit M, et al: Paradoxical rise in blood presure during ultrafiltration in dialysis patients. Nephrol Dial Transplant 10:1417-1420, 1995.

498. Grassi G, et al: Cardiopulmonary receptor modulation of plasma renin activity in normotensive and hypertensive subjects. Hypertension 11:92-99, 1988.

499. Abboud FM, et al: Carotid and cardiopulmonary baroreceptor control of splanchnic and forearm vascular resistance during venous pooling in man. J Physiol 286:173-184, 1979.

500. Julius S, et al: Cardiopulmonary mechanoreceptors and renin release in humans. Fed Proc 42:2703-2708, 1983.

501. Mancia G, Grassi G, Giannattasio C: Cardiopulmonary receptor reflex in hypertension. Am J Hypertens 1:249-255, 1988.

502. Mohanty PK, et al: Reflex vasoconstrictor responses to cardiopulmonary baroreceptor unloading, head-up tilt, and cold pressor testing in elderly mild- to-moderate hypertensives: Effect of clonidine. J Cardiovasc Pharmacol 10:135-137, 1987.

CHAPTER 48

Pathophysiology of Uremia

James L. Bailey and William E. Mitch

The search for the cellular mechanisms causing uremic symptoms continues, as no single factor has been isolated and proved to affect the function of multiple organs. P.A. Piorry coined the word urémie in 1847 to indicate problems caused by "contaminating the blood with urine".[1, 2] It is axiomatic that the basic abnormality is the presence of waste products that are not being eliminated by the kidney, but not all patients with renal failure are uremic. This is true because the ultimate source of most uremic toxins is dietary protein.[3, 4] Consequently, excessive dietary protein will induce uremia in patients with only modestly reduced renal function, and uremic symptoms are relieved when dietary protein is restricted (see Chapter 57). Normal adults can eat very large amounts of protein and even maintain high blood urea nitrogen (BUN) values with little or no symptoms.[5] Observations of such patients illustrate the complexity of determining which of the several substances disturb cellular metabolism and affect functions that are basic to many different cell types. Unfortunately, uremia is not studied easily using in vitro strategies because there is involvement of many organs yielding a constellation of symptoms (Table 48-1). Nevertheless, the central nervous system manifestations of uremia are reminiscent of intoxication, a strong argument in favor of considering uremia as a state of systemic intoxication.

UREMIC TOXINS

Toxins are defined as poisonous substances that are released as byproducts of the metabolic activities of a living organism. Such substances are produced by gastrointestinal bacteria.[6] In nephrology, however, the term "toxin" has a different connotation and is used to encompass all compounds that accumulate and cause metabolic abnormalities in patients with kidney disease. The strongest argument that unexcreted substances are uremic toxins rests on the prompt abatement of symptoms following institution of effective dialysis and its removal of low-molecular-weight substances. Based on these findings, Bergstrom proposed that a uremic toxin should satisfy the following criteria: (1) the chemical identity of the compound and its quantity in biologic fluids should be known; (2) its concentration in tissue or plasma from uremic patients should exceed that present in nonuremic subjects; (3) its concentration should correlate with specific uremic symptoms, and the symptom or symptoms should disappear when the concentration is reduced to normal; and (4) toxicity of the compound in tissue, cells, or a test system should be demonstrated at the concentration found in tissue or fluids from uremic patients.[7] These criteria have seldom been met, for several reasons. First, accurate quantitation of a compound in a fluid as chemically complex as plasma often requires accurate separation techniques.[8] Second, many nitrogen-containing compounds accumulate in renal failure, and the rate of accumulation of these substances, as well as the severity of symptoms, varies with dietary protein intake, suggesting that one or more toxins are derived from the metabolic products of protein. This is one explanation for the finding that adherence to a low-protein diet ameliorates many of these symptoms. However, the list of potential toxins is not confined to the products of the catabolism of dietary or endogenous protein. Some toxins result from bacterial metabolism, engendered by bacterial overgrowth in the intestines of patients with chronic renal failure (CRF).[9] Although there are aspects of the uremic syndrome that can be reproduced in experimental animals by administering an alleged toxin to the animal or adding it to an in vitro system (e.g., cerebral cortical slices or lymphocytes) to elicit specific metabolic responses, the metabolic change is often difficult to ascribe to a specific biochemical pathway. To complicate matters, combinations of compounds (e.g., urea, magnesium, acetoin, 2,3-butylene-glycol, sulfate, creatinine, T-cresol, and guanidine) impair oxidative metabolism in slices of cerebral cortex, but when studied separately each agent at the same concentration alone is nontoxic.[10] This makes it impossible to identify a specific toxin by correlating the severity of symptoms with the level of any one toxin. Third, compounds can be created through nonenzymatic modification of proteins. For example, carbamylation of hemoglobin

TABLE 48-1

Manifestations of the Uremic Syndrome

Neurologic

Central

   Daytime drowsiness and a tendency to sleep, which progresses to
      increasing obtundation and, eventually, coma
   Decreased attentiveness and performance of cognitive tasks
   Imprecise memory
   Slurred speech
   Asterixis and myoclonus
   Seizures
   Disorientation and confusion

Peripheral

   Sensorimotor peripheral neuropathy, often with burning dysesthesia
   Singultus (hiccup)
   Restless leg syndrome
   Increased muscle fatigability and muscle cramps

Cardiovascular

Accelerated atherosclerosis
Cardiomyopathy
Pericarditis

Pulmonary

Atypical pulmonary edema
Pneumonitis
Fibrinous pleurisy

Gastrointestinal

Anorexia progressing to nausea and vomiting
Stomatitis and gingivitis
Parotitis
Peptic ulcer diathesis
Gastritis and duodenitis
Enterocolitis
Pancreatitis
Ascites

Dermatologic

Pruritus
Dystrophic calcification
Changes in skin pigmentation

Hematologic

Anemia
Altered neutrophilic chemotaxis
Depressed lymphocyte function
Bleeding diathesis with platelet dysfunction

Endocrinologic

Secondary hyperparathyrodism
Carbohydrate intolerance due to insulin resistance
Type IV hyperlipidemia
Altered peripheral thyroxine metabolism
Testicular atrophy
Ovarian dysfunction with amenorrhea, dysmenorrhea, dysfunctional
   uterine bleeding, cystic ovarian disease

Ophthalmic

Conjunctival or corneal calcifications

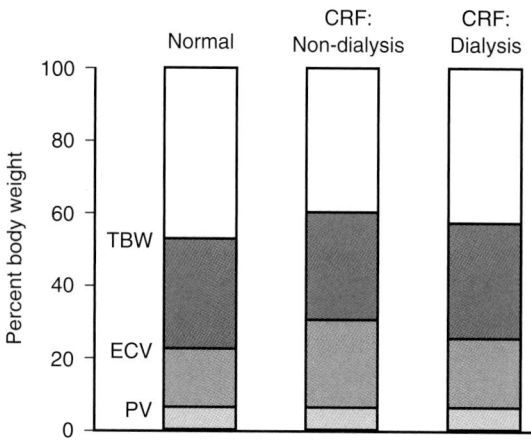

FIGURE 48-1. Diagrammatic representation of the distribution of body water as a percentage of body weight in normal subjects and in patients with chronic renal failure (CRF) not receiving dialysis or those receiving dialysis. Among patients not receiving dialysis, intracellular fluid volume (*dark shaded area*, calculated from the difference between total body water (TBW) and extracellular fluid volume) remains normal, yet there is an increase in the extracellular fluid volume (ECV) because of increases in the fluid volume (PV, *light blue area*) and more especially in the interstitial fluid volume (*medium blue area*). These apparent abnormalities in body water distribution are diminished in patients receiving regular dialysis. (From Mitch WE, Wilcox CS: Disorders of body fluids, sodium, and potassium in chronic renal failure. Am J Med 72:536, 1982.)

metabolism or provoking hormonal responses. Evidence for the latter will be discussed in the context of the "tradeoff hypothesis."

Considering the critical role of the kidney in regulating water balance, it is surprising that water intoxication is not more prevalent in patients with CRF.[14] When kidney function is rapidly lost, as in acute renal failure (ARF), hyponatremia frequently occurs, and water intoxication can mimic or exacerbate the central nervous system symptoms of uremia.[15] Besides water excess, a positive Na^+ balance aggravates hypertension and can cause pulmonary edema; the latter may be the major factor in the "pneumonitis" of uremia. Fortunately, the enormous reserve capacity of the damaged kidney generally maintains neutral Na^+ and water balance, even in advanced cases of renal insufficiency (Fig. 48-1).[14]

Metabolic Acidosis

Acidosis describes an abnormal state of reduced alkalinity of the blood and body tissues and fits most closely the definition of a uremic toxin.[7, 16] It generally accompanies uremia because the damaged kidney cannot sufficiently augment renal ammoniagenesis.[17] Reduced alkalinity of the blood and body tissues results. Acidosis also causes well-defined syndromes; in normal adults, acidosis can cause nausea, vomiting, anorexia, fatigue, exercise intolerance, and alterations in mental status.[18] It exacerbates renal osteodystrophy by accelerating skeletal mineral loss[19, 20] and contributes to the glucose intolerance of uremia by causing insulin resistance.[21]

Studies in rats established that metabolic acidosis also induces changes in nitrogen metabolism. These changes are important because they can cause loss of muscle mass and

or amino acids occurs in CRF patients at high serum levels of BUN.[11, 12] Likewise, Maillard reaction–mediated molecular damage to the extracellular matrix and other tissue proteins has been reported in uremia, perhaps as a consequence of accelerated oxidative injury.[13]

Electrolytes

Certain features of uremia can be related to the accumulation or depletion of inorganic ions, directly impairing cell can block the adaptive responses that are activated to maintain protein stores, including suppression of the breakdown of essential amino acids and protein (see Chapter 20). In skeletal muscle, the specific metabolic abnormalities induced by metabolic acidosis have been defined. Experimentally, acidosis stimulates the catabolism of essential amino acids in muscle by increasing branched-chain amino acid oxidation,[22] and accelerates protein catabolism.[23-25] Acidosis increases the activity of the enzyme branched-chain ketoacid dehydrogenase (BCKAD), which irreversibly degrades the essential branched-chain amino acids; the maximal activity of this enzyme is increased, as are the levels of messenger RNAs (mRNAs) encoding subunits of BCKAD.[26, 27] The implication of the latter is that acidosis increases the quantity of BCKAD, when actually, there is a greater fraction of the enzyme in its activated, dephosphorylated form in muscle. Presumably, the amount of the enzyme is not increased because there is accelerated breakdown of the BCKAD proteins in muscle.[23] Likewise, in chronically uremic rats with acidosis, rates of branched-chain amino acid oxidation are increased in muscle, and the levels of the corresponding branched-chain amino acids in plasma and in cellular water of muscle are lower, especially valine.[28] This is of interest because Bergstrom and colleagues[29] reported that the free valine concentration in muscle biopsies from dialysis patients is directly correlated with the predialysis bicarbonate. Moreover, they showed that the low levels of free isoleucine, leucine, and valine in muscle biopsies from acidotic hemodialysis patients were significantly increased by correcting the metabolic acidosis with sodium bicarbonate.[30]

Regarding protein degradation in muscle, induction of metabolic acidosis in rats fed ammonium chloride stimulates protein degradation.[23, 25, 31, 32] Similarly, acidosis-induced catabolism is also present in uremia; in uremic rats with metabolic acidosis, the rate of protein degradation in muscles is high but returns to control levels by feeding sodium bicarbonate.[24, 33]

Acceleration of the catabolism of essential amino acids and protein impairs the ability of the organism to adapt to dietary protein restriction and maintain neutral nitrogen balance (see Chapter 57). The consequences of metabolic acidosis, which include the stimulation of the activity of BCKAD and the degradation of protein, counteract the adaptive responses to dietary protein restriction and blunt the ability to achieve neutral nitrogen balance (i.e., the ability to reduce protein loss and suppress degradation of essential amino acids).[34, 35] From this formulation, it is not surprising that Papadoyannakis and Walls and their colleagues found improved nitrogen balance when chronically uremic, acidotic patients were treated with sodium bicarbonate.[36, 37]

Measuring the turnover of protein using the stochastic modeling technique and L-[^{13}C]leucine in humans has confirmed the catabolic effects of metabolic acidosis. Both ammonium chloride–induced acidemia in normal adults and the acidemia of CRF cause accelerated turnover of whole-body proteins and stimulation of amino acid oxidation,[38, 39] and sodium bicarbonate treatment blocks these responses in CRF patients. Using another strategy, Stein and co-workers[40] randomized peritoneal dialysis patients with mild acidosis to a standard (35 mM) or a higher (40 mM) lactate concentration in the dialysate. After 1 year, patients treated with 40 mM lactate had gained 2 kg and had evidence of more muscle mass.

The mechanism involves a suppression of protein degradation due to elimination of metabolic acidosis in continuous ambulatory peritoneal dialysis (CAPD) patients.[41] Recently, Pickering and colleagues[42] identified the biochemical mechanism that suppressed protein degradation. They provided evidence that the elimination of acidosis in CAPD patients reduced the activity of the ubiquitin-proteasome proteolytic pathway (see later) in muscle. Protein catabolism is also increased in hemodialysis patients who exhibit similar protein catabolism in response to acidosis and this is blocked when acidosis is eliminated.[43] In summary, metabolic acidosis blocks the adaptive responses the body can enlist to preserve nitrogen balance. Correction of metabolic acidosis resolves this malady, thereby fulfilling the criteria that acidosis is a uremic toxin.[7]

Aspects of the cellular mechanisms involved in the degradation of protein have been elucidated. In CRF rats, steady-state levels of corticosterone production increase, but this alone is insufficient to accelerate protein degradation.[24, 44] Likewise, increased protein degradation in muscle from predialysis patients is increased and is directly correlated with the serum cortisol level and inversely with serum HCO_3^-.[45] In dialysis patients, high serum cortisol is correlated with a poor nutritional status and poor prognosis.[46] These results indicate a role for glucocorticoids in stimulating protein degradation.

The signals causing protein degradation are complex as results from cell culture and adrenalectomized rats show that both glucocorticoids and acidosis are necessary to stimulate protein breakdown in muscle cells.[44, 47] Moreover, how acid activates protein breakdown is unknown. Although acidification of cultured kidney cells activates intracellular signaling pathways,[48] the hydrogen ion concentration in skeletal muscle of CRF rats is not significantly lower compared to normal rats, nor is the recovery of muscle pH from acidification different.[49] On the other hand, there is evidence that the activity of the Na^+/H^+ antiporter in thymocytes of CRF rats is impaired,[50] but whether this changes muscle metabolism is unknown.

Regarding the interaction between glucocorticoids and acidification, protein degradation in cultured myocytes is stimulated by acidification as long as glucocorticoids are available.[47] When adrenalectomized rats are made acidotic, muscle proteolysis is unchanged and does not increase unless the rats are given replacement doses of glucocorticoids.[23, 25] When adrenalectomized rats are given the same dose of glucocorticoids but are not acidotic, proteolysis is unchanged. There are parallel interactions among glucocorticoids, acidification, and the irreversible oxidation of branched-chain amino acids. Using cultured cells engineered to express or not express a glucocorticoid receptor, Wang and associates[51] showed that both acidification and glucocorticoids are required to stimulate BCKAD activity maximally. In adrenalectomized rats, both signals are required for stimulating branched-chain amino acid degradation.[25, 27]

What proteolytic pathway accounts for the acceleration in muscle protein degradation? There are four principal pathways: a lysosomal pathway; a calcium-activated system; an adenosine triphosphate (ATP)–dependent pathway involving ubiquitin; and an ATP-independent pathway. In response to metabolic acidosis, there is stimulation of the ATP-dependent, ubiquitin-proteasome proteolytic pathway in muscle.[32, 33] Inhibition of the three other pathways has little or no effect on accelerated protein degradation, but blocking the ATP-dependent pathway by depleting the muscle of ATP or using an inhibitor of the proteasome blocks the increase in muscle degradation.

This response is more complex than increasing flux through the ubiquitin-proteasome system; there also is a corresponding increase in mRNAs encoding various proteins required for protein degradation, just as there is increased BCKAD activity and higher levels of the mRNAs encoding components of BCKAD.[26, 32, 44] Specifically, muscle levels of mRNAs encoding ubiquitin and different subunits of the proteasome are increased. Ubiquitin, a protein present in all cells, is conjugated to cellular proteins that will be degraded and this targets them for degradation in the proteasome.[52] The higher levels of the mRNAs in turn are due to increased transcription of the respective genes.[33] This indicates that CRF initiates a program of protein degradation and these responses are blocked by correcting the metabolic acidosis (Fig. 48-2). These experimental results were duplicated in patients by Pickering and colleagues.[42] When they raised the serum HCO_3^- concentration of CAPD patients there was weight gain and an increase in the plasma levels of valine, leucine, and isoleucine, the branched-chain amino acids. There also was a decrease in the muscle levels of ubiquitin mRNA leading

to the conclusion that correction of serum HCO_3^- down-regulates branched-chain amino acid degradation and muscle proteolysis via the ubiquitin-proteasome pathway. Finally, acidosis also suppresses protein synthesis in muscle and in the liver (at least in the case of albumin), but this defect is not fully corrected by sodium bicarbonate.[24, 53, 54]

Besides metabolic acidosis, CRF causes insulin resistance,[55] and insulin is an important factor that suppresses protein degradation.[56, 57] Metabolic acidosis also causes insulin resistance.[21] Based on these findings, Mak[58] measured insulin sensitivity before and after 2 weeks of treatment with sodium bicarbonate tablets in hemodialysis patients and found significant increases in both venous blood pH and serum HCO_3^- levels. Moreover, the insulin insensitivity associated with acidosis was largely corrected. Insulin-induced responses of protein metabolism in CRF patients are blunted as insulin does not eliminate the higher rate of protein degradation.[59] This suggests that activation of the ATP-ubiquitin-proteasome–dependent proteolytic pathway in CRF will not be blocked solely by administering insulin.

The actions of other hormones change with acidosis (Table 48-2). Brungger and colleagues[60] reported that normal adults given an acid load have decreased thyroid hormone secretion despite a higher level of thyroid-stimulating hormone. There were no measurements of nitrogen balance or protein turnover, so it is unclear what role, if any, thyroid hormone plays in the muscle wasting that accompanies metabolic acidosis. In fact, the functional thyroid adaptations that occur in uremia might protect against accelerated protein degradation because administration of thyroid hormone to hypophysectomized rats stimulates the ubiquitin-proteasome pathway to degrade protein.[61]

Acidosis also interferes with the growth hormone–insulin-like growth factor-1 (IGF-1) axis.[62] Challa and colleagues[63, 64] showed that rats with metabolic acidosis exhibit suppressed growth hormone secretion and reduced expression of the IGF-1 receptor. There is also down-regulation of the negative modulators of the growth hormone receptor with increased expression of IGF binding protein-2 (IGFB-2) and IGF binding protein-4 (IGFB-4).[65] These types of responses

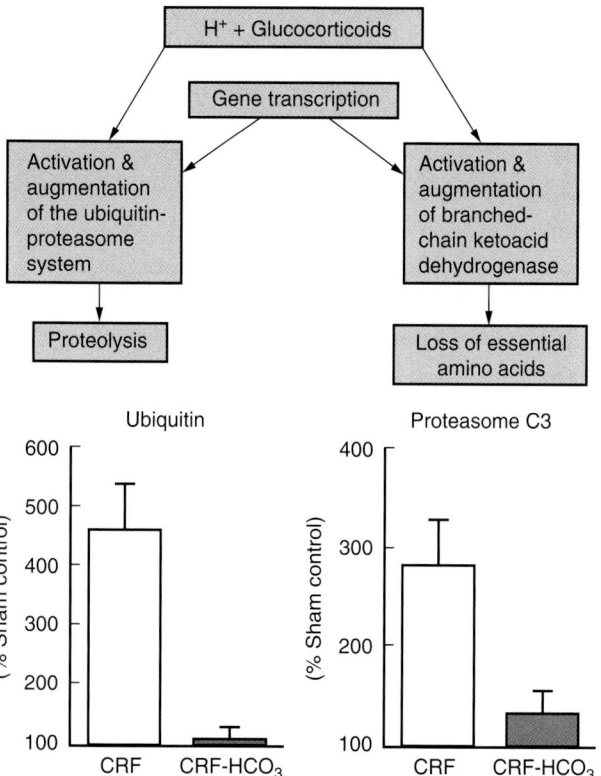

FIGURE 48-2. Metabolic acidosis activates the ubiquitin-proteasome proteolytic system, which in turn results in accelerated protein degradation. This process requires glucocorticoids and is augmented by activation of gene transcription, leading to increased levels of mRNAs for ubiquitin and subunits of the proteasome. Addition of sodium bicarbonate neutralizes the metabolic acidosis, and the pathway becomes quiescent. (From JL Bailey, Wang X, England BK, et al: The acidosis of chronic renal failure activates muscle proteolysis in rats by augmenting transcription of genes encoding proteins of the ATP-dependent ubiquitin-proteasome pathway. J Clin Invest 97:1447-1453, 1996.)

TABLE 48-2

Toxic Sequelae of Metabolic Acidosis

ORGAN	MECHANISM	SEQUELAE
Muscle	Proteolysis	Loss of lean body mass
	↑BCAA oxidation	
	↑Cortisol	
Bone	Inhibition of osteoblasts	Dissolution of bony matrix
	Stimulation of osteoclasts	Physicochemical dissolution of bone mineral
Hormonal	↑PTH level	Osteopenia
	↓Vitamin D_3	Osteomalacia
	↑Cortisol	Activation of catabolism
	↓Thyroxine	Hypometabolism
	↓Growth hormone	Stunted growth
	↓JGF-1 receptor	Stunted growth
	Insulin resistance	Activation of catabolism

BCAA, branched-chain amino acid;

PTH, parathyroid hormone;

IGF-1, insulin-like growth factor-1.

can contribute to impaired growth of long bones in CRF children and renal osteodystrophy in adult CRF patients because growth hormone administration to normal adults with experimental acidosis yields a blunted rise in circulating IGF-1. The latter observation may have clinical relevance as Ding and associates[66] found that administration of IGF-1 to rats with CRF did not correct the reported increases in protein degradation and impaired protein synthesis in muscle. The biochemical reason for this defect in the IGF-1 receptor signaling pattern was not identified, although the results indicate abnormalities similar to the insulin signaling defects in muscles of uremic rats.[67, 68]

Metabolic acidosis is buffered in the bone and this promotes dissolution of bone.[19] Besides the physiochemical effect of hydrogen ions on bone mineral, cell-mediated bone calcium resorption is stimulated and osteoblastic function is inhibited, including the genes that control bone matrix formation.[69, 70] Acidosis even affects parathyroid hormone (PTH) responses; following rapid correction of the metabolic acidosis of CRF there is significant suppression of circulating intact PTH and an increase in vitamin D_3 levels.[71, 72] It is even possible that these responses affect more than bone. Mak[73] gave sodium bicarbonate or sodium chloride to acidotic children treated by hemodialysis in a crossover study and found that correction of acidosis ameliorated hypertriglyceridemia without changing levels of high-density lipoprotein (HDL) and total cholesterol. The circulating level of vitamin D_3 increased after correction of the acidosis, suggesting a mechanistic role for vitamin D_3.

Trace Minerals

Metabolism of trace metals is often abnormal in uremia. Serum levels of vanadium and arsenic are high in CRF patients,[74, 75] and oxidized vanadium can inhibit adenosine triphosphatases (ATPases), including (Na^+,K^+-ATPase).[76, 77] Aluminum toxicity stemming from contaminated dialysate or administration of aluminum-containing phosphate-binding gels can exacerbate renal osteodystrophy; it also may cause confusion or even coma that can be mistakenly attributed to uremia.[78, 79] Finally, zinc deficiency has been implicated in causing testicular atrophy, abnormal taste, and other phenomena present in patients with uremia.[80]

Toxic Products of Protein Metabolism

For more than one hundred years, it has been known that dietary protein restriction decreases the BUN and the severity of uremic symptoms.[81] Because urea production is directly related to protein intake, it follows that the production of other metabolic products of protein rises when the BUN increases and vice versa (Table 48-3). The importance of urea as an index of uremic toxins was underscored by the results of the National Cooperative Dialysis Study, which prospectively compared the clinical outcome of various dialysis regimens directed at maintaining the BUN at various levels between dialyses (i.e., TACurea).[82] Patients with the higher TACurea values had more hospitalizations, more electroencephalogram abnormalities and neurobehavioral symptoms, such as impaired concentration, plus increased morbidity. These results confirm that accumulation of urea is tantamount to accumulation of other waste products derived from protein.

TABLE 48-3

Potentially Toxic Compounds That Accumulate in Renal Failure

Urea	Pyridine derivatives
Phenols	Guanidino compounds
Indoles	β_2-Microglobulin
Skatoles	Aliphatic amines
Hormones	Hippurate esters
Polyamines	Middle molecules
Trace elements	Aromatic amines
Serum proteinases	

As a corollary, removal of urea by dialysis also removes other waste products, albeit at different rates. This is the basis for judging the efficiency of dialysis by calculating urea removal (i.e., Kt/V).[83] Although the genesis of the symptoms of uremia is complicated, urea accumulation remains an excellent index of the accumulation of toxins (see Chapter 57).

An elegant demonstration of the toxic consequences of excess dietary protein was reported by Cotton and Knochel.[84] They measured abnormalities in the resting membrane potential of skeletal muscle fibers in patients with advanced uremia. Following 6 weeks of intensive dialysis, uremic symptoms had abated and the skeletal muscle resting membrane potentials (V_m) returned to normal (Fig. 48-3).[85, 86] During these measurements, the patients ate 1 g protein/kg/day and when the investigators reduced the frequency of their dialysis treatments, anorexia, nausea, and vomiting developed in four of six patients and the muscle membrane potential fell. The dialysis regimen was maintained but the diet was switched to 0.5 g/kg/day plus a supplement of essential amino acids. With the reduced amount of dietary protein, five of six patients had normal membrane potential

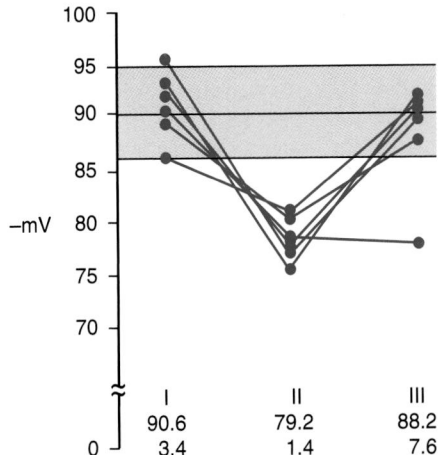

MEMBRANE POTENTIAL MEASUREMENT

FIGURE 48-3. Transmembrane electrical potential values in six patients with end-stage renal disease were almost all within normal limits (± 5.0) after they had undergone 6 hours of hemodialysis three times weekly for a long time (I). Successive reduction of dialysis time eventually resulted in a decline of membrane potential to abnormally low values (II). Although dialysis was continued at the same reduced rate, dietary protein intake was reduced from 1.0 to 0.5 g/kg/day, but the diet was supplemented with 6.5 g of mixed essential amino acids. In five patients, membrane potential returned to normal: the remaining patient did not comply with the diet (III).

values in skeletal muscle (the remaining patient did not comply with the dietary restriction) and in all patients, uremic symptoms resolved.[84]

The disappearance of uremic symptoms with initiation of dialysis and the observation that patients with declining kidney function tend to restrict dietary protein spontaneously[87, 88] have prompted several groups to recommend that patients begin dialysis early (i.e., at a higher level of clearance).[89, 90] Presumably, this suggestion arises from the severe biochemical abnormalities that can occur in patients with advancing kidney disease,[91] and the fact that these abnormalities are largely corrected by dialysis. Unfortunately, early dialysis is not associated with improved survival,[92] but fortunately, the biochemical abnormalities and even some of the cellular abnormalities described earlier can be corrected by attention to the diet (see Chapter 57). For these reasons, it is unwise to attribute the symptoms associated with CRF to malnutrition.[93] In fact, malnutrition is defined as abnormalities associated with an inadequate or abnormal diet and in uremia there are several easily identified reasons why cellular function can become abnormal. These may be aggravated by the accumulation of uremic toxins, but for the reasons discussed the cellular abnormalities will not be corrected by feeding more protein. Instead, this practice will simply raise the accumulation of uremic toxins.

Urea

The possibility that urea itself might be toxic was initially raised by Richard Bright in 1831.[94] This possibility has been tested but the results are inconclusive. Administration of urea to normal animals causes rapid but transient transmembrane shift in fluid and an osmotic diuresis, but the half-life of urea is short (7 hours), and it is difficult to sustain a high level of urea in animals or humans with normal kidney function.[95] Nephrectomized dogs, treated with peritoneal dialysis and a dialysate supplemented with urea, achieved BUN values between 173 and 224 mg/dL and developed weakness, anorexia, and decreased attentiveness.[96] Continued therapy was followed by vomiting, hemorrhagic diarrhea, hypothermia, and death. Regarding humans, Merrill and Hoigne[97] found no apparent toxicity when chronic dialysis patients were dialyzed against urea-supplemented dialysate. However, when Johnson and associates[98] gradually increased the urea concentration in the dialysate of stable long-term hemodialysis patients so that the BUN was sustained between 140 and 200 mg/dL for several weeks, most of the patients experienced malaise, weakness, lethargy, and a bleeding diathesis. One patient maintained a BUN above 130 mg/dL for more than 90 days, yet remained asymptomatic. However, when her BUN was raised above 190 mg/dL, she complained of lethargy, malaise, nausea, and vomiting, but never developed confusion, uremic fetor, or stomatitis. Although some symptoms of uremia, such as nausea, vomiting, malaise, and bleeding, may be due to urea intoxication, other uremic symptoms cannot be provoked by even high urea concentrations. Thus, urea does not fulfill the criteria for a uremic toxin, but seems to be clinically important at very high concentrations.

There are cellular abnormalities attributable to urea. Moeslinger and colleagues[99] demonstrated that urea suppresses inducible nitric oxide synthesis in mouse macrophages in a dose-dependent fashion. This is accompanied by macrophage proliferation and could be relevant to the development of atherosclerosis as the pathogenesis of this disorder includes proliferation of macrophages within atherosclerotic lesions. Urea may contribute to the central nervous system abnormalities of uremia because urea is converted to ammonia and carbon dioxide, principally by bacterial urease. The resulting ammonia diffuses across intestinal epithelia to portal blood and is reconverted to urea in the liver. If the process is inefficient, blood ammonia levels may rise and cause abnormalities. Fortunately, systemic blood ammonia levels are normal or minimally elevated in uremia.[100, 101] Urea can also be spontaneously decomposed to form ammonia or cyanate adducts. Cyanate can condense with NH_2-terminal amino and amide lysine groups on proteins to alter the tertiary structure of proteins; enzyme activity can change. This explains why CRF is associated with carbamoylation of hemoglobin.[102] The consequences of this process are not settled; protein carbamoylation has been reported to aggravate the uremic syndrome and may decrease the activity of insulin.[11, 12, 103]

Compounds besides urea can be channeled into more toxic compounds. For example, increased hepatic arginine levels could contribute to the production and accumulation of guanidino compounds in uremic patients (see following section) as the concentration of arginine is elevated in hepatocytes of CRF patients,[104] whereas CAPD patients can be arginine-deficient.[105] Another mechanism of waste nitrogen disposal involves the amino acid acylation reaction,[106] whereby amino acids are coupled to organic acids and rapidly excreted. As a result, nitrogen accumulation is reduced. For example, administration of sodium benzoate to CRF patients increased the synthesis of hippurate from glycine via the benzoyl coenzyme A (CoA) glycine transferase reaction.[107] This is of interest because hippurate is eliminated by both filtration and secretion and hence should remove more nitrogen. The administration of benzoate to CRF patients caused no change in either serum glycine or serine but a sharp decline in urea production.[107] Thus, nitrogen destined for urea must have been redirected toward synthesis of these nonessential amino acids that had been removed as hippurate.[106] This strategy has also been used to treat children with inherited disorders of urea cycle enzymes.[106, 108]

Guanidino-Containing Compounds

Guanidino compounds are strong organic bases that bear the amidino group N-C=NH; these compounds accumulate in the sera of uremic patients [109, 110] and at variable rates in tissues.[109] That there is a 100-fold difference in serum concentrations of a α-keto-δ-guanidinovaleric acid between humans and dogs makes it mandatory that results of experiments in animals be validated in humans.

As with all nitrogen-containing compounds, a high plasma level of a guanidino compound results from an increase in the production rate or a decrease in its renal or extrarenal clearance or both. In CRF patients in the steady state, urinary excretion of guanidino compounds is actually high even when protein intake is the same as that of control subjects.[110, 111] Because the extrarenal clearance of these compounds is negligible, it follows that CRF increases the production of guanidino compounds.

The biochemical pathways in which guanidino compounds are synthesized are largely unknown. Arginine can be converted into amidino groups in vivo, and urinary excretion of both methylguanidine (MG) and guanidinosuccinic acid (GSA) rise when dietary protein is increased, but whether this is attributable to an increase in arginine intake is unknown.[111, 114] There are other factors regulating their production; Kopple and associates[111] reported the course of three CRF patients with a constant protein intake who were found to have an increased excretion of GSA coincidental with a superimposed illness. Besides arginine intake, it has been reported that when rats with ARF were given exogenous creatinine, plasma and tissue levels of MG rose.[114] Although the kidney can synthesize a precursor of creatine from arginine and glycine, a biochemical pathway from creatine to arginine and glycine has never been documented. It is likely that most guanidine-containing compounds are synthesized in the liver because there is a high activity of glycine transamidinase[115] and a low rate of arginine export by hepatocytes.[116] In fact, arginine turnover in normal adults includes a relatively large nonexchangeable pool in the liver that could serve as a source of guanidino compounds,[117, 118] and perfusion of rat liver with L-[guanidino-^{14}C]arginine yields a progressive increase of ^{14}C-GSA.[119] Conversely, no ^{14}C-GSA release is detected if livers are perfused with D,L-[guanidino-^{14}C] canavanine. This is relevant because of the suggestion there is a "guanidine cycle." If creatinine were synthesized from canavanine, GSA could emerge as a byproduct (Fig. 48-4).[120] However, canavanine has never been isolated or identified in mammalian tissues. If the postulate is that canavanine arises from bacterial metabolism, GSA production should fall when broad-spectrum oral antibiotics are administered. This is not the case.[121] Regardless, ingestion of L-[guanidino-^{15}N] arginine by uremic patients yielded ^{15}N-MG at levels that initially exceeded that present in creatinine, consistent with

MG being a precursor of creatinine.[122] This result supports the hypothesis that arginine may be degraded to form MG and α-aminobutyric acid. Cohen[121] postulated that with a high serum creatinine or its immediate precursor, guanidinoacetic acid (GAA), there is decreased utilization of arginine to form GAA and hense increased availability of arginine to donate its amidino group to form other compounds, such as GSA, MG, γ-guanidinobutyric acid, and guanidinopropionic acid. Regardless of the mechanism, the concentration of guanidino compounds in tissue and plasma increases as renal function declines and their concentrations are best correlated with the amount of protein eaten.

Much of the controversy surrounding the importance of guanidino compounds as candidate uremic toxins is related to difficulties in measuring plasma and tissue concentrations, especially that of MG. Plasma levels as high as 8 to 10 mM can occur in uremic patients, but corresponding tissue levels have not been extensively studied so it is difficult to verify toxicity. MG has been detected in the cerebrospinal fluid of uremic patients, but not in normal subjects or experimental animal models of renal failure.[113] Giovannetti and co-workers[123] injected 12 normal dogs with 10 mg of MG thrice daily for 20 days. Weight loss and anemia developed in all dogs, and neurologic symptoms (hypertonus, myoclonus, and decreased nerve conduction velocity) became apparent in about half of the animals. Plasma MG levels in these dogs given large doses of MG far exceeded those present in patients. In vitro, high doses of MG cause autohemolysis and defects in erythrocyte metabolism and inhibit salivary and exocrine pancreatic secretion.[124, 125] Likewise, guanidinopropionic acid, guanidinoacetic acid, or γ-guanidinobutyric acid can cause autohemolysis of red blood cells, possibly related to inhibition of glucose-6-phosphate dehydrogenase.[126]

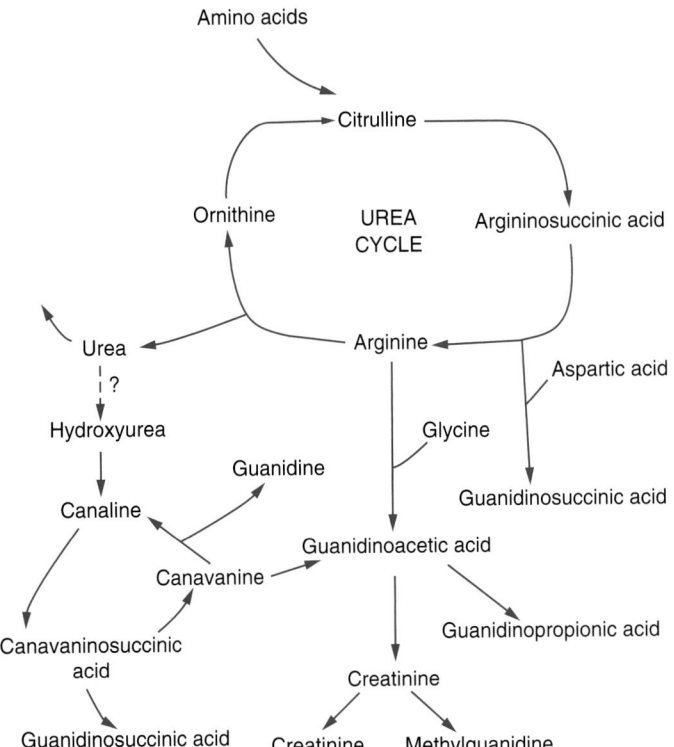

FIGURE 48-4. Proposed relationships between urea metabolism and the production of guanidino compounds. (From Kelly RA, Mitch WE: Creatinine, uric acid, and other nitrogenous waste products: Clinical implication of the imbalance between their production and elimination in uremia. Semin Nephrol 3:286, 1983.)

Clinically, plasma levels of these compounds in uremic patients can be shown to be inversely correlated with the erythrocyte glutathione concentration, suggesting they induce a loss of the protective effect of glutathione against hemolysis. Other guanidino compounds may have neurotoxic effects: guanidine and MG have been related to peripheral neuropathy, and γ-guanidinobutyric acid, taurocyamine, homoarginine and α-keto-δ-guanidinovaleric acid lower the seizure threshold of experimental animals. This may explain the observations that the seizure threshold is low in CRF patients.[127] De Deyn and co-workers[128, 129] measured the levels of guanidine compounds in serum, urine, and cerebrospinal fluid of nondialyzed patients with renal insufficiency and found that creatinine, guanidine, GSA, and MG were present in concentrations as much as 100-fold higher in the cerebrospinal fluid of uremic patients. In addition, they showed that these compounds can induce experimental convulsions at concentrations found in uremic brain. Not surprisingly the serum levels of MG and GSA were directly proportional to the BUN.[130] Based on biochemical and electrophysiologic measurements in vitro, they proposed that the central nervous system excitatory effects of uremic guanidino compounds could be explained by inhibition of depolarization at γ-aminobutyric acid (GABA) receptors, selective activation of N-methyl-D-aspartate (NMDA) receptors by GSA, and an intrinsic depolarizing response.[130, 131] Proof that these compounds cause uremic symptoms is not available but it is prudent to prevent CRF patients from eating excessive amounts of protein (see Chapter 57).

Besides the production of potential uremic toxins, abnormal arginine metabolism could change the NO pathway. NO is produced by the macula densa as well as by preglomerular and postglomerular resistance vessels and has an important role in controlling glomerular hemodynamics and filtration.[132, 133] For example, intrarenal administration of an NO inhibitor increases afferent arteriolar resistance slightly, with a small decrease in the single-nephron glomerular filtration rate (GFR) even though there is no change in systemic blood pressure. When NO synthesis is inhibited, medullary blood flow falls and Na^+ retention occurs with a resetting of the blood pressure–natriuresis relationship.[134, 135] Acute sodium loading stimulates NO synthesis as measured by increased nitrite excretion, but inhibition of NO synthesis blocks the natriuretic response to acute volume expansion. The mechanisms by which changes in NO regulate extracellular fluid volume and blood pressure include changes in the activity of specific ion transport processes, such as inhibition of H^+-ATPase activity,[136] Na^+ reabsorption,[137] plus antidiuretic hormone–stimulated osmotic water permeability in the cortical collecting duct[138] and Na^+/H^+ exchange,[139] as well as proximal tubular Na^+,K^+-ATPase activity.[140] These properties of NO may not point to a toxic effect but there is evidence that other compounds interfering with NO production can have toxic sequelae.

Compounds derived from arginine can inhibit NO synthase: asymmetric dimethylarginine (ADMA) inhibits this enzyme and some but not all investigators feel that ADMA accumulates in patients with impaired renal excretion.[141-143] In experimental animals, accumulation of this compound is associated with a concentration-dependent pressor and bradycardic response and vasoconstriction in mesenteric and hindquarter vessels.[144] In CRF patients, loss of the vasodilating properties

of NO (e.g., because of a high ADMA level) could aggravate hypertension and accelerate the progression of renal failure.[145, 146] A positive correlation between plasma levels of ADMA and mean arterial blood pressure has been noted and possibly an inverse relationship between progression of renal insufficiency and nitrate excretion.[147, 148] Besides changing hemodynamic responses, NO depletion may cause anorexia in hemodialysis patients as administration of N-nitro-L-arginine, an inhibitor of NO synthesis, reduced the food intake of rats.[149] Another possibility is that it raised the ornithine concentration because ornithine can inhibit protein ingestion in a dose-dependent manner.[150]

As might be expected from the molecular weight of ADMA (or similar compounds), hemodialysis could remove NO synthase inhibitors to improve NO synthesis, but this has been difficult to prove. For example, both MacAllistar and Anderstam and their colleagues[141, 143] found only a 20% reduction in ADMA concentrations during dialysis, whereas Kielstein and co-workers[142] reported a rise in serum ADMA levels immediately following dialysis, suggesting poor removal of ADMA compared to fluid losses (or release from intracellular stores). From these data, it is not surprising that the clearance of ADMA is lower than expected from its molecular weight, suggesting there is binding to plasma proteins or possibly adsorption to the dialyzer membrane. That plasma concentrations of ADMA are high in patients with peripheral vascular disease[151] and in patients with asymptomatic hypercholesterolemia with normal renal function[152] highlights why it is difficult to interpret changes in the plasma concentration of ADMA. It also points to a mechanism by which CRF could exacerbate an underlying disease process (e.g., arteriosclerosis). The variety of changes occurring via NO underscore the importance of a thorough understanding of the metabolism and potential toxicity of guanidino compounds.

Advanced Oxidation Products

Activated leukocytes and other phagocytic cells change the structure of proteins through the generation of reactive oxidation species such as hydrogen peroxide or hydroxyl radicals. Specific amino acid residues such as tyrosine undergo oxidation, with cross-linking, aggregation, or fragmentation of proteins following reactions with reactive oxygen species including advanced oxidation protein products (AOPP).[153, 155] Advanced oxidation products can be found even in the early stages of renal insufficiency but increase sharply with progressive loss of renal function. These products are at high concentrations in dialysis patients, forming protein aggregates, and there is a positive correlation between the levels of AOPP and inflammatory markers such as tumor necrosis factor-α (TNF-α) and its soluble receptor.[155] Because these compounds have been linked to the development of atherosclerosis, more information about their formation and fate should be forthcoming.

Products of Bacterial Metabolism

Uremic toxins can be synthesized by gut bacteria and absorption of bacterial products could be high because of increased permeability of the gastrointestinal mucosa.[156, 157] Products of tryptophan pyrolysis and heterocyclic amines, occurring as byproducts of bacterial metabolism and potential carcinogens, can be elevated in the plasma of uremic patients.[158, 159] For example, indole is derived from tryptophan through the action of intestinal flora and is further metabolized to indoxyl sulfate by the liver. Aliphatic amines are high in the plasma of uremic patients owing largely to production by gut bacteria[6]; monomethylamine is thought to be derived from the metabolism of creatinine through sarcosine, whereas bacterial metabolism of choline and lecithin produced tertiary methylamines, which are absorbed and oxidized or demethylated to form secondary methylamines that are excreted in urine or bile.[9] In uremic patients, secondary methylamines are high in blood, cerebrospinal fluid, and brain tissue, as well as in duodenal aspirates.[6, 160] This may reflect the greater density of bacteria in the small intestines of uremic patients or the higher choline levels in the plasma of uremic patients.[160, 161] Trimethylamine-*N*-oxide (TMAO) is readily absorbed from fish protein and is promptly excreted by normal adults, but accumulates in CRF patients.[162]

Experimentally, secondary methylamines can be shown to inhibit neuronal oxidative metabolism in vitro, but only at very high concentrations.[163] The evidence that secondary methylamines contribute to altered mental status in uremia is indirect: administration of nonabsorbable antibiotics to two patients with uremic encephalopathy resulted in a marked improvement in asterixis, myoclonus, mental alertness, and electroencephalographic abnormalities, coinciding with a decline in serum amine levels.[6]

Aromatic amines, resulting from bacterial metabolism of tyrosine, phenylalanine, or tryptophan, could contribute to uremic encephalopathy by serving as false neurotransmitters.[164, 165] Niwa has identified high levels of derivatives of hydroxyphenolic acids, including *p*-hydroxybenzoic acid and *p*-hydroxyphenylacetic acid and precursors of phenol and *p*-cresol, in the sera of hemodialysis patients; the levels were proportional to dietary protein intake.[166] Infusion of phenol or *p*-cresol into dogs results in a variety of neurologic symptoms, and conjugated phenols can inhibit ATPases and ion transport systems, leading to changes in intracellular ionic composition and abnormal cellular metabolism.[167] It is known that *p*-cresol can inactivate α-hydroxylase, a key enzyme in the transformation of dopamine to norepinephrine.[168] *p*-Cresol also blocks the synthesis of platelet-activating factor,[169] the production of free radicals by phagocytes,[170] and the methylation of arsenic.[171] It also impedes cell growth[172] and alters the permeability of the cell membrane.[173]

The plasma concentration of 3-carboxy-4-methyl-5-propyl-2-furnpropionic acid (CMPF) was found to correlate with the severity of neurologic abnormalities in uremic patients.[174] It also inhibits the deiodination of thyroxine (T_4) to triiodothyronine (T_3) in cultured hepatocytes,[175] blocks respiration in the isolated mitochondria,[176] and inhibits both hepatic glutathione *S*-transferase[177] and erythropoiesis.[178] Thus, like many of these nitrogen-containing waste products, CMPF can affect several metabolic pathways.

Another aromatic amino acid, tryptophan, has been touted as one of the major precursors of uremic toxins. Tryptophan undergoes deamination and decarboxylation by gut bacteria, yielding a variety of metabolites that include indole, indoxyl, skatole, skatoxyl, indican, and indoleacetic acid. Several of these compounds are high in the plasma of uremic subjects and can inhibit oxidative metabolism in brain slices.[179]

Moreover, patients with uremic encephalopathy have high concentrations of tryptophan, 5-hydroxyindoleacetic acid, and homovanillic acid in their cerebrospinal fluid.[180, 181] The pathogenic significance of this association is unclear, but 5-hydroxyindoleacetic acid is a precursor of the neurotransmitter serotonin, as well as indoxyl sulfate.[180, 181] In the liver, indoxyl sulfate is produced from indoles. Niwa fed uremic rats a proprietary resin that absorbs such compounds and found greatly reduced plasma and urinary levels of indoxyl sulfate, but more interestingly, there were improvements in several metabolic pathways even though the degree of azotemia was unchanged.[166] The administration of this resin was associated with increased food intake, leading to the suggestion that other toxins causing anorexia were removed. Like CMPF, indoxyl sulfate can inhibit the deiodination of T_4 to T_3 in cultured hepatocytes.[175]

Most if not all of the breakdown products of the aromatic amino acids have been shown to interfere with the binding of drugs to serum proteins and this could interfere with the action of the drugs. The inhibitory products include indoxyl sulfate,[182] hippuric acid,[183] *p*-cresol,[183] and 3-carboxy-4-methyl-5-propyl-2-furanpropionic acid.[42] In a different set of investigations, this group reported that oral administration of indole or indoxyl sulfate to uremic rats accelerates progression of glomerulosclerosis and of renal failure.[184] In summary, the degree to which gastrointestinal bacteria and their products contribute to the uremic syndrome is uncertain, and a taxonomic analysis of bacteria in the small intestine, as well as characterization of nitrogenous byproducts created by the bacteria, is needed.

Low-molecular-weight polyamines necessary for the synthesis of nucleic acid and cell growth[185] are synthesized or produced by intestinal bacteria. Putrescine, spermidine, and spermine are synthesized in mammalian tissues and cadaverine and putrescine are formed by intestinal bacteria in a reaction that decarboxylates lysine and ornithine.[186] Even these compounds can be toxic as in vitro experiments indicate that spermine can inhibit erythropoiesis, whereas in hemodialysis patients, the serum spermine levels vary inversely with the hematocrit.[187]

Homocyst(e)ine

Homocyst(e)ine, a sulfur-containing amino acid derived from the metabolism of methionine or cysteine, is rapidly oxidized to homocystine and cysteine-homocyst(e)ine, creating a special class of uremic toxins (Fig. 48-5). Homocyst(e)ine is found in the plasma and in erythrocytes and cells of the liver and other organs.[188-190] In plasma from CRF patients, the levels of sulfur-containing amino acids including homocyst(e)ine, are high; the mechanism for these abnormalities is unknown. Accumulation of homocyst(e)ine is a potentially severe complication because of the association between homocyst(e)ine levels and cardiovascular disease.[191] By convention, plasma or serum total homocysteine, named homocyst(e)ine, refers to the sum of homocyst(e)ine and its disulfide derivatives whether they exist in the bound or the free state (about 70% of homocyst(e)ine is bound to proteins and hence is not removed by dialysis). Studies in rats[192] and human[193] suggest that the kidney eliminates about 70% of the daily homocyst(e)ine burden daily and this indicates why homocyst(e)inemia levels are high in predialysis as well as renal

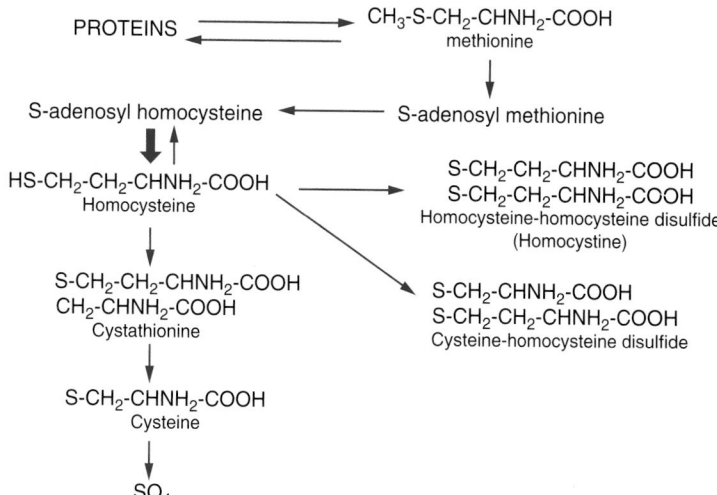

FIGURE 48-5. Metabolic scheme for homocysteine production in vivo.

transplant patients.[194, 195] Homocyst(e)ine is metabolized by reactions that include transsulfuration or remethylation. In transsulfuration, homocysteine is degraded to cystathione and then to cysteine and other sulfur-containing compounds, including glutathione, taurine, hydrogen sulfide, and sulfate. In remethylation, homocysteine is methylated through the action of methylenetetrahydrofolate reductase. Vitmin B_6 is a cofactor involved in transsulfuration and vitamin B_{12} is involved in remethylation. Treatment of homocysteine excess has included these two vitamins (see subsequent discussion).

The prototype of homocyst(e)ine toxicity is homocystinuria, an autosomal recessive disorder due to defective cystathione β-synthase, resulting in failure of the conversion (transulfuration) of homocysteine to cysteine. Homocystinuric patients have severe homocyst(e)inemia, and neurologic, ocular, skeletal, and vascular abnormalities that result in early death from myocardial infarction, stroke, or pulmonary embolism.[196] McCully and Wilson[197] proposed the "homocysteine theory of arteriosclerosis" because an elevated blood homocyst(e)ine level is correlated with premature cardiovascular disease in subjects without kidney disease. Moderately high levels of homocyst(e)ine are present in 12% to 47% of patients with coronary, cerebral, or peripheral vascular disease,[198] and the risk of death in men and women with coronary artery disease is highly correlated with the homocyst(e)ine level. In uremia, the fasting level of homocyst(e)ine in plasma is high in dialysis patients and there is a direct correlation between fasting plasma homocyst(e)ine and vascular complications.[199] It is postulated that homocysteine plays a role in the excessive cardiovascular risk associated with CRF.[191]

The water-soluble vitamins folic acid, vitamin B_6, and vitamin B_{12} are cofactors and substrates in the metabolism of methionine and homocyst(e)ine; all are removed with dialysis. Kang and colleagues first reported an inverse association between homocyst(e)ine and folic acid blood levels,[200] and there also is an inverse correlation with plasma vitamin B_6 levels.[201] The risk of carotid artery stenosis is associated with high levels of homocyst(e)ine and is inversely proportional to the intake of folic acid and vitamin B_{12}.[202] Based on these data, dialysis patients have two factors that raise homocyst(e)ine levels: Dialysis does not remove homocyst(e)ine

efficiently but does remove the water-soluble vitamins that are needed to metabolize this amino acid. The level of homocyst(e)ine can be raised by a diet restricted in the intake of green leafy vegetables, fruits, and legumes, because such diets are rich in folate and vitamin B_6. However, prolonged heating or boiling of foods (often encouraged in the diets of kidney patients to remove potassium) reduces the folate content, pointing to another reason why attention to the diet of CRF patients is so critical.

The U.S. Food and Drug Administration has issued regulations stipulating that cereal grains must be fortified with folic acid, but, there have been no controlled clinical trials to date demonstrating that lowering homocyst(e)ine levels reduces atherosclerotic event rates in patients with chronic renal disease or other cardiovascular risks. Moreover, Mezzano and colleagues have argued that inflammation, not hyperhomocyst(e)inemia, is related to oxidative stress and hemostatic and endothelial dysfunction in uremia.[203] They evaluated 64 CRF patients and healthy controls and found a significant correlation with homocyst(e)ine levels and serum creatinine, but no significant correlation between homocyst(e)ine levels and indices of oxidative stress such as advanced oxidation protein products, endothelial cell markers such as von Wilebrand factor, markers of intravascular thrombin generation such as thrombin-antithrombin complexes, or indices of activation of fibrinolysis such as plasmin-antiplasmin complexes. For these reasons, both the American Heart Association[204] and the American Society of Nephrology[205] advise that screening and treatment guidelines for homocyst(e)ine are premature and inappropriate. Treatment of hyperhomocyst(e)inemia has been attempted. In observation studies, users of multivitamin supplements have lower homocyst(e)ine levels and higher concentrations of folic acid and vitamin B_6 and B_{12} and a corresponding reduction in coronary artery disease,[206, 207] but a satisfactory folic acid dose for CRF patients has not been determined. Numerous reports[208] about the treatment of this group of patients using supraphysiologic doses of folic acid with and without vitamins B_6 and B_{12} have had disappointing results; more than 90% of treated patients still maintain hyperhomocyst(e)ine levels above 12.0 μmol/L at the end of treatment. Alternative agents such as the reduced form of 5-methyltetrahydrofolate or folinic acid, which is rapidly converted to 5-methyltetrahydrofolate, have also yielded disappointing results.[209-211] In the trials in which homocyst(e)ine levels are reduced by therapy, carotid artery stiffness remains,[212] although this may represent irreversible vascular damage. Currently, there is a randomized, placebo-controlled trial to lower homocyst(e)ine in transplant patients and hopefully the outcome here will reveal a benefit. Besides uremia, plasma levels of homocyst(e)ine are affected by polymorphisms in genes encoding enzymes involved in its metabolism. Frost and colleagues uncovered a common mutation at nucleotide position 677 of the gene coding for 5,10-methylenetetrahydrofolate reductase that predisposes individuals to low folate levels and high homocyst(e)ine levels.[182] There are other genetic polymorphisms and the impact of these defects on therapeutic efforts will have to be studied.[183] It may turn out that alternative approaches, such as chelation of homocyst(e)ine, are required for CRF patients.[213]

In summary, there is much confusion surrounding the identity of uremic toxins. Much of the available information is based on correlations between blood concentrations of a putative uremic toxin and the severity of symptoms that are difficult to quantitate. For example, the demonstration that uremic encephalopathy is reversed with broad-spectrum antibiotics may be related to modification of trytophan metabolites or to reduced aliphatic amines, or both, so which compound would be considered toxic is debatable. Regardless, certain principles have emerged: the degree of uremic toxicity is roughly related to protein intake; the most severe symptoms occur in the patients with the highest protein intake; and most symptoms decline in severity when dietary protein intake is reduced. Second, uremia must involve impairment of a fundamental cell function because there are abnormalities in multiple organs in patients with renal failure.

MIDDLE MOLECULE HYPOTHESIS

A discrepancy between the severity of symptoms and the degree of azotemia seems to be most marked in patients who are treated with maintenance peritoneal dialysis. Despite relatively high BUN and serum creatinine levels, these patients have only mild symptoms of uremia, and they are less prone than hemodialysis patients to develop peripheral neuropathy. Moreover, uremic neuropathy has been linked to accumulation of middle molecules; weighing between 500 and 3000 Ds, these poorly characterized substances are cleared more readily by peritoneal dialysis than by hemodialysis. The suggestion is that some large fraction of the toxic consequences of uremia is related to the accumulation of the middle molecules rather than accumulation of smaller molecules for which urea is a surrogate marker. The alternative explanation for the decreased occurrence of neuropathy among peritoneal dialysis patients is that they retain their endogenous kidney function for a longer period, permitting clearance of middle molecules by residual renal function.

For hemodialysis patients, the middle molecule hypothesis predicts that shortening the length of dialysis treatments will compromise removal of these compounds and place them at risk for the development of uremic symptoms despite sufficient clearance of smaller solutes. Interestingly, increasing the surface area of dialysis membranes will increase the elimination of middle molecules by raising the likelihood that these compounds will interact with pores in the membrane. Because the concentration gradients for middle molecules from blood to dialysate are less critical than the gradients for small molecules, dialysis with large surface area dialysis membranes should decrease the risk of uremic symptoms, including neuropathy. These hypotheses were tested in the National Cooperative Dialysis Study in which dialysis regimens were directed at removing more urea or more middle molecules.[82] Unfortunately, the results of that study did not provide a firm conclusion, as patients with high time-averaged BUN values (TACurea) did less well than groups with a low TACurea, and the high probability of developing clinical manifestations of uremia (approximately 60%) in those with Kt/V values between 0.4 and 0.8 declined sharply to 13% when Kt/V values were between 0.9 and 1.5.[214]

The middle molecule hypothesis cannot be simply discounted based on these results because the relationship between uremic symptoms and the higher BUN (i.e., TACurea) may simply reflect the fact that urea production closely reflects protein intake and thus the production of all protein-derived waste products, including the substance(s) causing uremic symptoms. At the same level of dialysis intensity, a high BUN means that there is accumulation of all nitrogen-containing waste products in addition to urea. Moreover, the results of the National Cooperative Dialysis Study did not exclude an additional, albeit small, benefit from removing middle molecules by dialysis. A more definitive assessment of the middle molecule hypothesis is being uncovered from the results of the HEMO study trial, which was specifically designed to examine the influence of middle molecules.

Undoubtedly, much of the controversy about the clinical importance of accumulating middle molecules stems from difficulties in identifying compounds present at low concentrations in fluid that is as chemically complex as plasma. On the other hand, there are indications that these compounds do cause some of the problems attributed to loss of kidney function. A fascinating report is that middle molecules might cause the poor appetite of uremia.[215, 216] Mamoun and colleagues examined feeding behavior in response to injection of plasma ultrafiltrates from uremic patients undergoing their first dialysis treatment and compared it to the feeding behavior occurring after injection of ultrafiltrates of plasma or urine from normal adults.[217] When the plasma ultrafiltrates from uremic patients or urine from normal adults were injected intraperitoneally into rats, their appetites fell sharply, whereas injections of normal saline or ultrafiltrates of plasma from normal adults did not alter feeding behaviour.[216] It was concluded that one or more factors eliminated by the kidney accumulate in the body fluids of patients with renal failure and suppress appetite.[216] Ultrafiltrate subfractions with molecular weights ranging between 1 and 5 kD and 5 and 10 kD (i.e., middle molecules) obtained from uremic patients were also shown to inhibit the hunger for carbohydrates and proteins in a dose-dependent manner.[217] Similar results occurred after direct injection of the middle molecule fractions into the lateral brain ventricles of rats, suggesting that specific brain receptors or neurotransmitters control feeding.[215] These results were site- and route-specific because intravenous injection of the same uremic ultrafiltrate subfractions had no effect on feeding behavior nor was the sexual behavior of the rats altered.[218] The authors concluded that middle molecules contained in plasma from uremic patients or from urine of normal adults act in both the brain and the splanchnic region to inhibit food intake and these responses inhibit eating behavior.[218] Whether these substances influence the appetite of patients remains to be elucidated, but these results point to a defined toxic effect of middle molecules.

Middle molecules have been implicated in the impairment of immune responses and abnormalities in lipoprotein metabolism associated with uremia. When middle molecule fractions from uremic serum were incubated with lymphocytes, cellular proliferation as measured by tritiated thymidine incorporation was inhibited by 50%. The mechanism could involve inhibition of interleukin-2 production because there was a decrease in this cytokine which stimulates T lymphocyte proliferation.[219] Middle molecules also cause polymorphonuclear leukocyte dysfunction in uremia. Horl and colleagues [220-223] report that serum samples containing middle molecules can inhibit chemotaxis, oxidative metabolism, intracellular bacterial killing, and other polymorphonuclear leukocyte functions.

Middle molecule fractions from serum of uremic patients directly inhibit apolipoprotein A-I (apo A-I) production in hepatoma cells.[224] Since apo A-I is the structural protein for HDL, this finding may provide insight into why lower HDL levels and a higher incidence of atherosclerotic vascular complications are common in hemodialysis patients. For example, Leypoldt and colleagues[225] reported that increased clearance of small and middle molecules is independently and inversely associated with the risk of mortality in chronic hemodialysis patients. They concluded that differences in mortality associated with the various types of dialysis membranes could be explained by differences in middle molecule removal.

What is the chemical identity of these molecules? Small polypeptides accumulate in the plasma of uremic patients; at least 38 ninhydrin-positive peptides have been isolated from dialysate, while peptide-bound, N-substituted amino acids are present in excess amounts in the plasma of uremic patients.[226] Abiko and associates isolated four peptides from the plasma of patients with severe uremia that were characterized as peptide fragments of plasma proteins that are eliminated or metabolized by the normal kidney.[227, 228] Similarly, Chu and colleagues identified six middle molecules weighing between 800 and 2015 Ds that accumulate in the serum of uremic patients but are excreted by healthy subjects.[229] Specific toxic responses to these peptides are unknown, although β_2-microglobulin, which accumulates in the plasma of patients with renal failure, is the major constituent of amyloid-like deposits that accumulate in dialysis-related secondary amyloidosis.[230]

A number of hormones or fragments of hormones accumulate in uremic patients, including PTH, These peptide fragments are identified by antibodies (eg., to PTH) so it is possible that fragments of PTH, as well as the intact PTH molecule, may contribute to toxic responses such as the pathogenesis of anemia,[231] platelet dysfunction,[232] encephalopathy,[233] neuropathy,[234] cardiomyopathy,[235] and glucose intolerance.[236] Whether these abnormalities are due to the effects of PTH or secondary to changes in the cell calcium content is being investigated.[237]

Despite this information, the middle molecule hypothesis has a number of shortcomings. First, the efficiency of correcting the uremic syndrome after initiating dialysis argues that the more rapid removal of low-molecular-weight solutes is pathophysiologically preeminent. Second, most solutes are of low molecular weight and are not in the molecular weight range of middle molecules.[237] Chemically identified solutes such as glucuronyl-O-hydroxyhippurate or ascorbic acid 2-sulfate,[181] phenylacetylglutamine,[238] and 3-carboxy-4-methyl-5-propyl-2-furanpropionic acid[239] with claims to causing toxic reponses are, in fact, below the middle molecule range of 500 to 3000 Ds. It may be more fitting to think of middle molecules as solutes that are cleared by the kidney or by the dialyzer at rates similar to that of compounds with a molecular weight between 500 and 3000 Ds. Unfortunately, that characterization blurs the distinction between dialyzability and elimination. For instance, MG is readily cleared through cuprophane dialysis membranes but during a dialysis session is removed poorly because of its large volume of distribution and slow release from its intracellular stores. Inorganic phosphorus has similar properties; although readily dialyzable, it is poorly removed by dialysis.

In summary, the middle molecule hypothesis remains controversial despite a great deal of research. The data suggest that middle molecules still have a potential for enhancing the morbidity associated with the uremic syndrome. Investigation of the hypothesis has led to improvements in dialysis membrane design, culminating in a high-flux dialysis membrane that yields improved clearances of both middle molecules and small solutes, but the contribution of these compounds is still unsettled.[218]

ENDOCRINE CONTRIBUTIONS TO THE UREMIC SYNDROME

Several types of abnormalities are proposed as mechanisms causing the dysfunctions of endocrine systems in uremia (Table 48-4). There can be inadequate production of hormones by the damaged kidneys as occurs in the case of erythropoietin or 1,25-dihydroxyvitamin D$_3$, resulting in anemia and osteomalacia respectively. Alternatively, metabolic clearance of peptide hormones can be impaired leading to prolongation of the hormone half-life and higher plasma levels of a hormone. Classically, this type of abnormality should decrease the production of the hormone through negative feedback mechanisms but since the hormone level remains high, there must be an additional defect in feedback responses. For example, Sievertsen and co-workers[240] found a high plasma prolactin level in 51 (70%) of 73 patients receiving maintenance hemodialysis. Their pharmacokinetic analysis of prolactin turnover revealed a prolonged half-life from reduced clearance plus increased pituitary secretion. Production is high because in uremia, there is decreased release of the inhibitor dopamine, yielding unresponsiveness to the inhibitory effects of dopamine on prolactin secretion from the pituitary.[241]

Uremia exerts toxic effects on gonad functions, resulting in deficiencies in steroid production with a lower activity of androgen-dependent hepatic cytochrome P-450 oxidases.[242, 243] Because these enzymes are important in the metabolism of

TABLE 48-4

Endocrine Dysfunction in Chronic Renal Failure

NATURE OF DEFECT	HORMONAL DEFECTS
Diminishsed production of renal hormones	Decreased erythropoietin production
	Decreased conversion of 25-hydroxyvitamin D_3 to 1,25-dihydroxyvitamin D_3
Hormonal hypersecretion to re-establish homeostasis	Hyperparathyroidism
	Secretion of the "natriuretic hormone"
Decreased metabolic clearance of hormones	Follicle-stimulating hormone, luteinizing hormone, prolactin, growth hormone, melanocyte-stimulating hormone, gastrin
Blunted feedback response causing increased hormone secretion	Luteinizing hormone, corticotropin, prolactin
Defective tissue conversion of prohormone to hormone	Thyroxine to triiodothyronine
	25-Hydroxyvitamin D_3 to 1,25-dihydroxyvitamin D_3
Decreased hormone production	Testosterone
End-organ unresponsiveness	Insulin, parathyroid hormone
Increased circulating inhibitors of hormones	Somatomedin inhibitory factor

From May RC, Mitch WE: Chronic renal failure. *In* Branch WT(ed): Office Practice of Medicine, 2nd ed. Philadelphia, WB Saunders, 1987, p 608.

many hormones and drugs, an enzyme deficiency state could contribute to uremic toxicity or at least raise susceptibility to the toxic effects of certain drugs. Another mechanism that interferes with hormone action is increased production of inhibitors that blunt hormone action. An example is the induction of proteins that bind IGF-1, thereby suppressing its activity by reducing the availability of free IGF-1.[244] Finally, uremia can induce resistance of target tissues to the hormone so there is a reduced response to the hormone. One of the most intensively studied end-organ resistance states to hormones that is associated with uremia is insulin resistance. Despite a prolongation in the half-life of insulin due to impaired removal of insulin by the damaged kidneys and a higher plasma level of insulin, CRF patients typically exhibit a higher blood sugar and intolerance to glucose loading.[55] In addition, there is decreased insulin-mediated glucose uptake by forearm tissues, and patients with renal failure metabolize less glucose in response to infused insulin than normal subjects.[245] The biochemical mechanism causing uremia-associated resistance to the action of insulin in muscle has been linked to abnormalities in insulin signaling, but it is not known which step(s) in the signaling pathway is abnormal Fig. 48-6.[67, 246]

In normal cells, activation of the insulin receptor following insulin binding requires phosphorylation of specific tyrosines in the β-subunit and this step stimulates the activity of a tyrosine kinase that phosphorylates other substrates.[247] In this case, the major substrate is the insulin-receptor substrate-1 (IRS-1) which after phosphorylation acts as a scaffold to bring together enzymes critical for subsequent insulin events, including phosphatidylinositol 3-kinase (PI3-K).[248] The PI3-K complex is a heterodimer composed of an 86-kD (p85) regulatory subunit and a 110-kD (p110) catalytic subunit. The p85 regulatory subunit can form stable high-affinity complexes with the p110 catalytic subunit, but the amount of these cellular complexes and the amounts of the subunits are differentially regulated by stimuli like glucocorticoids.[249, 250] For example, Giorgino and co-workers reported that stimulation of expression of the p85 subunit of PI3-K following glucocorticoid treatment was associated with reduced IRS-1-associated PI3-K activity.[251] They speculated that the excess of p85 competed with the p85-p110 complex for binding to phosphorylated IRS-1. The reduced amount of IRS-1 associated p110 catalytic subunit resulted in decreased PI3-K activity. This would partially explain the insulin resistance associated with glucocorticoid administration.

The relevance of these observations to the uremic state is that May and colleagues[124] found that glucocorticoid production was augmented in uremic rats. These observations led Bailey and colleagues[252] to investigate whether the activity of PI3-K in muscle is impaired in uremia. Their results are in line with the concept that there is impaired PI3-K activity in muscle, possibly related to an excess of the p85 subunit. He showed that the quantity of p85 in substantially increased in muscle of chronically uremic rats. Supraphysiologic doses of insulin can overcome the suppression of PI3-K activity and it is tempting to speculate that impairment of this pathway in linked to the excessive protein catabolism of chronic uremia. Additional factors associated with uremia that could aggravate insulin resistance include angiotensin II, TNF-α, and chronic insulin stimulation.[21, 253, 254] The relative contributions of these factors is unknown.

Another example of end-organ resistance to stimulation by a hormone is the growth hormone–IGF-1 axis; despite normal levels of circulating growth hormone and IGF-1, growth retardation is common in uremic children.[255] Growth hormone receptor binding to hepatocytes is similar in tissues from uremic and pair-fed control rats.[256] Which signaling steps become abnormal following binding has not been elucidated. Besides abnormalities in cell signaling pathways, resistance to the action of IGF-1 is thought to be in part due to the accumulation of circulating binding proteins that reduce the free fraction (i.e., the active fraction) of the hormone.[257] In the case of growth hormone, there are circulating proteins that bind growth hormone and these may be the result of fragments of receptors broken off from cell membranes.[258] Because these binding fragments may yield an estimate of total receptor numbers throughout the body, it may be that the growth hormone receptor number is low in uremia. In uremic children, IGF-1 receptor binding capacity and levels of IGFBs are both increased.[259]

The physiologic relevance of these changes was reported by Mak and Pak who isolated chondrocytes from bones of uremic rats and demonstrated that the growth responses of these chondrocytes to growth hormone, to IGF-1, or to insulin was blunted compared to responses measured in chondrocytes from normal rats.[260] Specificity in the involvement of the growth hormone–IGF-1 axis was present because they found that growth responses to other growth factors, such as fibroblast growth factor or transforming growth factor-β1 (TGF-β1), were normal. Based on these results, Schaefer and colleagues investigated whether a postreceptor defect in growth hormone signaling was the cause of growth hormone resistance in uremic rats.[258] When growth hormone binds to its receptor, phosphorylation of a tyrosine kinase (Janus-associated kinase 2 or JAK2) occurs.[261]

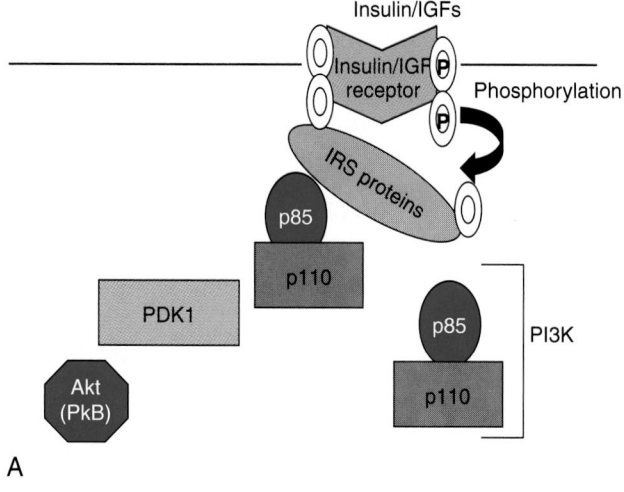

A

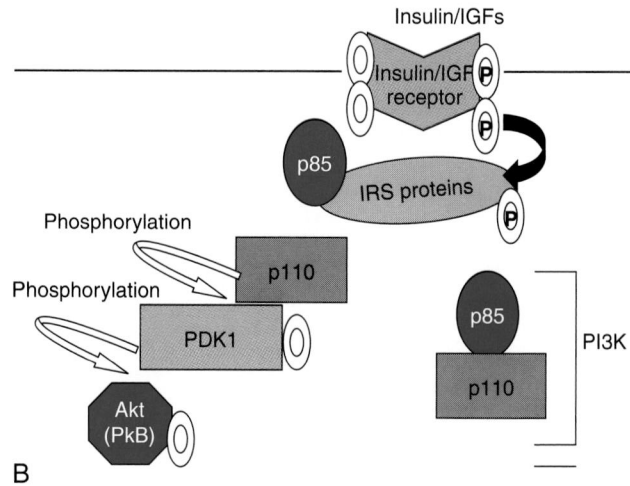

B

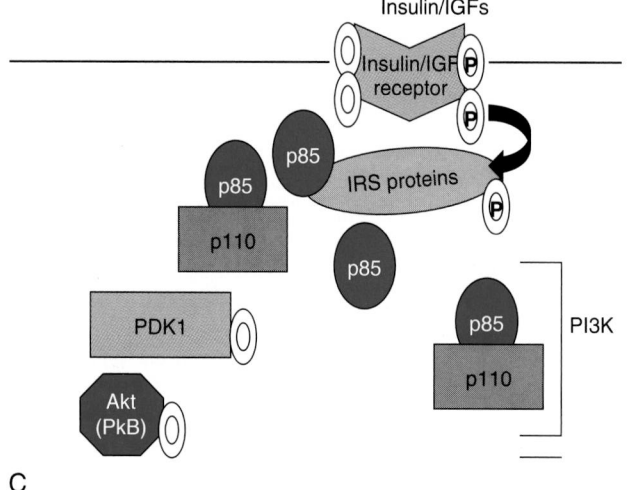

C

FIGURE 48-6. Schematic representation of the intracellular response to insulin. Insulin binding to its receptor results in autophosphorylation of the receptor on tyrosines. Subsequently, insulin-receptor substrates (IRS proteins) are phosphorylated resulting in phosphorylation of phosphatidylinositol-3-kinase (PI-3K). Following this step, "downstream" kinases, including PDK1 and Akt, are activated by phosphorylation leading to the multiple responses of insulin. Available information indicates that uremia impairs activation of PI-3K.

Subsequently, a group of molecules known as signal transducers and activators of transcription (STATs) are phosphorylated and translocate to the nucleus to regulate transcription or transactivation of growth hormone–dependent genes.[261] Schaefer and colleagues found a 75% reduction in phosphorylation of the JAK2, STAT1, SAT3, and STAT 5 protein in lysates of liver tissue isolated from uremic rats and a twofold increase in the corresponding suppressor protein (suppressor of cytokine signaling-2, or SOCS-2).[258] This leads to the conclusion that there is an impairment in the intracellular signal transduction pathway of growth hormone and this defect contributes to the growth hormone resistance found in patients with CRF.

Uremic patients are often intolerant of cold temperatures and have a lower body temperature; the incidence of goiters is also high. The development of a goiter could be related to the failure to excrete iodides, but even without a goiter, dialysis patients often have subnormal plasma levels of total T_4, T_3, and free thyroid hormones plus higher levels of thyroid-stimulating hormone (TSH), and decreased conversion of T_4 to T_3 in nonthyroid tissues.[262] This pattern is reminiscent of the euthyroid sick syndrome that is characterized by end-organ resistance to T_3. In uremia, the basal rate of oxygen

uptake is unaffected by uremia but does not rise normally after administration of T_3. There is documented impaired peripheral conversion of T_4 to T_3 in nonthyroid tissues, although the pituitary-hypothalamic axis appears to be intact. Thus, there is evidence of abnormal thyroid metabolism at several levels in uremia, including inefficient iodination of thyroid hormone precursors in the thyroid gland, depressed T_4-to-T_3 conversion in nonthyroid tissues, and a suppressed thermogenic response to T_3. It has been suggested that depressed T_4-to-T_3 conversion is related to circulating aromatic inhibitors such as indoxyl sulfate and 3-carboxy-4-methyl-5-propyl-2-furanpropionic acid.[175]

Conservation of body weight is dependent upon a complex interplay between energy expenditure and caloric intake and this interplay is subject to several neuroendocrine factors. Specific hormones act rapidly to regulate food intake at each meal or act more slowly to promote body fat stores (Fig. 48-7). Long-term regulators such as insulin and leptin are released into the bloodstream and inhibit food intake while increasing energy expenditure from body fat stores.[263] As fat stores decline, the levels of insulin and leptin decrease to conserve energy and there is a surge in appetite. In contrast, short-term regulatory factors rise and fall quickly in

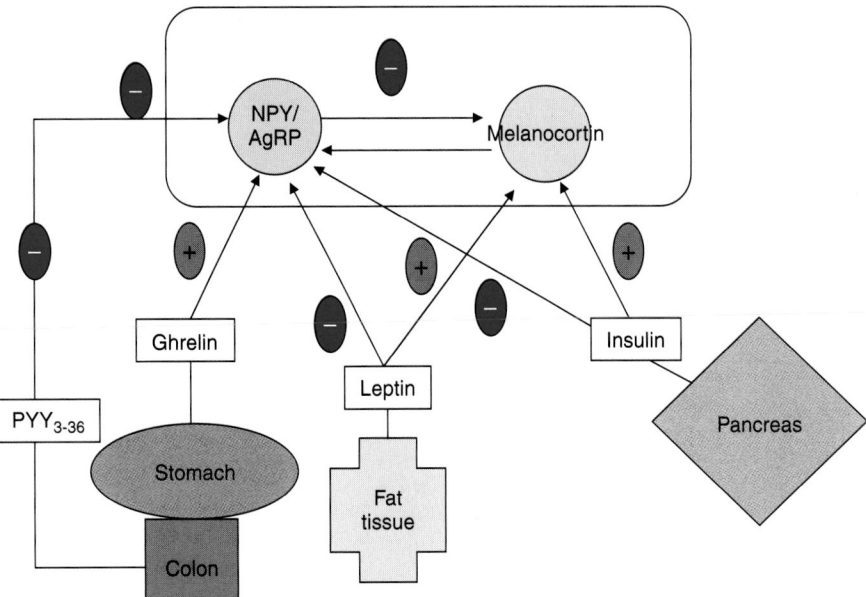

FIGURE 48-7. Hormonal and neural pathways regulating appetite. Appetite-suppressing hormones, leptin and PYY$_{3-36}$, decrease appetite by inhibiting neurons that produce neuropeptide Y (NPY) and agouti-related peptide (AgRP). Both leptin and insulin can also stimulate melanocortin-producing neurons to produce melanocortin, which can also inhibit NPY- and AgRP-producing neurons. Hormones that stimulate specific neurons that can suppress appetite are indicated by plus signs. The hormones that inhibit neurons that can stimulate appetite are indicated by minus signs.

the blood; ghrelin[264] stimulates appetite whenever the stomach is empty whereas cholecystokinin[265] suppresses appetite following a meal. There are also "intermediate" levels of control. For example, in response to food being eaten, PYY$_{3-36}$ is secreted by endocrine cells lining the distal small bowel and the result is inhibition of appetite for up to 12 hours.[266] PYY$_{3-36}$ circulates to the arcuate nucleus of the hypothalamus and is bound to two types of neurons that control food intake. One type of neuron stimulates the appetite by releasing neuropeptide Y; the other type of neuron produces melanocortin peptide to inhibit eating.[267, 268] The neuropeptide Y neurons also produce the agouti-related peptide[269] which blocks neuronal melanocortin receptors, resulting in stimulation of the appetite. It appears that there is an interplay between the two types of neurons such that when one is stimulated, the other is suppressed. PYY$_{3-36}$, like leptin and insulin, interacts with neurons that express neuropeptide Y and inhibit release of this hormone, as well as agouti-related peptide.[266]

Leptin and neuropeptide Y play important roles in determining food and energy expenditure. Leptin is produced in adipose cells,[263] in the placenta,[270] and in skeletal muscle,[263] and it serves as a signal to "inform" the brain, via a hypothalamus-mediated mechanism, of available energy stores. When fat stores are large, the level of leptin is high and acts to suppress appetite,[263] but changes in serum leptin levels can occur within hours of fasting and are out of proportion to corresponding changes in body fat.[271] Leptin is regulated by various hormones, including glucocorticoids,[272] insulin,[273] and proinflammatory cytokines[274] (e.g., interleukin-1 and TNF-α). Moreover, testosterone and thyroid hormones decrease leptin synthesis.[275] A decline in leptin levels yields a reciprocal increase in the production of neuropeptide Y by the hypothalamus which stimulates appetite. When body fat rises, leptin production, as well as melanocyte-stimulating hormone release, is stimulated.[268] Thus, there are multiple functional changes that should counteract obesity, including

a reduction in food intake because of decreased appetite plus an increase in energy expenditure. At a cellular level, leptin activates the PI3-K signal transduction pathway which is a key step in insulin signaling[276] and inhibits pancreatic insulin secretion[277] to suppress lipid accumulation in fat cells. Leptin also stimulates endothelial cell proliferation[278] and activates T cells,[279] and these properties may explain some of the problems associated with uremia; by promoting angiogenesis, leptin could improve energy expenditure through an increase in blood flow that facilitates heat loss and lipid oxidation, and a reduction in leptin may increase susceptibility to infection by reducing T cell activation.

Because it is a small peptide, leptin is largely cleared by the kidney and with kidney damage, there is reduced net leptin extraction, leading to a fourfold rise in plasma leptin levels in patients with advanced renal failure. The physiologically relevant fraction of circulating leptin is the free level and hence variation in the amount of leptin bound to proteins could affect its function. Nonobese individuals have as much as 46% of leptin in the bound form, whereas obese patients have less than 20% bound. In contrast, uremic patients have nearly all their circulating leptin in the free form. Despite intensive investigation, the role of leptin in regulating fat mass or lean body mass is unsettled. For example, higher serum leptin levels have been associated with reduced protein intake and inversely correlated with indices of nutritional status such as serum albumin and body mass index in dialysis patients.[280] In CAPD patients, serum leptin levels were found to rise progressively in those patients suffering weight loss over time, whereas dialysis patients with the highest leptin-to-fat mass ratios had lower protein intakes and lower body mass indices.[281, 282] In short, the role of leptin promoting anorexia and weight loss in uremic patients has not been proved because even peritoneal dialysis and hemodialysis patients with normal body mass indices have high serum leptin levels.[283] This pattern suggests there is dysregulation of the normal adipocyte-hypothalamic-leptin axis. Alternatively, high leptin levels may result from excessive leptin production that is stimulated by other hormones, such as insulin and glucocorticoids (both of which are elevated in uremia). Interestingly, restoration of renal function results in a decrease in serum plasma leptin concentrations to control levels.[284] This provides further evidence of a cause-and-effect relationship between impaired renal function and abnormal leptin metabolism.

Leptin also can stimulate TGF-α1 and type IV collagen production in glomerular endothelial cells, as well as their proliferation.[285] In mesangial cells exposed to leptin, there is increased glucose transport, type 1 collagen production, and sysnthesis of the TGF-α2 receptor.[286] Because leptin increases extracellular matrix production in both cell types, it has been suggested that the leptin-induced production of TGF-α1 by glomerular endothelial cells permits sensitized mesangial cells to secrete the collagen that accumulates as extracellular matrix. In support of this hypothesis, infusion of leptin into normal rats for 3 weeks fostered the development of focal glomerulosclerosis and resulted in proteinuria[285] (possibly related to production of reactive oxidation species). Besides these potentially pathologic consequences, leptin may even affect function of the normal kidney. For example, leptin can promote natriuresis and diuresis in rats,[287] but these responses are blunted in spontaneously hypertensive rats and are restored when sympathetic tone to the kidney is interrupted. These data were interpreted to suggest that leptin suppresses adrenergic activity to countermand natriuretic activity under normal conditions. Taken together, these data suggest that leptin may play a pathophysiologic role in the kidney.

The host of endocrine abnormalities present in uremia highlights the complex nature of defects in cellular metabolism that are induced by kidney failure. Specific mediators or toxins that cause these defects remain unknown, and exactly how intracellular signaling is impaired by uremia is unknown.

ION TRANSPORT ABNORMALITIES IN UREMIA

Abnormal regulation of ion transport could change the electrical potential of cell membranes as well as the intracellular ion composition. These changes in turn could affect the body's metabolism of substrates that require transmembrane ion gradients for their uptake or could activate specific pathways that change the metabolism of the cell.

Abnormal Active Sodium/Potassium Transport in Erythrocytes

In the 1960s, ion homeostasis in uremia was shown to be abnormal in 25% of patients with end-stage renal disease.[288] Red blood Cell (RBC) Na^+ content was high, whereas RBC Na^+,K^+-ATPase activity was reduced. The patients expressing these abnormalities were clinically more ill than patients with a normal RBC Na^+ content. The link to uremia was established when both the RBC Na^+ concentration and Na^+,K^+-ATPase activity were improved by hemodialysis, plus the finding that RBCs from normal subjects acquire a similar defect in active cation transport when they are incubated

in sera obtained from uremic patients.[289, 290] These original observations were extended when leukocytes and skeletal muscle from uremic subjects were studied.[86, 291] Because these abnormalities were found in a variety of organs, uremia could be characterized by a circulating inhibitor of Na^+,K^+-ATPase activity.

Virtually all reports suggest that the abnormalities in Na^+,K^+-ATPase activity improve with long-term, aggressive dialysis.[290, 292, 293] Reversibility of the defect suggests the following mechanisms: (1) accumulated toxins inhibit the Na^+ pump; (2) uremia could change the lipid composition of cell membranes, causing a secondary reduction in pump activity; (3) uremia could reduce the action of hormones that stimulate Na^+ pump activity (e.g., insulin); and (4) the Na^+ pump could be indirectly inhibited by changes in the activity of other ion transporters. None of these potential explanations is mutually exclusive.

Toxins as Endogenous Inhibitors of Na^+,K^+-ATPase

The mature RBC cannot respond to a higher intracellular Na^+ or to a circulating inhibitor by synthesizing additional pumps. This implies that circulating factors must change the activity of the Na^+ pump and is consistent with the finding that hemodialysis increases ouabain-sensitive ^{18}Rb influx without affecting ^3H-ouabain binding.[290] Kelly and colleagues[293] extended these observations and showed that hemodialysis-related changes in ouabain-sensitive Na^+ efflux are correlated with changes in intracellular Na^+ concentration.

Putative Na^+ pump inhibitors have been detected by measuring Na^+,K^+-ATPase activity in vitro or cross-reactivity with antibodies directed against cardiac glycosides.[294-296] Both ouabain and a compound with properties that are indistinguishable from digoxin have been isolated from human sources, but certain observations suggest that the uremic factor is not a cardiac glycoside.[297-299] For example, digoxin-like immunoreactive factors (DLIFs) are more highly protein-bound than digoxin or ouabain and second, the degree of Na^+ pump inhibition is not correlated with the natriuretic or pressor activities exerted by uremic factors.[299, 300] Finally, the synthetic pathways required to produce cardiac glycosides are specific to plant cells and have not been detected in mammalian cells.[301] Other types of molecules have been suggested. Gallice and colleagues[302] obtained ultrafiltrates of plasma from uremic patients and urine from normal subjects and were able to separate a non-ouabain-like inhibitor of the Na^+ pump. This inhibitor differed from ouabain because it bound to the Na^+,K^+-ATPase even when magnesium and sodium phosphate were not added. The inhibitor did not compete with potassium or ATP for binding to the enzyme but did compete with sodium. The authors concluded that the inhibitor acted intracellularly and that it was therefore different from ouabain or ouabain-like compounds which act extracellularly and compete with potassium for binding to the enzyme.

Abnormalities of Membrane Composition and Function

An important fraction of the digitalis-like activity found in normal human plasma is present in the polar lipid fraction and includes nonesterified fatty acids (NEFAs) and certain lysophospholipids,[303-307] suggesting that abnormalities in the plasma membrane of cells from uremic patients could change transmembrane cation flux. Kelly and colleagues[304] demonstrated that a large dialysis-induced decrease in the NEFA content of RBC membranes results in an immediate improvement in ouabain-sensitive Na^+ efflux. When there was at least a 10% drop in RBC NEFA, the improvement in Na^+ pump activity was highly correlated with the reduction in membrane NEFA content. Notably, simply incubating the RBCs of dialysis patients with delipidated albumin not only reduced membrane NEFA but also improved Na^+,K^+-ATPase activity. Reduced RBC membrane fluidity has been described in uremia; it was ascribed to a decline in the molar ratio of phosphatidylcholine to sphingomyelin.[308]

Hormonal Milieu and Erythropoiesis in Uremia

Decreased RBC Na^+ pump activity in uremia could be due to impaired synthesis of Na^+,K^+-ATPase. Cheng and associates[309] found that patients with CRF tended to have fewer Na^+ pumps in the youngest RBC cells. Uremia-induced impairment of protein synthesis or local factors that suppress protein synthesis or translocation of Na^+ pumps into the membrane could account for their findings. For example, insulin resistance could affect Na^+ pump activity.[310] Uremia also reduces the activity of thyroid hormone, mineralocorticoids, or catecholamines, and these changes affect active Na^+ and K^+ transport in other tissues.[308, 310-312] For example, thyroid hormone is a major endocrinologic factor influencing the synthesis of Na^+,K^+-ATPase as thyroid hormone induces the up-regulation of Na^+,K^+-ATPase pumps resulting in the more rapid clearance of K^+ from the plasma. Kubota and Ingbar[313] infused potassium into nephrectomized hyperthyroid rats and found that the expected increase in serum K^+ was smaller compared to a comparable infusion of potassium into euthyroid, nephrectomized rats. Conversely, hypothyroid nephrectomized rats became hyperkalemic more rapidly with the same intravenous dose of potassium.

Abnormalities in Other Erythrocyte Cation Transporters

Defects in bumetanide-sensitive $Na^+/K^+/2Cl^-$ cotransport, Na^+/Li^+ exchanger, and depressed Ca^{2+}-ATPase also have been detected in RBCs of patients with CRF. The clinical relevance of these findings is unknown but investigators have found virtually no $Na^+/K^+/2Cl^-$ activity associated with experimental chronic renal insufficiency.[292, 293] The link to uremia is found in the report of Kelly and colleagues[293] who reported that hemodialysis leads to an acute increase in $Na^+/K^+/2Cl^-$ cotransport rates. Abnormalities in Na^+/Li^+ transport have been associated with the development of hypertension, whereas changes in the kinetics of the Na^+/Li^+ exchanger are related to uremia-induced changes in a thiol group, and both defects are at least temporarily improved with hemodialysis.[314] Finally, Zidek and colleagues[315] observed that intracellular Ca^{2+} is high in RBCs from hemodialysis patients related to depression in both basal and maximal Ca^{2+}-ATPase activity.

Similar to other transport systems, the abnormalities could be reproduced in RBCs from normal subjects by incubating the cells in plasma from uremic patients. Lindner and colleagues[316] characterized a potential uremic toxin as a 3000-D, heat-stable, and protease-resistant dialyzable inhibitor from uremic plasma filtrates that directly inhibited the RBC membrane Ca^{2+} pump. This is of interest because Soldati and co-workers[317] demonstrated that voltage-sensitive Ca^{2+} influx is significantly reduced in RBCs from hemodialysis patients and the reduction was correlated with an increased incidence of ventricular arrhythmias. The authors concluded that myocardial dysfunction and ventricular excitability in uremic hemodialysis patients could be related to alterations of Ca^{2+} transport.

The marked ion transport abnormalities found in earlier reports depend on inadequate dialysis. This raises the possibility that the adequacy of dialysis could be assessed by examining Na^+,K^+-ATPase activity, but this would require prospective studies.

Abnormal Membrane Potential in Skeletal Muscle

Transmembrane ion flux has also been studied extensively in the skeletal muscle of uremic patients. Knochel and colleagues observed a significantly lower potential of the muscle membrane in patients with a creatinine clearance below 6 mL/minute.[86] The defect in Na^+ pump activity was accompanied by increased intracellular Na^+ and Cl^-, and a low K^+ concentration. Notably, the resting muscle membrane potential returned to normal with regular hemodialysis, or when a less frequent dialysis schedule was accompanied by a low-protein diet supplemented with essential amino acids.[84] Similar benefical changes in leukocyte Na^+,K^+-ATPase activity induced by dietary protein restriction were reported by Aparicio and colleagues.[318] They reported that impaired Na^+,K^+-ATPase activity was fully reversed by treating patients with a low-protein diet (0.3 g/kg/day) plus an amino acid–keto acid supplement. Thus, abnormalities in membrane ion flux result from the accumulation of dialyzable uremic toxins derived from dietary protein.

Abnormalities in Non-Ion Transporters

Recent work suggests that the urea transporter may be important in transporting urea in other organs besides the kidney.[319] In chronic renal insufficiency, there is loss of the urine concentrating ability which is thought to be largely due to a major reduction in the number of urea transporters per nephron segment.[320] Interestingly, changes in the expression of urea transporter appear to be organ-specific in uremia. For example, there is a marked reduction of urea transporters in the brain as well as the kidney.[320] On the other hand, there is up-regulation of urea transporters in the heart and liver.[321, 322] In the latter case, some of the changes in heart may be linked to hypertension, but the explanation for changes in urea transporter expression in liver is unknown. It is possible that these changes have clinical relevance. For example, a lower number of urea transporters in the brain of patients may contribute to the syndrome of brain edema occurring with the dialysis disequilibrium syndrome. An up-regulation of the urea transporter number in hepatocytes may allow these cells to increase ureagenesis and thereby reduce the accumulation of ammonium in patients with uremia.

ION TRANSPORT ABNORMALITIES IN EXPERIMENTAL UREMIA

Defective Na^+,K^+-ATPase activity and abnormalities associated with these defects were noted in several organs when rats with ARF were examined.[323] Fraser and colleagues[324] measured Na^+ transport in synaptosomes obtained from the cerebral cortex and found a substantial increase in Na^+ uptake into synaptosomes from acutely uremic rats relative to control animals. Moreover, both the initial and maximal rates of Na^+/Ca^{2+} exchange and Ca^{2+}-ATPase activity in cerebral cortex synaptosomes were higher in those isolated from acutely uremic rats compared to control rats.[325] As both pathways contribute to Ca^{2+} efflux from normal neurons, finding an enhanced extrusion rate could contribute to the finding that there is a higher extracellular concentration of Ca^{2+} in brain associated with ARF. In contrast to Ca^{2+}, Verkman and Fraser[326] detected no difference in the synaptosomal permeability to water or urea, indicating that the abnormalities in Ca^{2+} flux were not due simply to increased permeability but reflected an underlying abnormality in ion transport.

Intracellular changes in Ca^{2+} could also affect signaling processes in other organs. Massry and Smogorzewski[232] studied chronically uremic rats that had been subjected to parathyroidectomy or treated with verapamil to bring intracellular Ca^{2+} levels into the normal range. Among the abnormalities corrected by normalizing intracellular Ca^{2+} levels are impaired insulin secretion,[327] decreased Na^+,K^+-ATPase activity in cardiac myocytes,[328] adipocytes, and pancreatic islets,[235, 329, 330] and impaired cardiac function.[331] Although these experiments do not define the abnormality in signaling pathways caused by uremia, they provide evidence that defects in the maintenance of ion homeostasis contribute to the pathophysiology of uremia.

Inhibition of monovalent cation flux and accumulation of intracellular Ca^{2+} has been proposed as a cause of hypertension.[332] For example, inhibition of Na^+,K^+-ATPase activity in vascular smooth muscle cells of arteriolar resistance vessels could cause a rise in cytosolic Ca^{2+} by reducing Ca^{2+} efflux through the Na^+/Ca^{2+}-exchanger.[333] The hypothesis is that an Na^+,K^+-ATPase inhibitor causes enhanced smooth muscle vasoconstriction to contribute to the high prevalence of hypertension in CRF.[332]

Decreased Na^+,K^+-ATPase activity is present in other organs of uremic rats. Druml and colleagues[334] found decreased ouabain-sensitive ^{86}Rb influx in skeletal muscle and adipocytes from uremic rats. As expected, the intracellular Na^+ content was increased in both muscle and adipocytes, and there was reduced furosemide-sensitive $Na^+/K^+/2Cl^-$ cotransport. Surprisingly, the mechanism of decreased ^{86}Rb intake differed in the two tissues. The number of Na^+ pumps as assessed by ^3H-ouabain binding was reduced in proportion to the decline in Na^+ flux in adipocytes, but ^3H-ouabain binding was not affected by uremia in skeletal muscle. It was concluded that there is reduced Na^+ pump activity in skeletal muscle,

whereas the pump turnover rate in adipocytes was reduced by uremia. In support of this formulation, incubation of muscle from normal rats with uremic sera led to an immediate drop in ouabain-sensitive ^{86}Rb uptake. In contrast, adipocytes did not acquire loss of Na^+ pump function when exposed to uremic sera. The relevance of these observations is that impairment of Na^+ pump activity can affect the uptake of other compounds such as amino acids and, possibly, other nutrients.

Bonilla and colleagues[335] proposed that the mechanism responsible for decreased Na^+,K^+-ATPase activity in skeletal muscle involves suppressed synthesis of the Na^+ pump. They found a reduced level of the mRNAs encoding Na^+,K^+-ATPase subunits in proportion to the degree of inhibition of Na^+ pump activity. Greiber and colleagues[336] pursued this question by measuring the levels of Na^+,K^+-ATPase subunits by Western blot testing and the mRNAs encoding subunits in skeletal muscle, adipose tissue, and liver of chronically uremic rats. There was no consistent decrease in either the mRNAs or the protein content that could explain impaired Na^+,K^+-ATPase activity. These findings were confirmed by da Silva and colleagues.[337] Thus, endogenous inhibitors of Na^+ pump activity are the major mechanism accounting for impaired Na^+,K^+-ATPase activity and increased intracellular Na^+ in muscle of uremic animals.

There also are abnormalities of Na^+,K^+-ATPase in heart muscle.[334] In contrast to skeletal muscle, there were no abnormalities in ouabain-sensitive ^{86}Rb uptake or intracellular Na^+ in heart muscle of uremic rats. All was not normal, however, because ^3H-ouabain binding in the myocardium was reduced 45% in CRF.

Metabolic processes in bone and muscle are sensitive to metabolic acidosis. This is important because abnormalities in cation transport could extend to the mechanisms that regulate intracellular pH.[16] For example, there are changes in the function of the Na^+/H^+ antiporter, at least in thymocytes and hepatocytes of uremic rats.[50, 338] Although the resting intracellular pH in thymocytes of uremic rats was normal, there was decreased activity of the Na^+/H^+ antiporter in response to cell swelling, as well as decreased Na^+,K^+-ATPase activity.[50] On the other hand, no consistent defect in pH regulation can be detected in the muscles of uremic rats. Bailey and colleagues[49] used magnetic resonance techniques to measure the cell pH in muscles of anesthetized rats with acute or chronic metabolic acidosis or with the acidosis of CRF. There was a small but statistically significant lowering of muscle pH in rats with chronic, but not acute, induction of acidosis. Despite the presence of a number of metabolic abnormalities in muscle, there was no consistent defect in muscle cell pH of rats with chronic uremia. In addition, there was no difference in the recovery of muscle cell pH following induction of metabolic acidosis. For this reason, changes in muscle cell pH cannot be a direct signal causing muscle protein degradation in uremia (see earlier discussion).

In attempting to understand if there is pH regulation of kidney cells, cultured cells have been examined. In cultured kidney cells exposed to an acid environment, cell pH does decrease and there is activation of protein kinase pathways.[339] Activation of tubular cells by incubating them in acidified media was associated with increased phosphorylation of unidentified cytosolic proteins of the 65- and 120-kD size via a specific tyrosine kinase, c-Src. This same kinase functions as a proto-oncogene that is activated when mitosis is stimulated.[340] Although these reactions could be involved in stimulating the growth of kidney cells, observations from cultured cells will have to be confirmed in the intact organ. For example, there is evidence that intracellular pH of cultured muscle cells exposed to an acidified media falls, but as noted above, there is no detectable decrease in the muscle of rats with uremia.[47, 49, 341] For these reasons, it is unclear if the mechanisms identified in cultured kidney cells can be extrapolated to muscle.

The loss of kidney function is also characterized by changes in secretion of drugs by kidney tubule cells. This may contribute to some of the alterations in pharmacokinetics associated with renal failure. Experimentally, renal failure is likened to changes in ATP-dependent drug transporters, particularly P-glycoprotein in the renal tubules.[342] Because expression of specific P-glycoproteins in polarized epithelial cells can induce transport of both the small (type I) and bulky (type II) cationic drugs, changes in P-glycoprotein expression due to renal failure could also contribute to alterations in pharmacokinetics.[342] Similarly, loss of kidney function could affect the expression of the multidrug resistance protein-2 to cause drug resistance.[343] The transport of drugs from blood to urine involves the organic anion and cation transporters which utilize ATP or ion gradients to transport drugs (and other cations or anions) against a gradient and into the urine.[342-344] The influence of kidney failure on drug distribution in other organs may be linked to similar mechanisms, as Laouari and colleagues[345] reported that both multidrug resistance protein-2 and P-glycoprotein were expressed at a lower level in liver and kidney. They suggested this change was linked to an adaptive response to circulating toxins.

In summary, the functions of a number of transport systems are changed in response to uremia. The causes of defects in ion transport are multifactorial, but tissue-specific changes in Na^+-pump number and activity occur in conditions other than uremia.[311] Besides defining the mechanism causing changes in ion transport, a major question is whether any change contributes to the syndrome of uremia. The answer seems to be yes, because the decrease in ^3H-ouabain-sensitive ^{86}Rb influx rates in adipocytes is correlated directly with impaired Na^+-dependent amino acid uptake (Fig. 48-8),[294] and the defect in muscle Na^+,K^+-ATPase contributes to muscle fatigue.[86] Second, experimental evidence strongly links a high cellular Ca^{2+} concentration with metabolic disorders.[232] Finally, abnormal depolarization of the plasma membrane in skeletal muscle, and probably other tissues as well, suggests that many of the metabolic characteristics of the uremic syndrome might be direct consequences of a generalized defect in monovalent cation transport.

REFERENCES

1. Piorry PA: *In* Piorry PALD (ed): Traite des Alterations du Sang, chap 12. Paris, Bury and J.B. Balliere, 1840.
2. Richet G: Early history of uremia. Kidney Int 33:1013-1015, 1998.
3. Maroni BJ, Steinman T, Mitch WE: A method for estimating nitrogen intake of patients with chronic renal failure. Kidney Int 27:58-65, 1985.
4. Masud T, Manatunga A, Cotsonis G, Mitch WE: The precision of estimating protein intake of patients with chronic renal failure. Kidney Int 62:1750-1756, 2002.
5. Richards P, Brown CL: Urea metabolism in an azotemic woman with normal renal function. Lancet 2:207-209, 1975.
6. Simenhoff ML, Burke JF, Sankkonen JJ, et al: Amine metabolism and the small bowel in uremia. Lancet 2:818-822, 1976.
7. Bergstrom J: Why are dialysis patients malnourished? Am J Kidney Dis 26:229-241, 1995.
8. Schoots AC, Verheggen TPEM, DeVries PMJM, Evaeraerts FM: Ultraviolet absorbing organic ions in uremic serum separated by capillary zone electrophoresis and quantification of hippuric acid. Clin Chem 36:435-440, 1990.
9. Simenhoff ML, Saukkonen JJ, Burke JF, et al: Bacterial populations of the small bowel in uremia. Nephron 22:63-68, 1978.
10. Lascelles PT, Taylor WH: The effect upon tissue respiration in vitro of metabolites which accumulate in uremic coma. Clin Sci (Colch) 31:403-413, 1966.
11. Kraus LM, Miyamura S, Pecha BR, Kraus AP: Carbamylation of hemoglobin in uremic patients determined by antibody specific for homocitrulline (carbamylated e-N-lysine). Mol Immunol 28:459-463, 1991.
12. Kraus LM, Jones MR, Kraus AP: Essential carbamoyl-amino acids in vivo in patients with end-stage renal disease managed by continuous ambulatory peritoneal dialysis: Isolation, identification and quantitation. J Lab Clin Med 131:425-431, 1998.
13. Monnier VM, Sell DR, Nagaraj RH, et al: Maillard reaction–mediated molecular damage to extracellular matrix and other tissue proteins in diabetes, aging, and uremia. Diabetes 41 (suppl 2):36-41, 1992.
14. Mitch WE, Wilcox CS: Disorders of body fluids, sodium and potassium in chronic renal failure. Am J Med 72:536-550, 1982.
15. Bush A: The lungs in uremia. Semin Respir Med 9:273-282, 1988.
16. Bailey JL, Mitch WE: Metabolic acidosis as a uremic toxin. Semin Nephrol 16:160-166, 1996.
17. Goodman AD, Lemann J, Lennon EJ, Relman AJ: Production, excretion, and net balance of fixed acid in patients with renal acidosis. J Clin Invest 44:495-506, 1965.
18. Spriet LL, Matsos CG, Peters SJ, et al: Effects of acidosis on rat muscle metabolism and performance during heavy exercise. Am J Physiol 248:C337-C347, 1985.
19. Litzgow JR, Lemann J, Lennon EJ: The effect of treatment of acidosis on calcium balance in patients with chronic azotemic renal failure. J Clin Invest 46:280-286, 1967.

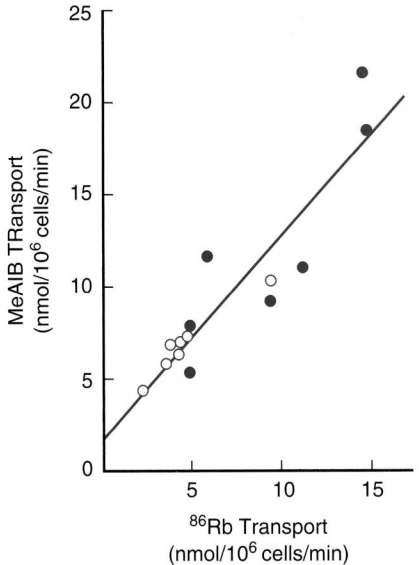

FIGURE 48-8. The rate of uptake of a nonmetabolized amino acid probe specific for the Na^+-dependent amino acid uptake pathway system **A**, MeAIB, is plotted against the ouabain-sensitive influx of ^{86}Rb into adipocytes from both uremic (*open circles*) and pair-fed, sham-operated control animals (*closed circles*). The correlation between these two parameters is highly significant ($r = .91$; $P < .001$). (From Druml W, Kelly RA, May RC, Mitch WE: Abnormal cation flux in uremia: Mechanism in adipocytes and skeletal muscle from uremic rats. J Clin Invest 81:1197, 1988.)

20. Bushinsky DA, Lam BC, Nespeca R, et al: Decreased bone bicarbonate content in response to metabolic, but not respiratory, acidosis. Am J Physiol 256:F530-F536, 1993.

21. DeFronzo RA, Beckles AD: Glucose intolerance following chronic metabolic acidosis in man. Am J Physiol 236:E328-E334, 1979.

22. May RC, Hara Y, Kelly RA, et al: Branched-chain amino acid metabolism in rat muscle: Abnormal regulation in acidosis. Am J Physiol 252:E712-E718, 1987.

23. May RC, Kelly RA, Mitch WE: Metabolic acidosis stimulation protein degradation in rat muscle by a glucocorticoid-dependent mechanism. J Clin Invest 77:614-621, 1986.

24. May RC, Kelly RA, Mitch WE: Mechanisms for defects in muscle protein metabolism in rats with chronic uremia: The influence of metabolic acidosis. J Clin Invest 79:1099-1103, 1987.

25. May RC, Bailey JL, Mitch WE, et al: Glucocorticoids and acidosis stimulate protein and amino acid catabolism in vivo. Kidney Int 49:679-683, 1996.

26. England BK, Greiber S, Mitch WE, et al: Rat muscle branched-chain ketoacid dehydrogenase activity and mRNAs increase with extracellular acidemia. Am J Physiol 268:C1395-C1400, 1995.

27. Price SR, Reaich D, Marinovic AC, et al: Mechanisms contributing to muscle wasting in acute uremia: Activation of amino acid catabolism. J Am Soc Nephrol 9:439-443, 1998.

28. Hara Y, May RC, Kelly RA, Mitch WE: Acidosis, not azotemia, stimulates branched-chain amino acid catabolism in uremic rats. Kidney Int 32:808-814, 1987.

29. Bergstrom J, Alvestrand A, Furst P: Plasma and muscle free amino acids in maintenance hemodialysis patients without protein malnutrition. Kidney Int 38:108-114, 1990.

30. Lofberg E, Wernerman J, Anderstam B, Bergstrom J: Correction of metabolic acidosis in dialysis patients increases branched-chain and total essential amino acid levels in muscle. Clin Nephrol 48:230-237, 1997.

31. May RC, Masud T, Logue B, et al: Chronic metabolic acidosis accelerates whole body proteolysis and leucine oxidation in awake rats. Kidney Int 41:1535-1542, 1992.

32. Mitch WE, Medina R, Greiber S, et al: Metabolic acidosis stimulates muscle protein degradation by activating the ATP-dependent pathway involving ubiquitin and proteasomes. J Clin Invest 93:2127-2133, 1994.

33. Bailey JL, Wang X, England BK, et al: The acidosis of chronic renal failure activates muscle proteolysis in rats by augmenting transcription of genes encoding proteins of the ATP-dependent, ubiquitin-proteasome pathway. J Clin Invest 97:1447-1453, 1996.

34. Motil KJ, Matthews DE, Bier DM, et al: Whole-body leucine and lysine metabolism: Response to dietary protein intake in young men. Am J Physiol 240:E712-E721, 1981.

35. Goodship THJ, Mitch WE, Hoerr RA, et al: Adaptation to low-protein diets in renal failure: Leucine turnover and nitrogen balance. J Am Soc Nephrol 1:66-75, 1990.

36. Papadoyannakis NJ, Stefanides CJ, McGeown M: The effect of the correction of metabolic acidosis on nitrogen and protein balance of patients with chronic renal failure. Am J Clin Nutr 40:623-627, 1984.

37. Williams B, Hattersley J, Layward E, Walls J: Metabolic acidosis and skeletal muscle adaptation to low protein diets in chronic uremia. Kidney Int 40:779-786, 1991.

38. Reaich D, Channon SM, Scrimgeour CM, Goodship THJ: Ammonium Chloride–induced acidosis increases protein breakdown and amino acid oxidation in humans. Am J Physiol 263:E735-E739, 1992.

39. Reaich D, Channon SM, Scrimgeour CM, et al: Correction of acidosis in humans with CRF decreases protein degradation and amino acid oxidation. Am J Physiol 265:E230-E235, 1993.

40. Stein A, Moorhouse J, Iles-Smith H, Baker R, et al: Role of an improvement in acid-base status and nutrition in CAPD patients. Kidney Int 52:1089-1095, 1997.

41. Graham KA, Reaich D, Channon SM, et al: Correction of acidosis in CAPD decreases whole body protein degradation. Kidney Int 49:1396-1400, 1996.

42. Pickering WP, Price SR, Bircher G, et al: Nutrition in CAPD: Serum bicarbonate and the ubiquitin-proteasome system in muscle. Kidney Int 61:1286-1292, 2002.

43. Graham KA, Reaich D, Channon SM, et al: Correction of acidosis in hemodialysis decreases whole-body protein degradation. J Am Soc Nephrol 8:632-637, 1997.

44. Price SR, England BK, Bailey JL, et al: Acidosis and glucocorticoids concomitantly increase ubiquitin and proteasome subunit mRNAs in rat muscle. Am J Physiol 267:C955-C960, 1994.

45. Garibotto G, Russo R, Sofia A, et al: Skeletal muscle protein synthesis and degradation in patients with chronic renal failure. Kidney Int 45:1432-1439, 1994.

46. Himmelfarb J, Holbrook D, McMonagle E, et al: Kt/V, nutritional parameters, serum cortisol, and insulin growth factor-I levels and patient outcome in hemodialysis. Am J Kidney Dis 24:473-479, 1994.

47. Isozaki Y, Mitch WE, England BK, Price SR: Interaction between glucocorticoids and acidification results in stimulation of proteolysis and mRNAs of proteins encoding the ubiquitin-proteasome pathway in BC3H-1 myocytes. Proc Natl Acad Sci U S A 93:1967-1971, 1996.

48. Yamaji Y, Moe OW, Miller RT, Alpern RJ: Acid activation of immediate early genes in renal epithelial cells. J Clin Invest 94:1297-1303, 1994.

49. Bailey JL, England BK, Long RC, et al: Experimental acidemia and muscle cell pH in chronic acidosis and renal failure. Am J Physiol 269:C706-C712, 1995.

50. Greiber S, O'Neill WC, Mitch WE: Impaired cation transport in thymocytes of rats with chronic uremia includes the Na^+/H^+ antiporter. J Am Soc Nephrol 5:1689-1696, 1995.

51. Wang X, Jurkovitz C, Price SR: Regulation of branched-chain ketoacid dehydrogenase flux by extracellular pH and glucocorticoids. Am J Physiol 272:C2031-C2036, 1997.

52. Mitch WE, Goldberg AL: Mechanisms of muscle wasting: The role of the ubiquitin-proteasome system. N Engl J Med 335:1897-1905, 1996.

53. Conley SB, Rose GM, Robson AM, Bier DM: Effects of dietary intake and hemodialysis on protein turnover in uremic children. Kidney Int 17:837-846, 1980.

54. Movilli E, Zani R, Carli O, et al: Correction of metabolic acidosis increases serum albumin concentration and decreases kinetically evaluated protein intake in hemodialysis patients: A prospective study. Nephrol Dial Transplant 13:1719-1722, 1998.

55. DeFronzo RA, Alvestrand A, Smith D, Hendler R: Insulin resistance in uremia. J Clin Invest 67:563-568, 1981.

56. Gelfand RA, Barrett EJ: Effect of physiologic hyperinsulinemia on skeletal muscle protein synthesis and breakdown in man. J Clin Invest 80:1-6, 1987.

57. Louard RJ, Fryburg DA, Gelfand RA, Barrett EJ: Insulin sensitivity of protein and glucose metabolism in human forearm skeletal muscle. J Clin Invest 90:2348-2354, 1992.

58. Mak RHK: Effect of metabolic acidosis on insulin action and secretion in uremia. Kidney Int 54:603-607, 1998.

59. Reaich D, Graham KA, Channon SM, et al: Insulin mediated changes in protein degradation and glucose utilization following correction of acidosis in humans with CRF. Am J Physiol 268:E121-E126, 1995.

60. Brungger M, Hulter HN, Krapf R: Effect of chronic metabolic acidosis on thyroid hormone homeostasis in humans. Am J Physiol 272:F648-F653, 1997.

61. Tawa NE, Goldberg AL: Protein and amino acid metabolism in muscle. In Engle AG, Franzini-Armstrong C (eds): Myology: Basic and Clinical. New York, 1994, pp 683-707.

62. Brungger M, Hulter HN, Krapf R: Effect of chronic metabolic acidosis on the growth hormone/IGF-1 endocrine axis: New cause of growth hormone insensitivity in humans. Kidney Int 51:216-221, 1997.

63. Challa A, Krieg RJ, Thabet MA, et al: Metabolic acidosis inhibits growth hormone secretion in rats: Mechanism of growth retardation. Am J Physiol 265:E547-E553, 1993.

64. Challa A, Chan W, Krieg RJ, et al: Effect of metabolic acidosis on the expression of insulin-like growth factor and growth hormone receptor. Kidney Int 44:1224-1227, 1993.

65. Green J, Maor G: Effect of metabolic acidosis on the growth hormone/IGF-1 endocrine axis in skeletal growth centers. Kidney Int 57:2258-2267, 2002.

66. Ding H, Gao X-L, Hirschberg R, et al: Impaired actions of insulin-like growth factor-1 on protein synthesis and degradation in skeletal muscle of rats with chronic renal failure: Evidence for a postreceptor defect. J Clin Invest 97:1064-1075, 1996.

67. Cecchin F, Ittoop O, Sinha MK, Caro JF: Insulin resistance in uremia: Insulin receptor kinase activity in liver and muscle from chronic uremic rats. Am J Physiol 254:E394-E401, 1988.

68. May RC, Clark AS, Goheer A, Mitch WE: Identification of specific defects in insulin-mediated muscle metabolism in acute uremia. Kidney Int 28:490-497, 1985.

69. Kraut JA, Mishler DR, Kurokawa K: Effect of colchicine and calcitonin on calcemic response to metabolic acidosis. Kidney Int 25:608-612, 1984.

70. Bushinsky DA, Frick KK: The effects of acid on bone. Curr Opin Nephrol Hypertens 9:369-379, 2000.

71. Lu K-C, Shieh S-D, Li B-L, et al: Rapid correction of metabolic acidosis in chronic renal failure: Effect on parathyroid hormone activity. Nephron 67:419-424, 1994.

72. Movilli E, Zani R, Carli O, et al: Direct effect of the correction of acidosis on plasma parathyroid hormone concentrations, calcium and phosphate in hemodialysis patients: A prospective study. Nephron 87:257-262, 2001.

73. Mak R: Effect of metabolic acidosis on hyperlipidemia in uremia. Pediatr Nephrol 13:891-893, 2002.

74. Bello-Ruess EN, Grady T, Mazundar E: Serum vanadium levels in chronic renal disease. Ann Intern Med 91:743 1978.

75. Zhang X, Cornelis R, DeKumpe J, et al: Accumulation of arsenic species in serum of patients with chronic renal disease. Clin Chem 42:1231-1237, 1996.

76. Balfour WE, Grantham JS, Glynn IM: Vanadate-stimulated natriuresis. Nature 275:768, 1978.

77. Clark AS, Mitch WE: Selectivity of the insulin-like actions of vanadate on glucose and protein metabolism in skeletal muscle. Biochem J 232:273-276, 1985.

78. Alfrey AC, LeGendre GR, Kaehny WD: The dialysis encephalopathy syndrome: Possible aluminum intoxication. N Engl J Med 294:184-189, 1976.

79. Plachot JJ, Cournot-Witmer G, Halpern S, et al: Bone ultrastructure and x-ray microanalysis of aluminum-intoxicated hemocdialysis patients. Kidney Int 25:796-803 1984.

80. Mahajan SK, Abbasi AA, Prasad AS, et al: Effect of oral zinc therapy on gonadal function in hemodialysis patients: A double-blind study. Ann Intern Med 97:357-361, 1982.

81. Beale LS: Kidney Diseases, Urinary Deposits and Calculous Disorders; their Nature and Treatment, 3rd ed. Phildelphia, Lindsay & Blakiston, 1869.

82. Lowrie EG, Laird NM, Parker TF, Sargent JA: The effect of hemodialysis prescription on patient morbidity. N Engl J Med 305:1176-1181, 1981.

83. Levine J, Bernard DB: The role of urea kinetic modeling, TACurea and Kt/V in achieving optimal dialysis: A critical reappraisal. Am J Kidney Dis 15:285-301, 1990.

84. Cotton JR, Knochel JP: Correction of uremic cellular injury with a protein-restricted, amino acid-supplemented diet. Am J Kidney Dis 5:233-238, 1985.

85. Bilbrey GL, Carter NW, White MG, et al: Potassium deficiency in chronic renal failure. Kidney Int 4:423-430, 1973.

86. Cotton JR, Woodward T, Carter NW, Knochel JP: Resting skeletal muscle membrane potential as an index of uremic toxicity. J Clin Invest 63:501-508, 1979.

87. Ikizler TA, Greene JH, Wingard RL, et al: Spontaneous dietary protein intake during progression of chronic renal failure. J Am Soc Nephrol 6:1386-1391, 1995.

88. Kopple JD, Levey AS, Greene T, et al: Effect of dietary protein restriction on nutritional status in the Modification of Diet in Renal Disease (MDRD) Study. Kidney Int 52:778-791, 1997.

89. Hakim RM, Lazarus JM: Initiation of dialysis. J Am Soc Nephrol 6:1319-1320, 1995.

90. Mehrotra R, Nolph KD: Treatment of advanced renal failure: Low-protein diets or timely initiation of dialysis. Kidney Int 58:1381-1388, 2000.

91. Hakim RM, Lazarus JM: Biochemical parameters in chronic renal failure. Am J Kidney Dis 9:238-247, 1988.

92. Traynor JP, Simpson K, Geddes CC, et al: Early initiation of dialysis fails to prolong survival in patients with end-stage renal failure. J Am Soc Nephrol 13:2125-2132, 2002.

93. Mitch WE: Malnutrition: A frequent misdiagnosis for hemodialysis patients. J Clin Invest 110:437-439, 2002.

94. Bright R: Richard Bright: Original Papers on Renal Diseases. London, Oxford University Press, 1937.

95. Walser M, Bodenlos LJ: Urea metabolism in man. J Clin Invest 38:1617-1622, 1959.

96. Grollman EF, Grollman A: Toxicity of urea and its role in the pathogenesis of uremia. J Clin Invest 38:749, 1959.

97. Merrill JP, LM, Hoigne R: Observations on the role of urea in uremia. Am J Med 14:519, 1953.

98. Johnson WJ, Hagge WH, Wagoner RD, et al: Effects of urea loading in patients with far-advanced renal failure. Mayo Clinic Proc 47:21-29, 1972.

99. Moeslinger T, Friedl R, Volv I, et al: Urea induces macrophage proliferation by inhibition of inducible nitric oxide synthesis. Kidney Int 56:581-588, 2002.

100. Walser M: Urea metabolism in chronic renal failure. J Clin Invest 53:1385-1392, 1974.

101. Tizianello A, DeFerrari G, Garibotto G, et al: Renal metabolism of amino acids and ammonia in subjects with normal renal function and in patients with chronic renal insufficiency. J Clin Invest 65:1162-1173, 1980.

102. Kwan JTC, Carr EC, Bending MR, Barron JL: Determination of carbamylated hemoglobin by high-performance liquid chromatography. Clin Chem 36:607-610, 1990.

103. Oimomi M, Hatanaka H, Yoshimura Y, et al: Carbamylation of insulin and its biological activity. Nephron 46:63-66, 1987.

104. Tizianello A, DeFerrari G, Garibotto G, Robaudo C: Amino acid metabolism and the liver in renal failure. Am J Clin Nutr 33:1354-1362, 1980.

105. Suh H, Peresleni T, Wadhwa N, et al: Amino acid profile and nitric oxide pathway in patients on continuous ambulatory peritoneal dialysis: L-Arginine depletion in acute peritonitis. Am J Kidney Dis 29:712-719, 1997.

106. Pimentel L, Brusilow SW, Mitch WE: Unexpected encephalopathy in chronic renal failure: Hyperammonemia complicating acute peritonitis. J Am Soc Nephrol 5:1066-1073, 1994.

107. Mitch WE, Brusilow SW: Benzoate-induced changes in glycine and urea metabolism in patients with chronic renal failure. J Pharmacol Exp Ther 222:572-576, 1982.

108. Brusilow SW, Horwich A: Urea cycle enzymes. *In* Scriver C, Beaudet A, Sly W, Valle D (eds): The Metabolic Basis of Inherited Disease. New York, McGraw-Hill, 1989, pp 624-664.

109. Marescau B, Deshumkh DR, Kockx M, et al: Guanidino compounds in serum, urine, liver, kidney, and brain of man and some ureotelic animals. Metabolism 41:526-532, 1992.

110. Ando A, Orita Y, Tsubakihara R, et al: The effect of low protein diet and surplus of essential amino acids on the serum concentrations and the urinary excretion of methyl-guanidine and guanidinosuccinic acid in chronic renal failure. Nephron 24:161-169, 1979.

111. Kopple JD, Gordon SI, Wang M, Swenseid ME: Factors affecting serum and urinary guanidinosuccinic acid levels in normal and uremic subjects. J Lab Clin Med 90:303-311, 1977.

112. Marescau B, DeDeyn PP, Qureshi IA, et al: The pathobiochemistry of uremia and hyperargininemia further demonstrates a metabolic relationship between urea and guanidinosuccinic acid. Metabolism 41:1021-1024, 1992.

113. Orita Y, Ando A, Tsubakihara Y: Tissue and blood cell concentration of methylguanidine in rats and patients with chronic renal failure. Nephron 27:35-39, 1981.

114. Yokozawa T, Fujitsuka N, Oura H: Studies on the precursor of methylguanidine in rats with renal failure. Nephron 58:90-94, 1991.

115. Brusilow S, Tinker T, Batshaw ML: Amino acid acylation: A mechanism of nitrogen excretion in inborn errors of urea synthesis. Science 207:659-661, 1980.

116. Windmueller HG, Spaeth AE: Source and fate of circulating citrulline. Am J Physiol 241:E473-E480, 1981.

117. Castillo L, DeRojas TC, Chapman TE, et al: Splanchnic metabolism of dietary arginine in relation to nitric oxide synthesis in normal adult man. Proc Natl Acad Sci U S A 90:193-197, 1993.

118. Castillo L, Chapman TE, Yu Y-M, et al: Dietary arginine uptake by the splanchnic region in adult humans. Am J Physiol 265:E532-E539, 1993.

119. Perez G, Rey A, Schiff E: The biosynthesis of guanidinosuccinic acid by perfused rat liver. J Clin Invest 57:807-809, 1976.

120. Kelly RA, Mitch WE: Creatinine, uric acid and other nitrogenous waste products: Clinical implication of the imbalance between their production and elimination in uremia. Semin Nephrol 3:286-294, 1983.

121. Cohen BD: Guanidinosuccinic acid in uremia. Arch Intern Med 126:846-850, 1970.

122. Orita Y, Tsubakihara Y, Ando A, et al: Effect of arginine or creatinine administration on the urinary excretion of methylguanidine. Nephron 22:328-336, 1978.

123. Giovannetti S, Balestri PL, Barsotti G: Methylguanidine in uremia. Arch Intern Med 131:709-713, 1973.

124. Giovannetti S, Dioni L, Balestri PL, Biagini M: Evidence that guanidines and some related compounds cause hemolysis in chronic uremia. Clin Sci (Colch) 34:141-148, 1968.

125. Wizeman V: Exocrine pancreatic function in chronic renal failure. Proc Eur Dial Transplant Assoc 13:585-593, 1977.

126. Shainkin-Kestenbaum R, Giatt Y, Berlyne GM: The toxicity of guanidino compounds in the rat blood cell in uremia and the effect of hemodialysis. Nephron 31:20-23, 1982.

127. Marescau B, Hiramatsu M, Mori A: α-Keto-*d*-guanidinovaleric acid induced electroencephalographic, epileptiform discharges in rabbits. Neurochem Pathol 1:203-211, 1983.

128. DeDeyn PP, Marescau B, Cuykens JJ, et al: Guanidino compounds in serum and cerebrospinal fluid of non-dialyzed patients with renal insufficiency. Clin Chim Acta 167:81-88, 1987.

129. Marescau B, Nagel G, Possemiers I, et al: Guanidino compounds in serum and urine of nondialyzed patients with chronic renal insufficiency. Metabolism 46:1024-1037, 1997.

130. DeDeyn PP, Macdonald RL: Guanidino compounds that are increased in cerebrospinal fluid and brain of uremic patients inhibit GABA and glycine responses on mouse neurons in cell culture. Ann Neurol 28:627-633, 1990.

131. D'Hooge R, DeDeyn PP, van de Vijver G, et al: Uraemic guanidino compounds inhibit γ-amino-butyric acid–evoked whole-cell currents in mouse spinal cord neurons. Neurosci Lett 265:83-86, 1999.

132. King AJ, Brenner BM: Endothelium-derived vasoactive factors and the renal vasculature. Am J Physiol 260:R653-R662, 1991.

133. Blantz RC, Lortie M, Vallon V, et al: Activities of nitric oxide in normal physiology and uremia. Semin Nephrol 16:144-150, 1996.

134. Fenoy FJ, Perrer P, Carbonell L, Garcia-Salom M: Role of nitric oxide on papillary blood flow and pressure natriuresis. Hypertension 25:408-414, 1995.

135. Mattson DL, Lu S, Nakanishi K, et al: Effect of chronic renal medullary nitric oxide inhibition on blood pressure. Am J Physiol 266:H1918-H1926, 1994.

136. Tojo A, Garg LC, Guzman NC, et al: Nitric oxide inhibits bafilomycin-sensitive H⁺-ATPase activity in rat cortical collecting duct. Am J Physiol 267:F509-F515, 1994.

137. Stoos BA, Garcia NH, Garvin JL: Nitric oxide inhibits sodium reabsorption in the isolated perfused cortical collecting duct. J Am Soc Nephrol 6:89-94, 1995.

138. Garcia NH, Stoos BA, Carretero OS, Garvin JL: Mechanism of the nitric oxide induced blockade of collecting duct permeability. Hypertension 27:679-683, 1996.

139. Roczniak A, Burns KD: Nitric oxide stimulates quanylate cyclase and regulates sodium transport in rabbit proximal tubule. Am J Physiol 270:F106-F115, 1996.

140. Guzman NJ, Fang MZ, Tang SS, et al: Autocrine inhibition of N⁺/K⁺-ATPase by nitric oxide in mouse proximal tubule epithelial cells. J Clin Invest 95:2083-2088, 1995.

141. MacAllister RJ, Rambausek MH, Vallance P, et al: Concentration of dimethyl-L-arginine in the plasma of patients with end-stage renal failure. Nephrol Dial Transplant 11:2449-2452, 1996.

142. Kielstein JT, Boger RH, Gode-Boger SM, et al: Asymmetric dimethylarginine plasma concentrations differ in patients with end-stage renal disease: Relationship to treatment method and atherosclerotic disease. J Am Soc Nephrol 10:594-600, 1999.

143. Anderstam B, Katzaraki K, Bergstrom J: Serum levels of NG, NG-dimethyl-L-arginine, a potential endogenous nitric oxide inhibitor in dialysis patients. J Am Soc Nephrol 8:1437-1442, 1997.

144. Gardiner SM, Kemp PA, Bennett R, et al: Regional and cardiac haemodynamic effects of NG, NG-dimethyl-L-arginine and their reversibility by vasodilators in conscious rats. Br J Pharmacol 110:1457-1464, 1993.

145. Reyes AA, Karl IE, Kissane J, Klahr S: L-Arginine administration prevents glomerular hyperfiltration and decreases proteinuria in diabetic rats. J Am Soc Nephrol 4:1039-1045, 1993.

146. Katoh T, Takahashi K, Klahr S, et al: Dietary supplementation with L-arginine ameliorates glomerular hypertension in rats with subtotal nephrectomy. J Am Soc Nephrol 4:1690-1694, 1994.

147. Miyazaki H, Matsuoka H, Cook JPUM, et al: Endogenous nitric oxide synthase inhibitor: A novel marker of atherosclerosis. Circulation 99:1141-1146, 1999.

148. Walser M: Urea metabolism in chronic renal failure. J Am Soc Nephrol 9:1544-1551, 1995.

149. Mamoun A-H, Soderstein P, Divino J, et al: Inhibition of nitric oxide (NO) attenuates ingestive behavior: Evidence for preference of ornithine pathway in uremia. J Am Soc Nephrol 8:S809, 1997.

150. Mamoun A-H, Bergstrom J, Soderstein P: Cholecystokinin octapeptide inhibits carbohydrate but not protein intake. Am J Physiol 273:R972-R980, 1987.

151. Boger RH, Bode-Boger SM, Thiele W, et al: Biochemical evidence for impaired nitric oxide synthesis in patients with peripheral arterial occlusive disease. Circulation 95:2068-2074, 1997.

152. Boger RH, Bode-Boger SM, Szuba T, et al: Asymmetric dimethylarginine (ADMA): A novel risk factor for endothelial dysfunction: Its role in hypercholesterolemia. Circulation 98:1842-1847, 1998.

153. Witko-Sarsat V, Descamps-Latscha B: Advanced oxidation protein products: Novel uraemic toxins and pro-inflammatory mediators in chronic renal failure? Nephrol Dial Transplant 12:1310-1312, 2002.

154. Watko-Sarsat V, Friedlander M, Khoa TN, et al: Advanced oxidation protein products as novel mediators of inflammation and monocyte activation in chronic renal failure. J Immunol 161:2524-2532, 1998.

155. Himmelfarb J, McMonagle E, McMenamin E: Plasma protein thiol oxidation and carbonyl formation in chronic renal failure. Kidney Int 58:2571-2578, 2000.

156. Magnusson M, Magnusson K, Sundqvist T, Denneberg T: Increased intestinal permeability to differently sized polyethylene glycols in uremic rats: Effects of low- and high-protein diets. Nephron 56:306-311, 1990.

157. Magnusson M, Magnusson K, Sundqvist T, Dennenberg T: Urinary excretion of differently sized polyethylene glycols after intravenous administration in uremic and control rats: Effects of low- and high-protein diets. Nephron 56:312-316, 1990.

158. Yanagisawa H, Wada O: Significant increase of IQ-type heterocyclic amines, dietary carcinogens in the plasma of patients with uremia just before induction of hemodialysis treatment. Nephron 52:6-10, 1989.

159. Manabe S, Suszuke M, Kusano E, et al: Elevation of levels of carcinogenic tryptophan pyrolysis products in plasma and red blood cells of patients with uremia. Clin Nephrol 37:28-33, 1992.

160. Simenhoff ML, Milne MD, Asatoor AM, Zilva JF: Retention of aliphatic amines in uremia. Clin Sci (Colch) 25:65-77, 1963.

161. Rennick B, Acara M, Hysert P, Mookerjee B: Choline loss during hemodialysis: Homeostatic control of plasma choline concentrations. Kidney Int 10:329-335, 1976.

162. Bell JD, Lee JA, Lee HA, et al: Nuclear magnetic resonance studies of blood plasma and urine from patients with chronic renal failure: Identification of trimethylamine-N-oxide. Biochim Biophys Acta 1096:101-107, 1991.

163. Young DS, Wooton IDP: The retention of amines as a factor in uremic toxaemia. Clin Chim Acta 9:503-505, 1964.

164. Noree L-O, Bergstrom J: Treatment of chronic uremic patients with protein-poor diet and oral supply of essential amino acids. Clin Nephrol 3:195-203, 1975.

165. Walser M, Hill SB: Free and protein-bound tryptophan in serum of untreated patients with chronic renal failure. Kidney Int 44:1366-1371, 1993.

166. Niwa T: Organic acids and the uremic syndrome: Protein metabolite hypothesis in the progression of chronic renal failure. Semin Nephrol 16:167-182, 1996.

167. Wardle EN: Phenols, phenolic acids and sodium-potassium ATPases. J Mol Med 3:319, 1978.

168. Goodhart PJ, DeWolf WE, Kruse LI: Mechanism based inactivation of dopamine β-hydroxylase by *p*-cresol and related alkyl phenols. Biochemistry 26:2576-2583, 1987.

169. Wratten ML, Tetta C, DeSmet R, et al: Uremic ultrafiltrate inhibits platelet-activating factor synthesis. Blood Purif 17:134-141, 1999.

170. Vanholder R, DeSmet R, Waterloos MA, et al: Mechanisms of uremic inhibition of phagocytic reactive species production: Characterization of the role of *p*-cresol. Kidney Int 47:510-517, 1995.

171. De Kemp J, Cornelis R, Vanholder R: In vitro methylation of arsenite by rabbit liver cytosol: Effect of metal ions, metal chelating agents, methyltransferase inhibitors and uremic toxins. Drug Chem Toxicol 22:613-628, 1999.

172. Yokoyama MT, Tabori C, Miller ER, Hogberg MG: The effects of antibiotics in the weanling pig diet on growth and the excretion of volatile phenolic and aromatic bacterial metabolites. Am J Clin Nutr 35:1417-1424, 1982.

173. Heipieper HJ, Keweloh H, Rehm HJ: Influence of phenols on growth and membrane permeability of free and immobilized *Escherichia coli*. Appl Environ Microbiol 57:1213-1217, 1991.

174. Costigan MG, Callahan CA, Lindup WE: Hypothesis: Is accumulation of furan dicarboxylic acid (3-carboxy-4-methyl-5-propyl-2-furanpropanoic acid) related to neurological abnormalities in patients with renal failure? Nephron 73:169-173, 1996.

175. Lim CF, Bernard BF, DeJong M, et al: A furan fatty acid and indoxyl sulfate are the putative inhibitors of thyroxine hepatocyte transport in uremia. J Clin Endocrinol Metab 76:318-324, 1993.

176. Niwa T, Aiuchi T, Nakaya K, et al: Inhibition of mitochondrial respiration by furancarboxylic acid accumulated in uremic serum in its albumin-bound and non-dialyzable form. Clin Nephrol 39:92-96, 1993.

177. Mabuchi H, Nakahashi H: Inhibition of hepatic glutathione *S*-transferases by a major endogenous ligand substance in uremic serum. Nephron 49:281-283, 1988.

178. Niwa T, Yazawa T, Kodama T, et al: Efficient removal of albumin-bound furancarboxylic acid, an inhibitor of erythropoiesis, by continuous ambulatory peritoneal dialysis. Nephron 56:241-245, 1990.

179. Byrd DJ, Berthold HW, Trefz KF, et al: Indolic tryptophan metabolism in uraemia. Proc Eur Dial Transplant Assoc 12:347-354, 1976.

180. Siassi F, Wang M, Chan W, Swenseid ME: Brain serotonin turnover in chronically uremic rats. Am J Physiol 232:E526-E528, 1977.

181. Niwa T, Miyazaki T, Hashimoto N, et al: Suppressed serum and urine levels of indoxyl sulfate by oral sorbent in experimental uremic rats. Am J Nephol 12:201-206, 1992.

182. Frosst P, Blom HJ, Milos R, et al: A candidate genetic risk factor for vascular disease: A common mutation in methylenetetrahydrofolate reductase. Nat Genet 10:111-113, 1995.

183. Weisberg I, Tran P, Christensen B, et al: A second genetic polymorphism in methylenetetrahydrofolate reductase (MTHFR) associated with decreased enzyme activity. Mol Genet Metab 64:169-172, 1998.

184. Niwa TIM: Indoxyl sulfate, a circulating uremic toxin, stimulates the progression of glomerular sclerosis. J Lab Clin Med 124:96-104, 1994.

185. Takami H, Nishioka K: Raised polyamines in erythrocytes from melanoma-bearing mice and patients with solid tumors. Br J Cancer 41:751-756, 1980.

186. Saito A, Takaji T, Chung TG, Ohta K: Serum levels of polyamines in patients with chronic renal failure. Kidney Int 24 (suppl 16): S234-S237, 1983.

187. Radtke HW, Rege AB, Lamarche MB, et al: Identification of spermine as an inhibitor of erythropoiesis in patients with chronic renal failure. J Clin Invest 67:1623-1629, 1981.

188. Christensen B, Refsum H, Vintermyr O, Ueland PM: Homocysteine export from cells cultured in the presence of physiological or superfluous levels of methionine: Methionine loading of non-transformed, proliferating and quiescent cells in culture. J Cell Physiol 146:52-62, 1991.

189. Finkelstein JD, Kyle WR, Harris BJ: Methionine metabolism in mammals: Regulation of homocysteine methyltransferases in rat tissues. Arch Biochem Biophys 146:84-92, 1971.

190. Malinow MR, Axthelm M, Meredith M, et al: Synthesis and transsulfuration of homocysteine in blood. J Lab Clin Med 123:421-429, 1994.

191. Gupta A, Robinson K: Hyperhomocysteinaemia and end stage renal disease. J Nephrol 10:77-84, 1997.

192. Bostom AG, Brosnan JT, Hall B, Nadeu MR, Selhub J: Net uptake of plasma homocysteine by the rat kidney in vivo. Atherosclerosis 116:59-62, 1995.

193. Guttormsen AB, Schneede J, Ueland PM, Refsum H: Kinetic basis of hyperhomocyst(e)inemia in patients with chronic renal failure. Kidney Int 52:495-502, 1997.

194. Bostom AG, Lathrop L: Hyperhomocysteinemia in end-stage renal disease: Prevalence, etiology, and potential relationship to arteriosclerotic outcomes. Kidney Int 52:10-20, 1997.

195. Kang SS, Wong PWK, Cook HY, Norusis M, Messer JV: Protein-bound homocyst(e)ine: A possible risk factor for coronary heart disease. J Clin Invest 77:1482-1486, 1986.

196. Mudd SH, Levy HLSF: Disorders in transsulfuration. *In* Scriver C, Beaudet, AL, Sly WS, Valle D (eds): The Metabolic and Molecular Basis of Metabolic Disease. New York, McGraw-Hill, 1995, pp 1279-1327.

197. McCully KS, Wilson RB: Homocysteine theory of arteriosclerosis. Atherosclerosis 22:215-227, 1975.

198. Kang SS, Wong PWK, Malinow MR: Hyperhomocyst(e)inemia as a risk factor for occlusive vascular disease. Annu Rev Nutr 12: 259-278, 1992.

199. Nygard O, Nordrehaug JE, Refsun H, et al: Plasma homocysteine levels and mortality in patients with coronary artery disease. N Engl J Med 337:230-236, 1997.

200. Kang SS, Wong PWK, Norusis M: Homocysteinemia due to folate deficiency. Metabolism 36:458-462, 1987.

201. Robinson K, Arheart K, Refsum H, et al, European COMAC Group: Low circulating folate and vitamin B$_6$ concentrations. Circulation 97:437-443, 1998.

202. Selhub J, Jacques PF, Bostom AG, et al: Association between plasma homocysteine concentrations and extracranial carotid-artery stenosis. N Engl J Med 332:286-299, 1995.

203. Mezzano D, Pais EO, Aranda E, et al: Inflammation not hyperhomocysteinemia is related to oxidative stress and hemostatic and endothelial dysfunction in uremia. Kidney Int 60: 1844-1850, 2001.

204. Malinow MR, Bostom AG, Krauss RM: Homocyst(e)ine, diet and cardiovascular disease: A statement for health care professionals from the Nutrition Committee, American Heart Association. Circulation 99:178-182, 1999.

205. Kasiske BL, Vasquez MA, Harmon WE, et al: Recommendations for the outpatient surveillance of renal transplant recipients. J Am Soc Nephrol 11:S1-S86, 2000.

206. Graham IM, Daly LE, Refsum HM, et al: Plasma homocysteine as a risk factor for vascular disease. JAMA 277:2781, 1997.

207. Malinow MR, Nieto FJ, Kruger WD, et al: The effects of folic acid supplementation on plasma total homocysteine are modulated by multivitamin use and methylenetetrahydrofolate reductase genotypes. Arterioscler Thromb Vasc Biol 17:1157-1162, 1997.

208. Shemin D, Bostom AG, Selhum J: Treatment of hyperhomocysteinemia in end-stage renal disease. Am J Kidney Dis 38:S91-S94, 2001.

209. Bostom AG, Shemin D, Bagley P, et al: Controlled comparison of L-5-methyltetrahydrofolate versus folic acid for the treatment of hyperhomocysteinemia in hemodialysis patients. Circulation 101: 2829-2832, 2000.

210. Yango A, Shemin D, Hsu N, et al: Folinic acid versus folic acid for the treatment of hyperhomocysteinemia in hemodialysis patients. Kidney Int 59:324-327, 2000.

211. Hauser A, Hagen W, Rehak PH, et al: Efficacy of folinic versus folic acid for the correction of hyperhomocysteinemia in hemodialysis patients. Am J Kidney Dis 37:758-765, 2001.

212. van Guldener C, Lambert J, Ter Wee PM, et al: Carotid artery stiffness in patients with end-stage renal disease: No effect of long-term homocysteine-lowering therapy. Clin Nephrol 53:33-41, 2000.

213. Graziano JH, Siris ES, Lolancono N, et al: 2,3-Dimercaptosuccinic acid as an antidote to lead poisoning. Clin Pharmacol 37:431-438, 1985.

214. Lowrie EG: Thoughts about judging dialysis treatment: Mathematics and measurements, mirrors in the mind. Semin Nephrol 16:242-262, 1996.

215. Bergstrom J: Anorexia in dialysis patients. Semin Nephrol 16: 222-229, 1996.

216. Anderstam B, Mamoun A-H, Bergstrom J, Sodersten P: Middle-sized molecule fractions isolated from uremic ultrafiltrate and normal urine inhibit ingestive behavior in the rat. J Am Soc Nephrol 7:2453-2460, 1996.

217. Mamoun AH, Anderstam B, Sodersten P, et al: Influence of peritoneal dialysis solutions with glucose and amino acids on ingestive behavior in rats. Kidney Int 49:1276-1282, 1996.

218. Mamoun AH, Sodersten P, Anderstam B, Bergstrom J: Evidence of splanchnic-brain signaling in inhibition of ingestive behaviour by middle molecules. J Am Soc Nephrol 10:309-314, 1999.

219. Severini G, Diana L, DiGiovannandrea R, Sagliaschi G: Influence of uremic middle molecules on in vitro stimulated lymphocytes and interleukin-2 production. ASAIO J 42:64-67, 1996.

220. Horl WH, Haag-Weber M, Georgopoulos A, Block LH: Physiochemical characterization of a polypeptide present in uremic serum that inhibits the biological activity of polymorphonuclear cells. Proc Natl Acad Sci U S A 87:6353-6357, 1990.

221. Haag-Weber M, Mai B, Horl WH: Isolation of a granulocyte inhibitory protein from uraemic patients with homology of β_2-microglobulin. Nephrol Dial Transplant 9:382-388, 1994.

222. Tschesche H, Kopp C, Horl WH, Hempelmann U: Inhibition of degranulation of polymorphonuclear leukocytes by angiogenin and its tryptic fragment. J Biol Chem 269:30274-30280, 1994.

223. Balke N, Holtkamp U, Horl WH, Hempelmann U: Inhibition of degranulation of human polymorphonuclear leukocytes by complement factor D. FEBS Lett 371:300-302, 1995.

224. Kamanna VS, Kashyap ML, Pai R, et al: Uremic serum subfraction inhibits apolipoprotein A-1 production by a human hepatoma cell line. J Am Soc Nephrol 5:193-200, 1994.

225. Leypoldt JK, Cheung AK, Carroll CE, et al: Effect of dialysis membranes and middle molecule removal on chronic hemodialysis patient survival. Am J Kidney Dis 33:349-355. 1999.

226. Lubash GD, Stenzel KH, Rubin AL: Nitrogenous compounds in hemodialysate. Circulation 30:848-852, 1964.

227. Abiko T, Kumikawa M, Ishizaki M, et al: Identification and synthesis of a tripeptide in coecum fluid of a uremic patient. Biochem Biophys Res Commun 83:357-364, 1978.

228. Abiko T, Kumikawa M, Higuchi H, Sekono H: Identification and synthesis of a heptapeptide in uremic fluid. Biochem Biophys Res Commun 84:184-194, 1978.

229. Chu J, Yuan Z, Liu X, et al: Separation of six uremic middle molecular compounds by high performance liquid chromatography and analysis by matrix-assisted laser desorption/ionization time-of-flight mass spectrometry. Clin Chim Acta 311:95-107, 2001.

230. Gejyo F, Homma N, Arakawa M: Long-term complications of dialysis: Pathogenic factors with special reference to amyloidosis. Kidney Int Suppl 43:S78-S82, 1993.

231. Maytes D, Bogin E, Ma A, et al: Effect of parathyroid hormone on erythropoiesis. J Clin Invest 67:1263-1269, 1981.

232. Massry SG, Smogorzewski M: Mechanisms through which parathyroid hormone mediates its deleterious effects on organ function in uremia. Semin Nephrol 14:219-231, 1994.

233. Akmal M, Goldstein DA, Multani S, Massry SG: Role of uremia, brain calcium, and parathyroid hormone on changes in electroencephalogram in chronic renal failure. Am J Physiol 246:F575-F586, 1984.

234. Akmal M, Massry SG: Role of parathyroid hormone in the decreased motor nerve conduction velocity of chronic renal failure. Proc Exp Biol Med 195:202-207, 1990.

235. Smogorzewski M, Galfayan V, Massry SG: High glucose concentration causes a rise in $[Ca^{2+}]_i$ of cardiac myocytes. Kidney Int 53:1237-1243, 1998.

236. Fadda GZ, Hajjar SM, Perna AF, et al: On the mechanism of impaired insulin secretion in chronic renal failure. J Clin Invest 87:255-261, 1991.

237. Shoots A, Mikkers F, Cramers C, et al: Uremic toxins and the elusive middle molecules. Nephron 38:1-8, 1984.

238. Motojima M, Nishijima F, Ikoma M, et al: Role for "uremic toxin" in the progressive loss of intact nephrons in chronic renal failure. Kidney Int 40:461-469, 1991.

239. Henderson SJ, Lindup WE: Interaction of 3-carboxy-4-methyl-5-propyl-2-furanpropanoic acid, an inhibitor of plasma protein binding in uremia, with human albumin. Biochem Pharmacol 40:2543-2548, 1990.

240. Sievertsen GD, Lim VS, Nakawatase C, Frohman LA: Metabolic clearance and secretion rates of human prolactin in normal subjects and in patients with chronic renal failure. J Clin Endocrinol Metab 50:846-852, 1980.

241. Adachi N, Lei B, Deshpande G, et al: Uremia suppresses central dopaminergic metabolism and impairs motor activity in rats. Intensive Care Med 27:1655-1660, 2001.

242. Lim VS, Fang VS: Gonadal dysfunction in uremic men: A study of the hypothalamo-pituitary-testicular axis before and after renal transplantation. Am J Med 58:655-662, 1975.

243. Ikemoto S, Imaoka S, Hayahara N, et al: Expression of hepatic microsomal cytochrome P450s as altered by uremia. Biochem Pharmacol 43:2407-2412, 1992.

244. Phillips LS, Fusco AC, Unterman TG, del Greco F: Somatomedin inhibitor in uremia. J Clin Endocrinol Metab 59:764-772, 1984.

245. Westervelt FB: Insulin effect in uremia. J Lab Clin Med 74:79-87, 1969.

246. Bak JF, Schmitz O, Sorensen SS, et al: Activity of insulin receptor kinase and glycogen synthase in skeletal muscle from patients with chronic renal failure. Acta Endocrinol 121:744-750, 1989.

247. White MF, Kahn CR: The insulin signaling system. J Biol Chem 269:1-4, 1994.

248. Saad MJA, Araki E, Miralpeix M, et al: Regulation of insulin receptor substrate-1 in liver and muscle of animal models of insulin resistance. J Clin Invest 90:1839-1849. 1992.

249. Folli F, Saad MJA, Kahn CR: Insulin receptor/IRS-1/PI 3-kinase signaling system in corticosteroid-induced insulin resistance. Diabetologia 33:185-192, 1996.

250. Rojas FA, Hirata AE, Saad MJA: Regulation of IRS-2 tyrosine phosphorylation in fasting and diabetes. Mol Cell Endocrinol 183:63-69, 2001.

251. Giorgino F, Pedrini MT, Matera L, Smith RJ: Specific increase in p85a expression in response to dexamethasone is associated with inhibition of insulin-like growth factor-1 stimulated phophatidylinositol 3-kinase activity in cultured muscle cells. J Biol Chem 272:7455-7463, 1997.

252. Baumgartner RN: Electrical impedance and total body electrical conductivity, In Roche AF, Heymsfield SB, Lohman TD (eds): Human Body Composition. Champaign. University of Illinois Press, 1996, pp 79-107.

253. Hotamisligil GS: The role of TNF-α and TNF receptors in obesity and insulin resistance. J Intern Med 245:621-625, 1999.

254. Folli F, Kahn CR, Hansen H, et al: Angiotensin II inhibits insulin signaling in aortic smooth muscle cells at multiple levels: A potential role for serine phosphorylation in insulin/angiotensin II crosstalk. J Clin Invest 100:2158-2169, 1997.

255. Fouque D, Peng SC, Kopple JD: Impaired metabolic response to recombinant insulin-like growth factor-I in dialysis patients. Kidney Int 47:876-883, 1995.

256. Villares SM, Goujon L, Maniar S, et al: Reduced food intake is the main cause of low growth hormone expression in uremic rats. Mol Cell Endocrinol 106:51-56, 1994.

257. Jones JI, Clemmons DR: Insulin-like growth factors and their binding proteins: Biological actions. Endocr Rev 16:3-34, 1995.

258. Schaefer F, Chen Y, Tsao T, et al: Impaired JAK-STAT signal transduction contributes to growth hormone resistance in chronic uremia. J Clin Invest 108:467-475, 2001.

259. Mak RHK: Renal disease, insulin resistance and glucose intolerance. Diabetes Rev 2:19-28, 1994.

260. Mak RHK, Pak YK: End-organ resistance to growth hormone and IGF-1 in epiphyseal chondrocytes of rats with chronic renal failure. Kidney Int 50:400-406, 1996.

261. Carter-Su C, Rui L, Herrington J: Role of the tyrosine kinase JAK2 in signal transduction by growth hormone. Pediatr Nephrol 14:550-557, 2000.

262. Kaptein EM, Feinstein EI, Nicoloff JT, Massry SG: Serum reverse triiodothyronine and thyroxine kinetics in patients with chronic renal failure. J Clin Endocrinol Metab 57:181-189, 1983.

263. Auwerx J, Staels B: Leptin. Lancet 351:737-742, 1998.

264. Cummings DE, Purnell JQ, Frayo S, Schmidova K, et al: A preprandial rise in plasma ghrelin levels suggests a role in meal initiation in humans. Diabetes 50:1714-1719, 2001.

265. Gibbs J, Young RC, Smith GP: Cholecystokinin decreases food intake in rats. J Comp Physiol Psychol 84:488-495, 1973.

266. Batterham RL, Cowley MA, Small CJ, et al: Gut hormone PYY(3-36) physiologically inhibits food intake. Nature 418:650-654, 2002.

267. Stanley BG, Kyrkouli SE, Lampert S, Leibowitz SF: Neuropeptide Y chronically injected into the hypothalamus: A powerful neurochemical inducer of hyperphagia and obesity. Peptides 7:1189-1192, 1986.

268. Fan W, Boston BA, Kesterson RA, et al: Role of melanocortinergic neurons in feeding and the agouti obesity syndrome. Nature 385:165-168, 1997.

269. Hahn TM, Breininger JF, Baskin DG, Schwartz MW: Coexpression of Agrp and NPY in fasting-activated hypothalamic neurons. Nature Neurosci 1:271-272, 1998.

270. Masuzaki H, Ogawa Y, Sagawa N, et al: Nonadipose tissue production of leptin: Leptin as a novel placenta-derived hormone in humans. Nat Med 3:1029-1033, 1997.

271. Kolaczynski JW, Considine RV, Ohannesian J, et al: Responses of leptin to short-term fasting and refeeding in humans: A link with ketogenesis but not ketones themselves. Diabetes 45:1511-1515, 1996.

272. Ahima RS, Flier JS: Leptin. Annu Rev Physiol 62:413-437, 2000.
273. Fruhbeck G, Salvador J: Relation between leptin and the regulation of glucose metabolism. Diabetologia 43:3-12, 2000.
274. Loffreda S, Yang SQ, Lin HZ, et al: Leptin regulates proinflammatory immune responses. FASEB J 12:57-65, 1998.
275. Wolf G, Chen SC, Han DC, Ziyadeh FJ: Leptin and renal disease. Am J Kidney Dis 39:1-11, 2002.
276. Berti L, Kellerer M, Capp E, Haring HU: Leptin stimulates glucose transport and glycogen synthesis in C2C12 myotubes: Evidence for a PI 3-kinase mediated effect. Diabetologia 40:606-609, 1997.
277. Barzilai N, Wang J, Massilon D, et al: Leptin selectively decreases visceral adiposity and enhances insulin action. J Clin Invest 100:3105-3110, 1997.
278. Sierra-Honigmann MR, Nath AK, Murakami C, et al: Biological action of leptin as an angiogenic factor. Science 281:1683-1686, 1998.
279. Lord GM, Matarese G, Howard JK, et al: Leptin modulates the T-cell immune response and reverses starvation-induced immunosuppression. Nature 394:897-901, 1998.
280. Johansen KL, Mulligan K, Tai V, Schambelan M: Leptin, body composition and indices of malnutrition in patients on dialysis. J Am Soc Nephrol 9:1080-1084, 1998.
281. Stenvinkel P, Lindholm B, Lonnqvist F, et al: Increases in serum leptin levels during peritoneal dialysis are associated with inflammation and a decrease in lean body mass. J Am Soc Nephrol 11:1303-1309, 2000.
282. Young GA, Woodrow G, Kendall S, et al: Increased plasma leptin/fat ratio in patients with chronic renal failure: A cause of malnutrition? Nephrol Dial Transplant 12:2318-2323, 1997.
283. Fontan MP, Rodriguez-Carmona A, Cordido F, Garcia-Buela J: Hyperleptinemia in uremic patients undergoing conservative management, peritoneal dialysis and hemodialysis: A comparative analysis. Am J Kidney Dis 34:824-831, 1999.
284. Landt M, Brennan DC, Parvin CA, et al: Hyperleptinemia of end-stage renal disease is corrected by renal transplantation. Nephrol Dial Transplant 13:2271-2275, 1998.
285. Wolf G, Hamann A, Han DC, et al: Leptin stimulates proliferation and TGF-β expression in renal glomerular endothelial cells: Potential role in glomerulosclerosis. Kidney Int 56:860-872, 1999.
286. Han DC, Isono M, Chen S, et al: Leptin stimulates type I collagen production in db/db mesangial cells: Glucose uptake and TGF-β type II receptor expression. Kidney Int 59:1315-1323, 2001.
287. Jackson EK, Li P: Human leptin has natriuretic activity in the rat. Am J Physiol 272:F333-F338, 1997.
288. Welt LG, Sachs JR, McManus TJ: An ion transport defect in erythrocytes from uremic patients. Trans Assoc Am Physicians 77:169-181, 1964.
289. Kaji DM, Kahn T: The Na^+/K^+ pump in chronic renal failure. Am J Physiol 252:F785-F793, 1987.
290. Izumo H, Izumo S, DeLuise M, Flier JS: Erythrocyte Na,K pump in uremia: Acute correction of a transport defect by hemodialysis. J Clin Invest 74:581-588, 1984.
291. Edmondson RPS, Hilton NF, Jones NF, et al: Leukocyte sodium transport in uremia. Clin Sci (Colch) 49:213-216, 1975.
292. Corry DB, Tuck ML, Brickman AS, et al: Sodium transport in red blood cells from dialyzed uremic patients. Kidney Int 20:1197-1202, 1986.
293. Kelly RA, Canessa ML, Steinman TI, Mitch WE: Hemodialysis and red cell cation transport in uremia: Role of membrane free fatty acids. Kidney Int 35:595-603, 1989.
294. Druml W, Kelly RA, May RC, Mitch WE: Abnormal cation transport in uremia: Mechanisms in adipocytes and skeletal muscle from uremic rats. J Clin Invest 81:1197-1203, 1988.
295. Kelly RA, O'Hara DS, Mitch WE, et al: Endogenous digitalis-like factors in hypertension and chronic renal insufficiency. Kidney Int 30:723-729, 1986.
296. Graves SW, Brown B, Valdes R: An endogenous digoxin-like substance in patients with renal impairment. Ann Intern Med 99:604-608,1983.
297. Hamlyn JM, Blaustein MP, Bova S, et al: Identification and characterization of a ouabain-like compound from human plasma. Proc Natl Acad Sci U S A 88:6259-6263, 1991.
298. Goto A, Yamada K: Purification of endogenous digitalis-like factors from normal human urine. Clin Exp Hypertens 20:531-556, 1998.
299. Graves SW, Williams GH: Endogenous digitalis-like natriuretic factors. Annu Rev Med 48:433-444, 1987.
300. Benaksas EJ, Murray ED, Rodgers CL, et al: Endogenous natriuretic factors I: Sodium pump inhibition does not correlate with natriuretic or pressor activities from uremic urine. Life Sci 52:1045-1054, 1993.
301. Goto A, Yamada K, Yagi N, et al: Physiology and pharmacology of endogenous digitalis-like factors. Pharmacol Rev 44:377-399, 1992.
302. Gallice PM, Kovacic HN, Brunet PJ, et al: A non-ouabain-like inhibitor of the sodium pump in uremic plasma ultrafiltrates and urine from healthy subjects. Clin Chim Acta 237:149-160, 1998.
303. Tamura M, Kuwano H, Kinoshita T, Inagami T: Identification of linoleic and oleic acids on endogenous Na^+K^+-ATPase inhibitors from acute volume-expanded hog plasma. J Biol Chem 260:9672-9677, 1985.
304. Kelly RA, O'Hara DS, Mitch WE, Smith TW: Identification of NaK-ATPase inhibitors in human plasma as nonesterified fatty acids and lysophospholipids. J Biol Chem 261:11704-11711, 1986.
305. Ludens JH, Clark MS, Ducharme DW, et al: Purification of an endogenous digitalis-like factor from human plasma for structural analysis. Hypertension 17:923-929, 1991.
306. Matthews WR, Ducharme DW, Hamlyn JM, et al: Mass spectral characterization of an endogenous digitalis-like factor from human plasma. Hypertension 17:930-935, 1991.
307. Tamura M, Harris TM, Higashimori K, et al: Lysophosphaditylcholines containing polyunsaturated fatty acids were found as Na^+,K^+-ATPase inhibitors in acutely volume-expanded hog. Biochemistry 26:2797-2806, 1987.
308. Komidori K, Kamada T, Yamashita T, et al: Erythrocyte membrane fluidity is decreased in uremic hemodialyzed patients. Nephron 40:185-188, 1985.
309. Cheng JT, Kahn T, Kaji DM: Mechanism of alteration of sodium potassium pump of erythrocytes from patients with chronic renal failure. J Clin Invest 74:1811-1820, 1984.
310. Lytton J: Insulin affects the sodium affinity of the rat adipocyte $(Na^+$-$K^+)$-ATPase. J Biol Chem 260:10075-10080, 1985.
311. Clausen T, Everts ME: Regulation of the Na,K-pump in skeletal muscle. Kidney Int 35:1-13, 1989.
312. Brown MJ, Brown DC, Murphy MB: Hypokalemia from beta$_2$ receptor stimulation by circulating epinephrine. N Engl J Med 309:1414-1419, 1983.
313. Kubota K, Ingbar SH: Influences of thyroid status and sympathoadrenal system on extrarenal potassium disposal. Am J Physiol 258:E428-E435, 1990.
314. Rutherford PA, Thomas TH, O'Kelly J, et al: Thiol group control of sodium-lithium countertransport kinetics in uraemia: Evidence of a membrane abnormality affected by haemodialysis. Nephron 72:184-188, 1996.
315. Zidek W, Rustemeyer T, Schluter W, et al: Isolation of an ultrafiltrable calcium-ATPase inhibitor from the plasma of uraemic patients. Clin Sci (Colch) 82:659-665, 1992.
316. Lindner A, Vanholder R, DeSmet R, et al: HPLC fractions of human uremic plasma inhibit the RBC membrane calcium pump. Kidney Int 51:1042-1052, 1997.
317. Soldati L, Adamo D, Manunta P, et al: Erythrocyte calcium influx is related to the severity of ventricular arrhythmias in uraemic patients. Nephrol Dial Transplant 16:85-90, 2001.
318. Aparicio M, Vincendeau P, Combe C, et al: Improvement of leucocytic Na^+K^+ pump activity in uremic patients on low protein diet. Kidney Int 40:238-242, 1991.
319. Sands JM: Regulation of urea transporter proteins in kidney and liver. Mt Sinai J Med 67:112-119, 2000.
320. Hu MC, Bankir L, Michelet S, et al: Massive reduction of urea transporters in remnant kidney and brain of uremic rats. Kidney Int 58:1202-1210, 2000.
321. Duchesne R, Klein JD, Velotta JB, et al: UT-A urea transporter protein in heart: Increased abundance during uremia, hypertension and heart failure. Circ Res 89:139-145, 2001.
322. Klein JD, Timmer RT, Rouillard, P, et al: UT-A urea transporter protein expressed in liver. Upregulation by uremia. J Am Soc Nephrol 10:2076-2083, 1999.
323. Guisado R, Arieff AI, Massry SG: Changes in the electroencephalogram in acute uremia: Effects of parathyroid hormone and brain electrolytes. J Clin Invest 55:738-745, 1975.

324. Fraser CL, Sarnacki P, Arieff AI: Abnormal sodium transport in synaptosomes from brain of uremic rats. J Clin Invest 75:2014-2023, 1985.

325. Fraser CL, Sarnacki P, Arieff AI: Calcium transport abnormality in uremic rat brain synaptosomes. J Clin Invest 76:7189-1795, 1985.

326. Verkman AS, Fraser CL: Water and nonelectrolyte permeability in brain synaptosomes isolated from normal and uremic rats. Am J Physiol 250:R306-R312, 1986.

327. Fadda GZ, Akmal M, Soliman AR, et al: Correction of glucose intolerance and the impaired insulin release of chronic renal failure by verapamil. Kidney Int 36:773-779, 1989.

328. Zhang Y-B, Smogorzewski M, Ni Z, Massry SG: Altered cytosolic calcium homeostasis in rat cardiac myocytes in CRF. Kidney Int 45:1113-1119, 1994.

329. Ni ZW, Smogorzewski M, Massry SG: Elevated cytosolic calcium of adipocytes in chronic renal failure. Kidney Int 47:1624-1649, 1995.

330. Hajjar SM, Fadda GZ, Thanakitcharu P, et al: Reduced activity of Na$^+$-K$^+$ ATPase of pancreatic islets in chronic renal failure: Role of secondary hyperparathyroidism. J Am Soc Nephrol 2:1355-1359, 1992.

331. Massry SG, Smogorzewski K: The heart in uremia. Sem Nephrol 16:214-221, 1996.

332. Blaustein MP: Sodium ions, calcium ions, blood pressure regulation and hypertension: A reassessment and a hypothesis. Am J Physiol 232:C165-C173, 1977.

333. Hout SJ, Pamnani MB, Clough DL, et al: Sodium-potassium pump activity in reduced renal mass hypertension. Hypertension 5:194-1100, 1983.

334. Druml W, Kelly RA, England BE, et al: Effects of acute and chronic uremia on active cation transport in rat myocardium. Kidney Int 38:1061-1067, 1990.

335. Bonilla S, Goecke IA, Bozzo S, et al: Effect of chronic renal failure on NaK-ATPase α_1 and α_2 mRNA transcription in rat skeletal muscle. J Clin Invest 88:2137-2141, 1991.

336. Greiber S, England BK, Price SR, et al: Na pump defects in chronic uremia cannot be attributed to changes in Na-K-ATPase mRNA or protein. Am J Physiol 266:F536-F542, 1994.

337. da Silva JCT, Shi X-J, Johns CA, et al: Experimental renal failure in the rat modulates cardiac Na,K-ATPase α_2 mRNA but not protein. J Am Soc Nephrol 5:27-35, 1994.

338. Michnowska M, Smogorzewski M, Massry SG: Impaired Na$^+$-H$^+$ exchanger activity of hepatocytes in chronic renal failure. J Am Soc Nephrol 8:929-934, 1997.

339. Yamaji Y, Tsuganezawa H, Moe OW, Alpern RJ: Intracellular acidosis activates c-Src. Am J Physiol 272:C886-C893, 1997.

340. Bagrodia S, Chackalaparampil I, Kmiecik TE, Shalloway D: Altered tyrosine 527 phosphorylation and mitotic activation of p60 c-src. Nature 349:172-175, 1991.

341. England BK, Chastain J, Mitch WE: Extracellular acidification changes protein synthesis and degradation in BC3H-1 myocytes. Am J Physiol 260:C277-C282, 1991.

342. Smit JW, Weert B, Schinkel AH, Meijer DF: Heterologous expression of various P-glycoporteins in polarized epithelial cells induces directional transport of small (type I) and bulky (type II) cationic drugs. J Pharmacol Exp Ther 286:321-327, 1998.

343. Konig J, Nies AT, Cui Y, et al: Conjugate export pumps of the multidrug resistance protein (MRP) family: Localization, substrate specificity, and MRP2 mediated drug resistance. Biochim Biophys Acta 146:377-394, 1999.

344. Pritchard JB, Miller DS: Renal secretion of organic anions and cations. Kidney Int 49:1649-1654, 1996.

345. Laouari D, Yang R, Veau C, et al: Two apical multidrug transporters, p-gp and MRP2, are differently altered in chronic renal failure. Am J Physiol 280:F636-F645, 2001.

CHAPTER 49

Hematologic Consequences of Renal Failure

Giuseppe Remuzzi, Arrigo Schieppati, and Luigi Minetti

ANEMIA OF RENAL FAILURE

Anemia associated with renal failure was first noted by Richard Bright in 1836 when he observed pallor in the development of Bright disease.[1] In 1907, Riesman[2] documented its hemorrhagic diathesis and cited the description of Morgagni (1682-1771) of epistaxis and hematemesis in a patient who "had the odor of urine on the breath." By 1922, Brown and Roth[3] had concluded that the anemia of chronic nephritis was due to decreased bone marrow production, and in 1957 Jacobson and co-workers[4] reported that the recently described erythroid growth factor was produced by the kidneys in response to anemia. This factor, erythropoietin (EPO), emerged as the principal regulator of erythropoiesis.

The anemia of renal failure is characterized by normocytic and normochromic red blood cells (RBCs); the reticulocyte count is low for the degree of anemia, and the erythroid bone marrow appears hypoplastic, without interference with leukopoiesis or megakaryocytopoiesis.[5] Anemia, initially mild and inconsequential, is virtually a constant feature of acute or chronic renal failure. However, as renal function progressively deteriorates, the hematocrit continues to decline and may reach concentrations as low as 15% to 20%. At that point, the patient usually experiences symptoms, and transfusions may be necessary. Before the introduction of recombinant human erythropoeitin (rhEPO), approximately one fourth of chronic uremic patients were dependent on blood transfusion. Anemia also contributes to the development of heart failure in chronic uremia.

Pathophysiology of Renal Anemia

The anemia of renal failure is a complex disorder determined by a variety of factors. Although the primary defect is decreased erythropoiesis, a number of other factors may play contributory roles. Some degree of hemolysis is frequently present, bleeding can occur, and a superimposed iron or folic acid deficiency can complicate the problem. In the past, attention was drawn to the potential direct effects of uremic waste products,[6] but the advent of dialysis put their significance into perspective. Toxic metabolites, the so-called uremic toxins, had been assumed to inhibit erythropoiesis either directly or by interfering with the actions of EPO and hematopoiesis-stimulating cytokines, but this is a controversial issue.[7, 8]

More recent studies tend to minimize an inhibiting role of substances previously suggested as erythropoiesis inhibitors, including polyamines such as spermine spermidine.[9] Concerning substances that accumulate in the serum of uremic patients, such as 5-propyl-2-furanpropionic acid and quinolinic acid,[10] final proof of their role as erythropoiesis inhibitors is lacking. There are reports of an inverse correlation between RBC survival time and serum blood urea nitrogen concentration.[11] The mechanisms leading to shortening of RBC half-life remain unclear.

The RBCs from uremic patients are probably intrinsically normal, because cross-transfusion studies have shown that RBCs from normal subjects have a shortened half-life after transfusion into uremic patients, whereas RBCs from uremic patients have a normal survival after transfusion into nonuremic recipients.[6, 12] However, the RBC life span may become nearly normal or even normal in carefully dialyzed patients.[13] Other than restoring erythropoiesis, rhEPO therapy brings back to normal erythrocyte survival and viability; it also increases the elasticity, deformability, and antioxidant enzymatic system of RBCs. Significantly higher levels of RBC superoxide dismutase and total glutathione peroxidase were found in hemodialysis (HD) patients 3 months after initiation of rhEPO treatment.[13, 14]

A relevant factor in shortening RBC survival is lipid peroxidation of the cell membrane, which may depend on the defective antioxidant activity of uremia or on the aging of circulating RBCs, as the membranes of young cells contain more antioxidant enzymes. The increased tendency to bleed, frequent blood sampling, occult blood loss, and blood loss during HD can be additional factors contributing to the anemia of renal failure.

Erythropoiesis

Erythropoiesis is the dynamic process of RBC production. After erythroid commitment of undifferentiated pluripotent hematopoietic stem cells, subsequent cellular divisions amplify the early erythroid progenitors, providing a proper quantity of cells for terminal differentiation into mature erythrocytes. The transformation of a multipotential stem cell into a mature RBC occurs in two morphologically distinct stages, of which only the first is responsive to EPO. The first stage includes stem cells (consisting of small mononuclear cells) that display a single glycophosphoprotein, CD34, on their surface,[15] and the progenitor cells are responsive to EPO. In the second, or precursor, stage, the cells appear as morphologically recognizable erythroblasts.

Erythropoiesis begins when the multipotential stem cell is stimulated by nonspecific cytokines, such as interleukin-3 (IL-3), insulin-like growth factor-1(IGF-1), and granulocyte-macrophage colony-stimulating factor (GM-CSF), to proliferate and transform into the unipotential erythroid-committed progenitor cell. The earliest of these progenitor cells—which keep the receptors for the cytokines while acquiring receptors for EPO—proliferate luxuriantly and produce colonies composed of many cells (burst-forming units–erythroid [BFU-E]). These latter—which lose the receptors for cytokines while experiencing an increase in receptors for EPO—in turn multiply and differentiate into CFU-E (colony-forming units–erythroid). From the CFU-E arise the hemoglobin-synthesizing precursor cells.[16] These latter profilerate and mature, and eventually reach the stage of mature RBCs, apparently without any influence from EPO but in the presence of adequate supplies of substrates, iron, vitamin B_{12}, and folic acid. The EPO receptor (a transmembrane protein with a molecular weight of 55,000 D that belongs to the cytokine receptor superfamily)[17] has been identified only on the surface of erythroid-committed progenitor cells. CFU-E is actually the key target cell for EPO, which indeed regulates RBC production.[18] The expansion of the BFU-E and CFU-E compartment, which is directly related to the EPO concentration in the medium, affects the size of the precursor cell stage, which, in turn, determines the size of mature cell mass and the erythropoietic response.[19]

Erythropoietin

In 1893, Miescher suggested that low oxygen pressure acted directly on the bone marrow to stimulate the production of RBCs. However, in 1906, Carnot and Deflandre produced an increase in RBC count by injecting serum from anemic rabbits into normal rabbits. They suggested that the serum contained a substance called *hémopoïétine* that was capable of stimulating the bone marrow. In 1943, Krumdieck[20] documented reticulocytosis in normal rabbits after injection of anemic serum. Bonsdorff and Jalavisto[21] induced erythropoiesis in rabbits with plasma derived from patients with congestive heart failure and coined the term *EPO*. A linkage between a humoral erythropoietic factor and hypoxia was fashioned by Riessmann[22] in 1950 with an ingenious experiment an parabiotic rats. He produced hypoxemia in one animal enclosed in a special breathing chamber containing 7.6% oxygen and augmented erythropoiesis in the parabiotic partner breathing normal air. Thus, hypoxemia

was shown to act indirectly through an intermediary substance. Erslev[23, 24] confirmed the presence of an erythropoietic factor in the blood of anemic animals, and Stohlman and colleagues[25] associated increased erythropoiesis and secondary polycythemia with regional hypoxia in a patient with patent ductus arteriosus. In 1957, Jacobson and associates[4] demonstrated that bilaterally nephrectomized animals subjected to bleeding failed to elaborate increased EPO. The following year, Gurney and co-workers[26] reported that patients with renal disease and anemia lacked erythropoietic-stimulating factor (ESF) in their plasma. In 1977, Miyake and co-workers[27] purified human EPO, and in 1986 Lai and colleagues[28] characterized its molecular structure. Several reviews summarize the current knowledge regarding the structure and function of EPO[18, 29] and its receptor.[17, 30] EPO is a sialylglycoprotein composed of 165 amino acids, 18 with an estimated molecular mass of 34,000 D.[29] The carbohydrate moiety, rich in sialic acid, is critical to in vivo reactivity in that the asialo form is rapidly sequestered in the liver.[31]

Serum concentrations of EPO normally range from 8 to 18 mU/mL (approximately 0.1 mg/mL, or 5 pmol/L) and, in anemia, may increase 100- to 1000-fold.[32] The cloning and sequencing of the EPO gene[33, 34] has provided probes for studying EPO synthesis and secretion; as the amounts of messenger RNA (mRNA) for EPO are highly sensitive to changes in tissue oxygenation, it appears that EPO synthesis is regulated primarily at the level of gene transcription.[35]

Studies have shown that hypoxia intially causes the production of a protein named *hypoxia-inducible factor* (HIF-1).[36] This factor binds to an oxygen-sensitive enhancer located immediately downstream from the transcription stop site of the gene for EPO (located on chromosome 7) and activates the transcription of the EPO gene. An in situ hybridization technique for EPO mRNA has shown that the site of production is extratubular, in the interstitial cells of the renal cortex near the base of the proximal tubule cells, and the rate of production appears to be correlated with the number of EPO mRNA-containing cells.[16] The in vitro experiments suggest that the same cell that perceives hypoxia may produce EPO. Oxygen deficiency may be sensed effectively in renal cortex, and reduced capillary flow also might induce increased EPO production (Fig. 49-1).

Anemia can develop relatively early in the course of chronic renal failure (at creatinine clearances between 20 and 35 mL/minute/1.73 m^2); the impairment of EPO production appears to parallel the progressive reduction of nephron mass,[37] and the plasma concentration of EPO becomes disproportionately low for the degree of reduction of hemoglobin concentration.[35] However, the oxygen-EPO-hemoglobin feedback loop is still operating, even if at a lower set-point. In chronic renal failure, indeed, the plasma EPO concentration declines after blood transfusion[38] and even though remaining inappropriate to the severity of anemia, measurably increases (up to fivefold) after hemorrhage or hypoxic crisis.[38] Detectable levels of plasma EPO have been noted also in anephric patients,[39] to confirm the experimental studies in rats after binephrectomy showing that a share (10%-15%, and probably less in humans) of serum EPO, indistinguishable from that produced by the kidney, is produced by hepatocytes and, possibly, macrophages.[40] In humans, the EPO gene has mapped sequences, other than those

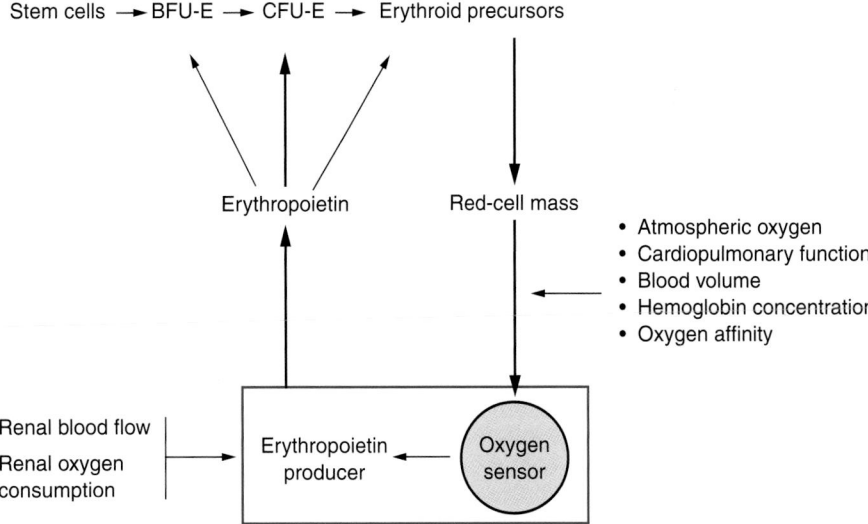

FIGURE 49-1. Feedback control of red blood cell (RBC) production by erythropoietin. The surface of maturing progenitor cells in bone marrow contains erythropoietin receptors that first disappear at the early precursor-cell stage. The receptors close a feedback loop, between a renal oxygen sensor and bone marrow progenitor cells, that ensures that under normal conditions the rate of RBC production matches the need for oxygen-carrying RBCs in the circulation. BFU-E, burst-forming units–erythroid; CFU-E, colony-forming units–erythroid. (Modified from Erslev AJ: Erythropoietin. N Engl J Med 324: 1339-1344, 1991. Copyright © 1991 Massachusetts Medical Society. All rights reserved.)

directing expression in the kidney, that control the hepatocyte-specific expression of EPO mRNA.[41]

The relationship between the degree of anemia, the supply of oxygen to the tissues, and the rate of production of EPO is quite broad, and it is assumed that other factors may play a role by interfering in either the production or the action of EPO. Cobalt, androgens, and insulin-derived growth factor seem to work as agonists, and inflammatory cytokines as antagonists. In autosomal dominant polycystic disease, the degree of anemia is less than, and the serum level of EPO greater than, those usually accounted for by increased serum creatinine concentration, as if cystic kidneys could maintain better EPO production despite renal failure. The percentage of dialysis patients who do not need treatment of anemia seems to be about 7%. Besides, when acquired polycystic kidney disease develops in HD patients, a significant spontaneous improvement of anemia may be observed. Cells containing EPO mRNA have been found in the walls of the cysts.

Recombinant Human Erythropoietin

The cloning and expression of the human EPO gene was achieved in 1984,[33] and by the end of 1986 the efficacy of rhEPO in reversing the anemia of uremia was established (see also Chapter 58).[42, 43] The first clinical trials of rhEPO were performed in England[42] and the United States.[43] The results were remarkable. Winearls and colleagues[42] gave rhEPO by intravenous bolus to nine patients three times per week and raised the mean hemoglobin concentration from 6.1 to 10.3 g/dL within 12 weeks. Eschbach and co-workers[43] gave rhEPO intravenously to 25 patients in doses ranging from 15 to 500 U/kg body weight and demonstrated a dose-dependent response (Fig. 49-2). Anephric transfusion–dependent patients responded equally well to rhEPO, and the need for transfusion was eliminated. Other clinical trials in the United States,[44] Europe,[45, 46] and Japan[47] confirmed these favorable results. Concerns that the effectiveness of

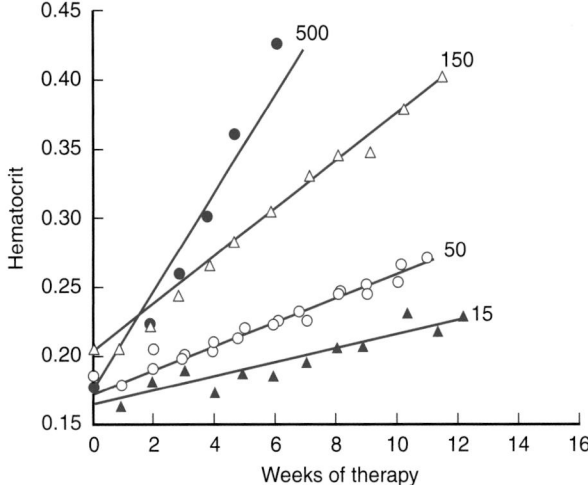

FIGURE 49-2. Slopes of the rates of increase in hematocrit associated with various doses of erythropoietin (IU/kg body weight) given three times per week. (From Eschbach JW, Egrie JC, Downing MR, et al: Correction of the anemia of end-stage renal disease with recombinant human erythropoietin: Results of a combined phase I and II clinical trial. N Engl J Med 316:73-78, 1987. Reprinted by permission of the New England Journal of Medicine. Copyright 1987 Massachusetts Medical Society.)

rhEPO might be dependent on concomitant HD were dispelled by the equally favorable results obtained with predialysis patients[44, 48, 49] and patients receiving continuous ambulatory peritoneal dialysis (CAPD).[50] A large multicenter trial reported in 1989[51] greatly expanded the number of favorable responses to rhEPO. By 1990,[52] an estimated 2000 patients had been treated, and a 1991 review placed at 175,000 the number of patients who had been treated with this remarkable drug.[37]

rhEPO contains the identical 165–amino acid sequence of isolated natural EPO, but the glycosylated moiety is different. There are two forms of rhEPO: epoetin alfa and epoetin beta. The first one is produced by genomic DNA (gDNA), the second one by complementary DNA (cDNA); they differ from each other in the oligosaccharide component. Both forms of rhEPO, epoetin alfa (39% oligosaccharide moiety) and epoetin beta (24% oligosaccharide moiety), are available for clinical use; they do not show any difference in pharmacokinetics and efficacy.[41] The half-life ranges from 4 to 13 hours after intravenous administration and is around 24 hours after subcutaneous administration. With the subcutaneous route, levels peak at 8 to 12 hours and decline slowly thereafter; maximum levels with subcutaneous administration are only about 10% of those achieved after the same intravenous dose. Both rhEPO preparations appear to be eliminated by primarily nonrenal routes.

Novel Erythropoiesis-Stimulating Protein (ARANESP)

Novel erythropoiesis stimulating protein (ARANESP) is a molecule that stimulates erythropoiesis by the same mechanism as erythropoietin.[53] ARANESP, also named *darbepoetin alpha,* contains five N-linked carbohydrate chains, two more than rhEPO,[54] and has an increased molecular weight and greater negative charge. ARANESP has an approximately three-fold serum half-life.[55] In peritoneal dialysis (PD) patients the mean half-life following a single dose of intravenous ARANESP was 25.3 hours as compared to 8.5 hours of rhEPO.[55] Subcutaneous administration of ARANESP is associated with a longer half-life, which is protracted to 48.8 hours.[5] This difference reflects both a slow absorption from the injection site and a slow elimination from the circulation. These pharmacokinetic properties suggest that ARANESP can be administered less frequently than rhEPO. Clinical studies in more than 1500 patients have concluded that ARANESP is as effective and safe as rhEPO in correcting uremic anemia.[56] The suggested initial dose of ARANESP is 0.45 µg/kg once a week either subcutaneously or intravenously. When the target hemoglobin level is reached, the maintenance dose of ARANESP is determined for the individual patient. To change from rhEPO to ARANESP, a rule of thumb is to divide the rhEPO dose by a factor of 200.[57]

MANAGEMENT OF RENAL ANEMIA

Treatment with Recombinant Erythropoietin

The 1996 U.S. Renal Data System Annual Report, which refers to 1993 data from the United States, shows that the mean hematocrit for rhEPO-treated dialysis patients was 30.2%, with 43% of patients having hematocrit values less than 30%.[58] A study conducted in a random sample of 1317 adult PD patients and 7310 adult in-center HD patients alive on December 31, 1995, showed that whereas 77% of PD and 93% of HD patients used rhEPO, 33% of PD and 37% of HD patients had a hematocrit less than 30%.[59] Thus, not all patients who could benefit are receiving the therapy, and of those who are, many are not being treated adequately (the routine clinical practice throughout the world is to maintain hematocrit at a level of 28%-33%)[60] (Table 49-1).

Renal anemia is rapidly corrected by rhEPO therapy, but the dose required can vary greatly.[61] Within the therapeutic range of approximately 50 to 300 IU/kg three times per week, the rate of hemoglobin increase, even if varying among patients, depends on the dose of rhEPO. Doses exceeding

TABLE 49-1

Guidelines for Treatment with Recombinant Human Erythropoietin (rhEPO) in Patients with Chronic Kidney Disease

Anemia workup should be initiated when
    Hemoglobin <11 g/dL (hematocrit <33%) in premenopausal women and prepubertal patients
    Hemoglobin <12 g/dL (hematocrit <37%) in adult males and postmenopausal women
Anemia workup should include a test for occult blood in the stool and measurement of iron parameters
    Serum iron
    Total iron binding capacity (TIBC)
    Transferrin saturation
    Ferritin
Patients with microcytic anemia and normal iron stores should be evaluated for aluminum toxicity and thalassemia.
Uncontrolled hypertension is a contraindication to the initiation of rhEPO therapy.
The hemoglobin level or hematocrit should be measured each week during induction of therapy and every 2 wk thereafter. Serum iron, TIBC, and serum ferritin should be measured monthly for 3 mo and every 2-3 mo thereafter.
The target range for hemoglobin (hematocrit) should be 11 g/dL (33%) to 12 g/dL (36%).

Adapted from Ad Hoc Committee for the National Kidney Foundation: Statement of the clinical use of recombinant erythropoietin in anemia of end-stage renal disease. Am J Kidney Dis 14:163-169, 1989; and National Kidney Foundation–K/DOQI-Clinical Practice Guidelines for Anemia of Chronic Kidney Disease, 2000. A M J Kidney Dis 37(suppl 1):S182-S238, 2001.

300 IU/kg three times per week do not enhance the erythropoietic response. Current recommendations[61] are to start with 50 to 100 IU/kg IV three times per week. With an intravenous dosage of 50 IU/kg three times per week, the rate of hemoglobin rise is approximately 1 g/dL every 4 weeks, and with 100 IU/kg three times per week it is 1.5 to 2.0 g/dL. Higher starting doses are employed when there is the need to rapidly increase the level of hemoglobin; however, a rate of hemoglobin rise of more than 3 g/dL in any 4-week period should be avoided because of the possible exacerbation of hypertension. During the correction phase, the dosage of rhEPO must be adjusted monthly until the target is attained; the response to any change of dosage requires 4 weeks to be completely assessed. Each time a dosage needs to be increased, the increment should not exceed 30 IU/kg three times per week. When the target hemoglobin is about to be reached, and in rapid responders, the dosage should be decreased by approximately 25 IU/kg three times per week to avoid overshooting the target. Thereafter, the dose should be titrated down gradually by making adjustments at convenient intervals (8 weeks).

In the maintenance phase, the minimal dosage of rhEPO able to maintain target hemoglobin levels must be sought; it has been suggested that the increased sensitivity to EPO of the progenitor cells and the gradual expansion of their compartment and that of erythroblasts could result from constant rhEPO therapy.[62] In general, the higher the target, the greater the maintenance dose. The median intravenous maintenance dose necessary for maintaining the target hemoglobin-hematocrit (Hb/Hct) value at approximately 12 g/dL (36%) is on average 75 IU/kg three times per week. However, some patients may first need 25 IU/kg three times per week, whereas others may require more than 200 IU/kg three times per week.

In some studies the subcutaneous administration of EPO appeared more effective and less expensive than the intravenous one,[63, 64] requiring on average a 32% smaller dose to achive the same target,[58, 63] but this was not confirmed by other studies.[65, 66] In CAPD patients, the intraperiotoneal route has been tested and found not to be cost-effective. There is waste of drug because absorption is scanty: the bioavailability of intraperitoneally given rhEPO is one-fifth to one-tenth that of a subcutaneous dose. In conclusion, both routes, intravenous and subcutaneous, are appropriate for patients on HD,[67] and the subcutaneous route is suited for CAPD or predialysis patients.

Predialysis

The timing of rhEPO treatment should not be dependent on whether the patient is already on dialysis.[44] In fact, rhEPO therapy could be started for patients with uncomplicated anemia of chronic renal disease before end-stage renal disease (ESRD) has developed.[68] As a matter of fact, rhEPO is increasingly used to treat the anemia of predialysis patients.[69-71] The progression of renal disease is not significantly altered, provided that hypertension is treated adequately. Optimal regimens, doses, and routes of administration are still under discussion. In most published sutdies, the rhEPO doses used in this setting were lower than those in dialysis patients, that is, 50 to 100 IU/kg/week subcutaneously.

In a study of 83 predialysis patients, correction of anemia (hematocrit $\geq 36\%$) occurred in 34 (79%) of the 43 treated patients, who enjoyed a significantly improved quality of life.[72]

Dialysis

There has long been an impression that removal of more small or middle "toxic" molecules results in higher hemoglobin. However, tha data are controversial. In the early years of dialysis, switching from twice-weekly to thrice-weekly HD resulted in improved erythropoiesis,[73] but the routine use of RBC transfusions, which suppress erythropoiesis, was discontinued at the same time. The National Cooperative Dialysis Study of 1983 noted that better removal of small molecules, with lower blood urea nitrogen levels, resulted in hegher hematocrit levels.[74] However, a prospective study of 6 months of reduced hemodialysis hours, three times a week, in which middle and small molecule clearances were decreased, disclosed no change in hematocrit levels.[75] A quantitative study of erythropoiesis, utilizing ferrokinetics, reticulocyte response, and transferrin receptor activity, noted that the erythropoietic response in hemodialysis subjects to 15, 50, or 150 IU/kg of EPO every other day for four doses was similar to the responses in normal subjects given the same dose of rhEPO.[76] Therefore, for these HD patients, there was no blunting in the action of rhEPO from the uremic solutes present in their circulation, and this finding suggests that more dialysis is not necessarily going to improve erythropoiesis.

This view has, however, been challenged by studies showing that 40% to 60% of U.S. patients undergoing HD who were receiving EPO had hematocrit values that did not rise above 30%, despite therapy with doses of EPO equivalent to those used in the original clinical trials.[71-81] This finding has been attributed to the effect of the intensity of dialysis on the response to EPO. Indeed in 135 randomly selected patients

undergoing HD and receiving intravenous EPO for at least 4 months, inadequate dialysis (indicated by a urea-reduction value <65%) was associated with a poor response to rhEPO (i. e., a low hematocrit). Increasing the level of dialysis in patients who were receiving inadequate dialysis results in an increase in the hematocrit.[82]

Analysis of a very large population of 2094 EPO-treated hemodialysis patients from the USRDS Dialysis Morbidity and Moratality Study (DMMS) showed that the effect of the delivered dose of dialysis on the response to rhEPO was evident only for those who were dialyzed with a synthetic dialyzer.[83] Apart from the specific effect of better removal of uremic toxins, an adequate dialysis may ameliorate the anemia as a consequence of improvements in RBC survival, blood coagulation, nutritional status, and well-being.

Transplant

With immediate kidney graft function, the EPO serum levels will double within 7 days after transplantation and will remain elevated until the anemia is corrected. The gradual increase of EPO is accompanied, after a lag period of 3 weeks, by a parallel increase in transferrin receptor levels (meaning erythroid marrow expansion), which, in turn, precedes by some weeks the hematocrit increase; within 4 months, EPO levels have reached the normal range, and the hematocrit is normalized. In some recipients, iron deficiency secondary to increased iron utilization may occur,[84] but it corrects spontaneously.[85]

In the first weeks after renal transplantation, some patients present with marked anemia due to blood loss, intercurrent inflammatory and infectious diseases, graft rejection, and still inadequate EPO production by the transplanted kidney.[86] The anemia associated with progressive chronic graft failure can be effectively treated with rhEPO, without significant alterations of renal function.

Post-transplant erythrocytosis (hemoglobin 16-17 g/dL) is not uncommon. It developed in 7.6% of 223 patients who received a kidney graft, and it was shown to be due to increased erythropoietic activity and was independent of the EPO plasma level and BFU-E sensitivity in vitro to increasing EPO concentrations.[87] Angiotensin-converting enzyme inhibitors (ACEIs) and losartan, an angiotensin II type 1 (AT_1) receptor antagonist, diminish post-transplant errhocytosis without altering EPO plasma levels.[88] It has been reported that ACEIs worsen the anemia caused by renal failure,[89] reduce the response to rhEPO in HD patients,[90, 91] and increase the need for rhEPO.[92, 93]

Studies on the erythroid differentation of CD34+ hematopoietic progenitor cells in culture have shown that angiotensin II, through activation of AT_1, enhances EPO-stimulated erythroid cell proliferation.[88] These findings suggest that angiotensin II may be one of the factors stimulating erythropoiesis. This issue has been clarified by in vitro demonstration that angiotensin II increased proliferation of early erythroid progenitors induced by EPO, an event completely abolished by the AT_1 receptor antagonist losartan.[88] Thus, activation of the AT_1 receptor with angiotensin II enhances EPO-stimulated erythroid proliferation.

On the other hand, erythroid differentiation from pluripotent hematopoietic stem cells may be directly blocked by ACE inhibition. Thus, a single oral dose of 50 mg of the

ACEI captopril, when administered to eight healthy subjects in a double-blind, placebo-controlled study, massively increased the plasma level of the tetrapeptide N-acetyl-seryl-aspartyl-lysyl-proline, a regulatory factor of hematopoiesis that reversibly prevents the recruitment of pluripotent hematopoietic stem cells and normal early progenitors into S phase.[94]

Side Effects

The incidence (number of events per patient-year) of some of the most frequently reported adverse events has been reported as follows: arterial hypertension (0.75), clotted vascular access (0.25), and hyperkalemia (0.11). The relationship of rhEPO therapy to seizures is uncertain. The real incidence of these events is difficult to ascertain, because seizures are not infrequent in the untreated dialysis population. However, the rate of seizures during the first 90 days of rhEPO therapy appears to be higher than that during the subsequent 90 days.[51] Strict control of the rate of hemoglobin rise (no more than 1.5 g/dL in any 4-week period) and close monitoring of the blood pressure appear warranted.

CLOTTING. Clotting of the vascular access and the artificial kidney are frequently reported.[95] In patients treated with either epoetin alfa or epoetin beta, increases in factor VIII, von Willebrand factor antigen, fibrinogen, and whole-blood platelet aggregation have been observed. These effects, together with other transient but significant changes occuring in tissue plasminogen activator antigen, plasminogen activator inhibitor, and antithrombin III, combined with reduction of fibrinolytic activity, all favor a tendency to thrombosis. Increased anticoagulation with heparin may be required. Other thrombotic events of concern are cerebrovascular accidents, transient ischemic attacks, and myocardial infarction. A statistically certain relationship has not been established between the rate of rise in hemoglobin and the incidence of thrombotic events. Neither higher hemoglobin concentrations nor higher rhEPO doses adversely affect the survival of a prosthetic arteriovenous access graft.

HYPERKALEMIA. Hyperkalemia reflects both less efficient dialysis (blood flow being equal, higher hematocrit means less plasma available for correction) and lesser compliance with dietary prescriptions (compliance should be reinforced in rhEPO-treated patients, who experience improved well-being and quality of life).

ARTERIAL HYPERTENSION. A new onset or worsening of hypertension is the most commonly reported side effect of rhEPO therapy in ESRD patients. In a review of 47 publications including 3428 patients, development or aggravation of preexisting hypertension was found in 785 of them (23%) during rhEPO treatment.[58] Increases in blood pressure have been reported more often during the first 90 days of therapy. The incidence reportedly varies between 1 in 4 and 1 in 3 patients. Hypertension was never observed in patients with anemia but no renal disease.[96] The following risk factors have been identified: preexisting hypertension, rapid correction of anemia, and high doses of rhEPO, whereas intravenous administration of rhEPO is not considered a risk factor. Serum EPO, even if within normal range, significantly correlated with systolic and diastolic blood pressure in patients with established essential hypertension but not in subjects with borderline hypertension; furthermore, EPO was inversely correlated with renal plasma flow in both groups.[97]

Enhanced vascular reactivity associated with an increased RBC mass is the plausible cause of rhEPO-induced hypertension. In uremic (five-sixths nephrectomized) rats the blood pressure response to rhEPO is enhanced compared to control animals.[98] Although rhEPO is not a direct vasoconstrictor, it does enhance vascular responsiveness to norepinephrine.[99] Acute administration of rhEPO in intact rats raised blood pressure and reduced renal plasma flow, in association with enhanced endothelin-1 release.[100] However in 32 patients on HD, levels of plasma endothelin-1 did not change with rhEPO treatment.[101] More recent findings have reported a direct action of rhEPO on vascular smooth muscle cells via a specific EPO receptor.[102] In cultured rat vascular smooth muscle cells, increasing rhEPO concentrations up to 6 to 8 U/mL caused parallel and significant increases in mRNA of renin, angiotensinogen, angiotensin II receptors, and angiotensin II–responsive growth factors. In this context, rhEPO-induced hypertension in the rat is associated with increased gene transcription of renin and angiotensinogen in the kidney and in vascular tissue. In most cases, arterial hypertension can be effectively managed by reducing dry body weight,[101] starting or increasing antihypertensive therapy, and reducing the dose of rhEPO. Regression of left ventricular hypertrophy and normalization of cardiac index and other hemodynamic and functional parameters are evident during treatment with rhEPO, and are maintained afterward, providing an adequate control of blood pressure.[96]

PURE RED CELL APLASIA. A most alarming side effect of EPO use is the development of antierythropoietin antibodies which is associated with severe transfusion-dependent anemia, caused by a pure red cell (bone marrow) aplasia. Only three cases were reported in the literature[103, 104] before the publication of the seminal work of Casadevall and colleagues in early 2002,[105] which described and characterized 13 patients with pure red cell aplasia who had developed antibodies able to block the formation of erythroid colonies by normal bone marrow cells. Following this report, in July 2002, the manufacturer of epoetin alfa issued a "Dear Doctor letter," warning that 141 suspected cases of pure red cell aplasia had been reported worldwide.[106] In 114 cases a bone marrow biopsy confirmed the erythroblastopenia. Of 80 patients whose serum was available for antibody testing, 66 were found positive for antierythropoeitin antibodies. Anemia developed, on average, 10 months post therapy initiation, with a range of 1 to 92 months. Although the data are too scanty for a firm conclusion, it seems that the incidence of pure red cell aplasia is higher in patients who are taking EPO subcutaneously than in those who are taking the drug intravenously. When pure red cell aplasia is suspected, EPO administration should be immediately interrupted. It is also recommended to avoid switching patients to another form of EPO or to darbopoietin, as the antierythropoietin antibodies cross-react with all commercially available recombinant erythropoietic products.[105] Immunosuppressive treatment was followed by disappearance of the antibodies in 16 of the cases described by Casadevall.[107]

Causes of Inadequate Response

Hyporesponsiveness to rhEPO has been defined as failure to achieve target hematocrit in the presence of adequate iron stores at a dose of 450 IU/kg/week intravenously, within 4 to 6 months,[58] or failure to maintain it subsequently at that dose.[108]

Several conditions have been associated with inadequate responses to rhEPO. Iron deficiency (both absolute and functional) is the most common cause.[64, 109-112] Other factors are inadequate dialysis; protein malnutrition; severe hyperparathyroidism; aluminium overload; underlying infectious, inflammatory, or malignant diseases; occult blood loss; and hemoglobinopathies (e.g., thalassemias) (Table 49-2).[112]

IRON DEFICIENCY

A suboptimal response to rhEPO most commonly results from failure of delivery of an adequate amount of iron to the erythron. Enhanced iron utilization due to rhEPO-induced RBC formation can quickly deplete iron stores previously reduced by poor iron absorption, occult gastrointestinal bleeding, or dialysis-related blood losses.[16] Treatment with rhEPO is, at this time, the most common cause of iron deficiency. Most treated patients become iron deficient[113] and therefore require more rhEPO to maintain the same rate of RBC production. If the iron balance is not restored by oral or parenteral iron replacement and iron deficiency worsens, an initial good response may then falter. The most accurate assessment of iron stores is given by staining the bone marrow aspirate for iron with Perl Prussian blue stain.[114]

In the absence of this reliable, but invasive, reference standard, iron status is commonly assessed by serum iron concentration, serum ferritin (SF), transferrin saturation (TfS), and RBC indices.[113] Serum iron concentration fluctuates during rhEPO administration, but SF, a protein secreted into the plasma by the reticuloendothelial cells under the regulation of intracellular iron concentration, is a good indicator of iron stores[105]; The TfS index (calculated according to the formula: saturation % = serum iron/total iron capacity)—that means transferrin-bound iron—appears to be even better (higher sensitivity and similar specificity).[114]

Iron deficiency secondary to the consumption of iron deposits by rhEPO-stimulated erythropoiesis may be concealed by the persistence of apparently adequate ferritin levels, but it is disclosed by both a TfS less than 20% and prompt erythropoietic response to intravenous administration of iron dextran. In a study on the early predictors of a response to rhEPO, the initial values of serum iron, TfS, mean corpuscular volume (MCV), and mean corpuscular hemoglobin concentration (MCHC) were significantly lower in the iron-responsive group than in the iron-nonresponsive one; furthermore, there was a strong inverse relationship between initial TfS and the change in hematocrit following iron therapy in patients hyporesponsive to rhEPO.[116]

TABLE 49-2

Causes of Inadequate Response to Recombinant Human Erythropoietin Therapy

1. Infection/inflammation
2. Chronic blood loss
3. Malnutrition: folate or vitamin B_{12} deficiency
4. Aluminum toxicity
5. Osteitis fibrosa
6. Hemoglobinopathies (e.g., α- and β-thalassemia, sickle cell anemia)
7. Malignancies
8. Hemolysis
9. Pure red cell aplasia

The failure to make enough iron available to meet the demands of enhanced erythropoiesis despite the presence of adequate iron stores, as reflected by the level of SF, has been defined as "functional iron deficiency" (compared to "absolute iron deficiency" or "iron storage deficiency"). The RBCs appear hypochromic (with MCHC <28 g/dL) when mobilization of iron from stores and its transport to the erythron become inadequate. A percentage of circulating hypochromic RBCs greater than 10% (normal range: <2.5% of circulating RBCs), in the presence of adequate iron stores and the absence of hemoglobinopathies or inflammatory diseases, should be diagnostic of functional iron deficiency.[117, 118]

Other more sophisticated tests for iron deficiency have been proposed: erythrocyte ferritin[119, 120]; hemoglobin content of reticulocytes (CHr); free erythrocyte protoporphyrin (FEP); and serum transferrin receptors (STr). A reduced erythrocyte ferritin level despite normal SF should suggest functional iron deficiency, a condition that measurement of both CHr and erythrocyte ferritin could help identify.[121] In 1364 stable HD patients, CHr was weakly but consistently correlated with TfS and SF. A CHr less than 26 pg at baseline should predict iron deficiency with a sensitivity of 100% and a specificity of 80%,[122] and more accurately than TfS, SF, or their combination.[123] The CHr/MHC ratio (mean hemoglobin content of mature RBCs) could, when increased, indicate the response to iron load and, when decreased, herald the acute onset of iron deficiency.[122] FEP levels measure the amount of protoporphyrin not incorporated into heme. Patients with an FEP of at least 90 mmol/mol heme were considered likely to be iron deficient. FEP and SF have been shown to have a similar reliability as predictors of iron deficiency. STr are released by erythroid progenitor cells under conditions of both enhanced erythropoiesis and reduced iron supply; their measurement could help to distinguish iron deficiency anemia from that associated with chronic diseases[124] and to predict the erythropoietic response to rhEPO.[125]

In any case, the primary goal is to ascertain whether an inadequate response to rhEPO is due to iron deficiency or other causes. By first replenishing and then maintaining iron stores, it is possible to achieve the target hematocrit with the lowest necessary dose of rhEPO.[126-128] In the presence of an adequate response to rhEPO, iron supplementation should be targeted at keeping the level of SF greater than 100 ng/mL, TfS more than 20%, and hypocrhomic RBCs less than 10%.[129] The intravenous route is mandatory in the presence of absolute or functional iron deficiency; oral iron supplementation is often unsuccessful,[130] because rapid replacement of the iron consumed is not well tolerated, and gastrointestinal absorption is diminished by the presence of phosphate binders or H_2 blockers. In the maintenance phase, oral iron alone can only rarely sustain the response to rhEPO,[131] as has been suggested by the experience on a national scale in the United States when iron dextran was unavailable for an extended time.[132] The intravenous administration of iron enhances the erythropoietic response despite apparently adequate iron stores.

The availability of new, well-tolerated, parenteral iron preparations—iron dextran, iron saccharate, and sodium ferric gluconate complex—is a factor promoting the use of the intravenous route in the maintenance phase of rhEPO therapy.[133] Supplementation of intravenous iron on a regular basis at a dose of 10 to 20 mg of iron saccharate at the end of each HD session[134] seems to be superior to bolus therapy[135] in maintaining target hematocrit while requiring significantly less rhEPO.[136, 137] Guidelines and treatment schedules for iron supplementation in predialysis, HD, and CAPD patients have been published.[58, 134, 138]

Resistance to rhEPO sometimes occurs in iron-overload (TrS >50%, and SF >500-1000 ng/mL), and ascorbate supplementation may prevent it.[139] Iron overload is treated by withholding iron, increasing rhEPO, and doing phlebotomy[58]; the administration of deferoxamine could improve hemosiderosis and maintain the response to rhEPO without iron administration.[130]

ALUMINUM OVERLOAD

In HD patients, aluminum toxicity may cause microcytic anemia despite normal iron deposits. Aluminum and iron utilize common pathways for intestinal absorption, transport in the plasma, and binding to transferrin; aluminum overload may interfere with iron utilization in the response to rhEPO.[140, 141] The sources of aluminum accumulation are primarily both gastrointestinal absorption from antacids used to bind dietary phosphorus and improperly processed water for dialysate. The best way of diagnosing aluminum overload is bone biopsy. Basal serum aluminum concentrations greater than 50 ng/mL and aluminium levels after the deferoxamine (an aluminum-binding agent) challenge test (a single dose of 500-1000 mg intravenously) higher than 175 ng/mL should indicate an aluminium accumulation great enough to interfere with the response to rhEPO. Treatment with intravenous deferoxamine should be able to improve not only the aluminium-induced microcytic anemia but also the normocytic anemia with questionable aluminum accumulation; it could also restore responsiveness to rhEPO.

During the last decade, water for dialysate has been properly processed, and aluminum salts have been widely replaced by calcium-containing phosphate binders, so at present lower serum aluminum levels are generally observed in the dialysis population. According to a report, iron-depleted rats should be more susceptible to aluminum accumulation.[142] As the introduction of rhEPO therapy has resulted in a higher incidence of iron depletion and this latter may substantially affect uptake, transport, and tissue distribution of aluminum, it has been suggested that in some patients toxic effects could take place despite the absence of overt aluminum overload.[143]

INFECTIOUS AND INFLAMMATORY CHRONIC DISEASES AND MALIGNANCIES

Erythropoiesis is negatively regulated by several macrophage-derived cytokines, including tumor necrosis factor-α (TNF-α), interleukin-I (IL-1) and IL-6, and transforming growth factor-β (TGF-β), all factors that are elevated in inflammatory processes. These cytokiness have inhibitory effects, either direct or mediated, on the erythroid progenitor cells (BFU-E and CFU-E); they may also impair iron metabolism by sequestering iron inside the macrophages ("inflammatory iron block").[144] Activated macrophages synthesize lactoferrin, a high-affinity iron-binding protein that may compete with transferrin for iron binding. As a consequence, the anemia that occurs with inflammation, infection, and malignancies is normocytic and normochromic in most cases, but not

uncommonly may be microcytic and hypochromic despite normal or raised levels of SF. This is due to the fact that, in addition to reflecting iron stores, ferritin is also an acute-phase protein. The measurement of the levels of zinc protoporphyrin, a metabolic intermediate generated in the erythroid cells by incorporation of zinc instead of iron, has been proposed as a marker of endogenous iron availability[145, 146]; it could be an indicator of functional iron deficiency following blockade of iron release from macrophages.[147] The association of chronic inflammatory disease with chronic renal failure gives rise to a therapeutic challenge, as the anemia may possibly become resistant to rhEPO at the usual dosage but may respond, at least partially, to high doses. In dialysis patients, the dose of rhEPO required to maintain the target hematocrit was found to be higher when baseline plasma fibrinogen and STr concentrations[148] and the serum C-reactive protein concentration[133] were also high. Both rhEPO dose and serum C-reactive protein were inversely correlated with serum albumin and serum iron levels, suggesting that the mechanisms by which inflammatory cytokines inhibit erythropoiesis are coupled to iron metabolism.[149] Hyporesponsiveness to rhEPO has been reported in HD patients with severe hyperparathyroidism[150]; a dramatic improvement has been observed after surgical parathyroidectomy.[150, 151] A direct toxic effect of parathyroid hormone (PTH) on erythropoietic bone marrow has been suggested,[152] but the osteitis fibrosa induced by hyperparathyroidism, with the consequent bone marrow fibrosis and reduction of the erythroid cell mass, appears to be the main cause of the poor response to rhEPO.[151]

Other Therapies

Blood transfusions do not represent an optimal therapy: the target hematocrit is markedly lower than that for rhEPO therapy, and they do not prevent or retard the development of heart disease. The risks of repeated blood transfusions are as follows: iron overload (suppression of erythroid marrow); blood-borne viral infections; and HLA immunization (production of cytotoxic antibodies to HLA antigens).

Androgens have been employed, with moderate success.[153] Their erythrogenic action appears to be mediated through increased EPO production.[154] Anephric patients do not, as a rule, benefit from administration of androgens. In a 6-month, prospective, randomized trial in 19 anemic chronic HD patients, comparing low-dose rhEPO (1500 IU, three times a week, intravenously) alone and in combination with nandrolone decanoate (100 mg/week intramuscularly), a stastically greater increase in hematocrit was observed in the latter group.[155]

Quality of Life

The correction of anemia with rhEPO has virtually eliminated the need for transfusion in most patients with the anemia of chronic renal failure. It has also improved the quality of life as measured by several different parameters. Exercise capacity and tolerance have been measurably increased,[156-158] and surveys of both objective and subjective quality-of-life indicators have shown significant improvement.[159-161] rhEPO has had a truly extraordinary impact on the treatment of the anemia of chronic renal failure.

SURVIVAL. The age-adjusted mortality rate for dialysis patients is 3.5 times that of the general population. The most common cause of death is cardiovascular disease. Anemia and hypertension are independent predictors of mortality; anemia is also independently predictive of heart failure. In a study on clinical and laboratory data of 21,899 HD patients collected in dialysis centers throught the United States in 1993, hemoglobin concentrations (Hb/Hct = 10/30) less than or equal to 8 g/dL were associated with a twofold increase in the odds of death when compared with concentrations of 10 to 11 g/dL; no improvement in the odds of death was observed for hemoglobin concentrations higher than 11g/dL.[162] Conversely, in another study, the relative risk of death was significantly decreased with hematocrit of 33% to 36%.[163] A review of the literature showed that, compared to higher Hb/Hct values, Hb/Hct values less than 11/33 are associated with increased morbidity and mortality.[53] In a study of 3111 adult HD patients in 17 prospective clinical trials, a reduction in mortality risk (of about 20% after 1 year on rhEPO therapy), in comparison with 246 untreated patients was observed, and in the long term the percentage of total mortality due to cardiovascular disease was reduced as well.[164]

Target Hematocrit

Significant relief of symptoms, with a low risk of side effects, has been observed when the Hb/Hct value in HD patients is between 9.5/29 and 11/33.[165] Additional improvements in the quality of life, cardiac function, physical work capacity, cognitive function, and sexual function have been reported at a hematocrit of 36% to 39%.[58] The benefits and risks of complete correction of anemia (hematocrit 38%-42%) and the optimal target concentration have not yet been established. Clinicians are reluctant to totally correct anemia in ESRD because (1) the morbidity of anemia is not well appreciated; (2) there is a bias that moderate anemia is acceptable for dialysis patients; (3) the principles of rhEPO therapy are not followed; (4) there is an inordinate amount of concern about the side effects of therapy; and (5) the cost of the treatment is high.[60]

As to the complete correction of anemia by rhEPO therapy, the improved deformability of RBCs counterbalances the increase in blood viscosity, and as a consequence the microcirculation is not impaired.[166] On the other hand, other data suggest that as a reslult of complete correction of anemia the increased blood viscosity is associated with reduced deformability of RBCs, and impaired brain microcirculation ensues.[167] Conversely, short-term studies have shown a significant improvement in brain function with a hematocrit of 42% compared with a hematocrit of 31%.[168] The safety of long-term maintenance of a normal hematocrit has been questioned, as a consequence, in part, by the early termination of the Normal Hematocrit Cardiac Trial, in which the patients randomly assigned to the normal hematocrit group presented with a higher mortality and a higher incidence of nonfatal myocardial infarction.[169]

EFFECT OF RENAL FAILURE ON HEMOSTASIS

Bleeding in uremia[170, 171] is more easily controlled since the introduction of dialysis. Ecchymoses and epistaxis are the major bleeding manifestations seen today, with gastrointestinal bleeding, hemopericardium, or subdural hematoma occuring only occcasionally.[172] However, the underlying bleeding diathesis remains. Uremic patients who undergo surgery or invasive procedures are always at risk for serious bleeding.

Causes of Uremic Bleeding

Over the past 20 years, research has partially clarified the nature of uremic bleeding. The pathogenesis is multifactorial, and the major defects involve platelet–vessel wall and platelet–platelet interactions. The skin bleeding time is the best predictor of clinical bleeding.[173-175] It depends on platelet number and function, vascular integrity, and the hematocrit and thus gives an excellent overall assessment of primary hemostasis.[164] The platelet count in uremia is usually normal,[176, 177] whereas platelet function is impaired. Dense granule content is decreased,[178, 179] and a storage pool defect with reduction in platelet adenosine diphosphate (ADP) and serotonin is present. Decreased subnormal platelet adenosine triphosphate (ATP) release in response to stimuli[168] indicates a defect in granule secretion.[180] Calcium content is increased in uremic platelets,[181] which also mobilize calcium abnormally in response to stimulation.[182] Elevation in platelet cyclic adenosine monophosphate (cAMP)[183] and abnormal calcium mobilization[182] drew attention to the possibility that PTH may play a role in uremic platelet dysfunction. This speculation was supported by the observation that PTH inhibits platelet aggregation in vitro.[184, 185] However, the bleeding time does not correlate with serum concentrations of intact PTH or PTH fragments.[186] This suggests that elevated PTH in renal failure patients is not likely to play a major role in the uremic platelet defect.

Several abnormalities of platelet-platelet interaction have also been reported in uremia. They include defective platelet aggregation in vitro in response to various stimuli[178, 187-189] and defective platelet thromboxane A$_2$ (TXA$_2$) production in response to endogenous and exogenous stimuli,[190, 191] not correctable by thrombin.[181] In a subpopulation of uremic patients, irreversible platelet aggregation does not occur in response to platelet-activating factor (PAF).[192, 193] This abnormality is independent of a plasma factor or factors but is probably due to the platelets' reduced capacity to form TXA$_2$ in response to PAF.

Experimental and clinical data suggested the possibility that the bleeding tendency in uremia is associated with excessive formation of nitric oxide,[194] a potent vasoactive molecule.[195] Plasma concentrations of the stable NO metabolites, nitrites and nitrates, were higher than normal in uremic rats with prolonged bleeding time.[196] Excessive formation of NO at systemic levels derives from vessels, as documented by increased NO synthase (NOS) activity and higher expression of both inducible NOS (iNOS) and endothelial NOS (eNOS) in the aorta of uremic animals.[196] Besides its vasoactive properties, NOS platelet aggregation in vitro and platelet adhesion to cultured endothelial cells.[197, 198] The in vivo counterpart of this activity is the prolongation of skin bleeding time observed in healthy volunteers given NO by inhalation.[199] The possibility that high systemic NO may play a role in the abnormal primary hemostasis in uremia is supported by the observation that *N*-monomethyl-L-arginine, a competitive inhibitor of NO synthesis, normalized the prolonged bleeding time in uremic rats.[194] In the same model, the shortening effect of conjugated estrogens on bleeding time,[200] abolished by L-arginine administration,[201] was associated with a complete normalization of plasma concentrations of NO metabolites and vascular expression of NOS isoenzymes.[202] Experimental findings were confirmed by human studies; thus, patients with chronic renal failure have a defective platelet aggregation associated with higher than normal platelet NO synthesis (Fig. 49-3A and B).[203] In addition, plasma from chronic hemodialyzed patients, unlike normal plasma, potently induced NO synthesis in human umbilical vein endothelial cells (HUVECs) (see Fig. 49-3C).

The same results have been obtained in cultured human microvascular endothelial cells exposed to uremic plasma.[204] The aforementioned findings suggested that substances accumulate in the plasma of uremic patients capable of up-regulating vascular NO synthesis. The stimulatory activity was attributed to cytokines such as TNF-α and IL-1β, which are potent inducers of the inducible isoform of NOS and circulate in increased amounts in the plasma of patients with chronic renal failure who either do not receive dialysis or are on maintenance HD.[203, 205-208]

Two adhesive proteins, fibrinogen and von Willebrand factor (vWF), and two adhesion receptors, glycoprotein (gp) Ib and the gpIIb-IIIa complex, play a vital role in the formation of platelet thrombi at the sites of injury.[209] Binding of gbIb to vWF is normal in uremic patients,[210] as is the surface expression of the receptor.[210, 211] In patients with chronic renal failure, a decrease in the total content of platelet gpIb has been documented,[211, 212] accompanied by an increase in soluble glycocalicin (a soluble proteolytic fragment of gpIb), and is probably due to proteolytic damage to membrane gpIb. The normal surface expression of this receptor and the total decrease in content account for a redistribution from the intraplatelet pool to the surface pool.[210, 211] The activation-dependent receptor function of the gpIIb-IIIa complex is defective in uremia, as shown by decreased binding of both vWF and fibrinogen to stimulated platelets.[210] The number of gpIIb-IIIa receptors expressed on the platelet membrane is normal. Removal of substances present in uremic plasma markedly improves the gpIIb-IIIa defect. Thus, a reversible abnormality of the activation-dependent binding activity of gpIIb-IIIa caused by a dialyzable toxic substance or substances,[210, 213] or due to receptor occupancy by fibrinogen fragments present in uremic plasma,[214] is probably a major component of the altered platelet function in uremia. The impaired gpIIb-IIIa activation in uremia may explain aggregation defects as well as reduced vWF-dependent adhesion and thrombus formation.[215-217]

The evidence that several dialyzable "toxins" (e.g., urea, creatinine, phenol, phenolic acids, or guanidinosuccinic acid) may possibly be involved in the genesis of uremic platelet dysfunction[218-220] is not compelling. Guanidinosuccinic acid, which accumulates in uremic plasma, inhibits the second wave of platelet aggregation to ADP when added to normal platelet-rich plasma.[219] Phenolic acid, at the concentrations found in uremic plasma, also impairs primary aggregation to ADP.[218] All these observations suggest that reducing the blood levels of these compounds may correct the abnormal hemostasis of patients with renal failure. However, no correlation has been found between bleeding time or platelet adhesion and the serum level of the dialyzable metabolites mainly accumulating in uremia.[220]

In an investigation of vWF and platelet adhesion with the use of blood from uremic patients with a bleeding tendency, evidence was found of both platelet and plasma abnormalities.[215] Quantitative and functional abnormalities of the vWF molecule, which promotes platelet adhesion and aggregation to subendothelial collagen,[221] have been reported. They may alter the platelet–vessel wall interaction and contribute to the hemorrhagic tendency of uremia.[222] Kazatchkine and associates[223] reported elevated vWF antigen levels but reduced ristocetin cofactor activity in uremic patients. However, other investigators have reported increased vWF functional activity.[224-226] Studies of the multimeric structure of vWF have not disclosed abnormalities.[227, 228] The observation that cryoprecipitate,[227] a plasma derivative rich in factor VIII and vWF, and desmopressin,[218] a synthetic derivative of antidiuretic hormone that releases autologous vWF from storage sites, significantly shorten the bleeding time of uremic patients suggests that a functional defect in the vWF-platelet interaction may indeed play a role in the abnormal hemostasis of these patients.

Platelet adhesion and aggregation in following systems[229, 230] are markedly potentiated by red RBCs. Erythrocytes enhance platelet function by releasing ADP,[231] by inactivating prostacyclin,[232] and by increasing platelet–vessel wall

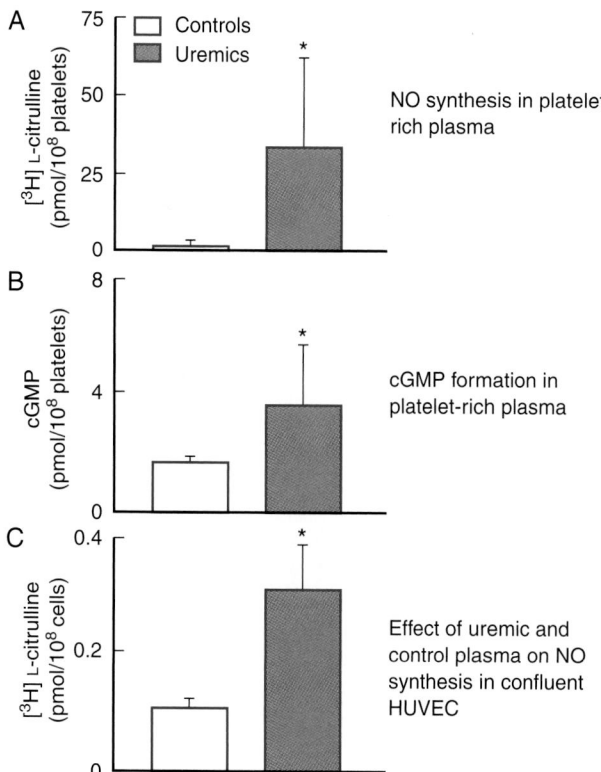

FIGURE 49-3. **A,** Conversion of [³H] L-arginine to [³H] L-citrulline in platelets from control subjects and uremic patients. **B,** Intracellular cyclic guanosine monophosphate in platelets from control subjects and uremic patients. **C,** Conversion of [³H] L-arginine to [³H] L-citrulline by human vascular endothelial cells (HUVEC) exposed to control or uremic plasma. (From Noris M, Benigni A, Boccardo P, et al: Enhanced nitric oxide synthesis in uremia: Implications for platelet dysfunction and dialysis hypotension. Kidney Int 44:445-450, 1993.)

contact by displacing platelets away from the axial flow and toward the vessel wall.[229] The independent role of anemia in the bleeding tendency of uremia has been extensively investigated. A significant negative correlation was found between bleeding time and packed cell volume (PCV) in 52 patients on chronic HD.[233] The bleeding time was longer than 270 seconds in 90% of patients with PCV less than 30% but in only 45% of patients with PCV greater than 30%. Despite a shorter bleeding time, a significant negative correlation between hematocrit and bleeding time was still demonstrable in 15 nonuremic anemic patients. These results were subsequently confirmed by other studies[234, 235] that found that anemia was the main determinant of the prolonged bleeding time in uremic patients. Uremic bleeding time has been shortened and symptomatic hemostatic improvement achieved by treatment with rhEPO.[236, 237] In one randomized study,[238] the bleeding time became normal in all patients on EPO as hematocrits increased to 27% to 32%. Thus, partial correction of anemia was sufficient to correct defective primary hemostasis in uremia.

Consequences of the Bleeding Tendency in Uremia

Gastrointestinal bleeding occurs with greater frequency and higher mortality in uremic patients than in the general population.[239, 240] Upper gastrointestinal bleeding is the second leading cause of death in acute renal failure.[241] The most common causes of bleeding are peptic ulcers, hemorrhagic esophagitis, gastritis, duodenitis, and gastric telangiectasias.[242-244] Angiodysplasia with gastrointestinal bleeding has been observed in the stomach, duodenum, jejunum, and colon.[245, 246] This abnormality, affecting the microcirculation of the gastrointestinal mucosa and submucosa, occurs most often in HD patients.[247] Finally, dialysis patients suffering from human immunodeficiency virus (HIV) nephropathy may have specific lesions, such as Kaposi sarcoma, cytomegalovirus colitis, and non-Hodgkin lymphoma,[248] that contribute to gastrointestinal bleeding.

Although now rare, hemorrhagic pericarditis with cardiac tamponade can occur in uremia.[249, 250] The clinical features of this condition include normal cardiac shadow, increased jugular venous distention with hypotension, shortness of breath, and a pericardial friction rub. Deaths due to hemorrhagic pericarditis have been reported to be as high as 3% to 5% among dialysis patients.[251, 252]

Subdural hematoma has been reported to occur in 5% to 15% of HD patients.[253] It usually overlies the frontal or parietal lobe and is bilateral in approximately 15% of cases. Headache, vomiting, seizures, hypertension, drowsiness, confusion, and coma are the usual symptoms. Head trauma, hypertension, and systemic anticoagulation are risk factors.[253] The prognosis is at least partly related to the stage of diagnosis, and the mortality rate may be as high as 90% in patients requiring emergency surgery. Anticoagulation during dialysis may be a major risk factor in causing bleeding in patients with fibrinous pleuritis.[254, 255] Spontaneous retroperitoneal bleeding is a rare complication in patients receiving chronic HD.[256, 257] Trauma, anticoagulation, and the presence of polycystic kidneys are predisposing factors. The symptoms and signs include sudden onset of pain in the abdomen, flank, back, or hip, with an associated drop in blood pressure. The hematocrit drops in the absence of any obvious blood loss.

Computed tomography is useful in the diagnosis of retroperitoneal bleeding. Spontaneous subcapsular hematoma of the liver is a newly recognized complication in uremia.[258] Typically, patients have right upper quadrant pain, fever, and sometimes elevated bilirubin and alkaline phosphate levels accompanied by a falling hematocrit.

Intraocular hemorrhage can also occur in uremia, and spontaneous hyphema has been reported during dialysis.[259] There is no visual loss, and the hemorrhage generally resolves without any therapy. Intraocular bleeding with only temporary visual loss has also been reported in a large percentage of transplant and dialysis patients after cataract surgery. Another risk of bleeding in uremic patients is associated with aspirin given to prevent vascular access thrombosis[260] or platelet activation on dialyzer membranes.[261] The beneficial effect of aspirin on vascular access thrombosis can be achieved with a moderate dose of aspirin (160 mg/day), which inhibits platelet TXA_2 generation without affecting vascular prostacyclin formation.[260] However, even a moderate dose of aspirin prolongs the bleeding time,[262] and this fact may explain the frequency of gastrointestinal bleeding in uremic patients.[246, 263] Thus, the use of aspirin in uremic patients treated with rhEPO to prevent the thrombotic complications associated with an increasing hematocrit is highly questionable.

Abnormalities of Coagulation and Fibrinolysis

Activated partial thromboplastin, prothrombin, and thrombin times are generally normal in uremia[223, 264-272]; fibrinogen and factor VIII:C are usually increased. Changes in the major natural inhibitors of coagulation have been found. Conflicting results regarding antithrombin III levels have been reported; in fact, previous reports demonstrated increased levels of this natural anticoagulant.[264, 273-275] Reduced levels of antithrombin III have been found in uremic patients.[276, 277] This evidence, together with the observed decrease in protein C anticoagulant activity with normal protein C amidolytic activity and antigen[278, 279] and decreased protein S,[280] may further contribute to the thrombotic tendency. Thrombin is continuously formed, as demonstrated by increased levels of the thrombin–antithrombin III complex,[211, 281-283] D dimer,[277, 281, 282, 284] and fibrinopeptide A.[281, 282, 285, 286] These findings suggest that a hypercoagulable state exists in chronic uremia. Contrasting results regarding the fibrinolytic system have been obtained. Previous reports described decreased fibrinolytic activity in uremia either absolutely[285, 287-292] or relative to the extent of activation of coagulation,[275] and this has been used as an explanation for the thrombotic tendency. Studies found, instead, activation of fibrinolysis in uremia, with an increase of plasmin-antiplasmin complexes[211, 284, 283] and fibrinogen and fibrin degradation products[211, 277, 281] as well as a decrease in the activity of plasminogen activator inhibitor in ESRD[201] and after HD sessions.[283, 294] These findings probably reflect a fibrinolytic response secondary to fibrin deposition, which may take place also if the overall fibrinolytic activity is depressed. These abnormalities of coagulation or fibrinolysis partially corrected by dialysis[287, 295] predispose the uremic patient to thrombosis rather than bleeding. Of interest, levels of protein C and its cofactor protein S are further and significantly decreased in association with EPO therapy, a finding that may contribute to the increased risk of vascular access thrombosis in patients receiving chronic EPO treatment.

Thrombotic Complications

Thrombosis of the arteriovenous shunt is a frequent occurrence in uremic patients undergoing HD. Plasma levels of lipoprotein(a), an independent risk factor for atherosclerotic cardiovascular disease, are markedly increased in chronic uremic patients either on HD[296, 297] or CAPD.[297] Because platelet aggregation plays a major role in thrombus formation, antiplatelet agents have been used, with encouraging results. Sulfinpyrazone, aspirin, or dipyridamole, singly or in combination, have proved useful in several studies.[298] Fibrinolytic agents, such as streptokinase[299, 300] or urokinase,[301] have produced contrasting results. More studies are needed to determine the most effective treatment for this complication.

Therapeutic Strategies

Although some investigators have found that both HD and PD partially improve the hemostatic abnormality of uremia, both forms of dialysis can potentially produce adverse effects on hemostasis (Table 49-3). For all patients with hemorrhagic complications or undergoing major surgery, the adequency of dialysis should be appropriately checked. It is also advisable to change the dialysis schedule for 1 or 2 months in patients who have experienced severe hemorrhages (such as major gastrointestinal bleeding, hemorrhagic pericarditis, subdural hematomas) or who have undergone recent cardiovascular surgery so that heparin can be avoided. Acute bleeding episodes may be treated with desmopressin at a dose of 0.3 μg/kg intravenously (added to 50 mL of saline over 30 minutes) or subcutaneously. Intranasal administration of this drug at a dose of 3 μg/kg is also effective and is well tolerated. The effect of desmopressin lasts only a few hours, a major limitation to its use in treating severe hemorrhage, and desmopressin appears to lose efficacy when repeatedly administered. Because the favorable effect of cryoprecipitate on bleeding time has not been uniformly observed, we do not recommend its use. The ideal treatment of persistent chronic bleeding should have a

TABLE 49-3

Guidelines for the Management of Hemorragic Complications of Uremia

For patients with hemorrhagic complications or undergoing major surgery, dialysis adequacy should be assessed.
Acute anemia should be promptly corrected and hematocrit should be increased to 30% or more, by infusion of packed red blood cells.
For long-term correction of anemia, erythropoietin is administered.
Acute bleeding episodes may be treated by intravenous infusion of desmopressin at a dose of 0.3 μg/kg body weight in 50 mL of saline over 30 min, or by subcutaneous injection at the same dose. Intranasal administration of desmopressin at a dose of 3 μg/kg body weight is also effective. The effect of desmopressin is short-lasting, and repeated doses are associated with loss of effect.
Persistent chronic bleeding may be effectively treated with intravenous infusion of conjugated estrogen. The usual dose schedule is 0.6 mg/kg body weight per day for 5 days.

long-lasting effect. Conjugated estrogen treatment given by intravenous infusion in a cumulative dose of 3 mg/kg as daily divided doses (e.g., 0.6 mg/kg for 5 consecutive days) is the most appropriate way of achieving long-lasting hemostatic competence. Severely anemic patients should receive blood or RBC transfusions to improve hematocrit values. RBC transfusions are hemostatically effective only when the hematocrit rises above 30%. As an alternative, bleeding in patients with renal failure and hematocrit less than 30% can be treated successfully with erythropoietin (see Table 49-1).

PD has been reported to cause platelet hyperreactivity, which in some cases may be related to hypoalbuminemia.[302] HD is accompanied by a transient form of platelet activation related to the interaction of platelets with artificial membranes[303-310] and vascular access itself.[311, 312] Dialysis patients have an accelerated platelet turnover,[313] supporting the concept that platelets are chronically activated by dialytic treatment. Repeated platelet activation on dialysis membranes may induce refractoriness to further platelet stimulation, possibly contributing to clinical bleeding that can occur at termination of the dialysis procedure. It has been documented that plasma levels of the potent NO inducers TNF-α and IL-1β rise during dialysis. IL-1 and TNF are generated in vivo by circulating monocytes during HD with complement-activating membranes.[195-198] Production of increased cytokines may also be triggered by intact endotoxin, endotoxin fragments, and other bacterial toxins that may cross the dialysis membranes,[312-314] and also by acetate-containing dialysate.[206-208, 314-317] As a result of massive release of cytokines during dialysis, there is an increase in NO synthesis (Fig. 49-4). Yokokawa and associates[318] found that uremic patients may occasionally have an increase in plasma levels of NO metabolites during HD. In addition, in a study it was found that plasma collected after HD appears to stimulate NO synthesis by cultured endothelial cells more than does plasma from the same patients before dialysis.[319] Thus, the capacity of the dialysis procedure to remove uremic toxins is negatively counterbalanced by its effects on platelet activation and NO synthesis.

In addition, heparin may also present a problem. "Regional" heparinization has been used to minimize the effects of systemic anticoagulation.[320-322] Heparin is given by constant infusion through the inlet line of the dialyzer. Simultaneously, protamine sulfate is infused into the outlet port before the blood returns to the patient. Even this schedule of heparin administration, however, may be associated with a high incidence of bleeding.[323] As an alternative, frequent injections of low-dose heparin can be given during dialysis to maintain a lower and more constant level.[324] Usually, 40 to 50 IU/kg of heparin is given at the beginning of HD, followed by 60% of the initial dose after 1 hour and 2 hours, and 30% of the initial dose after 3 hours.[314] The activated partial thromboplastin time (APTT) is measured hourly and should be maintained at 1.5 to 2.0 times the basal value. Patients at high risk for bleeding can use an ethylene–vinyl alcohol copolymer hollow-fiber dialysis membrane that does not require systemic anticoagulation, provided that blood flow is maintained at more than 200 mL/minute.[325] Low-molecular-weight heparin has been proposed as an alternative to unfractionated heparin in patients receiving chronic HD who are at high risk for bleeding.[326] Dermatan sulfate has been proposed[327] as an alternative to heparin, because it causes less

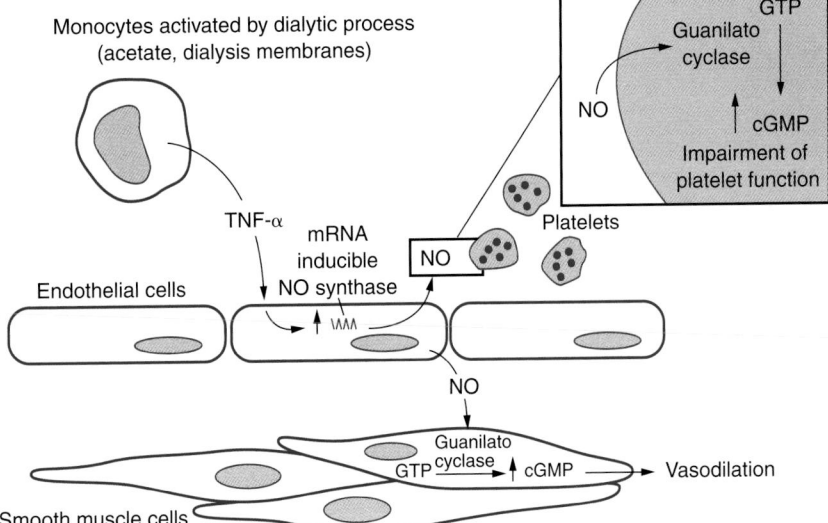

FIGURE 49-4. Proposed mechanism for NO-mediated disorders in uremia. The contact with dialysis membrane or acetate dialysis buffer activates circulating monocytes that release cytokines, such as tumor necrosis factor-α (TNF-α). TNF-α causes the transcription of inducible NO synthase messenger RNA in vascular endothelial cells that release a large amount of NO either in the circulation or within the vessel wall. NO enters target cells (platelets and smooth muscle cells), where it activates soluble guanylate cyclase, causing impairment of platelet function (hence bleeding tendency) and relaxation of smooth muscle cells (hence vasodilation).

bleeding than heparin in animal models. This may be due to its reduced effect on platelets.[328, 329] It also induced a moderate prolongation of APTT.[328, 330, 331] Effective doses ranged from 6 to 10 mg/kg body weight per dialysis session, depending on the type of dialyzer and the duration of the procedure.[328, 330-334] The dermatan sulfate dose can be given as a single predialysis bolus when the procedure is of short duration (4 hours); when the dialysis lasts for a longer period, a combined regimen (bolus plus infusion) is required. A comparative short-term clinical study has been performed on 10 hemodialyzed patients,[334] demonstrating that the DS dose can be individually titrated to suppress clot formation during HD as efficiently as does individualized heparin. Aspirin and dipyridamole analogs reduce fibrin and cellular deposition on the filter membrane but increase the risk of gastrointestinal bleeding.[261, 335] Prostacyclin shows some promise as an alternative.[336-338] Given in a continuous infusion during dialysis at a mean dose of 5 ng/kg/minute, prostacyclin completely inhibited platelet aggregation without causing bleeding.[326] However, it was associated with headache, flushing, tachycardia, and chest and abdominal pain, which required careful monitoring and a physician's supervision.[338-340] Thus, the use of prostacyclin should be limited to patients at high risk for hemorrhage. PD, when applicable, avoids the risk of bleeding associated with heparin or anticoagulants. Anemia can contribute to the prolongation of bleeding time in uremia.[233-235] The progressive increase in hematocrit associated with rhEPO therapy was accompanied by a significant decrease in the bleeding time (Fig. 49-5A).[237, 238, 341] No consistent changes were found in platelet number, platelet aggregability, or platelet TXA$_2$ formation.[227, 341] Several studies[342-344] observed a significant increase in the levels of vWF and ristocetin cofactor activity. In a study, 20 dialysis patients with prolonged bleeding time (average: 15 minutes) were randomly allocated to rhEPO or no specific treatment. EPO was given intravenously at the dose of 50 IU/kg three times a week; every 4 weeks the dose was increased by 25 IU/kg until bleeding time became normal. An EPO dosage of 150 to 300 IU/kg/week increased PCV to

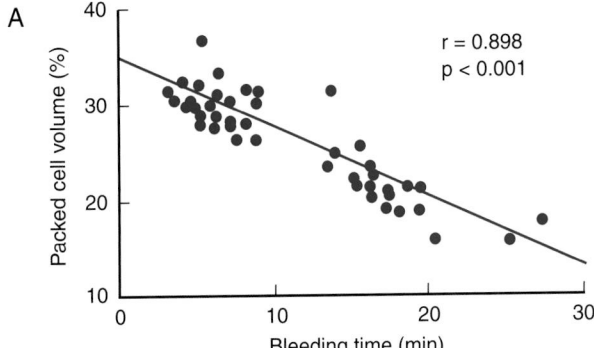

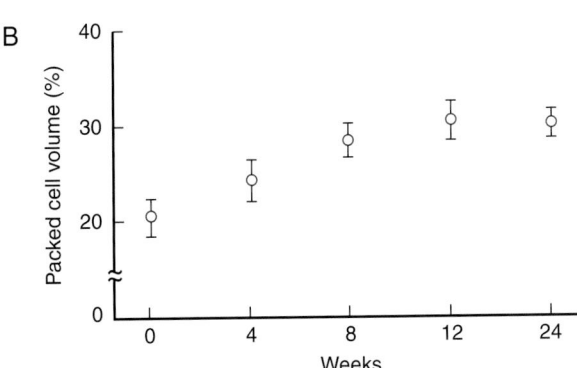

FIGURE 49-5. A, Correlation between bleeding time and packed cell volume in patients treated with erythropoietin. **B,** Effect of rhEPO therapy on packed cell volume and bleeding time in uremic patients. *Dotted area* indicates the threshold of packed cell volume to be reached for normalization of bleeding time values. (From Viganò G, Benigni A, Mendogni D, et al: Recombinant human erythropoietin to correct uremic bleeding. Am J Kidney Dis 18:44-49, 1991.)

a range of 27% to 32% and normalized bleeding times in all patients (see Fig. 49-5B). A significant negative correlation was found between PCV and bleeding time.[238] Thus, the correction of anemia with rhEPO may contribute significantly to the prevention and control of bleeding in uremic patients.

Cryoprecipitate is a plasma derivative rich in vWF, fibrinogen, and fibronectin that has traditionally been used in the treatment of hemophilia A, von Willebrand disease, hypofibrinogenemia, and dysfibrinogenemia. Cryoprecipitate corrects prolonged bleeding in uremic patients within 4 to 12 hours, and the effect lasts 24 to 36 hours.[237] The mechanism of action of cryoprecipitate is not known. A small rise in platelet levels of fibrinogen and vWF-related proteins were the only changes noted after cryoprecipitate infusion. Different preparations of cryoprecipitate, however, had different effects on bleeding time.[345] The poor reproducibility of results and the risk of disease transmission prompted the search for alternatives to cryoprecipitate.

Desmopressin (1-deamino-8-D-arginine-vasopressin)—a synthetic derivative of antidiuretic hormone—induces the release of autologous vWF from storage sites.[346] In a randomized, double-blind, crossover trial, desmopressin given intravenously at a dose of 0.3 mg/kg body weight in 50 mL of physiologic saline over a period of 30 minutes temporarily corrected the prolonged bleeding time in patients with chronic renal failure.[218] The shortening of bleeding time was significant 1 hour after the end of the infusion, and the effect lasted 6 to 8 hours. Desmopressin loses efficacy with repeated administration.[347] Desmopressin also can be given by the intranasal route,[348, 349] which is well tolerated and quite safe. At 10 to 20 times the intravenous dose (3 mg/kg) intranasal desmopressin shortens the bleeding time[348, 349] and decreases clinical bleeding. Desmopressin has also been given subcutaneously,[350] with the dose the same as that used for intravenous administration. Peak responses are achieved after a 30- to 90-minute delay when the subcutaneous route is employed. Adverse effects include facial flushing, mild transient headache, nausea, abdominal cramps, and mild tachycardia. Protein C anticoagulant activity decreases after desmopressin infusion.[351, 352] In one case report, an elderly uremic patient with atherosclerosis suffered a stroke immediately after desmopressin infusion.[353] Nonetheless, desmopressin is useful in the treatment of bleeding, and in the prevention of bleeding during surgery or invasive procedures.

The anecdotal observation of diminished gastrointestinal bleeding in uremic patients treated with conjugated estrogens, and the improved hemostasis in von Willebrand disease during pregnancy, led to investigations of the effect of estrogens on bleeding in uremia.[354-356] One oral dose of 25 mg of conjugated estrogen normalizes the bleeding time for 3 to 10 days, with no apparent ill effects.[354] A controlled study showed that conjugated estrogens, given intravenously at a cumulative dose of 3 mg/kg divided over 5 consecutive days, produced a long-lasting reduction in the bleeding time in uremic patients. At least 0.6 mg/kg of estrogen was needed to reduce the bleeding time,[356] and four or five infusions spaced 24 hours apart were needed to reduce the bleeding time by at least 50%. The effect of estrogens on bleeding time in an animal model of chronic uremia was completely reversed by the NO precursor L-arginine,[201] suggesting that the effect of estrogens might be mediated by changes in NO synthesis. Thus, estrogens may be a reasonable alternative to cryoprecipitate or desmopressin in the treatment of uremic bleeding, especially when a long-lasting effect is required.

EFFECT OF RENAL FAILURE ON GRANULOCYTES AND MONOCYTES

Renal failure is associated with an increased susceptibility to infections. This has stimulated research on the effect of uremia on leukocyte function. In cell-mediated defense against infectious agents, granulocytes and monocytes move by chemotaxis to the site of injury. Cells then phagocytose microorganisms through complex processes that include cell adhesion and the formation of oxygen free radicals (particularly H_2O_2) from O_2.

Many studies have found that leukocyte chemotaxis is impaired in uremia.[357-362] Impairment of chemotactic function may be associated with a circulating inhibitor of chemotaxis,[359, 352] decreased intracellular cyclic guanosine monophosphate–cyclic adenosine monophosphate ratio,[363, 364] or a plasma factor blocking granulocyte membrane receptors. Interestingly, the chemotactic activity of granulocytes is diminished further, rather than corrected, by HD.[365]

Studies of granulocyte phagocytosis and respiratory burst in uremia are conflicting. Abrutyn and co-workers[366] found normal phagocytic and bactericidal activities in uremic granulocytes, together with normal serum opsonizing activity for staphylococci. H_2O_2 formation and O_2 consumption during phagocytosis were also normal. Other investigators found depressed phagocytic activity[367] and respiratory burst.[368] Thus, reduced phagocytosis related to decreased expression of Fc receptors has been reported [369] on polymorphonuclear leukocytes from patients with chronic renal failure. H_2O_2 production by phorbol myristate acetate (PMA)–stimulated polymorphs was impaired, but normalized with HD. Because the subjects of the last-cited study had virtually no renal function, conflicting results might be reconciled by the speculation that uremic granulocytes retain the capacity to generate H_2O_2 until the very late stages of renal failure.

In another study,[370] reduced phagocytosis by granulocytes was associated with increased intracellular $[Ca^{2+}]$ and reduced ATP. The latter two findings suggest that the activity of the ATP-dependent Ca^{2+} pump is reduced in uremia. A possible explanation may be that elevated PTH levels augment leukocyte Ca^{2+}, which inhibits mitochondrial O_2 consumption and reduces ATP. A protein that inhibited chemotaxis, oxidative metabolism, and bacterial killing by granulocytes has been isolated from uremic serum.[371]

However, more recent studies suggested that uremia is associated with increased granulocyte activation. Thus, using the granulocytes from nondialyzed patients with varying degrees of renal insufficiency and from normal individuals, Ward and co-workers[372] compared the ability of these cells to phagocytose bacteria and produce a respiratory burst. Phagocytosis of opsonized bacteria did not differ between the two groups; however, uremic leukocytes demonstrated an enhanced oxidative burst,[372] as documented by a greater release of H_2O_2 in response to phagocytosis or stimuli by the chemoattractant f-MLP (N-formyl-methionylleucyl-phenylalanine). In a subsequent report,[373] the same group demonstrated that incubation of polymorphonuclear leukocytes from healthy control subjects with uremic plasma results in activation of oxidative burst, which would indicate that in uremic circulation a soluble factor is present that induces granulocyte priming. The preceding data are consistent with a previous report of Rhee and co-workers[374] that identified a low-molecular-weight factor (<1000 D) in the serum of patients with renal insufficiency that enhanced the oxidative burst activity of normal granulocytes.

HD has a profound effect on granulocyte kinetics. During the first 2 hours of HD, all patients develop peripheral neutropenia mediated by complement activation on the dialysis membrane[375] and sequestration of granulocytes in the lung. In the hours following HD, the release of neutrophils from the bone marrow and sites of sequestration produces rebound neutrophilia. Thus, pulmonary dysfunction occurring within the first hours of HD may be the result of endothelial injury caused by massive granulocyte adherence to pulmonary vessels. The normal interaction between dialysis membrane and plasma complement components is diminished as the dialyzer is reused.[376]

Several laboratories have studied the effects of HD on white blood cell integrins, a family of transmembrane glycoproteins that interact with endothelial cell ligands as well as with complement components.[377-379] Mac-1, an integrin primarily expressed on granulocytes and macrophages, is a receptor for C3b1[379-381] and is involved in the adhesion of white blood cells to dialysis membranes.[382-385] During cuprophane HD there is a rapid increase in the surface expression of Mac-1 associated with a consistent decrease in granulocyte counts.[386] By contrast, the use of hemophane or polysulfone membranes produced less Mac-1.[386] The findings that surface expression of Mac-1 remains elevated with cuprophane membranes, even when the granulocyte count normalizes, suggest that more than one molecule may be implicated in the mechanism of granulocytopenia during cellulose membrane dialysis. A new family of leukocyte adhesion molecules has been described, and the structure of one of them, LAM-1, has been elucidated.[387] LAM-1 is shed during leukocyte activation by chemotactic factors. LAM-1 shedding associated with decreased endothelial cell binding has also been exhibited by granulocytes harvested early during the first use of a cellulose dialysis membrane. This suggests that during cellulose HD, complement activation up-regulates Mac-1, producing cell adhesion and sequestration. This is followed by LAM-1 shedding. Possibly, the increased susceptibility to infection exhibited by HD patients is the consequence of "low" LAM-1 granulocytes and the loss of their capacity to transmigrate to sites of infection. This suggestion is concordant with the higher incidence of infection seen in patients receiving chronic cuprophane HD as compared to polysulfone HD.[388]

The study of the adhesive properties of circulating cells can be misleading, because the most adhesive cells are likely to adhere and be unobtainable for study. Up-regulation of Mac-1 during cuprophane HD was slower and less pronounced for monocytes than for granulocytes, even though the degree of monocytopenia during the first 15 minutes of HD was comparable to that observed for granulocytes. This may reflect a lesser amount of Mac-1 on monocytes[389] or the involvement of different molecules in monocyte adhesion. While there is little question that extracorporeal circulation causes a complement-dependent increase in the expression of phagocyte adhesion receptors, leading to cell aggregation and sequestration in the pulmonary vasculature, there is limited consensus regarding its effects on other aspects of phagocyte function.

Several studies have examined the impact of extracorporeal circulation on the production of oxygen radicals by polymorphonuclear leukocytes. Resting oxygen radical production is generally reported to be increased, compared to predialysis values, after a few minutes of dialysis when complement-activating membranes are used,[390-392] whereas stimulated oxygen radical production is decreased.[390, 391, 393, 394] These changes are absent with membranes that do not release active complement fragments into the blood.[391, 394] Cristol and associates[395] found increased oxygen radical production in polymorphonuclear leukocytes from patients during HD with cuprophane, but not during HD with polysulfone. Consistently, Himmelfarb and colleagues[396] documented that HD with complement-activating membrane resulted in a 3.2-fold increase in ex vivo granulocyte H_2O_2 production, 15 minutes after HD initiation, in comparison to both predialysis values and values with a non–complement-activating membrane. The close contact between granulocytes and vascular endothelium that occurs during the early phase of dialysis, owing to overexpression of adhesive molecules[395, 397] on circulating leukocytes, probably favors the aggression against endothelial cells by polymorphonuclear leukocyte–derived oxidants, resulting in vascular damage. Richard and co-workers[398] have demonstrated decreased intracellular antioxidant capability in chronic hemodialyzed patients, which would support this concept.

Monocytes are markedly activated by contact with dialysis membranes, as documented by transient increases in plasma levels of IL-1 and TNF[399] during HD.[206, 208, 400-402] Thus, within 5 minutes of cuprophane HD, monocytes initiate transcription of IL-1 and TNF in large amounts.[403] In addition, macrophage colony-stimulating factor (M-CSF)[404]—the growth factor for monocytes—accumulates in uremia and provides a further stimulus to the synthesis and secretion of IL-1 and TNF by monocytes. Candidate factors for monocyte activation during HD include complement activation, a component of dialysis buffer such as acetate,[317] but also bacterial and endotoxin contaminations, and the direct contact of monocytes with dialysis membrane.[318]

Because IL-1 and TNF up-regulate cell metabolism in different systems and increase the expression of genes encoding for various biologically active proteins,[405] the functional consequences of monocyte activation during HD may be of some importance. The possibility that cytokines released by activated monocytes might augment susceptibility to infections, immune dysfunction, and atherosclerosis has been investigated.[406] However, attempts to modify these abnormalities with IL-1 receptor antagonists or soluble TNF receptors have been inconclusive. Other studies indicated that IL-1 and TNF may mediate HD-associated hypotension.[407, 408] In 1992, the theory[409] was advanced that both chronic and acute hypotension during dialysis may be the consequence of cytokine-induced activation of NO synthesis by endothelial cells and macrophages (see Fig. 49-4). This possibility is consistent with recent data[193, 318] that NO production is elevated in patients receiving chronic HD.[410]

It has been known for many years that uremic patients suffer from an acquired form of immunodeficiency characterized by abnormal T cell proliferation in response to antigenic challenges. This defect could well be the consequence of monocyte dysfunction, as T cell activation is monocyte-dependent. The monocytes in uremic nonresponders to hepatitis B vaccination are unable to deliver to T lymphocytes the necessary signal required for triggering IL-2 synthesis. Consistently, exogenous IL-2 normalizes the proliferative response of uremic T lymphocytes. More recent studies[411, 412] have shown that purified IL-1, the monocyte-derived signal for T cell activation, is unable to normalize the T cell proliferative response. However, exogenous IL-2 eliminates the defect.[401] This observation is consistent with other studies[412, 413] that document reduced IL-2 production by uremic T cells.

Normal T cell activation is followed by the release of a soluble form of IL-2 receptor (IL-2R) into the circulation.[414] Uremic serum markedly inhibits the release of IL-2R.[412] Because the release of IL-2R is IL-2-dependent and is improved by dialysis, uremic serum may contain a "toxin" that inhibits IL-2 production.[412] IL-2 exerts its biologic effect by binding to a high-affinity receptor that consists of two different α- and β-polypeptide chains. The α-subunit is expressed de novo and is an index of lymphocyte activation.[415] The β-subunit is constitutively expressed on resting T cells.[416] Both subunits have low affinity for IL-2, but the association of the two generates a receptor complex—IL-2R—with high affinity for IL-2. This receptor complex mediates IL-2 binding and internalization, thus triggering IL-2-dependent T cell proliferation.[417] The normal proliferative response of activated lymphocytes to recombinant IL-2 in the presence of uremic serum[402] could be taken as indirect evidence that uremia does not inhibit IL-2 binding to its high-affinity receptors or IL-2 internalization.

Moreover, in the same set of experiments, uremic serum up-regulated cell surface expression of biologically active high-affinity IL-2R. Despite a deficient response of T cells from uremic patients to most pathogens and mitogens, these cells show clear signs of activation, such as an increased expression of the IL-2R α-subunit and IL-2R, and increased levels of soluble IL-2R into the circulation. Chronic dialysis with cuprophane membrane increased the expression of IL-2R α- and β-subunits but reduced the lymphocyte's expression of high-affinity receptors following stimulation with mitogens in vitro.[418] This abnormality is evident after 2 weeks of cuprophane membrane HD and persists thereafter.

The same phenomenon has been reported in other immunodeficiency states, such as acquired immunodeficiency syndrome (AIDS).[419] In cuprophane HD, this observation could be explained by the assumption that lymphocytes activated by contact with cuprophane membrane become refractory to subsequent stimulation. In fact, a study reported[420] that at the end of 2 weeks of dialysis with cuprophane membrane, the capacity of these cells to express, after in vitro stimulation, IL-2 and IL-2R was reduced in comparison to the respective baseline levels before HD with cuprophane was started. When a biocompatible (low-flux, low–complement-activating) membrane was used,[420] these levels increased and after 2 weeks approached those of normal control subjects. Normal T cell function has been reported also with polysulfone biocompatible membrane.[421]

These findings may explain some of the conflicting results in the measurement of cytokine levels in HD patients. A loss of capacity in inducing IL-2 gene expression was found in HD patients.[422] This may partially explain the fact that immunodeficiency is more severe in HD patients than in PD patients. However, further studies are needed to clarify the true clinical impact of reduced surface expression of IL-R on the immunodeficiency of uremic patients.

ACKNOWLEDGMENTS

The authors are grateful to Drs. Paola Boccardo, Miriam Galbusera, Marina Noris, and Norberto Perico for their invaluable cooperation. Ms. Laura Arioli helped to prepare the manuscript.

REFERENCES

1. Bright R: Cases and observations illustrative of renal disease accompanied with the secretion of albuminous urine. Guys Hosp Rep 1:338-400, 1836.
2. Riesman D: Hemorrhages in the course of Bright's disease, with especial reference to the occurrence of a hemorrhagic diathesis of nephritic origin. Am J Med Sci 134:709-716, 1907.
3. Brown GE, Roth GM: The anemia of chronic nephritis. Arch Intern Med 30:817-840, 1922.
4. Jacobson LO, Goldwasser E, Fried W, et al: Role of the kidney in erythropoiesis. Nature 179:633-634, 1957.
5. Callen IR, Limarzi LR: Blood and bone marrow studies in renal disease. Am J Clin Pathol 20:3-23, 1950.
6. Kaye M: The anemia associated with renal disease. J Lab Clin Med 52:83-100, 1958.
7. Delwiche F, Segal GM, Eschbach JW, et al: Hematopoietic inhibitors in chronic renal failure: Lack of in vitro specificity. Kidney Int 29:641-648, 1986.
8. Brunati C, Cappellini MD, DeFeo T, et al: Uremic inhibitors of erythropoiesis: A study during treatment with recombinant human erythropoietin. Am J Nephrol 12:9-13, 1992.
9. Segal GM, Stueve T, Adamson JW: Spermine and spermidine are non-specific inhibitors of in vitro hematopoiesis. Kidney Int 31:72-76, 1987.
10. Costigan MG, Yaqoob M, Lindup WE: Effects of haemodialysis and continuous ambulatory peritoneal dialysis on the plasma clearance of an albumin-bound furan dicarboxylic acid. Nephrol Dial Transplant 10:648-652, 1995.
11. Shaw AB: Haemolysis in chronic renal failure. BMJ 2:213-216, 1967.
12. Eschbach JW, Haley NR, Adamson JW: The anemia of chronic renal failure: Pathophysiology and effects of recombinant erythropoietin. Contrib Nephrol 78:24-36, 1990.
13. Erslev AJ, Besarb A: The rate and control of baseline red cell production in hematologically stable patients with uremia. J Lab Clin Med 126:283-286, 1995.
14. Cavdar C, Camsari T, Semin I, et al: Lipid peroxidation and antioxidant activity in chronic hemodialysis patients treated with recombinant human erythropoietin. Scad J Urol Nephrol 31:371-375, 1997.
15. Krause DS, Fackler MJ, Civin CI, et al: CD34: Structure, biology, and clinical utility. Blood 87:1-13, 1996.
16. Erslev AJ, Besarb A: Erythropoietin in the pathogenesis and treatment of the anemia of chronic renal failure. Kidney Int 51:662-630, 1997.
17. D'Andrea AD, Zon LI: Erythropoietin receptor: Subunit structure activation. J Clin Invest 86:681-687, 1990.
18. Jelkman W: Erythropoietin: Structure, control of production and function. Physiol Rev 72:449-489, 1992.
19. Erslev AJ: Clinical erythrokinetics: A critical review. Blood Rev 11:160-167, 1997.
20. Krumdieck N: Erythropoietic substance in the serum of anemic animals. Proc Soc Exp Biol Med 54:14-17, 1943.
21. Bonsdorff E, Jalavisto E: A humoral mechanism in anoxic erythrocytosis. Acta Physical Scand 16:150-170, 1948.
22. Reissmann KR: Studies on the mechanism of erythropoietic stimulation in parabiotic rats during hypoxia. Blood 5:372-380, 1950.
23. Erslev A: Humoral regulation of red cell production. Blood 8:349-357, 1953.
24. Erslev A: Physiologic control of red cell production. Blood 10:954-961, 1955.
25. Stohlman F Jr, Rath CE, Rose JC: Evidence for a humoral regulation of erythropoiesis. Blood 9:721-733, 1954.
26. Gurney CW, Jacobson LO, Goldwasser E: The physiologic and clinical significance of erythropoietin. Ann Intern Med 49:363-370, 1958.

27. Miyake T, Kung CK-H, Goldwasser E: Purification of human erythropoietin. J Biol Chem 252:5558-5564, 1977.

28. Lai P-H, Everett R, Wang F-F, et al: Structural characterization of human erythropoietin. J Biol Chem 261:3116-3121, 1986.

29. Krantz SB: Erythropoietin. Blood 77:419-434, 1991.

30. Youssoufian H, Longmore G, Neuman D, et al: Structure, function and activation of the erythroproietin receptor. Blood 81:2223-2236, 1993.

31. Spivak JL, Hogans BB: The in vivo metabolism of recombinant human erythropoietin in the rat. Blood 73:90-99, 1989.

32. Cotes PM: Immunoreactive erythropoietin in serum. Br J Haematol 50:427-438, 1982.

33. Jacobs K, Shoemaker C, Rudersdorf R, et al: Isolation and characterization of genomic and cDNA clones of human erythropoietin. Nature 313:806-810, 1985.

34. Lin FK, Suggs S, Lin CH, et al: Cloning and expression of the human erythropoietin gene. Proc Natl Acad Sci U S A 82:7580-7584, 1985.

35. Erslev AJ: Erythropoietin. N Engl J Med 324:1339-1334, 1991.

36. Semenza GL, Nejfelt MK, Chi SM, et al: Hypoxia-inducible nuclear factors bind to an enhancer element located 3' to the human erythropoietin gene. Proc Natl Acad Sci U S A 88:5680-5684, 1991.

37. Eschbach JW: Erythropoietin 1991—an overview. Am J Kidney Dis 18(suppl 1):3-9, 1991.

38. Walle AJ, Wong GY, Clemons GK, et al: Erythropoietin-hematocrit feedback circuit in the anemia of end-stage renal disease. Kidney Int 31:1205-1209, 1987.

39. Caro J, Brown S, Miller O, et al: Erythropoietin levels in uremic nephric and anephric patients. J Lab Clin Med 93:449-458,1979.

40. Erslev AL, Caro J, Kansu E, et al: Renal and extrarenal erythropoietin production in anaemic rats. Br J Haematol 45:65-72, 1980.

41. Fisher JW: Erythropoietin: Physiologic and pharmacologic aspects. Proc Soc Exp Biol Med 216:358-369, 1997.

42. Winearls CG, Oliver DO, Pippard MJ, et al: Effect of human erythropoietin derived from recombinant DNA on the anemia of patients maintained by chronic hemodialysis. Lancet 2:1175-1178, 1986.

43. Eschbach JW, Egrie JC, Downing MR, et al: Correction of the anemia of end-stage renal disease with recombinant human erythropoietin. N Engl J Med 316:73-78, 1987.

44. Stone WJ, Graber SE, Krantz SB, et al: Treatment of the anemia of predialysis patients with recombinant human erythropoietin: A randomized, placebo-controlled trial. Am J Med Sci 296:171-179, 1988.

45. Casati S, Passerini P, Campise MR, et al: Benefits and risks of protracted treatment with human recombinant erythropoietin in patients having haemodialysis. BMJ 295:1017-1020, 1987.

46. Bommer J, Kugel M, Schoeppe W, et al: Dose-related effects of recombinant human erythropoietin on erythropoiesis: Results of a multicenter trial in patients with end-stage renal disease. Contrib Nephrol 66:85-93, 1988.

47. Akizawa T, Koshikawa S, Takaku F, et al: Clinical effect of recombinant human erythropoietin on anemia associated with chronic renal failure: A multi-institutional study in Japan. Int J Artif organs 11:343-350, 1988.

48. Lim VS, DeGowin RL, Zavala D, et al: Recombinant human erythropoietin treatment in pre-dialysis patients: A double-blind placebo-controlled trial. Ann Intern Med 110:108-114, 1989.

49. Eschbach JW, Kelly MR, Haley NR, et al: Treatment of the anemia of progressive renal failure with recombinant human erythropoietin. N Engl J Med 321:158-163, 1989.

50. Steinhauer HB, Lubrich-Birkner I, Dreyling KW, et al: Effect of human recombinant erythropoietin on anemia and dialysis efficiency in patients undergoing continuous ambulatory peritoneal dialysis. Eur J Clin Invest 21:47-52, 1991.

51. Eschbach JW, Abdulhadi MH, Browne JK, et al: Recombinant human erythropoietin in anemic patients with end-stage renal disease: Results of a phase III multicenter clinical trial. Ann Intern Med 111:992-1000, 1989.

52. Adamson JW, Eschbach JW: Treatment of the anemia of chronic renal failure with recombinant human erythropoietin. Annu Rev Med 41:349-360, 1990.

53. Macdougall IC: An overview of the efficacy and safety of novel erythropoiesis stimulating protein (NESP). Nephrol Dial Transplant 16(suppl 3): 14-21, 2001.

54. Egrie JC, Browne JK: Development and characterization of novel erythropoiesis stimulating protein (NESP). Nephrol Dial Transplant 16(suppl 3):3-13, 2001.

55. Macdougall IC, Gray SJ, Elston O et al: Pharmacokinetics of novel erthropoiesis stimulating protein compared to epoetin alfa in dialysis patients. J Am Soc Nephrol 10:2392-2395, 1999.

56. Locatelli F, Olivares J, Walker R, et al: Novel erythropoiesis stimulating protein for treatment of anemia in chronic renal insufficiency. Kidney Int 60:741-747, 2001.

57. The NESP Usage Guideline Group: Practical guidelines for the use of NESP in treating renal anaemia. Nephrol Dial Transplant, 16(suppl 3): 22-28, 2001.

58. NKF-DOQI: Clinical practice guidelines: Treatment of anemia of chronic renal failure. Am J Kidney Dis 30(suppl 3):S192-S237, 1997.

59. Bailie G, Rocco M, Flanigan M, et al: 1996 ESRD peritoneal dialysis core indicators study (PD-CIS): Hematocrit (Hct) and blood pressure (BP) data [abstract]. J Am Soc Nephrol 8:215A, 1997.

60. Eschbach JW: The future of r-HuEPO. Nephrol Dial Transplant 10(suppl 2):96-109, 1995.

61. Linde T, Sandhagen B, Wickstrom B, et al: The required dose of erythropoietin during renal anaemia treatment is related to the degree of impairment in erythrocyte deformability. Nephrol Dial Transplant 12:2375-2379, 1997.

62. Beguin Y, Loo M, R'Zik S, et al: Quantitative assessment of erythropoiesis in haemodialysis patients demonstrates gradual expansion of erythroblasts during constant treatment with recombinant human erythropoietin. Br J Haematol 89:17-23, 1995.

63. Kaufman J, Reda D: Subcutaneous (SC) versus intravenous (IV) administration of recombinant human erythropoietin (rHuEPO) in hemodialysis (HD) patients (pts) [abstract]. J Am Soc Nephrol 8:196A, 1997.

64. Macdougall IC: How to get the best out of rHuEPO. Nephrol Dial Transplant 10(suppl 2): 85-91, 1995.

65. Sunder-Plassmann G, Horl WH (guest eds): Erythropoietin and iron. Kidney Int Suppl 69:S1-S137, 1999.

66. De Schoenmakere G, Lameire N, Dhondt AM, et al: The haematopoioeotic effect of recombinant human erythropoietin in haemodialysis is independent from the administration mode (IV or SC) [abstract]. J Am Soc Nephrol 8:155A, 1997.

67. Taylor JE, Belch JJF, Fleming LW, et al: Erythropoietin response and route of administration. Clin Nephrol 41:297-302, 1994.

68. Koene RAP, Frenken LAM: Starting r-HuEPO in chronic renal failure: When, why, and how? Nephrol Dial Transplant 10(suppl 2):35-42, 1995.

69. Koch KM, Koene RAP, Messinger D, et al: The use of epoetin beta in anemic predialysis patients with chronic renal failure. Clin Nephrol 44:201-208, 1995.

70. Besarab A, Ross RP, Nasca TJ: The use of recombinant human erythropoietin in predialysis patients. Curr Opin Nephrol Hypertens 4:155-161, 1995.

71. Lopez-Gomez JM, Jofre R, Moreno F, et al: rHuEPO before dialysis and in dialysed patients. Nephrol Dial Transplant 10(suppl 6):31-35, 1995.

72. Revicki DA, Brown RE, Feeny DH, et al: Health-related qualify of life associated with recombinant human erythropoietin therapy for pre-dialysis chronic renal disease patients. Am J Kidney Dis 25:548-554, 1995.

73. Eschbach JW, Adamson JW, Cook JD: Disorders of red blood cell production in uremia. Arch Intern Med 126:812, 1970.

74. Santiago GC, Rao TKS, Laird NM: Effect of dialysis therapy on the hematopoietic system: The National Cooperative Dialysis Study. Kidney Int Suppl 23:S-95-S-100, 1983.

75. Teschan PE, Ginn HE, Bourne JR, et al: A prospective study of renal dialysis. Trans Am Soc Artif Intern Organs 3:108, 1983.

76. Eschbach JW, Haley NR, Egrie JC, et al: A comparison of the responses to recombinant human erythropoietin in normal and uremic subjects. Kidney Int 43:407-416, 1992.

77. Powe NR, Griffiths RI, Greer JW, et al: Early dosing practices and effectiveness of recombinant human erythropoietin. Kidney Int 43:1125-1133, 1993.

78. Powe NR, Griffiths RI, de Lissovoy G, et al: Access to recombinant erythropoietin by Medicare-entitled dialysis patients in the first year after FDA approval. JAMA 268:1434-1440, 1992.

79. Raleigh NC: Southeastern Kidney Council 1992 Annual Report. Raleigh, NC, Southeastern Kidney Council, 1992.

80. Ifudu O, Mayers J, Matthew J, et al: Dismal rehabilitation in geriatric inner-city hemodialysis patients. JAMA 271:29-33, 1994.

81. Ifudu O, Paul H, Mayers JD, et al: Pervasive failed rehabilitation in center-based maintenance hemodialysis patients. Am J Kidney Dis 23:394-400, 1994.

82. Ifudu O, Feldman J, Friedman EA: The intensity of haemodialysis and the response to erythropoietin in patients with end-stage renal disease. N Engl J Med 334:420-425, 1996.

83. Young EW, Woods JD, Segieda GE, et al: Predictors of target hematocrit among erythropoietin-treated HD patients [abstract]. J Am Soc Nephrol 8:259A, 1997.

84. Miles AM, Markell MS, Daskalakis P, et al: Anemia following renal transplantation: Erythropoietin response and iron deficiency. Clin Transplant 11:313-315, 1997.

85. Beshara S, Birgegard G, Goch J, et al: Assessment of erythropoiesis following renal transplantation. Eur J Haematol 58:167-173, 1997.

86. Van Loo A, Vanholder R, Bernaert P, et al: Recombinant human erythropoietin corrects anaemia during the first weeks after renal transplantation: A randomized prospective study. Nephrol Dial Transplant 11:1815-1821, 1996.

87. Martin B, Bondia A, Martin M, et al: Study of sensitivity of BFU-E to EPO-rHu in posttransplantation renal erythrocytosis [abstract]. J Am Soc Nephrol 8:716A, 1997.

88. Mrug M, Stopka T, Julian BA, et al: Angiotensin II stimulates proliferation of normal early erythroid progenitors. J Clin Invest 100:3210-3214, 1997.

89. Walter J: Does captopril decrease the effect of human recombinant erythropoietin in haemodialysis patients? Nephrol Dial Transplant 8:1428-1431, 1993.

90. Vlahakos DV, Balodimus C, Papachristopoulos V, et al: Renin-angiotensin system stimulates erythropoietin secretion in chronic hemodialysis patients. Clin Nephrol 43:53-59, 1995.

91. Matsumura M, Nomura H, Koni I, et al: Angiotensin-converting enzyme inhibitors are associated with the need for increased recombinant human erythropoietin maintenance doses in hemodialysis patients: Risk of Cardiac Disease in Dialysis Patients Study Group. Nephron 77:164-168, 1997.

92. Dhondt AW, Vanholder RC, Ringoir SM: Angiotensin-converting enzyme inhibitors and higher erythropoietin requirement in chronic haemodialysis patients. Nephrol Dial Transplant 10:2107-2109, 1995.

93. Kurijama R, Kogure H, Itoh S, et al: Angiotensin converting enzyme inhibitor induced anemia in a kidney transplant recipient. Transplant Proc 28:1635, 1996.

94. Azizi M, Rousseau A, Ezan E, et al: Acute angiotensin-converting enzyme inhibition increases the plasma level of the natural stem cell regulator N-acetyl-seryl-aspartyl-lysyl-proline. J Clin Invest 97:839-844, 1996.

95. Eschbach JW: Hematological problems of renal failure. In Jacobs C, Kjellstrand CM, Koch KM, et al (eds): Replacement of Renal Function by Dialysis, 4th ed. Dordrecht, Netherlands, Kluwer Academic Publishers, 1996, pp 1059-1076.

96. Radermacher J, Koch KM: Treatment of renal anemia by erythropoietin substitution: The effects on the cardiovascular system. Clin Nephrol 44(suppl 1):S56-S60, 1995.

97. Langelfeld MR, Veelken R, Schobel HP, et al: Is endogenous erythropoietin a pathogenetic factor in the development of essential hypertension. Nephrol Dial Transplant 12:1115-1160, 1997.

98. Lacasse MS, Kingma I, Lariviere R, et al: Uremia enhances the blood pressure response to erythropoietin. Clin Exp Hypertens 19:389-401, 1997.

99. Bode-Boger SM, Boger RH, Kuhn M, et al: Recombinant human erythropoietin enhances vasoconstrictor tone via endothelin-1 and constrictor prostanoids. Kidney Int 50:1225-1261, 1996.

100. Tojo A, Doumoto M, Oka K, et al: Endothelin-mediated effect of erythropoietin on blood pressure and renal hemodynamics on hypertensive rats. Am J Physiol 270:R744-R748, 1996.

101. Lebel M, Kingma I, Grose JH, et al: Hemodynamic and hormonal changes during erythropoietin therapy in hemodialysis patients. J Am Soc Nephrol 9:97-104, 1998.

102. Ammarguellat F, Gogusev J, Drueke TB: Direct effect of erythropoietin on rat vascular smooth-muscle cell via a putative erythropoietin receptor, Nephrol Dial Transplant 11:687-692, 1996.

103. Bergrem H, Danielson BG, Eckardt KU, et al: A case of antierythropoietin antibodies following recombinant human erythropoietin treatment. In Bauer C, Kock KM, Scigalla P, Wieczorek

104. L (eds): Erythropoietin: Molecular Physiology and Clinical Application. New York, Marcel Dekker, 1993, pp 266-275.

104. Pece R, de la Torre M, Alcázar R, Urra JM: Antibodies against recombinant human erythropoietin in a patient with erythropoietin-resistant anemia. N Engl J Med 335:523-524, 1996.

105. Casadevall N, Nataf J, Viron B, et al: Pure red-cell aplasia and antierythropoietin antibodies in patients treated with recombinant erythropoietin. N Engl J Med 346:469-475, 2002.

106. Agence Française de Sécurité Sanitaire des Produits de Santé: Communiqué de presse. Available at http://agmed.sante.gouv.fr/htm/10/filcoprs/020704.htm as accessed September 2002.

107. Casadevall N. Antibodies against rHuEPO: Native and recombinant. Nephrol Dial Transplant 17(suppl 5):42-47, 2002.

108. Nissenson AR: Hyporesponsiveness to erythropoietin: Overview, 1996. Perit Dial Int 16:417-420, 1996.

109. Worral JC, Allen DA, Raftery MJ, et al: Impaired iron utilization and duration of hemodialysis are principal factors in erythropoietin resistance [abstract]. J Am Soc Nephrol 8:225A, 1997.

110. Macdougall IC: Poor response to erythropoietin. BMJ 310: 1424-1425, 1995.

111. Adamson J: Erythropoietin, iron metabolism, and red blood cell production. Semin Hematol 33(suppl 2):5-7, 1997.

112. Tarng DC, Huang TP, Chen TW, et al: Resistance to recombinant human erythropoietin treatment in thalassaemic patients on chronic hemodialysis: A real clinical entity? Nephrol Dial Transplant 11: 1893-1895, 1996.

113. Schwartz AB, Orquiza CS: The effects of recombinant human erythropoietin on mean corpuscular volume in patients with the anemia of chronic renal failure. Clin Nephrol 43:256-259, 1995.

114. Kalantar-Zadeh K, Hoffken B, Wunsch H, et al: Diagnosis of iron deficiency anemia in renal failure patients during the post-erythropoietin era. Am J Kidney Dis 26:292-299, 1995.

115. Barany P, Eriksson LC, Hultcrantz R, et al: Serum ferritin and tissue iron in anemic dialysis patients. Miner Electrolyte Metab 23:273-276, 1997.

116. Tarng DC, Chen TW, Huang TP: Iron metabolism indices for early prediction of the response and resistance to erythropoietin therapy in maintenance hemodialysis patients. Am J Nephrol 15:230-237, 1995.

117. Braun J, Lindner K, Schreiber M, et al: Percentage of hypochromic red blood cells as predictor of erythropoietic and iron response after i.v. iron supplementation in maintenance hemodialysis patients. Nephrol Dial Transplant 12:1173-1181, 1997.

118. Olmer M, Fossat Ch, Bouchouareb D, et al: Hypochromic red cells as a marker of functional iron deficiency in uremic dialyzed patients receiving r-HuEPO treatment [abstract]. J Am Soc Nephrol 8:206A, 1997.

119. Bandhari S, Owda AK, Kendall RG, et al: Red cell ferritin, a marker of iron deficiency in hemodialysis patients. Ren Fail 19:771-780, 1997.

120. Brunati C, Piperno A, Guastoni C, et al: Erythrocyte ferritin in patients on chronic hemodialysis treatment. Nephron 87:219-223, 1990.

121. Bhandari S, Norfolk D, Brownjohn A, et al: Evaluation of RBC ferritin and reticulocyte measurements in monitoring response to intravenous iron therapy. Am J Kidney Dis 30:814-821, 1997.

122. Fishbane S, Galgano C, Langley RC, et al: Reticulocyte hemoglobin content in the evaluation of iron status of hemodialysis patients. Kidney Int 52:217-222, 1997.

123. Mittman N, Sreedhara R, Mushnick R, et al: Reticulocyte hemoglobin content predicts functional iron deficiency hemodialysis patients receiving rHuEPO. Am J Kidney Dis 30:912-922, 1997.

124. Drueke TB, Barany P, Cazzola M, et al: Management of iron deficiency in renal anemia: Guidelines for the optimal therapeutic approach in erythropoietin-treated patients. Clin Nephrol 48:1-8, 1997.

125. Ahluwalia N, Skikne BS, Savin V, et al: Markers of masked iron deficiency and effectiveness of EPO therapy in chronic renal failure. Am J Kidney Dis 30:532-541, 1997.

126. Fishbane S, Kowalski EA, Imbriano LJ, et al: The evaluation of iron status in hemodialysis patients. J Am Soc Nephrol 7:2654-2657, 1996.

127. Sunder-Plassman G, Hoerl WH: Erythropoietin and iron. Clin Nephrol 47:141-157, 1997.

128. Nissenson AR: Achieving target hematocrit in dialysis patients: New concepts in iron management. Am J Kidney Dis 30:907-911, 1997.

129. Fishbane S, Maesaka JK: Iron management in end-stage renal disease. Am J Kidney Dis 29:319-333, 1997.

130. Lye WC, Chin S, Wong KC, et al: Prospective randomized comparison of three routes of iron administration during erythropoietin (rHuEPO) therapy in hemodialysis patients [abstract]. J Am Soc Nephrol 8:220A, 1997.

131. Markowitz GS, Kahn GA, Feingold RE, et al: An evaluation of the effectiveness of oral iron therapy in hemodialysis patients receiving recombinant human erythropoietin. Clin Nephrol 48:34-40, 1997.

132. Stivelman JC: Optimization of iron therapy in hemodialysis patients treated with rHuEPO. Semin Dial 7:288-292, 1994.

133. Fishbane S, Ungureanu VD, Maesaka JK, et al: The safety of intravenous iron dextran in hemodialysis patients. Am J Kidney Dis 28:529-534, 1996.

134. Sunder-Plassmann G, Horl WH: Importance of iron supply for erythropoietin therapy. Nephrol Dial Transplant 10:2070-2076, 1995.

135. Sakiewicz P, Paganini E: The use of iron in patients on chronic dialysis: Mistakes and misconceptions. J Nephrol 11:5-15, 1998.

136. Taylor JE, Peat N, Porter C, et al: Regular low-dose intravenous iron therapy improves response to erythropoietin in haemodialysis patients. Nephrol Dial Transplant 11:1079-1083, 1996.

137. Kausz A, Ahmad S, Sherrard D: Effectiveness of intravenous iron in hemodialysis patients: A randomized controlled trial [abstract]. J Am Soc Nephrol 8:220A, 1997.

138. Muirhead N, Bargman J, Burgess E, et al: Evidence-based recommendations for the clinical use of recombinant human erythropoietin. Am J Kidney Dis 26(suppl 1):S1-S24, 1995.

139. Gastaldello K, Vereerstraeten A, Nzame-Nze T, et al: Resistance of erythropoietin in iron-overloaded haemodialysis patients can be overcome by ascorbic acid administration. Nephrol Dial Transplant 10(suppl 6):44-47, 1995.

140. Grutzmacher P, Ehmer B, Messinger D, et al: Effect of aluminum overload on the bone marrow response to recombinant human erythropoietin. Contrib Nephrol 76:315-321, 1989.

141. Casati S, Castelnovo C, Campise M, et al: Aluminum interference in the treatment of hemodialysis with recombinant human erythropoietin. Nephrol Dial Transplant 5:441-443, 1990.

142. Cannata JB, Fernandez SI, Fernandez MMJ: The role of iron metabolism in absorption and cellular uptake of aluminum. Kidney Int 39:799-803, 1991.

143. Smans KA, Van Landeghem FG, D'Haese PC, et al: Is there a link between erythropoietin therapy and adynamic bone disease? Nephrol Dial Transplant 11:1248-1249, 1996.

144. Casadevall N: Cellular mechanism of resistance to erythropoietin. Nephrol Dial Transplant 10(suppl 6):27-30, 1995.

145. Fishbane S, Lynn RI: The utility of zinc protoporphyrin for predicting the need for intravenous iron therapy in hemodialysis patients. Am J Kidney Dis 25:426-432, 1995.

146. Baldus M, Salopek S, Moller M, et al: Experience with zinc protoporphyrin as a marker of endogenous iron availability in chronic hemodialysis patients. Nephrol Dial Transplant 11:486-491, 1996.

147. Braun J, Hammerschmidt M, Schreiber M, et al: Is zinc protoporphyrin an indicator of iron-deficiency erythropoiesis maintenance hemodialysis patients? Nephrol Dial Transplant 11:492-497, 1996.

148. Beguin Y, Loo M, R-Zik S, et al: Early prediction of response to recombinant human erythropoietin in patients with the anemia of renal failure by serum transferrin receptor and fibrinogen. Blood 82:2010-2016, 1993.

149. Barany P, Divino Filho JC, Bergstrom J: High C-reactive protein is a strong predictor of resistance to erythropoietin in hemodialysis patients. Am J Kidney Dis 29:565-568, 1997.

150. Fujita Y, Inoue S, Horiguchi S, et al: Excessive level of parathyroid hormone may induce the reduction of recombinant human erythropoietin effect on renal anemia. Miner Electrolyte Metab 21:50-54, 1995.

151. Rao DS, Shih M-S, Mohini R: Effect of serum parathyroid hormone and bone marrow fibrosis on the response to erythropoietin in uremia. N Engl J Med 328:171-175, 1993.

152. Urena P, Eckardt KU, Sarfati E, et al: Serum erythropoietin and erythropoiesis in primary and secondary hyperparathyroidism: Effect of parathyroidectomy. Nephron 59:384-393, 1991.

153. Teruel JL, Marcen R, Navarro-Antolin J, et al: Androgen versus erythropoietin for the treatment of anemia in hemodialyzed patients: A prospective study. J Am Soc Nephrol 7:140-144, 1996.

154. Yared K, Gagnon RF, Brox AG: Mechanism of action of androgen treatment on the anemia of experimental chronic renal failure [abstract]. J Am Soc Nephrol 8:633A, 1997.

155. Gaughan WJ, Liss KA, Dunn SR, et al: A 6-month study of low dose recombinant human erythropoietin alone and in combination with androgens for the treatment of anemia in chronic hemodialysis patients. Am J Kidney Dis 30:495-500, 1997.

156. Mayer G, Thum J, Cada EM, et al: Working capacity is increased following recombinant human erythropoietin treatment. Kidney Int 34:525-528, 1988.

157. Robertson HT, Haley NR, Guthrie MR, et al: Recombinant erythropoietin improves exercise capacity in anemic hemodialysis patients. Am J Kidney Dis 15:325-332, 1990.

158. Guthrie M, Cardenas D, Eschbach JW, et al: Effects of erythropoietin on strength and functional status of patients on hemodialysis. Clin Nephrol 39:97-102, 1993.

159. Evans RW, Rader B, Manninen DL: The quality of life of hemodialysis recipients treated with recombinant human erythropoietin. Cooperative Multicenter EPO Clinical Trial Group. JAMA 263:825-830, 1990.

160. Evans RW: Recombinant human erythropoietin and the quality of life of end-stage renal disease patients: A comparative study. Am J Kidney Dis 18(suppl 1):62-70, 1991.

161. McMahon LP, Dawborn JK: Subjective quality of life assessment in hemodialysis patients at different levels of hemoglobin following use of recombinant human erythropoietin. Am J Nephrol 12:162-169, 1992.

162. Madore F, Lowrie EG, Brugnara C, et al: Anemia in hemodialysis patients: Variables affecting this outcome predictor. J Am Soc Nephrol 8:1921-1929, 1997.

163. Collins A, Ma J, Ebben J: Patient survival is associated with hematocrit (HCT) level [abstract]. J Am Soc Nephrol 8:190A, 1997.

164. Mocks J, Franke W, Ehmer B, et al: Epoetin reduces mortality? Clinical trials in 3111 HD patients show a decreased CV risk [abstract]. J Am Soc Nephrol 8:222A, 1997.

165. Nagao K, Tsuchihashi K, Ura N, et al: Appropriate hematocrit levels of erythropoietin supplementary therapy in end-stage renal failure complicated by coronary artery disease. Can J Cardiol 13:747-753, 1997.

166. Hampl H, Paulitschke M, Lerche D, et al: Improved rheology of the newly generated RBC population as a result of rh erythropoietin-therapy (rhEPO) [abstract]. J Am Soc Nephrol 8:219A, 1997.

167. Metry G, Wikstrom B, Valind S, et al: Effect of normalization of hematocrit on brain circulation and metabolism in hemodialysis patients [abstract]. J Am Soc Nephrol 8:246A, 1997.

168. Nissenson AR: Optimal hematocrit for hemodialysis. Curr Opin Nephrol Hypertens 6:524-527, 1997.

169. Minetti L: Erythropoietin treatment in renal anemia: How high should the target hematocrit be? J Nephrol 10:117-119, 1997.

170. Morgagni GB: Opera Omnia Ex Typographia Remondiniana, Venezia, 1764.

171. Bright R: Reports of medical cases. London, 1827.

172. Watson AJ, Gimenez LF: The bleeding diathesis of uremia. Semin Dial 4:86-93, 1991.

173. Steiner RW, Coggins C, Carvalho ACA: Bleeding time in uremia: A useful test to assess clinical bleeding. Am J Hematol 7:107-117, 1979.

174. Lind SE: Prolonged bleeding time. Am J Med 77:305-312, 1984.

175. Kumar R, Ansell JE, Conoso RT, et al: Clinical trial of a new bleeding time device. Am J Clin Pathol 70:642-645, 1978.

176. Lindsay RM, Moorthy AV, Koens F, et al: Platelet function in dialyzed and non-dialyzed patients with chronic renal failure. Clin Nephrol 4:52-57, 1975.

177. Eknoyan G, Wacksman SJ, Glueck HI, et al: Platelet function in renal failure. N Engl J Med 280:677-681, 1969.

178. Di Minno G, Martinez J, McKean M, et al: Platelet dysfunction in uremia: Multifaceted defect partially corrected by dialysis. Am J Med 79:552-559, 1985.

179. Eknoyan G, Brown CH: Biochemical abnormalities of platelets in renal failure: Evidence for decreased platelet serotonin, adenosine diphosphate and Mg-dependent adenosine triphosphatase. Am J Nephrol 1:17-23, 1981.

180. Kyrle PA, Stockenhuber F, Brenner BM, et al: Evidence for an increased generation of prostacyclin in the microvasculature and an impairment of the platelet alpha granule release in chronic renal failure. Thromb Haemost 60:205-208, 1988.

181. Gura V, Creter D, Levi J: Elevated thrombocyte calcium content in uremia and its correction by alpha (OH) vitamin D treatment. Nephron 30:237-239, 1992.

182. Ware JA, Clark BA, Smith M, et al: Abnormalities of cytoplasmic Ca^{2+} in platelets from patients with uremia. Blood 73:172-176, 1989.

183. Vlachoyannis J, Schoeppe W: Adenylate cyclase activity and cAMP content of human platelets in uremia. Eur J Clin Invest 12:379-381, 1982.

184. Remuzzi G, Benigni A, Dodesini P, et al: Parathyroid hormone inhibits human platelet function. Lancet 2:1321-1323, 1981.

185. Benigni A, Livio M, Dodesini P, et al: Inhibition of human platelet aggregation by parathyroid hormone: Is cyclic AMP implicated? Am J Nephrol 5:243-247, 1985.

186. Viganò G, Gotti E, Comberti E, et al: Hyperparathyroidism does not influence the abnormal primary haemostasis in patients with chronic renal failure. Nephrol Dial Transplant 4:971-974, 1989.

187. Rabiner SF: Uraemic bleeding. In Spaet TH (ed): Progress in Hemostasis and Thrombosis. New York, Grune & Stratton, 1972, pp 233-250.

188. Remuzzi G, Benigni A, Dodesini P, et al: Platelet function in patients on maintenance hemodialysis: Depressed or enhanced? Clin Nephrol 17:60-63, 1982.

189. Zicker MB: Biological aspects of heparin action: Heparin and platelet function. Fed Proc 36:47-49, 1977.

190. Smith MC, Dunn MJ: Impaired platelet thromboxane production in renal failure. Nephron 29:133-137, 1981.

191. Remuzzi G, Benigni A, Dodesini P, et al: Reduced platelet thromboxane formation in uremia: Evidence for a functional cyclooxygenase defect. J Clin Invest 71:762-768, 1983.

192. Macconi D, Viganò G, Bisogno G, et al: Defective platelet aggregation in response to platelet-activating factor in uremia associated with low platelet thromboxane A$_2$ generation. Am J Kidney Dis 19:318-325, 1992.

193. Livio E, Benigni A, Remuzzi G: Coagulation abnormalities in uremia. Semin Nephrol 5:82-90, 1985.

194. Remuzzi G, Perico N, Zoja C, et al: Role of endothelium-derived nitric oxide in the bleeding tendency of uremia. J Clin Invest 86:1768-1771, 1990.

195. Ignarro LJ: Endothelium-derived nitric oxide: Actions and properties. FASEB J 3:31-36, 1988.

196. Aiello S, Noris M, Todeschini M, et al: Renal and systemic nitric oxide synthesis in rats with renal mass reduction. Kidney Int 52:171-181, 1997.

197. Marletta MA: Nitric oxide: Biosynthesis and biological significance. Trends Biochem Sci 14:488-492, 1989.

198. Moncada S, Higgs EA: Molecular mechanism and therapeutic strategies related to nitric oxide. FASEB J 9:1319-1330, 1995.

199. Hogman M, Frostell C, Arnberg H, et al: Bleeding time prolongation and NO inhalation. Lancet 341:1664-1665, 1993.

200. Viganò G, Zoja C, Corna D, et al: 17β-Estradiol is the most active component at the conjugated estrogen mixture active on uremic bleeding by a receptor mechanism. J Pharmacol Exp Ther 252:344-348, 1990.

201. Zoja C, Noris M, Corna D, et al: L-Arginine, the precursor of nitric oxide, abolishes the effect of estrogens on bleeding time in experimental uremia. Lab Invest 65: 479-483, 1991.

202. Bonazzola S, Noris M, Todeschini M, et al: 17β-Estradiol corrects abnormal primary hemostasis in uremic rats by limiting vascular endothelial expression of nitric oxide (NO) forming enzymes [abstract]. J Am Soc Nephrol 9:604A, 1998.

203. Noris M, Benigni A, Boccardo P, et al: Enhanced nitric oxide synthesis in uremia: Implications for platelet dysfunction and dialysis hypotension. Kidney Int 44:445-450, 1993.

204. Thuraisingham RC, Cramp HA, McMahon AC, et al: Increased superoxide and nitric oxide production results in peroxynitrite formation in uremic vasculature [abstract]. J Am Soc Nephrol 8:340A, 1997.

205. Descamps-Latscha B, Herbelin A, Nguyen AT, et al: Balance between IL-1β, TNF-α, and their specific inhibitors in chronic renal failure and maintenance dialysis. J Immunol 154:882-892, 1995.

206. Herbelin A, Nguyen AT, Zingraff J, et al: Influence of uremia and hemodialysis on circulating interleukin-1 and tumor necrosis factor α. Kidney Int 37:116-125, 1990.

207. Pereira BJG, Dinarello CA: Production of cytokines and cytokine inhibitory proteins in patients on dialysis. Nephrol Dial Transplant 9:60-71, 1994.

208. Luger A, Kovarik J, Stummvoll HK, et al: Blood-membrane interaction in hemodialysis leads to increased cytokine production. Kidney Int 32:84-88, 1987.

209. Lefkovits J, Plow EF, Topol EJ: Platelet glycoprotein IIb/IIIa receptors in cardiovascular medicine. N Engl J Med 332:1553-1559, 1995.

210. Benigni A, Boccardo P, Galbusera M, et al: Reversible activation defect of the platelet glycoprotein IIb-IIIa complex in patients with uremia. Am J Kidney Dis 22:668-676, 1993.

211. Mezzano D, Tagle R, Panes O, et al: Hemostatic disorder of uremia: The platelet defect, main determinant of the prolonged bleeding time, is correlated with indices of activation of coagulation and fibrinolysis. Thromb Haemost 76:312-321, 1996.

212. Sloand EM, Sloand JA, Prodouz K, et al: Reduction of platelet glycoprotein Ib in uraemia. Br J Haematol 77:375-381, 1991.

213. Gawaz MP, Dobos G, Spath M, et al: Impaired function of platelet membrane glycoprotein IIb-IIIa in end-stage renal disease. J Am Soc Nephrol 5:36-46, 1994.

214. Sreedhara R, Itagaki I, Hakim RM: Uremic patients have decreased shear-induced platelet aggregation mediated by decreased availability of glycoprotein IIb-IIIa receptors. Am J Kidney Dis 27:355-364, 1996.

215. Castillo R, Lozano T, Escolar G, et al: Defective platelet adhesion on vessel subendothelium in uremic patients. Blood 65:337-342, 1986.

216. Zwaginga JJ, Ijsseldijk MJW, Beeser-Visser N, et al: High von Willebrand factor concentration compensates a relative adhesion defect in uremic blood. Blood 75:1498-1508, 1990.

217. Escolar G, Cases A, Bastida E, et al: Uremic platelets have a functional defect affecting the interaction of von Willebrand factor with glycoprotein IIb-IIIa. Blood 76:1336-1340, 1990.

218. Rabiner SF, Molinas F: The role of phenol and phenolic acids on the thrombocytopathy and defective platelet aggregation of patients with renal failure. Am J Med 49:346-351, 1970.

219. Horowitz HI, Stein IM, Cohen BD, et al: Further studies on the platelet inhibitory effect of guanidinosuccinic acid and its role in uremic bleeding. Am J Med 49:336-345, 1970.

220. Remuzzi G, Livio E, Marchiaro G, et al: Bleeding in renal failure: Altered platelet function in chronic uraemia only partially corrected by haemodialysis. Nephron 22:347-353, 1978.

221. Ruggeri ZM, Zimmerman TS: von Willebrand factor and von Willebrand disease. Blood 70:895-904, 1987.

222. Gordge MP, Neild GH: Platelet function in uremia. Platelets 2:115-123, 1991.

223. Kazatchkine N, Sultan V, Caen JP, et al: Bleeding in renal failure: A possible cause. BMJ 2:612-615, 1976.

224. Nerrmann RP, Marshall LR, Hurst PE: Bleeding in renal failure: A possible cause. BMJ 1:1601-1602, 1977.

225. Remuzzi G, Livio M, Roncaglioni MC, et al: Bleeding in renal failure: Is von Willebrand factor implicated? BMJ 2:359-361, 1977.

226. Warrell RPJr, Hultin MB, Coller BS: Increased factor VIII/von Willebrand factor antigen and von Willebrand factor activity in renal failure. Am J Med 66:226-228, 1979.

227. Janson PA, Jubelirer SJ, Weinstein MJ, et al: Treatment of the bleeding tendency in uremia with cryoprecipitate. N Engl J Med 303:1318-1322, 1980.

228. Mannucci PM, Remuzzi G, Pusineri F, et al: Deamino-8-D-arginine vasopressin shortens the bleeding time in uremia. N Engl J Med 308:8-12, 1983.

229. Turitto VT, Weiss HJ: Red blood cells: Their dual role in thrombus formation. Science 207:541-543, 1980.

230. Sakariassen KS, Bolhuis PA, Sixma JJ: Platelet adherence to subendothelium of human arteries in pulsatile and steady flow. Thromb Res 19:547-559, 1980.

231. Gaarder A, Jonsen J, Lland S, et al: Adenosine diphosphate in red cells as a factor in the adhesiveness of human blood platelets. Nature 192:531-532, 1961.

232. Willems C, Stel HV, van Aken WG, et al: Binding and inactivation of prostacyclin (PGI$_2$) by human erythrocytes. Br J Haematol 54:43-52, 1983.

233. Livio M, Gotti E, Marchesi D, et al: Uraemic bleeding: Role of anemia and beneficial effect of red cell transfusions. Lancet 2: 1013-1015, 1982.

234. Fernandez F, Goudable C, Sie P, et al: Low hematocrit and prolonged bleeding time in uraemic patients: Effect of red cell transfusions. Br J Haematol 59:139-148, 1985.

235. Howard AD, Moore JJr, Welch PG, et al: Analysis of the quantitative relationship between anemia and chronic renal failure. Am J Med Sci 297:303-313, 1989.

236. Gordge MP, Leaker B, Patel A, et al: Recombinant human erythropoietin shortens the uraemic bleeding time without causing intravascular haemostatic activation. Thromb Res 57:171-182, 1990.

237. Moia M, Mannucci PM, Vizzotto L, et al: Improvement in the haemostatic defect of uraemia after treatment with recombinant human erythropoietin. Lancet 2:1227-1229, 1987.

238. Viganò G, Benigni A, Mendogni D, et al: Recombinant human erythropoietin to correct uremic bleeding. Am J Kidney Dis 18:44-49, 1991.

239. Eiser AR: Gastrointestinal bleeding in maintenance dialysis patients. Semin Dial 1:198-202, 1988.

240. Dinoso VP, Murthy SNS, Saris AL, et al: Gastric and pancreatic function in patients with end-stage renal disease. J Clin Gastroenterol 4:321-324, 1982.

241. Kleinknecht D, Jungers P, Chanard J, et al: Uremic and non-uremic complications in acute renal failure: Evaluation of early and frequent dialysis on prognosis. Kidney Int 1:190-196, 1972.

242. Shepherd AM, Stewart WK, Wormsley KG: Peptic ulceration in chronic renal failure. Lancet 1:1357-1359, 1973.

243. Margolis DM, Saylor JL, Geisse G, et al: Upper gastrointestinal disease in chronic renal failure: A prospective evaluation. Arch Intern Med 138:1214-1217, 1978.

244. Dave PB, Romeu J, Antonelli A, et al: Gastrointestinal telangiectasias: A source of bleeding in patients receiving hemodialysis. Arch Intern Med 144:1781-1783, 1984.

245. Boley SJ, Sammartano R, Adams A, et al: On the nature and aetiology of vascular ectasias of the colon: Degenerative lesions of aging. Gastroenterology 72:652-660, 1977.

246. Zuckerman GR, Cornette GL, Clouse RE, et al: Upper gastrointestinal bleeding in patients with chronic renal failure. Ann Intern Med 102:588-592, 1985.

247. Cunningham JT: Gastric telangiectasias in chronic hemodialysis patients: A report of six cases. Gastroenterology 81:1131-1133, 1981.

248. Doroty CC: Gastrointestinal bleeding in dialysis patients. Nephron 63:132-139, 1993.

249. Kumar S, Lesch M: Pericarditis in renal disease. Prog Cardiovasc Dis 22:357-369, 1980.

250. Rutsky EA, Rostand SG: Treatment of uremic pericarditis and pericardial effusion. Am J Kidney Dis 10:2-8, 1987.

251. Comty CM, Shapiro FL: Cardiac complications of regular dialysis therapy. *In* Mather J (ed): Replacement of Renal Function by Dialysis, 2nd ed. Dordrecht, Netherlands, Kluwer Academic Publishers, 1983, pp 33-70.

252. Drueke T, Le-Pailleur C, Zingraff J, et al: Uraemic cardiomyopathy and pericarditis. Adv Nephrol Necker Hosp 9:33-70, 1980.

253. Bechar M, Lakke JP, van der Hem GK, et al: Subdural hematoma during long-term hemodialysis. Arch Neurol 26:513-516, 1972.

254. Berger HW, Rammohan G, Neff MS, et al: Uraemic pleural effusion: A study in 14 patients on chronic dialysis. Ann Intern Med 83:362-364, 1975.

255. Galen MA, Steinberg SM, Lowrie FG, et al: Hemorrhagic pleural effusion in patients undergoing chronic dialysis. Ann Intern Med 82:359-361, 1975.

256. Bhasin HK, Dana CL: Spontaneous retroperitoneal hemorrhage in chronically hemodialyzed patients. Nephron 22:322-327, 1978.

257. Milutinovich J, Follette WC, Scribner BH: Spontaneous retroperitoneal bleeding in patients on chronic hemodialysis. Ann Intern Med 86:189-192, 1977.

258. Borra S, Kleinfeld M: Subcapsular liver hematomas in a patient on chronic hemodialysis. Ann Intern Med 93:574-575, 1980.

259. Slusher MN, Hamilton RW: Spontaneous hyphema during hemodialysis. N Engl J Med 293:561, 1975.

260. Harter HR, Burch JW, Majerus PW, et al: Prevention of thrombosis in patients on hemodialysis by low dose aspirin. N Engl J Med 301:577-579, 1979.

261. Lindsay RM, Ferguson D, Prentice CR, et al: Reduction of thrombus formation on dialyser membranes by aspirin and RA233. Lancet 2:1287-1290, 1972.

262. Livio M, Benigni A, Viganò G, et al: Moderate doses of aspirin and risk of bleeding in renal failure. Lancet 1:414-416, 1986.

263. Boyle JM, Johnston B: Acute upper gastrointestinal hemorrhage in patients with chronic renal disease. Am J Med 75:409-412, 1983.

264. Gross R, Nieth H, Mammen E: Blutungsbereitschaft und Gerinnungsstörungen bei Urämie. Klin Wochenschr 136:107-109, 1958.

265. Larsson SO: On coagulation and fibrinolysis in renal failure. Scand J Haematol 15(suppl):1-59, 1971.

266. Rabiner SF: Bleeding in uremia. Med Clin North Am 56:221-233, 1972.

267. Lewis J, Zucher MB, Ferguson JH: Bleeding tendency in uremia. Blood 11:1073-1076, 1956.

268. Rath CD, Mailliard JA, Schreiner GE: Bleeding tendency in uremia. N Engl J Med 257:808-811, 1957.

269. Cheney K, Bonnin JA: Haemorrhage, platelet dysfunction and other coagulation defects in uremia. Br J Haematol 8:215-222, 1962.

270. Panicucci F, Sagripanti A, Pinori E, et al: Comprehensive study of haemostasis in chronic uremia. Nephron 33:5-8, 1983.

271. Ruggeri ZM, Ponticelli C, Mannucci PM: Factor VIII and chronic renal failure. BMJ 1:1085, 1977.

272. Quereda C, Pardo A, Lamas S, et al: Lupus-like anticoagulant activity in end-stage renal disease. Nephron 49:39-44, 1988.

273. von Kaulla KN, von Kaula KN: Antithrombin III and diseases. Am J Clin Pathol 48:69-75, 1976.

274. Jorgensen KA, Stoffersen E: Antithrombin III in uremia. Scand J Urol Nephrol 13:299-303, 1979.

275. Tomura S, Nakamura Y, Deguchi F, et al: Coagulation and fibrinolysis in patients with chronic renal failure undergoing conservative treatment. Thromb Res 64:81-90, 1991.

276. Lai K-N, Yin JA, Yuen PMP, et al: Effect of hemodialysis on protein C, protein S, and antithrombin III levels. Am J Kidney Dis 17:38-42, 1991.

277. Vaziri ND, Gonzales ED, Wang J, et al: Blood coagulation, fibrinolytic, and inhibitory proteins in end-stage renal disease: Effect of hemodialysis. Am J Kidney Dis 23:828-835, 1994.

278. Sorensen PJ, Knudsen F, Nielsen AH, et al: Protein C assays in uremia. Thromb Res 54:301-310, 1989.

279. Faioni EM, Franchi F, Krachmalnicoff A, et al: Low levels of the anticoagulant activity of protein C in patients with chronic renal insufficiency: An inhibitor of protein C is present in uremic plasma. Thromb Haemost 66:420-425, 1991.

280. D'Angelo A, Vigano-D'Angelo SV, Esmon CT, et al: Acquired deficiencies of protein S: Protein S activity during oral anticoagulation, in liver disease and in disseminated intravascular coagulation. J Clin Invest 81:1445-1454, 1988.

281. Sagripanti A, Cupisti A, Baicchi U, et al: Plasma parameters of the prothrombotic state in chronic uremia. Nephron 63:273-278, 1993.

282. Ireland HA, Boisclair MD, Lane DA, et al: Hemodialysis and heparin: Alternative methods of measuring heparin and of detecting activation of coagulation. Clin Nephrol 35:26-34, 1991.

283. Reber G, Stoermann C, De Moerloose P, et al: Hemostatic disturbances by two hollow-fiber hemodialysis membranes. Int J Artif Organs 15:269-275, 1992.

284. Nakamura Y, Chida Y, Tomura S: Enhanced coagulation fibrinolysis in patients on regular hemodialysis treatment. Nephron 58:201, 1991.

285. Lane DA, Ireland H, Knight I, et al: The significance of fibrinogen derivatives in plasma in human renal failure. Br J Haematol 56:251-260, 1984.

286. Sultan Y, London GM, Goldfarb B, et al: Activation of platelets, coagulation and fibrinolysis in patients on long-term haemodialysis: Influence of cuprophane and polyacrylonitrile membranes. Nephrol Dial Transplant 5:362-378, 1990.

287. Bennett NB, Ogston D: Inhibitors of the fibrinolytic enzyme system in renal disease. Clin Sci (Colch) 39:549-557, 1970.

288. Ito T, Niwa T, Matsui E: Fibrinolytic activity in renal disease. Clin Chim Acta 36:145-151, 1972.

289. Homma T, Ichikawa T: Studies of fibrinolytic activity of uremic and long-term hemodialysis patients with special reference to fibrinolytic inhibitor. Biochem Exp Biol 15:229-236, 1979.

290. Canavese C, Stratta P, Pacitti A, et al: Impaired fibrinolysis in uremia: Partial and variable correction by four different dialysis regimens. Clin Nephrol 17:82-89, 1982.

291. Tomura S, Oono Y, Kuriyama R, et al: Plasma concentrations of fibrinopeptide A and fibrin peptide Bb15-42 in glomerulonephritis and the nephrotic syndrome. Arch Intern Med 145:1033-1035, 1985.

292. Nishimoto K, Yamagami S, Katoh Y, et al: Coagulation and fibrinolysis in chronic renal failure: Change in tissue-type plasminogen activator activity. ASAIO J 32:478-481, 1986.

293. Nakamura Y, Tomura S, Tachibana K, et al: Enhanced fibrinolytic activity during the course of hemodialysis. Clin Nephrol 38:90-96, 1992.

294. Speiser W, Wojta J, Korninger C, et al: Enhanced fibrinolysis caused by tissue plasminogen activator release in hemodialysis. Kidney Int 32:280-283, 1987.

295. Brommer EJP, Schicht I, Wijngaards G, et al: Fibrinolytic activators and inhibitors in terminal renal insufficiency and in anephric patients. Thromb Haemost 52:311-314, 1984.

296. Cressman MD, Heyka RJ, Paganini EP, et al: Lipoprotein(a) is an independent risk factor for cardiovascular disease in hemodialysis patients. Circulation 86:475-482, 1992.

297. Webb AT, Reaveley DA, O'Donnell M, et al: Lipoprotein(a) in patients on maintenance haemodialysis and continuous ambulatory peritoneal dialysis. Nephrol Dial Transplant 8:609-613, 1993.

298. Del Greco F, Soper WS, Krumlovsky FA, et al: Thrombosis of vascular access for haemodialysis. *In* Remuzzi G, Rossi EC (eds): Haemostasis and the Kidney. London, Butterworths, 1989, pp 303-308.

299. Rodkin RS, Bookstein JJ, Heeney DJ, et al: Streptokinase and transluminal angioplasty in the treatment of acutely thrombosed hemodialysis access fistulas. Radiology 149:425-428, 1983.

300. Young AT, Hunter DW, Castaneda-Zuniga WR, et al: Thrombosed synthetic hemodialysis access fistulas: Failure of fibrinolytic therapy. Radiology 154:639-642, 1985.

301. Mangiarotti G, Canavese C, Thea A, et al: Urokinase treatment for arteriovenous fistulae declotting in dialyzed patients. Nephron 36:60-64, 1984.

302. Sloand EM, Bern MM, Kaldany A: Effect on platelet function of hypoalbuminemia in peritoneal dialysis. Thromb Res 44:415-419, 1986.

303. Gawaz MP, Ward RA: Effects on hemodialysis on platelet derived thrombospondin. Kidney Int 40:257-265, 1991.

304. Hakim RM, Schafer AI: Hemodialysis-associated platelet activation and thrombocytopenia. Am J Med 78:575-580, 1958.

305. Deguchi N, Ohigashi T, Tazaki H, et al: Haemodialysis and platelet activation. Nephrol Dial Transplant 2:40-42, 1991.

306. Adler AJ, Berlyne GM: β-Thromboglobulin and platelet factor-4 during hemodialysis with polyacrylonitrile. Trans Am Soc Artif Intern Organs 4:100-102, 1981.

307. Reverter JC, Escolar G, Sanz C, et al: Platelet activation during hemodialysis measured through exposure of *p*-selectin: Analysis for flow cytometric and ultrastructural techniques. J Lab Clin Med 124:79-85, 1994.

308. Matsuda T, Takemoto Y, Kishimoto T, et al: Mechanistic aspects of cellular interactions with artificial dialyzer membrane surfaces. Biomater Artif Cells Artif Organs 18:579-584, 1990.

309. Akizawa T, Nishiyama H, Koshikawa S: Plasma β-thromboglobulin levels in chronic renal failure patients. Artif Organs 5:54-58, 1981.

310. Schmitt GW, Moake JL, Rudy CK, et al: Alterations in hemostatic parameters during hemodialysis with dialyzers of different membrane composition and flow design: Platelet activation and factor VIII–related von Willebrand factor during hemodialysis. Am J Med 83:411-418, 1987.

311. Dewanjee MK, Kapadvanjwala M, Cavagnaro CF, et al: In vitro and in vivo evaluation of the comparative thrombogenicity of cellulose acetate hemodialyzers with radiolabeled platelets. ASAIO J 40:49-55, 1994.

312. Windus DW, Santoro S, Royal HD: The effects of hemodialysis on platelet deposition in prosthetic graft fistulas. Am J Kidney Dis 26:614-621, 1995.

313. Himmelfarb J, Holbrook D, McMonagle E, et al: Increased reticulated platelets in dialysis patients. Kidney Int 51:834-839, 1997.

314. Lonnemann G, Bingel M, Floege J, et al: Detection of endotoxin-like interleukin-1-inducing activity during in vitro dialysis. Kidney Int 33:29-35, 1988.

315. Laude-Sharp M, Caroff M, Simard L, et al: Induction of IL-1 during hemodialysis: Transmembrane passage of intact endotoxins (LPS). Kidney Int 38:1089-1094, 1990.

316. Libby P, Ordonas JM, Auger KR: Endotoxin and tumor necrosis factor induce interleukin-1 gene expression in adult human vascular endothelial cells. Am J Pathol 124:179-185, 1986.

317. Bingel M, Koch KM, Lonnemann G, et al: Enhancement of in-vitro human interleukin-1 produced by sodium acetate. Lancet 1:14-16, 1987.

318. Yokokawa K, Mankus R, Saklayen MG, et al: Increased nitric oxide production in patients with hypotension during hemodialysis. Ann Intern Med 123:35-37, 1995.

319. Noris M, Todeschini M, Casiraghi F, et al: Effect of acetate, bicarbonate dialysis and acetate-free biofiltration on nitric oxide synthesis: Implications for dialysis hypotension. Am J Kidney Dis 32:115-124, 1998.

320. Gordon LA, Somon ER, Rukes JM, et al: Studies in regional heparinization. N Engl J Med 255:1063-1066, 1956.

321. Maher JF, Lapierre L, Schreiner GE, et al: Regional heparinization for hemodialysis. N Engl J Med 268:451-456, 1963.

322. Lindholm DD, Murray S: A simplified method of regional heparinization during hemodialysis according to a predetermined dosage formula. Trans Am Soc Artif Intern Organs 10:92-97, 1964.

323. Blaufox MD, Hampers CL, Merril JP: Rebound anticoagulation occurring after regional heparinization for hemodialysis. Trans Am Soc Artif Intern Organs 12:207-209, 1966.

324. Lohr YW, Schwab S: Minimizing hemorrhagic complications in dialysis patients. J Am Soc Nephrol 2:961-975, 1991.

325. Tolkoff-Rubin NE, Nardini J, Fang LST, et al: Successful hemodialysis of patients at high risk of hemorrhage using the Ex Val dialyzer. Dial Transplant 15:125-126, 1986.

326. Ljungberg B: A low molecular heparin fraction as an anticoagulant during hemodialysis. Clin Nephrol 25:15-20, 1985.

327. Nurmohamed MT, Hoek JA, Ten Cate JW, et al: A randomized cross-over study comparing the efficacy and safety of two dosages of dermatan sulfate and standard heparin in six chronic hemodialysis patients. Br J Haematol 76:23, 1990.

328. Ryan KE, Lane DA, Flynn A, et al: Antithrombotic properties of dermatan sulphate (MF 701) in hemodialysis for chronic renal failure. Thromb Haemost 68:563-569, 1992.

329. Fernandez F, Van Ryn J, Ofosu F, et al: The haemorrhagic and antithrombotic effects of dermatan sulphate. Br J Haematol 64:309-317, 1986.

330. Nurmohamed MT, Knipscheer HC, Stevens P, et al: Clinical experience with a new antithrombotic (dermatan sulfate) in chronic hemodialysis patients. Clin Nephrol 39:166-171, 1993.

331. Gianese F, Nurmohamed MT, Imbimbo BP, et al: The pharmacodynamic of dermatan sulphate MF 701 during haemodialysis for chronic renal failure. Br J Clin Pharmacol 35:335-339, 1993.

332. Lane DA, Ryan K, Ireland H, et al: Dermatan sulphate in haemodialysis. Lancet 339:334-335, 1992.

333. Nurmohamed MT, Knipscheer HC, Gianese F, et al: No clinically relevant accumulation of dermatan sulphte (DS) during chronic use in hemodialysis [abstract]. Thromb Haemost 69:1118, 1993.

334. Boccardo P, Melacini D, Rota S, et al: Individualized anticoagulation with dermatan sulphate for haemodialysis in chronic renal failure. Nephrol Dial Transplant 12:2349-2354, 1997.

335. Morring K, Sinn H, Schuler HW, et al: Comparative evaluation of iatrogenic sources of blood loss during maintenance dialysis. *In* Proceedings of the 13th Congress of the European Dialysis and Transplant Association, Vienna, 1976, p 233.

336. Turney JH, Williams LC, Fewell MR, et al: Platelet protection and heparin sparing with prostacyclin during regular therapy. Lancet 2:219-222, 1980.

337. Arze RS, Ward MK: Prostacyclin safer than heparin in hemodialysis. Lancet 2:50, 1981.

338. Zusman RM, Rubin RH, Cato AE, et al: Hemodialysis using prostacyclin instead of heparin as the sole antithrombotic agent. N Engl J Med 304:934-939, 1981.

339. Swartz RD, Flamenbaum W, Dubrow A, et al: Epoprostenol (PGI, prostacyclin) during high risk hemodialysis: Preventing further bleeding complications. J Clin Pharmacol 28:818-825, 1988.

340. Dubrow A, Flamenbaum W, Mittman N, et al: Safety and efficacy of epoprostenol (PGI$_2$) versus heparin H in hemodialysis HD. Trans Am Soc Artif Intern Organs 30:52-54, 1984.

341. Zwaginga JJ, Ijsseldijk MJW, de Groot PG, et al: Treatment of uraemic anemia with recombinant erythropoietin also reduces the defects in platelet adhesion and aggregation caused by uraemic plasma. Thromb Haemost 66:638-647, 1991.

342. Huraib S, Al-Momen Ak, Gader AMA, et al: Effect of recombinant human erythropoietin (rHuEpo) on the hemostatic system in chronic hemodialysis patients. Clin Nephrol 36:252-257, 1991.

343. Taylor JE, Belch JJF, McLaren M, et al: Effect of erythropoietin therapy and withdrawal on blood coagulation and fibrinolysis in hemodialysis patients. Kidney Int 44:182-190, 1993.

344. Ozsoylu S, Gürsel T: von Willebrand factor and rise in ristocetin co-factor with erythropoietin. Lancet 341:1221, 1993.

345. Triulzi DJ, Blumberg N: Variability in response to cryoprecipitate treatment for hemostatic defects in uremia. Yale J Biol Med 63:1-7, 1990.

346. Mannucci PM, Ruggeri ZM, Pareti FI, et al: 1-Deamino-8-D-arginine vasopressin: A new pharmacological approach to the management of haemophilia and von Willebrand's diseases. Lancet 1:869-872, 1977.

347. Canavese C, Salomone M, Pacitti A, et al: Reduced response of uraemic bleeding time to repeated doses of desmopressin. Lancet 1:867-868, 1985.

348. Shapiro MD, Kelleher SP: Intranasal deamino-8-D-arginine vasopressin shortens the bleeding time in uremia. Am J Nephrol 4:260-261, 1984.

349. Rydzewski A, Rowinski M, Mysliwiec M: Shortening of the bleeding time after intranasal administration of 1-deamino-8-D-arginine vasopressin to patients with chronic anemia. Folia Haematol (Leipz) 113:823-830, 1986.

350. Viganò G, Mannucci PM, Lattuada A, et al: Subcutaneous injection of desmopressin (DDAVP) shortens the bleeding time in uremia. Am J Hematol 31:32-35, 1989.

351. Aunsholt NA, Schmidt EB, Stoffersen E: 1-Deamino-8-D-arginine vasopressin lowers protein C activity in uremics. Nephron 53:6-9, 1989.

352. Akpolat T, Ozdemir O, Arik N, et al: Effect of desmopressin (DDAVP) on protein C and protein C inhibitors in uremia. Nephron 64:232-234, 1993.

353. Byrnes JJ, Larcada A, Moake JL: Thrombosis following desmopressin for uremic bleeding. Am J Hematol 28:63-65, 1988.

354. Liu YK, Kosfeld RE, Marcum SG: Treatment of uraemic bleeding with conjugated oestrogen. Lancet 2:887-890, 1984.

355. Livio M, Mannucci PM, Viganò GL, et al: Conjugated estrogens for the management of bleeding associated with renal failure. N Engl J Med 315:731-735, 1986.

356. Viganò G, Gaspari F, Locatelli M, et al: Dose-effect and pharmacokinetics of estrogens given to correct bleeding time in uremia. Kidney Int 34:853-858, 1988.

357. Salant DJ, Galver AM, Anderson R, et al: Depressed neutrophil chemotaxis in patients with chronic renal failure and after renal transplantation. J Lab Clin Med 88:536-545, 1976.

358. Clark RA, Hamory BH, Ford GH, et al: Chemotaxis in acute renal failure. J Infect Dis 126:460-463, 1972.

359. Baum J, Cestero RV, Freeman RB: Chemotaxis of the polymorphonuclear leukocyte and delayed hypersensitivity in uremia. Kidney Int suppl 7:S147-S153, 1975.

360. Bjorksten B, Mauer SM, Mills EL, et al: The effect of hemodialysis on neutrophil chemotactic responsiveness. Acta Med Scand 203:67-70, 1978.

361. Siriwatratananonta P, Sinsakul V, Stern K, et al: Defective chemotaxis in uremia. J Lab Clin Med 92:402-407, 1978.

362. Martin RR, Eknoyan G, Saenz C, et al: Effects of renal failure on leukotaxis. J Med 10:267-278, 1979.

363. Anderson R, Glover A, Koornhof HJ, et al: In vitro stimulation of neutrophil motility by levamisole: Maintenance of cGMP levels in chemotactically stimulated levamisole-treated neutrophils. J Immunol 117:428-432, 1976.

364. Hogan NA, Hill HR: Enhancement of neutrophil chemotaxis and alteration of levels of cellular cyclic nucleotides by levamisole. J Infect Dis 138:437-444, 1978.

365. Greene WH, Ray C, Mauer SM, et al: The effect of hemodialysis on neutrophil chemotactic responsiveness. J Lab Clin Med 88:971-974, 1976.

366. Abrutyn E, Solomons NW, Clair LST, et al: Granulocyte function in patients with chronic renal failure: Surface adherence, phagocytosis, and bactericidal activity in vitro. J Infect Dis 135:1-8, 1977.

367. Burleson RL: Reversible inhibition of phagocytosis in anephric uremic patients. Surg Forum 24:75-77, 1973.

368. Davidson WD, Tanaka KR: Effect of uremia on phagocytosis-stimulated glucose oxidation (PSGO) in human granulocytes. Clin Res 19:416, 1971.

369. Hirabayashi Y, Kobayashi T, Nishikawa A, et al: Oxidative metabolism and phagocytosis of polymorphonuclear leukocytes in patients with chronic renal failure. Nephron 49:305-312, 1988.

370. Alexiewicz JM, Smogorzewski M, Fadda GZ, et al: Impaired phagocytosis in dialysis patients: Studies on mechanisms. Am J Nephrol 11:102-111, 1991.

371. Horl WH, Haag-Weber M, Georgopoulos A, et al: Physicochemical characterization of a polypeptide present in uremic serum that inhibits the biological activity of polymorphonuclear cells. Proc Natl Acad Sci U S A 87:6353-6357, 1990.

372. Ward RA, McLeish KR: Polymorphonuclear leukocyte oxidative burst is enhanced in patients with chronic renal insufficiency. J Am Soc Nephrol 5:1697-1702, 1995.

373. McLeish KR, Klein JB, Lederer ED, et al: Azotemia, TNF-α, and LPS prime the human neutrophil oxidative burst by distinct mechanisms. Kidney Int 50:407-416, 1996.

374. Rhee MS, McGoldrick MD, Meuwissen HJ: Serum factor from patients with chronic renal failure enhances polymorphonuclear leukocyte oxidative metabolism. Nephron 42:6-13, 1986.

375. Craddock PR, Fehr J, Dalmasso AP, et al: Hemodialysis leukopenia: Pulmonary vascular leukostasis resulting from complement activation by dialyzer cellophane membranes. J Clin Invest 59:879-888, 1977.

376. Stroncek DF, Keshaviah P, Craddock PR, et al: Effect of dialyzer reuse on complement activation and neutropenia in hemodialysis. J Lab Clin Med 104:304-311, 1984.

377. Cohen MS, Elliott DM, Chaplinski T, et al: A defect in oxidative metabolism in human polymorphonuclear leukocytes that remain in circulation early in hemodialysis. Blood 60:1283-1289, 1982.

378. Skubitz KM, Craddock PR: Reversal of hemodialysis granulocytopenia and pulmonary leukostasis: A clinical manifestation of selective down-regulation of granulocyte responses to C5adesarg. J Clin Invest 67:1383-1391, 1981.

379. Larson RS, Springer TA: Structure and function of leukocyte integrins. Immunol Rev 114:181-217, 1990.

380. Arnaout MA: Leukocyte adhesion molecules deficiency: Its structural basis, pathophysiology and implications for modulating the inflammatory response. Immunol Rev 114:145-180, 1990.

381. Miller LJ, Bainton DF, Borregard N, et al: Stimulated mobilization of monocyte Mac-1 and p150,95 adhesion proteins from an intracellular vesicular compartment to the cell surface. J Clin Invest 80:535-544, 1987.

382. Roccatello D, Mazzucco G, Coppo R, et al: Functional changes of monocytes due to dialysis membranes. Kidney Int 35:622-631, 1989.

383. Arnaout MA, Hakim RM, Todd RF III, et al: Increased expression of an adhesion-promoting surface glycoprotein in the granulocytopenia of hemodialysis. N Engl J Med 312:457-462, 1985.

384. Jacobs AA, Ward RA, Wellhausen SR, et al: Polymorphonuclear leukocyte function during hemodialysis: Relationship to complement activation. Nephron 52:119-124, 1982.

385. Lundahl J, Hed J, Jacobson SH: Dialysis granulocytopenia is preceded by an increased surface expression of the adhesion-promoting glycoprotein Mac-1. Nephron 61:163-169, 1992.

386. Thylén P, Lundahl J, Fernvik E, et al: Mobilization of an intracellular glycoprotein (Mac-1) on monocytes and granulocytes during hemodialysis. Am J Nephrol 12:393-400, 1992.

387. Ord DC, Ernst TJ, Zhou LJ, et al: Structure of the gene encoding of the human leukocyte adhesion molecule-1 (TQ1, Leu-8) of lymphocytes and neutrophils. J Biol Chem 265:7760-7767, 1990.

388. Vanholder R, Ringoir S, Dhondt A, et al: Phagocytosis in uremic and hemodialysis patients: A prospective and cross sectional study. Kidney Int 39:320-327, 1991.

389. Thylen P, Lundahl Y, Fernvile E: Mobilization of an intracellular glycoprotein (Mac-1) on monocytes and granulocytes during hemodialysis. Am J Nephrol 12:393-400, 1992.

390. Himmelfarb J, Lazarus JM, Hakim R: Reactive oxygen species production by monocytes and polymorphonuclear leukocytes during dialysis. Am J Kidney Dis 17:271-276, 1991.

391. Descamps-Latscha B, Goldfarb B, Nguyen AT, et al: Establishing the relationship between complement activation and stimulation of phagocyte oxidative metabolism in hemodialyzed patients: A randomized prospective study. Nephron 59:279-285, 1991.

392. Trznadel K, Luciak M, Pawlicki L, et al: Superoxide anion generation and lipid peroxidation processes during hemodialysis with reused cuprophane dialyzers. Free Radi Biol Med 8:429-432, 1990.

393. Wissow LS, Greenberg RS, Burns RO, et al: Altered leukocyte chemiluminescence during hemodialysis. J Clin Immunol 1:262-265, 1981.

394. Markert M, Heierli C, Kuwahara T, et al: Dialyzed polymorphonuclear neutrophil oxidative metabolism during dialysis: A comparative study with 5 new and reused membranes. Clin Nephrol 29:129-136, 1988.

395. Cristol JP, Canaud B, Rabesandratana H, et al: Enhancement of reactive oxygen species production and cell surface markers expression due to haemodialysis. Nephrol Dial Transplant 9:389-394, 1994.

396. Himmelfarb J, Ault KA, Holbrook D, et al: Intradialytic granulocyte reactive oxygen species production: A prospective, crossover trial. J Am Soc Nephrol 4:178-186, 1993.

397. Kaupke CJ, Zhang J, Cesario T, et al: Effect of hemodialysis on leukocyte adhesion receptor expression. Am J Kidney Dis 27:244-252, 1996.

398. Richard MJ, Arnaud J, Jurkovitz C, et al: Trace elements and lipid peroxidation abnormalities in patients with chronic renal failure. Nephron 57:10-15, 1991.

399. Dinarello CA, Lonnemann G, Bingel M, et al: Biological consequences of monocyte activation during hemodialysis. *In* Koch KM, Streicher E (eds): Contribution to Nephrology, Basel, S Karger, 1987, p 1.

400. Descamps-Latscha B, Herbelin A, Nguyen AT, et al: Hemodialysis-membrane-induced phagocyte oxidative metabolism activation and interleukin-1 production. Life Support Syst 4:349-353, 1986.

401. Lonnemann G, Bingel M, Koch KM, et al: Plasma interleukin-1 activity in humans undergoing hemodialysis with regenerated cellulosic membranes. Lymphokine Res 6:63-70, 1987.

402. Bingel M, Lonnemann G, Koch KM, et al: Plasma interleukin-1 activity during hemodialysis: The influence of dialysis membranes. Nephron 50:273-276, 1988.

403. Dinarello CA: Interleukin-1 and interleukin-1 receptor antagonist production during haemodialysis: Which cytokine is a surrogate marker for dialysis-related complications? Nephrol Dial Transplant 10(suppl 3):25-28, 1995.

404. Lamperi S, Carozzi S: Monocyte-macrophage–mediated suppression of erythropoiesis in renal anemia. Nephrol Dial Transplant 2:86-92, 1987.

405. Dinarello CA: Interleukin-1 and interleukin-1 antagonism. Blood 77:1627-1652, 1991.

406. Dinarello CA: Interleukin-1 and tumor necrosis factor and their naturally occurring antagonists during hemodialysis. Kidney Int 42:S68-S77, 1992.

407. Henderson LW, Koch KM, Dinarello CA, et al: Hemodialysis hypotension. The interleukin hypothesis. Blood Purif 1:3-8, 1983.

408. Shaldon S, Deschodt G, Branger B, et al: Haemodialysis hypotension: The interleukin hypothesis restated. Proc Eur Dial Transplant Assoc 22:229-243, 1985.

409. Beasley D, Brenner BM: Role of nitric oxide in hemodialysis hypotension. Kidney Int Suppl 42:S96-S100, 1992.

410. Rysz J, Luciak M, Kedziora J, et al: Nitric oxide release in the peripheral blood during hemodialysis. Kidney Int 51:294-300, 1997.

411. Ladefoged J, Langhoff E: Accessory cell functions in mononuclear cell cultures from uremic patients. Kidney Int 37:126-130, 1990.

412. Donati D, Degiannis D, Raskova J, et al: Uremic serum effects on peripheral blood mononuclear cell and purified T lymphocyte responses. Kidney Int 42:681-689, 1992.

413. Beaurain G, Naret C, Marcon L, et al: In vivo T-cell preactivation in chronic uremic hemodialyzed and non-hemodialyzed patients. Kidney Int 36:636-644, 1989.

414. Rubin LA, Kurman CC, Fritz ME, et al: Soluble interleukin-2 receptors are released from activated human lymphoid cells in vitro. J Immunol 135:3172-3177, 1985.

415. Uchiyama T, Broder S, Waldman TA: A monoclonal antibody (anti-TAC) reactive with activated and functionally mature T cells. I. Production of anti-Tac monoclonal antibody and distribution of Tac (+) cells. J Immunol 126:1393-1397, 1981.

416. Dukovich M, Wano Y, Thyu L, et al: A second human IL-2 binding protein that may be a component of high affinity IL-2 receptors. Nature 327:518-522, 1987.

417. Reed JC, Robb RJ, Greene WC, et al: Effect of wheat germ agglutinin on the interleukin pathway of human T lymphocyte activation. J Immunol 134:314-323, 1985.

418. Zaoui P, Green W, Hakim RM: Hemodialysis with cuprophane membrane modulates interleukin-2 receptor expression. Kidney Int 39:1020-1026, 1991.

419. Gupta S: Interleukin-2 receptor and transferrin receptor expression on T cells and production of inteleukin-2 in patients with acquired immune deficiency syndrome (AIDS) and AIDS-related complex. Clin Immunol Immunopathol 38:93-100, 1986.

420. Zaoui P, Hakim RM: The effects of the dialysis membrane on cytokine release. J Am Soc Nephrol 4:1711-1718, 1994.

421. Degiannis D, Czarnecki M, Donati D, et al: Normal T lymphocyte function in patients with end-stage renal disease hemodialyzed with "high-flux" polysulfone membranes. Am J Nephrol 10:276-282, 1990.

422. Gerez L, Madar L, Shkolnik T, et al: Regulation of interleukin-2 and interferon-γ gene expression in renal failure. Kidney Int 40:266-272, 1991.

CHAPTER 50

Cardiovascular Aspects of Chronic Kidney Disease

Lawrence P. McMahon and Patrick S. Parfrey

BACKGROUND

Cardiovascular Disease

Cardiovascular disease is recognized as the predominant cause of death in patients with chronic kidney disease (CKD). The cardiac death rate in dialysis patients is reported to be between 104 and 157 per 1000 patient-years, with heart disease accounting for 40% to 45% of all deaths among both dialysis and transplantation patients worldwide.[1-4] Compared with that in the general population, the annual cardiovascular death rate in dialysis patients is higher for all age groups, and particularly for the young, whose mortality rate is up to 100 times higher than in the general population (Fig. 50-1).[5] Indices of morbidity are also high. The probability of having a myocardial infarction or angina requiring hospitalization in hemodialysis patents is 10% per year,[6] and such patients have been shown to have 1- and 5-year mortality rates of 60% and 90%, respectively. There is a similar probability of developing pulmonary edema requiring hospitalization or additional ultrafiltration. Evidence of disease, however, manifests well before the onset of dialysis,[7, 8] with approximately 35% of patients demonstrating clinical symptoms of heart failure by the time they require dialysis (Table 50-1).[7-10]

Most clinical consequences of cardiac disease result from cardiomyopathy or ischemic heart disease. Cardiomyopathy may manifest as an enlarged, dilated left ventricle (LV) with systolic dysfunction or as a hypertrophic ventricle with diastolic dysfunction, with or without myocardial ischemia (Fig. 50-2). Although symptoms of ischemic heart disease are most often attributable to the presence of critical coronary artery disease (CAD, defined as the presence of critical narrowing of the large coronary vessels due to atherosclerotic plaques), they may also result from nonatherosclerotic disease caused by small vessel disease and LV hypertrophy. Myocardial infarction and angina can result from decreased perfusion of the myocardium from either cause. It has also become evident that the structure of large arteries can be altered, not only by atherogenesis, but also by arteriosclerosis.[11]

Intramural vascular remodeling occurs as a consequence of sustained hemodynamic overload, with an increase in vessel stiffness and diameter. Persistent effects result in conduit vessel dilatation and hypertrophy, which have been shown to contribute adversely to LV structure and function and are strongly associated with an increased risk of death.[12-14]

The relative contribution of each of these disorders to cardiac dysfunction in CKD varies from patient to patient. However, in each patient there is a persistent and complex interplay of destructive vascular events and myocyte dysfunction that, if unrecognized, ultimately results in cardiac failure and death (see Fig. 50-2). Ischemic symptoms result from CAD or nonatherosclerotic ischemic disease. Arteriosclerosis contributes directly to ischemic symptoms, LV hypertrophy, and systolic dysfunction by increasing cardiac workload. CAD predisposes to diastolic dysfunction and to systolic failure. LV hypertrophy is almost always present in dilated cardiomyopathy, but it also causes diastolic dysfunction with or without normal systolic function.

Cardiac disease can also result from the development of valvular heart disease. Most valvular lesions observed in patients with CKD are acquired and develop from dystrophic calcifications of the valvular annulus and leaflets, particularly the aortic and mitral valves.[11] Such calcification is now known to be present far more frequently than previously recognized, with a prevalence of up to 55% for the aortic valves and 39% for the mitral valves.[15, 16] Once considered benign, aortic valve sclerosis is itself associated with an increased cardiovascular mortality in the general community.[17] In CKD, it is part of the spectrum of valvular disease and may sometimes evolve rapidly to hemodynamically significant stenosis.

Cardiovascular Disease and Stage of Chronic Kidney Disease

It is important to recognize that the time of presentation of cardiovascular disease depends not only on prevailing

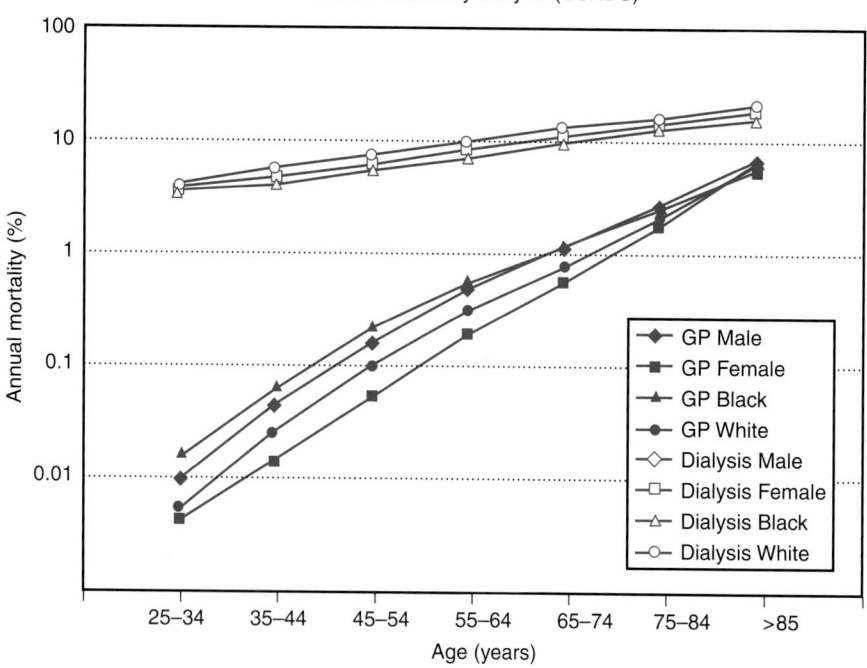

Cardiovascular Mortality in the General Population (NCHS) and in ESRD Treated by Dialysis (USRDS)

FIGURE 50-1. Annual cardiovascular disease mortality for patients undergoing dialysis, by age, gender, and race, compared with the general population (GP). ESRD, end-stage renal disease. (From Foley RN, Parfrey PS, Sarnak M: The clinical epidemiology of cardiovascular disease in chronic renal disease. Am J Kidney Dis 32[suppl]:S112-S115, 1998, with permission.)

cardiovascular abnormalities but also on the duration, severity, and type of renal disease. LV hypertrophy is already evident in 40% of patients with moderate renal insufficiency[8] and in 75% of those commencing dialysis.[7] Both forms of LV hypertrophy (concentric and eccentric) are associated with an increased mortality risk in dialysis patients.[18] Associated risk factors, including diabetes,

hypertension, tobacco use, and anemia, predispose to the much more rapid development of symptomatic cardiomyopathy.[19] Such patients display a higher incidence of cardiovascular abnormalities at an earlier stage of CKD and at a younger age, often becoming symptomatic or exhibiting significant morbidity well before reaching end-stage kidney function.

TABLE 50-1

Approximate Prevalence (%) of Cardiovascular Disease in the General Population and in Patients with Chronic Kidney Disease

POPULATION	CORONARY ARTERY DISEASE (SYMPTOMATIC)	LEFT VENTRICULAR HYPERTROPHY (ECHOCARDIOGRAM)	CARDIAC FAILURE (SYMPTOMATIC)
General population	5–12*	20†	5‡
Predialysis	NA	25–50‡‡	NA
Hemodialysis	42‖	75¶	40‖
Peritoneal dialysis	40‖	75¶	40‖
Renal transplantation	15**	50††	10§

NA, not available.

*Lower value refers to age 45–64 years; higher value, age >65 years. Data from the National Heart, Lung, and Blood Institute (NHLBI) Morbidity and Mortality Chartbook 1996.

†Data from Levy et al., N Engl J Med, 1990.

‡Age 60 years. Data from NHLBI Morbidity and Mortality Chartbook 1996.

§Data from Dialysis Morbidity and Mortality (Wave 2). USRDS Annual Data Report, 1997.

‖Data from Foley et al., Kidney Int, 1995.

¶Data from Kasiske, Am J Med, 1988.

**Data from Parfrey et al., Transplantation, 1995.

††Data from Rigatto et al., J Am Soc Nephrol, 2002.

‡‡Prevalence inversely proportional to reval function. Data from Levin et al., Am J Kidney Dis, 1996.

Adapted and reprinted with permission from Foley RN, Parfrey PS, Sarnak M: The clinical epidemiology of cardiovascular disease in chronic renal disease. Am J Kidney Dis 32(suppl):S112-S115, 1998.

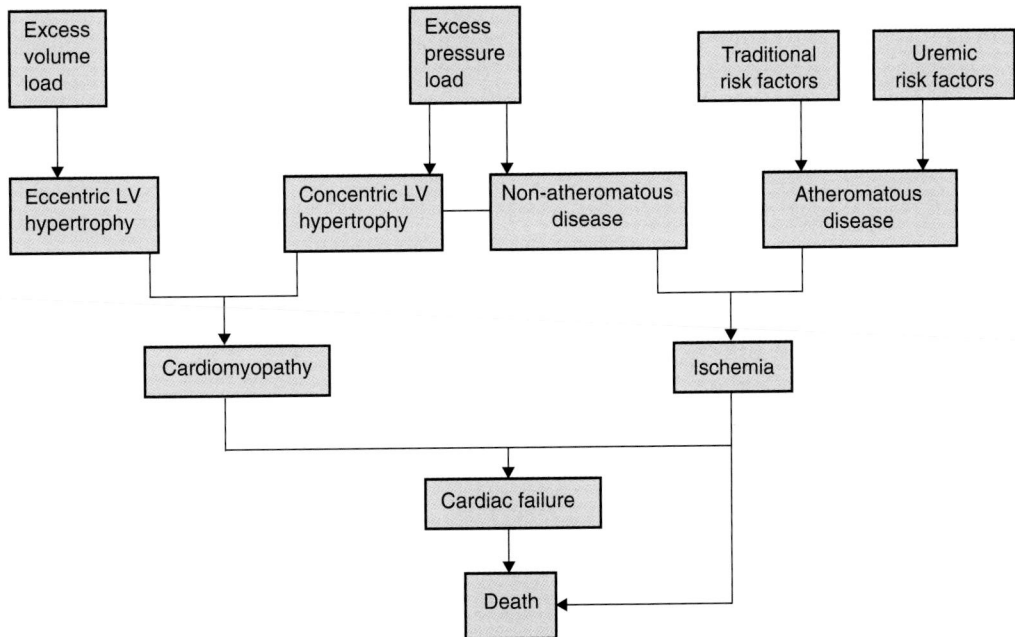

FIGURE 50-2. Cause of cardiac death in patients with chronic kidney disease. LV, left ventricular.

By the time of starting dialysis, only 15% of patients have a normal echocardiogram, and 15% already display systolic dysfunction (see Table 50-1).[7] The characteristic changes in LV geometry subsequently represent a progressive increase over time in both LV volume and LV mass, particularly during the first years,[18] and possibly more so in patients receiving peritoneal dialysis.[20, 21] As a result, the geometry of the heart changes from concentric LV hypertrophy with normal LV volumes to eccentric LV hypertrophy with dilatation, the end stage of this tendency being severe LV dilatation with systolic dysfunction (see Fig. 50-3B). LV growth and a decrease in myocardial contractility each contribute to the development of elevated LV pressures for a given volume, predisposing to symptomatic heart failure.[22]

Patients from the dialysis population historically have been selected as suitable candidates for renal transplantation by being relatively free from significant symptomatic cardiac disease. Although mortality rates for those undergoing transplantation are lower than for dialysis patients, they are still substantially higher than in the community, and cardiovascular disease remains the predominant cause of death.[3] There is evidence that systolic dysfunction, LV dilatation, and concentric hypertrophy improve after renal transplantation[23] and that further regression continues after the first year. Failure to regress is associated with markers of sustained hypertension.[24] Improvement in extracellular volume control, anemia, and calcium and phosphate abnormalities, as well as normalization of the uremic environment undoubtedly could account for the enhanced longevity after transplantation. However, the incidence of death—2.9% overall and approximately 1% for patients 35 to 44 years of age—remains too high.[4] With this in mind, it should be remembered that these patients remain subject to a wide variety of deleterious influences after transplantation, particularly diabetes, hypertension, and dyslipidemia. In addition, the effects of prior exposure (often prolonged) to the specific cardiovascular risk factors of CKD are not dissolved simply by restoration of normal renal function. Inexorable deterioration in renal function with the progression of time in most patients further complicates this picture.

The recently established staging of CKD by the Kidney Disease Outcome Quality Initiative (KDOQI) working party[25] is a clear and simple guide to assessing renal dysfunction. Although the staging of dialysis and transplantation patients is clear, many studies in the historical literature did not address the level of renal dysfunction in predialysis patients with precision. Hence, although the influence of cardiovascular disease in patients with CKD is manifested early and increases as renal function declines, the evidence for the stage at which this occurs is not well defined. For this reason, clinical studies (and patients) have been grouped in this chapter according to the more simplistic categories of predialysis, dialysis, and transplantation.

PATHOLOGY AND PATHOPHYSIOLOGY

Cardiac Disease

Left Ventricular Hypertrophy

PATHOPHYSIOLOGY

LV hypertrophy is an adaptive process that occurs in response to a long-term increase in myocardial work caused by LV pressure or volume overload; it results from the interactions among mechanical stimuli, locally generated growth factors, and vasoactive substances.

The work performed by the heart in each cardiac cycle (stroke work) is the product of LV pressure and stroke volume and is accordingly related to each. The heart rate multiplied by stroke work is the total work per minute performed by the heart. As stroke work increases, myocardial energy expenditure and oxygen consumption increase proportionately. LV tensile wall stress (σ), according to the law of Laplace, relates directly to the intraventricular pressure (P) generated and to the internal radius (r) of the ventricular cavity. It is inversely proportional to the ventricular wall thickness (θ), so that

$$\sigma = Pr/2\theta$$

Therefore, the wall tension at any given pressure increases with the radius, and vice versa. Conversely, as pressure or cavity volume (or both) is increased, there is an increase in wall thickness which reduces the systolic tension (and hence oxygen consumption) that must be developed by each myocyte. It is this wall remodeling that results in LV hypertrophy.

Biomechanical stress, such as that exerted by pressure or volume overload, has been found to be a powerful inducer of LV growth through the expression of embryonic and proto-oncogenes that encode growth factors and growth factor receptors.[26-29] It is intriguing that a common biochemical pathway appears to be responsible for the development of both compensatory hypertrophy and apoptosis. Stress-induced activation of gp130-dependent ligands, such as cardiotrophin 1, bind to their receptor, gp130-LIF (leukemic inhibitory factor), promoting downstream pathways inducing sarcomere formation and blocking apoptosis.[30] In the presence of gp130, the balance is shifted toward myocyte hypertrophy; in its absence, myocyte response is shifted to apoptosis, heralding the onset of heart failure.

The initial effects of LV hypertrophy are beneficial. As indicated previously, the energy-sparing effects of a stable parietal tensile stress permit the generation of higher intraventricular pressures without a large increase in wall stress. Such changes can be observed physiologically. For instance, cardiac hypertrophy is a normal response during late pregnancy, after prolonged training in athletes, and with normal growth from infancy to adulthood. In each of these cases, an appropriate relationship is maintained between the radius and wall thickness and the systolic pressure generated, so that the intrinsic performance of the myocardium is not altered. Chronic pressure or volume overload, or both, is also initially beneficial. Modifications in the heart structure, as described earlier, result in an increased work capacity while the parietal tensile stress is kept stable, thus sparing energy.[31]

Eventually, however, LV hypertrophy becomes maladaptive, with a sustained imbalance between energy expenditure and production, resulting in a chronic energy deficit and myocyte death.[29, 32] The pathogenesis of a reduced energy deficit is complex and appears to be related to a number of factors, including diminished myocardial capillary density,[33, 34] decreased coronary reserve with reduced subendocardial perfusion,[35, 36] and increased stiffness of the aorta and major conduit arteries.[37] Within the myocardium, overstretching of papillary muscles is coupled with oxidant stress, apoptosis, architectural rearrangement of myocytes, and impairment in force development of the myocardium.[38] There is also evidence that abnormal expression of proto-oncogenes promotes the development of, particularly, fibroblasts, with an increase in extracellular collagen matrix and hence the development of myocardial fibrosis.[29, 39]

The consequences of these alterations are electrophysiologic abnormalities and maintenance of systolic efficiency at the expense of impaired diastolic filling. Arrhythmias are caused partly by conduction aberrations secondary to fibrosis and partly by prolongation of the action potential due to a slower reuptake of calcium by the sarcoplasmic reticulum. The latter, together with fibrotic change and increased LV wall stiffness, contributes substantially to abnormal diastolic function. Eventually, in conditions of chronic and sustained overload, the deleterious effects of hypertrophy, increased LV chamber pressure, and fibrosis dominate, leading to the development of cardiomyopathy and LV failure.[29]

CLINICOPATHOLOGIC FEATURES

At autopsy, the hearts of dialysis patients are frequently enlarged, with grossly thickened walls and often a markedly dilated LV cavity. Light microscopic examination of the myocardium reveals hypertrophy of the myocytes and hyperplasia of the nonmyocytic components.[40] The coronary arteries are also enlarged and thickened, with evidence of atheromatous plaques and intramural calcification. These features represent the end stage of injurious and persistent forces in effect throughout the period of CKD.

The myocardial changes relate primarily to a combination of prolonged excessive pressure and volume loads and an attempt by the contracting myocytes to respond and adapt to the prevailing conditions, resulting in LV hypertrophy (Fig. 50-3A). Because myocytes are unable to replicate, they hypertrophy by producing more sarcomeres that can be deposited within the myocyte, either in series or in parallel. The resulting pathologic and clinical correlates are concentric and eccentric (and asymmetric) hypertrophy.[30]

The principal factors comprising pressure and volume overload in patients with CKD are known collectively as hemodynamic risk factors. Pressure overload results from sustained increases in LV afterload and includes predominantly hypertension, arteriosclerosis, and aortic stenosis. Volume overload embraces increased extracellular volume, anemia, and arteriovenous fistulas. These factors are rarely discrete, however, and one often contributes to the effects of another. An increase in extracellular volume, for instance, not only results in an increased volume load on the LV but also exacerbates underlying hypertension and contributes to reduced arterial compliance, each with subsequent effects on LV morphology (see Fig. 50-3B).

Concentric hypertrophy is considered an adaptive mechanism in response to chronic LV pressure overload. The parallel addition of new sarcomeres produces an increase in myocyte thickness. The increased LV mass is associated with increased thickness of both the interventricular septum and the LV free (or "posterior") wall. The overall volume of the ventricle remains normal, so that, relative to the LV end-diastolic diameter, wall thickness is increased. Eccentric hypertrophy is a mechanism of adaptation to states of chronic volume overload in which LV end-diastolic pressure tends to normalize at the expense of increased end-diastolic volume. LV volume overload induces the addition of new sarcomeres mainly in series, and myocytes grow longer. The increased LV mass is associated with an increased LV volume and some increase in LV posterior wall thickness;

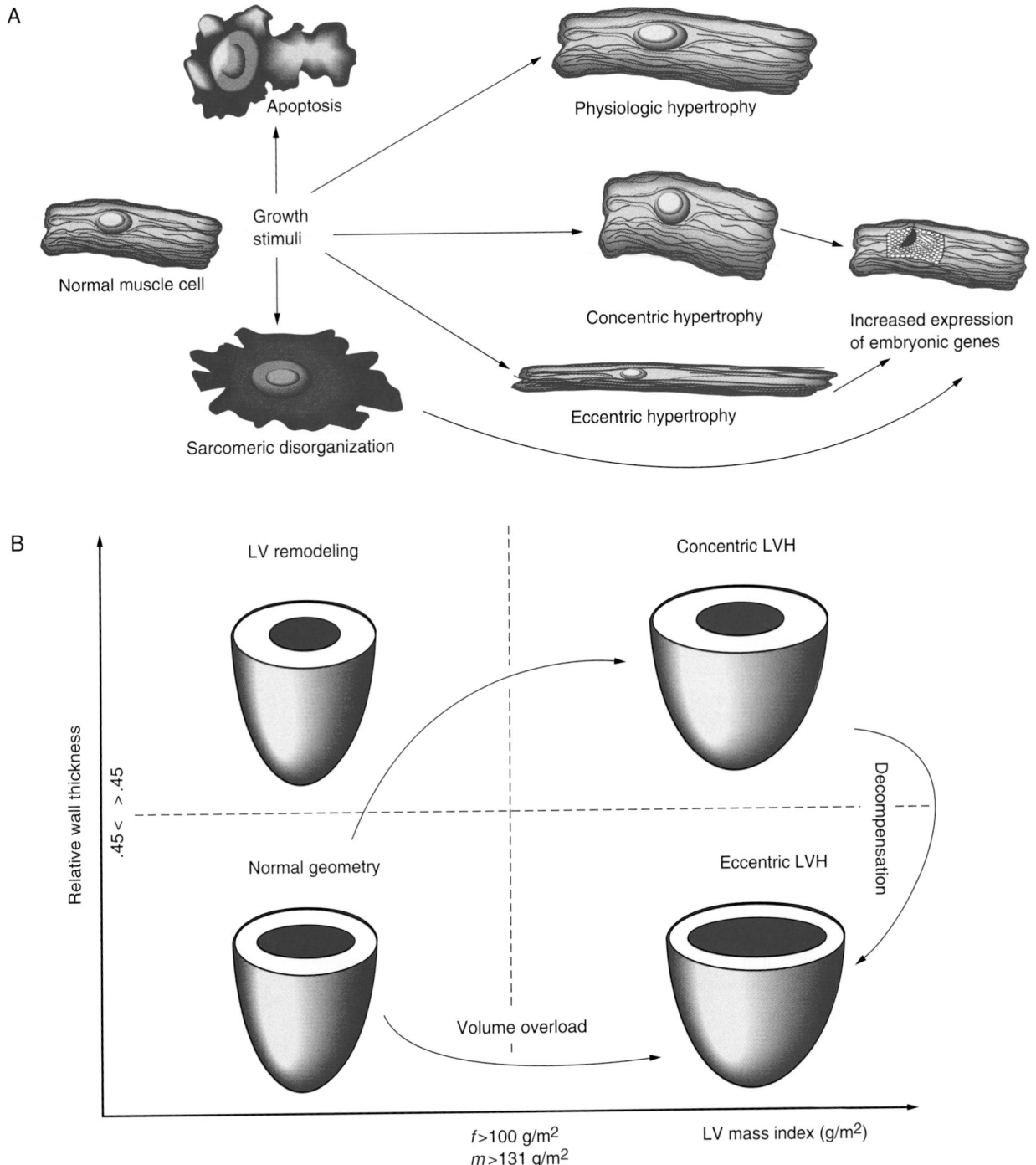

FIGURE 50-3. **A,** Morphology of ventricular myocytes in cardiac hypertrophy and failure. Concentric left ventricular hypertrophy (LVH) occurs in response to LV pressure overload, and eccentric LV hypertrophy in response to LV volume overload. Sarcomeric disorganization and apoptosis are additional characteristics of hypertrophic cardiomyopathies. (From Hunter JJ, Chien KR: Signaling pathways for cardiac hypertrophy and failure. N Engl J Med 341:1276, 1999, with permission.) **B,** Patterns of LV growth. An increase in LV mass index beyond gender-specific limits (i.e., *f*, female; *m*, male) is, by definition, LV hypertrophy *(right panels).* An increase in relative LV wall thickness (diastolic LV posterior wall and septal thickness divided by LV end-diastolic diameter) beyond a ratio of 0.45 is called concentric remodeling or hypertrophy *(upper panels).* An increase in LV mass despite normal relative wall thickness is called eccentric LV hypertrophy. The arrows indicate the most frequent pathophysiologic mechanisms. (From Schunkert H, Hense HW: A heart price to pay for anaemia. Nephrol Dial Transplant 16:445-448, 2001, with permission.)

however, the ratio of LV end-diastolic diameter to posterior wall thickness is lower than in concentric hypertrophy. Asymmetric hypertrophy is a variant of concentric hypertrophy whereby the septal wall is disproportionately thickened in relation to the posterior LV wall. This can result from an increased afterload, which exposes the septum to greater stress than the free wall,[41] or from stimulation of the sympathetic nervous system.[42]

In addition to the dominant influence of pressure and volume overload, humoral factors may also contribute to alterations in LV morphology and hence to LV hypertrophy. A number of these factors have now been defined, including cardiac natriuretic peptides, troponin, homocysteine, asymmetric dimethyl arginine, and endothelin, but whether they are markers of hypertrophy or significant factors in the pathogenic process remains to be demonstrated.[43-46] Raised sympathetic activity and catecholamine levels may also contribute either directly or indirectly to the pathologic process. A high sympathetic activity, for instance, is associated with sleep apnea and nocturnal hypoxia, which are in turn associated with cardiovascular complications in dialysis patients.[47-49]

Therefore, at all stages of disease, patients with CKD are exposed to variable but sustained conditions of volume and pressure overload which, in the setting of humoral and sympathetic imbalance, result in a combination of both concentric and eccentric hypertrophy, although the primary pattern of hypertrophy usually develops in accordance with the predominant initial mechanical stress.[7, 8, 19, 50] Initially, the hypertrophy is a balanced response to reduce the individual work of each muscle fiber, regulate cardiac efficiency, and improve the LV working capacity. However, with time, the

degree of hypertrophy relative to LV volume may prove inadequate,[51] predisposing to the development of sustained energy deficit and cell death. Diminished perfusion, malnutrition, hyperparathyroidism, perhaps inadequate dialysis, and other factors exacerbate the death of myocytes in chronic uremia. Such cell death in the presence of LV hypertrophy and continuing pressure and volume overload may ultimately be catastrophic, leading to further LV dilatation and eventually to systolic dysfunction. In the final stages of cardiomyopathy, hypoperfusion results when the maximally hypertrophied myocardium expends most of its energy of contraction in developing pre-ejection wall tension and is unable to transfer additional force into maintaining cardiac output during systole (Fig. 50-4).

Interstitial Fibrosis

The interstitium constitutes 25% of the normal myocardium, and it retains this proportion in even the largest hearts, through a proliferation of the cellular, vascular, and connective tissue elements normally present.[40] The causes of myocardial fibrosis relate to proliferation of fibroblasts within the interstitium, and in CKD there are numerous pathways

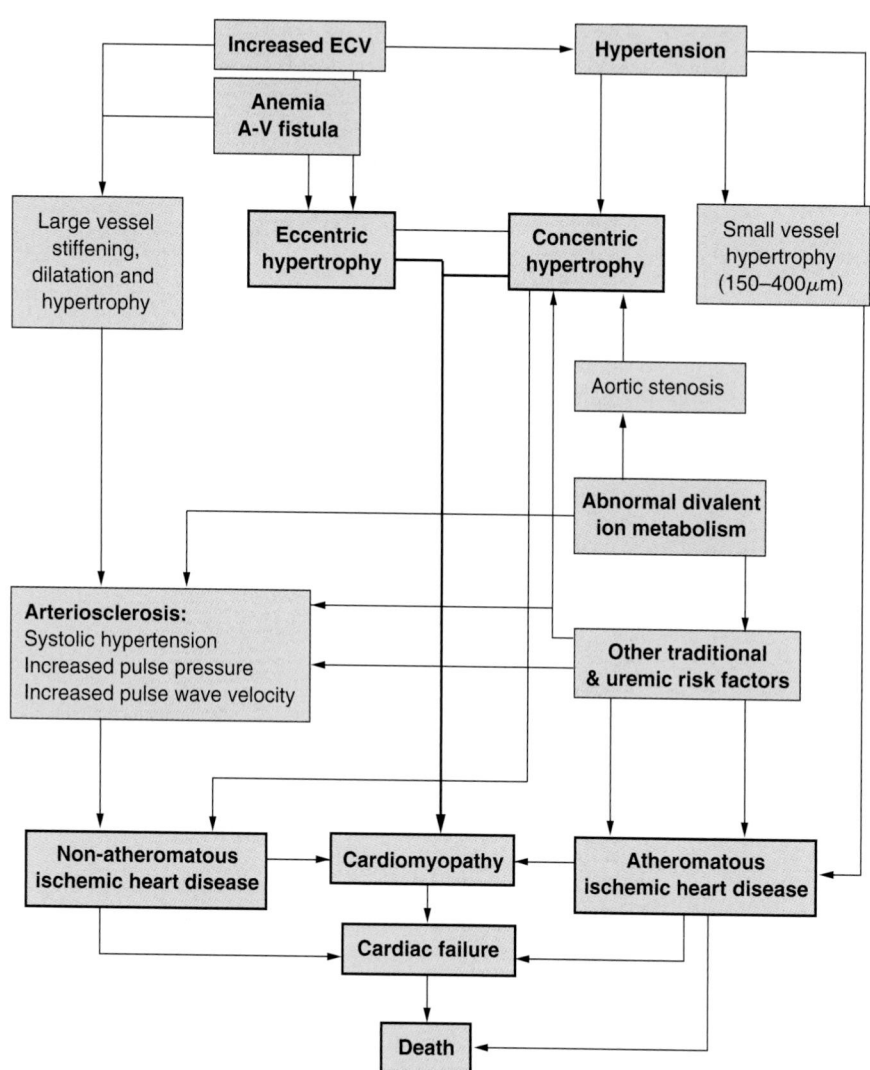

FIGURE 50-4. Cause of cardiac failure in chronic kidney disease and relationships between hemodynamic and other risk factors.

permitting a disproportionate degree of fibrosis particularly within the LV, often in a perivascular distribution.

Interstitial myocardial fibrosis is a prominent finding in CKD[52] and has been demonstrated at autopsy in uremic patients. From these and animal studies, it appears that uremia is an important factor related to intermyocardiocytic fibrosis, independent of hypertension, diabetes mellitus, anemia, heart weight, and dialysis procedure.[53] Clinical studies have shown also that the extent of myocardial fibrosis in dialysis patients is greater than in patients with diabetes mellitus or essential hypertension with similar LV mass.[53, 54] This is seen particularly in LV hypertrophy, more so in pressure than in volume overload, and is exacerbated by many factors, including male gender, senescence, ischemia, and effects of hormones such as catecholamines, angiotensin II, aldosterone, and transforming growth factors.[54, 55] Increasing evidence indicates also that abnormal proto-oncogene activation can result in a rapid increase in collagen synthesis and deposition of extracellular matrix.[53] An additional humoral factor contributing to myocardial fibrosis[53] appears to be hyperparathyroidism. Recent studies have demonstrated that parathyroid hormone (PTH) is a permissive factor in the genesis of cardiac interstitial fibrosis.[53] The extensive intramyocardial fibrosis in dialysis patients with elevated PTH could account for the attenuation of the hypertrophic response to pressure overload and the development of high-stress cardiomyopathy and cardiac failure.

Regardless of the inducing factors, because the cardiac myocytes remain normal in number, the proliferation of fibroblasts and increase in collagen matrix result in a marked imbalance in the myocyte-to-fibroblast ratio. An abnormal alignment of myocytes subsequently occurs, which may lead to abnormal interdigitation in systole and limitation of slippage during diastole.[56] The predominant clinical effects appear to relate to diastolic dysfunction and an increase in arrhythmias. In nonuremic patients with LV hypertrophy, a close correlation has been reported between impaired LV compliance measured invasively and interstitial fibrosis observed on endomyocardial biopsy.[57] Impaired diastolic

function appears to relate to the induction by fibrosis of a slower re-uptake of calcium by the sarcoplasmic reticulum, which results in a delayed relaxation phase of the cardiac cycle. Concurrent prolongation of the action potential causes a delay in depolarization, which in turn contributes to reentry tachycardias and severe arrhythmias, an effect that is augmented by fibrosis-induced conduction aberrations and by cardiac hypertrophy per se.[58-61]

Cardiac Failure

Table 50-2 indicates the prevalence of various comorbid conditions among North American dialysis patients, according to three studies with different approaches.

FUNCTIONAL ABNORMALITIES

Assessment of LV functional abnormalities in patients with CKD is often difficult. Absence of symptoms does not imply intact functional reserve regardless of the stage of disease. Dialysis patients in particular are prone to variations in fluid loading and humoral homeostasis during dialysis, and both may augment and reduce the capacity to detect underlying abnormalities in systolic and diastolic function.[62-66] Additional difficulties in differentiating abnormalities in LV function relate to assessing the common and often concurrent phenomena of preexisting heart disease and effects of prolonged hemodynamic overload. Primary myocardial dysfunction and pure volume overload can each manifest with acute pulmonary edema. Similar difficulties can be encountered when trying to distinguish clinically between systolic and diastolic dysfunction. In reality, as has been outlined for other conditions, multiple pathologic conditions are frequently present simultaneously, although usually one particular condition predominates in a clinical context.

DIASTOLIC DYSFUNCTION. Hemodialysis patients with LV hypertrophy often have some impairment in LV diastolic function[67] (Fig. 50-5). The degree of disturbance is probably more than that observed in patients with hypertensive

TABLE 50-2

Number of Patients with Comorbid Cardiac Conditions among Incident Dialysis Patients in the United States and Canada

COMORBID CONDITION	USA, 1996–1997 (N=2443)*	CANADA, 1994–1995 (N=822)†	CANADA, 1983–1991 (N=432)‡
Cardiac failure	36	35	31
Myocardial infarction	16	18	12
Angina	N/A	21	19
Peripheral vascular disease	20	17	8
Insulin-dependent diabetes	33	21	15
LV hypertrophy	N/A	N/A	74
LV dilatation	N/A	N/A	36
LV systolic dysfunction	N/A	N/A	15

LV, left ventricle; N/A, not available.

*USRDS special study, DMMS wave 2, retrospective chart extraction. U. S. Renal Data System: Patient characteristics at the start of ESRD: Data from the HCFA Medical Evidence Form. Am J Kidney Dis 34(suppl 1):S63-S73, 1999, with permission.

†11 centers, prospective evaluation by physician on starting dialysis. Data from Barrett BJ, Parfrey PS, Morgan J, et al: Prediction of early death in end-stage renal disease patients starting dialysis. Am J Kidney Dis 29:214-222, 1997.

‡Three centers, retrospective evaluation of patients, who survived 6 months on dialysis and entered prospective echocardiographic study. Data from Foley RN, Parfrey PS, Harnett JD, et al: Clinical and echocardiographic disease in patients starting end-stage renal disease therapy. Kidney Int 47:186-192, 1995.

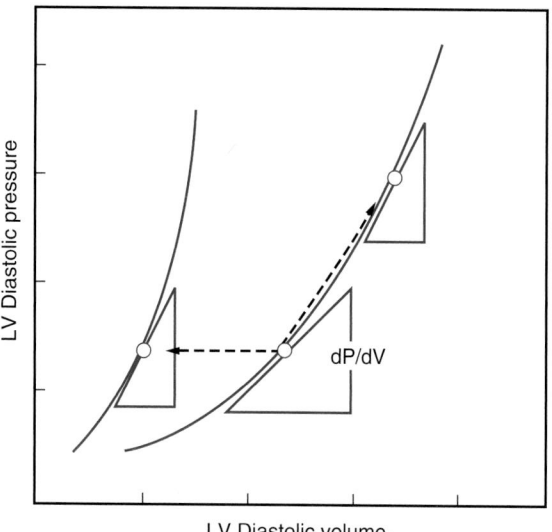

FIGURE 50-5. Compliance characteristics of left ventricular (LV) hypertrophy during diastolic filling. Normal myocardial compliance is defined by the curve on the right, which shows the relationship between LV end-diastolic volume and LV end-diastolic pressure. With (uremic) LV hypertrophy, myocardial compliance is decreased, and the pressure-volume relationship is shifted to the left, operating within a narrow range while maintaining similar resting end-diastolic pressures. Consequently, an increase in plasma volume leads to cardiac failure, and a decrease leads to hypotension. (From Palmer BF, Henrich WL: The effect of dialysis on left ventricular contractility. In: Parfrey PS, Harnet JD [eds]: Cardiac Dysfunction in Chronic Uremia. Boston, Kluwer Academic, 1992, with permission.)

heart disease but milder than in those with hypertrophic cardiomyopathy.[52, 54, 68] The abnormal ventricular filling in uremia results from increased LV stiffness caused by intramyocardial fibrosis and associated delayed relaxation. By virtue of an increase in LV stiffness, small changes in volume result in large changes in LV pressure, predisposing to symptomatic pulmonary edema.[9, 69] The reverse is also true: volume depletion results in a large fall in LV pressure with symptomatic hypotension and hemodynamic instability.[70] This is often the presenting feature of diastolic dysfunction.

SYSTOLIC DYSFUNCTION. Resting systolic function is usually normal or even increased in patients with advanced renal disease in the absence of antecedent cardiac disease.[71-73] However, decreased systolic function is frequently observed in patients in whom cardiac disease was present before the onset of dialysis therapy and in patients who have experienced prolonged and marked hemodynamic overload. Approximately 15% of patients have systolic dysfunction by the time they start dialysis.[7] Diminished myocardial contractility may also be a result of overload cardiomyopathy, in which the myocardium relies on Starling forces to maintain a normal output.[53] This manifestation of cardiomyopathy has a substantially worse prognosis than that for either concentric LV hypertrophy or LV dilatation with normal systolic function.[23] In dialysis patients, systolic dysfunction is strongly associated with the presence of ischemic heart disease or sustained biomechanical stress or both. However, it can also be a reversible manifestation of severe uremia, abating when the uremic environment is removed. Uremic serum has been found to reduce the force of contraction of cultured myocytes in a concentration-dependent manner.[74] Renal transplantation has also been shown to normalize systolic function in dialysis

patients with systolic dysfunction and subsequently to reduce but not normalize LV mass index,[75-77] although such improvement has not yet been shown to confer a survival benefit.[78]

SYMPTOMATIC CARDIAC FAILURE

LV failure is a clinical condition that can be defined as the inability of the heart to maintain sufficient output to meet metabolic demands at rest, or the ability to maintain such demands only at the expense of a sufficiently raised venous pressure to result in pulmonary edema. If left untreated, myocardial hypertrophy can be viewed as an early milestone in the clinical course of cardiac failure.[30] In a Canadian cohort study, 275 patients had serial echocardiograms on starting dialysis and after 1 year of dialysis therapy.[22] An increase in LV mass index was an independent risk factor for the development of subsequent heart failure (hazard ratio, 1.3 per each 20 g/m^2 increase), as was a reduction in fractional shortening (hazard ratio, 1.43 per 5% decrease). Both LV hypertrophy and LV dilatation will ultimately progress to dilated cardiomyopathy if pressure and volume overload are not appropriately managed. Conversely, there is some evidence of a reduction in LV hypertrophy and possibly in mortality if due attention is paid to these risk factors.[79, 80] Such effects may have important clinical consequences: diabetics, for instance, have been found to have a reduced hospitalization rate for congestive cardiac failure after successful renal transplantation.[81]

In cardiac failure, ventricular output is maintained at the expense of numerous mechanisms. These include an increase in both end-diastolic fiber length and end-diastolic volume (i.e., through the Frank-Starling mechanism), increased sympathetic activity, enhanced secretion of regulatory hormones (e.g., angiotensin II, arginine vasopressin, vasoactive endothelial hormones, brain and atrial natriuretic peptide), and the presence of ouabain-like substances which, through impairment of the sodium-potassium pump (Na$^+$,K$^+$-ATPase), result in enhanced contractility, albeit at the expense of impaired relaxation.[82, 83] In a circuit already coping with an elevated LV volume and pressure this can easily result, as previously seen, in a raised pulmonary capillary pressure. The clinical presentation then is one of symptomatic heart failure, with dyspnea and pulmonary venous congestion, ultimately resulting in acute pulmonary edema. This end-stage clinical manifestation of cardiac disease may result from systolic failure, usually caused by dilated cardiomyopathy or ischemia or both, or from diastolic dysfunction in association with LV hypertrophy. The latter is almost as frequent a cause of recurrent or persistent heart failure in dialysis patients as is dilated cardiomyopathy.[84]

Ischemic Heart Disease

ATHEROMATOUS ISCHEMIC HEART DISEASE

In humans, basal myocardial perfusion tends to remain constant regardless of the severity of coronary artery stenosis. During conditions requiring increased flow, a progressive relative decrease in perfusion occurs after the degree of stenosis is 40% or greater, and perfusion cannot increase above basal conditions when the stenosis is 80% or greater.[85] Therefore, stenosis progressively exhausts the coronary vasodilator reserve (defined as the ratio of maximal to basal coronary perfusion). Because the effective resistance, Ω, of the site of stenosis is proportional to the fourth power of the radius, r, ($\Omega \propto r^4$), small changes that are undetectable by arteriographic assessment can cause larger changes in resistance at the region of stenosis, particularly at more severe lesions.[86]

It appears that the uremic milieu or the prevailing comorbid condition (or both) provide the hemodynamic and metabolic perturbations that favor vascular wall damage. This results in a diffusion of lipids and monocytes into the arterial wall (with development of foam cell, fibroblast, and smooth muscle cell proliferation), expansion of the atheromatous plaque, and clot formation.

CAD, characterized by critical stenoses of the major coronary arteries, is highly prevalent in the CKD population, because of both the demographic characteristics of the patient population and their underlying disease states (e.g., hypertension, diabetes mellitus). Estimates of prevalence by the time patients reach the need for dialysis vary from 15%[7, 9] to 73%.[87] The wide range in prevalence most likely relates to whether a patient presents symptomatically or the condition is detected on screening, often for transplantation. It is estimated that more than 50% of patients, particularly diabetics, are asymptomatic.[87-89]

Both mechanical and humoral factors predispose to atheroma formation (Fig. 50-6). Arterial hypertension causes increased tensile stress, and shear stress alterations occur at internal vessel orifices and bifurcations. Both types of stress result in endothelial cell activation.[90] Changes in tensile and shear stress activate stretch- and flow-sensitive cationic channels, producing secretions of vasoactive and growth-regulating factors. Subsequent effects include alterations in cytokine migration, cellular apoptosis, and extracellular matrix synthesis. There is evidence of chronic in vivo endothelial activation and injury in uremia.[91, 92] Furthermore, compared with normal subjects, nondiabetic patients with chronic renal insufficiency have elevated concentrations of von Willebrand factor and fibrinogen, which most likely reflects endothelial activation.[93]

In addition to endothelial injury and activation, the vascular pathology of chronic uremia includes autocrine and endocrine sequelae from a diverse range of seemingly unrelated factors. These include (1) a propensity for atherogenic lipid profiles and dyslipidemias[94]; (2) a complex derangement of platelet function that increases bleeding time but is associated with high levels of prothrombotic factors[95]; (3) an increased oxidant stress because of increased production of reactive oxygen species (ROS) and diminished antioxidant

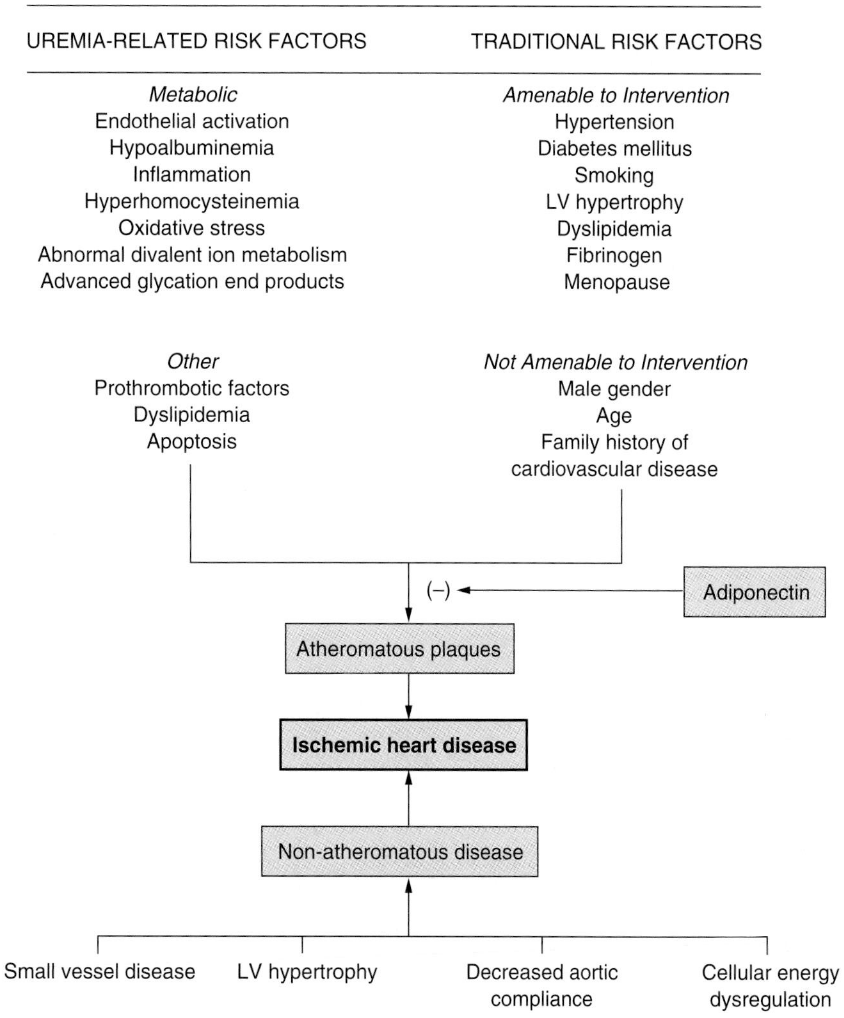

FIGURE 50-6. Cause of ischemic heart disease in dialysis patients. LV, left ventricular.

levels, which increases oxidative modification of lipids and enhances atherogenesis[96]; (4) hyperhomocysteinemia, which may have toxic effects on the endothelium and favor vascular thrombosis[97, 98]; (5) disturbances of glucose metabolism, which may be atherogenic through numerous metabolic anomalies and through hyperglycemia-induced irreversible modification of extracellular molecules such as advanced glycation end products[90]; and (6) dysregulation in the balance between proinflammatory cytokines and their inhibitors, which may contribute to a chronic immunoinflammatory disorder[99-101] through cytokine activation,[102] mediated in turn through the production of increased oxidant stress[103, 104] and acute phase reactants.[105]

Two factors have received particular attention recently in regard to their contribution to the development of atheroma in CKD: inflammation and vascular calcification.

Evidence from experimental and clinical studies has shown that inflammation in general, and C-reactive protein (CRP) specifically, may contribute directly to the pathogenesis of atherosclerosis and its complications both in the general community and in patients with CKD. CRP has been shown to bind to damaged cells, promoting activation of the complement system.[106] It displays calcium-dependent in vitro binding and aggregation of low-density lipoproteins (LDLs) and very-low-density lipoproteins (VLDLs),[107] and it is a potent stimulator of tissue factor by monocytes.[108] Epidemiologic studies support its pathogenetic role as a cardiovascular risk factor in the general community,[109-114] a situation that may be amenable to intervention by agents such as aspirin[115] and pravastatin.[116, 117] In CKD, the source of the (sometimes marked) elevation in CRP is uncertain. Potential sources include backfiltration of endotoxin during dialysis,[118] type of vascular access,[119] unrecognized infection, and bioincompatibility of peritoneal dialysate.[120] CRP levels have been shown to have a powerful predictive value for mortality in both hemodialysis and peritoneal dialysis patients[121] and to be an independent predictor of the number of atherosclerotic plaques and of intima-media thickness in carotid arteries of hemodialysis[122] and predialysis patients[123] respectively.

In one study, coronary atherosclerotic plaque morphology in patients with CKD was distinguished most readily by composition rather than by size or number. Calcium deposition in such plaques was extreme, and such deposits may contribute substantially to the high rate of complications seen in CKD.[124] Additional differences between CKD patients and nonuremic controls in this postmortem study included increased media thickness and a reduced lumen area. Such findings are entirely consistent with clinical assessment of CKD patients in recent years, in both coronary and larger peripheral vessels.[125-127] Markers of coronary and carotid calcification included longer duration of dialysis, hyperparathyroidism, estimates of calcium and phosphate load, CRP levels, elevated homocysteine levels, and age (although manifest calcification was evident in adults aged 20 and 30 years).[126, 127] Importantly, lesions progressed with time and persisted after transplantation.

The etiology of such changes almost certainly relates to the positive calcium and phosphate balance to which CKD patients are exposed, through both increased intake and inadequate excretion. Calcium-containing phosphate buffers, together with hyperparathyroidism, vitamin D use, and a

"closed" skeleton unable to buffer increased levels of calcium and phosphate, all undoubtedly contribute to vessel calcification. There is evidence also to suggest that raised plasma phosphate can alter the phenotype of smooth muscle cells from contractile to secretory, acting as one of a series of triggers permitting new bone formation in vessel walls.[128]

Although coronary artery calcification is predictive of subsequent coronary events in the general population, its clinical significance in patients with CKD is unknown. It is possible that the more generalized arterial calcification observed in dialysis patients is not predictive of atherosclerotic coronary events, but rather is a marker for arteriosclerosis and diminished vascular compliance and a risk factor for LV hypertrophy.

NONATHEROMATOUS ISCHEMIC HEART DISEASE

About 25% of dialysis patients with ischemic symptoms do not have critical CAD.[129] A significant percentage of predialysis and transplantation patients are similarly affected. It is likely that these symptoms result from microvascular disease and the underlying cardiomyopathy, in which a reduction in coronary vasodilator reserve and altered myocardial oxygen delivery and use predispose to ischemic symptoms (see Fig. 50-6). In dialysis patients, the presence of LV hypertrophy predisposes to nonatherosclerotic ischemic disease. Because LV hypertrophy is primarily a response to increased tensile stress requiring an overall increase in myocardial energy, as the demand for oxygen increases the coronary vasculature dilates above baseline. A further increase in myocardial oxygen requirement may not be met with an adequate increase in coronary flow, especially if there are pathologic changes in the large coronary arteries or in the small coronary vessels. Alterations in subendocardial perfusion are partly related to structural abnormalities of intramyocardial microvasculature and to abnormal structure and function of the aorta and major arteries.[90]

Small vessel smooth muscle hypertrophy and endothelial abnormalities have been described in LV hypertrophy that would further predispose to ischemia.[130] In uremic rats, Amann and colleagues showed diminished myocardial arteriolar diameter attributable to smooth muscle cell hyperplasia.[131] Myocyte-capillary mismatch, which has also been reported in the hearts of both rats and uremic patients, must increase the critical oxygen diffusion distance in the myocardium and expose the myocytes to the risk of hypoxia.[132, 133]

In dialysis patients, decreased arterial compliance may be associated with a decreased subendocardial viability index (an index of the propensity for myocardial ischemia) when altered hemodynamic forces exist in the absence of occlusive arterial lesions. This is in agreement with canine studies showing that aortic stiffening directly decreases subendocardial flow, despite an increase in mean coronary flow, and that chronic aortic stiffening reduces cardiac transmural perfusion and aggravates subendocardial ischemia.[134]

Susceptibility to myocardial ischemia may increase further as a result of dysregulation of high-energy phosphate compounds during ischemia. A reduced phosphocreatine–adenosine triphosphate ratio under hypoxic stress has been observed in the myocardium of uremic animals.[135] Hyperparathyroidism plays a critical role in the genesis of impaired energy production, transfer, and utilization by the myocardium[136] and therefore could increase susceptibility to ischemia.

Dialysis Hypotension

The pathophysiology of the clinical manifestation of dialysis hypotension is multifactorial and not fully understood. It may occur in the presence of systolic failure, diastolic dysfunction, or ischemic disease. In the last, it is usually associated with chest pain, whether atherosclerotic or nonatherosclerotic in origin. In dilated cardiomyopathy, hypotension during dialysis occurs only in patients who are unable to increase resting cardiac output in response to plasma volume depletion. Such patients usually have severe systolic failure, because the dialysis procedure actually improves myocardial performance in most patients with depressed LV function.[137-139] In one study, the predominant cause of dialysis-induced hypotension was found to be impaired myocardial reserve rather than ischemia. Those patients who were "hypotension-prone" demonstrated a reduced increment in cardiac index ($L \cdot min^{-1} \cdot m^{-2}$) on dobutamine-atropine stress echocardiography, compared with patients who were "hypotension-resistant," indicative of a markedly reduced myocardial reserve.[140]

LV hypertrophy may also be a contributing factor to dialysis hypotension. Because of diminished LV compliance, the relationship between LV end-diastolic pressure and volume is exaggerated (see Fig. 50-5).[69] As a result, during dialysis, relative hypovolemia may result in a disproportionately large decrease in LV end-diastolic pressure, which in turn leads to a decreased stroke volume and hypotension, if a compensatory increase in peripheral resistance does not occur. A high prevalence of LV hypertrophy among dialysis patients prone to dialysis hypotension has been reported.[140, 141]

Arrhythmias

In patients without renal failure, LV hypertrophy and coronary heart disease appear to be associated with an increased risk of arrhythmias. As outlined earlier, these cardiac diseases are among the most prevalent in dialysis patients. In addition, serum levels of electrolyte that can affect cardiac conduction, including potassium, calcium, magnesium, and hydrogen, are often abnormal or undergo rapid fluctuations during hemodialysis. For all these reasons, cardiac arrhythmias should be common in CKD; however, the presence of such factors also explains why their assessment and interpretation are difficult.

Arrhythmias and sudden death are of particular concern in patients undergoing dialysis. In cross-sectional studies of hemodialysis patients, atrial arrhythmias were present in 68% to 88%, ventricular arrhythmias in 56% to 76%, and premature ventricular complexes in 14% to 21% of the patients.[142-144] Older age, preexisting heart disease, LV hypertrophy, and digoxin therapy were associated with a higher prevalence and greater severity of cardiac arrhythmias. There is a considerable variation in the frequency and severity of arrhythmias during hemodialysis, as well as in the interdialytic period. Because of these factors, there is no consensus on the frequency of arrhythmias in these patients or their clinical significance.

CAD has been associated with a higher frequency of arrhythmias in some,[139, 145] but not all,[143, 144] studies of hemodialysis.

Neither has the association between coronary disease, LV hypertrophy, and fatal arrhythmias (sudden death) been clarified. There are also conflicting data about the effect of dialysis and of various dialysis compositions and dialysis protocols on the occurrence of rhythm disturbances. Some studies showed a higher incidence of premature ventricular contractions during dialysis or in the immediate postdialysis period,[142, 144] whereas in others no differences were observed.[143] Most atrial arrhythmias are of low clinical significance, although sustained, rate-related (fast or slow) impairment of LV filling can certainly produce hemodynamic consequences.

The majority of the premature ventricular contractions are unifocal and occur at a rate of less than 30 times per hour, but high-grade ventricular arrhythmias such as multiple premature ventricular contractions, ventricular couplets, and ventricular tachycardia were found in 27% of 92 patients with 24-hour Holter monitoring.[146] The finding of high-grade ventricular arrhythmias in the presence of CAD has been associated with an increased risk of cardiac mortality and sudden death.[139, 147] Whereas the choice of dialysis method, membrane, and buffer does not seem to have a direct effect on the incidence of arrhythmias,[148] dialysis-associated hypotension appears to be an important factor in precipitating high-grade ventricular arrhythmias, regardless of the type of dialysis.[148, 149]

Arrhythmias in peritoneal dialysis patients appear different from those in hemodialysis patients. Holter monitoring of cardiac rhythm in 21 such patients revealed a high frequency of atrial and/or ventricular premature beats.[150] There were no differences in type or frequency of extrasystoles between days on which dialysis was administered and days on which it was deliberately withheld. It seems that, in contrast to hemodialysis, peritoneal dialysis by itself is not responsible for provoking or aggravating arrhythmias. The arrhythmias seen in these patients are more often a reflection of the patient's age, underlying ischemic heart disease, or an association with LV hypertrophy.[151, 152]

A study[153] in which 27 peritoneal dialysis patients were compared with 27 hemodialysis patients revealed that severe cardiac arrhythmias occurred in 4% of the former and in 33% of the latter group. Patients in both groups were matched for age, sex, duration of treatment, and etiology of chronic renal failure. The lower frequency of LV hypertrophy, the maintenance of a relatively stable blood pressure, the absence of sudden hypotensive events, and the significantly lower incidence of hyperkalemia in patients undergoing peritoneal dialysis[154] may explain their lower incidence of severe arrhythmias.

The use of digoxin in hemodialysis patients has also raised concern regarding precipitation of arrhythmias, especially in the immediate postdialysis period, when both hypokalemia and relative hypercalcemia may occur.[145, 139, 155] Keller and associates[156] studied 55 patients in a crossover study of "on-and-off" digoxin and found no increase in the incidence of arrhythmias when patients were taking the drug.

Valvular Disease

Most valvular lesions observed in CKD patients are acquired and develop from dystrophic calcification of the valvular annulus and leaflets, particularly the aortic and mitral valves.[157]

The prevalence of aortic valve calcification in dialysis patients is as high as 55%,[16, 157] similar to that in the elderly general population, although it occurs 10 to 20 years earlier.[158-160] Aortic valve orifice stenosis in CKD evolves from valve sclerosis, which itself is now recognized generally to be associated with increased cardiovascular mortality.[17] In dialysis patients, the prevalence of aortic stenosis is between 3% and 13%.[161] It may sometimes evolve rapidly (within 6 months) to hemodynamically significant stenosis, with a worsening of LV hypertrophy and rapidly evolving symptomatology. Age, duration of dialysis, a raised phosphate level, and an elevated calcium phosphate product appear to be the most important risk factors for the development of aortic stenosis.[157, 162]

Mitral valve calcification is not as common as aortic valve disease in CKD and may have a different pathophysiology. In one study in which patients were evaluated by echocardiography, mitral annulus calcification was present in 45% of 92 hemodialysis patients (compared with 10% of age and gender–matched controls).[157] Other studies have found prevalences of 39% in hemodialysis patients, 18% in those undergoing peritoneal dialysis, 16% in predialysis patients, and 10% in the general population.[15, 163] Age and calcium phosphate product have been correlated with valve calcification, although in one study of 135 peritoneal dialysis patients with low PTH levels, a constant involvement of the posterior cusp, together with left atrial enlargement, was observed.[163] Valve calcification has also been associated with rhythm and cardiac conduction defects, valvular insufficiency, and peripheral vascular calcification. Although most studies have identified abnormalities in calcium phosphate metabolism as the predominant underlying risk factor, additional factors include specific involvement of the posterior cusp, left atrial dilatation, duration of dialysis, and duration of predialysis systolic hypertension.[15, 157, 159, 163, 164] Factors associated with decreased survival include severity of calcification, mitral regurgitation, and reduced LV function.[164]

Vascular Disease
Large Vessel Disease
ARTERIOSCLEROSIS

Increased cardiovascular morbidity and mortality have been correlated, either directly or indirectly, with various estimates of elevated LV afterload in patients with CKD, such as raised pulse pressure,[165-167] increased carotid wall thickness,[168] predialysis[166, 169] or 48-hour[170] mean systolic blood pressure (SBP) levels, elevated pulse wave velocity,[165] and absence of diurnal blood pressure variability.[171] Postulated etiologic factors include increased arterial wall stiffness,[165] raised sympathetic tone mediated by elevated noradrenaline levels,[66] primary hormonal aberrations associated with CKD (including adiponectin[48] and atrial or brain natriuretic peptides[65]), seasonal changes,[172] and autonomic dysregulation manifested by nocturnal hypoxia.[171]

Some of these factors have only recently been identified. Many, however, are related to two established components of LV afterload—hypertension and reduced arterial wall compliance—for which some studies exist. Before examining these topics, it is important to recognize the pathophysiologic similarities and differences by which they are characterized.

Hypertension has usually been attributed to a reduction in the caliber or number of muscular arteries (150 to 400 μm in diameter), which results in an increase in peripheral resistance. However, this approach does not acknowledge that blood pressure fluctuates during the cardiac cycle and that systolic and diastolic levels represent only the limits of this fluctuation.[173] Fourier analysis of the blood pressure curve can determine both its steady state (mean blood pressure) and oscillatory components (fluctuation about the mean).[173] The former is determined exclusively by cardiac output and peripheral resistance (with pressure and flow considered constant over time). The oscillatory component is determined by the pattern of LV ejection, the viscoelastic properties of large conduit arteries, and the intensity and timing of arterial wave reflection.[174] A faster pulse wave velocity is primarily associated with arterial stiffness, which, in CKD, is an acceleration of the normal aging process with vessel dilatation and a diffuse, nonocclusive medial and intimal wall hypertrophy (arteriosclerosis).[175] It has been correlated with shortened stature,[176] male gender, smoking, blood pressure, diabetes, volume overload, humoral imbalance, and age.[177, 178]

The clinical characteristics of hypertension depend on the predominant abnormality. Increased peripheral resistance is characterized principally by increased diastolic and mean blood pressures, whereas increased arterial stiffness and early wave reflections are indicated by increased systolic and widened pulse pressures. Because the peripheral resistance of most dialysis patients is within the normal range,[173] it is likely that effects from an accelerated pulse wave velocity contribute more significantly to cardiovascular morbidity than does an elevation in mean blood pressure. Increased systolic pressure and pulse pressure are observed in dialysis patients[179, 180] and are closely correlated with LV hypertrophy.[178, 181] Canine studies furthermore indicate that aortic stiffening directly decreases subendocardial blood flow owing to an increase in LV systolic stress and oxygen demand, despite an increase in mean coronary flow.[182, 183]

ATHEROMATOUS DISEASE

The pathology and pathogenesis of atheromatous disease in larger peripheral vessels were addressed earlier in the section on ischemic heart disease. Atherosclerotic plaques are primarily intimal, focal, and patchy, inducing occlusive lesions and compensatory focal enlargement of arterial diameters. Mechanical and humoral factors predispose to formation of atheroma, which has a predilection for such sites as bifurcations, bends, and areas of pronounced arterial tapering. Turbulence or low-average shear stress characterizes the latter sites over the cardiac cycle.[184, 185] Atherosclerosis is uncommon in sides where laminar shear stress is high, such as at flow dividers or on the inner sides of arteries downstream from dividers or on the outer wall of an arterial bend.

Small Vessel Disease
HYPERTENSION

The pathophysiology of hypertension in CKD has been covered extensively in other sections of this book. Several mechanisms are involved in the development of hypertension, each probably of varying significance at different stages of disease. At an early stage of CKD, the link between the kidney and hypertension is not clear. As dysfunction progresses, an increase in extracellular volume through salt and water retention becomes more important, although, to result in hypertension, it would seem that an increase in peripheral resistance is also required. Factors responsible for this development include enhanced sympathetic activity, activation of the renin-angiotensin system, and endothelial cell dysfunction.

Various functional abnormalities have been found in recent years within the endothelial cell in hypertensive patients with CKD. Reduced nitric oxide production,[186, 187] increased levels of endothelin-1,[188] and increased oxygen free radical activity[189] all support the notion of a primary endothelial role in hypertension in these patients. Additional potential influences include renal vasculopathy, which has been found to correlate with the presence of hypertension in CKD[190]; a permissive role of hyperparathyroidism for a hypertensive effect of intracellular calcium[191]; and low initial nephron number in association with reduced birthweight.[192]

DIABETES

The pathophysiology of diabetic vascular disease is complex and is also covered in other sections of this book. Through a combination of sustained chronic hyperglycemia, dyslipidemia, and insulin resistance, adverse and proatherogenic metabolic events, including increased oxidative stress, protein kinase C activation, and an increased activation of the receptor for advanced glycation end product (RAGE), are engendered. Four important destructive and interactive mechanisms result: (1) impaired endothelial cell function, mainly through an imbalance in vasoactive hormonal and paracrine factors[193, 194]; (2) vasoconstriction and smooth muscle hypertrophy[195, 196]; (c) increased production of inflammatory cytokines and cellular adhesion molecules[197-199]; and (4) a prothrombotic milieu through calcium-dependent platelet activation and increased expression of procoagulant clotting factors, including tissue factor and plasmin activator inhibitor 1.[200, 201] Subsequent profound effects on vessel morphology and function result which, in renal disease, are further complicated and exacerbated by increased exposure to traditional and uremic risk factors.

Posttransplantation diabetes (PTDM) is a complication of immunosuppression, particularly with the combination of steroids and calcineurin inhibitors. The incidence has been reported to be between 4% and 41%. The range is presumably affected by the lack of a standard definition for PTDM: some patients exhibit transient hyperglycemia, whereas others develop persistent diabetes. Steroids exert their effect largely by increasing peripheral insulin resistance. It has been hypothesized that, in high doses, calcineurin inhibitors are concentrated in the insulin-producing pancreatic beta cells, inhibiting insulin production. Tacrolimus may have a greater predisposition to the development of PTDM than does cyclosporine.[202] Additional risk factors include higher doses of calcineurin inhibitors in the first weeks after transplantation, age, ethnicity, a family history of diabetes, and previous rejection episodes.[203, 204] The condition is not benign; detrimental effects on patient and graft survival within 3 years have been reported, and one study demonstrated a stronger association between cardiovascular disease and PTDM than in pretransplantation diabetes.[205]

EPIDEMIOLOGY AND CARDIAC RISK FACTORS

Overview

Table 50-3 shows the potentially modifiable cardiovascular risk factors in CKD. Although studies are in progress, there is little information currently available on the mortality rate of predialysis patients. However, the predominant burden of ill health in CKD occurs during the period of dialysis. The survival of dialysis patients is worse than that of patients with colon or prostate cancer, resulting predominantly from an excessively high cardiovascular mortality rate. Figure 50-1 and Table 50-1 show the annual cardiovascular mortality rate by gender, race, and diabetic status in patients undergoing hemodialysis, peritoneal dialysis, and renal transplantation, compared with the general population. In hemodialysis patients the rate is 35 times higher than in the general population,[5] although there has been a decrease in mortality rate during the past decade.[206]

Overall annual adjusted death rates in patients waiting for renal transplantation and in transplant recipients decreased between 1989 and 1996.[206] The relative risk (RR) for patient

TABLE 50-3

Potentially Modifiable Cardiovascular Risk Factors in Chronic Kidney Disease, Identified by Cohort Studies

	PREDIALYSIS	RENAL TRANSPLANT			DIALYSIS			
	LVH	LVH	CHF	IHD	LVH	CHF	IHD	DEATH
Anemia	+	+	+	−	+	+	−	+
Hypertension	+	+	+	+	+	+	+	−
Hyperlipidemia	−	−	−	+	−	−	−	−
Smoking	−	−	−	+	−	+	+	+
Hypoalbuminemia	−	−	−	+	−	+	−	+
C-reactive protein	−	−	−	−	−	−	−	+
Homocysteine	−	−	−	−	−	−	−	+
Divalent ion abnormalities	−	−	−	−	−	−	−	+

CHF, congestive heart failure; IHD, ischemic heart disease; LVH, left ventricular hypertrophy.

death decreased by 23% in the former group and by 30% in the latter. Slope analysis of the cause-specific mortality rates for cardiovascular disease and for infection showed almost equivalent, linear decreases for both groups. These favorable trends probably represent equal advances in transplantation, dialysis, and general medical care.

Figure 50-7A shows the survival of patients starting dialysis according to their echocardiographic diagnosis. Those with systolic dysfunction had significantly worse survival than those with a normal echocardiogram through all time frames, whereas those with concentric LV hypertrophy and LV dilatation had significantly worse late survival, after 2 years on dialysis.[23] Confirmation that LV mass is a strong and independent predictor for survival and for cardiovascular events in dialysis patients was confirmed recently, as was the prognostic impact of the different types of hypertrophy.[65] Aortic and large artery stiffness is increased in dialysis and is associated with LV hypertrophy.[207] Aortic stiffness was an independent predictor of all-cause and cardiovascular mortality in French[181] and Japanese dialysis patients.[208]

Congestive heart failure has been consistently shown to be a strong independent risk factor for death (see Fig. 50-7B), whereas ischemic heart disease is not a significant risk factor for death when assessed independent of age, diabetes, and the presence of cardiac failure.[209] This suggests that the impact of ischemic heart disease exerts its effect through compromising LV pump function. In diabetes, however, both heart failure and ischemic heart disease are independent predictors of death.[210]

Other cardiovascular events in CKD are associated with a high mortality rate. After acute myocardial infarction in dialysis patients, the mortality rate was found to be 59% at 1 year and 90% by 5 years,[211] which may reflect the catastrophic effect of impaired perfusion in overload cardiomyopathy. In Japan, mortality after stroke in dialysis patients was 47% at 1 month and 64% at 1 year.[212] Survival after interventions for vascular disease in dialysis patients is also lowered. Median survival was 1.72 years after lower limb revascularization in dialysis patients, as opposed to 5.17 years after the same procedure in control subjects.[213] Lower limb amputation is also associated with a high mortality rate in the postoperative period.[214]

Uremia as an Independent Cardiac Risk Factor

There is little doubt that proteinuria is an independent, adverse cardiac risk factor.[215-217] It is also likely that the uremic state is cardiomyopathic because of its unique hemodynamic milieu. The latter conclusion is supported by numerous data. There is a higher rate of de novo symptomatic heart failure in renal transplant recipients than in the general population.[218] A high prevalence of cardiac failure on starting dialysis is recognized,[7, 9] and there is a high incidence of de novo cardiac failure in hemodialysis patients (13.6% over 2.2 years mean follow-up in the United States[219] and 17% over 3.4 years in Canada[209]). There is also an independent adverse effect of cardiac failure on subsequent mortality in those patients starting dialysis.[180]

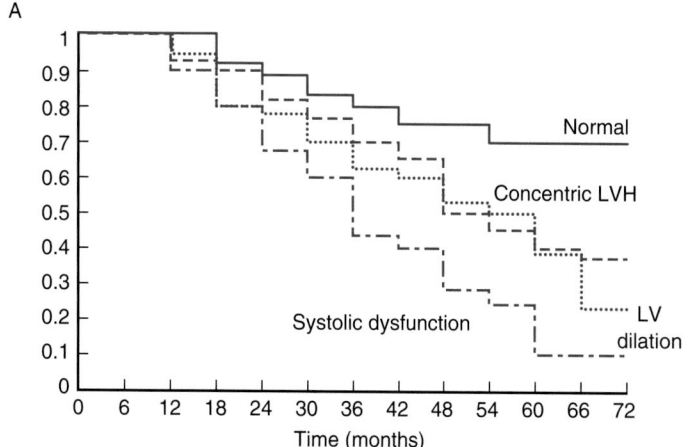

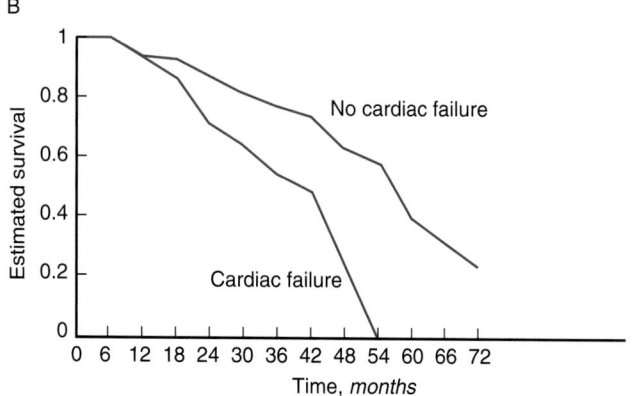

FIGURE 50-7. A, Survival of patients starting dialysis, comparing those with normal echocardiogram, concentric left ventricular (LV) hypertrophy, LV dilatation, and systolic dysfunction at baseline. (From Parfrey PS, Foley RN, Harnett JD, et al: Outcome and risk factors for left ventricular disorders in chronic uremia. Nephrol Dial Transplant 11:1280, 1996, with permission.) **B,** Survival of patients starting dialysis, comparing those with and without cardiac failure at baseline. (From Foley RN, Parfrey PS, Harnett JD, et al: Clinical and echocardiographic cardiovascular disease in patients starting dialysis therapy: Prevalence, associations, and prognosis. Kidney Int 47:189, 1995, with permission.)

The evidence for uremia as an independent risk factor for atherogenic disease is less certain. Longitudinal studies of community-derived cohorts, such as the Framingham study[215] and the First National Health and Nutritional Examination Survey, (NHANES I),[216] failed to identify renal insufficiency as an independent cardiac risk factor, although the converse was found with NHANES II.[220] In contrast, similar studies of cohorts with higher degrees of comorbidity, including elderly, hypertensive, and cardiac patients,[217, 221-223] consistently identified renal insufficiency as an independent predictor of an adverse cardiovascular outcome. It is clear that renal insufficiency is a marker for more advanced vascular disease with adverse cardiac outcomes. Whether it is also an independent cardiac risk factor is less clear.

After starting dialysis therapy, atheromatous event rates are much higher than before dialysis. The incidences of de novo coronary events, stroke, and peripheral vascular disease of U.S. hemodialysis patients, after 2.2 years of follow-up from the start of dialysis, were 10.2%, 2.2%, and 14%, respectively.[219]

One way to appraise the uncertainty of cardiovascular risk in this population is to derive prediction equations for atheromatous outcomes, with traditional risk factor "weightings," and compare the predictions in CKD cohorts with de novo cardiac event rates in the general population. The "weighted risk" projected by the Framingham coronary risk score was higher in hemodialysis patients[224] and in renal transplant recipients[225] than in the reference population, but it was probably insufficient to predict the increased incidence of cardiac disease in these groups. It is also possible that the variable ability to detect specific atherogenic factors in CKD may be because proatherogenic tendencies are balanced at least to some extent by an antiatherogenic effect. The adipocyte protein adiponectin, for example, seems to play a protective role in experimental models of vascular injury, perhaps because it suppresses the attachment of monocytes to endothelial cells. In one study of 227 hemodialysis patients, plasma adiponectin levels were 2.5 times higher than in normal subjects and were inversely predictive of cardiovascular outcome.[48] Adiponectin was also inversely related to levels of several metabolic risk factors, including insulin, triglycerides, and von Willebrand factor, and directly related to high-density lipoprotein (HDL)–cholesterol levels, in a manner consistent with the hypothesis that adiponectin is protective to the cardiovascular system.

The observed findings therefore can be explained by (1) the result of qualitatively or quantitatively different risk relationships theoretically associated with cardiac disease in CKD patients compared with the general population, (2) an independent contribution to outcome events by associated cardiomyopathic disease, or (3) greater proatherogenic than antiatherogenic uremia-related risk factor influences not addressed in the Framingham risk equation.

Traditional Risk Factors

Hypertension

Hypertension is prominent in all stages of CKD, with associated deleterious effects according to its degree and duration. It may be the result of high peripheral resistance with diastolic hypertension or the result of volume overload and arteriosclerosis with systolic hypertension and widened pulse pressures. Whatever the etiologic mechanism, hypertension is a risk factor for LV hypertrophy in patients with moderately severe CKD,[8] those undergoing renal transplantation,[24, 218] or those on dialysis.[180] It is also an independent risk factor for cardiac failure and for symptomatic ischemic heart disease in renal transplantation and in dialysis patients.[23, 24, 209, 218]

PREDIALYSIS. About 70% to 80% of patients with CKD have hypertension, and the prevalence increases as the glomerular filtration rate (GFR) declines. The level of SBP is correlated with GFR and proteinuria, and hypertension is more common in glomerular than in tubulointerstitial disease. Although more than 70% of patients are treated with antihypertensive agents, fewer than half achieve blood pressure levels lower than 140/90 mm Hg.[25, 226-230]

DIALYSIS. Up to 80% of patients starting hemodialysis and 50% of those starting peritoneal dialysis are hypertensive. It is frequently inadequately treated: the 1996 Core Indicators project reported that 53% of prevalent adult hemodialysis patients had predialysis SBP readings in excess of 150 mm Hg, and 17% had predialysis DBP readings of 90 mm Hg or more. The comparable rates in peritoneal dialysis patients were 29% and 18%, respectively.[231] More than 70% exceed the criteria of the Sixth Report of the Joint National Committee on Prevention, Detection, Evaluation and Treatment of High Blood Pressure (JNC VI).[232] In the Dialysis Morbidity and Mortality Study by U.S. Renal Data System (USRDS), hypertension was common and poorly controlled, with higher interdialytic weight gains, noncompliance with the dialysis regimen, and younger age being independent predictors of higher levels.[233-237] Despite strong evidence that high blood pressure is an independent risk factor for cardiac events in CKD, low blood pressure is associated with a higher risk of death in multiple studies of dialysis patients.[238-240] This is likely (but not proven) to be due to residual confounding from cardiac comorbidity that is associated with lower blood pressure.[241]

TRANSPLANTATION. Hypertension is common in the transplantation group, with an estimated prevalence of 50% to 90%. Apart from effects of vascular modelling during the period of dialysis, numerous concurrent factors after transplantation, including obesity, raised extracellular volume, medications, and renal dysfunction, may all contribute to hypertension in this patient group. The vasoconstrictive effects of calcineurin inhibitors in particular augment hypertension after transplantation.[218, 242-244]

Dyslipidemia

As with hypertension, the prevalence of dyslipidemia in patients with CKD is high. In early stages of disease, the prevalence varies according to renal function and the degree of proteinuria.[226, 245] As GFR falls, triglyceride levels increase and HDL-cholesterol falls. As proteinuria increases, total cholesterol, LDL-cholesterol and triglycerides all increase, while HDL-cholesterol decreases. Approximately 50% of hemodialysis patients and 70% of peritoneal dialysis patients have hyperlipidemia.[245] Hemodialysis patients characteristically demonstrate alterations from the general population only in their levels of triglycerides (elevated) and HDL-cholesterol (reduced). In peritoneal dialysis and transplantation patients, levels of total cholesterol, LDL-cholesterol, and triglycerides are usually higher than in the general population. In transplantation patients, this may be partly related to immunosuppression, with tacrolimus permitting a more favorable profile than that obtainable with cyclosporine, and sirolimus producing significant increases in both cholesterol and triglycerides.[246]

Monitoring and treatment of dyslipidemia are often inadequate. Only 8% to 18% of nondiabetic patients take lipid-lowering drugs before dialysis, and 4% to 10% of dialysis patients use 3-hydroxy-3-methylglutaryl coenzyme A (HMG-CoA) reductase inhibitors (statins).[226, 229, 230, 247] Fewer than 40% of transplantation patients and 60% of dialysis patients have their lipids measured during the course of a year.[248]

Few longitudinal studies have examined the relationship between lipid abnormalities and cardiac outcomes in CKD, although dyslipidemia has been linked to progression of renal disease. In predialysis patients, low HDL-cholesterol levels have been identified as an independent risk factor for cardiovascular events, and several studies have identified significant associations between various lipid abnormalities and cardiovascular events in transplantation patients.[225, 249, 250] Studies in dialysis patients have found a U-shaped relationship with either cardiovascular events or overall mortality: one 10-year prospective cohort study of 1167 Japanese hemodialysis patients demonstrated that patients with a serum cholesterol concentration between 200 and 220 mg/dL had the best outcome.[251] It is likely, however, that confounding factors such as concurrent malnutrition or inflammation explain these findings.[252] In 196 incident diabetic hemodialysis patients, higher than median serum cholesterol and higher LDL-cholesterol were associated with cardiovascular mortality.[253] Kasiske and co-workers[225] also reported significant associations between elevated cholesterol and triglycerides with low HDL-cholesterol levels and ischemic heart disease events in renal transplantation recipients.

Tobacco Use

Approximately 25% of predialysis patients and 50% of dialysis and transplantation patients do smoke or have smoked tobacco. This is now clearly linked to the progression of kidney disease, the development of cardiovascular disease, and mortality. At the start of dialysis therapy, smoking has been independently associated with de novo heart failure, peripheral vascular disease, and death.[219] In renal transplant recipients, the risks of cardiovascular disease, cerebrovascular disease, and death are increased with smoking.[225, 249, 250, 254-256]

Diabetes

Diabetes in patients with moderate to severe CKD predicts deterioration in cardiovascular state, regardless of the presence of cardiovascular disease at baseline.[257] Diabetic patients have more widespread CAD than do age- and sex-matched controls.[258] Some diabetic dialysis patients have impaired LV function despite normal coronary arteries, perhaps because of a diabetic cardiomyopathy.[259] Echocardiographic LV hypertrophy is probably a more frequent finding in hypertensive diabetic patients than in hypertensive nondiabetic patients.[260] In diabetic patients, this increased LV mass seems closely related to the level of blood pressure. A comparison of

the pathologic spectrum of patients with hypertensive, diabetic, and hypertensive-diabetic heart disease showed that the latter group had a significantly higher heart weight and a higher total fibrosis score than either of the other two groups.[261]

In one study of a cohort of dialysis patients who survived at least 6 months after the initiation of dialysis, 15% had insulin-dependent diabetes and 12% had non–insulin-dependent diabetes. On starting dialysis therapy, the prevalence of clinical manifestations of cardiac disease was significantly higher in diabetic than in nondiabetic patients. Only 11% of diabetic patients had normal echocardiographic dimensions, compared with 25% of nondiabetic patients, predominantly because of the prevalence of severe LV hypertrophy (34% versus 18%).[210] Among this group of incident diabetic dialysis patients, older age, LV hypertrophy, a history of smoking, ischemic heart disease, cardiac failure, and hypoalbuminemia were independently associated with mortality.[210] The excessive cardiac morbidity and mortality of diabetic compared with nondiabetic patients seem to be mediated via ischemic disease rather than progression of cardiomyopathy while during dialysis therapy. Echocardiographic determination of LV size and function was a good predictor of survival. Diabetic patients receiving dialysis therapy who had abnormal LV wall motion and abnormal LV internal diameter had the lowest mean survival time (8 months)—not matched in any subgroup defined by coronary anatomy, ventricular function, or clinical manifestation.[262]

Diabetes has also been found to be an independent risk factor for ischemic heart disease[24, 224, 250] and for cardiac failure[218] in renal transplant recipients.

Left Ventricular Hypertrophy

LV hypertrophy is a condition that is exceptionally common in CKD, being present in 75% of patients starting dialysis. After renal transplantation, two thirds of dialysis patients had substantial regression of hypertrophy, despite maintenance of blood pressure at similar levels before and after transplantation.[76] This implies that some factor or factors other than hypertension, probably associated with uremia, maintain LV hypertrophy. In dialysis patients, LV hypertrophy is a strong predictor of the subsequent development of heart failure and of ischemic heart disease.[23] In renal transplantation recipients, the electrocardiographic diagnosis of LV hypertrophy is also a strong predictor for the development of cardiac failure.[263]

Other Traditional Risk Factors

Other risk factors for cardiovascular disease are well defined in the general population (see Fig. 50-6); however, either there are insufficient data pertaining to their relevance in CKD (e.g., physical activity, menopause) or they are not amenable to change (e.g., age, gender).

Uremia-Related Risk Factors

Uremia-related risk factors can be classified into hemodynamic and metabolic types, some of which are peculiar to the uremic state and some magnified. Hemodynamic factors include anemia, increased extracellular volume, and arteriovenous fistulas. Metabolic factors include hypoalbuminemia, inflammation markers, hyperhomocysteinemia, oxidative stress, abnormal divalent ion metabolism (calcium and phosphate), dyslipidemia, thrombogenic factors, and others.

Hemodynamic Risk Factors

ANEMIA

In moderate to severe CKD before dialysis (GFR <50 mL/min), anemia is associated with LV growth.[8] In dialysis patients, it is associated with progressive LV dilatation and hypertrophy[18] and with development of de novo heart failure.[209] In renal transplant recipients, anemia is an independent risk factor for the development of electrocardiographically diagnosed LV hypertrophy[263] and of symptomatic heart failure.[24] In no group with CKD, however, has anemia been found to be a risk factor for ischemic heart disease.

INCREASED EXTRACELLULAR VOLUME

At all stages of CKD, sodium and water overload may cause plasma volume expansion, LV dilatation, and LV hypertrophy. However, the main group affected is dialysis patients. LV hypertrophy is more severe in long-term peritoneal dialysis patients than in hemodialysis patients.[21] This finding is associated with evidence of more pronounced volume expansion, hypertension, and hypoalbuminemia. Greater interdialytic weight gain is independently associated with higher blood pressure in hemodialysis patients,[264] and the latter is a risk factor for cardiac events. In 125 incident peritoneal dialysis patients, lower total sodium and fluid removal rates, in addition to higher blood pressure, comorbidity, lower serum creatinine levels, and higher residual renal function, were independent factors affecting survival.[265]

ARTERIOVENOUS FISTULAS

Blood flow in arteriovenous fistulas and grafts predisposes to LV volume overload. The only controlled study to demonstrate this clearly was one that examined 20 renal transplant recipients with a mean fistula flow of 1790 ± 648 mL/min.[266] Three to four months after fistula closure, LV end-diastolic diameter had decreased from 51.5 to 49.3 mm ($P < .01$) and LV mass index from 135 to 120 g/m^2 ($P < .01$).

ARTERIOSCLEROSIS

Increased pulse pressure and SBP are closely correlated with LV hypertrophy.[178, 181] Raised pulse pressure,[165-167] increased carotid wall thickness,[168] and elevated pulse wave velocity[165] have all been associated with an increased mortality. This was addressed more fully in an earlier section of this chapter.

MODE OF DIALYSIS THERAPY

Although Canadian and Italian cohorts in the 1980s and early 1990s found higher risks for death in peritoneal dialysis compared with hemodialysis patients,[36, 267] more recent comparative studies from the same groups found no difference in mortality.[268, 269] The hemodialysis state constitutes a condition of hemodynamic overload and metabolic perturbation that is lethal in its impact on the heart. However, the Lombardy study reported that the risk of de novo cardiovascular disease did not differ by treatment modality.[267] It is unclear whether further improvements in dialysis technology, such as daily or nocturnal dialysis, are necessary to diminish the uremic component of cardiac disease. Dialysis provides inadequate treatment of the uremic state, but the target quantity of dialysis, which may limit the contribution of so-called uremic toxins to cardiac dysfunction, is unknown. A current trial in the United States comparing two quantities of hemodialysis may be helpful in this regard.

Renal transplantation is the best model of what happens to the heart when uremia is treated properly. Although hypertension usually persists, as does the fistula and sometimes hypervolemia, anemia and the metabolic perturbation are usually corrected. Improvements in concentric LV hypertrophy and LV dilatation are seen, but the most striking observation is the improvement in systolic dysfunction.[76] It is not known which adverse risk factors characteristic of the uremic state have been corrected to produce this improvement in LV contractility. In a virtually complete national U.S. survey of diabetic dialysis patients, there was a significant decrease in the risk of hospitalization for cardiac failure among patients after renal transplantation compared with those still on the waiting list, even accounting for selection bias.[81] Carotid intima-media thickness (IMT), as a surrogate marker of cardiovascular risk, also has been shown to decrease independently of changes in LV mass after transplantation, although this is possibly associated with PTH levels.[77]

Metabolic Risk Factors

HYPOALBUMINEMIA

Hypoalbuminemia has been shown repeatedly to be a most potent predictor of outcome in dialysis patients. Hypoalbuminemia is associated with LV dilatation, which may reflect the impact of malnutrition in predisposing to myocyte death. It predisposes to de novo cardiac failure and to de novo ischemic heart disease.[270] It is more characteristic of peritoneal dialysis than of hemodialysis patients, and it may result from different mechanisms in patients treated by these different modalities. It is likely that the path to death is different in hemodialysis patients, because a higher proportion of this group develop cardiac failure, which predisposes to earlier death. A more marked inflammatory milieu is a possible explanation, as is a more unfavorable hemodynamic environment. In renal transplant recipients, hypoalbuminemia is an independent risk factor for the development of both de novo cardiac failure and ischemic heart disease,[218] a observation similar to that made in dialysis patients.[18]

INFLAMMATION

CRP is an acute phase reactant and a marker for inflammation. It has also become recognized as an important link in the development of atheroma in CKD. In one study, hemodialysis patients in the highest CRP quartile had a fivefold increased RR of cardiovascular death compared with those in the lowest quartile.[271] The association between CRP and death in dialysis patients has also been corroborated by other studies.[272, 273] Recently, high CRP levels in 240 peritoneal dialysis patients starting treatment were observed frequently and were found to correlate independently with an increased incidence of cardiovascular events.[274]

HYPERHOMOCYSTEINEMIA

The pathogenesis of atheroma formation by homocysteine remains obscure, although endothelial cell injury, oxidative stress, and a prothrombotic effect are likely.[275-277] Increased levels of homocysteine are a risk factor for cardiovascular disease in the general population[278, 279] and appear to be associated with further risk in patients with CKD.[280] Most hemodialysis patients have grossly elevated plasma homocysteine levels, but the absolute level is dependent on nutritional status, protein intake, and serum albumin.[281] Lower homocysteine levels in patients with cardiovascular disease appear to be related to the higher prevalence of malnutrition and hypoalbuminemia in affected patients.[281] Although one must be aware of the impact of survivor bias in longitudinal studies of prevalent dialysis patients, prospective studies have also demonstrated that hyperhomocysteinemia is an adverse prognostic factor for cardiovascular disease outcomes in dialysis patients.[280, 282, 283]

OXIDATIVE STRESS

Oxidative stress is said to occur when there is an imbalance between formation of ROS and antioxidant defense mechanisms. ROS (e.g., hydrogen peroxide [H_2O_2], free radicals such as superoxide [O_2^-], hydroxyl radical [OH]) are continuously formed in vivo and play an important role in host defense against tumor cells and pathogens.[284-286] A number of enzymatic and nonenzymatic defense mechanisms have evolved to "detoxify" ROS. The predominant nonenzymatic agents include vitamin E, vitamin C, selenium, and zinc. Superoxide dismutase and glutathione peroxidase are the main antioxidants. It is thought that oxidative stress is important in the formation of atheroma, because it generates lipid peroxidation products that are consistently found in atheromatous streaks and sclerotic lesions.[287, 288]

Compelling evidence indicates that oxidative stress is an important trigger in the complex chain of events leading to atherosclerosis in CKD.[289] Enhanced oxidative stress may be identified by an increase in the products of lipid peroxidation (e.g., malondialdehyde), a decrease in substances that enhance oxidative resistance (e.g., plasmalogen), or a decrease in reducing substances (e.g., glutathione). There is evidence for all of these in CKD.[288, 290] Dialysis may also contribute to oxidative stress through removal of antioxidants or stimulation of ROS by the use of incompatible dialysis components.

Markers of oxidative stress are particularly increased in CKD patients. One such marker, serum malondialdehyde, was significantly higher in hemodialysis patients with cardiovascular disease than in those without such disease.[291] Tight correlations have been observed between ROS and cardiac failure in patients with heart disease and between ROS and blood pressure levels in patients with CKD.[189, 292, 293]

ABNORMAL DIVALENT ION METABOLISM

There is substantial experimental and clinical evidence that the hyperparathyroid state and altered vitamin D status found in uremia contribute to cardiomyopathy, LV hypertrophy, LV fibrosis, atherosclerosis, myocardial ischemia, and vascular and cardiac calcification.[294]

Data from the USRDS have identified hyperphosphatemia and raised calcium-phosphate product as independent predictors of mortality.[163] Analysis of data from two national samples of prevalent hemodialysis patients identified strong relationships between elevated phosphate, calcium-phosphate product, and PTH on the one hand and death from cardiac causes, especially from CAD, and sudden death on the other hand.[295] Long-term survival in 12,000 dialysis patients was also found to be related to control of serum phosphate in addition to three other modifiable factors (dialysis dose, hematocrit, and compliance with the dialysis schedule).[296]

Increased prevalence and extent of coronary artery calcification, particularly in young dialysis patients, have been significantly associated with higher serum phosphate, calcium-phosphate product, and calcium intake.[126] Whether this calcification represents specific changes within atherosclerotic plaques or a stage associated with arteriosclerosis is not clear. The presence of vascular calcification in hemodialysis patients was associated in one study with increased stiffness of large-capacity, elastic-type arteries such as the aorta and common carotid artery.[125] The extent of arterial calcifications increased with the use of calcium-based phosphate binders.

A viable hypothesis is that disturbed divalent ion metabolism promotes vascular calcification, which produces noncompliant major vessels. This in turn predisposes to LV hypertrophy, cardiac disease, and subsequent death.

PROTHROMBOTIC FACTORS

Decreased platelet aggregation and increased bleeding time occur in patients with CKD, especially in those with chronic renal insufficiency and those undergoing hemodialysis.[95] Elevated levels of fibrinogen and other procoagulant factors are also observed in CKD. There is no evidence concerning the relationship of these abnormalities in platelet function and procoagulant activity to cardiac outcomes in CKD. In the general population, the percentage reduction of cardiac disease by aspirin use in patients with prior myocardial infarct, stroke, transient ischemic attacks, unstable angina, coronary bypass graft surgery, coronary angioplasty, atrial fibrillation, valvular heart disease, or peripheral vascular disease is approximately 25%.[297]

LIPOPROTEIN (A)

Although uremia has complex effects on lipoproteins and is associated with atherogenic dyslipidemias, the epidemiologic evidence to support an adverse impact is weak. Dialysis patients have higher levels of lipoprotein(a) and of low-molecular-weight apolipoprotein(a) isoforms than those in patients with normal renal function.[123] Evidence concerning the atherogenic potential of lipoprotein(a) has been reported from prospective studies in hemodialysis patients.[298, 299]

OTHER POTENTIAL RISK FACTORS

There is increasing evidence that circulating levels of apoptotic molecules (soluble Fas and soluble Fas ligand) may play an important clinical role in atherogenesis.[300, 301] Epidemiologic studies are now required to better define this relationship.

Carnitine insufficiency also has been associated with atherogenic risk, although elucidation through appropriate clinical longitudinal studies is currently lacking. Some patients appear to benefit from administration of carnitine, possibly through an improvement in erythrocyte Na^+,K^+-ATPase activity and prolonged red blood cell life span.[302, 303] It is an expensive compound, however, and further preliminary trials would appear wise before larger interventional studies are considered.

Summary

Current epidemiologic evidence supports the importance of the traditional cardiac risk factors in a predisposition to the excessive cardiovascular event rate in chronic uremia. Furthermore, the hemodynamic and metabolic perturbations characteristic of this state further predispose to cardiac hypertrophy and vascular disease, which magnify the cardiac risk in these patients.

MANAGEMENT

Diagnosis

Substantial developments in diagnostic techniques for the appraisal of cardiovascular disease have occurred in the last decade. These diagnostic tools can often be applied across the spectrum of CKD; they can be used to investigate both ischemic and cardiomyopathic disease, and they are limited by the same clinical considerations, both renal and cardiovascular. In a practical context, it is of course assumed that careful clinical assessment will always precede further diagnostic endeavors.

Cardiac Disease

ELECTROCARDIOGRAPHY

The increasing prevalence of LV hypertrophy as renal function worsens predisposes to abnormalities in resting and exercise electrocardiographic (ECG) findings in patients with CKD. In dialysis patients, minor incremental changes in the PR and QRS intervals, together with nonspecific ST-T wave changes, are frequently seen in the resting ECG. Changes may be more manifest during dialysis because of the substantial intracellular and extracellular electrolyte shifts, and a concurrent reduction in extracellular fluid levels has been found to alter the QRS amplitude.[304] However, in episodes of acute coronary ischemia (unstable angina and myocardial infarction), classic ECG changes seem to occur as expected.

Ambulatory ECG recordings have identified asymptomatic ST-T wave changes, particularly during and after dialysis.[305, 306] Whether this relates to underlying coronary ischemia or electrolyte shifts has not been determined. Exercise-related ECG changes should be interpreted with caution. Resting abnormalities, a restricted maximal pulse rate (autonomic neuropathy), and limited exercise capacity in patients with CKD may either mask or erroneously predict underlying ischemia.

BIOCHEMICAL MARKERS OF ISCHEMIA

Serial estimates of levels of standard myocardial enzymes (creatine phosphokinase and lactate dehydrogenase), when elevated, reliably diagnose acute myocardial infarction in CKD, although single estimates have poor specificity.[307]

Recently, attention has focused on the role of troponin levels in acute ischemia. The troponin complex regulates the contraction of striated muscle and consists of three subunits: troponin C, which binds to calcium ions; troponin I, which binds to actin and inhibits actin-myosin interactions; and troponin T, which binds to tropomyosin, thereby attaching the troponin complex to the thin filament. The presence of either troponin T or troponin I in the serum can be used to assess acute ischemia. Although each is present in both skeletal and cardiac muscle, they are encoded by different genes and retain immunologic specificity. They are considered more sensitive than cardiac enzymes for estimating severity of myocardial infarction,[308] and they have been shown to predict short-term cardiac mortality.[309] In CKD, despite concerns regarding impaired troponin clearance as renal function worsened, third-generation cardiac troponin T assays were found to be an independent predictor of death within 30 days across the whole spectrum of renal function in 7033 patients studied.[310]

ECHOCARDIOGRAPHY

Two-dimensional and M-mode echocardiographic studies provide a noninvasive assessment of LV structure and function, together with imaging of valves and pericardium. Systolic dysfunction, diagnosed by low fractional shortening or ejection fraction, can be determined, as can LV geometry and LV hypertrophy. The degree of hypertrophy can be identified by increased LV wall thickness or by calculating the LV mass index according to various formulas. Systolic failure is measured more accurately with the use of nuclear scintigraphy, as is the detection of regional wall abnormalities.

Although LV mass measurement using echocardiography is highly reproducible between observers, its measurement varies over the course of a hemodialysis session by as much as 25 g/m^2.[102] This occurs because LV internal diastolic diameter decreases as a result of fluid removal during the procedure. A concurrent decrease in LV wall thickness is not observed. Consequently, the LV mass index measured before dialysis is higher than that measured afterward, although the actual LV mass has not changed. Therefore, whenever possible, imaging should be carried out when the patient has achieved so-called dry weight—the weight below which hypotension or symptoms such as muscle cramps occur.

Diastolic LV function can be assessed noninvasively with the use of pulsed Doppler analysis of flow across the mitral valve during diastole. Normally, as the mitral valve opens, ventricular relaxation occurs, with a rapid increase in flow leading to an E (early) peak, followed by a later increase, the A (atrial) peak, which reflects atrial contraction. Assuming normal atrial function, the increased stiffness of the hypertrophic LV leads to a smaller E peak and a larger A peak, expressed conveniently as a decreased E/A ratio.

Dobutamine stress echocardiography is achieving recognition as a screening tool for ischemic heart disease in patients with CKD. It can also be used in patients with valvular disease or impaired systolic function to assess underlying systolic reserve. In the general population, the overall sensitivity and specificity for detection of CAD have been reported as 80% and 84%, respectively, with improved sensitivity as the number of affected vessels increases.[311] Sensitivity was comparable to that of exercise-related scintigraphic scanning in one study in patients with known CAD,[312] although it may be reduced in women and in the elderly.[311] In CKD, it has some inherent advantages over scintigraphy, particularly for those patients who are unable to exercise significantly. For dialysis patients, negative predictive values in excess of 95% have been reported with reasonable patient numbers and follow-up times.[313, 314]

NUCLEAR SCINTIGRAPHIC SCANNING

Nuclear scintigraphy can be used both for assessment of myocardial systolic function and for ischemia. The former method examines ejection fraction of the left and/or right ventricle and relies on gated analysis techniques. Care needs to be taken with regard to associated valve regurgitation, which, when present, can substantially confound functional estimates. If valve function is intact, accurate estimates of systolic function at rest and with exercise can be achieved.

The predominant role for nuclear scanning techniques, however, is in the assessment of myocardial ischemia, both as a screening tool in the workup for transplantation and in cases of diagnostic uncertainty. Exercise-based studies and dipyridamole to enhance vasodilatation are commonly employed, together with ^{99m}Tc-labeled thallium, methoxy-isobutylisonitrite (MIBI), or metaiodobenzylguanidine (MIBG). Inherent problems with scintigraphy need to be taken into consideration: blood pressure may be too high or too low to permit safe administration of a vasodilatory agent; high endogenous circulating levels of adenosine may blunt the efficacy of dipyridamole[315]; coronary flow reserve may be reduced due to LV hypertrophy and small vessel disease[313]; and symmetrical coronary disease or a blunted tachycardic response due to autonomic neuropathy, or both, can mask significant pathology.

Studies have shown a varying response to and reliability of scanning. One study of 80 patients reported a significantly increased mortality in those with, compared to those without, reversible ischemia. Fixed as opposed to reversible defects were predictive of future cardiac death but at a later period.[315] Dahan and colleagues[316] found positive and negative predictive values of 47% and 91%, respectively, for coronary events using comparative thallium scanning and coronary angiography in a study of 60 asymptomatic hemodialysis patients over 2.8 years. Other studies have shown a poor sensitivity and positive predictive value for mortality over time.[317, 313] It is likely that on-site expertise, together with the recognized testing limitations in patients with CKD described earlier, influences the utility of nuclear scanning and to some extent dictates interpretation and screening strategy for a particular center.

ELECTRON-BEAM ULTRAFAST COMPUTED TOMOGRAPHY–DERIVED CORONARY ARTERY CALCIFICATION

The relatively new technique of electron-beam ultrafast computed tomography (EBCT) relies on the principle that coronary artery calcification is a reliable surrogate for significant coronary atherosclerosis.[318] This is far from certain in patients with CKD. As has been discussed, widespread and severe vessel wall calcification is common in uremia owing to the combination of a highly positive net calcium balance, excessive use of vitamin D analogs, and a relatively

"closed" skeleton. Nonetheless, evidence is accumulating that increased calcium content per se is a poor prognostic sign.[16, 207, 319, 320] Of note, EBCT has been used recently to demonstrate a reduction in coronary artery calcification after treatment with the non–calcium-containing medication sevelamer, although subsequent effects on cardiovascular events or mortality were not defined.[321] The role of EBCT in evaluating risk or disease in patients undergoing transplantation also is unknown.

CORONARY ANGIOGRAPHY

The diagnosis of large vessel CAD can be problematic in patients with CKD for several reasons. Patients are frequently asymptomatic; they have a relatively high prevalence of nonatherosclerotic ischemia; and many who are at highest risk are unable to exercise sufficiently to facilitate noninvasive diagnosis. Despite the availability of newer diagnostic tools, as already discussed, the sensitivity and specificity of most techniques are limited, and the "gold standard" for diagnosis of CAD remains coronary angiography.[322]

In patients not receiving dialysis there is some risk of contrast nephropathy, and in all patients with CKD there is a risk of cholesterol embolization with angiography. Coronary angiography should be reserved for those patients with unstable angina/myocardial infarction on maximal therapy in whom coronary revascularization is a viable therapeutic modality.

For reasons of cost, access, demand, and possible deterioration in renal function, it is not possible to screen all patients with CKD by formal angiography. This is of particular significance for patients being evaluated for transplantation, and some effort has been directed to establishing guidelines to determine which patients are most at risk and hence may benefit from coronary catheterization. In one study, it was found that more than 60% of angiograms in 89 patients being assessed for transplantation could have been avoided by restricting angiography to diabetics and those patients with a history or symptoms of ischemic heart disease, without changing their place on the transplantation waiting list.[323] Most units now have a strategy (often a cascade algorithm) to determine which patients require more intensive cardiac workup in this context, usually stratified into diabetics and nondiabetics. The American Society of Transplant Physicians advocates screening all patients except those at lowest risk for ischemic heart disease,[322] a recommendation that acknowledges the high prevalence of asymptomatic CAD in the dialysis population.[87]

Vascular Disease

Several techniques are now available for the evaluation of peripheral blood vessels and blood flow. These include duplex ultrasonography and color-flow imaging, the ankle-brachial index test, venous plethysmography and brachial artery reactivity, magnetic resonance imaging and angiography, intravascular ultrasonography, and digital imaging.

DUPLEX ULTRASONOGRAPHY AND DOPPLER COLOR-FLOW IMAGING

Technical advances in ultrasonography have allowed reproducible measurements of blood vessels and blood flow in a wide variety of vessels.[324-326] The various vascular beds have typical waveforms, and alterations from normal indicate disease. General features of a diseased arterial segment include spectral broadening of the waveform signal, increased flow velocity at the site of vessel narrowing, and prestenotic waveform characteristics above a site of obstruction or poststenotic characteristics below it. Peak systolic velocity is the most reliable waveform measurement and the one least subject to interobserver variability.[327]

The assessment of large-vessel pulse wave velocity has become important in risk factor analysis and is correlated closely with pulse pressure.[14] It requires the use of Doppler ultrasound to measure the arterial flow tracing transcutaneously at two different, accessible arterial sites simultaneously (usually carotid and femoral). From this, the aortic pulse wave velocity, PWV, can be calculated simply by the following formula:

$$PWV = D/t$$

where D is the distance between the two recording sites and t is the difference in time. An increase in pulse wave velocity due to large vessel stiffening, as described earlier, is a potent predictor of mortality and can be affected favorably by the use of angiotensin-converting enzyme (ACE) inhibitors in particular.

ANKLE-BRACHIAL INDEX TEST

The most useful initial screening test for arterial disease of the lower extremities is the ankle-brachial index. It is determined by continuous-wave Doppler interrogation of blood pressure measurements in the ankle and arm. The index is determined by dividing ankle SBP by arm SBP. Measurements are usually taken at rest and after a standardized treadmill exercise. Completion of the protocol without pain virtually excludes the diagnosis of vascular claudication. A normal resting ankle-brachial index is 1 or 1.1. Progressive decrements indicate worsening, often multilevel, arterial stenosis. A resting ankle pressure of less than 50 mm Hg or an ankle-brachial index of less than 0.26 indicates severe, limb-threatening arterial compromise.[328] However, the hallmark of arterial insufficiency of the lower extremity is a decrease in the ankle-brachial index after exercise.

Potential problems of the ankle-brachial index test include changes in brachial pressure caused by upper-extremity vascular disease and calcification of blood vessels. Diabetics often display an increased ankle-brachial index due to arteriosclerosis and medial wall calcification. In this case, a toe SBP (versus arm SBP) index can be useful; normal values are greater than 0.6.

PLETHYSMOGRAPHY AND BRACHIAL ARTERY REACTIVITY

Recently, venous plethysmography and high-precision ultrasonography have been used in dialysis patients to assess postischemic forearm blood flow and brachial and radial artery reactivity to heat-induced peripheral dilatation. By combining plethysmographic data and assessment of IMT, pulse wave velocity, and LV mass, it has been possible to show that dialysis patients have a reduced postischemic vasodilatory capacity that correlates with large vessel stiffening, IMT, markers of endothelial cell activation, and LV mass index.[329, 330]

An initial suggestion was that endothelial dysfunction in these patients may be a factor influencing large vessel cardiovascular change. Large vessel compliance was improved by chronic ACE inhibition with perindopril, suggesting not only a causal link between endothelial cell activation and large vessel compliance but one amenable to treatment. Further studies will be of interest.

MAGNETIC RESONANCE IMAGING AND ANGIOGRAPHY

Magnetic resonance imaging and angiography are becoming widely used techniques for evaluating blood vessels. Magnetic resonance techniques are especially useful in evaluating arterial dissection and in characterizing vessel-wall morphology (including hematoma or thrombus). Some success has also been found in imaging renal and mesenteric vessels, which is an attractive option for patients in whom invasive investigation is relatively contraindicated, particularly those at high risk for cholesterol embolization or radiocontrast-induced nephropathy. Current limitations include the high cost of the study, patient dissatisfaction with the technique (especially the claustrophobia experienced during a scan), the need to ensure there is no indwelling metal hardware, and difficulty with patient positioning. Decreased scan times and more open design of the newer machines have lessened patient-related problems.

INTRAVASCULAR ULTRASONOGRAPHY

Intravascular ultrasonography is most widely used as an adjunct to peripheral vascular and coronary intervention and can characterize vessel and plaque morphology. Using high-frequency ultrasound transducers and imaging of the vessel lumen, this technique avoids some of the drawbacks of transcutaneous ultrasound, such as shadowing artifact from vessel-wall calcification and acoustic impedance from interposed tissues. Computerized, three-dimensional reconstruction techniques can be used to display a map or facsimile of the vessel lumen.

DIGITAL IMAGING

Digital imaging technology is an important advance in noninvasive imaging of the vascular system. The ability to store information in a digital format allows remote reading and serial comparisons of studies via telemedicine.[331] Theoretically, the patient's entire imaging history could be stored in this format and could be easily transferred to different imaging stations, despite differences in viewing equipment or software. Such an application has important clinical and research applications.

Treatment
Cardiac Disease
CARDIOMYOPATHY AND CARDIAC FAILURE

A reversible precipitating or aggravating factor is frequently found in patients with CKD who present with cardiac failure. Arrhythmias, underlying myocardial ischemia, anemia, uncontrolled hypertension, and the use of drugs that may adversely affect cardiac performance (particularly those associated with negative inotropic activity or tachycardia) can all precipitate a clinical presentation of cardiac failure.

In patients with CKD also, the synergistic and destructive effects of an increase in extracellular volume frequently coexist with cardiac failure and, in combination with myocardial dysfunction, precipitate the need for initiation of dialysis. Dialysis patients with severe myocardial impairment require ultrafiltration acutely, which is associated with less metabolic perturbation than acute dialysis is. Careful assessment of target weight is necessary, and more formal cardiac evaluation, according to the clinical context, is required, although echocardiography is often mandatory. For reasons outlined earlier, echocardiograms are most accurate when performed at the patient's dry weight, which may not be possible until several days after an acute admission. In diabetic dialysis patients, there is also some evidence that transplantation reduces the incidence of cardiac failure and associated hospitalization.[81] An approach to the treatment of LV disorders is shown in Figure 50-8.

PHARMACOTHERAPY. In a clinical setting, most patients with cardiac failure and CKD require numerous medications for appropriate control and treatment. Combination therapy is therefore the rule, and interactions among medications need careful consideration, particularly with regard to reductions in dose or frequency. Other issues, such as effects on comorbid conditions (e.g., diabetes, peripheral vascular disease, glaucoma, chronic airflow obstruction), compliance, and potential interactions with other drugs (e.g., immunosuppression, anticoagulants, statin therapy) can be important.

Loop diuretics are indispensable for achieving and maintaining euvolemia in all patients with cardiac failure, including those with CKD. Their effect is attenuated in patients with advanced renal failure, but not as severely as that of thiazide diuretics, which usually become ineffective with a GFR lower than 30 mL/min. However, the synergistic diuretic effect of loop diuretics and thiazides persists even at relatively advanced stages of renal insufficiency and can be a useful therapeutic option. The effects of aldosterone antagonists

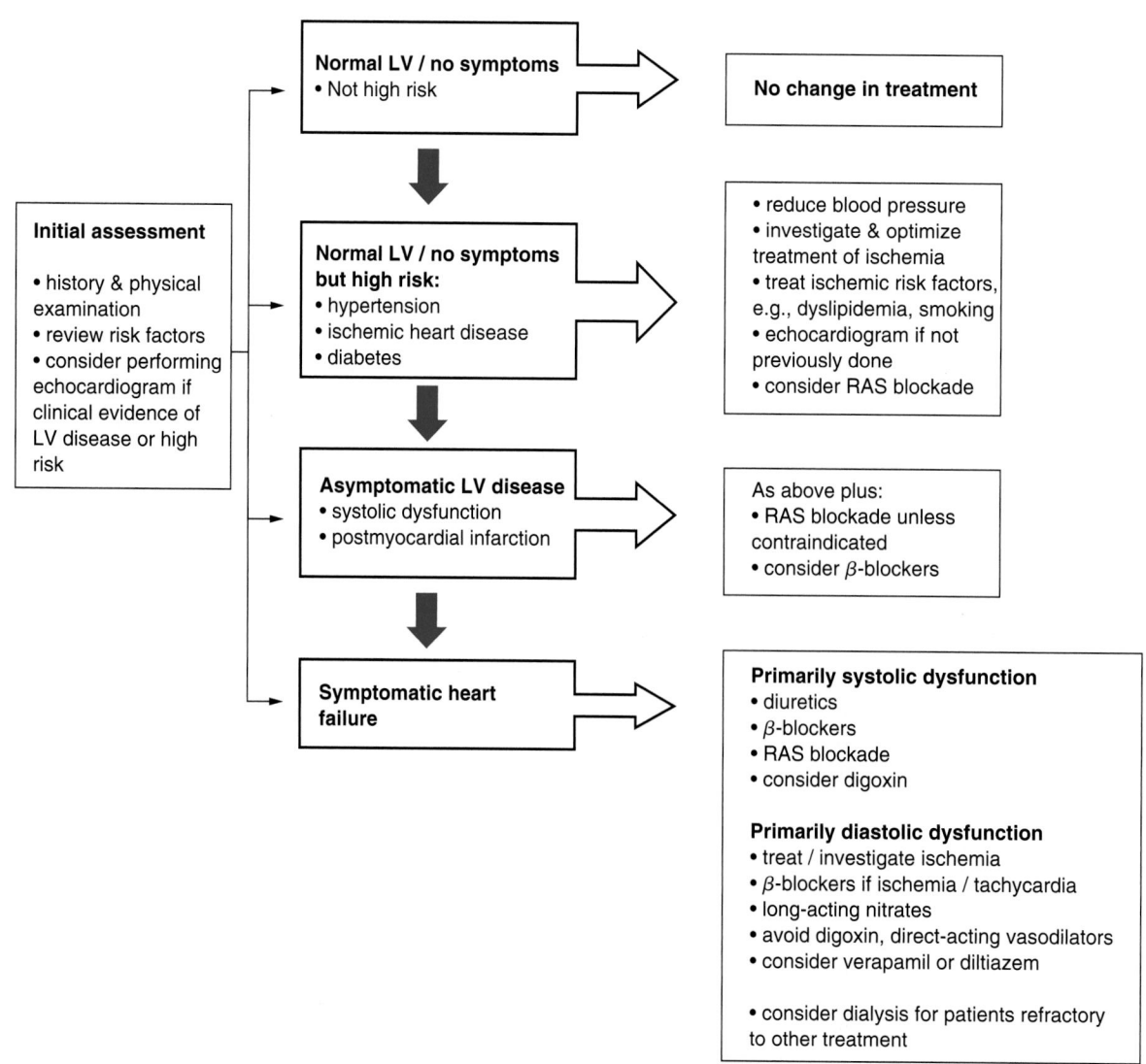

FIGURE 50-8. An approach to the treatment of left ventricular (LV) disorders and cardiac failure in patients with chronic kidney disease. RAS, renin-angiotensin system.

are unpredictable in patients with CKD. They exert a weak diuretic action, and perhaps the primary reason for consideration of their use resides in their recently reported benefit in cardiac disease or reduction in proteinuria in patients with CKD.[332, 333] Hyperkalemia in particular can result when these drugs are combined with blockade of the renin-angiotensin system or β-receptor antagonists in the setting of CKD. Dose reduction or avoidance is advised in such circumstances.

ACE inhibitors have clearly been shown to relieve symptoms, decrease morbidity, and improve survival in nonuremic individuals with heart failure.[334] It seems reasonable to extrapolate these results to the dialysis population and to recommend the use of these agents. The benefit of ACE inhibition is applicable to patients with diastolic and systolic dysfunction. ACE inhibitors should also be used to prevent cardiac failure in asymptomatic patients whose LV ejection fraction is less than 35%[335] and in post–myocardial infarction patients with an ejection fraction of 40% or less.[336] Although these drugs have not been as well studied in patients with CKD, it is reasonable to consider using them if there is no contraindication. It is unlikely that ACE inhibitors can produce a reduction in GFR generally in CKD, given the beneficial effects on renal function preservation observed in diabetics with the use of angiotensin receptor (AR) antagonists.[337-339] However, their effects in patients with a GFR lower than 25 mL/min is largely unknown, and, until better data are available, caution may be advisable in this group as well as in patients with severe renovascular disease, acute renal dysfunction, or posttransplantation status. Hyperkalemia in moderately advanced CKD and renal artery stenosis in a transplanted kidney are additional concerns requiring monitoring after treatment is started. Apart from renoprotection in diabetics, there is less information available for AR antagonists. They are probably as effective as ACE inhibitors for cardiac failure, but there is no evidence that the risk of serious side effects is any lower.

β-Receptor antagonists improve the prognosis of individuals with asymptomatic systolic dysfunction, regardless of whether they have had a myocardial infarction.[340] Comparable mortality-based trials have not been conducted in the dialysis population, but improvements in LV dimensions and fractional shortening have been demonstrated.[341] Chronic activation of the adrenergic nervous system is recognized in hemodialysis patients. It contributes to the development of LV hypertrophy, ischemia, and myocyte damage and exerts a maladaptive role in chronic heart failure.[342] In a meta-analysis of 22 trials in patients with mild to moderate heart failure, the odds ratio for death was 0.65 with β-receptor antagonists, and the odds ratio for hospitalization with heart failure was 0.64.[343] In more severe heart failure, carvedilol has also been proved efficacious.[344] However, it is possible that the positive role of the adrenergic system in supporting the failing circulation may be inappropriately blocked in some patients, causing intensification of heart failure.[345] In recommending increased use of β-receptor antagonists in dialysis patients, one should remember that the contraindications to their use (reactive airway disease, sinus-node dysfunction, and cardiac conduction abnormalities) occur frequently in this group of patients. Furthermore, the dose of some drugs (e.g., atenolol) often needs to be reduced according to the degree of renal impairment, and agents with intrinsic sympathomimetic activity appear to be detrimental and should not be used in patients with cardiac failure.

The use of digoxin is controversial. It relieves symptoms in subjects with heart failure but no renal disease, and clinical deterioration may occur when it is discontinued.[346] It has not been found to reduce mortality, however, and its use is associated with a variety of risks in patients with severe impairment of kidney function. These risks include a predisposition to toxicity because of impaired clearance as renal function declines and an increased risk of arrhythmia in association with hypokalemia, which can occur particularly during or after dialysis. Based on these results, it is reasonable to consider the use of digoxin for rate control in atrial fibrillation and for patients with substantial systolic dysfunction or symptoms despite the use of other agents, with or without atrial fibrillation. It should usually be avoided in subjects with diastolic dysfunction, because the increased contractility can exacerbate diastolic function, although cautious use in this group to control rapid atrial fibrillation is reasonable, particularly if β-receptor antagonists are contraindicated. Other inotropic agents, with the possible exception of dobutamine in intractable cases, are not recommended.

The treatment of diastolic dysfunction is less well defined. Attempts to eliminate the cause are usually the focus of therapy. This includes aggressive control of hypertension, treatment of anemia, and control of other factors responsible for the development of LV hypertrophy. Relatively contraindicated in systolic cardiac failure, the drugs of choice in diastolic failure are probably verapamil and diltiazem, which enhance LV diastolic relaxation.[347, 348] Other agents to consider include long-acting nitrates, which may be advantageous in some patients, and β-receptor antagonists, which are useful for treating concurrent ischemia and tachycardia. Excessive diuresis should be avoided, as should the use of digoxin, as previously mentioned, because of a probable increase in hypercontractility. Direct vasodilators, such as prazosin, hydralazine, or minoxidil, are generally contraindicated in this setting.[349]

ISCHEMIC HEART DISEASE

The treatment of both the acute (unstable angina and acute myocardial infarction) and the nonacute (stable angina and cardiac failure) presentations of CAD in patients with CKD is the same as in the general population.

PHARMACOTHERAPY. Patients with CKD and stable angina who have not had an infarct should be treated with standard antianginal agents for relief of symptoms. For those who have had an infarct, β-receptor blockade should be prescribed if tolerated, as should an ACE inhibitor for patients with LV dysfunction. To date there have been no studies of aspirin for either primary or secondary treatment of myocardial ischemia in the CKD or the dialysis population. Although the benefit of aspirin in nonuremic patients is substantial, the risk of complications, mainly bleeding, probably increases as renal function declines and effects of uremia increase. This was also the finding of a recent meta-analysis of aspirin therapy looking at more than 45,000 subjects in the general community.[350] Consequently, advocating widespread use of aspirin for the primary prevention of CAD cannot be recommended. Nevertheless, the benefits probably outweigh the risks for patients with acute presentations of ischemia and for those who are at high risk of the same. There are few data regarding the efficacy of clopidogrel in CKD, and further details regarding risks versus benefits are required before recommendations can be made.

CORONARY REVASCULARIZATION. Despite the relatively high incidence of asymptomatic ischemia in CKD, due presumably to autonomic disease associated with uremia or diabetes, there is no evidence to suggest that investigation and treatment in these patients results in improved mortality statistics. For patients who have had an infarction, angiography is indicated if there are symptoms of myocardial ischemia at rest or after minimal exertion, or if there is early, severe ischemia during a stress test. For other patients, coronary angiography should be limited to those with symptoms refractory to medical therapy. As in the general population, coronary arteriography should be reserved for patients in whom revascularization (angioplasty, stenting, or bypass grafting) would be undertaken if critical CAD were identified. This decision can be difficult, particularly in light of a recognized inability to predict life span in dialysis patients.[9] It should therefore be based on an assessment of the significance of the lesion, the operative risk, and overall life expectancy made by the cardiologist and nephrologist.

The initial success rate for coronary angioplasty for patients with CKD is greater than 90% in most published series. The restenosis rate in the general population is roughly 30% at 1 year. The rate in uremic patients is unclear because studies have been difficult to compare, although early studies in which repeat angiography was performed in all patients demonstrated poor results, with more than 80% restenosis in some series. One of the larger studies to assess clinical outcome in CKD patients analyzed a registry of more than 5000 patients undergoing coronary angioplasty.[351] Initial success was similar in all groups, but the 1 year mortality rate varied proportionately with renal function, with an increase from 18.3% in patients with a creatinine clearance of less than 30 mL/min to 1.5% if clearance was greater than 70 mL/min. Other reports have found similar results.[352-354]

Among hemodialysis patients, the in-hospital mortality rate for coronary artery bypass grafting (CABG) is 12.5%, or four times higher than in the general population.[355, 356] Hence, there is a consensus in favor of bypass surgery for left main or extensive three-vessel disease and in favor of angioplasty for single-vessel disease. In the remaining multivessel cases, it appears that clinical outcomes with angioplasty with stents are similar to those with CABG, but more repeat revascularization procedures are needed.[356] In view of the propensity for restenosis after angioplasty in dialysis patients,[357, 358] CABG is probably the revascularization procedure of choice, although angioplasty with stenting may be useful in single-vessel disease or in multivessel disease with culprit lesions. There are recent encouraging reports also of a substantial reduction in restenosis rate up to 6 months after stenting with the use of sirolimus-coated stents in high-risk patients.[359]

Although the prevalence of coronary artery disease is high among incident dialysis patients,[360] it is uncertain whether transplant recipients are at an increased risk of death from myocardial ischemia.[218, 361] There are few data regarding the outcome of revascularization procedures. However, case reports and small series suggest that transplanted patients with near-normal renal function have a perioperative mortality rate and a long-term survival rate that are close to those observed in the nondialysis population.[361-365]

In summary, the evidence suggests that patients with CKD in general are at higher risk for complications and have poorer long-term outcomes, regardless of the revascularization procedure used. It is not meaningful to compare clinical trials of angioplasty and CABG because of the marked inherent selection bias. Coronary artery stenting does appear to confer a benefit over angioplasty alone, and stents coated with immunosuppressive agents may have further advantages. Effectively, the decision for a particular procedure will rely on the specific cardiac and overall clinical condition of the patient, together with available resources.

ARRHYTHMIAS AND VALVULAR DISEASE

Specific and detailed management of cardiac arrhythmias is largely beyond the scope of this text. An awareness of the potential for and types of arrhythmias likely to be encountered is advocated and management should accord with general principles. Perhaps the most important practical consideration is to solicit cardiologic advice and support for patients with resistant or troublesome arrhythmias and/or poor cardiac function. The combination frequently coexists. Consideration of the renal metabolism of drugs (such as digoxin and β-receptor antagonists) in patients with impaired renal function is necessary, as is the disturbed homeostasis of monovalent and divalent ions in the CKD population. Hyperkalemia, hypocalcemia, hypomagnesemia, and hyponatremia can all potentially complicate the pathogenesis and treatment of cardiac arrhythmias.

In CKD patients with mitral or aortic valve disease, primary control of potentiating factors (listed previously), frequent monitoring once valve aperture is encroached, and appraisal of the individual patient and associated comordities once surgery is considered would appear, in the absence of evidence, to be a reasonable approach to treatment.

Vascular Disease

Discussion of much of the extensive vascular disease that patients with CKD experience is beyond the scope of this chapter. Diabetic patients in particular are prone to macrovascular and microvascular disease in most arterial beds from a relatively early stage of renal impairment. A variety of risk factors predisposes to vascular disease in these beds, as occurs in the coronary arterial tree.

CAROTID ARTERY DISEASE

Carotid ultrasonography has become a useful surrogate marker for large vessel vascular disease. It has become the mainstay of diagnosis of symptomatic and asymptomatic carotid disease and is used to assess both atherosclerotic plaques and IMT. However, interventional studies of carotid artery disease are limited. There are no reports of treatment and associated outcome of atheromatous plaque disease in CKD, and evaluation of IMT is at best a surrogate end point. No interventional studies attempting to reduce risk factor exposures have yet shown a clear benefit on IMT.[366, 367]

Further prospective interventional studies may clarify the significance and relevance of both carotid atheroma and IMT in relation to morbidity and mortality in CKD.

PERIPHERAL VASCULAR DISEASE

Peripheral vascular disease is an extremely debilitating and expensive comorbid cardiovascular complication among patients with CKD. It is present more commonly in patients undergoing dialysis, presumably because of the concentration of atherogenic risk factors in this group, though it is seen also in predialysis and transplantation groups. Its incidence appears to be increasing, with the 2000 USRDS report demonstrating an increase from 14.3% to 15.4% between 1995 and 1997 in incident dialysis patients. In transplantation, amputation for peripheral vascular disease is the most common vascular complication after renal transplantation, occurring in 13% to 25% of allograft recipients within 5 years after transplantation.[368] Peripheral vascular disease is more common in diabetics, and other risk factors include age (in nondiabetics only), hypertension, dyslipidemia, smoking, and CAD. Blacks may be at lower risk for the development of peripheral vascular disease.[369]

In the United Kingdom and in Sweden, reductions in limb amputation by up to 80% have been described after treatment in specialized multidisciplinary clinics.[370, 371] The cost–benefit ratio for such clinics is considerable. Specific treatment includes prevention, conservative management, and amputation. General measures of primary foot care are inadequately reinforced in most cases. Smoking cessation is theoretically important, although no studies to assess the benefits of cessation have been performed. Exercise is probably the best conservative measure available to relieve claudication symptoms, but it is of little benefit in advanced microvascular disease.

Medications are not frequently used in these patients. A randomized study of pentoxifylline showed no benefit in walking distance over placebo. Furthermore, levels accumulate in moderate renal impairment.[372] Cilostazol, a new cyclic adenosine monophosphate (cAMP) phosphodiesterase inhibitor, has improved claudication distances in randomized trials but has altered lipid binding in CKD and may not be safe.[373] The use of statins does not appear to be of benefit, in contrast to the situation with CAD, and there is no evidence pertaining to aspirin or other agents.

Angioplasty is suitable in some patients, although frequently the lesions are multiple and diffuse and involve small vessels. Recurrence of symptoms in non-CKD patients occurs early, and there are no trials examining effects in patients with CKD. Intermittent claudication is the most common reason for bypass surgery (73% in one study),[374] and evidence for appropriate intervention in CKD is lacking. Nonetheless, in dialysis patients, conservative therapy (amputation or autoamputation) has been advocated as a primary maneuver because of the high risk of primary failure of bypass surgery, symptom recurrence, and perioperative mortality.[375, 376]

A total of almost 36,000 amputations were performed in the United States Medicare Dialysis program between 1991 and 1994. The crude amputation rate for all patients on dialysis was 4.3/100 person-years, compared with 13.8/100 person-years for diabetic patients. The rate increased over the 3 years of the study. Survival after amputation was dismal,

with only 30% still alive after 2 years. The presence of gangrene, below-knee (compared with above-toe) amputation, and age older than 55 years were associated with a higher risk of death after amputation. Dossa and colleagues[377] recorded a hospital mortality rate of 7% and a 2-year survival rate of 79% in 375 predialysis patients; for dialysis patients, the comparable figures were 24% and 27%, respectively.

In each of these studies, the amputation rate in transplantation patients was significantly lower than for dialysis patients. Particular risk factors for the transplantation group included associated ischemic heart disease, undergoing dialysis before transplantation, and having an abnormal brachial-ankle index at the time of transplantation.[378]

Risk Factor Intervention

Table 50-4 lists pharmacologic and nonpharmacologic interventions to minimize cardiovascular disease risk in patients with CKD.

TRADITIONAL RISK FACTORS

Most individual cardiac risk factors are more prevalent in subjects with CKD, and they are commonly clustered in an individual. Hence, efforts to reduce cardiovascular disease risk, although dealt with separately here, usually require a multifaceted approach that addresses numerous risk factors simultaneously.

HYPERTENSION

Predialysis. ACE inhibitors or AR antagonists are considered the agents of first choice in most patients owing to

---

TABLE 50-4

Interventions to Minimize Cardiovascular Disease Risk in Patients with Chronic Kidney Disease

Nonpharmacologic Interventions

Stop tobacco use
Minimize excess extracellular fluid to target blood pressure <140/90 mm Hg
Awareness and prevention of inflammation and hypoalbuminemia
Dietary modification to target low-density lipoprotein cholesterol <100 mg/dL
Renal transplantation when appropriate
Coronary revascularization for secondary prevention of ischemic vascular disease

Pharmacologic Interventions

Drug therapy to target blood pressure <140/90 mm Hg
Epoetin and iron therapy to target hemoglobin concentration >110 g/L (upper limits not clearly defined)
Treatment with HMG-CoA reductase inhibitor (statin) therapy to target low-density lipoprotein cholesterol <100 mg/dL
Treat abnormal divalent ion levels to target serum calcium 9.2–9.6 mg/dL, serum phosphate 2.5–5.5 mg/dL, and intact parathyroid hormone 100–200 pg/mL
Anti-platelet agents in patients with coronary disease, vascular disease, or diabetes
Appropriate use of ACE inhibitors (or ARAs in predialysis patients) for treatment of proteinuria and arteriosclerosis
Use of ACE inhibitors and β-receptor antagonists in patients with known ischemic vascular disease

ACE, angiotensin-converting enzyme; ARA, angiotensin receptor antagonist; HMG-CoA, 3-hydroxy-3-methylglutaryl coenzyme A.

their documented benefit in delaying the progression of CKD in both diabetic and nondiabetic disease, particularly with associated proteinuria.[337-339, 379-383] Ramipril has improved cardiovascular disease outcomes in patients with decreased GFR and at least one cardiovascular disease risk factor in addition to either diabetes or manifest vascular disease.[217] Losartan has reduced hospitalization for heart failure in diabetics with overt nephropathy.[337] It appears that the beneficial impact of blockade of the renin-angiotensin system is more than can be accounted for by lowering of blood pressure alone.

Concerns with treatment, particularly as renal function deteriorates, relate to hyperkalemia, the potential for retarding functional improvement in association with acute renal dysfunction, and the use of these agents in patients with renovascular disease. Calcium channel blockers, particularly the dihydropyridines, have not compared well against ACE inhibitors and AR antagonists in reduction of proteinuria, delay in progression of renal function, or prevention of cardiovascular events.[338, 384, 385] The use of β-receptor antagonists, diuretics, and other vasodilators depends on the response to treatment and underlying comorbid conditions. The more common of these, cardiac failure and ischemic heart disease, were covered earlier in this chapter.

Treatment of hypertension should generally aim for blood pressure levels lower than 130/85 mm Hg for individuals with parenchymal disease, 125/75 mm Hg if there is proteinuria with excretion of more than 1 g/day of protein, and 130/80 mm Hg for patients with diabetes and proteinuria with excretion less than 1 g/day of protein.[232, 386-389] In some patients, particularly diabetics with moderate to advanced renal dysfunction, blood pressure can be highly resistant to intervention, requiring extensive combination treatment.

Dialysis. The goal of therapy in dialysis patients is maintenance of normal extracellular fluid volume, and there is evidence to suggest that a dialysis regimen with long, slow ultrafiltration is associated with normotension, regression of LV hypertrophy, and improved survival.[239, 390] A reasonable target blood pressure for antihypertensive treatment is less than 140/90 mm Hg before dialysis, unless the patient develops symptomatic hypotension or low blood pressure during or after dialysis. Patients whose blood pressure is higher than 140/90 mm Hg after achievement of dry weight should have antihypertensive drugs prescribed.

Selection of antihypertensive agents is best guided by the presence of associated comorbid conditions. In their absence, there are data supporting the effectiveness of ACE inhibitors, possibly through reduction in pulse wave velocity and arterial stiffness. For example, in two studies of hemodialysis patients ACE inhibitors were associated with regression of LV hypertrophy.[391, 392] However, there have been no large, randomized trials to support one agent over another. Hence, patients with reduced LV systolic function are likely to benefit from ACE inhibitors or AR antagonists, and patients with relatively intact LV function after myocardial infarction should be treated with β-receptor antagonists. Practical difficulties in this patient group in particular include associated cerebrovascular or coronary disease, advanced age, and cardiovascular instability in relation to ultrafiltration. In such situations, blood pressure requires individual targeting and some compromise on the optimal target.

Transplantation. Limited data are available concerning intervention in the transplantation group. Calcium channel blockers are widely used because they are well tolerated and because of their effects in counteracting calcineurin-mediated vasoconstriction. The use of ACE inhibitors or AR antagonists is probably justified in most patients, although issues relating to hyperkalemia, anemia, and uremia warrant consideration, particularly during the first 12 months after transplantation.[225, 393] The American Society of Transplantation recommends maintaining blood pressure below 140/90 mm Hg, lower if possible, in line with JNC VI for patients with kidney disease.[394]

DYSLIPIDEMIA. In short-term studies, statins have been recognized as being safe and efficient for patients with CKD, although their benefit in reducing cardiovascular outcomes has not yet been proved.[395-399] Advice therefore derives from trials in the general population, until results of ongoing multicenter trials in CKD[400-402] become available.

The National Kidney Foundation Task Force on Cardiovascular disease has recommended that the National Cholesterol Education Program (NCEP) Adult Treatment Panel General Population Guidelines for initial classification, treatment initiation, and target cholesterol levels for diet and drug therapy should be used for patients with CKD, because they are in the highest risk group for cardiac disease.[245] Patients with a serum cholesterol concentration higher than 200 mg/dL or an HDL-cholesterol concentration of 35 mg/dL or less should have a fasting lipid profile. LDL-cholesterol levels in excess of 100 mg/dL and 130 mg/dL or more indicate treatment initiation values for diet and drug therapy, respectively. Target LDL-cholesterol levels are below 100 mg/dL for each type of therapy. The statins are the most effective drugs to lower LDL-cholesterol in CKD and should be agents of first choice. Dose reduction should be instituted in combination with calcineurin inhibitors and may be required in individual patients as GFR declines. Fibric acid analogs are also effective, but dosage reduction is required due to reduced renal function. Failure to control LDL-cholesterol levels with statins is not uncommon. However, combination therapy in severe CKD is controversial because of the high risk of side effects. Elevated serum triglycerides or low HDL-cholesterol, in the absence of increased LDL-cholesterol, should be treated by diet and increased physical activity; drug therapy to reduce cardiac risk is not currently recommended.

There is some degree of uncertainty concerning the overall effects of lowering cholesterol in dialysis patients: the absolute risk of atheromatous CAD is unclear, the benefit of lowering LDL-cholesterol to less than 130 mg/dL is uncertain, and the long-term risk between hyperlipidemia and the risk of cardiac events is unknown.[403] On the other hand, it is possible that patients with high CRP levels and LDL-cholesterol levels lower 130 mg/dL could benefit from the anti-inflammatory effects of statins. Ongoing large-scale studies should help ascertain the risk and cost-benefit relationships, although it should be noted that one large trial in CKD patients was stopped because of concerns about the high incidence of myositis with cerivastatin. Conversely, in a recent retrospective analysis of 3716 incident dialysis patients, statin use was independently associated with a reduced risk of all-cause and cardiovascular mortality.[404]

SMOKING. There are no studies demonstrating that cessation of smoking improves the outcome of CKD at any stage. Nevertheless, it is reasonable to extrapolate data from the general population that indicates reduction of cardiovascular risk over time after smoking cessation.[405] Nicotine or bupropion therapy should be considered to help cessation, although the kidney metabolizes nicotine and the dosage may need to be reduced as GFR declines. Little information concerning bupropion is currently available.

DIABETES. Only limited data are available regarding the potential benefits of tight glycemic control in predialysis diabetic patients. At least two trials have demonstrated that strict glycemic control reduces microvascular but not necessarily macrovascular complications of type 1 and type 2 diabetes.[248, 406] In the dialysis group, monitoring is probably inadequate, with fewer than half of those with diabetes in the USA having an annual determination of hemoglobin HbA_{1c} and less than 10% having more than three estimates per year.[407] There is one report to suggest that tight glycemic control after transplantation may reduce the development of new diabetic changes in the transplanted kidney,[408] and one study indicated that transplantation in diabetics reduces the risk of hospitalization from cardiac failure.[81] All-cause mortality may also be reduced in type 1 diabetics with combined renal and pancreatic transplantation.[409]

In the absence of definitive evidence, the approach to treatment probably rests on data from the general population, taken in conjunction with the patient's specific condition. Tight glycemic control would seem an appropriate aim in predialysis patients, unless hypoglycemic episodes are troublesome or unpredictable. There is less support for near-euglycemic levels in dialysis patients because of the inability to influence renal function and the propensity for hypoglycemia due to glucose diffusion during dialysis. In transplantation patients, tight control may be difficult because of the hyperglycemic tendency of immunosuppressive agents, and in both dialysis and transplantation patients relative hypoglycemic unawareness may exist owing to advanced vascular disease, with the potential for serious effects. Therefore, an individual approach to therapy in such situations seems advisable.

OTHER TRADITIONAL RISK FACTORS. There are few objective data regarding treatment of other risk factors in this population. Exercise in predialysis patients has been shown to improve well-being and to increase muscle strength.[410, 411] Exercise may also favorably influence lipid profiles and blood pressure levels in dialysis patients.[412, 413] In the absence of contraindications, it would seem reasonable to encourage a graded exercise program from as early a stage as possible in patients with CKD, although cardiovascular assessment should be considered in high-risk patients.

UREMIA-RELATED RISK FACTORS

Uremia-related risk factors are also described in Figures 50-4 and 50-6 and Table 50-3.

ANEMIA. Results from the Australian Multicenter Predialysis Study shows a significant increase in LV mass in patients whose hemoglobin levels fell to less than 100 g/dL over 2 years, compared with those who were maintained with epoetin at near-physiologic levels. No adverse effects were observed.[414] In the short term in hemodialysis patients, hemoglobin normalization improves the hyperkinetic heart, as shown by a decrease in LV diameter and systolic hyperfunction.[73] In hemodialysis patients with concentric

LV hypertrophy normalization of hemoglobin prevented LV dilatation, but in patients with severe LV dilatation no regression was observed.[415] In hemodialysis patients with symptomatic heart disease, normalization of hemoglobin failed to improve mortality and was associated with an increased risk of vascular access loss.[416]

Anemia is clearly a risk factor for adverse cardiac events in dialysis patients, and some benefit may occur if anemia is treated or prevented before the development of severe cardiac disease. Trials to test this hypothesis are necessary. Correction of anemia is of little benefit for patients who are in the advanced phases of cardiac disease with severe LV dilatation or symptoms.

ARTERIOSCLEROSIS. Almost exclusively, it is the dialysis population that has been assessed in regard to outcome from intervention on arteriosclerosis (distinct from hypertension). Two studies are of note, both from the same group. London and colleagues[417] compared the effects of an ACE inhibitor (perindopril) with those of a calcium channel blocker (nitrendipine) in a double-blind, randomized trial involving 24 hemodialysis patients with LV hypertrophy over a period of 12 months. At baseline, each group displayed LV hypertrophy due predominantly to an increased LV end-diastolic diameter. Similar and significant changes were found in blood pressure, total peripheral resistance, aortic and arterial pulse wave velocities, and arterial wave reflections. After treatment, there was a significant decrease in LV mass in the perindopril-treated group only. It was also found that LV mass reductions were related not to changes in LV wall thickness but rather to a reduction in LV end-diastolic diameter. Animal studies[418, 419] and a prior controlled clinical study[420] reported similar effects, with improved arterial distensibility and reduced wall thickness in response to long-term treatment with both a dihydropyridine calcium channel blocker and an ACE inhibitor, but a reduction in LV mass was evident only with the ACE inhibitor.

A similar cohort of patients was examined for the effects of blood pressure changes on 150 patients undergoing dialysis over a mean of 51 months.[14] Independent predictors of cardiovascular mortality included no reduction in pulse wave velocity in response to a blood pressure decrease (RR, 2.59; 95% confidence interval [CI], 1.51 to 4.43); an increased LV mass (RR, 1.11 per 10 g increase in LV mass index; 95% CI, 1.03 to 1.19); age (RR, 1.69; 95% CI, 1.32 to 2.17); preexisting cardiovascular disease; and, importantly, lack of ACE inhibitor treatment (RR, 0.19; 95% CI, 0.14 to 0.43). These findings were consistent with earlier descriptive studies but for the first time suggested that there might be a survival advantage in reducing pulse wave velocity. Importantly, ACE inhibitors appeared also to have a favorable effect on survival in this patient group which was independent of blood pressure change.

INFLAMMATION. As has been discussed, the source of elevated CRP levels in patients with CKD is uncertain. Accordingly, attempts at reducing inflammation have been general, rather than specific, and sometimes unintentional.[112, 421-424] Both statins and aspirin have been studied in regard to their effects on reducing inflammation in CKD patients and in the general population. Aspirin has been shown to be of greatest benefit in patients with the highest CRP levels. A reduction in CRP with the use of statin therapy has now also been demonstrated in hemodialysis patients. The suggestion is that each agent modifies the inflammatory response beyond the effects for which it was designed. As discussed in another section, the use of these agents should be considered in patients who have evidence of, or are at high risk from, cardiovascular disease, bearing in mind an increased bleeding tendency with aspirin and a risk of myositis or liver functional abnormalities with statin therapy.

HYPERHOMOCYSTEINEMIA. A combination of high-dose folic acid, vitamin B_{12}, and vitamin B_6 lowers homocysteine levels by 25%, which may restore normal levels in patients with chronic renal insufficiency or in renal transplant recipients, but not in dialysis patients.[425] No trials have yet shown that lowering homocysteine levels improves cardiovascular outcome. Neither surrogate or event-related end points were improved or reduced in association with lowered homocysteine levels in three studies in dialysis patients.[366, 367, 426] A trial is currently in progress in renal transplant recipients to determine whether treatment of hyperhomocysteinemia using vitamin supplementation can prevent cardiovascular events.

Data currently do not support supplementation with vitamin B_6, vitamin B_{12}, or doses of folate greater than 5 to 10 mg per day. Administration of folinic acid may have a role, based on promising initial studies,[427] but further results are awaited. Screening for homocysteine levels also would appear to have only a limited role and currently cannot be advocated as part of a general management strategy.

OXIDATIVE STRESS. Although evidence of increased oxidative stress in CKD exists, there are no longitudinal studies examining the impact of oxidative stress on subsequent de novo cardiac events. One small, randomized study suggested there may be some clinical advantage in the use of antioxidants. Vitamin E supplementation (800 IU daily) was given to hemodialysis patients with cardiovascular disease and produced a significant reduction in myocardial infarction compared with controls[428]; however, there was no improvement in cardiovascular or total mortality, indicating the need for further study, possibly with higher doses of vitamin E.

On the basis of current evidence for dialysis patients, it is possible only to suggest replacement of vitamins C and E lost to dialysis or metabolism rather than increased intake for antioxidant purposes. The potential for systemic oxalate deposition with the use of vitamin C provides further strength for this approach. There are no data regarding treatment of oxidative stress for predialysis or transplantation patients.

ABNORMAL DIVALENT ION METABOLISM. Patients with CKD are in a substantial positive calcium balance from an early stage of disease. Attempts to minimize the calcium load in the context of PTH and phosphate control have a sound teleologic if not yet empirical base. The appropriate use of vitamin D analogs and phosphate binders is currently recommended to achieve target levels of divalent ions and related compounds. For serum calcium, the target concentration is between 9.2 and 9.6 mg/dL, and for serum phosphate it is 2.5 to 5.5 mg/dL, to achieve a calcium-phosphate product of less than 55 mg^2/dL. The target range for intact PTH levels is suggested to be between 100 and 200 pg/mL.[429]

Many noncalcium, nonaluminum phosphate binders have been suggested, the most attractive one being polyallylamine hydrochloride, marketed as Renagel (sevelamer hydrochloride). It is an effective, albeit costly, phosphate binder that is not associated with hypercalcemia. Calcimetic agents, which reduce PTH levels, are on the horizon. In view of the pathogenic effect of PTH on intracellular calcium accumulation in myocytes and vascular smooth muscle cells, calcium channel blockade is a rational therapeutic intervention to prevent cardiovascular disease.[294] Preliminary animal evidence suggesting that deposition of intramural calcium in a rat model with CKD may be prevented with the use of a molecule related to transforming growth factor-β, bone mineral protein-7 (BMP-7), requires confirmation and assessment of relevance in human disease.[430]

PROTHROMBOTIC FACTORS. In one large meta-analysis of non-CKD patients examining primary prevention of CAD, the absolute benefit of aspirin was 0.15% reduction per year in myocardial infarction, compared with an increased risk of 0.04% per year for major noncerebral hemorrhage (noncerebral bleeds resulting in death, transfusion, or surgery) and 0.18% per year for minor hemorrhage.[431]

Aspirin therapy probably worsens the platelet defect in CKD and increases the risk of bleeding. Despite these risks, patients with overt cardiovascular disease should probably be prescribed aspirin (81 mg/day) to reduce the risk of subsequent cardiovascular events. However, for renal patients without clinical cardiac disease, although they are at high risk for development of cardiac disease, it is not possible to recommend universal use. Individual treatment decisions must be based on considerations of patients' individual risks, likely benefits, and preferences.

MULTIPLE RISK FACTOR INTERVENTION

It is likely that underutilization of efficacious therapies occurs in CKD patients[432] and that optimal targets for treatment are not achieved.[433] The excellent results achieved in the STENO study of diabetic patients receiving intensive therapy[434] and in studies of heart failure managed in multidisciplinary clinics suggest that a similar approach in CKD patients would produce better outcomes than conventional health care delivery models do. The objective of enhancing appropriate utilization of interventions to slow progression of renal disease and to prevent cardiovascular disease requires a multifaceted, multidisciplinary approach that may not be feasible under current primary care provider models.

SUMMARY

The burden of cardiovascular disease in patients with CKD is high. Multiple traditional cardiac risk factors and potential uremia-related risk factors for cardiac disease exist. The impact of the latter on the development and progression of cardiac disease and the interrelationships among these factors are currently uncertain. Severe LV hypertrophy, dilated cardiomyopathy, and CAD occur frequently and predispose to cardiac failure, myocardial infarction and angina, arrhythmias, dialysis hypotension, and death.

Predominant cardiovascular risk factors identified in CKD populations include hypertension, anemia, hypoalbuminemia, divalent ion abnormalities, CRP, dyslipidemia, and LV hypertrophy. The efficacy of risk factor intervention has not been clearly established in these populations, although there is good evidence for blood pressure control, (partial) correction of anemia, treatment of dyslipidemia, cessation of tobacco use, correction of divalent ion abnormalities, and use of aspirin and statins in selected cases. Appropriate use of ACE inhibitors, AR antagonists, β-receptor antagonists, and coronary revascularization should be encouraged.

REFERENCES

1. The United States Renal Data System: Causes of death. Am J Kidney Dis 34(suppl 1):S87-S94, 1999.
2. Ojo AO, Hanson JA, Wolfe RA, Leichtman AB, et al: Long-term survival in renal transplant recipients with graft function. Kidney Int 57:307-313, 2000.
3. Herzog CA, Ma JZ, Collins AJ: Long-term survival of renal transplant recipients in the United States after acute myocardial infarction. Am J Kidney Dis 36:145-152, 2000.
4. Annual Report of the Australian and New Zealand Dialysis and Transplantation Association, 2001. Available at: http://www.anzdata. org.au.
5. Foley RN, Parfrey PS, Sarnak M: The clinical epidemiology of cardiovascular disease in chronic renal disease. Am J Kidney Dis 32(suppl):S112-S115, 1998.
6. Churchill DN, Taylor DW, Cook RJ, et al: Canadian Hemodialysis Morbidity Study. Am J Kidney Dis 19:214-234, 1992.
7. Foley RN, Parfrey PS, Harnett JD, et al: Clinical and echocardiographic disease in patients starting end-stage renal disease therapy. Kidney Int 47:186-192, 1995.
8. Levin A, Singer J, Thompson CR, et al: Prevalent left ventricular hypertrophy in the predialysis population: Identifying opportunities for intervention. Am J Kidney Dis 27:347-354, 1996.
9. Barrett BJ, Parfrey PS, Morgan J, et al: Prediction of early death in end-stage renal disease patients starting dialysis. Am J Kidney Dis 29:214-222, 1997.
10. The United States Renal Data System: Patient characteristics at the start of ESRD: Data from the HCFA Medical Evidence Form. Am J Kidney Dis 34(suppl 1):S63-S73, 1999.
11. London GM, Pannier B, Guerin AP, et al: Cardiac hypertrophy, aortic compliance, peripheral resistance, and wave reflection in end-stage renal disease: Comparative effects of ACE inhibition and calcium channel blockade. Circulation 90:2786-2796, 1994.
12. London GM, Guerin AP, Marchais SJ: Hemodynamic overload in end-stage renal disease patients. Semin Dialysis 12:77-83, 1999.
13. London GM, Pannier B, Guerin AP, et al: Alterations of left ventricular hypertrophy in and survival of patients receiving hemodialysis: follow-up of an interventional study. J Am Soc Nephrol 12:2759-2767, 2001.
14. Guerin AP, Blacher J, Pannier B, et al: Impact of aortic stiffness attenuation on survival of patients in end-stage renal failure. Circulation 103:987-992, 2001.
15. Mazzaferro S, Coen G, Bandini S, et al: Role of ageing, chronic renal failure and dialysis in the calcification of the mitral annulus. Abstract. Nephrol Dial Transplant 8:335-340, 1993.
16. London GM, Pannier B, Marchais SJ, Guerin AP: Calcification of the aortic valve in the dialyzed patient. J Am Soc Nephrol 11:778-783, 2000.
17. Otto CM, Lind BK, Kitzman DW, et al: Association of aortic-valve sclerosis with cardiovascular mortality and morbidity in the elderly. N Engl J Med 341:142-147, 1999.
18. Foley RN, Parfrey PS, Kent GM, et al: Long-term evolution of cardiomyopathy in dialysis patients. Kidney Int 54:1720-1725, 1998.
19. Levin A, Thompson CR, Ethier J, et al: Left ventricular mass index increase in early renal disease: Impact of decline in hemoglobin. Am J Kidney Dis 34:125-134, 1999.
20. Takeda K, Nakamoto M, Baba M, et al: Echocardiographic evaluation in long-term continuous ambulatory peritoneal dialysis compared with hemodialysis patients. Clin Nephrol 49:308-312, 1998.
21. Enia G, Mallamaci F, Benedetto FA, et al: Long-term CAPD patients are volume expanded and display more severe left ventricular hypertrophy than haemodialysis patients. Nephrol Dial Transplant 16:1459-1464, 2001.
22. Foley RN, Parfrey PS, Kent GM, et al: Serial change in echocardiographic parameters and cardiac failure in end-stage renal disease. J Am Soc Nephrol 11:912-916, 2000.
23. Parfrey PS, Foley RN, Harnett JD, et al: Outcome and risk factors for left ventricular disorders in chronic uraemia. Nephrol Dial Transplant 11:1277-1285, 1996.
24. Rigatto C, Foley RN, Kent GM, et al: Long-term changes in left ventricular hypertrophy after renal transplantation. Transplantation 70:570-575, 2000.
25. K/DOQI clinical practice guidelines for CKD: Evaluation, classification and stratification. Kidney Disease Outcome Quality Initiative. Am J Kidney Dis 39:S1-S246, 2002.
26. Mann DL, Gillam LD, Mich R, et al: Functional relation between infarct thickness and regional systolic function in the acutely and subacutely infarcted canine left ventricle. J Am Coll Cardiol 14:481-488, 1989.
27. Dzau VJ: The role of mechanical and humoral factors in growth regulation of vascular smooth muscle and cardiac myocytes. Curr Opin Nephrol Hypertens 2:27-32, 1993.
28. Katz AM: Cardiomyopathy of overload: A major determinant of prognosis in congestive heart failure. N Engl J Med 322:100-110, 1990.
29. Katz AM: The cardiomyopathy of overload: An unnatural growth response in the hypertrophied heart. Ann Intern Med 121:262-371, 1994.
30. Hunter JJ, Chien KR: Signaling pathways for cardiac hypertrophy and failure. N Engl J Med 341:1276-1283, 1999.
31. Levy D, Garrison RJ, Savage DD, et al: Prognostic implications of echocardiographically determined left ventricular mass in the Framingham Heart Study. N Engl J Med 322:1561-1566, 1990.
32. Cheng W, Li B, Kajstura J, et al: Stretch-induced programmed myocyte cell death. J Clin Invest 96:2247-2259, 1995.
33. Amann K, Breitbach M, Ritz E, Mall G: Myocyte/capillary mismatch in the heart of uremic patients. J Am Soc Nephrol 9:1018-1022, 1998.
34. Anversa P, Olivetti G, Melissari M, Loud AV: Stereological measurement of cellular and subcellular hypertrophy and hyperplasia in the papillary muscle of adult rat. J Mol Cell Cardiol 12:781-795, 1980.
35. Hofman JI: Transmural myocardial perfusion. Prog Cardiovasc Dis 29:429-464, 1987.
36. Brilla CG, Janicki JS, Weber KT: Impaired diastolic function and coronary reserve in genetic hypertension. Circ Res 69:107-115, 1991.
37. Watanabe H, Ohtsuka S, Kakihana M, Sugishita Y: Coronary circulation in dogs with an experimental decrease in aortic compliance. J Am Coll Cardiol 21:1497-1506, 1993.
38. Cheng W, Li B, Kajstura J, et al: Stretch-induced programmed myocyte cell death. J Clin Invest 96:2247-2259, 1995.
39. Weber KT: Cardiac interstitium in health and disease: The fibrillar collagen network. J Am Coll Cardiol 13:1637-1652, 1989.
40. Hutchins GM: Cardiac pathology in chronic renal failure. *In* Parfrey PS, Harnett JD (eds): Cardiac Dysfunction in Chronic Uremia. Boston, Kluwer Academic Publishers, 1992, p 85.
41. Heng MK, Janz RF, Jobin J: Estimation of regional stress in the left ventricular septum and free wall: An echocardiographic study suggesting a mechanism for asymmetric septal hypertrophy. Am Heart J 110:84-89, 1985.
42. Bernardi D, Bernini L, Cini C, et al: Asymmetric septal hypertrophy and sympathetic overactivity in normotensive hemodialyzed patients. Am Heart J 109:539-545, 1985.
43. Demuth K, Blacher J, Guerin AP, et al: Endothelin and cardiovascular remodelling in end-stage renal disease. Nephrol Dial Transplant 13:375-383, 1998.
44. Blacher J, Demuth K, Guerin AP, et al: Influence of biochemical alterations on arterial stiffness in patients with end-stage renal disease. Arterioscl Thromb Vasc Biol 18:535-541, 1998.
45. Zoccali C, Bode-Boger S, Mallamaci F, et al: Plasma concentration of asymmetrical dimethylarginine and mortality in patients with end-stage renal disease: A prospective study. Lancet 358:2113-2117, 2001.
46. Mallamaci F, Zoccali C, Parlongo S, et al: Troponin is related to left ventricular mass and predicts all-cause and cardiovascular mortality in hemodialysis patients. Am J Kidney Dis 40:68-75, 2002.
47. Bernardi D, Bernini L, Cini G, et al: Asymmetric septal hypertrophy and sympathetic overactivity in normotensive hemodialyzed patients. Am Heart J 109:539-545, 1985.
48. Zoccali C, Mallamaci F, Tripepi G, et al: Adiponectin, metabolic risk factors, and cardiovascular events among patients with end-stage renal disease. J Am Soc Nephrol 13:134-141, 2002.
49. Zoccali C, Mallamaci F, Tripepi G, et al: Norepinephrine and concentric hypertrophy in patients with end-stage renal disease. CREED Investigators. Hypertension 40:41-46, 2002.

50. Grossman W, Jones D, McLaurin LP: Wall stress and patterns of hypertrophy in the human left ventricle. J Clin Invest 56:56-64, 1975.

51. London GM, Fabiani F, Marchais SJ, et al: Uremic cardiomyopathy: an inadequate left ventricular hypertrophy. Kidney Int 31:973-980, 1987.

52. Mall G, Huther W, Schneider J, et al: Diffuse intermyocardiocytic fibrosis in uraemic patients. Nephrol Dial Transplant 5:39-44, 1990.

53. Amann K, Ritz E, Wiest G, et al: A role of parathyroid hormone for the activation of cardiac fibroblasts in uremia. J Am Soc Nephrol 4:1814-1819, 1994.

54. Amann K, Ritz E: Cardiac disease in chronic uremia: Pathophysiology. Adv Ren Replace Ther 4:212-224, 1997.

55. Weber KT, Brilla CG, Campbell SE, et al: Pathologic hypertrophy with fibrosis: The structural basis for myocardial failure. Blood Press 1:75-85, 1992.

56. Weber KT: Cardiac interstitium in health and disease: The fibrillar collagen network. J Am Coll Cardiol 13:1637-1644, 1989.

57. Hess OM, Schneider J, Koch R, et al: Diastolic function and myocardial structure in patients with myocardial hypertrophy. Circulation 63:360-366, 1981.

58. McLenachan JM, Henderson E, Dargie HJ: A possible mechanism of sudden death in hypertensive left ventricular hypertrophy. J Hypertens 5(suppl 5):630-634, 1987.

59. Keung EC: Calcium current is increased in isolated adult myocytes from hypertrophied rat myocardium. Circ Res 64:753-763, 1989.

60. Keller E, Moravec CS, Bond M: Altered subcellular Ca^{2+} regulation in papillary muscles from cardiomyopathic hamster hearts. Am J Physiol 268:H1875-H1883, 1995.

61. LeWinter MM, Decena B, Tischler MD: Abnormalities of myocardial relaxation and filling: Diastolic dysfunction. In Hosenpud JD, Greenberg BH (eds): Congestive Heart Failure, 2nd ed. Philadelphia, Lippincott Williams & Wilkins, 2000, pp 83-100.

62. Leunissen KM, Menheere PP, Cheriex EC, et al: Plasma alpha-human atrial natriuretic peptide and volume status in chronic haemodialysis patients. Nephrol Dial Transplant 4:382-386, 1989.

63. Nappi SE, Saha HH, Virtanen VK, et al: Hemodialysis with high-calcium dialysate impairs cardiac relaxation. Kidney Int 55:1091-1096, 1999.

64. Severi S, Cavalcanti S, Mancini E, Santoro A: Heart rate response to hemodialysis-induced changes in potassium and calcium levels. J Nephrol 14:488-496, 2001.

65. Zoccali C, Mallamaci F, Benedetto FA, et al: Cardiac natriuretic peptides are related to left ventricular mass and function and predict mortality in dialysis patients. CREED Investigators. J Am Soc Nephrol 12:1508-1515, 2001.

66. Zoccali C, Mallamaci F, Parlongo S, et al: Plasma norepinephrine predicts survival and incident cardiovascular events in patients with end-stage renal disease. Circulation 105:1354-1359, 2002.

67. Kramer W, Wizemann V, Lammlein G, et al: Cardiac dysfunction in patients on maintenance hemodialysis: II: Systolic and diastolic properties of the left ventricle assessed by invasive methods. Contrib Nephrol 52:97-109, 1986.

68. Fujimoto S, Kagoshima T, Hashimoto T, et al: Left ventricular diastolic function in patients on maintenance dialysis: Comparison with hypertensive heart disease and hypertrophic cardiomyopathy. Clin Nephrol 42:109-116, 1994.

69. Palmer BF, Henrich WL: The effect of dialysis on left ventricular contractility. In Parfrey PS, Harnett JD (eds): Cardiac Dysfunction in Chronic Uremia. Boston, Kluwer Academic, 1992, pp 171-198.

70. Ritz E, Rambausek M, Mall G, et al: Cardiac changes in uraemia and their possible relationship to cardiovascular instability on dialysis. Nephrol Dial Transplant 5(suppl 1):93-97, 1990.

71. Verbeelen D, Bossuyt A, Smitz J, et al: Hemodynamics of patients with renal failure treated with recombinant human erythropoietin. Clin Nephrol 31:6-11, 1989.

72. Cannella G, La Canna G, Sandrini M, et al: Renormalization of high cardiac output and of left ventricular size following long-term recombinant human erythropoietin treatment of anemic dialyzed uremic patients. Clin Nephrol 34:272-278, 1990.

73. McMahon LP, Mason K, Skinner SL, et al: Effects of haemoglobin normalization on quality of life and cardiovascular parameters in end-stage renal failure. Nephrol Dial Transplant 15:1425-1430, 2000.

74. Weusenee D, Low-Friedrich I, Richle M, et al: In vitro approach to "uremic cardiomyopathy." Nephron 65:392-400, 1993.

75. Burt RK, Gupta-Burt S, Suki W, et al: Reversal of left ventricular dysfunction after renal transplantation. Ann Intern Med 111:635-640, 1989.

76. Parfrey PS, Harnett JD, Foley RN, et al: Impact of renal transplantation on uremic cardiomyopathy. Transplantation 60:908-914, 1995.

77. De Lima JJ, Vieira ML, Viviani LF, et al: Long-term impact of renal transplantation on carotid artery properties and on ventricular hypertrophy in end-stage renal failure patients. Nephrol Dial Transplant 17:645-651, 2002.

78. McGregor E, Stewart G, Rodger RS, Jardine AG: Early echocardiographic changes and survival following renal transplantation. Nephrol Dial Transplant 15:93-98, 2000.

79. London GM, Pannier B, Guerin AP, et al: Alterations of left ventricular hypertrophy in and survival of patients receiving hemodialysis: Follow-up of an interventional study. J Am Soc Nephrol 12:2759-2767, 2001.

80. Foley RN, Parfrey PS, Kent GM, et al: Long-term evolution of cardiomyopathy in dialysis patients. Kidney Int 54:1720-1725, 1998.

81. Abbott KC, Hypolite IO, Hshieh P, et al: The impact of renal transplantation on the incidence of congestive heart failure in patients with end-stage renal disease due to diabetes. J Nephrol 14:369-376, 2001.

82. Periyasamy SM, Chen J, Cooney D, et al: Effects of uremic serum on isolated cardiac myocyte calcium cycling and contractile function. Kidney Int 60:2367-2376, 2001.

83. Abraham WT, Lowes BD, Ferguson DA, et al: Systemic hemodynamic, neurohormonal, and renal effects of a steady-state infusion of human brain natriuretic peptide in patients with hemodynamically decompensated heart failure. J Card Fail 4:37-44, 1998.

84. Parfrey PS, Harnett JD, Griffiths SM, et al: Congestive heart failure in dialysis patients. Arch Intern Med 148:1519-1525, 1988.

85. Uren MG, Melin JA, De Bruynr B, et al: Relation between myocardial blood flow and the severity of coronary-artery stenosis. N Engl J Med 330:1782-1788, 1994.

86. Gould KL, Lipscomb K: Effects of coronary stenosis on coronary flow reserve and resistance. Am J Cardiol 34:48-55, 1974.

87. Joki N, Hase H, Nakamura R, Yamaguchi T: Onset of coronary artery disease prior to initiation of haemodialysis in patients with end-stage renal disease. Nephrol Dial Transplant 12:718-723, 1997.

88. Koch M, Gradaus F, Schoebel FC, et al: Relevance of conventional cardiovascular risk factors for the prediction of coronary artery disease in diabetic patients on renal replacement therapy. Nephrol Dial Transplant 12:1187-1191, 1997.

89. Braun WE, Phillips DF, Vidt DG, et al: Coronary artery disease in 100 diabetics with end-stage renal failure. Transplant Proc 16:603-607, 1984.

90. London GM, Drueke TB: Atherosclerosis and arteriosclerosis in chronic renal failure. Kidney Int 51:1678-1695, 1997.

91. Gris J-C, Branger B, Vecina F, et al: Increased cardiovascular risk factors and features of endothelial activation and dysfunction in dialyzed uremic patients. Kidney Int 46:807-813, 1994.

92. Segarra A, Chacon P, Martinez-Eyarre C, et al: Circulating levels of plasminogen activator inhibitor type-1, tissue plasminogen activator, and thrombomodulin in hemodialysis patients: Biochemical correlations and role as independent predictors of coronary artery stenosis. J Am Soc Nephrol 12:1255-1263, 2001.

93. Haaber AB, Eidemak I, Jensen T, et al: Vascular endothelial cell function and cardiovascular risk factors in patients with chronic renal failure. J Am Soc Nephrol 5:1581-1584, 1995.

94. Shoji T, Ishimura E, Inaba M, et al: Atherogenic lipoproteins in end-stage renal disease. Am J Kidney Dis 38(suppl 1):S30-S33, 2001.

95. Culleton BF, Wilson PWF: Thrombogenic risk factors for cardiovascular disease in dialysis patients. Semin Dial 12:117-125, 1999.

96. Khaper N, Rigatto C, Seneviratne C, et al: Chronic treatment with propranolol induces antioxidant changes and protects against ischemia-reperfusion injury. J Mol Cell Cardiol 29:3335-3344, 1997.

97. Bostom AG, Lathrop L: Hyperhomocysteinemia in end-stage renal disease: Prevalence, etiology, and potential relationship to arteriosclerotic outcomes. Kidney Int 52:10-20, 1997.

98. Friedman AN, Bostom AG, Selhub J, et al: The kidney and homocysteine metabolism. J Am Soc Nephrol 12:2181-2189, 2001.

99. Pereira BJG, Shapiro L, King AJ, et al: Plasma levels of IL1-beta, TNF-alpha and their specific inhibitors in undialyzed chronic renal failure, CAPD and hemodialysis patients. Kidney Int 45:890-896, 1994.

100. Descamps-Latscha B, Herbelin A, Nguyen AT, et al: Balance between IL1-beta, TNF-alpha, and their specific inhibitors in chronic renal failure and maintenance dialysis: Relationships with activation markers of T cells, B cells, and monocytes. J Immunol 54:882-892, 1995.

101. Kaysen GA: The microinflammatory state in uremia: Causes and potential consequences. J Am Soc Nephrol 12:1549-1557, 2001.

102. Nilsson J: Cytokines and smooth muscle in atherosclerosis. Cardiovasc Res 27:1184-1190, 1993.

103. Sutherland WHF, Walker RJ, Ball MJ, et al: Oxidation of low density lipoproteins from patients with renal failure or renal transplants. Kidney Int 48:227-236, 1995.

104. Witzum JL, Steinberg D: Role of oxidized low density lipoprotein in atherogenesis. J Clin Invest 88:1785-1792, 1991.

105. Wanner C, Zimmermann J, Queschning T, Galle J: Inflammation, dyslipidemia, vascular risk factors in hemodialysis patients. Kidney Int 52(suppl 62):S53-S55, 1997.

106. Griselli M, Herbert J, Hutchinson WL, et al: C-reactive protein and complement are important mediators of tissue damage in acute myocardial infarction. J Exp Med 190:1733-1740, 1999.

107. Torzewski M, Klouche M, Hock J, et al: Immunohistochemical demonstration of enzymatically modified human LDL and its colocalization with the terminal complement complex in the early atherosclerotic lesion. Arterioscl Thromb Vasc Biol 18:369-378, 1998.

108. Cermak J, Key NS, Bach RR, et al: C-reactive protein induces human peripheral blood monocytes to synthesize tissue factor. Blood 82:513-520, 1993.

109. Berk BC, Weintraub WS, Alexander RW: Elevation of C-reactive protein in "active" coronary artery disease. Am J Cardiol 65:168-172, 1990.

110. Liuzzo G, Biasucci LM, Gallimore JR, et al: The prognostic value of C-reactive protein and serum amyloid a protein in severe unstable angina. N Engl J Med 331:417-424, 1994.

111. Mendall MA, Patel P, Ballam L, et al: C reactive protein and its relation to cardiovascular risk factors: A population based cross sectional study. BMJ 312:1061-1065, 1996.

112. Ridker PM, Cushman M, Stampfer MJ, et al: Inflammation, aspirin, and the risk of cardiovascular disease in apparently healthy men. [Erratum appears in N Engl J Med 337:356, 1997.] N Engl J Med 336:973-979, 1997.

113. Haverkate F, Thompson SG, Pyke SD, et al: Production of C-reactive protein and risk of coronary events in stable and unstable angina. European Concerted Action on Thrombosis and Disabilities Angina Pectoris Study Group. Lancet 349:462-466, 1997.

114. Koenig W, Rothenbacher D, Hoffmeister A, et al: Infection with *Helicobacter pylori* is not a major independent risk factor for stable coronary heart disease: Lack of a role of cytotoxin-associated protein A-positive strains and absence of a systemic inflammatory response. Circulation 100:2326-2331, 1999.

115. Kaysen GA, de Sain-van der Velden MG: New insights into lipid metabolism in the nephrotic syndrome. Kidney Int Suppl 71:S18-S21, 1999.

116. Ridker PM, Buring JE, Shih J, et al: Prospective study of C-reactive protein and the risk of future cardiovascular events among apparently healthy women. Circulation 98:731-733, 1998.

117. Ridker PM, Glynn RJ, Hennekens CH: C-reactive protein adds to the predictive value of total and HDL cholesterol in determining risk of first myocardial infarction. Circulation 97:2007-2011, 1998.

118. Panichi V, Migliori M, De Pietro S, et al: Plasma C-reactive protein in hemodialysis patients: A cross-sectional, longitudinal clinical survey. Blood Purif 18:30-36, 2000.

119. Kaysen GA, Stevenson FT, Depner TA: Determinants of albumin concentration in hemodialysis patients. Am J Kidney Dis 29:658-668, 1997.

120. Libetta C, De Nicola L, Rampino T, et al: Inflammatory effects of peritoneal dialysis: Evidence of systemic monocyte activation. Kidney Int 49:506-511, 1996.

121. Yeun JY, Levine RA, Mantadilok V, Kaysen GA: C-Reactive protein predicts all-cause and cardiovascular mortality in hemodialysis patients. Am J Kidney Dis 35:469-476, 2000.

122. Zoccali C, Benedetto FA, Maas R, et al, and CREED Investigators. Asymmetric dimethylarginine, C-reactive protein, and carotid intima-media thickness in end-stage renal disease. J Am Soc Nephrol 13:490-496, 2002.

123. Stenvinkel P, Heimburger O, Paultre F, et al: Strong association between malnutrition, inflammation, and atherosclerosis in chronic renal failure. Kidney Int 55:1899-1911, 1999.

124. Schwarz U, Buzello M, Ritz E, et al: Morphology of coronary atherosclerotic lesions in patients with end-stage renal failure. Nephrol Dial Transplant 15:218-223, 2000.

125. Guerin AP, London GM, Marchais SJ, Metivier F: Arterial stiffening and vascular calcifications in end-stage renal disease. Nephrol Dial Transplant 15:1014-1021, 2000.

126. Goodman WG, Goldin J, Kuizon BD, et al: Coronary-artery calcification in young adults with end-stage renal disease who are undergoing dialysis. N Engl J Med 342:1478-1483, 2000.

127. Oh J, Wunsch R, Turzer M, et al: Advanced coronary and carotid arteriopathy in young adults with childhood-onset chronic renal failure. Circulation 106:100-105, 2002.

128. Jono S, McKee MD, Murry CE, et al: Phosphate regulation of vascular smooth muscle cell calcification. Circ Res 87:E10-E17, 2000.

129. Rostand RG, Kirk KA, Rutsky EA: Dialysis ischaemic heart disease: Insights from coronary angiography. Kidney Int 25:653-659, 1984.

130. James TN: Morphologic characteristics and functional significance of focal fibromuscular dysplasia of small coronary arteries. Am J Cardiol 65:12G-22G, 1990.

131. Amann K, Neususs R, Ritz E, et al: Changes of vascular architecture independent of blood pressure in experimental uremia. Am J Hypertens 8:409-417, 1995.

132. Amann K, Wiest G, Zimmer G, et al: Reduced capillary density in the myocardium of uremic rats: A stereological study. Kidney Int 42:1078-1085, 1992.

133. Amann K, Breitbach M, Ritz E, Mall G: Myocyte/capillary mismatch in the heart of uremic patients. J Am Soc Nephrol 9:1018-1022, 1998.

134. Watanabe H, Ohtuska S, Kakihana M, Sugishita Y: Coronary circulation in dogs with an experimental decrease in aortic compliance. J Am Coll Cardiol 21:1497-1506, 1993.

135. Raine AEG, Seymour A-ML, Roberts AFC, et al: Impairment of cardiac function and energetics in experimental renal failure. J Clin Invest 92:2934-2940, 1993.

136. Massry SG, Smorgorzewski M: Mechanisms through which parathyroid hormone mediates its deleterious effects on organ function in uremia. Semin Nephrol 14:219-231, 1994.

137. Madsen BR, Alpert MA, Shiting RB, et al: Effect of hemodialysis on left ventricular performance: Analysis of echocardiographic subsets. Am J Nephrol 4:86-92, 1984.

138. Hung J, Harris PJ, Uren RF: Uremic cardiomyopathy: Effect of hemodialysis on left ventricular function in end-stage renal failure. N Engl J Med 302:547-551, 1980.

139. D'Elia JA, Weinrauch LA, Gleason RE, et al: Application of the ambulatory 24-hour electrocardiogram in the prediction of cardiac death in dialysis patients. Arch Intern Med 148:2381-2385, 1988.

140. Poldermans D, Man in 't Veld AJ, Rambaldi R, et al: Cardiac evaluation in hypotension-prone and hypotension-resistant hemodialysis patients. Kidney Int 56:1905-1911, 1999.

141. Ruffmann K, Mandelbaum A, Bommer J, et al: Doppler echocardiographic findings in dialysis patients. Nephrol Dial Transplant 5:426-431, 1990.

142. Kimura K, Tabei K, Asano J, Hosoda S: Cardiac arrhythmias in hemodialysis patients: A study of incidence and contributory factors. Nephron 53:201-207, 1989.

143. Wizemann V, Kramer W, Thormann J, et al: Cardiac arrhythmias in patients on maintenance hemodialysis: Causes and management. Contrib Nephrol 52:42-53, 1986.

144. Gruppo Emodialisi e Pathologia Cardiovasculari: Multicentre cross-sectional study of ventricular arrhythmias in chronically hemodialysed patients. Lancet 6:305-309, 1988.

145. Blumberg A, Hausermann M, Strub B, Jenzer HR: Cardiac arrhythmias in patients on maintenance hemodialysis. Nephron 33:91-95, 1983.

146. Niwa A, Taniguchi K, Ito H, et al: Echocardiographic and holter findings in 321 uremic patients on maintenance hemodialysis. Jpn Heart J 26:403-411, 1985.

147. Sforzini S, Latini R, Mingadi G, et al: Ventricular arrhythmias and four-year mortality in hemodialysis patients. Lancet 339:212-213, 1992.

148. Wizemann V, Kramer W, Funke T, Schütterle G: Dialysis-induced cardiac arrhythmias: Fact or fiction? Nephron 39:356-360, 1985.

149. Qellhorst E, Scheunemann B, Hildebrand U: Hemofiltration: An improved method of treatment for chronic renal failure. Contrib Nephrol 4:194-211, 1985.

150. Peer G, Korzets A, Hochhauzer E, et al: Cardiac arrhythmia during chronic ambulatory peritoneal dialysis. Nephron 45:192-195, 1987.

151. McLenachan JM, Dargie HJ: Ventricular arrhythmias in hypertensive left ventricular hypertrophy. Am J Hypertens 3:735-740, 1990.

152. Canziani ME, Saragosa MA, Draibe SA, et al: Risk factors for the occurrence of cardiac arrhythmias in patients on continuous ambulatory peritoneal dialysis. Perit Dial Int 13(suppl 2):S409-S411, 1993.

153. Canziani ME, Cendoroglo Neto M, Saragoça MA, et al: Hemodialysis versus continuous ambulatory peritoneal dialysis: Effects on the heart. Artif Organs 19:241-244, 1995.

154. Tzamaloukas A, Avasthi P: Temporal profile of serum potassium concentration in nondiabetic and diabetic outpatients on chronic dialysis. Am J Nephrol 7:101-109, 1987.

155. Morrison G, Michelson EL, Brown S, Morganroth J: Mechanism and prevention of cardiac arrhythmias in chronic hemodialysis patients. Kidney Int 17:811-819, 1980.

156. Keller F, Weinmann J, Schwarz A, et al: Effect of digitoxin on cardiac arrhythmias in hemodialysis patients. Klin Wochen 65:1081-1086, 1987.

157. Ribeiro S, Ramos A, Brandao A, et al: Cardiac valve calcification in haemodialysis patients: Role of calcium-phosphate metabolism. Nephrol Dial Transplant 13:2037-2040, 1998.

158. Maher ER, Young G, Smyth-Walsh B, et al: Aortic and mitral valve calcification in patients with end-stage renal disease. Lancet 2:875-877, 1987.

159. Braun J, Oldendorf M, Moshage W, et al: Electron beam computed tomography in the evaluation of cardiac calcification in chronic dialysis patients. Am J Kidney Dis 27:394-401, 1996.

160. Urena P, Malergue MC, Goldfarb B, et al: Evolutive aortic stenosis in hemodialysis patients: Analysis of risk factors. Nephrologie 20:217-225, 1999.

161. Raine AEG: Acquired aortic stenosis in dialysis patients. Nephron 68:159-168, 1994.

162. Rosenhek R, Binder T, Porenta G, et al: Predictors of outcome in severe, asymptomatic aortic stenosis. N Engl J Med 343:611-617, 2000.

163. Fernandez-Reyes MJ, Auxiliadora Bajo M, Robles P, et al: Mitral annular calcification in CAPD patients with a low degree of hyperparathyroidism: An analysis of other possible risk factors. Nephrol Dial Transplant 10:2090-2095, 1995.

164. Huting J: Predictive value of mitral and aortic valve sclerosis for survival in end-stage renal disease on continuous ambulatory peritoneal dialysis. Nephron 64:63-68, 1993.

165. Guerin AP, Blacher J, Pannier B, et al: Impact of aortic stiffness attenuation on survival of patients in end-stage renal failure. Circulation 103:987-992, 2001.

166. Tozawa M, Iseki K, Iseki C, Takishita S: Pulse pressure and risk of total mortality and cardiovascular events in patients on chronic hemodialysis. Kidney Int 61:717-726, 2002.

167. Klassen PS, Lowrie EG, Reddan DN, et al: Association between pulse pressure and mortality in patients undergoing maintenance hemodialysis. JAMA 287:1548-1555, 2002.

168. Benedetto FA, Mallamaci F, Tripepi G, Zoccali C: Prognostic value of ultrasonographic measurement of carotid intima media thickness in dialysis patients. J Am Soc Nephrol 12:2458-2564, 2001.

169. Nishikimi T, Minami J, Tamano K, et al: Left ventricular mass relates to average systolic blood pressure, but not loss of circadian blood pressure in stable hemodialysis patients: An ambulatory 48-hour blood pressure study. Hypertens Res Clin Exp 24:507-514, 2001.

170. Zoccali C, Mallamaci F, Tripepi G, et al: Prediction of left ventricular geometry by clinic, pre-dialysis and 24-h ambulatory BP monitoring in hemodialysis patients: CREED Investigators. J Hypertens 17:1751-1758, 1999.

171. Zoccali C, Benedetto FA, Tripepi G, et al: Nocturnal hypoxemia, night-day arterial pressure changes and left ventricular geometry in dialysis patients. Kidney Int 53:1078-1084, 1998.

172. Argiles A, Mourad G, Mion C: Seasonal changes in blood pressure in patients with end-stage renal disease treated with hemodialysis. N Engl J Med 339:1364-1370, 1998.

173. Nichols WW, O'Rourke MF: Vascular impedance. In McDonald's Blood Flow in Arteries: Theoretic, Experimental and Clinical Principles. Philadelphia, Lea & Febiger, 1990.

174. London GM, Marchais SJ, Guerin AP, et al: Cardiac hypertrophy and arterial alterations in end-stage renal disease: Hemodynamic factors. Kidney Int Suppl 41:S42-S49, 1993.

175. Anversa P, Olivetti G, Melissari M, Loud AV: Stereological measurement of cellular and subcellular hypertrophy and hyperplasia in the papillary muscle of adult rat. J Mol Cell Cardiol 12:781-795, 1980.

176. Marchais SJ, Guerin AP, Pannier BM, et al: Wave reflections and cardiac hypertrophy in chronic uremia: Influence of body size. Hypertension 22:876-883, 1993.

177. Savage T, Giles M, Tomson CV, Raine AE: Gender differences in mediators of left ventricular hypertrophy in dialysis patients. Clin Nephrol 49:107-112, 1998.

178. Greaves SC, Gamble GD, Collins JF, et al: Determinants of left ventricular hypertrophy and systolic dysfunction in chronic renal failure. Am J Kidney Dis 24:768-776, 1994.

179. de Lima JJ, Abensur H, Krieger EM, Pileggi F: Arterial blood pressure and left ventricular hypertrophy in haemodialysis patients. J Hypertens 14:1019-1024, 1996.

180. Harnett JD, Kent GM, Barre PE, et al: Risk factors for the development of left ventricular hypertrophy in a prospectively followed cohort of dialysis patients. J Am Soc Nephrol 4:1486-1490, 1994.

181. Blacher J, Guerin AP, Pannier B, et al: Impact of aortic stiffness on survival in end-stage renal disease. Circulation 99:2434-2439, 1999.

182. Buckberg GD, Towers B, Paglia DE, et al: Subendocardial ischemia after cardiopulmonary bypass. J Thorac Cardiovasc Surg 64:669-684, 1972.

183. Buckberg GD, Fixler DE, Archie JP, Hoffman JI: Experimental subendocardial ischemia in dogs with normal coronary arteries. Circ Res 30:67-81, 1972.

184. Asakura T, Karino T: Flow patterns and spatial distribution of atherosclerotic lesions in human coronary arteries. Circ Res 66:1045-1066, 1990.

185. Gibbons GH, Dzau VJ: The emerging concept of vascular remodeling. N Engl J Med 330:1431-1438, 1994.

186. Xiao S, Schmidt RJ, Baylis C: Plasma from ESRD patients inhibits nitric oxide synthase activity in cultured human and bovine endothelial cells. Acta Physiol Scand 168:175-179, 2000.

187. Schroder M, Riedel E, Beck W, et al: Increased reduction of dimethylarginines and lowered interdialytic blood pressure by the use of biocompatible membranes. Kid Int Suppl 78:S19-S24, 2001.

188. Surdacki A, Sulowicz W, Wieczorek-Surdacka E, Herman ZS: Effect of a hemodialysis session on plasma levels of endothelin-1 in hypertensive and normotensive subjects with end-stage renal failure. Nephron 81:31-36, 1999.

189. Vaziri ND, Ni Z, Zhang YP, et al: Depressed renal and vascular nitric oxide synthase expression in cyclosporine-induced hypertension. Kidney Int 54:482-491, 1998.

190. Schieppati A, Remuzzi G: Prevalence and significance of hypertension in systemic lupus erythematosus. Am J Kidney Dis 21(5 suppl 2):58-60, 1993.

191. Raine AE, Bedford L, Simpson AW, et al: Hyperparathyroidism, platelet intracellular free calcium and hypertension in chronic renal failure. Kidney Int 43:700-705, 1993.

192. van Hooft IM, Grobbee DE, Derkx FH, et al: Renal hemodynamics and the renin-angiotensin-aldosterone system in normotensive subjects with hypertensive and normotensive parents. N Engl J Med 324:1305-1311, 1991.

193. Johnstone MT, Creager SJ, Scales KM, et al: Impaired endothelium-dependent vasodilation in patients with insulin-dependent diabetes mellitus. Circulation 88:2510-2516, 1993.

194. Williams SB, Cusco JA, Roddy MA, et al: Impaired nitric oxide-mediated vasodilation in patients with non-insulin-dependent diabetes mellitus. J Am Coll Cardiol 27:567-574, 1996.

195. Hopfner RL, Gopalakrishnan V: Endothelin: Emerging role in diabetic vascular complications. Diabetologia 42:1383-1394, 1999.

196. Tesfamariam B, Brown ML, Deykin D, Cohen RA: Elevated glucose promotes generation of endothelium-derived vasoconstrictor prostanoids in rabbit aorta. J Clin Invest 85:929-932, 1990.

197. Schmidt AM, Stern D: Atherosclerosis and diabetes: The RAGE connection. Curr Atheroscler Rep 2:430-436, 2000.

198. Rosen P, Nawroth PP, King G, et al: The role of oxidative stress in the onset and progression of diabetes and its complications: A summary of a Congress Series sponsored by UNESCO-MCBN, the American Diabetes Association and the German Diabetes Society. Diabetes Metab Res Rev 17:189-212, 2001.

199. Zeiher AM, Fisslthaler B, Schray-Utz B, Busse R: Nitric oxide modulates the expression of monocyte chemoattractant protein 1 in cultured human endothelial cells. Circ Res 76:980-986, 1995.

200. Vinik AI, Leichter SB, Pittenger GL, et al: Phospholipid and glutamic acid decarboxylase autoantibodies in diabetic neuropathy. Diabetes Care 18:1225-1232, 1995.

201. Assert R, Scherk G, Bumbure A, et al: Regulation of protein kinase C by short term hyperglycaemia in human platelets in vivo and in vitro. Diabetologia 44:188-195, 2001.

202. Greenspan LC, Gitelman SE, Leung MA, et al: Increased incidence in post-transplant diabetes mellitus in children: A case-control analysis. Pediatr Nephrol 17:1-5, 2002.

203. von Kiparski A, Frei D, Uhlschmid G, et al: Post-transplant diabetes mellitus in renal allograft recipients: A matched-pair control study. Nephrol Dial Transplant 5:220-225, 1990.

204. Rao M, Jacob CK, Shastry JC: Post-renal transplant diabetes mellitus: A retrospective study. Nephrol Dial Transplant 7:1039-1042, 1992.

205. Vesco L, Busson M, Bedrossian J, et al: Diabetes mellitus after renal transplantation: Characteristics, outcome, and risk factors. Transplantation 61:1475-1478, 1996.

206. Meier-Kriesche H-U, Ojo AO, Port FK, et al: Survival improvements among patients with end-stage renal disease: Trends over time for transplant recipients and wait listed patients. J Am Soc Nephrol 12:1293-1296, 2001.

207. London GM, Marchais SJ, Safar ME, et al: Aortic and large artery compliance in end-stage renal failure. Kidney Int 37:137-142, 1990.

208. Shoji T, Emoto M, Shinohara K, et al: Diabetes mellitus, aortic stiffness, and cardiovascular mortality in end-stage renal disease. J Am Soc Nephrol 12:2117-2124, 2001.

209. Harnett JD, Foley RN, Kent GM, et al: Congestive heart failure in dialysis patients: Prevalence, incidence, prognosis, and risk factors. Kidney Int 47:884-890, 1995.

210. Foley RN, Culleton BF, Parfrey PS, et al: Cardiac disease in diabetic end-stage renal disease. Diabetologia 40:1307-1312, 1997.

211. Herzog CA, Ma JZ, Collins AJ: Poor long-term survival after acute myocardial infarction among patients on long-term dialysis. N Engl J Med 339:799-805, 1998.

212. Iseki K, Fukiyama K, for the Okawa Dialysis Study (OKIDS) Group: Clinical demographics and long-term prognosis after stroke in patients on chronic hemodialysis. Nephrol Dial Transplant 15:1808-1813, 2000.

213. Reddan DN, Marcus RJ, Owen WF Jr, et al: Long-term outcomes of revascularization for peripheral vascular disease in end-stage renal patients. Am J Kidney Dis 38:57-63, 2001.

214. Dossa CD, Shepard AD, Amos AM, et al: Results of lower extremity amputations in patients with end-stage renal disease. J Vasc Surg 20:14-19, 1994.

215. Culleton BF, Larson MG, Evans JC, et al: Prevalence and correlates of elevated serum creatinine levels: The Framingham Heart Study. Arch Intern Med 159:1785-1790, 1999.

216. Garg AX, Clark WF, Haynes RB, House AA: Moderate renal insufficiency and the risk of cardiovascular mortality: Results from the NHANES I. Kidney Int 61:1486-1494, 2002.

217. Mann JF, Gerstein HC, Pogue J, et al: Renal insufficiency as a predictor of cardiovascular outcomes and the impact of ramipril: The HOPE randomized trial. Ann Intern Med 134:629-636, 2001.

218. Rigatto C, Parfrey P, Foley R, et al: Congestive heart failure in renal transplant recipients: Risk factors, outcomes, and relationship with ischemic heart disease. J Am Soc Nephrol 13:1084-1090, 2002.

219. Foley RN, Herzog CA, Collins AJ: Smoking and cardiovascular outcomes in dialysis patients: The United States Renal Data System Wave 2 Study. Kidney Int 63:1462-1467, 2003.

220. Muntner P, He J, Hamm L, et al: Renal insufficiency and subsequent death resulting from cardiovascular disease in the United States. J Am Soc Nephrol 13:745-753, 2002.

221. Shulman NB, Fod CE, Hall WD, et al: Prognostic value of serum creatinine and effect of treatment of hypertension on renal function: Results from the Hypertension Detection and Follow-Up Program. Hypertension 13(suppl 1):S180-S193, 1989.

222. Fried LP, Kronmal RA, Newman AB, et al: Risk factors for 5-year mortality in older adults: The cardiovascular health study. JAMA 279:585-592, 1998.

223. Hemmelgarn BR, Ghali WA, Quan H, et al, for the APPROACH Investigators: Poor long-term survival after coronary angiography in patients with renal insufficiency. Am J Kidney Dis 37:64-72, 2001.

224. Longenecker JC, Coresh J, Powe NR, et al: Traditional cardiovascular disease risk factors in dialysis patients compared with the general population: The CHOICE Study. J Am Soc Nephrol 13:1918-1927, 2002.

225. Kasiske BL, Chakkera HA, Roel J: Explained and unexplained ischemic heart disease risk after renal transplantation. J Am Soc Nephrol 11:1735-1743, 2000.

226. Sarnak MJ, Coronado BE, Greene T, et al: Cardiovascular disease risk factors in chronic renal insufficiency. Clin Nephrol 57:327-335, 2002.

227. Coresh J, Wei GL, McQuillan G, et al: Prevalence of high blood pressure and elevated serum creatinine level in the United States: Findings from the third National Health and Nutrition Examination Survey (1988-1994). Arch Intern Med 161:1207-1216, 2001.

228. Borhani NO, Mercuri M, Borhani PA, et al: Final outcome results of the Multicenter Isradipine Diuretic Atherosclerosis Study (MIDAS): A randomized controlled trial. JAMA 276:785-791, 1996.

229. Shoji T, Emoto M, Tabata T, et al: Advanced atherosclerosis in pre-dialysis patients with chronic renal failure. Kidney Int 61:2187-2192, 2002.

230. Tonelli M, Astephen P, Andreou P, et al: Blood volume monitoring in intermittent hemodialysis for acute renal failure. Kidney Int 62:1075-1080, 2002.

231. Rocco MV, Flanigan MJ, Beaver S, et al: Report from the 1995 Core Indicators for Peritoneal Dialysis Study Group. Am J Kidney Dis 30:165-173, 1997.

232. The sixth report of the Joint National Committee on Prevention, Detection, Evaluation and Treatment of High Blood Pressure. Arch Intern Med 157:2413-2446, 1997.

233. Rahman M, Fu P, Sehgal AR, Smith MC: Interdialytic weight gain, compliance with dialysis regimen, and age are independent predictors of blood pressure in hemodialysis patients. Am J Kidney Dis 35:257-265, 2000.

234. Mailloux LU, Levey AS: Hypertension in patients with chronic renal disease. Am J Kidney Dis 32(5 suppl 3):S120-S141, 1998.

235. Salem MM: Hypertension in the hemodialysis population: A survey of 649 patients. Am J Kidney Dis 26:461-468, 1995.

236. Rocco MV, Yan G, Heyka RJ, et al, and HEMO Study Group. Risk factors for hypertension in chronic hemodialysis patients: Baseline data from the HEMO study. Am J Nephrol 21:280-288, 2001.

237. Mittal SK, Kowalski E, Trenkle J, et al: Prevalence of hypertension in a hemodialysis population. Clin Nephrol 51:77-82, 1999.

238. Foley RN, Parfrey PS, Harnett JD, et al: Impact of hypertension on cardiomyopathy, morbidity and mortality in end-stage renal disease. Kidney Int 49:1379-1385, 1996.

239. Zager PG, Nikolic J, Brown RH, et al: "U" curve association of blood pressure and mortality in hemodialysis patients. Kidney Int 54:561-569, 1998.

240. Port FK, Hulbert-Shearon TE, Wolfe RA, et al: Predialysis blood pressure and mortality risk in a national sample of maintenance hemodialysis patients. Am J Kidney Dis 33:507-517, 1999.

241. Coresh J, Longenecker JC, Miller ER 3rd, et al: Epidemiology of cardiovascular risk factors in chronic renal disease. J Am Soc Nephrol 9:S24-S30, 1998.

242. Aakhus S, Dahl K, Wideroe TE: Cardiovascular morbidity and risk factors in renal transplant patients. Nephrol Dial Transplant 14:648-654, 1999.

243. Warholm C, Wilczek H, Pettersson E: Hypertension two years after renal transplantation: Causes and consequences. Transplant Int 8:286-292, 1995.

244. Schwenger V, Zeier M, Ritz E: Hypertension after renal transplantation. Ann Transplant 6:25-30, 2001.

245. Kasiske BL: Hyperlipidemia in patients with chronic renal disease. Am J Kidney Dis 32(5 suppl 3):S142-S156, 1998.

246. Ligtenberg G, Hene RJ, Blankestijn PJ, Koomans HA: Cardiovascular risk factors in renal transplant patients: Cyclosporin A versus tacrolimus. J Am Soc Nephrol 12:368-373, 2001.

247. Seliger SL, Weiss NS, Gillen DL, et al: HMG-CoA reductase inhibitors are associated with reduced mortality in ESRD patients. Kidney Int 61:297-304, 2002.

248. Collins AJ, Li S, Ma JZ, Herzog C: Cardiovascular disease in end-stage renal disease patients. Am J Kidney Dis 38(4 suppl 1): S26-S29, 2001.

249. Jungers P, Massy ZA, Khoa TN, et al: Incidence and risk factors of atherosclerotic cardiovascular accidents in predialysis chronic renal

failure patients: A prospective study. Nephrol Dial Transplant 12:2597-2602, 1997.

250. Kasiske BL, Guijarro C, Massy ZA, et al: Cardiovascular disease after renal transplantation. J Am Soc Nephrol 7:158-165, 1996.

251. Iseki K, Yamazato M, Tozawa M, Takishita S: Hypocholesterolemia is a significant predictor of death in a cohort of chronic hemodialysis patients. Kidney Int 61:1887-1893, 2002.

252. Lowrie EG, Lew NL: Death risk in hemodialysis patients: The predictive value of commonly measured variables and an evaluation of death rate differences between facilities. Am J Kidney Dis 15:458-482, 1990.

253. Tschope W, Koch M, Thomas B, Ritz E: Serum lipids predict cardiac death in diabetic patients on maintenance hemodialysis: Results of a prospective study. The German Study Group Diabetes and Uremia. Nephron 64:354-358, 1993.

254. Held PJ, Port FK, Gaylin DS, et al: Comorbid conditions and correlations with mortality risk among 3,399 incident hemodialysis patients. Am J Kidney Dis 20:32-38, 1992.

255. Orth SR, Ritz E, Schrier RW: The renal risks of smoking. Kidney Int 51:1669-1677, 1997.

256. The United States Renal Data System: 1997 Annual Data Report in National Institutes of Health, National Institute of Diabetes and Digestive and Kidney Diseases, Baltimore, MD: USRDS, 1998.

257. Levin A, Djurdjev O, Barrett B, et al: Cardiovascular disease in patients with chronic kidney disease: Getting to the heart of the matter. Am J Kidney Dis 38:1398-1407, 2001.

258. Valsania P, Zarich SW, Kowalchuk GJ, et al: Severity of coronary artery disease in young patients with insulin-dependent diabetes mellitus. Am Heart J 122:695-699, 1991.

259. Galderisi M, Anderson KM, Wilson PWF, Levy D: Echocardiographic evidence for the existence of a distinct diabetic cardiomyopathy (the Framingham Heart Study). Am J Cardiol 68:85-90, 1991.

260. Grossman E, Shemesh E, Shamiss A, et al: Left ventricular mass in diabetes-hypertension. Arch Intern Med 152:1001-1004, 1992.

261. van Hoeven KH, Factor SM: A comparison of the pathological spectrum of hypertensive, diabetic, and hypertensive-diabetic heart disease. Circulation 82:848-855, 1990.

262. Weinrauch LA, D'Elia JA, Gleason RE, et al: Usefulness of left ventricular size and function in predicting survival in chronic dialysis patients with diabetes mellitus. Am J Cardiol 70:300-303, 1992.

263. Rigatto C, Foley RN, Jeffrey J, et al: Electrocardiographic left ventricular hypertrophy in renal transplant recipients: Prognostic value and impact of blood pressure and anemia. J Am Soc Nephrol 14:462-468, 2003.

264. Rahman M, Fu P, Sehgal AR, Smith MC: Interdialytic weight gain, compliance with dialysis regimen, and age are independent predictors of blood pressure in hemodialysis patients. Am J Kidney Dis 35:257-265, 2000.

265. Ates K, Nergizoglu G, Kevan K, et al: Effect of fluid and sodium removal on mortality in peritoneal dialysis patients. Kidney Int 60:767-776, 2001.

266. van Duijnhoven EC, Cheriex EC, Tordoir JH, et al: Effect of closure of the arteriovenous fistula on left ventricular dimensions in renal transplant patients. Nephrol Dial Transplant 16:368-372, 2001.

267. Locatelli F, Marcelli D, Conte F, et al: 1983-1992: Report on regular dialysis and transplantation in Lombardy. Am J Kidney Dis 25:196-205, 1995.

268. Murphy SW, Foley RN, Barrett BJ, et al: Comparative mortality of hemodialysis and peritoneal dialysis in Canada. Kidney Int 57:1720-1726, 2000.

269. Locatelli F, Marcelli D, Conte F, et al: Survival and development of cardiovascular disease by modality of treatment in patients with end-stage renal disease. J Am Soc Nephrol 12:2411-2417, 2001.

270. Foley RN, Parfrey PS, Harnett JD, et al: Hypoalbuminemia, cardiac morbidity, and mortality in end-stage renal disease. J Am Soc Nephrol 7:728-736, 1996.

271. Zimmermann J, Herrlinger S, Pruy A, et al: Inflammation enhances cardiovascular risk and mortality in hemodialysis patients. Kidney Int 55:648-658, 1999.

272. Iseki K, Tozawa M, Yoshi S, Fukiyama K: Serum C-reactive protein (CRP) and risk of death in chronic dialysis patients. Nephrol Dial Transplant 14:1956-1960, 1999.

273. Kumar VA, Craig M, Depner TA, Yeun JY: Extended daily dialysis: A new approach to renal replacement for acute renal failure in the intensive care unit. Am J Kidney Dis 36:294-300, 2000.

274. Ducloux D, Bresson-Vautrin C, Kribs M, et al: C-reactive protein and cardiovascular disease in peritoneal dialysis patients. Kidney Int 62:1417-1422, 2002.

275. Wall RT, Harlan JM, Harker LA, Striker GE: Homocysteine-induced endothelial cell injury in vitro: A model for the study of vascular injury. Thromb Res 18:113-121, 1980.

276. Heinecke JW, Rosen H, Suzuki LA, Chait A: The role of sulfur-containing amino acids in superoxide production and modification of low density lipoprotein by arterial smooth muscle cells. J Biol Chem 262:10098-100103, 1987.

277. Di Minno G, Davi G, Margaglione M, et al: Abnormally high thromboxane biosynthesis in homozygous homocystinuria: Evidence for platelet involvement and probucol-sensitive mechanism. J Clin Invest 92:1400-1406, 1993.

278. Bostom AG, Silbershatz H, Rosenberg IH, et al: Nonfasting plasma total homocysteine levels and all-cause and cardiovascular disease mortality in elderly Framingham men and women. Arch Intern Med 159:1077-1080, 1999.

279. Kark JD, Selhub J, Adler B, et al: Nonfasting plasma total homocysteine level and mortality in middle-aged and elderly men and women in Jerusalem. Arch Intern Med 131:321-330, 1999.

280. Bostom AG, Shemin D, Verhoef P, et al: Elevated fasting total plasma homocysteine levels and cardiovascular disease outcomes in maintenance dialysis patients: A prospective study. Arterioscl Thromb Vasc Biol 17:2554-2558, 1997.

281. Suliman ME, Qureshi AR, Barany P, et al: Hyperhomocysteinemia, nutritional status, and cardiovascular disease in hemodialysis patients. Kidney Int 57:1727-1735, 2000.

282. Moustapha A, Naso A, Nahlawi M, et al: Prospective study of hyperhomocysteinemia as an adverse cardiovascular risk factor in end-stage renal disease. Circulation 97:138-141, 1998.

283. Mallamaci F, Zoccali C, Tripepi G, et al: Hyperhomocysteinemia predicts cardiovascular outcomes in hemodialysis patients. Kidney Int 61:609-614, 2002.

284. Halliwell B, Gutteridge JM, Cross CE: Free radicals, antioxidants, and human disease: Where are we now? J Lab Clin Med 119:598-620, 1992.

285. Allen RC, Yevich SJ, Orth RW, Steele RH: The superoxide anion and singlet molecular oxygen: Their role in the microbicidal activity of the polymorphonuclear leukocyte. Biochem Biophys Res Commun 60:909-917, 1974.

286. Galle J: Oxidative stress in chronic renal failure. Nephrol Dial Transplant 16:2135-2137, 2001.

287. Tetta C, Biasioli S, Schiavon R, et al: An overview of haemodialysis and oxidant stress. Blood Purif 17:118-126, 1999.

288. Becker BN, Himmelfarb J, Henrich WL, Hakim RM: Reassessing the cardiac risk profile in chronic hemodialysis patients: A hypothesis on the role of oxidant stress and other non-traditional cardiac risk factors. J Am Soc Nephrol 8:475-486, 1997.

289. Tardif J-C: Insights into oxidative stress and atherosclerosis. Can J Cardiol 16(supp lD):2D-4D, 2000.

290. Stenvinkel P, Holmberg I, Heimburger O, Diczfalusy U: A study of plasmalogen as an index of oxidative stress in patients with chronic renal failure: Evidence of increased oxidative stress in malnourished patients. Nephrol Dial Transplant 13:2594-2600, 1998.

291. Boaz M, Matas Z, Biro A, et al: Serum malondialdehyde and prevalent cardiovascular disease in hemodialysis. Kidney Int 56:1078-1083, 1999.

292. Tsutsui T, Tsutamoto T, Wada A, et al: Plasma oxidized low-density lipoprotein as a prognostic predictor in patients with chronic congestive heart failure. J Am Coll Cardiol 39:957-962, 2002.

293. Singal PK, Kirshenbaum LA: A relative deficit in antioxidant reserve may contribute in cardiac failure. Can J Cardiol 6:47-49, 1990.

294. Rostand SG, Drueke TB: Parathyroid hormone, vitamin D, and cardiovascular disease in chronic renal failure. Kidney Int 56:383-392, 1999.

295. Block GA, Hulbert-Shearon TE, Levin NW, Port FK: Association of serum phosphorus and calcium × phosphate product with mortality risk on chronic hemodialysis: A national study. Am J Kidney Dis 31:607-617, 1998.

296. Okechukwu CN, Lopes AA, Stack AG, et al: Impact of years of dialysis therapy on mortality risk and the characteristics of longer term dialysis survivors. Am J Kidney Dis 39:533-538, 2002.

297. Hennekens CH, Dyken ML, Fuster V: Aspirin as a therapeutic agent in cardiovascular disease: A statement for healthcare professionals

from the American Heart Association. Circulation 96:2751-2753, 1997.

298. Kronenberg F, Neyer U, Lhotta K, et al: The low molecular weight apo(a) phenotype is an independent predictor for coronary artery disease in hemodialysis patients: A prospective follow-up. J Am Soc Nephrol 10:1027-1036, 1999.

299. Cressman MD, Heyka RJ, Paganini EP, et al: Lipoprotein(a) is an independent risk factor for cardiovascular disease in hemodialysis patients. Circulation 86:475-482, 1992.

300. Hebert MJ, Masse M, Vigneault N, et al: Soluble Fas is a marker of coronary artery disease in patients with end-stage renal disease. Am J Kidney Dis 38:1271-1276, 2001.

301. Masse M, Hebert MJ, Troyanov S, et al: Soluble Fas is a marker of peripheral arterial occlusive disease in haemodialysis patients. Nephrol Dial Transplant 17:485-491, 2002.

302. Labonia WD, Morelli OH Jr, Gimenez MI, et al: Effects of L-carnitine on sodium transport in erythrocytes from dialyzed uremic patients. Kidney Int 32:754-759, 1987.

303. Cristol JP, Bosc JY, Badiou S, et al: Erythropoietin and oxidative stress in hemodialysis: Beneficial effects of vitamin E supplementation. Nephrol Dial Transplant 12:2312-2317, 1997.

304. Ojanen S, Koobi T, Korhonen P, et al: QRS amplitude and volume changes during hemodialysis. Am J Nephrol 19:423-427, 1999.

305. Pochmalicki G, Jan F, Fouchard I, et al: [Frequency of painless myocardial ischemia during hemodialysis in 50 patients with chronic kidney failure]. Arch Mal Coeur Vaiss 83:1671-1675, 1990.

306. Kremastinos D, Paraskevaidis I, Voudiklari S, et al: Painless myocardial ischemia in chronic hemodialysed patients: A real event? Nephron 60:164-170, 1992.

307. George SK, Singh AK: Current markers of myocardial ischemia and their validity in end-stage renal disease. Curr Opin Nephrol Hypertens 8:719-22, 1999.

308. Jaffe AS, Ravkilde J, Roberts R, et al: It's time for a change to a troponin standard. Circulation 102:1216-1220, 2000.

309. Antman EM, Tanasijevic MJ, Thompson B, et al: Cardiac-specific troponin I levels to predict the risk of mortality in patients with acute coronary syndromes. N Engl J Med 335:1342-1349, 1996.

310. Aviles RJ, Askari AT, Lindahl B, et al: Troponin T levels in patients with acute coronary syndromes, with or without renal dysfunction. N Engl J Med 346:2047-2052, 2002.

311. Geleijnse ML, Fioretti PM, Roelandt JR: Methodology, feasibility, safety and diagnostic accuracy of dobutamine stress echocardiography. J Am Coll Cardiol 30:595-606, 1997.

312. Ho YL, Wu CC, Huang PJ, et al: Dobutamine stress echocardiography compared with exercise thallium-201 single-photon emission computed tomography in detecting coronary artery disease-effect of exercise level on accuracy. Cardiology 88:379-385, 1997.

313. Marwick TH, Cain P: Screening for coronary artery disease. Review. Med Clin North Am 83:1375-1402, 1999.

314. Reis G, Marcovitz PA, Leichtman AB, et al: Usefulness of dobutamine stress echocardiography in detecting coronary artery disease in end-stage renal disease. Am J Cardiol 75:707-710, 1995.

315. Le A, Wilson R, Douek K, et al: Prospective risk stratification in renal transplant candidates for cardiac death. Am J Kidney Dis 24:65-71, 1994.

316. Dahan M, Viron BM, Faraggi M, et al: Diagnostic accuracy and prognostic value of combined dipyridamole-exercise thallium imaging in hemodialysis patients. Kidney Int 54:255-262, 1998.

317. Boudreau RJ, Strony JT, duCret RP, et al: Perfusion thallium imaging of type I diabetes patients with end stage renal disease: Comparison of oral and intravenous dipyridamole administration. Radiology 175:103-105, 1990.

318. Stanford W, Thompson BH: Imaging of coronary artery calcification: Its importance in assessing atherosclerotic disease. Radiol Clin North Am 37:257-272, 1999.

319. Ganesh SK, Stack AG, Levin NW, et al: Association of elevated serum PO(4), Ca × PO(4) product, and parathyroid hormone with cardiac mortality risk in chronic hemodialysis patients. J Am Soc Nephrol 12:2131-2138, 2001.

320. Kimura K, Saika Y, Otani H, et al: Factors associated with calcification of the abdominal aorta in hemodialysis patients. Kidney Int Suppl 71:S238-S241, 1999.

321. Chertow GM, Burke SK, Raggi P: Treat to Goal Working Group: Sevelamer attenuates the progression of coronary and aortic calcification in hemodialysis patients. Kidney Int 62:245-252, 2002.

322. Murphy SW, Foley RN, Parfrey PS: Screening and treatment for cardiovascular disease in patients with chronic renal disease. Am J Kidney Dis 32(5 suppl 3):S184-S199, 1998.

323. Holley JL, Monaghan J, Byer B, Bronsther O: An examination of the renal transplant evaluation process focusing on cost and the reasons for patient exclusion. Am J Kidney Dis 32:567-574, 1998.

324. Fell G, Phillips DJ, Chikos PM, et al: Ultrasonic duplex scanning for disease of the carotid artery. Circulation 64:1191-1195, 1981.

325. Fronek A, Coel M, Berstein EF: Quantitative ultrasonographic studies of lower extremity flow velocities in health and disease. Circulation 53:957-960, 1976.

326. Carpenter JP, Lexa FJ, Davis JT: Determination of duplex Doppler ultrasound criteria appropriate to the North American Symptomatic Carotid Endarterectomy Trial. Stroke 27:695-699, 1996.

327. Winter-Warnars HA, van der Graaf Y, Mali WP: Interobserver variation in duplex sonographic scanning in the femoropopliteal tract. J Ultrasound Med 15:421-428; discussion 329-330, 1996.

328. Weitz JI, Byrne J, Clagett GP, et al: Diagnosis and treatment of chronic arterial insufficiency of the lower extremities: A critical review. [Erratum appears in Circulation 102:1074, 2000.] Circulation 94:3026-3049, 1996.

329. Pannier B, Guerin AP, Marchais SJ, et al: Postischemic vasodilation, endothelial activation, and cardiovascular remodeling in end-stage renal disease. Kidney Int 57:1091-109, 2000.

330. Joannides R, Bizet-Nafeh C, Costentin A, et al: Chronic ACE inhibition enhances the endothelial control of arterial mechanics and flow-dependent vasodilatation in heart failure. Hypertension 38:1446-1450, 2001.

331. Reiner BI, Siegel EL, Hooper F, et al: Picture archiving and communication systems and vascular surgery: Clinical impressions and suggestions for improvement. J Digit Imaging 9:167-171, 1996.

332. Pitt B, Zannad F, Remme WJ, et al: The effect of spironolactone on morbidity and mortality in patients with severe heart failure: Randomized Aldactone Evaluation Study Investigators. N Engl J Med 341:709-717, 1999.

333. Chrysostomou A, Becker G: Spironolactone in addition to ACE inhibition to reduce proteinuria in patients with chronic renal disease. N Engl J Med 345:925-926, 2001.

334. The SOLVD Investigators: Effect of enalapril on survival in patients with reduced left ventricular ejection fractions and congestive heart failure. N Engl J Med 325:293-302, 1991.

335. The SOLVD Investigators: Effect of enalapril on mortality and the development of heart failure in asymptomatic patients with reduced left ventricular ejection fractions. N Engl J Med 327:685-691, 1992.

336. Pfeffer MA, Braunwald E, Moye LA, et al: Effect of captopril on mortality and morbidity in patients with left ventricular dysfunction after myocardial infarction: Results of the survival and ventricular enlargement trial. The SAVE Investigators. N Engl J Med 327:669-677, 1992.

337. Brenner BM, Cooper ME, de Zeeuw D, et al: RENAAL Study Investigators: Effects of losartan on renal and cardiovascular outcomes in patients with type 2 diabetes and nephropathy. N Engl J Med 345:861-869, 2001.

338. Lewis EJ, Hunsicker LG, Clarke WR, et al: Collaborative Study Group: Renoprotective effect of the angiotensin-receptor antagonist irbesartan in patients with nephropathy due to type 2 diabetes. N Engl J Med 345:851-860, 2001.

339. Parving HH, Lehnert H, Brochner-Mortensen J, et al: Irbesartan in Patients with Type 2 Diabetes and Microalbuminuria Study Group: The effect of irbesartan on the development of diabetic nephropathy in patients with type 2 diabetes. N Engl J Med 345:870-878, 2001.

340. Hunt SA, Baker DW, Chin MH, et al, and American College of Cardiology/American Heart Association: ACC/AHA guidelines for the evaluation and management of chronic heart failure in the adult: Executive summary. A report of the American College of Cardiology/American Heart Association Task Force on Practice Guidelines (Committee to Revise the 1995 Guidelines for the Evaluation and Management of Heart Failure). J Am Coll Cardiol 38:2101-2113, 2001.

341. Hara Y, Hamada M, Shigematsu Y, et al: Beneficial effect of beta-adrenergic blockade on left ventricular function in haemodialysis patients. Clin Sci 101:219-225, 2001.

342. Bristow MR: β-Adrenergic receptor blockade in chronic heart failure. Circulation 101:558-569, 2000.

343. Brophy JM, Joseph L, Ronleau JL: β-Blockers in congestive heart failure: A Bayesian meta-analysis. Ann Intern Med 134:550-560, 2001.

344. Packer M, Coats AJ, Fowler MB, et al: Carvedilol Prospective Randomized Cumulative Survival Study Group: Effect of carvedilol on survival in severe chronic heart failure. N Engl J Med 344: 1651-1658, 2001.

345. Braunwald E: Expanding indications for beta-blockers in heart failure. N Engl J Med 344:1711-1712, 2001.

346. The Digitalis Investigation Group: The effect of digoxin on mortality and morbidity in patients with heart failure. N Engl J Med 336:525-533, 1997.

347. Dimitrow PP, Surdacki A, Dubiel JS: Verapamil normalizes the response of left ventricular early diastolic filling to cold pressor test in asymptomatic and mildly symptomatic patients with hypertrophic cardiomyopathy. Cardiovasc Drugs Ther 11:741-746, 1997.

348. Millaire A: [Diastolic cardiac failure: therapeutic modalities]. Arch Mal Coeur Vaiss 91:1365-1369, 1998.

349. Anonymous: Consensus recommendations for the management of chronic heart failure: On behalf of the membership of the advisory council to improve outcomes nationwide in heart failure. Am J Cardiol 83:1A-38A, 1999.

350. Sanmuganathan PS, Ghahramani P, Jackson PR, et al: Aspirin for primary prevention of coronary heart disease: Safety and absolute benefit related to coronary risk derived from meta-analysis of randomised trials. Heart 85:265-271, 2001.

351. Best PJ, Lennon R, Ting HH, et al: The impact of renal insufficiency on clinical outcomes in patients undergoing percutaneous coronary interventions. J Am Coll Cardiol 39:1113-1119, 2002.

352. Rubenstein MH, Harrell LC, Sheynberg BV, et al: Are patients with renal failure good candidates for percutaneous coronary revascularization in the new device era? Circulation 102:2966-2972, 2000.

353. Asinger RW, Henry TD, Herzog CA, et al: Clinical outcomes of PTCA in chronic renal failure: A case-control study for comorbid features and evaluation of dialysis dependence. J Invas Cardiol 13:21-28, 2001.

354. Herzog CA, Ma JZ, Collins AJ: Long-term outcome of dialysis patients in the United States with coronary revascularization procedures. Kidney Int 56:324-332, 1999.

355. Clough RA, Leavitt BJ, Morton JR, et al: The effect of comorbid illness on mortality outcomes in cardiac surgery. Arch Surg 137:428-432, 2002.

356. Serruys PW, Unger F, Sousa JE, et al: Arterial Revascularization Therapies Study Group: Comparison of coronary-artery bypass surgery and stenting for the treatment of multivessel disease. N Engl J Med 344:1117-1124, 2001.

357. Rinehart AL, Herzog CA, Collins AJ, et al: A comparison of coronary angioplasty and coronary artery bypass grafting in chronic dialysis patients. Am J Kidney Dis 25:281-290, 1995.

358. Koyanagi T, Nishida H, Kitamura M, et al: Comparison of clinical outcomes of coronary artery bypass grafting and percutaneous transluminal coronary angioplasty in renal dialysis patients. Ann Thorac Surg 61:1793-1796, 1996.

359. Morice MC, Serruys PW, Sousa JE, et al: RAVEL Study Group: Randomized Study with the Sirolimus-Coated Bx Velocity Balloon-Expandable Stent in the Treatment of Patients with de Novo Native Coronary Artery Lesions. A randomized comparison of a sirolimus-eluting stent with a standard stent for coronary revascularization. N Engl J Med 346:1773-1780, 2002.

360. Stack AG, Bloembergen WE: Prevalence and clinical correlates of coronary artery disease among new dialysis patients in the United States: A cross-sectional study. J Am Soc Nephrol 12:1516-1523, 2001.

361. De Meyer M, Wyns W, Dion R, et al: Myocardial revascularization in patients on renal replacement therapy. Clin Nephrol 36:147-151, 1991.

362. Christiansen S, Splittgerber FH, Marggraf G, et al: Results of cardiac operations in five kidney transplant patients. Thorac Cardiovasc Surg 45:75-77, 1997.

363. Hueb WA, Oliveira SA, Bittencourt D, et al: Coronary bypass surgery for patients with renal transplantation. Cardiology 73:151-155, 1986.

364. Defraigne JO, Meurisse M, Limet R: Valvular and coronary surgery in renal transplant patients. J Cardiovasc Surg 31:581-583, 1990.

365. Christiansen S, Claus M, Philipp T, Reidemeister JC: Cardiac surgery in patients with end-stage renal failure. Clin Nephrol 48:246-252, 1997.

366. Dierkes J, Domrose U, Ambrosch A, et al: Response of hyperhomocysteinemia to folic acid supplementation in patients with end-stage renal disease. Clin Nephrol 51:108-115, 1999.

367. van Guldener C, Lambert J, ter Wee PM, et al: Carotid artery stiffness in patients with end-stage renal disease: No effect of long-term homocysteine-lowering therapy. Clin Nephrol 53:33-41, 2000.

368. Manske CL, Wilson RF, Wang Y, Thomas W: Atherosclerotic vascular complications in diabetic transplant candidates. Am J Kidney Dis 29:601-607, 1997.

369. Cheung AK, Sarnak MJ, Yan G, et al: Atherosclerotic cardiovascular disease risks in chronic hemodialysis patients. Kidney Int 58:353-362, 2000.

370. Larsson J, Apelqvist J, Agardh CD, Stenstrom A: Decreasing incidence of major amputation in diabetic patients: A consequence of a multidisciplinary foot care team approach? Diabet Med 12:770-776, 1995.

371. Edmonds ME, Blundell MP, Morris ME, et al: Improved survival of the diabetic foot: The role of a specialized foot clinic. Q J Med 60:763-771, 1986.

372. Silver MR, Kroboth PD: Pentoxifylline in end-stage renal disease. Drug Intell Clin Pharm 21:976-978, 1987.

373. Pignone M, Phillips C, Mulrow C: Use of lipid lowering drugs for primary prevention of coronary heart disease: Meta-analysis of randomised trials. BMJ 321:983-986, 2000.

374. Wilson SE, White GH, Wolf G, Cross AP: Proximal percutaneous balloon angioplasty and distal bypass for multilevel arterial occlusion: Veterans Administration Cooperative Study No. 199. Ann Vasc Surg 4:351-355, 1990.

375. Edwards JM, Taylor LM Jr, Porter JM: Limb salvage in end-stage renal disease (ESRD): Comparison of modern results in patients with and without ESRD. Arch Surg 123:1164-1168, 1988.

376. Isiklar MH, Kulbaski M, MacDonald MJ, Lumsden AB: Infrainguinal bypass in end-stage renal disease: When is it justified? Semin Vasc Surg 10:42-48, 1997.

377. Dossa CD, Shepard AD, Amos AM, et al: Results of lower extremity amputations in patients with end-stage renal disease. J Vasc Surg 20:14-19, 1994.

378. Makisalo H, Lepantalo M, Halme L, et al: Peripheral arterial disease as a predictor of outcome after renal transplantation. Transplant Int 11(suppl 1):S140-S143, 1998.

379. Kasiske BL, Kalil RS, Ma JZ, et al: Effect of antihypertensive therapy on the kidney in patients with diabetes: A meta-regression analysis. Ann Intern Med 118:129-138, 1993.

380. Anonymous: Randomised placebo-controlled trial of effect of ramipril on decline in glomerular filtration rate and risk of terminal renal failure in proteinuric, non-diabetic nephropathy: The GISEN Group (Gruppo Italiano di Studi Epidemiologici in Nefrologia). Lancet 349:1857-1863, 1997.

381. Ruggenenti P, Perna A, Gherardi G, et al: Renoprotective properties of ACE-inhibition in non-diabetic nephropathies with non-nephrotic proteinuria. Lancet 354:359-364, 1999.

382. Maschio G, Alberti D, Janin G, et al: Effect of the angiotensin-converting-enzyme inhibitor benazepril on the progression of chronic renal insufficiency: The Angiotensin-Converting-Enzyme Inhibition in Progressive Renal Insufficiency Study Group. N Engl J Med 334:939-945, 1996.

383. Jafar TH, Schmid CH, Landa M, et al: Angiotensin-converting enzyme inhibitors and progression of nondiabetic renal disease: A meta-analysis of patient-level data. [Erratum appears in Ann Intern Med 137:299, 2002.] Ann Intern Med 135:73-87, 2001.

384. Agodoa LY, Appel L, Bakris GL, et al: African American Study of Kidney Disease and Hypertension (AASK) Study Group. Effect of ramipril vs amlodipine on renal outcomes in hypertensive nephrosclerosis: A randomized controlled trial. JAMA 285:2719-2728, 2001.

385. Estacio RO, Jeffers BW, Hiatt WR, et al: The effect of nisoldipine as compared with enalapril on cardiovascular outcomes in patients with non-insulin-dependent diabetes and hypertension. N Engl J Med 338:645-652, 1998.

386. Adler AI, Stratton IM, Neil HA, et al: Association of systolic blood pressure with macrovascular and microvascular complications of type 2 diabetes (UKPDS 36): Prospective observational study. BMJ 321:412-419, 2000.

387. Bakris GL, Williams M, Dworkin L, et al: Preserving renal function in adults with hypertension and diabetes: A consensus approach. National Kidney Foundation Hypertension and Diabetes Executive Committees Working Group. Am J Kidney Dis 36: 646-661, 2000.

388. Hansson L, Zanchetti A, Carruthers SG, et al: Effects of intensive blood-pressure lowering and low-dose aspirin in patients with hypertension: Principal results of the Hypertension Optimal Treatment (HOT) randomised trial. HOT Study Group. Lancet 351:1755-1762, 1998.

389. Estacio RO, Jeffers BW, Gifford N, Schrier RW: Effect of blood pressure control on diabetic microvascular complications in patients with hypertension and type 2 diabetes. Diabetes Care 23(suppl 2): B54-B64, 2000.

390. Charra B, Calemard E, Ruffet M, et al: Survival as an index of adequacy of dialysis. Kidney Int 41:1286-1291, 1992.

391. Cannella G, Paoletti E, Delfino R, et al: Regression of left ventricular hypertrophy in hypertensive dialyzed uremic patients on long-term antihypertensive therapy. Kidney Int 44:881-886, 1993.

392. Yusuf S, Sleight P, Pogue J, et al: Effects of an angiotensin-converting-enzyme inhibitor, ramipril, on cardiovascular events in high-risk patients: The Heart Outcomes Prevention Evaluation Study Investigators. N Engl J Med 342:145-153, 2000.

393. Klingbeil AU, Muller HJ, Delles C, et al: Regression of left ventricular hypertrophy by AT1 receptor blockade in renal transplant recipients. Am J Hypertens 13:1295-1300, 2000.

394. Kasiske BL, Vazquez MA, Harmon WE, et al: Recommendations for the outpatient surveillance of renal transplant recipients: American Society of Transplantation. J Am Soc Nephrol 11(suppl 15):S1-S86, 2000.

395. Saltissi D, Morgan C, Rigby RJ, Westhuyzen J: Safety and efficacy of simvastatin in hypercholesterolemic patients undergoing chronic renal dialysis. Am J Kidney Dis 39:283-290, 2002.

396. Harris KP, Wheeler DC, Chong CC: Atorvastatin in CAPD Study Investigators. Continuous ambulatory peritoneal dialysis: A placebo-controlled trial examining atorvastatin in dyslipidemic patients undergoing CAPD. Kidney Int 61:1469-1474, 2002.

397. Hufnagel G, Michel C, Vrtovsnik F, et al: Effects of atorvastatin on dyslipidaemia in uraemic patients on peritoneal dialysis. Nephrol Dial Transplant 15:684-688, 2000.

398. Holdaas H, Jardine AG, Wheeler DC, et al: Effect of fluvastatin on acute renal allograft rejection: A randomized multicenter trial. Kidney Int 60:1990-1997, 2001.

399. Arnadottir M, Eriksson LO, Germershausen JI, Thysell H: Low-dose simvastatin is a well-tolerated and efficacious cholesterol-lowering agent in ciclosporin-treated kidney transplant recipients: Double-blind, randomized, placebo-controlled study in 40 patients. Nephron 68:57-62, 1994.

400. Diercks GF, Janssen WM, van Boven AJ, et al: Rationale, design, and baseline characteristics of a trial of prevention of cardiovascular and renal disease with fosinopril and pravastatin in nonhypertensive, nonhypercholesterolemic subjects with microalbuminuria: The Prevention of REnal and Vascular ENdstage Disease Intervention Trial (PREVEND IT). Am J Cardiol 86:635-638, 2000.

401. Holdaas H, Fellstrom B, Holme I, et al: ALERT Study Group: Assessment of Lescol in Renal Transplantation. Effects of fluvastatin on cardiac events in renal transplant patients: ALERT (Assessment of Lescol in Renal Transplantation) study design and baseline data. J Cardiovasc Risk 8:63-71, 2001.

402. Wanner C, Krane V, Ruf G, et al: Rationale and design of a trial improving outcome of type 2 diabetics on hemodialysis: Die Deutsche Diabetes Dialyse Studie Investigators. Kidney Int Suppl 71:S222-S226, 1999.

403. Baigent C, Wheeler DC: Should we reduce blood cholesterol to prevent cardiovascular disease among patients with chronic renal failure? Nephrol Dial Transplant 15:1118-1119, 2001.

404. Seliger SL, Weiss NS, Gillen DL, et al: HMG-CoA reductase inhibitors are associated with reduced mortality in ESRD patients. Kidney Int 61:297-304, 2002.

405. Beto JA, Bansal VK: Interventions for other risk factors: Tobacco use, physical inactivity, menopause, and homocysteine. Am J Kidney Dis 32(5 suppl 3):S172-S183, 1998.

406. Anonymous: Intensive blood-glucose control with sulphonylureas or insulin compared with conventional treatment and risk of complications in patients with type 2 diabetes (UKPDS 33): UK Prospective Diabetes Study (UKPDS) Group. [Erratum appears in Lancet 354:602, 1999.]. Lancet 352:837-853, 1998.

407. Barbosa J, Steffes MW, Sutherland DE, et al: Effect of glycemic control on early diabetic renal lesions: A 5-year randomized controlled clinical trial of insulin-dependent diabetic kidney transplant recipients. JAMA 272:600-606, 1994.

408. Becker BN, Brazy PC, Becker YT, et al: Simultaneous pancreas-kidney transplantation reduces excess mortality in type 1 diabetic patients with end-stage renal disease. Kidney Int 57:2129-2135, 2000.

409. Tyden G, Bolinder J, Solders G, et al: Improved survival in patients with insulin-dependent diabetes mellitus and end-stage diabetic nephropathy 10 years after combined pancreas and kidney transplantation. Transplantation 67:645-648, 1999.

410. Lim VS, DeGowin RL, Zavala D, et al: Recombinant human erythropoietin treatment in pre-dialysis patients: A double-blind placebo-controlled trial. Ann Intern Med 110:108-114, 1989.

411. Clyne N, Jogestrand T: Effect of erythropoietin treatment on physical exercise capacity and on renal function in predialytic uremic patients. Nephron 60:390-396, 1992.

412. Goldberg AP, Geltman EM, Gavin JR 3rd, et al: Exercise training reduces coronary risk and effectively rehabilitates hemodialysis patients. Nephron 42:311-316, 1986.

413. Miller BW, Cress CL, Johnson ME, et al: Exercise during hemodialysis decreases the use of antihypertensive medications. Am J Kidney Dis 39:828-833, 2002.

414. McMahon LP, Roger SD, Schou M: Does early intervention and treatment with epoetin prevent left ventricular hypertrophy in chronic kidney disease? Abstract. J Am Soc Nephrol 13:440A, 2002.

415. Foley RN, Parfrey PS, Morgan J, et al: Effect of hemoglobin levels in hemodialysis patients with asymptomatic cardiomyopathy. Kidney Int 58:1325-1335, 2000.

416. Besarab A, Bolton WK, Browne JK, et al: The effects of normal as compared with low hematocrit values in patients with cardiac disease who are receiving hemodialysis and epoetin. N Engl J Med 339:584-590, 1998.

417. London GM, Pannier B, Guerin AP, et al: Cardiac hypertrophy, aortic compliance, peripheral resistance, and wave reflection in end-stage renal disease: Comparative effects of ACE inhibition and calcium channel blockade. Circulation 90:2786-2796, 1994.

418. Levy BI, Michel JB, Salzmann JL, et al: Effects of chronic inhibition of converting enzyme on mechanical and structural properties of arteries in rat renovascular hypertension. Circ Res 63:227-239, 1988.

419. Levy BI, Michel JB, Salzmann JL, et al: Remodeling of heart and arteries by chronic converting enzyme inhibition in spontaneously hypertensive rats. Am J Hypertens 4:240S-245S, 1991.

420. London GM, Marchais SJ, Guerin AP, et al: Salt and water retention and calcium blockade in uremia. Circulation 82:105-113, 1990.

421. Rubattu S, Ridker P, Stampfer MJ, et al: The gene encoding atrial natriuretic peptide and the risk of human stroke. Circulation 100:1722-1726, 1999.

422. Jialal I, Stein D, Balis D, et al: Effect of hydroxymethyl glutaryl coenzyme a reductase inhibitor therapy on high sensitive C-reactive protein levels. Circulation 103:1933-1935, 2001.

423. Musial J, Undas A, Gajewski P, et al: Anti-inflammatory effects of simvastatin in subjects with hypercholesterolemia. Int J Cardiol 77:247-253, 2001.

424. Chang JW, Yang WS, Min WK, et al: Effects of simvastatin on high-sensitivity C-reactive protein and serum albumin in hemodialysis patients. Am J Kidney Dis 39:1213-1217, 2002.

425. Bostom AG, Shemin D, Gohh RY, et al: Treatment of hyperhomocysteinemia in hemodialysis patients and renal transplant recipients. Kidney Int 17(suppl):S246-S252, 2001.

426. van Guldener C, Janssen MJ, Lambert J, et al: Folic acid treatment of hyperhomocysteinemia in peritoneal dialysis patients: No change in endothelial function after long-term therapy. Perit Dial Int 18:282-289, 1998.

427. Touam M, Zingraff J, Jungers P, et al: Effective correction of hyper-homocysteinemia in hemodialysis patients by intravenous folinic acid and pyridoxine therapy. Kidney Int 56:2292-2296, 1999.

428. Boaz M, Smetana S, Weinstein T, et al: Secondary prevention with antioxidants of cardiovascular disease in endstage renal disease (SPACE): Randomised placebo-controlled trial. Lancet 356: 1213-1218, 2000.

429. Block GA, Port FK: Re-evaluation of risks associated with hyperphosphatemia and hyperparathyroidism in dialysis patients: Recommendations for a change in management. Am J Kidney Dis 35: 1226-1237, 2000.

430. Gonzalez EA, Lund RJ, Martin KJ, et al: Treatment of a murine model of high-turnover renal osteodystrophy by exogenous BMP-7. Kidney Int 61:1322-1331, 2002.

431. Sanmuganathan PS, Ghahramani P, Jackson PR, et al: Aspirin for primary prevention of coronary heart disease: Safety and absolute benefit related to coronary risk derived from meta-analysis of randomised trials. Heart 85:265-271, 2001.

432. Tonelli M, Bohm C, Pandeya S, et al: Cardiac risk factors and the use of cardioprotective medications in patients with renal insufficiency. Am J Kidney Dis 37:484-489, 2001.

433. Ruilope LM, Salvetti A, Jamerson K, et al: Renal function and intensive lowering of blood pressure in hypertensive participants of the Hypertension Optimal Treatment (HOT) study. J Am Soc Nephrol 12:218-225, 2001.

434. Gaede P, Vedel P, Parving HH, Pedersen O: Intensified multifactorial intervention in patients with type 2 diabetes mellitus and microalbuminuria: The STENO type 2 randomised study. Lancet 353:617-622, 1999.

Neurologic Complications of Renal Insufficiency

Allen I. Arieff

Although technical advancements in dialysis therapy, improved immunosuppression with renal transplantation, and overall progress in medical management have resulted in improvement of both the duration and the quality of life in patients with end-stage renal disease (ESRD), this progress has introduced major drawbacks. The disorders introduced by extended longevity among patients with ESRD include amyloid-associated arthropathy[1] and myocardopathy,[2] increased frequency of leg amputation among diabetic subjects treated with hemodialysis,[3] more severe coronary artery disease,[4] and left ventricular hypertrophy, largely as a consequence of uremic anemia.[5, 6] Recent evidence suggests a common linkage of oxidative stress and carbonyl stress with increased cardiovascular morbidity and mortality.[7-9]

Patients with ESRD continue to manifest an increasing variety of neurologic disorders. Those with chronic renal failure (CRF) who have not yet received dialysis therapy may develop a symptom complex progressing from mild sensorial clouding to tremor, delirium and coma.[10] Even after the institution of otherwise adequate maintenance dialysis therapy, patients may continue to manifest more subtle nervous system dysfunction, such as impaired mentation, generalized weakness, and peripheral neuropathy.

The central nervous system (CNS) disorders of untreated renal failure have traditionally been referred to as uremic encephalopathy. In this chapter, I have attempted to introduce a new concept, that of a syndrome of CNS disorders that persists despite otherwise adequate hemodialysis.

This new disorder is called *dialysis-dependent encephalopathy* (Table 51-1).

The maintenance of life by dialysis treatment of patients with ESRD has itself been associated with the emergence of at least four previously well-described disorders of the CNS: (1) dialysis dysequilibrium syndrome (DDS), (2) dialysis dementia, (3) stroke, and (4) sexual dysfunction.[11, 12] DDS is

TABLE 51-1

Chronic Dialysis-Dependent Encephalopathy

Neuroimaging of uremic brain: generally unremarkable
Pathology of uremic brain: generally nonspecific
Pathophysiologic mechanisms
  Apoptosis
    Calcium ion
    Free radicals
    Glutamate
    Hypoxia
  Oxidative stress
    Advanced glycation end products
    Metabolism of lipids
    Metabolism of carbohydrates
    Inhibited by nitric oxide donors
  Inflammation
    Elevated C-reactive protein
    Elevated homocysteine
    Occult infection
    Occult inflammatory nidus

a consequence of the initiation of dialysis therapy in a minority of patients. Dialysis dementia is a progressive, usually fatal encephalopathy that can affect patients receiving chronic hemodialysis as well as children with CRF who have not been treated with dialysis. Cardiovascular disorders are the major cause of death in hemodialysis patients, accounting for 40% of deaths.[13] These disorders include myocardial infarction, cardiomyopathy, ischemic heart disease, and stroke.[14] The factors associated with uremia that lead to an increased incidence and mortality from stroke are not well known but are beginning to be understood, because they are similar to those factors that lead to myocardial infarction.[13-15]

In addition to the manifestations of neurologic dysfunction just described, which are specifically related to renal insufficiency, dialysis, or both, a number of other neurologic disorders occur with increased frequency in patients who have ESRD and are being treated with chronic hemodialysis. Subdural hematoma, acute stroke, certain electrolyte disorders (hyponatremia, hypernatremia, hyperkalemia, phosphate depletion, hypercalcemia), vitamin deficiencies, Wernicke encephalopathy, drug intoxication, hypertensive encephalopathy, and acute trace element intoxication must be considered in patients with CRF who manifest an altered mental state. In the recent past, renal transplantation was associated with a variety of nervous system infections and neoplasms, such as reticulum cell sarcoma and lymphoma, which were probably a direct result of immunosuppressive therapy then in use (azathioprine, prednisone). This situation appears to be altered with the current widespread use of other immunosuppressive regimens (mycophenolate mofetil, cyclosporin, tacrolimus, rapamycin, polyclonal antisera) for renal transplantation.[16, 17]

Patients with renal failure are also at risk for development of the same varieties of organic brain disease and metabolic encephalopathy that can affect the general population. Therefore, when a patient with ESRD presents with altered mental status, a thorough and complete evaluation is necessary.

ACUTE RENAL FAILURE

The clinical manifestations of acute renal failure (ARF) have been studied in several large patient series.[18-20] Abnormalities of mental status have been noted as early and sensitive indices of a neurologic disorder that progressed rapidly into disorientation and confusion.[21] Fixed attitudes, torpor, and other signs of toxic psychosis were common. When uremia is untreated and allowed to progress, coma often supervenes. Cranial nerve signs such as nystagmus and mild facial asymmetries are common but usually transient. There can be visual field defects and papilledema of the optic fundi. About half of the patients have dysarthria, and many have diffuse weakness and fasciculations. Marked variation of deep tendon reflexes is noted in most patients, often in an asymmetrical pattern. Progression of hyperreflexia, with sustained clonus at the patella or ankle, is common.[22] In contrast to patients with CRF, those with ARF do not generally have long histories of diabetes mellitus and do not tend to have the extensive cardiovascular damage that is found in so many patients with chronic ESRD.

Electroencephalogram in Patients with Acute Renal Failure

Electroencephalograms (EEGs) in patients with ARF[20] are usually grossly abnormal when the diagnosis of renal failure is first established. In most instances, the percentage of EEG power lower than 5 Hz and lower than 7 Hz, which are standard measurements of the percentage of EEG power devoted to abnormal (delta) slow wave activity, is more than 20 times the normal value. The percentage of EEG frequencies greater than 9 Hz and lower than 5 Hz is not affected by dialysis for 6 to 8 weeks, but it does return to normal with recovery of renal function. Similar findings have been shown in experimental animals with renal failure.[23] The EEG may worsen both during and for several hours after hemodialysis and up to 6 months after initiation of dialytic therapy.[24, 25] In patients with ARF, the EEG is abnormal within 48 hours after the onset of renal failure[20] and usually is not affected by dialysis within the first 3 weeks (Fig. 51-1). During this interval, patients with ARF have been shown to have elevated levels of parathyroid hormone (PTH) in plasma.[20, 26] Several months after return of renal function, plasma PTH levels also return to normal. Although there are many factors that contribute to uremic encephalopathy, investigators have shown no correlation between encephalopathy and any of the commonly measured indicators of renal failure (e.g., BUN, creatinine, bicarbonate, arterial pH, potassium).[20, 26, 27] On this basis, PTH has been postulated to be an important CNS system "uremic toxin."[26, 28]

UREMIC ENCEPHALOPATHY

Uremic encephalopathy is a metabolic encephalopathy that has much in common with other types, such as diabetic ketoacidosis, hepatic failure, hypoxia, carbon dioxide narcosis, and acute ethanol intoxication.[29, 30] The symptoms of uremic encephalopathy are shown in Table 51-2. Uremic encephalopathy is an acute or subacute organic brain syndrome that regularly occurs in patients with ARF or CRF when the glomerular filtration rate (GFR) declines to less than 10% of normal. As with other organic brain syndromes, these patients display variable disorders of consciousness, psychomotor behavior, thinking, memory, speech, perception, and emotion.[10, 18, 31]

The term *uremic encephalopathy* is used to describe the early appearance and dialysis responsiveness of the nonspecific neurologic symptoms of uremia. Other systemic abnormalities observed in patients with CRF are separable from uremic encephalopathy on the grounds that they tend to appear late in the progressive clinical course, infrequently produce symptoms, are detected in tissues and organs rather than as integrated whole-organism phenomena, and respond sluggishly and irregularly to dialysis procedures. The symptoms may include sluggishness and easy fatigue; daytime drowsiness and insomnia with a tendency toward sleep-inversion; itching; inability to focus or sustain attention or to perform mental (cognitive) tasks and manipulation; inability to manage ideas and abstractions; slurring of speech; anorexia, nausea, and vomiting (probably of CNS origin); restlessness; imprecise memory; diminished sexual interest and performance; volatile emotionality and withdrawal; myoclonus and

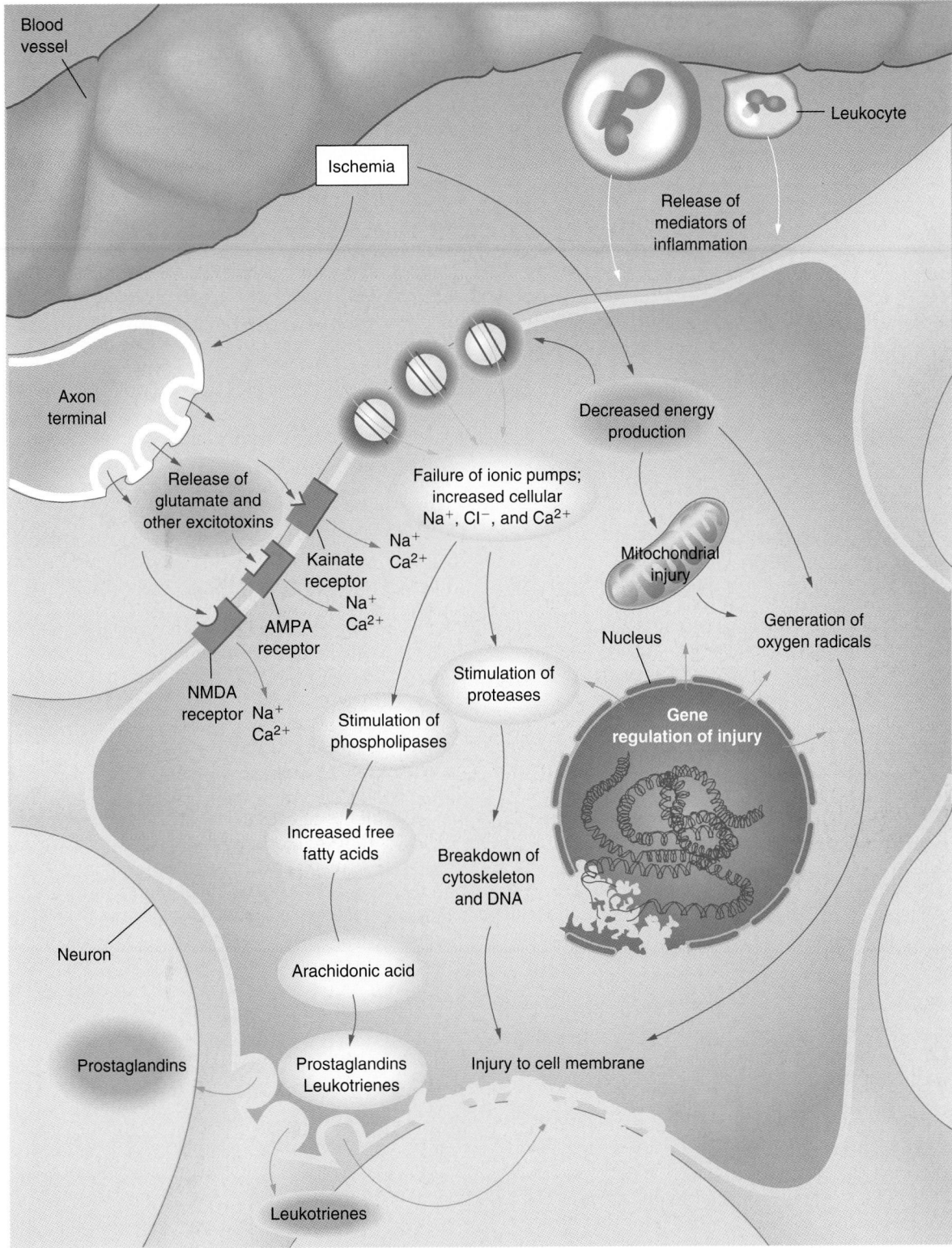

FIGURE 51-1. The molecular events initiated in brain tissue by acute cerebral ischemia. Interruption of cerebral blood flow results in decreased energy production, which in turn causes failure of ionic pumps, mitochondrial injury, activation of leukocytes (with release of mediators of inflammation), generation of oxygen radicals, and release of excitotoxins. Increased cellular levels of sodium, chloride, and calcium ions result in stimulation of phospholipases and proteases, followed by generation and release of prostaglandins and leukotrienes, breakdown of DNA and the cytoskeleton, and, ultimately, breakdown of the cell membrane. Alteration of genetic components regulates elements of the cascade to alter the degree of injury. AMPA, α-amino-3-hydroxy-5-methyl-4-isoxazole propionic acid; NMDA, *N*-methyl-D-aspartate. (From Brott T, Bogousslavsky J: Treatment of acute ischemic stroke. N Engl J Med 343:710-722, 2000.)

TABLE 51-2

Signs and Symptoms of Uremic Encephalopathy

Early Uremia

Anorexia
Malaise
Insomnia
Diminished attention span
Decreased libido

Moderate Uremia

Emesis
Decreased activity
Easy fatigability
Decreased cognition
Impotence

Advanced Uremia

Severe weakness and fatigue
Pruritus
Disorientation
Confusion
Asterixis
Stupor, seizures, coma (rare after 1990)

"restless legs"; "burning feet"; asterixis; hiccoughs; paranoid thought content; disorientation and confusion with bizarre behavior; hallucinosis, muttering, and mumbling; meningeal signs, nystagmus; vertigo and ataxia; transient pareses and aphasic episodes; and coma and convulsions.

Certain salient characteristics of the symptoms of uremic encephalopathy are especially noteworthy: They are caused by dysfunction of the nervous system and are manifested as cognitive, neuromuscular, somatosensory, and autonomic impairments; and their severity and overall rates of progression vary directly with the rate at which renal function deteriorates. Uremic symptoms are generally more severe and progress more rapidly in patients with ARF than in those with CRF. In more slowly progressive CRF, the number and severity of symptoms also typically vary cyclically, with intervals of acceptable well-being in an otherwise inexorable downhill course toward increasing disability. The symptoms are readily ameliorated by dialysis procedures and suppressed by maintenance dialysis regimens. They are also usually relieved entirely by restoration of renal function (e.g., after successful renal transplantation). Therefore, the encephalopathy of renal failure is important to recognize precisely because it is promptly and decisively treatable by clinical methods that are generally available.

The causes of uremic encephalopathy are multiple and complex. Brain oxygen utilization is diminished in patients with ESRD.[32] Although most such individuals have anemia, correction of the anemia only partially improves the impaired brain oxygen utilization.[32] However, since the widespread introduction of recombinant human erythropoietin (EPO) as a therapeutic agent in patients with ESRD treated with hemodialysis,[33] it is now clear that brain function and quality of life are improved by correction of the anemia with EPO.[34-37]

Diagnosis of Uremic Encephalopathy

The diagnosis of uremic encephalopathy in most patients is suspected if there is a constellation of clinical signs and symptoms that indicate renal or urologic disease or injury. However, the presenting symptoms of uremia, as mentioned earlier, are similar to those of many other encephalopathic states. Therefore, there is a risk of misdiagnosis and mistreatment. The differential diagnosis is even more complex, because patients with renal failure are subjected to other intercurrent illnesses that may also induce other encephalopathic effects. Moreover, if a drug or its metabolites with potential CNS toxicity are excreted or significantly metabolized by the kidney, the ensuing encephalopathic symptoms may not be entirely attributable to "uremia" but to the fact that the drug has reached toxic levels at ordinary dose rates. If levels of azotemia sometimes associated with uremic encephalopathy are present in the absence of associated illness, differentiation of the effects of drug versus renal failure can be very difficult. One or more dialysis treatments may both restore more normal body fluid composition and also reduce drug levels, so that the question remains moot while the patient recovers. Despite the possibilities that such multiple causes of encephalopathy might occur simultaneously, uremic encephalopathy may be successfully differentiated in most instances by means of the usual clinical and laboratory methods.

Role of Parathyroid Hormone

Although there are many factors that contribute to uremic encephalopathy, most investigators have shown no correlation between encephalopathy and any of the commonly measured indicators of renal failure. In recent years, there has been considerable discussion of the possible role of PTH as a uremic toxin. There is a substantial amount of evidence to suggest that PTH may exert adverse effects on the CNS.[20, 23, 26, 38]

PTH is known to have CNS effects in humans even in the absence of impaired renal function. Neuropsychiatric symptoms have been reported to be among the most common manifestations of primary hyperparathyroidism.[39-42] In uremic patients, both EEG changes and psychological abnormalities are improved by parathyroidectomy or medical suppression of PTH.[26] PTH, a high brain calcium content, or both are probably responsible, at least in part, for some of the encephalopathic manifestations of renal failure.

Uremic Encephalopathy in Patients with Hepatic Insufficiency

In patients who have advanced liver disease with hepatic insufficiency, it is often difficult to differentiate whether the cause of encephalopathy is hepatic or renal. Under normal conditions, protein and amino acids in the gastrointestinal tract are metabolized by colonic bacteria and mucosal enzymes to form ammonia.[43] Ammonia then enters the liver through the portal circulation, where it participates in the urea cycle to form urea. More than 90% of the urea produced is excreted in the urine, and the remainder enters the colon via hepatoportal recirculation. However, in patients with renal failure, the major route for elimination of urea is not available; therefore, there is an increase in blood urea. The amount of urea that enters the colon is increased because of the elevated plasma urea. Urea is then acted on by colonic bacteria and mucosal enzymes, leading to increased ammonia production, which may increase plasma ammonia levels. Plasma ammonia levels have been shown to correlate well with the severity of hepatic encephalopathy.[44]

If the patient with kidney failure also has some other form of hepatic insufficiency (e.g., hepatitis), this additional ammonia load may present a stress that cannot be adequately handled by the diseased liver. The result may be increased blood and CNS ammonia levels with development of encephalopathy.[43] Therefore, patients with liver damage and ESRD are at particular risk for development of encephalopathy, because both conditions act synergistically to increase blood ammonia. Ammonia can be readily removed from the blood by hemodialysis. The increased incidence of hepatitis C in the United States has led to a major increase in the number of dialysis patients with liver damage[45] and elevated ammonia levels.

It should also be noted that plasma urea and serum creatinine do not always adequately reflect renal function in patients with severe liver disease. Additionally, many patients who have liver disease, ascites, and normal plasma urea and creatinine values may in fact have severe renal functional impairment.[46-48] Among such individuals, differentiation of hepatic from uremic encephalopathy on clinical grounds is more difficult.

CHRONIC RENAL FAILURE

The incidence of ESRD in the United States is 180 cases per 1 million population,[49] or about 46,000 new cases per year.[50] There are currently 300,000 individuals in the United States with ESRD, 72% of whom are undergoing dialysis.[51] Among patients with ESRD treated with chronic hemodialysis, the mortality rate in the United States is 21% per year.[52] This figure is substantially higher than that of Japan and most European countries. Although it is unlikely that any one factor is responsible for the higher mortality rate in the United States, one important factor might be dialyzer reuse. Reuse of dialyzers in the United States is a common cost-containment procedure.[53] The opportunities for contamination, increased cytokine production, and infection associated with dialyzer reuse are substantial. In the United States, the most frequent causes of ESRD are diabetes, hypertension, glomerulonephritis, and polycystic kidney disease.[51] The neurologic manifestations reported in patients with CRF are numerous.[21]

Electroencephalogram in Patients with Chronic Renal Failure

EEG findings in patients with CRF are usually less severe than those observed in patients with ARF.[10] Several investigations have shown a good correlation between the percentage of EEG frequencies and power below 7 Hz and the decline of renal function as estimated by serum creatinine.[18, 31] After the initiation of dialysis, there may be an initial period of clinical stabilization during which time the EEG deteriorates (up to 6 months), but it then approaches normal values.[24] Still more improvement is seen in the EEG after renal transplantation.[31, 54]

Cognitive functions have also been shown to be impaired in uremia. These include sustained attention, selective attention, speed of decision making, short-term memory, and mental manipulation of symbols.[10]

The causes of the EEG abnormalities observed in uremic patients are probably multifactorial, but there is evidence that a very important element may be an effect of PTH on brain. In experimental animals with either ARF or CRF, many of the EEG abnormalities have been shown to be related to a direct effect of PTH on brain, which leads to an elevated brain content of calcium (Ca^{2+}).[23] Studies in patients with either ARF or CRF suggest a similar pathogenesis.[55, 56]

Psychological Testing in Patients with Chronic Renal Insufficiency

Several different types of psychological tests have been applied to subjects with CRF. These have been designed to measure the effects of dialysis, renal transplantation, or parathyroidectomy.[21, 26, 57]

The Trailmaking Test has been administered to a number of uremic subjects. In general, their performance was less effective than that of normal subjects. Improvement with practice limits repeated use of this test. The Continuous Memory Test correlates well with the degree of renal failure, as does the Choice Reaction Time. Scores in both tests improved with treatment by dialysis or renal transplantation. Similar but less impressive results are obtained with the Continuous Performance Test. Of all these tests, it appeared that the Choice Reaction Time best correlates with renal function and with improvement in the patient's condition as a result of dialysis or transplantation.[10, 58]

Patients with CRF who were maintained on dialysis were evaluated as to the possible effects of PTH on psychological function.[26] After establishment of baseline values, patients with CRF underwent parathyroidectomy for other medical reasons, such as for bone disease, soft tissue calcification, or persistent hypercalcemia unresponsive to medical management. In these patients, parathyroidectomy resulted in a significant improvement in several areas of psychological testing. They showed significant improvement in Raven's Progressive Matrices percentile scores and in the Visual Motor Index raw and percentage scores. These are tests of general cognitive function, nonverbal problem solving, and visual-motor or visual-spatial skills.[10, 58]

In addition, patients with CRF maintained on dialysis manifested significantly fewer errors on the Trailmaking Test and had significantly lower raw and T-score values on the Profile of Mood States Fatigue Scale postoperatively. In the latter, patients reported feeling significantly less fatigue, weariness, and inertia after undergoing surgery. Control subjects who underwent neck surgery for other reasons showed significant postoperative improvement in the Trailmaking Test but showed no change in any of the other tests.[26] Other studies have shown that there is intellectual impairment in most patients with CRF treated with dialysis.[59-61] In these studies, the procedures included the full Weschler Adult Intelligence Scale (WAIS), the Walton-Black Modified Word Learning Test (MWLT), and the Block Design Learning Test (BDLT).

The overall intellectual level, as measured by the WAIS full-scale IQ, did not differ significantly from normal. The patients' performance was due mainly to the digit symbol, block design, and picture arrangement subtests, all of which produced scores significantly below normal. The impairment of intellectual level as represented by the Weschler Deterioration Quotient was also outside the normal range. The data on verbal learning obtained with the MWLT and performance learning obtained with the BDLT did not indicate any gross learning abnormality. Cognitive data were compared with other information, such as age, sex, length of dialysis, and biochemical variables, by a multiple regression technique. The analysis suggested that, of the cognitive data, those obtained with the BDLT bore the strongest relation to duration of dialysis. Other studies have suggested that the WAIS full-scale IQ in dialysis patients is below that of the general population.[10] There appears to be a consensus, based on psychological testing, that CRF results in organic-like losses of intellectual function, particularly information-processing capacities.[59-61]

Biochemical Changes in Brain with Renal Insufficiency

To determine the possible causes of the EEG abnormalities and clinical manifestations observed in patients with renal insufficiency, in vivo biochemical studies have been carried out in brain of both patients and laboratory animals. Measurements have included brain intracellular pH and concentrations of Na^+, K^+, Cl^-, Al^{3+}, Ca^{2+}, Mg^{2+}, urea, adenine nucleotides (creatine phosphate, ATP, ADP, AMP), lactate, and sodium-potassium adenosine triphosphatase (Na^+,K^+-ATPase) enzyme activity.[20, 27, 62-68] In patients with ARF, the brain content of water, K^+, and Mg^{2+} is normal, that of Na^+ is modestly decreased, and that of Al^{3+} is slightly elevated.[20] However, cerebral cortex Ca^{2+} content is almost twice the normal value.[20, 26, 55] Similar findings were observed in dogs with ARF.[23, 66] Permeability of uremic rat brain to inert molecules (inulin, sucrose, other nonelectrolytes) is increased, whereas permeability to weak acids (sulfate, penicillin, and dimethadione) is normal to low.[67-70]

Alterations of cerebral metabolism that might be related to the changes in brain permeability have also been studied in animal brain.[38, 63, 70, 71] In several older studies, investigators attempted to evaluate the effects of uremia on the CNS using subcellular analysis. Early studies evaluated Na^+,K^+-ATPase activity in crude microsomal fractions obtained from brains of acutely uremic rats.[62, 64] There was a significantly decreased Na^+,K^+-ATPase activity in their preparation, and they suggested that this result was caused not by acidosis but by the uremic state itself.[62] On the other hand, an earlier study by Van den Noort and associates[64] found no significant difference in cationic ATPase activity in normal and uremic rat brains. In the brain of rats with ARF, creatine phosphate, adenosine triphosphate (ATP), and glucose were increased, but there were corresponding decreases in adenosine monophosphate (AMP), adenosine diphosphate (ADP), and lactate. Total brain adenine nucleotide content and Na^+,K^+-ATPase were normal to low. The uremic brain utilized less ATP and thus failed to produce ADP, AMP, and lactate at normal rates. The brain energy charge was normal, as was the redox state.[63] There was a corresponding decrease in brain metabolic rate, along with elevated glucose and low lactate levels.[63] Other studies of uremic brain have shown a decrease in cerebral oxygen consumption.[32] Patients with

chronic renal insufficiency (GFR <20 mL/min) have decreased brain uptake of glutamine and increased ammonia uptake. The relevance of these findings, in terms of neurotransmitters or other brain function, is unknown.[71]

In animals with either ARF or CRF, both urea concentration and osmolality are similar in brain, cerebrospinal fluid, and plasma. The solute content of brain in animals with ARF is such that essentially all of the increase in brain osmolality is due to an increase of brain urea concentration. However, in animals with CRF, about half of the increase in brain osmolality occurs because of the presence of undetermined solute (idiogenic osmoles), with the other half being attributed to an increase in the urea concentration.[38, 65]

In dogs with CRF, brain content of Na^+, K^+, Cl^-, and water were not different from control values. Similarly, the extracellular space was not different from control.[38] Calcium content was measured in eight parts of the brain in dogs who had CRF for 4 months. Calcium content was found to be normal in the subcortical white matter, pons, medulla, cerebellum, thalamus, and caudate nucleus. However, calcium was about 60% above control values in both cortical gray matter and hypothalamus. Magnesium content was normal in all eight parts of the brain, as was water content.[38] Other investigators have also found an elevated cerebral cortex calcium content in dogs with CRF.[72] In animals who have ARF and metabolic acidosis, the intracellular pH (pHi) of brain and skeletal muscle is normal.[67] In dogs with CRF, intracellular pH is normal in brain, liver, and skeletal muscle.[38] In patients with renal failure, intracellular pH has been reported to be normal in both skeletal muscle and leukocytes, as well as in the "whole body."[73-76] The pH of cerebrospinal fluid has also been shown to be normal in both patients and laboratory animals with renal failure.[38, 65, 67, 77] Therefore, despite the presence of extracellular metabolic acidemia in patients or laboratory animals with ARF or CRF, the intracellular pH is normal in brain, white cells, liver, and skeletal muscle.

More recently, guanidino compounds, such as methyl guanidine and guanidino succinic acid, have been shown to be neurotoxic and also to be present in several brain regions and cerebrospinal fluid of nondialyzed uremic patients at levels that have been shown to be experimental convulsants.[78, 79]

In general, then, studies of brain tissue from both intact animal models of uremia and humans with renal failure have revealed many different biochemical abnormalities associated with the uremic state. However, such investigations have not as yet revealed much about the fundamental mechanisms that might induce such abnormalities. Such studies may have to be done in isolated cell systems or subcellular systems from the brain. These systems have the advantage of permitting one to study isolated manifestations of the uremic state while removing the numerous potential confounding influences present in an in vivo model.

Cellular and Subcellular Studies

Studies have been carried out in neurons, synaptosomes, and glia of uremic rat brain.[66, 80, 81] Two different cytoskeletal proteins, both early indicators of brain injury, have been examined: glial fibrillary acidic protein (GFAP), which is specific to astrocytes, and microtubule-associated protein-2 (MAP-2), which localizes to neuronal cell bodies and dendrites. Loss of MAP-2 provides one of the earliest indications of neuronal degeneration. In uremic brain (12 hours of ARF), there was a diffuse increase in GFAP in cerebral cortex. Changes in MAP-2 immunoreactivity were observed in all regions of the cerebral cortex. These and other data suggest that there may be degenerative changes in neurons in brain of animals with only moderate azotemia.[82]

Studies by Fraser, Sarnacki, and Arieff[83, 84] in rat brain synaptosomes demonstrated abnormalities of both sodium and calcium transport and decreased Na+,K+-ATPase pump activity in the brains of rats with uremia.[83] Their findings suggested that these transport abnormalities may affect neurotransmitter release in the uremic state.[83, 84] This defect did not appear to be caused by the uremic environment at the time of study, because nerve cell membranes were washed and frozen before study. The defect observed in uremia appeared to result from a physical alteration of the neuronal membrane in acute uremia. These workers also demonstrated alterations of calcium transport in uremic rat brain.[85] Based on the relationship between extracellular calcium and the release of neurotransmitter substances in nerve terminals, they concluded that this defect may affect neurotransmitter release and information processing in the uremic state. In subsequent studies, the increase in calcium transport in uremia appeared to be PTH dependent.[83, 85]

Although calcium and sodium transport in synaptosomes appears to be influenced by uremia, not all transport processes are affected in this manner. Verkman and Fraser[70] evaluated water and urea transport in synaptosomes by stopped-flow light scattering technique and found no differences in either water or urea permeabilities in normal rats compared to rats with uremia. From these studies, they were also able to show that synaptosomal water and urea transport occurred by a lipid diffusive pathway and was not affected by uremia.[70]

CHRONIC DIALYSIS-DEPENDENT ENCEPHALOPATHY

Radiologic and Pathologic Examination of Uremic Brain

There does not currently exist a large prospective study of the radiology of uremic brain in humans.[86] Pathologic studies of brains of patients who died with CRF are old, and there has been no extensive study of uremic brain using more modern pathologic methods.[87, 88] Before 1974, subdural hemorrhages were believed to be very common in dialyzed subjects, and they were reported in about 1% to 3% of such autopsies. In addition, intracerebral hemorrhages were said to be present in about 6% of dialysis patients who died. Cerebral edema is not found in brain of patients or laboratory animals with CRF, by either biochemical or histologic criteria. Generalized but variable neuronal degeneration is often present, but its anatomic location is quite variable. Among patients who have died with uremia, there is some evidence of necrosis of the granular layer of the cerebral cortex. Small intracerebral hemorrhages and necrotic foci are seen in about 10% of uremic patients, and focal glial proliferation is found in about 2%.

Uremic patients are prone to several risk factors that have a tendency to be associated with a high incidence of stroke (Table 51-3). Such factors include diabetes mellitus, uremia, hyperparathyroidism, a smoking history, hypertension, elevated cholesterol and triglycerides, elevated C-reactive protein, atherosclerosis, hemodialysis therapy, and use of over-the-counter vasoactive drugs.[12, 89-94]

When uremic patients maintained on chronic dialysis suffer a possible stroke, computed tomography (CT) or magnetic resonance imaging (MRI) of the brain is likely to be carried out for diagnostic purposes. However, as yet, a series of such neuroimaging cases has not been assembled for research purposes. Therefore, nephrologists and neurologists are not generally aware of structural changes in the uremic brain. The few available studies suggest that brains of patients with uremia have a very high incidence of cerebral atrophy, which is disproportionately high for the age of the individuals studied.[95, 96] Earlier studies had also found a high incidence of cerebral atrophy among chronic hemodialysis patients.[97] There appears to be subtle brain damage that is not detectable by standard neuroimaging techniques or the EEG but is often manifested by deterioration of intellectual capability.[59, 60, 98]

It is currently not unusual for patients to survive on hemodialysis for 25 years.[99] However, among patients who have been undergoing hemodialysis for longer than 10 years, there is often mental deterioration, with markedly decreased intellectual capability, even without medical evidence of stroke.[27] The collective syndrome of *chronic dialysis-dependent encephalopathy* is a combination of probable organic mental disorders plus psychiatric disorders commonly associated with hemodialysis.[100] Although the exact etiology is unknown, the clinical manifestations are shown in Table 51-4.

TABLE 51-3

Important Risk Factors for Stroke

Diabetes mellitus
Uremia
Hyperparathyroidism
Smoking history
Hypertension
Elevated cholesterol
Elevated triglycerides
Elevated C-reactive protein
Atherosclerosis
Hemodialysis therapy
Elevated homocysteine

TABLE 51-4

Clinical Manifestations of Chronic Dialysis-Dependent Encephalopathy

Decreased intellectual capability
Impaired cognition
Chronic depression
Decreased capability of physical activity
Senility
Deterioration of vision
Suicidal behavior
Sexual dysfunction
Psychosis

The recent use of advanced neuroimaging techniques has led to increased understanding of the changes in uremic brain in humans.[86] Acute and subacute movement disorders have been observed in patients with ESRD.[101] These have been associated with bilateral basal ganglia and internal capsule lesions.[101, 102] Cerebral atrophy has been observed in chronic hemodialysis patients,[96] and it tends to worsen as dialysis therapy continues.[95, 103] Cerebral atrophy was previously thought to be associated with dialysis dementia, but this is apparently not the case.[104] ESRD has also been reported to lead to deterioration of vision.[105] Some cases are associated with uremic pseudotumor cerebri, and in these selected cases, surgical optic nerve fenestration may improve visual loss.[106]

There is probably a loss of neurons that is not detectable by techniques currently in common use. There are several well-studied pathophysiologic mechanisms that probably contribute to the potential loss of brain tissue in patients with chronic dialysis-dependent encephalopathy. The potential mechanisms are discussed later. There are at least three important biochemical processes that have recently been explored in depth and are likely contributors to the syndrome of chronic dialysis-dependent encephalopathy (see Table 51-1).

Biochemical Processes Contributing to Chronic Dialysis-Dependent Encephalopathy

Apoptosis

Apoptosis is a physiologically essential mechanism of cell death which, together with cell proliferation, is responsible for the precise regulation of cell numbers for a variety of cell populations during normal development.[107-109] It also serves as a defense mechanism to remove unwanted and potentially dangerous cells.[108, 110] The inappropriate activation or inhibition of apoptosis, however, is now thought to cause or contribute to a variety of diseases, including cancer, stroke, brain trauma, and several neurodegenerative diseases.[108, 111-113] Cell exposure to a number of pathologic entities that are present in the uremic state, such as free radicals, glutamate, hypoxia, and calcium ion (Ca^{2+}),[32, 66, 114, 115] can trigger both apoptosis and necrosis in the brain, two distinctly different types of cell death.[108] The outcome of cell survival or evolution of either type of cell death can depend on the intensity of the initial stimuli or a combination of type, intensity, and duration.[116-118] Uremic toxins can act by altering immune function and increasing viable neutrophils, which can inhibit apoptotic removal of such cells.[114]

A major cause of brain cell death by both apoptosis and necrosis is oxidative stress related to cerebral hypoxia/ischemia.[82, 119] It has been demonstrated that brain oxygen utilization is decreased in patients with ESRD.[32] In adults, cell death can occur by only two mechanisms, necrosis or apoptosis.[120] A number of processes are capable of initiating apoptosis, including free radical generation, glutamate excess, hypoxia, and calcium. All of these processes are present in the brain and cerebrospinal fluid of patients with advanced renal failure. In addition, diabetes, the most common cause of ESRD, increases neuronal cell death by apoptosis, suggesting that diabetes itself may be an important contributor to brain cell death in patients with ESRD.[121]

Death receptors are cell-surface receptors that transmit apoptotic signals initiated by specific death ligands. These death receptors belong to the tumor necrosis factor (TNF) receptor gene superfamily and also contain a "death domain."[122] Activation of these death receptors inappropriately by some factor present in uremia may lead to apoptotic brain cell death. In ischemic brain tissue, the contents of sodium and calcium are reduced, and this may activate apoptosis in neurons via activation of the N-methyl-D-aspartate (NMDA) receptor.[123]

Oxidative Stress

A constellation of reactive intermediates (electrophiles and free radicals) capable of damaging cellular constituents is generated during normal pathophysiologic processes.[124] The consequences of this damage include altered cell signaling, enhanced mutation rates, and accelerated neurodegeneration. In many cases, the initially generated reactive intermediates convert cellular constituents into second-generation reactive intermediates capable of inducing further damage. High levels of damage can lead to cell death through apoptosis or necrosis.[124]

Uremia is associated with progressive and irreversible alterations of proteins. Reactive carbonyl compounds are derived from the metabolism of lipids and carbohydrates and are known to accumulate in uremia.[125] Such compounds may play a major role in the development of uremic complications in the nervous system. The term "carbonyl stress" is a new form of uremic toxicity based on effects of such compounds.[8]

Advanced glycosylation (glycation) end products (AGEs) accumulate during the normal course of aging, and at accelerated rates in patients with diabetes and uremia. In animal models of ARF, AGEs accumulate much more rapidly than expected,[126] regardless of the plasma glucose concentration. They are deposited in several tissues, including skin, kidney, and blood vessels.[127] The generation of AGEs in uremic serum has been shown to be inhibited by the presence of nitric oxide (NO) donors,[128] and the inhibition appears to result from NO itself.[129] A link has been established between formation of AGEs, decreased production of NO, and endothelial dysfunction in atherosclerosis.[129] NO donors appear to be able to scavenge free radicals and suppress the formation of carbonyl compounds.

The deposition in tissues of AGEs has been linked to initiation of oxidative stress via generation of reactive oxygen species (ROS). Cardiovascular disease is the major cause of death and morbidity among patients with renal insufficiency and those maintained with chronic hemodialysis.[13, 130] In hemodialysis patients, there is overproduction of oxidants (ROS, reactive nitrogen species) compared with antioxidant defense mechanisms.[131] Several AGEs are important mediators of inflammation. There is also an important inverse relationship between nutritional status and extent of inflammation and arteriosclerosis.[132] Malnutrition is very common among dialysis patients with ESRD.[133] The activated reduced nicotinamide adenine dinucleotide phosphate (NADPH) oxidase complex catalyzes reduction of oxygen to superoxide anion and then to hydrogen peroxide, which can react with halides to produce ROS in patients with CRF.[134]

Among the mechanisms that may contribute to generation of oxidative stress and increasing atherogenesis is histoin-compatibility of the dialysis system, which may lead to increasing generation of ROS.[135] There is evidence that heparin[136] and addition of vitamin E to the dialysis membrane may help somewhat to alleviate generation of ROS.[137] Dehydroascorbic acid may also be cerebroprotective in cases of impending stroke.[138] The generation of oxidants does not result simply from an accidental disruption of aerobic metabolism, but rather from an active process that is crucial for the nonspecific immune defenses of the brain. Although these processes are essential for survival, they may be inappropriately activated to cause neurodegeneration.[82] Neurons are highly susceptible to oxidative stress, which can induce both neuronal necrosis and apoptosis. Oxidants may also have more subtle roles in compromising the integrity of the blood-brain barrier and in producing reactive changes in astrocytes that further propagate injury.[82] Oxidative stress also appears to provide a critical link between exposure to multiple environmental factors and genetic risk factors in the pathogenic mechanisms of neurodegeneration. Oxidative stress appears to be a major factor in the pathogenesis of many brain disorders characterized by neurodegeneration, including Parkinson disease, Alzheimer disease, and amyotrophic lateral sclersosis.[82] The toxicity is enhanced by inflammatory cells.

Inflammation

An outpouring of data recently has pointed to the presence of a chronic low-grade inflammatory condition as a major factor in atherosclerosis.[139] Plasma markers of inflammation, such as C-reactive protein (CRP), are strong independent predictors of future coronary events in apparently healthy and asymptomatic individuals,[140] particularly women.[132] Measurement of CRP has been proposed as a major marker for the presence of cardiovascular disease as well as chronic inflammation.[141] Preliminary data also suggest that CRP is most efficacious in predicting cardiovascular disease in women.[140] Increased plasma levels of CRP may also predict renal functional loss, particularly in patients with certain comorbid conditions, such as a high body mass index.[142] β-Blockers may lower CRP concentrations.[143] By using measurements of albumin and fibrinogen synthesis and interleukin-6 (IL-6) production, Caglar and associates[144] were able to demonstrate that hemodialysis itself induces an inflammatory state.

Although there are substantial data relating increased plasma levels of homocysteine to progressive atherosclerosis, some data suggest that the effects of homocysteine are in fact secondary to those of chronic inflammation.[145] Recent studies by Ayus and associates strongly suggest that a chronic inflammatory state in dialysis patients may lead to anemia, with resistance to EPO.[94, 146] In particular, Ayus and colleagues[147] demonstrated that the presence of an old clotted arteriovenous graft can be a nidus for hidden infection with resistant anemia. The infected, nonfunctioning graft may also give rise to other severe infectious complications, such as endocarditis, pneumonia, and brain abscess. Only surgical removal of the clotted and infected graft would eliminate the infection or ameliorate the anemia.[146, 148] Such nonfunctioning arteriovenous grafts may also occur in renal transplant recipients.[147]

Homocysteine

Homocysteine is derived by transmethylation of methionine. Methionine is an essential sulfur-containing amino acid that is derived from protein breakdown.[149] Homocysteine levels in plasma increase with declining GFR. Homocysteine is involved in the pathogenesis of atherosclerosis, and it is often elevated in ESRD. Homocysteine is important in the pathogenesis of arteriosclerosis in patients with ESRD who are being treated with hemodialysis, and it is therefore important in the development of stroke.[150] Increased plasma homocysteine levels are a predictor of cardiovascular mortality in patients with ESRD treated with hemodialysis.[151]

However, homocysteine may be a uremic neurotoxin for several different reasons. Homocysteine activates the coagulation system and has adverse affects on the endothelium and arterial wall. The mechanism may involve generation of ROS and a decrease in the bioavailability of NO,[152] which also leads to cerebral vasodilation.[153] The decreased bioavailability of NO results in increased generation of AGEs by uremic serum.[128, 129] Additionally, homocysteine acts as an agonist at the glutamate-binding site of the NMDA receptor, allowing excessive influx of Ca^{2+} and ROS generation, which can be major contributors to neuronal cell death.[154] The incidence of stroke is substantially increased in uremic individuals maintained on hemodialysis.[12] Homocysteine-induced oxidative stress may be only one of a number of mechanisms whereby increased arteriosclerosis is generated in uremic individuals.[152, 155, 156] Even in patients who have not suffered myocardial infarction, a high plasma homocysteine level is an important predictor of congestive heart failure.[157]

UREMIC NEUROTOXINS

Central Nervous System

The number of compounds retained by the body in patients with renal failure, either singly or in combination, is substantial.[133] Numerous studies have attempted to identify which of the many compounds that are elevated in uremic subjects are truly uremic toxins. Criteria established by Bergstrom and Furst for uremic toxins are as follows[158]: (1) The compound should be chemically identified and quantifiable in biologic fluids; (2) the concentration of the substance in plasma from uremic subjects should be higher than that found in subjects who do not have renal insufficiency; (3) the concentration of the substance in plasma should somehow correlate with specific uremic symptoms, and these should be alleviated with reduction of the substance to normal; (4) the toxic effects of the substance should be demonstrable at concentrations found in plasma from uremic patients. Uremic neurotoxins would imply retention of solutes that have specific detrimental effects on CNS or peripheral nervous system function.[159, 160]

There are at least three different types of uremic solutes that are potentially toxic and can be characterized[125]: (1) small, water-soluble compounds, such as urea and creatinine[159]; (2) middle molecules; and (3) protein-bound compounds. Most of the small, water-soluble compounds, such as urea and creatinine, are not particularly toxic and are easily removed by dialysis.

Guanidine Compounds

Guanidine compounds have been postulated to be "uremic toxins" for many years,[161] based on possible detrimental effects on the CNS. Recent studies have demonstrated that several guanidine compounds are present in uremic brain[79] and may be important in the etiology of uremic encephalopathy.[78] There are at least four guanidine compounds that are experimental convulsants; they appear to work by activation of NMDA receptors by guanidinosuccinic acid (GSA). Activation of the NMDA receptor is a major pathologic mechanism in the etiology of several types of brain damage, including head trauma[162] and stroke.[163, 164]

In addition, guanidine compounds have a depressant effect on mitochondrial function.[165] In brain of uremic patients, guanidine compounds were measured in 28 different regions.[79] Guanidinosuccinic acid levels were elevated up to 100 fold in uremic brain versus control brain, and levels increased with increasing extent of uremia. The concentrations of guanidinosuccinic acid in ureic brain were similar to those observed in normal animal brain after injection to blood levels that cause convulsions.[79] Guanidines inhibit neutrophil superoxide production, can induce seizures, and suppress the natural killer cell response to IL-2.[166] Other guanidines, which are arginine analogs, are competitive inhibitors of nitric oxide synthetase (NOS); they therefore impair removal of AGEs[128] and can lead to vasoconstriction, hypertension, ischemic glomerular injury, immune dysfunction, and neurologic changes.[166]

Middle molecules are large-molecular-weight compounds (300 to 12,000 D) that have in the past been believed responsible for some of the manifestations of uremia.[167] Despite the fact that at one time, dialysis membranes were designed with the specific intent of removing more middle molecules, evidence of their toxicity is generally lacking.[167-170] There has recently been a renewed interest in these molecules,[169, 171] but evidence of their toxicity is still conjectural.[166]

With established renal insufficiency, guanidines rapidly accumulate in blood, where their presence competitively inhibits NOS, impairs removal of AGEs,[128] and can lead to worsening hypertension, immune dysfunction,[114] and neurologic changes[166] such as stroke.[172]

Advanced Glycation End Products

AGEs can modify tissues, enzymes, and proteins and may play a role in the pathogenesis of dialysis-associated amyloidosis.[125] AGEs may also play a role in the pathogenesis of diabetic nephropathy.[173] AGEs are markedly elevated in plasma of patients with ESRD.[174] They react with vascular cells to inactivate endothelial NO and may increase the propensity of ESRD patients to develop hypertension. Current dialysis therapy is relatively ineffective in removal of AGEs, so that there is accumulation of AGEs in patients with ESRD, particularly those with diabetes mellitus.[174] The AGEs are "middle molecules" and have the potential to cause tissue damage leading to hypertension. Therefore, at least some middle molecules may actually be deleterious in patients with ESRD, and they are poorly removed with conventional dialysis.[174] There is evidence that angiotensin-converting enzyme (ACE) antagonists decrease the formation of AGEs.[175]

Protein-bound compounds (toxins) are not substantially removed by dialysis, and almost all are lipophilic.

Such compounds include polyamines such as spermine.[176] Spermine is postulated to be a uremic toxin and appears to react with the NMDA receptor, which affects calcium and sodium permeability in brain cells.[176] Stimulation of the NMDA receptor in brain is the final common pathway for brain cell death in a number of pathologic pathways.[163, 164] The uremic state is associated with increased oxidative stress, which results in protein oxidation products in plasma and cell membranes. There is eventual alteration of proteins with formation of oxidized amino acids, including glutamine and glutamate.[125] Such reactions may ultimately lead to stimulation of the NMDA receptor in brain, with brain cell damage or death.[15]

Peripheral Nervous System
Nerve Conduction and Uremic Toxins

A number of solutes are purported to impair peripheral nerve function. Several possible uremic toxins have been identified that appear to be correlated with depression of motor nerve conduction velocity (MNCV) in laboratory animals.[161, 177, 178] The MNCV has become a standard test for assessment of nerve function, although it has many flaws. Most studies do not take into account the facts that (1) depressed MNCV is a cyclic phenomenon, with abnormally low values seen one day and normal values the next[19]; (2) there is a day-to-day variation in MNCV that approaches 20%[179]; and (3) the finding of depressed MNCV in laboratory animals associated with high plasma levels of potential uremic neurotoxins has generally not been confirmed in human subjects with renal failure.[170, 180-182] Although it is possible to relate impairment in MNCV to levels in blood of various substances, the best correlation was obtained between reduced MNCV and a reduction in GFR (Table 51-5).

Parathyroid Hormone

It was suggested in the past that PTH is a peripheral nerve uremic neurotoxin, a theory based on a correlation between plasma PTH levels and MNCV in patients with CRF.[180] Some earlier studies suggested a possible effect of PTH on MNCV in the dog,[178] but these impressions have not been confirmed.[38] In patients who have hyperparathyroidism without uremia, PTH has no observable effect on peripheral nerve function.[183] In both patients and laboratory animals with ARF, the MNCV has been found to be normal (see Table 51-5).[20, 184, 185] In all studies of both patients and laboratory animals with CRF, the MNCV has not been shown to be affected by PTH.[38] Therefore, in both patients and laboratory animals with either ARF or CRF, or either primary or secondary hyperparathyroidism, no effect of PTH on nerve function can be demonstrated. In patients with CRF, there is no change in MNCV as a result of either recovery of renal function or chronic hemodialysis; there is also no effect of parathyroidectomy.[184] In addition, when patients begin dialysis therapy, MNCV either stabilizes or improves.[186] However, virtually all of these patients have elevated plasma PTH levels.[187]

Animal studies suggest that, in either ARF or CRF, changes in MNCV take longer than 6 months to develop and are probably not related to an effect of PTH. Mahoney and

TABLE 51-5

Relation between Nerve Function and Various "Uremic Neurotoxins"

PUTATIVE "UREMIC NEUROTOXIN"	CORRELATION COEFFICIENT WITH MNCV	OTHER COMMENTS	REF. NO.
PTH	0.09	No effect of PTH on motor nerve function	184
PTH	0.45	—	180
Urea	0.41	—	339
Creatinine	0.51		
GFR	0.68–0.84		
Urea	0.51	—	350
Creatinine	0.57		
Myoinositol	0.03	—	351
Myoinositol	0.67	—	182
Myoinositol	NA	Detrimental effect of myoinositol on nerve function	177
Middle molecules	NA	No in vivo evidence of MNCV impairment with renal failure	168
Middle molecules	NA	As above	167
Middle molecules	NA	As above	353
Methylguanidine	NA	Chronic injection Depressed MNCV in patients	161
Transketolase deficiency	NA	Deficiency related to impaired MNCV in patients	181
PTH	0.05	No effect of PTH on motor nerve function	38
PTH	NA	No effect of PTH on sensory nerve function	354

GFR, glomerular filtration rate; MNCV, motor nerve conduction velocity; NA, not available; PTH, parathyroid hormone.

associates[63] studied dogs with renal failure for periods of 3.5 days to 6 months. There was no change in the MNCV, and the MNCV was normal even after 6 months with GFR less than 22% of control.

Parathyroid Hormone in Uremic Encephalopathy

In patients dying with ARF or CRF, the calcium content in brain cerebral cortex is significantly elevated.[20, 23, 26] Dogs with ARF or CRF show increases of brain gray matter calcium and EEG changes similar to those seen in humans with ARF.[38, 63, 66] In dogs, both the EEG and brain calcium abnormalities can be prevented by parathyroidectomy. Conversely, these abnormalities can be reproduced by administration of PTH to normal animals while maintaining serum calcium and phosphate in the normal range. Therefore, PTH is essential to produce some of the CNS manifestations in the canine model of uremia.[23, 72] In addition, hyperparathyroidism in subjects with CRF is strongly associated with multiple types of cardiovascular disease, including myocardial infarction, congestive heart failure,[188] and stroke.[89]

PTH is known to have CNS effects in humans even in the absence of impaired renal function. Neuropsychiatric symptoms are reported to be among the most common manifestations of primary hyperparathyroidism.[39-42] Patients with primary hyperparathyroidism also have EEG changes similar to those observed in patients with ARF.[20, 189] The common denominator appears to be elevated plasma levels of PTH.[20, 23, 26, 66] In patients with ARF, the EEG is abnormal within 18 hours of the onset of renal failure and is generally not affected by dialysis for periods of up to 8 weeks.[20] In patients with either primary or secondary hyperparathyroidism, parathyroidectomy results in an improvement of both EEG and psychological testing, suggesting a direct effect of PTH on the CNS. Similarly, dialysis results in a decrement of brain (cerebral cortex) calcium toward normal

in both patients and laboratory animals with renal failure, concomitant with improvement of the EEG.[20, 23, 26, 66] In uremic patients, both EEG changes and psychological abnormalities are improved by parathyroidectomy or medical suppression of PTH.[26] PTH, a high brain calcium content, and abnormal calcium transport are probably responsible, at least in part, for some of the encephalopathic manifestations of renal failure.

The mechanisms by which PTH might impair CNS function are much better understood but are far from complete. The increased calcium content in such diverse tissues as skin, cornea, blood vessels, brain, and heart in patients with hyperparathyroidism suggests that PTH may somehow facilitate the entry of Ca^{2+} into such tissues. The finding of increased calcium in the brains of both dogs and humans with either acute or chronic renal disease and secondary hyperparathyroidism is consistent with the conception that the CNS dysfunction and EEG abnormalities found in ARF or CRF may be due in part to a PTH-mediated increase in brain calcium. Calcium is essential for the function of neurotransmission in the CNS as well as a number of intracellular enzyme systems. An increased brain calcium content could disrupt cerebral function by interfering with these processes.[55, 190]

NEUROLOGIC COMPLICATIONS OF END-STAGE RENAL DISEASE AND ITS THERAPY

Dialysis Dysequilibrium Syndrome

In patients with ESRD, there are several CNS disorders that may occur as a consequence of dialytic therapy. DDS is a clinical syndrome that occurs in patients being treated with hemodialysis. The syndrome was first described in 1962[191] and may include symptoms such as headache, nausea, emesis, blurring of vision, muscular twitching, disorientation, hypertension, tremors, and seizures.[192, 193] The syndrome has since been expanded to include milder symptoms, such as muscle cramps, anorexia, restlessness, and dizziness.[193-196] Although DDS has been reported in all age groups, it is more common among younger patients, particularly the pediatric age group.[197] The syndrome is most often associated with rapid hemodialysis of patients with ARF, but it also has occasionally been reported after maintenance hemodialysis of patients with CRF.[198-201] The pathogenesis of DDS has been extensively investigated and the findings summarized elsewhere.[65, 193, 202, 203] The symptoms are usually self-limited, but recovery may take several days.

It appears that present methods of dialysis have altered the clinical picture of DDS. Most reports of seizures, coma, and death were published before 1970. The symptoms of DDS as reported since the late 1970s have generally been mild, consisting of nausea, weakness, headache, fatigue, and muscle cramps. Almost all cases have occurred in patients undergoing their initial four hemodialyses. Sporadic reports of death associated with DDS do exist.[193] However, it is unclear whether in any case DDS was the actual cause of death, rather than some other neurologic complication associated with dialysis, such as acute stroke, subdural hematoma, subarachnoid hemorrhage, or hyponatremia.[193] A differential diagnosis of patients presenting with these symptoms is shown in Table 51-6. Recently, the diagnosis of DDS has become a "wastebasket" for a number of disorders that can occur in patients with renal failure and may affect the CNS.[193] It is important to recognize that the diagnosis of DDS should be one of exclusion.

DDS has been treated either by addition of osmotically active solute (glucose, glycerol, albumin, urea, fructose, NaCl, mannitol) to the dialysate, or by intravenous infusion of mannitol or glycerol. Because of the technical difficulties of adding osmolytes to the dialysate, this modality is seldom used. Usually, mannitol is given intravenously before the start of dialysis, to achieve blood levels of about 16 mmol/L. With the technique of *pure ultrafiltration,* the patient is subjected to ultrafiltration without dialysis.[204] The net result is loss of fluid without the need to undergo dialysis. Ultrafiltration followed by ordinary hemodialysis has not been associated with DDS.[205, 206] Additionally, DDS can be prevented by decreasing the time on dialysis and increasing the frequency of dialysis at the initiation of hemodialysis. Mannitol infusion accompanying the initial three hemodialyses has been successful in prevention of DDS.[195]

Administration of 50 mL of 25% mannitol both at the initiation of dialysis and after 2 hours of dialysis has generally been successful in preventing symptoms of DDS. The same effects can be obtained by addition of glycerol to the dialysate, but technical considerations render this option less popular.[196, 207]

Chronic peritoneal dialysis is currently in use worldwide. Different types of peritoneal dialysis are carried out either in-center, at home, or with a combination of ambulatory and home dialysis.[51] Patients undergo continuous low-volume peritoneal dialysis for as long as 24 hours per day.[208, 209] Symptoms of DDS have not presently been reported in patients using this mode of dialysis.

Dialysis Dementia

Dialysis dementia (also called dialysis encephalopathy) is a progressive, frequently fatal neurologic disease that was initially described in several reports between 1970 and 1973.[87, 210, 211] Existence of the syndrome was then independently confirmed worldwide by several different groups.[104, 212-222] In adults, the disease has been reported almost exclusively in patients being treated with chronic hemodialysis. The early literature focused on the distinctive neurologic findings.[210, 211, 213-215, 223] However, more recent reports from both Europe and the United States suggest that some forms of dialysis dementia represent part of a multisystem disease that may include encephalopathy, osteomalacic bone disease, proximal myopathy, and anemia.[27, 223-226]

The etiology has largely been elucidated.[227] Although an increase in brain aluminum content has been strongly implicated in some cases of dialysis dementia, the evidence is far less convincing in others. With current knowledge, it seems useful to subdivide dialysis dementia into three categories (Table 51-7): (1) an epidemic form that is related to contamination of the dialysate, often with aluminum; (2) sporadic cases in which aluminum intoxication is less likely to be a contributory factor; and (3) dementia associated with congenital or early childhood renal disease. This entity has been reported in several children who were never dialyzed or exposed to aluminum compounds. These early childhood cases may represent developmental neurologic defects

---

TABLE 51-6

Differential Diagnosis of Dialysis Disequilibrium Syndrome

Subdural hematoma
Uremia, per se
Acute cerebrovascular accident
Dialysis dementia
Cardiac arrhythmia
Malfunction of fluid-proportioning system
Hypoglycemia
Hypercalcemia
Hyponatremia

TABLE 51-7

Sungroups of Dialysis Dementia

Sporadic Endemic
No clear relation to aluminum intake
Worldwide distribution
No known therapy

Epidemic
Geographic clusters
Often related to aluminum (Al^{3+}) in dialysis water
Epidemic usually stops with treatment of water supply
Probably often related to other trace elements in water, such as tin, manganese, cobalt, magnesium, and iron

Childhood
May be secondary to effects of uremia on the immature brain
No clear association with aluminum administration

resulting from exposure of the growing brain to a uremic environment.[61]

Clinical Manifestations of Dialysis Dementia

The initial reports of dialysis dementia in the 1970s were soon followed by reports throughout the world.[228] These patients all had the endemic form and usually had been on chronic hemodialysis for longer than 2 years before the onset of symptoms. Early manifestations consisted of a mixed dysarthria-apraxia of speech with slurring, stuttering, and hesitancy. Personality changes, including psychoses, progressed to dementia, myoclonus, and seizures. Symptoms initially were intermittent and were often worse during dialysis, but generally became constant. In most cases, the disease progressed to death within 6 months. Speech disturbances were found in 90% of patients, affective disorders culminating in dementia in 80%, motor disturbances in 75%, and convulsions in 60% to 90%. In contrast to this fairly distinct clinical picture, brain histology has generally been normal or nonspecific.

Early in the disease, the EEG shows multifocal bursts of high-amplitude delta activity with spikes and sharp waves, intermixed with runs of more normal-appearing background activity. These EEG abnormalities may precede overt clinical symptoms by 6 months. As the disease progresses, the normal background activity also deteriorates to slow frequencies.[197] The EEG has been said to be pathognomonic, but a similar pattern may also be seen in other metabolic encephalopathies. The diagnosis depends on the presence of the typical clinical picture and is confirmed by the characteristic EEG pattern.[215] Magnetoencephalography (MEG) has been used in the evaluation of uremic patients[229] but not yet in the evaluation of patients with dialysis dementia.

Aluminum and Dialysis Dementia

Aluminum intoxication was first implicated in this disorder by Alfrey and associates.[218] Aluminum content of brain gray matter was elevated to 11 times the normal value in patients with dialysis dementia, compared with an increase of 3 times normal in patients on chronic hemodialysis without dialysis dementia. Aluminum content was also increased in bone and other soft tissues. Oral phosphate binders containing aluminum—$Al(OH)_3$ and $Al_2(CO_3)_2$—were originally suspected as the source of the aluminum.

Most of the aluminum in blood is bound to transferrin, and as a result blood contains very little free aluminum.[230] The brain contains few transferrin receptors, so that, normally, aluminum uptake into brain is negligible. Any free aluminum in blood, usually in the form of aluminum-citrate, can readily enter the CNS. Aluminum binding can be studied with the aluminum analog gallium.[231] Normally, there is an excess of gallium-binding sites in plasma, so that even in situations in which blood aluminum is increased, there is still almost no free aluminum in blood. In studies of gallium-transferrin binding in blood of patients with Alzheimer disease, Down syndrome, or renal failure treated with chronic hemodialysis, gallium binding to transferrin was significantly reduced in the first two groups.[230] However, gallium binding to transferrin was normal in patients with CRF treated with hemodialysis. In such patients, there was

accumulation of aluminum in those brain regions with high densities of transferrin receptors.[102]

The aforementioned findings involve studies in only small numbers of subjects with dialysis dementia ($n = 9$)[230, 232] or CRF treated with hemodialysis ($n = 5$). More such studies are needed before it can be conclusively stated that the distribution of aluminum in brain of patients with dialysis dementia is not similar to that in patients with Alzheimer disease. In patients with CRF without dialysis dementia, neurofibrillary changes are not present.[102, 103]

More recent studies have further added to our knowledge of the possible effects of aluminum on the CNS in patients with CRF. A possible pathophysiologic basis for detrimental effects of aluminum on the CNS was described by Altmann and associates.[233] Dihydropteridine reductase is an important enzyme in the synthesis of several important neurotransmitters, such as tyrosine and acetylcholine. Altmann's group found that erythrocyte levels of dihydropteridine reductase activity were less than the predicted values and correlated with the plasma aluminum concentration.[233] After treatment with desferrioxamine, erythrocyte dihydropteridine reductase activity levels doubled. Although brain levels of dihydropteridine reductase activity were not evaluated, it was suggested that high brain aluminum levels might lead to decreased availability of dihydropteridine reductase in the brain. It has been suggested that merely the presence of an increased body burden of aluminum has an adverse effect on overall mortality.[234] More specifically, an increased body aluminum burden (estimated by the desferrioxamine infusion test) has been associated with memory impairment and increased severity of myoclonus with decreased motor strength.[235]

Altmann and associates evaluated patients with CRF and apparently normal cerebral function.[233, 236] They found that these patients had abnormalities in six tests of psychomotor function, compared to a control group with similar IQ. Plasma aluminum levels were only mildly elevated (59 ± 9 μg/L). When 15 of these patients were treated for 3 months with desferrioxamine, anemia improved and the erythrocyte activity of dihydropteridine reductase rose significantly. Changes in erythrocyte dihydropteridine reductase activity correlated significantly with changes in psychomotor performance.[233, 236] Even at high blood Al levels, most Al is bound to transferrin[230] and therefore cannot bind to the cerebral transferrin receptors. It may be that patients who develop dialysis dementia have less transferrin binding capacity, less transferrin, or a greater density of transferrin receptors in the brain. These issues have not been studied to date.

Toxic Manifestations of Aluminum on the Central Nervous System

Aluminum may be potentially toxic in patients with CRF, possibly leading to both dialysis dementia and osteomalacia.[216, 217, 224-226] Most nephrologists would agree that the potential hazards of poor control of plasma phosphate are worse than the potential toxicity of aluminum accumulation from oral aluminum-containing antacids. However, studies have suggested that calcium carbonate (or acetate) may be more effective for the control of hyperphosphatemia than is aluminum hydroxide.[237, 238] More recently, sevelamer (Renagel), a polymeric phosphate binder, has come into wide use for control of phosphate in chronic dialysis patients.[239] Renagel, although expensive, has been found to be more effective than either calcium carbonate, calcium acetate, or aluminum hydroxide for the treatment of hyperphosphatemia in dialysis patients,[239] and it does not introduce aluminum into the body. However, aluminum is still the second most prevalent element in the earth's crust, and a substantial quantity will enter the body, even without administration of aluminum-containing antacids.[240-242]

Deionization of the water used to prepare dialysate has become a standard procedure and is a preventive measure for dialysis dementia.[243, 244] However, deionization may be beneficial by removing any number of other agents from dialysis water. Other trace elements in water can result in CNS toxicity, including cadmium, mercury, lead, manganese, copper, nickel, thallium, boron, and tin.[227] Among these potentially neurotoxic elements no one has measured brain content of cadmium, mercury, nickel, thallium, vanadium, or boron. Manganese was found to be increased in cortical white matter in the eight encephalopathic patients in whom it was measured.[222] These patients also had elevated aluminum levels in gray matter.

Most of the controversy over the etiology of dialysis dementia has involved sporadic cases. As noted previously, dialysate aluminum levels are not always elevated. The history of use of aluminum-containing antacids is no different in patients with dialysis dementia than in unaffected patients, and brain aluminum levels in patients with dialysis dementia generally overlap with those of unaffected patients.[227] The largest group of sporadic cases was reported from Nashville, Tennessee.[224] The reported incidence of dialysis dementia in the area is 5%, despite the use of deionized water for dialysate with aluminum levels lower than 5 µg/L. Osteomalacic bone disease was not clinically apparent in this group. Serum aluminum levels in the encephalopathic group were three to four times higher than in other dialyzed patients, despite equivalent prescribed doses of aluminum-containing phosphate binders. These results suggest greater absorption and/or retention of aluminum or other trace metal contaminants in this group of encephalopathic patients. No other metals were measured in the Nashville study.

The evidence available thus far indicates that aluminum is increased in the brain (cortical gray matter) of patients with dialysis dementia. However, the actual contribution of aluminum to the encephalopathy remains unclear. Aluminum content has been reported to be increased in the brain of patients with other disorders, including senile dementia and Alzheimer syndrome, and might actually be a nonspecific finding associated with dementia. Aluminum is also elevated in the brains of patients who have other disorders associated with altered blood-brain barrier. Such disorders, include renal failure, hepatic encephalopathy, and metastatic cancer. Other evidence suggests that brain aluminum content may increase as a function of the aging process. Therefore, blood-brain barrier abnormalities can result in increased brain aluminum content.[245]

Prevention and Treatment of Dialysis Dementia

Despite these unresolved questions, most past outbreaks of the epidemic form of dialysis dementia have been associated with high levels of aluminum in the dialysate.[216, 246, 247]

Lowering the dialysate aluminum to less than 20 µg/L, usually by deionization, appears to prevent onset of the disease in patients who are beginning dialysis. New cases may continue to appear among those patients who were previously exposed to dialysate with high aluminum content, although the course is milder and mortality is somewhat decreased. Among patients with overt disease, eliminating the source of aluminum has resulted in improvement in some but not all patients. Renal transplantation has generally not been helpful in patients with established dialysis dementia. Diazepam or clonazepam is useful in controlling seizure activity associated with the disease but becomes ineffective later on and does not alter the final outcome.[214] Because the treatment of dialysate water with deionization has become standard (in the United States, western Europe, and Israel), epidemic dialysis dementia has become increasingly rare.

Treatment of sporadic cases, in which the etiology is not clear, is more difficult. Every effort should be made to identify a treatable cause. Dialysis dementia must be differentiated from other metabolic encephalopathies such as hypercalcemia and hypophosphatemia, hyperparathyroidism, acute heavy metal intoxications, and structural neurologic lesions such as subdural hematoma (Table 51-8).[248] Because of the low incidence, the uncertain etiology, and the poor correlation of plasma with tissue aluminum levels, screening tests have not generally been employed.

The source of excess Al^{3+} in brain is not entirely clear. Some Al^{3+} apparently is absorbed after oral administration of aluminum-containing antacids.[37, 141] Significant absorption of oral aluminum can occur in patients with CRF, but the weight of evidence is against oral aluminum as an important source of aluminum in brain. The retention of Al^{3+} after oral administration of Al^{3+} salts is greater in patients with renal failure than in normal subjects.[249, 250] The typical daily dietary Al^{3+} intake is 10 to 100 mg,[242] although absorption is normally minimal. This quantity of dietary Al^{3+} is more than enough to account for the entire increase of brain Al^{3+} observed in patients with dialysis dementia. Among 22 such patients, the mean brain Al^{3+} content was 22 mg/kg

TABLE 51-8

Differential Diagnosis of Dialysis Dementia

Metabolic encephalopathies
Hypercalcemia
Hypophosphatemia
Hypoglycemia
Hyperosmolality
Hyponatremia
Symptomatic uremia
Drug intoxications
Trace metal intoxications
Hyperparathyroidism

Hypertensive encephalopathy

Dialysis disequilibrium

Structural lesions of the brain
Subdural hematoma
Normal-pressure hydrocephalus
Stroke

dry weight. The normal human brain weighs about 1500 g and is about 80% water, or 300 g dry weight. Therefore, the total increase in Al^{3+} content for the whole brain is less than 7 mg in patients with dialysis dementia. The entire increase of brain Al^{3+} in such patients can theoretically be accounted for by dietary aluminum.[251] The increase in body aluminum stores may also be, in part, the result of Al^{3+} contamination from other sources, such as Al^{3+} in dialysate water, dialysis system aluminum pipes, or aluminum leaked from anodes.[227]

Brain Lesions and Dialysis Dementia

There are a large number of children who have renal insufficiency and also require hospitalization with intravenous therapy. Such children may receive large quantities of intravenous aluminum (Al^{3+}) from contamination of intravenous solutions with aluminum salts.[252-257] Thus, even in the absence of hemodialysis therapy, children with CRF may receive large quantities of intravenous aluminum, which may explain the development of dialysis dementia in the absence of dialysis.[257] The location of the aluminum in brain of patients with dialysis dementia has not been well established. In Alzheimer disease, it initially appeared that the aluminum was localized only to the nuclear regions of neurofibrillary tangles.[258] More recent investigations revealed that in Alzheimer disease aluminum accumulates in at least four different sites: DNA-containing structures of the nucleus, protein moieties of neurofibrillary tangles, amyloid cores of senile plaques, and cerebral ferritin.[259-261]

Senile plaques and neurofibrillary tangles are diagnostic features of Alzheimer's disease.[262] It is not generally appreciated that in dialysis dementia, the brain also contains senile plaques and neurofibrillary tangles in most cases.[232] However, in dialysis dementia, aluminum was located not in the neurons but rather in glial cells and the walls of blood vessels.[243] As mentioned previously, these findings involved studies in small numbers of patients[230, 232]; more such studies are needed before it can be conclusively stated that the distribution of aluminum in brain of patients with dialysis dementia is not similar to that in patients with Alzheimer disease.

The source of the increased Al^{3+} in brain of patients with dialysis encephalopathy can theoretically be accounted for on the basis of increased Al^{3+} intake. However, it is unclear how the Al^{3+} enters brain in increased quantities. It may be that the increased body aluminum burdens in uremic subjects contribute to increased Al^{3+} content in the brains of such individuals. To clarify the role of oral ingestion of aluminum salts in the causation of increased brain Al^{3+} content, it would be instructive to examine brain tissue from patients without renal failure who had ingested large quantities of $AlOH_3$ (e.g., patients with chronic peptic ulcer disease). However, because such material is not likely to be available, studies in laboratory animals given large quantities of aluminum salts should provide similar information. In both rats and dogs receiving oral aluminum salts, there is a significant increment in brain Al^{3+} content.[221, 263, 264] Administration of PTH to rats receiving aluminum salts results in an additional increment of brain Al^{3+} content.[249, 264, 265] Therefore, in laboratory animals, both a chronic increase in oral Al^{3+} ingestion and PTH excess can lead to an increase of cerebral cortex Al^{3+}, even in the absence of renal failure.

Alternative Etiologies

Many other possible causes of dialysis dementia have been proposed, including other trace element contaminants,[211, 227, 264] normal-pressure hydrocephalus,[227] slow virus infection of the CNS,[168] and regional alterations in cerebral blood flow.[266] Some patients with dialysis dementia have altered cerebrospinal fluid dynamics that are at least suggestive of normal-pressure hydrocephalus.[267] Six patients with dialysis dementia were found to have normal cerebrospinal fluid dynamics but only mild dilatation of the cerebral ventricles.[267] In that study, however, control subjects (uremic patients treated with hemodialysis but without dialysis dementia) were not evaluated, and results of recent studies suggest that many patients who have ESRD without dialysis encephalopathy may also have ventricular dilatation with cerebral atrophy.[103] Furthermore, there is a generally poor correlation between ventricular dilatation, cerebral atrophy, and the presence of dementia.[268]

Slow virus infection of the nervous system is a possible etiology for dialysis dementia. The clinical manifestations resemble those of other slow virus infections, such as Kuru or Creutzfeldt-Jakob disease.[269, 270] In at least one instance, a slow virus (foamy virus) was isolated from the brain of patients who died with dialysis encephalopathy.[269]

In summary, dialysis dementia probably represents an end point in a disease with multiple causes. There are at least three subgroups, and in two of them the etiology of dialysis encephalopathy must be regarded as unknown. The possible role of aluminum or other trace element abnormalities is unclear. At this time, there is no known satisfactory treatment for patients with dialysis encephalopathy. Most patients reported in the literature have not survived, usually dying within 18 months from the time of diagnosis. The syndrome is not alleviated by increased frequency of dialysis, and usually not by renal transplantation.[223, 251] Definitive therapy must await a better understanding of the pathogenesis of this disorder. The use of deferoxamine to chelate aluminum or other trace elements is experimental and is currently under extensive investigation. There have been several reports of improvement in patients with dialysis dementia treated with deferoxamine,[267, 271] but these results have not been confirmed.

OTHER CENTRAL NERVOUS SYSTEM COMPLICATIONS OF DIALYSIS

In addition to dialysis dementia and DDS, several other neurologic disorders have been reported in patients being treated with dialysis. In most instances, patients have initially presented with headache, nausea, emesis, or hypotension; some have had seizures. Most of these patients were initially diagnosed with DDS, but others, particularly those with chronic subdural hematoma, were suspected of having dialysis dementia. The disorders include copper intoxications, subdural hematoma, muscle cramps, nonketotic hyperosmolar coma with hyperglycemia, cerebral embolus secondary to shunt declotting, acute cerebrovascular accident, depletion syndrome, malfunction of fluid proportioning system, excessive ultrafiltration with hypotension and seizures, hypoglycemia, and Wernicke encephalopathy.[38, 58]

In the past, cerebral complications were the second most frequent cause of death among patients being treated with hemodialysis.[272]

Subdural Hematoma

Subdural hematoma is currently an infrequent cause of death in patients maintained on chronic hemodialysis.[56] This condition may initially present with headache, drowsiness, nausea, and vomiting. If the patient loses consciousness or develops signs of increased intracranial pressure, a diagnosis of subarachnoid bleeding should be considered. Such episodes in uremic patients are usually fatal unless operated on. If the symptoms persist between hemodialysis, or progressively worsen, subdural hematoma is likely, particularly if the patient is taking anticoagulants. On physical examination, there is often evidence of localized neurologic disease; there may be signs of meningeal irritation, and somnolence and focal seizures may be observed. The diagnosis can usually be made by modern neuroimaging techniques (CT or MRI).[86, 273] Subarachnoid bleeding in hemodialysis patients is probably often related to anticoagulant excess.[274] The initial symptom when intracranial hemorrhage occurs is usually depression of sensorium: convulsions may follow, and the patients may lapse into coma.

Technical Dialysis Errors

Improper proportioning of dialysate, due to human or mechanical error, is still an important cause of neurologic abnormality in dialysis patients.[275] The usual effect of such mistakes is the production of hyponatremia or hypernatremia. Either of these abnormalities of body fluid osmolality can lead to seizures and coma, although different mechanisms are involved. In acute hypernatremia, there is excessive thirst, lethargy, irritability, seizures, and coma, with spasticity and muscle rigidity. In acute hyponatremia, there is weakness, fatigue, and dulled sensorium, which may also progress to seizures and coma, respiratory arrest, and death. Such symptoms developing soon after initiation of hemodialysis should alert the physician to the possibility of an error. A check of the dialysate osmolality or sodium concentration is the most rapid means of detecting this problem. Death has been reported as a consequence of either hypernatremia or hyponatremia.[276, 277]

About 1 L of fluid per hour can be removed by ultrafiltration hemodialysis, and about 300 mL/hr by peritoneal dialysis using hypertonic dialysate. Such a rate of fluid removal from the intravascular space may be faster than the rate at which fluid can be replaced from the interstitial compartment, and hypotension may develop. Symptoms of hypotension may include seizures, which, although actually caused by cerebrovascular insufficiency, may be mistaken for DDS, particularly in diabetic subjects.

Most of the neurologic complications of renal transplantation relate to secondary afflictions, such as infection and neoplasia. As already discussed, most of the neurologic complications of the uremic state tend to improve after renal transplantation. These include the neuropathy, encephalopathy, and EEG changes.[278-280]

Stroke
Mechanisms of Cell Damage with Stroke

Acute ischemic stroke (cerebrovascular accident, or CVA) is a condition in which a portion of the brain is acutely deprived of sufficient blood flow. The brain requires about 50 mL/min of blood that contains an adequate level of glucose and oxygen to function normally.[281] Acute ischemic stroke can be subdivided into three different mechanisms: decreased systemic perfusion, thrombosis, and embolism. Decreased systemic perfusion implies cardiopulmonary insufficiency (hypoxic ischemia), usually resulting from myocardial infarction, arrhythmia, or hemorrhage. Systemic hypoperfusion does not cause acute ischemic stroke and is discussed elsewhere.[282] Thrombosis refers to blockage of blood flow due to a localized in situ occlusive process within one or more blood vessels. The most common vascular pathology is atherosclerosis. Fibrous and muscular tissues overgrow in the subintima, and fatty materials form plaques that can encroach on the lumen. Next, platelets adhere to plaque crevices and form clumps that serve as nidi for the deposition of fibrin, thrombin, and clot.[281] Plaque rupture can activate the coagulation cascade, leading to formation of an occlusive thrombus. Another important possibility is acute hemorrhagic stroke, in which there is actual rupture of a vessel, with bleeding into the substance of the brain, followed by secondary tissue ischemia. Brain damage after occlusion of a blood vessel is mediated by several biochemical mechanisms.

Excessive amounts of glutamate in brain extracellular fluid initiate at least a part of the pathogenesis for brain damage in ischemic states.[282] Ischemia causes a release of glutamate into the cerebral extracellular space, leading to excitation of a subset of glutamate receptors, the NMDA receptor. Hypoxia increases excitation in neurons, particularly at the NMDA receptor, which in turn leads to an excessive influx of sodium ions and water.[164] Excitation, or increased synaptic activity, is an important factor in eventual cell death in hypoxic neurons.[162] The classic biochemical hypothesis, by which hypoxia/ischemia leads to a decrease of brain high-energy phosphate compounds with a secondary influx of sodium, chloride, and water into brain, is probably incorrect.

A point is eventually reached at which cerebral edema has occurred and cell viability is severely compromised. If the cellular damage continues, there follows an influx of calcium ions and a probable decrease in intracellular magnesium,[283] which is at some point followed by permanent neuronal damage. The actual event that leads to irreversible cell death in hypoxic brain is not entirely clear. A late event is the movement into hypoxic cells of calcium, and in certain types of cell injury, calcium overload is the actual pathogenetic mechanism.[284] There are a number of theoretical reasons why calcium overload may be detrimental to cells. An increase in free cytosolic calcium can activate calcium-dependent phospholipases, resulting in the breakdown of cell membranes and production of substances that are toxic to cells, such as free fatty acids and phospholipids.

Demographics of Stroke in Uremic Patients

From a clinical standpoint, cerebrovascular disease is a common cause of death in chronic hemodialysis patients,[55] and the three most frequent causes of death are heart attack, stroke, and infection.[12, 155, 285, 286] In the United States and western Europe (including Israel), cardiovascular disease is far more common in dialysis patients than in the rest of the population.[14, 287] Part of the reason may be that the major cause of ESRD in the United States is diabetes mellitus (27%), far more than in Europe (19%) or Japan (10%).[288, 289] Among the factors that contribute to the high incidence of stroke in patients with ESRD treated with hemodialysis are the high incidence of hypertension and smoking, both of which are higher in ESRD patients than in the rest of the population. Other factors are the large number of such patients who have diabetes mellitus and the accelerated arteriosclerosis in such patients.[290] In addition, uremic patients tend to have high cholesterol levels and a high incidence of obesity, and they tend to have a higher prevalence of cigarette smoking than in the rest of the population.[291, 292] There is a high incidence of chronic infection in dialysis patients, which leads to increased blood levels of atherogenic risk factors such as cytokines, which appear to contribute to the increased incidence of stroke in such patients.[94, 148, 293] The elevated cytokines are largely caused by the high incidence of chronic inflammatory conditions in chronic hemodialysis patients.[293]

Chronic Inflammation and Cardiovascular Disease

There is substantial recent evidence that chronic inflammation plays a role in the pathogenesis of cardiovascular disease.[172] Cytokines released from involved tissues stimulate the liver to synthesize acute phase proteins, including CRP. Increased levels of CRP and other cytokines constitute an independent risk factor for cardiovascular disease,[94] particularly in women.[294] AGEs can modify tissues, enzymes, and proteins and may play a role in the pathogenesis of dialysis-associated amyloidosis.[8, 125, 295] AGEs are markedly elevated in plasma of patients with ESRD,[8] particularly if they also have diabetes mellitus.[289] These AGEs react with vascular cells to inactivate endothelial NO and may increase the propensity of ESRD patients to develop arteriosclerosis and hypertension.[174]

There is evidence for increased cytokine production secondary to blood interaction with bioincompatible dialysis components. In particular, blood-dialyzer interaction can activate mononuclear cells, leading to production of inflammatory cytokines.[134] Synthetic high-flux dialyzer membranes are permeable to the proinflammatory cytokines and are capable of removing IL-1β, tumor necrosis factor-α (TNF-α), and IL-6, thus offering a potential therapeutic approach.[135] It is unclear whether cytokine removal by continuous renal replacement therapy can decrease the incidence of stroke.[296] The use of sorbents with continuous plasma filtration offers another possibility for a novel therapeutic approach.[296] Some of the cytokines, such as IL-1β, TNF-α, and IL-6, may induce an inflammatory state and are believed to play an important role in dialysis-related mortality.[293]

Recent prospective studies have demonstrated that patients with ESRD and higher blood levels of certain cytokines have a greater mortality and have a larger number of cardiovascular events. In fact, increased levels of markers of inflammation are associated with increased mortality and decline in function in elderly patients without ESRD.[297]

However, just the presence of renal failure, even with a GFR of 71 mL/min, results in an increased risk of myocardial infarction and death.[298] Contaminated dialysate water can result in absorption of pyogenic substances of bacterial origin into the dialysis membrane.[135] The consequence could be induction of an inflammatory response in certain dialysis patients. Substances of bacterial origin activate circulating mononuclear cells to produce proinflammatory cytokines. The cytokines include IL-1β, TNF-α, and IL-6, and they mediate the acute phase response, resulting in increased levels of acute phase proteins, including CRP.[135] The effects of dialysis reuse on cytokine production have not been evaluated but may be important, because reuse could theoretically lead to more contamination of dialysate.[135] Reactive carbonyl compounds and AGEs, which tend to modify proteins in a deleterious manner,[125] can be decreased by the use of a peritoneal dialysate containing icodextrin and amino acids instead of glucose.

The cardiovascular disease and cerebrovascular disease can lead to cerebral ischemia. Cerebral ischemia initiates a number of processes that can lead to progressive brain damage.[299] Cerebral ischemia can lead to activation in brain of free radicals, NMDA,[300] and apoptosis,[120] all potential mechanisms of brain damage in patients with hypoperfusion or stroke (see Fig. 51-1).[116, 117, 109] Anoxic injury to brain endothelial cells can increase production of NO, which can lead to free radical formation.[301, 302] Apoptosis, or programed cell death, is another mode of destruction of brain cells in stroke.[109] Glutamate activates the NMDA receptor complex and can also lead to later activation of apoptosis.[109] In general, the ischemic event of a stroke only serves to initiate the biochemical events that may lead to brain damage. Interventions that counter these biochemical events may decrease the brain damage associated with acute stroke.[119, 303]

Prevention of Stroke

Recent knowledge about the pathogenesis of stroke has led to a major expansion in the opportunities for prevention of stroke. Some of the simplest and most important strategies are shown in Table 51-9. High-grade carotid stenosis can lead to stroke, although the exact percentage of patients with carotid stenosis who will suffer stroke is not known. Screening patients who have renal failure for the presence of carotid stenosis can diagnose a substantial number of such patients, albeit at considerable cost. However, because of noninvasive diagnostic techniques such as duplex Doppler ultrasonography, screening for carotid stenosis involves essentially no morbidity.[119] Studies of the aortic arch for the presence of large atherosclerotic plaques (>4 mm thick) are an important predictor for the possibility of stroke in the future,[304] as is the presence of atrial fibrillation, both for initial strokes[92, 305] and for recurrent stroke.[306] Transient ischemic attacks are often associated with numbness, weakness, or partial blindness. Such symptoms occur in patients with ESRD, particularly if they also have diabetes mellitus. It is not generally appreciated that they are often the harbinger of stroke.[305] The presence of such a symptom complex should trigger a workup that includes evaluation of the carotids (ultrasound, CT, or MRI).

Migraine is a common clinical disorder, often characterized by an aura, headache, and autonomic dysfunction.[307] In patients with ESRD, headache is common, and the possible

TABLE 51-9

Strategies for Prevention of Stroke

Cessation of smoking
Daily exercise
Healthy diet (low fat, modest protein, high fiber)
Treatment and control of hypertension
Control of diabetes
Control of cholesterol, triglyceride, and homocysteine
Treatment of atrial fibrillation
Weight control

association with impending stroke may not be appreciated. Other common preventive measures include treatment of hypertension, cessation of smoking, lowering of plasma cholesterol, control of plasma glucose (in diabetic patients), weight loss, increased exercise, and decreased alcohol consumption.[292] Other possible preventive measures include dietary antioxidants, low-dose aspirin, and a decrease of intake of saturated fatty acids.[292] Until very recently, there was believed to be substantial evidence that administration of hormone replacement therapy in postmenopausal women was associated with a reduced risk of stroke.[292, 308] Such therapy often included other compounds that have estrogen-like effects.[309] Recent findings demonstrating that administration of estrogen to postmenopausal women may lead to an increased risk of breast cancer and thrombotic episodes have served to decrease the routine administration of such agents.[310] However, new drugs, now in the final stages of testing, have many of the beneficial effects of estrogens and fewer of the objectionable side effects.[309]

Although treatment of hypertension is known to decrease the incidence of stroke, not all antihypertensive agents are of equal efficacy. In general, only β-blockers, thiazide diuretics, and ACE inhibitors have been shown to reduce the incidence of stroke, whereas α-adrenergic blocking agents and calcium channel blockers may not.[311, 312]

Therapy for Stroke

Given the likely mechanisms of brain damage associated with stroke, a whole new field is opened for as far as potential therapeutic agents for decreasing such damage. Such agents include calcium channel blockers,[313, 314] inhibitors of NMDA receptors,[315] and agents that scavenge free radicals.[316] In many cases, acute stroke can be successfully treated, but only if physicians realize that stroke should be considered a medical emergency, wherein timely therapy can make the difference in functional survival of the brain.

Therapies for acute stroke that are now being administered in teaching hospitals in the United States start with acute neuroimaging in the emergency room. An initial CT scan usually reveals acute stroke and serves to differentiate occlusive from hemorrhagic stroke. If a nonhemorrhagic stroke is present, treatment prospects can be examined with magnetic resonance angiography (MRA), which is noninvasive. Contrast should not be administered to patients with impaired renal function, but it may be given to dialysis patients.[317] If acute stroke is diagnosed within the appropriate time window (within 3 hours after onset of symptoms), current treatments

may include intravenous thrombolytic therapy,[318] intraarterial thrombolytic therapy, antithrombotic and antiplatelet drugs, defibrinogenating agents, and neuroprotective drugs.[299, 319-321] Administration of the defibrinogenating agent ancrod to patients with acute ischemic stroke resulted in a better functional status after 3 months of follow-up.[321] Nizofenone can scavenge free radicals and inhibit glutamate release, and it may prove useful as a cerebroprotective agent.[299, 322]

Some cases of acute stroke are caused by dissection of the carotid or vertebral artery systems. These patients have lesions that are not amenable to dissolution of clot, because the obstructing lesion is in fact a hemorrhage in the arterial wall.[323, 324] Dissection of the carotid or vertebral artery system can be initiated by chiropractic manipulation of the cervical spine, and such maneuvers should probably be avoided in dialysis patients. In addition, some cases of apparent acute stroke in dialysis patients are caused by subdural hematoma, which must always be considered in the differential diagnosis of stroke in dialysis patients. Another potential cause of stroke is the use of over-the-counter medications (dietary supplements) containing ephedra (phenylpropanolamine).[90] Although recent publicity has related to deaths that may have been associated with the use of ephedra-containing products by athletes,[325] there have been many reports of stroke in ordinary individuals after use of such agents, often for weight control.[326]

SEXUAL DYSFUNCTION IN UREMIA

Pathogenesis of Uremic Sexual Dysfunction

Disturbances in sexual function are a common complication of CRF.[11, 327, 328] These complications include erectile dysfunction, decreased libido, and decreased frequency of intercourse.[329, 330] Studies in uremic rats showed that erectile impairment was associated with a disturbance in NOS gene expression.[328] Sexual dysfunction in men with ESRD treated with maintenance hemodialysis is common, and previously impotence was observed in at least 50% of such patients.[93] A number of abnormalities associated with renal failure appear to be important in the genesis of impotence. There are abnormalities in autonomic nervous system function,[329] impairment in arterial and venous systems of the penis (along with vascular pathology in other vascular beds), hypertension (many drugs used to treat hypertension cause secondary impotence), and other associated endocrine abnormalities.[331] Failure to treat patients with ACE inhibitors was an important factor in the development of erectile dysfunction.[330] There are also the associated effects of aging, with impotence observed in more than 50% of men older than 60 years of age who do not have renal failure.[332]

Therapy for Sexual Dysfunction in Uremia

There are a variety of approaches to the evaluation of impotency in uremic men.[333] Patients with ESRD have a high incidence of cardiovascular disease,[13] which impairs penile vessels along with those of the rest of the body.[287] The incidence of hypertension is also higher in ESRD patients than in the rest of the population, and hypertension is a major contributor to vascular disease.[13, 287] Many drugs used to treat hypertension can lead to impotence, including calcium channel blockers, thiazides, and guanethidine. The incidence of depression is high in patients with ESRD, and many drugs used to treat depression can lead to impotence, including phenothiazines, tricyclics, and fluoxetine. Although appreciation of the aforementioned abnormalities may increase understanding of these problems, until very recently there was little that could be done other than to discontinue certain drugs used to treat hypertension or depression.[93] There are now a number of drugs that can successfully treat impotence in hemodialysis patients.[334] Alprostadil was successful but had to be delivered transurethrally.[335] Sildenafil in particular can be administered orally and is highly effective, even in men who have cardiovascular disease[336] or uremia.[337, 338] Other treatments for impotence among men with ESRD include penile prostheses, direct injection of α-blocking agents or other vasodilators (e.g., papaverine, phentolamine, alprostadil) into the penis, and vacuum constrictive devices.[327, 334]

UREMIC NEUROPATHY

Clinical Manifestations

Peripheral neuropathy in patients with renal failure has been recognized for more than 100 years,[339] but it was not fully appreciated until the early 1960s.[186] Before the institution of chronic dialysis therapy, approximately 65% of patients with ESRD probably did not live long enough to develop clinically apparent neuropathy. Although existing data are difficult to evaluate, neuropathy is probably present in about 65% of patients with ESRD at the time of institution of dialysis.[340]

Many patients with CRF who are neurologically asymptomatic may exhibit abnormalities on physical examination. They may also have evidence of autonomic neuropathy, such as impotence and postural hypotension. Moreover, in patients who have renal insufficiency, abnormal nerve conduction may be present in the absence of symptoms or abnormal findings on physical examination. Additionally, alternations in nerve conduction do not necessarily indicate structural changes in the peripheral nerves. It is often overlooked that many patients with ESRD have autonomic dysfunction, which in turn results in impaired baroreceptor sensitivity, which can impair blood pressure regulation.[341]

The MNCV is a test that is frequently used to assess peripheral neuropathy. However, this test is somewhat unreliable, because there is a large normal variation in MNCV (up to 20% on a day-to-day basis),[179] and the test has very limited utility in detecting moderate impairment of peripheral nerve function. Sensory nerve conduction velocity (SNCV) is more sensitive than MNCV, but the test is painful and most patients do not permit repeated tests.

In general, there are two broad categories of peripheral neuropathy. These are described in terms of the pattern of involvement of the peripheral nervous system. First, there are processes that result in a bilaterally symmetrical disturbance of function that can be designated as polyneuropathies. Polyneuropathy tends to be associated with agents such as toxic substances, metabolic disorders (uremia, diabetes, deficiency states), and certain examples of immune reaction that act diffusely on the peripheral nervous system. The second category comprises isolated lesions of peripheral nerves (mononeuropathy) or multiple isolated lesions (multiple mononeuropathy). In severe symmetrical polyneuropathies, a generalized loss of peripheral nerve function may occur, and the impairment is usually maximal distally in the limbs. A mixed motor and sensory polyneuropathy with a distal distribution results in weakness and wasting that is most frequently observed peripherally in the arms and legs. There are also distal sensory changes of "glove and stocking" distribution. In those neuropathies that involve "dying back" of the axons from the periphery,[339] it is possible that the neurons that have the longest axons to maintain are the first to suffer.

Uremic neuropathy is a distal, symmetrical, mixed polyneuropathy. In general, motor and sensory modalities are both affected, and lower extremities are more severely involved than are the upper extremities. Clinically, uremic polyneuropathy cannot be distinguished from the neuropathies associated with certain other metabolic disorders, such as diabetes mellitus, chronic alcoholism, and various deficiency states. The occurrence of neuropathy bears no relation to the type of underlying disease process (i.e., glomerulonephritis or pyelonephritis). However, certain diseases that can lead to renal failure may simultaneously affect peripheral nerve function in a manner separate from the manifestations of uremia. Such diseases include amyloidosis, multiple myeloma, systemic lupus erythematosus, polyarteritis nodosa, diabetes mellitus, and hepatic failure.[186] The clinical manifestations of uremic neuropathy are characterized by several different stages. It appears that when GFR exceeds 12 mL/min, clinical evidence of neuropathy is generally absent.

Peripheral Nerves

The restless leg syndrome is a common early manifestation of CRF. Clinically, patients experience sensations in lower extremities such as crawling, prickling, and pruritus. The sensations are worse distally than proximally and are generally more prominent in the evening. The restless leg syndrome may initially be present in up to 40% of patients with CRF.[342] Another symptom experienced by patients with early uremic neuropathy is the burning foot syndrome, which is present in fewer than 10% of patients with CRF.[343] Rather than "burning," the actual symptoms consist of swelling sensations, constriction, and tenderness of the distal lower extremities.

The physical signs of peripheral nerve dysfunction often begin with loss of deep tendon reflexes, particularly knee and ankle jerks.[276, 277] Impaired vibratory sensation is also an early sign of uremic neuropathy. Loss of sensation in the lower leg is common and often takes the form of "stocking glove" anesthesia of the lower leg. The sensory loss includes pain, light touch, vibration, and pressure.

Metabolic Neuropathy

Uremic neuropathy is one of a group of central-peripheral axonopathies, also known as dying-back polyneuropathies, which were described by Spencer and Schaumberg.[344] The causes of such central-peripheral axonopathies involve many types of toxic compounds. These causes include neuropathies associated with diabetes, multiple myeloma, certain hereditary polyneuropathies, and uremia.[344] There is also an associated degeneration of the spinal cord, particularly involving posterior columns, as well as other portions of the CNS. Such findings are usually attributed to local CNS disease or to damage of spinal ganglion cells secondary to ascending peripheral nervous system damage. The clinical characteristics of such distal axonopathies, as described by Schaumberg and Spencer,[344] include the following:

1. *Insidious onset:* In most human toxic neuropathies, there is a steady, low-level exposure. Because only the distal portion of selected, scattered fibers are affected, the patient may still function well despite the axonal degeneration.
2. *Onset in legs:* Large and long axons are affected early, and fibers of the sciatic nerve are especially vulnerable.
3. *Stocking-glove sensory loss:* Degeneration in the distal axon proceeds toward the cell body, resulting in clinical signs in the feet and hands initially.
4. *Early loss of Achilles reflex:* Fibers to the calf muscles are of large diameter and among the first affected by many toxins, even when longer, smaller-diameter axons in the feet are spared.
5. *Moderate slowing of motor nerve conduction:* In demyelinating neuropathies, motor nerves or roots are diffusely affected; in axonal neuropathies, scattered motor fibers are often intact and motor nerve conduction velocity may appear normal or only slightly slow despite severe paresis.
6. *Normal cerebrospinal fluid protein content:* Pathologic changes are usually distal, and nerve roots are spared.
7. *Slow recovery:* Axonal regeneration (in contrast to remyelination) is slow, about 1 mm/day. Therefore, after institution of dialysis or renal transplantation, recovery of nerve function may take months or years.
8. *Residual disability:* Most toxic axonopathies are characterized by tract degeneration of long, large-diameter fibers in the CNS, concomitant with changes in the peripheral nervous system. Signs of lesions in the corticospinal and spinocerebellar pathways may not be clinically apparent if there is severe peripheral neuropathy. However, on recovery from the neuropathy, spasticity or ataxia may be observed.

It can readily be recognized that these features are similar to many descriptions of uremic neuropathy.[186, 339, 345] The cellular basis for distal axonopathies, however, remains unclear. Spencer and associates[346] emphasized that a number of chemically unrelated neurotoxic compounds and several types of metabolic abnormalities can cause strikingly similar patterns of distal symmetrical polyneuropathy in humans and animals. They suggested a possible common metabolic basis for many distal axonopathies. Neurotoxic compounds may deplete energy supplies in the axon by inhibiting nerve fiber enzymes required for the maintenance of energy synthesis. Resupply of enzymes from the neuronal soma may fail to meet the increased demand for enzyme replacement in the axon, causing the concentration of enzymes to decrease in distal regions. This could lead to a local blockade of energy-dependent axonal transport, which could then produce a series of pathologic changes culminating in distal nerve fiber

degeneration. Among uremic patients who also have diabetes mellitus, oxidative stress, including superoxide accumulation, and accumulation of AGEs appear to be major contributors to the development of uremic neuropathy.[3, 8, 125] In experimental diabetic neuropathy, there was a significant reduction in sonic hedgehog messenger RNA, which was substantially improved by treatment with sonic hedgehog-immunoglobulin G fusion protein.[347] Such an approach may be promising in the treatment of uremic neuropathy as well.

In addition to uremic neuropathy, uremic myopathy is a frequent cause of weakness, exercise limitation, and rapid-onset tiredness in dialysis patients.[348, 349] Later on, muscle wasting occurs, particularly in the limb muscles.

Uremic Toxins and Nerve Conduction

Several possible uremic toxins have been identified that appear to be correlated with depression of MNCV in laboratory animals.[161, 177, 178] However, studies of these toxins have not taken into account the limitations of MNCV testing (see earlier discussion). Although it is possible to relate impairment in MNCV with levels in blood of various substances, the best correlation was obtained between reduced MNCV and reduced GFR (see Table 51-5).

Parathyroid Hormone

Among the potential uremic neurotoxins is PTH.[28] This supposition ignores the criteria suggested by Bergstrom and Furst,[158] and is based instead on a possible correlation between plasma PTH levels and MNCV in patients with CRF.[180] Some earlier studies suggested a possible effect of PTH on MNCV in the dog,[178] but these early impressions have not been confirmed.[38, 184] In fact, if the early data in humans are critically examined, the correlation coefficient (r value) when MNCV is graphed against the PTH level is -0.45.[180] This means that $r^2 = 0.202$, and $1 - r^2 = 0.8$. Thus, for any change in MNCV, 80% of the change could *not* be due to an effect of PTH. Therefore, the original data are substantially flawed, further weakening the argument for an implied relationship between PTH and impaired nerve function in uremia. Other contradictions to this relationship were discussed earlier.

It has also been suggested, without adequate explanation and without confirmation, that either PTH or ARF results in an increase of nerve calcium content and that this might be related to impaired MNCV.[178] This postulate must now be considered as both unlikely and unproved. In dogs with renal failure for periods of 3.5 days to 4 months, there were no observed increases in nerve calcium content.[63] Nerve calcium values in dogs with ARF with or without parathyroidectomy also were not different and in fact actually fell significantly (versus control) in dogs with CRF.

ACKNOWLEDGMENT

This research in this manuscript was supported by a grant from the NIH, National Institute of Aging, Grant # AG-08575-02S1. The support of Doctors Charles Kleeman, Raul Guisado, Cosmo Fraser, Cynthia Mahoney, Jerry Cooper, and Virginia Lazarowitz is gratefully acknowledged. I wish to thank my wife Patricia N. Hale, J.D., for her inspirational support and intellectual assistance.

REFERENCES

1. Stone WJ: Beta 2-microglobulin-associated amyloidosis of end-stage renal disease. *In* Henrich WL (ed): Principles and Practice of Dialysis. Baltimore, Williams & Wilkins, 1994, pp 225-233.
2. Takayama F, Miyazaki S, Morita T, et al: Dialysis related amyloidosis of the heart in long-term hemodialysis patients. Kidney Int 59(suppl 78):S172-S176, 2002.
3. Feldman E: Oxidative stress and diabetic neuropathy: A new understanding of an old problem. J Clin Invest 111:431-433, 2003.
4. Kennedy R, Case C, Fathi R, et al: Does renal failure cause an atherosclerotic milieu in patients with end-stage renal disease? Am J Med 110:198-204, 2001.
5. Hsu C, McCulloch CE, Curhan GC: Epidemiology of anemia associated with chronic renal insufficiency among adults in the United States: Results from the Third Health and Nutrition Examination Survey. J Am Soc Nephrol 13:504-510, 2002.
6. Levin A: Anemia and left ventricular hypertrophy in chronic kidney disease populations. Kidney Int 61(suppl 80):S35-S38, 2002.
7. Himmelfarb J, Stenvinkel P, Ikizler TA, Hakim RM: The elephant in uremia: Oxidative stress as a unifying concept of cardiovascular disease in uremia. Kidney Int 62:1524-1538, 2002.
8. Miyata T, Sugiyama S, Saito A, Kirokawa K: Reactive carbonyl compounds related to uremic toxicity (carbonyl stress). Kidney Int 59 (suppl 78):S25-S31, 2001.
9. Vanholder R, De Smet R, Lameire N: Protein-bound uremic solutes: The forgotten toxins. Kidney Int 59(suppl 78):S266-S270, 2001.
10. Teschan PE, Arieff AI: Uremic and dialysis encephalopathies. *In* McCandless DW (ed): Cerebral Energy Metabolism and Metabolic Encephalopathy. New York, Plenum Press, 1985, pp 263-285.
11. Palmer BF: Sexual dysfunction in uremia. J Am Soc Nephrol 10:1381-1388, 1999.
12. Iseki K, Fukiyama K: Predictors of stroke in patients receiving chronic hemodialysis. Kidney Int 50:1672-1675, 1996.
13. Meeus F, Kourilsky O, Guerin AP, et al: Pathophysiology of cardiovascular disease in hemodialysis patients. Kidney Int 58(suppl 76):S140-S147, 2000.
14. Parfrey PS: Cardiac and cerebrovascular disease in chronic uremia. Am J Kidney Dis 21:77-80, 1993.
15. Wratten ML, Tetta C, Ursini F, Sevanian A: Oxidant stress in hemodialysis: Prevention and treatment strategies. Kidney Int 58(suppl 76):S126-S132, 2000.
16. Slomowitz LA, Wilkinson A, Hawkins R, Danovitch G: Evaluation of kidney function in renal transplant patients receiving long-term cyclosporine. Am J Kidney Dis 15:530-534, 1990.
17. Chan L, Wang W, Kam I: Outcomes and complications of renal transplantation. *In* Schrier RW, Gottschalk CW (eds): Diseases of the Kidney, Vol 3. Philadelphia, Lippincott Williams & Wilkins, 2001, pp 2871-2938.
18. Teschan PE, Ginn HE, Bourne JR, et al: Quantitative indices of clinical uremia. Kidney Int 15:676-697, 1979.
19. Locke SJ, Merrill JP, Tyler HR: Neurological complications of acute uremia. Arch Intern Med 108:519-530, 1961.
20. Cooper JD, Lazarowitz VC, Arieff AI: Neurodiagnostic abnormalities in patients with acute renal failure: Evidence for neurotoxicity of parathyroid hormone. J Clin Invest 61:1448-1455, 1978.
21. Fraser CL, Arieff AI: Nervous system manifestations of renal failure. *In* Schrier RW, Gottschalk CW (eds): Diseases of the Kidney, Vol 3. Philadelphia, Lippincott Williams & Wilkins, 2001, pp 2769-2794.
22. Moe SM, Sprague SM: Uremic encephalopathy. Clin Nephrol 42:251-256, 1994.
23. Guisado R, Arieff AI, Massry SG, et al: Changes in the electroencephalogram in acute uremia: Effects of parathyroid hormone and brain electrolytes. J Clin Invest 55:738-745, 1975.
24. Kiley JE, Woodruff MW, Pratt KI: Evaluation of encephalopathy by EEG frequency analysis in chronic dialysis patients. Clin Nephrol 5:245, 1976.
25. Basile C, Miller JD, Koles ZJ, Grace M: The effects on brain water and EEG in stable chronic uremia. Am J Kidney Dis 9:462-469, 1987.
26. Cogan MG, Covey C, Arieff AI: Central nervous system manifestations of hyperparathyroidism. Am J Med 65:963-970, 1978.
27. Fraser CL, Arieff AI: Nervous system complications in uremia. Ann Intern Med 109:143-153, 1988.
28. Slatopolsky E, Martin K, Hruska K: Parathyroid hormone metabolism and its potential as a uremic toxin. Am J Physiol 239:F1-F12, 1980.
29. Griggs RC, Satran R: Metabolic encephalopathy. *In* Rosenberg RN, Grossman RG (eds): Neurology/Neurosurgery. New York, Churchill-Livingstone, 1983, pp 651-653.
30. Adams RD, Victor M: The acquired metabolic disorders of the nervous system: Hypoxic-hypotensive encephalopathy. *In* Adams RD, Victor M (eds): Principles of Neurology. New York, McGraw-Hill, 1985, pp 788-791.
31. Teschan PE, Bourne JR, Reed RB: Electrophysiological and neurobehavioral responses to therapy: The National Cooperative Dialysis Study. Kidney Int 23:558, 1983.
32. Hirakata H, Yao H, Osato S, et al: CBF and oxygen metabolism in hemodialysis patients: Effects of anemia correction with recombinant human EPO. Am J Physiol 262(Renal Fluid Electrolyte Physiol 31):F737-F743, 1992.
33. Ifudu O, Feldman J, Friedman EA: The intensity of hemodialysis and the response to erythropoietin in patients with end-stage renal disease. N Engl J Med 334:420-425, 1996.
34. Nissenson AR: Epoetin and cognitive function. Am J Kidney Dis 20:21-24, 1992.
35. Kokot F, Wiecek A: Evidence that the anemia of renal failure participates in overall uremic toxicity. Kidney Int 52(suppl 62):S83-S86, 1997.
36. Grimm G, Stockenhuber F, Schneeweiss B, et al: Improvement of brain function in hemodialysis patients treated with erythropoietin. Kidney Int 38:480-486, 1990.
37. Moreno F, Sanz-Guajardo D, Lopez-Gomez J, et al: Increasing the hematocrit has a beneficial effect on quality of life and is safe in selected hemodialysis patients. J Am Soc Nephrol 11:335-342, 2000.
38. Mahoney CA, Arieff AI, Leach WJ, Lazarowitz VC: Central and peripheral nervous system effects of chronic renal failure. Kidney Int 24:170-177, 1983.
39. Crammer JL: Calcium metabolism and mental disorder. Psychol Med 7:557, 1977.
40. Gatewood JW, Organ CH, Mead BT: Mental changes associated with hyperparathyroidism. Psychiatry 123:129, 1975.
41. Heath H, Hodgson SF, Kennedy MA: Primary hyperparathyroidism: Incidence, morbidity, and potential impact in a community hospital. N Engl J Med 302:189-193, 1980.
42. Luxenberg J, Feigenbaum LZ, Aron JM: Reversible long-standing dementia with normocalcemic hyperparathyroidism. J Am Geriatr Soc 32:546-547, 1984.
43. Fraser CL, Arieff AI: Hepatic encephalopathy. N Engl J Med 313:865-873, 1985.
44. Ong JP, Aggarwal A, Kriegr D, et al: Correlation between ammonia levels and the severity of hepatic encephalopathy. Am J Med 114:188-193, 2003.
45. Kuhns M, Medina M, McNamara A: Detection of hepatitis C virus RNA in hemodialysis patients. J Am Soc Nephrol 4:1491-1496, 1994.
46. Takabatake T, Ohta H, Ishida Y, et al: Low serum creatinine levels in severe hepatic disease. Arch Intern Med 148:1313-1315, 1988.
47. Papadakis MA, Arieff AI: Unpredictability of clinical evaluation of renal function in cirrhosis. Am J Med 82:945-952, 1987.
48. Gines P, Jimenez W: Aquaretic agents: A new potential treatment of dilutional hyponatremia in cirrhosis. J Hepatol 24:506-512, 1996.
49. U. S. Renal Data System: Renal Data System Annual Report, 1996–1998. Bethesda, MD, National Institutes of Health, National Institute of Diabetes and Digestive and Kidney Diseases, 2000.
50. Lazarus JM, Denker BM, Owen WF: Hemodialysis. *In* Brenner BM (ed): The Kidney, Vol 2. Philadelphia, WB Saunders, 1996, pp 2424-2506.
51. Miles AM, Friedman EA: Center and home chronic hemodialysis: Outcome and complications. *In* Schrier RW, Gottschalk CW (eds): Diseases of the Kidney, Vol 3. Philadelphia, Lippincott Williams & Wilkins, 2001, pp 2807-2838.
52. Garg PP, Frick KD, Diener-West M, Powe NR: Effect of the ownership of dialysis facilities on patients' survival and referral for transplantation. N Engl J Med 341:1653-1660, 1999.
53. Depner TA: Dialysis therapy: Role of dialyzer membranes. *In* Massry SG, Glassock RJ (eds): Massry and Glassock's Textbook of Nephrology, Vol 1. Philadelphia, Lippincott Williams & Wilkins, 2001, pp 1512-1515.
54. Bowling PS, Bourn JR: Discriminant analysis of electroencephalograms recorded from renal patients. IEEE Trans Biomed Eng 25:12, 1978.
55. Mahoney CA, Arieff AI: Uremic encephalopathies: Clinical, biochemical and experimental features. Am J Kidney Dis 2:324-336, 1982.

56. Fraser CL, Arieff AI: Metabolic encephalopathy as a complication of acid base, and electrolyte disorders. *In* Arieff AI, DeFronzo RA (eds): Fluid, Electrolyte and Acid-Base Disorders. New York, Churchill Livingstone, 1995, pp 685-740.

57. Teschan PE, Ginn HE, Bourne JR, et al: A prospective study of reduced dialysis. ASAIO J 6:108, 1983.

58. Fraser CL, Arieff AI: Metabolic encephalopathy as a complication of renal failure: Mechanisms and mediators. *In* Matuschak GM (ed): New Horizons: The Science and Practice of Acute Medicine, Vol 2. Baltimore, Williams & Wilkins, 1994, pp 518-526.

59. Osberg JW, Meares GJ, McKee DC, Burnett GB: Intellectual functioning in renal failure and chronic dialysis. J Chronic Dis 35:445-457, 1982.

60. English A, Savage RD, Britton PG, et al: Intellectual impairment in chronic renal failure. Br Med J 1:888-890, 1978.

61. Greenberg MD: Brain damage in hemodialysis patients. Dial Transplant 7:238, 1978.

62. Minkoff L, Gaertner M, Darah C, et al: Inhibition of brain sodium-potassium ATPase in uremic rats. J Lab Clin Med 80:71-78, 1972.

63. Mahoney CA, Sarnacki P, Arieff AI: Uremic encephalopathy: Role of brain energy metabolism. Am J Physiol 247 (Renal Fluid Electrolyte Physiol 16):F527-F532, 1984.

64. Van den Noort S, Eckel RE, Brine K, Hrdlicka JT: Brain metabolism in uremic and adenosine-infused rats. J Clin Invest 47:2133-2142, 1968.

65. Arieff AI, Massry SG, Barrientos A, Kleeman CR: Brain water and electrolyte metabolism in uremia: Effects of slow and rapid hemodialysis. Kidney Int 4:177-187, 1973.

66. Arieff AI, Massry SG: Calcium metabolism of brain in acute renal failure: Effects of uremia, hemodialysis, and parathyroid hormone. J Clin Invest 53:387-392, 1974.

67. Arieff AI, Guisado R, Massry SG: Central nervous system pH in uremia and the effects of hemodialysis. J Clin Invest 58:306, 1977.

68. Perry TL, Yong VW, Kish SJ, et al: Neurochemical abnormalities in brain of renal failure patients treated by repeated hemodialysis. J Neurochem 45:1043-1048, 1985.

69. Fishman RA: Permeability changes in experimental uremic encephalopathy. Arch Intern Med 126:835-837, 1970.

70. Verkman AS, Fraser CL: Water and non-electrolyte permeability in brain synaptosomes isolated from normal and uremic rats. Am J Physiol 250:R306-R312, 1986.

71. Deferrari G: Brain metabolism of amino acids and ammonia in patients with chronic renal insufficiency. Kidney Int 20:505, 1981.

72. Akmal M, Goldstein DA, Multani S, Massry SG: Role of uremia, brain calcium and parathyroid hormone on changes in electroencephalogram in chronic renal failure. Am J Physiol 246(Renal, Fluid, Electrolyte Physiol 15):F575-F579, 1984.

73. Arieff AI: Neurological manifestations of uremia. *In* Brenner BM, Rector FC Jr (eds): The Kidney, Vol 2. Philadelphia, WB Saunders, 1986, pp 1731-1756.

74. Levin GE, Baron DN: Leucocyte intracellular pH in patients with metabolic acidosis or renal failure. Clin Sci (Colch) 52:325, 1977.

75. Maschio G, Bazzato G, Bertaglia E, et al: Intracellular pH and electrolyte content of skeletal muscle in patients with chronic renal acidosis. Nephron 7:481-487, 1970.

76. Tizianello A, Deferrari G, Gurreri G, Acquarone N: Effects of metabolic alkalosis, metabolic acidosis and uraemia on whole-body intracellular pH in man. Clin Sci (Oxford) 52:125-135, 1977.

77. Pauli HG, Vorburger C, Reubi F: Chronic derangements of cerebrospinal fluid acid base components in man. J Appl Physiol 17:993-998, 1962.

78. De Deyn PP, D'Hooge R, Van Bogaert P, Marescau B: Endogenous guanidino compounds as uremic neurotoxins. Kidney Int 59(suppl 78):S77-S83, 2002.

79. De Deyn PP, Marescau B, D'Hodge R, et al: Guanidino compound levels in brain regions of non-dialyzed uremic patients. Neurochem Int 27:227-237, 1995.

80. Sadowski RH, Haynes BD, He J, et al: Acute renal failure induces rapid glial and neuronal changes in the rat cerebral cortex. Kidney Int (in press).

81. Fraser CL, Sarnacki P: Parathyroid hormone mediates changes in calcium transport in uremic rat brain synaptosomes. Am J Physiol 254 (Renal Fluid Electrolyte Physiol 23):F837-F844, 1988.

82. Ischiropoulos H, Beckman JS: Oxidative stress and nitration in neurodegeneration: Cause, effect, or association. J Clin Invest 111: 163-169, 2003.

83. Fraser CL, Sarnacki P, Arieff AI: Calcium transport abnormality in uremic rat brain synaptosomes. J Clin Invest 76:1789-1795, 1985.

84. Fraser CL, Arieff AI: Abnormalities of transport in synaptosomes from uremic rat brain: Role of parathyroid hormone. J Gen Physiol 88:24, 1986.

85. Fraser CL, Sarnacki P, Budayr A: Evidence that parathyroid hormone-mediated calcium transport in rat brain synaptosomes is independent of cyclic adenosine monophosphate. J Clin Invest 81:982-988, 1988.

86. Arieff AI, Fraser CL, Rowley H, et al: Metabolic encephalopathy. *In* Kucharczyk J, Moseley M, Barkovich AJ (eds): Magnetic Resonance Neuroimaging, Vol 1. Boca Raton, FL, CRC Press, 1994, pp 319-349.

87. Siddiqui JY, Fitz AE, Lawton RL: Causes of death in patients receiving long-term hemodialysis. JAMA 212:1350, 1970.

88. Olsen S: The brain in uremia. Acta Psychiatr Scand 36(suppl 156): 1-128, 1961.

89. Sato Y, Kaji M, Metoki N, et al: Does compensatory hyperparathyroidism predispose to ischemic stroke? Neurology 60:626-629, 2003.

90. Kernan WN, Viscolli CM, Brass LM, Broderick JP: Phenyl-propanolamine and the risk of hemorrhagic stroke. N Engl J Med 343:1826-1832, 2000.

91. Bachelard HS: The molecular basis of coma and stroke. *In* Cohen RD, Lewis B, Alberti KGMM, Denman AM (eds): The Metabolic and Molecular Basis of Acquired Disease, Vol 2. Philadelphia and London, WB Saunders/Baillière Tindall, 1990, pp 1354-1380.

92. Amarenco P, Duyckaerts C, Tzourio C, et al: The prevalence of ulcerated plaques in the aortic arch in patients with stroke. N Engl J Med 326:221-225, 1992.

93. Massry SG, Smogorzewski MJ, Klahr S: Metabolic and endocrine dysfunctions in uremia. *In* Schrier RW, Gottschalk CW (eds): Diseases of the Kidney, Vol 3. Boston, Little, Brown, 1997, pp 2661-2698.

94. Kaysen GA: The microinflammatory state in uremia: Causes and potential consequences. J Am Soc Nephrol 12:1549-1557, 2001.

95. Savazzi GM, Cusamo F, Vinci S, Allegri L: Progression of cerebral atrophy in patients on regular hemodialysis treatment: Long-term follow-up with cerebral computed tomography. Nephron 69:29-33, 1995.

96. Savazzi GM: Pathogenesis of cerebral atrophy in uraemia. Nephron 49:94-103, 1988.

97. Papageorgiou C, Ziroyannis P, Vathylakis J: A comparative study of brain atrophy by computerized tomography in chronic renal failure and chronic hemodialysis. Acta Neurol Scand 66:378-384, 1982.

98. Fraser CL, Arieff AI: Neuropsychiatric complications of uremia. *In* Brady HR, Wilcox CS (eds): Therapy in Nephrology and Hypertension. Philadelphia, WB Saunders, 1999, pp 488-490.

99. Dean S, Allegretti C: 25 years of good health. Patient Line (FMC Medical Services) Winter:1-3, 2003.

100. Levy NB, Cohen LM: Central and peripheral nervous system in uremia: Psychiatric and psychosocial considerations. *In* Massry SG, Glassock RJ (eds): Massry and Glassock's Textbook of Nephrology, Vol 1. Philadelphia, Lippincott Williams & Wilkins, 2001, pp 1279-1282.

101. Okada J, Yoshikawa K, Matsuo H, Oouchi M: Reversible MRI and CT findings in uremic encephalopathy. Neuroradiology 33:524-526, 1991.

102. Wang HC, Brown P, Lees AJ: Acute movement disorders with bilateral basal ganglia lesions in uremia. Mov Disord 13:952-957, 1998.

103. Passer JA: Cerebral atrophy in end-stage uremia. Proc Clin Dial Transplant Forum 7:91, 1977.

104. Mahurkar SD, Myers L, Cohen J, Kamath RV, Dunea G: Electroencephalographic and radionucleotide studies in dialysis dementia. Kidney Int 13:306-315, 1978.

105. Korzets Z, Zeltzer E, Rathaus M, et al: Uremic optic neuropathy: A uremic manifestation mandating dialysis. Am J Nephrol 18:240-242, 1998.

106. Guy J, Johnston PK, Corbett JJ, et al: Treatment of visual loss in pseudotumor cerebri associated with uremia. Neurology 40:28-32, 1990.

107. Raff MC, Barrers BA, Burne JF, et al: Programmed cell death and the control of cell survival. Science 262:695-700, 1993.

108. Steller H: Mechanisms and genes of cellular suicide. Science 267:1445-1449, 1995.

109. Vexler ZS, Roberts TPL, Bollen AW, et al: Transient cerebral ischemia: Association of apoptosis induction with hypoperfusion. J Clin Invest 99:1453-1459, 1997.

110. Pittman RN, Wang S, DiBenedetto AJ, Mills JC: A system for characterizing cellular and molecular events in programmed neuronal cell death. J Neurosci 13:3669-3680, 1993.

111. Linnik MR, Zobrist R, Hatfield M: Evidence supporting a role for programmed cell death in focal cerebral ischemia in rats. Stroke 24:2002-2008, 1993.

112. Tominaga T, Kure S, Narisawa K, Yoshimoto T: Endonuclease activation following ischemic injury in the rat brain. Brain Res 608:21-26, 1993.

113. de la Monte SM: p53- and CD95-associated apoptosis in neurodegenerative diseases. Lab Invest 78:401-411, 1998.

114. Cohen, Rdnicki M, Horl WH: Uremic toxins modulate the spontaneous apoptotic cell death and essential functions of neutrophils. Kidney Int 59(suppl 78):S48-S52, 2001.

115. Aoyagi K, Shahrzad S, Ida S, Tomida C: Role of nitric oxide in the synthesis of guanidinosuccinic acid, an activator of the N-methyl-D-aspartate receptor. Kidney Int 59(suppl 78):537-547, 2001.

116. Coyle JT, Puttfarcken P: Oxidative stress, glutamate and neurodegenerative disorders. Science 262:689-695, 1993.

117. Bonfoco E, Krainc M, Ankarcrona M, et al: Apoptosis and necrosis. Proc Natl Acad Sci U S A 92:7162-7166, 1995.

118. Chen J, Graham P, Chan P, et al: Bcl-2 is expressed in neurons that survive focal ischemia in the rat. Neuroreport 6:394-398, 1995.

119. Lee JM, Grabb MC, Zipfel GJ, Choi DW: Brain tissue responses to ischemia. J Clin Invest 106:723-731, 2000.

120. Honig LS, Rosenberg RN: Apoptosis and neurologic disease. Am J Med 108:317-330, 2000.

121. Barber AJ, Lieth E, Khin SA, Antonetti DA: Neural apoptosis in the retina during experimental and human diabetes. J Clin Invest 102:783-791, 1998.

122. Ashkenazi A, Dixit VM: Death receptors: Signaling and modulation. Science 281:1305-1308, 1998.

123. Yu SP, Yeh CH, Strasser M, et al: NMDA receptor-mediated K$^+$ efflux and neuronal apoptosis. Science 284:336-338, 1999.

124. Marnett LJ, Riggins JN, West JD: Endogenous generation of reactive oxidants and electrophiles and their reactions with DNA and protein. J Clin Invest 111:583-593, 2003.

125. Miyata T, Kirokawa K, van Ypersele de Strihou C: Relevance of oxidative and carbonyl stress to long-term uremic complications. Kidney Int 58(suppl 76):S120-S125, 2000.

126. Sebekova K, Blazicek P, Syrova D, Krivosikova Z: Circulating advanced glycation end product levels in rats rapidly increase with acute renal failure. Kidney Int 59(suppl 78):S48-S62, 2001.

127. Schwedler S, Schinzel R, Vaith P, Wanner C: Inflammation and advanced glycation end product levels in uremia: Simple coexistence, potentiation or causal relationship? Kidney Int 59(suppl 78): S32-S36, 2001.

128. Asahi K, Ichimori K, Nakaawa H, Izuhara Y: Nitric oxide inhibits the formation of advanced glycation end products. Kidney Int 58:1780-1787, 2000.

129. Devuyst O, van Ypersele de Strihou C: Nitric oxide, advanced glycation end products, and uremia. Kidney Int 58:1814-1815, 2000.

130. Henry RMA, Kostense PJ, Bos G, Dekker JM: Mild renal insufficiency is associated with increased cardiovascular mortality: The Hoorn study. Kidney Int 62:1402-1407, 2002.

131. Loughrey CM, Young IS, Lightbody JH: Oxidative stress in haemodialysis. Q J Med 87:679-683, 1994.

132. Stenvinkel P, Wanner C, Metzger T, et al: Inflammation and outcome in end-stage renal failure: Does female gender constitute a survival advantage? Kidney Int 62:1791-1798, 2002.

133. May RC, Mitch WE: Pathophysiology of uremia. *In* Brenner BM (ed): The Kidney, Vol 2. Philadelphia, WB Saunders, 1996, pp 2148-2169.

134. Morena M, Cristol JP, Senecal L, Leray-Moragues H: Oxidative stress in hemodialysis patients: Is NADPH oxidase complex the culprit? Kidney Int 61(suppl 80):S109-S114, 2002.

135. Lonnemann G: Chronic inflammation in hemodialysis: The role of contaminated dialysate. Blood Purif 18:214-223, 2000.

136. Sela S, Shurtz-Swirski R, Shapiro G, et al: Oxidative stress during hemodialysis: Effect of heparin. Kidney Int 59(suppl 78): S159-S163, 2002.

137. Mydlik M, Derzsiova K, Racz O, Sipulova A: A modified dialyzer with vitamin E and antioxidant defense parameters. Kidney Int 59(suppl 78):S144-S147, 2002.

138. Huang J: Dehydroascorbic acid, a blood-brain barrier transportable form of vitamin C, mediates potent cerebroprotection in experimental stroke. Proc Natl Acad Sci U S A 98:11720-11724, 2001.

139. Ross R: Atherosclerosis: An inflammatory disease. N Engl J Med 340:115-126, 1999.

140. Rifai N, Buring JE, Lee IM, et al: Is C-reactive protein specific for vascular disease in women? Ann Intern Med 136:529-533, 2002.

141. Ridker PM, Hennekens CH, Buring JE, Rifai N: C-reactive protein and other markers of inflammation in the prediction of cardiovascular disease in women. N Engl J Med 342:836-843, 2000.

142. Stuveling EM, Hillege HL, Bakker SJL, Gans ROB: C-reactive protein is associated with renal function abnormalities in a non-diabetic population. Kidney Int 63:654-661, 2003.

143. Jenkins NP, Keevil BG, Hutchinson IV, Brooks NH: Beta-blockers are associated with lower C-reactive protein concentrations in patients with coronary artery disease. Am J Med 112:269-274, 2002.

144. Caglar K, Peng Y, Pupim LB, Flakoll PJ: Inflammatory signals associated with hemodialysis. Kidney Int 62:1408-1416, 2002.

145. Mezzano D, Pais EO, Aranda E, Panes O: Inflammation, not hyperhomocysteinemia, is related to oxidative stress and hemostatic and endothelial dysfunction in uremia. Kidney Int 60:1844-1850, 2001.

146. Nassar GM, Fishbane S, Ayus JC: Occult infection of old nonfunctioning arteriovenous grafts: A novel cause of erythropoietin resistance and chronic inflammation in hemodialysis patients. Kidney Int 61:S49-S54, 2002.

147. Nassar GM, Ayus JC: Infectious complications of old nonfunctioning arteriovenous grafts in renal transplant recipients: A case series. Am J Kidney Dis 40:832-836, 2002.

148. Ayus JC, Sheikh-Hamad D: Silent infection in clotted hemodialysis access grafts. J Am Soc Nephrol 9:1314-1317, 1998.

149. Van Guldener C, Stam F, Stehouwer CDA: Homocysteine metabolism in renal failure. Kidney Int 59(suppl 78):S234-S237, 2002.

150. Perna AF, Ingrosso D, Castaldo P, et al: Homocysteine and transmethylations in uremia. Kidney Int 59(suppl 78):S230-S233, 2002.

151. Mallamaci F, Zoccali C, Tripepi G, et al: Hyperhomocysteinemia predicts cardiovascular outcomes in hemodialysis patients. Kidney Int 61:609-614, 2002.

152. Massy ZA, Ceballos I, Chadefaux-Vekemens B, et al: Homocyst(e)ine, oxidative stress, and endothelium function in uremic patients. Kidney Int 59(suppl 78):S243-S245, 2002.

153. Meng W, Tobin JR, Busija DW: Glutamate-induced cerebral vasodilation is mediated by nitric oxide through N-methyl-D-asparate receptors. Stroke 26:857-863, 1995.

154. Lipton SA, Kim WK, Choi YB: Neurotoxicity associated with dual actions of homocysteine at the N-methyl-D-aspartate receptor. Proc Natl Acad Sci U S A 94:5923-5928, 1997.

155. Iseki K, Kinjo K, Kimura Y, et al: Evidence for a high risk of cerebral hemorrhage in chronic dialysis patients. Kidney Int 44:1086-1090, 1993.

156. Drueke T, Khoa TN, Massy ZA, et al: Role of oxidized low-density lipoprotein in the atherosclerosis of uremia. Kidney Int 59(suppl 78): S114-S119, 2002.

157. Vasan RS, Beiser A, D'Augostino RB, et al: Plasma homocysteine and risk for congestive heart failure in adults without prior myocardial infarction. JAMA 289:1251-1257, 2003.

158. Bergstrom J, Furst P: Uremic toxins. *In* Drukker W, Parsons FM, Maher JF (eds): Replacement of Renal Function by Dialysis. Boston, Martinus Nijhoff, 1983, pp 354-377.

159. Vanholder R: Low molecular weight uremic toxins. *In* Ronco C, Bellomo R (eds): Critical Care Nephrology. Hingham, MA: Kluwer Academic, 1998, pp 855-868.

160. Vanholder R: Pathogenesis of uremic toxicity. *In* Ronco C, Bellomo R (eds): Critical Care Nephrology. Hingham, MA: Kluwer Academic, 1998, pp 845-853.

161. Giovannetti S, Balestri PL, Barsotti G: Methylguanidine in uremia. Arch Intern Med 131:709-713, 1973.

162. Faden AI, Demediuk P, Panter SS, Vink R: The role of excitatory amino acids and NMDA receptors in traumatic brain injury. Science 244:798-800, 1989.

163. Lipton SA, Rosenberg PA: Excitatory amino acids as a final common pathway for neurologic disorders. N Engl J Med 330: 613-622, 1994.

164. Beal MF: Mechanisms of excitotoxicity in neurologic disease. FASEB J 6:3338-3344, 1992.

165. Davidoff F: Guanidine derivatives in medicine. N Engl J Med 289:141-146, 1973.

166. Dhondt A, Vanholder R, van Beisen W, Lameire N: The removal of uremic toxins. Kidney Int 58(suppl 76):S47-S59, 2000.

167. Scribner BH, Babb AL: Evidence for toxins of "middle" molecular weight. Kidney Int 7(suppl 3):S349-S353, 1975.

168. Man NK: An approach to "middle molecules" identification in artificial kidney dialysate, with reference to neuropathy prevention. Trans Am Soc Artif Intern Organs 19:320, 1973.

169. Kjellstrand CM, Arieff AI, Friedman EA, et al: Inadequacy of dialysis: Why patients are not well. Trans Am Soc Artif Intern Organs 25:518-520, 1979.

170. Scribner BH, Farrell PC, Milutinovic J: Evolution of the middle molecular hypothesis. Proc 5th Int Congr Nephrol, Mexico, 1972, vol 5, p 190.

171. Vanholder R, DeSmet R, Hsu C, et al: Uremic toxins: The middle molecule hypothesis revisited. Semin Nephrol 14:205-218, 1994.

172. Wanner C, Zimmermann J, Schwedler S, Metzger T: Inflammation and cardiovascular risk in dialysis patients. Kidney Int 61(suppl 80):S99-S102, 2002.

173. Makita Z, Radoff S, Rayfield EJ, et al: Advanced glycosylation end products in patients with diabetic nephropathy. N Engl J Med 325:836-842, 1991.

174. Haag-Weber M: AGE-modified proteins in renal failure. In Ronco C, Bellomo R (eds): Critical Care Nephrology. Hingham, MA: Kluwer Academic, 1998, pp 878-883.

175. Miyata T, van Ypersele de Strihou C, Ueda Y, et al: Angiotensin II receptor antagonists and angiotensin-converting enzyme inhibitors lower in vitro the formation of advanced glycation end products: Biochemical mechanisms. J Am Soc Nephrol 13:2478-2487, 2002.

176. Koenig H, Goldstone AD, Lu CY, Trout JJ: Polyamines: Transducers of osmotic signals at the blood-brain barrier. Proc Am Soc Neurochem 19:79, 1988.

177. Clements RSJ, DeJesus PVJ, Winegrad AI: Raised plasma-myoinositol levels in uraemia and experimental neuropathy. Lancet 1:1137-1141, 1973.

178. Goldstein DA, Chui LA, Massry SG: Effect of parathyroid hormone and uremia on peripheral nerve calcium and motor nerve conduction velocity. J Clin Invest 62:88-92, 1978.

179. McQuillen MP, Gorin FJ: Serial ulnar nerve conduction velocity measurements in normal subjects. J Neurol Neurosurg Psychiatry 32:144, 1969.

180. Avram MM, Feingold DA, Huatuco AH: Search for the uremic toxin: Decreased motor nerve conduction velocity and elevated parathyroid hormone in uremia. N Engl J Med 298:1000-1003, 1978.

181. Lonergan ET, Semar M, Sterzel RB, et al: Erythrocyte transketolase activity in dialyzed patients. N Engl J Med 284:1399-1403, 1971.

182. Reznek RH, Salway JG, Thomas PK: Plasma myoinositol concentrations in uraemic neuropathy. Lancet 1:675-676, 1977.

183. Mallette LE, Pattern BM, Engle WK: Neuromuscular disease in secondary hyperparathyroidism. Ann Intern Med 82:474, 1975.

184. Giulio SD, Chkoff N, Lhoste F, et al: Parathormone as a nerve poison in uremia. N Engl J Med 299:1134-1135, 1978.

185. Aurbach GD: Neuromuscular disease in primary hyperparathyroidism. Ann Intern Med 80:182, 1974.

186. Asbury AK: Uremic neuropathy. In Dyck PJ, Thomas PK, Lambert EH (eds): Peripheral Nerve Disorders, Vol 2. Philadelphia, WB Saunders, 1975, pp 220-252.

187. Arnaud CD: Hyperparathyroidism and renal failure. Kidney Int 4:89, 1973.

188. De Boer IH, Gorodetskaya I, Young B, et al: The severity of secondary hyperparathyroidism in chronic renal insufficiency is GRF-dependent, race dependent, and associated with cardiovascular disease. J Am Soc Nephrol 13:2762-2769, 2002.

189. Goldstein DA, Massry SG: The relationship between the abnormalities in EEG and blood levels of parathyroid hormone in dialysis patients. J Clin Endocrinol Metab 51:130, 1980.

190. Rasmussen H, Goodman DBP: Relationships between calcium and cyclic nucleotides in cell activation: Cellular calcium metabolism and calcium-mediated cellular processes. Physiol Rev 57:428, 1977.

191. Kennedy AC, Linton AL, Eaton JC: Urea levels in cerebrospinal fluid after hemodialysis. Lancet 1:410, 1962.

192. Arieff AI: Dialysis disequilibrium syndrome: Current concepts on pathogenesis. In Schreiner GE, Winchester JF (eds): Controversies in Nephrology, Vol 4. Washington, DC, George Washington University Press, 1982, pp 367-376.

193. Arieff AI: Dialysis disequilibrium syndrome: Current concepts on pathogenesis and prevention. Kidney Int 45:629-635, 1994.

194. Pagel MD, Ahmad S, Vizzo JE: Acetate and bicarbonate fluctuations and acetate intolerance during dialysis. Kidney Int 21:513, 1982.

195. Rodrigo F, Shideman J, McHugh R, et al: Osmolality changes during hemodialysis: Natural history, clinical correlations, and influence of dialysate glucose and intravenous mannitol. Ann Intern Med 86:554-561, 1977.

196. Van Stone JC, Carey J, Meyer R, Murrin C: Hemodialysis with glycerol containing dialysate. ASAIO J 2:119-123, 1979.

197. Grushkin CM, Korsch B, Fine RN: Hemodialysis in small children. JAMA 221:869, 1972.

198. de Peterson H, Swanson AG: Acute encephalopathy occurring during hemodialysis. Arch Intern Med 113:877, 1964.

199. Fukusige M, Tado O, Matsuki S, et al: Hemodialysis with kill-type artificial kidney: Clinical study on disequilibrium syndrome. Acta Urol Jap 17:89, 1971.

200. Mawdsley C: Neurological complications of hemodialysis. Proc R Soc Med 65:871, 1972.

201. Porte FK, Johnson WJ, Klass DW: Prevention of dialysis disequilibrium syndrome by use of high sodium concentration in the dialysate. Kidney Int 3:327, 1973.

202. Arieff AI, Leach W, Park R, Lazarowitz VC: Systemic effects of $NaHCO_3$ in experimental lactic acidosis in dogs. Am J Physiol 242:F586-F591, 1982.

203. Greca G, Dettori P, Biasoli S: Brain density studies in dialysis. Lancet 2:582, 1980.

204. Paganini EP: General application of continuous therapeutic techniques. In Henrich WL (ed): Principles and Practice of Dialysis. Baltimore, Williams & Wilkins, 1994, pp 98-110.

205. Kliger AS: Complications of dialysis: Hemodialysis, peritoneal dialysis and CAPD. In Arieff AI, DeFronzo RA (eds): Fluid, Electrolyte and Acid-Base Disorders. New York, Churchill Livingstone, 1985, pp 777-826.

206. Rouby JJ, Rottenbourg J, Durande JP: Hemodynamic changes induced by regular hemodialysis and sequential ultrafiltration hemodialysis: A comparative study. Kidney Int 17:801, 1980.

207. Arieff AI, Lazarowitz VC, Guisado R: Experimental dialysis disequilibrium syndrome: Prevention with glycerol. Kidney Int 14:270-278, 1978.

208. Burkart J: Adequacy of peritoneal dialysis. In Henrich WL (ed): Principles and Practice of Dialysis. Baltimore, Williams & Wilkins, 1994, pp 111-129.

209. Gutman RA, Blumenkrantz MJ, Chan YK: Controlled comparison of hemodialysis and peritoneal dialysis: Veterans Administration multicenter study. Kidney Int 26:459-470, 1984.

210. Mahurkar SD, Dkar SK, Salta R, et al: Dialysis dementia. Lancet 1:1412-1415, 1973.

211. Alfrey AC, Mishell J, Burks SR, et al: Syndrome of dysphaxia and multifocal seizures associated with chronic hemodialysis. Trans Am Soc Artif Intern Organs 18:257-261, 1972.

212. Barratt LJ, Lawrence JR: Dialysis-associated dementia. Aust N Z J Med 5:62-65, 1975.

213. Chokroverty S, Bruetman ME, Berger V, Reyes MG: Progressive dialytic encephalopathy. J Neurol Neurosurg Psychiatry 39:411-419, 1976.

214. Nadel AM, Wilson WP: Dialysis encephalopathy: A possible seizure disorder. Neurology 26:1130-1134, 1976.

215. Noriega-Sanchez A, Martinez-Maldonado M, Haiffe RM: Clinical and electroencephalographic changes in progressive uremic encephalopathy. Neurology 28:667-669, 1978.

216. Dunea G, Mahurkar SD, Mamdami B: Role of aluminum in dialysis dementia. Ann Intern Med 88:502-504, 1978.

217. Flendrig JA, Kruis H, Das HA: Aluminum and dialysis dementia. Lancet 1:1235, 1976.

218. Alfrey AC, LeGendre GR, Kaehny WD: The dialysis encephalopathy syndrome: Possible aluminum intoxication. N Engl J Med 294:184-188, 1976.

219. McDermott JR, Smith AI, Ward MK, et al: Brain aluminum concentration in dialysis encephalopathy. Lancet 1:901, 1978.

220. Parkinson ID: Fracturing dialysis osteodystrophy and dialysis encephalopathy. Lancet 1:406, 1979.

221. Arieff AI, Cooper JD, Armstrong D, Lazarowitz VC: Dementia, renal failure and brain aluminium. Ann Intern Med 90:741-747, 1979.

222. Cartier F, Allain P, Gary J, et al: Encephalopathie myoclonique progressive des dialyses: Role de l'eau utilisee pour l'hemodialyse. Nouv Presse Med 7:97-102, 1978.

223. Burks JS, Alfrey AC, Huddlestone J, et al: A fatal encephalopathy in chronic haemodialysis patients. Lancet 1:764-768, 1976.

224. Ward MK, Feest TG, Ellis HA, et al: Osteomalacia dialysis osteodystrophy: Evidence for a water-borne aetiological agent, probably aluminum. Lancet 1:841, 1978.

225. Pierides AM, Edwards WG Jr, Cullum UX Jr, et al: Hemodialysis encephalopathy with osteomalacic fractures and muscle weakness. Kidney Int 18:115, 1980.

226. Prior JC, Cameron EC, Knickerbocker WJ, et al: Dialysis encephalopathy and osteomalacic bone disease. Am J Med 72:33, 1982.

227. Arieff AI: Aluminum and the pathogenesis of dialysis dementia. Environ Geochem Health 12:89-93, 1990.

228. Fraser CL, Arieff AI: Nervous system manifestations of renal failure. *In* Schrier RW, Gottschalk CW (eds): Diseases of the Kidney, Vol 3. Boston, Little, Brown, 1993, pp 2789-2816.

229. Thodis E, Anninos PA, Pasadakis P, et al: Evaluation of CNS function in CAPD patients using magnetoencephalography (MEG). Adv Peritoneal Dial 8:181-184, 1992.

230. Farrar G, Altmann P, Welch S, et al: Defective gallium-transferrin binding in Alzheimer disease and Down syndrome: Possible mechanism for accumulation of aluminum in brain. Lancet 335:747-750, 1990.

231. Farrar G, Morton AP, Blair JA: The intestinal speciation of gallium: Possible models to describe the bioavailability of aluminum. *In* Bratter P, Schramel P (eds): Trace Element Analytical Chemistry in Medicine and Biology, Vol 5. Berlin, Walter de Gruyter, 1988, pp 343-347.

232. Brun A, Dictor M: Senile plaques and tangles in dialysis dementia. Acta Pathol Microbiol Scand 89(sect A):193-198, 1981.

233. Altmann P, Al-Salihi F, Butter K, et al: Serum aluminum levels and erythrocyte dihydropteridine reductase activity in patients on hemodialysis. N Engl J Med 317:80-84, 1987.

234. Chazan JA, Blonsky SL, Abuelo JG, Pezzullo JC: Increased body aluminum: An independent risk factor for patients undergoing long-term hemodialysis? Arch Intern Med 148:1817-1820, 1988.

235. Sprague SM, Corwin HL, Tanner CM, et al: Relationship of aluminum to neurocognitive dysfunction in chronic dialysis patients. Arch Intern Med 148:2169-2172, 1988.

236. Altmann P, Hamon C, Blair J, et al: Disturbance of cerebral function by aluminum in haemodialysis patients without overt aluminum toxicity. Lancet 2:7-12, 1989.

237. Emmett M, Sirmon MD, Kirkpatrick WG, et al: Calcium acetate control of serum phosphorus in hemodialysis patients. Am J Kidney Dis 17:544-550, 1991.

238. Mai ML, Emmett M, Sheikh MS, et al: Calcium acetate, an effective phosphorus binder in patients with renal failure. Kidney Int 36:690-695, 1989.

239. Slatopolsky EA: Renagel®, a nonabsorbed calcium- and aluminum-free phosphate binder, lowers serum phosphorus and parathyroid hormone. Kidney Int 55:299-307, 1999.

240. Perl DP, Good PF: Uptake of aluminum into central nervous system along nasal-olfactory pathways. Lancet 329:1028, 1989.

241. Rifat SL, Eastwood MR, McLachlan DRC, Corey PN: Effect of exposure of miners to aluminum powder. Lancet 336:1162-1165, 1990.

242. Campbell IR, Cass JF, Cholak J: Aluminum in the environment of man. AMA Arch Indust Health 15:359-361, 1957.

243. Good PF, Perl DP: A lasar microprobe mass analysis study of aluminum distribution in the cerebral cortex of dialysis encephalopathy. J Neuropathol Exp Neurol 47:321, 1988.

244. Collins AJ: High-flux, high-efficiency procedures. *In* Henrich WL (ed): Principles and Practice of Dialysis. Baltimore, Williams & Wilkins, 1994, pp 76-88.

245. Banks WA, Kastin AJ: Aluminium increases permeability of the blood-brain barrier to labelled DSIP and beta-endorphin: Possible implications for senile and dialysis dementia. Lancet 2:1227-1229, 1983.

246. Wing AJ: Dialysis dementia in Europe: Report from the registration committee of the EDTA. Lancet 1:190, 1980.

247. Berkseth RO, Shapiro FL: An epidemic of dialysis encephalopathy and exposure to high aluminum dialysate. *In* Schriener GE, Winchester JF (eds): Controversies in Nephrology. Georgetown, MD, Georgetown University Press, 1980, p 42.

248. Arieff AI: Effects of water, acid base, and electrolyte disorders on the central nervous system. *In* Arieff AI, DeFronzo RA (eds): Fluid, Electrolyte and Acid-Base Disorders, Vol 2. New York, Churchill Livingstone, 1985, pp 969-1040.

249. Graf H, Stummvoll HK, Messinger V: Aluminum removal by hemodialysis. Kidney Int 19:587-592, 1981.

250. Kaehny WD, Hegg AP, Alfrey AC: Gastrointestinal absorption of aluminum from aluminum-containing antacids. N Engl J Med 296:1389-1390, 1977.

251. Arieff AI, Mahoney CA: Pathogenesis of dialysis encephalopathy. Neurobehav Toxicol Teratol 5:641-644, 1983.

252. Sedman AB, Wilkening GN, Warady BA: Encephalopathy in childhood secondary to aluminum intoxication. J Pediatr 105:836-838, 1984.

253. Sedman AB, Klein GL, Merritt RJ, et al: Evidence of aluminum loading in infants receiving intravenous therapy. N Engl J Med 312:1337-1343, 1985.

254. Santos F, Massie MD, Chan JCM: Risk factors in aluminum toxicity in children with chronic renal failure. Nephron 42:189-195, 1986.

255. Salusky IB, Foley J, Nelson P, Goodman WG: Aluminum accumulation during treatment with aluminum hydroxide and dialysis in children and young adults with chronic renal disease. N Engl J Med 324:527-531, 1991.

256. Polinsky MS, Gruskin AB: Aluminum toxicity in childhood secondary to aluminum toxicity. J Pediatr 105:758-761, 1984.

257. Andreoli SP, Bergstein JM, Sherrard DJ: Aluminum intoxication from aluminum-containing phosphate binders in children with azotemia not undergoing dialysis. N Engl J Med 310:1079, 1984.

258. Perl DP, Brody AR: Alzheimer's disease: X-ray spectrometric evidence of aluminum accumulation in neurofibrillary tangle-bearing neurons. Science 208:297-299, 1980.

259. Kogeorgos J, Scholtz C: Neurofibrillary tangles in aluminum encephalopathy: A new finding. Neuropathol Appl Neurobiol 8:246, 1982.

260. Garruto RM, Fukatsu R, Yanagihara R, et al: Imaging of calcium and aluminum in neurofibrillary tangle-bearing neurons in parkinsonism-dementia of Guam. Proc Natl Acad Sci U S A 81:1875-1879, 1983.

261. Candy JM, McArthur FK, Oakley AE, et al: Aluminum accumulation in relation to senile plaque and neurofibrillary tangle formation in the brains of patients with renal failure. J Neurol Sci 107:210-218, 1992.

262. Katzman R: Alzheimer's disease. N Engl J Med 314:964-973, 1986.

263. Berlyne GM, Ben-Ari J, Pest D: Hyperaluminemia from aluminum resins in renal failure. Lancet 2:494, 1970.

264. Mayor GH, Sprague SM, Hourani MR, Sanchez TV: Parathyroid hormone-mediated aluminum deposition and egress in the rat. Kidney Int 17:40-44, 1980.

265. Cantin M, Genest J: The heart and the atrial natriuretic factor. Endocrinol Rev 6:107-127, 1985.

266. Mathew RJ, Rabin P, Stone WJ, Wilson WH: Regional cerebral blood flow in dialysis encephalopathy and primary degenerative dementia. Kidney Int 28:64-68, 1985.

267. Malluche HH, Smith AJ, Abreo K: The use of deferoxamine in the management of aluminum accumulation in bone in patients with renal failure. N Engl J Med 311:140, 1984.

268. Smith JS: The investigation of dementia: Results in 200 consecutive admissions. Lancet 1:824, 1981.

269. Gajdusek DC: Hypothesis: Interference with axonal transport of neurofilament as a common pathogenetic mechanism in certain diseases of the central nervous system. N Engl J Med 312:714-719, 1985.

270. Selkoe DJ: Cerebral aging and dementia. *In* Tyler HR, Dawson DM (eds): Current Neurology, Vol 1. Boston, Houghton Mifflin, 1978, pp 360-387.

271. Drueke T: Aluminum toxicity in chronic renal failure. J Nephrol 1:49-57, 1989.

272. Rotter W, Roettger P: Comparative pathologic-anatomic study of cases of chronic global renal insufficiency with and without preceding hemodialysis. Clin Nephrol 1:257, 1974.

273. Kucharczyk W, Brant-Zawadzki M, Norman D: Magnetic resonance imaging of the central nervous system: An update. West J Med 142:54-62, 1985.

274. Weber DL, Reagan T, Leeds M: Intracerebral hemorrhage during hemodialysis. N Y State J Med 72:1853, 1972.

275. Bleumle LW: Current status of chronic hemodialysis. Am J Med 44:749, 1968.

276. Smith RJ, Block MR, Arieff AI, et al: Hypernatremic, hyperosmolar coma complicating chronic peritoneal dialysis. Proc Clin Dial Transplant Forum 4:96-99, 1974.

277. Arieff AI: Central nervous system manifestations of disordered sodium metabolism. *In* Morgan DB (ed): Clinics in Endocrinology and Metabolism: Electrolyte Disorders, Vol 13(2). Philadelphia, WB Saunders, 1984, pp 269-294.

278. Bolton CF: Electrophysiologic changes in uremic neuropathy after successful renal transplantation. N Engl J Med 284:1170, 1976.

279. Bolton CF, Baltzan MA, Baltzan RB: Effects of renal transplantation on uremic neuropathy. N Engl J Med 26:1170, 1971.

280. Anderson RJ, Schafer LA, Olin DB: Infectious risk factors in the immunosuppressed host. Am J Med 54:453, 1973.

281. Caplan LR, Hacke W: Acute ischemic stroke. *In* Brandt T, Caplan LR, Dichgans J, et al (eds): Neurological Disorders: Course and Treatment. London, Academic Press, 2003, pp 327-347.

282. Griggs RC, Arieff AI: Hypoxia and the central nervous system. *In* Griggs RC, Arieff AI (eds): Metabolic Brain Dysfunction in Systemic Disorders. Boston, Little, Brown, 1992, pp 39-54.

283. Vink R, McIntosh TK, Demediuk P, et al: Decline in intracellular free Mg^{2+} is associated with irreversible tissue injury after brain trauma. J Biol Chem 263:757-761, 1988.

284. Cheung JY, Bonventre JV, Malis CD, Leaf A: Calcium and ischemic injury. N Engl J Med 314:1670-1676, 1986.

285. Iseki K, Kawazoe N, Osawa A: Survival analysis of dialysis patients in Okinawa, Japan (1971–1990). Kidney Int 43:404-409, 1993.

286. Mazzuchi N, Carbonell E, Fernandez-Caen J: Importance of blood pressure control in hemodialysis patient survival. Kidney Int 58: 2147-2154, 2000.

287. Rostand SG, Brunzell JD, Cannon RO, Victor RG: Cardiovascular complications in renal failure. J Am Soc Nephrol 2:1053-1062, 1991.

288. Held PJ, Brunner F, Okada M, Garcia JR: Five year survival for end stage renal disease patients in the USA, Europe and Japan, 1982–1987. J Am Soc Nephrol 15:451-457, 1990.

289. Breyer JA: Medical management of nephropathy in type I diabetes mellitus: Current recommendations. J Am Soc Nephrol 6:1523-1529, 1995.

290. Foley RN, Harnett JD, Parfrey PS: Cardiovascular complications of end-stage renal disease. *In* Schrier RW, Gottschalk CW (eds): Diseases of the Kidney, Vol 3. Boston, Little, Brown, 1997, pp 2647-2660.

291. Orth DN, Kovacs WJ: The adrenal cortex. *In* Wilson JD, Foster DW, Kronenberg HM, Larsen PR (eds): Williams Textbook of Endocrinology. Philadelphia, WB Saunders, 1998, pp 517-664.

292. Bronner L, Kanter DS, Manson JE: Primary prevention of stroke. N Engl J Med 333:1392-1400, 1995.

293. Zimmerman JS, Herringer JS: Inflammation enhances cardiovascular risk and mortality in hemodialysis patients. Kidney Int 55:648-658, 1999.

294. Tice JA, Browner W, Tracy RP, Cummings SR: The relation of C-reactive protein levels to total and cardiovascular mortality in older U.S. women. Am J Med 114:199-205, 2003.

295. Miyata T, Inagi R, Iida Y, et al: Involvement of β_2-microglobulin modified with advanced glycosylation end products in the pathogenesis of hemodialysis-associated amyloidosis. J Clin Invest 93: 521-528, 1994.

296. Ronco C, Brendolan A, Bellomo R: Current technology for continuous renal replacement therapies. *In* Ronco C, Bellomo R (eds): Critical Care Nephrology. Hingham, MA: Kluwer Academic, 1998, pp 1269-1308.

297. Cohen HJ, Harris T, Pieper CF: Coagulation and development of inflammatory pathways in the development of functional decline and mortality in the elderly. Am J Med 114:180-187, 2003.

298. Beddhu S, Allen-Brady K, Cheung AK, et al: Impact of renal failure on the risk of myocardial infarction and death. Kidney Int 62:1776-1783, 2002.

299. Brott T, Bogousslavsky J: Treatment of acute ischemic stroke. N Engl J Med 343:710-722, 2000.

300. Beal MF: Does impairment of energy metabolism result in excitotoxic neuronal death in neurodegenerative illnesses? Ann Neurol 31:119-130, 1992.

301. Kumar M, Liu GJ, Floyd RA, Grammas P: Anoxic injury of endothelial cells increases production of nitric oxide and hydroxyl radicals. Biochem Biophys Res Commun 219:497-501, 1996.

302. Kurose I, Wolf R, Grisham MH, et al: Microvascular responses to inhibition of nitric oxide production: Role of active oxidants. Circ Res 76:30-39, 1995.

303. Collins RC, Dobkin BH, Choi DW: Selective vulnerability of the brain: New insights into the pathophysiology of stroke. Ann Intern Med 110:992-1000, 1989.

304. The French Study of Aortic Plaques in Stroke Study Group. Atherosclerotic disease of the aortic arch as a risk factor for recurrent ischemic stroke. N Engl J Med 334:1216-1221, 1996.

305. Vidaillet H, Granada JF, Chyou PH, Maassen K: A population-based study of mortality among patients with atrial fibrillation or flutter. Am J Med 113:365-370, 2002.

306. Penado S, Cano M, Acha O, et al: Atrial fibrillation as a risk factor for stroke recurrence. Am J Med 114:206-210, 2003.

307. Goadsby PJ, Lipton RB, Ferari MD: Migraine: Current understanding and treatment. N Engl J Med 346:257-270, 2002.

308. Lieberman EH, Gerhard MD, Uehata A, et al: Estrogen improves endothelium-dependent, flow-mediated vasodilation in postmenopausal women. Ann Intern Med 121:936-941, 1994.

309. Riggs BL, Hartmann LC: Selective estrogen-receptor modulators: Mechanism of action and application to clinical practice. N Engl J Med 348:618-629, 2003.

310. Rossouw JE, Anderson GL, Prentice RL, et al: Risks and benefits of estrogen plus progestin in healthy post-menopausal women: Principal results from the Women's Health Initiative randomized controlled trial. JAMA 288:321-333, 2002.

311. Appel LJ: The verdict from ALLHAT. JAMA 288:3039-3041, 2002.

312. Major outcomes in high-risk hypertensive patients randomized to angiotensin-converting enzyme inhibitor or calcium channel blocker vs diuretic. The Antihypertensive and Lipid-Lowering Treatment to Prevent Heart Attack Trial (ALLHAT). JAMA 288:2981-2997, 2002.

313. Kucharczyk J, Mintorovitch J, Moseley ME, et al: Ischemic brain edema is reduced by a novel calcium and sodium channel entry blocker. Radiology 179:221-227, 1991.

314. Kucharczyk J, Chew W, Derugin N, Moseley ME: Nicardipine reduces ischemic brain injury: Magnetic resonance imaging/spectroscopy study in cats. Stroke 20:268-274, 1989.

315. Albers GW, Atkinson RP, Kelley RE, Rosenbaum DM: Safety, tolerability and pharmacokinetics of the NMDA antagonist dextrorphan in patients with acute stroke. Stroke 26:254-258, 1995.

316. Gress DR: Stroke: Revolution in therapy. West J Med 161:288-291, 1994.

317. Parfrey PS, Griffiths SM, Barrett BJ, et al: Contrast material-induced renal failure in patients with diabetes mellitus, renal insufficiency, or both: A prospective controlled study. N Engl J Med 320:143-149, 1989.

318. Study Group E: Thrombolytic therapy with streptokinase in acute ischemic stroke. N Engl J Med 335:145-150, 1996.

319. rt-PA Stroke Study Group N: Tissue plasminogen activator for acute ischemic stroke. N Engl J Med 333:1581-1587, 1995.

320. del Zoppo GJ: Acute stroke: On the threshold of a therapy. N Engl J Med 333:1632-1633, 1995.

321. Sherman DG, Atkinson RP, Chippendale T: Intravenous ancrod for treatment of acute ischemic stroke. JAMA 283:2395-2403, 2000.

322. Yasuda H, Nakajiima A: Brain protection against ischemic injury by nizofenone. Cerebrovasc Brain Metab Rev 5:264-268, 1993.

323. Schievink WI: Spontaneous dissection of the carotid and vertebral arteries. N Engl J Med 344:898-906, 2001.

324. Schievink WI, Mokri B, O'Fallon WM: Recurrent spontaneous cervical-artery dissection. N Engl J Med 330:393-397, 1994.

325. Chass M: Pitcher's autopsy points to ephedra as one factor. New York Times, March 14:C17, 2003.

326. Haller CA, Benowitz NL: Adverse cardiovascular and central nervous system events associated with dietary supplements containing ephedra alkaloids. N Engl J Med 343:1833-1838, 2000.

327. Droller MJ, Anderson JR, Beck JC: Impotence. JAMA 270:83-90, 1993.

328. Abdel-Gawad M, Huynh H, Brock GB: Experimental chronic renal failure-associated erectile dysfunction: Molecular alterations in nitric oxide synthetase pathway and IGF-I system. Mol Urol 3:117-125, 1999.

329. Campese VM, Romoff MS, Levitan D: Mechanisms of autonomic nervous system dysfunction in uremia. Kidney Int 20:246, 1981.

330. Rosas SE, Joffe M, Franklin E, Strom BL: Prevalence and determinents of erectile dysfunction in hemodialysis patients. Kidney Int 59:2259-2266, 2001.

331. Massry SG, Bellinghieri G: Sexual dysfunction. *In* Massry SG, Glassock RJ (eds): Textbook of Nephrology, Vol 2. Baltimore, Williams & Wilkins, 1995, pp 1416-1421.

332. Lamberts SWJ, van den Beld AW, van der Lely A: The endocrinology of aging. Science 278:419-424, 1997.

333. Campese VM, Liu CL: Sexual dysfunction in uremia. Contrib Nephrol 77:1-14, 1990.

334. Leland J: A pill for impotence? Newsweek Nov. 17:62-68, 1997.

335. Nathan HP, Hellstrom WJG, Kaiser FE: Treatment of men with erectile dysfunction with transurethral alprostadil. N Engl J Med 336:1-7, 1997.

336. Herrmann HC, Chang G, Klugherz BD, Mahoney PD: Hemodynamic effects of sildenafil in men with severe coronary artery disease. N Engl J Med 342:1622-1626, 2000.

337. Utiger RD: A pill for impotence. N Engl J Med 338:1458-1459, 1998.

338. Seibel I, De Figueiredo CEP, Teloken C, Moraes JF: Efficacy of oral sildenafil in hemodialysis patients with erectile dysfunction. J Am Soc Nephrol 13:2770-2775, 2002.

339. Nielsen VK: The peripheral nerve function in chronic renal failure: VI. Acta Med Scand 194:455-462, 1973.

340. Raskin NH, Fishman RA: Neurologic disorders in renal failure. N Engl J Med 294:143, 1976.

341. Robinson TG, Carr SJ: Cardiovascular autonomic dysfunction in uremia. Kidney Int 62:1921-1932, 2002.

342. Fernandez JP, McGinn JT, Hoffman RS: Cerebral edema from blood-brain glucose differences complicating peritoneal dialysis second membrane syndrome. N Y State J Med 68:677, 1968.

343. Schneck SA: Neuropathological features of human organ transplantation 1. J Neuropathol Exp Neurol 24:415, 1965.

344. Spencer PS, Schaumberg HH: Central peripheral distal axonopathy: The pathology of "dying-back" polyneuropathies. Prog Neuropathol 3:255, 1977.

345. Thomas PK, Hollinrake K, Lascelles RG: The polyneuropathy of chronic renal failure. Brain 94:761, 1971.

346. Spencer PS, Sabri MI, Schaumberg HH: Does a defect of energy metabolism in the nerve fiber underlie axonal degeneration in polyneuropathies? Ann Neurol 5:501, 1979.

347. Calcutt NA, Allendoerfer Kl, Mizisin AP, Middlemas A: Therapeutic efficacy of sonic hedgehog protein in experimental diabetic neuropathy. J Clin Invest 111:507-514, 2003.

348. Campistol JM: Uremic myopathy. Kidney Int 62:1901-1913, 2002.

349. Tyler HR: Neurologic disorders seen in the uremic patient. Arch Intern Med 126:781-786, 1970.

350. Blagg CR, Kemble F, Taverner D: Nerve conduction velocity in relationship to the severity of renal disease. Nephron 5:290, 1968.

351. Blumberg A, Esslen E, Burgi W: Myoinositol: A uremic neurotoxin? Nephron 21:186, 1978.

352. Kjellstrand CM, Petersen RJ, Evans RL, et al: Considerations of the middle molecular hypothesis: II. Neuropathy in nephrectomized patients. Trans Am Soc Artif Intern Organs 19:325, 1973.

354. Kanda F, Jinnai K, Tada K, Fujita T: Somatosensory evoked potentials in acute renal failure: Effect of parathyroidectomy. Kidney Int 38:1085, 1990.

CHAPTER 52

Renal Osteodystrophy

Kevin J. Martin, Esther A. González, and Eduardo Slatopolsky

Bone disease has been known for more than 60 years to be associated with chronic kidney disease.[1-4] There have been considerable advances in understanding the factors that lead to the abnormalities of metabolism of divalent ions, parathyroid hormone (PTH), and vitamin D that play an important part in the pathogenesis and maintenance of skeletal disorders such as hyperparathyroid bone disease. These findings have led to changes in clinical practice for patients with chronic kidney disease, such that the prevalence, distribution, clinical features, and course of the bone abnormalities have been constantly changing over this period of time. Additional forms of skeletal abnormalities, such as adynamic bone, have been recognized in recent years. Aluminum-associated bone disease, which became prevalent as a result of therapy directed at phosphate control, has now diminished in frequency. Considerable effort continues toward understanding the details of the abnormalities involved, and therapeutic strategies undergo constant evolution based on these new findings.

Renal osteodystrophy is the term used to describe the many different patterns of skeletal abnormalities that can occur in the course of chronic kidney disease. One abnormality, osteitis fibrosa, is a manifestation of the effects of high levels of PTH on bone and is associated with a high rate of bone turnover. A second abnormality, adynamic bone, is characterized by an extremely low bone turnover rate, as is the osteomalacia of aluminum accumulation. These patterns of bony abnormality may occur together, leading to the designation of mixed renal osteodystrophy,

a disorder with some signs of secondary hyperparathyroidism associated with mineralization defects. In addition, the skeleton may be affected by other processes associated with the management of end-stage renal disease (ESRD), such as amyloidosis, owing to or caused by the accumulation of β_2-microglobulin. The skeletal picture can also be influenced by other systemic effects on bone, such as postmenopausal osteoporosis or osteoporosis resulting from corticosteroid therapy. This chapter reviews current knowledge of the pathogenesis, clinical manifestations, and diagnostic tools related to the multiple abnormalities of bone associated with chronic kidney disease and offers therapeutic recommendations.

PATHOGENESIS OF RENAL OSTEODYSTROPHY

Secondary Hyperparathyroidism (High Bone Turnover Renal Osteodystrophy)

Hyperplasia of the parathyroid glands and increased levels of PTH in blood have been demonstrated to occur early in the course of chronic kidney disease with decreased renal function.[5, 6] Bone histology shows evidence of the effects of high levels of PTH in patients with mild to moderate chronic kidney disease.[7]

Many investigators have contributed to the identification of the factors that lead to overactivity of the parathyroid glands in chronic kidney disease. Whereas under normal circumstances the concentration of ionized calcium in blood is

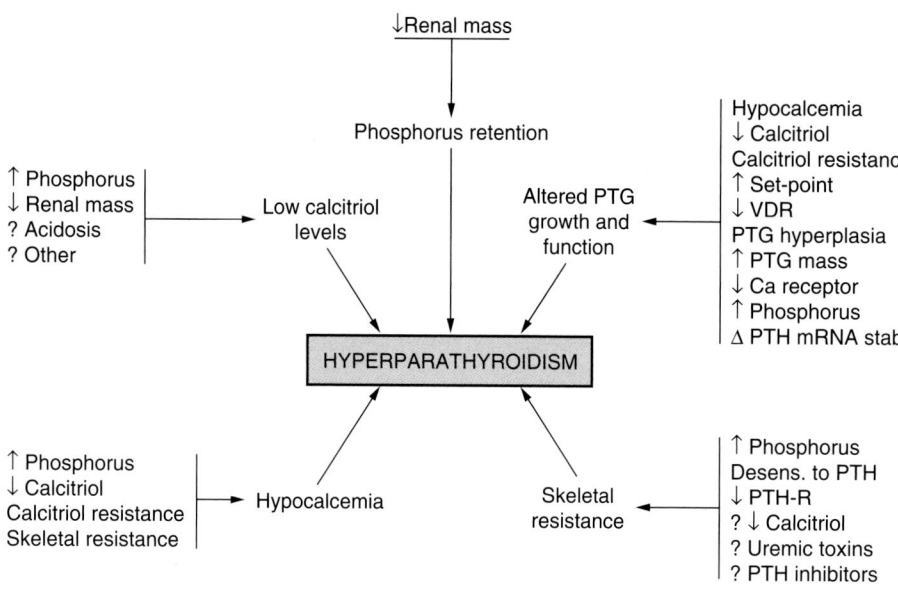

PTG: Parathyroid gland   VDR: Vitamin D receptor

FIGURE 52-1. The factors involved in the pathogenesis of secondary hyperparathyroidism. Note that multiple factors contribute to one or more categories. PTH, parathyroid hormone. (Modified from Martin KJ, González EA, Slatopolsky E: The parathyroids in renal disease. *In* Bilezikian JP, Marcus R, Levine MA [eds]: The Parathyroids: Basic and Clinical Concepts, 2nd ed. New York, Academic Press, 2001, pp 625-634, with permission.)

the principal determinant of the rate of PTH secretion, in the presence of kidney disease there is a constellation of factors that contribute to alter the regulation of PTH secretion. Figure 52-1 illustrates the principal factors involved in the pathogenesis of hyperparathyroidism in the setting of chronic kidney disease. These factors include the retention of phosphorus as renal function is reduced, decreased levels of calcitriol in blood as a consequence of decreased renal mass, intrinsic abnormalities of the parathyroid gland leading to abnormal PTH secretion and parathyroid cell growth, decreases in serum calcium, and skeletal resistance to the calcemic actions of PTH. Each of these abnormalities is considered separately here, but it is important to realize that they are closely interrelated; one or more of these factors may predominate at different degrees of renal insufficiency and could conceivably vary according to the particular type of kidney disease.

Role of Phosphorus Retention

The major role of phosphate retention as a factor in the pathogenesis of secondary hyperparathyroidism of renal insufficiency has been demonstrated by several studies over a number of years.[8-12] It was originally proposed that a decrease in the glomerular filtration rate (GFR) would lead to retention of phosphorus in blood, causing serum phosphorus to rise as a consequence of the decreased ability of the failing kidney to excrete phosphorus in the urine.[9, 10] This transient episode of hyperphosphatemia would give rise to a decrease in the levels of ionized calcium in the blood, which would then trigger an increase in the secretion of PTH in an effort to restore the serum calcium back to normal. The increase in PTH secretion would facilitate an increase in phosphorus excretion by decreasing phosphorus absorption in the proximal tubule and serve to restore the elevation in serum phosphorus back to normal. Thus, a new steady state would be achieved, but at the consequence of

maintaining a higher level of circulating PTH. The "trade-off" for the maintenance of normal concentrations of calcium and phosphorus was a necessarily higher level of PTH secretion.[13] Experimental support for this proposal for the genesis and maintenance of hyperparathyroidism was provided by several observations. It was shown that a diet high in phosphorus results in parathyroid hyperplasia.[14, 15] More compelling evidence was presented in a series of studies in experimental animals, in which it was demonstrated that a restriction of dietary phosphate in proportion to the decrease in GFR prevents the initial stimulus for the series of events outlined and thereby prevents the development of hyperparathyroidism and its attendant effects on bone in dogs with renal insufficiency (Fig. 52-2).[16] These observations were subsequently confirmed in studies in human subjects.[17]

Therefore, it is clear that phosphate retention plays an important role in the pathogenesis of hyperparathyroidism in renal failure. The studies mentioned did not define the mechanism by which this effect occurs. Indeed, several potential mechanisms need to be considered in this regard, including the original hypothesis of phosphorus-induced hypocalcemia. Phosphate-induced decreases in the levels of calcitriol may also play a role, and phosphorus may directly affect the parathyroid gland and influence the response of the skeleton to PTH. These many potential mechanisms by which phosphate may affect parathyroid function emphasize the point that the groups of pathogenetic factors outlined in Figure 52-1 are all closely interrelated and are not mutually exclusive.

PHOSPHATE RETENTION AND HYPOCALCEMIA

Studies in normal subjects demonstrated that an increase in serum phosphorus was associated with an increase in PTH secretion.[18] For example, an oral phosphate load led to an increase in serum phosphorus, a decline in the level of ionized calcium, and an increase in the levels of PTH in

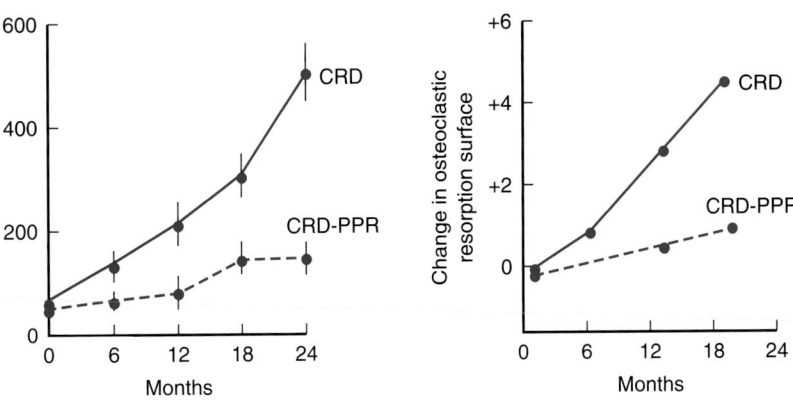

FIGURE 52-2. The effect of dietary restriction of phosphorus on levels of parathyroid hormone (PTH) *(left panel)* and on osteoclastic bone resorption *(right panel)* in experimental renal failure in dogs. CRD, chronic renal disease. (Modified from Rutherford WE, Bordier P, Marie P, et al: Phosphate control and 25-hydroxycholecalciferol administration in preventing experimental renal osteodystrophy in the dog. J Clin Invest 60:332-341, 1977, with permission.)

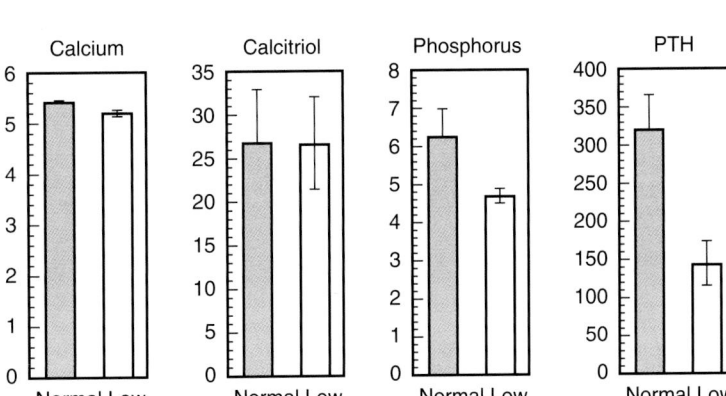

FIGURE 52-3. The effect of dietary phosphorus restriction on the levels of calcium, calcitriol, phosphorus, and parathyroid hormone (PTH) in dogs with renal failure. Despite the fact that there is no difference in the level of calcium or calcitriol, marked decreases in PTH occurred in response to the change in dietary phosphorus. (Modified from Lopez-Hilker S, Dusso AS, Rapp NS, et al: Phosphorus restriction reverses hyperparathyroidism in uremia independent of changes in calcium and calcitriol. Am J Physiol 259:F432-F437, 1990, with permission.)

normal subjects. Some investigators questioned whether this sequence of events occurs in early renal failure, because hyperphosphatemia is not seen in patients with early renal failure who have elevated PTH.[19, 20] In some patients, fasting levels of serum phosphorus may also be at the lower limits of normal. In addition, hypocalcemia is not demonstrable in many patients with chronic renal failure (CRF).[21] Other investigators could not demonstrate that intermittent hypocalcemia occurred after phosphate loading,[19] and, accordingly, it appears that the mechanism of the effect of phosphate retention may not be exerted exclusively through the induction of hypocalcemia. This concept led to further studies in experimental animals in which decreases in serum calcium were prevented after the induction of uremia by the administration of a diet that was high in calcium.[22] In these animals, hypocalcemia did not occur. In fact, serum calcium increased slightly, and yet the levels of PTH increased. Therefore, it was demonstrated clearly that hypocalcemia is not an essential part of the development of secondary hyperparathyroidism in CRF, and that other factors need consideration to understand the effects of phosphate retention on the pathogenesis of secondary hyperparathyroidism.

PHOSPHATE RETENTION AND CALCITRIOL

Because the rate of production of 1,25-dihydroxyvitamin D (calcitriol) is regulated by phosphorus, it is possible that phosphate retention leads to a decrease in the levels of calcitriol in blood.[23] In this regard, the effect of phosphorus restriction in preventing the development of hyperparathyroidism or in decreasing established hyperparathyroidism

could be explained by the changes in calcitriol. Studies in experimental animals have shown that the administration of calcitriol in amounts sufficient to prevent a fall in the levels of calcitriol in blood after reduction in renal mass is successful in preventing the development of hyperparathyroidism. These findings support the concept that decreases in calcitriol, as a consequence of phosphate retention or as a consequence of decreased renal mass, or both, is an important factor in the pathogenesis of secondary hyperparathyroidism.[24]

DIRECT EFFECTS OF PHOSPHORUS ON THE PARATHYROID GLAND

Studies in intact animals with CRF suggested that phosphate could affect parathyroid function independent of changes in serum calcium or calcitriol.[24] In these studies, dietary phosphorus was restricted in a progressive fashion, and dietary calcium levels were adjusted to maintain the levels of ionized calcium within the normal range. Calcitriol concentrations remained low and did not change, because the reduction in total renal mass limited any response to changes in dietary phosphorus. And yet, in these circumstances, with no change in the levels of ionized calcium or calcitriol, the changes in serum phosphate were associated with remarkable changes in the levels of PTH (Fig. 52-3). These data supported the possibility that dietary phosphorus (or the serum phosphorus concentration) affects the secretion of PTH in a direct or indirect fashion. Two groups of investigators successfully demonstrated, in studies in vitro, that changes in extracellular phosphorus concentrations are associated with significant changes in PTH secretion under circumstances in which the concentration of ionized calcium

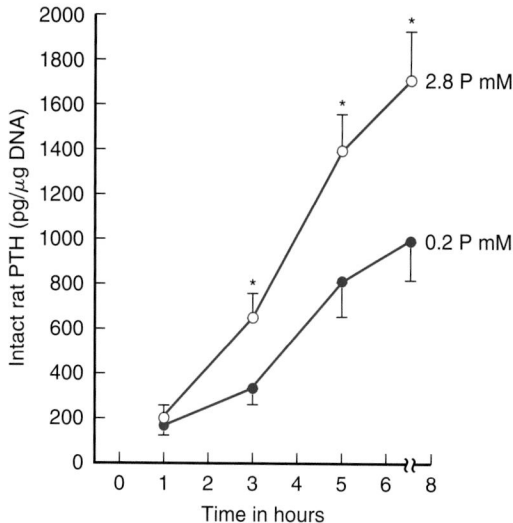

FIGURE 52-4. The direct effect of phosphorus on secretion of parathyroid hormone (PTH) demonstrated in intact rat parathyroid glands in vitro. (From Slatopolsky E, Finch J, Denda M, et al: Phosphorus restriction prevents parathyroid gland growth: High phosphorus directly stimulates PTH secretion in vitro. J Clin Invest 97:2534-2540, 1996, with permission.)

is unchanged (Fig. 52-4).[12, 25] These observations were confirmed in human parathyroid tissue in vitro,[26] and several investigators have provided clinical observations to confirm the correlation of serum phosphorus with levels of PTH.[27, 28]

The precise mechanism by which phosphorus affects PTH secretion is not well understood at the present time, although several lines of investigation are being actively pursued. Some investigators have reported that high-phosphorus diets result in an increased level of PTH messenger RNA (mRNA)[29]; others have not demonstrated any change.[12] These apparently contradictory results may be reconciled by the fact that the studies indicating an increase in PTH mRNA used thyroparathyroid tissue, rather than isolated parathyroid tissue. Parathyroid hyperplasia (an increase in the number of parathyroid cells) could lead to an increase in PTH mRNA in the total thyroparathyroid tissue, compared with the level of a control mRNA such as β-actin, which is present in both thyroid and parathyroid tissue, even if there were no increase in PTH mRNA per parathyroid cell. No such increase would be evident with the use of isolated parathyroid tissue.

Nuclear run-on studies have demonstrated that the effect of high phosphorus concentrations to increase PTH secretion appears to be a posttranscriptional one,[29] and these observations led to the investigation of an effect of phosphorus on regulation of the stability of PTH mRNA. Moallem and colleagues[30] demonstrated that parathyroid cytosolic proteins bind to the 3′-untranslated region (3′-UTR) of PTH mRNA. Using an in vitro RNA degradation assay, they showed that the 3′-UTR mediates the rapid degradation of PTH mRNA by parathyroid proteins from hypophosphatemic animals, whereas the PTH mRNA is stabilized by parathyroid proteins from hypocalcemic animals.[30] Parathyroid cytosolic proteins from uremic animals result in marked decreases in PTH mRNA degradation.[31] The increased PTH mRNA would facilitate increased PTH synthesis. Further studies have identified AUF1 as a protein involved in the regulation of PTH mRNA stability[32] and have determined the minimal protein-binding sequence in the 3′-UTR.[33]

Recently, Almaden and co-workers[34] demonstrated that high extracellular phosphate concentrations reduce the production of arachidonic acid by parathyroid tissue, an effect that was associated with an increase in PTH secretion. Other investigators showed that an increased release of arachidonic acid from parathyroid cells, or the addition of arachidonic acid to parathyroid tissue, is associated with the suppression of PTH secretion.[35] Further studies by Almaden and associates[36] evaluated the simultaneous effect of high intracellular calcium in parathyroid cells, achieved by the addition of the ionophore A23187 or the use of thapsigargin in the medium, and elevated phosphorus in the medium. Both agents increased cytosolic calcium and the release of arachidonic acid, with the consequent suppression of PTH, despite a high phosphorus concentration in the medium. On the other hand, it has been demonstrated that a high phosphate concentration stimulates PTH secretion, despite high extracellular calcium. These authors conclude that an elevation of cytosolic calcium levels stimulates the phospholipase A_2-arachidonic acid pathway and prevents the inhibition of arachidonic acid synthesis induced by high phosphorus concentrations.[36] It is not known at the present time how high phosphorus levels affect the regulation of intracellular calcium in parathyroid cells.

Phosphorus has also been found to affect the parathyroid gland in other important ways. It has been demonstrated that changes in dietary phosphorus content have a major effect on parathyroid cell growth. Studies using proliferating cell nuclear antigen (PCNA) staining of parathyroid tissue in rats showed that a high-phosphorus diet is associated with an acceleration of parathyroid gland growth, whereas a low-phosphorus diet prevents parathyroid hyperplasia.[37] Similar studies by Yi and colleagues[38] confirmed these findings. Studies in intact animals also showed that parathyroid hyperplasia is regulated by dietary phosphorus and contributed the important observation that parathyroid hyperplasia appears to begin very rapidly (within days) after the induction of renal insufficiency (Fig. 52-5).[39] A diet low in phosphorus prevents this increase in parathyroid growth.

The mechanism for the prevention of parathyroid growth by phosphorus restriction does not appear to involve the induction of apoptosis. The mechanism of the direct effect of phosphorus on parathyroid growth is not well understood, but it has been demonstrated that dietary phosphate induces changes in the cell cycle regulator, p21, and the expression of transforming growth factor-α (TGF-α) appears to be involved. In animals with renal failure, a low-phosphate diet is associated with an increase in the cyclin-dependent kinase inhibitor p21 at both mRNA and protein levels, and this is associated with the prevention of parathyroid hyperplasia.[40] Further studies have suggested a role for TGF-α, in that a high-phosphorus diet is associated with a marked increase in the expression of TGF-α after a few days of experimental renal failure. The increases in TGF-α in the parathyroid, induced by a high-phosphorus diet, parallel those of PCNA expression and are specific for the parathyroid, because there were no changes in hepatic or intestinal cell growth or TGF-α content.[40] Additional studies have emphasized the induction of TGF-α by a high-phosphorus diet in uremic animals. Three days after reducing the amount of

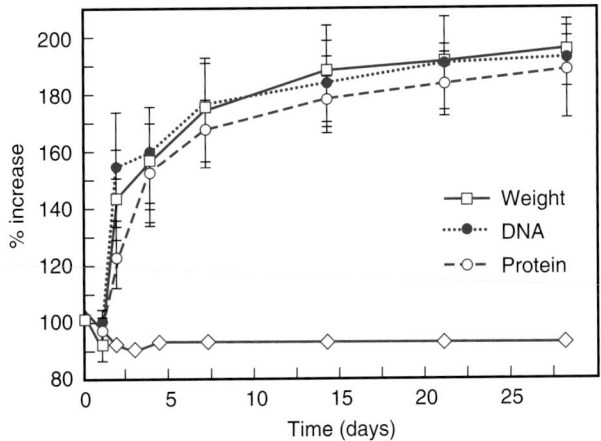

FIGURE 52-5. A high-phosphorus diet results in rapid increase in parathyroid gland weight, protein, and DNA in rats after the induction of renal failure. Note that the increase in parathyroid weight occurs within a few days after the onset of renal failure. The *diamonds* represent data from animals on a low-phosphate diet. (From Denda M, Finch J, Slatopolsky E: Phosphorus accelerates the development of parathyroid hyperplasia and secondary hyperparathyroidism in rats with renal failure. Am J Kidney Dis 28:596-602, 1996, with permission.)

phosphorus in the diet, the content of TGF-α in the parathyroid glands returned to normal levels. These changes in TGF-α are probably mediated through the epidermal growth factor (EGF) receptor, which, on activation, would lead to the activation of mitogen-activated protein kinase (MAPK) and the induction of cyclin-1 to drive the cell from the G_1 to the S phase of the cell cycle.[40]

How phosphorus mediates these effects on the parathyroid gland is not well understood at the present time, but it is of considerable interest that a type 3 phosphate transporter, PiT-1, is present in the parathyroid glands, and the levels of its mRNA appear to be regulated by changes in dietary phosphorus, as well as by changes in the levels of calcitriol in serum.[41] There is no evidence to date that this transporter serves to mediate the effects of phosphorus on PTH secretion, and further studies are clearly required to delineate the exact mechanisms whereby phosphorus affects the parathyroid glands. However, such studies are severely hampered by the lack of a parathyroid cell line, which is necessary to allow progress toward understanding of the molecular mechanisms by which phosphorus affects parathyroid function.

OTHER EFFECTS OF PHOSPHORUS

Phosphorus may also affect the development of hyperparathyroidism by indirectly affecting parathyroid function through contributions to the skeletal resistance of the calcemic actions of PTH (see later discussion).

Role of Decreased Synthesis of Calcitriol

The principal site for the production of calcitriol is the kidney; therefore, decreases in renal mass lead to a decrease in the ability of the kidney to produce calcitriol. Decreased production of calcitriol contributes to the development of secondary hyperparathyroidism. In the course of chronic

kidney disease, the levels of calcitriol in blood remain in the normal range until the GFR falls to less than 50% of normal.[42-45] Some investigators have described patients whose plasma levels of calcitriol were below normal with creatinine clearances between 50 and 80 mL/min.[20] Even though blood levels of calcitriol may be within the normal range, it is important to consider these values in the light of the ambient level of PTH. PTH levels may already be elevated at this stage of chronic kidney disease, and this normally would provide a stimulus to raise calcitriol levels above the normal range. Therefore, even normal levels of calcitriol may be inappropriately low in the presence of hyperparathyroidism. Studies by Ritz and colleagues[46] examined "calcitriol reserve" in patients with chronic kidney disease and found, in a group of subjects with a mean GFR of 70 mL/min, that the subjects' usual levels of calcitriol did not increase after injection of a pharmacologic dose of PTH to levels seen in normal subjects.[46]

It is possible that phosphate retention could contribute to counteracting the stimulatory actions of PTH on calcitriol production. Other factors present during the course of chronic kidney disease, such as metabolic acidosis, could also decrease the level of calcitriol and prevent the appropriate increase with higher levels of PTH. This area remains somewhat controversial, because acidosis has been reported to decrease, to increase, or not to change the levels of calcitriol in blood.[47-51] The effects of acidosis on calcitriol metabolism may be compounded by concurrent effects of acidosis on phosphate homeostasis.[52] An additional mechanism that could limit the production of calcitriol in the course of chronic kidney disease could be decreased delivery of the precursor 25-hydroxyvitamin D, bound to the circulating vitamin D–binding protein, to the proximal tubule uptake mechanism. This has been described to involve megalin, which is required for uptake of 25-hydroxy–bound vitamin D–binding protein into the cell, facilitating the delivery of the precursor to the 1-hydroxylase.[53] Such factors may certainly be relevant in advanced kidney disease. The consequences of low calcitriol in blood are direct effects on the parathyroid gland and effects on the intestine, where low calcitriol leads to impaired intestinal calcium absorption, thus contributing to hypocalcemia, which in turn could influence the function of the parathyroid glands.

In addition to decreases in calcitriol production, there is also evidence that uremia is associated with resistance to the actions of calcitriol. This could occur because of decreases in vitamin D receptor in target tissues[54-57] or from failure of the liganded vitamin D receptor to interact in a normal fashion with the vitamin D response element on DNA (VDRE). Reduced density and binding of vitamin D receptors has been observed in parathyroid glands of both animals and humans with renal failure.[54-57] Furthermore, it has been shown that ultrafiltrates of uremic plasma appear to reduce the interaction of the vitamin D receptor with DNA in vitro.[58] It has therefore been postulated that uremic toxins may reduce the biologic actions of calcitriol in renal failure by interfering with the normal actions of the vitamin D receptor. Additional studies have suggested that a possible mechanism for the impaired interaction of vitamin D receptor with DNA involves decreases in the levels of RXR, which is the necessary binding partner for the vitamin D receptor to form a functional heterodimer that interacts with the VDRE.[59]

Role of Altered Parathyroid Function

ROLE OF HYPOCALCEMIA

Hypocalcemia is a potent stimulus for PTH secretion and parathyroid growth. Although hypocalcemia can occur in patients with renal failure, it has clearly been shown from experimental studies that hypocalcemia is not essential for the development of hyperparathyroidism in this setting.[24] Indeed, clinical observations have suggested that hypocalcemia (corrected for serum albumin) is relatively uncommon in patients with CRF in the current era.[21] However, evidence has been obtained to indicate that there are intrinsic abnormalities in the hyperplastic parathyroid glands in renal failure which lead to abnormalities in the normal inverse sigmoid relationship between calcium and PTH secretion. Early studies suggested that adenylate cyclase activity in membranes prepared from hyperplastic parathyroid glands was less susceptible to inhibition by calcium than in membranes prepared from normal parathyroid tissue.[60] This phenomenon can also be demonstrated for calcium-regulated PTH secretion in vitro using dispersed cells from parathyroid glands of patients with renal failure.[61] Similar findings have been demonstrated in parathyroid adenomata. These observations suggest that there is an abnormality in the set point for calcium in hyperplastic parathyroid tissue; that is, a higher calcium concentration is required to decrease PTH secretion by 50% in the abnormal tissue. Several investigators have examined the calcium-PTH relationship in vivo in both primary and secondary hyperparathyroidism.[62-68] Although some have found that the set point for calcium is shifted to the right, others have not confirmed these observations.[65-67]

Recent studies have suggested that the set point may be altered by several factors, including the baseline serum calcium concentration, the rate of change in serum calcium, the size of the glands, and polymorphisms of the calcium-sensing receptor gene.[69-73] These differences may explain, at least in part, the apparently conflicting results that have been obtained. Other studies have focused on the potential mechanisms involved in the regulation of PTH secretion by calcium, and several investigators have shown that there appears to be decreased expression of the calcium receptor in parathyroid glands from uremic animals and patients.[74, 75] The decrease in calcium receptors could lead to increased PTH secretion, because the response of the parathyroid glands to calcium may be diminished as a result. However, recent work by Lewin and colleagues,[76] using a murine model of renal transplantation, showed that shortly after transplantation PTH returned to normal in the presence of reduced calcium receptors in the parathyroid gland. It is important to point out that these animals had normal levels of serum phosphorus. In addition, in studies by Ritter and co-workers[77] using uremic rats, when the diet was switched from high to low phosphorus, PTH levels normalized in 1 day but calcium receptor expression was not restored until 1 to 2 weeks later. These studies suggest that the level of expression of the calcium receptor may not directly influence the ambient levels of PTH.

ROLE OF CALCITRIOL

There is substantial evidence that calcitriol is a major regulator of PTH secretion. There is clear evidence that the vitamin D receptor is present in the parathyroid glands.[78] It has been demonstrated that calcitriol decreases PTH secretion in vitro,[79, 80] and the mechanism of this effect has been clarified by several investigators who demonstrated an effect at the level of transcription of the PTH gene.[81, 82] These studies have been confirmed in vivo.[83] Subsequent studies have extended these observations to identify a region in the 5' flanking region of the PTH gene that appears to mediate the inhibition of transcription of the PTH gene by calcitriol.[84-86]

In addition to the effect on PTH gene transcription, there are a number of other mechanisms by which calcitriol may directly and indirectly alter PTH secretion, as illustrated in Figure 52-6. In addition to the indirect effects of increasing intestinal calcium absorption and possibly improving skeletal resistance to PTH, the direct effects of calcitriol on parathyroid function are likely to play a role. In addition to a direct effect on PTH gene transcription, it has been demonstrated that calcitriol receptors in the parathyroid glands are reduced in patients with chronic kidney disease, compared with renal transplant recipients or patients with primary hyperparathyroidism.[54] Such observations have shown that a

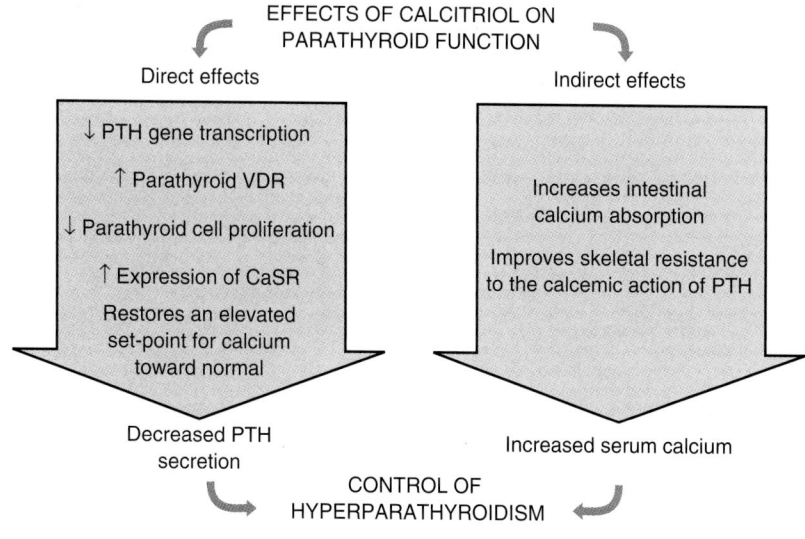

FIGURE 52-6. The multiple mechanisms by which calcitriol decreases secretion of parathyroid hormone (PTH). VDR, vitamin D receptor. (Modified from Martin KJ, González EA, Slatopolsky E: Renal osteodystrophy. *In* Becker KL [ed]: Principles and Practice of Endocrinology and Metabolism, 3rd ed. Philadelphia, Lippincott Williams & Wilkins, 2001, pp 603-610, with permission.)

decrease in VDR number may contribute to the pathogenesis of hyperparathyroidism by reducing the ability of calcitriol to inhibit the production of PTH. Other investigators also confirmed a decreased number of calcitriol receptors in the parathyroid glands of uremic animals.[55, 56] The converse has also been shown, in that administration of calcitriol leads to a dose-dependent increase in VDR in the parathyroid glands in experimental animals.[87] The data from a variety of investigators are all consistent with the view that calcitriol regulates its own receptor number in parathyroid cells.

An additional effect of calcitriol on parathyroid function may be an effect on parathyroid growth. Quiescent bovine parathyroid cells in culture with serum or serum substitute show an increase in tritiated thymidine incorporation, followed by an increase in cell number.[88] These changes were associated with an increase in c-*myc* and c-*fos* proto-oncogene mRNA levels. When calcitriol was added, the increase in c-*myc* mRNA levels was blocked and the expected increase in parathyroid cell growth failed to occur. These results demonstrate that calcitriol may directly modulate parathyroid cell proliferation by altering the expression of replication-associated oncogenes.

The antiproliferative effects of calcitriol appear to involve the induction of the cyclin-dependent kinase inhibitor p21 by a transcriptional mechanism that involves the vitamin D receptor. Cozzolino and colleagues[89] demonstrated in uremic rats that the administration of calcitriol, or the vitamin D analog, 19-nor-1,25-dihydroxyvitamin D_2, was effective in controlling parathyroid hyperplasia. In addition, the suppression of secondary hyperparathyroidism and parathyroid hyperplasia in these uremic animals was associated with enhanced expression of p21. Consistent with a role of p21 in parathyroid growth, it has been shown that patients with the more aggressive nodular form of parathyroid hyperplasia have the lowest p21 expression.[90] In addition, the effects of calcitriol or 19-nor-1,25-dihydroxyvitamin D_2 on p21 prevented the increase in parathyroid gland TGF-α and EGF receptor induced by a high-phosphate diet in uremic rats (Fig. 52-7;

see also Color Plate I).[89] There was a significant correlation between the reduction of parathyroid gland growth and reduction in TGF-α content. It is important to note that in experimental animals with established parathyroid hyperplasia, the administration of vitamin D or vitamin D analogs induces a growth arrest of the parathyroid tissue, but the enlarged glands do not return to normal size and no apoptosis is observed. These experimental observations might suggest that early treatment with calcitriol in patients with chronic kidney disease may be crucial to prevent growth of the parathyroid glands.

Although these effects of vitamin D on parathyroid growth and parathyroid function have been convincingly demonstrated, recent studies in vitamin D receptor knockout mice have shown that if serum concentrations of calcium and phosphorus are normalized by the use of a rescue diet, parathyroid hyperplasia does not occur.[91] Again, it is important to emphasize that there are multiple factors that play a role in the pathogenesis and maintenance of hyperparathyroidism in chronic kidney disease; although each factor can have direct effects, all of these mediators are closely interrelated.

ROLE OF ABNORMAL PARATHYROID GROWTH

The consequence of parathyroid growth is an extremely important factor in the disordered parathyroid function of renal failure. Although very enlarged parathyroid glands have been recognized for a long time, the studies of Fukuda and co-workers demonstrated that some glands resected at parathyroidectomy had numerous nodules.[57] Further studies demonstrated that staining for the vitamin D receptor was markedly decreased in these nodules, and that some of these nodules may undergo monoclonal expansions of parathyroid cells.[92] Further studies showed that these nodules also have marked decrease in the expression of the calcium receptor.[74, 75] These observations raised the issue of whether the loss of vitamin D receptor and calcium receptor leads to the accelerated growth or conversely, whether the accelerated growth is somehow associated with loss of the vitamin D and calcium receptors.

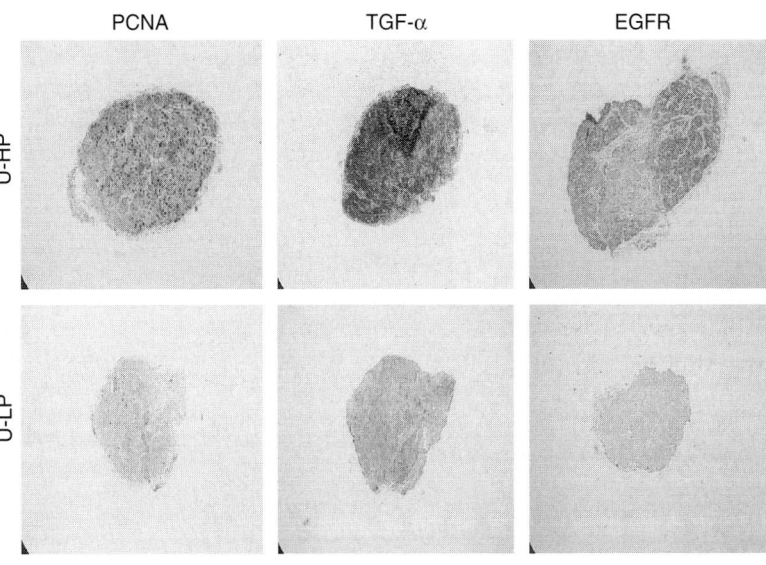

FIGURE 52-7. Dietary phosphorus regulation of parathyroid growth directly correlates with expression of transforming growth factor-α (TGF-α) and epidermal growth factor receptor (EGFR). High dietary phosphorus (HP) induces, and low dietary phosphorus (LP) prevents, increases in the expression of proliferating cell nuclear antigen (PCNA) as well as that of TGF-α and EGFR in uremic (U) rats. (See also Color Plate I.)

Uremia = 7 days

This issue was investigated by Ritter and associates,[93] using immunohistochemical techniques. These researchers demonstrated that parathyroid cell proliferation appears to precede loss of the calcium receptor in parathyroid glands from experimental animals. Evidence has also been presented that signaling at the calcium receptor may be involved in the regulation of parathyroid growth. Administration of the calcimimetic agent, NPS R-568, was shown to suppress and prevent the development of parathyroid hyperplasia in experimental animals with uremia.[94, 95] Additional studies have indicated that both calcitriol and phosphate may be involved in regulation of the expression of the calcium receptor in the parathyroid gland, and, accordingly, the role of the calcium receptor in the regulation of the parathyroid cell growth may be an important one.[96]

Skeletal Resistance to the Actions of Parathyroid Hormone

A decreased calcemic response to PTH in patients with CRF was described by Evanson in 1966.[97] This was confirmed by other investigators and extended by the observations that recovery from hypocalcemia induced by ethylenediamine tetra-acetic acid (EDTA) in patients with renal failure was delayed, compared with that in normal subjects.[97, 98] This phenomenon has been demonstrated in patients with early renal failure. The pathogenesis of the impaired calcemic response is multifactorial.

ROLE OF PHOSPHORUS RETENTION

That phosphorus retention plays a role in the decreased calcemic response to PTH was demonstrated by Sommerville and Kaye in an experimental model of acute uremia achieved by reinfusion of urine.[99] Removal of phosphate from this urine by zirconium oxide restored the calcemic response to PTH. Rats fed a low-phosphate diet also demonstrated an improvement in the calcemic response.[99] The effect of dietary phosphate restriction in improving the calcemic response to PTH has also been demonstrated in humans.[17] The mechanism of the effect of phosphorus is probably related to an effect of the ambient phosphorus concentration on the amount of calcium mobilized from the skeleton.

ROLE OF DECREASED LEVELS OF CALCITRIOL

Decreased levels of calcitriol have also been implicated in the pathogenesis of the impaired calcemic response to PTH in CRF. It has been shown that the calcemic response to PTH can be improved by the administration of calcitriol.[100] Not all investigators, however, have been able to confirm an effect of calcitriol on the calcemic response to PTH.[101, 102] In uremic dogs, the calcemic response to PTH was impaired, and treatment with calcitriol (0.5 μg/day for 7 days) did not change the calcemic response to PTH. However, after parathyroidectomy, the calcemic response was restored to normal.[102]

ROLE OF DOWN-REGULATION OF THE PTH RECEPTOR

In studies in isolated perfused bones from uremic dogs with renal failure, a decreased production of cyclic adenosine

monophosphate (cAMP) in response to PTH was demonstrated, and, importantly, this response could be restored to normal by parathyroidectomy.[103, 104] These observations suggest that the blunted end-organ response to PTH may result from desensitization of the PTH receptor adenylate cyclase complex. These observations have been extended by studies demonstrating that the expression of PTH receptor mRNA is decreased in bone from patients with CRF.[105] Similar findings have also been obtained in kidneys from animals with CRF[106-108] but did not change after parathyroidectomy.[109] These observations suggest that other factors in uremia may be involved in down-regulation of PTH receptor mRNA in addition to the effects of PTH itself in the regulation of its own receptor.

ROLE OF PARATHYROID HORMONE METABOLISM

In recent years, an additional mechanism for skeletal resistance to the actions of PTH has been elucidated. As discussed in detail later, second-generation PTH assays using two-site immunoradiometric techniques,[110] which were initially believed to be specific for the intact PTH (1-84) molecule, were found to also measure some NH_2-terminally truncated PTH fragments.[111-113] One such fragment, PTH (7-84), was shown in acute studies to blunt the calcemic effect of PTH,[114, 115] and further studies in vitro demonstrated that this fragment of PTH can inhibit bone resorption induced by a variety of stimulators of bone resorption (e.g., calcitriol, interleukin-11 [IL-11], prostaglandin E_2), in addition to PTH.[116] These circulating NH_2-terminally truncated PTH fragments may have effects on bone that oppose the well-described actions of PTH and therefore could contribute to the skeletal resistance to the calcemic effects of PTH.

Adynamic Bone and Osteomalacia (Low Bone Turnover Renal Osteodystrophy)

The low bone turnover skeletal disorders in patients with renal failure include adynamic bone, which is characterized by an extremely slow rate of bone formation, and osteomalacia, which is characterized by a slow rate of bone formation with marked defects in bone mineralization, reflected by an increased volume of nonmineralized bone matrix. Although the pathogenesis of the osteomalacic lesion has been clarified in detail, and most cases are due to aluminum accumulation, the pathogenesis of the non–aluminum-related adynamic bone disease is ill understood.

Adynamic Bone

In the last decade, adynamic bone disease has been found with increasing frequency. Although it has been reported in patients with chronic kidney disease before dialysis,[117, 118] most cases have been described in patients receiving dialytic therapy, and it appears to be especially prevalent among patients receiving peritoneal dialysis.[117-121] It is likely that the pathogenesis of adynamic bone includes a number of factors, as illustrated in Figure 52-8.[122] It also appears that a major factor involved in the decreased bone formation rate is a relative degree of hypoparathyroidism in this patient group. Although PTH levels are higher than in subjects with normal renal function, patients with adynamic bone disease

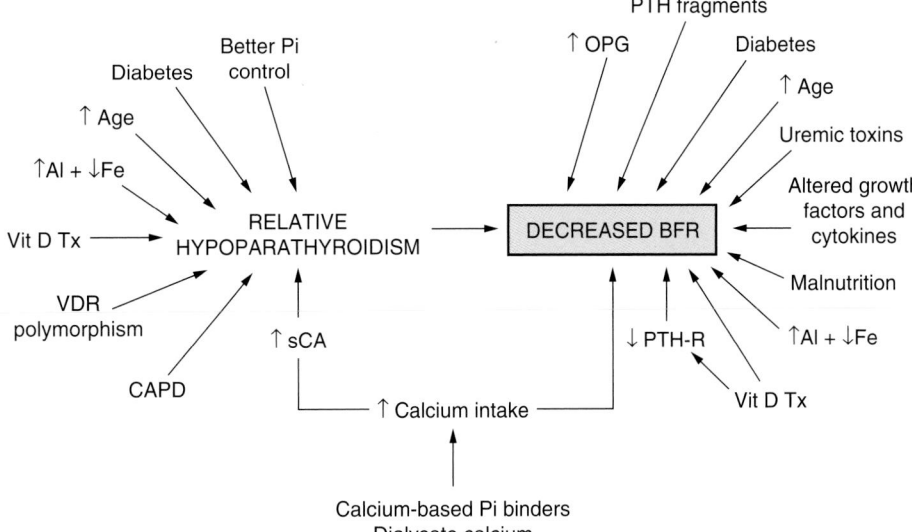

FIGURE 52-8. The pathogenesis of adynamic bone in renal failure. One set of factors serves to decrease secretion of parathyroid hormone (PTH), while several factors act to decrease the bone formation rate (BFR). For full description see text. OPG, osteoprotegrin; VDR, vitamin D receptor. (Modified from Couttenye MM, D'Haese PC, Verschoren WJ, et al: Low bone turnover in patients with renal failure. Kidney Int 56[suppl 73]:S70–S76, 1999, with permission.)

have significantly lower PTH values than patients with other types of renal osteodystrophy.[118-120, 123, 124] A variety of factors may contribute to this relative degree of hypoparathyroidism, such as better phosphate control with the use of calcium-containing phosphate binders, treatment with vitamin D, older age, and the presence of diabetes, which appears to be associated with low bone turnover even in the absence of renal failure.[122] Some of these factors have been associated with direct effects on bone. Furthermore, it is possible that other factors in the uremic environment, such as alterations in growth factors and cytokines, could directly contribute to decreased bone formation and decreased osteoblast function.[125]

Low Turnover Osteomalacia

Low turnover osteomalacia, in the setting of chronic renal disease, has been recognized for more than 30 years. Initially, it was identified in particular geographic areas and was often associated with dialysis dementia and microcytic anemia. After detailed investigation, substantial epidemiologic and experimental evidence indicated that aluminum was the cause of this low turnover osteomalacia, as well as of dialysis dementia. Further studies later implicated the ingestion of aluminum-containing phosphate binders as etiologic in cases of sporadic osteomalacia. The incidence of aluminum-related bone disease has decreased markedly in recent years, as water purification standards for hemodialysis have been improved and the use of aluminum-containing phosphate binders has decreased.

Although many patients with aluminum-related bone disease have osteomalacia, some also appear to have adynamic bone, in which osteoid seam width is not increased. This is probably related to the toxic effects of aluminum on osteoblast function, as well as the inhibitory effects of aluminum on the parathyroid gland.

Compared with adynamic bone disease, osteomalacia has now become much less common. This can be attributed to the fact that most cases of osteomalacia appear to be associated with aluminum deposition in bone; with decreasing use

of aluminum-based phosphate binders, this complication of therapy has decreased.[126, 127] The histologic features of osteomalacia are an increased area of osteoid, resulting from widened osteoid seams, and an increase in the fraction of the trabecular surface that is covered by osteoid. Cellular activity is low, and there is absence or paucity of osteoblasts and osteoclasts. The osteoblasts that remain continue to produce osteoid, which does not get mineralized. Although most cases of osteomalacia are due to aluminum accumulation, some cases are probably due to vitamin D deficiency, because it occurs during the course of CRF.[128] Osteomalacia has also been associated with metabolic acidosis and may represent a toxic effect of acidosis on osteoblast and osteoclast activity, as well as an inhibitory role on the calcification process.[129-131] Other abnormalities, such as hypophosphatemia, could play a role in osteomalacia.[132] It is possible that other trace elements (e.g., fluoride, strontium) may play a role.

Other Factors That May Affect the Skeleton in Chronic Renal Failure
Metabolic Acidosis

Metabolic acidosis probably makes a significant contribution to skeletal disease in patients with renal failure.[133-135] Acidosis may affect bone by liberation of bone mineral as hydrogen ions are buffered by bone carbonate. In addition, there is evidence that acidosis enhances osteoclast-mediated bone resorption and inhibits osteoblast-mediated bone formation,[129, 136-139] and it may alter the biologic effects of PTH[140, 141] or vitamin D,[52, 142] or both. Net bone mineral loss has been induced in vitro and in vivo during metabolic acidosis. Some studies in patients have suggested that correction of acidosis may prevent the progression of secondary hyperparathyroidism.[143] More recent studies have shown that metabolic acidosis appears to increase the expression of PTH/PTHrP receptor mRNA and protein as well as PTH signaling in osteoblast-like cells in vitro.[144] Data have also been presented indicating that acidosis influences the RANK/RANKL/OPG system (see later discussion).[145]

Therefore, because of the multiple effects of metabolic acidosis on bone, the presence of acidosis may play a role in determining the state of the skeleton throughout the course of chronic kidney disease, and these effects may persist even during the management of ESRD and dialysis.

Sex Steroids

There is substantial evidence that estrogen plays an important role in the regulation of skeletal function. These effects probably also contribute to the complex pathology of bone during renal failure, particularly because many patients are postmenopausal. Although this mechanism undoubtedly modifies the picture of the skeletal pathology in CRF, its precise role or the role of estrogen replacement therapy in the setting of renal osteodystrophy is ill defined at the present time.

Corticosteroids

It is well recognized that the use of glucocorticoids is associated with loss of bone and an increased risk of fracture.[146] In the course of chronic renal disease, many patients have received corticosteroid therapy, and its use complicates the manifestation of renal osteodystrophy. Glucocorticoid treatment usually results in a rapid loss of bone for the first few months, followed by a slower phase of steady bone loss. Although both cortical and cancellous bone are lost, the effects appear to be most evident in the axial skeleton and lead to fractures of the vertebrae or ribs as a presenting feature. Corticosteroid use may lead to osteonecrosis of the hip, which is a common finding in patients treated with glucocorticoids for renal transplantation. The principal feature of glucocorticoid-induced osteoporosis is a decrease in the bone formation rate with decreased thickness of the trabeculae, together with some increase in bone resorption.

Recent studies have detailed the mechanisms involved in steroid-induced osteoporosis. It has been demonstrated that there is a marked suppressive effect of glucocorticoids on osteoblastogenesis, as well as a promotion of apoptosis of both osteoblasts and osteocytes.[147, 148] Indeed, it has been proposed that apoptosis of osteocytes may be an important factor in the pathogenesis of osteonecrosis as a result of glucocorticoid therapy.[148] Therefore, prior glucocorticoid therapy may result in loss of bone mineral and decreased cellular activity of bone and may influence the integrated pattern of renal osteodystrophy in such patients.

Cytokines and Growth Factors

Although studies of the pathogenesis of renal bone disease have centered on perturbations in the PTH–vitamin D axis, several observations suggest that the spectrum of renal osteodystrophy cannot be explained solely on the basis of these hormonal abnormalities.[149-152] In patients with chronic kidney disease, the correlation between PTH levels and bone histology is less than perfect. In addition, a direct role of calcitriol in bone has recently been questioned, because vitamin D receptor knockout mice exhibit normal bone histology after correction of calcium and phosphorus levels.[153] Recent experiments have provided a great deal of information regarding the complex processes involved in the regulation

TABLE 52-1

Cytokine Systems That May Affect the Skeleton in Uremia

Activation of bone remodeling
IL-1
IL-1 receptor antagonist
Tumor necrosis factor-α

Osteoclast development and bone resorption
RANK/RANKL/OPG
IL-6
IL-6 receptors
IL-1
IL-1Ra

Osteoblast development and bone formation
IGF
IGFBPs
Bone morphogenetic proteins

IGF, insulin-like growth factor; IGFBPs, IGF binding proteins; IL, interleukin; OPG, osteoprotegrin; RANK, receptor activator of NK-κB; RANKL, receptor activator of NK-κB ligand.

of bone remodeling and have demonstrated that a variety of cytokines and growth factors are involved in the normal biology of bone cells. In uremia, there are alterations of several cytokines and growth factors, which are likely to contribute to abnormalities of bone remodeling (Table 52-1).[154-157]

Bone remodeling requires that bone resorption and subsequent bone formation take place in a coordinated fashion which involves the orderly development and activation of osteoclasts and osteoblasts (Fig. 52-9).[158-160] After activation of the remodeling cycle, osteoclasts and osteoblasts are stimulated to develop from their precursors in the bone marrow. Subsequently, a series of events leads to activation of osteoclastic bone resorption. After the resorption of a cavity of bone and detachment of osteoclasts from the bone surface, osteoblasts are attracted to the resorption site, where they lay down matrix that later becomes mineralized, thus completing the cycle.[161, 162] Each of these steps is regulated by a variety of factors that have the potential to be affected during the course of chronic kidney disease.[163-166]

Activation of bone remodeling is subject to regulation by several cytokine systems, including IL-1 and tumor necrosis factor-α (TNF-α). Abnormalities of these systems have been reported in uremic patients. For example, IL-1 has been found to be elevated in patients requiring dialysis.[167, 168] The levels of IL-1 receptor antagonist (IL-1Ra), an inhibitor of IL-1 actions, have also been found to be elevated in this patient population. In addition, Ferreira and co-workers[168, 169] demonstrated an inverse relationship between circulating levels of IL-1Ra and osteoblast surface. TNF-α also plays a role in the activation of bone remodeling, and high circulating levels of this cytokine have been described in uremic patients.[167]

Recent advances in the field of bone biology have enhanced the understanding of osteoclastogenesis and osteoclastic bone resorption.[163] The generation of osteoclasts in vitro is known to require close interaction with cells of the osteoblastic lineage, which produce a factor essential for osteoclast development and activity, known as receptor activator of NK-κB ligand (RANKL).[170, 171] As illustrated in

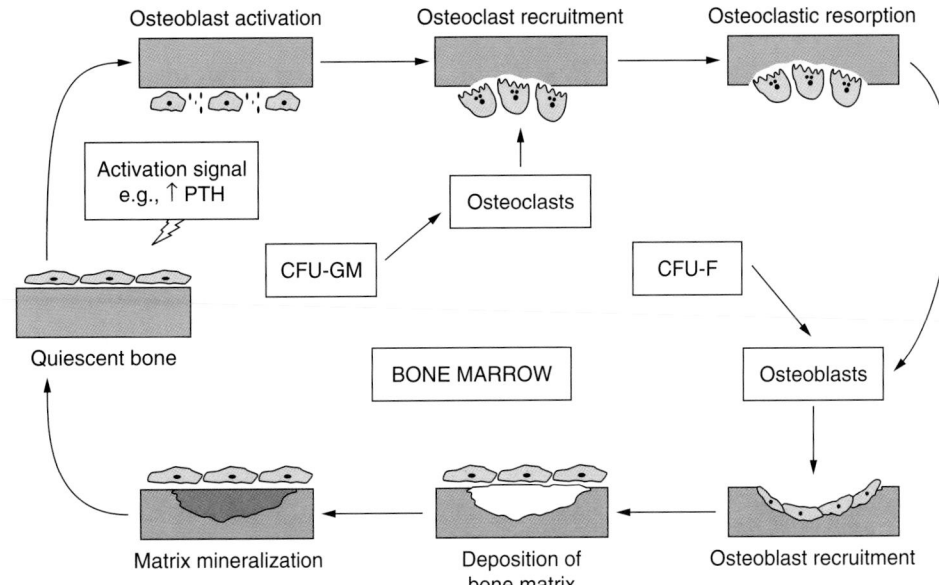

FIGURE 52-9. The bone remodeling cycle. For complete description, see text. CFU, colony-forming unit; PTH, parathyroid hormone. (From González E, Martin K: Bone cell response in uremia. Semin Dial 9:339-346, 1996, with permission.)

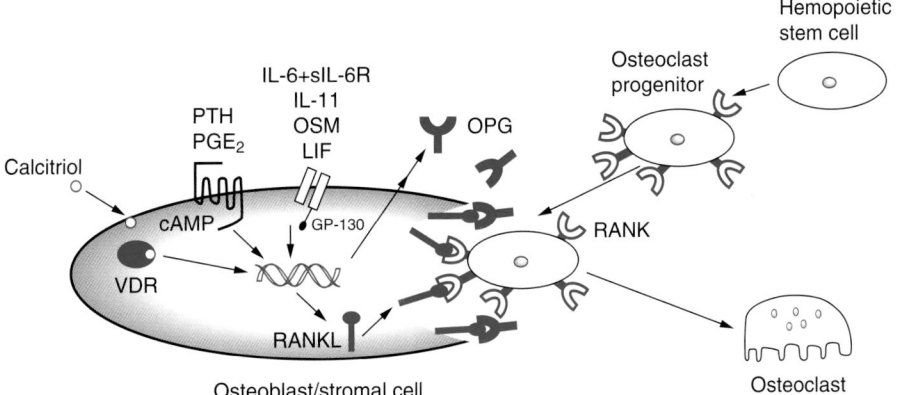

FIGURE 52-10. The role of the RANK/RANKL/OPG system in osteoclast development. The osteoblast or stromal cell expresses receptor activator of NF-κB ligand (RANKL), where it serves as a ligand for receptor activator of NF-κB (RANK), which is expressed on the osteoclast progenitor cell. The interaction between RANKL and RANK is essential for osteoclast development. Osteoprotegrin (OPG), secreted by the osteoblast/stromal cell, serves as a decoy receptor for RANKL and thus can regulate osteoclastogenesis. cAMP, cyclic adenosine monophosphate; PGE_2, prostaglandin E_2; PTH, parathyroid hormone; VDR, vitamin D receptor. (Modified from Nakagawa N, Kinosaki M, Yamaguchi K, et al: RANK is the essential signaling receptor for osteoclast differentiation factor in osteoclastogenesis. Biochem Biophys Res Commun 253:395-400, 1998, with permission.)

Figure 52-10, this ligand interacts with a receptor on the surface of osteoclast precursors, receptor activator of NF-κB (RANK), thus inducing the development and activity of mature osteoclasts.[170, 172-174] The actions of RANKL can be modified by osteoprotegrin (OPG), which is produced and secreted by osteoblastic cells. OPG can inhibit osteoclast development and activity by binding to RANKL, thus preventing the interaction of RANKL with its receptor on the osteoclast surface.[175-179] Disturbances of the RANK/RANKL/OPG system are likely to influence bone remodeling in uremia, because this system is regulated by the major calciotropic hormones, PTH and calcitriol, which are often abnormal in patients with chronic kidney disease.[180-182] Recent studies by Kazama and associates[183] reported increased circulating levels of OPG in patients with chronic kidney disease.[183] In the same study, the investigators demonstrated that concentrations of OPG in the serum of patients requiring dialysis were inhibited by osteoclast formation in vitro.

These findings suggest that OPG may contribute to the PTH resistance present in patients with chronic kidney disease. A role of OPG in renal osteodystrophy was also suggested by Haas and co-workers,[184] who found that OPG levels were significantly lower in patients undergoing hemodialysis with high bone turnover, compared with those who had normal or low bone turnover.

IL-6 is a potent bone-resorptive cytokine that has been implicated in a variety of states associated with increased bone resorption, such as osteoporosis, multiple myeloma, and Paget disease.[185-187] Although the effects of IL-6 in osteoclasts may be mediated by RANKL, recent studies point to RANKL-independent effects of IL-6.[188] Several abnormalities of the IL-6 system have been described in uremia. Circulating levels of IL-6 were reported to be increased in patients with chronic kidney disease, and a correlation has been demonstrated between serum IL-6 levels and markers of bone remodeling in patients with renal osteodystrophy.[189, 190]

The high levels of IL-6 may be due, at least in part, to the high levels of PTH found in this patient population, because PTH is a known regulator of IL-6.[191-194] Abnormalities of IL-6 receptors have also been reported in association with chronic kidney disease. Langub and collaborators[195] found increased expression of IL-6 receptor (IL-6R) mRNA in osteoclasts of patients with chronic kidney disease, and, interestingly, bone-resorbing activity correlated with the level of IL-6R mRNA. The levels of soluble IL-6R (sIL-6R), an enhancer of IL-6 actions, have also been reported to be elevated in uremia, and bone biopsy studies in patients requiring dialysis have demonstrated an inverse relationship between the sIL-6R:IL-6 ratio and osteoclast surface.[168, 196, 197] Other studies, involving patients dialyzed with the use of biocompatible membranes, found no differences in sIL-6R levels, compared with control subjects.[196, 198] Therefore, although the precise contribution of the multiple components of the IL-6 system to the abnormalities of bone remodeling encountered in patients with chronic kidney disease is not clear, the fact that the cytokine and its receptors are all affected by the uremic environment points towards a potential involvement of IL-6 in the pathogenesis of renal bone disease.

Another important bone-resorptive cytokine, IL-1, has also been implicated in disorders of increased bone resorption, including hypercalcemia of malignancy and postmenopausal osteoporosis.[199-201] IL-1 is known to influence the RANK/RANKL/OPG cytokine system, but it may also affect bone remodeling by other, independent pathways.[202-204] High circulating levels of IL-1 have been found in patients requiring dialysis.[167] In addition, patients with chronic kidney disease have been reported to have increased levels of circulating IL-1Ra, an endogenous antagonist of the IL-1 receptor.[169]

Osteoblasts, the bone-forming cells, derive from pluripotential mesenchymal stem cells after going through several stages of differentiation that are under the regulation of a multitude of systemic and local factors, including PTH, insulin-like growth factor (IGF), the bone morphogenetic proteins, fibroblast growth factor, TGF-β, and EGF.[159] The IGF system has been shown to play an important role in osteoblast development and activity.[205-208] IGF circulates bound to IGF-binding proteins (IGFBPs), which modify the effects of IGF on bone by either enhancing or blunting its actions. The skeletal expression of IGF as well as IGFBPs is regulated by a variety of factors, including the major calciotropic hormones PTH and calcitriol; because these hormone systems are affected by the uremic state, it is likely that abnormalities in the IGF system contribute to the pathogenesis of renal osteodystrophy.[205, 209-212] Andress and colleagues[213] have found increased levels of IGF-I in patients with chronic kidney disease; in addition, their findings suggested that the bone formation rate correlates with IGF-I levels.[213] Weinreich and co-workers, however, found no correlation between circulating levels of IGF peptides and serologic or histologic markers of renal osteodystrophy.[214] Recent studies by Jehle and associates demonstrated low levels of IGFBP-5, a stimulator of IGF actions, in patients with secondary hyperparathyroidism.[215] In addition, the level of IGFBP-5 correlated with biochemical markers and indices of bone formation.

The bone morphogenetic proteins (BMPs) play a central role in osteoblast development, and, importantly, BMP-7 is highly expressed in mouse kidney.[216-222] It is possible that BMP-7 deficiency may develop during the course of chronic kidney disease, which may lead to abnormal bone remodeling. A role for BMP-7 in the pathogenesis of renal osteodystrophy is supported by recent studies using a mouse model of renal bone disease, which demonstrated that BMP-7 administration prevents much of the histologic abnormalities characteristic of high-turnover osteodystrophy.[223] Interestingly, the marrow fibrosis characteristic of hyperparathyroid bone disease was virtually absent in animals treated with BMP-7, suggesting a role of impaired osteoblastic differentiation in the development of marrow fibrosis. In this regard, the EGF system has been suggested to play an important role in suppressing the osteoblast phenotype,[224, 225] and studies in osteoblastic cells have shown that PTH increases the expression of EGF receptors.[226, 227] Therefore, it is possible that excess PTH, by enhancing the EGF effect in osteoblastic cells, may indirectly prevent normal osteoblast differentiation, resulting in accumulation of collagen-producing osteoprogenitors, which may then give rise to marrow fibrosis.

CLINICAL SIGNS AND SYMPTOMS OF RENAL OSTEODYSTROPHY

Bone disease in patients with CRF is usually asymptomatic; symptoms appear only late in the course of renal failure, and they may be nonspecific at first and insidious in nature. By the time symptoms appear, significant biochemical abnormalities and severe histologic changes are usually present. Periarthritis and arthritis, pain or stiffness, and functional impairment of one or more joints are commonly encountered in patients with chronic kidney disease. Often, these symptoms are associated with significant hyperparathyroidism. X-ray studies may reveal characteristic changes of hyperparathyroidism or show calcium deposits (chondrocalcinosis in the affected joints). The principal differential diagnosis involves distinguishing this condition from pseudogout or gout. Anti-inflammatory agents usually provide symptomatic relief, but consideration should be given to the treatment of hyperparathyroidism. Erosive arthritis and effusions may be found with dialysis amyloidosis, and the joints involved are usually the metacarpophalangeal, interphalangeal, and wrist joints, as well as shoulders, hips, and knees.

Bone Pain

Although bone pain is not a prominent symptom of renal osteodystrophy in the present era, it can develop insidiously and may be present as nonspecific ache. The most severe bone pain occurs with osteomalacia, particularly when it is associated with aluminum deposition. The pain is usually vague and deep-seated. It may be diffuse or localized to the low back, hips, knees, and legs. It may also be prominent in joints. Back pain may represent vertebral collapse and fractures with minimal trauma, such as a fractured rib caused by coughing or even normal breathing. Physical findings are usually absent, but occasionally localized bone tenderness may be demonstrated.

Myopathy and Muscle Weakness

Weakness of the proximal muscles is a serious and debilitating problem, especially in patients with advanced renal failure.

The plasma levels of muscle enzymes are normal, and there are no specific characteristics on electromyography. Proximal muscle weakness can be associated with secondary hyperparathyroidism, phosphate depletion, and, potentially, vitamin D deficiency.[228, 229] Some clinical improvement has been demonstrated after vitamin D repletion. Other causes of muscle weakness can be found in the presence of chronic renal disease, including peripheral neuropathy, weakness from electrolyte disturbances, and possibly iron overload or carnitine deficiency.

Spontaneous Tendon Rupture

Spontaneous rupture of tendons has been noted in patients with long-standing renal disease undergoing dialysis, and it usually has been associated with evidence of severe secondary hyperparathyroidism.[230-232] The quadriceps or triceps tendons and the Achilles tendon have been most commonly described, but the condition may also involve extensor tendons of the fingers. The development of spontaneous tendon rupture should alert the clinician to inadequate control of secondary hyperparathyroidism, which, if present, should be treated.

Pruritus

Itching is a common symptom in patients with renal failure. It may reflect the presence of a high level of PTH, hypercalcemia, and a high calcium-phosphorus product (Ca × P), or

metastatic calcifications. In some patients, it improves or disappears rapidly after parathyroidectomy. The mechanism by which secondary hyperparathyroidism leads to pruritus is not fully understood. Increased levels of calcium in the skin have been reported in such patients, but the rapid improvement after surgery suggests that the calcium does not contribute to the itching, because it would take longer for calcium to decrease. Symptomatic relief can be provided by ultraviolet radiation, but a variety of other treatments have been suggested.

Metastatic and Extraskeletal Calcifications

Extraskeletal calcifications have been observed in patients with CRF for many years. In recent years, the potential clinical consequences of soft tissue calcification, particularly those involving the cardiovascular system, have received increased focus. Extraskeletal calcifications may occur either in damaged tissue (dystrophic calcification) or in apparently normal tissue. Examples of such calcification are shown in Figure 52-11, which illustrates calcification of the lung, shoulder joint, peripheral arteries, and coronary arteries. Calcification of the arterial system is a relatively common finding. Vascular calcification is in the form of hydroxyapatite, similar to that of normally calcifying tissues, such as bone. Amorphous calcium phosphate can be found in visceral tissues. It appears likely that extraskeletal calcification may be influenced by the state of bone turnover. Thus, as

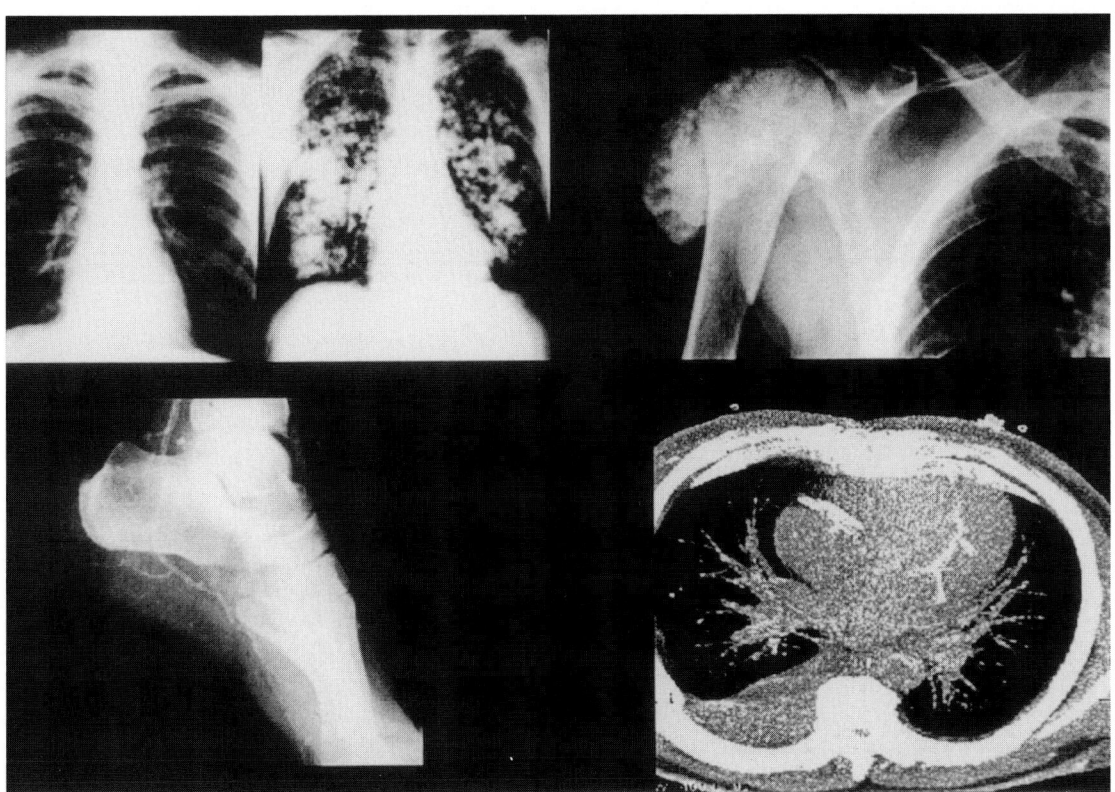

FIGURE 52-11. Extraskeletal calcifications in patients with chronic renal failure. *Upper left panel* shows severe calcification of the lungs. Severe calcification around the shoulder joint is evident in the *upper right panel*. The *lower left panel* shown calcification of the arterial system (an "auto-arteriogram"). The *lower right panel*, courtesy of Paulo Raggi, M.D., shows severe coronary artery calcification as demonstrated by electron-beam computed tomography (EBCT).

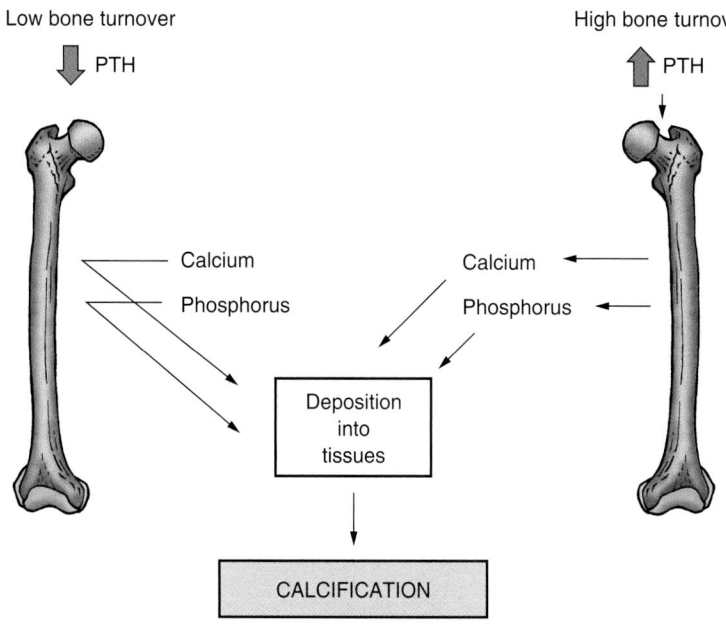

Low bone turnover

⬇ PTH

High bone turnover

⬆ PTH

Calcium   Calcium

Phosphorus   Phosphorus

Deposition into tissues

CALCIFICATION

FIGURE 52-12. The potential role of alterations in bone turnover on extraskeletal calcification. If bone turnover and bone matrix synthesis are low, as illustrated on the left, calcium and phosphate cannot be deposited in bone and therefore are available for deposition at nonskeletal sites. If bone turnover is high, as shown on the right, calcium and phosphorus are mobilized from bone and can then be deposited at extraskeletal sites. PTH, parathyroid hormone. (Adapted from diagrams from Sharon Moe, M.D., Indiana University.)

illustrated in Figure 52-12, if bone turnover is low and there is decreased matrix synthesis, mineral ions entering the bloodstream cannot be deposited in bone and therefore may be available for deposition in extraskeletal sites. Conversely, if bone turnover is high, as in severe hyperparathyroid bone disease, the mineral ions are mobilized from the skeleton and may be deposited in extraskeletal sites.

Clinical Manifestations

CALCIFICATION OF THE SKIN AND CALCIPHYLAXIS

Calcification in the skin may result in severe pruritus, which is believed to be associated with an elevated Ca × P value. Skin calcification may also be manifested as an acutely occurring skin necrosis, which can result in gangrene and has a poor prognosis. This syndrome, calciphylaxis, appears to occur as a result of arteriolar calcification; accordingly, it is often termed *calcific uremic arteriolopathy*. It often manifests with the development of painful areas on the lower extremities, trunk, or buttocks that become violaceous, mottled, and indurated and subsequently ulcerate (Fig. 52-13A; see also Color Plate II). The proximal lesions appear to be associated with the worst prognosis. If a skin biopsy is performed, calcification within the arterioles and fat necrosis may be evident (Fig. 52-13B; see also Color Plate II).

There appears to have been an increase in this syndrome recently, and it is not clear whether this is a real increase or represents an increase in recognition of this complication of chronic kidney disease.[233] In the original descriptions of calciphylaxis, Seyle described the condition in which tissues, which had been sensitized, responded to a challenge with this local calcification and inflammation.[234] Vitamin D and PTH were among the sensitizing agents, and the challenging agents were egg white and metallic salts, which included iron dextran. Because the current therapies for hyperparathyroidism include the prescription of calcium salts and vitamin D, it is important to consider these factors in the clinical presentations of this problem. Although this disorder had been associated with severe hyperparathyroidism,

many cases occur in the absence of hyperparathyroidism at the time of diagnosis. Many patients with this syndrome appear to be obese, and there is a high prevalence of diabetes.[235] The clinical appearance of these lesions is similar to that seen with warfarin skin necrosis, which suggests a role for altered coagulation, particularly in the protein C and protein S pathways, in the final manifestations of this problem.[236-238] Patients on dialysis with calciphylaxis have been noted to have decreased levels of protein C and protein S activity.[237, 238] Recent observations suggest that decreased levels of the calcification inhibitor Ahsg/Fetuin may play a role in the pathogenesis of calciphylaxis.[239]

OCULAR CALCIFICATION

Calcifications are often found in the cornea and conjunctiva and rarely give rise to symptoms. However, they may lead to complaints of dry or gritty eyes or erythema of the conjunctiva.

CALCIFICATION OF JOINTS

The periarticular structures are often involved in calcification in patients with renal failure. The articular cartilage may become calcified, which may lead to significant symptoms and is manifested as pseudogout. Calcification around the joint also may occur, often after trauma or degenerative changes in the joint. This is manifested as arthritis and may be associated with joint effusion. Calcification may be associated with tendon rupture. Larger areas of calcification may also occur in close proximity to a large joint; this is termed *tumoral calcinosis* (see Fig. 52-11). The lesion is usually pain free in the early stages, but as it continues to grow, it can give rise to significant symptoms. Such calcifications often regress after parathyroidectomy or control of the Ca × P is achieved.

CALCIFICATION OF THE CARDIOVASCULAR SYSTEM

Cardiovascular calcification is extremely common in patients with ESRD. Calcification of the cardiovascular system and

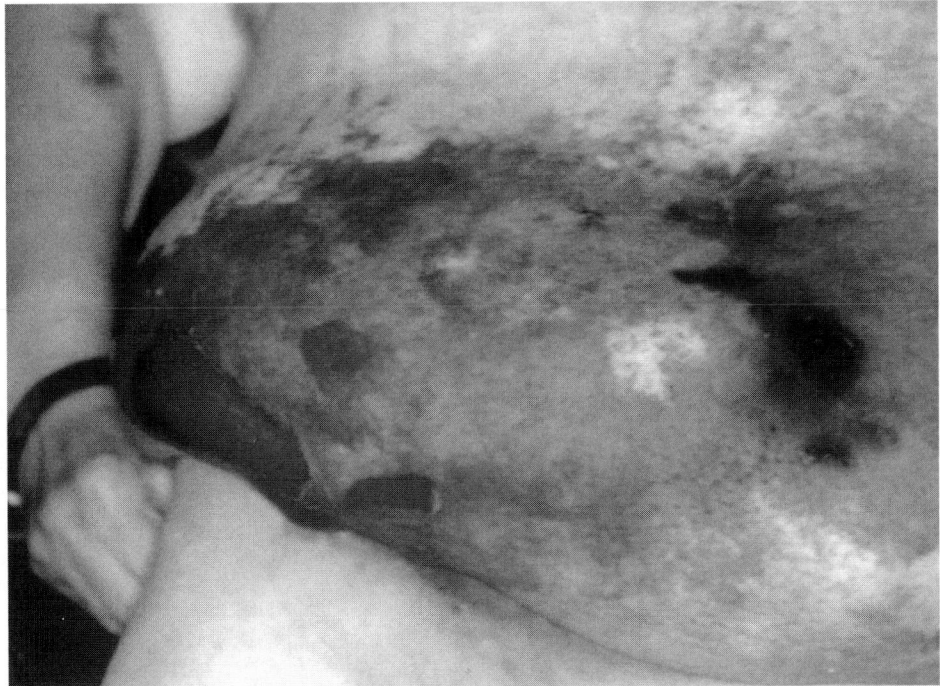

A

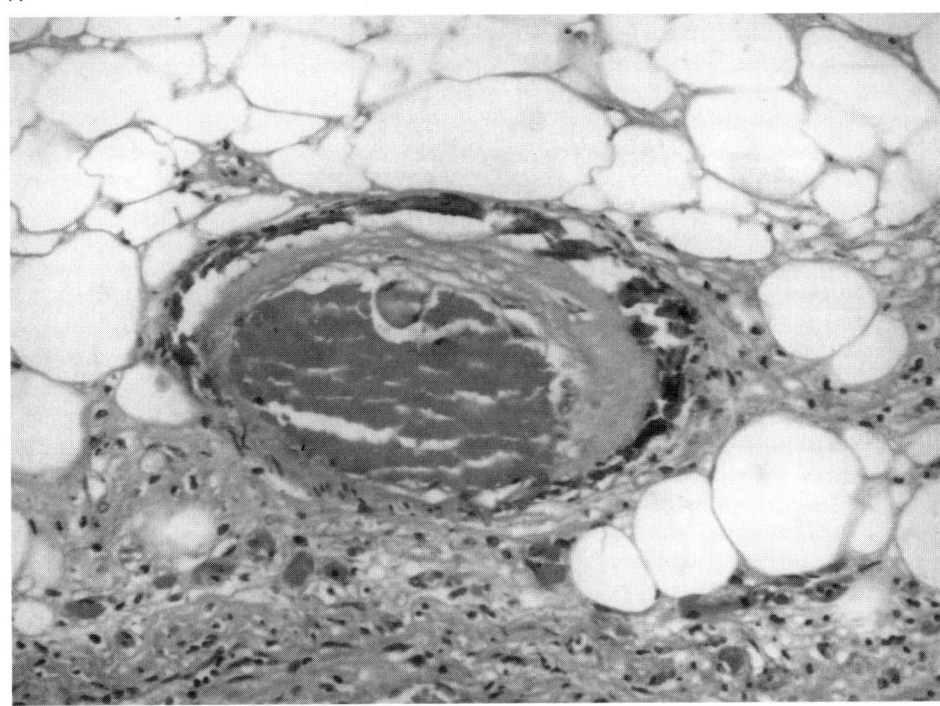

FIGURE 52-13. Calciphylaxis. **A,** Ulceration of the abdominal wall with a characteristic violaceous rash. **B,** Skin biopsy specimen with thrombosis of a calcified blood vessel. (From González EA, Martin KJ: Bone and mineral metabolism in chronic renal failure. *In* Johnson J, Feehally RJ [eds]: Comprehensive Clinical Nephrology. London, Mosby, 2000, pp 69.1-69.11, with permission.) (See also Color Plate II.)

B

heart may contribute to the higher mortality rate in this patient group by contributing to peripheral ischemia, impaired myocardial function, coronary artery disease, cardiac valvular dysfunction, sudden death, and other cardiovascular events such as stroke.[240] The calcification of the arteries, including coronary arteries, appears to be a medial calcification. The mitral and aortic valves often become calcified, and this condition can be associated with cardiac conduction defects, rupture of the cordae tendineae, and susceptibility to endocarditis. Vascular calcifications appear to be associated with

hyperphosphatemia and an elevated Ca × P value.[240-242] Valvular calcifications can often be seen on routine chest radiographs or echocardiograms, and calcification of large blood vessels is often manifest on radiographs of the abdomen or extremities (see Fig. 52-11). Calcification of coronary arteries is best visualized and quantitated by electron-beam computed tomography (EBCT), as illustrated in Figure 52-11.[243] Goodman and colleagues[244] studied a group of young patients between 5 and 29 years of age and found that several of those age 20 to 29 years had very high EBCT scores,

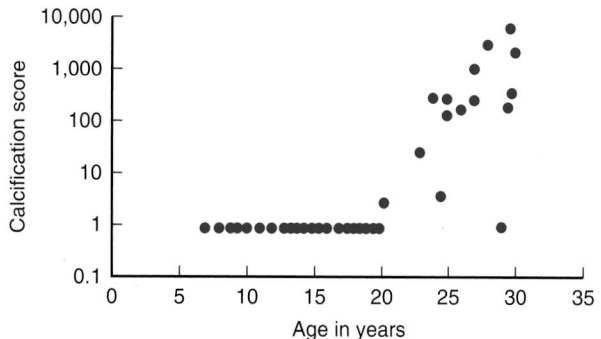

FIGURE 52-14. Coronary artery calcification scores by electron-beam computed tomography (EBCT) in young adults on hemodialysis. (From Goodman WG, Goldin J, Kuizon BD, et al: Coronary-artery calcification in young adults with end-stage renal disease who are undergoing dialysis. N Engl J Med 342:1478-1483, 2000, with permission.)

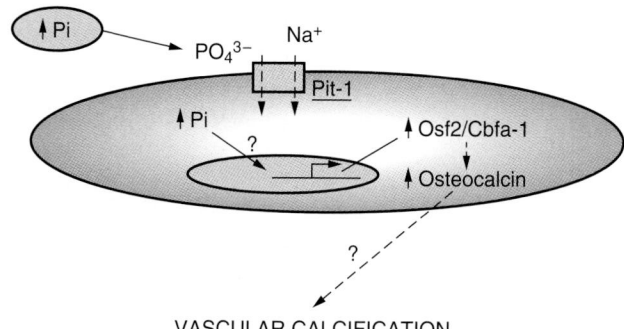

VASCULAR CALCIFICATION

FIGURE 52-15. Regulation of vascular smooth muscle cell calcification by phosphate. In human smooth muscle cells in vitro, a high-phosphate medium is associated with induction of the osteoblast specific genes, core binding factor α–subunit 1 (Cbfa-1) and osteocalcin and increases calcification. These effects are mediated by the sodium-dependent phosphate cotransporter, Pit-1. (Adapted from Giachelli CM, Jono S, Shioi A, et al: Vascular calcification and inorganic phosphate. Am J Kidney Dis 38: S34-S37, 2001, with permission.)

indicating severe coronary artery calcification (Fig. 52-14). The high EBCT scores were associated with high calcium intake and an elevated $Ca \times P$; in addition, these patients had significantly lower levels of alkaline phosphatase, consistent with a low bone turnover state, which may play a role in the pathogenesis of extraskeletal calcification (see previous discussion and Fig. 52-12). High-speed spiral CT is also useful for detecting coronary artery calcification. Ultrasonographic techniques measuring arterial stiffness also appear to be valuable for the assessment of vascular calcification.[245]

Uremic arterial calcification is a significant problem in this patient group, and there is active research in the area to define the mechanisms involved in this process. In recent years, it has been realized that vascular calcification is an active rather than a passive process. Numerous observations have demonstrated the presence of bone matrix proteins such as osteopontin, osteocalcin, osteonectin, and matrix-GLA-protein (MGP) in calcified vascular tissue.[246, 247] These data are supported by observations in experimental animals in which the MGP-null mouse,[248] the *klotho* mouse,[249] the OPG-null mouse,[250] and others showed enhanced susceptibility to vascular calcification.

Further studies have implicated phosphate as a key regulator of these processes. It has been shown that phosphorus leads to the expression of the osteoblast-differentiating markers, core binding factor α–subunit 1 (Cbfa-1) and osteocalcin, in human vascular smooth muscle cells. It also increases calcification of the cultures, as illustrated in Figure 52-15.[251, 252] This process appears to involve the type 3 phosphate transporter, Pit-1 (Glvr-1), and it can be inhibited by the phosphate transport inhibitor, phosphonoformic acid.[251] Active research continues to investigate the roles of PTH, PTH-related protein, $Ca \times P$, vitamin D, and cytokines, including TNF and TGF-β, in this process.

Dialysis-Associated Amyloidosis

Amyloid deposits in articular and periarticular tissues resulting in a disabling arthropathy have been recognized in patients who have been on dialysis for a long period.[253-259] This amyloid deposition has been demonstrated to be β$_2$-microglobulin. β$_2$-microglobulin can form amyloid fibrils without previous modification of its structure,[260-262] although

modification by advanced glycation products has been demonstrated in dialysis patients.[263] This may play a role in the pathogenesis of amyloidosis.[264]

Although amyloid deposits may be present for a number of years before the onset of symptoms, the clinical manifestations of β$_2$-microglobulin amyloidosis usually occur after 8 to 12 years on hemodialysis,[265] and it affects more than 50% of patients.[266] β$_2$-microglobulin amyloidosis often manifests clinically as carpal tunnel syndrome in addition to joint symptoms such as swelling around joints. It appears to be less of a problem in patients who are dialyzed with the use of biocompatible membranes,[267, 268] consistent with the idea that the synthesis of β$_2$-microglobulin may be increased after the release of cytokines associated with the contact of blood with dialysis membranes. The differential diagnosis of carpal tunnel syndrome in patients on dialysis includes β$_2$-microglobulin amyloidosis, edema as a consequence of vascular access, uremic neuropathy, and vitamin B$_6$ deficiency. Calcification of ligaments (calcium phosphate crystal deposition) should also be considered.

β$_2$-microglobulin arthropathy is usually insidious in onset and follows a progressive course. It usually manifests as chronic arthralgias, often bilateral, and frequently affecting the shoulders.[269, 270] This needs to be differentiated from cervical nerve root involvement by a destructive spondyloarthropathy. Shoulder involvement with β$_2$-microglobulin is best demonstrated by MRI, which shows thickening of the rotator tendons or subacromial bursa, or can demonstrate synovitis. Chronic tenosynovitis of the finger flexors are also frequently observed, as is chronic swelling of the knees, shoulders, wrists, fingers, and elbows.

Destructive arthropathies may also be part of the β$_2$-microglobulin amyloid syndrome.[271, 272] This is manifested by subchondral bone erosions, often in large joints such as hip or knee. Erosive lesions can also be present in the spine.[271, 273-275] These are often asymptomatic and remain undiagnosed for many years, but they can result in cervical pain. Such destructive spondyloarthropathies are often seen in the cervical spine and are best evaluated by CT or MRI, which can be helpful in differentiating this syndrome from discitis. Amyloid bone cysts may lead to pathologic fractures in patients undergoing hemodialysis.[276, 277]

The diagnosis of β_2-microglobulin amyloidosis is made by the characteristic histology, using Congo red, which can be followed with precise typing of the amyloid by immunohistochemistry.[278] β_2-microglobulin amyloid may be suspected when x-ray examination reveals subchondral bone cysts or erosions that increase in size or number over time and appear to have a symmetrical distribution.[278] Swelling of the periarticular soft tissue may also be seen. Some investigators have used serum amyloid P component scintigraphy and β_2-microglobulin scintigraphy, but these are not in routine clinical use.[279, 280]

BIOCHEMICAL FEATURES OF RENAL OSTEODYSTROPHY

The diagnosis of renal bone disease often presents a challenge because the clinical signs and symptoms are often nonspecific in nature, and by the time they are present, the disease has most likely already progressed into the advanced stages, when therapeutic intervention may be less effective. Although the histologic examination of undecalcified sections of bone remains the gold standard for the diagnosis of renal osteodystrophy, the fact that bone biopsy is an invasive technique has prevented its widespread application, and it is only used in a limited set of clinical situations. Imaging studies also have limited clinical utility for the diagnosis of renal osteodystrophy. Therefore, it becomes important to evaluate biochemical parameters related to bone and mineral metabolism early in the course of chronic kidney disease in order to provide a working diagnosis and to guide therapeutic interventions.

Figure 52-16 illustrates the general approach to assessment of the factors that contribute to the spectrum of skeletal abnormalities encountered in patients with chronic kidney disease. The uremic environment is associated with a variety of derangements that collectively contribute to the pathogenesis of secondary hyperparathyroidism. Early in the course of chronic kidney disease, phosphate retention plays a major role in the development of hyperparathyroidism. Calcitriol deficiency and hypocalcemia are also important in this regard. High circulating levels of PTH lead to a variety of effects that result in alterations in bone remodeling, giving rise to the classic lesion of hyperparathyroid bone disease known as osteitis fibrosa (a state of high bone turnover characterized by increased osteoblastic and osteoclastic activity as well as peritrabecular marrow fibrosis). The measurement of circulating levels of PTH therefore becomes important in the diagnosis and management of renal osteodystrophy.

PTH also plays a major role in divalent ion homeostasis, so the levels of serum calcium and phosphorus may also reflect PTH activity. PTH acts directly on cells of the osteoblastic lineage, which in turn interact with osteoclastic cells, affecting bone formation and bone resorption, respectively. The assessment of markers of osteoblastic and osteoclastic activity may be useful in the determination of PTH activity. For example alkaline phosphatase and osteocalcin may be useful as markers of osteoblastic bone formation. Similarly, PTH regulates a variety of factors secreted by osteoblastic cells, which in turn have effects on osteoclastic bone resorption. These include cytokines such as IL-6, IL-11, and OPG. Measurement of osteoclast markers released into the circulation, such as tartrate-resistant acid phosphatase, may also assess osteoclastic activity. Products of bone resorption can also be detected in the circulation and may be useful in the estimation of osteoclast activity.

A variety of other factors related to the uremic state may also influence bone histology and contribute to the spectrum of renal osteodystrophy. Metabolic acidosis results in demineralization of bone by several mechanisms involving buffering of hydrogen ions by bone carbonate, as well as alteration of the expression of a variety of genes in bone cells. Impaired bone mineralization in chronic kidney disease may also occur as a result of aluminum accumulation at the mineralization front, and the determination of serum aluminum levels provides a starting point in the evaluation of aluminum bone disease. β_2-microglobulin accumulates in patients with impaired renal function and may accumulate in bone and joint ligaments, giving rise to β_2-microglobulin amyloidosis. As stated earlier, the validity of the various biochemical parameters used in the diagnosis of renal osteodystrophy relies on the examination of bone histology.

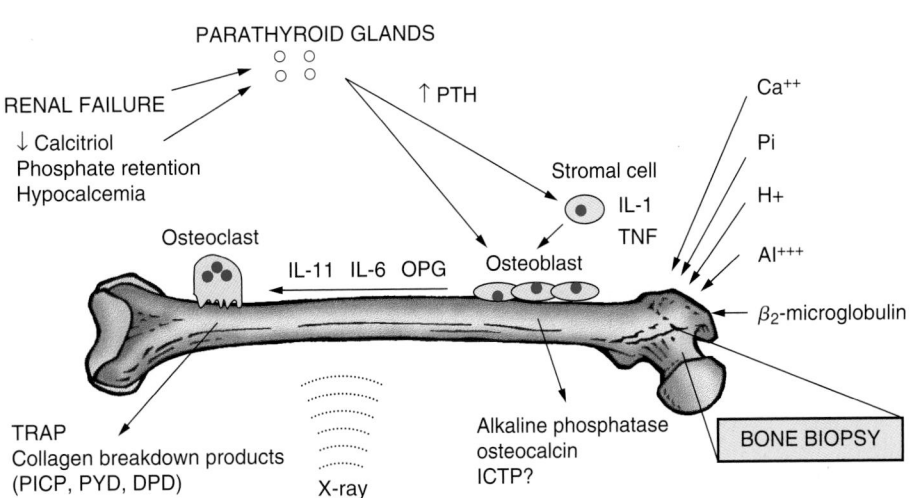

FIGURE 52-16. Diagrammatic representation of a framework for the assessment of various factors involved in renal osteodystrophy. DPD, lysylpyridinium; IL, interleukin; OPG, osteoprotegrin; PICP, type I procollagen COOH-terminal extension peptide; PTH, parathyroid hormone; PYD, hydroxylysylpyridinium; TNF, tumor necrosis factor; TRAP, tartrate-resistant acid phosphatase. (Modified from González EA, Martin KJ: Assessment of bone and joint diseases: Renal osteodystrophy. *In* Bilezikian JP [ed]: Dynamics of Bone and Cartilage Metabolism. New York, Academic Press, 1999, pp 561-569, with permission.)

Serum Calcium and Phosphorus Levels

Serum Phosphorus

In adults, the concentration of serum phosphorus is maintained between 3.0 and 4.5 mg/dL. The two major organs involved in the regulation of phosphorus homeostasis are the kidney and the gastrointestinal tract. Unlike the kidney, which continuously maintains phosphorus homeostasis, the intestine may provide intermittent phosphate loads depending on dietary intake. In the setting of chronic kidney disease, disturbances in phosphorus homeostasis may be expected. Indeed, a variety of factors related to the uremic environment contribute to alterations in both renal and intestinal handling of phosphorus, which may lead to abnormal serum phosphorus concentrations. For the most part, the levels of serum phosphorus remain normal to slightly decreased in the early stages of chronic kidney disease, and hyperphosphatemia does not usually become clinically evident until the GFR has decreased to 20% of normal due to the phosphaturic action of PTH.[21, 281] Control of hyperphosphatemia is of paramount importance in the management of chronic kidney disease, not only because it contributes to the development of secondary hyperparathyroidism but also because it has been associated with increased mortality.[240, 282]

Most of the intestinal absorption of phosphorus takes place in the duodenum and jejunum, but smaller amounts are also absorbed in the ileum and colon. Intestinal absorption of phosphorus involves both passive diffusion via the paracellular pathway and active transport via cell-mediated mechanisms.[283] The majority of intestinal phosphorus absorption occurs by passive diffusion, and therefore there is a linear relationship between net intestinal absorption of phosphorus and dietary phosphorus intake. A variety of hormonal and nonhormonal factors regulate the active component of intestinal phosphate absorption. Calcitriol is known to increase the intestinal absorption of phosphorus. In chronic kidney disease, calcitriol deficiency may result in increased fecal losses of phosphorus; however, because of the concomitant defect in renal handling of phosphorus, phosphorus retention prevails and clinically significant hypophosphatemia is rarely observed.[284, 285]

Urinary phosphate excretion may be modified by factors that affect either the filtered load or the tubular reabsorption of phosphate. Approximately 80% of the filtered load of phosphate is reabsorbed along the nephron. Between 60% and 70% of renal phosphate reabsorption takes place in the proximal tubule via specific cellular mechanisms. Although a significant fraction of filtered phosphate is reabsorbed between the early distal tubule and the final urine, the mechanisms involved are not well understood. Proximal tubular phosphate reabsorption is mostly transcellular and involves transport across the luminal membrane, translocation across the cell, and extrusion across the basolateral membrane. Cellular uptake of phosphate across the luminal membrane is mediated by the sodium-phosphate (Na/Pi) cotransporter, which is driven by the sodium gradient maintained by the sodium-potassium adenosine triphosphatase pump (Na^+, K^+,-ATPase) in the basolateral membrane. The mechanisms involved in the translocation of phosphate across the cell and its extrusion across the basolateral membrane remain poorly understood. A variety of hormonal, dietary, and metabolic factors are known to regulate tubular reabsorption of phosphate.

The major regulator of phosphate reabsorption in the kidney is PTH, which acts primarily in the proximal tubule. The actions of PTH are mediated by the PTH/PTHrP receptor.[286] PTH is known to decrease the expression of Na/Pi cotransporters at the cell surface by promoting their endocytosis and subsequent lysosomal degradation, thus promoting phosphaturia.[287, 288] Another factor that may play a role in renal phosphate handling during the course of chronic kidney disease is calcitriol deficiency. Although the precise mechanisms by which vitamin D_3 metabolites affect tubular phosphate reabsorption is not clear, the antiphosphaturic effect induced by these agents is likely to involve the Na/Pi cotransporter, because VDREs have been described in the promoter of the gene coding for the Na/Pi cotransporter.[289] The progressive reduction in GFR observed during the course of chronic kidney disease results in phosphate retention. However, hyperphosphatemia is not a prominent metabolic abnormality early in the course of chronic kidney disease,[21, 281] due to the phosphaturic action of PTH, because hyperparathyroidism is a common finding in this patient population.[9] In addition, calcitriol deficiency also promotes decreased phosphate reabsorption.

Hyperphosphatemia has a tendency to occur once the GFR has decreased to 20% of normal, because renal excretory capacity becomes inadequate to handle dietary intake of phosphorus. Hyperphosphatemia may also be observed in cases of severe hyperparathyroidism, as a result of the increased resorption of phosphorus from bone. Treatment of secondary hyperparathyroidism with vitamin D compounds may affect serum phosphorus levels directly by influencing phosphate handling by the intestine and kidney, as well as indirectly through the actions of PTH on bone remodeling. The increased levels of phosphorus observed as a result of increased bone resorption due to hyperparathyroidism may be significantly decreased, especially during the early stages of treatment with vitamin D, while rapid skeletal mineralization takes place. Subsequently, hyperphosphatemia may then result due to the effect of vitamin D compounds to increase intestinal absorption of phosphorus. Although hyperphosphatemia may result from increased bone resorption, monitoring of the serum phosphorus concentration is not very helpful in establishing the diagnosis of a specific type of renal osteodystrophy. However, control of hyperphosphatemia remains a crucial intervention in the setting of chronic kidney disease, because it may aggravate hyperparathyroidism by decreasing the levels of ionized calcium, decreasing the synthesis of calcitriol, and directly increasing PTH secretion and promoting the growth of parathyroid cells.

Serum Calcium

Total serum calcium concentration represents the sum of three fractions, namely ionized, complexed, and protein bound calcium. The ionized calcium, approximately 50% of total serum calcium, is the physiologically important fraction and can be measured directly. More commonly, the total calcium concentration is corrected for changes in serum protein. The major calciotropic hormones, PTH and calcitriol, maintain normal calcium homeostasis by the regulation of intestinal calcium absorption, renal calcium reabsorption, and calcium deposition and release from bone. Therefore, abnormalities of these two hormone systems, which are commonly encountered during the course of chronic kidney disease, are likely to result in alterations in serum calcium levels.

In advanced chronic kidney disease, the total serum calcium concentration may decrease below the normal range; however, this is not a universal finding.[21, 281] Hypocalcemia in chronic kidney disease may result from several mechanisms, including increased serum phosphorus concentration leading to the formation of calcium-phosphorus complexes, impaired calcitriol synthesis resulting in decreased intestinal absorption of calcium, and skeletal resistance to the actions of PTH and calcitriol. Other factors related to the uremic environment may lead to a decrease in ionized calcium. For example, advanced uremia is associated with the retention of various anions, resulting in increased complexed and therefore decreased ionized fraction of total serum calcium. Hemoconcentration after the hemodialysis procedure also results in increases in the protein-bound fraction.[21, 281] The parathyroid glands detect a decrease in ionized calcium via the calcium-sensing receptor on the cell surface and respond by increasing the secretion of PTH, which in turn exerts its actions in target organs to return the serum calcium concentration to the normal range.[290] Thus, PTH mobilizes calcium from bone, decreases renal tubular calcium excretion, and, by increasing the synthesis of calcitriol, increases intestinal calcium absorption. Regardless of the etiology of hypocalcemia, it is important to correct serum calcium concentration during the course of chronic kidney disease, because it is a very important stimulus for PTH secretion.

Hypercalcemia in patients with chronic kidney disease may be suggestive of low bone turnover osteodystrophy (osteomalacia and adynamic bone disease). In these patients, the hypercalcemia often becomes manifest after administration of low doses of vitamin D compounds or calcium supplements.[291] As a result of the low bone turnover, the excess calcium absorbed from the intestine may not be deposited in the bone, leading to the development of hypercalcemia.[292] Severe secondary hyperparathyroidism is also associated with hypercalcemia, as is persistent hyperparathyroidism after successful renal transplantation. Although elevations in serum calcium may suggest abnormal bone turnover, hypercalcemia in chronic kidney disease is often the result of therapeutic strategies used in the management of renal osteodystrophy. The intestinal absorption of calcium may increase after the administration of calcium-containing phosphate binders, since oral calcium administration increases calcium absorption by ionic diffusion. The effect of increasing serum calcium may be more pronounced when calcium salts are administered in conjunction with vitamin D compounds, because the latter increase calcium transport by the intestinal cells. Elevated serum calcium concentrations may suppress PTH secretion, leading to relative hypoparathyroidism, which may in turn contribute to the development of low-turnover osteodystrophy.

Numerous factors associated with the uremic environment have the potential to alter the concentrations of serum phosphorus and calcium. Although neither serum phosphorus nor serum calcium levels have diagnostic value with regard to the specific nature of the underlying bone disease, their interpretation in conjunction with measurements of PTH and biologic markers of bone turnover may provide clues as to the nature of the abnormalities of bone histology in chronic kidney disease.

Assay for Parathyroid Hormone

Accurate assessment of the activity of the parathyroid glands is essential for the monitoring and management of hyperparathyroidism. Accordingly, the identification of high bone turnover states resulting from hyperparathyroidism is of importance. It also becomes necessary to be able to monitor parathyroid activity accurately during the treatment phase, because oversuppression of the parathyroid glands may lead to an abnormally low bone turnover state.

The measurement of PTH in blood has evolved considerably in recent years.[293] After the introduction of an immunoassay for PTH in the early 1960s, there was a long period of difficulty in interpretation of the results, owing to different characteristics of the antisera used and the realization that PTH circulates not only in the form of the intact 84-amino-acid peptide but also as multiple fragments of the hormone, particularly from the middle and COOH-terminal regions of the PTH molecule.[294, 295] These PTH fragments arise from direct secretion from the parathyroid gland as well as from metabolism of PTH (1-84) by peripheral organs, especially liver and kidney, as diagrammed in Figure 52-17. For this

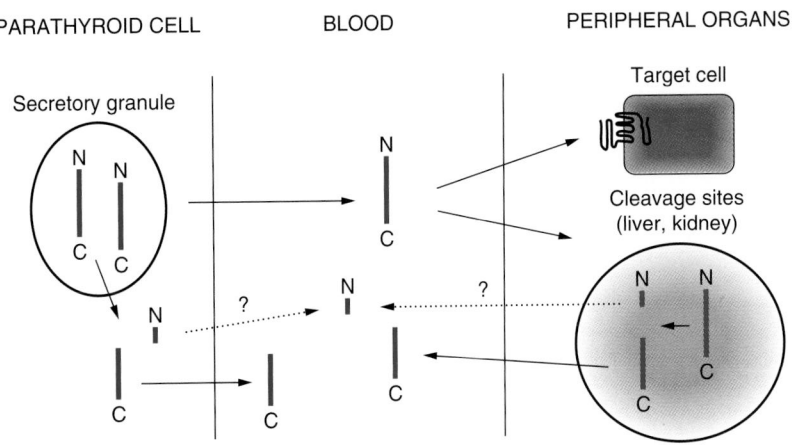

PARATHYROID CELL   BLOOD   PERIPHERAL ORGANS

FIGURE 52-17. Schematic diagram illustrating the metabolism of parathyroid hormone (PTH). PTH may undergo degradation within the parathyroid cell, and both the intact PTH (1-84) and PTH fragments may be secreted. In the circulation, intact PTH is delivered to and binds to specific receptors associated with the biologic effects of PTH. In addition, PTH (1-84) is cleaved by peripheral organs, especially the liver, and hormone fragments are returned to the circulation. (Modified from Potts JT Jr, Juppner H: Parathyroid hormone and parathyroid hormone-related peptide in calcium homeostasis, bone metabolism, and bone development: The proteins, their genes, and receptors. *In* Avioli LV, Krane SM [eds]: Metabolic Bone Disease, 3rd ed. New York, Academic Press, 1998, pp 51-94, with permission.)

reason, assays for PTH that were directed toward different parts of the PTH molecule yielded different results.[296] Clinical experience showed that assays directed toward the middle and COOH-terminal regions of the PTH molecule were most useful clinically, but such assays were somewhat problematic in the setting of kidney failure because COOH-terminal fragments, which depend on GFR for their removal from plasma, accumulate in the presence of decreased renal function.[297] As assay techniques became more refined, a new era of PTH measurement began with the use of two-site immunoradiometric assays (Fig. 52-18).[110, 298, 299] Such assays capture PTH peptides from plasma with a solid phase-coupled antibody, usually directed toward the COOH-terminal region of the PTH molecule, and the captured PTH peptides are detected with a second antibody directed toward a different region of the molecule, usually the NH$_2$ terminus. Such assays are now widely used. Further refinements have been instituted since the demonstration that such intact PTH assays detect more than a single species of PTH when serum is fractionated by high-performance liquid chromatography.[111] New assays have been developed in which the detection antibody recognizes the precise NH$_2$ terminus of the PTH molecule, so that only intact PTH (1-84) is measured.[113, 300]

The development of this assay has refined understanding of the measurement of PTH in serum and has initiated new interest in the nature and actions of other PTH peptides that are truncated at the NH$_2$ terminus, such as PTH (7-84). Large NH$_2$-terminally truncated PTH fragments can be found within the parathyroid gland, as PTH undergoes degradation after synthesis (see Fig. 52-17). This degradation of PTH within the parathyroid gland has been known for some time to be influenced by the levels of extracellular calcium.[301-303] Presumably, this regulated intracellular degradation of PTH makes it possible for the parathyroid gland to respond quickly when varying amounts of active hormone are required for a physiologic response. After secretion from the parathyroid gland, intact PTH is rapidly metabolized in peripheral tissues.[304-307] Intact PTH cleared from the blood is cleaved by endoproteases to a number of large fragments, which reenter the circulation, most of which appear to begin

with residues between 34 and 43 of the PTH peptide.[304, 306] Additional fragments from the NH$_2$-terminal region of PTH or middle-molecule fragments may also circulate and have the potential to accumulate when GFR is reduced. Recent studies have suggested that NH$_2$-terminally truncated PTH fragments may have biologic actions,[114-116] and although these peptides do not appear to interact at the classic PTH-1 receptor, emerging evidence indicates the likelihood of a receptor for COOH-terminal regions of PTH, where NH$_2$-terminally truncated fragments such as PTH (7-84) could have significant biologic effects.[308] Studies in vivo have shown that PTH (7-84) can blunt the calcemic response to PTH (1-84).[114, 115] Studies in vitro have shown that PTH (7-84) can decrease basal bone resorption and bone resorption stimulated by a variety of agonists, such as 1,25-dihydroxyvitamin D, IL-11, and prostaglandin E$_2$.[116] These data imply that circulation of such NH$_2$-terminally truncated PTH fragments in significant concentrations may modulate the effects of PTH in peripheral tissues. Preliminary studies in a selected group of patients demonstrated that the ratio between intact PTH (1-84) and NH$_2$-terminally truncated PTH fragments may have some diagnostic value,[309] although not all investigators have confirmed this finding at the present time.[310] Considerable heterogeneity in results is still possible, because the intact PTH assays, which measure total PTH as the sum of PTH and NH$_2$-terminally truncated fragments, vary considerably in their ability to detect peptides such as PTH (7-84). Further studies are required to define the diagnostic utility of the measurement of NH$_2$-terminally truncated PTH fragments. As the biologic effects of such fragments are elucidated, additional insights into the effects of PTH on peripheral tissues will be revealed.

Biologic Markers of Bone Formation
Total Alkaline Phosphatase

Total alkaline phosphatase in serum is the sum of five isoforms: hepatic, skeletal, renal, intestinal, and placental.[311-313] Most of the circulating total alkaline phosphatase in normal individuals is a combination of the bone and liver isoforms in approximately equal proportions. In chronic kidney disease, the contributions of hepatic, skeletal, and intestinal isoforms may be altered because of changes in their half-lives. Nonetheless, measurement of total alkaline phosphatase may provide an index of osteoblastic bone formation, because studies in uremic patients have demonstrated that increased total alkaline phosphatase in this patient population is often the result of increases in the bone-specific isoform.[314] Although high levels of alkaline phosphatase have been shown to correlate with PTH levels and histologic findings of hyperparathyroid bone disease, most studies examining the correlation of total alkaline phosphatase with levels of PTH and histologic parameters of bone formation have shown wide variation, and normal serum concentrations of total alkaline phosphatase have been described in uremic patients with overt osteitis fibrosa.

Total alkaline phosphatase may be useful in monitoring the progression of bone disease as well as the response to therapy.[315] In contrast to the case in high bone turnover states, elevations in total alkaline phosphatase are not a feature of low turnover osteodystrophy. Because liver disease is commonly associated with elevations in total alkaline

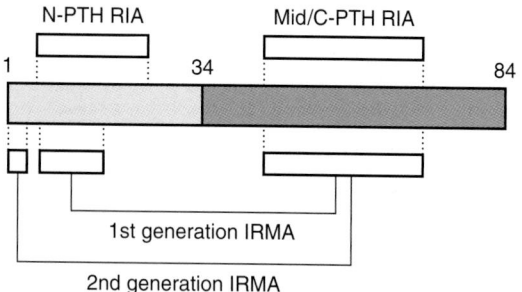

FIGURE 52-18. Diagram of the recognition sites on the full-length parathyroid hormone (PTH) molecule, PTH (1-84), as recognized by various PTH assays. In general, the NH$_2$-terminal and mid/COOH-terminal assays have given way to first-generation PTH immunoradiometric assays (IRMA) or immunochemiluminescent assays (ICMA), which are widely used as "intact" PTH assays. More recently, these assays have been refined to more precisely measure only the PTH (1-84) peptide by the use of a detection antibody for the exact NH$_2$ terminus of PTH. (From Juppner H, Potts JT Jr: Immunoassays for the detection of parathyroid hormone. J Bone Miner Res 17[suppl 2]:N81-N86, 2002, with permission.)

phosphatase and hepatitis C is frequently found in patients undergoing dialysis, it is important to rule out hepatic abnormalities when interpreting the levels of total alkaline phosphatase in this patient population. Because serum total alkaline phosphatase lacks sensitivity and specificity as a marker of bone formation in patients with chronic kidney disease, efforts have been made to develop measurements of the bone-specific isoform in an attempt to increase the diagnostic value of the test.

Bone-Specific Alkaline Phosphatase

In bone, alkaline phosphatase is made by cells of the osteoblastic lineage; although its exact physiologic role remains unclear, alkaline phosphatase participates in the process of mineralization and bone formation. Pyrophosphate is a potent inhibitor of the bone mineralization process, and bone-specific alkaline phosphatase enhances mineralization by catalyzing the hydrolysis of pyrophosphate, which also provides a high phosphate concentration at the osteoblastic surface.[316, 317] The role of bone-specific alkaline phosphatase in the mineralization process has been supported by studies demonstrating that cells normally lacking the gene for alkaline phosphatase acquire mineralizing capability after transfection with its complementary DNA.[316, 317] The development of monoclonal antibodies specific for bone alkaline phosphatase has allowed the opportunity to evaluate its usefulness as an index of bone formation.[318]

Urena and colleagues[319] studied 42 patients on hemodialysis and demonstrated that bone-specific alkaline phosphatase is a better correlate than PTH or total alkaline phosphatase with regard to histomorphometric parameters of bone formation and bone resorption. These investigators found that a level of bone-specific alkaline phosphatase greater than 20 ng/mL had a sensitivity and specificity of 100% and a positive predictive value of 84% for the diagnosis of high-turnover bone disease. Levels of bone-specific alkaline phosphatase greater than 20 ng/mL combined with PTH levels greater than 200 pg/mL had a positive predictive value of 94% for the diagnosis of high-turnover bone disease. Furthermore, because of the high specificity of the test, levels of bone-specific alkaline phosphatase greater than 20 ng/mL allow for the formal exclusion of low-turnover bone disease (Fig. 52-19). Bone biopsy studies by Couttenye and associates[320] including 103 patients on hemodialysis showed that bone-specific alkaline phosphatase levels had a higher predictive value for adynamic bone disease than did osteocalcin levels. Coen and co-workers[321] studied 41 patients on hemodialysis and found that a level of bone-specific alkaline phosphatase lower than 12.9 ng/mL had a sensitivity of 100%, a specificity of 94%, and a positive predictive value of 72% for the diagnosis of low-turnover bone disease.[321] Therefore, measurements of bone-specific alkaline phosphatase may be helpful in the diagnosis of both high- and low-turnover renal osteodystrophy, especially when examined in conjunction with PTH levels.[319-325]

Osteocalcin

Osteocalcin, also known as bone Gla protein, BGP or bone γ-carboxy-glutamic acid–containing protein, is the most abundant noncollagenous protein present in the bone matrix.[319-325]

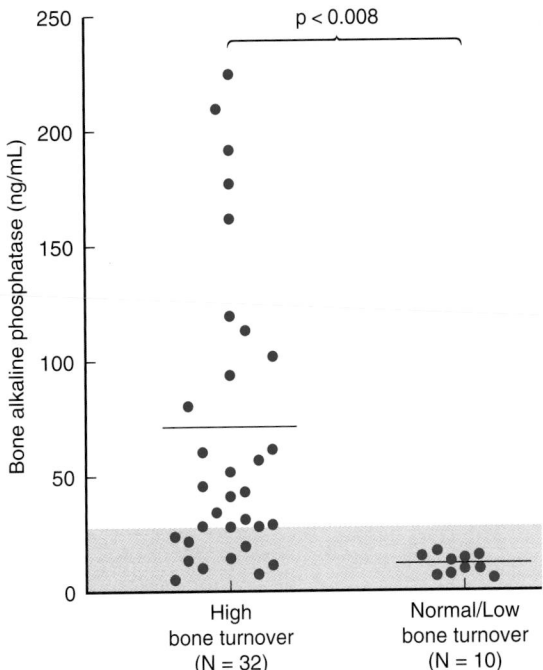

FIGURE 52-19. Values for bone-specific alkaline phosphatase in patients with high bone turnover, compared with values obtained in patients whose bone turnover was normal or low. (From Urena P, Hruby M, Ferreira A, et al. Plasma total versus bone alkaline phosphatase as markers of bone turnover in hemodialysis patients. J Am Soc Nephrol 7:506-512, 1996, with permission.)

γ-Carboxylation of osteocalcin depends on the presence of vitamin K. Decreases in the carboxylated fraction have been described in states of vitamin K deficiency and have been associated with decreased bone mass and increased fracture risk.[326-329] Osteocalcin is produced only by osteoblasts and odontoblasts, and it is a phenotypic marker for the osteoblast differentiation process. Transgenic animals lacking the osteocalcin gene demonstrated increased bone formation rates,[330-332] suggesting a role for osteocalcin as an inhibitor of bone formation. Osteocalcin levels have been shown to reflect bone formation; however, because osteocalcin is released from both osteoblasts and bone matrix, it is thought to be a less specific marker for bone formation than bone-specific alkaline phosphatase. Unlike total alkaline phosphatase, however, osteocalcin levels are not affected by the presence of extraskeletal disorders.[333]

There are several difficulties when considering the use of osteocalcin levels in the setting of renal bone disease. Osteocalcin levels are increased in patients with chronic kidney disease because of decreased renal clearance.[334] In addition, a variety of osteocalcin fragments of unknown function accumulate in uremic plasma and are also detected by the antibodies directed toward the intact molecule. Nonetheless, plasma osteocalcin levels have been shown to have good sensitivity in differentiating high- from low-turnover renal osteodystrophy. Malluche and associates[335] studied 30 patients on dialysis and found a correlation between osteocalcin levels and histologic parameters of bone turnover. Osteocalcin levels were superior to total alkaline phosphatase and PTH levels in differentiating adynamic bone disease from hyperparathyroid bone disease.[335] Studies by

Charhon and colleagues[336] demonstrated that osteocalcin levels lower than 4 nmol/L have a specificity of 100% for the diagnosis of adynamic bone disease; however, the sensitivity was only 17%.[336] Although osteocalcin levels have been shown to correlate with histologic parameters of bone formation in patients undergoing either hemodialysis or peritoneal dialysis, they do not add to the predictive value of PTH levels in this regard.[335, 337-339] In terms of monitoring the treatment of renal osteodystrophy, osteocalcin levels have been shown to exhibit a biphasic response after the administration of calcitriol to patients with secondary hyperparathyroidism. An initial increase is followed by a decrease in the levels of osteocalcin after the intravenous administration of calcitriol.[340] Although plasma osteocalcin levels have been shown to correlate with bone histomorphometric parameters, the correlations are weaker than those observed with bone-specific alkaline phosphatase or PTH levels.[319, 341] A better understanding of the role of osteocalcin and its fragments on bone physiology, together with the development of more specific assays, may improve the value of osteocalcin levels in the diagnosis of renal bone disease.[342, 343]

Procollagen Propeptides

Ninety percent of bone extracellular matrix is composed of type I collagen. Osteoblasts produce type I procollagen, which is then cleaved extracellularly at both NH_2 and COOH termini to give rise to the collagen molecule. The collagen molecules form fibrils that are incorporated into the bone matrix. As its name implies, type I procollagen COOH-terminal extension peptide (PICP) results from excision of the COOH terminus from type I procollagen. Because PICP undergoes hepatic degradation, circulating levels are not altered in the setting of impaired renal function. Because the production of PICP takes place while osteoblasts are engaged in the process of bone formation, circulating levels of PICP have the potential to be useful markers of osteoblastic activity and thus of bone formation. Coen and co-workers[344] studied patients with chronic kidney disease before the initiation of maintenance dialysis and found increased circulating levels of PICP. However, there was no correlation between the increased levels of PICP and either biochemical or histomorphometric parameters of bone turnover. In patients on maintenance hemodialysis, Hamdy and colleagues[345] found good correlation between the levels of PICP and those of bone-specific alkaline phosphatase, osteocalcin, and PTH, as well as histomorphometric parameters of bone formation.[345] Other investigators have not found the levels of PICP to be useful in the diagnosis of specific types of renal osteodystrophy in patients on dialysis.[319, 341, 346, 347] Similar to the case with total alkaline phosphatase, PICP levels may be altered in patients with liver disease, adding to the difficulty of interpretation of circulating PICP levels in patients on dialysis, since hepatitis C is a frequent finding in this patient population. Therefore, the use of PICP levels in the diagnosis of renal osteodystrophy awaits further investigation.

Biologic Markers of Bone Resorption
Collagen Breakdown Products

The mechanical force of bone tissue is provided by type I collagen. The type I collagen molecule has a variety of intermolecular and intramolecular cross-links that account for the tensile strength of type I collagen fibers.[348, 349] Two pyridinoline cross-links of collagen, namely, hydroxylysylpyridinium (PYD) and lysylpyridinium (DPD), have been studied in detail. PYD and DPD are found in bone and cartilage and are released into the circulation during the process of osteoclastic bone resorption. PYD and DPD are renally excreted, and the serum levels are very low to undetectable in normal individuals.[350-352] The excretion of these molecules in the urine has been used as a marker of bone resorption in a variety of metabolic bone diseases. Studies that included patients with impaired renal function have suggested that the excretion of PYD and DPD was not altered; however, the patients studied were not on dialysis, and their creatinine clearance rates were greater than 10 mL/min.[353, 354] Ibrahim and colleagues[355] examined circulating levels of PYD and DPD in patients on hemodialysis and on peritoneal dialysis and found that the levels were 50 to 100 times higher than those found in normal subjects. In addition, both cross-links were found to be dialyzable, because the levels decreased after the dialysis procedure and they could be detected in the dialysate. Urena and co-workers[341] studied 37 patients on hemodialysis and found that the highest circulating levels of PYD corresponded to the patients with high-turnover bone disease. In their study, the levels of PYD were superior in terms of correlating with bone histology, compared with PTH or osteocalcin, and were similar to the levels of bone-specific alkaline phosphatase in this regard. Therefore, pyridinoline cross-links of collagen have the potential to be useful biochemical markers in the diagnosis of renal bone disease.

Tartrate-Resistant Acid Phosphatase

Acid phosphatases are produced by a variety of cells including osteoclasts. The bone-specific acid phosphatase, also known as tartrate-resistant acid phosphatase (TRAP), has been evaluated as a potential biochemical marker of bone resorption.[356-360] It appears that TRAP is not specific for osteoclasts, because cells of the osteoblastic lineage have also been found to have significant TRAP activity.[361] Studies in patients with impaired renal function demonstrated correlations of serum TRAP activity with plasma total alkaline phosphatase as well as PTH levels.[362] However, studies in dialysis patients did not support the use of this marker as a predictor of the underlying form of bone disease.[321] Therefore, the value of serum TRAP in the diagnosis of renal osteodystrophy remains to be determined. Recent studies have identified TRAP-5b as the osteoclast-specific isoform, and future studies involving patients with chronic kidney disease are needed to evaluate the value of this new marker in renal bone disease.[360, 363]

Type I Collagen Cross-Linked COOH-Terminal Telopeptide

Type I collagen cross-linked COOH-terminal telopeptide (ICTP) is a collagen derivative released during bone resorption. Therefore, circulating levels of ICTP have the potential to be useful as an index of bone resorption. Indeed, studies in patients with a variety of metabolic bone diseases have described good correlations between ICTP levels and histomorphometric parameters of bone resorption.[364, 365]

Other studies, however, have not found ICTP levels to be of value as an index of bone resorption.[365, 366] Because the elimination rate of ICTP depends on the GFR, increased levels are expected in patients with impaired renal function. Studies in patients on hemodialysis performed by Mazzaferro and associates[367] found that circulating levels of ICTP correlated with serum concentrations of total alkaline phosphatase, bone-specific alkaline phosphatase, and PTH, as well as with bone histomorphometry. Other studies in patients on hemodialysis did not find ICTP levels to be useful in this regard.[341] Based on these findings, measurements of serum concentrations of ICTP do not seem to be of value in the diagnosis of renal osteodystrophy.

Aluminum Levels and the Deferoxamine Test

The prevalence of aluminum-related bone disease has decreased in recent years; however, aluminum overload continues to be a problem. A 1998 study showed that approximately two thirds of patients from Portugal and Spain with biopsy evidence of adynamic bone disease had significant aluminum accumulation in the bone surface.[368] The measurement of basal serum aluminum levels is of limited diagnostic value in identifying patients with aluminum-related bone disease, because these levels are affected by recent aluminum load and are less indicative of aluminum toxicity.[369] D'Haese and colleagues[370] found that a serum aluminum level of 60 μg/L had a sensitivity of 82% and a specificity of 86% for detecting aluminum-related bone disease. Serum aluminum levels may fall rapidly over the course of a few months after discontinuation of aluminum-containing phosphate binders; therefore, the incidence of false-negative results may increase from 30% to 90% after cessation of aluminum intake.[370]

Because aluminum is deposited in several organs including bone, brain, heart, and liver, the measurement of the increment in serum aluminum level after a standardized infusion of deferoxamine has been used to assess tissue stores of aluminum and to identify patients who are at high risk for aluminum-related bone disease.[369] However, the deferoxamine test has been shown not to be a reliable indicator of aluminum-related bone disease in the absence of determinations of PTH levels.[371-373] In addition, the presence of other metals (e.g., iron) may affect the results of the test.[374]

Pei and co-workers[373] analyzed the deferoxamine test in conjunction with PTH levels in both hemodialysis and peritoneal dialysis patients. An increment of plasma aluminum of more than 150 μg/L after the infusion of deferoxamine (40 mg/kg) in the presence of PTH levels lower than 200 pg/mL had a positive predictive value of 95% for aluminum-related bone disease. More recently, lower doses of deferoxamine have been used for the evaluation of aluminum-related bone disease. D'Haese and colleagues[371] also evaluated the deferoxamine test in conjunction with PTH levels.[371] In this study, an increase in serum aluminum level by more than 50 μg/L after the infusion of deferoxamine (5 mg/kg) and a PTH level greater than 650 pg/mL were consistent with aluminum overload but not with aluminum-related bone disease. On the other hand, the same increment in serum aluminum level accompanied by a PTH level lower than 650 pg/mL was likely to indicate the presence of aluminum-related bone disease. The combination of an increment in

serum aluminum of greater than 50 μg/L and an intact PTH level of less than 150 pg/mL offered the greatest risk of aluminum-related bone disease, with a sensitivity and specificity of 87% and 95%, respectively.

In addition to the PTH levels, iron status can affect the deferoxamine test.[372] Patients with iron deficiency (serum ferritin <100 μg/L) may have increased serum aluminum levels despite a low aluminum burden as indicated by the deferoxamine test.[375] Conversely, patients with iron overload (serum ferritin >1000 μg/L) may have low serum aluminum levels (<30 μg/L) in the presence of a positive deferoxamine test and significant accumulation of aluminum in bone.[376]

Therefore, the noninvasive assessment of aluminum-related bone disease is rather complex. Random levels of serum aluminum have poor diagnostic value. The increment of serum aluminum concentration after the infusion of a standardized dose of deferoxamine, when interpreted in conjunction with PTH and ferritin levels, is a useful aid in the diagnosis of aluminum-related bone disease. However, because of the potential toxicity of treating aluminum-related bone disease with deferoxamine, the confirmation of bone aluminum burden by bone biopsy may still be necessary before the initiation of therapy, especially in uncertain or mixed cases.

β₂-Microglobulin

β_2-microglobulin accumulates in the serum of patients with impaired renal function and is the major component of amyloid deposits encountered in osteoarticular tissues in this patient population. There is evidence to suggest that serum β_2-microglobulin levels may be useful as a marker of bone remodeling.[377-379] Ferreira and associates[380] studied patients on hemodialysis and found higher serum levels of β_2-microglobulin in patients with high-turnover bone disease compared with patients with normal or low bone turnover. In addition, the same study reported that the levels of β_2-microglobulin correlated with the levels of osteocalcin, bone-specific alkaline phosphatase, and PYD; however, there was no correlation between β_2-microglobulin levels and PTH concentrations in serum. The value of β_2-microglobulin levels as an index of bone turnover awaits further studies.

Cytokines and Growth Factors

Although the major calciotropic hormones, PTH and calcitriol, play important roles in the pathogenesis of renal osteodystrophy, it is likely that additional systemic and local factors are also involved in this process. The uremic state is associated with a multitude of abnormalities in different growth factors as well as cytokine systems involved in the regulation of bone remodeling.[154-157] IL-6 is a very important bone-resorbing cytokine that has been implicated in states of increased bone resorption.[185-187] Circulating levels of IL-6 are reportedly increased in uremic patients, which may be partially explained by the facts that PTH stimulates the synthesis of IL-6 and secondary hyperparathyroidism is commonly present in patients with CRF.[189-194] Circulating levels of IL-6 have been shown to correlate with markers of bone remodeling in patients with renal bone disease.[189, 190]

IL-1, another cytokine with bone-resorptive characteristics, has also been associated with clinical disorders characterized by increased bone resorption. IL-1 levels are reported to be elevated in dialysis patients.[189, 190] The actions of IL-1 are modulated by an endogenous antagonist, the IL-1 receptor antagonist (IL-1Ra), and patients on dialysis have been found to have increased levels of circulating IL-1Ra.[169] These findings suggest that, within a single cytokine system, the uremic milieu may alter both stimulatory and inhibitory components, and that the final impact on bone depends on the relative contributions of these alterations.

The RANK/RANKL/OPG system plays a crucial role in osteoclastogenesis and osteoclast development.[163] OPG has an inhibitory effect on bone resorption and was recently evaluated as a potential marker for the diagnosis of renal osteodystrophy in patients on dialysis. Kazama and colleagues[183] found increased levels of OPG in patients with chronic kidney disease, which suggests a potential role of OPG in the skeletal resistance to PTH observed in this patient population. Haas and coworkers[184] examined bone biopsies from 26 patients on hemodialysis and found that OPG levels were significantly lower in patients with high bone turnover, compared with those with normal or low bone turnover. Patients with high-turnover bone disease also had significantly higher levels of PTH. In addition, the combination of low levels of OPG with high levels of PTH was consistent with the diagnosis of high bone turnover in 88% of the patients; conversely, the combination of high levels of OPG with low levels of PTH was accurate in establishing the diagnosis of low-turnover osteodystrophy in 72% of the patients.[184]

In addition to its effects on osteoclasts, the uremic environment has the potential to affect factors responsible for osteoblast development and activity, which can have an impact on bone remodeling. Dialysis patients have been found to have increased levels of IGF-I, and a positive correlation between plasma IGF levels and bone formation rate has also been reported.[213] Most of the circulating IGF is bound by IGFBPs, which can either enhance or inhibit the actions of IGF. Jehle and associates[215] found that patients with secondary hyperparathyroidism had low serum levels of IGFBP-5 (a stimulatory IGFBP). Furthermore, serum levels of IGFBP-5 correlated with biochemical and histologic parameters of bone formation in patients with renal osteodystrophy. Therefore, components of the IGF system may have the potential to serve as markers of bone turnover in patients with chronic kidney disease.

RADIOGRAPHIC FEATURES OF RENAL OSTEODYSTROPHY

The sensitivity of radiography for the evaluation of renal osteodystrophy is limited. Considerable amounts of bone mineral can be lost before there is obvious radiologic change. In addition, the radiograph reflects chronic changes in the bone and does not necessarily indicate skeletal activity at the time of the examination. The radiologic features do not correlate well with histologic appearance. Therefore, routine use of skeletal radiographs for screening of bone disease in patients with CRF has limited value.

Hyperparathyroid Bone Disease

One of the principal radiologic features of secondary hyperparathyroidism is evidence of bone resorption, which occurs mainly in the subperiosteal area but can also be seen at other sites. The earliest lesions often appear in the middle phalanges of the second or third digits (Fig. 52-20). As the lesions progress, the erosions may extend along the bone and involve other sites. These erosions are asymptomatic but are occasionally associated with synovitis or symptoms of joint pain. Subperiosteal erosions may also be seen in the tibia, the neck of the femur, the humerus, the pelvic bones, and the distal ends of the clavicles (Fig. 52-21). Bone resorption in the skull produces a mottled, lucent appearance commonly associated with areas of osteosclerosis, giving the appearance of a "pepper-pot skull" (see Fig. 52-21). These erosions usually do not heal rapidly after therapy for high-turnover bone disease, and remineralization may be extremely slow, even after successful therapy for the underlying metabolic abnormality.

Hyperparathyroidism can also be associated with cystic lesions of bone that may represent brown tumors (osteoclastomas). These may be accompanied by pain, and there is a need to distinguish these lesions from malignant tumors, metastases, or cysts associated with amyloidosis. With correction of the underlying metabolic abnormality, these cystic areas may be replaced by areas of sclerosis. Alteration of trabecular volume of spongy bone may lead to osteosclerosis. This is generally apparent in vertebrae, pelvis, skull, clavicle, humerus, and proximal and distal femur and tibia. These areas of osteosclerosis in the spine lead to the characteristic "rugger-jersey" appearance on lateral view (see Fig. 52-21). Osteosclerosis also contribute to the salt-and-pepper appearance of the skull.

Osteomalacia

The pathognomonic feature of osteomalacia in adults is pseudofractures or Looser zones. These are straight bands of radiolucency that are usually perpendicular to the long axis of the bone. They may be bilateral, and they are sometimes associated with a small, poorly mineralizing callus. Pseudofractures may also be seen in the pubic rami, scapulae, or ribs. Spontaneous stress fractures occur in the metatarsals and ribs and are often painful. Deformities of the long bones, characteristic of rickets, may also be seen, especially in children and young adults. The features of secondary hyperparathyroidism may also be associated with these features of osteomalacia.

Osteopenia

A common radiographic feature of renal bone disease is decreased bone mineral density. This is a nonspecific finding that can be seen in either high- or low-turnover bone disease. Osteopenia may result in fractures, particularly in the vertebrae; crush fractures can result in deformities of the vertebrae.

Metastatic Calcification

Radiographs may reveal extraskeletal calcifications in patients with CRF. This may be manifested in organs such as the heart, lungs, and skeletal muscle. Metastatic calcification is more commonly observed in large blood vessels such as the aorta, iliac, and femoral arteries and in the arteries of

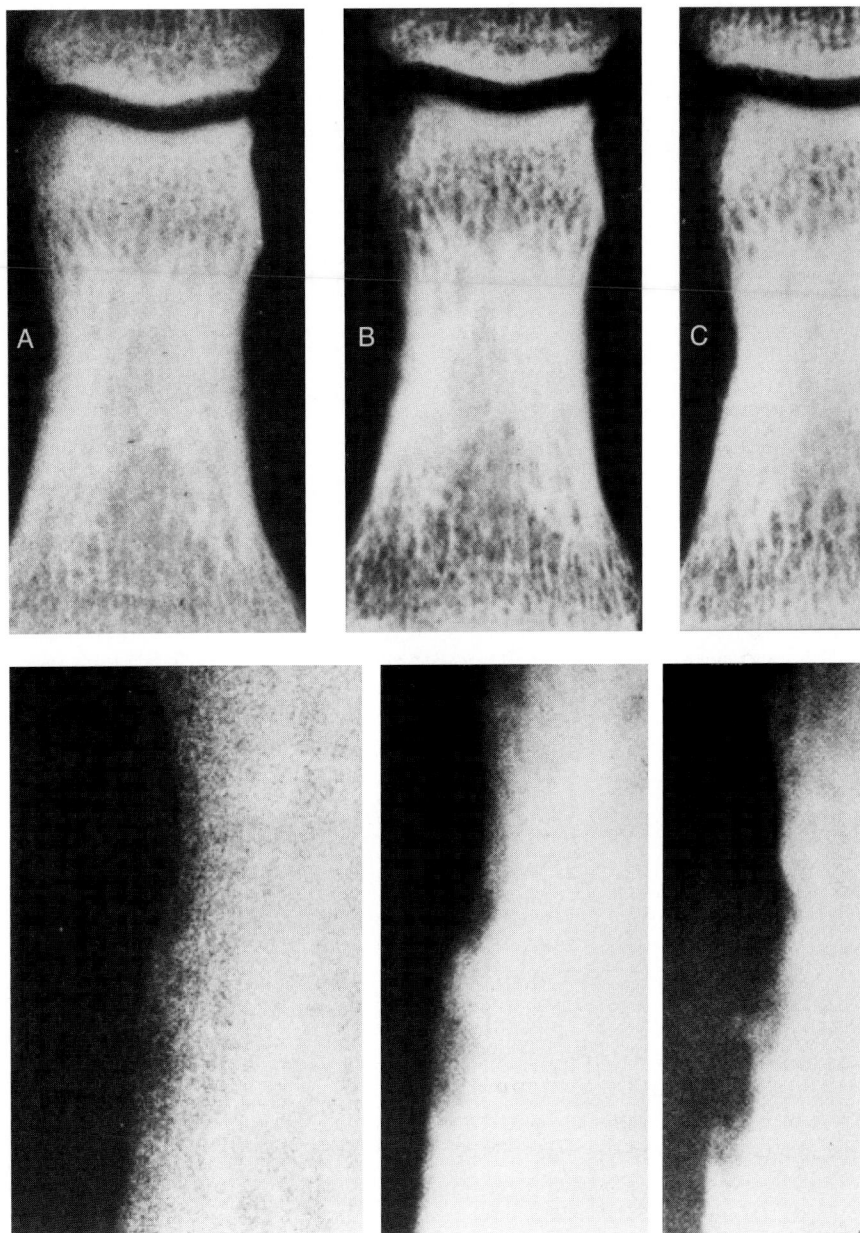

FIGURE 52-20. Serial magnified radiographs of the index finger in a patient on peritoneal dialysis. The upper panels of **A, B,** and **C** are magnification ×3, and the corresponding lower panels are ×12. The high magnification of panel **B** shows subperiosteal resorption, which progresses to periosteal resorption in panel **C.** (From Meema HE, Meema S: Microradioscopic quantitation of periosteal resorption in secondary hyperparathyroidism of chronic renal failure. Clin Orthop 130:297-302, 1978, with permission.)

the extremities (Fig. 52-22). Calcification can also be found in periarticular sites such as the hips or shoulders.

Dialysis-Related Amyloidosis

The radiologic features of dialysis-related amyloidosis are present long before the onset of symptoms. They are usually manifested as bone cysts, and periarticular cystic bone lesions may be seen in the wrist or tarsal bone, femoral or humeral head, distal radius, acetabulum, pubic symphysis, or tibial plateau (Fig. 52-23). These lesions are characteristic but are not pathognomonic for dialysis-related amyloidosis, and they need to be differentiated from other cystic lesions. Amyloid-related cysts often involve the large synovial joints, and subchondral cysts are more characteristic of amyloidosis. These cysts may also be demonstrated

by CT or MRI, techniques that can be useful to evaluate the extent of disease, particularly in the spine and femoral neck.

Destructive Spondyloarthropathy

Spondyloarthropathy, usually affecting the cervical spine, may be seen in patients who have been on dialysis for a prolonged period. There is a reduction in the disc space with destruction or sclerosis of the adjacent vertebral end-plates. These findings need to be distinguished from infective osteomyelitis, and other imaging techniques (e.g., MRI) may be helpful in this regard.

Quantitative Measurements of Bone Mineral Content

Dual x-ray absorptiometry (DEXA) is a noninvasive method used for the quantification of bone mineral density that has

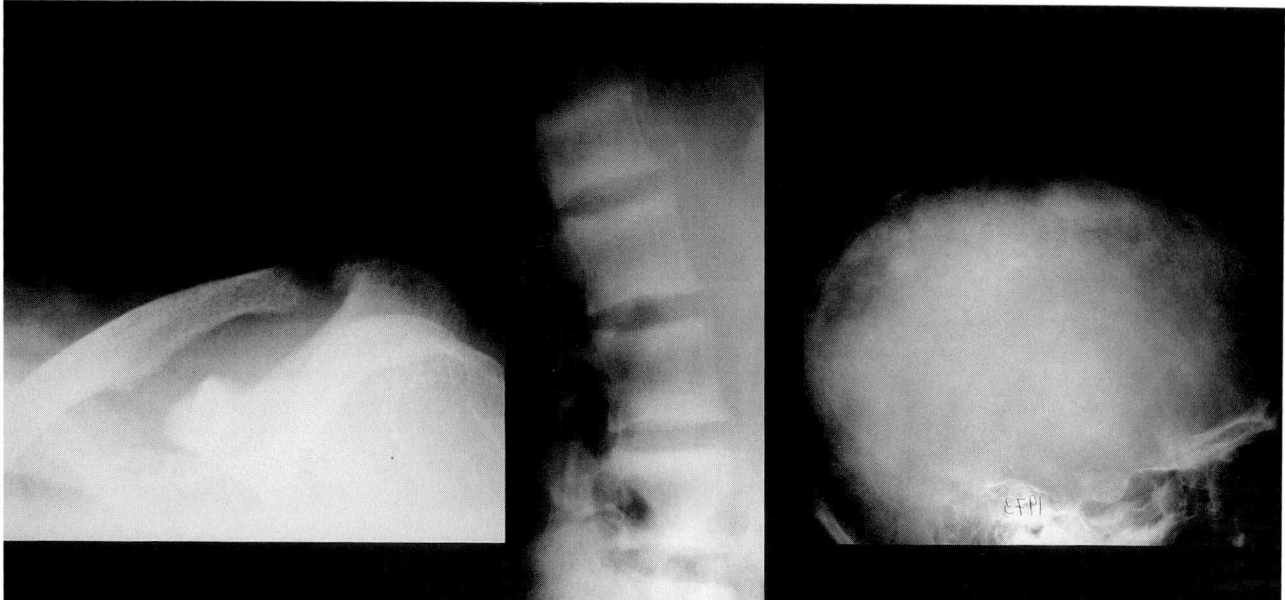

FIGURE 52-21. The characteristic skeletal radiographic findings of renal osteodystrophy. The *left panel* shows severe erosion of the distal clavicle as a result of secondary hyperparathyroidism. The *middle panel* shows an example of "rugger-jersey spine." The *right panel* shows a "pepper-pot skull" with areas of erosion and patchy osteosclerosis. (Images courtesy of David Rubin, M.D., Washington University, St. Louis, MO.)

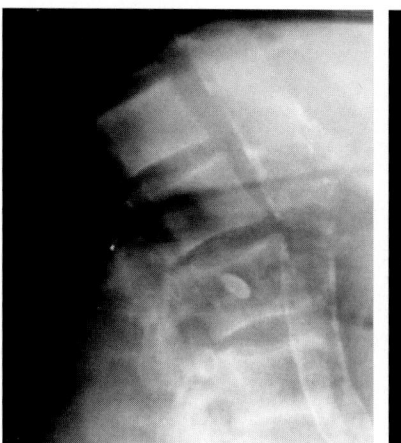 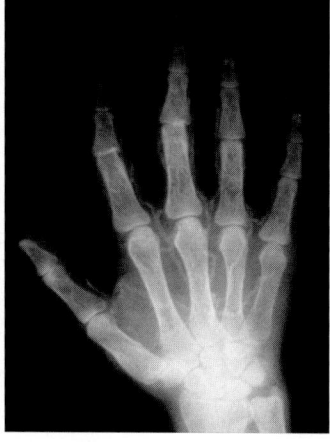

FIGURE 52-22. Radiograph illustrating severe arterial calcification in the arteries of the hand *(right panel)* and severe aortoiliac calcification *(left panel)*.

been shown to be a strong predictor of bone strength in patients without renal disease.[381, 382] Several investigators have reported decreased bone mineral density in patients who require dialysis.[383-386] Ha and co-workers[387] studied 24 patients with various degrees of chronic kidney disease and correlated the findings obtained by DEXA with biochemical markers of bone turnover. They found decreased bone mineral density in patients with chronic kidney disease, compared with control subjects, and they were able to demonstrate an inverse correlation between bone mineral density and alkaline phosphatase, PTH, and urine deoxypyridinoline. Rix and colleagues[388] studied 113 patients with chronic kidney disease (GFR ranging from 83 to 16 mL/min) and found that bone mineral density decreased with decreasing renal function. There was a negative correlation between bone mineral density and the degree of hyperparathyroidism. In addition, bone mineral density was significantly lower in patients with

diabetic nephropathy, compared with patients whose kidney disease resulted from other causes.[388] The type of dialysis modality may also affect bone mineral density, as was suggested by Hampson and associates,[389] who found that patients on hemodialysis had lower bone mineral density than on peritoneal dialysis.

Although data on the use of bone mineral density to discriminate among the various types of renal osteodystrophy remain inconclusive, recent studies suggest a potential for DEXA as a tool to evaluate renal bone disease. Gerakis and colleagues[390] performed simultaneous bone biopsies and DEXA in 62 patients on hemodialysis. There was an inverse relation between bone mineral density and serum PTH, osteocalcin, and alkaline phosphatase. Furthermore, bone mineral density was lower in patients with hyperparathyroid bone disease than in those with adynamic bone disease, and there was a negative correlation between bone mineral density

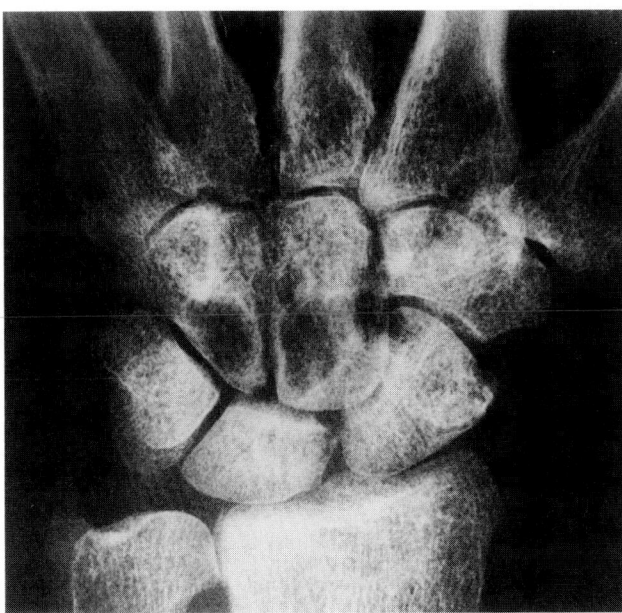

FIGURE 52-23. Multiple cystic areas in the wrist bones are a result of dialysis-associated amyloidosis. (From Fenves AZ, Emmett M, White MG, et al: Carpal tunnel syndrome with cystic bone lesions secondary to amyloidosis in chronic hemodialysis patients. Am J Kidney Dis 7:130-134, 1986, with permission.)

and histomorphometric indices of bone turnover.[390] The use of DEXA as a diagnostic tool in renal osteodystrophy appears to be rather limited, because it is only a measure of bone mineral density and does not provide information regarding bone structure or bone cell activity.

Evaluation of bone by quantitative ultrasonography allows for the assessment of bone elasticity and architecture in addition to bone mineral density. Montagnani and co-workers studied 98 patients on hemodialysis and found that ultrasound parameters were significantly lower in the hemodialysis patients than in control subjects.[390a] Arici and associates[391] performed quantitative ultrasonography in 39 hemodialysis patients and compared the findings with those obtained by DEXA on the same patients. The values obtained by quantitative ultrasonography were markedly reduced in the patients on dialysis compared with control subjects. In addition, there was a significant association between the quantitative ultrasound parameters and the DEXA findings.[391] Although quantitative ultrasonography may have potential applications as a tool in the assessment of renal osteodystrophy, future studies are needed to establish its usefulness in this regard.

Quantitative CT is a technique that evaluates apparent volumetric bone mineral density and can distinguish between the trabecular and cortical components of bone. Spinal quantitative CT has been shown to be useful in detecting bone loss and predicting fracture risk in patients with normal renal function.[392, 393] Lechleitner and co-workers[394] studied 45 patients on hemodialysis and found reduced bone mineral density of the spine assessed with quantitative CT. Follow-up quantitative CT performed in 14 patients 1 year after the initial study revealed no change in trabecular bone of the spine and increased cortical bone mineral density.[394] A recent study using peripheral quantitative CT in 10 women on hemodialysis found that there was decreased bone mineral

density that primarily affected cortical bone.[395] Further evaluation of this technique in patients with renal osteodystrophy is necessary before its clinical application can be established.

HISTOLOGIC FEATURES OF RENAL OSTEODYSTROPHY

Bone biopsy is the gold standard for the classification and diagnosis of renal osteodystrophy. Because it is an invasive technique, it is not in widespread clinical use and considerable efforts have been made to try to find noninvasive, biochemical correlates of bone histology for clinical management. However, if a diagnosis cannot be made with the use of noninvasive parameters, a bone biopsy should be considered. Analysis of the static and dynamic histomorphometric parameters leads to a pathologic classification of renal bone disease. The characteristic features of osteitis fibrosa and adynamic bone are listed in Table 52-2. The dynamic parameters are defined by the administration of tetracycline at intervals separated by 2 to 3 weeks. The tetracycline is rapidly incorporated into bone and can be visualized by microscopy with polarized light, allowing for calculation of the bone formation rate. Normal bone is illustrated in Figure 52-24A (see also Color Plate III).

In states of hyperparathyroidism, the bone formation rate is high, whereas in the low bone turnover disorders, osteomalacia or adynamic bone disease, bone formation is low. The histologic features of hyperparathyroidism or osteitis fibrosa are characterized by increased rate of bone formation, increased bone resorption, extensive osteoclastic and osteoblastic activity, and progressive increase in endosteal peritrabecular fibrosis (see Fig. 52-24B and Color Plate III). High osteoblast activity is manifested by an increase in unmineralized bone matrix. The number of osteoclasts is also increased in osteitis fibrosa, as is the total resorption surface. There may be numerous dissecting cavities through which the osteoclasts tunnel into individual trabeculae. In osteitis fibrosa, the alignment of strands of collagen in the bone matrix has an irregular woven pattern that contrasts with the normal parallel

TABLE 52-2

Histologic Features of Renal Osteodystrophy

Osteitis fibrosa
Increased bone turnover
Increased number of osteoblasts
Increased osteoblastic activity
Increased bone formation rate
Increased osteoid (often woven)
Increased osteoclast number
Increased osteoclast activity
Increased bone resorption
Endosteal fibrosis
Marrow fibrosis

Adynamic bone
Decreased bone turnover
Decreased number of osteoblasts
Decreased osteoblastic activity
Decreased bone formation rate
Normal or decreased osteoid
Decreased number of osteoclasts
Decreased osteoclastic activity

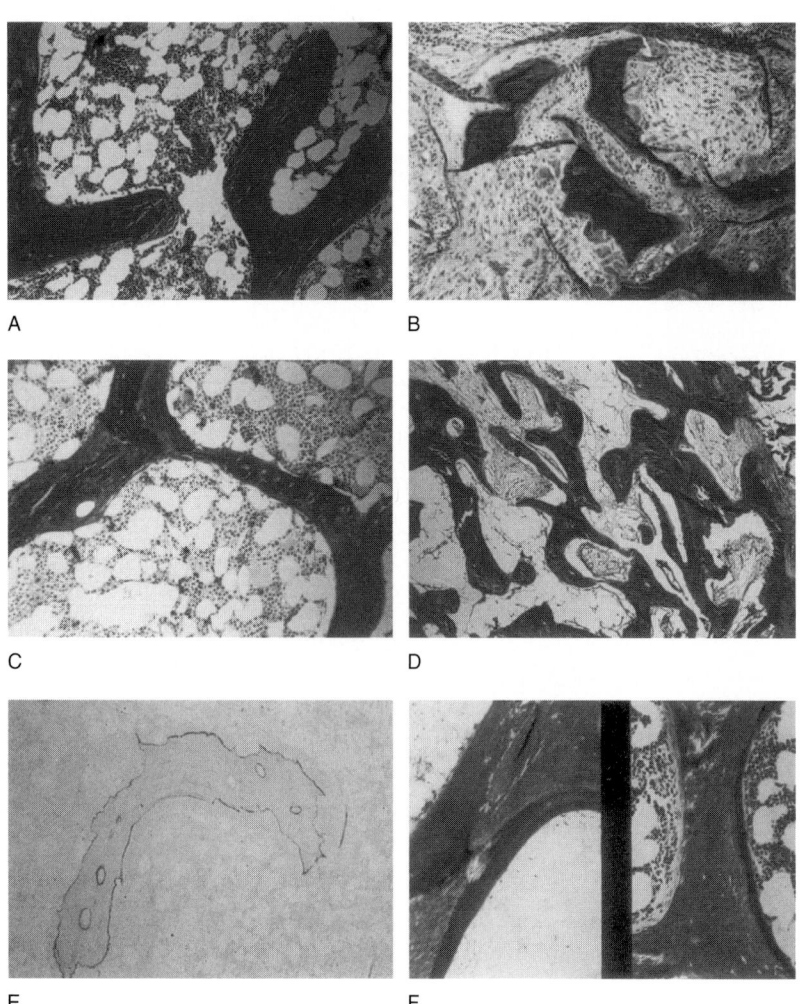

A

B

C

D

E

F

FIGURE 52-24. The characteristic histologic features of renal osteodystrophy. **A,** Normal trabecular bone. Modified Masson stain results in the mineralized matrix staining blue. There is little osteoid present. **B,** Osteitis fibrosa. There is excess osteoid (stained red) lined by osteoblasts surrounding the trabeculae (stained blue). There are numerous multinucleated osteoclasts, and there is marrow fibrosis. **C,** Osteomalacia. There is excess osteoid (stained red) and little osteoblastic activity. **D,** Osteosclerosis. There is loss of distinction between cortical and trabecular bone, and wide osteoid seams are evident. **E,** Staining for aluminum, demonstrating a red band at the junction of the trabecular bone and the wide osteoid seams (the mineralization front). **F,** A higher-power view of the findings in aluminum-induced osteomalacia *(left)* and resolution of the findings after therapy with deferoxamine *(right)*. (**A-D** and **F,** Courtesy of S. L. Teitelbaum, M.D.; **E,** courtesy of D. J. Sherrard, M.D.) (See also Color Plate III.)

alignment of strands of collagen in the lamellar bone. This disorganized collagen structure in woven bone may render the bone physically vulnerable in response to stress.

Osteomalacia is characterized by an excess of unmineralized osteoid, manifested as wide osteoid seams and a markedly decreased mineralization rate (see Fig. 52-24C and Color Plate III). The presence of increased unmineralized osteoid per se does not necessarily indicate a mineralizing defect, because increased quantities of osteoid appear in conditions associated with high rates of bone formation when mineralization lags behind the increased synthesis of matrix. Other features of osteomalacia include the absence of cell activity and the absence of endosteal fibrosis. Special staining for the presence of aluminum can demonstrate that osteomalacic renal bone disease has large deposits of aluminum at the mineralization front—that is, at the interface between trabecular bone and osteoid (see Fig. 52-24E, F and Color Plate III). The degree of osteomalacia correlates closely with bone aluminum content.

Osteosclerosis, illustrated in Figure 52-24D (see also Color Plate III), may be encountered in some biopsy specimens and is manifested by loss of the distinction between cortical and trabecular bone.

Adynamic bone disease is characterized histologically by features similar to those of osteomalacia, with a major difference being the absence of large osteoid seams. Biopsies from patients with adynamic bone disease appear to have markedly deficient cellular activity and decreased number of both osteoblasts and osteoclasts. It appears that this is essentially a disorder of decreased bone formation, accompanied by a secondary decrease in bone mineralization.

Mixed uremic osteodystrophy has features of secondary hyperparathyroidism together with evidence of a mineralization defect. There is more osteoid than expected, and tetracycline labeling uncovers a concomitant mineralization defect.

Recent advances in histologic techniques have demonstrated that additional information may be acquired by supplementing the static and dynamic parameters described with newer techniques, such as in situ hybridization or immunohistochemistry.[195] It is hoped that the application of such work can lead to a new horizon in the analysis of bone cell activity in patients with renal failure.

PREVENTION AND MANAGEMENT OF RENAL OSTEODYSTROPHY

The objectives for the management of abnormal divalent ion metabolism and bone disease in patients with kidney failure are as follows:

1. To maintain the blood levels of calcium and phosphorus as close to normal as possible

2. To prevent the development of parathyroid hyperplasia, or, if secondary hyperparathyroidism has already developed, to suppress the secretion of PTH
3. To prevent extraskeletal deposition of calcium
4. To prevent or reverse the accumulation of substances such as aluminum and iron, which can adversely affect the skeleton

The specific treatment used and the intensity of treatment vary with the stage of kidney insufficiency and with the presence or absence of overt bone disease and cardiovascular calcifications. General guidelines for the management of renal osteodystrophy are summarized in Table 52-3.

Management of Phosphorus

Phosphorus retention in patients with CRF plays a key role in the pathogenesis of secondary hyperparathyroidism, osteitis fibrosa, metastatic calcifications, and calciphylaxis.[242, 282, 396] Studies in experimental renal failure in dogs have shown that restriction of dietary phosphorus in proportion to the decrease in GFR can prevent or reverse secondary hyperparathyroidism independent of the level of serum

TABLE 52-3

Guidelines for the Management of Renal Osteodystrophy

Begin management early in the course of renal disease
Monitor PTH; if elevated, evaluate vitamin D status
    Measure 25(OH)D levels
    Supplement if 25(OH)D is <30 ng/mL
    Ergocalciferol 50,000 U once a week × 4, then once per month
If PTH is elevated and the levels of 25(OH)D are normal, begin dietary phosphate restriction within limits of adequate protein intake
Phosphate binders with meals (maintain serum phosphorus at 3.5-5.5 mg/dL)
    Calcium acetate, calcium carbonate (limit calcium intake to <2 g/day)
    Magnesium carbonate (if no dialysis, may need to decrease dialysate magnesium)
    Sevelamer hydrochloride
    Aluminum-based phosphate binders (monitor for toxicity)
Ensure adequate calcium intake
    If on non–calcium-containing phosphate binder and/or using dialysate calcium of 2.5 mEq/L, give calcium supplement
Treat acidosis
Consider vitamin D sterols
    In chronic renal failure, low-dose calcitriol or alphacalcidol (monitor closely for toxicity)
    If on dialysis, oral or intravenous vitamin D sterols with close monitoring for toxicity
        Calcitriol
        1α-$(OH)D_3$ or 1α-$(OH)D_2$
        Paricalcitol
    Desired range for intact PTH 150-300 pg/mL; preliminary estimates for the range for PTH (1-84) assays are 50-60% lower.
Consider parathyroidectomy for severe hyperparathyroidism with the following:
    Hypercalcemia
    Persistent hyperphosphatemia
    Failure to respond to therapy with vitamin D sterols and phosphate binders
    Persistently elevated calcium-phosphate product leading to metastatic calcification
    Transplantation candidate with living related donor
    Calciphylaxis

PTH, parathyroid hormone.

calcium and $1,25$-$(OH)_2D_3$.[16, 22] Therefore, control of dietary phosphate absorption during the course of chronic kidney disease is essential for the prevention of the above-described abnormalities.

The dietary intake of phosphorus depends primarily on the intake of meat and dairy products. The dietary phosphorus intake can be lowered in proportion to the decrease in GFR in patients with mild renal insufficiency. Dietary phosphorous intake can be reduced by restricting the intake of dairy products and by rigid adherence to a low-phosphate diet. In patients with advanced chronic kidney disease or ESRD, it is very difficult to lower phosphorus intake in proportion to the reduced GFR simply by dietary manipulation. The new Kidney Disease Outcome Quality Initiative (K/DOQI) recommendations suggest 1.2 g of protein per kilogram of body weight for patients maintained on hemodialysis and 1.4 g for patients maintained on continuous ambulatory peritoneal dialysis. Such protein intake makes it difficult to restrict the amount of phosphorus in the diet to less than 1200 mg/day. Because 60% to 70% of phosphorus is absorbed, approximately 5000 mg of phosphorus per week enters the extracellular fluid. Most hemodialysis patients are dialyzed three times per week, with roughly 800 mg of phosphorus removed per treatment.[397] Therefore, most well-nourished patients are in positive phosphorus balance, approximately 300 to 500 mg/day on the average. Consequently, more than 90% of dialysis patients use phosphate binders to reduce the amount of phosphorus absorbed and achieve a normal serum phosphorus concentration (3.5 to 4.5 mg/dL or 1.2 to 1.5 mM/L). Recent data from studies by Mucsi and associates[398] showed that not only do patients on nocturnal dialysis (6- to 8-hour sessions, 6 to 7 nights per week) require no phosphate binders, but phosphorus must be added to the dialysate or the ingestion of phosphate must be increased to prevent the development of hypophosphatemia.

In the 1960s and 1970s, the most commonly used phosphate binder contained aluminum; in the 1980s and 1990s, aluminum was replaced by calcium. Aluminum causes neurologic, skeletal, and hematologic toxicity in ESRD patients, whereas calcium can lead to hypercalcemia in some patients and to soft tissue and cardiovascular calcification. In the past 10 years, numerous publications have shown an increase in the vascular tree and mitral and aortic valve calcifications in patients with ESRD receiving calcium salts as phosphate binders.[244, 399, 400] Similarly, significantly stiffness of the arterial wall has been demonstrated as a complication in patients receiving large amounts of calcium salts.[401, 402]

Block and collaborators[242, 282] demonstrated that the Ca × P value and the serum phosphorus concentration are associated with increased mortality. Until recently, it was accepted that a Ca × P of 70 mg^2/dL^2 was a relatively safe level, but these authors demonstrated increased mortality when the Ca × P exceeded 60 mg^2/dL^2. When the Ca × P was greater than 70 mg^2/dL^2, mortality was increased by 35%. Therefore, it is critical to control serum phosphorus within the range of 3.5 to 5.5 mg/dL and to attempt to maintain a Ca × P of less than 55 mg^2/dL^2. At the same time, it is important that the total amount of calcium ingested by the patient (dietary calcium plus calcium-containing phosphate binders) is no greater than 2 g/day, because high calcium intake has been associated with cardiovascular complications.[403, 404]

Aluminum as a Phosphate Binder

Aluminum-containing compounds that bind phosphorus in the intestinal tract include aluminum hydroxide and aluminum carbonate gels, which are available in liquid, tablet, or capsule form. Capsules are less effective than liquid gels in binding phosphorus, but patient compliance is easier to achieve with capsules than with either the liquid or the tablets. However, as described previously, the use of large amounts of aluminum for long periods is associated with significant pathology. For example, osteomalacia is a frequent complication of this treatment because aluminum deposits at the mineralization front in the skeleton and prevents the normal calcification of osteoid tissue. In addition, aluminum may affect the central nervous system, causing varying degrees of encephalopathy. The hematologic system is also affected, and aluminum intoxication is usually accompanied by microcytic anemia. It is also critical to emphasize that citrate greatly increases the absorption of aluminum in the small intestine.[405-407] Citric acid, which is present in a number of fruits, also increases the absorption of aluminum. The serum aluminum level in dialysis patients should be less than 20 µg/L.

Calcium Carbonate as a Phosphate Binder

It has been shown that calcium carbonate can reduce the intestinal absorption of phosphate. Clarkson and co-workers[408] reported decreased absorption of phosphorus in the gastrointestinal tract in patients whose calcium carbonate ingestion was high. Subsequently, many investigators have demonstrated the effectiveness of calcium carbonate as a phosphate binder.[409-419] Transient episodes of hypercalcemia have frequently been observed during therapy with calcium carbonate, and the administration of large amounts of calcium carbonate could increase the risk of hypercalcemia and extraskeletal cardiovascular calcification.

In the United States, most patients undergo hemodialysis with dialysate containing 2.5 mEq/L of calcium, and some use dialysate containing 3.0 mEq/L of calcium. Several investigators have attempted to decrease the incidence of hypercalcemic episodes by reducing the amount of calcium in the dialysate. Slatopolsky and associates[417] evaluated the effect of the long-term administration of calcium carbonate (mean dose, 10.5 g/day, range, 2.5 to 18 g/day) in conjunction with a dialysate with reduced calcium (2.5 mEq/L) in the management of hyperphosphatemia in 20 patients undergoing maintenance hemodialysis. They confirmed the effectiveness of calcium carbonate as a phosphate binder. Moreover, the development of hypercalcemia was minimized by reducing the calcium concentration of the dialysate from 3.25 to 2.5 mEq/L. It is important to emphasize that when patients use a dialysate concentration of 2.5 mEq/L and do not ingest additional calcium or receive calcitriol, hypocalcemia may develop and may result in progressive secondary hyperparathyroidism. Therefore, the use of such a dialysate should be restricted to patients who demonstrate compliance with ingestion of the prescribed doses of calcium.

If calcium carbonate is prescribed as a phosphate binder it must be ingested with the meal, both to increase its efficiency as a phosphate binder and to minimize the absorption of calcium and the risk of hypercalcemia. It is recommended that a dietitian determine the total amount of phosphorus ingested over a 24-hour period and at each individual meal, because there is both individual and meal-to-meal variability in any given patient. To prevent the development of hypercalcemia, it is important that the amount of calcium carbonate prescribed be in proportion to the amount of phosphorus ingested at each meal.

Calcium Acetate as a Phosphate Binder

Sheik and coworkers[420] demonstrated that calcium acetate may bind phosphorus more efficiently than calcium carbonate or calcium citrate. They found that calcium acetate bound 1.04 ± 0.2 mg of phosphorus per milligram of calcium absorbed, which was better than either calcium carbonate (0.57 ± 0.5 mg/mg calcium absorbed) or calcium citrate (0.47 ± .05 mg/mg calcium absorbed). In a crossover study, Delmez and colleagues[421] investigated the effects of calcium carbonate and calcium acetate in a group of 20 patients maintained on hemodialysis. They found that calcium acetate allowed control of PTH, calcium, and phosphorus levels similar to that achieved with calcium carbonate, but with only half the amount of elemental calcium ingested in the form of calcium acetate (349 ± 25 versus 699 ± 75 mmol/day; $P < .001$). However, the overall incidence of hypercalcemia was the same with each formulation. Calcium acetate is soluble in both alkaline and acid media, and its solubility is not pH dependent. On the other hand, calcium carbonate dissolves only in acid media, and proton pump inhibitors or H_2-receptor antagonists may limit its efficiency.

Calcium Citrate as a Phosphate Binder

Calcium citrate has also been shown to be an effective phosphate-binding agent, but it increases aluminum absorption.[422] Therefore, calcium citrate should not be given to patients with renal failure, especially if there is a possibility that they may also ingest aluminum-containing drugs.

Magnesium as a Phosphate Binder

Another phosphate-binding agent, magnesium hydroxide, was reported to be of benefit by several investigators.[423-426] Delmez and colleagues[427] performed a prospective, randomized, crossover study to evaluate whether the chronic use of $MgCO_3$ would allow for a reduction in the dose of calcium carbonate ($CaCO_3$). They compared the use of $MgCO_3$ combined with half the usual dose of $CaCO_3$, versus $CaCO_3$ alone given in the usual dose. The administration of $MgCO_3$ (465 ± 52 mg of elemental Mg) allowed for a decrease in the amount of elemental Ca ingested from 2.9 ± 0.4 to 1.2 ± 0.2 g/day ($P < .0001$). If these studies are confirmed, the use of $MgCO_3$ may be considered in selected patients who are prone to development of hypercalcemia during treatment with vitamin D compounds and calcium salts. It should be pointed out that the magnesium concentration in the dialysate should be lowered (0.6 mg/dL) while magnesium-containing phosphate binders are administered, so that hypermagnesemia is prevented.

Sevelamer Hydrochloride as a Phosphate Binder

Recently, new phosphate binders have been developed. One of them, sevelamer hydrochloride (Renagel) is now widely available.[428] This phosphate binder is completely resistant to intestinal digestion and is not absorbed in the gastrointestinal tract. Studies have shown that this agent can effectively and safely lower the serum phosphate concentration without changing the serum calcium level (Fig. 52-25).[429] Long-term studies have shown a decrease in low-density lipoprotein and an increase in high-density lipoprotein cholesterol in patients treated with sevelamer (Fig. 52-26).[429] The mechanism may be similar to that of cholestyramine (i.e., binding of bile salts). Recently, Chertow and colleagues[404] published the results of a multicenter study performed in Europe and the United States comparing the effects of sevelamer versus calcium carbonate or calcium acetate on calcifications affecting the cardiovascular system. The study population was divided into two groups with 50 to 55 patients in each group. One group received sevelamer, and the other received calcium salts (calcium carbonate or calcium acetate) for a period of 52 weeks. The calcium content in coronary arteries and aorta was assessed by EBCT. Both calcium salts and sevelamer controlled Ca × P, but patients receiving calcium salts became hypercalcemic more

frequently (16%, compared with 5% in the sevelamer-treated group). More importantly, EBCT at study completion demonstrated that the increase in mean calcium score in coronary arteries and aorta was greater in the subjects treated with calcium than in those treated with sevelamer (Fig. 52-27). This study strongly suggests that calcium load is an important factor associated with vascular calcification. Because cardiovascular mortality in dialysis patients is 50% to 60%, alterations in mineral metabolism are critical, as are inflammatory processes, hypertension, and alterations in lipid metabolism. The control of phosphorus is crucial; not only do increases in Ca × P increase soft tissue calcification but, as discussed earlier, phosphorus per se increases the expression of transcription factor Cbfa-1.[251] This factor has been shown to induce the differentiation of arterial smooth muscle cells into osteoblast-like cells that secrete osteocalcin, thus promoting the process of calcification (see Fig. 52-15).

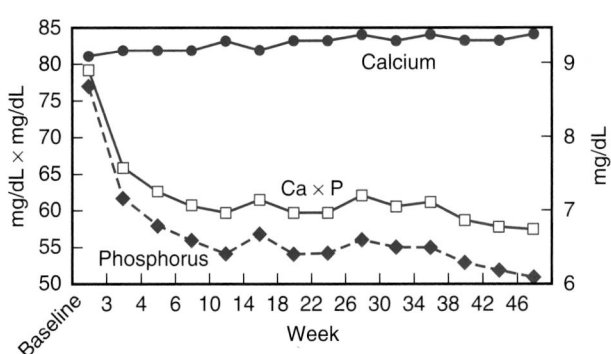

FIGURE 52-25. Long-term effect of sevelamer hydrochloride on the levels of serum calcium and phosphorus and the calcium-phosphate product in patients on hemodialysis. (Modified from Chertow GM, Burke SK, Dillon MA, Slatopolsky E: Long-term effects of sevelamer hydrochloride on the calcium × phosphate product and lipid profile of haemodialysis patients. Nephrol Dial Transplant 14:2907-2914, 1999, with permission.)

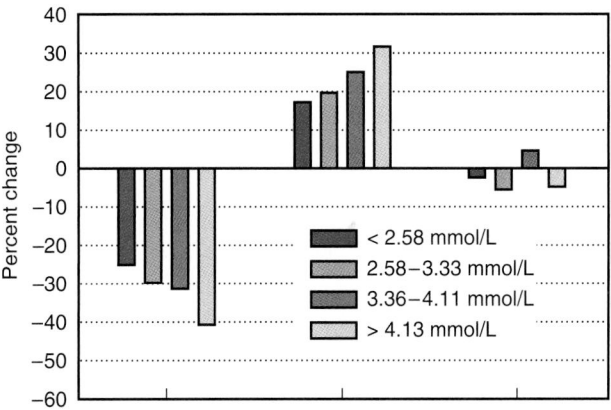

FIGURE 52-26. The effect of sevelamer hydrochloride on serum lipids. Shown from left to right are the percent changes in the levels of low-density lipoprotein (LDL) cholesterol, high-density lipoprotein (HDL) cholesterol, and triglycerides in patients on hemodialysis, stratified by initial LDL concentration. (From Chertow GM, Burke SK, Dillon MA, Slatopolsky E: Long-term effects of sevelamer hydrochloride on the calcium × phosphate product and lipid profile of haemodialysis patients. Nephrol Dial Transplant 14:2907-2914, 1999, with permission.)

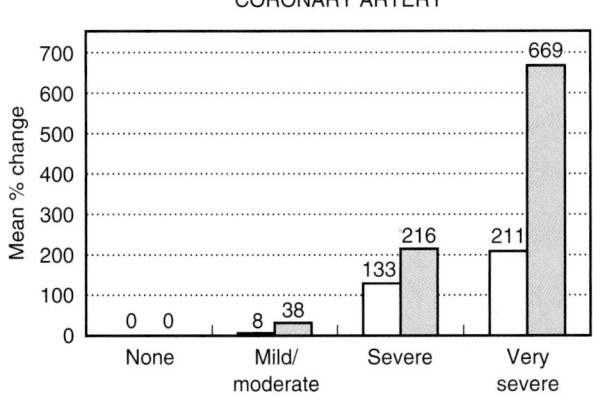

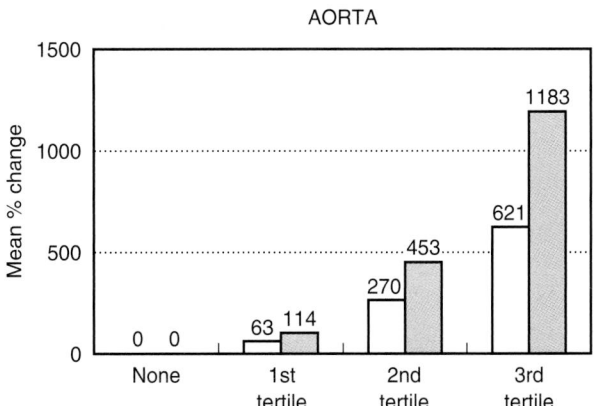

FIGURE 52-27. The change in coronary artery and aortic calcification scores as determined by electron-beam computed tomography (EBCT) in patients on hemodialysis treated with calcium acetate *(shaded bars)* or sevelamer hydrochloride *(open bars)*. The increase in calcification was greater in the calcium-treated patients regardless of whether the initial calcification was mild/moderate, severe, or very severe. (From Chertow GM, Burke SK, Raggi P: Sevelamer attenuates the progression of coronary and aortic calcification in hemodialysis patients. Kidney Int 62:245-252, 2002, with permission.)

Lanthanum Carbonate as a Phosphate Binder

Lanthanum carbonate is a trivalent cation that binds phosphate at all pH levels to form lanthanum phosphate, which is insoluble. Hutchison[430] demonstrated that the phosphate-binding capacity of lanthanum is similar to that of aluminum in vitro. Studies in patients maintained on hemodialysis or continuous ambulatory peritoneal dialysis demonstrated that lanthanum carbonate can reduce serum phosphate to approximately 5.0 mg/dL. However, significant concentrations of lanthanum (0.1 to 0.8 ng/L) were found in blood. Further long-term studies in dialysis patients are necessary to determine the potential toxic effects of lanthanum accumulation.

Goals of Therapy

The goal of therapy with phosphate binders is to reduce serum phosphorus to normal or near-normal levels. The acceptable predialysis level for serum phosphorus is 3.5 to 5.5 mg/dL (ideally, 3.5 to 4.5 mg/dL). In patients with creatinine clearances lower than 30 mL/min, dietary phosphorus should be restricted to approximately 800 mg/day. Serum phosphorus should be monitored at least once a month to permit appropriate dosage adjustment. If the serum phosphorus level drops below 3.5 mg/dL or stays above the desired range, the dose of phospate binders should be decreased or increased, respectively.

The fall in serum phosphorus that occurs with dietary phosphorus restriction and treatment with phosphate binders is sometimes associated with a rise in serum calcium. If this rise is adequate, blood levels of iPTH often decrease. Such a fall in serum iPTH can allow for better maintenance of normal serum phosphorus levels, because high PTH levels contribute to elevated serum phosphorus concentrations in uremic patients by increasing mobilization from bone.

To prevent phosphate depletion, it is important to keep the serum phosphate from falling below normal levels. Some uremic patients (fewer than 10%) do not require phosphate-binding agents, and overzealous use of phosphate binders can produce hypophosphatemia and phosphate depletion, which can aggravate bone disease and even lead to osteomalacia.

Management of Calcium

Dietary Calcium Supplements

Impaired calcium absorption exists in patients with advanced renal failure, including those undergoing dialysis, and their diets generally contain suboptimal quantities of calcium. Oral calcium supplements are usually necessary in such patients. The dietary intake of calcium usually ranges from 400 to 600 mg/day. Studies of net intestinal calcium absorption suggest that a natural or positive calcium balance can be achieved in uremic patients if calcium carbonate, calcium citrate, or calcium acetate is added to increase the total intake to approximately 1.5 g of elemental calcium per day.

The time at which calcium supplements should be added during the course of chronic kidney disease is uncertain. Coburn and colleagues[431] found normal intestinal calcium absorption in patients with serum creatinine levels lower than 2.5 mg/dL, whereas Werner and colleagues[432] found reduced intestinal calcium absorption in patients with GFRs

of 20 to 50 mL/min. Patients with advanced renal failure who are given dietary supplements of calcium may be more likely to develop hypercalcemia than normal persons, because they lack the mechanisms for increased urinary calcium excretion if calcium absorption increases more than expected.

Treatment with oral calcium supplements is not without risk. Calcium supplements should be given cautiously to patients with marked hyperphosphatemia because of the risk of increasing $Ca \times P$ and predisposing the patient to extraskeletal and cardiovascular calcifications. Hypercalcemia is more common in patients whose serum phosphorus levels are decreased to less than 2 to 3 mg/dL. Most uremic patients with moderate to advanced kidney failure and mild hypercalcemia are asymptomatic. However, these patients can develop pruritus and an acute increase in blood pressure associated with hypercalcemia, in addition to the more common symptoms of nausea, anorexia, vomiting, mental confusion, and lethargy.

In patients with advanced renal failure who have creatinine clearances lower than 10 mL/min and in patients undergoing regular dialysis, calcium supplementation may be recommended to provide a maximum of 1.5 g of elemental calcium per day. The calcium supplements should be taken in several small doses throughout the day, rather than in one or two large doses. Also, ingestion of calcium supplements with meals that are high in phosphate should be limited if the goal is to augment intestinal absorption of calcium rather than to bind calcium phosphate in the intestine. The monitoring of serum calcium and phosphorus at biweekly or monthly intervals is important because of the variability in response of individual patients to a given amount of calcium. If the serum calcium levels exceed the upper limit of normal, the amount of supplemental calcium should be discontinued.

Dialysate Calcium Concentration

The level of calcium in the dialysate can affect serum calcium levels in patients treated with maintenance hemodialysis. Predialysis iPTH levels vary inversely with plasma calcium levels in dialysis patients who use a dialysate with a calcium concentration lower than 3.0 mEq/L for longer than 6 months. From this information, it was generally recommended in the past that the dialysate calcium concentration be 3.0 to 3.5 mEq/L. However, these data were obtained from patients who ingested aluminum-containing phosphate-binding agents. In uremic patients who use calcium carbonate or acetate as a phosphate binder or who use vitamin D preparations, there is considerable risk of hypercalcemia with the use of dialysate containing calcium concentrations between 3.0 and 3.5 mEq/L. Studies have shown that use of a dialysate with a calcium concentration of 2.5 mEq/L is safe in patients who are taking calcium salts and vitamin D compounds.[433]

Use of Vitamin D Sterols

As discussed earlier, decreases in calcitriol production play a major role in the generation and maintenance of secondary hyperparathyroidism and, accordingly, the use of vitamin D sterols is a rational approach to its treatment. Because hyperparathyroidism begins relatively early in the course of chronic kidney disease, it is important to assess patients for vitamin D deficiency. Relatively large amounts of vitamin D–binding protein may be lost in the urine of proteinuric patients, and this, coupled with poor dietary intake and lack of exposure to sunlight, may result in vitamin D deficiency. The overall vitamin D status is best assessed with measurements of 25-hydroxyvitamin D; if values are found to be less than 30 ng/mL, supplementation should be undertaken. Although it would be desirable to administer vitamin D, such as ergocalciferol, at a dose of 1000 to 2000 U/day, such preparations are not readily available in the United States; accordingly, a reasonable dose would be 50,000 U taken once a month.

As chronic kidney disease progresses, hyperparathyroidism becomes more severe despite efforts to control phosphorus, and the use of active vitamin D sterols has a role as part of the treatment regimen, if toxicity can be avoided. The occurrence of hypercalcemia or aggravation of hyperphosphatemia (or both) by the use of active vitamin D sterols may well be detrimental to residual renal function, so these drugs should be used with caution and monitored closely. Several investigators have indicated that these active vitamin D sterols can be used safely, and it is desirable to restrict the dosage of calcitriol or α-calcidol to 0.25 to 0.50 μg/day.[434, 435] In patients who require dialysis, because monitoring of calcium, phosphate, and PTH can be accomplished with increased frequency, active vitamin D sterols can be used effectively to control hyperparathyroidism. Several vitamin D sterols have been used in this regard, such as calcitriol, the synthetic prohormones 1-α-hydroxyvitamin D_3 and 1-α-hydroxyvitamin D_2, and, more recently, vitamin D analogs that offer the potential of lesser toxicity.

Use of Calcitriol

Calcitriol, 1,25-dihydroxyvitamin D_3, is the most active metabolite of vitamin D and has been demonstrated to have direct effects on the parathyroid gland by suppressing the synthesis and secretion of PTH and by limiting parathyroid cell growth. Calcitriol has been administered orally or intravenously for the treatment of secondary hyperparathyroidism. In the United States, the majority of use is by intravenous injection, and its efficacy in suppressing PTH in patients with secondary hyperparathyroidism has been well established. The principal toxicities of calcitriol result from its potent effects of increasing intestinal absorption of calcium and phosphate and its potential to mobilize calcium and phosphate from bone. Hypercalcemia, hyperphosphatemia, or both is a common complication of such therapy that may limit its use at doses that effectively suppress PTH levels. The hypercalcemic toxicity of calcitriol is aggravated by the concomitant use of large doses of calcium-containing phosphate-binding antacids. The advent of non–calcium-containing phosphate binders may facilitate the use of vitamin D sterols in this patient group.

Although in the United States most calcitriol therapy is administered by intermittent intravenous injection, oral therapy can also be used, and some investigators have administered oral calcitriol in an intermittent fashion (oral pulse) with good results.[436, 437] Such a regimen is especially useful for patients on peritoneal dialysis. Several investigators have examined the relative efficacy of oral and intravenous calcitriol, and although both decrease the levels of PTH in

general, it appears that intravenous administration is somewhat more effective and may have lesser toxicity.[438, 439] Calcitriol has also been administered by the intraperitoneal route in patients on peritoneal dialysis, with good clinical effect.[440]

Vitamin D Prohormones

1-α-Hydroxyvitamin D_3, or α-calcidol, is widely used outside the United States for the control of hyperparathyroidism. This vitamin D sterol becomes hydroxylated in the 25 position by the hepatic 25-hydroxylase, resulting in the production of 1,25-dihydroxyvitamin D_3. This sterol has been shown to be active in patients with chronic kidney disease, and it has been used both orally and intravenously with good clinical effect, similar to that of calcitriol. α-Calcidol has also been used for patients in the early phases of chronic kidney disease, and it appears to have been successful in the prevention of bone disease in this patient group.

1-α-Hydroxyvitamin D_2 is a similar prohormone based on the vitamin D_2 structure, which also requires hydroxylation in the 25 position in the liver before it becomes an active vitamin D sterol. In experimental animals, this vitamin D sterol was shown to be less toxic than its vitamin D_3 counterpart when administered at high doses.[441] The mechanism of this decrease in toxicity is not understood, because the stimulation of calcium transport and phosphate transport by 1-α-hydroxyvitamin D_2 is not different from that of its D_3 counterpart.[441, 442] However, at high doses there may be metabolism to 1,24-dihydroxyvitamin D_2, which appears to have lower calcemic activity compared with calcitriol.[443, 444] In therapeutic doses, there appears to be little evidence that this sterol is less calcemic or phosphatemic than its vitamin D_3 counterpart. 1-α-Hydroxyvitamin D_2 has been approved for the treatment of secondary hyperparathyroidism and has been used in both oral and intravenous forms.[438, 445] PTH levels are lowered effectively with 1-α-hydroxyvitamin D_2, and intravenous administration appears to be associated with lesser increases in serum calcium and phosphate than is the oral administration.[438] Hypercalcemia and hyperphosphatemia were encountered in a significant proportion of the blood samples obtained during this clinical trial, and there appeared to be a more frequent occurrence of these complications with oral administration.[438]

Vitamin D Analogs

In an effort to utilize the effects of vitamin D on the parathyroid gland and to minimize the toxicities of such therapy, structural alterations of the vitamin D molecule were undertaken to develop vitamin D analogs that retain the effects on the parathyroid but have lesser effects on calcium and phosphate metabolism. Such analogs would be relatively selective for parathyroid effects and would therefore be more useful therapeutic agents. There is substantial evidence that structural alterations of the vitamin D molecule can result in some selectivity of action in various test systems in vitro, such that the calcemic and phosphatemic effects of the sterol can be dissociated from the other effects of vitamin D on many cellular functions. Currently, there is substantial experimental and clinical evidence for the efficacy of three such vitamin D analogs, which have been approved for the treatment of secondary hyperparathyroidism. These are

22-oxa-1-α, 25-dihydroxyvitamin D₃   1-α, 25-dihydroxyvitamin D₃   19-nor-1-α, 25-dihydroxyvitamin D₃

26,27-F₆,1-α, 25-dihydroxyvitamin D₃   1-α, hydroxyvitamin D₃   1-α, hydroxyvitamin D₂

FIGURE 52-28. The structure of vitamin D sterols used for the management of secondary hyperparathyroidism in renal failure. Structural differences from calcitriol are shown in the shaded areas.

19-nor-1,25-dihydroxyvitamin D_2, 22-oxacalcitriol (OCT), and falecalcitriol. The structure of these sterols is shown in Figure 52-28.

22-OXACALCITRIOL

OCT differs from calcitriol by the substitution of an oxygen at the 22 position. This structural modification appears to reduce the affinity of OCT for the vitamin D receptor, as well as for vitamin D–binding protein. Decreased affinity for vitamin D–binding protein results in rapid clearance from the circulation and this may be a mechanism to account for the relatively low calcemic and phosphatemic effects of OCT.[446-448] When administered in vivo, this vitamin D sterol is effective in decreasing PTH secretion, an effect that is maintained for a long period. The mechanism for the differences in duration of effect in the parathyroid glands, compared with intestine and bone, are not understood at the present time. Studies in animal models with experimental renal failure demonstrated the efficacy of OCT in suppressing PTH with minimal changes in serum calcium and found this agent to be clearly less calcemic than calcitriol.[449] This vitamin D analog was also successful in reversing abnormalities in bone formation, including the appearance of woven osteoid and fibrosis, and bone turnover did not appear to change.[450, 451] This vitamin D analog is now available and used in Japan.

19-NOR-1,25-DIHYDROXYVITAMIN D₂

19-Nor-1,25-dihydroxyvitamin D_2, or paricalcitol, which lacks the exocyclic carbon at position 19, has been studied extensively and has been demonstrated to suppress PTH secretion in vitro as potently as calcitriol does. Studies in experimental animals have shown that this vitamin D analog is effective in suppressing PTH levels with markedly less hypercalcemia and hyperphosphatemia than occurs with calcitriol. Indeed, paricalcitol is approximately 10 times less active than calcitriol in mobilizing calcium or phosphate from bone (Fig. 52-29).[452]

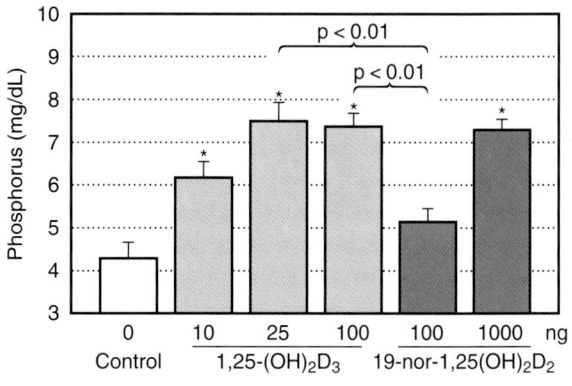

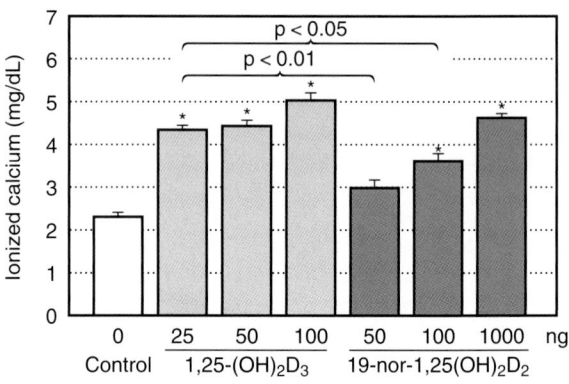

* = p < 0.01 vs. control

FIGURE 52-29. Comparison of the effects of 1,25-(OH)₂D₃ and 19-nor-1,25-(OH)₂D₂ on the levels of serum phosphorus *(top panel)* and serum calcium *(bottom panel).* A 10-fold greater dose of 19-nor-1,25-(OH)₂D₂ was required to achieve the same increment in calcium or phosphorus as occurred with 1,25-(OH)₂D₃. (From Finch JL, Brown AJ, Slatopolsky E: Differential effects of 1,25-dihydroxy-vitamin D3 and 19-nor-1,25-dihydroxy-vitamin D2 on calcium and phosphorus resorption in bone. J Am Soc Nephrol 10:980-985, 1999, with permission.)

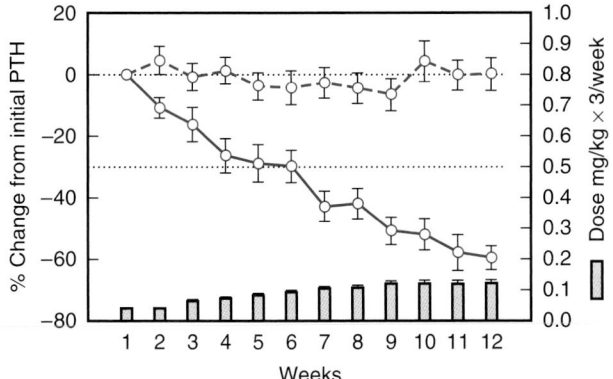

FIGURE 52-30. The effect of 19-nor-1,25-(OH)$_2$D$_2$ administered intravenously three times per week *(solid line)*, compared with placebo *(dashed line)*, on the levels of intact parathyroid hormone (PTH) in patients on hemodialysis. (From Martin KJ, González EA, Gellens M, et al: 19-Nor-1-a-25-dihydroxyvitamin D$_2$ [paricalcitol] safely and effectively reduces the levels of intact PTH in patients on hemodialysis. J Am Soc Nephrol 9:1427-1432, 1998, with permission.)

In addition, the vitamin D receptor did not appear to be up-regulated in the intestine of these experimental animals, in contrast to the effects seen with calcitriol. This vitamin D analog is in widespread clinical use among patients on hemodialysis in the United States, and it has been demonstrated to be very effective in suppressing PTH levels (Fig. 52-30).[453-455] Although paricalcitol has less calcemic potential than calcitriol, hypercalcemia can still occur during therapy, and it appears to occur when PTH is suppressed markedly to levels that are considered to be at or below the desired target range, which is consistent with overtreatment.[456] With increasing experience in its use and frequent monitoring of PTH levels, these toxicities can be minimized.

The mechanism of the lesser calcemic and phosphatemic effects of paricalcitol has not been defined at the present time. Studies in patients demonstrate that the findings in experimental animals of PTH suppression, as well as less calcemic and phosphatemic effects, appear to be reasonably concordant. Therefore, although three times more paricalcitol than calcitriol is required to achieve equivalent suppression of PTH in animals, studies in patients indicate that a ratio of 3 to 4 is required.[454, 456] Similarly, whereas paricalcitol is 10 times less calcemic and phosphatemic than calcitriol in animals, studies in patients with ESRD on a very low-calcium diet, have shown that at least 8 times more paricalcitol is required to achieve a similar increment in serum calcium, presumably representing mobilization of calcium from bone.[457] Finally, Sprague and colleagues[455] were able to demonstrate less severe hyperphosphatemia in patients treated with paricalcitol compared with calcitriol. Importantly, recent studies indicate a 16% decrease in mortality among patients treated with paricalcitol compared with calcitriol.[458] The exact mechanism for this effect is not clear at the present time.

OTHER ANALOGS

Falecalcitriol is an analog in which the hydrogens at carbon 26 and 27 have been substituted with fluorine atoms. This vitamin D analog has greater activity than calcitriol and is considerably more calcemic and more potent in calcifying epiphyseal cartilage in rats.[459] The increased potency is probably a result of the decreased metabolism of this sterol. In patients with CRF, falecalcitriol was effective in decreasing PTH and appeared to be somewhat more effective than α-calcidol in suppressing hyperparathyroidism.[460] This sterol is available for use in Asia. Other vitamin D analogs are currently under investigation for the treatment of hyperparathyroidism as well as for a variety of other applications in skeletal and nonskeletal disorders.

Parathyroidectomy

Surgical removal of parathyroid tissue should be considered for patients with severe hyperparathyroidism manifested by very high levels of PTH (e.g., intact PTH >800 pg/mL), who have hypercalcemia and/or hyperphosphatemia or an elevated Ca × P that is resistant to or precludes medical therapy. Several surgical procedures have been described, including subtotal parathyroidectomy, subtotal parathyroidectomy with parathyroid tissue autotransplantation, and total parathyroidectomy. If autotransplantation is undertaken, it is advisable to avoid nodular areas of the gland and to use the smallest gland.[461-464] This is to avoid excessive proliferation of the parathyroid cells, which may lead to parathyromatosis. The use of stereomicroscopic techniques may be of value in tissue selection.[461, 462] All of these approaches result in satisfactory reductions in PTH.

Total parathyroidectomy is not widely used and is not recommended for patients who might undergo renal transplantation. There is a risk of inducing a low bone turnover state if total parathyroidectomy is achieved. However, in the studies of Kaye and Ljutic and their colleagues, total removal of all PTH-producing tissue was uncommon.[465, 466] If total parathyroidectomy is attempted, it is advisable to cryopreserve parathyroid tissue so that it may be reimplanted if necessary. Persistent hyperparathyroidism after surgery is probably due to a missed gland, which has been reported in 8% to 25% of cases.[467-469] Preoperative imaging of parathyroids by technetium 99m-sestamibi, CT, MRI, or ultrasonography is not routinely performed by most surgeons and is usually reserved for reoperation.

Even after initially successful surgery, the recurrence of hyperparathyroidism may be 20% to 30% after 5 years.[470, 471] Postoperatively, it is imperative to monitor the levels of calcium closely (e.g., every 6 hours for a few days), and a calcium infusion should be given, if necessary, to maintain the levels of ionized calcium between 1.1 and 1.3 mM. Patients may require high doses of oral calcium supplementation (up to 4 g of elemental calcium or higher per day). Calcitriol should be continued either orally or intravenously, and up to 5 μg/day may be required to normalize serum calcium. Phosphate supplementation may be necessary if hypophosphatemia occurs.

Nonsurgical Parathyroid Ablation

A minimally invasive approach to parathyroid ablation has been pioneered by investigators from Japan using percutaneous injection of ethanol into parathyroid tissue localized by high-resolution ultrasound with color Doppler (known as percutaneous ethanol injection therapy, or PEIT).[472, 473] The reduction in functioning parathyroid tissue by this technique appears to be satisfactory and allows control of residual parathyroid activity with standard therapy. The recurrence rate and long-term follow-up results have been described for only small numbers of patients, and the consequences of the ethanol injection (e.g., fibrosis) are not well defined should parathyroid surgery become necessary later.

Integrated Management of Renal Osteodystrophy

Based on the pathophysiologic principles outlined previously, it is clear that hyperparathyroidism begins early in the course of renal insufficiency, and, accordingly, monitoring of parathyroid activity should begin when the GFR is initially decreased (Fig. 52-31). If PTH levels are elevated, it is reasonable to evaluate vitamin D status by measurement of 25-hydroxyvitamin D levels; if the result is less than 30 ng/mL, vitamin D supplementation should be prescribed to provide 1000 to 2000 U/day or 50,000 units once a month. The degree of elevation in PTH before active therapy is begun and the lower limit of PTH that is desired are somewhat uncertain in early to moderate renal insufficiency. It seems reasonable that, at a GFR of 50 to 80 mL/min, a target range from the upper half of the normal range to 50% above the upper limit of normal in the intact PTH assay would be appropriate. Values above this range should be treated to prevent parathyroid growth. After vitamin D status is demonstrated to be adequate, dietary phosphorus restriction should be instituted, and the effect on PTH levels should be monitored. If this does not result in a satisfactory decrease in PTH, phosphate binders should be prescribed with meals, and the resultant effect on PTH should be monitored. Initially, calcium-containing salts (e.g., 1.5 g of elemental calcium per day) can be used because the calcium load can be handled by the kidneys, but if large doses are required, consideration should be given to non–calcium-containing phosphate binders. If acidosis is present, it should be treated with sodium bicarbonate. If PTH levels remain elevated despite these measures, the use of vitamin D sterols should be considered. Calcitriol or 1-α-hydroxyvitamin D_3 may be used in initial doses of 0.25 to 0.5 µg/day, respectively, with the patient monitored closely for hypercalcemia. Increased doses should be used with appropriate

caution, and dosing two to three times per week may be considered. As renal failure advances, these measures need to be intensified. PTH values may be tolerated up to twice the upper limit of normal as GFR becomes less that 20 mL/min.

Considerably more data are available for the management of patients once dialysis is required. In this situation, consideration should be given to the use of higher doses of vitamin D sterols, because monitoring is easier in the dialysis setting. Adequate control of serum levels of phosphorus continues to be of paramount importance, and every effort should be made to achieve predialysis values no higher than 5.5.mg/dL, with calcium values in the lower half of the normal range if possible. Target values for PTH are now believed to range from 150 to 300 pg/mL in the intact PTH assay and 30% to 50% lower than this when using assays that are specific for PTH (1-84). Ongoing investigations of correlations of PTH values with bone biopsy will refine these targets as more information becomes available. Consideration should be given to the choice of dialysate calcium in light of the total calcium intake of the patient. In the future, there is hope that a new class of agents, the calcimimetics, may offer an additional approach to the control of hyperparathyroidism and parathyroid growth.[474]

With regard to the prevention and management of aluminum-related bone disease, it is important to avoid aluminum exposure. The water used for dialysis should be monitored for aluminum content, and aluminum-containing phosphate binders as well as citrate-containing compounds should be avoided.[405, 422] In patients with severe hyperparathyroidism and significant aluminum accumulation in bone, aluminum removal should be considered before parathyroidectomy, because aluminum accumulation may increase rapidly after removal of the parathyroid glands.[475] Chelation therapy with deferoxamine has been used for many years; however, this therapy is associated with significant side effects, and regimens using low-dose deferoxamine are advisable.[372]

Management of Calciphylaxis

The management of calciphylaxis remains a difficult problem (Table 52-4). Attempts should be made to lower the Ca × P value. Serum phosphorus may be lowered by the use of

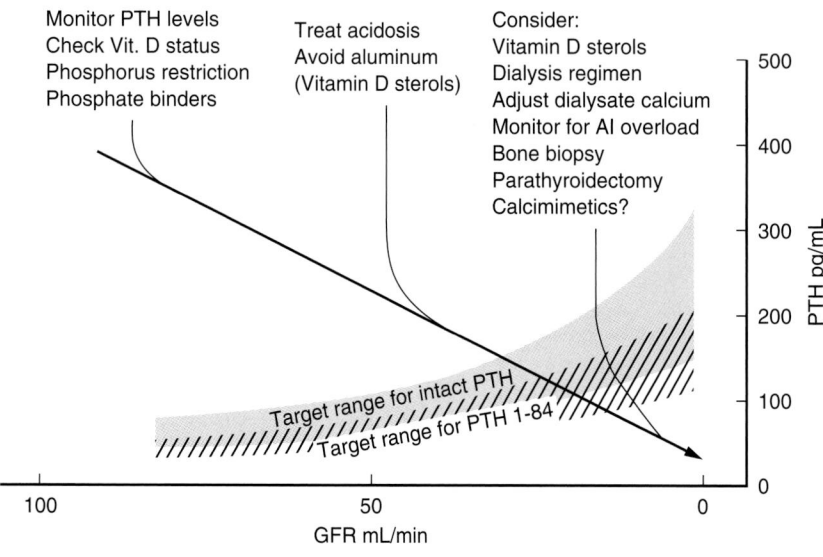

FIGURE 52-31. Diagrammatic representation of the treatment options for prevention and management of renal osteodystrophy throughout the course of renal insufficiency. Target ranges for intact parathyroid hormone (PTH) and for PTH (1-84) are shown by the shaded and hatched areas, respectively. GFR, glomerular filtration rate. (Modified from González EA, Martin KJ: Bone and mineral metabolism in chronic renal failure. *In* Johnson J, Feehally RJ [eds]: Comprehensive Clinical Nephrology. London, Mosby, 2000, pp 69.1-69.11, with permission.)

TABLE 52-4

Guidelines for the Treatment of Calciphylaxis

Lower serum phosphorus (at least to the lower limit of normal)
  Use non–calcium-containing phosphate binders
  Intensify dialysis (consider daily dialysis)
Lower serum calcium
  Avoid calcium-containing compounds
  Use low dialysate calcium (1-2 mEq/L)
Avoid vitamin D compounds
Parathyroidectomy if PTH >300 pg/mL
Treat infections
Consider the following:
  Hyperbaric oxygen
  Glucocorticoids
  Cimetidine
  Bisphosphonates

TABLE 52-5

Factors Influencing Post-transplantation Bone Disease

Severity and type of underlying renal osteodystrophy
Renal function after transplantation
Persistent hyperparathyroidism
Immunosuppressive regimen
Menopausal status
Systemic illness
Nutritional status
Gender

non–calcium-containing phosphate binders and by intensifying hemodialysis so as to increase removal of phosphorus. Calcium supplements and vitamin D compounds should be avoided, because they are known risk factors for the development of calciphylaxis.[476-478] In addition, the use of dialysate containing a low calcium concentration has been recommended.[479] Parathyroidectomy should be considered only in cases in which PTH levels are elevated.[480, 481] Aggressive control of infections with local care and antibiotic therapy is central in the management of calciphylaxis. Other measures that have been described in the management of this disorder include hyperbaric oxygen, glucocorticoids, cimetidine, and bisphosphonates.[478, 482, 483]

Management of Dialysis-Associated Amyloidosis

The options for management of dialysis-associated amyloidosis are rather limited. The use of biocompatible, high-flux dialysis membranes may be useful to delay the development of this disorder by removing β_2-microglobulin.[484] Hemofiltration may be more effective than hemodialysis in this regard.[485] Renal transplantation controls the symptoms of dialysis-associated amyloidosis, which may be related to the use of immunosuppressive agents, and it also stops the progression of this disorder.[486]

BONE DISEASE AFTER RENAL TRANSPLANTATION

Although many of the abnormalities of mineral ion homeostasis associated with chronic kidney disease are corrected by renal transplantation, bone disease continues to be a problem. Studies of recipients of renal transplants have demonstrated a threefold increase in fracture rates, compared with patients undergoing maintenance dialysis.[487] The nature of the skeletal abnormalities in transplant recipients is a combination of the underlying bone disease present at the time of transplantation and the subsequent influence of a variety of factors associated with transplantation (Table 52-5). Post-transplantation bone disease develops in the background of the entire spectrum of renal osteodystrophy, ranging from hyperparathyroid bone disease to adynamic bone. After transplantation, the skeleton is exposed to a variety of immunosuppressive agents that have the potential to affect bone

metabolism. In addition, renal transplantation may result in partial recovery of renal function, in which case many of the factors responsible for the development of renal osteodystrophy remain operative and continue to affect the skeleton. Therefore, the renal transplant recipient is affected by a multitude of factors that have the potential to give rise to a wide spectrum of skeletal pathology.

Persistent Hyperparathyroidism after Renal Transplantation

Successful renal transplantation results in the correction of phosphate excretory capacity as well as the restoration of calcitriol production by the transplanted kidney. These changes result in elimination of the major stimuli for excess PTH synthesis and parathyroid gland proliferation that are present during the course of chronic kidney disease. However, studies have demonstrated that the levels of PTH may remain elevated after renal transplantation even in patients who achieve adequate renal function.[488, 489] The reason for persistent hyperparathyroidism in this setting is thought to be related to advanced parathyroid gland hyperplasia already present at the time of transplantation. The hyperplastic glands are less likely to be suppressible owing to down-regulation of both calcium and vitamin D receptors, especially in the case of nodular hyperplasia.[57, 74, 75] Furthermore, significant apoptosis of hyperplastic parathyroid glands appears to occur very slowly, if at all, adding to the difficulty in controlling advanced hyperparathyroidism after renal transplantation even in the setting of normal renal function.[490, 491]

Effect of Immunosuppressive Agents on the Skeleton

Glucocorticoid therapy is well known to be associated with bone loss. Histologically, glucocorticoid-induced osteoporosis is characterized by a decreased bone formation rate, decreased trabecular wall thickness, and death of portions of bone. Glucocorticoid excess may have both direct and indirect effects on the skeleton. Glucocorticoids have been shown to suppress BMP-2 and Cbfa-1, which are important factors involved in osteoblastogenesis.[492, 493] In addition, glucocorticoids increase osteoblast and osteocyte apoptosis.[147] Other aspects of osteoblast function may also be affected by glucocorticoids, because they have been shown to impair the synthesis of IGFs, osteocalcin, and type I collagen.[494, 495] Osteoclasts may also be affected by glucocorticoids, and there is evidence to suggest that these agents may decrease osteoclastogenesis and prolong osteoclast survival.[496] The mechanism explaining increased osteoclast survival may relate to the demonstration that glucocorticoids inhibit OPG and increase the expression of RANKL.[160, 497] Based on these findings, it has been suggested that the rapid bone loss induced by glucocorticoids may result from increased osteoclast survival mediated by RANKL.[498] With chronic glucocorticoid exposure there is a decreased bone formation rate and decreased trabecular thickness, which may be explained in terms of the toxic effects of glucocorticoids on osteoblasts; in addition, the decreased bone turnover may be linked to the effects of steroids to inhibit osteoclastogenesis. Recent findings suggest that osteocyte apoptosis may be involved in the pathogenesis of glucocorticoid-induced osteonecrosis.[148] In addition to the direct effects of glucocorticoids in bone cells, a variety of systemic effects induced by these agents may also affect bone metabolism. Glucocorticoids decrease intestinal calcium absorption and increase urinary calcium excretion, which may result in negative calcium balance and secondary hyperparathyroidism.[499]

There is accumulating evidence to suggest that cyclosporine may have deleterious effects on the skeleton,[500, 501] although the process by which cyclosporine contributes to bone disease remains somewhat controversial. Studies in vivo have shown that cyclosporine administration results in osteopenia associated with increased bone formation and bone resorption,[501, 502] whereas studies in vitro have demonstrated that cyclosporine inhibits bone resorption.[503, 504] The contribution of cyclosporine to the pathogenesis of bone disease after renal transplantation has been difficult to separate from that of glucocorticoids. Tacrolimus has also been shown to cause bone loss in animal and human studies.[501, 505]

Bone Mineral Loss and Bone Histology after Renal Transplantation

The early post-transplantation period is associated with remarkable bone loss. Julian and colleagues[506] reported a 6.8% decrease in vertebral bone mineral density 6 months after renal transplantation, compared with baseline. During the subsequent 12 months, bone mineral density continued to decrease, but at a much slower rate than that observed during the initial 6 months. Other investigators subsequently obtained similar results, and a variety of factors, such as steroid dose, PTH levels, decreased GFR, acidosis, gender, menopausal status, hypovitaminosis D, and systemic disease, were found to influence bone mineral density in this patient population.[507-513] The fact that the timing of the greatest rate of bone loss corresponds to the period of greater immunosuppression suggests a major contribution of immunosuppressive agents to the rapid loss of bone mineral that occurs early after renal transplantation.

Histologic studies have shown a wide range of bone lesions in patients undergoing renal transplantation; as expected, the nature and course of bone disease after renal transplantation is highly influenced by the preexisting renal osteodystrophy and the immunosuppressive regimen. Pierides and co-workers[514] studied transplant recipients and found that 45% of them had osteomalacia and 55% had osteitis fibrosa. After 2 years, there was complete resolution of osteomalacia, but approximately 50% of the patients with osteitis fibrosa still had evidence of bone disease. Slow resolution of osteitis fibrosa after successful renal transplantation was also reported by Carroll and associates,[515] who found that

resolution of the bone lesion took at least 4 years. Julian and colleagues[506] performed serial bone histomorphometric studies in patients undergoing renal transplantation before initiating dialysis and found that at the time of transplantation there was evidence of mild hyperparathyroid bone disease, which had resolved 6 months later.

The type of immunosuppression has also been shown to influence bone histology after renal transplantation. In the same study, Julian and colleagues[506] found that, 6 months after transplantation, the lesions of osteitis fibrosa had been replaced by a low bone turnover state that may have been related to steroid use. Cueto-Manzano and colleagues[516] found that steroid-based immunosuppressive regimens are likely to result in mixed uremic osteodystrophy, whereas cyclosporine use is associated with either adynamic bone or high-turnover osteodystrophy. More recently, Monier-Faugere and co-workers[517] performed a bone biopsy study of 57 patients who had received a kidney transplant 5 years earlier. They found a high incidence of low bone volume, low bone turnover, and osteomalacia. In addition, both prednisone dose and length of time after transplantation correlated negatively with bone volume and low bone turnover. Carlini and co-workers[518] also studied bone disease after long-term renal transplantation. They examined bone biopsy specimens in 25 men who had received a renal transplant 7.5 years earlier and found features of mixed bone disease with features of high bone turnover, altered bone formation, and delayed mineralization.

Therefore, the nature of the bone disease after renal transplantation has been difficult to assess, because it is highly dependent on the type and severity of the underlying renal osteodystrophy. Information on bone histomorphometry is not easily obtainable in recipients of cadaveric transplants, because the timing of the surgery does not allow for bone labeling so that dynamic parameters of bone histomorphometry can be assessed. Although these parameters can be assessed in the case of living related transplant recipients, the information obtained is representative of only a limited patient population, because these patients are usually transplanted promptly and therefore tend to have a much milder form of bone disease.

Management of Bone Disease after Renal Transplantation

Very little information is available to guide the management of post-transplantation bone disease. Steroid therapy is widely used early after renal transplantation, and interventions to prevent the effects of steroids on bone have been studied in this patient population. Treatment of steroid-induced osteoporosis with oral calcium and calcitriol appears to be effective in patients with rheumatic disorders; however, Cueto-Manzano and colleagues[519] recently studied the use of this regimen in transplant recipients and found no significant effect on bone loss after 1 year of therapy.

Bisphosphonates are powerful agents with anti–bone-resorptive properties that have been used to prevent steroid-induced bone loss in patients with normal renal function.[520, 521] Studies by Fan and associates[380] examined the effect of pamidronate on steroid-induced bone loss in renal transplant recipients. These investigators studied 26 male patients who were randomly assigned to receive either placebo or two

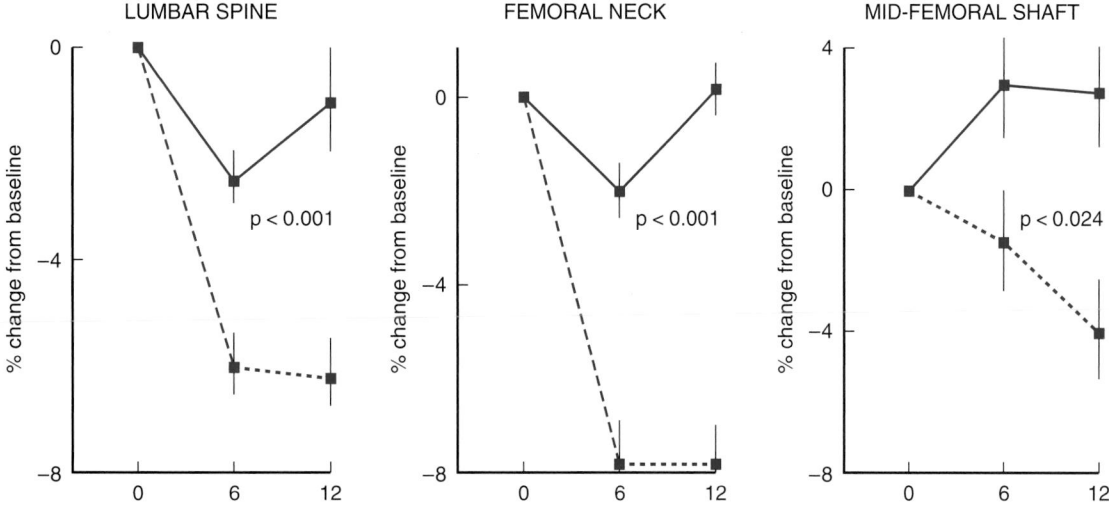

FIGURE 52-32. The effect of the bisphosphonate, ibandronate, on bone mineral density after renal transplantation. (From Grotz W, Nagel C, Poeschel D, et al: Effect of ibandronate on bone loss and renal function after kidney transplantation. J Am Soc Nephrol 12:1530-1537, 2001, with permission.)

doses of intravenous pamidronate (0.5 mg/kg), one at the time of transplantation and another 1 month later. They found a 6% decrease in vertebral bone mineral density in the placebo group 12 months after transplantation whereas no change occurred in the pamidronate-treated patients. More recently, Grotz and co-workers[522] reported the results of a prospective, randomized, controlled trial involving the use of ibandronate in 80 transplant recipients. Forty patients received 1 mg intravenous ibandronate immediately before transplantation, followed by three doses of 2 mg each, at 3, 6, and 9 months after transplantation. The results demonstrated that ibandronate prevented bone loss, spinal deformities, and loss of height during the first year after transplantation (Fig. 52-32). Bisphosphonates have also been found to be beneficial in the late post-transplantation period.[523] Therefore, it appears that bisphosphonates may offer protection against the bone loss that occurs after kidney transplantation; however, their use is not recommended in patients with low bone turnover states. A potential mechanism for the therapeutic effect of bisphosphonates on glucocorticoid-induced osteoporosis is the ability of these agents to prevent osteoblast apoptosis.[524]

REFERENCES

1. Albright F, Drake TG, Sulkowitch HW: Renal osteitis fibrosa cystica: Report of case with discussion of metabolic aspects. Johns Hopkins Medical Journal 60:377, 1937.
2. Follis RHJ, Jackson DA: Renal osteomalacia and osteitis fibrosa in adults. Johns Hopkins Medical Journal 72:232, 1943.
3. Pappenheimer AM, Wilens SL: Enlargement of the parathyroid glands in renal disease. Am J Pathol 11:73, 1935.
4. Pappenheimer AM: Effect of an experimental reduction of kidney substance upon parathyroid glands and skeletal tissue. J Exp Med 64:965, 1936.
5. Reiss E, Canterbury JM, Kanter A: Circulating parathyroid hormone concentration in chronic renal insufficiency. Arch Intern Med 124:417-422, 1969.
6. Arnaud CD: Hyperparathyroidism and renal failure. Kidney Int 4:89-95, 1973.
7. Malluche H, Ritz E, Lange H: Bone histology in incipient and advanced renal failure. Kidney Int 9:355-362, 1976.
8. Slatopolsky E, Caglar S, Pennell JP, et al: On the pathogenesis of hyperparathyroidism in chronic experimental renal insufficiency in the dog. J Clin Invest 50:492-499, 1971.

9. Slatopolsky E, Caglar S, Gradowska L, et al: On the prevention of secondary hyperparathyroidism in experimental chronic renal disease using "proportional reduction" of dietary phosphorus intake. Kidney Int 2:147-151, 1972.
10. Slatopolsky E, Bricker NS: The role of phosphorus restriction in the prevention of secondary hyperparathyroidism in chronic renal disease. Kidney Int 4:141-145, 1973.
11. Slatopolsky E, Delmez JA: Pathogenesis of secondary hyperparathyroidism. Am J Kidney Dis 23:229-236, 1994.
12. Slatopolsky E, Finch J, Denda M, et al: Phosphorus restriction prevents parathyroid gland growth: High phosphorus directly stimulates PTH secretion in vitro. J Clin Invest 97:2534-2540, 1996.
13. Bricker NS: On the pathogenesis of the uremic state: An exposition of the "trade-off hypothesis." N Engl J Med 286:1093-1099, 1972.
14. Laflamme GH, Jowsey J: Bone and soft tissue changes with oral phosphate supplements. J Clin Invest 51:2834-2840, 1972.
15. Jowsey J, Reiss E, Canterbury JM: Long-term effects of high phosphate intake on parathyroid hormone levels and bone metabolism. Acta Orthop Scand 45:801-808, 1974.
16. Rutherford WE, Bordier P, Marie P, et al: Phosphate control and 25-hydroxycholecalciferol administration in preventing experimental renal osteodystrophy in the dog. J Clin Invest 60:332-341, 1977.
17. Llach F, Massry SG: On the mechanism of secondary hyperparathyroidism in moderate renal insufficiency. J Clin Endocrinol Metab 61:601-606, 1985.
18. Reiss E, Canterbury JM, Bercovitz MA, Kaplan EL: The role of phosphate in the secretion of parathyroid hormone in man. J Clin Invest 49:2146-2149, 1970.
19. Portale AA, Booth BE, Halloran BP, Morris RCJ: Effect of dietary phosphorus on circulating concentrations of 1,25-dihydroxyvitamin D and immunoreactive parathyroid hormone in children with moderate renal insufficiency. J Clin Invest 73:1580-1589, 1984.
20. Wilson L, Felsenfeld A, Drezner MK, Llach F: Altered divalent ion metabolism in early renal failure: Role of 1,25(OH)2D. Kidney Int 27:565-573, 1985.
21. Martinez I, Saracho R, Montenegro J, Llach F: The importance of dietary calcium and phosphorous in the secondary hyperparathyroidism of patients with early renal failure. Am J Kidney Dis 29:496-502, 1997.
22. Lopez-Hilker S, Dusso AS, Rapp NS, et al: Phosphorus restriction reverses hyperparathyroidism in uremia independent of changes in calcium and calcitriol. Am J Physiol 259:F432-F437, 1990.
23. Tanaka Y, Deluca HF: The control of 25-hydroxyvitamin D metabolism by inorganic phosphorus. Arch Biochem Biophys 154:566-574, 1973.
24. Lopez-Hilker S, Galceran T, Chan YL, et al: Hypocalcemia may not be essential for the development of secondary hyperparathyroidism in chronic renal failure. J Clin Invest 78:1097-1102, 1986.

25. Almaden Y, Canalejo A, Hernandez A, et al: Direct effect of phosphorus on PTH secretion from whole rat parathyroid glands in vitro. J Bone Miner Res 11:970-976, 1996.

26. Almaden Y, Hernandez A, Torregrosa V, et al: High phosphate level directly stimulates parathyroid hormone secretion and synthesis by human parathyroid tissue in vitro. J Am Soc Nephrol 9:1845-1852, 1998.

27. Fournier AE, Arnaud CD, Johnson WJ, et al: Etiology of hyperparathyroidism and bone disease during chronic hemodialysis: II. Factors affecting serum immunoreactive parathyroid hormone. J Clin Invest 50:599-605, 1971.

28. Indridason OS, Pieper CF, Quarles LD: Predictors of short-term changes in serum intact parathyroid hormone levels in hemodialysis patients: Role of phosphorus, calcium, and gender. J Clin Endocrinol Metab 83:3860-3866, 1998.

29. Kilav R, Silver J, Naveh-Many T: Parathyroid hormone gene expression in hypophosphatemic rats. J Clin Invest 96:327-333, 1995.

30. Moallem E, Kilav R, Silver J, Naveh-Many T: RNA-protein binding and post-transcriptional regulation of parathyroid hormone gene expression by calcium and phosphate. J Biol Chem 273:5253-5259, 1998.

31. Yalcindag C, Silver J, Naveh-Many T: Mechanism of increased parathyroid hormone mRNA in experimental uremia: Roles of protein RNA binding and RNA degradation. J Am Soc Nephrol 10:2562-2568, 1999.

32. Sela-Brown A, Silver J, Brewer G, Naveh-Many T: Identification of AUF1 as a parathyroid hormone mRNA 3'-untranslated region-binding protein that determines parathyroid hormone mRNA stability. J Biol Chem 275:7424-7429, 2000.

33. Kilav R, Silver J, Naveh-Many T: A conserved cis-acting element in the parathyroid hormone 3'-untranslated region is sufficient for regulation of RNA stability by calcium and phosphate. J Biol Chem 276:8727-8733, 2001.

34. Almaden Y, Canalejo A, Ballesteros E, et al: Effect of high extracellular phosphate concentration on arachidonic acid production by parathyroid tissue in vitro. J Am Soc Nephrol 11:1712-1718, 2000.

35. Bourdeau A, Souberbielle JC, Bonnet P, et al: Phospholipase-A2 action and arachidonic acid metabolism in calcium-mediated parathyroid hormone secretion. Endocrinology 130:1339-1344, 1992.

36. Almaden Y, Canalejo A, Ballesteros E, et al: Regulation of arachidonic acid production by intracellular calcium in parathyroid cells: Effect of extracellular phosphate. J Am Soc Nephrol 13:693-698, 2002.

37. Naveh-Many T, Rahamimov R, Livni N, Silver J: Parathyroid cell proliferation in normal and chronic renal failure rats: The effects of calcium, phosphate, and vitamin D. J Clin Invest 96:1786-1793, 1995.

38. Yi H, Fukagawa M, Yamato H, et al: Prevention of enhanced parathyroid hormone secretion, synthesis and hyperplasia by mild dietary phosphorus restriction in early chronic renal failure in rats: Possible direct role of phosphorus. Nephron 70:242-248, 1995.

39. Denda M, Finch J, Slatopolsky E: Phosphorus accelerates the development of parathyroid hyperplasia and secondary hyperparathyroidism in rats with renal failure. Am J Kidney Dis 28:596-602, 1996.

40. Dusso AS, Pavlopoulos T, Naumovich L, et al: p21 (WAF1) and transforming growth factor-alpha mediate dietary phosphate regulation of parathyroid cell growth. Kidney Int 59:855-865, 2001.

41. Tatsumi S, Segawa H, Morita K, et al: Molecular cloning and hormonal regulation of PiT-1, a sodium-dependent phosphate cotransporter from rat parathyroid glands. Endocrinology 139:1692-1699, 1998.

42. Mason RS, Lissner D, Wilkinson M, Posen S: Vitamin D metabolites and their relationship to azotaemic osteodystrophy. Clin Endocrinol 13:375-385, 1980.

43. Christiansen C, Christensen MS, Melsen F, et al: Mineral metabolism in chronic renal failure with special reference to serum concentrations of 1,25(OH)2D and 24,25(OH)2D. Clin Nephrol 15:18-22, 1981.

44. Juttmann JR, Buurman CJ, De Kam E, et al: Serum concentrations of metabolites of vitamin D in patients with chronic renal failure (CRF): Consequences for the treatment with 1-alpha-hydroxy-derivatives. Clin Endocrinol 14:225-236, 1981.

45. Tessitore N, Venturi A, Adami S, et al: Relationship between serum vitamin D metabolites and dietary intake of phosphate in patients with early renal failure. Miner Electrolyte Metab 13:38-44, 1987.

46. Ritz E, Seidel A, Ramisch H, et al: Attenuated rise of 1,25 (OH)2 vitamin D3 in response to parathyroid hormone in patients with incipient renal failure. Nephron 57:314-318, 1991.

47. Gafter U, Kraut JA, Lee DB, et al: Effect of metabolic acidosis in intestinal absorption of calcium and phosphorus. Am J Physiol 239: G480-G484, 1980.

48. Bushinsky DA, Favus MJ, Schneider AB, et al: Effects of metabolic acidosis on PTH and 1,25(OH)2D3 response to low calcium diet. Am J Physiol 243:F570-F575, 1982.

49. Kraut JA, Gordon EM, Ransom JC, et al: Effect of chronic metabolic acidosis on vitamin D metabolism in humans. Kidney Int 24:644-648, 1983.

50. Bushinsky DA, Riera GS, Favus MJ, Coe FL: Response of serum 1,25(OH)2D3 to variation of ionized calcium during chronic acidosis. Am J Physiol 249:F361-F365, 1985.

51. Langman CB, Bushinsky DA, Favus MJ, Coe FL: Ca and P regulation of 1,25(OH)2D3 synthesis by vitamin D-replete rat tubules during acidosis. Am J Physiol 251:F911-F918, 1986.

52. Krapf R, Vetsch R, Vetsch W, Hulter HN: Chronic metabolic acidosis increases the serum concentration of 1,25-dihydroxyvitamin D in humans by stimulating its production rate: Critical role of acidosis-induced renal hypophosphatemia. J Clin Invest 90:2456-2463, 1992.

53. Nykjaer A, Dragun D, Walther D, et al: An endocytic pathway essential for renal uptake and activation of the steroid 25-(OH) vitamin D3. Cell 96:507-515, 1999.

54. Korkor AB: Reduced binding of [3H]1,25-dihydroxyvitamin D3 in the parathyroid glands of patients with renal failure. N Engl J Med 316:1573-1577, 1987.

55. Merke J, Hügel U, Zlotkowski A, et al: Diminished parathyroid 1,25(OH)2D3 receptors in experimental uremia. Kidney Int 32:350-353, 1987.

56. Brown AJ, Dusso A, Lopez-Hilker S, et al: 1,25-(OH)2D receptors are decreased in parathyroid glands from chronically uremic dogs. Kidney Int 35:19-23, 1989.

57. Fukuda N, Tanaka H, Tominaga Y, et al: Decreased 1,25-dihydroxyvitamin D3 receptor density is associated with a more severe form of parathyroid hyperplasia in chronic uremic patients. J Clin Invest 92:1436-1443, 1993.

58. Patel SR, Ke HQ, Vanholder R, et al: Inhibition of calcitriol receptor binding to vitamin D response elements by uremic toxins. J Clin Invest 96:50-59, 1995.

59. Sawaya BP, Koszewski NJ, Qi Q, et al: Secondary hyperparathyroidism and vitamin D receptor binding to vitamin D response elements in rats with incipient renal failure. J Am Soc Nephrol 8:271-278, 1997.

60. Bellorin-Font E, Martin KJ, Freitag JJ, et al: Altered adenylate cyclase kinetics in hyperfunctioning human parathyroid glands. J Clin Endocrinol Metab 52:499-507, 1981.

61. Brown EM, Brennan MF, Hurwitz S, et al: Dispersed cells prepared from human parathyroid glands: Distinct calcium sensitivity of adenomas vs. primary hyperplasia. J Clin Endocrinol Metab 46:267-275, 1978.

62. Felsenfeld AJ, Jara A, Pahl M, et al: Differences in the dynamics of parathyroid hormone secretion in hemodialysis patients with marked secondary hyperparathyroidism. J Am Soc Nephrol 6:1371-1378, 1995.

63. Felsenfeld AJ, Rodriguez M, Dunlay R, Llach F: A comparison of parathyroid-gland function in haemodialysis patients with different forms of renal osteodystrophy. Nephrol Dial Transplant 6:244-251, 1991.

64. Malberti F, Corradi B, Pagliari B, et al: The sigmoidal parathyroid hormone-ionized calcium curve and the set point of calcium in hemodialysis and continuous ambulatory peritoneal dialysis. Perit Dial Int 13(suppl 2):S476-S479, 1993.

65. Goodman WG, Belin T, Gales B, et al: Calcium-regulated parathyroid hormone release in patients with mild or advanced secondary hyperparathyroidism. Kidney Int 48:1553-1558, 1995.

66. Messa P, Vallone C, Mioni G, et al: Direct in vivo assessment of parathyroid hormone-calcium relationship curve in renal patients. Kidney Int 46:1713-1720, 1994.

67. Ramirez JA, Goodman WG, Gornbein J, et al: Direct in vivo comparison of calcium-regulated parathyroid hormone secretion in normal volunteers and patients with secondary hyperparathyroidism. J Clin Endocrinol Metab 76:1489-1494, 1993.

68. Khosla S, Ebeling PR, Firek AF, et al: Calcium infusion suggests a "set-point" abnormality of parathyroid gland function in familial benign hypercalcemia and more complex disturbances in primary hyperparathyroidism. J Clin Endocrinol Metab 76:715-720, 1993.

69. De Cristofaro V, Colturi C, Masa A, et al: Rate dependence of acute PTH release and association between basal plasma calcium and set point of calcium-PTH curve in dialysis patients. Nephrol Dial Transplant 16:1214-1221, 2001.

70. Borrego MJ, Felsenfeld AJ, Martin-Malo A, et al: Evidence for adaptation of the entire PTH-calcium curve to sustained changes in the serum calcium in haemodialysis patients. Nephrol Dial Transplant 12:505-513, 1997.

71. Indridason OS, Heath H 3rd, Khosla S, et al: Non-suppressible parathyroid hormone secretion is related to gland size in uremic secondary hyperparathyroidism. Kidney Int 50:1663-1671, 1996.

72. Yokoyama K, Shigematsu T, Tsukada T, et al: Calcium-sensing receptor gene polymorphism affects the parathyroid response to moderate hypercalcemic suppression in patients with end-stage renal disease. Clin Nephrol 57:131-135, 2002.

73. Pahl M, Jara A, Bover J, et al: The set point of calcium and the reduction of parathyroid hormone in hemodialysis patients. Kidney Int 49:226-231, 1996.

74. Gogusev J, Duchambon P, Hory B, et al: Depressed expression of calcium receptor in parathyroid gland tissue of patients with hyperparathyroidism. Kidney Int 51:328-336, 1997.

75. Kifor O, Moore FD Jr, Wang P, et al: Reduced immunostaining for the extracellular Ca2+-sensing receptor in primary and uremic secondary hyperparathyroidism [see comments]. J Clin Endocrinol Metab 81: 1598-1606, 1996.

76. Lewin E, Garfia B, Recio FL, et al: Persistent downregulation of calcium-sensing receptor mRNA in rat parathyroids when severe secondary hyperparathyroidism is reversed by an isogenic kidney transplantation. J Am Soc Nephrol 13:2110-2116, 2002.

77. Ritter CS, Martin DR, Lu Y, et al: Reversal of secondary hyperparathyroidism by phosphate restriction restores parathyroid calcium-sensing receptor expression and function. J Bone Miner Metab (in press).

78. Brumbaugh PF, Hughes MR, Haussler MR: Cytoplasmic and nuclear binding components for 1alpha25-dihydroxyvitamin D3 in chick parathyroid glands. Proc Natl Acad Sci U S A 72:4871-4875, 1975.

79. Chertow BS, Baylink DJ, Wergedal JE, et al: Decrease in serum immunoreactive parathyroid hormone in rats and in parathyroid hormone secretion in vitro by 1,25-dihydroxycholecalciferol. J Clin Invest 56:668-678, 1975.

80. Cantley LK, Russell J, Lettieri D, Sherwood LM: 1,25-Dihydroxyvitamin D3 suppresses parathyroid hormone secretion from bovine parathyroid cells in tissue culture. Endocrinology 117:2114-2119, 1985.

81. Silver J, Russell J, Sherwood LM: Regulation by vitamin D metabolites of messenger ribonucleic acid for preproparathyroid hormone in isolated bovine parathyroid cells. Proc Natl Acad Sci U S A 82:4270-4273, 1985.

82. Russell J, Lettieri D, Sherwood LM: Suppression by 1,25(OH)$_2$D$_3$ of transcription of the pre-proparathyroid hormone gene. Endocrinology 119:2864-2866, 1986.

83. Silver J, Naveh-Many T, Mayer H, et al: Regulation by vitamin D metabolites of parathyroid hormone gene transcription in vivo in the rat. J Clin Invest 78:1296-1301, 1986.

84. Okazaki T, Igarashi T, Kronenberg HM: 5′-Flanking region of the parathyroid hormone gene mediates negative regulation by 1,25-(OH)$_2$ vitamin D$_3$. J Biol Chem 263:2203-2208, 1988.

85. Demay MB, Kiernan MS, DeLuca HF, Kronenberg HM: Sequences in the human parathyroid hormone gene that bind the 1,25-dihydroxyvitamin D3 receptor and mediate transcriptional repression in response to 1,25-dihydroxyvitamin D3. Proc Natl Acad Sci U S A 89:8097-8101, 1992.

86. Mackey SL, Heymont JL, Kronenberg HM, Demay MB: Vitamin D receptor binding to the negative human parathyroid hormone vitamin D response element does not require the retinoid x receptor. Mol Endocrinol 10:298-305, 1996.

87. Naveh-Many T, Marx R, Keshet E, et al: Regulation of 1,25-dihydroxyvitamin D3 receptor gene expression by 1,25-dihydroxyvitamin D3 in the parathyroid in vivo. J Clin Invest 86:1968-1975, 1990.

88. Kremer R, Bolivar I, Goltzman D, Hendy GN: Influence of calcium and 1,25-dihydroxycholecalciferol on proliferation and proto-oncogene expression in primary cultures of bovine parathyroid cells. Endocrinology 125:935-941, 1989.

89. Cozzolino M, Lu Y, Finch J, et al: p21WAF1 and TGF-alpha mediate parathyroid growth arrest by vitamin D and high calcium. Kidney Int 60:2109-2117, 2001.

90. Tokumoto M, Hirakawa M, Kazuhiko T, et al: Diminished expression of cyclin-dependent kinase inhibitor p21 and vitamin D receptor in nodular hyperplasia in secondary hyperparathyroidism. J Am Soc Nephrol 11:584A, 2000.

91. Li YC, Amling M, Pirro AE, et al: Normalization of mineral ion homeostasis by dietary means prevents hyperparathyroidism, rickets, and osteomalacia, but not alopecia in vitamin D receptor-ablated mice. Endocrinology 139:4391-4396, 1998.

92. Arnold A, Brown MF, Urena P, et al: Monoclonality of parathyroid tumors in chronic renal failure and in primary parathyroid hyperplasia. J Clin Invest 95:2047-2053, 1995.

93. Ritter CS, Finch JL, Slatopolsky EA, Brown AJ: Parathyroid hyperplasia in uremic rats precedes down-regulation of the calcium receptor. Kidney Int 60:1737-1744, 2001.

94. Wada M, Furuya Y, Sakiyama J, et al: The calcimimetic compound NPS R-568 suppresses parathyroid cell proliferation in rats with renal insufficiency: Control of parathyroid cell growth via a calcium receptor. J Clin Invest 100:2977-2983, 1997.

95. Wada M, Nagano N, Furuya Y, et al: Calcimimetic NPS R-568 prevents parathyroid hyperplasia in rats with severe secondary hyperparathyroidism. Kidney Int 57:50-58, 2000.

96. Brown AJ, Ritter CS, Finch JL, Slatopolsky EA: Decreased calcium-sensing receptor expression in hyperplastic parathyroid glands of uremic rats: Role of dietary phosphate. Kidney Int 55:1284-1292, 1999.

97. Evanson JM: The response to the infusion of parathyroid extract in hypocalcaemic states. Clin Sci (Colch) 31:63-75, 1996.

98. Massry SG, Coburn JW, Lee DB, et al: Skeletal resistance to parathyroid hormone in renal failure: Studies in 105 human subjects. Ann Intern Med 78:357-364, 1973.

99. Somerville PJ, Kaye M: Evidence that resistance to the calcemic action of parathyroid hormone in rats with acute uremia is caused by phosphate retention. Kidney Int 16:552-560, 1979.

100. Massry SG, Tuma S, Dua S, Goldstein DA: Reversal of skeletal resistance to parathyroid hormone in uremia by vitamin D metabolites: Evidence for the requirement of 1,25(OH)2D3 and 24,25(OH)2D3. J Lab Clin Med 94:152-157, 1979.

101. Somerville PJ, Kaye M: Resistance to parathyroid hormone in renal failure: Role of vitamin D metabolites. Kidney Int 14:245-254, 1978.

102. Galceran T, Martin KJ, Morrissey JJ, Slatopolsky E: Role of 1,25-dihydroxyvitamin D on the skeletal resistance to parathyroid hormone. Kidney Int 32:801-807, 1987.

103. Olgaard K, Schwartz J, Finco D, et al: Extraction of parathyroid hormone and release of adenosine 3′,5′-monophosphate by isolated perfused bones obtained from dogs with acute uremia. Endocrinology 111:1678-1682, 1982.

104. Olgaard K, Arbelaez M, Schwartz J, et al: Abnormal skeletal response to parathyroid hormone in dogs with chronic uremia. Calcif Tiss Int 34:403-407, 1982.

105. Picton ML, Moore PR, Mawer EB, et al: Down-regulation of human osteoblast PTH/PTHrP receptor mRNA in end-stage renal failure. Kidney Int 58:1440-1449, 2000.

106. Ureña P, Kubrusly M, Mannstadt M, et al: The renal PTH/PTHrP receptor is down-regulated in rats with chronic renal failure. Kidney Int 45:605-611, 1994.

107. Ureña P, Ferreira A, Morieux C, et al: PTH/PTHrP receptor mRNA is down-regulated in epiphyseal cartilage growth plate of uraemic rats. Nephrol Dial Transplant 11:2008-2016, 1996.

108. Tian J, Smogorzewski M, Kedes L, Massry SG: PTH-PTHrP receptor mRNA is downregulated in chronic renal failure. Am J Nephrol 14:41-46, 1994.

109. Ureña P, Mannstadt M, Hruby M, et al: Parathyroidectomy does not prevent the renal PTH/PTHrP receptor down-regulation in uremic rats. Kidney Int 47:1797-1805, 1995.

110. Nussbaum SR, Zahradnik RJ, Lavigne JR, et al: Highly sensitive two-site immunoradiometric assay of parathyrin, and its clinical utility in evaluating patients with hypercalcemia. Clin Chem 33:1364-1367, 1987.

111. Lepage R, Roy L, Brossard JH, et al: A non-(1-84) circulating parathyroid hormone (PTH) fragment interferes significantly with intact PTH commercial assay measurements in uremic samples. Clin Chem 44:805-809, 1998.

112. Gao P, Scheibel SJ, D'Amour P, Cantor T: Measuring the biologically active or authentic whole-parathyroid hormone (PTH) with a novel immunoradiometric assay without cross reaction to the PTH (7-84) fragment. J Bone Miner Res 14:S446, 1999.

113. Gao P, Scheibel S, D'Amour P, et al: Development of a novel immunoradiometric assay exclusively for biologically active whole parathyroid hormone 1-84: Implications for improvement of accurate assessment of parathyroid function. J Bone Miner Res 16:605-614, 2001.

114. Nguyen-Yamamoto L, Rousseau L, Brossard JH, et al: Synthetic carboxyl-terminal fragments of parathyroid hormone (PTH) decrease ionized calcium concentration in rats by acting on a receptor different from the PTH/PTH-related peptide receptor. Endocrinology 142: 1386-1392, 2001.

115. Slatopolsky E, Finch J, Clay P, et al: A novel mechanism for skeletal resistance in uremia. Kidney Int 58:753-761, 2000.

116. Divieti P, John MR, Juppner H, Bringhurst FR: Human PTH-(7-84) inhibits bone resorption in vitro via actions independent of the type 1 PTH/PTHrP receptor. Endocrinology 143:171-176, 2002.

117. Torres A, Lorenzo V, Hernandez D, et al: Bone disease in predialysis, hemodialysis, and CAPD patients: Evidence of a better bone response to PTH. Kidney Int 47:1434-1442, 1995.

118. Hernandez D, Concepcion MT, Lorenzo V, et al: Adynamic bone disease with negative aluminium staining in predialysis patients: Prevalence and evolution after maintenance dialysis. Nephrol Dial Transplant 9:517-523, 1994.

119. Hutchison AJ, Whitehouse RW, Boulton HF, et al: Correlation of bone histology with parathyroid hormone, vitamin D3, and radiology in end-stage renal disease. Kidney Int 44:1071-1077, 1993.

120. Sherrard DJ, Hercz G, Pei Y, et al: The spectrum of bone disease in end-stage renal failure: An evolving disorder. Kidney Int 43:436-442, 1993.

121. Malluche H, Faugere MC: Renal bone disease 1990: An unmet challenge for the nephrologist. Kidney Int 38:193-211, 1990.

122. Couttenye MM, D'Haese PC, Verschoren WJ, et al: Low bone turnover in patients with renal failure. Kidney Int 56(suppl 73):S70-S76, 1999.

123. Cohen-Solal ME, Sebert JL, Boudailliez B, et al: Non-aluminic adynamic bone disease in non-dialyzed uremic patients: A new type of osteopathy due to overtreatment? Bone 13:1-5, 1992.

124. Coen G, Mazzaferro S, Ballanti P, et al: Renal bone disease in 76 patients with varying degrees of predialysis chronic renal failure: A cross-sectional study. Nephrol Dial Transplant 11:813-819, 1996.

125. Gonzalez EA: The role of cytokines in skeletal remodelling: Possible consequences for renal osteodystrophy. Nephrol Dial Transplant 15:945-950, 2000.

126. González E, Martin K: Aluminum and renal osteodystrophy: A diminishing clinical problem. Trends Endocrinol Metab 3:371-375, 1992.

127. Malluche HH, Monier-Faugere MC: Uremic bone disease: Current knowledge, controversial issues, and new horizons. Miner Electrolyte Metab 17:281-296, 1991.

128. Ghazali A, Fardellone P, Pruna A, et al: Is low plasma 25-(OH)vitamin D a major risk factor for hyperparathyroidism and Looser's zones independent of calcitriol? Kidney Int 55:2169-2177, 1999.

129. Krieger NS, Sessler NE, Bushinsky DA: Acidosis inhibits osteoblastic and stimulates osteoclastic activity in vitro. Am J Physiol 262:F442-F448, 1992.

130. Kraut JA, Mishler DR, Singer FR, Goodman WG: The effects of metabolic acidosis on bone formation and bone resorption in the rat. Kidney Int 30:694-700, 1986.

131. Coen G, Manni M, Addari O, et al: Metabolic acidosis and osteodystrophic bone disease in predialysis chronic renal failure: Effect of calcitriol treatment. Miner Electrolyte Metab 21:375-382, 1995.

132. Clarke BL, Wynne AG, Wilson DM, Fitzpatrick LA: Osteomalacia associated with adult Fanconi's syndrome: Clinical and diagnostic features. Clin Endocrinol (Oxf) 43:479-490, 1995.

133. Kraut JA: The role of metabolic acidosis in the pathogenesis of renal osteodystrophy. Adv Ren Replace Ther 2:40-51, 1995.

134. Kleeman CR: The role of chronic anion gap and/or nonanion gap acidosis in the osteodystrophy of chronic renal failure in the predialysis era: A minority report. Miner Electrolyte Metab 20:81-96, 1994.

135. Bushinsky DA: The contribution of acidosis to renal osteodystrophy. Kidney Int 47:1816-1832, 1995.

136. Frick KK, Jiang L, Bushinsky DA: Acute metabolic acidosis inhibits the induction of osteoblastic egr-1 and type 1 collagen. Am J Physiol 272:C1450-C1456, 1997.

137. Frick KK, Bushinsky DA: Chronic metabolic acidosis reversibly inhibits extracellular matrix gene expression in mouse osteoblasts. Am J Physiol 275:F840-F847, 1998.

138. Frick KK, Bushinsky DA: In vitro metabolic and respiratory acidosis selectively inhibit osteoblastic matrix gene expression. Am J Physiol 277:F750-F755, 1999.

139. Bushinsky DA: Stimulated osteoclastic and suppressed osteoblastic activity in metabolic but not respiratory acidosis. Am J Physiol 268:C80-C88, 1995.

140. Martin KJ, Freitag JJ, Bellorin-Font E, et al: The effect of acute acidosis on the uptake of parathyroid hormone and the production of adenosine 3',5'-monophosphate by isolated perfused bone. Endocrinology 106:1607-1611, 1980.

141. Bushinsky DA, Nilsson EL: Additive effects of acidosis and parathyroid hormone on mouse osteoblastic and osteoclastic function. Am J Physiol 269:C1364-C1370, 1995.

142. Cunningham J, Bikle DD, Avioli LV: Acute, but not chronic, metabolic acidosis disturbs 25-hydroxyvitamin D3 metabolism. Kidney Int 25:47-52, 1984.

143. Lefebvre A, de Vernejoul MC, Gueris J, et al: Optimal correction of acidosis changes progression of dialysis osteodystrophy. Kidney Int 36:1112-1118, 1989.

144. Disthabanchong S, Martin KJ, McConkey CL, Gonzalez EA: Metabolic acidosis up-regulates PTH/PTHrP receptors in UMR 106-01 osteoblast-like cells. Kidney Int 62:1171-1177, 2002.

145. Frick KK, Bushinsky DA: Metabolic acidosis stimulates expression of rank ligand RNA. J Am Soc Nephrol 13:576A, 2002.

146. Manolagas SC, Weinstein RS: New developments in the pathogenesis and treatment of steroid-induced osteoporosis. J Bone Miner Res 14: 1061-1066, 1999.

147. Weinstein RS, Jilka RL, Parfitt AM, Manolagas SC: Inhibition of osteoblastogenesis and promotion of apoptosis of osteoblasts and osteocytes by glucocorticoids: Potential mechanisms of their deleterious effects on bone. J Clin Invest 102:274-282, 1998.

148. Weinstein RS, Nicholas RW, Manolagas SC: Apoptosis of osteocytes in glucocorticoid-induced osteonecrosis of the hip. J Clin Endocrinol Metab 85:2907-2912, 2000.

149. González EA, Martin KJ: Renal osteodystrophy: Pathogenesis and management. Nephrol Dial Transplant 10(suppl 3):13-21, 1995.

150. Slatopolsky E, Brown A, Dusso A: Pathogenesis of secondary hyperparathyroidism. Kidney Int Suppl 73:S14-S19, 1999.

151. Wang M, Hercz G, Sherrard DJ, et al: Relationship between intact 1-84 parathyroid hormone and bone histomorphometric parameters in dialysis patients without aluminum toxicity. Am J Kidney Dis 26:836-844, 1995.

152. Malluche H, Monier-Faugere M: The role of bone biopsy in the management of patients with renal osteodystrophy. J Am Soc Nephrol 4:1631-1642, 1994.

153. Amling M, Priemel M, Holzmann T, et al: Rescue of the skeletal phenotype of vitamin D receptor-ablated mice in the setting of normal mineral ion homeostasis: Formal histomorphometric and biomechanical analyses. Endocrinology 140:4982-4987, 1999.

154. Disthabanchong S, Gonzalez EA: Regulation of bone cell development and function: Implication for renal osteodystrophy. J Investig Med 49:240-249, 2001.

155. Hory B, Drüeke TB: The parathyroid-bone axis in uremia: New insights into old questions. Curr Opin Nephrol Hypertens 6:40-48, 1997.

156. Hruska K: New concepts in renal osteodystrophy. Nephrol Dial Transplant 13:2755-2760, 1998.

157. Monier-Faugere MC, Malluche HH: Role of cytokines in renal osteodystrophy. Curr Opin Nephrol Hypertens 6:327-332, 1997.

158. Baron R, Neff L, Tran Van P, et al: Kinetic and cytochemical identification of osteoclast precursors and their differentiation into multinucleated osteoclasts. Am J Pathol 122:363-378, 1986.

159. Lian JB, Stein GS, Canalis E, et al: Bone formation: Osteoblast lineage cells, growth factors, matrix proteins, and the mineralization process. In Favous MJ (ed): Primer on the Metabolic Bone Diseases and Disorders of Mineral Metabolism, 4th ed. Philadelphia, Lippincott Williams & Wilkins, 1999, pp 14-29.

160. Hofbauer LC: Osteoprotegerin ligand and osteoprotegerin: Novel implications for osteoclast biology and bone metabolism. Eur J Endocrinol 141:195-210, 1999.

161. Parfitt AM: Osteonal and hemi-osteonal remodeling: The spatial and temporal framework for signal traffic in adult human bone. J Cell Biochem 55:273-286, 1994.

162. Väänänen HK: Mechanism of bone turnover. Ann Med 25:353-359, 1993.

163. Hofbauer LC, Khosla S, Dunstan CR, et al: The roles of osteoprotegerin and osteoprotegerin ligand in the paracrine regulation of bone resorption. [Review.] J Bone Miner Res 15:2-12, 2000.

164. Karsenty G: The central regulation of bone remodeling. Trends Endocrinol Metab 11:437-439, 2000.

165. Goldring SR, Goldring MB: Cytokines and skeletal physiology. Clin Orthop 324:13-23, 1996.

166. Weryha G, Leclere J: Paracrine regulation of bone remodeling. Horm Res 43:69-75, 1995.

167. Herbelin A, Nguyen AT, Zingraff J, et al: Influence of uremia and hemodialysis on circulating interleukin-1 and tumor necrosis factor alpha. Kidney Int 37:116-125, 1990.

168. Ferreira A, Simon P, Drueke TB, Deschamps-Latscha B: Potential role of cytokines in renal osteodystrophy. [Letter.] Nephrol Dial Transplant 11:399-400, 1996.

169. Moutabarrik A, Nakanishi I, Namiki M, Tsubakihara Y: Interleukin-1 and its naturally occurring antagonist in peritoneal dialysis patients. Clin Nephrol 43:243-248, 1995.

170. Lacey DL, Timms E, Tan HL, et al: Osteoprotegerin ligand is a cytokine that regulates osteoclast differentiation and activation. Cell 93:165-176, 1998.

171. Yasuda H, Shima N, Nakagawa N, et al: Osteoclast differentiation factor is a ligand for osteoprotegerin/osteoclastogenesis-inhibitory factor and is identical to TRANCE/RANKL. Proc Natl Acad Sci U S A 95:3597-3602, 1998.

172. Nakagawa N, Kinosaki M, Yamaguchi K, et al: RANK is the essential signaling receptor for osteoclast differentiation factor in osteoclastogenesis. Biochem Biophys Res Commun 253:395-400, 1998.

173. Kong YY, Yoshida H, Sarosi I, et al: OPGL is a key regulator of osteoclastogenesis, lymphocyte development and lymph-node organogenesis. Nature 397:315-323, 1999.

174. Quinn JM, Elliott J, Gillespie MT, Martin TJ: A combination of osteoclast differentiation factor and macrophage-colony stimulating factor is sufficient for both human and mouse osteoclast formation in vitro. Endocrinology 139:4424-4427, 1998.

175. Tan KB, Harrop J, Reddy M, et al: Characterization of a novel TNF-like ligand and recently described TNF ligand and TNF receptor superfamily genes and their constitutive and inducible expression in hematopoietic and non-hematopoietic cells. Gene 204:35-46, 1997.

176. Simonet WS, Lacey DL, Dunstan CR, et al: Osteoprotegerin: A novel secreted protein involved in the regulation of bone density [see comments]. Cell 89:309-319, 1997.

177. Tsuda E, Goto M, Mochizuki S, et al: Isolation of a novel cytokine from human fibroblasts that specifically inhibits osteoclastogenesis. Biochem Biophys Res Commun 234:137-142, 1997.

178. Kwon BS, Wang S, Udagawa N, et al: TR1, a new member of the tumor necrosis factor receptor superfamily, induces fibroblast proliferation and inhibits osteoclastogenesis and bone resorption. FASEB J 12:845-854, 1998.

179. Emery JG, McDonnell P, Burke MB, et al: Osteoprotegerin is a receptor for the cytotoxic ligand TRAIL. J Biol Chem 273:14363-14367, 1998.

180. Tsukii K, Shima N, Mochizuki S, et al: Osteoclast differentiation factor mediates an essential signal for bone resorption induced by 1 alpha,25-dihydroxyvitamin D3, prostaglandin E2, or parathyroid hormone in the microenvironment of bone. Biochem Biophys Res Commun 246:337-341, 1998.

181. Lee SK, Lorenzo JA: Parathyroid hormone stimulates TRANCE and inhibits osteoprotegerin messenger ribonucleic acid expression in murine bone marrow cultures: Correlation with osteoclast-like cell formation. Endocrinology 140:3552-3561, 1999.

182. Horwood NJ, Elliott J, Martin TJ, Gillespie MT: Osteotropic agents regulate the expression of osteoclast differentiation factor and osteoprotegerin in osteoblastic stromal cells. Endocrinology 139:4743-4746, 1998.

183. Kazama JJ, Shigematsu T, Yano K, et al: Increased circulating levels of osteoclastogenesis inhibitory factor (osteoprotegerin) in patients with chronic renal failure. Am J Kidney Dis 39:525-532, 2002.

184. Haas M, Leko-Mohr Z, Roschger P, et al: Osteoprotegerin and parathyroid hormone as markers of high-turnover osteodystrophy and decreased bone mineralization in hemodialysis patients. Am J Kidney Dis 39:580-586, 2002.

185. Jilka RL, Hangoc G, Girasole G, et al: Increased osteoclast development after estrogen loss: Mediation by interleukin-6. Science 257:88-91, 1992.

186. Klein B, Wijdenes J, Zhang XG, et al: Murine anti-interleukin-6 monoclonal antibody therapy for a patient with plasma cell leukemia. Blood 78:1198-1204, 1991.

187. Roodman GD, Kurihara N, Ohsaki Y, et al: Interleukin 6: A potential autocrine/paracrine factor in Paget's disease of bone. J Clin Invest 89:46-52, 1992.

188. Adebanjo OA, Moonga BS, Yamate T, et al: Mode of action of interleukin-6 on mature osteoclasts: Novel interactions with extracellular Ca2+ sensing in the regulation of osteoclastic bone resorption. J Cell Biol 142:1347-1356, 1998.

189. Herbelin A, Ureña P, Nguyen AT, et al: Elevated circulating levels of interleukin-6 in patients with chronic renal failure. Kidney Int 39:954-960, 1991.

190. Montalbán C, García-Unzueta MT, De Francisco AL, Amado JA: Serum interleukin-6 in renal osteodystrophy: Relationship with serum PTH and bone remodeling markers. Hormone Metab Res 31:14-17, 1999.

191. Löwik CW, van der Pluijm G, Bloys H, et al: Parathyroid hormone (PTH) and PTH-like protein (PLP) stimulate interleukin-6 production by osteogenic cells: A possible role of interleukin-6 in osteoclastogenesis. Biochem Biophys Res Commun 162:1546-1552, 1989.

192. Pollock JH, Blaha MJ, Lavish SA, et al: In vivo demonstration that parathyroid hormone and parathyroid hormone-related protein stimulate expression by osteoblasts of interleukin-6 and leukemia inhibitory factor. J Bone Miner Res 11:754-759, 1996.

193. Onyia JE, Libermann TA, Bidwell J, et al: Parathyroid hormone (1-34)-mediated interleukin-6 induction. J Cell Biochem 67:265-274, 1997.

194. Huang YF, Harrison JR, Lorenzo JA, Kream BE: Parathyroid hormone induces interleukin-6 heterogeneous nuclear and messenger RNA expression in murine calvarial organ cultures. Bone 23:327-332, 1998.

195. Langub MC Jr, Koszewski NJ, Turner HV, et al: Bone resorption and mRNA expression of IL-6 and IL-6 receptor in patients with renal osteodystrophy. Kidney Int 50:515-520, 1996.

196. Memoli B, Postiglione L, Cianciaruso B, et al: Role of different dialysis membranes in the release of interleukin-6-soluble receptor in uremic patients. Kidney Int 58:417-424, 2000.

197. Le Meur Y, Lorgeot V, Aldigier JC, et al: Whole blood production of monocytic cytokines (IL-1B, IL-6, TNF-α, sIL-6R, IL-1Ra) in hemodialysed patients. Nephrol Dial Transplant 14:2420-2426, 1999.

198. Disthabanchong S, González EA, Martin KJ: Soluble IL-6 receptor in chronic hemodialysis patients. J Am Soc Nephrol 11:562A, 2000.

199. Pacifici R, Rifas L, McCracken R, et al: Ovarian steroid treatment blocks a postmenopausal increase in blood monocyte interleukin 1 release. Proc Natl Acad Sci U S A 86:2398-2402, 1989.

200. Pacifici R, Rifas L, Teitelbaum S, et al: Spontaneous release of interleukin 1 from human blood monocytes reflects bone formation in idiopathic osteoporosis. Proc Natl Acad Sci U S A 84:4616-4620, 1987.

201. Fiore CE, Falcidia E, Foti R, et al: Differences in the time course of the effects of oophorectomy in women on parameters of bone metabolism and interleukin-1 levels in the circulation. Bone Miner 20:79-85, 1993.

202. Jimi E, Nakamura I, Duong LT, et al: Interleukin 1 induces multinucleation and bone-resorbing activity of osteoclasts in the absence of osteoblasts/stromal cells. Exp Cell Res 247:84-93, 1999.

203. Hofbauer LC, Lacey DL, Dunstan CR, et al: Interleukin-1beta and tumor necrosis factor-alpha, but not interleukin-6, stimulate osteoprotegerin ligand gene expression in human osteoblastic cells. Bone 25:255-259, 1999.

204. O'Brien CA, Gubrij I, Lin SC, et al: STAT3 activation in stromal/osteoblastic cells is required for induction of the receptor activator of NF-kappaB ligand and stimulation of osteoclastogenesis by gp130-utilizing cytokines or interleukin-1 but not 1,25-dihydroxyvitamin D3 or parathyroid hormone. J Biol Chem 274:19301-19308, 1999.

205. Conover CA, Rosen C: The role of insulin-like growth factors and binding proteins in bone cell biology. *In* Bilezikian JP, Raisz LG, Rodan GA (eds): Principles of Bone Biology. San Diego, Academic Press, 2002, pp 801-815.

206. Canalis E, McCarthy T, Centrella M: Isolation and characterization of insulin-like growth factor I (somatomedin-C) from cultures of fetal rat calvariae. Endocrinology 122:22-27, 1988.

207. Jones JI, Clemmons DR: Insulin-like growth factors and their binding proteins: Biological actions. Endocr Rev 16:3-34, 1995.

208. Andress DL, Birnbaum RS: Human osteoblast-derived insulin-like growth factor (IGF) binding protein-5 stimulates osteoblast mitogenesis and potentiates IGF action. J Biol Chem 267:22467-22472, 1992.

209. Canalis E, Centrella M, Burch W, McCarthy TL: Insulin-like growth factor I mediates selective anabolic effects of parathyroid hormone in bone cultures. J Clin Invest 83:60-65, 1989.

210. McCarthy TL, Centrella M, Canalis E: Parathyroid hormone enhances the transcript and polypeptide levels of insulin-like growth factor I in osteoblast-enriched cultures from fetal rat bone. Endocrinology 124:1247-1253, 1989.

211. McCarthy TL, Centrella M, Canalis E: Cyclic AMP induces insulin-like growth factor I synthesis in osteoblast-enriched cultures. J Biol Chem 265:15353-15356, 1990.

212. Pfeilschifter J, Laukhuf F, Müller-Beckmann B, et al: Parathyroid hormone increases the concentration of insulin-like growth factor-I and transforming growth factor beta 1 in rat bone. J Clin Invest 96:767-774, 1995.

213. Andress DL, Pandian MR, Endres DB, Kopp JB: Plasma insulin-like growth factors and bone formation in uremic hyperparathyroidism. Kidney Int 36:471-477, 1989.

214. Weinreich T, Zapf J, Schmidt-Gayk H, et al: Insulin-like growth factor 1 and 2 serum concentrations in dialysis patients with secondary hyperparathyroidism and adynamic bone disease. Clin Nephrol 51:27-33, 1999.

215. Jehle PM, Ostertag A, Schulten K, et al: Insulin-like growth factor system components in hyperparathyroidism and renal osteodystrophy. Kidney Int 57:423-436, 2000.

216. Urist MR. Bone: Formation by autoinduction. Science 150:893-899, 1965.

217. Gitelman SE, Kobrin MS, Ye JQ, et al: Recombinant Vgr-1/BMP-6-expressing tumors induce fibrosis and endochondral bone formation in vivo. J Cell Biol 126:1595-1609, 1994.

218. Reddi AH: Cell biology and biochemistry of endochondral bone development. Collagen Rel Res 1:209-226, 1981.

219. Thies RS, Bauduy M, Ashton BA, et al: Recombinant human bone morphogenetic protein-2 induces osteoblastic differentiation in W-20-17 stromal cells. Endocrinology 130:1318-1324, 1992.

220. Gimble JM, Morgan C, Kelly K, et al: Bone morphogenetic proteins inhibit adipocyte differentiation by bone marrow stromal cells. J Cell Biochem 58:393-402, 1995.

221. Beresford JN, Bennett JH, Devlin C, et al: Evidence for an inverse relationship between the differentiation of adipocytic and osteogenic cells in rat marrow stromal cell cultures. J Cell Sci 102:341-351, 1992.

222. Ozkaynak E, Schnegelsberg PN, Oppermann H: Murine osteogenic protein (OP-1): High levels of mRNA in kidney. Biochem Biophys Res Commun 179:116-123, 1991.

223. Gonzalez EA, Lund RJ, Martin KJ, et al: Treatment of a murine model of high-turnover renal osteodystrophy by exogenous BMP-7. Kidney Int 61:1322-1331, 2002.

224. Yoneda T: Local regulators of bone. In Bilezikian JP, Raisz LG, Rodan GA (eds): Principles of Bone Biology. San Diego, Academic Press, 1996, pp 729-738.

225. Chien HH, Lin WL, Cho MI: Down-regulation of osteoblastic cell differentiation by epidermal growth factor receptor. Calcif Tissue Int 67:141-150, 2000.

226. Drake MT, Baldassare JJ, McConkey CL, et al: Parathyroid hormone increases the expression of receptors for epidermal growth factor in UMR 106-01 cells. Endocrinology 134:1733-1737, 1994.

227. Gonzalez EA, Disthabanchong S, Kowalewski R, Martin KJ: Mechanisms of the regulation of EGF receptor gene expression by calcitriol and parathyroid hormone in UMR 106-01 cells. Kidney Int 61:1627-1634, 2002.

228. Baker LR, Ackrill P, Cattell WR, et al: Iatrogenic osteomalacia and myopathy due to phosphate depletion. Br Med J 3:150-152, 1974.

229. Mallette LE, Patten BM, Engel WK: Neuromuscular disease in secondary hyperparathyroidism. Ann Intern Med 82:474-483, 1975.

230. Lotem M, Robson MD, Rosenfeld JB: Spontaneous rupture of the quadriceps tendon in patients on chronic haemodialysis. Ann Rheum Dis 33:428-429, 1974.

231. Lotem M, Berheim J, Conforty B: Spontaneous rupture of tendons: A complication of hemodialyzed patients treated for renal failure. Nephron 21:201-208, 1978.

232. De Franco P, Varghese J, Brown WW, Bastani B: Secondary hyperparathyroidism, and not beta 2-microglobulin amyloid, as a cause of spontaneous tendon rupture in patients on chronic hemodialysis. Am J Kidney Dis 24:951-955, 1994.

233. Angelis M, Wong LL, Myers SA, Wong LM: Calciphylaxis in patients on hemodialysis: A prevalence study. Surgery 122:1083-1089; discussion 1089-1090, 1997.

234. Seyle H: Calciphylaxis. Chicago, University of Chicago Press, 1962.

235. Bleyer AJ, Choi M, Igwemezie B, et al: A case control study of proximal calciphylaxis [see comments]. Am J Kidney Dis 32:376-383, 1998.

236. Comp PC, Elrod JP, Karzenski S: Warfarin-induced skin necrosis. Semin Thromb Hemost 16:293-298, 1990.

237. Kant KS, Glueck HI, Coots MC, et al: Protein S deficiency and skin necrosis associated with continuous ambulatory peritoneal dialysis. Am J Kidney Dis 19:264-271, 1992.

238. Mehta RL, Scott G, Sloand JA, Francis CW: Skin necrosis associated with acquired protein C deficiency in patients with renal failure and calciphylaxis. Am J Med 88:252-257, 1990.

239. Westenfeld R, Heiss A, Ketteler M, et al: Calciphylaxis is linked to systemic deficiency of the calcification inhibitor ahsg/fetuin. J Am Soc Nephrol 13:461A, 2002.

240. Ganesh SK, Stack AG, Levin NW, et al: Association of elevated serum PO(4), Ca × PO(4) product, and parathyroid hormone with cardiac mortality risk in chronic hemodialysis patients. J Am Soc Nephrol 12:2131-2138, 2001.

241. London GM, Pannier B, Marchais SJ, Guerin AP: Calcification of the aortic valve in the dialyzed patient. J Am Soc Nephrol 11:778-783, 2000.

242. Block GA, Port FK: Re-evaluation of risks associated with hyperphosphatemia and hyperparathyroidism in dialysis patients: Recommendations for a change in management. Am J Kidney Dis 35:1226-1237, 2000.

243. Raggi P: Imaging of cardiovascular calcifications with electron beam tomography in hemodialysis patients. Am J Kidney Dis 37:S62-S65, 2001.

244. Goodman WG, Goldin J, Kuizon BD, et al: Coronary-artery calcification in young adults with end-stage renal disease who are undergoing dialysis. N Engl J Med 342:1478-1483, 2000.

245. London GM, Blacher J, Pannier B, et al: Arterial wave reflections and survival in end-stage renal failure. Hypertension 38:434-438, 2001.

246. Parhami F, Bostrom K, Watson K, Demer LL: Role of molecular regulation in vascular calcification. J Atheroscler Thromb 3:90-94, 1996.

247. Giachelli CM: Ectopic calcification: Gathering hard facts about soft tissue mineralization. Am J Pathol 154:671-675, 1999.

248. Luo G, Ducy P, McKee MD, et al: Spontaneous calcification of arteries and cartilage in mice lacking matrix GLA protein. Nature 386:78-81, 1997.

249. Kuro-o M, Matsumura Y, Aizawa H, et al: Mutation of the mouse klotho gene leads to a syndrome resembling ageing. Nature 390:45-51, 1997.

250. Bucay N, Sarosi I, Dunstan CR, et al: Osteoprotegerin-deficient mice develop early onset osteoporosis and arterial calcification. Genes Devel 12:1260-1268, 1998.

251. Jono S, McKee MD, Murry CE, et al: Phosphate regulation of vascular smooth muscle cell calcification. Circ Res 87:E10-E17, 2000.

252. Giachelli CM, Jono S, Shioi A, et al: Vascular calcification and inorganic phosphate. Am J Kidney Dis 38:S34-S37, 2001.

253. Kenzora JE: Dialysis carpal tunnel syndrome. Orthopedics 1:195-203, 1978.

254. Bardin T: Dialysis related amyloidosis. J Rheumatol 14:647-649, 1987.

255. Bardin T, Zingraff J, Shirahama T, et al: Hemodialysis-associated amyloidosis and beta-2 microglobulin: Clinical and immunohistochemical study. Am J Med 83:419-424, 1987.

256. Bardin T, Zingraff J, Kuntz D, Drueke T: Dialysis-related amyloidosis. Nephrol Dial Transplant 1:151-154, 1986.

257. Bardin T, Kuntz D, Zingraff J, et al: Synovial amyloidosis in patients undergoing long-term hemodialysis. Arthritis Rheum 28:1052-1058, 1985.

258. Drueke TB, Zingraff J, Noel LH, et al: Amyloidosis and dialysis: Pathophysiological aspects. Contrib Nephrol 62:60-66, 1988.

259. Zingraff JJ, Noel LH, Bardin T, et al: Beta 2-microglobulin amyloidosis in chronic renal failure. N Engl J Med 323:1070-1071, 1990.

260. Connors LH, Shirahama T, Skinner M, et al: In vitro formation of amyloid fibrils from intact beta 2-microglobulin. Biochem Biophys Res Commun 131:1063-1068, 1985.

261. Campistol JM, Sole M, Bombi JA, et al: In vitro spontaneous synthesis of beta 2-microglobulin amyloid fibrils in peripheral blood mononuclear cell culture. Am J Pathol 141:241-247, 1992.

262. Ono K, Uchino F: Formation of amyloid-like substance from beta-2-microglobulin in vitro—Role of serum amyloid P component: A preliminary study. Nephron 66:404-407, 1994.

263. Miyata T, Oda O, Inagi R, et al: Beta 2-microglobulin modified with advanced glycation end products is a major component of hemodialysis-associated amyloidosis. J Clin Invest 92:1243-1252, 1993.

264. Hou FF, Chertow GM, Kay J, et al: Interaction between beta 2-microglobulin and advanced glycation end products in the development of dialysis-related amyloidosis. Kidney Int 51:1514-1519, 1997.

265. Stein G, Schneider A, Thoss K, et al: Beta-2-microglobulin-derived amyloidosis: Onset, distribution and clinical features in 13 hemodialysed patients. Nephron 60:274-280, 1992.

266. Kessler M, Netter P, Azoulay E, et al: Dialysis-associated arthropathy: A multicentre survey of 171 patients receiving haemodialysis for over 10 years. The Co-operative Group on Dialysis-Associated Arthropathy. Br J Rheumatol 31:157-162, 1992.

267. Vandenbroucke JM, Jadoul M, Maldague B, et al: Possible role of dialysis membrane characteristics in amyloid osteoarthropathy. Lancet 1:1210-1211, 1986.

268. van Ypersele de Strihou C, Jadoul M, Malghem J, et al: Effect of dialysis membrane and patient's age on signs of dialysis-related amyloidosis. The Working Party on Dialysis Amyloidosis. Kidney Int 39:1012-1019, 1991.

269. Konishiike T, Hashizume H, Nishida K, et al: Shoulder pain in long-term haemodialysis patients: A clinical study of 166 patients. J Bone Joint Surg Br 78:601-605, 1996.

270. Katz GA, Peter JB, Pearson CM, Adams WS: The shoulder-pad sign: A diagnostic feature of amyloid arthropathy. N Engl J Med 288: 354-355, 1973.

271. Kuntz D, Naveau B, Bardin T, et al: Destructive spondylarthropathy in hemodialyzed patients: A new syndrome. Arthritis Rheum 27:369-375, 1984.

272. Bardin T, Kuntz D: The arthropathy of chronic haemodialysis. Clin Exp Rheumatol 5:379-386, 1987.

273. Kaplan P, Resnick D, Murphey M, et al: Destructive noninfectious spondyloarthropathy in hemodialysis patients: A report of four cases. Radiology 162:241-244, 1987.

274. Menard HA, Langevin S, Levesque RY: Destructive spondyloarthropathy in short term chronic ambulatory peritoneal dialysis and hemodialysis. J Rheumatol 15:644-647, 1988.

275. Cruz A, Gonzalez T, Balsa A, et al: Destructive spondyloarthropathy in longterm CAPD and hemodialysis. J Rheumatol 16:1169-1170, 1989.

276. DiRaimondo CR, Casey TT, DiRaimondo CV, Stone WJ: Pathologic fractures associated with idiopathic amyloidosis of bone in chronic hemodialysis patients. Nephron 43:22-27, 1986.

277. Campistol JM, Sole M, Munoz-Gomez J, et al: Pathological fractures in patients who have amyloidosis associated with dialysis: A report of five cases. J Bone Joint Surg Am 72:568-574, 1990.

278. Bardin T: Dialysis-associated amyloidosis. *In* Drüeke T, Salusky I (eds): The Spectrum of Renal Osteodystrophy. New York, Oxford, 2001, pp 285-307.

279. Floege J, Nonnast-Daniel B, Gielow P, et al: Specific imaging of dialysis-related amyloid deposits using 131I-beta-2-microglobulin. Nephron 51:444-447, 1989.

280. Nelson SR, Hawkins PN, Richardson S, et al: Imaging of haemodialysis-associated amyloidosis with 123I-serum amyloid P component. Lancet 338:335-339, 1991.

281. Kates D, Sherrard D, Andress D: Evidence that serum phosphate is independently associated with serum PTH in patients with chronic renal failure. Am J Kidney Dis 30:809-813, 1997.

282. Block GA, Hulbert-Shearon TE, Levin NW, Port FK: Association of serum phosphorus and calcium × phosphate product with mortality risk in chronic hemodialysis patients: A national study. Am J Kidney Dis 31:607-617, 1998.

283. Walton J, Gray TK: Absorption of inorganic phosphate in the human small intestine. Clin Sci (Lond) 56:407-412, 1979.

284. Walling MW, Hartenbower DL, Coburn JW, Norman AW: Effects of 1 alpha,25-, 24R,25-, and 1 alpha,24R,25-hydroxylated metabolites of vitamin D3 on calcium and phosphate absorption by duodenum from intact and nephrectomized rats. Arch Biochem Biophys 182:251-257, 1977.

285. Wiegmann TB, Kaye M: Malabsorption of calcium and phosphate in chronic renal failure: 32P and 45Ca studies in dialysis patients. Clin Nephrol 34:35-41, 1990.

286. Abou-Samra AB, Juppner H, Force T, et al: Expression cloning of a common receptor for parathyroid hormone and parathyroid hormone-related peptide from rat osteoblast-like cells: A single receptor stimulates intracellular accumulation of both cAMP and inositol trisphosphates and increases intracellular free calcium. Proc Natl Acad Sci U S A 89:2732-2736, 1992.

287. Traebert M, Roth J, Biber J, et al: Internalization of proximal tubular type II Na-P(i) cotransporter by PTH: Immunogold electron microscopy. Am J Physiol Ren Physiol 278:F148-F154, 2000.

288. Keusch I, Traebert M, Lotscher M, et al: Parathyroid hormone and dietary phosphate provoke a lysosomal routing of the proximal tubular Na/Pi-cotransporter type II. Kidney Int 54:1224-1232, 1998.

289. Taketani Y, Miyamoto K, Tanaka K, et al: Gene structure and functional analysis of the human Na+/phosphate co-transporter. Biochem J 324:927-934, 1997.

290. Garrett JE, Capuano IV, Hammerland LG, et al: Molecular cloning and functional expression of human parathyroid calcium receptor cDNAs. J Biol Chem 270:12919-12925, 1995.

291. Boyce BF, Fell GS, Elder HY, et al: Hypercalcaemic osteomalacia due to aluminium toxicity. Lancet 2:1009-1013, 1982.

292. Kurz P, Monier-Faugere MC, Bognar B, et al: Evidence for abnormal calcium homeostasis in patients with adynamic bone disease. Kidney Int 46:855-861, 1994.

293. Martin KJ, Gonzalez EA: The evolution of assays for parathyroid hormone. Curr Opin Nephrol Hypertens 10:569-574, 2001.

294. Canterbury JM, Reiss E: Multiple immunoreactive molecular forms of parathyroid hormone in human serum: 1. Proc Soc Exp Biol Med 140:1393-1398, 1972.

295. Habener JF, Segre GV, Powell D, et al: Immunoreactive parathyroid hormone in circulation of man. Nat New Biol 238:152-154, 1972.

296. Martin KJ, Hruska K, Freitag JJ, et al: Clinical utility of radioimmunoassays for parathyroid hormone. Miner Electrolyte Metab 3:283-290, 1980.

297. Martin KJ, Hruska KA, Lewis J, et al: The renal handling of parathyroid hormone: Role of peritubular uptake and glomerular filtration. J Clin Invest 60:808-814, 1977.

298. Brown RC, Aston JP, Weeks I, Woodhead JS: Circulating intact parathyroid hormone measured by a two-site immunochemiluminometric assay. J Clin Endocrinol Metab 65:407-414, 1987.

299. Kao PC, van Heerden JA, Grant CS, et al: Clinical performance of parathyroid hormone immunometric assays. Mayo Clin Proc 67: 637-645, 1992.

300. Brossard JH, Lepage R, Gao P, et al: A new commercial whole-PTH assay free of interference by non-(1-84) parathyroid hormone fragments in uremic samples. J Bone Miner Res 14:S444, 1999.

301. Sherwood LM, Mayer GP, Ramberg CF Jr, et al: Regulation of parathyroid hormone secretion: Proportional control by calcium, lack of effect of phosphate. Endocrinology 83:1043-1051, 1968.

302. Chu LL, MacGregor RR, Anast CS, et al: Studies on the biosynthesis of rat parathyroid hormone and proparathyroid hormone: Adaptation of the parathyroid gland to dietary restriction of calcium. Endocrinology 93:915-924, 1973.

303. Habener JF, Kemper B, Potts JT Jr: Calcium-dependent intracellular degradation of parathyroid hormone: A possible mechanism for the regulation of hormone stores. Endocrinology 97:431-441, 1975.

304. Segre GV, D'Amour P, Hultman A, Potts JT Jr: Effects of hepatectomy, nephrectomy, and nephrectomy/uremia on the metabolism of parathyroid hormone in the rat. J Clin Invest 67:439-448, 1981.

305. Bringhurst FR, Stern AM, Yotts M, et al: Peripheral metabolism of PTH: Fate of biologically active amino terminus in vivo. Am J Physiol 255:E886-E893, 1988.

306. Bringhurst FR, Segre GV, Lampman GW, Potts JT Jr: Metabolism of parathyroid hormone by Kupffer cells: Analysis by reverse-phase high-performance liquid chromatography. Biochemistry 21:4252-4258, 1982.

307. Martin KJ, Hruska KA, Freitag JJ, et al: The peripheral metabolism of parathyroid hormone. N Engl J Med 301:1092-1098, 1979.

308. Divieti P, Inomata N, Chapin K, et al: Receptors for the carboxyl-terminal region of PTH(1-84) are highly expressed in osteocytic cells. Endocrinology 142:916-925, 2001.

309. Monier-Faugere MC, Geng Z, Mawad H, et al: Improved assessment of bone turnover by the PTH-(1-84)/large C-PTH fragments ratio in ESRD patients. Kidney Int 60:1460-1468, 2001.

310. Coen G, Bonucci E, Ballanti P, et al: PTH 1-84 and PTH "7-84" in the noninvasive diagnosis of renal bone disease. Am J Kidney Dis 40:348-354, 2002.

311. Goldstein DJ, Rogers C, Harris H: A search for trace expression of placental-like alkaline phosphatase in non-malignant human tissues: Demonstration of its occurrence in lung, cervix, testis and thymus. Clin Chim Acta 125:63-75, 1982.

312. Seargeant LE, Stinson RA: Evidence that three structural genes code for human alkaline phosphatases. Nature 281:152-154, 1979.

313. Weiss MJ, Henthorn PS, Lafferty MA, et al: Isolation and characterization of a cDNA encoding a human liver/bone/kidney-type alkaline phosphatase. Proc Natl Acad Sci U S A 83:7182-7186, 1986.

314. Pierides AM, Skillen AW, Ellis HA: Serum alkaline phosphatase in azotemic and hemodialysis osteodystrophy: A study of isoenzyme patterns, their correlation with bone histology, and their changes in response to treatment with 1alphaOHD3 and 1,25(OH)2D3. J Lab Clin Med 93:899-909, 1979.

315. Cannella G, Bonucci E, Rolla D, et al: Evidence of healing of secondary hyperparathyroidism in chronically hemodialyzed uremic patients treated with long-term intravenous calcitriol. Kidney Int 46:1124-1132, 1994.

316. Fishman WH: Alkaline phosphatase isozymes: Recent progress. Clin Biochem 23:99-104, 1990.

317. Fishman WH: Recent developments in alkaline phosphatase research. Clin Chem 38:2484, 1992.

318. Hill CS, Wolfert RL: The preparation of monoclonal antibodies which react preferentially with human bone alkaline phosphatase and not liver alkaline phosphatase. Clin Chim Acta 186:315-320, 1990.

319. Urena P, Hruby M, Ferreira A, et al. Plasma total versus bone alkaline phosphatase as markers of bone turnover in hemodialysis patients. J Am Soc Nephrol 7:506-512, 1996.

320. Couttenye MM, D'Haese PC, Van Hoof VO, et al: Low serum levels of alkaline phosphatase of bone origin: A good marker of adynamic bone disease in haemodialysis patients. Nephrol Dial Transplant 11:1065-1072, 1996.

321. Coen G, Ballanti P, Bonucci E, et al: Bone markers in the diagnosis of low turnover osteodystrophy in haemodialysis patients. Nephrol Dial Transplant 13:2294-2302, 1998.

322. Ferreira A: Biochemical markers of bone turnover in the diagnosis of renal osteodystrophy: What do we have, what do we need? Nephrol Dial Transplant 13(suppl 3):29-32, 1998.

323. Jarava C, Armas JR, Salgueira M, Palma A: Bone alkaline phosphatase isoenzyme in renal osteodystrophy. Nephrol Dial Transplant 11(suppl 3):43-46, 1996.

324. Goodman WG, Ramirez JA, Belin TR, et al: Development of adynamic bone in patients with secondary hyperparathyroidism after intermittent calcitriol therapy. Kidney Int 46:1160-1166, 1994.

325. Pei Y, Hercz G, Greenwood C, et al: Risk factors for renal osteodystrophy: A multivariant analysis. J Bone Miner Res 10:149-156, 1995.

326. Kohlmeier M, Saupe J, Shearer MJ, et al: Bone health of adult hemodialysis patients is related to vitamin K status. Kidney Int 51:1218-1221, 1997.

327. Kohlmeier M, Saupe J, Schaefer K, Asmus G: Bone fracture history and prospective bone fracture risk of hemodialysis patients are related to apolipoprotein E genotype. Calcif Tissue Int 62:278-281, 1998.

328. Szulc P, Chapuy MC, Meunier PJ, Delmas PD: Serum undercarboxylated osteocalcin is a marker of the risk of hip fracture: A three year follow-up study. Bone 18:487-488, 1996.

329. Vermeer C, Jie KS, Knapen MH: Role of vitamin K in bone metabolism. Annu Rev Nutr 15:1-22, 1995.

330. Ducy P, Desbois C, Boyce B, et al: Increased bone formation in osteocalcin-deficient mice. Nature 382:448-452, 1996.

331. Ingram RT, Park YK, Clarke BL, Fitzpatrick LA: Age- and gender-related changes in the distribution of osteocalcin in the extracellular matrix of normal male and female bone. Possible involvement of osteocalcin in bone remodeling. J Clin Invest 93:989-997, 1994.

332. Slovik DM, Gundberg CM, Neer RM, Lian JB: Clinical evaluation of bone turnover by serum osteocalcin measurements in a hospital setting. J Clin Endocrinol Metab 59:228-230, 1984.

333. Gundberg CM, Hauschka PV, Lian JB, Gallop PM: Osteocalcin: Isolation, characterization, and detection. Methods Enzymol 107:516-544, 1984.

334. Delmas PD, Wilson DM, Mann KG, Riggs BL: Effect of renal function on plasma levels of bone Gla-protein. J Clin Endocrinol Metab 57:1028-1030, 1983.

335. Malluche HH, Faugere MC, Fanti P, Price PA: Plasma levels of bone Gla-protein reflect bone formation in patients on chronic maintenance dialysis. Kidney Int 26:869-874, 1984.

336. Charhon SA, Delmas PD, Malaval L, et al: Serum bone Gla-protein in renal osteodystrophy: Comparison with bone histomorphometry. J Clin Endocrinol Metab 63:892-897, 1986.

337. Qi Q, Monier-Faugere MC, Geng Z, et al: Predictive value of serum parathyroid hormone levels for bone turnover in patients on chronic maintenance dialysis. Am J Kidney Dis 26:622-631, 1995.

338. Gerakis A, Hutchison AJ, Apostolou T, et al: Biochemical markers for non-invasive diagnosis of hyperparathyroid bone disease and adynamic bone in patients on haemodialysis. Nephrol Dial Transplant 11:2430-2438, 1996.

339. Coen G, Mazzaferro S, Bonucci E, et al: Bone GLA protein in predialysis chronic renal failure: Effects of 1,25(OH)2D3 administration in a long-term follow-up. Kidney Int 28:783-790, 1985.

340. Cannella G, Bonucci E, Rolla D, et al: Evidence of healing of secondary hyperparathyroidism in chronically hemodialyzed uremic patients treated with long-term intravenous calcitriol. Kidney Int 46:1124-1132, 1994.

341. Urena P, Ferreira A, Kung VT, et al: Serum pyridinoline as a specific marker of collagen breakdown and bone metabolism in hemodialysis patients. J Bone Miner Res 10:932-939, 1995.

342. Ylikoski A, Hellman J, Matikainen T, et al: A dual-label immunofluorometric assay for human osteocalcin. J Bone Miner Res 13:1183-1190, 1998.

343. Minisola S, Rosso R, Romagnoli E, et al: Serum osteocalcin and bone mineral density at various skeletal sites: a study performed with three different assays. J Lab Clin Med 129:422-429, 1997.

344. Coen G, Ballanti P, Mazzaferro S, et al: Procollagen type 1 C-terminal extension peptide, PTH and 1,25(OH)2D3 in chronic renal failure. Bone 14:415-420, 1993.

345. Hamdy NA, Risteli J, Risteli L, et al: Serum type I procollagen peptide: A non-invasive index of bone formation in patients on haemodialysis? Nephrol Dial Transplant 9:511-516, 1994.

346. Hoshino H, Kushida K, Takahashi M, et al: Short-term effect of parathyroidectomy on biochemical markers in primary and secondary hyperparathyroidism. Miner Electrolyte Metab 23:93-99, 1997.

347. Parfitt AM, Simon LS, Villanueva AR, Krane SM: Procollagen type I carboxy-terminal extension peptide in serum as a marker of collagen biosynthesis in bone: Correlation with iliac bone formation rates and comparison with total alkaline phosphatase. J Bone Miner Res 2:427-436, 1987.

348. Eyre DR, Koob TJ, Van Ness KP: Quantitation of hydroxypyridinium crosslinks in collagen by high-performance liquid chromatography. Anal Biochem 137:380-388, 1984.

349. Prockop DJ, Kivirikko KI, Tuderman L, Guzman NA: The biosynthesis of collagen and its disorders [first of two parts]. N Engl J Med 301:13-23, 1979.

350. Seibel MJ, Woitge H, Scheidt-Nave C, et al: Urinary hydroxypyridinium crosslinks of collagen in population-based screening for overt vertebral osteoporosis: Results of a pilot study. J Bone Miner Res 9:1433-1440, 1994.

351. Robins SP, Black D, Paterson CR, et al: Evaluation of urinary hydroxypyridinium crosslink measurements as resorption markers in metabolic bone diseases. Eur J Clin Invest 21:310-315, 1991.

352. Kamel S, Brazier M, Neri V, et al: Multiple molecular forms of pyridinoline cross-links excreted in human urine evaluated by chromatographic and immunoassay methods. J Bone Miner Res 10:1385-1392, 1995.

353. McLaren AM, Isdale AH, Whiting PH, et al: Physiological variations in the urinary excretion of pyridinium crosslinks of collagen. Br J Rheumatol 32:307-312, 1993.

354. Robins SP, Woitge H, Hesley R, et al: Direct, enzyme-linked immunoassay for urinary deoxypyridinoline as a specific marker for measuring bone resorption. J Bone Miner Res 9:1643-1649, 1994.

355. Ibrahim S, Mojiminiyi S, Barron JL: Pyridinium crosslinks in patients on haemodialysis and continuous ambulatory peritoneal dialysis. Nephrol Dial Transplant 10:2290-2294, 1995.

356. Cheung CK, Panesar NS, Haines C, et al: Immunoassay of a tartrate-resistant acid phosphatase in serum. Clin Chem 41:679-686, 1995.

357. Chamberlain P, Compston J, Cox TM, et al: Generation and characterization of monoclonal antibodies to human type-5 tartrate-resistant acid phosphatase: Development of a specific immunoassay of the isoenzyme in serum. Clin Chem 41:1495-1499, 1995.

358. Kraenzlin ME, Lau KH, Liang L, et al: Development of an immunoassay for human serum osteoclastic tartrate-resistant acid phosphatase. J Clin Endocrinol Metab 71:442-451, 1990.

359. Halleen J, Hentunen TA, Hellman J, Vaananen HK: Tartrate-resistant acid phosphatase from human bone: Purification and development of an immunoassay. J Bone Miner Res 11:1444-1452, 1996.

360. Halleen JM, Ylipahkala H, Alatalo SL, et al: Serum tartrate-resistant acid phosphatase 5b, but not 5a, correlates with other markers of bone turnover and bone mineral density. Calcif Tissue Int 71:20-25, 2002.

361. Lau KH, Onishi T, Wergedal JE, et al: Characterization and assay of tartrate-resistant acid phosphatase activity in serum: Potential use to assess bone resorption. Clin Chem 33:458-462, 1987.

362. Seabrook RN, Bailyes EM, Price CP, et al: The distinction of bone and liver isoenzymes of alkaline phosphatase in serum using a monoclonal antibody. Clin Chim Acta 172:261-266, 1998.

363. Halleen JM, Alatalo SL, Suominen H, et al: Tartrate-resistant acid phosphatase 5b: A novel serum marker of bone resorption. J Bone Miner Res 15:1337-1345, 2000.

364. Eriksen EF, Charles P, Melsen F, et al: Serum markers of type I collagen formation and degradation in metabolic bone disease: Correlation with bone histomorphometry. J Bone Miner Res 8:127-132, 1993.

365. Hassager C, Jensen LT, Podenphant J, et al: The carboxy-terminal pyridinoline cross-linked telopeptide of type I collagen in serum as a marker of bone resorption: The effect of nandrolone decanoate and hormone replacement therapy. Calcif Tissue Int 54:30-33, 1994.

366. Garnero P, Shih WJ, Gineyts E, et al: Comparison of new biochemical markers of bone turnover in late postmenopausal osteoporotic women in response to alendronate treatment. J Clin Endocrinol Metab 79:1693-1700, 1994.

367. Mazzaferro S, Pasquali M, Ballanti P, et al: Diagnostic value of serum peptides of collagen synthesis and degradation in dialysis renal osteodystrophy. Nephrol Dial Transplant 10:52-58, 1995.

368. Diaz Lopez JB, Jorgetti V, Caorsi H, et al: Epidemiology of renal osteodystrophy in Iberoamerica. Nephrol Dial Transplant 13(suppl 3): 41-45, 1998.

369. Milliner DS, Nebeker HG, Ott SM, et al: Use of the deferoxamine infusion test in the diagnosis of aluminum-related osteodystrophy. Ann Intern Med 101:775-779, 1984.

370. D'Haese PC, Clement JP, Elseviers MM, et al: Value of serum aluminium monitoring in dialysis patients: A multicentre study. Nephrol Dial Transplant 5:45-53, 1990.

371. D'Haese PC, Couttenye MM, Goodman WG, et al: Use of the low-dose desferrioxamine test to diagnose and differentiate between patients with aluminium-related bone disease, increased risk for aluminium toxicity, or aluminium overload. Nephrol Dial Transplant 10:1874-1884, 1995.

372. D'Haese PC, Couttenye MM, De Broe ME: Diagnosis and treatment of aluminium bone disease. Nephrol Dial Transplant 11(suppl 3):74-79, 1996.

373. Pei Y, Hercz G, Greenwood C, et al: Non-invasive prediction of aluminum bone disease in hemo- and peritoneal dialysis patients. Kidney Int 41:1374-1382, 1992.

374. Cannata JB, Fernandez-Martin JL, Diaz-Lopez B, et al: Influence of iron status in the response to the deferoxamine test. J Am Soc Nephrol 7:135-139, 1996.

375. Huang JY, Huang CC, Lim PS, et al: Effect of body iron stores on serum aluminum level in hemodialysis patients. Nephron 61:158-162, 1992.

376. Vanuytsel JL, D'Haese PC, Couttenye MM, De Broe ME: Higher serum aluminium concentrations in iron-depleted dialysis patients. Nephrol Dial Transplant 7:177, 1992.

377. Zofkova I, Kancheva RL, Bendlova B: Effect of 1,25(OH)2 vitamin D3 on circulating insulin-like growth factor-I and beta 2 microglobulin in patients with osteoporosis. Calcif Tissue Int 60:236-239, 1997.

378. Ripoll E, Arribas I, Relea P, et al: Beta-2-microglobulin in diseases with high bone remodeling. Calcif Tissue Int 57:272-276, 1995.

379. Rico H, Ripoll E, Revilla M, et al: Beta 2-microglobulin in postmenopausal osteoporosis. Calcif Tissue Int 53:78-80, 1993.

380. Fan SL, Almond MK, Ball E, et al: Pamidronate therapy as prevention of bone loss following renal transplantation. Kidney Int 57:684-690, 2000.

381. Melton LJ 3rd, Atkinson EJ, O'Fallon WM, et al: Long-term fracture prediction by bone mineral assessed at different skeletal sites. J Bone Miner Res 8:1227-1233, 1993.

382. Black DM, Cummings SR, Genant HK, et al: Axial and appendicular bone density predict fractures in older women. J Bone Miner Res 7:633-638, 1992.

383. Rickers H, Christensen M, Rodbro P: Bone mineral content in patients on prolonged maintenance hemodialysis: A three year follow-up study. Clin Nephrol 20:302-307, 1983.

384. Stein MS, Packham DK, Ebeling PR, et al: Prevalence and risk factors for osteopenia in dialysis patients. Am J Kidney Dis 28:515-522, 1996.

385. Gabay C, Ruedin P, Slosman D, et al: Bone mineral density in patients with end-stage renal failure. Am J Nephrol 13:115-123, 1993.

386. Chan TM, Pun KK, Cheng IK: Total and regional bone densities in dialysis patients. Nephrol Dial Transplant 7:835-839, 1992.

387. Ha SK, Park CH, Seo JK, et al: Studies on bone markers and bone mineral density in patients with chronic renal failure. Yonsei Med J 37:350-356, 1996.

388. Rix M, Andreassen H, Eskildsen P, et al: Bone mineral density and biochemical markers of bone turnover in patients with predialysis chronic renal failure. Kidney Int 56:1084-1093, 1999.

389. Hampson G, Vaja S, Evans C, et al: Comparison of the humoral markers of bone turnover and bone mineral density in patients on haemodialysis and continuous ambulatory peritoneal dialysis. Nephron 91:94-102, 2002.

390. Gerakis A, Hadjidakis D, Kokkinakis E, et al: Correlation of bone mineral density with the histological findings of renal osteodystrophy in patients on hemodialysis. J Nephrol 13:437-443, 2000.

390a. Montagnani A, Gonnelli S, Cepollaro C, et al: Quantitative ultrasound in the assessment of skeletal status in uremic patients. J Clin Densitom 2:389-395, 1999.

391. Arici M, Erturk H, Altun B, et al: Bone mineral density in haemodialysis patients: A comparative study of dual-energy X-ray absorptiometry and quantitative ultrasound. Nephrol Dial Transplant 15:1847-1851, 2000.

392. Ito M, Hayashi K, Kawahara Y, et al: The relationship of trabecular and cortical bone mineral density to spinal fractures. Invest Radiol 28:573-580, 1993.

393. Pacifici R, Rupich R, Griffin M, et al: Dual energy radiography versus quantitative computer tomography for the diagnosis of osteoporosis. J Clin Endocrinol Metab 70:705-710, 1990.

394. Lechleitner P, Krimbacher E, Genser N, et al: Bone mineral densitometry in dialyzed patients: Quantitative computed tomography versus dual photon absorptiometry. Bone 15:387-391, 1994.

395. Tsurusaki K, Ito M, Hayashi K: Differential effects of menopause and metabolic disease on trabecular and cortical bone assessed by peripheral quantitative computed tomography (pQCT). Br J Radiol 73:14-22, 2000.

396. Slatopolsky E, Brown A, Dusso A: Role of phosphorus in the pathogenesis of secondary hyperparathyroidism. Am J Kidney Dis 37 (1 Suppl 2):S54-S57, 2001.

397. Hou SH, Zhao J, Ellman CF, et al: Calcium and phosphorus fluxes during hemodialysis with low calcium dialysate. Am J Kidney Dis 18:217-224, 1991.

398. Mucsi I, Hercz G, Uldall R, et al: Control of serum phosphate without any phosphate binders in patients treated with nocturnal hemodialysis. Kidney Int 53:1399-1404, 1998.

399. Braun J, Oldendorf M, Moshage W, et al: Electron beam computed tomography in the evaluation of cardiac calcification in chronic dialysis patients. Am J Kidney Dis 27:394-401, 1996.

400. Moe SM, O'Neill KD, Duan D, et al: Medial artery calcification in ESRD patients is associated with deposition of bone matrix proteins. Kidney Int 61:638-647, 2002.

401. Guerin AP, London GM, Marchais SJ, Metivier F: Arterial stiffening and vascular calcifications in end-stage renal disease. Nephrol Dial Transplant 15:1014-1021, 2000.

402. Guerin AP, Blacher J, Pannier B, et al: Impact of aortic stiffness attenuation on survival of patients in end-stage renal failure. Circulation 103:987-992, 2001.

403. Goodman WG, Goldin J, Kuizon BD, et al: Coronary-artery calcification in young adults with end-stage renal disease who are undergoing dialysis. N Engl J Med 342:1478-1483, 2000.

404. Chertow GM, Burke SK, Raggi P: Sevelamer attenuates the progression of coronary and aortic calcification in hemodialysis patients. Kidney Int 62:245-252, 2002.

405. Molitoris BA, Froment DH, Mackenzie TA, et al: Citrate: A major factor in the toxicity of orally administered aluminum compounds. Kidney Int 36:949-953, 1989.

406. Kirschbaum BB, Schoolwerth AC: Acute aluminum toxicity associated with oral citrate and aluminum-containing antacids. Am J Med Sci 297:9-11, 1989.

407. Coburn JW, Mischel MG, Goodman WG, Salusky IB: Calcium citrate markedly enhances aluminum absorption from aluminum hydroxide. Am J Kidney Dis 17:708-711, 1991.

408. Clarkson EM, McDonald SJ, De Wardener HE: The effect of a high intake of calcium carbonate in normal subjects and patients with chronic renal failure. Clin Sci 30:425-438, 1966.

409. Bro S, Rasmussen RA, Handberg J, et al: Randomized crossover study comparing the phosphate-binding efficacy of calcium ketoglutarate versus calcium carbonate in patients on chronic hemodialysis. Am J Kidney Dis 31:257-262, 1998.

410. Tan CC, Harden PN, Rodger RS, et al: Ranitidine reduces phosphate binding in dialysis patients receiving calcium carbonate. Nephrol Dial Transplant 11:851-853, 1996.

411. Osler P, Raniga P, Farrington K: Effect of omeprazole on the phosphate-binding capacity of calcium carbonate. Nephron 69:89-90, 1995.

412. Pflanz S, Henderson IS, McElduff N, Jones MC: Calcium acetate versus calcium carbonate as phosphate-binding agents in chronic haemodialysis. Nephrol Dial Transplant 9:1121-1124, 1994.

413. Sperschneider H, Gunther K, Marzoll I, et al: Calcium carbonate (CaCO3): An efficient and safe phosphate binder in haemodialysis patients? A 3-year study. Nephrol Dial Transplant 8:530-534, 1993.

414. Oettinger CW, Oliver JC, Macon EJ: The effects of calcium carbonate as the sole phosphate binder in combination with low calcium dialysate and calcitriol therapy in chronic hemodialysis patients. J Am Soc Nephrol 3:995-1001, 1992.

415. Malberti F, Surian M, Poggio F, et al: Efficacy and safety of long-term treatment with calcium carbonate as a phosphate binder. Am J Kidney Dis 12:487-491, 1988.

416. Slatopolsky E, Weerts C, Stokes T, et al: Alternative phosphate binders in dialysis patients: calcium carbonate. Semin Nephrol 6(4 suppl 1):35-41, 1986.

417. Slatopolsky E, Weerts C, Lopez-Hilker S, et al: Calcium carbonate as a phosphate binder in patients with chronic renal failure undergoing dialysis. N Engl J Med 315:157-161, 1986.

418. Taber TE, Hegemen TF, York S: Calcium carbonate as a phosphate binder in hemodialysis patients. ASAIO Trans 32:127-129, 1986.

419. Hercz G, Kraut JA, Andress DA, et al: Use of calcium carbonate as a phosphate binder in dialysis patients. Miner Electrolyte Metab 12:314-319, 1986.

420. Sheikh MS, Maguire JA, Emmett M, et al: Reduction of dietary phosphorus absorption by phosphorus binders: A theoretical, in vitro, and in vivo study. J Clin Invest 83:66-73, 1989.

421. Delmez JA, Tindira CA, Windus DW, et al: Calcium acetate as a phosphorus binder in hemodialysis patients. J Am Soc Nephrol 3:96-102, 1992.

422. Nestel AW, Meyers AM, Paiker J, Rollin HB: Effect of calcium supplement preparation containing small amounts of citrate on the absorption of aluminium in normal subjects and in renal failure patients. Nephron 68:197-201, 1994.

423. Fournier A, Moriniere P: Magnesium hydroxide is a useful complementary aluminum-free phosphate binder to moderate doses of oral calcium in uremic patients on chronic hemodialysis. Clin Nephrol 29:319, 1988.

424. Chanard J, Roujouleh H, Bernieh B, et al: Long-term use of magnesium hydroxide [Mg(OH)2] as a phosphate binder in patients on hemodialysis. Clin Nephrol 29:216-217, 1988.

425. Moriniere P, Vinatier I, Westeel PF, et al: Magnesium hydroxide as a complementary aluminium-free phosphate binder to moderate doses of oral calcium in uraemic patients on chronic haemodialysis: Lack of deleterious effect on bone mineralisation. Nephrol Dial Transplant 3:651-656, 1988.

426. Oe PL, Lips P, van der Meulen J, et al: Long-term use of magnesium hydroxide as a phosphate binder in patients on hemodialysis. Clin Nephrol 28:180-185, 1987.

427. Delmez JA, Kelber J, Norword KY, et al: Magnesium carbonate as a phosphorus binder: A prospective, controlled, crossover study. Kidney Int 49:163-167, 1996.

428. Chertow GM, Burke SK, Lazarus JM, et al: Poly[allylamine hydrochloride] (RenaGel): A noncalcemic phosphate binder for the treatment of hyperphosphatemia in chronic renal failure. Am J Kidney Dis 29:66-71, 1997.

429. Chertow GM, Burke SK, Dillon MA, Slatopolsky E: Long-term effects of sevelamer hydrochloride on the calcium x phosphate product and lipid profile of haemodialysis patients. Nephrol Dial Transplant 14:2907-2914, 1999.

430. Hutchison AJ: Calcitriol, lanthanum carbonate, and other new phosphate binders in the management of renal osteodystrophy. Perit Dial Int 19(suppl 2):S408-S412, 1999.

431. Coburn JW, Koppel MH, Brickman AS, Massry SG: Study of intestinal absorption of calcium in patients with renal failure. Kidney Int 3:264-272, 1973.

432. Werner E, Malluche HH, Kutschera J, et al: Intestinal calcium absorption and whole-body calcium retention in various stages of renal insufficiency. Calcif Tissue Res 21(suppl):210-215, 1976.

433. Slatopolsky E, Weerts C, Norwood K, et al: Long-term effects of calcium carbonate and 2.5 mEq/liter calcium dialysate on mineral metabolism. Kidney Int 36:897-903, 1989.

434. Hamdy NA, Kanis JA, Beneton MN, et al: Effect of alfacalcidol on natural course of renal bone disease in mild to moderate renal failure. BMJ 310:358-363, 1995.

435. Ritz E, Kuster S, Schmidt-Gayk H, et al: Low-dose calcitriol prevents the rise in 1,84-iPTH without affecting serum calcium and phosphate in patients with moderate renal failure (prospective placebo-controlled multicentre trial). Nephrol Dial Transplant 10:2228-2234, 1995.

436. Martin KJ, Ballal HS, Domoto DT, et al: Pulse oral calcitriol for the treatment of hyperparathyroidism in patients on continuous ambulatory peritoneal dialysis: Preliminary observations. Am J Kidney Dis 19:540-545, 1992.

437. Tsukamoto Y, Nomura M, Takahashi Y, et al: The "oral 1,25-dihydroxyvitamin D3 pulse therapy" in hemodialysis patients with severe secondary hyperparathyroidism. Nephron 57:23-28, 1991.

438. Maung HM, Elangovan L, Frazao JM, et al: Efficacy and side effects of intermittent intravenous and oral doxercalciferol (1alpha-hydroxyvitamin D(2)) in dialysis patients with secondary hyperparathyroidism: a sequential comparison. Am J Kidney Dis 37:532-543, 2001.

439. Indridason OS, Quarles LD: Oral versus intravenous calcitriol: Is the route of administration really important? Curr Opin Nephrol Hypertens 4:307-312, 1995.

440. Salusky IB, Goodman WG, Horst R, et al: Pharmacokinetics of calcitriol in continuous ambulatory and cycling peritoneal dialysis patients. Am J Kidney Dis 16:126-132, 1990.

441. Sjoden G, Smith C, Lindgren U, DeLuca HF: 1 alpha-Hydroxyvitamin D2 is less toxic than 1 alpha-hydroxyvitamin D3 in the rat. Proc Soc Exp Biol Med 178:432-436, 1985.

442. Sjoden G, Lindgren JU, DeLuca HF: Antirachitic activity of 1 alpha-hydroxyergocalciferol and 1 alpha-hydroxycholecalciferol in rats. J Nutr 114:2043-2046, 1984.

443. Knutson JC, Hollis BW, LeVan LW, et al: Metabolism of 1 alpha-hydroxyvitamin D2 to activated dihydroxyvitamin D 2 metabolites decreases endogenous 1 alpha, 25-dihydroxyvitamin D 3 in rats and monkeys. Endocrinology 136:4749-4753, 1995.

444. Mawer EB, Jones G, Davies M, et al: Unique 24-hydroxylated metabolites represent a significant pathway of metabolism of vitamin D2 in humans: 24-Hydroxyvitamin D2 and 1,24- dihydroxyvitamin D2 detectable in human serum. J Clin Endocrinol Metab 83:2156-2166, 1998.

445. Frazao JM, Elangovan L, Maung HM, et al: Intermittent doxercalciferol (1alpha-hydroxyvitamin D(2)) therapy for secondary hyperparathyroidism. Am J Kidney Dis 36:550-561, 2000.

446. Dusso AS, Negrea L, Gunawardhana S, et al: On the mechanisms for the selective action of vitamin D analogs. Endocrinology 128:1687-1692, 1991.

447. Okano T, Tsugawa N, Masuda S, et al: Protein-binding properties of 22-oxa-1 alpha,25-dihydroxyvitamin D3, a synthetic analogue of 1 alpha,25-dihydroxyvitamin D3. J Nutr Sci Vitaminol (Tokyo) 35:529-533, 1989.

448. Brown AJ, Finch J, Grieff M, et al: The mechanism for the disparate actions of calcitriol and 22-oxacalcitriol in the intestine. Endocrinology 133:1158-1164, 1993.

449. Brown AJ, Ritter CR, Finch JL, et al: The noncalcemic analogue of vitamin D, 22-oxacalcitriol, suppresses parathyroid hormone synthesis and secretion. J Clin Invest 84:728-732, 1989.

450. Tsukamoto Y, Hanaoka M, Matsuo T, et al: Effect of 22-oxacalcitriol on bone histology of hemodialyzed patients with severe secondary hyperparathyroidism. Am J Kidney Dis 35:458-464, 2000.

451. Monier-Faugere MC, Geng Z, Friedler RM, et al: 22-Oxacalcitriol suppresses secondary hyperparathyroidism without inducing low bone turnover in dogs with renal failure. Kidney Int 55:821-832, 1999.

452. Finch JL, Brown AJ, Slatopolsky E: Differential effects of 1,25-dihydroxy-vitamin D3 and 19-nor-1,25-dihydroxy-vitamin D2 on calcium and phosphorus resorption in bone. J Am Soc Nephrol 10:980-985, 1999.

453. Martin KJ, González EA, Gellens M, et al: 19-Nor-1-a-25-Dihydroxyvitamin D2 (paricalcitol) safely and effectively reduces

the levels of intact PTH in patients on hemodialysis. J Am Soc Nephrol 9:1427-1432, 1998.

454. Llach F, Yudd M: Paricalcitol in dialysis patients with calcitriol-resistant secondary hyperparathyroidism. Am J Kidney Dis 38(5 suppl 5):S45-S50, 2001.

455. Sprague SM, Lerma E, McCormmick D, et al: Suppression of parathyroid hormone secretion in hemodialysis patients: Comparison of paricalcitol with calcitriol. Am J Kidney Dis 38(5 suppl 5):S51-S56, 2001.

456. Martin KJ, Gonzalez EA, Gellens ME, et al: Therapy of secondary hyperparathyroidism with 19-nor-1alpha,25-dihydroxyvitamin D2. Am J Kidney Dis 32(2 suppl 2):S61-S66, 1998.

457. Coyne DW, Grieff M, Ahya S, et al: Differential potencies of 1,25(OH)$_2$D$_3$ and 19-nor-1,25(OH)$_2$D$_2$ on bone resorption in hemodialysis patients. J Am Soc Nephrol 11:574A, 2000.

458. Teng M, Wolf M, Lowrie E, et al: Survival of patients undergoing hemodialysis with paracalcitol or calcitriol therapy. N Engl J Med 349:446-456, 2003.

459. Tanaka Y, DeLuca HF, Kobayashi Y, Ikekawa N: 26,26,26,27,27,27-Hexafluoro-1,25-dihydroxyvitamin D3: A highly potent, long-lasting analog of 1,25-dihydroxyvitamin D3. Arch Biochem Biophys 229:348-354, 1984.

460. Akiba T, Marumo F, Owada A, et al: Controlled trial of falecalcitriol versus alfacalcidol in suppression of parathyroid hormone in hemodialysis patients with secondary hyperparathyroidism. Am J Kidney Dis 32:238-246, 1998.

461. Neyer U, Hoerandner H, Haid A, et al: Total parathyroidectomy with autotransplantation in renal hyperparathyroidism: Low recurrence after intra-operative tissue selection. Nephrol Dial Transplant 17:625-659, 2002.

462. Niederle B, Horandner H, Roka R, Woloszczuk W: Morphologic and functional studies to prevent graft-dependent recurrence in renal osteodystrophy. Surgery 106:1043-1048, 1989.

463. Niederle B, Roka R, Brennan MF: The transplantation of parathyroid tissue in man: Development, indications, technique, and results. Endocr Rev 3:245-279, 1982.

464. Wells SA Jr, Stirman JA Jr, Bolman RM 3rd, Gunnells JC: Transplantation of the parathyroid glands: Clinical and experimental results. Surg Clin North Am 58:391-402, 1978.

465. Kaye M, Rosenthall L, Hill RO, Tabah RJ: Long-term outcome following total parathyroidectomy in patients with end-stage renal disease. Clin Nephrol 39:192-197, 1993.

466. Ljutic D, Cameron JS, Ogg CS, et al: Long-term follow-up after total parathyroidectomy without parathyroid reimplantation in chronic renal failure. QJM 87:685-692, 1994.

467. Kessler M, Avila JM, Renoult E, Mathieu P: Reoperation for secondary hyperparathyroidism in chronic renal failure. Nephrol Dial Transplant 6:176-179, 1991.

468. Edis AJ, Levitt MD: Supernumerary parathyroid glands: Implications for the surgical treatment of secondary hyperparathyroidism. World J Surg 11:398-401, 1987.

469. Meakins JL, Milne CA, Hollomby DJ, Goltzman D: Total parathyroidectomy: Parathyroid hormone levels and supernumerary glands in hemodialysis patients. Clin Invest Med 7:21-25, 1984.

470. Tominaga Y, Tanaka Y, Sato K, et al: Recurrent renal hyperparathyroidism and DNA analysis of autografted parathyroid tissue. World J Surg 16:595-602; discussion 602-603, 1992.

471. Gagne ER, Urena P, Leite-Silva S, et al: Short- and long-term efficacy of total parathyroidectomy with immediate autografting compared with subtotal parathyroidectomy in hemodialysis patients. J Am Soc Nephrol 3:1008-1017, 1992.

472. Kitaoka M, Fukagawa M, Ogata E, Kurokawa K: Reduction of functioning parathyroid cell mass by ethanol injection in chronic dialysis patients. Kidney Int 46:1110-1117, 1994.

473. Fukagawa M, Kitaoka M, Tominaga Y, et al: Selective percutaneous ethanol injection therapy (PEIT) of the parathyroid in chronic dialysis patients: The Japanese strategy. Japanese Working Group on PEIT of Parathyroid, Tokyo, Japan. Nephrol Dial Transplant 14:2574-2577, 1994.

474. Goodman WG: Calcimimetic agents and secondary hyperparathyroidism: Treatment and prevention. Nephrol Dial Transplant 17:204-207, 2002.

475. de Vernejoul MC, Marchais S, London G, et al: Increased bone aluminum deposition after subtotal parathyroidectomy in dialyzed patients. Kidney Int 27:785-791, 1985.

476. Zacharias JM, Fontaine B, Fine A: Calcium use increases risk of calciphylaxis: A case-control study. Perit Dial Int 19:248-252, 1999.

477. Campistol JM, Almirall J, Martin E, et al: Calcium-carbonate-induced calciphylaxis. Nephron 51:549-550, 1989.

478. Fine A, Zacharias J: Calciphylaxis is usually non-ulcerating: Risk factors, outcome and therapy. Kidney Int 61:2210-2217, 1992.

479. Lipsker D, Chosidow O, Martinez F, et al: Low-calcium dialysis in calciphylaxis. Arch Dermatol 133:798-799, 1997.

480. Budisavljevic MN, Cheek D, Ploth DW: Calciphylaxis in chronic renal failure. J Am Soc Nephrol 7:978-982, 1996.

481. Chan YL, Mahony JF, Turner JJ, Posen S: The vascular lesions associated with skin necrosis in renal disease. Br J Dermatol 109:85-95, 1983.

482. Vassa N, Twardowski ZJ, Campbell J: Hyperbaric oxygen therapy in calciphylaxis-induced skin necrosis in a peritoneal dialysis patient. Am J Kidney Dis 23:878-881, 1994.

483. Elamin EM, McDonald AB: Calcifying panniculitis with renal failure: A new management approach. Dermatology 192:156-159, 1996.

484. Sethi D, Gower PE: Dialysis arthropathy, beta 2-microglobulin and the effect of dialyser membrane. Nephrol Dial Transplant 3:768-772, 1988.

485. Schiffl H, D'Agostini B, Held E: Removal of beta 2-microglobulin by hemodialysis and hemofiltration: A four year follow up. Biomater Artif Cells Immobilization Biotechnol 20:1223-1232, 1992.

486. Campistol JM: Dialysis-related amyloidosis after renal transplantation. Semin Dial 14:99-102, 2001.

487. Grotz WH, Mundinger FA, Gugel B, et al: Bone fracture and osteodensitometry with dual energy X-ray absorptiometry in kidney transplant recipients. Transplantation 58:912-915, 1994.

488. Pietschmann P, Vychytil A, Woloszczuk W, Kovarik J: Bone metabolism in patients with functioning kidney grafts: Increased serum levels of osteocalcin and parathyroid hormone despite normalisation of kidney function. Nephron 59:533-536, 1991.

489. Parfitt AM: Hypercalcemic hyperparathyroidism following renal transplantation: Differential diagnosis, management, and implications for cell population control in the parathyroid gland. Miner Electrolyte Metab 8:92-112, 1982.

490. Parfitt AM: The hyperparathyroidism of chronic renal failure: A disorder of growth. Kidney Int 52:3-9, 1997.

491. Drueke TB, Zhang P, Gogusev J: Apoptosis: Background and possible role in secondary hyperparathyroidism. Nephrol Dial Transplant 12:2228-2233, 1997.

492. Chang DJ, Ji C, Kim KK, et al: Reduction in transforming growth factor beta receptor I expression and transcription factor CBFa1 on bone cells by glucocorticoid. J Biol Chem 273:4892-4896, 1998.

493. Centrella M, Rosen V, Wozney JM, et al: Opposing effects by glucocorticoid and bone morphogenetic protein-2 in fetal rat bone cell cultures. J Cell Biochem 67:528-540, 1997.

494. Kasperk C, Schneider U, Sommer U, et al: Differential effects of glucocorticoids on human osteoblastic cell metabolism in vitro. Calcif Tissue Int 57:120-126, 1995.

495. Canalis E: Inhibitory actions of glucocorticoids on skeletal growth: Is local insulin-like growth factor I to blame? Endocrinology 139:3041-3042, 1998.

496. Weinstein RS, Chen JR, Powers CC, et al: Promotion of osteoclast survival and antagonism of bisphosphonate-induced osteoclast apoptosis by glucocorticoids. J Clin Invest 109:1041-1048, 2002.

497. Sasaki N, Kusano E, Ando Y, et al: Glucocorticoid decreases circulating osteoprotegerin (OPG): Possible mechanism for glucocorticoid induced osteoporosis. Nephrol Dial Transplant 16:479-482, 2001.

498. Manolagas SC: Birth and death of bone cells: Basic regulatory mechanisms and implications for the pathogenesis and treatment of osteoporosis. Endocr Rev 21:115-137, 2000.

499. Lane NE, Lukert B: The science and therapy of glucocorticoid-induced bone loss. Endocrinol Metab Clin North Am 27:465-483, 1998.

500. Epstein S, Shane E, Bilezikian JP: Organ transplantation and osteoporosis. Curr Opin Rheumatol 7:255-261, 1995.

501. Cvetkovic M, Mann GN, Romero DF, et al: The deleterious effects of long-term cyclosporine A, cyclosporine G, and FK506 on bone mineral metabolism in vivo. Transplantation 57:1231-1237, 1994.

502. Schlosberg M, Movsowitz C, Epstein S, et al: The effect of cyclosporin A administration and its withdrawal on bone mineral metabolism in the rat. Endocrinology 124:2179-2184, 1989.

503. Stewart PJ, Green OC, Stern PH: Cyclosporine A inhibits calcemic hormone-induced bone resorption in vitro. J Bone Miner Res 1:285-291, 1986.

504. Klaushofer K, Hoffmann O, Stewart PJ, et al: Cyclosporine A inhibits bone resorption in cultured neonatal mouse calvaria. J Pharmacol Exp Ther 243:584-590, 1987.

505. Park KM, Hay JE, Lee SG, et al: Bone loss after orthotopic liver transplantation: FK 506 versus cyclosporine. Transplant Proc 28: 1738-1740, 1996.

506. Julian BA, Laskow DA, Dubovsky J, et al: Rapid loss of vertebral mineral density after renal transplantation. N Engl J Med 325:544-550, 1991.

507. Casez JP, Lippuner K, Horber FF, et al: Changes in bone mineral density over 18 months following kidney transplantation: The respective roles of prednisone and parathyroid hormone. Nephrol Dial Transplant 17:1318-1326, 2002.

508. Heaf J, Tvedegaard E, Kanstrup IL, Fogh-Andersen N: Bone loss after renal transplantation: Role of hyperparathyroidism, acidosis, cyclosporine and systemic disease. Clin Transplant 14:457-463, 2000.

509. Wolpaw T, Deal CL, Fleming-Brooks S, et al: Factors influencing vertebral bone density after renal transplantation. Transplantation 58:1186-1189, 1994.

510. Almond MK, Kwan JT, Evans K, Cunningham J: Loss of regional bone mineral density in the first 12 months following renal transplantation. Nephron 66:52-57, 1994.

511. Grotz WH, Mundinger FA, Gugel B, et al: Bone mineral density after kidney transplantation: A cross-sectional study in 190 graft recipients up to 20 years after transplantation. Transplantation 59: 982-986, 1995.

512. Grotz WH, Mundinger FA, Rasenack J, et al: Bone loss after kidney transplantation: A longitudinal study in 115 graft recipients. Nephrol Dial Transplant 10:2096-2100, 1995.

513. Pichette V, Bonnardeaux A, Prudhomme L, et al: Long-term bone loss in kidney transplant recipients: A cross-sectional and longitudinal study. Am J Kidney Dis 28:105-114, 1996.

514. Pierides AM, Ellis HA, Peart KM, et al: Assessment of renal osteodystrophy following renal transplantation. Proc Eur Dial Transplant Assoc 11:481-487, 1975.

515. Carroll RN, Williams ED, Aung T, et al: The effects of renal transplantation on renal osteodystrophy. Proc Eur Dial Transplant Assoc 10:446-454, 1973.

516. Cueto-Manzano AM, Konel S, Hutchison AJ, et al: Bone loss in long-term renal transplantation: Histopathology and densitometry analysis. Kidney Int 55:2021-2029, 1999.

517. Monier-Faugere MC, Mawad H, Qi Q, et al: High prevalence of low bone turnover and occurrence of osteomalacia after kidney transplantation. J Am Soc Nephrol 11:1093-1099, 2000.

518. Carlini RG, Rojas E, Weisinger JR, et al: Bone disease in patients with long-term renal transplantation and normal renal function. Am J Kidney Dis 36:160-166, 2000.

519. Cueto-Manzano AM, Konel S, Freemont AJ, et al: Effect of 1,25-dihydroxyvitamin D3 and calcium carbonate on bone loss associated with long-term renal transplantation. Am J Kidney Dis 35:227-236, 2000.

520. Cummings SR, Black DM, Nevitt MC, et al: Bone density at various sites for prediction of hip fractures. The Study of Osteoporotic Fractures Research Group. Lancet 341:72-75, 1993.

521. Gallacher SJ, Fenner JA, Anderson K, et al: Intravenous pamidronate in the treatment of osteoporosis associated with corticosteroid dependent lung disease: An open pilot study. Thorax 47:932-986, 1992.

522. Grotz W, Nagel C, Poeschel D, et al: Effect of ibandronate on bone loss and renal function after kidney transplantation. J Am Soc Nephrol 12:1530-1537, 2001.

523. Giannini S, Dangel A, Carraro G, et al: Alendronate prevents further bone loss in renal transplant recipients. J Bone Miner Res 16: 2111-2117, 2001.

524. Plotkin LI, Weinstein RS, Parfitt AM, et al: Prevention of osteocyte and osteoblast apoptosis by bisphosphonates and calcitonin. J Clin Invest 104:1363-1374, 1999.

525. Martin KJ, Gonzalez EA, Slatopolsky E: The parathyroids in renal disease. *In* Bilezikian JP, Marcus R, Levine MA (eds): The Parathyroids: Basic and Clinical Concepts, 2nd ed. New York, Academic Press, 2001, pp 625-634.

526. Martin KJ, Gonzalez EA, Slatopolsky E: Renal osteodystrophy. *In* Becker KL (ed): Principles and Practice of Endocrinology and Metabolism, 3rd ed. Philadelphia, Lippincott Williams & Wilkins, 2001, pp 603-610.

527. González E, Martin K: Bone cell response in uremia. Semin Dial 9:339-346, 1996.

528. Gonzalez EA, Martin KJ: Bone and mineral metabolism in chronic renal failure. *In* Johnson J, Feehally RJ (eds): Comprehensive Clinical Nephrology. London, Mosby, 2000, pp 69.1-69.11.

529. Gonzalez EA, Martin KJ: Assessment of bone and joint diseases: Renal osteodystrophy. *In* Bilezikian JP (ed): Dynamics of Bone and Cartilage Metabolism. New York, Academic Press, 1999, pp 561-569.

530. Potts JT Jr, Juppner H: Parathyroid hormone and parathyroid hormone-related peptide in calcium homeostasis, bone metabolism, and bone development: The proteins, their genes, and receptors. *In* Avioli LV, Krane SM (eds): Metabolic Bone Disease, 3rd ed. New York, Academic Press, 1998, pp 51-94.

531. Juppner H, Potts JT Jr: Immunoassays for the detection of parathyroid hormone (PTH). J Bone Miner Res 17(suppl 2):N81-N86, 2002.

532. Meema HE, Meema S: Microradioscopic quantitation of periosteal resorption in secondary hyperparathyroidism of chronic renal failure. Clin Orthop 130:297-302, 1978.

533. Fenves AZ, Emmett M, White MG, et al: Carpal tunnel syndrome with cystic bone lesions secondary to amyloidosis in chronic hemodialysis patients. Am J Kidney Dis 7:130-134, 1986.

CHAPTER 53

Effect of Aging on Renal Function and Disease

Devasmita Choudhury, Dominic S. C. Raj, and Moshe Levi

Although the aging kidney maintains the day-to-day internal milieu, renal reserve in the aging kidney is challenged in the face of physiologic and pathophysiologic perturbations. The structural and functional impact of biologic aging on the kidney is most evident when stresses of intercurrent insults, including infections, immunologic processes, drugs, toxins, or other organ failure, affect the patient. Donor kidneys demonstrate this change: Kidneys older than 55 years of age are more likely to fail from chronic allograft nephropathy.[1-5]

Recent Census Bureau estimates suggest a growing population of elderly (older than 65 years of age), from 35 million in the year 2000 to 54 million by the year 2010.[6] The prevalence of moderate to severe renal failure is 20.6% in this population, and even in the absence of diabetes and hypertension it is 10.8%.[6] Furthermore a decrease in kidney function is an independent risk factor for both cardiovascular disease and all-cause mortality in the general population.[6] In addition, the prevalence of end-stage renal disease (ESRD) is five times higher in the elderly than in young adults.[7] In fact, a greater number of elderly subjects are dominating dialysis registries in both the United States and Europe.[7, 8] Therefore increasing our insight by understanding the anatomic, physiologic, and pathologic changes of aging in the kidney is important to prevent disastrous outcomes in elderly patients. Various new molecular probes and techniques have furthered our ability to investigate and increase understanding of basic mechanisms involving renal senescence. Current understanding of the interactions among aging, renal function, and renal disease is reviewed in this chapter.

ANATOMY AND STRUCTURE OF THE AGING KIDNEY

Both the mass and the weight of the kidney progressively decline with advancing age. Size and volume of older postmortem kidneys are smaller, as evaluated by intravenous urography and computed tomography.[9, 10] A parallel decrease in kidney weight occurs, from 250 to 270 g during young adulthood to 180 to 200 g by 90 years of age.[11] However, when the change in renal mass and weight are adjusted for a concurrent decrease in body surface area with aging, the changes in the kidney appear to be age appropriate.[12]

Histologic evaluation of the aging kidney reveals glomerulosclerosis and tubulointerstitial fibrosis. Ischemia of the cortical glomeruli is prevalent, with glomerular number decreasing by 30% to 50% by age 70.[13] Medullary glomeruli appear to be relatively spared. Glomerular obsolescence is characterized by loss of glomerular tuft lobulation, an increase in mesangial volume of 8% to 12%, and progressive capillary collapse with obliteration.[14] A significant decrease in glomerular and peritubular capillary density correlates (Fig. 53-1) with reduced expression of proangiogenic vascular endothelial growth factor and increased expression of antiangiogenic factor, thrombospondin-1 in aged (24-month-old) Sprague-Dawley rats, compared with younger (3-month-old) rats,[15] suggesting possible impaired angiogenesis in aging kidneys. There is thickening and wrinkling of the basement membranes of both glomeruli and tubules, with eventual reduction and simplification of the vascular channels.[16, 17] Redistribution of blood flow favors the renal medulla as blood is shunted from the afferent to the efferent arterioles of the juxtamedullary glomeruli (Fig. 53-2).[18] Blood flow is maintained to the medulla via the arteriolar vera recta, which remain intact.[17, 19] Scarring occurs as hyaline deposits in residual glomeruli and the Bowman space with little to no cellular response. Histologic changes seem to correlate with changes at the molecular level. Telomere length, as investigated by Southern blotting of terminal restriction fragments, shortens in an age-dependent fashion in the renal cortex faster than in the renal medulla.[20] Because telomeres can act as a mitotic clock reflecting replicate senescence of the cell,[21-23] critical telomere shortening in the renal cortex of the

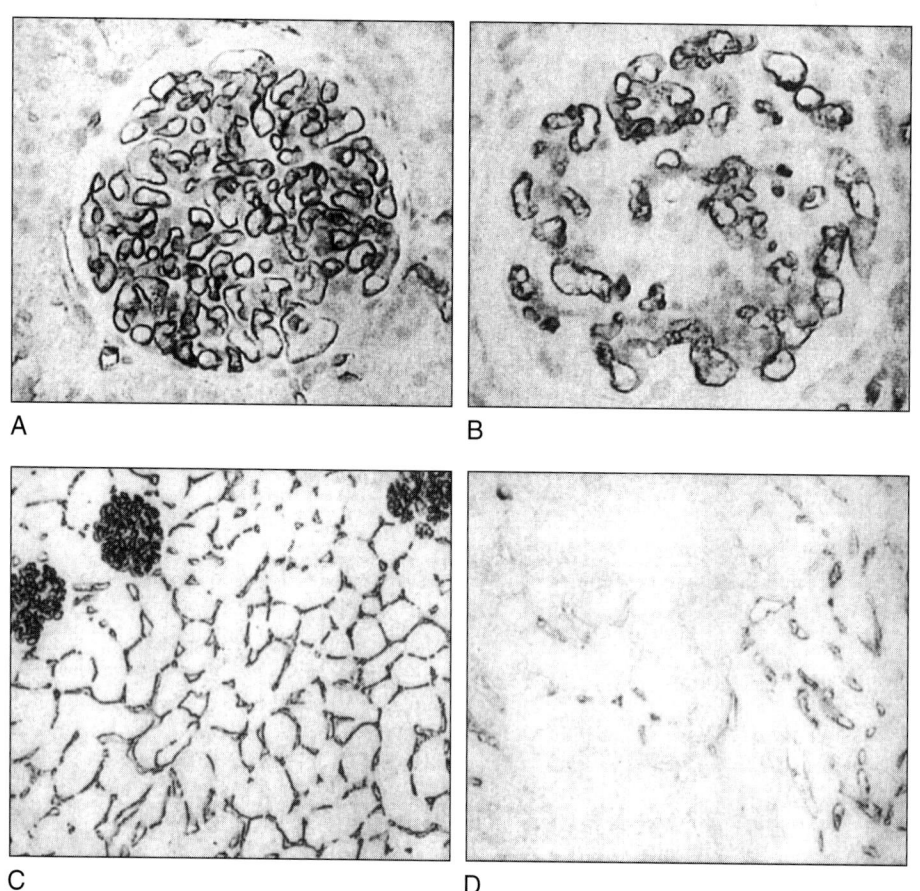

FIGURE 53-1. Glomerular and peritubular capillary immunostaining in young kidneys (**A** and **C**) and in aging kidneys (**B** and **D**). Glomerular capillary loops stained with RECA-1 in young rats are well preserved (**A**), whereas glomerular hypertrophy and decreased capillary loop numbers are observed in aging rats (**B**). Photomicrographs also show normal peritubular capillary architecture by JG-12 staining in a young rat (**C**) and focal and patchy loss in peritubular capillary staining by JG-12 in aging rats (**D**). RECA-1, rat endothelial cell antigen-1. (Reprinted with permission from Kang DH, Anderson S, Kim YG, et al: Impaired angiogenesis in the aging kidney: Vascular endothelial growth factor and thrombospondin-1 in renal disease. Am J Kidney Dis 37:601-611, 2001.)

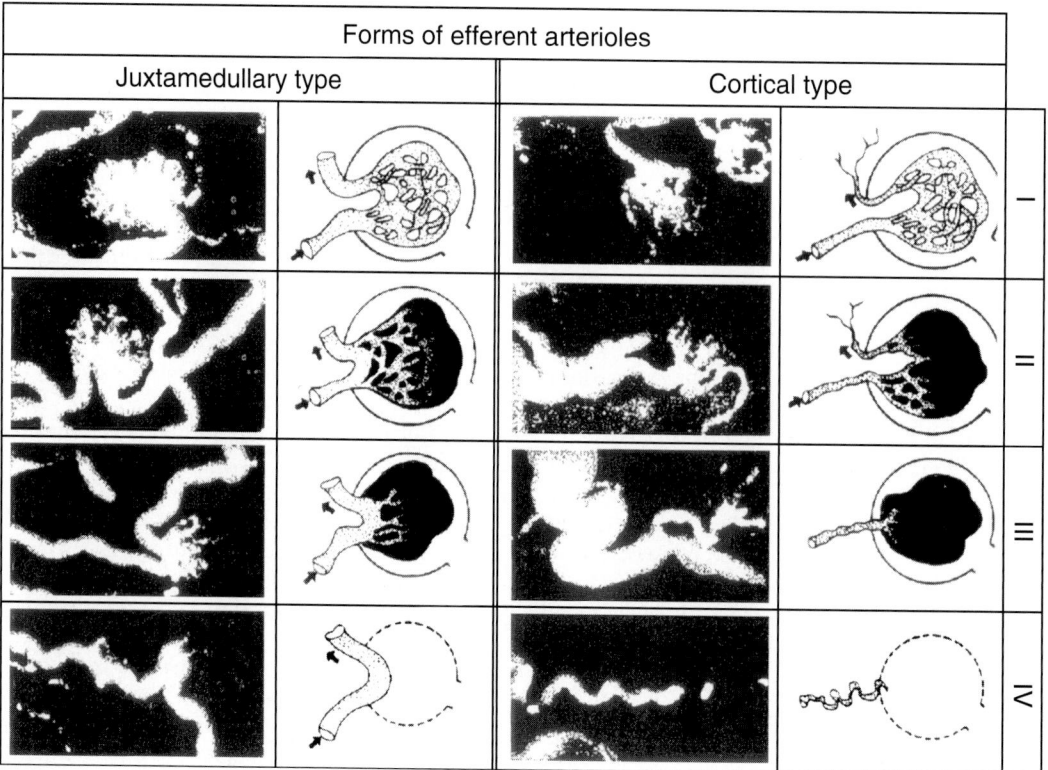

FIGURE 53-2. Progressive (stage I through IV) vascular simplification and glomerular degeneration of the cortical and juxtamedullary arteriole-glomerular units with corresponding microangiograms. (Reprinted with permission from Takazakura E, Sawabu N, Handa A, et al: Intrarenal vascular changes with age and disease. Kidney Int 2:224-230, 1972.)

aged kidney raises the possibility that in some renal cell populations this may be a limiting factor and may contribute to some features seen in the senescent kidney.[20]

Renal tubules also decrease in size and number as they atrophy to form distal diverticula. These outpouchings may represent the earliest formation of acquired cysts as seen in aged kidneys (Fig. 53-3).[24] Bacteria and debris can collect in these diverticula and may predispose to infection and pyelonephritis.[25]

Evaluation of changes in the renal extracellular matrix of aging rats suggests that tubulointerstitial fibrosis actually precedes the development of focal glomerulosclerosis or tubular atrophy.[26, 27] Furthermore, tubulointerstitial fibrosis in aging is an active process associated with interstitial inflammation, fibroblast activation, and accelerated apoptosis of cells in areas of fibrosis.[28] Focal tubular cell proliferation, myofibroblast activation, macrophage infiltration, increased immunostaining for the adhesive proteins osteopontin and intracellular adhesion molecule-1, and collagen IV deposition are found in aged rats. Age-related increases in types I and IV collagen and fibronectin messenger RNA (mRNA) expression were also found in 24- and 30-month-old rats. Ischemia from peritubular capillary injury with altered endothelial nitric oxide synthase (eNOS) expression triggers this inflammation. Collagen I mRNA was up-regulated in aging Sprague-Dawley rats in association with histologic evidence of collagen I accumulation and progressive fibrosis.[29] Collagen I protein accumulation also increased significantly with age in human renal autopsy tissue and correlated with the extent of interstitial fibrosis, indicating that collagen I is a key component of age-related development of interstitial fibrotic lesions; however,

the same was not observed for collagen IV.[30] Interestingly, changes in mRNA levels of the collagen proteins were opposite to that of the tissue protein accumulation (Fig. 53-4). Because degradation is accomplished by different metalloproteinases (MMPs), including MMP-3, MMP-9 for collagen IV and MMP-8, MMP-13 for collagen I, aging may affect the activity of these proteinases differently, leading to accumulation of one and not the other.[30]

Changes in the aging intrarenal vasculature occur independently of hypertension or other renal disease. Walls of the larger renal vessels undergo variable sclerotic changes that are made worse by hypertension.[16] Donor biopsies from healthy elderly individuals show increased arteriosclerosis of intrarenal vessels and interlobular and arcuate arteries, compared with younger kidneys.[31] Smaller vessels are spared, with fewer than 20% of senescent kidneys from nonhypertensive subjects displaying arteriolar changes.[16] Results of pyelography and angiography on postmortem kidneys of normotensive subjects older than 50 years of age suggest that loss of renal cortical tissue in the elderly may be related more to changes in the renal vasculature than to age alone.[32]

GLOMERULOSCLEROSIS AND TUBULOINTERSTITIAL FIBROSIS IN AGING: MEDIATORS AND POTENTIAL STRATEGIES FOR MODULATION

Although it is evident from histologic studies that aging is associated with glomerulosclerosis and tubulointerstitial fibrosis, the rate of sclerosis may vary depending on specific etiologic factors more recently identified by animal models

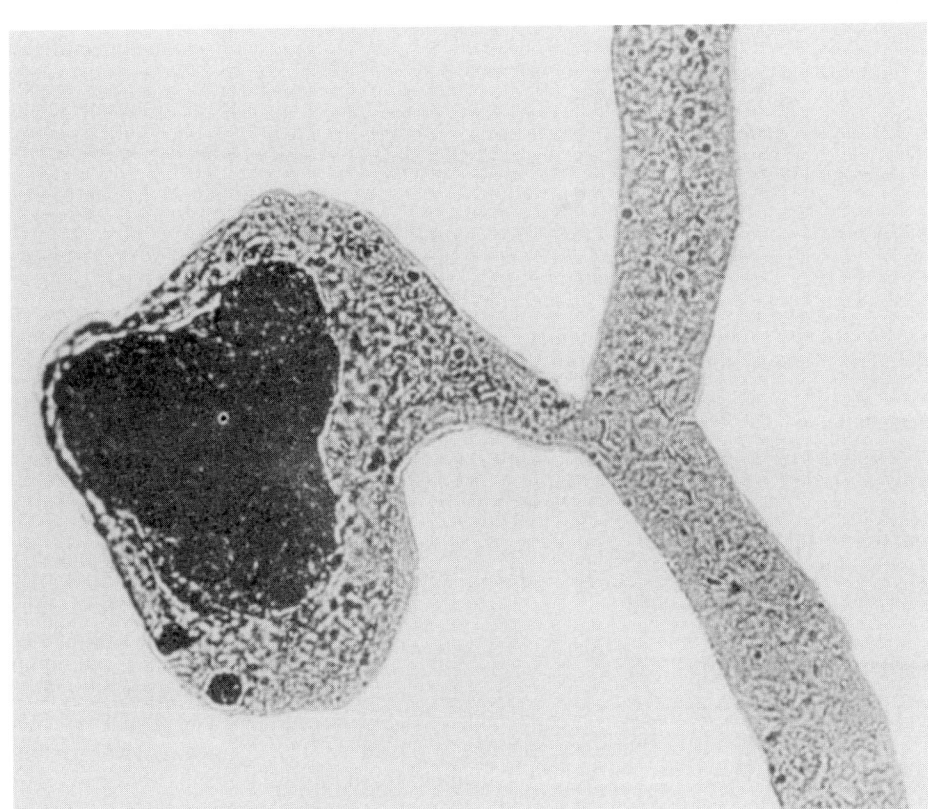

FIGURE 53-3. Microdissection of collecting tubule and associated diverticulum showing continuity between tubular lumen and diverticulum. (Reprinted with permission from Baert L, Steg A: Is the diverticulum of the distal and collecting tubules a preliminary stage of the simple cyst in the adult? J Urol 113:707-710, 1977.)

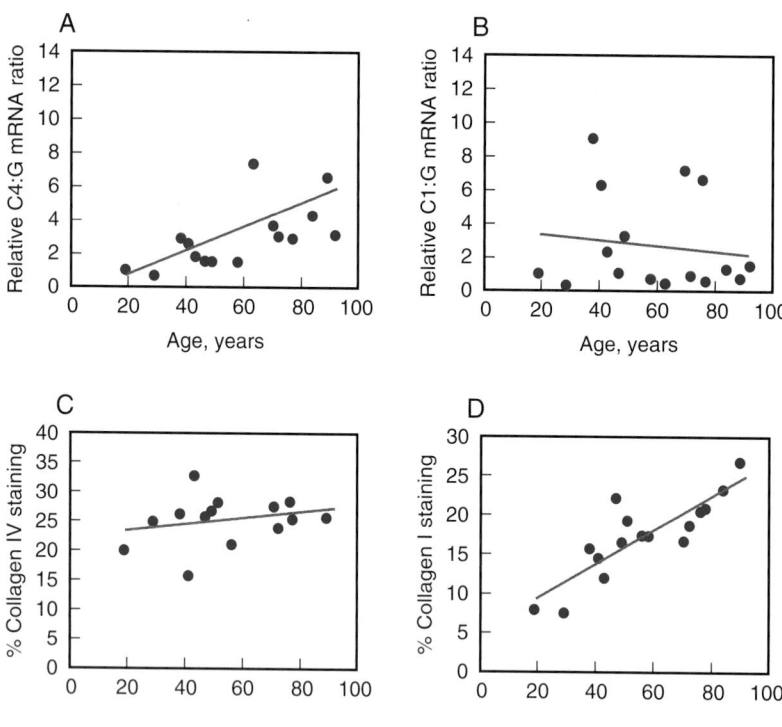

FIGURE 53-4. Effect of age on the ratio of collagen α1 (IV) messenger RNA (mRNA) to glyceraldehyde-3-phosphate dehydrogenase (GAPDH) mRNA (C4:G mRNA ratio) (**A**) and on the C1:G mRNA ratio (**B**). The C4:G mRNA ratio and the Cl:G mRNA ratio in cortical tissue from kidneys taken from healthy individuals (19 to 92 years old) at autopsy were assessed by real-time polymerase chain reaction. Each panel shows mRNA ratios relative to the mRNA ratio in the youngest kidney. Data are presented as means of duplicate measurements. Effect of age on collagen IV accumulation (**C**) and on collagen I accumulation (**D**). Cryostat sections (4 μm) from cortical tissue of the autopsied kidneys were immunohistochemically stained with collagen IV antibodies and collagen I antibodies, respectively. The surface area stained was quantified by digital image analysis at ×20 magnification. Results for each kidney are shown as the percentage of surface staining relative to the total surface area of five microscopic fields in a section. (Reprinted with permission from Eikmans M, Baeld HJ, de Heer E, Bruijn JA: Effect of age and biopsy site on extracellular matrix mRNA and protein levels in human kidney biopsies. Kidney Int 60:974-981, 2001.)

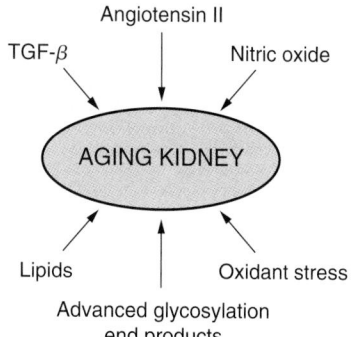

FIGURE 53-5. Factors associated with the pathogenesis of age-related glomerulosclerosis and decline in renal function. TGF-β, transforming growth factor-β.

of aging (Fig. 53-5), including angiotensin II, transforming growth factor-β (TGF-β), nitric oxide (NO), advanced glycosylation end products (AGE), oxidative stress, and lipids. These pathophysiologic factors are also evident in diabetic nephropathy, with the process more accelerated than that seen with normal aging. How these factors interplay may help explain why two thirds of 254 healthy elderly individuals had a decrease in creatinine clearance and one third had no absolute change in creatinine clearance during longitudinal follow-up over 23 years.[33] The ability to modulate these factors may result in prevention of the progressive age-related decline in renal function.

Role of Angiotensin II

Known primarily for its vasoactive effects on the renal vasculature and glomerular hemodynamics, angiotensin II mediates diverse biologic effects on the kidney, including proximal tubular transport of sodium and water,[34, 35] glomerular and tubular growth,[36-40] decrease in NO synthesis,[41] immunomodulation, growth factor induction, and accumulation of extracellular matrix proteins, all of which may modulate glomerulosclerosis and tubulointerstitial fibrosis. Intraglomerular hypertension mediated by angiotensin II–induced preferential efferent arteriolar vasoconstriction to maintain filtration pressure in aging nephrons has been implicated in age-dependent glomerular damage.[42] Increased renal plasma flow (RPF) and glomerular filtration rate (GFR) caused by angiotensin-converting enzyme inhibitors (ACEIs), as noted previously, provides indirect evidence supporting this mechanism of glomerulosclerosis.[43] Decreased intrarenal vascular resistance (RVR) and intracapillary pressure decreased protein leak in aging rodents treated with ACEI.[44] In addition, chronic ACEI decreased postprandial hyperfiltration, thereby decreasing the filtered load delivered to the kidney.[45] ACEI may also play a role to modify the size selectivity of the glomerular capillaries or change the negative charge distribution within the glomerular barrier.[44, 46] Glomerular diameter, mesangial area, and total glomerulosclerosis were markedly decreased in ACEI-treated aged mice, compared with age- and sex-matched untreated mice (Fig. 53-6).[46-50]

Beneficial effects of angiotensin antagonism are mediated by both hemodynamic and nonhemodynamic mechanisms. Angiotensin II induces growth-promoting profibrotic cytokines. It stimulates collagen type IV transcription in medullary collecting tubule cells[51] via endogenous synthesis and autocrine action of TGF-β,[52] and it promotes monocyte-macrophage influx, stimulating mRNA and protein expression of the chemokine RANTES in endothelial cells.[53] Angiotensin II inhibition of NO induces transcription of the proinflammatory chemokine, monocyte chemoattractant protein-1 (MCP-1). With similar blood pressure control, enalapril-treated aged rats had significant reduction in tubulointerstitial fibrosis and α smooth muscle cell-actin when compared with nifedipine-treated aged rats or untreated

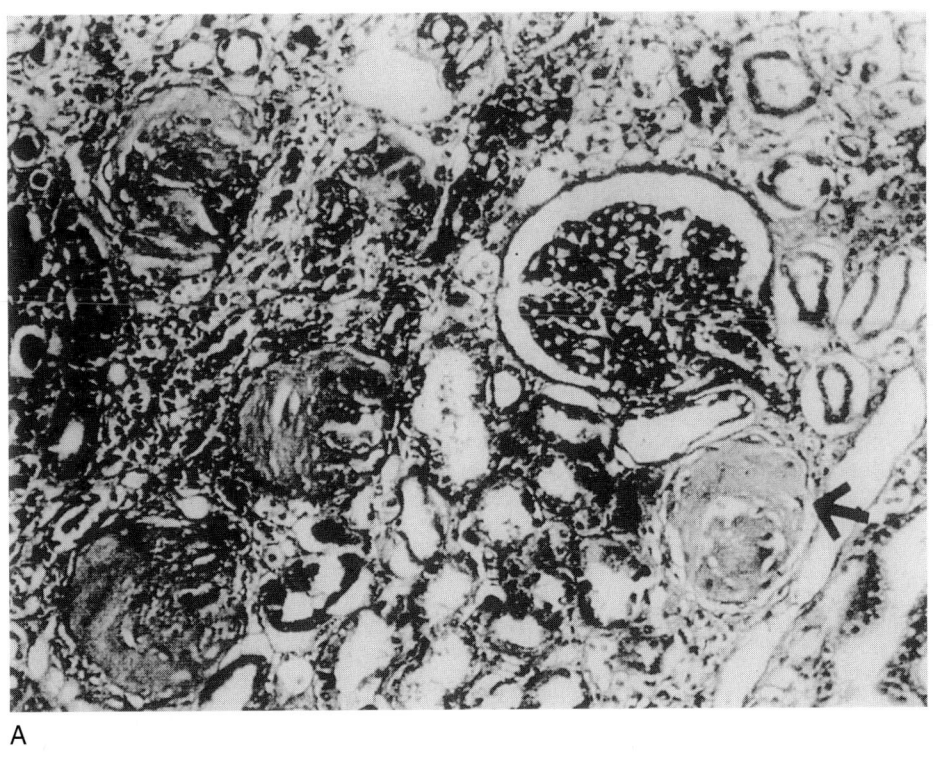

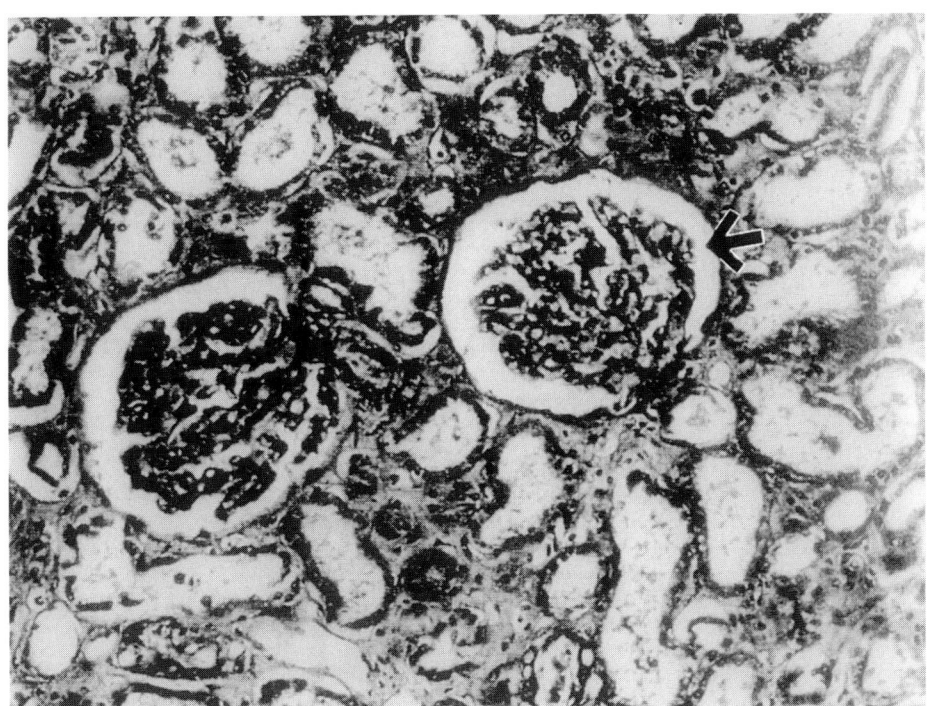

FIGURE 53-6. Angiotensin-converting enzyme inhibitor (Enalapril) decreases glomerulosclerosis in aged mice. **A,** Animals treated with placebo; **B,** animal treated with enalapril. (Reprinted with permission from Ferder L, Inserra F, Romano L, et al: Decreased glomerulosclerosis in aging by angiotensin-converting enzyme inhibitors. J Am Soc Nephrol 5:1147-1152, 1994.)

aged rats.[54] Furthermore, angiotensin II may promote matrix accumulation by stimulating secretion of plasminogen activator inhibitor-1 (PAI-1) from the endothelium.[55] Because PAI-1 inhibits tissue plasminogen activator and urokinase-plasminogen activator, increased PAI-1 levels can lead to decreased proteolysis and fibrinolysis and increased matrix accumulation.[56] Regression of age-related glomerular and vascular sclerosis and decreased collagen content were found in rats treated with angiotensin II antagonists.[57]

A recently identified gene, *klotho,* and its protein product have been associated with suppression of premature aging and arteriosclerosis. This gene appears to be primarily expressed in the kidney. Angiotensin II appears to down-regulate this gene expression. Adenovirus-mediated mouse *klotho* gene transfer into male Sprague-Dawley rats ameliorated angiotensin II–mediated renal morphologic damage. Furthermore angiotensin II inhibition by the angiotensin II receptor blocker losartan, and not by other antipressor agents such as hydralazine, reversed *klotho* mRNA downregulation.[58] Taken together, these experimental data imply beneficial effects of angiotensin II antagonism in elderly patients with age-related renal functional decline, although further conclusive data in humans are necessary.

Role of Transforming Growth Factor-β

Ample evidence associates TGF-β with renal scarring, such as that found with the structural changes that accompany age-related renal decline. TGF-β, an active modulator of tissue repair, can be stimulated by a myriad of factors in the aging kidney, including increased angiotensin II activity, abnormal glucose metabolism, platelet-derived growth factors, hypoxic or oxidative stress, mesangial stretch, and increased levels of AGE. Renal fibrosis seen with aging may be the result of normal or pathologic tissue repair, or both. The response to injury is wound healing. In the face of persistent injury, this response can lead to tissue fibrosis. TGF-β stimulates gene transcription and production of collagen III, IV, and I, as well as production of fibronectin, tenascin, osteonectin, osteopontin, thrombospondin, and matrix glycoaminoglycans.[59] In addition, TGF-β inhibits collagenase and stimulates the synthesis of MMP inhibitors.[60] The net result is the accumulation of extracellular matrix proteins with subsequent glomerulosclerosis and tubulointerstitial fibrosis.[60-63] TGF-β mRNA abundance and TGF-β immunostaining are increased in the renal interstitium of aged rats (Fig. 53-7).[27, 64] Furthermore, the renal protective effects of long-term angiotensin II antagonism are associated with TGF-β down-regulation resulting in decreased interstitial fibrosis.[64] Increased expression of TGF-β probably mediates, in part, age-related sclerosis, although specific proof is still lacking. Future use of TGF-β–neutralizing agents (e.g., decorin) that antagonize TGF-β action, or antisense oligonucleotides that specifically inhibit TGF-β expression in models of age-related renal sclerosis, may establish a more definite role for TGF-β in mediating age-related renal dysfunction.

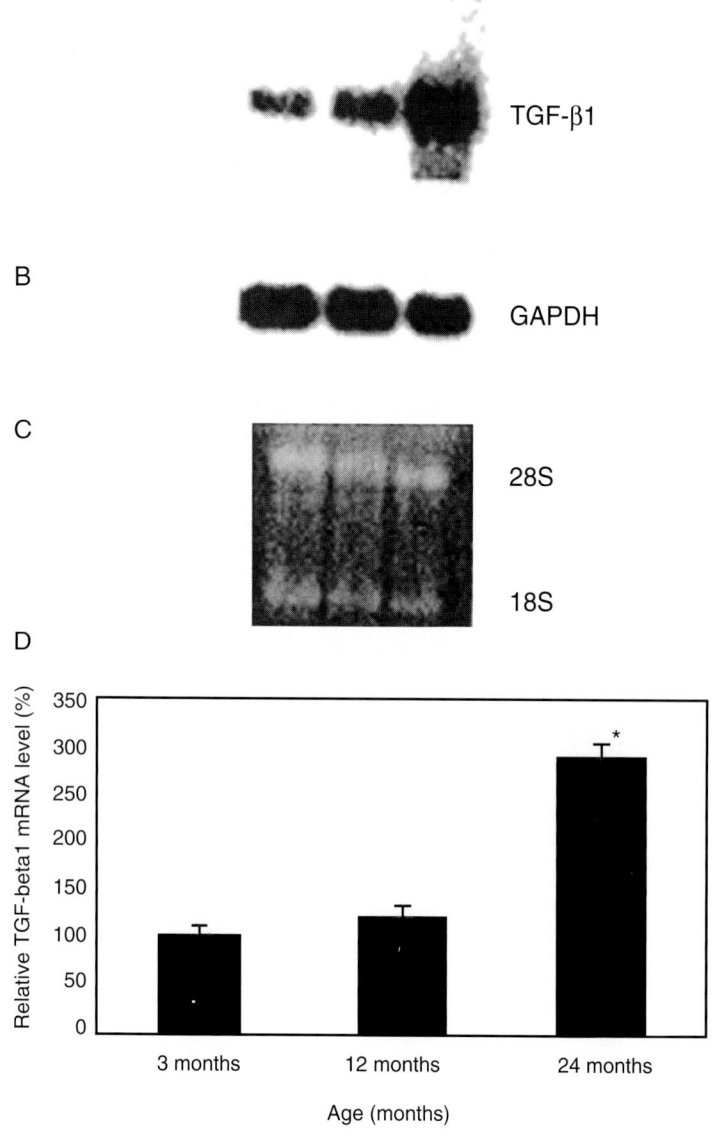

FIGURE 53-7. Northern blot analysis of transforming growth factor-β1 (TGF-β1) messenger RNA (mRNA) expression in renal cortex in aging. Total RNA isolated from 3-, 12-, and 24-month-old rats (lanes 1, 2, and 3, respectively) was electrophoresed, blotted onto a nylon membrane, and then probed for TGF-β1 (**A**) and for glyceraldehyde-3-phosphate dehydrogenase (GAPDH) (**B**). **C,** 28S and 18S rRNA. **D,** Quantitative expression of TGF-β1 mRNA abundance after correcting for GAPDH signal. *$P < .05$ versus 3 and 12 months ($n = 3$). (Reprinted with permission from Ding G, Franki N, Kapsai AA, et al: Tubular cell senescence and expression of TGF-β and p21WAF1/CIP1 in tubulointerstitial fibrosis of aging rats. Exp Mol Pathol 70:43-53, 2001.)

Role of Nitric Oxide

In addition to maintaining renal perfusion in the aging kidney (discussed later), the role of NO as an interactive chemokine in ameliorating fibrosis is becoming more evident. NO inhibits the transcription factor family NFκB, which, in the presence of reactive oxygen intermediates, stimulates MCP-1 and promotes influx of monocyte-macrophages, causing inflammation injury.[65, 66] Therefore NO acts in the negative feedback loop to decrease inflammation and subsequent fibrosis. Levels of NO are decreased in aged rats, as noted by decreased urinary excretion of stable NO oxidation products (nitrites and nitrates).[67, 68] In addition, there is decreased expression of eNOS in the peritubular capillaries of aged rats.[69] Decreased eNOS expression and NO levels can lead to the chronic tubulointerstitial ischemia and tubulointerstitial fibrosis seen with aging.[69] Long-term dietary supplementation of aged rats with L-arginine resulted in significant increases in RPF and GFR and decreases in proteinuria and glomerulosclerosis (Fig. 53-8).[70] In addition, dietary L-arginine supplementation resulted in significant decreases in kidney collagen and N-ε-(carboxymethyl) lysine accumulation.[71] The causes for the age-related decrease in eNOS are not known, but potential causes include increased angiotensin II activity, increased levels of AGE, hypoxia or oxidative stress, and perhaps dietary protein intake.[68, 72-75] Treatment of aged rats with angiotensin II antagonists or dietary protein restriction (or both) resulted in significant increases and normalization of urinary NO excretion.[68]

Role of Advanced Glycosylation End Products

Cross-links of glycoxidated proteins, lipids, and nucleic acids (AGE) slowly accumulate and produce damage to the vascular and renal tissue with aging.[76, 77] In the presence of hyperglycemia, these end products accumulate more rapidly and accelerate tissue damage.[78] These glycated proteins decrease vascular elasticity, induce endothelial cell permeability, and increase monocyte chemotactic activity via AGE-receptor ligand binding, which stimulates macrophage activation and secretion of cytokines and growth factors. AGE accumulation in the vascular endothelium and basement membrane results in defective NO vasodilatation, possibly due to chemical inactivation of endothelium-derived relaxing factor.[79-83] Similar perturbations of the vascular endothelium are evident in diabetic patients and those with age-related vasculopathy. Both biochemical assays and immunohistochemical studies have demonstrated increased levels of AGE and AGE-receptor (RAGE) in aged kidneys of animals. In the kidney, there is increased mesangial matrix with mesangial AGE deposition, increased basement thickening, increased vascular permeability, and induction of platelet-derived growth factor and TGF-β, resulting in glomerulosclerosis and tubulointerstitial fibrosis.[79] Several factors contribute to accumulation of AGE and RAGE, including (1) a decline in GFR with age; (2) increased oxidative stress associated with age, causing oxidative modification of glycated proteins and accumulation of N-ε-(carboxymethyl) lysine; and (3) age-related insulin resistance, resulting in abnormal glucose metabolism and glycation of proteins. Recent studies also suggest that lifelong consumption of AGE-enriched food substances and smoking may also result in

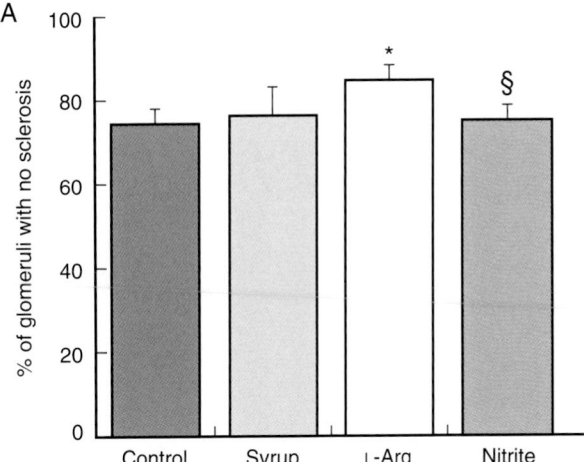

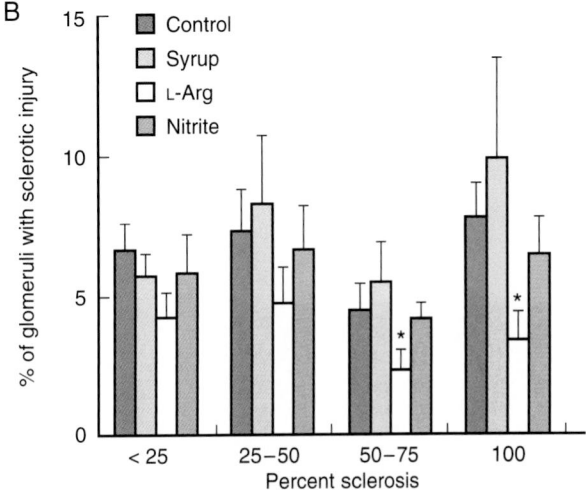

FIGURE 53-8. Morphologic examination of kidneys from aging rats. **A,** Average percentage of glomeruli per kidney with no sclerosis. *$P < .05$, compared with untreated controls; §$P < .05$, nitrite-treated versus L-arginine–treated groups. **B,** Average percentage of glomeruli per kidney with graded sclerotic injury. *$P < .05$, L-arginine–treated rats versus other groups. (Reprinted with permission from Reckelhoff JF, Kellum JA, Racusen LC, et al: Long-term dietary supplementation with L-arginine prevents age-related reduction in renal function. Am J Physiol 272:R1768-R1774, 1997.)

increased AGE loads and increased AGE accumulation in tissues.[84, 85]

Further evidence for AGE's significant role in age-related renal and cardiovascular disease comes from animal studies in aged rats and rabbits treated with aminoguanidine.[86, 87] Long-term aminoguanidine treatment in aged rats markedly diminished glomerulosclerosis and proteinuria[86] (Fig. 53-9), as well as age-related arterial stiffening and cardiac hypertrophy.[88] Reversal of the AGE-associated increase in vascular permeability, prevention of defective vasodilatory response to acetylcholine and nitroglycerin, and prevention of mononuclear cell migratory activity was seen in the subendothelial and periarteriolar spaces in various tissues of rats and rabbits treated with aminoguanidine.[87] Caloric restriction may also have some role to increase life span and lessen the renal lesions noted in aged animals. Calorie restriction by 60% from the ad libitum diet intake in female Brown-Norway rats

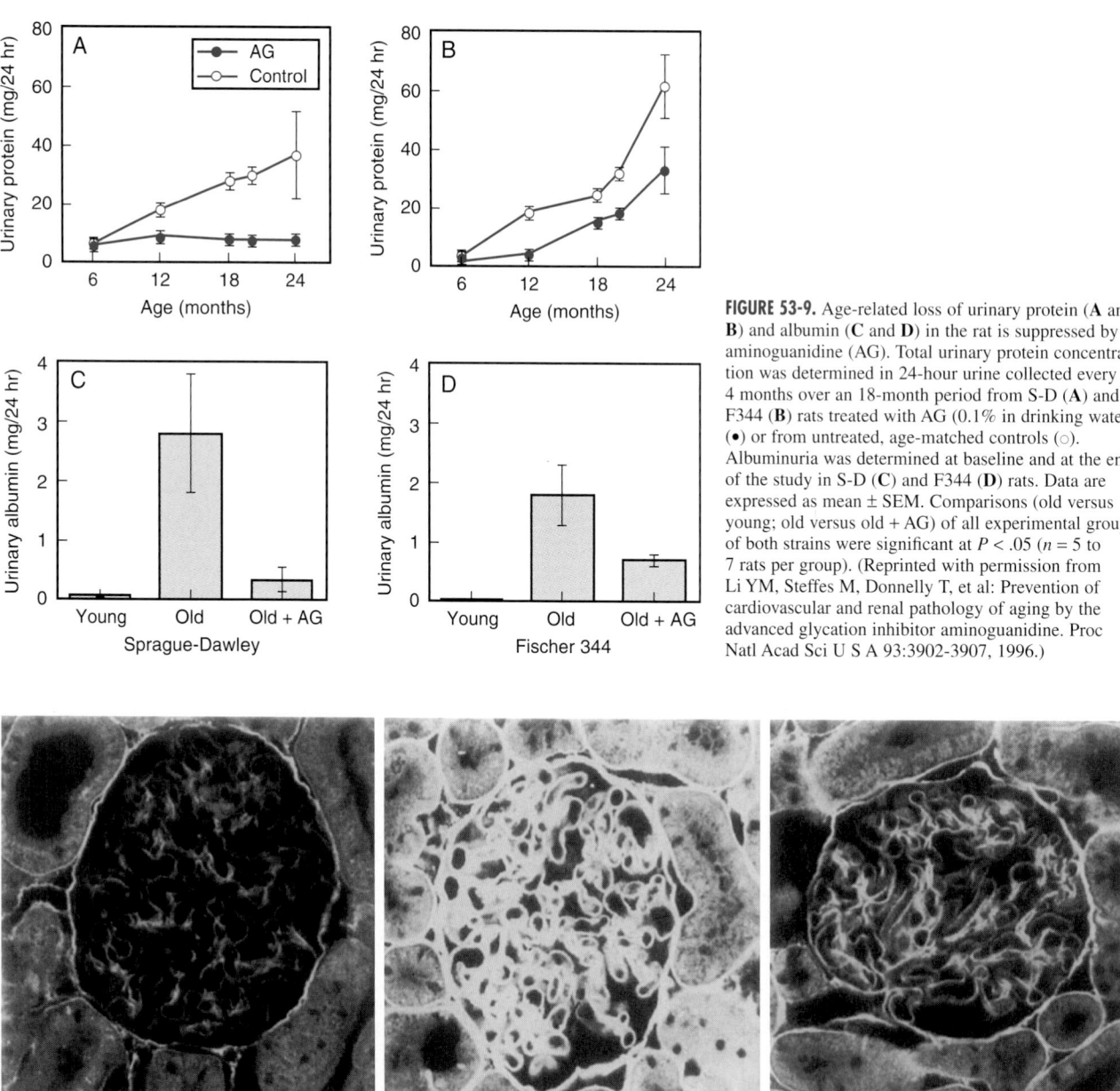

FIGURE 53-9. Age-related loss of urinary protein (**A** and **B**) and albumin (**C** and **D**) in the rat is suppressed by aminoguanidine (AG). Total urinary protein concentration was determined in 24-hour urine collected every 4 months over an 18-month period from S-D (**A**) and F344 (**B**) rats treated with AG (0.1% in drinking water) (●) or from untreated, age-matched controls (○). Albuminuria was determined at baseline and at the end of the study in S-D (**C**) and F344 (**D**) rats. Data are expressed as mean ± SEM. Comparisons (old versus young; old versus old + AG) of all experimental groups of both strains were significant at $P < .05$ ($n = 5$ to 7 rats per group). (Reprinted with permission from Li YM, Steffes M, Donnelly T, et al: Prevention of cardiovascular and renal pathology of aging by the advanced glycation inhibitor aminoguanidine. Proc Natl Acad Sci U S A 93:3902-3907, 1996.)

FIGURE 53-10. Immunolocalization of advanced glycosylation end products (AGE) in the renal cortex of 10-month-old (**A**) and 30-month-old (**B**) female WAG/Rij rats fed ad libitum and 30-month-old animals food-restricted by 30% (**C**). AGE localized predominantly in extracellular matrix. Increased AGE accumulation was evident in tubular basement membranes, mesangial matrix, glomerular basement membranes, and the Bowman capsule between 10 to 30 months in rats fed ad libitum. Such accumulation was mostly prevented in food-restricted animals. Magnification, ×350. (Reprinted with permission from Teillet L, Verbeke P, Gouraud S, et al: Food restriction prevents advanced glycation end products accumulation and retards kidney aging in lean rats. J Am Soc Nephrol 11:1488-1497, 2000.)

attenuated the burden of AGE and other major oxidatively modified glycated proteins N-ε-(carboxymethyl) lysine and pentosidine.[89, 90] Similarly, 30-month-old lean WAG/Rij rats restricted to reduced caloric intake at 30% less than the ad libitum diet (7 g/day) also showed marked decrease in collagen AGE content in kidneys, glomeruli, and abdominal aorta, compared with nonrestricted 30-month-old rats (Fig. 53-10).[91]

Cumulative evidence of AGE-associated acceleration of diabetes and age-associated vasculopathy and the possibility of treatment with aminoguanidine has led to clinical trials in humans. Results of these trials may change the progression of both diabetic and age-related changes in glomerulosclerosis.

Role of Oxidative Stress

With aging, an increase in free radical production or antioxidant enzyme deficiency, or both, can lead to lipid peroxidation and oxidative stress resulting in tissue injury.[92-95] Increased levels of oxidized amino acids in urine indicated increased oxidized protein levels in the skeletal muscle of aged rats.[96] As indicators of lipid oxidative damage, levels of

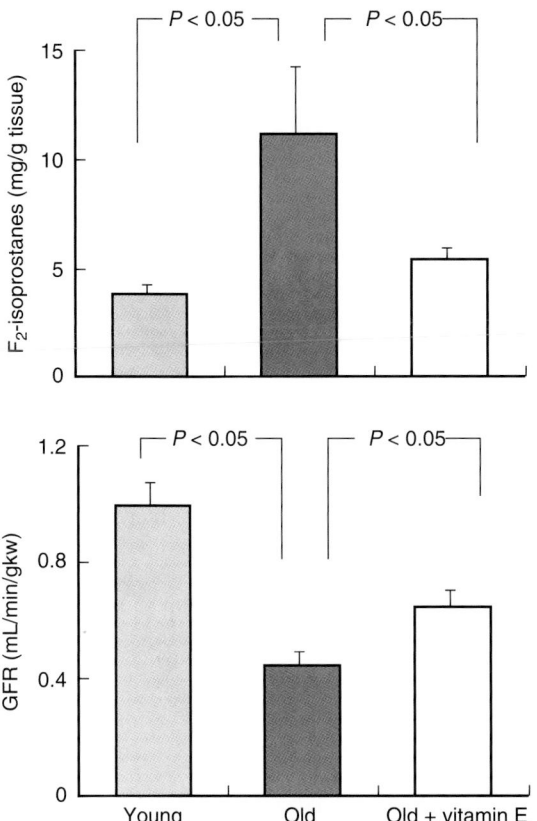

FIGURE 53-11. *(Top)* F_2-isoprostane levels in kidneys from young rats, aged 2 to 3 months, and old rats, aged 22 months, given either a control diet or a diet high in vitamin E. *(Bottom)* Effect of a high–vitamin E diet on glomerular filtration rate (GFR) in old animals. (Redrawn with permission from Reckelhoff JF, Kanji V, Racusen LC, et al: Vitamin E ameliorates enhanced renal lipid peroxidation and accumulation of F2-isoprostanes in aging kidneys. Am J Physiol 274:R767-R774, 1998.)

reactive oxygen species and of thiobarbituric acid reactive substance (TBARS) are increased in the aged kidney,[97] whereas antioxidant enzyme activities are decreased in aged rat kidneys.[92] Other markers for oxidative stress and lipid peroxidation, including increased formation of isoprostanes, AGE, and RAGE and increased induction of heme oxygenase,[98] are also present in aged rats. Furthermore, treatment of these rats with antioxidants such as high vitamin E diet attenuated these changes, with significant improvements noted in RPF and GFR and decreased glomerulosclerosis (Fig. 53-11).[98] Some studies have shown that angiotensin II stimulates superoxide production by activating membrane-bound NADH/NADPH oxidase, and ACEI can increase the activity of antioxidant enzymes.[99, 100] Ongoing studies also indicate that increased extracellular mesangial matrix synthesis resulting from TGF-β induction by reactive oxygen species in cultured mesangial cells and aged rats can be blocked with the antioxidant taurine or by treatment with ACE inhibitors.[101] Aging-associated oxidative stress also appears to enhance the cellular-signaling mitogen-activated protein kinase (MAPK) pathways, including extracellular signal-related kinases (ERK), c-Jun NH_2-terminal kinases (JNK), and the p38 MAPK in the rat kidney.[102] Calorie restriction has been shown to suppress age-related oxidative stress.[103] Furthermore, calorie restriction suppressed age-related increases in activation of MAPK in the aging rat

kidney, perhaps suggesting the need for dietary discrimination in the prevention of age-associated renal disease.

Role of Lipids

Age-related accumulation of cholesterol occurs in several tissues, including the kidney,[104-111] and may play an important role in the progression of glomerulosclerosis and proteinuria in a number of disease states, including diabetes.[111-115] Furthermore, in the presence of oxidative stress and AGE with aging, increased levels of modified low-density lipoproteins (LDL) lipoprotein(a) may occur.[116-118] These lipid products have been associated with increased oxygen radical formation, increased expression of growth factors such as platelet-derived growth factor and TGF-β, inhibition of NO synthesis, migration and adherence of monocytes, and growth of mesangial cells and vascular cells, effects that play an important pathogenic role in renal disease progression.

Lipoxidation stress induced by high-cholesterol feeding in type 2 diabetic rats has been shown to result in glomerulosclerosis and tubulointerstitial fibrosis.[119] Rats with streptozotocin-induced diabetes treated with 3-hydroxy-3-methylglutaryl–coenzyme A (HMG-CoA) reductase inhibitors for 12 months had significant improvement in urinary albumin excretion and glomerular volume, compared with untreated rats.[120] Other studies have shown a decrease in proteinuria and partial preservation of GFR in diabetic and nondiabetic patients with long-term administration of HMG-CoA reductase inhibitors (statins) and/or peroxisome proliferator activated receptor-α (PPAR-α) agonists (fibrates).[121-123] Similar trials may be important in aged individuals.

RENAL PLASMA FLOW AND GLOMERULAR FILTRATION RATE

In addition to anatomic changes, functional changes occur in the aging renal vasculature and contribute to decreased renal blood flow. Para-aminohippurate (PAH) clearances of 600 mL/min/1.73 m^2 at age 20 to 29 years drop to 300 mL/min/1.73 m^2 by age 80 to 89 years, a change of approximately 10% per decade.[124, 125] Xenon washout scans in healthy kidney donors between ages 17 to 76 years demonstrated preferential decrease in cortical blood flow and preservation of medullary flow with age, paralleling histologic changes of loss of selective cortical vasculature.[126]

Whether this change in RPF is affected by possible age-related changes in cardiac output is not clearly established, because some studies have shown an age-related decrease in cardiac output, whereas other carefully designed studies have not shown such change.[127, 128] There may be a small but definite decrease in the renal fraction of the cardiac output.[129] This decrease in the ratio of RPF to cardiac output may reflect the change in anatomic and vascular responsiveness observed with renal aging.

An altered functional response of the renal vasculature in aged humans and animals may be an underlying factor in the decreased RPF and change in filtration fraction noted in progressive renal aging. Whereas RPF increases, as measured by PAH clearances, the vasodilatory response to intravenous infusion of vasorelaxants such as pyrogen[125] or atrial natriuretic peptide (ANP)[130] and intra-arterial acetylcholine[126] is blunted in elderly subjects, compared with their younger counterparts. Similarly, amino acid infusion results in an increase in GFR and filtration fraction, whereas RPF remains unchanged.[131] However, when combined amino acid and dopamine was infused into elderly (compared with younger) healthy kidney donors to achieve maximal vasorelaxation of the renal bed, there was significant increase in both RPF and GFR; filtration fraction was unchanged in both groups, although the response was less in the older donors (Fig. 53-12).[31]

Impaired vasorelaxation may be the result of defective intracellular signaling.[132] An exaggerated vasoconstrictive response is seen with stimulation of the renal sympathetic system, which may result from an inadequate response of cyclic adenosine monophosphate (cAMP) to β-adrenergic agonists or altered response of cyclic guanosine monophosphate (cGMP) to ANP.[133, 134] Other mediators of vasorelaxation, including vasodilatory prostacyclin (PGI$_2$), are also decreased in aged human vascular cells and aged rat kidneys, compared with the vasoconstrictive thromboxanes.[135, 136] Aging humans are also noted to excrete the less vasodilatory natriuretic prostaglandins, PGE$_2$.[137]

Interestingly, inhibition of angiotensin II results in a preserved or exaggerated vasodilatory response in the elderly,[138, 139] suggesting a greater role for angiotensin II–mediated vasoconstriction of the aged renal vasculature. This is further demonstrated by significant increases in RPF and GFR in aged rats treated with ACEIs and angiotensin receptor blockers.[43] The vasoconstrictive response to intra-arterial angiotensin is identical in both young and older human subjects.[126] A blunted vasodilatory capacity with appropriate vasoconstriction may indicate that the aged kidney is in a state of renal vasodilatation to compensate for underlying glomerular sclerotic damage.

Intravenous glycine infusion in progressively aged groups of Sprague-Dawley rats mimics the change in RPF seen in humans and correlates histologically with progressive glomerulosclerosis.[140] N-nitro-L-arginine-methyl-ester (L-NAME), an L-arginine analog that competitively inhibits the formation of endothelium-derived relaxing factor, causes a marked increase in the vasoconstrictive response with a significant increase in RVR and a decrease in RPF in aged

Sprague-Dawley rats, compared with their younger counterparts.[141] In vivo micropuncture of young and aged Sprague-Dawley rats also revealed no age-related change in the magnitude of the pressor and vasoconstrictive response in angiotensin II infusion. Angiotensin II caused increased arteriolar resistance in both preglomerular and efferent vessels and decreased RPF and glomerular plasma flow. This was accompanied by a rise in the glomerular hydraulic pressure gradient and increased filtration fraction in both young and older rats. However, the glomerular capillary ultrafiltration coefficient (K$_f$) decreased in the older rats, leading to a fall in GFR and in the single-nephron glomerular filtration rate (SNGFR). In contrast, there was no change in K$_f$, GFR, or SNGFR in the younger rats. An angiotensin II–dependent decrease in K$_f$ via contraction of glomerular mesangial cells, with a subsequent decrease in filtration surface area, is thought to be a possible explanation for the finding.[142]

Despite a linear decrease in RPF with age, filtration fraction appears to increase. Because juxtamedullary nephrons have a higher filtration fraction than cortical nephrons do, a combination of preserved medullary flow and decreased cortical RPF may explain this observation.

A decrease in nephron mass is expected with senescence of the kidney. However, the rate of decline in GFR in aging individuals can vary depending on methods of measurements, race, gender, genetic variance, and other underlying risk factors for renal dysfunction. Lewis and Alving[143] noted a drop in urea clearance as early as 1938, and this was later confirmed by inulin, creatinine, and iothalamate clearances.[124, 144] Creatinine clearance drops linearly, from 140 mL/min/1.73 m^2 during the third and fourth decade to 97 mL/min/1.73 m^2 by age 80 years, a rate of decline of 0.8 mL/min/1.73 m^2 per year.[145] Iohexol clearance indicates a decrease of 1.0 mL/min/1.73 m^2 per year.[146] Inulin clearances, while slightly greater than 100 mL/min/1.73 m^2 in healthy, normotensive elderly subjects without renal disease who have a normal dietary protein intake of 1 g/kg/day, were still lower than younger counterparts.[147] Lew and Bosch[148] also pointed out a drop in GFR with age. At the same time, they noted variability of creatinine clearance measurements in relation to protein intake.

Despite variation in creatinine clearance measurements in relation to protein intake, the GFR of aged individuals is

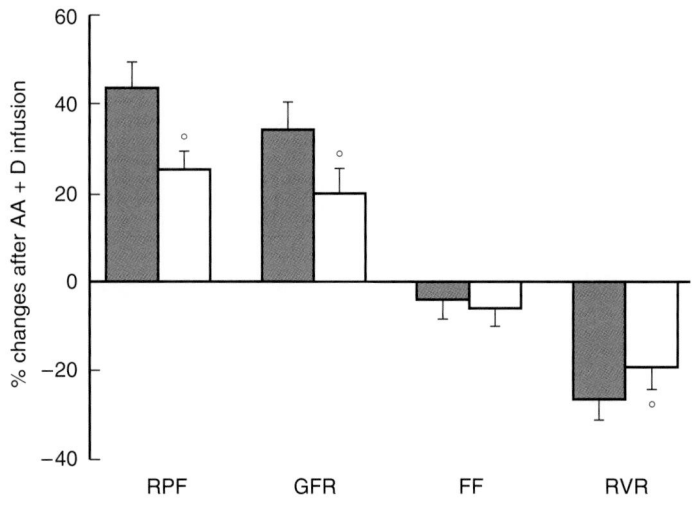

FIGURE 53-12. Percent changes in renal plasma flow (RPF), glomerular filtration rate (GFR), filtration fraction (FF), and renal vascular resistance (RVR) in younger *(shaded bars)* and older *(clear bars)* subjects ($P < .05$ for the difference in the changes between the two groups). (Reprinted with permission from Fuiano G, Sund S, Mazza G, et al: Renal hemodynamic response to maximal vasodilating stimulus in healthy older subjects. Kidney Int 59:1052-1058, 2001.)

lower than that of younger subjects. Although a drop in GFR is measured, a parallel rise in serum creatinine concentration (S_{Cr}) is not seen, because muscle mass, from which creatinine is derived, concomitantly decreases with age. Clinically, this translates to an overestimation of GFR in the elderly. The importance of this fact lies in interpreting clearance values during medication dosing and in assessing the risk of the aged kidney for ischemic, toxic, or metabolic events from the S_{Cr} alone. Commonly used formulas either underestimate or overestimate GFR in the elderly (Table 53-1).[149-152] Data analysis from the Third National Health and Nutrition Examination Survey (NHANES III) of 15,625 individuals aged 20 years and older, examining S_{Cr} and GFR calculation using the Crockcroft-Gault equation in relation to earlier inulin clearance data from Davies and Shock, demonstrates this relationship (Fig. 53-13). Although it is cumbersome, a more accurate formula derived from the Modification of Diet in Renal Disease (MDRD) study may be useful in assessing creatinine clearance in the elderly.[152] Regardless of which formula is used to estimate GFR, when using drugs that are known to be dependent on the kidney for excretion or metabolism, appropriate dose adjustment, followed by serial drug concentration monitoring, is strongly recommended.

Some have recommended routine measurement of creatinine clearance values. Again, variability in the collection may occur because of diet or other factors. Radionuclide clearance measurements with technetium 99m-labeled diethylenetriamine-pentacetic acid (^{99m}Tc-DTPA)[125]-iothalamate or radiocontrast clearance with single-injection iohexol x-ray fluorescence analysis may be considered.[144] Expense, exposure to radioactive substance, and test availability may be limiting factors.

Whether differences in gender have a significant effect on the rate of GFR decline in the aged is not clear. Some have suggested a more gradual decline in women than in men, but prospective cross-sectional human studies have not borne out this difference.

Racial and genetic differences do seem, however, to affect declining GFR in the elderly. African-American subjects showed a greater declining slope in creatinine clearance with increasing age compared with white Americans, which in part may result from genetic variance.[153] Increased nephrosclerosis as a cause for worsening renal function was also noted in elderly subjects of Japanese origin, compared with that for elderly white Americans.[11]

Comparative analyses of GFR, RPF, and RVR in elderly subjects with normotension, hypertension, or heart failure and younger subjects were notable for worsening hemodynamics and increased RVR in all the elderly groups but especially in those with heart failure.[147] In this study, elderly hypertensives did not show a significant decline in GFR compared with elderly normotensives, although when elderly hypertensives not requiring treatment were compared separately with those who had a history of drug treatment for hypertension, the latter group had a lower GFR and a higher RVR.[147] Other studies have also noted age-related decline in renal function among hypertensives.[154, 155] A possible role for intraglomerular hypertension hastening renal functional impairment in the elderly hypertensive patient has been suggested.[156, 157] Older, spontaneously hypertensive

TABLE 53-1

Commonly Used Formulas to Estimate Glomerular Flow Rate (GFR)

1. Creatinine clearance (mL/min/1.73 m^2) = $(1.33 - 0.64) \times$ age*
2. Creatinine clerance (ml/min)

$$= \frac{(140 - \text{age}) \times \text{weight (kg)}}{72 \times \text{serum creatinine (mg/dl)}^a}$$

3. GFR = $170 \times [P_{cr}]^{-0.999} \times [\text{age}]^{-0.0176} \times [0.762 \text{ if patient is female}] \times [1.180 \text{ if patient is black}] \times [\text{SUN}]^{-0.0170} \times [\text{alb}]^{+0.318}$

*15% less in females.

Formula 1 from Rowe JW, Andrew R, Tobin JD, et al: Age-adjusted standards for creatinine clearance. Ann Intern Med 84:567–569, 1976. Formula 2 from Cockcroft DW, Gault MH: Prediction of creatinine clearance from serum creatinine. Nephron 16:31–41, 1976. Formula 3 from Levey AS, Bosch J, Lewis JB, et al: A more accurate method to estimate glomerular filtration rate from serum creatinine: A new prediction equation. Ann Intern Med 130:461–470, 1999.

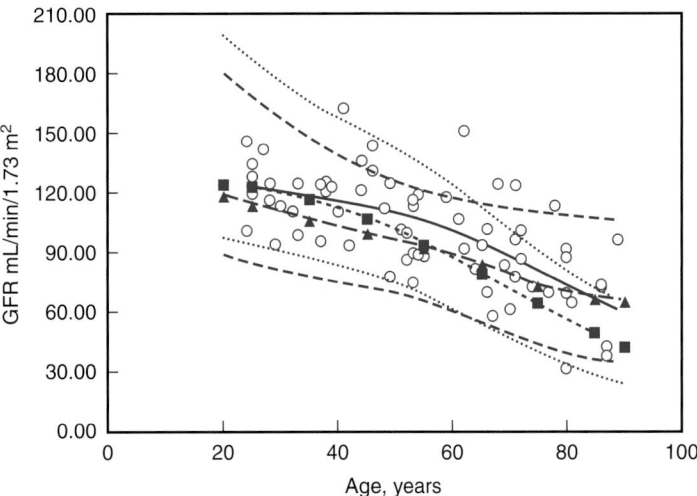

○ Inulin clearance in healthy men (Davies & Shock 1950)
—▲— NHANES III GFR calculation (median, 5th, 95th %iles)
--■-- NHANES III Cockroft-Gault (median, 5th, 95th %iles)

FIGURE 53-13. Percentiles of glomerular filtration rate (GFR) and Cockcroft-Gault creatinine clearance (CCr) by age, plotted on the same graph as data by Davies and Shock[124] on inulin clearance in healthy men. Percentiles are calculated using a fourth-order polynomial weighted quantile regression. The solid line shows a polynomial regression to the inulin data. Dashed lines without symbols show the 5th and 95th percentiles for GFR estimates. (Reprinted with permission from Coresh J, Astor BC, Greene T, et al: Prevalence of chronic kidney disease and decreased kidney function in the US population: Third National Health and Nutrition Examination Survey. Am J Kidney Dis 41:1-12, 2003.)

rats have a rise in blood pressure and a functional decrease in preglomerular RVR that leads to glomerular hypertension predating the appearance of significant vascular or glomerular injury.[157] Other risk factors leading to progressive renal dysfunction, including atherosclerosis of systemic and renal vasculature, diabetes mellitus, and abnormal lipid metabolism, may also play an important role in the functional decline of GFR in the elderly. In a recent study, impaired glucose tolerance in the presence of essential hypertension was found to result in an age-associated decline in GFR.[158]

RENAL TUBULAR FUNCTION

Anatomic, hemodynamic, and hormonal changes in the aged kidney affect crucial physiologic functions that maintain homeostasis of fluids and electrolytes, acid-base balance, and volume and water balance. Under normal conditions, the aging kidney is able to maintain homeostasis. Under stress, however, the adaptive response of the kidney to maintain homeostasis is impaired.

Sodium Conservation

The aged kidney conserves sodium less efficiently under conditions of sodium deprivation. When sodium restriction is imposed on healthy elderly subjects, it takes almost twice as long for the aged kidney to decrease urinary sodium excretion as it does in younger control subjects. The half-time to decrease urinary sodium excretion with an abrupt decrease in sodium intake to 10 mmol/day was 30.9 hours in subjects older than 60 years of age, compared to 17.6 hours in subjects younger than 30 years of age (Fig. 53-14).[159] Decreased distal tubular reabsorption may be at fault, as demonstrated by clearance studies.[160] Several factors may be playing a role in the age-related change in distal sodium conservation ability. It is possible that age-induced renal interstitial scarring, decreased nephron number, and increased medullary flow may increase solute load per nephron, as has been observed in patients with chronic renal failure.

Changes in the levels of hormones that regulate sodium excretion (e.g., renin, angiotensin, aldosterone), and in the response to these hormones, also occur during the process of aging. Concentrations of both plasma renin and aldosterone have been found to decrease with aging in healthy elderly subjects. Basal plasma renin concentration or activity is decreased by 30% to 50% despite normal levels of renin substrate. Despite maneuvers to stimulate renin secretion, including upright position, 10 mEq/day sodium intake, furosemide administration, and air jet stress, age-related differences in plasma renin activity are further amplified (Fig. 53-15).[161-171] Studies in rats showed a decrease in juxtamedullary single-nephron renin content[167] and down-regulation of renin mRNA abundance (Fig. 53-16) and renal ACE levels.[172] Another study found a 56% decrease in type 1 angiotensin II receptor mRNA expression in aged rats.[173]

Prehemorrhage and posthemorrhage plasma renin content was significantly decreased in older (15 months) versus younger (3 months) rats (see Fig. 53-14).[172] Sodium-deprived aged rats showed a blunted rise in plasma renin activity with delayed fall in urinary sodium excretion, despite a drop in mean arterial pressure.[174] Measurements of

plasma renin substrate concentrations in normal aging adults showed decreased conversion of inactive to active renin.[170] Therefore, both decreased renin synthesis and impaired renin release may in part be responsible for reduced active renin content in the elderly.

Similarly, plasma aldosterone decreases in parallel with aging. There is a 30% to 50% decrease in supine plasma aldosterone levels in elderly versus younger subjects. This becomes exaggerated with upright posture, sodium restriction, and furosemide administration (see Fig. 53-15).[171, 175-177] That this aldosterone deficiency is more likely to be related to a renin-angiotensin deficiency and not to an intrinsic adrenal defect is evident when infusion of adrenocorticotropic hormone in elderly subjects produces a normal aldosterone and cortisol response.[171] The sluggish renal response to dietary sodium restriction seen in the elderly can be reproduced by ACE inhibition and blockade of the renin-angiotensin-aldosterone system.[178] Because aldosterone infusion results in marked improvement in sodium reabsorption in the elderly, tubular insensitivity seems a less likely cause of impaired sodium excretion, further supporting a deficiency in the renin-angiotensin aldosterone mechanism.[179] These data seem to suggest that deficiency of renin-angiotensin or of aldosterone, or both, may be an important factor underlying the inability of the elderly to appropriately conserve sodium in the face of sodium deprivation.

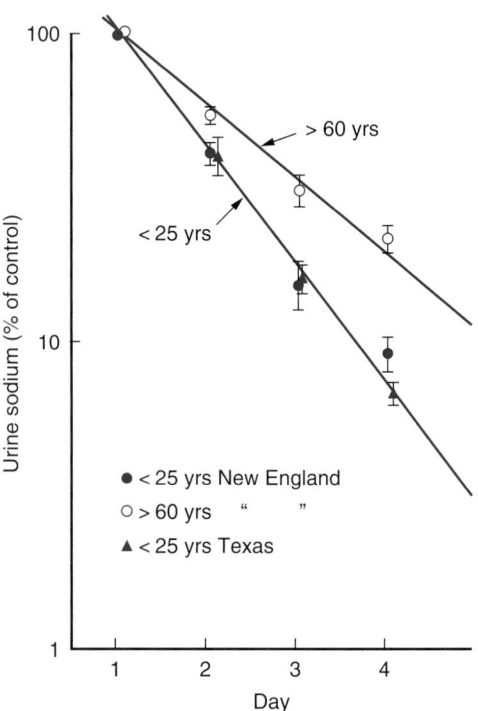

FIGURE 53-14. Response of urinary sodium excretion to restriction of sodium intake in normal humans. The mean half-time ($t_{1/2}$) for eight subjects older than 60 years of age was 30.9 ± 2.8 hours, exceeding the mean half-time of 17.6 ± 0.7 hours for subjects younger than 25 years of age ($P < .01$). When the younger subjects were separated according to geographic area, the mean half-time for the Texas group (>17.9 ± 0.7 hours) was similar to that of the New England group (>15.6 ± 1.4 hours; $P < .3$). (Reprinted with permission from Epstein M, Hollenberg N: Age as a determinant of renal sodium conservation in normal man. J Lab Clin Med 87:411-417, 1976.)

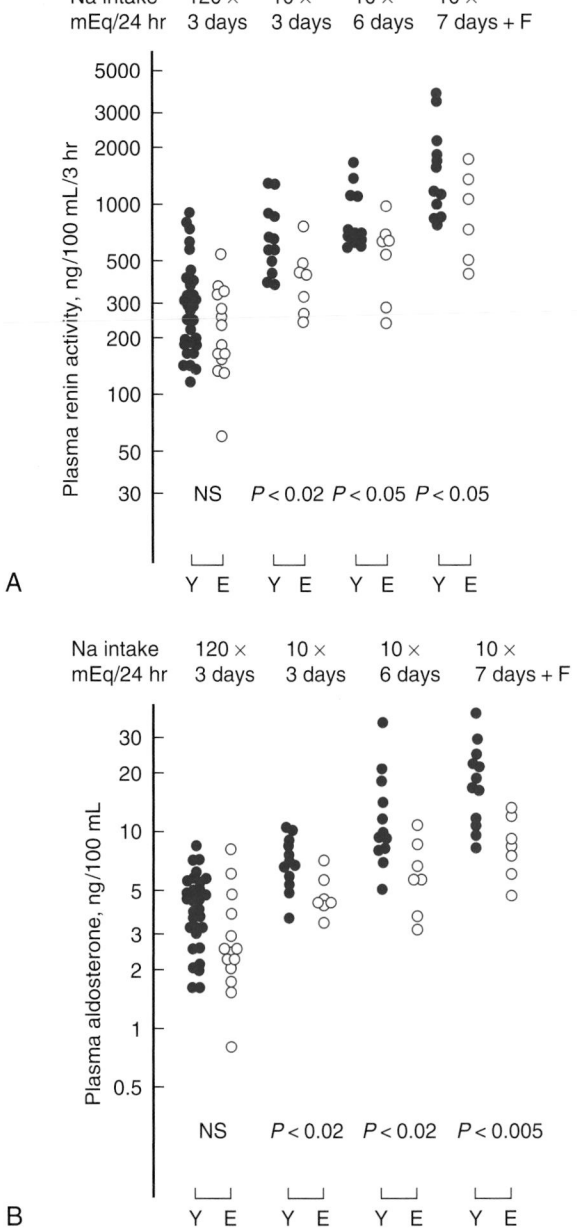

FIGURE 53-15. Distribution of individual supine plasma renin concentrations (**A**) and aldosterone values (**B**) before and during progressive sodium depletion in young (Y) and elderly (E) healthy subjects. Values indicating statistical significance refer to differences between young and elderly subjects. Plasma renin activity values are those obtained with incubation at pH 5.7. (Reprinted with permission from Weidmann P, De Chatel R, Schiffmann A, et al: Interrelations between age and plasma renin, aldosterone, and cortisol, urinary catecholamines, and the body sodium/volume state in normal man. Klin Wochenschr 55:725-733, 1977.)

Sodium Excretion

Natriuretic ability of the aged kidney appears to be blunted in response to sodium loading or volume expansion.[180-182] With a 2-L normal saline load, individuals older than 40 years of age excrete less sodium than younger adults matched for size, sex, and race[153, 183] (Fig. 53-17). Similarly, aged Sprague-Dawley rats given blood volume expansion excrete significantly less sodium, especially when factored for body weight.[182] Age also influences circadian variation in sodium excretion in the

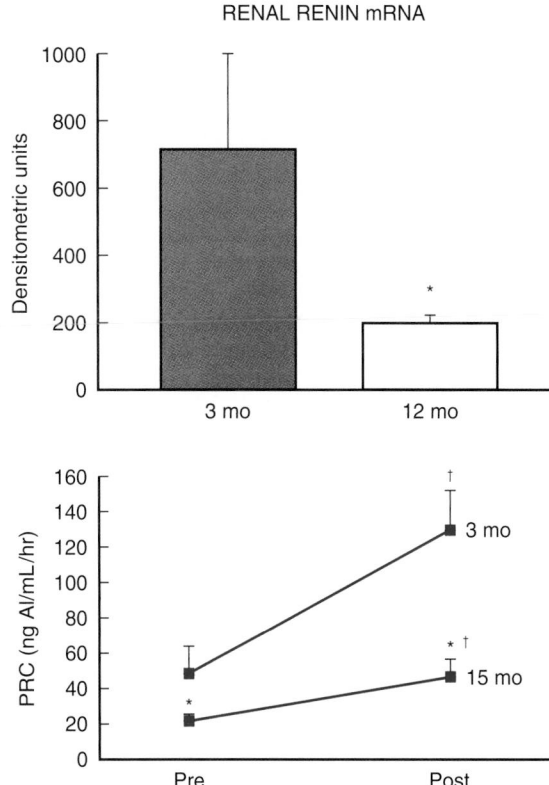

FIGURE 53-16. Northern blot analysis of renin messenger RNA (mRNA). *Top,* Renal renin mRNA is significantly decreased in older (12 months) versus younger (3 months) rats (*, $P < .05$). *Bottom,* Prehemorrhage (Pre) and posthemorrhage (Post) values for plasma renin content (PRC) revealed significantly lower levels in older rats, as well as a smaller increase after hemorrhage (*, $P < .05$), compared with younger rats in same period. (†, $P < .05$ versus prehemorrhage). (Reprinted with permission from Jung FF, Kennefick TM, Ingelfinger JR, et al: Down-regulation of the intrarenal renin-angiotensin system in the aging rat. J Am Soc Nephrol 5:1573-1580, 1995.)

elderly, with a greater percentage of the sodium load being excreted at night.[183] This may contribute to the nocturia observed in elderly individuals. Because sodium excretion is affected by GFR, an age-associated decline in GFR may play a significant a role in limiting sodium excretion.

Emerging studies, however, suggest that aging may affect changes in renal response to ANP, an important factor in the control of Na excretion. ANP is released from atrial myocytes in response to atrial stretch or volume loading. In the kidney, ANP acts via specific cell-surface receptors on renal microvasculature and tubular epithelium to induce hyperfiltration, inhibit sodium reabsorption, and suppress renin release. The interaction of ANP with the cell-surface receptor results in activation of plasma membrane–associated guanylate cyclase to convert MgGTP to cGMP. The latter then phosphorylates intracellular proteins to result in physiologic actions, including inhibition of luminal membrane sodium channels. Proteases in atrial tissue and serum are capable of cleaving the stored 126-amino-acid prohormone (proANP), converting it to the biologically active 28-amino-acid peptide ANP.[1-28] ANP is rapidly degraded, but its serum half-life may be prolonged by selective blockade of degradative enzymes or clearance receptors.[184] Elevated basal ANP levels have been found in healthy elderly to be three to five times those of the healthy young.[181, 185, 186] With high salt intake, head-out body water immersion, and saline loading, ANP secretion is stimulated to a greater extent in elderly compared with younger subjects.[181, 185, 187, 188] With low salt intake, however, ANP levels are similar to those of the younger comparison group. Therefore, ANP secretion in response to increased salt intake and volume loading appears to remain intact.

Some have suggested that increased basal ANP levels may result from decreased metabolic clearance, increased half-life, and a larger volume of distribution in the elderly.[189-192] It appears less likely that decreased GFR in the aged contributes significantly to high plasma ANP levels, given that patients with advanced chronic renal failure do not have significantly elevated ANP levels compared to normal.[193] However, the renal proximal tubule brush border membrane, which is rich in degradative enzymes (endopeptidases), plays a major role in peptide degradation.[184] Infusion of inhibitors of endopeptidases such as phosphoramidon in rats with reduced renal mass increased ANP levels in parallel with increases in urinary cGMP (ANP second messenger) and urinary salt excretion.[194] Renal neutral endopeptidase inhibition by candoxatril in 12 patients with New York Heart Association class II congestive heart failure significantly increased ANP and cGMP levels as well as urinary sodium excretion without changes in renal hemodynamics.[195] Endopeptidase inhibition significantly decreases metabolic clearance and prolongs the half-life of ANP in this population. The metabolic clearance in elderly subjects was decreased in comparison with younger subjects at similar low ANP infusion rates.[192, 196] Perhaps with aging the number or quality of brush border membrane degradative enzymes changes, resulting in decreased metabolic clearance. This possibility needs further investigation.

Several investigators have proposed that higher ANP levels possibly represent a homeostatic adaptation to the reduced sensitivity in the kidney.[180, 182, 197] Although incremental increases in ANP infusion result in progressive increases in urinary sodium excretion in the young, elderly subjects do not continue to significantly increase their sodium excretion beyond a physiologic ANP infusion of 2 ng/kg/min (Fig. 53-18). Therefore, renal response to ANP appears to be blunted in the aged kidney. Other investigators have noted that baseline levels of cGMP (ANP second messenger) show no change with age.[181, 188] However, with exogenous administration of low-dose ile-ANP, cGMP increased significantly in plasma and urine of healthy elderly subjects.[192]

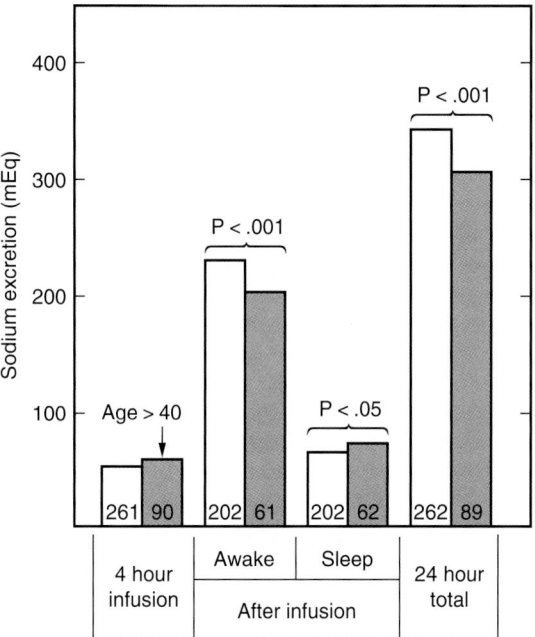

FIGURE 53-17. Comparisons of urinary sodium excretion in younger subjects *(clear bars)* and in older subjects *(shaded bars)* after 2 L intravenous normal saline. Normal subjects older than 40 years of age excrete a sodium load more slowly than do younger subjects. Numbers at the base of the bars represent the number of subjects in each group. (Reprinted with permission from Luft FC, Grim CE, Fineberg NS, et al: Effects of volume expansion and contraction in normotensive whites, blacks, and subjects of different ages. Circulation 59:643-650, 1979.)

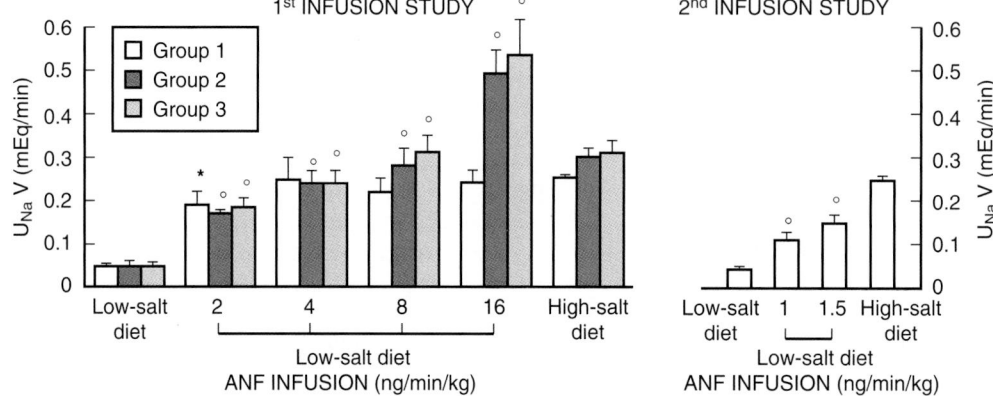

FIGURE 53-18. Urinary sodium excretion ($U_{Na}V$) with a low-salt diet (in basal condition and during infusion of atrial natriuretic peptide [ANP]) and with a high-salt diet in young (group 1), middle-aged (group 2), and elderly (group 3) subjects. The columns represent means and the bars SE. °, $P < .05$ versus other steps and low-salt diet; *, $P < .01$ versus low-salt diet. (Reprinted with permission from Leasco D, Ferrara N, Landino P, et al: Effects of age on the role of atrial natriuretic factor in renal adaptation to physiologic variations of dietary salt intake. J Am Soc Nephrol 7:1045-1051, 1996.)

Despite the increase in cGMP levels after ANP infusion, an increase in sodium excretion is not seen.[192] This suggests that the defect may be at the post-cGMP effector mechanism.

Because ANP can suppress the renin-angiotensin-aldosterone system and inhibit sodium reabsorption, simultaneous measurements of plasma renin activity and plasma aldosterone concentration during ANP infusion studies were done. The results suggested that the natriuretic property of ANP is different from the property of inhibition of sodium reabsorption via suppression of the renin-angiotensin-aldosterone system. Each of these properties of ANP is influenced differently by age.[180, 181, 192]

Renal Concentrating Capacity

Studies in the elderly have clearly demonstrated impaired renal concentrating ability in comparison with younger subjects (Fig. 53-19).[143, 198-201] Appropriate maximal water conservation under hyperosmolar and water-deprived conditions depends on an intact osmoreceptor and volume receptor sensitivity for arginine vasopressin (AVP) release as well as intact collecting tubule response to AVP in the face of maximal medullary tonicity. In the elderly, a combination of processes may be affected, leading to a defect in water conservation.

AVP release appears to be intact in the elderly in response to both osmotic stimulation and volume pressure stimulation, although the extent of the response depends on the type of stimulus. The osmoreceptor sensitivity to AVP release appears to be enhanced in the elderly. The hypothalamic-neurohypophyseal response to hypertonic saline in Long-Evans rats indicates increased AVP release in response to osmotic stimuli.[202, 203] Similarly, there was heightened osmoreceptor sensitivity in elderly subjects receiving a 3% saline infusion over 2 hours.[204] Basal circulating AVP levels were also increased in elderly subjects after 24 hours of water deprivation.[205-208] Plasma AVP levels measured under

conditions of water deprivation at 9 hours[209] and 14 hours[210] appeared to suggest, respectively, a level that was lower or only slightly higher than in the younger group. It may be that increased AVP response in the elderly depends on maximal osmoreceptor stimulation, as seen with prolonged water deprivation or hypertonic saline infusion. Some studies suggest that baroreceptor-mediated AVP release from volume-pressure changes such as an acute assumption of upright posture decreases with age,[211] as does the oropharyngeal inhibition of AVP release in response to drinking and cold liquids.[207] However, AVP levels increased significantly in 24 healthy elderly subjects aged 65 to 80 years who underwent a 60-degree head-up tilt stimulation, compared with 24 subjects aged 20 to 34 years of age.[212]

With AVP release reasonably intact, possibilities for an intrarenal defect in urinary concentrating ability have been investigated. Intrarenal resistance to AVP has been postulated as a possible cause for decreased urinary concentrating ability of the aged kidney. Despite AVP infusion to healthy elderly, reduced concentrating capacity was not corrected.[213] Rowe and colleagues suggested a "washout" of the medullary tonicity in the face of increased medullary blood flow in the aged kidney. In their study of 98 healthy community-dwelling volunteers (ages 20 to 79 years), a significant decrease in urine osmolality and increase in solute excretion and osmolar clearance after 12 hours of overnight dehydration was found, independent of changes in creatinine clearance.[201] This may also be explained by impaired solute transport in the ascending loop of Henle leading to inadequate medullary tonicity. Water diuresis in elderly subjects demonstrates decreased sodium chloride transport in the ascending loop of Henle, supporting this possibility.[160, 214] However, data in aging rats are more suggestive of an AVP resistance in the collecting tubules. Maximal urinary concentration despite 40 hours of dehydration and exogenous AVP was impaired in aged rats. Though solute-free water formation was normal (C_{H_2O}/GFR as a function of V/GFR), solute-free water reabsorption ($T_c H_2O$/GFR as a function of C Osm/GFR) was impaired. Inner medullary solute content was identical in old and young rats. Therefore, ascending limb solute transport appears to be intact, whereas collecting tubule water transport is diminished.[215]

An age-related decrease in cAMP generation in response to AVP was also found in inner medullary slices of both rats and mice.[216, 217] Maximum cAMP levels in older animals were less in comparison to younger animals (Fig. 53-20).[216, 217] In fact, older mice required a greater threshold dose of AVP to initiate a significant increase in cAMP.[217] Down-regulation of AVP receptors with subsequent decreased cAMP response in the face of chronically elevated levels of AVP has been suggested[203]; however, no change in receptor number or affinity for AVP has been found.[218] A postreceptor mechanism may be playing a role. The abundance of expression of stimulatory guanine nucleotide-binding protein (Gs) is decreased in aging kidneys.[219] This may suggest a possible impairment in adenosine triphosphate (ATP)-stimulated adenylate cyclase activity and cAMP levels. In vitro perfusion studies with cholera toxin and forskolin on freshly isolated cortical collecting tubules (CCT) of young (3 months), middle-aged (2 to 3 years), and old (4 to 5 years) rabbits showed that the ability of Gs to stimulate adenylate cyclase was severely compromised in collecting tubules

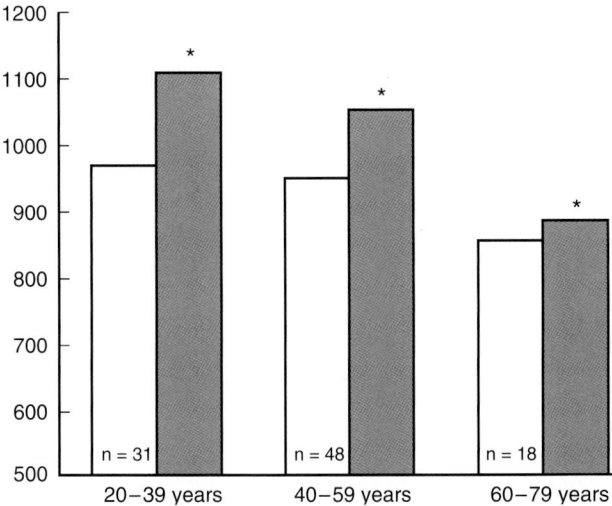

FIGURE 53-19. The effect of age on urine osmolality in response to 12 hours of water deprivation. The number of individuals in each group is noted at the base of each bar. Urine osmolality decreases significantly with age after water deprivation. Clear bars, pretreatment values; shaded bars, post-treatment values; *, $P < .05$. (Reprinted with permission from Rowe J, Shock N, DeFronzo R: The influence of age on the renal response to water deprivation in man. Nephron 17:270-278, 1976.)

from old animals. Infusion of cholera toxin, known to ADP-ribosylate the G proteins, thereby stimulating adenylate cyclase and generation of cAMP, resulted in only 32% stimulation in epithelia from old rabbit CCT compared with CCT from young controls. Infusion of forskolin, a potent stimulator of adenylate cyclase at the level of the catalytic unit and also G protein interaction, yielded significantly lower adenylate cyclase stimulation (12% that of young controls) in cultures from old rabbits. Gs proteins with the catalytic subunit of adenylate cyclase may be responsible for the age-associated decline in CCT response to AVP.[220]

AVP regulates collecting duct water channels, aquaporin-2 (AQP-2), by down regulating V2 receptors on the basolateral membrane. Northern blot analysis of V2 receptor mRNA and AQP-2 mRNA in dehydrated young and old rats found similar degrees of down-regulation of V2 receptor

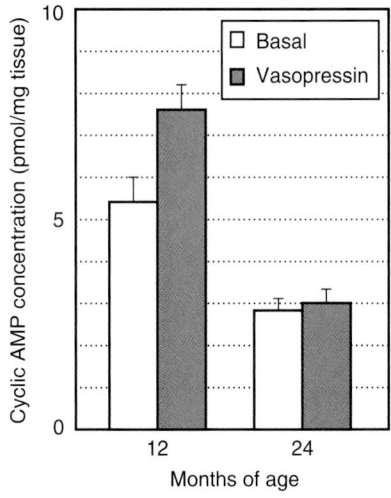

FIGURE 53-20. Cyclic adenosine monophosphate (AMP) concentration in renal papillary slices before and after stimulation by vasopressin (5 mU/mL). Cyclic AMP increased significantly after vasopressin infusion in 12-month-old rats (by 2.81 ± 0.62 pmol/mg of tissue, $n = 10$) compared with 24-month-old rats (0.25 ± 0.21 pmol/mg tissue, $n = 9$) ($P < .05$ in paired analysis). Each bar represents mean $\pm$ SEM. (Redrawn with permission from Beck N, Yu B: Effect of aging on urinary concentrating mechanisms and vasopressin-dependent cAMP in rats. Am J Physiol 243:F121-F125, 1982.)

mRNA in both young and old rats. However, AQP-2 mRNA expression in old rats in response to dehydration was significantly less than in young rats (Fig. 53-21).[221] In situ hybridization of AQP-2 mRNA confirmed this finding.[221] A more recent study reported decreased expression of AQP-2 and AQP-3 in the medullary collecting duct of 30-month-old female WAG/Rij rats compared with 10-month-old female counterpart, whereas papillary cAMP content measured by ELISA in these normally hydrated animals was not significantly different between the two groups (Fig. 53-22).[222] Whether gender played a role in these findings is not clear. Taken together, these results seem to suggest that decreased expression of AQP-2 and AQP-3 in older rats is independent of changes in circulating AVP and intracellular cAMP[222] and in part may explain the low water permeability in the inner medullary collecting duct and the decrease in urine concentrating ability seen with aging.

Recent studies have also detected a decreased expression of urea transporters, UT-A1 and UT-B1, in the renal medulla and decreased papillary osmolality in older rats, whether food restricted or on ad libitum diet (Fig. 53-23).[223] Chronic infusion of deamino-8-D arginine vasopressin (DDAVP), however, increased papillary urea accumulation and improved urine osmolality and flow rates in 30-month-old compared with 10-month-old WAG/Rij female rats in the face of upregulation of urea transporters.[224] This may be an additive factor leading to decreased concentrating ability in the elderly. Further studies are needed to clarify the role of urea transporters in the aged kidney.

Renal Diluting Capacity

With aging, the ability to achieve minimal urinary dilution decreases.[199, 225-227] During water diuresis subjects aged 77 to 88 years decreased their urine osmolality to 92 mOsm/kg H$_2$O. This is significantly higher than in younger subjects (17 to 40 years), who were able to achieve a urine osmolality of 52 mOsm/kg H$_2$O. Solute-free water clearance dropped from 16.2 mL/min to 5.9 mL/min in old versus young individuals. Appropriate urinary dilution occurs if filtered fluid delivered distally undergoes appropriate solute extraction from the ascending loop of Henle with adequate AVP suppression in

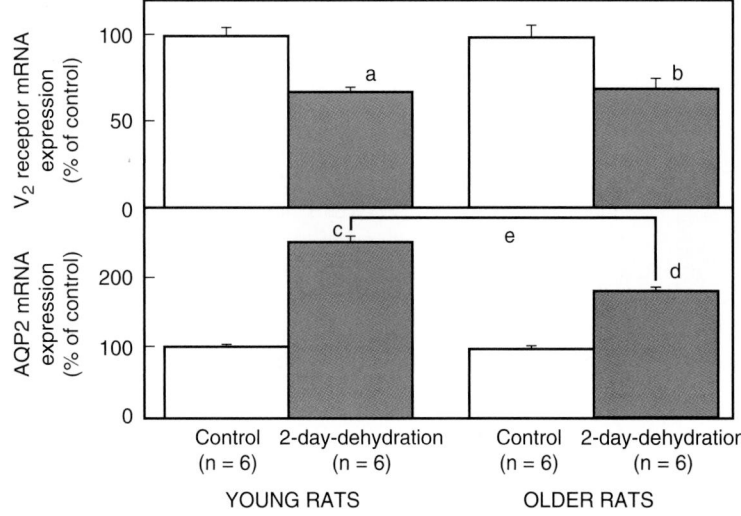

FIGURE 53-21. Changes in expression of vasopressin-2 (V$_2$) receptor messenger RNA (mRNA) and aquaporin-2 (AQP2) mRNA after dehydration, as measured by Northern blot hybridization. The expression of mRNA after dehydration is presented as the mean percentage change from control $\pm$ SE. a, $P < .005$ versus young control group; b, $P < .05$ versus older control group; c, $P < .01$ versus young control group; d, $P < .001$ versus older control group; e, $P < .01$ between young and older rats after dehydration for 2 days. (Reprinted with permission from Terashima Y, Kondo K, Inaguki A, et al: Age associated decrease in response of rat aquaporin-2 gene expression to dehydration. Life Sci 62: 873-882, 1998.)

A

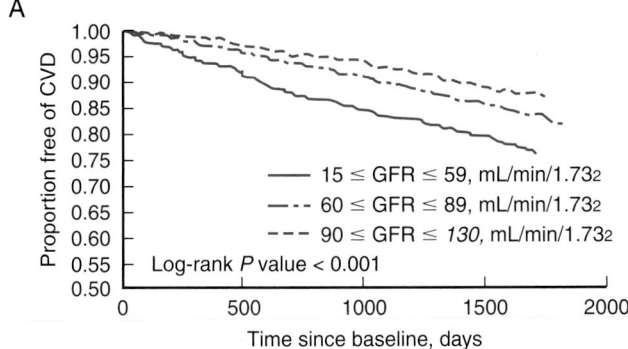

B

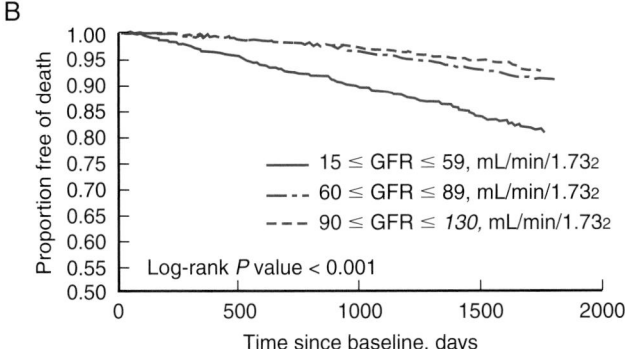

FIGURE 53-22. Semiquantitative analysis of aquaporin (AQP) expression in aging kidney. (Values are means ± SE, *n* = 4–7). Western blot staining for AQP2 and AQP3 in 10- and 30-month-old rat kidney outer and inner medulla integrated densitometry expressed as percent staining of 10-month-old animals (*, *P* < .05). CVD, cardiovascular disease; GFR, glomerular filtration rate. (Redrawn with permission from Preisser L, Teillet L, Aliotti S, et al: Downregulation of aquaporin-2 and -3 in aging kidney is independent of V_2 vasopressin receptor. Am J Physiol Renal Physiol 279:F144-F152, 2000.)

93 years of age), with urinary ammonia accounting for less of the total acid excretion than in younger subjects. When glutamine was given, the increases in ammonium excretion occurred as rapidly in old subjects as in young subjects and with equal magnitude. Phosphate excretion increased, and titratable acid accounted for a significantly greater percentage of total acid excretion. However, when acid excretion was factored for GFR, a decrease in renal tubular mass rather than a specific tubular defect was believed to be the cause for decreased acid excretion. On the other hand, Agarwal and Cabebe[230] found that ammonium loading in older patients resulted in reduced ammonium excretion and ability to reach minimal pH even after correction for GFR, suggesting an intrinsic tubular defect (Fig. 53-25). Whether this defect is the result of an anatomic or a functional defect (such as impairment in the renin-angiotensin-aldosterone axis, which is frequently encountered in the aged) is not clear. Statistical significance was not reached for titratable acid. Studies in senescent rats fed equivalent amounts of NH_4Cl confirmed findings of a deficiency in the absolute amount of ammonium excreted after an acid load. This accounted for the more severe acidemia in the older rats (pH from 7.40 to 7.09) compared with younger controls (pH from 7.43 to 7.32).[231] Renal proximal tubular apical brush border membrane vesicle transport studies revealed that sodium-hydrogen exchange activity (Na/H exchange), a major regulator of proximal tubular acidification, was similarly enhanced by the acid load in adult and aged rats.[231] Phosphate transport was reduced to the same extent in both adult and aged rats. This suggests that impaired ammonium excretion may also mediate the age-related impairment in renal adaptation to metabolic acidosis, even when compensating mechanisms appear to be intact.[231]

Although a subtle degree of metabolic acidosis exists in the elderly,[229] neither serum bicarbonate concentration nor pH is found to be outside the normal range. Bone demineralization and muscle wasting, complications of chronic metabolic acidosis, are common in the elderly. Underlying metabolic acidosis regulates mobilization of calcium and alkali from bone and inhibits renal calcium reabsorption, leading to calcium removal from the body. Increased protein intake increases endogenous acid production. Acidosis-induced enhanced muscle breakdown is mediated by activation of an ATP-dependent pathway involving ubiquitin and proteasome.[232] Despite eubicarbonatemia, increased protein intake, often found in industrialized nations, in conjunction with aging and impaired acid excretion, may be associated with a negative calcium balance, osteoporosis, and increased incidence of fractures as well as muscle wasting, as seen with aging.[233] Studies in postmenopausal women have suggested improvement in nitrogen balance[234] and calcium balance[235] with potassium bicarbonate administration. Whether bicarbonate supplementation could be an important intervention in the elderly to prevent complications of chronic subtle metabolic acidosis remains to be investigated.

MINERAL AND ELECTROLYTE BALANCE

Osmolar Disorders

Disorders of osmolality are commonly seen in the elderly.[236-240] Subtle changes in conservation and excretion of both water

the face of water loading and hypoosmolality. The decline in GFR with aging may be contributing to the decrease in the ability to excrete free water. However some investigators have found that, despite correction for GFR, solute-free water clearance is decreased in older subjects.[225] Whether adequate AVP suppression occurs with water loading or hypoosmolality or appropriate solute extraction occurs in the ascending loop of Henle remains to be investigated.

Acid-Base Balance

Although homeostatic maintenance of acid-base balance appears to be adequate in the elderly, acid loading demonstrates an impaired ability to excrete the acid load in the elderly. An age-related decline in renal mass and GFR has been associated with this change.[228] In healthy subjects, when endogenous acid production was held constant by a steady-state acid diet in a research setting, a progressively worsening low-grade metabolic acidosis was observed with age (Fig. 53-24).[229] The changes in GFR with age correlated significantly with decreases in blood pH and in plasma HCO_3. A decrease in plasma HCO_3 was accompanied by a reciprocal increase in plasma chloride concentration, similar to that found with early renal disease or renal tubular acidosis.[229] Earlier studies by Adler and associates[228] had shown decreased excretion of an oral ammonium load in elderly subjects (72 to

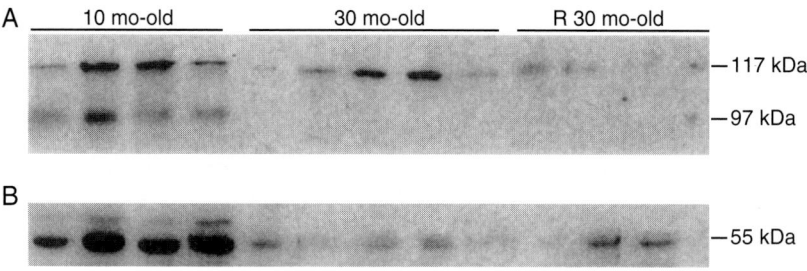

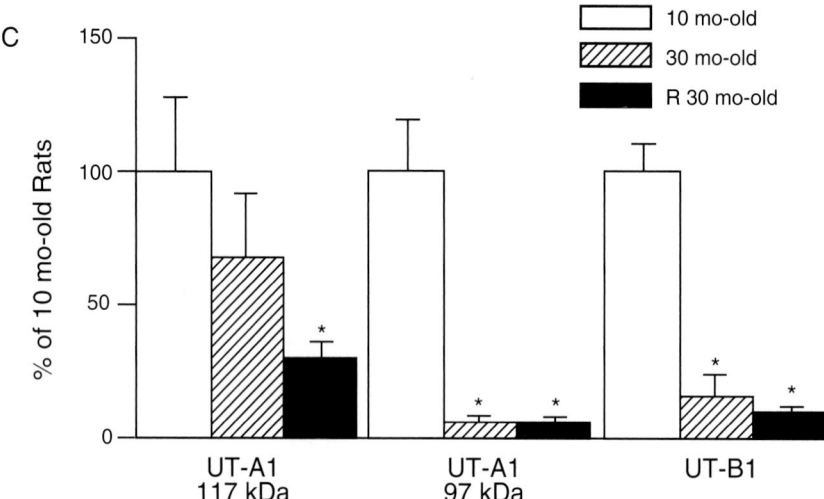

FIGURE 53-23. Immunoblotting of urea transporters UT-A1 (**A**) and UT-B1 (**B**) in kidney inner medulla of 10- and 30-month-old rats fed ad libitum and 30-month-old food-restricted rats. Each lane was loaded with 15 μg protein and probed with polyclonal antibodies raised against UT-A1 and UT-A2 (0.5 μ/mL) or UT-B1 (1:2000 serum). Density quantification (**C**) showed a markedly decreased expression of both UT-A1 and UT-B1 in senescent rats fed ad libitum or food restricted, compared with adult rats. Values are means ± SE for 4 to 5 rats and are expressed as a percentage of the value for 10-month-old rats. No significant difference was observed between 30-month-old rats fed ad libitum and food-restricted rats. *, $P < .05$ versus 10-month-old rats. (Reprinted with permission from Combet S, Teillet L, Geelen G, et al: Food restriction prevents age-related polyuria by vasopressin-dependent recruitment of aquaporin-2. Am J Physiol Renal Physiol 281: F1123-F1131, 2001.)

and solute, added to underlying factors such as medications, infections, and emotional disability, can predispose the elderly to hyponatremia or hypernatremia.

Hyponatremia

Hyponatremia occurred in 11.3% of geriatric hospital inpatients over a 10-month period and was found to be as high as 22.5% in a chronic disease facility.[237, 240] Enhanced osmotic AVP release, along with impaired diluting ability, predisposes elderly persons to a higher incidence of hyponatremia.[241] Idiopathic syndrome of inappropriate antidiuretic hormone secretion (SIADH) has been reported in a subset of ambulatory geriatric clinic patients.[242] Thiazide diuretics, implicated in 20% to 30% of the hyponatremia cases in elderly patients, further impair an already existing renal dilution defect (Fig. 53-26).[237, 239, 240, 243, 244] A role for deficient prostaglandin synthesis in the elderly has also been suggested in the increased susceptibility to thiazide-induced hyponatremia, because water diuresis is impaired when prostaglandin synthesis is inhibited.[243] Thiazide diuretics administered in combination with other medications, such as sulfonylurea compounds, chlorpropamide, tolbutamide, or nonsteroidal anti-inflammatory drugs (NSAIDs) that potentiate peripheral AVP action, can act in synergy to impair water excretion. Medications that stimulate the nonosmotic release of AVP or potentiate the renal tubular effects of AVP also act in synergy with impaired diluting ability and should be used in the elderly with extreme caution (Table 53-2).

An osmotic shift of water from the extracellular to the intracellular space occurs with hyponatremia. This leads to a myriad of signs and symptoms, including apathy, disorientation, lethargy, muscle cramps, anorexia, nausea, agitation, depressed deep tendon reflexes, pseudobulbar palsy, and seizures.[245] Recognition and appropriate institution of therapy is important to avoid severe neurologic sequelae including central pontine myelinolysis.

Hypernatremia

Similarly, impaired renal concentrating and sodium-conserving ability may increase susceptibility to hypernatremia in the elderly. Under normal physiologic conditions, thirst and fluid intake defend against hypernatremia and volume depletion. However, both of these defense mechanisms are impaired in the healthy elderly subjects (Fig. 53-27).[207, 246] Further impairment of fluid intake in geriatric patients with a depressed level of consciousness or immobility and ability to access free water can lead to lethal hypernatremic states, with mortality rates ranging from 46% to 70%.[236, 238] Acute increase in the serum sodium concentration to more than 160 mEq/L is associated with a 75% mortality rate.

Because elderly persons are prone to hypernatremia with impaired ability to conserve water or solute in combination with a decreased thirst and decreased fluid intake, use of medications that further inhibit renal tubular action of AVP (e.g., lithium, demeclocycline) or medications that cloud the sensorium and decrease the thirst mechanism (e.g., sedatives, major tranquilizers) should be avoided. The use of

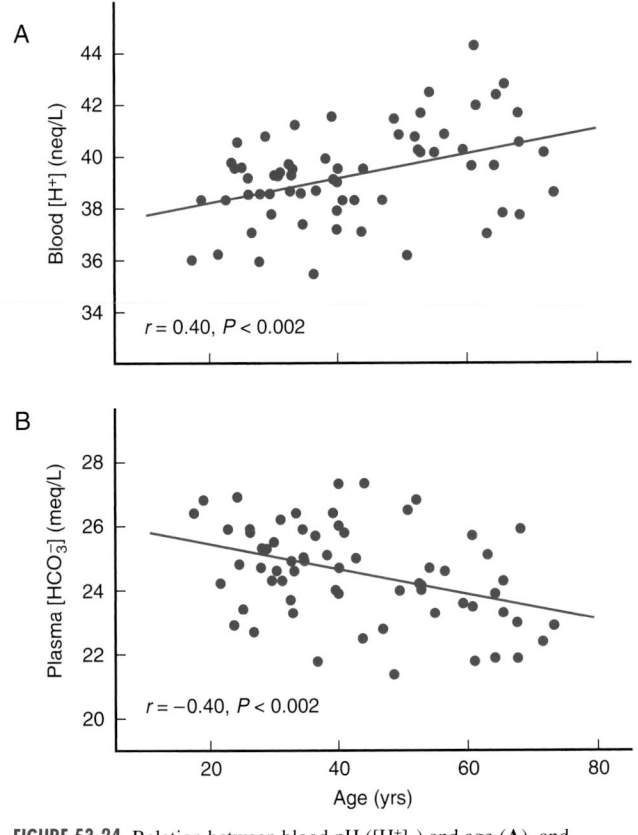

FIGURE 53-24. Relation between blood pH ([H⁺]ᵦ) and age (**A**), and between plasma bicarbonate concentration ([HCO₃⁻]ₚ) and age (**B**), in normal adult humans (*n* = 64). Each data point represents the mean steady-state value in a subject eating a constant diet. Regression equations: $[H^+]_b = 0.045 \times age + 37.2$; $[HCO_3^-]_p = -0.038 \times age + 26.0$. (Reprinted with permission from Frassetto L, Morris RC Jr, Sebastian A: Effect of age on blood acid-base composition in adult humans: Role of age-related renal functional decline. Am J Physiol 271:F1112-F1114, 1996.)

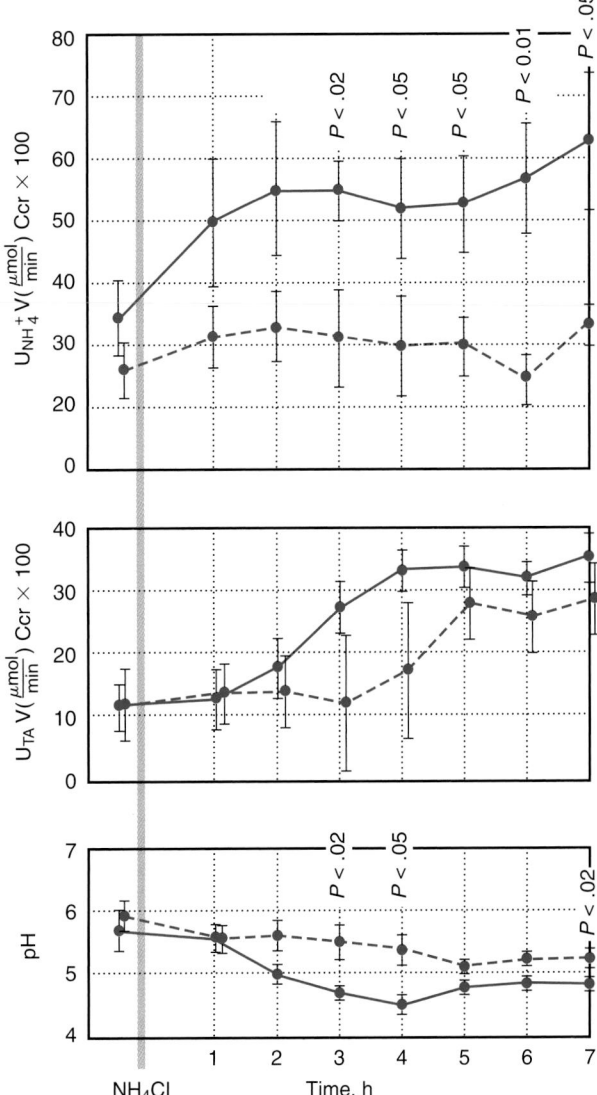

FIGURE 53-25. Acid excretion in young and elderly subjects. Comparison of urinary excretion of ammonium (Uₙₕ₄V), excretion of titratable acid (UₜₐV) corrected for glomerular filtration rate (creatinine clearance × 100), and urinary pH in young (group 1, *solid line*) and aged subjects (group 3, *dashed line*). Mean values (± SEM) along with probability values of the difference between the two groups are shown. (Reprinted with permission from Agarwal BN, Cabebe FG: Renal acidification in elderly subjects. Nephron 26:291-295, 1980.)

osmotic diuretics, external feedings containing high protein and glucose, and bowel cathartics should be monitored. Elderly patients with systemic illnesses, infections, dementia, fever, or neurologic disorders that impair AVP release are at high risk for dehydration. Cellular dehydration can lead to severe neurologic sequelae, including obtundation, stupor, coma, seizures, and death. Therefore, cautious monitoring of elderly patients, especially those who are debilitated and those who are receiving medications that affect tubular conservation of water or solute or affect sensorium, is warranted (see Table 53-2).

Potassium Balance

With advancing age and loss of muscle mass, there are decreases in total body potassium[247] and total exchangeable potassium. This effect is more pronounced in women than in men. Plasma renin and aldosterone levels also decrease with age.[169, 177] Because potassium excretion in the distal tubule is enhanced by the presence of aldosterone, relative hypoaldosteronism predisposes the elderly to hyperkalemia. Healthy elderly subjects, aged 65 to 85 years, had lower basal plasma aldosterone and blunted aldosterone response to potassium infusion compared with younger subjects, aged

20 to 35 years (Fig. 53-28).[248] Potassium-loading studies in aging rats demonstrate a defect in both renal and extrarenal potassium adaptation. When intravenous KCl infusion was administered to young and old rats on a normal diet, the efficiency of potassium excretion was similar.[249] However, with high-potassium feeding, the efficiency of potassium excretion seen with young rats was absent in older rats.[249] The rise in plasma potassium was also higher after KCl infusion in the aged rats on high-potassium intake, compared with younger rats. KCl infusion after bilateral nephrectomy revealed that older rats on a high-potassium diet were unable to decrease the serum potassium, compared with the younger rats.[249] Activity of the sodium-potassium exchange pump (Na⁺,K⁺-ATPase) was also markedly reduced (by 38%) in the medulla

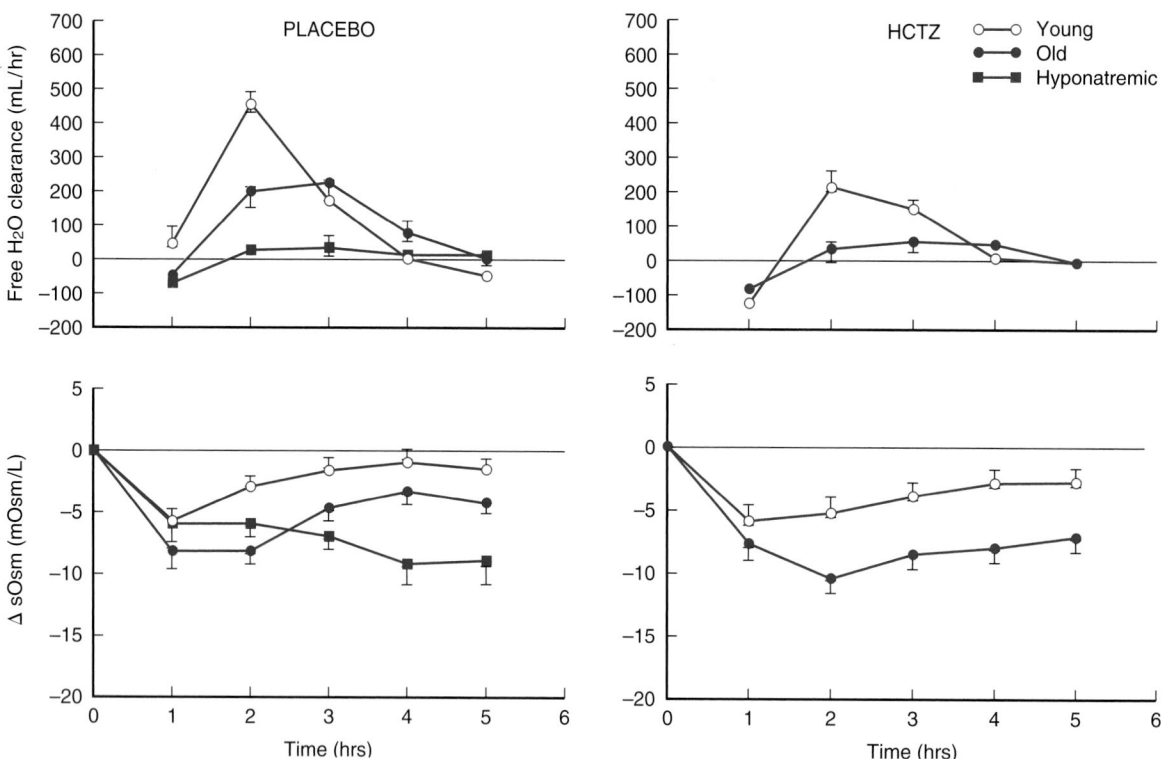

FIGURE 53-26. Free water clearance (CH_2O) and change in serum osmolality ($\Delta sOsm$, in units of mOsm/kg H_2O) after a water load with placebo versus hydro-chlorothiazide (HCTZ) in young subjects, old subjects, and old subjects with a history of thiazide-induced hyponatremia. CH_2O and the decline in sOsm were significantly less in the old than in the young ($P < .05$ by analysis of variance [ANOVA]). This difference was magnified after the use of HCTZ. Those subjects with a history of hyponatremia had lower CH_2O and a lower decline in sOsm than did the healthy elderly ($P < .05$ by ANOVA). (Reprinted with permission from Clark BA, Shannon RP, Rosa RM, et al: Increased susceptibility to thiazide-induced hyponatremia in the elderly. J Am Soc Nephrol 5:1106-1111, 1994.)

TABLE 53-2

Mechanisms by which Drugs Can Lead to Impaired Water Metabolism

INHIBIT ADH RELEASE	INHIBIT PERIPHERAL ACTION OF ADH	POTENTIATE ADH RELEASE
Fluphenazine	Lithium	Nicotine
Haloperidol	Colchicine	Vincristine
Promethazine	Vinblastine	Histamine
Morphine (low doses)	Demeclocycline	Morphine (high doses)
Alcohol	Glyburide	Epinephrine
Carbamazepine	Methoxyflurane	Cyclophosphamide
Norepinephrine	Acetohexamide	Angiotensin
Cisplatinum	Propoxyphene	Bradykinin
Clonidine	Loop diuretics	
Glucocorticoids		

ADH, antidiuretic hormone.

of the older rats compared with younger rats.[249] These findings suggest that mechanisms protecting against acute hyperkalemia after potassium loading may not be affected by aging in rats, but renal and extrarenal potassium adaptation may be blunted.[249] Whether these findings apply to human aging remains to be determined. No effect of aging was found with insulin-mediated potassium uptake in humans.[250] However, exercise-induced elevation of plasma potassium in both

healthy young and elderly subjects suggests that there may be an impaired response of the β-adrenergic–induced increase in the adenylate cyclase system, resulting in decreased activity of the Na^+,K^+-ATPase pump in skeletal muscle.[251]

A renal acidification defect in addition to decreased activity of the renin-angiotensin-aldosterone system may be an important cause for the increased incidence of type 4 renal tubular acidosis (RTA) or syndrome of hyporeninemic hypoaldosteronism in the elderly.[252] Also, given possible problems with chronic potassium adaptation with aging, medications that inhibit the renin-angiotensin-aldosterone system, such as ACEIs, heparin, cyclosporine, tacrolimus, β-blockers, and NSAIDs, may increase the risk of hyperkalemia in the elderly. Similarly, sodium channel blocking agents such as trimethoprim and pentamidine and potassium-sparing diuretics such as amiloride, triamterene, and spironolactone can add to underlying defects in potassium excretion in the elderly (Fig. 53-29).[253-255]

Calcium Balance

Renal tubular reabsorption of calcium appears to be unaffected with aging despite impaired calcium metabolism. Urinary calcium excretion and reabsorption remain appropriate under conditions of either increased and decreased dietary calcium in aged rats.[256] In addition, there is no change in the absolute filtered load or in proximal reabsorption of calcium per nephron between young and aged rats.[257]

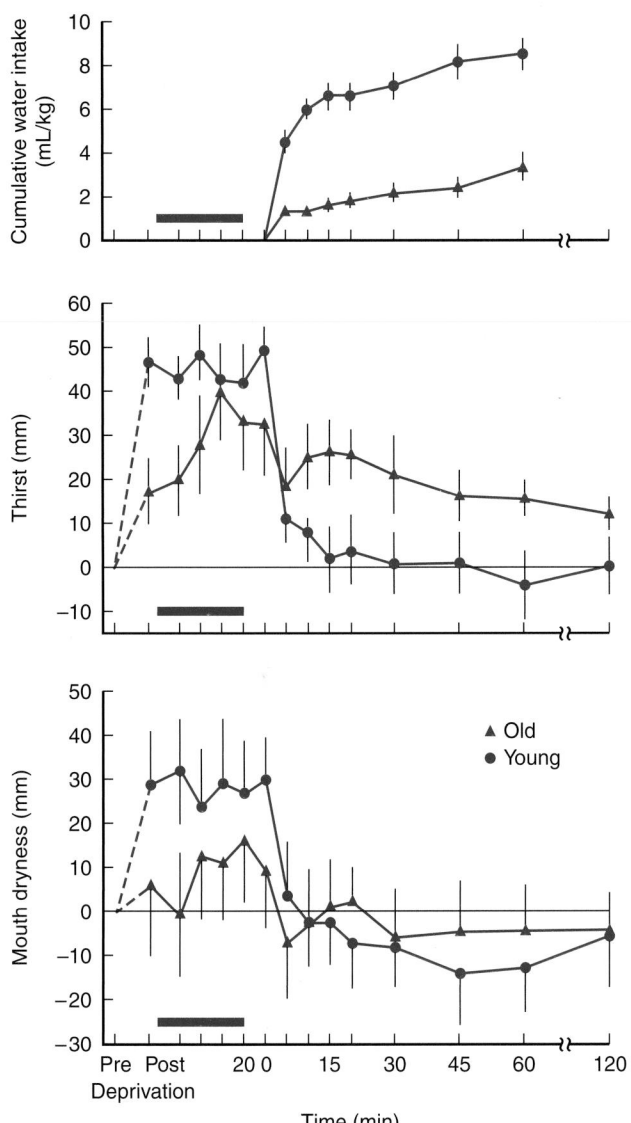

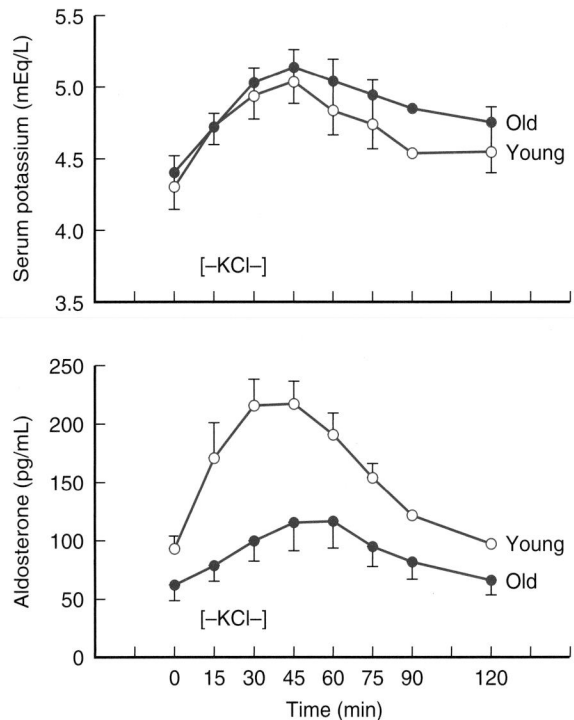

FIGURE 53-28. Serum potassium and aldosterone levels before, during, and after infusion of potassium chloride (0.5 mEq/kg body weight over 45 minutes) in six healthy young and six healthy elderly men. Changes in serum potassium levels were similar, but elderly subjects had lower aldosterone responses (*P* < .005 by analysis of variance). (Reprinted with permission from Mulkerrin E, Epstein FH, Clark BA: Aldosterone responses to hyperkalemia in healthy elderly humans. J Am Soc Nephrol 6:1459-1462, 1995.)

FIGURE 53-27. Cumulative water intake and changes in thirst and mouth dryness in old (*n* = 7) and young (*n* = 7) subjects. Symbols and bars represent mean values ± SEM. Changes in thirst and mouth dryness were measured on a visual-analog rating scale. The hatched rectangle represents the single-blind sham infusion. (Reprinted with permission from Phillips PA, Phil D, Rolls BJ, et al: Reduced thirst after water deprivation in healthy elderly men. N Engl J Med 311:753-759, 1984.)

Aging is associated with decreased intestinal calcium reabsorption, which seems to correlate with decreased 1-α-hydroxylase activity, decreased levels of 1,25-dihydroxy-cholecalciferol (1,25(OH)$_2$D$_3$), and increased basal parathyroid hormone (PTH) levels. The 1,25(OH)$_2$D$_3$–dependent calcium-binding protein declines with age in parallel with the age-related decline in calcium absorption.[256, 258] Other studies suggested that the rate of renal 1,25(OH)$_2$D$_3$ production with PTH infusion was initially lower in healthy elderly versus young subjects; however, the final concentration of 1,25(OH)$_2$D$_3$ was not different in the two groups. Urinary cAMP and fractional phosphorus excretion also increased similarly in both groups, suggesting that the renal response to PTH infusion with aging is intact.[259] The same investigators found that calcium regulation of PTH release may be altered with aging when they studied the effect of calcium gluconate infusion and sodium ethylenediamene tetraacetic acid (NaEDTA) infusion in relation to PTH response. Their observations led them to conclude that the age-related increase in serum concentration of PTH reflects an increase in both the set point for calcium and the number of parathyroid cells. Whether the cell surface G protein–coupled calcium-sensing receptor (CaSR), which may be the underlying reason for the altered set point for PTH seen in both primary and secondary hyperparathyroidism of uremia, plays a role in the increase in set point for PTH release seen with aging awaits further investigation.[260]

Phosphate Balance

Metabolic balance and clearance studies in humans and in rats revealed an age-related decrement in renal tubular reabsorption of phosphate.[104, 260-267] The impairment in renal tubular phosphate occurs in addition to an age-related decrement in intestinal phosphate absorption.[268] Furthermore, renal tubular adaptation to a low-phosphate diet is also impaired in aged rats.[104, 261, 264, 268] Despite increased levels of serum PTH activity,[269, 270] the impairment in renal phosphate transport is independent of endogenous PTH activity, because parathyroidectomy in aged rats results in a significant improvement but not normalization of renal tubular reabsorption of phosphate.[261, 264, 265]

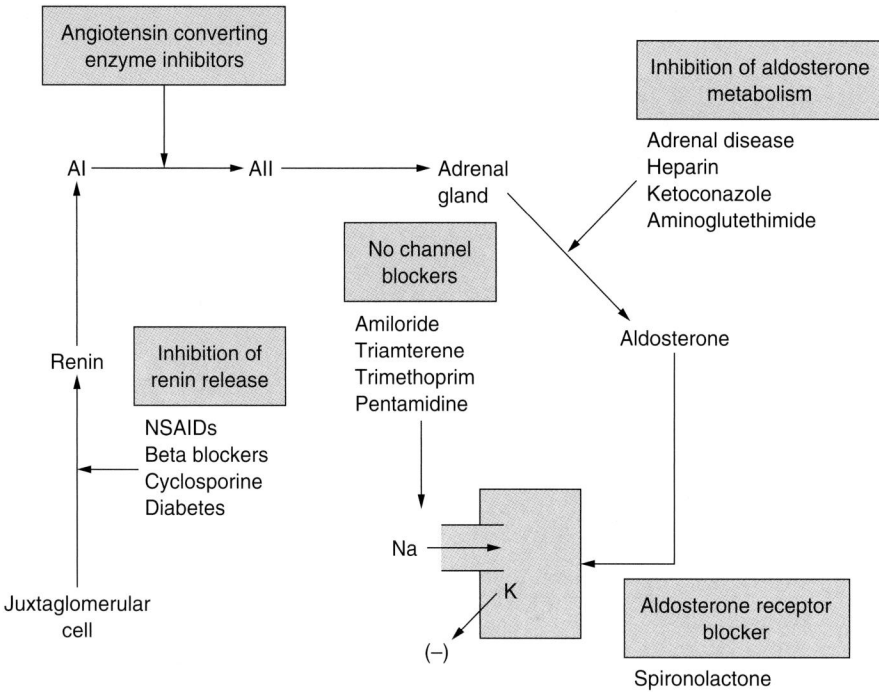

FIGURE 53-29. Site of action of various pharmacologic agents and disease states that can further impair activity of the renin-angiotensin-aldosterone axis and exacerbate hyperkalemia in aged individuals with progressive decline in renin and aldosterone levels. AI, angiotensin; AII, angiotensin II; NSAIDs, nonsteroidal anti-inflammatory drugs.

A similar age-related impairment in phosphate transport has also been demonstrated in primary cultures of renal tubule cells from young and adult rats.[271] In agreement with the in vivo studies,[264] the decrease in phosphate transport is mediated by a decrease in the maximum velocity (Vmax) of sodium gradient–dependent phosphate transport (Na/Pi cotransport). Furthermore, adaptation to a low phosphate concentration in the culture medium is also significantly impaired in renal tubular cells cultured from old compared to young adult rats.

In aged rats, the decrease in the proximal tubular Na/Pi cotransport was associated with decreases in type IIa Na/Pi cotransporter protein and mRNA levels.[272] In fact, immunohistochemistry revealed a marked decrease in the expression of type IIa Na/Pi cotransporter protein at the level of the apical brush border membrane.[272]

An additional factor that may play a role in the decrease in Na/Pi cotransport is the age-related increase in membrane cholesterol content.[104, 273-276] In brush border membrane isolated from young adult rats, in vitro enrichment with cholesterol to similar levels measured in aged rats simulated the age-related impairment in the Vmax of Na/Pi cotransport.[277] In opossum kidney cells with renal proximal tubular cell characteristics, direct alterations in cell cholesterol content per se was shown to modulate Na/Pi cotransport activity by causing alterations in the expression of the apical membrane type II Na/Pi cotransport protein.[278] This suggests that the age-related increase in membrane cholesterol could also play an important role in the age-related decrease in Na/Pi cotransport.

The role of impaired $1,25(OH)_2D_3$ metabolism in the age-related impairment in renal and intestinal phosphate transport also deserves to be determined, because in vitamin D–deficient animals administration of $1,25(OH)_2D_3$ results in significant improvements in renal[279-281] and intestinal[279]

phosphate transport. Of interest, the stimulatory effects of $1,25(OH)_2D_3$ on phosphate transport are also paralleled by significant alterations in brush border membrane lipid composition and fluidity.[282, 283] It is therefore quite possible that similar lipid-modulating effects of $1,25(OH)_2D_3$ in the aged might also result in significant improvements in renal and intestinal transport of phosphate (and calcium).

CLINICAL RENAL DISEASES IN THE AGED

Acute Renal Failure

Susceptibility to acute renal failure (ARF) in the elderly may be more common given the underlying compromise of renal function with aging. ARF was found to be 3.5 times more common in patients older than 70 years of age than in those younger than 70 years when 437 prospective ARF patients were studied over a 9-year period in Spain.[284] The increased prevalence of systemic diseases such as atherosclerosis, hypertension, diabetes, heart failure, and malignancy in a growing elderly population necessitates various medical and surgical interventions that can further exacerbate common causes of ARF, including prerenal or volume depletion, sepsis, acute interstitial nephritis, nephrotoxin-induced glomerular and tubular dysfunction, and obstruction. Specifically, more common in elderly persons with generalized atherosclerosis is cholesterol embolization, which can occur spontaneously or secondary to invasive procedures that manipulate the arterial vasculature. Less common, but not to be overlooked, are acute vasculitis and rapidly progressive glomerulonephritis, which may lead to significant morbidity and ESRD in the elderly.

Volume loss from vomiting, diarrhea, overzealous diuretic use, bleeding, or decreased renal perfusion due to drug- or sepsis-induced vasodilatation or low cardiac output frequently leads to prerenal azotemia in the elderly. In two prospective studies noting prevalence of renal failure, a prerenal etiology was found in more than 50% of elderly patients.[284, 285] Underlying impaired ability to concentrate urine, regulate thirst, and retain sodium in the aged may contribute to the high prevalence. In addition, age-related decreases in baseline RPF and GFR impairments in autoregulation of RPF and renal functional reserve may render the kidney more susceptible to prerenal failure. Hemodynamic alterations with the use of prostaglandin inhibitors (NSAIDs) or angiotensin II antagonists, including ACEIs and angiotensin II receptor blockers (ARBs), or α-adrenergic blockers, commonly used for the treatment of rheumatologic, cardiovascular, or genitourinary disorders in the elderly, can further compromise renal vasoregulatory mechanisms. With appropriate intervention, including adequate and careful volume replacement, discontinuation of exacerbating medications, and improvement of cardiac output, renal recovery is expected.

Most instances of prerenal failure are potentially reversible with volume replacement; others lead to acute tubular necrosis (ATN). Sixty percent of elderly patients with prerenal azotemia recovered renal function in one study.[285] Evolution to ATN is more common in the elderly than in younger patients (23% versus 15%).[286] Moreover, urinary indices, such as the fractional excretion of sodium (FE_{Na}), that are traditionally used to evaluate the possibility of a prerenal etiology of ARF in the elderly should be interpreted with caution. Elderly patients with volume depletion may not have the capacity to conserve adequate tubular sodium to achieve an FE_{Na} lower than 1. Therefore, an elevated FE_{Na} may exist in the face of hypoperfusion from the preexisting tubular defect.[287]

Complications of major surgery account for approximately 30% of cases of ARF. Hypotension during or after surgery, postoperative fluid loss due to gastrointestinal fistulous drainage, arrhythmia, and myocardial infarction are common postoperative complications in the elderly that may result in ARF.

Vasodilatation and hypotension from infection and sepsis with subsequent ARF often complicates the hospital course in elderly patients. Infection, and especially gram-negative septicemia, accounts for 30% of cases of ARF in the elderly. Gram-negative infections are frequently associated with endotoxin-induced renovascular vasoconstriction, which in susceptible individuals can result in ATN. Frequently, these patients have multiorgan dysfunction or perioperative sepsis with an increased catabolic rate, which carries a poor prognosis in the elderly.[288-290] Hemodynamic instability, along with the need for complicated nephrotoxic antibiotic regimens such as the use of aminoglycosides or amphotericin, can prolong renal dysfunction. Antibiotic dosing needs to be carefully monitored in elderly patients. GFR estimation may be unreliable with the use of S_{Cr} alone, or formulas based on S_{Cr}, because of the decrease in bulk muscle mass with aging. Further renal tubular and biochemical alterations with aging may enhance the toxic effects of antibiotics such as aminoglycosides on renal tubules. Age is a well-known risk factor for aminoglycoside-induced nephrotoxicity.[291]

Similarly, various common infections (staphylococci, streptococci, legionella, cytomegalovirus, human immunodeficiency virus), as well as common antibiotics (β-lactams, sulfonamides) and a myriad of other medications, may cause interstitial inflammation and interstitial nephritis.[292] Tubulointerstitial inflammation with activated macrophages releases degradative enzymes and may result in the loss of intact basement membranes, which will hamper regeneration of the tubular segment. The fall in GFR may result from a loss of functioning nephrons and failure of the remaining nephrons to compensate with hyperfiltration.[292]

Medications such as NSAIDs and angiotensin II antagonists not only compromise renal vasoregulating mechanisms that maintain GFR in the elderly but also may cause interstitial inflammation and acute interstitial nephritis. Presentation can be typical, with pyuria and worsening ARF, or atypical, with nephrotic-range proteinuria. Renal biopsy has shown both a minimal change lesion and membranous lesions with NSAIDs,[293] especially propionic acid derivatives, and membranous lesions with the ACEI captopril.

Acute and prolonged vasoconstriction from radiocontrast infusion can significantly impair renal function in the elderly.[294] With radiocontrast-induced renal failure, the initial increased osmotic load delivered to the macula densa may also trigger tubuloglomerular feedback, inducing renin release and reduction in GFR.[295]

Experimental studies in aging rats indicate that the aging kidney has a greater propensity for ischemic and toxic ARF.[296-300] Renal artery occlusion produced a greater decline in renal function in older compared with younger rats, as well as slower recovery.[301, 302] Glomerulosclerosis may not be the primary factor leading to ischemic renal failure in aging rats. In fact, when histologic variations between young and old rats were minimized by low-protein feeding, renal artery clamping led to a significant decrease in GFR and RPF and an increase in RVR in older compared with younger rats (Fig. 53-30).[301] RVR increased with age in euvolemic men given a constant sodium intake of 240 mEq/day, and the response to orthostatic change in RVR was blunted.[303] Studies using blood oxygenation level–dependent magnetic resonance imaging in nine female volunteers between 59 and 79 years of age showed inability to improve medullary oxygenation with water diuresis, compared to younger subjects,

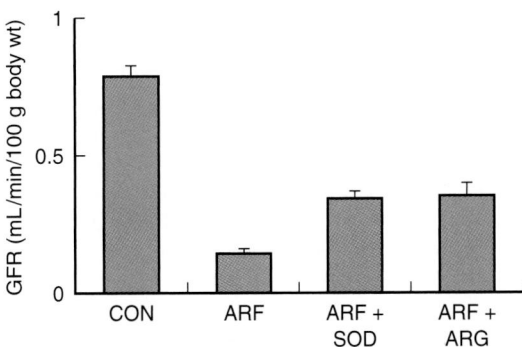

FIGURE 53-30. Change in glomerular filtration rate (GFR) in aged (18-month-old) rats measured under basal conditions (CON); 1 day after acute renal failure (ARF); with super oxide dismutase infusion 1 day after ARF (ARF + SOD); and with pretreatment with L-arginine and ARF (ARF + ARG). (Redrawn with permission from Sabbatini M, Sansone G, Uccello F, et al: Functional versus structural changes in the pathophysiology of acute ischemic renal failure in aging rats. Kidney Int 45: 1355-1361, 1994.)

suggesting a possible predisposition to hypoxic renal injury in older patients.[304] Oxygen free radicals can be generated during hemodynamically mediated ischemic ARF.[305] When exogenous superoxide dismutase, a free radical scavenger, was infused to ischemic aged rats, renal hemodynamics significantly improved (see Fig. 53-30).[301]

Some have suggested that ischemic aged rats may also have impaired NO production or reduced intrarenal NO levels, which may predispose to renal failure.[301] NO is released tonically by vascular endothelium[306] to induce active vasodilatation and also to oppose vasoconstriction and thereby maintain blood pressure.[67] Basal tonically produced NO appears to have a pronounced role in maintenance of renal perfusion in aging.[67, 307] NO production appears to be reduced with aging in isolated conduit arteries.[308-310] Studies in aging rats have found a 40% decrease in serum levels of the nitric oxide synthase (NOS) substrate L-arginine.[310] Similar findings have been noted in aging humans.[311] However, a recent study in aging Sprague-Dawley rats showed that gene expression regulating renal arginine synthesis and small-intestinal synthesis of citrulline (precursor of arginine) is unchanged or is up-regulated in older rats compared with younger rats.[312] This suggests that decreased NO may not be related to decreased substrate but to other changes in the NO biosynthetic pathway. The maximum percent change in plasma cGMP, a marker for NO production, decreased with aging in normotensive Japanese individuals given L-arginine infusion.[313] Older healthy subjects, despite a significant fall in blood pressure while consuming a low-sodium diet, showed an age-related decline in urinary nitrate and nitrite and urinary cGMP, reflecting an age-dependent reduction in clearance.[314] It may be that renal endothelial NO production is maximized in normal aged individuals in order to maintain stable renal function. This appears to be consistent with a blunted vasodilatory response seen in the elderly.[126]

Measurements of NO production in the face of renal ischemia have yet to be performed in human subjects. When older rats were pretreated with L-arginine feeding 7 days before renal artery occlusion, there was marked improvement in GFR and RPF and a decrease in RVR (see Fig. 53-30). L-NAME, an NOS inhibitor, given to older rats fed L-arginine, abolished the renal hemodynamic response seen with L-arginine and super oxide dismutase.[301] Whether normal or high-protein feeding would have altered these responses is speculative, given that rats fed a high-protein diet develop an age-related decline in NO excretion, as measured by urinary nitrite and nitrate excretion (NO_x), whereas protein-restricted aged rats maintain urinary NO_x excretion comparable to controls (Fig. 53-31).[68] L-Arginine supplementation in drinking water of aged animals appears to limit structural changes that occur in the aging glomerular basement membrane.[70, 71] It remains to be seen whether NO is in some way related to the beneficial effects of a low-protein diet on age-related glomerulosclerosis.

The endogenous NOS inhibitor and L-arginine analog, N(G),N(G')-asymmetric dimethylarginine (ADMA), has recently been found to be significantly elevated in aged (20-month-old) Sprague-Dawley rats, compared with adult (6-month-old) rats in the face of similar levels of L-arginine.[315] Similarly, ADMA levels were found to increase with age in humans.[316] Increased ADMA levels can decrease NO

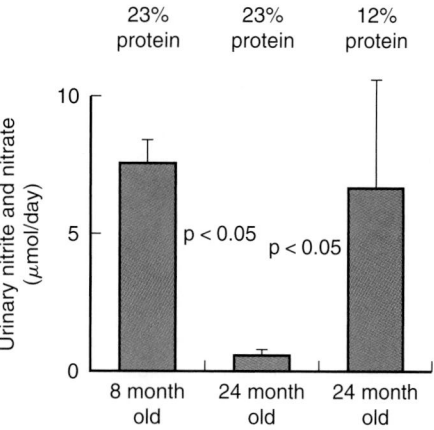

FIGURE 53-31. Urinary excretion of nitrite and nitrate in control (8-month-old) rats, aged (24-month-old) rats fed a 23% protein diet, and aged rats fed a 12% protein diet. (Redrawn with permission from Sabbatini M, Sansone G, Uccello F, et al: Functional versus structural changes in the pathophysiology of acute ischemic renal failure in aging rats. Kidney Int 45:1355-1361, 1994.)

synthesis in the endothelial cells and lead to decreased nitrite content and decreased NOS activity, as seen in aging, thus impairing endothelium-dependent vasodilation[315] and predisposing the aged kidney to ischemia.

Alterations in the metabolism and biochemistry of aging tubular cells may also be playing a role in mediating age-related enhancement of ischemic renal injury.[300] When uptake of PAH and tetraethylammonium (TEA) was assessed in renal cortical slices after periods of in vitro anoxia, uptake was impaired to a greater extent in older than in younger rats.[300]

Atheroembolic renal disease may be a complication after intra-arterial cannulation, especially in elderly patients with generalized atherosclerosis. Spontaneous cholesterol embolization may also occur,[314] although it is more commonly seen after manipulation of the arterial vasculature for radiographic or surgical intervention such as carotid, coronary, renal, or abdominal angiography; aortic surgery; or percutaneous transluminal angioplasty of coronary or renal arteries. Use of anticoagulants or fibrinolytic treatment in patients with diffuse atherosclerosis has also been found to trigger cholesterol emboli.[317] Renal failure is irreversible and progressive and may or may not be associated with other systemic findings of cholesterol embolization such as purpura, livido reticularis of the abdominal and lumbar wall and/or lower extremities, Hollenhorst plaques with retinal ischemia, gastrointestinal bleeding, pancreatitis, myocardial infarction, cerebral infarction, and distal ischemic necrosis of the toes.[318] Laboratory evidence for cholesterol embolization, including eosinophilia, eosinophiluria, and low complement levels, is frequently absent. No specific therapy is available for reversal of this disease entity. The benefits and risks of angiographic procedures in elderly patients with widespread atherosclerotic disease must be weighed carefully, and excessive anticoagulation must be avoided in these patients.

Symptomatic obstructive uropathy in the face of progressively rising blood urea nitrogen and creatinine levels can be a common presentation in elderly men with prostatic hypertrophy.[319] Ureteric obstruction in women commonly arises from pelvic tumors of the uterus or cervix. Other retroperitoneal or pelvic neoplasms, such as lymphoma, bladder carcinoma, and rectal tumors, can also present as ARF in the geriatric population. However, typical symptoms of urinary tract obstruction, such as urinary frequency and voiding difficulty with stopping and starting micturition, may not always be apparent in the elderly. Prolonged presence of obstruction may manifest with irreversible renal function. Careful review of medications (e.g., anticholinergic agents) and studies such as postvoid residual and renal ultrasonography may be necessary, followed by prompt urologic intervention. Infected residual urine may potentiate impairments in tubular function, RBF, and GFR caused by obstruction.

Although elderly persons may be at higher risk for development of ARF[284] and renal recovery may take longer,[320] age per se is not an important determinant of survival in patients with ARF[285, 321] and should not be used as a discriminating factor in therapeutic decisions concerning ARF.[288, 322] Most elderly patients respond well to treatment of ARF with dialysis. Therefore, prompt management, with dialysis support as necessary to alleviate uremic symptoms and prevent uremic complications such as infection, congestive heart failure, myocardial infarction, and bleeding, is recommended in elderly patients with ARF.

Renal Vascular Disorders

Atherosclerotic renovascular disease is an important cause of hypertension and leads to progressive ischemic renal failure and ESRD in up to 15% of patients.[323, 324] Atheromatous involvement of the renal vasculature may present as renal artery stenosis, as complex intrarenal lesions with multiple stenosis of intrarenal vasculature, or as cholesterol embolism. New onset of hypertension or progressive azotemia in the elderly, especially in the presence of other underlying risk factors for generalized atherosclerosis, obviates the need to consider atherosclerotic renal disease in this population.[325, 326] The natural history of atheromatous renal disease is progressive occlusion of the major renal arteries, especially when luminal narrowing is greater than 75% by angiogram.[327, 328] Angiographic progression of renal artery stenosis was present in almost 50% of 237 patients monitored by Rimmer and Gennari.[329] Mean GFR declined by 4 mL/min in 51 patients with bilateral atherosclerotic renovascular disease who were monitored for a median period of 52 months.[330] Varying degrees of stenosis may be present in one or more renal arteries. Azotemic patients with high-grade renal artery stenosis in a solitary kidney or unilateral renal artery occlusion and contralateral stenosis are at highest risk for progressive renal failure.[328, 331] Bilateral renal artery stenosis was associated with a crude mortality rate of 45% at 60 months in one study.[330]

Smoking has emerged as an independent risk factor in the progression of macrovascular and microvascular renal disease in the elderly. Thirty smokers older than 55 years of age without other risk factors for vascular disease had significant decrease in RPF as measured by radionuclide study and increased endothelin-1 (ET-1) concentration, compared with 24 age- and gender-matched nonsmokers.[332] Smoking has been reported as a predictor of renal artery stenosis[333] as well as a factor increasing the risk of developing ESRD.[334] In a multivariate "best fit" model adjusted for gender, race, weight, baseline S_{Cr}, and age of nondiabetic elderly patients

older than 65 years of age in the Cardiovascular Health Study Cohort, the number of cigarettes smoked per day was independently associated with an increase in S_{Cr}.[335] Both norepinephrine and epinephrine are released as a result of smoking.[336] In addition, smoking interferes with metabolism of prostacyclin and thromboxane A_2 in the endothelium[337-340] and with vascular response to acetylcholine,[341] NO, and ET-1.[342, 343] ET-1 levels are increased in active smokers.[344] A potent vasoconstrictor with mitogenic and atherogenic activity on vascular smooth muscle, ET-1 may be important in mediating the renal arteriolar thickening noted in pathologic studies.[345-347] Up-regulation of renal ET-1 protein has also been noted in the kidneys of healthy aging rodents.[348]

Various methods have been used to help in the diagnosis of significant atherosclerotic renovascular disease. An increase in S_{Cr} with the addition of angiotensin II antagonists (ACEI or ARB) may provide a clinical clue to the consideration for bilateral atherosclerotic renovascular disease or unilateral atherosclerotic stenosis in a solitary functional kidney.[349] The decrease in GFR results from inhibition of the autoregulatory vasoconstrictive action of angiotensin II on the efferent arteriole, which maintains glomerular filtration in light of decreased glomerular perfusion.[350] Renal scintigraphy using ^{99}Tc-DTPA or technetium-mercaptoacetythiglycine (^{99}Tc-MAG3) before and after administration of an ACEI can be a useful tool to increase clinical suspicion for a significant functional unilateral renal artery stenosis.[351, 352] Duplex ultrasound scanning of the renal arteries in some centers may provide noninvasive visualization of stenosis in the main renal arteries as well as blood flow velocity data to determine the significance of the stenosis with high sensitivity and specificity.[353] Alternatively, magnetic resonance angiography is being used in some centers to visualize the renal arteries noninvasively. In addition, CO_2 angiography is often used in the presence of decreased GFR. However, investigation with contrast angiography remains the gold standard, because the renal vasculature can be visualized in completeness, including the smaller intrarenal branches. Atheromatous narrowing of the distal branches of the renal arteries and microvasculature may also cause hypertension and ischemic renal failure.[354]

Arterial cannulation and contrast injection of diffuse atherosclerotic vessels can lead to cholesterol embolization or contrast-induced nephropathy, or both. An acute reversible rise in S_{Cr} within 1 to 4 days after contrast administration can be attributed to the contrast dye. Irreversible and often progressive renal failure that occurs 1 to 4 weeks after arterial contrast injection may be secondary to renal cholesterol embolization with or without systemic manifestations. Cholesterol crystals lodge in arteries with diameters of 100 to 200 μm or smaller, including glomerular tufts.[355] Histologically, clear biconvex clefts with surrounding inflammatory reaction can be seen, because the lipid material is dissolved by tissue fixation.[356] Blood pressure control, supportive management, and avoidance of further nephrotoxic insults are recommended in the face of cholesterol embolization or intrarenal atheromatous disease.

Percutaneous transluminal angioplasty (PTA) or surgical revascularization should be considered when technically possible to preserve renal function and improve blood pressure control in patients with significant atherosclerotic renal artery disease. Occasionally, the presence of collateral circulation may protect the renal parenchyma from ischemic injury despite progressive occlusive disease.[357, 358] Several cases have suggested reversibility of renal failure with angioplasty and/or surgical revascularization of renal artery stenosis.[358-362] However, a S_{Cr} of 3 mg/dL or higher predicted poor outcome after technically successful PTA, with two thirds of the patients in this group either showing no improvement in blood pressure, requiring dialysis within months after the procedure, or dying.[363] These patients were noted to have a higher incidence of bilateral renal artery occlusion or high-grade stenosis of a solitary functioning kidney.[363] Lesions amenable to angioplasty are more commonly unilateral, nonostial, and technically feasible to approach. Angioplasty may need to be repeated in at least 20% of cases with recurrence.[326] Some investigators are considering intravascular stent placement.[364] However, a S_{Cr} of 2 mg/dL or higher may be a poor prognostic indicator after stent revascularization.[365] Revascularization is more commonly recommended for ostial, bilateral, or totally occluding lesions.[326]

Acute Glomerulonephritis

Acute glomerulonephritis in the elderly results most commonly from rapidly progressive glomerulonephritis (RPGN). Severe crescentic involvement, usually affecting more than 50% of the glomeruli, is seen histologically. Clinically, a rapid decline in renal function associated with active nephritic urine sediment (hematuria, pyuria, red blood cell casts, and moderate to severe proteinuria) is seen. The pathogenesis is believed to be immune mediated, although clear-cut evidence for immunologic injury is absent in many cases. Immunohistologic presentation in the kidney is of three major types: type 1, presence of antiglomerular basement membrane antibody; type 2, with granular immune deposits; and type 3, with no immune deposits,[366] although circulating anti-neutrophilic cytoplasmic antibodies may be present. Type 2 and type 3 histologic patterns are more commonly found in elderly patients with RPGN.[367, 368] Of 19 patients with crescentic glomerulonephritis in a biopsy series of 115 elderly patients, 9 had evidence for granular immunoglobulin G (IgG) deposition on immunofluorescence, 6 patients had no immune deposits, and 3 had evidence of antiglomerular basement membrane disease.[369] In another study, 8 of 10 elderly patients with RPGN had antineutrophil cytoplasm antibody (ANCA)–positive sera, although no immune deposits were found.[370] Pauci-immune crescentic glomerulonephritis was the diagnosis in 79 (31.2%) of 259 biopsies for ARF in adults aged 60 years or older.[371]

In one series of 40 and another series of 60 patients with crescentic glomerulonephritis, the average or median age was greater than 60 years.[372, 373] In general, the prognosis for elderly patients with RPGN is poor despite success of treatment in small, uncontrolled series.[367, 372, 374] The risk-benefit ratio for treatment with pulse steroids, cyclophosphamide, and or plasmapheresis for RPGN in elderly patients must be individualized given the side effect profile of available treatment options.

Diffuse proliferative poststreptococcal acute glomerulonephritis in the elderly occurs in association with streptococcal infections of the throat and skin[373, 375-377] and generally carries a favorable prognosis. In patients older than 55 years

of age, up to a 22.6% incidence of poststreptococcal glomerulonephritis has been reported.[373, 378]

Nephrotic Syndrome

The presentation of marked proteinuria, edema, and hypertension frequently leads to assessment by renal biopsy in the elderly. Thirty percent of patients in the Medical Research Council Glomerulonephritis Registry from 1978 to 1990 were biopsied for nephrotic syndrome.[379] Membranous glomerulopathy (36.6%) was the most common histologic finding, followed by minimal change disease (11%) and renal amyloidosis (10.7%). Other reviews from countries including the United States, France, Israel, England, Japan, and Korea corroborate this data.[369, 380-389] Cumulative data are shown in Table 53-3. Of 545 elderly patients with primary nephrotic syndrome, 54% were noted to have membranous glomerulonephritis, 19% with minimal change, 10% with mesangial proliferative, and 9% with membranoproliferative glomerulonephritis.[371, 377-383, 385, 388, 389] Minimal change disease in the elderly is associated with a higher risk for ARF, more severe proteinuria, and a lower albumin level than in younger patients.[390] Systemic amyloidosis, usually of the AL type, is found frequently in elderly patients with nephrotic syndrome. Paraproteinemia may be found in 40% to 68% of patients presenting with nephrotic syndrome secondary to primary amyloidosis.[391] All elderly patients who present with unexplained nephrotic syndrome should undergo serum and urine protein electrophoresis. Those with abnormal findings should undergo bone marrow aspiration to rule out multiple myeloma. Abdominal fat pad aspiration examined with Congo red stain may also be useful in the diagnosis of primary amyloidosis. Kidney biopsy specimens in elderly patients with unexplained proteinuria should be routinely stained with Congo red and examined under electron microscopy for amyloid fibrils. Treatment with melphalan and prednisone may delay the progression to ESRD.

Glomerulosclerosis has been reported to be present in 7% of the renal biopsies of the elderly. Glomerulosclerosis in the elderly resembles the focal segmental glomerulosclerosis seen more commonly in younger age groups. Juxtamedullary glomeruli are frequently affected, with positive immunofluorescence for IgM and the third component of complement (C3). This pathology is often seen as an end result of other glomerulopathies and secondary advanced systemic diseases such as hypertension and diabetes,[392] where hyperfiltration of functioning glomeruli may hasten the process of glomerulosclerosis.[36, 393] Juxtamedullary glomeruli may be more affected, given the significantly higher filtration fraction in comparison with superficial cortical nephrons. Glomerular ischemia from renovascular disease may lead to adaptive glomerular enlargement and segmental sclerosing lesions with nephrotic proteinuria in the elderly.[394] Interestingly, normal, healthy aging rats have shown histology similar to that seen in human glomerulosclerosis with IgM and C3 deposition and proteinuria.[395-400]

The histopathology of nephrotic syndrome is unpredictable given only clinical data. With the greater number of aged individuals being referred for renal replacement therapy, renal biopsies in elderly patients with proteinuria have

TABLE 53-3

Histologic Lesions in 545 Elderly Patients with Primary Nephrotic Syndrome

AUTHORS	MINIMAL CHANGE	MEMBRANOUS GLOMERULO-NEPHRITIS	MESANGIAL PROLIFERATIVE GLOMERULONEPHRITIS	MEMBRANO-PROLIFERATIVE GLOMERULONEPHRITIS	GLOMERULO-SCLEROSIS	CHRONIC GLOMERULO-NEPHRITIS
Fawcett et al., 1971	6	5	—	4	16	5
Huriet et al., 1975	4	2	—	6	—	—
Moorthy and Zimmerman, 1980	9	15	7	2	1	—
Ishimuto et al., 1981	1	6	—	2	7	—
Lustig et al., 1982	2	16	—	2	3	—
Zech et al., 1982	19	31	2	4	—	3
Kingswood et al., 1984	2	16	11	3	—	—
Murphy et al., 1987	2	2	—	2	—	—
Sato et al., 1987	7	30	12	7	1	—
Johnston et al., 1992	35	116	18	—	5	—
Ozono et al., 1994	6	26	—	8	—	—
Shin et al., 2001	14	27	—	8	6	1
Total	**107 (19%)**	**292 (54%)**	**50 (9%)**	**48 (9%)**	**39 (7%)**	**9 (2%)**

increased in the hope of early diagnosis and possible intervention. A retrospective review of idiopathic membranous nephropathy in the elderly revealed no evidence of improved outcome with prednisone therapy in 33 of 74 patients who received treatment. The rate of decline in renal function was not different in comparison to a younger group, but the incidence of chronic renal failure was much worse. This may have been secondary to a decreased renal functional reserve in the elderly.[401] Others have reported partial or complete remission of nephrotic syndrome and protection from renal failure in patients with idiopathic membranous disease treated with prednisone and cytotoxic agents.[402] Therefore, the use of steroid and cytotoxic treatment needs to be considered cautiously and individualized in elderly patients with idiopathic membranous nephropathy. The outcome of treatment of proliferative glomerulonephritis was highly variable. However, because up to 19% of elderly patients present with minimal change disease, which has a more favorable response and remission rate with corticosteroids, a complete workup including renal biopsy should be performed for the elderly patient with nephrotic syndrome.

Nephrotic syndrome may coexist or precede a malignancy.[403] Between 7% and 20% of patients with nephrotic syndrome have an associated malignancy.[387, 404] The association between membranous lesions and malignancy is presumed to be mediated by immune complexes composed in part of tumor-associated antigens.[404] Solid tumors of the lung, colon, rectum, kidney, breast, and stomach have been most commonly associated with membranous glomerulopathy. Therefore, a thorough history, physical examination, and basic screening for an underlying malignancy should be done in elderly patients presenting with nephrotic syndrome.

Chronic Renal Failure

Progression of age-dependent medical diseases often leads to the chronic renal failure late in life. NHANES III data suggest that 6.6 million persons older than 60 years of age have a GFR of less than 60 mL/min/1.73 m².[405] Long-standing diabetes, hypertension, chronic glomerulonephritis, ischemic atherosclerotic renovascular disease, and obstructive nephropathy are common diagnoses of chronic renal failure in the elderly. In the community-based longitudinal cohort study of patients older than 65 years of age known as the Cardiovascular Health Study, the level of GFR was an independent risk factor for de novo cardiovascular disease and all-cause mortality (Fig. 53-32).[406] Clinical progression of chronic renal failure in the elderly frequently manifests as a decompensated preexisting medical illness such as congestive heart failure, gastrointestinal bleeding, hypertension, or dementia rather than frank symptoms of uremia per se. Evidence for progression may not always be evident from laboratory findings, because gradual loss of muscle mass in the elderly uremic patient may result in no significant change in the S_{Cr}. The actual renal reserve is usually lower than that estimated by the S_{Cr}.

Advanced renal failure with no identifiable reversible causes such as obstruction or renal artery stenosis in necessitates dialysis support before disabling symptoms of uremia and organ dysfunction become irreversible. Older patients become symptomatically uremic at lower levels of S_{Cr} than do younger patients and hence require earlier initiation of dialysis. Also, manifestation of uremia may be subtle and atypical in elderly patients (e.g., unexplained worsening of congestive cardiac failure, behavioral changes). Age itself should not be the sole criterion for exclusion from dialysis. In the absence of major extrarenal organ dysfunction, elderly patients adjust fairly well to dialysis. Increasing numbers of elderly patients are being accepted for renal replacement therapy, with 55% of ESRD patients older than 60 years of age.[407-409] Longevity of older dialysis patients is not markedly reduced, although it is not as favorable as for younger patients. A recent 10-year review of octogenarians on hemodialysis suggests a 24-month median survival time.[410] Elderly ESRD patients are more often treated with short

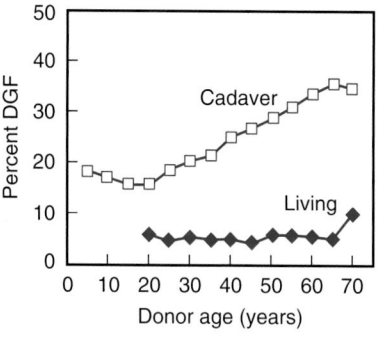
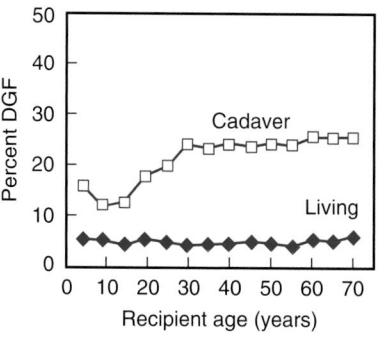

FIGURE 53-32. Effect of donor age on delayed graft function (DGF) of first transplants (1996–2000). (Reprinted with permission from Cecka JM: The UNOS renal transplant registry. Clin Transplant 1-18, 2001.)

dialysis and are more likely to die from it.[411, 412] These patients are at increased risk for silent ischemia during hypotensive episodes, which is common during short hemodialysis.[413]

Elderly patients with significant cardiovascular disease often do well with chronic ambulatory peritoneal dialysis (CAPD).[408, 414-417] No major difference has been found in the incidence of peritonitis, type of infectious organism, or likelihood of technique failure between elderly and younger CAPD patients.[408, 418] In fact, elderly patients may have less need for catheter replacement than younger CAPD patients do.[408, 418]

Neither mode of dialysis therapy, hemodialysis or peritoneal dialysis, has been demonstrated to be clearly superior to the other in the elderly.[419-421] Variability in patient selection and underlying comorbid conditions (e.g., diabetes, cardiovascular disease, malignancy, peripheral vascular disease) affect patient survival and contribute to conflicting studies.[408] One study looking at an historical prospective national sample from 1986 to 1987 of diabetic and nondiabetic Medicare-insured ESRD patients suggested that elderly diabetic subjects may have a lower survival rate with CAPD versus hemodialysis.[422] However, controlled trials are lacking to assess actual mortality among diabetic CAPD patients.

The mode of renal replacement therapy should be individualized in elderly patients, taking into consideration underlying medical and psychosocial factors. For instance, CAPD may be the choice for those patients with widespread vascular disease and inability to maintain a patent vascular access, or for those with significant hemodynamic instability during hemodialysis. Similarly, hemodialysis may be preferred for those patients with deconditioning or a home situation that prevents appropriate self-care dialysis. The socialization that is available at in-center hemodialysis units may be an important factor for elderly patients who live alone or are depressed. Comorbid conditions such as vascular disease, infection, malnutrition, and malignancy, as well as withdrawal from dialysis therapy, have contributed to mortality in elderly patients with ESRD.

Age alone does not preclude denial for renal transplantation. Many elderly, medically eligible patients have undergone successful renal transplantation.[423, 424] Donor age is more significant in determining delayed graft function than recipient age (see Fig. 53-32).[4] A decision analytic model comparing cadaveric transplantation with hemodialysis suggested that well-selected elderly patients younger than 70 years of age with few comorbidities may have significant quality-adjusted life expectancy gains of 1.1 years with

transplantation.[425] In fact, elderly patients older than 60 years of age with well-matched demographics for comorbidities undergoing rigorous screening with anticipated 5-year survival rates in excess of 80% had substantial survival advantage over patients with ESRD undergoing dialysis. The preoperative 1-, 3-, and 5-year survival rates were 98%, 95%, and 90%, respectively, for elderly patients undergoing transplantation, compared with 92%, 62%, and 27% for those on dialysis.[426] Post-transplantation 1-year patient survival and allograft survival rates are similar between young and elderly patients. The major cause of allograft loss in the post-transplantation elderly is patient death from cardiovascular disease or infection.[424, 427] A retrospective analysis of adult patients in the U.S. Renal Data System and United Network for Organ Sharing (UNOS) Renal Transplant Scientific Registry between 1988 to 1997 noted age as an independent factor increasing the relative risk of death from infection in elderly patients after transplantation.[428] This analysis also confirmed previous data indicating a decrease in acute rejection in older transplant recipients.[429] Therefore, underlying comorbid conditions, such as significant cardiovascular disease and ability to tolerate immunosuppressive therapy in light of "biologic age," should be assessed carefully when considering renal transplantation in an elderly patient.[429]

URINARY TRACT INFECTION

Infection of the urinary tract is an important and significant problem in the aging population. Various factors contribute to the increased prevalence of urinary tract infections in the elderly. These include altered bladder function and defenses, "immune senescence," changes in pelvic musculature, prostate size, and concomitant illnesses such as cerebrovascular accident or dementia which may lead to poor hygiene, impaired mobility, and neurogenic bladder dysfunction.[430, 431] Decreased prostate secretions in elderly men can predispose to lower urinary tract infections, as can prostatic microcalculi, which can harbor bacteria and act as a nidus for prostate infections.[432] Postmenopausal women have decreased estrogen levels; this changes the pH of the vaginal secretions, allowing for vaginal colonization of bacteria and subsequent cystitis.[433] Intravaginal estrogen administration may prevent recurrent urinary tract infections in these women.[434]

Asymptomatic bacteriuria has been found in 20% of healthy men older than 65 years of age, and the prevalence increases to 25% among both men and women who live in extended care facilities.[435] Bacteriuria has also been noted in 30% to 50% of older hospitalized patients and more than 35% of the aged admitted to nursing homes.[436] Creatinine clearance is decreased in elderly persons with bacteriuria compared with those without bacteriuria.[227, 437] Chronic pyelonephritis with glomerulosclerosis may contribute to this loss of renal function, although the mechanism is not clear. Decreased survival with chronic bacteriuria may be related to underlying associated illnesses predisposing to bacteriuria.[438] Treatment of asymptomatic bacteriuria has not resulted in improved survival.[439, 440] Treatment of asymptomatic bacteriuria in the absence of renal or other urologic abnormalities is not necessary, because the prevalence of treatment failure and relapse is high.[441] Benefits of chronic suppressive therapy need yet to be determined, because long-term antibiotic therapy may lead to the emergence of resistant gram-negative organisms.[442, 443]

RENAL CYSTS

There is an age-related increase in development of simple renal cysts. Incidental renal cysts are being recognized more commonly with increased use of sonography and computed tomography of the abdomen for various other diagnoses. Ectasia, diverticula, and microscopic cysts of the distal renal tubule are found by microdissection of adult and elderly kidneys (>50 years of age) and comparison with 20-year-old kidneys. Morphologically, these seem to progress to large cysts in the normal kidneys of adults. At least one renal cyst is found on postmortem examination in more than half of patients older than 50 years of age.[444] A recent sonographic study in 729 patients revealed a 22.1% prevalence of an acquired renal cyst in patients 70 years and older, whereas those in the age group from 15 to 29 years had 0% prevalence.[445] Frequently, these acquired cysts are simple, painless, and asymptomatic, although symptoms of abdominal or lumbar pain, hematuria, secondary infection, and renin-dependent hypertension have been associated. Simple acquired asymptomatic cysts, which have a thin, smooth wall and clear, fluid-filled space with no internal echoes, usually require no treatment. Cysts that are filled with debris or have internal echoes, are thick walled, or occur in association with a possible renal mass are considered complicated. Complicated cysts need to be investigated by cyst puncture, angiography, or surgical exploration as indicated.

ACKNOWLEDGMENT

The authors wish to thank Ms. Regina Easley for her secretarial expertise for preparation of the manuscript, Dallas Veterans Affairs Medical Library for providing prompt and unrelenting help, and Dallas Veterans Affairs Medical Media Service for preparation of figures and tables.

REFERENCES

1. Prommool S, Jhangri GS, Cockfield SM, et al: Time dependency of factors affecting renal allograft survival. J Am Soc Nephrol 11: 565-573, 2000.
2. Terasaki PI, Gjertson DW, Cecka JM, et al: Significance of the donor age effect on kidney transplants. Clin Transplant 11:366-372, 1997.
3. Kasiske BL, Snyder J: Matching older kidneys with older patients does not improve allograft survival. J Am Soc Nephrol 13:1067-1072, 2002.
4. Cecka JM: The UNOS renal transplant registry. Clin Transplant 1-18, 2001.
5. Asderakis A, Dyer P, Augustine T, et al: Effect of cold ischemic time and HLA matching in kidneys coming from "young" and "old" donors: Do not leave for tomorrow what you can do tonight. Transplantation 72:674-678, 2001.
6. Coresh J, Astor BC, Greene T, et al: Prevalence of chronic kidney disease and decreased kidney function in the adult US population: Third National Health and Nutrition Examination Survey. Am J Kidney Dis 41:1-12, 2003.
7. United State Renal Data System. 1999 Annual Data Report. Bethesda, MD: National Institutes of Health, 1999:31.
8. Gomez Campdera FJ, Luno J, Garcia de Vinuesa S, et al: Renal vascular disease in the elderly. Kidney Int Suppl 68:S73-S77, 1998.
9. Gourtsoyiannis N, Prassopoulos P, Cavouras D, et al: The thickness of the renal parenchyma decreases with age: A CT study of 360 patients. AJR Am J Roentgenol 155:541-544, 1990.
10. McLachlan M, Wasserman P: Changes in sizes and distensibility of the aging kidney. Br J Radiol 54:488-491, 1981.
11. Tauchi H, Tsuboi K, Okutomi J: Age changes in the human kidney of the different races. Gerontologia 17:87-97, 1971.
12. Kasiske BL, Umen AJ: The influence of age, sex, race, and body habitus on kidney weight in humans. Arch Pathol Lab Med 110:55-60, 1986.
13. Moore RA: The total number of glomeruli in the normal human kidney. Anat Rec 48:153, 1958.
14. Sorensen FH: Quantitative studies of the renal corpuscles IV: Determination of normal values in various age categories, and an analysis of the possible influence of physiological degrees of arteriolosclerosis. Acta Pathol Microbiol Scand [A] 85:356-366, 1977.
15. Kang DH, Anderson S, Kim YG, et al: Impaired angiogenesis in the aging kidney: Vascular endothelial growth factor and thrombospondin-1 in renal disease. Am J Kidney Dis 37:601-611, 2001.
16. Lindeman RD, Goldman R: Anatomic and physiologic age changes in the kidney. Exp Gerontol 21:379-406, 1986.
17. McManus JFA, Lupton CH Jr: Ischemic obsolescence of renal glomeruli. Lab Invest 9:413, 1960.
18. Takazakura E, Sawabu N, Handa A, et al: Intrarenal vascular changes with age and disease. Kidney Int 2:224-230, 1972.
19. MacCallum DB: The bearing of degenerating glomeruli on the problem of the vascular supply of the mammalian kidney. Am J Anat 65:69, 1939.
20. Melk A, Ramassar V, Helms LM, et al: Telomere shortening in kidneys with age. J Am Soc Nephrol 11:444-453, 2000.
21. Harley CB, Futcher AB, Greider CW: Telomeres shorten during ageing of human fibroblasts. Nature 345:458-460, 1990.
22. Harley CB, Vaziri H, Counter CM, et al: The telomere hypothesis of cellular aging. Exp Gerontol 27:375-382, 1992.
23. Johnson FB, et al: Molecular biology of aging. Cell 96:291-302, 1999.
24. Baert L, Steg A: Is the diverticulum of the distal and collecting tubules a preliminary stage of the simple cyst in the adult? J Urol 118: 707-710, 1977.
25. Darmady EM, Offer J, Woodhouse MA: The parameters of the ageing kidney. J Pathol 109:195-207, 1973.
26. Abrass CK, Adcox MJ, Raugi GJ: Aging-associated changes in renal extracellular matrix. Am J Pathol 146:742-752, 1995.
27. Ding G, Franki N, Kapasi AA, et al: Tubular cell senescence and expression of TGF-beta1 and p21(WAF1/CIP1) in tubulointerstitial fibrosis of aging rats. Exp Mol Pathol 70:43-53, 2001.
28. Thomas SE, Anderson S, Gordon KL, et al: Tubulointerstitial disease in aging: Evidence for underlying peritubular capillary damage, a potential role for renal ischemia. J Am Soc Nephrol 9:231, 1988.
29. Gagliano N, Arosio B, Santambrogio D, et al: Age-dependent expression of fibrosis-related genes and collagen deposition in rat kidney cortex. J Gerontol A Biol Sci Med Sci 55:B365-B372, 2000.
30. Eikmans M, Baelde HJ, de Heer E, et al: Effect of age and biopsy site on extracellular matrix mRNA and protein levels in human kidney biopsies. Kidney Int 60:974-981, 2001.
31. Fuiano G, Sund S, Mazza G, et al: Renal hemodynamic response to maximal vasodilating stimulus in healthy older subjects. Kidney Int 59:1052-1058, 2001.
32. Griffiths GJ, Robinson KB, Cartwright GO, et al: Loss of renal tissue in the elderly. Br J Radiol 49:111-117, 1976.
33. Lindeman RD, Tobin J, Shock NW: Longitudinal studies on the rate of decline in renal function with age. J Am Geriatr Soc 33:278-285, 1985.

34. Schuster VL, Kokko JP, Jacobson HR: Angiotensin II directly stimulates sodium transport in rabbit proximal convoluted tubules. J Clin Invest 73:507-515, 1984.

35. Cogan MG: Angiotensin II: A powerful controller of sodium transport in the early proximal tubule. Hypertension 15:451-458, 1990.

36. Norman J, Badie-Dezfooly B, Nord EP, et al: EGF-induced mitogenesis in proximal tubular cells: Potentiation by angiotensin II. Am J Physiol 253:F299-F309, 1987.

37. Norman JT: The role of angiotensin II in renal growth. Ren Physiol Biochem 14:175-185, 1991.

38. Wolf G, Neilson EG: Angiotensin II induces cellular hypertrophy in cultured murine proximal tubular cells. Am J Physiol 259:F768-F777, 1990.

39. Maric C, Aldred GP, Antoine AM, et al: Effects of angiotensin II on cultured rat renomedullary interstitial cells are mediated by AT1A receptors. Am J Physiol 271:F1020-F1028, 1996.

40. Wolf G, Ziyadeh FN, Zahner G, et al: Angiotensin II is mitogenic for cultured rat glomerular endothelial cells. Hypertension 27:897-905, 1996.

41. Wolf G, Ziyadeh FN, Schroeder R, et al: Angiotensin II inhibits inducible nitric oxide synthase in tubular MCT cells by a posttranscriptional mechanism. J Am Soc Nephrol 8:551-557, 1997.

42. Anderson S, Brenner BM: Effects of aging on the renal glomerulus. Am J Med 80:435-442, 1986.

43. Baylis C: Renal responses to acute angiotensin II inhibition and administered angiotensin II in the aging, conscious, chronically catheterized rat. Am J Kidney Dis 22:842-850, 1993.

44. Heudes D, Michel O, Chevalier J, et al: Effect of chronic ANG I-converting enzyme inhibition on aging processes: I. Kidney structure and function. Am J Physiol 266:R1038-R1051, 1994.

45. Corman B, Chami-Khazraji S, Schaeverbeke J, et al: Effect of feeding on glomerular filtration rate and proteinuria in conscious aging rats. Am J Physiol 255:F250-F256, 1988.

46. Remuzzi A, Puntorieri S, Battaglia C, et al: Angiotensin converting enzyme inhibition ameliorates glomerular filtration of macromolecules and water and lessens glomerular injury in the rat. J Clin Invest 85:541-549, 1990.

47. Zoja C, Remuzzi A, Corna D, et al: Renal protective effect of angiotensin-converting enzyme inhibition in aging rats. Am J Med 92:60S-63S, 1992.

48. Anderson S, Rennke HG, Zatz R: Glomerular adaptations with normal aging and with long-term converting enzyme inhibition in rats. Am J Physiol 267:F35-F43, 1994.

49. Michel JB, Heudes D, Michel O, et al: Effect of chronic ANG I-converting enzyme inhibition on aging processes: II. Large arteries. Am J Physiol 267:R124-R135, 1994.

50. Ferder L, Inserra F, Romano L, et al: Decreased glomerulosclerosis in aging by angiotensin-converting enzyme inhibitors. J Am Soc Nephrol 5:1147-1152, 1994.

51. Wolf G, Killen PD, Neilson EG: Intracellular signaling of transcription and secretion of type IV collagen after angiotensin II-induced cellular hypertrophy in cultured proximal tubular cells. Cell Regul 2:219-227, 1991.

52. Wolf G, Zahner G, Schroeder R, et al: Transforming growth factor beta mediates the angiotensin-II-induced stimulation of collagen type IV synthesis in cultured murine proximal tubular cells. Nephrol Dial Transplant 11:263-269, 1996.

53. Wolf G, Ziyadeh FN, Thaiss F, et al: Angiotensin II stimulates expression of the chemokine RANTES in rat glomerular endothelial cells: Role of the angiotensin type 2 receptor. J Clin Invest 100:1047-1058, 1997.

54. Inserra F, Romano LA, de Cavanagh EM, et al: Renal interstitial sclerosis in aging: Effects of enalapril and nifedipine. J Am Soc Nephrol 7:676-680, 1996.

55. Vaughan DE, Lazos SA, Tong K: Angiotensin II regulates the expression of plasminogen activator inhibitor-1 in cultured endothelial cells: A potential link between the renin-angiotensin system and thrombosis. J Clin Invest 95:995-1001, 1995.

56. Fogo AB: The role of angiotensin II and plasminogen activator inhibitor-1 in progressive glomerulosclerosis. Am J Kidney Dis 35:179-188, 2000.

57. Ma LJ, Nakamura S, Whitsett J, et al: Regression of glomerulosclerosis in aging by angiotensin II type I receptor antagonist (AIIRA) is linked to inhibition of plasminogen activator-1 (PAI-1). Abstract. J Am Soc Nephrol 10:576A, 1999.

58. Mitani H, Ishizaka N, Aizawa T, et al: In vivo klotho gene transfer ameliorates angiotensin II-induced renal damage. Hypertension 39:838-843, 2002.

59. Roberts AB, McCune BK, Sporn MB: TGF-beta: Regulation of extracellular matrix. Kidney Int 41:557-559, 1992.

60. Wolf G: Link between angiotensin II and TGF-beta in the kidney. Miner Electrolyte Metab 24:174-180, 1998.

61. Noble NA: Angiotensin II in renal fibrosis: Should TGF-B rather than blood pressure be the therapeutic target? Semin Nephrol 17:455, 1997.

62. Peters H, Noble NA, Border WA: Transforming growth factor-beta in human glomerular injury. Curr Opin Nephrol Hypertens 6:389-393, 1997.

63. Frishberg Y, Kelly CJ: TGF-beta and regulation of interstitial nephritis. Miner Electrolyte Metab 24:181-189, 1998.

64. Ruiz-Torres MP, Bosch RJ, O'Valle F, et al: Age-related increase in expression of TGF-beta1 in the rat kidney: Relationship to morphologic changes. J Am Soc Nephrol 9:782-791, 1998.

65. Wolf G: Molecular mechanisms of angiotensin II in the kidney: Emerging role in the progression of renal disease—Beyond haemodynamics. Nephrol Dial Transplant 13:1131-1142, 1998.

66. Satriano JA, Shuldiner M, Hora K, et al: Oxygen radicals as second messengers for expression of the monocyte chemoattractant protein, JE/MCP-1, and the monocyte colony-stimulating factor, CSF-1, in response to tumor necrosis factor-alpha and immunoglobulin G: Evidence for involvement of reduced nicotinamide adenine dinucleotide phosphate (NADPH)-dependent oxidase. J Clin Invest 92:1564-1571, 1993.

67. Hill C, Lateef AM, Engels K, et al: Basal and stimulated nitric oxide in control of kidney function in the aging rat. Am J Physiol 272:R1747-R1753, 1997.

68. Sonaka I, Futami Y, Maki T: L-Arginine–nitric oxide pathway and chronic nephropathy in aged rats. J Gerontol 49:B157-B161, 1994.

69. Thomas SE, Anderson S, Gordon KL, et al: Tubulointerstitial disease in aging: Evidence for underlying peritubular capillary damage—A potential role for renal ischemia. J Am Soc Nephrol 9:231-242, 1998.

70. Reckelhoff JF, Kellum JA Jr, Racusen LC, et al: Long-term dietary supplementation with L-arginine prevents age-related reduction in renal function. Am J Physiol 272:R1768-R1774, 1997.

71. Radner W, Hoger H, Lubec B, et al: L-Arginine reduces kidney collagen accumulation and N-epsilon-(carboxymethyl)lysine in the aging NMRI-mouse. J Gerontol 49:M44-M46, 1994.

72. Nakayama I, Kawahara Y, Tsuda T, et al: Angiotensin II inhibits cytokine-stimulated inducible nitric oxide synthase expression in vascular smooth muscle cells. J Biol Chem 269:11628-11633, 1994.

73. Arima S, Ito S, Omata K, et al: High glucose augments angiotensin II action by inhibiting NO synthesis in vitro microperfused rabbit afferent arterioles. Kidney Int 48:683-689, 1995.

74. Hogan M, Cerami A, Bucala R: Advanced glycosylation endproducts block the antiproliferative effect of nitric oxide: Role in the vascular and renal complications of diabetes mellitus. J Clin Invest 90:1110-1115, 1992.

75. McQuillan LP, Leung GK, Marsden PA, et al: Hypoxia inhibits expression of eNOS via transcriptional and posttranscriptional mechanisms. Am J Physiol 267:H1921-H1927, 1994.

76. Verbeke P, Perichon M, Borot-Laloi C, et al: Accumulation of advanced glycation endproducts in the rat nephron: Link with circulating AGEs during aging. J Histochem Cytochem 45:1059-1068, 1997.

77. Schleicher ED, Wagner E, Nerlich AG: Increased accumulation of the glycoxidation product N(epsilon)-(carboxymethyl)lysine in human tissues in diabetes and aging. J Clin Invest 99:457-468, 1997.

78. Raj DS, Choudhury D, Welbourne TC, et al: Advanced glycation end products: A nephrologist's perspective. Am J Kidney Dis 35:365-380, 2000.

79. Vlassara H: Advanced glycosylation in nephropathy of diabetes and aging. Adv Nephrol Necker Hosp 25:303-315, 1996.

80. Bucala R, Tracey KJ, Cerami A: Advanced glycosylation products quench nitric oxide and mediate defective endothelium-dependent vasodilatation in experimental diabetes. J Clin Invest 87:432-438, 1991.

81. Saenz de Tejada I, Goldstein I, Azadzoi K, et al: Impaired neurogenic and endothelium-mediated relaxation of penile smooth muscle from diabetic men with impotence. N Engl J Med 320:1025-1030, 1989.

82. McVeigh GE, Brennan GM, Johnston GD, et al: Impaired endothelium-dependent and independent vasodilation in patients with type 2 (non-insulin-dependent) diabetes mellitus. Diabetologia 35:771-776, 1992.

83. Gascho JA, Fanelli C, Zelis R: Aging reduces venous distensibility and the venodilatory response to nitroglycerin in normal subjects. Am J Cardiol 63:1267-1270, 1989.

84. He C, Sabol J, Mitsuhashi T, et al: Dietary glycotoxins: Inhibition of reactive products by aminoguanidine facilitates renal clearance and reduces tissue sequestration. Diabetes 48:1308-1315, 1999.

85. Cerami C, Founds H, Nicholl I, et al: Tobacco smoke is a source of toxic reactive glycation products. Proc Natl Acad Sci U S A 94: 13915-13920, 1997.

86. Li YM, Steffes M, Donnelly T, et al: Prevention of cardiovascular and renal pathology of aging by the advanced glycation inhibitor aminoguanidine. Proc Natl Acad Sci U S A 93:3902-3907, 1996.

87. Vlassara H, Fuh H, Makita Z, et al: Exogenous advanced glycosylation end products induce complex vascular dysfunction in normal animals: A model for diabetic and aging complications. Proc Natl Acad Sci U S A 89:12043-12047, 1992.

88. Corman B, Duriez M, Poitevin P, et al: Aminoguanidine prevents age-related arterial stiffening and cardiac hypertrophy. Proc Natl Acad Sci U S A 95:1301-1306, 1998.

89. Cefalu WT, Bell-Farrow AD, Wang ZQ, et al: Caloric restriction decreases age-dependent accumulation of the glycoxidation products, N epsilon-(carboxymethyl)lysine and pentosidine, in rat skin collagen. J Gerontol A Biol Sci Med Sci 50:B337-B341, 1995.

90. Novelli M, Masiello P, Bombara M, et al: Protein glycation in the aging male Sprague-Dawley rat: Effects of antiaging diet restrictions. J Gerontol A Biol Sci Med Sci 53:B94-B101, 1998.

91. Teillet L, Verbeke P, Gouraud S, et al: Food restriction prevents advanced glycation end product accumulation and retards kidney aging in lean rats. J Am Soc Nephrol 11:1488-1497, 2000.

92. Xia E, Rao G, Van Remmen H, et al: Activities of antioxidant enzymes in various tissues of male Fischer 344 rats are altered by food restriction. J Nutr 125:195-201, 1995.

93. Oppenheim RW: Related mechanisms of action of growth factors and antioxidants in apoptosis: An overview. Adv Neurol 72:69-78, 1997.

94. Papa S, Skulachev VP: Reactive oxygen species, mitochondria, apoptosis and aging. Mol Cell Biochem 174:305-319, 1997.

95. Beckman KB, Ames BN: The free radical theory of aging matures. Physiol Rev 78:547-581, 1998.

96. Leeuwenburgh C, Hansen PA, Holloszy JO, et al: Oxidized amino acids in the urine of aging rats: Potential markers for assessing oxidative stress in vivo. Am J Physiol 276:R128-R135, 1999.

97. Ruiz-Torres P, Lucio J, Gonzalez-Rubio M, et al: Oxidant/antioxidant balance in isolated glomeruli and cultured mesangial cells. Free Radic Biol Med 22:49-56, 1997.

98. Reckelhoff JF, Kanji V, Racusen LC, et al: Vitamin E ameliorates enhanced renal lipid peroxidation and accumulation of F2-isoprostanes in aging kidneys. Am J Physiol 274:R767-R774, 1998.

99. Ushio-Fukai M, Zafari AM, Fukui T, et al: p22phox is a critical component of the superoxide-generating NADH/NADPH oxidase system and regulates angiotensin II-induced hypertrophy in vascular smooth muscle cells. J Biol Chem 271:23317-23321, 1996.

100. de Cavanagh EM, Inserra F, Ferder L, et al: Superoxide dismutase and glutathione peroxidase activities are increased by enalapril and captopril in mouse liver. FEBS Lett 361:22-24, 1995.

101. Cruz CI, Ruiz-Torres P, del Moral RG, et al: Age-related progressive renal fibrosis in rats and its prevention with ACE inhibitors and taurine. Am J Physiol Renal Physiol 278:F122-F129, 2000.

102. Kim HJ, Jung KJ, Yu BP, et al: Influence of aging and calorie restriction on MAPKs activity in rat kidney. Exp Gerontol 37: 1041-1053, 2002.

103. Yu BP: Aging and oxidative stress: Modulation by dietary restriction. Free Radic Biol Med 21:651-668, 1996.

104. Levi M, Jameson DM, van der Meer BW: Role of BBM lipid composition and fluidity in impaired renal Pi transport in aged rat. Am J Physiol 256:F85-F94, 1989.

105. Cohen BM, Zubenko GS: Aging and the biophysical properties of cell membranes. Life Sci 37:1403-1409, 1985.

106. Eisenberg S, Stein Y, Stein O: Phospholipases in arterial tissue: IV. The role of phosphatide acyl hydrolase, lysophosphatide acyl hydrolase, and sphingomyelin choline phosphohydrolase in the regulation of phospholipid composition in the normal human aorta with age. J Clin Invest 48:2320-2329, 1969.

107. Hegner D: Age-dependence of molecular and functional changes in biological membrane properties. Mech Ageing Dev 14:101-118, 1980.

108. Hegner D, Platt D, Heckers H, et al: Age-dependent physiochemical and biochemical studies of human red cell membranes. Mech Ageing Dev 10:117-130, 1979.

109. Hubbard RE, Garratt CJ: The composition and fluidity of adipocyte membranes prepared from young and adult rats. Biochim Biophys Acta 600:701-704, 1980.

110. Rivnay B, Bergman S, Shinitzky M, et al: Correlations between membrane viscosity, serum cholesterol, lymphocyte activation and aging in man. Mech Ageing Dev 12:119-126, 1980.

111. Yechiel E, Barenholz Y: Relationships between membrane lipid composition and biological properties of rat myocytes: Effects of aging and manipulation of lipid composition. J Biol Chem 260: 9123-9131, 1985.

112. Ravid M, Rachmani R: Cholesterol as a predictor of progression in diabetic renal disease. Contrib Nephrol 120:39-47, 1997.

113. Greco BA, Breyer JA: Cholesterol as a predictor of progression in nondiabetic chronic renal disease. Contrib Nephrol 120:48-61, 1997.

114. Neverov NI, Kaysen GA, Tareyeva IE: Effect of lipid-lowering therapy on the progression of renal disease in nondiabetic nephrotic patients. Contrib Nephrol 120:68-78, 1997.

115. Cheng IK, Lam KS, Janus ED, et al: Treatment of hyperlipidaemia in patients with non-insulin-dependent diabetes mellitus with progressive nephropathy. Contrib Nephrol 120:79-87, 1997.

116. Wanner C, Greiber S, Kramer-Guth A, et al: Lipids and progression of renal disease: Role of modified low density lipoprotein and lipoprotein(a). Kidney Int Suppl 63:S102-S106, 1997.

117. Kamanna VS, Roh DD, Kirschenbaum MA: Hyperlipidemia and kidney disease: Concepts derived from histopathology and cell biology of the glomerulus. Histol Histopathol 13:169-179, 1998.

118. Wu ZL, Liang MY, Qiu LQ: Oxidized low-density lipoprotein decreases the induced nitric oxide synthesis in rat mesangial cells. Cell Biochem Funct 16:153-158, 1998.

119. Dominguez JH, Tang N, Xu W, et al: Studies of renal injury III: Lipid-induced nephropathy in type II diabetes. Kidney Int 57:92-104, 2000.

120. Kim SI, Han DC, Lee HB: Lovastatin inhibits transforming growth factor-beta1 expression in diabetic rat glomeruli and cultured rat mesangial cells. J Am Soc Nephrol 11:80-87, 2000.

121. Lam KS, Cheng IK, Janus ED, et al: Cholesterol-lowering therapy may retard the progression of diabetic nephropathy. Diabetologia 38:604-609, 1995.

122. Tonolo G, Ciccarese M, Brizzi P, et al: Reduction of albumin excretion rate in normotensive microalbuminuric type 2 diabetic patients during long-term simvastatin treatment. Diabetes Care 20:1891-1895, 1997.

123. Fried LF, Orchard TJ, Kasiske BL: Effect of lipid reduction on the progression of renal disease: A meta-analysis. Kidney Int 59:260-269, 2001.

124. Davies D, Shock N: Age changes in glomerular filtration rate, effective renal plasma flow, and tubular excretory capacity in adult males. J Clin Invest 29:496, 1950.

125. McDonald R, Solomon D, Shock N: Aging as a factor in the renal hemodynamic changes induced by a standardized pyrogen. J Clin Invest 30:457, 1951.

126. Hollenberg NK, Adams DF, Solomon HS, et al: Senescence and the renal vasculature in normal man. Circ Res 34:309-316, 1974.

127. Danziger RS, Tobin JD, Becker LC, et al: The age-associated decline in glomerular filtration in healthy normotensive volunteers: Lack of relationship to cardiovascular performance. J Am Geriatr Soc 38: 1127-1132, 1990.

128. Manyari DE, Patterson C, Johnson D, et al: Left ventricular diastolic function in a population of healthy elderly subjects: An echocardiographic study. J Am Geriatr Soc 33:758-763, 1985.

129. Lee TD Jr, Lindeman RD, Yiengst MJ, et al: Influence of age on the cardiovascular and renal responses to tilting. J Appl Physiol 21: 55-61, 1966.

130. Mulkerrin EC, Brain A, Hampton D, et al: Reduced renal hemodynamic response to atrial natriuretic peptide in elderly volunteers. Am J Kidney Dis 22:538-544, 1993.

131. Clark B: Biology of renal aging in humans. Adv Ren Replace Ther 7:11-21, 2000.

132. Fliser D, Zeier M, Nowack R, et al: Renal functional reserve in healthy elderly subjects. J Am Soc Nephrol 3:1371-1377, 1993.

133. Lakatta EG: Cardiovascular regulatory mechanisms in advanced age. Physiol Rev 73:413-467, 1993.

134. Moritoki H, Yoshikawa T, Hisayama T, et al: Possible mechanisms of age-associated reduction of vascular relaxation caused by atrial natriuretic peptide. Eur J Pharmacol 210:61-68, 1992.

135. Sato I, Kaji K, Morita I, et al: Augmentation of endothelin-1, prostacyclin and thromboxane A2 secretion associated with in vitro ageing in cultured human umbilical vein endothelial cells. Mech Ageing Dev 71:73-84, 1993.

136. Rathaus M, Greenfeld Z, Podjarny E, et al: Altered prostaglandin synthesis and impaired sodium conservation in the kidneys of old rats. Clin Sci (Lond) 83:301-306, 1992.

137. Kuhlik A, Elahi D, Epstein FH, et al: Decline in urinary excretion of dopamine and PGE2 with age. Geriatr Nephrol Urol 5:79, 1995.

138. Naeije R, Fiasse A, Carlier E, et al: Systemic and renal haemodynamic effects of angiotensin converting enzyme inhibition by zabicipril in young and in old normal men. Eur J Clin Pharmacol 44:35-39, 1993.

139. Hollenberg NK, Moore TJ: Age and the renal blood supply: Renal vascular responses to angiotensin converting enzyme inhibition in healthy humans. J Am Geriatr Soc 42:805-808, 1994.

140. Baylis C, Fredericks M, Wilson C, et al: Renal vasodilatory response to intravenous glycine in the aging rat kidney. Am J Kidney Dis 15:244-251, 1990.

141. Tank JE, Vora JP, Houghton DC, et al: Altered renal vascular responses in the aging rat kidney. Am J Physiol 266:F942-F948, 1994.

142. Zhang XZ, Qiu C, Baylis C: Sensitivity of the segmental renal arterioles to angiotensin II in the aging rat. Mech Ageing Dev 97:183-192, 1997.

143. Lewis WH, Alving AS: Changes with age in the renal function in adult men. Am J Physiol 123:500, 1938.

144. Baracskay D, Jarjoura D, Cugino A, et al: Geriatric renal function: Estimating glomerular filtration in an ambulatory elderly population. Clin Nephrol 47:222-228, 1997.

145. Rowe JW, Andres R, Tobin JD, et al: The effect of age on creatinine clearance in men: A cross-sectional and longitudinal study. J Gerontol 31:155-163, 1976.

146. Back SE, Ljungberg B, Nilsson-Ehle I, et al: Age dependence of renal function: Clearance of iohexol and p-amino hippurate in healthy males. Scand J Clin Lab Invest 49:641-646, 1989.

147. Fliser D, Franek E, Joest M, et al: Renal function in the elderly: Impact of hypertension and cardiac function. Kidney Int 51:1196-1204, 1997.

148. Lew SW, Bosch JP: Effect of diet on creatinine clearance and excretion in young and elderly healthy subjects and in patients with renal disease. J Am Soc Nephrol 2:856-865, 1991.

149. Goldberg TH, Finkelstein MS: Difficulties in estimating glomerular filtration rate in the elderly. Arch Intern Med 147:1430-1433, 1987.

150. Rowe JW, Andres R, Tobin JD: Letter: Age-adjusted standards for creatinine clearance. Ann Intern Med 84:567-569, 1976.

151. Cockcroft DW, Gault MH: Prediction of creatinine clearance from serum creatinine. Nephron 16:31-41, 1976.

152. Levey AS, Bosch JP, Lewis JB, et al: A more accurate method to estimate glomerular filtration rate from serum creatinine: A new prediction equation. Modification of Diet in Renal Disease Study Group. Ann Intern Med 130:461-470, 1999.

153. Luft FC, Fineberg NS, Miller JZ, et al: The effects of age, race and heredity on glomerular filtration rate following volume expansion and contraction in normal man. Am J Med Sci 279:15-24, 1980.

154. Lindeman RD, Tobin JD, Shock NW: Association between blood pressure and the rate of decline in renal function with age. Kidney Int 26:861-868, 1984.

155. Wollom GL, Gifford RW Jr: The kidney as a target organ in hypertension. Review. Geriatrics 31:71, 1976.

156. Brenner BM: Nephron adaptation to renal injury or ablation. Am J Physiol 249:F324-F337, 1985.

157. Tolbert EM, Weisstuch J, Feiner HD, et al: Onset of glomerular hypertension with aging precedes injury in the spontaneously hypertensive rat. Am J Physiol Renal Physiol 278:F839-F846, 2000.

158. Ribstein J, Du Cailar G, Mimran A: Glucose tolerance and age-associated decline in renal function of hypertensive patients. J Hypertens 19:2257-2264, 2001.

159. Epstein M, Hollenberg NK: Age as a determinant of renal sodium conservation in normal man. J Lab Clin Med 87:411-417, 1976.

160. Macias Nunez JF, Garcia Iglesias C, Bonda Roman A, et al: Renal handling of sodium in old people: A functional study. Age Ageing 7:178-181, 1978.

161. Anderson GH Jr, Springer J, Randall P, et al: Effect of age on diagnostic usefulness of stimulated plasma renin activity and saralasin test in detection of renovascular hypertension. Lancet 2:821-824, 1980.

162. Bauer JH: Age-related changes in the renin-aldosterone system: Physiological effects and clinical implications. Drugs Aging 3:238-245, 1993.

163. Baylis C, Engels K, Beierwaltes WH: Beta-adrenoceptor-stimulated renin release is blunted in old rats. J Am Soc Nephrol 9:1318-1320, 1998.

164. Crane MG, Harris JJ: Effect of aging on renin activity and aldosterone excretion. J Lab Clin Med 87:947-959, 1976.

165. Cugini P, Murano G, Lucia P, et al: The gerontological decline of the renin-aldosterone system: A chronobiological approach extended to essential hypertension. J Gerontol 42:461-465, 1987.

166. Hall JE, Coleman TG, Guyton AC: The renin-angiotensin system: Normal physiology and changes in older hypertensives. J Am Geriatr Soc 37:801-813, 1989.

167. Hayashi M, Saruta T, Nakamura R, et al: Effect of aging on single nephron renin content in rats. Ren Physiol 4:17-21, 1981.

168. Hayduk K, Krause DK, Kaufmann W, et al: Age-dependent changes of plasma renin concentration in humans. Clin Sci Mol Med Suppl 45(suppl 1):273S-278S, 1973.

169. Noth RH, Lassman MN, Tan SY, et al: Age and the renin-aldosterone system. Arch Intern Med 137:1414-1417, 1977.

170. Tsunoda K, Abe K, Goto T, et al: Effect of age on the renin-angiotensin-aldosterone system in normal subjects: Simultaneous measurement of active and inactive renin, renin substrate, and aldosterone in plasma. J Clin Endocrinol Metab 62:384-389, 1986.

171. Weidmann P, de Chatel R, Schiffmann A, et al: Interrelations between age and plasma renin, aldosterone and cortisol, urinary catecholamines, and the body sodium/volume state in normal man. Klin Wochenschr 55:725-733, 1977.

172. Jung FF, Kennefick TM, Ingelfinger JR, et al: Down-regulation of the intrarenal renin-angiotensin system in the aging rat. J Am Soc Nephrol 5:1573-1580, 1995.

173. Lu X, Li X, Li L, et al: Variation of intrarenal angiotensin II and angiotensin II receptors by acute renal ischemia in the aged rat. Ren Fail 18:19-29, 1996.

174. Jover B, Dupont M, Geelen G, et al: Renal and systemic adaptation to sodium restriction in aging rats. Am J Physiol 264:R833-R838, 1993.

175. Flood C, Gherondache C, Pincus G, et al: The metabolism and secretion of aldosterone in elderly subjects. J Clin Invest 46:961-966, 1967.

176. Hegstad R, Brown RD, Jiang NS, et al: Aging and aldosterone. Am J Med 74:442-448, 1983.

177. Weidmann P, De Myttenaere-Bursztein S, Maxwell MH, et al: Effect on aging on plasma renin and aldosterone in normal man. Kidney Int 8:325-333, 1975.

178. Mimran A, Ribstein J, Jover B: Aging and sodium homeostasis. Kidney Int Suppl 37:S107-S113, 1992.

179. Luft FC, Weinberger MH, Grim CE: Sodium sensitivity and resistance in normotensive humans. Am J Med 72:726-736, 1982.

180. Leosco D, Ferrara N, Landino P, et al: Effects of age on the role of atrial natriuretic factor in renal adaptation to physiologic variations of dietary salt intake. J Am Soc Nephrol 7:1045-1051, 1996.

181. Ohashi M, Fujio N, Nawata H, et al: High plasma concentrations of human atrial natriuretic polypeptide in aged men. J Clin Endocrinol Metab 64:81-85, 1987.

182. Pollack JA, Skvorak JP, Nazian SJ, et al: Alterations in atrial natriuretic peptide (ANP) secretion and renal effects in aging. J Gerontol A Biol Sci Med Sci 52:B196-B202, 1997.

183. Luft FC, Grim CE, Fineberg N, et al: Effects of volume expansion and contraction in normotensive whites, blacks, and subjects of different ages. Circulation 59:643-650, 1979.

184. Brenner BM, Ballermann BJ, Gunning ME, et al: Diverse biological actions of atrial natriuretic peptide. Physiol Rev 70:665-699, 1990.

185. Haller B, Zust H, Shaw S, et al: Effects of posture and aging on circulating atrial natriuretic peptide levels in man. J Hypertens 5:551, 1987.

186. McKnight JA, Roberts G, Sheridan B, et al: Aging and atrial natriuretic factor. J Hum Hypertens 4:53, 1990.

187. Tajima F, Sagawa S, Iwamoto J, et al: Renal and endocrine responses in the elderly during head-out water immersion. Am J Physiol 254:R977, 1988.

188. Tan AC, Hoefnagels WH, Swinkels LM, et al: The effect of volume expansion on atrial natriuretic peptide and cyclic guanosine monophosphate levels in young and aged subjects. J Am Geriatr Soc 38:1215, 1990.

189. Clark BA, Elahi D, Shannon RP, et al: Influence of age and dose on the end-organ responses to atrial natriuretic peptide in humans. Am J Hypertens 4:500-507, 1991.

190. Jansen TL, Tan AC, Smits P, et al: Hemodynamic effects of atrialnatriuretic factor in young and elderly subjects. Clin Pharmacol Ther 48:179, 1990.

191. Ohashi J, Fujjo N, Nawata H, et al: Pharmacokinetics of synthetic alpha-human atrial natriuretic polypeptide in normal men: Effect of aging. Regul Pept 19:265, 1987.

192. Or K, Richards AM, Espiner EA, et al: Effect of low dose infusions of ile-atrial natriuretic peptide in healthy elderly males: Evidence for a postreceptor defect. J Clin Endocrinol Metab 76:1271-1274, 1993.

193. Rascher W, Tulassay T, Lang RE: Atrial natriuretic peptide in plasma of volume overloaded children with chronic renal failure. Lancet 2:303, 1985.

194. Lafferty HM, Gunning ME, Silva P, et al: Enkephalinase inhibition increases plasma atrial natriuretic peptide levels, glomerular filtration rate, and urinary sodium excretion in rats with reduced renal mass. Circ Res 65:640-646, 1989.

195. Kimmelstiel CD, Perrone R, Kilcoyne L, et al: Effects of renal neutral endopeptidase inhibition on sodium excretion, renal hemodynamics and neurohormonal activation in patients with congestive heart failure. Cardiology 87:46, 1996.

196. Gillies AH, Crozier IG, Nicholls MG, et al: Effect of posture on clearance of atrial natriuretic peptide from plasma. J Clin Endocrinol Metab 65:1095, 1987.

197. Tonolo G, Soro A, Scardaccio V, et al: Correlates of atrial natriuretic factor in chronic renal failure. J Hypertens 7:S238, 1989.

198. Lindeman RD, Lee TD Jr, Yiengst MJ: Influence of age, renal disease, hypertension, diuretics, and calcium on the antidiuretic responses to suboptimal infusions of vasopressin. J Lab Clin Med 68:206, 1966.

199. Lindeman RD, Van Buren H, Maisz L: Osmolar renal concentrating ability in healthy young men and hospitalized patients without renal disease. N Engl J Med 262:1306, 1960.

200. Meyer BR: Renal function in aging. J Am Geriatr Soc 37:791, 1989.

201. Rowe JW, Shock N, DeFronzo RA: The influence of age on the renal response to water deprivation in man. Nephron 17:270, 1976.

202. Handelmann GE, Sayson SC: Neonatal exposure to vasopressin decreases binding sites in the adult kidney. Peptides 5:1217, 1984.

203. Miller M: Increased vasopressin secretion: an early manifestation of aging in the rat. J Gerontol 42:3, 1987.

204. Helderman JH, Vestal RE, Rowe JW, et al: The response of arginine vasopressin to intravenous ethanol and hypertonic saline in man: The impact of aging. J Gerontol 33:39, 1978.

205. Kirkland J: Plasma arginine vasopressin in dehydrated elderly patients. Clin Endocrinol 20:451, 1984.

206. Phillips PA, Bretherton M, Risvanis J, et al: Effects of drinking on thirst and vasopressin in dehydrated elderly men. Am J Physiol 264:R877, 1993.

207. Phillips PA, Phil D, Rolls BJ, et al: Reduced thirst after water deprivation in healthy elderly men. N Engl J Med 311:753, 1984.

208. Rendeau E, de Lima J, Caillens H, et al: High plasma antidiuretic hormone in patients with cardiac failure: Influence of age. Miner Electrolyte Metab 8:267, 1982.

209. Faull C, Holmes C, Baylis P: Water balance in elderly people: Is there a deficiency of vasopressin? Age Ageing 22:114, 1993.

210. Li C, Hsieh S, Nagai I: The response of plasma arginine vasopressin to 14h water deprivation in the elderly. Acta Endocrinol (Copenh) 105:314, 1984.

211. Rowe JW, Minaker KL, Sparrow D, et al: Age-related failure of volume-pressure-mediated vasopressin release. J Clin Endocrinol Metab 54:661-664, 1982.

212. Ishikawa S, Fujita N, Fujisawa G, et al: Involvement of arginine vasopressin and renal sodium handling in pathogenesis of hyponatremia in elderly patients. Endocr J 43:101-108, 1996.

213. Miller JH, Shock NW: Age differences in the renal tubular response to antidiuretic hormone. J Gerontol 8:446, 1953.

214. Macias Nunez JF, Garcia Iglesias C, Tabernero Romo JM, et al: Renal management of sodium under indomethacin and aldosterone in the elderly. Age Ageing 9:165-172, 1980.

215. Bengele HH, Mathias RS, Perkins JH, et al: Urinary concentrating defect in the aged rat. Am J Physiol 240:F147-F150, 1981.

216. Beck N, Yu BP: Effect of aging on urinary concentrating mechanism and vasopressin-dependent cAMP in rats. Am J Physiol 243:F121-F125, 1982.

217. Goddard C, Davidson YS, Moser BB, et al: Effect of ageing on cyclic AMP output by renal medullary cells in response to arginine vasopressin in vitro in C57BL/Icrfat mice. J Endocrinol 103:133-139, 1984.

218. Davidson YS, Davies I, Goddard C: Renal vasopressin receptors in ageing C57BL/Icrfat mice. J Endocrinol 115:379-385, 1987.

219. Liang CT, Barnes J, Hanai H, et al: Decrease in Gs protein expression may impair adenylate cyclase activation in old kidneys. Am J Physiol 264:F770-F773, 1993.

220. Wilson PD, Dillingham MA: Age-associated decrease in vasopressin-induced renal water transport: A role for adenylate cyclase and G protein malfunction. Gerontology 38:315-321, 1992.

221. Terashima Y, Kondo K, Inagaki A, et al: Age-associated decrease in response of rat aquaporin-2 gene expression to dehydration. Life Sci 62:873-882, 1998.

222. Preisser L, Teillet L, Aliotti S, et al: Downregulation of aquaporin-2 and -3 in aging kidney is independent of V^2 vasopressin receptor. Am J Physiol Renal Physiol 279:F144-F152, 2000.

223. Combet S, Teillet L, Geelen G, et al: Food restriction prevents age-related polyuria by vasopressin-dependent recruitment of aquaporin-2. Am J Physiol Renal Physiol 281:F1123-F1131, 2001.

224. Combet S GN, Berthonaud V, et al: Correction of age-related polyuria by dDAVP: Molecular analysis of aquaporins and urea transporters. Am J Physiol Renal Physiol 284:F199-F208, 2003.

225. Crowe MJ, Forsling ML, Rolls BJ, et al: Altered water excretion in healthy elderly men. Age Ageing 16:285-293, 1987.

226. Davis FB, Van Son A, Davis PJ, et al: Urinary diluting capacity in elderly diabetic subjects. Exp Gerontol 21:407-412, 1986.

227. Dontas AS, Marketos SG, Papanayiotou PC: Mechanisms of renal tubular defects in old age. Postgrad Med J 48:295, 1972.

228. Adler S, Lindeman RD, Yiengst MJ, et al: Effect of acute acid loading on urinary acid excretion by the aging human kidney. J Lab Clin Med 72:278-289, 1968.

229. Frassetto LA, Morris RC Jr, Sebastian A: Effect of age on blood acid-base composition in adult humans: Role of age-related renal functional decline. Am J Physiol 271:F1114-F1122, 1996.

230. Agarwal BN, Cabebe FG: Renal acidification in elderly subjects. Nephron 26:291-295, 1980.

231. Rajendra P, Kinsella JL, Sacktor B: Renal adaptation to metabolic acidosis in senescent rats. Am J Physiol 255:F1183, 1988.

232. Mitch WE, Medina R, Grieber S, et al: Metabolic acidosis stimulates muscle protein degradation by activating the adenosine triphosphate-dependent pathway involving ubiquitin and proteasomes. J Clin Invest 93:2127-2133, 1994.

233. Alpern RJ, Sakhaee K: The clinical spectrum of chronic metabolic acidosis: Homeostatic mechanisms produce significant morbidity. Am J Kidney Dis 29:291-302, 1997.

234. Frassetto LA, Morris RC Jr, Sebastian A: Potassium bicarbonate improves nitrogen balance in postmenopausal women. Abstract. J Am Soc Nephrol 6:308, 1995.

235. Sebastian A, Morris RC Jr: Improved mineral balance and skeletal metabolism in postmenopausal women treated with potassium bicarbonate. N Engl J Med 331:279, 1994.

236. Himmelstein DU, Jones AA, Woolhandler S: Hypernatremic dehydration in nursing home patients: An indicator of neglect. J Am Geriatr Soc 31:466-471, 1983.

237. Kleinfeld M, Casimir M, Borra S: Hyponatremia as observed in a chronic disease facility. J Am Geriatr Soc 27:156-161, 1979.

238. Snyder NA, Feigal DW, Arieff AI: Hypernatremia in elderly patients: A heterogeneous, morbid, and iatrogenic entity. Ann Intern Med 107:309-319, 1987.

239. Shannon RP, Minaker KL, Rowe JW: Aging and water balance in humans. Semin Nephrol 4:346, 1984.

240. Sunderam SG, Mankikar GD: Hyponatremia in the elderly. Age Ageing 12:77, 1983.

241. Beck LH, Lavizzo-Morey R: Geriatric hyponatremia. Ann Intern Med 107:768, 1987.

242. Miller M, Hecker MS, Friedlander DA, et al: Apparent idiopathic hyponatremia in an ambulatory geriatric population. J Am Geriatr Soc 44:404-408, 1996.

243. Clark BA, Shannon RP, Rosa RM, et al: Increased susceptibility to thiazide-induced hyponatremia in the elderly. J Am Soc Nephrol 5:1106-1111, 1994.

244. Hochman I, Cabili S, Peer G: Hyponatremia in internal medicine ward patients: Causes, treatment and prognosis. Isr J Med Sci 25:73-76, 1989.

245. Arieff AI, Guisado R: Effects on the central nervous system of hypernatremic and hyponatremic states. Kidney Int 10:104-116, 1976.

246. Miller PD, Krebs RA, Neal BJ, et al: Hypodipsia in geriatric patients. Am J Med 73:354-356, 1982.

247. Allen TH, Anderson EC, Langham WH: Total body potassium and gross body composition in relation to age. J Gerontol 15:348, 1960.

248. Mulkerrin E, Epstein FH, Clark BA: Aldosterone responses to hyperkalemia in healthy elderly humans. J Am Soc Nephrol 6:1459-1462, 1995.

249. Bengele HH, Mathias R, Perkins JH, et al: Impaired renal and extrarenal potassium adaptation in old rats. Kidney Int 23:684-690, 1983.

250. Minaker KL, Rowe JW: Potassium homeostasis during hyperinsulinemia: Effect of insulin level, beta-blockade, and age. Am J Physiol 242:E373-E377, 1982.

251. Ford GA, Blaschke TF, Wiswell R, et al: Effect of aging on changes in plasma potassium during exercise. J Gerontol 48:M140-M145, 1993.

252. DeFronzo RA: Hyperkalemia and hyporeninemic hypoaldosteronism. Kidney Int 17:118-134, 1980.

253. Meier DE, Myers WM, Swenson R, et al: Indomethacin-associated hyperkalemia in the elderly. J Am Geriatr Soc 31:371-373, 1983.

254. Mor R, Pitlik S, Rosenfeld JB: Indomethacin- and Moduretic-induced hyperkalemia. Isr J Med Sci 19:535-537, 1983.

255. Walmsley RN, White GH, Cain M, et al: Hyperkalemia in the elderly. Clin Chem 30:1409-1412, 1984.

256. Armbrecht HJ, Zenser TV, Gross CJ, et al: Adaptation to dietary calcium and phosphorus restriction changes with age in the rat. Am J Physiol 239:E322-E327, 1980.

257. Corman B, Roinel N: Single-nephron filtration rate and proximal reabsorption in aging rats. Am J Physiol 260:F75-F80, 1991.

258. Armbrecht HJ, Zenser TV, Bruns ME, et al: Effect of age on intestinal calcium absorption and adaptation to dietary calcium. Am J Physiol 236:E769-E774, 1979.

259. Halloran BP, Lonergan ET, Portale AA: Aging and renal responsiveness to parathyroid hormone in healthy men. J Clin Endocrinol Metab 81:2192-2197, 1996.

260. Portale AA, Lonergan ET, Tanney DM, et al: Aging alters calcium regulation of serum concentration of parathyroid hormone in healthy men. Am J Physiol 272:E139-E146, 1997.

261. Caverzasio J, Murer H, Fleisch H, et al: Phosphate transport in brush border membrane vesicles isolated from renal cortex of young growing and adult rats: Comparison with whole kidney data. Pflugers Arch 394:217-221, 1982.

262. Corman B, Michel JB: Glomerular filtration, renal blood flow, and solute excretion in conscious aging rats. Am J Physiol 253:R555-R560, 1987.

263. Corman B, Pratz J, Poujeol P: Changes in anatomy, glomerular filtration, and solute excretion in aging rat kidney. Am J Physiol 248:R282-R287, 1985.

264. Kiebzak GM, Sacktor B: Effect of age on renal conservation of phosphate in the rat. Am J Physiol 251:F399-F407, 1986.

265. Lee DB, Yanagawa N, Jo O, et al: Phosphaturia of aging: Studies on mechanisms. Adv Exp Med Biol 178:103-108, 1984.

266. Naafs MA, Fischer HR, Koorevaar G, et al: The effect of age on the renal response to PTH infusion. Calcif Tissue Int 41:262-266, 1987.

267. Haramati A, Mulroney S, Sacktor B: Age-related decrease in the tubular capacity for phosphate reabsorption in the rat. Abstract. Kidney Int 31:349, 1987.

268. Armbrecht HJ, Gross CJ, Zenser TV: Effect of dietary calcium and phosphorus restriction on calcium and phosphorus balance in young and old rats. Arch Biochem Biophys 210:179-185, 1981.

269. Marcus R, Madvig P, Young G: Age-related changes in parathyroid hormone and parathyroid hormone action in normal humans. J Clin Endocrinol Metab 58:223-230, 1984.

270. Wiske PS, Epstein S, Bell NH, et al: Increases in immunoreactive parathyroid hormone with age. N Engl J Med 300:1419-1421, 1979.

271. Chen ML, King RS, Armbrecht HJ: Sodium-dependent phosphate transport in primary cultures of renal tubule cells from young and adult rats. J Cell Physiol 143:488-493, 1990.

272. Sorribas V, Lotscher M, Loffing J, et al: Cellular mechanisms of the age-related decrease in renal phosphate reabsorption. Kidney Int 50:855-863, 1996.

273. Grinna LS: Age related changes in the lipids of the microsomal and the mitochondrial membranes of rat liver and kidney. Mech Ageing Dev 6:197-205, 1977.

274. Grinna LS, Barber AA: Age-related changes in membrane lipid content and enzyme activities. Biochim Biophys Acta 288:347-353, 1972.

275. Pratz J, Corman B: Age-related changes in enzyme activities, protein content and lipid composition of rat kidney brush-border membrane. Biochim Biophys Acta 814:265-273, 1985.

276. Pratz J, Ripoche P, Corman B: Cholesterol content and water and solute permeabilities of kidney membranes from aging rats. Am J Physiol 253:R8-R14, 1987.

277. Levi M, Baird BM, Wilson PV: Cholesterol modulates rat renal brush border membrane phosphate transport. J Clin Invest 85:231-237, 1990.

278. Zajicek H, Wang H, Widerkehr M, et al: Cholesterol modulates Na/Pi cotransport in OK cells. Abstract. J Am Soc Nephrol 8:570A, 1997.

279. Brandis M, Harmeyer J, Kaune R, et al: Phosphate transport in brush-border membranes from control and rachitic pig kidney and small intestine. J Physiol 384:479-490, 1987.

280. Kurnik BR, Hruska KA: Effects of 1,25-dihydroxycholecalciferol on phosphate transport in vitamin D-deprived rats. Am J Physiol 247:F177-F184, 1984.

281. Liang CT, Barnes J, Cheng L, et al: Effects of 1,25-(OH)$_2$D$_3$ administered in vivo on phosphate uptake by isolated chick renal cells. Am J Physiol 242:C312-C318, 1982.

282. Brasitus TA, Dudeja PK, Eby B, et al: Correction by 1-25-dihydroxycholecalciferol of the abnormal fluidity and lipid composition of enterocyte brush border membranes in vitamin D-deprived rats. J Biol Chem 261:16404-16409, 1986.

283. Tsutsumi M, Alvarez U, Avioli LV, et al: Effect of 1,25-dihydroxyvitamin D3 on phospholipid composition of rat renal brush border membrane. Am J Physiol 249:F117-F123, 1985.

284. Pascual J, Orofino L, Liano F, et al: Incidence and prognosis of acute renal failure in older patients. J Am Geriatr Soc 38:25-30, 1990.

285. McInnes EG, Levy DW, Chaudhuri MD, et al: Renal failure in the elderly. Q J Med 64:583-588, 1987.

286. Macias-Nunez JF, Lopez-Novoa JM, Martinez-Maldonado M: Acute renal failure in the aged. Semin Nephrol 16:330-338, 1996.

287. Zarich S, Fang LS, Diamond JR: Fractional excretion of sodium: Exceptions to its diagnostic value. Arch Intern Med 145:108-112, 1985.

288. Gentric A, Cledes J: Immediate and long-term prognosis in acute renal failure in the elderly. Nephrol Dial Transplant 6:86-90, 1991.

289. Klouche K, Cristol JP, Kaaki M, et al: Prognosis of acute renal failure in the elderly. Nephrol Dial Transplant 10:2240-2243, 1995.

290. Santacruz F, Barreto S, Mayor MM, et al: Mortality in elderly patients with acute renal failure. Ren Fail 18:601-605, 1996.

291. Moore RD, Smith CR, Lipsky JJ, et al: Risk factors for nephrotoxicity in patients treated with aminoglycosides. Ann Intern Med 100:352-357, 1984.

292. Michel DM, Kelly CJ: Acute interstitial nephritis. J Am Soc Nephrol 9:506-515, 1998.

293. Kleinknecht D: Interstitial nephritis, the nephrotic syndrome, and chronic renal failure secondary to nonsteroidal anti-inflammatory drugs. Semin Nephrol 15:228-235, 1995.

294. Rich MW, Crecelius CA: Incidence, risk factors, and clinical course of acute renal insufficiency after cardiac catheterization in patients 70 years of age or older: A prospective study. Arch Intern Med 150:1237-1242, 1990.

295. Porter GA: Radiocontrast-induced nephropathy. Nephrol Dial Transplant 9:146-156, 1994.

296. Beierschmitt WP, Keenan KP, Weiner M: Age-related increased susceptibility of male Fischer 344 rats to acetaminophen nephrotoxicity. Life Sci 39:2335-2342, 1986.

297. Goldstein RS, Pasino DA, Hook JB: Cephaloridine nephrotoxicity in aging male Fischer-344 rats. Toxicology 38:43-53, 1986.

298. Goldstein RS, Tarloff JB, Hook JB: Age-related nephropathy in laboratory rats. FASEB J 2:2241-2251, 1988.

299. Kyle ME, Kocsis JJ: The effect of age on salicylate-induced nephrotoxicity in male rats. Toxicol Appl Pharmacol 81:337-347, 1985.

300. Miura K, Goldstein RS, Morgan DG, et al: Age-related differences in susceptibility to renal ischemia in rats. Toxicol Appl Pharmacol 87:284-296, 1987.

301. Sabbatini M, Sansone G, Uccello F, et al: Functional versus structural changes in the pathophysiology of acute ischemic renal failure in aging rats. Kidney Int 45:1355-1361, 1994.

302. Zager RA, Alpers CE: Effects of aging on expression of ischemic acute renal failure in rats. Lab Invest 61:290-294, 1989.

303. Adachi T, Kawamura M, Owada M, et al: Effect of age on renal functional and orthostatic vascular response in healthy men. Clin Exp Pharmacol Physiol 28:877-880, 2001.

304. Prasad PV, Epstein FH: Changes in renal medullary pO2 during water diuresis as evaluated by blood oxygenation level-dependent magnetic resonance imaging: Effects of aging and cyclooxygenase inhibition. Kidney Int 55:294-298, 1999.

305. Paller MS, Hoidal JR, Ferris TF: Oxygen free radicals in ischemic acute renal failure in the rat. J Clin Invest 74:1156-1164, 1984.

306. Moncada S, Palmer RM, Higgs EA: Nitric oxide: Physiology, pathophysiology, and pharmacology. Pharmacol Rev 43:109-142, 1991.

307. Tan D, Cernadas MR, Aragoncillo P, et al: Role of nitric oxide-related mechanisms in renal function in ageing rats. Nephrol Dial Transplant 13:594-601, 1998.

308. Kung CF, Luscher TF: Different mechanisms of endothelial dysfunction with aging and hypertension in rat aorta. Hypertension 25:194-200, 1995.

309. Luscher TF, Bock HA: The endothelial L-arginine/nitric oxide pathway and the renal circulation. Klin Wochenschr 69:603-609, 1991.

310. Reckelhoff JF, Kellum JA, Blanchard EJ, et al: Changes in nitric oxide precursor, L-arginine, and metabolites, nitrate and nitrite, with aging. Life Sci 55:1895-1902, 1994.

311. Sarwar G, Botting HG, Collins M: A comparison of fasting serum amino acid profiles of young and elderly subjects. J Am Coll Nutr 10:668-674, 1991.

312. Mistry SK, Greenfeld Z, Morris SM Jr, et al: The "intestinal-renal" arginine biosynthetic axis in the aging rat. Mech Ageing Dev 123:1159-1165, 2002.

313. Higashi Y, Oshima T, Ozono R, et al: Aging and severity of hypertension attenuate endothelium-dependent renal vascular relaxation in humans. Hypertension 30:252-258, 1997.

314. Cronin RE: Renal failure following radiologic procedures. Am J Med Sci 298:342-356, 1989.

315. Xiong Y, Yuan LW, Deng HW, et al: Elevated serum endogenous inhibitor of nitric oxide synthase and endothelial dysfunction in aged rats. Clin Exp Pharmacol Physiol 28:842-847, 2001.

316. Miyazaki H, Matsuoka H, Cooke JP, et al: Endogenous nitric oxide synthase inhibitor: a novel marker of atherosclerosis. Circulation 99:1141-1146, 1999.

317. Gupta BK, Spinowitz BS, Charytan C, et al: Cholesterol crystal embolization-associated renal failure after therapy with recombinant tissue-type plasminogen activator. Am J Kidney Dis 21:659-662, 1993.

318. Smith MC, Ghose MK, Henry AR: The clinical spectrum of renal cholesterol embolization. Am J Med 71:174-180, 1981.

319. Feest TG, Round A, Hamad S: Incidence of severe acute renal failure in adults: Results of a community based study. BMJ 306:481-483, 1993.

320. Arora P, Kher V, Kohli HS, et al: Acute renal failure in the elderly: Experience from a single centre in India. Nephrol Dial Transplant 8:827-830, 1993.

321. Druml W, Lax F, Grimm G, et al: Acute renal failure in the elderly, 1975-1990. Clin Nephrol 41:342-349, 1994.

322. Pascual J, Liano F, Ortuno J: The elderly patient with acute renal failure. J Am Soc Nephrol 6:144-153, 1995.

323. Scoble JE, Maher ER, Hamilton G, et al: Atherosclerotic renovascular disease causing renal impairment: A case for treatment. Clin Nephrol 31:119-122, 1989.

324. Scoble JE, Sweny P, Stansby G, et al: Patients with atherosclerotic renovascular disease presenting to a renal unit: An audit of outcome. Postgrad Med J 69:461-465, 1993.

325. Harding MB, Smith LR, Himmelstein SI, et al: Renal artery stenosis: Prevalence and associated risk factors in patients undergoing routine cardiac catheterization. J Am Soc Nephrol 2:1608-1616, 1992.

326. Group W: Detection, evaluation, and treatment of renovascular hypertension: Final report. Working Group on Renovascular Hypertension. Arch Intern Med 147:820-829, 1987.

327. Jacobson HR: Ischemic renal disease: An overlooked clinical entity? Kidney Int 34:729-743, 1988.

328. Schreiber MJ, Pohl MA, Novick AC: The natural history of atherosclerotic and fibrous renal artery disease. Urol Clin North Am 11:383-392, 1984.

329. Rimmer JM, Gennari FJ: Atherosclerotic renovascular disease and progressive renal failure. Ann Intern Med 118:712-719, 1993.

330. Baboolal K, Evans C, Moore RH: Incidence of end-stage renal disease in medically treated patients with severe bilateral atherosclerotic renovascular disease. Am J Kidney Dis 31:971-977, 1998.

331. Connolly JO, Higgins RM, Walters HL, et al: Presentation, clinical features and outcome in different patterns of atherosclerotic renovascular disease. QJM 87:413-421, 1994.

332. Gambara G, Budakovic A, Baggio B, et al: Cigarette smoking is associated with altered hemodynamics. Nephrol Dial Transplant 11:A72, 1996.

333. Appel RG, Bleyer AJ, Reavis S, et al: Renovascular disease in older patients beginning renal replacement therapy. Kidney Int 48:171-176, 1995.

334. Klag MJ, Whelton PK, Randall BL, et al: End-stage renal disease in African-American and white men: 16-year MRFIT findings. JAMA 277:1293-1298, 1997.

335. Bleyer AJ, Shemanski LR, Burke GL, et al: Tobacco, hypertension, and vascular disease: Risk factors for renal functional decline in an older population. Kidney Int 57:2072-2079, 2000.

336. Cryer PE, Haymond MW, Santiago JV, et al: Norepinephrine and epinephrine release and adrenergic mediation of smoking-associated hemodynamic and metabolic events. N Engl J Med 295:573-577, 1976.

337. Orth SR, Ritz E, Schrier RW: The renal risks of smoking. Kidney Int 51:1669-1677, 1997.

338. Nadler JD, Velasco JS, Horton R: Cigarette smoking inhibits prostacyclin formation. Lancet 1:1248, 1976.

339. Wennmalm A, Bethin G, Grastrom EF, et al: Relation between tobacco use and urinary excretion of thromboxane A2 and prostacyclin metabolites in young men. Circulation 83:1698, 1991.

340. Baggio B, Budakovic A, Gambaro G: Cardiovascular risk factors, smoking and kidney function. Nephrol Dial Transplant 13:2-5, 1998.

341. Nitenberg A, Antony I, Foult JM: Acetylcholine-induced coronary vasoconstriction in young, heavy smokers with normal coronary arteriographic findings. Am J Med 95:71-77, 1993.

342. Celermajer DS, Sorensen KE, Georgakopoulos D, et al: Cigarette smoking is associated with dose-related and potentially reversible impairment of endothelium-dependent dilation in healthy young adults. Circulation 88:2149-2155, 1993.

343. Kiowski W, Linder L, Stoschitzky K, et al: Diminished vascular response to inhibition of endothelium-derived nitric oxide and enhanced vasoconstriction to exogenously administered endothelin-1 in clinically healthy smokers. Circulation 90:27-34, 1994.

344. Haak T, Jungmann E, Raab C, et al: Elevated endothelin-1 levels after cigarette smoking. Metabolism 43:267-269, 1994.

345. Kohan DE: Endothelins in the kidney: Physiology and pathophysiology. Am J Kidney Dis 22:493-510, 1993.

346. Black HR, Zeevi GR, Silten RM, et al: Effect of heavy cigarette smoking on renal and myocardial arterioles. Nephron 34:173-179, 1983.

347. Oberai B, Adams CW, High OB: Myocardial and renal arteriolar thickening in cigarette smokers. Atherosclerosis 52:185-190, 1984.

348. Barton M, Lattmann T, d'Uscio LV, et al: Inverse regulation of endothelin-1 and nitric oxide metabolites in tissue with aging: Implications for the age-dependent increase of cardiorenal disease. J Cardiovasc Pharmacol 36:S153-S156, 2000.

349. van de Ven PJ, Beutler JJ, Kaatee R, et al: Angiotensin converting enzyme inhibitor-induced renal dysfunction in atherosclerotic renovascular disease. Kidney Int 53:986-993, 1998.

350. Anderson WP, Woods RL: Intrarenal effects of angiotensin II in renal artery stenosis. Kidney Int Suppl 20:S157-S167, 1987.

351. Erbsloh-Moller B, Dumas A, Roth D, et al: Furosemide-131I-hippuran renography after angiotensin-converting enzyme inhibition for the diagnosis of renovascular hypertension. Am J Med 90:23-29, 1991.

352. Prigent A: The diagnosis of renovascular hypertension: The role of captopril renal scintigraphy and related issues. Eur J Nucl Med 20:625-644, 1993.

353. Olin JW, Piedmonte MR, Young JR, et al: The utility of duplex ultrasound scanning of the renal arteries for diagnosing significant renal artery stenosis. Ann Intern Med 122:833-838, 1995.

354. Bleyer AJ, Chen R, D'Agostino RB Jr, et al: Clinical correlates of hypertensive end-stage renal disease. Am J Kidney Dis 31:28-34, 1998.

355. Meyrier A: Renal vascular lesions in the elderly: Nephrosclerosis or atheromatous renal disease? Nephrol Dial Transplant 11(suppl 9):45-52, 1996.

356. Kassirer JP: Atheroembolic renal disease. N Engl J Med 280:812-818, 1969.

357. Morris GC Jr, Heider CF, Moyer JH: The protective effect of subfiltration arterial pressure on the kidney. Surg Forum 6:623, 1995.

358. Schlanger LE, Haire HM, Zuckerman AM, et al: Reversible renal failure in an elderly woman with renal artery stenosis. Am J Kidney Dis 23:123-126, 1994.

359. Beraud JJ, Calvet B, Durand A, et al: Reversal of acute renal failure following percutaneous transluminal recanalization of an atherosclerotic renal artery occlusion. J Hypertens 7:909-911, 1989.

360. Flye MW, Anderson RW, Fish JC, et al: Successful surgical treatment of anuria caused by renal artery occlusion. Ann Surg 195:346-353, 1982.

361. O'Donohoe MK, Donohoe J, Corrigan TP: Acute renal failure of renovascular origin: Cure by aortorenal reconstruction after 25 days of anuria. Nephron 56:92-93, 1990.

362. Ramsay AG, D'Agati V, Dietz PA, et al: Renal functional recovery 47 days after renal artery occlusion. Am J Nephrol 3:325-328, 1983.

363. Sandy DT, Vidt DG, Geisinger MA, et al: Serum creatinine prior to angioplasty (PTRA): A predictor of clinical success in atherosclerotic disease. J Am Soc Nephrol 6:648, 1995.

364. Kuhn FP, Kutkuhn B, Torsello G, et al: Renal artery stenosis: Preliminary results of treatment with the Strecker stent. Radiology 180:367-372, 1991.

365. Dorros G, Jaff M, Dorros I, et al: Renal dysfunction is a poor prognosticator of patient survival after Palmaz stent revascularization for renal artery stenosis. Abstract. J Am Coll Cardiol 29:486A, 1997.

366. Couser WG: Idiopathic rapidly progressive glomerulonephritis. Am J Nephrol 2:57-69, 1982.

367. Furci L, Medici G, Baraldi A, et al: Rapidly progressive glomerulonephritis in the elderly: Long-term results. Contrib Nephrol 105: 98-101, 1993.

368. Jeffrey RF, Gardiner DS, More IA, et al: Crescentic glomerulonephritis: experience of a single unit over a five year period. Scott Med J 37:175-178, 1992.

369. Moorthy AV, Zimmerman SW: Renal disease in the elderly: Clinicopathologic analysis of renal disease in 115 elderly patients. Clin Nephrol 14:223-229, 1980.

370. Bergesio F, Bertoni E, Bandini S, et al: Changing pattern of glomerulonephritis in the elderly: A change of prevalence or a different approach? Contrib Nephrol 105:75-80, 1993.

371. Haas M, Spargo BH, Wit EJ, et al: Etiologies and outcome of acute renal insufficiency in older adults: A renal biopsy study of 259 cases. Am J Kidney Dis 35:433-447, 2000.

372. Bindi P, Mougenot B, Mentre F, et al: Necrotizing crescentic glomerulonephritis without significant immune deposits: A clinical and serological study. Q J Med 86:55-68, 1993.

373. Melby PC, Musick WD, Luger AM, et al: Poststreptococcal glomerulonephritis in the elderly: Report of a case and review of the literature. Am J Nephrol 7:235-240, 1987.

374. Donadio JV Jr: Treatment and clinical outcome of glomerulonephritis in the elderly. Contrib Nephrol 105:49-57, 1993.

375. Abrass CK: Glomerulonephritis in the elderly. Am J Nephrol 5: 409-418, 1985.

376. Arieff AI, Anderson RJ, Massry SG: Acute glomerulonephritis in the elderly. Geriatrics 26:74-84, 1971.

377. Montoliu J, Darnell A, Torras A, et al: Acute and rapidly progressive forms of glomerulonephritis in the elderly. J Am Geriatr Soc 29: 108-116, 1981.

378. Washio M, Oh Y, Okuda S, et al: Clinicopathological study of poststreptococcal glomerulonephritis in the elderly. Clin Nephrol 41:265-270, 1994.

379. Johnston PA, Brown JS, Davison AM: The nephrotic syndrome in the elderly: Clinicopathologic correlations in 317 patients. Geriatr Nephrol Urol 2:85, 1992.

380. Fawcett IW, Hilton PJ, Jones NF, et al: Nephrotic syndrome in the elderly. Br Med J 2:387-388, 1971.

381. Ishimoto F, Shibasaki T, Nakano M, et al: [Nephrotic syndrome in the elderly—a clinicopathological study (author's transl)]. Nippon Jinzo Gakkai Shi 23:1251-1261, 1981.

382. Kingswood JC, Banks RA, Tribe CR, et al: Renal biopsy in the elderly: Clinicopathological correlations in 143 patients. Clin Nephrol 22:183-187, 1984.

383. Lustig S, Rosenfeld JB, Ben-Bassat M, et al: Nephrotic syndrome in the elderly. Isr J Med Sci 18:1010-1013, 1982.

384. Murphy PJ, Wright G, Rai GS: Nephrotic syndrome in the elderly. J Am Geriatr Soc 35:170-173, 1987.

385. Ozono Y, Harada T, Yamaguchi K, et al: Nephrotic syndrome in the elderly: Clinicopathological study. Nippon Jinzo Gakkai Shi 36: 44-50, 1994.

386. Sato H, Saito T, Furuyama T, et al: Histologic studies on the nephrotic syndrome in the elderly. Tohoku J Exp Med 153:259-264, 1987.

387. Zech P, Colon S, Pointet P, et al: The nephrotic syndrome in adults aged over 60: Etiology, evolution and treatment of 76 cases. Clin Nephrol 17:232-236, 1982.

388. Shin J, Pyo H, Kwon Y, et al: Renal biopsy in elderly patients: Clinicopathological correlation in 117 Korean patients. Clin Nephrol 56:19-26, 2001.

389. Huriet C, Rauber G, Kessler Cuny G: Le syndrome nephrotique apres 60 ans, considerations etiologique d'apres une seri de 25 cas. Ann Med Nancy 14:1021, 1975.

390. Nolasco F, Cameron JS, Heywood EF, et al: Adult-onset minimal change nephrotic syndrome: A long-term follow-up. Kidney Int 29: 1215-1223, 1986.

391. Kyle RA, Greipp PR: Amyloidosis (AL): Clinical and laboratory features in 229 cases. Mayo Clin Proc 58:665-683, 1983.

392. D'Agati V: The many masks of focal segmental glomerulosclerosis. Kidney Int 46:1223-1241, 1994.

393. Hostetter TH, Rennke HG, Brenner BM: The case for intrarenal hypertension in the initiation and progression of diabetic and other glomerulopathies. Am J Med 72:375-380, 1982.

394. Thadhani R, Pascual M, Nickeleit V, et al: Preliminary description of focal segmental glomerulosclerosis in patients with renovascular disease. Lancet 347:231-233, 1996.

395. Baylis C, Fredericks M, Leypoldt J, et al: The mechanisms of proteinuria in aging rats. Mech Ageing Dev 45:111-126, 1988.

396. Bolton WK, Sturgill BC: Spontaneous glomerular sclerosis in aging Sprague-Dawley rats: II. Ultrastructural studies. Am J Pathol 98: 339-356, 1980.

397. Bolton WK, Benton FR, Maclay JG, et al: Spontaneous glomerular sclerosis in aging Sprague-Dawley rats. Am J Pathol 85:277, 1976.

398. Couser WG, Stilmant MM: The immunopathology of the aging rat kidney. J Gerontol 31:13-22, 1976.

399. Meyer TW, Lawrence WE, Brenner BM: Dietary protein and the progression of renal disease. Kidney Int Suppl 16:S243-S247, 1983.

400. Yumura W, Sugino N, Nagasawa R, et al: Age-associated changes in renal glomeruli of mice. Exp Gerontol 24:237-249, 1989.

401. Zent R, Nagai R, Cattran DC: Idiopathic membranous nephropathy in the elderly: A comparative study. Am J Kidney Dis 29:200-206, 1997.

402. Ponticelli C, Altieri P, Scolari F, et al: A randomized study comparing methylprednisolone plus chlorambucil versus methylprednisolone plus cyclophosphamide in idiopathic membranous nephropathy. J Am Soc Nephrol 9:444-450, 1998.

403. Eagen JW: Glomerulopathies of neoplasia. Kidney Int 11:297-303, 1977.

404. Donadio JV Jr: Treatment of glomerulonephritis in the elderly. Am J Kidney Dis 16:307-311, 1990.

405. Kidney Disease Outcome Quality Initiative (K/DOQI) clinical practice guidelines for chronic kidney disease: Evaluation, classification, and stratification. Am J Kidney Dis 39(2 suppl 2):S1-S246, 2002.

406. Manjunath G, Tighiouart H, Coresh J, et al: Level of kidney function as a risk factor for cardiovascular outcomes in the elderly. Kidney Int 63:1121-1129, 2003.

407. Agodoa LY, Eggers PW: Renal replacement therapy in the United States: Data from the United States Renal Data System. Am J Kidney Dis 25:119-133, 1995.

408. Nissenson AR: Dialysis therapy in the elderly patient. Kidney Int Suppl 40:S51-S57, 1993.

409. Port FK: Morbidity and mortality in dialysis patients. Kidney Int 46:1728-1737, 1994.

410. Peri UN, Fenves AZ, Middleton JP: Improving survival of octogenarian patients selected for haemodialysis. Nephrol Dial Transplant 16:2201-2206, 2001.

411. Lowrie EG, Lew NL: Death risk in hemodialysis patients: The predictive value of commonly measured variables and an evaluation of death rate differences between facilities. Am J Kidney Dis 15: 458-482, 1990.

412. Wizemann V, Kramer W: Short-term dialysis-long term complications: Ten year experience with short duration renal replacement therapy. Blood Purif 5:193-201, 1987.

413. Capuano A, Sepe V, Cianfrone P, et al: Cardiovascular impairment, dialysis strategy and tolerance in elderly and young patients on maintenance haemodialysis. Nephrol Dial Transplant 5:1023-1030, 1990.

414. Gorban-Brennan N, Kliger AS, Finkelstein FO: CAPD therapy for patients over 80 years of age. Perit Dial Int 13:140-141, 1993.

415. Ismail N, Hakim RM, Oreopoulos DG, et al: Renal replacement therapies in the elderly: Part 1. Hemodialysis and chronic peritoneal dialysis. Am J Kidney Dis 22:759-782, 1993.

416. Vlachojannis J, Kurz P, Hoppe D: CAPD in elderly patients with cardiovascular risk factors. Clin Nephrol 30:S13-S17, 1988.

417. Williams AJ, Nicholl JP, el Nahas AM, et al: Continuous ambulatory peritoneal dialysis and haemodialysis in the elderly. Q J Med 74: 215-223, 1990.

418. Wolcott DL, Nissenson AR: Quality of life in chronic dialysis patients: A critical comparison of continuous ambulatory peritoneal dialysis (CAPD) and hemodialysis. Am J Kidney Dis 11:402-412, 1988.

419. Balaskas EV, Yuan ZY, Gupta A, et al: Long-term continuous ambulatory peritoneal dialysis in diabetics. Clin Nephrol 42:54-62, 1994.

420. Lunde NM, Port FK, Wolfe RA, et al: Comparison of mortality risk by choice of CAPD versus hemodialysis among elderly patients. Adv Perit Dial 7:68-72, 1991.

421. Maiorca R, Vonesh EF, Cavalli P, et al: A multicenter, selection-adjusted comparison of patient and technique survivals on CAPD and hemodialysis. Perit Dial Int 11:118-127, 1991.

422. Held PJ, Port FK, Turenne MN, et al: Continuous ambulatory peritoneal dialysis and hemodialysis: Comparison of patient mortality with adjustment for comorbid conditions. Kidney Int 45:1163-1169, 1994.

423. Cantarovich D, Baranger T, Tirouvanziam A, et al: One-hundred and five cadaveric kidney transplants with cyclosporine in recipients more than 60 years of age. Transplant Proc 25:1323, 1993.

424. Ismail N, Hakim RM, Helderman JH: Renal replacement therapies in the elderly: Part II. Renal transplantation. Am J Kidney Dis 23:1-15, 1994.

425. Jassal SV, Krahn MD, Naglie G, et al: Kidney transplantation in the elderly: A decision analysis. J Am Soc Nephrol 14:187-196, 2003.

426. Johnson DW, Herzig K, Purdie D, et al: A comparison of the effects of dialysis and renal transplantation on the survival of older uremic patients. Transplantation 69:794-799, 2000.

427. Nyberg G, Nilsson B, Hallste G, et al: Renal transplantation in elderly patients: Survival and complications. Transplant Proc 25:1062-1063, 1993.

428. Meier-Kriesche HU, Ojo A, Hanson J, et al: Increased immunosuppressive vulnerability in elderly renal transplant recipients. Transplantation 69:885-889, 2000.

429. Becker BN, Ismail N, Becker YT, et al: Renal transplantation in the older end stage renal disease patient. Semin Nephrol 16:353-362, 1996.

430. Gardner ID: The effect of aging on susceptibility to infection. Rev Infect Dis 2:801-810, 1980.

431. Sant GR: Urinary tract infection in the elderly. Semin Urol 5:126-133, 1987.

432. Garibaldi RA, Nurse BA: Infections in the elderly. Am J Med 81:53-58, 1986.

433. Parsons CL, Schmidt JD: Control of recurrent lower urinary tract infection in the postmenopausal woman. J Urol 128:1224-1226, 1982.

434. Raz R, Stamm WE: A controlled trial of intravaginal estriol in postmenopausal women with recurrent urinary tract infections. N Engl J Med 329:753-756, 1993.

435. Garibaldi RA, Brodine S, Matsumiya S: Infections among patients in nursing homes: Policies, prevalence, problems. N Engl J Med 305:731-735, 1981.

436. Kaye D: Urinary tract infections in the elderly. Bull N Y Acad Med 56:209-220, 1980.

437. Dontas AS, Kasviki-Charvati P, Papanayiotou PC, et al: Bacteriuria and survival in old age. N Engl J Med 304:939-943, 1981.

438. Nordenstam GR, Brandberg CA, Oden AS, et al: Bacteriuria and mortality in an elderly population. N Engl J Med 314:1152-1156, 1986.

439. Abrutyn E, Mossey J, Berlin JA, et al: Does asymptomatic bacteriuria predict mortality and does antimicrobial treatment reduce mortality in elderly ambulatory women? Ann Intern Med 120:827-833, 1994.

440. Nicolle LE, Bjornson J, Harding GK, et al: Bacteriuria in elderly institutionalized men. N Engl J Med 309:1420-1425, 1983.

441. Stamm WE, Hooton TM: Management of urinary tract infections in adults. N Engl J Med 329:1328-1334, 1993.

442. Abrutyn E, Boscia JA, Kaye D: The treatment of asymptomatic bacteriuria in the elderly. J Am Geriatr Soc 36:473-475, 1988.

443. Boscia JA, Abrutyn E, Kaye D: Asymptomatic bacteriuria in elderly persons: Treat or do not treat? Ann Intern Med 106:764-766, 1987.

444. Kissane JM: The morphology of renal cystic disease. Perspect Nephrol Hypertens 4:31-63, 1976.

445. Ravine D, Gibson RN, Donlan J, et al: An ultrasound renal cyst prevalence survey: Specificity data for inherited renal cystic diseases. Am J Kidney Dis 22:803-807, 1993.

Management of the Patient with Renal Failure

Diuretics

Christopher S. Wilcox

This chapter reviews the mechanisms of action, physiologic adaptation, adverse effects, and clinical uses of diuretics. The major transport targets for diuretic drugs have been defined and their genes cloned.[1, 2] The effects of disease on diuretic kinetics are discussed because this predicts the required dosage modifications. Loop diuretics and thiazides are the most widely used diuretics, and the physiologic adaptations to their prolonged use are described. Diuretic resistance, its management, and the major adverse effects of therapy are discussed. This provides a framework for the design of strategies to maximize the desired actions while minimizing the unwanted effects. The chapter concludes with a discussion of the practical use of diuretics in the treatment of specific clinical conditions. Diuretics have been recently reviewed.[1-7]

Other chapters discuss the treatment of hypertension by diuretic drugs (Chapters 45, 47, and 55), diuretic-induced changes in potassium excretion (Chapters 10 and 21), acid-base disturbances (Chapters 20 and 25), divalent cation excretion and nephrolithiasis (Chapters 12, 15, and 39), the syndrome of inappropriate antidiuretic hormone (SIADH) secretion (Chapters 8 and 13), and acute renal failure (ARF) (Chapter 27). Diuretics have been reviewed extensively.[1-3, 5-10]

INDIVIDUAL CLASSES OF DIURETICS

The major sites of action of diuretics and the fraction of filtered Na^+ reabsorbed at the corresponding nephron segments are summarized in Figure 54-1.

Carbonic Anhydrase Inhibitors

SITES AND MECHANISMS OF ACTION. Carbonic anhydrase is found in erythrocytes, kidney, gut, ciliary body, choroid plexus, and glial cells. Carbonic anhydrase IV and XIV are expressed on the luminal border of the cells of the proximal and thick ascending limb (TAL) of the loop of Henle, and carbonic anhydrase IV is also expressed on α-intercalated cells of the collecting ducts (CDs).[11] The first administration of a carbonic anhydrase inhibitor (CAI) causes a brisk alkaline diuresis. The excretion of Na^+,K^+,

HCO_3^-, and PO_4^{2-} increases, whereas titratable acid and NH_4^+ decrease sharply. Excretion of Ca^{2+} is little altered. There is substantial kaliuresis due to the presence of nonreabsorbable HCO_3^- and high flow rates in the distal nephron. However, hypokalemia is uncommon, because acidosis partitions K^+ out of cells.

CAIs block the catalytic dehydration of luminal carbonic acid at the brush border of the proximal tubule, decrease the intracellular generation of H^+ required for countertransport with Na^+, and decrease the peritubular capillary fluid uptake.[12] The natriuretic efficacy of acetazolamide and furosemide is additive, which confirms their independent mechanisms of action.[13] CAIs also are weak inhibitors of reabsorption in the TAL.[14]

There are several reasons why the natriuretic response to a CAI is not as profound as might be anticipated for a drug acting on the proximal tubule, where the bulk of filtered Na^+ is reabsorbed (see Fig. 54-1). First, carbonic anhydrase is required for reabsorption of HCO_3^-, whereas about two thirds of the proximal Na^+ reabsorption is accompanied by Cl^-. Second, some proximal HCO_3^- reabsorption persists even after apparently full inhibition of carbonic anhydrase.[15] Third, some of the HCO_3^- that is delivered from the proximal tubule can be reabsorbed at more distal sites.[15] Fourth, the metabolic acidosis that develops limits the filtered load to HCO_3^- and thereby curtails the natriuresis.[16] Fifth, the increased delivery of filtered Na^+ to the macula densa elicits a tubuloglomerular feedback (TGF)-induced reduction in the glomerular filtration rate (GFR).[17]

Most diuretics have some CAI action.[18] This contributes to the weak inhibition of proximal reabsorption by furosemide and chlorothiazide and to the relaxation of vascular smooth muscle cells by high-dose furosemide.[18]

PHARMACOKINETICS. Acetazolamide (Diamox) is readily absorbed. It is eliminated with a half-life ($t_{1/2}$) of 13 hours by tubular secretion, which is diminished during hypoalbuminemia.[19] Methazolamide (Neptazane) has less plasma protein binding, a longer $t_{1/2}$, and greater lipid solubility, all of which favor penetration into aqueous humor and cerebrospinal fluid (CSF). It has less renal effect and therefore is preferred for treatment of glaucoma.

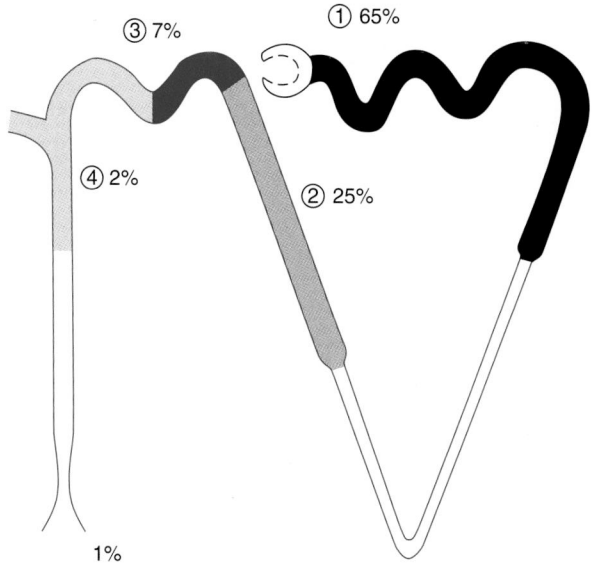

③ 7%

① 65%

④ 2%

② 25%

1%

1. Carbonic anhydrase inhibitors
   Osmotic diuretics

2. Loop diuretics
   Osmotic diuretics
   Mercurials

3. Thiazides

4. Potassium-sparing diuretics
   Aldosterone antagonists

FIGURE 54-1. Nephron diagram showing the primary sites of diuretic action and the approximate fraction of filtered sodium reabsorbed at each.

CLINICAL INDICATIONS. The use of CAIs as diuretics is limited by their transient action, the development of metabolic acidosis, and a spectrum of adverse effects. They can be used with $NaHCO_3$ infusion to cause an alkaline diuresis that increases the excretion of weakly acidic drugs (e.g., salicylates and phenobarbital) or acidic metabolites (urate). Chloride-responsive metabolic alkalosis is best treated by administering Cl^- with K^+ or Na^+. However, if this produces unacceptable extracellular volume (ECV) expansion, acetazolamide (250-500 mg/day) and KCl can be used to increase HCO_3^- excretion.

Metabolic alkalosis due to loop diuretics or thiazides can depress respiration further in patients with chronic respiratory acidosis. This provides a rationale for a CAI. Indeed, the administration of acetazolamide to such subjects can reduce their partial pressure of arterial carbon dioxide ($Paco_2$) and improve their partial pressure of arterial oxygen (Pao_2). Since both $Paco_2$ and bicarbonate tension (P_{HCO_3}) decrease, there is little change in blood pH.[20, 21] However, a reduction in P_{HCO_3} limits the buffer capacity of blood. Further hypercapnia can produce a dangerous fall in blood pH. Moreover, CAIs can increase the $Paco_2$ during metabolic acidosis or exercise and can cause ventilation-perfusion imbalance.[22] Careful surveillance is required when CAIs are administered to such patients.

When used to treat glaucoma, CAIs diminish the transport of HCO_3^- and Na^+ by the ciliary process, thereby reducing the intraocular pressure.[23] CAIs also limit formation of CSF[24] and endolymph.[25]

Acute mountain sickness is characterized by headache, nausea, drowsiness, insomnia, shortness of breath, dizziness, and malaise after an abrupt ascent. Acetazolamide improves the performance of mountaineers. It is useful in a dose of 125 mg twice daily as prophylaxis against mountain sickness, probably through stimulating respiration and diminishing cerebral blood flow.[26] In established mountain sickness, it improves oxygenation and pulmonary gas exchange.[27] It can stimulate ventilation in patients with central sleep apnea.[28]

CAIs are effective in prophylaxis of hypokalemic periodic paralysis because they diminish the influx of K^+ into cells.[29] Paradoxically, they are also useful in the treatment of hyperkalemic periodic paralysis.[30]

ADVERSE EFFECTS. Patients may complain of weakness, lethargy, abnormal taste, paresthesia, gastrointestinal distress, malaise, and decreased libido. These symptoms can be diminished by $NaHCO_3$, but this increases the risk of nephrocalcinosis and nephrolithiasis.[31] Overall, symptomatic metabolic acidosis develops in half of glaucoma patients treated with CAIs.[32]

Elderly patients or those with diabetes mellitus or chronic renal insufficiency (CRI) can develop a serious metabolic acidosis.[32] An alkaline urine favors partitioning of renal ammonia into blood rather than its elimination in urine. An increase in blood ammonia may precipitate encephalopathy in patients with liver failure.[33]

Acetazolamide increases the risk of nephrolithiasis by more than 10-fold.[34] CAIs occasionally cause allergic reactions, hepatitis, and blood dyscrasias.[35] They can cause osteomalacia when used with phenytoin or phenobarbital.[36]

Osmotic Diuretics

SITES AND MECHANISMS OF ACTION. Mannitol is freely filtered but poorly reabsorbed.[37] In the water-permeable nephron segments of the proximal nephron and the thin limbs of the loop of Henle, fluid reabsorption concentrates filtered mannitol sufficiently to diminish tubular fluid reabsorption. Ongoing Na^+ reabsorption lowers the tubular fluid $[Na^+]$ and creates a gradient for back-flux of reabsorbed Na^+ into the tubule. Increased distal flow stimulates K^+ secretion.

Mannitol is a hypertonic solute that abstracts water from cells. The increase in total renal blood flow (RBF) relates in part to hemodilution and a decrease in blood hematocrit and viscosity. Mannitol increases medullary blood flow and decreases the medullary solute gradient, thereby preventing urinary concentration. The rise in renal plasma flow and fall in plasma colloid osmotic pressure can increase the GFR.[38]

PHARMACOKINETICS AND DOSAGE. During intravenous infusion, mannitol is distributed in the ECV. It is filtered freely at the glomerulus. Consequently, the $t_{1/2}$ for plasma clearance depends on the GFR. The $t_{1/2}$ can be prolonged from 1 to 36 hours in advanced renal failure.[39] It can be infused intravenously in daily doses of 50 to 200 g as a 15% or 20% solution or 1.5 to 2.0 g/kg of 20% mannitol over 30 to 60 minutes to treat raised intraocular or intracranial pressure.[37]

CLINICAL INDICATIONS. Mannitol has been evaluated for the prophylaxis of ARF. The rationale includes its ability to expand the ECV, block TGF, maintain GFR, increase

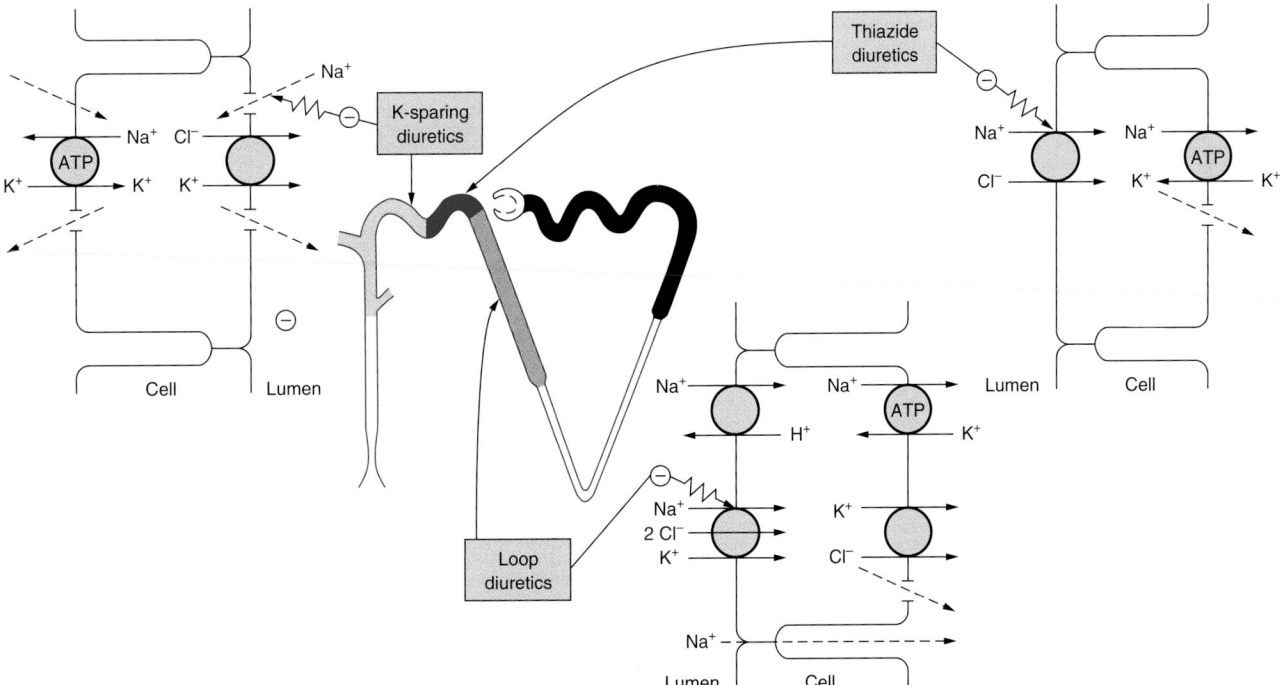

FIGURE 54-2. Cell diagram of the transport mechanisms of the thick ascending limb of the loop of Henle, the early distal convoluted tubule, and the principal cells of the collecting ducts, showing the major sites of action of loop diuretics, thiazides, and distal agents, respectively. ATP, adenosine triphosphate.

tubule fluid flow, prevent tubule obstruction from shed cell constituents or crystals, reduce renal edema, redistribute blood flow from the outer cortex to the relatively hypoxic inner cortex and outer medulla, and scavenge oxygen radicals.[37, 38] Mannitol is reported to decrease the incidence of ARF in selected high-risk settings, including mismatched blood transfusion and shock,[40] myoglobinuria,[41] and rhabdomyolysis.[37] It can protect against ARF in cadaveric kidney transplant recipients.[37] and those receiving cisplatin.[42] However, in a controlled trial of mannitol prophylaxis in patients with mild chronic renal failure, it was less effective than hydration alone with 0.074 M NaCl at 2 mL/minute in preventing contrast-associated nephropathy.[43] Although none of the treated patients developed acute tubular necrosis, this trial has reduced enthusiasm for the prophylactic use of mannitol. Ligation of the common bile duct of the rat to produce obstructive jaundice increases the severity of renal failure following renal artery clamping; this effect is prevented by mannitol infusion.[44] Two controlled trials have confirmed the high incidence of postoperative ARF in patients with obstructive jaundice; both trials reported that a mannitol infusion, begun before surgery and maintained until postoperative day 1 or 2, reduced the incidence of ARF.[44, 45] However, a randomized, controlled trial found no benefit of mannitol on postoperative renal function or survival in patients undergoing biliary tract surgery.[46] Conger[47] concluded that, apart from the prophylaxis of ARF in kidney transplantation, there is no clear evidence that mannitol, or any diuretic, is effective in prevention or treatment of ARF. The use of diuretics to convert oliguric to nonoliguric ARF is discussed later (see "Clinical Uses of Diuretics"; "Nonedematous Conditions": "Acute Renal Failure").

A trial of mannitol therapy for cerebral edema complicating hepatic failure demonstrated a markedly improved survival of 47%, compared with only 6% in the control group.[48] Mannitol is recommended for management of severe head injury.[49] It is more effective than loop diuretics or hypertonic saline in reducing brain water content.[50] Mannitol can reverse the dialysis disequilibrium syndrome.

ADVERSE EFFECTS. The effects of mannitol on plasma electrolyte concentrations are complicated. The osmotic abstraction of cell water initially causes hyponatremia and hypochloremia. Later, when the excess extracellular fluid (ECF) is excreted, the decrease in cell water concentrates K^+ and H^+ within cells, which increases the gradient for their diffusion into the ECF, leading to hyperkalemic acidosis. These electrolyte changes are normally rapidly corrected by the kidney, provided that renal function is adequate. Later, hypernatremic dehydration may develop if free water is not provided, because urinary concentrating ability is inhibited.

Expansion of ECV, hemodilution, and hyperkalemic metabolic acidosis occur in patients with renal failure who cannot eliminate the drug. Circulatory overload, pulmonary edema, central nervous system depression, and severe hyponatremia require urgent hemodialysis.[51] Doses above 200 g/day can cause renal vasoconstriction and ARF.[37]

Loop Diuretics

SITES AND MECHANISMS OF ACTION. The prime action of loop diuretics occurs from the luminal aspect of the TAL[52] (Fig. 54-2). An electroneutral $Na^+/K^+/2Cl^-$ cotransporter, termed NKCC2, is located in the luminal membrane of the TAL.[53, 54] A high K^+ conductance allows complete recycling of K^+ across the luminal membrane.[55] The energy for transport is provided indirectly via the basolateral Na^+,K^+-ATPase, which maintains a low intracellular $[Na^+]$.

The complementary DNA (cDNA) for NKCC2 has been cloned.[56] It is expressed on the apical membranes of medullary and cortical TALs and macula densa segments.[57] The abundance of NKCC2 is increased by prolonged infusion of saline or furosemide.[57] A closely related gene, NKCCl, encodes a protein that is widely expressed in transporting epithelia.[53] It is implicated in uptake and secretion of Cl^{-56} and NH_4^+ at the basolateral membrane of the medullary CDs.[58]

Hormones that stimulate cyclic adenosine monophosphate (cAMP), such as arginine vasopressin (AVP), enhance TAL reabsorption and should enhance the response to loop diuretics. In contrast, those that stimulate cyclic guanosine monophosphate (cGMP), such as nitric oxide and atrial natriuretic peptide (ANP), or those that increase intracellular $[Ca^{2+}]$, such as 20-hydroxyeicosatetraenoic acid (20-HETE), or that activate the Ca^{2+} (polyvalent cation)-sensing protein[59] inhibit TAL reabsorption and reduce the response to loop diuretics.[60, 61] These hypotheses await clinical trial.

The rat TAL also transports NH_4^{+} [62] that can substitute for K^+ on the $Na^+/K^+/2Cl^-$ cotransporter. In the rat, there is a luminal Na^+/H^+ countertransporter that contributes to tubular fluid acidification. Loop diuretics block the luminal entry of Na^+, but not the peritubular exit via the Na^+,K^+-ATPase, and thereby reduce the intracellular $[Na^+]$ sufficiently to promote luminal Na^+ uptake via the Na^+/H^+ countertransport process. This explains why furosemide stimulates acid excretion in the rat.[63] In contrast, furosemide does not change net acid excretion or urine pH in normal human subjects.[64]

Loop diuretics reduce proximal fluid reabsorption modestly. This has been ascribed to a weak CAI action. However, furosemide depresses proximal reabsorption in tubules perfused with HCO_3^--free solutions.[65] Moreover, bumetanide, which is a much less potent inhibitor of carbonic anhydrase, also impairs proximal fluid reabsorption.[66]

Furosemide exerts two contrasting effects on reabsorption in the superficial distal tubule. Increased delivery to the unsaturated distal tubule reabsorption process increases Na^+ reabsorption.[63] However, Velazquez and Wright perfused rat distal tubules in vivo to obviate the confounding effects of altered delivery.[67] They concluded that furosemide, but not bumetanide, was a weak inhibitor of the thiazide-sensitive Na^+/Cl^- cotransporter (NCC). Loop diuretics also inhibit NaCl transport in short descending limbs of the loop of Henle[68] and CDs.[69] Although the TAL is clearly the major site of action of loop diuretics, actions at other nephron segments contribute to the natriuresis by blunting the expected increase in reabsorption in the proximal tubule (in response to volume depletion) and the distal nephron (in response to increased load).

Reabsorption of solute from the water-impermeable TAL segments dilutes the tubule fluid and concentrates the interstitium. Inhibition of this process by loop diuretics impairs both free water excretion during water loading and free water reabsorption during dehydration.[70]

Loop diuretics increase the fractional excretion of Ca^{2+} by up to 30%.[71] Two mechanisms have been identified. First, loop diuretics decrease the lumen-positive transepithelial potential that promotes paracellular Ca^{2+} reabsorption from the lumen. Second, they decrease the reabsorption of Ca^{2+} by a $NaCl^-$ independent process[72] (Fig. 54-3).

The loop of Henle is the major nephron segment for reabsorption of Mg^{2+}.[73] Loop diuretics can increase fractional Mg^{2+} excretion by more than 60% [74] by diminishing voltage-dependent paracellular transport[73] (see Fig. 54-3).

Loop diuretics initially increase urate excretion by inhibition of proximal urate transport.[75] However, there is a succeeding reduction in urate clearance that is largely secondary to volume depletion, which enhances proximal fluid and urate reabsorption.[76] Unlike most diuretics, the plasma urate is reduced by tienilic acid[77] and indacrinone.[78] Tienilic acid inhibits urate uptake into proximal tubule brush border membranes.[75] Indacrinone inhibits both the reabsorption and the secretion of urate by the proximal tubule.[79]

The total RBF is maintained or increased and the GFR is little changed during administration of loop diuretics to normal subjects.[80] However, there is a marked redistribution of blood flow from the inner to the outer cortex.[81] The fall in papillary plasma flow is dependent on angiotensin II (AII).[82] Furosemide increases the renal generation of prostaglandins (PGs).[83] Blockade of cyclooxygenase prevents

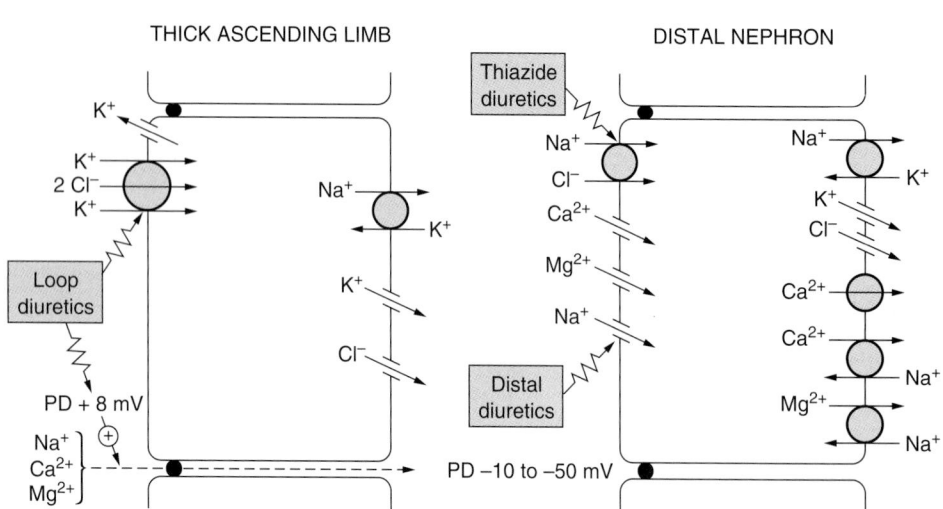

FIGURE 54-3. Cell diagram of effects of diuretics on Ca^{2+} and Mg^{2+} transport.

furosemide-induced renal vasodilation.[84] Furosemide blocks the TGF response that constricts the afferent arteriole.[85] Thus, after loop diuretic administration, AII contributes to the medullary vasoconstriction, while PGs and interruption of TGF contribute to the cortical vasodilation.

Furosemide dilates veins[86] by an endothelium-dependent hyperpolarizing action[87] via CAI.[88]

PHARMACOKINETICS AND DIFFERENCES BETWEEN DRUGS. Furosemide is well absorbed; its bioavailability averages 50% but is highly variable.[89] Between 91% and 99% is bound to albumin, for which it competes with other acidic drugs. Approximately half of an oral dose is eliminated unchanged by the kidneys. Loop diuretics, thiazides, and CAIs are secreted avidly by a probenecid-sensitive organic anion transporter type 1 (OAT1) mechanism in the S2 segment of the proximal tubule (Fig. 54-4).[90, 91]

Approximately 50% of furosemide is eliminated by metabolism to the inactive glucuronide. Only the unmetabolized and secreted fraction is available to inhibit NaCl reabsorption. In contrast, bumetanide and torasemide are metabolized in the liver.[92-94] The bioavailability of torasemide is significantly greater than that of furosemide and its duration of action is approximately twice as long,[95] but clinically relevant differences in salt-depleting action are not evident.[96]

In patients with chronic renal insufficiency (CRI) the elimination of furosemide, unlike bumetanide or torasemide,[95] is greatly reduced because its metabolism to the inactive glucuronide occurs in the kidney, whereas metabolic inactivation of bumetanide and torasemide occurs mainly in the liver and therefore they are unaffected by uremia.[8] This prolongs the $t_{1/2}$ of furosemide in CRI, leading to drug accumulation. However, the fraction of a dose excreted unchanged in patients with CRI is greater for furosemide, leading to an enhanced natriuretic response (Fig. 54-5). There is therefore a tradeoff when selecting a loop diuretic in CRI: furosemide can accumulate and cause ototoxicity at high dose, whereas

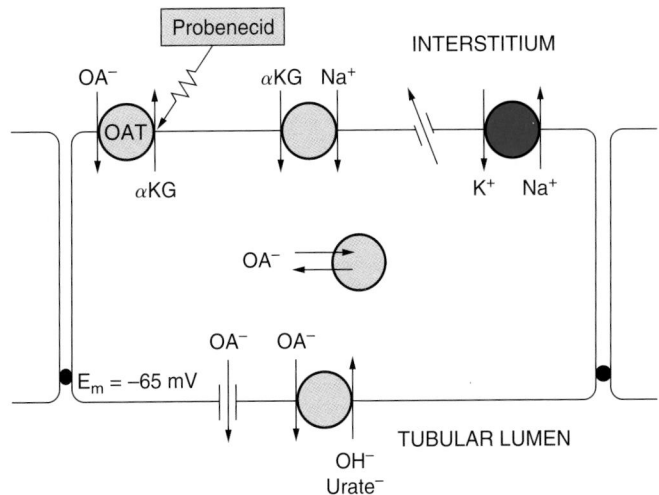

FIGURE 54-4. Cell diagram of the S2 segment of the proximal tubule showing secretion of organic anions (OA), such as diuretics. Peritubular uptake by an organic anion transporter (OAT) is in exchange for α-ketoglutarate (αKG). Organic anions can be sequestered in intracellular organelles. Luminal secretion can be via a voltage-dependent pathway or in exchange for luminal hydroxyl (OH⁻) or urate. (After Wilcox CS: New insights into diuretic use in patients with chronic renal disease. J Am Soc Nephrol 13:798-805, 2002.)

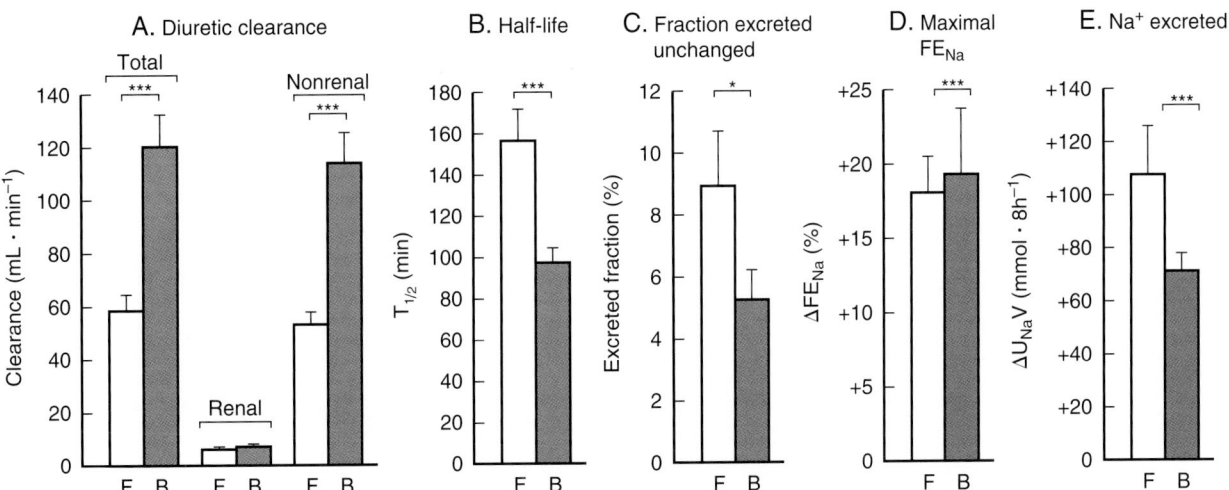

FIGURE 54-5. Comparison of the pharmacokinetics and dynamics of furosemide (F, 160 mg; metabolically inactivated in the kidney) and bumetanide (B, 4 mg; metabolically inactivated in the liver) in 10 subjects with chronic renal insufficiency (mean creatinine clearance 12 ± 2 mL/minute). Significance of difference: *, $P < .05$; ***, $P < .005$. (Redrawn from data in Voelker JR, Cartwright-Brown D, Anderson S, et al: Comparison of loop diuretics in patients with chronic renal insufficiency. Kidney Int 32:572-578, 1987.)

bumetanide retains its metabolic inactivation but is therefore somewhat less potent.

Renal clearance of the active form of loop diuretics falls in proportion to the creatinine clearance.[97] CAIs, thiazides, and loop diuretics are bound strongly to plasma albumin, which limits filtration. They gain access to tubular fluid almost exclusively by probenecid-inhibitable proximal secretion. Recent studies have characterized this weak organic anion (OA⁻) transport process. Four isoforms of an OAT have been cloned and are expressed in the kidney.[91, 98] Peritubular uptake by an OAT is a tertiary active process (see Fig. 54-4). Energy derives from the basolateral Na⁺,K⁺-ATPase that provides a low intracellular [Na⁺] that drives an uptake of Na⁺ coupled to α-ketoglutarate (αKG⁻) to maintain a high intracellular level of αKG⁻. This in turn drives a basolateral OA⁻/αKG⁻ countertransporter. OAT translocates diuretics into the proximal tubule cell where they can be sequestered in intracellular vesicles. They are secreted across the luminal membrane by a voltage-driven OA⁻ transporter[99] and by a countertransporter in exchange for urate or OH⁻.[98] There is competition both for peritubular uptake[91] and for luminal secretion[99] with other OA⁻, including urate that accumulates in uremia. Metabolic acidosis depolarizes the membrane potential (E_m) of proximal tubule cells,[100] which decreases OA⁻ secretion,[99] which explains why diuretic secretion is enhanced by alkalosis.[101] Therefore, the increased plasma levels of OA⁻ and urate and the metabolic acidosis of CRIs impair proximal tubule secretion of diuretics, and hence impair their delivery to their active sites in the nephron.

Proximal secretion of active furosemide is potentiated by albumin.[102] In the rabbit, an equal fraction of administered furosemide is taken up by a probenecid-sensitive mechanism into the S1 segment of the proximal tubule, where it is conjugated and excreted as the inactive glucuronide[103] (Fig. 54-6). Unlike the uptake and secretion of active furosemide by the S2 segment, uptake and metabolism by the S1 segment is enhanced by a fall in albumin concentration. Therefore, a low serum albumin concentration enhances furosemide metabolism,[104] yet decreases tubular secretion of active diuretic.[102.] The consequences of this are described later (see "Clinical Uses of Diuretics": "Nephrotic Syndrome").

There is normally a sigmoidal relationship between natriuresis and the log of the excretion of loop diuretic (Fig. 54-7). Inhibition of proximal secretion with probenecid increases the plasma diuretic concentration but does not perturb the relationship between natriuresis and diuretic excretion.[105] Thus, the natriuresis is related to the urinary, but not the plasma, diuretic concentration. The administration of indomethacin or other nonsteroidal anti-inflammatory drugs (NSAIDs) reduces the responsiveness of the tubule to furosemide.[106] This is due predominantly to reduced generation of PGE_2, because a natriuretic response to furosemide can be restored in indomethacin-treated rats by infusion of PGE_2.[107] A reduced dietary salt intake and repeated administration of furosemide during salt restriction[108] both diminish the renal tubular response to furosemide (see Fig. 54-7).

Most loop diuretics are water-soluble weak acids (pK_a ranges from 3.5-4.1),[109] Indacrinone and tienilic acid are uricosuric.[75, 78]

New loop diuretics, such as torasemide,[94] azosemide,[110] tripamide,[111] and piretanide,[112] resemble furosemide.[113] Slow-release forms are more effective in reducing blood pressure and treating edema.[114] Indacrinone has two enantiomers; one is a potent loop diuretic, but both are uricosuric.[115] Torasemide has a more prolonged action,[93] but this does

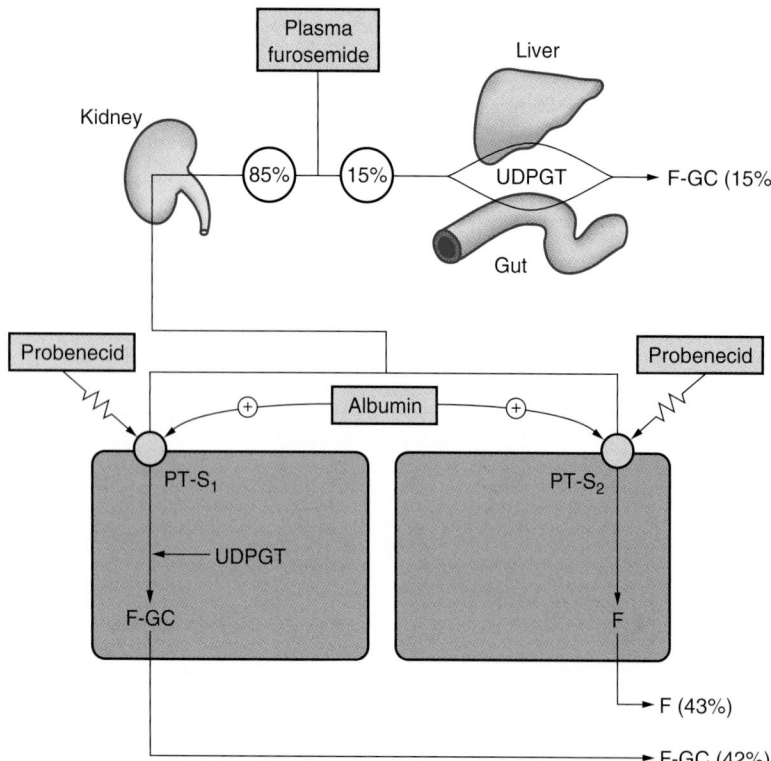

FIGURE 54-6. Diagrammatic representation of the disposition of intravenous furosemide and the effects of hypoalbuminemia or probenecid in normal or hypoalbuminemic rabbits. After intravenous furosemide, 15% is metabolized by uridine diphosphate glucoronyl transferase (UDPGT) in the liver and gut to the inactive furosemide gluconide (F-GC). Of the remainder, 85% is transported by the kidney. Some 42% is taken up in the Sl segment of the proximal tubule (PT-S₁) and metabolized to the inactive gluconide while the remainder is taken up by the S2 segment (PT-S₂) and secreted in active form into the lumen. Both uptake processes are inhibited by probenecid. Plasma albumin concentration facilitates uptake and secretion by PT-S₂ but inhibits uptake and metabolism by PT-S₁. (Drawn from data in Pichette V, Geadah D, du Souich P: The influence of moderate hypoalbuminemia on the renal metabolism and dynamics of furosemide in the rabbit. Br J Pharmacol 119:885, 1996.)

little[94] or nothing[116] to improve efficacy in patients with cirrhosis and ascites. However, longer-acting loop diuretics induce less neurohumoral stimulation in patients with congestive heart failure (CHF).[117] Bumetanide and torasemide are more completely absorbed (>80%) than furosemide. Therefore, changing from intravenous to oral dosing requires a doubling of dose of furosemide, but not of bumetanide or torasemide. Moreover, there is considerable variation in furosemide absorption, both between patients and over time,[118] which is accentuated by food intake.[119] This pharmacokinetic variability of furosemide leads to a less predictable effectiveness in patients with CHF who were found in a controlled trial to have fewer hospitalizations and better quality of life if randomized to torasemide.[120]

CLINICAL INDICATIONS. These are described under "Clinical Uses of Diuretics."

ADVERSE EFFECTS. These are discussed under "Adverse Effects of Diuretics."

Thiazides

SITES AND MECHANISMS OF ACTION. The major site of action of thiazide diuretics is the early distal convoluted tubule, where they block 40% of coupled reabsorption of Na$^+$ and Cl$^-$ (see Fig. 54-2).[67, 121, 122] Thiazides do not augment K$^+$ secretion directly.[121, 123] The water-soluble thiazides (e.g., chlorothiazide and hydrochlorothiazide) inhibit carbonic anhydrase.[124]

The thiazide-sensitive Na$^+$/Cl$^-$ cotransporter (TSC) is expressed in the distal convoluted tubule (DCT)[125, 126] and the connecting tubule.[125] Patients with Gitelman syndrome have a loss-of-function mutation in the TSC and an impaired response to a thiazide.[127]

Mineralocorticosteroids, glucocorticosteroids,[128] and estrogens[129] enhance thiazide binding and tubular actions.

In the absence of AVP, reabsorption of NaCl from the early DCT dilutes the tubular fluid. Therefore, thiazides impair maximal urinary dilution, but not maximal urinary concentration,[130] thereby predisposing to hyponatremia.

Three mechanisms have been identified for the thiazide-induced reduction in Ca^{2+} excretion (see Fig. 54-3). First, blockade of luminal NaCl entry reduces the tubule cell [Na$^+$] sufficiently to enhance the basolateral Na$^+$/Ca^{2+} exchange.[131]

Second, thiazides can stimulate Ca^{2+} permeability.[132] Third, thiazides can stimulate proximal reabsorption of Ca^{2+} in response to ECV depletion.[133] Thiazides produce a sustained reduction in renal Ca^{2+} excretion, which is accompanied by a small rise in serum Ca^{2+} concentration (S$_{Ca}$).[134] The reduction in Ca^{2+} excretion can counteract osteoporosis (see under "Clinical Use of Diuretics": "Osteoporosis").

Excretion of Mg^{2+} is enhanced during prolonged therapy[135] (see Fig. 54-3). K$^+$ depletion depolarizes the DCT luminal membrane and blocks Mg^{2+} uptake. Therefore, the Mg^{2+} depletion that can occur during chronic thiazide administration may be augmented by K$^+$ depletion.[135]

Thiazides reduce urate clearance secondary to ECV depletion[76] and competition for tubular uptake.[90]

Thiazides cause vasorelaxation by enhancement of calcium-activated K$^+$ channels.[136] Indapamide is a calcium channel antagonist.[136]

PHARMACOKINETICS AND DIFFERENCES BETWEEN DRUGS. Thiazides are readily absorbed. They are extensively bound to plasma proteins. They are eliminated largely by secretion by the S2 segment of the proximal tubule.[90] The t$_{1/2}$ is prolonged in renal failure and in the elderly, which reduces natriuretic efficacy.[137] The more lipid-soluble drugs (e.g., bendroflumethiazide and polythiazide) are more potent, have a more prolonged action, and are more extensively metabolized.[138] Chlorthalidone has a particularly prolonged action.[138] Indapamide is sufficiently metabolized to limit accumulation in renal failure.[138]

Thiazides can inhibit proximal carbonic anhydrase.[139]

CLINICAL INDICATIONS. These are described under "Clinical Uses of Diuretics."

ADVERSE EFFECTS. These are described under "Adverse Effects of Diuretics."

Distal Potassium-Sparing Diuretic Agents

Distal K$^+$-sparing diuretics comprise those that directly inhibit luminal Na$^+$ entry (e.g., amiloride and triamterene) and competitive antagonists of aldosterone (e.g., spironolactone and eplerenone).

SITES AND MECHANISMS OF ACTION. Distal K$^+$-sparing diuretics act on the principal cells in the late DCT and initial connecting tubule and the cortical CD, where

RENAL RESPONSE TO FUROSEMIDE IN HUMANS: EFFECTS OF INDOMETHACIN, SALT RESTRICTION, AND REPEATED FUROSEMIDE ADMINISTRATION

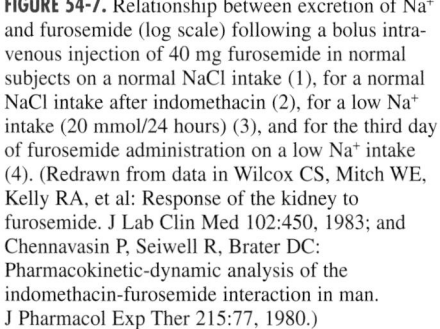
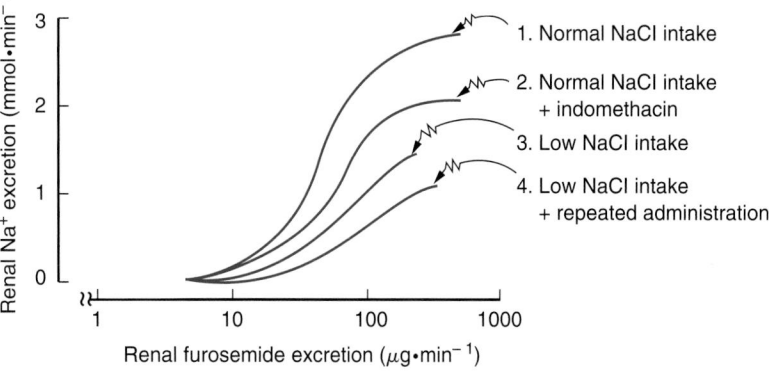

FIGURE 54-7. Relationship between excretion of Na$^+$ and furosemide (log scale) following a bolus intravenous injection of 40 mg furosemide in normal subjects on a normal NaCl intake (1), for a normal NaCl intake after indomethacin (2), for a low Na$^+$ intake (20 mmol/24 hours) (3), and for the third day of furosemide administration on a low Na$^+$ intake (4). (Redrawn from data in Wilcox CS, Mitch WE, Kelly RA, et al: Response of the kidney to furosemide. J Lab Clin Med 102:450, 1983; and Chennavasin P, Seiwell R, Brater DC: Pharmacokinetic-dynamic analysis of the indomethacin-furosemide interaction in man. J Pharmacol Exp Ther 215:77, 1980.)

1. Normal NaCl intake
2. Normal NaCl intake + indomethacin
3. Low NaCl intake
4. Low NaCl intake + repeated administration

they inhibit luminal Na$^+$ entry (see Fig. 54-2).[122, 140] The fall in cellular [Na$^+$] diminishes basolateral Na$^+$,K$^+$-ATPase.[122] This reduces cellular [K$^+$], which, together with hyperpolarization of the apical membrane, diminishes the electrochemical gradient for K$^+$ and H$^+$ secretion.[122, 140] The genes for the amiloride-sensitive Na$^+$ channel have been cloned.

Trimethoprim and pentamidine have amiloride-like actions and can cause hyperkalemia.[141] Trimethoprim-induced hyperkalemia can be prevented by increasing distal Na$^+$ delivery with saline infusion or furosemide[142] or by urinary alkalinization, which converts trimethoprim to an inactive, electroneutral compound.[143]

These drugs cause a modest natriuresis. Their more important actions are to reduce the excretion of K$^+$ and net acid, especially when distal secretion is augmented by aldosteronism.[144] Amiloride and triamterene reduce the excretion of Ca^{2+} and Mg^{2+}.[74, 135]

PHARMACOKINETICS. Triamterene is well absorbed. It is rapidly hydroxylated to metabolites that retain diuretic actions.[145] The drug and its metabolites are secreted by the OAT pathway in the proximal tubule[7] (see Fig. 54-4), with half-lives of 3 to 5 hours. Triamterene and its active metabolites accumulate in patients with cirrhosis because of decreased biliary secretion,[146] and in the elderly,[137, 145] and in those with renal disease[137] because of decreased renal excretion.

Amiloride is incompletely absorbed. It is secreted into the tubular fluid.[147] Its duration of action is approximately 18 hours. It accumulates in renal failure[148] and may worsen renal function.[149]

Spironolactone is readily absorbed. It is bound to plasma proteins. It is metabolized to active compounds (canrenones), which are further metabolized by cytochrome P-450IIIA.[150] It enters distal renal tubules from the plasma.[151] Spironolactone has a t$_{1/2}$ of 20 hours. It takes 10 to 48 hours to become maximally effective.[152] During fludrocortisone administration, spironolactone (25-100 mg) causes dose-dependent natriuresis and reduction in kaliuresis.[153] Increasing the dose produces little further benefit.[154]

CLINICAL INDICATIONS. Distal K$^+$-sparing agents are used primarily or as K$^+$-sparing agents in patients with hypokalemic alkalosis.[155] Amiloride can prevent amphotericin-induced hypokalemia and hypomagnesemia.[156]

ADVERSE EFFECTS AND DRUG INTERACTIONS. The risk of hyperkalemia is dose-dependent and increases considerably in patients with renal failure or in those receiving K$^+$ supplements, angiotensin-converting enzyme inhibitors (ACEIs), angiotensin receptor blockers (ARBs), NSAIDs, β-blockers, heparin, or ketoconazole.[144] Impaired net acid excretion can cause metabolic acidosis,[157] which worsens hyperkalemia.

Amiloride and triamterene accumulate in renal failure[145, 148] and triamterene accumulates in cirrhosis.[146] Therefore, these drugs should be avoided in these situations.

Triamterene occasionally precipitates in the urinary collecting system and causes obstruction.[158] It can cause ARF when given with indomethacin.[159] Spironolactone can cause gastrointestinal distress and antiandrogenic effects (e.g., impotence, loss of libido, gynecomastia, or postmenopausal bleeding).[160, 161] Gynecomastia is dose-related.[161] A related drug, eplerenone, causes less gynecomastia.

DOPAMINERGIC AGONISTS. In low doses (1-3 μg/kg/minute) dopamine is natriuretic, owing primarily to a modest increase in the GFR and reduction in proximal reabsorption attributed to a cAMP-induced inhibition of the Na$^+$/H$^+$ antiporter.[162] Fenoldopam is a selective dopamine type 1 (DA1) receptor agonist with little cardiac stimulation.[163] Unfortunately, studies in patients with CHF or alcoholic cirrhosis have shown only modest natriuresis.[163] Ibopamine has a modest effect, but less than furosemide, in patients with CHF.[164]

At higher doses, the pressor response to dopamine might be beneficial in patients with hypotensive shock,[165] but it has little or no renal effect in critically ill or septic patients.[166] Controlled trials have failed to detect an improved outcome in patients given dopamine.[162, 165] Renal-dose dopamine for the treatment of ARF lacks efficacy, is expensive, and can cause cardiac arrhythmias.[167]

ADENOSINE TYPE I RECEPTOR ANTAGONISTS. Aminophylline is an adenosine receptor antagonist that inhibits NaCl reabsorption in the proximal tubule and diluting segments and causes a modest increase in GFR.[168] Aminophylline (400 mg intravenously) produces an additional natriuresis in patients with CHF receiving optimal doses of loop diuretics.[169] Highly selective adenosine I (A$_1$) receptor antagonists are natriuretic,[170, 171] antihypertensive,[172] and potentiate furosemide-induced natriuresis in normal humans[173] and in patients with diuretic-resistant CHF.[173] A$_1$ antagonists disrupt glomerulotubular balance and TGF, thereby decreasing proximal reabsorption and increasing GFR.[170]

VASOPRESSIN ANTAGONISTS. Nonpeptide, orally active vasopressin V$_2$ receptor antagonists cause free water diuresis without appreciable natriuresis in water-deprived human subjects.[174] They increase urine volume, free water clearance, and serum sodium concentration (S$_{Na}$) in hyponatremic patients with SIADH.[175] These agents improve cardiac hemodynamics in animal models of cardiac failure.[176]

ADAPTATION TO DIURETIC THERAPY

Diuretics entrain a set of homeostatic mechanisms that limit their fluid-depleting actions and contribute to diuretic resistance and adverse effects.

Diuretic Braking Phenomenon

The first dose of a diuretic normally produces a reassuring diuresis. However, in normal subjects a new equilibrium is attained within 1 day when body weight stabilizes and daily fluid and electrolyte excretion no longer exceeds intake.[108]

The patterns of Na$^+$ excretion during 3 days of loop diuretic administration to normal human subjects are shown in Figure 54-8.[108, 177, 178] During a high Na$^+$ intake (280 mmol/24 hours), furosemide causes a large negative Na$^+$ balance over the ensuing 6 hours (dark blue in Fig. 54-8A) followed by 18 hours when Na$^+$ excretion is reduced well below intake (postdiuresis salt retention), which results in positive Na$^+$ balance (medium blue in Fig. 54-8A) that is quantitatively equivalent to the preceding period of negative Na$^+$ balance. The natriuresis caused by the third daily dose of furosemide is strictly comparable to the first dose and also is followed by a restoration of Na$^+$ balance. Consequently, at high levels of Na$^+$ intake, subjects regain neutral Na$^+$ balance within 24 hours of each dose of furosemide and

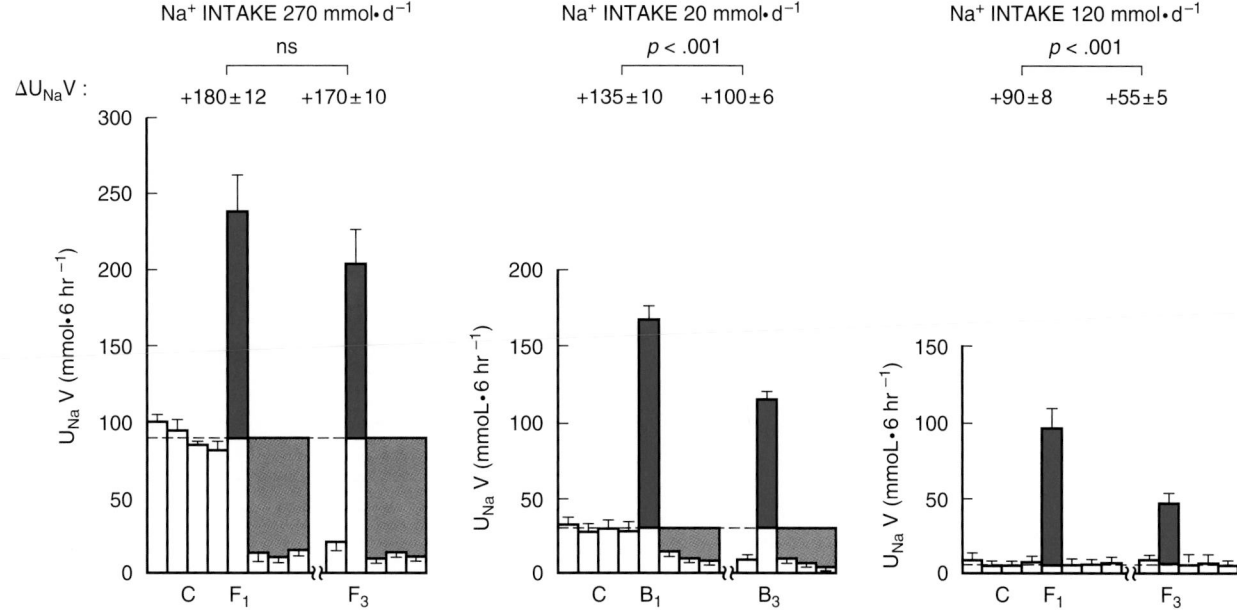

FIGURE 54-8. Effects of dietary salt intake on diuretic braking phenomenon showing renal Na^+ excretion (mmol/6 hours) for 24 hours before and after the first (F_1) and third (F_3) daily doses of furosemide (40 mg intravenously) or bumetanide (B, 1 mg intravenously) in groups of 8 to 10 normal subjects equilibrated to fixed daily Na^+ intakes. The average level of Na^+ intake (mmol/6 hours) is shown by the *broken horizontal line*. Negative Na^+ balance is indicated by the *dark blue* and positive Na^+ balance by the *medium blue*. The mean ± SEM values for diuretic-induced increases in Na^+ excretion above baseline values for 6 hours after the administration of the diuretic are shown at the top. (Redrawn from data in Wilcox CS, Mitch WE, Kelly RA, et al: Response of the kidney to furosemide. J Lab Clin Med 102:450, 1983.)

maintain their original body weight. A similar diuretic braking phenomenon occurs during established furosemide therapy.[80]

During severe dietary Na^+ restriction (20 mmol/24 hours), the first dose of furosemide produces a blunted natriuresis (see Fig. 54-8C). Although renal Na^+ excretion reverts abruptly to low levels after each diuresis, Na^+ balance cannot be restored because of the low level of dietary Na^+ intake. Consequently, virtually all the Na^+ lost during the diuretic phase is represented as negative Na^+ balance for the day. Unlike the high-salt protocol, tolerance manifests as a 40% reduction in the natriuretic response to the drug over 3 days. However, despite a blunted initial response and the development of tolerance, all subjects lose Na^+ and body weight.

A loop diuretic given during an Na^+ intake of 120 mmol/24 hours (equivalent to a "no added salt" diet) leads to Na^+ loss that is curtailed by a combination of postdiuretic renal salt retention and diuretic tolerance (see Fig. 54-8B).[179]

Furosemide kinetics and GFR are unchanged over 3 days of furosemide administration. What, then, mediates diuretic tolerance? During a low NaCl intake, the relationship between natriuresis and furosemide excretion is shifted to the right by the third day of diuretic administration (see Fig. 54-7), indicating a blunting of diuretic responsiveness.

One month of furosemide therapy for hypertension reduces the natriuretic response to a test dose of furosemide by 18%.[80] This tolerance cannot be ascribed to aldosterone, nor to a fall in plasma or ECV, because tolerance to furosemide is not prevented by spironolactone and does not develop during thiazide therapy, which causes similar reductions in body fluids. In fact, the natriuretic response to a test dose of a thiazide is augmented during furosemide therapy. Thus, tolerance to furosemide is class-specific and is dependent on increased NaCl reabsorption at a downstream, thiazide-sensitive nephron site.

Furosemide activates the renin-angiotensin-aldosterone (RAA) axis[178] and sympathetic nervous system.[178] However, postdiuretic Na^+ retention is not blunted by doses of an ACEI which prevents any changes in plasma AII or aldosterone concentrations,[178, 180, 181] or by prazosin, which blocks adrenergic receptors even when given in combination.[177] A natriuretic calcium entry blocker does not modify postdiuretic Na^+ retention.[179]

Micropuncture studies have shown that the blunted natriuretic response to furosemide during repeated administration can be attributed to three factors: a reduced NaCl delivery to the site of furosemide action; a limited inhibition of NaCl reabsorption by furosemide in the loop of Henle; and an enhanced ability of the distal tubule to reabsorb the extra NaCl load delivered during furosemide's upstream action.[182]

Rats receiving prolonged infusions of loop diuretics have considerable structural hypertrophy of the DCT, connecting tubule, and intercalated cells of the CD[183-185] that are partially dependent on AII.[186] The DCT and CD have a large increase in messenger RNA (mRNA) for insulin-like growth factor–binding protein-1[187] and increased Na^+,K^+-[188] and H^+-ATPase.[183] The Na^+,K^+-ATPase activity of rat cortical CD segments increases abruptly following an increase in cellular [Na^+], owing to mobilization of a latent pool of enzyme.[189] There is doubling of NCC expression in the distal tubules of rats adapted to diuretics that is partially dependent on hyperaldosteronism.[190] Microperfusion studies of rats adapted to prolonged diuretic infusion have shown enhanced, aldosterone-independent distal Na^+ and Cl^- absorption and K^+ secretion.[191] Therefore, diuretics induce structural and functional adaptations of downstream nephron segments, apparently in response to increased rates of NaCl delivery and to some extent on RAA axis activation. Nephronal adaptation could explain the inappropriate renal Na+ retention that can persist for up to 2 weeks after abrupt cessation of diuretic therapy.[192]

Normal subjects eliminate a modest (100 mmol) NaCl load over 2 days.[193] However, when challenged with the same NaCl load delivered after administration of bumetanide during simultaneous infusion of sufficient fluid, Na+,K+, and Cl− to prevent any losses, the elimination of the load is prevented. Thus, diuretics can entrain an ECV-independent NaCl retention apparent when distal delivery is enhanced, as during high NaCl intake.

Even a single dose of loop diuretic causes a Cl− depletion "contraction" alkalosis.[64] In a study of normal subjects with a mild metabolic alkalosis produced by equimolar substitution of NaHCO₃ for NaCl, bumetanide-induced natriuresis was reduced during alkalosis despite enhanced delivery of bumetanide to the urine (Fig. 54-9).[101] This implies a profound defect in tubular responsiveness to the diuretic. Several mechanisms may contribute. First, the Na+/K+/2Cl− cotransporter has affinities for Na+, K+, and Cl− of 7.0, 1.3, and 67 mM, respectively. Thus, the [Cl−] of tubular fluid may be sufficiently low during Cl− depletion alkalosis to limit reabsorption by this transporter and thereby to limit the responsiveness to loop diuretics. Second, alkalosis causes glycosylation of the bumetanide-sensitive cotransporter that could alter its transport function.[57] Third, thiazide-sensitive cotransporters in the rat DCT are increased by 40% during NaHCO₃ administration.[194]

There are several clinical implications from these studies. First, dietary salt intake must be restricted, even in subjects receiving powerful loop diuretics, to obviate postdiuretic salt retention and to ensure the development of a negative NaCl balance. Second, during prolonged diuretic administration, subjects may be particularly responsive to another class of diuretic. Third, diuretic therapy should not be stopped abruptly unless dietary salt intake is effectively curtailed, because the adaptive mechanisms limiting salt excretion persist for days after diuretic use. Fourth, selection of a diuretic with a prolonged action, or more frequent administration of the diuretic, will enhance NaCl loss by limiting the time available for postdiuretic salt retention. Indeed, a continuous infusion of a loop diuretic is more effective than the same dose given as a bolus injection in volunteers,[195] in patients with cardiac disease,[196] and in those with chronic renal failure[197] despite a similar delivery of diuretic to the urine. Fifth, prevention or reversal of diuretic-induced metabolic alkalosis may enhance diuretic efficacy.

There are similar patterns of furosemide-induced K+ loss followed by renal K+ retention[198] associated with an increase in the transtubular K+ gradient.[199] In contrast, loop diuretics induce ongoing renal K+ losses during severe salt restriction due to hyperaldosteronism[198] that can be countered by distal, K+-sparing diuretics.[199]

Humoral and Neuronal Modulators of the Response to Diuretics

RENIN-ANGIOTENSIN-ALDOSTERONE AXIS. Diuretic therapy increases plasma renin activity and serum aldosterone concentrations (SACs). The initial increase in renin with loop diuretics is independent of volume depletion or the sympathetic nervous system (SNS) and is related to inhibition of NaCl reabsorption at the macula densa.[200] Loop diuretics also stimulate renal prostacyclin release, which promotes renin secretion.[201] Later, renin secretion is dependent on ECV depletion and the SNS.

Patients treated with diuretics and salt restriction for poorly compensated edema often have sufficient activation of the RAA axis to limit the clearance of edema.[202] In a study of patients with CHF, ACE inhibition potentiated the diuretic and natriuretic responses to furosemide despite a fall in blood pressure.[203] However, severe volume depletion and azotemia can complicate overzealous therapy with ACEIs, particularly in patients with CHF receiving high doses of diuretics or in those with stenosis of both renal arteries or the artery to a single or dominant kidney.[204, 205] Thus, the combination of diuretics and ACEIs can be highly effective but requires careful surveillance.

When the RAA axis is stimulated by severe dietary salt restriction, further diuretic-induced increases in SAC can promote renal K+ losses.[206] ACEIs counter diuretic-induced increases in SAC and blunt diuretic-induced hypokalemia.[198]

PROSTAGLANDINS. PGE₂ acting on luminal E₂ prostaglandin type 4 (EP₄) receptors inhibits NaCl reabsorption via the Na+,K+,2Cl− cotransporter [207] and inhibits free water and Na+ absorption in the CDs via changes in cAMP (Fig. 54-10).[208]

Loop diuretics, thiazides, triamterene, and spironolactone increase PGs substantially.[209] Inhibition of PG synthesis

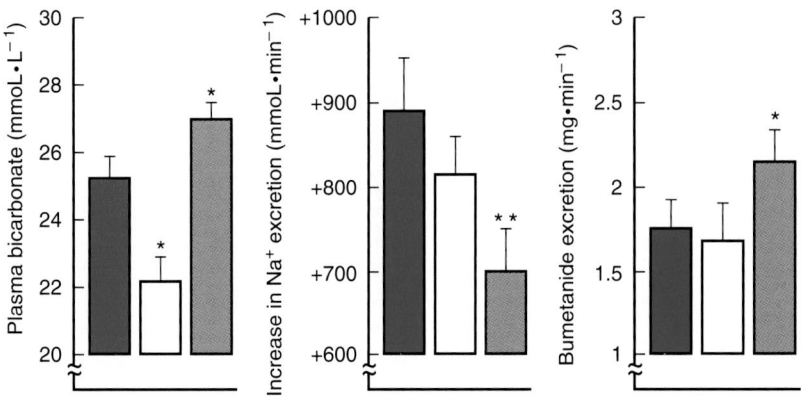

FIGURE 54-9. Mean ± SEM values for plasma bicarbonate concentration, increase in Na+ excretion with bumetanide (1 mg intravenously), and rate of bumetanide excretion in normal subjects (n = 8) after equilibration to equivalent diets containing 100 mmol/24 hours of NaCl (control, *dark blue boxes*), NH₄Cl (mild metabolic acidosis, *open boxes*), or NaHCO₃ (mild metabolic alkalosis, *medium blue boxes*). Compared with control: *$P < .05$; **$P < .01$. (Redrawn from Loon NR, Wilcox CS: Mild metabolic alkalosis impairs the natriuretic response to bumetanide in normal human subjects. Clin Sci (Colch) 94:287, 1998.)

by NSAIDs (e.g., indomethacin) can diminish the natriuresis and diuresis induced by furosemide,[210] hydrochlorothiazide,[211] spironolactone,[209] or triamterene.[212] Microperfusion of the loop segment with PGE_2[107] restores the response to furosemide in indomethacin-treated rats. Indomethacin also blunts furosemide-induced renal[213] and capacitance vessel vasodilation[214] and stimulation of renin.[215] The blunting of furosemide-induced natriuresis by NSAIDs is potentiated by salt depletion [216] and is prominent in edematous patients.[210, 217] Recent studies in rats indicate that cyclooxygenase-2 (COX-2) blockers also may impair the response to furosemide (Fig. 54-11).

Loop diuretics also increase the excretion of the thromboxane A_2 (TXA_2) metabolite TXB_2. Inhibition of TXA_2 synthesis or receptors in the rat increases furosemide diuresis[218] and diminishes the renal vasodilation.[219] Thus, TXA_2 may antagonize the actions of loop diuretics.

ARGININE VASOPRESSIN. AVP increases after administration of furosemide to rats[220] or to water-deprived subjects[221]

but not to those allowed access to water.[222] This may be a response to a reduced blood volume. Plasma AVP is increased in many edematous states, such as CHF,[223] especially in those who develop hyponatremia during thiazide treatment.[176, 224] AVP stimulates K^+ secretion in the rat distal tubule.[225] Diuretic-induced AVP release contributes to hypokalemia, because the kaliuretic response to furosemide is reduced by 40% in subjects whose AVP release is suppressed by a water load.[206] AVP also offsets furosemide-induced reduction in peripheral vascular resistance.[220, 226]

CATECHOLAMINES AND SYMPATHETIC NERVOUS SYSTEM. The first dose of furosemide increases the heart rate and plasma catecholamine concentrations.[101, 177] However, blockade of α_1-adrenergic-receptors with prazosin does not modify the response to furosemide or the ensuing renal salt retention[177] but blockade of β-adrenergic-receptors blunts the renin release.[200]

Short-term, furosemide-induced ECV depletion in the conscious rat activates baroreceptor-induced increases in

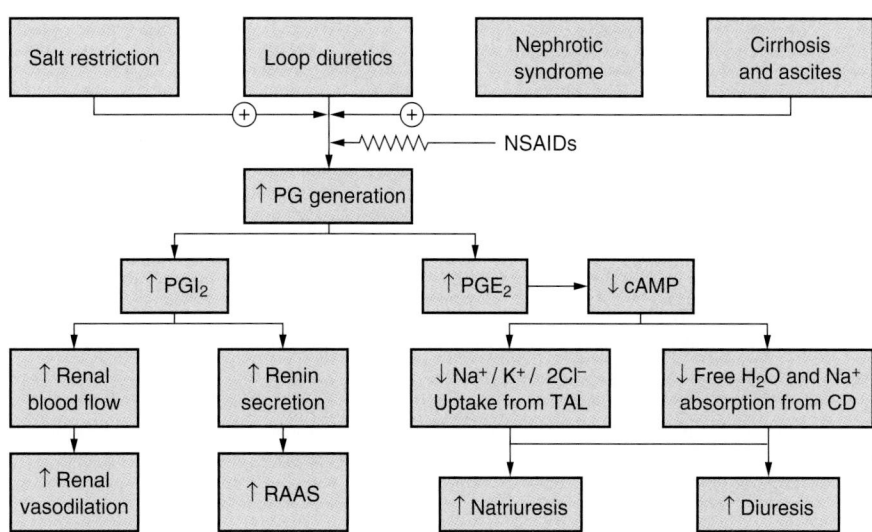

FIGURE 54-10. Flow diagram showing some effects of loop diuretics that are facilitated by prostaglandin (PG) release. These are potentiated in subjects who are salt-depleted or have edema due to the nephrotic syndrome or cirrhosis and ascites in whom nonsteroidal anti-inflammatory drugs (NSAIDs) cause marked blunting of diuretic actions. Generation of prostacyclin (PGI_2) causes renal vasodilation but stimulates renin release, leading to activation of the renin-angiotensin-aldosterone system (RAAS). Generation of PGE_2 inhibits guanyl cyclase and cyclic adenosine monophosphate (cAMP), which inhibit the $Na^+/K^+/2Cl^-$ cotransporter in the thick ascending limb (TAL) at the loop of Henle and reduce free water and Na^+ absorption from the collecting ducts (CD). These effects of PGs promote the natriuretic and diuretic actions of loop diuretics.

EFFECTS OF COX-2 INHIBITION ON RENAL
RESPONSE TO FUROSEMIDE IN THE RAT

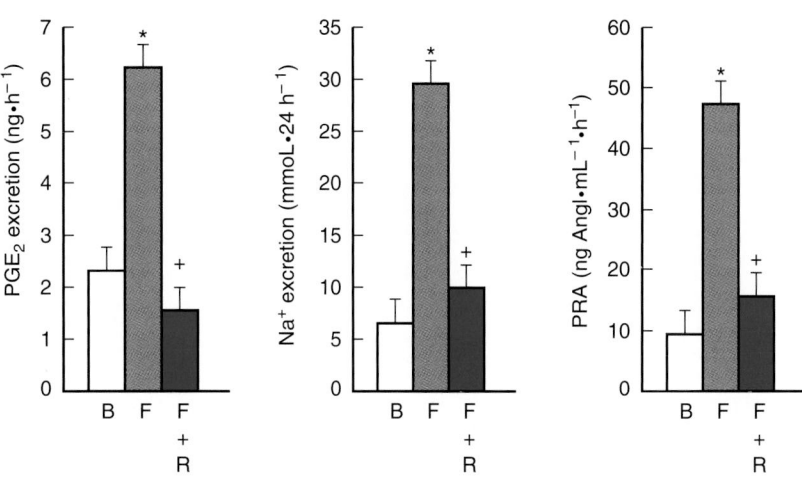

FIGURE 54-11. Mean ± SEM values for excretion of prostaglandin E_2 and sodium, and for plasma renin activity (PRA) of groups of rats studied before (B), after 7 days of furosemide (F, 12 mg/day) or after furosemide and 5 days of rofecoxib (F + R, 10 mg/day). Compared to B: *, $P < .05$; compared to F: t, $P < .05$. (Drawn from data in Kammerl MC, Nüsing RM, Richthammer W, et al: Inhibition of COX-2 counteracts the effects of diuretics in rats. Kidney Int 60:1684-1691, 2001.)

plasma norepinephrine[227] and muscle and renal sympathetic nerve activity that stabilizes the blood pressure.[228] Although chronic sympathectomy[229] or blockade of α-adrenergic-receptors[227, 230] blunts the increase in proximal fluid reabsorption that follows furosemide diuresis, this is offset by enhanced distal reabsorption so that natriuresis is unimpaired. Thus, the renal sympathetic nerves or circulating catecholamines contribute to the circulatory and proximal nephron adaptation to diuretic-induced fluid loss, yet they are not normally required for maintenance of Na^+ homeostasis during diuretic therapy.

ATRIAL NATRIURETIC PEPTIDE. Diuretics are often used to treat patients who have an expanded blood volume and elevated levels of ANP. Administration of furosemide to dogs with CHF reduces ANP levels.[231] Infusion of ANP in this dog model promotes furosemide-induced natriuresis and blunts the activation of the RAA axis and the fall in GFR. Thus, a fall in ANP may contribute to postdiuretic renal NaCl retention.[231]

NITRIC OXIDE AND KININS. Furosemide releases nitric oxide (NO) and PGs from cultured endothelial cells.[232] Administration of a bradykinin B_2 receptor antagonist blunts furosemide-induced diuresis, natriuresis, and reduction in renal vascular resistance.[233]

Diuretic Resistance

Diuretic resistance implies an inadequate clearance of edema despite a full dose of diuretic[5] (Table 54-1). The principal causes are summarized in Table 54-1. The first step is to select the appropriate target response (e.g., a specific body weight) and to ensure that the edema is due to inappropriate renal NaCl and fluid retention rather than to lymphatic or venous obstruction (Fig. 54-12). The next step is to exclude noncompliance, severe blood volume depletion, or concurrent NSAID use.[234] Thereafter, dietary NaCl intake should be quantitated. In the steady state, dietary Na^+ intake can be assessed from measurements of 24-hour Na^+ excretion.

TABLE 54-1

Common Causes of Diuretic Resistance

CAUSE	EXAMPLE
Incorrect diagnosis	Venous or lymphatic edema
Inappropriate NaCl or fluid intake	
Inadequate drug reaching tubule lumen in active form:	
Noncompliance	
Dose inadequate or too infrequent	
Poor absorption	Uncompensated CHF
Decreased renal blood flow	CHF, cirrhosis of liver, elderly
Decreased functional renal mass	ARF, CRI, elderly
Proteinuria	Nephrotic syndrome
Inadequate renal response:	
Low GFR	ARF, CRI
Decreased effective ECV	Edematous conditions
Activation of RAA axis	Edematous conditions
Nephron adaptation	Prolonged diuretic therapy
NSAIDs	Indomethacin, aspirin

ARF, acute renal failure; CHF, congestive heart failure; CRI, chronic renal insufficiency; ECV, extracellular fluid volume; GFR, glomerular filtration rate; NSAIDs, nonsteroidal anti-inflammatory drugs; RAA, renin-angiotensin-aldosterone.

For patients with mild edema or hypertension, a "no added salt" diet may be sufficient to reduce daily Na^+ intake to 100 to 120 mmol. For patients with diuretic resistance, the help of a dietitian is usually necessary to reduce daily Na^+ intake to 80 to 100 mmol. The next step is to double the dose or, better, to give two daily doses of the diuretic. Furosemide or bumetanide act for only 3 to 6 hours. Two divided doses, by interrupting postdiuretic salt retention, produce a greater response than the same total dose given once daily. Concurrent disease may impair the absorption of the diuretic. Thus a more bioavailable diuretic, such as torasemide, may be preferable.

Diuretic resistance is often accompanied by a pronounced metabolic alkalosis.[101] This may be reversed by KCl or by adding a distal K^+-sparing diuretic. Severe metabolic acidosis may also impair diuretic responsiveness.[235]

A progressive increase in diuretic dosage may produce an inadequate reduction in body fluids because of activation of NaCl-retaining mechanisms. ACEIs can sometimes restore a diuresis in resistant patients with CHF,[202] but a fall in blood pressure often limits the response. Adaptive changes in downstream nephron segments during prolonged diuretic therapy[80, 185] provide a rational basis for combining diuretics (see the following section).

If there is no response, the patient probably should be admitted for a trial of intravenous loop diuretic infusion or ultrafiltration.[236]

Diuretic Combinations

Full doses of diuretics acting on the same transport mechanism are less than additive, whereas diuretics acting on a separate mechanism may be synergistic.[5, 237]

LOOP DIURETICS AND THIAZIDES. A loop diuretic and a thiazide (e.g., hydrochlorothiazide or metolazone) are synergistic in normal subjects and in those with edema or renal insufficiency.[5, 237-241] Metolazone is equivalent to bendrofluazide in enhancing NaCl and fluid losses in furosemide-resistant subjects with CHF or the nephrotic syndrome.[242] During prolonged furosemide therapy, the responsiveness to a thiazide is augmented.[80] Patients with advanced chronic renal failure (GFR <30 mL/min) who are unresponsive to thiazide alone have a marked natriuresis when the thiazide is added to loop diuretic therapy,[240] probably by blockade of enhanced distal tubular Na^+ reabsorption.[243] However, such combination therapy should be initiated under close surveillance because of a high incidence of hypokalemia, excessive ECV depletion, and azotemia.[244]

LOOP DIURETICS OR THIAZIDES AND DISTAL POTASSIUM-SPARING DIURETICS. Amiloride or triamterene increases furosemide natriuresis only modestly but curtails the excretion of K^+ and net acid[63] and preserves total body K^+.[245, 246] Distal K^+-sparing agents are generally contraindicated in renal failure because they may cause severe hyperkalemia and acidosis.

ADVERSE EFFECTS OF DIURETICS

Although diuretic therapy is generally well tolerated, there is a spectrum of adverse effects.[247] A Medical Research Council (MRC) trial showed the following adverse effects occurred more frequently with thiazide than placebo: impaired

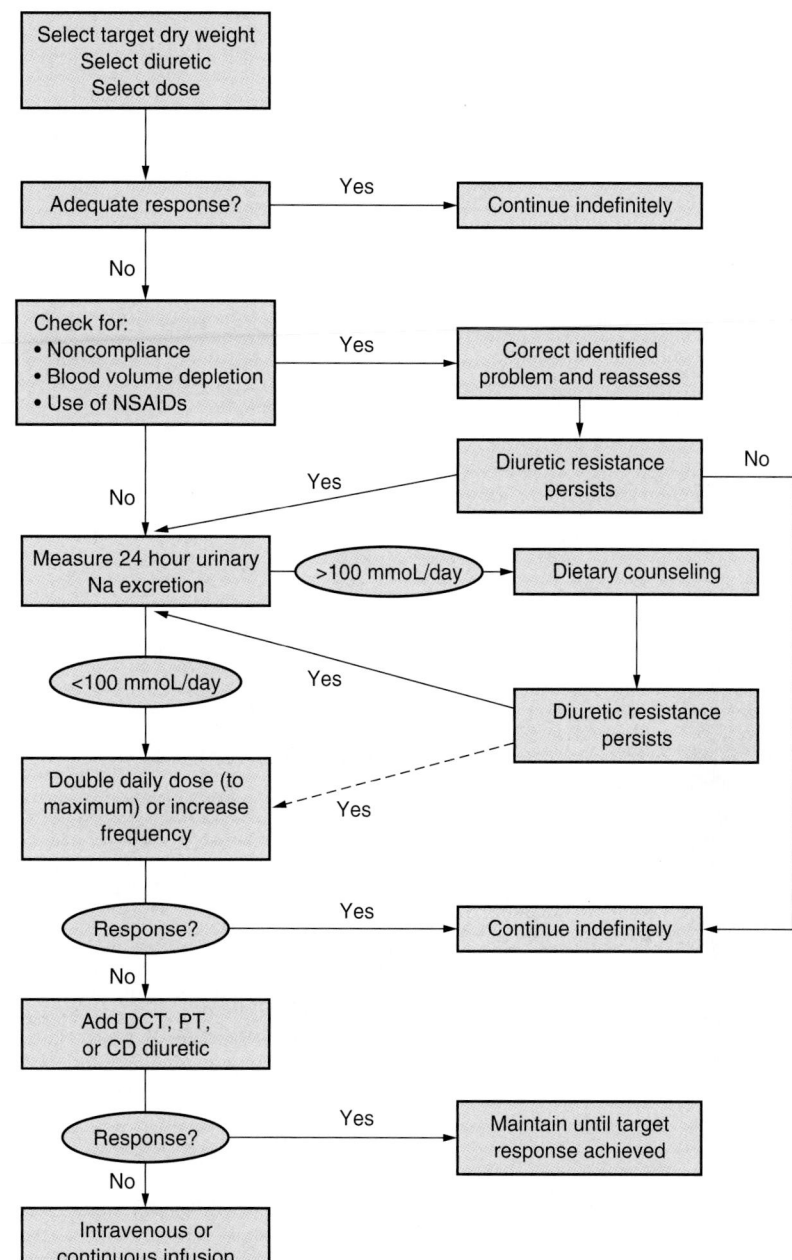

FIGURE 54-12. Diagrammatic representation of an approach to the management of a patient with resistance to a loop diuretic. CD, collecting duct diuretic (e.g., amiloride, triamterene, or spironolactone). DCT, distal convoluted tubule diuretic (e.g., thiazide); PT, proximal tubule diuretic (e.g., acetazolamide). (From Ellison DH, Wilcox CS: Diuretics: Use in edema and the problem of resistance. *In* Brady HR, Wilcox CS (eds): Therapy in Nephrology and Hypertension, 2nd ed. London, Elsevier Science Publishing Co, 2003.)

glucose tolerance, gout, impotence, lethargy, nausea, dizziness, headache, and constipation.[247] However, the withdrawal rate of those receiving a thiazide was similar to that for a β-blocker, and the dose of thiazide was higher than that used currently.

Fluid and Electrolyte Abnormalities

EXTRACELLULAR VOLUME DEPLETION AND AZOTEMIA. Diuretics normally do not decrease the GFR.[80, 248] However, renal failure can be precipitated by vigorous diuresis in patients with impaired renal function, severe edema, or cirrhosis and ascites. A rise in the ratio of blood urea nitrogen to creatinine suggests ECV depletion. This change can be ascribed to decreased renal urea clearance because of increased urea reabsorption in the distal nephron[249] and to increased urea appearance due to increased arginine uptake by the liver with metabolism by arginase.[250-252]

HYPONATREMIA. Two mechanisms can be identified. The first, illustrated in a self-experiment by McCance[253] (Fig. 54-13) of severe salt depletion by a salt-free diet and forced perspiration shows that the loss of the first 2 L of body fluid occurs isotonically. However, further obligated NaCl losses are not accompanied by corresponding fluid losses, leading to progressive hyponatremia. This is likely a consequence of AVP release in response to severe plasma volume depletion.[254] Despite salt depletion, the degree of hyponatremia is mild.

The second mechanism is illustrated in the study of Clark and colleagues.[255] They showed that older age and thiazide

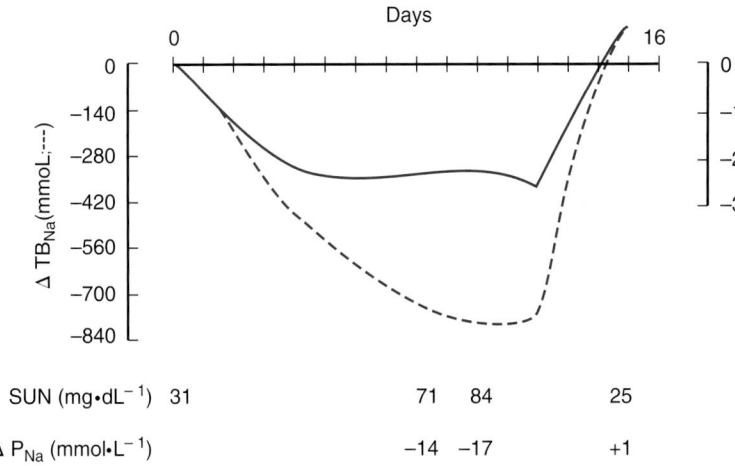

FIGURE 54-13. Data from normal volunteers subjected to progressive salt depletion over 12 days (followed by 3 days of salt repletion) caused by a zero salt intake and forced perspiration. Results shown are for changes in total body Na^+, body weight and plasma sodium concentration, and serum urea nitrogen. (Drawn from data in McCance RA: Experimental sodium chloride deficiency in man. Proc R Soc Lond B Biol Sci 119:245-268, 1936.)

diuretics are additive in impairing maximal free water excretion following a water load (Fig. 54-14). This effect is relatively specific for thiazides, which inhibit urinary dilution specifically, whereas loop diuretics inhibit urinary concentration and dilution.[256] Indeed, thiazides are 12-fold more likely than loop diuretics to cause hyponatremia.[257] Thiazide-induced hyponatremia usually entails an inappropriate fluid intake and an expanded total body water.[257-259] Estradiol enhances the expression of the thiazide-sensitive cotransporters in the DCT.[260] This may explain why 80% of thiazide-induced hyponatremia occurs in females,[261] most of whom are elderly.[262]

Hyponatremia can develop during rechallenge with a thiazide.[258, 263] It often develops within the first 2 weeks of thiazide therapy.[257, 263] Mild, asymptomatic hyponatremia can be treated by withdrawing diuretics, restricting the daily intake of free water to 1.0 to 1.5 L, restoring any K^+ and Mg^{2+} losses, and replenishing NaCl if the patient is clearly volume-depleted.[257] Severe, symptomatic hyponatremia complicated by seizures is an emergency requiring intensive treatment. The ideal management remains controversial.[261, 264, 265] Central pontine myelinolysis has been related to overcorrection of hyponatremia[264] or to a rapid corrective of S_{Na} by over 12 to 20 mmol/L in the first 24 hours.[261, 265, 266]

In one series, eight elderly patients with severe diuretic-induced hyponatremia (average S_{Na}= 110 mmol/L) and neurologic manifestations received 3% NaCl at 35 to 50 mL/hour and 20 mg furosemide intravenously after 6 and 24 hours of infusion. The S_{Na} was corrected over an average of 29 hours to 132 mmol/L at a rate of 0.8 mmol/L/hour. Seven patients recovered from their neurologic deficit, and none died from hyponatremia.[267] However, there is a high rate of permanent neurologic damage in patients with severe, symptomatic hyponatremia due to thiazide therapy that has been corrected slowly over 18 to 56 hours.[263] For symptomatic patients, some recommend an initial rate of infusion of 3% NaCl at 2 mL/kg/hour for 3 hours. This must be reduced sharply when the S_{Na} has increased by 6 to 8 mEq/L or if symptoms have abated.[257]

A survey of the members of the American Society of Nephrology identified 56 patients with severe hyponatremia.[268] Complications were correlated with the chronicity of hyponatremia and a high rate of correction of S_{Na} in the first

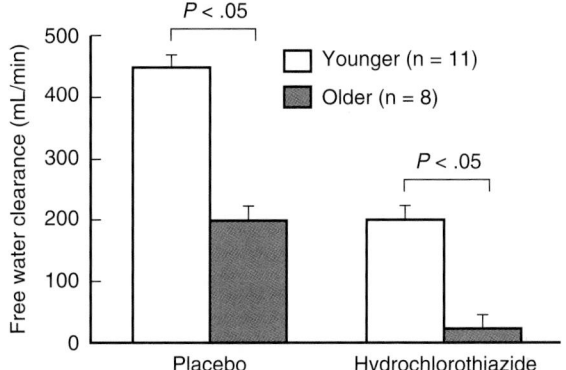

FIGURE 54-14. Mean ± SEM values for positive free water clearance during water loading. Data shown compare values in younger (*open boxes*) and older (*blue boxes*) normal volunteers given placebo or hydrochlorothiazide. Note that older age and thiazide diuretics both impair free water excretion. (Redrawn from Clark BA, Shannon RP, Rosa RM, Epstein FH: Increased susceptibility to thiazide-induced hyponatremia in the elderly. J Am Soc Nephrol 5:1106, 1994.)

48 hours. No neurologic complications were observed among patients corrected by less than 12 mmol/L/24 hours, or by less than 18 mmol/L/48 hours, or where the average rate of correction was less than 0.55 mmol/L/hour. In practice, the risks of ongoing hyponatremia must be balanced against those of too rapid correction.[269]

HYPOKALEMIA. Furosemide inhibits the coupled reabsorption of $Na^+/K^+/2Cl^-$ at the luminal border of the TAL. A luminal K^+ conductance provides for rapid secretion of reabsorbed K^+ and thereby completes a futile cycle. The outcome is little net K^+ retrieval from tubular fluid in the loop of Henle.[140] Thiazides inhibit the coupled reabsorption of Na^+/Cl^- in the early DCT. Therefore, hypokalemia with these agents cannot be ascribed to their direct effects on K^+ transport.

Four mechanisms have been identified that increase renal K^+ elimination during therapy with thiazides or loop diuretics. First, flow-dependent K^+ secretion by the distal nephron provides a universal mechanism for increased K^+ secretion in response to diuretics that act more proximally.[140, 270] Normally, a flow-dependent increase in K^+ secretion during increased

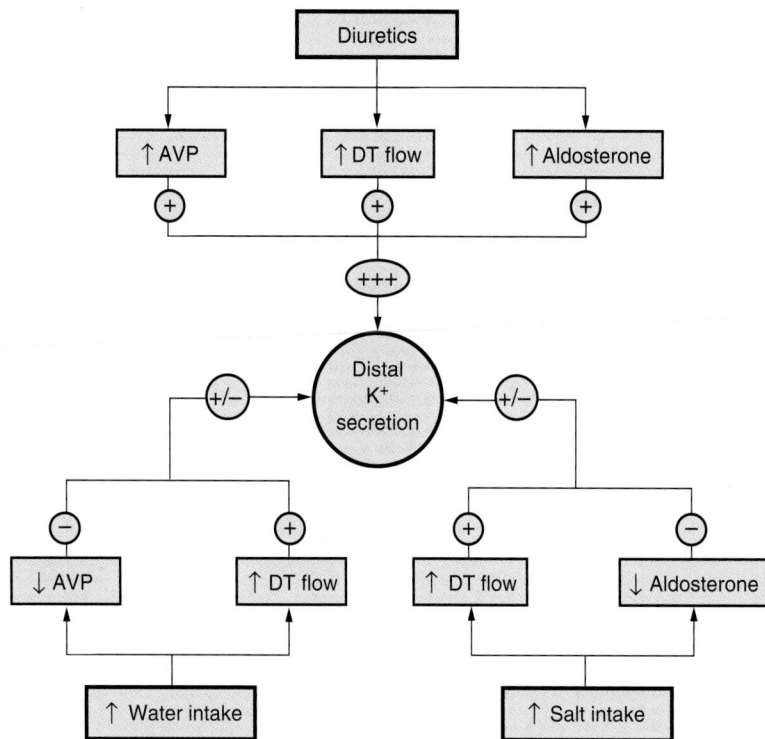

FIGURE 54-15. Contrasting effects of increased water or salt intakes with diuretic action on potassium secretion by the distal nephron. AVP, arginine vasopressin; DT, distal tubule. (From Wilcox CS: Metabolic and adverse effects of diuretics. Semin Nephrol 19:557-568, 1999.)

water intake is offset by a fall in AVP concentration that diminishes distal K$^+$ secretion (Fig. 54-15). Diuretic therapy is unusual because it combines increased distal tubule flow with increased AVP release due to nonosmotic stimulation. Indeed, inhibition of AVP release in normal human subjects undergoing a furosemide diuresis inhibits the kaliuresis.[206] Nonosmotic AVP release is common in edematous subjects.[271, 272] Enhanced release of AVP and enhanced distal tubule fluid delivery combine to promote ongoing K$^+$ losses during diuretic therapy for edema.

Aldosterone promotes distal K$^+$ secretion, especially during increases in distal flow, and provides a further mechanism for K$^+$ secretion.[123, 140, 225, 273] Renin release and aldosterone secretion in normal subjects are inhibited by salt loading. This is accompanied by enhanced distal tubule flow. Therefore, the effects of flow and aldosterone on distal K$^+$ secretion are normally counterbalanced during changes in salt intake just as are the effects of flow and AVP induced by changes in water intake (see Fig. 54-15). However, during diuretic therapy, enhanced secretions of aldosterone and AVP occur during periods of diuretic-induced increase in distal flow, thereby accounting for the importance of aldosterone and AVP in promoting K$^+$ loss with diuretics.[206] Simulation to aldosterone secretion produced by a very low NaCl diet of 20 mEq/day enhances furosemide-induced kaliuresis and prevents post-diuretic renal K$^+$ reclamation.[206]

Lastly, diuretic-induced alkalosis enhances distal secretion of K$^+$.[140]

The serum K$^+$ concentration (S$_K$) of patients not receiving KCl supplements falls by an average of 0.3 mmol/L with furosemide and by 0.6 mmol/L with thiazides.[274] Although this represents a fall in S$_K$ of approximately 20%, numerous studies have shown that the fall in total body K$^+$ is either unmeasurable or averages less than 5%.[273, 274] Diuretic-induced

hypokalemia is associated with small[275] or unmeasurable[276] reductions in intracellular [K$^+$] or [Mg^{2+}] of blood monocytes or skeletal muscle. Moreover, in normal subjects receiving daily doses of loop diuretics, there is no detectable change in K$^+$ balance despite a reproducible fall in S$_K$ of about 0.5 mmol/L.[206] This implies that the primary cause of hypokalemia during thiazide administration is a redistribution of K$^+$ into cells. There is consistent mild metabolic alkalosis during initiation of furosemide or thiazide therapy which increases the serum HCO$_3^-$ concentrate by 2 to 3 mmol/L[64, 101] which could redistribute extracellular K$^+$ into cells. A subgroup that develops significant hypokalemia with thiazides experiences a small, but significant, negative K$^+$ balance during initiation of therapy, in contrast to normokalemic patients who maintain their K$^+$ balance.[277]

Mild diuretic-induced hypokalemia (S$_K$ 3.0-3.5 mmol/L) increases the frequency of ventricular ectopy.[278, 279] However, there has been disagreement about the clinical significance of this finding. Some authors have shown that thiazide-induced hypokalemia does not pose a risk of clinically significant cardiac dysrhythmia even in large populations of hypertensive patients.[280, 281] In contrast, others report a dose-dependent risk of cardiac arrest in patients receiving thiazides which is prevented by therapy with a K$^+$-sparing diuretic such as amiloride.[282]

Adverse effects of hypokalemia are clearly important in certain circumstances. First, severe hypokalemia (S$_K$ < 3.0 mmol/L) is associated with a doubling of serious ventricular dysrhythmias, muscular weakness, and rhabdomyolysis.[276] It requires treatment. Second, mild hypokalemia can precipitate dangerous dysthythmias in patients with cardiac dysfunction due to left ventricular hypertrophy, coronary ischemia, CHF, prolonged QT interval, anoxia, or ischemia, and in patients with a known dysrhythmia. Third, hypokalemia enhances the toxicity of cardiac glycosides by pharmacokinetic and dynamic effects. Hypokalemia diminishes renal tubule secretion of digoxin, thereby prolonging the $t_{1/2}$ for elimination and increasing steady-state serum levels. It also enhances the binding of digoxin to cardiac Na^+,K^+-ATPase, and thereby exaggerates its actions on the heart. Fourth, hypokalemia stimulates renal ammoniagenesis. This is dangerous for patients with cirrhosis and ascites who are prone to develop hepatic encephalopathy due to hyperammonemia. Moreover, the accompanying diuretic-induced alkalosis partitions ammonia into tissues, including the brain, thereby further predisposing to encephalopathy. Fifth, catecholamines partition K^+ into cells and lower S_K. Myocardial infarction provokes sufficient catecholamine release to lower S_K by approximately 0.5 mmol/L.[283] A steeper fall in S_K occurs in patients who have received prior thiazide therapy. Sixth, hypokalemia impairs insulin release and predisposes to hyperglycemia.[284] Seventh, hypokalemia limits the antihypertensive action of thiazides.[285] In a placebo-controlled study of hypokalemic subjects receiving thiazide diuretics, coadministration of KCl that restored S_K reduced blood pressure significantly.[285] Diuretic-induced hypokalemia can be easily prevented. Clearly, the adverse consequences can be clinically significant. Therefore, it is prudent to prevent even mild degrees of hypokalemia.

Hypokalemia can be prevented by increasing intake of K^+ with Cl^- (Fig. 54-16). The normal daily dietary K^+ intake is 40 to 80 mmol. Therefore, to increase this by 50% requires 20 to 40 mmol K^+ daily. Moreover, in the presence of alkalosis, hyperaldosteronism, or Mg^{2+} depletion, hypokalemia is quite unresponsive to dietary KCl. A more effective, convenient, and predictable strategy is to prescribe a combined therapy with a distal K^+-sparing agent such as amiloride or triamterene. This prevents falls in S_K during short- or long-term hydrochlorothiazide therapy.[286] It also prevents diuretic-induced alkalosis and provides further natriuresis and antihypertensive efficacy. An alternative strategy is to administer an ACEI or an ARB or an aldosterone antagonist to counter angiotensin-induced hyperaldosteronism that promotes distal K^+ secretion. The further fall in blood pressure and the beneficial cardiovascular actions of these agents are further advantages. While spironolactone therapy is logical, its adverse effects during long-term therapy limit its acceptability.[287]

HYPERKALEMIA. Diuretics acting in the CDs decrease K^+ secretion and predispose to hyperkalemia.[123, 288] Amiloride and triamterene blunt luminal Na^+ entry into CD cells, thereby diminishing intracellular $[Na^+]$. A fall in cellular $[Na^+]$ inhibits the basolateral Na^+,K^+-ATPase that accumulates K^+ in the cytoplasm for tubular secretion. Moreover, blunting of luminal Na^+ entry diminishes the lumen-negative membrane potential, thereby diminishing the electrical gradient for secretion of K^+ and H^+. Recently, trimethoprim and pentamidine have been identified as amiloride-like agents that inhibit K^+ secretion in the CDs. Trimethoprim increases serum K^+ reproducibly in patients receiving high-dose trimethoprim-sulfamethoxazole (Bactrim) therapy for acquired immunodeficiency syndrome (AIDS).[141] This can be prevented by increases in distal Na^+ delivery with saline infusion or furosemide[142] or by alkalinization of the urine which converts trimethoprim to an uncharged, inactive compound.[143]

HYPOMAGNESEMIA. Loop diuretics inhibit Mg^{2+} reabsorption in the TAL[71, 74] by reducing the transepithelial voltage (R_m) that drives Mg^{2+} and Ca^{2+} paracellularly (see Fig. 54-3).[289] Thiazides first enhance Mg^{2+} uptake in the DCT but, during prolonged therapy, there is enhanced renal Mg^{2+} excretion[135] attributed to a fall in cellular $[Na^+]$ that stimulates basolateral Na^+/Mg^{2+} and Na^+/Ca^{2+} exchange.[289] Distal K^+-sparing agents[171] and spironolactone[290] diminish Mg^{2+} excretion. During prolonged therapy with thiazides and loop diuretics, serum Mg^{2+} concentration (S_{Mg}) falls by 5% to 10%. Diuretic-induced hyponatremia and hypokalemia cannot be reversed fully until any Mg^{2+} deficit is replaced.[291] Mg^{2+}-depleted rats secrete K^+ inappropriately into the distal tubule, independent of aldosterone.[292] Associated symptoms of hypomagnesemia include depression, muscular weakness,

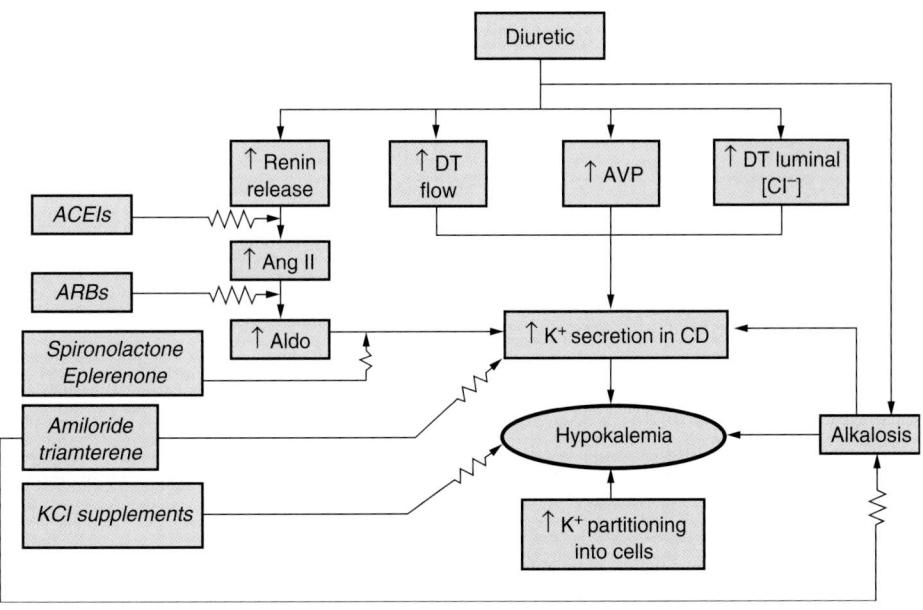

FIGURE 54-16. Diagrammatic representation of mechanisms that partition K^+ into cells or increase K^+ excretion by the collecting ducts (CDs) during therapy with a thiazide or loop diuretic, and strategies for prevention or treatment with angiotensin-converting enzyme inhibitors (ACEIs), angiotensin receptor blockers (ARBs), aldosterone antagonists (e.g., spironolactone), distal K^+-retaining diuretics (amiloride or triamterene), or KCl supplements. Diuretics stimulate the renin-angiotensin-aldosterone (RAA) axis, increase distal tubule flow, increase release of arginine vasopressin (AVP), increase the chloride concentration of distal tubule (DT) fluid, and generate a metabolic alkalosis, all of which enhance K^+ secretion in the collecting ducts.

and atrial fibrillation. These are corrected by administration of magnesium oxide or sulfate.[291]

HYPERCALCEMIA. Thiazides increase the serum concentrations of total and ionized calcium (S_{Ca}). During established thiazide treatment, parathyroid hormone (PTH) concentrations are inversely related to ionized S_{Ca}.[293] The increased S_{Ca} can be ascribed primarily to enhanced Ca^{2+} reabsorption in the early DCT[106] (see Fig. 54-3). Persistent hypercalcemia should prompt a search for a specific cause, for example, an adenoma of the parathyroid glands.[293] Loop diuretics and saline infusion are given to treat hypercalcemia.

ACID-BASE CHANGES. Metabolic alkalosis induced by thiazides or loop diuretics is an important adverse factor in patients with hepatic cirrhosis and ascites, in whom the alkalosis may provoke hepatic coma by partitioning ammonia into the brain, and in those with underlying pulmonary insufficiency, in whom the alkalosis diminishes ventilation.[294] The generation of metabolic alkalosis with loop diuretics is due to a contraction of the extracellular HCO_3^- space by the excretion of a relatively HCO_3^--free urine.[64, 295] The maintenance of metabolic alkalosis involves increased net acid excretion in response to hypokalemia-induced ammoniagenesis and mineralocorticoid excess during continued Na^+ delivery and reabsorption at the distal nephron sites of H^+ secretion.[296] Diuretic-induced metabolic alkalosis is best managed by administration of Cl^- as KCl, but a distal K^+-sparing diuretic,[297] or occasionally a CAI, should be considered.[20] Metabolic alkalosis impairs the natriuretic response to loop diuretics[101] (see Fig. 54-9) and may thereby contribute to diuretic resistance.

CAIs produce metabolic acidosis. Spironolactone and distal K^+-sparing diuretics can cause hyperkalemic metabolic acidosis, especially in elderly patients, those with renal impairment or cirrhosis, and those receiving KCl supplements.

Metabolic Abnormalities

HYPERGLYCEMIA. Diuretic therapy, especially with thiazides, impairs carbohydrate tolerance and occasionally precipitates diabetes mellitus.[247, 298] The increase in blood glucose concentration is greatest during initiation of therapy. In one study, hydrochlorothiazide given to patients with non-insulin-dependent diabetes mellitus increased the fasting serum glucose concentration by 31% at 3 weeks. This was attributed to decreased hepatic glucose utilization.[299] Hyperglycemia persists, but is reversed rapidly after diuretic discontinuation even following 14 years of thiazide therapy.[300] The increase in blood glucose provoked by thiazides is worsened by concurrent β-adrenergic-receptor blockade.[299]

Furosemide can inhibit glucose uptake into rat isolated adipocytes by directly inactivating a carrier protein.[301] However, the dose required is high. Thiazides impair glucose uptake into muscle[275, 302] and liver.[299] This effect is more pronounced during initiation of therapy. It has been ascribed to a diuretic-induced reduction in cardiac output with reflex activation of the SNS and catecholamine secretion leading to reductions in hepatic glucose uptake, muscle blood flow, and muscle glucose uptake (Fig. 54-17). During sustained thiazide therapy, there is decreased insulin release which can be corrected by reversal of hypokalemia with KCl hypomagnesemia with magnesium oxide or administration of spironolactone.[303-309] Experimental K^+ deficiency causes

glucose intolerance and impairs insulin secretion in the absence of diuretics.[310] Hydrochlorothiazide and ACEIs have opposite effects on glucose disposal attributed to opposing effects on S_K.[302] The increase in serum glucose levels that occurs with thiazide therapy is more pronounced in obese patients and correlates with a fall in intracellular $[K^+]$ or $[Mg^{2+}]$.[311] It can be prevented by reducing the thiazide dosage[284] or by KCl replacement.[309] Therefore, care should be taken to monitor blood glucose during thiazide therapy, particularly in obese or diabetic patients.

Thiazide-induced hyperglycemia should be anticipated and prevented. Measures include coadministration of a distal, K^+-sparing diuretic, spironolactone, ACEI, or ARB, prescribing extra KCl, or reducing the thiazide dosage. Thiazide diuretics are not contraindicated in patients with diabetes. Indeed, diuretics produce an even greater reduction in the absolute risk for cardiovascular events in hypertensive patients who are diabetic.[312] Therefore, diabetes mellitus is an indication for close surveillance and attention to coadministration of agents designed to prevent hypokalemia.[313] (see Fig. 54-16).

HYPERLIPIDEMIA. Administration of loop diuretics or thiazides increases the plasma concentrations of total cholesterol, triglycerides, and low-density lipoprotein (LDL) cholesterol, but reduces high-density lipoprotein (HDL) cholesterol. Therefore, it raises the LDL/HDL cholesterol ratio. These changes average 5% to 20% during initiation of therapy.[314] The mechanism is uncertain, but may relate to ECV depletion because severe dietary NaCl restriction has similar metabolic effects,[315] whereas increasing NaCl intake lowers serum cholesterol.[308] Alternatively, it may relate to hypokalemia because this impairs insulin secretion.[309, 311] However, studies of patients treated with thiazides have not shown a benefit of addition of spironolactone.[308] Importantly, most studies have shown that serum cholesterol returns to baseline over 3 to 12 months of thiazide therapy.[314] In fact, when combined with lifestyle management, 4 years of thiazide therapy for hypertension is associated with a modest improvement in lipid profile.[316] A study of 4081 middle-aged men with hyperlipidemia showed no effect of diuretic therapy for 1 year on any plasma lipid parameter. Overall, the beneficial cardiovascular effects of antihypertensive therapy are substantial.[317]

HYPERURICEMIA. Prolonged thiazide therapy for hypertension increases the serum urate concentration by approximately 35%. Renal urate clearance falls because of competition for secretion between urate and the diuretic,[75] and ECV depletion–induced urate reabsorption[76] (see Fig. 54-4). Hyperuricemia is dose-related and can lead to gout. A very long-term outcome analysis of 3693 patients showed no adverse effects of diuretic-induced hyperuricemia in hypertensive subjects who did not have gout.[318] However, recent studies have correlated raised serum urate with cardiovascular death rate.[319-321]

Other Adverse Effects

IMPOTENCE. In the MRC trial of 15,000 hypertensive subjects, impotence was much higher in those receiving a thiazide.[247] In the Treatment of Mild Hypertension Study erection problems were twice as high in those receiving a thiazide.[322] Impotence often responds to sulfinadryl.

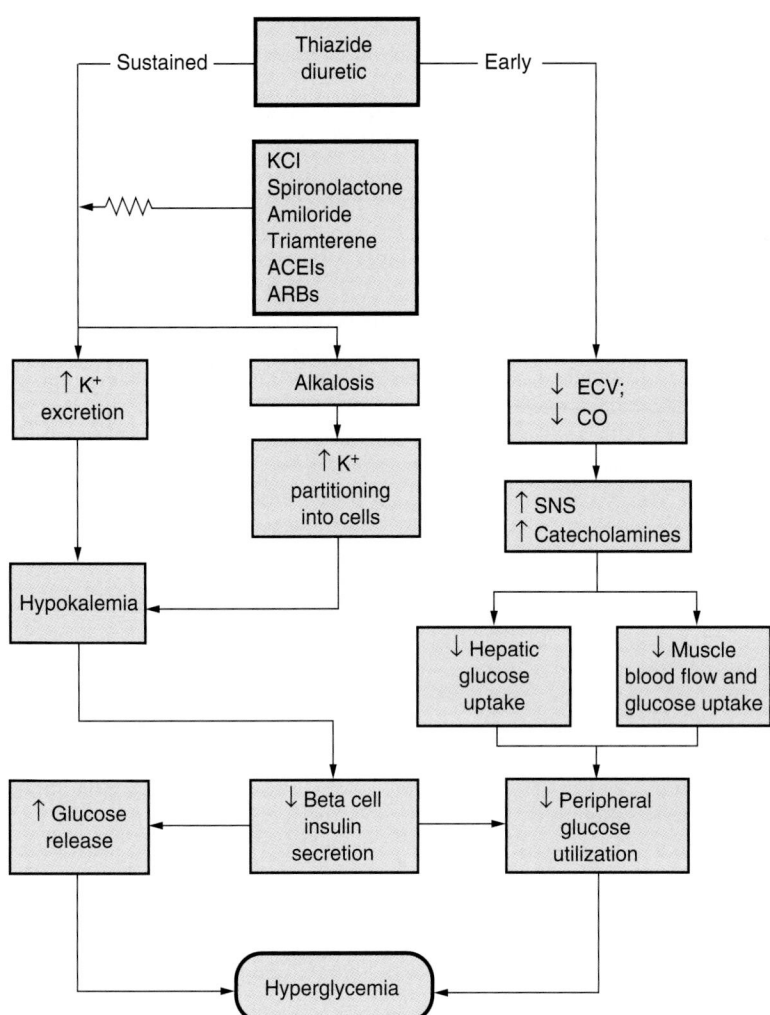

FIGURE 54-17. Hypothesis for the hyperglycemic actions of thiazide diuretics. ACEI, angiotensin-converting enzyme inhibitor; ARB, angiotensin receptor blocker; ECV, extracellular fluid volume; SNS, sympathetic nervous system. (From Wilcox CS: Metabolic and adverse effects of diuretics. Semin Nephrol 19:557-568, 1999.)

OTOTOXICITY. Loop diuretics inhibit the Na+/K+/2Cl⁻ cotransporter[323] and can thereby cause deafness that may occasionally be permanent.[324] The risk is greater with ethacrynic acid and when combined with another ototoxic drug (e.g., an aminoglycoside), during high-dose bolus intravenous therapy in patients with renal failure where plasma levels are increased, and in hypoalbuminemic subjects.[325] In a crossover trial, no ototoxicity was noted in patients with severe CHF when given an infusion of 250 to 2000 mg of furosemide over 8 hours, whereas reversible deafness occurred in 25% when the same dose was given as a bolus.[326]

HAZARDS IN PREGNANCY AND NEWBORNS. Diuretics do not prevent preeclampsia. There is little effect on perinatal mortality.[327] Thiazides can be maintained during pregnancy in those whose hypertension has been controlled by them. They can be used in pregnancy to treat pulmonary edema.[328]

Intensive therapy with loop diuretics for neonates with respiratory distress syndrome increases the prevalence of patent ductus arteriosus because of increased PG generation,[329] cholelithiasis, secondary hyperparathyroidism, bone disease, and drug fever.[330] Prolonged furosemide therapy in preterm infants can cause renal calcification.[331] Diuretics can be transferred from the mother to the infant in breast

milk[332] and can cause serious fluid and electrolyte abnormalities in the infant.[333]

B VITAMIN DEFICIENCY. Diuretics increase the excretion of water-soluble vitamins.[334] Long-term diuretic therapy for CHF[335] or hypertension[336] reduces folate and vitamin B₁ (thiamine) levels[335] and increases plasma homocysteine. Thiamine can improve left ventricular function in patients with CHF treated with furosemide.[337]

DRUG ALLERGY. A reversible photosensitivity dermatitis occurs rarely during thiazide or furosemide therapy.[338, 339] High-dose furosemide in renal failure can cause bullous dermatitis.[340] Diuretics may cause a more generalized dermatitis, sometimes with eosinophilia, purpura, or blood dyscrasia. Occasionally, they cause a necrotizing vasculitis. Cross-sensitivity can occur with other sulfonamide drugs. Acute allergic reactions to sulfonamides are mediated via immunoglobulin E, whereas delayed-onset hypersensitivities are mediated by antibodies to specific protein epitopes.[341] Severe necrotizing pancreatitis is a rare complication.[342]

Acute interstitial nephritis with fever, skin rash, and eosinophilia may develop abruptly some months after initiation of therapy with a thiazide or, less often, furosemide.[343, 344] Ethacrynic acid is chemically dissimilar from other loop diuretics and can be a substitute.

MALIGNANCY. There is a 50% increased risk of renal cell carcinoma associated with prolonged diuretic use.[345, 346] However, this has been attributed to associated hypertension.[347] The risk for colon cancer is also increased modestly by thiazides.[348]

ADVERSE DRUG INTERACTIONS. Hyperkalemia in patients receiving distal K^+-sparing diuretics can be precipitated by concurrent therapy with KCl, ACEIs, ARBs, heparin, ketoconazole, trimethoprim, or pentamidine. Therefore, these drugs should not normally be prescribed in combination, especially in patients with impaired renal function or diabetes. Loop diuretics and aminoglycosides potentiate ototoxicity and nephrotoxicity.[324, 349] Diuretic-induced hypokalemia increases digitalis toxicity fourfold.[350] Plasma lithium concentrations increase during thiazide therapy because of increased proximal lithium reabsorption.[351] NSAIDs may impair the diuretic, natriuretic, antihypertensive, and venodilating responses to diuretics and predispose to renal vasoconstriction and a fall in GFR (see Fig. 54-10 and "Adaptation to Diuretic Therapy"). Used together, indomethacin and triamterene may precipitate renal failure.[352]

CLINICAL USES OF DIURETICS

Edematous Conditions

The first aim of treatment of edema is to reverse the primary cause by restoration of hemodynamics and cardiac output in patients with cardiac failure (e.g., use of vasodilators or elimination of cardiac depressant drugs); by improving hepatic funtion in patients with cirrhosis and ascites (e.g., stopping alcohol intake); or by diminishing proteinuria in patients with the nephrotic syndrome (e.g., administration of ACEIs or ARBs).

Low-dose diuretic therapy doses not alter the GFR. However, overzealous diuresis can decrease the cardiac output, blood pressure, and renal function, and stimulate the RAA axis, the SNS, PG, and AVP, all of which may compromise the desired hemodynamic and renal responses.[353] Therefore, diuretic therapy for edema should be initiated with the lowest effective dose. Additional drugs can be used to counteract unwanted actions. For example, ACEIs or ARBs can prevent the expression of an activated RAA axis and enhance fluid losses, yet diminish K^+ depletion (see Fig. 54-16). The use of a second diuretic can produce a synergistic action, whereas the use of a distal K^+-sparing agent may counteract unwanted hypokalemia, alkalosis, or Mg^{2+} depletion (see "Adaptation to Diuretic Therapy").

Dietary Na^+ intake should be monitored and restricted to 100 to 120 mmol/24 hours in patients with mild edema. Increasingly severe restrictions of dietary salt to 80 to 100 mmol/24 hours are required for patients with refractory edema.

Some resistance to diuretic therapy should be anticipated in all patients with renal CRI and those with more than mild edema (Fig. 54-18).

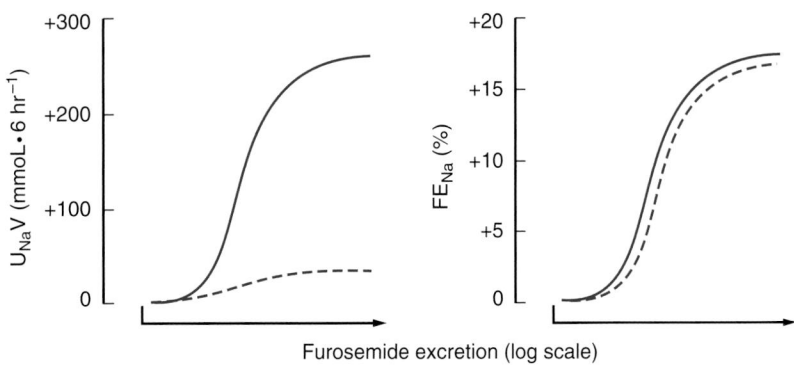

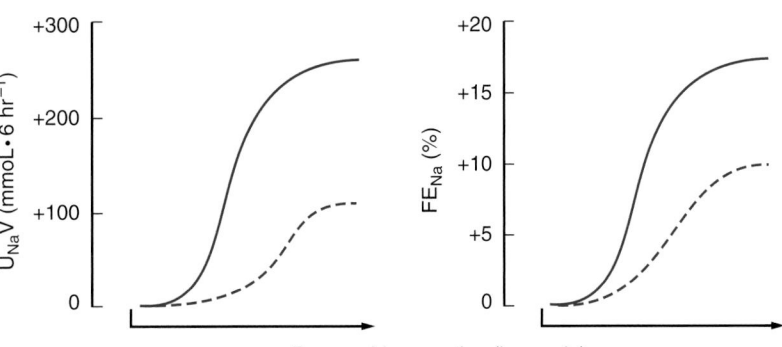

FIGURE 54-18. Effects of chronic renal insufficiency (**A**) or uncompensated edema (**B**) on the relationship between the absolute and fractional sodium excretion and the quantity of furosemide delivered to the urine in healthy controls (*continous lines*) or patients (*broken lines*). CHF, congestive heart failure.

Cardiac Failure

The therapeutic approach for cardiac failure depends on the cause of the left ventricular dysfunction.[354]

ACUTE ISCHEMIC LEFT VENTRICULAR FAILURE. Patients with acute myocardial infarction require the rapid establishment of coronary reperfusion (e.g., by thrombolysis or percutaneous transluminal coronary angioplasty) and treatment of arrhthymias. The aim of concomitant treatment is to counter the increase in left ventricular end-diastolic pressure, the decrease in cardiac output, and the accumulation of pulmonary edema. Judicious use of diuretics may be beneficial. In one study, intravenous furosemide for left ventricular failure (LVF) complicating acute myocardial infarction reduced the left ventricular filling pressure from 20 to 15 mm Hg within 5 to 15 minutes and increased the venous capacitance by 50%.[355] This rapid venodilation is blocked by NSAIDs[214] and ACEIs.[356] The ensuing diuresis reduces left ventricular end-diastolic pressure further.

A study of first-line therapy for 48 patients with acute LVF following myocardial infarction compared the response to intravenous furosemide with a venodilator (isosorbide dinitrate), an arteriolar dilator (hydralazine), or a positive inotrope (prenalterol).[357] The venodilator and furosemide both reduced left ventricular filling pressure while maintaining the cardiac index and heart rate. The authors concluded that the best first-line agent was furosemide or a venodilator but that these should be combined with an arteriolar vasodilator.

One study randomized 110 patients with acute LVF to high-dose isosorbide dinitrate (3 mg intravenously every 5 minutes) or to high-dose furosemide (80 mg intravenously every 15 minutes).[358] An adverse end point occurred more frequently in those randomized to furosemide (46%) than to nitrate (25%). The authors cautioned against the use of high-dose furosemide in acute LVF.

Although intravenous furosemide decreases left ventricular filling pressure in patients with LVF, the shape of the Frank-Starling ventricular function curve predicts little change in cardiac output at elevated filling pressures. However, ischemia can lead to diastolic dysfunction. In this setting, diuretic-induced volume losses can reduce cardiac output occasionally to the point of hypotension and shock.[353, 359-361] Accordingly, intravenous diuretics should not be used in patients with cardiogenic shock and must be used carefully in those with acute LVF, especially when diastolic dysfunction is suspected.

DECOMPENSATED CHRONIC CONGESTIVE HEART FAILURE. Acute decompensation often results from an imbalance in the neurohumoral systems that regulate cardiac and renal function.[362] Therefore, it is rational to target these mechanisms with selective therapy. These patients often respond to intravenous vasodilators, which counteract the efffects of baroreceptor-dependent increases in sympathetic tone, AII and aldosterone, endothelin, and AVP.[176, 290] Venodilation and diuresis evoked by intravenous furosemide may be useful. However, in a study of 15 patients with severe decompensated CHF, intravenous furosemide led to an abrupt increase in systemic vascular resistance and blood pressure and a decrease in the cardiac index.[353] Over the next 2 hours, a diuresis occurred that decreased the left ventricular filling pressure and right atrial pressure and reversed the adverse hemodynamic changes. The authors concluded that intravenous furosemide had activated neural and humoral

mechanisms of vasoconstriction that had contributed to acute pump dysfunction. In contrast, other studies in patients with severe heart failure show that neurohumoral activation with diuretics decreases rapidly with improvement in central filling pressure.[363] Moreover, longer-acting loop diuretics, such as torasemide[364] or azosemide[365] produce less neurohumoral activation and may be preferable.

CHRONIC STABLE CONGESTIVE HEART FAILURE. Diuretics are extremely useful in the long-term management of chronic, stable CHF. Avid renal NaCl and fluid retention leads to pulmonary edema that limits ventilation and to cardiac dilation that limits cardiac function. This can create a spiral of decreasing oxygenation and cardiac output. In a study of 13 patients with severe edema due to CHF, furosemide therapy increased stroke volume by 15% and decreased peripheral vascular resistance despite reducing body weight by an average of 10 kg.[359] In another study, combined therapy with a diuretic and a vasodilator reduced left and right atrial volumes, corrected atrioventricular valvular regurgitation, and improved stroke volume by 64%.[357] A loop diuretic improves congestive symptoms and pulmonary capillary wedge pressure similarly to a cardiac glycoside.[366] Clearly, this is effective therapy for CHF. On the other hand, because the failing heart has a decreased capacity to regulate its contractility in response to changes in venous return, if diuretic therapy is too abrupt or severe, patients suffer from a decreased effective blood volume (orthostatic hypotension, weakness, fatigue, decreased exercise ability, and prerenal azotemia). Therefore, salt-depleting therapy requires continual reassessment and judicious use of other measures (e.g., vasodilators, ACEIs, or ARBs).

A meta-analysis of diuretic trials for CHF concluded that the odds ratio was reduced to 0.25 for mortality and 0.31 for hospitalization for those randomized to diuretics.[367] These remarkable data strongly support the use of diuretics in CHF.

Diuretics are also useful in the treatment of heart failure due to cor pulmonale,[368] primary pulmonary hypertension,[369] or coronary artery disease.[370] They should be used cautiously in those with diastolic dysfunction.[361]

A recent study has shown that patients with CHF have an improved outcome if randomized to spironolactone (25-50 mg/day), even if they are receiving concurrent ACEI therapy.[371] Spironolactone is recommended for CHF.[372]

Diuretic kinetics are impaired in decompensated CHF.[373-376] The absolute absorption of diuretics is normal in patients with decompensated CHF, but may be markedly delayed.[373] There is a decreased plasma clearance because of a decreased RBF.[373] Together, these can limit the peak diuretic concentration in the tubular fluid to the foot of the dose-response curve, and thereby diminish the response.[373]

There is impaired diuretic responsiveness in patients with advanced CHF, as shown by a shift to the right in the natriuresis/excretion relationship of diuretics.[375] (see Fig. 54-17). Thus, resistance should be anticipated in patients with severe CHF and the diuretic dosage increased accordingly.

Mild CHF often responds to dietary Na^+ restriction (100-120 mmol/day) and low doses of a thiazide diuretic. As cardiac failure progresses, larger, more frequent doses of loop diuretics and tighter control of dietary salt (80-100 mmol/day) are required. For the refractory patient, the addition of a second diuretic acting at the proximal tubule (e.g., acetazolamide) or a downstream site (e.g., a thiazide) can produce a dramatic diuresis, even in individuals with impaired renal function.[377] Many resistant patients with advanced CHF have a satisfactory diuresis after addition of spironolactone (25-100 mg/day).[378] Spironolactone also reduces K^+ and Mg^{2+} losses, cardiac norepinephrine uptake, and arrhythmias.[290] In resistant patients, admission to the hospital for an escalating continuous intravenous infusion of furosemide (20-160 mg/day as needed) reduces weight by 13 kg and improves symptoms.[379] Nevertheless, as patients progress through this treatment strategy, the risks of volume depletion, azotemia, and electrolyte abnormalities increase sharply. Therefore, patients with diuretic resistance require close monitoring.

Decompensated CHF stimulates the RAA axis and AVP,[353] predisposing these patients to hypokalemia, hypomagnesemia, hyponatremia, and arrhythmias. Hypokalemia potentiates the binding of digitalis to cardiac myocytes,[380] decreases its renal elimination,[381] and enhances its cardiac toxicity.[382] Therefore, hypokalemia and hypomagnesemia should be anticipated and prevented in patients with cardiac failure receiving digitalis, glycosides and diuretics (see "Adverse Effects of Diuretics").

RIGHT VENTRICULAR FAILURE. The requirement for diuretic therapy in patients with pure right heart failure or cor pulmonale is not compelling. A decrease in venous return induced by vigorous diuresis may worsen right heart function. Furosemide administration increases AII-induced hypoxic pulmonary vascular resistance.[383] Therefore, the emphasis should be on reversal of chronic hypoxemia.

Cirrhosis of the Liver

A reduction in serum albumin and an increase in portal venous pressure partition plasma water into the peritoneum.[354] Such patients with "underfill edema" have a reduced effective blood volume, which stimulates renin, aldosterone, AVP, and norepinephrine.[384] Diuretic therapy may lead to hypotension, azotemia, and electrolyte dysfunction. In contrast, those with a primary renal NaCl retention have "overflow edema"[385] and a normal or increased plasma volume[386] (Fig. 54-19).

Cirrhotic dogs given furosemide have only a transient fall in plasma volume because all the fluid lost by the diuresis could be accounted for by a reduction in the volume of ascites.[387] The furosemide diuresis reduced central venous pressure and increased the plasma protein concentration sufficiently to partition ascitic fluid back into the vascular space, thereby preventing any contraction of the plasma volume.

Studies in patients with cirrhosis demonstrate increases in proximal reabsorption in response to a diminished effective arterial blood volume.[388] Patients with cirrhosis and ascites have an increased natriuretic response to a thiazide, yet a markedly diminished response to ethacrynic acid. This finding suggests that there is also enhanced reabsorption at the distal, thiazide-sensitive nephron sites.[389] Thus, diuretics acting on the distal nephron and spironolactone are rational for cirrhosis.[390-392]

Ascitic fluid is largely cleared by lymphatics. Diuretics increase thoracic duct lymph flow by increasing lymph production by the small intestine and peritoneum[393, 394] and by increasing AII which augments lymphatic pulsations.[395] Thus, diuretics decrease ascites formation by decreasing the venous and portal hydraulic pressures, concentrating the plasma

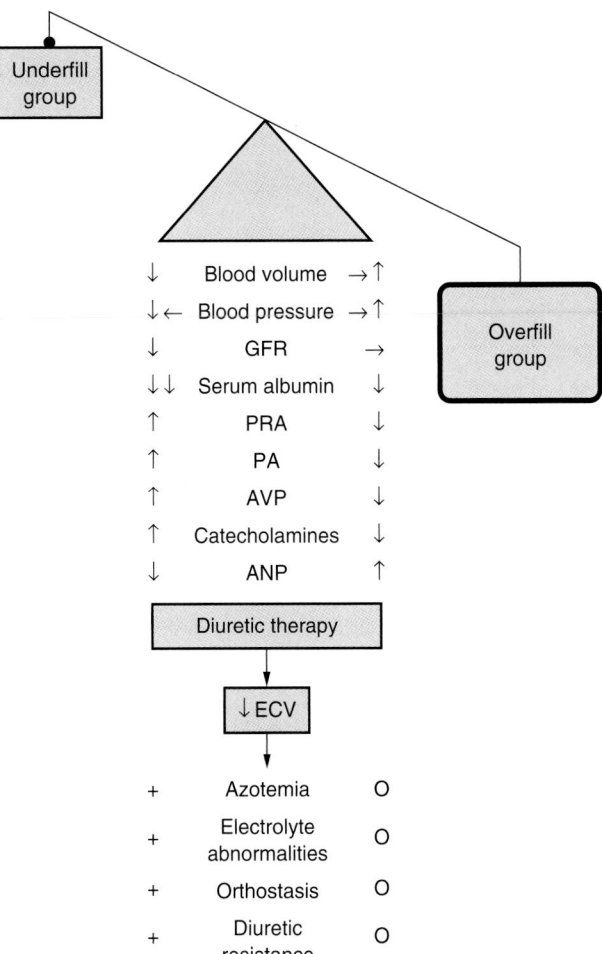

FIGURE 54-19. Comparison of clinical and biochemical characteristics and responses in patients with nephrotic syndrome and underfill vs. overfill edema. ANP, atrial natriuretic peptide; AVP, arginine vasopressin; ECV, extracellular fluid volume; GFR, glomerular filtration rate; PA, plasma aldosterone; PRA, plasma renin activity. (Redrawn from Schrier RW, Fassett RG: A critique of the overfill hypothesis of sodium and water retention in the nephrotic syndrome. Kidney Int 53:1111, 1998.)

proteins,[396] and increasing ascites absorption into the plasma[280] and the lymph.[393]

Patients with peripheral edema may tolerate a diuresis of 1 to 3 kg/day.[397] However, as the daily ascites drainage is limited to 300 to 900 mL,[398] the maximum daily weight loss in nonedematous patients should not exceed 0.3 to 0.5 kg. A study of patients with ascites and edema showed that initially a daily diuretic-induced weight loss of 1 to 3 kg did not perturb the plasma volume or renal function.[397] However, the same diuretic regimen maintained after the peripheral edema had cleared, or given to nonedematous patients, led to a 24% reduction in plasma volume and a high prevalence of hyponatremia, alkalosis, and azotemia. Thus a diuretic prescription that is initially safe must be reviewed continuously.

Patients with mild cirrhosis of the liver have a normal or reduced natriuretic response to furosemide with little change in diuretic kinetics.[9] However, in those with advanced disease, furosemide absorption is slowed,[399] its volume of distribution is increased because of hypoalbuminemia and an expanded ECV, and its elimination is delayed because of hypoalbuminemia that limits proximal tubule diuretic secretion and a low RBF that limits renal clearance.[9]

Loop diuretic resistance in early cirrhosis is largely due to decreased responsiveness to the drug which correlates with an elevated serum aldosterone.[390] With the development of ascites, a further decrease in natriuretic response correlates with decreased delivery of furosemide to the urine[400] and with further stimulation of the RAA axis.[390]

Patients with cirrhosis who fail to respond to a large bolus dose of furosemide (80 mg intravenously) usually have an inadequate response to combined therapy with furosemide (80 mg/day) plus metolazone (2.5 mg/day) and spironolactone (200 mg/day) and therefore have refractory ascites.[401] The traditional concept that paracentesis is dangerous in such patients has been challenged by controlled trials that have shown that it is more effective than diuretic therapy in relieving ascites and reducing hospital stay but that it does not influence the mortality.[402] Even repeated, large-volume paracenteses (4-6 L/day) are safe if intravenous albumin (40 g with each procedure) is administered.[402-404] Indeed, in patients who have pitting edema, large-volume paracentesis alone does not normally induce renal or circulatory dysfunction or electrolyte abnormalities or a fall in plasma volume.[405] Intravenous albumin is recommended with paracentesis to prevent plasma volume depletion, unless there is a reservoir of available peripheral edema.

Mild edema can be treated by dietary restriction of Na^+ (100 mmol/day) and free water (1.5 L/day) if the S_{Na} falls below 130 mmol/L. Patients with more severe ascites require stricter reduction of salt and fluid intake, bed rest, and close monitoring. Bed rest blunts the activation of the RAA axis and SNS in patients with cirrhosis or cardiac failure and increases the response to bumetamide.[406] Such patients may respond to spironolactone (25-100 mg/day). More severe diuretic resistance requires paracentesis or increasing doses of a loop diuretic (e.g., furosemide 20-40 mg twice daily, initially under observation (Fig. 54-20).

The salt-depleting action of spironolactone in cirrhosis correlates with elevated serum aldosterone concentrations but is diminished in patients with a low GFR or S_{Na}.[392] Even malignant ascites may respond to spironolactone or combined diuretic therapy,[407] provided that the ascites is due to hepatic metastases.[408] In a randomized comparison of spironolactone with furosemide in nonazotemic cirrhotic patients, 19 of 20 responded favorably to spironolactone, whereas only 11 of 21 responded favorably to furosemide.[390] Even in those who did not have a significant diuresis, the S_K was reduced by furosemide but increased by spironolactone. Resistant patients have been given up to 600 mg/day of spironolactone,[409] but the adverse effects of spironolactone and its antiandrogenic actions are dose-related.[161] Patients with cirrhosis and ascites cannot normally tolerate ACEIs or ARBs because of a fall in blood pressure.[410]

The most common problems with furosemide in cirrhosis are electrolyte disturbances and volume depletion.[411, 412] Hypokalemia is related to preexisting K^+ depletion and hyperaldosteronism. It can be countered by the use of spironolactone or distal K^+-sparing agents. However, patients with cirrhosis can develop hyperkalemic metabolic acidosis with spironolactone.[413]

Diuretic resistance is common in advanced cirrhosis. In addition to the usual causes (see Table 54-1), it may herald the development of infection, bleeding, or a critical fall in cardiac output.[414] Patients who are refractory and disabled by recurrent paracentesis may respond to body compression,[415] a transjugular intrahepatic portosystemic shunt,[416] or a saphenoperitoneal shunt.[417]

Nephrotic Syndrome

Renal albumin losses and reduced hepatic synthesis in the nephrotic syndrome eventually lead to hypoalbuminemia. The ensuing fall in plasma oncotic pressure increases the flux of fluid into the interstitial spaces, leading to underfill edema.[418, 419] Additionally, a primary renal salt retention can lead to overfill edema.[5, 6, 420] This distinction is important for understanding the response to diuretic therapy[421] (see Fig. 54-18). Patients with minimal-change disease often have a contracted plasma volume and a stimulated RAA axis, whereas those with diabetes and hypertension usually have an expanded plasma volume and a suppressed RAA axis.[422] Micropuncture studies of sodium-retaining animal models of the nephrotic syndrome[423, 424] demonstrate pronounced NaCl reabsorption in the distal nephron and TAL. The proteinuric kidney of a rat model of unilateral nephrotic syndrome has an enhanced Na^+ reabsorption in the CDs[425] and a diminished response to ANP.[426] Hyperaldosteronism reinforces NaCl reabsorption at these sites. Renin and aldosterone levels are highly variable in patients with the nephrotic syndrome.[427] A reduction in serum aldosterone produced by an ACEI does not usually induce a diuresis.[427]

Furosemide kinetics contribute to resistance in patients with the advanced nephrotic syndrome.[9] Hypoalbuminemia decreases the binding of furosemide to plasma proteins and thereby increases its volume of distribution.[428] Whereas one study reported that premixing furosemide with 25 g of albumin prior to intravenous injection enhanced the diuresis of patients with the nephrotic syndrome,[429] this has not been confirmed.[430-432] Indeed, two studies have shown that patients with a serum albumin of 2 g/100 dL can deliver normal quantities of furosemide into the urine.[428, 433] Iso-oncotic plasma volume expansion with albumin in patients with the nephrotic syndrome fails to induce negative NaCl balance[434] or to enhance the response to furosemide.[430] Albumin is not generally recommended for treatment of resistant nephrotic syndrome.[430, 435]

A more logical approach to diuretic resistance is to limit albuminuria with an ACEI or ARB or both, which also may combat the associated coagulopathy, dyslipidemia, edema, and progressive loss of renal function.

The secretion of CAIs[19] and loop diuretics[103] by the S2 segment of the proximal tubule is dependent on albumin. However, in the rabbit, the uptake of loop diuretics into the S1 portion of the proximal tubule where furosemide is inactivated by glucuronidation is inhibited by albumin[104, 436] (see Fig. 54-6). Albumin infusion into nephrotic patients does indeed increase renal furosemide excretion, whereas hypoalbuminemia enhances its metabolic clearance.[437]

The interaction of furosemide with its receptor in the lumen of the TAL is restricted by binding to filtered albumin.[438] Addition of albumin to the tubular perfusate of the loop of Henle attenuates the response to perfused furosemide because of binding to albumin and is reversed by coperfusion with warfarin, which displaces it from its albumin binding site.[439, 440]

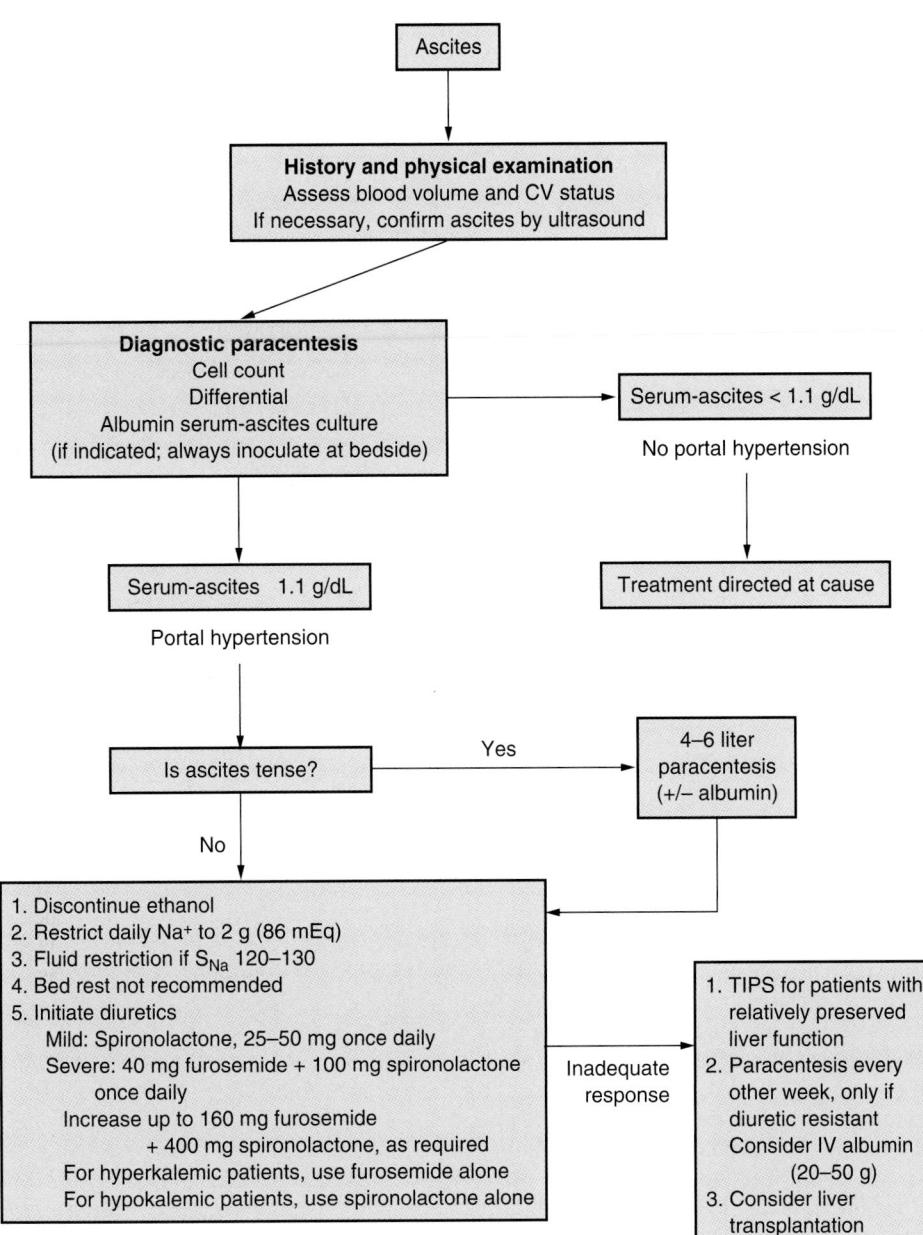

FIGURE 54-20. Treatment algorithm for management of fluid retention in patients with hepatic cirrhosis and ascites. (From Ellison DH, Wilcox CS: Diuretics: Use in edema and the problem of resistance. *In* Brady HR, Wilcox CS (eds): Therapy in Nephrology and Hypertension, 2nd ed. London, Elsevier Science, 2003.)

However, Agarwal and colleagues[441] found that displacing furosemide from albumin by coadministration of sulfisoxazole did not affect natriuresis in patients with the nephrotic syndrome. This study is not definitive as these patients did not have diuretic resistance.

Animal studies demonstrate six mechanisms that could impair the responsiveness to loop diuretics in patients with the nephrotic syndrome (Table 54-2). Clinical studies confirm that they have an impaired tubular response to loop diuretics (see Fig. 54-18).

Nephrotic edema is best managed by dietary salt and fluid restriction. Most patients respond initially to a loop diuretic when required. There is a variable stimulation of the RAA axis and a poor diuretic response to ACEIs, but spironolactone is effective in some patients.[419] Decreasing renal function[221] or administration of indomethacin[210] causes marked resistance to loop diuretics in patients wih the nephrotic syndrome.

The combination of a thiazide diuretic with furosemide dissipates edema but at the expense of marked kaliuresis.[442]

With advancing nephrotic syndrome, the maintenance of plasma volume is compromised by hypoalbuminemia. Diuretic therapy then causes renal function to deteriorate. Nevertheless, diuretic therapy reduces the ECV more than it does the plasma volume.[414]

Idiopathic Edema

Idiopathic edema affects women predominantly. It causes fluctuating salt retention and edema, exacerbated by orthostasis.[443] The effects of diuretic withdrawal during controlled salt intake were studied in 10 such patients.[444] Although their body weight increased by 0.5 to 5.0 kg within 2 to 8 days, seven returned to their original weight by 3 weeks without reinstituting diuretics. The authors

TABLE 54-2

Some Identified Mechanisms and Their Possible Solutions for Limited Response to Loop Diuretics in Patients with the Nephrotic Syndrome

LIMITATION OF RESPONSE	MECHANISM	POTENTIAL SOLUTION
Decreased renal diuretic delivery	Decreased albumin increases V_D and reduces renal delivery	Premix diuretic with albumin in syringe
Decreased tubular secretion of active diuretic	Decreased albumin limits proximal secretion	Reduce albuminuria with ACEI or ARB
Increased renal metabolism of furosemide	Decreased albumin increases tubular uptake and glucuronidization	Consider bumetanide or torasemide which are hepatically metabolized
Decreased blockade of tubular NaCl reabsorption	Filtered albumin binds free drug	Reduce albuminuria with ACEI or ARB
Enhanced NaCl reabsorption in downstream segments	Functional and structural adaptation in distal nephron	Coadministration with thiazide or K^+-sparing diuretic
Enhanced reabsorption in the collecting ducts	ANP resistance	Increase dose of diuretic

ACEI, angiotensin-converting enzyme inhibitor; ANP, atrial natriuretic peptide; ARB, angiotensin receptor blocker; V_D, volume of distribution.

concluded that diuretic abuse could cause idiopathic edema. However, this has been challenged.[445] Patients are best treated by salt restriction.

Nonedematous Conditions

HYPERTENSION. This is discussed in Chapters 45, 47, and 55.

ACUTE RENAL FAILURE. Diuretics can be used to treat edema[446] or to convert patients to nonoliguric ARF. A single large intravenous dose of furosemide (200-1000 mg) given to patients with oliguric ARF produces a sustained diuresis (>500 mL/24 hours) in only 8% to 22% of patients.[10, 447, 448] However, a sustained diuresis can be provoked in most patients given 1 g furosemide orally three times daily but this very large dose produced deafness in two patients, which was permanent in one,[448] and therefore cannot be recommended. Furosemide therapy for ARF does not reduce mortality,[47, 448, 449] but can reduce the need for dialysis by diminishing hyperkalemia, acidosis, or fluid overload.[447, 450] According to one protocol, patients are given two doses of 50 mL of 25% mannitol at 30-minute intervals. If the urine volume remains below 40 mL/hour, crescendo intravenous doses of a loop diuretic are used (e.g., bumetanide, 2 mg, with doubling of the dose at 30-minute intervals to a maximum of 10 mg).[451] A hepatically metabolized diuretic (e.g., bumetanide or torasemide) is less cumulative than furosemide, which is metabolized by the kidney (see Fig. 54-5). Thus bumetanide and torasemide may cause less ototoxicity.

CHRONIC RENAL INSUFFICIENCY. In order to maintain salt and water balance, the fractional reabsorption of NaCl and fluid by the renal tubules is reduced in proportion to the fall in GFR. The renal clearance of loop diuretics falls in parallel with the GFR because of a decreased renal mass and the accumulation of organic acids that compete for proximal secretion.[452] Thus CRI limits the response to diuretics by reducing the absolute rate of NaCl reabsorption in the kidney that is the target for the diuretic, and reducing diuretic delivery to the urine. However, the maximal increase in fractional excretion of Na^+ produced by furosemide is maintained quite well in CRI[5, 453, 454] (see Fig. 54-18). This is explained by the adaptive changes in transport that occur in CRI. Although CRI decreases the reabsorption of NaCl and fluid of the

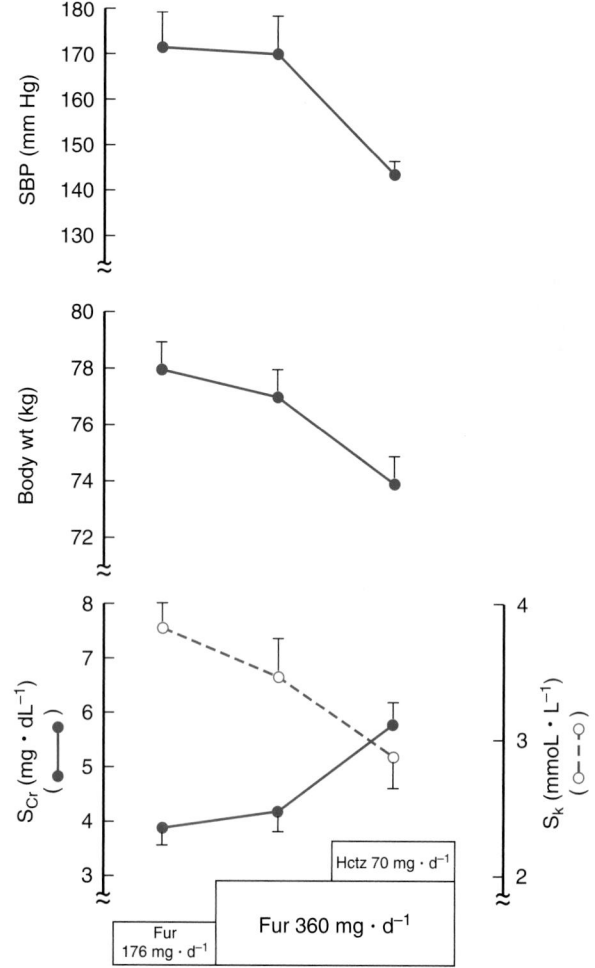

FIGURE 54-21. Mean ± SEM values in eight azotemic patients with resistant hypertension showing systolic blood pressure (SBP), body weight, serum creatinine, and blood urea nitrogen. Subjects were studied while receiving high-dose furosemide (Fur) alone (mean 176 mg/day), after doubling the furosemide dose, and after addition of hydrochlorothiazide (mean dose 70 mg/day). (Drawn from data in Wollam GL, Tarazi RC, Bravo EL, et al: Diuretic potency of combined hydrochlorothiazide and furosemide therapy in patients with azotemia. Am J Med 72:929-938, 1982.)

TABLE 54-3

Ceiling Doses (in mL) of Loop Diuretics

CONDITION	FUROSEMIDE		BUMETANIDE	TORASEMIDE
	IV	PO	IV or PO	IV or PO
Chronic renal insufficiency				
Moderate (GFR 20-50 mL·min^{-1})	80-160	160	6	50
Severe (GFR <20 mL·min^{-1})	200	240	10	100
Nephrotic syndrome with normal GFR	120	240	3	50
Cirrhosis with normal GFR	40-80	80-160	1	20
CHF with normal GFR	40-80	80-160	1	20

CHF, congestive heart failure; GFR, glomerular filtration rate; IV, intravenous; PO, oral.

Data from references 5, 7, 8.

TABLE 54-4

Some Identified Mechanisms and Their Possible Solutions for Limited Response to Loop Diuretics in Patients with Renal Insufficiency

LIMITATION OF RESPONSE	POTENTIAL MECHANISM	POTENTIAL SOLUTION
Decreased renal diuretic delivery	Decreased RBF	Optimize BP and body fluids to restore RBF
Decreased basal fractional NaCl reabsorption	Limits effects of less active diuretics	Select a loop diuretic
Decreased proximal tubule diuretic secretion	Competition with urate and organic anions for basolateral uptake by OAT	Correct uremic milieu and hyperuricemia
	Acidosis impairs secretion	Correct acidosis
	Competition with drugs for tubular secretion by OAT	Avoid co-dosing with probenecid, NSAIDs, β-lactam and sulfonamide antibiotics, valproic acid, methotrexate, cimetidine, and antivirals
Maintained metabolic, but decreased renal clearance (furosemide only)	Hepatic metabolism of bumetanide and torasemide preserved	Avoid furosemide to prevent accumulation and ototoxicity
Enhanced NaCl reabsorption in downstream segments	Enhanced distal tubule fluid and NaCl delivery Enhanced TSC expression	Use thiazide or metolazone with loop diuretic in resistant patients

BP, blood pressure; OAT, organic anion transporter; NSAIDs, nonsteroidal anti-inflammatory drugs; RBF, renal blood flow; TSC, thiazide-sensitive Na$^+$/Cl$^-$ cotransporter.

proximal nephron, there is enhanced fractional reabsorption in the loop segment, distal tubule, and CDs[455] with a relative increase of three- to fourfold per residual nephron in the expression of the Na$^+$/K$^+$/2Cl$^-$ transporter in the TAL and the NCC in the DCT[456] that are the targets for loop diuretics and thiazides, respectively. This may explain why loop diuretics retain some efficacy even in patients with advanced CRI. Torasemide has the greatest oral bioavailability in chronic renal failure.[94] For refractory patients, a loop diuretic infusion (e.g., bumetanide, 1 mg/hour for 12 hours) produces a greater natriuresis and less myalgia than two bolus injections.[196] An observational study showed that patients with autosomal dominant polycystic kidney disease lost GFR twice as fast if they were receiving diuretics, compared to ACEIs.[457] Thiazides when used alone become relatively ineffective in patients with a moderate-to-severe degree of CRI (creatinine clearance <35 mL·min^{-1}), although high doses of thiazide diuretics such as metolazone do retain some efficacy in even quite advanced CRI.[458] When used in combination with a loop diuretic that increases NaCl delivery and reabsorption at the distal tubule, larger doses of thiazides are effective in patients with moderate azotemia.[244] However, these benefits are bought at the cost of a sharp further rise in the serum creatinine and blood urea nitrogen concentrations, and a high incidence of hypokalemia and electrolyte disorders[244] (Fig. 54-21). Moreover, high plasma levels of furosemide can cause ototoxicity.[459] For these reasons, it is preferable to use escalating doses of loop diuretics up to the ceiling dose in patients with CRI (Table 54-3), and to reserve combined loop and thiazide diuretic therapy for the occasional highly resistant patients. The mechanisms of impaired diuretic response in CRI are outlined in Table 54-4. Maximum ceiling doses of loop diuretics have been established[5, 453, 454] and are shown in Table 54-3.

RENAL TUBULAR ACIDOSIS. Furosemide increases the distal delivery of NaCl and fluid and stimulates aldosterone secretion and phosphate elimination which enhance acid elimination.[460] Furosemide increases renal acid excretion in patients with distal renal tubular acidosis.[461] Patients with type IV renal tubular acidosis can be managed with diuretics or mineralocorticoid therapy depending on their blood pressure.[462]

HYPERCALCEMIA. Ca^{2+} excretion is increased by osmotic or loop diuretics but decreased by thiazides and distal agents. Hypercalcemia activates the Ca^{2+} (polyvalent cation)-sensing protein[59, 463] that inhibits fluid and NaCl reabsorption in the TAL and impairs renal concentration. The ensuing ECV depletion further limits Ca^{2+} excretion by reducing the GFR and enhancing proximal fluid and Ca^{2+} reabsorption. Therefore, the initial therapy for hypercalcemia is volume expansion with saline. Thereafter, an infusion of a loop diuretic (e.g., 80-120 mg of furosemide every 1 to 2 hours) causes the loss of approximately 80 mg of Ca^{2+} per dose. Fluid and electrolytes should be replaced quantitatively.[464]

NEPHROLITHIASIS. Thiazides reduce stone formation in hypercalciuric and even normocalciuric patients by reducing excretion of Ca^{2+} and oxalate.[465] Some patients continue to form stones and require additional citrate therapy.[466] Ca^{2+} excretion can be enhanced by addition of amiloride[467] or a low-salt diet. $KHCO_3$ produces a greater reduction in Ca^{2+} excretion than KCl when given with hydrochlorothiazide.[468]

OSTEOPOROSIS. Bone cells express an NaCl cotransporter[469] which, when blocked by a thiazide, enhances bone Ca^{2+} uptake.[470] Thiazides inhibit osteocalcin, an osteoblast-specific protein that retards bone formation[471] and inhibits bone reabsorption in vitro.[472] Thiazides augment bone mineralization independent of PTH.[473] Thus, thiazides may promote bone mineralization both by reducing renal Ca^{2+} excretion and by direct effects on bone. Indeed, thiazide therapy is associated with an increase in bone mineral density and a reduction in hip fractures in elderly persons.[474] In a placebo-controlled trial in postmenopausal women,[475] hydrochlorothiazide (50 mg/day) slowed cortical bone loss significantly. Surprisingly, despite opposite effects on Ca^{2+} excretion, a thiazide and a loop diuretic both enhance bone formation in postmenopausal women, at least in the short term.[476]

DIABETES INSIPIDUS. Thiazides can reduce urine flow by about 50% in patients with central or nephrogenic diabetes insipidus.[477] Antidiuresis is related to a decreased GFR, enhanced water reabsorption in the proximal and distal nephron,[478, 479] and an increase in papillary osmolarity.[480]

REFERENCES

1. Giebisch G: Distal nephron effects of diuretics. *In* Puschett J, Greenberg A (eds): Diuretics III: Chemistry, Pharmacology, and Clinical Applications, New York, Elsevier Science Publishing Co, 1990, pp 667-677.
2. Greger R: Loop diuretics. *In* Greger RF, Knauf H, Mutschler E (eds): Diuretics. New York, Springer-Verlag, 1995, pp 221-274.
3. Bleich M, Greger R: Mechanism of action of diuretics. Kidney Int 51:S11-S15, 1997.
4. Rose BD: Diuretics. Kidney Int 39:336-352, 1981.
5. Ellison DH, Wilcox CS: Diuretic resistance. *In* Brady HR, Wilcox CS (eds): Therapy in Nephrology and Hypertension. Philadelphia, WB Saunders Co, 1999, pp 665-674.
6. Unwin RJ, Capasso G, Wilcox CS: Therapeutic use of diuretics. *In* Brady HR, Wilcox CS (eds): Therapy in Nephrology and Hypertension, Philadelphia, WB Saunders Co, 1998, pp 654-664.
7. Brater DC: Pharmacology of diuretics. Am J Med Sci 319:38-50, 2000.
8. Swan SK, Brater DC: Clinical pharmacology of loop diuretics and their use in chronic renal insufficiency. J Nephrol 6:118-123, 1993.
9. Brater DC: Use of diuretics in cirrhosis and nephrotic syndrome. Semin Nephrol. 19:575-580, 1999.
10. Wilcox CS: New insights into diuretic use in patients with chronic renal disease. J Am Soc Nephrol 13:798-805, 2002.
11. Kaunisto K, Parkkila S, Rajaniemi H, et al: Carbonic anhydrase XIV: Luminal expression suggests key role in renal acidification. Kidney Int 61:2111-2118, 2002.
12. Ichikawa I, Kon V: Role of peritubular capillary forces in the renal action of carbonic anhydrase inhibitor. Kidney Int 30:828-835, 1986.
13. Ellison DH, Karlsen FM: Intensive diuretic therapy: High doses, combinations and constant infusions. *In* Seldin DW, Giebisch G (eds): Diuretic Agents: Clinicial Physiology and Pharmacology, San Diego, Academic Press, 1997, pp 281-300.
14. Unwin RJ, Walter SJ, Giebisch G, et al: Localization of diuretic effects along the loop of Henle: An in vivo microperfusion study in rats. Clin Sci (Colch) 98:481-488, 2000.
15. Cogan MG, Maddox DA, Warnock DG, et al: Effect of acetazolamide on bicarbonate reabsorption in the proximal tubule of the rat. Am J Physiol 237:F447-454, 1979.
16. Maren TH: Carbonic anhydrase inhibition. IV: The effects of metabolic acidosis on the response to Diamox. Bull Johns Hopkins Hosp 98:159, 1956.
17. Leyssac PP, Karlsen FM, Holstein-Rathlou NH, Skott O: On determinants of glomerular filtration rate after inhibition of proximal tubular reabsorption. Am J Physiol 266:R1544-R1550, 1994.
18. Puscas I, Coltau M, Baican M, et al: The inhibitory effect of diuretics on carbonic anhydrase. Res Commun Mol Pathol Pharmacol 105:213-236, 1999.
19. Taft DR, Sweeney KR: The influence of protein binding on the elimination of acetazolamide by the isolated perfused rat kidney: Evidence of albumin-mediated tubular secretion. J Pharmacol Exp Ther 274:752-760, 1995.
20. Miller PD, Berns AS: Acute metabolic alkalosis perpetuating hypercarbia. A role for acetazolamide in chronic obstructive pulmonary disease. JAMA 238:2400-2401, 1977.
21. Bear R, Goldstein M, Phillipson E, et al: Effect of metabolic alkalosis on respiratory function in patients with chronic obstructive lung disease. Can Med Assoc J 117:900-903, 1977.
22. Swenson ER, Robertson HT, Hlastala MP: Effects of carbonic anhydrase inhibition on ventilation-perfusion matching in the dog lung. J Clin Invest 92:702-709, 1993.
23. Maren TH: Carbonic anhydrase: General perspective and advances in glaucoma research. Drug Dev Res 10:255, 1987.
24. Vogh BP: The relation of choroid plexus carbonic anhydrase activity to cerebrospinal fluid formation: Study of three inhibitors in cat with extrapolation to man. J Pharmacol Exp Ther 213:321-331, 1980.
25. Brookes GB, Hodge RA, Booth JB, Morrison AW: The immediate effects of acetazolamide in Meniere's disease. J Laryngol Otol 96:57-72, 1982.
26. Larson EB, Roach RC, Schoene RB, Hornbein TF: Acute mountain sickness and acetazolamide. Clinical efficacy and effect on ventilation. JAMA 248:328-332, 1982.
27. Grissom CK, Roach RC, Surnquist FH, Hackett PH: Acetazolamide in the treatment of acute mountain sickness: Clinical efficacy and effect on gas exchange. Ann Intern Med 116:461-465, 1992.
28. White DP, Zwillich CW, Pickett CK, et al: Central sleep apnea. Improvement with acetazolamide therapy. Arch Intern Med 142:1816-1819, 1982.
29. Griggs RC, Engel WK, Resnick JS: Acetazolamide treatment of hypokalemic periodic paralysis. Prevention of attacks and improvement of persistent weakness. Ann Intern Med 73:39-48, 1970.
30. McArdle B: Adynamia episodica hereditaria and its treatment. Brain 85:121, 1962.
31. Parfitt AM: Acetazolamide and sodium bicarbonate induced nephrocalcinosis and nephrolithiasis: Relationship to citrate and calcium excretion. Arch Intern Med 124:736-740, 1969.
32. Heller I, Halevy J, Cohen S, Theodor E: Significant metabolic acidosis induced by acetazolamide. Not a rare complication. Arch Intern Med 145:1815-1817, 1985.
33. Webster LT, Davidson CS: Production of impending hepatic coma by a carbonic anhydrase inhibitor, Diamox. Proc Soc Exp Biol Med 91:27-31, 1956.
34. Kass MA, Kolker AE, Gordon M, et al: Acetazolamide and urolithiasis. Ophthalmology 88:261-265, 1981.
35. Krivoy N, Ben-Arieh Y, Carter A, Alroy G: Methazolamide-induced hepatitis and pure RBC aplasia. Arch Intern Med 141:1229-1230, 1981.
36. Mallette LE: Acetazolamide-accelerated anticonvulsant osteomalacia. Arch Intern Med 137:1013-1017, 1977.
37. Better OS, Rubinstein I, Winaver JM, Knochel JP: Mannitol therapy revisited (1940-1997). Kidney Int 52:886-894, 1997.
38. Warren SE, Blantz RC: Mannitol. Arch Intern Med 141:493-497, 1981.
39. Cloyd JC, Snyder BD, Cleeremans B, et al: Mannitol pharmacokinetics and serum osmolality in dogs and humans. J Pharmacol Exp Ther 236:301-306, 1986.

40. Byrne JJ: Shock. N Engl J Med 275:659-660, 1966.
41. Eneas JF, Schoenfeld PY, Humphreys MH: The effect of infusion of mannitol–sodium bicarbonate on the clinical course of myoglobinuria. Arch Intern Med 139:801-805, 1979.
42. Ostrow S, Egorin MJ, Hahn D, et al: High-dose cisplatin therapy using mannitol versus furosemide diuresis: Comparative pharmacokinetics and toxicity. Cancer Treat Rep 65:73-78, 1981.
43. Solomon R, Werner C, Mann D, et al: Effects of saline, mannitol and furosemide on acute decreases in renal function induced by radiocontrast agents. N Engl J Med 331:1416-1420, 1994.
44. Dawson JL: Jaundice and anoxic renal damage: Protective effect of mannitol. BMJ 1:810-811, 1964.
45. Untura A: Incidence and prophylaxis of acute postoperative renal failure in obstructive jaundice. Rev Med Chir Soc Med Iasi 83:247, 1979.
46. Gubern JM, Sancho JJ, Simo J, Sitges-Serra A: A randomized trial on the effects of mannitol on postoperative renal function in patients with obstructive jaundice. Surgery 103:39-44, 1988.
47. Conger JD: Interventions in clinical acute renal failure: What are the data? Am J Kidney Dis 26:565-576, 1995.
48. Canalese J, Gimson AE, Davis C, et al: Controlled trial of dexamethasone and mannitol for the cerebral oedema of fulminant hepatic failure. Gut 23:625-629, 1982.
49. Vukic M, Negovetic L, Kovac D, et al: The effect of implementation of guidelines for the management of severe head injury on patient treatment and outcome. Acta Neurochir 141:1203-1208, 1999.
50. Toung TJ, Hurn PD, Traystman RJ, Bhardwaj A: Global brain water increases after experimental focal cerebral ischemia: Effect of hypertonic saline. Crit Care Med 30:644-649, 2002.
51. Borges HF, Hocks J, Kjellstrand CM: Mannitol intoxication in patients with renal failure. Arch Intern Med 142:63-66, 1982.
52. Burg M, Stoner L: Renal tubular chloride transport and the mode of action of some diuretics. Annu Rev Physiol 38:37-45, 1976.
53. Hannaert P, Alvarez-Guerra M, Pirot D, et al: Rat NKCC2/NKCC1 cotransporter selectivity for loop diuretic drugs. Naunyn Schmiedebergs Arch Pharmacol 365:193-199, 2002.
54. Isenring P, Forbush B: Ion transport and ligand binding by the Na-K-Cl cotransporter, structure-function studies. Comp Biochem Physiol A Mol Integr Physiol 130:487-497, 2001.
55. Greger R, Schlatter E: Properties of the lumen membrane of the cortical thick ascending limb of Henle's loop of rabbit kidney. Pflugers Arch 396:315-324, 1983.
56. Hebert SC, Gamba G, Kaplan M: The electroneutral Na^+-(K^+)-Cl^- cotransport family. Kidney Int 49:1638-1641, 1996.
57. Ecelbarger CA, Terris J, Hoyer JR, et al: Localization and regulation of the rat renal Na^+-K^+-$2Cl^-$ cotransporter, BSC-1. Am J Physiol 271(3 pt 2): F619-F628, 1996.
58. Glanville M, Kingscote S, Thwaites DT, et al: Expression and role of sodium, potassium, chloride cotransport (NKCC1) in mouse inner medullary collecting duct (mIMCD-K2) epithelial cells. Pflugers Arch 443:123-131, 2001.
59. Riccardi D, Hall AE, Chattopadhyay N, et al: Localization of the extracellular Ca^{2+}/(polyvalent cation)-sensing protein in rat kidney. Am J Physiol 274:F611-F622, 1998.
60. Bailly C: Transducing pathways involved in the control of NaCl reabsorption in the thick ascending limb of Henle's loop. Kidney Int Suppl 53:S-29-S-35, 1998.
61. Dong J, Delamere NA: Protein kinase C inhibits Na^+-K^+-$2Cl^-$ cotransporter activity in cultured rabbit nonpigmented ciliary epithelium. Am J Physiol 267:C1553-C1560, 1994.
62. Good DW, Knepper MA, Burg MB: Ammonia and bicarbonate transport by thick ascending limb of rat kidney. Am J Physiol 247:F35-F44, 1984.
63. Duarte CG, Chomety F, Giebisch G: Effect of amiloride, ouabain, and furosemide on distal tubular function in the rat. Am J Physiol 221: 632-640, 1971.
64. Wilcox CS, Loon NR, Kanthawatana S, et al: Generation of alkalosis during furosemide infusion: Roles of contraction and acid excretion. J Nephrol 2:81-87, 1991.
65. Radtke HW, Rumrich G, Kinne-Saffran E, Ullrich KJ: Dual action of acetazolamide and furosemide on proximal volume absorption in the rat kidney. Kidney Int 1:100-105, 1972.
66. Puschett JB, Sylk D, Teredesai PR: Uncoupling of proximal sodium bicarbonate from sodium phosphate transport by bumetanide. Am J Physiol 235:F403-F408, 1978.
67. Velazquez H, Wright FS: Effects of diuretic drugs on Na, Cl, and K transport by rat renal distal tubule. Am J Physiol 250:F1013-F1023, 1986.
68. Jung KY, Endou H: Furosemide acts on short loop of descending thin limb, but not on long loop. J Pharmacol Exp Ther 253:1184-1188, 1990.
69. Wilson DR, Honrath U, Sonnenberg H: Furosemide action on collecting ducts: Effect of prostaglandin synthesis inhibition. Am J Physiol 244:F666-F673, 1983.
70. Earley LE, Friedler RM: Renal tubular effects of ethacrynic acid. J Clin Invest 43:1495, 1964.
71. Quamme GA: Effect of furosemide on calcium and magnesium transport in the rat nephron. Am J Physiol 241:F340-F347, 1981.
72. Suki WN, Rouse D, Ng RC, Kokko JP: Calcium transport in the thick ascending limb of Henle. Heterogeneity of function in the medullary and cortical segments. J Clin Invest 66:1004-1009, 1980.
73. Quamme GA: Control of magnesium transport in the thick ascending limb. Am J Physiol 256:F197-F210, 1989.
74. Ryan MP, Devane J, Ryan MF, Counihan TB: Effects of diuretics on the renal handling of magnesium. Drugs 28:167-181, 1984.
75. Roch-Ramel F, Guisan B, Diezi J: Effects of uricosuric and antiuricosuric agents on urate transport in human brush-border membrane vesicles. J Pharmacol Exp Ther 280:839-845, 1997.
76. Weinman EJ, Eknoyan G, Suki WN: The influence of the extracellular fluid volume on the tubular reabsorption of uric acid. J Clin Invest 55:283-291, 1975.
77. Lau K, Stote RM, Goldberg M, Agus ZS: Mechanisms of the uricosuric effect of the diuretic tienilic acid (ticrynafen) in man. Clin Sci Mol Med 53:379-386, 1977.
78. Tobert JA, Cirillo VJ, Hitzenberger G, et al: Enhancement of uricosuric properties of indacrinone by manipulation of the enantiomer ratio. Clin Pharmacol Ther 29:344-350, 1981.
79. Weinman EJ, Knight TF, Mckenzie R, Eknoyan G: Dissociation of urate from sodium transport in the rat proximal tubule. Kidney Int 10:295-300, 1976.
80. Loon NR, Wilcox CS, Unwin RJ: Mechanism of impaired natriuretic response to furosemide during prolonged therapy. Kidney Int 36: 682-689, 1989.
81. Epstein M, Hollenberg NK, Guttmann RD, et al: Effect of ethacrynic acid and chlorothiazide on intrarenal hemodynamics in normal man. Am J Physiol 220:482-487, 1971.
82. Spitalewitz S, Chou SY, Faubert PF, Porush JG: Effects of diuretics on inner medullary hemodynamics in the dog. Circ Res 51:703-710, 1982.
83. Gerber JG: Role of prostaglandins in the hemodynamic and tubular effects of furosemide. Fed Proc 42:1707-1710, 1983.
84. Gerber JG, Nies AS: Furosemide-induced vasodilation: Importance of the state of hydration and filtration. Kidney Int 18:454-459, 1980.
85. Wright FS, Schnermann J: Interference with feedback control of glomerular filtration rate by furosemide, triflocin, and cyanide. J Clin Invest 53:1695-1708, 1974.
86. Pickkers P, Dormans TPJ, Russel FGM, et al: Direct vascular effects of furosemide in humans. Circulation 96:1847-1852, 1997.
87. Pourageaud F, Bappel-Gozalbes C, Marthan R, Freslon JL: Role of EDHF in the vasodilatory effect of loop diuretics in guinea-pig mesenteric resistance arteries. Br J Pharmacol 131:1211-1219, 2000.
88. Puscas I, Coltau M, Baican M, et al: Vasodilatory effect of diuretics is dependent on inhibition of vascular smooth muscle carbonic anhydrase by a direct mechanism of action. Drugs Exp Clin Res 25:271-279, 1999.
89. Benet LZ: Pharmacokinetics/pharmacodynamics of furosemide in man: A review. J Pharmacokinet Biopharm 7:1-27, 1979.
90. Bartel C, Wirtz C, Brandle E, Greven J: Interaction of thiazide and loop diuretics with the basolateral para-aminohippurate transport system in isolated S_2 segments of rabbit kidney proximal tubules. J Pharmacol Exp Ther 266:972-977, 1993.
91. Uwai Y, Saito H, Hashimoto Y, Inui KI: Interaction and transport of thiazide diuretics, loop diuretics, and acetazolamide via rat renal organic anion transporter rOAT1. J Pharmacol Exp Ther 295:261-265, 2000.
92. Brater DC: Disposition and response to bumetanide and furosemide. Am J Cardiol 57:20A-25A, 1986.
93. Brater DC, Leinfelder J, Anderson SA: Clinical pharmacology of torasemide, a new loop diuretic. Clin Pharmacol Ther 42:187-192, 1987.

94. Dunn CJ, Fitton A, Brogden R: Torasemide: An update of its pharmacological properties and therapeutic efficacy. Drugs 49:121-142, 1995.

95. Blose JS, Adams KF, Patterson JH: Torsemide: A pyridine-sulfonylurea loop diuretic. Ann Pharmacother 29:396-402, 1995.

96. Brunner G, Von Bergmann K, Häcker W, von Mollendorff E: Comparison of diuretic effects and pharmacokinetics of torasemide and furosemide after a single oral dose in patients with hydropically decompensated cirrhosis of the liver. Arzneimittelforschung 38:176-179, 1998.

97. Rose HJ, O'Malley K, Pruitt AW: Depression of renal clearance of furosemide in man by azotemia. Clin Pharmacol Ther 21:141-145, 1976.

98. Sweet DH, Bush KT, Nigam SK: The organic anion transporter family: From physiology to ontogeny and the clinic. Am J Physiol 281:F197-F205, 2001.

99. Krick W, Wolff NA, Burckhardt G: Voltage-driven *p*-aminohippurate, chloride, and urate transport in porcine renal brush-border membrane vesicles. Pflugers Arch 441:125-132, 2000.

100. Cemerikic D, Wilcox CS, Giebisch G: Intracellular potential and K^+ activity in rat kidney proximal tubular cells in acidosis and K^+ depletion. J Membr Biol 69:159-165, 1982.

101. Loon NR, Wilcox CS: Mild metabolic alkalosis impairs the natriuretic response to bumetanide in normal human subjects. Clin Sci (Colch) 94:287-292, 1998.

102. Besseghir K, Mosig D, Roch-Ramel F: Facilitation by serum albumin of renal tubular secretion of organic ions. Am J Physiol 256:F475-F484, 1989.

103. Pichette V, Geadah D, du Souich P: The influence of moderate hypoalbuminaemia on the renal metabolism and dynamics of furosemide in the rabbit. Br J Pharmacol 119:885-890, 1996.

104. Schali C, Roch-Ramel F: Transport and metabolism of [³H]morphine in isolated, nonperfused proximal tubular segments of the rabbit kidney. J Pharmacol Exp Ther 233:811-815, 1982.

105. Chennavasin P, Seiwell R, Brater DC, Liang WM: Pharmacodynamic analysis of the furosemide-probenecid interaction in man. Kidney Int 16:187-195, 1979.

106. Chennavasin P, Seiwell R, Brater DC: Pharmacokinetic-dynamic analysis of the indomethacin-furosemide interaction in man. J Pharmacol Exp Ther 215:77-81, 1980.

107. Kirchner KA, Martin CJ, Bower JD: Prostaglandin E_2 but not I_2 restores furosemide response in indomethacin-treated rats. Am J Physiol 250:F980-F985, 1986.

108. Wilcox CS, Mitch WE, Kelly RA, et al: Response of the kidney to furosemide: I. Effects of salt intake and renal compensation. J Lab Clin Med 102:450-458, 1983.

109. Imbs JL, Schmidt M, Giesen-Crouse E: Pharmacology of loop diuretics: State of the art. Adv Nephrol Necker Hosp 16:137-158, 1987.

110. Brater DC, Day B, Anderson S, Seiwell R: Azosemide kinetics and dynamics. Clin Pharmacol Ther 34:454-458, 1983.

111. Brater DC, Anderson S: Sites of action of tripamide. Clin Pharmacol Ther 34:79-85, 1983.

112. Marsh JD, Smith TW: Piretanide: A loop-active diuretic. Pharmacology, therapeutic efficacy and adverse effects. Pharmacotherapy 4:170-180, 1984.

113. Gutsche HU, Muller-Ott K, Brunkhorst R, Niedermayer W: Dose-related effects of furosemide, bumetanide, and piretanide on the thick ascending limb function in the rat. Can J Physiol Pharmacol 61:159-165, 1983.

114. Donnelly R: Clinical implications of indapamide sustained release 1.5 mg in hypertension. Clin Pharmacokinet 37(suppl 1): 21-32, 1999.

115. Fanelli GM, Bohn DL, Scriabine A, Beyer KH: Saluretic and uricosuric effects of (6,7-dichloro-2-methyl=1-oxo-2-phenyl-5-indanyloxy) acetic acid (MK-196) in the chimpanzee. J Pharmacol Exp Ther 200:402-412, 1977.

116. Abecasis R, Guevara M, Miguez C, et al: Long-term efficacy of torsemide compared with frusemide in cirrhotic patients with ascites. Scand J Gastroenterol 36:309-313, 2001.

117. Tsutsui T, Tsutamoto T, Maeda K, Kinoshita M: Comparison of neurohumoral effects of short-acting and long-acting diuretics in patients with chronic congestive heart failure. J Cardiovasc Pharmacol 38 (suppl 1):S81-S85, 2001.

118. Murray MD, Haag KM, Black PK, et al: Variable furosemide absorption and poor predictability of response in elderly patients. Pharmacotherapy 17:98-106, 1997.

119. Kramer WG: Effect of food on the pharmacokinetics and pharmacodynamics of torsemide. Am J Ther 2:499-503, 1995.

120. Murray MD, Ferguson JA, Bennett SJ: Fewer hospitalizations for heart failure by using a completely and predictably absorbed loop diuretic [abstract]. J Gen Intern Med 13(suppl 1):18, 1998.

121. Ellison DH, Velazquez H, Wright FS: Thiazide-sensitive sodium chloride cotransport in early distal tubule. Am J Physiol 253:F546-F554, 1987.

122. Gesek FA, Friedman PA: Sodium entry mechanisms in distal convoluted tubule cells. Am J Physiol 268:F89-F98, 1995.

123. Velazquez H, Wright FS: Control by drugs of renal potassium handling. Annu Rev Pharmacol Toxicol 26:293-309, 1986.

124. Maren TH: The general physiology of reactions catalyzed by carbonic anhydrase and their inhibition by sulfonamides. Ann N Y Acad Sci 429:568-579, 1984.

125. Obermuller N, Bernstein P, Velazquez H, et al: Expression of the thiazide-sensitive Na-Cl cotransporter in rat and human kidney. Am J Physiol 296:F900-F910, 1995.

126. Plotkin MD, Kaplan MR, Verlander JW, et al: Localization of the thiazide sensitive Na-Cl cotransporter, rTSCl, in the rat kidney. Kidney Int 50:174-183, 1996.

127. Colussi G, Rombola G, Brunati C, De Ferrari ME: Abnormal reabsorption of Na^+/Cl^- by the thiazide-inhibitable transporter of the distal convoluted tubule in Gitelman's syndrome. Am J Nephrol 17:103-111, 1997.

128. Velazquez G, Bartiss A, Bernstein P, Ellison DH: Adrenal steroids stimulate thiazide-sensitive NaCl transport by rat renal distal tubules. Am J Physiol 270:F211-F219, 1996.

129. Chen Z, Vaughn DA, Fanestil DD: Influence of gender on renal thiazide diuretic receptor density and response. J Am Soc Nephrol 5:1112-1119, 1994.

130. Seldin DW, Eknoyan G, Suki WN, Rector FC: Localization of diuretic action from the pattern of water and electrolyte excretion. Ann N Y Acad Sci 139:328-343, 1966.

131. Costanzo LS, Windhager EE: Calcium and sodium transport by the distal convoluted tubule of the rat. Am J Physiol 235:F492-F506, 1978.

132. Brunette MG, Harvey N, Mailloux J, et al: The hypocalciuric effect of thiazides: Study of the mechanisms. *In* Puschett J, Greenberg A (eds): Diuretics III: Chemistry, Pharmacology, and Clinical Applications. New York, Elsevier Science Publishing Co, 1990, pp 225-227.

133. Porter RH, Cox BG, Heaney D, et al: Treatment of hypoparathyroid patients with chlorthalidone. N Engl J Med 298:577-581, 1978.

134. Giles TD, Sander GE, Roffidal LE, et al: Comparative effects of nitrendipine and hydrochlorothiazide on calciotropic hormones and bone density in hypertensive patients. Am J Hypertens 5:875-879, 1992.

135. Dai L-J, Friedman PA, Quamme GA: Cellular mechanism of chlorothiazide and cellular potassium depletion on Mg^{2+} uptake in mouse distal convoluted tubule cells. Kidney Int 51:1008-1017, 1996.

136. Calder JA, Schachter M, Sever PS: Ion channel involvement in the acute vascular effects of thiazide diuretics and related compounds. J Pharmacol Exp Ther 265:1175-1180, 1993.

137. Muhlberg W, Mutschler E, Hofner A, et al: The influence of age on the pharmacokinetics and pharmacodynamics of bemetizide and triamterene: A single and multiple dose study. Arch Gerontol Geriatr 32:265-273, 2001.

138. Welling PG: Pharmacokinetics of the thiazide diuretics. Biopharm Drug Dispos 7:501-535, 1986.

139. Suki WN, Dawoud F, Eknoyan G, Martinez-Maldonado M: Effects of metolazone on renal function in normal man. J Pharmacol Exp Ther 180:6-12, 1972.

140. Giebisch G: Renal potassium transport: Mechanisms and regulation. Am J Physiol 274:F817-F833, 1998.

141. Velazquez H, Perazella MA, Wright FS, Ellison DH: Renal mechanism of trimethoprim-induced hyperkalemia. Ann Intern Med 119:296-301, 1993.

142. Reiser IW, Chou SY, Brown MI, Porush JG: Reversal of trimethoprim-induced antikaliuresis. Kidney Int 50:2063-2069, 1996.

143. Schreiber M, Schlanger LE, Chen CB, et al: Antikaliuretic action of trimethoprim is minimized by raising urine pH. Kidney Int 49:82-87, 1996.

144. Brater DC: Clinical utility of the potassium-sparing diuretics. Hosp Formul Manage 19:79, 1984.

145. Mutschler E, Gilfrich HJ, Knauf H, et al: Pharmacokinetics of triamterene. Clin Exp Hypertens A 5:249-269, 1983.

146. Villeneuve JP, Rocheleau F, Raymond G: Triamterene kinetics and dynamics in cirrhosis. Clin Pharmacol Ther 35:831-837, 1984.

147. Somogyi AA, Hovens CM, Muirhead MR, Bochner F: Renal tubular secretion of amiloride and its inhibition by cimetidine in humans and in an animal model. Drug Metab Dispos 17:190-196, 1989.

148. Knauf H, Mohrke W, Mutschler E: Delayed elimination of triamterene and its active metabolite in chronic renal failure. Eur J Clin Pharmacol 24:453-456, 1983.

149. Lynn KL, Bailey RR, Swainson CP, et al: Renal failure with potassium-sparing diuretics. N Z Med J 98:629-633, 1985.

150. Cook CS, Hauswald C, Oppermann JA, Schoenhard GL: Involvement of cytochrome P-450IIIA in metabolism of potassium canrenoate to an epoxide: Mechanism of inhibition of the epoxide formation by spironolactone and its sulfur-containing metabolite. J Pharmacol Exp Ther 266:1-7, 1993.

151. Rahn KH: Clinical pharmacology of diuretics. Clin Exp Hypertens A 5:157-166, 1983.

152. McInnes GT: Relative potency of amiloride and spironolactone in healthy man. Clin Pharmacol Ther 31:472-477, 1982.

153. McInnes GT, Clarke JM, Shelton JR: Dose-response relationships for spironolactone in combination with a potassium wasting diuretic. Clin Pharmacol Ther 33:35-43, 1983.

154. McInnes GT, Perkins RM, Shelton JR, Harrison IR: Spironolactone dose-response relationships in healthy subjects. Br J Clin Pharmacol 13:513-518, 1982.

155. Schombelan M, Sebastian A, Biglieri EG, et al: Amelioration of hypokalemia by amiloride in diverse syndromes associated with renal potassium wasting. Kidney Int 21:157, 1982.

156. Wazny LD, Brophy DF: Amiloride for the prevention of amphotericin B–induced hypokalemia and hypomagnesemia. Ann Pharmacother 34:94-97, 2000.

157. Hulter HN, Licht JH, Glynn RD, et al: Pathophysiology of chronic renal tubular acidosis induced by administration of amiloride. J Lab Clin Med 95:637-653, 1980.

158. Ettinger B: Excretion of triamterene and its metabolite in triamterene stone patients. J Clin Pharmacol 25:365-368, 1985.

159. Favre L, Glasson P, Vallotton MB: Reversible acute renal failure from combined triamterene and indomethacin: A study in healthy subjects. Ann Intern Med 96:317-320, 1982.

160. Potter C, Willis D, Sharp HL, Scharzenberg SJ: Primary and secondary amenorrhea associated with spironolactone therapy in chronic liver disease. J Pediatr 121:141-143, 1992.

161. De Gasparo M, Whitebread SE, Preiswerk G, et al: Antialdosterones: Incidence and prevention of sexual side effects. J Steroid Biochem 32:223-227, 1989.

162. Jose PA, Felder RA: What can we learn from the selective manipulation of dopaminergic receptors about the pathogenesis and treatment of hypertension? Curr Opin Nephrol Hypertens 5:447-451, 1996.

163. Singer I, Epstein M: Potential of dopamine D-1 agonists in the management of acute renal failure. Am J Kidney Dis 31:743-755, 1998.

164. Andrews R, Charlesworth A, Evans A, Cowley AJ: A double-blind cross-over comparison of the effects of a loop diuretic and a dopamine receptor agonist as first-line therapy in patients with mild congestive heart failure. Eur Heart J 18:852-857, 1997.

165. Bellomo R, Cole L, Ronco C: Hemodynamic support and the role of dopamine. Kidney Int 53:S71-S74, 1998.

166. Duke GJ, Bersten AD: Dopamine and renal salvage in the critically ill. Anaesth Intensive Care 20:277-302, 1992.

167. Denton MD, Chertow GM, Brady HR: "Renal-dose" dopamine for the treatment of acute renal failure: Scientific rationale, experimental studies and clinical trials. Kidney Int 50:4-14, 1996.

168. Brater DC, Kaojaren S, Chennavasin P: Pharmacodynamics of the diuretic effects of aminophylline and acetazolamide alone and combined with furosemide in normal subjects. J Pharmacol Exp Ther 227:92-97, 1983.

169. Sigurd B, Olesen KH: Comparative natriuretic and diuretic efficacy of theophylline ethylenediamine and of bendroflumethiazide during long-term treatment with the potent diuretic bumetanide. Acta Med Scand 203:113-119, 1978.

170. Wilcox CS, Welch WJ, Schreiner GF, Belardinelli L: Natriuretic and diuretic actions of a highly selective adenosine A$_1$ receptor antagonist. J Am Soc Nephrol 10:714-720, 1999.

171. Yao K, Kusaka H, Sano J, et al: Diuretic effects of KW-3902, a novel adenosine A$_1$-receptor antagonist, in various models of acute renal failure in rats. Jpn J Pharmacol 64:281-288, 1994.

172. Kost CK, Herzer WA, Rominski BR, et al: Diuretic response to adenosine A(1) receptor blockade in normotensive and spontaneously hypertensive rats: Role of pertussis toxin–sensitive G-proteins. J Pharmacol Exp Ther 292:752-760, 2000.

173. Welch WJ: Adenosine A1 receptor antagonists in the kidney: Effects in fluid-retaining disorders. Curr Opin Pharmacol 2:165-170, 2002.

174. Shimuzu K: Aquaretic effects of the non-peptide V$_2$ antagonist OPC-31260 in hydropenic humans. Kidney Int 48:220-226, 1995.

175. Sato T, Ishikawa S, Abe K, et al: Acute aquaresis by nonpeptide arginine vasopressin (AVP) antagonist OPC-31260 improves hyponatremia in patients with syndrome of inappropriate secretion of antidiuretic hormone (SIADH). J Clin Endocrinol Metab 82:1054-1057, 1997.

176. Nishikimi T, Kawano Y, Saito Y, Matsuoka H: Effect of long-term treatment with selective vasopressin V$_1$ and V$_2$ receptor antagonist on the development of heart failure in rats. J Cardiovasc Pharmacol 27:275-282, 1996.

177. Wilcox CS, Guzman NJ, Mitch WE, et al: Na$^+$, K$^+$, and BP homeostasis in man during furosemide: Effects of prazosin and captopril. Kidney Int 31:135-141, 1987.

178. Kelly RA, Wilcox CS, Mitch WE, et al: Response of the kidney to furosemide. II. Effect of captopril on sodium balance. Kidney Int 24:233-239, 1983.

179. Wilcox CS, Loon NR, Ameer B, Limacher MC: Renal and hemodynamic responses to bumetanide in hypertension. Effects of nitrendipine. Kidney Int 36:719-725, 1989.

180. Nowack R, Fliser D, Richter J, et al: Effects of angiotensin-converting enzyme inhibition on renal sodium handling after furosemide injection. Clin Invest 71:622-627, 1993.

181. Bak M, Shalmi M, Petersen JS, et al: Effects of angiotensin-converting enzyme inhibition on renal adaptations to acute furosemide administration in conscious rats. J Pharmacol Exp Ther 266:33-40, 1993.

182. Shirley DG, Walter SJ, Unwin RJ: Mechanism of the impaired natriuretic response to frusemide during sodium depletion: A micropuncture study in rats. Clin Sci 91:299-305, 1996.

183. Kim J, Welch WJ, Cannon JK, et al: Immunocytochemical response of type A and type B intercalated cells to increased sodium chloride delivery. Am J Physiol 262:F288-F302, 1992.

184. Kaissling B, Stanton BA: Adaptation of distal tubule and collecting duct to increased sodium delivery. I. Ultrastructure. Am J Physiol 255:F1256-F1268, 1988.

185. Kaissling B, Bachmann S, Kriz W: Structural adaptation of the distal convoluted tubule to prolonged furosemide treatment. Am J Physiol 248:F374-F381, 1985.

186. Beck FX, Ohno A, Muller E, et al: Inhibition of angiotensin-converting enzyme modulates structural and functional adaptation to a loop diuretic induced diuresis. Kidney Int 51:36-43, 1997.

187. Kobayashi S, Clemmons DR, Nogami H, et al: Tubular hypertrophy due to work load induced by furosemide associated with increases of IGF-1 and IGFBP-1. Kidney Int 47:818-828, 1995.

188. Scherzer P, Wald H, Popovtzer MM: Enhanced glomerular filtration and Na$^+$-K$^+$-ATPase with furosemide administration. Am J Physiol 252:F910-F915, 1987.

189. Barlet-Bas C, Khadouri C, Marsy S, Doncet A: Enhanced intracellular sodium concentration in kidney cell recruits a latent pool of Na-K-ATPase whose size is modulated by corticosteroids. J Biol Chem 15:7799-7803, 1990.

190. Garg LC, Kapturczak M: Renal compensatory response to hydrochlorothiazide changes Na-K-ATPase in distal nephron. *In* Puschett JB, Greenberg A (eds): Diuretics II: Chemistry, Pharmacology, and Clinical Applications. New York, Elsevier Science, pp 188-194, 1987.

191. Stanton BA, Kaissling B: Adaptation of distal tubule and collecting duct to increased Na delivery. II. Na$^+$ and K$^+$ transport. Am J Physiol 255:F1269-F1275, 1988.

192. DeWardener HE: Idiopathic edema: Role of diuretic abuse. Kidney Int 19:881, 1981.

193. Almeshari K, Ahlstrom NG, Capraro FE, Wilcox CS: A volume-independent component to post-diuretic sodium retention in man. J Am Soc Nephrol 3:1878-1883, 1993.

194. Fanestil DD, Vaughn DA, Blakely P: Metabolic acid-base influences on renal thiazide receptor density. Am J Physiol 272:R2004-R2008, 1997.

195. van Meyel JJ, Smits P, Russel FG, et al: Diuretic efficiency of furosemide during continuous administration versus bolus injection in healthy volunteers. Clin Pharmacol Ther 51:440-444, 1992.

196. Copeland JG, Campbell DW, Plachetka JR, et al: Diuresis with continuous infusion of furosemide after cardiac surgery. Am J Surg 146:796-799, 1983.

197. Rudy DW, Voelker JR, Greene PK, et al: Loop diuretics for chronic renal insufficiency: A continuous infusion is more efficacious than bolus therapy. Ann Intern Med 115:360-366, 1991.

198. Johnson CI, McGrath BP, Matthews PG: Interaction between captopril and hydrochlorothiazide in hypertension. Med J Aust 2:18, 1979.

199. Haris A, Rado JP: Patterns of potassium wasting in response to step-wise combinations of diuretics in nephrotic syndrome. Int J Clin Pharmacol Ther 37:332-340, 1999.

200. Imbs JL, Schmidt M, Velly J, Schwartz J: Comparison of the effect of two groups of diuretics on renin secretion in the anaesthetized dog. Clin Sci Mol Med 52:171-182, 1977.

201. Wilson TW, Loadholt CB, Privitera PJ, Halushka PV: Furosemide increases urine 6-keto-prostaglandin $F_{1\alpha}$: Relation to natriuresis, vasodilation, and renin release. Hypertension 4:634-641, 1982.

202. Dzau VJ, Colucci WS, Williams GH, et al: Sustained effectiveness of converting-enzyme inhibition in patients with severe congestive heart failure. N Engl J Med 302:1373-1379, 1980.

203. Goof JM, Brady AJB, Noormohamed FH, et al: Effect of intense angiotensin II suppression on the diuretic response to furosemide during chronic ACE inhibition. Circulation 90:220-224, 1994.

204. Wilcox CS, Williams CM, Smith TB, et al: Diagnostic uses of angiotensin-converting enzyme inhibitors in renovascular hypertension. Am J Hypertens 1:344S-349S, 1988.

205. Murphy BF, Whitworth JA, Kincaid-Smith P: Renal insufficiency with combinations of angiotensin converting enzyme inhibitors and diuretics. BMJ 285:844-845, 1986.

206. Wilcox CS, Mitch WE, Kelly RA, et al: Factors affecting potassium balance during frusemide administration. Clin Sci (Colch) 67:195-203, 1984.

207. Kaji DM, Chase HS, Eng JP, Diaz J: Prostaglandin E_2 inhibits Na-K-2Cl cotransport in medullary thick ascending limb cells. Am J Physiol 271:C354-C361, 1996.

208. Sakairi Y, Jacobson HR, Noland TD, Breyer MD: Luminal prostaglandin E receptors regulate salt and water transport in rabbit cortical collecting duct. Am J Physiol 269:F257-F265, 1995.

209. Kramer HJ, Dusing R, Stinnesbeck B, et al: Interaction of conventional and antikaliuretic diuretics with the renal prostaglandin system. Clin Sci (Colch) 59:67-70, 1980.

210. Tiggeler RG, Koene RA, Wijdeveld PG: Inhibition of frusemide-induced natriuresis by indomethacin in patients with the nephrotic syndrome. Clin Sci Mol Med 52:149-151, 1977.

211. Kirchner KA, Brandon S, Mueller RA, et al: Mechanism of attenuated hydrochlorothiazide response during indomethacin administration. Kidney Int 31:1097-1103, 1987.

212. Favre L, Glasson P, Riondel A, Vallotton MB: Interaction of diuretics and non-steroidal anti-inflammatory drugs in man. Clin Sci (Colch) 64:407-415, 1983.

213. Data JL, Rane A, Gerkens J, et al: The influence of indomethacin on the pharmacokinetics, diuretic response and hemodynamics of furosemide in the dog. J Pharmacol Exp Ther 206:431-438, 1978.

214. Johnston GD, Hiatt WR, Nies AS, et al: Factors modifying the early nondiuretic vascular effects of furosemide in man. The possible role of renal prostaglandins. Circ Res 53:630-635, 1983.

215. Frolich JC, Hollifield JW, Dormois JC, et al: Suppression of plasma renin activity by indomethacin in man. Circ Res 39:447-452, 1976.

216. Kover G, Tost H: The effect of indomethacin on kidney function: Indomethacin and furosemide antagonism. Pflugers Arch 372:215-220, 1977.

217. Planas R, Arroyo V, Rimola A, et al: Acetylsalicylic acid suppresses the renal hemodynamic effect and reduces the diuretic action of furosemide in cirrhosis with ascites. Gastroenterology 84:247-252, 1983.

218. Melki TS, Foegh ML, Ramwell PW: Implication of thromboxane in frusemide diuresis in rats. Clin Sci (Colch) 71:647-650, 1986.

219. Wilson TW, Badahman AH, Kaushal RD: Thromboxane synthase inhibition enhances furosemide-induced renal vasodilation. Clin Invest Med 16:372-378, 1993.

220. DiPette DJ, Rogers AH: Compensatory pressor role of vasopressin following acute diuresis. J Hypertens 24:633-637, 1988.

221. Danielsen H, Pedersen EB, Madsen M, Jensen T: Abnormal renal sodium excretion in the nephrotic syndrome after furosemide: Relation to glomerular filtration rate. Acta Med Scand 217:513-518, 1985.

222. Baylis PH, DeBeer FC: Human plasma vasopressin response to potent loop-diuretic drugs. Eur J Clin Pharmacol 20:343, 1981.

223. Goldsmith SR, Francis GS, Cowley AW, et al: Increased plasma arginine vasopressin levels in patients with congestive heart failure. J Am Coll Cardiol 1:1385-1390, 1983.

224. Ghose RR: Plasma arginine vasopressin in hyponatraemic patients receiving diuretics. Postgrad Med J 61:1043-1046, 1985.

225. Field MJ, Stanton BA, Giebisch GH: Influence of ADH on renal potassium handling: A micropuncture and microperfusion study. Kidney Int 25:502-511, 1984.

226. Schmitt SL, Taylor K, Schmidt R, et al: The role of volume depletion, antidiuretic hormone and angiotensin II in the furosemide-induced decrease in mesenteric conductance in the dog. J Pharmacol Exp Ther 219:407-414, 1981.

227. Petersen JS, Shalmi M, Abildgaard U, et al: Renal effects of α-adrenoceptor blockade during furosemide diuresis in conscious rats. Pharmacol Toxicol 70:3-12, 1992.

228. Petersen JS, DiBona GF: Reflex control of renal sympathetic nerve activity during furosemide diuresis in rats. Am J Physiol 266:R537-R545, 1994.

229. Petersen JS, Shalmi M, Lam HR, Christensen S: Renal response to furosemide in conscious rats: Effects of acute instrumentation and peripheral sympathectomy. J Pharmacol Exp Ther 258:1-7, 1991.

230. Petersen JS, Shalmi M, Abildgaard U, Christensen S: Alpha-1 blockade inhibits compensatory sodium reabsorption in the proximal tubules during furosemide-induced volume contraction. J Pharmacol Exp Ther 258:42-48, 1991.

231. Fett DL, Cavero PG, Burnett JC: Low-dose atrial natriuretic factor and furosemide in experimental acute congestive heart failure. J Am Soc Nephrol 4:162-167, 1993.

232. Wiemer G, Fink E, Linz W, et al: Furosemide enhances the release of endothelial kinins, nitric oxide and prostacyclin. J Pharmacol Exp Ther 271:1611-1615, 1994.

233. Madeddu P, Glorioso N, Parpaglia PP, et al: Kinin antagonist blunts the diuretic effect of furosemide in deoxycorticosterone-treated rats. Agents Actions Suppl 38:156-162, 1992.

234. Brater DC, Anderson S, Baird B, Campbell WB: Effects of ibuprofen, naproxen, and sulindac on prostaglandins in men. Kidney Int 27:66-73, 1985.

235. Greenberg A, Ray SM, Shahawy M, et al: Influence of pH on the natriuretic response to bumetanide and furosemide. In Puschett J, Greenberg A (eds): Diuretics III: Chemistry, Pharmacology, and Clinical Applications. Elsevier Science Publishing Co, 1990, pp 154-159.

236. Davenport A: Ultrafiltration in diuretic-resistant volume overload in nephrotic syndrome and patients with ascites due to chronic liver disease. Cardiology 96:190-195, 2001.

237. Ellison DH: The physiologic basis of diuretic synergism: Its role in treating diuretic resistance. Ann Intern Med 144:886-894, 1991.

238. Brater DC, Pressley RH, Anderson SA: Mechanisms of the synergistic combination of metolazone and bumetanide. J Pharmacol Exp Ther 233:70-74, 1985.

239. Knauf H, Mutschler E: Diuretic effectiveness of hydrochlorothiazide and furosemide alone and in combination in chronic renal failure. J Cardiovasc Pharmacol 26:394-400, 1995.

240. Fliser D, Schroter M, Neubeck M, Ritz E: Coadministration of thiazides increases the efficacy of loop diuretics even in patients with advanced renal failure. Kidney Int 46:482-488, 1994.

241. Nakahama H, Orita Y, Yamazaki M, et al: Pharmacokinetic and pharmacodynamic interactions between furosemide and hydrochlorothiazide in nephrotic patients. Nephron 49:223-227, 1988.

242. Channer KS, McLean KA, Lawson-Matthew P, Richardson M: Combination diuretic treatment in severe heart failure: A randomised controlled trial. Br Heart J 71:146-150, 1994.

243. Jonassen TEN, Gronbeck L, Shalmi M, et al: Supra-additive natriuretic synergism between bendroflumethiazide and furosemide in rats. J Pharmacol Exp Ther 275:558-565, 1995.

244. Wollam GL, Tarazi RC, Bravo EL, Dustan HP: Diuretic potency of combined hydrochlorothiazide and furosemide therapy in patients with azotemia. Am J Med 72:929-938, 1982.

245. Jeunemaitre X, Charru A, Chatellier G, et al: Long-term metabolic effects of spironolactone and thiazides combined with potassium-sparing agents for treatment of essential hypertension. Am J Cardiol 62:1072-1077, 1988.

246. Schapel GJ, Edwards KDG, Robinson J: Potassium-sparing effect of amiloride in a diuretic factorial study in man. Clin Exp Pharmacol Physiol 2:277-287, 1975.

247. Greenberg G: Adverse reactions to bendrofluazide and propranolol for the treatment of mild hypertension. Report of Medical Research Council Working Party on Mild to Moderate Hypertension. Lancet 2:539-543, 1981.

248. Blantz RC: Pathophysiology of pre-renal azotemia. Kidney Int 53:512-523, 1998.

249. Canton AD, Fuiano G, Conte G, et al: Mechanism of increased plasma urea after diuretic therapy in uraemic patients. Clin Sci (Colch) 68:255-261, 1985.

250. Kamm DE, Genin M, Kuchmy B, Hollander J: Diuretic-induced azotemia: Unmasking the role of increased peripheral catabolism through evisceration-hepatectomy. Kidney Int 16:S58-S60, 1983.

251. Thomas RD, Newill A, Morgan DB: The cause of the raised plasma urea of acute heart failure. Postgrad Med J 55:10-14, 1979.

252. Kitiyakara C, Chabrashvili T, Jose P, et al: Effects of dietary salt intake on plasma arginine. Am J Physiol 280:R1069-R1075, 2001.

253. McCance RA: Experimental sodium chloride deficiency in man. Proc R Soc Lond B Biol Sci 119:245-268, 1936.

254. Zhang X, Hense HW, Riegger GA, Schunkert H: Association of arginine vasopressin and arterial blood pressure in a population-based sample. J Hypertens 17:319-324, 1999.

255. Clark BA, Shannon RP, Rosa RM, Epstein FH: Increased susceptibility to thiazide-induced hyponatremia in the elderly. J Am Soc Nephrol 5:1106-1111, 1994.

256. Szatalowicz VL, Miller PD, Lacher JW, et al: Comparative effect of diuretics on renal water excretion in hyponatraemic oedematous disorders. Clin Sci (Colch) 62:235-238, 1982.

257. Spital A: Diuretic-induced hyponatremia. Am J Nephrol 19:447-452, 1999.

258. Friedman E, Shadel M, Halkin H, Fartel Z: Thiazide-induced hyponatremia. Reproducibility by single dose rechallenge and an analysis of pathogenesis. Ann Intern Med 110:24-30, 1989.

259. Kennedy RM, Earley LE: Profound hyponatremia resulting from a thiazide-induced decrease in urinary diluting capacity in a patient with primary polydipsia. JAMA 282:1185-1186, 1970.

260. Verlander JW, Tran TM, Zhang L, et al: Estradiol enhances thiazide-sensitive NaCl cotransporter density in the apical plasma membrane of the distal convoluted tubule in ovariectomized rats. J Clin Invest 101:1661-1669, 1998.

261. Sonnenblick M, Friedlander Y, Rosin AJ: Diuretic-induced severe hyponatremia. Review and analysis of 129 reported patients. Chest 103:601-606, 1993.

262. Booker JA: Severe symptomatic hyponatremia in elderly outpatients: The role of thiazide therapy and stress. J Am Geriatr Soc 32:108-113, 1984.

263. Ashraf N, Locksley R, Arieff AI: Thiazide-induced hyponatremia associated with death or neurologic damage in outpatients. Am J Med 70:1163-1168, 1981.

264. Ayus JC, Krothapalli RK, Arieff AI: Changing concepts in treatment of severe symptomatic hyponatremia. Rapid correction and possible relation to central pontine myelinolysis. Am J Med 78:897-902, 1985.

265. Halterman RK, Berl T: Therapy of dysnatremic disorders. *In* Brady HR, Wilcox CS (eds): Therapy in Nephrology and Hypertension. Philadelphia, WB Saunders Co, 1998, pp 257-269.

266. Sterns RH: "Slow" correction of hyponatremia: A break with tradition? Kidney 23:1-5, 1991.

267. Ashouri OS: Severe diuretic-induced hyponatremia in the elderly. A series of eight patients. Arch Intern Med 146:1355-1357, 1986.

268. Sterns RH, Cappuccio JD, Silver SM, Cohen EP: Neurologic sequelae after treatment of severe hyponatremia: A multicenter perspective. J Am Soc Nephrol 4:1522-1530, 1994.

269. Berl T: Treating hyponatremia: What is all the controversy about? [see comments]. Ann Intern Med 113:417-419, 1990.

270. DuBose T: Effect on acid-base balance. *In* Eknoyan G, Martinez-Maldonado M (eds): The Physiological Basis of Diuretic Therapy in Clinical Medicine. Orlando, FL, Grune & Stratton, 1986, p 125.

271. Anderson RJ, Chung HM, Kluge R, Schrier RW: Hyponatremia: A prospective analysis of its epidemiology and the pathogenetic role of vasopressin. Ann Intern Med 102:164-168, 1985.

272. Packer M, Medina N, Yushak M: Correction of dilutional hyponatremia in severe chronic heart failure by converting-enzyme inhibition. Ann Intern Med 100:782-789, 1984.

273. Wilcox CS: Diuretics and potassium. *In* Hoffman JF, Giebisch G (eds): Current Topics in Membrane and Transport. Orlando, FL, Academic Press, 1987, pp 250-331.

274. Morgan DB, Davidson C: Hypokalaemia and diuretics: An analysis of publications. BMJ 280:905-908, 1980.

275. Bergstrom J, Hultman E: The effect of thiazides, chlorthalidone and furosemide on muscle electrolytes and muscle glycogen in normal subjects. Acta Med Scand 180:363-376, 1966.

276. Siegel D, Hulley SB, Black DM, et al: Diuretics, serum and intracellular electrolyte levels, and ventricular arrhythmias in hypertensive men. JAMA 267:1083-1089, 1992.

277. Papademetriou V, Price M, Johnson E, et al: Early changes in plasma and urinary potassium in diuretic-treated patients with systemic hypertension. Am J Cardiol 54:1015-1019, 1984.

278. Freis ED, Papademetriou V: How dangerous are diuretics? Drugs 30:469-474, 1985.

279. Holland OB, Nixon JV, Kuhnert L: Diuretic-induced ventricular ectopic activity. Am J Med 70:762-768, 1981.

280. Levy M: Physiological factors constraining the mobilization of ascites. *In* Puschett J, Greenberg A (eds): Diuretics III: Chemistry, Pharmacology, and Clinical Applications, Elsevier Science, 1990, pp 376-382.

281. Robertson JWK, Isles CG, Brown I, et al: Mild hypokalaemia is not a risk factor in treated hypertensives. J Hypertens 4:603-608, 1986.

282. Siscovick DS, Raghunathan TE, Psaty B, et al: Diuretic therapy for hypertension and the risk of primary cardiac arrest. N Engl J Med 330:1852-1857, 1994.

283. Rosa RM, Silva P, Young JB, et al: Adrenergic modulation of extrarenal potassium disposal. N Engl J Med 302:431-434, 1980.

284. Weinberger MH: Mechanisms of diuretic effects on carbohydrate tolerance, insulin sensitivity and lipid levels. Eur Heart J 13:5-9, 1992.

285. Krishna GG, Miller E, Kapoor S: Increased blood pressure during potassium depletion in normotensive men. N Engl J Med 320:1177-1182, 1989.

286. Maronde RF, Milgrom M, Vlachakis N, Chan L: Response of thiazide-induced hypokalemia to amiloride. JAMA 249:237-241, 1983.

287. Jeunemaitre X, Chatellier G, Kreft-Jais C, et al: Efficacy and tolerance of spironolactone in essential hypertension. Am J Cardiol 60:820-825, 1987.

288. Hropot M, Fowler N, Karlmark B, Giebisch G: Tubular action of diuretics: Distal effects on electrolyte transport and acidification. Kidney Int 28:477-489, 1985.

289. Dai LJ, Ritchie G, Kerstan D, et al: Magnesium transport in the renal distal convoluted tubule. Physiol Rev 81:51-84, 2001.

290. Barr CS, Lang CC, Hanson J, et al: Effects of adding spironolactone to an angiotensin-converting enzyme inhibitor in chronic congestive heart failure secondary to coronary artery disease. Am J Cardiol 76:1259-1265, 1995.

291. Dyckner T, Wester PO: Effects of magnesium infusions in diuretic induced hyponatraemia. Lancet 1:585-586, 1981.

292. Quamme GA: Renal magnesium handling: New insights in understanding old problems. Kidney Int 52:1180-1195, 1997.

293. Suki WN: Effects of diuretics on calcium metabolism. Adv Exp Med Biol 151:493-500, 1982.

294. Brijker F, Heijdra YF, van den Elshout FJ, Folgering HT: Discontinuation of furosemide decreases $PaCO_2$ in patients with COPD. Chest 121:377-382, 2002.

295. Cannon PJ, Heineman HO, Albert MS, et al: "Contraction" alkalosis after diuresis of edematous patients with ethacrynic acid. Ann Intern Med 62:979-990, 1965.

296. Wagner CA, Geibel JP: Acid-base transport in the collecting duct. J Nephrol 15(suppl 5):S112-S127, 2002.

297. Levine DZ, Iacovitti M, Buckman S, et al: Distal tubule unidirectional HCO_3^- reabsorption in vivo during acute and chronic metabolic alkalosis in the rat. Am J Physiol 266:F919-F925, 1994.

298. Fruman BL: Impairment of glucose intolerance produced by diuretics and other drugs. Pharmacol Ther 12:613, 1981.

299. Dornhorst A, Powell SH, Pensky J: Aggravation by propranolol of hyperglycaemic effect of hydrochlorothiazide in type II diabetics without alteration of insulin secretion. Lancet 1:123-126, 1985.

300. Murphy MB, Lewis PJ, Kohner E, et al: Glucose intolerance in hypertensive patients treated with diuretics: A fourteen-year follow-up. Lancet 2:1293-1295, 1982.

301. Jacobs DB, Mookerjee BK, Jung CY: Furosemide inhibits glucose transport in isolated rat adipocytes via direct inactivation of carrier proteins. J Clin Invest 74:1679-1685, 1984.

302. Pollare T, Lithell H, Berne C: A comparison of the effects of hydrochlorothiazide and captopril on glucose and lipid metabolism in patients with hypertension. N Engl J Med 321:868-873, 1989.

303. Paolisso G, Di Maro G, Cozzolino D, et al: Chronic magnesium administration enhances oxidative glucose metabolism in thiazide treated hypertensive patients. Am J Hypertens 5:681-686, 1992.

304. Paolisso G, Gambardella A, Balbi V, et al: Effects of magnesium and nifedipine infusions on insulin action, substrate oxidation, and blood pressure in aged hypertensive patients. Am J Hypertens 6:920-926, 1993.

305. Haenni A, Andersson PE, Lind L, et al: Electrolyte changes and metabolic effects of lisinopril/bendrofluazide treatment: Results from a randomized, double-blind study with parallel groups Am J Hypertens 7:615-622, 1994.

306. Rapoport MI, Hurd HF: Thiazide-induced glucose intolerance treated with potassium. Ann Intern Med 113:405-408, 1964.

307. Grunfeld C, Chappell DA: Hypokalemia and diabetes mellitus. Am J Med 75:553-554, 1983.

308. Ames RP: Hyperlipidemia in hypertension: Causes and prevention. Am Heart J 122:1219-1224, 1991.

309. Helderman JH, Elahi D, Andersen DK, et al: Prevention of the glucose intolerance of thiazide diuretics by maintenance of body potassium. Diabetes 32:106-111, 1983.

310. Rowe JW, Tobin JD, Rosa RM, Andres R: Effect of experimental potassium deficiency on glucose and insulin metabolism. Metabolism 29:498-502, 1980.

311. Siegel D, Saliba P, Haffner S: Glucose and insulin levels during diuretic therapy in hypertensive men. Hypertension 23:688-694, 1994.

312. Curb JD, Pressel SL, Culter JA: Effects of diuretic-based antihypertensive treatment on cardiovascular disease risk in older diabetic patients with isolated systolic hypertension. JAMA 276:1886-1892, 1996.

313. Schmitz O, Hermansen K, Nielsen OH, et al: Insulin action in insulin-dependent diabetics after short-term thiazide therapy. Diabetes Care 9:631-636, 1986.

314. Ames RP: The effects of antihypertensive drugs on serum lipids and lipoproteins. II. Non-diuretic drugs. Drugs 32:335-357, 1986.

315. Ruppert M, Overlack A, Kolloch R, et al: Neurohormonal and metabolic effects of severe and moderate salt restriction in non-obese normotensive adults. J Hypertens 11:743-749, 1993.

316. Grimm RH, Flack JM, Grandits GA: Antihypertensive drugs had either a neutral or beneficial effect on lipids. JAMA 275:1549-1556, 1996.

317. Manttari M, Tenkanen L, Manninen V, et al: Antihypertensive therapy in dyslipidemic men: Effects on coronary heart disease incidence and total mortality. Hypertension 25:47-52, 1995.

318. Langford HG, Blaufox MD, Borhani NO, et al: Is thiazide-induced uric acid elevation harmful? Analysis of data from the Hypertension Detection and Follow-up Program. Arch Intern Med 147:645-649, 1987.

319. Fang J, Alderman MH: Serum uric acid and cardiovascular mortality the NHANES I epidemiologic follow-up study, 1971-1992, National Health and Nutrition Examination Survey. JAMA 283:2404-2410, 2000.

320. Wong KY, Macwalter RS, Fraser HW, et al: Urate predicts subsequent cardiac death in stroke survivors. Eur Heart J 23:788-793, 2002.

321. Verdecchia P, Schillaci G, Reboldi G, et al: Relation between serum uric acid and risk of cardiovascular disease in essential hypertension. Hypertension 36:1072-1078, 2000.

322. Grimm RH, Grandits GA, Prineas RJ, et al: Long-term effects on sexual function of five antihypertensive drugs and nutritional hygienic treatment in hypertensive men and women. Treatment of Mild Hypertension Study (TOMHS). Hypertension 29:8-14, 1997.

323. Delpire E, Lu J, England R, et al: Deafness and imbalance associated with inactivation of the secretory Na-K-2Cl co-transporter. Nat Genet 22:192-195, 1999.

324. Rybak LP: Ototoxicity of loop diuretics. Otolaryngol Clin North Am 26:829-844, 1993.

325. Rybak LP, Whitworth C, Scott V: Furosemide ototoxicity is enhanced in analbuminemic rats. Arch Otolaryngol Head Neck Surg 119:758-761, 1993.

326. Dormans TP, Gerlag PG: Combination of high-dose furosemide and hydrochlorothiazide in the treatment of refractory congestive heart failure. Eur Heart J 17:1867-1874, 1996.

327. Collins R, Yusuf S, Peto R: Overview of randomised trials of diuretics in pregnancy. BMJ 290:19-23, 1985.

328. Davison JM: Edema in pregnancy. Kidney Int 51:S90-S96, 1997.

329. Green TP, Thompson TR, Johnson DE, Lock JE: Furosemide promotes patent ductus arteriosus in premature infants with the respiratory-distress syndrome. N Engl J Med 308:743-748, 1983.

330. Prandota J: Clinical pharmacology of furosemide in children: A supplement. Am J Ther 8:275-289, 2001.

331. Hufnagle KG, Khan SN, Penn D, et al: Renal calcifications: A complication of long-term furosemide therapy in preterm infants. Pediatrics 70:360-363, 1982.

332. Mulley BA, Parr GD, Pau WK, et al: Placental transfer of chlorthalidone and its elimination in maternal milk. Eur J Clin Pharmacol 13:129-131, 1978.

333. Bailie MD, Linshaw MA, Stygles VG: Diuretic pharmacology in infants and children. Pediatr Clin North Am 217:231-240, 1981.

334. Lubetsky A, Winaver J, Seligmann H, et al: Urinary thiamin excretion in the rat: Effects of furosemide, other diuretics and volume load. J Lab Clin Med 134:232-237, 1999.

335. Suter PM, Haller J, Hany A, Vetter W: Diuretic use: A risk for subclinical thiamine deficiency in elderly patients. J Nutr Health Aging 4:69-71, 2000.

336. Morrow LE, Grimsley EW: Long-term diuretic therapy in hypertensive patients: Effects on serum homocysteine, vitamin B6, vitamin B12, and red blood cell folate concentrations. South Med J 92:866-870, 1999.

337. Shimon I, Almog S, Vered Z, et al: Improved left ventricular function after thiamine supplementation in patients with congestive heart failure receiving long-term furosemide therapy. Am J Med 98:484-490, 1995.

338. Addo HA, Ferguson J, Frain Bell W: Thiazide-induced photosensitivity: A study of 33 subjects. Br J Dermatol 116:749-760, 1987.

339. Diffey BL, Langtry J: Phototoxic potential of thiazide diuretics in normal subjects. Arch Dermatol 125:1355-1358, 1989.

340. Heydenreich G, Pindborg T, Schmidt H: Bullous dermatosis among patients with chronic renal failure on high dose frusemide. Acta Med Scand 202:61-64, 1977.

341. Cribb AE, Pohl LR, Spielberg SP, Leeder JS: Patients with delayed-onset sulfonamide hypersensitivity reactions have antibodies recognizing endoplasmic reticulum luminal proteins. J Pharmacol Exp Ther 282:1064-1072, 1997.

342. Eckhauser ML, Dokler M, Imbembo AL: Diuretic-associated pancreatitis: A collective review and illustrative cases. Am J Gastroenterol 82:865-870, 1987.

343. Lyons H, Pinn VW, Cortell S, et al: Allergic interstitial nephritis causing reversible renal failure in four patients with idiopathic nephrotic syndrome. N Engl J Med 288:124-128, 1973.

344. Magil AB, Ballon HS, Cameron EC, Rae A: Acute interstitial nephritis associated with thiazide diuretics. Clinical and pathologic observations in three cases. Am J Med 69:939-943, 1980.

345. Grossman E, Messerli FH, Goldbourt U: Antihypertensive therapy and the risk of malignancies. Eur Heart J 22:1343-1352, 2001.

346. Grossman E, Messerli FH, Goldbourt U: Does diuretic therapy increase the risk of renal cell carcinoma? Am J Cardiol 83:1094, 2002.

347. Shapiro JA, Williams MA, Weiss NS, et al: Hypertension, antihypertensive medication use, and risk of renal cell carcinoma. Am J Epidemiol 149:521-530, 1999.

348. Tenenbaum A, Grossman E, Fisman EZ, et al: Long-term diuretic therapy in patients with coronary disease: Increased colon cancer-related mortality over a 5-year follow-up. J Hum Hypertens 15:373-379, 2001.

349. Lawson DH, Macadam RF, Singh MH, et al: Effect of furosemide on antibiotic-induced renal damage in rats. J Infect Dis 126:593-600, 1972.

350. Shapiro S, Slone D, Lewis GP, Jick H: The epidemiology of digoxin toxicity. A study in three Boston hospitals. J Chronic Dis 22: 361-371, 1969.

351. Petersen V, Hvidt S, Thomsen K, Schon M: Effect of prolonged thiazide treatment on renal lithium clearance. BMJ 3:143-145, 1974.

352. Weinberg MS, Quigg RJ, Salant DJ, Bernard DB: Anuric renal failure precipitated by indomethacin and triamterene. Nephron 40:216-218, 1983.

353. Francis GS, Siegel RM, Goldsmith SR, et al: Acute vasoconstrictor response to intravenous furosemide in patients with chronic congestive heart failure. Ann Intern Med 103:1-6, 1985.

354. Schrier RW, Gurevich AK, Cadnapaphornchai MA: Pathogenesis and management of sodium and water retention in cardiac failure and cirrhosis. Semin Nephrol 21:157-172, 2001.

355. Dikshit K, Vyden JK, Forrester JS, et al: Renal and extrarenal hemodynamic effects of furosemide in congestive heart failure after acute myocardial infarction. N Engl J Med 288:1087-1090, 1973.

356. Johnston GD, Nicholls DP, Leahey WJ, Finch MB: The effects of captopril on the acute vascular responses to frusemide in man. Clin Sci 65:359-363, 1983.

357. Verma SP, Silke B, Hussain M, et al: First-line treatment of left ventricular failure complicating acute myocardial infarction: A randomised evaluation of immediate effects of diuretic, venodilator, arteriodilator, and positive inotropic drugs on left ventricular function. J Cardiovasc Pharmacol 10:38-46, 1987.

358. Cotter G, Metzkor E, Kaluski E, et al: Randomised trial of high-dose isosorbide dinitrate plus low-dose furosemide versus high-dose furosemide plus low-dose isosorbide dinitrate in severe pulmonary oedema. Lancet 351:389-393, 1998.

359. Wilson JR, Reichek N, Dunkman WB, Goldberg S: Effect of diuresis on the performance of the failing left ventricle in man. Am J Med 70:234-239, 1981.

360. Silke B: Central hemodynamic effects of diuretic therapy in chronic heart failure. Cardiovasc Drugs Ther 7:45-53, 1993.

361. Chatterjee K: Primary diastolic heart failure. Am J Geriatr Cardiol 11:178-187, 2002.

362. Martin PY, Schrier RW: Sodium and water retention in heart failure: Pathogenesis and treatment. Kidney Int 51:S57-S61, 1997.

363. Johnson W, Omland T, Hall C, et al: Neurohormonal activation rapidly decreases after intravenous therapy with diuretics and vasodilators for class IV heart failure. J Am Coll Cardiol 39:1623-1629, 2002.

364. Noe LL, Vreeland MG, Pezzella SM, Trotter JP: A pharmacoeconomic assessment of torsemide and furosemide in the treatment of patients with congestive heart failure. Clin Ther 21:854-866, 1999.

365. Tomiyama H, Nakayama T, Watanabe G, et al: Effects of short-acting and long-acting loop diuretics on heart rate variability in patients with chronic compensated congestive heart failure. Am Heart J 137:543-548, 1999.

366. Bauer U, Haerer W, Fehske KJ, et al: Hemodynamic effects of piretanide and methyldigoxin in congestive heart failure: Long-term results of a placebo-controlled randomized double blind study. *In* Puschett J, Greenberg A (eds): Diuretics III: Chemistry, Pharmacology and Clinical Applications. New York, Elsevier Science Publishing Co, 1990, pp 316-321.

367. Faris R, Flather M, Purcell H, et al: Current evidence supporting the role of diuretics in heart failure: A meta-analysis of randomised controlled trials. Int J Cardiol 82:149-158, 2002.

368. Romano PM, Peterson S: The management of cor pulmonale. Heart Dis 2:431-437, 2000.

369. De Backer TL, Smedema JP, Carlier SG: Current management of primary pulmonary hypertension. BioDrugs 15:801-817, 2001.

370. Serro-Azul JB, de Paula RS, Gruppi C, et al: Effects of chlorthalidone and diltiazem on myocardial ischemia in elderly patients with hypertension and coronary artery disease. Arq Bras Cardiol 76:268-272, 2001.

371. Pitt B, Zannad F, Remme WJ, et al: The effect of spironolactone on morbidity and mortality in patients with severe heart failure. N Engl J Med 341:709-717, 1999.

372. Chavey WE II, Blaum CS, Bleske BE, et al: Guideline for the management of heart failure caused by systolic dysfunction: Part II. Treatment. Am Fam Physician 64:1045-1054, 2001.

373. Vasko MR, Cartwright DB, Knochel JP, et al: Furosemide absorption is altered in decompensated congestive heart failure. Ann Intern Med 102:314-318, 1985.

374. Brater DC, Seiwell R, Anderson S, et al: Absorption and disposition of furosemide in congestive heart failure. Kidney Int 22:171-176, 1982.

375. Brater DC, Day B, Burdette A, Anderson S: Bumetanide and furosemide in heart failure. Kidney Int 26:183-189, 1984.

376. Cook JA, Smith DE, Cornish LA, et al: Kinetics, dynamics, and bioavailability of bumetanide in healthy subjects and patients with congestive heart failure. Clin Pharmacol Ther 44:487-500, 1988.

377. Knauf H: Functional state of the nephron and diuretic dose-response rationale for low dose combination therapy. Cardiology 84(suppl 2): 18-26, 1994.

378. van Vliet AA, Donker AJ, Nauta JJ, Verhengt FW: Spironolactone in congestive heart failure refractory to high-dose loop diuretic and low-dose angiotensin-converting enzyme inhibitor. Am J Cardiol 71:21A-28A, 1993.

379. van Meyel JJM, Smits P, Dormans T, et al: Continuous infusion of furosemide in the treatment of patients with congestive heart failure and diuretic resistance. J Intern Med 235:329-334, 1994.

380. Steiness E: Digoxin toxicity compared with myocardial digoxin and potassium concentration. Br J Pharmacol 63:233-237, 1978.

381. Steiness E: Suppression of renal excretion of digoxin in hypokalemic patients. Clin Pharmacol Ther 23:511-514, 1978.

382. Steiness E, Olesen KH: Cardiac arrhythmias induced by hypokalaemia and potassium loss during maintenance digoxin therapy. Br Heart J 38:167-172, 1976.

383. Keily DG, Cargill RI, Lipworth BJ: Effects of furosemide and hypoxia on the pulmonary vascular bed in man. Br J Clin Pharmacol 43:309-313, 1997.

384. Bichet D, Szatalowicz V, Chaimovitz C, Schrier RW: Role of vasopressin in abnormal water excretion in cirrhotic patients. Ann Intern Med 96:413-417, 1982.

385. Lopez Novoa JM, Rengel MA: A micropuncture study of salt and water retention in chronic experimental cirrhosis. Am J Physiol 232:F315-F318, 1977.

386. Lieberman FL, Denison EK, Reynolds TB: The relationship of plasma volume, portal hypertension, ascites and renal sodium retention in cirrhosis: The overflow theory of ascites formation. Ann N Y Acad Sci 170:202-212, 1970.

387. Levy M, Richard C: Mobilization of ascites in cirrhotic dogs following furosemide or mannitol diuresis. Am J Physiol 235:F12-F21, 1978.

388. Diez J, Simon MA, Prieto J: Analysis of segmental tubular Na$^+$ handling: A rational approach to the use of spironolactone in cirrhotic patients with ascites. *In* Puschett J, Greenberg A (eds): Diuretics III: Chemistry, Pharmacology and Clinical Applications. New York, Elsevier Science Publishing Co, 1990, pp 394-395.

389. Earley LE, Martino JA: Influence of sodium balance on the ability of diuretics to inhibit tubular reabsorption. A study of factors that influence renal tubular sodium reabsorption in man. Circulation 42:323-334, 1970.

390. Perez-Ayuso RM, Planas AR, Gaya J, et al: Randomized comparative study of efficacy of furosemide versus spironolactone in nonazotemic cirrhosis with ascites: Relationship between the diuretic response and the activity of the renin-aldosterone system. Gastroenterology 84:961-968, 1983.

391. Thompson EJ, Torres E, Grosberg SJ, Martinez-Maldonado M: Effect of triamterene on potassium excretion in cirrhotic patients receiving furosemide. Clin Pharmacol Ther 21:392-394, 1977.

392. Bernardi M, Servadei D, Trevisani F, et al: Importance of plasma aldosterone concentration on the natriuretic effect of spironolactone in patients with liver cirrhosis and ascites. Digestion 31:189-193, 1985.

393. Henriksen JH, Schlichting P: Increased extravasation and lymphatic return rate of albumin during diuretic treatment of ascites in patients with liver cirrhosis. Scand J Clin Lab Invest 41:589-599, 1981.

394. McCaffrey C, Levy M: Effect of furosemide on thoracic duct lymph flow in the dog. Am J Physiol 238:F363-F371, 1980.

395. Szwed AJ, Maxwell DR, Kleit SA, Hamburger RJ: Angiotensin II, diuretics, and thoracic duct lymph flow in the dog. Am J Physiol 244:705-708, 1973.

396. Rector WGJ: Ascites kinetics in cirrhosis: Effects of rapid volume expansion and diuretic administration. J Lab Clin Med 111:166-172, 1988.

397. Pockros PJ, Reynolds TB: Rapid diuresis in patients with ascites from chronic liver disease: The importance of peripheral edema. Gastroenterology 90:1827-1833, 1986.

398. Shear L, Ching S, Gabuzda GJ: Compartmentalization of ascites and edema in patients with hepatic cirrhosis. N Engl J Med 282:1391-1396, 1970.

399. Fredrick MJ, Pound DC, Hall SD, et al: Furosemide absorption in patients with cirrhosis. Clin Pharmacol Ther 9:241-247, 1991.

400. Pinzani M, Daskalopoulos G, Laffi G, et al: Altered furosemide pharmacokinetics in chronic alcoholic liver disease with ascites contributes to diuretic resistance. Gastroenterology 92:294-298, 1987.

401. Spahr L, Villeneuve JP, Tran HK, Pomier-Layrargues G: Furosemide-induced natriuresis as a test to identify cirrhotic patients with refractory ascites. Hepatology 33:28-31, 2001.

402. Gines P, Arroyo V, Quintero E, et al: Comparison of paracentesis and diuretics in the treatment of cirrhotics with tense ascites. Results of a randomized study. Gastroenterology 93:234-241, 1987.

403. Gines A, Fernandez-Esparrach G, Monescillo A: Randomized trial comparing albumin, dextron 70 and polygeline in cirrhotic patients with ascites treated by paracentesis. Gastroenterology 111:1102-1110, 1998.

404. Garcia N, Sanyal AJ: Ascites. Curr Treat Options Gastroenterol 4:527-537, 2001.

405. Kao HW, Rakov NE, Savage E, Reynolds TB: The effect of large volume paracentesis on plasma volume—a cause of hypovolemia? Hepatology 5:403-407, 1985.

406. Ring-Larsen H, Henriksen JH, Wilken C, et al: Diuretic treatment in decompensated cirrhosis and congestive heart failure: Effect of posture. BMJ 292:1351-1353, 1986.

407. Greenway B, Johnson PJ, Williams R: Control of malignant ascites with spironolactone. Br J Surg 69:441-442, 1982.

408. Pockros PJ, Esrason KT, Nguyen C, et al: Mobilization of malignant ascites with diuretics is dependent on ascitic fluid characteristics. Gastroenterology 103:1302-1306, 1992.

409. Campra JL, Reynolds TB: Effectiveness of high-dose spironolactone therapy in patients with chronic liver disease and relatively refractory ascites. Am J Dig Dis 23:1025-1030, 1978.

410. Pariente EA, Bataille C, Bercoff E, Lebrec D: Acute effects of captopril on systemic and renal hemodynamics and on renal function in cirrhotic patients with ascites. Gastroenterology 88:1255-1259, 1985.

411. Gregory PB, Broekelschen PH, Hill MD, et al: Complications of diuresis in the alcoholic patient with ascites: A controlled trial. Gastroenterology 73:534-538, 1977.

412. Naranjo CA, Pontigo E, Valdenegro C, et al: Furosemide-induced adverse reactions in cirrhosis of the liver. Clin Pharmacol Ther 25:154-160, 1979.

413. Gabow PA, Moore S, Schrier RW: Spironolactone-induced hyperchloremic acidosis in cirrhosis. Ann Intern Med 90:338-340, 1979.

414. Epstein M: Therapeutic strategies in the management of ascites. In Puschett J, Greenberg A (eds): Diuretics III: Chemistry, Pharmacology, and Clinical Applications, Elsevier Science Publishing Co, 1990, pp 383-393.

415. Uemura M, Matsumoto M, Tsujii T, et al: Effects of "body compression" on parameters related to ascites formation: Therapeutic trial in cirrhotic patients. J Gastroenterol 34:75-82, 1999.

416. Wong W, Liu P, Blendis L, Wong F: Long-term renal sodium handling in patients with cirrhosis treated with transjugular intrahepatic portosystemic shunts for refractory ascites. Am J Med 106:315-322, 1999.

417. Vadeyar HJ, Doran JD, Charnley R, Ryder SD: Saphenoperitoneal shunts for patients with intractable ascites associated with chronic liver disese. Br J Surg 86:882-885, 2002.

418. Orth SR, Ritz E: The nephrotic syndrome. N Engl J Med 338:1202-1211, 1998.

419. Schrier RW, Fassett RG: A critique of the overfill hypothesis of sodium and water retention in the nephrotic syndrome. Kidney Int 53:1111-1117, 1998.

420. De Santo NG, Pollastro RM, Saviano C, et al: Nephrotic edema. Semin Nephrol 21:262-268, 2001.

421. Vande Walle JG, Donckerwolcke RAMG, van Isselt JW, et al: Volume regulation in children with early relapse of minimal-change nephrosis with or without hypovolaemic symptoms. Lancet 346:148-152, 1995.

422. Meltzer JI, Keim HJ, Laragh JH, et al: Nephrotic syndrome: Vasoconstriction and hypervolemic types indicated by renin-sodium profiling. Ann Intern Med 91:688-696, 1979.

423. Bernard DB, Alexander EA, Couser WG, Lennsky NG: Renal sodium retention during volume expansion in experimental nephrotic syndrome. Kidney Int 14:478-485, 1978.

424. Kirchner KA, Voelker JR, Brater DC: Tubular resistance to furosemide contributes to the attenuated diuretic response in nephrotic rats. J Am Soc Nephrol 2:1201-1207, 1992.

425. Ichikawa I, Rennke HG, Hoyer JR, et al: Role for intrarenal mechanisms in the impaired salt excretion of experimental nephrotic syndrome. J Clin Invest 71:91-103, 1983.

426. Humphreys MH: Mechanisms and management of nephrotic edema. Kidney Int 45:266-281, 1994.

427. Brown EA, Markandu ND, Sagnella GA, et al: Evidence that some mechanism other than the renin system causes sodium retention in nephrotic syndrome. Lancet 2:1237-1240, 1982.

428. Keller E, Hoppe-Seyler G, Schollmeyer P: Disposition and diuretic effect of furosemide in the nephrotic syndrome. Clin Pharmacol Ther 32:442-449, 1982.

429. Inoue M, Okajima K, Itoh K, et al: Mechanism of furosemide resistance in analbuminemic rats and hypoalbuminemic patients. Kidney Int 32:198-203, 1987.

430. Akcicek F, Yalniz T, Basci A, et al: Diuretic effect of frusemide in patients with nephrotic syndrome: Is it potentiated by intravenous albumin [see comments]? BMJ 310:162-163, 1995.

431. Chalasani N, Gorski JC, Horlander JC, et al: Effects of albumin/furosemide mixtures on responses to furosemide in hypoalbuminemic patients. J Am Soc Nephrol 12:1010-1016, 2001.

432. Fliser D, Zurbruggen I, Mutschler E, et al: Coadministration of albumin and furosemide in patients with the nephrotic syndrome. Kidney Int 55:629-634, 1999.

433. Rane A, Villeneuve JP, Stone WJ, et al: Plasma binding and disposition of furosemide in the nephrotic syndrome and in uremia. Clin Pharmacol Ther 24:199-207, 1978.

434. Ribelink TJ, Bijlsma JA, Koomans HA: Iso-oncotic volume expansion in the nephrotic syndrome. Clin Sci (Colch) 84:627-632, 1993.

435. Mees EJD: Does it make sense to administer albumin to the patient with nephrotic oedema? Nephrol Dial Transplant 11:1224-1226, 1996.

436. Pichette V, du Souich P: Role of the kidneys in the metabolism of furosemide: Its inhibition by probenecid. J Am Soc Nephrol 7:345-349, 1996.

437. Sjostrom PA, Odlind BG, Beermann BA, et al: Pharmacokinetics and effects of frusemide in patients with the nephrotic syndrome. Eur J Pharmacol 37:173-180, 1989.

438. Green TP, Mirkin BL: Furosemide disposition in normal and proteinuric rats: Urinary drug-protein binding as a determinant of drug excretion. J Pharmacol Exp Ther 218:122-127, 1981.

439. Kirchner KA, Voelker JR, Brater DC: Binding inhibitors restore furosemide potency in tubule fluid containing albumin. Kidney Int 40:418-424, 1991.

440. Kirchner KA, Voelker JR, Brater DC: Intratubular albumin blunts the response to furosemide—A mechanism for diuretic resistance in the nephrotic syndrome. J Pharmacol Exp Ther 252:1097-1101, 1990.

441. Agarwal R, Gorski JC, Sundblad K, Brater DC: Urinary protein binding does not affect response to furosemide in patients with nephrotic syndrome. J Am Soc Nephrol 11:1100-1105, 2000.

442. Garin EH: A comparison of combinations of diuretics in nephrotic edema. Am J Dis Child 141:769-771, 1987.

443. Streeten DH: Idiopathic edema. Pathogenesis, clinical features, and treatment. Endocrinol Metab Clin North Am 24:531-547, 1995.

444. MacGregor GA, Markandu ND, Roulston JE, et al: Is "idiopathic" edema idiopathic? Lancet 1:397-400, 1979.

445. Young JB, Brownjohn AM, Lee MR: Diuretics and idiopathic oedema. Nephron 43:311-312, 1986.

446. Andreucci M, Federico S, Andreucci VE: Edema and acute renal failure. Semin Nephrol 21:251-256, 2001.

447. Minuth AN, Terrell JB, Suki WN: Acute renal failure: A study of the course and prognosis of 104 patients and of the role of furosemide. Am J Med Sci 271:317-324, 1976.

448. Brown CB, Ogg CS, Cameron JS: High dose frusemide in acute renal failure: A controlled trial. Clin Nephrol 15:90-96, 1981.

449. Kleinknecht D, Ganeval D, Gonzalez Duque LA, Fermanian J: Furosemide in acute oliguric renal failure. A controlled trial. Nephron 17:51-58, 1976.

450. Sirivella S, Gielchinsky I, Parsonnet V: Mannitol, furosemide, and dopamine infusion in postoperative renal failure complicating cardiac surgery. Ann Thorac Surg 69:501-506, 2000.

451. Narins RG, Chusid P: Diuretic use in critical care. Am J Cardiol 57:26A-32A, 1986.

452. Rose HJ, O'Malley K, Pruitt AW: Depression of renal clearance of furosemide in man by azotemia. Clin Pharmacol Ther 21:141-146, 1977.

453. Brater DC, Anderson SA, Brown Cartwright D: Response to furosemide in chronic renal insufficiency: Rationale for limited doses. Clin Pharmacol Ther 40:134-139, 1986.

454. Voelker JR, Cartwright Brown D, Anderson S, et al: Comparison of loop diuretics in patients with chronic renal insufficiency. Kidney Int 32:572-578, 1987.

455. Buerkert J, Martin D, Prasad J, et al: Response of deep nephrons and the terminal collecting duct to a reduction in renal mass. Am J Physiol 236:F454-F464, 1979.

456. Kwon TH, Frokiaer J, Fernandez-Llama P, et al: Altered expression of Na transporters NHE-3, NaPi-II, Na-K-ATPase, BSC-1, and TSC in CRF rat kidneys. Am J Physiol 277:F257-F270, 1999.

457. Ecder T, Edelstein CL, Fick-Brosnahan GM, et al: Diuretics versus angiotensin-converting enzyme inhibitors in autosomal dominant polycystic kidney disease. Am J Nephrol 21:98-103, 2001.

458. Dargie HJ, Allison ME, Kennedy AC, Gray MJ: High dosage metolazone in chronic renal failure. BMJ 4:196-198, 1972.

459. Humes HD: Insights into ototoxicity. Analogies to nephrotoxicity. Ann N Y Acad Sci 884:15-18, 1999.

460. Wilcox CS, Granges F, Kirk G, et al: Effects of saline infusion on titratable acid generation and ammonia secretion. Am J Physiol 247:F506-F519, 1984.

461. Rastogi SP, Crawford C, Wheeler R, et al: Effect of furosemide on urinary acidification in distal renal tubular acidosis. J Lab Clin Med 104:271-282, 1984.

462. Schambelan M, Sebastian A, Hulter HN: Mineral corticoid excess and deficiency syndromes. *In* Brenner BM, Stein JH (eds): Contemporary Issues in Nephrology: Acid-Base and Potassium Homeostasis, vol 2, 2nd ed. New York, Churchill Livingstone, 1978, p 232.

463. Sands JM, Naruse M, Baum M, et al: Apical extracellular calcium/polyvalent cation–sensing receptor regulates vasopressin-elicited water permeability in rat kidney inner medullary collecting duct. J Clin Invest 99:1399-1405, 1997.

464. Suki WN, Yium JJ, Von Minden M, et al: Acute treatment of hypercalcemia with furosemide. N Engl J Med 283:836-840, 1970.

465. Borghi L, Meschi T, Guerra A, Novarini A: Randomized prospective study of a nonthiazide diuretic, indapamide, in preventing calcium stone recurrences. J Cardiovasc Pharmacol 22:S78-S86, 1993.

466. Pak CYC, Peterson R, Sakhaee K, et al: Correction of hypocitraturia and prevention of stone formation by combined thiazide and potassium citrate therapy in thiazide-unresponsive hypercalciuric nephrolithiasis. Am J Med 79:284-288, 1985.

467. Leppla D, Browne R, Hill K, Pak CY: Effect of amiloride with or without hydrochlorothiazide on urinary calcium and saturation of calcium salts. J Clin Endocrinol Metab 57:920-924, 1983.

468. Frassetto LA, Nash E, Morris RC, Sebastian A: Comparative effects of potassium chloride and bicarbonate on thiazide-induced reduction in urinary calcium excretion. Kidney Int 58:748-752, 2000.

469. Barry ELR, Gesek FA, Kaplan MR, et al: Expression of the sodium-chloride cotransporter in osteoblast-like cells: Effects of thiazide diuretics. Am J Physiol 272:C109-C116, 1997.

470. Aubin R, Menard P, Lajeunesse D: Selective effect of thiazides on the human osteoblast-like cell line MG-63. Kidney Int 50:1476-1482, 1996.

471. Lajeunesse D, Delalandre A, Guggino SE: Thiazide diuretics affect osteocalcin production in human osteoblasts at the transcription level without affecting vitamin D3 receptors. J Bone Miner Res 15:894-901, 2000.

472. Lalande A, Roux S, Denne MA, et al: Indapamide, a thiazide-like diuretic, decreases bone resorption in vitro. J Bone Miner Res 16:361-370, 2001.

473. Sigurdsson G, Franzson L: Increased bone mineral density in a population-based group of 70-year-old women on thiazide diuretics, independent of parathyroid hormone levels. J Intern Med 250:51-56, 2001.

474. Cauley JA, Cummings SR: Thiazide diuretics preserve bone mass and reduce the risk of fractures in elderly women: A prospective study. J Bone Miner Res 4:216-217, 1989.

475. Reid IR, Ames RW, Orr-Walker BJ, et al: Hydrochlorothiazide reduces loss of cortical bone in normal postmenopausal women: A randomized controlled trial. Am J Med 109:362-370, 2000.

476. Rejnmark L, Vestergaard P, Heickendorff L, et al: Effects of thiazide- and loop-diuretics, alone or in combination, on calcitropic hormones and biochemical bone markers: A randomized controlled study. J Intern Med 250:144-153, 2001.

477. Crawford JD, Kennedy GC: Chlorothiazide in diabetes insipidus. Nature 183:891, 1959.

478. Spannow J, Thomsen K, Petersen JS, et al: Influence of renal nerves and sodium balance on the acute antidiuretic effect of bendroflumethiazide in rats with diabetes insipidus. J Pharmacol Exp Ther 282:1155-1162, 1997.

479. Gronbeck L, Marples D, Nielsen S, Christensen S: Mechanism of antidiuresis caused by bendroflumethiazide in conscious rats with diabetes insipidus. Br J Pharmacol 123:737-745, 1998.

480. Shirley DG, Walter SJ, Laycock JF: The antidiuretic effect of chronic hydrochlorothiazide treatment in rats with diabetes insipidus: Renal mechanisms. Clin Sci (Colch) 63:533-538, 1982.

CHAPTER 55

Antihypertensive Drugs

Matthew R. Weir, Donna S. Hanes, and David K. Klassen

This chapter is divided into three major sections. The first section reviews the pharmacology of the nondiuretic antihypertensive drugs in order to provide clinicians with a complete overview of how to employ these therapies safely in practice (Table 55-1). The first section also discusses the individual drug classes and highlights the class mechanism of action, class members, class renal effects, and class efficacy and safety. Individual similarities and differences both within and between classes are addressed.

The second section reviews clinical decision making with regard to the selection of antihypertensive therapy, blood pressure goals, considerations about choosing the first agent or using fixed-dose combination therapy, and how to deal with refractory hypertension.

The third section reviews the pharmacology of the parenteral and oral drugs available for the treatment of hypertensive urgencies and emergencies and discusses clinical considerations in the acute reduction of blood pressure.

PHARMACOLOGY OF THE NONDIURETIC ANTIHYPERTENSIVE DRUGS

Angiotensin-Converting Enzyme Inhibitors

Class Mechanisms of Action

The angiotensin-converting enzyme (ACE) inhibitors inhibit the activity of ACE, which converts the inactive decapeptide angiotensin I (AI) to the potent hormone angiotensin II (AII). Because AII plays a crucial role in maintaining and regulating blood pressure by vasoconstriction and renal sodium and water retention, the ACE inhibitors are powerful tools for targeting multiple pathways that contribute to hypertension. ACE inhibitors directly reduce the circulating and tissue

levels of AII, blocking the potent vasoconstriction induced by the hormone (Table 55-2).[1-4] The resulting decrease in peripheral vascular resistance is not accompanied by changes in cardiac output or glomerular filtration rate (GFR); heart

TABLE 55-1

Pharmacology of Nondiuretic Antihypertensive Drugs

Angiotensin-converting enzyme inhibitors
  Sulfhydryl
  Carboxyl
  Phosphinyl
Angiotensin II type 1 receptor antagonists
  Biphenyl tetrazoles
  Nonbiphenyl tetrazoles
  Nonheterocyclics
β-Adrenergic and α_1- and β-adrenergic antagonists
  Nonselective β-adrenergic antagonists
  Nonselective β-adrenergic antagonists with partial agonist activity
    β_1-Selective adrenergic antagonists
    β_1-Selective adrenergic antagonists with partial agonist activity
    Nonselective β-adrenergic and α_1-adrenergic antagonists
Calcium antagonists
Direct-acting vasodilators
  Benzothiazepines
  Dihydropyridines
  Diphenylalkylamines
  Tetralines
Central α_2-adrenergic agonists
Central and peripheral adrenergic-neuronal blocking agents
Moderately selective peripheral α_1-adrenergic antagonists
Peripheral α_1-adrenergic antagonists
Peripheral adrenergic-neuronal blocking agents
Selective aldosterone receptor antagonists
Tyrosine hydroxylase inhibitors
Vasopeptidase inhibitors

TABLE 55-2

Antihypertensive Mechanism of Action of Angiotensin-Converting Enzyme Inhibitors

↓Peripheral vascular resistance
↓Vasodilatory bradykinins
Enhance vasodilatory prostaglandin synthesis
Improve nitric oxide–mediated endothelial function
Reverse vascular hypertrophy
↓Aldosterone secretion
Induce natriuresis
Augment renal blood flow
Blunt SNS activity and pressor responses
Inhibit NE and AVP release
Inhibit baroreceptor reflexes
↓Endothelin-1 levels
Inhibit thirst

AVP, arginine vasopressin; NE, norepinephrine; SNS, sympathetic nervous system.

rate is unchanged or may be reduced in patients whose baseline heart rate is higher than 85 beats/min.[5-7]

Reduction in systemic and local levels of AII also leads to effects beyond vasodilation that contribute to the antihypertensive efficacy of ACE inhibitors (see Table 55-1).[8] Additional mechanisms include (1) inhibition of the breakdown of vasodilatory bradykinins catalyzed by ACE or kininase II (the hypotensive action of ACE inhibitors is blocked by bradykinin antagonists)[9]; (2) enhancement of vasodilatory prostaglandin synthesis induced by elevated bradykinins[10]; (3) improvement of nitric oxide–mediated endothelial function[11, 12]; (4) reversal of vascular hypertrophy[13, 14]; (5) decrease in aldosterone secretion that causes natriuresis or attenuates the compensatory increase in sodium retention that accompanies a fall in blood pressure[15]; (6) augmentation of renal blood flow to induce natriuresis[8, 16-18]; (7) blunting of sympathetic nervous system activity[19, 20] through presynaptic modulation of norepinephrine release[21]; (8) inhibition of postjunctional pressor responses to norepinephrine or AII[22]; (9) inhibition of central AII-mediated sympathoexcitation, norepinephrine synthesis, and AVP release[23-25]; (10) inhibition of centrally controlled baroreceptor reflexes, which results in increased baroreceptor sensitivity[26-28]; (11) decrease in vasoconstrictor endothelin-1 levels[29]; and (12) possibly inhibition of thirst.[30]

Class Members

There are currently more than 15 ACE inhibitors in clinical use. Each drug has a unique structure that determines its potency, tissue receptor binding affinity, metabolism, and prodrug compound, but they remarkably similar clinical effects (Table 55-3).[8, 31] The drugs are classified into either sulfhydryl, carboxyl, or phosphinyl categories on the basis of the ligand that binds to the ACE-zinc moiety.[31, 32]

SULFHYDRYL ANGIOTENSIN-CONVERTING ENZYME INHIBITORS

Alacepril is an investigational ACE inhibitor currently in use in Japan.[33] The optimal dose appears to be 50 mg/day, with ranges from 12.5 to 100 mg being effective for hypertension (see Table 55-3). After absorption, alacepril is rapidly

hydrolyzed in the liver to desacetylalacepril and then to captopril. The onset of action is 1 hour (Table 55-4).[32] Peak concentrations of captopril are achieved in 3 hours and last for 24 hours. The bioavailability is 70%. Alacepril is 100% metabolized in the liver into an intermediate that is converted into captopril, the active metabolite. The elimination of captopril is 1.9 hours and is markedly reduced in renal failure.[33] Renal excretion eliminates up to 70%. Alacepril is dialyzable, and doses should be reduced in renal failure.

Captopril is a sulfhydryl-containing ACE inhibitor that is available in tablets of 12.5, 25, 50, and 100 mg (see Tables 55-3 and 55-4).[34-38] The usual starting dose in hypertension is 25 mg two to three times daily (see Table 55-2) and can be titrated at 1- to 2-week intervals.[34] Captopril has 75% bioavailability, with peak onset occurring within 1 hour.[33-35] The half-life is 2 hours; with chronic administration, the hemodynamic effects are maintained for 3 to 8 hours and are dose related.[35, 36] Food may decrease captopril absorption by up to 54% but is clinically insignificant.[39] Thirty percent of captopril is protein bound, but the amount decreases with decreasing renal function.[40] Captopril is partially metabolized in the liver into an inactive captopril–cysteine disulfide compound; 95% of the parent compound and metabolites are eliminated in the urine within 24 hours. The elimination half-life increases markedly in patients with creatinine clearances less than 20 mL/min. Initial dosages should be reduced and smaller increments used for titration. Hemodialysis removes approximately 35% of the dose.[40]

CARBOXYL ANGIOTENSIN-CONVERTING ENZYME INHIBITORS

Benazepril hydrochloride is a long-acting, non–sulfhydryl-containing, carboxyl ACE inhibitor that is available as 10- or 20-mg tablets alone or in combination with amlodipine. The usual initial dose is 10 mg daily, with maintenance doses of 20 to 40 mg daily. Some patients respond better to twice-daily dosing (see Tables 55-3 and 55-4).[36, 41-43] The onset of action occurs in 2 to 6 hours; maximal antihypertensive responsiveness occurs in 2 weeks. Bioavailability is 37% and is unaffected by food. Benazepril is a prodrug that is rapidly and almost completely bioactivated in the liver into the active benazeprilat compound, which is 200 times more potent than benazepril.[41] The elimination half-life of benazeprilat is 22 hours. Benazeprilat is excreted primarily in the urine by tubular secretion; nonrenal and bile elimination accounts for most of the inactive metabolites and contributes to clearance of benazeprilat in patients with renal failure.[34] Dialysis does not remove benazepril, but initial doses should be reduced to 10 and 5 mg in patients with creatinine clearances less than 60 and 30 mL/min, respectively.

Cilazapril is a nonsulfhydryl prodrug of the long-acting ACE inhibitor cilazaprilat.[34, 36] The usual dose is 2.5 to 10 mg daily or in divided doses. The oral bioavailability approaches 75%.[44, 45] After absorption, cilazapril is rapidly deesterified in the liver to its active metabolite, cilazaprilat. There is no further metabolism of cilazaprilat. The initial antihypertensive response occurs in 1 to 2 hours, peaks at 6 hours, and lasts for 8 to 12 hours.[46] Elimination of the active metabolite is biphasic, with a terminal half-life of 30 to 50 hours. Renal excretion accounts for 53% of the clearance, and doses should be reduced by 25% to 50% in renal failure.

TABLE 55-3

Pharmacodynamic Properties of Angiotensin-Converting Enzyme Inhibitors

DRUG GENERIC (TRADE) NAME	PEAK RESPONSE (H)	DURATION OF RESPONSE (H)	INITIAL DOSE (MG)	USUAL DOSE (MG)	MAXIMUM DOSE (MG)	INTERVAL
Alacepril (Cetapril)	3	24	12.5	12.5-100	100	qd
Captopril (Capoten)	1-2	6-12	12.5	12.5-50	150	bid/tid
Benazepril (Lotensin)	2-6	24	10	10-20	40	qd
Enalapril (Vasotec)	4-8	12-24	5	10-40	40	qd/bid
Moexipril (Univasc)	3-6	24	7.5	7.5-30	30	qd/bid
Quinapril (Accupril)	2	24	5	20-80	30	qd
Ramipril (Altace)	3-6	24	2.5	2.5-20	40	qd/bid
Trandolapril (Mavik)	2-12	24	1	2-4	8	qd
Fosinopril (Monopril)	2-7	24	5	5-40	40	qd/bid
Cilazipril (Dynorm)	6	8-10	2.5	2.5-10	10	qd/bid
Perindopril (Aceon)	3-7	24	4	4-8	8	qd
Spirapril (SCH 33844)	3-6	24	6	6	6	qd
Zofenopril (SQ 26991)	—	—	30	30-60	60	qd
Lisinopril (Zestril, Prinivil)	6-8	24	10	20-40	40	qd
Imidipril (TA 6366)	5-6	24	10	10-40	40	qd

Enalapril maleate is a nonsulfhydryl prodrug of the long acting ACE inhibitor enalaprilat.[34, 36] The oral preparations are available in tablets of 2.5, 5, 10, and 20 mg (see Tables 55-3 and 55-4). The initial dose of enalapril is 5 mg once daily. The usual daily dose is 10 to 40 mg, singly or in divided doses. The oral bioavailability approaches 73%. Initial responses occur in 1 hour, and the peak serum levels of enalaprilat are achieved in 3 to 4 hours. Enalapril undergoes biotransformation in the liver into the active compound, enalaprilat. Enalapril is excreted primarily in the urine with an elimination half-life of 1.3 hours. Enalaprilat has an elimination half-life of up to 35 hours, which is prolonged by renal failure. Doses should be reduced by 25% to 50% in patients with end-stage renal disease (ESRD).

Imidapril is the nonsulfhydryl prodrug of the long-acting ACE inhibitor imidaprilat. The usual daily dose is 10 to 40 mg (see Table 55-3). The oral bioavailability is approximately 40%. The time to peak concentration of imidaprilat is 3 to 10 hours (see Table 55-4). The peak response occurs in 5 to 6 hours and lasts for 24 hours.[47] Imidapril is hydrolyzed in the liver into the active diacid imidaprilat, and both compounds are excreted primarily in the urine and bile. The elimination half-life of the metabolites is 10 to 19 hours.[48] No dose adjustments are necessary in patients with renal failure. It has a unique advantage over other ACE inhibitors in causing a lower incidence of cough.[49]

Lisinopril is a nonsulfhydryl lysine analog of enalaprilat.[34, 36, 50-52] The initial dose is 10 mg/day, and the usual daily dose is 20 to 40 mg (see Tables 55-3 and 55-4). The bioavailability is 6% to 60%[52] and is not affected by food. The initial antihypertensive response occurs in 1 hour, peaks at 6 hours, and lasts for 24 hours. The maximal effect may not be seen for 24 hours. The elimination half-life is 12 hours. Lisinopril is not metabolized and is exclusively eliminated unchanged in the kidneys. Lisinopril is dialyzable, and patients may require supplemental doses. The initial dose should be

reduced to 2.5 to 7.5 mg/day in patients with moderate to advanced renal failure.

Moexipril hydrochloride is the nonsulfhydryl prodrug of the ACE inhibitor moexiprilat. The usual daily dose is 7.5 to 30 mg in single or divided doses (see Table 55-3).[34, 36, 53] The oral bioavailability of moexipril as moexiprilat is 13% to 22%, and absorption is impaired by food, particularly high-fat meals. Peak plasma concentrations occur at 1.5 hours; the peak response occurs at 3 to 6 hours and lasts 24 hours (see Table 55-4). After absorption, moexipril is rapidly converted in the liver to moexiprilat, which is 1000 times more potent than the parent compound.[53] The elimination half-life of moexiprilat is 2 to 10 hours. Both parent and active compounds and subsequent inactive metabolites are excreted in the feces (50%) and urine. Dosage should be reduced by 50% in renal failure.

Perindopril is a nonsulfhydryl prodrug of the long-acting ACE inhibitor perindoprilat.[34, 36] The usual daily dose is 4 to 8 mg (see Table 55-3). The initial response is seen in 1.5 hours[54] and peaks at 3 to 7 hours (see Table 55-4). A single dose has a duration of action of 24 hours. The bioavailability of perindopril is 75% and is slowed by food. Perindopril undergoes extensive first-pass hepatic metabolism into the active metabolite, perindoprilat. The elimination half-life of perindoprilat is 3 to 10 hours. Renal excretion accounts for 75% of the clearance of the parent drug and metabolites. Dosage should be reduced by 75% and 50% in patients with creatinine clearances less than 50 and 10 mL/min, respectively.[55]

Quinapril hydrochloride is a nonsulfhydryl, ethyl ester prodrug of the ACE inhibitor quinaprilat.[34, 36, 56, 57] The initial dose is 10 mg, and the usual daily dose is 20 to 80 mg and should be adjusted at 2-week intervals (see Table 55-3). Twice-daily therapy may provide a more sustained blood pressure reduction. The onset of action occurs in 1 hour; the peak response occurs in 2 hours and lasts for 12 to 24 hours

TABLE 55-4

Pharmacokinetic Properties of Angiotensin-Converting Enzyme Inhibitors

ACTIVE DRUG METABOLISM	EXCRETION*	BIOAVAILABILITY % METABOLITES	AFFECTED BY FOOD	PEAK BLOOD LEVEL (H)	ELIMINATION HALF LIFE	ABSORPTION
Alacepril U(70)	— Captopril	70	—	1	1.9	L
Captopril U	60-75 Inactive	75	Yes	1	2	K
Benazepril F/U	35 Benazeprilat	>37	No	2-6	22	L/K
Enalapril F/U	55-75 Enalaprilat	73	—	3-4	11-35	L/K
Lisinopril U	25 Enalaprilat	6-60	—	1	12	K
Moexepril F(50)/U	>20 Moexeprilat	13-22	Yes	1.5	2-10	L/K
Quinapril U(50)	60 Quinaprilat	50	Yes	1	25	K
Ramipril F/U	50-60 Ramiprilat	60	—	2-4	13-17	L/K
Trandolapril F(66)/U	70 Trandalaprilat	10	No	2-12	16-24	L/K
Fosinopril L/K/I	36 F/U Fosinoprilat	36	—	1	12	
Cilazapril U(52)	— Cilazaprilat	57-76	No	1-2	30-50	K
Spirapril F(60)/U(40)	— Spiraprilat	50	Yes	1	33-41	L
Perindopril F/U(75)	— Perindoprilat	75	Yes	1.5	3-10	L
Imidapril U	— Imidaprilat	40	—	3-10	10-19	L
Zofenopril F(26)/U(69)	>80 Zofenoprilat	96	Yes	5	5	K

*Excretion values in parentheses are percentages.

F, feces; I, intestine; K, kidney; L, liver; U, urine.

(see Table 55-4). Bioavailability is 50% and is delayed by food. After absorption, quinapril is extensively metabolized in the liver into the active metabolite, quinaprilat, and several inactive compounds. Renal excretion by way of filtration and active tubular secretion accounts for 50% of the clearance. The elimination half-life is biphasic with a terminal half-life of 25 hours. Quinapril is not dialyzable. The dose should be reduced by 25% to 50% in patients with renal failure.

Ramipril is a potent, nonsulfhydryl prodrug of the ACE inhibitor ramiprilat.[34, 36, 58-60] Ramipril capsules are available in 1.25, 2.5 or 5 mg. The initial daily dose is 2.5 mg (see Table 55-3). The usual daily dose is 2.5 to 20 mg and can be titrated by doubling the current dose at 2- to 4-week intervals. Ramipril is well absorbed from the gastrointestinal tract with a bioavailability of 60%; peak concentrations are achieved in 1 hour (see Table 55-4). Peak response occurs in 2 hours and lasts for 24 hours. Ramipril is extensively metabolized by saponification in the liver into the active metabolite, ramiprilat. The elimination half-life of the active compound is 13 to 17 hours and is prolonged with renal failure to almost 50 hours.[61] The dosage should be reduced by 50% to 75% in patients with a creatinine clearance less than 50 mL/min.

Spirapril hydrochloride is a nonsulfhydryl prodrug of the ACE inhibitor spiraprilat[34, 62] that has been approved for hypertension in the United States but has not been marketed. The initial and usual daily dose is 6 mg (see Table 55-3).[63] The initial response occurs in 1 hour, and the peak response occurs in 3 to 6 hours. The time to peak concentration is approximately 1 hour (see Table 55-4).[64] The bioavailability is 50% and is slowed by high-fat meals. Spirapril is rapidly deesterified in the liver into spiraprilat. The elimination half-life of spiraprilat is 33 to 41 hours.[65] The metabolites are excreted in the urine (40%) and feces (60%). Dose adjustment is indicated only in severe renal failure.

Trandolapril is a nonsulfhydryl, ethyl ester prodrug of the ACE inhibitor trandolaprilat.[34, 36, 66] It is available in tablets of 1, 2, and 4 mg or in combination with verapamil. The usual starting dose is 1 to 2 mg/day and is frequently higher in blacks (see Table 55-3). Trandolapril is only 10% bioavailable, and absorption is not affected by food (see Table 55-4).[67] Trandolapril undergoes extensive first-pass hepatic metabolism by cleavage of the ethyl group into the active diacid trandolaprilat and inactive glucuronide conjugates. Trandolaprilat is further metabolized into inactive compounds. Peak serum concentrations of trandolaprilat occur within 2 to 12 hours; the duration of action is 24 hours but may reach up to 6 weeks.

The elimination half-life of trandolaprilat is 16 to 24 hours. Sixty-six percent of the metabolites are excreted in the feces. The remaining metabolites are excreted in a dose-dependent manner by the kidney and are related to creatinine clearance. The recommended starting dose with creatinine clearance less than 30 mL/min is 0.5 mg.

Zofenopril is an investigational ACE inhibitor. The effective dose for the treatment of hypertension is 30 to 60 mg/day (see Table 55-3).[68] It is well absorbed from the gastrointestinal tract, with a bioavailability of 96% (see Table 55-4).[69] It is partially metabolized in the liver by hydrolysis into the active compound, zofenoprilat.[69, 70] The time to peak response and duration are unknown. Zofenopril is cleared both hepatically (26%) and renally (69%), with an elimination half-life of 5 hours.[70] The need for dosage adjustment in renal failure is unknown.

PHOSPHINYL ANGIOTENSIN-CONVERTING ENZYME INHIBITOR

Fosinopril sodium is a nonsulfhydryl prodrug of the long-acting ACE inhibitor fosinoprilat.[34, 36, 71-74] The usual daily dose is 5 to 40 mg (see Table 55-3). Maximal effects may not occur until 4 weeks. The initial response occurs in 1 hour, the peak response occurs in 2 to 7 hours, and the duration of response is 24 hours and is prolonged in ESRD (see Table 55-4).[74] Bioavailability of fosinopril is approximately 36%. Eighty percent of fosinopril is hydrolyzed in the liver and intestines into the active compound, fosinoprilat, the remainder into inactive metabolites. The elimination half-life of fosinoprilat is 11.5 to 12 hours. All metabolites are excreted in both the urine and feces. Hepatic biliary clearance increases significantly as renal function declines. Thus, dosage needs to be reduced by 25% in patients with ESRD.[74]

Class Renal Effects

There has been considerable interest in the ability of the ACE inhibitors to protect the kidney from the unrelenting deterioration that occurs with hypertension and renal insufficiency. The ACE inhibitors have vast hemodynamic and non-hemodynamic effects that afford such protection (Table 55-5). In patients with hypertension, the ACE inhibitors have the ability to restore the pressure-natriuresis relationship to normal, allowing sodium balance to be maintained at a lower arterial blood pressure.[75] In the setting of restricted sodium intake, the response is exaggerated. The mechanism responsible for this effect is direct inhibition of proximal, and possibly distal, tubule sodium reabsorption.[76] The natriuretic effect is unlikely to be due to inhibition of aldosterone because it is immediate.[8] The increase in renal excretory capacity plays a major role in the long-term antihypertensive activity of the drugs. Clinically, the increase in sodium excretion is transitory because the reduction in arterial pressure returns sodium excretion to normal. However, the maintenance of normal sodium excretion at lower arterial pressures correlates with increased excretion in the setting of hypertension.[75] After several days, both inhibition of AII and aldosterone contribute to the natriuresis.[8, 77-79] The long-term effects on water excretion are less certain. ACE inhibitors induce an initial increase in free water clearance, but there are no long-term changes in total body weight, plasma, or extracellular fluid volume.[80] The decrease in aldosterone caused by ACE inhibition also

TABLE 55-5

Potential Renoprotective Effects of Antiotensin-Converting Enzyme Inhibitors

Restore pressure-natriuresis relationship to normal
Inhibit tubule sodium resorption
Decrease arterial pressure
Decrease aldosterone production
Decrease proteinuria
Improve altered lipid profiles
Decrease renal blood flow
Decrease filtration fraction
Decrease renal vascular resistance
Reduce scarring and fibrosis
Attenuate oxidative stress and free radicals

correlates with decreased potassium excretion,[78] particularly in patients with impaired renal function. The antikaliuretic effect appears to be transient but can be exacerbated by concomitant administration of potassium-sparing diuretics, supplements, and nonsteroidal anti-inflammatory drugs (NSAIDs) and should be monitored rigorously.

The effects of ACE inhibitors on angiotensin peptide levels depend on the responsiveness of renin secretion.[81, 82] All ACE inhibitors decrease AII, increase angiotensin 1-7 (a potential vasodilator), and increase plasma renin. When renin shows little increase in response to ACE inhibition, the levels of AII and its metabolites decrease markedly, with little change in the levels of AI. Large increases in renin levels in response to ACE inhibition also increase the levels of AI and its metabolites. The increased levels of AI can produce higher levels of AII by uninhibited ACE and other pathways, thereby blunting the effect of reduced AII.[82] This phenomenon is referred to as *ACE escape* and may contribute to reduced ACE inhibitor efficacy when used chronically.[6] Consequently, ACE inhibitors with the greatest potency in suppressing AII at the level of the tissue may be the most important determinant of renal protection.[8]

The importance of tissue ACE specificity remains controversial. It is clear that local inhibition of ACE in the vascular wall and renal vessels contributes to the antihypertensive activity of the drugs. ACE inhibitor–induced changes in blood pressure correlate with the degree of renin-angiotensin system (RAS) inhibition in both plasma and tissues. The ACE inhibitors with the greatest tissue specificity, however, are associated with prolonged activity at the tissue level even after the serum ACE levels return to normal. Consequently, they are more efficacious at once-daily dosing. Other potential renoprotective effects noted in experimental models include attenuation of oxidative stress,[83, 84] scavenging of free radicals, and attenuation of lipid peroxidation.[85] The clinical importance of these effects is under investigation.

Insofar as the degree of proteinuria correlates best with the rate of decline of renal function and a decrease in proteinuria correlates better with renal function outcome than lowering blood pressure, reduction of proteinuria can have a substantial impact.[86] All ACE inhibitors decrease urinary protein excretion[86-93] in normotensive and hypertensive patients with renal disease of various origins.[94-97] Individual response rates vary from a rise of 31% to a fall of 100% and are strongly influenced by drug dose and changes in dietary sodium. There is a clear dose-response relationship between increasing doses and reduction of proteinuria that is not dependent on changes in blood pressure, renal plasma flow, or GFR. Furthermore, the effect of ACE inhibitors on reduction of proteinuria is abolished with high salt intake.[98]

In normotensive diabetics, studies demonstrate that ACE inhibitors can normalize GFR, markedly reduce the progression of renal disease, and normalize microalbuminuria.[99] The effect is noted in the first month of therapy and is maximal at 14 months. Several mechanisms account for the reduction in urinary protein excretion: a decrease in glomerular capillary hydrostatic pressure, a decrease in mesangial uptake and clearance of macromolecules, and improved glomerular basement membrane permselectivity.[8, 100] The ACE inhibitors have superior antiproteinuric efficacy compared with other classes of antihypertensive agents, with the exception of angiotensin receptor blockers (ARBs). The antiproteinuric effect is additive with the ARBs and does not depend on changes in creatinine clearance, GFR, or blood pressure.[86, 101] Clinical trials also demonstrate a superior renoprotective effect of ACE inhibitors in blacks, once thought not to benefit from this class. In the African American Study of Kidney Disease, hypertensive patients with proteinuria greater than 300 mg/day had a much slower rate of progression of kidney disease when treated with an ACE inhibitor than with a dihydropyridine calcium antagonist (CA).[102]

ACE inhibitors also ameliorate the deranged lipid profile in patients with nephrotic range protein, which may affect the rate of progression of renal failure.[103, 104] However, up to 0.7% of patients treated with captopril may develop proteinuria with total urinary protein excretion exceeding 1 g/day.[35, 36] About 90% of affected patients have evidence of prior renal disease or received doses in excess of 150 mg/day, or both. The nephrotic syndrome occurred in one fifth of proteinuric patients. In most cases, proteinuria subsides within 6 months whether or not captopril is continued, with no residual change in GFR. Renal biopsy specimens reveal a membranous nephropathy. The sulfhydryl group of captopril is thought to invoke an immune complex–mediated nephropathy similar to that which occurs with penicillamine.[105-108]

Evidence suggests that the majority of the vasoconstrictor action of AII is confined to the efferent arteriole. ACE inhibitors preferentially dilate the efferent arteriole by reducing the systemic and intrarenal levels of AII. The effect is a reduction in intraglomerular capillary pressure. ACE inhibitors uniformly increase renal blood flow, decrease filtration fraction, have variable to no effect on GFR, decrease renal vascular resistance, reduce urinary protein excretion, and impair microvasculatory autoregulation,[16-18, 93, 109-112] in patients with hypertension. In patients with nondiabetic glomerular renal damage, acute ACE inhibitor administration causes a decrease of renal perfusion, glomerular filtration, and pressure and an increase of afferent resistances.[113, 114] Long-term administration is associated with a decrease in renal perfusion, with a tendency to higher filtration fraction and lower afferent resistances. Marked improvement in GFR occurs and is sustained for up to 3 years.[17, 76-78, 115, 116] However, many patients with impaired renal function exhibit a reversible fall in GFR with ACE inhibitor therapy that is

not detrimental. Numerous studies demonstrate that the GFR declines initially because of the hemodynamic changes, but the long-term reduction in perfusion pressure is renoprotective. Type 1 diabetic patients with the greatest initial decline in GFR have the slowest rate of loss of renal function over time.[117] It should be emphasized that ACE inhibitors should not be withdrawn immediately if an increase in serum creatinine is noted; a 20% to 30% decline in GFR can be expected, and close monitoring is warranted.

A genetically inherited trait of disordered regulation of the RAS by the kidney and the adrenal gland contributes to the pathogenesis of hypertension in approximately 45% of patients.[118] Such patients have sodium-sensitive hypertension, abnormalities in the renal vascular responses to changes in sodium intake and AII, blunted decrements of renin release in response to saline or AII, and accentuated vasodilator responses to ACE inhibition[118, 119]; they have been termed *nonmodulators*. In these patients, ACE inhibition not only increases renal blood flow substantially more than it does in normal subjects but also restores to normal the renal vascular and adrenal responses to AII, renin release, renal sodium handling, and blood pressure.[120]

In patients with an activated RAS, ACE inhibitors cause a decrease in GFR and can precipitate acute renal failure. Patients with severe bilateral renal artery stenosis, unilateral renal artery stenosis of a solitary kidney, severe hypertensive nephrosclerosis, volume depletion, congestive heart failure, cirrhosis, or a transplanted kidney are at high risk for renal deterioration with ACE inhibitors.[80, 121-126] These patients typically have a precipitous drop in blood pressure and deterioration of renal function when treated with ACE inhibitors. In these states of reduced renal perfusion related to low effective arterial circulating volume or flow reduced by an obstructed artery, the maintenance of renal blood flow and GFR is highly dependent on increased efferent arteriolar vasoconstriction mediated by AII. Interruption of the increased tone causes a critical reduction in perfusion pressure and can lead to dramatic reductions in GFR and urinary flow, worsening of renal ischemia, and, in selected cases, anuria.[127] The hemodynamic effect is reversible with cessation of therapy and forms the basis for the use of the captopril-plasma renin activity (PRA) challenge test and renography in the diagnosis of renal artery stenosis.[128, 129] In unilateral renal artery stenosis, ACE inhibitors cause a significant decline in GFR that is compensated by an increase in renal blood flow to the contralateral kidney. Clinically, no significant change is measured in total GFR, but increases in plasma renin activity and reduced or delayed uptake on renography are seen. If this condition is undiagnosed, continued ACE inhibitor therapy may potentiate ischemia to the stenotic kidney.[8, 130]

Class Efficacy and Safety

ACE inhibitors are recommended for initial monotherapy in patients with mild, moderate, and severe hypertension[131] regardless of age, race, or gender.[2, 3, 5, 76] They are effective in diabetic patients, obese patients, and patients with renal transplants.[132-134] They are safe to use in patients with mild, moderate, and severe renal insufficiency but are underutilized.[135] In general, patients with high-renin hypertension and chronic renal parenchymal disease respond particularly well, presumably because they have inappropriately high intrarenal renin and AII levels. Black hypertensives have been found to respond less well to lower doses than whites, but higher doses are as effective.[136, 137] In most studies, ACE inhibitors elicit an adequate response in 40% to 60% of patients. An immediate fall in blood pressure occurs in 70% of patients. The enhanced efficacy of ACE inhibitors in the presence of salt restriction is paralleled by the additive effects of diuretic therapy. The addition of low-dose hydrochlorothiazide (HCTZ) enhances the efficacy more than 80%, normalizing blood pressure in another 20% to 25% of patients.[138-141] Addition of the diuretic is more effective than increasing the dose of ACE inhibitor.[140, 141]

Neither the duration nor the degree of blood pressure lowering is predicted by the effect on blood ACE or AII levels, and all ACE inhibitors appear to have comparable efficacy. The response may, in part, be due to interindividual variability of the ACE genotype. The activity of ACE is partially dependent on the presence or absence of a 287-base-pair element in intron 16, and this insertion-deletion (ID) polymorphism accounts for 47% of the total phenotypic variation in plasma ACE. DD subjects have the highest, ID subjects have intermediate, and II subjects have the lowest concentrations. Genotype also influences tissue ACE activity, but the clinical implications are under investigation.[142]

ACE inhibitors are indicated as first-line therapy in hypertensive patients with heart failure and systolic dysfunction, those with type 1 diabetes and proteinuria, patients after myocardial infarction with reduced systolic function, and patients with left ventricular dysfunction.[117, 143] ACE inhibitors reduce ventricular hypertrophy independent of the blood pressure lowering.[144] All patients with diabetes and no evidence of nephropathy should be given ACE inhibitors for cardiovascular risk reduction.[145, 146] Clinical studies showed that ACE inhibitors improve endothelial dysfunction and cardiac and vascular remodeling, retard the progression of atherosclerosis, improve arterial distensibility, and reduce the risk of myocardial ischemia and infarction, stroke, and cardiovascular death in primary and secondary prevention[145, 147-149] trials. They are also associated with improved exercise performance in patients with hypertension and intermittent claudication, reduced pain perception, reduced perioperative myocardial ischemia, and prolonged survival of arteriovenous polytetrafluoroethylene grafts.[150-152]

ACE inhibitors are contraindicated in patients with known renovascular hypertension or hypersensitivity to ACE inhibitors. ACE inhibitors may cause fetal or neonatal injury or death when used during the second and third trimesters of pregnancy.[36, 153, 154] Exposure to ACE inhibitors limited to the first trimester has not been associated with injury. If a patient becomes pregnant during treatment, the ACE inhibitor should be discontinued and alternative treatment found; termination of pregnancy is not warranted. A potential increased risk for renal cancer in patients treated with ACE inhibitors has not been substantiated and probably reflects a correlation between hypertension and kidney cancer.[155]

Overall, ACE inhibitors are well tolerated and have relatively neutral metabolic effects. ACE inhibitors are associated with 8% to 11% reductions in low-density lipoprotein (LDL)-cholesterol and triglycerides and 5% increases in high-density lipoprotein (HDL)-cholesterol.[156] They do not cause perturbations of serum sodium or uric acid. ACE inhibitors reduce the levels of plasminogen activator inhibitor-1 and may improve fibrinolysis.[157] Hyperkalemia greater than 5.8 mmol/L rarely requires discontinuation of therapy and occurs in 2% of patients.[36] It is more likely to develop in patients with renal insufficiency or diabetes or those taking potassium-sparing drugs. The effects on glucose metabolism are variable. They have no adverse effect on serum glucose,[158, 159] may improve glucose tolerance by augmenting the insulin secretory response to glucose,[159] and may help ameliorate obesity and hyperinsulinemia.[160] Many of the ACE inhibitors need dose adjustment in the presence of renal dysfunction (Table 55-6).

There are few class side effects, and they may occur with all ACE inhibitors. The newer agents appear to have a lower incidence of side effects, possibly because of the lack of the sulfhydryl moiety found in captopril. The most common side effect of ACE inhibitors is a dry, hacking, nonproductive, and often intolerable cough that is reported in up to 20% of patients.[161-163] The cough is thought to be secondary to hypersensitivity to bradykinins, which are inactivated by ACE; increases in prostaglandins; and accumulation of substance P, a potent bronchoconstrictor.[8, 164, 165] The cough can begin initially or many months after therapy,[166] is more common in women, and may disappear spontaneously.[166] It may be more common in patients with bronchial hyperreactivity, but ACE inhibitors are safe in asthmatics.[167] NSAIDs and sodium cromoglycate have been reported to improve the cough.[168, 169]

Angioedema is a rare but potentially life-threatening complication of ACE inhibitor therapy. It occurs in less than 0.2% of patients within hours of the first dose of ACE inhibitor or after prolonged use.[163, 170, 171] Understanding of the mechanism of ACE inhibitor–induced angioedema is evolving and involves several components: tissue accumulation of bradykinin and inhibition of C1 esterase activity.[162, 171, 172] Susceptible individuals typically have defects in non-ACE, non–kininase I pathways of bradykinin degradation, such as the aminopeptidase P–dipeptidyl peptidase IV or the carboxypeptidase N pathway, or both.[171-173] Swelling confined to the face, mucous membranes, and lips usually resolves with discontinuation of therapy. Involvement of the glottis and larynx requires management of the airway, epinephrine, H_2-blockers, corticosteroids, or fresh-frozen plasma.[36, 162, 174]

First-dose hypotension, with reduction of blood pressure up to 30%, has been reported with all ACE inhibitors with a frequency of up to 2.5% of patients. Hypotension occurs more commonly in volume-depleted states,[175, 176] patients with high-renin hypertension, and those with systolic heart failure. The hypotension is usually well tolerated but may be associated with syncope.[177] In elderly patients, ACE inhibitor therapy more frequently causes nocturnal hypotension.[178] The accompanying increase in plasma norepinephrine may explain the low incidence of orthostatic symptoms.[178] In high-risk patients, therapy should be initiated with lower doses and preferably after discontinuation of diuretics. Rebound hypertension has not been reported with discontinuation of ACE inhibitors.

Side effects related to the chemical structure are more frequently seen with the sulfhydryl-containing captopril than

TABLE 55-6

Antihypertensive Drugs Requiring Dose Modification* in Renal Insufficiency: Estimated Glomerular Filtration Rate (Creatinine Clearance)

DRUG	>50 ML/MIN	10–15 ML/MIN	<10 ML/MIN	DIALYSIS†
Angiotensin-Converting Enzyme Inhibitors				
Alacepril	No change	50%	25%	(H) 50%
Benazepril	No change	50%	25%	Negligible
Captopril	No change	50%	25%	(H) 50%
Cilazepril	No change	50%	25%	(H) 50%
Enalapril	No change	50%	25%	(H) 50%
Fosinopril	No change	No change	75%	
Imidipril	No change	No change	—	—
Lisinopril	No change	50%	25%	(H) 50%
Moexipril	No change	50%	25%	—
Perindopril	No change	75%	50%	—
Quinapril	No change	50%	25%	—
Ramipril	No change	50%	25%	—
Spirapril	No change	No change	50%	—
Trandolapril	No change	50%	25%	—
Zofenopril	No change	—	—	—
Angiotensin Receptor Blockers				
Candesartan	No change	No change	No change	Negligible
Eprosartan	No change	No change	50%	Negligible
Irbesartan	No change	No change	—	Negligible
Losartan	No change	No change	No change	Negligible
Olmesartan	No change	—	—	
Telmisartan	No change	No change	No change	Negligible
Valsartan	No change	No change	No change	—
β-Adrenergic Antagonists				
Nadolol	No change	50%	25%	(H) 50%
Carteolol	No change	50%	25%	—
Penbutolol	No change	No change	50%	Negligible
Pindolol	No change	No change	50%	Negligible
Atenolol	No change	50%	25%	(H) 50%
Betaxolol	No change	No change	50%	(H) 50%
Bisoprolol	No change	50%	25%	Negligible
Acebutolol	No change	50%	30%–50%	(H) 50%
Celiprolol	No change	50%	Avoid	—
Nebivolol	No change	50%	—	—
Calcium Antagonists				
Diltiazem	No change	No change	No change	Negligible
Verapamil	No change	No change	No change	Negligible
Nifedipine	No change	No change	No change	Negligible
Amlodipine	No change	No change	No change	Negligible
Felodipine	No change	No change	No change	Negligible
Isradipine	No change	No change	No change	Negligible
Manidipine	No change	No change	No change	Negligible
Nicardipine	No change	No change	No change	Negligible
Nisoldipine	No change	No change	No change	Negligible
Lacidipine	No change	No change	No change	Negligible
Lercanidipine	—			
Ca Central α_2-Adrenergic or Imidazole I_1-Agonists				
Methyldopa	No change	No change	50%	(H) 50%
Clonidine	No change	50%	25%	Negligible
Moxonidine	No change	50%	—	—
Rilmenidine	No change	50%	25%	—
Peripheral Adrenergic-Neuronal Blocking Agents				
Guanethidine	No change	No change	50% (avoid)	—
Guanadrel	No change	50%	25% (avoid)	—
Direct-Acting Vasodilators				
Hydralazine	No change	No change	75%‡	Negligible
Minoxidil	No change	50%	50%	(H and P) 50%
Tyrosine Hydroxylase Inhibitor				
Metyrosine	No change	50%	25%	—

Continued

TABLE 55-6

Antihypertensive Drugs Requiring Dose Modification* in Renal Insufficiency: Estimated Glomerular Filtration Rate (Creatinine Clearance)—Cont'd

DRUG	>50 ML/MIN	10–15 ML/MIN	<10 ML/MIN	DIALYSIS†
Selective Aldosterone Receptor Antagonists				
Eplerenone	Dosage adjustment in renal failure unknown Caution in regard to hyperkalemia			
Vasopeptidase Inhibitors				
Omapatrilat	No dosage adjustment is necessary in renal failure. Limited pharmacokinetic studies in patients with mild to severe renal insufficiency suggest that no dose adjustment in required.[34]			

*Percent of total dose given.

†Replacement dose at end of dialysis (% of dose prescribed for patient with GFR< 10 mL/min).

‡Slow acetylators.

H, hemodialysis; P, peritoneal dialysis.

with the other agents. Dysgeusia appears to be related to the binding of zinc by the ACE inhibitors. Approximately 2% to 4% of patients experience a diminution or loss of taste sensation that is associated with a metallic taste. It is usually self-limited and resolves in 2 to 3 months even with continued therapy. It may be severe enough to interfere with nutrition and cause weight loss.[179] Cutaneous reactions are manifest as a nonallergic, pruritic maculopapular eruption that appears during the first few weeks of therapy; they may be associated with a fever or arthralgias and may disappear even with continuation of the ACE inhibitor.[35] Leukopenia and anemia have been reported with ACE inhibitor therapy. Neutropenia (<1000 neutrophils/mm³) with myeloid hypoplasia occurs almost exclusively in patients with renal insufficiency, immunosuppression, collagen vascular diseases, or autoimmune diseases. It is associated with systemic and oral cavity infections common with agranulocytosis. Neutropenia occurs within 3 months of therapy and generally resolves 2 weeks after therapy is discontinued.[36] Although usually reversible, it may be fatal.[180]

Anaphylactoid reactions ranging from mild pruritus to bronchospasm and cardiopulmonary collapse have been reported in hemodialysis patients treated with ACE inhibitors who are dialyzed with high-flux polyacrylonitrile, cellulose acetate, or cuprophane membranes or patients receiving apheresis with dextran sulfate membranes.[8, 179, 181, 182] The frequency of reactions is unknown, but they occur within the first few minutes of treatment. Such membranes should be avoided in patients receiving ACE inhibitors.

Significant drug interactions with ACE inhibitors are few. AII stimulates the production of vasodilatory prostaglandins. Aspirin inhibits the production of vasodilator and antithrombotic prostaglandins. Theoretically, either agent may antagonize the effectiveness of the other. Studies show that aspirin doses of 100 mg/day or less do not negate the effects of ACE.[183-185] Concomitant use of ACE inhibitors and cyclosporine may exacerbate renal hypoperfusion.[36] Concomitant use of ACE inhibitors with trimethoprim may exaggerate hyperkalemia. Finally, ACE inhibitors

have been demonstrated to interfere with the response to erythropoietin. Hemodialysis and renal transplant patients receiving erythropoietin frequently require higher doses to maintain adequate hematocrits.[186, 187] Consequently, ACE inhibitors can be used effectively to reduce post-transplantation erythrocytosis.[188]

Angiotensin II Type I Receptor Antagonists
Class Mechanisms of Action

The AII receptor blockers (ARBs) allow more specific and complete blockade of the RAS than the ACE inhibitors because they circumvent all pathways that lead to the formation of AII. For example, AI is metabolized not only by ACE to form AII but also by chymase, cathepsin G, tissue plasminogen activator (t-PA), and other enzymes.[189-194] AII can be formed at sites other than those in the systemic circulation such as the brain, kidney, and heart.[189] Furthermore, long-term ACE inhibitor therapy is associated with a return of AII levels to baseline, possibly contributing to reduced efficacy. The ARBs selectively antagonize AII directly at the AT1 receptor regardless of the source of production. Because AII plays a crucial multifactorial role in maintaining and regulating blood pressure, blockade of the AT1 receptor with ARBs is a powerful tool for targeting multiple pathways that contribute to hypertension.

Like ACE inhibitors, ARBs directly block the vasoconstricting action of AII and cause a decrease in peripheral vascular resistance.[195-198] The hypotensive effect is not accompanied by changes in cardiac output, heart rate, or GFR.[195-198] Interruption of the binding of AII at the tissue level also leads to other effects beyond vasodilation that contribute to the antihypertensive effect (see Table 55-4).[8] Additional mechanisms include (1) augmentation of renal blood flow and reduction of aldosterone release to induce natriuresis and attenuate the compensatory increase in sodium retention that accompanies a fall in blood pressure,[8] (2) direct depression of tubule sodium reabsorption,[199, 200]

(3) improvement of nitric oxide–mediated endothelial function,[201] (4) reversal of vascular hypertrophy,[201] (5) blunting of sympathetic nervous system activity and presynaptic noradrenaline release,[202, 203] (6) inhibition of postjunctional pressor responses to NE or AII, (7) inhibition of central AII-mediated sympathoexcitation and vasopressin release,[204-208] (8) inhibition of centrally controlled baroreceptor reflexes,[202, 209] (9) inhibition of central nervous system norepinephrine synthesis,[207] (10) inhibition of thirst mechanisms,[30, 210-212] and possibly inhibition of RAS-mediated actions on endothelin-1.[213] The antihypertensive action of ARBs is dependent on activation of the RAS and is associated with clinically insignificant increases in circulating levels of AII.[196] ARBs also increase bradykinin levels by antagonizing AII at its type I receptor and diverting AII to its counterregulatory type 2 receptor, which potentiates vasodilation.[214, 215] ARBs also increase the level of other angiotensin peptides, including angiotensin 1-7, AIII, and AIV, which can act on their respective receptors to modulate vasoconstriction, renal blood flow, and vascular hypertrophy.[216-230]

Class Members

The ARB class is composed of peptide and nonpeptide analogs that vary in structure, mechanism of receptor inhibition, metabolism, and potency. There are currently seven drugs in clinical use. Many of the newer drugs arose from modification of losartan, the first biologically active ARB oral agent. They are categorized according to the substitution of carboxylic and other moieties into several groups: the biphenyl tetrazoles (derivatives of losartan), nonbiphenyl tetrazoles, and nonheterocyclic compounds.[8, 195] They are also classified according to their ability to antagonize AII. The competitive (surmountable) antagonists shift the dose-response curve for AII-mediated contraction to the right without depressing the maximal response to AII. The noncompetitive (insurmountable) antagonists also depress the maximal response to AII. The variable effects of ARBs are mediated by differences in the interaction with allosteric binding sites on the receptor, dissociation of the drug-receptor complex, removal of the agonists from tissues, or the ability to modulate the amount of internalized receptors.[231-234]

BIPHENYL TETRAZOLE DERIVATIVES

Candesartan cilexetil is an esterified prodrug imidazole that is rapidly and completely converted into the active 7-carboxylic acid candesartan (CV 11974) in the intestinal wall.[34, 36] Candesartan is a selective, nonpeptide ARB noncompetitive (insurmountable) blocker with the highest receptor binding affinity with a slow detachment rate from the receptor (Table 55-7).[233] Consequently, the effects are long lasting and unlikely to be overcome by the up-regulation of AII that commonly accompanies AT1 receptor blockade. The initial dose is 16 mg daily, and the usual daily dose is 8 to 32 mg in one or two divided doses (Table 55-8). The oral bioavailability is 15% and is unaffected by meals (Table 55-9). The initial antihypertensive response occurs in 2 to 4 hours, peaks at 6 to 8 hours, and lasts 24 hours.[234, 235] Radioreceptor assays demonstrate the presence of candesartan at the receptor site for periods longer than predicted from plasma half-life analysis, which correlates with the clinical observation of a sustained effect beyond 24 hours.[236] Maximal response is achieved in 4 weeks. The terminal half-life of candesartan is approximately 9 hours and is not affected by renal failure. No unchanged parent compound is detected in the serum or urine. The active metabolite is excreted by biliary secretion into the feces (67%) and renal excretion (33%). Candesartan is not dialyzable.

Eprosartan is a nonpeptide, selective ARB that was modified to resemble AII more closely. It is a noncompetitive antagonist with a high affinity for the AT1 receptor (see Table 55-7).[34, 36] The initial daily dose is 200 mg (see Table 55-8). The usual daily dose is 200 to 400 mg. The bioavailability is 13% (see Table 55-9). Eprosartan is rapidly absorbed, but absorption is delayed by food. The initial response occurs in 4 hours and lasts for 24 hours. Eprosartan is only 20% metabolized into inactive metabolites that are excreted in the urine (7%) and the feces (70%).[237] The elimination half-life is 6 hours. Doses should be reduced by 50% in patients with renal failure.

Irbesartan is a nonpeptide specific imidazolinone derivative of losartan that acts as a noncompetitive AT1 receptor blocker with a very high receptor binding affinity (see Table 55-7).[34, 36] The initial dose is 150 mg daily. The usual daily dose is 150 to 300 mg. The bioavailability of irbesartan is 60% to 80%.[238, 239] The initial response occurs in 2 hours. The peak response is bimodal; in hypertensive

TABLE 55-7

Pharmacokinetic Interactions between AT₁ Receptor Blockers and the Receptor

AT₁ RECEPTOR RECEPTOR ANTAGONIST	DISSOCIATION RATE	AFFINITY	TYPE OF AT₁, ANTAGONISM
Candesartan cilexetil (Candesartan)	Slow	280	Noncompetitive
Irbesartan	Slow	5	Noncompetitive
Valsartan	Slow	10	Noncompetitive
Telmisartan	Slow	10	Noncompetitive
Losartan	Fast	50	Competitive
(E3174)	Slow	10	Noncompetitive
Eprosartan	Fast	100	Competitive

TABLE 55-8

Pharmacodynamic Properties of Angiotensin Receptor Blockers

DRUG GENERIC (TRADE) NAME AND PEAK RESPONSE (H)	DURATION OF RESPONSE (H)	INITIAL DOSE (MG)	USUAL DOSE (MG)	MAXIMUM DOSE (MG)	INTERVAL
Eprosartan (Teveten) 4	24	200	200-400	400	qd/bid
Irbesartan (Avapro) 4-6, 14	24	150	150-300	300	qd
Losartan (Cozaar) 6	12-24	50	50-100	100	qd/bid
Valsartan (Diovan) 4-6	24	80	80-160	300	qd
Candesartan (Atacand) 6-8	24	8	8-32	32	qd
Telmisartan (Micardis) 3-6	24	40	40-80	80	qd
Olmesartan (Benicar) 1.4-2.8	24	20	20-40	40	qd

TABLE 55-9

Pharmacokinetic Properties of Angiotensin Receptor Blockers

ACTIVE DRUG METABOLISM	EXCRETION*	BIOAVAILABILITY (%) METABOLITES	AFFECTED BY FOOD	PEAK BLOOD LEVEL (H)	ELIMINATION HALF LIFE	ABSORPTION
Eprosartan F(70)/U(7)	>80 Inactive	13	No	4	6	L
Irbesartan F(65)/U(20)	>80 Inactive	60-80	No	1.5-2	10-14	L/K
Losartan F(60)/U(40)	>80 Active	25	No	1	4-9	L/K
Valsartan F(83)/U(13)	>80 Inactive	25	Yes	2-4	6-9	L/K
Candesartan I/L/K	F(67)/U(33)	15 None	No	2-4	9	
Telmisartan F	— Inactive	42	Yes	0.5-1	24	L
Olmesartan F(50)/U(50)	— Active	26	No	1	12-18	I

*Excretion values in parentheses are percentages.

F = feces; I = intestine; K = kidney; L = liver; U = urine.

patients, peak responses occur in 4 to 6 hours and 14 hours, corresponding to the peak increases in plasma renin activity and AII levels.[36] With continuous dosing, the maximal effect may not be seen for up to 6 weeks. The duration of action is 24 hours. Irbesartan is metabolized by N-glucuronidation into inactive metabolites. It does not induce or inhibit isoenzymes normally associated with drug metabolism. The inactive metabolites are cleared by renal (20%) and fecal excretion (65%), with an elimination half-life of 10 to 14 hours. Irbesartan is not dialyzable.

Losartan potassium is the prototype ARB. The tetrazole moiety on the biphenyl ring accounts for its oral activity and duration of action. It was the first orally active agent and is a competitive, nonpeptide selective AT1 receptor inhibitor with moderate receptor binding affinity (see Table 55-7).[8, 34, 36, 195, 240] The usual starting dose is 50 mg once daily (see Table 55-8). Dose adjustments should be made at weekly intervals. The antihypertensive efficacy may be improved with divided doses. The usual daily dose is 50 to 100 mg. The potassium contents of the 25-, 50-, and 100-mg tablets are 0.054, 0.108, and 0.216 mEq, respectively. The oral bioavailability of losartan is 25% and is unaffected by food (see Table 55-9). The initial response occurs in 1 hour, peaks at 6 hours, and lasts for 24 hours. Fourteen percent of losartan is metabolized in the liver by the cytochrome P450-2C9 and P450-3A4 oxidation system into the active metabolite E-3174. The E-3174 5–carboxylic acid compound is up to 40 times as potent as losartan and acts as a reversible noncompetitive AT1 receptor blocker. The E-3174 component accounts for the long duration of action.[240] The elimination half-lives of the parent compound and E-3174 are 1.5 to 2 hours and 4 to 9 hours, respectively. Only 5% of losartan is recovered unchanged in the urine, supporting extensive metabolism and biliary secretion. Sixty percent of radiolabeled losartan is recovered in the feces, the remainder in the urine. Neither the parent drug nor metabolites are removed by dialysis.

Olmesartan medoxomil is a selective, nonpeptide ARB prodrug that is rapidly and completely bioactivated by hydrolysis to olmesartan during absorption from the gastrointestinal tract.[241, 242] The initial dose is 20 mg, and the usual dose is 20 to 40 mg daily (see Table 55-8). The absolute bioavailability is 26% and is not affected by food (see Table 55-9). The peak plasma concentration is reached in 1 hour. The blood pressure–lowering effect lasts for 24 hours and reaches a maximum at 2 weeks. Olmesartan is eliminated in a biphasic manner with a terminal half-life of 13 hours. Following conversion to the active drug upon absorption, there is no further metabolism. Approximately 35% to 50% of the absorbed dose is eliminated in the urine, the remainder in the feces by biliary excretion. Dosing and pharmacokinetics have not been studied in dialysis patients.

NONBIPHENYL TETRAZOLE DERIVATIVES

Telmisartan incorporates a carboxylic acid as the biphenyl acidic group. Telmisartan is a nonpeptide, noncompetitive ARB with high specificity and receptor affinity.[34, 36, 243] The usual starting dose is 40 mg, and the usual daily dose is 40 to 80 mg. The initial response occurs in 3 hours and is dose dependent (see Table 55-9). The duration of action is 24 hours but may be up to 7 days after discontinuation of the drug.[36] Telmisartan is rapidly absorbed, with a dose-dependent bioavailability of 42%. Women typically achieve plasma levels two to three times higher than those of men, but this is not associated with differences in blood pressure response. Less than 3% of the drug is metabolized in the liver into inactive compounds. The parent and metabolites are excreted in the feces by biliary excretion with an elimination half-life of 24 hours. Telmisartan is not dialyzable, and dose adjustment is not necessary in patients with renal disease.

NONHETEROCYCLIC DERIVATIVES

Valsartan is a nonheterocyclic ARB in which the imidazole of losartan is replaced by an acetylated amino acid.[34, 36, 244, 245] Valsartan is a noncompetitive antagonist with high specificity and receptor binding affinity (see Table 55-7). The initial starting dose is 80 mg once daily (see Table 55-8). The usual dose is 80 to 16 mg daily. The maximal blood pressure response is achieved after 4 weeks of therapy (see Table 55-9). The initial response occurs in 2 hours, peaks at 4 to 6 hours, and lasts 24 hours. The bioavailability is 25% and is not affected by food. Valsartan does not undergo significant metabolism.

The parent and a few inactive metabolites are excreted in the feces (83%) by biliary secretion and in the urine (13%). The elimination half-life is 6 to 9 hours and is not affected by renal failure.

Class Renal Effects

Intrarenal AII receptors are widely distributed in the afferent and efferent arterioles, glomerular mesangial cells, the inner stripe of the outer medulla, medullary interstitial cells,[148, 246, 247] and on the luminal and basolateral membranes of the proximal and distal tubule cells, collecting ducts, podocytes, and macula densa cells.[248-250] The majority of receptors are of the AT1 subclass. Circulating and predominantly locally produced AII interacts with the receptors; the complex is internalized and AII is released into the intracellular compartment, where it exerts its effects. Studies suggest that the majority of renal interstitial AII is formed at sites not readily accessible to ACE inhibition or is formed by non-ACE pathways.[236]

ARBs antagonize the binding of AII and cause a number of intrarenal changes. The overall renal hemodynamic responses of AT1 receptor blockade are variable depending on the counteracting influences of the decrease in arterial pressure.[251-253] Decreases in systemic arterial pressure by ARBs may be associated with compensatory activation of the intrarenal sympathetic nervous system, resulting in decreased renal function.[244, 254] This effect is more pronounced during sodium-depleted states because activation of the RAS helps to maintain arterial and renal pressure.[245] In contrast, direct intrarenal infusions of ARBs cause an increase in sodium excretion.[255] The enhanced sodium excretion has been shown to be due to direct inhibition of sodium reabsorption by the proximal tubules but may also be due to hemodynamic changes in medullary blood flow and tubule absorption in distal nephron segments.[256] Because AII blockade enhances the ability of the kidneys to excrete sodium, sodium balance can be maintained at lower arterial pressures. AII blockade also reduces tubuloglomerular feedback sensitivity[257] by decreasing macula densa transport of sodium chloride to the afferent arteriole. This leads to increased delivery of sodium chloride to the distal segments for excretion without compensatory changes in GFR.

In addition to the natriuretic and diuretic actions, acute administration of some ARBs has been observed to induce reversible kaliuresis in salt-depleted normotensive subjects in the absence of changes in GFR.[258] However, chronic AII receptor blockade does not cause appreciable changes in urinary electrolyte excretion or volume. The kaliuretic effect may be due to specific intrinsic pharmacologic effects of the losartan molecule.[36]

Another property unique to the losartan molecule is induction of uricosuria. This effect is not seen with ACE inhibitors or other ARBs, including the active metabolite of losartan, E3174, and does not appear to be related to inhibition of the RAS.[259-261] Losartan has a greater affinity for the urate/anion exchanger than other antagonists and causes inhibition of urate reabsorption in the proximal tubule.[262] The uricosuria is associated with a concomitant decrease in serum uric acid in normal subjects, hypertensive subjects, and patients with renal disease and kidney transplants.[259, 263, 264]

The effect occurs within 4 hours of drug administration and is dose dependent. Long-term administration reduces uric acid levels by approximately 0.4 mg/dL.[265] The clinical implications of this effect are unknown. Concerns that increased uric acid supersaturation might perpetuate renal uric acid deposition have not been borne out clinically, as losartan simultaneously increases urinary pH, which protects against crystal nucleation.[266, 267] Conversely, the decrease in serum uric acid might be beneficial, as it has been suggested that hyperuricemia is a risk factor for renal disease progression and coronary artery disease.

Hypertensive patients treated with ARBs, with normal or impaired renal function, exhibit renal responses similar to or slightly greater than the responses of those treated with ACE inhibitors.[196, 268, 269] In addition to decreases in systolic and diastolic blood pressure, patients demonstrate increases in renal blood flow and decreases in filtration fraction and renal vascular resistance with no substantial changes in GFR.[270] These effects are probably a result of combined decreases in both pre- and postglomerular resistances. It has been suggested that elevated intrarenal AII levels in the presence of AT1 receptor blockade stimulates AT2 receptors, which can increase preglomerular vasodilator actions of bradykinin, cyclic guanosine monophosphate, and nitric oxide.[271, 272] ACE inhibitors can potentiate this effect.[271] The clinical importance of this finding has yet to be established. AII blockade may significantly reduce GFR in underperfused kidneys. Patients with low perfusion pressures, dehydration, or renal artery stenosis may experience severe decreases in GFR, but less severe decreases than with ACE inhibitors.[129, 273, 274] Under conditions of overperfusion, such as with hypertension associated with glomerulosclerosis and nephron loss or diabetes, AII blockade is protective. Such patients often have a suboptimal suppression of the RAS. The lowering of efferent arteriole resistance reduces intraglomerular hydrostatic pressure, attenuating the progression of renal injury, and increases renal sodium excretory capacity. In concert with the reduction in systemic arterial pressure, these actions provide more renal protection than other classes of antihypertensive agents despite equivalent reductions of blood pressure.[275-280]

In healthy and hypertensive patients, ARBs produce dose-dependent increases in circulating AII levels and plasma renin activity,[281-283] presumably as a consequence of withdrawal of the negative feedback of AII on renal release and synthesis of renin. The increases occur at the peak plasma drug levels and persist up to 24 hours; they remain elevated with chronic administration. Decreases in plasma levels of aldosterone have been reported but are variable. In normal subjects, the decreases coincide with the peak interval of ARB activity; in hypertensive patients with a fixed sodium diet, there are no significant changes in aldosterone from baseline.[8, 258] Indeed, ARBs suppress the AII-mediated adrenal cortical release of aldosterone, but these effects appear to be quantitatively less important than the intrarenal suppression of AII action. Long-term AT1 receptor blockade does not appear to induce aldosterone escape.[284] Minor decreases in plasma aldosterone may contribute, in part, to the natriuretic action of the ARBs but do not appear to have significant antikaliuretic effects.

Urinary protein excretion is significantly decreased with ARBs[36] and parallels findings with ACE inhibitors.

Antiproteinuric effects have been described in diabetic and nondiabetic patients and those with renal transplants.[285] The time course of the antiproteinuric effect has a slow onset, and the dose-response curves differ from those of the antihypertensive effects: the maximal effect occurs at 3 to 4 weeks.[91] Currently, the peak of the dose-response curve has not been determined. Whether the antiproteinuric effects are equivalent to or better than those of ACE inhibitors remains to be determined. They do appear to have additive and similar hemodynamic and antiproteinuric effects.[86] In a number of trials, ACE I therapy or ARB therapy reduced proteinuria by up to 40%. Combined therapy resulted in a 70% reduction of proteinuria with no further changes in blood pressure.[286, 287] Such findings suggest that the mechanism of the antiproteinuric effect may differ between the two classes. It is currently recommended that patients receiving ACE inhibitor therapy with persistent hypertension or proteinuria should be treated with angiotensin receptor antagonist therapy.[288] This combination appears to reduce intrarenal AII and transforming growth factor β (TGF-β) levels more than high doses of either agent alone.[289, 290]

Clinical trials have demonstrated superior clinical antiproteinuric effects of the ARBs compared with conventional treatment. In patients with diabetic nephropathy, ARBs reduced macroscopic proteinuria up to 28% and could revert microscopic proteinuria to baseline in one third of patients.[278-280, 291] Long-term renoprotection with these agents substantially retards the progression of renal disease. Patients with diabetic nephropathy and more than 900 mg/dL protein per day receiving ARBs had a 20% reduction in the risk of composite end points (doubling of serum creatinine, developing ESRD, or death).[278, 279] The risk of doubling of the serum creatinine was 33% lower in the ARB arm than in the placebo group and 37% lower than in the amlodipine arm. These effects were independent of changes in blood pressure. Thus, the ARBs should be the foundation of therapy in patients with type 2 diabetes and nephropathy.[292]

Like the ACE inhibitors, ARBs have multiple nonhemodynamic effects that may contribute to renoprotection. These include antiproliferative actions on the vasculature and mesangium, inhibition of TGF-β,[236, 290, 293] inhibition of atherogenesis[294, 295] and vascular deterioration,[296] improved superoxide production and nitric oxide bioavailability,[297, 298] reduction of collagen formation, reduced mesangial matrix production, improved vascular wall remodeling, decreased vasoconstrictor effects of endothelin-1,[298] improved endothelial function,[296] reduction of oxidative stress, and protection from calcineurin inhibitor injury. The clinical importance of these effects is under investigation.

Class Efficacy and Safety

All AT1 receptor blockers have been demonstrated to lower blood pressure effectively and safely in patients with mild, moderate, and severe hypertension regardless of age, gender, or race.[8, 299-303] They are indicated as first-line monotherapy or add-on therapy for hypertension and are comparable in efficacy to ACE inhibitor therapy.[304-306] They are safe and effective in patients with renal insufficiency, diabetes, heart failure, renal transplants, coronary artery disease (CAD), and left ventricular hypertrophy (LVH)[304, 307] and have been shown to protect against hypertensive end-organ damage, such as LVH, stroke, ESRD, and possibly diabetes.[278, 279, 308-312] Although they may not be the most efficacious agents in terms of blood pressure reduction in blacks, they are equally or more efficacious in offering target organ protection and arresting disease progression than agents that do not inhibit the RAS. Moreover, the antihypertensive activity is not attenuated by high-salt diets in blacks.[306] In most patients, the ARBs offer blood pressure lowering comparable to that of all other classes, with an improved tolerability profile.[313] ARBs provide effective control over a 24-hour period and are suitable for once-daily dosing.[314] Response rates vary from 40% to 60%. They do not affect the normal circadian blood pressure variation.[315] The long onset of action of 4 to 6 weeks avoids the first-dose hypotension and rebound hypertension commonly seen with other drugs. There is a dose-dependent response with newer agents, and losartan and valsartan have a relatively flat dose-response curve.[316, 317] Candesartan, irbesartan, and olmesartan may have the greatest efficacy with a longer duration of action because of their noncompetitive binding nature.[318, 319]

The addition of thiazide diuretics potentiates the therapeutic effect and increases response rates to 70% to 80% and is more effective than increasing the dose of ARB.[137] The ARBs may also abrogate the adverse metabolic effects of thiazides.[312] Combination of ARBs and ACE inhibitors is safe and additive in reducing blood pressure and effectively suppressing sympathetic activity.[320, 321] Combination therapy with dihydropyridines has additive effects in reducing blood pressure and is well tolerated.[322] ARBs are contraindicated in patients with known renovascular hypertension and may cause fetal or neonatal death when used during the second and third trimesters of pregnancy.[323]

Overall, the ARBs have neutral metabolic effects and are superior to other classes with respect to tolerability. They do not cause hyper- or hyponatremia, and hyperkalemia is rare. In clinical trials, hyperkalemia occurs in less than 1.5% of patients and is comparable to that observed with ACE inhibitor therapy. It is more likely to develop in patients with renal insufficiency or diabetes or in those taking potassium-sparing drugs. ARBs have no effect on serum lipids in hypertensive patients but may improve the abnormal lipoprotein profile of patients with proteinuric renal disease.[103] ARBs have variable effects on serum glucose and insulin sensitivity in hypertensive patients.[324, 325] Reports of deleterious effects on beta cell function in chronic hemodialysis patients require further investigation.[326] In contrast, a clinical trial comparing losartan-based therapy with a β-blocker in patients with hypertension and LVH demonstrated a 25% reduced risk for the development of diabetes in the losartan group. The mechanism for this effect has not been defined.[308, 327] Increased liver transaminases are occasionally reported, but the effects are usually transient despite continued therapy.[36]

Clinically relevant side effects are not observed more frequently than in placebo-treated patients. Because ARBs do not interfere with kinin metabolism, cough is rare. This is a major clinical advantage of the use of ARBs.[328] The incidence of cough in patients with a history of ACE inhibitor–induced cough is no greater than in those receiving placebo.[329] Similarly, the incidence of angioedema and facial swelling

is no greater than with placebo, but they can occur.[330, 331] The most frequent side effects are headache (14%), dizziness (2.4%), and fatigue (2%), which occur at rates lower than those with placebo.[332] ARB therapy not only does not worsen sexual activity but may improve it.[333] Like ACE inhibitors, ARBs may cause minor decreases in serum hemoglobin; they may lower the hematocrit effectively in post-transplantation erythrocytosis.[188, 334] Drug interactions are uncommon, but as with ACE inhibitors, NSAIDS may blunt the natriuretic effect of ARBs.[335] Acute reversible renal failure has been reported with AII receptor blockade therapy in salt-depleted patients. Thus, therapy should not be instituted in hypovolemic patients or in the setting of active diuresis.

β-Adrenergic Antagonists
Mechanisms of Action

β-adrenergic blocking drugs can be classified on the basis of their pharmacologic and pharmacokinetic differences. These drugs differ in their selectivity for β subtypes, the presence or absence of partial agonist activity, and membrane-stabilizing activity. These drugs exert their effects by attenuation of sympathetic stimulation through competitive antagonism of catecholamines at the β-adrenergic receptor.[336, 337] In addition to β-blockade properties, certain drugs have antihypertensive effects mediated through several different mechanisms including α₁-adrenergic blocking activity, β_2-adrenergic agonist activity, and perhaps effects on nitric oxide–dependent vasodilator action. Partial agonist activity is a property of certain β-adrenergic blockers that results from a small degree of direct stimulation of the receptor by the drug, which occurs at the same time that receptor occupancy blocks access of strongly stimulating catecholamines.[338, 339] Whether the presence of partial agonist activity is advantageous or disadvantageous remains unclear.[340] Drugs with partial agonist activity slow resting heart rate less than drugs that lack this pharmacologic effect.[341, 342] The exercise-induced increase in heart rate is similarly blocked by both groups of drugs.[341, 343, 344] However, β-adrenergic blockers with nonselective partial agonist activity may reduce peripheral vascular resistance and cause less atrial ventricular conduction depression than drugs without partial agonist activity. The specificity of partial agonist activity for β_1- or β_2-receptors may also have a role in the antihypertensive response to a given drug. Membrane-stabilizing activity is a specific electrophysiologic property that results in quinidine-like effects.[345] The height and rate of rise of the intracardiac action potential are observed to be reduced without reduction of the overall duration of the resting potential. These effects occur at drug concentrations well above therapeutic levels and can be manifest clinically with β-blocker intoxication.[345] This membrane-stabilizing effect is not thought to be responsible for a direct negative inotropic effect of β-blockers.

β-Adrenergic receptor blockers may be nonspecific and stimulate both β_1- and β_2-adrenergic receptors, or they may be relatively specific for β_1-adrenergic receptors. β_1-Receptors are found predominantly in heart, adipose, and brain tissue, whereas β_2-receptors predominate in the lung, liver, smooth muscle, and skeletal muscle.[346-349] Many tissues, however, have both β_1- and β_2-receptors, including the heart, and it is important to realize that the concept of a cardioselective drug is only relative.

β-Adrenergic blockers can also be classified by their different pharmacokinetic properties. They may differ significantly in gastrointestinal absorption, first-pass hepatic metabolism, protein binding, lipid solubility, penetration into the central nervous system, and hepatic or renal clearance. β-Blockers eliminated primarily by hepatic metabolism have a relatively short plasma half-life; however, the duration of the clinical pharmacologic effect does not correlate well with plasma half-life in many of these drugs. Water-soluble drugs eliminated by the kidney may have longer half-lives. Bioavailability varies greatly.

Overall, the precise mechanism of the antihypertensive effect of β-adrenergic blockers remains incompletely understood.[350] β_1-Adrenergic receptor blockade has generally been considered responsible for the blood pressure–lowering effect; however, β_2-receptor blockade has an independent antihypertensive effect.[351] Inhibition of β_1-adrenergic receptors in the juxtaglomerular cells within the kidney may inhibit renin release.[352, 353] A direct action on the central nervous system with reduction in central nervous system sympathetic outflow may also be involved.[354-356] Attenuation of cardiac pressor stimuli related to β-blockade may result in baroreceptor resetting. In additional, adrenergic neuron output may be blocked because of inhibition of β_2-adrenergic receptors at the vascular wall.[357-359]

Class Members

The β-adrenergic antagonists are classified and reviewed on the basis of the following subclasses: nonselective β-adrenergic antagonism, nonselective β-adrenergic antagonism with partial agonist activity, β_1-selective adrenergic antagonism, β_1-selective adrenergic antagonism with partial agonist activity, and nonselective β-adrenergic antagonism with α_1-adrenergic antagonism or other mechanisms (Table 55-10).

NONSELECTIVE β-ADRENERGIC ANTAGONISTS

Nadolol is a nonselective β-adrenergic blocking agent without membrane-stabilizing or partial agonist activity[360-363] (Table 55-11). It has low lipid solubility. The average adult dose is 40 to 80 mg given once daily, with a maximum daily dose of 320 mg. Oral absorption averages 20% to 40%. The drug is about 30% protein bound. Elimination half-life is 20 to 24 hours with peak serum concentrations measured 2 to 4 hours after a dose (Table 55-12). Nadolol is not appreciably metabolized, and elimination occurs predominantly in the urine and feces. Dose adjustment is indicated in patients with renal failure. Dosage intervals should be increased to 24 to 36 hours, 24 to 48 hours, and 40 to 60 hours in patients with creatinine clearances of 30 to 50 mL/min per 1.73 m^2, 10 to 30 mL/min per 1.73 m^2, and less than 10 mL/min per 1.73 m^2, respectively. Dose adjustment is not necessary in hepatic insufficiency. Hemodialysis reduces the serum concentration of nadolol, but specific recommendations for dosage during dialysis are not available.

Propranolol is a noncardioselective β-adrenergic blocker[364-369] (see Tables 55-11 and 55-12). It has no partial adrenergic activity and has moderate to high membrane-stabilizing activity. The usual daily dosage range is 80 to 320 mg. It may be administered as a single daily dose if a long-acting preparation is used. Propranolol is lipophilic, with almost complete absorption and extensive first-pass hepatic metabolism. Peak concentrations are reached 1 to 3 hours after administration of a standard formulation and about 6 hours after administration of a long-acting formulation. Respective plasma half-lives are 3 to 4 hours and 10 hours. The drug is metabolized by the liver. The major metabolite, 4-hydroxypropranolol, has β-adrenergic blocking activity. Renal excretion is less than 1%. Adjustment in renal failure is not necessary. Patients with liver disease may require variable dosage adjustments and more frequent monitoring.

Timolol is a nonselective β-adrenergic blocking agent without membrane-stabilizing or partial adrenergic activity[370-373]

TABLE 55-10

Pharmacodynamic Properties of β-Adrenergic Antagonists

DRUG	β_1-SELECTIVITY	PARTIAL AGONIST ACTIVITY	MEMBRANE-STABILIZING ACTIVITY	α-ADRENERGIC ANTAGONIST
Nadolol	0	0	0	
Propranolol	0	0	+	
Carteolol	0	+	0	
Penbutolol	0	+	0	
Pindolol	0	+	+	
Labetalol	0	+	0	+
Carvedilol	0	0	+	+
Atenolol	+	0	0	
Metoprolol	+	0	0	
Betaxolol	+	0	+	
Acebutolol	+	+	+	
Celiprolol	+	0	0	+
Bisoprolol	+	0	0	
Nebivolol	+	0	0	

TABLE 55-11

Pharmacokinetic Properties of β-Adrenergic Antagonists

DRUG	BIOAVAILABILITY (%)	AFFECTED BY FOOD	PEAK BLOOD LEVEL (H)	ELIMINATION HALF-LIFE (H)	METABOLISM	EXCRETION*	ACTIVE METABOLITES
Nadolol	20-40	No	2-4	20-24	—	U/F	—
Propranolol	16-60	Yes	—	3-4	L	—	—
Timolol	50-90	—	—	2-4	L	U(20)	—
Carteolol	84	Yes	—	5-8.5	L	—	—
Penbutolol	100	No	—	17-24	L	U	—
Pindolol	95	No	2	3-11	L	U(40)	—
Atenolol	40-60	Yes	—	14-16	—	U/F	—
Metoprolol	50	—	1.5-2	3-7	L	U	—
Betaxolol	78-90	No	2-6	12-22	L	U	—
Bisoprolol	90	—	2.3	9.6	L	U	—
Acebutolol	90	No	2-3	3-8	L	U	—

*Excretion values in parentheses represent percentages.

F, feces; L, liver; U, urine.

TABLE 55-12

Pharmacodynamic Properties of β-Adrenergic Antagonists

DRUG	INITIAL DOSE (MG)	USUAL DOSE (MG)	MAXIMUM DOSE (MG)	INTERVAL	PEAK RESPONSE (H)	DURATION OF RESPONSE (H)
Nadolol	40	40-80	320	qd	—	—
Propranolol	40	80-320	640	bid	—	—
Timolol	10	20-40	60	bid	—	—
Carteolol	2.5	2.5-10	60	qd	6	24
Penbutolol	20	20-40	80	qd-bid	2	20-24
Pindolol	5	10-40	60	qd-bid	—	24
Atenolol	25	50-100	200	qd	3	24
Metoprolol	12.5-50	100-200	450	qd-bid	1	3-6
Betaxolol	10	10-40	40	qd	3	23-25
Bisoprolol	2.5	5-20	40	qd	2-4	24
Acebutolol	400	400-800	1200	qd	3	24

(see Tables 55-11 and 55-12). It has low to moderate lipid solubility. The recommended initial dose of timolol in the treatment of hypertension is 10 mg twice daily. The maintenance dose generally ranges from 20 to 40 mg daily. No dosage adjustment is necessary in patients with renal failure. Because timolol undergoes extensive hepatic metabolism, patients with liver disease may require a dosage adjustment and frequent monitoring. Absorption is 90% with approximately 50% first-pass metabolism. The half-life is 2 to 4 hours. It is not removed by dialysis.

NONSELECTIVE β-ADRENERGIC ANTAGONISTS WITH PARTIAL AGONIST ACTIVITY

Carteolol is a long-acting nonselective β-adrenergic blocker.[374, 375] It has moderate partial agonist activity. There is no membrane-stabilizing activity. It has low lipid solubility. Recommended dosing is 2.5 to 10 mg daily (see Tables 55-11 and 55-12). Doses up to 60 mg/day have been utilized. Oral absorption is approximately 84%. Carteolol is eliminated primarily by the kidney with a half-life of 5 to 8.5 hours. Dosage adjustment should be made for decreased renal function. The recommended dosing interval is 72 hours for creatinine clearances less than 20 mL/min per 1.73 m², and 48 hours for creatinine clearances between 20 and 60 mL/min per 1.73 m².

Penbutolol is a nonselective β-adrenergic blocking agent with no membrane-stabilizing activity.[374, 376-381] It has low partial agonist activity (see Tables 55-11 and 55-12). The drug is highly lipid soluble. Usually, doses are 20 to 40 mg given either as a single dose or divided twice daily. Bioavailability is near 100%. Protein binding ranges from 80% to 98%. The elimination half-life is 17 to 26 hours. Hepatic metabolism to inactive metabolites occurs with subsequent renal elimination. Plasma levels peak 1.5 to 3 hours after dosing. The optimal antihypertensive effect is seen at an average of 14 days after initiation of therapy. Dosage adjustments for patients with renal insufficiency are not recommended, but adjustment may be required for patients with hepatic insufficiency.

Pindolol is a nonselective β-adrenergic blocking agent with high partial agonist activity.[382-386] There is no membrane-stabilizing activity (see Tables 55-11 and 55-12). It is moderately lipid soluble. The usual adult oral dose is 5 mg twice daily with incremental increases by 10 mg every 3 to 4 weeks. The maximum daily recommended dose is 60 mg. Absorption is 95% with peak plasma concentrations at about 2 hours. Protein binding is 40% to 60%. Half-life is 3 to 4 hours. Approximately 40% of a dose of pindolol is excreted unchanged in the urine; 60% is metabolized in the liver. The drug half-life increases modestly in patients with renal impairment. Dosage adjustments do not appear be necessary. Dosage adjustments may be necessary in patients with severely impaired hepatic function and in patients with concomitant cirrhosis and renal failure.

β$_1$-SELECTIVE ADRENERGIC ANTAGONISTS

Atenolol is a long-acting β$_1$-selective adrenergic blocking agent (see Tables 55-11 and 55-12). It has no membrane-stabilizing action or partial agonist activity.[373, 387-391] The usual dose is 50 to 100 mg once daily. Atenolol is incompletely absorbed from the gastrointestinal tract. It is poorly bound to serum proteins. It is not metabolized by the liver and is eliminated approximately 50% by the kidneys and 50% excreted in the feces. The elimination half-life is 6 to 14 hours. Doses greater than 100 mg/day are unlikely to produce additional benefit. The time required to achieve the optimal antihypertensive effect is 1 to 2 weeks. In anephric patients, the half-life may be extended to more than 100 hours. Alternatively, the dosing interval can be increased. Patients with moderate renal insufficiency should have the dose interval increased to 48 hours, and for patients with advanced renal disease dosing intervals should be increased to 96 hours. Atenolol is not significantly metabolized by the liver, and no dosage adjustment is necessary in patients with hepatic disease. The drug is removed by dialysis and a maintenance dose should be given after a dialysis treatment.

Metoprolol is a β$_1$-selective adrenergic blocker.[392, 393] It has weak membrane-stabilizing activity (see Tables 55-11 and 55-12). There is no partial agonist activity. It has moderate lipid solubility. Onset of therapeutic effect occurs within 1 hour after oral administration. It is 12% protein bound. Penetration into the central nervous system does occur. The elimination half-life is 3 to 5 hours. Extensive hepatic metabolism occurs, and 3% to 10% of the drug is excreted unchanged in the urine. The initial oral dose is 12.5 to 50 mg either once or twice daily, increasing to 100 to 200 mg twice daily. Sustained-released preparations may be substituted as a once-daily dose.

Betaxolol is a long-acting β$_1$-selective adrenergic blocking agent.[394, 395] It has weak membrane-stabilizing activity (see Tables 55-11 and 55-12). There is no partial agonist activity. It has low lipid solubility. Betaxolol is well absorbed orally, producing peak serum levels in 2 to 6 hours. The elimination half-life is 12 to 22 hours. The usual oral dose for hypertension is 10 to 40 mg once daily. Therapy is typically started at a dose of 10 mg once daily. The majority of patients respond to 20 mg once daily. The time to achieve the optimal antihypertensive effect is approximately 1 to 2 weeks. Renal dysfunction results in a decrease in betaxolol clearance. Titration should begin at 5 mg once daily in those

with severe renal impairment. The reported elimination half-life in uremic patients is 14 to 28 hours. The drug is 50% to 60% protein bound. It is metabolized predominantly in the liver with excretion of up to 80% by the kidney. Approximately 15% of the dose is recovered unchanged in the urine.

Bisoprolol is a long-acting β$_1$-selective adrenergic blocking agent.[396, 397] There is no membrane-stabilizing or partial agonist activity (see Tables 55-11 and 55-12). The usual oral dose is 2.5 to 20 mg given once daily. Dosing adjustments are required in patients with hepatic or renal dysfunction. Oral bioavailability is 90%. Peak plasma concentrations occur 2.3 hours after administration. The half-life is 9.6 hours. Hepatic metabolism occurs with renal excretion of metabolites; however, 50% of the drug is excreted by the kidney unchanged. In patients with renal failure, the initial oral dose should be 2.5 mg once daily with careful monitoring in dose titration. The maximum recommended dose of bisoprolol in patients with renal failure is 10 mg/day. Patients with severe renal dysfunction should have dose reduction. Similar dose reduction is also required for patients with hepatic insufficiency.

β$_1$-SELECTIVE ADRENERGIC ANTAGONISTS WITH PARTIAL ADRENERGIC ACTIVITY

Acebutolol is a β$_1$-selective adrenergic blocking agent.[398-401] It has low membrane-stabilizing activity as well as partial agonist activity (see Tables 55-11 and 55-12). Doses of 400 to 1200 mg/day are effective in hypertension. Acebutolol is 90% absorbed from the gastrointestinal tract. Drug is metabolized to diacetolol, an active metabolite, with the parent compound being excreted both renally and in bile. Diacetolol is excreted mainly by the kidneys. The drug half-life is from 3 to 8 hours. It is not prolonged in renal failure. However, the half-life of diacetolol is prolonged in renal dysfunction. Dose reduction of 50% to 75% is recommended for patients with advanced renal insufficiency.

NONSELECTIVE β-ADRENERGIC ANTAGONISTS WITH α-ADRENERGIC ANTAGONISM OR OTHER MECHANISMS OF ANTIHYPERTENSIVE ACTION

Labetalol is a nonselective β-adrenergic blocking agent.[402-405] It also possesses selective α-adrenergic blocking activity (Tables 55-13 and 55-14). It has no membrane-stabilizing activity. It does have weak partial agonist activity. The blocking of β$_1$- and β$_2$-adrenergic receptors is approximately equivalent. In addition, labetalol is highly selective for postsynaptic α$_1$-adrenergic receptors. After an oral dose, the ratio of α$_1$- to β-blocking potency is approximately 1:3. With intravenous administration, the β-blocking potency seems more prominent. Labetalol has moderate lipid solubility. The usual initial doses in hypertension are 100 mg orally twice daily, increasing gradually to a maintenance dose of 200 to 400 mg twice daily. Labetalol is rapidly absorbed from the gastrointestinal tract. Maximum effect is seen in about 3 hours. The drug is metabolized in the liver with 50% to 60% of a dose excreted in the urine (5% unchanged) and the remainder in the bile. The serum half-life is 5 to 8 hours. Dosing adjustment is not required for any degree of renal failure. Chronic liver disease has been demonstrated to decrease the first-pass metabolism of labetalol, thus increasing bioavailability of the drug. Dosage reduction is

TABLE 55-13

Pharmacokinetic Properties of β-Adrenergic Antagonists with Vasodilatory Properties

DRUG	BIOAVAILABILITY (%)	AFFECTED BY FOOD	PEAK BLOOD LEVEL (H)	ELIMINATION HALF-LIFE (H)	METABOLISM	EXCRETION*	ACTIVE METABOLITES
Labetalol	25-40	Yes	1-2	5-8	L	U (50-60)	—
Carvedilol	25-35	No	1-1.5	6-8	L	F	—
Celiprolol	30-70	Yes	—	5-6	—	F/U	—
Nebivolol	12-96	No	2.4-3.1	8-27	L	—	—

*Excretion values in parentheses represent percentages.
F, feces; L, liver; U, urine.

TABLE 55-14

Pharmacodynamic Properties of β-Adrenergic Antagonists

DRUG	INITIAL DOSE (MG)	USUAL DOSE (MG)	MAXIMUM DOSE (MG)	INTERVAL	PEAK RESPONSE (H)	DURATION OF RESPONSE (H)
Labetalol	100	200-800	1200-2400	bid	3	8-12
Carvedilol	6.25	12.5-25	50	bid	4-7	24
Celiprolol	200	200-600	—	qd	—	—
Nebivolol	5	5	—	qd	6	24

required in these patients to avoid excessive decreases in heart rate and supine blood pressure.

Carvedilol is a nonselective β-adrenergic blocking agent with peripheral α_1-blocking activity.[406, 407] It has moderate membrane-stabilizing activity but no partial agonist activity (see Tables 55-13 and 55-14). It is highly lipid soluble. It is approximately equipotent in blocking β_1- and β_2-adrenergic receptors. Carvedilol is highly selective for postsynaptic α_1-adrenergic receptors. The ratio of α_1- to β_1-blocking activity is estimated to be 1:7.6. For the treatment of hypertension, an initial oral dose of 6.25 mg twice daily is recommended and may be increased to 12.5 to 25 mg twice daily if needed. Peak serum levels of carvedilol are observed 1 to $1^1/2$ hours after oral administration. The drug is extensively metabolized in the liver and excreted by the feces. Only small amounts of unchanged carvedilol are excreted in the urine. The half-life of the drug is 6 to 8 hours. Dosing adjustments are not required for patients with renal insufficiency. Carvedilol is extensively metabolized in the liver, and dose reductions are suggested for patients with hepatic insufficiency.

Celiprolol is a β-blocker with several unique properties.[408-412] It is a β_1-adrenergic blocking agent with α_2-receptor blocking activity (see Tables 55-13 and 55-14). Celiprolol also causes vasodilatation through β_2-receptor stimulation and a subsequent decrease in systemic vascular resistance. In contrast to other β-blockers, celiprolol does not appear to induce bronchospasm or have negative inotropic effects. Celiprolol has no membrane-stabilizing activity. It does have moderate partial agonist activity. The initial dose of celiprolol is 200 mg once daily. This can be increased to 400 to 600 mg once daily. Bioavailability is 30% to 70%. Renal excretion is 35% to 42%. Drug half-life is 5.1 to 5.8 hours.

A 50% dose reduction is suggested in patients with a creatinine clearance of 15 to 40 mL/min per 1.73 m². It is not recommended for patients with a creatinine clearance of less than 15 mL/min per 1.73 m².

Nebivolol is a long-acting β_1-selective adrenergic antagonist[413-419] (see Tables 55-13 and 55-14). The compound is a 1:1 racemic mixture of two enantiomers, D-nebivolol and L-nebivolol. The actions of nebivolol are unique and unlike those of other β-blocking agents. These are attributed to the individual effects of the isomers. The β_1-adrenergic blocking effects are related to the d-isomer, whereas the L-isomer is essentially devoid of β-blocking properties at therapeutic doses. When administered alone, the L-isomer does not produce significant effects on blood pressure; however, the antihypertensive effects of the D-isomer are enhanced by the presence of the L-isomer. The hypotensive effects of the racemic mixture are associated with a decrease in peripheral vascular resistance. The mechanism by which the L-isomer enhances the hypotensive effects of the D-isomer is unclear. It has been suggested that L-nebivolol may potentiate the effects of endothelium-derived relaxing factor and induce decreases in blood pressure and peripheral vascular resistance. It has also been suggested that the L-isomer may inhibit norepinephrine actions at the presynaptic β-receptors. The initial oral dose is 5 mg once daily. Peak antihypertensive effects occur after 6 hours. The drug is metabolized in the liver. Both rapid and slow metabolizers have been identified. Bioavailability varies from 12% to 96%. Only small amounts of an oral dose are excreted unchanged in the urine. The half-life of nebivolol is 8 hours in rapid metabolizers and 27 hours in slow metabolizers. Reduced initial doses are recommended for patients with renal insufficiency.

Renal Effects of β-Adrenergic Blockers

Both α- and β-adrenergic receptors in the kidney mediate vasoconstriction and vasodilatation in renin secretion. β-Adrenergic blockers might be expected to influence renal blood flow and GFR through their effects on cardiac output and blood pressure in addition to direct effects on intrarenal adrenergic receptors.[420] β-Adrenergic receptors have been localized to the juxtaglomerular apparatus in autoradiographic studies. β_2-Receptors predominate in the kidney. The degree of specificity of β-adrenergic blockers for β_1- and β_2-receptors might be expected to influence the effect on renal function, as might the degree of intrinsic partial agonist activity. In general, the acute administration of a β-adrenergic blocker usually results in reduction of GFR and effective renal plasma flow.[421] This effect is independent of whether the drug has a β_1-selectivity or intrinsic partial agonist activity.

An exception is nadolol, which has been shown in some studies to increase renal plasma flow in glomerular filtration with intravenous administration; however, oral administration may result in decrements in blood flow and GFR.[422] β_1-Selective drugs, when administered orally, tend to produce smaller reductions in GFR and renal plasma flow. The degree of reduction in GFR and renal plasma flow is modest and probably not of great clinical significance in most cases.[376, 423, 424]

The chronic use of propranolol has been characterized by a 10% to 20% decrement in renal plasma flow and GFR.[425, 426] The fractional excretion of sodium has been observed to decrease by up to 20% to 40% in some studies of the acute renal effects of β-blockade. Combined α- and β-blockade with labetalol has shown little effect on renal hemodynamics. Dilevalol, which has β_2-agonist activity in addition to β-adrenergic blocking properties, has not shown significant effects on renal function at either peak or trough drug levels.[427] In patients with impaired kidney function, some dosage adjustment is necessary (see Table 55-7).

β-Adrenergic antagonist therapy is usually associated with suppression of plasma renin activity. Long-term effects are, however, less well defined. The degree of partial agonist activity may have a direct effect on renin secretion regardless of the degree of β_1-selectivity of the adrenergic blocking agent, although not all studies have been consistent.[343] The exercise-induced rise in plasma renin activity has been shown to be suppressed by β-blockade.[428]

Efficacy and Safety of β-Adrenergic Antagonists

β-Adrenergic antagonists are effective first on therapy for the treatment of mild to moderate hypertension. The Sixth Report of the Joint National Committee on Prevention, Detection, Evaluation, and Treatment of High Blood Pressure (JNC VI) recommended a β-blocker or diuretic as appropriate initial therapy for hypertension.[131, 429] This recommendation was based on numerous randomized clinical trials showing a reduction in mortality and morbidity with these agents. The Medical Research Council trials have found no overall differences in outcome between a thiazide diuretic and propranolol as initial therapy. In the STOP-Hypertension-II Trial, over 6000 elderly patients with hypertension were randomly assigned to receive therapy with a β-blocker or diuretic, an ACE inhibitor, or a dihydropyridine

calcium channel blocker. The degree of blood pressure control at baseline and at 4½ years of follow-up and the combined end point of fatal and nonfatal stroke or myocardial infarction and other cardiovascular mortality were the same in the three groups. The United Kingdom Prospective Diabetes Study (UKPDS) found that atenolol was as effective as captopril in lowering blood pressure in patients with type 2 diabetes.[430]

In the past, it was generally thought that the degree of β_1-selctivity or partial agonist activity conveyed no specific advantage in lowering of blood pressure.[338, 339, 431-434] Some more recent studies have suggested, however, that β_1-selective blockers may have a slightly greater antihypertensive effect than nonselective agents. This may be in the range of 2 to 3 mm Hg. It may be that β_2-blockade in some fashion blunts the antihypertensive effects of β_1-blockade. β_2 partial agonist activity may mediate peripheral vasodilator effects that could contribute to the antihypertensive action. A β_1-selective antagonist with partial agonist activity at the β_1-receptor may result in less hypotensive effect. The magnitude and clinical significance of these differences are unclear.

β-Adrenergic antagonists are effective therapy for patients in all age groups.[435, 436] Data from the Veterans Affairs Cooperative Study Group on antihypertensive agents have shown that patients older than 60 years had an antihypertensive response to atenolol that was comparable to that of patients treated with diltiazem, HCTZ, or captopril.[435-438] The response was, however, less in elderly black patients. Additional studies have suggested that β-adrenergic blockers may be less efficacious in black than in white patients when compared with therapy with calcium channel blockers and diuretics.[435, 436, 439] As a group, the drugs are useful in black patients with significant reductions in blood pressure, particularly with more highly β_1-selective agents. β-Adrenergic blockers have been used to treat women with hypertension in the third trimester of pregnancy, although birth weights have been observed to be decreased. β-Adrenergic blockers are generally avoided in early pregnancy.[440, 441] Labetalol with α- and β-adrenergic blocking characteristics is, however, commonly used in pregnancy.

Messerli and colleagues[442] examined 10 trials involving over 16,000 elderly patients randomly assigned to diuretics or β-blockers, or both. Diuretic therapy was associated with superior reduction in cerebrovascular events, fatal stroke, cardiovascular mortality, and all-cause mortality. In this analysis, β-blockers in elderly patients were effective in reducing cerebrovascular events and heart failure. This meta-analysis was complicated by the concurrent use of diuretics and β-blockers in 52% to 60% of patients. Others have suggested that β-blockers are suitable first-line therapy for elderly patients with hypertension. This is based on evidence that β-adrenergic blockers are effective for primary prevention of stroke, myocardial infarction, and sudden death. At present, β-blockers appear to be effective for many hypertensive elderly patients, particularly those with comorbid conditions and tachycardia.[443, 444] They may be somewhat less effective than diuretics or CAs as first-line therapy.

β-Adrenergic antagonists have been shown to have important effects on outcome in patients with coronary artery disease.[445, 446] The use of a β-blocker following an acute myocardial infarction has been shown to reduce morbidity and mortality in multiple trials. In patients with a Q wave or non–Q wave myocardial infarction, a reduction in mortality of up to 40% has been observed. Despite the clear evidence of benefit, β-blockers have been underutilized in this setting. When prescribed, they are often used in doses considerably lower than those proved to be effective in the clinical trials. Up to 80% to 90% of patients with acute myocardial infarction have no contraindications for β-blocker therapy. Despite this, a substantially lower number of patients have received such treatment. In a survey of postinfarction β-blockade usage involving over 200,000 patients it was found that survival benefit from β-blockade was apparent regardless of systolic blood pressure, age, or ejection fraction.[446] Patients with chronic obstructive pulmonary disease, which is commonly regarded as a contraindication to β-blockade, also had a significant decrease in the risk of death when treated with a β-blocker.[446] Other studies have shown a 20% reduction in total mortality and a 32% to 50% reduction in sudden death with β-blocker therapy in patients who have suffered a myocardial infarction.[445] For hypertensive patients with a previous myocardial infarction, β-adrenergic antagonists may be the drugs of choice for antihypertensive therapy.[131, 445, 447] β-Adrenergic antagonists have also been documented to reduce LVH.[131, 431, 448, 449]

Small doses of β-adrenergic blockers used in conjunction with diuretics and ACE inhibitors have been shown to improve the prognosis in patients with heart failure.[450] Patients with coexisting heart failure and hypertension are an appropriate population for use of β-adrenergic antagonists.[451, 452] The Cardiac Insufficiency Bisoprolol Study II demonstrated a 20% reduction in mortality in patients with moderate heart failure.[453] Hospitalizations for heart failure were reduced by 36% and sudden death was reduced by 44%. Overall mortality in the 2647 patients randomly assigned in this study was lower in the group receiving β-adrenergic blockade. Similar results were observed in a large randomized intervention trial utilizing metoprolol in patients with congestive heart failure. Over the long term, β-adrenergic blockers improve exercise tolerance, left ventricular geometry, and left ventricular structure and reduce myocardial oxygen demand. β-Blockers lower mortality in heart failure largely by reducing the incidence of sudden death. This effect may result from damping of the underlying neurohormonal activation.[454-456] It is also possible that protection from hypokalemia may be involved in the decreased incidence of sudden death. Whether β-adrenergic blockers have a role in the primary prevention of cardiac disease in hypertensive patients is less clear than their role in patients with preexisting cardiac disease, in whom the benefits are quite clear.[457-459] Retrospective studies have suggested that β-blockade reduces the incidence of fatal and nonfatal heart and cerebrovascular disease. Meta-analysis has shown β-blockade to be significantly associated with a reduced risk of stroke and congestive heart failure.[457]

Agents with β₁-selectivity may have a relative therapeutic advantage over nonselective β-adrenergic antagonists in the treatment of patients with bronchospastic airway disease, peripheral vascular disease, or diabetes mellitus.[338, 431, 460-469] Bronchoconstriction is mediated in part by β₂-adrenergic receptors in the airways. β-Blockade with nonselective agents can lead to increased airway resistance. This is less likely to occur in agents with β₁-selectivity. β₁-Selectivity is relative, however, and may be less apparent at higher doses. Patients with severe bronchospastic airway disease should

not receive β-blockers.[462, 464, 470] In patients with mild to moderate disease, β₁-selective agents may be used cautiously. Symptoms of peripheral vascular disease may be exacerbated by β-blocker therapy. Cold extremity and absent pulses have been described in patients with severe disease. Raynaud's phenomenon has been reported with nonselective β-blockade.[462-464] Blockade of β₂-receptor–mediated skeletal muscle vasodilatation as well as decreased cardiac output may contribute to vascular insufficiency. Drugs with β₁-selectivity and partial agonist activity may have a relative advantage in patients with underlying significant peripheral vascular disease. However, a meta-analysis of studies involving patients with mild to moderate vascular disease showing no exacerbation of symptoms with β-adrenergic blockade.

Central nervous system symptoms of sedation, sleep disturbance, depression, and visual hallucinations have been reported with β-adrenergic blockade.[462-464, 471, 472] Placebo-controlled studies have, however, suggested that depression and memory are not affected. Symptoms may be more common with lipid-soluble β-blockers. Sexual dysfunction has been reported but is less of a problem with β₁-selective non–lipid-soluble agents.[473-477] Changes in cognitive function, both improvement and worsening, have been reported; however, there is no clear mechanism by which the symptoms may arise. Constipation, diarrhea, nausea, or indigestion may occasionally occur with β-blockers.[462-464, 478] These symptoms are probably less common with β₁-selective agents.

β-Adrenergic receptors have important effects on glucose metabolism.[462, 464, 479, 480] β-Adrenergic stimulation increases both glycogenolysis and gluconeogenesis from amino acids and glycerol. It also inhibits glucose utilization in the periphery. Resting insulin levels tend to be unchanged, but peripheral insulin sensitivity is reduced. These effects result in impaired glucose tolerance and increased blood sugar in some diabetic patients. β-Blockade can result in blunting the effects of epinephrine secretion resulting from hypoglycemia. This may result in hypoglycemia unawareness. Nonselective β-adrenergic blockers have also been reported to cause severe hypoglycemia in both diabetic and nondiabetic patients.[480] The mechanisms of this effect are unclear. Nonselective β-adrenergic blockers and to a lesser degree β₁-selective agents have been associated with the rise is serum potassium. Suppression of aldosterone and inhibition of β₂-linked sodium-potassium membrane transport skeletal muscle have been proposed as possible mechanisms. This effect is probably of limited clinical importance in patients with normal renal function and in patients not taking other medications that may effect serum potassium levels.

β-Adrenergic blocking agents can affect lipid levels.[481, 482] Chronic use of β-adrenergic blockers has been associated with an increase in triglyceride levels and decrease in HDL-cholesterol. β-Blockers with increased β₁-selectivity or with partial agonist activity appear to have less effect on the lipid profile. Nonselective β-blockers without partial agonist activity may decrease HDL-cholesterol up to 20%, and increases in triglycerides of up to 50% have been reported. The effects of β-blockade on lipid metabolism are attributed primarily to modulation of lipoprotein lipase activity. Very low density lipoprotein (VLDL)-cholesterol and triglyceride metabolism are retarded in the setting of unopposed α-adrenergic stimulation of the lipoprotein lipase activity.

Decreased VLDL metabolism results in decreases in HDL-cholesterol.

Abrupt withdrawal of β-adrenergic blockers may be associated with overshoot hypertension and worsening angina in patients with coronary artery disease.[483-486] Myocardial infarction has been reported. These withdrawal symptoms may be due to increased sympathetic activity, which is a reflection of possible adrenergic receptor up-regulation during chronic sympathetic blockade. Gradual tapering of β-blockers decreases the risk of withdrawal. Withdrawal symptoms have been reported more commonly with abrupt discontinuation of relatively short-acting drugs. Withdrawal symptoms are relatively unusual with longer acting agents.

Calcium Antagonists
Mechanisms of Action

CAs have emerged as an important therapeutic class of medications for a variety of cardiovascular disorders.[487, 488] Initially introduced in the 1970s as antianginal agents, they are now widely advocated as first-line therapy for hypertension.[131] The pharmacologic effects of these drugs are related to their ability to attenuate cellular calcium uptake.[489-496] CAs do not directly antagonize the effects of calcium, but they inhibit the entry of calcium or its mobilization from intracellular stores.

Calcium channels have binding sites for both activators and antagonists. The voltage-dependent L-type calcium channel is a multimeric complex composed of alpha 1, alpha 2, omega, beta, and gamma subunits.[497] These channels appear to have different binding sites for the various CAs located on the alpha 1 subunit and are regulated by voltage-dependent as well as receptor-dependent events involving protein phosphorylation and G protein coupling resulting from, for example, β-adrenergic stimulation.[498-502] Each class of CA is quantitatively and qualitatively unique, possessing differential sensitivity and selectivity for binding pharmacologic receptors as well as the slow calcium channel in various vascular tissues. Even within the dihydropyridine class, there is considerable pharmacologic variability.[503] This differential selectivity of action has important clinical implications for the use of these drugs and explains why the CAs vary considerably in their effects on regional circulatory beds, sinus and atrioventricular (AV) nodal function, and myocardial contractility. It further explains the diversity of indications for clinical use, ancillary effects, and side effects.

CAs represent ideal antihypertensive agents because they uniformly lower peripheral vascular resistance in patients regardless of race, salt sensitivity, age, or comorbid conditions. There are at least three mechanisms whereby they lower blood pressure. First, CAs reduce peripheral vascular resistance by attenuating the calcium-dependent contractions of vascular smooth muscle.[491] The contraction of vascular smooth muscle is dependent on the total cytosolic calcium concentration, regulated by two distinct mechanisms. Depolarization of vascular smooth muscle tissue is dependent on the inward flux of calcium through voltage-sensitive L-type and T-type calcium channels. Hypertensive patients have an abnormal influx of calcium, promoting increased peripheral vascular resistance.[489, 490] Calcium released from the sarcoplasmic reticulum in response to

extracellular calcium influx is a non–voltage dependent pathway. Cytosolic calcium binds to calmodulin, initiating a sequence of cellular events that promotes the interaction between actin and myosin, resulting in smooth muscle contraction. Therefore, the importance of the calcium channels is due to their pivotal role of linking cell membrane electrical activity to biologic responses. Calcium influxes through L-type channels from extracellular sources and intracellular sources are both attenuated by CAs.[492, 504, 505]

Second, CAs decrease vascular responsiveness to AII and the synthesis and secretion of aldosterone.[495, 506-508] They also interfere with α_2-adrenergic receptor–mediated vasoconstriction and possibly α_1-adrenergic receptor–mediated vasoconstriction.[493, 494, 509-511] The maximal vasodilatory response measured by forearm blood flow appears to be inversely related to the patient's plasma renin activity and AII concentration. Thus, it is possible that there is a greater influence of the calcium influx–dependent vasoconstriction in patients with low-renin hypertension, such as blacks, explaining the clinical observation that CAs are often more potent than other agents in such groups.

Finally, the CAs may induce a mild diuresis. It is well known that, in particular, the dihydropyridines reduce preglomerular resistance and maintain or increase the GFR[496, 512-514] because of their preferential vasodilatory action on the renal afferent arteriole. Subsequently, decreased tubule sodium reabsorption and improved renal blood flow and natriuresis are observed. With isradipine, the sodium excretion rate correlates with the reduction in blood pressure.[515]

Antihypertensive activity has not uniformly been demonstrated to be secondary to changes in nitric oxide release. The vasorelaxant properties of nifedipine and verapamil appear to be nitric oxide independent, whereas those of amlodipine are partly NO dependent.[516, 517] This effect of amlodipine is thought to be mediated by inhibition of local ACE and increases in vasodilatory bradykinins.[517]

Class Members

Despite their shared mechanism of action, the CAs are a very heterogeneous group of compounds. They differ with respect to pharmacologic profile, chemical structure, pharmacokinetic profile, tissue specificity, receptor binding, clinical indications, and side effect profile. Two primary subtypes are distinguished on the basis of their behavior: dihydropyridines and nondihydropyridines. The nondihydropyridines are further divided into two classes: benzothiazepines (diltiazem) and diphenylalkylamines (verapamil). The distinctly different pharmacologic effects are summarized in Table 55-15.

Although all CAs vasodilate coronary and peripheral arteries, the dihydropyridines are the most potent. Insofar as this subclass of CAs are membrane-active drugs, they exert a greater effect on the peripheral vessels than myocardial cells, which depend less heavily on the external calcium influx than vessels.[492, 518] Their potent vasodilatory action prompts a rapid compensatory increase in sympathetic nervous activity, mediated by baroreceptor reflexes creating a neutral or positive inotropic stimulus.[519] Longer acting dihydropyridines, however, do not appear to activate the sympathetic nervous system.[520] They also elicit greater activation of the renin-angiotensin-aldosterone system (RAAS). In contrast,

TABLE 55-15

Pharmacodynamic Properties of Calcium Antagonists

DRUG GENERIC (TRADE) NAME	MAXIMAL HYPOTENSIVE RESPONSE (H)	DURATION OF HYPOTENSIVE RESPONSE (H)	FIRST DOSE (MG)	USUAL DAILY DOSE (MG)	MAXIMAL DAILY DOSE (MG)
Diltiazem (Cardizem)	2.5-4	8	60	60-120 tid/qid	480
Diltiazem SR (Cardizem SR)	6	12	180	120-240 bid	480
Diltiazem CD (Cardizem CD)	—	24	180	240-280 qd	480
Diltiazem XR (Dilacor XR)	3-6	24	180	180-480 qd	480
Diltiazem ER (Tiazac)	6-10	24	180	180-480 qd	480
Amlodipine (Norvasc)	—	24	5	5-10 qd	10
Felodipine (Plendil ER)	2-5	24	5	5-10 qd	20
Isradipine (DynaCirc)	2-3	12	2.5	2.5-5 bid	20
Isradipine CR (DynaCirc CR)	2	7-18	5	5-20 qid	20
Nicardipine (Cardene)	1-2	8	20	20-40 tid	120
Nicardipine SR (Cardene SR)	2-6	12	30	30-60 bid	120
Nifedipine (Procardia, Adalat)	0.5-1	4-6	10	10-30 tid/qid	120
Nifedipine GITS (Procardia XL)	4-6	24	30	30-90 qd	120
Nifedipine ER (Adalat CC)	2-4	24	30	30-90 qd	120
Nisoldipine (Sular)	—	24	20	20-40 qd	60
Verapamil (Calan, Isoptin)	6-8	8	80	80-120 tid	480
Verapamil SR (Calan SR, Isoptin SR)	—	12-24	90	90-240 bid	480
Verapamil SR pellet (Verelan)	—	24	120	24-480 qd	480
Verapamil COER-24 (Covera-HS)	>4-5	24	180	180-480 qHS	480

CD, controlled diffusion; COER, controlled-onset extended release; GITS, gastrointestinal therapeutic system; SR, sustained release; XR and ER, extended release.

the nondihydropyridines are moderately potent arterial vasodilators but directly decrease AV nodal conduction and have negative inotropic and chronotropic effects, not abrogated by the reflex increase in sympathetic tone. Because of their negative inotropic action, they are contraindicated in patients with systolic heart failure. They are also more effective at reducing stress-induced cardiovascular responses than the dihydropyridines.[521]

A clinically useful classification system for the CAs categorizes them by their duration of action into short-acting and long-acting agents (to be given once daily) (Table 55-16). This schema is helpful because the short-acting agents are no longer recommended for the treatment of hypertension as the powerful stimulation of the sympathetic nervous system by the vasodilation may predispose patients to angina, myocardial infarction, and stroke.[522] The long-acting drugs are commonly divided into three generations. First-generation agents such as nifedipine have shorter half-lives and require multiple daily doses. Second-generation agents are those manipulated to provide modified or sustained release, requiring once-daily dosing. The third-generation agents have intrinsically longer plasma or receptor half-lives, possibly related to greater lipophilicity.[523]

BENZOTHIAZEPINES

Diltiazem hydrochloride is the prototype of the benzothiazepine CAs. Diltiazem is 98% absorbed from the gastrointestinal tract, but because of extensive first-pass hepatic metabolism, the bioavailability is only 40% compared with intravenous dosing[36] (see Tables 55-25 and 55-16). Diltiazem is extensively metabolized in the liver by O-deacetylation or N-demethylation. Several metabolites exist: deacetyldiltiazem represents up to 45% and retains 25% to 50% activity of the parent compound; N-desmethyldiltiazem accounts for 20% but has little clinical activity. In vivo, the competitively inhibited liver isoenzyme CYP2D6 is the most important metabolic pathway, which probably accounts for the substantial proportion of drug interactions that occur with diltiazem.[524] The remainder of metabolites are unidentified but may reach concentrations exceeding that of diltiazem and have half-lives up to 20 hours. Only 4% of the unchanged drug is excreted in the urine. Renal excretion accounts for 35%, with the remainder excreted in the feces. Rates of elimination are slower in elderly persons and those with chronic liver disease but unchanged with renal insufficiency.

Oral forms of diltiazem have been modified to improve delivery and currently include tablets, sustained-release (SR) capsules, controlled-diffusion (CD) capsules, Geomatrix extended-release (XR) capsules, extended-release (ER) capsules, and buccoadhesive formulations.[36, 525-531] The usual starting dose in tablet form is 180 mg/day in three divided doses and may be titrated to a total dose of 480 mg/day (see Table 55-15). Peak hypotensive effect is achieved in 2.5 to 4 hours, and the maximum antihypertensive effects occur in up to 14 days. After tablet absorption, diltiazem is rapidly and widely distributed, with up to 93% being protein bound.[532]

The SR tablet release rate varies with the size of the matrix.[533] Therefore, the long-acting preparations should not be divided. The usual daily dose is 120 to 240 mg, and peak response usually occurs in 6 hours. The CD capsules are

TABLE 55-16

Pharmacokinetic Properties of Calcium Antagonists

DRUGS	ORAL ABSORPTION (%)	FIRST PASS EFFECT	BIOAVAILABILITY (%)	PEAK BLOOD LEVEL	ELIMINATION HALF-LIFE (H)	METABOLISM/ EXCRETION	PROTEIN BINDING	ACTIVE METABOLITES
Diltiazem	98	50%	40	2-3 h	4-6	Liver/feces and urine	77-93	Yes
Diltiazem SR	>80	50%	35	6-11 h	5-7	Liver/feces and urine	77-93	Yes
Diltiazem CD	95	Extensive	35	10-14 h	5-8	Liver/feces and urine	77-93	Yes
Diltiazem XR	95	Extensive	41	4-6 h	5-10	Liver/feces and urine	95	Yes
Diltiazem ER	93	Extensive	40-60	4-6 h	10	Liver/feces and urine	95	Yes
Amlodipine	>90	Minimal	88	6-12 h	30-50	Liver/urine	>95	Yes
Felodipine	>90	Extensive	13-18	2.5-5 h	11-16	Liver/urine	>95	No
Isradipine	>90	Extensive	15-25	1-2 h	8	Liver/feces and urine	>95	No
Isradipine CR	>90	Extensive	15-25	7-18 h	—	Liver/feces and urine	>95	No
Nicardipine	>90	Extensive	35	0.5-2 h	8.6	Liver/feces and urine	>95	No
Nicardipine SR	>90	Extensive	30	1-4 h	—	Liver/feces and urine	>95	No
Nifedipine	>90	20%–30%	60	<30 min	2	Liver/urine	98	Yes
Nifedepine GITS	>90	25%–35%	86	6 h	—	Liver/urine	98	Yes
Nifedipine ER	>90	25%–35%	89	2.5-5 h; 6-12	7	Liver/urine	98	Yes
Nisoldipine	>85	Extensive	4-8	6-12 h	10-22	Liver/feces and urine	99	No
Verapamil	>90	70%–80%	20-35	1-2 h	2.8-7.4	Liver/feces and urine	85-95	Yes
Verapamil SR	>90	70%–80%	20-35	5-6 h	4-12	Liver/feces and urine	85-95	Yes
Verapamil SR Pellet	>90	70%–80%	20-35	7-9 h	12	Liver/feces and urine	85-95	Yes
Verapamil COER-24/CODAS	>90	70%–80%	20-35	11 h	—	Liver/feces and urine	85-95	Yes

CD, controlled-diffusion; COER, controlled-onset extended release; GITS, gastrointestinal therapeutic system; SR, sustained release; XR and ER, extended release.

composed of two types of diltiazem beads: 40% of the beads release the drug within 12 hours, and the remaining 60% release the drug over the next 12 hours.[36] The usual daily dose is 240 to 480 mg. Approximately 95% of the drug is absorbed, peak plasma levels occur in 10 to 14 hours, and the plasma half-life is 5 to 8 hours but increases with increasing dose. The XR capsules contain a degradable swellable controlled-release matrix that slowly releases the drug over 24 hours. The usual daily dose is 180 to 480 mg. Ninety-five percent of the drug is absorbed, and the absolute bioavailability is 41%. Onset of action occurs in 3 to 6 hours, and the half-life ranges from 5 to 10 hours. The ER capsules contain prolonged liberation microgranules that dissolve at a constant rate. Peak blood levels are achieved after 4 to 6 hours, and bioavailability is 93%. The usual daily dose is 180 to 480 mg, with an elimination half-life of up to 10 hours. A buccoadhesive formulation has been developed to bypass the effects of the hepatic first-pass metabolism and improve bioavailability.[531] The dissolution and diffusion of the buccoadhesive hydrophilic matrices of diltiazem polymers provide reliable delivery for up to 10 hours. The optimal use of this vehicle is under investigation.

DIPHENYLALKYLAMINE

Verapamil hydrochloride, the oldest CA, is the prototype diphenylalkylamine derivative. Verapamil inhibits membrane transport of calcium in myocardial cells, particularly the AV node, and smooth muscle cells, rendering it antiarrhythmic, antihypertensive, and a negative inotrope. It is available for oral administration in film-coated tablets containing 40, 80, or 120 mg of racemic verapamil HCl[36] (see Table 55-15). The usual daily dose is 80 to 120 mg three times per day. The time to peak concentration is 1 to 2 hours. The onset of action is achieved in 6 to 8 hours, and the maximal antihypertensive response is achieved within 1 to 4 weeks. The elimination half-life of verapamil ranges from 2.8 to 7.4 hours but increases with chronic administration and in elderly patients with renal insufficiency (see Table 55-16).

The SR caplets are available in scored 120-, 180-, and 240-mg forms. The usual antihypertensive dose is equivalent to the total daily dose of immediate-release tablets and can be given as 240 to 480 mg/day. Adequate antihypertensive response may be improved by divided twice-daily dosing. Maximum plasma levels occur in 5 to 6 hours and are delayed by concomitant food absorption. The half-life is 4 to 12 hours.

The SR pellet-filled verapamil capsules are gel-coated capsules with an onset of action of 7 to 9 hours that is not affected by food. Peak concentrations are approximately 65% of those of immediate-release tablets, but the trough concentrations are 30% higher. The plasma half-life is 12 hours, and the usual daily dose is 240 to 480 mg.

The controlled-onset, extended-release (COER) and chronotherapeutic oral drug absorption system (CODAS) tablets have unique pharmacologic properties and deliver verapamil 4 to 5 hours after ingestion. A delay coating is inserted between the outer semipermeable membrane and the active inner drug core. As the delay coating expands in the gastrointestinal tract, the pressure causes drug from the inner core to be released through laser-drilled holes in the outer membrane. This makes it ideal for nighttime dosing by providing maximal plasma levels in the early morning hours from 6 AM to noon and minimizing nighttime diurnal blood pressure variations.[534, 535] A promising buccal drug formulation of 40 mg that significantly improves the bioavailability of verapamil and results in fewer metabolites is under investigation.[536]

Gastrointestinal absorption of verapamil exceeds 90%; however, it is extensively metabolized in the liver by N-dealkylation and O-demethylation and only 10% to 30% reaches the systemic circulation. Of the 13 known metabolites of verapamil, norverapamil is the only one with cardiovascular activity; it has 20% of the potency of the parent compound. Renal excretion accounts for 70% of clearance and occurs within 5 days. The remainder is excreted in the feces. Clearance is fourfold higher for the S-verapamil enantiomer than the R-enantiomer and decreases with increasing age and decreasing weight.[537] With chronic administration, there is a significant increase in bioavailability, possibly as a result of saturation of hepatic enzymes.[538] Dose adjustment is necessary with hepatic but not renal failure; however, verapamil should be used with caution in patients who ingest large amounts of grapefruit juice or those with renal insufficiency taking concurrent AV nodal blocking agents.[539]

A novel CA, AH-1058, is currently under investigation. It is a cyproheptadine-related compound that preferentially binds to phenylalkylamine and benzothiazepine receptors in cardiac cells. It exerts negative dromotropic and chronotropic and weak coronary vasodilator effects. It has very little effect on the peripheral vasculature and thus is anticipated to be useful for conditions in which selective inhibition of ventricular calcium channels is warranted (i.e., arrhythmias).[540] The clinical usefulness of this compound remains to be determined.

DIHYDROPYRIDINES

Nifedipine is a dihydropyridine CA that causes decreased peripheral resistance with no clinically significant depression of myocardial function. It has no tendency to prolong AV conduction, prolong sinus node recovery, or slow sinus rate. This is a result of the reflex sympathetic stimulation triggered by vasodilation. Clinically, there is usually a small increase in heart rate and cardiac index. The labeling for immediate-release nifedipine capsules has been revised to recommend against using this dosage form for the treatment

of chronic hypertension.[36] In elderly persons, the immediate-release form has been associated with a greater than threefold increase in mortality compared with other antihypertensive agents, including other calcium channel blockers.[541] In most patients, immediate-release nifedipine causes a modest hypotensive effect that is well tolerated. However, in occasional patients the hypotensive effect is profound and has resulted in myocardial infarction, stroke, and death. This effect appears to be more pronounced in patients taking concomitant β-blockers. Consequently, its use should be reserved for short periods but not in the setting of acute syndromes.[36] The usual adult dose is 10 to 20 mg three times daily and can be titrated weekly (see Table 55-15). Nifedipine is rapidly and fully absorbed, and drug levels are detectable within 10 minutes of ingestion. Peak levels are achieved within 30 minutes and the half-life is 2 hours. The bioavailability approaches 60% and is unaffected by the route of administration. There is no clinical advantage to bite-and-swallow or bite-and-hold sublingually.

Nifedipine is extensively metabolized in the liver into at least two inactive metabolites and then excreted in the urine. Eighty-three percent of the population are reported to metabolize the drug rapidly; the other 17% are slow-metabolizers. The clinical significance of this finding is unknown.[542] Nifedipine is 98% protein bound, so the dose should be adjusted in patients with hepatic insufficiency or severe malnutrition.

The extended-release tablets of nifedipine are available in 30-, 60-, and 90-mg doses. These tablets consist of an outer semipermeable membrane surrounding an active drug core. The core is composed of an inner active drug layer surrounded by an osmotically active, inert layer that forces dissolution of the drug core as it swells from gastrointestinal juice absorption. The drug is then slowly and steadily released over 16 to 18 hours. This method of delivery is referred to as the gastrointestinal therapeutic system or GITS formulation.[543] The extended-release form should not be bitten or divided. The time to peak concentration is 6 hours, and plasma levels remain steady for 24 hours. With chronic administration, full therapeutic drug levels are achieved in 30 hours. The bioavailability of the extended-release tablet is 86% compared with immediate-release forms, and tolerance does not develop.[544] Eighty percent of the metabolites are excreted in the urine. The remainder is excreted in the feces with the outer semipermeable membrane shell. The usual adult maintenance dose is 30 to 90 mg/day. Conversion from the immediate-release form to extended-release tablets can be done on an equal milligram basis.

A similar extended-release formulation is composed of a coat and a core (CC).[36] The outer layer contains a slow-release form of nifedipine; the inner core is a fast-release preparation. The bioavailability of the CC formulation is 89% compared with the immediate-release form. Peak concentrations are reached within 2.5 to 5 hours, and there is a second peak after 6 to 12 hours as the inner core is released. With administration in this way, the half-life is extended from 2 to 7 hours. The usual daily dose is 30 to 90 mg and should be titrated by 30-mg increments in 7 to 14 days for maximal effect. Because of the unique delivery system, which provides a rapid-release core, peak plasma concentrations are not always reliable.[34, 36] Ingestion of three 30-mg tablets simultaneously, but not two, results in a 29% higher peak plasma concentration than a single 90-mg tablet. Consequently, two tablets may be substituted for 60 mg, but substitution of 30-mg tablets to make 90 mg is not recommended.[34, 36]

Amlodipine besylate is unique among the dihydropyridine CAs. It appears to bind to both dihydropyridine and nondihydropyridine sites to produce peripheral arterial vasodilation without significant activation of the sympathetic nervous system.[545] The parent compound has substantially slower, but more complete, absorption than others in the class, with a bioavailability up to 88%[546] (see Table 55-16). After ingestion, amlodipine is almost completely absorbed and widely distributed. Peak plasma concentrations are achieved in 6 to 12 hours, and the clinical response can be detected at 24 hours.[547] Mean peak serum levels are linear, age independent, and achieved after 7 to 8 days of chronic dosing.[36, 547, 548] The elimination half-life is long, ranging from 30 to 50 hours, and is prolonged in elderly people.[547, 548] The long half-life permits once-daily dosing, and the hypotensive response may last up to 5 days.[549] Ninety percent of amlodipine is metabolized in the liver by oxidation to the inactive pyridine analog. Ten percent is excreted unchanged; the metabolites are excreted primarily in the urine, but no dose adjustment is necessary with renal impairment. The minimum effective dose is 2.5 mg, particularly in elderly patients.[509] Most patients require a dose of 5 to 10 mg/day.

Felodipine is a dihydropyridine CA that is administered in extended-release tablets of 2.5, 5, and 10 mg[36] (see Table 55-15). Felodipine is almost completely absorbed from the gastrointestinal tract with a time to peak concentration of 2 to 5 hours. The mean systemic availability varies between only 13% and 18% as a result of extensive first-pass hepatic metabolism.[550] Bioavailability is influenced by food. Large meals and the flavonoids in grapefruit juice increase the bioavailability by approximately 50%.[551] The elimination half-life is triphasic. The mean half-life of the initial distribution phase is 4.8 minutes, and the mean half-lives of the second and third phases are 1.5 and 9.1 hours, respectively.[552] The overall half-life is 11 to 16 hours. Felodipine is metabolized in the liver into at least six inactive metabolites. Seventy percent of the metabolites are excreted in the urine, the remainder in the feces. The usual daily dose is 2.5 to 10 mg, and titration can be instituted at 2-week intervals. The dose should be adjusted for hepatic, but not renal, insufficiency.

Isradipine is a dihydropyridine CA that is effective alone or in combination with other antihypertensive agents for the treatment of mild to moderate hypertension[36, 553] (see Table 55-15). Isradipine is rapidly and almost completely absorbed after oral administration. Extensive first-pass hepatic metabolism reduces bioavailability to less than 25%. The initial hypotensive effect occurs within 1 hour and peaks at 2 to 3 hours for the regular release form. The drug is active for 12 hours; however, the full antihypertensive response does not occur until 14 days. The usual daily dose is 2.5 to 5 mg two to three times daily. The onset of action of the SR formulation is achieved in 2 hours and lasts for 7 to 18 hours. The usual daily dose of the CR tablet is 5 to 20 mg. Isradipine is extensively protein bound. The elimination half-life is biphasic with a terminal half-life of 8 hours. Isradipine is metabolized into at least six pyridine derivatives that have no biologic activity. Sixty percent to 65% are excreted into the urine, the remainder in the feces. Dosage adjustment is unnecessary in renal or liver failure.

Manidipine is a second-generation dihydropyridine CA structurally related to nifedipine.[554-556] The usual adult dose is 10 to 20 mg once daily. Dosage should be adjusted at 2-week intervals. Manidipine is 36% to 60% absorbed after oral administration. It is highly protein bound and extensively metabolized in the liver. Sixty-three percent of the drug is excreted in the feces. The peak plasma concentration occurs after 2 to 3.5 hours, with an elimination half-life of 5 to 8 hours. Dose adjustment is not necessary in renal failure.

Nicardipine hydrochloride is a dihydropyridine CA available as 20- and 40-mg immediate-release gelatin capsules or 30-, 45-, and 60-mg SR capsules.[36, 557] The usual daily dose is 20 to 40 mg three times for the immediate-release form and 30 to 60 mg twice daily for the SR preparation. When converting to the SR form, the previous daily total of immediate-release drug should be administered on a twice-daily regimen but may not be predictive of eventual response. Titration should be instituted no sooner than 3 days. Nicardipine is well absorbed orally but has only 35% systemic bioavailability because of extensive first-pass hepatic metabolism; protein binding is greater than 95%. The time to peak concentration is 30 minutes to 2 hours for immediate-release capsules and 1 to 4 hours for SR forms. The elimination half-life is 8.6 hours. Nicardipine is 100% oxidized in the liver to inactive pyridine metabolites. There is no evidence of microsomal enzyme induction. Metabolites are excreted primarily in the urine and feces. The parent compound is not dialyzable. Dose adjustments are necessary in hepatic, but not renal, insufficiency.

Nisoldipine is a dihydropyridine CA formulated as extended-release tablets of 10, 20, 30, and 40 mg (see Table 55-15).[36, 558] The initial starting dose is 20 mg and the usual maintenance dose is 20 to 40 mg given once daily, which can be titrated at weekly intervals. Bioavailability of nisoldipine drug is low and variable (4% to 8%). The coat-core design allows a full 24-hour effect after oral administration. Eighty percent of the dose is contained in the outer coat, which is slowly absorbed in the stomach and upper intestine. The inner core releases the remaining drug in the lower intestine. The drug reaches therapeutic concentrations in 6 to 12 hours, and absorption is slowed by high-fat meals. The elimination half-life ranges from 10 to 22 hours. Nisoldipine is metabolized by dehydrogenation in the liver and intestine. Variable hepatic blood flow induced by the drug probably contributes to its pharmacokinetic variability. Eighteen known metabolites exist, possessing 10% of the parent activity. Seventy-five percent of the metabolites are excreted in the urine, the remainder in the feces. Dose adjustments are necessary with hepatic, but not renal, impairment.

Lacidipine is a second-generation dihydropyridine CA available in tablet form. It is reported to be unusually potent and long acting, possibly because it diffuses deeper into lipid bilayer membranes. A unique attribute of this drug appears to be its greater vascular selectivity, but the clinical relevance of this remains unclear.[559] The usual dose is 4 to 6 mg once daily and should be titrated at 2- to 4-week intervals.[560] Bioavailability is only 2% to 9% because of extensive first-pass hepatic metabolism. The peak serum levels of lacidipine are achieved in 1 to 1.5 hours. The duration of action is 12 to 24 hours. The elimination half-life is 12 to 19 hours. The parent compound is converted 100% by the liver into inactive fragments that are excreted primarily in the feces (70%) and the kidney. Dose adjustment is necessary in elderly persons and in patients with hepatic, but not renal, impairment.

Lercanidipine is a novel dihydropyridine CA whose molecular design imparts greater solubility within the arterial cellular membrane bilayer, conferring a 10-fold higher vascular selectivity than that of amlodipine.[561] In contrast to amlodipine, it has a relatively short half-life but a long-lasting effect at the receptor and membrane level and is associated with significantly less peripheral edema.[562, 563] It is administered at a starting dose of 10 mg and increased to 20 mg as needed. It has a gradual onset of action and the effects last for 24 hours.[564, 565] Lercanidipine is unique among dihydropyridines in that it also appears to dilate the efferent renal arteriole.[566]

Class Renal Effects

The potential benefits of CAs in acute and chronic kidney disease have been well described. There are multiple mechanisms whereby they alter or protect renal function, notably as natriuretics, vasodilators, and antiproteinuric agents (Table 55-17). All CAs exert natriuretic and diuretic effects. Experimental studies and studies in humans with hypertension indicate that the increase in sodium excretion is, in part, independent of vasodilatory action or changes in GFR, renal blood flow, or filtration fraction.[8, 567, 568] This effect is probably the result of changes in renal sodium handling that can potentiate the antihypertensive vascular effect. In normal subjects, CAs acutely increase sodium excretion from 10% to 240%, frequently in the absence of changes in blood pressure.[569] In hypertensive subjects, acute administration of CAs uniformly increases sodium excretion 1.1- to 3.4-fold, the magnitude of which is not related to the decrement in blood pressure.[570]

The natriuretic effect appears to persist in the long term. Chronic administration of CAs to hypertensive patients results in a cumulative sodium deficit that is abruptly reversed with discontinuation of the drug.[571] Natriuresis frequently occurs 3 to 6 hours after the morning dose,[572-574] and the net negative sodium balance levels off after the first 2 to 3 days of administration but persists for the duration of therapy.[575] There are no significant changes in long-term body weight, potassium, urea nitrogen, catecholamines, or GFR, all of which would be expected to change in the setting of natriuresis.[8] Moreover, stimulation of renin release and aldosterone does not occur to an appreciable degree. It has been postulated that the natriuresis induced by CAs increases distal sodium delivery to the macula densa, suppressing renin release. Because AII mediates aldosterone synthesis by way of cytosolic calcium messengers, CAs blunt this response as well.[576-578]

The mechanism whereby CAs induce natriuresis appears to be direct inhibition of renal tubule sodium and water absorption. Dihydropyridines increase urinary flow rate and sodium excretion without changes in the filtered water and sodium load.[579] Studies suggest that CAs may diminish sodium uptake at the amiloride-sensitive sodium channels.[580] Inhibition of water reabsorption occurs distal to the late distal tubule.[581] Proximal tubule sodium reabsorption may be inhibited by higher doses.[582] One possible mediator of this effect is atrial natriuretic peptide. In human studies, CAs augmented atrial natriuretic peptide release and potentiated its action at the level of the kidney.[583, 584] Other potential mediators are under investigation. What magnitude the natriuretic effects contribute to the antihypertensive response is unknown, but in contrast to those related to other vasodilators, the changes attenuate the expected adaptive changes in sodium handling.

The renal hemodynamic effects of CAs are variable and depend primarily on which vasoconstrictors modulate renal vascular tone.[585] Experimentally, CAs improve GFR in the presence of the vasoconstrictors norepinephrine and AII and others by preferentially attenuating afferent arteriolar resistance.[586, 587] The efferent arteriole appears to be refractory to these vasodilatory effects. Patients with primary hypertension appear to be more sensitive to the renal hemodynamic effects of CAs than normotensive subjects, and this effect is more pronounced with advancing kidney disease.[588-590] Acute administration of CA results in little change or augmentation of the GFR and renal plasma flow, no change in the filtration fraction, and reduction of renal vascular resistance. Chronic administration is not associated with significant changes in renal hemodynamics. The response is maximal in the presence of AII, which selectively causes postglomerular vasoconstriction. Clinically significant changes are counteracted by the reduction in renal perfusion pressure coincident with reduction of blood pressure.

The long-term effects of CAs on renal function are controversial and variable. In hypertensive patients, the effects on renal hemodynamics vary. Some patients exhibit no change in GFR, whereas others have an exaggerated increase in GFR and renal plasma flow.[585] Even normotensive patients with a family history of hypertension have an exaggerated hemodynamic response.[591]

The antiproteinuric effects of CAs are also controversial and variable with respect to the class of drug and the level of

TABLE 55-17

Renal Effects of Calcium Antagonists

CLASS	Na EXCRETION	GLOMERULAR FILTRATION RATE	FILTRATION FRACTION	RENAL BLOOD FLOW	RENAL VASCULAR RESISTANCE	PROTEINURIA
Dihydropyridines	↑	↑ to ↔	—	↑ to ↔	↓	↑
Diltiazem	↑	↑ to ↔	—	↑ to ↔	↓	—↓
Verapamil	↑	↑ to ↔	—	↑ to ↔	↓	↓

blood pressure reduction achieved.[592, 593] Some dihydropyridines may increase protein excretion by up to 40%. It is not clear whether this is a result of hemodynamic vasodilation at the afferent arteriole resulting in increased glomerular capillary pressure, as CAs directly impair renal autoregulation, changes in glomerular basement membrane permeability, or increased intrarenal AII.[112, 594, 595] In contrast, felodipine, diltiazem, and verapamil do not appear to have this effect and may lower protein excretion, possibly by also decreasing efferent arteriolar tone and glomerular pressure. The clinical implications remain to be determined.

Large clinical trials underscore the controversy. In blacks with hypertension and mild to moderate renal insufficiency with proteinuria greater than 1 g/day, renoprotection with an ACE inhibitor far exceeded any effect of the dihydropyridine calcium channel blocker amlodipine, with which renal function deteriorated.[594, 596] This effect was independent of blood pressure reduction and was more evident in proteinuric patients; it was also suggestive in patients with baseline proteinuria less than 300 mg/day. Hypertensive patients with diabetic nephropathy also fared considerably worse with amlodipine therapy than with an ARB.[278] Patients experienced higher rates of progression of renal disease and all-cause mortality in the amlodipine and placebo group. This effect was also independent of blood pressure levels achieved. However, coadministration of amlodipine with an ARB does not abrogate the protective effect on kidney function.[279] It is postulated that selective dilation of the afferent arteriole favors an increase in glomerular capillary pressure that perpetuates renal disease progression.

CAs have many nonhemodynamic effects that may also afford renoprotection (Table 55-18). In addition to lowering blood pressure, they act as free radical scavengers; retard renal growth and kidney weight[597-600]; reduce the entrapment of macromolecules in the mesangium[601]; attenuate the mitogenic actions of platelet-derived growth factor and platelet-activating factor[599]; block mitochondrial overload of calcium[602]; decrease lipid peroxidation; decrease glomerular basement membrane thickness; augment the antioxidant activities of superoxide dismutase, catalase, and glutathione peroxidase; inhibit metalloproteinase-1 and collagenolytic activity; suppress the expression of the angiogenic growth factors vascular endothelial growth factor, basic fibroblast growth factor, TGF-β, and endothelial nitric oxide synthase[603]; and prevent renal cortical remodeling and scarring (see Table 55-18).[585, 604-606]

Because of their renal hemodynamic effects and inhibition of calcium-mediated injury, the CAs have the ability to attenuate various types of kidney damage, including radiocontrast-induced nephropathy and hypoperfusion ischemic injury such as occurs during cardiac surgery.[607, 608] In experimental models, pretreatment with CA variably preserved GFR and renal blood flow.[609] The clinical effectiveness of this class of drugs in these settings requires further evaluation.

CAs represent an important treatment option for renal transplant recipients. Administration of CAs in the renal allograft perfusate and to renal allograft recipients reduces initial graft nonfunction by attenuating ischemic and reperfusion injury[610] and preserves long-term renal function by protecting against cyclosporine nephrotoxicity and, possibly, by contributing to immunomodulation.[611, 612] Cyclosporine

TABLE 55-18

Renal Protective Mechanisms of Calcium Antagonists

↓ Blood pressure
↓ Proteinuria
Free radical scavengers
↓ Kidney growth
↓ Mesangial molecule entrapment
Attenuate antigenic PDGF and PAF
Block mitochondrial calcium overload
↓ Lipid peroxidation
↓ GBM thickness
Augment antioxidant effects of SOD/catalase and GTP
Inhibit collagenic activity
Suppress angiogenic growth factors: VCGF, bFGF, TGF-beta and eNOS
Prevent renal cortical remodeling
Ameliorate cyclosporine toxicity
Block thromboxane- and endothelin cyclosporine-induced vasoconstriction

bFGF, basic fibroblast growth factor; eNOS, endothelial nitric oxide synthase; GTP, glutathione peroxidase; GBM, glomerular basement membrane; PAF, platelet-activating factor; PDGF, platelet-derived growth factor; SOD, superoxide dismutase; TGF-β, transforming growth factor β.

causes direct tubule injury and induces intrarenal vasoconstriction. The thromboxane- and endothelin-induced vasoconstriction of the afferent arteriole stimulated by cyclosporine is reversed by CA.[613, 614] Conversely, the CAs have been reported to enhance cyclosporine-induced apoptosis of renal tubule cells,[615] suggesting that their benefits might be hemodynamically mediated.

Class Efficacy and Safety

All CAs are considered initial antihypertensive agents and appear to be equally efficacious and safe.[131] Approximately 70% to 80% of patients in stage I and II respond to monotherapy. Up to 50% of unselected patients respond to monotherapy. In contrast to other vasodilators, the CAs attenuate the reflex increase of neurohormonal activity that accompanies reduction in blood pressure, and in the long term they inhibit or do not change sympathetic activity.[545, 616] The CAs are effective in young, middle-aged, and elderly patients with "white coat," mild, moderate, or severe hypertension.[617-620] CAs are equally efficacious in men and women, patients with a high or low plasma renin activity regardless of dietary salt intake, and black and white patients.[621, 622] They are effective and safe in patients with hypertension and coronary artery disease[623] and ESRD.[624] The long-acting agents produce sustained systolic and diastolic blood pressure reductions of 16 to 28 mm Hg and 14 to 17 mm Hg, respectively, with no appreciable development of tolerance.

Among the different classes, the dihydropyridines appear to be the most powerful at reducing blood pressure but may also be associated with greater activation of baroreceptor reflexes.[625] Dihydropyridines induce a shift in sympathovagal balance that favors sympathetic predominance compared with nondihydropyridines.[521] In general, however, when compared with other vasodilators, CAs attenuate the reflex increase in sympathetic activity (increased heart rate, cardiac index, and plasma norepinephrine levels and renin activity).

Verapamil and to a lesser extent diltiazem exert greater effects on the heart and less vasoselectivity. They typically reduce heart rate, slow AV conduction, and depress contractility (Table 55-19). The second- and third-generation CAs consist of pharmacologically manipulated formulations whose half-lives are progressively longer.[523]

CAs are contraindicated in patients with severely depressed left ventricular function (except perhaps amlodipine), hypotension, sick sinus syndrome (unless a pacemaker is in place), second- or third-degree heart block, and atrial arrhythmias associated with an accessory pathway.[36] They should not be used as first-line antihypertensive agents in patients with heart failure, patients after myocardial infarction, those with unstable angina, or blacks with proteinuria greater than 300 mg/day.[596] Conversely, CAs are indicated, and may be preferred, in patients with metabolic disorders such as diabetes, peripheral vascular disease, and stable ischemic heart disease. They may also be ideal agents for elderly hypertensive patients because they tend to lower the risk of stroke more than other classes.[626]

The CAs are generally well tolerated and are not associated with significant perturbations of glycemic balance or sexual dysfunction. The rapid antihypertensive action of CAs may encourage compliance. Orthostatic changes do not occur because venoconstriction remains intact. Side effects are usually transient and are the direct result of vasodilation. Hypotension is most common with intravenous administration. The most common side effect of the dihydropyridines is peripheral edema. It is dose related and thought to be the result of uncompensated precapillary vasodilation, causing increased intracapillary hydrostatic pressure. The edema is not responsive to diuretics but improves or resolves with the addition of an ACE inhibitor, which preferentially vasodilates postcapillary beds and reduces intracapillary hydrostatic pressure.[612] Other side effects related to vasodilation include headache, nausea, dizziness, and flushing, and occur three times more commonly in women.[627] The nondihydropyridines verapamil and isradipine more commonly cause constipation and nausea. The gastrointestinal effects are directly related to inhibition of calcium-dependent smooth muscle contraction: reduced peristalsis and relaxation of the lower esophageal sphincter.[628] Another common side effect of the dihydropyridines is gingival hyperplasia, which is exacerbated in patients taking concomitant cyclosporine.

Nifedipine, primarily, causes a gingival inflammatory B cell infiltrate stimulated by bacterial plaque and increased sulfated glycosaminoglycans, immunoglobulins, and folic acid, creating growth of the gingiva.[629] This can be controlled with regular periodontal treatment and reversed with discontinuation of the drug.[630]

The CAs are notable among antihypertensive agents because of their metabolic neutrality. Insofar as calcium influx across beta cell membranes helps to regulate insulin release, CAs might predispose to low insulin levels. Only in very high concentrations do CAs reduce insulin secretion.[631] At usual therapeutic levels, CAs have no effect on serum glucose, insulin secretion, or insulin sensitivity in nondiabetic and diabetic subjects.[632-634] They do not increase triglycerides or cholesterol and do not reduce HDL-cholesterol.[632] CAs do not precipitate hyponatremia, hyper- or hypokalemia, or hyperuricemia. Therefore, they are ideal agents for patients with dysmetabolic syndromes or diabetes. Initial trials indicated that CAs were more efficacious in blacks and elderly persons or those with low-renin hypertension. However, they have been demonstrated to be equally efficacious in young and old patients, black and white patients, diabetic patients, and obese patients.[635, 636] In elderly patients with hypertension or coronary artery disease, verapamil may cause more bradycardia than other agents, but second- or third-degree heart block is not seen.[623] In elderly patients receiving chronic ACE inhibitor therapy, the addition of verapamil can reverse ACE-induced increases in creatinine safely without further lowering blood pressure.[637] CAs are safe and effective in elderly patients with stage I isolated systolic hypertension and can reduce progression to higher stages of hypertension.[638] The latter may be a result of their ability to correct altered arteriole resistance structure and endothelial function.[639]

Properties beyond their antihypertensive actions make the CAs particularly useful in certain clinical situations. CAs not only lower arterial pressure but also have variable effects on cardiac function. All CAs are vasodilators and increase coronary blood flow.[640, 641] With the exception of the short-acting dihydropyridines, most CAs reduce heart rate, improve myocardial oxygen demand, improve ventricular filling, diminish ventricular arrhythmias, reduce myocardial ischemia, and conserve contractility,[642-645] making them ideal for patients with angina or diastolic dysfunction.[623] Acutely, they improve diastolic relaxation; administered chronically, they reduce left ventricular wall thickness[646, 647] and may prevent the development of hypertrophy.[648] This may be crucial in

TABLE 55-19

Hemodynamic Effects of Calcium Antagonists

	ARTERIOLAR DILATION	CORONARY DILATION	CARDIAC AFTERLOAD	CARDIAC CONTRACTILITY	MYOCARDIAL O$_2$ DEMAND	CARDIAC OUTPUT	AV CONDUCTION	SA AUTO-MATICITY	HEART RATE ACUTE/ CHRONIC	ACTIVATION OF BARORECEPTOR REFLEXES
Dihydropyridines	↑↑↑	↑↑↑	↓↓	↔	↓	↑↔	↔	↔	↑/↑	↑↔
Diltiazem	↑↑	↑↑↑	↓	↓	↓	↔	↓	↓↓	↓/↓↔	↔
Verapamil	↑↑	↑↑	↓	↓↓	↓	↔	↓↓	↓	↓/↓↔	↔

hypertensive patients insofar as LVH is one of the strongest blood pressure–independent predictors of cardiovascular morbidity and mortality.[649-651] Verapamil may also be used for secondary cardioprotection to reduce reinfarction rates in patients intolerant of β-blockers unless they have concomitant heart failure.[652, 653] The blood pressure–independent inhibition of atherogenesis by CAs may be another indication to use a CA, particularly in high-risk patients such as those with diabetes and ESRD.[514, 654]

In general, the antihypertensive effects of CAs are enhanced more in combination with β-blockers or ACE inhibitors than with diuretics. Perhaps this effect reflects the fact that CAs already have diuretic activity that cannot be further mobilized. In combination with ACE inhibitors, response rates approach 70% of those in patients with stage 1 to 3 hypertension.[655] It is theorized that this particular combination, particularly with dihydropyridines and an ACE inhibitor, maximizes pre- and postcapillary vasodilation to lower peripheral vascular resistance. The combined use of CAs with β-blockers is more problematic (Table 55-20). The combination of dihydropyridine CA with β-blockers is efficacious and even desirable in selected patients. The CAs have the potential to blunt the adverse effects associated with β-blockade, such as vasoconstriction, and the β-blockers have the ability to attenuate the increased sympathetic stimulation induced by CA vasoconstriction. Concomitant therapy with β-blockers and nondihydropyridine CAs is potentially more dangerous, as they may have additive effects on suppressing heart rate, AV node conduction, and cardiac contractility. This combination may be particularly dangerous in patients with ESRD.

Drug interactions are not uncommon (see Table 55-20). Concurrent use of a CA and amiodarone exacerbates sick sinus syndrome and AV block.[656] Diltiazem, verapamil, and nicardipine have been shown to increase cyclosporine, including the microemulsion formulation, tacrolimus, and sirolimus levels by 25% to 100% by inhibiting the cytochrome p4503A4

isoenzyme, which metabolizes the calcineurin inhibitors.[657] This interaction may be clinically useful to reduce the dosage and cost associated with cyclosporine or tacrolimus therapy. Frequent monitoring of calcineurin inhibitor levels is recommended. In contrast, nifedipine and isradipine have no effect on these concentrations and can be used safely. Diltiazem is a potent inhibitor of CYP3A4, which is responsible for metabolism of methylprednisolone. Coadministration of diltiazem and methylprednisolone resulted in a greater than 2.5-fold increase in the steroid blood level and enhanced adrenal suppressive responses.[658] Coadministration of diltiazem also increased nifedipine levels by 100% to 200%.[514, 659] This combination has additive antihypertensive efficacy and appears to be safe.[660] Concomitant administration of nifedipine, diltiazem, nicardipine, and verapamil with the digitalis glycosides resulted in up to a 50% increase in serum digoxin concentrations. This effect is the result of reduced renal clearance of digoxin and appears to be dose dependent.[661, 662]

Several issues regarding the inherent safety of CAs have come under scrutiny. CAs may be associated with an increased risk of gastrointestinal hemorrhage, particularly in elderly persons.[663] Diltiazem inhibits platelet aggregation in vitro, but the clinical relevance of this finding has not been substantiated.[664] Nonetheless, it is prudent to use caution when coadministering CAs with NSAIDs, as NSAIDs may exacerbate the risk of bleeding and may antagonize the antihypertensive effects of CAs.[665-667] A similar concern regarding the possible relationship between CAs and cancer has not been substantiated.[668] The safety of CAs in treating cardiovascular diseases remains controversial. There is clear evidence that CAs reduce cardiovascular mortality and morbidity, particularly stroke; however, short-acting agents such as nifedipine have been associated with a small increased risk for myocardial infarction in meta-analyses[457, 669] when compared with other agents. It is speculated that the disadvantageous activation of the renin-angiotensin and sympathetic nervous

TABLE 55-20

Drug-Drug Interactions with Calcium Antagonists

CALCIUM ANTAGONIST	INTERACTING DRUG	RESULT
Verapamil	Digoxin	↑ Digoxin levels by 50%–90%
Diltiazem	Digozin	↑ Digoxin level by 40%
Verapamil	β-Blockers	↑ AV nodal blockade, hypotension, bradycardia, asystole
Verapamil, diltiazem	Cyclosporine/tacrolimus and sirolimus	↑Cyclosporine levels by 25%–100%
Verapamil, diltiazem	Cimetidine	↑Verapamil and diltiazem levels by decreased metabolism
Verapamil	Rifampin/phenytoin	↓ Verapamil levels by enzyme induction
Dihydropyridines	Amiodarone	Exacerbate sick sinus syndrome and AV nodal blockade
Dihydropyridines	α-Blockers	Excessive hypotension
Dihydropyridines	Propranolol	Increased propranolol levels
Dihydropyridines	Cimetidine	Increased area under the curve and plasma levels of calcium antagonist
Nicardipine	Cyclosporine	↑ Cyclosporine levels by 40%–50%
Amlodipine	Cyclosporine	↑ Cyclosporine levels by 10%
Felodipine	Flavinoids	↑ Bioavailability by 50%
Diltiazem	Methylprednisone	↑ Methylprednisone 0.5-fold
Nifedipine	Diltiazem	↑ Nifedipine levels 100%–200%

TABLE 55-21

Receptor Binding of Centrally Acting Antihypertensives

DRUG	RECEPTOR
Clonidine	$\alpha_2 + I_1$
α-Methyldopa	α_2
Guanabenz	α_2
Guanfacine	α_2
Rilmenidine	$I_1 > \alpha_2$
Moxonidine	$I_1 > \alpha_2$

α_2, α_2-adrenergic receptor; I_1, imidazole receptor.

system induced by the short-acting agents may predispose to myocardial ischemia. Currently, there is no evidence to prove the existence of either additional beneficial or detrimental effects of CAs on coronary disease events, including fatal or nonfatal myocardial infarctions and other deaths from coronary heart disease. Because of a potential risk, however, as well as simplicity and improved compliance, longer acting agents should be considered over short-acting CAs for the treatment of hypertension.[670]

Central Adrenergic Agonists
Mechanisms of Action

Central adrenergic agonists act by crossing the blood-brain barrier and have a direct effect on α_2-adrenergic receptors located in the midbrain and brainstem.[671-677] Binding to the more recently described imidazole (I_1 subtype) receptors within the brain may also play a role in the inhibition of central sympathetic output.[676-684] Drugs in this class may bind to either the α-adrenergic receptors or the imidazole receptors with some degree of specificity, or they may bind to both receptors (Table 55-21). The side effect profile of a specific agent may be related to the specificity of its binding. In addition to decreasing total sympathetic outflow, binding to these receptors results in increases in vagal activity. Vasodepressor barrier reflexes are also enhanced. A reduction in catecholamine release and turnover as evidenced by decreased biochemical markers of noradrenergic activity such

as plasma norepinephrine levels correlated with the magnitude of blood pressure decreases.[685-691]

Clonidine is a stimulant of both α-adrenergic receptors and imidazole receptors. More selective imidazole receptor stimulants such as moxonidine and rilmenidine activate the I_1 receptors. Stimulation of both the α_2 and I_1 receptors in the central nervous system reduces activity of the sympathetic nervous system. Stimulation of both receptors is probably mediated through the same neuronal pathways.[684] The classical α_2-receptor agonists such as clonidine and α-methyldopa (acting through its active metabolite α-methylnoradrenaline) results in vasodilatation in the resistance vessels and hence a reduction in peripheral vascular resistance. As a result, blood pressure is reduced. In spite of the vasodilator action, reflex tachycardia generally does not occur; this is probably the result of peripheral sympathetic inhibition.

Studies have shown that the selective I_1 receptor agonists moxonidine and rilmenidine are predominantly arterial vasodilators, resulting in a reduction in peripheral vascular resistance.[680, 681] The effects of these drugs are also caused by inhibition of the sympathetic outflow, resulting in lowering of plasma noradrenaline levels. Moxonidine is associated with the reduction in plasma renin activity. The central α_2-adrenergic agonists may also stimulate peripheral α_2-adrenergic receptors. This effect predominates at high drug concentrations. These receptors mediate vasoconstriction, and this may result in a paradoxical increase in blood pressure.[673-675] Overall, these drugs generally result in a decrease in peripheral vascular resistance, a slowing of heart rate, and either no change or a mild decrease in cardiac output.[692-697] Orthostatic hypotension is generally not a feature of these drugs. The pharmacokinetic and pharmacodynamic properties of these drugs are shown in Tables 55-22 and 55-23.

Class Members

Methyldopa is a methyl-substituted amino acid that is active after conversion to an active metabolite.[675, 691, 698, 699] This active metabolite, α-methylnorepinephrine, accumulates in the central nervous system and is selective for α_2-adrenergic receptors. The initial dose of methyldopa in hypertension is 250 mg two to three times daily. It may be increased at intervals of not less than 2 days until a therapeutic response is achieved. The usual maintenance dose is 500 mg to 2 g in

TABLE 55-22

Pharmacokinetic Properties of Central Adrenergic Agonists

DRUG	BIOAVAILABILITY (%)	AFFECTED BY FOOD	PEAK BLOOD LEVEL (H)	ELIMINATION HALF-LIFE (H)	METABOLISM	EXCRETION*	ACTIVE METABOLITES
Clonidine	50	—	—	7-16	L	F (30-50) U (24)	Methyldopa-o-sulfite
α-Methyldopa	65-96	—	1.5-5	6-23	L	F (22) U (65)	—
Guanabenz	75	—	2-5	7-10	L	F (16) U (40-75)	—
Guanfacine	80	—	1.4	17	L	U (90)	—
Rilmenidine	80-90	No	0.5	2-3	L	U (90)	—
Moxonidine	100	No	2	5.5	L	U (90)	—

*Excretion values in parentheses represent percentages.

F, feces; L, liver; U, urine.

TABLE 55-23

Pharmacodynamic Properties of Central Adrenergic Agonists

DRUG	INITIAL DOSE (MG)	USUAL DOSE (MG)	MAXIMUM DOSE (MG)	INTERVAL	PEAK RESPONSE (H)	DURATION OF RESPONSE (H)
α-Methyldopa	250	250-300	3000	bid-qid	3-6	24-48
Clonidine	0.1	0.2-0.6	1.2	bid	2-4	6-10
Guanabenz	4	16-32	96	bid	2-4	6-8
Guanfacine	1	1-3	6	qd-bid	6	24
Moxonidine	0.2-0.3	0.2-0.4	0.6	bid	1.5-4	48-72
Rilmenidine	1	1-2	—	qd-bid	1-2	10-12

2 to 4 doses. Maximum recommended daily dose is 3 g. Initial response occurs within 3 to 6 hours after a dose. Peak response is at 6 to 9 hours. Bioavailability is 25% to 50%. The drug is approximately 50% metabolized by the liver. Drug half-life is increased in renal failure. Excretion in the urine is largely in the form of an inactive metabolite. The dosing interval should be increased to every 12 to 24 hours in patients with severe renal failure. Approximately 60% of methyldopa is removed with hemodialysis. A supplemental dose is recommended after a dialysis treatment.

Clonidine is a central-acting α-adrenergic agonist.[675, 678, 679, 700-702] The usual oral dose is 0.1 mg twice daily adjusted as necessary in 0.1- to 0.2-mg increments. Usual maintenance dose is 0.2 to 0.6 mg once daily in two divided doses. Total doses above 1.2 mg daily are usually not associated with a greater effect. Beyond selectivity the onset of activity is 30 to 60 minutes after an oral dose. Peak antihypertensive activity occurs within 2 to 4 hours. The duration of the antihypertensive effect is 6 to 10 hours. Oral bioavailability ranges from 65% to 96%. The half-life of the absorbed drug is 6 to 23 hours. Hepatic metabolism to inactive metabolites is followed by renal excretion. Transdermal patches are available and may be applied on a once-weekly basis. The drug half-life with the transdermal patch is approximately 20 hours after removal of the patch. With a transdermal patch, steady-state drug levels are reached within approximately 3 days. Dosage adjustment is not needed for patients with any degree of renal dysfunction including severe renal failure. Approximately 5% of clonidine body stores are removed after a 5-hour dialysis treatment.

Guanabenz is an orally active central α₂-adrenergic agonist.[675, 703-705] The usual starting dose for treatment of hypertension is 4 mg twice daily. Dosages may be increased to 4 to 8 mg/day at 1- to 2-week intervals. Doses as high as 96 mg/day have been used. Bioavailability is approximately 75%. The usual onset of antihypertensive activity occurs within 60 minutes and the activity lasts approximately 10 to 12 hours. The drug is highly protein bound and extensively metabolized. Less than 1% of unchanged drug is excreted in urine. The half-life of the drug is 7 to 10 hours. Dose adjustment in renal failure is not necessary. It appears that dose reductions may be necessary in patients with severe hepatic insufficiency. Because of extensive protein binding, drug removal by dialysis or peritoneal dialysis is minimal.

Guanfacine is a centrally acting antihypertensive drug with actions similar to those of clonidine.[675, 706-711] Effective doses are 1 to 3 mg daily. Oral bioavailability is approximately

80%. Peak levels are noted between 1 and 4 hours. The drug half-life is approximately 17 hours. The drug is 70% protein bound. The drug is metabolized in the liver, with renal excretion of 40% to 75% as unchanged drug. Limited data are available on dosing in renal failure; however, dosage adjustments do not appear warranted. Nonrenal elimination of the drug is believed to be important in patients with renal failure. It is unclear whether dosing adjustments are required in patients with significant liver disease.

Moxonidine is a central imidazole I_1 and α₂-receptor agonist.[679, 712, 713] Oral bioavailability is reported to be 89%. Serum concentration peaks are reached within 30 to 180 minutes. Ninety percent of the dose is excreted through the urine within 24 hours. Fifty percent of this is as unchanged drug. The average half-life is 2.2 to 2.3 hours. For the treatment of hypertension the starting dose is 0.2 to 0.4 mg/day. The dose may be increased after several weeks to 0.2 to 0.3 mg twice daily. The maximum daily dose is 0.6 mg. Moxonidine has 600-fold greater selectivity at the imidazole receptor compared with the α₂-receptor. This results in fewer central side effects such as dry mouth and sedation compared with those of clonidine. Drug clearance is delayed in renal impairment. Single doses of 0.2 mg and a maximum daily dose of 0.4 mg should not be exceeded.

Rilmenidine is a centrally acting imidazole receptor and α₂-adrenergic receptor agonist.[679, 682, 714-718] Rilmenidine appears to bind preferentially to central imidazole I_1 receptors in the brainstem. At higher doses, rilmenidine can bind and activate central α₂-adrenergic receptors. The relative affinity of binding of rilmenidine to imidazole receptors in comparison with α₂-adrenergic receptors is 2.5 times higher than that of clonidine. Antihypertensive effects occur within 1 hour after a single 1-mg dose. The duration of action is 10 to 12 hours. Peak concentration after oral dosing is at approximately 2 hours. Steady-state plasma levels are reached by day 3. Rilmenidine is eliminated primarily unchanged in the urine. In chronic renal failure, clearance of the drug is decreased. The usual oral dose is 1 mg once or twice daily. Dose reductions are required for patients with renal dysfunction. Patients with advanced renal disease should have the dose decreased to 1 mg every other day. Dose adjustments for patients with hepatic insufficiency are probably not needed.

Renal Effects of Central α₂-Adrenergic Agonists

Central α₂-agonists and imidazole I_1 agonists have little if any clinically important effect on renal plasma flow or GFR in hypertensive patients.[719] The central adrenergic agonists also have little effect on the renin-angiotensin-aldosterone axis. Moxonidine has been reported to both decrease and increase plasma renin activity. It has no significant effect on epinephrine levels, AII levels, aldosterone levels, or atrial natriuretic peptide levels. Similarly, other adrenergic agonists with the possible exception of guanfacine do not have effects on the RAS. The fractional excretion of sodium is unchanged. Body fluid composition and weight are not altered. A water diuresis may be associated with guanabenz, through inhibition of central release of vasopressin or altered renal responsiveness to vasopressin.[720-722] These agents may result in decreased renal vascular resistance mediated by a decrease in preglomerular capillary resistance related to decreased levels of circulating catecholamines. Some dosage adjustment is required for patients with renal disease (see Table 55-6).

Antihypertensive Efficacy and Safety

The antihypertensive efficacy of clonidine and α-methyldopa has been confirmed in large numbers of patients and analyzed in clinical trials. Similarly, the antihypertensive efficacy of moxonidine and rilmenidine has been demonstrated in large numbers of hypertensive patients. These agents have been shown to be effective monotherapy for hypertension.[675, 692-695, 723-732] Additive effects are associated with addition of a diuretic.[723-727] They have been shown to be effective in both young and old patients, and the effects do not differ in racial groups.[729, 733-736] There are no significant effects on carbohydrate tolerance.[480, 675, 697, 737, 738]

The central α$_2$-adrenergic agonists appear to be neutral with respect to lipid metabolism. There may be a decrease in total cholesterol, LDL, and HDL. These agents may also be of benefit in patients with congestive heart failure. Congestive heart failure is associated with activation of neurohumoral and neuroendocrine compensatory mechanisms that may be unfavorable.[739] Central α$_2$-adrenergic agonists may play a role in abrogation of these factors.[739-741] This may include activation of the sympathetic nervous system as well as the RAAS. Treatment with rilmenidine has been shown to reverse LVH and improve arterial compliance. This effect was associated with a reduction in plasma atrial natriuretic peptide levels. Stimulation of α$_2$-adrenergic receptors in the central nervous system induces several side effects of these drugs including sedation and drowsiness. The most common side effect related to α$_2$-adrenergic activation is dry mouth related to a decrease in salivary flow. This is due to a centrally mediated inhibition of cholinergic transmission. Clonidine in high doses may precipitate a paradoxical hypertensive response related to stimulation of postsynaptic vascular α$_2$-adrenergic receptors.[671-673, 675] Methyldopa has been associated with a positive direct Coombs test with or without hemolytic anemia.[675, 742, 743] The α$_2$-adrenergic agonists are associated with sexual dysfunction and may produce gynecomastia in men and galactorrhea in both men and women.[743]

Abrupt cessation of α$_2$-adrenergic blockers may result in rebound hypertension. This occurs 18 to 36 hours after cessation of short-acting agents.[673, 697, 744-751] Patients may have tachycardia, tremor, anxiety, headache, nausea, and vomiting. This syndrome may be related to down-regulation of the α$_2$-adrenergic receptors in the central nervous system associated with chronic therapy. Concurrent use of β-adrenergic blockers may amplify this syndrome. The agents that have specificity for the I$_2$ receptor appear to have significantly fewer central nervous system effects such as dry mouth and drowsiness. These effects may be mediated by α$_2$ stimulation. Rebound hypertension secondary to abrupt withdrawal has not been associated with moxonidine or rilmenidine.

Central and Peripheral Adrenergic Neuronal Blocking Agents
Mechanisms of Action and Class Member

Reserpine, a rauwolfia alkaloid, reduces blood pressure by lowering the activity of central and peripheral noradrenergic neurons. Reserpine blocks noradrenaline and dopamine uptake into storage granules of noradrenergic neurons. The result is noradrenaline depletion.[752] A similar effect is seen in central dopaminergic and serotoninergic neurons. In doses currently used for hypertension, the major effect of reserpine is in the central nervous system. Reserpine results in a rapid reduction in cardiac output, heart rate, and peripheral vascular resistance. Enhanced vagal activity may be involved as well. Tolerance to the antihypertensive effects of reserpine does not occur.

Reserpine is used in initial doses of 0.1 to 0.25 mg daily.[753-756] Approximately 40% of an oral dose is absorbed. The half-life is 50 to 100 hours. Extensive hepatic metabolism occurs; 1% is recovered as unchanged compound in the urine. Maximal clinical effect is observed 2 to 3 weeks after initiation of therapy. No dosage adjustment is necessary for patients with renal insufficiency. Dosage supplementation is not required after hemodialysis.

Renal Effects

GFR and renal plasma flow are not affected by reserpine therapy. Renal vascular resistance may be reduced, perhaps mediated through decreased sympathetic stimulation of vascular α-adrenergic receptors.[353, 719] Significant effects on the RAAS have not been observed. Renal handling of sodium and potassium is unchanged.

Efficacy and Safety

Reserpine has been shown to be effective therapy as a single agent or in combination with HCTZ.[755-761] This has been observed in numerous large and small trials including the Veterans Administration Cooperative Study, the Hypertension Detection and Follow-up Program, and the Multiple Risk Factor Intervention Trial. The antihypertensive action has compared favorably in many studies with that of methyldopa. Reserpine used in combination with a diuretic has shown comparable efficacy to combinations of β-blockers and diuretics. In these studies, the dose of reserpine was between 0.1 and 0.3 mg daily. This is many times lower than the doses used in the 1960s that led to a reputation of a poor side effect profile. The most common side effect of reserpine is nasal congestion, which is reported in 6% to 20% of patients. Unlike other side effects, it does not appear to decrease with lower doses of drug, and it is felt to be related to cholinergic effects of the drug.[742, 743, 762] Increased gastric motility and gastric acid secretion can occur; however, the incidence of dyspepsia or peptic ulcer disease with reserpine is not greater than that with other antihypertensive drug treatments. Inability to concentrate, sedation, sleep disturbance, and depression have been reported.[742, 743, 762, 763] Other side effects include weight gain, increased appetite, and sexual dysfunction.[473, 474, 742, 743, 762, 763]

Direct-Acting Vasodilators
Mechanisms of Action

The direct-acting vasodilators reduce systolic and diastolic blood pressure by decreasing peripheral vascular resistance. The drugs act directly on vascular smooth muscle with selective vasodilatation of the arteriolar resistance vessels and have little or no effect on the venous capacitance vessels.[764-769] There is no effect on the functioning of carotid or aortic baroreceptors. The vasodilating effects have thought to involve inhibition of calcium uptake to the cells. Decreases in arterial pressure are associated with a fall in peripheral resistance and a reflex increase in cardiac output. Sodium and water retention is promoted secondary to the stimulation of renin release and possibly by direct effects on renal tubules. The arteriolar dilatation produced by these drugs causes a decrease in cardiac afterload, and the absence of venodilation leads to an increase in venous return to the heart, producing an elevated preload. These combined effects result in increased cardiac output. The pharmacokinetic and pharmacodynamic properties of these drugs are shown in Tables 55-24 and 55-25.

Class Members

Hydralazine is a direct-acting arteriole vasodilator.[770-772] Initial oral doses in hypertension should be 10 mg four times daily increasing to 50 mg four times daily over several weeks. Patients may require doses of up to 300 mg/day. Dosing can be changed to twice daily for maintenance. The drug may also be used as an intravenous bolus injection or as a continuous infusion. Oral absorption is 50% to 90% of the dose. The drug is up 90% protein bound. The elimination half-life is 1.5 to 8 hours and varies with acetylation rate in the liver. Both slow and fast acetylators have been described. Onset of action is approximately 1 hour. Patients with mild to moderate renal insufficiency should have the dosing interval increased to every 8 hours. In severe renal failure, the dose interval should increase to every 8 to 24 hours. No dosage supplement is required following hemodialysis or peritoneal dialysis (see Table 55-6).

Minoxidil is a direct vasodilator.[773-777] It is more potent than hydralazine and induces a more marked activation of adrenergic drive. For severe hypertension the initial recommended dose is 5 mg as a single daily dose, increasing to 10 to 20 or 40 mg in single or divided doses. Minoxidil is usually used in conjunction with salt restriction and diuretics to prevent fluid retention. Concomitant therapy with a β-adrenergic blocking agent is often required to control tachycardia related to minoxidil use. Onset of the antihypertensive effect occurs within 30 to 60 minutes. Peak response is at 4 to 8 hours. The drug is 90% metabolized by the liver. The glucuronide metabolite has reduced pharmacologic effects but does accumulate in patients with ESRD. Renal excretion is 90%. Dosage adjustments may be required in patients with renal failure, although the mean daily doses required to control blood pressure have been reported to be similar in patients with normal renal function and those with renal failure (see Table 55-6).

Renal Effects of Direct-Acting Vasodilators

Hydralazine and minoxidil both increase secretion of renin as a result of enhanced synthetic stimulation of the juxtaglomerular cells in the kidney.[353] This is associated with

TABLE 55-24

Pharmacokinetic Properties of Direct-Acting Vasodilators

DRUG	BIOAVAILABILITY (%)	AFFECTED BY FOOD	PEAK BLOOD LEVEL (H)	ELIMINATION HALF-LIFE (H)	METABOLISM	EXCRETION*	ACTIVE METABOLITES
Hydralazine	20-50	No	1-2	1.5-8	L	U (3-14) F (3-12)	—
Minoxidil	90-100	—	1	4.2	L	U (90) F (3)	Glucuronide

*Excretion values in parentheses represent percentages.
F, feces; L, liver; U, urine.

TABLE 55-25

Pharmacodynamic Properties of Direct-Acting Vasodilators

DRUG	INITIAL DOSE (MG)	USUAL DOSE (MG)	MAXIMUM DOSE (MG)	INTERVAL	PEAK RESPONSE (H)	DURATION OF RESPONSE (H)
Hydralazine	10	200-400	400	bid-qid	1	3-8
Minoxidil	2.5	10-20	40	qd-qid	4-8	10-12

elevations of AII and aldosterone.[778] Chronic use is associated with return of plasma aldosterone levels to baseline.[779, 780] Retention of salt and water may be due to direct drug effects on the proximal convoluted tubule. Renal vascular resistance is decreased in relation to relaxation of resistance vessels. GFR and renal plasma flow are preserved.

Efficacy and Safety

Although minoxidil has been used to treat mild to moderate hypertension, it is commonly reserved for severe or intractable hypertension.[781] When added to a diuretic and a β-blocker, minoxidil is generally well tolerated. Hypertrichosis is common. Pericarditis and pericardial infusions have been described.[742, 782, 783] An increase in left ventricular mass has been reported. This may be due to adrenergic hyperactivity. Similar findings have been observed with hydralazine. Apart from adrenergic activation and fluid retention, chronic treatment with hydralazine has been associated with the development of systemic lupus erythematosus.[784-789] Generally, the syndrome occurs early in therapy, but it can occur after many years of treatment. A positive antinuclear antibody titer is used to confirm a clinical diagnosis of lupus. It has been estimated that between 6% and 10% of patients receiving doses of hydralazine of 400 mg/day or higher for more than 6 months develop hydralazine-induced lupus. It occurs most frequently in women and rarely in blacks. This syndrome occurs primarily in slow acetylators. The syndrome is reversible when hydralazine is discontinued but may require months for complete clearing of symptoms.

Moderately Selective Peripheral α₁-Adrenergic Antagonists
Mechanisms of Action

The nonselective agents phentolamine and phenoxybenzamine have an occasional role in hypertension management. Phentolamine is utilized parenterally, and the longer acting agent phenoxybenzamine has been used orally for the management of hypertension associated with pheochromocytoma. Phenoxybenzamine is a moderately selective peripheral α₁-adrenergic antagonist.[790] Its specificity for the α₁-adrenergic receptor is 100 times greater than that for the α₂-adrenergic receptor. Nonspecific α₁-adrenergic receptor antagonists are no longer used in the treatment of essential hypertension.

Class Members

Phenoxybenzamine is a long-acting α-adrenergic blocking agent.[790-793] This agent irreversibly and covalently binds to the α-receptors only. β-Receptors and the parasympathetic system are not affected by phenoxybenzamine. Total peripheral resistance is lower than cardiac output and is increased by phenoxybenzamine. Phenoxybenzamine is also believed to inhibit the uptake of catecholamines into both adrenergic nerve terminals and extraneural tissues. The usual oral dose of phenoxybenzamine for pheochromocytoma is 10 mg twice daily, gradually increasing every other day to doses ranging between 20 and 40 mg two or three times a day. The final dose should be determined by blood pressure response. Phenoxybenzamine may be administered with a β-blocking

agent if tachycardia becomes excessive during therapy. The pressor effects of a pheochromocytoma must be controlled by α-blockade before β-blockers are initiated. With oral use the pheochromocytoma symptoms are decreased after several days. Oral bioavailability is 20% to 30%. The drug is extensively metabolized by the liver. Administration of phenoxybenzamine to patients with renal impairment should be done cautiously. Specific dosage recommendations are not available.

Phentolamine is an α-adrenergic blocking agent that produces peripheral vasodilatation in cardiac stimulation with a resulting fall in blood pressure in most patients. The drug is used parenterally. The usual dose is 5 mg repeated as needed. The onset of activity with intravenous dosing is immediate. Drug is not absorbed well orally. Half-life is 19 minutes. The drug is metabolized by the liver with 10% excreted in the urine as unchanged drug.

Renal Effects

Phenoxybenzamine has no clear effect on the renin-angiotensin-aldosterone axis.[353, 794] Blood volume and body weight are not altered. Salt and water retention does not occur. GFR and effective renal plasma flow would be expected to increase. Renal vascular resistance probably decreases in proportion to the degree of blockade of α-adrenergic receptors.

Efficacy and Safety

Phenoxybenzamine is used primarily as an agent to counteract the excessive α-adrenergic tone associated with pheochromocytoma.[791-793] Tachycardia may result from α-adrenergic blockade, which unmasks β-adrenergic effects with epinephrine-secreting tumors. This may be controlled with concurrent use of a β-adrenergic antagonist. α-Adrenergic blockade must be initiated prior to β-adrenergic blockade to avoid paradoxical hypertension. Side effects of phenoxybenzamine are sedation, weakness, nasal congestion, hypertension, and tachycardia.

Peripheral α₁-Adrenergic Antagonists
Mechanisms of Action

Drugs of this class are selective for the postsynaptic α₁-adrenergic receptor.[671, 795-801] The affinity of these drugs for the α₂-receptor is very low. The initial studies with these drugs suggested that there might be a direct vasodilator action on vascular smooth muscle; however, subsequent studies demonstrated that the sympatholytic activity alone was responsible for the antihypertensive effects.[671] Because of the selective α₁ action, there is no interference with the negative feedback control mechanisms mediated by the prejunctional α₂-receptors. As a result, the reflex tachycardia associated with blockade of the presynaptic α₂-receptor is decreased substantially.[794, 802-804] With these drugs, the increases in arteriolar and venous tone mediated by norepinephrine released from sympathetic nerve terminals and acting at the α₁-adrenergic receptor located postjunctionally in the blood vessel wall are blunted. The pharmacokinetic and pharmacodynamic properties of these drugs are shown in Tables 55-26 and 55-27.

TABLE 55-26

Pharmacokinetic Properties of Peripheral α₁-Adrenergic Antagonists

DRUG	BIOAVAILABILITY (%)	AFFECTED BY FOOD	PEAK BLOOD LEVEL (H)	ELIMINATION HALF-LIFE (H)	METABOLISM	EXCRETION*	ACTIVE METABOLITES
Doxazosin	62-69	No	2-5	9-22	L	F (63-65) U (1-9)	—
Prazosin	—	No	1-3	2-4	L	F	—
Terazosin	90	Yes	1	12	L	F (55-60) U (10)	—

*Excretion values in parentheses represent percentages.
F, feces; L, liver; U, urine.

TABLE 55-27

Pharmacodynamic Properties of Peripheral α₁-Adrenergic Antagonists

DRUG	INITIAL DOSE (MG)	USUAL DOSE (MG)	MAXIMUM DOSE (MG)	INTERVAL	PEAK RESPONSE (H)	DURATION OF RESPONSE (H)
Doxazosin	1	8	16	qd-qid	4-8	24
Prazosin	1	6-15	20	bid-qid	½-1½	10
Terazosin	1	5	20	qd-bid	3	24

Class Members

Doxazosin is a selective long-acting α₁-adrenergic antagonist.[805, 806] Its structure is similar to that of prazosin and terazosin. The initial antihypertensive dose is 1 mg daily. This can be titrated up to a maximum of 16 mg daily. The drug is between 60% and 70% absorbed. Maximal antihypertensive effect is seen 4 to 8 hours after a single dose. The drug is highly plasma protein bound and extensively metabolized. The majority of the administered dose is excreted in the feces. The estimated half-life is from 9 to 22 hours. Doxazosin pharmacokinetics are not altered in patients with renal impairment. The drug should be used with caution in patients with advanced liver dysfunction.

Prazosin is a selective α₁-adrenergic antagonist structurally related to doxazosin and terazosin.[801, 807-809] Oral dosing is 3 to 20 mg/day. A first-dose phenomenon with postural hypertension resulting in palpitations, tachycardia, and potentially syncope has been associated with prazosin. This can be minimized by limiting the initial dose to 1 mg at bedtime. Full therapeutic effects are seen within 4 to 8 weeks after initiation of therapy. Peak serum levels are reached 1 to 3 hours after an oral dose. The drug is 97% protein bound. The elimination half-life is 2 to 4 hours. There is extensive hepatic metabolism followed by renal excretion of a very small amount of unchanged drug. Dosage adjustment is not required for patients with renal failure. Patients with significant liver disease may require a dose adjustment and more frequent monitoring.

Terazosin is a selective long-acting α₁-adrenergic antagonist. It has structural similarities to prazosin and doxazosin.[810-812] The initial dose is 1 mg orally at bedtime with titration to 5 mg daily. Doses of 10 to 20 mg orally have been given. Peak serum levels following oral administration occur within 1 hour. The half-life is approximately 12 hours.

Terazosin is extensively metabolized in the liver and eliminated primarily through the biliary tract. Renal insufficiency does not affect the pharmacokinetics of terazosin and dosage adjustment is not required. Patients with severe hepatic insufficiency may require dosage adjustments.

Renal Effects

GFR and renal blood flow are maintained during long-term treatment with prazosin.[719] In some studies there was a slight increase in renal blood flow. Renal vascular resistance may be reduced, perhaps mediated by a reduction in preglomerular capillary resistance related to inhibition of α₁-mediated vasoconstriction. Urinary protein excretion has been reported to be reduced. The RAAS is not significantly affected by specific α₁-adrenergic antagonists.[353, 719] The extracellular fluid volume has been reported to be increased, and the fractional excretion may be decreased. Doxazosin has been reported to enhance renin release at rest but does not modify the renin response to exercise. No dosage adjustment is necessary in patients with renal disease.

Efficacy and Safety

Comparative clinical studies of the efficacy of α₁-adrenergic blockers have shown that the antihypertensive responses are similar to those of other antihypertensives.[437, 798-800, 813-820] This conventional viewpoint has come under criticism with results of a large study in which patients receiving doxazosin as their initial antihypertensive drugs were found to have poorer blood pressure control than those receiving a chlorthalidone-based treatment.[821] In this study, patients receiving doxazosin had no difference in the primary outcomes of fatal coronary heart disease or nonfatal myocardial infarction but did have higher rates of stroke and congestive heart failure.[822] Prazosin treatment has been shown to increase insulin sensitivity. There is, however, no significant clinical difference in carbohydrate tolerance.[479] There are potentially beneficial effects of α_1-blockers on lipid metabolism.[437, 481, 823, 824] These drugs have been consistently shown to result in a modest reduction in total and LDL-cholesterol and a small increase in HDL-cholesterol. This metabolic benefit may be linked to the beneficial effect on insulin responsiveness leading to increased peripheral glucose uptake.

Use of α-blockers has been associated with regression of LVH. Whether this is a result of effective blood pressure reduction or a specific pharmacologic property of these drugs remains to be established. The most important side effect of α_1-adrenergic receptor blockers is the first-dose effect.[742, 799, 800, 825-828] This is a result of orthostatic hypotension resulting in lightheadedness, palpitations, and occasional syncope. It is related to the drug effect on the venous capacitance vessels resulting in venous dilatation and inadequate venous return. It may occur with peak drug levels 30 to 90 minutes after the first dose. It can be minimized by initiating therapy with a small dose taken at bedtime. This effect can be exacerbated in patients with underlying autonomic insufficiency. α_1-Adrenergic antagonists are also used for symptomatic treatment of prostatic hypertrophy. Prostatic smooth muscle has significant α_1-adrenal receptors. Blockade of these receptors results in smooth muscle relaxation within the prostate.[800, 829, 830]

The nonselective agents phentolamine and phenoxybenzamine have an occasional role in hypertension management. Phentolamine is utilized parenterally and the longer acting agent phenoxybenzamine has been used orally for the management of hypertension associated with pheochromocytoma. Phenoxybenzamine is a moderately selective peripheral α_1-adrenergic antagonist.[790] Its specificity for the α_1-adrenergic receptor is 100 times greater than that for the α_2-adrenergic receptor. Nonspecific α_1-adrenergic receptor antagonists are no longer used in the treatment of essential hypertension.

Selective Aldosterone Receptor Antagonists
Class Mechanism and Class Member

Potassium-sparing diuretics are discussed in the previous chapter, including spironolactone, a nonselective aldosterone receptor antagonist. However, eplerenone is a selective aldosterone receptor antagonist that is the first in its class to be evaluated for its antihypertensive and cytoprotective properties. It may have antihypertensive effects distinct from its diuretic properties.

Eplerenone is a 9α, 11α epoxy derivative of spironolactone, which is currently undergoing late-stage clinical testing in the treatment of hypertension, heart failure, and myocardial infarction. It is approximately 24 times less potent in blocking mineralocorticoid receptors than spironolactone. However, it is substantially more selective than spironolactone and has little agonist activity for estrogen and progesterone receptors.[831-833] Therefore, it is associated with a lower incidence of gynecomastia, breast pain, and impotence in men and diminished libido and menstrual irregularities in women. Time to peak concentration is 1 to 2 hours. No

significant accumulation occurs with multiple-dose administration. It appears well absorbed, but absolute (oral versus intravenous) data are not available. Specific data on protein binding and metabolism are unavailable. Its elimination half-life is 3.5 to 5.0 hours.

The mineralocorticoid receptor forms part of the steroid/thyroid/retinoid/orphan-receptor family of nuclear transactivating factors.[834] When unbound, these receptors are in an inactive multiprotein complex of chaperones. Upon binding aldosterone, the chaperones are released and the receptor hormone complex is translocated into the nucleus, where it binds to hormone response elements on DNA and interacts with transcription initiation complexes, which ultimately modulates gene expression.[835] In the kidney, mineralocorticoid receptors are located primarily in the epithelial cells of the distal nephron. These receptors bind physiologic glucocorticoids and mineralocorticoids with similar affinity. Activation of mineralocorticoid receptors by aldosterone results in activation of epithelial sodium channels, which leads to a rapid increase in sodium and water reabsorption and promotes the tubule secretion of potassium.[836, 837] A persistent increase in sodium balance does not occur despite continued stimulation of mineralocorticoid receptor by aldosterone.[837] The mechanism of this escape phenomenon has not been fully elucidated.

There is evidence that indicates the presence of biologic activity of mineralocorticoid receptors in nonepithelial tissues.[838] These receptors have been identified in blood vessels of the heart and the brain and may be involved in vascular injury and repair responses.[839-841] It has been reported that aldosterone mediates fibrosis and collagen formation through up-regulation of AII receptor responsiveness.[838] Aldosterone increases sodium influx in vascular smooth muscle and inhibits norepinephrine uptake in vascular smooth muscle and myocardial cells.[842, 843] It also directly participates in vascular smooth muscle cell hypertrophy. Consequently, clinical trials have been started to validate the hypothesis that aldosterone receptor antagonism may inhibit vascular, myocardial, and renal injury.

Class Renal Effects

Selective aldosterone receptor antagonism may have benefits for the kidney independent of its effects on blood pressure. Both experimental and clinical studies have demonstrated that AII is probably the primary mediator of the RAAS that is associated with progression of renal disease.[844-846] The relative importance of aldosterone within this cascade has been the subject of experimental and clinical studies. Hyperaldosteronism and adrenal hypertrophy are common observations in remnant kidney models and correlate with progressive loss of renal function.[847] Investigators demonstrated that hypertension, proteinuria, and structural injury were less prevalent in the subtotally nephrectomized rats that underwent adrenalectomy despite large doses of replacement glucocorticoids.[848] Other investigators have demonstrated that aldosterone infusion could reverse the renal protective effects of the ACE inhibitor in stroke-prone spontaneously hypertensive rats.[849] Interestingly, in this model, the renal injury induced by aldosterone was independent of blood pressure increases, suggesting a toxic tissue effect of aldosterone. Other experimental studies indicated that aldosterone receptor antagonism can prevent the development of proteinuria.[850]

Despite having no observable effects on glomerular hemodynamics, selective aldosterone receptor antagonism therapy may provide an incremental opportunity to protect the kidney in addition to ACE inhibitor or AII receptor blocker therapy by inhibiting the effects of aldosterone that persist despite therapy with these drugs.

Class Efficacy and Safety

Eplerenone lowers blood pressure in a dose-dependent fashion when administered at 25, 50 or 200 mg twice daily.[851] Changes in blood pressure were greater with twice-daily dosing (50 mg twice a day = −11.7 mm Hg systolic reduction) as opposed to a single daily dose (100 mg daily = −7.9 mm Hg systolic blood pressure reduction) in 24-hour ambulatory measurements.[851]

Clinical trials also demonstrated that eplerenone has antihypertensive activity that is additive with that of either an ACE inhibitor or AII receptor blocker.[852] Additional reductions in blood pressure were 6.0 mm Hg systolic with the ACE inhibitor and 6.6 mm Hg with the AII receptor blocker. Another clinical trial demonstrated that in diabetic hypertensive patients with microalbuminuria, adding eplerenone to ACE inhibitor therapy was capable of reducing proteinuria more than the ACE inhibitor alone independent of blood pressure reduction.[853]

The advantage of eplerenone over spironolactone in clinical practice is probably related to fewer endocrine side effects because of more selective aldosterone receptor antagonism.

Tyrosine Hydroxylase Inhibitor
Mechanisms of Action

Metyrosine, the only drug in this class, blocks the rate-limiting step in the biosynthetic pathway of catecholamines. Metyrosine inhibits tyrosine hydroxylase, the enzyme responsible for conversion of tyrosine to dihydroxyphenylalanine.[854-857] This inhibition results in decreased levels of endogenous catecholamines. In patients with pheochromocytomas resulting in excessive production of norepinephrine and epinephrine, metyrosine reduces catecholamine biosynthesis by up to 80%. This results in a decrease in total peripheral vascular resistance. Heart rate and cardiac output increase because of the vasodilatation.

Class Members

The recommended initial dose of metyrosine is 250 mg four times a day orally. This may be increased by 250 to 500 mg every day until a maximum of 4 g/day is given. Following oral absorption, metyrosine is eliminated primarily unchanged in the urine. The half-life is 7.2 hours. Dosage reduction is appropriate in patients with renal failure.

Renal Effects

Little information is available on the renal affects of metyrosine. On the basis of its mechanism of action, which would be to counteract the renal effects of excessive circulating catecholamines, renal plasma flow and glomerular

filtration would probably increase. Renal vascular resistance would be expected to decrease. Some dosage adjustment is necessary in patients with renal disease (see Table 55-6).

Efficacy and Safety

Metyrosine is used in the preoperative or intraoperative management of pheochromocytoma.[793, 855-859] Hypertension and reflex tachycardia may result from vasodilatation. These effects can be minimized by volume expansion. Side effects include sedation, changes in sleep patterns, and extrapyramidal signs.[855, 857] Metyrosine crystals have been noted in the urine in patients receiving high doses. Patients should maintain a general fluid intake; occasional patients have been noted to have diarrhea.

Vasopeptidase Inhibitors

Omapatrilat (BMS-186716) is the first of the new class of agents termed vasopeptidase inhibitors. Others are in development including sampatrilat,[860] fasidotril,[861] and M100-240, but none has progressed as far in clinical development as omapatrilat.

Class Mechanism of Action and Class Member

Omapatrilat is an orally active, long-acting selective competitive inhibitor of neutral endopeptidase (NEP) and ACE with similar K_i values for both NEP (8.9 nM) and ACE (6.0 nM). As a result of this combined activity, omapatrilat potentiates multiple endogenous vasodilatory peptides, including natriuretic peptides (atrial, brain, and calcium-activated neutral proteases), bradykinin, and adrenomedullin while also inhibiting the generation of the vasoconstrictive peptide AII.[862-864] Vasopeptidase inhibitors are metalloproteinases that bind zinc, which is found in both NEP and ACE.[862] This provides its level of activity. Combined ACE and NEP inhibition should theoretically have greater antihypertensive potency than inhibition of either enzyme alone. In part, this stems from the ability of AII to neutralize the vasodilatory properties of NEP.

Omapatrilat has an oral bioavailability of about 30%. It may be given with or without food, and its protein binding is approximately 80%. It has a large volume of distribution (1800 L), suggesting extensive tissue penetration. Time to maximum concentration after an oral dose is about 2 hours. Its effective half-life is 14 to 19 hours.[865, 866]

The drug is metabolized in the liver by S-methylation, amide hydrolysis, S-oxidation, and glucoronidation.[865, 866] There are no substantial concentrations of active metabolites in the plasma. The majority of the metabolites are excreted in the urine, with less than 1% as unchanged drug. Cytochrome P-450 enzymes are not involved in the metabolism of omapatrilat, nor does this chemical affect P-450 isoenzymes including CYP-1A2, CYP-3A4, CYP-2C9, CYP-2C19, and CYP-2D6.[865, 866] Omapatrilat has no known interaction with other medications.

Class Renal Effects

Vasopeptidase inhibitors that combine the dual effects of ACE and NEP inhibition offer substantial promise for renal protection in that they provide not only an excellent strategy for reducing blood pressure but also reduction of glomerular capillary pressure and proteinuria.[867, 868] Experimental studies have indicated that dual ACE-NEP inhibition may offer a greater opportunity to attenuate progressive renal disease then ACE inhibition alone.[867, 868]

Taal and colleagues[867] studied the renal protective efficacy of the vasopeptidase inhibitor omapatrilat versus the ACE inhibitor enalapril in male Munich-Wistar rats subjected to 5/6 nephrectomy. In their initial studies, they started the pharmacotherapies on day 2 after surgery and noted that the agents were equally effective in normalizing blood pressure and preventing glomerulosclerosis after a period of 12 weeks. Micropuncture studies demonstrated a greater reduction of glomerular capillary pressure with omapatrilat compared with enalapril despite similar mean arterial pressures. These interesting observations stimulated the investigators to study whether these glomerular hemodynamic differences might be associated with chronic renoprotective efficacy. In the next set of experiments, they subjected the same type of rats to 5/6 nephrectomy and then delayed treatment until 4 weeks after surgery, when the animals had developed full-blown hypertension and proteinuria. After 20 weeks of treatment, both omapatrilat- and enalapril-treated rats exhibited less glomerulosclerosis than nontreated control rats, but only the difference between omapatrilat-treated and control rats was significant. With prolonged follow-up, the omapatrilat-treated rats demonstrated a substantially slower increase in proteinuria compared with the enalapril-treated rats.

On the basis of this experimental study, it was concluded that omapatrilat afforded greater long-term renoprotection than enalapril when the doses of the drugs were adjusted to yield equivalent reductions of systolic blood pressure. Similarly, Cao and colleagues[868] performed a 12-week study in 5/6 nephrectomized rats comparing low and high doses of a vasopeptidase inhibitor, ACE inhibitor, or no treatment. In the groups receiving low and high doses of vasopeptidase inhibitor, omapatrilat, blood pressure reduction was greater than in the ACE inhibitor or no-treatment group. Proteinuria was reduced in a dose-dependent manner by the vasopeptidase inhibitor and was greater than with the ACE inhibitor alone. Although there was no difference in renal function after 12 weeks of study, the vasopeptidase inhibitor–treated animals tended to have lower kidney weight and lower kidney/body weight ratios. The authors concluded that the reduction in kidney weight represents an antitrophic effect of the vasopeptidase inhibitor.

Clinical studies have also demonstrated that vasopeptidase inhibition with omapatrilat provides an important opportunity to reduce blood pressure and proteinuria in patients with type 2 diabetes. In a head-to-head clinical trial comparing omapatrilat (20 to 80 mg) versus amlodipine (2.5 to 10 mg), similar levels of blood pressure were achieved with the monotherapies, but only omapatrilat provided statistically significant reductions in proteinuria.[869] Longer term studies are needed to demonstrate that the antihypertensive effect coupled with the antiproteinuric effect will provide evidence of renoprotection in humans. Whether the dual ACE-NEP inhibition will provide greater renoprotection then ACE inhibition alone, independent of changes in systemic blood pressure, needs to be explored in long-term clinical trials.

Class Efficacy and Safety

Clinical trials with omapatrilat have demonstrated a dose-dependent efficacy in reducing systolic and diastolic blood pressure (10 to 80 mg).[870] Reductions in systolic blood pressure are more substantial with fully titrated omapatrilat (20 to 80 mg daily) than with fully titrated lisinopril (10 to 40 mg daily)[871, 872] or amlodipine (5 to 10 mg daily).[872, 873] Moreover, clinical studies have demonstrated that omapatrilat has a more substantial monotherapeutic antihypertensive effect than lisinopril in salt-sensitive hypertensive patients.[874, 875] These studies suggest that combined ACE-NEP inhibition may provide more antihypertensive efficacy than ACE inhibition alone. Of note are the interesting observations of Campese and colleagues,[874] who demonstrated that omapatrilat significantly increased urinary excretion of natriuretic peptide and cyclic guanosine monophosphate in salt-sensitive hypertensive patients compared with lisinopril. These investigators theorized that the hormonal profiles of the vasopeptidase inhibitor facilitated better control of diastolic and systolic blood pressure than ACE inhibition alone in salt-sensitive hypertension.

Omapatrilat is effective when combined with HCTZ for additional reduction of blood pressure. A study evaluated 274 subjects with mild to severe hypertension (stage 1 to 3 diastolic blood pressure elevation) and demonstrated the utility of adding omapatrilat to patients receiving HCTZ whose blood pressure was not sufficiently controlled with the diuretic alone.[876]

Omapatrilat may also have promise as a new treatment strategy in congestive heart failure.[877, 878] Short-term studies demonstrate a dose response, with omapatrilat producing substantial reductions in pulmonary capillary wedge pressure, systolic blood pressure, and systemic vascular resistance.[879-881] There is also experimental evidence of less acute activation of renin and aldosterone production with omapatrilat coupled with a diuretic compared with an ACE inhibitor coupled with a diuretic.[882] In the Inhibition of Metallo Protease by BMS-186716 in a Randomized Exercise and Symptoms Study in Subjects with Heart Failure (IMPRESS) trial, omapatrilat was compared with lisinopril in relation to exercise tolerance and morbidity in patients with heart failure.[883] The investigators noted that there was a trend in favor of omapatrilat on the combined end point or death or admission to hospital for worsening of heart failure ($P = .052$) and a significant benefit of omapatrilat in the composite end point of death, hospital admission, or discontinuation of study treatment for worsening of heart failure ($P = .035$). Omapatrilat also improved New York Heart Association class more than lisinopril in patients who started with classes III and IV but not in patients with class II and resulted in reduced hospitalization costs.[884] The investigators concluded that omapatrilat could have some advantages over lisinopril in the treatment of patients with congestive heart failure. The more recently completed Omapatrilat Versus Enalapril Randomized Trial of Utility in Reducing Events (OVERTURE) also demonstrated important new opportunities with omapatrilat as a treatment strategy in patients with congestive heart failure.[885]

Despite the marked promise for omapatrilat for the treatment of both hypertension and congestive heart failure and its unique therapeutic features, the approval of the drug has been delayed by the Food and Drug Administration because in the New Drug Application, 44 instances of angioedema occurred among more than 6000 patients who were treated, including 4 cases that were severe enough to require intubation. The increased frequency of angioedema is thought to be related to increased bradykinin concentration.[162, 886-888] Bradykinin is probably the mediator of angioedema associated with ACE inhibitors, and it can rise more than 10-fold during acute attacks of angioedema associated with ACE inhibition.[162, 886-888] The inhibition of ACE and NEP by omapatrilat reduces the inactivation of bradykinin. Thus, there may be larger increases in kinins associated with dual ACE-NEP inhibition to explain the increase incidence of angioedema.

The Omapatrilat Cardiovascular Treatment Assessment Versus Enalapril (OCTAVE) trial was conducted to more carefully elucidate both efficacy and safety differences between omapatrilat and the ACE inhibitor enalapril.[889] More than 25,000 patients were randomly assigned to one therapy or the other. Approximately 9300 patients were untreated hypertensives, 11,200 were patients with treated stage 1 hypertension, and approximately 4300 patients had treated stage 2 hypertension. Patients received titrated doses of omapatrilat from 10 to 80 mg and could then have adjunctive therapy. Patients receiving enalapril had doses titrated from 5 to 40 mg/day and then could have adjunctive therapy. Target blood pressure was less than 140/90 mm Hg. For all three groups of patients enrolled in the clinical trial, there was on average a 3 mm Hg greater reduction in systolic blood pressure with omapatrilat compared with enalapril ($P < .001$). In addition, fewer patients receiving omapatrilat required adjunctive antihypertensive therapy in order to achieve goal blood pressure. Thus, omapatrilat provided consistently greater effectiveness across all groups of patients whether used as an initial treatment or as an add-on antihypertensive therapy. In addition, it provided more blood pressure reduction than a full dose of an ACE inhibitor whether used alone or in combination with other antihypertensive drugs.

Although most common adverse events were similar in both groups, there were significantly more cases of angioedema in the omapatrilat group (274 out of 12,609 patients) versus enalapril (86 out of 12,557). Only two patients in the omapatrilat group developed airway compromise. One required treatment with epinephrine and the other mechanical airway protection. The overall incidence of angioedema in the omapatrilat group was 2.17% versus 0.68% in the enalapril group. Interestingly, the highest frequency of angioedema occurred in black patients, who had a threefold greater risk of angioedema with omapatrilat compared with enalapril. In nonblack patients, the incidence of angioedema was still greater with omapatrilat but similar to the incidence of angioedema in blacks seen with enalapril. Another interesting observation was that current smokers had a greater risk for angioedema with omapatrilat or enalapril.

Although omapatrilat provides substantial opportunity for facilitating better blood pressure control and hemodynamic benefits in patients with congestive heart failure, particularly with fewer episodes of renal dysfunction, it also carries a higher risk of life-threatening angioedema than ACE inhibitors alone. Consequently, the risk/benefit ratio of this therapy must be more carefully assessed in each individual patient when it becomes available on the market.

SELECTION OF ANTIHYPERTENSIVE DRUG THERAPY

Goal Blood Pressure Selection

Numerous factors confound the treatment of high blood pressure. The treatment is often delayed many years because the disease process is frequently asymptomatic. Consequently, it is not uncommon to have subclinical or even clinically evident target organ damage at the initiation of treatment. Moreover, the mechanistic underpinnings of high blood pressure are not well elucidated, and frequently the use of pharmacotherapy is simply based on what brings the "numbers" down and not necessarily what may be well tolerated or what may be best for preventing the development of cardiovascular disease or renal disease.

The whole purpose of treating blood pressure elevation is to prevent the development of cardiovascular events. In that sense, blood pressure is nothing more than one of many surrogate markers of risk contributing to cardiovascular disease. Consequently, the word "hypertension" is a nebulous concept. A factual definition of hypertension would be the level of blood pressure at which there is a greater net attributable risk for cardiovascular disease. Thus, the optimal goal blood pressure for different patients may be somewhat different depending on coexistent cardiovascular risk factors. The treatment of high blood pressure is much more complex than we once assumed it to be, and the estimation of goal blood pressure needs to be carefully individualized for each patient.

Clinicians must ask themselves three major questions: How low should you go? What drugs should you use? What are the best strategies for facilitating the attainment of goal blood pressure?

The question of how low you should go is not an easy one to answer as there are so many different aspects of patients' care that require consideration. Observational data indicate the advantages of lower systolic and diastolic blood pressure, preferably below 120/80 mm Hg.[890, 891] This was defined as optimal in JNC VI simply because it was the level of blood pressure least likely to be associated with development of cardiovascular events.[131] However, treated blood pressures at the same levels as observed blood pressures may not provide the same cardiovascular risk reduction. This may be particularly important when treating blood pressure to lower goals as recommended for patients with target organ damage or diabetes.[131] Consequently, more effort is needed to study the advantages of treated blood pressures below 140/90 mm Hg, which has been the traditional "gold standard."

Whether one should treat the systolic, diastolic, or pulse pressure is another important consideration. This is particularly true when one considers the vast number of patients with isolated systolic hypertension who have been traditionally assumed to have normal blood pressure because their diastolic pressure was below 90 mm Hg. Interventional trials demonstrate the advantage of lowering systolic blood pressure.[892-896] In fact, evidence from three large clinical trials on the treatment of isolated systolic hypertension indicates a consistent benefit related to reduction in congestive heart failure, myocardial infarction, and stroke with control of systolic blood pressure to an intermediate goal of less than 160 mm Hg and preferably a final goal of less than 140 mm Hg.[892-894]

Epidemiologic data have also demonstrated the importance of pulse pressure (systolic – diastolic blood pressure) in predicting cardiovascular events.[897-899] It correlates directly with the risk of myocardial infarction and the development of LVH. Because the measurement of diastolic blood pressure is frequently difficult in older patients with vascular disease, the exact assessment of pulse pressure may not always be possible. Consequently, relying on the systolic blood pressure may give the clinician a more realistic opportunity to gauge the adequacy of antihypertensive therapy. It is important to realize that the treatment of systolic blood pressure may provide one of the most important opportunities to provide cardiovascular risk reduction, particularly in patients with lower diastolic pressures who have a wider pulse pressure.

Decision making about identifying goal blood pressure should focus primarily on the patient's age, target organ damage, and associated cardiovascular risk factors. In JNC VI, the recommendation to chose a goal of less than 130/85 mm Hg was suggested for patients with heart disease, kidney disease, or diabetes because these patients had already manifested target organ damage or had risk factors that markedly increased their risk for cardiovascular events. Unfortunately, these recommendations are not always adhered to, as many of these patients have multiple medical problems that require pharmacotherapy, and the addition of medications to intensify treatment of high blood pressure is viewed as untenable.

Decisions about which drug or drugs should be employed for a given patient require careful consideration and individualization. As discussed later, this may depend on age, gender, race, obesity, and associated cardiovascular or renal disease. Clinical trials in patients with vascular disease, heart disease, or kidney disease have demonstrated the important therapeutic advantage of drugs that block the RAAS, either the ACE inhibitor[102, 117, 900-904] or the AII receptor blocker,[278-280, 905-907] to prevent progression of cardiac or renal disease as part of a multidrug regimen to lower blood pressure. These drugs should be part of every antihypertensive regimen in patients with heart disease or kidney disease unless there are specific contraindications. Although these drugs provide important risk reduction opportunities, they are not a substitute for achieving control of blood pressure.

Fixed-Dose Combination Therapy

With the shift in emphasis for treatment from the diastolic to both the systolic and diastolic blood pressure[131] and the lower blood pressure goals being recommended, particularly in patients with target organ damage, there is a substantial increase in the complexity of medical regimens. Most available antihypertensive drugs, when appropriately dosed, reduce systolic blood pressure about 8 to 10 mm Hg. Therefore, the number of drugs needed to reach goal blood pressure can probably be predicted by dividing the number 10 into the difference between current and goal systolic blood pressure. In many patients, this may require three or four drugs. Ideally, medications that are long acting, capable of being taken once daily, and well tolerated and preferably work well with other medications to facilitate blood pressure control should be employed. In addition, there has been a marked increase in the number of fixed-dose combination antihypertensive drugs that are available in the marketplace,

in large part to facilitate compliance by reducing the complexity of the antihypertensive regimen (Table 55-28).

Drugs that block the RAAS system, such as ACE inhibitors, AII receptor blockers, or β-blockers, can be prescribed with a low dose of HCTZ (6.25 or 12.5 mg).[24] The advantage of the low-dose HCTZ is that it nearly doubles the antihypertensive effects of the parent drug without adding any toxicity to the regimen.[908] Fixed-dose combinations of an ACE inhibitor and calcium channel blocker are also available. Clinical studies have demonstrated that these drugs are also additive in their ability to lower diastolic and systolic blood pressure.[909] Moreover, there is good clinical evidence that the ACE inhibitor antagonizes the development of pedal edema, which is not uncommonly seen with the calcium channel blocker.[910] Fixed-dosed combinations, although not recommended in the JNC VI[131] report as a routine first-line approach for the treatment of hypertension, are likely to receive more attention in future consensus reports as part of a simplification strategy to facilitate better blood pressure control, particularly in patients whose systolic blood pressure is 15 to 20 mm Hg or more from the desired goal.[137, 911-915]

Considerations for physicians about how to consolidate and simplify pharmacotherapy for the control of blood pressure are of great interest given the complexity of the current multidrug regimens that many patients require. Giving four drugs in two pills is possible with available fixed-dose combinations. This is an important goal as many patients frequently require 8 to 10 medications for control of their various medical problems, including diabetes, dyslipidemia, and angina. High blood pressure is a disease that is largely asymptomatic, and consequently the therapeutic approach should be simple, effective, and well tolerated.

Choosing Appropriate Agents

This section of the chapter considers initial therapy in various types of patients depending on age, gender, race, obesity, and coexistent cardiovascular or renal disease. These considerations are primarily generalizations based on clinical experience and should not be viewed as rigorous guidelines. Because each patient is different, variation in the approach is frequently necessary.

The major considerations for initial therapy in older patients (Table 55-29) should take into account the major pathophysiologic problem, which is an increase in peripheral vascular resistance. With associated proximal aortic stiffening, there are frequently an increase in systolic blood pressure, a decrease in diastolic pressure, and a wider pulse pressure.[898, 916-918] There are also an associated reduction in cardiovascular baroreceptor reflex function, greater blood pressure lability, and consequent propensity for orthostasis.[919] Older patients also tend to have hypertrophic cardiomyopathy with impaired diastolic function, which may impair cardiac output.[920, 921]

Ideal therapeutic strategies for these patients are vasodilators, preferably a low dose of HCTZ, 12.5. to 25 mg/day.[918] Thiazide diuretics function primarily as vasodilators and have minimal long-term effects on blood volume.[922, 923] In low doses, they are well tolerated and cause minimal problems related to glycemia control, potassium homeostasis, and cholesterol metabolism.[924, 925] They are particularly effective

TABLE 55-28

Fixed-Dose Combination Therapy

CLASS	COMBINATION	TRADE NAME
β-Adrenergic blockers and diuretics	Atenolol 50-100 mg/chlorthalidone 25 mg	Tenoretic
	Bisoprolol 2.5-10 mg/HCTZ 6.25	Ziac*
	Metoprolol 50-100 mg/HCTZ 25-50 mg	Lopressor HCT
	Nadolol 40-80 mg/bendroflumethiazide 5 mg	Corzide
	Propranolol 40-80 mg/HCTZ 25 mg	Inderide
	Propranolol ER 80-160 mg/HCTZ 50 mg	Inderide LA
	Timolol 10 mg/HCTZ 25 mg	Timolide
ACEIs and diuretics	Benazepril 5-20 mg/HCTZ 6.25 mg-25 mg	Lotensin HCT
	Captopril 25-50 mg/HCTZ 15-25 mg	Capozide*
	Enalapril 5-10 mg/HCTZ 12.5-25 mg	Vaseretic
	Lisinopril 10-20 mg/HCTZ 12.5-25 mg	Zestoretic; Prinzide
Angiotensin II receptor blocker and diuretic	Losartan 50 mg/HCTZ 12.5 mg	Hyzaar
	Losartan 50-100 mg/HCTZ 12.5-25 mg	
	Valsartan 80-160 mg/HCTZ 12.5	Diovan HCT
	Valsartan 80-160 mg/HCTZ 12.5-25 mg	
	Irbesartan 150-200 mg/HCTZ 12.5	
	Telmisartan 80-160 mg/HCTZ 12.5	
	Candesartan 16-32 mg/HCTZ 12.5	
Calcium antagonists and ACEIs	Amlodipine 2.5-10 mg/benazepril 10-20 mg	Lotrel
	Diltiazem 180 mg/enalapril 5 mg	Teczem
	Felodipine 5 mg/enalapril 5 mg	Lexxel
	Verapamil 180-240 mg/trandolapril 1-4 mg	Tarka
Other combinations	Clonidine HCl 0.1-0.3 mg/chlorthalidone 15 mg	Combipres
	Deserpidine 0.25-0.5	Enduronyl (Forte)
	Guanethidine 10 mg/HCTZ 25 mg	Esimil
	Hydralazine 25-100/HCTZ 25-50 mg	Apresazide
	Hydralazine 25 mg/reserpine 0.1 mg/HCTZ 15 mg	Ser-Ap-Es; Unipres; Tri-Hydroserpine
	Methyldopa 250 mg/chlorothiazide 150-250 mg	Aldoclor
	Methyldopa 250-500 mg/HCTZ 30-50 mg	Aldoril
	Prazosin 1-5 mg/polythiazide 0.5 mg	Minizide
	Rauwolfia 50 mg/bendroflumethiazide 4 mg	Rauzide
	Reserpine 0.125 mg/chlorthalidone 25 mg	Demi-Regroton
	Reserpine 0.125 mg/chlorothiazide 250-500 mg	Diupres
	Reserpine 0.125 mg/HCTZ 25-50 mg	Hydropres; Hydroserpine
	Reserpine 0.125 mg/hydroflumethiazide 50 mg	Salutensin (-Demi)
	Reserpine 0.25 mg/polythiazide 2 mg	Renese-R
	Reserpine 0.1 mg/trichlormethiazide 2-4 mg	Metatensin

*Approved for initial therapy of hypertension.

ACEI, angiotensin-converting enzyme inhibitor; ER, extended release; HCT, HCTZ; hydrochlorothiazide; LA, long acting.

Adapted from Joint National Committee on Prevention, Detection, Evaluation and Treatment of High Pressure: The sixth report. Arch Intern Med 157:2413-2446, 1997.

in controlling systolic blood pressure.[918, 926] Their biologic half-life extends well beyond their pharmacologic half-life.

Thiazide diuretics also facilitate vasodilation with other therapeutic classes, particularly those that block the RAAS.[908] They can be utilized together as fixed-dose combinations.

Calcium channel blockers are also useful vasodilators in older patients. They are much better tolerated in the lower half of their dosing range and are quite effective even in the presence of a high-salt diet, perhaps owing to their natriuretic effects[927] or intrinsic vasodilatory effects.[928, 929] α-Blockers may be useful in older men with benign prostatic hypertrophy because they facilitate prostatic urethral relaxation and improve urinary stream.[930] ACE inhibitors and AII receptor blockers are also effective vasodilators in older patients. They are well tolerated, and their efficacy is enhanced with low-dose thiazide diuretic therapy.[908] β-Blockers may impair baroreceptor responses in older patients and worsen orthostasis and should be used with caution.

Older patients have a greater likelihood of orthostasis than younger patients. As many as 18% of untreated elderly patients with hypertension may have a decrease of systolic blood pressure greater than 20 mm Hg after standing for 1 to 3 minutes.[931] Older patients may also have pseudohypertension, which may interfere with a true determination of blood pressure.[932] Consequently, three position blood pressures should always be employed during initiation and titration of medications. If recumbent blood pressures remain elevated, short-acting medications taken before bedtime such as clonidine or captopril may be useful in controlling blood pressure overnight.

Treatment of isolated systolic hypertension in older patients frequently requires multiple drugs. Regardless of the agents that are utilized, a slow careful titration approach is recommended, preferably not more frequently than every 3 months. A careful assessment of the metabolic and excretory routes of the drugs as well as possible drug-drug interactions

TABLE 55-29

Considerations for Initial Therapy in Older Patients

CLINICAL OBSERVATIONS	PHARMACOLOGIC CONSIDERATIONS
Decreased vascular compliance and ↑ peripheral vascular resistance	Vasodilation (e.g., HCTZ, ACEI, ARB, CCB, α-blockers)
Isolated systolic hypertension and wide pulse pressure	Vasodilation (e.g., HCTZ, CCB)
Reduction of cardiovascular baroreflex function with blood pressure lability	Avoid sympatholytics and volume depletion. Use β-blockers cautiously
Orthostatic hypotension	Consider using short-acting meds (<8 h duration) at bedtime during recumbency
Reduced metabolic capability	Adjust all medications for renal/hepatic function—start at half dose
Prostatic hypertrophy	α-Blockers
More than 20 mm Hg from systolic goal	Fixed-dose combination (ACEI/HCTZ, ARB/HCTZ, ACEI/CCB, BB/HCTZ)

HCTZ, thiazide diuretic; ACEI, angiotensin-converting enzyme inhibitor; ARB, angiotensin II receptor blocker; CCB, calcium channel blocker.

is recommended because older patients frequently have impaired metabolic function.

Differences in gender (Table 55-30) may be important with regard to the selection of antihypertensive therapy.[627] Men and women benefit equally with more intensive control of blood pressure resulting in a reduction in risk of cardiovascular events.[933] In general, men have a decreased resting heart rate, a longer left ventricular injection fraction time, and an increased pulse pressure when stressed compared with women.[934, 935] Women tend to have reduced peripheral vascular resistance and greater blood volume than men.[934] They also have a lower likelihood of coronary disease before menopause. However, when menopause occurs or in the presence of diabetes, women assume the same risk for coronary disease as men.[936]

Vasodilation is always a good choice for treatment, as elevated peripheral vascular resistance is almost always involved in blood pressure elevation regardless of gender. Thiazide diuretics, ACE inhibitors, AII receptor blockers, and calcium channel blockers are all effective treatments. Many patients require two or more of these drugs, and fixed-dose combinations can be used.

Women should avoid the use of ACE inhibitors and AII receptor blockers in pregnancy because of their possible teratogenic effects. Calcium channel blockers may delay labor. Optimal therapy in a pregnant woman should remain α-methyldopa, hydralazine, or β-blockers as they have a proven safety record with minimal risk of teratogenic effects.

In women with osteoporosis, thiazide diuretics are ideal agents because they antagonize calciuria and facilitate bone mineralization.[937-941]

Women experience more cough with ACE inhibitors and more pedal edema with calcium channel blockers compared with men.[942, 943] These differences in side effects may require adjustment in dose or switching medications. Interestingly, despite differences in the underlying pathophysiologic mechanisms of high blood pressure between genders, there does not appear to be a substantial difference in response rate to similar doses of commonly used antihypertensive drugs.

Race may play a role in choice of antihypertensive agents (Table 55-31). Blacks frequently present with high blood pressure at an earlier age and have more substantial elevations in blood pressure and earlier development of target organ damage than similar demographically matched white

TABLE 55-30

Considerations for Initial Therapy Based on Gender

CLINICAL OBSERVATIONS	PHARMACOLOGIC CONSIDERATIONS
Men have ↓ resting heart rate, longer LVEF time, ↑stressed pulse pressure compared with women	Vasodilation (e.g., HCTZ, ACEI, ARB, CCB)
Women have ↓ TPR and ↓ blood volume compared with men	Vasodilation, heart rate reduction, may need diuresis (HCTZ, ACE inhibitor, ARB, β-blocker, CCB)
Postmenopausal women more frequently have CAD with atypical chest pain	Antianginal; heart rate reduction (β-blocker, CCB)
Osteoporosis	Antagonize calciuria (HCTZ)
Pregnancy	Avoid teratogenic drugs (ACEI, ARB). Avoid drugs that may cause ureteroplacental insufficiency (loop diuretics). Optimal choices: α-methyldopa, hydralazine, β-blocker
Women report more pedal edema with CCB and cough with ACEI than men	Adjust dose or discontinue drug
More than 20 mm Hg systolic goal	Fixed-dose combination (ACEI/HCTZ, BB/HCTZ, ARB/HCTZ, ACEI/CCB)

ACEI, angiotensin-converting ezyme inhibitor; ARB, angiotensin II receptor blocker; CCB, calcium channel blocker; HCTZ, thiazide diuretic; CAD, coronary artery disease; HR, heart rate; LVEF, left ventricular ejection fraction; TPR, total peripheral resistance.

TABLE 55-31

Considerations for Initial Therapy in Black Patients

CLINICAL OBSERVATIONS	PHARAMACOLOGIC CONSIDERATIONS
High peripheral vascular resistance with associated reduction in cardiac output	Vasodilation (e.g., HCTZ, ACEI, CCB, ARB)
Salt sensitivity	Natriuresis (HCTZ, ACE inhibitor, ARB, CCB). Reduce salt intake
Variable increase in blood volume (perhaps greater in some patients relative to ↑ peripheral vascular resistance)	Natriuresis, diuresis (HCTZ; if creatinine >2.0, loop diuretic)
More than 20 mm Hg from systolic goal	Fixed-dose combination therapy (ACEI/HCTZ, BB/HCTZ, ARB/HCTZ, ACEI/CCB)

ACEI, angiotensin-converting ezyme inhibitor; ARB, angiotensin II receptor blocker; BB, β-blocker; CCB, calcium channel blocker; HCTZ, thiazide diuretic.

counterparts.[439, 944-946] Racial differences in the response to antihypertensive medications have been demonstrated in numerous clinical trials.[439] The mechanisms for these differences are not yet elucidated but appear to be independent of dietary salt or potassium.[928] Some investigators have suggested possible genetic differences in renal sodium handling, yet this has not been conclusively demonstrated in clinical trials. Despite this observation, blacks frequently display blood pressure salt sensitivity.[947, 948] A careful assessment of the dose response of different medication classes, adjusting for differences in dietary sodium consumption and body mass index between races, has not been performed.

In general, thiazide diuretics and calcium channel blockers have been demonstrated to have more robust antihypertensive properties in lower doses in blacks than other commonly used therapeutic classes.[928, 929, 949] Drugs that block the RAAS are effective in blacks, but higher doses are frequently required in order to achieve the same level of blood pressure as seen in nonblacks.[950] As in most population groups, elevated peripheral vascular resistance contributes to blood pressure elevation. Some investigators have suggested that blacks have a modest volume component contributing to blood pressure elevation that may also contribute to antihypertensive drug resistance.[947, 948] It is not uncommon for multiple drugs to be required to reach goal blood pressure given the greater degree of blood pressure elevation and somewhat different patterns in the antihypertensive responses.[147, 911] Consequently, fixed-dose combinations may prove to be most useful in this population group as part of the strategy to simplify the approach.

Hispanic and Asian Americans do not appear to have different hypertensive responses to commonly used drugs compared with white Americans.[439, 928] Consequently, there do not appear to be any reasons to treat these ethnic groups differently from whites.

Obese hypertensive patients frequently have other medical problems that complicate their hypertensive management (Table 55-32).[951] They tend to have a hyperdynamic circulation, increased peripheral vascular resistance, expanded plasma volume, and, like blacks, tend to have greater sensitivity to the influence of dietary salt in raising blood pressure.[952-954]

β-Blockers may be helpful in diminishing sympathoadrenal drive. Vasodilators, such as HCTZ and ACE inhibitors, ARBs, and calcium channel blockers, are useful for reducing peripheral vascular resistance. Combinations of these drugs may also be helpful. Because of the tendency toward expanded plasma volume, thiazide diuretics can be helpful as they provide both an opportunity to cause vasodilation and mild volume reduction.[922, 923] Frequently, these patients require multiple drugs to achieve blood pressure goals, and simplification strategies are important. Given the increased frequency of cardiovascular risk clustering phenomena in these patients, drug therapies that are metabolically neutral are ideal. One also should use β-blockers carefully as they may increase the likelihood of weight gain and may compromise glucose tolerance.[955]

Patients with hypertension and cardiac disease need tailored approaches, as the medications used to control blood pressure are all quite different with regard to their effects on the heart (Table 55-33). In patients with coronary artery disease, it is important to remember that the majority of coronary

TABLE 55-32

Considerations for Initial Therapy in Obese Hypertensive Patients

CLINICAL OBSERVATIONS	PHARMACOLOGIC CONSIDERATIONS
Hyperdynamic circulation	Reduce heart rate and sympathoadrenal outflow (β-blocker)
Increased peripheral vascular resistance	Vasodilation (e.g., HCTZ, ACEI, ARB, CCB)
Salt sensitivity	Natriuresis (HCTZ, ACEI, ARB, CCB). Reduce salt intake
Expanded plasma volume	Diuresis (HCTZ). Reduce salt intake
Hypoventilation	Sleep study to evaluate the need for positive-pressure ventilation at night
More than 20 mm Hg from systolic goal	Fixed-dose combination (ACEI/HCTZ, BB/HCTZ, ARB/HCTZ, ACEI/CCB)

ACEI, angiotensin-converting ezyme inhibitor; ARB, angiotensin II receptor blocker; BB, β-blocker; CCB, calcium channel blocker; HCTZ, thiazide diuretic.

TABLE 55-33

Considerations for Initial Therapy in Patients with Heart Diesease

CLINICAL OBSERVATIONS	PHARMACOLOGIC CONSIDERATIONS
Angina	Reduce heart rate and induce coronary vasodilation (reduce heart rate 20% or 60–65 bpm). (β-blocker, nitrates, CCB)
Left ventricular hypertrophy	Reduce systolic blood pressure (HCTZ, ACEI, CCB, ARB). Avoid nonspecific vasodilator or therapies that result in reflex ↑ heart rate
Systolic dysfunction	Reduce afterload and preload natriuresis (ACEI, HCTZ, ARB). Antineurohormonal agents, β-blocker, spironolactone
Diastolic dysfunction	Improve myocardial compliance, reduce heart rate, avoid volume depletion (β-blocker, CCB, ACEI, ARB, avoid loop diuretics)
Myocardial infarction	Reduce heart rate (β-blocker, ACEI)
More than 20 mm Hg from systolic goal	Fixed-dose combination therapy (ACEI/HCTZ, BB/HCTZ, ARB/HCTZ, ACEI/CCB)

ACEI, angiotensin-converting enzyme inhibitor; ARB, angiotensin II receptor blocker; BB, β-blocker; CCB, calcium channel blocker; HCTZ, thiazide diuretic.

artery perfusion occurs during diastole. Hence, pharmacotherapy should be targeted toward slowing heart rate in order to enhance perfusion during diastole. β-Blockers and heart rate–lowering calcium channel blockers, such as nondihydropyridines, would be ideal in this respect.[956, 957]

LVH is evidence of the chronicity and magnitude of blood pressure elevation. All drugs that lower blood pressure except the direct-acting vasodilators effectively cause LVH to regress.[958] Thus, most antihypertensives can be useful in this regard. Some trials indicate that drugs that block the RAAS may be more effective in reducing LVH than other drugs.[958] A large-scale clinical trial demonstrated that the ARB losartan was more effective in reducing overall cardiovascular morbidity and mortality (primarily related to reduction in the incidence of stroke) in patients with hypertension and LVH than a β-blocker–based antihypertensive regimen.[905]

If patients have dyspnea, it is important to use an echocardiogram to distinguish between diastolic and systolic dysfunction. The treatment of diastolic dysfunction should include therapies that facilitate ventricular relaxation and reduce heart rate (β-blockers and calcium channel blockers). With systolic dysfunction, drugs that block the RAAS are more suitable to provide both preload and afterload reduction and diminish sympathoadrenal response.[959] β-Blockers

are also helpful in these patients in addition to ACE inhibitor therapy.[960] Diuretic therapy should be used to adjust blood volume as necessary.

In patients with kidney disease (Table 55-34), blood pressure control is more complex to manage in that they not only have an increased vascular resistance but also frequently have increased blood volume contributing to the hypertensive process.[961-963] Understandings about renal autoregulation provide some insight into appropriate levels of blood pressure control and the relative importance of different kinds of antihypertensive drugs in preserving renal function.

The glomerular circulation operates optimally at one half to two thirds of the systemic blood pressure.[964] Preglomerular vasoconstriction is necessary to step systemic pressure down to glomerular capillary pressure levels that are optimal for filtration yet low enough to avoid mechanical injury to the filtering apparatus.[965, 966] The efferent glomerular arteriole also serves an important purpose. It vasoconstricts during situations of diminished effective arterial blood volume to maintain adequate pressure for glomerular filtration.[967] With the development of vascular disease, the afferent glomerular arteriole does not vasoconstrict properly, allowing transmission of systemic blood pressure into the glomerulus. A clinical clue that could indicate failure of autoregulation is the

TABLE 55-34

Considerations for Initial Therapy in Patients with Renal Disease*

CLINICAL OBSERVATIONS	PHARMACOLOGIC CONSIDERATIONS
Increased blood volume (common in glomerular diseases)	Reduce blood volume (HCTZ, loop diuretic if creatinine >2.0)
Decreased blood volume (common in tubular diseases)	May need salt supplementation
Increased peripheral vascular resistance	Vasodilation (ACEI, CCB, ARB)
Proteinuria	Reduce proteinuria (ACEI, ARB, NDCCB) (blood pressure systolic ≤125 mm Hg if more than 1 g/day
Diabetes with proteinuria	Control blood pressure and glycemia (ACEI if type 1, ARB if type 2 (blood pressure systolic <130 mm Hg)
More than 20 mm Hg from systolic goal	Fixed-dose combination therapy (ACEI/HCTZ, BB/HCTZ, ACEI/CCB, ARB/HCTZ) Use of HCTZ depends on renal function

*All medications adjusted according to renal function.

NDCCB, nondihydropyridine calcium channel blocker; ACEI, angiotensin-converting enzyme inhibitor; ARB, angiotensin II receptor blocker; BB, β-blocker; CCB, calcium channel blocker; HCTZ, thiazide diuretic.

presence of microalbumin or protein in the urine. Under these circumstances, systemic blood pressure should be reduced more substantially to minimize the risk of mechanical injury to the glomerulus. In JNC VI, recommended systolic blood pressure was less than 130 mm Hg in patients with renal disease and less than 125 mm Hg if there was evidence of clinical proteinuria (more than 1 g per 24 hours).[131] It is possible that even lower pressures may be necessary for optimal delay of progression of renal disease, particularly in the presence of proteinuria and in patients with diabetes.

Drugs that block the RAS such as ACE inhibitors[102, 117, 904, 907] and ARBs[278-280] provide a more consistent opportunity to reduce progression of renal disease as part of an intensive blood pressure–lowering strategy compared with other commonly used antihypertensive drugs. The benefit of these drugs resides, in part, in their effects to facilitate efferent glomerular arteriolar dilation by antagonizing the effects of AII as they lower blood pressure.[968] Thus, there is a more consistent reduction in both systemic and glomerular capillary pressure. Additional medications can be added to these drugs to facilitate better blood pressure control and also help reduce glomerular capillary pressure and proteinuria. Sufficient diuretics to control blood volume should also be employed. When the serum creatinine reaches 2 mg/dl, volume reduction is more amenable to the use of loop diuretics as opposed to thiazides, which are more effective as peripheral vasodilators.

Some investigators have questioned the safety of using calcium channel blockers in patients with kidney disease given their preferential effects on dilating the afferent glomerular arteriole.[102] Some studies have demonstrated that they can increase proteinuria despite lowering blood pressure.[969] However, if these drugs are given with either ACE inhibitors or ARBs, which dilate the efferent glomerular arteriole, there is no clinical evidence that they are detrimental and worsen progression of renal disease. If anything, lower blood pressure achieved with these drugs in combination may provide a better opportunity to protect against the loss of kidney function.

Antiproteinuric strategies should be considered in patients with kidney disease as reduction in proteinuria with specific antihypertensive drugs, such as ACE inhibitors or ARBs, is beneficial in retarding progression of renal disease.[970]

Refractory Hypertension

Refractory hypertension is a term used to characterize high blood pressure that fails to respond to what the clinician feels is an adequate antihypertensive regimen (Table 55-35).[971-973] Thus, the definition can vary substantially from clinician to clinician. There are a variety of factors that interfere with the ability of what is deemed to be appropriate antihypertensive therapy to normalize blood pressure. Perhaps most important is nonadherence to therapy. Noncompliance is common and is one of the most serious problems that interfere with attaining goal blood pressure. It has many sources, including inadequate education, poor clinician-patient relationship, lack of understanding about side effects, and the complexity of multidrug regimens. The health care provider should make every effort to establish whether or not compliance with therapy is part of the problem before pursuing other potential explanations for refractory hypertension. If noncompliance

TABLE 55-35

Causes of Refractory Hypertension

Pseudoresistance
  1. "White-coat hypertension" or office elevations
  2. Pseudohypertension in older patients
  3. Use of small cuff on very obese arm
Nonadherence to therapy
Volume overload
Drug-related causes
  1. Doses too low
  2. Wrong type of diuretic
  3. Inappropriate combinations
  4. Drug actions and interactions
    Sympathiomimetics
    Nasal decongestants
    Appetite suppressants
    Cocaine
    Caffeine
    Oral contraceptives
    Adrenal steroids
    Licorice (may be found in chewing tobacco)
    Cyclosporine, tacrolimus
    Epoetin
    Antidepressants
    Nonsteroidal anti-inflammatory drugs
Concomitant conditions
  1. Obesity
  2. Sleep apnea
  3. Ethanol intake of >1 oz (30 mL) per day
  4. Anxiety, hyperventilation
Secondary causes of hypertension
  Renovascular hypertension
  Primary aldosteronism
  Pheochromocytoma
  Hypothyroidism
  Hyperthyroidism
  Hyperparathyroidism
  Aortic coarctation
  Renal disease

is eliminated, a methodologic approach can be used to help diagnose the cause of refractory hypertension and then correct it.

Pseudohypertension may also be a cause of refractory hypertension.[974] This is most commonly observed in older hypertensive patients who have hardened atherosclerotic arteries, which are not easily compressible. This interferes with auscultatory measurements of blood pressure. It is also known as the Osler phenomenon.[932] Because of the conformational changes of the vessels, greater apparent pressure is required to compress the sclerotic vessel than the intra-arterial blood pressure requires.

Another common cause of pseudohypertension is improper measurement. This occurs when the blood pressure is taken with an inappropriately small cuff in people with large arm circumference. Because of the substantial proportion of hypertensive patients who are obese, it is critical to have the appropriate cuff size for determining auscultatory pressure. The bladder within the cuff should encircle at least 80% of the arm in order to provide an accurate determination.

Some clinicians may view white coat hypertension as a cause of refractory hypertension. This is an area of contentious debate in that elevated office readings despite lower home readings still provide important predictive value for the development of cardiovascular events. Some clinical studies indicate that patients with so-called white coat hypertension also have LVH and may not have an appropriate nocturnal dip in blood pressure.[975-977]

Volume overload is an important and common cause of refractory hypertension.[978] It may be related to excessive salt intake or inability of the kidney to excrete an appropriate salt and water load because of either endocrine abnormalities or intrinsic renal disease.

Increasing dietary salt offsets the antihypertensive activities of all antihypertensive medications.[928] Some patients are more salt sensitive than others. Salt sensitivity is common in patients of African American descent. It is also a more common problem in patients with renal disease and congestive heart failure. A careful clinical examination coupled with judicious use of either thiazide or loop diuretics (depending on the level of renal function) is critical in achieving ideal blood volume in order to restore the antihypertensive efficacy of most classes of drugs. It is also appropriate to consider educating the patient about avoiding foods that are rich in salt content, such as processed foods.

Drug-related causes of refractory hypertension are common and need to be carefully assessed in each patient. Perhaps the most common drugs that cause refractory hypertension are over-the-counter preparations of sympathomimetics such as nasal decongestants, appetite suppressants, and NSAIDs.[979] In addition, oral contraceptives,[980] immunosuppressants such as cyclosporine, and even some antidepressants can raise blood pressure. Caffeine, licorice, and even erythropoietin may also raise blood pressure. Unfortunately, patients may not always recognize over-the-counter preparations as a medication. Therefore, careful questioning specifically focusing on these types of medications should be routine during the evaluation for refractory hypertension. In addition, ethanol, cigarettes, and cocaine can be complicating factors that interfere with the ability of medications to lower blood pressure.[981]

Some medications may interfere with the antihypertensive activity of other drugs. For example, NSAIDs interfere with the antihypertensive activity of diuretics and ACE inhibitors.[982] Interestingly, only the antihypertensive effects of calcium channel blockers appear to be immune to the effects of NSAIDs.[983] Drug-drug interactions that can interfere in drug absorption, metabolism, or the pharmacodynamics of concomitantly administered drugs can also interfere with antihypertensive activity.

Concomitant medical conditions can also interfere with the ability of medications to control blood pressure. Obesity is an often overlooked cause of refractory hypertension because it is commonly associated with the obesity hypoventilation syndrome, obstructive sleep apnea.[984] Nighttime ventilation techniques such as continuous positive airway pressure enhance the control of blood pressure.[984]

Secondary causes of hypertension might also be considered as a cause of refractory hypertension. These can be divided into two groups: either renal parenchymal and renal vascular or endocrine. Renal parenchymal and renal vascular diseases are not uncommon (90% of the total). A chemistry profile and urinalysis facilitate diagnosis of renal disease, whereas a renal vascular assessment with a Doppler or direct imaging technique determines whether renal vascular hypertension is present. Additional endocrine abnormalities include hyperaldosteronism, pheochromocytoma, or hypo- or hyperthyroidism and hyperparathyroidism; rarely, aortic coarctation can be a cause of refractory hypertension.[982]

Strategies to control blood pressure in patients with refractory hypertension should first deal with issues related to compliance, simplifying the medical regimen, and being sure that side effects are not playing a role. Subsequently, one can evaluate the medications and try to choose those that work well with one another to facilitate a nearly additive antihypertensive response. Most drugs reduce systolic blood pressure by approximately 8 to 10 mm Hg. Consequently, it is not unusual for patients who are 40 or 50 mm Hg from goal systolic blood pressure to require four or five medications or possibly even more.

One should also be careful to be sure that volume excess is controlled and that there are no drug-drug interactions or clinical situations that would promote diuretic resistance such as excessive salt intake, impaired drug bioavailability, impaired diuretic secretion by the proximal tubule, increased protein binding in the tubule lumen, or reduced GFR. Both pseudohypertension and secondary causes of hypertension should be eliminated as possibilities. True refractory hypertension is unusual, and a methodologic approach should be taken to help facilitate blood pressure control in these patients because lack of control puts these patients at greater risk for cardiovascular complications.

DRUG TREATMENT OF HYPERTENSIVE URGENCIES AND EMERGENCIES

It is important to distinguish between hypertensive urgency and emergency (Table 55-36). These terms are used loosely in clinical practice with a great deal of overlap. The distinction between the two is important because the management approach is substantially different.

TABLE 55-36

Hypertensive Emergencies

Hypertensive encephalopathy*
Acute aortic dissection*
  Central nervous system bleeding*
  Intracranial hemorrhage
  Thrombotic cerebrovascular accident
  Subarachnoid hemorrhage
Acute left ventricular failure refractory to conventional medical therapy*
Myocardial ischemia or infarction associated with persistent chest pain*
Accelerated or malignant hypertension[†]
Toxemia of pregnancy: eclampsia*
Renal failure or insufficiency[†]
Hypertension associated with hyperadrenergic states*
  Pheochromocytoma
  Interaction between monoamine oxidase inhibitors and tyramine-
    containing foods
  Interaction between an α-adrenergic agonist and a nonselective
    β-adrenergic antagonist
  After abrupt withdrawal of clonidine or guanabenz
  After severe body burns
  Neurogenic hypertension
Hypertension in the surgical patient[†]
  Associated with postoperative bleeding
  After open heart or vascular surgery
  Preceding emergency surgery
  After kidney transplantation
Hypertension in the diabetic patient with retinal hemorrhage*

*Considered by some authors to be a true hypertensive emergency.
[†]Considered by some authors to be a hypertensive urgency.

A hypertensive emergency is a clinical syndrome in which marked elevation in blood pressure results in ongoing target organ damage in the body. This can be manifested by encephalopathy, retinal hemorrhage, papilledema, acute myocardial infarction, stroke, or acute renal dysfunction. Any delay in control of blood pressure may lead to irreversible sequelae, including death.

These syndromes are unusual but require immediate hospitalization in an intensive care unit, with careful and judicious use of intravenous vasodilators to lower systolic and diastolic blood pressure cautiously to approximately 140/90 mm Hg.

Hypertensive urgencies are clinical situations in which a patient may have marked elevation in blood pressure (greater than 200/130 mm Hg) yet no evidence of ongoing target organ damage. These patients can be treated with rapid-onset drugs such as captopril or clonidine and be observed cautiously with long-acting medications on an outpatient basis as progressive restoration of more appropriate blood pressure level is attained. Thus, the history and physical examination are the critical factors in delineating the difference between these two syndromes. The decision about whether to hospitalize the patient in an intensive care unit and use intravenous medication or to observe the patient carefully and use oral medications to facilitate better blood pressure control depends in large part on the presence or absence of ongoing target organ injury.

A variety of different antihypertensive therapeutic classes are effective in the treatment of hypertensive emergencies. These drugs can be given parenterally and include the direct-acting vasodilators, diazoxide, hydralazine, nitroprusside, and nitroglycerine; the β_1-selective adrenergic antagonist esmolol; the α- and β-adrenergic antagonist labetalol; the central adrenergic methyldopa; the ganglionic blocking agent trimethaphan; the ACE inhibitor enalaprilat; the peripheral α-adrenergic blocker phentolamine; the calcium channel blocker nicardipine; and the dopamine D_1-like receptor agonist fenoldopam mesylate.

Parenteral Drugs, Direct-Acting Vasodilators

Diazoxide is a benzothiadiazine drug that is used primarily in the treatment of acute hypertensive emergencies.[985-998] It is a pure arterial dilator. The "minibolus" (1 mg/kg administered at intervals of 5 to 15 minutes) and the continuous infusion of diazoxide have become the preferred methods of administration to avoid excessive reduction in blood pressure. Diazoxide acts rapidly, and the blood pressure effect persists up to 12 hours. It has a plasma half-life of 17 to 31 hours, 20% is eliminated unchanged in the urine, and the remainder undergoes hepatic metabolism to inactive metabolites. In renal disease, the plasma half-life is prolonged, and dose reduction is required.

Because diazoxide relaxes smooth muscle at peripheral arterioles, reduction in blood pressure is accompanied by an increase in cardiac output and heart rate, which in susceptible patients can provoke cardiac ischemia. Concurrent administration of a β-adrenergic antagonist controls these reflex vasodilatory responses. Transient hyperuricemia and hyperglycemia occur in the majority of patients. Consequently, the blood glucose level should be monitored. Salt and water retention also occurs, and concurrent diuretic administration is often required. Diazoxide and its metabolites are removed

by hemodialysis and peritoneal dialysis, but clearance is relatively low because of its extensive protein binding.

Hydralazine is a direct-acting vasodilator and may be given intramuscularly as a rapid intravenous bolus injection (Table 55-37). It acts rapidly, and the blood pressure effect persists up to 6 hours.[770] It is less potent that diazoxide, and the blood pressure response is less predictable. It may also cause a reflex increase in heart rate and sodium and water retention.

Sodium nitroprusside is the most potent of the parenteral vasodilators.[991-1003] Nitroprusside acts on the excitation-contraction coupling of vascular smooth muscle by interfering with the intracellular activation of calcium. Unlike diazoxide and hydralazine, nitroprusside dilates both arteriolar resistance and venous capacitance vessels. It has the advantages of being immediately effective when given as an infusion and of having an extremely short duration of action, which permits minute-to-minute adjustments in blood pressure control (see Table 55-37). Disadvantages of nitroprusside therapy include (1) the need for intra-arterial blood pressure monitoring, (2) the need for the drug to be prepared fresh every 4 hours, (3) the need to protect the solution from light during infusion, and (4) the potential for toxic effects from metabolic side products. Nitroprusside is not excreted intact. It is rapidly metabolized to cyanide and thiocyanate through a reaction with hemoglobin, which yields methemoglobin and an unstable intermediate that dissociates to release cyanide. The major elimination pathway of cyanide is conversion in the liver and kidney to thiocyanate. Back-conversion of thiocyanate to cyanide may occur. Thiocyanate is largely excreted in the urine; it has a plasma half-life of 1 week in normal subjects and accumulates in renal insufficiency.

Toxic concentrations of cyanide or thiocyanate may occur if nitroprusside infusions are given for more than 48 hours or at infusion rates greater than 2 mg/kg/min; the maximal dose rate of 10 mg/kg/min should not last more than 10 minutes. Toxic manifestations include air hunger, hyperreflexia, confusion, and seizures. Lactic acidosis and venous hyperoxemia are laboratory indicators of cyanide intoxication. The appearance of drug unresponsiveness may reflect an increase in the concentration of free cyanide. The drug should be promptly discontinued and levels of cyanide measured. Nitroprusside is hemodialyzable.

Intravenous nitroglycerin produces, in a dose-related manner, dilation of both arterial and venous beds.[991-996] At lower doses, its primary effect is on preload; at higher infusion rates, afterload is reduced. Nitroglycerin may also dilate both epicardial coronary vessels and their collaterals, increasing blood supply to ischemic regions. Effective coronary perfusion is maintained provided that blood pressure does not fall excessively or heart rate does not increase significantly. Nitroglycerin has an immediate onset of action but is rapidly metabolized to dinitrates and mononitrates (see Table 55-37). Because nitroglycerin is absorbed by many plastics, dilution should be performed only in glass parenteral solution bottles. Nitroglycerin is also absorbed by polyvinyl chloride tubing; non–polyvinyl chloride intravenous administration sets should be used.

Patients with normal or low left ventricular filling pressure or pulmonary wedge pressure may be hypersensitive to the effects of nitroglycerin. Therefore, continuous monitoring of blood pressure, heart rate, and pulmonary capillary wedge pressure must be performed to assess the correct dose.

TABLE 55-37

Parenteral Drugs Used in the Treatment of Hypertensive Emergencies

DRUG	DOSAGE (MAXIMAL)	ONSET OF ACTION	PEAK EFFECT	DURATION OF ACTION
Direct-Acting Vasodilators				
Diazoxide	7.5-30 mg/min infusion or 1 mg/kg bolus q5-15 min (300 mg)	1-5 min	30 min	4-12 h
Hydralazine	0.5-1.0 mg/min infusion or 10-50 mg intramuscularly	1-5 min	10-80 min	3-6 h
Nitroglycerine	5-100 µg/min infusion	1-2 min	2-5 min	3-5 min
Nitroprusside	0.25-10 µg/kg/min infusion	Immediate	1-2 min	2-5 min
β_1-Adrenergic Antagonist				
Esmolol	250-500 µg/min × 1(loading dose), then 50-100 µg/kg/min × 4 (maintenance); maintenance dose may be increase to maximum 300 mg/kg/min	1-2 min	5 min	10-30 min
α_1- and β-Adrenergic Antagonist				
Labetalol	2 mg/min infusion or 0.25 mg/kg	5 min	10 min	3-6 h
Central α_2-Agonist				
Methyldopa	250-500 mg bolus every 6 hr (2 g)	2-3 h	3-5 h	6-12 h
Ganglionic Blockers				
Trimethaphan	0.5-10 mg/min infusion bolus over 2 min (300 mg)	Immediate	1-2 min	5-10 min
Angiotensin-Converting Enzyme Inhibitor				
Enalaprilat	0.625-5.0 mg bolus over 5 min q6h	5-15 min	1-4 h	6 h
Peripheral α-Adrenergic Antagonist				
Phentolamine	0.5-1.0 mg/min infusion or 2.5-5.0 mg bolus	Immediate	3-5 min	10-15 min
Calcium Antagonist				
Nicardipine	5-15 mg/h	5-10 min	45 min (~50%)	50 h
Dopamine D_1-Like Receptor Agent				
Fenoldopam	0.01-1.6 µg/min constant infusion	5-15 min	30 min	5-10 min

Intravenous nitroglycerin may be the drug of choice in the treatment of the patient with moderate hypertension associated with coronary ischemia because it provides collateral coronary vasodilation, a property not seen with the other direct-acting arteriolar vasodilators. The principal side effects are headache, nausea, and vomiting. Tolerance may develop with prolonged use.

β_1-Selective Adrenergic Antagonist

Esmolol hydrochloride is a short-acting β_1-selective adrenergic antagonist.[1004, 1005] Esmolol hydrochloride concentrate for injection must be diluted to a final concentration of 10 mg/mL. Extravasation of esmolol hydrochloride may cause serious local irritation and skin necrosis. Esmolol shares all of the toxic potential of the β_1-adrenergic antagonists previously discussed.

After intravenous injection of a loading dose of 250 to 500 mg/kg and then infusion of a maintenance dose ranging from 50 to 100 mg/kg/min, steady-state blood concentrations are achieved within 5 minutes (see Table 55-37). Efficacy should be assessed after the 1-minute loading dose and 4 minutes of maintenance infusion. If an adequate therapeutic effect is observed (as assessed by blood pressure and heart rate response), the maintenance infusion should be maintained. If an adequate therapeutic effect is not observed, the same loading dose can be repeated for 1 minute followed by an increased maintenance rate of infusion.

Esmolol has pharmacologic actions similar to those of other β_1-selective adrenergic antagonists; it produces negative chronotropic and inotropic activity. It has been used to prevent or treat hemodynamic changes induced by surgical events, including increases in systolic and diastolic blood pressure and double product heart rate times systolic blood pressure. Esmolol may be particularly useful for the treatment of postoperative hypertension and hypertension associated with coronary insufficiency.[991-996] Esmolol is hydrolyzed rapidly in blood, and negligible concentrations are present 30 minutes after discontinuance. Because the kidneys eliminate the deesterified metabolite of esmolol, the drug should be used cautiously in patients with renal insufficiency.

α_1- and β-Adrenergic Antagonists

The α_1- and β-adrenergic antagonist labetalol chloride may be given by either repeated intravenous injection or slow continuous infusion[991-998, 1006-1009] (see Table 55-37). The maximal blood pressure–lowering effect is within 5 minutes of the first injection. The drug should be administered to patients in the supine position to avoid symptomatic postural hypotension. The adverse side effects of labetalol have been discussed previously. It has been proved to be safe and useful in hypertensive urgencies and emergencies in pregnant women.[1010, 1011]

Central α₂-Adrenergic Agonist

Methyldopate hydrochloride is a central α_2-adrenergic agonist that may be administered intravenously as a bolus infusion (see Table 55-37). It has a delayed onset of action and peak effect, and its effect on blood pressure is unpredictable.[1012-1014] The adverse side effects of methyldopa have been discussed previously.

Ganglionic Blocking Agent

Trimethaphan camsylate is a ganglionic blocking agent; it blocks transmission of impulses at both sympathetic and parasympathetic ganglia by occupying receptor sites and by stabilizing the postsynaptic membranes against the action of acetylcholine liberated from presynaptic nerve endings.[1015] Peripheral vascular resistance is decreased, heart rate is usually increased, and cardiac output is decreased because of venous dilation and peripheral pooling of blood. Trimethaphan is used exclusively for the treatment of hypertensive emergencies.[991-996] It has an immediate onset of action when administered as a continuous infusion (see Table 55-37). The resulting dramatic reduction of blood pressure requires intra-arterial monitoring. The main disadvantage is that the drug must be administered with the patient supine to avoid profound postural hypotension. It has been shown to be useful for acute blood pressure reduction in patients with acute aortic dissection. Other disadvantages include (1) the potential for tachyphylaxis after sustained infusion (48 hours), (2) the appearance of side effects associated with parasympathetic and sympathetic blockade, and (3) histamine release.

Angiotensin-Converting Enzyme Inhibitor

Enalaprilat, the active metabolite of the oral ACE inhibitor enalapril, is administered as a slow intravenous infusion for 5 minutes (see Table 55-37) in an intravenous dose that is approximately one fourth of an oral dose. Onset of action occurs within 15 minutes, and the maximal effect is within 1 to 4 hours.[1016-1019] The duration of action is about 6 hours. Adverse effects of enalapril have been discussed previously. In patients with renal insufficiency, the initial dose should be no more than 0.625 mg.

α-Adrenergic Antagonist

Phentolamine mesylate is a nonselective α-adrenergic antagonist used primarily in the treatment of hypertension associated with pheochromocytoma.[790, 791] It has a rapid onset of action when administered intravenously as either a bolus or a continuous infusion (see Table 55-37). The duration of action is 10 to 15 minutes. It has a plasma half-life of 19 minutes; approximately 13% of a single dose appears in the urine as unchanged drug. Adverse effects include those associated with nonselective α-adrenergic blockade, as discussed previously.

Calcium Antagonists

Nicardipine hydrochloride, a dihydropyridine CA, is administered by slow continuous infusion at a concentration of 0.1 mg/mL; each 1-mL ampule (25 mg) should be diluted with 240 mL of a compatible intravenous fluid (not including sodium bicarbonate or lactated Ringer injection), resulting in 250 mL of solution at a concentration of 0.1 mg/mL. There is a dose-dependent decrease in blood pressure.[998, 1020-1022] Onset of action is within minutes; 50% of the ultimate decrease occurs in 45 minutes, but a final steady state does not occur for about 50 hours (see Table 55-7). Discontinuation of infusion is followed by a 50% offset of action in 30 minutes, but gradually decreasing antihypertensive effects exist for about 50 hours. Adverse effects of nicardipine have been discussed previously. It has been shown to be safe and effective in pediatric hypertensive emergencies.[998, 1020-1022]

Dopamine D₁-like Receptor Agonist

Fenoldopam mesylate, a dopamine D_1–like receptor agonist, is formulated as a solution to be diluted for intravenous infusion for acute hypertensive treatment.[1023-1025] It is a rapid-acting vasodilator by functioning as an agonist for dopamine D_1-like receptors and has moderate affinity for α_2-adrenoreceptors.[1026]

Fenoldopam is a racemic mixture in which the *R*-isomers are responsible for the biologic activity. It has vasodilatory effects on coronary, renal, mesenteric, and peripheral arteries in experimental studies; however, not all vascular beds respond uniformly. In humans, it has been shown to increase renal blood flow in both hypertensive and normotensive subjects.[1027, 1028]

It comes in 1-mL ampules that contain 10 mg of fenoldopam and is diluted for administration as a constant infusion at a rate of 0.01 to 1.6 mg/kg/min (see Table 55-37). It produces steady-state plasma concentrations proportional to its infusion rate. Elimination half-life is 5 minutes, and steady-state concentrations are reached within 20 minutes.[1027, 1028]

Clearance of the active compound is not altered by ESRD or hepatic disease. About 90% of infused fenoldopam is eliminated in urine and 10% in feces. Elimination is largely by conjugation, not involving cytochrome P-450 enzymes. There are no data on drug-drug interactions.

Side effects include reflex increase in heart rate, increase in intraocular pressure, headache, flushing, nausea, and hypotension.

Rapid-Acting Oral Drugs

A more gradual, progressive reduction in systemic blood pressure may be achieved after the oral administration of drugs having rapid absorption.[1029, 1030] These include (1) the α_1- and β-adrenergic antagonist labetalol, (2) the central α_2-adrenergic agonist clonidine,[1031-1033] (3) the CAs diltiazem and verapamil,[1034, 1035] (4) the ACE inhibitors captopril and enalapril, (5) the postsynaptic α_1-adrenergic antagonist prazosin,[1036] and (6) a combination of oral therapies. The doses and pharmacodynamic effects of rapid-acting oral drugs used commonly in the treatment of hypertensive emergencies are given in Table 55-38. Note that rapid-acting oral dihydropyridine CAs such as sublingual nifedipine are no longer recommended as they may cause large and

TABLE 55-38

Rapid-Acting Oral Drugs Used in the Treatment of Hypertensive Emergencies

DRUG	DOSAGE (MAXIMAL)	ONSET OF ACTION	PEAK EFFECT	DURATION OF ACTION
α_1- and β-Adrenergic Antagonist				
Labetalol	100-400 mg q12h (2400 mg)	1-2 h	2-4 h	8-12 h
Central α_2-Agonist				
Clonidine	0.2 mg initially, then 0.1 mg/h (0.8 mg)	30-60 min	2-4 h	6-8 h
Calcium Antagonist				
Diltiazem	30-120 mg q8h (480 mg)	<15 min	2-3 h	8 h
Verapamil	80-120 mg q8h (480 mg)	<60 min	2-3 h	8 h
Angiotensin-Converting Enzyme (ACE) Inhibitors				
Captopril	12.5-25 mg qh (150 mg)	<15 min	1 h	6-12 h
Enalapril	2.5-10 mg q6h (40 mg)	<60 min	4-8 h	12-24 h
α_1-Adrenergic Antagonist				
Prazosin	1-5 mg q2h (20 mg)	<60 min	2-4 h	6-12 h

unpredictable reductions in blood pressure with resultant ischemic events.[1037]

Clinical Considerations in the Acute Reduction of Blood Pressure

The acute reduction of blood pressure carries the risk of impairing blood supply to vital structures such as the brain and the heart. Consequently, every effort should be made to avoid excessive reduction of blood pressure. The risk of overreduction of blood pressure in a rapid fashion was evidenced in a review published by Grossman and colleagues[1037] linking the use of sublingual nifedipine capsules with stroke and heart attack in hypertensive subjects. Because this approach is variable and rapid, clinicians were unable to set a lower limit of blood pressure achieved with therapy.

Cerebral blood flow is normally carefully autoregulated such that sufficient perfusion is maintained during lower levels of blood pressure and perfusion is diminished during states of chronic hypertension to avoid cerebral edema.[1038-1040] With chronic hypertension, the short-term, rapid reduction of blood pressure may decrease cerebral blood flow sufficiently to precipitate ischemia and infarction.[1041-1043] This may be particularly important in patients with atherosclerotic disease of the cerebral blood vessels in whom there may be areas of uneven cerebral perfusion. Although drugs that do penetrate the blood-brain barrier, such as hydralazine, sodium nitroprusside, and nicardipine, dilate cerebral vessels and may lessen the likelihood of ischemia, intrinsic vascular disease may render some areas more ischemic than others with blood pressure reduction. In addition, potent cerebral vasodilators could conceivably cause a rise in intracranial pressure, creating the potential for cerebral edema and possible herniation.

Sudden drops in blood pressure can also interfere with coronary perfusion during diastole and result in myocardial ischemia, infarction, or arrhythmia.[1037, 1044, 1045] In addition, rapid reduction of blood pressure may result in a reflex increase in heart rate, which would also interfere with coronary perfusion during diastole. For these reasons, careful, cautious, and controlled reduction in blood pressure is necessary in these patients. For most hypertension emergencies, a parenteral drug such as sodium nitroprusside is ideal. However, if the patient has coronary disease, intravenous nitroglycerin or esmolol, or both, is a useful approach as they can induce coronary dilation or slow heart rate, respectively. Intravenous nicardipine could also be used as it facilitates coronary vasodilation. Patients with acute aortic dissection are best treated with a β-adrenergic antagonist plus nitroprusside or a ganglionic blocker such as trimethaphan. Patients with hypertensive encephalopathy or central nervous system hemorrhage may be best treated with drugs that do not cause cerebral vasodilation such a hydralazine, nitroprusside, nicardipine, or fenoldopam. Fenoldopam may be helpful in patients with kidney diseases, as it maintains renal blood flow.

REFERENCES

1. Gavras H, Brunner HR, Laragh JH, et al: An angiotensin converting-enzyme inhibitor to identify and treat vasoconstrictor and volume factors in hypertensive patients. N Engl J Med 291:817-821, 1974.
2. Johnston CI, Millar JA, McGrath BP, Matthews PG: Long-term effects of captopril (SQ14 225) on blood-pressure and hormone levels in essential hypertension. Lancet 2:493-496, 1979.
3. Fouad FM, Tarazi RC, Bravo EL, Textor SC: Hemodynamic and antihypertensive effects of the new oral angiotensin-converting-enzyme inhibitor MK-421 (enalapril). Hypertension 6:167-174, 1984.
4. Jackson B, Cubela R, Johnston C: Angiotensin converting enzyme (ACE), characterization by ^{125}I-MK351A binding studies of plasma and tissue ACE during variation of salt status in the rat. J Hypertens 4:759-765, 1986.
5. Fagard R, Amery A, Lijnen P, Reybrouck T: Haemodynamic effects of captopril in hypertensive patients: comparison with saralasin. Clin Sci (Lond) 57(suppl 5):131s-134s, 1979.
6. Ujhelyi MR, Ferguson RK, Vlasses PH: Angiotensin-converting enzyme inhibitors: Mechanistic controversies. Pharmacotherapy 9:351-362, 1989.
7. Pierdomenico SD, Bucci A, Lapenna D, et al: Heart rate in hypertensive patients treated with ACE inhibitors and long-acting dihydropyridine calcium antagonists. J Cardiovasc Pharmacol 40:288-295, 2002.
8. Bauer JH, Reams GP: Antihypertensive drugs. *In* Brenner BM (ed): The Kidney, 6th ed. Philadelphia, WB Saunders, 2000, pp 2253-2297.

9. Bao G, Gohlke P, Qadri F, Unger T: Chronic kinin receptor blockade attenuates the antihypertensive effect of ramipril. Hypertension 20: 74-79, 1992.

10. Quilley J, Duchin KL, Hudes EM, McGiff JC: The antihypertensive effect of captopril in essential hypertension: Relationship to prostaglandins and the kallikrein-kinin system. J Hypertens 5:121-128, 1987.

11. Hirooka Y, Imaizumi T, Masaki H, et al: Captopril improves impaired endothelium-dependent vasodilation in hypertensive patients. Hypertension 20:175-180, 1992.

12. O'Driscoll G, Green D, Maiorana A, et al: Improvement in endothelial function by angiotensin-converting enzyme inhibition in non–insulin-dependent diabetes mellitus. J Am Coll Cardiol 33:1506-1511, 1999.

13. Mombouli JV, Nephtali M, Vanhoutte PM: Effects of the converting enzyme inhibitor cilazaprilat on endothelium-dependent responses. Hypertension 18:II22-II29, 1991.

14. Nakamura M, Funakoshi T, Yoshida H, et al: Endothelium-dependent vasodilation is augmented by angiotensin converting enzyme inhibitors in healthy volunteers. J Cardiovasc Pharmacol 20:949-954, 1992.

15. Gavras H, Gavras I, Textor S, et al: Effect of angiotensin converting enzyme inhibition on blood pressure, plasma renin activity and plasma aldosterone in essential hypertension. J Clin Endocrinol Metab 46:220-226, 1978.

16. Romero JC, Ruilope LM, Bentley MD, et al: Comparison of the effects of calcium antagonists and converting enzyme inhibitors on renal function under normal and hypertensive conditions. Am J Cardiol 62:59G-68G, 1988.

17. Bauer JH, Reams GP: Renal effects of angiotensin converting enzyme inhibitors in hypertension. Am J Med 81:19-27, 1986.

18. Brunner HR, Waeber B, Nussberger J: Renal effects of converting enzyme inhibition. J Cardiovasc Pharmacol 9(suppl 3):S6-S14, 1987.

19. Eikenburg DC: Effects of captopril on vascular noradrenergic transmission in SHR. Hypertension 6:660-665, 1984.

20. Richer C, Doussau MP, Giudicelli JF: Influence of captopril and enalapril on regional vascular alpha-adrenergic receptor reactivity in SHR. Hypertension 6:666-674, 1984.

21. Antonaccio MJ, Kerwin L: Pre- and postjunctional inhibition of vascular sympathetic function by captopril in SHR. Implication of vascular angiotensin II in hypertension and antihypertensive actions of captopril. Hypertension 3:I54-I62, 1981.

22. Cline WH Jr: Enhanced in vivo responsiveness of presynaptic angiotensin II receptor–mediated facilitation of vascular adrenergic neurotransmission in spontaneously hypertensive rats. J Pharmacol Exp Ther 232:661-669, 1985.

23. Bonjour JP, Malvin RL: Stimulation of ADH release by the renin-angiotensin system. Am J Physiol 218:1555-1559, 1970.

24. Ferrario CM, Gildenberg PL, McCubbin JW: Cardiovascular effects of angiotensin mediated by the central nervous system. Circ Res 30:257-262, 1972.

25. Fukiyama K: Central action of angiotensin and hypertension—increased central vasomotor outflow by angiotensin. Jpn Circ J 36:599-602, 1972.

26. Philips M: Functions of angiotensin in the central nervous system. Annu Rev Physiol 49:413-435, 1987.

27. Unger T, Badoer E, Ganten D: Brain angiotensin: Pathways and pharmacology. Abstract. Circulation 77(suppl I):I40-I54, 1988.

28. Ganten D, Paul M, Lang RE: The role of neuropeptides in cardiovascular regulation. Cardiovasc Drugs Ther 5:119-130, 1991.

29. Hlubocka Z, Umnerova V, Heller S, et al: Circulating intercellular cell adhesion molecule-1, endothelin-1 and von Willebrand factor—Markers of endothelial dysfunction in uncomplicated essential hypertension: the effect of treatment with ACE inhibitors. J Hum Hypertens 16:557-562, 2002.

30. Yamamoto T, Shimizu M, Morioka M, et al: Role of angiotensin II in the pathogenesis of hyperdipsia in chronic renal failure. JAMA 256:604-608, 1986.

31. Salvetti A: Newer ACE inhibitors. A look at the future. Drugs 40:800-828, 1990.

32. Mizuno K, Hashimoto S, Kunii N, et al: Acute effects of the new oral angiotensin converting enzyme inhibitor 1-(D-3-acetylthio-2-methylpropanoyl)-L-prolyl-L-phenylalanine (Alacepril) in essential hypertension. Res Commun Chem Pathol Pharmacol 49:175-187, 1985.

33. Ogihara T, Nakamaru M, Higaki J, et al: Pharmacodynamics and pharmacokinetics of a new orally active angiotensin-I–converting enzyme inhibitor, alacepril (DU-1219), in normal subjects and hypertensive patients. Curr Ther Res 41:492-508, 1987.

34. Micromedex Health Care Series, Vol 114. Greenwood Village, Co, Thomson Micromedex, 2002.

35. Heel RC, Brogden RN, Speight TM, Avery GS: Captopril: A preliminary review of its pharmacological properties and therapeutic efficacy. Drugs 20:409-452, 1980.

36. Physicians' Desk Reference, 56th ed. Montvale, NJ, 2002.

37. Ader R, Chatterjee K, Ports T, et al: Immediate and sustained hemodynamic and clinical improvement in chronic heart failure by an oral angiotensin-converting enzyme inhibitor. Circulation 61:931-937, 1980.

38. Tarazi RC, Fouad FM, Ceimo JK, Bravo EL: Renin, aldosterone and cardiac decompensation: Studies with an oral converting enzyme inhibitor in heart failure. Am J Cardiol 44:1013-1018, 1979.

39. Salvetti A, Pedrinelli R, Magagna A, et al: Influence of food on acute and chronic effects of captopril in essential hypertensive patients. J Cardiovasc Pharmacol 7(suppl 1):S25-S29, 1985.

40. Sica DA, Gehr TW, Fernandez A: Risk-benefit ratio of angiotensin antagonists versus ACE inhibitors in end-stage renal disease. Drug Saf 22:350-360, 2000.

41. Fogari R, Zoppi A, Tettamanti F, et al: Evaluation by 24-hour ambulatory blood pressure monitoring of efficacy of benazepril 20 mg plus hydrochlorothiazide 25 mg fixed combination as compared to captopril 50 mg (corrected) plus hydrochlorothiazide 25 mg fixed combination in treating mild to moderate hypertension: A double-blind, within-patient, placebo-controlled study. J Cardiovasc Pharmacol 24:687-693, 1994.

42. Balfour JA, Goa KL: Benazepril. A review of its pharmacodynamic and pharmacokinetic properties, and therapeutic efficacy in hypertension and congestive heart failure. Drugs 42:511-539, 1991.

43. Shionoiri H, Ueda S, Minamisawa K, et al: Pharmacokinetics and pharmacodynamics of benazepril in hypertensive patients with normal and impaired renal function. J Cardiovasc Pharmacol 20:348-357, 1992.

44. Williams PE, Brown AN, Rajaguru S, et al: A pharmacokinetic study of cilazapril in elderly and young volunteers. Br J Clin Pharmacol 27(suppl 2):211S-215S, 1989.

45. Williams PE, Brown AN, Rajaguru S, et al: The pharmacokinetics and bioavailability of cilazapril in normal man. Br J Clin Pharmacol 27(suppl 2):181S-188S, 1989.

46. Kleinbloesem CH, van Brummelen P, Francis RJ: Clinical pharmacology of cilazapril. Am J Med 87:45S-49S, 1989.

47. Vandenburg MJ, Mackay EM, Dews I, et al: Dose finding studies with imidapril—A new ACE inhibitor. Br J Clin Pharmacol 37:265-272, 1994.

48. Harder S, Thurmann PA, Ungethum W: Single dose and steady state pharmacokinetics and pharmacodynamics of the ACE-inhibitor imidapril in hypertensive patients. Br J Clin Pharmacol 45:377-380, 1998.

49. Hosoya K, Ishimitsu T: Protection of the cardiovascular system by imidapril, a versatile angiotensin-converting enzyme inhibitor. Cardiovasc Drug Rev 20:93-110, 2002.

50. Kostis JB: Angiotensin-converting enzyme inhibitors. Emerging differences and new compounds. Abstract. Am J Hypertens 2:57-64, 1989.

51. Gomez HJ, Cirillo VJ, Moncloa F: The clinical pharmacology of lisinopril. J Cardiovasc Pharmacol 9(suppl 3):S27-S34, 1987.

52. Van Schaik BA, Geyskes GG, van der Wouw PA, et al: Pharmacokinetics of lisinopril in hypertensive patients with normal and impaired renal function. Eur J Clin Pharmacol 34:61-65, 1988.

53. Grass GM, Morehead WT: Evidence for site-specific absorption of a novel ACE inhibitor. Pharm Res 6:759-765, 1989.

54. Bussien JP, d'Amore TF, Perret L, et al: Single and repeated dosing of the converting enzyme inhibitor perindopril to normal subjects. Clin Pharmacol Ther 39:554-558, 1986.

55. Aronoff GR, Bernes JS, Brier ME: Drug Prescribing in Renal Failure: Dosing Guidelines for Adults. American College of Physicians, Philadelphia, 1999.

56. Blum RA, Olson SC, Kohli RK, et al: Pharmacokinetics of quinapril and its active metabolite, quinaprilat, in patients on chronic hemodialysis. J Clin Pharmacol 30:938-942, 1990.

57. Halstenson CE, Opsahl JA, Rachael K, et al: The pharmacokinetics of quinapril and its active metabolite, quinaprilat, in patients with various degrees of renal function. J Clin Pharmacol 32:344-350, 1992.

58. Kindler J, Schunkert H, Gassmann M, et al: Therapeutic efficacy and tolerance of ramipril in hypertensive patients with renal failure. J Cardiovasc Pharmacol 13(suppl 3):S55-S58, 1989.

59. Schunkert H, Kindler J, Gassmann M, et al: Pharmacokinetics of ramipril in hypertensive patients with renal insufficiency. Eur J Clin Pharmacol 37:249-256, 1989.

60. De Leeuw PW, Birkenhager WH: Short- and long-term effects of ramipril in hypertension. Am J Cardiol 59:79D-82D, 1987.

61. Shionoiri H, Miyakawa T, Yasuda G, et al: Pharmacokinetics of a single dose of ramipril in patients with renal dysfunction: Comparison with essential hypertension. J Cardiovasc Pharmacol 10(suppl 7): S145-S147, 1987.

62. Anonymous: Spirapril hydrochloride. In Phase III Drug Profiles 4: 16-24, 1994.

63. Schmidt J, Kraul H: Clinical experience with spirapril in human hypertension. J Cardiovasc Pharmacol 34(suppl 1):S25-S30, 1999.

64. Hayduk K, Kraul H: Efficacy and safety of spirapril in mild-to-moderate hypertension. J Cardiovasc Pharmacol 34(suppl 1):S19-S23, 1999.

65. Grass P, Gerbeau C, Kutz K: Spirapril: Pharmacokinetic properties and drug interactions. Blood Press Suppl 2:7-13, 1994.

66. Wiseman LR, McTavish D: Trandolapril. A review of its pharmaco-dynamic and pharmacokinetic properties, and therapeutic use in essential hypertension. Drugs 48:71-90, 1994.

67. Peters DC, Noble S, Plosker GL: Trandolapril. An update of its pharmacology and therapeutic use in cardiovascular disorders. Drugs 56: 871-893, 1998.

68. Borghi C, Ambrosioni E, Magnani B: Effects of the early administration of zofenopril on onset and progression of congestive heart failure in patients with anterior wall acute myocardial infarction. The SMILE Study Investigators. Survival of Myocardial Infarction Long-term Evaluation. Am J Cardiol 78:317-322, 1996.

69. DeForrest JM, Waldron TL, Krapcho J, et al: Preclinical pharmacology of zofenopril, an inhibitor of angiotensin I converting enzyme. J Cardiovasc Pharmacol 13:887-894, 1989.

70. Cleophas TJ, vanMaurum R, van der Wall EF: Properties of the ACE inhibitor zofenopril. Perfusions 15:38-43, 2002.

71. Duchin KL, Waclawski AP, Tu JI, et al: Pharmacokinetics, safety, and pharmacologic effects of fosinopril sodium, an angiotensin-converting enzyme inhibitor in healthy subjects. J Clin Pharmacol 31:58-64, 1991.

72. Hui KK, Duchin KL, Kripalani KJ, et al: Pharmacokinetics of fosino-pril in patients with various degrees of renal function. Clin Pharmacol Ther 49:457-467, 1991.

73. Guthrie R: Fosinopril: An overview. Am J Cardiol 72:22H-24H, 1993.

74. Sica DA, Cutler RE, Parmer RJ, Ford NF: Comparison of the steady-state pharmacokinetics of fosinopril, lisinopril and enalapril in patients with chronic renal insufficiency. Clin Pharmacokinet 20: 420-427, 1991.

75. Hall JE: Angiotensin converting enzymes inhibition: Renal effects and their role in reducing arterial pressure. In MacGregor GA, Sever PS (eds): Current Advances in ACE Inhibition. London, Churchill Livingstone, 1989.

76. Atlas SA, Case DB, Sealey JE, et al: Interruption of the renin-angiotensin system in hypertensive patients by captopril induces sus-tained reduction in aldosterone secretion, potassium retention and natriuresis. Hypertension 1:274-280, 1979.

77. Hollenberg NK, Swartz SL, Passan DR, Williams GH: Increased glomerular filtration rate after converting-enzyme inhibition in essen-tial hypertension. N Engl J Med 301:9-12, 1979.

78. Hollenberg NK, Meggs LG, Williams GH, et al: Sodium intake and renal responses to captopril in normal man and in essential hyperten-sion. Kidney Int 20:240-245, 1981.

79. Larochelle P, Gutkowska J, Schiffrin E, et al: Effect of enalapril on renin, angiotensin converting enzyme activity, aldosterone and prostaglandins in patients with hypertension. Clin Invest Med 8:197-201, 1985.

80. Reams GP, Bauer JH, Gaddy P: Use of the converting enzyme inhibitor enalapril in renovascular hypertension. Effect on blood pres-sure, renal function, and the renin-angiotensin-aldosterone system. Hypertension 8:290-297, 1986.

81. Mooser V, Nussberger J, Juillerat L, et al: Reactive hyperreninemia is a major determinant of plasma angiotensin II during ACE inhibition. J Cardiovasc Pharmacol 15:276-282, 1990.

82. Campbell DJ: Bioactive angiotensin peptides other than angiotensin II. In Epstein M, Brunner H (eds): Angiotensin II Receptor Antagonists. Philadelphia, Hanley & Belfus, 2001, pp 9-27.

83. de Cavanagh EM, Inserra F, Toblli J, et al: Enalapril attenuates oxida-tive stress in diabetic rats. Hypertension 38:1130-1136, 2001.

84. Liu X, Engelman RM, Rousou JA, et al: Attenuation of myocardial reperfusion injury by sulfhydryl-containing angiotensin converting enzyme inhibitors. Cardiovasc Drugs Ther 6:437-443, 1992.

85. Gansewoort RT, de Zeeuw D, de Jong PE: Is the antiproteinuric effect of ACE inhibition mediated by interference in the renin-angiotensin system? Kidney Int 45:861-867, 1994.

86. Kasiske BL, Kalil RS, Ma JZ, et al: Effect of antihypertensive ther-apy on the kidney in patients with diabetes: A meta-regression analy-sis. Ann Intern Med 118:129-138, 1993.

87. ter Wee PM, Epstein M: Angiotensin-converting enzyme inhibitors and progression of nondiabetic chronic renal disease. Arch Intern Med 153:1749-1759, 1993.

88. Bauer JH, Reams GP, Hewett J, et al: A randomized, double-blind, placebo-controlled trial to evaluate the effect of enalapril in patients with clinical diabetic nephropathy. Am J Kidney Dis 20:443-457, 1992.

89. Heeg JE, de Jong PE, van der Hem GK, de Zeeuw D: Reduction of proteinuria by angiotensin converting enzyme inhibition. Kidney Int 32:78-83, 1987.

90. Heeg JE, de Jong PE, van der Hem GK, de Zeeuw D: Efficacy and variability of the antiproteinuric effect of ACE inhibition by lisino-pril. Kidney Int 36:272-279, 1989.

91. Gansevoort RT, de Zeeuw D, de Jong PE: Dissociation between the course of the hemodynamic and antiproteinuric effects of angiotensin I converting enzyme inhibition. Kidney Int 44:579-584, 1993.

92. Heeg JE, de Jong PE, van der Hem GK, de Zeeuw D: Angiotensin II does not acutely reverse the reduction of proteinuria by long-term ACE inhibition. Kidney Int 40:734-741, 1991.

93. Leoncini G, Martinoli C, Viazzi F, et al: Changes in renal resistive index and urinary albumin excretion in hypertensive patients under long-term treatment with lisinopril or nifedipine GITS. Nephron 90:169-173, 2002.

94. Herlitz H, Edeno C, Mulec H, et al: Captopril treatment of hyper-tension and renal failure in systemic lupus erythematosus. Nephron 38:253-256, 1984.

95. Hommel E, Parving HH, Mathiesen E, et al: Effect of captopril on kidney function in insulin-dependent diabetic patients with nephropathy. Br Med J (Clin Res Ed) 293:467-470, 1986.

96. Reams GP, Bauer JH: Effect of enalapril in subjects with hyperten-sion associated with moderate to severe renal dysfunction. Arch Intern Med 146:2145-2148, 1986.

97. Lagrue G, Robeva R, Laurent J: Antiproteinuric effect of captopril in primary glomerular disease. Nephron 46:99-100, 1987.

98. Navis G, de Jong PE, Donker AJ, et al: Moderate sodium restriction in hypertensive subjects: Renal effects of ACE-inhibition. Kidney Int 31:815-819, 1987.

99. Apperloo AJ, de Zeeuw D, de Jong PE: A short-term antihyperten-sive treatment–induced fall in glomerular filtration rate predicts long-term stability of renal function. Kidney Int 51:793-797, 1997.

100. de Zeeuw D, Heeg JE, Stelwagen T, et al: Mechanism of the antipro-teinuric effect of angiotensin-converting enzyme inhibition. Contrib Nephrol 83:160-165, 1990.

101. Ferrari P, Marti HP, Pfister M, Frey FJ: Additive antiproteinuric effect of combined ACE inhibition and angiotensin II receptor blockade. J Hypertens 20:125-130, 2002.

102. Agodoa LY, Appel L, Bakris GL, et al: Effect of ramipril vs amlodip-ine on renal outcomes in hypertensive nephrosclerosis: A random-ized controlled trial. JAMA 285:2719-2728, 2001.

103. Sakemi T, Baba N: Effects of antihypertensive drugs on the progression of renal failure in hyperlipidemic Imai rats. Nephron 63:323-329, 1993.

104. Keilani T, Schlueter WA, Levin ML, Batlle DC: Improvement of lipid abnormalities associated with proteinuria using fosinopril, an angiotensin-converting enzyme inhibitor. Ann Intern Med 118: 246-254, 1993.

105. Hoorntje SJ, Kallenberg CG, Weening JJ, et al: Immune-complex glomerulopathy in patients treated with captopril. Lancet 1: 1212-1215, 1980.

106. Case DB, Atlas SA, Mouradian JA, et al: Proteinuria during long-term captopril therapy. JAMA 244:346-349, 1980.

107. Sunderrajan S, Luger A, Bauer JH: Captopril-induced membranous glomerulopathy. South Med J 76:1294-1296, 1983.

108. Textor SC, Gephardt GN, Bravo EL, et al: Membranous glomerulopa-thy associated with captopril therapy. Am J Med 74:705-712, 1983.

109. Bauer JH, Reams GP: The effects of antihypertensive therapy on renal function. In Kaplan NM, Brenner BM, Laragh JN (eds): Perspectives on Hypertension, Vol 3, New Therapeutic Strategies for Hypertension. New York, Raven Press, 1989, pp 253-287.

110. Bauer JH, Reams GP: Renal protection in essential hypertension: How do angiotensin-converting enzyme inhibitors compare with calcium antagonists? J Am Soc Nephrol 1:580-587, 1990.

111. Ichihara A, Inscho EW, Imig JD, et al: Role of renal nerves in afferent arteriolar reactivity in angiotensin-induced hypertension. Hypertension 29:442-449, 1997.

112. Mackie FE, Meyer TW, Campbell DJ: Effects of antihypertensive therapy on intrarenal angiotensin and bradykinin levels in experimental renal insufficiency. Kidney Int 61:555-563, 2002.

113. Guidi E, Minetti EE, Cozzi MG: Acute and long-term effects of ACE inhibition on renal haemodynamics in glomerular and interstitial nephropathies. J Renin Angiotensin Aldosterone Syst 3:40-45, 2002.

114. Doucet J, Richard V, Mulder P, et al: Effects of combination of low doses of angiotensin-converting enzyme inhibitor and diuretics on renal function in spontaneously hypertensive rats: Comparison between acute and chronic treatment. J Renin Angiotensin Aldosterone Syst 2:107-111, 2001.

115. Simon G, Morioka S, Snyder DK, Cohn JN: Increased renal plasma flow in long-term enalapril treatment of hypertension. Clin Pharmacol Ther 34:459-465, 1983.

116. Reams GP, Bauer JH: Long-term effects of enalapril monotherapy and enalapril/hydrochlorothiazide combination therapy on blood pressure, renal function, and body fluid composition. J Clin Hypertens 2:55-63, 1986.

117. Lewis EJ, Hunsicker LG, Bain RP, Rohde RD: The effect of angiotensin-converting-enzyme inhibition on diabetic nephropathy. The Collaborative Study Group. N Engl J Med 329:1456-1462, 1993.

118. Hollenberg NK, Moore T, Shoback D, et al: Abnormal renal sodium handling in essential hypertension. Relation to failure of renal and adrenal modulation of responses to angiotensin II. Am J Med 81:412-418, 1986.

119. Hollenberg NK, Williams GH: Sensitivity to sodium and nonmodulation of renal and adrenal responsiveness to angiotensin II: Implications for the pathogenesis of essential hypertension. *In* Zanchetti A, Tarazi R (eds): Handbook of Hypertension, Vol 8. New York, Elsevier, 1986, pp 520-552.

120. Dluhy RG, Smith K, Taylor T, et al: Prolonged converting enzyme-inhibition in non-modulating hypertension. Hypertension 13:371-377, 1989.

121. Hricik DE: Captopril-induced renal insufficiency and the role of sodium balance. Ann Intern Med 103:222-223, 1985.

122. Curtis JJ, Luke RG, Whelchel JD, et al: Inhibition of angiotensin-converting enzyme in renal-transplant recipients with hypertension. N Engl J Med 308:377-381, 1983.

123. Murphy BF, Whitworth JA, Kincaid-Smith P: Renal insufficiency with combinations of angiotensin converting enzyme inhibitors and diuretics. Br Med J (Clin Res Ed) 288:844-845, 1984.

124. Wenting GJ, Tan-Tjiong HL, Derkx FH, et al: Splint renal function after captopril in unilateral renal artery stenosis. Br Med J (Clin Res Ed) 288:886-890, 1984.

125. Bender W, La France N, Walker WG: Mechanism of deterioration in renal function in patients with renovascular hypertension treated with enalapril. Hypertension 6:I193-I197, 1984.

126. Jackson B, McGrath BP, Matthews PG, et al: Differential renal function during angiotensin converting enzyme inhibition in renovascular hypertension. Hypertension 8:650-654, 1986.

127. Levenson DJ, Dzau VJ: Effects on angiotensin-converting enzyme inhibition on renal hemodynamics in renal artery stenosis. Kidney Int Suppl 20:S173-S179, 1987.

128. Muller FM, Sealy JE, Case DB, et al: The captopril test for identifying renovascular disease in hypertensive patients. Am J Med 80:633-644, 1986.

129. Hricik DE, Dunn MJ: Angiotensin-converting enzyme inhibitor–induced renal failure: Causes, consequences, and diagnostic uses. J Am Soc Nephrol 1:845-858, 1990.

130. Hricik DE, Browning PJ, Kopelman R, et al: Captopril-induced functional renal insufficiency in patients with bilateral renal-artery stenoses or renal-artery stenosis in a solitary kidney. N Engl J Med 308:373-376, 1983.

131. Sixth Report of the Joint National Committee on Prevention, Detection, Evaluation, and Treatment of High Blood Pressure (JNC VI). Arch Intern Med 158:2413-2113, 1997.

132. Lin J, Valeri AM, Markowitz GS, et al: Angiotensin converting enzyme inhibition in chronic allograft nephropathy. Transplantation 73:783-788, 2002.

133. Midtvedt K, Hartmann A, Foss A, et al: Sustained improvement of renal graft function for two years in hypertensive renal transplant recipients treated with nifedipine as compared to lisinopril. Transplantation 72:1787-1792, 2001.

134. Midtvedt K, Hartmann A, Holdaas H, Fauchald P: Efficacy of nifedipine or lisinopril in the treatment of hypertension after renal transplantation: A double-blind randomised comparative trial. Clin Transplant 15:426-431, 2001.

135. Hsu CY, Bates DW, Kuperman GJ, Curhan GC: Blood pressure and angiotensin converting enzyme inhibitor use in hypertensive patients with chronic renal insufficiency. Am J Hypertens 14:1219-1225, 2001.

136. Materson BJ: Adverse effects of angiotensin-converting enzyme inhibitors in antihypertensive therapy with focus on quinapril. Am J Cardiol 69:46C-53C, 1992.

137. Weir MR, Smith DH, Neutel JM, Bedigian MP: Valsartan alone or with a diuretic or ACE inhibitor as treatment for African American hypertensives: Relation to salt intake. Am J Hypertens 14:665-671, 2001.

138. Weinberger MH: Comparison of captopril and hydrochlorothiazide alone and in combination in mild to moderate essential hypertension. Br J Clin Pharmacol 14(suppl 2):127S-131S, 1982.

139. Vlasses PH, Rotmensch HH, Swanson BN, et al: Comparative antihypertensive effects of enalapril maleate and hydrochlorothiazide, alone and in combination. J Clin Pharmacol 23:227-233, 1983.

140. Townsend RR, Holland OB: Combination of converting enzyme inhibitor with diuretic for the treatment of hypertension. Arch Intern Med 150:1175-1183, 1990.

141. Holland OB, von Kuhnert L, Campbell WB, Anderson RJ: Synergistic effect of captopril with hydrochlorothiazide for the treatment of low-renin hypertensive black patients. Hypertension 5:235-239, 1983.

142. Mayer G: ACE genotype and ACE inhibitor response in kidney disease: A perspective. Am J Kidney Dis 40:227-235, 2002.

143. Ambrosioni E, Borghi C, Magnani B: The effect of the angiotensin-converting-enzyme inhibitor zofenopril on mortality and morbidity after anterior myocardial infarction. The Survival of Myocardial Infarction Long-Term Evaluation (SMILE) Study Investigators. N Engl J Med 332:80-85, 1995.

144. De Rosa ML, Cardace P, Rossi M, et al: Comparative effects of chronic ACE inhibition and AT1 receptor blocked losartan on cardiac hypertrophy and renal function in hypertensive patients. J Hum Hypertens 16:133-140, 2002.

145. Garg J, Bakris GL: Angiotensin converting enzyme inhibitors or angiotensin receptor blockers in nephropathy from type 2 diabetes. Curr Hypertens Rep 4:185-190, 2002.

146. Lonn E: Angiotensin-converting enzyme inhibitors and angiotensin receptor blockers in atherosclerosis. Curr Atheroscler Rep 4:363-372, 2002.

147. Assessment of perindopril's efficacy on arterial distensibility in mild to moderate hypertension. J Med Assoc Thai 84:1006-1014, 2001.

148. Zhuo JL, Mendelsohn FA, Ohishi M: Perindopril alters vascular angiotensin-converting enzyme, AT(1) receptor, and nitric oxide synthase expression in patients with coronary heart disease. Hypertension 39:634-638, 2002.

149. Emanueli C, Salis MB, Stacca T, et al: Ramipril improves hemodynamic recovery but not microvascular response to ischemia in spontaneously hypertensive rats. Am J Hypertens 15:410-415, 2002.

150. Culy CR, Jarvis B: Quinapril: A further update of its pharmacology and therapeutic use in cardiovascular disorders. Drugs 62:339-385, 2002.

151. Guasti L, Zanotta D, Diolisi A, et al: Changes in pain perception during treatment with angiotensin converting enzyme-inhibitors and angiotensin II type 1 receptor blockade. J Hypertens 20:485-491, 2002.

152. Gradzki R, Dhingra RK, Port FK, et al: Use of ACE inhibitors is associated with prolonged survival of arteriovenous grafts. Am J Kidney Dis 38:1240-1244, 2001.

153. Burrows RF, Burrows EA: Assessing the teratogenic potential of angiotensin-converting enzyme inhibitors in pregnancy. Aust NZ J Obstet Gynaecol 38:306-311, 1998.

154. Cunniff C, Jones KL, Phillipson J, et al: Oligohydramnios sequence and renal tubular malformation associated with maternal enalapril use. Am J Obstet Gynecol 162:187-189, 1990.

155. Friis S, Sorensen HT, Mellemkjaer L, et al: Angiotensin-converting enzyme inhibitors and the risk of cancer: A population-based cohort study in Denmark. Cancer 92:2462-2470, 2001.

156. Manzato E, Capurso A, Crepaldi G: Modification of cardiovascular risk factors during antihypertensive treatment: A multicentre trial with quinapril. J Int Med Res 21:15-25, 1993.

157. Pahor M, Franse LV, Deitcher SR, et al: Fosinopril versus amlodipine comparative treatments study: A randomized trial to assess effects on plasminogen activator inhibitor-1. Circulation 105:457-461, 2002.

158. Pollare T, Lithell H, Berne C: A comparison of the effects of hydrochlorothiazide and captopril on glucose and lipid metabolism in patients with hypertension. N Engl J Med 321:868-873, 1989.

159. Santoro D, Natali A, Palombo C, et al: Effects of chronic angiotensin converting enzyme inhibition on glucose tolerance and insulin sensitivity in essential hypertension. Hypertension 20:181-191, 1992.

160. Ortlepp JR, Breuer J, Eitner F, et al: Inhibition of the renin-angiotensin system ameliorates genetically determined hyperinsulinemia. Eur J Pharmacol 436:145-150, 2002.

161. Morice AH, Lowry R, Brown MJ, Higenbottam T: Angiotensin-converting enzyme and the cough reflex. Lancet 2:1116-1118, 1987.

162. Israili ZH, Hall WD: Cough and angioneurotic edema associated with angiotensin-converting enzyme inhibitor therapy. A review of the literature and pathophysiology. Ann Intern Med 117:234-242, 1992.

163. Gavras H, Gavras I: Angiotensin converting enzyme inhibitors. Properties and side effects. Hypertension 11:II37-II41, 1988.

164. Gavras I: Bradykinin-mediated effects of ACE inhibition. Kidney Int 42:1020-1029, 1992.

165. Yeo WW, Maclean D, Richardson PJ, Ramsay LE: Cough and enalapril: Assessment by spontaneous reporting and visual analogue scale under double-blind conditions. Br J Clin Pharmacol 31:356-359, 1991.

166. Reisin L, Schneeweiss A: Spontaneous disappearance of cough induced by angiotensin-converting enzyme inhibitors (captopril or enalapril). Am J Cardiol 70:398-399, 1992.

167. Overlack A: ACE inhibitor–induced cough and bronchospasm. Incidence, mechanisms and management. Drug Saf 15:72-78, 1996.

168. Fogari R, Zoppi A, Tettamanti F, et al: Effects of nifedipine and indomethacin on cough induced by angiotensin-converting enzyme inhibitors: A double-blind, randomized, cross-over study. J Cardiovasc Pharmacol 19:670-673, 1992.

169. Keogh A: Sodium cromoglycate prophylaxis for angiotensin-converting enzyme inhibitor cough. Lancet 341:560, 1993.

170. Chu TJ, Chow N: Adverse effects of ACE inhibitors. Ann Intern Med 118:314, 1993.

171. Adam A, Cugno M, Molinaro G, et al: Aminopeptidase P in individuals with a history of angio-oedema on ACE inhibitors. Lancet 359:2088-2089, 2002.

172. Hedner T, Samuelsson O, Lunde H, et al: Angio-oedema in relation to treatment with angiotensin converting enzyme inhibitors. BMJ 304:941-946, 1992.

173. Lefebvre J, Murphey LJ, Hartert TV, et al: Dipeptidyl peptidase IV activity in patients with ACE-inhibitor–associated angioedema. Hypertension 39:460-464, 2002.

174. Karim MY, Masood A: Fresh-frozen plasma as a treatment for life-threatening ACE-inhibitor angioedema. J Allergy Clin Immunol 109:370-371, 2002.

175. Sedman AJ, Posvar E: Clinical pharmacology of quinapril in healthy volunteers and in patients with hypertension and congestive heart failure. Angiology 40:360-369, 1989.

176. McMurray J, Matthews DM: Consequences of fluid loss in patients treated with ACE inhibitors. Postgrad Med J 63:385-387, 1987.

177. Kantola I, Terent A, Kataja M, Breig-Asberg E: ACE-inhibitor therapy with spirapril increases nocturnal hypotensive episodes in elderly hypertensive patients. J Hum Hypertens 15:873-878, 2001.

178. Williams LS, Hill D, Davis J, Lowenthal DT: Effects of fosinopril or sustained-release verapamil on blood pressure and serum catecholamine concentrations in elderly hypertensive men. Am J Ther 7:3-9, 2000.

179. Verresen L, Waer M, Vanrenterghem Y, Michielsen P: Angiotensin-converting-enzyme inhibitors and anaphylactoid reactions to high-flux membrane dialysis. Lancet 336:1360-1362, 1990.

180. el Makri A, Larabi MS, Kechrid C, et al: Fatal bone-marrow suppression associated with captopril. Br Med J (Clin Res Ed) 283:277-278, 1981.

181. Tielemans C, Madhoun P, Lenaers M, et al: Anaphylactoid reactions during hemodialysis on AN69 membranes in patients receiving ACE inhibitors. Kidney Int 38:982-984, 1990.

182. Brunet P, Jaber K, Berland Y, Baz M: Anaphylactoid reactions during hemodialysis and hemofiltration: Role of associating AN69 membrane and angiotensin I-converting enzyme inhibitors. Am J Kidney Dis 19:444-447, 1992.

183. Nawarskas JJ, Spinler SA: Update on the interaction between aspirin and angiotensin-converting enzyme inhibitors. Pharmacotherapy 20:698-710, 2000.

184. Zanchetti A, Hansson L, Leonetti G, et al: Low-dose aspirin does not interfere with the blood pressure–lowering effects of antihypertensive therapy. J Hypertens 20:1015-1022, 2002.

185. Ahmed A: Interaction between aspirin and angiotensin-converting enzyme inhibitors: Should they be used together in older adults with heart failure? J Am Geriatr Soc 50:1293-1296, 2002.

186. Le Meur Y, Lorgeot V, Comte L, et al: Plasma levels and metabolism of AcSDKP in patients with chronic renal failure: Relationship with erythropoietin requirements. Am J Kidney Dis 38:510-517, 2001.

187. Hayashi K, Hasegawa K, Kobayashi S: Effects of angiotensin-converting enzyme inhibitors on the treatment of anemia with erythropoietin. Kidney Int 60:1910-1916, 2001.

188. Remuzzi G, Perico N: Routine renin-angiotensin system blockade in renal transplantation? Curr Opin Nephrol Hypertens 11:1-10, 2002.

189. Campbell DJ: Circulating and tissue angiotensin systems. J Clin Invest 79:1-6, 1987.

190. Dzau VJ: Circulating versus local renin-angiotensin system in cardiovascular homeostasis. Circulation 77:I4-I13, 1988.

191. Johnson CI: Renin-angiotensin system: A dual tissue and hormonal system for cardiovascular control. J Hypertens 10:S13-S26, 1992.

192. Urata H, Nishimura H, Ganten D, et al: Angiotensin converting enzyme independent pathways of angiotensin II formation in human tissues and cardiovascular diseases. Blood Press Suppl 2:22-28, 1996.

193. Urata H, Nishimura H, Gamten D: Mechanisms of angiotensin II formation in humans. Eur Heart J 16:79-85, 1995.

194. Hollenberg MK, Fisher ND, Price DA: Pathways for angiotensin II generation in intact human tissue: Evidence from comparative pharmacologic interruption of the renin system. Hypertension 32:387-392, 1998.

195. Timmermans PB, Wong PC, Chui AT: Angiotensin II receptors and angiotensin receptor antagonists. Pharmacol Rev 45:205-251, 1993.

196. Bauer JH, Reams GP: The angiotensin II type 1 receptor antagonists. A new class of antihypertensive drugs. Arch Intern Med 155:1361-1368, 1995.

197. Wexler RR, Greenlee WJ, Irvin JD, et al: Nonpeptide angiotensin II receptor antagonists: the next generation in antihypertensive therapy. J Med Chem 39:625-656, 1996.

198. Fridman K, Andersson OK, Wysocki M, et al: Acute effects of candesartan cilexetil (the new angiotensin II antagonist) on systemic and renal haemodynamics in hypertensive patients. Eur J Clin Pharmacol 54:497-501, 1998.

199. Cogan MG: Angiotensin II: A powerful controller of sodium transport in the early proximal tubule. Hypertension 15:451-458, 1990.

200. Cervenka L, Wang CT, Mitchell KD, Navar LG: Proximal tubular angiotensin II levels and renal functional responses to AT1 receptor blockade in nonclipped kidneys of Goldblatt hypertensive rats. Hypertension 33:102-107, 1999.

201. Schiffrin EL: Vascular changes in hypertension in response to drug treatment: Effects of angiotensin receptor blockers. Can J Cardiol 18(suppl A):15A-18A, 2002.

202. Hughes J, Roth RH: Evidence that angiotensin enhances transmitter release during sympathetic nerve stimulation. Br J Pharmacol 41:239-255, 1971.

203. Imai Y, Abe K, Seino M, et al: Captopril attenuates pressor responses to norepinephrine and vasopressin through depletion of endogenous angiotensin II. Am J Cardiol 49:1537-1539, 1982.

204. Esler M: Differentiation in the effects of the angiotensin II receptor blocker class on autonomic function. J Hypertens 20(suppl 5):S13-S19, 2002.

205. Balt JC, Mathy MJ, Nap A, et al: Effect of the AT1-receptor antagonists losartan, irbesartan, and telmisartan on angiotensin II–induced facilitation of sympathetic neurotransmission in the rat mesenteric artery. J Cardiovasc Pharmacol 38:141-148, 2001.

206. Thrasher TN: Circumventricular organs, thirst and vasopressin secretion. In Schrier RW (ed): Vasopressin. New York, Raven Press, 1985, pp 311-318.

207. Zhang J, Leenen FH: Peripheral administration of AT1 receptor blockers and pressor responses to central angiotensin II and sodium. Can J Physiol Pharmacol 79:861-867, 2001.

208. Zhang J, Leenen FH: AT(1) receptor blockers prevent sympathetic hyperactivity and hypertension by chronic ouabain and hypertonic saline. Am J Physiol 280:H1318-H1323, 2001.

209. Heesch CM, Crandall ME, Turbek JA: Converting enzyme inhibitors cause pressure-independent resetting of baroreflex control of sympathetic outflow. Am J Physiol 270:R728-R737, 1996.

210. Phillips PA, Rolls BJ, Ledingham JG: Angiotensin-II induced thirst and vasopressin release in man. Clin Sci 68:669-674, 1995.

211. Robinson MM, Evered MD: Pressor action of intravenous angiotensin II reduces drinking response in rats. Am J Physiol 252:R754-R759, 1987.

212. Rogers PW, Kurtzman NA: Renal failure, uncontrollable thirst, and hyperreninemia. Cessation of thirst with bilateral nephrectomy. JAMA 225:1236-1238, 1973.

213. Rossi GP, Sacchetto A, Cesari M, Pessina AC: Interactions between endothelin-1 and the renin-angiotensin-aldosterone system. Cardiovasc Res 43:300-307, 1999.

214. Siragy HM, de Gasparo M, El Kersh M, Carey RM: Angiotensin-converting enzyme inhibition potentiates angiotensin II type 1 receptor effects on renal bradykinin and cGMP. Hypertension 38:183-186, 2001.

215. Carey RM, Howell NL, Jin XH, Siragy HM: Angiotensin type 2 receptor–mediated hypotension in angiotensin type-1 receptor–blocked rats. Hypertension 38:1272-1277, 2001.

216. Shibasaki Y, Mori Y, Tsutumi Y, et al: Differential kinetics of circulating angiotensin IV and II after treatment with angiotensin II type 1 receptor antagonist and their plasma levels in patients with chronic renal failure. Clin Nephrol 51:83-91, 1999.

217. Chappell MC, Pirro NT, Sykes A, Ferrario CM: Metabolism of angiotensin-(1-7) by angiotensin-converting enzyme. Hypertension 31:362-367, 1998.

218. Menard J, Campbell DJ, Azizi M, Gonzales MF: Synergistic effects of ACE inhibition and Ang II antagonism on blood pressure, cardiac weight, and renin in spontaneously hypertensive rats. Circulation 96:3072-3078, 1997.

219. Campbell DJ, Kladis A, Valentijn AJ: Effects of losartan on angiotensin and bradykinin peptides and angiotensin-converting enzyme. J Cardiovasc Pharmacol 26:233-240, 1995.

220. Ferrario CM: Angiotensin I, angiotensin II and their biologically active peptides. J Hypertens 20:805-807, 2002.

221. Kono T, Oseko F, Shimpo S, et al: Biological activity of des-asp1-angiotensin II (angiotensin III) in man. J Clin Endocrinol Metab 41:1174-1177, 1975.

222. Blair-West JR, Coghlan JP, Denton DA, et al: The effect of the heptapeptide (2-8) and hexapeptide (3-8) fragments of angiotensin II on aldosterone secretion. J Clin Endocrinol Metab 32:575-578, 1971.

223. Patel JM, Martens JR, Li YD, et al: Angiotensin IV receptor–mediated activation of lung endothelial NOS is associated with vasorelaxation. Am J Physiol 275:L1061-L1068, 1998.

224. Coleman JK, Krebs LT, Hamilton TA, et al: Autoradiographic identification of kidney angiotensin IV binding sites and angiotensin IV–induced renal cortical blood flow changes in rats. Peptides 19:269-277, 1998.

225. Champion HC, Czapla MA, Kadowitz PJ: Responses to angiotensin peptides are mediated by AT1 receptors in the rat. Am J Physiol 274:E115-E123, 1998.

226. Brosnihan KB, Li P, Tallant EA, Ferrario CM: Angiotensin-(1-7): A novel vasodilator of the coronary circulation. Biol Res 31:227-234, 1998.

227. Simoes-e-Silva AC, Baracho NC, Passaglio KT, Santos RA: Renal actions of angiotensin-(1-7). Braz J Med Biol Res 30:503-513, 1997.

228. Fontes MA, Silva LC, Campagnole-Santos MJ, et al: Evidence that angiotensin-(1-7) plays a role in the central control of blood pressure at the ventro-lateral medulla acting through specific receptors. Brain Res 665:175-180, 1994.

229. Paula RD, Lima CV, Khosla MC, Santos RA: Angiotensin-(1-7) potentiates the hypotensive effect of bradykinin in conscious rats. Hypertension 26:1154-1159, 1995.

230. Li P, Chappell MC, Ferrario CM, Brosnihan KB: Angiotensin-(1-7) augments bradykinin-induced vasodilation by competing with ACE and releasing nitric oxide. Hypertension 29:394-400, 1997.

231. Robertson MJ, Barnes JC, Drew GM, et al: Pharmacological profile of GR117289 in vitro: A novel, potent and specific non-peptide angiotensin AT1 receptor antagonist. Br J Pharmacol 107:1173-1180, 1992.

232. Wienen W, Hauel N, van Meel JC, et al: Pharmacological characterization of the novel nonpeptide angiotensin II receptor antagonist, BIBR 277. Br J Pharmacol 110:245-252, 1993.

233. Ojima M, Inada Y, Shibouta Y, et al: Candesartan (CV-11974) dissociates slowly from the angiotensin AT1 receptor. Eur J Pharmacol 319:137-146, 1997.

234. Vauquelin G, Fierens F, Vanderheyden P: Distinction between surmountable and insurmountable angiotensin II AT1 receptor antagonists. In Epstein M, Brunner H (eds): Angiotensin II Receptor Antagonists. Philadelphia, Hanley & Belfus, 2001, p 105.

235. Malerczyk C, Fuchs B, Belz GG, et al: Angiotensin II antagonism and plasma radioreceptor-kinetics of candesartan in man. Br J Clin Pharmacol 45:567-573, 1998.

236. Nishiyama A, Seth DM, Navar LG: Renal interstitial fluid angiotensin I and angiotensin II concentrations during local angiotensin-converting enzyme inhibition. J Am Soc Nephrol 13:2207-2212, 2002.

237. Ilson BE, Martin DE, Boike SC, Jorkasky DK: The effects of eprosartan, an angiotensin II AT1 receptor antagonist, on uric acid excretion in patients with mild to moderate essential hypertension. J Clin Pharmacol 38:437-441, 1998.

238. Ruilope L: Human pharmacokinetic/pharmacodynamic profile of irbesartan: A new potent angiotensin II receptor antagonist. J Hypertens 15:S15-S20, 1997.

239. Vachharajani NN, Shyu WC, Greene DS: Effects of food on the pharmacokinetics of irbesartan/hydrochlorothiazide. Clin Drug Invest 16:399-404, 1998.

240. Ohtawa M, Takayama F, Saitoh K, et al: Pharmacokinetics and biochemical efficacy after single and multiple oral administration of losartan, an orally active nonpeptide angiotensin II receptor antagonist, in humans. Br J Clin Pharmacol 35:290-297, 1993.

241. Ichikawa S, Takayama Y: Long-term effects of olmesartan, an Ang II receptor antagonist, on blood pressure and the renin-angiotensin-aldosterone system in hypertensive patients. Hypertens Res 24:641-646, 2001.

242. Neutel JM: Clinical studies of CS-866, the newest angiotensin II receptor antagonist. Am J Cardiol 87:37C-43C, 2001.

243. Wienen W, Entzeroth M: Effects on binding characteristics and venal function of the novel, nonpeptide angiotensin-II antagonist Bibr-277 in the rat. J Hypertens 12:119-128, 1994.

244. DiBona GF, Jones SY, Sawin LL: Angiotensin receptor antagonist improves cardiac reflex control of renal sodium handling in heart failure. Am J Physiol 274:H636-H641, 1998.

245. Jover B, Saladini D, Nafrialdi N, et al: Effect of losartan and enalapril on renal adaptation sodium restriction in rat. Am J Physiol 267:F281-F288, 1994.

246. Mendelsohn FA, Dunbar M, Allen A, et al: Angiotensin II receptors in the kidney. Fed Proc 45:1420-1425, 1986.

247. Paxton WG, Runge M, Horaist C, et al: Immunohistochemical localization of rat angiotensin II AT1 receptor. Am J Physiol 264:F989-F995, 1993.

248. Douglas JG: Angiotensin receptor subtypes of the kidney cortex. Am J Physiol 253:F1-F7, 1987.

249. Harrison-Bernard LM, Navar LG, Ho MM, et al: Immuno-histochemical localization of ANG II AT1 receptor in adult rat kidney using a monoclonal antibody. Am J Physiol 273: F170-F177, 1997.

250. Miyata N, Park F, Li XF, Cowley AW Jr: Distribution of angiotensin AT1 and AT2 receptor subtypes in the rat kidney. Am J Physiol 277:F437-F446, 1999.

251. Braam B, Navar LG, Mitchell KD: Modulation of tubuloglomerular feedback by angiotensin II type 1 receptors during the development of Goldblatt hypertension. Hypertension 25:1232-1237, 1995.

252. Cervenka L, Wang CT, Navar LG: Effects of acute AT1 receptor blockade by candesartan on arterial pressure and renal function in rats. Am J Physiol 274:F940-F945, 1998.

253. Cervenka L, Navar LG: Renal responses of the nonclipped kidney of two-kidney/one-clip Goldblatt hypertensive rats to type 1 angiotensin II receptor blockade with candesartan. J Am Soc Nephrol 10(suppl 11):S197-S201, 1999.

254. Takishita S, Muratani H, Sesoko S, et al: Short-term effects of angiotensin II blockade on renal blood flow and sympathetic activity in awake rats. Hypertension 24:445-450, 1994.

255. Peng Y, Knox FG: Comparison of systemic and direct intrarenal angiotensin II blockade on sodium excretion in rats. Am J Physiol 269:F40-F46, 1995.

256. Knox FG, Burnett JC Jr, Kohan DE, et al: Escape from the sodium-retaining effects of mineralocorticoids. Kidney Int 17:263-276, 1980.

257. Navar LG, Inscho EW, Majid SA, et al: Paracrine regulation of the renal microcirculation. Physiol Rev 76:425-536, 1996.

258. Burnier M, Brunner HR: Angiotensin II receptor antagonists and the kidney. Curr Opin Nephrol Hypertens 3:537-545, 1994.

259. Gansevoort RT, de Zeeuw D, Shahinfar S: Effects of the angiotensin II antagonist losartan in hypertensive patients with renal disease. J Hypertens 12(suppl)S37-S42, 1994.

260. Boike S, Ilson B, Audet P: The angiotensin II receptor antagonist SK&F 108566 does not increase uric acid excretion in healthy men. J Am Soc Nephrol 4:530, 1993.

261. Puig JG, Mateos F, Buno A, et al: Effect of eprosartan and losartan on uric acid metabolism in patients with essential hypertension. J Hypertens 17:1033-1039, 1999.

262. Edwards RM, Trizna W, Stack EJ, Weinstock J: Interaction of non-peptide angiotensin II receptor antagonists with the urate transporter in rat renal brush-border membranes. J Pharmacol Exp Ther 276:125-129, 1996.

263. Tsunoda K, Abe K, Hagino T, et al: Hypotensive effect of losartan, a nonpeptide angiotensin II receptor antagonist, in essential hypertension. Am J Hypertens 6:28-32, 1993.

264. Nakashima M, Uematsu T, Kosuge K, Kanamaru M: Pilot study of the uricosuric effect of DuP-753, a new angiotensin II receptor antagonist, in healthy subjects. Eur J Clin Pharmacol 42:333-335, 1992.

265. Schaefer KL, Porter JA: Angiotensin II receptor antagonists: The prototype losartan. Ann Pharmacother 30:625-636, 1996.

266. Burnier M, Rutschmann B, Nussberger J, et al: Salt-dependent renal effects of an angiotensin II antagonist in healthy subjects. Hypertension 22:339-347, 1993.

267. Shahinfar S, Simpson RL, Carides AD, et al: Safety of losartan in hypertensive patients with thiazide-induced hyperuricemia. Kidney Int 56:1879-1885, 1999.

268. Shaw W, Snavely D, Shaninfar S: Safety and efficacy of losartan in hypertensive patients with renal impairment. J Am Soc Nephrol 5:567, 1994.

269. Doig JK, McFadyen R, Sweet CS: Hemodynamic and renal response to losartan during salt depletion or salt repletion. J Hypertens 11:S419-S420, 1993.

270. Buter H, Navis G, de Zeeuw D, de Jong PE: Renal hemodynamic effects of candesartan in normal and impaired renal function in humans. Kidney Int Suppl 63:S185-S187, 1997.

271. Siragy HM, Carey RM: Protective role of the angiotensin AT2 receptor in a renal wrap hypertension model. Hypertension 33:1237-1242, 1999.

272. Delles C, Jacobi J, John S, et al: Effects of enalapril and eprosartan on the renal vascular nitric oxide system in human essential hypertension. Kidney Int 61:1462-1468, 2002.

273. Textor SC, Tarazi RC, Novick AC, et al: Regulation of renal hemodynamics and glomerular filtration in patients with renovascular hypertension during converting enzyme inhibition with captopril. Am J Med 76:29-37, 1984.

274. Cooper ME, Webb RL, de Gasparo M: Angiotensin receptor blockers and the kidney: Possible advantages over ACE inhibition? Cardiovasc Drug Rev 19:75-86, 2001.

275. Anderson S, Rennke HG, Brenner BM: Therapeutic advantage of converting enzyme inhibitors in arresting progressive renal disease associated with systemic hypertension in the rat. J Clin Invest 77:1993-2000, 1986.

276. Perico N, Amuchastegui CS, Malanchini B, et al: Angiotensin-converting enzyme inhibition and calcium channel blockade both normalize early hyperfiltration in experimental diabetes, but only the former prevents late renal structural damage. Exp Nephrol 2:220-228, 1994.

277. Bohlen L, de Court, Weidmann P: Comparative study of the effect of ACE-inhibitors and other antihypertensive agents on proteinuria in diabetic patients. Am J Hypertens 7:84S-92S, 1994.

278. Lewis EJ, Hunsicker LG, Clarke WR, et al: Renoprotective effect of the angiotensin-receptor antagonist irbesartan in patients with nephropathy due to type 2 diabetes. Irbesartan Diabetic Nephropathy Trial (IDNT). N Engl J Med 345:851-860, 2001.

279. Brenner BM, Cooper ME, de Zeeuw D, et al: Effects of losartan on renal and cardiovascular outcomes in patients with type 2 diabetes and nephropathy (RENAAL). N Engl J Med 345:861-869, 2001.

280. Parving HH, Lehnert H, Brochner-Mortensen J, et al: The effect of irbesartan on the development of diabetic nephropathy in patients with type 2 diabetes. Irbesartan Microalbuminuria Type II Diabetes in Hypertensive Patients (IRMA II). N Engl J Med 345:870-878, 2001.

281. Christen Y, Waeber B, Nussberger J: Dose-response relationships following oral administration of DuP 753 to normal humans. Am J Hypertens 4:350S-353S, 1991.

282. Munafo A, Christen Y, Nussberger J: Drug concentration response relationships in normal volunteers after oral administration of losartan, an angiotensin II receptor antagonist. Clin Pharmacol Ther 51:513-521, 1992.

283. Ogihara T, Nagano M, Mikami H: Effects of the angiotensin II receptor antagonist, TCV-116, on BP and the renin-angiotensin system in healthy subjects. Clin Ther 16:74-86, 1994.

284. Li S, Wu P, Zhong S, et al: Effects of long-term enalapril and losartan therapy of hypertension on cardiovascular aldosterone. Horm Res 55:293-297, 2001.

285. Ersoy A, Dilek K, Usta M, et al: Angiotensin-II receptor antagonist losartan reduces microalbuminuria in hypertensive renal transplant recipients. Clin Transplant 16:202-205, 2002.

286. Russo D, Pisani A, Balletta MM, et al: Additive antiproteinuric effect of converting enzyme inhibitor and losartan in normotensive patients with IgA nephropathy. Am J Kidney Dis 33:851-856, 1999.

287. Kuriyama S, Tomonari H, Abe A, et al: Augmentation of antiproteinuric effect by combined therapy with angiotensin II receptor blocker plus Ca channel blocker in a hypertensive patient with IgA glomerulonephritis. J Hum Hypertens 5:371-373, 2002.

288. Taal MW, Brenner BM: Combination ACEI and ARB therapy: Additional benefit in renoprotection? Curr Opin Nephrol Hypertens 11:377-381, 2002.

289. Komine N, Khang S, Wead LM, et al: Effect of combining an ACE inhibitor and an angiotensin II receptor blocker on plasma and kidney tissue angiotensin II levels. Am J Kidney Dis 39:159-164, 2002.

290. Agarwal R, Siva S, Dunn SR, Sharma K: Add-on angiotensin II receptor blockade lowers urinary transforming growth factor-beta levels. Am J Kidney Dis 39:486-492, 2002.

291. Doggrell SA: Class benefits of AT(1) antagonists in type 2 diabetes with nephropathy. Expert Opin Pharmacother 3:625-628, 2002.

292. Sica DA, Barkris GL: Type 2 diabetes: RENAAL and IDNT—The emergence of new treatment options. J Clin Hypertens (Greenwich) 1:52-57, 2002.

293. Inigo P, Campistol JM, Lario S, et al: Effects of losartan and amlodipine on intrarenal hemodynamics and TGF-beta(1) plasma levels in a crossover trial in renal transplant recipients. J Am Soc Nephrol 12:822-827, 2001.

294. Ferrario CM, Smith R, Levy P, Strawn W: The hypertension-lipid connection: Insights into the relation between angiotensin II and cholesterol in atherogenesis. Am J Med Sci 323:17-24, 2002.

295. Ferrario CM: Use of angiotensin II receptor blockers in animal models of atherosclerosis. Am J Hypertens 15:9S-13S, 2002.

296. Schiffrin EL, Park JB, Intengan HD, Touyz RM: Correction of arterial structure and endothelial dysfunction in human essential hypertension by the angiotensin antagonist losartan. Circulation 101:1653-1659, 2000.

297. Brosnan MJ, Hamilton CA, Graham D, et al: Irbesartan lowers superoxide levels and increases nitric oxide bioavailability in blood vessels from spontaneously hypertensive stroke-prone rats. J Hypertens 20:281-286, 2002.

298. Taddei S, Virdis A, Ghiadoni L, et al: Effects of antihypertensive drugs on endothelial dysfunction: Clinical implications. Drugs 62:265-284, 2002.

299. McIntyre M, Caffe SE, Michalak RA, Reid JL: Losartan, an orally active angiotensin (AT1) receptor antagonist: A review of its efficacy and safety in essential hypertension. Pharmacol Ther 74:181-194, 1997.

300. Markham A, Goa KL: Valsartan. A review of its pharmacology and therapeutic use in essential hypertension. Drugs 54:299-311, 1997.

301. Brown MJ: Irbesartan treatment in hypertension. Hosp Med 59:808-811, 1998.

302. McClellan KJ, Goa KL: Candesartan cilexetil. A review of its use in essential hypertension. Drugs 56:847-869, 1998.

303. Okereke CE, Messerli FH: Efficacy and safety of angiotensin II receptor blockers in elderly patients with mild to moderate hypertension. Am J Geriatr Cardiol 10:42-49, 2001.

304. Hannedouche T, Chanard J, Baumelou B: Evaluation of the safety and efficacy of telmisartan and enalapril, with the potential addition of frusemide, in moderate-renal failure patients with mild-to-moderate hypertension. J Renin Angiotensin Aldosterone Syst 2:246-254, 2001.

305. Wienen W, Richard S, Champeroux P, Audeval-Gerard C: Comparative antihypertensive and renoprotective effects of telmisartan and lisinopril after long-term treatment in hypertensive diabetic rats. J Renin Angiotensin Aldosterone Syst 2:31-36, 2001.

306. Weir MR, Weber MA, Neutel JM, et al: Efficacy of candesartan cilexetil as add-on therapy in hypertensive patients uncontrolled on background therapy: A clinical experience trial. ACTION Study Investigators. Am J Hypertens 14:567-572, 2001.

307. Weir MR: Are drugs that block the renin-angiotensin system effective and safe in patients with renal insufficiency? Am J Hypertens 12:195S-203S, 1999.

308. Dahlof B, Devereux RB, Kjeldsen SE, et al: Cardiovascular morbidity and mortality in the Losartan Intervention For Endpoint reduction in hypertension study (LIFE): A randomised trial against atenolol. Lancet 359:995-1003, 2002.

309. Mutlu H, Ozhan H, Okcun B, et al: The efficacy of valsartan in essential hypertension and its effects on left ventricular hypertrophy. Blood Press 11:53-55, 2002.

310. Fournier A, Oprisiu R, Andrejak M, et al: Age-adjusted stroke incidence increase: Could angiotensin AT1 receptor antagonists enhance stroke prevention? Stroke 33:881-882, 2002.

311. Lindholm LH, Ibsen H, Borch-Johnsen K, et al: Risk of new-onset diabetes in the Losartan Intervention For Endpoint reduction in hypertension study. J Hypertens 20:1879-1886, 2002.

312. Ohnishi K, Kohno M, Yukiiri K, et al: Influence of the angiotensin II receptor antagonist losartan on diuretic-induced metabolic effects in elderly hypertensive patients: Comparison with a calcium channel blocker. Int J Clin Pharmacol Ther 39:417-422, 2001.

313. Ross SD, Akhras KS, Zhang S, et al: Discontinuation of antihypertensive drugs due to adverse events: A systematic review and meta-analysis. Pharmacotherapy 21:940-953, 2001.

314. Elliott HL: Angiotensin II antagonists: Efficacy, duration of action, comparison with other drugs. J Hum Hypertens 12:271-274, 1998.

315. Heuer HJ, Schondorfer G, Hogemann AM: Twenty-four hour blood pressure profile of different doses of candesartan cilexetil in patients with mild to moderate hypertension. J Hum Hypertens 11(suppl 2):S55-S56, 1997.

316. Ikeda LS, Harm SC, Arcuri KE, et al: Comparative antihypertensive effects of losartan 50 mg and losartan 50 mg titrated to 100 mg in patients with essential hypertension. Blood Press 6:35-43, 1997.

317. Pool JL, Guthrie RM, Littlejohn TW III, et al: Dose-related antihypertensive effects of irbesartan in patients with mild-to-moderate hypertension. Am J Hypertens 11:462-470, 1998.

318. Unger T: Differences among angiotensin II type 1 receptor blockers: Characteristics of candesartan cilexetil. Blood Press Suppl 1:14-18, 2000.

319. Oparil S, Williams D, Chrysant SG, et al: Comparative efficacy of olemesartan, losartan, valsartan and irbesartan in the control of essential HTN. J Clin Hypertens (Greenwich) III:283-291, 2001.

320. Rossing K, Christensen PK, Jensen BR, Parving HH: Dual blockade of the renin-angiotensin system in diabetic nephropathy: A randomized double-blind crossover study. Diabetes Care 25:95-100, 2002.

321. Sakata K, Yoshida H, Obayashi K, et al: Effects of losartan and its combination with quinapril on the cardiac sympathetic nervous system and neurohormonal status in essential hypertension. J Hypertens 20:103-110, 2002.

322. Morgan T, Anderson A: A comparison of candesartan, felodipine, and their combination in the treatment of elderly patients with systolic hypertension. Am J Hypertens 15:544-549, 2002.

323. Pryde PG, Sedman AB, Nugent CE, et al: Angiotensin-converting enzyme inhibitor fetopathy. J Am Soc Nephrol 3:1575-1582, 1993.

324. Laakso M, Karjalainen L, Lempiainen-Kuosa P: Effects of losartan on insulin sensitivity in hypertensive subjects. Hypertension 28:392-396, 1996.

325. Moan A, Hoieggen A, Seljeflot I, et al: The effect of angiotensin II receptor antagonism with losartan on glucose metabolism and insulin sensitivity. J Hypertens 14:1093-1097, 1996.

326. Fishman S, Rapoport MJ, Weissgarten J, et al: The effect of losartan on insulin resistance and beta cell function in chronic hemodialysis patients. Ren Fail 23:685-692, 2001.

327. Sica DA, Weber M: The Losartan Intervention for Endpoint reduction (LIFE) trial—Have angiotensin-receptor blockers come of age? J Clin Hypertens (Greenwich) 4:301-305, 2002.

328. Hernandez-Hernandez R, Sosa-Canache B, Velasco M, et al: Angiotensin II receptor antagonists role in arterial hypertension. J Hum Hypertens 16(suppl 1):S93-S99, 2002.

329. Chan P, Tomlinson B, Huang TY, et al: Double-blind comparison of losartan, lisinopril, and metolazone in elderly hypertensive patients with previous angiotensin-converting enzyme inhibitor–induced cough. J Clin Pharmacol 37:253-257, 1997.

330. Chiu AG, Krowiak EJ, Deeb ZE: Angioedema associated with angiotensin II receptor antagonists: Challenging our knowledge of angioedema and its etiology. Laryngoscope 111:1729-1731, 2001.

331. Acker G, Greenberg A: Angioedema induced by the angiotensin II blocker losartan. N Engl J Med 333:1572, 1995.

332. Neutel JM, Smith DHG: Dose response and antihypertensive efficacy of the AT1 receptor antagonist telmisartan in patients with mild to moderate hypertension. Adv Ther 15:206-217, 1998.

333. Fogari R, Zoppi A, Poletti L, et al: Sexual activity in hypertensive men treated with valsartan or carvedilol: A crossover study. Am J Hypertens 14:27-31, 2001.

334. Ducloux D, Fournier V, Bresson-Vautrin C, Chalopin JM: Long-term follow-up of renal transplant recipients treated with losartan for post-transplant erythrosis. Transplant Int 11:312-315, 1998.

335. Fricker AF, Nussberger J, Meilenbrock S, et al: Effect of indomethacin on the renal response to angiotensin II receptor blockade in healthy subjects. Kidney Int 54:2089-2097, 1998.

336. Black JW, Duncan WA, Shanks RG: Comparison of some properties of pronethalol and propranolol. Br J Pharmacol 25:577-591, 1965.

337. Paterson JW, Conolly ME, Dollery CT: The pharmacodynamics and metabolism of propranolol in man. Pharmacol Clin 2:127-133, 1970.

338. Fitzgerald JD: The applied pharmacology of beta-adrenoceptor antagonists (beta blockers) in relation to clinical outcomes. Cardiovasc Drugs Ther 5:561-576, 1991.

339. Fitzgerald JD: Do partial agonist beta-blockers have improved clinical utility? Cardiovasc Drugs Ther 7:303-310, 1993.

340. Man in 't Veld, Schalekamp MA: Haemodynamic consequences of intrinsic sympathomimetic activity in relation to changes in plasma renin activity and noradrenaline during beta-blocker therapy for hypertension. Postgrad Med J 59(suppl 3):140-158, 1983.

341. McDevitt DG, Brown CH, Carruthers SG, Shanks RG: Influence of intrinsic sympathomimetic activity and cardioselectivity on beta-adrenoceptor blockade. Clin Pharmacol Ther 21:556-566, 1997.

342. Man in 't Veld AJ, Schalekamp MA: How intrinsic sympathomimetic activity modulates the haemodynamic responses to beta-adrenoceptor antagonists. A clue to the nature of their antihypertensive mechanism. Br J Clin Pharmacol 13:245S-257S, 1982.

343. Man in 't Veld AJ, Schalekamp MA: Effects of 10 different beta-adrenoceptor antagonists on hemodynamics, plasma renin activity, and plasma norepinephrine in hypertension: The key role of vascular resistance changes in relation to partial agonist activity. J Cardiovasc Pharmacol 5(suppl 1):S30-S45, 1983.

344. Franz IW, Behr U, Ketelhut R: Resting and exercise blood pressure with atenolol, enalapril and a low-dose combination. J Hypertens Suppl 5:S37-S41, 1987.

345. Frishman W: Clinical pharmacology of the new beta-adrenergic blocking drugs. Part 1. Pharmacodynamic and pharmacokinetic properties. Am Heart J 97:663-670, 1979.

346. Lands AM, Luduena FP, Buzzo HJ: Differentiation of receptors responsive to isoproterenol. Life Sci 6:2241-2249, 1967.

347. Lands AM, Arnold A, McAuliff JP, et al: Differentiation of receptor systems activated by sympathomimetic amines. Nature 214:597-598, 1967.

348. Carlsson E: On the classification and distribution of beta-adrenoceptors. Acta Pharmacol Toxicol (Copenh) 44(suppl 2):17-20, 1979.

349. Minneman KP, Molinoff PB: Classification and quantitation of beta-adrenergic receptor subtypes. Biochem Pharmacol 29:1317-1323, 1980.

350. Prichard BN, Owens CW: Mode of action of beta-adrenergic blocking drugs in hypertension. Clin Physiol Biochem 8(suppl 2):1-10, 1990.

351. Vincent HH, Man in't Veld AJ, Boomsma F, et al: Is beta 1-antagonism essential for the antihypertensive action of beta-blockers? Hypertension 9:198-203, 1987.

352. Buhler FR, Laragh JH, Baer L, et al: Propranolol inhibition of renin secretion. A specific approach to diagnosis and treatment of renin-dependent hypertensive diseases. N Engl J Med 287:1209-1214, 1972.

353. Keeton TK, Campbell WB: The pharmacologic alteration of renin release. Pharmacol Rev 31:81-227, 1981.

354. Day MD, Roach AG: Central alpha- and beta-adrenoceptors modifying arterial blood pressure and heart rate in conscious cats. Br J Pharmacol 51:325-333, 1974.

355. Garvey HL, Ram N: Centrally induced hypotensive effects of beta-adrenergic blocking drugs. Eur J Pharmacol 33:283-294, 1975.

356. Hollifield JW, Sherman K, Zwagg RV, Shand DG: Proposed mechanisms of propranolol's antihypertensive effect in essential hypertension. N Engl J Med 295:68-73, 1976.

357. Stjarne L, Brundin J: Beta2-adrenoceptors facilitating noradrenaline secretion from human vasoconstrictor nerves. Acta Physiol Scand 97:88-93, 1976.

358. Weinstock M: The presynaptic effect of beta-adrenoceptor antagonists on noradrenergic neurones. Life Sci 19:1453-1466, 1976.

359. Jackson EK, Campbell WB: Inhibition of angiotensin II potentiation of sympathetic nerve activity by beta-adrenergic antagonists. Hypertension 2:90-96, 1980.

360. Herrera J, Vukovich RA, Griffith DL: Elimination of nadolol by patients with renal impairment. Br J Clin Pharmacol 7(suppl 2):227S-231S, 1979.

361. Dreyfuss J, Griffith DL, Singhvi SM, et al: Pharmacokinetics of nadolol, a beta-receptor antagonist: Administration of therapeutic single- and multiple-dosage regimens to hypertensive patients. J Clin Pharmacol 19:712-720, 1979.

362. Heel RC, Brogden RN, Pakes GE, et al: Nadolol: A review of its pharmacological properties and therapeutic efficacy in hypertension and angina pectoris. Drugs 20:1-23, 1980.

363. Frishman WH: Nadolol: A new beta-adrenoceptor antagonist. N Engl J Med 305:678-682, 1981.

364. Nies AS, Shand DG: Clinical pharmacology of propranolol. Circulation 52:6-15, 1975.

365. Holland OB, Kaplan NM: Propranolol in the treatment of hypertension. N Engl J Med 294:930-936, 1976.

366. McAinsh J, Baber NS, Smith R, Young J: Pharmacokinetic and pharmacodynamic studies with long-acting propranolol. Br J Clin Pharmacol 6:115-121, 1978.

367. Leahey WJ, Neill JD, Varma MP, Shanks RG: Comparison of the efficacy and pharmacokinetics of conventional propranolol and a long acting preparation of propranolol. Br J Clin Pharmacol 9:33-40, 1980.

368. Wood AJ, Vestal RE, Spannuth CL, et al: Propranolol disposition in renal failure. Br J Clin Pharmacol 10:561-566, 1980.

369. Fagan TC, Walle T, Corns-Hurwitz R, et al: Time course of development of the antihypertensive effect of propranolol. Hypertension 5:852-857, 1983.

370. Tocco DJ, Duncan AE, Delauna FA, et al: Physiological disposition and metabolism of timolol in man and laboratory animals. Drug Metab Dispos 3:361-370, 1975.

371. Else OF, Sorenson H, Edwards IR: Plasma timolol levels after oral and intravenous administration. Eur J Clin Pharmacol 14:431-434, 1978.

372. Lowenthal DT, Pitone JM, Affrime MB, et al: Timolol kinetics in chronic renal insufficiency. Clin Pharmacol Ther 23:606-615, 1978.

373. Frishman WH: Drug therapy: Atenolol and timolol, two new systemic beta-adrenoceptor antagonists. N Engl J Med 306:1456-1462, 1982.

374. Frishman WH, Covey S: Penbutolol and carteolol: Two new beta-adrenergic blockers with partial agonism. J Clin Pharmacol 30:412-421, 1990.

375. Amemiya M, Tabei K, Furuya H, et al: Pharmacokinetics of carteolol in patients with impaired renal function. Eur J Clin Pharmacol 43:417-421, 1992.

376. Bailey RR, Carlson RV, Walker RJ, Swainson CP: Effect of oral penbutolol on renal haemodynamics of hypertensive patients with renal insufficiency. NZ Med J 98:683-685, 1985.

377. Mucklow JC, Kuhn S: The comparative beta-adrenoceptor blocking effects of penbutolol, atenolol and sustained-release metoprolol in healthy volunteers. Eur J Clin Pharmacol 27:269-273, 1984.

378. Ohman KP, Asplund J, Landahl S, Liander B: Penbutolol (Hoe 893d) in primary hypertension. Blood pressure effects, tolerance and plasma concentrations. Eur J Clin Pharmacol 22:95-99, 1982.

379. van der MJ, Reijn E, Heidendal GA, et al: Comparison of the effects of penbutolol and propranolol on glomerular filtration rate in hypertensive patients with impaired renal function. Br J Clin Pharmacol 22:469-474, 1986.

380. Vedin JA, Wilhelmsson C, Maass L, Peterson LE: Pharmacodynamic and pharmacokinetic study of oral and intravenous penbutolol. Eur J Clin Pharmacol 25:529-534, 1983.

381. Bernard N, Cuisinaud G, Pozet N, et al: Pharmacokinetics of penbutolol and its metabolites in renal insufficiency. Eur J Clin Pharmacol 29:215-219, 1985.

382. Ohnhaus EE, Heidemann H, Meier J, Maurer G: Metabolism of pindolol in patients with renal failure. Eur J Clin Pharmacol 22:423-428, 1982.

383. Aellig WH: Clinical pharmacology of pindolol. Am Heart J 104:346-356, 1982.

384. Schwarz HJ: Pharmacokinetics of pindolol in humans and several animal species. Am Heart J 104:357-364, 1982.

385. Meier J: Pharmacokinetic comparison of pindolol with other beta-adrenoceptor-blocking agents. Am Heart J 104:364-373, 1982.

386. Frishman WH: Drug therapy. Pindolol: A new beta-adrenoceptor antagonist with partial agonist activity. N Engl J Med 308:940-944, 1983.

387. Heel RC, Brogden RN, Speight TM, Avery GS: Atenolol: A review of its pharmacological properties and therapeutic efficacy in angina pectoris and hypertension. Drugs 17:425-460, 1979.

388. McAinsh J, Holmes BF, Smith S, et al: Atenolol kinetics in renal failure. Clin Pharmacol Ther 28:302-309, 1980.

389. Kirch W, Kohler H, Mutschler E, Schafer M: Pharmacokinetics of atenolol in relation to renal function. Eur J Clin Pharmacol 19:65-71, 1981.

390. Ishizaki T, Oyama Y, Suganuma T, et al: A dose ranging study of atenolol in hypertension: Fall in blood pressure and plasma renin activity, beta-blockade and steady-state pharmacokinetics. Br J Clin Pharmacol 16:17-25, 1983.

391. Wadworth AN, Murdoch D, Brogden RN: Atenolol. A reappraisal of its pharmacological properties and therapeutic use in cardiovascular disorders. Drugs 42:468-510, 1991.

392. Brogden RN, Heel RC, Speight TM, et al: Metoprolol: A review of its pharmacological properties and therapeutic efficacy in hypertension and angina pectoris. Drugs 14:321-348, 1979.

393. Koch-Weser J: Drug therapy: Metoprolol. N Engl J Med 301:698-703, 1979.

394. Beresford R, Heel RC: Betaxolol. A review of its pharmacodynamic and pharmacokinetic properties, and therapeutic efficacy in hypertension. Drugs 31:6-28, 1986.

395. Frishman WH, Tepper D, Lazar EJ, Behrman D: Betaxolol: A new long-acting beta 1-selective adrenergic blocker. J Clin Pharmacol 30:686-692, 1990.

396. Leopold G, Pabst J, Ungethum W, Buhring KU: Basic pharmacokinetics of bisoprolol, a new highly beta 1-selective adrenoceptor antagonist. J Clin Pharmacol 26:616-621, 1986.

397. Johns TE, Lopez LM: Bisoprolol: Is this just another beta-blocker for hypertension or angina? Ann Pharmacother 29:403-414, 1995.

398. Kirch W, Kohler H, Berggren G, Braun W: The influence of renal function on plasma levels and urinary excretion of acebutolol and its main N-acetyl metabolite. Clin Nephrol 18:88-94, 1982.

399. Smith RS, Warren DJ, Renwick AG, George CF: Acebutolol pharmacokinetics in renal failure. Br J Clin Pharmacol 16:253-258, 1983.

400. Ryan JR: Clinical pharmacology of acebutolol. Am Heart J 109:1131-1136, 1985.

401. Giacomini JC, Thoden WR: Ancillary pharmacologic properties of acebutolol: Cardioselectivity, partial agonist activity, and membrane-stabilizing activity. Am Heart J 109:1137-1144, 1985.

402. Wallin JD, O'Neill WM Jr: Labetalol. Current research and therapeutic status. Arch Intern Med 143:485-490, 1983.

403. MacCarthy EP, Bloomfield SS: Labetalol: A review of its pharmacology, pharmacokinetics, clinical uses and adverse effects. Pharmacotherapy 3:193-219, 1983.

404. McNeil JJ, Louis WJ: Clinical pharmacokinetics of labetalol. Clin Pharmacokinet 9:157-167, 1984.

405. van Zwieten PA: An overview of the pharmacodynamic properties and therapeutic potential of combined alpha- and beta-adrenoceptor antagonists. Drugs 45:509-517, 1993.

406. Dunn CJ, Lea AP, Wagstaff AJ: Carvedilol. A reappraisal of its pharmacological properties and therapeutic use in cardiovascular disorders. Drugs 54:161-185, 1997.

407. Tomlinson B, Bompart F, Graham BR, et al: Vasodilating mechanism and response to physiological pressor stimuli of acute doses of carvedilol compared with labetalol, propranolol and hydralazine. Drugs 36(suppl 6):37-47, 1988.

408. Capone P, Mayol R: A placebo-controlled double-blind multicenter study of celiprolol in the treatment of mild and moderate hypertension. J Cardiovasc Pharmacol 8(suppl 4):S119-S121, 1986.

409. Milne RJ, Buckley MM: Celiprolol. An updated review of its pharmacodynamic and pharmacokinetic properties, and therapeutic efficacy in cardiovascular disease. Drugs 41:941-969, 1991.

410. Dunn CJ, Spencer CM: Celiprolol. An evaluation of its pharmacological properties and clinical efficacy in the management of hypertension and angina pectoris. Drugs Aging 7:394-411, 1995.

411. Silke B, Rosenthal F, Taylor S: A randomized double-blind study of atenolol and celiprolol in mild to moderate hypertension. J Cardiovasc Pharmacol 8(suppl 4):S122-S126, 1986.

412. Taylor SH, Beattie A, Silke B: Celiprolol in the treatment of hypertension: A comparison with propranolol. J Cardiovasc Pharmacol 8(suppl 4):S127-S131, 1986.

413. Chan TY, Woo KS, Nicholls MG: The application of nebivolol in essential hypertension: A double-blind, randomized, placebo-controlled study. Int J Cardiol 35:387-395, 1992.

414. De Cree J, Cobo C, Geukens H, Verhaegen H: Comparison of the subacute hemodynamic effects of atenolol, propranolol, pindolol, and nebivolol. Angiology 41:95-105, 1990.

415. McNeely W, Goa KL: Nebivolol in the management of essential hypertension: A review. Drugs 57:633-651, 1999.

416. Van Bortel LM, de Hoon JN, Kool MJ, et al: Pharmacological properties of nebivolol in man. Eur J Clin Pharmacol 51:379-384, 1997.

417. McNeely W, Gao KL: Nebivolol in the management of essential hypertension: a review. Drugs 57:633-651, 1999.

418. Van Bortel LM, Breed JG, Joosten J, et al: Nebivolol in hypertension: A double-blind placebo-controlled multicenter study assessing its antihypertensive efficacy and impact on quality of life. J Cardiovasc Pharmacol 21:856-862, 1993.

419. Van de WA, Janssens W, Van Neuten J, et al: Pharmacological and hemodynamic profile of nebivolol, a chemically novel, potent, and selective beta 1-adrenergic antagonist. J Cardiovasc Pharmacol 11:552-563, 1988.

420. Wilkinson R: Beta-blockers and renal function. Drugs 23:195-206, 1982.

421. Zech P, Pozet N, Labeeuw M, et al: Acute renal effects of beta-blockers. Am J Nephrol 6(suppl 2):15-19, 1986.

422. Valvo E, Gammaro L, Bedogna V, et al: Effects of nadolol on systemic and renal hemodynamics in patients with renoparenchymal hypertension and various degrees of renal function. Int J Clin Pharmacol Ther Toxicol 24:202-206, 1986.

423. Paillard F, Lantz B, Leviel F, Ardaillou R: Renal hemodynamic effects of tertatolol in essential hypertension. Am J Nephrol 6(suppl 2):40-44, 1986.

424. Salvetti A, Leonetti G, Bernini GP, et al: Antihypertensive and renal effects of tertatolol, a new beta-blocking agent, in hypertensive patients. Am J Nephrol 6(suppl 2):45-49, 1986.

425. Epstein M, Oster JR: Beta blockers and renal function: A reappraisal. J Clin Hypertens 1:85-99, 1985.

426. Beaufils M: Alterations in renal hemodynamics during chronic and acute beta-blockade in humans. Am J Hypertens 2:233S-236S, 1989.

427. Cook ME, Wallin JD, Clifton GG, Poland M: Renal function effects of dilevalol, a nonselective beta-adrenergic blocking drug with beta-2 agonist activity. Clin Pharmacol Ther 43:393-399, 1988.

428. Taverner D, Mackay IG, Craig K, Watson ML: The effects of selective beta-adrenoceptor antagonists and partial agonist activity on renal function during exercise in normal subjects and those with moderate renal impairment. Br J Clin Pharmacol 32:387-391, 1991.

429. Frishman WH, Burris JF, Mroczek WJ, et al: First-line therapy option with low-dose bisoprolol fumarate and low-dose hydrochlorothiazide in patients with stage I and stage II systemic hypertension. J Clin Pharmacol 35:182-188, 1995.

430. UK Prospective Diabetes Study Group: Tight blood pressure control and risk of macrovascular and microvascular complications in type 2 diabetes: UKPDS 38. Br Med J 317:703-713, 1998.

431. McAreavey D, Vermeulen R, Robertson JI: Newer beta blockers and the treatment of hypertension. Cardiovasc Drugs Ther 5:577-587, 1991.

432. Frishman W, Silverman R: Clinical pharmacology of the new beta-adrenergic blocking drugs. Part 2. Physiologic and metabolic effects. Am Heart J 97:797-807, 1979.

433. Koch-Weser J, Frishman WH: Beta-adrenoceptor antagonists: New drugs and new indications. N Engl J Med 305:500-506, 1981.

434. Frishman WH: Clinical significance of beta 1-selectivity and intrinsic sympathomimetic activity in a beta-adrenergic blocking drug. Am J Cardiol 59:33F-37F, 1987.

435. Materson BJ, Reda DJ, Cushman WC, et al: Single-drug therapy for hypertension in men. A comparison of six antihypertensive agents with placebo. The Department of Veterans Affairs Cooperative Study Group on Antihypertensive Agents. N Engl J Med 328:914-921, 1993.

436. Materson BJ, Reda DJ, Cushman WC: Department of Veterans Affairs single-drug therapy of hypertension study. Revised figures and new data. Department of Veterans Affairs Cooperative Study Group on Antihypertensive Agents. Am J Hypertens 8:189-192, 1995.

437. Neaton JD, Grimm RH Jr, Prineas RJ, et al: Treatment of Mild Hypertension Study. Final results. Treatment of Mild Hypertension Study Research Group. JAMA 270:713-724, 1993.

438. Philipp T, Anlauf M, Distler A, et al: Randomised, double blind, multicentre comparison of hydrochlorothiazide, atenolol, nitrendipine, and enalapril in antihypertensive treatment: Results of the HANE study. HANE Trial Research Group. BMJ 315:154-159, 1997.

439. Jamerson K, DeQuattro V: The impact of ethnicity on response to antihypertensive therapy. Am J Med 101:22S-32S, 1996.

440. Rubin PC, Butters L, Clark DM, et al: Placebo-controlled trial of atenolol in treatment of pregnancy-associated hypertension. Lancet 1:431-434, 1983.

441. Magee LA, Elran E, Bull SB, et al: Risks and benefits of beta-receptor blockers for pregnancy hypertension: Overview of the randomized trials. Eur J Obstet Gynecol Reprod Biol 88:15-26, 2000.

442. Messerli FH, Grossman E, Goldbourt U: Are beta-blockers efficacious as first-line therapy for hypertension in the elderly? A systematic review. JAMA 279:1903-1907, 1998.

443. Buhler FR, Burkart F, Lutold BE, et al: Antihypertensive beta blocking action as related to renin and age: A pharmacologic tool to identify pathogenetic mechanisms in essential hypertension. Am J Cardiol 36:653-669, 1975.

444. Beard K, Bulpitt C, Mascie-Taylor H, et al: Management of elderly patients with sustained hypertension. BMJ 304:412-416, 1992.

445. Kendall MJ, Lynch KP, Hjalmarson A, Kjekshus J: Beta-blockers and sudden cardiac death. Ann Intern Med 123:358-367, 1995.

446. Gottlieb SS, McCarter RJ, Vogel RA: Effect of beta-blockade on mortality among high-risk and low-risk patients after myocardial infarction. N Engl J Med 339:489-497, 1998.

447. 1993 guidelines for the management of mild hypertension. Memorandum from a World Health Organization/International Society of Hypertension meeting. Guidelines Subcommittee of the WHO/ISH Mild Hypertension Liaison Committee. Hypertension 22:392-403, 1993.

448. Bonow RO, Udelson JE: Left ventricular diastolic dysfunction as a cause of congestive heart failure. Mechanisms and management. Ann Intern Med 117:502-510, 1992.

449. Gottdiener JS, Reda DJ, Massie BM, et al: Effect of single-drug therapy on reduction of left ventricular mass in mild to moderate hypertension: Comparison of six antihypertensive agents. The Department of Veterans Affairs Cooperative Study Group on Antihypertensive Agents. Circulation 95:2007-2014, 1997.

450. Lechat P, Packer M, Chalon S, et al: Clinical effects of beta-adrenergic blockade in chronic heart failure: A meta-analysis of double-blind, placebo-controlled, randomized trials. Circulation 98:1184-1191, 1998.

451. Sackner-Bernstein JD, Mancini DM: Rationale for treatment of patients with chronic heart failure with adrenergic blockade. JAMA 274:1462-1467, 1995.

452. Cohn JN: Beta-blockers in heart failure. Eur Heart J 19(suppl F):F52-F55, 1998.

453. The Cardiac Insufficiency Bisoprolol Study II (CIBIS-II): A randomised trial. Lancet 353:9-13, 1999.

454. Packer M: The neurohormonal hypothesis: A theory to explain the mechanism of disease progression in heart failure. J Am Coll Cardiol 20:248-254, 1992.

455. Podlowski S, Luther HP, Morwinski R, et al: Agonistic anti–beta1-adrenergic receptor autoantibodies from cardiomyopathy patients reduce the beta1-adrenergic receptor expression in neonatal rat cardiomyocytes. Circulation 98:2470-2476, 1998.

456. Mann DL, Kent RL, Parsons B, Cooper G: Adrenergic effects on the biology of the adult mammalian cardiocyte. Circulation 85:790-804, 1992.

457. Psaty BM, Smith NL, Siscovick DS, et al: Health outcomes associated with antihypertensive therapies used as first-line agents. A systematic review and meta-analysis. JAMA 277:739-745, 1997.

458. Staessen JA, Wang JG, Birkenhager WH, Fagard R: Treatment with beta-blockers for the primary prevention of the cardiovascular complications of hypertension. Eur Heart J 20:11-24, 1999.

459. Schmieder RE, Langenfeld MR, Gatzka CD, et al: Impact of alpha- versus beta-blockers on hypertensive target organ damage: Results of a double-blind, randomized, controlled clinical trial. Am J Hypertens 10:985-991, 1997.

460. Deacon SP, Barnett D: Comparison of atenolol and propranolol during insulin-induced hypoglycaemia. Br Med J 2:272-273, 1976.

461. Lager I, Blohme G, Smith U: Effect of cardioselective and non-selective beta-blockade on the hypoglycaemic response in insulin-dependent diabetics. Lancet 1:458-462, 1979.

462. Frishman W, Silverman R, Strom J, et al: Clinical pharmacology of the new beta-adrenergic blocking drugs. Part 4. Adverse effects. Choosing a beta-adrenoreceptor blocker. Am Heart J 98:256-262, 1979.

463. Cruickshank JM: The clinical importance of cardioselectivity and lipophilicity in beta blockers. Am Heart J 100:160-178, 1980.

464. Frishman WH: Beta-adrenergic receptor blockers. Adverse effects and drug interactions. Hypertension 11:II21-II29, 1988.

465. Astrom H: Comparison of the effects on airway conductance of a new selective beta-adrenergic blocking drug, atenolol, and propranolol in asthmatic subjects. Scand J Respir Dis 56:292-296, 1975.

466. Decalmer PB, Chatterjee SS, Cruickshank JM, et al: Beta-blockers and asthma. Br Heart J 40:184-189, 1978.

467. Tattersfield AE: Beta adrenoceptor antagonists and respiratory disease. J Cardiovasc Pharmacol 8(suppl 4):S35-S39, 1986.

468. Tsukiyama H, Otsuka K, Higuma K: Effects of beta-adrenoceptor antagonists on central haemodynamics in essential hypertension. Br J Clin Pharmacol 13:269S-278S, 1982.

469. Frishman W, Kostis J, Strom J, et al: Clinical pharmacology of the new beta-adrenergic blocking drugs. Part 6. A comparison of pindolol and propranolol in treatment of patients with angina pectoris. The role of intrinsic sympathomimetic activity. Am Heart J 98:526-535, 1979.

470. McDevitt DG: Pharmacologic aspects of cardioselectivity in a beta-blocking drug. Am J Cardiol 59:10F-12F, 1987.

471. Kostis JB, Rosen RC: Central nervous system effects of beta-adrenergic-blocking drugs: The role of ancillary properties. Circulation 75:204-212, 1987.

472. Gengo FM, Huntoon L, McHugh WB: Lipid-soluble and water-soluble beta-blockers. Comparison of the central nervous system depressant effect. Arch Intern Med 147:39-43, 1987.

473. Reichgott MJ: Problems of sexual function in patients with hypertension. Cardiovasc Med 4:149-154, 1979.

474. Moss HB, Procci WR: Sexual dysfunction associated with oral antihypertensive medication: A critical survey of the literature. Gen Hosp Psychiatry 4:121-129, 1982.

475. Croog SH, Levine S, Testa MA, et al: The effects of antihypertensive therapy on the quality of life. N Engl J Med 314:1657-1664, 1986.

476. Croog SH, Levine S, Sudilovsky A, et al: Sexual symptoms in hypertensive patients. A clinical trial of antihypertensive medications. Arch Intern Med 148:788-794, 1988.

477. Grimm RH Jr, Grandits GA, Prineas RJ, et al: Long-term effects on sexual function of five antihypertensive drugs and nutritional hygienic treatment in hypertensive men and women. Treatment of Mild Hypertension Study (TOMHS). Hypertension 29:8-14, 1997.

478. Jacob H, Brandt LJ, Farkas P, Frishman W: Beta-adrenergic blockade and the gastrointestinal system. Am J Med 74:1042-1051, 1983.

479. Houston MC: The effects of antihypertensive drugs on glucose intolerance in hypertensive nondiabetics and diabetics. Am Heart J 115:640-656, 1988.

480. Pandit MK, Burke J, Gustafson AB, et al: Drug-induced disorders of glucose tolerance. Ann Intern Med 118:529-539, 1993.

481. Kasiske BL, Ma JZ, Kalil RS, Louis TA: Effects of antihypertensive therapy on serum lipids. Ann Intern Med 122:133-141, 1995.

482. Madu EC, Reddy RC, Madu AN, et al: Review: The effects of antihypertensive agents on serum lipids. Am J Med Sci 312:76-84, 1996.

483. Houston MC: Abrupt cessation of treatment in hypertension: Consideration of clinical features, mechanisms, prevention and management of the discontinuation syndrome. Am Heart J 102:415-430, 1981.

484. Watanabe AM: Recent advances in knowledge about beta-adrenergic receptors: Application to clinical cardiology. J Am Coll Cardiol 1:82-89, 1983.

485. Frishman WH: Beta-adrenergic blocker withdrawal. Am J Cardiol 59:26F-32F, 1987.

486. Houston MC, Hodge R: Beta-adrenergic blocker withdrawal syndromes in hypertension and other cardiovascular diseases. Am Heart J 116:515-523, 1988.

487. Antman EM, Stone PH, Muller JE, Braunwald E: Calcium channel blocking agents in the treatment of cardiovascular disorders. Part I: Basic and clinical electrophysiologic effects. Ann Intern Med 93:875-885, 1980.

488. Buhler FR: Calcium antagonists. In Largh JH, Brenner BM (eds): Hypertension: Pathophysiology, Diagnosis and Management. New York, Raven Press, 1990, p 2169.

489. Muiesan G, Agabiti-Rosei E, Castellano M, et al: Antihypertensive and humoral effects of verapamil and nifedipine in essential hypertension. J Cardiovasc Pharmacol 4(suppl 3):S325-S329, 1982.

490. Middlemost SJ, Sack M, Davis J, et al: Effects of long-acting nifedipine on casual office blood pressure measurements, 24-hour ambulatory blood pressure profiles, exercise parameters and left ventricular mass and function in black patients with mild to moderate systemic hypertension. Am J Cardiol 70:474-478, 1992.

491. Wysocki M, Persson B, Bagge U, Andersson OK: Flow resistance and its components in hypertensive men treated with the calcium antagonist isradipine. Eur J Clin Pharmacol 43:463-468, 1992.

492. Braunwald E: Mechanism of action of calcium-channel-blocking agents. N Engl J Med 307:1618-1627, 1982.

493. Pedrinelli R, Panarace G, Salvetti A: Calcium entry blockade and adrenergic vascular reactivity in hypertensives: Differences between nicardipine and diltiazem. Clin Pharmacol Ther 49:86-93, 1991.

494. Pedrinelli R, Taddei S, Salvetti A: Calcium entry blockade and alpha-adrenergic vascular reactivity in human beings: Differences between nicardipine and verapamil. Clin Pharmacol Ther 45:285-290, 1989.

495. Donati L, Buhler FR, Beretta-Piccoli C, et al: Antihypertensive mechanism of amlodipine in essential hypertension: Role of pressor reactivity to norepinephrine and angiotensin II. Clin Pharmacol Ther 52:50-59, 1992.

496. Krishna GG, Riley LJ Jr, Deuter G, et al: Natriuretic effect of calcium-channel blockers in hypertensives. Am J Kidney Dis 18:566-572, 1991.

497. Krizanova O, Lory P, Schwartz A: Structure-function studies of the voltage-dependent Ca channels. In Godraind T, Govani S, Poole HR (eds): Calcium Antagonists: Pharmacology and Clinical Research. Dordrecht, Kluwer Academic Publishers, 1993, pp 1-8.

498. Hosey MM, Lazdunski M: Calcium channels: Molecular pharmacology, structure and regulation. J Membr Biol 104:81-105, 1988.

499. Hess P: Calcium channels in vertebrate cells. Annu Rev Neurosci 13:337-356, 1990.

500. Tsien RW, Bean BP, Hess P, et al: Mechanisms of calcium channel modulation by beta-adrenergic agents and dihydropyridine calcium agonists. J Mol Cell Cardiol 18:691-710, 1986.

501. Brown AM, Birnbaumer L: Ionic channels and their regulation by G protein subunits. Annu Rev Physiol 52:197-213, 1990.

502. Brown AM: Presented at the 5th International Symposium on Calcium Antagonists: Pharmacology and Clinical Research, 1991, Houston.

503. Kelly JG, O'Malley K: Clinical pharmacokinetics of calcium antagonists. An update. Clin Pharmacokinet 22:416-433, 1992.

504. Toro L, Stefani E: Ca^{2+} and K^+ current in cultured vascular smooth muscle cells from rat aorta. Pflugers Arch 408:417-419, 1987.

505. Opie LH: Calcium channel antagonists, Part I: Fundamental properties: mechanisms, classification, sites of action. Cardiovasc Drugs Ther 1:411-430, 1987.

506. Rea RF, Hamdan M: Baroreflex control of muscle sympathetic nerve activity in borderline hypertension. Circulation 82:856-862, 1990.

507. Cohn JN: Sympathetic nervous system activity and the heart. Am J Hypertens 2:353S-356S, 1989.

508. Lederballe Pedersen OL, Christensen NJ, Ramsch KD: Comparison of acute effects of nifedipine in normotensive and hypertensive man. J Cardiovasc Pharmacol 2:357-366, 1980.

509. Frick MH, McGibney D, Tyler HM: Amlodipine: A double-blind evaluation of the dose-response relationship in mild to moderate hypertension. J Cardiovasc Pharmacol 12(suppl 7):S76-S78, 1988.

510. Lund-Johansen P, Omvik P, White W, et al: Long-term haemodynamic effects of amlodipine at rest and during exercise in essential hypertension. Cardiology 80(suppl 1):37-45, 1992.

511. Wood AJ: Calcium antagonists. Pharmacologic differences and similarities. Circulation 80:IV184-IV188, 1989.

512. Ohta Y, Higuchi N, Emura S, et al: Quantitative analysis of antiatherosclerotic effect of nifedipine in cholesterol-fed rabbits. Cardiovasc Drugs Ther 4(suppl 5):1021-1026, 1990.

513. Koibuchi Y, Sakai S, Miura S, et al: Suppression of atherogenesis in cholesterol-fed rabbits treated with nilvadipine, a new vasoselective calcium entry blocker. Atherosclerosis 79:147-155, 1989.

514. Willis AL, Nagel B, Churchill V, et al: Antiatherosclerotic effects of nicardipine and nifedipine in cholesterol-fed rabbits. Arteriosclerosis 5:250-255, 1985.

515. Held PH, Yusuf S, Furberg CD: Calcium channel blockers in acute myocardial infarction and unstable angina: An overview. BMJ 299: 1187-1192, 1989.

516. Nakamura M, Arakawa N, Yoshida H, et al: Nitric oxide plays an insignificant role in direct vasodilator effects of calcium channel blockers in healthy humans. Heart Vessels 16:105-110, 2002.

517. Xu B, Xiao-hong L, Lin G, et al: Amlodipine, but not verapamil or nifedipine, dilates rabbit femoral artery largely through a nitric oxide– and kinin-dependent mechanism. Br J Pharmacol 136: 375-382, 2002.

518. Braunwald E: Calcium-channel blockers: Pharmacologic considerations. Am Heart J 104:665-671, 1982.

519. Lefrandt JD, Heitmann J, Sevre K, et al: The effects of dihydropyridine and phenylalkylamine calcium antagonist classes on autonomic function in hypertension: The VAMPHYRE study. Am J Hypertens 14:1083-1089, 2001.

520. Siche JP, Baguet JP, Fagret D, et al: Effects of amlodipine on baroreflex and sympathetic nervous system activity in mild-to-moderate hypertension. Am J Hypertens 14:424-428, 2001.

521. Lefrandt JD, Heitmann J, Sevre K, et al: Contrasting effects of verapamil and amlodipine on cardiovascular stress responses in hypertension. Br J Clin Pharmacol 52:687-692, 2001.

522. Grossman E, Messerli FH: Effect of calcium antagonists on plasma norepinephrine levels, heart rate, and blood pressure. Am J Cardiol 80:1453-1458, 1997.

523. Messerli FH: Calcium antagonists in hypertension: From hemodynamics to outcomes. Am J Hypertens 15:94S-97S, 2002.

524. Molden E, Asberg A, Christensen H: Desacetyl-diltiazem displays severalfold higher affinity to CYP2D6 compared with CYP3A4. Drug Metab Dispos 30:1-3, 2002.

525. Smith MS, Verghese CP, Shand DG, Pritchett EL: Pharmacokinetic and pharmacodynamic effects of diltiazem. Am J Cardiol 51: 1369-1374, 1983.

526. Hermann P, Rodger SD, Remones G, et al: Pharmacokinetics of diltiazem after intravenous and oral administration. Eur J Clin Pharmacol 24:349-352, 1983.

527. McAllister RG Jr, Hamann SR, Blouin RA: Pharmacokinetics of calcium-entry blockers. Am J Cardiol 55:30B-40B, 1985.

528. Halperin AK, Cubeddu LX: The role of calcium channel blockers in the treatment of hypertension. Am Heart J 111:363-382, 1986.

529. Buckley MM, Grant SM, Goa KL, et al: Diltiazem. A reappraisal of its pharmacological properties and therapeutic use. Drugs 39: 757-806, 1990.

530. Prisant LM, Bottini B, DiPiro JT, Carr AA: Novel drug-delivery systems for hypertension. Am J Med 93:45S-55S, 1992.

531. Singh B, Ahuja N: Development of controlled-release buccoadhesive hydrophilic matrices of diltiazem hydrochloride: Optimization of bioadhesion, dissolution, and diffusion parameters. Drug Dev Ind Pharm 28:431-442, 2002.

532. Bloedow DC, Piepho RW, Nies AS, Gal J: Serum binding of diltiazem in humans. J Clin Pharmacol 22:201-205, 1982.

533. Costa P, Sousa Lobo JM: Divisibility of diltiazem matrix sustained-release tablets. Pharm Dev Technol 6:343-351, 2001.

534. Nguyen BN, Parker RB, Noujedehi M, et al: Effects of COER-verapamil on circadian pattern of forearm vascular resistance and blood pressure. J Clin Pharmacol 40:1480-1487, 2000.

535. Smith DH, Neutel JM, Weber MA: A new chronotherapeutic oral drug absorption system for verapamil optimizes blood pressure control in the morning. Am J Hypertens 14:14-19, 2001.

536. Sawicki W, Janicki S: Pharmacokinetics of verapamil and its metabolite norverapamil from a buccal drug formulation. Int J Pharm 238:181-189, 2002.

537. Gupta S, Modi NB, Sathyan G, et al: Pharmacokinetics of controlled-release verapamil in healthy volunteers and patients with hypertension or angina. Biopharm Drug Dispos 23:17-31, 2002.

538. Shand DG, Hammill SC, Aanonsen L, Pritchett EL: Reduced verapamil clearance during long-term oral administration. Clin Pharmacol Ther 30:701-706, 1981.

539. Fuhr U, Muller-Peltzer H, Kern R, et al: Effects of grapefruit juice and smoking on verapamil concentrations in steady state. Eur J Clin Pharmacol 58:45-53, 2002.

540. Takahara A, Sugiyama A, Yoshimoto R, Hashimoto K: AH-1058: A novel cardioselective Ca^{2+} channel blocker. Cardiovasc Drug Rev 19:279-296, 2001.

541. Pahor M, Psaty BM, Alderman MH, et al: Health outcomes associated with calcium antagonists compared with other first-line antihypertensive therapies: A meta-analysis of randomised controlled trials. Lancet 356:1949-1954, 2000.

542. Kleinbloesem CH, van Brummelen P, van de Linde JA, et al: Nifedipine: Kinetics and dynamics in healthy subjects. Clin Pharmacol Ther 35:742-749, 1984.

543. Chung M, Reitberg DP, Gaffney M, Singleton W: Clinical pharmacokinetics of nifedipine gastrointestinal therapeutic system. A controlled-release formulation of nifedipine. Am J Med 83:10-14, 1987.

544. Grundy JS, Foster RT: The nifedipine gastrointestinal therapeutic system (GITS). Evaluation of pharmaceutical, pharmacokinetic and pharmacological properties. Clin Pharmacokinet 30:28-51, 1996.

545. Binggeli C, Corti R, Sudano I, et al: Effects of chronic calcium channel blockade on sympathetic nerve activity in hypertension. Hypertension 39:892-896, 2002.

546. Faulkner JK, McGibney D, Chasseaud LF, et al: The pharmacokinetics of amlodipine in healthy volunteers after single intravenous and oral doses and after 14 repeated oral doses given once daily. Br J Clin Pharmacol 22:21-25, 1986.

547. Donnelly R, Meredith PA, Miller SH, et al: Pharmacodynamic modeling of the antihypertensive response to amlodipine. Clin Pharmacol Ther 54:303-310, 1993.

548. Abernethy DR: An overview of the pharmacokinetics and pharmacodynamics of amlodipine in elderly persons with systemic hypertension. Am J Cardiol 73:10A-17A, 1994.

549. Leonetti G, Rupoli L, Chianca R, et al: Acute, chronic and postwithdrawal antihypertensive and renal effects of amlodipine in hypertensive patients. J Hypertens Suppl 9:S394-S395, 1991.

550. Edgar B, Hoffmann KJ, Lundborg P, et al: Absorption, distribution and elimination of felodipine in man. Drugs 29(suppl 2):9-15, 1985.

551. Edgar B, Bailey D, Bergstrand R, et al: Acute effects of drinking grapefruit juice on the pharmacokinetics and dynamics of felodipine—And its potential clinical relevance. Eur J Clin Pharmacol 42:313-317, 1992.

552. Edgar B: Clinical Pharmacokinetics of Felodipine. Thesis. University of Goteborg, 1988.

553. Fitton A, Benfield P: Isradipine. A review of its pharmacodynamic and pharmacokinetic properties, and therapeutic use in cardiovascular disease. Drugs 40:31-74, 1990.

554. Aoi Y, Yamachika S: Effects of a new Ca antagonist, manidipine-HCl, on circadian rhythm of BP and renal function in hypertensive patients. Clin Rep 23:3230-3238, 1989.

555. Arakawa K, Kaneko Y, Iimura O: Efficacy and safety or manidipine HCl in patients with essential HTN: A dose-finding study in monotherapy and combined therapy with thiazide diuretics or beta-blocking agents. J Pharmacol Ther 17:2681-2712, 1989.

556. Atarashi K, Takagi M, Minami M, et al: Effects of manidipine and delapril on glucose and lipid metabolism in hypertensive patients with non–insulin-dependent diabetes mellitus. Blood Press Suppl 3:130-134, 1992.

557. Sorkin EM, Clissold SP: Nicardipine. A review of its pharmacodynamic and pharmacokinetic properties, and therapeutic efficacy, in the treatment of angina pectoris, hypertension and related cardiovascular disorders. Drugs 33:296-345, 1987.

558. Mitchell J, Frishman W, Heiman M: Nisoldipine: A new dihydropyridine calcium-channel blocker. J Clin Pharmacol 33:46-52, 1993.

559. Micheli D, Ratti E, Toson G: Pharmacology of lacidipine, a vascular-selective Ca antagonist. J Cardiovasc Pharmacol 17(suppl 4): S1-S8, 1991.

560. Rizzini P, Castello C, Salvi S, Recchia G: Efficacy and safety of lacidipine, a new long-lasting calcium antagonist, in elderly hypertensive patients. J Cardiovasc Pharmacol 17(suppl 4):S38-S43, 1991.

561. Angelico P, Guarneri L, Leonardi A, Testa R: Vascular-selective effect of lercanidipine and other 1,4-dihydropyridines in isolated rabbit tissues. J Pharm Pharmacol 51:709-714, 1999.

562. Herbette LG, Vecchiarelli M, Sartani A, Leonardi A: Lercanidipine: Short plasma half-life, long duration of action and high cholesterol tolerance. Updated molecular model to rationalize its pharmacokinetic properties. Blood Press Suppl 2:10-17, 1998.

563. Fogari R, Malamani GD, Zoppi A: Comparative effect of lercanidipine and nifedipine gastrointestinal therapeutic system on ankle volume and subcutaneous interstitial pressure in hypertensive patients: A double-blind, randomized parallel-group study. Curr Ther Res 61:850-862, 2000.

564. Epstein M: Lercanidipine: A novel dihydropyridine calcium-channel blocker. Heart Dis 3:398-407, 2001.

565. Ram CV: Usefulness of lercanidipine, a new calcium antagonist, for systemic hypertension. Am J Cardiol 89:214-215, 2002.

566. Sabbatini M, Leonardi A, Testa R, et al: Effect of calcium antagonists on glomerular arterioles in spontaneously hypertensive rats. Hypertension 35:775-779, 2000.

567. Epstein M: Implications for renal protection. Am J Hypertens 4:482S-486S, 1991.

568. Dietz JR, Davis JO, Freeman RH, et al: Effects of intrarenal infusion of calcium entry blockers in anesthetized dogs. Hypertension 5:482-488, 1983.

569. Wallia R, Greenberg A, Puschett JB: Renal hemodynamic and tubular transport effects of nitrendipine. J Lab Clin Med 105:498-503, 1985.

570. Epstein M, DeMicheli AG, Forster H: Natriuretic effects of Ca antagonists in humans: A review of experimental evidence and clinical data. Cardiovasc Drug Rev 9:399-413, 1985.

571. MacGregor GA, Prerahouse JB, Cappuccio FB: Nifedipine, diuretics and Na balance. J Hypertens 5(suppl):S127-S131, 1987.

572. Hulther UL, Katzman PL: Renal effects of acute and long-term treatment with felodipine in essential HTN. J Hypertens 6:231-237, 1988.

573. Krusell LR, Jespersen LT, Christensen CK, et al: Acute natriuresis induced by inhibition of proximal tubular reabsorption of sodium and water in hypertensives following acute calcium entry blockade with nifedipine. J Cardiovasc Pharmacol 10(suppl 10):S162-S163, 1987.

574. Krusell LR, Jespersen LT, Schmitz A, et al: Repetitive natriuresis and blood pressure. Long-term calcium entry blockade with isradipine. Hypertension 10:577-581, 1987.

575. Leonetti G, Gradnik R, Terzoli L, et al: Effects of single and repeated doses of the calcium antagonist felodipine on blood pressure, renal function, electrolytes and water balance, and renin-angiotensin-aldosterone system in hypertensive patients. J Cardiovasc Pharmacol 8:1243-1248, 1986.

576. Shima S, Kawashima Y, Hirai M: Studies on cyclic nucleotides in the adrenal gland. VIII. Effects of angiotensin on adenosine 3',5'-monophosphate and steroidogenesis in the adrenal cortex. Endocrinology 103:1361-1367, 1978.

577. Fakunding JL, Chow R, Catt KJ: The role of calcium in the stimulation of aldosterone production by adrenocorticotropin, angiotensin II, and potassium in isolated glomerulosa cells. Endocrinology 105:327-333, 1979.

578. Fakunding JL, Catt KJ: Dependence of aldosterone stimulation in adrenal glomerulosa cells on calcium uptake: Effects of lanthanum nd verapamil. Endocrinology 107:1345-1353, 1980.

579. DiBona GF: Effects of felodipine on renal function in animals. Drugs 29(suppl 2):168-175, 1985.

580. Marunaka Y, Niisato N: Effects of Ca^{2+} channel blockers on amiloride-sensitive Na^+ permeable channels and Na^+ transport in fetal rat alveolar type II epithelium. Biochem Pharmacol 63:1547-1552, 2002.

581. DiBona GF, Sawin LL: Renal tubular site of action of felodipine. J Pharmacol Exp Ther 228:420-424, 1984.

582. Katzman PL, DiBona GF, Hokfelt B, Hulthen UL: Acute renal tubular and hemodynamic effects of the calcium antagonist felodipine in healthy volunteers. J Am Soc Nephrol 2:1000-1006, 1991.

583. Gaillard CA, Koomans HA, Rabelink TJ, et al: Opposite effects of enalapril and nitrendipine on natriuretic response to atrial natriuretic factor. Renal function evaluated with clearance studies in humans. Hypertension 13:173-180, 1989.

584. Rappelli A, Dessi-Fulgheri P, Madeddu P, Glorioso N: Studies on the natriuretic effect of nifedipine in hypertensive patients: Increase in levels of plasma atrial natriuretic factor without participation of the renal kallikrein-kinin system. J Hypertens Suppl 5:S61-S65, 1987.

585. Epstein M: Ca antagonists and the kidney: Implications for renal protection. In Epstein M (ed): Calcium Antagonists in Clinical Medicine. Philadelphia, Hanley & Belfus, 1992, p 309.

586. Loutzenhiser R, Epstein M: Effects of calcium antagonists on renal hemodynamics. Am J Physiol 249:F619-F629, 1985.

587. Epstein M, Loutzenhiser R: Renal hemodynamic effects of Ca antagonists. In Epstein M, Loutzenhiser R (eds): Calcium Antagonists and the Kidney. Philadelphia, Hanley & Belfus, 1990, pp 33-74.

588. Sunderrajan S, Reams G, Bauer JH: Long-term renal effects of diltiazem in essential hypertension. Am Heart J 114:383-388, 1987.

589. Reams GP, Lau A, Hamory A, Bauer JH: Amlodipine therapy corrects renal abnormalities encountered in the hypertensive state. Am J Kidney Dis 10:446-451, 1987.

590. Sunderrajan S, Reams G, Bauer JH: Renal effects of diltiazem in primary hypertension. Hypertension 8:238-242, 1986.

591. Blackshear JL, Garnic D, Williams GH, et al: Exaggerated renal vasodilator response to calcium entry blockade in first-degree relatives of essential hypertensive subjects. Hypertension 9:384-389, 1987.

592. Demarie BK, Bakris GL: Effects of different calcium antagonists on proteinuria associated with diabetes mellitus. Ann Intern Med 113:987-988, 1990.

593. Bakris GL: Effects of diltiazem or lisinopril on massive proteinuria associated with diabetes mellitus. Ann Intern Med 112:707-708, 1990.

594. Isshiki T, Amodeo C, Messerli FH, et al: Diltiazem maintains renal vasodilation without hyperfiltration in hypertension: Studies in essential hypertension man and the spontaneously hypertensive rat. Cardiovasc Drugs Ther 1:359-366, 1987.

595. Brunner FP, Hermle M, Thiel G: Verapamil in contrast to enalapril aggravates hyperfiltration despite lowered BP in rats with reduced renal mass. Abstract. Proceedings of the Tenth International Congress of Nephrology, 1987, p 497.

596. Sica DA, Douglas JG: The African American Study of Kidney Disease and Hypertension (AASK): New findings. J Clin Hypertens (Greenwich) 3:244-251, 2001.

597. Dworkin LD: Effects of Ca channel blockers on experimental glomerular injury. J Am Soc Nephrol 1:S21-S27, 1990.

598. Dworkin LD: Impact of calcium entry blockers on glomerular injury in experimental hypertension. Cardiovasc Drugs Ther 4:1325-1330, 1990.

599. Sweeney C, Shultz P, Raij L: Interactions of the endothelium and mesangium in glomerular injury. J Am Soc Nephrol 1:S13-S20, 1990.

600. Raij L, Keane WF: Glomerular mesangium: Its function and relationship to angiotensin II. Am J Med 79:24-30, 1985.

601. Keane WF, Raij L: Relationship among altered glomerular barrier permselectivity, angiotensin II, and mesangial uptake of macromolecules. Lab Invest 52:599-604, 1985.

602. Schwertschlag U, Schrier RW, Wilson P: Beneficial effects of calcium channel blockers and calmodulin binding drugs on in vitro renal cell anoxia. J Pharmacol Exp Ther 238:119-124, 1986.

603. Jesmin S, Sakuma I, Hattori Y, et al: Long-acting calcium channel blocker benidipine suppresses expression of angiogenic growth factors and prevents cardiac remodelling in a type II diabetic rat model. Diabetologia 45:402-415, 2002.

604. Mandarim-de-Lacerda CA, Pereira LM: Renal cortical remodelling by NO-synthesis blockers in rats is prevented by angiotensin-converting enzyme inhibitor and calcium channel blocker. J Cell Mol Med 5:276-283, 2001.

605. Kedziora-Kornatowska K, Szram S, Kornatowski T, et al: The effect of verapamil on the antioxidant defence system in diabetic kidney. Clin Chim Acta 322:105-112, 2002.

606. Wada Y, Kato S, Okamoto K, et al: Diltiazem, a calcium antagonist, inhibits matrix metalloproteinase-1 (tissue collagenase) production and collagenolytic activity in human vascular smooth muscle cells. Int J Mol Med 8:561-566, 2001.

607. Yavuz S, Ayabakan N, Goncu T, Ozdemir A: Effect of combined dopamine and diltiazem on renal function after cardiac surgery. Med Sci Monit 8:I45-I50, 2002.

608. Bergman AS, Odar-Cederlof I, Westman L, et al: Diltiazem infusion for renal protection in cardiac surgical patients with preexisting renal dysfunction. J Cardiothorac Vasc Anesth 16:294-299, 2002.

609. Wang YX, Jia YF, Chen KM, Morcos SK: Radiographic contrast media induced nephropathy: Experimental observations and the protective effect of calcium channel blockers. Br J Radiol 74:1103-1108, 2001.

610. Frei U, Margreiter R, Harms A, et al: Preoperative graft reperfusion with a calcium antagonist improves initial function: Preliminary results of a prospective randomized trial in 110 kidney recipients. Transplant Proc 19:3539-3541, 1987.

611. Rodicio JL: Calcium antagonists and renal protection from cyclosporine nephrotoxicity: Long-term trial in renal transplantation patients. J Cardiovasc Pharmacol 35:S7-11, 2000.

612. Weir MR: Clinical benefits of Ca antagonists in renal transplant recipients. In Epstein M (ed): Calcium Antagonists in Clinical Medicine. Philadelphia, Hanley & Belfus, 1992, p 391.

613. Loutzenhiser R, Epstein M, Horton C, Sonke P: Reversal of renal and smooth muscle actions of the thromboxane mimetic U-44069 by diltiazem. Am J Physiol 250:F619-F626, 1986.

614. Kon V, Sugiura M, Inagami T, et al: Role of endothelin in cyclosporine-induced glomerular dysfunction. Kidney Int 37: 1487-1491, 1990.

615. Cheng CH, Hsieh CL, Shu KH, et al: Effect of calcium channel antagonist diltiazem and calcium ionophore A23187 on cyclosporine A–induced apoptosis of renal tubular cells. FEBS Lett 516:191-196, 2002.

616. Tsuda K, Tsuda S, Nishio I, Masuyama Y: Role of dihydropyridine-sensitive calcium channels in the regulation of norepinephrine release in hypertension. J Cardiovasc Pharmacol 38(suppl 1):S27-S31, 2001.

617. Buhler FR, Kiowski W: Calcium antagonists in hypertension. J Hypertens Suppl 5:S3-10, 1987.

618. Moser M: Calcium entry blockers for systemic hypertension. Am J Cardiol 59:115A-121A, 1987.

619. Ram CV: Calcium antagonists as antihypertensive agents are effective in all age groups. J Hypertens 11:166-173, 1988.

620. Zing W, Ferguson RK, Vlasses PH: Calcium antagonists in elderly and black hypertensive patients. Therapeutic controversies. Arch Intern Med 151:2154-2162, 1991.

621. Cubeddu LX, Aranda J, Singh B, et al: A comparison of verapamil and propranolol for the initial treatment of hypertension. Racial differences in response. JAMA 256:2214-2221, 1986.

622. Kiowski W, Buhler FR, Fadayomi MO, et al: Age, race, blood pressure and renin: predictors for antihypertensive treatment with calcium antagonists. Am J Cardiol 56:81H-85H, 1985.

623. White WB, Johnson MF, Anders RJ, et al: Safety of controlled-onset extended-release verapamil in middle-aged and older patients with hypertension and coronary artery disease. Am Heart J 142: 1010-1015, 2001.

624. Kestenbaum B, Gillen DL, Sherrard DJ, et al: Calcium channel blocker use and mortality among patients with end-stage renal disease. Kidney Int 61:2157-2164, 2002.

625. Opie LH, Yusuf S, Kubler W: Current status of safety and efficacy of calcium channel blockers in cardiovascular diseases: A critical analysis based on 100 studies. Prog Cardiovasc Dis 43:171-196, 2000.

626. Morgan TO, Anderson AI, MacInnis RJ: ACE inhibitors, beta-blockers, calcium blockers, and diuretics for the control of systolic hypertension. Am J Hypertens 14:241-247, 2001.

627. Hanes DS, Weir MR, Sowers JR: Gender considerations in hypertension pathophysiology and treatment. Am J Med 101:10S-21S, 1996.

628. Blackwell JN, Holt S, Heading RC: Effect of nifedipine on oesophageal motility and gastric emptying. Digestion 21:50-56, 1981.

629. Ellis JS, Seymour RA, Monkman SC, Idle JR: Gingival sequestration of nifedipine in nifedipine-induced gingival overgrowth. Lancet 339:1382-1383, 1992.

630. Bullon P, Machuca G, Armas JR, et al: The gingival inflammatory infiltrate in cardiac patients treated with calcium antagonists. J Clin Periodontol 28:897-903, 2001.

631. Dominic JA, Miller RE, Anderson J, McAllister RG Jr: Pharmacology of verapamil. II. Impairment of glucose tolerance by verapamil in the conscious dog. Pharmacology 20:196-202, 1980.

632. Trost BN, Weidmann P: Effects of calcium antagonists on glucose homeostasis and serum lipids in non-diabetic and diabetic subjects: A review. J Hypertens Suppl 5:S81-104, 1987.

633. Pollare T, Lithell H, Morlin C, et al: Metabolic effects of diltiazem and atenolol: Results from a randomized, double-blind study with parallel groups. J Hypertens 7:551-559, 1989.

634. Tentorio A, Ghilardi G, Pedroncelli A, et al: Insulin secretion and glucose tolerance in non-insulin dependent diabetic patients after chronic nifedipine treatment. Eur J Clin Pharmacol 36:311-313, 1989.

635. Andren L, Hoglund P, Dotevall A, et al: Diltiazem in hypertensive patients with type II diabetes mellitus. Am J Cardiol 62:114G-120G, 1988.

636. Speders S, Sosna J, Schumacher A: Efficacy and tolerability of isoptin SR in essential hypertension: Results of phase IV study under practice conditions. Hockdruck 8:3-14, 1988.

637. Bitar R, Flores O, Reverte M, et al: Beneficial effect of verapamil added to chronic ACE inhibitor treatment on renal function in hypertensive elderly patients. Int Urol Nephrol 32:165-169, 2000.

638. Black HR, Elliott WJ, Weber MA: One-year study of felodipine or placebo for stage 1 isolated systolic hypertension. Hypertension 38:1118-1123, 2001.

639. Schiffrin EL, Pu Q, Park JB: Effect of amlodipine compared to atenolol on small arteries of previously untreated essential hypertensive patients. Am J Hypertens 15:105-110, 2002.

640. De Servi S, Ferrario M, Ghio S, et al: Effects of diltiazem on regional coronary hemodynamics during atrial pacing in patients with stable exertional angina: Implications for mechanism of action. Circulation 73:1248-1253, 1986.

641. Emanuelsson H, Holmberg S: Mechanisms of angina relief after nifedipine: A hemodynamic and myocardial metabolic study. Circulation 68:124-130, 1983.

642. Walsh RA, O'Rourke RA: Direct and indirect effects of calcium entry blocking agents on isovolumic left ventricular relaxation in conscious dogs. J Clin Invest 75:1426-1434, 1985.

643. Messerli FH, Nunez BD, Nunez MM, et al: Hypertension and sudden death. Disparate effects of calcium entry blocker and diuretic therapy on cardiac dysrhythmias. Arch Intern Med 149:1263-1267, 1989.

644. Pearson AC, Pasierski T, Labovitz AJ: Left ventricular hypertrophy: Diagnosis, prognosis, and management. Am Heart J 121:148-157, 1991.

645. Novo S, Abrignani MG, Novo G, et al: Effects of drug therapy on cardiac arrhythmias and ischemia in hypertensives with LVH. Am J Hypertens 14:637-643, 2001.

646. Szlachcic J, Tubau JF, Vollmer C, Massie BM: Effect of diltiazem on left ventricular mass and diastolic filling in mild to moderate hypertension. Am J Cardiol 63:198-201, 1989.

647. Diamond JA, Krakoff LR, Goldman A, et al: Comparison of two calcium blockers on hemodynamics, left ventricular mass, and coronary vasodilatory in advanced hypertension. Am J Hypertens 14:231-240, 2001.

648. Semsarian C, Ahmad I, Giewat M, et al: The L-type calcium channel inhibitor diltiazem prevents cardiomyopathy in a mouse model. J Clin Invest 109:1013-1020, 2002.

649. Casale PN, Devereux RB, Milner M, et al: Value of echocardiographic measurement of left ventricular mass in predicting cardiovascular morbid events in hypertensive men. Ann Intern Med 105: 173-178, 1986.

650. Koren MJ, Devereux RB, Casale PN, et al: Relation of left ventricular mass and geometry to morbidity and mortality in uncomplicated essential hypertension. Ann Intern Med 114:345-352, 1991.

651. Kannel WB, Gordon T, Castelli WP, Margolis JR: Electro cardio-graphic left ventricular hypertrophy and risk of coronary heart disease. The Framingham study. Ann Intern Med 72:813-822, 1970.

652. Yusuf S, Held P, Furberg C: Update of effects of calcium antagonists in myocardial infarction or angina in light of the second Danish Verapamil Infarction Trial (DAVIT-II) and other recent studies. Am J Cardiol 67:1295-1297, 1991.

653. Danish Study Group: Secondary prevention with verapamil after myocardial infarction. The Danish Study Group on Verapamil in Myocardial Infarction. Am J Cardiol 66:33I-40I, 1990.

654. Lichtlen PR, Hugenholtz PG, Rafflenbeul W, et al: Retardation of angiographic progression of coronary artery disease by nifedipine. Results of the International Nifedipine Trial on Antiatherosclerotic Therapy (INTACT). INTACT Group Investigators. Lancet 335: 1109-1113, 1990.

655. DeQuattro V, Lee D: Fixed-dose combination therapy with trandolapril and verapamil SR is effective in primary hypertension. Trandolapril Study Group. Am J Hypertens 10:138S-145S, 1997.

656. Marcus FI: Drug interactions with amiodarone. Am Heart J 106: 924-930, 1983.

657. Bottiger Y, Sawe J, Brattstrom C, et al: Pharmacokinetic interaction between single oral doses of diltiazem and sirolimus in healthy volunteers. Clin Pharmacol Ther 69:32-40, 2001.

658. Varis T, Backman JT, Kivisto KT, Neuvonen PJ: Diltiazem and mibefradil increase the plasma concentrations and greatly enhance the adrenal-suppressant effect of oral methylprednisolone. Clin Pharmacol Ther 67:215-221, 2000.

659. Ohashi K, Tateishi T, Sudo T, et al: Effects of diltiazem on the pharmacokinetics of nifedipine. J Cardiovasc Pharmacol 15:96-101, 1990.

660. Toyosaki N, Toyo-oka T, Natsume T, et al: Combination therapy with diltiazem and nifedipine in patients with effort angina pectoris. Circulation 77:1370-1375, 1988.

661. Clarke WR, Horn JR, Kawabori I, Gurtel S: Potentially serious drug interactions secondary to high-dose diltiazem used in the treatment of pulmonary hypertension. Pharmacotherapy 13:402-405, 1993.

662. North DS, Mattern AL, Hiser WW: The influence of diltiazem hydrochloride on trough serum digoxin concentrations. Drug Intell Clin Pharm 20:500-503, 1986.

663. Pahor M, Guralnik JM, Furberg CD, et al: Risk of gastrointestinal haemorrhage with calcium antagonists in hypertensive persons over 67 years old. Lancet 347:1061-1065, 1996.

664. Shinjo A, Sasaki Y, Inamasu M, Morita T: In vitro effect of the coronary vasodilator diltiazem on human and rabbit platelets. Thromb Res 13:941-955, 1978.

665. Das UN: Modification of anti-hypertensive action of verapamil by inhibition of endogenous prostaglandin synthesis. Prostaglandins Leukot Med 9:167-169, 1982.

666. Harvey PJ, Wing LM, Beilby J, et al: Effect of indomethacin on blood pressure control during treatment with nitrendipine. Blood Press 4:307-312, 1995.

667. Minuz P, Pancera P, Ribul M, et al: Amlodipine and haemodynamic effects of cyclo-oxygenase inhibition. Br J Clin Pharmacol 39:45-50, 1995.

668. Effects of calcium antagonists on the risks of coronary heart disease, cancer and bleeding. Ad Hoc Subcommittee of the Liaison Committee of the World Health Organisation and the International Society of Hypertension. J Hypertens 15:105-115, 1997.

669. Furberg CD, Psaty BM, Meyer JV: Nifedipine. Dose-related increase in mortality in patients with coronary heart disease. Circulation 92:1326-1331, 1995.

670. Van Zwietan PA, Hansson L, Epstein M: Slowly acting calcium antagonists and their merits. Blood Press 6:78-80, 2002.

671. Langer SZ, Cavero I, Massingham R: Recent developments in noradrenergic neurotransmission and its relevance to the mechanism of action of certain antihypertensive agents. Hypertension 2:372-382, 1980.

672. Reid JL: Alpha-adrenergic receptors and blood pressure control. Am J Cardiol 57:6E-12E, 1986.

673. Dollery CT: Advantages and disadvantages of alpha 2-adrenoceptor agonists for systemic hypertension. Am J Cardiol 61:1D-5D, 1988.

674. Louis WJ, Jarrott B, Conway EL: Sites of actions of alpha 2 agonists in the brain and periphery. Am J Cardiol 61:15D-17D, 1988.

675. Oster JR, Epstein M: Use of centrally acting sympatholytic agents in the management of hypertension. Arch Intern Med 151:1638-1644, 1991.

676. van Zwieten PA, Chalmers JP: Different types of centrally acting antihypertensives and their targets in the central nervous system. Cardiovasc Drugs Ther 8:787-799, 1994.

677. Prichard BN: Clinical experience with moxonidine. In van Zwieten PA, Hamilton CA, Julius S, Prichard BN (eds): The I1-Imidazoline Receptor Agonist Moxonidine: A New Antihypertensive, 2nd ed. London, Royal Society of Medicine Press, 1996, pp 49-77.

678. Molderings GJ, Michel MC, Gothert M, et al: [Imidazole receptors: site of action of a new generation of antihypertensive drugs. Current status and future prospects]. Dtsch Med Wochenschr 117:67-71, 1992.

679. van Zwieten PA: Central imidazoline (I1) receptors as targets of centrally acting antihypertensives: Moxonidine and rilmenidine. J Hypertens 15:117-125, 1997.

680. Bousquet P, Esler M: I1-agents in high blood pressure and cardioprotection management: the contribution of rilmenidine. J Hypertens 16:S1-S62, 1998.

681. Prichard BN: Clinical pharmacology of moxonidine. In van Zwieten PA, Hamilton CA, Julius S, Prichard BN (eds): The I1-Imidazoline Receptor Agonist Moxonidine: A New Antihypertensive, 2nd ed. London, Royal Society of Medicine Press, 1996, pp 31-47.

682. Bousquet P, Feldman J: Drugs acting on imidazoline receptors: A review of their pharmacology, their use in blood pressure control and their potential interest in cardioprotection. Drugs 58:799-812, 1999.

683. van Zwieten PA, Peters SL: Central I1-imidazoline receptors as targets of centrally acting antihypertensive drugs. Clinical pharmacology of moxonidine and rilmenidine. Ann NY Acad Sci 881: 420-429, 1999.

684. Szabo B: Imidazoline antihypertensive drugs: A critical review on their mechanism of action. Pharmacol Ther 93:1-35, 2002.

685. Hokfelt B, Hedeland H, Dymling JF: Studies on catecholamines, renin and aldosterone following Catapresan (2-(2,6-dichlorphenylamine)-2-imidazoline hydrochloride) in hypertensive patients. Eur J Pharmacol 10:389-397, 1970.

686. Hokfelt B, Hedeland H, Hansson BG: The effect of clonidine and penbutolol, respectively on catecholamines in blood and urine, plasma renin activity and urinary aldosterone in hypertensive patients. Arch Int Pharmacodyn Ther 213:307-321, 1975.

687. Campese VM, Romoff M, Telfer N, et al: Role of sympathetic nerve inhibition and body sodium-volume state in the antihypertensive action of clonidine in essential hypertension. Kidney Int 18:351-357, 1980.

688. Manhem P, Paalzow L, Hokfelt B: Plasma clonidine in relation to blood pressure, catecholamines, and renin activity during long-term treatment of hypertension. Clin Pharmacol Ther 31:445-451, 1982.

689. Farsang C, Kapocsi J, Vajda L, et al: Reversal by naloxone of the antihypertensive action of clonidine: Involvement of the sympathetic nervous system. Circulation 69:461-467, 1984.

690. Sullivan PA, De Q, V, Foti A, Curzon G: Effects of clonidine on central and peripheral nerve tone in primary hypertension. Hypertension 8:611-617, 1986.

691. Bobik A, Jennings G, Jackman G, et al: Evidence for a predominantly central hypotensive effect of alpha-methyldopa in humans. Hypertension 8:16-23, 1986.

692. Sannerstedt R, Varnauskas E, Werko L: Hemodynamic effects of methyldopa (Aldomet) at rest and during exercise in patients with arterial hypertension. Acta Med Scand 171:75-82, 1962.

693. Weil MH, Barbour BH, Chesne RB: Alpha-methyldopa for the treatment of hypertension. Circulation 28:165-174, 1963.

694. Onesti G, Schwartz AB, Kim KE, et al: Antihypertensive effect of clonidine. Circ Res 28(suppl 2):53-69, 1971.

695. Onesti G, Bock KD, Heimsoth V, et al: Clonidine: A new antihypertensive agent. Am J Cardiol 28:74-83, 1971.

696. Brest AN: Hemodynamic and cardiac effects of clonidine. J Cardiovasc Pharmacol 2(suppl 1):S39-S46, 1980.

697. Houston MC: Clonidine hydrochloride: Review of pharmacologic and clinical aspects. Prog Cardiovasc Dis 23:337-350, 1981.

698. Myhre E, Stenbaek O, Rugstad HE, et al: Pharmacokinetics of methyldopa in renal failure and bilaterally nephrectomized patients. Scand J Urol Nephrol 16:257-263, 1982.

699. Myhre E, Rugstad HE, Hansen T: Clinical pharmacokinetics of methyldopa. Clin Pharmacokinet 7:221-233, 1982.

700. Pettinger WA: Drug therapy: Clonidine, a new antihypertensive drug. N Engl J Med 293:1179-1180, 1975.

701. Hulter HN, Licht JH, Ilnicki LP, Singh S: Clinical efficacy and pharmacokinetics of clonidine in hemodialysis and renal insufficiency. J Lab Clin Med 94:223-231, 1979.

702. Lowenthal DT: Pharmacokinetics of clonidine. J Cardiovasc Pharmacol 2(suppl 1):S29-S37, 1980.

703. Baum T, Shropshire AT, Rowles G, et al: General pharmacologic actions of the antihypertensive agent 2,6-dichlorobenzylidene aminoguanidine acetate (WY-8678). J Pharmacol Exp Ther 171: 276-287, 1970.

704. Meacham RH, Emmett M, Kyriakopoulos AA, et al: Disposition of ^{14}C-guanabenz in patients with essential hypertension. Clin Pharmacol Ther 27:44-52, 1980.

705. Weber MA, Drayer JI: Centrally acting antihypertensive agents: A brief overview. J Cardiovasc Pharmacol 6(suppl 5):S803-S807, 1984.

706. Weiss YA, Lavene DL, Safar ME, et al: Guanfacine kinetics in patients with hypertension. Clin Pharmacol Ther 25:283-293, 1979.

707. Dollery CT, Davies DS: Centrally acting drugs in antihypertensive therapy. Br J Clin Pharmacol 10(suppl 1):5S-12S, 1980.

708. Saameli K, Jerie P, Scholtysik G: Guanfacine and other centrally acting drugs in antihypertensive therapy, pharmacological and clinical aspects. Clin Exp Hypertens A 4:209-219, 1982.

709. Sorkin EM, Heel RC: Guanfacine. Drugs 31:310-366, 1986.

710. Scholtysik G: Animal pharmacology of guanfacine. Am J Cardiol 57:13E-17E, 1986.

711. Kiechel JR: Pharmacokinetics of guanfacine in patients with impaired renal function and in some elderly patients. Am J Cardiol 57:18E-21E, 1986.

712. Schachter M: Moxonidine: A review of safety and tolerability after seven years of clinical experience. J Hypertens 17(suppl 3):S37-S39, 1999.

713. Messerli F: Moxonidine: A new and versatile antihypertensive. J Cardiovasc Pharmacol 35:S53-S56, 2000.

714. United Kingdom Working Party on Rilmenidine: Rilmenidine in mild-to-moderate essential hypertension. Curr Ther Res 1:194-211, 1990.

715. Aparicio M, Dratwa M, el Esper N, et al: Pharmacokinetics of rilmenidine in patients with chronic renal insufficiency and in hemodialysis patients. Am J Cardiol 74:43A-50A, 1994.

716. Luccioni R, Lambert M, Ambrosi P, Scemama M: Dose-effect relationship of rilmenidine after chronic administration. Eur J Clin Pharmacol 45:157-160, 1993.

717. Pillion G, Fevrier B, Codis P, Schutz D: Long-term control of blood pressure by rilmenidine in high-risk populations. Am J Cardiol 74:58A-65A, 1994.

718. Trimarco B, Rosiello G, Sarno D, et al: Effects of one-year treatment with rilmenidine on systemic hypertension-induced left ventricular hypertrophy in hypertensive patients. Am J Cardiol 74:36A-42A, 1994.

719. Bauer JH: Adrenergic blocking agents and the kidney. J Clin Hypertens 1:199-221, 1985.

720. Strandhoy JW, Morris M, Buckalew VM, Jr: Renal effects of the antihypertensive, guanabenz, in the dog. J Pharmacol Exp Ther 221:347-352, 1982.

721. Gehr M, MacCarthy EP, Goldberg M: Natriuretic and water diuretic effects of central alpha 2-adrenoceptor agonists. J Cardiovasc Pharmacol 6(suppl 5):S781-S786, 1984.

722. Goldberg M, Gehr M: Effects of alpha-2 agonists on renal function in hypertensive humans. J Cardiovasc Pharmacol 7(suppl 8): S34-S37, 1985.

723. Dollery CT, Harrington M: Methyldopa in hypertension. Clinical and pharmacological studies. Lancet 1:759-763, 1962.

724. Bayliss RI, Harvey-Smith EA: Methyldopa in the treatment of hypertension. Lancet 1:763-768, 1962.

725. Yeh BK, Nantel A, Goldberg LI: Antihypertensive effect of clonidine. Its use alone and in combination with hydrochlorothiazide and guanethidine in the treatment of hypertension. Arch Intern Med 127:233-237, 1971.

726. Mroczek WJ, Davidov M, Finnerty FA Jr: Prolonged treatment with clonidine: Comparative antihypertensive effects alone and with a diuretic agent. Am J Cardiol 30:536-541, 1972.

727. Garrett BN, Kaplan NM: Clonidine in the treatment of hypertension. J Cardiovasc Pharmacol 2(suppl 1):S61-S71, 1980.

728. Thananopavarn C, Golub MS, Eggena P, et al: Clonidine, a centrally acting sympathetic inhibitor, as monotherapy for mild to moderate hypertension. Am J Cardiol 49:153-158, 1982.

729. McMahon FG, Ryan JR, Jain AK, et al: Guanabenz in essential hypertension. Clin Pharmacol Ther 21:272-277, 1977.

730. Walker BR, Deitch MW, Schneider BE, et al: Long-term therapy of hypertension with guanabenz. Clin Ther 4:217-228, 1981.

731. Safar ME, Loria Y, Weiss YA, Boutier JR Jr: Antihypertensive effects and plasma levels of guanfacine in man. J Clin Pharmacol 22: 385-390, 1982.

732. Fillingim JM, Blackshear JL, Strauss A, Strauss M: Guanfacine as monotherapy for systemic hypertension. Am J Cardiol 57:50E-54E, 1986.

733. MacFarlane JP: Methyldopa in the elderly hypertensive. Curr Med Res Opin 7:63-67, 1982.

734. Thananopavarn C, Golub MS, Sambhi MP: Clonidine in the elderly hypertensive. Monotherapy and therapy with a diuretic. Chest 83:410-411, 1983.

735. Douchamps J, Papalexion P, Semadeni S, Herchuelz A: Antihypertensive effect of guanfacine in the elderly. Curr Ther Res 38:984-989, 1985.

736. Traub YM: Comparison of oxprenolol vs methyldopa as second-line antihypertensive agents in the elderly. Arch Intern Med 148:77-80, 1988.

737. Swislocki A: Insulin resistance and hypertension. Am J Med Sci 300:104-115, 1990.

738. Weber MA: Transdermal antihypertensive therapy: Clinical and metabolic considerations. Am Heart J 112:906-912, 1986.

739. Gavras I, Manolis AJ, Gavras H: The alpha2-adrenergic receptors in hypertension and heart failure: Experimental and clinical studies. J Hypertens 19:2115-2124, 2001.

740. Stefanadis C, Manolis A, Dernellis J, et al: Acute effect of clonidine on left ventricular pressure-volume relation in hypertensive patients with diastolic heart dysfunction. J Hum Hypertens 15:635-642, 2001.

741. Palkhiwala SA, Yu A, Frishman WH: Imidazoline receptor agonist drugs for treatment of systemic hypertension and congestive heart failure. Heart Dis 2:83-92, 2000.

742. Husserl FE, Messerli FH: Adverse effects of antihypertensive drugs. Drugs 22:188-210, 1981.

743. Engelman K: Side effects of sympatholytic antihypertensive drugs. Hypertension 11:II30-II33, 1988.

744. Hansson L, Hunyor SN, Julius S, Hoobler SW: Blood pressure crisis following withdrawal of clonidine (Catapres, Catapresan), with special reference to arterial and urinary catecholamine levels, and suggestions for acute management. Am Heart J 85:605-610, 1973.

745. Weber MA: Discontinuation syndrome following cessation of treatment with clonidine and other antihypertensive agents. J Cardiovasc Pharmacol 2(suppl 1):S73-S89, 1980.

746. Metz S, Klein C, Morton N: Rebound hypertension after discontinuation of transdermal clonidine therapy. Am J Med 82:17-19, 1987.

747. Ram CV, Holland OB, Fairchild C, et al: Withdrawal syndrome following cessation of guanabenz therapy. J Clin Pharmacol 19: 148-150, 1978.

748. Bauer JH, Burch RN: Comparative studies: Guanabenz versus propranolol as first-step therapy for the treatment of primary hypertension. Cardiovasc Rev Rep 4:329-339, 1983.

749. Zamboulis C, Reid JL: Withdrawal of guanfacine after long-term treatment in essential hypertension. Observations on blood pressure and plasma and urinary noradrenaline. Eur J Clin Pharmacol 19: 19-24, 1981.

750. Jerie P: Long-term evaluations of therapeutic efficacy and safety of guanfacine. Am J Cardiol 57:55E-59E, 1986.

751. Rupp H, Maisch B, Brilla CG: Drug withdrawal and rebound hypertension: Differential action of the central antihypertensive drugs moxonidine and clonidine. Cardiovasc Drugs Ther 10(suppl 1): 251-262, 1996.

752. Weber MA, Drayer JI: Antihypertensive agents that act in the central nervous system. Cardiovasc Rev Rep 3:255-270, 1982.

753. Maass AR, Jenkins B, Shen Y, Tannenbaum P: Studies on absorption, excretion and metabolism of ^{3}H-reserpine in man. Clin Pharmacol Ther 10:366-371, 1970.

754. Zsoter TT, Johnson GE, DeVeber GA, Paul H: Excretion and metabolism of reserpine in renal failure. Clin Pharmacol Ther 14:325-330, 1973.

755. Participating Veterans Administration Medical Centers: Low doses v standard dose of reserpine. A randomized, double-blind, multiclinic trial in patients taking chlorthalidone. JAMA 248:2471-2477, 1982.

756. Lederle FA, Applegate WB, Grimm RH Jr: Reserpine and the medical marketplace. Arch Intern Med 153:705-706, 1993.

757. Moyer JH: Cardiovascular and renal hemodynamic response to reserpine (Serpasil), and clinical results of using this agent for the treatment of hypertension. Ann NY Acad Sci 59:82-94, 1954.

758. Krogsgaard AR: The effect of reserpine on the electrolyte and fluid balance in man. Acta Med Scand 69:127-132, 1957.

759. Reusch CS: The cardiorenal hemodynamic effects of antihypertensive therapy with reserpine. Am Heart J 64:643-649, 1962.

760. Veterans Administration Cooperative Study Group on Antihypertensive Agents: Effects of treatment on morbidity in hypertension. II. Results in patients with diastolic blood pressure averaging 90 through 114 mm Hg. JAMA 213:1143-1152, 1970.

761. Fraser HS: Reserpine: A tragic victim of myths, marketing, and fashionable prescribing. Clin Pharmacol Ther 60:368-373, 1996.

762. Pottash AL, Black HR, Gold MS: Psychiatric complications of antihypertensive medications. J Nerv Ment Dis 169:430-438, 1981.

763. Curb JD, Borhani NO, Blaszkowski TP, et al: Long-term surveillance for adverse effects of antihypertensive drugs. JAMA 253: 3263-3268, 1985.

764. Chidsey CA III, Gottlieb TB: The pharmacologic basis of antihypertensive therapy: The role of vasodilator drugs. Prog Cardiovasc Dis 17:99-113, 1974.

765. Page LT, Yager HM, Sidd JJ: Drugs in the management of hypertension. Part III. Am Heart J 92:252-259, 1976.

766. Tarazi RC: Vasodilators in hypertension: Spectrum of action and counteractions. Cardiovasc Med 3:1125-1131, 1978.

767. Khayyal M, Gross F, Kreye VA: Studies on the direct vasodilator effect of hydralazine in the isolated rabbit renal artery. J Pharmacol Exp Ther 216:390-394, 1981.

768. Lipe S, Moulds RF: In vitro differences between human arteries and veins in their responses to hydralazine. J Pharmacol Exp Ther 217:204-208, 1981.

769. DuCharme DW, Freyburger WA, Graham BE, Carlson RG: Pharmacologic properties of minoxidil: A new hypotensive agent. J Pharmacol Exp Ther 184:662-670, 1973.

770. Koch-Weser J: Hydralazine. N Engl J Med 295:320-322, 1976.

771. Shepherd AM, McNay JL, Ludden TM, et al: Plasma concentration and acetylator phenotype determine response to oral hydralazine. Hypertension 3:580-585, 1981.

772. Ludden TM, McNay JL Jr, Shepherd AM, Lin MS: Clinical pharmacokinetics of hydralazine. Clin Pharmacokinet 7:185-205, 1982.

773. Zins GR, Martin WB: The clinical pharmacology of minoxidil. *In* Velasco M (ed): Proceedings of the Second International Symposium on Arterial Hypertension. Amsterdam, Excerpta Medica, 1979, pp 72-79.

774. Lowenthal DT, Affrime MB: Pharmacology and pharmacokinetics of minoxidil. J Cardiovasc Pharmacol 2(suppl 2):S93-106, 1980.

775. Pettinger WA: Minoxidil and the treatment of severe hypertension. N Engl J Med 303:922-926, 1980.

776. Campese VM: Minoxidil: A review of its pharmacological properties and therapeutic use. Drugs 22:257-278, 1981.

777. Halstenson CE, Opsahl JA, Wright CE, et al: Disposition of minoxidil in patients with various degrees of renal function. J Clin Pharmacol 29:798-802, 1989.

778. Zins GR: Alteration in renal function during vasodilator therapy. *In* Wesson LG, Fanelli GM (eds): Recent Advances in Renal Physiology and Pharmacology. Baltimore, University Park Press, 1974, pp 165-186.

779. Grim CE, Luft FC, Grim CM, et al: Rapid blood pressure control with minoxidil: Acute and chronic effects on blood pressure, sodium excretion, and the renin-aldosterone system. Arch Intern Med 139:529-533, 1979.

780. Pratt JH, Yager CJ, Grim CE, Parkinson CA: Increased aldosterone metabolic clearance in hypertensive patients treated with minoxidil: An effect of greater hepatic perfusion. J Cardiovasc Pharmacol 2(suppl 2):S236-S241, 1980.

781. Reams GP, Bauer JH: The effect of triple drug therapy on renal function in patients with essential hypertension. J Clin Pharmacol 29:803-808, 1989.

782. Pettinger WA, Mitchell HC: Side effects of vasodilator therapy. Hypertension 11:II34-II36, 1988.

783. Martin WB, Spodick DH, Zins GR: Pericardial disorders occurring during open-label study of 1,869 severely hypertensive patients treated with minoxidil. J Cardiovasc Pharmacol 2(suppl 2):S217-S227, 1980.

784. Koch-Weser J: Vasodilator drugs in the treatment of hypertension. Arch Intern Med 133:1017-1027, 1974.

785. Perry HM Jr: Late toxicity to hydralazine resembling systemic lupus erythematosus or rheumatoid arthritis. Am J Med 54:58-72, 1973.

786. Bing RF, Russell GI, Thurston H, Swales JD: Hydralazine in hypertension: Is there a safe dose? Br Med J 281:353-354, 1980.

787. Litwin A, Adams LE, Zimmer H, Hess EV: Immunologic effects of hydralazine in hypertensive patients. Arthritis Rheum 24:1074-1078, 1981.

788. Perry HM Jr: Possible mechanisms of the hydralazine-related lupus-like syndrome. Arthritis Rheum 24:1093-1105, 1981.

789. Cameron HA, Ramsay LE: The lupus syndrome induced by hydralazine: A common complication with low dose treatment. Br Med J (Clin Res Ed) 289:410-412, 1984.

790. Weiner N: Drugs that inhibit adrenergic nerves and block adrenergic receptors. In Gilman AG, Goodman LS, Rall TW, Murad F (EDS): The Pharmacological Basis of Therapeutics, 7th ed. New York, Macmillan, 1985, pp 181-214.

791. Wheeler MH, Chare MJ, Austin TR, Lazarus JH: The management of the patient with catecholamine excess. World J Surg 6:735-747, 1982.

792. Stenstrom G, Haljamae H, Tisell LE: Influence of pre-operative treatment with phenoxybenzamine on the incidence of adverse cardiovascular reactions during anaesthesia and surgery for phaeochromocytoma. Acta Anaesthesiol Scand 29:797-803, 1985.

793. Hull CJ: Phaeochromocytoma. Diagnosis, preoperative preparation and anaesthetic management. Br J Anaesth 58:1453-1468, 1986.

794. Mulvihill-Wilson J, Gaffney FA, Pettinger WA, et al: Hemodynamic and neuroendocrine responses to acute and chronic alpha-adrenergic blockade with prazosin and phenoxybenzamine. Circulation 67:383-393, 1983.

795. Graham RM: Selective alpha 1-adrenergic antagonists: therapeutically relevant antihypertensive agents. Am J Cardiol 53:16A-20A, 1984.

796. Davey M: Mechanism of alpha blockade for blood pressure control. Am J Cardiol 59:18G-28G, 1987.

797. van Zwieten PA: Basic pharmacology of alpha-adrenoceptor antagonists and hybrid drugs. J Hypertens Suppl 6:S3-11, 1988.

798. Cubeddu LX: New alpha 1-adrenergic receptor antagonists for the treatment of hypertension: Role of vascular alpha receptors in the control of peripheral resistance. Am Heart J 116:133-162, 1988.

799. Luther RR: New perspectives on selective alpha 1 blockade. Am J Hypertens 2:729-735, 1989.

800. Khoury AF, Kaplan NM: Alpha-blocker therapy of hypertension. An unfulfilled promise. JAMA 266:394-398, 1991.

801. Reid JL, Vincent J: Clinical pharmacology and therapeutic role of prazosin and related alpha-adrenoceptor antagonists. Cardiology 73:164-174, 1986.

802. Lund-Johansen P: Hemodynamic changes at rest and during exercise in long-term prazosin therapy for essential hypertension. Postgrad Med Spec No 45-52, 1975.

803. Koshy MC, Mickley D, Bourgiognie J, Blaufox MD: Physiologic evaluation of a new antihypertensive agent: Prazosin HCl. Circulation 55:533-537, 1977.

804. Mancia G, Ferrari A, Gregorini L, et al: Effects of prazosin on autonomic control of circulation in essential hypertension. Hypertension 2:700-707, 1980.

805. Taylor SH: Pharmacotherapeutic stature of doxazosin and its role in coronary risk reduction. Am Heart J 116:1735-1747, 1988.

806. Taylor SH: Clinical pharmacotherapeutics of doxazosin. Am J Med 87:2S-11S, 1989.

807. Koch-Weser J, Graham RM, Pettinger WA: Drug therapy. Prazosin. N Engl J Med 300:232-236, 1979.

808. Stanaszek WF, Kellerman D, Brogden RN, Romankiewicz JA: Prazosin update. A review of its pharmacological properties and therapeutic use in hypertension and congestive heart failure. Drugs 25:339-384, 1983.

809. Lameire N, Gordts J: A pharmacokinetic study of prazosin in patients with varying degrees of chronic renal failure. Eur J Clin Pharmacol 31:333-337, 1986.

810. Kyncl JJ: Pharmacology of terazosin. Am J Med 80:12-19, 1986.

811. Sonders RC: Pharmacokinetics of terazosin. Am J Med 80:20-24, 1986.

812. Jungers P, Ganeval D, Pertuiset N, Chauveau P: Influence of renal insufficiency on the pharmacokinetics and pharmacodynamics of terazosin. Am J Med 80:94-99, 1986.

813. Ames RP, Chrysant SG, Gonzalez F, et al: Effectiveness of doxazosin in systemic hypertension. Am J Cardiol 64:203-208, 1989.

814. Dauer AD: Terazosin: An effective once-daily monotherapy for the treatment of hypertension. Am J Med 80:29-34, 1986.

815. Davey MJ: The pharmacological basis for the use of alpha 1-adrenoceptor antagonists in the treatment of essential hypertension. Br J Clin Pharmacol 21(suppl 1):5S-8S, 1986.

816. Deger G: Comparison of the safety and efficacy of once-daily terazosin versus twice-daily prazosin for the treatment of mild to moderate hypertension. Am J Med 80:62-67, 1986.

817. Fernandes M, Smith IS, Weder A, et al: Prazosin in the treatment of hypertension. Clin Sci Mol Med Suppl 2:181s-184s, 1975.

818. Hayduk K: Efficacy and safety of doxazosin in hypertension therapy. Am J Cardiol 59:35G-39G, 1987.

819. Okun R: Effectiveness of prazosin as initial antihypertensive therapy. Am J Cardiol 51:644-650, 1983.

820. Taylor SH, Grimm RH Jr: New developments in the role of alpha1-adrenergic receptors in cardiovascular disease. Am Heart J 119:655-662, 1990.

821. Major cardiovascular events in hypertensive patients randomized to doxazosin vs chlorthalidone: The antihypertensive and lipid-lowering treatment to prevent heart attack trial (ALLHAT). ALLHAT Collaborative Research Group. JAMA 283:1967-1975, 2000.

822. Davis BR, Cutler JA, Furberg CD, et al: Relationship of antihypertensive treatment regimens and change in blood pressure to risk for heart failure in hypertensive patients randomly assigned to doxazosin or chlorthalidone: Further analyses from the Antihypertensive and Lipid-Lowering treatment to prevent Heart Attack Trial. Ann Intern Med 137:313-320, 2002.

823. Kinoshita M, Shimazu N, Fujita M, et al: Doxazosin, an alpha1-adrenergic antihypertensive agent, decreases serum oxidized LDL. Am J Hypertens 14:267-270, 2001.

824. Pool JL: Effects of doxazosin on serum lipids: A review of the clinical data and molecular basis for altered lipid metabolism. Am Heart J 121:251-259, 1991.

825. Graham RM, Thornell IR, Gain JM, et al: Prazosin: The first-dose phenomenon. Br Med J 2:1293-1294, 1976.

826. Nicholson JP, Resnick LM, Pickering TG, et al: Relationship of blood pressure response and the renin-angiotensin system to first-dose prazosin. Am J Med 78:241-244, 1985.

827. Rosendorff C: Prazosin: Severe side effects are dose-dependent. Br Med J 2:508, 1976.

828. Turner AS: Prazosin in hypertension. Br Med J 2:1257-1258, 1976.

829. Lepor H: The emerging role of alpha antagonists in the therapy of benign prostatic hyperplasia. J Androl 12:389-394, 1991.

830. Wilde MI, Fitton A, Sorkin EM: Terazosin. A review of its pharmacodynamic and pharmacokinetic properties, and therapeutic potential in benign prostatic hyperplasia. Drugs Aging 3:258-277, 1993.

831. de Gasparo M, Joss U, Ramjoue HP, et al: Three new epoxyspirolactone derivatives: Characterization in vivo and in vitro. J Pharmacol Exp Ther 240:650-656, 1987.

832. de Gasparo M, Whitebread SE, Preiswerk G, et al: Antialdosterones: Incidence and prevention of sexual side effects. J Steroid Biochem 32:223-227, 1989.

833. Delyani JA: Mineralocorticoid receptor antagonists: The evolution of utility and pharmacology. Kidney Int 57:1408-1411, 2000.

834. Mangelsdorf DJ, Thummel C, Beato M, et al: The nuclear receptor superfamily: The second decade. Cell 83:835-839, 1995.

835. Pratt WB: The role of heat shock proteins in regulating the function, folding, and trafficking of the glucocorticoid receptor. J Biol Chem 268:21455-21458, 1993.

836. Bhargava A, Fullerton MJ, Myles K, et al: The serum- and glucocorticoid-induced kinase is a physiological mediator of aldosterone action. Endocrinology 142:1587-1594, 2001.

837. Granger JP, Kassab S, Novak J, et al: Role of nitric oxide in modulating renal function and arterial pressure during chronic aldosterone excess. Am J Physiol 276:R197-R202, 1999.

838. Rocha R, Stier CT Jr: Pathophysiological effects of aldosterone in cardiovascular tissues. Trends Endocrinol Metab 12:308-314, 2001.

839. Lombes M, Alfaidy N, Eugene E, et al: Prerequisite for cardiac aldosterone action. Mineralocorticoid receptor and 11 beta-hydroxysteroid dehydrogenase in the human heart. Circulation 92:175-182, 1995.

840. Roland BL, Krozowski ZS, Funder JW: Glucocorticoid receptor, mineralocorticoid receptors, 11 beta-hydroxysteroid dehydrogenase-1 and -2 expression in rat brain and kidney: In situ studies. Mol Cell Endocrinol 111:R1-R7, 1995.

841. Takeda Y, Miyamori I, Inaba S, et al: Vascular aldosterone in genetically hypertensive rats. Hypertension 29:45-48, 1997.

842. Christ M, Douwes K, Eisen C, et al: Rapid effects of aldosterone on sodium transport in vascular smooth muscle cells. Hypertension 25:117-123, 1995.

843. Alzamora R, Michea L, Marusic ET: Role of 11beta-hydroxysteroid dehydrogenase in nongenomic aldosterone effects in human arteries. Hypertension 35:1099-1104, 2000.

844. Ibrahim HN, Rosenberg ME, Hostetter TH: Role of the renin-angiotensin-aldosterone system in the progression of renal disease: A critical review. Semin Nephrol 17:431-440, 1997.

845. Remuzzi G, Ruggenenti P, Benigni A: Understanding the nature of renal disease progression. Kidney Int 51:2-15, 1997.

846. Epstein M: Aldosterone as a mediator of progressive renal dysfunction: Evolving perspectives. Intern Med 40:573-583, 2001.

847. Greene EL, Kren S, Hostetter TH: Role of aldosterone in the remnant kidney model in the rat. J Clin Invest 98:1063-1068, 1996.

848. Quan ZY, Walser M, Hill GS: Adrenalectomy ameliorates ablative nephropathy in the rat independently of corticosterone maintenance level. Kidney Int 41:326-333, 1992.

849. Gavras H, Brunner HR, Laragh JH, et al: Malignant hypertension resulting from deoxycorticosterone acetate and salt excess: Role of renin and sodium in vascular changes. Circ Res 36:300-309, 1975.

850. Rocha R, Chander PN, Khanna K, et al: Mineralocorticoid blockade reduces vascular injury in stroke-prone hypertensive rats. Hypertension 31:451-458, 1998.

851. Weinberger MH, Roniker B, Krause SL, Weiss RJ: Eplerenone, a selective aldosterone blocker, in mild-to-moderate hypertension. Am J Hypertens 15:709-716, 2002.

852. Krum H, Nolly H, Roniker B, et al: Coadministration of eplerenone with an angiotensin-converting enzyme inhibitor or an angiotensin II blocker in patients with mild to moderate hypertension. Eur Heart J (Suppl) 22:612, 2001.

853. Epstein M, Buckalew V, Martinez F, et al: Antiproteinuric efficacy of eplerenone, enalapril, and eplerenone/enalapril combination in diabetic hypertensives with microalbuminuria Abstract. Am J Hypertens 15:24A, 2002.

854. Engelman K, Jequier E, Udenfriend S, Sjoerdsma A: Metabolism of alpha-methyltyrosine in man: Relationship to its potency as an inhibitor of catecholamine biosynthesis. J Clin Invest 47:568-576, 1968.

855. Engelman K, Horwitz D, Jequier E, Sjoerdsma A: Biochemical and pharmacologic effects of alpha-methyltyrosine in man. J Clin Invest 47:577-594, 1968.

856. Jones NF, Walker G, Ruthven CR, Sandler M: Alpha-methyl-*p*-tyrosine in the management of phaeochromocytoma. Lancet 2:1105-1109, 1968.

857. Brogden RN, Heel RC, Speight TM, Avery GS: alpha-Methyl-*p*-tyrosine: A review of its pharmacology and clinical use. Drugs 21:81-89, 1981.

858. Green KN, Larsson SK, Beevers DG, et al: Alpha-methyltyrosine in the management of phaeochromocytoma. Thorax 37:632-633, 1982.

859. Hauptman JB, Modlinger RS, Ertel NH: Pheochromocytoma resistant to alpha-adrenergic blockade. Arch Intern Med 143:2321-2323, 1983.

860. Norton GR, Woodiwiss AJ, Hartford C, et al: Sustained antihypertensive actions of a dual angiotensin-converting enzyme neutral endopeptidase inhibitor, sampatrilat, in black hypertensive subjects. Am J Hypertens 12:563-571, 1999.

861. Laurent S, Boutouyrie P, Azizi M, et al: Antihypertensive effects of fasidotril, a dual inhibitor of neprilysin and angiotensin-converting enzyme, in rats and humans. Hypertension 35:1148-1153, 2000.

862. Robl JA, Sun CQ, Stevenson J, et al: Dual metalloprotease inhibitors: Mercaptoacetyl-based fused heterocyclic dipeptide mimetics as inhibitors of angiotensin-converting enzyme and neutral endopeptidase. J Med Chem 40:1570-1577, 1997.

863. Levin ER, Gardner DG, Samson WK: Natriuretic peptides. N Engl J Med 339:321-328, 1998.

864. Burnett JC Jr: Vasopeptidase inhibition: A new concept in blood pressure management. J Hypertens Suppl 17:S37-S43, 1999.

865. Sica DA, Liao W, Gehr TW, et al: Disposition and safety of omapatrilat in subjects with renal impairment. Clin Pharmacol Ther 68:261-269, 2000.

866. Malhotra BK, Iyer RA, Soucek KM, et al: Oral bioavailability and disposition of (^{14}C)omapatrilat in healthy subjects. J Clin Pharmacol 41:833-841, 2001.

867. Taal MW, Nenov VD, Wong W, et al: Vasopeptidase inhibition affords greater renoprotection than angiotensin-converting enzyme inhibition alone. J Am Soc Nephrol 12:2051-2059, 2001.

868. Cao Z, Burrell LM, Tikkanen I, et al: Vasopeptidase inhibition attenuates the progression of renal injury in subtotal nephrectomized rats. Kidney Int 60:715-721, 2001.

869. Weir MR, Levy E, for the Omapatrilat Study Group: A comparative study of the antiproteinuric effect of omapatrilat and amlodipine in hypertensive patients with type 2 diabetes. Abstract. J Am Soc Nephrol 13:650A, 2002.

870. Weber MA, Chang PI, Reeves RA, et al: Antihypertensive dose response of omapatrilat, a vasopeptidase inhibitor, in mild to moderate hypertension. Abstract. Am J Hypertens 12:122A, 1999.

871. Asmar R, Fredebohm W, Senftleber I, et al: Omapatrilat compared with lisinopril in treatment of hypertension as assessed by ambulatory blood pressure monitoring. Abstract. Am J Hypertens 2000:143A, 2002.

872. Black HR, Chang PI, Reeves RA, et al: Monotherapy treatment success rate of omapatrilat, a vasopeptidase inhibitor, compared with lisinopril and amlodipine in mild to moderate hypertension. Abstract. Am J Hypertens 12:26A, 1999.

873. Ruilope LM, Palatini P, Grossman E, et al: Randomized double-blind comparison of omapatrilat with amlodipine in mild-to-moderate hypertension. Abstract. Am J Hypertens 13:134A-135A, 2000.

874. Campese VM, Lasseter KC, Ferrario CM, et al: Omapatrilat versus lisinopril: Efficacy and neurohormonal profile in salt-sensitive hypertensive patients. Hypertension 38:1342-1348, 2001.

875. Trippodo NC, Robl JA, Asaad MM, et al: Effects of omapatrilat in low, normal, and high renin experimental hypertension. Am J Hypertens 1998:11-363, 1998.

876. Ferdinand KC: Advances in antihypertensive combination therapy: Benefits of low-dose thiazide diuretics in conjunction with omapatrilat, a vasopeptidase inhibitor. J Clin Hypertens(Greenwich) 3:307-312, 2001.

877. Trippodo NC, Fox M, Monticello TM, et al: Vasopeptidase inhibition with omapatrilat improves cardiac geometry and survival in cardiomyopathic hamsters more than does ACE inhibition with captopril. J Cardiovasc Pharmacol 34:782-790, 1999.

878. Thomas CV, McDaniel GM, Holzgrefe HH, et al: Chronic dual inhibition of angiotensin-converting enzyme and neutral endopeptidase during the development of left ventricular dysfunction in dogs. J Cardiovasc Pharmacol 32:902-912, 1998.

879. McClean DR, Ikram H, Garlick AH, et al: The clinical, cardiac, renal, arterial and neurohormonal effects of omapatrilat, a vasopeptidase inhibitor, in patients with chronic heart failure. J Am Coll Cardiol 36:479-486, 2000.

880. Klapholz M, Thomas I, Eng C, et al: Effects of omapatrilat on hemodynamics and safety in patients with heart failure. Am J Cardiol 88:657-661, 2001.

881. McClean DR, Ikram H, Mehta S, et al: Vasopeptidase inhibition with omapatrilat in chronic heart failure: Acute and long-term hemodynamic and neurohumoral effects. J Am Coll Cardiol 39:2034-2041, 2002.

882. Cataliotti A, Boerrigter G, Chen HH, et al: Differential actions of vasopeptidase inhibition versus angiotensin-converting enzyme inhibition on diuretic therapy in experimental congestive heart failure. Circulation 105:639-644, 2002.

883. Rouleau JL, Pfeffer MA, Stewart DJ, et al: Comparison of vasopeptidase inhibitor, omapatrilat, and lisinopril on exercise tolerance and morbidity in patients with heart failure: IMPRESS randomised trial. Lancet 356:615-620, 2000.

884. Eisenstein EL, Nelson CL, Simon TA, et al: Vasopeptidase inhibitor reduces inhospital costs for patients with congestive heart failure: Results from the IMPRESS trial. Inhibition of Metallo Protease by BMS-186716 in a Randomized Exercise and Symptoms Study in Subjects With Heart Failure. Am Heart J 143:1112-1117, 2002.

885. Packer M, Califf RM, Konstam MA, et al: Comparison of Omapatrilat and Enalapril in Patients With Chronic Heart Failure: The Omapatrilat Versus Enalapril Randomized Trial of Utility in Reducing Events (OVERTURE). Circulation 106:920-926, 2002.

886. Pellacani A, Brunner HR, Nussberger J: Plasma kinins increase after angiotensin-converting enzyme inhibition in human subjects. Clin Sci (Lond) 87:567-574, 1994.

887. Nussberger J, Cugno M, Amstutz C, et al: Plasma bradykinin in angio-oedema. Lancet 351:1693-1697, 1998.

888. Agostoni A, Cicardi M, Cugno M, et al: Angioedema due to angiotensin-converting enzyme inhibitors. Immunopharmacology 44:21-25, 1999.

889. Kostis J, Black H, Packer M, et al. The Octave Study Group, Comparative efficacy and safety of omapatrilat in treated or untreated hypertensive patients: Results of the Omapatrilat Cardiovascular Treatment Assessment Versus Enalapril (OCTAVE) trial. Am J Hypertens (in press).

890. National High Blood Pressure Education Program Working Group report on primary prevention of hypertension. Arch Intern Med 153:186-208, 1993.

891. Vasan RS, Larson MG, Leip EP, et al: Impact of high-normal blood pressure on the risk of cardiovascular disease. N Engl J Med 345:1291-1297, 2001.

892. SHEP Cooperative Research Group: Prevention of stroke by antihypertensive drug treatment in older persons with isolated systolic hypertension. JAMA 265:3255-3264, 1991.

893. Staessen JA, Fagard R, Thijs L, et al: Randomised double-blind comparison of placebo and active treatment for older patients with isolated systolic hypertension. The Systolic Hypertension in Europe (Syst-Eur) Trial Investigators. Lancet 350:757-764, 1997.

894. Wang JG, Staessen JA, Gong L, Liu L: Chinese trial on isolated systolic hypertension in the elderly. Systolic Hypertension in China (Syst-China) Collaborative Group. Arch Intern Med 160:211-220, 2000.

895. Amery A, Birkenhager W, Brixko P: Mortality and morbidity results from the European Working party on High Blood Pressure in the Elderly Trial. Lancet 1:1349-1354, 1985.

896. MRC Working Party: Medical Research Council trial of treatment of hypertension in older adults: Principal results. BMJ 304:405-412, 1992.

897. Benetos A, Safar M, Rudnichi A, et al: Pulse pressure: A predictor of long-term cardiovascular mortality in a French male population. Hypertension 30:1410-1415, 1997.

898. Franklin SS, Gustin W, Wong ND, et al: Hemodynamic patterns of age-related changes in blood pressure. The Framingham Heart Study. Circulation 96:308-315, 1997.

899. Franklin SS, Khan SA, Wong ND, et al: Is pulse pressure useful in predicting risk for coronary heart disease? The Framingham heart study. Circulation 100:354-360, 1999.

900. The CONSENSUS Trial Study Group: Effects of enalapril on mortality in severe congestive heart failure: Result of the Cooperative North Scandinavian Enalapril Survival Study (CONSENSUS). N Engl J Med 316:1429-1435, 1987.

901. The SOLVD Investigators: Effects of enalapril on mortality and the development of heart failure in asymptomatic patients with reduced left ventricular ejection fractions. N Engl J Med 325:685-691, 1992.

902. Pfeffer MA, Braunwald E, Moye LA, et al: Effect of captopril on mortality and morbidity in patients with left ventricular dysfunction after myocardial infarction. Results of the survival and ventricular enlargement trial. The SAVE Investigators. N Engl J Med 327:669-677, 1992.

903. The AIRE Study Investigators: Effect of ramipril on mortality and morbidity of survivors of acute myocardial infarction with clinical evidence of heart failure. Lancet 342:821-828, 1993.

904. The GISEN Group: Randomized placebo-controlled trial of effect of ramipril on decline in glomerular filtration rate and risk of terminal renal failure in proteinuric, non-diabetic nephropathy. Lancet 349:1857-1863, 1997.

905. Lindholm LH, Ibsen H, Dahlof B, et al: Cardiovascular morbidity and mortality in patients with diabetes in the Losartan Intervention For Endpoint reduction in hypertension study (LIFE): A randomised trial against atenolol. Lancet 359:1004-1010, 2002.

906. Cohn JN, Tognoni G, for the Val-HeFT Investigators: Effects of the angiotensin receptor blocker valsartan on morbidity and mortality in heart failure: The Valsartan Heart Failure Trial (Val-HeFT). Circulation 102:2672-2676, 2000.

907. Jafar TH, Schmid CH, Landa M, et al: Angiotensin-converting enzyme inhibitors and progression of nondiabetic renal disease. A meta-analysis of patient-level data. Ann Intern Med 135:73-87, 2001.

908. Neutel JM, Black HR, Weber MA: Combination therapy with diuretics: An evolution of understanding. Am J Med 101:61S-70S, 1996.

909. Weir MR: Effects of low dose combination therapy with amlodipine/benazepril on systolic blood pressure. Cardiovasc Rev Rep 20:368-374, 2002.

910. Weir MR, Rosenberger C, Fink JC: Pilot study to evaluate a water displacement technique to compare effects of diuretics and angiotensin converting enzyme inhibitors to alleviate lower extremity edema due to dihydropyridine calcium antagonists. Am J Hypertens 14:968, 2001.

911. Weir MR: The role of multiple drug therapies for controlling hypertension in African Americans. J Clin Hypertens (Greenwich) 123:99-108, 2000.

912. Epstein M, Bakris G: Newer approaches to antihypertensive therapy. Use of fixed-dose combination therapy. Arch Intern Med 156:1969-1978, 1996.

913. Wei C, Song H, Papadimitriou J, et al: Increase transforming growth factor-β1 and its receptors in human renal tissue with rejection. Abstract. J Am Soc Nephrol A3354:722A, 1997.

914. Weir MR: When initial antihypertensive monotherapy fails: Potential benefits of fixed-dose angiotensin-converting enzyme inhibitor/calcium antagonist combination therapy. South Med J 93:548-556, 2000.

915. Messerli FH, Weir MR, Neutel JM: Combination therapy of amlodipine/benazepril versus monotherapy of amlodipine in a practice-based setting. Am J Hypertens 15:550-556, 2002.

916. Smulyan H, Safar ME: Systolic blood pressure revisited. J Am Coll Cardiol 29:1407-1413, 1997.

917. Nichols WW, Nicolini FA, Pepine CJ: Determinants of isolated systolic hypertension in the elderly. J Hypertens 10:S73-S77, 1992.

918. Applegate WB, Sowers JR: Elevated systolic blood pressure: Increased cardiovascular risk and rationale for treatment. Am J Med 101:3S-9S, 1996.

919. Ooi WL, Barrett S, Hossain M, et al: Patterns of orthostatic blood pressure change and their clinical correlates in a frail, elderly population. JAMA 277:1299-1304, 1997.

920. Sagie A, Benjamin EJ, Galderisi M, et al: Echocardiographic assessment of left ventricular structure and diastolic filling in elderly subjects with borderline isolated systolic hypertension (the Framingham Heart Study). Am J Cardiol 72:662-665, 1993.

921. Nicolino A, Ferrara N, Longobardi G, et al: Left ventricular diastolic filling in elderly hypertensive patients. J Am Geriatr Soc 41:217-222, 1993.

922. Conway J, Lauwers P: Hemodynamic and hypotensive effects of long-term therapy with chlorothiazide. Circulation 21:21-27, 1960.

923. Jones B, Nanra RS: Double-blind trial of antihypertensive effect of chlorothiazide in severe renal failure. Lancet 2:1258-1260, 1979.

924. Neutel JM: Metabolic manifestations of low-dose diuretics. Am J Med 101:71S-82S, 1996.

925. Weir MR, Moser M: Diuretics and beta-blockers: Is there a risk for dyslipidemia? Am Heart J 139:174-183, 2000.

926. Flack JM, Cushman WC: Evidence for the efficacy of low-dose diuretic monotherapy. Am J Med 101:53S-60S, 1996.

927. Romero JC, Raij L, Granger JP, et al: Multiple effects of calcium entry blockers on renal function in hypertension. Hypertension 10:140-151, 1987.

928. Weir MR, Chrysant SG, McCarron DA, et al: Influence of race and dietary salt on the antihypertensive efficacy of an angiotensin-converting enzyme inhibitor or a calcium channel antagonist in salt-sensitive hypertensives. Hypertension 31:1088-1096, 1998.

929. Weir MR, Hall PS, Behrens MT, Flack JM: Salt and blood pressure responses to calcium antagonism in hypertensive patients. Hypertension 30: 422-427, 1997.

930. Hedlund H, Andersson KE, Ek A: Effects of prazosin in patients with benign prostatic obstruction. J Urol 130:275-278, 1983.

931. Applegate WB, Davis BR, Black HR, et al: Prevalence of postural hypotension at baseline in the Systolic Hypertension in the Elderly Program (SHEP) cohort. J Am Geriatr Soc 39:1057-1064, 1991.

932. Messerli FH, Ventura HO, Amodeo C: Osler's maneuver and pseudo-hypertension. N Engl J Med 312:1548-1551, 1985.

933. Gueyffier F, Boutitie F, Boissel JP, et al for the INDANA Investigators: Effect of antihypertensive drug treatment on cardiovascular outcomes in women and men: A meta-analysis of individual patten data from randomized, controlled trials. Ann Intern Med 126:761-767, 1997.

934. Messerli FH, Garavaglia GE, Schmeider R: Disparate cardiovascular findings in men and women with essential hypertension. Ann Intern Med 107:158-163, 1987.

935. Stoney CM, Davis MC, Matthews KA: Sex differences in physiological responses to stress and coronary heart disease: A causal link? Psychophysiology 24:127-131, 1987.

936. Lerner DJ, Kannel WB: Patterns of coronary heart disease morbidity and mortality in the sexes. A 26-year follow-up of the Framingham population. Am Heart J 1:383-390, 1986.

937. Hiedrich FE, Stergachis A, Gross KM: Diuretic drug use and the risk for hip fracture. Ann Intern Med 115:1-6, 1991.

938. Morton DJ, Barrett-Connor EL, Edelstein SL: Thiazides and bone mineral density in elderly men and women. Am J Epidemiol 139:1107-1115, 1994.

939. Wasnich R, Davis J, Ross P, Vogel J: Effect of thiazide diuretics on rates of bone mineral loss: A longitudinal study. BMJ 301:1303-1305, 1990.

940. Ray WA: Thiazide diuretics and osteoporosis: Time for a clinical trial. Ann Intern Med 115:64-65, 1991.

941. Jones G, Nguyen T, Sambrook PN, Eisman JA: Thiazide diuretics and fracture: Can meta-analysis help? J Bone Miner Res 10:106-111, 1995.

942. Os I, Bratland B, Dahlof B, et al: Female preponderance for lisinopril-induced cough in hypertension. Am J Hypertens 7:1012-1015, 1994.

943. Weir MR: Antihypertensive combination therapy. Drugs Today 34: 5-9, 1998.

944. Hall WD, Ferrario CM, Moore MA, et al: Hypertension-related morbidity and mortality in the southeastern United States. Am J Med Sci 313:195-206, 1997.

945. Burt VL, Whelton P, Roccella EJ, et al: Prevalence of hypertension in the US adult population: Results from the third National Health and Nutrition Examination Survey, 1988-1991. Hypertension 25:305-313, 1995.

946. Klag MJ, Whelton PK, Randall BL, et al: End-stage renal disease in African-American and white men: 16-year MRFIT findings. JAMA 277:1293-1298, 1997.

947. Luft FC, Grim CE, Fineberg NS, Weinberger MC: Effects of volume expansion and contraction in normotensive whites, blacks, and subjects of different ages. Circulation 59:643-650, 1979.

948. Luft FC, Rankin LI, Bloch R, et al: Cardiovascular and humoral responses to extremes of sodium intake in normal black and white men. Circulation 60:706, 2002.

949. Saunders E, Weir MR, Kong BW, et al: A comparison of the efficacy and safety of a beta-blocker, a calcium channel blocker, and a converting enzyme inhibitor in hypertensive blacks. Arch Intern Med 150:1707-1713, 1990.

950. Weir MR, Gray JM, Paster R, Saunders E: Differing mechanisms of action of angiotensin-converting enzyme inhibition in black and white hypertensive patients. Hypertension 26:124-130, 1995.

951. Bakris GL, Weir MR, Sowers JR: Therapeutic challenges in the obese diabetic patients with hypertension. Am J Med 101:513-517, 1996.

952. Messerli FJ, Sundgaard-Riise K, Reisin E, et al: Obesity and essential hypertension: Hemodynamics, intravascular volume, sodium excretion and plasma renin activity. Ann Intern Med 74:808-813, 1983.

953. Messerli FH, Sundgaard-Riise K, Reisin E, et al: Disparate cardiovascular effects of obesity and arterial hypertension: Hemodynamics, intravascular volume, sodium excretion and plasma renin activity. Am J Med 74:808-813, 1983.

954. Sowers JR, Whitfield LA, Catania RA, et al: Role of the sympathetic nervous system in blood pressure maintenance in obesity. J Clin Endocrinol Metab 54:1181-1185, 1982.

955. Gress TW, Nieto FJ, Shahar E, et al: Hypertension and antihypertensive therapy as risk factors for type 2 diabetes mellitus. N Engl J Med 342:905-912, 2000.

956. Cuocolo A, Sax FL, Brush FL, et al: Left ventricular hypertrophy and impaired diastolic filling in essential hypertension. Circulation 81:978-986, 1990.

957. Bonow RO, Dilsizian V, Rosing DR, et al: Verapamil-induced improvement in left ventricular diastolic filling and increased exercise tolerance in patients with hypertrophic cardiomyopathy: Short- and long-term effects. Circulation 72:853-864, 1985.

958. Schmieder RE, Klingbell MP: Reversal of left ventricular hypertrophy in essential hypertension. JAMA 275:1507-1513, 1996.

959. Garg R, Yusuf S for the Collaborative Group on ACE Inhibitor Trials: Overview of randomized trials of angiotensin-converting enzyme inhibitors on mortality and morbidity in patients with heart failure. JAMA 273:1450-1456, 1995.

960. Packer M, Bristow MR, Cohn JN, et al: The effect of carvedilol on morbidity and mortality in patients with chronic heart failure. U.S. Carvedilol Heart Failure Study Group. N Engl J Med 334: 1349-1355, 1996.

961. Brown MA, Whitworth JA: Hypertension in human renal disease. J Hypertens 10:701-712, 1992.

962. Koomans HA, Roos JC, Boer P, et al: Salt sensitivity of blood pressure in chronic renal failure. Evidence for renal control of body fluid distribution in man. Hypertension 4:190-197, 1982.

963. Beretta-Piccoli C, Weidmann P, Schiffl H, et al: Enhanced cardiovascular pressor reactivity to norepinephrine in mild renal parenchymal disease. Am J Med 61:739-747, 1976.

964. Navar LG, Burke TJ, Robinson RR, Clapp JR: Distal tubular feedback in the autoregulation of single nephron glomerular filtration rate. J Clin Invest 53:516-525, 1974.

965. Casellas D, Moore LC: Autoregulation of intravascular pressure in preglomerular juxtamedullary vessels. Am J Physiol 264: F315-F321, 1993.

966. Takenaka T, Harrison-Bernard LM, Inscho EW, et al: Autoregulation of afferent arteriolar blood flow in juxtamedullary nephrons. Am J Physiol 267:F879-F887, 1994.

967. Yared A, Kon V, Ichikawa I: Mechanism of preservation of glomerular perfusion and filtration during acute extracellular fluid volume depletion. Importance of intrarenal vasopressin-prostaglandin interaction for protecting kidneys from constrictor action of vasopressin. J Clin Invest 75:1477-1487, 1985.

968. Weir MR, Dworkin LD: Antihypertensive drugs, dietary salt and renal protection: How low should you go, and with which therapy? Am J Kidney Dis 32:1-22, 1998.

969. Kloke HJ, Branten AJ, Huysmans FT, Wetzels JF: Antihypertensive treatment of patients with proteinuric renal diseases: Risks or benefits of calcium channel blockers? Kidney Int 53:1559-1573, 1998.

970. Jafar TH, Stark PC, Schmid CH, et al: Proteinuria as a modifiable risk factor for the progression of non-diabetic renal disease. Kidney Int 60:1131-1140, 2001.

971. Alderman MH, Budner N, Cohen H, et al: Prevalence of drug resistant hypertension. Hypertension 11:II-71-II-75, 1988.

972. Yakovlecitch M, Black HR: Resistant hypertension in a tertiary care clinic. Arch Intern Med 151:1786-1792, 1991.

973. Swales JD, Bing RF, Heagerty A, et al: Treatment of refractory hypertension. Lancet 1:894-896, 1982.

974. Zuschke CA, Prettyjohn FS: Pseudohypertension. South Med J 88:1185-1190, 1995.

975. Vedercchia P, Schillaci F, Zampi I, Portellati C: White coat hypertension. Hypertension 20:555-562, 1992.

976. Glen SK, Elliott HL, Curzio JL, et al: White-coat hypertension as a cause of cardiovascular dysfunction. Lancet 348:654-657, 1996.

977. Cavallini MC, Roman MI, Pickering TG, et al: Is white coat hypertension associated with arterial disease or left ventricular hypertrophy? Hypertension 26:413-419, 1995.

978. Dustan HP, Tarazi RC, Bravo EL: Dependence of arterial pressure on intravascular volume in treated hypertensive patients. N Engl J Med 286:861-866, 1972.

979. Fierro-Carrion GA, Ram CV: Nonsteroidal anti-inflammatory drugs (NSAIDs) and blood pressure. Am J Cardiol 80:775-776, 1997.

980. Lip GY, Beevers M, Churchill D, Beevers DG: Hormone replacement therapy and blood pressure in hypertensive women. J Hum Hypertens 8:491-494, 1994.

981. Tuomilehto J, Enlund H, Salonen JT, Nissinen A: Alcohol, patient compliance and blood pressure control in hypertensive patients. Scand J Soc Med 12:177-181, 1984.

982. Vidt PG: Resistant hypertension. In Oparil S, Weber MA (eds): Hypertension: A Companion to Brenner and Rector's The Kidney. Philadelphia, WB Saunders, 2000, pp 564-572.

983. Houston MC, Weir M, Gray J, et al: The effects of nonsteroidal anti-inflammatory drugs on blood pressures of patients with hypertension controlled by verapamil. Arch Intern Med 155:1049-1054, 1995.

984. Richert A, Ansarin K, Baran AS: Sleep apnea and hypertension: Pathophysiologic mechanisms. Semin Nephrol 22:71-77, 2002.

985. Koch-Weser J: Diazoxide. N Engl J Med 294:1271-1273, 1976.

986. Mroczek WJ, Leibel BA, Davidov M, Finnerty FA Jr: The importance of the rapid administration of diazoxide in accelerated hypertension. N Engl J Med 285:603-606, 1971.

987. Ram CV, Kaplan NM: Individual titration of diazoxide dosage in the treatment of severe hypertension. Am J Cardiol 43:627-630, 1979.

988. Garrett BN, Kaplan NM: Efficacy of slow infusion of diazoxide in the treatment of severe hypertension without organ hypoperfusion. Am Heart J 103:390-394, 1982.

989. Ogilvie RI, Nadeau JH, Sitar DS: Diazoxide concentration-response relation in hypertension. Hypertension 4:167-173, 1982.

990. Huysmans FT, Thien T, Koene RA: Acute treatment of hypertension with slow infusion of diazoxide. Arch Intern Med 143:882-884, 1983.

991. Deal JE, Barratt TM, Dillon MJ: Management of hypertensive emergencies. Arch Dis Child 67:1089-1092, 1992.

992. Murphy C: Hypertensive emergencies. Emerg Med Clin North Am 13:973-1007, 1995.

993. Abdelwahab W, Frishman W, Landau A: Management of hypertensive urgencies and emergencies. J Clin Pharmacol 35:747-762, 1995.

994. Grossman E, Ironi AN, Messerli FH: Comparative tolerability profile of hypertensive crisis treatments. Drug Saf 19:99-122, 1998.

995. Rosenow DJ, Russell E: Current concepts in the management of hypertensive crisis: Emergencies and urgencies. Holist Nurs Pract 15:12-21, 2001.

996. Elliot WJ: Hypertensive emergencies. Crit Care Clin 17:435-451, 2001.

997. Groshong T: Hypertensive crisis in children. Pediatr Ann 25:368-396, 1996.

998. Tenney F, Sakarcan A: Nicardipine is a safe and effective agent in pediatric hypertensive emergencies. Am J Kidney Dis 35:E20, 2000.

999. Tuzel IH: Sodium nitroprusside: A review of its clinical effectiveness as a hypotensive agent. J Clin Pharmacol 14:494-503, 1974.

1000. Ahearn DJ, Grim CE: Treatment of malignant hypertension with sodium nitroprusside. Arch Intern Med 133:187-191, 1974.

1001. Palmer RF, Lasseter KC: Drug therapy. Sodium nitroprusside. N Engl J Med 292:294-297, 1975.

1002. Cottrell JE, Casthely P, Brodie JD, et al: Prevention of nitroprusside-induced cyanide toxicity with hydroxocobalamin. N Engl J Med 298:809-811, 1978.

1003. Schulz V, Gross R, Pasch T, et al: Cyanide toxicity of sodium nitroprusside in therapeutic use with and without sodium thiosulfate. Klin Wochenschr 60:1393-1400, 1982.

1004. Gorczynski RJ: Basic pharmacology of esmolol. Am J Cardiol 56:3F-13F, 1985.

1005. Gray RJ, Bateman TM, Czer LS, et al: Use of esmolol in hypertension after cardiac surgery. Am J Cardiol 56:49F-56F, 1985.

1006. Cumming AMM, Brown JJ, Lever AF: Intravenous labetalol in the treatment of severe hypertension. Br J Clin Pharmacol 13:93S-96S, 1982.

1007. Wilson DJ, Wallin JD, Vlachakis ND, et al: Intravenous labetalol in the treatment of severe hypertension and hypertensive emergencies. Am J Med 75:95-102, 1983.

1008. LeBel M, Langlois S, Belleau LJ, Grose JH: Labetalol infusion in hypertensive emergencies. Clin Pharmacol Ther 37:615-618, 1985.

1009. Vlachakis ND, Maronde RF, Maloy JW, et al: Pharmacodynamics of intravenous labetalol and follow-up therapy with oral labetalol. Clin Pharmacol Ther 38:503-508, 1985.

1010. Vermillion ST, Scardo JA, Newman RB, Chauhan SP: A randomized, double-blind trial of oral nifedipine and intravenous labetalol in hypertensive emergencies of pregnancy. Am J Obstet Gynecol 181:858-861, 1999.

1011. Scardo JA, Vermillion ST, Newman RB, et al: A randomized, double-blind, hemodynamic evaluation of nifedipine and labetalol in preeclamptic hypertensive emergencies. Am J Obstet Gynecol 181:862-866, 1999.

1012. Ferguson RK, Vlasses PH: Hypertensive emergencies and urgencies. JAMA 255:1607-1613, 1986.

1013. Calhoun DA, Oparil S: Treatment of hypertensive crisis. N Engl J Med 323:1177-1183, 1990.

1014. Ram CV: Management of hypertensive emergencies: Changing therapeutic options. Am Heart J 122:356-363, 1991.

1015. Taylor P: Ganglionic stimulating and blocking agents. In Gilman G, Goodman LS, Rall TW, Murad F (eds): The Pharmacological Basis of Therapeutics, 7th ed. New York, Macmillan, 1985, pp 215-221.

1016. Hirschl MM, Binder A, Bur A, et al: Clinical evaluation of different doses of intravenous enalaprilat in patients with hypertensive crises. Arch Intern Med 155:2217-2223, 1995.

1017. Hirschl MM, Binder M, Bur A, et al: Impact of the renin-angiotensin-aldosterone system on blood pressure response to intravenous enalaprilat in patients with hypertensive crises. J Hum Hypertens 11:177-183, 1997.

1018. DiPette DJ, Ferraro JC, Evans RR, Martin M: Enalaprilat, an intravenous angiotensin-converting enzyme inhibitor, in hypertensive crises. Clin Pharmacol Ther 38:199-204, 1985.

1019. Reams GP, Lal SM, Whalen JJ, Bauer JH: Enalaprilat: An intravenous substitute for oral enalapril therapy. Humoral and pharmacokinetic effects. J Clin Hypertens 2:245-253, 1986.

1020. Wallin JD, Fletcher E, Ram CV, et al: Intravenous nicardipine for the treatment of severe hypertension. A double-blind, placebo-controlled multicenter trial. Arch Intern Med 149:2662-2669, 1989.

1021. Michael J, Groshong T, Tobias JD: Nicardipine for hypertensive emergencies in children with renal disease. Pediatr Nephrol 12:40-42, 1998.

1022. Temple ME, Nahata MC: Treatment of pediatric hypertension. Pharmacotherapy 20:140-150, 2000.

1023. Trissel LA, Zhang Y, Baker MB: Stability of fenoldopam mesylate in two infusion solutions. Am J Health Syst Pharm 59:846-848, 2002.

1024. Cooper ZA, Mihm FG: Blood pressure control with fenoldopam during excision of a pheochromocytoma. Anesthesiology 91:558-560, 1999.

1025. Oparil S, Aronson S, Deeb GM, et al: Fenoldopam: A new parenteral antihypertensive: Consensus roundtable on the management of perioperative hypertension and hypertensive crises. Am J Hypertens 12:653-664, 1999.

1026. Han G, Kryman JP, McMillin PJ, et al: A novel transduction mechanism mediating dopamine-induced vascular relaxation: Opening of BKCa channels by cyclic AMP–induced stimulation of the cyclic GMP–dependent protein kinase. J Cardiovasc Pharmacol 34:619-627, 1999.

1027. Taylor AA, Shepherd AM, Polvino W, et al: Prolonged fenoldopam infusions in patients with mild to moderate hypertension: Pharmacodynamic and pharmacokinetic effects. Am J Hypertens 12:906-914, 1999.

1028. Taylor AA, Mangoo-Karim R, Ballard KD, et al: Sustained hemodynamic effects of the selective dopamine-1 agonist, fenoldopam, during 48-hour infusions in hypertensive patients: A dose-tolerability study. J Clin Pharmacol 39:471-479, 1999.

1029. Catapano MS, Marx JA: Management of urgent hypertension: A comparison of oral treatment regimens in the emergency department. J Emerg Med 4:368, 1986.

1030. Gales MA: Oral antihypertensives for hypertensive urgencies. Ann Pharmacother 28:353-358, 1994.

1031. Cohen IM, Katz MA: Oral clonidine loading for rapid control of hypertension. Clin Pharmacol Ther 24:11-15, 1978.

1032. Anderson RJ, Hart GR, Crumpler CP, et al: Oral clonidine loading in hypertensive urgencies. JAMA 246:848-850, 1981.

1033. Karachalios GN: Hypertensive emergencies treated with oral clonidine. Eur J Clin Pharmacol 31:227-229, 1986.

1034. Houston MC: Treatment of hypertensive urgencies and emergencies with nifedipine. Am Heart J 111:963-969, 1986.

1035. Bauer JH, Reams GP: The role of calcium entry blockers in hypertensive emergencies. Circulation 75:V174-V180, 1987.

1036. Hayes JM: Rapid control of serious high blood pressure with single large oral doses of prazosin. Med J Aust 1:31-32, 1980.

1037. Grossman E, Messerli FH, Grodzicki T, Kowey P: Should a moratorium be placed on sublingual nifedipine capsules given for hypertensive emergencies and pseudoemergencies? JAMA 276: 1328-1331, 1996.

1038. Strandgaard S, Olesen J, Skinhoj E, Lassen NA: Autoregulation of brain circulation in severe arterial hypertension. Br Med J 1: 507-510, 1973.

1039. Strandgaard S: Autoregulation of cerebral blood flow in hypertensive patients. Abstract. Circulation 53:720-727, 1976.

1040. Strandgaard S: Autoregulation of cerebral circulation in hypertension. Abstract. Acta Neurol Scand 57(suppl 66):1-82, 1978.

1041. Barry DI, Lassen NA: Cerebral blood flow autoregulation in hypertension and effects of antihypertensive drugs. J Hypertens Suppl 2:S519-S526, 1984.

1042. Reed G, Devous M: Cerebral blood flow autoregulation and hypertension. Am J Med Sci 289:37-44, 1985.

1043. Bertel O, Marx BE, Conen D: Effects of antihypertensive treatment on cerebral profusion. Abstract. Am J Med 82(suppl 3B):29-36, 1987

1044. Jariwalla AG, Anderson EG: Production of ischaemic cardiac pain by nifedipine. Br Med J 1:1181-1182, 1978.

1045. Yagil Y, Kobrin I, Leibel B, Ben Ishay D: Ischemic ECG changes with initial nifedipine therapy of severe hypertension. Am Heart J 103:310-311, 1982.

Specific Pharmacologic Approaches to Clinical Renoprotection

Gerjan Navis, Paul E de Jong, and Dick de Zeeuw

SPECIFIC PHARMACOLOGIC INTERVENTION: A RISK FACTOR–BASED APPROACH

In many patients with chronic renal disease, progressive loss of renal function occurs despite the absence of any overt activity of the underlying renal disorder. This progressive nature of chronic renal disease has been well recognized for more than half a century. As early as 1942, Ellis suggested hypertension to be a main determinant of chronic loss of renal function, irrespective of the initial cause of the renal damage.[1] Since then, the hypothesis that common mechanisms account for the progressive loss of renal function in many renal conditions was fueled by numerous observations, including the linear deterioration in renal function that occurs in many patients regardless of their initial renal disease, as well as the similarity in histopathologic abnormalities in end-stage kidneys with different underlying diseases. Furthermore, a main line of evidence is provided by the fact that the risk factors for progressive loss of renal function tend to be similar for different renal disorders. Accordingly, it is currently assumed that the rate of progression is determined by three main factors: the activity of the primary disease process, adaptive alterations in the kidney, and local and systemic sequelae of the renal disorder.[2, 3] Systemic and glomerular hypertension, proteinuria, and metabolic abnormalities such as hyperlipidemia are assumed to be common mediators in the pathophysiology of focal glomerulosclerosis, the alleged final common pathway of progressive renal damage,[4] as depicted in Figure 56-1. In many renal conditions, hypertension, proteinuria, and metabolic abnormalities are simultaneously present. This clustering of risk factors is presumably of prime importance for renal outcome inasmuch as many experimental and clinical data suggest that the mutual interaction of risk factors accelerates progressive renal damage. To prevent progressive loss of renal function, as a matter of clinical common sense, any prevailing primary damaging factors should be eliminated first. When disease-specific factors are accessible to intervention, such as in analgesic abuse[5] or obstructive nephropathy,[6] progression may indeed be halted by elimination of these factors. In malignant hypertension, if adequately treated, recovery of renal function may even be possible.[7] In diabetes, strict metabolic control can reverse early hyperfiltration and retard the progression in diabetic renal function loss.[8]

In a large proportion of renal patients, however, no disease-specific factors accessible to intervention can be identified. This lack of specific factors prompted the development of additional treatment strategies aimed at ameliorating non–disease-specific, common renal risk factors for preventing progressive loss of renal function. Specific modes of intervention are available for several risk factors, as depicted in Figure 56-1. Demonstration of a renoprotective benefit of a specific intervention for a certain risk factor has a dual impact. It not only represents an advancement in terms of patient care but also augments pathophysiologic insight by providing evidence for a causal role of that risk factor in progressive loss of renal function, thereby enabling further improvements in therapy.

The major effort of the last decades was directed at evaluating the long-term renoprotective efficacy of two main intervention strategies: pharmacologic intervention aimed at reduction of blood pressure and dietary intervention aimed at reduction of protein intake. Recent trials, including hard end points, have provided important new insight. Most importantly, it has been shown that the rate of loss of renal function can be effectively retarded in diabetic as well as nondiabetic patients and the need for renal replacement therapy postponed. Moreover, the importance of proteinuria as a

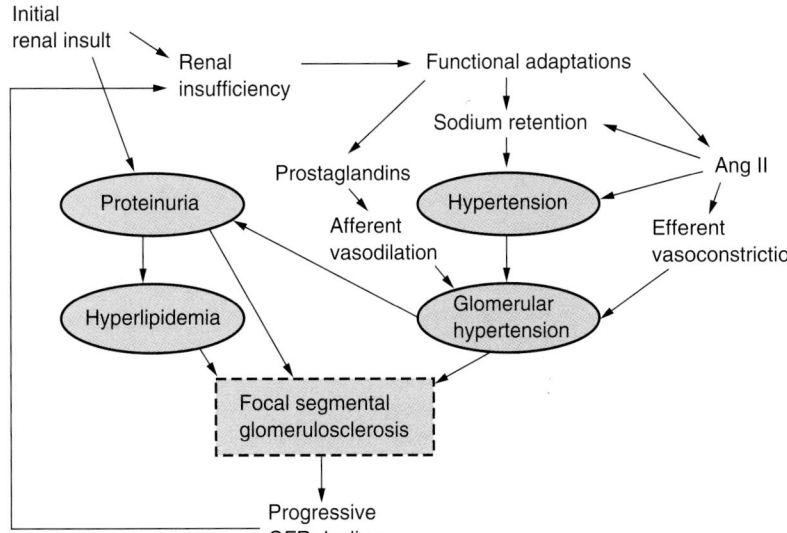

FIGURE 56-1. Outline of the alleged mechanisms of progressive loss of renal function; also depicted is the interaction between different mediators of progressive focal segmental glomerulosclerosis. The possibilities for clinical intervention with specific risk mediators are indicated as well. Genetic factors—not depicted—may modify any of the elements shown in this scheme. Ang II, angiotensin II; GFR, glomerular filtration rate.

promoter of progressive renal damage—and consequently, the need for reduction of proteinuria as a prerequisite for renoprotection—stands out as a consistent finding. Therefore, it is argued that improvement in renoprotective efficacy may be obtained by considering reduction of proteinuria as an independent treatment target—in addition to the reduction in blood pressure. Finally, recent trials have provided substantial evidence for the importance of blocking the renin-angiotensin-aldosterone system (RAAS) as a mode of intervention with specific renoprotective properties beyond blood pressure control.

In this chapter we review the current insights into the role of common risk factors for progressive loss of renal function in humans, the results of interventions directed against these risk factors, and therapeutic options for specific pharmacologic intervention, and we discuss the implications for clinical management of renal patients with an emphasis on optimization of renoprotective therapy.

RISK FACTORS FOR LOSS OF RENAL FUNCTION AND RENOPROTECTIVE BENEFIT OF SPECIFIC INTERVENTION

Hypertension

Whereas malignant hypertension has for decades been recognized to lead to rapid loss of renal function, the role of less severe hypertension in progressive renal damage is less well defined. Epidemiologic data on patients entering dialysis suggest a substantial role for hypertension, with hypertensive nephrosclerosis being the second most common cause of end-stage renal failure, surpassed only by diabetes.[9] Among patients with a diagnosis of hypertensive nephrosclerosis, however, only 6% had a history of malignant hypertension, a finding that strongly suggests a causal role for less severe hypertension in the development of end-stage renal failure.[10] Strikingly, whereas the incidence of cardiac and cerebral hypertensive end-organ damage is decreasing, the number of patients entering dialysis with a diagnosis of

hypertensive renal damage is steadily increasing, thus emphasizing its importance for the renal population.[11]

Morphologic studies support a causal role for hypertension in eliciting structural renal damage. Autopsy data in young accident victims from different countries have shown a correlation between the prevalence of nephrosclerosis and hypertension in the respective countries.[12] Moreover, the severity of nephrosclerosis was closely correlated with blood pressure records in autopsy series,[13, 14] as well as with renal biopsy results in essential hypertensives.[15] In African Americans with hypertensive nephrosclerosis, the severity of glomerulosclerosis correlated with blood pressure.[16] Finally, in a small series of proteinuric hypertensives, a primary renal disorder was present in only a minority of the patients, thus suggesting that the segmental glomerular lesions or the global sclerosis (or both) in the remainder of the patients might be due to hypertension per se.[17]

Clinical data support the role of blood pressure as a renal risk factor in several populations. A large epidemiologic screening investigation, the Okinawa study, found blood pressure to be a predictor of end-stage renal disease in the general population. Specifically, diastolic blood pressure was found to be associated with end-stage renal disease after 10 years of follow-up in this community-based study.[18] Blood pressure was also a strong predictor of end-stage renal failure during 16 years of follow-up in 332,544 middle-aged men in the Multiple Risk Factor Intervention Trial (MRFIT).[19] Remarkably, the association with increased renal risk was already apparent with a systolic blood pressure of 127 mm Hg and a diastolic pressure of 82 mm Hg, values well within the normotensive range. Longitudinal studies of selected samples of the general population[20, 21] have found an association between blood pressure and rate of the age-related decline in renal function. Yet these population studies do not explain the role of blood pressure as a cause of end-stage renal failure. The prevalence of end-stage renal failure is very low,[18] and moreover, in longitudinal studies the observed rate of renal function loss was very slow. In hypertensive subjects, creatinine clearance fell by only 0.92 ± 0.32 mL/min/yr versus 0.75 ± 0.12 mL/min/yr in normotensive subjects,[20] and even in subjects with evidence of renal or urinary tract disease, the rate of loss of renal function was just 1.1 ± 0.23 mL/min/yr. Other studies have also found a well-preserved glomerular filtration rate (GFR) in hypertensives in spite of long-standing hypertension.[22-24] Nonetheless, in these studies the age-related decline in renal blood flow was consistently more pronounced in hypertensives, and furthermore, even in the normotensive range, effective renal blood flow is inversely related to blood pressure.[25] Thus, a pressure-associated reduction in renal blood flow appears to be consistently present in different studies and in different populations, but these renal effects do not invariably lead to loss of renal function. This notion is consistent with the wide range of changes in the slope of creatinine clearance over time reported by the MRFIT intervention trial.[26]

The data just presented support the role of blood pressure as a renal risk factor. Importantly, this increased risk is also apparent in the normotensive range.[19] Because the development of renal failure is very rare, however, the impact of blood pressure on long-term renal function apparently depends on the concomitant presence of other renal risk factors, specific renal susceptibility to hypertensive renal damage, or a combination of these features. Several predictors of loss of renal function have been identified in hypertensive populations, including racial factors such as an increased risk in African Americans, impaired glucose tolerance, increased uric acid levels, and elevated serum creatinine.[27-29] In accord with experimental data,[30] the latter strongly suggests that previous renal damage is associated with an enhanced susceptibility to hypertensive renal damage. Genetic factors other than ethnicity may also be involved in the susceptibility to hypertensive renal damage, as suggested by an association between the deletion polymorphism of the angiotensin-converting enzyme (ACE) gene and hypertensive nephrosclerosis.[31-33] In patients with renal disease, hypertension is common, as reviewed in Chapter 47. Its prevalence appears to increase with deteriorating renal function, with some 90% of patients entering dialysis being hypertensive.[34] High blood pressure is consistently associated with a poor renal outcome. In diabetic patients, the development of hypertension is closely associated with the transition from normoalbuminuria to microalbuminuria,[35] with subsequent progression to overt proteinuria, and with progressive loss of renal function.[36-38] Morphologic studies of nephropathy in patients with insulin-dependent diabetes mellitus (IDDM) have found an association between the severity of renal structural lesions and blood pressure, without, however, establishing a cause-and-effect relationship.[39, 40] In nondiabetic renal disease, high blood pressure is likewise associated with a poor long-term renal outcome across a spectrum of renal disorders.[41-44] Moreover, blood pressure predicted subsequent loss of renal function in glomerular disorders,[45, 46] as well as in adult polycystic kidney disease.[47] Even though high blood pressure has been the leading paradigm for explaining progressive loss of renal function for many years, the number of studies supporting its role as an independent renal risk factor is relatively small. In several studies, blood pressure failed to be recognized as an independent determinant of loss of renal function because of a predominant effect of proteinuria.[6, 42, 48] The relative impact of blood pressure, disease activity, and concomitant risk factors (e.g., proteinuria) on loss of renal

function has proved hard to ascertain[49] and may vary between different study populations.

Blood Pressure Reduction

Antihypertensive therapy has been the cornerstone of renoprotective intervention for decades. Reduced blood pressure was associated with a more favorable course of long-term renal function in diabetic as well as nondiabetic patients in many studies.[41, 43, 48-53] Until recently, however, the evidence for renoprotection provided by a reduction in blood pressure was debated. First, the evidence relied mainly on studies in which both the response of blood pressure to treatment and the long-term course of renal function might reflect the aggressiveness of the underlying renal condition per se. Moreover, as reviewed by Oldrizzi and colleagues,[43] a number of studies failed to show a relationship between the reduction in blood pressure and the rate of progression.[54-61] Finally, nonspecific trial-related effects such as more frequent follow-up and better patient compliance were argued to account for part of the renoprotective benefit.[62] Several factors, such as the level of blood pressure reduction obtained and differences in patient characteristics, were suggested to be responsible for the discrepancies.[43]

Evidence for the renoprotective effect of a reduction in blood pressure is supported by studies investigating the long-term renal effects of more aggressive blood pressure control. In essential hypertensives, more effective stabilization of renal function was obtained by stepped care, with a blood pressure level of 129/86 mm Hg, than by referred care, with a blood pressure level of 139/90 mm Hg.[27] A small prospective study in patients with hypertensive nephrosclerosis (mostly black males) found that an initial period of aggressive blood pressure reduction was followed by an improvement in long-term renal function.[63] The recent African American Study of Kidney Disease (AASK) in black patients with hypertensive nephrosclerosis, however, found no added benefit for a target mean arterial pressure (MAP) below 92 mm Hg versus 102 to 107 mm Hg.[64] A major contribution to the role of aggressive blood pressure reduction in renal patients was provided by the Modification of Diet in Renal Disease (MDRD) study.[65] This prospective trial in 840 nondiabetic patients (GFR of 13 to 55 mL/min) studied the renoprotective benefit of a target MAP of 92 versus 98 mm Hg. For subjects older than 60 years, a target level of 107 mm Hg was compared with 113 mm Hg. Additional therapy included dietary protein restriction in half the patients. For the study population as a whole, the more aggressive blood pressure regimen resulted in a difference in MAP of 4.7 mm Hg, which was not associated with a more favorable course of renal function during the 3 years of follow-up. However, subgroup analysis revealed that this seeming lack of renoprotective benefit was explained by an uneven distribution of benefit over the patient population. Proteinuria, the specific diagnosis, and race all had an effect on the renoprotective benefit of blood pressure reduction. Baseline proteinuria was a potent determinant of the benefit of a reduction in blood pressure, with a greater renoprotective benefit of the lower blood pressure goal noted in patients with higher baseline proteinuria (Fig. 56-2).

In diabetic nephropathy, the importance of aggressive blood pressure reduction for preservation of renal function

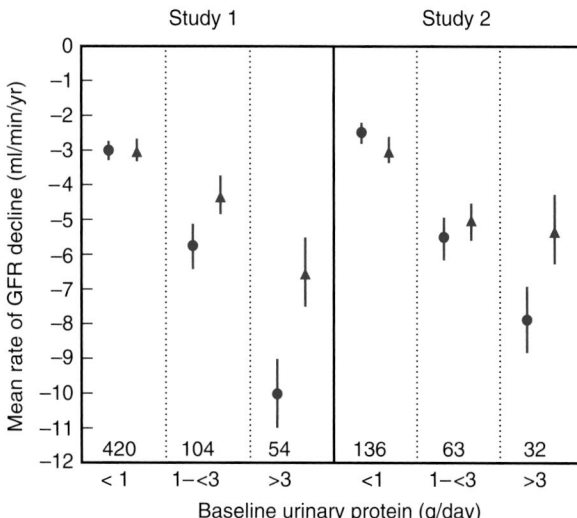

FIGURE 56-2. Decline in glomerular filtration rate (GFR) from baseline to 3 years of follow-up, according to baseline proteinuria and blood pressure group from the Modification of Diet in Renal Disease (MDRD) Study. *Closed circles* represent the low blood pressure target groups. Study 1 *(left panel)* refers to 585 patients with a baseline GFR of 25 to 55 mL/min; study 2 *(right panel)* includes 255 patients with a baseline GFR of 13 to 24 mL/min. (Reprinted, by permission, from Klahr S, Levey AS, Beck GJ, et al: The effect of dietary protein restriction and blood pressure control on the progression of chronic renal disease. N Engl J Med 330:877-884, 1994.)

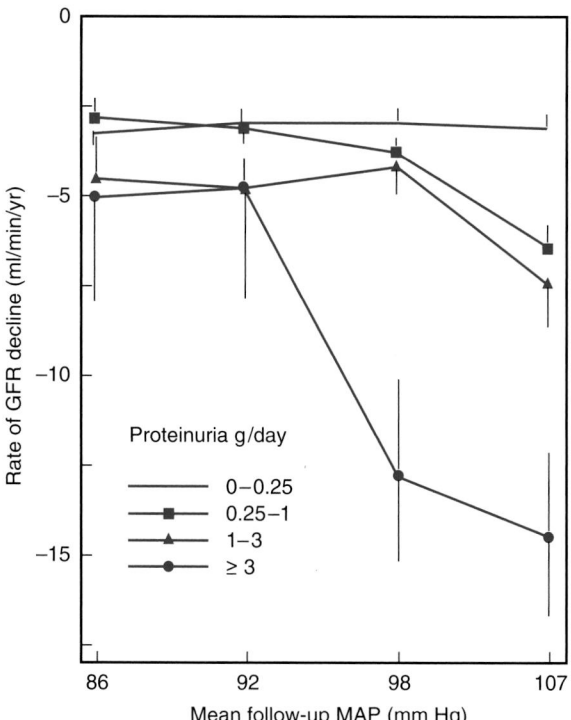

FIGURE 56-3. Mean rate of decline in glomerular filtration rate (GFR) and blood pressure (mean arterial pressure [MAP]) during follow-up in the Modification of Diet in Renal Disease (MDRD) Study for patients stratified according to baseline proteinuria. (Adapted with permission from Peterson JC, Adler S, Burkart JM, et al: Blood pressure control, proteinuria and the progression of renal disease. Ann Intern Med 123:754-762, 1995.)

has been extensively demonstrated in observational studies.[53, 66] Trials comparing ACE inhibitors with conventional antihypertensive agents in IDDM,[67] as well as in non-insulin-dependent diabetes mellitus (NIDDM),[68] found that loss of renal function was ameliorated more effectively in the treatment groups with the lower blood pressure, specifically, those assigned to ACE inhibition. Although non–pressure-related effects of ACE inhibitors are likely to be involved in renoprotection as well, the association between blood pressure reduction and the protection obtained against loss of renal function is strong, a finding corroborated by similar results with AT1 receptor blockade.[69, 70]

Target Blood Pressure

The insight on target blood pressure for renoprotection in nondiabetic renal disease has been greatly increased by the MDRD trial. These data demonstrated that the renoprotective benefit of lower blood pressure depends on the severity of proteinuria, with additional differences explained by racial factors.[71, 72] In patients with proteinuria of 1 to 3 g/day, a MAP of 98 mm Hg (corresponding to 135/80 mm Hg) provided additional renoprotection, whereas such additional benefit was absent in patients with protein loss of less than 1 g/day. Moreover, in patients with proteinuria greater than 3 g/day, additional benefit was demonstrated for an even lower target blood pressure—a MAP of 92 mm Hg (125/75 mm Hg) (Fig. 56-3). Ethnic factors had an impact on the benefit of a given blood pressure level. In black subjects, the difference in overall loss of renal function during 3 years of follow-up between those assigned to the usual (107 mm Hg) versus the low target level (92 mm Hg) was 11.8 mL/min, whereas in

whites it was 0.3 mL/min (not significant). The difference between black and white subjects was due to the patients with a MAP above 98 mm Hg. Prospective data from the AASK trial, however, showed no added benefit of a target below 92 mm Hg in blacks with hypertensive nephrosclerosis.[64]

For diabetic patients, the importance of a low target blood pressure for renoprotection has been increasingly emphasized. Even though no formal trials comparing different target levels have been performed, the recommendation for a target blood pressure below 120 to 130 systolic and 80 to 85 mm Hg diastolic for microalbuminuric patients[74] finds substantial support.[75, 76]

From the data available thus far, no signs of a J curve are apparent. In fact, when comparing the rate of decline in renal function between several controlled studies, it appears that the rate of decline in renal function displays a linear relationship with the level of blood pressure obtained during the study (Fig. 56-4).[75] Although the evidence from such combined data is clearly of an indirect nature, this analysis appears to support a target blood pressure not exceeding 130/85 mm Hg and suggests that stabilization of renal function would require a target MAP of 95 mm Hg, which corresponds to approximately 120/80 mm Hg.

Along with the recognition that target blood pressures need to be lower than in the past comes the challenge of actually achieving these target pressures. The effort needed in recent trials to obtain the lower target blood pressure is illustrated in Figure 56-5. Multiple antihypertensive

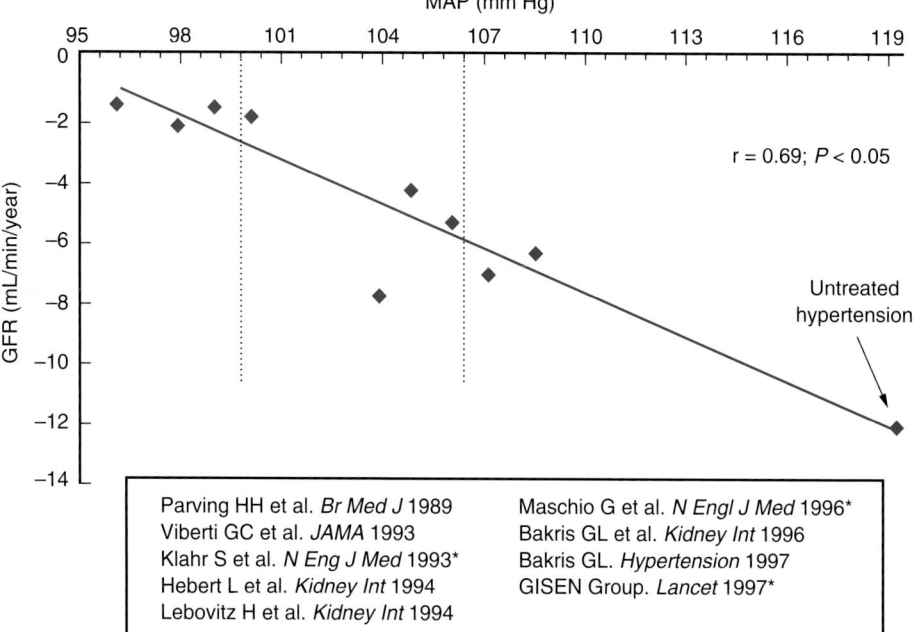

FIGURE 56-4. Relationship between achieved blood pressure control and the rate of renal function decline in different clinical trials involving diabetic and nondiabetic patients. GFR, glomerular filtration rate; MAP, mean arterial pressure. (Adapted with permission from Bakris GL, Williams M, Dworkin L, et al: The National Kidney Foundation Hypertension and Diabetes Executive Committees Working Group. Preserving renal function in adults with hypertension and diabetes: A consensus approach. Am J Kidney Dis 36:646-661, 2000.)

Parving HH et al. *Br Med J* 1989
Viberti GC et al. *JAMA* 1993
Klahr S et al. *N Eng J Med* 1993*
Hebert L et al. *Kidney Int* 1994
Lebovitz H et al. *Kidney Int* 1994

Maschio G et al. *N Engl J Med* 1996*
Bakris GL et al. *Kidney Int* 1996
Bakris GL. *Hypertension* 1997
GISEN Group. *Lancet* 1997*

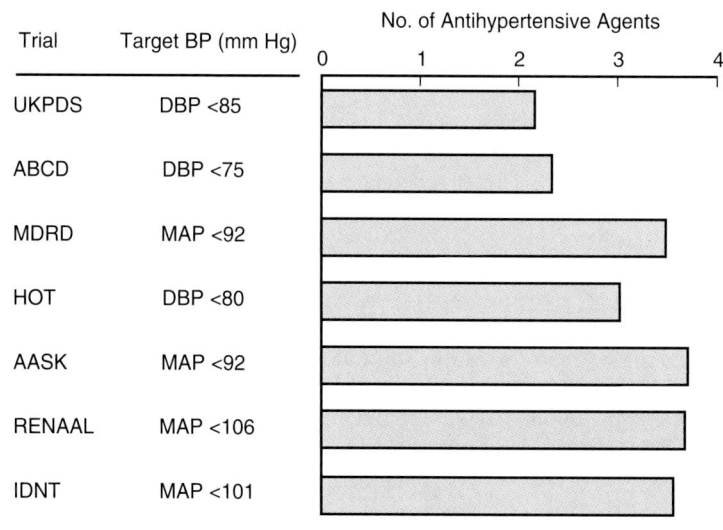

FIGURE 56-5. Average number of antihypertensives needed to achieve lower blood pressure (BP) goals in the available trials that randomized for lower blood pressure targets. (Adapted from Bakris GL, Williams M, Dworkin L, et al: The National Kidney Foundation Hypertension and Diabetes Executive Committees Working Group. Preserving renal function in adults with hypertension and diabetes: A consensus approach. Am J Kidney Dis 36:646-661, 2000.)

agents were needed to obtain the target pressure in different patient populations, with an average of three different agents required.[75]

Glomerular Hypertension

In healthy kidneys, glomerular pressure is well autoregulated by the unique position of the glomerular capillaries between a preglomerular and a postglomerular resistance vessel. A series of animal studies from the 1980s showed that glomerular hyperfiltration of remnant nephrons, associated with glomerular hypertrophy, occurs as a renal adaptive response to loss of functional renal mass, as discussed

extensively in Chapter 43. Briefly, such hyperfiltration serves to maintain the short-term overall GFR but appears to accelerate progressive renal damage by exposure of the glomerular capillaries to elevated hydrostatic pressure.[77] Hyperfiltration is predominantly mediated by preglomerular vasodilation, which leads to enhanced transmission of systemic blood pressure to the glomerular capillaries. The resulting impairment in autoregulation has been shown to be associated with increased renal vulnerability to hypertensive renal damage in rats with reduced renal mass.[30] Preglomerular tone can also be reduced by high protein intake, which may contribute to the accelerating effect of high protein intake on progression of renal failure.[78]

In humans, no direct data on glomerular capillary pressure are available. Nevertheless, indirect data suggest that hyperfiltration is involved in loss of renal function in several human renal conditions. Diabetic nephropathy in IDDM provides perhaps the most convincing case with its well-documented typical biphasic course consisting of an elevated GFR and filtration fraction preceding progressive loss of renal function.[79, 80] Thus, in IDDM hyperfiltration appears to be a primary phenomenon rather than a compensatory response to nephron loss. Morphologic studies have demonstrated an association between hyperfiltration and glomerular hypertrophy in IDDM.[81] Data are less consistent in NIDDM, presumably because of the greater heterogeneity of this population. Nonetheless, early hyperfiltration[82-84] and glomerular hypertrophy[85] were reported in a subset of NIDDM as well.

In nondiabetic renal parenchymal disease, on the other hand, hyperfiltration is notoriously hard to demonstrate because patients usually come to medical attention only after the development of renal damage. Thus, hyperfiltration in remnant nephrons, if present, cannot be established by the available methods because they measure only total GFR. Interestingly, a recent observation in children and adolescents with autosomal dominant polycystic kidney disease (ADPKD) suggests that hyperfiltration precedes the decline in renal function in this condition.[86] Nevertheless, long-term follow-up in kidney donors indicates that in healthy kidneys, a substantial compensatory elevation in GFR may persist for decades without inducing renal damage.[87] However, it may be relevant in this respect that obesity, which is known to induce hyperfiltration,[88] increases the risk for long-term renal damage after uninephrectomy.[89]

Fogo and co-workers found that glomerular hypertrophy in minimal change disease predicts later progression to focal glomerulosclerosis, thus providing some support for a role of glomerular hypertrophy and perhaps hyperfiltration in this condition in humans.[90, 91] In essential hypertension, an elevated GFR with an elevated filtration fraction is present in a subset of patients with newly diagnosed disease.[92, 93] Interestingly, in this population hyperfiltration is associated with left ventricular hypertrophy, which suggests that it may reflect a generalized propensity for the development of hypertensive target organ damage. Whether early hyperfiltration predicts loss of renal function in patients with essential hypertension is not yet clear.[94] Finally, recent epidemiologic data from the general population have revealed a biphasic pattern of GFR that is strikingly similar to that in diabetes in its association with albuminuria. This pattern is illustrated in Figure 56-6, which shows that in subjects with albuminuria in the high-normal range, a higher filtration rate is observed, whereas in subjects with higher rates of albumin excretion, the GFR tends to be lower.[95]

The prognostic impact of an elevated GFR in nondiabetic subjects, however, is thus far unknown, but longitudinal studies addressing this question are currently under way.

Reduction of Glomerular Pressure

In experimental studies, a reduction in elevated glomerular capillary pressure rather than a reduction in systemic blood pressure closely correlates with protection against the development of focal glomerulosclerosis in several renal conditions.[96, 97] Thus, a reduction in glomerular pressure appears to afford renoprotection in addition to a reduction in systemic blood pressure. Indirect data suggest that a reduction in intraglomerular hydrostatic pressure may be relevant to the outcome of renoprotective interventions in humans as well. In nondiabetic and diabetic renal disease, the early renal hemodynamic response (but not the response of systemic blood pressure) to antihypertensive therapy was shown to predict its long-term renoprotective efficacy. A slight drop in GFR at the onset of treatment—which may indicate a reduction in glomerular hydrostatic pressure—predicts a favorable long-term course of renal function, thus suggesting that a reduction in glomerular pressure may play a role in long-term renoprotection in humans (Fig. 56-7).[98, 99] The predictive value of the early renal hemodynamic response is independent of the mode of intervention because it occurs with ACE inhibition as well as with β-blockade and, moreover, it was also observed during nonpharmacologic intervention consisting of a low-protein diet.[100] Although these data strongly suggest that a reduction in glomerular pressure plays a causal role in renoprotection, the evidence is not conclusive because alternatively, these relationships might also reflect

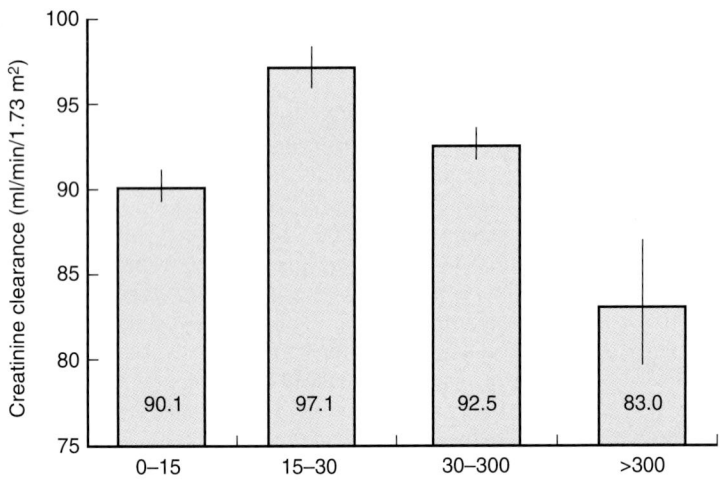

FIGURE 56-6. Creatinine clearance in 7728 subjects from the Prevention of Renal and Vacular End Stage Disease (PREVEND) cohort according to albuminuria categories: 0 to 15, 15 to 30, 30 to 300, and over 300 mg/24 hr. Numbers in the *bars* represent the age- and gender-adjusted mean of creatinine clearance (mL/min/1.73 m²). (Adapted from Pinto-Sietsma S-J, Janssen WMT, Hillege HJ, et al: Urinary albumin excretion is associated with renal functional abnormalities in a non-diabetic population. J Am Soc Nephrol 11:1882-1888, 2000.)

the overall responsiveness of the renal condition to intervention and thus be an epiphenomenon. Finally, the observed relationship between renal hemodynamic response and long-term renoprotection may not be equally relevant in all renal conditions because it could not be demonstrated in NIDDM.[101, 102]

Proteinuria

A pathogenetic role for proteinuria in progressive loss of renal function is suggested by many experimental studies involving renal damage of diverse origin. In ablation models, proteinuria is closely associated with glomerular hypertension, presumably reflecting the severity of hypertension-induced renal damage. Studies in experimental nephrotic syndrome caused by puromycin nucleoside or doxorubicin (Adriamycin) have demonstrated that in these models, proteinuria precedes progressive glomerulosclerosis in the absence of glomerular hypertension.[103] Taken together with studies on the tubulotoxicity of the components of proteinuric urine, these studies provide evidence that proteinuria as such can be an independent pathogenetic factor in progressive renal structural damage.

In humans, the severity of proteinuria appears to correlate well with the severity of glomerular sclerotic lesions in such diverse renal conditions[104] as IgA nephropathy,[105] preeclampsia,[106] diabetic nephropathy,[85] human immunodeficiency virus–induced nephropathy,[107] crescentic glomerulonephritis,[108] unilateral agenesis or surgical removal of renal tissue,[109, 110] reflux nephropathy,[111] and hypertensive nephropathy,[112] as reviewed elsewhere.[113] Moreover, proteinuria consistently predicts the subsequent rate of loss of renal function in many renal conditions[6, 42, 114, 115] and is the best predictor of end-stage renal failure.[116] This relationship has been found not only in populations with renal conditions of diverse origin—where it might reflect differences in prognosis between different disorders—but also in homogeneous populations such as those with IgA nephropathy,[117] diabetic nephropathy,[74, 118] membranous glomerulopathy,[119, 120] atherosclerotic renal disease,[121] and immune-mediated renal disease such as Wegener granulomatosis.[122] Remarkably, the association between proteinuria and the rate of progression is present not only in conditions in which proteinuria might reflect the severity or activity of a primary glomerular disorder but also in chronic pyelonephritis[6] and vesicoureteral reflux.[123, 124] Thus, proteinuria, once present, is a major risk factor for progressive loss of renal function across a spectrum of renal disorders. This consistent relationship fueled the hypothesis that proteinuria is a key factor in a vicious circle of non–disease-specific factors that account for progressive renal function loss.[4] Because many patients progress toward end-stage renal failure without significant proteinuria, however, its impact relative to disease-specific factors may vary between different populations. Jungers and colleagues[125] as well as Williams and associates[6] reported that both proteinuria and the underlying disorder were independent determinants of the rate of progression, whereas Wight and co-authors reported that differences in the progression rate between different renal disorders—except for polycystic kidney disease—were no longer apparent after correction for proteinuria.[44]

Reduction of Proteinuria

Intervention studies support a pathogenetic role of proteinuria in progressive loss of renal function in experimental as well as human renal disease. In comparative studies, antihypertensive regimens associated with a better reduction in proteinuria provided better renoprotection in both diabetic[67, 126] and nondiabetic nephropathy.[65, 127-130] This finding may not be limited to overt proteinuria or hypertension because studies of patients with NIDDM have revealed that the association between the reduction in albuminuria and the long-term course of renal function was also present in normotensive, normoalbuminuric patients.[68] The association between a reduction in proteinuria and renal prognosis applies not only to antihypertensive treatment but also to remission of proteinuria attained spontaneously,[106, 107] by immunosuppressive treatment,[131] or by the nonsteroidal anti-inflammatory drug (NSAID) indomethacin.[132]

Interestingly, in individual patients, the course of long-term renal function correlates with the antiproteinuric response to therapy.[133] In patients with an effective antiproteinuric response that results in lower residual proteinuria during treatment, the long-term course of renal function is more favorable than in patients with a less pronounced antiproteinuric response, as shown in many studies.[42, 68, 134-142] For clinical purposes, it is important that this correlation already be apparent early after the start of therapy to allow early distinction between patients who will benefit from the intervention and those in whom the intervention will not be effective for long-term renoprotection—specifically, patients who need additional therapy. Of note, with the exception of the MDRD study, such a predictive value was not present for the blood

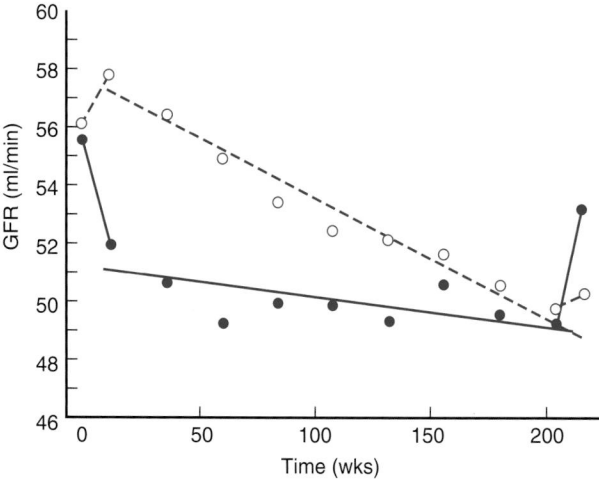

FIGURE 56-7. Time course of glomerular filtration rate (GFR) before, during, and after withdrawal of antihypertensive therapy in renal patients. *Closed circles* and *continuous lines* are patients who initially showed a distinct fall in GFR (*n* = 20). *Open circles* and *broken lines* are patients in whom the GFR did not fall at the start of therapy (*n* = 20). After withdrawal of therapy, a rise in GFR occurs in patients with an initial drop only, thus demonstrating the functional nature of the initial drop in GFR. Interestingly, withdrawal of treatment reveals that the GFR is better preserved in patients with an initial drop. (Used with permission from Apperloo AJ, de Zeeuw D, de Jong PE: A short-term antihypertensive treatment induced fall in glomerular filtration rate predicts long term stability of renal function. Kidney Int 51:793-797, 1997.).

pressure response, thus supporting an independent role of proteinuria. The predictive value is present in both diabetic and nondiabetic patients and appears to be independent of the severity of baseline proteinuria or albuminuria (Fig. 56-8). It also appears to be independent of the mode of therapy because it was found in studies with different antihypertensive regimens, as well as in populations treated with a single regimen. Moreover, the predictive value was also present with nonpharmacologic reduction of proteinuria by a low-protein diet.[100] Animal experiments have shown that the efficacy of the initial reduction in proteinuria also predicts protection against the development of structural renal damage (i.e., focal glomerulosclerosis).[143] In humans, however, similar data on protection against renal structural damage are not available.

The consistent relationship between residual proteinuria and long-term renal prognosis demonstrates first and foremost that a reduction in proteinuria is a prerequisite for renoprotection; moreover, this relationship supports the hypothesis that proteinuria plays a causal role in progressive loss of renal function. Additional support is provided by the correlation between residual proteinuria during treatment and the rate of progression.[137] However, the evidence is not conclusive. A valid assessment of the severity of renal damage before

intervention—which might determine both the antiproteinuric response and the subsequent rate of renal function loss—is difficult to obtain in humans. Uncontrolled, retrospective data in human transplant recipients suggest that pretreatment renal interstitial damage is a determinant of the antiproteinuric efficacy of ACE inhibition,[144] a finding supported by prospective animal data.[145] Moreover, it is hard to envisage how a reduction in normoalbuminuria to even lower levels, as reported by Ravid and colleagues,[68] in itself would exert a renoprotective effect. Finally, perhaps the most important piece of evidence that is lacking are studies deliberately attempting to improve antiproteinuric efficacy to assess whether it would afford additional renoprotection. In studies evaluating the renoprotective potential of antihypertensive agents, either a fixed dose was used or treatment was titrated to obtain a target blood pressure level. In the study of El Nahas and associates on the renoprotective potential of protein restriction, standardized regimens were also used rather than titrating for given target criteria.[100] In view of the consistent relationship between a reduction in proteinuria and renoprotection, as well as the absence of a J-shaped curve for proteinuria, exploration of the renoprotective potential of a treatment regimen titrated to obtain a maximally effective

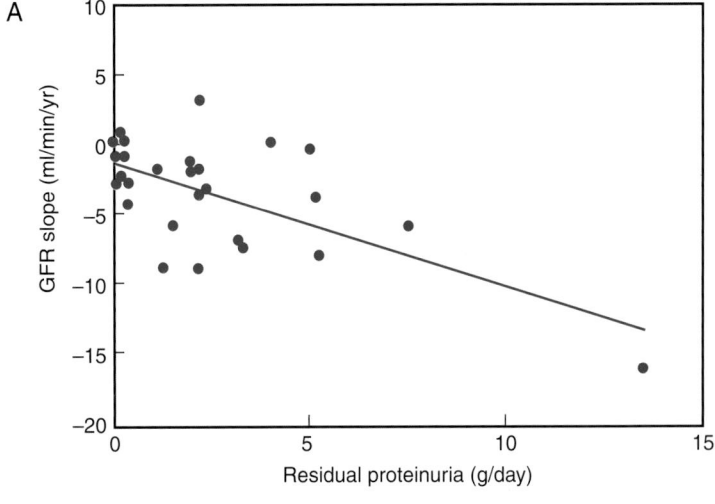

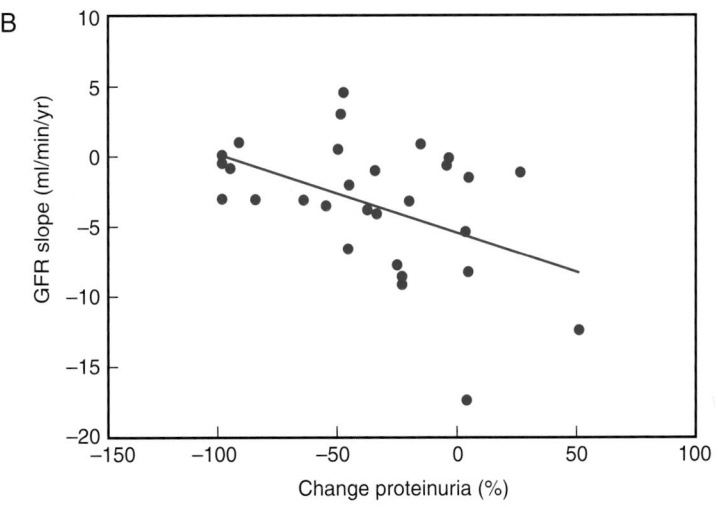

FIGURE 56-8. A, Correlation between residual proteinuria after stabilization of the antiproteinuric response (x axis) and rate of subsequent renal function loss (glomerular filtration rate [GFR] slope, y axis): $r = 0.62$, $P < .0004$; $r = 0.43$, $P < .025$ if the right-side outlier is omitted. **B,** The correlation between the reduction in proteinuria from pretreatment values (percent change in proteinuria; x axis) and rate of subsequent renal function loss (GFR slope, y axis) in the same patients; $r = 0.47$, $P < .011$. (Adapted with permission from Apperloo AJ, de Zeeuw D, de Jong PE: Short-term antiproteinuric response to antihypertensive therapy predicts long-term GFR decline in patients with non-diabetic renal disease. Kidney Int Suppl 45:174-178, 1994.)

reduction in proteinuria might be a fruitful approach to improve renoprotection.

Hyperlipidemia

Hyperlipidemia aggravates renal damage in experimental renal disease of diverse origin.[146] Because dyslipidemia is common in renal disease, lipid nephrotoxicity was hypothesized to be involved in the progression of renal damage.[147, 148] This association may be particularly relevant in proteinuric renal disease because first, proteinuria induces a distinct dyslipidemia[149] and, second, experimental data indicate that glomerular leakage of lipoproteins elicits a sequence of intrarenal pathophysiologic processes likely to be involved in progressive glomerular and interstitial sclerosis.[150] A permissive role for previous renal damage in lipid nephrotoxicity is suggested by the limited potency of hyperlipidemia to initiate renal damage in normal kidneys in most animal models as opposed to diseased kidneys,[151, 152] with the exception of certain genetic models of renal damage such as the obese Zucker rat.[153] Hyperlipidemia may also affect the renal prognosis in an indirect way, by modifying response to therapy. In Adriamycin-induced nephrosis, a high pretreatment cholesterol level was reported to predict a poor antiproteinuric response to ACE inhibitors, independent of the pretreatment proteinuria.[154] Whether this association is due to a causal effect of the hyperlipidemia or whether it is just a marker of resistance to therapy, however, remains to be investigated.

In humans, rare forms of primary hyperlipidemia, such as lecithin-cholesterol acyltransferase (LCAT) deficiency[155] and elevated apolipoprotein E (apo E) levels,[156] have been shown to elicit renal lesions, thereby allowing one to delineate the nephrotoxic potential of individual lipoproteins. On the other hand, the common forms of primary hyperlipidemia do not appear to initiate overt renal disease in normal kidneys.[157, 158] Nevertheless, in dyslipidemic men, the age-related decline in renal function was more rapid in subjects with an elevated ratio of low- to high-density cholesterol.[159] This association was apparent only when hypertension was simultaneously present, thus suggesting an interaction between hypertension and hyperlipidemia. The latter assumption is also supported by morphologic findings in hypertensive African-American subjects, in whom the severity of glomerulosclerosis correlated not only with blood pressure and the reciprocal of serum creatinine but also with serum cholesterol.[16]

A role for lipids in promoting renal damage in overt kidney disease in humans is supported by several lines of evidence. Morphologic studies in renal patients have revealed glomerular deposition of lipids and lipid-loaded macrophages in various renal disorders.[160] Mesangial accumulation of apo B and apo E was found in renal patients with diverse underlying disorders; its association with the presence of proteinuria, hyperlipidemia, and more severe mesangial hypercellularity and glomerular sclerosis may reflect its pathophysiologic significance.[161, 162] Several clinical studies have found that hyperlipidemia is associated with a faster rate of renal function loss in renal patients. In nondiabetic nephropathy, patients with hyperlipidemia progressed at a faster rate than did patients without hyperlipidemia.[163] A higher plasma cholesterol concentration was associated

with a faster progression rate in several studies.[137, 164] Samuelsson and colleagues[165] highlighted the importance of the lipoprotein profile when they reported an association between elevated levels of low-density lipoprotein (LDL) cholesterol and apo B and the subsequent progression rate; nephrotoxicity was suggested to be linked to a specific lipoprotein, possibly triglyceride-rich apo B.[166] The association between a reduced apo A-I/apo B ratio (but not total cholesterol) and the rate of progression is in line with the assumption of a role for specific lipoproteins.[167] A secondary analysis from the MDRD study identified high-density lipoprotein (HDL) cholesterol as a predictor of the rate of decline in renal function, thereby supporting the relevance of the lipid profile. Proportional hazards analysis has revealed that controlling for the higher HDL levels in premenopausal women eliminated the difference in progression rate in favor of this subgroup.[168] In IDDM nephropathy, the rate of progression was found to be associated with higher serum cholesterol[169-172] and apo B levels[173] in several studies. In NIDDM, an association of the rate of progression with serum cholesterol[102, 174] or triglycerides[175] was reported, but not all studies confirm this finding.[176, 177]

Whether the association between hyperlipidemia and the rate of progression reflects a causal role of lipid nephrotoxicity or, alternatively, the poor prognosis associated with proteinuria is still uncertain because in studies reporting hyperlipidemia to be associated with a poor renal outcome, proteinuria was usually more severe in hyperlipidemic patients.[163] Additional data on lipoprotein profiles would be highly useful because they can already be abnormal early in the course of renal disease, without hyperlipidemia being detected on routine laboratory investigation.[178]

Reduction of Lipids

In experimental renal disease, pharmacologic reduction of elevated serum lipids ameliorates the severity of progressive renal damage in different disease models.[151, 179] In humans, the number of well-controlled studies reporting on the renal effects of specific antihyperlipidemic therapy is small, and data appear to be conflicting. An overview of studies on the effect of treatment with hydroxymethylglutaryl–coenzyme A (HMG-CoA) reductase inhibitors on renal function and proteinuria in different renal conditions is presented in Table 56-1.[180-196] The effect on the lipid profile in these studies was relatively uniform, with a reduction in total cholesterol, LDL-cholesterol, and apo B. A reduction in proteinuria was found in several studies, but no effect was demonstrated in others, however. The positive studies have in common a relatively high baseline proteinuria and a relatively long follow-up. The latter may be relevant inasmuch as data on the time course provided by Rayner and co-workers[181] showed a very gradual onset of the antiproteinuric effect, with a reduction in the urinary albumin-creatinine ratio that does not reach statistical significance until after a year of treatment. The rate of loss of renal function was not affected in any study, but it should be noted that the power to detect such a change was low for all studies, not only because of the number of patients but also because of the duration of follow-up. Interestingly, in well-regulated, proteinuric hypertensives with normal lipid profiles, 6-month treatment with pravastatin reduced the proteinuria by half—with only

TABLE 56-1

Renal Effects of Antihyperlipidemic Therapy by HMG-CoA Reductase Inhibitors

INTERVENTION AND DESIGN	PATIENT CATEGORY OF PROTEINURIA	N	FOLLOW-UP (MO)	EFFECT ON LIPIDS*	RENAL EFFECT*	REF
Simvastatin, open	NDRD U_{alb}, 5.8 g/day	7	48	Chol ↓ LDL ↓	Albuminuria ↓ Creatinine =	180
Lovastatin, placebo controlled	MGP prot/creat ratio: 0.52 g/mmol	9/8	24	Chol ↓ LDL ↓	prot/creat ratio: ↓/= GFR decline: −1.27/−1.28 mL/min/mo	181
Lovastatin, open	NDRD U_{prot}, 6.41 g/day	14	6	Chol ↓ LDL ↓ Apo B ↓	Proteinuria = GFR = Rise in GFR in subgroup	182
Lovastatin, open vs. control	NDRD U_{prot}, 11.85 g/day	20	12-30	Chol ↓ LDL ↓ Apo B ↓	Proteinuria ↓↓	183
Simvastatin, open	NDRD U_{prot}, 10 g/day	16	3	Chol ↓ LDL ↓ Apo B ↓	Proteinuria = Creatinine =	184
Lovastatin, open	NDRD U_{prot}, 8.6 g/day	7	24	Chol ↓ LDL ↓ Apo B ↓	Proteinuria ↓ Renal function stable	185
Lovastatin, open	NDRD U_{alb}, 5.6 g/day	13	1, 5	Chol ↓ LDL ↓ Apo B ↓	Proteinuria = Renal function =	186
Lovastatin, placebo controlled	NDRD U_{alb}, 4 g/day	5/5	1, 5	Chol ↓/= LDL ↓/=	Proteinuria = Creatinine =	187
Simvastatin, double blind, placebo controlled	NDRD U_{prot}, 5.9 g/day	15/15	6	Chol ↓ LDL ↓ Apo B ↓	Proteinuria =/= GFR decline not different	188
Pravastatin, open	NIDDM alb/creat ratio: 49 mg/g	12	3	Chol ↓ LDL ↓	alb/creat ratio ↓	189
Simvastatin, double blind, placebo controlled	NIDDM U_{alb}, 18.4 μg/min	8/10	9	Chol ↓/= LDL ↓/= Apo B ↓/=	Albuminuria =/= GFR =/=	190
Lovastatin, open	IDDM U_{prot}, 5.9 g/day	10	3	Chol LDL	Proteinuria = Creatinine clearance =	191
Simvastatin, double blind, placebo controlled	IDDM U_{alb}, 698 mg/day	14/12	3	Chol ↓/= LDL ↓/= Apo B ↓/=	Albuminuria =/= GFR =/= U_{prot} ↑ in both groups	192
Lovastatin, single blind, placebo controlled	NIDDM U_{prot}, 0.81 g/day	16/18	24	Chol ↓/= LDL ↓/= HDL =/↑ Lp(a) =/= Apo B ↓/=	Serum creatinine: stable in statin group only	193
Pravastatin, prospective, crossover	IDDM Incipient nephropathy	20	3	Chol ↓ LDL ↓ Apo B ↓	Albuminuria = Serum creatinine =	195
Simvastatin, double blind, crossover	NIDDM Microalbuminuria	19	24	Chol ↓/= LDL ↓/=	Albuminuria ↓	196
Pravastatin	Normolipemic hypertension Proteinuria: 0.3-3 g/day	31/32	6	Chol ↓/= LDL ↓/=	U_{prot} ↓ in pravastatin group Serum creatinine stable	194

*Effect in statin group or in statin group/control group, if applicable.

alb/creat, albumin/creatinine; Chol, cholesterol; GFR, glomerular filtration rate; HDL, high-density lipoprotein; HMG-CoA, hydroxymethylglutaryl–coenzyme A; IDDM, insulin-dependent diabetes mellitus; LDL, low-density lipoprotein; Lp(a), lipoprotein (a); MGP, membranous glomerulopathy; NDRD, nondiabetic renal disease; NIDDM, non-insulin-dependent diabetes mellitus; prot/creat, protein/creatinine.

slight effects on the lipid profile. This effect was also noted in patients in whom the antihypertensive regimen included an AT1 receptor blocker, thus indicating an additive antiproteinuric potential of the statin.[194] The antiproteinuric effect of different antihyperlipidemic drugs was also addressed in a recent meta-analysis that included 13 prospective controlled trials with a total of 392 patients treated with different classes of antihyperlipidemic agents; the results supported a tendency toward a reduction in proteinuria by reducing lipids.[197]

Taken together, these findings suggest that pharmacologic treatment of hyperlipidemia may have renoprotective potential in humans but that treatment needs to be prolonged. Data on cardiovascular disease suggest that the nonlipid effects of HMG-CoA reductase inhibitors may also provide protection against target organ damage. However, more solid data are required, especially on the long-term outcome of renal function, to substantiate the possible renoprotective benefit in humans provided by specific antihyperlipidemic treatments—or by HMG-CoA reductase inhibition as such.

Genetic Factors

Until recently, the relevance of genetic factors for progressive renal disease was largely limited to single-gene renal disorders with mendelian inheritance, such as polycystic kidney disease or Alport disease. Several lines of evidence have nevertheless supported a role for genetic factors in multifactorial renal conditions as well. Animal data have clearly demonstrated a role for genetic differences in susceptibility to the development of progressive renal function loss and glomerulosclerosis in response to various renal insults.[198] In humans, the familial clustering of diabetic nephropathy[199] and the association of several renal disorders (e.g., membranous glomerulopathy,[200] IgA nephropathy,[201] and focal segmental sclerosis[202]) with distinct HLA patterns suggested that susceptibility to the development of these disorders was subject to genetic influences.

A role for genetic factors in modifying the course of renal function loss is suggested by the remarkably constant individual progression rate as opposed to the large interindividual differences in the rate of progression, even for subjects suffering from the same underlying disorder.[203] Ethnic differences in renal risk also suggest a role for genetic factors. A greatly increased risk for end-stage renal failure as a result of hypertension or diabetes (or both) is consistently reported for African, Native, and Mexican Americans,[9] as well as Indian subjects in the United Kingdom.[204] The relative contribution of environmental factors, such as socioeconomic status and limited access to medical care,[205] and truly genetic factors to the renal risk in ethnic minorities is the subject of current studies.

The recent advancements in molecular genetics provide great potential to elucidate the role of normal genetic variability in the likelihood of acquiring renal disease, the course of renal function loss, and response to therapy. Polymorphisms for many genes are present in the normal population, and exploration of their role in renal disease is only starting. Thus far, attention has focused mainly on a common insertion/deletion (I/D) polymorphism for the ACE gene. An association between the DD genotype and progression of renal function loss was reported in renal disorders of diverse origin,[206] IgA nephropathy,[207, 208] diabetic nephropathy,[209, 210] ADPKD,[211] graft loss after renal transplantation,[212] and nephrosclerosis in hypertensive subjects.[31, 32, 33, 213] However, the number of conflicting studies is considerable as well—as reviewed elsewhere[214]—and the number of different potential gene-gene and gene-environment interactions that may modulate the phenotype is tremendous. To deal with this complexity, it has been argued that in multifactorial disease in humans, the most fruitful approach for the moment might be to focus on the functional consequences of genetic variations (i.e., the molecular and physiologic phenotype) as a first step toward gaining insight regarding their impact in health and disease.

ACE levels in serum[215] and cardiac[216] and renal tissue[217] are higher in DD homozygotes, thus suggesting that under certain circumstances, the availability of angiotensin II might be increased in the DD genotype. This finding is supported by the enhanced conversion of angiotensin II in isolated human blood vessels.[218] In vivo, the responses of blood pressure[219] and renal vascular resistance[220] to angiotensin I were reported to be enhanced in DD homozygotes as well. A role for an altered RAAS phenotype is suggested by the interaction of an ACE (I/D) polymorphism with a 235 MT polymorphism of the angiotensinogen gene in diabetic[221] and nondiabetic nephropathy.[222]

Pharmacogenetics

An effect of genetic factors on response to therapy has long been recognized. Genetic factors were known to account for differences in drug metabolism, such as slow versus rapid acetylation of hydralazine and isoniazid.[223] Not until recently, however, has the development in genetic techniques allowed knowledge of the genetic determinants of response to therapy to expand beyond the array of pharmacokinetics to pharmacodynamics. Several genetic polymorphisms are associated with individual differences in therapeutic benefit from, for instance, diuretic therapy[224] and prevention of coronary restenosis by statin therapy.[225] These developments may have the potential to provide a novel basis to design individual treatment strategies by identifying responders and nonresponders before therapy by their genetic profile.[226] Promising as this may be, it should be noted that the response to pharmacologic intervention in multifactorial processes such as renal disease is complex. Drug response is definitely a complex phenotype. Variations in pathophysiologic factors and compensatory responses—all subject to polygenic regulation, as well as environmental factors—are relevant to the eventual therapeutic benefit.

With respect to response to therapy in renal patients, most attention has focused on the ACE genotype and the response to ACE inhibition. In view of the higher ACE levels in the DD genotype, one might expect that these subjects either would be particularly susceptible to ACE inhibition, would require higher doses of ACE inhibitors to obtain effective RAAS blockade, or would particularly benefit from AT1 blockade (i.e., circumventing the higher ACE levels). The latter assumption, however, was recently refuted.[227] The relationship between ACE genotype and response to ACE inhibition was tested in several post hoc analyses of clinical studies, but the results were conflicting. The blood pressure and proteinuria response in the DD genotype was reported to be better, similar, or worse than in the I/D and II genotypes.[208, 228-232] Differences in genetic or environmental background, gene-gene interactions, gene-environment interactions, or a combination of these factors may be involved in these discrepancies. Interaction with gender was observed in the Ramipril Efficacy in Nephropathy (REIN) population, in which resistance to ACE inhibition was shown in the II and I/D genotypes in men only.[233] Interaction with high dietary sodium intake has also been reported inasmuch as high sodium intake appears to evoke differences in the response of blood pressure and proteinuria to ACE inhibitors in patients with different ACE (I/D) genotypes.[234] The latter—if confirmed—would be of therapeutic interest because it might provide a strategy to circumvent genotype-associated treatment resistance by dietary sodium restriction. These post hoc data in proteinuric patients are supported by prospective data in normal subjects, in whom the exaggerated renal hemodynamic response to angiotensin I in DD homozygotes was apparent during a 200-mmol but not a 50-mmol sodium intake in the same subjects.[220] If volume loading unmasks the phenotype in patients with the DD genotype, it would be logical to expect a gene-gene interaction with genetic factors that affect volume status, such as the α-adducin polymorphism. Indeed, the ACE (I/D) genotype and the α-adducin genotype appeared to exert a synergistic effect on the response to volume expansion in humans.[235] These data demonstrate the complexity of the pathophysiologic consequences of normal genetic variation, but they also show that the impact of genetic variation can fruitfully be studied by starting from logical physiologic hypotheses.

Regarding the impact of genetic variation on response to therapy, well-documented studies are needed to assess the relative impact of genetic versus phenotypic determinants of response to therapy and identify contextual factors (other genes, but also factors such as gender and sodium intake) that allow alleged candidate genes to modulate the response to therapy. Obviously, modifiable contextual factors such as sodium intake deserve specific attention because they may help overcome the adverse effects of a specific genetic makeup on the response to therapy.

Miscellaneous

OBESITY. Massive obesity has long been known to be associated with focal glomerulosclerosis.[236] Less extreme obesity is now increasingly being recognized as a renal risk factor in diverse conditions such as uninephrectomy,[89] IgA nephritis,[237] and renal transplantation.[238] The mechanism underlying the renal risk of obesity is not well characterized and may relate to its association other renal risk factors such as hypertension, diabetes mellitus, and lipid abnormalities. Hyperfiltration may be involved in obesity-associated renal risk,[239] but its interaction with hypertension, glucose tolerance, and sodium intake[240] needs further study. Recent data have shown an association between higher body mass index (BMI) and an unfavorable renal hemodynamic profile, with a higher filtration fraction noted in normotensive subjects in whom the BMI did not exceed 30, thus suggesting that the renal effects of excess weight may be more widespread than assumed thus far.[241] Specific obesity-related mechanisms, such as the role of leptin, are currently under investigation.[242] For therapeutic purposes, it is important that a study of morbidly obese, proteinuric patients with diverse glomerular disorders found that weight loss (reduction of BMI from 37.1 to 32.6) by ingestion of a hypocaloric diet resulted in a reduction in proteinuria (2.9 to 0.4 g/day) that correlated with weight loss. This finding was similar to the efficacy of captopril in the control of proteinuria in obese patients without weight reduction.[243] The renal effects of weight loss in less extreme obesity have not been investigated thus far.

SMOKING. An increasing body of evidence indicates that cigarette smoking is associated with an increased rate of loss of renal function, as reviewed elsewhere.[244] The effect appears to be particularly prominent in diabetic nephropathy, but it is also apparent in nondiabetic renal disease. Obviously, the most important intervention measure is to quit smoking.

PHARMACOLOGIC APPROACHES

Antihypertensive Treatment

It has been firmly established in experimental and human renal disease that reduction of blood pressure per se is of prime importance to renoprotection. In renal patients, blood pressure reduction can be achieved with all of the currently available classes of antihypertensive agents, as illustrated by the meta-analysis data in Figure 56-9.[245] Whether the choice of a particular antihypertensive agent matters for long-term renoprotection, independent of the reduction in blood pressure achieved, has long been a matter of debate. Animal studies first provided evidence for class-specific renoprotective effects in addition to the effects on blood pressure for ACE inhibitors, AT1 blockers, and selected calcium channel blockers (CCBs). Comparative studies of ACE inhibitors suggested class-specific renoprotective properties of RAAS blockade beyond blood pressure control in humans as well, although the differences in blood pressure control achieved between ACE inhibitors and control treatment in many studies have long hampered definitive conclusions. Recent meta-analyses of ACE inhibitors, however, support a renoprotective effect of RAAS blockade beyond blood pressure control in nondiabetic and diabetic patients[130, 246]; this finding is supported by recent data on the renoprotective effects of AT1 blockade.[69, 70]

Angiotensin-Converting Enzyme Inhibitors

Animal studies from the 1980s showed that ACE inhibitors attenuate loss of renal function more effectively than do other antihypertensives with a similar effect on blood pressure.[96] ACE inhibitors inhibit cleavage of the decapeptide angiotensin I to angiotensin II, one of the main effector hormones of the RAAS. In addition, they inhibit the inactivation of bradykinin, as well as the breakdown of many other peptides. Several hemodynamic and nonhemodynamic mechanisms have been postulated to be involved in their renoprotective action.

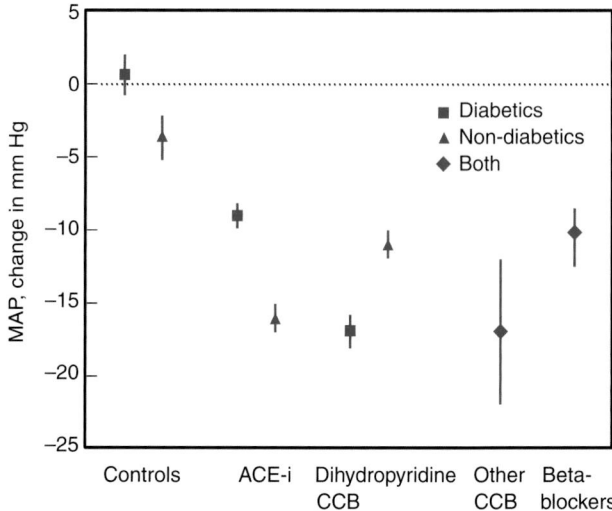

FIGURE 56-9. Meta-analysis data on the unadjusted effects of different classes of antihypertensives on blood pressure in renal patients. Data are given as pooled weighted means and 95% confidence intervals for controlled and uncontrolled studies. Groups were pooled by therapy and, when there were at least two studies of each, by diabetes status. ACE, angiotensin-converting enzyme; CCB, calcium channel blocker; MAP, mean arterial pressure. (From Maki DD, Ma JZ, Louis TA, Kasiske BL: Long-term effects of antihypertensive agents on proteinuria and renal function. Arch Intern Med 155:1073-1080, 1995. Copyright 1995, American Medical Association.)

Apart from the fall in blood pressure, the hemodynamic effects include a reduction in glomerular pressure by a vasodilator effect on efferent arterioles. Reduction of proteinuria (see the next paragraph also) with a concomitant reduction in the trafficking of macromolecules through the mesangium[247] is assumed to be an important renoprotective mechanism.[4] In addition, angiotensin II stimulates various growth factors and inflammatory cytokines involved in the processes of glomerular and interstitial sclerosis.[248] Attenuation of the angiotensin II–induced processes of cell growth and repair and extracellular matrix formation may therefore contribute to the renoprotection. Inhibition of angiotensin II formation may not be the sole mechanism of action of ACE inhibitors. Decreased bradykinin breakdown may play a role in specific experimental models,[249] but this finding does not appear to be uniform.[250] Studies in the spontaneously hypertensive rat,[251] as well as humans with essential hypertension,[252] suggest that the increased availability of smaller angiotensins such as the heptapeptide angiotensin[1-7] may play a role in the effects of ACE inhibitors, but their impact in renal disease remains to be seen.

In humans, the long-term renoprotective action of ACE inhibitors has been the subject of several clinical trials. Comparative studies have found more effective attenuation of long-term renal function loss by ACE inhibition than by other antihypertensives.[127, 253] Meta-analysis data[254] support the greater renoprotective efficacy of ACE inhibition—in association with a greater reduction in blood pressure as well as proteinuria.[130] In 11 randomized controlled trials that included a total of 1860 nondiabetic patients, the relative risk for end-stage renal disease was 0.69 (95% confidence interval, 0.51 to 0.94) with ACE inhibition versus control antihypertensive treatment (Fig. 56-10). The more effective renoprotection afforded by ACE inhibitors could not be completely attributed to their antihypertensive and antiproteinuric effects. Recent data from the AASK trial—showing similar blood pressure, but better renoprotection with ramipril than with amlodipine in proteinuric African Americans with hypertensive nephropathy—further support a nonpressor renoprotective effect of ACE inhibition.[64]

Patient characteristics are relevant to the benefit of ACE inhibition. Post hoc data from the ACE Inhibitor Protection in Renal Insufficiency (AIPRI) study, for instance, show that in patients with polycystic kidneys, ACE inhibition fails to reduce the rate of loss of renal function.[127] The overall renal risk appears to be a determinant of the outcome of comparative studies: studies favoring ACE inhibition tend to be ones in which renal risk (rate of loss of renal function or baseline proteinuria) is highest. Van Essen and colleagues, for instance, found a similar low rate of progression with enalapril and atenolol (−1.92 versus −1.32 mL/min/yr).[255] Hannedouche and associates, however, found a difference in favor of enalapril, with loss of renal function amounting to −3.96 mL/min/yr versus −6.84 mL/min/yr with β-blockade.[253] The importance of a priori renal risk is supported by the REIN study; patients with proteinuria greater than 3 g/day demonstrated a benefit of ACE inhibition that was already

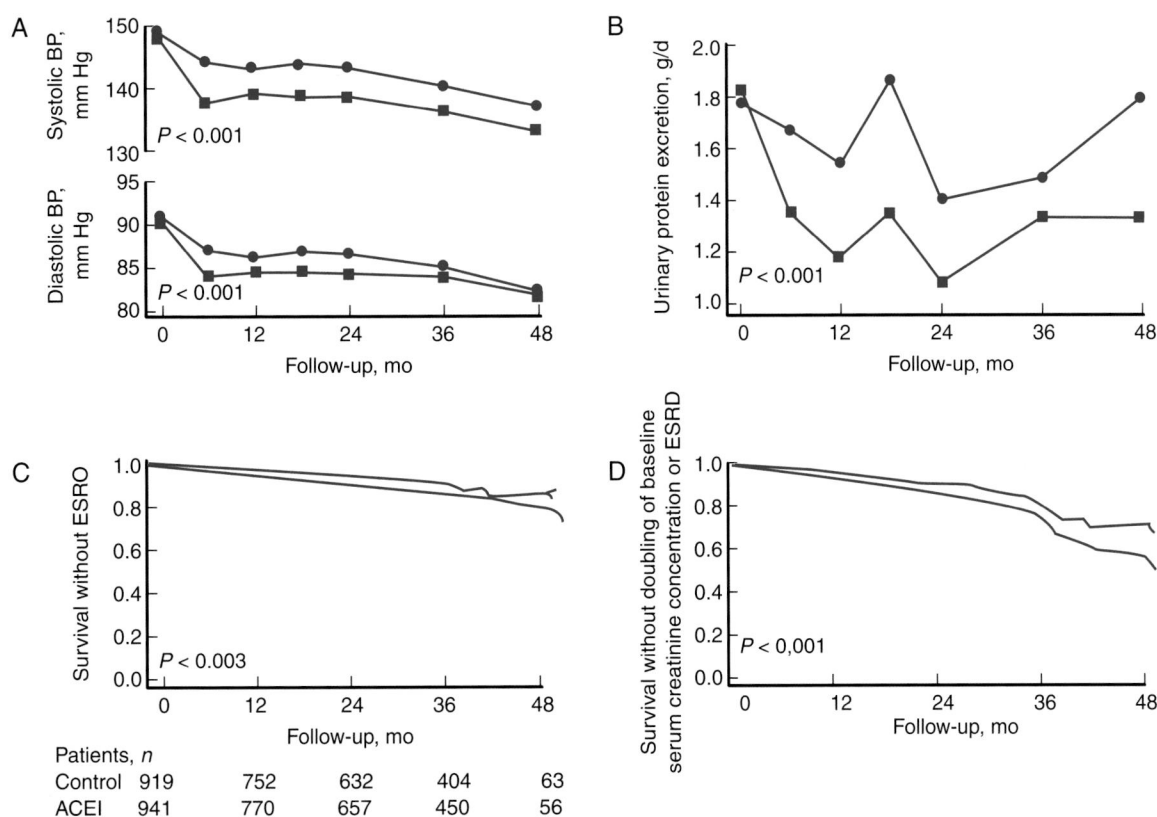

FIGURE 56-10. Meta-analysis data on blood pressure (BP) (**A**), urinary protein excretion (**B**), survival without end-stage renal disease (ESRD) (**C**), or the combined outcome of doubling of the baseline serum creatinine concentration or ESRD (**D**) during follow-up in patients treated by angiotensin-converting enzyme (ACE) inhibition *(squares)* and controls *(circles)*. (Reproduced with permission from Jafar TH, Schmid CH, Landa M, et al: Angiotensin converting enzyme inhibitors and progression of nondiabetic disease. A meta-analysis of patient-level data. Ann Intern Med 135:73-87, 2001.)

apparent after only 1 year of treatment, with the rate of loss of renal function being −6.36 mL/min/yr with ramipril versus −10.56 mL/min/yr in controls. Interestingly, the REIN data show that the renoprotective benefit of ACE inhibition is proportional to the baseline proteinuria,[129] as apparent from Figure 56-11. The greater advantage of ACE inhibitors over control treatment in more severely proteinuric patients was confirmed by recent meta-analysis data and explained by a greater absolute reduction in proteinuria.[130] Nevertheless, patients with less severe proteinuria also benefit from ACE inhibition, as shown by the reduction in hard end points (initiation of dialysis) in patients with proteinuria of 1 to 3 g/day.[256] This benefit appears to be related to the antiproteinuric effects of the ACE inhibitor regimen, as suggested by the association between reduction in proteinuria and stabilization of renal function in patients from the control group who were switched to the ACE inhibitor regimen after completion of the original study.[257] This stabilization has been argued to reflect true regression of the renal disorder and has raised hope that ACE inhibitor–based regimens will allow one to not only postpone but perhaps altogether prevent end-stage renal disease, at least in some patients.[258]

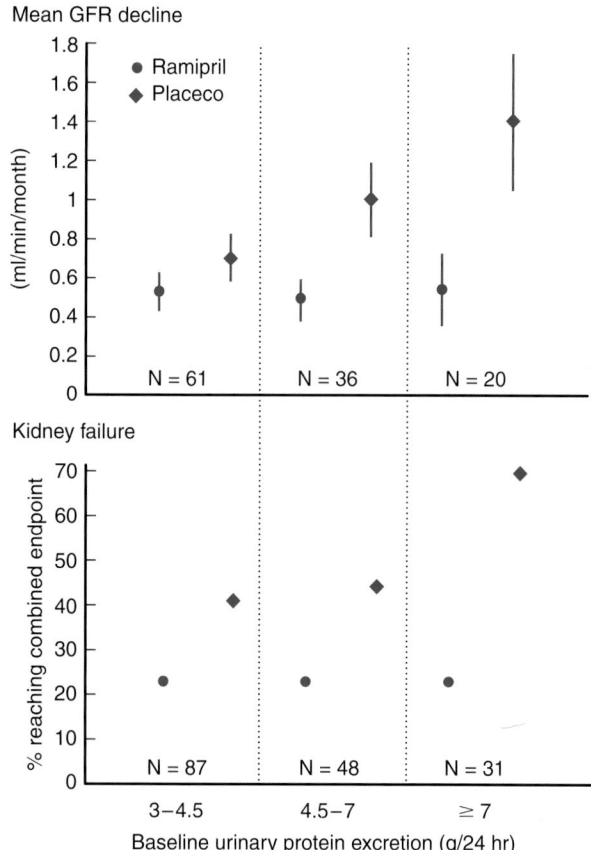

FIGURE 56-11. Rate of decline in glomerular filtration rate (GFR) *(upper panel)* and risk of progression of nephropathy *(lower panel;* combined end point: doubling of baseline serum creatinine and end-stage renal failure) for patients grouped according to baseline proteinuria and receiving ramipril *(circles)* or placebo *(diamonds).* (From The GISEN Group: Randomised placebo-controlled trial of effect of ramipril on decline in glomerular filtration rate and risk of terminal renal failure in proteinuric, non-diabetic nephropathy. Lancet 349:1857-1863, 1997. © by the Lancet Ltd., 1997.)

It is of clinical importance to note that the absolute reduction in hard end points was largest in patients with the lowest GFR at entry.[259]

In diabetic patients with overt nephropathy, ACE inhibition attenuated the long-term rate of renal function loss in IDDM more effectively than placebo did.[67] ACE inhibition attenuated the progression of incipient nephropathy (as apparent from microalbuminuria) to overt nephropathy in normotensive IDDM patients[260-262] as well as NIDDM patients,[174, 264] independent of its effects on blood pressure,[246] with a tendency for better preservation of renal function.[263] Interestingly, ACE inhibition also appears to be able to induce regression toward normoalbuminuria in subjects with microalbuminuria.[246] ACE inhibition reduced the rate of loss of renal function in a population of relatively young, normotensive, normoalbuminuric NIDDM patients.[68] Importantly, ACE inhibition reduced not only the risk for nephropathy but also overall mortality and cardiovascular events in diabetic patients with high cardiovascular risk.[265]

ACE inhibitors are generally considered to be a fairly homogeneous class of drugs, apart from their kinetic properties. Nevertheless, animal data suggest that the effects on renal tissue may not necessarily be similar for all ACE inhibitors. In the meta-analysis by Maki and co-workers,[245] no long-term renoprotection was demonstrated for lisinopril, as opposed to enalapril and captopril, thus suggesting differences in renoprotective potential between ACE inhibitors. However, studies comparing the renoprotective efficacy of different ACE inhibitors are not available and are unlikely to be conducted in the near future. Data from essential hypertensive patients nevertheless suggest that extrapolation of renal findings from one ACE inhibitor to another may be unwarranted inasmuch as lisinopril exerted less pronounced renal hemodynamic effects than enalapril did in spite of similar effects on systemic blood pressure.[266]

All in all, ACE inhibitors are particularly effective in reducing the long-term loss of renal function. In addition to their antihypertensive potency, this benefit is due to their antiproteinuric effects and possibly also additional specific renoprotective effects. This renoprotective potential is most readily apparent in high-risk renal populations, such as patients with overt proteinuria and blacks with hypertensive nephrosclerosis.[267]

AT1 Receptor Blockers

In light of the importance of RAAS blockade for the renoprotective properties of ACE inhibition, it would be logical to assume that the renoprotective efficacy of specific AT1 receptor blockers would mimic that of ACE inhibitors. Indeed, in animal as well as human studies, AT1 receptor blockade results in all the "classic" actions of RAAS blockade, such as a reduction in blood pressure and renal vasodilation with a predominant effect on efferent arterioles.[268, 269] Moreover, AT1 receptor blockade reduces proteinuria and was shown to provide protection against structural renal damage in several animal models.[270] Nonetheless, in comparative studies between ACE inhibitors and AT1 receptor blockers, differences in renoprotective efficacy have also been reported, with somewhat less extensive effects of AT1 receptor blockade.[271, 272] It may be relevant that AT1 receptor blockers, unlike ACE inhibitors, induce a large increase in angiotensin II levels while leaving the other receptor subtype, the AT2 receptor, unblocked.[273] The precise function of the AT2 receptor remains to be explored further, but some evidence indicates that this receptor subtype affects processes of cell proliferation[274] and apoptosis,[275] presumably in an interaction with the AT1 receptor.[276] The impact of these differential effects on the AT1 and the AT2 receptor subtype for long-term renoprotection is as yet unclear.

In patients with essential hypertension, as well as renal patients, AT1 receptor blockers induce a gradual fall in blood pressure that is associated with a renal hemodynamic profile similar to that achieved by ACE inhibitors,[277-279] in addition to an antiproteinuric effect (see later).

The renoprotective profile of this class was recently substantiated by a series of landmark studies, the Irbesartan Microalbuminuria in Type 2 Diabetes (IRMAII)[280] and the Irbesartan Diabetic Nephropathy Trial (IDNT),[70] which investigated irbesartan, and the RENAAL trial (Reduction in Endpoints in Non–Insulin Dependent Diabetes Mellitus with the Angiotensin II Antagonist Losartan),[69] which investigated losartan. The IRMA trial showed that irbesartan dose-dependently protected hypertensive patients with type 2 diabetes from progression from the microalbuminuric state to overt nephropathy during a 2-year follow-up. The RENAAL study and the IDNT showed that AT1 blockade provided added renoprotective potential when compared with placebo plus conventional (non–ACE-inhibiting, non–AT1-blocking) antihypertensives in type 2 diabetic subjects with overt nephropathy; the protection was significant in terms of the rate of loss of renal function and the development of end-stage renal disease, as shown in Figure 56-12. This regimen leads to an estimated postponement of the need for dialysis of approximately 2 years.

Interestingly, the IDNT study also had a comparative arm in which CCBs were administered. CCBs resulted in an identical blood pressure but worse renal outcome than in the AT1 receptor blocker arm, thus supporting the nonpressor renoprotective effects of AT1 receptor blockade. Taken together, these studies indicate that in addition to the protective effect of a reduction in blood pressure, additional renoprotective benefit in this population appears to be conferred by inhibiting the RAAS. This renoprotective effect again appears to be linked to the reduction in proteinuria.

Calcium Channel Blockers

CCBs are effective antihypertensive agents in renal patients. Their renoprotective effects, however, have been questioned because disparate effects on renal function have been found with CCBs. CCBs are a relatively heterogeneous class of drugs that inhibit different types of calcium channels with different intrarenal distribution.[281] A main distinction can be made between dihydropyridine (such as nifedipine) and non-dihydropyridine (such as verapamil and diltiazem) CCBs. Differences in renal effects have been described between different CCB subclasses as well as within subclasses. In experimental renal disease, both protective[282, 283] and detrimental effects on the development of renal damage[284-286] were reported for CCBs. Differential effects on autoregulation may play a role in these discrepancies inasmuch as nifedipine was shown to impair afferent arteriolar autoregulatory vascular tone, thereby leading to increased transmission of systemic blood pressure to the glomerular capillary bed,[287] whereas non-dihydropyridines leave autoregulation intact. The nonhemodynamic renoprotective effects of nifedipine,

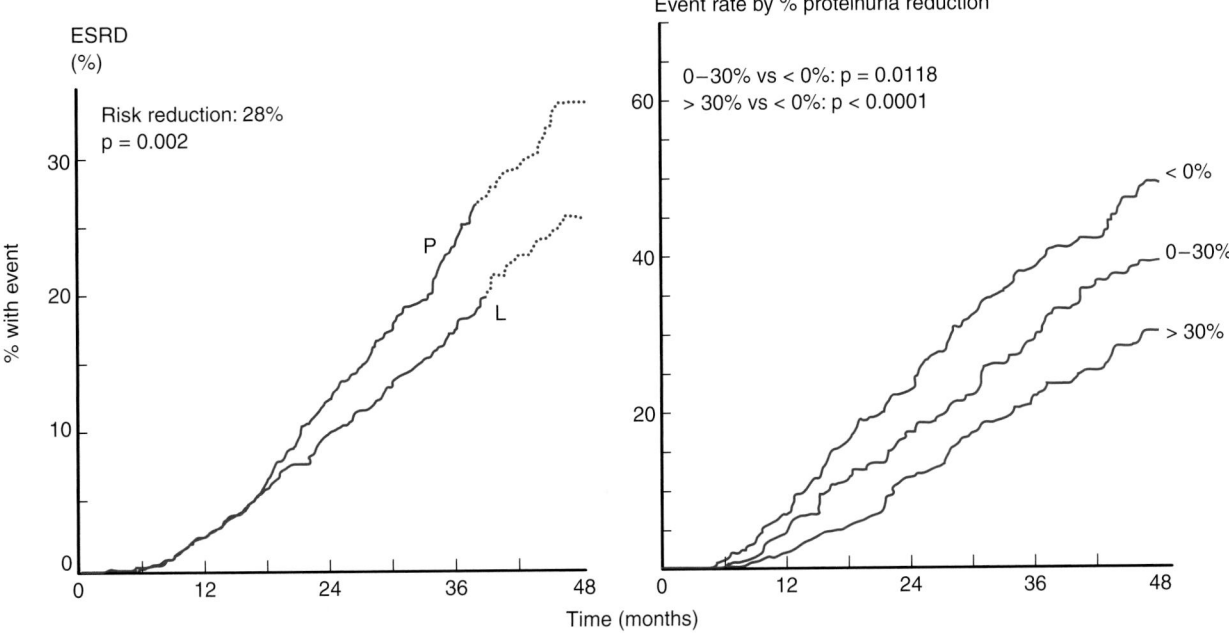

FIGURE 56-12. A Kaplan-Meier curve of the risk for end-stage renal disease (ESRD) in the RENAAL trial *(left panel)* with losartan (L) versus placebo (P) shows a difference in favor of the losartan group, and the cumulative risk (doubling of serum creatinine, ESRD, death) grouped by the initial antiproteinuric response to therapy (losartan or placebo, *right panel*) shows that the reduction in proteinuria is associated with a reduction in risk. (Adapted from Brenner BM, Cooper ME, de Zeeuw D, et al: Effects of losartan on renal and cardiovascular outcomes in patients with type 2 diabetes and nephropathy. N Engl J Med 345:861-869, 2001; and de Zeeuw D, Navis GJ: Optimizing the RAAS intervention treatment strategy in diabetic and non-diabetic nephropathy: The potential of exploring the mechanisms of response variability. *In* Mogensen CE [ed]: Diabetic Nephropathy in Type 2 Diabetes. London, Science Press, 2002, pp 103-116.)

such as attenuation of glomerular hypertrophy,[288] may thus be counteracted by the deleterious effects of increased glomerular pressure because the severity of the renal structural damage during nifedipine treatment appears to be closely related to systemic blood pressure.[251] Furthermore non-dihydropyridines improve glomerular membrane permeability characteristics,[289] whereas dihydropyridines appear to leave the permeability characteristics unaffected.[290] One study with the dihydropyridine CCB manidipine suggests that disparate outcomes may be due to the deleterious renal effects of a higher than optimal—renoprotective—dose,[291] but these findings require further confirmation.[292] Differences in renal effects may be related to sodium status. Because sodium status appears to modify the efficacy of CCBs, failure to control for sodium intake may account for differences in study outcomes. Moreover, some evidence suggests that sodium status may differentially affect the renal effects of different CCBs.[293] Finally, genetic factors may account for part of the differences in response to CCBs.[294]

In humans, most studies have addressed diabetic patients—with RAAS blockade being a comparator regimen. In a 6-year follow-up of 52 NIDDM patients, non-dihydropyridine CCBs and lisinopril were equally effective in reducing blood pressure and retarding the rate of renal function loss, whereas β-blockade was less effective in both respects.[295] In African Americans with NIDDM, verapamil more effectively reduced the rate of renal function loss than β-blockade did despite similar effects on blood pressure during a 5-year follow-up.[296] A 3-year follow-up of hypertensive NIDDM patients found a similar well-controlled blood pressure and a similar rate of decline in GFR with the long-acting dihydropyridines amlodipine and cilazapril.[297] In hypertensive IDDM patients, a prospective 4-year follow-up study showed similar protection against a decline in GFR by lisinopril and the long-acting dihydropyridine nisoldipine.[298] An older study that investigated incipient nephropathy in IDDM and NIDDM found no difference between nifedipine and perindopril[299] during a 1-year follow-up. A more recent 3-year follow-up, however, in 25 normotensive, microalbuminuric IDDM patients showed that perindopril was more effective than placebo and nifedipine in reducing albuminuria toward normal, whereas renal function fell significantly with nifedipine, but not with perindopril or placebo.[300] Similar albuminuria and renal function were reported with perindopril and nitrendipine in a 1-year follow-up of patients with incipient nephropathy,[301] and likewise, no significant differences were found between ramipril and nitrendipine in a 2-year prospective comparison of 51 subjects with nephropathy and NIDDM.[302] The recent IDNT findings—in 1715 patients with nephropathy caused by NIDDM with a mean follow-up of 2.6 years—provide important data: better reduction of the risk for end-stage renal disease or doubling of serum creatinine was achieved with irbesartan, 300 mg, than with similar blood pressure achieved with the comparator drug, amlodipine, 10 mg.

In nondiabetic patients, an older study found that blood pressure and the rate of progression were similar for nifedipine and captopril at 2 years of follow-up.[303] However, during the third year more patients receiving nifedipine entered dialysis, thus weakening the authors' claim that nifedipine exerted a renoprotective effect. In the AASK trial, ramipril provided better renoprotection than amlodipine did at similar blood pressure levels in African Americans with hypertensive nephrosclerosis; the difference in the rate of loss of renal function even prompted premature termination of the trial.[64] Thus, the presently available large trials favor RAAS blockade–based regimens over CCB-based regimens. Comparing CCBs with placebo—not usually warranted in renal populations—provides an additional perspective: in older subjects with systolic hypertension, active therapy with the CCB nitrendipine resulted in a reduction in proteinuria and serum creatinine when compared with placebo.[304] All in all, it would be cautious to assume that the renoprotective properties of dihydropyridines are closely linked to their antihypertensive properties and that a renoprotective benefit can be expected only in patients in whom blood pressure is rigorously controlled.

β-Blockers

Experimental data on β-blockade as a mode of renoprotection are almost entirely lacking because β-blockers fail to reduce blood pressure in rats. In humans, on the other hand, the antihypertensive efficacy of β-blockers has been well documented for decades. Moreover, in essential hypertension, β-blockade has been shown not only to affect blood pressure as an intermediate parameter but also to reduce mortality. In renal patients, β-blockers are generally effective in reducing blood pressure. By virtue of this long-standing experience, in comparative studies of the renoprotective potential of newer classes of drugs, β-blockers are often part of the so-called conventional antihypertensive regimen, mostly in combination with diuretics. No studies are available to support specific renoprotection by β-blocker–based antihypertensive treatment. β-blockers were reported to be less effective than ACE inhibitors for long-term renoprotection in nondiabetic patients,[253, 305] as well as in African American NIDDM patients.[296] However, other well-controlled studies have found a similar rate of loss of renal function with β-blockers and ACE inhibitors in diabetic[306-308] and nondiabetic patients.[255] This finding suggests that β-blockers are useful for long-term renoprotection, possibly by virtue of their effects on blood pressure.

Diuretics

In essential hypertension, diuretics have been shown to reduce not only blood pressure but also the incidence of mortality from cardiovascular causes.[309] In many renal patients diuretics are required for effective blood pressure control. Accordingly, diuretics are part of the therapeutic regimen in many studies. Nonetheless, it has been argued that surprisingly, their long-term renoprotective effect in humans has not been established.[310] Retrospective data in hypertensive renal patients suggested that the use of diuretics may be associated with more rapid loss of renal function,[41] and prospective data in elderly hypertensive patients do not support a long-term renoprotective effect.[304] Experimental data suggest that diuretic treatment may lack renoprotective effects in specific models of experimental renal disease,[311] as opposed to dietary sodium restriction.[312] Although this issue deserves further exploration, for the moment, diuretics are indispensable in renoprotective intervention in view of the importance of control of volume status and blood pressure in patients with overt renal disease. This point is clearly illustrated by data from Buter and colleagues, in which the poor therapeutic efficacy of ACE inhibition during high sodium intake was restored by adding hydrochlorothiazide.[313]

Whether different diuretics are equivalent for renoprotection is unknown. The specific cardioprotective effects of aldosterone blockade by spironolactone suggest that this issue may be relevant to renal patients as well. Although spironolactone appears to have added antiproteinuric efficacy on top of ACE inhibition, it is unclear whether this finding reflects specific aldosterone blockade or just its effect on volume control.[314] Of note, in renal patients the combination of RAAS blockade and aldosterone blockade will require close consideration of safety issues in light of the risk of development of hyperkalemia.

Antiproteinuric Treatment

Reduction of proteinuria can be obtained by pharmacologic treatment, by dietary intervention, and by a combination of the two.

Pharmacologic measures to reduce proteinuria can be categorized as symptomatic or causal treatment—specifically, treatment aimed at reduction of proteinuria as such or aimed at intervention for the underlying condition. A causal intervention is available for some specific conditions. Minimal change disease is the typical proteinuric disorder in which a causal approach (i.e., steroid therapy) is undisputedly the first-choice therapy because total and often permanent remission can be obtained. This approach may also apply to the related condition of glomerular tip lesions. For other conditions such as focal glomerulosclerosis and membranous glomerulopathy, the results of causal therapy are more equivocal, and both causal and symptomatic regimens have been recommended. Conditions initially responsive to causal approaches, such as immunologically mediated glomerular disorders, may become unresponsive when the renal disorder takes a chronic course. Such altered responsiveness to therapy presumably reflects a shift in the determinants of renal damage, with a decreased impact of the primary disease-specific factors. Causal therapy usually involves potent immunosuppressive regimens. Thus, a careful workup, including renal morphologic data and an assessment of the previous course of the disease and circulating parameters of disease activity, is required to estimate the potential therapeutic benefit of a causal approach for the individual patient. Causal therapeutic regimens are discussed extensively in Chapter 55 of this volume.

For many proteinuric patients, a causal approach is not available or does not exert the intended benefit. For these patients, symptomatic antiproteinuric therapy is warranted. Pharmacologic treatment can elicit a symptomatic reduction in proteinuria by lowering systemic blood pressure and inducing class-specific renal effects.

ACE inhibitors consistently reduce albuminuria and proteinuria more effectively than conventional antihypertensive treatment does, even when the effect on blood pressure is similar,[315-317] as illustrated in Figure 56-10. The antiproteinuric effect may be partly due to a reduction in systemic and glomerular pressure. However, the antiproteinuric effect is more gradual than the hemodynamic effects,[318] which suggests that gradual improvement in glomerular permselectivity

contributes to the reduction in proteinuria as well.[319] In diabetic patients, an antiproteinuric effect as well as preservation of renal structural characteristics[320] was found in the absence of an effect on blood pressure, thus supporting specific renal effects as well.[321] The antiproteinuric effect of ACE inhibitors occurs irrespective of previous patient characteristics such as the specific diagnosis, renal function, pretreatment blood pressure, and severity of proteinuria—with a greater absolute reduction observed in subjects with the highest baseline proteinuria.

AT1 receptor blockers have been shown to reduce albuminuria and proteinuria in many recent studies.[32, 67, 269, 323-334] The absolute reduction in proteinuria—as apparent from Figure 56-13—is largest in patients with the highest pretreatment proteinuria, which is in accord with similar findings with ACE inhibitors. The magnitude of the antiproteinuric response is more or less similar to that for ACE inhibitors—provided that adequate doses are given. The same holds true when comparing groups of patients receiving the two different regimens; moreover, a remarkably strong correlation between the response to ACE inhibition and AT1 receptor blockade is also observed for individual patients,[335] as shown in Figure 56-14. This correlation reflects the fact that blockade of the renin-angiotensin system is the main mechanism of the therapeutic efficacy of ACE inhibitors and AT1 receptor blockers. However, alternatively, it could indicate that responsiveness to antiproteinuric therapy is an individual characteristic—as supported by an analogous correlation with the antiproteinuric effect of NSAIDs.[335] Evidence for renal responsiveness as an individual characteristic is discussed in more detail later.

Specific *renin inhibition* reduces proteinuria. Although clinical use of this class of drugs has been hampered by their poor bioavailability, their antiproteinuric effect supports the assumption that blockade of the RAAS as such provides a mechanism for reduction of proteinuria.[336]

CCBs can reduce proteinuria, but distinct differences in renal effects are apparent between dihydropyridine CCBs (such as nifedipine, nicardipine, and nitrendipine) and non-dihydropyridine CCBs (such as verapamil and diltiazem). The latter were reported to reduce proteinuria in patients with NIDDM similar to ACE inhibitors[337] and better than β-blockers, thus supporting specific renal effects of this subclass of CCBs in this population.[338] Dihydropyridine CCBs, in contrast, are less effective in reducing proteinuria for a given reduction in blood pressure and can even lead to an increase in proteinuria.[339, 340] This effect is particularly apparent when no effective blood pressure control is obtained and may be due to the impairment in autoregulatory afferent vascular tone induced by this subclass of CCBs. Nonetheless, attenuation of albuminuria during long-term treatment with nifedipine, similar to ACE inhibition, has also been reported.[341] Data on the antiproteinuric effect of non-dihydropyridine CCBs have thus far largely been derived from studies in NIDDM, with the exception of a study in nondiabetic proteinuric patients, in which it was found that the reduction in proteinuria by verapamil (−12%) was significantly less than with trandolapril (−51%).[342] In this study, verapamil did not reduce blood pressure, thus suggesting that a reduction in blood pressure may be a prerequisite for the antiproteinuric effect of verapamil.

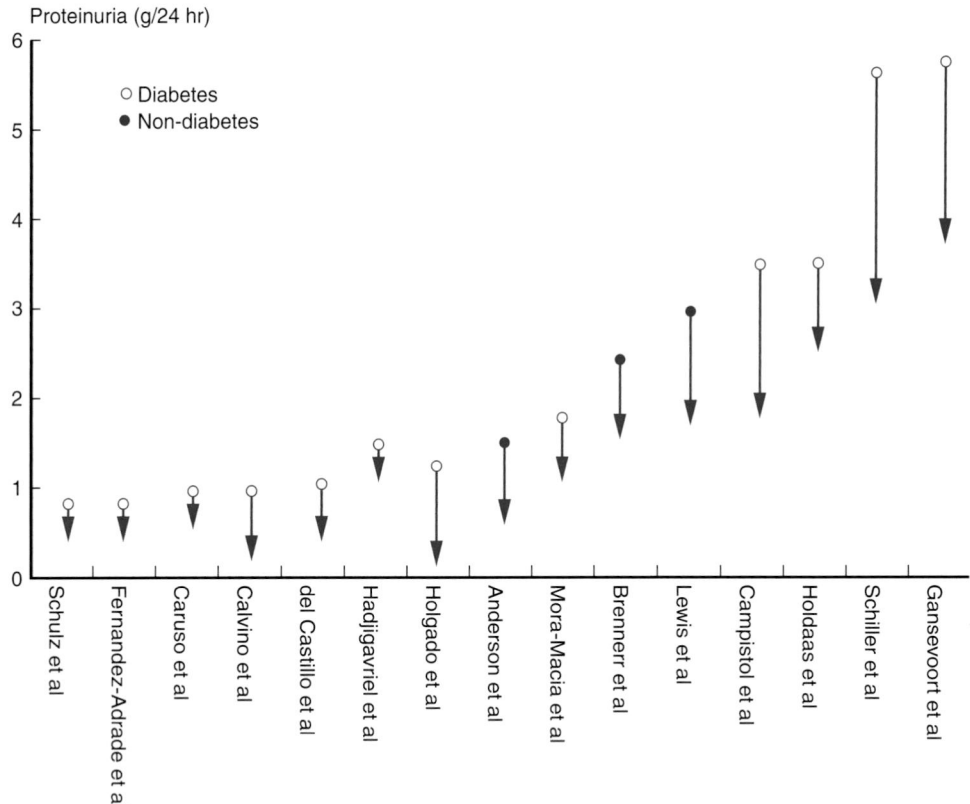

FIGURE 56-13. The antiproteinuric effect of AT1 receptor blockade in different studies involving diabetic and nondiabetic patients. The albuminuria data from Anderson and colleagues were converted to proteinuria by using the formula from the authors (prot = 1.4 × alb). The albumin/creatinine data from Brenner and associates were converting to proteinuria per 24 hours by using a formula from the authors (prot = 8.658 × [alb (mg)/creat (mg)] 0.793). (Adapted from de Zeeuw D, Navis GJ: Optimizing the RAAS intervention treatment strategy in diabetic and non-diabetic nephropathy: The potential of exploring the mechanisms of response variability. *In* Mogensen CE [ed]: Diabetic Nephropathy in Type 2 Diabetes. London, Science Press, 2002, pp 103-116.)

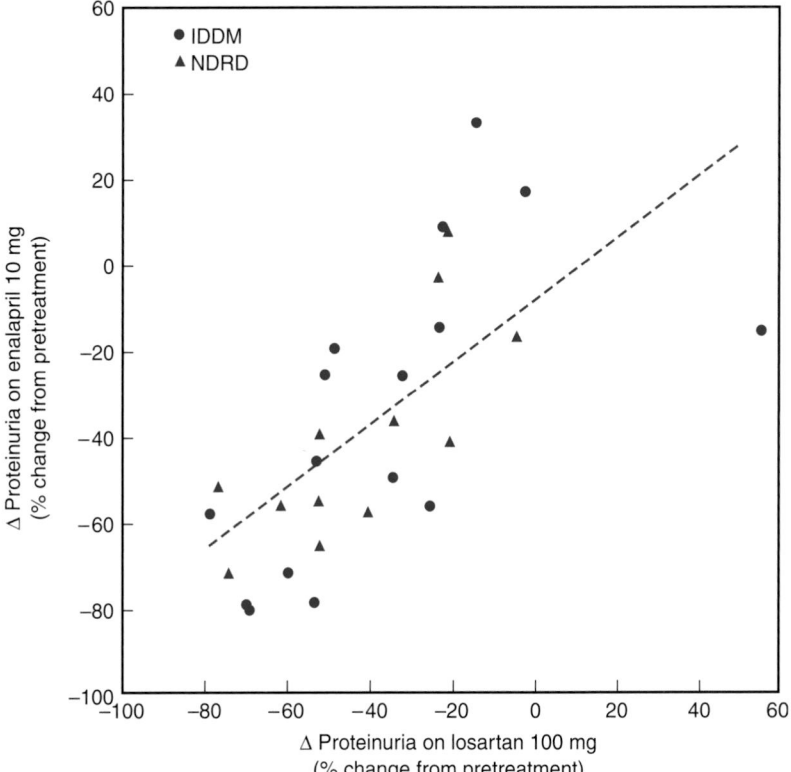

FIGURE 56-14. Antiproteinuric effect of the angiotensin-converting enzyme inhibitor enalapril and the AT1 receptor blocker losartan administered to the same patient. Close correlation is observed between the effect of the two interventions in the same patient, whether the proteinuria is due to nondiabetic renal disease (NDRD, *triangles*) or insulin-dependent diabetes mellitus (IDDM, *circles*). (Adapted with permission from Bos H, Andersen S, Rossing P, et al: The role of patient factors in therapy resistance to antiproteinuric intervention in non-diabetic and diabetic nephropathy. Kidney Int Suppl 75:32-37, 2000.)

The effect of *β-blockers* on proteinuria varies between different studies and tends to be small.[343-345] Pooled data from comparative studies indicate a slight reduction in proteinuria that appears to be related to the decrease in blood pressure achieved.[245, 316, 317]

Few controlled data on the effects of *diuretics* as monotherapy are available. One study reported a reduction in albuminuria with indapamide in patients with NIDDM,[346] but others did not find any effects with hydrochlorothiazide[347] and chlorthalidone.[348]

The number of controlled studies on the effect of *other antihypertensives* on proteinuria is very limited as well. No effect on proteinuria was found with α-methyldopa in overt proteinuria.[349] The α-blocker doxazosin was reported to reduce microalbuminuria in essential hypertensives.[350]

NSAIDs reduce proteinuria without affecting blood pressure. The antiproteinuric efficacy of different NSAIDs is proportional to their effect on renal prostaglandin production.[351] The reduction in proteinuria by NSAIDs is associated with a reduction in GFR that is presumed to reflect reduced glomerular hydrostatic pressure as a result of afferent vasoconstriction.

COMBINATION THERAPY. When combining agents with a different mechanism of action, an additive effect may be anticipated. In addition, pharmacologic treatment of proteinuria should be combined with dietary measures to obtain the full therapeutic benefit. Options for combination treatment to reduce proteinuria are discussed later.

Antihyperlipidemic Treatment

The dyslipidemia in renal patients is highly variable and may vary with the underlying renal disorder, in particular, the presence of proteinuria, as well as with previous abnormalities in the lipid profile. Therefore, an individual approach tailored to the specific lipid profile abnormalities has been advocated for renal patients. Similar to nonrenal patients, dietary intervention combined with specific pharmacologic therapy is the cornerstone of lipid correction. In proteinuric patients, moreover, symptomatic reduction of proteinuria exerts a lipid-lowering effect as well.

HMG-CoA reductase inhibitors effectively reduce total cholesterol, LDL-cholesterol, apo B, and triglycerides in renal patients with and without proteinuria. The effect on HDL-cholesterol appears to be highly variable between patients. As a result, the slight increase in HDL-cholesterol that is noted in several studies more often than not lacks statistical significance.[181, 182, 188, 352] Pooled data in a large meta-analysis nevertheless support improved HDL during statin therapy in renal patients.[353] The discrepancies regarding HDL may also be due to differential effects on HDL subtypes; for instance, Warwick and colleagues found unchanged total HDL and HDL3 associated with an increase in HDL2.[354] Lipoprotein (a) [Lp(a)] levels do not appear to be affected by HMG-CoA reductase inhibitors, neither in nonrenal patients[355] nor in patients with diabetic nephropathy.[356-358] On the whole, HMG-CoA reductase inhibitors seem to be better tolerated than other pharmacologic interventions.

Fibric acid derivatives appear to be the most effective agents for reducing triglyceride levels in renal patients. Their efficacy in reducing total cholesterol and LDL-cholesterol, however, seems to be limited.

The efficacy of bile sequestrants on total cholesterol and LDL-cholesterol is variable. Of note, these agents appear to increase triglyceride levels in proteinuric patients. The latter is in accord with findings in other populations and limits their use in patients with high triglyceride levels.

In nonrenal patients, the new nicotinic acid derivative acipimox was shown to be a useful adjunct to HMG-CoA reductase inhibition in that a combination of the two was shown to reduce Lp(a) levels.[359] The efficacy and safety of this combination in renal patients, however, have not been investigated.

Interestingly, symptomatic antiproteinuric treatment leads to improvement of the lipid profile of proteinuric patients.[360] The effect appears to be proportional to the efficacy of proteinuria reduction and is independent of the mode of reduction of proteinuria, as was observed with ACE inhibition,[361, 362, 363] AT1 receptor blockade,[364] and indomethacin therapy (Fig. 56-15).[365] Interestingly, reduction of proteinuria is also associated with a reduction in Lp(a) that is proportional to the reduction in proteinuria,[361, 366] which may be of prognostic relevance for the reduction in cardiovascular risk.

In patients with proteinuria caused by diabetic nephropathy, the hyperlipidemia may be related not only to the proteinuric state but also to metabolic abnormalities inherent in patients with impaired glucose tolerance, or it may be related to primary lipid abnormalities predisposing to the development of diabetic nephropathy. However, data on the effect of a reduction in proteinuria on lipids in diabetic patients are scarce. Hebert and co-workers found that remission of nephrotic-range proteinuria (from 5 to 0.9 g/day) in eight IDDM patients was associated with a reduction in total cholesterol whereas no effect on cholesterol occurred in patients (*n* = 95) in whom the proteinuria remained in the nephrotic range (*n* = 95; from 6.2 to 5.1 g/day).[367] In NIDDM patients, a reduction in proteinuria from 6.8 to 1.7 g/day, achieved by the combination of lisinopril and verapamil, resulted in a reduction in

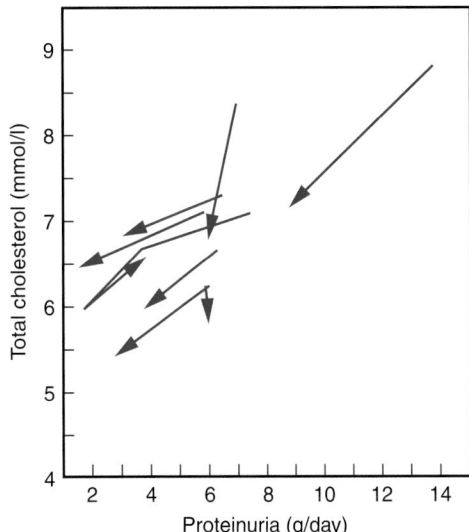

FIGURE 56-15. Relationship between reduction in proteinuria and reduction in total cholesterol (mean values per study) during antiproteinuric treatment in different studies. (Adapted from Navis GJ, Buter H, de Jong PE, et al: Effect of antiproteinuric treatment on the lipid profile in non-diabetic renal disease. Contrib Nephrol 120:88-96, 1997.)

total cholesterol from 7.6 to 6.5 mmol/L.[337] In this study the smaller reductions in proteinuria by monotherapy with lisinopril (to 2.5 g/day) or verapamil (to 2.9 g/day) did not alter total cholesterol. In NIDDM patients with albuminuria in the non-nephrotic range, ACE inhibition appears to reduce albuminuria without an effect on cholesterol,[368, 369] although a slight reduction in cholesterol has been reported in one study.[370] Taken together, the findings in diabetic patients seem to indicate that symptomatic reduction of proteinuria needs to be substantial to exert an effect on total cholesterol. However, in microalbuminuric IDDM, reduction of albuminuria by losartan was associated with a slight decrease in total cholesterol, very low density lipoprotein cholesterol, LDL-cholesterol, and apo-B levels, without any effect on Lp(a).[371] Clearly, more data are needed to better explore this issue. Moreover, the effect of a reduction in proteinuria on specific lipoproteins remains to be explored altogether.

RISK FACTOR PROFILE IN RENAL PATIENTS

Clustering of Renal Risk Factors

Renal risk factors can be identified in most renal patients, and several risk factors are often simultaneously present. In light of the evidence for synergism between different renal risk factors, this simultaneous presence has considerable clinical impact. Proteinuria in particular appears to cluster with hypertension, as well as with metabolic risk factors. An association between proteinuria, hypercholesterolemia, and hypertension is present in nondiabetic[139, 372] as well as diabetic nephropathy.[37] The mechanism underlying the clustering of hypertension and proteinuria is not entirely clear. Both hypertension and proteinuria may be related to the nature or the activity of the underlying renal disorder, but a causal interaction may be involved, such as aggravation of the proteinuria by the higher blood pressure or, the other way round, the pressor effect of proteinuria-associated sodium retention. The association between proteinuria and hypertension bears particular relevance because of the enhanced renal susceptibility to hypertensive renal damage in proteinuric patients. Furthermore, the clustering of proteinuria with hyperlipidemia may be important as well in view of the experimental evidence that hyperlipidemia is involved in renal damage, particularly in proteinuric kidneys.[151, 152]

Concordance of Renal and Cardiovascular Risk Factors

The main clinical and demographic factors associated with an increased renal risk are also well-established risk factors for cardiovascular morbidity and mortality. This concordance may reflect the similarity of the pathophysiologic pathways of progressive glomerulosclerosis and interstitial sclerosis with the process of atherosclerosis.[373]

Renal patients have a particularly high risk for cardiovascular morbidity and mortality, not only after the development of end-stage renal disease[374] but also early in the disease.[27] The increased risk is attributed, first, to risk factors also present in the nonrenal population, such as demographic factors, hypertension, hyperlipidemia, and smoking. In addition, factors specific for renal disorders are involved.

Proteinuria has been shown to be a particularly potent cardiovascular risk factor. Experimental and clinical data also suggest the involvement of many other factors, such as accumulation of uremic toxins, hyperhomocysteinemia, advanced glycosylation end products, and elevated fibrinogen, but their relative contribution still requires better delineation. A greater a priori cardiovascular susceptibility may also be involved, as suggested by the evidence for common genetic determinants of renal and cardiovascular target organ damage.[375] The grim clinical consequences of the dual risk associated with this risk factor profile were demonstrated for the diabetic population by Krolewski and associates.[170] Among 439 IDDM patients with nephropathy, rapid loss of renal function occurred in approximately a third of the patients. Strikingly, cardiovascular mortality in these progressors was twofold to threefold higher than in patients with stable or slowly deteriorating function. The concordance of cardiac and renal risk in IDDM is also supported by the predictive value of an abnormal electrocardiogram for deterioration in renal function.[172]

The impact of proteinuria as a cardiovascular risk factor is reflected by the fivefold to sixfold increased risk for myocardial infarction in nephrotic patients as opposed to the normal population.[376] The high prevalence of established cardiovascular risk factors in this population is likely to play an important role in this high cardiovascular risk. In a large population of nondiabetic nephrotic patients, at least one cardiovascular risk factor was present in 99% of the patients, with two risk factors in 68% and three risk factors present in 25%.[377] Hyperlipidemia is usually proportional to the severity of the proteinuria, with a particularly atherogenic lipid profile including an elevation of the highly atherogenic Lp(a).[378] Endothelial dysfunction may constitute an important pathway of the enhanced cardiovascular risk in proteinuria. Distinct impairment in endothelial function was found in proteinuric patients as opposed to nonproteinuric renal patients.[379] An interaction between hyperlipidemia and hypoalbuminemia may be involved because recent in vitro studies have found that albumin ameliorates the vasculotoxic effects of oxidized LDL.[380] Interestingly, a reduction in proteinuria by ACE inhibition was found to be associated with a reduction in von Willebrand factor, which may indicate reversibility of proteinuria-associated endothelial dysfunction.[381]

Glomerular protein leakage is a consistent predictor of cardiovascular mortality in the renal population, in IDDM[382] and NIDDM,[383, 384] in the general population,[385] in selected subgroups from the general population such as the MRFIT cohort,[386] and in patients with primary hypertension.[115] Remarkably, increased cardiovascular risk is present not only in overtly proteinuric individuals but also in microalbuminuric diabetic and nondiabetic subjects.[383, 387] This finding elicited the hypothesis that microalbuminuria is a marker of generalized endothelial dysfunction.[388] An unfavorable metabolic risk factor profile (albeit less prominent than in overt proteinuria) was reported in microalbuminuric essential hypertensive patients, thus demonstrating that clustering of cardiovascular risk factors is not limited to overt renal disease and nephrotic-range proteinuria.[389, 390] The predictive value of microalbuminuria for progressive renal damage in diabetic patients raises the intriguing possibility that microalbuminuria may be a renal risk factor in the nondiabetic population as well. Thus, it might serve to identify hypertensive patients with an increased risk for loss of renal function. This hypothesis was fueled by the presence of renal abnormalities—an abnormal renal vasoconstrictor response to high sodium intake—in microalbuminuric hypertensives,[343] which has been suggested to reflect a propensity to glomerular hypertension and progressive loss of renal function,[391] but the latter remains to be proved.

Feasibility of an Integrated Approach to Cardiorenal Protection

Specific renoprotection and reduction of the high cardiovascular risk are both important therapeutic targets that preferably require an integrated approach in the management of renal patients. In view of the concordance of risk factors for renal and cardiovascular risk, specific intervention in any of the renal risk factors may have the potential to reduce cardiovascular risk as well. Moreover, because both proteinuria and impaired renal function are powerful cardiovascular risk factors, it could be argued that effective renoprotection provides cardiovascular protection as well!

The feasibility of a single intervention to reduce a dual risk would be a major advantage in establishing an integrated approach for overall risk reduction. Data from the Heart Outcomes Prevention Evaluation (HOPE) and the MICRO-HOPE study, which showed a reduction in renal as well as cardiovascular risk with the use of ramipril in patients at high cardiovascular risk,[265] may prove to be a paradigmatic example of such an approach. It is important to realize, however, that the optimal regimens for reducing renal and cardiovascular risk may not be entirely similar with respect to the preferred class of drug, optimal dose, and optimal target blood pressure for risk reduction.

CLINICAL MANAGEMENT

A Framework for Renoprotective Intervention

Many pharmacologic agents useful for renoprotective interventions are currently available. To put these therapeutic options into effect for a fruitful strategy to prevent progressive renal disease, one must consider who should be treated, what the treatment aims are, what treatment should be given, how the treatment effect should be monitored, and how treatment should be adjusted when the therapeutic aims are not met. An overall framework for renoprotective intervention is outlined in Table 56-2. As noted previously, renal and

cardiovascular risk are closely intertwined, and most patients at risk for loss of renal function will eventually die of cardiovascular causes. Treatment aims should therefore also explicitly entail an overall reduction in cardiovascular risk. Results from recent trials have demonstrated that loss of renal function can be effectively retarded. To this end, however, aggressive and costly therapy is required and must be continued for years, if not lifelong. A risk factor–based approach may serve to properly identify patients likely to benefit from such aggressive treatment while alleviating the burden of treatment in those at low risk. An analysis of intervention in essential hypertension emphasizes that the reduction in risk achieved is largest in high-risk patients.[392] Stated the other way around, no risk, no risk reduction. This principle apparently applies to renoprotective intervention as well. Data from the MDRD trial[65] and the REIN study[129] and recent meta-analysis data[130] demonstrate that proteinuria—the principal determinant of renal risk—is also a main determinant of renoprotective benefit. Moreover, improvement in the rate of loss of renal function by antihypertensive treatment directly correlates with the rate of renal function loss before intervention, with a larger treatment benefit observed in patients with rapid loss of renal function before intervention.[393]

Primary Prevention

Because renal disease often has an insidious and asymptomatic course, many renal patients come to medical attention late in the course of the disease, which would suggest that for renal disease, primary prevention is impracticable. However, the two main causes of end-stage renal failure are hypertension and diabetes. In these populations, primary prevention of renal function loss appears to be feasible.

PRIMARY PREVENTION OF RENAL FUNCTION LOSS IN HYPERTENSION

Because of its high prevalence, hypertension is a main cause of renal failure, but in only a minority of the hypertensive population will renal failure eventually develop. Risk factors for loss of renal function in hypertensive patients are summarized in Table 56-3. The main preventive measure is effective blood pressure reduction.[309] It has been noted that formal evidence for improvement in overall mortality has been obtained only for β-blockade and diuretics, but more recent data have shown low mortality with ACE inhibitors and CCBs as well.[394] ACE inhibition was more effective than CCBs in proteinuric African Americans with hypertensive nephropathy,[64] but at present, no data are available to

---

TABLE 56-2

A Framework for Renoprotective Intervention

Identify patients at risk for renal function loss
Establish individual overall risk profile
Intervention: pharmacologic and nonpharmacologic measures for overall risk reduction
Monitor therapeutic efficacy: blood pressure and proteinuria
Optimize therapy
If therapy resistant, consider causes and re-evaluate treatments.

TABLE 56-3

Risk Factors for Renal Function Loss in Hypertensive patients

Proteinuria/albuminuria
Elevated serum creatinine
Impaired glucose tolerance
Hyperuricemia
Urinary tract problems
Hyperlipidemia
Genetic factors

substantiate a specific renal advantage of any particular class of antihypertensive agents for hypertensive patients in the absence of overt renal disease or proteinuria (or both).[395] Accordingly, in uncomplicated hypertension, ACE inhibitors, CCBs, diuretics, α-blockers, and AT1 receptor blockers may be used as a first line of therapy. The preferred choice of drug for the individual patient can thus be guided by specific indications and contraindications as a result of comorbid conditions such as coronary artery disease, heart failure, peripheral vascular disease, gout, and chronic obstructive pulmonary disease.

No conclusive data are available to decide whether the target blood pressure should be similar for a reduction in renal, cardiovascular, and cerebrovascular risk. Systolic blood pressure less than 140 mm Hg has been recommended to prevent loss of renal function in essential hypertension.[396] In the hypertensive population, microalbuminuria is a marker of increased cardiovascular risk[341] and thus can serve to identify patients who will benefit from intensive blood pressure control supplemented by specific intervention for additional risk factors such as hyperlipidemia. It is reasonable to assume that this strategy may also apply to renoprotective benefit, but this issue awaits the results of ongoing research.

PRIMARY PREVENTION IN DIABETES

Increasing evidence supports the efficacy of primary measures for preventing or postponing diabetic nephropathy. In IDDM, both improved glycemic control[8] and aggressive blood pressure control have clearly been shown to be effective in primary prevention.[397] Recent studies have demonstrated that primary prevention is feasible in NIDDM as well: antihypertensive treatment with ACE inhibitors provides primary prevention of nephropathy,[68] intensified glycemic control appears to be effective in the prevention of nephropathy,[398] and finally, treatment with the AT1 receptor blocker irbesartan dose-dependently prevented progression from microalbuminuria to overt albuminuria.[280]

In the natural history of diabetes, the onset of overt nephropathy is preceded by the appearance of low levels of albumin in urine accompanied by a slight rise in blood pressure within the so-called normotensive range, as discussed in detail in Chapter 38 of this volume. The presence of microalbuminuria, defined as an excretion rate of 30 to 300 mg/day or 20 to 200 μg/min, is a strong predictor of subsequent progression to overt nephropathy[399-402] in IDDM. The different definitions of microalbuminuria, screening procedures, confounding factors, and confirmatory procedures have been reviewed elsewhere.[74] In spite of such differences, microalbuminuria stands out as an initial prognostic sign that should guide the start and subsequent monitoring of renoprotective intervention therapy.[74, 403]

Accordingly, the first step in primary prevention of nephropathy in diabetic patients is screening for microalbuminuria on a yearly basis,[74, 403, 404] although more frequent screening has also been advocated.[405] Because microalbuminuria seldom develops in IDDM of short duration, screening should start 5 years after diagnosis. For children, screening can be postponed until after puberty. In NIDDM, a larger proportion of patients may have microalbuminuria at the time of diagnosis or shortly thereafter; thus, screening of patients with NIDDM should start at the time of diagnosis.

In addition, blood pressure should be monitored at least annually in IDDM and NIDDM. A blood pressure of 140/90 or higher in subjects younger than 60 years or 160/90 in those older than 60 years should prompt the institution of antihypertensive treatment with a target pressure under 130/85 mm Hg.

It is agreed by now that pharmacologic intervention should start when the presence of microalbuminuria has been established,[74, 404] irrespective of blood pressure.[246] Based on the evidence available, ACE inhibitors can be recommended as first-choice agents in IDDM and AT1 receptor blockers in NIDDM. Whether one of these classes has a specific advantage over the other is uncertain, but it is unlikely that comparative studies will become available. It should be recollected that in NIDDM—with similar rigorous blood pressure control—regimens based on β-blockers and ACE inhibitors provided a similar reduction in renal and cardiovascular risk, thus suggesting that class differences become less relevant during strict blood pressure control.[308] In IDDM as well, the importance of rigorous blood pressure control, rather than class-specific drug properties, has been emphasized.[406] Monitoring of therapy should entail monitoring of microalbuminuria as well as blood pressure, with a goal of stabilization and eventually reduction of microalbuminuria and a blood pressure less than 120 to 130/80 to 85 mm Hg.[75] If the response to therapy is insufficient, a diuretic should be added. Whether primary prevention should extend to normotensive, normoalbuminuric patients is not well established. Although ACE inhibitors exerted a beneficial effect on albuminuria and a decline in GFR in a population of relatively young and lean normotensive, normoalbuminuric NIDDM patients,[68] it is not clear whether these results similarly apply to the typical obese elderly NIDDM patient. In normotensive normoalbuminuric IDDM, ACE inhibitors reduce albuminuria.[407] However, the prognostic significance of normoalbuminuria is unknown, and data on the effect of a decline in renal function are awaited.[408]

Adjunctive therapy should entail strict glycemic control. Whether restriction of dietary protein will contribute to prevention of nephropathy in microalbuminuric diabetics has not been established. Primary prevention should also address overall cardiovascular risk, in particular in NIDDM.

Secondary Prevention

In patients with established renal disease, primary causal factors for ongoing renal damage, if present, should first be eliminated as effectively as possible. Such factors include obstructive uropathy, urinary tract infections and analgesic abuse, and poor glycemic control in diabetic patients.

In established renal disease, the renal benefit of rigorous blood pressure control is supported by many studies. Reduction of blood pressure to below 130/80 mm Hg has been recommended for renal patients.[75] Based on observational studies, a similar low blood pressure level has been recommended for patients with diabetic nephropathy.[74, 397, 403] For proteinuric patients, the target blood pressure should be even lower. In patients with proteinuria greater than 1 g/day, additional renal benefit is obtained by blood pressure reduction to 135/80 mm Hg, and for proteinuria over 3 g/day, additional benefit is obtained by blood pressure reduction to 125/75 mm Hg. Achievement of such low blood pressure levels in renal patients was shown to be feasible as well as safe.[409]

The MDRD data highlight the importance of proteinuria as a renal risk factor that should guide therapy. Even if blood pressure is in the so-called normotensive range, the presence of proteinuria should prompt the institution of therapy. In light of the consistent predictive value of a reduction in proteinuria for subsequent renoprotection, not only a reduction in blood pressure but also a reduction in proteinuria should be a main target of renoprotective intervention. Consequently, proteinuria as well as blood pressure should be monitored as discussed in the next section.

Whereas any of the currently available antihypertensives may reduce blood pressure in renal patients, the proven renoprotective efficacy of ACE inhibitors renders them first-choice agents in patients at high risk for deterioration of renal function, such as nondiabetic patients with overt proteinuria and patients with diabetic nephropathy. In NIDDM, the renoprotective efficacy of AT1 blockers has now been established, and thus AT1 blockers are first-choice drugs. In patients without proteinuria, notably those with polycystic kidneys and tubulointerstitial disease, other classes of drugs, such as β-blockers and CCBs, may also be used as first-line drugs. Cardiovascular comorbidity can provide additional considerations. Impaired sodium excretion with volume overload is common in renal patients. Accordingly, for optimal blood pressure control in renal patients, correction of volume status by dietary sodium restriction or diuretics, or both, is crucial, as discussed in the next section. Although diuretics are often required as adjunctive therapy in renal patients, their renoprotective efficacy has not been well established.[41, 395]

In addition to dietary sodium restriction, adjunctive therapy in subjects with overt proteinuria should preferably entail dietary protein restriction. Even though conflicting study outcomes have generated controversy on the benefit of protein restriction, a large meta-analysis supports the renoprotective benefit of protein restriction in nondiabetic as well as diabetic subjects.[410] In this respect it should be noted that post hoc analysis of the MDRD study showed that adherence to the diet was a determinant of the renoprotective benefit.[411] In proteinuric patients, moreover, dietary protein restriction optimizes the antiproteinuric effect of ACE inhibition.

Additional measures in renal patients should entail control of prevalent cardiorenal risk factors. The main measures are discontinuation of smoking and control of hyperlipidemia. In proteinuric patients, reduction of proteinuria—by pharmacologic intervention supplemented by restriction of dietary protein and cholesterol—is a prerequisite for improvement of the lipoprotein profile, including a reduction in Lp(a). Nonetheless, specific antihyperlipidemic therapy is required in many renal patients. HMG-CoA reductase inhibitors are effective for this purpose and may be combined with fibric acid derivates in patients with high triglycerides. The combination of HMG-CoA reductase inhibitors and newer nicotinic acid derivatives yielded promising results in nonrenal patients by reducing Lp(a), but data in renal patients are not yet available.

Monitoring of Renoprotective Therapy

Usually, chronic loss of renal function is a gradual process that takes years or decades to lead to end-stage renal failure. This gradual deterioration in renal function has implications for monitoring the efficacy of renoprotective interventions. The limitations of creatinine-based monitoring of renal function are well known.[412] Data from the MDRD study, in which it was demonstrated that tubule creatinine secretion is affected by the diagnosis, class of antihypertensive drug, and diet, underline the importance of accurate GFR measurements by clearance of specific tracers.[413] Even with specific tracers, however, the intratest variability in GFR measurement is considerable,[414] and large study populations or prolonged follow-up, or both, are needed. Reduction of the intratest and intertest coefficient of variation for GFR, by correcting for voiding errors, can substantially reduce the error of the slope of decline in GFR.[415] Frequent measurements can further improve the accuracy of GFR slope calculations, thus alleviating the need for large populations in clinical trials.

A slight reduction in GFR at the onset of antihypertensive therapy predicts better long-term renoprotection.[98, 99] This drop presumably reflects functional hemodynamic changes—such as a drop in glomerular capillary pressure—that are favorable in the long run. Data from the MDRD trial showed the onset of dietary protein restriction to be associated with a slight initial drop in GFR as well. In clinical trials, therefore, comparison of GFR slopes should preferably be based on the GFR slope at completion of the titration phase of the renoprotective regimen. For individual patients, the implication is that a drop in GFR at the onset of treatment is a favorable prognostic sign, provided that it is relatively modest and not progressive. However, when the drop in GFR is substantial or the clinical condition is compatible with renal artery stenosis, it is important to exclude renal artery stenosis, especially when the treatment includes ACE inhibition or AT1 receptor blockade.

In individual patients, even with sophisticated and frequent measurements, the rate of decline in GFR is usually too slow to monitor and titrate renoprotective therapy. Titration based on intermediate parameters predicting future loss of renal function provides a feasible alternative. Whereas blood pressure should obviously be monitored, proteinuria (or albuminuria) is the best predictor of future loss of renal function[416] and thus reflects the renoprotective efficacy of the regimen. Proteinuria can therefore guide adjustment of therapy. Accordingly, it can be inferred that titration for reduction of proteinuria will allow better long-term renoprotection, but thus far no controlled studies are available on this issue.

Optimizing Response to Therapy

Despite recent advances, chronic renal disease is still essentially a progressive condition, as reflected by the increasing number of patients entering dialysis programs. For better prevention of end-stage renal failure, several strategies are needed, including early identification of patients at risk for progressive loss of renal function, monitoring of the response to therapy, and optimization of renoprotective intervention by an integrated regimen of pharmacologic and nonpharmacologic measures.

As outlined earlier, it is of great clinical importance that the long-term renoprotective efficacy of an intervention can be predicted from its effects on proteinuria and blood

TABLE 56-4

Circumvention of Treatment Resistance in Renoprotective Intervention

General measures	Check and, if necessary, improve compliance
Dietary measures	Restrict dietary sodium to 50 mEq/day
	Restrict dietary protein in proteinuric patients
Pharmacologic measures	Consider dose-response evaluation for proteinuria separately
	Add a diuretic
	Add another antihypertensive/consider dual RAAS blockade
	Add indomethacin*

*Only when close clinical and laboratory monitoring is feasible.
RAAS, renin-angiotensin-alderosterone system.

pressure—which allows proper adjustment of therapy. Several dietary and pharmacologic measures are available for that purpose and can (and usually need to) be applied simultaneously. A stepped approach to optimize the response to therapy is summarized in Table 56-4.

Sodium Status

The disturbed sodium and volume homeostasis in most renal patients leads to expanded extracellular volume and hypertension—effects particularly prominent in advanced renal failure[417] and proteinuric patients. In specific patient categories such as African Americans and microalbuminuric diabetic patients, impaired sodium handling may be an early phenomenon.[389, 418] Blood pressure is often sodium sensitive in renal patients, and correction of volume expansion by sodium restriction or diuretic therapy, or both, is often required to obtain effective blood pressure control. Sodium overload is associated not only with higher blood pressure but also with specific renal effects. In experimental renal disease,

sodium overload induces glomerular hypertrophy by hemodynamic as well as direct, nonhemodynamic growth-promoting effects.[419, 420] In patients with hypertension, high sodium intake is associated with increased glomerular protein leakage[421] and, in susceptible individuals, with renal vasoconstriction and an elevated filtration fraction.[389, 422]

Sodium status is a main determinant of the efficacy of antihypertensive therapy. The role of volume factors in resistance to treatment with older antihypertensives (which tended to induce sodium retention) is well established. However, also for newer classes of drugs that do not induce sodium retention themselves, volume status affects the response to therapy. This dependence of response on volume status applies particularly to all RAAS-blocking drugs: ACE inhibitors,[423] AT1 receptor blockers,[424] and renin inhibitors.[425] Sodium restriction enhances the effects of ACE inhibition on blood pressure, renal hemodynamics, and proteinuria. It increases the top of the dose-response curve; specifically, a more pronounced maximal response can be obtained during sodium depletion.[143, 426] An increase in sodium intake from 50 to 200 mEq/day annihilated the antiproteinuric effect of ACE inhibition almost completely, with less prominent blunting of the blood pressure response.[349] Cross-sectional data demonstrating a correlation between the antiproteinuric efficacy of ACE inhibition and urinary sodium excretion in nondiabetic as well as diabetic nephropathy support these intervention data.[427] Blunting of the therapeutic effect of ACE inhibition during liberal sodium intake could be overcome by addition of the diuretic hydrochlorothiazide (Fig. 56-16).[313] The effect of sodium status on antiproteinuric efficacy may be partly related to its concomitant effects on blood pressure, but the intrarenal effects of sodium status may be important as well, as suggested by the prominent effect of sodium restriction on proteinuria in contrast to its relatively modest effect on blood pressure.

For CCBs, the interaction with sodium status appears to be more heterogeneous. In essential hypertension, CCBs were found to be less effective during a low-sodium diet.[428, 429]

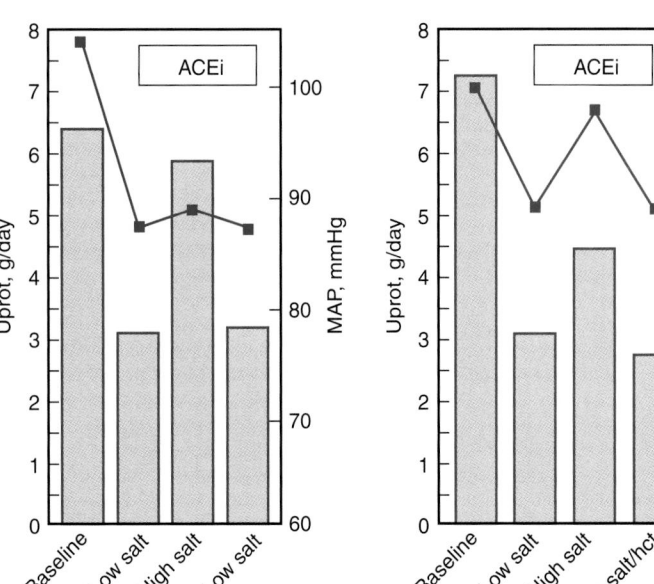

FIGURE 56-16. Effect of sodium status on the response of proteinuria *(bars)* and blood pressure (mean arterial pressure [MAP], *lines*) to angiotensin-converting enzyme (ACE) inhibition. The *left panel* shows the effect of ACE inhibition in comparison to pretreatment values during a low- and high-salt diet, with almost complete blunting of the antiproteinuric effect noted during the high-salt diet. The *right panel* shows the effect of a shift from low to high salt intake during chronic ACE inhibition, with the subsequent addition of hydrochlorothiazide (hct). (Adapted from Heeg JE, de Jong PE, van der Hem GK, de Zeeuw D: Reduction of proteinuria by angiotensin converting enzyme inhibition. Kidney Int 32:78-83, 1987; and Buter H, Hemmelder MH, Navis GJ, et al: Blunting of the antiproteinuric efficacy of ACE inhibition by high sodium intake can be restored by hydrochlorothiazide. Nephrol Dial Transplant 13:1682-1685, 1998.)

However, this finding may not apply similarly to renal patients. Sodium restriction was found to be required for an optimal antiproteinuric response to the non-dihydropyridine agent diltiazem (but not for nifedipine)[427, 430] in NIDDM. Accordingly, sodium restriction may be a specific renal intervention because high sodium intake blunted the antiproteinuric effect without affecting blood pressure.

It is not completely clear whether the renoprotective effect of correction of sodium status by diuretics is equivalent to dietary sodium restriction. Animal data suggest that sodium restriction exerts more effective renoprotection than diuretic therapy does,[313] but similar data in humans are lacking.

Protein Intake

The renoprotective potential of dietary protein restriction has been extensively evaluated in experimental animals and humans, as reviewed in Chapter 43. In addition, protein intake can modulate the antiproteinuric effect of ACE inhibition. A rise in protein intake from 0.3 to 1 g/kg/day in enalapril-treated patients led to a rise in proteinuria from 1.7 to 3 g/day.[431] In patients with moderately severe proteinuria (pretreatment value of 7.4 g/day), restriction of protein intake from a calculated value of 1.31 to 0.81 g/kg/day reduced proteinuria to 6.3 g/day, with a further reduction to 3.4 g/day after the addition of lisinopril.[363] In severe proteinuria, institution of protein restriction during lisinopril therapy resulted in a reduction in calculated intake from 1.3 to 0.87 g/kg/day with a reduction in proteinuria from 8.8 to 5.9 g/day. Thus, the effects of ACE inhibition and dietary protein restriction appear to be additive regarding a reduction in proteinuria. No additive effects were observed for blood pressure and renal hemodynamics.

Dose Titration for Proteinuria

In view of the importance of proteinuria, it may be surprising that few data are available on dose-response curves for proteinuria with the use of ACE inhibitors or AT1 receptor blockers. Usually, doses are based on dose-response data for blood pressure. Nonetheless, the dose-response curves for blood pressure and proteinuria are not necessarily similar. Nonhypotensive doses of an ACE inhibitor can reduce proteinuria,[432, 144] and a progressive antiproteinuric effect with doses of lisinopril of up to 20 mg/day was found in normotensive subjects with IgA nephropathy in whom the maximal reduction in blood pressure was already achieved at 5 mg/day.[433] Because a reduction in proteinuria is an independent treatment target, these data prompt study of the antiproteinuric potential of doses of ACE inhibitors higher than needed for maximal blood pressure reduction or for achieving recommended target blood pressure values.

Laverman and co-authors reported a progressive reduction in proteinuria with increasing doses of lisinopril of 10, 20, and 40 mg/day in subjects with nondiabetic nephropathy.[434] Because no plateau phase was observed for the antiproteinuric response, it was suggested that a further dose increase might result in a further reduction in proteinuria. Studies addressing this issue are currently under way. With regard to AT1 receptor blockade, the optimal antiproteinuric effect of losartan was obtained at a higher dose than needed for the maximal blood pressure response in nondiabetic as well as

diabetic nephropathy.[435, 334] An uncontrolled study with candesartan found that increasing the dose up to 96 (!) mg was associated with a progressive reduction in proteinuria independent of blood pressure control.[436] These data again indicate that the responses of blood pressure and proteinuria are not always concordant. A common trend across these studies seems to be that in subjects with normal blood pressure, an antiproteinuric effect can be obtained with doses that do not or only slightly affect blood pressure.

For a balanced view of the renoprotective potential of supramaximal doses of ACE inhibitors or AT1 receptor blockers, further studies in different populations are needed, as well as research on the issue of tolerability. The benefits of high-dose ACE inhibitor or AT1 receptor blocker monotherapy should also be weighed against those of dual blockade of the RAAS (see the next section). For the moment, controlled studies to support specific dose recommendations for long-term renoprotection are lacking. However, the treatment targets—blood pressure control *plus* optimal reduction of proteinuria—should guide titration of therapy. If proteinuria persists despite good blood pressure control, increasing the dose is worth a try, although it may not be invariably effective.[437]

Combination Therapy

Combinations of drugs with different mechanisms of action can exert additive effects. Many renal patients require a combination of different antihypertensives for effective blood pressure control.[75] With regard to renal protection, several combinations are of specific interest as judged by their effect on intermediate renal parameters. First, as noted earlier, during ACE inhibition, cotreatment with diuretics can overcome the effects of high sodium intake on blood pressure and proteinuria. Next, the combination of ACE inhibition and the NSAID indomethacin exerts an additive effect on proteinuria without affecting blood pressure.[365] A similar additive effect was found for AT1 receptor blockade and indomethacin.[438] Thus, combination therapy provides a way to overcome resistance to antiproteinuric efficacy. Monitoring of renal function and serum potassium is warranted when using this combination[439] because it can result in a substantial fall in the GFR. The reduction in GFR correlates with a further reduction in proteinuria and is presumably due to functional reduction of filtration pressure because it is reversible after withdrawal of indomethacin. RAAS blockade combined with an NSAID can also result in pronounced hyperkalemia because of the combined effects of a drop in GFR and decreased aldosterone as a result of the RAAS blockade and the direct tubule effects of indomethacin; such hyperkalemia may prompt dietary potassium restriction or treatment with resin exchangers. Finally, the sodium-retaining effects of indomethacin warrant control of sodium status because sodium retention may offset the beneficial effects. Thus, this combination should be used only by experienced practitioners. Whether selective cyclooxygenase-2 inhibitors will turn out to have a similar profile remains to be established.

Experimental data support an additive renoprotective effect of ACE inhibitors and non-dihydropyridine CCBs.[440] In patients with NIDDM, an additive effect of ACE inhibition and verapamil was reported.[337] In nondiabetic patients, the antiproteinuric effect of the combination of a 2-mg dose of trandolapril with verapamil equaled the effect of 4-mg of trandolapril, which may indicate an additive effect as well.[342]

In light of the different levels of RAAS blockade, a case may be made for combining ACE inhibitors with other RAAS blockers, such as AT1 receptor blockers[441, 442] and renin inhibitors.[443] In renal populations, several studies thus far have reported that combined therapy with an ACE inhibitor and an AT1 receptor blocker exerts a more effective antiproteinuric response than either does as monotherapy in diabetic as well as nondiabetic nephropathy.[434, 444-446] However, a study in primarily black diabetic patients found no added effect of losartan, 50 mg, combined with lisinopril, 40 mg.[447] Dose considerations may be relevant. In studies reporting an added effect of dual blockade, the doses used were deliberately chosen to be submaximal—with the rationale of possibly inducing fewer side effects than with the drugs used separately. Thus, the efficacy of dual blockade could be due to more effective RAAS blockade as such; however, efficacy might also have been achieved with a higher dose of either drug. For the purpose of maximal reduction in proteinuria, it would also be relevant to assess whether dual blockade, at optimal doses of both drugs, would result in a further reduction in proteinuria. Studies of Agarwal[447] and Laverman and colleagues[434] considered the dose issue and showed that adding a relatively low dose of losartan to an adequate dose of lisinopril (40 mg) does not result in enhanced efficacy, as shown in Figure 56-17. On the other hand, adding lisinopril to an optimal antiproteinuric dose of losartan further reduced proteinuria. All in all, the available data suggest an enhanced potential of dual blockade over monotherapy, but

this additive effect may not apply to all conditions. Optimal dosing schedules, also in relation to other optimizing measures such as volume control, will have to be developed further.

Finally, it would be relevant whether dual RAAS blockade might improve the response to therapy in individuals resistant to monotherapy. Thus far, no human studies have addressed this issue, but recent animal data show that resistance to ACE inhibition is not circumvented by combined therapy at adequate doses or by supramaximal doses of ACE inhibitors.[448] This finding suggests that the potential of rigorous blockade of the renin-angiotensin system to overcome resistance to therapy is limited and that multidrug regimens, with combined intervention in different pathways of renal damage, should be explored to further improve renoprotection. In this respect, animal data suggest a role for combination with statins,[449] mycophenolate mofetil,[450] or adrenergic blockade, but thus far no data are available in humans.

Time Course

In nondiabetic patients, the reduction in proteinuria takes several weeks to achieve a maximum, which should be taken into account when titrating for optimal reduction of proteinuria. In microalbuminuric IDDM, on the other hand, the time course of reduction in albuminuria parallels the reduction in blood pressure, with maximal responses already taking place in the first week of treatment,[451] which may reflect the greater renal impact of blood pressure in these patients. The lack of similar data on other antihypertensives or on diabetics with overt nephropathy for the moment precludes recommendation of

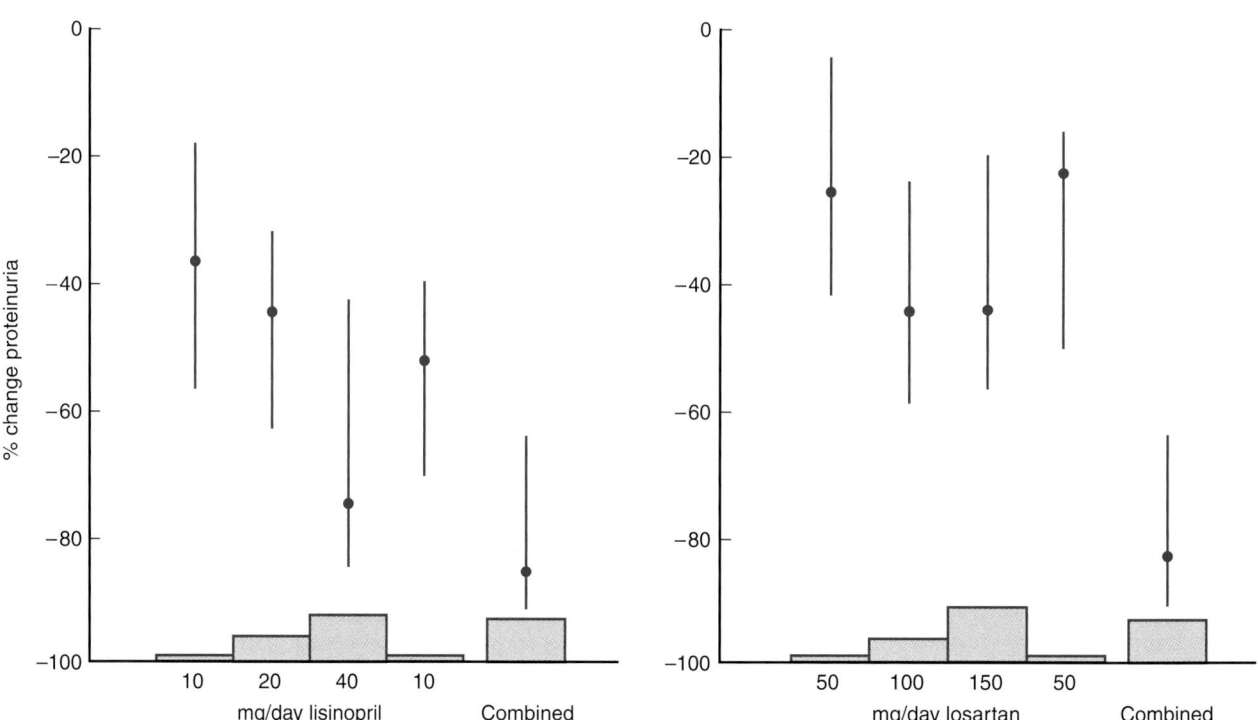

FIGURE 56-17. Antiproteinuric effect of increasing doses of lisinopril followed by dual renin-angiotensin-aldosterone system (RAAS) blockade by adding losartan to the maximally effective dose of lisinopril *(left panel),* as well as increasing doses of losartan followed by combined therapy with lisinopril added to the maximally effective dose of losartan. (Adapted with permission from Laverman GD, Navis GJ, Henning RH, et al: Dual renin-angiotensin system blockade at optimal doses for proteinuria. Kidney Int 62:1020-1025, 2002.)

a fixed schedule for the time course of titration. The diurnal pattern of response to therapy also shows dissociation between reduction of blood pressure and proteinuria. Whereas chronic treatment with either the long-acting ACE inhibitor trandolapril or the renin inhibitor remikiren exerted effective blood pressure control for 24 hours, proteinuria was reduced only during the daytime (Fig. 56-18).[452] The mechanism underlying nocturnal resistance to a reduction in proteinuria and its impact on the long-term renal prognosis are not yet clear. Its occurrence during treatment with long-acting agents suggests a pharmacodynamic rather than a pharmacokinetic interaction. Interestingly, preliminary data suggest that an alternative dosing schedule consisting of dosing in the evening results in improved antiproteinuric efficacy, but these data still await further confirmation.

Individual Patient Factors in Response to Therapy: New Perspective to Improve Renoprotection?

For improvement of the response to therapy, thus far we have focused on options proven to be effective at the group level. However, for almost any intervention, within-group differences in response by far exceed the differences between the treatment groups, be it different classes of drugs, different doses or diet, or combinations of these factors. Thus, even for interventions providing evidence-based renoprotection at the group level, therapeutic efficacy is insufficient in a substantial proportion of patients. A focus on the mechanisms underlying individual differences in response may therefore allow new perspectives to improve therapeutic efficacy in poor responders.

Studies of essential hypertension in which different interventions were used in individual patients have shown that the blood pressure response to different classes of antihypertensive agents is individually determined.[453] Renal responsiveness to antihypertensive therapy is individually determined as well. For ACE inhibition as well as AT1 receptor blockade, the renal vasodilator response varies greatly between patients. Studying the same patient twice under different conditions reveals the individual pattern of responsiveness,[454] as shown in Figure 56-18. The left panel, which depicts the renal response to ACE inhibition during low and liberal sodium intake in essential hypertension,[455] shows that potentiation of the response by a low-sodium diet does not affect the ranking of patients. Data on IDDM patients (right panel) show that shifting from ACE inhibition to AT1 blockade does not alter the individual ranking either.[456] Thus, the range of responses is large, and neither potentiation of the response by low sodium intake nor shift to another class of RAAS blockade makes poor responders catch up with good responders (Fig. 56-19). Importantly, individual responsiveness is a main factor in the renoprotective efficacy of antiproteinuric intervention as well, as shown earlier (see Fig. 56-14).[335] Whereas both ACE inhibition and AT1 blockade are effective at the group level, individual responses range from an almost complete reduction in proteinuria to absence of a response. Importantly, neither the switch from ACE inhibition to AT1 receptor blockade nor doubling of the doses could make poor responders catch up with good responders. Moreover, measures that significantly improved antiproteinuric responses at the group level (i.e., protein restriction and diuretic therapy) did not make poor responders catch up either, as reviewed elsewhere (Fig. 56-20).[457]

Thus, because individual factors are the main determinants of the response to renoprotective intervention, exploration of the mechanisms underlying individual differences in response should be undertaken. Disease-specific factors may be relevant, as suggested by the lack of benefit of ACE inhibitors in polycystic kidney disease[65, 127] and tubulointerstitial disease[127]; however, large differences in response occur between patients with the same renal condition that cannot be accounted for by the type of renal disease. The extent of pretreatment renal damage is likely to be involved, as suggested by retrospective data in transplant recipients[144] and prospective data in animal studies.[145] If prospectively confirmed in humans, such findings would prompt the institution of treatment as early as possible! Race[458] as well as nonethnic genetic factors are relevant to the response to therapy. Familial factors (thus far unidentified) appear to modulate the blood pressure response to ACE inhibition in hypertension.[459] Genetic polymorphisms can affect the response to therapy as well, as discussed earlier,[224, 225] so better identification of genetic determinants of the response to therapy may in the future have an impact on the preferred choice of therapy by allowing earlier identification of

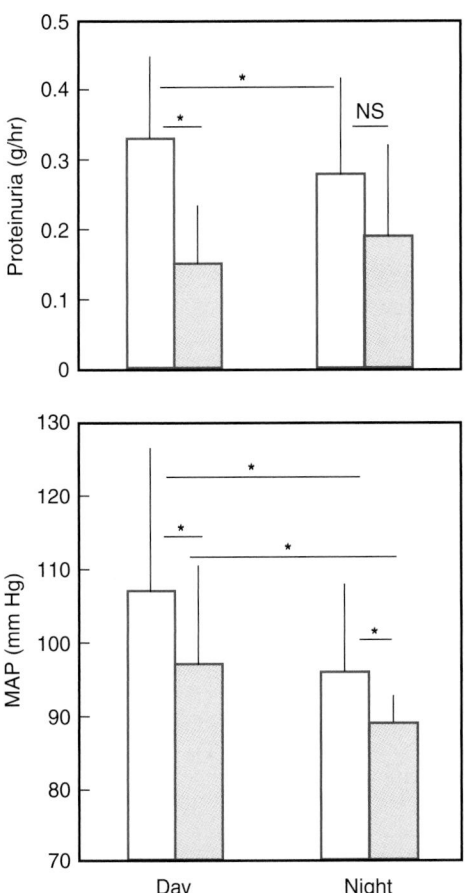

FIGURE 56-18. Daytime and nighttime values for proteinuria *(upper panel)* and mean arterial pressure (MAP, *lower panel*) during placebo *(open bars)* and trandolapril *(blue bars)* treatment. (from Buter H, Hemmelder M, van Paassen P, et al: Is the reduction of proteinuria by RAAS blockade less effective during the night? Nephrol Dial Transplant 12[suppl 2]: 53-56, 1997.)

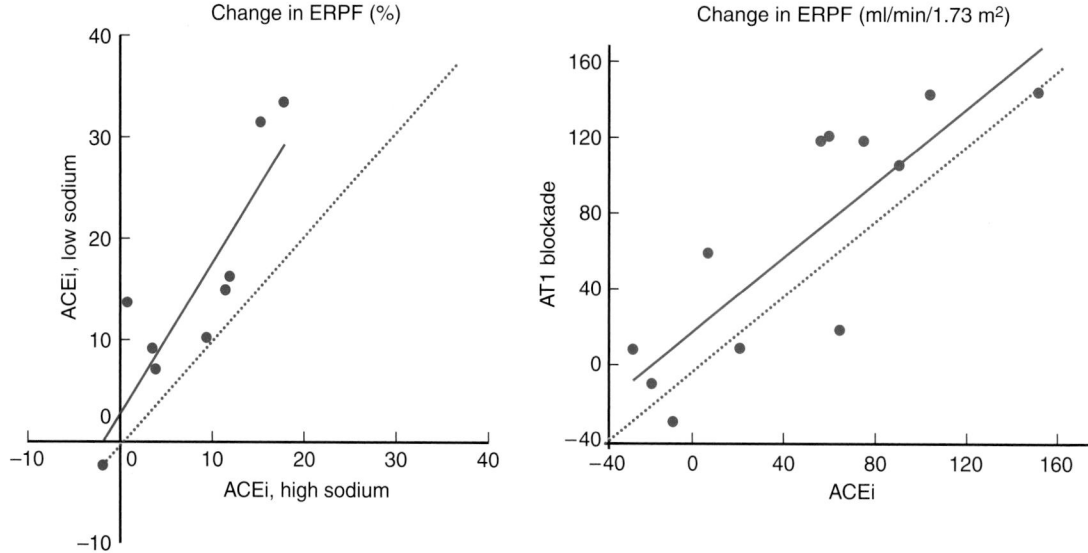

FIGURE 56-19. Individual responses of effective renal plasma flow (ERPF) to blockade of the renin-angiotensin-aldosterone system (RAAS) in essential hypertension *(left panel)* and insulin-dependent diabetes mellitus (IDDM) *(right panel)*. Regression lines *(continuous)* and lines of identity *(dotted)* are also given. The data show that between-patient differences persist when the patient is studied a second time, irrespective of whether the other intervention leaves the overall magnitude of the response unchanged *(right panel)* or when the overall response is potentiated *(left panel)*. (Adapted from Navis GJ, de Jong PE, Donker AJM, et al: Moderate sodium restriction in hypertensive subjects: Renal effects of ACE-inhibition. Kidney Int 31:815-819, 1987; and Lansang MC, Price DA, Laffel LM, et al: Renal vascular responses to captopril and to candesartan in patients with type 1 diabetes mellitus. Kidney Int 59:1432-1438, 2001.)

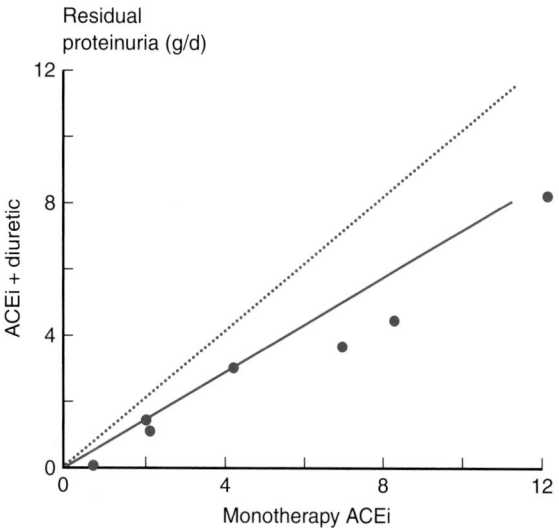

FIGURE 56-20. Individual data on residual proteinuria during angiotensin-converting enzyme inhibitor (ACEi) monotherapy, during high sodium intake (*x* axis), and after addition of the diuretic hydrochlorothiazide (*y* axis). The regression line *(continuous line)* and the line of identity *(dotted line)* are given as well. (Adapted from Buter H, Hemmelder MH, Navis GJ, et al: Blunting of the antiproteinuric efficacy of ACE inhibition by high sodium intake can be restored by hydrochlorothiazide. Nephrol Dial Transplant 13:1682-1685, 1998; and Laverman GD, de Zeeuw D, Navis GJ: Between-patient differences in the renal response to renin-angiotensin system intervention: Clue to optimizing renoprotective therapy? J Renin Angiotensin Aldosterone Syst 3:205-213, 2002.)

responders versus nonresponders. However, unraveling of the underlying mechanisms, intermediate phenotypes, and interaction with environmental factors[220] is even more important. Such information will help overcome genetically determined resistance to therapy, as illustrated by correction of the poor antihypertensive response to ACE inhibitors in blacks by cotreatment with a diuretic, which was determined by taking into account the intermediate phenotype of sodium sensitivity.

CONCLUSIONS AND FUTURE PROSPECTS

Major advances have marked the prevention of progressive loss of renal function over the last decade. A reduction in hard end points, specifically, the need for dialysis, was obtained with ACE inhibitors in nondiabetic nephropathy and with AT1 receptor blockers in type 2 diabetic nephropathy. These studies underline the potency of RAAS blockade as a renoprotective intervention and the reduction of proteinuria as a treatment target. Nevertheless, chronic renal failure is still a progressive condition in many patients. The insight obtained has provided several guidelines to enhance the renoprotective efficacy of the available therapeutics. First, it has been shown that aggressive interventional therapy improves the prognosis in high-risk patients. In view of the predictive value of a reduction in proteinuria for long-term renoprotection, titrating for antiproteinuric effect seems promising. In this respect, the dose-response curve for renoprotection with specific classes of drugs, as well as combinations of different classes of drugs, deserves consideration. Because systemic sequelae of proteinuria such as hyperlipidemia may play a potentiating role in proteinuria-induced renal damage, specific antihyperlipidemic treatment may be a useful adjunct to reduction of blood pressure and proteinuria.

Identification of patients likely to benefit from such an aggressive approach is warranted. Importantly, proteinuria is not only a main determinant of renal risk but also a determinant of the benefit that can be obtained from intervention. Further elucidation of individual determinants of renal risk and responsiveness to therapy may allow new perspectives to improve the prognosis of patients with renal disease.

REFERENCES

1. Ellis A: Natural history of Bright's disease; clinical, histological and experimental observations. The vicious circle in Bright's disease. Lancet 2:72-76, 1942.
2. Klahr S, Schreiner G, Ichikawa I: The progression of renal disease. N Engl J Med 318:1657-1666, 1988.
3. Narins RG, Cortes P: The role of dietary protein restriction in progressive azotemia [editorial]. N Engl J Med 330:929-930, 1994.
4. Remuzzi G, Bertani T: Is glomerulosclerosis a consequence of altered glomerular permeability to macromolecules? Kidney Int 38:384-394, 1990.
5. Hauser AC, Derfler K, Balcke P: Progression of renal insufficiency in analgesic nephropathy: Impact of drug abuse. J Clin Epidemiol 44:53-56, 1991.
6. Williams PS, Fass G, Bone JM: Renal pathology and proteinuria determine progression in untreated mild/moderate chronic renal failure. Q J Med 67:343-354, 1988.
7. Isles GC, McLay A, Boulton-Jones JM: Recovery in malignant hypertension presenting as acute renal failure. Q J Med 212:439-452, 1984.
8. The effect of intensive treatment of diabetes on the development and progression of long-term complications in insulin-dependent diabetes mellitus. The Diabetes Control and Complications Trial Research Group. N Engl J Med 329:977-986, 1993.
9. Agodoa L, Jones C, Held P: End stage renal disease in the USA: Data from the United States Renal Data System. Am J Nephrol 16:7-16, 1996.
10. Perneger TV, Whelton PK, Klag ML: History of hypertension in patients treated for end-stage renal disease. J Hypertens 15:451-456, 1997.
11. US Renal Data System: Excerpts of renal failure and hypertensive nephrosclerosis. Am J Kidney Dis 34(suppl 1):1-176, 1999.
12. Tracy RE, Malcom GR, Oalmann MC, et al: Renal microvascular features of hypertension in Japan, Guatemala and the United States. Arch Pathol Lab Med 116:50-55, 1992.
13. Tracy RE, Tabares Toca V: Nephrosclerosis and blood pressure. I: Rising and falling patterns in lengthy records. Lab Invest 34:20-29, 1974.
14. Tracy RE, Velez-Duran M, Heigle T, Oalmann MC: Two variants of nephrosclerosis separately related to age and blood pressure. Am J Pathol 131:270-282, 1988.
15. Katafuchi R, Takebayashi S: Morphometrical and functional correlations in benign nephrosclerosis. Clin Nephrol 28:238-243, 1987.
16. Fogo A, Breyer JA, Smith MC, et al: Accuracy of diagnosis of hypertensive nephrosclerosis in African Americans: A report from the African American Study of Kidney Disease (AASK) Trial. AASK Pilot Study Investigators. Kidney Int 51:244-252, 1997.
17. Harvey JM, Howie AJ, Lee SJ, et al: Renal biopsy findings in hypertensive patients with proteinuria. Lancet 340:1435-1436, 1992.
18. Iseki K, Iseki C, Ikemiya Y, Fukiyama K: Risk of developing end-stage renal disease in a cohort of mass screening. Kidney Int 49:800-805, 1996.
19. Klag MJ, Whelton PK, Randall BL, et al: Blood pressure and end stage renal disease in men. N Engl J Med 334:13-18, 1996.
20. Lindeman RD, Tobin J, Shock NW: Association between blood pressure and the rate of decline in renal function with age. Kidney Int 26:861-868, 1984.
21. Perneger TV, Nieto FJ, Whelton PK, et al: A prospective study of blood pressure and serum creatinine. Results from the "Clue study and the ARIC study. JAMA 269:488-493, 1993.
22. Schmieder RE, Schachtinger H, Messerli FH: Accelerated decline in renal perfusion with aging in essential hypertension. Hypertension 23:351-357, 1994.
23. London GM, Safar ME, Sassard JE, et al: Renal and systemic hemodynamics in sustained essential hypertension. Hypertension 6:743-754, 1984.
24. Fliser D, Franek E, Joest M, et al: Renal function in the elderly: Impact of hypertension and cardiac function. Kidney Int 51:1196-1204, 1997.
25. Kimura G, London GM, Safar ME, et al: Glomerular hypertension in renovascular hypertensive patients. Kidney Int 39:966-972, 1991.

26. Walker WG, Neaton JD, Cutler JA, et al: Renal function change in hypertensive members of the Multiple Risk Factor Intervention Trial. JAMA 268:3085-3091, 1992.
27. Shulman NB, Ford CE, Hall WD, et al: Prognostic value of serum creatinine and effect of treatment of hypertension on renal function. Hypertension 13(suppl 1):80-93, 1989.
28. Perry HM Jr, Miller JP, Fornoff JR, et al: Early predictors of 15-year end-stage renal disease in hypertensive patients. Hypertension 25:587-594, 1995.
29. Walker WG, Neaton JD, Cutler JA, et al: Renal function change in hypertensive members of the Multiple Risk Factor Intervention Trial. JAMA 268:3085-3091, 1992.
30. Bidani AK, Schwartz MM, Lewis EJ: Renal autoregulation and vulnerability to hypertensive injury in remnant kidney. Am J Physiol 252:F1003-F1010, 1987.
31. Kario K, Kanai N, Nishiuma S, et al: Hypertensive nephropathy and the gene for angiotensin-converting enzyme. Arterioscler Thromb Vasc Biol 17:252-256, 1997.
32. Pontremoli R, Sofia A, Tirotta A, et al: The deletion polymorphism of the angiotensin I–converting enzyme gene is associated with target organ damage in essential hypertension. J Am Soc Nephrol 7:2550-2558, 1996.
33. Mallamaci F, Zuccala A, Zoccali C, et al: The deletion polymorphism of the angiotensin-converting enzyme is associated with nephroangiosclerosis. Am J Hypertens 13:433-437, 2000.
34. Brown MA, Whitworth JA: Hypertension in human renal disease. J Hypertens 10:701-712, 1992.
35. Poulsen PL, Hansen KW, Mogensen CE: Ambulatory blood pressure in the transition from normo to microalbuminria: A longitudinal study in IDDM: Diabetes 43:1248-1253, 1994.
36. Hasslacher C, Ritz E, Terpstra J, et al: Natural history of nephropathy in type I diabetes. Hypertension 7(suppl 2):74-78, 1985.
37. Mogensen CE, Christensen CK: Blood pressure changes and renal function in incipient and overt diabetic nephropathy. Hypertension 7(suppl 2):64-73, 1985.
38. Rossing P, Hommel E, Smidt U, Parving H-H: Impact of blood pressure and albuminuria on the progression of diabetic nephropathy in IDDM patients. Diabetes 42:715-719, 1993.
39. Harris RD, Steffes MW, Bilous RW, et al: Global glomerular sclerosis and glomerular arteriolar hyalinosis in insulin dependent diabetes. Kidney Int 40:107-114, 1991.
40. Mauer SM, Sutherland DER, Steffes MW: Relationship of blood pressure to nephropathology in insulin-dependent diabetes mellitus. Kidney Int 41:736-740, 1992.
41. Brazy PC, Fitzwilliam JF: Progressive renal disease: Role of race and antihypertensive medications. Kidney Int 37:1113-1119, 1990.
42. Locatelli F, Marcelli D, Comelli M, et al: Proteinuria and blood pressure as causal components of progression to end-stage renal failure. Nephrol Dial Transplant 11:461-467, 1996.
43. Oldrizzi L, Rugiu C, de Biase V, Maschio G: The place of hypertension among the risk factors for renal function in chronic renal failure. Am J Kidney Dis 21(suppl 2):119-123, 1993.
44. Wight JP, Salzano S, Brown CB, El Nahas AM: Natural history of chronic renal failure: A reappraisal. Nephrol Dial Transplant 7:379-383, 1992.
45. Orofino L, Quereda C, Lamas S, et al: Hypertension in primary chronic glomerulonephritis: An analysis of 288 biopsied patients. Nephron 45:22-26, 1987.
46. Rambausek M, Rhien C, Waldherr R, et al: Hypertension in chronic idiopathic glomerulonephritis: An analysis of 311 biopsied patients. Eur J Clin Invest 19:176-180, 1989.
47. Gonzalo A, Gallego A, Rivera M, et al: Influence of hypertension on early renal insufficiency in autosomal dominant polycystic kidney disease. Nephron 72:225-230, 1996.
48. Stenvinkel P, Alvestrand A, Bergström J: Factors influencing progression in patients with chronic renal failure. J Intern Med 226:183-188, 1989.
49. Walker WG: Hypertension-related renal injury: A major contributor to end stage renal disease. Am J Kidney Dis 22:164-173, 1993.
50. Alvestrand A, Gutierrez A, Bucht H, Bergström J: Reduction of blood pressure retards the progression of chronic renal failure in man. Nephrol Dial Transplant 3:624-631, 1988.
51. Hannedouche T, Albouze G, Chauveau P, et al: Effects of blood pressure and antihypertensive treatment on progression of advanced renal failure. Am J Kidney Dis 21(5 suppl 2):131-137, 1993.

52. Mogensen CE: Long term antihypertensive treatment inhibiting progression of diabetic nephropathy. BMJ 285:685-689, 1982.

53. Parving H-H, Andersen AR, Smidt UM, Svendsen PA: Early aggressive antihypertensive treatment reduces rate of decline in kidney function in diabetic nephropathy. Lancet 1:1175-1179, 1983.

54. Pohl JF, Thurston H, Swales JD: Hypertension with renal impairment. Influence of intensive therapy. Q J Med 43:569-581, 1974.

55. Mitchell HC, Graham RM, Pettinger WA: Renal function during long term treatment of hypertension with minoxidil. Comparison of benign and malignant hypertension. Ann Intern Med 93:676-681, 1980.

56. Oldrizzi L, Rugio C, Maschio G: Hypertension and progression of renal failure in patients on protein-restricted diet. Contrib Nephrol 54:134-143, 1987.

57. Vetter K, Lindenau K, Kripki F, Frohling PT: Influence of hypertension on the rate of progression of chronic renal failure. Scand J Urol Nephrol Suppl 108:21-23, 1988.

58. Shimamatsu K, Onoyama K, Harada A, Kumagai H: Effect of blood pressure on the progression rate of renal impairment in chronic glomerulonephritis. J Clin Hypertens 5:239-244, 1985.

59. Hannedouche T, Chauveau P, Fehrat A, et al: Effect of moderate protein restriction on the rate of renal function loss in chronic renal failure. Kidney Int Suppl 27:91-95, 1989.

60. Madhavan S, Stockwell D, Cohen H, Alderman MH: Renal function during antihypertensive treatment. Lancet 345:749-751, 1995.

61. Alberti D, Locatelli F, Graziani G, et al: Hypertension and chronic renal insufficiency: The experience of the Northern Italian Cooperative Study Group. Am J Kidney Dis 21:124-130, 1993.

62. Bergström J, Alvestrand A, Bucht H, Gutierrez A: Progression of chronic renal failure in man is retarded with more frequent clinical follow-ups and blood pressure control. Clin Nephrol 25:1-6, 1986.

63. Pettinger WA, Lee HC, Reisch J, Mitchell HC: Long term improvement in renal function after short term strict blood pressure control hypertensive nephrosclerosis. Hypertension 13:766-772, 1989.

64. Wright JT, Bakris G, Grenne T, et al: African American Study of Kidney Disease and Hypertension Study Group. Effect of blood pressure lowering and antihypertensive drug class on progression of hypertensive kidney disease: Results from the AASK trial. JAMA 288:2421-2431, 2002.

65. Klahr S, Levey AS, Beck GJ, et al: The effect of dietary protein restriction and blood pressure control on the progression of chronic renal disease. Modification of Diet in Renal Disease Study Group. N Engl J Med 330:877-884, 1994.

66. Parving H-H, Andersen AR, Smidt UM, et al: Effect of antihypertensive treatment on kidney function in diabetic nephropathy. BMJ 294:1443-1447, 1987.

67. Lewis EJ, Hunsicker LG, Bain RP, et al: The effect of angiotensin-converting enzyme inhibition on diabetic nephropathy. N Engl J Med 329:1456-1462, 1993.

68. Ravid M, Brosh D, Levi Z, et al: Use of enalapril to attentuate decline in renal function in normotensive normo-albuminuric patients with type 2 diabetes mellitus. Ann Intern Med 128:983-988, 1998.

69. Brenner BM, Cooper ME, de Zeeuw D, et al: Effects of losartan on renal and cardiovascular outcomes in patients with type 2 diabetes and nephropathy. N Engl J Med 345:861-869, 2001.

70. Lewis EJ, Hunsicker LG, Clarke WR, et al: Renoprotective effects of the angiotensin-receptor antagonist irbesartan in patients with nephropathy due to type 2 diabetes. N Engl J Med 345:851-860, 2001.

71. Peterson JC, Adler S, Burkart JM, et al: Blood pressure control, proteinuria and the progression of renal disease. The Modification of Diet in Renal Disease Study. Ann Intern Med 123:754-762, 1995.

72. Hebert LA, Kusek JA, Green T, et al: Effects of blood pressure control on progressive renal disease in blacks and whites. The Modification of Diet in Renal Disease Study Group. Hypertension 30:428-435, 1997.

73. Wright JT Jr, Kusek JW, Toto RD, et al: Design and baseline characteristics of participants in the African American study of Kidney Disease and Hypertension (AASK) Pilot Study. Control Clin Trials 17(suppl):3-13, 1996.

74. Mogensen CE, Keane WF, Bennett PH, et al: Prevention of diabetic renal disease with special reference to microalbuminuria. Lancet 346:1080-1084, 1995.

75. Bakris GL, Williams M, Dworkin L, et al: The National Kidney Foundation Hypertension and Diabetes Executive Committees Working Group. Preserving renal function in adults with hypertension and diabetes: A consensus approach. Am J Kidney Dis 36:646-661, 2000.

76. Parving H-H, Smidt UM, Hommel E, et al: Effective antihypertensive therapy postpones renal insufficiency in diabetic nephropathy. Am J Kidney Dis 22:188-195, 1993.

77. Hostetter TH, Olson JL, Rennke HG, et al: Hyperfiltration in remnant nephrons. A potentially adverse response to renal ablation. Am J Physiol 241 F85-F83, 1981.

78. Zatz R, Meyer TW, Rennke HG, Brenner BM: Predominance of hemodynamic rather than metabolic factors in the pathogenesis of diabetic glomerulopathy. Proc Natl Acad Sci U S A 82:5963-5967, 1985.

79. Mogensen CE, Hansen KW, Nielsen S, et al: Monitoring diabetic nephropathy: Glomerular filtration rate and abnormal albuminuria in diabetic renal disease—reproducibility, progression, and efficacy of antihypertensive intervention. Am J Kidney Dis 22:174-187, 1993.

80. Parving H-H, Kastrup H, Smidt UM, et al: Impaired autoregulation of glomerular filtration rate in type I (insulin-dependent) diabetic patients with nephropathy. Diabetologia 27:547-552, 1984.

81. Hirose K, Tsuchida H, Osterby R, Gundersen HJ: A strong correlation between glomerular filtration rate and filtration surface in diabetic kidney hyperfunction. Lab Invest 43:434-437, 1980.

82. Vedel P, Obel J, Nielsen FS, et al: Glomerular hyperfiltration in microalbuminuric NIDDM patients. Diabetologia 39:1584-1589, 1996.

83. Nowack R, Raum E, Blum W, Ritz E: Renal hemodynamics in recent onset type II diabetes. Am J Kidney Dis 20:342-347, 1992.

84. Vora JP, Dolben J, Dean JD, et al: Renal hemodynamics in newly presenting non-insulin dependent diabetes meliitus. Kidney Int 41:829-835, 1992.

85. Gambara V, Mecca G, Remuzzi G, Bertani T: Heterogeneous nature of renal lesions in type II diabetes. J Am Soc Nephrol 3:1458-1466, 1993.

86. Weller GS, Filler G: Patients with APKD hyperfiltrate early in their disease: An indication for ACE-inhibitors [abstract]? J Am Soc Nephrol 13:264, 2002.

87. Talseth T, Fauchald P, Skrede S, et al: Long-term blood pressure and renal function in kidney donors. Kidney Int 29:1072-1076, 1986.

88. Anastasio P, Spitali L, Frangiosa A, et al: Glomerular filtration rate in severely overweight normotensive humans. Am J Kidney Dis 35:1144-1148, 2000.

89. Praga M, Hernandez E, Herrero JC, et al: Influence of obesity on the appearance of proteinuria and renal insufficiency after unilateral nephrectomy. Kidney Int 58:2111-2118, 2000.

90. Fogo A, Hawkins EP, Berry PL, et al: Glomerular hypertrophy in minimal change predicts subsequent progression to focal glomerular sclerosis. Kidney Int 38:115-123, 1990.

91. Baker L, Dahelm S, Goldfarb S, et al: Hyperfiltration and renal disease in glycogen storage disease. Kidney Int 35:1345-50, 1989.

92. du Cailar G, Ribstein J, Mimran A: Glomerular hyperfiltration and left ventricular mass in mild never-treated essential hypertension. J Hypertens 9(suppl 6):158-159, 1991.

93. Schmieder RE, Messerli FH, Garavaglia G, Nunez B: Glomerular hyperfiltration indicates early target organ damage in essential hypertension. JAMA 264:2775-2780, 1990.

94. Schmieder RE, Veelken R, Gatzka CD, et al: Predictors for hypertensive nephropathy: Results of a 6-year follow-up study. J Hypertens 13:357-365, 1995.

95. Pinto-Sietsma S-J, Janssen WMT, Hillege HJ, et al: Urinary albumin excretion is associated with renal functional abnormalities in a non-diabetic population. J Am Soc Nephrol 11:1182-1888, 2000.

96. Anderson SA, Rennke HG, Brenner BM: Therapeutic advantage of converting enzyme inhibitors in arresting progressive renal disease associated with systemic hypertension in rats. J Clin Invest 77: 1993-2000, 1986.

97. Dworkin LD, Grosser M, Feiner HD, et al: Renal vascular effects of anithypertensive therapy in uninephrectomized spontaneously hypertensive rats. Kidney Int 35:790-798, 1989.

98. Apperloo AJ, de Zeeuw D, de Jong PE: A short-term antihypertensive treatment induced fall in glomerular filtration rate predicts long term stability of renal function. Kidney Int 51:793-797, 1997.

99. Hansen HP, Rossing P, Tarnow L, et al: Increased glomerular filtration rate after withdrawal of long-term antihypertensive therapy in diabetic nephropathy. Kidney Int 47:1726-1731, 1994.

100. El Nahas AM, Masters-Thomas A, Brady SA, et al: Selective effect of low protein diets in chronic renal diseases. BMJ 289:1337-1341, 1984.

101. Hansen HP, Nielsen FS, Rossing P, et al: Kidney function after withdrawal of long-term antihypertensive therapy in diabetic nephropathy. Kidney Int Suppl 63:49-53, 1997.

102. Ravid M, Savin H, Jurtin I, et al: Long term stabilizing effect of angiotensin-converting enzyme inhibition on plasma creatinine and on proteinuria in normotensive type II diabetic patients. Ann Intern Med 118:577-581, 1993.

103. Fogo A, Yoshida Y, Glick AD, et al: Serial micropuncture analysis of glomerular function in two rat models of glomerular sclerosis. J Clin Invest 82:322-330, 1988.

104. Howie AJ, Lee SJ, Green NJ, et al: Different clinicopathological types of segmental sclerosing glomerular lesions in adults. Nephrol Dial Transplant 8:590-599, 1993.

105. Kroker BP, Dawson DV, Sanfilipppo F: IgA nephropathy. Correla tion of clinical and histological features. Lab Invest 48:19-24, 1983.

106. Nagai Y, Arai H, Washisawa Y, et al: FGS-like lesions in pre-ecclampsia. Clin Nephrol 36:134-140, 1991.

107. d'Agati V, Suh J, Carbone L, et al: Pathology of HIV associated nephropathy: A detailed morphologic and comparative study. Kidney Int 35:1358-1370, 1989.

108. Ferrario F, Tadros MT, Napodano P, et al: Critical reevaluation of 41 cases of "idiopathic" crescentic glomerulonephritis. Clin Nephrol 41:1-9, 1994.

109. Novick AC, Gephardt G, Guz B, et al: Long term follow-up after partial removal of a solitary kidney. N Engl J Med 325:1059-1062, 1991.

110. Kiprov DD, Colvin RB, McCluskey RT: Focal and segmental glomerulosclerosis and proteinuria associated with unilateral agenesis. Lab Invest 46:275-281, 1982.

111. El Khatib MT, Becker GJ, Kincaid-Smith P: Morphological aspects of reflux nephropathy. Kidney Int 32:261-266, 1987.

112. Harvey JM, Howie AJ, Lee SJ, et al: Renal biopsy findings in hypertensive patients with proteinuria. Lancet 340:1435-1436, 1992.

113. Perna A, Remuzzi G: Abnormal permeability to proteins and glomerular lesions: A meta-analysis of experimental and clinical studies. Am J Kidney Dis 27:34-41, 1996.

114. Mallick NP, Short CD, Hunt LP: How far since Ellis? Nephron 46:113-124, 1987.

115. Samuelsson O, Wilhelmsen L, Elmfeldt D, et al: Predictors of cardiovascular morbidity in treated hypertension: Results from the primary preventive trial in Göteborg, Sweden. J Hypertens 3:167-176, 1985.

116. Ruggenenti P, Perna A, Mosconi L, et al: Urinary protein excretion rate is the best predictor of ESRF in non-diabetic proteinuric chronic nephropathies. "Gruppo Italiano di Studi Epidemiologici in Nefrologia" (GISEN). Kidney Int 53:1209-1216, 1998.

117. Beukhof JR, Kardaun O, Schaafsma W, et al: Toward individual prognosis of IgA nephropathy. Kidney Int 29:549-556, 1986.

118. Breyer JA, Bain RP, Evans JK, et al: Predictors of the progression of renal insufficiency in patients with insulin-dependent diabetes and overt diabetic nephropathy. The Collaborative Study Group. Kidney Int 50:1651-1658, 1996.

119. Donadio JV Jr, Torres VE, Velosa JA, et al: Idiopathic membranous glomerulopathy: The natural history of untreated patients. Kidney Int 33:708-715, 1988.

120. Hunt LP, Short CD, Mallick NP: Prognostic indicators in patients presenting with nephrotic syndrome. Kidney Int 34:382-388, 1988.

121. Halimi J-M, Ribstein J, Du Cailar G, et al: Albuminuria predicts renal functional outcome after intervention in atheromatous renovascular disease. J Hypertens 13:1335-1342, 1995.

122. Franssen CFM, Stegeman CA, Oost-Kort WW, et al: Determinants of renal outcome in anti-myeloperoxidase–associated crescentic glomerulonephritis. J Am Soc Nephrol 9:1915-1923, 1998.

123. Kincaid-Smith P, Becker G: Reflux nephropathy and chronic atrophic glomerulonephritis: A review. J Infect Dis 138:774-780, 1978.

124. Zuchelli P, Gaggi R: Reflux nephropathy in adults. Nephron 57:2-9, 1991.

125. Jungers P, Hannedouche T, Itakura Y, et al: Progression to end-stage renal failure in non-diabetic kidney diseases: A multivariate analysis of determinant factors. Nephrol Dial Transplant 10:1353-1360, 1995.

126. Bjorck S, Mulec H, Jonson SA, et al: Contrasting effects of enalapril and metoprolol on proteinuria in diabetic nephropathy. BMJ 300:904-907, 1990.

127. Maschio G, Alberti D, Janin G, et al: Effect of the angiotensin converting enzyme inhibitor benazepril on the progression of chronic renal insufficiency. N Engl J Med 334:939-945, 1996.

128. Kamper AL, Strandgaard S, Leyssac PP: Effect of enalapril on progression of chronic renal failure. Am J Hypertens 5:423-430, 1992.

129. The GISEN group: Randomized placebo-controlled trial of effect of ramipril on decline in glomerular filtration rate and progression to terminal renal failure in proteinuric, non-diabetic nephropathy. Lancet 349:1857-1863, 1997.

130. Jafar TH, Schmid CH, Landa M, et al: Angiotensin converting enzyme inhibitors and progression of nondiabetic disease. A meta-analysis of patient-level data. Ann Intern Med 135:73-87, 2001.

131. Idelson BA, Smithlime N, Smith GW, Harrington JT: Prognosis in steroid treated idiopathic nephrotic syndrome. Ann Intern Med 137:891-896, 1977.

132. Vriesendorp R, Donker AJM, de Zeeuw D: Effects of non-steroidal anti-inflammatory drugs on proteinuria. Am J Med 81(supp 2B):84-93, 1986.

133. Wapstra FH, Navis GJ, de Jong PE, de Zeeuw D: Short term and long term antiproteinuric response to inhibition of renin angiotensin axis in patients with non-diabetic renal disease; prediction of GFR decline. Exp Nephrol 4(suppl 1):47-52, 1996.

134. El Nahas AM, Masters-Thomas A, Brady SA, et al: Selective effect of low protein diets in chronic renal diseases. BMJ 289:1337-1341, 1984.

135. Praga M, Hernández E, Montoyo C, et al: Long-term beneficial effects of angiotensin-converting enzyme inhibition with nephrotic proteinuria. Am J Kidney Dis 20:240-248, 1992.

136. Gansevoort RT, de Zeeuw D, de Jong PE: Long-term benefits of the antiproteinuric effect of ACE-inhibition in non-diabetic renal disease. Am J Kidney Dis 2:202-206, 1993.

137. Apperloo AJ, de Zeeuw D, de Jong PE: Short-term antiproteinuric response to antihypertensive therapy predicts long-term GFR decline in patients with non-diabetic renal disease. Kidney Int Suppl 45:174-178, 1994.

138. The GISEN Group: Randomised placebo-controlled trial of effect of ramipril on decline in glomerular filtration rate and risk of terminal renal failure in proteinuric, non-diabetic nephropathy. Lancet 349:1857-1863, 1997.

139. Peterson JC, Adler S, Burkart JM, et al: Blood pressure control, proteinuria and the progression of renal disease. The Modification of diet in Renal Disease Study Group. Ann Intern Med 123:754-762, 1995.

140. Kamper A-L, Strandgaard S, Leyssac PP: Late outcome of a controlled trial of enalapril treatment in progressive chronic renal failure. Hard end-points and influence of proteinuria. Nephrol Dial Transplant 10:1182-1188, 1995.

141. Rossing P, Hommel E, Smidt UM, Parving H-H: Reduction in albuminuria predicts diminished progression in diabetic nephropathy. Kidney Int Suppl 45:145-149, 1994.

142. Rossing P, Hommel E, Smidt UM, Parving HH: Reduction in albuminuria predicts a beneficial effect on diminishing the progression of human diabetic nephropathy during antihypertensive treatment. Diabetologia 37:511-516, 1994.

143. Wapstra FH, van Goor H, Navis GJ, et al: Antiproteinuric effect predicts renal protection by angiotensin-converting enzyme inhibition in rats with established Adriamycin nephrosis. Clin Sci 90:393-401, 1996.

144. Lufft V, Kliem V, Hamkens A, et al: Antiproteinuric efficacy of fosinopril after renal transplantation is determined by the extent of vascular and tubulointerstitial damage. Clin Transplant 12:409-415, 1998.

145. Kramer AM, Laverman GD, van Goor H, Navis GJ: Interindividual differences in antiproteinuric response to ACEi in established Adriamycin nephrosis are predicted by pre-treatment renal damage. J Pathol 201:160-167, 2003.

146. Kasiske BL, O'Donnell MP, Schmits PG, et al: Renal injury of diet-induced hypercholesterolemia in rats. Kidney Int 37:880-891, 1990.

147. Keane WF, Kasiske B, O'Donnell MP, Kin Y: The role of altered lipid metabolism in the progression of renal disease. Am J Kidney Dis 17(suppl):38-42, 1991.

148. Moorhead JF: Lipids and pathogenesis of kidney disease. Am J Kidney Dis 17:65-70, 1991.

149. Joven J, Villabona C, Vilella Masana L, et al: Abnormalities of lipoprotein metabolism in patients with the nephrotic syndrome. N Engl J Med 323:579-584, 1990.

150. Keane WF, Raij L: Relationship among altered glomerular barrier permselectivity, angiotensin II and mesangial uptake of macromolecules. Lab Invest 53:599-604, 1985.

151. Kasiske DL, O'Donnell MP, Schmitz PC, et al: Effects of reduced renal mass on tissue lipids and renal injury in hyperlipemic rats. Kidney Int 35:40-47, 1989.

152. de Boer E, Navis GJ, Tiebosch ATM, et al: Systemic factors are involved in the pathogenesis of proteinuria-induced glomerulosclerosis in Adriamycin nephrotic rats. J Am Soc Nephrol, 10: 2359-2366, 1999.

153. Kasiske BL, O'Donnell MP, Cleary MP, Keane WF: Treatment of hyperlipidemia reduces glomerular injury in obese Zucker rats. Kidney Int 33:667-672, 1990.

154. Bos H, Henning RH, de Jong PE, et al: Do severe systemic sequelae of proteinuria modulate the antiproteinuric response to chronic ACE-inhibition? Nephrol Dial Transplant 17:793-797, 2002.

155. Ohta Y, Yamamoto S, Tsuchida H, et al: Nephropathy of familial lecithin-cholesterol acyl transferase deficiency: Report of a case. Am J Kidney Dis 7:41-46, 1986.

156. Saito T, Sato H, Kudo K, et al: Lipoprotein glomerulopathy: Glomerular lipoprotein thrombi in a patient with hyperlipoproteinemia. Am J Kidney Dis 13:148-153, 1989.

157. Keane WF, St Peter JV, Kasiske BL: Is the aggressive mangement of hyperlipidemia in nephrotic syndrome mandatory? Kidney Int Suppl 42:134-141, 1992.

158. Smellie WSA, Warwick GL: Primary hyperlipidemia is not associated with increased urinary albumin excretion. Nephrol Dial Transplant 6:398-401, 1991.

159. Manttari M, Alikoski T, Manninine V: Effects of hypertension and dyslipidemia on the decline in renal function. Hypertension 26:670-675, 1995.

160. Lee HS, Lee JS, Koh HI, Ko KW: Intraglomerular lipid deposition in routine biopsies. Clin Nephrol 36:67-75, 1991.

161. Sato H, Suzuki S, Kobayshi H, et al: Immunohistochemical localization of apolipoproteins in the glomeruli in renal disease: Specifically apoB and apoE: Clin Nephrol 36:127-133, 1991.

162. Sato H, Suzuki S, Ueno M, et al: Localization of apolipoprotein(a) and B-100 in various renal diseases. Kidney Int 43:430-435, 1993.

163. Maschio G, Oldrizzi L, Rugiu C, et al: Factors affecting progression of renal failure in patients on long term dietary protein restriction. Kidney Int Suppl 22:49-52, 1987.

164. Samuelsson O, Aurell M, Knight-Gibson C, et al: Apolipoprotein-B containing lipoproteins and the progression of renal insuffiency. Nephron 63:279-285, 1993.

165. Samuelsson O, Mulec H, Knight-Gibson C, et al: Lipoprotein abnormalities are associated with an increased rate of renal insufficiency. Nephrol Dial Transplant 12:1908-1915, 1997.

166. Attman P-O, Samuelsson O, Alaupovic P: Progression of renal failure; role of apoB-containing lipoproteins. Kidney Int Suppl 63: 98-101, 1997.

167. Capelli P, Evangelista M, Bonomini M, et al: Lipids and the progression of chronic renal failure. Nephron 62:31-35, 1992.

168. Coggins CH, Breyer Lewis JH, Caggiula AW, et al: Differences between women and men with chronic renal disease. Nephrol Dial Transplant 13:1430-1437, 1998.

169. Parving H-H, Rossing P, Hommel E, Smidt UM: Angiotensin converting enzyme inhibition in diabetic nephropathy: Ten years experience. Am J Kidney Dis 26:99-107, 1995.

170. Krolewski AS, Warram JH, Christlieb AR: Hypercholesterolemia. A determinant of renal function loss and deaths in IDDM patients with nephropathy. Kidney Int Suppl 45:125-131, 1994.

171. Mulec H, Johnson S-A, Björck S: Relation between serum cholesterol and diabetic nephropathy. Lancet 335:1536-1538. 1990.

172. Breyer JA, Bain RP, Evans JK, et al: Predictors of the progression of renal insufficiency in patients with insulin-dependent diabetes and overt diabetic nephropathy. The Collaborative Study Group. Kidney Int 50:1651-1658, 1996.

173. Mulec H, Johnsen SA, Wiklund O, Björck S: Cholesterol: A renal risk factor in diabetic nephropathy? Am J Kidney Dis 22:196-201, 1993.

174. Ravid M, Savin H, Jurtin I, et al: Long term stabilizing effect of angiotensin-converting enzyme inhibition on plasma creatinine and on proteinuria in normotensive type II diabetic patients. Ann Intern Med 118:577-581, 1993.

175. Hasslacher C, Bostedt-Kiesel A, Kempe HP, Wahl P: Effect of metabolic factors and blood pressure on kidney function in proteinuric

176. type 2 (non-insulin-dependent) diabetic patients. Diabetologia 36:1051-1056, 1995.

176. Jerums G, Allen TJ, Salamandris C, et al: Relationship of progressively increasing albuminuria to apolipoprotein (a) and blood pressure in type 2 (non-insulin dependent) diabetic patients. Diabetologia 36:1037-1044, 1993.

177. Yokota C, Kimura G, Inenaga T, Kawano Y: Risk factors for progression of diabetic nephropathy. Am J Nephrol 15:488-492, 1995.

178. Samuelsson O, Attman P-O, Knight-Gibson C, et al: Lipoprotein abnormalities without hyperlipidemia in moderate renal insufficiency. Nephrol Dial Transplant 9:1580-1585, 1994.

179. Diamond JR, Hanchak NA, McCarter MD, Karnovsky MJ: Cholestyramine resin ameliorates chronic aminonucleoside nephrosis. Am J Clin Nutr 51:606-611, 1990.

180. Rabelink AJ, Hené RJ, Erkelens DW, et al: Partial remission of nephrotic syndrome in patients on long term simvastatin. Lancet 335:1045-1046, 1990.

181. Rayner BL, Byrne MJ, van Zyl Smit R: A prospective clinical trial comparing the treatment of idiopathic membranous nephropathy and nephrotic syndrome with simvastatin and diet, versus diet alone. Clin Nephrol 46:219-224, 1996.

182. Chan PCK, Robinson JD, Yeung WC, et al: Lovastatin therapy in glomerulonephritis patients with hyperlipidemia and heavy proteinuria. Nephrol Dial Transplant 7:93-99, 1992.

183. Neverov NI, Kaysen GA, Tareyeva IE: Effect of lipid-lowering therapy on the progression of renal disease in nondiabetic nephrotic patients. Contrib Nephrol 120:68-78, 1997.

184. Warwick GL, Packard CJ, Murray L, et al: Effect of simvastatin on plasma lipid and lipoprotein concentration and low-density lipoprotein metabolism in the nephrotic syndrome. Cli Sci 82:701-708, 1992.

185. Prata MM, Nogueira AC, Pinto JR, et al: Long-term effect of lovastatin on lipoprotein profile in patients with primary nephrotic syndrome. Clin Nephrol 41:277-283, 1994.

186. Kasiske BL, Velosa JA, Halstenson CE, et al: The effects of lovastatin in hyperlipemic patients with the nephrotic syndrome. Am J Kidney Dis 15:8-15, 1990.

187. Golper TA, Illingwirth DR, Morris CD, Bennett WM: Lovastatin in the treatment of multifactorial hyperlipidemia associated with proteinuria. Am J Kidney Dis 13:312-320, 1989.

188. Thomas ME, Harris KPG, Ramaswamy C, et al: Simvastatin for hypercholesterolemic patients with nephrotic syndrome or significant proteinuria. Kidney Int 44:1124-1129, 1993.

189. Shoyi J, Nishizawa Y, Toyokawa A, et al: Decreased albuminuria by pravastatin in hyperlipidemic diabetics. Nephron 59:664-665, 1991.

190. Nielsen S, Schmitz O, Møller N, et al: Renal function and insulin sensitivity during simvastatin treatment in type 2 (non-insulin-dependent) diabetic patients with microalbuminuria. Diabetologia 36:1079-1086, 1993.

191. Biesenbach G, Zagornik J: Lovastatin in the treatment of hypercholesterolemia in nephrotic syndrome due to diabetic nephropathy stage IV-V. Clin Nephrol 37:274-279, 1992.

192. Hommel E, Andersen P, Gall M, et al: Plasma lipoproteins and renal function during simvastatin treatment in diabetic nephropathy. Diabetologia 35:447-451, 1992.

193. Lam KSL, Cheng IKP, Janus ED, Pang RWC: Cholesterol lowering therapy may retard the progression of diabetic nephropathy. Diabetologia 38:604-609, 1995.

194. Lee T-M, Su S-F, Tsai C-H: Effect of pravastatin on proteinuria in patients with well-controlled hypertension. Hypertension 40:67-73, 2002.

195. Zhang A, Vertommen J, van Gaal L, de Leeuw I: Effects of pravastatin on lipid levels, in vitro oxidizability of non-HDL lipoproteins and microalbuminuria in IDDM. Diabetes Res Clin Pract 29:189-94, 1995.

196. Tonolo G, Ciccarese M, Brizzi P, et al: Reduction of albumin excretion rate in normotensive microalbuminuric type 2 diabetic patients during long-term simvastatin treatment. Diabetes Care 20:1891-1895, 1997.

197. Fried LF, Orchard TJ, Kasiske BL: Effect of lipid reduction on the progression of renal disease: A meta-analysis. Kidney Int 59: 260-269, 2001.

198. Grond J, Beukers JYB, Schilthuis MS, et al: Analysis of renal structural and functional features in two rat strains with a different susceptibility to glomerular slcerosis. Lab Invest 54:77-83, 1986.

199. Seaquist ER, Goetz FC, Rich S, Barbosa J: Familial clustering of diabetic kidney disease: Evidence for genetic susceptibility to diabetic nephropathy. N Engl J Med 320:1161-1165, 1989.

200. Klouda PT, Manos J, Acheson EJ, et al: Strong association between idiopathic membranous glomerulopathy and HLA-DRW3. Lancet 2:770-771, 1979.

201. Egido J, Julian BA, Wyatt RJ: Genetic factors in primary IgA nephropathy. Nephrol Dial Transplant 2:134-142, 1987.

202. Glicklich D, Haskell L, Senitzer D, Weis RA: Possible genetic predisposition to idiopathic focal and segmental glomerulosclerosis. Am J Kidney Dis 12:26-30, 1988.

203. Mitch WE, Buffington G, Lemaan J, Walser M: Progression of renal failure: A simple method of estimation. Lancet 2:1326-1331, 1976.

204. Pazanias M, Eastwood JB, MacRae KD, Phillips ME: Racial origin and primary renal diagnosis in 771 patients with end stage renal disease. Nephrol Dial Transplant 6:931-935, 1991.

205. Perneger TV, Whelton PK, Klag MJ: Race and end-stage renal disease. Arch Intern Med 155:1201-1208, 1995.

206. van Essen GG, Rensma PL, de Zeeuw D, et al: Association between angiotensin-converting enzyme gene polymorphism and failure of renoprotective therapy. Lancet 347:94-95, 1996.

207. Harden PN, Geddes C, Rowe PA, et al: Polymorphism in angiotensin converting enzyme gene and progression of IgA nephropathy. Lancet 345:1540-1542, 1995.

208. Yoshida H, Kuriyama S, Atsumi Y, et al: Role of the deletion polymorphism of the angiotensin converting enzyme gene in the progression and therapeutic responsiveness of IgA nephropathy. J Clin Invest 96:2162-2169, 1995.

209. Parving H-H, Jacobsen P, Tarnow L, et al: Effect of deletion polymorphism of angiotensin converting enzyme gene on progression of diabetic nephropathy during inhibition of angiotensin converting enzyme: Observational follow-up study. BMJ 313:591-594, 1996.

210. Yoshida H, Kuriyama S, Atsumi Y, et al: Angiotensin I converting enzyme gene polymorphism in non-insulin dependent diabetes mellitus. Kidney Int 50:657-664, 1996.

211. Baboolal K, Ravine D, Daniels J, et al: Association of the angiotensin I converting enzyme gene deletion polymorphism with early onset of ESRF in PKD1 adult polycystic kidney disease. Kidney Int 52:607-613, 1997.

212. Broekroelofs J, Stegeman CA, Navis GJ, et al: Is donor or recipient ACE genotype associated with long-term graft survival after renal transplantation? J Am Soc Nephrol 9:2075-2081, 1998.

213. Fernandez-LLama P, Poch E, Oriola J, et al: Angiotensin converting enzyme gene I/D polymorphism in essential hypertension and nephroangiosclerosis. Kidney Int 53:1743-1747, 1998.

214. Boonstra AH, de Jong PE, de Zeeuw D, Navis GJ: Genetic markers for angII in renal disease. Semin Nephrol 21:580-592, 2001.

215. Rigat B, Hubert C, Alhenc Gelas F, et al: An insertion/deletion polymorphism in the angiotensin converting enzyme gene accounting for half of the variance of serum enzyme levels. J Clin Invest 86:1343-1346, 1990.

216. Danser JAH, Schalekamp MADH, Bax WA, et al: Angiotensin converting enzyme in the human heart. Effect of the deletion/insertion polymorphism. Circulation 92:1387-1388, 1995.

217. Mizuiri S, Yoshikawa H, Tanegashima M, et al: Renal ACE immunohistochemical localization in NIDDM patients with nephropathy. Am J Kidney Dis 31:301-307, 1998.

218. Buikema H, Pinto YM, Rooks G, et al: The deletion polymorphism of the angiotensin converting enzyme gene is related to phenoptypic differences in human arteries. Eur Heart J 17:787-794, 1996.

219. Ueda S, Elliot HL, Morton JJ, Connel JM: Enhanced pressor response to angiotensin I in normtensive men with the deletion genotype (DD) for angiotensin-converting-enzyme. Hypertension 25:1266-1269, 1995.

220. van der Kleij FGH, de Jong PE, Henning RH, et al: Enhanced responses of blood pressure, renal function and aldosterone to angiotensin I in DD genotype are blunted by low sodium intake. J Am Soc Nephrol 13:1025-1033, 2002.

221. Marre M, Jeunemaitre X, Gallois Y, et al: Contribution of genetic polymorphism in the renin-angiotensin system to the development of renal complications in insulin-dependent diabetes. J Clin Invest 99:1585-1595, 1997.

222. Pei Y, Scholey J, Thai K, et al: Association of angiotensinogen gene T235 variant with progression of immunoglobulin A nephropathy in Caucasian patients. J Clin Invest 100:814-820, 1997.

223. Veseij ES, Penno MB: Assessment of methods to identify sources of interindividual pharmacokinetic variations. Clin Pharmacol 8:378-409, 1983.

224. Cusi D, Barlassina C, Azzani T, et al: Polymorphism of alpha-adducin and salt-sensitivity in patients with essential hypertension. Lancet 349:1353-1357, 1997.

225. Kuivenhoven JA, Jukema JW, Zwinderman AH, et al: The role of a common variant of the cholersteryl ester transfer protein gene in the progression of coronary atherosclerosis. The Regression Growth Evaluation Statin Study Group. N Engl J Med 338:86-93, 1998.

226. Marshall A: Laying the foundations of personalized medicine. Nat Biothechnol 15:954-957, 1997.

227. Andersen S, Tarnow L, Cambien F, et al: Renoprotective effects of losartan in diabetic nephropathy: Interaction with ACE insertion/deletion genotype? Kidney Int 62:192-198, 2002.

228. Moriyama T, Kitamara H, Ochi S, et al: Association of angiotensin I converting enzyme gene polymorphism with susceptibility to antiproteinuric effect of angiotensin I converting enzyme inhibitors in patients with proteinuria. J Am Soc Nephrol 6:1674-1678, 1995.

229. Jacobsen P, Rossing K, Rossing P, et al: Angiotensin-converting enzyme gene polymorphism and ACE inhibition in diabetic nephropathy. Kidney Int 53:1002-1006, 1998.

230. van der Kleij FGH, Navis GJ, Gansevoort RT, et al: ACE genotype does not determine the short term renal response to ACE inhibition in proteinuric patients. Nephrol Dial Transplant 12(suppl 2):42-46, 1997.

231. Penno G, Chaturvaedi N, Talmud PJ, et al: Effect of angiotensin converting enzyme (ACE) gene polymorphism on progression of renal disease and the influence of ACE inhibition in IDDM patients: Findings from the EUCLID Randomized Controlled Trial. EURODIAB Controlled Trial of Lisinopril in IDDM. Diabetes 47:1507-1511, 1998.

232. Perna A, Ruggenenti P, Testa A, et al: ACE genotype and ACE inhibitors induced renoprotection in chronic proteinuric nephropathies. Kidney Int 57:274-281, 2000.

233. Ruggenenti P, Perna A, Zoccali C, et al: Chronic proteinuric nephropathies II: Outcomes and response to treatment in a prospective cohort of 352 patients: Differences between men and women in relation to the ACE gene polymorphism. Gruppo Italiano di Studi Epidemiologici in Nefrologia (Gisen). J Am Soc Nephrol 11:88-96, 2000.

234. van der Kleij FGH, Schmidt A, Navis GJ, et al: ACE I/D polymorphism and short term response to ACE inhibition: Effect of sodium status. Kidney Int Suppl 63:23-26, 1997.

235. Barlassina C, Schork N, Manunta P, et al: Synergistic effect of alpha-adducin and ACE genes in causing blood pressure changes with body sodium and volume expansion. Kidney Int 57:1083-1090, 2000.

236. Kambham N, Markowitz GS, Valeri AM, et al: Obesity-related glomerulopathy: An emerging epidemic. Kidney Int 59:1498-1509, 2001.

237. Bonnet F, Deprele C, Sassolas A, et al: Excessive body weight as a new independent risk factor for clinical and pathological progression in primary IgA nephritis. Am J Kidney Dis 37:720-724, 2001.

238. Meier-Kriesche HU, Arndorfer JA, Kaplan B: The impact of body mass index on renal transplant outcomes: A significant independent risk factor for graft failure and patient death. Transplantation 15:70-74, 2002.

239. Ribstein J, Du Cailar G, Mimran A: Combined renal effects of overweight and hypertension. Hypertension 26:610-615, 1995.

240. Porter L, Hollenberg NK: Obesity, salt intake and renal perfusion in healthy humans. Hypertension 32:144-148, 1998.

241. Bosma RJ, Homan van der Heide JJ, Oosterop EJ, et al: Body mass index is associated with altered renal hemodynamics in non-obese healthy subjects. Kidney Int 2003 (in press).

242. Wolf G, Chen S, Cheol Han D, Ziadeh FN: Leptin and renal disease. Am J Kidney Dis 39:1-11, 2002.

243. Praga M, Hernandez E, Andres A, et al: Effects of body weight loss and captopril treatment on proteinuria associated with obesity. Nephron 70:35-41, 1995.

244. Orth SR, Ritz E, Schrier RW: The renal risks of smoking. Kidney Int 51:1669-1677, 1997.

245. Maki DD, Ma JZ, Louis TA, Kasiske BL: Long-term effects of antihypertensive agents on proteinuria and renal function. Arch Intern Med 155:1073-1080, 1995.

246. Should all patients with type 1 diabetes mellitus and micro-albuminuria receive angiotensin-converting enzyme inhibitors? A meta-analysis of individual patient data. Ann Intern Med 134:370-379, 2001.

247. Keane WF, Raij L: Relationship among altered glomerular barrier permselectivity, angiotensin II and mesangial uptake of macromolecules. Lab Invest 52:599-604, 1985.

248. Wolf G: Angiotensin as a renal growth promoting factor. Adv Exp Med Biol 377:225-236, 1995.

249. Kon V, Fogo A, Ichikawa I: Bradykinin causes selective efferent arteriolar dilation during angiotensin I converting enzyme inhibition. Kidney Int 44:545-550, 1993.

250. Wapstra FH, Navis GJ, de Jong PE, de Zeeuw D: Chronic angiotensin II-infusion, but not bradykinin blockade abolishes the antiproteinuric response to ACE-inhibition in established Adriamycin nephrosis. J Am Soc Nephrol 11:490-496, 2000.

251. Iyer SN, Chappell MC, Averill DB, et al: Vasodepressor actions of angiotensin (1-7) unmasked during combined treatment with lisinopril and losartan. Hypertension 31:699-705, 1998.

252. Luque M, Martin P, Martell N, et al: Effects of captopril related to increased levels of prostacyclin and angiotensin (1-7) in essential hypertension. J Hyptens 14:799-805, 1996.

253. Hannedouche T, Landais P, Goldfarb B, et al: Randomised controlled trial of enalapril and beta-blockers in non-diabetic chronic renal failure. BMJ 309:833-837, 1994.

254. Giatras I, Lau J, Levey A: Effect of angiotensin converting enzyme inhibitors on the progression of nondiabetic renal disease: A meta-analysis of randomized trials. Angiotensin-Converting-Enzyme Inhibition and Progressive Renal Disease Study Group. Ann Intern Med 127:337-345, 1997.

255. van Essen GG, Apperloo AJ, Rensma PL, et al: Are ACE inhibitors superior to beta-blockers in retarding progressive function decline? Kidney Int Suppl 63:58-62, 1997.

256. Ruggenenti P, Perna A, Gherardi G, et al: Renoprotective properties of ACE-inhibition in non-diabetic nephropathies with non-nephrotic proteinuria. Lancet 354:359-364, 1999.

257. Ruggenenti P, Perna A, Benini R: In chronic nephropathies prolonged ACE inhibition can induce remission: Dynamics of time-dependent changes in GFR. Investigators of the GISEN Group. Gruppo Italiano di Studi Epidemiologici in Nefrologia. J Am Soc Nephrol 10:997-1006, 1999.

258. Ruggenenti P, Schieppati A, Remuzzi G: Progression, remission, regression of chronic renal diseases. Lancet 357:1601-1608, 2001.

259. Ruggenenti P, Perna A, Remuzzi G: ACE inhibitors to prevent end-stage renal disease: When to start and why possibly never to stop: A post-hoc analysis of the REIN trial results. Ramipril Efficacy in Nephropathy. J Am Soc Nephrol 12:2832-2837, 2001.

260. Viberti GC, Mogensen CE, Groop LC, et al: Effect of captopril on the progression to clinical proteinuria in patients with insulin-dependent diabetes mellitus and microalbuminuria. European Microalbuminuria Captopril Study Group. JAMA 271:275-279, 1994.

261. Laffel LMB, McGill JB, Gans DJ: The beneficial effect of angiotensin converting enzyme inhibition with captopril on diabetic nephropathy in normotensive IDDM patients with microalbuminuria. North American Microalbuminuria Study Group. Am J Med 99:497-504, 1995.

262. Captopril reduces the risk of nephropathy in IDDM patients with microalbuminuria. The Microalbuminuria Captopril Study Group. Diabetologia 39:587-593, 1996.

263. Mathiesen ER, Hommel E, Giese J, Parving H-H: Efficacy of captopril in postponing nephropathy in normotensive insulin dependent diabetic patients with microalbuminuria. BMJ 303:81-87, 1991.

264. Ravid M, Lang R, Rachmani R, Lishner M: Long-term renoprotective effect of angiotensin converting enzyme inhibition in non-insulin dependent diabetes mellitus. Arch Intern Med 156:286-289, 1996.

265. Effects of ramipril on cardiovascular and microvascular outcomes in people with diabetes mellitus: Results of the HOPE and MICRO-HOPE study; Heart Outcomes Prevention Evaluation Study Investigators. Lancet 355:253-260, 2000.

266. Apperloo AJ, de Zeeuw D, de Jong PE: Discordant effects of enalapril and lisinopril on systemic and renal hemodynamics. Clin Pharmacol Ther 56:647-658, 1994.

267. Navis GJ, de Zeeuw D, de Jong PE: ACE inhibitors: Panacea for progressive renal disease [editorial]? Lancet 349:1852-1853, 1997.

268. Keiser JA, Bjork FA, Hodges JC, Taylor DG: Renal hemodynamic and excretory responses to PD 123319 and Losartan, nonpeptide

269. AT1 and AT2 subtype specific angiotensin II ligands. J Pharmacol Exp Ther 262:1154-1160, 1992.

269. Remuzzi A, Fassi A, Sangalli F, et al: Prevention of renal injury in diabetic MWF rats by angiotensin II antagonism. Exp Nephrol 6:28-28, 1998.

270. Remuzzi A, Malanchine B, Battaglia C, et al: Comparison of the effects of angiotensin converting enzyme inhibition and angiotensin II receptor blockade on the evolution of spontaneous glomerular injury in male MWF/Ztm rats. Exp Nephrol 4:19-25, 1996.

271. Morrisey JJ, Klahr S: Differential effects of ACE and AT1 receptor inhibition on chemoattractant and adhesion molecules. Am J Physiol 274:F580-F586, 1998.

272. Klahr S, Morrissey JJ: Comparative study of ACE inhibitors and angiotensin II receptor antagonists in interstitial scarring. Kidney Int Suppl 63:111-114, 1997.

273. Chung O, Unger T: Unopposed stimulation of the angiotensin AT2 receptor in the kidney. Nephrol Dial Transplant 13:537-540, 1998.

274. Stoll M, Steckelings UM, Paul M, et al: The angiotensin II AT2 receptor mediates inhibition of cell proliferation in coronary endothelial cells. J Clin Invest 95:651-657, 1995.

275. Yamada T, Horiuchi M, Dzau VJ: Angiotensin II type 2 receptor mediates programmed cell death. Proc Natl Acad Sci U S A 93: 156-160, 1996.

276. Nakajima M, Hutchinson HG, Fujinaga M, et al: The angiotensin II subtype 2 (AT2) receptor antagonizes the growth effects of the AT1 receptor: Gain-of-function study using gene transfer. Proc Natl Acad Sci U S A 92:10663-10667, 1995.

277. Gansevoort RT, de Zeeuw D, de Jong PE: Is the antiproteinuric effect of ACE inhibition mediated by interference in the renin-angiotensin system? Kidney Int 45:861-867, 1994.

278. Buter H, Navis GJ, de Zeeuw D, de Jong PE: Renal hemodynamic effects of candesartan in impaired and normal renal function. Kidney Int Suppl 63:185-187, 1997.

279. Burnier M, Roch-Ramel F, Brunner HR: Renal effects of angiotensin II receptor blockade in normotensive subjects. Kidney Int 49: 1787-1790, 1996.

280. Parving H-H, Lehnert H, Brochner-Mortensen J, et al: The effect of irbesartan on the development of diabetic nephropathy in patients with type 2 diabetes. N Engl J Med 345:870-878, 2001.

281. Tarif N, Bakris G: Preservation of renal function; the spectrum of effects by clacium channel blockers. Nephrol Dial Transplant 12:2244-2250, 1997.

282. Goligorsky MS, Chaimovits C, Rapoport J, et al: Calcium metabolism in uremic nephrocalcinosis: Preventive effect of verapamil. Kidney Int 27:774-779, 1985.

283. Harris DCH, Hammond WS, Burke TJ, Schrier RW: Verapamil protects against progression of experimental chronic renal failure. Kidney Int 31:41-46, 1987.

284. Jackson B, Johnston CI: The contribution of systemic hypertension to progression of chronic renal failure in the rat remnant kidney: Effect of treatment with an angiotensin converting enzyme inhibitor or a calcium inhibitor. J Hypertens 6:495-501, 1988.

285. Brunner FP, Thiel G, Hermle M, et al: Long term enalapril and verapamil in rats with reduced renal mass. Kidney Int 36:969-977, 1989.

286. Jyothirmayi GN, Reddi AS: Effect of diltiazem on glomerular heparan sulfate and albuminuria in diabetic rats. Hypertension 21:795-802, 1993.

287. Griffin KA, Picken MM, Bidani AK: Deleterious effects of calcium channel blockade on pressure transmission and glomerular injury in rat remnant kidneys. J Clin Invest 96:793-800, 1995.

288. Dworkin LD, Benstein JA, Parker M, et al: Calcium antagonists and converting enzyme inhibitors reduce renal injury by different mechanisms. Kidney Int 43:808-814, 1993.

289. Bakris GL, Smith AC: Effects of sodium intake on albumin excretion in patients with diabetic nephropathy treated with long-acting calcium antagonists. Ann Intern Med 125:201-203, 1996.

290. Anderson SA, Rennke HG, Brenner BM, et al: Nifedipine versus fosinopril in uninpehrectomized rats. Kidney Int 41:891-817, 1992.

291. Kobayashi S, Hishida A: Effects of a calcium antagonist, manidipine, on progressive renal injury associated with mild hypertension in remnant kidneys. J Lab Clin Med 125:572-580, 1995.

292. Bidani AK, Griffin KA: Calcium channel blockers and renal protection: Is there an optimal dose? J Lab Clin Med 125:553-555, 1995.

293. Bakris GL, Weir ML: Salt intake and reductions in arterial pressure: Is there a direct link? Am J Hypertens 9(suppl):200-206, 1996.

294. Vincent M, Samani NJ, Gaugier D, et al: A pharmacogenomic approach to blood pressure in Lyon hypertensive rats. A chromosome 2 locus influences the response to calcium antagonist. J Clin Invest 100:2000-2006, 1997.

295. Bakris GL, Copley JB, Vicknair N, et al: Calcium channel blockers versus other antihypertensives on progression of NIDDM associated nephropathy. Kidney Int 50:1641-1650, 1996.

296. Bakris GL, Mangrum A, Copley JB, et al: Calcium channel or beta-blockade on progression of diabetic renal disease in African-American. Hypertension 29:773-780, 1997.

297. Velussi M, Brocco E, Frigato F, et al: Effects of cilazapril and amlodipine on kidney function in hypertensive NIDDM. Diabetes 45:216-222, 1996.

298. Tarnow L, Rossing P, Jensen C, et al: Long term renoprotective benefit of nisoldipine and lisinopril in type 1 diabetic nephropathy. Diabetes Care 23:1725-1730, 2000.

299. Jerums G, Allen TJ, Tsalamandris C, Cooper ME: Angiotensin converting enzyme inhibition and calcium channel blockade in incipient diabetic nephropathy. Kidney Int 41:904-911, 1992.

300. Jerums G, Allen TJ, Campbell DJ, et al: Long term comparison between perindopril and nifedipine in normotensive patients with type 1 diabetes and microalbuminuria. Am J Kidney Dis 37:890-899, 2001.

301. Kopf D, Schmitiz H, Beyer J, et al: A double-blind study of perindopril and nitrendipine in incipient diabetic nephropathy. Diabetes Nutr Metab 14:245-252, 2001.

302. Fogari R, Zoppi A, Corradi L, et al: Long term effects of ramipril and nitrendipine on albuminuria in hypertensive patients with type II diabetes and impaired renal function. J Hum Hypertens 13:47-53, 1999.

303. Zucchelli P, Zuccala A, Borghi M, et al: Long term comparison between captopril and nifedipine in the progression of renal insufficiency. Kidney Int 42:452-458, 1992.

304. Voyaki SM, Staessen JA, Thijs L, et al: Follow-up of renal function in treated and untreated older patients with isolated systolic hypertension. Systolic Hypertension in Europe (Syst-Eur) Trial Investigators. J Hypertens 19:511-519, 2001.

305. Rekola A, Bergstrand A, Bucht H: Deterioration rate in IgA nephropathy: Comparison of a converting enzyme inhibitor and beta-blocking agents. Nephron 59:57-60, 1991.

306. Nielsen FS, Rossing P, Gall MA, et al: Long term effect of lisinopril and atenolol on kidney function in hypertensive NIDDM subjects with diabetic nephropathy. Diabetes 46:1182-1188, 1997.

307. Elving LD, Wetzels JFM, van Lier HJJ, et al: Captopril and atenolol are equally effective in retarding progression of diabetic nephropathy. Diabetologia 37:604-609, 1994.

308. UK Prospective Diabetes Study Group: Efficacy of atenolol and enalapril in reducing risk of macrovascular and microvascular complications in type 2 diabetes" UKPDS 39. BMJ 317:713-720, 1998.

309. The sixth report of the Joint National Committee on prevention, detection, evaluation and treatment of high blood pressure. Arch Intern Med 157:2413-2445, 1997.

310. Susic D, Frohlich ED: Nephroprotective effect of antihypertensive drugs in essential hypertension. J Hypertens 16:555-567, 1998.

311. Ono H, Ono Y, Frohlich ED: Hydrochlorothiazide exacerbates nitric oxide blockade nephrosclerosis with glomerular hypertension in spontaneously hypertensive rats. J Hypertens 14:823-828, 1996.

312. Benstein JA, Feiner HD, Parker M, Dworkin LD: Superiority of salt restriction over diuretics in reducing renal hypertrophy and injury in uninephrectomized SHR: Am J Physiol 258:F1675-F1681, 1990.

313. Buter H, Hemmelder MH, Navis GJ, et al: Blunting of the antiproteinuric efficacy of ACE inhibition by high sodium intake can be restored by hydrochlorothiazide. Nephrol Dial Transplant 13:1682-1685, 1998.

314. Chrysostomou A, Becker G: Spironolactone in addition to ACE inhibition to reduce proteinuria in patients with chronic renal disease. N Engl J Med 345:925-926, 2001.

315. Heeg JE, de Jong PE, van der Hem GK, de Zeeuw D: Reduction of proteinuria by angiotensin converting enzyme inhibition. Kidney Int 32:78-83, 1987.

316. Weidmann P, Schneider M, Böhlen L: Therapeutic efficacy of different antihypertensive drugs in human diabetic nephropathy: An updated meta-analysis. Nephrol Dial Transplant 10(suppl 9):39-45, 1995.

317. Kasiske BL, Kalil RSN, Ma JZ, et al: Effect of antihypertensive therapy on the kidney in patients with diabetes: A meta-regression analysis. Ann Intern Med 118:129-138, 1993.

318. Gansevoort RT, de Zeeuw D, de Jong PE: Dissociation between the course of the hemodynamic and antiproteinuric effects of angiotensin-I converting enzyme inhibition. Kidney Int 44:579-584, 1993.

319. Remuzzi A, Pertiucci E, Ruggenenti P, et al: Angiotensin converting enzyme inhibition improves glomerular size-selectivity in IgA nephropathy. Kidney Int 39:1267-1273, 1991.

320. Nankervis A, Nicholls K, Kilmartin G, et al: Effects of perindopril on renal histomorphometry in diabetic subjects with microalbuminuria: A 3-year placebo-controlled study. Metabolism 47(suppl 1):12-15, 1998.

321. Rudberg S, Aperia A, Freyschuss U, Persson B: Enalapril reduces microalbuminuria in young normotensive type I (insulin-dependent) diabetic patients irrespective of its hypotensive effect. Diabetologia 33:470-476, 1990.

322. de Zeeuw D, Navis GJ: Optimizing the RAAS intervention treatment strategy in diabetic and non-diabetic nephropathy: The potential of exploring the mechanisms of response variability. In Mogensen CE (ed): Diabetic Nephropathy in Type 2 Diabetes. London, Science Press, 2002, pp 103-116.

323. Schulz E, Beck J, Pedersen EB, et al: Tolerability and antihypertensive efficacy of losartan vs captopril in patients with mild to moderate hypertension and impaired renal function A randomized, double-blind, parallel study. Clin Drug Invest 19:183-194, 2000.

324. Fernandez-Andrade C, Russo D, Iversen B, et al: Comparison of losartan and amlodipine in renally impaired hypertensive patients. Kidney Int Suppl 68:120-124, 1998.

325. Caruso D, D'isanto F, Del Piano C, Caruso G: Losartan versus amlodipine in double blind study in hypertensive patients with diabetic nephropathy. J Human Hypertens 13(suppl 3):5, 1999.

326. Calvino J, Lens XM, Romero R, Sanchez GD: Long-term antiproteinuric effect of losartan in renal transplant recipients treated for hypertension. Nephrol Dial Transplant 15:82-86, 2000.

327. DelCastillo D, Campistol JM, Guirado L, et al: Efficacy and safety of losartan in the treatment of hypertension in renal transplant recipients. Kidney Int Suppl 68:135-139, 1998.

328. Hadjigavriel M, Kyriakides G: Efficacy and safety of losartan in renal transplant recipients. Transplant Proc 31:3300-3301, 1999.

329. Holgado R, Del Castillo D: Angiotensin II type I (AT1) receptor antagonists in the treatment of hypertension after renal transplantation. Nephrol Dial Transplant 16(suppl 6):1-4, 2001.

330. Mora-Macia J, Cases A, Calero F, Barcelo P: Effect of angiotensin II receptor blockade on renal disease progression in patients with non-diabetic chronic renal failure. Nephrol Dial Transplant 16(suppl 6): 1-3, 2001.

331. Campistol JM, Inigo P, Jimenez W, et al: Losartan decreases plasma levels of TGF-beta 1 in transplant patients with chronic allograft nephropathy. Kidney Int 56:714-719, 1999.

332. Holdaas H, Hartmann A, Berg KJ, et al: Renal effects of losartan and amlodipine in hypertensive patients with non-diabetic nephropathy. Nephrol Dial Transplant 13:3096-3102, 1998.

333. Schiller A, Ivan V, Gluhovschi L, et al: Short-term therapy with AII receptor blocker losartan. Cardiac and renal effects in patients with essential hypertension and hypertension of glomerular origin [abstract]. Nephrol Dial Transplant 14(suppl 9):63, 1999.

334. Andersen S, Rossing P, Juhl TR, et al: Optimal dose for losartan in renoprotection in diabetic nephropathy. Nephrol Dial Transplant 17:1413-1418, 2002.

335. Bos H, Andersen S, Rossing P, et al: The role of patient factors in therapy resistance to antiproteinuric intervention in non-diabetic and diabetic nephropathy. Kidney Int Suppl 75:32-37, 2000.

336. van Paassen P, de Zeeuw D, Navis GJ, de Jong PE: Renal and systemic effects of continued treatment with renin inhibitor remikiren in hypertensive patients with normal and impaired renal function. Nephrol Dial Transplant 15:637-643, 2000.

337. Bakris GL, Barnhill BW, Sadler R: Treatment of arterial hypertension in diabetic humans: Importance of therapeutic selection. Kidney Int 41:912-919, 1992.

338. Slataper R, Vicknair N, Sadler R, Bakris GL: Comparative effects of different antihypertensive treatments on progression of diabetic renal disease. Arch Intern Med 153:973-980, 1993.

339. Mimran A, Insua A, Ribstein J, et al: Contrasting effects of captopril and nifedipine in normotensive patients with incipient diabetic nephropathy. J Hypertens 6:919-923, 1988.

340. Demarie BK, Bakris GL: Effect of different calcium antagonists on proteinuria associated with diabetes mellitus. Ann Intern Med 113:987-988, 1990.

341. Comparison between perindopril and nifedipine in hypertensive and normotensive diabetic patients with microalbuminuria. Melbourne Diabetic Nephropathy Study Group. BMJ 302:210-216, 1992.

342. Hemmelder MH, de Zeeuw D, de Jong PE: Antiproteinuric efficacy of verapamil in comparison to trandolapril in non-diabetic renal disease. Nephrol Dial Transplant 14:98-104, 1999.

343. Apperloo AJ, de Zeeuw D, Sluiter HE, de Jong PE: Differential effects of enalapril and atenolol on proteinuria and renal hemodynamics in non-diabetic renal disease. BMJ 303:821-824, 1991.

344. Björk S, Mulec H, Johnson SA, et al: Renal protective effect of enalapril in diabetic nephropathy. BMJ 304:339-343, 1992.

345. Erley CM, Harrere U, Krämer BK, Risler T: Renal hemodynamics and reduction of proteinuria by a vasodilating beta-blocker versus and ACE inhibitor. Kidney Int 41:1297-1303, 1992.

346. Flack JR, Molyneaux L, Willey K, Yue DK: Regression of microalbuminuria: Results of a controlled study, indapamide versus captopril. J Cardiovasc Pharmacol 22(suppl 6):75-77, 1993.

347. Hallab M, Gallois Y, Chatellier G, et al: Comparison of reduction in microalbuminuria by enalapril and hydrochlorothiazide in normotensive patients with insulin dependent diabetes mellitus. BMJ 306:175-181, 1993.

348. Stornello M, Valvo EV, Scapatello L: Comparative effects of enalapril, atenolol and chlorthalidone on blood pressure and kidney function of diabetic patients affected by arterial hypertension and persistent proteinuria. Nephron 58:52-57, 1991.

349. Heeg JE, de Jong PE, van der Hem GK, de Zeeuw D: Efficacy and variability of the antiproteinuric effect of lisinopril. Kidney Int 36:272-279, 1989.

350. Erley CM, Haefele U, Heyne N, et al: Microalbuminuria in essential hypertension. Reduction by different antihypertensive drugs. Hypertension: 21:810-815, 1993.

351. Vriesendorp R, Donker AJM, de Zeeuw D: Effects of non-steroidal anti-inflammatory drugs on proteinuria. Am J Med 81(suppl 2B):84-93, 1986.

352. Rabelink A, Erkelens D, Hené R, et al: Effect of simvastatin and cholestyramine on lipoprotein profile in hyperlipidemia of nephrotic syndrome. Lancet 2:1335-1337, 1988.

353. Massy ZA, Ma JZ, Louis TA, Kasiske BL: Lipid lowering therapy in patients with renal disease. Kidney Int 48:188-198, 1995.

354. Warwick GL, Packard CJ, Murray L, et al: Effect of simvastatin on plasma lipid and lipoprotein concentration and low-density lipoprtoein metabolism in the nephrotic syndrome. Cli Sci 82:701-708, 1992.

355. Kostner GM, Gavish D, Leopold B, et al: HMG-CoA reductase inhibitors lower LDL cholesterol without reducing Lp(a) levels. Circulation 80:1313-1319, 1989.

356. Lam KSL, Cheng IKP, Janus ED, Pang RWC: Cholesterol lowering therapy may retard the progression of diabetic nephropathy. Diabetologia 38:604-609, 1995.

357. Hommel E, Andersen P, Gall M, et al: Plasma lipoproteins and renal function during simvastatin treatment in diabetic nephropathy. Diabetologia 35:447-451, 1992.

358. Shoyi J, Nishizawa Y, Toyokawa A, et al: Decreased albuminuria by pravastatin in hyperlipidemic diabetics. Nephron 59:664-665, 1991.

359. Hoogerbrugge N, Jansen H, de Heide L, et al: The additional effects of acipimox to simvastatin in the tretament of combined hyperlipidemia. J Intern med 241:151-155, 1997.

360. Navis GJ, Buter H, de Jong PE, et al: Effect of antiproteinuric treatment on the lipid profile in non-diabetic renal disease. Contrib Nephrol 120:88-96, 1997.

361. Gansevoort RT, Heeg JE, Dikkeschei FD, et al: Symptomatic antiproteinuric treatment decreases serum lipoprotein (a) concentration in patients with glomerular proteinuria. Nephrol Dial Transplant 9:244-250, 1994.

362. Praga M, Hernandez E, Montoyo C, et al: Long term beneficial effects of angiotensin converting enzyme inhibition in patients with nephrotic syndrome. Am J Kidney Dis 20:240-248, 1992.

363. Gansevoort RT, de Zeeuw D, de Jong PE: Additive antiproteinuric effect of ACE-inhibition and a low protein diet in human renal disease. Nephrol Dial Transplant 10:497-504, 1995.

364. de Zeeuw D, Gansevoort RT, de Jong PE: Angiotensin II antagonism improves the lipoprotein profile in patients with nephrotic syndrome. J Hypertens 13(suppl 1):53-58, 1995.

365. Heeg JE, de Jong PE, Vriesendorp R, de Zeeuw D: Additive antiproteinuric effect of the NSAID indomethacin and the ACE-inhibitor lisinopril. Am J Nephrol 10(suppl):94-97, 1990.

366. Keilani T, Schlueter WA, Levin ML, Batlle DC: Improvement of lipid abnormalities associated with proteinuria using fosinopril, an angiotensin converting enzyme inhibitor. Ann Intern Med 118:246-254, 1993.

367. Hebert LA, Bain RP, Verme D, et al: Remission of nephrotic range proteinuria in type I diabetics. Kidney Int 46:1688-1693, 1994.

368. Nielsen FS, Rossing P, Gall M-A, et al: Impact of lisinopril and atenolol on kidney function in hypertensive NIDDM subjects with diabetic nephropathy. Diabetes 43:1108-1113, 1994.

369. Romero R, Salinas I, Lucas A, et al: Renal function changes in microalbuminuric normotensive type II diabetic patients treated with angiotensin converting enzyme inhibitors. Diabetes Care 16:597-600, 1993.

370. Ravid M, Neumann L, Lishener M: Plasma lipids and the progression of nephropathy in diabetes mellitus type II: Effect of ACE inhibitors. Kidney Int 47:907-910, 1995.

371. Buter H, van Tol A, Navis GJ, et al: Angiotensin II receptor antagonist treatment lowers plasma total and very low plus low density lipoprotein cholesterol in type 1 diabetic patients with albuminuria without affecting plasma cholesterol esterification and cholesteryl ester transfer. Diabet Med 17:550-552, 2000.

372. Kuster S, Mehls O, Seidel C, Ritz E: Blood pressure in minimal change and other types of nephrotic syndrome. Am J Nephrol 10(suppl 1):76-80, 1990.

373. Diamond JR: Analogous pathobiological mechanisms in glomerulosclerosis and atherosclerosis. Kidney Int Suppl 31:39-34, 1991.

374. Ritz E, Koch M: Morbidity and mortality due to hypertension in patients with renal failure. Am J Kidney Dis 21:113-118, 1993.

375. Staessen JA, Wang JG, Ginocchio G, et al: The deletion/insertion polymorphism of the angiotensin converting enzyme gene and cardiovascular-renal risk. J Hypertens 15:1579-1592, 1997.

376. Ordonez JD, Hiatt RA, Killebrew EJ, Fireman BH: The increased risk of coronary heart disease associated with the nephrotic syndrome. Kidney Int 44:638-642, 1993.

377. Radhakrishan J, Appel AS, Valeri A, Appel GB: The nephrotic syndrome, lipids and risk factors for cardiovascular disease. Am J Kidney Dis 22:135-142, 1993.

378. Wanner C, Rader D, Bartens W, et al: Elevated plasma lipoprotein (a) in patients with the nephrotic syndrome. Ann Intern Med 119:263-269, 1993.

379. Stroes ESG, Joles JA, Chang PC, et al: Impaired endothelial function in patients with nephrotic range proteinuria. Kidney Int 48:544-550, 1995.

380. Vuong TD, de Kimpe S, de Roos R, et al: Albumin restores lysophosphatidylcholine induced inhibition of vasodilation in rat aorta. Kidney Int 60:1088-1096, 2001.

381. Hernandez E, Toledo T, Alamo C, et al: Elevation of von Willebrand factor levels in patients with IgA nephropathy: effect of ACE inhibition. Am J Kidney Dis 30:397-403, 1997.

382. Borch-Johnsen K, Andersen PK, Deckert T: The effect of proteinuria on relative mortality in type 1 (insulin-dependent) diabetes mellitus. Diabetologia 28:590-596, 1985.

383. Mogensen CE: Microalbuminuria predicts clinical proteinuria and early mortality in maturity onset diabetes. N Engl J Med 310:356-360, 1984.

384. Gall M-A, Borch-Johnsen K, Hougaard P, et al: Albuminuria and poor glycemic control predict mortality in NIDDM. Diabetes 44:1303-1309, 1994.

385. Kannel WB, Stampfer MJ, Castelli WP, Verter J: The prognostic significance of proteinuria: The Framingham study. Am Heart J 108:1347-1352, 1984.

386. Grimm RH Jr, Svendsen KH, Kasiske B, et al: Proteinuria is a risk factor for mortality over 10 years of follow-up. The MRFIT Research Group. Multiple Risk Factor Intervention Trial. Kidney Int Suppl 63:10-14, 1997.

387. Yudkin JS, Forrest RD, Jackson CA: Microalbuminuria as predictor of vascular disease in non-diabetic subjects. Lancet 2:530-533, 1988.

388. Deckert T, Feldt-Rasmussen B, Borch-Johnsen K, et al: Albuminuria reflects widespread vascular damage. The Steno hypothesis. Diabetologia 32:219-226, 1989.

389. Bigazzi R, Bianchi S, Baldari D, et al: Microalbuminuria in salt-sensitive patients. A marker for renal and cardiovascular risk factors. Hypertension 23:195-199, 1994.

390. Bianchi S, Bigazzi R, Valtriani C, et al: Elevated serum insulin levels in patients with essential hypertension and microalbuminuria. Hypertension 23:681-687, 1994.

391. Kimura G, Frem GJ, Brenner BM: Renal mechanisms of salt sensitivity in hypertension. Curr Opin Nephrol Hypertens 3:1-12, 1994.

392. Ramsay EL: The hypertension detection and follow-up program: 17 years on. JAMA 277:167-170, 1997.

393. Van der Kleij FGH, Navis GJ, Kistemaker TJ, et al: Benefit of renoprotective therapy in chronic renal failure: Impact of pre-study renal function decline and ACE I/D polymorphism. J Am Soc Nephrol 9:A0418, 1998.

394. Hansson L, Zanchetti A, Carruthers SG, et al: Effects of intensive blood pressure lowering and low-dose aspirin in patients with hypertension. Results of the Hypertension Optimal Treatment (HOT) randomised trial. Lancet 351:1755-1763, 1998.

395. Susic D, Frohlich ED: Nephroprotective effect of antihypertensive drugs in essential hypertension. J Hypertens 16:555-567, 1998.

396. 1995 Update of the Working Group Reports on Chronic Renal Failure and Renovascular Hypertension. National High Blood Pressure Education Program Working Group. Arch Intern Med 156:1938-1947, 1996.

397. Parving H-H: The use of antihypertensive agents in prevention and treatment of diabetic nephropathy. Curr Opin Nephrol Hypertens 3:292-300, 1994.

398. Kawazu S, Tomomo S, Shimizu M, et al: The relationship between early diabetic nephropathy and control of plasma glucose in non-insulin dependent diabetes mellitus. The effect of glycemic control on the development and progression of diabetic nephropathy in an 8-year follow-up. J Diabetes Complications 8:13-17, 1994.

399. Parving HH, Oxenbøll B, Svendsen PA, et al: Early detection of patients at risk of developing diabetic nephropathy. Acta Endocrinol (Copenh) 100:550-555, 1982.

400. Viberti GC, Hill RD, Jarrett RJ, et al: Microalbuminuria as a predictor of clinical nephropathy in insulin dependent diabetes mellitus. Lancet 1:1430-1432, 1982.

401. Mogensen CE, Christensen CK: Predicting diabetic nephropathy in insulin-dependent patients. N Engl J Med 311:89-93, 1984.

402. Mathiesen ER, Oxenbøll B, Johansen K, et al: Incipient nephropathy in type I (insulin dependent) diabetes. Diabetologia 26:406-410, 1984.

403. American Diabetes Association: Diabetic nephropathy. Position Statement. Diabetes Care 20(suppl 1):24-27, 1997.

404. Bennett PH, Haffner S, Kasiske BL, et al: Screening and management of microalbuminuria in patients with diabetes mellitus: Recommendations of the Scientific Advisory Board of the National Kidney Foundation from an ad hoc committee of the Council on Diabetes Mellitus of the National Kidney Foundation. Am J Kidney Dis 25:107-112, 1995.

405. Mogensen CE: Management of early nephropathy in diabetic patients: With emphasis on microalbuminuria. Annu Rev Med 46:79-94, 1995.

406. Parving HH, Jacobsen P, Rossing K, et al: Benefits of long-term antihypertensive treatment on prognosis in diabetic nephropathy. Kidney Int 49:1778-1782, 1996.

407. Euclid Study Group: Randomized placebo-controlled trial of lisinopril in normotensive patients with insulin-dependent diabetes and normoalbuminuria or microalbuminuria. Lancet 349:1787-1792, 1997.

408. Wang PH: When should ACE inhibitors be given to normotensive patients with IDDM. Lancet 349:1782-1783, 1997.

409. Lazarus JM, Bourgoignie JJ, Buckalew VM, et al: Achievement and safety of a low blood pressure goal in chronic renal disease. The Modification of Diet in Renal Disease Study Group. Hypertension 29:641-650, 1997.

410. Pedrini MT, Levey AS, Lau J, et al: The effect of dietary protein restriction on the progression of diabetic and non-diabetic renal diseases: A meta-analysis. Ann Intern Med 124:627-632, 1996.

411. Levey AS, Adler S, Caggiula AW, et al: Effects of dietary protein restriction on the progression of advanced renal disease in the Modification of Diet in Renal Disease Study. Am J Kidney Dis 27:652-663, 1996.

412. Walser MM, Drew HH, LaFrance LD: Creatinine measurements often yield false estimates in chronic renal failure. Kidney Int 34:412-418, 1988.

413. Effects of diet and antihypertensive therapy on creatinine clearance and serum creatinine concentration in the Modification of Diet in Renal Disease Study. J Am Soc Nephrol 4:556-565, 1996.

414. Levey AS, Green T, Schluchter MD, et al: Glomerular filtration rate in clinical trials. Modification of Diet in Renal Disease Study Group and the Diabetes Control and Complications Trial Research Group. J Am Soc Nephrol 4:1159-1171, 1993.

415. Apperloo AJ, de Zeeuw D, de Jong PE: Precision of GFR determinations for long term slope calculations is improved by simultaneous infusion of ^{125}I-iothalamate and ^{131}I-hippuran. J Am Soc Nephrol 7:567-572, 1996.

416. Mathiesen ER, Feldt-Rasmussen B, Hommel E, et al: Stable glomerular filtration rate in normotensive IDDM patients with stable microalbuminuria. Diabetes Care 26:286-289, 1997.

417. Koomans HA, Roos JC, Boer P, et al: Salt sensitivity of blood pressure in chronic renal failure. Evidence for renal control of body fluid volume distribution. Hypertension 4:190-192, 1982.

418. Strojek K, Grzeszczak W, Lacha B, et al: Increased prevalence of salt sensitivity of blood pressure in IDDM with and without microalbuminuria. Diabetologia 38:1443-1448, 1995.

419. Dworkin LD, Benstein JA, Tolbert E, Feiner HD: Salt restriction inhibits renal growth and stabilizes renal injury in rats with established renal disease. J Am Soc Nephrol 7:437-442, 1996.

420. Allen TJ, Waldron MJ, Casley D, et al: Salt restriction reduces hyperfiltration, renal enlargement and albuminuria in experimental diabetes. Diabetes 46:19-24, 1997.

421. Weir MR, Dengel DR, Behrens MT, Goldberg AP: Salt induced increases in systolic pressure affect renal hemodynamics. Hypertension 25:1339-1344, 1995.

422. van Paassen P, de Zeeuw D, Navis GJ, de Jong PE: Does the renin-angiotensin system determine the renal and systemic hemodynamic response to sodium in patients with essential hypertension? Hypertension 27:202-205, 1996.

423. Navis GJ, de Jong PE, Donker AJM, et al: Moderate sodium restriction in hypertensive subjects: Renal effects of ACE-inhibition. Kidney Int 31:815-819, 1987.

424. Burnier M, Rutschman B, Nussberger J, et al: Salt-dependent renal effects of an angiotensin II antagonist in healthy subjects. Hypertension 22:339-347, 1993.

425. Denolle T, Luo P, Guyene TT, et al: Acute effects of a pseudo-tetrapeptidase renin-inhibitor on blood pressure and renin-angiotensin system of sodium repleted and sodium depleted patients. Arzneimittelforschung 43:255-259, 1993.

426. Philipp T, Letzel H, Arens HJ: Dose-finding study of candesartan cilexetil plus hydrochlorothiazide in patients with mild to moderate hypertension. J Hum Hypertens 11(suppl 2):67-68, 1997.

427. Jerums G, Allen TJ, Tsalamandris C, Cooper ME: Angiotensin converting enzyme inhibition and calcium channel blockade in incipient diabetic nephropathy. Kidney Int 41:904-911, 1992.

428. Morgan T, Anderson A, Wilson D, et al: Paradoxical effect of sodium restriction on blood pressure in people on slow-channel calcium blocking drugs. Lancet 1:793, 1986.

429. Weinberger MH: The relationship of sodium balance and concomitant diuretic therapy to blood pressure response with calcium channel entry blockers. Am J Med 90(suppl 5a):15-20, 1991.

430. Weir MR: The influence of dietary salt on the antiproteinuric effect of calcium channel blockers. Am J Kidney Dis 29:800-805, 1997.

431. Ruilope LM, Casal MC, Praga M, et al: Additive antiproteinuric effect of converting enzyme inhibition and a low protein intake. J Am Soc Nephrol 3:1307-1311, 1992.

432. Rudberg S, Aperia A, Freyschuss U, Persson B: Enalapril reduces microalbuminuria in young normotensive type 1 (insulin-dependent) diabetic patients irrespective of its hypotensive effect. Diabetologia 33:470-476, 1990.

433. Palla R, Panichi V, Finato V, et al: Effect of increasing doese of lisinopril on proteinuria of normotensive patients with IgA nephropathy and normal renal function. Int J Clin Pharmacol Res 14:35-43, 1994.

434. Laverman GD, Navis GJ, Henning RH, et al: Dual renin-angiotensin system blockade at optimal doses for proteinuria. Kidney Int 62:1020-1025, 2002.

435. Laverman GD, de Jong PE, Henning RH, et al: Dose-response of losartan in proteinuric renal disease. Am J Kidney Dis 38:1381-1384, 2001.

436. Weinberg MS, Weinberg AJ, Cord R, Zappe DH: The effect of high-dose angiotensin II receptor blockade beyond maximal recommended doses in reducing urinary protein secretion. J Renin Angiotensin Aldosterone Syst 2(suppl 1):196-198, 2001.

437. Haas M, Leko-Mohr Z, Erler C, Mayer G: Antiproteinuric versus antihypertensive effects of high-dose ACE inhibitor therapy. Am J Kidney Dis 40:458-463, 2002.

438. Perico N, Remuzzi A, Sangalli F, et al: The antiproteinuric effect of angiotensin antagonism in human IgA nephropathy is potentiated by indomethacin. J Am Soc Nephrol 9:2308-2317, 1998.

439. Navis GJ, Faber HJ, de Zeeuw D, de Jong PE: ACE-inhibitors and the kidney: A risk-benefit assessment. Drug Saf 15:200-211, 1996.

440. Bakris GL, Griffin KA, Picken MM, Bidani AK: Combined effects of an angiotensin converting enzyme inhibitor and a calcium antagonist on renal injury. J Hypertens 15:1181-1185, 1997.

441. Azizi M, Chatelier G, Guyene TT, et al: Additive effects of combined angiotensin-converting enzyme inhibition and angiotensin II antagonism on blood pressure and renin release in sodium-depleted normotensives. Circulation 92:825-834, 1995.

442. Richer C, Bruneval P, Menard J, Giudicelli JF: Additive effects of enalapril and losartan in (mRen-2) 27 transgenic rats. Hypertension 31:692-698, 1998.

443. Fossa AA, Weinberg LJ, Barber RL, et al: Synergistic effect on reduction in blood pressure with co-administration of the renin-inhibitor CP 80,794, and the angiotensin converting enzyme inhibitor captopril. J Cardiovasc Pharmacol 20:75-82, 1992.

444. Mogensen CE, Neldam S, Tikkanen I, et al: Randomised controlled trial of dual blockade of renin-angiotensin system in patients with hypertension, microalbuminuria, and non–insulin dependent diabetes: The candesartan and lisinopril microalbuminuria (CALM) study. BMJ 321:1440-1444, 2000.

445. Russo D, Pisani A, Balletta MM, et al: Additive antiproteinuric effect of converting enzyme inhibitor and losartan in normotensive patients with IgA nephropathy. Am J Kidney Dis 33:851-856, 1999.

446. Russo D, Minutolo R, Pisana A, et al: Coadministration of losartan and enalapril exerts additive antiproteinuric effect in IgA nephropathy. Am J Kidney Dis 38:18-25, 2001.

447. Agarwal R: Add-on angiotensin receptor blockade with maximized ACE-inhibition. Kidney Int 59:2282-2289, 2001.

448. Bos H, Henning RH, de Jong PE, et al: Addition of AT1 receptor blockade fails to overcome resistance to ACE inhibition in Adriamycin nephrosis. Kidney Int 61:473-480, 2002.

449. Zoja C, Corna D, Rottoli D, et al: Effect of combining ACE inhibitor and statin in severe experimental nephropathy. Kidney Int 61:1635-1645, 2000.

450. Remuzzi G, Zoja C, Gagliardini E, et al: Combining an antiproteinuric approach with mycophenolate mofetil fully suppresses progressive nephropathy of experimental animals. J Am Soc Nephrol 10:1542-1549, 1999.

451. Buter H, Navis GJ, Dullaart RPF, et al: Time course of the antiproteinuric and renal haemodynamic responses to losartan in micro-albuminuric IDDM: Nephrol Dial Transplant 16:771-775, 2001.

452. Buter H, Hemmelder M, van Paassen P, et al: Is the reduction of proteinuria by RAAS blockade less effective during the night? Nephrol Dial Transplant 12(suppl 2):53-56, 1997.

453. Dickerson JEC, Hingorani AD, Ashby MJ, et al: Optimisation of antihypertensive treatment by crossover rotation of four major classes. Lancet 353:2008-2013, 1999.

454. Navis G, de Jong P, Donker AJ, et al: Diuretic effects of angiotensin-converting enzyme inhibition: Comparison of low and liberal sodium diet in hypertensive patients. J Cardiovasc Pharmacol 9:743-748, 1987.

455. Navis GJ, de Jong PE, Donker AJM, et al: Moderate sodium restriction in hypertensive subjects: Renal effects of ACE-inhibition. Kidney Int 31:815-819, 1987.

456. Lansang MC, Price DA, Laffel LM, et al: Renal vascular responses to captopril and to candesartan in patients with type 1 diabetes mellitus. Kidney Int 59:1432-1438, 2001.

457. Laverman GD, de Zeeuw D, Navis GJ: Between-patient differences in the renal response to renin-angiotensin system intervention: Clue to optimizing renoprotective therapy? J Renin Angiotensin Aldosterone Syst 3:205-213, 2002.

458. Weir MR, Saunders E: Differing mechanisms of action of angiotensin converting enzyme inhibition in black and white hypertensive patients. Hypertension 26:124-130, 1995.

459. Hollenberg NK, Anzalone DA, Falkner B, et al: Familial factors in the antihypertensive response to lisinopril. Am J Hypertens 14:218-223, 2000.

CHAPTER 57

Nutritional Therapy in Renal Disease

William E. Mitch and Mackenzie Walser

ASSESSMENT OF RENAL FUNCTION

Renal Plasma Flow and GFR in Normal Adults

Measurements of renal function made without the use of creatinine or cystatin C levels are considered first.

From the literature Wesson[1] compiled measurements of renal plasma flow (RPF) and glomerular filtration rate (GFR, expressed as mL/min/1.73 m^2) from a total of 488 normal men and 188 normal women. The ranges were extremely wide (threefold to fivefold). Means in younger men and women were 655 and 600 mL/min/1.73 m^2 for RPF and 130 and 120 mL/min/1.73 m^2 for GFR, respectively.

Some of the factors that account for this wide variation are considered in the following sections.

Effect of Race

Price and associates[2] compared renal function in normal African Americans with age-matched whites. GFRs were similar, but RPF was slightly, but significantly lower in African Americans. Major differences were seen in the intrarenal renin system: African Americans showed a sevenfold greater vasodilator response to captopril and a significantly smaller vasoconstrictor response to angiotensin II—a response that was accentuated after angiotensin-converting enzyme (ACE) inhibition. Plasma renin activity was not different. The results indicate that the intrarenal renin system is chronically activated in African Americans in comparison to whites.

Effect of Body Size in Adults

Traditionally, GFR and RPF have been "corrected" or "indexed" for body size by expressing these measurements per 1.73 m^2 of body surface area (BSA), as first suggested by McIntosh and co-workers.[3] It is generally presumed that this correction allows more appropriate comparisons not only of individual values but also of means of different groups.

These assumptions have repeatedly been shown to be invalid. In monitoring individual patients, uncorrected GFR values are generally more useful, in part because an indexed GFR depends on surface area, which is slightly different at each visit as a result of weight variation. More to the point, Dooley and Poole[4] found no correlation between GFR and BSA in 122 adults with cancer. In addition, progressive changes in weight can make a corrected GFR appear to change progressively in the opposite direction, even when the uncorrected GFR is constant. An example is shown in Figure 57-1. Furthermore, the precision of replicate measurements of GFR—or the precision of the standard error of the estimate of GFR about the regression of GFR on time (a measure of progression)—will be underestimated if the variability in weight is included in the calculation.[5] Thus, the only rationale for using corrected GFR in an individual patient is to determine whether the GFR is within normal limits. From a practical point of view, this information is relatively unimportant because renal disease can exist with a GFR within or outside the normal range. Hence, in monitoring individual patients, correction of GFR for body size is not only unnecessary but undesirable.

Nevertheless, consideration must be given to an alternative that arose when GFR measurements were first derived from the plasma disappearance curve of a tracer administered in a single injection. This slope—usually expressed as the corresponding half life ($t_{1/2}$)—is the quotient of the GFR divided by the volume of distribution of the tracer, which approximates the extracellular fluid volume for many tracers. Hence, the slope contains a built-in correction for body size. The same may be said for single-sample methods, which typically have less error than slope-intercept methods.[6] Blake and colleagues[5] found that the year-to-year variability (about the regression line) of $t_{1/2}$ was less than the year-to-year variability in GFR in a group of patients with chronic renal disease. Thus, monitoring patients by sequential measurement of $t_{1/2}$ yields greater precision than does sequential measurement of uncorrected GFR. In children, Peters and associates[7] maintain that the optimal normalization variable for GFR is extracellular fluid volume. Singer[8] and Singer and Morton[9] give arguments for using the metabolic rate. More information is provided in Chapter 24.

In comparing groups of subjects, some correction for body size is clearly mandatory. Turner and Reilly[10] have shown that indexing the RPF of normal adults for surface area leads to negative dependency on surface area and fails to eliminate the positive dependency of GFR on surface area. They recommend that regression be used to define the normal relationships between RPF, GFR, and BSA to yield expressions that are gender, age, and BSA independent, and they formulated equations based on their sample of 78 normal men and 78 normal women, as shown in Table 57-1. Age in the subjects in Table 57-1 varied from 20 to 50 years. No attempt was made to determine the age dependence of the results. Different regressions were reported for RPF and GFR when estimated as clearances by infusion techniques. Thus, Table 57-1 shows that for a man with 1.73 m^2 of surface area, the predicted RPF is $(141 \times 1.73) + 359$, or 603 mL/min, and the predicted GFR is $(69 \times 1.73) - 17$, or 102 mL/min.

Schmieder and co-workers[11] reported observations in normal subjects, including obese persons, but limited their measurements to RPF. They found that RPF varied with height but not with surface area. Age was also an important determinant, but the coefficients of these regressions were not provided. Opposite findings were reported almost simultaneously by Ribstein and colleagues.[12] Obese individuals had increased GFR and RPF, whether expressed without correction or per meter of height. However, Anastasio and co-workers[13] report that GFR/height is not different from normal in severely overweight subjects.

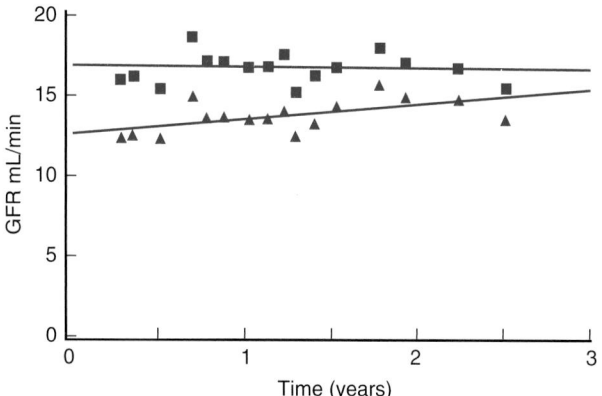

FIGURE 57-1. Sequential glomerular filtration rates in an obese woman expressed as mL/min (■) and as mL/min/1.73 m^2 (▲) during a 2-year period in which she lost 20% of her body weight. The expression of results in terms of surface area leads to the improbable conclusion that renal function is improving. (Redrawn from Walser M: Progression of chronic renal failure in man. Kidney Int 37:1195-1210, 1990. Used with permission from Kidney International.)

TABLE 57-1

Regression of Renal Plasma Flow and Glomerular Filtration

	MEN		WOMEN	
	Slope	Intercept	Slope	Intercept
RPF on BSA (mL/min)	141	359	125	325
GFR on BSA (mL/min)	69	−17	50	17

BSA, body surface area; GFR, glomerular filtration rate; RPF, renal plasma flow.
From Turner SJ, Reilly SL: Fallacy of indexing renal and systemic hemodynamic measurements for body surface area. Am J Physiol 268:R978-R988, 1995.

Curiously, none of these authors expresses renal hemodynamic data in relation to the square of height; yet body mass index is defined as weight/height[2]. Thus, ideal body weight is calculated as ideal body mass index times height[2]. According to Tokunaga and associates,[14] the body mass index value associated with the lowest morbidity is 22 kg/m[2]. Hence, ideal body weight is 22 × height[2]. It is therefore logical to express renal hemodynamic data in relation to height[2]. Because the average height[2] of adults is approximately 3 m[2], dividing measured GFR or RPF by (height[2]/3) yields values appropriately indexed for body size.

Effect of Age

Techniques for assessing renal function in children are limited by the difficulty of obtaining multiple blood samples or timed urine samples. Various techniques (other than blood creatinine measurements, see later) have been considered. Piepsz and associates[15] recommend single injection of either ^{51}Cr-ethylenediaminetetraacetic acid (EDTA) or ^{99m}Tc-diethylenetriamine pentaacetic acid (DTPA), followed by one or two blood samples. Various ways to calculate the results have been recommended. For single-sample estimations of GFR, Hamilton and associates[16, 17] attempted to identify a correction for body size that would yield an age-independent solution applicable to children as well as adults. They found that correction of measured plasma activity gave better results than did correction of the final GFR estimate. Swinkels and associates[18] recommend a seven-sample method in the 4 hours following inulin injection, with no urine samples. Delpassand and colleagues[19] maintain that after ^{99m}Tc-DTPA injection, a dual-detector gamma camera, which calculates the geometric mean of results from the two kidneys, yields results in children that are closely correlated with results calculated from multiple blood samples.

In adults, GFR declines with age older than 40 years in approximately two thirds of persons, especially if they are hypertensive[20] (even without frank kidney disease).[21] In the remaining third, the GFR remains constant or increases with age.[22] About two thirds of elderly subjects who are not in heart failure or receiving diuretics (even if hypertensive) have GFRs within the range of younger subjects.[23] Kidneys of persons dying of causes other than kidney disease examined at autopsy show a progressive, though extremely variable increase in the fraction of glomeruli that are sclerotic.[24]

Effect of Protein Intake on GFR and the Age-Related Decline in GFR

Increased dietary protein, a single meat meal, or infusion of amino acids leads to an increased GFR. The mechanism of this response has not been fully defined but may involve hormones (see later) and may in part be attributable to concomitant changes in sodium intake.[25] This relationship makes it difficult to define the limits of normal renal hemodynamics, as well as the effect of aging. Indeed, some of the apparent decrease in renal function with aging is attributable to a spontaneous decrease in protein intake in older persons.[26] The response to protein complicates the interpretation of studies of the effect of protein-restricted diets and progression: the acute decline in GFR that ensues when commencing such diets needs to be taken into account when determining the long-term effect on progression of chronic renal failure (CRF) (see later).

In rats, the development of CRF with age is nearly universal.[27, 28] The predominant lesion is glomerulosclerosis. Because this process is apparently attenuated by protein restriction,[29] Anderson and Brenner[30] suggested that the high-protein intake of Western societies plays a central role in the decline in renal function with age and suggested that restriction of dietary protein might prevent this decline.

This recommendation cannot be supported in normal adults for several reasons.[31] First, in rats, caloric restriction is more effective than protein restriction in retarding the age-associated decline in renal function.[32] Caloric restriction without protein restriction markedly retarded the progression of glomerulosclerosis. Unfortunately, the earlier studies indicating that protein restriction retarded renal damage failed to monitor food intake.

Second, protein restriction tends to lower the GFR rather than increase it. Lew and Bosch[33] recorded the dependence of creatinine clearance on spontaneous protein intake in two groups of subjects aged 22 to 50 years and 55 to 88 years. In both groups a similar pronounced dependence of clearance on protein intake was demonstrated; in the older subjects, a lower intercept was seen that corresponded to the effect of age on GFR. Older subjects consume less protein than younger subjects do.[34]

Third, Tobin and Spector[35] measured creatinine clearance in 198 normal men on two occasions 10 to 18 years apart and correlated the decline in clearance with estimates of protein intake. No relationship was detected, nor was any evidence found that high intake of protein causes a progressive reduction in renal function.

Fourth, the progressive decline in renal function in rats initiated by partial nephrectomy[36] may be unique to this species. In dogs with 75% nephrectomy, the GFR does not decline progressively with time in the ensuing 4 years, regardless of whether protein intake is high or low.[37] In baboons after subtotal nephrectomy, renal failure did not occur over a period of 5 years with either an 8% protein or a 25% protein diet.[38] The GFR, measured as inulin clearance, increased sharply in the baboons fed 25% protein, and this difference tended to disappear with time (curiously, creatinine clearances did not decrease with time in either group). Even in baboons fed 8% protein, a slow decline in GFR with time was seen (5% per year). Proteinuria did not differ between the two groups and did not progress. In human kidney donors, mild proteinuria is seen and the incidence of hypertension may be increased, but progressive renal failure rarely if ever occurs, and no correlation can be found between protein intake and proteinuria.[39, 40] Kidney donors are not generally advised to restrict their protein intake.[41] From these reports, it is clear that dietary protein restriction, rather than preventing the decline in renal function with age, is its major cause.

It is also clear that sequential GFR measurements must be interpreted in the light of protein intake. Thus, when studying the effect of protein restriction on progression of CRF, the initial decline in GFR caused by protein restriction, which apparently takes several weeks to stabilize,[42] must be taken into account.

Estimation of GFR from Creatinine Measurements and the Use of Cimetidine to Inhibit Creatinine Secretion

Creatinine measurements have traditionally been used to assess renal function because creatinine comes closer to being an ideal filtration marker than any other endogenous substance does, with the exception of cystatin C (see later). Because of the varying extent of tubule secretion of creatinine, creatinine clearance may be approximately equal to GFR or may be as much as twice the GFR; this error varies between individuals and even within a single individual. Consequently, estimation of renal function from creatinine levels in blood or in blood and urine, without cimetidine pretreatment, should be abandoned, as has been repeatedly recommended (with little effect).

Noting that cimetidine administration virtually eliminates creatinine secretion, Olsen and associates[43] and Roubenoff and colleagues[44] suggested that cimetidine administration could improve the utility of creatinine clearance. Indeed, it is possible to obtain an accurate estimate of GFR by measuring creatinine clearance (usually from three 30- to 50-minute urine collections) after administering cimetidine. The dosage of cimetidine is considered later. This procedure yields far more accurate estimates of GFR than does simply predicting the GFR from the plasma or serum creatinine concentration, even when demographic variables are taken into account[45] (as in the widely used formula of Cockcroft and Gault[45a]). The alkaline picrate method for determination of creatinine, still widely used in the United States, is not ideal for this purpose; both enzymatic and high-performance liquid chromatographic (HPLC) creatinine methods give more reliable results. Table 57-2 summarizes comparisons of this procedure with measured GFR. The average standard error of prediction is 4 mL/min, or 14% of the GFR.

TABLE 57-2

Results of Published Studies in Which the GFR Has Been Measured with Radioisotopes and Simultaneously Estimated as Creatinine Clearance after Pretreatment with Cimetidine, Arranged in Order (Approximately) of Increasing Estimation Error

AUTHOR	RANGE OF GFRs OF PATIENTS	NUMBER	RMSE	CV
van Olden[46]	2-10	9	0.5	18
Zaltzman[47]	2-45	17	1.2	7
Hilbrands[48]	40-80	6	?	7
	16-40	5	?	21
van Acker[49]	12-60	14	1.5	4
Hellerstein[50]	12-150	53	7	8
Olsen[43]	18-72	9	?	12
Roubenoff[44]	22-87	13	6	11
Ixkes[51]	22-121	19	7	10
Serdar[52]	20-120	27	?4	10
Shemesh[53]	?	12	?	21
Hirata-Dulas[54]	11-120	16	?	24
Marcen[55]	20-110	32	?	35
Mean			4	14

CV, RMSE/mean GFR or standard deviation of the ratio: estimated GFR/measured GFR; GFR, glomerular filtration rate; RMSE, standard deviation of the difference between estimated and measured GFR.

The total dosage of cimetidine has varied from 0.8 g[56] to 3.2 g,[44] administered at the start of the procedure[47] or continuously for as many as 3 days beforehand.[50] Van Acker and co-workers[49] reported that 1.2 g can achieve complete suppression of creatinine secretion in some patients, even though 0.4 g had not been completely effective. Although some workers[57] have recommended limiting creatine intake beforehand to reduce creatinine production, limitation of creatine intake seems unnecessary because there should not be any relationship between creatinine production and creatinine clearance. In fact, it has been shown that creatinine output is unaffected by cimetidine.[58]

It is important to remember that cimetidine administration increases the serum creatinine concentration for several days. This effect was in fact the observation that alerted investigators to this phenomenon and at first led to concern that cimetidine might aggravate renal insufficiency. In actuality, the GFR is unaffected.

Can the GFR be accurately estimated from serum creatinine alone after cimetidine administration? Kemperman and associates compared a Cockcroft-Gault estimate of GFR from the serum creatinine level after administration of cimetidine with a radioisotopic estimate of GFR in diabetic patients[59] and renal transplant recipients[60] and found close correspondence. They emphasized the importance of avoiding the alkaline picrate method for determination of creatinine, which is nevertheless still widely used.

Estimation of GFR from Cystatin C Concentration

Another endogenous substance whose serum concentration may be used to estimate the GFR is cystatin C, a low-molecular-weight protein produced by all cells. Cystatin C is filtered freely through the glomerulus but is almost completely reabsorbed and catabolized in the proximal tubule. Several studies have shown that the reciprocal serum cystatin C concentration is more closely correlated with the GFR (in patients with renal failure) than is the reciprocal serum creatinine concentration.[61-72] However, some discrepancies have been reported: for example, pregnancy alters the relationship between GFR and the serum cystatin C level.[73] In children, cystatin C levels may offer no improvement over creatinine levels in estimating the GFR.[74, 75] In addition, infants younger than 18 months tend to exhibit higher cystatin C levels.[76] Further study will be needed to resolve the role of cystatin C in estimating renal function.[77, 78]

Estimation of GFR from Other Substances

Beta$_2$-microglobulin is filtered by the glomeruli and reabsorbed by the proximal tubule, where it is metabolized. Its serum concentration may be more sensitive to an early decline in GFR than the serum creatinine level is.[79] Other candidates include beta-trace protein[80] and tryptophan glycoconjugate.[81]

Methods of Quantitating GFR after Injection of a Marker Substance

Methods can be grouped into (1) those that assess blood clearance from either the disappearance curve after a bolus injection or the steady-state plasma level at the end of a prolonged constant infusion; (2) those that calculate renal uptake of the marker substance; (3) those that determine, in addition to plasma concentration, urinary radioactivity by counting over the bladder; and (4) those that require measurement of urinary as well as plasma concentrations. The first technique yields total plasma clearance, which is assumed to be insignificantly greater than renal clearance (an assumption often invalidated). Total plasma clearance after bolus injection is calculated as the quotient of the tracer dose divided by the area under the plasma curve; after a constant infusion, total plasma clearance is the infusion rate divided by the final plasma concentration. Several prerequisites are necessary for the use of plasma clearance as a measure of GFR: (1) plasma clearance must be constant during the period of sampling (likely to be a problem with prolonged infusion); (2) measurements must be continued until monoexponential extrapolation to infinity is valid; and (3) extrarenal clearance of the marker must be negligible, especially in patients with severe renal failure—in such patients, all plasma clearance techniques tend to become unreliable because extrarenal clearance becomes a larger fraction of total clearance.

To avoid the necessity of sampling the entire plasma disappearance curve, several simplifications have been proposed, including the use of a single sample obtained several hours after injection. All such methods suffer from inaccuracy, particularly at low GFRs.[76, 82-87] Multiple-sample techniques, conversely, can yield consistent results[84, 88-91] despite some contribution from extrarenal clearance. Ultrafiltration of plasma before measurement may be advisable because of protein binding of the marker substance.

The single-sample method is said to be feasible in children; obviously, its practicality is greater.[92, 93] A better method in children may be the constant-infusion technique, in which a nonradioactive marker, such as iothalamate, is infused subcutaneously for many hours and a sample taken at the end of the infusion.[94-97] However, extrarenal clearance of the marker and diurnal variation in GFR both contribute to error.[98]

When a timed urine collection is measured, detection of incomplete bladder emptying becomes crucial. The coefficient of variation of sequential GFR determinations is often used as an estimate of the reliability of urine collections, but incomplete voiding in one period is likely to be followed by excessive voiding in the next. In this case, the reliability of sequential GFRs on different days may in fact bear little relationship to the coefficient of variation of the three periods on a given day.[99]

One way to deal with the problem of incomplete voiding is to set an arbitrary lower limit of urine flow, below which clearances are judged unacceptable. A better method is based on the observation that plasma and urinary clearance of ^{131}I-hippuran is indistinguishable when urine collection is complete.[100, 101] Thus, a correction for incomplete bladder emptying can be obtained by comparing the renal and plasma clearance of ^{131}I-hippuran infused simultaneously with a GFR marker substance. This correction, applied to urinary clearance of the GFR marker substance, reduces both the intratest and intertest variation in GFR measurements in patients with renal disease.[101] Another approach is to count over the bladder after the injection of a gamma-emitting isotope and correct for incomplete bladder emptying.[102]

In a logical extension of this approach, Bianchi and colleagues[103] report that counting over the bladder in patients told not to void at all (after the initial discarded sample) gives satisfactory clearance results. One technique that appears promising but has apparently not been used yet for clearance determinations is measurement of residual urine in the bladder by ultrasound; this method of measuring the volume of urine in the bladder is evidently quite accurate.[104]

Any GFR-measuring technique that involves water loading entails the danger of water intoxication. Nausea and vomiting are powerful stimuli to vasopressin release, which may affect the GFR and increase the likelihood of water intoxication. Severe headache and even convulsions may ensue.

Recently, a number of nonradioactive markers have been shown to be equally acceptable for measuring the GFR, provided that the dose is low enough to avoid nephrotoxicity. Such markers include iothalamate,[105, 106] iohexol,[107-110] iodixanol,[111] iopromide,[112] and others.

Many studies have appeared in which the clearances of two or more markers are compared in subjects with or without renal insufficiency. In general, these reports show that urinary clearance is more reliable than plasma clearance and that differences in urinary clearance as estimated by different markers are minor.

In normal children, the GFR can be estimated as $0.45 \times$ Ht/[Cr], where height is expressed in centimeters and serum creatinine in milligrams per deciliter.[112a] The constant in this formula was reported to be 0.33 in preterm infants, 0.45 in full-term infants, 0.55 in girls, and 0.70 in boys.[112b] In Nigeria, a value of 0.45 gave the best prediction.[112c] Leger and co-workers[113] proposed the following expression: GFR = 56.7 Wt + 0.142 Ht^2/[Cr], where Wt is in kilograms, Ht in centimeters, and [Cr] in micromoles per liter. This expression produces larger errors when the GFR declines.[114]

MEASUREMENT OF PROGRESSION

As recently as 25 years ago, no method was available to measure progression in quantitative terms. Now, several techniques, each with advantages and disadvantages, may be used. In choosing between methods, it should be remembered that comparing estimates of the rate of progression by two or more techniques gives a biased correlation because of measurement error. Beck and co-workers[115] present a method for overcoming this problem.

Rate of Change in Reciprocal Serum or Plasma Creatinine Concentration

In most patients whose renal failure is progressive, a plot of the reciprocal serum or plasma creatinine concentration [Cr]$^{-1}$ against time yields a straight line,[116] as has been repeatedly confirmed.[117] In a fraction of patients, however, such is not the case. Shah and Levey[118] used "breakpoint analysis"[119] to determine whether statistically significant changes in slope were present in 77 patients; they found that two slopes gave a better fit than one slope did to the observations in 32% of the patients and that the slopes of the two lines were significantly different in 51% of the patients. Conversely, Coresh and associates[120] found significant breakpoints in only 19% of a series of 67 patients studied to determine the projected dates of initiation of dialysis. Even when no breakpoints are present, the slopes of $[Cr]^{-1}$ versus time may give misleading information regarding the rate or even the existence of progression.[117, 121, 122] In view of these potential problems, $[Cr]^{-1}$ slopes should be used only for screening purposes in an investigation of methods of slowing progression; as clinical tools, these shortcomings should be kept in mind.

Another major problem with using $[Cr]^{-1}$ slopes as measures of progression is their susceptibility to large artifacts when the meat content of the diet is reduced. The resulting fall in creatinine production lowers $[Cr]$ and thus increases $[Cr]^{-1}$ independently of any change in clearance.

Rate of Change in Creatinine Clearance

Unless cimetidine is administered beforehand, creatinine clearance (2 hour or 24 hour), as noted earlier, is a very crude indicator of GFR. It is not surprising, therefore, that the slope of sequential changes in creatinine clearance is poorly correlated with the slope of sequential measurements of GFR,[123-125] so poorly, in fact, that it is almost useless.

Rate of Change in GFR

The best method for quantifying progression is determining the change in GFR despite the susceptibility of GFR to dietary influences.[126] When the interval during which progression is to be assessed is known, GFR measurements should be bunched at the beginning and end of this interval to minimize statistical error. Statistical aspects of measuring progression are complex.[115]

At least four GFR determinations are almost always necessary, but slower rates of progression will still be undetectable, particularly when the GFR is relatively high.[123, 127] Patients first seen with relatively high GFRs may need to be monitored for years, with multiple GFR determinations, to establish a statistically significant rate of progression. The advent of cimetidine-enhanced creatinine clearance (see earlier) makes such determinations a practical possibility, for clinical care as well as for research purposes.

CHARACTERIZATION OF PROGRESSION

Linearity

A definitive study of the linearity of the decline in GFR in CRF patients (other than from creatinine measurements) apparently has not been reported. In a series of 21 patients with diffuse proliferative lupus nephritis monitored for up to 5 years, Buckheit and colleagues[128] reported that no patients exhibited a linear decline in GFR (half had no decline at all). They suggest that therapeutic trials in patients with chronic glomerular disease should include "quantitative assessment of changes in glomerular morphology." Yet they also note that "renal biopsy is an invasive procedure and cannot be performed safely at frequent intervals," thus dismissing their own suggestion. It seems that the use of sequential GFR measurements and the implied or explicit assumption that they decline linearly with time are both inescapable, no matter how faulty.

Another way (besides the eigenvalue regression technique used by Buckheit and colleagues[128]) to ascertain the linearity (or nonlinearity) of the decline in GFR is breakpoint analysis.[119] In the only study that we have been able to identify in which this technique has been applied to serial GFR measurements,[129] a significant breakpoint was found in only 1 of 12 patients. Unfortunately, at least eight GFRs are generally required to detect a significant breakpoint. More conventional tests for curvilinearity, such as quadratic regression, have occasionally been applied[127] and have generally shown significant acceleration of progression in about a quarter of patients. A thorough study of this question is awaited.

An important question is whether the rate of decline in GFR tends to decrease or increase as renal failure progresses. Plots that have been published showing mean GFR versus time in groups of patients usually appear to be linear.[127, 130-137]

Quadratic regression revealed curvilinearity in 26% of one small series,[127] with acceleration more common than deceleration. However, in a small group of patients treated by nutritional therapy beyond the level of severity at which dialysis is usually started, it was found that some progressed much more slowly than they had previously.[138] Because the dietary regimen was the same as it had been before in these patients, it is evident that progression may slow dramatically near the end stage in some patients.

Distribution of Progression Rates

It has been stated that "once GFR falls below approximately 25% of normal, a relentless progression to end-stage renal failure inevitably ensues."[139] However, several reports have been published in which patients with less severe degrees of renal failure scarcely progressed at all. For example, Sawicki[140] observed inulin clearances for 2 years in 66 patients with insulin-dependent diabetes and CRF; the GFR improved in 51%, deteriorated in 39%, and remained stable in 10%. Toto and associates[141] monitored 87 nondiabetic hypertensive subjects with initial GFRs of less than 70 mL/min/1.73 m^2 for an average of 40 months. Blood pressure was well controlled. Mean GFR slopes were less than 1 mL/min/yr and did not differ significantly from zero, even though nine patients experienced either a doubling of serum creatinine or a 50% decline in GFR. Fink and colleagues[142] examined serial serum creatinine values from 3874 patients whose initial value was 1.4 mg/dL or greater for a median of 4 years. About half progressed. Rottey and associates[143] monitored 83 patients with initial serum creatinine values of 2 to 5 mg/dL for a mean of 67 months. Again, only about half progressed, especially those with more pronounced proteinuria.

Doubtless, some of these examples of arrested progression are attributable to good control of blood pressure and blood glucose, smoking cessation, and so forth; these results raise concern about the use of GFR slopes. We have reported numerous examples of patients with more severe renal failure whose progression has apparently ceased during treatment with a very low protein diet supplemented by keto acids[133, 144, 145] or, in one striking example,[133] essential amino acids (Fig. 57-2). More recently, Walser and Hill[138] reported 12 patients whose GFRs declined by an average of only 1.07 mL/min/yr, starting at an average GFR of less than 10 mL/min. At this level of severity, even such a slow loss of renal function is enough to necessitate dialysis before long.

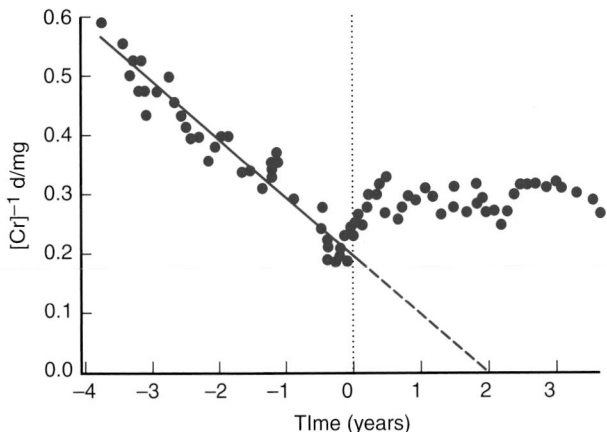

FIGURE 57-2. Sequential values for reciprocal serum creatinine concentration, [Cr]$^{-1}$, in one patient with chronic renal failure of unknown etiology. At time zero, a low-protein diet plus essential amino acids, 10 g/day, was started. Soon after the last point shown, he died immediately following open heart surgery. (Redrawn from Walser M, Drew HH, LaFrance ND: Reciprocal creatinine slopes often give erroneous estimates of progression of chronic renal failure. Kidney Int 36[suppl 27]:81-85, 1989. Used with permission from Kidney International.)

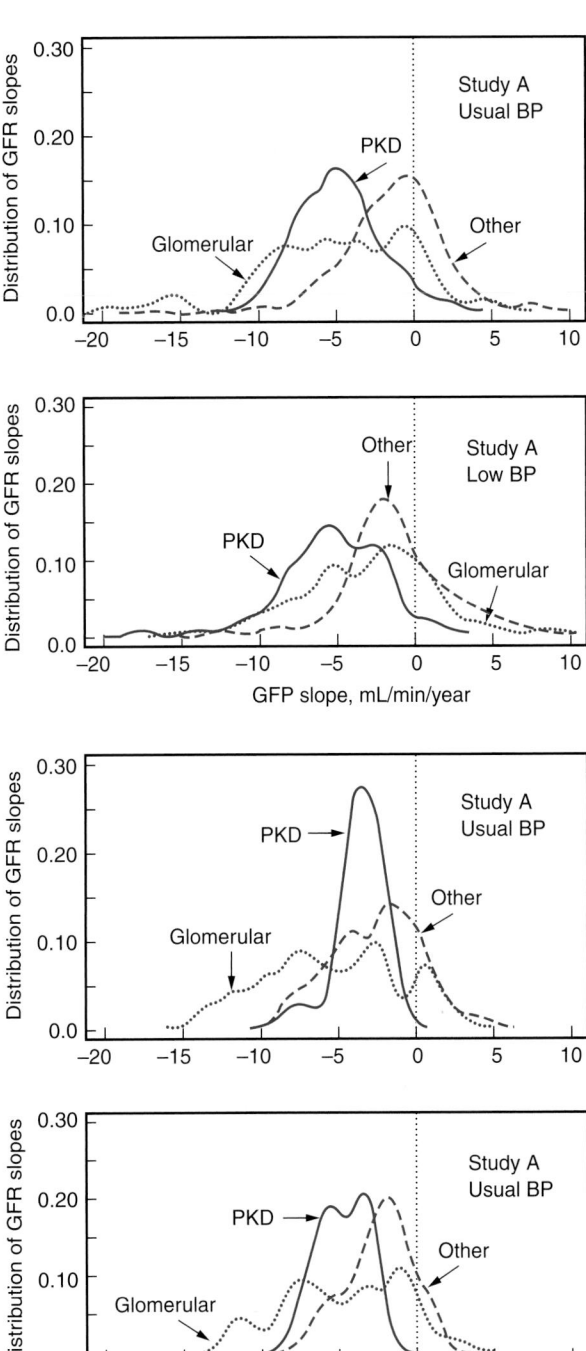

FIGURE 57-3. Glomerular filtration rate (GFR) slopes as a function of kidney disease diagnoses in patients treated in the National Institutes of Health Modification of Diet in Renal Disease Study. Patients are grouped according to the initial level of GFR and disease, as well as treatment category. The *upper panel* consists of patients with an initial GFR of 25 to 55 mL/min/1.73 m^2 and a mean blood pressure (BP) goal of 107 mm Hg (usual BP) or less than 92 mm Hg (low BP) during therapy. The *lower panel* is the same information for patients with an initial GFR of 13 to 24 mL/min/1.73 m^2. (Redrawn from Hunsicker LG, Adler S, Caggiula A, et al: Predictors of the progression of renal disease in the Modification of Diet in Renal Disease Study. Kidney Int 51:1908-1919, 1997. Used with permission from Kidney International.)

The largest published series of progression rates (excluding those based on creatinine measurements) was the operational phase of the Modification of Diet in Renal Disease (MDRD) Study, the results of which are presented in Figure 57-3.[146] Progression rates are depicted separately for study A (initial GFRs, 25 to 55 mL/min/1.73 m^2), for study B (initial GFRs, 13 to 24 mL/min/1.73 m^2), and for subjects randomized to a low target mean blood pressure (<93 mm Hg) or "usual" mean blood pressure (<108 mm Hg). Patients with glomerular disease showed a wider distribution of progression rates than other diagnostic groups did. At the other extreme, patients with polycystic kidney disease tended to progress at less variable rates; they also seldom improved and exhibited more rapid progression, on average, than other groups did. In all diagnostic groups, the most rapid individual progression rates were 15 to 20 mL/min/yr.

Multivariate analysis[146] has revealed that five factors are predictive of faster progression: (1) more proteinuria, (2) the presence of polycystic kidney disease, (3) lower serum transferrin, (4) higher mean arterial pressure, and (5) lower serum high-density lipoprotein (HDL) cholesterol. Still, these factors together accounted for only 34% of the observed variability in progression rates. Others also report that proteinuria is an important correlate of progression of CRF.[134, 147-158] Short stature and male gender have likewise been reported to be predictors of CRF progression in diabetics.[159] Benigni and Remuzzi[160] and others have suggested that passage of protein through the glomerular barrier and reabsorption with accumulation of protein in the proximal tubule cells can damage these cells and lead to infiltration of macrophages and T lymphocytes into the renal interstitium. In support of this concept, Zoja and colleagues[161] reported that incubation of proximal tubule cells with protein induces the production of RANTES, a chemokine with potent chemotactic activity for monocytes/macrophages and T lymphocytes. Wang and associates[162] have found that exposure to protein stimulates the expression of monocyte chemoattractant protein-1, probably at the level of translation as well as transcription, by proximal tubule cells. Cooper and colleagues[163] offer a different explanation for the damaging effect of proteinuria: as urine pH decreases below 6, iron is dissociated from transferrin and exists in tubule fluid in a soluble, labile state that can cause free radical damage to tubule cells. If this hypothesis is correct, alkalization of the urine should slow progression in proteinuric states.

Pathologic Correlates of Progression

Fioretto and co-workers[164] performed renal biopsies on 11 patients with insulin-dependent diabetes and nephropathy on two occasions some 6 years apart. The median albumin excretion rate during this interval increased from 12 to 19 mg/day. The dominant pathologic change at this stage was mesangial expansion; interstitial expansion was not observed. Rudberg and Osterby[165] performed biopsies on the kidneys of 17 diabetic adolescents and correlated the rate of fall in GFR in these subjects (the GFR had previously been measured in the normoalbuminuric state 2 to 5 years earlier) with glomerular structural abnormalities. They found that progression was most rapid in those with previous hyperfiltration (as has been reported before) and was correlated with basement membrane thickness, interstitial volume fraction, mean capillary diameter, and hemoglobin A_{1c} concentration. Buckheit and associates[128] conducted an extensive study of 21 patients with lupus nephritis and the nephrotic syndrome who were being treated with total lymphoid irradiation. GFRs were measured one to two times yearly for up to 5 years. The single-nephron ultrafiltration coefficient (K_f) of the remaining glomeruli rose in nonprogressors but not in progressors. GFR was strongly related to K_f in all patients and inversely related to glomerular oncotic pressure in progressors. Twelve patients had two renal biopsies. In progressors but not in nonprogressors, serial morphometric analysis revealed increasing global glomerulosclerosis.

Improvement in renal function can occur in association with resolution of glomerular pathology in rats with glomerulosclerosis given ACE inhibitors.[166]

DETERMINING THE EFFECT OF TREATMENT ON PROGRESSION

Survival Curves and Other End Point Analysis Methods

The simplest technique of assessing progression of CRF is a comparison of survival curves, nonsurvival being defined as progression to a defined end point, such as the beginning of dialysis. This technique is applicable for comparing the outcome of groups of patients randomly assigned to control and experimental treatments. It requires prolonged follow-up (at least 4 years) and has the advantage of avoiding the assumption of linearity. Furthermore, when the start of renal replacement therapy is the end point, the results have clear practical implications. A problem that arises is that criteria for renal replacement have not been standardized.

A more practical approach is use of the time to doubling of the serum creatinine concentration. Again, many patients may not reach this end point within a feasible interval.

According to Gretz[167] and Rossing,[168] at least 70% must reach this end point to allow proper evaluation. Another problem is that analysis after completion of the study may reveal that therapeutic efficacy is demonstrable only for certain ranges of initial serum creatinine.[168, 169]

Exclusion of Nonprogressors

As noted, a substantial fraction of CRF patients do not progress, even when their renal insufficiency is severe. It makes little sense to include such patients in a study of techniques or therapies intended to slow progression. The problem with making significant progression an entry criterion is "regression to the mean": the rate of progression after the last measurement that established the existence of progression will generally be slower by chance alone.

Responses to this problem have varied. First, nonprogressors can be included, which was done in the operational phase[137] (but not the feasibility phase)[170] of the MDRD Study. Progression before randomization was not measured. Some 15% of the patients did not progress, no matter which diet they were assigned to; hence, the power of the study to detect a significant effect of diet on progression was reduced accordingly. Second, nonprogressors can be excluded and regression to the mean can be balanced between treatment groups by randomization.[144, 170] Third, nonprogressors can be excluded but all patients nevertheless subjected to the same number of prerandomization GFRs, arbitrarily determined in advance. This last approach apparently has not been used.

"Intention to Treat" Analysis

Inclusion of noncompliant patients introduces yet another problem. They cannot readily be excluded from the analysis because such exclusion may introduce bias; those who fail to comply may progress at a different rate or respond differently to treatment (on average) from those who comply. When the proportion of noncompliant patients is large, this approach yields an essentially meaningless result. If a quantitative measure of compliance is available (such as serum alloisoleucine level as an index of compliance with the keto acid prescription[171]), comparison of outcomes in relation to this measure will be more persuasive than comparison of groups by intention to treat. Often, it will be possible to assign some probability to the possibility that bias has been introduced—in this example, the probability that patients compliant with the keto acid prescription are inherently slower progressors.

Crossovers

Some of these problems can be circumvented by crossover designs. Such designs are inherently more efficient because the variability between patients of changes in the progression rate in response to treatment is almost certain to be less than the variability in progression rates among patients. Depending on the crossover design chosen, errors caused by regression to the mean are minimized. Patients who drop out are excluded, although it is important to ascertain that dropout is not more frequent in subjects receiving one treatment than in subjects receiving the other. Unless compliance differs between the two treatments, these problems are also minimized.

Several new problems are introduced, however. First, carryover effects may occur; the effect of one treatment on progression may persist after the treatment is withdrawn, for an uncertain interval. Second, in a progressive disorder, with design AB (where A is one treatment and B is the other), severity will generally be greater during B than A, and there may be a relationship between severity and slope or between severity and response to treatment. If patients are randomized to the sequence AB or the sequence BA (design AB/BA), this potential error is reduced but may not be eliminated. A better design is ABA/BAB. If progression is linear, the mean severity during treatment A will probably be nearly the same as the mean severity during treatment B. As pointed out by Jones and Kenward,[172] AAB/BAA is preferable if carryover is a concern; however, their comments were not addressed to a progressive disorder. Third, unfortunately, crossover studies can never establish long-term outcomes.

Pilot Studies

The enormous expense of a full-scale trial to establish the efficacy (or lack thereof) of an agent purported to slow progression of CRF makes it imperative to obtain adequate justification before proceeding. Studies in animals will rarely, if ever, be sufficient for this purpose; a large number of agents have been reported to slow progression significantly in rats, but few of them have been deemed worthy of study in humans. The question of how to design a pilot clinical trial that could provide the justification for a full-scale clinical trial is a major concern, as yet scarcely addressed.

ROLE OF SPECIFIC DIETARY CONSTITUENTS IN RENAL DISEASE

Energy Intake

Patients entering dialysis therapy have a high incidence of anthropometric abnormalities, including decreased body weight.[173, 174] Kopple and colleagues note that these findings could result from inadequate uptake of energy.[175, 176] Because the energy requirement is determined by the amount expended during daily activities, the best method of determining energy needs is to measure energy expended during average activity and add the value to the resting energy expenditure (REE). The usual method to obtain this measurement is by indirect calorimetry measured over relatively brief periods and then extrapolating the result to 24 hours; the REE is then multiplied by a factor to account for the individual's activities. The 1981 FAO/WHO/UNU recommendation for energy used a database of approximately 11,000 REE determinations in healthy subjects.[177] It should be recognized that the regression equations used to derive the energy requirements published in this report led to considerable variability. In addition, the estimated REE from indirect calorimetry depends on the consistency and accuracy of the estimated time spent on various physical activities. Moreover, the issue of adaptation to different caloric intake must be taken into account. Healthy subjects adapt to decreased nutrient intake by decreasing the value of REE.[178] In semistarved adults, the REE decreased about 15% over a period of 3 weeks; ultimately, lean body mass was lost.[177]

This adaptation raises another issue, the relationship between an adequate amount of dietary calories and protein[176]: well-nourished adults can achieve energy balance with only half the usual caloric intake, but only if activity is decreased; even in this case, lean body mass may decrease.

Energy Requirements of Uremic Patients

Few evaluations of the caloric requirements of CRF patients or their capacity to adapt to a reduced-calorie intake have been published. Monteon and co-workers examined the energy expenditure of normal and CRF subjects during rest and exercise.[179] No difference was noted between the groups; when caloric intake was reduced, energy expenditure did not fall in either group, thus indicating that CRF patients do not have any special ability to adapt to a low-calorie intake. Consequently, if energy intake is inadequate, calorie malnutrition and negative nitrogen balance could develop in uremic subjects, especially when protein intake is restricted. Monteon and co-workers[179] also concluded that the energy expenditure of dialysis patients is not different from that of normal subjects. This conclusion is controversial because Ikizler and colleagues[180] noted that 10 hemodialysis patients had a 7% higher than expected level of energy expenditure on both dialysis and nondialysis days. The latter finding suggests that uremia per se increases energy expenditure. In this case, metabolic factors impairing energy utilization (e.g., insulin resistance) would contribute to insufficient energy for maintaining body mass. In fact, uremia as well as metabolic acidosis per se causes insulin resistance and would impair energy utilization.[181, 182] Interestingly, institution of a low-protein diet in the treatment of CRF patients substantially ameliorates insulin resistance. Rigalleau and associates[183] examined the insulin responses of CRF patients eating 0.3 g of protein per kilogram per day plus a supplement of essential amino acids and keto acids and found that plasma glucose and insulin levels were significantly lower. They also noted an improvement in glucose oxidation and nonoxidative disposal (mainly glycogen synthesis) and concluded that the low-protein diet increased energy production. They suggested that caloric intake be raised in such patients. In the MDRD Study, the initial values of energy intake were below the recommended levels of 30 to 35 kcal/kg/day.[184] During the study (average duration, 2.2 years), energy intake declined despite intensive dietary counseling and ranged from a high value of 26.7 to a low value of 21 kcal/kg/day. Even though only small changes occurred in body weight, other anthropometry measures, and serum proteins, the low values of energy intake are worrisome.

Hyne and colleagues[185] reported that the nitrogen balance of uremic patients fed a diet of 20 g of high-quality protein per day improved as caloric intake was raised. Although the patients remained in negative nitrogen balance when caloric intake was raised to 55 kcal/kg/day, the results are reminiscent of the findings of Rose,[186] in which a higher caloric intake is required to achieve nitrogen balance in normal subjects fed diets containing barely adequate amounts of essential amino acids. It is quite clear, however, that CRF patients do not ingest the prescribed amount of calories.[175] Even with intensive interactions with dieticians in the MDRD Study, energy intake was significantly below the prescribed level.[184] In less rigorously controlled conditions, the energy intake of

CRF patients with renal insufficiency as low as a creatinine clearance of 10 mL/min was below the recommended level of 30 to 35 kcal/kg/day.[187] The cause of the lower level of caloric intake is unclear but is likely to be associated with the anorexia of chronic uremia.[188] As discussed in Chapter 48, anorexia in CRF patients has several potential causes, including the accumulation of an anorectic factor.[188] The contribution of low levels of energy intake in producing abnormalities in nutritional status is unclear.[175] For example, Bergstrom and associates[189] studied patients in renal failure who were eating 16 to 20 g/day of protein supplemented with essential amino acids given orally or intravenously and found little or no change in nitrogen balance as energy intake was varied between 22 and 50 kcal/kg/day. These data suggest that caloric intake is not so critical if both nitrogen and essential amino acid intake is adequate. Conversely, Kopple and co-workers[190] systematically addressed the question of how calories affect protein conservation when protein intake is minimal. They fed six chronically uremic patients a constant, minimal protein intake of 0.55 to 0.6 g/kg/day and measured nitrogen balance while caloric intake was varied from 15 to 45 kcal/kg/day (Fig. 57-4). Extrapolation of their measurements indicates that nitrogen equilibrium can be achieved by most patients given 35 kcal/kg/day. These results suggest that the energy requirements of predialysis patients are similar to those of normal subjects despite abnormalities in glucose and possibly lipid metabolism. Unfortunately, the number of CRF patients with careful measurements of caloric requirements and the impact of varying calories on nitrogen balance are quite small. Based on the available data,[190] it is advisable to attempt to increase the caloric intake of CRF patients to 35 kcal/kg/day if they are eating a protein-restricted diet and if they are below ideal body weight. For overweight patients, calories should be restricted.

Salt Intake

As CRF progresses, the kidney adapts by increasing sodium excretion per nephron, facilitated in part by the action of atrial natriuretic peptide and other natriuretic peptides, whose release increases as extracellular volume tends to expand. In addition, renal hypoperfusion develops, along with an attendant increase in the filtration fraction. As renal failure becomes more severe, these hemodynamic changes play an increasingly important role.[25] Hyperaldosteronism is often present; yet aldosterone levels can be stimulated further by posture or by volume depletion.[191] Sodium excretion eventually diminishes, and edema and hypertension develop. At this point, administration of diuretics and salt restriction are necessary. As noted in the section on nitrogenous excretory products, a high serum uric acid level is another factor that could contribute to hypertension.[192] Results from experiments in rats suggest that a high uric acid level not only contributes to salt-sensitive hypertension but also could cause arteriolar damage in the kidney and other organs.[193-195]

In subjects with hypertension, but not in normotensive individuals, the GFR may[196] or may not[197] vary with salt intake, independently of the renin-angiotensin system. In CRF patients with hypertension, blood pressure is typically salt sensitive (see Chapter 47). Proteinuria also responds to salt restriction.[198] The antiproteinuric effect of ACE inhibitors or angiotensin II blockers and of nondihydropyridine calcium channel blockers is enhanced by salt restriction, in part because of a decrease in the filtration fraction.[198-203]

In rats with experimental diabetes, salt restriction acutely reduces hyperfiltration, renal enlargement, and albuminuria[204] and may paradoxically increase the GFR[205]; chronic salt loading may paradoxically decrease the GFR.[206] In patients with insulin-dependent diabetes, salt restriction exacerbates hyperfiltration.[207] In non-insulin-dependent diabetes melitus (NIDDM), salt restriction impairs insulin sensitivity.[208] Because the degree of proteinuria is correlated with the rate of progression,* it follows that salt restriction may also contribute to slowing of progression. Retrospective clinical studies support this inference.[25] Aldosterone has been postulated to play a major role in the progression of CRF,[212] based in part on studies in experimental animals.[213, 214] If this theory is correct, spironolactone could be useful to slow progression.

Protein Intake
Acute Effects of Protein or Amino Acids on Renal Hemodynamics

As noted earlier, excess dietary protein or intravenous infusion of amino acids leads to increases in GFR and RPF of 11% to 24%.[215, 216] Renal vascular resistance decreases.

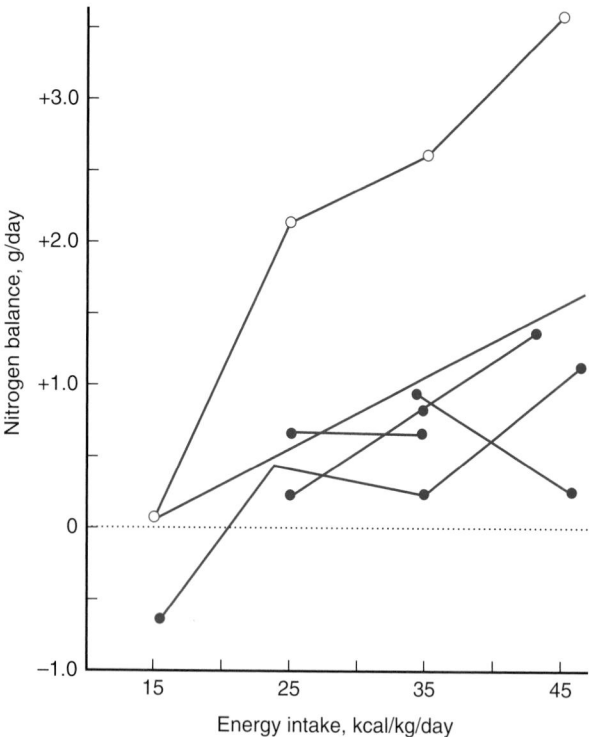

FIGURE 57-4. Correlation between nitrogen balance and energy intake in six clinically stable, nondialyzed, chronically uremic patients. (From Kopple JD, Monteon FJ, Shaib JK: Effect of energy intake on nitrogen metabolism in nondialyzed patients with chronic renal failure. Kidney Int 29:734-742, 1986. Used with permission from Kidney International.)

*See references 134, 147, 148, 150, 151, 153-157, 207, 209-211.

This increment in GFR has been called functional renal reserve, although it is not apparent what, if any function it serves. It is seen in children[217] and in the elderly[218] and may or may not be detected in hypertensive subjects.[219] Soy protein does not induce this response.[220] Hyperfiltering diabetics exhibit a markedly blunted renal reserve, unless they are ingesting a low-protein diet.[221-224] Non-hyperfiltering diabetics, however, respond normally to a protein challenge and may exhibit an exaggerated response to amino acid infusion,[225] unless the GFR has fallen.[226, 227] Indomethacin treatment prevents this response in normal subjects, but not in diabetics[228] unless they have received glucagon injections sufficient to restore normal glucagon levels.[222] Heart failure blunts the response, but enalapril treatment restores it.[229]

Both intrarenal and extrarenal mechanisms are probably involved. Evidence for intrarenal mechanisms, such as tubuloglomerular feedback and tubule reabsorption of amino acids and NaCl, was summarized by Woods.[230] Levels of many hormones increase in response to protein loads, including insulin, glucagon, corticosteroids, growth hormone, brain-gut peptides, vasopressin, atrial natriuretic peptide, and dopamine,[231] but nonrenal hormones, at least, do not appear to be essential for the response.[232-234] Mediators produced within the kidney that are likely to be involved include prostaglandins, kinins, angiotensin II, and nitric oxide.

Angiotensin II appears to play an important role in mediating this response through its inhibitory effect on proximal tubule reabsorption and activation of the tubuloglomerular feedback system.[219] In normal subjects, captopril eliminates the response, but nifedipine does not.[235] Renal reserve is attenuated in subjects with essential hypertension who are receiving ACE inhibitors.[236] In diabetics, however, captopril increases the response to amino acid infusion, but salt loading does not increase the response further.[237] Administration of a kinin receptor antagonist abolishes the response.[238] Nitric oxide probably plays a critical role[239] because administration of L-nitro-arginine methyl ester, an inhibitor of nitric oxide biosynthesis, abolishes it.[240]

Renal nerves also play a role because renal denervation abolishes the renal reserve.[241] Dietary phosphorus restriction abolishes the response to oral protein loads but not the response to intravenous amino acids.[242] Although it was initially hoped that the persistence of this response could exclude the presence of harmful hyperfiltration, it was found that neither unilateral renal agenesis[215] nor CRF[215, 230, 243, 244] blunted the response.

Acute Effects of Protein or Amino Acid Loads on Proteinuria

Protein loads in subjects with either microalbuminuria or macroalbuminuria increase the excretion of beta$_2$-microglobulin, retinol-binding protein, and IgG, as well as the excretion of albumin.[215, 245] Even in normal subjects, protein loads increase the excretion of proteins with a molecular radius near 55 Å.[246] In type 2 diabetics, a chicken-based diet reduces albuminuria when compared with a meat-based diet.[247] In nephrotic patients, proteinuria increases following a meat meal, before or after nifedipine pretreatment, but not after captopril or indomethacin pretreatment.[248] In children with reflux nephropathy, amino acid infusion augments the excretion of albumin, as well as beta$_2$-microglobulin.[249]

Effects of Variations in Dietary Protein Intake on Renal Hemodynamics

As noted by King and Levey,[250] the variation in GFR with dietary protein intake is seen in all animal species studied, but it is least pronounced in humans, in whom it varies from nonsignificant to approximately 20%. The time dependence of this effect has not been examined systematically, but indirect evidence suggests that the response may require months to reach its maximal effect. RPF changes in parallel, but clear-cut structural alterations such as glomerular and tubule hypertrophy, hyperplasia, or both, are also observed in the kidney, at least in rats.

Effects of Variations in Dietary Protein Intake on Albuminuria

In non-nephrotic patients, many studies have documented that protein restriction reduces proteinuria.[148, 251-258] This response and the antiproteinuric effect of ACE inhibition are additive.[259] Studies in rats with Heymann nephritis suggest that high-protein diets aggravate proteinuria by both angiotensin-independent and angiotensin-dependent mechanisms.[260, 261] The response to protein restriction may fail to occur in some diabetics without renal failure,[262, 263] particularly if they do not exhibit hyperfiltration.[262] On the other hand, diabetics who spontaneously consume relatively high amounts of protein (especially animal protein) are more likely to exhibit microalbuminuria according to one study,[264] but not another.[265] Diabetics adapt poorly to protein restriction,[256, 266] and diabetics with nephropathy may have adverse responses to diets containing 0.6 g/kg of protein,[256] so care must be exercised when recommending a reduction in protein intake. According to Aparicio and associates,[148] a reduction in proteinuria does not occur in patients in whom progression continues unabated. Furthermore, changing from moderate protein intake to high protein intake (3.5 g/kg) failed to augment proteinuria in type 1 diabetics.[267]

The role of dietary protein restriction in nephrotic syndrome is considered later.

Nutritional Effect of Protein Restriction in Experimental Renal Failure

Meireles and associates[268] fed rats with CRF diets that had a protein content varying from 8% to 30% and measured growth and feed efficiency. The lowest protein intake led to the highest efficiency of utilization of protein for growth, but 17% protein was the most efficient in terms of utilization of energy for growth. Thirty percent protein diets caused anorexia.

Effects of Dietary Protein Restriction on Progression of Chronic Renal Disease

During the past decade, a number of studies, some better controlled than others, have indicated that protein restriction may slow progression, but in a few studies, no such response was found. Three meta-analyses of these reports have appeared. The first[269] included six randomized controlled trials[150, 270-273a] for analysis of the frequency of renal death (start of dialysis or death of the patient) in control versus treated groups. A total of 890 patients were monitored for at least 1 year, half of whom received a low-protein diet. One hundred fifty-six renal deaths occurred, 61 in the low-protein group and 95 in the control group, for an odds ratio of 0.54 with a 95% confidence interval of 0.37 to 0.79. The authors concluded that the data strongly support the effectiveness of low-protein diets in delaying the onset of end-stage renal disease.

The second study[274] selected five randomized controlled studies that included 1413 patients with nondiabetic kidney disease[137, 150, 271-273] and five studies that included 108 patients with type 1 diabetic nephropathy.[255, 256, 275-277] Again, the meta-analysis indicated a significantly reduced risk of renal death in the nondiabetics. In the diabetics, protein restriction significantly slowed the increase in proteinuria or the rate of decline in GFR or creatinine clearance. The authors concluded that protein restriction slows the progression of both diabetic and nondiabetic renal disease. One of the studies included in this analysis[273] exemplifies the problems of compliance in interpreting such trials: protein intake estimated from 24-hour urea excretion scarcely differed between experimental and control groups (by only 0.16 g/kg). Not surprisingly, progression rates in the two groups of this study did not differ.

A third meta-analysis by Kasiske and co-workers[278] analyzed 24 studies by including 11 in which randomization was not performed; instead, a prospective, but not randomly allocated control group was used, or else an evaluation period preceded the treatment period in the same patients. In the randomized trials, the average effect of protein restriction was to slow progression by only 0.53 mL/min/yr, or about 10%; when the study of Locatelli and colleagues,[273] mentioned previously as showing minimal or no compliance, was excluded, this average effect rose to 0.66 mL/min/yr. When nonrandomized and smaller trials were included, greater effects were found, thus suggesting bias. Hence, these three meta-analyses have led to somewhat varying conclusions.

It should be noted that two of these meta-analyses[274, 278] included the operational phase of the MDRD Study,[137] which has been viewed by some as having disproven the hypothesis that protein restriction slows progression. This interpretation is clearly incorrect. In a secondary analysis of these results in patients with more advanced disease,[42, 279] it was found that a 0.2-g/kg/day reduction in protein intake was associated with a 1.15-mL/min/yr slower rate of decline in GFR, corresponding to a 41% prolongation of the time to end-stage renal disease. To quote Levey and colleagues,[279] "...the balance of evidence is more consistent with the hypothesis of a beneficial effect of protein restriction than with the contrary hypothesis."

Controversial results continue to be reported; for example, a study from Denmark[280] documented a reduced risk of end-stage renal disease in diabetic patients randomized to mild protein restriction (0.89 g/kg), whereas a report from Italy[281] found no slowing of progression with a 0.6-g/kg protein diet. Type 2 diabetics whose proteinuria diminishes are more likely to exhibit slowed progression.[282] In a recent study of patients with all types of renal failure, a low-protein diet, especially if combined with a soy protein isolate, slowed progression.[283]

Combe and colleagues[284] documented the role of compliance in achieving retardation of progression by protein restriction. The controversy concerning intention-to-treat analysis, mentioned earlier, is relevant here.

In patients with autosomal dominant polycystic kidney disease, Choukroun and co-workers[285] could find no effect of protein restriction on progression by multiple regression analysis. However, in the MDRD Study, protein restriction was marginally associated with slower progression in polycystic patients with more advanced disease.[286]

Effect of Protein Restriction in Children with Chronic Renal Disease

Growth retardation is a major problem in children with CRF and has many causes.[287, 288] Total body nitrogen is characteristically reduced,[289] but the pubertal growth spurt may be normal.[290] In children, no beneficial effect of mild protein restriction (to 0.8 to 1.1 g/kg) on progression has been found when sequential creatinine clearances was used as a measure of progression (see earlier).[291-293]

Possible Mediators of the Effect of Dietary Protein on Progression

Angiotensin II

Generated within the kidney, angiotensin II modulates glomerular hemodynamics by preferentially constricting efferent arterioles, and it stimulates the growth of renal vascular and glomerular cells. However, angiotensin II is not a necessary factor in the induction of renal growth by dietary protein.[294] Angiotensin promotes the synthesis of matrix molecules, thereby contributing to glomerular sclerosis and interstitial fibrosis.[295] Dietary protein restriction reduces plasma renin activity, and ACE inhibition reduces proteinuria.[294] Thus, renal levels of angiotensin II may be increased by dietary protein. In support of this possibility, renin mRNA in the kidney is increased in rats fed a high-protein diet.[296, 297] The vasoconstrictor responses of the renal microcirculation to exogenous angiotensin II in rats were reduced by feeding a high-protein diet, but not if the animals were pretreated with captopril.[298]

Transforming Growth Factor-β

Evidence from many sources indicates that transforming growth factor-β (TGF-β) plays a major role in mediating renal sclerosis.[299] Angiotensin II increases the synthesis and decreases the degradation of TGF-β, and ACE blockade suppresses it.[300] Protein restriction reduces TGF-β in rats with puromycin-induced nephrosis.[301] In rats with experimental glomerulonephritis, glomerular production of TGF-β is reduced by a low-protein diet, even with the addition of enalapril or losartan.[302] Urinary excretion of TGF-β is elevated in diabetic patients, but no more than in those with nephropathy.[303]

Eicosanoids

High-protein diets increase the urinary excretion of 6-keto-prostaglandin $F_{1\alpha}$ in normal subjects,[304] as well as the in vitro production of eicosanoids by rat renal medullary tubules.[305]

Glucocorticoids

Dietary protein stimulates cortisol production,[306-308] whereas protein-restricted diets reduce cortisol levels.[309] Proteinuria in nephrotic patients is increased acutely by glucocorticoid administration,[310-312] even though remission may be induced by long-term treatment. Adrenalectomy reduces proteinuria in several animal models of renal disease.[313] High doses of glucocorticoids amplify glomerular injury in rats with ablative nephropathy[314] and induce glomerular proteinuria in mice.[315] Walser and Ward[316] reported that 24-hour excretion of 17-hydroxyglucocorticoids was correlated with the rate of progression in CRF patients from various causes; further study showed that free cortisol excretion was similarly correlated with progression.[127, 155] Walser and Hill[317] administered ketoconazole (an inhibitor of cortisol synthesis) to a small number of patients with CRF of various types, along with a low dose (2.5 mg/day) of prednisone (to prevent pituitary "escape"), in a randomized crossover design. Progression (measured by sequential GFR determinations) slowed in patients with glomerulopathies, interstitial nephritis, or diabetic nephropathy, but it accelerated in patients with polycystic kidney disease. Surprisingly, proteinuria did not change. In rats with ablative nephropathy, the antiglucocorticoid RU-486 reduced hyperfiltration in superficial nephrons, but it did not alter proteinuria or glomerulosclerosis.[318]

Insulin-like Growth Factor-1

In rats, dietary protein restriction reduces hepatic insulin-like growth factor-1 (IGF-1) mRNA levels and plasma concentration of IGF-1; opposite effects are seen in the colon.[319] In adult CRF patients, however, a 40% reduction in dietary protein had no effect on serum levels of IGF-1 or its binding proteins.[320]

Insulin

As summarized in Chapter 48, insulin resistance and hyperinsulinemia are evident even in early renal failure.[321-323] Protein restriction improves the insulin sensitivity of endogenous glucose production; that is, postabsorptive insulin concentrations decrease with no change in postabsorptive glucose turnover rates.[324]

Role of Vegetable versus Animal Protein

Substitution of vegetable protein for animal protein in normal subjects decreases renal hemodynamics.[325] D'Amico and colleagues[326-329] fed nephrotic patients a low-fat, vegetarian, soy protein diet for 2 months and observed highly significant decreases in serum lipids and proteinuria. As they noted, it could not be determined whether the change in protein quality, protein quantity, or fat intake was responsible for these effects. Jibani and associates[330] observed a reduction in microalbuminuria after substituting vegetable protein for animal protein in diabetics with early nephropathy. Kontessis and co-workers[220] fed normal individuals either an animal protein diet or a vegetable protein diet for 3 weeks in random order. GFR, RPF, and fractional clearance of albumin were all greater with the animal protein diet. They also gave acute loads of protein from these two sources and noted that

plasma glucagon and 6-ketoprostaglandin $F_{1\alpha}$ rose more after the meat load. In nonproteinuric diabetics fed these two diets,[331] similar results were seen: plasma valine and lysine were significantly higher with the meat diet. Soroka and colleagues[332] fed a soy-based, low-protein diet and an animal-based, low-protein diet, in random order, for 6 months each to CRF patients. GFRs remained constant, as did nutritional status and proteinuria. The vegetarian diet was associated with lower protein and phosphate intake. Thus, the evidence suggests that vegetarian diets may be advantageous in chronic renal disease.

Role of "Low-Antigen" Diet

Ferri and co-workers[333] prescribed a diet containing 1 g/kg of protein but with no eggs, dairy products, or gluten and only occasional turkey or lamb in place of other meats, poultry, or fish to 21 patients with IgA nephropathy and proteinuria (up to 3 g/day) but normal or nearly normal GFR. By 1 month, proteinuria had decreased markedly in 17 of the 21 patients and remained minimal for at least 5 months (Fig. 57-5). Renal biopsy generally did not show histologic improvement.

Effects of Individual Amino Acids in the Diet
Arginine

As a substrate for nitric oxide synthesis, arginine has the potential to influence many physiologic processes. L-Arginine supplementation prevents the development of hypertension and nephrosclerosis in the salt-sensitive Dahl/Rapp strain of rats.[334, 335] Dietary supplementation with arginine ameliorated ablative nephropathy and diabetic nephropathy

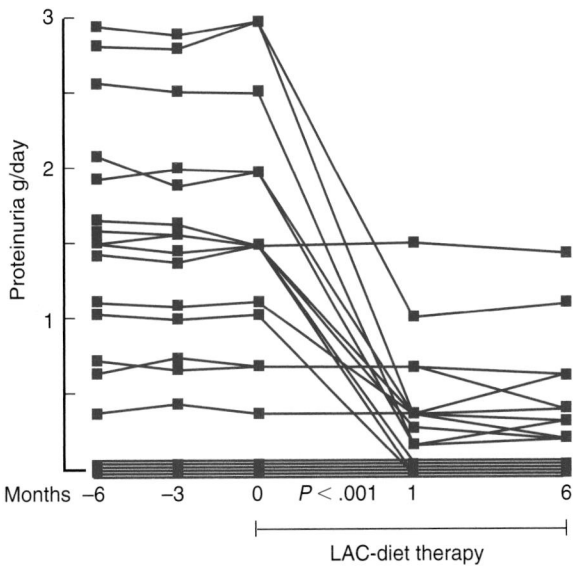

FIGURE 57-5. Twenty-four-hour proteinuria before/after a low-antigen content (LAC) diet in 21 IgA nephropathy patients. Values at −6, −3, 0, 1, and 6 months are expressed as the mean of at least three consecutive determinations. (From Ferri C, Puccini R, Longombardo G, et al: Low-antigen-content diet in the treatment of patients with IgA nephropathy. Nephrol Dial Transplant 8:1193-1198, 1993.)

in rats; it also reduced the renal hypertrophy induced by a high-protein diet.[336-338] Partial inhibition of arginase, induced by administration of a manganese-free diet, slowed the progression of renal failure after subtotal nephrectomy.[339, 340] Dietary arginine supplementation for only 3 days improved renal function in rats with bilateral ureteral obstruction or puromycin aminonucleoside–induced nephrosis.[341] A role of angiotensin II as well as nitric oxide in these responses was suggested by Ashab and associates.[342] They reported that ablative nephropathy (in the rat) was characterized by a reduction in nitrate plus nitrite excretion that was reversed by arginine or captopril administration; no additive benefit was observed when both were administered. They concluded that CRF, at least in the rat, is a low nitric oxide production state. Other evidence suggests that the vascular and hormonal effects of arginine administration might involve nonstereospecific responses, as opposed to the substrate effects on nitric oxide production (which should be stereospecific).[343] Moreover, there is also the problem of the arginine paradox: the intracellular arginine concentration is substantially above the K_m of nitric oxide synthase (NOS), so it is difficult to understand how arginine is serving only as a substrate. In addition, unexplained interactions also occur among glutamine, arginine, and endothelial cell nitric oxide production.[344] Finally, some of these responses could be linked to inhibition of ACE by arginine.[345] Both ACE inhibitors and angiotensin receptor blockers may enhance arginine-induced vasodilatation.[346] Dietary L-arginine (but not D-arginine) protected rats from cyclosporine nephrotoxicity, whereas inhibitors of nitric oxide biosynthesis aggravated it.[347, 348]

Oral or intravenous administration of arginine to normal subjects causes diuresis, lowers blood pressure,[349] and may induce microalbuminuria[350-352]; urinary cyclic adenosine monophosphate (cAMP) decreases. Creatinine excretion increases,[353] but little or no change in GFR occurs. In patients with heart failure, 15 g/day of oral arginine reduces endothelin levels and augments the diuretic response to saline loading.[351] In rats with renal ischemia, arginine infusion induces both beneficial and harmful effects.[354]

In contrast to these reports, Narita and associates[355, 356] suggested that the beneficial effects of low-protein diets in renal failure might be attributable to *reduced* intake of arginine. Dietary restriction of arginine ameliorated antithymocyte serum–induced glomerulonephritis, probably because the metabolism of arginine to polyamines and proline, as well as to nitric oxide, was up-regulated in this model of renal failure.[357] Oral arginine in children with CRF and endothelial dysfunction did not induce improvement.[358] A possible explanation of these discordant roles of nitric oxide in renal disease may be that iNOS is chronically stimulated by cytokines whereas acutely responsive cNOS activity may be depressed.[359] Further work will be needed to resolve these contradictory findings regarding the role of dietary arginine in progression of CRF.

Tryptophan

Kaysen and Kropp[360] reported in 1983 that dietary supplementation with tryptophan prevents the development of hypertension and proteinuria in seven-eighths nephrectomized rats. Further studies of tryptophan supplementation and progression do not appear to have been reported.

The keto acid/amino acid supplement used in the feasibility phase of the MDRD Study, as opposed to that used in the operational phase, was tryptophan free.[361, 362] This difference could be relevant because of a correlation between the rate of progression and the serum free tryptophan concentration[127]; the keto acid supplement used in the feasibility phase appeared to slow progression, whereas that used in the operational phase did not (see later). Profound hypotryptophanemia appeared in some of the patients in the feasibility study[363] and may have contributed to their slower progression.

In a series of reports, Japanese workers[364-367] have documented that indoxyl sulfate, a tryptophan metabolite, is nephrotoxic. Its removal by an orally administered sorbent slows progression of renal failure in patients ingesting a low-protein diet, at least as evidenced by sequential measurements of serum creatinine. A major problem with this scheme is that oral tryptophan administration, rather than increasing indoxyl sulfate levels, leads to a significant decrease in the urinary excretion of indoxyl sulfate.[368] Hence, it is not possible to attribute the purported slowing of progression induced by protein restriction to a lower intake of tryptophan with a resultant reduction in indoxyl sulfate production.

Effects of Modifications in Dietary Lipids

Many abnormalities of plasma lipids have been observed in CRF, and some of them clearly play a role in progression (see Chapter 50).[369-372] Whether progression can be slowed by dietary or pharmacologic modification of lipid levels is less clear. In rats with subtotal nephrectomy, a dietary supplement of linoleic acid did not protect against progression.[373] However, a study of dialysis patients indicated that those who ate fish tended to survive longer.[374] In diabetics with hyperlipidemia and nephropathy, statin treatment reduces proteinuria[372] and may slow progression.[375] However, a pronounced reduction in plasma total and low-density lipoprotein (LDL) cholesterol and triglycerides by statin therapy failed to alter albuminuria or the rate of progression to renal failure in children with steroid-resistant nephrotic syndrome.[376]

SUPPLEMENTED VEGETARIAN DIET. Whether based on soy protein and whether supplemented by essential amino acids, keto analogs, or both, protein-restricted vegetarian diets repeatedly have been reported to improve the lipid abnormalities associated with CRF.[329, 377, 378] It has not been established that progression is slowed by these maneuvers, however.

UNSATURATED FAT–ENRICHED DIET. According to Nielsen and co-workers,[379] feeding a diet containing 60% of its fat as monounsaturated fat had no effect on albuminuria in microalbuminuric patients with NIDDM. Conversely, Cappelli and associates[380] gave 3.4 g/day of polyunsaturated fatty acids for a year to half of a group of 20 CRF patients. When compared with the control group, treated patients exhibited lower circulating levels of lipids and cytokines, less proteinuria, and slower progression.

FISH OIL. The addition of fish oil to a vegetarian soy diet in nephrotic patients failed to exert additional effects on plasma lipids or proteinuria.[329] However, fish oil supplementation slows the rate of loss of renal function in IgA nephropathy.[381, 382] Manitius and co-workers[383] reported that serum concentrations of arachidonic acid and HDL increased in response to fish oil whereas urinary excretion of

N-acetyl-β-glucosaminidase and serum LDL decreased in 13 glomerulopathic patients with proteinuria and normal renal function; GFR and proteinuria were unaltered.

Effect of Gum

Dietary supplementation with gum arabic fiber (50 g/day) increases fecal nitrogen and lowers serum urea nitrogen (SUN) concentration in CRF patients, without altering nitrogen balance.[384] Fifteen grams per day of guar gum improves glycemic control and serum lipid levels in NIDDM patients.[385]

Effect of Dietary Antioxidants

There are good theoretical reasons to suppose that dietary supplementation with antioxidants should prove beneficial in CRF,[386] and two studies in rats have supported this view.[387, 388] As yet, no clinical trials of such treatment appear to have been reported.

Effect of Iron Supplements

Iron deficiency was common in CRF patients, both those undergoing dialysis and predialysis patients, even before the advent of erythropoietin therapy. The deficiency resulted from increased external losses, decreased availability of the body's store of iron, and (perhaps) defective intestinal iron absorption.[389] Erythropoietin treatment has exacerbated this problem because the need for iron to synthesize hemoglobin reduces body iron stores. Iron deficiency is in fact the main cause of resistance to erythropoietin treatment.[390] Other nutritional deficiencies, such as folic acid and vitamin B_{12}, can also impair the response to erythropoietin.[391] Unfortunately, no clear guidelines are available to establish the need for iron supplementation, although low levels of serum ferritin (<100 mg/dL), transferrin undersaturation (<20%), and low serum iron (<80 mg/dL) are all suggestive of iron deficiency. Each of these three measures of iron stores can be affected by diurnal variation and by the presence of inflammation. Clearly, some patients are unable to mobilize iron stores, as evidenced by normal or elevated ferritin levels despite transferrin undersaturation. Oral iron preparations include ferrous fumarate, ferrous sulfate (including slow-release forms and a wax-matrix form), ferrous gluconate, an iron-polysaccharide complex, and carbonyl iron. Only a few comparative studies of these different preparations have been reported; in one such study, ferrous fumarate was the most effective.[392] Intravenous therapy with iron dextran was reported earlier to be associated with life-threatening reactions in approximately 0.7% of subjects,[389] but subsequent studies have found it to be safe.[393] However, some evidence indicates that iron-induced oxidative stress may play a role in the development of arteriosclerosis in end-stage patients.[394, 395] An iron hydroxide–sucrose complex used in Europe did not cause a single life-threatening reaction during 8100 patient-years of treatment with approximately 160,000 ampules; five to seven reactions consisting of rapidly reversible hypotension and seven generalized skin reactions developed.[396] A sodium ferric gluconate complex is also efficacious,[397, 398] especially if given continuously,[399] and is relatively safe.[393, 400-403] Subcutaneous administration is effective and permits the dosage to be reduced. Oral administration of ferrous sulfate is just as effective in repleting iron stores in predialysis patients, but it causes more gastrointestinal symptoms.[404]

Initially, authorities were concerned that progression of renal insufficiency might be accelerated by erythropoietin administration. However, such has not proved to be the case[405]; in fact, slower progression during erythropoietin treatment has been noted in some studies.[406, 407] Such patients may respond to erythropoietin without supplemental iron.[408]

As an alternative to erythropoietin, androgens may be used in anemic hemodialysis patients at lower cost and apparently with comparable efficacy[409, 410]; iron supplementation is nevertheless necessary.

Effect of Calcium Supplements and Dietary Phosphorus

In early renal failure, serum calcitriol falls, and secondary hyperparathyroidism is nearly universal. As renal failure progresses, a reduction in parathyroid expression of vitamin D receptor as well as calcium receptor renders these glands resistant to both calcitriol and calcium. Dietary phosphorus further increases parathyroid hyperplasia in addition to parathyroid hormone (PTH) synthesis and secretion.[411]

In subtotally nephrectomized rats, dietary phosphorus restriction is more effective than protein restriction in ameliorating renal insufficiency.[412]

Calcium supplementation is widely used, both to reduce phosphate absorption and to raise serum calcium levels, but it can easily be overdone. Calcium acetate at a dose of 507 mg/day had no effect in predialysis patients, but 1521 mg/day reduced both PTH and 1,25-dihydroxyvitamin D concentrations and increased lumbar bone mineral density.[413]

Dietary Treatment of Nephrotic Syndrome

Current recommendations for nutritional therapy in patients with nephrotic syndrome[414] include moderate protein restriction (0.8 to 1.0 g/kg/day) and a soy vegetarian diet. The evidence for a special effect of soy protein comes from studies in rats; in animals with spontaneous hypercholesterolemia, in whom glomerular injury typically develops, Sakemi and colleagues[415] showed that soy protein, added to a conventional casein-based diet, did not have the ability to attenuate glomerular injury, but it was less harmful than additional casein.

Many studies have reported that dietary protein restriction reduces proteinuria in nephrotic syndrome. Fourteen studies published up to 1996 were summarized at that time.[416] Protein intake in the control period was usually about 1.2 g/kg; in the treatment period, it was restricted to 0.5 to 0.8 g/kg. The diet generally led to some decrease in proteinuria and some increase in serum albumin concentration, but none of the 202 patients exhibited normalization of serum albumin levels or a reduction in proteinuria to subnephrotic values. In a more recent study,[417] a low-protein diet was associated with a slight increase in serum albumin (6%), but albumin synthesis (which was more than twice normal) decreased.

In contrast to these findings, Walser and co-authors[416] reported that more severe protein restriction (to 0.3 g/kg) plus a supplement of essential amino acids (10 to 20 g/day) led to complete remission of nephrotic syndrome in a small number of cases. Sistani and Walser[418] recently reported the results of administering this regimen to a larger number of nephrotic patients. In 39 of them who complied with the diet, proteinuria decreased by half; surprisingly, the decrease was most pronounced in those with the largest degree of proteinuria (>4.0 g/day); no change occurred in those with 0.5 to 4.0 g/day of proteinuria. Serum albumin levels in the former group rose to normal at 1 year. Similar results were reported in preliminary form from Japan.[419]

These results are the opposite of conventional wisdom, which holds that protein-restricted diets should not be used in patients with pronounced proteinuria. On the contrary, it is only when proteinuria is pronounced that this regimen is effective. Obviously, dietary treatment of this type, though arduous for the patient, entails few risks, especially when compared with immunosuppressive drugs or high doses of steroids—therapies that are often used in such patients.

TURNOVER OF NITROGENOUS EXCRETORY PRODUCTS IN CHRONIC UREMIA

To maintain health, adults must remain in protein balance, with protein synthesis equaling protein degradation. In contrast, growing children must have a positive protein balance, with protein synthesis exceeding protein degradation. Because it is technically difficult to measure protein synthesis and degradation,[420, 421] nitrogen balance is frequently calculated and the results are assumed to be equivalent to protein balance. Nitrogen balance is calculated as the difference between the intake and excretion of nitrogen in subjects with normal kidney function, but in patients with kidney disease, another term must be added, the accumulation of nitrogen-containing products in body fluids. These nitrogenous products are not converted into body protein, and their accumulation is undoubtedly the cause of the symptoms of uremia because reducing their accumulation, either by restricting dietary protein or by dialysis, is associated with symptomatic improvement. Because of the enormous excretory capacity of the kidney, uremic symptoms from accumulation of these products is unusual until renal function is reduced to below 30% of normal. In summary, the hallmark of chronic uremia is the accumulation of nitrogenous waste products in body fluids. Because these waste products arise from catabolism of dietary protein and body protein stores, CRF is an example of a state of protein intolerance.

Once produced, a waste product has three fates: it is excreted, accumulates in body fluids, or is degraded. This relationship is the basis for a useful method of calculating the severity of uremia, the steady-state concentration of blood urea nitrogen (BUN).[422] It is calculated by rearranging the clearance formula so that production of urea minus its degradation divided by urea clearance yields the steady-state BUN for that patient. The calculation assumes that urea clearance is independent of the plasma concentration, which is reasonable for CRF subjects. The usefulness of calculating steady-state SUN is that it precisely expresses the severity of renal impairment in relation to the nitrogenous waste products that require excretion. The amount of waste products to be excreted is directly proportional to the amount of dietary and endogenous protein being catabolized because urea is the major end product of protein breakdown.

Moreover, the steady-state concentration of any nitrogen-containing waste product produced during protein catabolism will rise in blood as SUN increases.[423-426] Examples of waste nitrogen compounds important to consider in the treatment of CRF patients will be discussed.

Urea

It has been known since the classic report of Folin that urea nitrogen excretion by normal subjects varies directly with protein intake.[427] The refinement is that urea nitrogen is the major product of protein degradation, and hence, the urea nitrogen appearance rate calculated as the sum of urea excreted and accumulated varies directly with protein intake. The practical importance of this relationship is that it yields the intake of nitrogen (principally protein) in subjects with and without renal disease.[423-426] For dialysis patients, the same relationship between urea turnover and protein intake has been labeled "urea generation" or the "protein catabolic rate" by Sargent and co-workers.[428] They pointed out that urea generation by dialysis patients is calculated as the sum of urea excreted and removed by dialysis plus changes in the body pool of urea. This value is the same as the urea appearance rate and, hence, closely parallels protein in the diet.[428, 429] Designation of this value as the protein catabolic rate, however, is incorrect because it does not measure total protein catabolism. Rates of protein catabolism are far greater: the nitrogen flux occurring during the daily processes of protein synthesis and degradation amounts to 45 to 55 g of nitrogen per day, which is equivalent to 280 to 350 g of protein or more than 1 kg of muscle.[430, 431] More accurately, the protein catabolic rate is an estimate of protein intake because it is calculated by adding urea generation (i.e., urea appearance) to an estimate of non-urea nitrogen excretion (see later discussion) and multiplying the sum by 6.25 to convert nitrogen to its protein equivalent. The principle of conservation of mass indicates that the difference between the net nitrogen arising from the difference between whole-body protein synthesis and degradation plus dietary nitrogen must equal waste nitrogen production. However, the implication that the protein catabolic rate is a measure of whole-body protein catabolism is incorrect.

Urea Production and Degradation

To calculate rates of urea production and degradation, plasma disappearance of ^{14}C- or ^{15}N-urea must be measured. Interestingly, the rate of urea production exceeds the steady-state rate of urea excretion in both normal and uremic subjects. This difference is due to degradation of urea by bacterial urease in the gastrointestinal tract, and such degradation results in the formation of ammonia and carbon dioxide.[432-434] The rate of urea degradation in normal subjects eating a diet of about 90 g protein per day averages 3.6 g/day of nitrogen, thus indicating that only a fourth of the urea produced from dietary protein is degraded by intestinal bacteria. Apparently, urea arrives in the intestinal tract by secretion with gastrointestinal fluids, and the ammonia generated from urea is absorbed by passive, nonionic diffusion into portal blood for transport to the liver.[435, 436] The fate of ammonia nitrogen derived from urea has been extensively evaluated (see discussion later).

Another means of evaluating urea degradation is to express it as extrarenal urea clearance, defined as the rate of degradation divided by the plasma concentration of urea; the extrarenal urea clearance of normal subjects averages about 24 L/day.[432, 433, 437-439] If extrarenal clearance were unchanged in patients with high BUN values, a considerable amount of ammonia would be generated. Although an increased quantity of bacteria are found in the upper intestines of CRF patients,[440] careful measurements of urea degradation indicate that the quantity of ammonia arising from urea is not significantly different from that in normal subjects.[441-443] Accordingly, the extrarenal clearance of urea in CRF patients is greatly reduced in comparison to that of normal subjects and is not correlated with renal urea clearance.[443] Robson[442] found that the average extrarenal urea clearance of patients with CRF was 4.5 L/day; in patients being treated with low-protein diets supplemented with amino acids or their α-keto or α-hydroxy analogs, we found that it averages less than 4 L/day,[443, 444] which means that the amount of nitrogen available from urea degradation is not as large as originally thought. The most likely explanation for this finding is that chronic uremia induces a change in the gut mucosa that in some way limits the access of urea to bacterial urease. Regardless, the results obtained in patients with stable CRF do not exclude the possibility that a rapid elevation in plasma urea, as occurs in patients with acute renal failure, might increase the rate of urea degradation.[445]

Details of urea metabolism are critical for understanding the nutritional principles of treating patients with kidney disease because a goal is to minimize urea nitrogen production (or urea appearance). One factor that can change urea metabolism is diuretic therapy. Diuretics can cause volume depletion, thereby resulting in depressed urea clearance because of a secondary increase in the reabsorption of urea.[446] Kato and Sands provided insight into the molecular basis for this observation from studies of perfused tubules of rats treated with furosemide.[447] They found induction of urea transporters leading to urea reabsorption in the early segment of the inner medullary collecting duct, as well as suppression of urea secretion from the more distal collecting duct. Both processes had characteristics of active transport systems. Another factor influencing urea metabolism relates to sodium depletion. If sufficiently severe, sodium depletion causes urea appearance to rise in both animals and humans.[446, 448] The mechanism for stimulation of urea production by sodium depletion is unknown, but apparently, it does not require glucocorticoids.[448]

Creatinine

Creatinine is formed from the nonenzymatic dehydration of creatine and creatine phosphate. The turnover rate of the creatine pool is only 1.7% per day[256]; this low turnover rate means that a change in the rate of creatinine production does not reach a new steady state for 41 days.[449] Because the major pool of creatine is in muscle and because creatinine is excreted almost completely (see later discussion), the rate of creatinine excretion has been used as an index of lean body mass. Unfortunately, considerable variation exists in creatinine excretion that cannot explained by collection error,[45] so an average of 3 consecutive days of creatinine excretion is required for any reasonably precise estimate of lean body mass.[450-453]

Besides variations in lean body mass, meat in the diet changes creatinine excretion[452, 453]; when a diet is creatine free, creatinine excretion falls about 15%.[453] The fact that creatinine excretion does not decrease even more with these diets may be due to stimulation of creatine (and ultimately, creatinine) production by low-protein or low-creatine diets.[454, 455]

The most important factor affecting creatinine excretion in normal subjects, besides dietary creatine/creatinine and lean body mass, is age.[450] In order of descending importance, factors determining the relationship of age and creatinine excretion are (1) a lower lean body mass and hence muscle as a fraction of weight (aging is associated with increased body fat) and (2) a presumed decrease in meat intake with aging.[453] Creatinine excretion is also decreased in CRF patients who have high levels of serum creatinine.[456] This decrease has been attributed to a loss of lean body mass, but in patients with advanced CRF, it is far out of proportion to any possible change in their lean body mass.[449] In fact, when measured by isotope dilution, creatinine production in CRF patients was found to be virtually the same as the rates predicted for normal subjects of the same age, sex, and weight.[457] Thus, the explanation for decreased creatinine excretion in CRF must be degradation of creatinine.[458]

The first definitive evidence for creatinine degradation was reported by Jones and Burnett,[459] who measured the disappearance of ^{14}C-labeled creatinine administered to uremic patients by injection or by mouth. They estimated that as much as 66% of the creatinine produced was degraded, and they detected radioactivity in products of creatinine metabolism such as sarcosine, *N*-methylhydantoin, creatine, and carbon dioxide. We also examined the fate of ^{14}C-creatinine injected into CRF patients and found that creatinine degradation was positively correlated with the serum creatinine concentration.[457] We found that creatinine, like urea, can be recycled, and it forms creatine. Based on measured degradation rates, we calculated a low extrarenal creatinine clearance (average, 0.039 L/kg/day), which explains why creatinine metabolism is an important route of elimination only when the serum creatinine concentration is high. The low extrarenal clearance also may explain why creatinine degradation has not been detected previously in humans or animals with normal renal creatinine clearance.[460, 461]

It is likely that intestinal bacteria degrade creatinine because intestinal flora obtained from experimental animals that are being fed creatinine or from the intestines of normal subjects or CRF patients degrade creatinine readily.[462, 463] Conversely, creatinine metabolism in uremic subjects was not suppressed by the oral administration of antibiotics, even though the dose was sufficient to inhibit urea degradation.[457]

The physiologic importance of creatinine degradation and the decline in creatinine excretion occurring with protein-restricted diets is that creatinine excretion cannot be used as an index of lean body mass in CRF patients. The complex interrelationships among dietary creatine/creatinine, creatine production and turnover, and creatinine degradation emphasize the hazards of making judgments about lean body mass from changes in creatinine excretion.[184]

Uric Acid

The fractional clearance of uric acid rises markedly at GFR values below 15 mL/min, with the ratio of urate excreted to the GFR raised about fivefold because of increased secretion and reduced reabsorption.[464] Besides this adaptation, the steady-state level of uric acid excretion by patients with advanced renal failure also changes by falling to about 100 to 300 mg/day (normal rates, 400 to 600 mg/day).[465] From the preceding discussion, the fact that a serum uric acid level above 10 mg/dL is unusual in such patients must mean that uric acid production is sharply reduced or that extensive extrarenal degradation of uric acid occurs.[458, 466] Both possibilities are likely because a protein-restricted diet is generally associated with lower purine intake and evidence has shown that protein intake may drop spontaneously in patients with advancing renal insufficiency.[187, 467, 468] In addition to decreased uric acid production, it is likely that degradation of uric acid occurs. Sorensen and colleagues reported that intravenously injected, radiolabeled uric acid could not be completely recovered in the urine of either normal subjects or CRF patients and calculated that extrarenal urate clearance accounts for as much as 65% of the uric acid produced by patients with renal insufficiency.[469-472] Intestinal bacteria are probably responsible for uric acid degradation because the fraction of urate degraded is reduced from 22% to 3% after the oral administration of neomycin and streptomycin.[472]

Many compounds produced during the degradation of uric acid (e.g., ammonia, urea, allantoin) are also excreted by the kidney. Consequently, extrarenal urate clearance (as well as the extrarenal clearance of other compounds) does not necessarily eliminate nitrogen; it may simply lead to the accumulation of other compounds.[473] Nonetheless, degradation of urate must contribute to the fact that CRF patients have a low incidence of gouty arthritis or renal urate deposits.[474] Uric acid crystals surrounded by inflammatory cells and fibrous tissue may be found in the renal medulla of nongouty patients with long-standing progressive renal insufficiency, but they are unusual, and long-term allopurinol therapy does not significantly slow the progression of chronic renal insufficiency in patients with hyperuricemia.[475] Recently, another role for uric acid has been proposed.[192] Johnson and colleagues point out that humans have a higher serum uric acid level than other primates or animals do, presumably because of a mutation in uricase (the enzyme that initiates degradation of uric acid). Experimentally, a higher uric acid level is associated with the development of hypertension, and this hypertension in turn seems to be of the "salt-sensitive" type.[192] These authors have extended their studies to determine whether uric acid has other adverse effects. The experimental model is to administer oxonic acid to rats to block uricase activity and raise the serum uric acid level to about 2 mg/dL. This increased uric acid results in progressive renal insufficiency[193] that can be linked to the development of glomerular hypertrophy[194] and to pathologic changes in the arterioles of the kidney.[195] All these changes are substantially ameliorated by administering allopurinol or a uricosuric diuretic. Viewed in this light, it is interesting to note that Fessel[476] excluded patients with severe hypertension in his analysis of the outcome of high levels of uric acid. He examined the clinical course of 113 patients with asymptomatic hyperuricemia and 168 patients with gout, some of whom had mild renal insufficiency. He concluded that unless serum uric acid exceeded 10 mg/dL in women or 13 mg/dL in men, high uric acid alone will not affect residual renal function. Thus, the question remains of whether this problem

(and its consequences) develops in patients with hypertension because of a high serum uric acid.

Other problems associated with a high serum uric acid concentration do not appear to be common in patients with kidney failure. For example, uric acid stones are uncommon; they occurred in only 1.0% to 2.6% of 113 patients with normal renal function and asymptomatic hyperuricemia who were monitored for 8 or more years.[476] Likewise, in nongouty patients with renal insufficiency and hyperuricemia, uric acid stones are rare. Based on these data, allopurinol should not be prescribed for patients with CRF unless they have a history of gouty arthritis or biopsy-proven gouty nephropathy or unless the serum uric acid level is excessively high.[477] It remains to be tested whether allopurinol therapy will be useful in treating the hypertension that so commonly occurs in patients with renal insufficiency.[192]

Ammonia

Loss of renal mass reduces the capacity to excrete ammonia, even in response to metabolic acidosis (see Chapter 11). The major source of blood ammonia is bacterial degradation of urea, as well as amino acids, peptides, and protein in the intestine; in addition, glutamine is degraded to ammonia in the small intestinal mucosa.[478-480] Ammonia transported from the intestine to the liver is readily converted to urea, so blood ammonia levels in patients with renal insufficiency should not be elevated. Although a slightly high blood ammonia level has been reported,[481] the mechanisms for this finding and its clinical importance are unknown. Moreover, isolated cases of hyperammonemia have occurred in CRF patients who have apparently normal liver function.[482] The mechanisms causing hyperammonemia in these cases include partial defects in urea cycle enzymes or other inherited disorders,[483, 484] high-dose chemotherapy,[485] and infections.[482, 486] Urease-producing bacteria in urinary bladders or intestinal abscesses can also cause clinically important hyperammonemia, especially if venous blood from the infected area drains into the vena cava and bypasses the liver.

Other Nitrogenous Compounds in Urine

The difference between total urinary nitrogen and the sum of urea, uric acid, and creatinine nitrogen in urine is termed unmeasured nitrogen and includes peptides and protein.[423, 426, 487] In patients without proteinuria, it is small and measures only 6.2 mg/kg/day when total urinary nitrogen is 10.3 g/day.[427] In patients with proteinuria, albumin clearance as a fraction of the GFR varies from 0.3% to 3.0% or more.[488] In general, protein clearance falls as the GFR decreases, but the amount excreted depends on factors other than the degree of glomerular damage.[160, 489, 490] For example, raising dietary protein increases proteinuria in nephrotic patients,[491] and dietary protein restriction (see later) can reduce proteinuria.[489, 492-494] Drugs also affect the degree of proteinuria; it falls when blood pressure is reduced, especially with ACE inhibitors.[495]

Fecal Nitrogen

Patients with CRF commonly have occult intestinal blood loss. In one study, the average blood loss was 6 mL/day; this amount may be difficult to detect by the guaiac technique.[496] Regardless, whenever urea appearance is found to exceed protein nitrogen intake, gastrointestinal bleeding must be considered. Other causes of a change in fecal nitrogen identified in normal adults include variation in dietary roughage, fermentable carbohydrates, and nitrogen.[384, 497-501] Consequently, it has been suggested that dietary factors could play an important role in the amount of nitrogen excreted as feces. Kopple and colleagues[424] examined rates of nitrogen excretion in nondialysis CRF patients and concluded that fecal nitrogen was correlated with protein intake. In contrast, Maroni and associates[423] had reported that fecal nitrogen varied with body weight rather than the diet. This possibility was examined in 52 adult, nondialysis patients eating various types of diets while nitrogen balance was being measured.[426] No significant relationship was found between dietary nitrogen and fecal nitrogen excretion.

Total Non-Urea Nitrogen Excretion

Non-urea nitrogen consists of the nitrogen in feces plus the nitrogen excreted in urine in all other forms besides urea (i.e., urinary creatinine, uric acid, ammonium, peptides). Maroni and colleagues found that the average non-urea nitrogen excretion of CRF patients who were in neutral or nearly neutral nitrogen balance while eating diets containing as much as 94 g/day of protein or low-protein diets supplemented with keto acids was 0.031 g/kg/day of nitrogen.[423] This value was derived from nitrogen balance measurements in 19 nondialyzed CRF patients consuming 34 to 94 g of protein per day. When a non-urea nitrogen excretion value of 0.031 g N/kg/day was used, the estimated nitrogen balance did not differ statistically from the measured nitrogen balance. Interestingly, 0.031 g/kg/day of nitrogen (Fig. 57-6) is similar to the value for non-urea urinary nitrogen plus fecal nitrogen excreted by normal subjects or dialysis patients.[502-504] Thus, the proposal was to estimate protein intake as the sum of urea nitrogen appearance plus an estimate of non-urea nitrogen excretion (i.e., 0.031 g N/kg/day).

Because of the ease of this calculation, others have examined the relationship between dietary protein and nitrogen excretion. Kopple and associates[424] reported a correlation between fecal nitrogen and nitrogen intake. This finding suggests that total non-urea nitrogen excretion should increase with dietary protein intake, but Kopple and co-workers found no relationship between non-urea nitrogen excretion and dietary nitrogen (or body weight). Based on correlations between the components of nitrogen balance, they concluded that non-urea nitrogen excretion was the same for all patients, and they proposed that dietary protein would be equal to 1.204 times the urea appearance value plus 1.74 g nitrogen per day. Kopple and co-workers also found that total nitrogen excretion was correlated more closely with urea appearance than with nitrogen intake and then concluded that urea appearance should not be used to estimate dietary nitrogen and hence protein intake. Instead, urea appearance should be used to estimate total nitrogen excretion. Although the sum of urea and non-urea nitrogen excretion is, indeed, total nitrogen excretion, the conclusion that dietary protein cannot be estimated was disappointing. Consequently, Masud and colleagues re-examined these relationships by using the results of nitrogen balance measurements performed on 52 CRF patients ingesting different levels of dietary protein.[426] The results differed from those of Kopple and colleagues.[424] Neither fecal nitrogen nor non-urea nitrogen was correlated with dietary nitrogen, but non-urea nitrogen excretion was significantly correlated with body weight. Again, the average daily excretion of non-urea nitrogen was found to be 0.031 g nitrogen per kilogram body weight per day. These relationships were found when all 80 nitrogen balance studies were examined or when the analysis was restricted to a subgroup of patients who had had no previous investigation of the components of non-urea nitrogen excretion. Finally, Masud and associates evaluated the accuracy of the method of estimating dietary protein. A slightly lower error in estimating protein intake was found when using the original formula derived by Maroni and colleages versus that of Kopple and co-workers.[423, 424] The finding of similar results is probably related to the fact that body weight of the patients did not vary widely. In this case, the intercept of a regression analysis will yield similar information as that based on body weight.[426] These relationships are discussed because of the necessity of assessing protein intake in CRF patients to ensure that the diet is adequate but not excessive. Note that these relationships are based on the assumption that the patient is in neutral nitrogen balance (i.e., that nitrogen excretion equals nitrogen intake) and do not apply to hypercatabolic patients or patients receiving hyperalimentation or "totally digestible" diets.[505, 506]

Skin Nitrogen Losses

In otherwise normal adults, nitrogen loss from the skin and other unmeasured sources averages 0.5 g nitrogen per day. This amount should be used when calculating nitrogen balance. However, the concentration of urea in sweat is proportional to the plasma urea concentration,[507] and increased losses of nitrogen might occur in uremic individuals during periods of heavy perspiration.

In summary, nitrogen excretion by normal and uremic subjects can be divided into urea nitrogen and non-urea nitrogen.

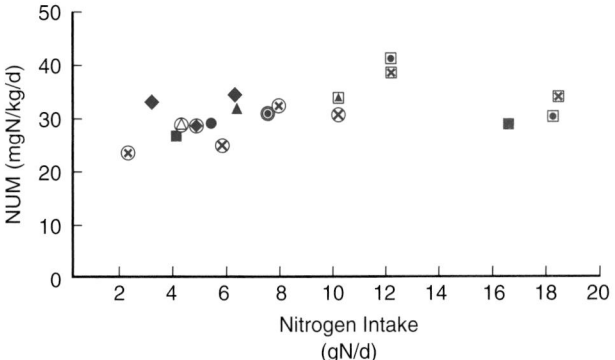

FIGURE 57-6. Calculated values of total non-urea nitrogen excretion (NUN) in normal subjects (▲, ●, ■) and patients with chronic renal failure being treated with nutritional therapy (♦, ⊗, ◎, ◇, ◉) or by hemodialysis or continuous ambulatory peritoneal dialysis (⊠, ▢). (From Maroni BJ, Steinman TI, Mitch WE: A method for estimating nitrogen intake of patients with chronic renal failure. Kidney Int 27:58, 1985. Used with permission from Kidney International.)

Production of urea nitrogen is closely related to protein intake; excretion of non-urea nitrogen is more closely related to weight. These relationships can be used to estimate dietary protein intake, with the caveat that the patient should be in neutral or nearly neutral nitrogen balance and not receiving intravenous hyperalimentation.

ASSESSMENT OF PROTEIN STORES IN CHRONIC RENAL FAILURE

In CRF patients, the requirement to minimize the accumulation of nitrogenous waste products must be balanced against the need to supply enough essential amino acids in the diet to prevent loss of body protein. The optimal diet, then, is one in which protein synthesis equals protein breakdown. In this case, the urea appearance rate is minimal. Degradation of amino acids will be minimal because they are used to synthesize protein, and when protein synthesis equals protein degradation, body protein stores are maintained and nitrogen balance is zero. As discussed, it is difficult to measure daily rates of protein synthesis and breakdown, which are high and subject to change by several factors, including an insufficient diet.[431, 508-510] Because protein turnover is high, even a small increase in protein breakdown or a decrease in protein synthesis persisting for several weeks can cause a marked loss of lean body mass. The "gold standard" for evaluating whether protein stores are being maintained is nitrogen balance. Unfortunately, measurement of nitrogen balance is difficult and requires careful measurement of the food eaten and all routes of nitrogen excretion.[511] It also does not provide rates of protein turnover and, hence, rarely gives insight into mechanisms that cause loss of protein stores. However, other assessments are associated with problems. For example, hypoalbuminemia is a frequently cited index of malnutrition, but albumin stores are affected by many factors, including inflammation, acidosis, and diet.[512-514] In short, uncovering a mechanism for loss of protein stores is complicated and requires repeated evaluation.

Nitrogen Balance

Nitrogen balance is equal to the difference between nitrogen intake and excretion, plus the accumulation of nonprotein nitrogen (principally urea). The $t_{1/2}$ of urea disappearance in a normal human is about 7 hours, so even a large load of urea is mostly excreted within a day. It follows that in normal subjects, any change in the urea pool can be ignored during measurement of daily nitrogen balance. In CRF patients, the $t_{1/2}$ of urea may be markedly prolonged, so the BUN concentration and body pool of urea nitrogen may not be stable for a prolonged period after a change in dietary protein. For this reason, the accumulation or loss of urea nitrogen in the body must be taken into account when the nitrogen balance of CRF patients is measured. Fortunately, the concentration of urea is equal throughout most of body water, so changes in the urea nitrogen pool can be calculated by assuming that the urea space is equivalent to 60% of body weight, the average body water in nonedematous uremic patients.[423, 130] When body water in liters is multiplied by the SUN in grams per liter, the result is the size of the urea nitrogen pool. Note that the precision of measuring BUN can dominate the nitrogen

balance calculation if only two measurements are made. For example, a change in BUN from 140 to 150 mg/dL, which may be within the laboratory error of measuring BUN, represents about 4 g of nitrogen in a 70-kg person. Because both a change in weight and a change in BUN can affect the calculation, it is more accurate to estimate the urea space on a given day and then calculate daily values of the urea pool as SUN times body water plus any change in weight to derive an average change in size of the urea pool. This calculation assumes that water accounts for all changes in weight during short periods (i.e., that dry weight, or body weight minus body water, remains constant). The daily rate of change in the urea nitrogen pool can be calculated by linear regression or other curve-fitting techniques.[428, 429]

It is more precise to measure the urea space by using ^{15}N- or ^{14}C-labeled urea.[442-444] This method avoids the error of assuming that all uremic subjects have the same fraction of body weight that is body water and the observation that the urea space occasionally exceeds body water or even body weight.[442, 515] Measurement of the urea space in patients with advanced renal failure does not require correction for losses of the label in urine because the excess urea excretion seen in normal subjects during equilibration of labeled urea does not occur to an appreciable extent.[442]

Other sources of nonprotein nitrogen that accumulate in CRF patients, such as creatinine, can be ignored because even a large increase in serum creatinine affects retained nitrogen minimally. For example, when serum creatinine rises from 10 to 15 mg/dL, it will increase nitrogen retention only 0.3 g in a 70-kg person.[457] Changes in the pool of other nonprotein nitrogenous compounds are not commonly measured because their volumes of distribution are not known. However, after extensive trauma, the loss of tissue glutamine nitrogen may amount to several grams. Calculating this change is difficult because of the large number of assumptions required.[516]

Urea Nitrogen Appearance Rate

Because the principal nonprotein source for nitrogen in the body is urea, it is important to assess how urea accumulation and excretion are changing when evaluating protein stores. To accomplish this task, the urea nitrogen appearance rate is calculated as the sum of urinary excretion plus accumulation (positive or negative) in the body pool of urea nitrogen. It should be calculated from several consecutive 24-hour urine collections, daily determinations of weight and SUN, and measurement of the urea space with the use of labeled urea,[443, 444] or 60% of weight in nonedematous subjects.[423] Knowledge of the urea appearance rate is critical when treating CRF patients because it provides a quantitative measurement of the parameter that nutritional therapy seeks to minimize: a minimal urea appearance value is associated with the most efficient use of dietary protein. Taylor and associates[517] fed low-protein diets containing different amounts of calories to normal young men and women. Their data reveal a correlation of $r = -0.87$ between the calculated fraction of dietary protein used for protein synthesis and urea excretion (which is equal to urea appearance in normal subjects). Cottini and associates[425] found that a diet containing 3 to 4 g/day of nitrogen was associated with neutral nitrogen balance in CRF patients (Fig. 57-7). Clearly, interpretation of

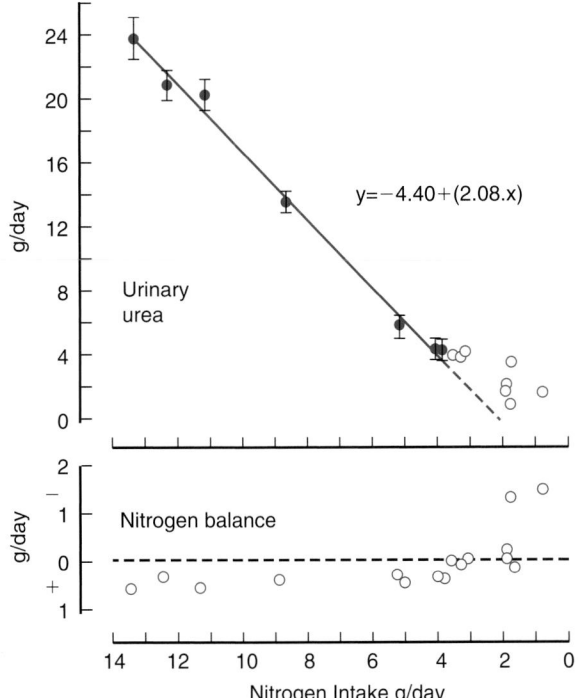

FIGURE 57-7. Nitrogen balance and urinary urea as a function of nitrogen intake in chronically uremic subjects fed varying quantities of dietary protein. All subjects receiving less than 4 g of nitrogen per day were in neutral or negative nitrogen balance, and urea excretion tends to plateau at a low value. In subjects receiving more than 4 g of nitrogen per day, urea nitrogen is equal to the increment in nitrogen intake above the amount required to achieve neutral nitrogen balance. (From Cottini EP, Gallina DK, Dominguez JM: Urea excretion in adult humans with varying degrees of kidney malfunction fed milk, egg, or an amino acid mixture: Assessment of nitrogen balance. J Nutr 102:11, 1973.)

the urea nitrogen appearance of CRF patients requires some knowledge of nitrogen intake because of the close relationship between nitrogen intake and urea appearance.

Serum Albumin

The concentration of serum albumin is frequently cited as an index of the adequacy of the diet, with a low value being equated with malnutrition. However, the serum albumin concentration is the result of a balance between synthesis and degradation of albumin, losses of albumin as in nephrotic syndrome, and dilution of albumin. When careful measurements of albumin turnover were made in hemodialysis patients, it was found that serum albumin was correlated with body weight and estimates of protein intake (i.e., normalized protein catabolic rate), thus suggesting that variation in albumin synthesis was an important factor controlling serum albumin.[512] Because albumin synthesis was also correlated with plasma volume, the association with body weight may have reflected the response to dilution more than to dietary inadequacy. Apparently, the more important determinant of serum albumin was related to variation in albumin catabolism, and variation in catabolism was correlated with evidence of inflammation (metabolic acidosis was not evaluated in this study, but this factor is also known to reduce serum albumin).[513] Hence, albumin stores were being lost through

degradation and external losses. In summary, serum albumin is affected by several factors. Concluding that a low serum albumin concentration is simply due to a low-protein diet can be very misleading. For example, patients in the MDRD Study who were prescribed the lowest amount of dietary protein had an increase in their serum albumin on average.[184] Second, nonacidotic patients eating very low protein diets supplemented with keto acids and essential amino acids over periods of a year or more had normal serum albumin values and plasma volume.[138, 518-520] Besides the difficulty of determining a cause for a low serum albumin level, other problems are encountered with reliance on serum albumin as an index of protein stores. Serum albumin responds relatively slowly to changes in protein stores because of a $t_{1/2}$ of about 20 days. Plasma albumin levels in malnourished patients are only slowly restored to normal during protein refeeding.[521]

Investigators have expressed widespread interest in documenting that inflammation is a major cause of the morbidity and mortality of CRF patients, including those being treated by dialysis. This interest has arisen for two reasons: Kaysen and co-workers[261, 512] showed that albumin synthesis falls sharply in subjects with inflammatory illnesses (i.e., albumin functions as a "negative" acute-phase reactant). Second, evidence of inflammation seems to be an important index of arteriosclerosis, a problem experienced by many CRF patients.[522] Regarding the association of inflammation and hypoalbuminemia, the initial studies revealed an association between the presence of hypoalbuminemia in dialysis patients and higher serum levels of the acute-phase reactant proteins amyloid A and C-reactive protein (CRP).[523] However, the finding that serum acute-phase reactant proteins are associated with a low serum albumin level cannot be considered a cause-effect relationship. More recently, Kaysen and colleagues reported that a high CRP level in 1 month did not predict a decrease in serum albumin in the subsequent month. Because of the long $t_{1/2}$ of albumin, they also examined the relationships between serum albumin and longer-lived acute-phase reactant proteins.[514] It was found that high serum levels of the longer-lived acute-phase reactant proteins ceruloplasmin and α_1-acid glycoprotein did predict a lower serum albumin level in the succeeding month. It was concluded that inflammation is a cause of low serum albumin levels.

Qureshi and associates[174] reported high levels of CRP in many of the patients whom they studied in a cross-sectional evaluation of hemodialysis patients, and they noted a relationship between hypoalbuminemia and higher levels of CRP. They equated the high level of CRP with inflammation and suggested a link between this inflammation and cardiovascular disease in dialysis patients. Others have confirmed these findings and emphasized the correlations between biochemical evidence of inflammation and atherosclerosis in dialysis patients.[524] The causes of inflammation and the association with atherosclerosis are unclear but could be related to the accumulation of advanced glycosylation proteins,[525] infection in the dialysis access,[526] or the dialysis procedure per se.[527] Even when some of these problems are not present, CRF patients are at risk for inflammation because they have high circulating levels of inflammatory cytokines[528, 529] and evidence of accelerated atherosclerosis.[522] Shoji and colleagues[530] examined 110 patients with a variety of diseases causing kidney disease; diabetics were excluded. They found increased thickening of the intima and media of the carotid vessels that was not related to age, gender, blood pressure, or smoking, thus suggesting that other factors associated with kidney disease accelerate atherosclerosis. Whether this factor is inflammation has not been settled. Other have suggested that another cause of accelerated atherosclerosis is accumulation of homocysteine,[531, 532] which carries an especially bad prognosis in patients with coronary artery disease.[532, 533] Treatment of this disorder is administration of vitamin B_6 and folinic acid (see Chapter 48), but it is only partially successful.[534, 535] On the other hand, some evidence indicates that inflammation in patients with kidney disease is a more important factor causing accelerated atherosclerosis.[536]

Serum Transferrin, Prealbumin, Complement, and Insulin-like Growth Factor-1

Some researchers[537, 538] have suggested that serum transferrin is more reliable than albumin as an estimate of protein nutrition because transferrin is more sensitive to protein deficiency and has a shorter $t_{1/2}$ ($\approx$10 days). The transferrin concentration in milligrams per deciliter is interconverted with total iron-binding capacity (TIBC) in micrograms per deciliter by multiplying TIBC by 0.7. A slightly greater degree of precision is obtained by using the formula transferrin $-1.0900 \times (\text{TIBC} - 63)$.[539] Unfortunately, serum transferrin levels, like serum albumin, change with factors other than nutritional status. Serum transferrin may rise when iron stores are depleted and diminish by as much as 50% with chronic inflammatory disorders such as malignant tumors, rheumatoid arthritis, and infections. Erythropoietin treatment causes no significant change in serum transferrin levels, at least in dialysis patients, nor any major change in nutritional status and no change or minimal improvement in serum albumin, anthropometry, and muscle protein content.[540-542] Left ventricular hypertrophy has a tendency to regress with erythropoietin, an important consideration in view of the excessive amount of cardiovascular disease in patients with kidney disease.[543, 544] Based on these data, in patients with hypertension or left ventricular hypertrophy (or both), a persuasive case for its use can be made. However, no persuasive reason can be found to use erythropoietin in predialysis patients solely to improve indices that have been used to monitor nutritional status.

The serum concentration of prealbumin also has been touted as an index of nutritional status.[545] It has a $t_{1/2}$ of about 2 days and therefore changes more rapidly with variations in nutritional status. However, the problem of other factors causing changes in serum albumin (e.g., inflammation) undoubtedly applies to serum prealbumin. When compared with serum albumin and transferrin, prealbumin concentrations in hemodialysis patients appeared to have a special advantage because they were more highly correlated with complications (at a level below 0.3 g/L, a higher incidence of complications was observed, including infections and mortality).[546] Results from other studies of hemodialysis[547] or chronic ambulatory peritoneal dialysis (CAPD) patients[548] concur; however, the usefulness of prealbumin as a nutritional marker has not been extensively evaluated in predialysis patients.

Abnormalities of most of the components of serum complement occur in patients with chronic uremia, especially an increase in C4.[549] Some of these changes may be due to

protein malnutrition because parenteral administration of essential amino acids for a month reportedly corrected most of them.[549]

IGF-1, the major hormone that mediates the effects of growth hormone, has been studied in uremic patients for three reasons. First, administration of growth hormone is associated with a remarkable improvement in the growth of children and in the nutritional status of hemodialysis and CAPD patients.[550-553] Second, IGF-1 administration has been proposed as a means of augmenting renal function in CRF patients.[554] Finally, administration of IGF-1 has also been proposed as a means of inhibiting the catabolism of muscle protein.[555] Indeed, some evidence has indicated that acute administration of IGF-1 can improve muscle protein synthesis in normal or uremic patients,[556, 557] but responsiveness in hemodialysis patients appears to be reduced, possibly because of a postreceptor defect in the action of IGF-1.[558, 559] This area of research is complicated because the action of IGF-1 is influenced by the concentration of IGF-binding proteins, as well as by circulating levels of amino acids.[320, 557, 560, 561] Evidence also indicates that IGF-1 levels are influenced by nutritional status. A diet containing an insufficient amount of protein reduces IGF-1 levels, as does the presence of chronic malnutrition.[560, 561] Down-regulation of the IGF-1 response may be blunted in uremic patients because IGF-1 levels change minimally when protein intake is reduced by as much as 40%.[320] Besides changes in nutritional status, serum IGF-1 levels fall with acute starvation[562] and in response to acidosis.[563, 564] Finally, it has been demonstrated that a low serum IGF-1 level is associated with a poor outcome in hemodialysis patients.[565] Clearly, more work is needed to understand the metabolic implications of variations in serum IGF-1 levels.

Anthropometrics

Evaluation of anthropometry in CRF patients is complicated because most reports are based on a single evaluation and the measurements are compared with those found in various groups of normal healthy adults.[566] For these and other reasons, the interpretation of abnormal values is questionable. For example, normal values of serum proteins have been reported, even though anthropometric changes were compatible with loss of muscle mass.[567] Kopple[173] and Bergstrom[568] concluded that virtually all cross-sectional studies of dialysis patients have found a high incidence of anthropometric abnormalities suggestive of malnutrition. Assigning the cross-sectional abnormalities to malnutrition[569] plus the observation that the average protein intake of predialysis patients decreases with advancing renal insufficiency[184, 187] has led some to suggest that dialysis should be initiated early to avoid malnutrition and improve the prognosis.[570-572] Several problems are encountered if one accepts these results as a reason for initiating dialysis. First, despite the average decrease in dietary protein that occurred in patients enrolled in the MDRD Study, the largest evaluation of the effects of dietary protein restriction, serum albumin increased even though other indices of protein stores decreased, and only two patients had to stop the trial because of concern about their nutritional status.[184] Second, the long-term results of patients eating low-protein diets indicate that body weight, serum proteins, and blood biochemistry levels are well maintained even when renal function is very impaired.[138, 518-520] This finding indicates that treatment with a well-planned diet does not cause malnutrition, nor does it lead to strikingly abnormal values in blood biochemical levels.[573] Finally, a recent analysis of the influence of "early" dialysis on mortality led to the conclusion that this practice does not reverse the excessive mortality associated with dialysis.[574] Instead, patients who began dialysis at lower levels of kidney function tended to have less mortality even after correcting for age, gender, body weight, diabetes, leukocyte count, dialysis type, or dialysis access. These data indicate the potential problems with reliance on anthropometrics to assess the effectiveness of nutritional therapy, especially with only a single measurement in a cross-sectional analysis of nutritional status.

Free Plasma Amino Acid and Keto Acid Levels

Patients with chronic uremia have many abnormalities in plasma amino acids, including an increase in 3-methylhistidine and 1-methylhistidine, apparently caused by reduced renal clearance of these amino acids. In addition, valine and, to a lesser extent, leucine and isoleucine values are subnormal.[575-577] Generally, these abnormalities were observed in fasting patients, but Garibotto and colleagues reported that similar changes occur after a meal.[578] At least two mechanisms account for the low levels of these branched chain amino acids (BCAAs). If protein intake is low, it undoubtedly contributes to low plasma levels, but it is unlikely that decreased absorption plays a role based on measurements of the uptake of dietary BCAAs by splanchnic tissue.[579] In fact, when groups of rats with experimental CRF were given different levels of dietary protein from minimal amounts to an excess, BCAA levels in blood became most abnormal in those fed the highest level of protein,[268] which suggests that a principal cause of the low BCAA levels in CRF is accelerated catabolism. All three BCAAs are irreversibly decarboxylated by the same enzyme, branched chain keto acid dehydrogenase (BCKAD), and several factors, including metabolic acidosis and glucocorticoids, stimulate the activity of BCKAD in skeletal muscle.[580-583] The accelerated catabolism of BCAAs in acidotic uremic patients explains why dialysis patients exhibit a correlation between plasma bicarbonate levels and the free valine content in skeletal muscle.[584, 585] Additional support for this conclusion is that correction of metabolic acidosis significantly raises the level of all three BCAAs in the muscle of hemodialysis patients.[586]

Other plasma amino acid abnormalities include an increased citrulline concentration, which has been attributed to impaired conversion of citrulline to arginine by the diseased kidney. However, measurements made in rats with subtotal nephrectomy indicate that the mechanism for a high citrulline level is probably more complex.[587-589] Also found are unexplained increases in cystine, homocysteine, and aspartate; decreased tyrosine, a result of impaired hydroxylation of phenylalanine[590-592]; and high glycine and a low or low-normal serine level, perhaps related to diminished production of serine from glycine by the diseased kidney.[593] Whether this last abnormality contributes to the high glycine levels is unknown.[594] The free tryptophan level is normal but total tryptophan is low because of reduced plasma protein binding.[595] Threonine and lysine decrease for unknown reasons.

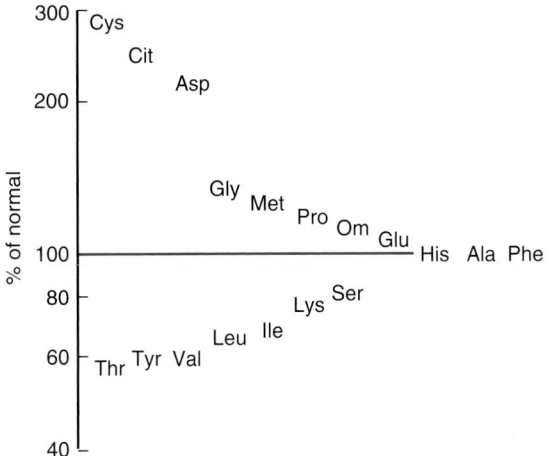

FIGURE 57-8. Plasma amino acids in patients with chronic renal failure treated by protein restriction alone. Results are calculated as percentages of normal values. A logarithmic scale is used, so decreases are emphasized as much as increases. The most abnormal values are shown on the *left*. Statistical significance cannot be evaluated in view of the variety of sources of the data. Note that not all essential amino acids are subnormal.

Thus, the essential amino acids, with some exceptions, tend to be reduced in plasma, whereas some of the nonessential amino acids tend to be increased (Fig. 57-8). This pattern is reminiscent of that seen in patients with protein malnutrition,[596] but it cannot be explained solely on this basis because the abnormalities occur with what appears to be adequate protein intake. Moreover, many of the same abnormalities persist after a large meal of meat.[578] It has been shown that the low levels of BCAAs, the essential/nonessential and valine/glycine ratios, and the degree of increase in cystine, citrulline, and methylhistidines all correlate with the GFR.[597] Evidence is increasing that concentrations of sulfur-containing amino acids (i.e., methionine, cysteine, cystine, taurine, homocysteine) are very abnormal in uremic patients, but the mechanisms accounting for these abnormalities have not been defined.[598, 599] In addition, some evidence indicates that binding of homocysteine to albumin is related to the high cysteine levels and that abnormalities in the intracellular levels of free sulfur-containing amino acids influence the plasma levels.[598, 599] After an intravenous load of amino acids in uremic subjects, removal of valine and phenylalanine is subnormal, but histidine removal is increased.[600] How such removal relates to the high plasma levels of histamine found in uremic patients (especially those with pruritus) is unknown.[601]

Because of the complexity of these abnormalities, it has been difficult to evaluate dietary requirements for individual amino acids on the basis of plasma amino acid levels. In general, the severity of amino acid abnormalities is correlated with the degree of renal insufficiency and uremic symptoms.[597] In addition, the abnormalities tend to worsen when protein intake is inadequate (e.g., a direct correlation exists between the valine-to-glycine ratio and protein intake).[602] An additional problem in interpreting plasma amino acid levels is that uremia alters the distribution of amino acids between cells and extracellular fluid.[603-606] The difference in

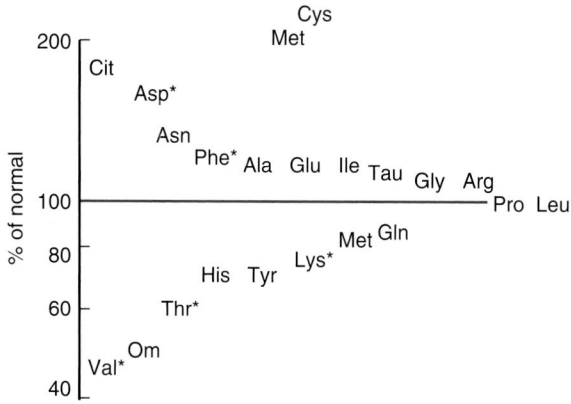

FIGURE 57-9. Intracellular free amino acid concentrations in the muscle of chronically uremic patients treated by protein restriction alone. A logarithmic scale is used, so decreases are emphasized as much as increases. *Asterisks* indicate statistically significant differences. (Data from Bergström J, Fürst P, Norée L-O, et al: Intracellular free amino acids in muscle tissue of patients with chronic uraemia: Effect of peritoneal dialysis and infusion of essential amino acids. Clin Sci Mol Med 54:51-60, 1978.)

distribution was not found in studies of erythrocytes or cerebrospinal fluid.[607, 608] The pattern in plasma is not an accurate reflection of the pattern within muscle in nondialysis, CRF patients (Fig. 57-9); of the BCAAs, only valine is clearly subnormal, whereas both ornithine and histidine are low. These investigators later found somewhat different results in another group of nondialysis CRF patients: not only was the valine concentration low, but leucine, isoleucine, threonine, lysine, and arginine levels were also low.[575] Divino Filho and colleagues[609] used the same techniques to compare levels of amino acids in plasma and in the intracellular space of erythrocytes and muscle. They concluded that the normal values of the BCAAs valine, isoleucine, and leucine in muscle were due to the absence of acidosis. Not only does acidification stimulate the degradation of BCAAs in metabolites of amino acids, including those containing sulfur,[610, 611] but a number of small peptides and amines (including polyamines, guanidines, and other nitrogenous compounds) also accumulate in blood.[458] Generally, the concentrations of these metabolites decrease when protein intake is reduced (see Chapter 48).

Plasma levels of branched-chain keto acids in CRF patients are low.[612-616] This finding has been correlated with the degree of metabolic acidosis (presumably because of activation of BCKAD) and impaired GFR.[580, 612, 616] Gastrointestinal absorption of branched-chain keto acids is unimpaired by CRF.[616] The nutritional efficiency of branched-chain keto acids in uremic animals is equal to[617] or greater than[618] that in normal animals.

NITROGEN CONSERVATION IN UREMIA

Nitrogen Requirements

Nutritional requirements for dietary protein are based primarily on short-term nitrogen balance measurements made while patients with moderate physical activity were ingesting a sufficient amount of calories.[177, 619] Most investigators agree that in the absence of a complicating illness or condition

(e.g., metabolic acidosis or inflammation), the nitrogen requirements of CRF patients are not substantially different from those of normal subjects.[510, 619]

Dietary regimens containing only the minimal daily protein requirement (i.e., 0.6 g/kg/day) or even a lower amount (i.e., about 0.3 g/kg/day) plus a supplement of essential amino acids or their nitrogen-free analogs (keto acids) are sufficient to achieve nitrogen balance and will maintain normal indices of nutrition during long-term therapy.[518, 620, 621] These diets require sufficient caloric intake to use dietary protein efficiently.[190]

As a measure of nutritional adequacy, nitrogen balance has limitations,[498, 566] so other methods have been developed, such as measuring the turnover of labeled amino acid during constant infusion of it. For this purpose, the most widely used is the leucine turnover technique; it can detect the inadequacy of a nutrient before clinical evidence of any deficit is apparent. It also provides insight into potential mechanisms because it measures protein synthesis, protein degradation, and the oxidation of leucine (an example of an essential amino acid). Finally, it can provide insight into the metabolic responses activated by changes in dietary protein. Leucine is the amino acid most frequently used because irreversible degradation of this essential amino acid is relatively easy to measure and the mechanisms activated to degrade leucine have been studied extensively. The initial step in leucine degradation in all cells is transamination followed by irreversible decarboxylation of α-ketoisocaproate, the resulting α-keto acid. Thus, if leucine is labeled in the 1 carbon position, its degradation results in the release of labeled CO_2, and expiration of the labeled CO_2 plus the enrichment of leucine or its keto acid (α-ketoisocaproate) by labeled leucine (or labeled α-ketoisocaproate) in plasma can then be used to calculate rates of whole-body leucine oxidation, protein synthesis, and protein degradation.[518, 585, 622-624]

Metabolic responses activated by an increase or decrease in dietary protein have been identified with the leucine turnover technique. For example, the major response to a meal containing more protein than needed for protein balance is a sharp increase in the rate of amino acid oxidation (Fig. 57-10). Conversely, when dietary protein is lowered, amino acid oxidation falls (Fig. 57-11), thereby leading to more efficient utilization of dietary amino acids for protein synthesis.[421, 518, 621] Because amino acid catabolism results in the release of nitrogen and progressive destruction of the carbon skeleton of the amino acid, it is understandable that a low-protein diet will decrease amino acid oxidation and reduce urea production. This concept is based on the finding that the nitrogen released during catabolism of the amino acid is converted to urea. The decrease in amino acid oxidation in response to a low-protein diet has been denoted as adaptation; Young has defined dietary protein adequacy as intake that maintains long-term neutral nitrogen balance with successful adaptation (a decrease in amino acid oxidation) but no reduction in protein synthesis or degradation.[625] However, when protein intake or the intake of an essential amino acid is so low that protein balance cannot be achieved, the capacity for amino acid oxidation does not continue to decrease. Instead, both protein synthesis and degradation fall. The ability to achieve protein balance will be inadequate, thus leading to progressive loss of lean body mass.[566, 625, 626] In short, the amount of protein in the diet determines the

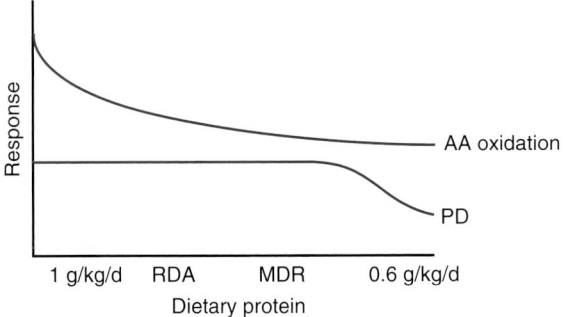

FIGURE 57-10. Hypothetic scheme of the metabolic changes permitting successful adaptation to dietary protein restriction. The initial response to lowering dietary protein is a reduction in the oxidation of amino acids (AA oxidation). Amino acid oxidation declines progressively as protein intake is reduced from an excess (>1 g/kg/day) to the recommended daily allowance (RDA) and even further to the minimal daily requirement (MDR) of 0.6 g/kg/day. In contrast, protein degradation (PD) changes minimally until protein intake is reduced to or below the minimal daily requirement. At this level, amino acid oxidation does not decrease further, but protein degradation falls. These considerations apply only to otherwise normal subjects. In catabolic conditions, responses can be blunted or blocked and the ability to preserve body protein stores is lost.

metabolic processes that produce a change in protein balance, and these changes are detected most easily after a meal. Certain conditions that impair the ability to adapt to a lower protein intake have been identified.[431] However, the signals that result in the metabolic responses to changes in protein intake have not been identified.

Only a few studies have evaluated the metabolic responses to dietary protein restriction in CRF patients. Goodship and co-workers studied nonacidotic patients with an average

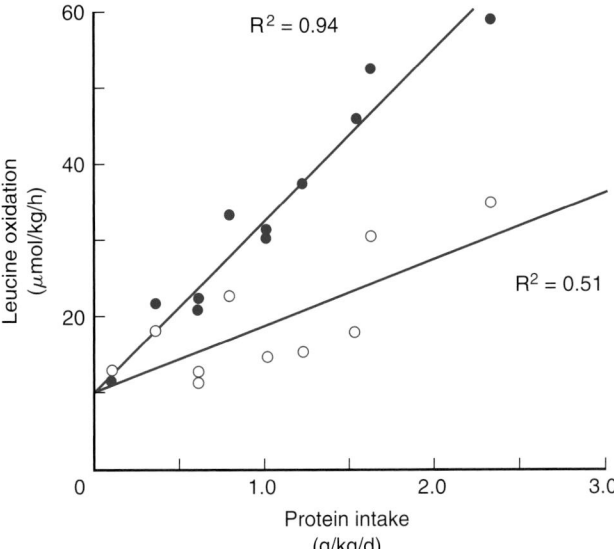

FIGURE 57-11. Relationships between different levels of dietary protein and rates of leucine oxidation in normal subjects and chronic renal failure patients during fasting (*open circles*) and feeding (*closed circles*). A significant correlation is seen between the amount of dietary protein and leucine oxidation during both fasting and feeding, indicative of the adaptive response to changes in dietary protein. (From Tom K, Young VR, Chapman T, et al: Long-term adaptive responses to dietary protein restriction in chronic renal failure. Am J Physiol 268:E668-E677, 1995.)

serum creatinine level of 5 mg/dL by measuring both short-term nitrogen balance and whole-body amino acid oxidation and protein turnover (i.e., leucine turnover) after an overnight fast and during a meal.[622] When the subjects were fed protein at 1 g/kg/day, nitrogen balance was neutral or positive and the values of amino acid oxidation and protein synthesis and degradation were indistinguishable from values measured in normal subjects. However, when dietary protein was reduced to the minimal daily requirement of 0.6 g/kg/day, both patients and normal subjects were in negative nitrogen balance. The reason why nitrogen balance was negative is not known but may have been related to an inadequate time to adapt to the lower protein intake.[621] Regardless, values of amino acid oxidation and protein turnover when normal subjects and CRF patients ate a low-protein diet changed to the same degree in both groups, thus indicating that metabolic responses were intact in these CRF patients who had no evidence of metabolic acidosis.

Masud and colleagues examined this question, but with another type of low-protein diet that contained only 0.3 g/kg/day of protein plus equimolar supplements of essential amino acids or keto acids.[621] The GFR averaged 19 mL/min, and none of the eight patients were acidotic. They were fed both the keto acid or essential amino acid regimens consecutively for at least 2 weeks before measurements were made to allow time for adaptation to the new diet. With either the essential amino acid or the keto acid regimen, patients were in neutral nitrogen balance and exhibited virtually identical changes in amino acid oxidation and protein turnover during feeding and fasting. As might be predicted from the relationships shown in Figure 57-10, the rates of leucine oxidation during fasting and feeding found by Masud and colleagues were about 50% lower than those measured in CRF patients ingesting 0.6 or 1.0 g/kg/day of protein. These results prove that very low protein regimens are a powerful stimulus to conserve dietary amino acids. The only difference between the keto acid and essential amino acid regimens was that with keto acids, patients achieved neutral nitrogen balance despite a 15% lower intake of nitrogen. The finding of neutral nitrogen balance as opposed to negative balance with the standard, low-protein diet containing 0.6 g/kg/day of protein is especially interesting. Presumably, the longer period of adaptation accounts for the difference, but neutral balance has been documented by just changing from a low-protein diet to a keto acid–based regimen.[627] This finding suggests either that the period of the initial low-protein diet was sufficient to achieve adaptation or that the keto acidregimen exerts a beneficial effect on protein turnover. In fact, the keto acid of leucine will suppress protein breakdown in isolated muscle and in starving obese individuals.[628, 629]

The ability to adapt to a reduced protein intake extends to patients with nephrotic syndrome. Maroni and colleagues[509] reported rates of leucine turnover in CRF patients with varying degrees of proteinuria. The patients were studied while eating two diets: a standard amount of protein (0.8 g/kg/day) or an excess of protein (1.6 g/kg/day). With both diets, the patients and control subjects were found to be in neutral or slightly positive nitrogen balance. The major adaptive response activated to achieve nitrogen balance was a change in the rate of amino acid oxidation. As can be seen in Figure 57-12, it was found that leucine oxidation decreased in proportion to net protein intake. Thus, metabolic processes were regulated

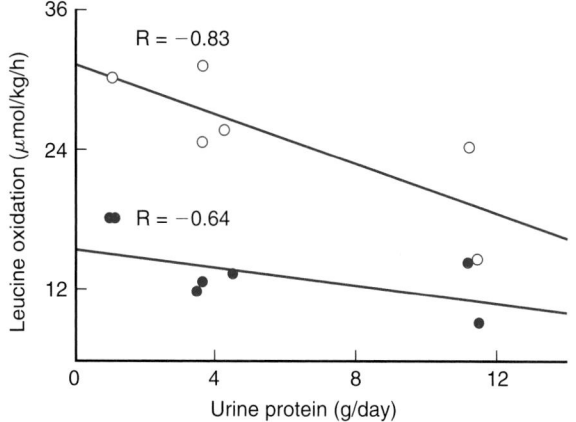

FIGURE 57-12. Relationships between rates of urinary protein loss and leucine oxidation during fasting *(open circles)* and feeding *(closed circles)* while nephrotic patients consumed a protein-restricted diet. A significant correlation is seen during feeding. (Reproduced from Maroni BJ, Staffeld C, Young VY, et al: Mechanisms permitting nephrotic patients to achieve nitrogen equilibrium with a protein-restricted diet. J Clin Invest 99:2479-2487, 1997 by copyright permission of the American Society for Clinical Investigation.)

precisely in proportion to the intake of protein even when the responses were complicated by urinary loss of protein. The metabolic basis for this remarkable result is not known.

FACTORS CAUSING INCREASED NITROGEN REQUIREMENTS

Metabolic Acidosis

Results from experimental animals and patients suggest that metabolic acidosis is a major factor causing excessive catabolism of amino acids and protein in CRF patients. The metabolic changes induced by metabolic acidosis would block the ability of the body to adapt to a decrease in protein intake (see earlier discussion). In addition, the responses activated by metabolic acidosis can act independently to decrease protein stores. As discussed in Chapter 48, metabolic acidosis activates specific pathways that increase the degradation of BCAAs (i.e., BCKAD) and protein (i.e., the ubiquitin-proteasome system) in muscle; these catabolic responses to acidosis include activation of transcription of the genes encoding components of these pathways. Although the abnormalities in cellular signaling that activate these pathways have not been completely defined, aspects of practical and therapeutic importance have been uncovered. First, when dietary protein is restricted, the likelihood of metabolic acidosis developing is reduced because the intake of fixed acid is lower. As expected, metabolic acidosis does not develop in CRF patients eating low-protein diets for prolonged periods.[138, 519] Second, patients with acidosis experience an increase in the degradation of BCAAs and lower levels of these amino acids in muscle.[584, 586] Third, correction of metabolic acidosis in predialysis patients, as well as those treated by hemodialysis or CAPD, sharply decreases the degradation of protein.[585, 623, 624] Finally, long-term therapy with higher levels of lactate buffer in the peritoneal dialysate results in weight gain and improved anthropometric indices

of muscle mass; this type of treatment is also associated with a decrease in the levels of mRNA encoding ubiquitin in muscle.[630, 631] The latter results are consistent with those from experiments in animal models of uremia and indicate that acidosis activates the ubiquitin-proteasome pathway to degrade protein in muscle. In summary, metabolic acidosis will block the ability of the body to adapt to a low-protein diet and preserve protein stores.

The relevance of these data to nutritional therapy was examined recently.[268] In this experiment, groups of rats with experimental CRF were fed low-protein diets of 6% protein, adequate diets of 17% protein, or an excess of protein (30%). The most efficient use of protein for growth was achieved with 8% protein, and those fed 17% grew at the highest rate. CRF rats fed 30% protein had suppressed growth and acidosis.

The mechanisms accelerating the activity of catabolic pathways in acidotic patients are poorly understood. One obvious cause could be a decrease in muscle cell pH leading to activation of cellular signaling processes.[431] To examine this question, Bailey and colleagues[632] measured the pH in muscle of rats by using nuclear magnetic resonance techniques. Rats were made acidotic by the intravenous infusion of acid, by feeding an acidified diet, and by creation of CRF. In all cases, serum bicarbonate and blood pH fell sharply, but the pH in muscle did not change in rats infused with acid or in rats with CRF; a small decrease in muscle cell pH was noted in rats fed acid for 5 days. To determine whether recovery of muscle cell pH was abnormal, these investigators examined the return of pH after exercise of the muscle. No difference in the recovery of muscle cell pH was found in CRF rats despite the accelerated degradation of amino acids and protein in muscle.[581, 633, 634] For these reasons, a change in cell pH cannot be implicated as the sole signal stimulating catabolic reactions.

Another potential mechanism involves glucocorticoids. These hormones can cause catabolism: high doses of glucocorticoids suppress protein synthesis, and supraphysiologic doses accelerate muscle protein breakdown.[635-637] May and associates[638] noted that rats with metabolic acidosis and normal renal function have accelerated protein degradation in muscle and increased rates of glucocorticoid production, measured as high rates of urinary corticosterone excretion. They then showed that chronically uremic rats with or without metabolic acidosis also have high rates of corticosterone excretion, but that only those with acidosis have increased muscle protein breakdown.[633, 634] These results suggest that metabolic acidosis and glucocorticoids could be linked to muscle protein degradation. Experimentally, there is also reason to believe that an interaction between acidification and glucocorticoids stimulates the activity of BCKAD to break down BCAAs.[639] Based on studies of adrenalectomized rats summarized in Chapter 48, it is clear that glucocorticoids are necessary for the catabolic effects of acidosis on protein and amino acid catabolism.[640-642]

Besides stimulating amino acid and protein degradation, accumulation of acid aggravates bone disease in patients with renal insufficiency (see Chapter 52). Mechanisms for the adverse effects of metabolic acidosis on bone metabolism include a direct action on bone to dissolve calcium and a more indirect action that stimulates osteoclastic activity.[643, 644] Other, more indirect effects on metabolism are also caused by acidosis. Patients with chronic kidney disease and acidosis are at risk for responding adversely to each of these consequences of acidosis. Acidosis impairs the action of growth hormone to stimulate the release of IGF-1, the major mediator of growth hormone action. Acidosis also reduces thyroid hormones and can stimulate PTH release. To avoid all these problems, acidosis in patients with renal insufficiency should be vigorously treated by sodium bicarbonate supplements.

Abnormal Carbohydrate Metabolism

In rats with acute renal failure, protein degradation in perfused or incubated muscle is increased. This defect is closely related to abnormalities in insulin-mediated carbohydrate metabolism in muscle.[645, 646] Additional evidence for a link to carbohydrate metabolism was presented by Holliday and associates,[647] who noted that chronically uremic rats fail to suppress protein catabolism in response to caloric deprivation as efficiently as normal animals do. Harter and co-workers[648] suggested that the accelerated muscle proteolysis in chronic uremia may be linked to diminished responsiveness to insulin, just as in acute uremia. This group found that insulin was less effective in inhibiting amino acid release from the incubated muscle of uremic rats when the animals were fed high-protein diets, and hence, they had more severe consequences of uremia. The response to insulin was more nearly normal in rats with kidney damage if they were fed lower amounts of dietary protein. Experimentally, insulin deficiency results in substantial activation of the ubiquitin-proteasome system such that it leads to excessive protein degradation in muscle and enhanced transcription of the genes that encode components of the ubiquitin-proteasome system.[649] In this model of acute diabetes, metabolic acidosis and increased glucocorticoid production are also present. However, in adrenalectomized rats, Mitch and colleagues carefully tested the relationships among acidemia, glucocorticoids, and protein degradation in muscle.[650] They found that acidosis does not play a role in accelerating muscle protein catabolism whereas glucocorticoids are critical for activating the ubiquitin-proteasome pathway to degrade muscle protein. The responses are reversed rapidly by administering insulin even though the blood level of glucose is not fully corrected. These results suggest that the resistance to insulin occurring in CRF might play an important role in activating catabolic pathways (see Chapter 48).

A potentially important factor that impairs protein metabolism and causes loss of protein stores in patients with kidney damage is the sedentary lifestyle of many patients. For example, exercise can augment the magnitude of the response to insulin. Davis and co-workers[651, 652] found that exercise training in chronically uremic rats increased the sensitivity of muscle to insulin, thereby improving glucose uptake, glycolysis, and the ability to suppress protein breakdown. The mechanisms by which these beneficial responses occur and the magnitude of the change in patients with kidney disease have not been established.

At least some evidence indicates that glucagon and glucagon-like peptides may participate in stimulation of muscle catabolism. Bilbrey and associates demonstrated that plasma glucagon levels are high in uremic subjects and do not decrease normally in response to hyperglycemia.[653] The influence of high levels of glucagon on protein metabolism has been tested in fasting obese subjects.[654] In this experiment,

doses of glucagon sufficient to increase the plasma concentration to about 200 pg/mL paradoxically decreased the urinary urea concentration but increased urinary ammonia. On the other hand, others find that large doses of glucagon in humans increase urea excretion.[655] No convincing mechanisms can explain these observations, and experimentally, muscle proteolysis is unaffected by glucagon, except at levels as high as 10 mg/mL.[656] Thus, the role of hyperglucagonemia in augmenting nitrogen requirements in uremia is uncertain.

More convincing data suggest that defective metabolism of fatty acids is associated with stimulation of protein breakdown in muscle. Li and Wassner[657] found no abnormalities in the muscle protein turnover of rats with mild to moderately severe chronic uremia after feeding. However, when the rats were fasted, breakdown of myofibrillar muscle protein occurred, but no change in protein synthesis. They also found that the degree of accelerated muscle protein breakdown was inversely correlated with body fat stores. Coupled with the evidence that defects in glucose metabolism in muscle are correlated with stimulation of protein breakdown, it is tempting to ascribe these problems to a defect in energy metabolism. Unfortunately, such a mechanism does not reveal how the ubiquitin-proteasome pathway is stimulated to degrade protein.[634]

External Losses of Protein

Digestion of the protein after gastrointestinal bleeding will lead to the reabsorption of amino acids, which in turn will augment urea production while depleting body stores of hemoglobin and plasma proteins.[496] The impact of nephrotic syndrome on body protein stores is discussed subsequently.

Altered Electrolyte Balance

In patients with advanced renal insufficiency, defects in ion transport have been demonstrated in blood cells, as well as an increase in intracellular sodium in muscle (see Chapter 48). In CRF rats, several defects in cation transport develop in skeletal muscle and adipocytes.[658] Although the absence of a change in muscle cell pH in CRF rats has been documented,[632] it is still possible that an acute affect of acidification or other types of transport abnormalities change the intracellular ionic milieu and stimulate abnormal metabolic pathways. Notably, potassium deficiency is often observed in CRF patients despite the presence of a normal or increased serum potassium concentration.[659] This finding is interesting because both potassium deficiency[660, 661] and hyperkalemia[662] are intertwined with abnormalities in intracellular acid/base changes, as well as with abnormalities in the metabolic responses to insulin or IGF-1. It is possible that these abnormalities could increase nitrogen catabolism, but such an association has not been convincingly demonstrated.

Hyperparathyroidism

Besides the toxic effects of PTH on bone, PTH administration was reported to augment urea production in normal subjects and in patients with hypoparathyroidism.[663] Some, but not all investigators[664, 665] find that PTH increases the rate of protein degradation in isolated muscle. It is also possible that hyperparathyroidism may be associated with an increase in muscle protein degradation in vivo by inhibiting the release of insulin. This possibility is raised because lack of insulin can clearly stimulate protein degradation in muscle.[649, 666] Thus, it is possible that secondary hyperparathyroidism may increase nitrogen requirements in patients with CRF.

FACTORS DECREASING THE REQUIREMENT FOR NITROGEN

The principal factor that decreases the requirement for nitrogen is the ability of the body to adapt to restriction of dietary protein (see earlier discussion). The signals and mechanisms accounting for these adaptive responses have not been identified, but they are sufficient to produce neutral nitrogen balance and maintain body stores of protein during the long-term treatment of CRF patients eating low-protein diets, as long as they do not have any complicating disease or disorder.[138, 518-520]

Reuse of Urea Nitrogen

Based on results obtained during initial studies of the efficacy of low-protein diets, it was concluded that certain metabolic pathways would permit utilization of the nitrogen in urea or ammonia for the synthesis of amino acids.[667] Indeed, urea or ammonia can provide a source of nonspecific nitrogen for growth in animals.[668-672] However, the evidence that this hypothetic scheme is correct in humans is conflicting. For example, the fact that ^{15}N can be detected in the protein of subjects given ^{15}N-urea or ammonia salts[673-676] does not prove that ammonium nitrogen is important in maintaining protein synthesis because the label could appear in amino acids via reversible reactions in which ammonia participates (e.g., the glutamate dehydrogenase reaction), followed by subsequent transamination reactions between glutamate and various keto acids contained in the carbon skeletons of amino acids.[441] The net reaction is no increase in the quantity of amino acids produced. Moreover, in CRF patients, some reports indicate that ammonia utilization for protein synthesis is not nutritionally important. Varcoe and associates[437] examined the rate of incorporation of labeled urea nitrogen into the albumin of uremic patients in comparison to the rate determined in normal subjects. They concluded that although the amount of urea nitrogen used in albumin synthesis might be greater in uremic subjects, it was still too small to be considered nutritionally significant. We examined the hypothesis by using another strategy. Because the urea nitrogen reutilization hypothesis depends on release of nitrogen from urea, we suppressed urea degradation to ammonia in CRF patients who were being treated with low-protein diets or very low protein diets plus keto acids. Oral doses of neomycin or kanamycin were administered, and rates of urea production and degradation were measured with isotopic techniques. The results were compared with the rates before antibiotic administration.[444, 677] We did not find any increase in urea nitrogen appearance despite an 85% average reduction in urea degradation. If urea nitrogen is being used to synthesize amino acids and urea degradation to ammonia is blocked, the amount of urea appearing in urine and body fluids should increase. Consequently, we concluded that the ammonium derived from degradation is simply recycled back into urea.[444] We also found that nitrogen balance

in these same patients improved despite removing the source of nitrogen from urea degradation (evidently because of a decrease in fecal nitrogen, which improved nitrogen balance).[677] Clearly, if ammonium were an important source of nitrogen for patients eating protein-restricted diets, nitrogen balance should have worsened. These studies demonstrate that urea nitrogen degradation does not contribute importantly to protein conservation in uremia. Still, the so-called nonspecific nitrogen requirement of normal subjects can be met by the administration of urea or ammonia salts to normal and malnourished adults,[678-682] so it is possible that uremic patients may be able to use urea nitrogen to a minor extent for the synthesis of protein. To date, convincing evidence that it plays an important role in nitrogen conservation is lacking.

Vitamins and Trace Elements in Uremia

Vitamins and trace elements are micronutrients that are necessary for energy production from food, for maintenance of organ function, and for cell growth and protection (e.g., from oxygen free radicals). The diet of patients with kidney disease is often limited because of anorexia[188, 568] or as part of therapy for advancing renal insufficiency.[683] Such dietary limitation jeopardizes the intake of micronutrients, and supplemental water-soluble vitamins are thus frequently recommended for uremic patients.[684] The loss of kidney function or the loss of micronutrients by patients with proteinuria can also affect daily requirements for specific micronutrients. In addition, some evidence has shown decreased intestinal absorption of micronutrients, impaired cellular metabolism, circulating inhibitors, or increased losses (at least during dialysis treatment).[684] All these factors could change the requirements for micronutrients. For these reasons and because of methodologic difficulties in measuring micronutrients, neither the minimal nor the recommended daily intake of vitamins has been extensively studied in patients with kidney disease. This lack of study has led investigators to use the recommended allowances for normal subjects. Problems with this practice have not been carefully evaluated, but some reports have documented levels of vitamin intake that are below the recommended daily allowance (RDA). Moreover, supplementation of certain vitamins seems to lead to an improvement in biochemical indices. Unfortunately, very few studies have documented the benefits of giving patients supplements of water-soluble vitamins. For example, long-term vitamin B_6 and folate supplementation has improved responses to erythropoietin.[685, 686] At the same time, questions regarding the need to prescribe water-soluble vitamins to all patients have not been resolved; data obtained from hemodialysis patients monitored for 1 year after discontinuing vitamin supplementation revealed that the average concentrations of folate, niacin, and vitamins B_1, B_6, B_{12}, and C were normal in whole blood and erythrocytes.[687] Initially, the levels of several vitamins decreased significantly, but these values stabilized and were within the normal range by 6 months. Presumably, the dietary content of vitamins was sufficient to maintain normal levels.

Accelerated loss of vitamin B_1 (thiamine) can occur during intensive diuretic therapy or dialysis. If the diet is severely restricted, a patient will be at risk for thiamine deficiency. Unfortunately, the cardiovascular and neurologic symptoms of thiamine deficiency may mimic some of the complications of CRF, such as the heart failure related to hypertension or the central nervous symptoms associated with advanced uremia. To circumvent this problem, a daily supplement containing the RDA of thiamine is recommended.

Riboflavin is used in the coenzymes flavin mononucleotide and flavin adenine dinucleotide, and these coenzymes participate in numerous metabolic pathways of energy utilization. Riboflavin is found in meat and dairy products, which are often restricted in CRF patients, but also in green leafy vegetables, which are not restricted. Because it is a water-soluble vitamin and the symptoms of riboflavin deficiency (sore throat, stomatitis, glossitis) may be mistaken for uremic symptoms, a supplement containing the RDA is recommended.

Folic acid is found in fruits and vegetables, but cooking can destroy the vitamin. It is involved in the synthesis of nucleic acids and in carbon transfer reactions, including those involved in the metabolism of amino acids (such as homocysteine).[684] The use of folate and vitamin B_6 to treat high plasma homocysteine levels is discussed in Chapter 48. Folate deficiency can accompany a highly restrictive diet and reduce the effectiveness of erythropoietin therapy, as well as many metabolic reactions. For these reasons, a supplement containing the RDA is recommended.

Vitamin B_6 (pyridoxine) is another compound critical for the metabolism of amino acids because it is involved in transaminase-catalyzed reactions that transfer nitrogen. It is contained in meat, vegetables, and cereal, and with restricted diets, deficiency may develop with symptoms of peripheral neuropathy. Because peripheral neuropathy is also a complication of advanced uremia, a supplement containing the RDA is recommended to avoid misdiagnosis of the cause of neuropathy.[684]

Vitamin B_{12} is necessary for the transfer of methyl groups and in the synthesis of nucleic acids. The major sources of vitamin B_{12} are meat and diary products, but a deficiency state is unusual. This vitamin is stored in the liver and is protein bound, and gastrointestinal absorption of it is carefully regulated. In dialysis patients, vitamin B_{12} can be removed and thus a supplement containing the RDA is recommended, but for CRF patients, the likelihood of a deficiency state developing is low.[684]

Vitamin C (ascorbic acid) is necessary as an antioxidant and is involved in the hydroxylation of proline during the formation of collagen. It is contained in meat, dairy products, and most vegetables, so a deficiency state is unusual. Symptoms of vitamin C deficiency are subtle and similar to those of advanced uremia (poor wound healing, periodontal disease). Deficiency states can develop in dialysis patients when their diet is inadequate. High doses of vitamin C are metabolized to oxalate and can increase plasma oxalate levels along with precipitation of oxalate in soft tissues (including the kidney). For this reason, vitamin C supplements should not contain more than the RDA.

The remaining water-soluble vitamins, biotin, niacin, and pantothenic acid, have been studied even less than the foregoing vitamins. Consequently, there is little reason to recommend a supplement unless a specific syndrome develops. Biotin functions as a coenzyme in bicarbonate-dependent carboxylation reactions and is produced by intestinal microorganisms, so a deficiency state is unusual. Niacin (nicotinic acid) is an essential component of the nicotinamide adenine dinucleotide phosphate coenzyme. It is synthesized from the essential amino acid tryptophan, and a deficiency state with diarrhea, dermatitis, or increased triglycerides can develop. Niacin supplements have been used to treat hyperlipidemic conditions such as a high LDL content. Supplements containing niacin can be associated with flushing symptoms. Pantothenic acid is involved in the function of coenzyme A and, hence, in the metabolism of fatty acids, steroid hormones, and cholesterol. Because so little work has been conducted on the efficacy and consequences of prescribing these vitamins, a supplement is recommended only for deficiency-related syndromes.

Dialysis can impose special requirements for vitamin intake. For example, hemodialysis patients often have elevated blood oxalate levels, and if they are given vitamin C, the serum oxalate concentration will rise.[688] One report contained a history of a hemodialysis patient who took 2.6 g of vitamin C daily for 7 years and was found to have excessive bone oxalate deposits.[689] Recently, extensive interest has arisen regarding the accumulation of homocysteine by patients with kidney disease; homocysteine levels are high in dialysis patients and could contribute to the development of arteriosclerosis in these patients.[690, 691] In theory, supplements of vitamin B_6 and folic acid could help reduce homocysteine levels,[692] but at least when standard doses are given to hemodialysis patients, this practice has not been successful (see Chapter 48). The experience with CRF patients who are not receiving dialysis is too limited to recommend that they receive these vitamins.

In summary, evidence indicates that vitamin intake by reasonably nourished hemodialysis patients is often insufficient to meet the RDAs for normal subjects.[693] In addition, there is evidence that the requirements for vitamin B_6 and folate may be increased in uremia, especially in patients receiving erythropoietin therapy.[685, 686] Thus, the practice of prescribing a water-soluble vitamin supplement for hemodialysis patients may be useful and probably does little harm. However, in view of the reports that peripheral neuropathy and hyperoxalemia can occur with high doses of pyridoxine and vitamin C, respectively, "megavitamin" therapy should be avoided.[688, 694]

The requirements for fat-soluble vitamins are even more difficult to establish than the requirements for water-soluble vitamins. It has also been suggested that fat-soluble vitamins may participate in some of the complications of kidney failure. For these reasons, fat-soluble vitamins should be given only to patients with a well-defined indication, and supplements providing all vitamins should not be prescribed to avoid the dangers of toxicity. For example, vitamin A (retinol) levels are generally increased in the plasma of CRF patients because plasma levels of retinol-binding protein are high in uremia.[684] Although the level of unbound or free retinol in plasma may be normal, it is likely that tissue levels are normal or increased. The danger associated with providing supplemental vitamin A is that it is suspected of being a contributor to anemia, dry skin, pruritus, and even hepatic dysfunction in uremic patients. For example, vitamin A skin and hepatic toxicity was reported in three CRF patients who were given parenteral nutrition that contained a multivitamin supplement (including 1500 mg of vitamin A).[695] Toxicity resolved with discontinuance of the vitamin supplement. Obviously, vitamin A should be removed from parenteral nutrition solutions used to treat patients with renal failure.

Requirements for vitamin E, another fat-soluble vitamin, are also not established. Vitamin E has the potential to suppress responses to oxidative injury to cells, and because oxidative injury could play a role in the progression of renal failure, vitamin E has been given to experimental models of CRF. It was reported that vitamin E supplements reduce the degree of injury in rats with experimental IgA nephropathy or glomerulosclerosis after subtotal nephrectomy or diabetes.[696-699] However, no evidence has been presented for a similar benefit in patients with progressive CRF. Can inadequate intake of vitamin E (or other antioxidants such as selenium) cause clinical problems? One group reported that the water supply of a dialysis unit containing excess chloramine was associated with oxidant-induced hemolytic anemia.[700] Vitamin E levels in the patients were low, and after removing chloramine, plasma levels of vitamin E became normal, thus suggesting that the vitamin E in these patients functioned as an antioxidant to protect them from hemolysis. Other reports have suggested that a low vitamin E level in erythrocytes is associated with lipid peroxidation and that oxidant stress may in part be responsible for an increased red cell turnover in uremia.[701] Fortunately, in the few reports that are available, plasma vitamin E levels are normal in uremic patients. Because the clinical conditions described are not clearly reversed by vitamin E supplements, we do not recommend supplemental vitamin E therapy.

Recommendations for supplemental vitamin D are complex (see Chapter 52). Plasma calcitriol invariably decreases as renal insufficiency progresses, and this decline plays an important role in the pathogenesis of secondary hyperparathyroidism. Although concern has been expressed that the use of vitamin D might accelerate the rate of loss of renal function in predialysis patients, even in the absence of overt hypercalcemia,[702] a double-blind prospective trial uncovered no adverse influence of $1,25(OH)_2D_3$ on renal function during a 12-month follow-up period.[703] Still, for CRF patients receiving $1,25(OH)_2D_3$ therapy, renal function, serum calcium, and phosphorus should be monitored closely.

Recommendations for providing trace element supplements for uremic patients are controversial for several reasons: it is very difficult to determine whether body stores are sufficient, insufficient, or excessive, and it is difficult to prove that symptoms are reversed solely by the administration of trace elements.[684] Based on postmortem studies, the distribution of trace elements in different tissues of uremic patients is abnormal, but it is not clear that these abnormalities are clinically important. For example, plasma and leukocyte zinc are reported to be decreased, and decreases in zinc may be associated with endocrine abnormalities such as high plasma prolactin levels.[704] One report suggested that zinc absorption was low in hemodialysis patients and that iron tablets or aluminum hydroxide inhibited zinc absorption.[705] Still, it is difficult to assign the entire problem of the high prolactin levels found in kidney failure patients to a low zinc level. On the other hand, a zinc supplement has been reported to increase B lymphocyte counts, granulocyte motility, and taste and sexual dysfunction.[684]

Aluminum-containing antacids have been used to control serum phosphorus, but they can be associated with the development of bone disease (see Chapter 52). Administration of aluminum-based antacids to critically ill patients has led to high plasma levels, especially in those with renal insufficiency. Aluminum should not be given without routine monitoring.[706] Moreover, when stable CRF patients were given an aluminum load, the degree of renal insufficiency determined the accumulation of aluminum; it was also noted that excess aluminum may be associated with reduced serum iron stores, and these reduced stores may contribute to resistance to erythropoietin administration.[707, 708] Finally, some reports have described specific toxic reactions caused by contamination of the dialysate with trace elements. Examples include nickel,[709] cobalt,[710] and chromium.[711, 712]

In conclusion, the dietary requirements for trace elements are not well defined in patients with renal failure. Unless specific indications are present, supplemental trace elements should not be given. An exception would be patients receiving long-term parenteral or enteral nutrition. In addition, it would seem prudent to monitor dialysis water and the peritoneal dialysate closely for excessive concentrations of trace elements. Because the kidney is the principal route of excretion, supplementation is not recommended to avoid the accumulation of trace elements in patients with renal failure.

TECHNIQUES OF NUTRITIONAL THERAPY

Rationale for Nutritional Therapy

Uncertainty about the benefits of dietary therapy in slowing progression has obscured a long-established point: protein restriction ameliorates the signs and symptoms of renal failure. This observation, which dates back at least as far as 1869,[713] has repeatedly been confirmed. Yet only a small minority of CRF patients receive instruction on a low-protein diet as the end stage approaches.[714] Some of the reasons that protein restriction is not routinely used have been discussed by Giovannetti.[715] None of them are valid, and in our view, every symptomatic CRF patient should receive instruction from a skilled dietitian. With few exceptions, patients should receive a trial of a protein-restricted diet before initiating dialysis.[683] Optimal protein intake is about 0.3 g/kg—a difficult goal to reach. If protein intake is successfully reduced below 0.6 g/kg, a supplement of essential amino acids should be provided.

Arguments against protein restriction that have been put forward, for example, by Mehrotra and Nolph,[572] obscure this issue in several ways: first and foremost, they ignore the disadvantages of dialysis. Apart from the major inconvenience of dialysis and its adverse psychological impact, mortality after initiation of dialysis[716] is at least 10 times greater than predialysis mortality. The latter has never been reported to be greater than 3% per annum[137, 138, 519] (although prolongation of the predialysis period too far would obviously lead to far greater mortality). These government mortality figures alone should give pause to those who advocate earlier dialysis. Second, they fail to consider the use of supplements of essential amino acids (or, when available—which they are not at present in the United States—keto analogs of essential amino acids). As Rose[186] and others showed many decades ago, nitrogen balance is neutral or positive in normal subjects in the total *absence* of dietary protein when essential amino acids are provided in appropriate quantities and proportions. Such mixtures are readily available as tablets or as flavored powder. Third, Mehrotra and Nolph[572] and others with similar views perpetuate (without data) the myth that "Initiation of chronic dialysis is as successful [as protein restriction] in ameliorating the symptoms and the metabolic abnormalities associated with uremia." It has been demonstrated many times that predialysis subjects who have been neglected (as many are) and are therefore hypoalbuminemic and acidotic (among other problems) exhibit improvement in these parameters when dialysis is begun. Typically, predialysis patients are malnourished and also show signs of chronic inflammation.[524] What has *not* been demonstrated is improvement in signs and symptoms when dialysis is begun in well-nourished patients—as carefully treated predialysis patients can be. In one small study from Stockholm that compared symptoms in 28 uremic patients before and after starting dialysis,[717] fatigue, lack of energy, and functional disability in work all *worsened* after dialysis commenced, although disability in recreation and pastime decreased. These patients, in contrast to the majority of patients in the United States, entered dialysis with normal average levels of serum albumin and bicarbonate. Thus, what little evidence is available does not support the notion that dialysis improves uremic symptoms. Moreover, no evidence has shown that early dialysis reduces dialysis mortality.[574]

Decreases in some sophisticated nutritional parameters have occurred in association with the ingestion of low-protein diets,[718] but these abnormalities are of minor clinical significance and pale in the light of the mortality data summarized earlier.

Why is protein restriction so effective in reducing signs and symptoms? A full explanation of this observation is as yet lacking. However, some points can be made. First, any reduction in protein intake is accompanied by a proportionately greater reduction in SUN concentration, with which symptoms are at least weakly correlated,[719, 720] because the rate of excretion of nitrogen in forms other than urea is relatively insensitive to nitrogen intake.[426] If a very low protein diet plus supplemental amino acids or keto acids is used, SUN may fall to nearly normal levels despite severe renal failure.[31] Second, most of the signs and symptoms of CRF are attributable to the retention of products of protein catabolism, except for anemia and dyslipidemia. Third, protein intake, at least in the United States, averages well above the requirement, so considerable restriction is feasible. However, a complete explanation of the clinical benefit of protein restriction in CRF remains elusive.

Compliance

The success or failure of nutritional therapy depends largely on patient compliance.[284, 520, 721] Low-protein diets are difficult to adhere to, and their limited use is probably attributable chiefly to difficulties in obtaining compliance. Some of the problems that are troublesome with such diets are their relatively high cost, the need for special low-protein products, the time required for separate cooking of meals, poor palatability, monotony, and the required changes in lifestyle for the patient and family. Indeed, the cooperation of family members is essential to success. Close cooperation of two professionals, the nephrologist and the dietitian, is also critical. Remarkably, the near absence of high-protein foods from such diets rarely poses a problem in achieving compliance,

perhaps because such foods are intuitively avoided by symptomatic patients. Support groups or e-mail groups composed of patients in whom similar diets are prescribed can be very useful. Some patients become enthusiasts, develop new recipes, and proselytize others.[722]

According to Rosman and Donker-Willenborg,[723] the most important factors determining compliance are (1) dedication of the dietitian, as well as an involved physician; (2) ongoing and consistent communication among patient, physician, and dietitian; (3) the personal, social, and geographic circumstances of the patient (rural patients were more compliant than urban patients); and (4) the availability of good dietary exchange lists, preferably on the Internet.

Compliance is a particularly troublesome problem in evaluating the efficacy of any dietary regimen. If a significant proportion of subjects assigned to the more restrictive diet fail to comply (or if some subjects assigned to the less restrictive diet tend to emulate the more restrictive group), a slower rate of progression could be caused by the diet or could reflect inherently less rapidly progressive disease in the more compliant subjects. In other words, more rapidly progressive renal failure may be associated a priori with a tendency to be noncompliant. Just why this might be so is not clear, but it has been demonstrated, for example, that participation in a clinical trial may by itself slow progression, at least as measured by $[Cr]^{-1}$ slopes.[724] Numerous studies have now been conducted in which the rate of progression with a variety of regimens (measured by reliable methods) is faster in noncompliant patients.[284, 520] If an analysis by intention to treat had been used in such studies (see earlier), one might have concluded that no significant effect on progression occurred. Thus, it is often advisable to use both intention-to-treat and secondary analyses (which take compliance into consideration) in interpreting such data.

Comparison of Different Regimens

When supplements of essential amino acids or their keto analogs are not provided, it is important to be certain that intake of these carbon skeletons is adequate to ensure that protein metabolism is not impaired. Unfortunately, the requirements of CRF patients for each of the individual essential amino acids have not been examined quantitatively. Amino acids whose circulating levels are particularly low in such patients include the BCAAs, threonine, and tyrosine. Protein-restricted diets that contain insufficient amounts of high-quality protein may not provide enough of these amino acids. Hence, a substantial proportion of high-quality protein is desirable.

A few comparative studies have been conducted on the effects of different dietary regimens in CRF patients. Di Landro and associates[725] compared the outcome of 3 years' treatment with a diet containing 0.6 g/kg of protein in 44 patients with a diet containing 0.3 g/kg of protein plus a supplement of essential amino acids and keto analogs in 46 patients. Progression, estimated from $[Cr]^{-1}$ slopes, was significantly slower in the latter group; PTH levels increased in the first group, but decreased in the second; and serum cholesterol remained elevated in the first group, but fell to normal in the second. Teplan and associates[726] randomized patients with renal failure, all of whom were prescribed a low-protein diet (0.6 g/kg) plus erythropoietin, to receive in addition a supplement of a keto acid–amino acid mixture at 0.1 g/kg; controls received no supplement. Another control group received no erythropoietin.[727] They were monitored for 1 to 3 years. The GFR fell more in controls; in those receiving the supplement, serum BCAA levels increased, as did serum albumin; proteinuria decreased. The serum concentration of free radicals declined. Ayli and associates[728] switched 18 patients with CRF from a diet containing 0.8 g/kg of protein to one containing 0.4 g/kg, supplemented with a mixture of keto acids and amino acids. The GFR fell less in the second period, and LDL-cholesterol decreased.

Herselman and co-workers[729] randomly assigned 22 CRF patients to a diet containing 0.6 g/kg of protein or a diet containing 0.4 g/kg supplemented with 0.14 g/kg of essential amino acids. The intake of protein plus supplements achieved scarcely differed between the two groups (0.73 versus 0.63 g/kg). After 9 months, the two groups did not differ significantly with respect to progression (as assessed by $[Cr]^{-1}$ slopes), with both exhibiting significant slowing in comparison to the control period. Biochemical parameters did not differ between the groups. Interestingly, changes in protein intake were inversely correlated with changes in serum albumin concentration ($P = .029$).

The primary results of the operational phase of the MDRD Study were inconclusive with regard to differing effects of various levels of protein restriction on progression.[137] In the 255 patients with advanced renal disease, no clear-cut benefit ($P = .07$) was achieved with a very low protein diet (0.28 g/kg) supplemented with a mixture of amino acids and keto acids versus a low-protein diet. Secondary analysis of these results,[42] however, suggested that lower protein intake was associated with slower progression in both the low-protein and very low protein diets. Each reduction of 0.2 g/kg in protein intake was associated with a slowing in GFR decline by 1.15 mL/min/yr, or approximately 30%. Lower protein intake was also associated with a delay in the onset of renal failure ($P = .001$). No benefit could be attributed to the keto acid supplement. In 585 patients with less severe renal failure, no significant difference was observed in the overall rate of progression between patients assigned to a low-protein diet (0.58 g/kg) and those assigned to a usual-protein diet (1.3 g/kg). However, the low-protein diet led to a decline in GFR during the first few months, followed by a slower rate of decline ($P < .01$) thereafter. Longer follow-up would therefore be necessary to determine whether protein restriction was beneficial in the long term in this group. In the secondary analysis,[42] no correlation was found between GFR decline and protein intake achieved.

In the feasibility phase of the MDRD Study,[362] 66 patients with more advanced renal failure were randomly assigned to a low-protein diet (0.575 g/kg), a very low protein diet (0.28 g/kg) supplemented with a mixture of essential amino acids, or the same very low protein diet supplemented by a mixture of keto acids and amino acids. This mixture differed substantially from that used in the operational phase, but it was the same as that used previously by Mitch, Walser, and associates.[133, 144, 145, 627, 730] The average follow-up was 14 months. Progression was significantly slower by intention-to-treat analysis in the group assigned to the keto acid–based supplement than in those assigned to the essential amino acid supplement ($P = .028$) despite the same protein intake (Fig. 57-13). The rate of progression in those assigned to the

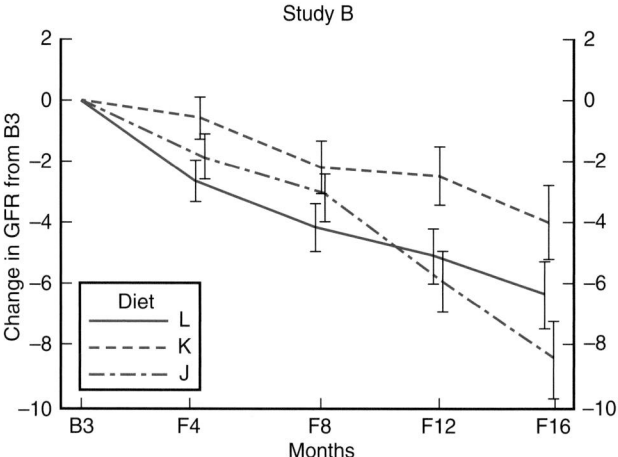

FIGURE 57-13. Mean (±SE) change in glomerular filtration rate (milliliters per minute) in patients with advanced renal failure in the feasibility phase of the Modification of Diet in Renal Disease Study. Progression on diet K (very low protein plus keto acids) is slower than progression on diet J (very low protein plus essential amino acids) or diet L (moderately low protein without a supplement).

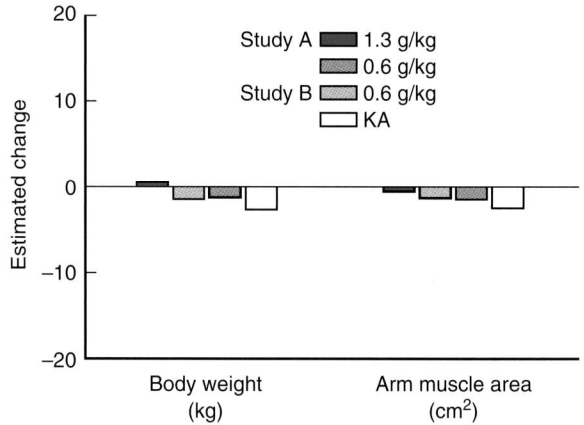

FIGURE 57-14. Projected changes over 3.2 years in body weight in kilograms and arm muscle area in square centimeters in patients participating in the Modification of Diet in Renal Disease Study. Patients with glomerular filtration rates (GFRs) between 24 and 55 mL/min/1.73 m² (study A) were fed 1.3 g protein/kg/day or 0.6 g protein/kg/day; patients in study B (GFRs between 13 and 24 mL/min/1.73 m²) were fed 0.6 g protein/kg/day or 0.3 g protein/kg/day plus a mixture of keto acids. (Data from Kopple JD, Levey AS, Greene T, et al: Effect of dietary protein restriction on nutritional status in the Modification of Diet in Renal Disease (MDRD) Study. Kidney Int 52:778-791, 1997.)

unsupplemented diet was intermediate. The explanation for the change in supplement composition between the two phases of the MDRD Study is discussed by Walser.[361]

Parameters of nutritional status scarcely differed between the diet assignments of the MDRD Study. In the feasibility phase, serum albumin and transferrin levels declined in a few patients, but they did not become subnormal; no patient became malnourished, even though mean energy intake fell below recommended values. In the full-scale trial,[184] patients assigned to the low-protein or very low protein diet lost about 2 kg and showed a slight decrease in other anthropometric parameters during the first 4 months only, probably because of reduced energy intake (Fig. 57-14). Serum albumin

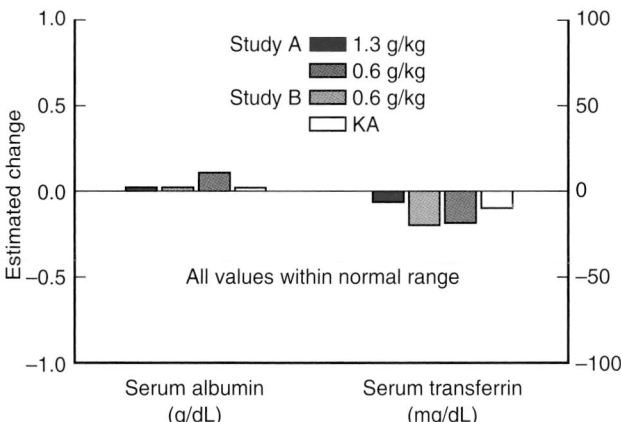

FIGURE 57-15. Projected changes over 3.2 years in serum albumin (grams per deciliter) and serum transferrin (milligrams per deciliter) in patients participating in the Modification of Diet in Renal Disease Study. The dietary-induced changes were small and serum albumin increased. (Data from Kopple JD, Levey AS, Greene T, et al: Effect of dietary protein restriction on nutritional status in the Modification of Diet in Renal Disease (MDRD) Study. Kidney Int 52:778-791, 1997.)

TABLE 57-3

Composition of Three Mixtures of Ketoacids and Amino Acids Used in the Treatment of Chronic Renal Failure*

	"EE" † (mg/kg/day)	"RKAP "‡ (mg/kg/day)	"KETOSTERIL"§ (mg/kg/day)
(L)-Ornithine	43.3	64.9	0
(L)-Lysine	47.9	34.7	22.5
(L)-Histidine	9.6	10.5	8.1
Ketoisocaproate	36.6	39.7	21.7
(R,S)-ketomethylvalerate	27.5	30.9	14.4
Ketoisovalerate	25.4	29.5	18.4
Phenylpyruvate	0	0	14.6
(L)-Tyrosine	56.5	49.1	6.4
(L)-Threonine	27.9	14.1	11.4
(L)-Tryptophan	0	0.8	5.0
Calcium	0.7	0.7	10.7
(D,L)-Hydroxymethyl-thiobutyrate	5.1	5.1	12.7

*Compositions are given as quantities present after hydrolysis of calcium salts and/or mixed salts formed between basic amino acids and keto acids.

†Used in the feasibility phase of the MDRD Study[362] and in earlier work.[133, 144, 145, 627, 730]

‡Used in the operational phase of the MDRD Study[137] and in a clinical trial sponsored by Ross Laboratories, reported only in abstract form.[733]

§From Meisinger and Strauch.[734]

levels rose, but transferrin levels fell in patients assigned to the low-protein or very low protein diets (Fig. 57-15). However, the average serum protein values were within the normal range.[184] A progressive decline in creatinine excretion was observed in the low-protein groups and was probably related to reduced meat intake or increasing degradation of creatinine.[457] Loss of skeletal muscle mass could not have contributed in a major way to the reduction in urinary creatinine excretion because arm muscle area remained the same or decreased only slightly. Importantly, the frequency of hospitalization and the number of patients reaching "stop points" for nutritional reasons did not differ among the groups.

Nutritional parameters in the three different diet groups of the feasibility phase of the MDRD Study were not compared. In other studies,[133, 144, 731] the effects of essential amino acid supplements to very low protein diets were compared with the effects of keto acid–based supplements; in general, more pronounced improvement in metabolic parameters has been found in those receiving keto acids. Clearly, the keto analogs of the essential amino acids are effective dietary substitutes for the corresponding amino acids, as has been reported previously. No toxicity or side effects associated with keto acid ingestion have been reported after the calcium salts were replaced with salts of basic amino acids; previously, indigestion and hypercalcemia occurred in some patients.[732]

The composition of some of the mixtures of amino acids and keto acids that have been used is shown in Table 57-3. They vary considerably, not only in the proportion of keto acids to amino acids, but also in the proportions of the individual components.

The most important conclusions to be drawn from the work summarized in this chapter are first, that dietary therapy reduces signs and symptoms and should be tried in every case of symptomatic CRF, and second, that this therapy is nutritionally safe. Arguments presented against these conclusions are tenuous: the progressive reduction in voluntary protein intake observed as patients approach end-stage renal failure, considered in light of the increasing prevalence

of hypoalbuminemia with its attendant ominous implications for dialysis patients,[735] has led to the suggestion that increasing protein intake can prevent complications.[571] However, the inference that encouraging a high-protein diet will counteract hypoproteinemia is not borne out by experimental evidence. On the contrary, protein-restricted diets, especially those supplemented with essential amino acids or keto acids, improve protein nutrition while ameliorating uremic symptoms, whereas a more "nearly normal" diet has the opposite effects. Thus, hypoalbuminemia can be prevented by prescribing a well-designed, low-protein diet. The suggestion that such diets will induce protein malnutrition has been repeatedly disproved.[519, 736-738] The largest study of this question, the MDRD Study, established unequivocally that low-protein diets as well as supplemented very low protein diets are nutritionally safe. Indeed, the only groups whose serum albumin levels changed in the MDRD Study were those who received the supplemented very low protein diets; in these patients, serum albumin rose.

REFERENCES

1. Wesson LG. Renal function. *In* Wesson LG (ed): Physiology of The Human Kidney. New York, Grune & Stratton, 1969.
2. Price DA, Fisher ND, Osei SY, et al: Renal perfusion and function in healthy African-Americans. Kidney Int 59:1037-1043, 2001.
3. McIntosh JF, Moller R, Van Slyke DD: Studies of urea excretions, III. The influence of body size on urea output. J Clin Invest 6:467-496, 1928.
4. Dooley MJ, Poole SG: Poor correlation between body surface area and glomerular filtration rate. Cancer Chemother Pharmacol 46:523-526, 2000.
5. Blake GM, Roe D, Lazarus CR: Long-term precision of glomerular filtration rate measurements using ⁵¹Cr-EDTA plasma clearance. Nucl Med Commun 18:776-784, 1997.
6. De Sadeleer C, Piepsz A, Ham HR: Influence of errors in sampling time and in activity measurements on the single sample clearance determination. Nucl Med Commun 22:429-432, 2001.

7. Peters AM, Gordon I, Sixt R: Normalization of glomerular filtration rate in children—body surface area, body weight or extracellular fluid volume. J Nucl Med 35:438-444, 1994.

8. Singer MA: Of mice and men and elephants: Metabolic rate sets glomerular filtration rate. Am J Kidney Dis 37:164-178, 2001.

9. Singer MA, Morton AR: Mouse to elephant: Biological scaling and Kt/V. Am J Kidney Dis 35:306-309, 2000.

10. Turner ST, Reilly SL: Fallacy of indexing renal and systemic hemodynamic measurements for body surface area. Am J Physiol 268:R978-R988, 1995.

11. Schmieder RE, Beil AH, Weihprecht H, Messerli FH: How should renal hemodynamic data be indexed in obesity. J Am Soc Nephrol 5:1709-1713, 1995.

12. Ribstein J, du Cailar G, Mimran A: Combined renal effects of overweight and hypertension. Hypertension 26:610-615, 1995.

13. Anastasio P, Spitali L, Frangiosa A, et al: Glomerular filtration rate in severely overweight normotensive humans. Am J Kidney Dis 35:1144-1148, 2000.

14. Tokunaga K, Matsuzawa Y, Kotanik K, et al: Ideal body weight estimated from the body mass index with the lowest morbidity. Int J Obesity 15:1-5, 1991.

15. Piepsz A, Colarinha P, Godon I, et al: Guidelines for glomerular filtration rate determination in children. Eur J Nucl Med 28:BP31-BP36, 2001.

16. Hamilton D, Miola UJ: Body surface area correction in single-sample methods of glomerular filtration rate determination in children. Nucl Med Commun 20:273-278, 1999.

17. Hamilton D, Riley P, Miola U, et al: Total plasma clearance of ^{51}Cr-EDTA: Variation with age and sex in normal adults. Nucl Med Commun 21:187-192, 2000.

18. Swinkels DW, Hendriks JC, Nauta J, de Jong MC: Glomerular filtration rate by single-injection inulin clearance: Definition of a workable protocol for children. Ann Clin Biochem 37:60-66, 2000.

19. Delpassand ES, Homayoon K, Madden TP, et al: Determination of glomerular filtration rate using a dual-detector gamma camera and the geometric mean of renal activity: Correlation with the Tc-99m DTPA clearance method. Clin Nucl Med 25:259-262, 2000.

20. Lindeman RD, Tobin JD, Shock NW: Association between blood pressure and the rate of decline in renal function with age. Kidney Int 26:861-868, 1984.

21. Lindeman RD, Tobin J, Shock NW: Longitudinal studies on the rate of decline in renal function with age. J Am Geriatr Soc 33:278-285, 1985.

22. Lindeman RD: Overview: Renal physiology and pathophysiology of aging. Am J Kidney Dis 16:275-282, 1990.

23. Fliser D, Feranek E, Joest M, et al: Renal function in the elderly: Impact of hypertension and cardiac function. Kidney Int 51:1196-1204, 1997.

24. Friedman SA, Raizner AE, Rosen H, et al: Functional defects in the aging kidney. Ann Intern Med 76:41-45, 1972.

25. Cianciaruso B, Bellizzi V, Minutolo R, et al: Renal adaptation to dietary sodium restriction in moderate renal failure resulting from chronic glomerular disease. J Am Soc Nephrol 7:306-313, 1996.

26. Kimmel PL, Lew SQ, Bosch JB: Nutrition, ageing and GFR: Is age-associated decline inevitable? Nephrol Dial Transplant 11(suppl 9):85-88, 1996.

27. Coleman GL, Barthold W, Osbaldiston GW, et al: Pathological changes during aging in barrier-reared Fischer 344 male rats. J Gerontol 32:258-278, 1977.

28. Hayashida M, Yu BP, Masoro EJ, et al: An electron microscopic examination of age-related changes in the rat kidney: The influence of diet. Exp Gerontol 32:258-278, 1986.

29. Masoro EJ, Yu BP: Diet and nephropathy [editorial]. Lab Invest 60:165-167, 1989.

30. Anderson S, Brenner BM: The aging kidney: Structure, function, mechanisms, and therapeutic implications. J Am Geriatr Soc 35:590-593, 1987.

31. Walser M: Dietary proteins and their relationship to kidney disease. *In* Liepa GU, Beitz DC, Beynen AC, Gorman MA (eds): Dietary Proteins in Health and Disease. Champaign, IL, American Oil Chemists Society Monograph, 1992, pp 168-178.

32. Tapp DC, Wortham WG, Addison JF, et al: Food restriction retards body growth and prevents end-stage renal pathology in remnant kidneys of rats regardless of protein intake. Lab Invest 60:184-195, 1989.

33. Lew SQ, Bosch JP: Effect of diet on creatinine clearance and excretion in young and elderly healthy subjects and in patients with renal disease. J Am Soc Nephrol 2:856-865, 1991.

34. Kerr GR, Sul Lee E, Lam M-KM, et al: Relationships between dietary and biochemical measures of nutritional status in NHANES I data. Am J Clin Nutr 35:294-308, 1982.

35. Tobin J, Spector D: Dietary protein has no effect on future creatinine clearance [abstract]. Gerontologist 26:59, 1986.

36. Brenner BM, Meyer TW, Hostetter TH: Dietary protein intake and the progressive nature of kidney disease: The role of hemodynamically mediated glomerular injury in the pathogenesis of progressive glomerular schlerosis in aging, renal ablation, and intrinsic renal disease. N Engl J Med 307:652-659, 1982.

37. Bovee KC: Influence of dietary protein on renal function in dogs. J Nutr 121(suppl):128-139, 1991.

38. Bourgoignie JJ, Gavellas G, Sabnis SG, Antonovych TT: Effect of protein diets on the renal function of baboons (*Papio hamadryas*) with remnant kidneys: A 5-year follow-up. Am J Kidney Dis 23:199-204, 1994.

39. Hakim RM, Goldszer RC, Brenner BM: Hypertension and proteinuria: Long-term sequelae of uninephrectomy in humans. Kidney Int 25:930-936, 1984.

40. Rocher LL, Swartz RD: Kidney donors and protein intake [letter]. Ann Intern Med 107:427, 1987.

41. Bay WH, Hebert LA: The living donor in kidney transplantation. Ann Intern Med 106:719-727, 1987.

42. Levey AS, Adler S, Caggiula AW, et al: Effects of dietary protein restriction on the progression of moderate renal disease in the Modification of Diet in Renal Disease Study. J Am Soc Nephrol 7:2616-2626, 1996.

43. Olsen NV, Ladefoged SD, Feldt-Rasmussen B, et al: The effects of cimetidine on creatinine excretion, glomerular filtration rate and tubular function in renal transplant recipients. Scand J Clin Lab Invest 49:155-159, 1989.

44. Roubenoff R, Drew H, Moyer M, et al: Oral cimetidine improves the accuracy and precision of creatinine clearance in lupus nephritis. Ann Intern Med 113:501-506, 1990.

45. Walser M: Assessing renal function from creatinine measurements in adults with chronic renal failure. Am J Kidney Dis 32:23-31,1998.

45a. Cockcroft DW, Gault MH: Prediction of creatinine clearance from serum creatinine. Naphron 16:31-41, 1976.

46. van Olden RW, Krediet RT, Struijk DG, Arisz L: Measurement of residual renal function in patients treated with continuous ambulatory peritoneal dialysis. J Am Soc Nephrol 7:745-750, 1996.

47. Zaltzman JS, Whiteside C, Cattran DC, et al: Accurate measurement of impaired glomerular filtration using single-dose oral cimetidine. Am J Kidney Dis 27:504-511, 1996.

48. Hilbrands LB, Artz MA, Wetzels JFM, Koene RAP: Cimetidine improves the reliability of creatinine as a marker of glomerular filtration. Kidney Int 40:1171-1176, 1991.

49. van Acker BAC, Koomen GCM, Koopman MG, et al: Limitations of creatinine during cimetidine as a filtration marker in renal disease. J Am Soc Nephrol 3:322, 1992.

50. Hellerstein S, Berenbom M, Alon US, Warady BA: Creatinine clearance following cimetidine for estimation of glomerular filtration rate. Pediatr Nephrol 12:49-54, 1998.

51. Ikxes MCJ, Koopman MG, van Acker BAC, et al: Cimetidine improves GFR—estimation by the Cockcroft and Gault formula. Clin Nephrol 47:229-236, 1997.

52. Serdar MA, Kurt I, Ozcelik F, et al: A practical approach to glomerular filtration rate measurements: Creatinine clearance estimation using cimetidine. Ann Clin Lab Sci 31:265-273, 2001.

53. Shemesh O, Golbetz H, Kriss JP, Myers BD: Limitations of creatinine as a filtration marker in glomerulopathic patients. Kidney Int 28:830-838, 1985.

54. Hirata-Dulas CAL, Halstenson CE, Kasiske BL: Improvement in the accuracy and precision of creatinine clearance as a measure of glomerular filtration rate with oral cimetidine in renal transplant recipients. Clin Transplant 7:552-558, 1993.

55. Marcen R, Serrano P, Teruel JL, et al: Oral cimetidine improves the accuracy of creatinine clearance in transplant patients on cyclosporine. Transplant Proc 26:2624-2625, 1994.

56. Dubb JW, Stote RM, Familiar RG, et al: Effect of cimetidine on renal function. Clin Pharm Ther 24:76-83, 1978.

57. Payne RB: Creatinine clearance with cimetidine for measurement of GFR. Lancet 341:187, 1993.

58. Hellerstein S, Simon SD, Berenbom M, et al: Creatinine excretion rates for renal clearance studies. Pediatr Nephrol 16:637-643, 2001.

59. Kemperman FA, Silberbusch J, Slaats EH, et al: Follow-up GFR estimated from plasma creatinine administration in patients with diabetes mellitus type 2. Clin Nephrol 54:255-260, 2000.

60. Kemperman FA, Surachno J, Krediet RT, Arisz L: Cimetidine improves prediction of the glomerular filtraton rate by the Cockcroft-Gault formula in renal transplant recipients. Transplantation 15:770-774, 2002.

61. Tian S, Kusano E, Ohara T, et al: Cystatin C measurement and its practical use in patients with various renal diseases. Clin Nephrol 48:104-108, 1997.

62. Plebani M, Dallamico R, Mussap M, et al: Is serum cystatin C a sensitive marker of glomerular filtration rate (GFR): A preliminary study on renal transplant patients. Ren Fail 20:303-309, 1998.

63. Helin I, Axenram M, Grubb A: Serum cystatin C as a determinant of glomerular filtration rate in children. Clin Nephrol 49:221-225, 1998.

64. Newman DJ, Thakkar H, Edwards RG, et al: Serum cystatin C measured by automated immunoassay: A more sensitive marker of changes in GFR than serum creatinine. Kidney Int 47:312-318, 1995.

65. Nilsson-Ehle P, Grubb A: New markers for the determination of GFR: Iohexol clearance and cystatin C serum concentration. Kidney Int 47(suppl 47):17-19, 1994.

66. Norlund L, Fex G, Lanke J, et al: Reference intervals for the glomerular filtration rate and cell-proliferation markers: Serum cystatin C and serum beta 2-microglobulin/cystatin C-ratio. Scand J Clin Lab Invest 57:463-470, 1997.

67. Tan GD, Lewis AV, James TJ, et al: Clinical usefulness of cystatin C for the estimation of glomerular filtration rate in type I diabetes: Reproducibility and accuracy compared with standard measures and iohexol clearance. Diabetes Care 25:2004-2009, 2002.

68. Dharnidharka VR, Kwon C, Stevens G: Serum cystatin C is superior to serum creatinine as a marker of kidney function: A meta-analysis. Am J Kidney Dis 40:221-226, 2002.

69. Kazama JJ, Kutsuwada K, Ataka K, et al: Serum cystatin C reliably detects renal dysfunction in patients with various renal diseases. Nephron 91:13-20, 2002.

70. Shimizu-Tokiwa A, Kobata M, Io H, et al: Serum cystatin C is a more sensitive marker of glomerular function than serum creatinine. Nephron 92:224-226, 2002.

71. Nitta K, Hayashi R, Honda K, et al: Serum cystatin C concentration as a marker of glomerular filtration rate in patients with various renal diseases. Intern Med 41:931-935, 2002.

72. Risch L, Blumberg A, Huber A: Rapid and accurate assessment of glomerular filtration rate in patients with renal transplants using serum cystatin C. Nephrol Dial Transplant 14:1991-1996, 1999.

73. Strevens H, Wide-Swensson D, Torffvit O, Grubb A: Serum cystatin C for assessment of glomerular filtration rate in pregnant and non-pregnant women. Indications of altered filtration process in pregnancy. Scand J Clin Lab Invest 62:141-147, 2002.

74. Krieser D, Rosenberg AR, Kainer G, Daya N: The relationship between serum creatinine, serum cystatin C and glomerular filtration rate in pediatric renal transplant recipients: A pilot study. Pediatr Transplant 6:392-395, 2002.

75. Hjorth L, Wiebe T, Karpman D: Correct evaluation of renal glomerular filtration rate requires clearance assays. Pediatr Nephrol 17:847-851, 2002.

76. Harmoinen A, Ylinen E, Ala-Houhala M, et al: Reference intervals for cystatin C in pre- and full-term infants and children. Pediatr Nephrol 15:105-108, 2000.

77. Filler G, Priem F, Lepage N, et al: Beta-trace protein, cystatin C, beta(2)-microglobulin, and creatinine compared for detecting impaired glomerular filtration rates in children. Clin Chem 48:729-736, 2002.

78. Oddoze C, Morange S, Portugal H, et al: Cystatin C is not more sensitive than creatinine for detecting renal impairment in patients with diabetes. Am J Kidney Dis 38:310-316, 2001.

79. Bianchi C, Donadio C, Tramonti G, et al: Reappraisal of serum beta 2-microglobulin as a marker of GFR. Ren Fail 23:419-429, 2001.

80. Giessing M: Beta-trace protein as indicator of glomerular filtration rate. Urology 54:940-941, 1999.

81. Takahira R, Yonemura K, Yonekawa O, et al: Tryptophan glycoconjugate as a novel marker of renal function. Am J Med 110:192-197, 2001.

82. Rydstrom M, Tengstrom B, Cederquist I, Ahlmen J: Measurement of glomerular filtration rate by single-injection, single-sample techniques, using ^{51}Cr-EDTA or iohexol. Scand J Urol Nephrol 29:135-139, 1995.

83. Frennby B, Sterner G, Almen T, et al: The use of iohexol clearance to determine GFR in patients with severe chronic renal failure: A comparison between different clearance techniques. Clin Nephrol 43:35-46, 1995.

84. Piepsz A, Ham HR: How good is the slope of the second exponential for estimating Cr-51-EDTA renal clearance. Nucl Med Commun 18:139-141, 1997.

85. Gaspari F, Guerini E, Perico N, et al: Glomerular filtration rate determined from a single plasma sample after intravenous iohexol injection: Is it reliable? J Am Soc Nephrol 7:2689-2693, 1996.

86. Li Y, Lee HB, Blaufox MD: Single-sample methods to measure GFR with technetium-99m-DTPA. J Nucl Med 38:1290-1295, 1997.

87. Itoh K, Tsuhima S, Tsukamoto E, Tamaki N: Accuracy of plasma sample methods for determination of glomerular filtration rate with ^{99m}Tc-DTPA. Ann Nucl Med 16:39-44, 2002.

88. Lundqvist S, Hietala SO, Groth S, Shodin JG: Evaluation of single sample clearance calculations in 902 patients: A comparison of multiple and single sample techniques. Acta Radiol 38:68-72, 1997.

89. Sambataro M, Thomaseth K, Pacini G, et al: Plasma clearance of ^{51}Cr-EDTA provides a precise and convenient technique for measurement of glomerular filtration rate in diabetic humans. J Am Soc Nephrol 7:118-127, 1996.

90. Gaspari F, Perico N, Remuzzi G: Measurement of glomerular filtration rate. Kidney Int 52(suppl 63):151-154, 1997.

91. Gaspari F, Perico N, Matalone M, et al: Precision of plasma clearance of iohexol for estimation of GFR in patients with renal disease. J Am Soc Nephrol 9:310-313, 1998.

92. Fleming JS, Waller DG: Feasibility of estimating glomerular filtration rate in children using single-sample adult technique. J Nucl Med 38:1665-1667, 1997.

93. Ham HR, Piepsz A: Feasibility of estimating glomerular filtration rate in children using single-sample adult technique. J Nucl Med 37:1805-1808, 1996.

94. Al-Uzri A, Holliday MA, Gambertoglio JG, et al: An accurate practical method for estimating GFR in clinical studies using a constant subcutaneous infusion. Kidney Int 41:1701-1706, 1992.

95. Holliday MA, Heilbron D, Al-Uzri A, et al: Serial mearsurement of GFR in infants using the continuous iothalamate infusion technique. Kidney Int 43:893-898, 1993.

96. Cole BR, Giangiacomo J, Ingelfinger JR, Robson AM: Measurement of renal function without urine collection. A critical evaluation of the constant-infusion technic for determination of inulin and para-aminohippurate. N Engl J Med 287:1109-1114, 1972.

97. Sharma AK, Mills MS, Grey VL, Drummond KN: Infusion clearance of subcutaneous iothalamate versus standard renal clearance. Pediatr Nephrol 11:711-713, 1997.

98. Hellerstein S, Berenbom M, Alon U, Warady BA: The renal clearance and infusion clearance of inulin are similar but not identical. Kidney Int 44:1058-1061, 1993.

99. Perrone RD, Steinman TI, Beck GJ, et al: Utility of radioisotopic filtration markers in chronic renal insufficiency: Simultaneous comparison of ^{125}I-iothalamate, ^{169}Yb-DPTA, ^{99m}Tc-DTPA and inulin. Am J Kidney Dis 16:224-235, 1990.

100. Apperloo AJ, De Zeeuw D, Donker AJ, De Jong PE: Precision of glomerular filtration rate determinations for long-term slope calculations is improved by simultaneous infusion of ^{125}I-iothalamate and ^{131}I-hippuran. J Am Soc Nephrol 7:567-572, 1996.

101. Donker AJ, van der Hem GK, Sluiter WJ, Beekhuis H: A radioisotope method for simultaneous determination of the glomerular filtration rate and the effective renal plasma flow. Neth J Med 20:97-130, 1977.

102. Fotopoulos A, Blaufox MB, Lee HB, Lynn R: Effects of residual urine on apparent renal clearance in patients with reduced function. Nuclear Med Commun 3:224-235, 1992.

103. Bianchi C, Donadio C, Tramonti G, et al: A reappraisal of the bladder cumulative method as a reliable technique for the measurement of glomerular filtration rate. Ren Fail 20:257-265, 1998.

104. Schott-Baer FD, Reaume L: Accuracy of ultrasound estimates of urine volume. Urol Nurs 21:193-195, 2001.

105. Isaka Y, Fujiwara Y, Yamamoto S, et al: Modified plasma clearance technique using nonradioactive iothalamate for measuring GFR. Kidney Int 42:1006-1011, 1992.

106. Gaspari F, Mosconi L, Vigano G, et al: Measurement of GFR with a single intravenous injection of nonradioactive iothalamate. Kidney Int 41:1081-1084, 1992.

107. Krutzen E, Back SE, Nilsoon-Ehle I, Nilsoon-Ehle P: Plasma clearance of a new contrast agent iohexol: A method for the assessment of glomerular filtration rate. J Lab Clin Med 104:955-961, 1984.

108. Frennby B, Sterner G, Almen T, et al: Clearance of iohexol, Cr51-EDTA and endogenous creatinine for determination of glomerular filtration rate in pigs with reduced renal function—a comparison between different clearance techniques. Scand J Clin Lab Invest 57: 241-252, 1997.

109. Gaspari F, Perico N, Ruggenenti P, et al: Plasma clearance of nonradioactive iohexol as a measure of glomerular filtration rate. J Am Soc Nephrol 6:257-263, 1995.

110. Pucci L, Bandinelli S, Pilo M, et al: Iohexol as a marker of glomerular filtration rate in patients with diabetes: Comparison of multiple and simplified sampling protocols. Diabet Med 18:116-120, 2001.

111. Kjaersgaard P, Jakobsen JA, Nossen JO, Berg KJ: Determination of glomerular filtration rate with Visipaque in patients with severely reduced renal function. Eur Radiol 6:865-871, 1996.

112. Erley CM, Bader BD, Berger ED, et al: Plasma clearance of iodine contrast media as a measure of glomerular filtration rate in critically ill patients. Crit Care Med 29:1544-1550, 2001.

112a. Schwartz GH, Feld LG, Langford DJ: A simple estimate of glomerular filtration rate in full-term infants during the first year of life. J Pediatr 104:849-854, 1998.

112b. Schwartz GJ, Brion LP, Spitzer A: The use of plasma creatinine concentration for estimating glomerular filtration rate in infants, children, and adolescents. Pediatr Clin North Am 34:571-590, 1987.

112c. Gbadegesin RA, Adeyemo AA, Asinobi AO, Osimasi K: Inaccuracy of the Schwartz formula in estimating glomerular filtration rate in Nigerian children. Ann Trop Pediatr 17:179-185, 1997.

113. Leger F, Bouissou F, Coulias Y, et al: Estimation of glomerular filtration rate in children. Pediatr Nephrol 17:903-9007, 2002.

114. Seikaly MG, Browne R, Bajaj G, Arant BS: Limitations to body length/serum creatinine ratio as an estimator of glomerular filtration in children. Pediatr Nephrol 10:709-711, 1996.

115. Beck GJ, Berg RL, Coggins CH, et al: Design and statistical issues of the Modification of Diet in Renal Disease Trial. Control Clin Trials 12:566-586, 1991.

116. Mitch WE, Buffington GA, Lemann J, Walser M: A simple method of estimating progression of chronic renal failure. Lancet 2:1326-1328, 1976.

117. Mitch WE: Measuring the rate of progression of renal insufficiency. In Mitch WE (ed): The Progressive Nature of Renal Disease. New York, Churchill Livingstone, 1992, pp 203-222.

118. Shah BV, Levey AS: Spontaneous changes in the rate of decline in reciprocal serum creatinine: Errrors in predicting the progression of renal disease from extrapolation of the slope. J Am Soc Nephrol 2:1186-1191, 1992.

119. Jones RH, Molitoris BA: A statistical method for determining the breakpoint of two lines. Anal Biochem 141:287-290, 1984.

120. Coresh J, Walser M, Hill S: Survival on dialysis among chronic renal failure patients treated with a supplemented low-protein diet before dialysis. J Am Soc Nephrol 6:1379-1385, 1995.

121. Walser M, Drew HH, LaFrance ND: Reciprocal creatinine slopes often give erroneous estimates of progression of chronic renal failure. Kidney Int 36 (suppl 27):81-85, 1989.

122. Maroni BJ, Mitch WE: Role of nutrition in prevention of the progression of renal disease. Annu Rev Nutr 17:435-455, 1997.

123. Levey AS, Gassman JJ, Hall PM, Walker WG: Assessing the progression of renal disease in clinical studies: Effects of duration of follow-up and regression to the mean. J Am Soc Nephrol 1:1087-1094, 1991.

124. Mathillas O, Attman PO, Aurell M, et al: Conflicting measurements in chronic renal failure. Contrib Nephrol 53:71-73, 1986.

125. Walser M, Drew HH, LaFrance ND: Creatinine measurements often yield false estimates of progression in chronic renal failure. Kidney Int 34:412-418, 1988.

126. Bosch JP: Renal reserve: A functional view of glomerular filtration rate. Semin Nephrol 15:381-385, 1995.

127. Walser M: Progression of chronic renal failure in man. Kidney Int 37:1195-1210, 1990.

128. Buckheit JB, Olshen RA, Blouch K, Myers BD: Modeling of progressive glomerular injury in humans with lupus nephritis. Am J Physiol 273:F158-F169, 1997.

129. Walser M, Hill S, Ward L: Progression of chronic renal failure on substituting a ketoacid supplement for an amino acid supplement. J Am Soc Nephrol 2:1178-1185, 1992.

130. Rehling M, Moller ML, Thamdrup B, et al: Simultaneous measurement of renal clearance and plasma clearance of ^{99m}Tc-labelled diethylenetriaminepenta-acetate, ^{51}Cr-labelled ethylenediaminetetra-acetate and inulin in man. Clin Sci 66:613-619, 1984.

131. Viberti GC, Bilous RW, Mackintosh BS, Keen H: Monitoring glomerular function in diabetic nephropathy. Am J Med 74:256-264, 1983.

132. Mogensen CE: Renal function changes in diabetes. Diabetes 25:872-877, 1976.

133. Walser M, LaFrance ND, Ward L, VanDuyn MA: Progression of chronic renal failure in patients given ketoacids following amino acids. Kidney Int 32:123-128, 1987.

134. Bergstrom J, Alvestrand A, Bucht H, Gutierrez A: Stockholm clinical study on progression of chronic renal failure—an interim report. Kidney Int 36(suppl 27):110-114, 1989.

135. Nyberg G, Blohme G, Norden G:. Constant glomerular filtration rate in diabetic nephropathy. Acta Med Scand 219:67-72, 1986.

136. Franz KA, Reubi FC: Rate of functional deterioration in polycystic kidney disease. Kidney Int 23:523-526, 1983.

137. Klahr S, Levey AS, Beck GJ, et al: The effects of dietary protein restriction and blood-pressure control on the progression of chronic renal failure. N Engl J Med 330:878-884, 1994.

138. Walser M, Hill S: Can renal replacement be deferred by a supplemented very-low protein diet? J Am Soc Nephrol 10:110-116, 1999.

139. Mackenzie HS, Brenner BM: Current strategies for retarding progression of renal disease. Am J Kidney Dis 31:161-170, 1998.

140. Sawicki PT: Stabilization of glomerular filtration rate over 2 years in patients with diabetic nephropathy under intensified therapy regimens. Nephrol Dial Transplant 12:1890-1899, 1997.

141. Toto RD, Mitchell HC, Smith RD, et al: "Strict" blood pressure control and progression of renal disease in hypertensive nephrosclerosis. Kidney Int 48:851-859, 1995.

142. Fink JC, Salmanullah M, Blahut SA, et al: The inevitability of renal function loss in patients with hypercreatininemia. Am J Nephrol 21:386-389, 2001.

143. Rottey S, Vanholder R, DeSchoenmakere G, Lameire N: Progression of renal failure in patients with compromised renal function is not always present: Evaluation of underlying disease. Clin Nephrol 54:1-10, 2000.

144. Walser M, Hill SB, Ward L, Magder L: A crossover comparison of progression of chronic renal failure: Ketoacids versus amino acids. Kidney Int 43:933-939, 1993.

145. Mitch WE, Walser M, Steinman TL, et al: The effect of keto acid–amino acid supplement to a restricted diet on the progression of chronic renal failure. N Engl J Med 311:623-629, 1984.

146. Hunsicker LG, Adler S, Caggiula A, et al: Predictors of the progression of renal disease in the Modification of Diet in Renal Disease Study. Kidney Int 51:1908-1919, 1997.

147. Rossing P, Hommel E, Smidt UM, Parving HH: Impact of arterial blood pressure and albuminuria on the progression of diabetic nephropathy in IDDM patients. Diabetes 42:715-719, 1993.

148. Aparicio M, Potaux L, Bouchet JL, et al: Proteinuria and progression of renal failure in patients on a low-protein diet. Nephron 51:292-293, 1989.

149. Cameron JS: Proteinuria and progression in human glomerular diseases. Am J Nephrol 10(suppl 1):81-87, 1990.

150. Rosman JB, Ter Wee PM: Relationship between proteinuria and response to low protein diets early in chronic renal failure. Blood Purif 7:52-57, 1989.

151. Williams PS, Fass G, Bone JM: Renal pathology and proteinuria determine progression in untreated mild/moderate chronic renal failure. Q J Med 67:343-354, 1988.

152. Stenvinkel P, Alvestrand A, Bergstrom J: Factors influencing progression in patients with chronic renal failure. J Intern Med 226: 183-188, 1989.

153. Nyberg G, Blohme G, Norden G: Constant glomerular filtration rate in diabetic nephropathy. Correlation to blood pressure and blood glucose control. Acta Med Scand 219:67-72, 1986.

154. Gall MA, Nielsen FS, Smidt UM, Parving HH: The course of kidney function in type-2 (non-insulin-dependent) diabetic patients with diabetic nephropathy. Diabetologia 36:1071-1078, 1993.

155. Walser M: Weighted least squares regression analysis of factors contributing to progression of chronic renal failure. Contrib Nephrol 75:127-133, 1989.

156. Wright JP, Salzano S, Brown CB, El Nahas AM: Natural history of chronic renal failure: A reappraisal. Nephrol Dial Transplant 7:379-383, 1992.

157. Locatelli F, Alberti D, Graziani G, et al: Factors affecting chronic renal failure progression: Results from a multicentre trial. Miner Electrolyte Metab 18:295-302, 1992.

158. Jungers P, Hannedouche T, Itakura Y, et al: Progression rate to end-stage renal failure in non-diabetic kidney diseases: A multivariate analysis of determinate factors. Nephrol Dial Transplant 10:1353-1360, 1995.

159. Jacobsen P, Rossing K, Tarnow L, et al: Progression of diabetic nephropathy in normotensive type 1 diabetic patients. Kidney Int 71(suppl):101-105, 1999.

160. Benigni A, Remuzzi G: Glomerular protein trafficking and progression of renal disease to terminal uremia. Semin Nephrol 16:151-159, 1996.

161. Zoja C, Donadelli R, Colleoni S, et al: Protein overload stimulates RANTES production by proximal tubular cells depending on NF-κB activation. Kidney Int 53:1608-1615, 1998.

162. Wang Y, Chen J, Chen L, et al: Induction of monocyte chemoattractant protein-1 in proximal tubules by urinary protein. J Am Soc Nephrol 8:1537-1545, 1997.

163. Cooper MA, Buddington B, Miller NL, Alfrey AC: Urinary iron speciation in nephrotic syndrome. Am J Kidney Dis 25:314-319, 1995.

164. Fioretto P, Kim Y, Mauer M: Diabetic nephropathy as a model of reversibility of established renal lesions. Curr Opin Nephrol Hypertens 7:489-494, 1998.

165. Rudberg S, Osterby R: Decreasing glomerular filtration rate—an indicator of more advanced diabetic glomerulopathy in the early course of microalbuminuria in IDDM adolescents. Nephrol Dial Transplant 12:1149-1154, 1997.

166. Ikoma M, Kawamura T, Kakinuma Y, et al: Cause of variable therapeutic efficiency of angiotensin converting enzyme inhibitors on glomerular lesions. Kidney Int 40:195-202, 1991.

167. Gretz NM: How to assess the rate of progression of chronic renal failure in children? Pediatr Nephrol 8:499-504, 1994.

168. Rossing P: Doubling of serum creatinine: Is it sensitive and relevant? Nephrol Dial Transplant 13:244-246, 1998.

169. Lewis EJ, Hunsicker LG, Bain RP, Rhode RR: The effect of angiotensin-converting-enzyme inhibition on diabetic nephropathy. N Engl J Med 329:1456-1462, 1993.

170. MDRD Study Group: The Modification of Diet in Renal Disease Study: Design, methods and results from the feasibility study. Am J Kidney Dis 20:18-33, 1992.

171. Ponto KH, Anderson PA, Kies CV: Plasma alloisoleucine: Analytical method and clearance in ketoacid-supplemented normals. Kidney Int 36(suppl 27):177-183, 1989.

172. Jones B, Kenward MG: Design and analysis of cross-over trials. *In* Monographs on Statistics and Applied Probability. New York, Chapman & Hall, 1989.

173. Kopple JD: Causes of catabolism and wasting in acute or chronic renal failure. *In* Robinson RR (ed): Nephrology. New York, Springer-Verlag, 1984, pp 1498-1514.

174. Qureshi AR, Alvestrand A, Danielsson A, et al: Factors predicting malnutrition in hemodialysis patients: A cross-sectional study. Kidney Int 53:773-782, 1998.

175. Kopple JD, Gao X-L, Oing P-Y: Diet protein and urea and total nitrogen appearance in chronic renal failure patients. Kidney Int 52:486-494, 1997.

176. Kopple JD: Protein-energy malnutrition in maintenance dialysis patients. Am J Clin Nutr 65:1544-1557, 1997.

177. Energy and protein requirements. Report of a joint FAO/WHO/UNU Expert Consultation. World Health Organ Tech Rep Ser 724:1-206, 1985.

178. Leibel RL, Rosenbaum M, Hirsch J: Changes in energy expenditure resulting from altered body weight. N Engl J Med 332:621-628, 1995.

179. Monteon FJ, Laidlaw SA, Shaib JK, Kopple JD: Energy expenditure in patients with chronic renal failure. Kidney Int 30:741-747, 1986.

180. Ikizler TA, Wingard RL, Sun M, et al: Increased energy expenditure in hemodialysis patients. J Am Soc Nephrol 7:2646-2653, 1996.

181. Smith D, DeFronzo RA: Insulin resistance in uremia mediated by postbinding defects. Kidney Int 22:54-62, 1982.

182. DeFronzo RA, Beckles AD: Glucose intolerance following chronic metabolic acidosis in man. Am J Physiol 236:E328-E334, 1979.

183. Rigalleau V, Combe C, Blanchetier V, et al: Low protein diet in uremia: Effects on glucose metabolism and energy production rate. Kidney Int 51:1222-1227, 1997.

184. Kopple JD, Levey AS, Greene T, et al: Effect of dietary protein restriction on nutritional status in the Modification of Diet in Renal Disease (MDRD) Study. Kidney Int 52:778-791, 1997.

185. Hyne BB, Fowell E, Lee HA: The effect of caloric intake on nitrogen balance in chronic renal failure. Clin Sci 43:679-687, 1972.

186. Rose WC: The amino acid requirements of adult man. Fed Proc 8:546-552, 1949.

187. Ikizler TA, Greene JH, Wingard RL, et al: Spontaneous dietary protein intake during progression of chronic renal failure. J Am Soc Nephrol 6:1386-1391, 1995.

188. Bergstrom J: Anorexia in dialysis patients. Semin Nephrol 16:222-229, 1996.

189. Bergstrom J, Furst P, Ahlberg M, Noree L-O: The role of dietary and energy intake in chronic renal failure. *In* Canzler VH (ed): Topical Questions in Nutritional Therapy in Nephrology and Gastroenterology. Stuttgart, Germany, Georg Thieme Verlag, 1978, pp 1-16.

190. Kopple JD, Monteon FJ, Shaib JK: Effect of energy intake on nitrogen metabolism in nondialyzed patients with chronic renal failure. Kidney Int 29:734-742, 1986.

191. Berl T, Katz FH, Henrich WL, De et al: Role of aldosterone in the control of sodium excretion in patients with advanced chronic renal failure. Kidney Int 14:228-235, 1978.

192. Watanabe S, Kang D-H, Feng L, et al: Uric acid, hominoid evolution and the pathogensis of salt-sensitivity. Hypertension 40:355-360, 2002.

193. Kang D-H, Nakagawa T, Feng L, et al: A role for uric acid in the progression of renal disease. J Am Soc Nephrol 13:2888-2898, 2002.

194. Nakagawa T, Mazzali M, Kang D-H, et al: Hyperuricemia causes glomerular hypertrophy in the rat. Am J Nephrol 23:2-7, 2003.

195. Mazzali M, Kanellis J, Han H, et al: Hyperuricemia induces a primary renal arteriolopathy in rats by a blood pressure–independent mechanism. Am J Physiol 282:F991-F997, 2002.

196. Mallamaci F, Leonardis D, Bellizzi V, Zoccali C: Does high salt intake cause hyperfiltration in patients with essential hypertension? J Hum Hypertens 10:157-161, 1996.

197. Dengel DR, Glodberg AP, Mayuga RS, et al: Insulin resistance, elevated glomerular filtration fraction, and renal injury. Hypertension 28:127-132, 1996.

198. Bakris GL, Weir MR: Salt intake and reductions in arterial pressure and proteinuria: Is there a direct link? Am J Hyperten 9(suppl):200-206, 1996.

199. Bigazzi R, Bianchi S, Baldari D, et al: Microalbuminuria in salt-sensitive patients. A marker for renal and cardiovascular risk factors. Hypertension 23:195-199, 1994.

200. Bank N, Lahorra G, Aynedjian HS, Wilkes BM: Sodium restriction corrects hyperfiltration of diabetes. Am J Physiol 254:F668-F676, 1988.

201. Weir MR: The influence of dietary salt on the antiproteinuric effect of calcium channel blockers. Am J Kidney Dis 29:800-803, 1997.

202. Campese VM, Parise M, Karubian F, Bigazzi R: Abnormal renal hemodynamics in black salt sensitive patients with hypertension. Hypertension 18:805-821, 1991.

203. Heeg JE, De Jong PE, van der Hem GK, De Zeeuw D: Efficacy and variability of the antiproteinuric effect of ACE inhibition by lisinopril. Kidney Int 36:272-279, 1989.

204. Allen TJ, Waldron MJ, Casley D, et al: Salt restriction reduces hyperfiltration, renal enlargement and albuminuria in experimental diabetes. Diabetes 46:119-124, 1997.

205. Vallon V, Wead LM, Blantz RC: Renal hemodynamics and plasma and kidney angiotensin II in established diabetes mellitus in rats: Effect of sodium and salt restriction. J Am Soc Nephrol 5:1761-1767, 1995.

206. Vallon V, Kirschenmann D, Wead LM, et al: Effect of chronic salt loading on kidney function in early and established diabetes mellitus in rats. J Lab Clin Med 130:76-82, 1997.

207. Schmitz A: Microalbuminuria, blood pressure, metabolic control, and renal involvement: Longitudinal studies in white non-insulin-dependent diabetic patients. Am J Hypertens 10(suppl S):189-197, 1997.

208. Petrie JR, Morris ASD, Minamisawa K, et al: Dietary sodium restriction impairs insulin sensitivity in noninsulin-dependent diabetes mellitus. J Clin Endocrinol Metab 83:1552-1557, 1998.

209. Ruggenenti P, Perna A, Mosconi L, et al: Urinary protein excretion rate is the best independent predictor of ESRF in non-diabetic proteinuric chronic nephropathies. Kidney Int 53:1209-1216, 1998.

210. Burton C, Harris KP: The role of proteinuria in the progression of chronic renal failure. Am J Kidney Dis 27:765-775, 1996.

211. Hellerstein S, Alon U, Warady BA: Creatinine for estimation of glomerular filtration rate. Pediatr Nephrol 6:507-511, 1992.

212. Ibrahim HN, Rosenberg ME, Greene EL, et al: Aldosterone is a major factor in the progression of renal disease. Kidney Int Suppl 63:115-119, 1997.

213. Quan ZY, Walser M, Hill GS: Adrenalectomy ameliorates ablative nephropathy in the rat independently of corticosterone maintenance level. Kidney Int 41:326-333, 1992.

214. Greene EL, Kren S, Hostetter TH: Role of aldosterone in the remnant kidney model in the rat. J Clin Invest 98:1063-1068, 1996.

215. de Santo NG, Anastasio P, Spitali L, et al: Renal reserve is normal in adults born with unilateral renal agenesis and is not related to hyperfiltration or renal failure. Miner Electrolyte Metab 23:283-286, 1995.

216. Thomsen K, Nielsen CB, Flyvbjerg A: Effects of glycine on glomerular filtration rate and segmental tubular handling of sodium in conscious rats. Clin Exp Pharmacol Physiol 29:449-454, 2002.

217. Anastasio P, Santoro D, Spitali L, et al: Renal functional reserve in children. Semin Nephrol 18:454-460, 1995.

218. Fliser D, Ritz E, Franek E: Renal reserve in the elderly. Semin Nephrol 15:463-467, 1995.

219. Gabbai FB: Renal reserve in patients with high blood pressure. Semin Nephrol 15:482-487, 1995.

220. Kontessis P, Jones S, Dodd R, et al: Renal, metabolic and hormonal responses to ingestion of animal and vegetable proteins. Kidney Int 38:136-144, 1990.

221. Jones SL, Kontessis P, Wiseman M, et al: Protein intake and blood glucose as modulators of GFR in hyperfiltering diabetic patients. Kidney Int 41:1620-1628, 1992.

222. Fioretto P, Trevisan R, Valerio A, et al: Impaired renal response to a meat meal in insulin-dependent diabetes: Role of glucagon and prostaglandins. Am J Physiol 258:F675-F683, 1990.

223. Brouhard BH, LaGrone L: Effect of dietary protein restriction on functional renal reserve in diabetic nephropathy. Am J Med 89:427-431, 1990.

224. Guizar JM, Kornhauser C, Malacara JM, et al: Renal functional reserve in patients with recently diagosed type 2 diabetes mellitus with and without microalbuminuria. Nephron 87:223-230, 2001.

225. Tuttle KR, Puhlman MF, Cooney SK, Short RA: Effects of amino acids and glucagon on renal hemodynamics in type 1 diabetes. Am J Physiol 282:F103-F112, 2002.

226. Pinto JR, Bending JJ, Dodds RA, Viberti GC: Effect of low protein diet on the renal response to meat ingestion in diabetic nephropathy. Eur J Clin Invest 21:175-183, 1991.

227. Sackmann H, Tran-Van T, Tack I, et al: Renal functional reseve in IDDM patients. Diabetologia 41:86-93, 1998.

228. Fioretto P, Trevisan R, Giorato C, et al: Type I insulin-dependent diabetic patients show an impaired renal hemodynamic response to protein intake. J Diabetes Complications 2:27-29, 1988.

229. Juncos LI, Juncos LA, Ferrer MC, et al: Abnormal renal vasodilatation to an amino acid infusion in congestive heart failure: Normalization by enalapril. Am J Kidney Dis 33:43-51, 1999.

230. Woods LL: Intrarenal mechanisms of renal reserve. Semin Nephrol 15:386-395, 1995.

231. Ter Wee PM: Renal effects of intravenous amino acid administration in humans with and without renal disease: Hormonal correlates. Semin Nephrol 15:426-432, 1995.

232. Nair KS, Pabico RC, Truglia JA, et al: Mechanism of glomerular hyperfiltration after a protein meal in humans: Role of hormones and amino acids. Diabetes Care 17:711-715, 1994.

233. Thomas DM, Coes GA, Williams JD: Dopamine does not mediate protein-induced hyperfiltration. Exp Nephrol 2:294-298, 1994.

234. de Santo NG, Capasso G, Anastasio P, et al: Brain-gut peptides and the renal hemodynamic response to an oral protein load: A study of gastrin, bombesin, and glucagon in man. Ren Physiol Biochem 15:53-56, 1992.

235. Bohler J, Woitas R, Keller E, et al: Effect of nifedipine and captopril on glomerular hyperfiltration in normotensive man. Am J Kidney Dis 20:132-139, 1992.

236. Tietze IN, Sorensen SS, Ivarsen PR, et al: Impaired renal haemodynamic response to amino acid infusion in essential hypertension during angiotensin converting enzyme inhibitor treatment. J Hypertensn 15:551-560, 1997.

237. Lopes de Faria JB, Friedman R, de Cosmo S, et al: Renal functional response to protein loading in type 1 (insulin-dependent) diabetic patients on normal or high salt intake. Nephron 76:411-417, 1997.

238. Jaffa AA, Vio CP, Silva RH, et al: Evidence for renal kinins as mediators of amino acid–induced hyperperfusion and hyperfiltration in the rat. J Clin Invest 89:1460-1468, 1992.

239. King AJ: Nitric oxide and the renal hemodynamic response to proteins. Semin Nephrol 15:405-414, 1995.

240. El Sayed AA, Haylor J, El Nahas AM: Involvement of renal autocoids in the direct effects of mixed amino acids on the kidney. Miner Electrolyte Metab 18:117-119, 1992.

241. Muhlbauer B, Spohr F, Schmidt R, Osswald H: Role of renal nerves and endogenous dopamine in amino acid–induced glomerular hyperfiltration. Am J Physiol 273:F144-F140, 1997.

242. Kraus ES, Cheng L, Sikorski I, Spector DA: Effect of phosphorus restriction on renal response to oral and intravenous protein loads in rats. Am J Physiol 264:F752-F759, 1993.

243. de Santo NG, Anastasio P, Spitali L, et al: The renal hemodynamic response to an oral protein load is normal in IgA nephropathy. Nephron 76:406-410, 1997.

244. Bach D, Mrowka H, Schauseil S, Grabensee B: Renal functional reserve in patients with IgA glomerulopathy. Ren Fail 16:617-627, 1994.

245. Hotz P, Mujyabwami F, Roels H, et al: Effect of oral protein load on urinary protein excretion in workers exposed to cadium and to lead. Am J Ind Med 29:195-200, 1996.

246. Narita R, Kitazto H, Koshimura J, et al: Effects of protein meals on the urinary excretion of various plasma proteins in healthy subjects. Nephron 81:398-405, 1999.

247. Gross JL, Zelmanovitz T, Moulin CC, et al: Effect of a chicken-based diet on renal function and lipid profile in patients with type 2 diabetes: A randomized crossover trial. Diabetes Care 25:645-651, 2003.

248. Garini G, Mazzi A, Buzio C, et al: Renal effects of captopril, indomethacin and nifedipine in nephrotic patients after an oral protein load. Nephrol Dial Transplant 11:628-634, 1996.

249. Coppo R, Porcellini MG, Gianoglio B, et al: Glomerular permselectivity to macromolecules in reflux nephropathy: Microalbuminuria during acute hyperfiltration due to aminoacid infusion. Clin Nephrol 40:299-307, 1993.

250. King AJ, Levey AS: Dietary protein and renal function. J Am Soc Nephrol 3:1723-1737, 1993.

251. Levine SE, D'Elia JE, Bistrian B, et al: Protein-restricted diet in diabetic nephropathy. Nephron 52:55-61, 1989.

252. Wiseman MJ, Bognetti E, Dodds R, et al: Changes in renal function in response to protein restricted diet in type 1 (insulin-dependent) diabetic patients. Diabetologia 30:154-159, 1998.

253. Evanoff GV, Thompson CS, Brown J, Weinman EJ: The effect of dietary protein restriction on the progression of diabetic nephropathy: A 12-month follow-up. Arch Intern Med 147:492-495, 1987.

254. Cohen D, Dodds R, Viberti G: Effect of protein restriction in insulin dependent diabetics at risk of nephropathy. BMJ 294:795-800, 1987.

255. Walker JD, Dodds RA, Murrells TJ, et al: Restriction of dietary protein and progression of renal failure in diabetic nephropathy. Lancet 2:1411-1414, 1989.

256. Brodsky IG, Robbins DC, Hiser E, et al: Effects of low-protein diets on protein metabolism in insulin-dependent diabetes mellitus patients with early nephropathy. J Clin Endocrinol Metab 75:351-357, 1992.

257. Sugimoto T, Kikkawa R, Haneda M, Shigeta Y: Effect of dietary protein restriction on proteinuria in non-insulin-dependent diabetic patients with nephropathy. J Nutr Sci Vitaminol 37(suppl):87-92, 1996.

258. Dullaart RP, Beusekamp BJ, Meijer S, et al: Long-term effects of protein-restricted diet on albuminuria and renal function in IDDM patients without clinical nephropathy and hypertension. Diabetes Care 16:483-492, 1993.

259. Gansevoort RT, De Zeeuw D, De Jong PE: Additive antiproteinuric effect of ACE inhibition and a low-protein diet in human renal disease. Nephrol Dial Transplant 10:497-504, 1995.

260. Kaysen GA, Webster S, Albander H, et al: High-protein diets augment albuminuria in rats with Heymann nephritis by angiotensin II–dependent and –independent mechanisms. Miner Electrolyte Metab 24:238-245, 1998.

261. Kaysen GA: Biological basis of hypoalbuminemia in ESRD: J Am Soc Nephrol 9:2368-2376, 1998.

262. Percheron C, Colette C, Astre C, Monnier L: Effects of moderate changes in protein intake on urinary albumin excretion in type I diabetic patients. Nutrition 11:345-349, 1995.

263. Kalk WJ, Osler C, Constable J, et al: Influence of dietary protein on glomerular filtration and urinary albumin excretion in insulin-dependent diabetes. Am J Clin Nutr 56:169-173, 1992.

264. Toeller M, Buyken A, Heitkamp G, et al: Protein intake and urinary albumin excretion rates in the EURODIAB IDDM complications study. Diabetologia 40:1219-1226, 1997.

265. Jameel N, Pugh JA, Mitchell BD, Stern MP: Dietary protein intake is not correlated with clinical proteinuria in NIDDM. Diabetes Care 15:178-183, 1992.

266. Hoffer LJ: Adaptation to protein restriction is impaired in insulin-dependent diabetes mellitus. J Nutr 128(suppl):333-336, 1998.

267. Kupin WL, Cortes P, Dumler F, et al: Effect on renal function of change from high to moderate protein intake in type I diabetic patients. Diabetes 36:73-79, 1987.

268. Meireles CL, Price SR, Pereira AML, et al: Nutrition and chronic renal failure in rats: What is an optimal dietary protein? J Am Soc Nephrol 10:2367-2373, 1999.

269. Fouque D, Laville M, Boissel JP, et al: Controlled low protein diets in chronic renal insufficiency: Meta-analysis. BMJ 304:216-220, 1992.

270. Jungers P, Chauveau PH, Lebkiri B, et al. Treatment of advanced chronic uremia with ketoanalogues of essential amino acids: A 4-year experience. Presse Med 16:1039, 1987.

271. Ihle BU, Becker GJ, Whitworth JA, et al: The effect of protein restriction on the progression of renal insufficiency. N Engl J Med 321:1773-1777, 1989.

272. Williams PS, Stevens ME, Fass G, et al: Failure of dietary protein and phosphate restriction to retard the rate of progression of chronic renal failure: A prospective, randomized, controlled trial. Q J Med 81:837-855, 1991.

273. Locatelli F, Alberti D, Graziani G, et al: Prospective, randomised, multicentre trial of effect of protein restriction on progression of chronic renal insufficiency. Lancet 337:1299-1304, 1991.

273a. Malvy D, Maingourd C, Pengloan J, et al: Effects of severe protein restriction with ketoanalogues in advanced renal failure. J Am Coll Nutr 8:481-486, 1999.

274. Pedrini MT, Levey AS, Lau J, et al: The effect of dietary protein restriction on the progression of diabetic and nondiabetic renal diseases: A meta-analysis. Ann Intern Med 124:627-632, 1996.

275. Mirtallo JM, Schneider PJ, Mavko K, et al: A comparison of essential and general amino acid infusions in the nutritional support of patients with compromised renal function. JPEN J Parenter Enteral Nutr 6:109-113, 1982.

276. Zeller KR, Whittaker E, Sullivan L, et al: Effect of restricting dietary protein on the progression of renal failure in patients with insulin-dependent diabetes mellitus. N Engl J Med 324:78-83, 1991.

277. Ciavarella A, DiMizio G, Stefoni S, et al: Reduced albuminuria after dietary protein restriction in insulin-dependent diabetic patients with clinical nephropathy. Diabetes Care 10:407-413, 1987.

278. Kasiske BL, Lakatua JDA, Ma JZ, Louis TA: A meta-analysis of the effects of dietary protein restriction on the rate of decline in renal function. Am J Kidney Dis 31:954-961, 1998.

279. Levey AS, Greene T, Beck GJ, et al: Dietary protein restriction and the progression of chronic renal disease: What have all the results of the MDRD Study shown? J Am Soc Nephrol 10:2426-2439, 1999.

280. Hansen HP, Tauber-Lassen E, Jensen BR, Parving HH: Effect of dietary protein restriction on prognosis in patients with diabetic nephropathy. Kidney Int 62:220-228, 2002.

281. Meloni C, Morosetti M, Suraci C, et al: Severe dietary protein restriction in overt diabetic nephropathy: Benefits or risks? J Ren Nutr 12:96-101, 2002.

282. Okada T, Matsumoto H, Nakao T, et al: Effect of dietary protein restriction and influence of proteinuria on progression of type 2 diabetic renal failure. Nippon Jinzo Gakkai Shi 42:365-373, 2000.

283. Riabov SI, Kucher AG, Grogor'eva ND, et al: [Effects of different variants of low-protein diet on progression of chronic renal failure and indices of nutritional status in predialysis stage.] Ter Arkh 73:10-15, 2001.

284. Combe C, Deforges-Lasseur C, Caix J, et al: Compliance and effects of nutritional treatment on progression and metabolic disorders of chronic renal failure. Nephrol Dial Transplant 8:412-418, 1993.

285. Choukroun G, Itakura Y, Albouze G, et al: Factors influencing progression of renal failure in autosomal dominant polycystic kidney disease. J Am Soc Nephrol 6:1634-1642, 1995.

286. Klahr S, Breyer JA, Beck GJ, et al: Dietary protein restriction, blood pressure control, and the progression of polycystic kidney disease. J Am Soc Nephrol 5:2037-2047, 1995.

287. Rees L, Rigden SP, Ward GM: Chronic renal failure and growth. Arch Dis Child 64:573-577, 1989.

288. Uauy RD, Hogg RJ, Brewer ED, et al: Dietary protein and growth in infants with chronic renal insufficiency: A report from the Southwest Pediatric Nephrology Study Group and the University of California, San Francisco. Pediatr Nephrol 8:45-50, 1994.

289. Baur LA, Knight JF, Crawford BA, et al: Total body nitrogen in children with chronic renal failure and short stature. Eur J Clin Nutr 48:433-441, 1994.

290. Polito C, La Manna A, Iovene A, Stabile D: Pubertal growth in children with chronic renal failure on conservative treatment. Pediatr Nephrol 9:734-736, 1995.

291. Kist-van Holthe tot Echten JE, Nauta J, Hop WC, et al: Protein restriction in chronic renal failure. Arch Dis Child 68:371-375, 1993.

292. Wingen AM, Fabian-Bach C, Schaefer F, Hehls O: Randomised multicentre study of a low-protein diet on the progression of chronic renal failure in children. European Study Group of Nutritional Treatment of Chronic Renal Failure in Childhood. Lancet 349:1117-1123, 1997.

293. Wingen AM, Fabian-Bach C, Mehls O: Multicentre randomized study on the effect of a low-protein diet on the progression of renal failure in childhood: One-year results. European Study Group for Nutritional Treatment of Chronic Renal Failure in Childhood. Miner Electrolyte Metab 18:303-308, 1992.

294. Hostetter TH: Progression of renal disease and renal hypertrophy. Annu Rev Physiol 57:263-278, 1995.

295. Hilgers KF, Mann JFE: Role of angiotensin II in glomerular injury: Lessons from experimental and clinical studies. Kidney Blood Press Res 19:254-262, 1996.

296. Correa-Rotter R, Hostetter TH, Rosenberg ME: Effect of dietary protein on renin and angiotensinogen gene expression after renal ablation. Am J Physiol 262:F631-F638, 1992.

297. Rosenberg ME, Chmielewski D, Hostetter TH: Effect of dietary protein on rat renin and angiotensinogen expression. J Clin Invest 85:1144-1149, 1990.

298. Inman SR, Stowe NT, Nally JV, et al: Dietary protein does not alter intrinsic reactivitiy of renal microcirculation to angiotensin II in rodents. Am J Physiol 268:F302-F308, 1995.

299. Kitamura M, Fine LG: Evidence for TGF-beta–mediated defense of the glomerulus: A blackguard molecule rehabilitated. Exp Nephrol 6:1-6, 1998.

300. Nobel NA, Border WA: Angiotensin II in renal fibrosis: Should TGF-β rather than blood pressure be the therapeutic target? Semin Nephrol 17:455-466, 1997.

301. Eddy AA: Protein restriction reduces transforming growth factor-beta and interstitial fibrosis in nephrotic syndrome. Am J Physiol 266:F884-F893, 1994.

302. Peters H, Border WA, Noble NA: Angiotensin II blockade and low-protein diet produce additive therapeutic effects in experimental glomerulonephritis. Kidney Int 57:1493-1501, 2000.

303. Fagerudd JS, Groop PH, Honkanen E, et al: Urinary excretion of TGF-beta 1, PDGF-BB and fibronectin in insulin-dependent diabetes mellitus patients. Kidney Int Suppl 63:195-197, 1997.

304. Daniels BS, Hostetter TH: Effects of dietary protein intake on vasoactive hormones. Am J Physiol 258:F1095-F1100, 1990.

305. Yanagisawa H, Wada O: Effects of dietary protein on eicosanoid production in rat renal tubules. Nephron 78:179-186, 1998.

306. Follenius M, Branderberger G, Hetter B: Diurnal cortisol peaks and their relationship to meals. J Clin Endocrinol Metab 55:757-761, 1982.

307. Slag MF, Ahmed M, Gannon MC, Nuttal FQ: Meal stimulation of cortisol secretion: A protein induced effect. Metabolism 30:1104-1108, 1981.

308. Schteingart DE, Conn JW: Dietary protein and corticosteroid secretion. Acta Diabetol Lat 9(suppl 1):328-346, 1972.

309. Anderson KE, Rosner W, Khan MS, et al: Diet-hormone interrelationships in the rat. Life Sci 40:1761-1768, 1987.

310. Wetzels JFM, Gerlag PGG, Sluiter HE, et al: Prednisone-induced fluctuations of proteinuria in patients with the nephrotic syndrome. Nephron 44:344-350, 1986.

311. Heymann W, Grupe WE: Increase in proteinuria due to steroid medication in chronic renal disease. Pediatrics 74:356-363, 1987.

312. Dowdle E, Saunders SJ: The acute effect of hydrocortisone sodium succinate on the proteinuria of the nephrotic syndrome. S Afr J Lab Clin Med 3:39-47, 1957.

313. Pessina AC, Peart WS: Renin induced proteinuria and the effects of adrenalectomy I: Haemodynamic changes in relation to function. Proc R Soc Lond B 180:43-60, 1972.

314. Garcia DL, Rennke HG, Brenner BM, Anderson S: Chronic gluco-corticoid therapy amplifies glomerular injury in rats with renal ablation. J Clin Invest 80:867-874, 1987.

315. Chen A, Sheu LF, Ho YS, et al: Administration of dexamethasone induces proteinuria of glomerular origin in mice. Am J Kidney Dis 31:443-452, 1998.

316. Walser M, Ward L: Progression of chronic renal failure is related to glucocorticoid production. Kidney Int 34:859-866, 1988.

317. Walser M, Hill S: Effect of ketoconazole plus low-dose prednisone on progression of chronic renal failure. Am J Kidney Dis 29:503-513, 1997.

318. Cardoso LR, Oliveira AV, Santos OF, et al: Effect of the antigluco-corticoid RU-486 on glomerular hemodynamics in remnant nephrons. Exp Nephrol 5:217-224, 1997.

319. Qu ZS, Chow JC, Ling PR, et al: Tissue-specific effects of chronic dietary protein restriction and gastrostomy on the insulin-like growth factor-1 pathway in the liver and colon of adult rats. Metabolism 46:691-697, 1997.

320. Fouque D, Le Bouc Y, Laville M, et al: Insulin-like growth factor-1 and its binding proteins during a low-protein diet in chronic renal failure. J Am Soc Nephrol 6:1427-1433, 1995.

321. Eidemak I, Feldt-Rasmussen B, Kanstrup IL, et al: Insulin resistance and hyperinsulinaemia in mild to moderate progressive chronic renal failure and its association with aerobic work capacity. Diabetologia 38:565-572, 1995.

322. Alvestrand A: Carbohydrate and insulin metabolism in renal failure. Kidney Int Suppl 62:48-52, 1997.

323. Fliser D, Pacini G, Engelleiter R, et al: Insulin resistance and hyper-insulinemia are already present in patients with incipient renal disease. Kidney Int 53:1343-1347, 1998.

324. Rigalleau V, Blanchetier V, Combe C, et al: A low-protein diet improves insulin sensitivity of endogenous glucose production in predialytic uremic patients. Am J Clin Nutr 65:1512-1516, 1997.

325. Kitazato H, Fujita H, Shimotomai T, et al: Effects of chronic intake of vegetable protein added to animal or fish protein on renal hemo-dynamics. Nephron 90:31-36, 2002.

326. D'Amico G, Gentile MG: Effect of dietary manipulation on the lipid abnormalities and urinary protein loss in nephrotic patients. Miner Electrolyte Metab 18:203-206, 1992.

327. D'Amico G, Gentile MG, Manna GDW, et al: Effect of vegetarian soy diet on hyperlipidaemia in nephrotic syndrome. Lancet 339:1131-1134, 1992.

328. D'Amico G, Gentile MG: Influence of diet on lipid abnormalities in human renal disease. Am J Kidney Dis 22:151-157, 1993.

329. Gentile MG, Fellin G, Cofano F, et al: Treatment of proteinuric patients with a vegetarian soy diet and fish oil. Clin Nephrol 40:315-320, 1993.

330. Jibani MM, Bloodworth LL, Foden E, et al: Predominantly vegetarian diet in patients with incipient and early clinical diabetic nephropathy: Effects on albumin excretion rate and nutritional status. Diabet Med 1991 8:949-953.

331. Kontessis PA, Bossinakou I, Sarika L, et al: Renal, metabolic, and hormonal responses to proteins of different origin in normotensive, nonproteinuric type I diabetic patients. Diabetes Care 18:1233, 1995.

332. Soroka N, Silverberg DS, Greenland M, et al: Comparison of a vegetable-based (SOYA) and an animal-based low-protein diet in predialysis chronic renal failure patients. Nephron 79:173-180, 1998.

333. Ferri C, Puccini R, Longombardo G, et al: Low-antigen-content diet in the treatment of patients with IgA nephropathy. Nephrol Dial Transplant 8:1193-1198, 1993.

334. Chen PY, Sanders PW: L-Arginine abrogates salt-sensitive hypertension in Dahl/Rapp rats. J Clin Invest 88:1559-1567, 1991.

335. Chen PY, St. John PL, Kirk KA, et al: Hypertensive nephrosclerosis in the Dahl/Rapp rat: Initial sites of injury and effect of dietary L-arginine supplementation. Lab Invest 68:174-181, 1993.

336. Reyes AA, Purkerson ML, Karl I, Klahr S: Dietary supplementation with L-arginine ameliorates the progression of renal disease in rats with subtotal nephrectomy. Am J Kidney Dis 20:168-176, 1992.

337. Reyes AA, Karl IE, Kissane J, Klahr S: L-Arginine administration prevents glomerular hyperfiltration and decreases proteinuria in diabetic rats. J Am Soc Nephrol 4:1039-1045, 1993.

338. Reyes AA, Klahr S: Dietary supplementation of L-arginine amelio-rates renal hypertrophy in rats fed a high-protein diet. Proc Soc Exp Biol Med 206:157-161, 1994.

339. Pisani A, Uccello F, Cesaro A, et al: Progression of chronic renal failure in remnant rats: Role of arginase inhibition. G Ital Nefrol 19:278-285, 2002.

340. Sabbatini M, Pisani A, Uccello F, et al: Arginase inhibition slows the progression of renal failure in rats with renal ablation. Am J Physiol Renal Physiol 284:F680-F687, 2003.

341. Reyes AA, Porras BH, Chasalow FI, Klahr S: L-Arginine decreases the infiltration of the kidney by macrophages in obstructive nephropathy and puromycin-induced nephrosis. Kidney Int 45:1346-1354, 1994.

342. Ashab I, Peer G, Blum M, et al: Oral administration of L-arginine and captopril in rats prevents chronic renal failure by nitric oxide production. Kidney Int 47:1515-1521, 1995.

343. MacAllister RJ, Whitley GStJ, Vallance P: Effects of guanidino and uremic compounds on nitric oxide pathways. Kidney Int 45:737-742, 1994.

344. Arnal J-F, Munzel T, Venema RC, et al: Interactions between L-arginine and L-glutamine change endothelial NO production: An effect independent of NO synthase substrate availability. J Clin Invest 95:2565-2572, 1995.

345. Higashi Y, Oshima T, Ono N, et al: Intravenous administration of L-arginine inhibits angiotensin-converting enzyme in humans. J Clin Endocrinol Metab 80:2198-2202, 1995.

346. Komers R, Komersova K, Ruzickova J, Pelikanova T: Intravenous administration of L-arginine inhibits angiotensin-converting enzyme in humans. J Hypertens 18:51-59, 2000.

347. Andoh TF, Gardner MP, Bennett WM: Protective effects of dietary L-arginine supplementation on chronic cyclosporine nephrotoxicity. Transplantation 64:1236-1240, 1997.

348. Yang CW, Kim YS, Kim J, et al: Oral supplementation of L-arginine prevents chronic cyclosporine nephrotoxicity in rats. Exp Nephrol 6:50-56, 1998.

349. Higashi Y, Oshima T, Ozono R, et al: Effect of L-arginine infusion on systemic and renal hemodynamics in hypertensive patients. Am J Hypertens 12:8-15, 1999.

350. Bello E, Caramelo C, Lopez MD, et al: Induction of microalbuminuria by L-arginine infusion in healthy individuals: An insight into the mechanisms of proteinuria. Am J Kidney Dis 33:1018-1025, 1999.

351. Watanabe G, Tomiyama H, Doba N: Effects of oral administration of L-arginine on renal function in patients with heart failure. J Hypertens 18:229-234, 2000.

352. Herlitz H, Jungersten LU, Wikstrand J, Widgren BR: Effect of L-arginine infusion in normotensive subjects with and without a family history of hypertension. Kidney Int 56:1838-1845, 1999.

353. Bello E, Caramelo C: Increase of tubular secretion of creatinine by L-arginine: Mechanism of practical significance in the assessment of renal function based on creatinine clearance. Nefrologia 20:517-522, 2000.

354. Tome LA, Yu L, de Castro I, et al: Beneficial and harmful effects of L-arginine on renal ischemia. Nephrol Dial Transplant 14:1139-1145, 1999.

355. Narita I, Border WA, Ketteler M, et al: L-Arginine may mediate the therapeutic effects of low protein diets. Proc Natl Acad Sci USA 92:4552-4556, 1995.

356. Narita I, Border WA, Ketteler M, Noble NA: Nitric oxide mediates immunologic injury to kidney mesangium in experimental glomerulonephritis. Lab Invest 72:17-24, 1995.

357. Ketteler M, Ikegaya N, Brees DK, et al: L-Arginine metabolism in immune-mediated glomerulonephritis in the rat. Am J Kidney Dis 28:878-887, 1996.

358. Bennett-Richards KJ, Kattenhorn M, Donald AE, et al: Oral L-arginine does not improve endothelial dysfunction in children with chronic renal failure. Kidney Int 62:1372-1378, 2002.

359. Blantz RC, Lortie M, Vallon V, et al: Activities of nitric oxide in normal physiology and uremia. Semin Nephrol 16:144-150, 1996.

360. Kaysen GA, Kropp J: Dietary tryptophan supplementation prevents proteinuria in the seven-eighths nephrectomized rat. Kidney Int 23:473-479, 1983.

361. Walser M: Do ketoacid-supplemented diets slow progression of chronic renal failure? A review of published studies. In Andreucci VE, Fine LG (eds): International Yearbook of Nephrology. New York, Oxford University Press, 1996, pp 119-126.

362. Teschan PE, Beck GJ, Dwyer JT, et al: Effect of a ketoacid-aminoacid–supplemented very low protein diet on the progression of advanced renal disease: A reanalysis of the MDRD Feasibility Study. Clin Nephrol 50:273-283, 1998.

363. Walser M, Ward L, Hill S: Hypotryptophanemia in patients with chronic renal failure on nutritional therapy. J Am Soc Nephrol 2:247, 1991.

364. Owada P, Nakao M, Koike J, et al: Effects of oral adsorbent AST-120 on the progression of chronic renal failure—a randomized controlled study. Kidney Int Suppl 63:188-190, 1997.

365. Miyazaki T, Ise M, Seo H, Niwa T: Indoxyl sulfate increases the gene expression of TGF-beta-1, TIMP-1 and Pro-alpha-1 collagen in uremic rat kidneys. Kidney Int 52(suppl 62):15-22, 1997.

366. Miyazaki T, Ise M, Hirata M, et al: Indoxyl sulfate stimulates renal synthesis of transforming gorwth factor-beta-1 and progression of renal failure. Kidney Int 52(suppl 63):211-214, 1997.

367. Niwa T, Tsukushi S, Ise M, et al: Indoxyl sulfate and progression of renal failure—effects of a low-protein diet and oral sorbent on indoxyl sulfate production in uremic rats and undialyzed uremic patients. Miner Electrolyte Metab 23:179-184, 1997.

368. Niwa T, Ise M, Miyazaki T: Progression of glomerular sclerosis in experimental uremic rats by administration of indole, a precursor of indoxyl sulfate. Am J Nephrol 14:207-212, 1994.

369. Keane WF, Guijarro C: Lipids and progressive renal failure. Contrib Nephrol 118:17-23, 1996.

370. Samuelsson O, Mulec H, Knight-Givson C, et al: Lipoprotein abnormalities are associated with increased rate of progression of human chronic renal insufficiency. Nephrol Dial Transplant 12:1908-1915, 1997.

371. Attman PO, Samuelsson O, Alaupovic P: Progression of renal failure—role of apolipoprotein B–containing lipoproteins. Kidney Int 52(suppl 63):98-101, 1997.

372. Krolewski AS, Warram JH, Christlieb AR: Hypercholesterolemia—a determinant of renal function loss and deaths in IDDM patients with nephropathy. Kidney Int 45(suppl 45):125-131, 1994.

373. Gregorio SM, Lemos CC, Caldas ML, Bregman R: Effect of dietary linoleic acid on the progression of chronic renal failure in rats. Braz J Med Biol Res 35:573-579, 2002.

374. Kutner NG, Clow PW, Zhang R, Aviles X: Association of fish intake and survival in a cohort of incident dialysis patients. Am J Kidney Dis 39:1018-1024, 2002.

375. Lam KSL, Cheng JKP, Janus ED, Pang RW: Cholesterol-lowering therapy may retard the progression of diabetic nephropathy. Diabetologia 38:604-609, 1995.

376. Sanjad SA, Alabbad A, Alshorafa S: Management of hyperlipidemia in children with refractory nephrotic syndrome—the effect of statin therapy. J Pediatr 130:470-474, 1997.

377. Monzani G, Bergesio F, Ciuti R, et al: Lp(a) levels—effects of progressive chronic renal failure and dietary manipulation. J Nephrol 10:41-45, 1997.

378. Bernard S, Fouque D, Laville M, Zech P: Effects of low-protein diet supplemented with ketoacids on plasma lipids in adult chronic renal failure. Miner Electrolyte Metab 22:143-146, 1996.

379. Nielsen S, Hermansen K, Rasmussen OW, et al: Urinary albumin excretion rate and 24-h ambulatory blood pressure in NIDDM with microalbuminuria: Effects of a monounsaturated-enriched diet. Diabetologia 38:1069-1075, 1995.

380. Cappelli P, Diliberato L, Stuard S, et al: N-3 polyunsaturated fatty acid supplementation in chronic progressive renal disease. J Nephrol 10:157-162, 1997.

381. Hamazaki T, Nakazawa R, Tateno S, et al: Effects of fish oil rich in eicosapentaenoic acid on serum lipids in hyperlipidemic hemodialysis patients. Kidney Int 26:81-84, 1984.

382. Donadio JV, Grande JP, Begstralh EJ, et al: The long-term outcome of patients with IgA nephropathy treated with fish oil in a controlled trial. J Am Soc Nephrol 10:1772-1777, 1999.

383. Manitius J, Sulikowska B, Fox J, et al: The effect of dietary enrichment with fish-oil on urinary excretion of *N*-acetyl-beta-D-glucosaminidase and renal function in proteinuric patients with primary glomerulopathies. Int Urol Nephrol 29:489-495, 1997.

384. Bliss DZ, Stein TP, Schleifer CR, Settle RG: Supplementation with gum arabic fiber increases fecal nitrogen excretion and lowers serum urea nitrogen concentration in chronic renal failure patients consuming a low-protein diet. Am J Clin Nutr 63:392-398, 1996.

385. Groop PH, Aro A, Stenman S, Groop L: Long-term effects of guar gum in subjects with non-insulin-dependent diabetes mellitus. Am J Clin Nutr 58:513-518, 1993.

386. Frank J, Biesalski HK: Involvement of reactive oxygen species in the progression of renal disease and the significance of antioxidants in therapy. Nieren- und Hochdruckkrankheiten 26:342-347, 1997.

387. Lee HS, Jeong JY, Kim BC, et al: Dietary antioxidant inhibits lipoprotein oxidation and renal injury in experimental focal segmental glomerulosclerosis. Kidney Int 51:1151-1159, 1996.

388. Craven PA, DeRubertis FR, Kagan VE, et al: Effects of supplementation with vitamin C or E on albuminuria, glomerular TGF-β and glomerular size in diabetes. J Am Soc Nephrol 8:1405-1414, 1997.

389. Fishbane S, Maesaka JK: Iron management in end-stage renal disease. Am J Kidney Dis 29:319-333, 1997.

390. Drueke TB, Barany P, Cazzola M, et al: Management of iron deficiency in renal anemia: Guidelines for the optimal therapeutic approach in erythropoietin-treated patients. Clin Nephrol 48:1-8, 1997.

391. Sanders HN, Rabb HA, Bittle P, Ramirez G: Nutritional implications of recombinant human erythropoietin therapy in renal disease. J Am Diet Assoc 94:1023-1029, 1994.

392. Wingard RL, Parker RA, Ismail N, Hakim RM: Efficacy of oral iron therapy in patients receiving recombinant human erythropoietin. Am J Kidney Dis 25:433-439, 1995.

393. Anuradha S, Singh NP, Agarwal SK: Total dose infusion iron dextran therapy in predialysis chronic renal failure patients. Ren Fail 24:207-213, 2002.

394. Drueke T, Witko-Sarsat V, Massy Z, et al: Iron therapy, advanced oxidation protein products and carotid artery intima-media thickness in end-stage renal disease. Circulation 106:2212-2217, 2002.

395. Zager RA, Johnson AC, Hanson SY, Wasse H: Parenteral iron formulations: A comparative toxicologic analysis and mechanisms of cell injury. Am J Kidney Dis 40:90-103, 2002.

396. Hoigne R, Breymann C, Kiinzi UP, Brunner F: Parenteral iron therapy—problems and possible solutions. Schweiz Med Wochenschr 128:528-535, 1998.

397. Taylor JE, Peat N, Porter C, Morgan AG: Regular low-dose intravenous iron therapy improves response to erythropoietin in haemodialysis patients. Nephrol Dial Transplant 11:1079-1083, 1996.

398. Panesar A, Agarwal R: Safety and efficacy of sodium ferric gluconate complex in patients with chronic kidney disease. Am J Kidney Dis 40:924-931, 2002.

399. Bolanos L, Castro P, Falcon TG, et al: Continuous intravenous sodium ferric gluconate improves efficacy in the maintenance phase of EPOrHu administration in hemodialysis patients. Am J Nephrol 22:67-72, 2002.

400. Jain AK, Bastani B: Safety profile of a high dose ferric gluconate in patients with severe chronic renal insufficiency. J Nephrol 15:681-683, 2002.

401. Michael B, Coyne DW, Fishbane S, et al: Sodium ferric gluconate in hemodialysis patients: Adverse reactions compared to placebo and iron dextran. Kidney Int 61:1830-1839, 2002.

402. Hoen B, Paul-Cauphin A, Kessler M: Intravenous iron administration does not significantly increase the risk of bacteremia in chronic hemodialysis patients. Clin Nephrol 57:457-461, 2002.

403. Yee J, Besarab A: Iron sucrose: The oldest iron therapy becomes new. Am J Kidney Dis 40:1111-1121, 2002.

404. Stoves J, Inglis H, Newstead CG: A randomized study of oral vs intravenous iron supplementation in patients with progressive renal insufficiency treated with erythropoietin. Nephrol Dial Transplant 16:967-974, 2001.

405. Albertazzi A, Di Liberato L, Daniele F, et al: Efficacy and tolerability of recombinant human erythropoietin treatment in pre-dialysis patients: Results of a multicenter study. Int J Artif Organs 21:12-18, 1998.

406. Krmar RT, Gretz N, Klare B, et al: Renal function in predialysis children with chronic renal failure treated with erythropoietin. Pediatr Nephrol 11:69-73, 1997.

407. Kuriyama S, Tomonari H, Yoshida H, et al: Reversal of anemia by erythropoietin therapy retards the progression of chronic renal failure, especially in nondiabetic patients. Nephron 77:176-185, 1997.

408. Trivedi HS, Brooks BJ: Erythropoietin therapy in pre-dialysis patients with chronic renal failure: Lack of need for parenteral iron. Am J Nephrol 23:78-85, 2003.

409. Teruel JL, Marcen R, Navarro-Antolin J, et al: Androgen versus erythropoietin for the treatment of anemia in hemodialyzed patients: A prospective study. J Am Soc Nephrol 7:140-144, 1996.

410. Navarro JF: Another use of androgens—treatment of anemia of end-stage renal disease. J Clin Endocrinol Metab 82:3176, 1997.

411. Slatopolsky E, Brown A, Dusso A: Role of phosphorus in the pathogenesis of secondary hyperparathyroidism. Am J Kidney Dis 37(suppl):54-57, 2001.

412. Koizumi T, Murakami K, Nakayama H, et al: Role of dietary phosphorus in the progression of renal failure. Biochem Biophys Res Commun 295:917-921, 2002.

413. Phelps KR, Stern M, Slingerland A, et al: Metabolic and skeletal effects of low and high doses of calcium acetate in patients with preterminal chronic renal failure. Am J Nephrol 22:445-454, 2002.

414. Yeun JY, Kaysen GA: The nephrotic syndrome: Nutritional consequences and dietary management. In Mitch WE, Klahr S (eds): Handbook of Nutrition and the Kidney. Philadelphia, Lippincott-Raven, 2002, pp 178-190.

415. Sakemi T, Ikeda Y, Shimazu K: Effect of soy portein added to casein diet on the development of glomerular injury in spontaneous hypercholesterolemic male Imai rats. Am J Nephrol 22:548-554, 2002.

416. Walser M, Hill S, Tomalis EA: Treatment of nephrotic adults with a supplemented, very low-protein diet. Am J Kidney Dis 28:354-364, 1996.

417. Giordano M, DeFeo P, Lucidi P, et al: Effects of dietary protein restriction on fibrinogen and albumin metabolism in nephrotic patients. Kidney Int 60:235-242, 2001.

418. Sistani S, Walser M: The effect of an essential amio acid–supplemented, very low protein diet on proteinuria. J Am Soc Nephrol 11:98A, 2000.

419. Ideura T, Yoshimura A, Shimazui M: Effect of a very low protein diet in nephrotic syndrome. Wien Klin Wochenschr 110:61, 1997.

420. Matthews DE, Motil KS, Rohrbaugh DR, et al: Measurements of leucine metabolism in man from a primed continuous infusion of [1-13C]leucine. Am J Physiol 238:E473-E479, 1980.

421. Motil KJ, Matthews DE, Bier DM, et al: Whole-body leucine and lysine metabolism: Response to dietary protein intake in young men. Am J Physiol 240:E712-E721, 1981.

422. Walser M, Coulter AW, Dighe S, Crantz FR: The effect of ketoanalogues of essential amino acids in severe chronic uremia. J Clin Invest 52:678-690, 1973.

423. Maroni BJ, Steinman T, Mitch WE: A method for estimating nitrogen intake of patients with chronic renal failure. Kidney Int 27:58-65, 1985.

424. Kopple JD, Gao X, Qing DP: Dietary protein, urea nitrogen appearance and total nitrogen appearance in chronic renal failure and CAPD patients. Kidney Int 52:486-494, 1997.

425. Cottini EP, Gallina DL, Dominguez JM: Urea excretion in adult humans with varying degrees of kidney malfunction fed milk, egg or an amino acid mixture: Assessment of nitrogen balance. J Nutr 103:11-19, 1973.

426. Masud T, Manatunga A, Cotsonis G, Mitch WE: The precision of estimating protein intake of patients with chronic renal failure. Kidney Int 62:1750-1756, 2002.

427. Folin O: Laws governing the clinical composition of urine. Am J Physiol 13:67-115, 1905.

428. Sargent J, Gotch F, Borah M, et al: Urea kinetics: A guide to nutritional management of renal failure. Am J Clin Nutr 31:1696-1702, 1978.

429. Borah MF, Schoenfeld PY, Gotch FA, et al: Nitrogen balance during intermittent dialysis therapy of uremia. Kidney Int 14:491-500, 1978.

430. Young VR: Some metabolic and nutritional considerations of dietary protein restriction. In Mitch WE (ed): Contemporary Issues in Nephrology: The Progressive Nature of Renal Disease. New York, Churchill Livingstone, 1986, pp 263-283.

431. Mitch WE, Goldberg AL: Mechanisms of muscle wasting: The role of the ubiquitin-proteasome system. N Engl J Med 335:1897-1905, 1996.

432. Walser M, Bodenlos LJ: Urea metabolism in man. J Clin Invest 38:1617-1622, 1959.

433. Jones EA, Smallwood RA, Craigie A, Rosenoer VM: The enterohepatic circulation of urea nitrogen. Clin Sci 37:825-836, 1969.

434. Wilson DR, Ing TS, Metcalfe-Gibson A, Wrong OM: The chemical composition of faeces in uremia, as revealed by in vivo faecal dialysis. Clin Sci 35:197-207, 1968.

435. Down PF, Agostini L, Murison J, Wrong OM: The interrelations of faecal ammonia, pH and bicarbonate: Evidence of colonic absorption of ammonia by non-ionic diffusion. Clin Sci 43:101-109, 1972.

436. Gibson JA, Park NJ, Sladen GE, Dawson AM: The role of the colon in urea metabolism in man. Clin Sci 50:51-59, 1976.

437. Varcoe R, Halliday D, Carson ER, et al: Efficiency of utilization of urea nitrogen for albumin synthesis by chronically uremic and normal man. Clin Sci Mol Med 48:379-390, 1975.

438. Long CL, Jeevandanam M, Kinney JM: Metabolism and recycling of urea in man. Am J Clin Nutr 31:1367-1382, 1987.

439. Murdaugh HV: Urea metabolism during low protein intake: Studies in man and dog. In Schmidt-Nielson B (ed): Urea and the Kidney. Amsterdam, Excerpta Medica, 1970, pp 471-477.

440. Simenhoff ML, Burke JF, Sankkonen JJ, et al: Amine metabolism and the small bowel in uremia. Lancet 2:818-822, 1976.

441. Walser M: Determinants of ureagenesis with particular reference to renal failure. Kidney Int 17:709-721, 1980.

442. Robson AM: Urea Metabolism in Chronic Renal Failure [thesis]. University of Newcastle upon Tyne, England, 1964.

443. Walser M: Urea metabolism in chronic renal failure. J Clin Invest 53:1385-1392, 1974.

444. Mitch WE, Lietman PS, Walser M: Effects of oral neomycin and kanamycin in chronic renal failure: I. Urea metabolism. Kidney Int 11:116-122, 1977.

445. Wolpert E, Phillips SF, Summerskill WHJ: Transport of urea and ammonia production in the human colon. Lancet 2:1387-1390, 1971.

446. Dal Canton A, Fuiano G, Conte G, et al: Mechanism of increased plasma urea after diuretic therapy in uraemic patients. Clin Sci 68:255-261, 1985.

447. Kato A, Sands JM: Active sodium-urea counter-transport is inducible in the basolateral membrane of rat renal initial inner medullary collecting ducts. J Clin Invest 102:1008-1015, 1998.

448. Kamm DE, Wu L, Kuchmy BL: Contribution of the urea appearance rate to diuretic-induced azotemia in the rat. Kidney Int 32:47-56, 1987.

449. Mitch WE, Walser M: A proposed mechanism for reduced creatinine excretion in severe chronic renal failure. Nephron 21:248-259, 1978.

450. Walser M: Creatinine excretion as a measure of protein nutrition in adults of varying age. JPEN J Parenter Enteral Nutr 11(suppl):73-77, 1987.

451. Forbes GB, Bruining GS: Urinary creatinine excretion and lean body mass. Am J Clin Nutr 29:1359-1366, 1978.

452. Fuller NJ, Elia M: Factors influencing the production of creatinine: Implications for the determination and interpretation of urinary creatine and creatinine in man. Clin Chim Acta 175:199-210, 1988.

453. Heymsfield SB, Arteaga C, McManus C, et al: Measurement of muscle mass in humans: Validity of the 24-hour urinary creatinine method. Am J Clin Nutr 37:478-498, 1983.

454. Walker JB: Metabolic control of creatine biosynthesis. J Biol Chem 235:2357-2361, 1960.

455. Van Pilsum JF, Canfield TM: Transamidinase activities in vitro of kidneys from rats fed diets supplemented with nitrogen-containing compounds. J Biol Chem 237:2574-2577, 1962.

456. Goldman R: Creatinine excretion in renal failure. Proc Soc Exp Biol Med 85:446-448, 1954.

457. Mitch WE, Collier VU, Walser M: Creatinine metabolism in chronic renal failure. Clin Sci 58:327-335, 1980.

458. Kelly RA, Mitch WE: Creatinine, uric acid and other nitrogenous waste products: Clinical implication of the imbalance between their production and elimination in uremia. Semin Nephrol 3:286-294, 1983.

459. Jones JD, Burnett PC: Creatinine metabolism in humans with decreased renal function: Creatinine deficit. Clin Chem 20:1204-1212, 1974.

460. Mackenzie CG, duVigneaud V: Biochemical stability of methyl group of creatine and creatinine. J Biol Chem 185:185-189, 1950.

461. Dominguez R, Pomerone E: Recovery of creatinine after ingestion and after intravenous injection in man. Proc Soc Exp Biol Med 58:26-28, 1945.

462. Jones JD, Burnett PD: Implication of creatinine and gut flora in the uremic syndrome: Induction of "creatinase" in colon contents of the rat by dietary creatinine. Clin Chem 18:280-284, 1972.

463. Owens CWI, Albuquerque ZP, Tomlinson GM: In vitro metabolism of creatinine, methylamine and amino acids by intestinal contents of normal and uremic subjects. Gut 20:568-574, 1979.

464. Danovitch GM, Weinberger J, Berlyne GM: Uric acid in advanced renal failure. Clin Sci 43:331-341, 1972.

465. Emmerson BT, Row PG: An evaluation of the pathogenesis of the gouty kidney. Kidney Int 8:65-74, 1975.

466. Emmerson BT: Abnormal urate excretion associated with renal and systemic disorders, drugs and toxins. In Kelley WN, Weiner IM (eds): Uric Acid, Handbook of Experimental Pharmacology. Berlin, Springer Verlag, 1978, p 287.

467. Clifford AJ, Riumallo JA, Young VR, et al: Effect of oral purines on serum and urinary uric acid of normal, hyperuricemic and gouty humans. J Nutr 106:428, 1976.

468. Lewis HB, Doisy EA: Studies in uric acid metabolism. I. The influence of high protein diets on the endogenous uric acid elimination. J Biol Chem 36:1-7, 1978.

469. Sorensen LB, Levinson DJ: Origin and extrarenal elimination of uric acid in man. Nephron 14:7-20, 1975.

470. Benedict JD, Forsham PH, Stetten DW: The metabolism of uric acid in the normal and gouty human studied with the aid of isotopic uric acid. J Biol Chem 181:183-193, 1949.

471. Sorensen LB: Degradation of uric acid in man. Metabolism 8:687-703, 1959.

472. Sorensen LB: Extrarenal disposal of uric acid. *In* Kelley WN, Weiner IM (eds): Uric Acid, Handbook of Experimental Pharmacology. Berlin, Springer-Verlag, 1978, p 325.

473. Mitch WE: Effects of intestinal flora on nitrogen metabolism in patients with chronic renal failure. Am J Clin Nutr 31:1594-1600, 1978.

474. Richet G: Some aspects of uric acid metabolism in chronic renal failure. *In* Berlyne GM (ed): Nutrition in Renal Disease. Edinburgh, Churchill Livingstone, 1968, p 133.

475. Rosenfeld JF: Effect of long-term allopurinol administration on serial GFR in normotensive and hypertensive subjects. *In* Sperling O, DeVries A, Wyngaarden JB (eds): Purine Metabolism in Man: Biochemistry and Pharmacology of Uric Acid Metabolism. New York, Plenum, 1974, pp 581-596.

476. Fessel WJ: Renal outcomes of gout and hyperuricemia. Am J Med 67:74-81, 1979.

477. Reif MC, Constantine A, Levitt MF: Chronic gouty nephropathy: A vanishing syndrome? N Engl J Med 304:535-536, 1981.

478. Vince A, Down PF, Murison J, et al: Generation of ammonia from non-urea sources in a fecal incubation system. Clin Sci Mol Med 51:313-322, 1976.

479. Windmueller HG, Spaeth AE: Uptake and metabolism of glutamine by the small intestine. J Biol Chem 249:5070, 1974.

480. Weber FL Jr, Maddrey WC, Walser M: Amino acid metabolism of dog jejunum before and during absorption of ketoanalogues. Am J Physiol 232:E263-E269, 1977.

481. Defarrari G, Garibotto G, Robaudo C, et al: Brain metabolism of amino acids and ammonia in patients with chronic renal insufficiency. Kidney Int 20:505-510, 1981.

482. Pimentel L, Brusilow SW, Mitch WE: Unexpected encephalopathy in chronic renal failure: Hyperammonemia complicating acute peritonitis. J Am Soc Nephrol 5:1066-1073, 1994.

483. Brusilow SW, Horwich A: Urea cycle enzymes. *In* Scriver C, Beaudet A, Sly W, Valle D (eds): The Metabolic Basis of Inherited Disease. New York, McGraw-Hill, 1989, pp 624-664.

484. Watson AJ, Karp JE, Walker WG, et al: Transient idiopathic hyperammonaemia in adults. Lancet 2:1271-1274, 1985.

485. Mitchell RB, Wagner JE, Karp JE, et al: Syndrome of idiopathic hyperammonemia after high-dose chemotherapy: Review of nine cases. Am J Med 85:662-667, 1988.

486. Drayna CJ, Titcomb CP, Varma RR, Soergel KH: Hyperammonemic encephalopathy caused by infection in a neurogenic bladder. N Engl J Med 304:766-768, 1981.

487. Deuel HF, Sandiford I, Sandiford K, Boothby WM: A study of the nitrogen minimum: The effect of sixty-three days of a protein-free diet on the nitrogen partition products in the urine and on the heat production. J Biol Chem 76:391-406, 1928.

488. Lavender S, Bennett J, Morse PF, Polak A: Albumin and creatinine clearances in renal disease. Clin Sci Mol Med 46:775-784, 1974.

489. Remuzzi A, Perticucci E, Battaglia C, et al: Low-protein diet and glomerular size-selective function in membranous glomerulopathy. Am J Kidney Dis 18:317-322, 1991.

490. Chan AYM, Cheng ML, Keil LC, Myers BD: Functional response of healthy and diseased glomeruli to a large, protein-rich meal. J Clin Invest 81:245-254, 1988.

491. Kaysen GA, Gambertoglio J, Jimenez I, et al: Effect of dietary protein intake on albumin homeostasis in nephrotic patients. Kidney Int 29:572-577, 1986.

492. D'Amico G, Remuzzi G, Maschio G, et al: Effect of dietary proteins and lipids in patients with membranous nephropathy and nephrotic syndrome. Clin Nephrol 35:237-242, 1991.

493. Don BR, Kaysen GA, Hutchison FN, Schambelan M: The effect of angiotensin-converting enzyme inhibition and dietary protein restriction in the treatment of proteinuria. Am J Kidney Dis 17:10-17, 1991.

494. Rosenberg ME, Salahudeen AK, Hostetter TH: Dietary protein and the renin-angiotensin system in chronic renal allograft rejection. Kidney Int 42 suppl 52):102-106, 1995.

495. Remuzzi G, Bertani T: Pathophysiology of progressive nephropathies. N Engl J Med 339:1448-1456, 1998.

496. Rosenblatt SG, Drake S, Fadem S, et al: Gastrointestinal blood loss in patients with chronic renal failure. Am J Kidney Dis 1:232-236, 1982.

497. Wrick KL, Robertson JB, Van Soest PJ, et al: The influence of dietary fiber source on human intestinal transit and stool output. J Nutr 113:1464-1479, 1983.

498. Hegsted M: Assessment of nitrogen requirements. Am J Clin Nutr 31:1669-1677, 1978.

499. Mitchell HH, Bert MH: The determination of metabolic fecal nitrogen. J Nutr 52:483-497, 1954.

500. Calloway DH, Margen S: Variation in endogenous nitrogen excretion and dietary nitrogen utilization as determinants of human protein requirements. J Nutr 101:205-216, 1971.

501. Hegsted DM, Tsongas AG, Abbott DB, Stare FJ: Protein requirements of adults. J Lab Clin Med 31:261-284, 1946.

502. Calloway DH: Nitrogen balance of men with marginal intakes of protein and energy. J Nutr 105:914-923, 1975.

503. Zanni E, Calloway DH, Zezulka AY: Protein requirements of elderly men. J Nutr 109:513-534, 1979.

504. Steffee WP, Goldsmith RS, Pencharz PB, et al: Dietary protein intake and dynamic aspects of whole body nitrogen metabolism in adult humans. Metabolism 25:281-297, 1976.

505. Loder PB, Kee AJ, Horsburgh R, et al: Validity of urinary urea nitrogen as a measure of total urinary nitrogen in adult patients requiring parenteral nutrition. Crit Care Med 17:309-312, 1989.

506. Konstantinides FN, Konstantinides NN, Li JC, et al: Urinary urea nitrogen: Too insensitive for calculating nitrogen balance studies in surgical clinical nutrition. JPEN J Parenter Enteral Nutr 15:189-193, 1991.

507. Koralnik O, Scholz H: Le gradient de l'azote ureique entre le sueur et le plasma. Proc Eur Dial Transplant Assoc 5:110, 1968.

508. Reaich D, Graham KA, Channon SM, et al: Insulin mediated changes in protein degradation and glucose utilization following correction of acidosis in humans with CR F: Am J Physiol 268:E121-E126, 1995.

509. Maroni BJ, Staffeld C, Young VR, et al: Mechanisms permitting nephrotic patients to achieve nitrogen equilibrium with a protein-restricted diet. J Clin Invest 99:2479-2487, 1997.

510. Kopple JD, Coburn JW: Metabolic studies of low protein diets in uremia: I. Nitrogen and potassium. Medicine (Baltimore) 52:583-594, 1973.

511. Rand WM, Scrimshaw NS, Young VR: Conventional ("long-term") nitrogen balance studies for protein quality evaluation in adults: Rationale and limitations. *In* Bodwell CE, Adkins JS, Hopkins DT (eds): Protein Quality in Humans: Assessment and In Vitro Estimation. Westport, CT, AVI Publishing, 1981, pp 61-97.

512. Kaysen GA, Dubin JA, Muller HG, et al: Relationships among inflammation nutrition and physiologic mechanisms establishing albumin levels in hemodialysis patients. Kidney Int 61:2240-2249, 2002.

513. Movilli E, Zani R, Carli O, et al: Correction of metabolic acidosis increases serum albumin concentration and decreases kinetically evaluated protein intake in hemodialysis patients: A prospective study. Nephrol Dial Transplant 13:1719-1722, 1998.

514. Kaysen GA, Dubin JA, Muller HG, et al: Levels of α-1 acid glycoprotein and ceruloplasmin predict future albumin levels in hemodialysis patients. Kidney Int 60:2360-2366, 2001.

515. Blackmore WP: Urea distribution in renal failure. J Clin Pathol 16:235-243, 1963.

516. Walser M: Misinterpretation of nitrogen balances when glutamine stores fall or are replenished. Am J Clin Nutr 53:1337-1338, 1991.

517. Taylor YSM, Scrimshaw NS, Young VR: The relationship between serum urea levels and dietary nitrogen utilization in young men. Br J Nutr 32:407-411, 1974.

518. Tom K, Young VR, Chapman T, et al: Long-term adaptive responses to dietary protein restriction in chronic renal failure. Am J Physiol 268:E668-E677, 1995.

519. Aparicio M, Chauveau P, dePrecigout V, et al: Nutrition and outcome on renal replacement therapy of patients with chronic renal failure treated by a supplemented very low protein diet. J Am Soc Nephrol 11:719-727, 2000.

520. Aparicio M, Chauveau P, Combe C: Low protein diets and outcome of renal patients. J Nephrol 14:433-439, 2001.

521. Waterlow JC: The assessment of protein nutrition and metabolism in the whole animal with special reference to man. *In* Munro HN (ed): Mammalian Protein Metabolism. New York, Academic Press, 1969.

522. Levey AS, NKF Task Force on Cardiovascular Disease: Controlling the epidemic of cardiovascular disease in chronic renal disease: What do we know? What do we need to know? Where do we go from here? Am J Kidney Dis 32(Suppl 3):1-199, 1998.

523. Kaysen GA, Rathore V, Shearer GC, Depner TA: Mechanisms of hypoalbuminemia in hemodialysis patients. Kidney Int 48:510-516, 1995.

524. Stenvinkel P, Heimburger O, Paultre F, et al: Strong association between malnutrition, inflammation and atherosclerosis in chronic kidney failure. Kidney Int 55:1899-1911, 1999.

525. Witko-Sarsat V, Descamps-Latscha B: Advanced oxidation protein products: Novel uraemic toxins and pro-inflammatory mediators in chronic renal failure? Nephrol Dial Transplant 12:1310-1312, 2002.

526. Nassar GM, Ayus JC: Infectious complications of the dialysis access. Kidney Int 60:1-13, 2001.

527. Hakim RM, Breillatt J, Lazarus JM, Port F: Complement activation and hypersensitivity reactions to dialysis membranes. N Engl J Med 311:878-882, 1984.

528. Herbelin A, Nguyen AT, Zingraff J, et al: Influence of uremia and hemodialysis on circulating interleukin-1 and tumor necrosis factor a. Kidney Int 37:116-127, 1990.

529. Herbelin A, Urena P, Nguyen AT, et al: Elevated circulating levels of interleukin-6 in patients with chronic renal failure. Kidney Int 39:954-960, 1991.

530. Shoji T, Emoto M, Tabata T, et al: Advanced atherosclerosis in predialysis patients with chronic renal failure. Kidney Int 61:2187-2192, 2002.

531. Graham IM, Daly LE, Refsum HM, et al: Plasma homocysteine as a risk factor for vascular disease. JAMA 2772775.:2781, 1997.

532. Selhub J, Jacques PF, Bostom AG, et al: Association between plasma homocysteine concentrations and extracranial carotid-artery stenosis. N Engl J Med 332:286-299, 1995.

533. Nygard O, Nordrehaug JE, Refsun H, et al: Plasma homocysteine levels and mortality in patients with coronary artery disease. N Engl J Med 337:230-236, 1997.

534. Bostom AG, Shemin D, Bagley P, et al: Controlled comparison of L-5-methyltetrahydrofolate versus folic acid for the treatment of hyperhomocysteinemia in hemodialysis patients. Circulation 101:2829-2832, 2000.

535. Touam M, Zingraff J, Jungers P, et al: Effective correction of hyperhomocysteinemia in hemodialysis patients by intravenous folic acid and pyridoxine therapy. Kidney Int 56:2292-2296, 1999.

536. Mezzano D, Pais EO, Aranda E, et al: Inflammation not hyperhomocysteinemia is related to oxidative stress and hemostatic and endothelial dysfunction in uremia. Kidney Int 60:1844-1850, 2001.

537. Ooi BS, Darocy AF, Pollak VE: Serum transferrin levels in chronic renal failure. Nephron 9:200-208, 1972.

538. Wardle EN, Kerr DNS, Ellis HA: Serum transferrin levels in chronic renal failure. Clin Nephrol 3:114-118, 1975.

539. Markowitz H, Fairbans VF: Transferrin assay and total iron binding capacity. Mayo Clinic Proc 58:827-828, 1983.

540. Eschbach JN, Abdulhadi MH, Brown JK, et al: Recombinant human erythropoietin in uremic patients with end-stage renal disease. Ann Intern Med 111:992-1000, 1989.

541. Barany P, Pettersson E, Ahlberg M, et al: Nutritional assessment on anemic hemodialysis patients treated with recombinant human erythropoietin. Clin Nephrol 35:270-279, 1991.

542. Toigo G, Situlin R, Vasile A, et al: Effects of erythropoietin administration on nutritional state and erythrocyte metabolism in maintenance hemodialysis patients. Contrib Nephrol 98:79-88, 1992.

543. Levin A, Singer J, Thompson CR, et al: Prevalent left ventricular hypertrophy in the predialysis population: Identifying opportunities for intervention. Am J Kidney Dis 27:347-354, 1996.

544. Dahlof B, Pennert K, Hansson L: Reversal of left ventricular hypertrophy in hypertensive patients: A meta-analysis of 109 treatment studies. Am J Hypertens 5:95-110, 1992.

545. Avram MM, Mittman N: Malnutrition in uremia. Semin Nephrol 14:238-244, 1994.

546. Cano N, Fernandez JP, LaCombe P, et al: Statistical selection of nutritional parameters in hemodialyzed patients. Kidney Int 37(suppl 22):178-180, 1987.

547. Sreedhara R, Avram MM, Blanco M, et al: Prealbumin is the best nutritional predictor of survival in hemodialysis and peritoneal dialysis. Am J Kidney Dis 28:937-942, 1996.

548. Avram MM, Goldwasser P, Erroa M, Fein PA: Predictors of survival in continuous ambulatory peritoneal dialysis. The importance of prealbumin and other nutritional and metabolic markers. Am J Kidney Dis 23:91-98, 1994.

549. Kult J, Richter U, Scheitza E, et al: Storungen im Komplementsystem bei Niereninsuffizienz und ihre Beeinflussung durch Aminosauren-substitution. Dtsch Med Wochenschr 99:339-342, 1974.

550. Mehls O, Haffner D: Treatment of growth retardation in uraemic children. Nephrol Dial Transplant 10(suppl):80-89, 1995.

551. Mehls O, Ritz E, Hunziker EB, et al: Role of growth hormone in growth failure in uremia. Kidney Int 34:118-126, 1988.

552. Ikizler TA, Wingard RL, Breyer JA, et al: Short-term effects of recombinant human growth hormone in CAPD patients. Kidney Int 46:1178-1183, 1994.

553. Ikizler TA, Wingard RL, Flakoll PJ, et al: Effects of recombinant human growth hormone on plasma and dialysate amino acid profiles in CAPD patients. Kidney Int 50:229-234, 1996.

554. Miller SB, Moulton M, O'Shea M, Hammermann MR: Effects of IGF-1 on renal function in end-stage chronic renal failure. Kidney Int 46:210-207, 1994.

555. Ziegler TR, Gatzen C, Wilmore DW: Strategies for attenuating protein-catabolic responses in the critically ill. Annu Rev Med 45:459-480, 1994.

556. Fryburg DA, Jahn LA, Hill SA, et al: Insulin and insulin-like growth factor-1 enhance human skeletal muscle protein anabolism during hyperaminoacidemia by different mechanisms. J Clin Invest 96:1722-1729, 1995.

557. Garibotto G, Barreca A, Russo R, et al: Effects of recombinant human growth hormone on muscle protein turnover in malnourished hemodialysis patients. J Clin Invest 99:97-105, 1997.

558. Fouque D, Peng SC, Kopple JD: Impaired metabolic response to recombinant insulin-like growth factor-I in dialysis patients. Kidney Int 47:876-883, 1995.

559. Ding H, Gao X-L, Hirschberg R, et al: Impaired actions of insulin-like growth factor-1 on protein synthesis and degradation in skeletal muscle of rats with chronic renal failure: Evidence for a postreceptor defect. J Clin Invest 97:1064-1075, 1996.

560. Oster MH, Fielder PJ, Levin N, Cronin MJ: Adaptation of the growth hormone and insulin-like growth factor-1 axis to chronic and severe calorie or protein malnutrition. J Clin Invest 95:2258-2265, 1995.

561. Thissen JP, Ketelslergers JM, Underwood LE: Nutritional regulation of the insulin-like growth factors. Endocr Rev 15:80-101, 1994.

562. Le Roith D: Insulin-like growth factors. N Engl J Med 336:633-640, 1997.

563. Brungger M, Hulter HN, Krapf R: Effect of chronic metabolic acidosis on the growth hormone/IGF-1 endocrine axis: New cause of growth hormone insensitivity in humans. Kidney Int 51:216-221, 1997.

564. Bereket A, Wilson TA, Kolasa AJ, et al: Regulation of the insulin-like growth factor system by acute acidosis. Endocrinology 137:2238-2245, 1996.

565. Himmelfarb J, Holbrook D, McMonagle E, et al: Kt/V, nutritional parameters, serum cortisol, and insulin growth factor-1 levels and patient outcome in hemodialysis. Am J Kidney Dis 24:473-479, 1994.

566. Maroni BJ: Requirements for protein, calories, and fat in the predialysis patient. *In* Mitch WE, Klahr S (eds): Handbook of Nutrition and the Kidney. Philadelphia, Lippincott-Raven, 1998, pp 144-165.

567. Lucas PA, Meadows JH, Roberts DE, Coles GA: The risks and benefits of a low protein–essential amino acid–keto acid diet. Kidney Int 29:995-1003, 1986.

568. Bergstrom J: Why are dialysis patients malnourished? Am J Kidney Dis 26:229-241, 1995.

569. Mitch WE: Malnutrition: A frequent misdiagnosis for hemodialysis patients. J Clin Invest 110:437-439, 2002.

570. Hakim RM, Lazarus JM: Initiation of dialysis. J Am Soc Nephrol 6:1319-1320, 1995.

571. Clinical practice guidelines for peritoneal dialysis adequacy. Am J Kidney Dis 30(suppl 2):70-73, 1997.

572. Mehrotra R, Nolph KD: Treatment of advanced renal failure: Low-protein diets or timely initiation of dialysis. Kidney Int 58:1381-1388, 2000.

573. Hakim RM, Lazarus JM: Biochemical parameters in chronic renal failure. Am J Kidney Dis 9:238-247, 1988.

574. Traynor JP, Simpson K, Geddes CC, et al: Early initiation of dialysis fails to prolong survival in patients with end-stage renal failure. J Am Soc Nephrol 13:2125-2132, 2002.

575. Alvestrand A, Furst P, Bergstrom J: Plasma and muscle free amino acids in uremia: Influence of nutrition with amino acids. Clin Nephrol 18:297-305, 1982.

576. Kopple JD, Swenseid MD: Nitrogen balance and plasma amino acid levels in uremic patients fed an essential amino acid diet. Am J Clin Nutr 27:806-812, 1974.

577. Young GA, Keogh JB, Parson FM: Plasma amino acids and protein levels in chronic renal failure and changes caused by oral supplements of essential amino acids. Clin Chim Acta 61:205-213, 1975.

578. Garibotto G, DeFerrari G, Robaudo C, et al: Effects of a protein meal on blood amino acid profile in patients with chronic renal failure. Nephron 64:216-225, 1993.

579. DeFerrari G, Garibotto G, Robauso C, et al: Splanchnic exchange of amino acids after amino acid ingestion in patients with chronic renal insufficiency. Am J Clin Nutr 48:72-83, 1988.

580. May RC, Hara Y, Kelly RA, et al: Branched-chain amino acid metabolism in rat muscle: Abnormal regulation in acidosis. Am J Physiol 252:E712-E718, 1987.

581. Hara Y, May RC, Kelly RA, Mitch WE: Acidosis, not azotemia, stimulates branched-chain amino acid catabolism in uremic rats. Kidney Int 32:808-814, 1987.

582. England BK, Greiber S, Mitch WE, et al: Rat muscle branched-chain ketoacid dehydrogenase activity and mRNAs increase with extracellular acidemia. Am J Physiol 268(Cell Physiol 37):C1395-C1400, 1995.

583. Liao DF, Duff JL, Daum G, et al: Angiotensin II stimulates MAP kinase kinase kinase activity in vascular smooth muscle cells: Role of Raf. Circ Res 79:1007-1014, 1996.

584. Bergstrom J, Alvestrand A, Furst P: Plasma and muscle free amino acids in maintenance hemodialysis patients without protein malnutrition. Kidney Int 38:108-114, 1990.

585. Reaich D, Channon SM, Scrimgeour CM, et al: Correction of acidosis in humans with CRF decreases protein degradation and amino acid oxidation. Am J Physiol 265:E230-E235, 1993.

586. Lofberg E, Wernerman J, Anderstam B, Bergstrom J: Correction of metabolic acidosis in dialysis patients increases branched-chain and total essential amino acid levels in muscle. Clin Nephrol 48:230-237, 1997.

587. Chan W, Wang M, Kopple JD, Swenseid ME: Citrulline levels and urea cycle enzymes in uremic rats. J Nutr 104:678-683, 1974.

588. Jansen A, Lewis S, Cattell V, Cook HT: Arginase is a major pathway of L-arginine metabolism in nephritic glomeruli. Kidney Int 42:1107-1112, 1992.

589. Hecker M, Sessa WC, Harris HJ, et al: The metabolism of L-arginine and its significance for the biosynthesis of endothelium-derived relaxing factor: Cultured endothelial cells recycle L-citrulline to L-arginine. Proc Natl Acad Sci U S A 87:8612-8616, 1990.

590. Young GA, Parsons FM: Impairment of phenylalanine hydroxylation in chronic renal insufficiency. Clin Sci Mol Med 45:89-92, 1973.

591. Wang M, Vhymeister I, Swenseid ME, Kopple JD: Phenylalanine hydroxylase and tyrosine aminotransferase activity in chronically uremic rats. J Nutr 105:122-127, 1975.

592. Letteri JM, Scipione RA: Phenylalanine metabolism in chronic renal failure. Nephron 13:365-371, 1974.

593. Tizianello A, DeFerrari G, Garibotto G, et al: Renal metabolism of amino acids and ammonia in subjects with normal renal function and in patients with chronic renal insufficiency. J Clin Invest 65:1162-1173, 1980.

594. Mitch WE, Chesney RW: Amino acid metabolism by the kidney. Miner Electrolyte Metab 9:190-202, 1983.

595. Walser M, Hill SB: Free and protein-bound tryptophan in serum of untreated patients with chronic renal failure. Kidney Int 44:1366-1371, 1993.

596. Edozien JC: The free amino acids of plasma and urine in kwashiorkor. Clin Sci 31:153-166, 1966.

597. Dalton RN, Chantler C: The relationship between BCAA and alpha-ketoacids in blood in uremia. Kidney Int 24(suppl 16):61-66, 1983.

598. Suliman ME, Anderstam B, Bergstrom J: Evidence of taurine depletion and accumulation of cysteinesulfinic acid in chronic dialysis patients. Kidney Int 50:1713-1717, 1996.

599. Suliman ME, Anderstam B, Lindholm B, Bergstrom J: Total, free, and protein-bound sulphur amino acids in uremic patients. Nephrol Dial Transplant 12:2332-2338, 1997.

600. Druml W, Fischer M, Liebisch B, et al: Elimination of amino acids in renal failure. Am J Clin Nutr 60:418-423, 1994.

601. Stockenhuber F, Kurz RW, Sertl K, et al: Increased plasma histamine levels in uremic pruritus. Clin Sci 79:477-482, 1990.

602. Pechar J, Malek P, Dobersky P, et al: Influence of protein intake and renal function on plamsa amino acids in patients with renal impairment and after kidney transplantation. Nutr Metab 22:278-287, 1978.

603. Odedra BR, Bates PC, Millward DJ: Time course of the effect of catabolic doses of corticosterone on protein turnover in rat skeletal muscle and liver. Biochem J 214:617-627, 1983.

604. Shear L: Internal redistribution of tissue protein synthesis in uremia. J Clin Invest 48:1252-1257, 1969.

605. Bergstrom J, Furst P, Noree L-O, Vinnars E: Intracellular free amino acids in muscle tissue of patients with chronic uraemia: Effect of peritoneal dialysis and infusion of essential amino acids. Clin Sci Mol Med 54:51-60, 1978.

606. Ganda OP, Aoki TT, Soeldner JS, et al: Hormone-fuel concentrations in anephric subjects. J Clin Invest 57:1403-1411, 1976.

607. Pye IF, McGale EHF, Stonier C: Studies of cerebrospinal fluid and plasma amino acids in patients with steady-state chronic renal failure. Clin Chim Acta 92:65-72, 1979.

608. Jontofsohn R, Trivisas G, Katz N, Kluthe R: Amino acid content of erythrocytes in uremia. Am J Clin Nutr 31:1956-1960, 1978.

609. Divino Filho JC, Barany P, Stehle P, et al: Free amino-acid levels simultaneously collected in plasma, muscle and erythrocytes of uraemic patients. Nephrol Dial Transplant 12:2339-2348, 1997.

610. Wilcken DEL, Gupta VJ, Reddy SG: Accumulation of sulphur-containing amino acids including cystine-homocystine in patients on maintenance hemodialysis. Clin Sci 58:427-430, 1980.

611. Gejyo F, Ito G, Kinoshita Y: Identification of N-monoacetylcystine in uremic plasma. Clin Sci 60:331-334, 1981.

612. Garibotto G, Paoletti E, Fiorini F, et al: Peripheral metabolism of branched-chain keto acids in patients with chronic renal failure. Miner Electrolyte Metab 19:25-31, 1993.

613. Mochizuki T: The effect of metabolic acidosis on amino and keto acid metabolism in chronic renal failure. Jpn J Nephrol 33:213-224, 1991.

614. Langer K, Frohling PT, Diederich J, et al: Plasma amino and ketoacids in chronic renal failure. Contrib Nephrol 65:55-59, 1989.

615. Schauder P, Matthaei D, Henning HV, et al: Blood levels of branched-chain amino acids and alpha-ketoacids in uremic patients given keto analogues of essential amino acids. Am J Clin Nutr 33:1660-1666, 1980.

616. Walser M, Jarskog FL, Hill SB: Branched-chain keto acid metabolism in patients with chronic renal failure. Am J Clin Nutr 50:807-813, 1989.

617. Laouari D, Rocchiccioli F, Dodu C, et al: Conversion efficiency of two branched-chain alpha ketoanalogs in normal and uremic rats. Kidney Int 32(suppl 22):186-190, 1987.

618. Tungsanga K, Kang CW, Walser M: Utilization of alpha-ketoisocaproate for protein synthesis in uremic rats. Kidney Int 30:891-894, 1986.

619. Mitch WE: Requirements for protein, calories, and fat in the pre-dialysis patient. *In* Mitch WE, Klahr S (eds): Handbook of Nutrition and the Kidney. Philadelphia, Lippincott, Williams & Wilkins, 2002, pp 144-165.

620. Alvestrand A, Ahlberg M, Furst P, Bergstrom J: Clinical results of long-term treatment with a low protein diet and a new amino acid preparation in patients with chronic uremia. Clin Nephrol 19:67-73, 1983.

621. Masud T, Young VR, Chapman T, Maroni BJ: Adaptive responses to very low protein diets: The first comparison of ketoacids to essential amino acids. Kidney Int 45:1182-1192, 1994.

622. Goodship THJ, Mitch WE, Hoerr RA, et al: Adaptation to low-protein diets in renal failure: Leucine turnover and nitrogen balance. J Am Soc Nephrol 1:66-75, 1990.

623. Graham KA, Reaich D, Channon SM, et al: Correction of acidosis in hemodialysis decreases whole-body protein degradation. J Am Soc Nephrol 8:632-637, 1997.
624. Graham KA, Reaich D, Channon SM, et al: Correction of acidosis in CAPD decreases whole body protein degradation. Kidney Int 49:1396-1400, 1996.
625. Young VR: 1987 McCollum award lecture. Kinetics of human amino acid metabolism: Nutritional implications and some lessons. Am J Clin Nutr 46:709-725, 1987.
626. McNurlan MA, Garlick PJ: Influence of nutrient intake on protein turnover. Diabetes Metab Rev 5:165-189, 1989.
627. Mitch WE, Abras E, Walser M: Long-term effects of a new ketoacid–amino acid supplement in patients with chronic renal failure. Kidney Int 22:48-53, 1982.
628. Mitch WE, Clark AS: Specificity of the effect of leucine and its metabolities on protein degradation in skeletal muscle. Biochem J 222:579-586, 1984.
629. Mitch WE, Walser M, Sapir DG: Nitrogen-sparing induced by leucine compared with that induced by its keto-analogue, alpha-ketoisocaproate, in fasting obese man. J Clin Invest 67:553-562, 1981.
630. Stein A, Moorhouse J, Iles-Smith H, et al: Role of an improvement in acid-base status and nutrition in CAPD patients. Kidney Int 52:1089-1095, 1997.
631. Pickering WP, Price SR, Bircher G, et al: Nutrition in CAPD: Serum bicarbonate and the ubiquitin-proteasome system in muscle. Kidney Int 61:1286-1292, 2002.
632. Bailey JL, England BK, Long RC, et al: Experimental acidemia and muscle cell pH in chronic acidosis and renal failure. Am J Physiol 269:C706-C712, 1995.
633. May RC, Kelly RA, Mitch WE: Mechanisms for defects in muscle protein metabolism in rats with chronic uremia: The influence of metabolic acidosis. J Clin Invest 79:1099-1103, 1987.
634. Bailey JL, Wang X, England BK, et al: The acidosis of chronic renal failure activates muscle proteolysis in rats by augmenting transcription of genes encoding proteins of the ATP-dependent, ubiquitin-proteasome pathway. J Clin Invest 97:1447-1453, 1996.
635. Tomas FM, Munro HN, Young VR: Effects of glucocorticoid administration and the rate of muscle protein breakdown in vivo in rats, as measured by urinary excretion of N-methylhistidine. Biochem J 178:139-146, 1979.
636. Odedra BR, Millward DJ: Effect of corticosterone treatment on muscle protein turnover in adrenalectomized rats and diabetic rats maintained on insulin. Biochem J 204:663-672, 1982.
637. Quan ZY, Walser M: The effect of corticosterone administration at varying levels on leucine oxidation and whole body protein synthesis and breakdown in adrenalectomized rats. Metabolism 40:1263-1267, 1992.
638. May RC, Kelly RA, Mitch WE: Metabolic acidosis stimulates protein degradation in rat muscle by a glucocorticoid-dependent mechanism. J Clin Invest 77:614-621, 1986.
639. Wang X, Jurkovitz C, Price SR: Regulation of branched-chain ketoacid dehydrogenase flux by extracellular pH and glucocorticoids. Am J Physiol 272:C2031-C2036, 1997.
640. May RC, Bailey JL, Mitch WE, et al: Glucocorticoids and acidosis stimulate protein and amino acid catabolism in vivo. Kidney Int 49:679-683, 1996.
641. Price SR, England BK, Bailey JL, et al: Acidosis and glucocorticoids concomitantly increase ubiquitin and proteasome subunit mRNAs in rat muscle. Am J Physiol 267:C955-C960, 1994.
642. Isozaki Y, Mitch WE, England BK, Price SR: Interaction between glucocorticoids and acidification results in stimulation of proteolysis and mRNAs of proteins encoding the ubiquitin-proteasome pathway in BC3H-1 myocytes. Proc Natl Acad Sci U S A 93:1967-1971, 1996.
643. Bushinsky DA: The contribution of acidosis to renal osteodystrophy. Kidney Int 47:1816-1832, 1995.
644. Bushinsky DA, Lam BC, Nespeca R, et al: Decreased bone bicarbonate content in response to metabolic, but not respiratory, acidosis. Am J Physiol 265:F530-F536, 1993.
645. May RC, Clark AS, Goheer A, Mitch WE: Identification of specific defects in insulin-mediated muscle metabolism in acute uremia. Kidney Int 28:490-497, 1985.
646. Clark AS, Mitch WE: Muscle protein turnover and glucose uptake in acutely uremic rat: Effects of insulin and the duration of renal insufficiency. J Clin Invest 72:836-845, 1983.

647. Holliday MA, Chantler CA, MacDonnell R, Keiges J: Effect of uremia on nutritionally-induced variations in protein metabolism. Kidney Int 11:236-245, 1977.
648. Harter HR, Karl IE, Klahr S, Kipnis DM: Effects of reduced renal mass and dietary protein intake on amino acid release and glucose uptake by rat muscle in vitro. J Clin Invest 64:513-523, 1979.
649. Price SR, Bailey JL, Wang X, et al: Muscle wasting in insulinopenic rats results from activation of the ATP-dependent, ubiquitin-proteasome pathway by a mechanism including gene transcription. J Clin Invest 98:1703-1708, 1996.
650. Mitch WE, Bailey JL, Wang X, et al: Evaluation of signals activating ubiquitin-proteasome proteolysis in a model of muscle wasting. Am J Physiol 276:C1132-C1138, 1999.
651. Davis TA, Klahr S, Karl IE: Glucose metabolism in muscle of sedentary and exercised rats with azotemia. Am J Physiol 252:F138-F145, 1987.
652. Davis TA, Klahr S, Karl IE: Insulin-stimulated protein metabolism in chronic azotemia and exercise. Am J Physiol 253:F164, 1987.
653. Bilbrey GL, Falonna GR, White MG, Knochel JP: Hyperglucagonemia of renal failure. J Clin Invest 53:841-847, 1974.
654. Aoki TT, Muller WA, Brennan MF, Cahill GF: Effect of glucagon on amino acid and nitrogen metabolism in fasting man. Metabolism 23:805-814, 1974.
655. Salter JM, Ezrin C, Laidlaw JC, Gronall AG: Metabolic effects of glucagon in human subjects. Metabolism 9:753-768, 1960.
656. Clark AS, Kelly RA, Mitch WE: Systemic response to thermal injury in rats: Increased protein degradation and altered glucose utilization in muscle. J Clin Invest 74:888-897, 1984.
657. Li JB, Wassner SJ: Protein synthesis and degradation in skeletal muscle of chronically uremic rats. Kidney Int 29:1136-1143, 1986.
658. Druml W, Kelly RA, May RC, Mitch WE: Abnormal cation transport in uremia: Mechanisms in adipocytes and skeletal muscle from uremic rats. J Clin Invest 81:1197-1203, 1988.
659. Bilbrey GL, Carter NW, White MG, et al: Potassium deficiency in chronic renal failure. Kidney Int 4:423-430, 1973.
660. Spergel G, Bleicher JJ, Goldberg M, et al: The effect of potassium on the impaired glucose tolerance on chronic uremia. Metabolism 16:581, 1967.
661. Hsu FW, Tsao T, Rabkin R: The IGF-1 axis in kidney and skeletal muscle of K deficient rats. Kidney Int 52:363-370, 1997.
662. Santeusanio F, Faloona GR, Knochel JP, Unger RH: Evidence for a role of endogenous insulin and glucagon in the regulation of potassium homeostasis. J Lab Clin Med 81:809-817, 1973.
663. Landau RL, Kappas A: Anabolic hormones in hyperparathyroidism: With observations on the general catabolic influence of parathyroid hormone in man. Ann Intern Med 62:1223-1233, 1965.
664. Garber AJ: Effect of parathyroid hormone on selected aspects of protein and amino acid metabolism in the rat. J Clin Invest 71:1806-1821, 1983.
665. Wassner SJ, Li JB: Lack of an acute effect of parathyroid hormone within skeletal muscle. Int J Pediatr Nephrol 8:15-20, 1987.
666. Akmal M, Massry SG, Goldstein DA, et al: Role of parathyroid hormone in the glucose intolerance of chronic renal failure. J Clin Invest 75:1037-1044, 1985.
667. Giordano C: Use of exogenous and endogenous urea for protein synthesis in normal and uremic subjects. J Lab Clin Med 62:231-246, 1963.
668. Underhill RP, Goldschmidt S: Studies on the metabolism of ammonium salts. III: The utilization of ammonium salts with a non-nitrogenous diet. J Biol Chem 15:341-355, 1913.
669. Rittenberg D, Schoenheimer R, Keston AS: Studies on protein metabolism. IX: The utilization of ammonia by normal rats on a stock diet. J Biol Chem 128:603, 1939.
670. Sprinson DB, Rittenberg D: The rate of utilization of ammonia for protein synthesis. J Biol Chem 180:707, 1949.
671. Lardy HA, Feldott G: The net utilization of ammonium nitrogen by the growing rat. J Biol Chem 179:509, 1949.
672. Rose WC, Smith LC, Womack M, Shane M: The utilization of the nitrogen of ammonium salts, urea, and certain other compounds in the synthesis of non-essential amino acids in vivo. J Biol Chem 181:307-316, 1949.
673. Richards P, Metcalfe-Gibson A, Ward EE, et al: Utilization of ammonia nitrogen for protein synthesis in man, and the effect of protein restriction and uraemia. Lancet 2:845-848, 1967.

674. Giordano C, de Pascale C, Balestrieri C, et al: Incorporation of urea ^{15}N in amino acids of patients with chronic renal failure on low nitrogen diet. Am J Clin Nutr 21:394-404, 1968.

675. Furst P: ^{15}N-studies in severe renal failure. I: Influence of amino acid administration on the nitrogen metabolism. Scand J Clin Lab Invest 30:299, 1972.

676. Read WWC, McLaren DS, Tchalian M, Nassar S: Studies with ^{15}N-labelled ammonia and urea in the malnourished child. J Clin Invest 48:1143-1149, 1969.

677. Mitch WE, Walser M: Effects of oral neomycin and kanomycin in chronic uremic patients. II. Nitrogen balance. Kidney Int 11:123-127, 1977.

678. Rose WC, Wixom RL: The amino acid requirements of man. XVI. The role of the nitrogen intake. J Biol Chem 217:997-1004, 1955.

679. Huang PC, Young VR, Cholakos B, Scrimshaw NS: Determination of the minimum dietary essential amino acid–to–total nitrogen ratio for beef protein fed to young men. J Nutr 90:416-422, 1966.

680. Watts JH, Tolber B, Ruff WL: Nitrogen balances for young adult males fed two sources of non-essential nitrogen at two levels of total nitrogen intake. Metabolism 13:172, 1964.

681. Clark HE, Yess NJ, Vermillion EJ, et al: Effect of certain factors in nitrogen retention and lysine requirements of adult human subjects. III: Source of supplementary nitrogen. J Nutr 79:131-139, 1963.

682. Tripathy K, Klahr S, Lotero H: Utilization of exogenous urea nitrogen in malnourished adults. Metabolism 19:253-262, 1970.

683. Walser M, Mitch WE, Maroni BJ, Kopple JD: Should protein be restricted in predialysis patients? Kidney Int 55:771-777, 1999.

684. Masud T: Trace elements and vitamins in renal disease. *In* Mitch WE, Klahr S (eds): Nutrition and the Kidney. Philadelphia, Lippincott, Raven, 2002, pp 233-252.

685. Mydlik M, Derzsiova K, Zemberova E: Metabolism of vitamin B$_6$ and its requirement in chronic renal failure. Kidney Int 52 (suppl 62): 56-59, 1997.

686. Pronai W, Riegler-Keil M, Silberbauer K, Stockenhuber F: Folic acid supplementation improves erythropoietin response. Nephron 71: 395-400, 1995.

687. Ramirez G, Chen M, Boyce HW, et al: Longitudinal follow-up of chronic hemodialysis patients without vitamin supplementation. Kidney Int 30:99-106, 1986.

688. Ono K: Secondary hyperoxalemia caused by vitamin C supplementation in regular hemodialysis patients. Clin Nephrol 26:239-243, 1986.

689. Ott SM, Andress DL, Sherrard DJ: Bone oxalate in a long-term hemodialysis patient who ingested high doses of vitamin C: Am J Kidney Dis 8:450-454, 1986.

690. Friedman JE, Dohm GL, Elton CW, et al: Muscle insulin resistance in uremic humans: Glucose transport, glucose transporters, and insulin receptors. Am J Physiol 261:E87-E94, 1991.

691. Robinson K, Gupta A, Dennis V, et al: Hyperhomocysteinemia confers an independent increased risk of atherosclerosis in end-stage renal disease and is closely linked to plasma folate and pyridoxine concentrations. Circulation 94:2473-2478, 1996.

692. Malinow MR, Nieto FJ, Kruger WD, et al: The effects of folic acid supplementation on plasma total homocysteine are modulated by multivitamin use and methylenetetrahydrofolate reductase genotypes. Arterioscler Thromb Vasc Biol 17:1157-1162, 1997.

693. Rocco MV, Poole D, Poindexter P, et al: Intake of vitamins and minerals in stable hemodialysis patients as determined by 9-day food food records. J Ren Nutr 7:17-24, 1997.

694. Schaumburg H, Kaplan J, Winderbank A, et al: Sensory neuropathy from pyridoxine abuse: A new megavitamin syndrome. N Engl J Med 309:445-489, 1983.

695. Gleghorn EE, Eisenberg LD, Hack S, et al: Observations of vitamin A toxicity in three patients with renal failure receiving parenteral alimentation. Am J Clin Nutr 44:107-112, 1986.

696. McCullough PA, Wolyn R, Rocher LL, et al: Acute renal failure after coronary intervention: Incidence, risk factors and relationship to mortality. Am J Med 103:368-375, 1997.

697. Hahn S, Kuemmerle NB, Chan W, et al: Glomerulosclerosis in the remnant kidney is modulated by dietary alpha-tocopherol. J Am Soc Nephrol 9:2089-2095, 1998.

698. Koya D, Lee IK, Ishii H, et al: Prevention of glomerular dysfunction in diabetic rats by treatment with D-alpha-tocopherol. J Am Soc Nephrol 8:426-435, 1997.

699. Douillet C, Tabib A, Bost M, et al: A selenium supplement associated or not with vitamin E delays early renal lesions in experimental diabetes in rats. Proc Soc Exp Biol Med 211:323-331, 1996.

700. Cohen JD, Viljoen M, Clifford D, et al: Plasma vitamin E levels in a chronically hemolyzing group of dialysis patients. Clin Nephrol 25:42-47, 1986.

701. Taccone-Gallucci M, Giardini O, Ausiello C, et al: Vitamin E supplementation in hemodialysis patients: Effects on peripheral blood mononuclear cells lipid peroxidation and immune response. Clin Nephrol 25:81-86, 1986.

702. Christiansen C, Rodbro P, Christiansen MS, et al: Deterioration of renal function during treatment of chronic renal failure with 1,25-dihydroxycholecalciferol. Lancet 2:700-703, 1978.

703. Laurence RI, Baker SM, Abrams L, et al: 1,25(OH)$_2$D$_3$ administration in moderate renal failure: A prospective double-blind trial. Kidney Int 35:661-669, 1989.

704. Caticha O, Norato DY, Tambascia MA, et al: Total body zinc depletion and its relationship to the development of hyperprolactinemia in chronic renal insufficiency. J Endocrinol Invest 19:441-448, 1996.

705. Abu-Hamdan DK, Mahajan SK, Migdal SD, et al: Zinc tolerance test in uremia: Effect of ferrous sulfate and aluminum hydroxide. Ann Intern Med 104:50-52, 1986.

706. Ittel TH, Gladziwa U, Muck W, Sieberth HG: Hyperaluminaemia in critically ill patients: Role of antacid therapy and impaired renal function. Eur J Clin Invest 21:93-102, 1991.

707. Lin JL, Leu ML: Aluminum-containing agents may be toxic in predialysis chronic renal insufficiency patients. J Intern Med 240:243-248, 1996.

708. Nesse A, Garbossa G, Stripeikis J, et al: Aluminium accumulation in chronic renal failure affects erythropoiesis. Nephrology 3:347-351, 1997.

709. Hopfer SM, Linden JV, Crisostomo MC, et al: Hypernickelemia in hemodialysis patients. Trace Elements Med 2:68-73, 1985.

710. Clyne N, Lins LE, Pehrsson SK: Serum cobalt in relation to cardiac performance in patients with chronic renal failure. Trace Elements Med 2:44-49, 1985.

711. Wallaeys B, Cornelis R, Mees L, Lameire N: Trace elements in serum, packed cells, and dialysate of CAPD patients. Kidney Int 30:599-604, 1986.

712. Eknoyan G: Chronic tubulointerstitial nephropathies. *In* Schrier RW, Gottschalk CW (eds): Diseases of the Kidney. Boston, Little, Brown, 1997,: pp 1983-2015.

713. Beale LS: Kidney Diseases, Urinary Deposits and Calculous Disorders; Their Nature and Treatment, 3 ed. Phildelphia, Lindsay & Blakiston, 1869.

714. Shakeel M, Curtis JJ, Wade S: Dietary instruction for protein restriction in predialysis patients [abstract]. J Am Soc Nephrol 9:161, 1998.

715. Giovannetti S: Dietary treatment of chronic renal failure: Why is it not used more frequently? Nephron 40:1-12, 1985.

716. Division of Kidney, Urologic and Hematologic Diseases, NIDDK, NIH: USRDS 2002 Annual Data Report: Atlas of end-Stage Renal Disease in the United States. Bethesda, MD, National Institutes of Health, 2003.

717. Klang B, Clyne N: Well-being and functional ability in uraemic patients before and after having started dialysis treatment. Scand J Caring Sci 11:159-166, 1997.

718. Chauveau P, Barthe N, Rigalleau V, et al: Outcome of nutritional status and body composition of uremic patients on a very low protein diet. Am J Kidney Dis 34:500-507, 1999.

719. Walser M, Thorpe B: Coping with kidney disease: A twelve step program to help you avoid dialysis. John Wiley & Sons (in press).

720. Mazhari R, Walser M: Dependence of the symptoms of chronic renal disease on biochemical changes [abstract]. J Am Soc Nephrol 10:81, 2001.

721. Mitch WE: Dietary therapy in uremia: The impact on nutrition and progressive renal failure. Kidney Int 57(suppl):38-43, 2000.

722. Ahlstrom TP: The Kidney Patient's Book, New Treatment, New Hope. Delran, NJ, Great Issues Press, 1991.

723. Rosman JB, Donker-Willenborg MA: Dietary compliance and its assessment in the Groningen trial on protein restriction in chronic renal failure. Contrib Nephrol 81:95-101, 1990.

724. Bergstrom J, Alvestrand A, Bucht H, Gutierrez A: Progression of chronic renal failure in man is retarded with more frequent clinical follow-ups and better blood pressure control. Clin Nephrol 25:1-6, 1986.

725. Di Landro D, Dattilo GA, Romagnoli GF: Comparative outcome of patients on a conventional low protein diet versus a supplemented diet in chronic renal failure. Contrib Nephrol 81:201-207, 1990.

726. Teplan V, Schuck O, Votruba M, et al: Metabolic effect of ketoacid–amino acid supplementation in patients with chronic renal insufficiency receiving a low-protein diet and recombinant human erythropoietin. Wien Klin Wochenschr 113:661-669, 2001.

727. Teplan V, Schuck O, Knotek A, et al: Effect of low-protein diet supplemented with ketoacids and erythropoietin in chronic renal failure: A long-term metabolic study. Ann Transplant 6:47-53, 2001.

728. Ayli MD, Ayli M, Ensari C, et al: Effect of low-protein diet supplemented with ketoacids on progression of disease in patients with chronic renal failure. Nephron 84:288-289, 2000.

729. Herselman MG, Albertse EC, Lombard CJ, et al: Supplemented low-protein diets—are they superior in chronic renal failure. S Afr Med J 85:361-365, 1995.

730. Abras E, Walser M: Nitrogen utilization in uremic patients fed by continuous nasogastric infusion. Kidney Int 22:392-397, 1982.

731. Teplan V, Schuck O, Ndavornikova H, et al: Metabolic characteristics of patients with chronic renal failure in long-term diet therapy and substitution with keto analogs of essential amino acids. Z Urol Nephrol 83(2):89-96, 1990.

732. Walser M: Keto-analogues of essential amino acids in the treatment of chronic renal failure. Kidney Int 13(suppl):180, 1978.

733. Cockram D, Weis J, Geraghty M, et al: Amino acid analogue (KA) supplementation does not delay disease progression in CRF patients [abstract 29]. Paper presented at the 7th International Congress on Nutrition and Metabolism in Renal Disease, Stockholm, 1994.

734. Meisinger E, Strauch M: The influence of two different essential amino acid/keto analogue preparations on the clinical status of patients with chronic renal failure. Z Ernahrungswiss 24:96-104, 1985.

735. Lowrie EG, Lew NL: Death risk in hemodialysis patients: The predictive value of commonly measured variables and an evaluation of the death rate differences among facilities. Am J Kidney Dis 15:458-482, 1990.

736. Tzekov VD, Tilkian EE, Pandeva SM, et al: Low protien diet and ketosteril in predialysis patients with renal failure. Folia Med (Plovdiv) 42:34-37, 2000.

737. Walser M: Is there a role for protien restriction in the treatment of chronic renal failure. Blood Purif 18:304-312, 2000.

738. Malvy D, Maingourd C, Pengloan J, et al: Effects of severe protein restriction with ketoanalogues in advanced renal failure. J Am Coll Nutr 8:481-486, 1999.

CHAPTER 58

Erythropoietin Therapy in Renal Disease and Renal Failure

John C. Stivelman, Steven Fishbane, and Allen R. Nissenson

CHARACTERIZATION OF THE ANEMIA OF CHRONIC KIDNEY DISEASE AND END-STAGE RENAL DISEASE

Anemia occurs in the majority of patients with chronic kidney disease (CKD).[1] This anemia is hypoproliferative and characterized by a normocytic, normochromic appearance of the red blood cells (RBCs).[2] The increased fragility and shortened life span of the RBCs may be manifested by occasional spiked-appearing cells on microscopy.[3] Although the bone marrow has been described as normal in patients with advanced kidney disease, the expected increase in hematopoietic activity that would be anticipated in the face of anemia is not present,[4] thus suggesting either inhibition or inadequate stimulation of erythropoiesis. The former suggestion, in which hypoproliferative anemia is attributed to an inhibitory effect of retained uremic solutes on bone marrow, was based on a number of in vitro studies showing that erythropoietic stem cells at various stages of maturation could have their development arrested if incubated with uremic serum.[5, 6] A small number of in vivo studies added evidence in support of this relationship,[7] but although a variety of inhibitors may play a modulating role in the anemia of renal disease, including polyamines and parathyroid hormone (PTH), their relative clinical importance appears to be minimal.

A multitude of evidence suggests, however, that inadequate stimulation of erythropoiesis is the primary lesion in the genesis of this anemia.[8] Although the failing kidney produces erythropoietin, its capacity to do so is both qualitatively and quantitatively impaired.[8, 9] Not only is native erythropoietin necessary for erythropoiesis to proceed normally, but it also plays an important role in the ability of the RBC progenitor to produce hemoglobin through its effect on erythron transferrin uptake.[10] In vitro, a reduction in intracellular iron stores stimulates erythropoietin production, whereas an increase in intracellular iron suppresses it.[11]

Erythropoietin has also been shown to stimulate transferrin receptor expression in erythroid cells, increase plasma iron turnover, and augment transferrin uptake by bone marrow precursors.[11]

The formation of heme in the presence of erythropoietin stimulation, in turn, is critically dependent on an adequate availability of iron and appropriate uptake of iron by the erythrocyte progenitor.[12] When CKD is present, with its associated inadequate quantities of native erythropoietin and significant decrease in RBC mass, iron utilization is decreased and iron is stored in greater quantities in the reticuloendothelial system, where it may reside for months to years.[13] The administration of recombinant human erythropoietin (rHuEPO), however, accelerates erythropoiesis, thereby increasing the demand for iron, and alters the relationship between iron stores and iron in erythrocytes. The need to incorporate iron into new erythrocytes may thus often exceed the ability of the reticuloendothelial system to release iron, and absolute or functional iron deficiency may result. Consequently, regular administration of iron is essential to keep up with the needs of accelerated erythropoiesis in an erythropoietin-treated patient.[14] It is clear that to maintain any given target hemoglobin level in a patient with CKD, an appropriate balance between administered rHuEPO and iron is needed at a higher level of iron turnover than before rHuEPO stimulation.[13]

MOLECULAR MECHANISMS OF ERYTHROPOIETIN ACTION

Erythropoietin is a glycoprotein essential for the normal production of RBCs in mammalian species. The molecular events that result in an increase in RBC mass have recently been reviewed.[15] Current evidence suggests that the cellular events that occur after native erythropoietin secretion or the administration of rHuEPO are the same. The activity of erythropoietin is initiated by binding to its receptor (EPOR). In the absence of EPOR in knockout mice, severe anemia results.[16, 17] EPOR has been cloned and is one of a superfamily of cytokine receptors with a single membrane-spanning domain.[18] EPOR is expressed in a number of cells and organs, with the colony-forming unit—erythroid (CFU-E)/proerythroblast being the primary target erythroid cell. Although the receptor is expressed in the blast-forming unit—erythroid (BFU-E), the number of receptors is greatest in CFU-E, which contains over 1000 per cell. The number of receptors gradually declines with increasing levels of erythroid cell maturation.[19] In addition, EPOR is expressed on the placenta, endothelium, megakaryocytes, and a variety of other cells, although it is unknown whether this distribution has any functional significance. Erythropoietin acting through the EPOR is essential to minimize apoptosis (programmed cell death) of CFU-E and thus promotes terminal differentiation of this cell line.[20]

Erythropoietin binds to the p66 chain of the EPOR, which becomes homodimerized on activation.[21] Homodimerization in turn induces the production of JAK2 tyrosine kinase, and JAK2 subsequently phosphorylates the tyrosine residues located on the intracellular domain of the receptor. This cascade is essential for RBC production, as demonstrated in studies of mice lacking JAK2.[22] The result of tyrosine phosphorylation is attraction of a variety of other intracellular proteins that bind to the EPOR, including Ras/mitogen-activated kinase, which is essential for cell proliferation, and STATs 1, 2, and 5, which are transcriptional factors, among other nonreceptor tyrosine kinases.[23-25]

Activation of the erythropoietin gene after binding of erythropoietin to the EPOR takes place through mechanisms that have not been fully elucidated. A variety of transcription factors are expressed in increased numbers after EPO/EPOR binding, and a plethora of proto-oncogenes have been shown to subsequently be activated.[26-28] Which of the transcription factors is most critical for this sequence to occur is unknown.

One of the purported regulators of erythropoietin activity is the intracellular calcium concentration. Binding of erythropoietin to its receptor leads to an increase in intracellular calcium,[29-31] and numerous cell culture studies have shown the modulating effect of calcium concentration on erythroid colony development.[32, 33] The effect of erythropoietin as a calcium ionophore is modulated through its effects on a voltage-independent ion channel,[34] a process dependent on tyrosine phosphorylation. The precise role of intracellular calcium in erythroid cell proliferation at the molecular level is undergoing intensive investigation at the present time. Possible mechanisms include stimulation of the phosphorylation of transcription factors, stimulation of proto-oncogenes, or effects on endonucleases that can induce breaks in chromosomal DNA.[35] Currently, however, no evidence has shown that medications affecting calcium channels, such as certain antihypertensive agents, have an impact on the response of patients to rHuEPO.

The expression and ultimate production of erythropoietin are stimulated by a variety of hypoxic conditions,[36, 37] a phenomenon recently demonstrated in patients with CKD.[38] An essential mediator of this response is the recently recognized transcription factor hypoxia inducible factor (HIF-α).[39] HIF-α, produced in a variety of cell types, normally degrades rapidly but stabilizes in a hypoxic environment.[40, 41] This factor binds to the oxygen-sensitive enhancer section of the erythropoietin gene. HIF-α has three isoforms, with HIF-2α being the form most likely to be active in the kidney.[42] Stabilization of HIF leads to enhanced transcriptional activity with resultant up-regulation of the erythropoietin gene and increased synthesis of the hormone.

TREATMENT OF ANEMIA IN CHRONIC KIDNEY DISEASE AND END-STAGE RENAL DISEASE WITH ERYTHROPOIETIN AND IRON

Historical Evolution of Erythropoietin Isolation; Studies Resulting in the Use of rHuEPO for Human Disease

Anemia was first recognized as a common accompaniment of kidney disease by Richard Bright, who noted in 1836 that "… after a time, the healthy color of the countenance fades" in affected patients.[43] Although the cause of the pale appearance of such patients was unknown, over the subsequent 60 years the notion that decreased blood oxygen tension stimulated RBC production gradually gained acceptance.[44] Considerable debate ensued, however, over the mechanism of hematopoietic stimulation, specifically, whether it was a direct effect or mediated by a hormone.[45] Although factors that stimulated erythropoiesis had previously been isolated from the urine and plasma of anemic humans and animals,[44] by the late 1950s, studies by Reissmann,[46] Erslev,[47] and Jacobson and co-workers[48] clearly demonstrated that a putative stimulator of RBC production did indeed exist and was located in the kidney. After studies showing that urine erythropoietin levels correlated inversely with changes in oxygen transport,[49] isolated perfused kidney experiments[50] provided irrefutable evidence of the source of this potent hormone, which was ultimately purified by Miyake and colleagues from the urine of patients with aplastic anemia in 1977.[51] At present, the peritubular capillary endothelial cell and peritubular fibroblast appear to be responsible for its synthesis within the kidney.[52-54]

The pioneering work of Eschbach and Adamson in the 1970s and 1980s demonstrated that the lack of an adequate quantity of erythropoietin is the predominant cause of renal anemia. Initially working with sheep, these investigators demonstrated that erythropoietin-rich plasma infused into normal and uremic sheep induced identical erythropoietic responses.[55] Chronic administration resulted in correction of anemia.[56] Subsequent studies in a hemodialysis patient, who received erythropoietin isolated from a patient with secondary polycythemia, reported a positive reticulocyte and ferrokinetic response, the first to be demonstrated in a uremic human. These studies were followed by isolation of the gene for native erythropoietin by Lin and colleagues[57, 58] in 1985, its cloning in the Chinese hamster ovary cell, and ultimately, the development of rHuEPO in 1986. Positive clinical trials of this agent shortly thereafter by Eschbach and associates reinforced the finding that deficiency of native erythropoietin was the primary cause of the anemia of renal disease and that this deficiency could be reversed by administration of the recombinant form of the protein.[59, 60]

The impact of this research cannot be understated: it is estimated that, over 95 percent of patients in the United States with end-stage renal disease (ESRD) receive replacement therapy with some form of recombinant erythropoietin. Transfusion dependence in ESRD has virtually been eliminated by this therapy,[60] its infectious sequelae thereby reduced, and the quality of life of patients with CKD and ESRD markedly enhanced.

Demographics of Patients at Risk for Anemia and Selection for Treatment

The third cycle of the National Health and Nutritional Examination Survey (NHANES) suggests that a significant reservoir of renal disease exists within the United States. In the report of these data in the recently issued Kidney Disease Outcome Quality Initiative (K/DOQI) clinical practice guidelines for CKD, the number of patients with CKD and glomerular filtration rates (GFRs) ranging from 30 to 59 mL/min/1.73 m^2 (GFR per Modification of Diet in Renal Disease [MDRD] equation; serum creatinine per NHANES III) is estimated at 7.6 million; those with GFRs of 15 to 29 mL/min/1.73 m^2, approximately 400,000; and the number of patients with GFRs less than 15 mL/min/1.73 m^2, about 300,000.[61] The risk of anemia developing in such populations as a function of falling GFR is illustrated in Figure 58-1.[61] Recent K/DOQI meta-analyses correlating GFR with the onset of anemia reveal both wider variability and higher values of GFR than could be inferred from previous anemia treatment guidelines.[14] Whereas the initial National Kidney Foundation K/DOQI anemia guidelines specified a serum creatinine value of 2.0 mg/dL as the benchmark to initiate investigation of anemia in the absence of a GFR correlation,[14] the more recent CKD guidelines recommend surveillance testing for its presence in all patients with renal disease at a GFR of less than 60 mL/min/1.73 m^2.[61]

U.S.,[14] European,[62] and Canadian[63] evidence-based guidelines for treatment of anemia link initiation of evaluation of anemia to a depressed hemoglobin value (<11 g/dL for premenopausal females, <12 g/dL for adult men and postmenopausal women in the U.S. and European guidelines; <11 g/dL for males and postmenopausal women in the Canadian guidelines).[14, 62, 63] The baseline workup in patients with CKD and anemia before further erythropoietic therapy should include, at a minimum, a hemogram with erythrocyte indices, reticulocyte count, transferrin saturation or percent hypochromic RBCs, and serum ferritin.[14, 62, 63] The additional use of C-reactive protein as a baseline screening tool for the presence of underlying inflammation, a potential cause of a poor response, has enjoyed widespread acceptance overseas and is increasingly being used in the United States. Any suggestion of iron deficiency should be followed by studies to exclude occult blood loss. Clinical suspicion of either a primary hematologic disorder or one known to induce a delayed or diminished response (see later) to initial therapy should prompt further evaluation, including an assessment of water-soluble vitamin concentrations, differential leukocyte count, and exclusion of hemolytic states, paraproteinemia, aluminum intoxication, and high-turnover bone disease.[14, 62, 63] Thorough pursuit of any poorly defined ongoing or new illness may unmask an important impediment to effective treatment.

Although the major evidence-based guidelines recommend consideration of hematopoietic treatment for patients with renal disease and a hemoglobin concentration of less than 11 to 12 g/dL, such guidelines beg the broader, unresolved physiologic issue of whether treatment should in fact begin before anemia evolves[64] in order to limit patient vulnerability to the potential end-organ sequelae of prolonged anemia in the predialysis period[65] (also discussed at length later in the section "Therapeutic Goals and Benefits: Target Hemoglobin Issues"). Even given optimal patient eligibility for treatment, however, early inception of care before initiation of renal replacement therapy depends critically on its accessibility, which within the United States remains complicated by regulatory issues related to reimbursement for home versus on-site treatment, and on geographic variation in hemoglobin levels at which payment for rHuEPO is authorized (see the later section on pharmacoeconomic issues in treatment).

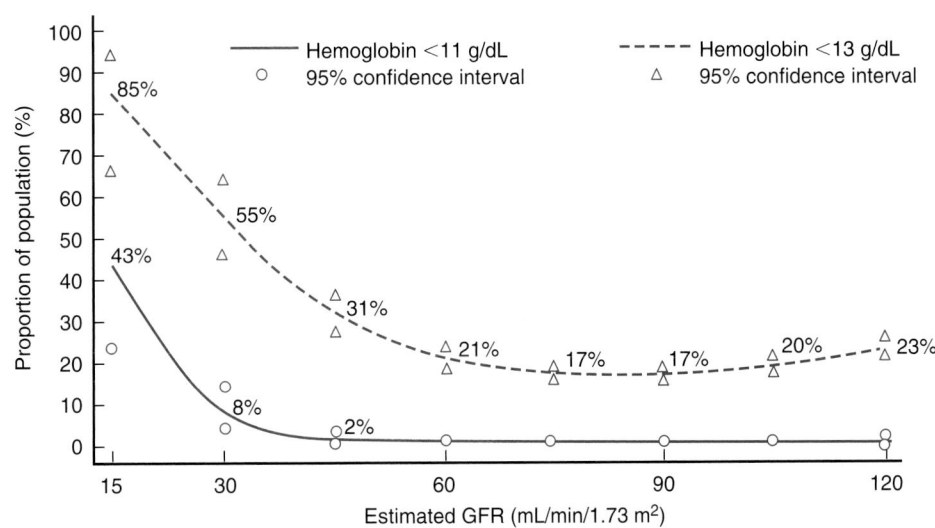

FIGURE 58-1. Adjusted prevalence of low hemoglobin by glomerular filtration rate (GFR) (NHANES III) in adults and predicted prevalence of a hemoglobin concentration less than 11 and 13 g/dL in adult participants 20 years and older in NHANES III, 1988 to 1994. Values are adjusted to the age of 60 years by polynomial regression. Ninety-five percent confidence intervals are shown at selected levels of estimated GFR. (Adapted from National Kidney Foundation: K/DOQI clinical practice guidelines for chronic kidney disease: Evaluation, classification, and stratification. Kidney Disease Outcome Quality Initiative. Am J Kidney Dis 39(2)[suppl 1]:1-246, 2002.)

Evidence-Based Erythropoietin Treatment
rHuEPO and Darbepoetin Alfa

Several forms of rHuEPO are available for the treatment of patients with anemia related to chronic renal failure, ESRD, and other nonrenal disorders by either the intravenous or subcutaneous route. Epoetin alfa and beta (165 amino acids)[66] are glycoproteins produced through recombination of the human erythropoietin gene with the Chinese hamster ovary cell.[57, 58] These rHuEPO molecules differ modestly in that the beta form contains quantitatively more basic sialic acid residues, which may confer slightly higher in vivo/in vitro activity.[67] The half-time ($t_{1/2}$) of epoetin alfa is between 4 and 12 hours when administered intravenously and is prolonged to approximately 25 hours by subcutaneous injection.[68, 69] Comparative pharmacokinetic studies in normal males have demonstrated that the beta form has a slightly larger volume of distribution, a 20% longer terminal elimination $t_{1/2}$ after intravenous administration, and delayed subcutaneous absorption when compared with the alfa form,[70] although these differences do not appear to be reflected in any substantive difference in clinical efficacy.[67] A third rHuEPO molecule, omega, produced in baby hamster kidney cells, has become available for clinical trials and possesses slightly different glycosylation and hydrophilicity characteristics.[71, 72]

Further investigation into the biologic properties of native human erythropoietin and rHuEPO has revealed a direct relationship between its in vivo activity, $t_{1/2}$, and sialic acid carbohydrate content. Affinity for receptor binding varies inversely with this specific carbohydrate content.[73] Such properties suggested a mechanism for enhancing both the duration of action and the biologic efficacy of this hormone inasmuch as increased glycosylation is postulated to slow metabolic clearance.[74] To this end, in the late 1990s a hyperglycosylated rHuEPO analog with five N-linked carbohydrate chains (rHuEPO contains three), designated darbepoetin alfa (also "novel erythropoiesis-stimulating protein," or "NESP"), was synthesized and has been used in extensive clinical trials in which it has been approved for patient care.[75-78] In a double-blind randomized crossover study of peritoneal dialysis patients, Macdougall and colleagues[75] showed dramatic prolongation of the mean $t_{1/2}$ for intravenous darbepoetin when compared with intravenous rHuEPO (25.3 versus 8.5 hours) despite comparable volumes of distribution (52.4 versus 47.8 mL/kg). In six patients in whom darbepoetin was administered subcutaneously, the mean terminal elimination $t_{1/2}$ increased to 48.8 hours. Despite these properties, darbepoetin and rHuEPO are identical with respect to their effect on intracellular signaling and mechanism of action, and they appear to have the same efficacy whether administered subcutaneously or intravenously.[79, 80]

In the last several years, a variety of safety and efficacy trials investigating the use of darbepoetin have addressed correction of anemia at varying doses, routes, and frequency of administration in predialysis, peritoneal dialysis, and hemodialysis patients; maintenance of stable hemoglobin concentrations in the setting of conversion from rHuEPO to darbepoetin therapy at a decreased dosing frequency; and long-term maintenance of hemoglobin levels.[75-81] Taken together, these studies suggest that the initial dose of darbepoetin should be 0.45 to 0.75 U/kg, that therapy can be switched from twice- to three-times-weekly or weekly rHuEPO administration to weekly or even alternate-week darbepoetin with successful maintenance of hemoglobin levels, and that darbepoetin is equally effective as rHuEPO in maintaining hemoglobin levels in dialysis patients with less frequent dosing. The side effect profile of darbepoetin therapy is comparable to that of rHuEPO, and no antibody formation has been noted.[81]

Dose, Route of Administration, Titration, and Monitoring

Since human trials with rHuEPO began in 1985 a large body of literature has evolved in which a wide spectrum of safe, effective treatment strategies have been described. Organization and evaluation of these studies have been enhanced by the coincident growth of evidence-based medical practice in nephrology, as exemplified by the American, European, and Canadian evidence-based practice guidelines[14, 62, 63] for the treatment of anemia in renal disease. These efforts have helped refine effective dosing and monitoring of rHuEPO therapy.

A variety of regimens are effective in raising hemoglobin to target levels (see "Therapeutic Goals and Benefits: Target Hemoglobin Issues"), the route of delivery of which may vary according to the clinical setting and the modality of renal replacement therapy. Patients with CKD and those undergoing peritoneal dialysis almost uniformly receive rHuEPO or darbepoetin by subcutaneous injection; hemodialysis patients may receive treatment by subcutaneous injection or intravenous infusion. Assuming adequate iron stores, an overview of available evidence-based guidelines suggests comparable initiating doses of rHuEPO (80 to 120 U/kg/wk subcutaneously, 120 to 180 U/kg/wk intravenously per K/DOQI,[14] 50 to 150 U/kg/wk subcutaneously or intravenously per European best-practice guidelines,[62] and 100 to 200 U/kg/wk per Canadian guidelines[63]), delivered as doses divided twice or three times per week. Once-weekly dosing of rHuEPO by the subcutaneous route[14, 79] (but less so by the intravenous route[79]) is supportable with the present available evidence. The primary treatment regimen in the United States, three-times-weekly intravenous administration to hemodialysis patients at the doses noted earlier, is at present effective, but as might be inferred from the differences in $t_{1/2}$ between the subcutaneous and intravenous routes, far less efficient use of rHuEPO is achieved with this regimen (among 36 studies involving 2028 patients, the rHuEPO dose needed to maintain a hematocrit of 33% varied between 0% and 68% lower than that required intravenously).[14] The reasons for the widespread preference for this route of administration, particularly given the recommendations of all best-practice guidelines for subcutaneous injection, may relate in large part to use of the intravenous route in the initial trials to optimize response, to greater patient acceptance of this route of administration, and secondarily, to pharmacoeconomic issues in hormone utilization (see "Pharmacoeconomic and ESRD Program–Related Issues in rHuEPO Treatment," later). Successful darbepoetin therapy has been achieved with both subcutaneous and intravenous routes at the dose range noted previously, and it maintains target hemoglobin levels at frequencies of once-weekly or even every-other-week administration—the latter in patients with previous rHuEPO treatment.[80, 81] Intraperitoneal administration in peritoneal dialysis patients has been examined for those who cannot tolerate either subcutaneous or intravenous administration; such administration requires a dry abdomen or the presence of minimal dialysate for optimal absorption,[14] and the risk of peritonitis may be increased, particularly in children receiving therapy by this route.[82]

Suggested safe rates of hemoglobin correction range from 1 to 2 g/dL/mo and should be less than 2.0 to 3.0 g/dL/mo.[14, 62, 63] Concern has been raised regarding blood pressure control with more rapid rates of correction,[60] potential induction of access clotting, and prolonged oscillation of hemoglobin values around the desired target causing a delay in attaining stable levels.[14] Patients with a slow initial response over the first month of treatment may have rHuEPO increased by up to 50%.[14, 62, 63] A dose reduction of 25% or extension of the interval between doses (the latter in particular for subcutaneous administration) is appropriate titration for patients experiencing rapid increases in hemoglobin. A stable hemoglobin concentration occurs when the rate of rHuEPO-generated erythrocyte entry into the circulation equals the rate of exit of these cells from the circulation at senescence. Thus, frequent changes in dose and, in particular, discontinuation of treatment, which results in cessation of erythrocyte entry at rHuEPO-stimulated rates while egress at that rate continues, may cause wide fluctuations in response to therapy, especially when administration of rHuEPO is started and stopped repetitively.[14, 83]

The frequency of monitoring rHuEPO therapy, particularly in the United States, reflects a fusion of rational practices and permissible reimbursement for performance of laboratory evaluations. After treatment has begun, provided that iron stores and essential cofactors are either adequate or being replenished, hemoglobin should be checked weekly or biweekly.[14, 62] After a stable hemoglobin concentration is attained, it should be checked at least monthly, with follow-up at shorter intervals (weekly or biweekly) for dosage changes,[14, 62, 63] instability such as intercurrent illnesses, or hospitalization. Iron stores should be evaluated a minimum of every 3 months by measurement of transferrin saturation and ferritin, with evaluations timed appropriately around periods of iron repletion[14, 84] to avoid artifactually elevated values. More frequent evaluation of iron stores is reasonable but may also be limited by reimbursement allowances.

Potential Adverse Effects of Treatment

At the time of release of rHuEPO for use in CKD and ESRD patients, many expressed concern regarding the development of a variety of serious potential complications of therapy, including worsening hypertension (occasionally in accelerated form), seizures, impaired solute clearance (particularly potassium), and an increased frequency of thrombotic events at (but not confined to) vascular access sites. Due attention has been devoted to all these concerns, and few have materialized over time as major clinical issues in the routine use of rHuEPO.

Changes in blood pressure regulation, either de novo hypertension or increasing antihypertensive medication requirements, are a frequent concomitant of treatment that occurred in an estimated 23% of patients in the largest meta-analysis.[14] Although a rising erythrocyte mass resulting in an increase in peripheral resistance not matched by a comparable decrease in cardiac output has been suggested to reverse the anemia-induced vasodilation in hemodialysis patients,[85] its role as the primary contributor to this phenomenon has been questioned recently.[86, 87] Several mechanisms, taken together, may play a role in increasing vascular reactivity in the setting of rHuEPO treatment, including a diminished effect of nitric oxide (diminished synthesis or resistance), release of endothelin and vasoconstrictor prostanoids,[62] elevation of cytosolic free calcium in smooth muscle cells,[86, 87] and a trophic effect of rHuEPO on endothelial cell growth.[86] Discrete roles for sensitivity to catecholamines or involvement of the renin-angiotensin system appear less probable.[86]

Worsening blood pressure control in patients undergoing therapy should be managed with a reduction in extracellular fluid volume (assuming that hemoglobin is not seriously out of the target range), initiation or an increase in antihypertensive medications, or in rare instances, a decrease in rHuEPO dose. The risk of precipitating seizures in patients being treated with rHuEPO, apart from that associated with hypertensive encephalopathy, has not appeared to be increased with appropriate attention to dosing and titration guidelines, and a previous history of seizures should not preclude treatment with rHuEPO.[14]

Initial concerns at the time of rHuEPO's introduction that increases in red cell mass, changes in blood rheology, and the use of high-efficiency/flux dialyzers with short dialysis times might result in worsening azotemia and hyperkalemia[59, 88-90] have not materialized as clinically significant issues. The incidence of reported hyperkalemia, in particular, has been minimal, with only 12 episodes in 1167 patients noted by the K/DOQI.[14] Although decrements in solute clearance have been reported with successful treatment,[88, 89, 91] they are small (10% to 15%), and when the delivered dialysis dose is closely monitored, shortfalls in delivered Kt/V can be investigated and rectified prospectively.[92]

Additional concern has centered on the relationship between rHuEPO treatment and enhanced thrombotic tendencies, particularly in vascular access sites. Although both platelet and endothelial function improve as hemoglobin increases in response to rHuEPO,[62] reviews of 26 studies involving over 4000 rHuEPO-treated patients with mean hematocrit values of 34% (targets less than 36%) have revealed an average clotting incidence of only 7.5%.[14, 62] Few controlled studies exist, and at present, there does not appear to be any added risk of thrombosis in rHuEPO-treated patients with either grafts or fistulas, save possibly in those with higher hemoglobin concentrations (>12.0 g/dL; see discussion of normalization of hemoglobin later). Data from the U.S. normalization of hematocrit trial demonstrate a higher rate of both fistula and graft thrombosis in patients randomized to the higher hemoglobin group (hemoglobin, 13 g/dL), although no correlation between the hemoglobin concentration attained, rHuEPO dose, and access thrombosis was observed[93]; of note, however, is the fact that the overall thrombosis rate in both groups was elevated when compared with the European experience.[62] At present, no consistent findings demonstrate a clear advantage to one or another form of antiplatelet therapy in maintaining access patency in patients receiving rHuEPO, and as yet no studies have been performed to address this issue in patients with a normalized hemoglobin concentration.

Evidence-Based Iron Treatment

Oral Iron

Erythropoietin therapy is most successful when adequate iron stores are present.[94] To achieve this goal in patients with kidney disease, therapeutic iron supplementation is often necessary by either the oral or parenteral route. Oral supplementation of iron offers the benefits of simplicity, low cost, and safety, but its efficacy is limited. K/DOQI guidelines recommend that when oral iron is used in adults, 200 mg of elemental iron should be administered daily in two to three divided doses.[14]

A variety of different oral iron drugs are available (Table 58-1). Most are iron salts, the most widely used being ferrous sulfate. All these agents cause gastrointestinal side effects, including dyspepsia, constipation, and bloating,[95] and little evidence is available to differentiate between them on the basis of efficacy or tolerability. As such, it is reasonable to choose an agent based primarily on cost.

The efficacy of oral iron in patients with kidney disease has been rigorously studied only in the subset of patients treated by hemodialysis, and the results have been disappointing in this population. Macdougall and colleagues found that during the initiation of erythropoietin treatment, oral iron was no more effective than no iron treatment.[96] Similarly, Wingard and associates treated 46 hemodialysis patients with oral iron and found that after 6 months, most patients had a hematocrit of less than 30% and declining iron stores.[97] Markowitz and co-workers studied 49 hemodialysis patients and found no difference in efficacy between oral iron and placebo.[98] Fudin and associates studied 39 iron-deficient subjects at the initiation of hemodialysis and found no difference in subsequent hemoglobin levels between oral iron therapy and no iron.[99] Taken together, these studies indicate that oral iron does not have demonstrable efficacy for iron supplementation in hemodialysis patients. In contrast, in patients with renal insufficiency who are not yet undergoing dialysis and in those being treated by peritoneal dialysis, ongoing iron losses are far less than what hemodialysis patients experience. Accordingly, they have less of a need for iron supplementation and may derive greater benefit from oral iron treatment. Few published data, however, support this assumption.

The reasons for failure of oral iron treatment in hemodialysis patients are multiple. First, it is generally thought that compliance with oral iron therapy is poor, although published data evaluating this phenomenon are limited. Factors having an impact on compliance with these agents include frequent gastrointestinal side effects,[95] the need to take the medication on an empty stomach, the obligatory intake of more than two pills per day with most supplements to achieve adequate elemental iron intake,[100] and incomplete education of the patient regarding the purpose and goals of iron therapy. It should be noted, however, that even in the studies reported earlier in which compliance was generally encouraged and monitored, oral iron efficacy was poor. A second factor explaining the poor efficacy of oral iron may relate to diminished gastrointestinal iron absorption in hemodialysis patients,[101] and finally, if oral iron is taken at the same time as food, phosphate binders, or other medications that directly interfere with its absorption, adequate intake will not be achieved.[102]

The efficacy of oral iron in patients with kidney disease may be enhanced through several simple practices: first, the dose should provide at least 200 mg of elemental iron per day[14] (for ferrous sulfate, this goal would be achieved by taking approximately three 325-mg tablets per day); second, iron administration should occur between meals[103, 104] and should be spaced at least 1 hour apart from the ingestion of phosphate binders, which may also interfere with iron absorption; and third, because iron is absorbed proximally in the gastrointestinal tract, delayed-release iron supplements should be avoided.[105]

Intravenous Iron

Because of the poor efficacy of oral iron when used for hemodialysis patients, intravenous iron is frequently administered. Three such agents are widely available, iron dextran, iron sucrose, and ferric gluconate. The efficacy of intravenous iron has been widely studied in hemodialysis patients, and a substantial body of literature has evolved in which it has consistently been demonstrated that treatment results in higher hemoglobin levels or a reduced erythropoietin dose requirement, or both.[96, 99, 106-111] Besarab and co-workers used intravenous iron dextran to raise the transferrin saturation of hemodialysis patients to 30% to 50%. The rHuEPO dose requirements for these patients decreased by 40% in comparison to control patients.[111] Macdougall and colleagues studied iron treatment in hemodialysis patients at the initiation of rHuEPO treatment. Patients treated with intravenous iron had a significant increase in mean hemoglobin, from 7.3 ± 0.8 to 11.9 ± 1.2 g/dL. This increase was also significantly greater than the final mean hemoglobin concentration with oral iron or no iron treatment.[96]

Two strategies for administering intravenous iron to hemodialysis patients are in common use. The first entails surveillance for the presence of iron deficiency every 3 months and, if detected, treatment with a short, repletive course of intravenous iron. Typically 1000 mg can be given in divided doses over a period of 2 to 3 weeks. Patients will generally demonstrate a significant improvement in responsiveness to rHuEPO thereafter. Many, however, will remain iron deficient,[110] so assessment of iron stores should be repeated after completing such a course of treatment. A second strategy is to anticipate iron deficiency by administering small weekly doses to maintain stable iron stores. Weekly doses

TABLE 58-1

Oral Iron Supplements

IRON SUPPLEMENT	TABLET SIZE (mg)	AMOUNT OF ELEMENTAL IRON (mg)	AVERAGE MONTHLY WHOLESALE COST (200 mg/day)
Ferrous gluconate	325	35	$5.08
Ferrous sulfate	325	65	$2.29
Ferrous fumarate	325	108	$1.63
Polysaccharide-iron complex	150	150	$7.12

Data from National Kidney Foundation: K/DOQI clinical practice guidelines for anemia of chronic kidney disease, 2000. Am J Kidney Dis 37(suppl 1):182-238, 2001.

of 12.5 to 100 mg of intravenous iron may improve responsiveness to rHuEPO. The potential advantage of such an approach lies in linking iron replacement temporally with ongoing iron losses. Assessment of iron stores should be performed quarterly, however, to ensure the adequacy of this approach. It is unclear whether these two treatment approaches have any important differences in safety or efficacy; few published studies have compared these strategies, and those reported have had conflicting results.[112, 113] In patients being treated by peritoneal dialysis or those with CKD who are not yet undergoing dialysis, iron deficiency develops less frequently than in hemodialysis patients because the former patients do not sustain the chronic ongoing losses of iron experienced by those on hemodialysis.[114, 115] Iron still plays a central role in the maintenance of responsiveness to rHuEPO,[116] however, and deficiency states refractory to oral iron replacement develop not infrequently during the course of treatment.[117] When these patients become iron deficient, a course of oral iron should be attempted. If it is not successful in repleting iron stores, intravenous iron can be administered. Because of the inconvenience of needing to obtain sequential intravenous access in these patients, a larger infusion of iron is often used; for example, 200 to 1000 mg of diluted iron dextran may be infused over a 2-hour period.[14] Such an approach appears to be effective and well tolerated.[113, 118]

Several forms of intravenous iron are available, three of which are most commonly used: iron dextran, iron sucrose, and ferric gluconate. Because each has different attributes, they will be discussed separately. Iron dextran has been used for several decades. Its structure is analogous to that of the storage protein ferritin, with both having a dense core of iron oxyhydroxide surrounded by a stabilizing shell.[94] In iron dextran, the shell is composed of dextran chains consisting of variably sized glucose polymers. Although iron dextran is clearly effective, its safety profile remains an issue in that a recent meta-analysis found that severe adverse reactions occur in approximately 0.6% of patients treated.[119] Moreover, it has been estimated that 31 deaths from iron dextran–related anaphylaxis occurred in the United States between 1976 and 1996.[120] Anaphylactic reactions are believed to be related to the drug's dextran component because non–iron-containing dextrans, when used as volume expanders, have been associated with similar reaction rates.[121, 122] The mechanism of iron dextran–related anaphylaxis is incompletely understood but may be related to direct release of vasoactive mediators by mast cells.[123] One approach that has been used successfully to block dextran-induced anaphylaxis is hapten inhibition with smaller dextran molecules.[124]

Ferric gluconate and iron sucrose are newer forms of intravenous iron in the American marketplace that were approved by the Food and Drug Administration (FDA) in 1999 and 2000, respectively, although both agents have been in use in Europe and elsewhere for decades. Rather than possessing a dense core of iron hydroxide, such as iron dextran does, these agents have polynuclear iron centers. The cores are surrounded by carbohydrate, primarily sucrose and gluconate (a salt of crystalline gluconic acid) for iron sucrose and ferric gluconate, respectively. Because these agents do not contain a dextran moiety, they appear to have a far lower risk of anaphylaxis than iron dextran does. Michael and colleagues recently studied over 2500 hemodialysis patients

and reported that after single-dose exposure to ferric gluconate, no statistically significant difference could be found in the rate of serious adverse reactions when compared with placebo. Moreover, the rate of such reactions was reduced 93% in comparison to iron dextran.[119] Although data from large studies are not available for iron sucrose, it is likely that it too has a more favorable safety profile than iron dextran does.[125]

Both iron sucrose and ferric gluconate can be administered without the need for a test dose and by slow intravenous push.[126, 127] Too few studies have directly compared these two agents with one another to be able to reach any conclusions regarding their relative safety and efficacy. At present, it would seem reasonable to conclude that both are probably as effective as iron dextran and that both have a much lower risk for immediate, severe reactions.

Evidence-Based Iron Monitoring

The K/DOQI anemia guidelines recommend that during the initiation of rHuEPO treatment, iron status be tested every month in patients not receiving ongoing iron repletion. Once rHuEPO dosing and iron maintenance have stabilized, the guidelines recommend monitoring every 3 months.[14] Iron assessment in patients with kidney disease has most frequently been performed with two tests, serum ferritin and transferrin saturation. Two other laboratory evaluations, the percentage of hypochromic red cells (PHR) and the reticulocyte hemoglobin content (CHr), may in fact offer greater overall utility.

Serum ferritin is an indirect measure of storage iron and has been thought to reflect iron deficiency in hemodialysis patients when its concentration is less than 100 ng/mL.[14] The diagnostic value of serum ferritin, however, is limited by its behavior as a potent acute-phase reactant.[127] Clinical settings may arise in which ferritin values may be quite high even in the presence of iron deficiency, such as in hemodialysis patients, in whom the test has a sensitivity of only 41% to 54%.[129, 130] Given its low sensitivity, iron deficiency cannot be excluded by the presence of a "normal" serum ferritin value.

Percent transferrin saturation (TSAT) assesses the availability of circulating iron, calculated as TSAT = (serum iron ÷ total iron-binding capacity) × 100. K/DOQI guidelines recommend using a value of less than 20% as an indicator of iron deficiency in patients with kidney disease.[14] This test, though reasonably sensitive, has a specificity in hemodialysis patients of only 61% to 63%.[129, 130] As a result, low values of transferrin saturation cannot reliably make the diagnosis of iron deficiency. Because of the poor specificity of transferrin saturation and the poor sensitivity of serum ferritin, it is not surprising that concurrently measured specimens often paradoxically suggest iron deficiency by transferrin saturation and iron overload by serum ferritin (such discordant results are frequently due to the effects of inflammation[131, 132] or functional iron deficiency).[94] Both tests are further limited by their high variability. Recently, the coefficient of variation for both tests was found to be high.[133] These limitations in the predictive value of serum ferritin and transferrin saturation mandate that the results of these tests not be used reflexively in guiding iron treatment, but that clinical judgment be used to correlate the results with the patient's clinical status.

PHR has been found to be a useful measure of iron status in patients undergoing hemodialysis.[134] Tessitore and co-workers recently found that the test had the greatest utility of any test for the diagnosis of iron deficiency in hemodialysis patients. When the PHR was over 6%, its efficiency was 89.6%, thus indicating excellent discriminative ability.[135] The test has one important limitation: it is affected by changes in erythrocyte mean corpuscular volume (MCV). When samples are stored or shipped, the MCV may be significantly altered.[136] In the United States, most laboratory samples for hemodialysis patients are shipped to central locations, a factor that might explain the inconsistent results of PHR in several studies[137, 138] and potentially limit its usefulness.

CHr is a direct measure of iron status at the level of the reticulocyte. Because it is a measure of content instead of concentration, it is unaffected by changes in cell volume. In addition, because reticulocytes circulate for only approximately 24 hours,[139] test results can indicate very acute changes in iron status. Studies have generally found that the test is an accurate measure of iron status in hemodialysis patients.[135, 137, 138, 140] Recently, Fishbane and colleagues found CHr to be more cost-effective for iron management than serum ferritin and transferrin saturation are. Importantly, the test was found to have far less variability than noted with other iron monitoring tests.[133] Generally, a CHr value of less than 29 to 30 pg indicates a need for more intensive iron treatment.

Functional Iron Deficiency

Given the poor sensitivity of serum ferritin and the low specificity of transferrin saturation, the clinician may often face the dilemma of interpreting transferrin saturation values suggesting iron deficiency (TSAT <20%) along with accompanying serum ferritin values indicating iron sufficiency or even overload (ferritin >300 to 1200 ng/mL). This physiologic phenomenon reflects "functional iron deficiency," which exists primarily as a sequela of rHuEPO treatment. During the supraphysiologic burst of RBC production after a pharmacologic dose of rHuEPO, the small circulating iron pool (0.1% of total body iron) may occasionally be insufficient to supply the stimulated erythron (as would be reflected by the aforementioned laboratory data suggesting low circulating but normal or high iron reserves). Thus, even in the face of normal iron stores, iron-deficient erythropoiesis may ensue, with further iron repletion often required for normal erythropoiesis to resume.[141] In addition to a rapid response to rHuEPO treatment, recent studies have also shown that acute or chronic inflammation may be partially responsible for this phenomenon[142, 143] by promoting iron sequestration in the reticuloendothelial system and thereby rendering it unavailable to erythrocyte precursors[144] (see "Inflammation" in the section "Delayed or Diminished Response to rHuEPO Treatment"). The disjunction between TSAT and ferritin values thus reflects the transient unavailability of substrate for proper cellular maturation. Regrettably, laboratory tools to differentiate functional iron deficiency from reticuloendothelial blockade are not immediately available; the use of CHr may offer some promise in resolving these issues in the future.

Evidence-Based Approach to Iron Safety

The human body is critically dependent on adequate circulating and tissue iron stores to ensure the normal function of a variety of cellular and subcellular processes. Free circulating iron, however, is a potent oxidizing agent highly toxic to lipid membranes through its catalytic effect on the production of hydroxyl radicals in the presence of hydrogen peroxide and superoxide.[145] To ensure an adequate, but safe supply of iron, storage and transport complexes such as ferritin and transferrin sequester it from free circulation in the blood and concentrate it within tissue parenchyma or the reticuloendothelial system. Although mechanisms for iron handling are highly regulated, treatment with intravenous iron has the potential to either bypass or overwhelm these safety systems. It is therefore important that treatment be administered safely and its results closely monitored.

IRON OVERLOAD. Several complications may occur with inattentive intravenous iron use. Iron overload may ensue if iron is administered indiscriminately and serum ferritin is allowed to rise to high levels. Parenchymal damage to organ systems similar to what is seen in hereditary hemochromatosis may result.[146] Although it is unlikely that iron overload to this degree will occur in hemodialysis patients as a result of iron treatment since the advent of rHuEPO, given that this therapy gains its efficacy from consumption of iron stores, the K/DOQI recommendation to withhold iron treatment when the serum ferritin concentration is higher than 800 ng/mL or the TSAT is greater than 50% nonetheless provides a reasonable safeguard for repetitive therapy.[14]

RISK OF INFECTION. The relationship of iron treatment to the risk of infection is incompletely understood. Bacteria and other organisms are reliant on the availability of iron for a variety of metabolic processes, including virulence, and several studies in animals have clearly demonstrated that iron administration can promote infections[147, 148] (as has, by inference, the historical experience with deferoxamine and precipitation of bizarre bacterial and fungal infections in dialysis patients).[149, 150] Dialysis patients, at baseline, have a high risk of infection by virtue of the underlying immunosuppressive state of their disease and the nature of the appliances and repetitive procedures required to perform either hemodialysis or peritoneal dialysis.[151] The role of iron exposure as a compounding risk factor in this complicated setting is both unclear and difficult to study, but some studies have shown an association between the serum ferritin concentration and the risk of infection. Kessler and colleagues found that the rate of infection was greatly increased when serum ferritin was over 1000 ng/mL.[152] In a subsequent analysis, this group found that a serum ferritin level higher than 500 ng/mL was a risk factor for infection.[153] Similarly, Tielemans and associates found an increased risk when serum ferritin was greater than 500 ng/mL.[154] The relationship between high serum ferritin and risk of infection in these studies might indicate that high levels of iron storage are causally linked to the risk of infection. However, a confounding issue in these studies remains the behavior of serum ferritin as a potent acute-phase reactant[128]; the high serum ferritin concentrations may simply reflect the presence of or predisposition for infection rather than indicating causality. Of note, in a well-designed prospective multicenter European study, no relationship was found between serum ferritin and the risk of infection.[151] Further research in this area is clearly needed.

Another path for investigating the relationship between iron and infection in hemodialysis patients is via analysis of supplemental iron administration. Canziani and co-workers found an increased risk of infection in patients who received a greater number of intravenous iron doses.[155] In an elegant series of experiments, Parkkinenl and colleagues found that iron sucrose injection resulted in free iron in the circulation, thereby creating conditions that strongly supported the growth of *Staphylococcus epidermidis* in vitro.[156] Jean and co-workers found that the cumulative intravenous iron dose was a predictor of risk for bacteremia in hemodialysis patients with tunneled catheters.[157] In contrast, Hoen and associates recently analyzed data from a large multicenter study and found no association between intravenous iron dosing and risk for bacteremia.[158] Given the conflicting results in the present literature, it is difficult to reach evidenced-based conclusions that could aid in practice. Until further data become available, the risk of infection should be considered in clinical decision making related to intravenous iron administration. It would seem reasonable, based on current knowledge, to avoid intravenous iron treatment during episodes of acute infection.

OXIDATIVE STRESS. A second potential, but poorly understood issue in the long-term safety of repetitive iron infusion is related to iron-mediated oxidative injury to tissues or vessels. As noted, under certain conditions, iron causes the oxidation of various biomolecules, including proteins, DNA, and lipids.[159] The capacity for intravenously administered iron to catalyze "free iron" reactions may depend on whether—and to what degree—iron is bound to its drug vehicle: iron bound in drugs may be less available for oxidative interaction with cells than free iron is. If the affinity of iron for its vehicle is low, free iron could potentially appear in serum or plasma. Parkkinen and colleagues have recently reported this finding with therapeutic doses of iron sucrose. After the injection of 100 mg iron sucrose, 7 of 12 subjects had free iron detectable in plasma.[156] Kooistra and colleagues also studied 10 hemodialysis patients receiving two 100-mg doses of iron sucrose and found a significant increase in free iron in the circulation.[160] Recently, Rooyakkers and associates found that injection of iron sucrose into healthy volunteers caused release of free iron into the circulation, a significant reduction in flow-mediated vascular dilatation, and generation of superoxide radicals.[161] Although these findings raise concern about the long-term safety of intravenous iron injections, the clinical importance of such phenomena requires further elucidation.

In another recent study, Zager and colleagues found that iron dextran, oligosaccharide, gluconate, and sucrose all led to substantial lipid peroxidation in vitro. In this study, cellular toxicity and death, however, occurred almost exclusively with iron sucrose (and to a far lesser degree with ferric gluconate). Iron sucrose induced severe cellular depletion of adenosine triphosphate, an effect that was not ouabain sensitive. Interestingly, the cell death was clearly dissociated from the pro-oxidant effects of the drugs.[162]

The clinical importance of these findings, however, still remains to be demonstrated. The doses of iron used were suprapharmacologic, and all studies were performed in vitro.[162] Furthermore, it is not clear whether these effects are specific to one form of iron or apply to other intravenous iron agents as well (in fact, all three drugs caused oxidative changes), and at present, no in vivo studies have compared the frequency of the appearance of either free iron or its consequences with the three currently available forms of parenteral iron. It appears that the carbohydrate and dextran forms of iron can affect cellular metabolism in a deleterious way, and all forms therefore require judicious use. Clearly, the issues raised by this area of increasing investigative focus signal a need for further attention.

The potential role of iron in accelerating cardiovascular disease has been proposed on the basis of the ability of iron to cause lipid oxidation and lipid peroxidation in vessel walls. This link was first proposed by Sullivan in 1981, who suggested that iron deficiency might provide a measure of protection against atherosclerotic disease.[163] Because of the high prevalence of cardiac disease in patients with kidney disease[164] and the frequent use of iron supplementation, any relationship between the two is of potential clinical relevance. Unfortunately, few published reports have addressed this subject specifically in patients with kidney failure, so knowledge must be extrapolated from studies in other populations. In one such study, Salonen and co-workers analyzed the risk for myocardial infarction in 1931 middle-aged Finnish men. They found that a serum ferritin level higher than 200 ng/mL was an independent risk factor for cardiac disease, with an odds ratio of 2.2.[165] In contrast, Magnusson and associates studied over 2000 men and women and found no association between serum ferritin and cardiac risk.[166] Indeed, results from the literature have been mixed, with more negative than positive studies.[165-174] Given the complexity of this subject and its implications for long-standing dual therapy with iron and rHuEPO, further research in this area is needed.

DELAYED OR DIMINISHED RESPONSE TO rHuEPO TREATMENT

In the 1989 multicenter phase III trial of rHuEPO, 97% of patients responded to intravenous treatment with an increase in hematocrit to a target of 35% ± 3% within 12 weeks of initiation of therapy; starting doses were either 150 or 300 U/kg per treatment, with subsequent dose reduction to 75 U/kg per treatment titrated to maintain a stable target value. The median maintenance dose of rHuEPO was 75 U/kg (225 U/kg/wk, range of 37.5 to 1575 U/kg/wk).[60] As a result of this trial and a literature review appearing in the evidence-based U.S. K/DOQI anemia guidelines, a threshold definition of rHuEPO resistance was proposed—namely, an inability to reach the target hematocrit over a period of 4 to 6 months given adequate iron stores at a dose of 450 U/kg/wk administered intravenously (300 U/kg/wk subcutaneously) or failure to maintain the hematocrit subsequently at that dose.[14] European guidelines[62] use lower limits, 300 U/kg/wk, because most patients receive rHuEPO by subcutaneous injection.

IRON DEFICIENCY. The most frequently encountered source of an inadequate response to rHuEPO is iron deficiency,[14] which evolves as a consequence of either iron loss, iron consumption by the growing erythron in an appropriate response to rHuEPO treatment,[14, 94] or of lesser importance, inadequate gastrointestinal absorption of oral iron. Proper detection of iron deficiency, particularly in the setting of hemodialysis, requires appreciation of potential losses occurring at the patient's interface with the dialysis machine, as well as processes intrinsic to the patient. In patients during the predialytic stages of CKD or in those receiving peritoneal dialysis, the aforementioned issues are relevant to a far lesser degree because of the absence of extracorporeal circulation and repetitive systemic anticoagulation. Blood loss associated with the dialysis procedure may be phlebotomy related as a result of inadequate blood return from the dialyzers or tubing, suboptimal heparinization, hematoma formation from poor access cannulation, loss of dialysis equipment from insufficient anticoagulation, or excessive access bleeding after dialysis. Iron loss from other sources may also be inferred clinically from an inability to raise iron stores in the face of repeated courses of therapy or from a progressive increase in rHuEPO requirements (see "Functional Iron Deficiency"). Of importance, several forms of iron loss may occur simultaneously. In patients who have adequate iron stores as defined by appropriate transferrin saturation and serum ferritin concentrations, however, other contributors to treatment resistance are noteworthy and discussed in the following paragraphs.

SECONDARY HYPERPARATHYROIDISM. Several studies, most from the pre-rHuEPO era, have investigated whether PTH exerts a direct inhibitory effect on erythroid proliferation, with indeterminate conclusions.[175-178] Experience with rHuEPO treatment since its availability, however, suggests a more complex relationship between PTH excess and response to rHuEPO. A correlation exists between rHuEPO requirements and the degree of marrow fibrosis, osteoclastic and eroded surfaces seen on bone biopsy specimens, and PTH levels.[179] This correlation has been underscored by the transnational analysis of medical practices in the Dialysis Outcomes and Practice Patterns Study (DOPPS), which has demonstrated a clear relationship between hemoglobin concentration and local practices related to the treatment of high-turnover bone disease; the study suggested improved outcomes with aggressive management of PTH excess, maintenance of eucalcemia, and good nutritional status.[180] Parathyroidectomy or acceleration of rHuEPO treatment (or both) often overcomes this particular block to an adequate response.[14, 62, 181-184] Given the frequency of iron deficiency, inflammatory insults, and the confounding effects of other subtle causes of a poor response, however, hyperparathyroidism per se must remain a modest contributor to this phenomenon.[185] The effect of non–aluminum-related low-turnover bone disease on responsiveness to rHuEPO is unclear, although one finding suggests that efficacy might be enhanced.[186]

One report suggests a possible role for vitamin D in improving erythropoiesis apart from its effect on PTH levels or serum calcium.[187] The effects of vitamin D as a growth factor in enhancing the response to rHuEPO, apart from effects on PTH and marrow fibrosis, require further investigation. Overall, effective management of high-turnover disease, whether by surgical or biochemical intervention,[180, 188] may have a beneficial effect on the efficacy of rHuEPO treatment.

ALUMINUM TOXICITY. Aluminum toxicity has been seen with decreasing frequency because of major improvements in water purification, widespread application of Association for the Advancement of Medical Instrumentation (AAMI) standards, diminishing use of aluminum-containing phosphate binders, and the availability of non–aluminum-containing agents. Mechanisms for this disorder have been ascribed variably to interference with enzymatic insertion of iron into the heme moiety at closure of the tetrapyrrole ring (or with heme synthesis itself) and competition between aluminum and iron for binding to transferrin before substrate delivery to erythropoietic elements.[189-191] Increasing rHuEPO dosing has in general proved effective in overcoming initial disruptions in erythropoiesis,[14, 192, 193] as has aluminum exclusion or, when necessary, deferoxamine treatment of bone or central nervous system disease. The hope that rHuEPO treatment might function as a physiologic probe to uncover subclinical aluminum intoxication has not been realized.

HEMOGLOBINOPATHIES AND HEMOLYTIC ANEMIA. The original promise of replacement therapy, particularly for sickle cell disease, has remained unfulfilled.[194-196] The initial high-dose therapy was approached optimistically in the hope of increasing fetal hemoglobin synthesis, which has not been seen as a common response to treatment—nor, however, has the induction of hyperhemolytic states, which was also an initial concern in the treatment of these patients.[194] Increasing rHuEPO requirements have been reported in conjunction with induction of slow hemolysis as a result of chloramine excess,[197, 198] responding to its removal with appropriate carbon treatment of city water, and anti-N_{form} antibody production after subclinical formaldehyde exposure.[199] Hemolysis related to lipid peroxidation manifested as resistance to rHuEPO has recently raised the more general issue of the role of oxidative stress as a modulator of the response to rHuEPO and the role of anemia in general in patients with ESRD.[200]

FOLATE AND VITAMIN B$_{12}$ DEFICIENCY. The absence of essential cofactors for hemoglobin synthesis is an impediment to an optimal response to rHuEPO. Though a less likely source of resistance to rHuEPO, particularly in patients receiving appropriate vitamin supplementation or ingesting a reasonable diet, an unexplained poor response should prompt an evaluation of the availability of sufficient cofactor.[201-203]

MULTIPLE MYELOMA. B cell dyscrasias have shown a variable erythropoietic response to therapy with rHuEPO over a wide range of doses.[204-206] Although relapse and lesion transformation have been reported in both dialysis and nondialysis patients with multiple myeloma managed with cytokine therapy,[204, 207, 208] they are rare, and the use of rHuEPO is not contraindicated in patients with renal disease that is myeloma related.[14]

INFLAMMATION. Extensive experience over the last decade in the direct patient care setting has demonstrated the critical impact of inflammation on response to rHuEPO[209] and has necessitated vigilance in detecting the often minor insults that may serve as root causes of resistance to treatment, in addition to obvious infections, malignancies, and connective tissue disorders. Concomitantly, an extensive literature has also convincingly demonstrated that an inflammatory state chronically underlies the vascular disease and catabolic processes attendant on ESRD.[209-211] It appears certain that resistance to rHuEPO—and possibly a component of the anemia of CKD as well—is a manifestation of both acute, intermittent, *and* chronic, continuous inflammatory dyscrasias.

In states of active inflammation (such as infectious processes, surgical insults, malignancies), iron metabolism is directly altered, and access to iron from the reticuloendothelial system by hematopoietic cells is blocked as a result of enhanced iron uptake by activated macrophages.[212] Ferritin synthesis increases, and gastrointestinal absorption of iron decreases. In addition to reticuloendothelial blockade, a variety of interactions between cytokines and marrow elements can impair the response to rHuEPO. On the basis of experimental evidence in both animals and humans,[213-217] the presence of sufficient quantities of several proinflammatory cytokines at the marrow level, particularly tumor necrosis factor-α (TNF-α), interleukin-1 (IL-1) or IL-6, and interferon-γ (IFN-γ), are thought to impair the growth of erythroid progenitor cells, decrease the local response to erythropoietin, and increase IFN production—a hypothesized mechanism for resistance to rHuEPO in this setting.[212] Of equal or perhaps greater importance is that these mediators may represent a linkage between inflammation, poor response to rHuEPO, and the larger syndrome of malnutrition, wasting, and increased risk of mortality seen in dialysis patients. In this regard, Barany and colleagues[210] and Gunnell and associates[218] have demonstrated clear associations between hypoalbuminemia, elevations in C-reactive protein, and an elevated rHuEPO dose, thus suggesting that these convergent pathogenic processes are potentially associated with poor outcomes.

CARNITINE DEFICIENCY. L-Carnitine is an essential cofactor for transmitochondrial transport of fatty acids for oxidation, and it is depleted by hemodialysis.[219] A role for carnitine in maintaining erythrocyte membrane integrity, improving deformability, and thereby increasing red cell survival has been postulated. Data accrued over the last several years (including a meta-analysis reviewing 18 randomized controlled trials[220]) have shown modest efficacy of L-carnitine therapy in improving red cell osmotic fragility[221, 222] and erythrocyte survival time[223] and either raising hemoglobin levels or reducing rHuEPO requirements[220-223] for treatment of anemia. Variable benefit has been shown for dyslipidemia or improvement in any specific abnormal lipid fraction.[220, 224] New regulatory requirements for drug reimbursement in the United States now permit L-carnitine use only for rHuEPO-resistant anemia without other apparent cause and for refractory intradialytic hypotension.[225]

ANGIOTENSIN-CONVERTING ENZYME INHIBITION. A relationship between treatment with angiotensin-converting enzyme inhibitors and decreasing hemoglobin levels has been known for many years from observations drawn from the treatment of both post-transplant erythrocytosis[226] and CKD. Since the advent of rHuEPO treatment, a variety of reports have offered divided opinions regarding whether these drugs impede the response to treatment (yes[227-230]; no,[231-233] in a series of retrospective and prospective crossover studies). One recent report[227] has shown that plasma levels of *N*-acetyl-seryl-aspartyl-lysyl-proline (AcSDKP), a physiologic inhibitor of erythropoiesis that is degraded in vivo by angiotensin-converting enzyme, are elevated in patients with impaired clearance and those with ESRD. Treatment with angiotensin-converting enzyme inhibitors results in

increases in AcSDKP in both populations, more so in dialysis patients. In these individuals, the weekly rHuEPO dose correlated with AcSDKP levels, thus suggesting its possible role as an inhibitor of erythropoiesis.

EFFECT OF DELIVERED DIALYSIS DOSE AND MEMBRANE. A few reports have previously suggested that an improved response to rHuEPO is associated with a higher dialysis dose or the use of biocompatible membranes.[234, 235] The biologic basis for these observations remains uncertain at present inasmuch as patients in the most aggressively dialyzed cohort ever reported (average Kt/V of 1.67) do not augment their hematocrit beyond an average of 28.1% without rHuEPO.[236] Additionally, it is unclear whether the improvements published are related to the delivered dose or the choice of biocompatible membranes. The discrete effects of intermittent dialysis and the choice of membrane on response to rHuEPO therefore remain inconclusive. Several reports of daily therapies, whether nocturnal[237, 238] or short daily dialysis,[238-242] however, have revealed no consistent effect on response to rHuEPO (improved response with increased hemoglobin[236, 237, 240]; modest improvement to no change[239, 240, 242]). As these therapies gain wider acceptance, the relationship between progressive increases in small- and middle-molecule clearance and responsiveness to rHuEPO will gain clearer focus.[243]

ANTI-rHuEPO ANTIBODIES. Though reported only three times from the availability of rHuEPO until 1998, from 1998 to 2001 Casadevall and colleagues noted 21 patients[244, 245] in whom pure red cell aplasia developed in the setting of rHuEPO treatment. These patients possessed antibody that neutralized rHuEPO and inhibited erythroid colony formation from normal marrow. Immunosuppressive treatment or discontinuation of rHuEPO treatment resulted in the disappearance of antibody in the large majority of reported cases. In these reports, 19 patients were treated with epoetin alfa and one with epoetin beta. The reasons for their evolution are unknown at this time and remain a source of ongoing inquiry.

INDIVIDUAL PATIENT MARROW SENSITIVITY TO rHuEPO. After the initial availability of rHuEPO in the United States, Uehlinger and co-authors described a quantitative method of assessing individual responsiveness to treatment.[246] Although such an expression has not proved to be a stable index of responsiveness to therapy on a large scale over the ensuing decade, it is increasingly apparent that wide biologic variability in response exists among patients who can attain appropriate target hemoglobin levels, assuming the presence of adequate iron stores, and that individual patients may have repetitive waxing and waning of responsiveness in various clinical settings. A recent retrospective analysis from a large, stable dialysis population in Seattle[247] revealed that most patients exhibiting resistance to rHuEPO (i.e., those who required >500 U/kg/wk rHuEPO or failed to achieve a hematocrit >30%) over a fixed interval did so reversibly when the resistance was precipitated by treatable inflammatory lesions, infections, iron deficiency, or ultimately discovered causes. Additionally, many of the patients who were "resistant" by virtue of requiring doses higher than 500 U/kg/wk did in fact achieve the target hematocrit. Of note, Brier and Aronoff[248] alluded to similar variability in the "normal" response, thus suggesting that present regulatory efforts to confine rHuEPO reimbursement to a narrow range of hemoglobin levels (11 to 12 g/dL) fail because of the wide variability in normal responses. Revisiting the definition of "normal" response given a broadening dosage spectrum will be necessary as further evidence-based guidelines for therapy evolve.

THERAPEUTIC GOALS AND BENEFITS: TARGET HEMOGLOBIN ISSUES

Current medical practice regarding target hemoglobin levels in patients with CKD is derived from the National Kidney Foundation K/DOQI clinical practice guidelines, which were first published in 1997[249] and recently updated.[14] After an exhaustive review of the literature, the work group determined the target hemoglobin concentration to be 11.0 to 12.0 g/dL, with lower levels associated with adverse outcomes. The upper limit was based on the lack of sufficient evidence to support the benefits or define the potential risks of higher hemoglobin levels. Similar efforts in Canada resulted in recommendations for a target hemoglobin concentration of 10.5 to 11.5 g/dL,[250] whereas the European Working Party published best-practice guidelines suggesting that hemoglobin should be maintained above 11 g/dL, with individualization to optimize outcomes.[62] Of note is the fact that the latter recommendations do not include an upper limit for the target.

From an organ system perspective, one may define the optimal hemoglobin concentration as the level that maximizes oxygen delivery to body tissues. Of additional importance are the clinical consequences and manifestations of that level, as well as adverse consequences, if any. Considerable debate regarding the most appropriate target hemoglobin level in this context has taken place since development of the various treatment guidelines, with many opinions being published, generally in the form of editorials or literature reviews.[251-259] In addition, an increasing body of literature has been published in which this issue has been addressed, with a focus on the benefits and risks of increasing hemoglobin toward or up to normal levels in CKD patients.

MORTALITY. The relationship between hemoglobin concentration and mortality has been reported in several studies, but variations in both study populations and the degree of study design rigor make it difficult to draw generalizable conclusions.[93, 260-263] Interest in this area was stimulated by studies suggesting that the hemoglobin concentration was an independent predictor of mortality in hemodialysis patients.[264] Cross-sectional analysis of a large administrative database from a national dialysis chain found increased mortality (relative risk [RR], 1.45) when the hematocrit was 35% to 40% as opposed to the reference range of 30% to 35%.[260] Although this study included adjustments for case mix and certain laboratory values, the very low correlation coefficient makes an association between hematocrit level and survival questionable. A larger cross-sectional study was published by investigators using administrative data from the Health Care Financing Administration (HCFA).[261] When compared with patients who had a hematocrit of 30% to 33%, those with a hematocrit of 33% to 36% had a significantly decreased likelihood of death (RR, 0.9). No mortality benefit was found for patients with a hematocrit greater than 36%, although the number of patients in this category was small. A follow-up study from the same group, with a larger number of patients in the hematocrit range of 36% to 39%, found no survival benefit for this group.[262] A final, nonrandomized clinical trial from Spain reported no deaths over a 6-month period in a group of hemodialysis patients whose hematocrit was raised from a baseline mean of 31% to a mean of 38.5%.[263]

The only randomized controlled trial of the impact of normalization of hemoglobin on survival was carried out in a subset of hemodialysis patients with cardiac disease, defined as ischemic heart disease or congestive heart failure.[93] Patients were randomized to a hematocrit of 30% ± 3% or 42% ± 3%. The planned duration of the study was 3 years after enrollment of the last patient. After 29 months, at the time of the third interim data analysis, higher mortality was observed in the higher hematocrit group, and although this higher mortality was not significantly different statistically from the mortality in the lower hematocrit group, the independent safety monitoring committee recommended halting the study. A total of 1233 patients were included in the intent-to-treat analysis, which showed a relative risk of death or first myocardial infarction of 1.3 for the higher versus the lower hematocrit group, although this finding did not reach statistical significance. Of note, however, was a decrease in mortality rate at higher hematocrit in both hematocrit groups when a cross-sectional post hoc analysis of mortality based on the average achieved hematocrit was performed—a finding that could potentially be confounded by survivor effects. Interpretation of this study is further complicated by lower values for Kt/V and more frequent use of intravenous iron in the higher hematocrit group. As pointed out in a recent editorial by Macdougall and Ritz,[265] this study has many issues that make it difficult to understand the implications of its findings, including the enrollment of only "high-risk" cardiac patients, lack of correlation between achieved hematocrit and mortality (survivor effect), the use of predialysis hematocrit values, the use of hematocrit rather than hemoglobin concentration, and the fact that the excess mortality seen was not related to cardiovascular causes.

HOSPITALIZATION. Assessment of the relationship between hematocrit level and hospitalization has been hampered by the lack of sufficient data on other patient characteristics that may influence this complication. In an analysis of a large administrative database[266] in which a Cox proportional hazards method was used to account for differences in patient characteristics, patients in the 33% to 36% hematocrit category had a lower risk of hospitalization than did patients with lower hematocrit levels. It is of note that patients with a hematocrit less than 30% had a 14% to 30% *increased* risk of hospitalization. In a subsequent study using more recent data,[262] hospitalization rates were 16% to 22% lower, depending on cause, in patients with hematocrit values greater than 36% than in those with lower hematocrit values. A study from Spain[263] reported a 58% reduction in the total number of hospitalizations and a 69% reduction in length of stay in patients after normalization of the hematocrit. It is unclear whether these results from observational studies represent a causal relationship between low hematocrit and increased risk of hospitalization or simply whether a low hematocrit indicates sicker patients at increased risk.

BRAIN AND COGNITIVE FUNCTION. Studies in dogs have documented that the optimal hematocrit for maximizing body oxygen consumption is one in the normal range.[267, 268] Similar findings have been reported in normal volunteers subjected to hemodilution.[269] Partial correction of anemia has been shown to improve brain electrophysiology, as measured by event-related electrophysiology.[270-272] Similar improvements in cognitive function have been found with partial correction of anemia as well; such improvements were identified with instruments that measure visual, conceptual, and vasomotor tracking, auditory-verbal learning, symbol-digit modality, and trail making, among many others.[273-275] More recent studies have shown that normalization of the hematocrit leads to even greater improvement in objective measures of brain function, as determined by electrophysiologic techniques.[276] Twenty chronic hemodialysis patients were studied by electroencephalographic frequency analysis before and after correction of anemia from a mean hematocrit of 31.6% to a mean hematocrit of 42.8%. Significant improvement in electrophysiologic parameters was seen at the higher hematocrit, and a significant correlation was observed between the incremental improvement in these parameters and the rise in hematocrit. Additional research on sleep disorders in ESRD patients, the SLEEPO study, demonstrated significant improvements in sleep patterns and daytime sleepiness when the hematocrit was normalized.[277] The mechanism by which brain function improves with normalization of the hematocrit is unknown, but it may be related to optimization of oxygen delivery to the brain and metabolism.[278, 279] In seven ESRD patients, full correction of anemia led to an increased oxygen supply to the brain and increased oxygen extraction by brain tissue.[278] In an additional study from Japan, five hemodialysis patients underwent positron emission tomography before and after normalization of the hematocrit. A minimal hematocrit of 35% was found to be necessary to maximize oxygen delivery and brain metabolism.[279] Finally, it should be noted that all the studies described used rHuEPO to increase the hemoglobin concentration. It has recently been found that erythropoietin is able to cross the blood-brain barrier in rats and ameliorate the extent of brain injury after a variety of insults.[280] Such studies raise the question of whether the improvements in brain and cognitive function seen after improvement and normalization of hemoglobin levels in ESRD patients are related entirely to its rise or may in part reflect a direct effect of rHuEPO.

QUALITY OF LIFE/EXERCISE CAPACITY. Considerable evidence demonstrates that partial correction of anemia improves the quality of life of ESRD patients.[281-284] More recent studies have shown that normalization of hemoglobin improves the quality of life to an even greater extent.[93, 263, 285, 286] In cardiac patients enrolled in the normalization of hematocrit study,[93] quality of life was assessed by using the Medical Outcomes Study Short-Form Health Survey[287]; as the hematocrit increased, quality of life improved, although few details of the analysis are provided. The Spanish study used the Sickness Impact Profile (SIP) and the Karnofsky Scale in patients before and after normalization of the hematocrit.[263] Highly significant improvement in scores on the SIP and the Karnofsky scale was documented, although the generalizability of these findings could be questioned because patients were excluded from the study if they were diabetic, were older than 65 years, or

had a variety of common comorbidities (severe hypertension, stroke, ischemic heart disease). A prospective, randomized, double-blind crossover study in 14 hemodialysis patients assessed the benefits of full reversal of anemia in stable hemodialysis patients.[285] The total score and psychosocial dimension score were significantly better when the hemoglobin was normalized. Similar findings were reported by Painter and colleagues, who found an improvement in exercise capacity when normalization of hematocrit was combined with exercise training.[286] The latter, however, remained below normal, thus suggesting that the poor exercise capacity in dialysis patients cannot be fully explained by either anemia or deconditioning. These results confirm earlier findings by other investigators[287-289] and implicate a role for uremia per se or local abnormalities in electrolyte metabolism related to uremia in this clinical abnormality. It is known that Na^+,K^+-ATPase activity is impaired in uremic rats.[290-292] Erythropoietin has also been shown to enhance the activity of this enzyme.[293] It is possible that increasing the hemoglobin concentration to normal may be responsible for the improved K^+ regulation and exercise performance reported by McMahon and colleagues.[289]

CARDIOVASCULAR DISEASE. Although it is well established that anemia is an independent risk factor associated with left ventricular hypertrophy (LVH), left ventricular dilation (LVD), and increased cardiac mortality[294-296] and that partial correction of anemia is beneficial in these areas,[297-299] it is less clear whether these adverse outcomes could be further minimized by normalization of hemoglobin. A randomized controlled trial from Canada evaluated the impact of normalizing the hemoglobin concentration on the degree of LVH or LVD present at baseline in a group of hemodialysis patients.[300] After 40 weeks, echocardiography revealed no significant regression of LVH or improvement in left ventricular cavity volume in patients with baseline LVD. However, a significant decrease in the development of LVD was observed in patients who had LVH at baseline. These findings suggest that normalization of hemoglobin may prevent increases in LVD in susceptible patients. A smaller study from Germany confirmed that normalization of hemoglobin can lead to preservation of normal left ventricular dimensions or reverse LVH in hemodialysis patients.[301] Studies in patients with mild to moderate CKD have also shown the hemoglobin level to be an independent and modifiable risk factor for abnormal left ventricular growth.[296] For each 0.5-g/dL decrease in hemoglobin, the risk of abnormal left ventricular growth increased by 32%. In a separate study from Japan in CKD patients not on dialysis, normalization of hematocrit (40%) was more effective than partial correction of anemia (hematocrit of 30%) in leading to regression of LVH.[302] Of interest is a study in patients without kidney disease, but with severe congestive heart failure and anemia (hemoglobin <12 g/dL).[303] Raising hemoglobin levels toward the normal range with rHuEPO led to an increase in the left ventricular ejection fraction, a fall in New York Heart Association class, and a decrease in the hospitalization rate. Whether such outcomes would also be seen in patients with CKD and congestive heart failure remains to be studied.

KIDNEY FUNCTION. When rHuEPO was introduced into practice, a single study in rats raised concern that correction of anemia might lead to an accelerated loss of renal function in CKD patients.[304] Subsequent studies in humans with CKD, however, failed to show any effect of anemia treatment on the rate of progression of renal failure,[305-308] and these findings were confirmed in a rigorous study using the remnant kidney model.[309] A more recent prospective clinical trial suggests that partial correction of anemia with rHuEPO can retard the progression of renal disease, particularly in nondiabetics.[310] Patients with mild to moderate CKD (serum creatinine ranging from 2.0 to 4.0 mg/dL) and a hematocrit less than 30% were randomized to maintain their baseline hematocrit or receive treatment with rHuEPO. The latter group had a baseline average hematocrit of 27.0%, which rose to 32.1% over the course of the study. Other aspects of medical management were identical in the two patient groups. Serum creatinine doubled in 84% of the CKD patients who remained anemic versus only 52% of those whose anemia was treated with rHuEPO. Jungers and colleagues measured the rate of decline of creatinine clearance in CKD patients maintained anemic (hemoglobin ≈10 g/dL) and compared them with patients whose anemia was treated with rHuEPO (hemoglobin ≈11.3 g/dL).[311] The latter group of patients had a significantly slower rate of decline in renal function when compared with the former group. Most recently, the RENAAL study (Reduction in Endpoints in Non–Insulin Dependent Diabetes Mellitus with the Angiotensin II Antagonist Losartan), a prospective, long-term clinical trial of type 2 diabetics with nephropathy (n = 1513; serum creatinine, 1.9 ± 0.5 mg/dL; albumin/creatinine ratio, 7.1 ± 1.0 mg/g; follow-up, average of 3.4 years), evaluated the baseline hemoglobin concentration as a risk factor for a poor renal outcome. In this analysis, the baseline hemoglobin concentration was independently associated with a poor renal outcome, either time to ESRD or time to the combined end point of ESRD or doubling of serum creatinine from the baseline value. After adjustment for covariates, each quartile (reference hemoglobin >13.8 g/dL) showed an increased risk for a poor outcome when compared with the reference group, thus suggesting that prevention or amelioration of anemia may lessen the risk for progression to ESRD in these patients.[312]

BLOOD RHEOLOGY/HEMOSTASIS/OXIDATIVE EFFECTS. Data on the potential effects of normalization of hemoglobin on vascular access clotting are limited (generic coagulation-related issues related to rHuEPO treatment are reviewed elsewhere in this contribution). Besarab and associates found a significant increase in vascular access thrombosis, in autologous arteriovenous fistulas as well as synthetic grafts, in patients randomized to a higher hemoglobin concentration.[93] In the Spanish study of hemoglobin normalization, however, no such increase in access clotting was observed.[263] The effects of normalization of hemoglobin on blood rheology and hemostasis have only recently been examined.[313-315] Thirty-nine patients with normal hematocrit (42%) were studied, but no significant changes in RBC aggregation or deformability were observed during a hemodialysis session.[313, 314] In a study from Sweden, hemostatic parameters (prothrombin complex test, activated partial thromboplastin time, platelet aggregation and retention, von Willebrand factor antigen, antithrombin, protein C, total and free protein S, activated protein C resistance, factor V-Leiden mutation, D-dimers, plasminogen activator inhibitor-1, and prothrombin fragments 1 and 2) were examined in a group of CKD patients before and after normalization of hemoglobin with rHuEPO.[315] The only statistically significant finding was a

transient decrease in total levels of protein S. Finally, complete correction of anemia in hemodialysis patients has been associated with a significant increase in whole-blood antioxidant capacity, indicative of a positive effect on free radical metabolism.[316]

It is clear that the base of evidence to adequately assess the benefits and risks of normalization of hemoglobin in CKD patients is still insufficient. Although considerable data continue to build and suggest that such an approach might lead to improved patient outcomes, the high cost of treatment and the possible complications of therapy have not been thoroughly assessed. At present it seems prudent to base the treatment of most patients on guideline recommendations from the National Kidney Foundation or the Canadian or European guideline groups, given the clear improvement in a wide variety of outcomes with progressive increases in hemoglobin.[14, 62, 63, 249, 250] Individualization of treatment, however, remains the cornerstone of the art of medicine and should be applied to the treatment of anemia so that patients who might benefit from normalization of hemoglobin are so treated.[317-320]

PHARMACOECONOMIC AND ESRD PROGRAM–RELATED ISSUES IN rHuEPO TREATMENT

After approval of rHuEPO by the U.S. FDA in 1989, the HCFA (now the Center for Medicare and Medicaid Services [CMS]), an agency in the Department of Health and Human Services, was responsible for developing an appropriate policy for its reimbursement. Several key issues in this regard immediately became apparent and have been addressed in numerous publications,[321-325] along with additional discussions regarding the pharmacoeconomics of rHuEPO therapy.[326-332] These issues and their resolution in subsequent policy have had a direct bearing on the day-to-day use of rHuEPO and have shaped standard practice in the correction of anemia.

Several alternative payment approaches are available for the use of any pharmaceutical given during dialysis, including a fixed rate per treatment independent of the dose used, inclusion in the composite rate (the payment that CMS offers as a flat reimbursement for the cost of each dialysis treatment), and payment according to a fee schedule.[322] The initial approach to payment for rHuEPO was a fixed rate per treatment, with $40 paid to dialysis facilities for a dose of 10,000 U or less and $70 paid for a dose *greater* than 10,000 U.[321] These payments were to cover the cost of the medication, but not its administration, which according to the CMS was already being addressed by the facility composite rate for dialysis treatments. At that time the list price to wholesalers was stated to be $10 per 1000 U.[321] The fixed payment per treatment in this fashion created the possibility of encouraging providers to limit dosing because even a single unit of rHuEPO would be reimbursed at $40. In the first year of Medicare coverage for rHuEPO, Medicare paid $144,000,000 for this therapy to dialysis providers,[333] but hemoglobin levels remained below recommended targets, and lower than expected rHuEPO doses were provided.[323] Providers explained that because Medicare paid only 80% of the allowed charges ($32 or $56, respectively, depending on the dose administered), it did not cover administration costs, and because a slower rise in hemoglobin was medically desirable, they used lower than anticipated doses. Medicare, however, thought that this practice resulted in a large profit margin for providers and that it was this profit margin, not the quality of care, that was the primary driver for the providers. This policy was further complicated by the fact that patients had to have a hematocrit less than 30% for reimbursable therapy to be initiated and that no payment would be made if it exceeded 36%. Finally, because self-administration of medications is not reimbursable by Medicare, home dialysis patients had to receive rHuEPO in the physician's office or dialysis center.

Starting in January 1991, this payment policy was changed. Payment was made on a per-unit basis linked to a fee schedule, with an initial approved rate of $11 per 1000 U administered.[324] The actual cost of acquisition by providers varied, depending on contractual arrangements with the manufacturer. This policy created conflicting incentives, with overuse encouraged on the one hand under the assumption that acquisition costs were less than reimbursement amounts, whereas the need to avoid excessively high hematocrit levels, which would result in no reimbursement, encouraged underuse. A careful analysis of the effects of the payment change showed that in the 6 months after its implementation, the dose of rHuEPO increased over 14%, the hematocrit increased just 0.2% to 0.3%, and the allowed charges for rHuEPO rose.[324] In addition, patients treated at for-profit facilities had lower rHuEPO doses before the change in policy and higher doses after the change in policy than patients in non-profit facilities did.[324] These findings illustrate the important influence of payment policy on clinical practice in this area.

Subsequent payment policy decisions again demonstrated their powerful influence on clinical practice with introduction of the initial hematocrit management audit (HMA) system by the CMS in 1996.[325] In response to concerns regarding lack of payment for rHuEPO if the hematocrit exceeded 36% and as an acknowledgement of the biologic variability in hematocrit values among patients, as well as fluctuations in an individual patient over time, the CMS implemented the use of a 3-month rolling average hematocrit exceeding 36.5% as the trigger to deny payment for rHuEPO for the entire month of treatment. The effect of this policy was both predictable and chilling. Providers concerned about lack of payment for rHuEPO began to reduce dosing to be certain that the hematocrit remained within limits. Average doses fell, as did the average hematocrit. The fraction of patients with severe anemia (hematocrit <30%) rose concomitantly.[334] In response to clear evidence of the negative impact of this policy and after considerable input from providers, the policy was changed. The 3-month rolling average hematocrit remained, but a level of 37.5% was set as the upper limit, and unlike the previous policy of withholding payment if the upper limit was exceeded, under the new policy, payment would still be made, but a "post-payment review" could be undertaken at the discretion of the local insurance carrier contracted to pay the claims on behalf of Medicare. The result of this policy revision has been a steady rise in rHuEPO doses and mean hematocrit. Despite this improvement, however, it is clear that significant variability still remains in the hemoglobin levels achieved in dialysis patients,[335] which has been attributed to differences in the

target hemoglobin range and perception of the threshold for action, variability in anemia management approaches, and intrapatient variability.[335]

Payment policy for pharmaceuticals is best framed in the context of pharmacoeconomics, namely, what are the overall costs and benefits of a particular agent? Such an analysis is often difficult and has been particularly so for rHuEPO.[326] Although the direct costs of acquisition and administration are not difficult to quantify, the "costs" of other benefits and complications of rHuEPO therapy are more challenging to understand. For example, a complete pharmacoeconomic analysis of this hormone would consider the decrease in transfusion requirements and androgens with anemia treatment, improved quality of life, value of the lack of sensitization and delay in kidney transplantation, decrease in hospitalizations, and improved survival (the last of which includes more ongoing costs of dialysis and overall medical care).[327-330] The costs of parenteral iron, additional antihypertensives, and procedures to clear vascular access clotting must also be considered. When such studies were performed by Powe and colleagues[330] in the early years of experience with rHuEPO, they found that the total cost for treating with rHuEPO versus blood transfusions or androgens was substantial, highly sensitive to the dose of rHuEPO, moderately sensitive to response rates to rHuEPO and reduction in cardiovascular morbidity, and slightly sensitive to transfusion rates, among other factors. When a more rigorous analysis was performed by the same group[331] in which dialysis patients who received rHuEPO were compared with those who did not, they found that rHuEPO treatment was associated with a decrease in readmissions, overall admissions, hospital days, and cost to the hospital, thus suggesting that overall, Medicare may realize substantial savings when anemia is appropriately treated with rHuEPO.

Recent experience has underscored the validity of this assumption. During the 1990s, doses of rHuEPO began to rise, as did average hemoglobin levels. This trend accelerated after the publication of clinical practice guidelines on the management of anemia in which a target hemoglobin of 11 to 12 g/dL was recommended.[14, 249] An analysis of data from CMS claims files showed that patients with hematocrits ranging from 33% to 36% had lower Medicare-allowable expenditures per month than did those with hematocrits ranging from 30% to 33%.[332] Patients with hematocrits less than 30% had even higher expenditures. These findings suggested that treatment of anemia with rHuEPO could result in overall cost savings, primarily by decreasing hospitalization rates. These findings were expanded in a more recent cohort of patients.[336] Patients undergoing hemodialysis in 1996 to 1998 were studied and their medical costs evaluated, with a focus on patients with a hematocrit greater than 36%. Patients with a hematocrit greater than 36% had a 16% to 22% lower hospitalization rate than did those in the reference range (hematocrit of 33% to 36%). In addition, expenditures were 8.3% to 8.5% lower in patients in the higher hematocrit group. Whether the lower expenditures were causally related to the higher hematocrit achieved cannot be determined by an epidemiologic study of this nature, but additional studies in this area are certainly warranted.

Total Medicare expenditures for rHuEPO in 1999 exceeded $1 billion and have nearly doubled since 1995, and costs for adjunctive therapy with intravenous iron have increased by

65% over this same period.[337] As alluded to earlier, one approach to lowering the costs of rHuEPO is to administer the drug subcutaneously because of its significant dose-sparing effect in achieving equivalent hemoglobin levels.[14, 249, 250, 338] It has been estimated that this approach alone could save Medicare up to $144 million annually.[339] Of the many barriers to this approach at present, most recently concern has been expressed over the possible appearance of neutralizing antibodies to rHuEPO, which though uncommon, seem to be more likely when subcutaneous rather than intravenous administration is used.[244, 340]

A major driver of current patterns of rHuEPO use is related to the overall structure of the payment system to dialysis facilities for ESRD services, an area of great interest and concern to regulators and providers.[341-343] Composite rate payment, which began in 1983, was designed to include all nursing services, supplies, equipment, and drugs associated with a single dialysis session.[341] The amount of the payment has been modified only minimally since that time despite numerous technologic changes in the delivery of dialysis care and increasing costs of providing safe and adequate treatment. The composite rate payment does not include, however, payment for certain injectable medications (e.g., rHuEPO, iron, vitamin D), many laboratory tests, and blood and blood products. Recent analyses by the Medicare Payment Advisory Commission (Medpac), an independent federal body established by statute in 1997 to advise Congress on Medicare-related issues, clearly show that the current composite rate payment is inadequate to cover the cost of providing dialysis treatments for most facilities.[342] The financial viability of the facilities thus becomes dependent to a significant extent on the excess revenue generated from injectable drugs, most importantly, rHuEPO, for which acquisition costs are still considerably lower than the current allowable reimbursement rate (although only 80% of the latter is actually paid by Medicare). Medpac found that payment-to-cost ratios for composite rate services for in-center and home dialysis ranged from 0.86 to 1.00, depending on the size of the facility, profit status, and location, thus indicating that at best, facilities were able to break even (large facilities), but smaller, nonprofit, and rural facilities were losing considerable sums based only on the composite rate. When separately billable drugs were included in the analysis, payment-to-cost ratios rose and ranged from 0.97 to 1.07, with the same facility characteristics predictive of the level.[342] As is apparent from this analysis, facilities have an incentive to maximize the use of injectable drugs, including rHuEPO, thereby driving therapy that could preferentially recommend intravenous versus subcutaneous administration and conservative use of parenteral iron, with both approaches leading to higher rHuEPO use for a given target hemoglobin level.

It is of interest that when the payment for dialysis services includes injectable drugs in a bundled or case rate approach, their use decreases because they become a cost rather than a revenue generator (J.D. Dickmeyer, M.D., personal communication, August 2002). Medpac has recommended that such an approach be explored for the Medicare ESRD program,[341, 342] and a study is currently under way to better understand the implications of such an approach. It is clear that the payment system, no matter how it is constructed, has in the past and will in the future drive medical practice.[343] It is therefore essential to have an ongoing assessment of relevant outcomes of anemia management to ensure that current medical practice remains focused on the highest quality of care for patients.

REFERENCES

1. Eschbach JW, Adamson JW: Anemia of end-stage renal disease (ESRD). Kidney Int 28:1-5, 1985.
2. Loge JP, Lange RD, Moore CV: Characterization of the anemia associated with chronic renal insufficiency. Am J Med 24:4-18, 1958.
3. Weed R: The red cell membrane in hemolytic disorders. Semin Hematol 7:249-258, 1970.
4. Pasternak A, Wahlberg P: Bone marrow in acute renal failure. Acta Med Scand 4:33-45, 1967.
5. Radtke HW, Rege AB, Lamarche B, et al: Identification of spermine as an inhibitor of erythropoiesis in patients with chronic renal failure. J Clin Invest 67:1623-1629, 1981.
6. Massry SG: Is parathyroid hormone an uremic toxin? Nephron 19;125-130, 1977.
7. Erslev AJ, Besarab A: The rate and control of baseline red cell production in hematologically stable patients with uremia. J Lab Clin Med 126:283-286, 1995.
8. Eschbach JW: The anemia of chronic renal failure: Pathophysiology and the effects of recombinant erythropoietin. Kidney Int 35:134-148, 1989.
9. McGonigle RJ, Wallin JD, Shadduck RK, Fisher JW: Erythropoietin deficiency and inhibition of erythropoiesis in renal insufficiency. Kidney Int 25:437-444, 1984.
10. Brittenham GM: Hematology II: Red blood cell function and disorders of iron metabolism. *In* Dale DC, Federman DD (eds): Medicine. New York, Scientific American, 1996, pp 1-18.
11. Spivak JL: Iron and the anemia of chronic disease. Oncology 16:25-33, 2002.
12. Papayannopoulou T, Finch CA: Radioiron measurements of red cell maturation. Blood Cells 1:535-544, 1975.
13. Besarab A, Frinak S, Yee J: An indistinct balance: The safety and efficacy of parenteral iron therapy. J Am Soc Nephrol 10:2029-2043, 1999.
14. National Kidney Foundation: K/DOQI Clinical Practice Guidelines for Anemia of Chronic Kidney Disease, 2000. Am J Kidney Dis 37(suppl 1):182-238, 2001.
15. Cheung JY, Miller BA: Molecular mechanisms of erythropoietin signaling. Nephron 87:215-222, 2001.
16. Kieran MW, Perkins AC, Orkin SH, Zon LI: Thrombopoietin rescues in vitro erythroid formation from mouse embryos lacking the erythropoietin receptor. Proc Natl Acad Sci U S A 93:9126-9131, 1996.
17. Lin CH, Lim SK, D'Agati VG, Costantini F: Differential effects of an erythropoietin receptor gene disruption on primitive and definitive erythropoiesis. Genes Dev 10:154-164, 1996.
18. Noguchi CT, Bae KS, Chin K, et al: Cloning of the human erythropoietin receptor gene. Blood 78:2548-2556, 1991.
19. Broudy VC, Lin N, Brice N, et al: Erythropoietin receptor characteristics on primary human erythroid cells. Blood 77:2583-2590, 1991.
20. Wu H, Liu X, Jaenisch R, Lodish HF: Generation of committed erythroid BFU-E and CFU-E progenitors does not require erythropoietin or the erythropoietin receptor. Cell 83:59-67, 1995.
21. Fisher JW: Erythropoietin: Physiology and pharmacology update. Exp Biol Med 228:1-14, 2003.
22. Neubauer H, Cumano A, Muller M, et al: Jak2 deficiency defines an essential developmental checkpoint in definitive hematopoiesis. Cell 93:397-409, 1998.
23. Carroll MP, Spivak JL, McMahon M, et al: Erythropoietin induces Raf-1 activation is required for erythropoietin-mediated proliferation. J Biol Chem 266:14964-14969, 1991.
24. Fujitani Y, Hibi M, Fukada Y, et al: An alternative pathway for STAT activation that is mediated by the direct interaction between JAK and STAT. Oncogene 14:751-761, 1997.
25. Nagata Y, Kiefer F, Watanabe T, Todokoro K: Activation of hematopoietic progenitor kinase-1 by erythropoietin. Blood 93:3347-3354, 1999.
26. Weiss MJ, Keller G, Orkin SH: Novel insights into erythroid development revealed through in vitro differentiation of GATA-1 embryonic stem cell. Genes Dev 8:1184-1197, 1994.

27. Condorelli G, Vitelli L, Valtieri M, et al: Coordinate expression and developmental role of Id2 protein and TAL-E2A heterodimer in erythroid progenitor differentiation. Blood 86:164-175, 1995.
28. Bondurant MC, Yamashita T, Muta K, et al: *c-myc* expression affects proliferation but not terminal differentiation or survival of explanted erythroid progenitor cells. J Cell Physiol 168:255-263, 1996.
29. Misti J, Spivak LJ: Erythropoiesis in vitro. Role of calcium. J Clin Invest 64:1573-1579, 1979.
30. Mladenovic J, Kay NE: Erythropoietin induces rapid increases in intracellular free calcium in human bone marrow cells. J Lab Clin Med 112:23-27, 1988.
31. Miller BA, Cheung JY, Tillotson DL, et al: Erythropoietin stimulates a rise in intracellular-free calcium concentration in single BFU-E derived erythroblasts at specific stages of differentiation. Blood 73:1188-1194, 1989.
32. Sawyer ST, Krantz SB: Erythropoietin stimulates $^{45}Ca^{2+}$ uptake in Friend virus–infected erythroid cells. J Biol Chem 259:2769-2774, 1984.
33. Gillo B, Ma Y-S, Marks AR: Calcium influx in induced differentiation of murine erythroleukemia cells. Blood 81:783-792, 1993.
34. Cheung JY, Elensky MB, Brauneis U, et al: Ion channels in human erythroblasts. Modulation by erythropoietin. J Clin Invest 90:1850-1856, 1992.
35. Schaefer A, Magocsi M, Stocker U, et al: Ca^{2+}/calmodulin-dependent and -independent down-regulation of c-myb mRNA levels in erythropoietin-responsive murine erythroleukemia cells. The role of calcineurin. J Biol Chem 271:13484-13490, 1996.
36. Ge RL, Witkowski S, Zhang Y, et al: Determinants of erythropoietin release in response to short-term hypobaric hypoxia. J Appl Physiol 92:2361-2367, 2002.
37. Levine BD: Intermittent hypoxic training: Fact and fancy. High Alt Med Biol 3:177-193, 2002.
38. Bosman DR, Osborne CA, Marsden JT, et al: Erythropoietin response to hypoxia in patients with diabetic autonomic neuropathy and non-diabetic chronic renal failure. Diabet Med 19:65-69, 2002.
39. Ema M, Taya S, Yokotani N, et al: A novel bHLH-PAS factor with close sequence similarity to hypoxia-inducible factor 1α regulates the VEGF expression and is potentially involved in lung and vascular development. Proc Natl Acad Sci U S A 94:4273-4278, 1997.
40. Ivan M, Kondo K, Yang H, et al: HIFα targeted for VHL-mediated destruction by proline hydroxylation: Implications for O_2 sensing. Science 292:464-468, 2001.
41. Epstein ACR, Gleadle JM, McNeill LA, et al: *C. elegans* EGL-9 and mammalian homologs define a family of dioxygenases that regulate HIF by prolyl hydroxylation. Cell 107:43-54, 2001.
42. Rosenberger C, Mandriota S, Jurgensen JS, et al: Expression of hypoxia-inducible factor-1alpha and -2alpha in hypoxic and ischemic rat kidneys. J Am Soc Nephrol 13:1721-1732, 2002.
43. Bright R: Cases and observations, illustrative of renal disease accompanied with the secretion of albuminous urine. Guys Hosp Rep 1:338-400, 1836.
44. Erslev AJ: The discovery of erythropoietin. ASAIO J 39:89-92, 1993.
45. Eschbach JW: The history of renal anaemia (anaemia and erythropoietin). Nephrology 4:279-287, 1998.
46. Reissmann KR: Studies on the mechanism of erythropoietic stimulation in parabiotic rats during hypoxia. Blood 5:372-380, 1950.
47. Erslev AJ: Humoral regulation of red cell production. Blood 8:349-357, 1953.
48. Jacobson LO, Goldwasser E, Fried W, Pizak L: Role of the kidney in erythropoiesis. Nature 179:633-634, 1957.
49. Adamson JW: The erythropoietin/hematocrit relationship in normal and polycythemic man: Implications for marrow regulation. Blood 32:597-609, 1968.
50. Erslev AJ: Renal biogenesis of erythropoietin. Am J Med 58:25-30, 1975.
51. Miyake T, Kung CK-H, Goldwasser E: Purification of human erythropoietin. J Biol Chem 252:5558-5564, 1977.
52. Koury ST, Bondurant MC, Koury MJ: Localization of erythropoietin synthesizing cells in murine kidneys by in situ hybridization. Blood 71:524-527, 1988.
53. Lacombe C, DaSilva J-L, Bariety J, et al: Peritubular cells are the site of erythropoietin synthesis in the murine hypoxic kidney. J Clin Invest 81:620-623, 1988.
54. Eckardt K-U: Erythropoietin production in liver and kidneys. Curr Opin Nephrol Hypertens 5:28-34, 1996.

55. Eschbach JW, Adamson JW, Anderson RG, Dennis MB Jr: Anemia of chronic renal failure: studies of marrow regulation in the uremic sheep. Trans Am Soc Artif Intern Organs 18:295-300, 1972.
56. Eschbach JW, Mladenovic J, Garcia JF, et al: The anemia of chronic renal failure in sheep. Response to erythropoietin-rich plasma in vivo. J Clin Invest 74:434-441, 1984.
57. Lin FK, Suggs S, Lin CH, et al: Cloning and expression of the human erythropoietin gene. Proc Natl Acad Sci U S A 82:7580-7584, 1985.
58. Egrie JC, Strickland TW, Lane J, et al: Characterization and biological effects of recombinant human erythropoietin. Immunobiology 72:213-224, 1986.
59. Eschbach JW, Egrie JC, Downing MR, et al: Correction of the anemia of end-stage renal disease with recombinant human erythropoietin. Results of a combined phase I and II clinical trial. N Engl J Med 316:73-78, 1987.
60. Eschbach JW, Abdulhadi MH, Browne JK, et al: Recombinant human erythropoietin in anemic patients with end-stage renal disease. Results of a phase III multicenter clinical trial. Ann Intern Med 111:992-1000, 1989.
61. National Kidney Foundation: K/DOQI clinical practice guidelines for chronic kidney disease: Evaluation, classification, and stratification. Kidney Disease Outcome Quality Initiative. Am J Kidney Dis 39(2)[suppl 1]:1-246, 2002.
62. European best practice guidelines for the management of anaemia in patients with chronic renal failure. Working Party for European Best Practice Guidelines for the Management of Anaemia in Patients with Chronic Renal Failure. Nephrol Dial Transplant 14(suppl 5):1-50, 1999.
63. Clinical practice guidelines for management of anemia coexistent with chronic renal failure. Canadian Society of Nephrology. J Am Soc Nephrol 10(suppl 13):292-296, 1999.
64. Macdougall I: Present and future strategies in the treatment of renal anemia. Nephrol Dial Transplant 16(suppl 5):50-55, 2001.
65. Besarab A, Levin A: Defining a renal anemia management period. Am J Kidney Dis 36(suppl 3):13-23, 2000.
66. Egrie J: The cloning and production of recombinant human erythropoietin. Pharmacotherapy 10(suppl 2):3-8, 1990.
67. Storring PL, Tiplady RJ, Gaines Das RE, et al: Epoetin alfa and beta differ in their erythropoietin isoform compositions and biological properties. Br J Haematol 100:79-89, 1998.
68. Macdougall IC, Roberts DE, Coles GA, Williams JD: Clinical pharmacokinetics of epoetin (recombinant human erythropoietin) Clin Pharmacokinet 20(2):99-113, 1991.
69. Salmonson T: Pharmacokinetic and pharmacodynamic studies on recombinant human erythropoietin. J Urol Nephrol 29(suppl 1):1-66, 1990.
70. Halstenson CE, Macres M, Katz SA, et al: Comparative pharmacokinetics and pharmacodynamics of epoetin alfa and epoetin beta. Clin Pharmacol Ther 50:702-712, 1991.
71. Sikole A, Spasovski G, Zafirov D, Polenakovic M: Epoetin omega for treatment of anemia in maintenance hemodialysis patients. Clin Nephrol 57:237-245, 2002.
72. Bren A, Kandus A, Varl J, Buturovic J, Ponikvar R, Kveder R, Primozic S, Ivanovich P: A comparison between epoetin omega and epoetin alfa in the correction of anemia in hemodialysis patients: A prospective, controlled crossover study, Artif Organs 26(2):91-97, 2002.
73. Egrie JC, Browne JK: Development and characterization of novel erythropoiesis stimulating protein (NESP). Nephrol Dial Transplant 16(suppl 3):3-13, 2001.
74. Macdougall IC: Darbepoetin alfa: A new therapeutic agent for renal anemia. Kidney Int Suppl 80:55-61, 2002.
75. Macdougall IC, Gray SJ, Elston O, et al: Pharmacokinetics of novel erythropoiesis stimulating protein compared with epoetin alfa in dialysis patients. J Am Soc Nephrol 10:2392-2395, 1999.
76. Locatelli F, Olivares J, Walker R, et al: Novel erythropoiesis stimulating protein for treatment of anemia in chronic renal insufficiency. Kidney Int 60:741-747, 2001.
77. Nissenson A: Novel erythropoiesis stimulating protein for managing the anemia of chronic kidney disease. Am J Kidney Dis 38:1390-1397, 2001.
78. Nissenson A, Swan S, Lindberg JS, et al: Randomized, controlled trial of darbepoetin alfa for the treatment of anemia in hemodialysis patients. Am J Kidney Dis 40:110-118, 2002.
79. Macdougall IC, Matcham J, Gray SJ: Correction of anaemia with darbepoetin alfa in patients with chronic kidney disease receiving dialysis. Nephrol Dial Transplant 18:576-581, 2003.

80. Locatelli F, Canaud B, Giacardy F, et al: Treatment of anaemia in dialysis patients with unit dosing of darbepoetin alfa at a reduced dose frequency relative to recombinant human erythropoietin (rHuEPO). Nephrol Dial Transplant 18:362-369, 2003.

81. Macdougall IC: An overview of the efficacy and safety of novel erythropoiesis stimulating protein (NESP). Nephrol Dial Transplant 16(suppl 3):14-21, 2001.

82. Kausz AT, Watkins SL, Hansen C, et al: Intraperitoneal erythropoietin in children on peritoneal dialysis: A study of pharmacokinetics and efficacy. Am J Kidney Dis 34:651-656, 1999.

83. Eschbach JW, Haley NR, Adamson JW: The use of recombinant erythropoietin in the treatment of the anemia of chronic renal failure. N Y Acad Sci 554:225-230, 1989.

84. Besarab A, Kaiser JW, Frinak S: A study of parenteral iron regimens in hemodialysis patients. Am J Kidney Dis 34(1):21-28, 1999.

85. Neff MS, Kim KE, Persoff M, et al: Hemodynamics of uremic anemia. Circulation 43:876-883, 1971.

86. Vaziri ND: Mechanism of erythropoietin-induced hypertension. Am J Kidney Dis 33:821-828, 1999.

87. Sunder-Plassman G, Horl WH: Effect of erythropoietin on cardiovascular diseases. Am J Kidney Dis 38(suppl 1):20-25, 2001.

88. Shinaberger JH, Miller JH, Gardner PW: Erythropoietin alert: Risks of high hematocrit hemodialysis. ASAIO Trans 34:179-184, 1988.

89. Movilli E, Cancarini GC, Mombelloni S, et al: The role of hematocrit in efficiency of dialysis. Blood Purif 8(4):183-189, 1990.

90. Schaefer RM, Schaefer L: Treatment with erythropoietin and loss of dialyser clearance. Nephrol Dial Transplant 11(suppl 2):81-82, 1996.

91. Delano BG, Lundin AP, Galonsky R, et al: Dialyzer urea and creatinine clearances are not significantly altered in erythropoietin treated maintenance hemodialysis patients. ASAIO Trans 36:36-39, 1990.

92. Lim VS, Flanigan MJ, Fangman J: Effect of hematocrit on solute removal during high efficiency hemodialysis. Kidney Int 7:1557-1562, 1990.

93. Besarab A, Bolton WK, Browne JK, et al: The effects of normal as compared with low hematocrit values in patients with cardiac disease who are receiving hemodialysis and epoetin. N Engl J Med 339:584-590, 1998.

94. Fishbane S, Maesaka JK: Iron management in end-stage renal disease. Am J Kidney Dis 29:319-333, 1997.

95. Hallberg L, Ryttinger L, Solvell L: Side-effects of oral iron therapy. A double-blind study of different iron compounds in tablet form. Acta Med Scand Suppl 459:3-10, 1966.

96. Macdougall IC, Tucker B, Thompson J, et al: A randomized controlled study of iron supplementation in patients treated with erythropoietin. Kidney Int 50:1694-1699, 1996.

97. Wingard RL, Parker RA, Ismail N, Hakim RM: Efficacy of oral iron therapy in patients receiving recombinant human erythropoietin. Am J Kidney Dis 25:433-439, 1995.

98. Markowitz GS, Kahn GA, Feingold RE, et al: An evaluation of the effectiveness of oral iron therapy in hemodialysis patients receiving recombinant human erythropoietin. Clin Nephrol 48:34-40, 1997.

99. Fudin R, Jaichenko J, Shostak A, et al: Correction of uremic iron deficiency anemia in hemodialyzed patients: A prospective study. Nephron 79:299-305, 1998.

100. Eisen SA, Miller DK, Woodward RS, et al: The effect of prescribed daily dose frequency on patient medication compliance. Arch Intern Med 150:1881-1884, 1990.

101. Donnelly SM, Posen GA, Ali MA: Oral iron absorption in hemodialysis patients treated with erythropoietin. Clin Invest Med 14:271-276, 1991.

102. Monsen ER, Cook JD: Food iron absorption in human subjects. IV: The effects of calcium and phosphate salts on the absorption of nonheme iron. Am J Clin Nutr 29:1142-1148, 1976.

103. Grebe G, Martinez-Torres C, Layrisse M: Effect of meals and ascorbic acid on the absorption of a therapeutic dose of iron as ferrous and ferric salts. Curr Ther Res Clin Exp 17:382-397, 1975.

104. Brise H, Hallberg L: Iron absorption studies. Acta Med Scand 171:1-5, 1962.

105. Baird IM, Walters RL, Sutton DR: Absorption of slow-release iron and effects of ascorbic acid in normal subjects and after partial gastrectomy. BMJ 4:505-508, 1974.

106. Fishbane S, Frei GL, Maesaka J: Reduction in recombinant human erythropoietin doses by the use of chronic intravenous iron supplementation. Am J Kidney Dis 26:41-46, 1995.

107. Sunder-Plassmann G, Horl WH: Importance of iron supply for erythropoietin therapy. Nephrol Dial Transplant 10:2070-2076, 1995.

108. Taylor JE, Peat N, Porter C, Morgan AG: Regular low-dose intravenous iron therapy improves response to erythropoietin in haemodialysis patients. Nephrol Dial Transplant 11:1079-1083, 1996.

109. Fishbane S, Mittal SK, Maesaka JK: Beneficial effects of iron therapy in renal failure patients on hemodialysis. Kidney Int Suppl 69:67-70, 1999.

110. Fishbane S, Lynn RI: The efficacy of iron dextran for the treatment of iron deficiency in hemodialysis patients. Clin Nephrol 44:238-240, 1995.

111. Besarab A, Amin N, Ahsan M, et al: Optimization of epoetin therapy with intravenous iron therapy in hemodialysis patients. J Am Soc Nephrol 11:530-538, 2000.

112. Kato A, Hamada M, Suzuki T, et al: Effect of weekly or successive iron supplementation on erythropoietin doses in patients receiving hemodialysis. Nephron 89:110-112, 2001.

113. Bolanos L, Castro P, Falcon TG, et al: Continuous intravenous sodium ferric gluconate improves efficacy in the maintenance phase of EPOrHu administration in hemodialysis patients. Am J Nephrol 22:67-72, 2002.

114. Milman N, Christensen TE, Bartels U, Pedersen NS: Iron status in patients undergoing regular peritoneal dialysis. Dan Med Bull 27:291-295, 1980.

115. Milman N, Christensen TE, Pedersen NS, Visfeldt J: Serum ferritin and bone marrow iron in non-dialysis, peritoneal dialysis and hemodialysis patients with chronic renal failure. Acta Med Scand 207:201-205, 1980.

116. Jonnalagadda V, Bloom EJ, Raja RM: Importance of iron saturation for erythropoietin responsiveness in chronic peritoneal dialysis. Adv Perit Dial 13:113-115, 1997.

117. Ahsan N, Groff JA, Waybill MA: Efficacy of bolus intravenous iron dextran treatment in peritoneal dialysis patients receiving recombinant human erythropoietin. Adv Perit Dial 12:161-166, 1996.

118. Auerbach M, Witt D, Toler W, et al: Clinical use of the total dose intravenous infusion of iron dextran. J Lab Clin Med 111:566-570, 1998.

119. Michael B, Coyne DW, Fishbane S, et al: Sodium ferric gluconate complex in hemodialysis patients: Adverse reactions compared to placebo and iron dextran. Kidney Int 61:1830-1839, 2002.

120. Faich G, Strobos J: Sodium ferric gluconate complex in sucrose: Safer intravenous iron therapy than iron dextrans. Am J Kidney Dis 33:464-470, 1999.

121. Ring J, Messmer K: Incidence and severity of anaphylactoid reactions to colloid volume substitutes. Lancet 1:466-469, 1977.

122. Fishbane S, Ungureanu VD, Maesaka JK, et al: The safety of intravenous iron dextran in hemodialysis patients. Am J Kidney Dis 28:529-534, 1996.

123. Novey HS, Pahl M, Haydik I, Vaziri ND: Immunologic studies of anaphylaxis to iron dextran in patients on renal dialysis. Ann Allergy 72:224-228, 1994.

124. Ljungstrom KG, Renck H, Hedin H, et al: Hapten inhibition and dextran anaphylaxis. Anaesthesia 43:729-732, 1988.

125. Charytan C, Levin N, Al-Saloum M, et al: Efficacy and safety of iron sucrose for iron deficiency in patients with dialysis-associated anemia: North American clinical trial. Am J Kidney Dis 37:300-307, 2001.

126. Package insert: Ferrlecit, sodium ferric gluconate complex in sucrose injection. 62.5 mg/5 mL.

127. Package insert: Venofer iron sucrose injection.

128. Rogers JT, Bridges KR, Durmowicz GP, et al: Translational control during the acute phase response. Ferritin synthesis in response to interleukin-1. J Biol Chem 265:14572-14578, 1990.

129. Fishbane S, Kowalski EA, Imbriano LJ, Maesaka JK: The evaluation of iron status in hemodialysis patients. J Am Soc Nephrol 7:2654-2657, 1996.

130. Kalantar-Zadeh K, Hoffken B, Wunsch H, et al: Diagnosis of iron deficiency anemia in renal failure patients during the post-erythropoietin era. Am J Kidney Dis 26:292-299, 1995.

131. Rahmati MA, Craig RG, Homel P, et al: Serum markers of periodontal disease status and inflammation in hemodialysis patients. Am J Kidney Dis 40:983-989, 2002.

132. Owen WF, Lowrie EG: C-reactive protein as an outcome predictor for maintenance hemodialysis patients. Kidney Int 54:627-636, 1998.

133. Fishbane S, Shapiro W, Dutka P, et al: A randomized trial of iron deficiency testing strategies in hemodialysis patients. Kidney Int 60:2406-2411, 2001.

134. Macdougall IC: What is the most appropriate strategy to monitor functional iron deficiency in the dialysed patient on rhEPO therapy? Merits of percentage hypochromic red cells as a marker of functional iron deficiency. Nephrol Dial Transplant 13:847-849, 1998.

135. Tessitore N, Solero GP, Lippi G, et al: The role of iron status markers in predicting response to intravenous iron in haemodialysis patients on maintenance erythropoietin. Nephrol Dial Transplant 16:1416-1423, 2001.

136. Olivieri O, de Franceschi L, de Gironcoli M, et al: Potassium loss and cellular dehydration of stored erythrocytes following incubation in autologous plasma: Role of the KCl cotransport system. Vox Sang 65:95-102, 1993.

137. Cullen P, Soffker J, Hopfl M, et al: Hypochromic red cells and reticulocyte haemglobin content as markers of iron-deficient erythropoiesis in patients undergoing chronic haemodialysis. Nephrol Dial Transplant 14:659-665, 1999.

138. Fishbane S, Galgano C, Langley RC Jr, et al: Reticulocyte hemoglobin content in the evaluation of iron status of hemodialysis patients. Kidney Int 52:217-222, 1997.

139. Groom AC, Song SH, Campling B: Clearance of red blood cells from the vascular bed of skeletal muscle with particular reference to reticulocytes. Microvasc Res 6:51-62, 1973.

140. Mittman N, Sreedhara R, Mushnick R, et al: Reticulocyte hemoglobin content predicts functional iron deficiency in hemodialysis patients receiving rHuEPO. Am J Kidney Dis 30:912-922, 1997.

141. Schaefer RM, Bahner U: Iron metabolism in rhEPO-treated hemodialysis patients. Clin Nephrol 53(suppl):65-68, 2000.

142. Nassar GM, Fishbane S, Ayus JC: Occult infection of old nonfunctioning arteriovenous grafts: A novel cause of erythropoietin resistance and chronic inflammation in hemodialysis patients. Kidney Int Suppl 80:49-54, 2002.

143. Gunnell J, Yeun JY, Depner TA, Kaysen GA: Acute-phase response predicts erythropoietin resistance in hemodialysis and peritoneal dialysis patients. Am J Kidney Dis 33:63-72, 1999.

144. Fuchs D, Hausen A, Reibnegger G, et al: Immune activation and the anaemia associated with chronic inflammatory disorders. Eur J Haematol 46(2):65-70, 1991.

145. Peterson DA, Gerrard JM: Evidence that the peroxidase of the fatty acid cyclooxygenase acts via a Fenton type reaction. Prostaglandins Leukot Med 12:73-76, 1983.

146. Moirand R, Adams PC, Bicheler V, et al: Clinical features of genetic hemochromatosis in women compared with men. Ann Intern Med 127:105-110, 1997.

147. Bullen JJ, Ward CG, Wallis SN: Virulence and the role of iron in *Pseudomonas aeruginosa* infection. Infect Immun 10:443-450, 1974.

148. Rogers HJ, Bullen JJ, Cushnie GH: Iron compounds and resistance to infection. Further experiments with *Clostridium welchii* type A in vivo and in vitro. Immunology 19:521-538, 1970.

149. Lin SH, Shieh SD, Lin YF, et al: Fatal *Aeromonas hydrophila* bacteremia in a hemodialysis patient treated with deferoxamine. Am J Kidney Dis 27:733-735, 1996.

150. Boelaert JR, Fenves AZ, Coburn JW: Deferoxamine therapy and mucormycosis in dialysis patients: Report of an international registry. Am J Kidney Dis 18:660-667, 1991.

151. Hoen B, Paul-Dauphin A, Hestin D, Kessler M: EPIBACDIAL: A multicenter prospective study of risk factors for bacteremia in chronic hemodialysis patients. J Am Soc Nephrol 9:869-876, 1998.

152. Kessler M, Hoen B, Mayeux D, et al: Bacteremia in patients on chronic hemodialysis. A multicenter prospective survey. Nephron 64:95-100, 1993.

153. Hoen B, Kessler M, Hestin D, Mayeux D: Risk factors for bacterial infections in chronic haemodialysis adult patients: A multicentre prospective survey. Nephrol Dial Transplant 10:377-381, 1995.

154. Tielemans CL, Lenclud CM, Wens R, et al: Critical role of iron overload in the increased susceptibility of haemodialysis patients to bacterial infections. Beneficial effects of desferrioxamine. Nephrol Dial Transplant 4:883-887, 1989.

155. Canziani ME, Yumiya ST, Rangel EB, et al: Risk of bacterial infection in patients under intravenous iron therapy: Dose versus length of treatment. Artif Organs 25:866-869, 2001.

156. Parkkinen J, von Bonsdorff L, Peltonen S, et al: Catalytically active iron and bacterial growth in serum of haemodialysis patients after i.v. iron-saccharate administration. Nephrol Dial Transplant 15:1827-1834, 2000.

157. Jean G, Charra B, Chazot C, et al: Risk factor analysis for long-term tunneled dialysis catheter–related bacteremias. Nephron 91:399-405, 2002.

158. Hoen B, Paul-Dauphin A, Kessler M: Intravenous iron administration does not significantly increase the risk of bacteremia in chronic hemodialysis patients. Clin Nephrol 57:457-461, 2002.

159. Welch KD, Davis TZ, Van Eden ME, Aust SD: Deleterious iron-mediated oxidation of biomolecules. Free Radic Biol Med 32:577-583, 2002.

160. Kooistra MP, Kersting S, Gosriwatana I, et al: Nontransferrin-bound iron in the plasma of haemodialysis patients after intravenous iron saccharate infusion. Eur J Clin Invest 32(suppl 1):36-41, 2002.

161. Rooyakkers TM, Stroes ES, Kooistra MP, et al: Ferric saccharate induces oxygen radical stress and endothelial dysfunction in vivo. Eur J Clin Invest 32(Suppl 1):9-16, 2002.

162. Zager RA, Johnson AC, Hanson SY, Wasse H: Parenteral iron formulations: A comparative toxicologic analysis and mechanisms of cell injury. Am J Kidney Dis 40:90-103, 2002.

163. Sullivan JL: Iron and the sex difference in heart disease risk. Lancet 1:1293-1294, 1981.

164. Parfrey PS, Foley RN: The clinical epidemiology of cardiac disease in chronic renal failure. J Am Soc Nephrol 10:1606-1615, 1999.

165. Salonen JT, Nyyssonen K, Korpela H, et al: High stored iron levels are associated with excess risk of myocardial infarction in eastern Finnish men. Circulation 86:803-811, 1992.

166. Magnusson MK, Sigfusson N, Sigvaldason H, et al: Low iron-binding capacity as a risk factor for myocardial infarction. Circulation 89:102-108, 1994.

167. Salonen JT, Nyyssonen K, Salonen R: Body iron stores and the risk of coronary heart disease. N Engl J Med 331:1159, 1994.

168. Klipstein-Grobusch K, Koster JF, Grobbee DE, et al: Serum ferritin and risk of myocardial infarction in the elderly: The Rotterdam Study. Am J Clin Nutr 69:1231-1236, 1999.

169. Tuomainen TP, Punnonen K, Nyyssonen K, Salonen JT: Association between body iron stores and the risk of acute myocardial infarction in men. Circulation 97:1461-1466, 1998.

170. Marniemi J, Jarvisalo J, Toikka T, et al: Blood vitamins, mineral elements and inflammation markers as risk factors of vascular and non-vascular disease mortality in an elderly population. Int J Epidemiol 27:799-807, 1998.

171. Kiechl S, Willeit J, Egger G, et al: Body iron stores and the risk of carotid atherosclerosis: Prospective results from the Bruneck study. Circulation 96:3300-3307, 1997.

172. Aronow WS, Ahn C: Three-year follow-up shows no association of serum ferritin levels with incidence of new coronary events in 577 persons aged > or = 62 years. Am J Cardiol 78:678-679, 1996.

173. Manttari M, Manninen V, Huttunen JK, et al: Serum ferritin and ceruloplasmin as coronary risk factors. Eur Heart J 15:1599-1603, 1994.

174. Frey GH, Krider DW: Serum ferritin and myocardial infarct. W V Med J 90:13-15, 1994.

175. Meytes D, Bogin E, Ma A, et al: Effect of parathyroid hormone on erythropoiesis. J Clin Invest 67:1263-1269, 1981.

176. Delwiche F, Garrity MJ, Powell JS, et al: Effect of parathyroid hormone on erythropoiesis. J Lab Clin Med 102:613-620, 1983.

177. Komatsuda A, Hirokawa M, Haseyama T, et al: Human parathyroid hormone does not influence human erythropoiesis in vitro. Nephrol Dial Transplant 13:2088-2091, 1998.

178. Basile C, Lacour B, Drueke T, et al: Parathyroid function and erythrocyte production in the rat. Miner Electrolyte Metab 7:197-206, 1982.

179. Rao DS, Shih MS, Mohini R: Effect of serum parathyroid hormone and bone marrow fibrosis on the response to erythropoietin in uremia. N Engl J Med 328:171-175, 1993.

180. Akiba T, Satayathum S, Akizawa T, et al: Effect of mineral metabolism management practices on hemoglobin concentration among hemodialysis patients in the dialysis outcomes and practice patterns study (DOPPS) [abstract]. J Am Soc Nephrol 13:425, 2002.

181. Rault R, Magnone M: The effect of parathyroidectomy on hematocrit and erythropoietin dose in patients on hemodialysis. ASAIO J 42:M901-M903, 1996.

182. Mandolfo S, Malberti F, Farina M, et al: Parathyroidectomy and response to erythropoietin in anemic patients with chronic renal failure. Nephrol Dial Transplant 13:2708-2709, 1998.

183. Gallieni M, Corsi C, Brancaccio D: Hyperparathyroidism and anemia in renal failure. Am J Nephrol 20:89-96, 2000.

184. Mohammed AK, Yee J, Frinak S, et al: Erythropoiesis and bone healing following parathyroidectomy in hemodialysis patients [abstract]. J Am Soc Nephrol 13:219, 2002.

185. Drueke TB, Eckardt K-U: Role of secondary hyperparathyroidism in erythropoietin resistance of chronic renal failure patients. Nephrol Dial Transplant 17(suppl 5):28-31, 2002.

186. Kcomt J, Sotelo C, Raja R: Influence of adynamic bone disease on responsiveness to recombinant human erythropoietin in peritoneal dialysis patients. Adv Perit Dial 16:294-296, 2000.

187. Albitar S, Genin R, Fen-Chong M, et al: High-dose alfacalcidol improves anaemia in patients on haemodialysis. Nephrol Dial Transplant 12:514-518, 1997.

188. Goicoechea M, Vazquez MI, Ruiz MA, et al: Intravenous calcitriol improves anaemia and reduces the need for erythropoietin in haemodialysis patients. Nephron 8:23-27, 1998.

189. Huber C, Frieden E: The inhibition of ferroxidase by trivalent and other metal ions. J Biol Chem 245:3979, 1970.

190. Mladenovic J: Aluminum inhibits erythropoiesis in vitro. J Clin Invest 81:1661-1665, 1988.

191. Trapp G: Plasma aluminum is bound to transferrin. Life Sci 33: 311-316, 1983.

192. Muirhead N, Hodsman AB, Hollomby DJ, Cordy PE: The role of aluminium and parathyroid hormone in haemodialysis patients. Nephrol Dial Transplant 6:342-345, 1991.

193. Grutzmacher P, Ehmer B, Messinger D, et al: Effect of aluminum overload on the bone marrow response to recombinant human erythropoietin. Contrib Nephrol 76:315-321, 1989.

194. Tomson CR, Edmunds ME, Chambers K, et al: Effect of recombinant human erythropoietin on erythropoiesis in homozygous sickle-cell anemia and renal failure. Nephrol Dial Transplant 7:817-821, 1992.

195. Steinberg MH: Erythropoietin in anemia of renal failure in sickle cell disease [letter]. N Engl J Med 324:1369-1370, 1991.

196. Roger SD, Macdougall IC, Thuraisingham RC, Raine AE: Erythropoietin in anemia of renal failure in sickle disease [letter]. N Engl J Med 325:1175-1176, 1991.

197. Fluck S, McKane W, Cairns T, et al: Chloramine-induced haemolysis presenting as erythropoietin resistance. Nephrol Dial Transplant 14:1687-1691, 1999.

198. Richardson D, Bartlett C, Goutcher E, et al: Erythropoietin resistance due to dialysate chloramine: The two-way traffic of solutes in haemodialysis. Nephrol Dial Transplant 14:2625-2627, 1999.

199. Ng, YY, Chow MP, Lyou JY, et al: Resistance to erythropoietin: Immunohemolytic anemia induced by residual formaldehyde in dialyzers. Am J Kidney Dis 21:213-216, 1993.

200. Gallucci MT, Lubrano R, Meloni C, et al: Red blood cell membrane lipid peroxidation and resistance to erythropoietin therapy in hemodialysis patients. Clin Nephrol 52:239-245, 1999.

201. Zachee P, Chew SL, Daelemans R, Lins RL: Erythropoietin resistance due to vitamin B_{12} deficiency; case report and retrospective analysis of B_{12} levels after erythropoietin treatment. Am J Nephrol 12:188-191, 1992.

202. Klemm A, Sperschneider H, Lauterbach H, Stein G: Is folate and vitamin B_{12} supplementation necessary in chronic hemodialsis patients with EPO treatment [letter]? Clin Nephrol 42:343-345, 1994.

203. Ono K, Hisasue Y: Is folate supplementation necessary in hemodialysis patients on erythropoietin therapy? Clin Nephrol 38:290-292, 1992.

204. Caillette A, Barreto S, Giminez E, et al: Is erythropoietin treatment safe and effective in myeloma patients receiving hemodialysis? Clin Nephrol 40:176-178, 1993.

205. Taylor JK, Mactier RA, Stewart WK, Henderson IS: Effect of erythropoietin on anaemia in patients with myeloma receiving hemodialysis. BMJ 301:476-477, 1990.

206. Ruedin P, Pechere Bertschi A, Chapuis B, et al: Safety and efficacy of recombinant human erythropoietin treatment of anaemia associated with multiple myeloma in haemodialyzed patients. Nephrol Dial Transplant 8:315-318, 1993.

207. Roger S, Russell NH, Morgan AG: Effect of erythropoietin in patients with myeloma. BMJ 301:667, 1990.

208. Olujohungbe A, Handa S, Holmes J: Does erythropoietin accelerate malignant transformation in multiple myeloma? Postgrad Med J 73:163-164, 1997.

209. Macdougall IC: Poor response to erythropoietin: Practical guidelines on investigation and management. Nephrol Dial Transplant 10:607-614, 1995.

210. Barany P, Divino Filho JC, Bergstrom J: High C-reactive protein is a strong predictor of resistance to erythropoietin in hemodialysis patients. Am J Kidney Dis 29:565-568, 1997.

211. Caglar K, Hakim RM, Ikizler TA: Approaches to the reversal of malnutrition, inflammation, and atherosclerosis in end-stage renal disease. Nutr Rev 60:378-387, 2002.

212. Stenvinkel P, Barany P: Anaemia, rHuEPO resistance, and cardiovascular disease in end-stage renal failure; links to inflammation and oxidative stress. Nephrol Dial Transplant 17(suppl 5):32-37, 2002.

213. Trey JE, Kushner I: The acute phase response and the hematopoietic system: The role of cytokines. Crit Rev Oncol Hematol 21:1-18, 1995.

214. Jurado RL: Iron, infections, and anemia of inflammation. Clin Infect Dis 25:888-895, 1997.

215. Feelders RA, Vreugdenhil G, Eggermont AM, et al: Regulation of iron metabolism in the acute-phase response: Interferon gamma and tumour necrosis factor alpha induce hypoferraemia, ferritin production and a decrease in circulating transferrin receptors in cancer patients. Eur J Clin Invest 28:520-527, 1998.

216. Allen DA, Breen C, Yaqoob MM, Macdougall IC: Inhibition of CFU-E colony formation in uremic patients with inflammatory disease: Role of IFN-gamma and TNF-alpha. J Invest Med 47:204-211, 1999.

217. Means RT Jr: Advances in the anemia of chronic disease. Int J Hematol 70:7-12, 1999.

218. Gunnell J, Yeun JY, Depner TA, Kaysen GA: Acute-phase response predicts erythropoietin resistance in hemodialysis and peritoneal dialysis patients. Am J Kidney Dis 33:63-72, 1999.

219. Ahmad S: L-Carnitine in dialysis patients. Semin Dial 14:209-217, 2001.

220. Hurot JM, Cucherat M, Haugh M, Fouque D: Effects of L-carnitine supplementation in mantenance hemodialysis patients: A systematic review. J Am Soc Nephrol 13:708-714, 2002.

221. Labonia WD: L-Carnitine effects on anemia in hemodialyzed patients treated with erythropoietin. Am J Kidney Dis 26:757-764, 1995.

222. Wang Y, Wang M: The effect of L-carnitine supplementation on anemia in maintenance hemodialysis patients [abstract]. J Am Soc Nephrol 13:581, 2002.

223. Kletzmayr J, Mayer G, Legenstein E, et al: Anemia and carnitine supplementation in hemodialyzed patients. Kidney Int Suppl 69: 93-106, 1999.

224. Guarnieri G, Situlin R, Biolo G: Carnitine metabolism in uremia. Am J Kidney Dis 38(4 suppl 1):63-67, 2001.

225. Department of Health and Human Services, Center for Medicare and Medicaid Services: Program Memorandum for Intermediaries/Carriers. Levocarnitine for use in the treatment of carnitine deficiency in ESRD patients. Transmittal AB-02-165, change request 2438, November 8, 2002.

226. Gaston RS, Julian BA, Curtis JJ: Posttransplant erythrocytosis: An enigma revisited. Am J Kidney Dis 24:1-11, 1994.

227. Le Meur Y, Lorgeot V, Comte L, et al: Plasma levels and metabolism of AcSDKP in patients with chronic renal failure: Relationship with erythropoietin requirements. Am J Kidney Dis 38:510-517, 2001.

228. Naito M, Kawashima A, Takanashi M, et al: Effects of angiotensin II and angiotensin-converting enzyme inhibitors on burst forming units-erythroid in chronic hemodialysis patients [abstract]. J Am Soc Nephrol 13:583, 2002.

229. Albitar S, Genin R, Fen-Chong M, et al: High dose enalapril impairs the response to erythropoietin treatment in haemodialysis patients. Nephrol Dial Transplant 13:1206-1210, 1998.

230. Navarro JF, Macia ML, Mora-Fernandez C, et al: Effects of angiotensin-converting enzyme inhibitors on anemia and erythropoietin requirements in peritoneal dialysis patients. Adv Perit Dial 13:257-259, 1997.

231. Cruz DN, Perazella MA, Abu-Alfa AK, Mahnensmith RL: Angiotensin-converting enzyme inhibitor therapy in chronic hemodialysis patients: Any evidence of erythropoietin resistance? Am J Kidney Dis 28:535-540, 1996.

232. Abu-Alfa AK, Cruz D, Perazella MA, et al: ACE inhibitors do not induce recombinant human erythropoietin resistance in hemodialysis patients. Am J Kidney Dis 35:1076-1082, 2000.

233. Saudan P, Halabi G, Perneger T, et al: Use of ACE inhibitors or angiotensin II receptors blockers is not associated with erythropoietin resistance in dialysis patients [abstract]. J Am Soc Nephrol 13:443, 2002.

234. Ifudu O, Feldman J, Friedman EA: The intensity of hemodialysis and the response to erythropoietin in patients with end-stage renal disease. N Engl J Med 334:420-425, 1996.

235. Ifudu O, Uribarri J, Rajwani I, et al: Adequacy of dialysis and differences in hematocrit among dialysis facilities. Am J Kidney Dis 36:1166-1174, 2000.

236. Charra B, Calemard E, Ruffet M, et al: Survival as an index of adequacy in dialysis. Kidney Int 41:1286-1291, 1992.

237. Pierratos A: Nocturnal home haemodialysis: An update on a 5-year experience. Nephrol Dial Transplant 14:2835-2840, 1999.

238. Klarenbach S, Heidenheim AP, Leitch R, Lindsay RM: Reduced requirement for erythropoietin with quotidian hemodialysis therapy. ASAIO J 48:57-61, 2002.

239. Vos PF, Zilch O, Kooistra MO: Clinical outcome of daily dialysis. Am J Kidney Dis 37(1 suppl 2):99-102, 2001.

240. Fagugli RM, De Smet R, Buoncristiani U, et al: Behavior of non–protein-bound and protein-bound uremic solutes during daily dialysis. Am J Kidney Dis 40:2339-347, 2002.

241. Galland R, Traeger J, Arkouche W, et al: Short daily hemodialysis and nutritional status. Am J Kidney Dis 37(1 suppl 2):95-98, 2001.

242. Kooistra MP, Vos J, Koomans HA, Vos PF: Daily home hemodialysis in the Netherlands: Effects on metabolic control, haemodynamics, and quality of life. Nephrol Dial Transplant 13:2853-2860, 1998.

243. Mohr PE, Neumann PJ, Franco SJ, et al: The case for daily dialysis: Its impact on costs and quality of life. Am J Kidney Dis 37:777-789, 2001.

244. Casadevall N, Nataf J, Viron B, et al: Pure red-cell aplasia and antierythropoietin antibodies in patients treated with recombinant erythropoietin. N Engl J Med 346:469-475, 2002.

245. Casadevall N: Antibodies against rHuEPO: Native and recombinant. Nephrol Dial Transplant 17(suppl 5):42-47, 2002.

246. Uehlinger DE, Gotch F, Sheiner LB: A pharmacodynamic model of erythropoietin therapy for uremic anemia. Clin Pharmacol Ther 51:176-189, 1992.

247. Eschbach JW, Varma A, Stivelman JC: Is it time for a paradigm shift? Is erythropoietin deficiency still the main cause of renal anaemia? Nephrol Dial Transplant 17(suppl 5):2-7, 2002.

248. Brier ME, Aronoff GR, Medical Review Board: Hemoglobin goals and the natural variability in the erythropoietin response [abstract]. J Am Soc Nephrol 13:628, 2002.

249. NKF-DOQI Work Group: NKF-DOQI clinical practice guidelines for the treatment of anemia of chronic renal failure. Am J Kidney Dis 30(suppl 3):192-240, 1997.

250. Muirhead N, Bargman J, Burgess E, et al: Evidence-based recommendations for the clinical use of recombinant human erythropoietin. Am J Kidney Dis 26(suppl 1):1-24, 1995.

251. Walls J: Haemoglobin—is more better? Nephrol Dial Transplant 10(suppl 2):56-61, 1995.

252. Williams C: Haemoglobin—is more better? Nephrol Dial Transplant 10(suppl 2):8-55, 1995.

253. Nissenson AR, Besarab A, Bolton WK, et al: Target haematocrit during erythropoietin therapy. Nephrol Dial Transplant 12:1813-1816, 1997.

254. Ritz E, Amann K: Optimal haemoglobin during treatment with recombinant human erythropoietin. Nephrol Dial Transplant 13(suppl 2):16-22, 1998.

255. Jacobs C: Normalization of haemoglobin: Why not? Nephrol Dial Transplant 14(suppl 2):75-79, 1999.

256. Ritz E, Schwenger V: The optimal target hemoglobin. Semin Nephrol 20:382-386, 2000.

257. Eckardt K-U: Target hemoglobin in patients with renal failure. Nephron 89:135-143, 2001.

258. Stevens L, Stigant C, Levin A: Should hemoglobin be normalized in patients with chronic kidney disease? Semin Dial 15:8-13, 2002.

259. Gomez JM, Carrera F: What should the optimal target hemoglobin be? Kidney Int Suppl 80:39-43, 2002.

260. Lowrie EG, Huang WH, Lew NL, Lin Y: The relative contribution of measured variables to death risk among hemodialysis patients.

In Friedman EA (ed): Death on Hemodialysis. Dordrecht, The Netherlands, Kluwer, 1994, pp 121-141.

261. Ma JZ, Ebben J, Xia H, Collins, AJ: Hematocrit level and associated mortality in hemodialysis patients. J Am Soc Nephrol 10:610-619, 1999.

262. Collins AJ, Li S, St Peter W, et al: Death, hospitalization, and economic associations among incident hemodialysis patients with hematocrit values of 36 to 39%. J Am Soc Nephrol 12:2465-2473, 2001.

263. Moreno F, Sanz-Guajardo D, Lopez-Gomez JM, et al: Increasing the hematocrit has a beneficial effect on quality of life and is safe in selected hemodialysis patients. J Am Soc Nephrol 11:335-342, 2000.

264. Foley RN, Parfrey PS, Harnett JD, et al: The impact of anemia on cardiomyopathy, morbidity, and mortality in end-stage renal disease. Am J Kidney Dis 28:53-61, 1996.

265. Macdougall IC, Ritz E: The normal haematocrit trial in dialysis patients with cardiac disease: Are we any the less confused about target hemoglobin? Nephrol Dial Transplant 13:3030-3033, 1998.

266. Xia H, Ebben J, Ma JZ, Collins AJ: Hematocrit levels and hospitalization risks in hemodialysis patients. J Am Soc Nephrol 10:1309-1316, 1999.

267. Crowell JW, Frod RG, Lews VM: Oxygen transport in hemorrhagic shock as a function of the hematocrit ratio. Am J Physiol 196:1033-1038, 1959.

268. Jan KM, Chien S: Effect of hematocrit variations on coronary hemodynamics and oxygen utilization. Am J Physiol 233:106-113, 1977.

269. Hino A, Ueda S, Mizukawa N, et al: Effect of hemodilution on cerebral hemodynamics and oxygen metabolism. Stroke 23:423-426, 1992.

270. Grimm G, Stockenhuber F, Schneeweiss B, et al: Improvement of brain function in hemodialysis patients treated with erythropoietin. Kidney Int 38:480-486, 1990.

271. Marsh JT, Brown WS, Wolcott D, et al: rHuEPO treatment improves brain and cognitive function of anemic dialysis patients. Kidney Int 39:151-163, 1991.

272. Sagales T, Gimeno V, Planella MJ, et al: Effects of rHuEPO on Q-EEG and event-related potentials in chronic renal failure. Kidney Int 44:1109-1115, 1993.

273. Nissenson AR: Recombinant human erythropoietin: Impact on brain and cognitive function, exercise tolerance, sexual potency, and quality of life. Semin Nephrol 9(suppl 2):25-31, 1989.

274. Nissenson AR: Neurobehavioral effects of recombinant human erythropoietin. Nefrologia 10(suppl 2):47-50, 1990.

275. Temple RM, Deary IJ, Winney RJ: Recombinant erythropoietin improves cognitive function in patients maintained on chronic ambulatory peritoneal dialysis. Nephrol Dial Transplant 10:1733-1738, 1995.

276. Pickett JL, Theberge DC, Brown WS, et al: Normalizing hematocrit in dialysis patients improves brain function. Am J Kidney Dis 33:1122-1130, 1999.

277. Benz RL, Pressman MR, Hovick ET, Peterson DD: A preliminary study of the effects of correction of anemia with recombinant human erythropoietin therapy on sleep, sleep disorders, and daytime sleepiness in hemodialysis patients (The SLEEPO Study). Am J Kidney Dis 34:1089-1095, 1999.

278. Metry G, Wikstrom B, Valind S, et al: Effect of normalization of hematocrit on brain circulation and metabolism in hemodialysis patients. J Am Soc Nephrol 10:854-863, 1999.

279. Hirakata H, Kanai H, Fukuda K, et al: Optimal hematocrit for the maximum oxygen delivery to the brain with recombinant human erythropoietin in hemodialysis patients. Clin Nephrol 53:354-361, 2000.

280. Brines ML, Ghezzi P, Keenan S, et al: Erythropoietin crosses the blood-brain barrier to protect against experimental brain injury. Proc Natl Acad Sci U S A 97:10526-10531, 2000.

281. Canadian Erythropoietin Study Group: Association between recombinant human erythropoietin and quality of life and exercise capacity of patients receiving hemodialysis. BMJ 300:573-578, 1990.

282. Laupacis A, Wong C, Churchill D: The use of generic and specific quality-of-life measures in hemodialysis patients treated with erythropoietin. The Canadian Erythropoietin Study Group. Control Clin Trials 12(suppl 4):68-179, 1991.

283. McMahon LP, Dawborn JK: Subjective quality of life assessment in hemodialysis patients at different levels of hemoglobin following use of recombinant human erythropoietin. Am J Nephrol 12:162-169, 1992.

284. Moreno F, Aracil FJ, Perez R, Valderrabano F: Controlled study on the improvement of quality of life in elderly hemodialysis patients after correcting end-stage-renal disease–related anemia with erythropoietin. Am J Kidney Dis 27:548-556, 1996.

285. McMahon LP, Mason K, Skinner SL, et al: Effects of haemoglobin normalization on quality of life and cardiovascular parameters in end-stage renal failure. Nephrol Dial Transplant 15:1425-1430, 2000.

286. Painter P, Moore G, Carlson L, et al: Effects of exercise training plus normalization of hematocrit on exercise capacity and health-related quality of life. Am J Kidney Dis 39:257-265, 2002.

287. McHorney CA, Ware JE Jr, Raczek AE: The MOS 36-item short form health survey (SF-36). II: Psychometric and clinical tests of validity in measuring physical and mental health constructs. Med Care 31:247-263, 1993.

288. Suzuki M, Tsutsui M, Yokoyama A, Hirasawa Y: Normalization of hematocrit with recombinant human erythropoietin in chronic hemodialysis patients does not fully improve their exercise tolerance abilities. Artif Organs 19:1258-1261, 1995.

289. McMahon LP, McKenna MJ, Sangkabutra T, et al: Physical performance and associated electrolyte changes after haemoglobin normalization: A comparative study in haemodialysis patients. Nephrol Dial Transplant 14:1182-1187, 1999.

290. Bonilla S, Goecke IA, Bozzo S, et al: Effect of chronic renal failure on Na+, K+ ATPase alpha 1 and alpha 2 mRNA transcription in rat skeletal muscle. J Clin Invest 88:2137-2141, 1991.

291. Renaud JM, Gramolini A, Light P, Comtois A: Modulation of muscle contractility during fatigue and recovery by ATP sensitive potassium channel. Acta Physiol Scand 156:203-212, 1996.

292. Lewis NP, Macdougall I, Willis N, et al: Effects of the correction of renal anemia by erythropoietin on physiological changes during exercise. Eur J Clin Invest 23:423-427, 1993.

293. Wald M, Gutnisky A, Borda E, Sterin-Borda L: Erythropoietin modified the cardiac action of ouabain in chronically anaemic-uraemic rats. Nephron 71:190-196, 1995.

294. Harnett JD, Kent GM, Barre PE, et al: Risk factors for the development of left ventricular hypertrophy in a prospective cohort of dialysis patients. J Am Soc Nephrol 4:1486-1490, 1994.

295. Parfrey PS, Foley RN, Harnett JD, et al: Outcome and risk factors for left ventricular disorders in chronic uremia. Nephrol Dial Transplant 11:1277-1285, 1996.

296. Levin A, Singer J, Thompson CR, et al: Prevalent left ventricular hypertrophy in the predialysis population: Identifying opportunities for intervention. Am J Kidney Dis 27:347-354, 1996.

297. Silberberg J, Racine N, Barre P, Sniderman AD: Regression of left ventricular hypertrophy in dialysis patients following correction of anemia with recombinant human erythropoietin. Can J Cardiol 6:31-37, 1990.

298. Cannella G, La Canna G, Sandrini M, et al: Reversal of left hypertrophy following recombinant human erythropoietin treatment of anaemic dialysed uremic patients. Nephrol Dial Transplant 6:31-37, 1991.

299. Foley RN, Parfrey PS, Morgan J: Regression of left ventricular hypertrophy after partial correction of anemia with erythropoietin in patients on hemodiaysis: A prospective study. Clin Nephrol 35:280-387, 1991.

300. Foley RN, Parfrey PS, Morgan J, et al: Effect of hemoglobin levels in hemodialysis patients with asymptomatic cardiomyopathy. Kidney Int 58:1325-1335, 2000.

301. Berweck S, Hennig L, Sternber C, et al: Cardiac mortality prevention in uremic patients. Therapeutic strategies with particular attention to complete correction of renal anemia. Clin Nephrol 53(suppl 1):80-85, 2000.

302. Hayashi T, Suzuki A, Shoji T, et al: Cardiovascular effect of normalizing the hematocrit level during erythropoietin therapy in predialysis patients with chronic renal failure. Am J Kidney Dis 35:250-256, 2000.

303. Silverberg DS, Wexler D, Blum M, et al: The use of subcutaneous erythropoietin and intravenous iron for the treatment of the anemia of severe, resistant congestive heart failure improves cardiac and renal function and functional cardiac class and markedly reduces hospitalizations. J Am Coll Cardiol 35:1737-1744, 2000.

304. Garcia DL, Anderson S, Rennke HG, Brenner BM: Anemia lessens and its prevention worsens glomerular injury and hypertension in rats with reduced renal mass. Proc Natl Acad Sci U S A 85:6142-6146, 1988.

305. Abraham PA, Opsahl JA, Rachael KM, et al: Renal function during erythropoietin therapy for anemia in predialysis chronic renal failure patients. Am J Nephrol 10:128-136, 1990.

306. Lim VS, Fangman J, Flanigan MJ, et al: Effect of recombinant human erythropoietin on renal function in humans. Kidney Int 37:131-136, 1990.

307. The US recombinant human erythropoietin predialysis study group. Double-blind, placebo-controlled study of the therapeutic use of recombinant human erythropoietin for anemia associated with chronic renal failure in predialysis patients. Am J Kidney Dis 18:50-59, 1991.

308. Roth D, Smith RD, Schulman G: Effects of recombinant human erythropoietin on renal function in chronic renal failure predialysis patients. Am J Kidney Dis 24:777-784, 1994.

309. Bellizzi V, Sabbatini M, Fuiano G, et al: The impact of early normalization of haematocrit by erythropoietin on renal damage in the remnant kidney model. Nephrol Dial Transplant 13:2210-2215, 1998.

310. Kuriyama S, Tomonari H, Hoshida H, et al: Reversal of anemia by erythropoietin therapy retards the progression of chronic renal failure, especially in nondiabetic patients. Nephron 77:176-185, 1997.

311. Jungers P, Choukroun G, Oualim Z, et al: Beneficial influence of recombinant human erythropoietin therapy on the rate of progression of chronic renal failure in predialysis patients. Nephrol Dial Transplant 16:307-312, 2001.

312. Mohanram A, Zhang J, Shahinar S, et al: Anemia is an independent risk factor for progression to end stage renal disease in type 2 diabetics with nephropathy: Results from the reduction in endpoints in non–insulin dependent diabetes mellitus with the angiotensin II antagonist losartan (RENAAL) trial [abstract]. J Am Soc Nephrol 13:8, 2002.

313. Ludat K, Paulitschke M, Riedel E, Hampl H: Complete correction of renal anemia by recombinant human erythropoietin. Clin Nephrol 53(suppl 1):42-49, 2000.

314. Paulitschke M, Ludat K, Riedel E, Hampl H: Long-term effects of rhEPO therapy on erythrocyte rheology in dialysis patients with different target hematocrits. Clin Nephrol 53(suppl 1):36-41, 2000.

315. Christensson AG, Danielson BG, Lethagen SR: Normalization of hemoglobin concentration with recombinant erythropoietin has minimal effect on blood haemostasis. Nephrol Dial Transplant 16:313-319, 2001.

316. Ludat K, Sommerburg O, Grune T, et al: Oxidation parameters in complete correction of renal anemia. Clin Nephrol 53(suppl 1):30-35, 2000.

317. Macdougall IC: Meeting the challenges of a new millennium: Optimizing the use of recombinant human erythropoietin. Nephrol Dial Transplant 13(suppl 2):23-27, 1998.

318. Macdougall IC: Individualizing target haemoglobin concentrations—tailoring treatment of renal anaemia. Nephrol Dial Transplant 16(suppl 7):9-14, 2001.

319. Muirhead N: A rationale for an individualized haemoglobin target. Nephrol Dial Transplant 17(suppl 6):2-7, 2002.

320. Ritz E: Optimizing clinical benefits: Shaping the future of renal anaemia with epoetin. Nephrol Dial Transplant 17(suppl 1):1-73, 2002.

321. Sisk JE, Gianfrancesco FD, Coster JM: Recombinant erythropoietin and medicare payment. JAMA 266(2):247-252, 1991.

322. Sisk JE, Gianfrancesco FD, Coster JM: Medicare payment options for recombinant erythropoietin therapy. Am J Kidney Dis 18:93-97, 1991.

323. Abraham PA: Health care payment policies: Lessons from erythropoietin. Am J Kidney Dis 22:596-597, 1993.

324. Powe NR, Griffiths RI, Anderson GF, et al: Medicare payment policy and recombinant erythropoietin. Am J Kidney Dis 22:557-567, 1993.

325. Wish JB: Can evidence drive the development of a sound national EPO reimbursement policy? Am J Kidney Dis 41:254-258, 2003.

326. Whittington R, Barradell LB, Benfield P: Epoetin: A pharmacoeconomic review of its use in chronic renal failure and its effects on quality of life. Pharmacoeconomics 3:45-82, 1993.

327. Harris DCH, Chapman JR, Stewart JH, et al: Low dose erythropoietin in maintenance haemodialysis: Improvement in quality of life and reduction in true cost of haemodialysis. Aus N Z J Med 21:693-700, 1991.

328. Sheingold SH, Churchill DN, Muirhead N, Laupacis A: Recombinant human erythropoietin: Factors to consider in cost-benefit analysis. Am J Kidney Dis 17:86-92, 1991.

329. Stevens M, Summerfield GP, Hall AA, et al: Cost benefits to low dose subcutaneous erythropoietin in patients with anemia of end stage renal disease. BMJ 304: 474-477, 1992.

330. Powe NR, Giffiths RI, Bass EB: Cost implications to Medicare of recombinant erythropoietin therapy for the anemia of end-stage renal disease. J Am Soc Nephrol 3:160-167, 1993.

331. Powe NR, Griffiths RI, Watson AJ, et al: Effect of recombinant erythropoietin on hospital admissions, readmission, length of stay, and costs of dialysis patients. J Am Soc Nephrol 4:1455-1465, 1994.

332. Collins A, Li S, Ebben J, et al: Hematocrit levels and associated Medicare expenditures. Am J Kidney Dis 36:282-293, 2000.

333. Griffiths RI, Powe NR, Greer J, et al: A review of the first year of Medicare coverage of erythropoietin. Health Care Finance Rev 15(3):83-102, 1994.

334. Health Care Financing Administration: 1998 Annual Report, End Stage Renal Disease Core Indicators Project. Baltimore, MD, Department of Health and Human Services, Health Care Financing Administration, Health Standards and Quality Bureau, 1998.

335. Lacson E, Ofsthun N, Lazarus JM: Effect of variability in anemia management on hemoglobin outcomes in ESRD. Am J Kidney Dis 41:111-124, 2003.

336. Collins AJ, Li S, St. Peter W, et al: Death, hospitalization, and economic associations among incident hemodialysis patients with hematocrit values of 36 to 39%. J Am Soc Nephrol 12:2465-2473, 2001.

337. United States Renal Data System: USRDS 2001 Annual Data Report. Bethesda, MD, National Institutes of Health, National Institute of Diabetes and Digestive and Kidney Diseases, 2001.

338. Kaufman JS, Reda DJ, Fye CL, et al: Subcutaneous compared with intravenous epoetin in patients receiving hemodialysis. Department of Veterans Affairs Cooperative Study Group on Erythropoietin in Hemodialysis Patients. N Engl J Med 339:578-583, 1998.

339. Hynes DM, Stroupe KT, Greer JW, et al: Potential cost savings of erythropoietin administration in end-stage renal disease. Am J Med 112:169-175, 2002.

340. Gershon SK, Luksenburg H, Cote TR, Braun MM: Pure red-cell aplasia and recombinant erythropoietin. N Engl J Med 346:1584-1586, 2002.

341. Medicare Payment Advisory Commission: End-stage renal disease payment policies in traditional Medicare. *In* MedPac Report to the Congress: Medicare Payment Policy. Washington, DC, MedPac, 2001, pp 121-138.

342. Medicare Payment Advisory Commission: Assessing payment adequacy and updating payments in traditional Medicare: Outpatient dialysis services. *In* MedPac Report to the Congress: Medicare Payment Policy. Washington, DC, MedPac, 2002, pp 99-108.

343. Renal Physicians Association/American Society of Nephrology Task Force on the ESRD Payment System: RPA/ASN white paper on the ESRD payment system. July 20, 2002. Available at www.renalmd.org., August 2002.

CHAPTER 59

Hemodialysis

Gerald Schulman and Jonathan Himmelfarb

THE HEMODIALYSIS POPULATION

Demographics

For more than 300,000 patients in the United States who have reached end-stage renal disease (ESRD), hemodialysis has become a routine therapy. However, it should not be forgotten that this lifesaving treatment has been routinely applied for ESRD only for the past 30 years. Beginning with the successful experiments by Abel and colleagues,[1] it was shown that when blood was circulated through numerous collodion tubes surrounded by a jacket containing dialysis fluid, substances diffused from the blood to the dialysate. The investigators also demonstrated that the composition of the dialysate fluid was a major determinant of what was removed or retained during the procedure. Based on these findings, Kolff developed the rotating drum artificial kidney, which rapidly found use in treating patients with acute renal

failure.[2] Pioneering physicians such as Merrill, Scribner, and Schreiner successfully supported patients through the oligoanuric phase of acute renal failure. Teschan introduced hemodialysis to the battlefield during the Korean War.

Successful application of labor-intensive and technically demanding hemodialysis to acute renal failure was accomplished in the acute care setting. However, adaptation of the acute procedure to the management of permanent, irreversible renal failure required the intersection of a number of medical and social developments that led to the creation of an infrastructure capable of supporting the current ESRD program. A major issue was finding a method of reliably and repeatedly entering the patient's circulation to perform the treatment. The use of an external bridge or shunt connected to an artery and vein in the wrist was championed by Scribner for use in acute renal failure and could be used in treating chronic renal failure, although with great difficulty because of infection and repeated episodes of clotting. It was then demonstrated that an internal connection between the radial artery and distal cephalic vein in the wrist (i.e., Cimino fistula) could be hemodynamically tolerated. The vein returning blood under high pressure eventually became "arterialized" and allowed repeated access to the circulation. Internal connections between suitable veins and arteries that were not near each other were accomplished with the use of bovine venous grafts or artificial tubing. Mass production of disposable devices for the treatment, such as dialyzers, tubing, and easily reconstituted dialysate, was also required to enable the widespread application of maintenance hemodialysis.

The last of the necessary pieces required for delivery of dialysis was the will of the nation to allow a sufficient portion of its health care funding to be dedicated to treating for an indefinite period a chronic, unremitting process such as ESRD. Until such a decision was made, hemodialysis for ESRD was an expensive and inefficient procedure. Often, it was made available by the decision of a selection committee who chose only the young who were free of comorbid conditions. Employment and level of education were important criteria for selection. However, after much debate in the lay and medical communities, in 1973, the U.S. Congress passed the law entitling Medicare patients to dialysis and transplantation treatments.[3] Perhaps as a legacy of the restrictive acceptance policies before entitlement, the initial estimate of the numbers of patients who would enter the ESRD program was low. This legislation eventually evolved to provide care for patients with ESRD irrespective of means, education, employment, or other medical conditions. The ESRD entitlement legislation represents a landmark providing life-sustaining therapy, and no similar program has been proposed for any other chronic disorder.

Incidence and Prevalence of Hemodialysis Patients in the United States

The United States Renal Data Survey (USRDS), the annual registry of the ESRD patients of the United States, indicates that as of December 31, 1999, the annual incidence of hemodialysis patients is 259.8 per 1 million people.[3] This represents 71,426 patients per year. Figure 59-1 demonstrates that the incidence is not uniform across the nation.

The highest incidences appear across the South and West. These areas correspond to regions of the nation having a high incidence of patients with diabetes, the most common cause of ESRD. These regions have high numbers of black and Hispanic American patients, with ESRD incidences of 843.1 per 1 million people and 582.5 per 1 million people, respectively. Figure 59-2 shows that the increasing numbers of patients are reaching ESRD due to diabetes and, to a lesser extent, hypertension. The incidence due to glomerulonephritis and cystic disease has remained constant over several years.

The prevalence of ESRD patients treated with hemodialysis is 758.8 per 1 million people. The prevalence rate for blacks with ESRD is approximately four times that of the general population and 6.5-fold the rate for whites. More than 40% of the ESRD patients have been diagnosed with diabetes, 28% with hypertension, 11.6% with glomerulonephritis, and 4.7% with cystic or other urologic conditions.

International Comparisons

The highest prevalence rate for ESRD is found in Japan, with a rate of nearly 1600 patients per 1 million people; the United States follows with a rate of 1200 patients per

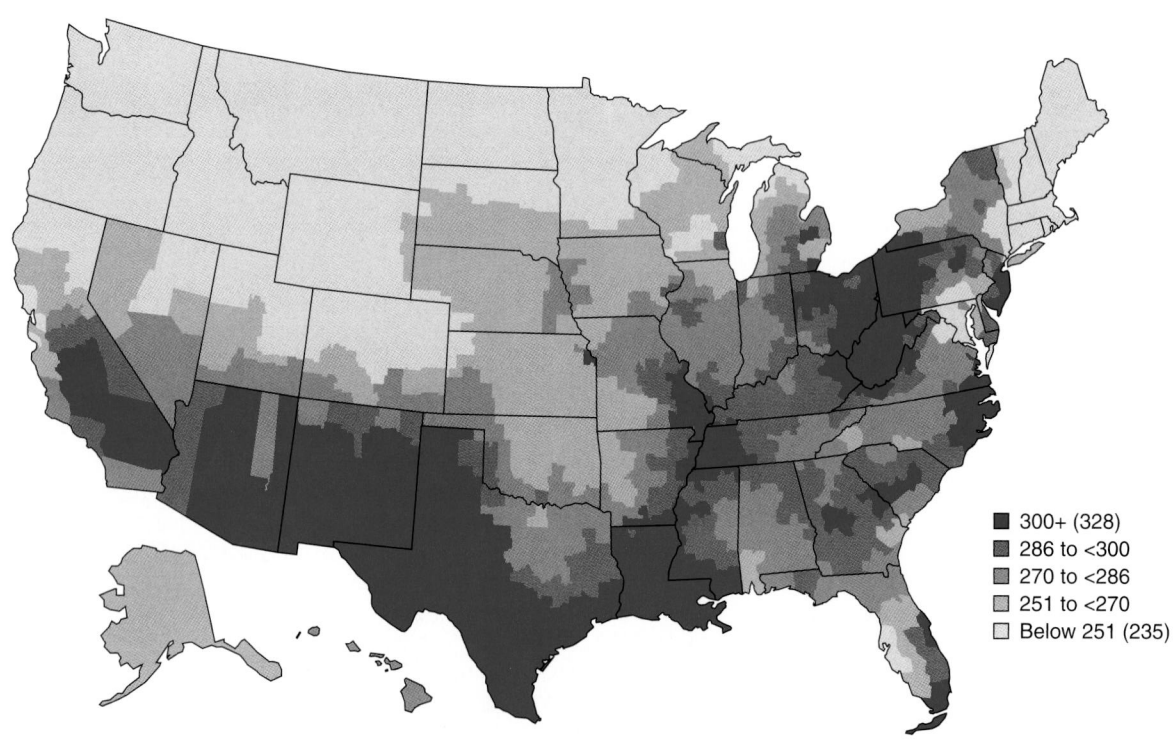

FIGURE 59-1. Incidence of hemodialysis patients in the United States.

1 million people. These high numbers reflect the policies of these nations to open access to this therapy and nearly universal care for patients with ESRD. The prevalence rates average 600 to 800 patients per 1 million people for most of Western Europe and 550 to 600 patients per 1 million people in Chile, Norway, Finland, Hungary, and the United Kingdom. There are wide differences in access to treatment, allocation to the various modalities of treatment, and methods of reimbursement between nations that account for the wide ranges of prevalence.

Outcomes: Morbidity and Mortality of Hemodialysis Patients in the United States

Figure 59-3 shows that over the years, the number of comorbid diseases in patients at initiation of therapy has increased. Patients initiated on hemodialysis have more comorbidities than patients who are initiated on peritoneal dialysis. Hemodialysis patients are more likely to have cardiovascular disease (i.e., congestive heart failure, ischemic heart disease, or myocardial infarction), cerebral vascular disease, peripheral vascular disease, and chronic lung disease. An important exception is that a higher percentage of insulin-dependent diabetics are initiated on peritoneal dialysis. These differences in the population must be taken into account when comparing the two modalities.

The number of hospitalizations and hospital days per patient-year serve as indices of patient morbidity. In 1999, a total of 1937 admissions for hemodialysis occurred per 1000 patient-years. Hospital days per patient-year for hemodialysis patients averaged 13.9 days in the year 2000. These rates have remained fairly stable over the past 5 years. Admission rates per patient-year at risk are significantly influenced by patient vintage. For all incident and prevalent hemodialysis patients, admission rates are highest for those with less than 1 year on dialysis. Admission rates decrease as the number of years on hemodialysis increases. For incident patients, the risk for a first hospitalization was greater for patients with the lowest hematocrits (<30%) and lowest hemodialysis dose (urea reduction ratio <60%). Admissions for cardiovascular and infectious complications also negatively correlated with hematocrit level and hemodialysis dose. Clinical indicators of care influence patient outcomes.

In 1999, 66,964 patients enrolled in the ESRD program died. This represented an annual mortality rate of 182 per 1000 patient-years at risk for the ESRD population. For hemodialysis patients and peritoneal dialysis patients, the mortality rates were 247 and 231 per 1000 patient-years at risk, respectively. In the past decade, a modest decline in the mortality rate has occurred in all age groups, except in the youngest group (i.e., 0 to 19 years old). Cardiovascular disease and infections account for most deaths. The mortality rates associated with hemodialysis are striking and indicate that the life expectancy of patients entering into hemodialysis is markedly shortened. At age 60, a healthy person can expect to live for more than 20 years, whereas the life expectancy of a 60-year-old patient starting hemodialysis is closer to 5 years.

A recurrent controversy is whether peritoneal or hemodialysis represents a superior form of depuration. The question is difficult to answer with certainty because selection for the two therapies is not random and subject to selection bias. In the past 5 years, the number of patients receiving peritoneal dialysis has remained fairly stable at 20,000 to 27,000, whereas the hemodialysis population has continued to increase. In 1999, only 10% of the dialysis population was treated by peritoneal dialysis.[4] Figure 59-4 demonstrates that in the first year of treatment for ESRD, survival of peritoneal dialysis patients is superior to that of hemodialysis patients. However, in subsequent years, the survival rate is greater for patients receiving hemodialysis. The reasons for

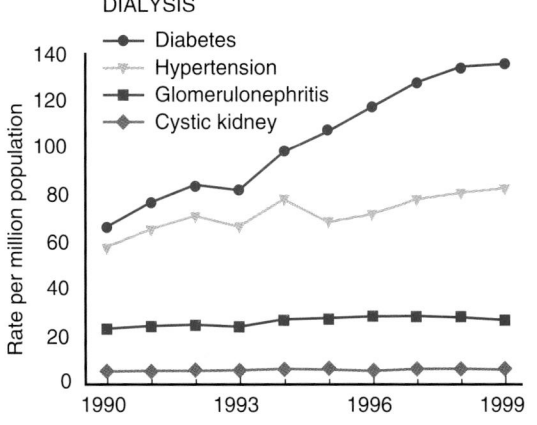

FIGURE 59-2. Causes of end-stage renal disease in the United States.

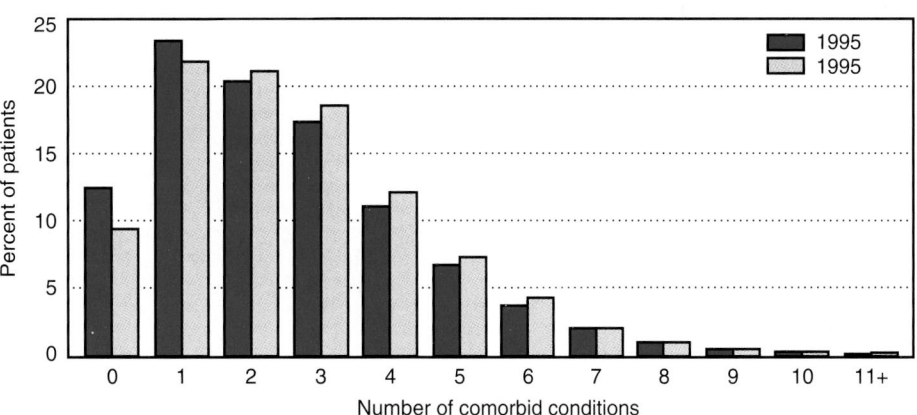

FIGURE 59-3. Increasing comorbid conditions in the end-stage renal disease population.

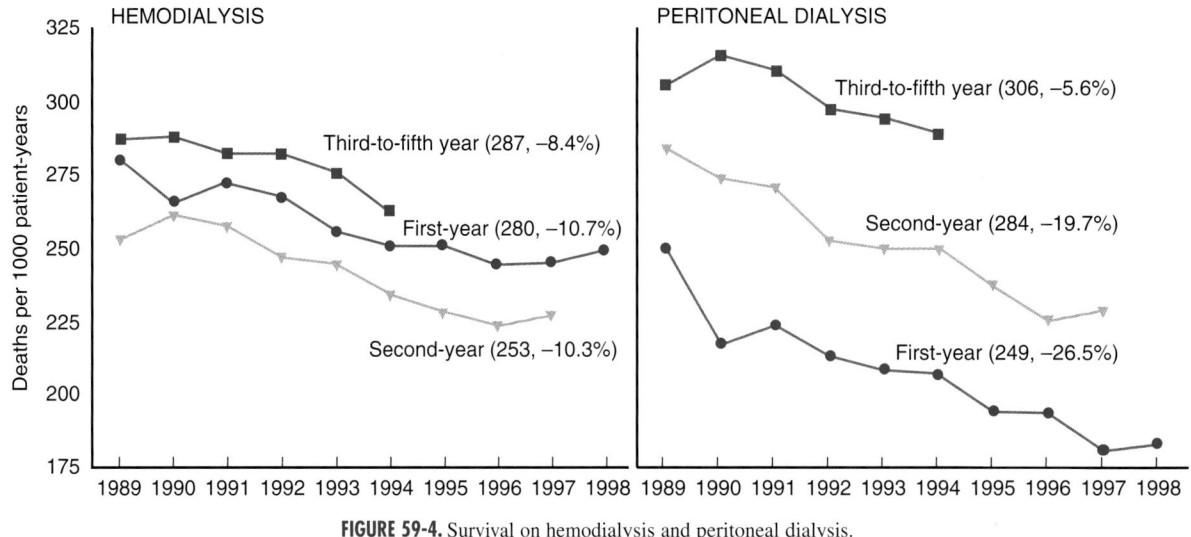

FIGURE 59-4. Survival on hemodialysis and peritoneal dialysis.

TABLE 59-1

Classification of Chronic Kidney Disease

STAGE	DESCRIPTION	GFR (mL/min/1.73m²)	ACTION
1	Injury, not acute, with preserved GFR	>90	Diagnose and treat, slow progression, ?comorbid conditions, decrease cardiovascular risk
2	Mild kidney damage	60–89	Estimate rate of progression
3	Moderate	30–59	Treat complications, ESRD education
4	Severe	15–29	Prepare for ESRD treatment
5	Kidney failure	<15	Initiate ESRD treatment

GFR, glomerular filtration rate.

Data from National Kidney Foundation: K/DOQI clinical practice guidelines for chronic kidney disease: Evaluation, classification and stratification. Am J Kidney Dis 39: S1-S266, 2002.

this finding have not been established. Loss of residual (native) kidney function, which correlates with mortality for peritoneal dialysis patients, has been suggested as a factor. Nevertheless, there are many issues of lifestyle that outweigh gross survival statistics in choosing one modality over the other.

TRANSITION FROM CHRONIC KIDNEY DISEASE TO HEMODIALYSIS

The knowledge that many patients enter into treatment for ESRD with comorbid conditions, particularly cardiac and vascular complications, and have a strikingly higher mortality rate than that of the general population led to the realization that these conditions often begin much earlier, at a time when chronic renal insufficiency has just been identified. In patients who are at risk for a progressive, inexorable decline in glomerular filtration, measures should be undertaken as early as possible to correct the common abnormalities associated with chronic kidney disease (CKD) to reduce comorbidity and allow a smooth transition to hemodialysis. To this end, the National Kidney Foundation has created the Kidney Disease Outcomes Quality Initiative (K/DOQI) clinical practice guidelines for CKD, a term chosen to be readily understood by patients and physicians.[5] Regardless of the primary cause,

CKD is categorized as one of five stages based on the glomerular filtration rate (GFR) and an action plan (Table 59-1).

Cardiovascular risk factors should be assessed as early as possible, and treatment should be instituted to prevent complications. Education should be provided sufficiently early so that permanent vascular access can be ready for use when the patient reaches ESRD. This is particularly important if the patient chooses hemodialysis. A Cimino fistula offers a number of advantages, including lower rates of thrombosis and infection. However, the veins arising from the fistula often require a number of months to become sufficiently enlarged and thickened so that they can be easily cannulated and provide adequate blood flow. There is also a chance that a fistula will not develop and that an entirely new alternative access plan will have to be developed. This can be a time-consuming process that, if not initiated early enough, may result in the patient reaching ESRD before the access site is mature. The undesirable consequence is the need for a percutaneous catheter, with its much higher risks of infection, thrombosis, and poor function, to bridge the interval between treatment initiation and the creation of a working, permanent access. Whenever possible, in patients with documented progression, a working, permanent hemodialysis access should be in place by the time the GFR falls below 20/mL/minute.

MANAGEMENT OF CHRONIC KIDNEY DISEASE

Reducing Comorbidity

In K/DOQI, 15 guidelines have been promulgated regarding the evaluation, classification, and management of CKD. These guidelines are aimed at correcting or modifying the common abnormalities that are found as renal disease progresses to reduce comorbidity in the ESRD population. Optimal pre-ESRD management includes strategies aimed at preventing or slowing progression by identifying those who have CKD and initiating appropriate care with dietary management, blood pressure and glycemic control, and blockade of the rennin-angiotensin-aldosterone system; preventing complications of uremia such as anemia, renal osteodystrophy, and malnutrition; and preparing the patient for the advent of ESRD with education concerning the available treatment modalities, planning for the creation of a permanent access for hemodialysis to avoid the use of temporary catheters, and planning for hemodialysis initiation before major symptoms of uremia arise.

Comorbid conditions that often coexist in patients suffering from renal disease must also be treated. The measures undertaken to treat the complications of CKD often modify the course of these comorbid conditions. Examples of this phenomenon include regression of left ventricular hypertrophy when erythropoietin is used to treat the anemia associated with renal failure and the suggestion that the calcium content in the vasculature partly depends on the type of phosphate binder used in the treatment of osteodystrophy.

Multiple lines of evidence suggest that the patient's health status at the time of initiation of dialysis affects subsequent morbidity and mortality. Protein intake often falls spontaneously as renal function deteriorates.[6] This can lead to a loss of muscle mass and lower serum albumin levels. The serum albumin level at treatment initiation of is a powerful predictor of subsequent mortality. Patients beginning hemodialysis with an albumin level of 3.0 to 3.5 g/dL have a 20% greater annual mortality rate than patients with an albumin level of 3.5 to 4.0 g/dL. Cardiovascular diseases, the greatest cause of mortality in the hemodialysis population, most often begin long before dialysis is initiated. Untreated or inadequately treated anemia may lead to worsened left ventricular hypertrophy and exacerbation of angina as the patient approaches ESRD.[7-10]

The best approach to treating complications of uremia and comorbid conditions is to identify patients early. Unfortunately, susceptible populations are not always screened for the presence of renal disease.[11] Agents such as angiotensin-converting enzyme (ACE) inhibitors are not always used, and the level of blood pressure control achieved is suboptimal. Education of patients with CKD is often lacking. This leads to little dietary instruction, poor planning for the creation of dialysis access, and failure of patients to avoid potential nephrotoxins.

Initiation of Hemodialysis

Common indications for initiation of hemodialysis in acute renal failure include uncontrolled hypertension, pulmonary edema, acidosis, hyperkalemia, pericarditis, encephalopathy, and elevated levels of blood urea nitrogen (BUN) and creatinine. These indications should never be reasons for initiating

chronic maintenance hemodialysis. Occasionally, a patient presents with manifestations of the acute uremic syndrome because of lack of prior medical attention or denial. However, the goal for the patients is a smooth transition from CKD to ESRD.

Referral to Nephrologists

Input from a nephrologist should be obtained after CKD has been identified. The frequency of visits increases as renal function declines. There is emerging evidence that referral to nephrology influences the time at which dialysis is initiated and subsequent outcome. In patients who are followed by nephrologists, dialysis is initiated at a creatinine concentration as much as 4 mg/dL lower than that of patients who have had no medical care. Multiple lines of evidence support the finding that the timing of referral to the nephrologist influences outcome and cost of dialytic therapy.[12-16]

Patients referred to nephrology less than 1 month before requiring dialysis are more likely to be hypertensive and have congestive heart failure, have marked abnormalities in their serum laboratory values, have lower serum albumin levels, and have markedly longer periods of initial hospitalization. Cost of treating the late referrals is sixfold greater than for patients referred earlier in their course. Each of four studies demonstrates increased mortality after dialysis has started in patients who were referred to nephrology late in their course. It is important to encourage referral to nephrology early in the course of chronic renal failure to prevent complications of uremia.

Starting Hemodialysis

Hemodialysis should be initiated at a level of residual renal function above which the major symptoms of uremia usually supervene. Among the criteria for initiating dialysis recognized by the funding entity for dialysis in the United States are residual creatinine clearances of 15 mL/minute and 10 mL/minute for diabetics and nondiabetics, respectively. K/DOQI guidelines suggest that dialysis should be initiated at a creatinine clearance between 9 and 14 mL/minute.[5] The determination of an adequate dose of hemodialysis is discussed subsequently. With current hemodialysis technology, thrice-weekly sessions of 5 hours each can achieve the equivalent urea clearance of approximately 20 mL/minute in a 70-kg individual.

The government guidelines of creatinine clearances of 15 mL/minute and 10 mL/minute or of serum creatinine concentrations of 6 mg/dL and 8 mg/dL for diabetics and nondiabetics, respectively, are reasonable criteria for initiating hemodialysis. It may be necessary to initiate patients even earlier in their course if they have otherwise uncorrectable symptoms or signs of renal failure such as nausea and vomiting, weight loss, intractable congestive heart failure, or hyperkalemia. After the creatinine clearance falls below 20 mL/minute the patients should be periodically questioned regarding symptoms related to nutrition: loss of appetite; nausea or vomiting, or both, especially in the morning due to overnight retention of uremic toxins in the gut; and unintended weight loss. These are very often the earliest markers of uremia. Asterixis, restless leg syndrome, and a reversal of the sleep-wake cycle are early neurologic manifestations of uremia. If alternative explanations for these symptoms and signs cannot be discerned, they should be considered as indications for initiating dialysis.

VASCULAR ACCESS

History

The use of hemodialysis for the treatment of patients with acute renal failure was introduced by Kolff in 1943 with temporary access to the circulation.[17] However, the development of maintenance hemodialysis therapy for the treatment of ESRD requires repeated access to the circulation. This was not feasible until the introduction of the external arteriovenous Quinton-Scribner shunt in 1960.[18] The Quinton-Scribner shunt was made of silastic tubing connected to a Teflon cannula. The Quinton-Scribner shunt developed frequent problems with thrombosis and infection, and it typically functioned for only a period of months. In 1966, Brescia, Cimino, and others developed the endogenous arteriovenous fistula, which remains the access of choice for maintenance hemodialysis today.[19] The unfeasibility of developing functional native arteriovenous fistulas in all patients led to the development of interpositional bridge grafts in the late 1960s and 1970s. Initial graft biomaterials consisted of autogenous saphenous veins, bovine carotid arteries, and human umbilical veins. In the late 1970s, synthetic bridge grafts made of expanded polytetrafluoroethylene (ePTFE) were introduced.[20, 21] The ePTFE grafts can be placed in most patients, are usable within weeks of surgical placement, and are relatively easy to cannulate. The ePTFE grafts remain the most frequently used graft biomaterial today and continue to be the type of permanent dialysis access most frequently placed in the United States.

Although the relative advantages and disadvantages of each type of permanent dialysis access are discussed further, it is clear that native vein arteriovenous fistulas are preferable to all other vascular access options. Current clinical practice guidelines recommend the radiocephalic primary arteriovenous fistula as the access of choice, followed by the brachial-cephalic primary arteriovenous fistula. Patients with CKD should be referred for a surgical attempt to create a primary arteriovenous fistula when the creatinine clearance falls below 25 mL/minute, when the serum creatinine level is greater than 4 mg/dL, or within 1 year of the anticipated need for maintenance dialysis therapy.

The use of catheters for hemodialysis access also parallels the history of dialysis itself. In 1961, Shaldon and colleagues first described femoral artery catheterization for hemodialysis access.[22] In 1979, Uldall and associates first reported the use of guidewire exchange techniques and subclavian vein puncture for placement of temporary dialysis catheters.[23] In the late 1980s, the use of surgically implanted, tunneled, cuffed, double-lumen catheters was introduced.[24] Subcutaneous vascular ports were introduced as an alternative to the cuffed, tunneled catheter.[25] Although the major use of catheters for hemodialysis access is as a bridging device to allow time for maturation of a more permanent access or for patients who need only temporary vascular access, catheters are increasingly being used for permanent vascular access in patients for whom all other options have been exhausted.[26]

Although there have been impressive technical improvements in hemodialysis vascular access, none of the available types of vascular access meet the performance characteristics required for "perfect" vascular access (see Table 59-1). Vascular access continues to be referred to as the "Achilles heel" of the hemodialysis procedure.[27] Vascular access complications are responsible for considerable cost, morbidity, and mortality in the patient population on maintenance hemodialysis.

Epidemiology

The rapid growth of end-stage renal failure programs in the United States and worldwide has been accompanied by a tremendous increase in dialysis vascular access–associated morbidity and cost.[27] The creation, maintenance, and replacement of vascular access in hemodialysis patients is recognized as a major source of morbidity and cost within the U.S. ESRD Program, with estimates that costs probably exceed $1 billion within the Medicare program on an annual basis.

There is compelling evidence that there are large differences in patterns of vascular access usage between Europe and the United States. The Dialysis Outcomes and Practice Patterns Study (DOPPS) compared vascular access use and survival in Europe and the United States.[28] Native arteriovenous fistulas were used by 80% of European patients, compared with 24% of prevalent dialysis patients in the United States. Arteriovenous fistula use was significantly associated with male gender, younger age, lower body mass index, absence of diabetes mellitus, and a lack of peripheral vascular disease. However, even after adjusting for these risk factors, the odds ratio for arteriovenous fistula use in Europe versus the United States was 21. Enormous facility variation also occurs in the United States, with the prevalence of arteriovenous fistulas ranging from 0% to 87%.[28] A follow-up study from DOPPS suggests that predialysis care by a nephrologist does not account for substantial variations in the proportion of patients commencing dialysis with an arteriovenous fistula and that the time to fistula cannulation after creation also varies greatly between countries.[29] Practice pattern variations in vascular access care are not entirely associated with patient-related factors; the processes of care also influence these variations.

The importance of vascular access care has been emphasized by data from the USRDS demonstrating that adjusted relative mortality risk is substantially higher for patients with central venous catheters than for arteriovenous fistulas in diabetic and nondiabetic patient populations.[30] For diabetic patients, the use of arteriovenous grafts is also associated with significantly higher mortality risk compared with arteriovenous fistulas; infectious and cardiovascular causes are implicated in these cases.

Data from Medicare and the USRDS indicate that the prevalence of arteriovenous fistula use is increasing in the United States. The increase in fistula placement coincides with the publication of K/DOQI guidelines in 1997. However, the K/DOQI clinical practice guideline recommending that an autologous fistula be placed in 40% of prevalent hemodialysis patients is not being met. The use of tunneled catheters as the primary means of hemodialysis access appears to be rising.[31] Considerable challenges remain in attempting to optimize vascular access practice patterns in the future.

Arteriovenous Fistula

Creation of a native vein fistula requires that an anastomosis be made between an adequate artery and vein in close proximity to each other. The most commonly used site is at the wrist, where the cephalic vein is connected to the radial artery (i.e., Brescia-Cimino fistula). The original operation described by Brescia and colleagues[19] was a side-to-side, artery-to-vein anastomosis. However, the end-to-side configuration is preferred by many surgeons today because there is a lower incidence of venous hypertension in the hand.[32] A radial-cephalic fistula can also be fashioned more distally in the anatomic snuff-box.[33] Although radial-cephalic fistulas are preferred when feasible, several reports suggest that, when an aggressive approach is undertaken, a high percentage of radial-cephalic fistulas fail to mature or develop thrombosis. Failure of radial-cephalic fistula maturation is especially prevalent in female, diabetic, and older hemodialysis patients.[34]

An alternative to the radial-cephalic fistula is to use the veins of the upper arm to create a brachiocephalic fistula or a brachiobasilic fistula. Because the basilic vein in the upper arm generally lies under deep fascia, use of this vein for an arteriovenous fistula requires that the vein be dissected and transposed into a more convenient subcutaneous position.[35] The brachial artery can also be anastomosed to a perforating vein, joining the superficial and deep venous system just below the elbow crease (i.e., Gracz fistula).[36] Compared with brachiocephalic fistulas, transposed brachiobasilic fistulas are more likely to mature, but have a higher long-term thrombosis rate.[37] Better patency for upper arm fistulas compared with lower arm fistulas or arteriovenous grafts has been reported, supporting the trend toward creation of upper arm arteriovenous fistulas as the access of choice in patients with poor forearm venous anatomy.[37, 38]

Several strategies are being used to increase the prevalence of functioning arteriovenous fistulas in the U.S. dialysis population.[39] It has been suggested that systematic use of preoperative ultrasonographic imaging can increase the success rate in the surgical placement of arteriovenous fistulas.[40, 41] Arterial and venous anatomy should be examined, and the cephalic vein should be examined from the wrist to the cephalic-subclavian junction. The vein should be at least 2.5 mm in diameter at the point of anastomosis to increase arteriovenous fistula success. Another successful strategy for increasing arteriovenous fistula prevalence involves ligation of tributary veins when arteriovenous fistulas fail to mature promptly. Surgical and endovascular techniques have been used. Whether the short-term use of antiplatelet agents after arteriovenous fistula creation can reduce early fistula thrombosis and increase the number of functioning arteriovenous fistulas is under study.

Arteriovenous Grafts

Dialysis arteriovenous grafts made of ePTFE continue to be the most frequently placed type of permanent dialysis access in the United States, accounting for up to 80% of all accesses, depending on geographical region. Compared with bovine carotid artery graft biomaterial, ePTFE grafts appear to have fewer complications and allow easier management of infection by a potential surgical excision of the infected graft segment. The ePTFE grafts have the advantage of low early thrombosis rate, surgical ease of placement, and a relatively short time between access creation and successful cannulation. However, short-term advantages are more than outweighed by the long-term increased risk for infection and thrombosis.[27, 42] Unfortunately, the 1- and 2-year primary patency rates for ePTFE grafts are a dismal 50% and 25%, respectively.[43] Graft thrombosis accounts for 80% of all vascular access dysfunction, and in more than 90% of thrombosed grafts, venous stenosis at or distal to the graft vein anastomosis is detected.[44] The underlying pathology for the development of venous stenosis is venous neointimal hyperplasia with exuberant vascular smooth muscle cell proliferation, neoangiogenesis within the neointima and adventitia, and an inflammatory macrophage cell layer lining the ePTFE graft material.[45, 46] Immunohistochemical studies have revealed the presence of vascular growth factors, cytokines, byproducts of oxidative stress, and inflammatory proteins within the intimal hyperplastic lesions obtained from hemodialysis patients.[46, 47] These studies suggest that specific pathophysiologic processes lead to venous stenoses in hemodialysis patients with arteriovenous grafts that may be amenable to pharmacologic inhibitory approaches.[48]

Vascular Access Monitoring and Surveillance

A significant advance in the care of hemodialysis patients with arteriovenous fistulas and grafts is the recognition that physiologic monitoring of access function can frequently identify incipient access failure before thrombosis. Vascular access monitoring is based on the premise that identification of high-risk patients for access thrombosis, coupled with elective correction of stenotic lesions, can decrease the incidence of vascular access failure and improve patient outcomes. Schwab and associates[49] initially demonstrated that intradialytic dynamic venous pressure monitoring of arteriovenous grafts had utility in the detection of graft-associated stenosis. Available hemodialysis vascular access monitoring techniques include physical examination,[50] static and dynamic venous pressure monitoring,[49, 51] vascular access blood flow monitoring,[52-59] vascular access imaging,[60-62] and measurement of access recirculation. Implementation of comprehensive vascular access surveillance programs has achieved access thrombosis rates lower than those targeted by current clinical practice guidelines. In a nonrandomized study, instituting a vascular access blood flow monitoring program substantially decreased graft thrombosis rates and reduced the number of hospital days, missed outpatient dialysis treatments, and the use of dialysis catheters because of thrombotic events.[52] Although venous stenoses developed less frequently and at a slower rate in patients with native arteriovenous fistulas compared with arteriovenous grafts, it has been suggested that vascular access blood flow monitoring has utility in this patient population as well.[63] Although almost all available data suggest considerable utility for vascular access monitoring and surveillance, there are no published randomized trials comparing results of monitoring with no monitoring.

Cuffed Venous Catheters

It has been suggested that the use of cuffed venous catheters is "a conundrum" because patients "hate living with them but can't live without them."[64] Cuffed, tunneled dialysis catheters have the advantage of immediate usability and relatively easy placement. Cuffed, tunneled catheters can be used as a permanent vascular access for patients who have exhausted all options for placement of an arteriovenous fistula or graft.[26] However, the high infections and thrombotic complications associated with catheter use and the epidemiologic data suggesting higher mortality in patients using catheters make the trend toward increased prevalence of catheter use in the U.S. dialysis population a disconcerting one.

Noncuffed, temporary catheters are suitable for acute vascular access for less than 3 weeks. They should be inserted immediately before use, and real-time, ultrasound-guided venous puncture is recommended for catheter insertion. Temporary catheters are most suitable for patients with acute renal failure, for the treatment of poisoning, in the intensive care unit setting for continuous renal replacement therapy, and as a short-term bridge until more permanent access can be placed. Tunneled, cuffed catheters are employed when more permanent vascular access will not be available for at least 3 weeks, in patients with such substantial comorbidity that there is a short life expectancy, and in patients with no remaining sites for permanent dialysis access.

The most frequent serious complication of venous catheter use is infection. The importance of sepsis as a cause of mortality in ESRD patients is emphasized by data demonstrating a 100- to 300-fold higher sepsis mortality in all dialysis patients compared with the general population.[65] In many studies, the frequency of catheter-associated bloodstream infection is approximately two to four episodes per 1000 patient-catheter days.[66] In contrast, the frequency of bacteremias associated with the use of arteriovenous fistulas is approximately 0.05 per patient-year. The data strongly emphasize the serious morbidity and mortality associated with catheter-related bacteremia in hemodialysis patients. Attempting to treat catheter-related bacteremia with antibiotics without catheter removal is unsuccessful in most patients. It has been suggested that catheter salvage can be obtained by installation of an antibiotic lock solution into the catheter lumen to eradicate luminal biofilms in addition to a 3-week course of appropriate systemic antibiotics. However, even this approach is successful in only about 50% of the cases.[67] An accepted strategy for the treatment of catheter-related bacteremia involves removal of the catheter with delayed replacement until defervescence in patients with severe clinical symptoms, catheter exchange by guidewire in patients with minimal symptoms and normal-appearing tunnel and exit site, and catheter replacement by guidewire with creation of a new tunnel in patients with exit site or tunnel infection.[68-70] Using this strategy, cure rates of more than 80% have been reported.[68] In all cases, patients should be treated with at least 3 weeks of systemic antibiotic therapy.[64, 68] However, even employing these conservative strategies, 15% to 20% of patients with catheter-related bacteremias experience complicated infections, including osteomyelitis, discitis, endocarditis, and septic arthritis. Catheter-related bacteremia due to *Staphylococcus aureus* is particularly associated with metastatic infection. Several preliminary studies suggest that the use of mupirocin ointment at the catheter exit site may decrease the incidence of *S. aureus*–associated bacteremias.

Venous catheters are also subject to frequent episodes of thrombosis requiring thrombolytic therapy or replacement of the catheter. A prospective, randomized, placebo-controlled trial of minidose warfarin for the prevention of dialysis catheter malfunction did not demonstrate a significant effective of warfarin on thrombosis-free catheter survival.[71] The long-term use of cuffed venous catheters may also lead to the development of right atrial thrombi. In one report, intravascular ultrasound prospectively identified the presence of right atrial thrombi in 22% of hemodialysis patients with indwelling venous catheters.[72] Further research is required to identify to what extent this poses a risk for hemodialysis patients. The use of cuffed venous catheters also predisposes patients to the development of central venous stenosis. Because subclavian vein stenosis may preclude the subsequent successful placement of ipsilateral arteriovenous fistulas or grafts, the use of subclavian venous catheters is generally contraindicated in dialysis patients unless used as a last resort.[73-78]

Treatment of Vascular Access Dysfunction

When an arteriovenous fistula or arteriovenous graft thromboses, thrombectomy must be performed, or a new dialysis access site must be created. Thrombectomy can be performed by endovascular or surgical techniques and must be accompanied by correction of the underlying pathophysiology leading to thrombosis (frequently a venous stenosis). When native arteriovenous fistulas thrombose early, technical factors are often responsible. Successful surgical revision has been reported in 14% to 90% of cases. Late thrombotic occlusion of autologous fistulas is usually due to outflow stenosis, and surgical approaches are less successful. Endovascular treatment of thrombosed autologous fistulas is generally reported to have a higher success rate than surgical techniques, but should not be attempted when there is suspected infection in the access. When arteriovenous grafts thrombose, similar success is reported with surgical and endovascular techniques. In all cases, attention must be directed to searching for and dilating or bypassing stenoses, including central venous lesions. Unfortunately, primary patency rates after graft thrombosis has occurred are dismal, generally in the range of 20% to 40% at 1 year.[79-82]

The poor results for arteriovenous fistulas and grafts that occurred after thrombosis led to successful implementation of surveillance and monitoring strategies. Stenotic lesions detected can in most cases undergo prophylactic percutaneous transluminal angioplasty with surgical revision reserved for recurrent stenoses or for long stenoses not amenable to percutaneous techniques. Clinical practice guidelines strongly support the judicious use of angioplasty and stents to preserve access function. However, although this approach has been documented to result in an approximately twofold to threefold decrease in the incidence of access thrombosis, the primary patency rate for arteriovenous grafts after angioplasty is approximately 60% at 6 months and 40% at 12 months in the best studies.[80, 83-85] There are no randomized, controlled trials demonstrating further efficacy or reduced costs associated with this approach.

Pharmacologic Prevention of Vascular Access Failure

Given the high cost of morbidity associated with vascular access failure, effective pharmacologic prevention of vascular access dysfunction and failure would likely have clinical utility and be cost-effective.[48] There are few randomized clinical trials of drug therapy to prevent hemodialysis vascular access dysfunction. Two separate pilot double-blind, randomized, prospective trials have suggested that fish oils or dipyridamole may be effective in reducing ePTFE graft thrombosis.[86, 87] A multicenter Veterans' Administration Cooperative Trial comparing a combination of clopidogrel plus aspirin versus placebo was discontinued prematurely due to an increase in bleeding complications in the active treatment group.[88] Several studies have suggested that short-term use of antiplatelet agents may reduce early thrombosis after native arteriovenous fistula placement. Retrospective analysis has suggested that the use of ACE inhibitors and calcium entry blockers may prolong survival of dialysis grafts.[89, 90] Because of the importance of this clinical and biologic problem, the National Institutes of Health developed a Dialysis Access Consortium, which is conducting multicenter, prospective, randomized, clinical trials of pharmacologic agents designed to reduce the vascular access failure rate for arteriovenous grafts and fistulas.

ARTIFICIAL PHYSIOLOGY: GENERAL PRINCIPLES OF HEMODIALYSIS

The differences between native and artificial kidneys are germane to this discussion. There are 1 to 2 million functioning elements or nephrons in the two native kidneys. The artificial kidney, in its hollow-fiber format, contains 8000 to 10,000 fibers and provides a surface area for exchange as high as 1.8 to 2 m^2. The proximal tubule of the nephron is 40 μm in diameter and is 14 mm long, and each hollow fiber is about 200 μm in diameter and more than 25 cm long. In addition to being influenced by diffusive and convective forces, the tubules perform a myriad of biochemical processes on the fluid that is filtered at the glomerulus whereas depuration in the artificial kidney is solely dependent on the physical forces of diffusion and convection across a semipermeable membrane.

Clearance

Definitions and Principles

The physiologist uses the concept of clearance to describe the net result of the transport functions of the kidney. The clearance of a substance is the amount removed from plasma, divided by the average plasma concentration over the time of measurement. Clearance is expressed in moles or weight of the substance per volume per time. It can be thought of as the volume of plasma that can be completely cleared of the substance in a unit of time. Clearance is also a useful concept when describing the process of dialysis.

The goals of dialysis are straightforward: to remove accumulated fluid and toxins. With respect to toxins, the goal is to maintain their concentrations below the levels at which they produce uremic symptoms. However, the toxic levels of retained substances are not used as performance measures for dialysis because their identities are unknown. Instead, performance of dialysis is judged by clearance. If the generation of a substance is fixed, its clearance (i.e., removal rate from plasma/plasma concentration) then becomes a measure

of its concentration levels in the patient. The principles and the calculation of clearance are the same for all substances removed by dialysis.

Dialysis relies on the mass transfer across semipermeable membranes. The hemodialysis membranes separate the blood and dialysate compartments. Diffusion, convection, and ultrafiltration across the membrane are properties that are integral to the dialysis procedure. Diffusion describes the movement of solutes from one compartment to another, relying on a concentration gradient between the two compartments. This is the principal mechanism for toxin removal during hemodialysis. Convective transport involves the movement of solutes by bulk flow in association with fluid removal. Convective clearance is the mechanism of toxin removal by the depurative process known as hemofiltration. It is not dependent on concentration gradients and the magnitude of its contribution to clearance is directly related to the ultrafiltration rate. Mass solute removal across the dialyzer is a function of effective blood flow (Q_B) and differences between the afferent and efferent concentrations of solute, traditionally labeled as "arterial" and "venous" (C_A and C_V). The definition of diffusive dialyzer clearance (K), similar to creatinine clearance in the normal kidney, is calculated as:

$$K = (Q_B)(C_A - C_V)/C_A$$

In the equation, $(Q_B)(C_A - C_V)$ represents the amount of solute removal and C_A is the driving force. This formula describes diffusive clearance when *single-pass* hemodialysis circuits, in which the blood side is always in contact with fresh dialysate that is continuously being generated, are employed. Older systems employed discrete batches of dialysate that were recirculated. The result of these configurations is that concentrations of the removed toxins rise in the dialysate. The consequence is that the driving force to diffusion decreases. In this case, the driving force is described by $C_A - D_I$, in which D_I is the concentration of the removed substance in the dialysate. Instead of clearance, the term dialysance is used:

$$D = (Q_B)(C_A - C_V)/(C_A - D_I).$$

The efficiency of recirculated hemodialysis systems is inferior to single-pass systems because the driving force for diffusion is continuously being dissipated by the appearance in the dialysate of the substances being removed. Systems employing single-pass dialysate circuits are almost universally employed.

These equations, however, neglect the contribution of convection. This phenomenon is directly related to ultrafiltration and involves the bulk movement of fluid across dialyzer membranes. The driving force for ultrafiltration is the hydrostatic pressure gradient across the membrane, the transmembrane pressure (TMP). With ultrafiltration, blood flow leaving the dialyzer (Q_{Bo}) is less than blood flow entering the dialyzer (Q_{Bi}). The difference between these values represents ultrafiltration (Q_{uf}). This can be incorporated into the previous equation to yield a more precise definition of clearance:

$$(Q_{Bo}) = (Q_{Bi}) - (Q_{uf})$$
$$K = [Q_{Bi}(C_A) - (Q_{Bo} - Q_{uf})(C_V)]/C_A$$
$$= [(Q_{Bi})(C_A - C_V) + (Q_{uf})(C_V)]/C_A$$

True clearance should be calculated by using the concentration in the aqueous compartment of blood and the concentration of solute in that compartment. Because solutes diffusing out of blood appear in the dialysate, it is possible to calculate clearance for solutes not present in the incoming dialysate (e.g., urea) as follows:

$$K = Q_{Do} (C_{Do})/C_A$$

In this equation, C_{Do} and Q_{Do} are the concentrations of solute in the dialysate outlet and the effluent dialysate flow, respectively. Although this equation provides a simple concept for determining clearance, the necessity of measuring low concentrations of any substance in the dialysate increases the error of measurement. The most accurate measurement of dialyzer clearance is achieved when "blood-side" and "dialysate-side" clearances are obtained, ensuring mass balance.

Factors Influencing Clearance

Several variables affect clearance by the dialyzer (Table 59-2). The physical and chemical properties of the substance to be removed and its distribution in the body are toxin-related variables. The procedure-related variables include the permeability of the membrane to toxins of various sizes (flux), its hydraulic permeability, the membrane surface area, dialysis time, blood and dialysate flow rates and dialysate composition.

The size and charge of the molecule are important intrinsic physical features governing its removal. If the molecule is charged, its behavior is governed by the Donnan equilibrium. The cation concentration on the blood side of the membrane is higher because of the presence of plasma proteins that are negatively charged (Fig. 59-5).

In the case of sodium, the dialysate-side concentration of sodium should be approximately 3 mEq/L less than the blood-side concentration to prevent net transfer of sodium from dialysate to the patient. The lower the molecular weight of the substance, the greater its rate of movement across the membrane or flux (J). Other factors such as binding of the toxin to plasma proteins, a large volume of distribution or delayed transfer of the substance from the intracellular pool to the intravascular space results in decreased clearance. An important example of the latter principle involves phosphorus. In Figure 59-6, phosphorus

is rapidly removed from the intravascular compartment and the patients actually become hypophosphatemic during the hemodialysis treatment. However, there is a rebound in the postdialysis interval with phosphorus levels rapidly returning to predialysis levels. Although phosphorus is a relatively small molecule, hemodialysis alone is not sufficient to control its level.

As the molecular weight of the substance increases, the properties of the dialysis membrane become increasingly important factors with regard to clearance. The association of J with clearance of the toxin is given in the following formula:

$$J = A(\Delta C/R)$$

In this equation, A is the surface area of the membrane in the dialyzer, ΔC is the concentration gradient between blood and dialysate, and R represents resistance to diffusivity of the substance across the membrane and the thickness of the membrane.

Removal of low-molecular-weight substances follows first-order kinetics. The efficiency of the removal of substances depends on the concentration of the toxin in the blood. Blood and dialysate flow rates are the most important variables for clearance of the small molecular substances. Clearance of higher-molecular-weight substances depends on membrane porosity, surface area, and dialysis time.

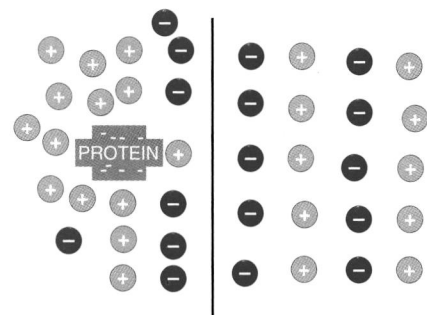

FIGURE 59-5. Consequences of the Donnan equilibrium.

TABLE 59-2

Factors Influencing Clearance by the Dialyzer

| TOXIN RELATED | PROCEDURE RELATED (IN ORDER OF IMPORTANCE) | |
	Low-Molecular-Weight Toxin	High-Molecular-Weight Toxin
Size	Dialysate composition*	Flux
Charge	Blood flow	Time
Protein binding	Dialysate flow	Membrane surface area
Volume of distribution	Membrane surface area	Blood flow
	Time	Dialysate flow
	Flux	Dialysate composition*

*For potassium, calcium, sodium, and total CO_2, this factor is not applicable.

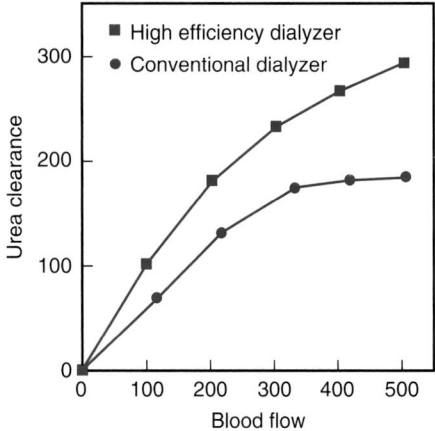

FIGURE 59-6. Clearance as a function of dialyzer type.

To increase the clearance of low-molecular-weight substances, mere engineering issues must be addressed. Dialyzers with larger surface areas or hollow-fiber geometry that permit higher blood flows to be used without promoting turbulence can be constructed. Two large dialyzers can be connected in series or in parallel configurations to increase the clearance of low-molecular-weight toxins. High-efficiency dialysis can be accomplished in patients with low to average body surface areas (i.e., body surface area bears a direct relationship to the volume of distribution of substances such as urea or creatinine) without major increases in dialysis time. However, multiple lines of evidence are emerging that lengthening dialysis time leads to better blood pressure control, nutritional status, and phosphorus management. The rate at which fluid can be safely mobilized from the various body compartments without producing hemodynamic instability also places limits on how short the treatment can be. These issues are dealt with in subsequent sections.

Hemodialysis Membranes: Effects and Characteristics

In place of glomeruli and tubules that have the ability to perform active transport, the point of exchange for hemodialysis is the membrane in the dialyzer. The surface area, surface charge, and pore size are properties of the membrane that directly govern the molecules that can diffuse from blood to the dialysate. These variables determine mass transfer coefficient (K_oA) of the membrane for a given solute. The relationship between K_oA and clearance (K) of a solute is a function the blood (Q_B) and dialysate (Q_D) flow rates, as described by the following equation:

$$K_oA = (Q_B/1 - Q_B/Q_D) \, Log[(1 - K/Q_D)/(1 - K/Q_B)].$$

The classic view of membranes as inert structures providing solely fluid, ion, and molecular transport is obsolete. Modern dialysis membranes display numerous physical and adsorptive properties that also contribute to the degree to which blood components are activated by the membranes. Membranes that produce little interaction with blood components such as white blood cells and the humoral components of plasma are described as being biocompatible. The structural compounds comprising the dialysis membranes may be their simplest distinguishing feature, dividing dialyzers into cellulosic, semisynthetic, and synthetic membranes. Although in decline, cellulose and its derivatives, cuprophane and cellulose acetate, continue to be the most commonly used membranes for dialysis worldwide. Cellulose extracted from cotton fibers is dissolved in sodium hydroxide and regenerated, and the membrane is then formed in an acid bath. Cuprophane is generated with an ammonium solution of copper hydroxide. Copper-ammonia-cellulose complexes are extruded into an acid bath, producing a membrane with cuprammonium radicals. This modification yields greater diffusion and ultrafiltration capabilities for cuprophane membranes compared with straight cellulose. Increasing glycerin content in membranes (average content for cuprophane is 5%) also affects these characteristics, as does membrane acetylation yielding greater solute and flux capacities to the membrane. The side groups of the cellulosic membranes activate the complement system through the alternate pathway, resulting in the repeated generation of the anaphylatoxins C3a and C5a.[91]

Synthetic membranes differ from cellulose-based dialyzers in several ways. All cellulose membranes have hydroxyl radicals at the surface that increase their hydrophilicity (i.e., membrane wetability). Techniques that mask hydroxyl radicals enhance hydrophobicity and increase protein adsorption.[92] Most synthetic membranes are thicker than less permeable cellulosic membranes. Membrane permeability is inversely proportional to membrane thickness and directly proportional to the membrane's intrinsic diffusion coefficient. However, synthetic membranes also display greater intrinsic diffusion coefficients and maintain their thickness when wet. Cuprophane and cellulose acetate membranes swell when wet.[93, 94] A number of synthetic membranes also strongly bind blood proteins, causing decreases in their filtration efficiency.

Membranes can be symmetrical or asymmetrical. The smooth "skin" side interacts with blood for asymmetrical membranes. Asymmetry, obtained by altering membrane precipitation during manufacturing allows for greater diffusive permeability.[95] Asymmetrical membranes are very useful for hemofiltration. Polyacrylonitrile (PAN) and polysulfone (PS) membranes are commonly used asymmetrical membranes. Polymethylmethacrylate (PMMA) membranes also manifest many of these characteristics. PAN, polyamide (PA), and PMMA membranes have low hydrophilicity and appreciable protein adsorption. Cellulose-based membranes have greater hydrophilicity and less adsorptive capacity.[95] Surface charge of the membranes also differs, which affects the sieving of charged solutes.[96]

Biocompatibility of Dialysis Membranes

During hemodialysis, patients may experience a number of reactions that are a direct consequence of establishing the extracorporeal circuit. The number and severity of these reactions define the degree of dialysis biocompatibility. In the broadest sense, all aspects of the treatment such as dialysate composition and temperature, the nature of the anticoagulant, or whether clearance is achieved predominantly by diffusion or convection, influence biocompatibility. However, it is the biocompatibility of the membrane surface itself that is most important and has been most closely studied. It is also important to remember that because hemodialysis is a repetitive process, even low-grade or minor membrane-induced reactions at each treatment can eventually lead to important clinical manifestations.

The initial observation that transient neutropenia occurred during hemodialysis was made a quarter of a century ago.[97] It was later determined that complement activation through the alternative pathway, with generation of the anaphylatoxins C3a and C5a, was responsible for the decline in neutrophils shortly after initiation of hemodialysis.[98]

In this context, cellulosic hemodialysis membranes react with blood coursing through them. Free hydroxyl groups on cellulosic membranes activate complement through the alternative pathway. Membrane modifications that favor binding of factor H and inhibit binding of factor B (e.g., replacing hydroxyl groups with acetate side groups or diethylaminoethyl radicals) may ameliorate complement activation.[95, 99] Complement activation is reduced as membrane hydrophobicity increases.[100] Surface charge further influences biocompatibility. Surfaces with a negative charge may interact with the Hageman factor and the contact pathway (kallikrein-kinin), activating the contact pathway and generating bradykinin.[101-103] This may lead to severe adverse reactions in patients dialyzed against PAN membranes (specifically AN69) while concomitantly receiving ACE inhibitors.[104] ACE inhibitors prevent bradykinin degradation. Reused cellulosic membranes have also been implicated in these acute reactions.[105] Conceivably, reuse alters membrane characteristics, favoring bradykinin generation, although this has not yet been proved.

The effect of the format of the membrane is also significant. Format refers to the structure of the dialyzer rather than the nature of membrane. Dialyzers may be formatted as hollow-fiber or parallel-plate devices. The same membrane type may produce alterations in neutrophils (e.g., release of proteolytic enzymes) that differ depending on whether the

membrane in the artificial kidney is formatted as hollow fibers or parallel plates.[106]

The adsorptive capacity of a membrane can affect its biocompatibility. PAN membranes bind vasoactive materials, including C3a, C5a, and bradykinin, to a greater extent than cuprophane.[107, 108] The ability to adsorb potentially harmful substances may confer distinct advantages to certain membranes. However, beneficial substances may be removed, and protein adsorption may alter the characteristics of the membrane.

Blood-Membrane Interactions

All humoral and cellular components in blood can potentially interact with the dialysis membrane (Fig. 59-7). Interactions involving cellulosic membranes are associated with the greatest

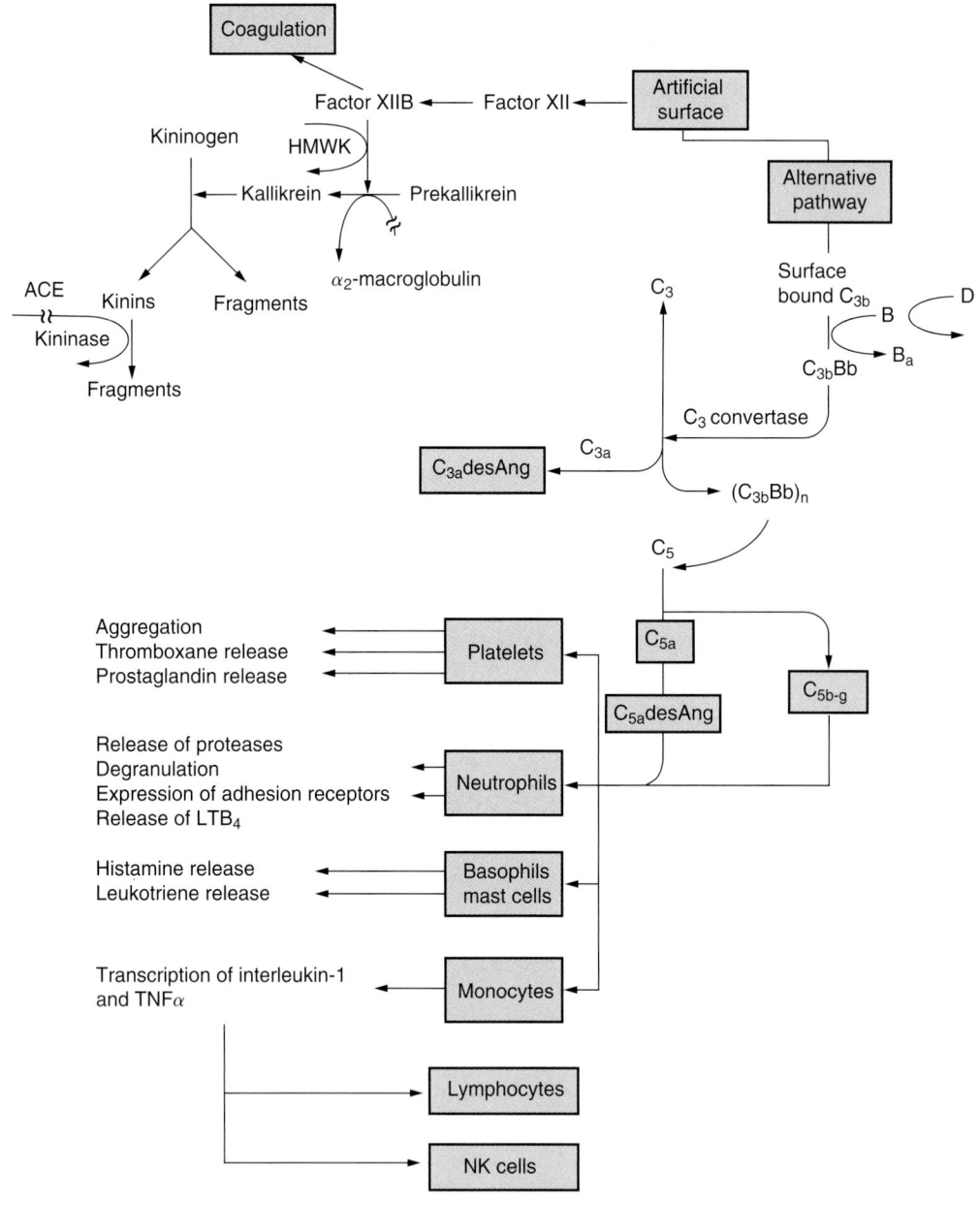

FIGURE 59-7. Pathways of blood and dialysis membrane interactions. LTB_4, leukotriene B_4; NK, natural killer; PMMA, polymethylmethacrylate; $TNF\alpha$, tumor necrosis factor α.

degree of complement activation. Generation of C3a and C5a is ultimately responsible for the clinical sequelae of blood-membrane interactions, including contraction of vascular smooth muscle, increased vascular permeability, and formation of the membrane attack complex (C5b-C9). Complement generation also results in neutrophil activation. Release of enzymes such as lactoferrin, production of reactive oxygen species, synthesis of arachidonic metabolites, expression of adhesion receptors, and increases in monocyte cytokine gene transcription are all consequences of complement activation.[109]

The coagulation pathway is activated to some degree by dialyzer membrane surfaces. Anticoagulation during dialysis blunts this response. Cellular components of blood are also affected by hemodialysis membranes. Abnormal leukocyte function has been reported in chronic hemodialysis patients, with complement-activating membranes inducing a greater degree of leukocyte dysfunction, defects in chemotaxis, and alterations in oxidative metabolism.[110-112] Peripheral blood mononuclear cells and monocytes harvested from patients chronically exposed to cuprophane membranes produce decreased concentrations of interleukin-1 (IL-1), tumor necrosis factor (TNF), decreased levels of interleukin-2 (IL-2) receptor expression, and variable degrees of natural killer cell activity dysfunction.[113-116]

Cytokines, such as IL-1, IL-2, and TNF are thought to mediate some of the adverse reactions that are seen after hemodialysis with cuprophane membranes.[117] The paradox associated with this conclusion is that the performance index of in vitro cytokine generation by cells after they have been exposed to cellulosic membranes and then harvested from the peripheral circulation, is downgraded at baseline and after endotoxin stimulation. It may be that repetitive insults are sufficient to produce adverse effects or that neutrophils and mononuclear cells produce tissue-level down-regulation of cytokine production.[114]

Platelets also react with dialysis-membrane surfaces, but less information is available about whether platelet function is affected by complement activation or other parameters of bio-compatibility. Survival of red blood cells is significantly decreased in hemodialysis patients, although the cause for this is multifactorial. Red blood cells from hemodialysis patients appear to be more susceptible to the membrane attack complex (C5b-C9) compared with red blood cells from normal individuals.[118] The significance of these reactions is only partially understood at present. The extent to which any given membrane has been examined with respect to activation of each of the blood components differs (Fig. 59-8 and Table 59-3). Operationally, the lack of complement activation and early neutropenia during hemodialysis should serve as useful indices of biocompatible membranes.

Membrane Permeability

Just as the glomeruli restrict the passage of substances based on surface charge and size, the dialysis membrane also limits the passage of material based on these same physical properties. The nephrologist has the option of regulating what is removed by selecting among the membrane based on its permeability to small and larger substances. Dialyzers are classified as conventional, high-efficiency, or high-flux devices. There is some imprecision surrounding these definitions. The blood flow and the length of treatment employed when using these dialyzers should not be part of the definition. Nor should urea clearance be used in the definition because clearance or dialysance varies with blood flow.

TABLE 59-3

Comparative Biocompatibility

PARAMETER	RELATIVE ORDER
Heparin consumption	Cuprophane > PS = PMMA
Complement activation	Cuprophane > Cellulose acetate > PC > PAN
Leukopenia	Cuprophane > Cellulose acetate > PC > PAN = PMMA
Granulocyte elastase	Cuprophane = PMMA > PS = PAN
Granulocyte adherence	Cuprophane > PS = PAN

PS, polysulfone; PMMA, polymethylmethacrylate; PC, polyetherpolycarbonate; PAN, polyacrylonitrile.

Data from Mujaijsk R, Ivanovich P: Membranes for extracorporeal therapy. *In* Maher JF (ed): Replacement of Renal Function by Dialysis. Dordrecht, Kluwer Academic Publishers, 1989, pp 181-188.

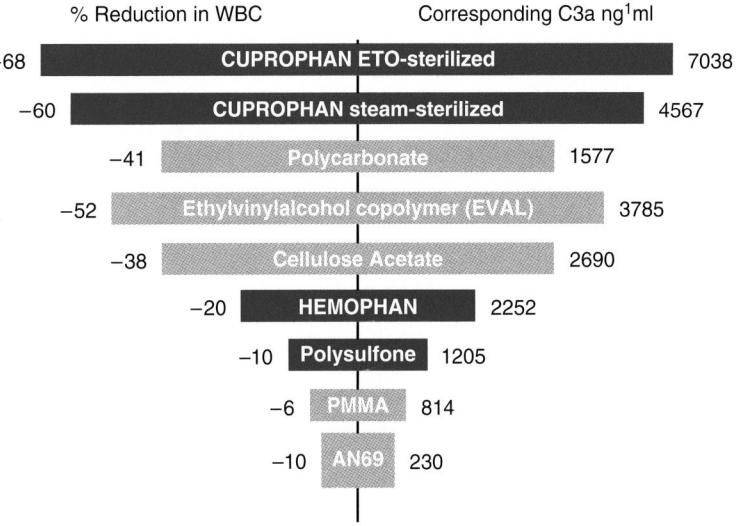

FIGURE 59-8. Range of changes in the parameters of various dialysis membranes. WBC, white blood cell.

TABLE 59-4

Comparison of Dialyzers

DIALYZER	KoA$_{urea}$ (mL/min)	ULTRAFILTRATION COEFFICIENT	HYDROPHOBIC/HYDROPHILIC	MEMBRANE STRUCTURE
Conventional	<450	<10 mL/mm Hg/hr	Hydrophilic	Symmetrical
High-efficiency	>450	10–19 mL/mm Hg/hr	Intermediate	Intermediate
High-flux	>450	>15 mL/mm Hg/hr	Hydrophobic	Asymmetrical

Instead, the dialyzer should be defined by the urea mass transfer coefficient (K_oA_{urea}), the ultrafiltration coefficient, and the degree of hydrophobicity or hydrophilicity of its membrane (Table 59-4). The latter parameter governs the permeability of the membrane to large-molecular-weight substances, its degree of biocompatibility, and its ability to adsorb plasma proteins and peptides to its surface.

The conventional dialyzer has a membrane that is homogeneous, permits effective small solute clearance, but its clearance of middle molecules (300 to 1500 daltons [D]) is relatively low. Urea clearance at a blood flow of 300 mL/minute is less than 200 mL/minute (see Fig. 59-6). The relatively low hydraulic permeability of many of the membranes permit treatment with a dialysis machine that does not have an ultrafiltration controller. These membranes are cellulose-based and contain nucleophilic groups that permit complement activation unless they have been chemically modified. The blood flow and membrane structural limitations on urea mass transfer preclude their use in high-efficiency hemodialysis. High-efficiency and high-flux dialyzers have membranes with a K_oA_{urea} of more than 450 mL/minute. Under standard operating conditions of a blood flow of 400 mL/minute, the urea clearance can be in excess of 250 mL/minute (see Fig. 59-6).

In addition to having a high K_oA_{urea}, the high-flux membranes are constructed with pores that permit the passage of molecules exceeding 10,000 D or more with a clearance as high as 40 mL/minute. Significant binding of protein and peptides from the blood may occur with these membranes. When the high-flux membrane is chemically modified, hydraulic permeability as well as the permeability to large-molecular-weight substances is reduced, creating a high-efficiency membrane. The final result is that with respect to low-molecular-weight substances, high-flux and high-efficiency dialyzers have similar performance characteristics. They differ in their ability to remove high-molecular-weight substances.

There are several reasons to use high-efficiency and high-flux dialyzers (Table 59-5). Both dialyzers have low-molecular-weight substance clearance rates far in excess of conventional dialyzers. They are useful in large patients with high urea volumes to ensure delivery of an adequate level of therapy. The high-flux dialyzers also clear higher-molecular-weight substances, including substances proved to produce toxicity such as beta$_2$-microglobulin (11,800 D). The surfaces of these membranes are more biocompatible and cause less activation of complement and less neutropenia and immune cell dysfunction during dialysis. However, the primary motivation behind the use of the efficient dialyzers often is the facilitation of shorter dialysis times.

TABLE 59-5

Reasons to Use High-Efficiency Dialyzers

LMW clearance	Ensure adequate dialysis in large patients
HMW clearance	Clearance of HMW substances such as β$_2$-microglobulin (high flux)
Biocompatibility	Reduced complement activation, less morbidity and mortality
Short dialysis	Improved lifestyle while receiving adequate therapy

HMW, high molecular weight; LMW, low molecular weight.

COMPONENTS OF THE EXTRACORPOREAL CIRCUIT

The point of exchange between blood and dialysate in the hemodialysis circuit is the artificial kidney. The machine is designed to deliver blood and properly constituted dialysate to the artificial kidney, where diffusive and convective may occur. This requires that blood and dialysate be delivered at accurate rates. The machine is also invested with a number of on-line monitors to ensure that acceptable ranges of chemical content, temperature, and circuit pressures are continuously present.

Blood Circuit

Blood in the extracorporeal circuit is contained within tubing that is connected to the venous and arterial sides of a patient's access (Fig. 59-9).

Needles are inserted into the patient's blood access, and blood tubing is connected to the needle hubs. Blood is withdrawn from the arterial segment by the blood pump and pumped through the dialyzer back to the patient through the venous segment of tubing. Inadvertent entry of air into the dialysis circuit, air embolism, is a potentially lethal complication and is likeliest to occur between the vascular access site and the blood pump. Air can enter the dialysis circuit from areas around the arterial needle, through leaky or broken tubing or tubing connections, and through the saline infusion set. Air traps are located in the blood tubing to trap air and prevent air from entering the patient's circulation. Air detectors are linked to a relay switch that automatically clamps the venous blood line and shuts off the blood pump if air is detected. If air embolism is suspected, the venous line leading back to the patient should be clamped. The patient should immediately be placed on the left side and in the Trendelenburg position. This tends to sequester the air in the right ventricle of the heart, preventing its propagation into the pulmonary circulation and allowing it to be reabsorbed.

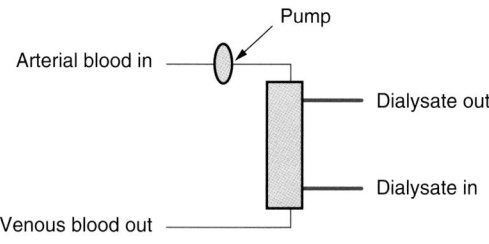

FIGURE 59-9. The dialysis circuit.

Blood pumps used for hemodialysis (HD) are roller pumps that use the principles of peristaltic pumping to move blood through tubing. A compressible part of the tubing (the pump segment) is occluded between rollers and a curved rigid track. Elastic recoil refills the pump tubing after the roller has passed over it. The flow rate of the blood pump is dependent on the stroke volume, the speed of rotation of the rollers, and the volume of the pump segment. The blood flow rate displayed on the dialysis machine is based on these three parameters, rather than an actual value from a blood flow probe. This can lead to significantly higher values for the displayed blood flow compared with the true blood flow rate. Incomplete occlusion of the pump segment due to a pump maladjustment leads to a reduced volume of blood with each pump rotation. This is a common cause of overestimation of blood flow and hence clearance. Careful maintenance of the pump is essential to ensure that the prescribed dialysis dose is actually delivered to the patient.

Pressure monitors are usually located proximal to the blood pump and immediately distal to the dialyzer. The proximal monitor (i.e., arterial monitor) guards against excessive suction on the vascular access site by the blood pump, and the distal monitor (i.e., venous monitor) gauges the resistance to blood return to the venous side of the vascular access. Some machines place the arterial monitor distal to the blood pump and proximal to the dialyzer to detect clotting in the dialyzer and more precisely estimate pressure in the dialyzer blood compartment. To prevent blood clotting in the dialyzer, an anticoagulant such as heparin is often infused into the circuit. A peristaltic pump or syringe pump delivers the anticoagulant into blood in the circuit through a T-tube or T-fitting usually located between the blood pump and the dialyzer.

A blood leak detector is usually placed in the dialysis circuit in the dialysate outflow line. If a blood leak develops through the dialysis membrane, then blood leaking into the dialysate is sensed by the blood leak detector and the appropriate alarm is activated.

Dialysate Circuit

Another major function of the hemodialysis machine is to deliver dialysate to the circuit. In some large dialysis units, dialysate is made as a batch and stored in tanks. The dialysate is then simply delivered to each dialysis station and connected to the machine. In other cases, water that has been treated to remove most elements is sent to the hemodialysis machine and then mixed with a dialysate concentrate. The water and concentrated dialysate then are properly proportioned by the machine so that dialysate with proper concentrations of electrolytes enters the dialyzer.

There are two properties of the dialysate that require constant monitoring: conductivity and temperature. A proportioning system dilutes a concentrated dialysate with water. If this system malfunctions, patient blood can be exposed to a hyperosmolar dialysate resulting in hypernatremia, or a hypo-osmolar dialysate leading to hyponatremia and hemolysis. The primary solutes in the dialysate are electrolytes. The concentration of the dialysate is reflected by the concentration of electrolytes and their electrical conductivity. Appropriate proportioning of water and the dialysate is monitored by a meter measuring conductivity of the product dialysate fed into the dialyzer.

A temperature monitor prevents complications related to overheated dialysate. Cool dialysate can be uncomfortable for the patient and is dangerous when the patient is unconscious, but otherwise may have therapeutic value in preventing hypotension. Overheated dialysate ($>42°C$), however, can lead to hemolysis. If the conductivity or the temperature is outside the normal range, a bypass valve diverts the dialysate around the dialyzer and directly to a drain.

Variations in the Extracorporeal Circuit
Continuous Renal Replacement Therapy

Continuous renal replacement therapy (CRRT) is a form of extracorporeal clearance therapy used in the treatment of acute renal failure. It is used in place of standard hemodialysis and requires an intensive care setting for its implementation. There are several techniques that fall under CRRT. They are similar to one another with respect to the extracorporeal circuit and to the general principles of exchange:

> Slow continuous ultrafiltration (SCUF)
> Continuous arteriovenous or venovenous hemofiltration (CAVH or CVVH)
> Continuous arteriovenous or venovenous hemodialysis (CAVHD or CAVVHD)
> Continuous arteriovenous or venovenous hemodiafiltration (CAVHDF or CVVHDF)

The arteriovenous configuration indicates that an artery and a vein are entered to remove and return blood in the extracorporeal circuit whereas the venovenous configuration indicates that blood is removed and returned through venous access, such as a catheter. Arteriovenous procedures can be performed using an external shunt, connecting an artery to a vein. The use of arteriovenous access allows arterial pressure to propel blood through the extracorporeal circuit without the absolute need of a blood pump, although a blood pump can be used. The venovenous procedures require a blood pump to be used. The disadvantage of arteriovenous procedures is that a large artery must be cannulated for a long period of time. An occasional patient with an existing arteriovenous fistula or graft may undergo CRRT. Although the blood in an A-V graft is under arterial pressure, a blood pump is still required because the blood must also be returned to the high-pressure system. In general, the low-molecular-weight substance clearance rates of the continuous therapies approximate the volume of fluid removed or the dialysate flow rate (Table 59-6).

CAVH, CVVH, and SCUF are all variations on the depurative process of hemofiltration (see "Artificial Physiology: General Principles of Hemodialysis"). In hemofiltration,

TABLE 59-6

Comparisons of Clearance by Extracorporeal Therapies

	CAVH	CVVH	CAVHD	CAVHDF	CVVHD	CVVHF	PD	IHD
Filtrate (L/day)	14	24	7	14	7	19	12	3-4
Dialysate flow	0	0	1	1	1	1	1-3	3-4
Replacement	12	22	5	12	5	17	0	0
K_{urea} (mL/min)	10	17	22	27	22	30	8.5	180

AV, arteriovenous; C, continuous; H, hemofiltration; HD, hemodialysis; I, intermittent; VV, venovenous.

Data from Conger J: Dialysis and related therapies. Semin Nephrol 11:533-540, 1998.

removal of fluid and waste occur by entirely by convection or bulk flow. Transmembrane pressure governs the amount of fluid and dissolved waste being ultrafiltered across the membrane. Blood flow through the extracorporeal circuit ranges between 150 and 200 mL/minute. With the usual parameters for blood flow and transmembrane pressure the ultrafiltration rate, as much as 40 L/day can be removed. The fluid removed is replaced with a balanced electrolyte solution at a rate that is less than the rate of fluid removed and governed by the desired amount of excess volume that is to be removed from the patient. For instance, a patient with acute renal failure after surgery may have an expanded volume and be receiving parenteral nutrition and medications amounting to an intake of more than 4 L/day. If 40 L/day is ultrafiltered, the physician may want to set the replacement rate at only 35 L/day to begin to correct volume expansion.

At high ultrafiltration rates, replacement fluid must be infused before the filter (i.e., predilution) to prevent excessive hemoconcentration in the filter. Excessive hemoconcentration poses a risk for clotting of the filter. Although infusing replacement fluid before filtering prevents clotting, it also reduces the efficiency of the clearance, because the urea concentration in the blood flowing into the filter is diluted by the replacement fluid. For low-molecular-weight substances, continuous hemofiltration is less efficient than continuous hemodialysis or continuous hemodiafiltration. For substances of higher molecular weight, convective clearance is superior to hemodialysis.

SCUF is a form of limited hemofiltration that provides slow, continuous ultrafiltration in volume-overloaded patients who are resistant to diuretics or who are hemodynamically unstable. The desired volume to be removed is calculated and removed over the entire day. Patients with massive volume overload and marginal blood pressures can be treated. No replacement fluid is required, but clearances are very low with this technique ($\approx$3.5 mL/min) and SCUF cannot be used to provide total renal replacement therapy.

CAVHD or CVVHD employs diffusion to replace renal function. Blood flow rate through the extracorporeal circuit is similar to that for continuous hemofiltration. Dialysate is run through the filter at 1 to 2 L/hour. This results in a urea clearance of 17 to 34 mL/minute, because the outflow dialysate is more than 90% saturated with urea at the blood flow rates employed. The clinician can further increase the clearance of urea by combining hemofiltration to the continuous hemodialysis procedure.

The technology permits any of these treatments to be implemented with the same machine. The tubing that directs the circuit path of blood, dialysate, or replacement fluid is

TABLE 59-7

Comparison of IHD, CVVHD, and EDD

INTERMITTENT HEMODIALYSIS	CVVHD	EDD
180 mL/min	22 mL/min	75 mL/min
43.2 L/treatment	31.7 L/treatment	36 L/treatment
(4 hr)	(24 hr)	(8 hr)

CVVHD, continuous venovenous hemodialysis; EDD, extended daily dialysis.

merely configured to provide the desired form of therapy. The available machines provide pressure monitors and pumps for the fluid pathway. However, unlike the machines used for intermittent hemodialysis that can take a dialysate concentrate and proportion it with ultrapure water, the dialysate and the replacement fluid are not generated by the machine. Prepackaged dialysate or hemofiltration replacement fluid or fluid provided by the hospital pharmacy must be used. Some of the newer hemodialysis machines have the software that permits their use for CAVHD or CVVHD. The software permits dialysate to be proportioned so that the lower dialysate flow rates associated with the continuous therapies may be applied to the treatment.

Extended Daily Dialysis

An alternative form of therapy has been suggested for the management of the unstable patient with acute renal failure.[119] A conventional hemodialysis machine is used to perform hemodialysis six or seven times each week at low blood and dialysate flows, such as blood flow of 100 to 200 mL/minute and dialysate flow of 300 mL/minute. Each treatment lasts 6 to 8 hours. The urea clearance of extended daily dialysis (EDD) can exceed that of the continuous therapies (Table 59-7).

EDD is less labor intensive than the continuous therapies. The continuous therapies often require a 1:1 ratio of nurses to patients because of the need to monitor fluid balance and change the replacement fluid. EDD employs the proportioning system of the hemodialysis machine and does not require the continuous presence of dialysis personnel at the bedside. EDD also allows the patient to more easily be available for diagnostic test and therapeutic procedures, because the treatment lasts for only 6 to 8 hours. Delivered therapy through EDD may be superior to continuous therapy due to fewer interruptions and clotting of the extracorporeal circuit associated with the former therapy.[119] EDD generally requires less heparin than the continuous therapies. Because it is easily implemented and similar to conventional intermittent hemodialysis, it is accepted by nursing staff and remains under control of nephrologists.

On-line Monitoring

Dialysis machines function as more than just dialysis delivery systems. Built-in monitors assess the physical and chemical characteristics of the dialysate, and they record and store data ranging from patient blood pressure and heart rate to treatment-related parameters (blood and dialysate flows, arterial and venous pressures, temperature), medication data, measures of delivered dialysis dose, plasma volume, thermal energy loss, and even dialysis access recirculation. Computerized medical information systems have been linked with dialysis delivery systems to provide information networks that can control treatments at individual patient stations while maintaining information and treatment records for future use. Real-time information regarding treatment parameters and patient information also can be recorded with other monitors during dialysis treatments. It is possible to integrate data, such as comparing present and past dialysis treatments, into a real-time display to help gauge therapy, change prescription and ultrafiltration goals, and generate better immediate assessment of a patient's and unit's overall status.[120, 121] Such on-line monitoring that allows sensors from the machine to change treatment parameters has been called a biofeedback system (Fig. 59-10). Automatic biofeedback systems have the potential to reduce adverse events such as hypotension, monitor the state of the hemodialysis access, and increase the efficiency of the hemodialysis treatment (Table 59-8).

Much effort has been devoted to applying technologic advances to improving measures of dialysis adequacy based on removal of low-molecular-weight substances. Data from numerous studies during the past decade suggest that the dose of dialysis greatly influences mortality and morbidity

in ESRD patients. A standard measure of the dose of dialysis is the Kt/V urea index, in which K = urea clearance, t = treatment time, and V = volume of urea distribution. When Gotch and Sargent analyzed data from the National Cooperative Dialysis Study,[48] they determined that values of less than 0.8 were associated with increased rates of patient morbidity. Additional studies have suggested that increasing Kt/V to values of more than 1.2 to 1.4 may improve patient survival.[122, 123] Urea kinetic modeling is therefore an easy tool for assessing the adequacy of dialysis.

Traditionally, this technique has required multiple blood samples, accurate assessment of blood and dialysate flows and treatment times, and mathematical calculations, simplified somewhat by custom-designed software. On-line systems that accurately measure urea kinetics are feasible. They measure urea concentration in dialysate effluent and determine urea kinetic parameters from a concentration- and time-dependent profile.[124, 125] This does not require blood sampling and has the additional advantage of providing a Kt/V based on whole-body urea clearance (i.e., two-pool

TABLE 59-8

On-line Features of the Hemodialysis Machine

PARAMETER	CONSEQUENCE
Blood pressure	Changes in ultrafiltration rate, sodium modeling
Plasma volume by hemoglobin	Changes in ultrafiltration rate, sodium modeling
Thermal energy loss/gain	Change in dialysate temperature
Transient change in dialysate sodium	Measurement of Kt/V
Transient change in hemoglobin	Access blood flow, recirculation, cardiac output
Transient change in temperature	Access recirculation

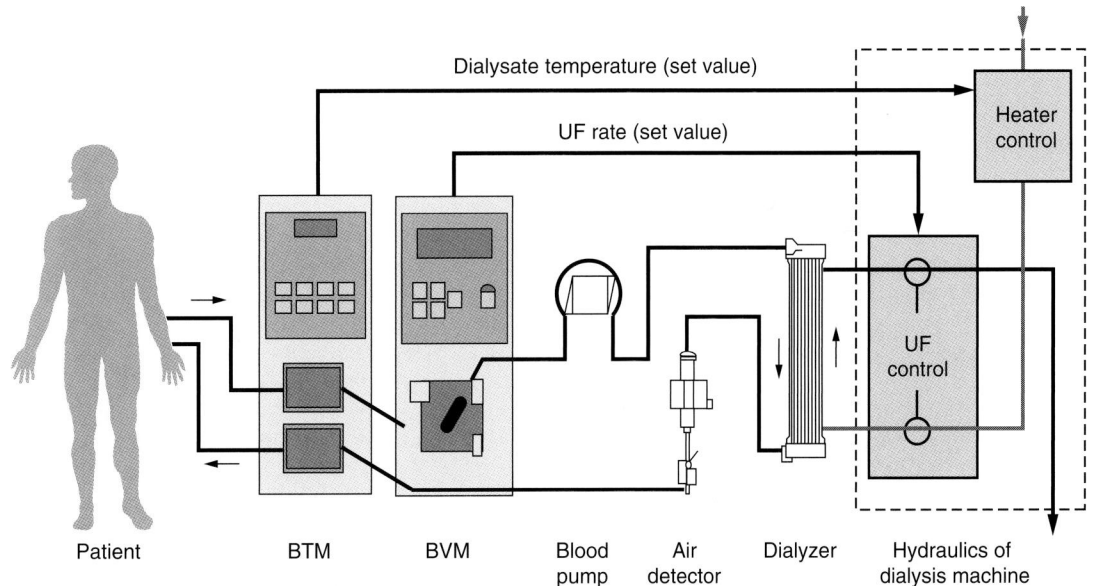

FIGURE 59-10. Integrated hemodialysis circuit and feedback system. BTM, ; BVM, ; UF, ultrafiltration.

model of urea kinetics) rather than traditional single-pool kinetics. Efforts to enhance the accuracy and simplicity of this system and other on-line urea monitoring devices are ongoing.

A variation employs sodium clearance in place of changes in urea concentration to simplify the measurement of on-line Kt/V. Sodium clearance across the dialyzer is almost identical to urea clearance. Sodium concentration or dialysate conductivity can be used as a surrogate for urea. Sodium concentration, as a function of dialysate conductivity, is measured by sensors located before and after the dialyzer. Dialysis time, prescribed Kt/V and the patient's urea volume, determined from a kinetic modeling session and not from anthropometrics, are entered into the machine. Clearance is measured by increasing the dialysate sodium concentration for a short period. This causes sodium to move from dialysate into the blood. By measuring the change in conductivity of the dialysate associated with its passage through the dialyzer, sodium clearance is determined and Kt/V can be calculated. Multiple measurements of Kt/V during the treatment allow the clinician to determine whether the prescribed goal can be reached. Common problems that prevent the goal from being reached include reduced actual blood flow or dialysate flow, reduced dialyzer performance, and access recirculation.

Other monitoring systems have been developed and used to measure access flow and function during dialysis and to make accurate determinations of circulating blood volume during the dialytic procedure. Single- and dual-sensor systems using saline injections and sound velocity dilution calibration have been investigated as a method for accurately determining access flow during hemodialysis.[126] Similar efforts have led to noninvasive optical hematocrit monitoring to continually measure hematocrit during dialysis to better determine circulating blood volume.[127] The measurement is based on the principle that as blood volume changes in one direction, hematocrit changes in the opposite direction. A rise in hematocrit is related to a decrease in plasma volume.

The measurement of on-line blood volume with these devices can identify patients who are not near their estimated dry weight. In 18% of hemodialysis patients, a less than 5% decrease in blood volume was noted during routine hemodialysis sessions. In subsequent treatments, increased volume was successfully removed without hypotensive episodes.[128] The patients were able to have intradialytic fluid removal intentionally increased by 47% (average 0.8 L). The change in blood volume can be determined noninvasively during hemodialysis with these devices.[129] A critical hematocrit can be determined with these devices above which hypotension can be reliably predicted in 75% of patients.[130] These devices provide an added on-line safety measure to the treatment.

Dialysate Composition

One of the major aims of hemodialysis is the restoration of normal ion concentrations. As such, the levels of individual ions in the dialysate can be set to their desired plasma levels; however, in some instances dialysate levels are set for the *diffusible* fraction of the ion found in plasma. Dialysis solutions have undergone substantial changes because of the inception of hemodialysis, and are discussed in detail in a following section.

Water Used in Hemodialysis

Hemodialysis patients are exposed to as much as 600 liters of dialysis water a week, and to all its potential contaminants. Although water treatment systems (WTS) used by dialysis centers produce high-quality water for safe dialysis, WTS are susceptible to malfunction or to user error. Technical advances such as high-flux and high-efficiency dialysis, reuse, and bicarbonate dialysate have heightened awareness about water safety.

Hazards Associated with Dialysis Water

Numerous reports of patient injury or death have been linked to improperly treated or inadequately monitored water used for hemodialysis. High levels of aluminum sulfate in dialysate water have been linked to bone disease (osteomalacia and aplastic bone disease) and dialysis-associated encephalopathy (dialysis dementia).[131-133] Limiting aluminum levels in dialysate water to 10 μg/L has resulted in a continued decline in the incidence and case-fatality rate of dialysis dementia.[134, 135]

Chloramines, used as bactericidal agents in treatment of municipal water, denature hemoglobin by oxidation and inhibition of the hexose monophosphate shunt. Chloramine exposure during dialysis has been associated with hemolysis, Heinz-body hemolytic anemia, and methemoglobinemia.[136-138] There are other compounds with adverse effects in dialysis patients. Sodium azide, used frequently with glycerine as a preservative for WTS ultrafilters, has been associated with hypotension.[139] Fluoride, even at the recommended level of 1 mg/L, can cause osteomalacia and bone disease as well cardiac death.[140, 141] Excess calcium and magnesium in dialysate water have been linked to the "hard water syndrome"—a constellation of symptoms, including nausea, vomiting, weakness, flushing, and fluctuations in blood pressure.[142, 143] Untoward effects have also been reported with nitrates (i.e., methemoglobinemia with cyanosis and hypertension), copper (i.e., hemolytic anemia), and zinc in excess concentrations in dialysate water.[144-147] Formaldehyde toxicity resulting from improper disinfectant use and leaching from sediment filters has caused hemolytic anemia and death.[148, 149]

Essential Components of Water Purification

The efficiency of a WTS depends on the capacity of the system, the nature of the water supply, variations in quality of municipal water, and the quality of product water. *Temperature-blending valves* mix incoming hot and cold water to provide an optimum water temperature for downstream components. Most reverse osmosis (RO) membranes work with greatest efficacy at 77°F. Water temperature less than 77°F reduces the flow rate of the RO system, and water temperature higher than 100°F may damage RO membranes. *Filters* remove particulate matter from the water. Sand filters remove particles of 25 to 100 μm; cartridge filters extract particles of 1 to 100 μm; and submicron filters remove particles as small as 0.25 μm. In general, 5-μm filters are generally accepted as adequate protection for equipment and water treatment.

Water softeners, often sodium-containing cation-exchange resins, can remove calcium, magnesium, and other polyvalent cations from the feedwater. Because calcium and magnesium are removed from water in exchange for sodium, the amount of sodium released can be problematic. Removing calcium and magnesium prevents these ions from depositing on the RO system with resulting malfunction. Granular activated-carbon (GAC) filters absorb chlorine, chloramines, and other organic substances from the water. Carbon filters are porous with a high affinity for organic material. GAC filters can be contaminated with bacteria if they are not serviced properly or exchanged frequently. The size of the activated carbon bed depends on the empty bed contact time (EBCT). EBCT is calculated as follows:

$$EBCT = (V)\ (7.48\ \text{gallons/ft}^3)/Q$$

In this equation, V = carbon volume required in cubic feet, Q = water flow rate in gallons/min); EBCT differs for different substances. Recommended EBCT values are 6 minutes for chlorine removal and 10 minutes for chloramine removal. The Food and Drug Administration recommends that two GAC-filled tanks be used in series, with each tank having an EBCT of 3 to 5 minutes.

RO applies high hydrostatic pressure to a solution across a semipermeable membrane to prepare a purified solvent. RO rejects 90% to 99% of monovalent and divalent ions and microbiologic contaminants, producing water safe for dialysis. An RO device is often used as pretreatment to deionization, as an economic measure to provide longer service life for the deionization system. Subsequent deionization of permeate (product) RO water is usually unnecessary. Deionization removes all types of cations and anions. The cation exchange resin exchanges hydrogen ions (H^+) for other cations; the anion exchange resin exchanges hydroxyl ions (OH^-) for other anions. Deionization efficacy is determined by measuring the resistivity of the effluent. Resistivity varies with temperature; therefore, resistivity monitors must be temperature compensated. When the deionization system is exhausted, previously adsorbed ions can elute into the effluent, causing ion-related toxicities.[150]

Microbiology of Hemodialysis Systems

Water used by HD centers is usually obtained from the community water supply. Community water treatment can reduce bacteria and the concentration of endotoxins in the water; however, the dialysis WTS (apart from ultraviolet light) can still become contaminated with bacteria and endotoxins.[151, 152] The primary microbial contaminants in dialysis fluids are water bacteria, gram-negative bacteria, and nontuberculous mycobacteria (Table 59-9).

Nontuberculous mycobacteria in particular are problematic. They do not produce endotoxins, but they are more resistant to germicides than gram-negative bacteria and they are infectious, especially in the setting of inadequately disinfected dialyzers.[153-156] They can survive and multiply in RO-treated water or deionized water that contains little organic matter. The Centers for Disease Control and Prevention (CDC) documented that nontuberculous mycobacteria were present in the water of 83% of dialysis centers surveyed in 1984.[154]

Sterilization destroys microorganisms, including highly resistant bacterial spores. Disinfection, in contrast, eliminates all but the highly resistant microorganisms.[157, 158] Disinfection

TABLE 59-9

Naturally Occurring Water Bacteria Commonly Found in Hemodialysis Systems

GRAM-NEGATIVE BACTERIA	NONTUBERCULOUS MYCOBACTERIA
Pseudomonas	Mycobacterium chelonei
Flavobacterium	Mycobacterium fortuitum
Acinetobacter	Mycobacterium gordonae
Alcaligenes	Mycobacterium scrofulaceum
Xanthomonas	Mycobacterium avium
Serratia	Mycobacterium abscessus
Achromobacter	Mycobacterium intracellularis
Aeromonas	

can be high-level, intermediate, or low, depending on the germicidal activity. High-level disinfection inactivates all microorganisms except bacterial spores. Low-level disinfection reduces the bacterial population to a "safe" level. WTS disinfection generally uses low-level disinfection. High-level disinfection is more often used for dialyzer reprocessing.

Pyrogenic Reactions during Hemodialysis

Pyrogenic reactions often develop during or after dialysis treatment, with an incident rate of 0.5% to 12%.[145, 146] A pyrogenic reaction can be defined as chills (or rigors) or fever (oral temperature above 37.8°C [100°F]), or both, in a previously afebrile patient with no recorded signs or symptoms of infection before dialysis.[148, 159] Hypotension is sometimes also included in the definition. Other signs of a pyrogenic reaction are headache, myalgia, nausea, and vomiting. The symptoms usually begin 30 to 60 minutes into the dialysis treatment and stop shortly after, unless they are extreme. There appears to be little difference in pyrogenic reaction rates between different hemodialysis modalities.[146, 159]

Three lines of evidence implicate endotoxin in the pathogenesis of a pyrogenic reaction: (1) antiendotoxin antibodies in dialysis patients; (2) *Limulus* lysate reactivity in plasma from patients experiencing a pyrogenic reaction; and (3) an association of a pyrogenic reaction with fluids contaminated with gram-negative bacteria.[160-164] It is unlikely that microorganisms cross intact dialyzer membranes because of their diameter of the pores. Rather, it is the endotoxins or other pyrogenic substances that probably gain access to the patient's bloodstream across the dialysis membrane.[163, 165] Some of these substances are bacterial pyrogens released by gram-negative bacteria,[159] including lipopolysaccharides (LPS), its subunit, layer A, other LPS fragments, peptidoglycans, muramylpeptides, exotoxins, and exotoxin fragments.[166]

Assays for determining the permeability of pyrogens include the *Limulus* amebocyte lysate (LAL) assay, the mononuclear cell (MNC) assay, radiolabeled LPS fragments, and neutrophil activation. Many bacterial substances, like endotoxin fragments, are small enough to penetrate tight cellulosic membranes. These fragments go undetected in the LAL assay. Measuring in vitro cytokine production by MNCs may be more sensitive and specific, allowing detection of these low-molecular-weight substances.[167-169]

The inability to detect passage of endotoxin across intact dialyzer membranes during conventional or high-flux dialysis suggests that additional factors are probably involved in a pyrogenic reaction. Bacterial products such as endotoxins induce human MNC production of IL-1 and TNF-α.[170-172] Experimental data suggest that cultured MNC increase IL-1 production in response to LPS, LPS fragments, or plasma proteins in the dialysate.[172, 173] Moreover, LPS-like fragments can cross dialyzer membranes.[173] Plasma must be present on the blood side for cytokine induction. LPS-binding proteins, complement, and other plasma proteins can be activated by regenerated cellulosic membranes and amplify MNC cytokine production.[173-176] Evidence also suggests that endotoxin fragments can cross intact hemodialysis membranes and induce MNC cytokine production, particularly in the presence of plasma.

Severe pyrogenic reactions in hemodialysis patients appear to correlate with the extent of bacterial contamination in the dialysate. Studies have suggested that up to 35% of all water samples and 19% of all dialysate samples in the United States do not comply with AAMI standards (<200 colony forming units [CFU]/mL of water, 2000 CFU/mL in dialysate). Presumably, bacteria adhere to and grow in the dialysis tubing, releasing endotoxin and endotoxin fragments into the dialysate.

Changing dialysis practices has had an impact on pyrogenic reactions. Pyrogenic reactions have been reported with higher frequency in association with dialyzer reuse. Theoretically, use of RO and membrane integrity monitoring should lead to a decrease in the incidence of a pyrogenic reaction.[177] The use of bicarbonate and high-flux dialysis has been linked with a higher risk for pyrogenic reaction. In dialysis units that used bicarbonate dialysis, a higher frequency of pyrogenic reactions occurred only in centers that also performed high-flux dialysis. Centers that prepared their own bicarbonate dialysate also were more likely to report pyrogenic reactions than centers that used commercially prepared bicarbonate dialysate. The method for preparing bicarbonate dialysate entails potential contamination.[176] Acetate dialysate is prepared from a single concentrate at a concentration that prohibits bacterial growth (4.8 M). However, bicarbonate dialysate must be prepared from two concentrates: an acid concentrate with a pH of 2.8 that is not conducive to bacterial growth and a 1.2 M bicarbonate concentrate with a neutral pH. Bicarbonate concentrates can support halotolerant, endotoxin-producing, gram-negative organisms. As many as 10^5 to 10^6 CFU/mL can develop in liquid bicarbonate in as few as 10 days after dialysate preparation. Because of this, active quality assurance should be exercised to use liquid bicarbonate concentrate (LBC) as soon as possible after manufacture or receipt by the dialysis center. Tanks and distribution lines containing stored LBC should be disinfected at least twice weekly.

Dialyzer reuse practices have been associated with pyrogenic reactions independent of high-flux dialyzer use. Manual dialyzer reprocessing has been associated with higher incidence of PR compared with automated reprocessing. Manual reprocessing can allow defects in dialyzer membranes to go undetected because testing for integrity of the membrane is generally not performed with this technique.

Several outbreaks of patient infections and pyrogenic reactions have been reported in HD patients.[178-181] Many of these involved substandard reprocessing or poor water quality. Inadequate mixing of germicide, or the use of a new germicide

(e.g., chlorine dioxide) has been implicated in several of these outbreaks.[182, 183] Errors in the design and maintenance of a WTS were responsible for pyrogenic reactions and gram-negative bacteremia in another center.[183] Damage to RO membranes contributed to this outbreak, leading to the recommendation of a thorough inspection for RO damage whenever the RO system removes less than 90% to 95% of total dissolved solids. Although HD has been safely conducted outside the hospital or dialysis center setting, fatal endotoxemia occurred in dialysis patients at summer camp, illustrating the importance of dialysis WTS in different environmental conditions.[184]

The formaldehyde content used for disinfection also may be important for the frequency of pyrogenic reactions. Formaldehyde (2%) does not effectively or reproducibly eradicate mycobacterial organisms within 36 hours.[172] If the concentration of formaldehyde is increased to 4%, mycobacteria cannot survive at room temperature beyond 24 hours.[185] However, there is increasing evidence that lower concentrations of formaldehyde (e.g., 1%) can be effective if the dialyzers are kept at a temperature of 37°C to 40°C.[186]

Water Quality Standards for Hemodialysis

Microbiologic samples should be assayed by the spread-plate or membrane-filtration technique. Internal fluid pathways should be disinfected weekly, the RO unit monthly. Aqueous formaldehyde (1% to 2%), glutaraldehyde, or chlorine-based disinfectants should be used to disinfect internal fluid pathways. Hot water (>80°C [176°F]) is an alternative that avoids hazards associated with chemical germicides.

Low-level disinfection is adequate for WTS components. High-level disinfection is mandatory for dialyzer reprocessing. When reprocessing hemodialyzers, monitoring of water requires more stringent criteria; the water used for dialysate, for rinsing, reprocessing, and disinfecting the dialyzers should contain less than 5 endotoxin units/mL (1 ng/mL).

Dialyzers can be treated with reverse ultrafiltration and sodium hypochlorite bleach (<1%) or cleaned with hydrogen peroxide (3%) and peracetic acid (2%) and then tested for leaks. Dialyzers can then undergo disinfection or sterilization with instillation of germicides into the blood and dialysate compartments for at least 24 hours. Three commonly used agents are formaldehyde (4%), peracetic acid–hydrogen peroxide–acetic acid mixture (Renalin), and glutaraldehyde (Diacide). However, even 1% solutions of formaldehyde may have excellent germicidal efficacy when dialyzers are incubated at 40°C for 24 hours.[187] Heat sterilization at 105°C for 20 hours for reprocessing certain PS membranes has been successful.[188]

There are other clinical concerns about reprocessing of dialyzers. High residual formaldehyde levels in the dialyzer previously predisposed to anti-N-like antibody formation, with resulting episodes of hemolysis and early transplant failure.[189] However, no such reports have appeared because the use of more sensitive methods to detect residual formaldehyde. Potential anaphylactoid reactions have also been noted in patients taking ACE inhibitors who undergo HD with dialyzers that were reprocessed with Renalin or bleach.[105] These reactions probably reflect the characteristic of the membrane rather than the sterilant. Increased mortality associated with manual dialyzer reprocessing using Renalin and glutaraldehyde has been reported.[190, 191] A direct causative link between these germicides and increased patient mortality remains to be established.

THE DIALYSIS PRESCRIPTION

The goal of hemodialysis in patients with ESRD is to restore the body's intracellular and extracellular fluid environment toward the body composition of healthy individuals with functioning kidneys to the extent possible. On a biophysical level, the use of hemodialysis as renal replacement therapy is accomplished by solute removal from the blood into the dialysate, as exemplified by intradialytic removal of potassium, urea, and phosphorus, as well as the addition of solute from the dialysate into the blood, as is exemplified by bicarbonate and calcium. An additional goal of the dialysis procedure is the elimination of excess water volume from the patient through ultrafiltration. The prescription for an individual hemodialysis session must take into account an examination and physiologic assessment of individual patient needs to achieve these goals. The variables in the hemodialysis procedure that may be manipulated by the physician on the basis of clinical assessment (Table 59-10) include the following:

1. Choosing the type of dialyzer
2. Establishing blood and dialysate flows
3. Prescribing the time for the dialysis procedure
4. Prescribing the dialysate composition
5. Determining the frequency of the dialysis procedure
6. Determining the intensity of anticoagulation of the extracorporeal circuit

The separate components of the dialysis prescription are inter-related, and must be integrated to meet the unique nature of the patient and clinical circumstances.

The principles that underlie the hemodialysis procedure are in practice simple. Blood and dialysate are circulated on opposites sides of a semipermeable membrane, thereby permitting the passage of solutes elevated as a consequence of renal failure but restricting the transfer of blood proteins and cellular elements. The device containing the semipermeable membrane is the hemodialyzer. Removal of water occurs by control of the hydrostatic pressure gradient across the semipermeable membrane and may be augmented by increasing the osmolality of the dialysate fluid.

TABLE 59-10

Components of the Dialysis Prescription

Dialyzer (membrane, configuration, surface area)
Time
Blood flow rate
Dialysate flow rate
Ultrafiltration rate
Dialysate composition
Dialysate temperature
Anticoagulation
Intradialytic medications
Dialysis frequency

Dialyzer Choice

In making a decision about the choice of dialyzer, the three most critical determinants are its capacity for solute clearance, capacity for ultrafiltration or fluid removal, and the nature of dialyzer membrane interactions with components of the blood and their potential clinical sequelae, referred to as *biocompatibility*. The ideal hemodialysis membrane would have high clearance of low- and middle-molecular-weight uremic toxins, negligible loss of vital solutes, adequate ultrafiltration in an effort to maximize efficiency, and reduce adverse metabolic effects from the hemodialysis procedure. Additional characteristics of the ideal dialyzer would be a low blood volume compartment, beneficial biocompatibility effects, high reliability, and low cost. In evaluating dialyzer solute clearance characteristics, urea is the solute most often used because of its relevance to kinetic models of dialysis adequacy. A detailed examination of the relationship of urea kinetic modeling to the delivery of adequate dialytic therapy is discussed later. In clinical practice, physicians typically rely on industry-derived determinations of in vitro dialyzer clearance of low- and middle-molecular-weight solutes. Frequently Gibbs-Donnan effects, membrane adsorption of solute, protein binding of solute, and solute aggregation are not taken into account in determining in vitro dialyzer clearances.

A further complication in evaluating solute clearance by different dialyzers is the variable relationship between the diffusive and convective clearance of a solute. As described mathematically in an earlier section, solutes that are larger than 300 D have relatively lower diffusive clearance values compared with smaller solutes such as urea and potassium. Clearance of larger solutes from the blood depends primarily on convective rather than diffusive clearance. In clinical circumstances in which large volumes of ultrafiltrate are generated, simple comparisons of diffusive solute characteristics (K values) of large-molecular-weight solutes can be misleading.

The capacity for fluid removal by a dialyzer is described by its ultrafiltration coefficient. Similar to the information provided for the diffusive clearance of a particular solute by a specific dialyzer, each dialyzer model also has a determined ultrafiltration coefficient. Because these values are also typically derived in vitro, similar limitations describe their application in the in vivo situation. It is not unusual for the ultrafiltration coefficient in vivo to vary by 10% to 20% in either direction.

Virtually all of the commercial dialyzers available in the United States are configured as large cylinders packed with hollow fibers, known as *hollow-fiber dialyzers*. Blood flows within the hollow fibers, and dialysate flows outside and around these fibers, generally in a countercurrent fashion whereby dialysate flow is in opposite direction to blood flow. Hollow-fiber dialyzers are generally noncompliant with fixed blood volumes. In parallel plate dialyzers, which are a less frequently used physical configuration, multiple sheets of flat dialysis membranes are stacked in a layered configuration, with separation of blood and dialysate compartments. The blood compartment of parallel plate dialyzers is more compliant and therefore varies more with transmembrane pressure. Parallel plate dialyzers generally require a larger blood volume compartment than hollow-fiber dialyzers. Hollow-fiber dialyzers have blood volume compartments of about 50 to 150 mL.

The biomaterials of the hollow-fiber dialyzer dictate its clearance characteristics, ultrafiltration characteristics, and biocompatibility. Coupled with the development of dialysis delivery systems with ultrafiltration controllers, the dialysis industry has developed dialyzers with a wide array of solute clearance and ultrafiltration coefficients. Dialyzers with urea clearances of 50 to 250 mL/minute (usually calculated for a blood flow of 200 to 300 mL/min), and ultrafiltration coefficients of approximately 2 to 65 mL/mm Hg/hour are readily available.

As the hemodialysis procedure constitutes an extracorporeal circulation, of necessity blood must be removed from the vascular space and come into contact with dialysis membrane biomaterials. The interaction of soluble and cellular elements of the blood with the dialysis membrane can result in activation of protein-mediated humoral cascades, as well as activation of several types of circulating cells, many of which have been described earlier.

A humoral pathway frequently activated by the dialysis membrane is the clotting cascade. Thrombus formation from extracorporeal thrombogenesis occurs when thrombin adsorbs to the dialyzer membrane in an enzymatically active form, thereby becoming a site for platelet adhesion and further thrombin deposition.[192] The use of anticoagulants to reduce active thrombin deposition on dialysis membranes is discussed later. Attempts to limit dialyzer membrane thrombogenicity by ionic bonding of heparin to the dialyzer membrane surface have been complicated by a resulting tendency for more pronounced complement activation.[193]

An additional consideration in the prescription of the dialysis membrane is whether the intent is for the membrane to be reused. Dialyzer reprocessing for reuse of disposable dialyzers has been widely practiced in the United States, largely due to financial constraints. Dialyzer reuse may be performed manually or with an automated rinsing device. Sterility during reprocessing is maintained by the use of a chemical disinfectant (e.g., peracetic acid, glutaraldehyde, formaldehyde) or through heat sterilization. After reprocessing, dialyzer adequacy is assessed indirectly by measuring the volume of the dialysis fiber bundle in the blood compartment (i.e., fiber bundle volume) and by pressurizing the dialyzer to evaluate the structural integrity of the fibers (i.e., pressure test). For a dialyzer to have acceptable reuse parameters, the fiber bundle volume must be greater than 80% of the initial value, the in vitro ultrafiltration rate must be greater than 20% of the manufacturer's stated value, and the dialyzer should not leak at a pressure that is within 20% of the maximal operating pressure. The safety of dialyzer reuse practices has been closely scrutinized, and data concerning the practice have been controversial.[191] Data suggest that, overall, facilities that reuse dialyzers have a risk-adjusted mortality that is similar to that of facilities that do not reuse dialyzers.[194] Most nephrologists believe that patients are not placed at increased risk if strict infection control precautions and quality assurance measures are implemented in dialyzer reprocessing.[195]

Anticoagulation for Hemodialysis

Interaction of plasma with the dialysis membrane produces activation of the clotting cascade, characterized by the development of thrombosis in the extracorporeal circuit, thrombin deposition in dialyzer hollow fibers, and resulting dialyzer dysfunction.[196] Dialyzer thrombogenicity is determined by dialysis membrane composition, surface charge, surface area, and configuration. The rate of blood flow through the dialyzer, the ultrafiltration rate prescribed (due to hemoconcentration), and the length, diameter, and composition of blood lines all affect thrombogenicity. Several patient-specific variables influence thrombogenicity and determine anticoagulation requirements during hemodialysis. They include acquired and inherited coagulopathies, neoplasia, malnutrition, hemoglobin concentration, and the presence or absence of congestive heart failure.

The most widely used anticoagulant for dialysis is heparin.[197] Heparin is easy to administer, has a low cost, and has a relatively short biologic half-life. For most patients, heparin is administered systemically during the dialysis procedure as a single bolus or incrementally during the dialysis treatment. For patients at high risk for bleeding, heparin is occasionally administered as regional anticoagulation, in which only the extracorporeal dialyzer circuit is anticoagulated by administering heparin into the arterial line and protamine into the venous line.[198-200] From a practical standpoint, the time constraints of dialysis limit the ability to monitor heparin efficacy through the partial thromboplastin time (PTT). In routine hemodialysis practice, the intensity of anticoagulation is not measured, but in some circumstances, the activated clotting time (ACT) is used. In this assay, whole blood is mixed with an activator of the extrinsic clotting cascade, and the time necessary for blood to first congeal is measured.

A simple method of heparin administration is the systemic administration of 50 to 100 U/kg of heparin at the initiation of dialysis, frequently followed by a bolus of 100 U/hour. When ACT is being measured, the target ACT is approximately 50% above baseline values. In fractional anticoagulation, a smaller initial bolus of heparin is administered (10 to 50 U/kg), followed by an infusion of 500 to 1000 U/hour. Fractional heparinization can be used to achieve less intensive anticoagulation where the target ACT is maintained at 25% (fractional) or 15% (tight fractional) above the baseline value. These approaches are generally reserved for patients at higher risk for bleeding complications.

Regional heparinization can be effective in preventing extracorporeal thrombogenesis with minimal systemic anticoagulation, but is labor-intensive and prone to error when used by less experienced personnel.[199, 200] In regional anticoagulation, the extracorporeal circuit alone is anticoagulated by administering 500 to 750 U/hour into the arterial line (often with an initial 500 unit bolus at the initiation of dialysis) and by the parallel administration of protamine into the venous line. The use of regional anticoagulation requires frequent checks of the ACT from the arterial and venous lines with adjustments of the heparin and protamine infusion rates to maintain the ACT for the patient at baseline while the ACT in the dialysis circuit is prolonged 10 seconds or longer. Because heparin has a longer half-life than protamine, additional protamine should be given at the end of the dialysis procedure to prevent a rebound heparin bleeding risk.[201, 202] Because of these difficulties, regional anticoagulation is rarely employed. As an alternative to regional anticoagulation for patients at high risk for bleeding, dialysis may be performed without any anticoagulation. Using the saline flush technique, hemodialysis is initiated at a high blood flow rate to reduce thrombogenicity, and the dialyzer is flushed every 15 to 60 minutes with 50 mL of saline.[203, 204] This technique is not likely to be successful in hypercoagulable patients, when high blood flow rates are not attainable, and in dialysis in which a high ultrafiltration rate is required.

For patients at high risk for serious adverse events from hemorrhage, guidelines for anticoagulation must be based on comorbid conditions, and the risk for thrombosis of the extracorporeal circuit becomes a secondary consideration. Under these circumstances, the following guidelines are recommended:

1. Patients who are bleeding, are at significant risk for bleeding, have a baseline major thrombostatic defect, or are within 7 days of a major operative procedure or within 14 days of intracranial surgery should undergo dialysis without heparin or by regional anticoagulation.
2. Patients who are within 72 hours of a biopsy of a visceral organ should undergo dialysis without heparin or by regional anticoagulation.
3. Patients who are more than 7 days past a major surgery or 72 hours past a biopsy can have dialysis by fractional heparinization. If they have previously received fractional heparinization, they can be considered for systemic anticoagulation.
4. Patients with pericarditis should have dialysis without heparin or by regional anticoagulation.
5. Patients who have undergone minor surgical procedures within the previous 72 hours should have dialysis by fractional anticoagulation.
6. Patients anticipated to undergo a major surgical procedure within 8 hours of hemodialysis should undergo dialysis without heparin or with tight fractional anticoagulation. If they are within 8 hours of a minor procedure, fractional anticoagulation is appropriate.

Blood and Dialysate Flow

The clearance of a solute during the hemodialysis procedure may functionally be defined as the volumetric removal of the solute from the patient, as expressed mathematically earlier. The blood flow and dialysate flow rates are critical elements of the dialysis prescription that can be altered to modify solute clearance. However, as blood and dialysate flow rates increase, resistance and turbulence within the dialyzer also increase. As a result, increases in nonlinear flow within hollow fibers occur, leading to a decline in the clearance per unit flow of blood or dialysate.[205] The resulting flow-limited mass transfer indicates that solute clearance can approach an asymptotic rate as blood flow or dialysate flow increases. The flow-limited mass transfer and membrane-limited mass transfer (defined by the specific dialyzer and the solute being measured) together determine clearance characteristics. A similar relationship is obtained for solute clearance and dialysate flow rate. Studies by Sigdell and Tersteegen demonstrated that the practical upper limit of effective dialysate flow was twice the blood flow rate, beyond which the gain in solute removal is minimal.[206] As a consequence, the use of high dialysate flow rates to enhance solute removal should be confined to clinical circumstances in which the

achievable blood flow rate is in excess of 300 mL/minute. In addition to the prescribed blood and dialysate flow rate, convective mass transport that occurs with ultrafiltration also influences solute removal, thereby adding complexity to predictions of actual solute clearance.[207-210]

In clinical practice, the efficacy of angioaccess may affect solute clearance obtained at a given prescribed blood flow rate. Access blood flow is a function of pressure and resistance. When blood is pumped out of the access into the dialyzer, a lower resistance circuit is created that generally results in an increase in total access blood flow. The increased blood flow increases pressure in the venous drainage of the access during dialysis. Should venous outflow be restricted, there is an increased likelihood of backflow (called *recirculation*) from the venous to the arterial side of the access. Backflow or recirculation is also facilitated by greater negative pressure at the arterial needle at higher blood pump speeds when there is impaired arterial flow. During recirculation, "dialyzed" blood reenters the dialytic circuit, thereby decreasing the efficiency of solute clearance.[211] Recirculation also increases when dialysis needles are placed close within the dialysis access.

Recirculation is diagnosed when the concentration of a dialyzable solute in arterial line blood is lower than that of systemic blood, indicating that there has been mixing of dialyzed "venous" blood with blood entering the dialyzer. The fractional recirculation (R) is calculated using this formula:

$$R = Cs - Ca/Cs - Cv$$

In this equation, Cs, Ca, and Cv are the concentrations (C) of the measured solute in systemic (s), arterial line (a), and venous (v) blood.

Recirculation has traditionally been measured by simultaneous measurement of a solute (usually BUN) from the arterial line, and from a peripheral blood source during the dialysis procedure. In traditional recirculation measurements, the source for the "systemic blood" sample was to draw blood from a vein in the contralateral arm. However, this approach is inaccurate and tends to overestimate recirculation.[212] A major problem with this approach is that there may be disequilibrium between a peripheral venous sample and the arterial sample before use of the dialyzer. Although normally there is a minimal difference in urea concentration between arterial and venous blood, during the dialysis procedure, blood leaving the dialyzer returns to the central veins, gets oxygenated in the pulmonary circulation, and is then delivered to the systemic circulation. Urea rapidly equilibrates across a gradient between the intracellular compartments and the arterial blood with a lower BUN, leading to a higher peripheral BUN concentration compared with the arterial BUN concentration. The resulting arteriovenous disequilibrium has also been called *cardiopulmonary recirculation* and can result in an overestimation of recirculation.[213] Cardiopulmonary recirculation is increased with high-efficiency dialysis (due to more blood with lower BUN concentration entering the circuit) and in low cardiac output states (in which dialyzed blood constitutes a greater proportion of the cardiac output). Another form of urea compartmentalization called *venovenous disequilibrium* occurs when peripheral vasoconstriction leads to a decrease in blood flow and a lower amount of total urea removal from the tissue bed.[214, 215] In principle, obtaining a peripheral arterial sample for measuring systemic urea concentration would overcome the inherent problems of arteriovenous and venovenous disequilibrium but is not practical during the hemodialysis procedure setting.

A more accurate approach to determine recirculation than the traditional three-needle method is to obtain the systemic sample from the arterial side of the dialyzer under conditions in which there is minimal reflux of blood that has already been dialyzed. However, timing of the peripheral arterial sample collection is important. If dialyzer blood flow is stopped to obtain the systemic sample, delays after stopping flow can increase the value of BUN as arterial and venous compartments equilibrate. Conversely, rapid sample collection may result in contamination with recirculated blood. A recommended alternative to stopping flow entirely is the low blood flow technique. With this procedure, after arterial line and venous line samples are obtained during dialysis, the blood flow is abruptly reduced to 50 mL/minute, with the dialysate flow off, and a peripheral sample is obtained from the arterial line after 150% of the volume from the needle to the sample point has been cleared (usually between 20 and 30 seconds).[216]

To more accurately measure recirculation, newer techniques have been developed that do not rely on withdrawal of blood for sampling solute concentrations. Instead, an indicator is infused and measurement of disappearance of the indicator and lack of reappearance on the arterial side can be used to estimate recirculation.[217] Saline has been used as an indicator with monitoring of hematocrit changes. Similarly, a bolus of cold fluid can be used with an accurate blood temperature monitor. Studies using indicator techniques demonstrate that recirculation is rare unless the blood pump is set at a higher rate of speed than vascular access blood flow.[218]

Dialysis Time

The clearance of any of a solute, such as urea, can be increased by lengthening the dialysis treatment. Because the typical dialysis prescription emphasizes optimal blood and dialysate flows and the selection of dialyzers with large mass transfer coefficient characteristics, the duration of dialysis is often the sole variable that can be used to augment solute clearance during an individual dialysis session. However, because diffusive solute clearance depends on solute concentration on the blood side, the efficiency of solute removal declines over the course of the dialysis procedure. From the standpoint of total solute removal, there are frequently "diminishing returns" in increasing the length of the dialysis procedure. The relationship of dialysis time to dialysis adequacy is further discussed in the section on dialysis adequacy in this chapter.

The duration of the dialysis procedure may also be important in achieving adequate volume homeostasis. A longer duration of the dialysis procedure allows for a lower net ultrafiltration rate per hour for a given targeted ultrafiltration goal over the course of the procedure. This may result in fewer intradialytic symptoms such as hypotension and cramping (see "Complications of Dialysis"). Data from Charra and colleagues in Tassin, France, indicate that the use of long dialysis with slow rates of ultrafiltration, coupled with the use of a low-sodium diet, allows for an excellent volume homeostasis and blood pressure control, frequently without the use of antihypertensive medications.[219] Patients undergoing long hemodialysis treatments with slow ultrafiltration rates are reported to have excellent long-term survival.[220]

Dialysate Composition

When blood comes into contact with dialysate across a semipermeable dialysis membrane, a bidirectional diffusive process takes place by which solutes tend to reach similar concentrations on both sides of the dialysis membrane. In hemodialysis, a countercurrent flow configuration is used for blood and dialysate flow to maintain concentration gradient as a driving force for solute transport throughout the length of the dialysis membrane. The composition of dialysate is crucial in achieving the desired blood purification to achieve body fluid and electrolyte homeostasis. Physical and microbiologic characteristics of dialysate are also critical in the dialysis procedure. In addition to influencing the final concentration of blood solute at the end of the dialysis procedure, dialysate composition can influence intermediary protein, carbohydrate, and lipid metabolism, affect systemic vasomotor tone, cardiac contractility and rhythm, pulmonary gas exchange, and bone turnover. The selection of dialysis solute concentrations is a critical component of the dialysis procedure.

In the early days of dialysis, dialysate was individualized and batched for a treatment session. For example, in Kolff's pioneering treatments, a batch of dialysate was prepared in advance and placed in the wooden slats where the drum was rotating. Kolff bubbled carbon dioxide or oxygen through the dialysate to adjust the pH of the solution. Kolff also added glucose to the dialysate to achieve osmotic ultrafiltration.[17] In 1949, Alwall applied negative pressure to the dialysate solution to increase ultrafiltration.[221] When early coil-type dialyzers were available, the dialyzer was completely immersed in a fixed volume of dialysate, which had to be changed every few hours.[222]

The modern era of dialysis began with the development of central delivery systems in which dialysate composition could be standardized. Dialysate is provided as a liquid or a powdered concentrate in commercial formulations that are diluted with prepared water and a fixed ratio to yield the final solute concentration. In central delivery systems, this portioning of the dialysate is done in a central retaining facility, and the reconstituted dialysate is provided from a storage tank to the individual dialysis machines. Individualized prescribing of dialysate concentration became possible after 1976 when dialysis machines that are equipped with bedside proportioning systems for dialysate became available. Dialysate is reconstituted with prepared water on entry into the dialysis machine immediately before entering the dialyzer, allowing for personalization of the dialysate composition.[223] Appropriate proportioning of the dialysate concentration and water is ensured by the use of on-line measurements of dialysate conductivity before its entry into the dialyzer.

Sodium

Sodium concentration is the major determinant of tonicity of extracellular fluids. Because sodium readily crosses dialysis membranes, sodium dialysate concentration plays a crucial role in determining cardiovascular stability during hemodialysis. Historically, the dialysate sodium concentration was maintained at hyponatric levels (130 to 135 mEq/L) to favor diffusive sodium loss during the dialysis procedure.[224-226] The use of hyponatric dialysate prevented interdialytic hypertension, exaggerated thirst, and excessive interdialytic weight gain.[227] However, the use of hyponatric dialysate, by inducing an interdialytic decline in plasma osmolality, favors fluid shifts from the extracellular to the intracellular space, thereby exacerbating the plasma-volume–depleting effects of hemodialysis. As a result, the intravascular space became dehydrated, and the intracellular space became overhydrated. The osmolar changes and fluid shifts resulted in a high incidence of dialysis disequilibrium, characterized by headaches, nausea, vomiting, and in severe cases, seizures.[228, 229] Interdialytic hypotension and cramps frequently resulted from the decline in intravascular volume. As a consequence, hyponatric dialysate has largely been abandoned, with the result of a reduction in interdialytic hemodynamic instability and an improvement in interdialytic patient well-being. Today, it is standard to have a dialysate sodium concentration similar to the plasma sodium concentration.

In an effort to further reduce dialysis disequilibrium, intradialytic hypotension, and dialysis-related symptomatology, particularly after the introduction of high-efficiency hemodialysis, the prescription of high sodium dialysate has become a common practice.[230-232] Unfortunately, an increase in the dialysate sodium concentration frequently results in polydipsia, increased interdialytic weight gain, and increased interdialytic hypertension, thereby offsetting the beneficial effects of increased intradialytic hemodynamic stability.[233] The influence of interdialytic weight gain on blood pressure determination is controversial. In some studies, a positive correlation has been identified between intradialytic weight gain and blood pressure, but other studies have shown no relationship.

In an effort to achieve greater intradialytic hemodynamic stability using higher dialysate sodium activity while minimizing potential effects on interdialytic hypertension and weight gain, a number of studies have evaluated the strategy of varying the dialysate sodium concentration over the course of a dialysis session using variable dilution proportioning systems. These techniques, described as sodium modeling or sodium ramping, have been espoused as a means of individualizing the hemodialysis session to optimize blood pressure support.[234, 235] Sodium modeling is often performed in a step fashion, in which the initial dialysate sodium concentration is greater than or equal to 145 mEq/L and, during the second half of the dialysis session, is abruptly reduced, or it may be reduced as a linear gradient over the course of the dialysis session (i.e., linear sodium modeling).

Although sodium modeling can reduce the frequency of hypotension during dialysis, it is unclear whether this technique offers any advantage over a fixed dialysate sodium concentration of 140 to 145 mEq/L.[235, 236] It has been suggested that plasma sodium concentrations may be high in patients who undergo sodium modeling immediately after dialysis, resulting in increased interdialytic weight gains.[237] In the absence of more compelling data, it seems reasonable to use higher dialysate sodium or sodium modeling in patients prone to intradialytic hypotension and to use dialysate sodium concentrations in patients similar to plasma sodium concentrations not predisposed to intradialytic hypotension.

Potassium

Unlike sodium, which is largely distributed in the extracellular space, only 1% to 2% of the 3000 to 3500 mEq of potassium is present in the extracellular space. In patients with ESRD, potassium tends to accumulate in the plasma during the interdialytic interval, and life-threatening plasma potassium concentrations can result. Dialysis is important in the maintenance of a normal or near-normal serum potassium concentration in ESRD patients, and the removal of excess potassium is achieved by use of a dialysate potassium concentration lower than that of plasma concentration.

The rate of potassium removal during dialysis is largely a function of the predialysis potassium concentration. However, the flux of potassium from the intracellular compartment to the extracellular space is frequently not in equilibrium with the mass transfer of potassium across the dialysis membrane to the dialysate compartment.[238] After the completion of a standard hemodialysis session, there is an increase in the plasma potassium concentration of approximately 30% over 4 to 5 hours due to ongoing movement of potassium from the intracellular to the extracellular space.[239]

The efficacy of intradialytic potassium removal is highly variable, difficult to predict, and influenced by dialysis-specific and patient-specific factors. In a study that controlled dialysis-specific components of the dialysis procedure (dialysate composition, dialyzer type and surface area, blood and dialysate flow rate, and duration of dialysis), interpatient potassium removal varied by approximately 70%, whereas intrapatient potassium removal varied by 20% with the same dialysis prescription.[240] During hemodialysis, approximately 70% of the removed potassium is derived from the intracellular compartment. However, the volume of distribution of potassium is not constant. Paradoxically, the greater the total body potassium content, the lower the volume of distribution.[239] As a consequence, the fractional decline in the plasma potassium concentration during hemodialysis is proportionately greater when there is a higher predialysis potassium concentration. Most of the cardiac morbidity that arises from dialysate potassium concentration occurs during the first half of the dialysis session.[241] It is the rapidity of the fall in plasma potassium concentration rather than the absolute plasma potassium level that determines the risk for interdialytic cardiac arrhythmias.

As a further complication in attempting to model potassium removal during dialysis, the movement of potassium between the intracellular and extracellular spaces is partially controlled by a number of factors that are simultaneously modified during the dialysis procedure. The transcellular distribution of potassium is influenced by plasma hydrogen ion concentration, because extracellular alkalosis shifts potassium into cells, and acidosis causes potassium to efflux from cells. Hyperinsulinemia promotes cellular potassium uptake, as do β-adrenergic catecholamines. Changes in plasma tonicity can also affect the transcellular distribution of potassium.

The selection of a dialysate potassium concentration is empirical and guided by patient-specific factors. Generally, a dialysate potassium concentration of 1 to 3 mEq/L is used in most patients. Patients who have excessive potassium loads from diet, medications, hemolysis, tissue breakdown, or gastrointestinal bleeding may require a lower dialysate potassium concentration. Low dialysate potassium concentrations should be used with caution, however, as an analysis has found an association between the use of low dialysate potassium with sudden cardiac death in outpatient hemodialysis patients.[242]

Calcium

Patients with ESRD are susceptible to hyperphosphatemia, hypocalcemia, secondary and tertiary hyperparathyroidism, and hypovitaminosis D. As a consequence, positive intradialytic calcium balance may be desired as an adjunct therapy for control of metabolic bone disease. In the setting of renal failure, more than 60% of plasma calcium is not protein bound and is capable of diffusible equilibrium during dialysis.[243] Assuming an additional conductance of calcium across the dialysis membrane due to convective losses, a dialysis calcium concentration of 3.5 mEq/L (7.0 mg/dL) is necessary to prevent intradialytic calcium losses.[244] For many years, a dialysate calcium concentration of 3.5 mEq/L was relatively standard. However, with the use of calcium-containing salts and phosphorous binders and with the aggressive use of vitamin D analogs, many dialysis facilities employ a standard dialysate calcium concentration of 2.5 to 3.0 mEq/L in an effort to prevent interdialytic hypercalcemia.

The dialysate calcium concentration may also affect hemodynamic stability during the hemodialysis procedure.[245] Left ventricular contractility has been demonstrated to be proportional to serum ionized calcium concentration during hemodialysis.[230] Several prospective crossover trials have demonstrated higher interdialytic mean arterial pressure with higher dialysate calcium concentrations.[246, 247] An increase in intradialytic electrocardiographic QT dispersion can also be reduced by increasing the dialysate calcium concentration.[248]

Magnesium

Similar to potassium, the serum magnesium concentration is a poor determinant of total body magnesium stores. Only approximately 1% of total body magnesium content is present in the extracellular fluid, and only 60% of extracellular magnesium is free and diffusible.[249] Magnesium flux that occurs during hemodialysis is difficult to predict, despite knowledge of the serum and dialysate magnesium concentrations. The ideal serum magnesium concentration in patients with ESRD and the appropriate dialysate magnesium concentration are unresolved. Many centers use a dialysate magnesium concentration of 1 mEq/L.

Buffers

Correction of uremic metabolic acidosis is a goal of the hemodialysis procedure. Hemodialysis therapy cannot remove large quantities of free hydrogen ion, because the low concentration in the blood prevents the development of a large gradient to support mass transfer. As hydrogen ions are produced, they are rapidly buffered by plasma bicarbonate and other body buffers. In hemodialysis, correction of acidosis is largely achieved by using a dialysate with a higher concentration of alkaline equivalents than are present in

the blood, promoting flux of base from the dialysate into the blood. Base transfer across the dialysis membrane has been achieved using bicarbonate- or acetate-containing dialysate.

Historically, Kolff and later Scribner used dialysate bicarbonate as a buffer, bubbling carbon dioxide through the dialysate to lower pH to prevent precipitation of calcium and magnesium salts.[17] Because of the instability of bicarbonate in aqueous solution at neutral pH in the presence of divalent cations, in 1964, Mion introduced acetate as a base equivalent in dialysate.[250] Acetate-containing dialysate was biochemically more stable and also avoided frequent bacterial contamination problems that result when bicarbonate is used as a buffer. Acetate-containing dialysate solutions became the clinical standard of practice worldwide for more than 20 years. However, in the 1980s, the introduction of high-efficiency dialysis led to reports of cardiovascular instability and intradialytic hypotension due to the slow conversion of acetate into bicarbonate with acetate dialysate. Under these circumstances, acetate accumulation contributes to nausea, vomiting, headache, fatigue, decreased myocardial contractility, peripheral vasodilatation, and arterial hypoxemia.[227, 234-236, 251] Adverse metabolic and hemodynamic effects associated with acetate dialysate have led to its virtual replacement as a buffer with bicarbonate.

The introduction of single patient proportioning systems that permit mixing of two separate dialysate concentrations (separately containing sodium bicarbonate and an acid concentrate with divalent cations) close to the entry point of the final dialysate into the dialyzer allowed the widespread reintroduction of bicarbonate as a dialysate buffer in the late 1970s and 1980s. A small amount of acetic acid (3 to 6 mEq/L) is present in the acid concentrate and serves to titrate some of the bicarbonate to carbonic acid and carbon dioxide, thereby controlling the pH of the final dialysate. Dialysate bicarbonate concentrations of 30 to 35 mEq/L are commonly used. Higher dialysate bicarbonate concentrations are sometimes used to fully correct metabolic acidosis due to the adverse effects of metabolic acidosis on protein catabolism and nutritional status in maintenance hemodialysis patients. Variable proportioning of bicarbonate (i.e., bicarbonate modeling) is also sometimes employed to individualize bicarbonate delivery to hemodialysis patients.

Unlike acetate buffer dialysate, liquid bicarbonate concentrate and reconstituted bicarbonate-containing dialysate can support the growth of gram-negative bacteria, filamentous fungi, and yeast. Because of the propensity of bicarbonate-containing dialysate to support bacterial growth, strict guidelines exist for the acceptable limits of bacterial growth and for the presence of lipopolysaccharide in the dialysate and dialyzer reuse system. Further reductions in dialysate bacterial colony–forming units beyond standards set by the Association for the Advancement of Medical Instrumentation (AAMI) have been advocated and are achievable by installation of membrane filters on each dialysis machine at the point where the dialysate leaves the dialysis machine before entering the patient's dialyzer.

Chloride

Chloride is the major anion in dialysate. Dialysate chloride concentration is defined by the prescribed concentration of cations and anionic buffers in the dialysate to maintain electrical neutrality.

Glucose

In the early 1960s, high glucose concentrations in dialysis fluid were used to provide osmotic pressure for water removal. However, advances in hydraulic ultrafiltration and the demonstration that high dialysate glucose (>320 mg/dL) increased the risk for hyperosmolar syndrome, postdialysis hyperglycemia and hyponatremia rendered the use of high dialysate glucose obsolete.[252] Contemporary dialysis fluids range from glucose-free to slightly hyperglycemic (≤200 mg/dL).[253] Most non–insulin-dependent diabetic patients tolerate well dialysis with glucose-free dialysate, despite losing 25 to 30 g of glucose across the dialyzer. However, this glucose loss may potentiate hypoglycemia and adversely affect hemodialysis catabolism, raising levels of free amino acids during dialysis and increasing the intradialytic protein catabolic rate.[60-64] Ketogenesis and gluconeogenesis are usually sufficient to maintain serum glucose in the physiologic range despite reductions in plasma insulin, lactate, and pyruvate. In contrast, physiologic dialysate glucose (200 mg/dL) has few adverse effects other than aggravating hypertriglyceridemia.[65] Dialysate glucose can affect potassium removal, the risk for dialysis disequilibrium syndrome, and postdialysis fatigue. In general, an optimal dialysate glucose concentration is 100 to 200 mg/dL for most patients. However, in diabetic patients, insulin doses may require adjustment to account for this dialysis-imposed "glucose clamp," in which levels of plasma glucose may be kept constant during dialysis due to the concentration in the dialysate.

Dialysate Temperature

Although not strictly reflecting dialysate composition, prescription of the dialysate temperature can be an important component of the dialysis prescription. Dialysate temperature is generally maintained between 36.5°C and 38°C at the inlet of the dialyzer. Heat exchangers and temperature monitors are built into dialysis machines. In cases in which temperature monitor failure has occurred, severe hemolysis has been reported.[254, 255]

Body temperature is determined by the balance between heat production through metabolism and heat losses from the body surface and through respiration. Although hemodialysis does not lead to direct heat transfer from the extracorporeal circulation to the patient, patient temperatures do increase during hemodialysis with conventional dialysate temperatures of 37°C. An increase in body temperature during dialysis can occur due to an increase in heat generation as a response to pyrogens in the dialysate. Ultrafiltration-induced volume contraction during hemodialysis results in peripheral vasoconstriction, which limits peripheral heat loss and raises core body temperature. Eventually, there is a reflex dilatation of peripheral blood vessels, which allows heat escape but reduces peripheral vascular resistance, resulting in an intradialytic fall in blood pressure. This led to the suggestion (originally by Maggiore) that lowering dialysate solution temperature might permit increased hemodynamic stability in hypotension-prone dialysis patients.[256] Numerous studies have confirmed that dialysate temperature is an important determinant of intradialytic blood pressure.[257-263] Lower dialysate temperature may also increase cardiac contractility, improve oxygenation, increase venous tone, and reduce complement activation during dialysis.

The introduction of blood temperature monitors with accuracy to greater than 0.05°C and temperature control modes with which arterial temperatures are monitored and dialysate temperatures are adjusted by negative feedback loops has allowed the delivery of isothermic hemodialysis. Careful thermal balance studies using these devices have demonstrated that heat accumulation during dialysis is directly related to ultrafiltration rate, suggesting that peripheral vasoconstriction in response to diminished blood volume is an important cause of heat accumulation during dialysis.[264] The provision of isothermic dialysis is associated with more hemodynamic stability than low temperature dialysate, suggesting that this may become a standard approach to reducing hemodialysis-induced hypotension.[265]

Ultrafiltration Rate

In addition to its use in comparing the ultrafiltration performance of individual dialyzers, the ultrafiltration coefficient is used to calculate the quantity of pressure that must be exerted across the dialysis membrane (i.e., transmembrane pressure) to generate a given volume of ultrafiltrate per unit time during a single dialysis session. The net pressure across the dialyzer membrane is determined by combining the hydraulic pressure, osmotic pressure, and oncotic pressure across the membrane. Because the hydraulic pressure is substantially higher than the osmotic or oncotic pressure, the net pressure gradient is approximated by the difference between blood and dialysate hydraulic pressure. For most available dialyzers, the hydraulic pressure can be calculated from the arithmetic mean of the inlet and outlet pressures. The effective pressure required for achieving a particular fluid loss during dialysis is described as the transmembrane pressure (TMP) and is calculated by the following formula:

$$\text{TMP} = \text{Desired weight loss/Ultrafiltration coefficient} \times \text{Dialysis time}$$

The performance of ultrafiltration during hemodialysis has been greatly simplified with the development of dialysis machines that possess ultrafiltration control systems. Ultrafiltration with these machines is remarkably precise. Use of ultrafiltration control systems is critical when hemodialysis is performed with high-efficiency or high-flux dialyzers due to their massive ultrafiltration capacities.

During hemodialysis, ultrafiltration and diffusive clearance are typically performed simultaneously. However, it is possible to temporally segregate the two procedures by a modification of the dialysis procedure that has been described as sequential ultrafiltration/clearance.[266, 267] Sequential ultrafiltration/clearance is accomplished by first ultrafiltering to the desired ultrafiltrate volume removal, followed by the performance of diffusive clearance without ultrafiltration. During the initial ultrafiltration phase, dialysate is not circulated through the dialyzer, preventing diffusive clearance. During the second phase, net obligate ultrafiltration losses are balanced by the infusion of saline. Sequential ultrafiltration/clearance is designed to reduce intradialytic hemodynamic instability by separating intravascular volume losses due to ultrafiltration from intravascular volume losses due to movement of fluid into the interstitium and intracellular spaces after a decrease in plasma osmolality. Sequential ultrafiltration/clearance has the disadvantage of decreasing net diffusive clearance unless dialysis time is substantially increased. Data also suggest that the strategy of sequential ultrafiltration or clearance is less effective in maintaining intradialytic hemodynamic stability than other maneuvers such as sodium modeling or the use of low temperature dialysate.[268]

Prescription of the ultrafiltration rate in maintenance hemodialysis patients is generally based on an assessment of estimated dry weight. *Dry weight* is defined as the lowest weight a patient can tolerate without the development of signs or symptoms of intravascular hypovolemia.[269] Tolerance of the ultrafiltration rate during hemodialysis is largely determined by the rate of vascular refilling to ensure that intravascular volume depletion does not occur.[270] Monitoring of blood volume changes during dialysis may provide further insight into prescribing an ultrafiltration rate, and blood volume changes have been associated with blood pressure changes, hypotensive events, and hydration status during hemodialysis.[271] Relative changes in circulating blood volume can be estimated in real time by continuously monitoring the hematocrit during dialysis.[272] The observed real time changes in relative blood volume can be used to adjust ultrafiltration rates in an effort to reduce interdialytic hypotensive events. However, there are limited data suggesting that this approach in and of itself can enhance the achievement of estimated dry weight while reducing intradialytic symptoms.

An additional approach to balancing the need for intradialytic hemodynamic stability with the achievement of estimated dry weight involves the use of variable ultrafiltration rates during the hemodialysis procedure, known as ultrafiltration modeling. Ultrafiltration modeling has been introduced as an available component in some commercially available dialysis machines. Few or no data suggest that the use of ultrafiltration modeling can significantly reduce intradialytic complications.[273] However, several studies suggest that combining sodium and ultrafiltration profiling may reduce the slope of the blood volume curve during dialysis and significantly reduce hemodialysis-related symptoms.[274] Eventually, the development of biofeedback loops whereby continuous variation in sodium and ultrafiltration modeling is combined with assessment of blood volume and cardiac output changes may significantly improve hemodynamic stability during dialysis.[275]

HEMODIALYSIS ADEQUACY

Dialysis is a lifesaving treatment for more than 300,000 patients with ESRD in the United States and well over 1 million patients worldwide. Despite this enviable record extending over more than a quarter of a century of treatment, the annual mortality rate of dialysis patients in the United States over the past decade remains in excess of 20%.[276] Multiple lines of evidence implicate inadequate dialysis prescriptions and underdelivery of the prescribed dose of dialysis as central factors responsible for the high mortality.[123, 277-281] This section examines the evidence supporting the use of quantitative assessment of dialysis adequacy as an outcome measure and as a method of improving the care of patients with ESRD.

Historical Perspective

It is instructive to review the evolution of the methods that have been employed to determine the adequacy of the dose of hemodialysis. A physician may pose a question regarding adequate dialytic therapy that is similar to the one asked by Dr. Henry Stubb centuries ago concerning the practice of blood transfusions: "What regulation shall we have for the operation? Shall a man transfuse (*dialyze*) he knows not what, to correct he knows not what, God knows how?"[282]

The maintenance of homeostasis and of fluid balance and the elimination of toxins generated from dietary protein catabolism and other sources are chief functions of the kidneys. The accumulation of toxins results in the manifestations of uremic syndrome. In chronic renal failure, uremic symptoms are worsened by excessive protein intake and may be ameliorated by restriction of protein intake. This clearly indicates that nitrogenous compounds are central in the pathogenesis of uremia. However, a quandary exists about which specific substance or combinations of compounds produce symptoms. This makes the task of assessing treatment adequacy by indexing the dose of dialysis to a simple plasma level or removal rate of particular compound difficult. Easily measured substances, such as urea or creatinine, are themselves not major toxins. The plasma levels of these substances are influenced by many factors beyond clearance by the artificial kidney. Generation rates and removal rates and volume of distribution must be used to describe the fate of the substance being used to describe the efficiency of the treatment.

Low-Molecular-Weight Substances and Middle Molecules

The use of compounds like urea to judge adequacy rests on the assumption that the clearance rate of low-molecular-weight solutes correlates with well-being. Conversely, the observation that the severity of peripheral neuropathy could be mitigated by long treatment sessions with the Kiil dialyzer, a relatively inefficient device with respect to urea but one with a large-surface-area membrane. Long dialysis time and large membrane surface area are characteristics that enhance the removal of higher-molecular-weight substances. The finding that these features improved neuropathy led to the square meter–hour hypothesis.[283] This hypothesis holds that solutes with molecular weights in the range of 300 to 12,000 D, called *middle molecules*, play a role in the pathogenesis of the uremic syndrome.[284]

The subject of middle molecules as uremic toxins has been reviewed.[285] Compounds resulting from protein catabolism as well as peptides such as parathyroid hormone (PTH) and beta$_2$-microglobulin are among the larger solutes that are retained in renal failure. The latter two high-molecular-weight substances have been assigned roles as mediators of uremic toxicity.[286-291] Vanholder has suggested that low molecular weight may also behave as middle molecules by virtue of their physical properties such as charge, steric configurations or ability to bind to plasma proteins, or because of their high generation rates.[285] These properties result in a reduction in their clearance rate by dialysis that would not have been predicted by size alone. Candidates for this designation include methylguanidine, indoxyl sulfate, hippuric acid, and inorganic phosphate. However, Teschan and the results of the National Cooperative Dialysis Study (NCDS) have suggested that a low-molecular-weight compound, urea, can serve as a legitimate surrogate for uremic toxins.[292, 293]

The attributes of an ideal marker of the adequacy of dialysis have been suggested by Vanholder[285] and are listed in Table 59-11. No single marker meets all of the requirements. There are unresolved issues that preclude the use of middle molecules to determine adequacy. PTH secretion does not directly depend on the dialysis treatment. Many putative uremic toxins are not routinely measured in a clinical chemistry laboratory. Levels of these substances have never been indexed to measures of well-being. The use of hemodialysis membranes with high permeability and the implementation of longer dialysis times would be required to enhance the removal of substances with high molecular weight, if these substances determine uremic toxicity. Yet, no evidence has been forthcoming to conclusively substantiate that long hemodialysis sessions with high-flux membranes improves patient survival independently of changes attributable to the simultaneously enhanced removal of low-molecular-weight substances (Table 59-12).

The National Cooperative Dialysis Study

The NCDS was initiated in 1976. The study applied pharmacokinetic principles to urea concentrations as they varied during the intradialytic and interdialytic periods of the hemodialysis session.[294] For the purposes of analysis, a single-pool volume of distribution for urea was assumed. Developed by Sargent and Gotch, changes in serum urea concentrations are measured over time, so that "average" concentration of urea for the treatment session can be expressed as the timed average urea concentration (TAC_{urea}). From the intradialytic curve, the index related to the elements of the dialysis treatment and the size of the patient or Kt/V can be calculated and from the interdialytic curve urea generation can be determined, as seen in Figure 59-11.

The NCDS was a multicenter prospective, randomized 2 × 2 factorial trial (Table 59-13). The study participants were hemodialysis patients randomized to one of four groups based on short or long dialysis treatment times and high and low TAC_{urea}. Based on the design, groups I and III received a higher level of dialysis delivered over a longer or shorter time, respectively; groups II and IV received a lower level of dialysis delivered over a longer or shorter time, respectively. The goals were achieved by manipulation of dialyzer size and T_D. If groups I and III have a good outcome, this would suggest that the dose of hemodialysis could be indexed to low-molecular-weight compounds such as urea.

Two measures of outcome were analyzed: subjects who withdrew from the study for medical reasons or death (F1), and those who withdrew from the study for hospitalization within the first 6 months of the experimental phase (F2). Of 160 randomized patients, approximately 50% completed the study protocol. Group IV (i.e., high TAC, short dialysis time) was discontinued before the study was completed because of excessive hospitalizations and medical withdrawal.

The TAC_{urea}, the index of dialysis adequacy used in the analysis of the primary outcome of the NCDS, was the best predictor of failure. A much weaker but statistically significant relation was found for dialysis time; short time was associated with a greater incidence of F2 failure. Not all adverse medical events or hospitalizations were those commonly associated with too little dialysis, such as episodes of volume overload, hyperkalemia, or pericarditis.

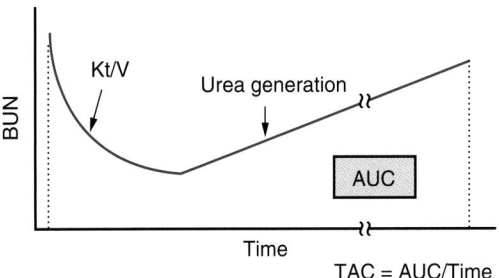

FIGURE 59-11. The hemodialysis cycle and elements of kinetic modeling. AUC, area under the curve.

TABLE 59-11

Ideal Marker of Dialysis Adequacy

Retained in renal failure
Eliminated by dialysis
Proven dose-related toxicity
Generation and elimination representative of other toxins
Easily measured

TABLE 59-12

Factors Affecting Dialyzer Clearance

SMALL MOLECULES*	LARGE MOLECULES*
Blood flow	Membrane
Dialysate flow	Dialysis time
Surface area	Surface area
Dialysis time	Blood and dialysate flows
Membrane	

*In order of decreasing importance.

TABLE 59-13

Design of the National Cooperative Dialysis Study

	INTENSIVE	LESS INTENSIVE
Long duration	Group I	Group II
	TAC = 51.3 ± 1.1 mg/dL	TAC = 87 ± 1.4 mg/dL
	T_D = 269 min	T_D = 271 min
Short duration	Group III	Group IV
	TAC = 54.1 ± 1.1 mg/dL	TAC = 89.6 ± 1.2 mg/dL
	T_D = 199 min	T_D = 194 min

Although only three patients died during the actual study, an additional 13 died during a 12-month follow-up after withdrawal from the study. Ten were assigned to groups II and IV. In many instances, these patients were returned to a higher level of therapy at the completion of the study, yet the adverse effects of what was shown to be an inadequate level of therapy were difficult to correct. The NCDS suggested that removal of small molecules strongly predicted morbidity and that urea kinetic modeling (i.e., determination of TAC) could be used to index the level of therapy delivered, despite the fact that urea does not fulfill all the criteria listed in Table 59-11.

The primary results of the NCDS were expressed in terms of TAC$_{urea}$; this index serves as a global parameter of interdialysis and intradialysis events. The value of TAC$_{urea}$ is influenced by many variables: dialyzer size, ultrafiltration, blood and dialysate flow rates, dialysis time, patient size, residual renal function, and rate of urea generation. The former six factors are important intradialytic variables, and the latter three are important interdialytic variables. When dialysis dose and residual renal function remain constant, TAC$_{urea}$ is influenced to the greatest extent by the interdialytic variable of urea generation rate (see Fig. 59-11). Poor protein intake associated with a low urea generation rate tends to lower TAC$_{urea}$ and masks a simultaneously inadequate dialysis dose. A relatively normal TAC would result from the combination of poor dialysis and low urea generation. This is similar to the finding that very low predialysis urea values are actually associated with high mortality rates.[295] Using TAC alone as an index of adequacy of treatment may be hazardous. The physician must be careful to interpret the TAC with the knowledge of the urea generation of the actual delivered dose of dialysis.

Subsequent analysis of the NCDS suggested that it would be informative to separately analyze the components of the dialysis cycle (see Fig. 59-11). The dimensionless term, Kt/V, describes aspects directly related to the hemodialysis treatment factored by the volume of urea distribution in the patient.[296] Morbidity could be indexed to this term. The advantage of using Kt/V as a marker of adequacy is that it allows the clinician to focus on the elements of the intradialytic period. This is the part of the dialysis cycle that is amenable to manipulation of the prescription: blood and dialysate flow, ultrafiltration rate, size of the artificial kidney and dialysis time in the case of hemodialysis, or dialysate volume in the case of peritoneal dialysis. The initial analysis of data from the NCDS indicated that a Kt/V greater than 0.8 was associated with a good outcome.

By design, the prescriptions in the NCDS were manipulated to achieve high or low TAC$_{urea}$ goals for the study. The TAC$_{urea}$ covers the entire dialysis cycle, and it is influenced by urea generation, an index of dietary protein intake in the stable hemodialysis patient (see Fig. 59-11). For the TAC goal to be reached, the dialysis dose (Kt/V) was partially determined by the subject's protein intake (i.e., urea generation). The implication of this design is that adequacy in the NCDS has been defined by Kt/V levels that have been interpreted in the context of protein intake of the subject (Fig. 59-12).

Although the initial interpretation from the NCDS suggested that there was little to be gained by increasing Kt/V to values beyond 0.8 to 1.0, subsequent analysis of the data indicates that the relationship between morbidity and Kt/V

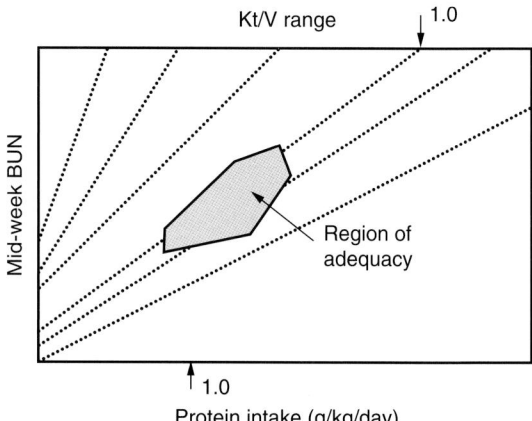

FIGURE 59-12. Relationship between Kt/V (standard measure of the dose of dialysis) and protein intake in the National Cooperative Dialysis Study. K, urea clearance; t, treatment time; V, volume of urea distribution.

may be continuous, with improved outcome found at higher doses of Kt/V.[297]

Assessment of Dialysis Adequacy and Derivatives of the National Cooperative Dialysis Study Outcome Measures

Since the conclusion of the NCDS, the principles of urea kinetic modeling have been applied to the assessment of the adequacy of hemodialysis and peritoneal dialysis. The impetus behind this practice has been the suggestion that improving the clearance of low-molecular-weight substances would impact favorably on the unacceptably high mortality rate experienced by dialysis patients in the United States. Subsequently, three retrospective and observational studies provided further evidence that patient outcome correlated with the dose of hemodialysis as measured by Kt/V.[123, 280, 281] A 5% and 7% decrease in the relative risk of mortality can be demonstrated for each 0.1% increase in Kt/V in nondiabetics and diabetics, respectively.[282] In all of these studies, patient survival improved as Kt/V was increased (Fig. 59-13).

The benefits of high levels of hemodialysis delivered by conventional cellulosic membranes over extremely long sessions of 6 to 8 hours has resulted in remarkable survival statistics.[298] In patients achieving a mean Kt/V of 1.67 delivered in this fashion, the 10-year survival rate ranges from 88% for patients initiating hemodialysis at 35 years of age or younger to 64% for patients older than 65 years of age. The 15-year survival for all patients in this dialysis center is 55%. These studies, along with data gathered from other dialysis registries, provide strong circumstantial evidence that Kt/V$_{urea}$, an index of removal of low-molecular-weight substances, is a predictor of mortality for hemodialysis patients.

The principles of urea kinetic modeling have also been applied to peritoneal dialysis as well.[299] The CANUSA Study has demonstrated that the expected 2-year survival on peritoneal dialysis is 78% with a weekly Kt/V of 2.1, whereas the 2-year survival falls to 67% at a weekly Kt/V of 1.5. Just as with hemodialysis, an increase of 0.1 unit of Kt/V per week is associated with a decrease in the relative risk of death of 5% in peritoneal dialysis patients.

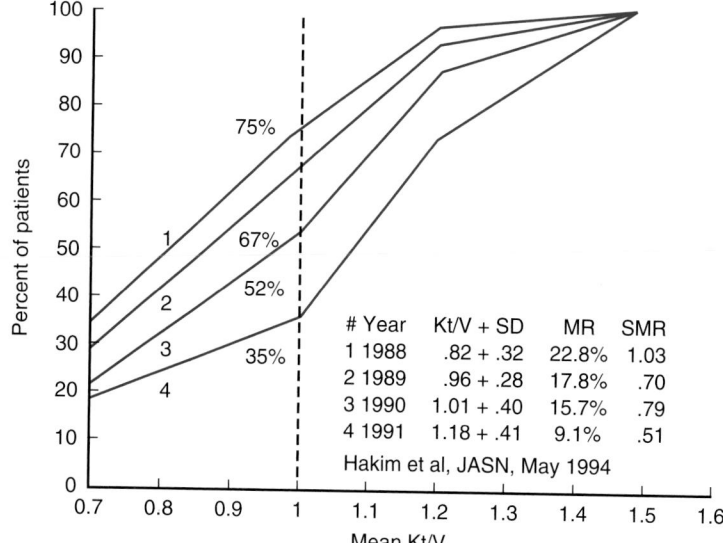

FIGURE 59-13. Improvement in the standardized mortality rate (SMR) as Kt/V (standard measure of the dose of dialysis) is increased over 4 years. The percentage of patients receiving higher doses of dialysis was increased during each year of the study. K, urea clearance; t, treatment time; V, volume of urea distribution.

#	Year	Kt/V + SD	MR	SMR
1	1988	.82 + .32	22.8%	1.03
2	1989	.96 + .28	17.8%	.70
3	1990	1.01 + .40	15.7%	.79
4	1991	1.18 + .41	9.1%	.51

Hakim et al, JASN, May 1994

The compelling evidence from these studies has served to make urea kinetic modeling a key outcome measure in the United States. They are part of the evidence use by the K/DOQI guidelines for determining the adequacy of hemodialysis and peritoneal dialysis.[300, 301] It is likely that documentation of the dose of dialysis delivered to ESRD patients will be mandated by governmental regulatory agencies and may be tied to reimbursement for treatment. Quality assurance programs in most dialysis centers already use kinetic modeling as part of the assessment of the care delivered to the patients.

Dialysis Adequacy: Applicability and Limitations of the National Cooperative Dialysis Study

The NCDS remains the only prospective study conducted to examine *hemodialysis* outcome indexed to clearance of low-molecular-weight substances. The remaining studies, which are described later in this chapter, are retrospective and observational. The same is true for studies that have been used to support the application of Kt/V_{urea} to determine adequate levels of peritoneal dialysis. The improvement in outcome for dialysis patients that occurred after the application of the principles of urea kinetic modeling is the ultimate proof that the clearance of low-molecular-weight substances has had a very important impact on survival. Nevertheless, the limitations of the NCDS should also be appreciated to understand unresolved issues regarding kinetic modeling.

The subjects eligible to enter the NCDS differed substantially from the current hemodialysis population. They were younger, compliant, and free of comorbid conditions. Only 20% of the current hemodialysis population would meet the NCDS entry criteria.[302] The follow-up period of the study was short. The influence of factors, such as age and comorbid conditions, that occur over a longer period of time could not be assessed by the NCDS. The NCDS was able to define a dose of dialysis below which an unacceptable number of complications occur but it was not designed to define an optimal level of dialysis beyond which no further improvement was realized.

Technical advances in dialysis delivery have also occurred since the NCDS was completed. The methods employed in that study may not be generalizable to our current practice. Biocompatible, synthetic, high-efficiency or high-flux dialyzers have largely replaced low-flux cellulose dialyzers used in the NCDS. Acetate-buffered dialysate has been universally replaced with bicarbonate-buffered dialysate. Hemodialysis treatments have been more stable with the use of dialysate with higher sodium concentration and with volumetric machines capable of changing ultrafiltration rate and sodium concentration during the treatment.

Increasing evidence points to nutrition as an important independent determinant of survival in dialysis patients.[303] In the NCDS, the level of protein intake influenced the dialysis dose. By design, the levels of dialysis determined by Kt/V and protein intake were *interdependent* rather than *independent* variables.

The dose of dialysis in the study was adjusted by alterations in blood flow, the dialyzer size, and length of time. Time was an independent variable in the design. Dialyzer surface area and time influence middle molecule clearance and the clearance of low-molecular-weight substances. Longer dialysis time and dialyzers of greater surface areas introduced a confounding variable, enhanced middle molecule clearance, when these techniques were used to increase Kt/V_{urea}. Group IV (i.e., short time, low Kt/V) fared most poorly of all groups, and it remains possible that reduced middle molecule clearance played a role in this outcome.

The National Cooperative Dialysis Study and Dialysis Time

The effect of the length of the dialysis treatment on outcome was not determined in the NCDS and it is yet to be included as an independent variable in any study of the dialysis prescription. The issue remains unsettled because time was partially confounded with the effects of Kt/V_{urea}; an increase or a decrease in time was one of the methods used to change the TAC to meet the goals assigned to the study participants.

The practice of using large-surface-area dialyzers at blood flows of more than 400 mL/minute and at dialysate flows of 600 to 800 mL/minute allows a Kt/V to be reached far in excess of values in NCDS groups I or III in many patients without increasing time. Many small to medium-sized individuals reach high levels of dialysis in times that are shorter than those employed in group III.

Whether time is an important factor remains to be proved. Increased time may have a direct effect or it may be a surrogate marker for the removal of larger substances with high flux. A decrease in cardiovascular instability and greater ease of ultrafiltration to a dry weight that is associated with a reduction or absence in the requirement of antihypertensive medications might be outcomes associated with increased dialysis time. In this regard, it should be remembered that the best survival statistics for hemodialysis patients, not withstanding somewhat favorable demographic features of the population, have been reported in a group of patients undergoing long, slow hemodialysis of 6 to 8 hours' duration against cellulosic membranes. Although this form of treatment is associated with very high Kt/V$_{urea}$, analysis of the data suggests that excellent blood pressure control *without the need of antihypertensive medication* is central to the favorable outcome experienced by the patients.

The superior control of hypertension with long dialysis is also supported by the experience from daily nocturnal hemodialysis.[304, 305] Preliminary studies show that fluid balance is better maintained and that fewer antihypertensive agents are required to maintain normotension. The control of phosphorus appears to be excellent with nocturnal hemodialysis. Given the developing evidence that accelerated vascular calcification occurs in patients on dialysis, likely due to the use of calcium-containing phosphate binders, nocturnal dialysis may eventually be shown to reduce cardiovascular morbidity associated with ESRD. This would be an effect of high-dose dialysis that is disassociated from urea kinetics. In this regard, despite its relatively low molecular weight, phosphorus behaves much more like a large-molecular-weight substance that depends on the length of treatment rather than on blood and dialysate flow.

Long dialysis times would be more forgiving of errors such as poor needle placement or incorrect or unachievable blood flow rates that lead to disparities between prescribed and delivered levels of dialysis. The optimal length of dialysis time needs to be defined by further investigation.

Effect of Dialysis with High-Efficiency and High-Flux Dialysis

In the NCDS, cellulosic membranes with a low-molecular-weight solute cutoff were exclusively used. The introduction of high-efficiency and high-flux membranes has added more complexity to the quantification of hemodialysis. The kinetic modeling used in the NCDS and in most of the observational studies assumed that urea would instantly equilibrate across all body fluid compartments: the single-pool model. This model did not account for the finding of an immediate, rapid increase in the postdialysis urea level that occurs at the termination of dialysis. This rapid rise, called urea rebound is caused by three factors: dialysis access recirculation, cardiopulmonary recirculation, and urea compartmentalization.[214, 306, 307] The first two phases

occur within 2 minutes after termination of hemodialysis. The rebound that results from urea compartmentalization occurs over 60 minutes. It is caused by a delay in urea equilibration between tissue stores and blood. This delay results from slower than expected removal of urea from the intracellular fluid compartment.[308-311] Alternatively, reduced perfusion of regions of the body containing high amounts of urea could explain the delay in equilibration.[306] Rebound is enhanced under conditions of high-efficiency dialysis and lower access blood flow during hypotension and in states of low cardiac output.[312-314] Single-pool Kt/V may overestimate the equilibrated Kt/V by more than 0.2 unit.[314] An equation that allows the equilibrated Kt/V to be estimated from single-pool Kt/V has been developed[315]:

$$\text{Equilibrated Kt/V} = \text{Single-pool Kt/V} - 0.6 \times \text{K/V} + 0.03$$

The HEMO Study

Although multiple lines of evidence indicate that kinetic modeling is an important index of dialysis adequacy and that the degree of removal of low-molecular-weight substances correlates with survival, these relationships have not been proved by prospective studies. It is important to confirm the impression of the observational studies that high doses of dialysis have a favorable impact on patient outcome. The time, effort, and costs associated with providing high doses of dialysis are substantial. The K/DOQI guidelines have already made recommendations regarding a dose of dialysis below which poor patient outcomes are likely to occur. Prospective data regarding the effects of increasing Kt/V to very high levels are lacking. Consequently, the National Institutes of Health initiated a multicenter, prospective, randomized trial to assess the impact of the dialysis prescription on morbidity and mortality of hemodialysis patients.[316, 317]

The study design consisted of a 2×2 factorial design that assessed the effect of hemodialysis dose and membrane flux on outcome. In this study, an equilibrated Kt/V of 1.05 was compared with an equilibrated Kt/V of 1.45, comparable on average to single-pool Kt/V of 1.25 and 1.65, respectively. The effect on mortality and morbidity of high-flux versus low-flux dialyzers was compared. All-cause mortality is the primary outcome and morbidity assessed from hospitalization, time to hospitalization for cardiovascular and infectious causes, and time to a decline in serum albumin concentration are secondary outcome measures. The design called for a concurrent sample size of 900 patients from 15 clinical centers with replacement of those participants who died or dropped out.

In the group of control subjects randomized to the usual hemodialysis dose arm, the achieved single-pool Kt/V was 1.32 ± 0.09, and the achieved equilibrated Kt/V was 1.16 ± 0.08; in the subjects randomized to the high-dose arm, the achieved values were 1.71 ± 0.11, and 1.53 ± 0.09, respectively. Dialyzer flux, based on the clearance of beta$_2$-microglobulin clearance, was 3 ± 7 mL/minute in the low-flux group and 34 ± 11 mL/minute in the high-flux group. The primary outcome, death from any cause, was not influenced by the dialysis dose or the dialyzer flux assignment: the relative risk of death in the high-dose group compared with the usual-dose group was 0.96 (95% confidence interval [CI], 0.84 to 1.10; $P = .53$), and the relative risk of death in the high-flux group compared with the low-flux group was 0.92 (95% CI: 0.81 to 1.06; $P = .23$). The main secondary outcomes, including first hospitalization for cardiac causes or infection or all-cause mortality, declines in albumin or all-cause mortality, and all hospitalization not related to vascular access problems, also did not differ between the dose and the flux groups.[316]

The effects of hemodialysis dose and flux intervention were also adjusted for a series of prespecified baseline factors of age, gender, race, years on dialysis, presence or absence of diabetes, score for coexisting conditions excluding diabetes, and albumin level. For the entire study population of 1846 randomized patients, all of the prespecified covariates were independent predictors of death. Older age (per 10-year increment), male gender, white race, presence of diabetes, longer time on dialysis (per 1-year increment), higher baseline Index of Coexisting Disease and lower baseline albumin level were associated with higher mortality in all patients, independently of their randomization.

When subgroup analysis was performed based on these prespecified baseline factors, interactions with the primary treatment interventions were detected. Females randomized to the high-dose hemodialysis group had a lower risk of mortality. Subjects with a longer length of time on hemodialysis *at entry into the study* had a lower mortality rate if they were allocated to the high-flux arm of the study. The reasons for these subgroup outcomes are not completely clear. For instance, lower body weight versus dose does not explain the improved outcome among female subjects. When length of time in the study is added to the baseline length of time on dialysis, the benefit of flux disappears.

Although the data from the subgroup analyses are interesting and suggest further avenues for inquiry, the primary results indicate that within the conventional schedule of thrice-weekly hemodialysis, neither an increased dose of dialysis nor the use of a high-flux membrane improves survival, reduces the hospitalization rate, or maintains a higher serum albumin level than a standard hemodialysis dose and the use of high-flux membranes. The results from the Hemodialysis (HEMO) Study should reassure nephrologists that if the current K/DOQI guidelines are achieved, adequate therapy is being delivered to their patients who are receiving thrice-weekly therapy. However, the study should not be interpreted as sanctioning a minimal dose of hemodialysis. It is prudent to provide a margin above a minimal dose to protect the patient from receiving less dialysis than intended due to factors that result in lower than intended blood flows, poor blood pump calibration, poor access function, or premature treatment termination. In particular, the HEMO Study should not be used as a justification to reduce hemodialysis time. Time and its interaction with flux were not independent interventions in this study. Dialysis time itself is an important factor in blood pressure control and in avoiding hypotension in patients.[219] It is not possible to conclude from the HEMO Study that minimizing time while maintaining an "acceptable" Kt/V is justified.

It is also apparent from the HEMO Study that the current 22% gross mortality rate for hemodialysis patients in the United States cannot be influenced by changing the dose of thrice-weekly treatments. Nondialytic therapies must be directed against processes such as inflammation and accelerated cardiovascular disease that lead to the mortality seen in the ESRD population. The processes that result in cardiovascular disease, the leading cause of mortality in dialysis patients, originate long before the patient is started on dialysis. Therapeutic interventions must begin when the patient is identified with early CKD.

ALTERNATIVE CHRONIC HEMODIALYSIS PRESCRIPTIONS

The HEMO Study can only be applied to thrice-weekly hemodialysis, as is practiced in the United States. There is increasing interest in different treatment times and frequency designed to improve outcome. Although the removal of low-molecular-weight substances has been validated as a method to index dose of dialysis, it is also possible that improved clearance of larger substances can influence mortality and morbidity rates.[283-285] The failure of the HEMO Study to show a benefit of high-flux dialyzers does not conclusively eliminate the potential benefits of the removal of high-molecular-weight substances. The removal of high-molecular-weight substances depends on porosity and on the length of the dialysis treatment. It is possible to argue that for the full benefit of these membranes to be realized, longer treatment times than those employed in the HEMO study are required.

Factors that influence the hemodialysis treatment include patient acceptance, the need for delivery of an adequate treatment (i.e., dialysis time, blood and dialysate flow, dialyzer size, and frequency), and economics.[318] The evolution of reimbursement has been a major stimulus for the movement away from earlier hemodialysis regimens consisting of more than three treatments per week. However, observational data have suggested a beneficial effect on survival of increasing low-molecular-weight substances, as measured by Kt/V or URR.[123, 280, 281] The remarkable patient survival of patients undergoing conventional, thrice-weekly, low-flux hemodialysis but for 8 hours per session has been reported from Tassin, France.[319] Efforts to improve survival and rehabilitation of patients with ESRD have led to a renewed interest in alternative hemodialysis schedules. The alternative schedules result in treatments that are longer or more frequent than the standard 2.5 to 5 hours per session, thrice-weekly, intermittent hemodialysis (IHD) that is widely practiced.

Nutritional status is an important predictor of outcome in ESRD patients. Nutritional indices (Table 59-14) such as serum albumin, cholesterol, and creatinine concentration have been demonstrated to be associated with survival in cross-sectional analysis in hemodialysis patients.[295] Nutritional status of patients can be improved by increasing the dose of conventional hemodialysis and by using biocompatible membranes.[320] It should not be surprising that daily hemodialysis treatments have also been found to affect nutrition. However, the full impact of these modalities of treatment has yet to be described.

Daily Dialysis and Outcome

There are several alternative methods to conventional IHD (defined previously). In Tassin, slow, long hemodialysis is given thrice weekly, with blood flow rates of 200 to 250 mL/minute and T_D of 6 to 8 hours. Short, daily hemodialysis (DHD) is characterized by five to seven treatments

TABLE 59-14

Nutritional Indices

Plasma markers
    Albumin
    Prealbumin
    Blood urea nitrogen
    Creatinine/creatinine index
    Cholesterol
    Insulin-like growth factor-1
    Transferrin
    Total lymphocyte count
Body composition
    Subjective global assessment (SGA)
    Anthropometric measures
    Dual energy x-ray absorptiometry (DEXA)
    Bioelectrical impedance analysis (BIA)
    Total neutron activation
Nutrition prescription
    Dietary interview/diary
    Normalized protein equivalent of nitrogen appearance (nPNA)
    Resting energy expenditure

per week, each lasting 1.5 to 2.5 hours, and by the use of high-flux biocompatible membranes at blood flow rates higher than 400 mL/minute and dialysate flow rates of 500 to 800 mL/minute. Nocturnal hemodialysis (NHD) is also performed five to seven times per week, with each treatment lasting 6 to 8 hours and using biocompatible membranes at blood flow rate of 200 to 300 mL/minute and dialysate flows of 200 to 300 mL/minute. The single-pool Kt/V values are 1.2 to 1.8 with conventional IHD, 1.6 to 1.8 with IHD as practiced in Tassin, 0.2 to 0.8 with DHD, and 0.9 to 1.2 with NHD.[321]

The experience of groups who have practiced long IHD (6 to 8 hours) or who have markedly increased the intensity of standard length IHD by the introduction of high-efficiency dialyzers is an improvement in the nutritional status of the patients. Dietary protein intake (DPI) is reported to be as high as 1.3 ± 0.42 g/kg/day and serum albumin is 4.2 ± 0.5 g/dL. In contrast, the DPI is 1.0 ± 0.3 g/kg/day and the serum albumin averages 3.8 ± 0.3 in patients undergoing conventional IHD.[319] Against this backdrop, the nutritional status of patients undergoing DHD can be compared.

Nocturnal Hemodialysis

Although the number of patients studied has been rather limited, multiple lines of evidence that compare the status of patients on conventional IHD with their status on NHD have been remarkably consistent. Neutron activation analysis, an extremely accurate method to measure total body nitrogen (TBN), demonstrates a significant increase in TBN in 18 of 24 patients after they were switched from IHD to NHD. The observation period spanned 12 to 30 months. The change in TBN was from 1.43 ± 0.38 kg to 1.89 ± 0.60 kg.[322]

In one study, initially involving five patients, 8 weeks after changing from IHD to NHD, significant increases in nitrogen intake, caloric intake, and sodium intake were observed. The protein catabolic rate increased from 1.07 ± 0.12 g/kg/day to 1.27 ± 0.20 g/kg/day.[323] In studies of a small number of patients from two different groups, no

differences were documented in albumin levels. The abnormal plasma and intracellular amino acid profiles found in patients receiving IHD were altered on changing to NHD. After 1 year on NHD, total amino acid, essential and nonessential amino acid, and branched chain amino acid levels increased significantly.[324] However, a number of aberrations persisted such as abnormal ratios of essential to nonessential amino acids: tyrosine to phenylalanine and valine to glycine.

A remarkable and unprecedented feature of NHD is the change in the management of renal osteodystrophy and phosphate control.[305] NHD results in the removal of more than 160 mmol of phosphate each week. This is more than double the removal seen with conventional IHD. This results in a serum phosphate level of 6.0 mg/dL with IHD falling to 3.9 mg/dL, despite an increase in phosphate intake. All patients were able to discontinue the use of phosphate binders entirely. Some patients actually require the addition of phosphate to the dialysate.

Short Daily Hemodialysis

Experience with 10 patients enrolled in the DHD arm of an ongoing clinical trial, the London, Ontario Daily/Nocturnal Hemodialysis Study, indicates that this form of therapy is associated with a significant improvement in protein catabolic rate and serum albumin levels.[318] The protein catabolic rate increased from 1.0 g/kg/day to 1.7 g/kg/day, and albumin levels increased from 38.6 g/L to 40.8 g/L at the end of 18 months. No significant change was observed in a control group of patients undergoing IHD.

In another study of five patients, nutritional parameters were compared before and after a switch to DHD. Significant improvement occurred in the levels of urea, creatinine, total carbon dioxide, and albumin and in dry weight.[325] The weekly sum of Kt/V was unchanged but the investigators did not express dose as stdKt/V.

Outcome Studies
Nocturnal Hemodialysis

Much of what has been described concerning daily dialysis modalities involves changes in biochemical parameters, quality of life, response to erythropoietin, and dose of dialysis. Because these modalities are new and the number of patients enrolled is relatively low, there have been very few outcome studies of daily dialysis. One report describes the use of NHD in four young patients with growth retardation and failure to thrive on peritoneal dialysis with treatments lasting 7 to 8 hours, six times weekly.[326] NHD was performed from 5 to 55 months. Treatment was accepted by the patients and resulted in improved nutritional status and increased bone length and mineralization. Improved quality of life and the chance for catch-up growth were features of the treatment.

Nocturnal Hemodialysis and Short Daily Dialysis: Comparative Effects on Nutrition

The two daily dialysis regimens are not equivalent. NHD requires long treatment times of 7 to 8 hours at relatively low blood and dialysate flows whereas DHD employs short treatment times of 1.5 to 2.5 hours at high blood flow rates.

Single treatment Kt/V with NHD is greater than with DHD but standard Kt/V based on low-molecular-weight substance removal is similar. The removal of high-molecular-weight substances is greater with NHD. Although estimated dry weight and protein catabolic rate increase with both modalities, an increased albumin level is more often seen with DHD. The control of phosphate is better with NHD. NHD is better adapted to the home, whereas DHD could easily be performed at home or in the medical center. The clinical and economic practicality of applying each of these modalities to large groups of patients awaits a randomized clinical trial.

ALTERNATIVE APPROACHES TO QUANTIFICATION OF DIALYSIS

The use of Kt/V_{urea} in determining adequacy of dialysis is based on mathematical models and is supported by clinical experience. However, a number of paradoxical observations have led some to question the validity of Kt/V_{urea} as the best index of judging adequacy. One paradox is that the curve relating dialysis dose and survival is J shaped.[327] Low dialysis dose is associated with high mortality, and mortality declines with increased doses of dialysis, but mortality again trends upward at the highest levels of dialysis. A second observation is that survival of black Americans on dialysis is better than that of white Americans, despite the finding that the latter group generally receives a higher dose of dialysis.[328-330] These observations do not necessarily invalidate the practice of indexing adequacy against low-molecular-weight substances. Rather, the issue is whether Kt/V_{urea} is the best measure of low-molecular-weight solute removal.

A common feature that may explain these observations is related to patient size.[331] At the same $K \times t$, the smaller individuals are more likely to receive higher Kt/V_{urea} than larger individuals because their urea volume is smaller. Black Americans tend to have a body mass than whites.[330, 332, 333] A low body mass is an independent risk factor for death in dialysis patients.[281, 333-336] V, the urea volume, may be an independent variable of survival because it tends to vary directly with body mass. When the work of dialysis, $K \times t$, is divided by V, a parameter that may also correlate with survival, in the computation of Kt/V, "these elements may offset each other, producing a complex quantity that does not reflect a true relationship between dialysis exposure and clinical outcome."[331] Proponents of this concept have demonstrated that, when patient survival is examined as a function of Kt, the J-shaped curve disappears, and mortality declines over the entire range of Kt.

Further analysis along these lines provides clarification of this complex relationship. From the USRDS database, 9165 prevalent patients treated between 1990 and 1995 were studied. A Cox proportional hazards model, adjusting for patient characteristics, was used to calculate the relative risk for death. Hemodialysis dose (i.e., equilibrated Kt/V) and various indices of body size (e.g., body mass index, body weight and volume) were found to be independently inversely related to mortality (Fig. 59-14).

Mortality was lower in patients with larger body size or volume and decreased as a function of hemodialysis dose. The relationship between Kt/V and declining mortality is valid but patient size must also be considered. The implication of this analysis is that the indices of body size may be surrogates for nutritional status. Nutritional status is clearly an important predictor of survival.

Urea Reduction Ratio and Solute Removal Index

There are alternative methods to the quantification of the dose of hemodialysis: urea reduction ratio (URR) (i.e., predialysis BUN − postdialysis BUN/predialysis BUN) and solute removal index (SRI), based on dialysate urea measurements (i.e., total dialysate urea in grams × 100/predialysis BUN × V). URR depends exclusively on the changes that occur in urea levels during intermittent hemodialysis. The urea removed by convection is not accounted for by URR. Although URR has been shown to correlate with survival in a fashion similar to Kt/V and is recognized by K/DOQI guidelines as a valid index of hemodialysis adequacy, Kt/V is a more precise index. Unlike URR, Kt/V also permits rational adjustments to the dialysis prescription to be made. The URR cannot be used to judge the adequacy of peritoneal dialysis because urea levels are essentially in a steady state (URR ≈ 0).

The SRI measures the *amount* of urea removed rather than the *fractional change* in urea. It is not influenced by compartmental distribution of urea. However, the measurement of dialysate urea requires special techniques and it is not routinely done. There have been few studies validating SRI as an index of adequacy.

The NCDS was designed to prospectively determine which determinants of the dialysis prescription had an impact on patient outcome. The study was able to validate urea removal, a surrogate for low-molecular-weight substances, as an index of morbidity. Based on urea kinetics, *minimum level* of hemodialysis below which increased morbidity resulted was a key finding that has stood the test of time. More importantly, the NCDS provided the stimulus for

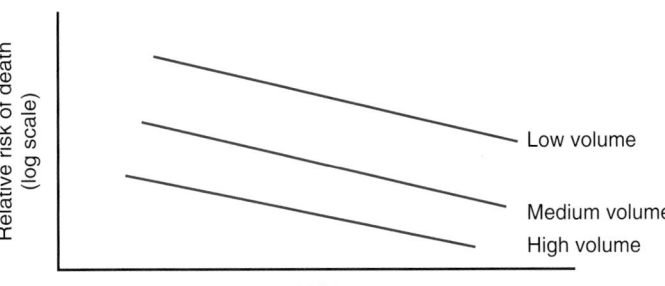

FIGURE 59-14. Risk of death as a function of urea volume and dialysis dose.

a large number of observational studies that has resulted in the recommendations of the K/DOQI guidelines. The validity of these recommendations is supported by the findings of the HEMO Study.

Standard Measure of the Dose of Dialysis: Kt/V

There are no established criteria for evaluating HD dose for intensive HD therapies such as DHD or NHD; two dose measures based on serum urea concentrations have been proposed: equivalent renal clearance (EKR) and standard Kt/V (stdKt/V). The EKR concept equalizes the time-averaged concentration of urea for different therapies; weekly EKR normalized by urea distribution volume (EKRt/V) is approximately equivalent to summing the EKt/V for each individual HD treatment during the week. This dose measure has been criticized by some because it does not explain why patients treated by continuous ambulatory peritoneal dialysis (CAPD) and conventional HD have similar outcomes but different EKR values for urea. Gotch has argued that EKR is not an appropriate dose measure because it does not account for the first-order nature of HD therapy.[337] Although the time-averaged weekly urea clearance or Kt/V is doubled by doubling the clearance of a set number of treatments per week or by doubling the number of treatments per week while leaving the clearance per treatment unchanged, the total solute removal is not the same. As the frequency of hemodialysis increases, the peak levels of urea decline, yet solute removal per session is greater because urea is cleared by first-order kinetics, which are concentration dependent.

It has been proposed that dialysis dose might be better expressed as standard Kt/V (stdKt/V), a dose measure that combines treatment dose with treatment frequency and allows for various intermittent therapies to be compared with continuous therapy. The stdKt/V can be defined as the continuous removal rate divided by the average peak concentration. In the steady state, the continuous removal rate for urea is equal to its generation rate (G_{urea}), producing the stdKt/V = G_{urea}/average peak urea concentration. As treatment frequency or length, or both, increases, peak concentration approaches the mean concentration found in continuous therapies. In this calculation, regimens that result in the same mean prehemodialysis serum urea concentrations during the week would have equivalent stdKt/V values (Fig. 59-15).

Because the weekly stdKt/V during intermittent therapy is based on peak urea concentration rather than mean urea concentration found during continuous therapy, it is lower than the sum of the intermittent single-pool Kt/V treatments per week.

Other issues also must be addressed. The small differences in time did not permit any conclusions to be made with respect to the importance of the removal of middle molecule in outcome. The poor outcome of group IV in the NCDS suggested that further examination of this question was necessary. The importance of the removal of higher-molecular-weight substances or related substances, such as phosphorus, that are associated with them has also been suggested by the studies of very long hemodialysis and nocturnal dialysis. The interaction between body size and dose of dialysis has also pointed out the complexity in interpreting the relationship between urea kinetics and survival.

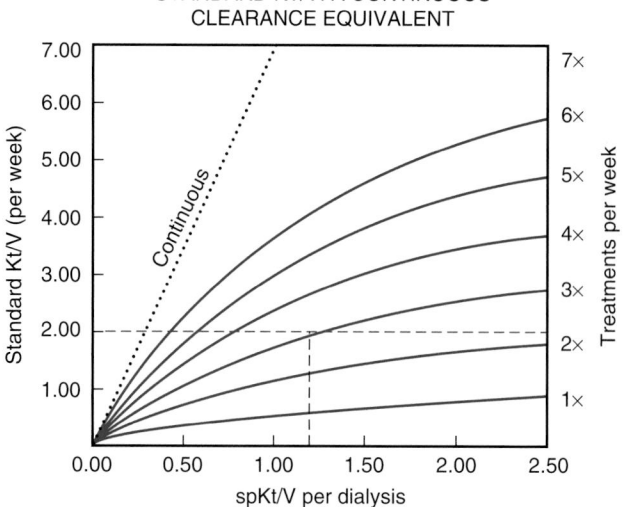

FIGURE 59-15. Relationship between intermittent hemodialysis (spKt/V) performed one to seven times each week and standard Kt/V per week. A thrice-weekly treatment providing a single-pool Kt/V of 1.2/treatment is equivalent to a regimen providing a single-pool Kt/V of 0.5 five times each week. K, urea clearance; t, treatment time; V, volume of urea distribution.

MANAGEMENT OF THE MAINTENANCE HEMODIALYSIS PATIENT

Uremic Syndrome

The uremic syndrome is a complex phenomenon involving dysfunction of a number of organ systems in the body attributable to the retention of myriad solutes normally secreted by healthy kidneys. Increased attention is being focused on identification of specific uremic toxins and on characterization of the biochemical and pathophysiologic processes that they contribute to the uremic syndrome.[338] Many of the effects of uremia on organ system function and how organ systems adapt to compromised renal function are the topics of discussion of other chapters in this textbook. The following section focuses on abnormalities attributable to uremia that persist in the dialysis patient or that are potentially accentuated by the hemodialysis procedure. Although the effects of uremia on specific organ systems are generally considered as an isolated phenomenon, multiple interactions between organ systems occur in the adaptation to uremic toxicity. For example, the influence of uremic toxicity on gastrointestinal tract function may exacerbate malnutrition by decreasing nutrient intake. Worsening nutritional status may affect endocrine function and increase the risk for infectious and cardiovascular complications. Hormonal abnormalities associated with uremia may similarly affect intermediary metabolism hematopoietic function. Alterations in lipid and carbohydrate metabolism may also adversely affect the development of atherosclerosis and cardiovascular complications.

Although many of the organ system abnormalities attributable to uremia may be improved with the institution of maintenance hemodialysis therapy, it must also be recognized that hemodialysis may actually potentiate or worsen other uremic complications. Gastrointestinal bleeding may be potentiated by the use of anticoagulation during hemodialysis. The hemodialysis procedure may induce a more catabolic state through amino acid losses and contribute to malnutrition. Similarly, treatments designed to prevent one uremic complication may potentiate another, such as suppression of secondary hyperparathyroidism leading to adynamic bone disease.

Because of the complexities of the relationships between uremia, renal replacement therapy, and various organ functions, nephrologists who take care of maintenance dialysis patients must be knowledgeable about the numerous ramifications that result from the loss of renal function. The nephrologist caring for the maintenance hemodialysis patient is practicing "anephric" internal medicine. The following section describes frequently occurring medical management problems in the maintenance hemodialysis patient.

Anemia

In healthy individuals, the kidney produces up to 80% of circulating erythropoietin, accounting for the pivotal role of the kidney in regulating erythropoiesis.[339] The pathogenesis of anemia in renal failure is described in detail in Chapter 49. In this section, emphasis is placed on describing factors specific to the management of anemia in maintenance hemodialysis patients and the interactions of hemodialysis and erythropoietic therapy. The first clinical trials of recombinant human erythropoietin in maintenance hemodialysis patients began in 1985, and erythropoietin received U.S. Food and Drug Administration (FDA) approval in June of 1989.[340] The target maintenance hematocrit for patients in the initial phase I/II clinical trials was 35% to 40% (i.e., at the lower range of normal values). A target hematocrit of 35% was used in the subsequent phase III multicenter clinical trials. From the outset of these clinical trials, it was apparent that erythropoietin would be a highly effective agent in the maintenance hemodialysis population, with a resulting dramatic decrease in required erythrocyte transfusions.[292] In the early trials, exacerbation of hypertension and on occasion the development of seizures was observed with the use of erythropoietin, probably as a consequence of the rapidity with which hematocrit was increased. In subsequent studies with a slower rate of rise of increase in hematocrit, only modest increases in the level of hypertension have been observed.[341]

The use of erythropoietin leads to improvement in cardiac hemodynamics, with studies demonstrating a decrease in left ventricular hypertrophy, improvement in oxygen-releasing capacity, enhanced exercise capability, and reduction in intradialytic hypotension.[342-348] Improvements of physical performance, work capacity, quality of life, sexual function, and cognitive capacity have also been demonstrated.[349-354] The decrease in erythrocyte transfusions associated with the use of erythropoietin has led to a beneficial decrease in the frequency of transfusion-associated hepatitis and a decreased human leukocyte antigen (HLA) presensitization for renal transplantation.

In the years before the introduction of erythropoietin, erythrocyte transfusions were used to replace blood losses and treat the anemia of CKD. In many dialysis patients, repeated erythrocyte transfusions led to a high frequency of iron overload manifested as hemosiderosis and hemochromatosis,

with subsequent hepatic, cardiac, and muscle dysfunction.[355, 356] Deferoxamine was often administered for treatment of iron overload, but was associated with severe complications, including propensity to increased infection.[357] Treatment of anemia with erythropoietin has virtually eliminated this syndrome by minimizing transfusion requirements in the dialysis population.

The appropriate dose and route of administration of erythropoietin remain somewhat controversial. Erythropoietin therapy is indicated for all patients undergoing maintenance hemodialysis who present with or develop a predialysis hemoglobin level of less than 11 g/dL. In many studies, subcutaneous administration of erythropoietin has more favorable pharmacodynamic characteristics than intravenous administration despite incomplete bioavailability of erythropoietin after subcutaneous administration.[358] Greater potency is achieved because of a prolonged half-life after subcutaneous compared with intravenous erythropoietin administration. At least 36 published studies involving more than 2000 patients comparing subcutaneous to intravenous administration reveal that, on average, the dose of erythropoietin required to maintain a stable hematocrit is approximately 30% lower (range, 0% to 68%).[359] In aggregate, patients respond better to subcutaneous than intravenous erythropoietin, but in some studies, up to 23% of patients require more erythropoietin on switching from an intravenous to subcutaneous route. The intravenous route of administration remains the predominant mode of erythropoietin administration in hemodialysis patients due to patient preference, convenience, and the lack of patient discomfort. When erythropoietin is administered subcutaneously, it is recommended that the site of injection be rotated with each administration.

When selecting an initial dose of erythropoietin, the goal is to achieve the target hemoglobin within a 2- to 4-month period through the induction of a slow, steady increase in the hemoglobin. It is not possible to accurately predict the fraction of patients who will respond adequately to any given dose of erythropoietin, and it is necessary to monitor individual patients' responses to optimize the dosing of erythropoietin therapy. Clinical practice guidelines recommend that, for initial subcutaneous erythropoietin administration, the dose should be 50 to 120 units/kg/week, administered in two or three doses per week. Data from two multicenter trials suggest that for pediatric patients younger than 5 years of age, a higher dose of erythropoietin may be required, and initial subcutaneous doses should be 300 units/kg/week. If the initial route of erythropoietin administration is intravenous, therapy should be initiated with 120 to 180 units/kg/week, given in three divided doses. For hemodialysis patients who are being switched from intravenous to subcutaneous administration of erythropoietin after achieving a target hemoglobin, it is recommended that the initial weekly subcutaneous erythropoietin dose be two thirds of the weekly intravenous dose.

Several protocols have been described for adjusting the dose of erythropoietin until a target hemoglobin and stable erythropoietin dose have been achieved. Hemoglobin or hematocrit levels should be checked within the first 2 weeks of initiating erythropoietin therapy or changing erythropoietin dose with the general goal of a 1% rise in hematocrit (or 0.33 g/dL rise in hemoglobin) per week. If the rate of increase in hemoglobin exceeds 3 g/dL per month or if the hemoglobin exceeds the target range, it is common to reduce the weekly dose of erythropoietin by approximately 25%. If the hemoglobin is not rising after initiating erythropoietin therapy, then a review for potential causes of erythropoietin resistance should be undertaken.

Optimal target hemoglobin concentrations for maintenance hemodialysis patients remain controversial. The original target hematocrit recommended in 1989 by the FDA was 33%, which was widened in 1994 to a target range of 30% to 36%. An extensive review as part of the DOQI and K/DOQI Clinical Practice Guidelines recommended a target hemoglobin of 11 to 12 g/dL. However, many of the initial physiologic and quality of life studies in hemodialysis patients used erythropoietin to achieve target hematocrit values above 36%. Virtually all of these studies demonstrated that with increased hematocrit, there were marked improvements in physiologic measures, including oxygen use, cardiac function, cognitive and brain electrophysiologic function, and sexual function. These studies led some investigators to advocate that normalization of hematocrit (or to a hemoglobin of 14 g/dL) might be beneficial in maintenance hemodialysis patients.

Several published studies have examined the consequences of targeting a normalized hemoglobin and hematocrit in hemodialysis patients. In the largest study, 1233 patients known to have cardiovascular disease (i.e., congestive heart failure or ischemic heart disease) were randomized to a target hematocrit of 42% versus 30%.[360] The study was terminated prematurely due to a trend for a higher incidence of nonfatal myocardial infarction or death in the normal hematocrit group. A randomized, prospective Canadian trial examined the effect of normalizing hematocrit on left ventricular geometry in hemodialysis patients with known cardiomyopathy. This study, although relatively underpowered in design, did not demonstrate significant benefits in left ventricular remodeling associated with normalizing hematocrit.[361] Quality of life did improve in this study with no apparent excess mortality in the normal hematocrit group. A Spanish cooperative study conducted a 6-month prospective trial on the effect of normalized hematocrit on patient quality of life in nondiabetic hemodialysis patients without known symptomatic cardiovascular disease.[362] In this study, quality of life scores and functional status improved significantly, hospitalization rates declined significantly, and no deaths were reported among the 156 patients. In an effort to shed light on the divergent results of published randomized clinical trials, observational data on incident U.S. patients with Medicare insurance between 1996 and 1998 have been examined.[363] The all-cause relative risk of death was higher in patients with hematocrits less than 33 but was similar in the 33-to-36, 36-to-39, and greater than 39 hematocrit groups. The relative risks for hospitalization were lower in the 36-to-39 group and greater than 39 hematocrit group compared with the reference 33-to-36 hematocrit group.

In evaluating the differing results of observational studies and randomized clinical trials, it is important to take into account the relative strengths and weaknesses of each individual study, as well as the type of study. All of the randomized clinical trials of hematocrit normalization have studied prevalent hemodialysis patients, for whom the length of time on dialysis (vintage) may ameliorate the cardiovascular benefits that could accrue from hemoglobin normalization. However, available observational studies are subject to selection bias and may not sufficiently account for confounding variables that could contribute to erythropoietin resistance. The current clinical practice guidelines seem prudent, especially for U.S. hemodialysis patients, who have a high prevalence of cardiovascular comorbidity. Selected patients with low cardiovascular risks may achieve additional quality of life and hospitalization benefits if hemoglobin levels are normalized.

Independent of administration of exogenous erythropoietin, the initiation of hemodialysis has been demonstrated to partially correct the anemia of chronic renal failure and to improve erythrocyte survival.[364, 365] This effect may be masked if erythropoietin is used in CKD before the initiation of dialysis. Studies have also demonstrated that inadequate dialysis may contribute to erythropoietin resistance. However, several components of the hemodialysis procedure may contribute to higher erythropoietin requirements. Blood loss occurring through the dialyzer or dialyzer lines or as a consequence of repeated phlebotomy can contribute to lower hemoglobin levels.[366] Hemolysis can rarely occur as a complication of the hemodialysis procedure due to kinking of dialysis tubing, other mechanical factors, thermal erythrocyte injury, dialysate contamination, or to changes in osmolarity from technical errors.[367] The two most important factors that may contribute to erythropoietin resistance in the maintenance dialysis population are chronic inflammation and iron deficiency (discussed later).

Other conditions can exacerbate the anemia of chronic renal disease and lead to erythropoietin resistance. Aluminum intoxication, now relatively rare in the maintenance dialysis population, can lead to microcytic hypochromic anemia in addition to inducing osteomalacia and dementia. Although unusual, deficiencies of folic acid or vitamin B_{12} can cause macrocytic anemia in the dialysis population.[368] Macrocytosis is often observed in patients who are responding vigorously to erythropoietin because reticulocytes have a larger mean corpuscular volume than mature erythrocytes.

Endogenous erythropoietin is a heavily glycosylated protein, and the glycosylation is essential for its biologic activity. Commercially available recombinant erythropoietin (Epoetin) is produced by recombinant methods in Chinese hamster ovary cells. There are differences in the glycosylation of recombinant Epoetin compared with native erythropoietin, primarily involving the sialic acid composition of the oligosaccharide groups. Until 2002, there were only three cases in which anti-erythropoietin antibodies were reported to have developed after the administration of Epoetin. In 2002, 13 cases in which patients with chronic renal failure developed severe transfusion-dependent anemia after an initial hematologic response to Epoetin were reported.[196] In all cases, this was due to the development of pure red cell aplasia in association with neutralizing anti-erythropoietin antibodies. Since this publication, numerous other cases, predominantly from Europe, of pure red cell aplasia developing after Epoetin therapy have been reported. The etiologic factors contributing to increased recognition of this clinical problem are under intense investigative scrutiny.

Darbepoetin alfa, a novel erythrocyte-stimulating protein, has also been developed for the treatment of anemia associated with chronic renal failure and has received FDA approval. Darbepoetin alfa is a glycoprotein with a three-fold longer terminal half-life than recombinant human erythropoietin in hemodialysis patients, thereby allowing it to be administered less frequently with similar clinical efficacy.[369] In clinical trials, an equivalent number of patients receiving darbepoetin alfa and recombinant human erythropoietin achieved a targeted increase in hemoglobin.[370, 371] A similar frequency of adverse events, withdrawals and deaths have been reported in clinical trials between patients receiving darbepoetin alfa and recombinant human erythropoietin. Darbepoetin alfa is likely to eventually be used in a substantial number of hemodialysis patients because of its longer half-life and less frequent need for administration.

With the introduction of erythropoietin therapy, there was concern that an increased hematocrit would cause a reduction in relative plasma volume, thereby having an adverse effect on solute clearance during hemodialysis. Clinical studies have not validated this concern. The slight decrease in dialyzer clearance associated with increasing the hematocrit has at most a minor effect on dialysis efficiency, which can be overcome by an appropriate change in the dialysis prescription. An additional concern with increasing the hematocrit is that improved platelet function and correction of the bleeding time that occur with correction of anemia would increase the potential for vascular access thrombosis. Several studies have suggested that there may be an increase in the frequency of arteriovenous fistula or graft thrombosis with higher hemoglobin levels.[372] This effect was notably seen in the large U.S. Normalization of Hematocrit Trial.[360] The clinical practice guidelines do not recommend an increased heparin dose or increase surveillance of hemodialysis accesses when patients are treated with erythropoietin.

The routine use of erythropoietic agents has increased the extent to which iron deficiency, rather than iron overload, is the norm for maintenance hemodialysis patients. Iron deficiency is among the most common causes of erythropoietin resistance. Iron deficiency likely develops due to ongoing blood losses and due to an increased rate of erythrocyte turnover in maintenance hemodialysis patients. Although oral iron can be used, generally speaking, oral iron preparations are relatively ineffective and poorly tolerated in the hemodialysis population.[373] Gastrointestinal distress and impaired iron absorption can adversely affect oral intake and also potentially increase the propensity to malnutrition. As a consequence, the provision of intravenous iron has become a common practice in the maintenance hemodialysis population.[374-376] However, concern has been raised that administration of large doses of parenteral iron may contribute to morbidity and mortality in hemodialysis patients due to infectious or cardiovascular causes. Concern has arisen because of observational data suggesting that the administration of higher doses of iron is associated with high rates of hospitalization and from post hoc analysis of the U.S. Normalization of Hematocrit results.[360, 377]

Iron is a growth factor for bacteria, and staphylococci express a cell wall transferrin binding protein that can function as a transferrin receptor, thereby facilitating bacterial iron uptake. Iron administration can inhibit in vitro phagocytic cell function. However, in evaluating the potential infectious risks of iron therapy, the largest prospective multicenter study evaluating risk factors for bacteremia in hemodialysis patients did not find that the serum ferritin level or the extent to iron administration were significant risk factors for bacteremia. There are no prospective clinical data to support theoretical concerns that intravenous iron administration may contribute to infection.

In the U.S. Normalization of Hematocrit Trial, patients randomized in the normal hematocrit group received a higher amount of intravenous iron than the lower hematocrit group, which led to the post hoc hypothesis that iron administration could have been responsible for excess cardiovascular mortality. Four hundred and sixty-four of 615 patients in the low hematocrit group received intravenous iron compared with 526 of 618 patients in the normal hematocrit group. Free iron in the plasma has the potential to increase oxidative stress and thereby contribute to cardiovascular mortality. However, serum transferrin and ferritin are potent binders of free iron, such that it rarely appears in the plasma except when excessive doses of iron are given over rapid time intervals. Lipid peroxidation in response to intravenous iron has been demonstrated with measurement of plasma esterified F_2-isoprostane levels, which are a sensitive measure of lipid peroxidation.[378] Investigators have also demonstrated that administration of high dose α-tocopherol before hemodialysis can attenuate increases in lipid peroxidation induced by the administration of intravenous iron.[379] Although there is speculation that iron administration may be cardiotoxic, perhaps through increased oxidative stress, there are no prospective clinical trials that have compared differences in intravenous iron administration strategies that have shown any difference in cardiovascular or other clinical outcomes.[380]

Until recently, the only FDA-approved source of parenteral iron in the United States was iron dextran. Dextran binds relatively tightly to iron, which allows slower dissociation and less potential for free iron toxicity. However, iron dextran administration is associated with anaphylactoid reactions in some patients due to the development of anti-dextran antibodies. Life-threatening anaphylactoid reactions have been reported to occur in up to 0.7% of iron dextran-treated hemodialysis patients and at least 30 deaths have been attributed to iron dextran reactions. In the United States, two forms of parenteral iron, iron sucrose and iron gluconate complex, have received FDA approval. The use of iron sucrose and iron gluconate complex is associated with substantially lower rates of adverse drug events than iron dextran.[381, 382] Iron sucrose and iron gluconate have been safely administered to patients who have had adverse drug events when receiving iron dextran.[383, 384] The newer iron preparations are coming into widespread clinical use in the U.S. hemodialysis patient population.

Cardiovascular Disease

Morbidity and mortality from cardiovascular disease are greatly increased in patients on maintenance hemodialysis therapy. Recognition that cardiovascular mortality is greater than 100-fold higher in hemodialysis patients under 45 years of age compared with the general population, and at least 5-fold higher at every age group has led to a resurgence of interest in this seemingly intractable problem.[385] Cardiovascular mortality continues to account for more than 50% of deaths in hemodialysis patients. Cardiac mortality can arise from arrhythmia, cardiomyopathy, and ischemic heart disease. In dealing with the high prevalence of cardiovascular disease in the maintenance hemodialysis population, nephrologists must rely heavily on the involvement of cardiologists. However, there are also important differences in pathophysiology, pharmacology, and prognosis between hemodialysis patients and patients in the general population with cardiovascular disease. It is important for nephrologists to remain aware of disease-specific factors that influence the care of cardiac problems in the hemodialysis patient population.

The first reports of accelerated atherosclerosis in dialysis patients originated in the 1970s from Scribner and colleagues based on their Seattle experience.[386, 387] The presence of angiographically confirmed atherosclerotic coronary arterial disease in the hemodialysis population varies with the study population reported. Overall, reports vary from 24% prevalence in young nondiabetic patients on hemodialysis undergoing evaluation for renal transplantation, to as high as 85% in diabetic hemodialysis patients older than 45 years of age.[388] Although the nature and distribution of coronary atherosclerotic lesions in the dialysis population have not been intensely studied, there is a much greater frequency of complex calcified atheroma, similar to the disease process seen in diabetic patients with coronary disease.[389] Postmortem examination of coronary atherosclerotic disease in dialysis and control patients confirms more calcified plaques in patients with ESRD. Coronary plaques in dialysis patients are also characterized by increased medial thickness.[390]

Traditional atherogenic factors that are highly prevalent in the hemodialysis population include dyslipidemia and hypertension.[391] Lp(a), an atherogenic lipoprotein, consists of a low-density-lipoprotein (LDL) cholesterol particle that is covalently bonded to apolipoprotein (a), a glycoprotein with genetic size polymorphism. Lp(a) level is negatively associated with APO(a) isoform size and is elevated in dialysis patients. Prospective studies of Lp(a) in atherosclerotic coronary vascular disease have yielded conflicting results.[392-394] However, an inception cohort study of incident dialysis patients followed prospectively demonstrated that small apolipoprotein (a) size predicts mortality, even with multiple adjustments for demographics, comorbidity, cause of renal failure, and congestive heart failure.[395] The association of APO(a) size with cardiovascular outcomes was greater for black than white patients.

An area of considerable controversy in evaluating atherosclerotic risk in hemodialysis patients concerns homocysteine metabolism. Hyperhomocystinemia is highly prevalent in hemodialysis patients, and serum homocysteine concentrations have been correlated with cardiovascular risk in the general population.[396] Hyperhomocystinemia may contribute to a prothrombotic state by reducing endothelial dysfunction. Early studies in the hemodialysis population also suggested that plasma homocysteine concentration is associated with cardiovascular risk. However, increased plasma homocysteine concentration was actually associated with a reduced overall mortality in hemodialysis patients in two prospectively published cohort studies.[397] Because plasma homocysteine levels in renal failure may be affected by dietary protein intake, it has been suggested that higher plasma homocysteine levels may be a surrogate for enhanced nutrition in hemodialysis patients. In recent trials, neither the use of folic acid nor folinic acid has been successful in decreasing plasma homocysteine levels to normal levels. The contribution of hyperhomocystinemia to cardiovascular risk in hemodialysis patients is speculative, and in the absence of

B vitamin deficiency, no effective therapy exists to significantly lower plasma levels. It is also possible that the simultaneous elevation of plasma fibrinogen, lipoprotein(a), and homocysteine levels synergistically contribute to a prothrombotic state in hemodialysis patients.

There has been a surge of interest in how the development of a persistent microinflammatory state, which is a frequent accompaniment to renal failure, can contribute to atherosclerotic complications.[398] Plasma levels of C-reactive protein (CRP) as a marker of acute phase inflammatory reactions have been demonstrated in prospective cross-sectional studies and in cohort studies to be powerful predictors of cardiovascular and all-cause mortality in hemodialysis patients.[399-401] Hypoalbuminemia is also associated with elevated CRP levels, likely as a negative acute phase reactant. The strong association between atherosclerosis, elevated CRP levels, and hypoalbuminemia has led to the term malnutrition, inflammation, and atherosclerosis (MIA) syndrome to describe this microinflammatory process.[402] The inverse relationship between serum albumin and prealbumin with CRP levels also applies to other acute phase proteins, including serum amyloid(a), fibrinogen, and proinflammatory cytokines.[398] Plasma levels of the proinflammatory cytokine interleukin-6 (IL-6) have similarly been associated with the presence and subsequent rapid progression of underlying atherosclerosis in hemodialysis patients.[403] High plasma IL-6 levels also predict subsequent cardiovascular and all-cause mortality.[404] This has led to the suggestion that atherosclerosis in the hemodialysis population may be driven by phagocytic cell activation with increased production of proinflammatory cytokines.

The cause of increased microinflammation in hemodialysis patients is still incompletely defined and likely multifactorial. Data make it clear that loss of kidney function predisposes patients to inflammation, because patients with moderate-to-severe CKD have elevated plasma levels of CRP and IL-6.[405] Dialysis-specific factors may also predispose to acute phase inflammation. Subclinical and overt infection occur commonly among hemodialysis patients and may contribute to a proinflammatory state. Vascular access infections, particularly when catheters are used as the source of vascular access, are common (see "Vascular Access"). Even old, clotted prosthetic grafts that do not exhibit signs of active inflammation may be an important source of occult infection and inflammation in individual cases.[406] Bioincompatibility due to blood-membrane interactions during the hemodialysis procedure may also contribute to persistence of the microinflammatory state.[407]

Oxidative stress is also highly prevalent in hemodialysis patients and may contribute to an acceleration of atherogenesis.[408] Oxidation of LDL, particularly in the subendothelial space, leads to uptake of oxidized LDL by monocytes-macrophages, and conversion into foam cells, the earliest stage in the atherosclerotic process. Numerous studies using multiple separate biomarkers of oxidative stress status have identified CKD in ESRD as states of increased oxidative stress. Oxidative stress may occur in hemodialysis patients directly as a result of loss of renal clearance of oxidants, and by increased production through activated phagocytic cells. Myeloperoxidase catalyzed oxidants, including hypochlorous acid, have been postulated to contribute to excess oxidant production in dialysis patients. The potential importance of increased oxidative stress as a contributor to cardiovascular disease is emphasized by the Secondary Prevention with Antioxidants of Cardiovascular Disease in End-Stage Renal Disease (SPACE) study.[409] In this study, administration of the antioxidant α-tocopherol as a secondary prevention agent reduced cardiovascular events in a cohort of hemodialysis patients by approximately 50% compared with placebo, although there was no difference in all-cause mortality. A similar result has been reported with the use of the thiol containing antioxidant *N*-acetylcysteine.[410]

Several additional cardiovascular correlates have been implicated in mortality in hemodialysis patients. The pulse pressure, or the difference between systolic and diastolic blood pressure, appears to have considerably more predictive power than the systolic or diastolic blood pressure alone in hemodialysis patients for adverse events.[411-413] QT dispersion, which is defined as the difference in duration between the shortest and longest QT intervals on an electrocardiogram, is a measure of regional heterogeneity in myocardial repolarization. Corrected QT interval dispersion can predict adverse cardiovascular outcomes in hemodialysis patients.[248, 414] Nocturnal hypoxemia may also be an important predictor of cardiovascular complications in hemodialysis patients.[415] Asymmetrical dimethylarginine, an endogenous nitric oxide inhibitor that accumulates in uremia, correlates with carotid atherosclerosis and has been associated with subsequent cardiovascular mortality in hemodialysis patients.[416]

There are myriad traditional and nontraditional risk factors that appear to have an importance in predicting cardiovascular events in the hemodialysis population, and the enormous atherosclerotic cardiovascular disease burden. It is surprising that there has been a paucity of secondary cardiovascular prevention trials in hemodialysis patients. A study was initiated to examine the effects of Cerivastatin, an HMG-CoA reductase inhibitor, on cardiovascular events and mortality in hemodialysis patients, but was discontinued due to safety considerations with this medication. Two randomized clinical trials examining the effect of other statins in hemodialysis patients are reportedly under way in Europe at this time. There have been no prospective, randomized, controlled trials examining the efficacy of antiplatelet agents reported in the hemodialysis population. Similarly, prospective, randomized studies using ACE inhibitors or angiotensin receptor blockers have not been reported. Adequately powered randomized clinical trials for secondary prevention of cardiovascular disease in hemodialysis patients remains a high priority for improving the outcomes of these patients.

Treatment of underlying atherosclerotic coronary artery disease in the hemodialysis population is complicated by the occasional discordance between symptoms of angina pectoris and active coronary artery disease. Several studies suggest that the prevalence of angina significantly exceeds the prevalence of large-vessel coronary artery disease. Angina in the absence of large-vessel coronary artery disease may occur due to left ventricular hypertrophy, intracardiac fibrosis, intramyocardial coronary artery disease, abnormal endothelial vasomotor function and cardiac autonomic neuropathy.[417-421] Subendocardial myocardial perfusion in diastole may also be adversely affected by decreased aortic compliance in hemodialysis patients. Conversely, the presence of severe coronary artery disease without symptomatology is also common in hemodialysis patients. In one

report, 75% of diabetic patients with angiographically significant coronary disease had no symptoms.[422] Similar findings have also been identified in nondiabetic hemodialysis patients.[423, 424] The lack of anginal symptoms in nondiabetic patients may be explained by uremic autonomic neuropathy or by a low level of physical activity in many hemodialysis patients.[425]

There are conflicting reports about which screening tests have the best sensitivity and specificity in hemodialysis patients.[388, 426] Ambulatory electrocardiographic recordings have not been well studied in hemodialysis patients. Exercise electrocardiography is often limited by abnormal resting electrocardiograms and by markedly reduced exercise tolerance. There are conflicting reports on the usefulness of nuclear medicine studies in comparison with stress echocardiography. Relatively high sensitivity and specificity have been reported for dipyridamole-exercise thallium imaging. Similar positive and negative predictive values have been reported in several studies using dobutamine stress echocardiography.[427]

Determining optimal therapeutic options, including revascularization strategies, for hemodialysis patients must be based on observational data because controlled long-term studies have not been performed. However, data from U.S. hemodialysis patients strongly suggest that patients do not receive therapies that are routine in the management of acute coronary syndromes in patients without renal disease. Fewer hemodialysis patients with acute myocardial infarction in the United States receive thrombolytic therapy.[428, 429] This practice exists despite the overall 1-year mortality rate being extraordinarily high after acute myocardial infarction in dialysis patients.[430, 431] A number of studies have suggested that coronary artery bypass graft (CABG) surgery may be associated with improved survival compared with percutaneous transluminal coronary angioplasty (PTCA) in dialysis patients.[432] Unfavorable outcomes in hemodialysis patients after PTCA compared with CABG surgery include increased coronary restenosis and an increase in cardiovascular events.[433] Using USRDS data, it has been projected that long-term survival of dialysis patients is more favorable after CABG than after PTCA, a result that has been independently confirmed. In a comparison of PTCA, coronary artery stenting, and CABG, the 2-year, all-cause survival rate was 56% for CABG patients, 48% for PTCA, and 48% for stent patients. In particular, diabetic patients receiving a CABG had a better outcome than those receiving stents or PTCA.[432] In nondiabetic ESRD patients, there was an advantage for stents compared with PTCA. Whether drug-eluting stents, brachytherapy, or newer revascularization approaches can increase clinical utility in hemodialysis patients has yet to be determined.

In addition to atherosclerosis, alterations in left ventricular geometry are common in hemodialysis patients. Left ventricular hypertrophy and left ventricular dilatation are found in 75% of patients at the start of dialysis and have been found to be independent risk factors for mortality.[434, 435] Alterations in left ventricular geometry result from chronic volume and pressure overload, often in association with metabolic and neurohumoral abnormalities. Anemia, hypoalbuminemia, and an increase in systolic blood pressure have all been found to contribute to the development of left ventricular hypertrophy.[436] Increased cardiac output and decreased peripheral vascular resistance associated with arteriovenous fistulas may also contribute to the development of cardiomyopathy.[410] Of importance in hemodialysis patients, left ventricular alterations tend to progress over time in most patients. In some studies, left ventricular hypertrophy can undergo regression with vigorous treatment of hypertension using ACE inhibitors or by means of treatment of anemia with erythropoietin. However, the finding that correction of anemia can induce partial regression of left ventricular hypertrophy was challenged in a prospective, randomized trial involving normalization of hemoglobin in patients with asymptomatic cardiomyopathy.[361] Hemodialysis patients who respond to aggressive treatment of hypertension and anemia with a regression of left ventricular hypertrophy have been shown to have better long-term survival than nonresponders. Nonresponders to medical management tend to have increased aortic stiffness and may also have a higher degree of microinflammation as evidenced by elevated CRP levels.[434, 437]

Vascular Calcification

In addition to a high prevalence of atherosclerosis, hemodialysis patients are also subject to excess vascular calcification and cardiac valvular calcification. In the general population, coronary artery calcification correlates with and predicts cardiovascular mortality. In hemodialysis patients, histologic and radiographic evidence of vascular calcification is more striking than in the general population and is even observed in young patients.[438, 439] However, whether the findings of excessive arterial calcification using imaging techniques such as electron beam computed tomography in dialysis patients represents evidence of atherosclerosis or a different process involving medial calcification is not yet entirely clear. Examination of the epigastric arteries of dialysis patients undergoing renal transplantation demonstrates excessive medial artery calcification that is associated with bone matrix protein deposition and disorganization of vascular smooth muscle cells.[440] Elevated serum phosphorus and the calcium $\times$ phosphorous product are risk factors for excessive vascular calcification in addition to increased mortality in hemodialysis patients.[441-443] Cardiac valvular calcification is also associated with a high calcium $\times$ phosphorous product, but it is additionally associated with biomarkers of inflammation, including CRP, low serum albumin levels, and high fibrinogen levels.[444]

The association of a high calcium $\times$ phosphorous product with progressive vascular calcification suggests that the use of non–calcium-containing phosphorous binders may reduce propensity for aortic and other vascular calcification.[445] In a randomized, placebo-controlled study, the use of sevelamer, a non–calcium-containing phosphorous binder, was found to be less likely to cause progressive coronary and aortic calcification than calcium-containing phosphorous binders.[446]

Calciphylaxis

The pathogenesis and treatment of uremic metabolic bone disease are discussed in detail in Chapter 52 and therefore are not discussed further in this chapter. Calciphylaxis, a small-vessel vasculopathy with some clinical and histopathologic features suggestive of hyperparathyroidism and vascular calcification, is discussed briefly. Calciphylaxis is a vasculopathy

largely confined to patients with renal insufficiency. Ischemia of the skin and subcutaneous tissues is the most common clinical presentation, leading to necrotizing skin ulcers that heal poorly, subcutaneous nodules of infarction, and areas of poor wound healing. The most common sites of involvement are subcutaneous tissue with increased adipose content, including the breast, abdominal wall, and thighs.[447-451] The overall prognosis for calciphylaxis is poor, and death from sepsis is extremely common.[452]

Risk factors for the development of calciphylaxis appear to include obesity, type 2 diabetes mellitus, and white race.[453] Much attention has also focused on the purported role of elevated serum calcium, serum phosphorus, and PTH level in patients who develop calciphylaxis.[440] In particular, sustained hyperphosphatemia may be a risk factor for calciphylaxis. However, phosphorus and calcium $\times$ phosphorous products in patients who develop calciphylaxis often overlap those of patients without calciphylaxis. Controversy exists about whether hypercalcemia alone can contribute to the development of calciphylaxis. A case report identifies a patient with hypercalcemia due to primary hyperparathyroidism who rapidly developed calciphylaxis skin lesions.[454] However, in two case series, the time-averaged serum calcium concentrations in hemodialysis patients who developed calciphylaxis were no different from those of patients who did not develop calciphylaxis.[452, 455]

Confusion exists in distinguishing vascular calcification associated with a high calcium $\times$ phosphorous product from calciphylaxis. At the risk of overgeneralizing, the relatively common vascular calcification associated with an elevated calcium $\times$ phosphorous product in hemodialysis patients largely involves medial calcification, whereas calciphylaxis appears to be an endovascular calcification involving the intima. The role of PTH hormone in the pathogenesis of calciphylaxis also remains controversial. In early animal experiments, Selye suggested that PTH might be a sensitizing agent for the development of calciphylaxis. In most but not all reported cases of calciphylaxis, serum PTH levels are elevated.[456, 457] Vitamin D analogs were similarly used as sensitizers in Selye's model of calciphylaxis, and some evidence suggests that high levels of $1\text{-}25\text{-}0(OH)_2$-vitamin D_3 can cause media wall calcification.

Several other risk factors for the development of calciphylaxis have been hypothesized. Protein calorie malnutrition, use of warfarin, vitamin K deficiency, and protein C or protein S deficiency have been postulated as potentially having an etiologic role in the development of calciphylaxis. Calciphylaxis is generally diagnosed clinically by the presence of subcutaneous and cutaneous nodules, necrotic lesions, and eschar with hyperesthesia of the skin. Tissue biopsy can confirm the diagnosis of calciphylaxis by demonstrating calcification of small arterioles or venules. However, skin biopsies in calciphylaxis are not always recommended because of a high likelihood of poor healing at the biopsy site. Low transcutaneous oxygen can be helpful in identifying calciphylaxis skin lesions.[455]

Unfortunately, treatment outcomes for patients with calciphylaxis are poor. Because of the sporadic nature of the disease, there are only anecdotal case reports of successful treatment modalities. Strategies that have been suggested include the discontinuation of calcium-containing phosphorous binders, subtotal parathyroidectomy, and hyperbaric oxygen therapy. For patients on warfarin, it may be appropriate to attempt to use a different type of anticoagulant, and a search for hypercoagulable states that may mimic calciphylaxis should be undertaken in appropriate cases. Careful attention to analgesia, avoidance of trauma, and wound care are essential to promote survival in patients with calciphylaxis.

Nutrition

Protein calorie malnutrition has been shown to be highly prevalent and associated with increased morbidity and mortality in maintenance hemodialysis patients.[43, 458] Alterations in nutritional status due to uremia per se as well as from the hemodialysis procedure may predispose the ESRD patient to multiple nutritional complications (Table 59-15). A comprehensive review of nutritional therapy in renal disease is provided in Chapter 57. This section focuses specifically on nutritional evaluation and therapy in the hemodialysis unit.

Optimal monitoring of protein-energy nutritional status for maintenance hemodialysis patients requires that several different parameters be measured for the assessment of different aspects of nutritional status. There is no single biochemical marker or clinical measure that can provide a complete overview of protein energy nutritional status. A combination of measures of protein and energy intake, biochemical measures of visceral protein pools, and anthropometric measures of body compositions are complementary in the assessment of nutritional status.

In hemodialysis patients, relatively simple biochemical measures reflecting the visceral protein stores, such as serum albumin, creatinine, and BUN, as well as more complex, less readily available measures such as transferrin, prealbumin, and insulin-like growth factor-1 (IGF-1) have been proposed as nutritional indices. The serum albumin is the most extensively examined nutritional index in virtually all patient populations due to ready availability of its measurement and association with clinical outcomes. Serum albumin levels are closely affected by the level of dietary protein intake, but it must be recognized that, in hemodialysis patients, inflammation and dietary protein intake exert competing effects on serum albumin concentration.[401] The serum albumin is also a negative acute phase reactant and its serum concentration decreases abruptly and sharply in response to stress and inflammation.[398, 459] Taken in isolation, the serum albumin may not necessarily reflect visceral nutritional status in acutely ill patients.

In addition to the serum albumin, the BUN and serum creatinine concentrations are also considered simple markers of nutritional status. Urea is the metabolic end product of

dietary protein intake, and the BUN is a composite measure of protein intake, volume of distribution of urea, as well as renal and dialyzer urea clearance. The serum creatinine level is a reflection of the total body muscle mass and reflects dietary intake and clearance. The creatinine index or creatinine synthetic rate can be estimated if dialysate and urinary creatinine losses are known by using the body weight and change in the serum creatinine concentration over time. However, some questions remain about the validity of the creatinine index because formulas used for the derivation of the creatinine index rely on constant values derived from individuals without renal disease. The use of BUN and creatinine as nutritional indices in dialysis patients may properly be viewed as a "one-tailed test" in that low values should raise suspicion for malnutrition, whereas high values may be related to good nutrition but may also be related to inadequate dialysis.

Similar to the serum albumin level, the serum prealbumin concentration can be used as a marker of nutritional status. Serum prealbumin has a shorter half-life (1 to 2 days) than serum albumin, and it may be a better marker to determine early response to a nutritional therapeutic intervention. Prealbumin is a serum transport protein that has a smaller body pool than serum albumin, but the major route of excretion of prealbumin is through the kidneys, and serum concentrations of prealbumin may be falsely elevated in patients on hemodialysis. Serum prealbumin can also function as a negative acute phase reactant. Some data suggest that the prealbumin level may be an even better prognostic indicator than albumin levels in hemodialysis patients.[460]

IGF-1 can also be a nutritional index in hemodialysis patients.[461] IGF-1 is a growth factor that is structurally related to insulin and is produced primarily within the liver. Ninety-five percent of plasma IGF-1 is protein bound, and there are limited daily fluctuations in serum concentrations. Several studies suggest that serum IGF-1 concentrations may have a better correlation with body composition than serum albumin and transferrin.[462] However, the level of IGF-1 at which malnutrition is significant has not been established in hemodialysis patients.

Analysis of body composition also provides important nutritional assessment information for hemodialysis patients. Anthropometric studies are easy to perform but unfortunately unreliable in the hemodialysis setting. More sophisticated body composition tools such as prompt neutron activation analysis or dual energy x-ray absorptiometry (DEXA) have reported utility as nutritional measures in hemodialysis patients but require expensive equipment and are available only in specialized centers.[463, 464] Bioelectrical impedance analysis (BIA) has also been proposed as useful for body composition analysis in hemodialysis patients.[465] Although there was a good correlation of total body water and lean body mass between BIA and DEXA in healthy subjects, the variation in hemodialysis patients may be large. The true utility of BIA as a measure of body composition in hemodialysis patients remains to be established.

Subjective global assessment is a proposed methodology for evaluating nutritional status of hemodialysis patients. Subjective global assessment is a simple technique based on objective and subjective aspects of physical examination and the medical history. Subjective global assessment was initially developed for evaluation of nutritional status in patients

TABLE 59-15

Factors Causing Malnutrition

Inadequate protein or calorie intake
Increased energy expenditure
Metabolic acidosis
Hormonal alterations
Comorbidities or hospitalizations
Dialytic nutrient losses
Dialysis-induced catabolism
Infection

undergoing elective surgery but has subsequently been applied to other patient populations. The use of subjective global assessment has been well studied in peritoneal dialysis patients, with fewer data available for hemodialysis patients.

Dietary protein intake assessment through dietary interviews and diaries can provide important information concerning protein energy and other nutrient intake. Three-day dietary record reviews and dietary interviews by qualified staff are recommended for accurate information. The protein equivalent of total nitrogen appearance (PNA), or protein catabolic rate, can also be used to assess dietary protein intake.[466] The total nitrogen appearance rate is the sum of nitrogen losses in dialysate, urine, and feces in addition to a measure of the interdialytic increment in total body urea nitrogen content. Because the nitrogen content of protein is relatively constant at 16%, the protein equivalent of total nitrogen appearance can be estimated by multiplying the nitrogen appearance rate by 6.25. The PNA is generally normalized to body weight, and is highly correlated with the urea nitrogen appearance rate.[467] However, it must be recognized that the PNA approximates protein intake only when patients are in neutral nitrogen balance. When dietary protein intake is high, the PNA may underestimate protein intake due to increased unmeasured nitrogen losses.

There are a number of potential causes for malnutrition in hemodialysis patients (see Table 59-15). These factors are discussed in more detail in Chapter 59. Because of the propensity for protein calorie malnutrition in maintenance hemodialysis patients, the recommended dietary protein for stable patients is 1.2 g/kg of body weight per day. At least 50% of dietary protein should be of high biologic value. The recommended daily energy intake is 35 kcal/kg of body weight per day for patients who are younger than 60 years of age and 30 to 35 kcal/kg of body weight per day for individuals 60 years of age or older, according to the clinical practice guidelines. Given the high prevalence of protein energy malnutrition and the important prognostic consequences of this in hemodialysis patients, it is recommended that all hemodialysis patients have initial intensive nutritional counseling with a development of a plan of care for nutritional management with regular and routine subsequent dietary and nutritional evaluation and follow-up.

Institution of maintenance dialysis may have complex effects on protein and energy balance.[468, 469] Early studies using low-flux dialyzers have documented a loss of 5 to 8 g of free amino acids during each hemodialysis session. With the use of high-flux dialysis membranes, these losses further increase by approximately 30% due to the larger surface area and higher blood flow used.[470] These losses may be increased when a glucose-free dialysate is used due to the stimulation of gluconeogenesis. There may be an increase in amino acid and albumin losses with the reprocessing of high-flux dialyzers by an increase in membrane porosity.[471] Amino acid losses during dialysis also stimulate a catabolic process that increases catabolism for hours after the dialysis procedure has ended.[472-474]

Despite the potential adverse effects of the hemodialysis procedure on nutritional parameters, several studies demonstrate that there are improvements in nutritional parameters after initiation of maintenance hemodialysis for the treatment of uremia. The serum albumin, prealbumin, normalized protein catabolic rate, BIA-derived reactants, and phase angle all improve after the initiation of hemodialysis therapy.[393, 475, 476] Similarly, the serum creatinine level has been demonstrated to rise by 12% in the first year of hemodialysis in the stable patient cohort. Correction of uremic symptomatology and an increase in dietary protein and calorie intake presumably explain the improvement in nutritional status. It has also been shown that the use of erythropoietin with a rise in hemoglobin results in an improvement in appetite along with a greater sense of well-being.[477, 478]

For hemodialysis patients who sustain inadequate nutrient intake for extended periods or develop indices of protein energy malnutrition, nutritional support may be indicated. For patients with an intact functional intestinal tract, the enteral route of nutritional support is favored. Oral nutritional supplementation during hemodialysis can contribute to increases in serum albumin, serum prealbumin, and subjective global assessment scores.[479-482] For patients unable to tolerate enteral feeding or unable to use nutrients provided by the intestinal tract, total parenteral nutrition or intradialytic parenteral nutrition can be considered. There have been few large-scale prospective studies of intradialytic parenteral nutrition for malnourished hemodialysis patients. Some studies have demonstrated efficacy in increasing serum albumin and other markers of nutritional status, but interdialytic parenteral nutrition is expensive and provides insufficient calories and protein to support long-term needs due to the limitations on its administration only during hemodialysis sessions.[430]

It has been proposed that many hemodialysis patients may have L-carnitine deficiency and may benefit from carnitine supplementation.[483] L-Carnitine is a naturally occurring substance that shuttles fatty acids into the mitochondria for β-oxidation. L-Carnitine is critical for energy production in cardiac and skeletal muscle tissue that depends on fatty acid oxidation. Because carnitine is water soluble and readily dialyzed, plasma concentrations of carnitine decline by as much as 75% with hemodialysis. The decrease in plasma carnitine concentration is quickly corrected by transport of carnitine from muscle and other tissues, which may lead to tissue carnitine deficiency. It has been proposed that L-carnitine supplementation would be beneficial in hemodialysis patients to improve a variety of metabolic abnormalities, including hypertriglyceridemia, hypercholesterolemia, anemia, and exercise tolerance.[484] The extent of clinical benefit to be derived from L-carnitine administration to hemodialysis patients is controversial. L-Carnitine administration may have the greatest clinical utility in the treatment of erythropoietin-resistant anemia. L-Carnitine is not recommended for routine use in hemodialysis patients, albeit selected individuals who have not responded adequately to standard therapies may be appropriate candidates for L-carnitine administration.

The concentration in the body of many trace elements depends on the degree of renal failure. The serum concentrations of trace elements, with the exceptions of selenium and zinc, tend to be elevated in hemodialysis patients. It has been proposed that trace element accumulation may contribute to uremic toxicity and that only selenium and zinc should be considered for supplementation in dialysis patients. Selenium deficiency has been associated with cardiovascular disease because selenium functions as a cofactor in antioxidant enzyme function. Studies have documented decreased concentrations of selenium in hemodialysis patients, probably resulting from inadequate dietary intake. However, whether selenium supplementation can lead to clinical benefit in dialysis patients is not well defined. Similarly, low concentrations of zinc have been reported in hemodialysis patients. Zinc deficiency may be associated with anorexia and impotence; however, the potential beneficial effects of supplemental zinc therapy have not been confirmed in hemodialysis patients.[485]

Supplementation of water-soluble vitamins is recommended for hemodialysis patients.[486, 487] B vitamin and folic acid supplementation may be required for optimal metabolism of homocysteine. Because folic acid is abundant in foodstuffs that are frequently restricted in dialysis patients due to the concomitant presence of high potassium, folic acid supplementation is recommended.[488] Several studies have suggested that there may be a role for vitamin C supplementation to prevent oxidative injury and to aid in iron metabolism. With the exception of vitamin D, the lipid-soluble vitamins have not been depleted in hemodialysis patients. Vitamin A or beta carotene supplements should be avoided due to potential toxicity in hemodialysis patients.[489] Vitamin E may have clinical benefit in reducing cardiovascular complications in hemodialysis patients (see "Cardiovascular Disease").[409] The metabolism of vitamin D and its supplementation are discussed in Chapter 52.

Infection and Immunity

Infection is the second leading cause of death in hemodialysis after cardiovascular diseases. The mortality rate due to infection in ESRD patients is approximately 12% to 22%.[490] Septicemia accounts for more than 75% of these infectious deaths. Overall, the annual percentage of mortality attributed to sepsis in dialysis patients is approximately 100- to 300-fold higher than in the general population, a stark portrayal of how serious infectious risks are for these patients.[65]

Older age and the presence of diabetes mellitus are independent risk factors for septicemia in longitudinal and cohort study analyses of incident ESRD patients in the USRDS.[491] For hemodialysis patients, low serum albumin levels, temporary vascular access, and the reprocessing of dialyzers are also associated with increased risk.[492-494] Dialysis patients who develop an episode of septicemia have twice the risk of death from any cause and a fivefold to ninefold increased risk of death from septicemia.

Several clinical and treatment-related characteristics make hemodialysis patients particularly susceptible to septicemia. The repeated disruption of dermal integrity to gain vascular access for hemodialysis increases infection risk. In patients with catheters for vascular access, there was risk of infection within and around the indwelling catheter's lumen. Clinical data confirm that central venous catheters are a major source of bacterial colonization and infection in hemodialysis patients compared with patients using arteriovenous grafts or arteriovenous fistulas.[492] There is increasing recognition that dialysis catheter bacterial colonization leads to bacterial adherence and biofilm formation. Biofilms, which are microbial communities attached to surfaces, develop resistance to phagocytes and to antibiotics. Biofilms eventually become covered with a dense layer of matrix material, rendering resistance to antibiotic penetration.[495]

Most infections in hemodialysis patients are caused by common catalase-producing bacteria such as *Staphylococcus* species, rather than opportunistic infections.[492, 493] The pattern of infectious organisms in hemodialysis patients is similar to that seen in patients with chronic granulomatous disease, in which phagocytic cells lack capability to produce reactive oxygen species. In this context, a number of studies have documented alterations in granulocyte function in patients with uremia on hemodialysis. Although the number and morphology of granulocytes are generally normal, defects in granulocyte chemotaxis, adherence, phagocytic capability, and reactive oxygen species production have all been demonstrated.[496, 497] Nutritional deficiencies and iron exposure may contribute to phagocytic cell dysfunction.[498] The use of bioincompatible hemodialysis membranes leads to recurrent leukocyte and complement activation, with long-term use contributing to phagocytic cell dysfunction. Data from the USRDS suggest that chronic use of unmodified cellulosic membranes is associated with an increase in infectious mortality.[499]

There is increasing concern about the development of antibiotic resistance in hemodialysis patients. The frequent occurrence of methicillin-resistant *S. aureus* infections over time has led to the frequent use of vancomycin to treat suspected and proven septicemia. A CDC survey in 1996 and 1997 demonstrated that approximately 5% of hemodialysis patients are administered vancomycin over the course of a month, and 30% of dialysis facilities reported having patients with known vancomycin-resistant *Enterococcus* (VRE) infections.[500] A valence study at 49 hospitals revealed that receipt of hemodialysis or peritoneal dialysis was an independent risk factor for VRE bacteremia.[501] Strains of *S. aureus* with intermediate sensitivity to vancomycin are being reported.

Viral infections are also common in hemodialysis patients. In the early days of dialysis, multiple blood product transfusions predisposed many patients to hepatitis B infections. The availability and use of erythropoietin has reduced the number of transfusions in dialysis patients. Coupled with the availability of the hepatitis B vaccine, the frequency of hepatitis B has decreased markedly in hemodialysis patients. According to the CDC, during the period from 1976 to 2000, the incidence of hepatitis B infection among hemodialysis patients decreased from 4.4% to 0.05%.[500] During the same period, the prevalence of hepatitis B surface antigen positivity among hemodialysis patients declined from 7.8% to 0.9%. Hemodialysis patients may acquire hepatitis B infection from community sources, from transmission in hemodialysis centers due to inadequate infection control precautions, or from accidental breaks in infection control technique.

The hepatitis C virus (HCV) was cloned in 1989 and identified as the leading cause of parentally transmitted, non-A, non-B hepatitis. HCV infection has become the most important cause of liver disease among hemodialysis patients and is a major concern for hemodialysis staff. The prevalence of anti-HCV antibody positivity in hemodialysis units has varied from 5% to 40%.[502, 503] Data suggest that the incidence of hepatitis C infection in hemodialysis units is declining worldwide, including in the United States, over the past decade. Many patients with anti-HCV antibodies do not exhibit hepatic enzyme abnormalities, and serum ALT levels are elevated in only a minority of hemodialysis patients with anti-HCV antibodies or with detectable HCV RNA.[504]

The clinical course of HCV infection in hemodialysis patients tends to be chronic and indolent with a characteristic fluctuating course and multiple peaks and troughs in ALT levels.[505] Molecular genotyping of HCV by protein catabolic rate and nucleotide sequencing of the viral genome have unequivocally demonstrated nosocomial transmission of HCV within the dialysis unit. Current recommendations are that hemodialysis patients should be considered a high-risk population for HCV infection and should undergo periodic screening. Isolation of HCV carriers within the hemodialysis unit is not recommended beyond standard universal precautions. Although most hemodialysis patients with HCV infection remain asymptomatic over a long period, identified patients should be instructed to avoid additional hepatic toxins, including alcohol consumption and potentially hepatotoxic medications. HCV-positive patients should undergo vaccination against hepatitis A and B. Antiviral therapy with interferon-α is recommended for selected categories of HCV-infected hemodialysis patients.[506]

HIV infection appears to be increasing in hemodialysis patients. During the period of 1985 to 2000, the percentage of centers reporting that dialysis care is being provided for patients with HIV infection has increased from 11% to 37%. Because few dialysis centers routinely test for HIV infection, these figures are likely underestimates of the true rate of HIV infection. According to the CDC, in 2000, 1.5% of hemodialysis patients had HIV infection, and 0.4% had acquired immunodeficiency syndrome.[500] HIV-positive hemodialysis patients are treated with highly active antiretroviral therapy.

Given the increased susceptibility to infections and the high associated mortality in hemodialysis patients, it is notable that many of the types of deaths are caused by infections that are preventable with vaccines. The incidence of pneumonia in dialysis patients has been reported to be as high as 4.9 episodes per 1000 patient-months, and 53% of these are caused by *Streptococcus pneumoniae*. The Advisory Committee on Immunization Practices recommended hepatitis B, pneumococcal, and influenza vaccines for hemodialysis patients.[507]

Patients on hemodialysis should receive 3 doses of recombinant hepatitis B vaccine as early in the course of renal disease as possible. The recommended dosage for adults on hemodialysis is 20 to 40 μg of Recombivax HB or Engerix-B given intramuscularly in the deltoid. Only 50% to 75% of adult patients develop protective antibody levels against hepatitis B surface antigen after 3 doses of vaccine, compared with more than 90% of healthy adults. Revaccination with up to 3 additional doses is recommended for those hemodialysis patients who do not develop protective antibody levels. Anti-HBs testing is recommended 1 to 2 months after vaccination of hemodialysis patients to demonstrate protective antibody levels. Additional postvaccination testing is recommended annually. A booster dose is recommended if the anti-HBs titer falls below 10 mU/mL.

A single dose of the 23-valent pneumococcal polysaccharide vaccine is recommended intramuscularly or subcutaneously for all dialysis patients greater than 2 years of age.[507] More than 75% of dialysis patients have an adequate response to the vaccine, although antibody levels are considerably lower than in the general population. Revaccination is recommended 3 years after the previous dose for children and after at least 5 years in adults. The influenza vaccine is recommended annually for hemodialysis patients because of an increased risk for influenza-related mortality. Household members and health care workers in contact with hemodialysis patients should also be vaccinated annually to decrease influenza transmission rates. The influenza vaccine is also recommended for children on hemodialysis.

Vaccines routinely administered in childhood (i.e., measles, mumps, and rubella vaccines; varicella vaccine; inactivated polio virus vaccine; diphtheria, tetanus, and pertussis vaccine; and *Haemophilus influenzae* type B conjugate vaccine) are generally recommended for children on hemodialysis.[507] Oral polio virus vaccine, which is no longer available in the United States, is not recommended because of a theoretical risk of producing paralytic polio. An *S. aureus* vaccine has been demonstrated to have efficacy in reducing these infections in hemodialysis patients, although it is neither commercially available nor FDA approved.

COMPLICATIONS OF HEMODIALYSIS

Chronic hemodialysis is directly responsible for the maintenance of life for more than 300,000 patients in the United States. Years have been added to the lives of patients who, without this remarkable intervention, would have died of renal failure. Although the benefits of this therapy are unquestioned, many complications have been associated with hemodialysis. Many of the complications are immediate, occurring during or shortly after the dialysis procedure itself, whereas other complications have become apparent only after several years of maintenance hemodialysis. These late complications are responsible for considerable morbidity associated with ESRD and contribute to the 22%/year U.S. mortality rate for patients with renal failure.

Hemodialysis has evolved into a relatively safe procedure, with an estimated 1 death in 75,000 treatments as a result of technical error. However, an extensive list of complications is related to this treatment, some of which are potentially life threatening. The age of the patient; the presence of underlying medical conditions such as diabetes mellitus, coronary artery disease, or congestive heart failure; and the patient's degree of compliance with a complex medical regimen necessary in end-stage disease have a great influence on the frequency and severity of adverse events.

Hypotension

Hypotension is the most common acute complication of hemodialysis.[508] Many dialytic and patient-related factors influence blood pressure during the treatment. The incidence of hypotension in the dialysis population ranges between 15% and 30%. The frequency varies with the age and sex of the patient, with the greatest number of episodes being seen in older patients and in women.

The hemodynamic response to hemodialysis must be reviewed for an understanding of the pathogenesis of hypotension.[509] The dialysis procedure can be considered to be made up of two separable processes: convection and diffusion. Convection refers to the movement of fluid and solute brought about by pressure across the dialysis membrane (i.e., transmembrane pressure). The higher the transmembrane pressure, the greater is the rate of convection.

The process of removing fluid by hydraulic forces is called *ultrafiltration*. During isolated ultrafiltration, a progressive increase in total systemic vascular resistance maintains blood pressure as fluid is removed. When diffusion is added to ultrafiltration (i.e., the usual dialysis treatment, which is a combination of ultrafiltration and diffusion), thermal energy can be transferred from the heated dialysate to the patient, stimulating vasodilatation and increased blood flow to the skin. As a consequence, vasoconstriction is less effective, and maintenance of central blood volume may be impaired during fluid removal. Cardiac output and blood pressure must be maintained by an increase in heart rate and in some instances by an increase in myocardial contractility. However, the large burden of cardiovascular disease in the hemodialysis population often limits the ability of the heart to respond appropriately to the stress of fluid removal. These inherently different responses to ultrafiltration and diffusion greatly influence maintenance of blood pressure during hemodialysis.

In addition to factors related to the method of exchange, dialysis patients often have abnormalities in autonomic function. The afferent arm of the baroreceptor reflex is believed to be blunted in hypotension-prone hemodialysis patients, and such patients do not mount reflex vasoconstriction during hypotensive episodes.[74] Although the efferent arm of this reflex pathway, which involves sympathetic output, is believed to be normal or even overactive in patients with chronic renal failure, this limb of the pathway has also been shown to fail in patients prone to hypotension during hemodialysis.[510]

Ultrafiltration Rate

During ultrafiltration, a protein-free ultrafiltrate of plasma is removed from the intravascular space. The resultant rise in plasma oncotic pressure causes fluid to move from the interstitial and intracellular spaces to replenish plasma volume. Hypotension results when the rate of intravascular volume depletion exceeds the rate of refilling of this space, especially if total peripheral resistance cannot compensate for the loss of intravascular volume. Whereas total peripheral resistance increases during isolated ultrafiltration, this compensatory response is attenuated when diffusion is added to the process. During combined ultrafiltration and diffusion when vasoconstriction is not evident, the ability to remove volume during hemodialysis is primarily dependent on the ability to refill the intravascular space.

Very large interdialytic weight gains cannot easily be removed during a typical treatment (usually lasting between 3.5 and 4 hours), even in the presence of volume overload, because the refilling of intravascular space is time dependent. Frequent hypotension in such individuals is probable with ultrafiltration rates in excess of 1.5 L/hour, and the incidence of hypotension generally is an exponential function of the rate of fluid removal.

Hypotension can occur when the weight of the patient is at or below his or her "estimated dry weight" when volume shifts no longer are able to compensate for intravascular depletion and maintain blood pressure. The estimated dry weight of a patient may be defined as that weight below which the patient develops symptomatic hypotension, *in the absence of edema and excessive interdialytic weight gains*. The assessment of volume status by physical examination can be augmented by measuring inferior vena cava diameter by echocardiography.[511] A narrow or collapsing inferior vena cava suggests volume depletion. A patient experiencing hypotension with these findings can benefit from an increase in dry weight.

Dialysate Composition

The composition of the dialysate can influence blood pressure in several ways. Sodium and calcium concentrations, the nature of the buffer (i.e., bicarbonate or acetate), and the temperature of the dialysis fluid are among the factors that influence the frequency of hypotension during dialysis.

The process of diffusion also leads to a decline in plasma osmolality because of removal of solutes from the patient. The magnitude of the fall in effective plasma osmolality ranges between 10 and 25 mOsm/kg. The fall in plasma osmolality creates an osmotic gradient between the plasma and the interstitial and intracellular spaces. Fluid moves from the plasma into cells and the interstitium, resulting in a reduction in plasma volume. This intravascular volume loss is superimposed on volume removed by ultrafiltration, and its magnitude can be as much as 1 to 1.5 liters during the treatment. This shift is opposed by an increase in oncotic pressure induced by ultrafiltration. Increases in the concentration of sodium, the principal osmotic agent in the dialysate, reduce this osmotic gradient. The frequency of hypotension reported at a dialysate sodium concentration of 140 mEq/L is substantially lower than the frequency at 130 mEq/L. A similar effect can be seen with mannitol administration during hemodialysis. However, chronic mannitol administration can lead to its accumulation in hemodialysis patients and should be avoided.

Dialysate with a sodium concentration of 130 mEq/L has been used in the past, in part because of the fear that dialysate with higher tonicity would stimulate thirst, leading to greater interdialytic weight gains and hypertension. Although weight gains may be somewhat greater with higher sodium concentrations, this additional fluid weight gain can usually be successfully removed. An increase in interdialytic hypertension has not been a major problem at the higher sodium concentration, and the use of dialysate with a sodium concentration of 140 mEq/L is common.

The calcium concentration of the dialysate has also been shown to affect myocardial contractility. Higher calcium concentrations in the dialysate, up to a concentration of 3.5 mEq/L, have been associated with improved contractility, independent of the nature of other factors in the dialysate. However, with the increasing use of calcium salts to prevent hyperphosphatemia, hypercalcemia is seen more often when the calcium concentration of dialysate is this high.

The buffer used to replenish bicarbonate lost during the interdialytic interval has also been clearly implicated in the pathogenesis of hypotension during hemodialysis. Historically, the principal buffer employed had been acetate. The use of acetate as a buffer was to reduce the potential of calcium precipitation (as calcium carbonate) when bicarbonate was used as the buffer. Acetate is a peripheral vasodilator and may also predispose to hypotension by reducing myocardial contractility. Hypoxemia during dialysis is exacerbated by acetate-buffered dialysate (discussed later) and contributes to hypotension.

Acetate is metabolized by skeletal muscle into bicarbonate. As much as 300 mmol/hour of acetate can be transferred from the dialysate to the patient. This rate is near the maximum capacity for conversion to bicarbonate. It is not surprising that the greatest number of adverse effects of acetate occur in individuals with reduced muscle mass, such as the elderly and women. As the technology for delivery of bicarbonate dialysate has improved, the use of acetate-based dialysate has dramatically declined in recent years, and this has resulted in a significant improvement in the rates of hypotension during dialysis.

Dialysate temperature has been shown to affect blood pressure during hemodialysis. Dialysate cooled to 35°C reduces the frequency of hypotensive episodes because vasoconstriction is potentiated at this temperature. Cooling of the dialysate to 35°C has been reported to be tolerated by the patient and often results in a more stable treatment.

Theoretically, vasoactive substances may be removed during the treatment. However, during hemodialysis, the changes in plasma norepinephrine levels or potassium concentration, for instance, have not been shown to play an important role in dialysis-induced hypotension.

Extracorporeal Volume

In the past, the volume of blood required to prime the extracorporeal circuit as well as the compliance of the dialyzer were two other potential causes of hypotension. The blood volume of coil dialyzers, rarely in use anymore, and, to a lesser extent, of parallel-plate dialyzers increases as transmembrane pressure increases. Hollow-fiber dialyzers are much less compliant, and their widespread use has reduced the potential for hypotension from this cause. Nevertheless, the blood volume needed to establish the extracorporeal circuit (including the dialyzer and blood lines) may still be as high as 200 mL.

Bioincompatibility of Membranes

During contact between blood and the dialysis membrane, various vasoactive substances are generated. Some of these have the potential to produce pulmonary hypertension and systemic hypotension. A particular clustering of events, including hypotension, which occur very early (within one-half hour) after the initiation of hemodialysis are discussed under the subject of first-use syndrome.

Medication

Patients undergoing hemodialysis are often receiving antihypertensive agents or other medications that can interfere with the normal hemodynamic response to ultrafiltration. β-Adrenergic receptor blockers reduce myocardial contractility and also exert a negative chronotropic effect. Such agents, by preventing a compensatory increase in the heart rate, interfere with a major defense supporting blood pressure during dialysis. Verapamil can be expected to exert a similar effect. Vasodilators can prevent vasoconstriction in response to ultrafiltration.

The development of several antihypertensive agents formulated to be administered orally as a single daily dose or by a transdermal delivery system (nifedipine and clonidine,

respectively) has reduced the incidence of drug-induced hypotension. These agents are generally well tolerated and may often be used on dialysis days because high peak levels are avoided. Nitroglycerin ointment can often aggravate the propensity for hypotension by inducing peripheral vasodilatation.

Other Factors Producing Hypotension

The foregoing discussion addressed factors inherent in the treatment that can produce hypotension. The health of the patient is another important variable that directly influences the frequency of hypotension. Patients at increased risk for hypotension are those who have arrhythmias, which can often be exacerbated by hemodialysis; those with poor cardiac function or pericarditis; or those with autonomic dysfunction, such as diabetic patients. The last two problems may prevent adequate changes in cardiac output or peripheral resistance to compensate for fluid removed during hemodialysis.

Management

The first step in the approach to hypotension is to determine whether hypotension occurs early or late in the treatment period. In a previously stable patient who is free of edema and signs of congestive heart failure, in whom hypotension occurs late in the treatment, the most common cause is that the patient's dry weight has been underestimated. Reducing the amount of ultrafiltration during hemodialysis, effectively raising the postdialysis dry weight, corrects the hypotension. In contrast, the patient with excessive intradialytic weight gains may become hypotensive before the dry weight is achieved because the rate at which fluid can be mobilized to refill the intravascular space is limited. In this instance, dialysis time or frequency may need to be increased for removal of all necessary fluid at a tolerable rate.

Whenever possible, doses of short-acting antihypertensive medication should not be administered at least 4 hours before the hemodialysis treatment. Many of the long-acting blood pressure medications can be taken at bedtime to avoid peak concentrations during dialysis. In patients with frequent hypotension early into the treatment, pericarditis with tamponade must be suspected.

A multifaceted approach often can prevent hypotension. The use of bicarbonate dialysate with a sodium concentration of 140 mEq/L is helpful. Sodium modeling and ultrafiltration modeling can be applied to the treatment.[79] The newer dialysis machines have programs that permit the dialysate sodium or the ultrafiltration rate, or both, to be automatically changed during the treatment. The dialysate sodium level can be gradually altered during the treatment from an initial concentration of 150 mEq/L to 140 mEq/L. Fluid is more easily mobilized from the intracellular space with sodium modeling. Most dialysis machines allow dialysate temperature to be easily lowered to 35°C. At this dialysate temperature, thermal energy is transferred from the patient to the dialysate, and the resultant vasoconstriction raises blood pressure.[512] Many membranes can produce less reaction during contact with the blood. Reuse of cuprophane membranes (with formaldehyde, but not bleach) also increases the biocompatibility of the membrane. For patients with persistent hypotension or autonomic insufficiency, the oral α_1-adrenergic agonist midodrine can be prescribed. A dose of 5 to 10 mg given 30 to 60 minutes before hemodialysis is effective in reducing the incidence of hypotension.[512]

Hypotension is treated by placing the patient in the Trendelenburg position, administering a 100 to 200 mL normal saline bolus, and reducing the ultrafiltration rate, at least temporarily. Alternatives to saline are occasional mannitol and albumin administration. Supplemental oxygen also may be useful to improve hypoxemia and cardiac contractility in some patients.

Cramps

Muscle cramps occur in as many as 20% of dialysis treatments. Although their pathogenesis is uncertain, cramps are known to be more frequent when ultrafiltration rates are high and when dialysate with low sodium concentration is employed, an indication that cramps are caused by acute extracellular volume contraction.

Reducing ultrafiltration rates can improve cramps. Bolus administration of normal saline (200 mL), small volumes (5 mL) of 23% hypertonic saline, or 50% dextrose in water ($D_{50}W$) is effective in treating cramps. In nondiabetic patients $D_{50}W$ is especially useful, particularly near the conclusion of the dialysis treatment, because as glucose is metabolized, hyperosmolality and intravascular volume expansion in the postdialysis period are avoided. The pain resulting from very severe cramps may be alleviated by administration of agents such as diazepam but at the risk of increased hypotension.

Quinine sulfate, an agent that increases the refractory period and excitability of skeletal muscle, is effective in preventing cramping if administered 1 to 2 hours before dialysis commences. Patients using quinine must be observed for the development of thrombocytopenia. This agent was temporarily banned by the FDA in 1994 because of this complication. Alternatives to quinine in preventing cramps include vitamin E and carnitine.[513-515] In patients with excessive weight gains, dialysis time must be increased to prevent cramps during attempts to achieve the patient's dry weight.

Dialysis Disequilibrium Syndrome

Dialysis disequilibrium refers to a constellation of symptoms, many of which are nonspecific, including nausea and vomiting, restlessness, headaches, and fatigue during hemodialysis or in the immediate postdialysis period. Severe disequilibrium may result in life-threatening emergencies, including seizures, coma, and arrhythmias. These symptoms are believed to arise from rapid rates of change in solute concentration and pH during hemodialysis in the central nervous system. A transient gradient may be created between plasma and cerebrospinal fluid (CSF) urea concentration, leading to increased concentration of water in the brain. A fall in CSF pH also may contribute to cerebral edema. During dialysis, there is a rapid correction of arterial pH, an increase in plasma bicarbonate, and therefore a rise in arterial Pco_2. The rise in plasma Pco_2 is accompanied by an increase in CSF Pco_2 because carbon dioxide is freely diffusible. However, bicarbonate is slower to enter the CSF. The net result is a decrease in CSF pH. It is possible that an increase in hydrogen ion concentration contributes to the increase in brain cell osmolality (i.e., idiogenic osmoles), which causes an increase in brain edema.

Dialysis disequilibrium is most commonly seen in situations in which the initial solute concentrations are very high and the rate at which they decline is rapid. This syndrome therefore is seen most commonly and in its severest form during the first few hemodialysis sessions experienced by the patient. Milder symptoms may occur in patients in chronic maintenance hemodialysis particularly if noncompliant behavior has resulted in missed or shortened treatments. The overall incidence is in the range of 10% and 20% of treatments. In particular, the shorter treatment times that are possible because of dialyzers of high clearance (high-efficiency and high-flux dialyzers) may lead to symptoms in smaller individuals who have low urea volumes.

During the initiation of a new patient to hemodialysis, measures that reduce the rate of osmolar change are helpful. The use of smaller-surface-area dialyzers and reduced rates of blood flow and maintaining the direction of flow of dialysate in the same direction as blood flow (rather than the customary countercurrent configuration) are measures that can be employed to lower solute clearance rates and reduce symptoms. A high dialysate sodium level (e.g., 145 mg/L) may also be helpful. For severe headache, seizures, or obtundation, the dialysis procedure should be immediately terminated. Intravenous administration of mannitol or diazepam is useful in treating seizures caused by disequilibrium.

Mild symptoms may be treated less intensively. In general, because patients are often seen before the onset of uremic symptoms, their initiation on dialysis may be planned to avoid these symptoms. Daily dialysis for 3 to 4 days with gradual increases in dialysis time and blood flow often prevents symptoms and signs of disequilibrium. An initial dose of dialysis equivalent to Kt/V of 0.3 on the first day, 0.6 on the second day, 0.9 on the third day, and 1.4 on the fourth day should be used during initiation.

Arrhythmias and Angina

Patients with ESRD frequently have several predisposing factors for arrhythmias; there is a high prevalence of left ventricular hypertrophy and valvular sclerosis. Because of disordered calcium and phosphate metabolism, the conduction system may be affected by calcific deposits. Coronary artery disease is common in the dialysis population, and pericardial effusions are frequently revealed by echocardiography. Superimposed on these organic problems are the rapid changes in electrolyte concentrations inherent in efficient hemodialysis. It is not surprising that hemodialysis may provoke cardiac arrhythmias. Ventricular ectopic activity, including nonsustained ventricular tachycardia, is seen most frequently in patients who are taking digoxin, particularly when dialysate potassium concentration is less than 2.0 mEq/L. Supraventricular tachycardic and atrial fibrillation also can be precipitated by hypotension and coronary ischemia.[516]

The physician must attempt to strike a balance between the need to remove potassium that accumulates during the interdialytic period and the exigency to avoid low serum potassium levels that produce arrhythmias. In patients taking digoxin or who have myocardial dysfunction, the use of a dialysate with a potassium concentration of 3.0 mEq/L may reduce the frequency of arrhythmia. The acute therapy for arrhythmias during hemodialysis is similar to that for patients with normal renal function, but appropriate dose adjustments must be made for those drugs normally removed by the kidney.[517, 518] A reassessment of the need for digoxin should also be considered. Digoxin is often started before dialysis is started, in an attempt to improve cardiac contractility and lessen congestive heart failure. After initiation of dialysis, patients' vascular volume status can often be well controlled by adjustments to this estimated dry weight, and digoxin can be discontinued.

Occasional episodes of atrial fibrillation after dialysis also occur in some patients at the end of dialysis. In many cases, these are self-limited episodes that last 1 to 2 hours, with controlled ventricular rate and no signs or symptoms of ischemia. Neither digoxin nor anticoagulation is definitely indicated in these cases because the risk of subsequent more serious arrhythmias, with concomitant digoxin and hypokalemia, may be greater.

Angina frequently occurs during dialysis. Coronary artery disease is common in the dialysis population. The anemia associated with chronic renal failure adds to the risk of episodes of angina. Increases in heart rate frequently accompany ultrafiltration during diffusive clearance (see "Hypotension"), making angina a likely event in patients with coronary artery disease. There is often a need to withhold β-blockers immediately before the hemodialysis treatment. Tachyarrhythmias and hypotension can also precipitate angina. Supplemental oxygen should be administered if angina occurs, and decreasing blood flow also may be helpful. If hypotension is not present, sublingual nitroglycerin may be given, but the patient should be in the recumbent position.

Hypoxia

Hypoxia occurs during hemodialysis and is influenced by the nature of the buffer used in the dialysate and by the type of membrane in the artificial kidney. The arterial Pco_2 ($Paco_2$) in acetate-buffered dialysate is low, creating a diffusion gradient from blood to dialysate. Because carbon dioxide is removed from the blood into the dialysate, there is a decrease in the respiratory drive. Hypoventilation and hypoxia result. In contrast to the low $Paco_2$ of acetate-buffered dialysate, the $Paco_2$ of bicarbonate-buffered dialysate is nearly 100 mm Hg, leading to the net transfer of carbon dioxide into the blood from dialysate. Respiratory drive is stimulated to a degree with bicarbonate-buffered dialysate, reducing hypoxia.

The second factor influencing the magnitude of hypoxia that occurs during dialysis is the type of membrane used. Hypoxia is noted when patients are dialyzed against a biocompatible membrane such as cellulosic membranes. The activation of complement, leading to generation of other mediators such as thromboxane, alters pulmonary function and produces hypoxia. The use of more biocompatible membranes lowers the magnitude of the hypoxia. The effect of buffer lasts throughout the entire dialysis session, whereas the membrane effect is most pronounced within the first hour of the treatment. This corresponds to the period when there is the greatest activation of the complement system.[519]

In stable patients who are free of cardiorespiratory problems, the fall in $Paco_2$ can be tolerated without adverse symptoms. In patients with compromised cardiac or pulmonary function or in those who have strong reactions to the dialysis membrane, clinically significant hypoxia may occur, necessitating the use of supplemental oxygen.

Hypoglycemia

Carbohydrate metabolism is quite abnormal in patients with chronic renal failure. Although there is a peripheral resistance to the effects of insulin in uremia, the half-life of insulin is significantly prolonged when the GFR is less than 20 mL/minute. The effect of a given dose of insulin is enhanced after dialysis is instituted because an improvement in peripheral responsiveness to insulin occurs after hemodialysis has been initiated.

The implication of the foregoing is that a diabetic patient who takes a usual dose of insulin may experience hypoglycemia when undergoing dialysis against a bath with a fixed glucose concentration (i.e., glucose clamp) and too low for the amount of insulin being administered. It is frequently necessary to decrease the dose of insulin on dialysis days to prevent hypoglycemic episodes. Diabetic patients should not be dialyzed against a bath that has a glucose concentration of less than 100 mg/dL.

Hemorrhage

The uremic environment produces impaired platelet functioning, changes in capillary permeability, and anemia, all of which can impair hemostasis. There also may be increased blood loss from the gastrointestinal tract because of gastritis or angiodysplasia, lesions associated with renal failure.

The initiation of hemodialysis is reported to partially correct the defects responsible for the platelet dysfunction and capillary permeability that occur in uremia. However, patients undergoing hemodialysis still have a higher risk of hemorrhagic events because of repeated exposure to heparin. Heparin is used to prevent clotting in the extracorporeal circuit. Although strategies have been developed to dialyze patients without systemic anticoagulation, these techniques are time consuming and require greater supervision than is practical in the setting of an outpatient chronic hemodialysis center.

Acute bleeding episodes can occur at many sites; gastrointestinal blood loss, subdural and retroperitoneal hematomas, and the development of a hemopericardium may be life threatening. Patients with acute inflammatory pericarditis, those who have had trauma or who have had recent surgery, or who have an underlying coagulopathy or thrombocytopenia are at particular risk for developing hemorrhagic complications during hemodialysis.

In addition to acute bleeding episodes, patients undergoing hemodialysis are exposed to chronic, low-grade episodes of blood loss with each dialysis treatment. Between 5 and 10 mL of residual blood remains in the artificial kidney and tubing even after thorough rinsing. There may be blood loss as needles are inserted and removed and as repeated blood tests are performed on the patients. Estimates of loss of between 5 and 50 mL of blood per dialysis treatment have been made.

Prevention of bleeding episodes requires identification of patients who are at increased risk. In hospitalized patients, regional anticoagulation, a technique by which citrate is infused as blood leaves the patient and calcium is infused as blood returns to the patient, permits anticoagulation of blood only when it is in the extracorporeal circuit. If the patient is closely supervised, the use of heparin-free dialysis may be useful. In this case, blood coagulation of the extracorporeal circuit is prevented by maintenance of high blood flows (>300 mL/minute) and frequent flushes of saline into the extracorporeal circuit. There is a suggestion that low hematocrit in itself predisposes to bleeding. The use of erythropoietin to increase hematocrit may lessen the risk of bleeding. Attention to iron stores and iron supplementation is therefore important in these patients. The use of low-molecular-weight heparin compounds should be avoided in patients with ESRD. Massive hemorrhage has been described with repeated use of these compounds in dialysis patients.

First-Use Syndrome or Blood-Membrane Interaction

The membrane interposed between the blood and dialysate should not be considered an inert material. Numerous reactions, involving the activation of the complement pathway and the coagulation cascade, as well as the formed elements of blood, occur during contact of the blood with the dialysis membrane.

First-Use Syndrome

Most chronic hemodialysis units reuse their dialyzers. The first-use syndrome refers to a symptom complex encountered when a new dialyzer made of cuprophane, a cellulosic material, is employed. The symptoms associated with the first use of a dialyzer appear early, usually within the first half-hour after the commencement of the treatment. One group of symptoms resembles an anaphylactic reaction, with urticaria, angioedema, and wheezing. A severe reaction is associated with profound hypotension and cardiac arrest.

Many patients who have suffered from this reaction have elevated levels of immunoglobulin E (IgE) directed against serum proteins that have interacted with ethylene oxide, a sterilizing agent used in the manufacture of dialyzers. The hollow fibers of the artificial kidney are embedded in a potting compound that may be a reservoir for residual ethylene oxide even if the dialyzer is flushed before its use.[173]

Complement activation also has been implicated in some of these reactions. Very high rates of complement activation have been demonstrated in patients who have had reactions during the first use of cellulosic dialyzers. The response of their plasma to zymosan, an activator of complement, through an alternative pathway is also exaggerated.

The full anaphylactoid response occurs rarely (1 of 60,000 exposures to new dialyzers). Much more frequent is the host of nonspecific symptoms, such as coughing, sneezing, pruritus, and back pain, that occur early in the treatment with a new dialyzer. The frequency is reduced when dialyzers are reused. The attenuated reaction in this instance is likely to be attributable to coating of the membrane with serum proteins during the first use. Protein is fixed to the membrane by formaldehyde, which is used as a sterilant in many reuse procedures. A reused dialyzer can be shown to produce symptoms if the protein coat is removed by bleach in the reuse process. Noncellulosic membranes, such as polyacrylonitrile, polysulfone, or polymethylmethacrylate,

do not cause large amounts of complement to be released into the circulation, and they appear to be better tolerated as well.

Anaphylactoid reactions have been reported when patients taking ACE inhibitors undergo hemodialysis using polyacrylonitrile (AN69) membranes or other reused membranes of various kinds. These reactions occur despite the fact that the biocompatibility profile of these membranes, at least with respect to complement activation, is superior to that of new cuprophane membranes. Evidence indicates that AN69, because of its negative surface charge, is capable of generating bradykinin by activation of Hageman factor and the kallikrein-kininogen pathway. ACE is a potent kinase responsible for degrading bradykinin. ACE inhibition may lead to higher bradykinin levels and to the unopposed action of this substance. Bradykinin-induced hypotension and bronchoconstriction result. The role of reuse in these occurrences is uncertain, but possibly the character of several membrane surfaces is altered by the reuse procedure.

Treatment of mild forms of this syndrome is symptomatic, but anaphylactoid reactions need to be treated with epinephrine and steroids. Blood in the extracorporeal circuit should not be returned to the patient. The use of biocompatible membranes, reuse programs, the avoidance of ACE inhibitor when AN69 membranes are used, and dialyzers constructed without the potting compound can significantly lessen the frequency of these reactions.

Other Interactions

Cellulosic membranes produce a wide variety of reactions after they interact with blood to produce complement activation, as has been discussed. The consequences of complement activation, as well as the elaboration of other mediators of inflammation, extend beyond the first-use syndrome. Activated complement can produce neutropenia and activation of neutrophils. It is not unusual for the white blood cell count to fall by as much as 70% within the first 20 minutes of dialysis. This decline is followed by a rebound during the remainder of the treatment, making a white blood cell count obtained after the commencement of dialysis very difficult to interpret. Neutrophils initially activated by contact with the dialysis membrane become less responsive to chemotactic agents and also demonstrate reduced phagocytic ability. Neutrophil function is poorest in patients chronically exposed to new cellulosic membranes. The clinical significance of this may be important, given the morbidity and mortality in patients on dialysis brought about by infection. Infection accounts for at least 30% of the deaths of patients undergoing hemodialysis.

Platelets, monocytes, and lymphocytes also interact with membranes. The potential consequences of repeated exposure of blood to new cellulosic membranes and the benefits of more biocompatible membranes and the benefits of more biocompatible membranes such as polyacrylonitrile, polysulfone, and polymethylmethacrylate are discussed later.

Problems with Dialysate Composition and Integrity of the Extracorporeal Circuit

Among the most important requirements during hemodialysis are the constant monitoring of the composition and the temperature of the dialysate and of the safety of the extracorporeal circuit. Water treatment before dialysate is reconstituted, and the alarm features on the dialysis machine are integral components to ensure safe treatments.

During each hemodialysis treatment, the patient's blood is exposed to 120 to 200 liters of dialysate across the membrane. Dialysate must therefore receive the same consideration as we give to drugs we administer. Given the magnitude of the exposure to water used in dialysate, even small amounts of trace elements or organic material may be harmful on repeated contact. Chloramine, used in water treatment, and copper have been associated with anemia, and aluminum has been associated with severe osteomalacia and fatal encephalopathy. Outbreaks of infection caused by agents such as *Mycobacterium chelonei* have been reported with improper reuse techniques or ineffective maintenance of the WTS. Bicarbonate-buffered dialysate has the potential to become contaminated by gram-negative organisms, and even if they cannot cross an intact dialysis membrane, endotoxin fragments and other bacterial products can induce pyrogenic reactions, particularly when highly permeable synthetic membranes are used.

To prevent toxicity, water must be treated before it reaches the patient. Strict guidelines exist for water treatment and dialyzer reuse. The use of a properly configured WTS consisting of carbon beds to remove organic material, filters, reverse osmosis and deionization to remove trace metals and other material such as chloramines, and ultraviolet light eliminates water-borne risks. It is also essential that periodic surveillance cultures be obtained at various points of the water and dialysate circuit. The entire water circuit also should be disinfected on a regular basis.

THE FUTURE OF RENAL REPLACEMENT THERAPY

Despite the many technical advances that have occurred over the past 5 decades in the delivery of hemodialysis and associated care, morbidity and mortality rates remain high for hemodialysis patients. The ever-increasing numbers of patients in the United States and worldwide who are developing ESRD also present a challenge to health care providers and systems to optimize treatment outcomes in the most cost-effective manner. The reported results of the HEMO Study, in which increasing the delivered dialysis dose or using high-flux dialyzer membranes did not improve mortality, suggest that further research and new approaches will be required to improve overall mortality rates for hemodialysis patients.

In the future, there will undoubtedly be further technical advances to support the delivery of hemodialysis. A number of on-line monitoring devices that provide physiologic data in real time during the hemodialysis session have been used. In the future, integrated systems simultaneously measuring multiple physiologic parameters with built-in feedback loops controlling many features of the dialysis prescription and treatment will undoubtedly be developed. Artificial intelligence programs may also assist in the development of more patient-specific dialytic therapy.[520] There will likely be further technologic improvements in the biocompatibility of dialysis membranes, dialysate, and water use for dialysis treatment. We anticipate that there will be technologic improvements in vascular access for hemodialysis such that

the success rate for vascular access will be higher and the complication rate (especially thrombogenicity and infection) will be lower. The lack of significant technologic breakthroughs in vascular access care because the development of the autogenous fistula and prosthetic bridge graft more than 30 years ago has limited improvement in this area.

Despite more than 30 years of the ESRD program in the United States, there has not been a published randomized clinical trial demonstrating that any pharmacologic agent can lower mortality rates in the dialysis population. Despite the high morbidity, mortality, and cost associated with the care of hemodialysis patients, there have been few adequately powered pharmaceutical studies published. Targeting cardiovascular complications, which are extraordinarily common in this patient population, will undoubtedly happen and may result in identification of successful therapeutic agents. There is also much interest in performing clinical trials of hemodialysis more frequently than three times per week, which has been known for decades to be inherently "unphysiologic."[521] Uncontrolled observational cohorts of patients receiving more frequent hemodialysis appear to experience substantial clinical improvements. We anticipate that randomized trials will demonstrate that these improvements in cohort studies are the result of the therapy and not due to patient selection bias or other factors.

As far back as the inception of maintenance hemodialysis therapy for the treatment of ESRD, it was recognized that hemodialysis attempts to recapitulate glomerular filtration but not replace renal tubule function.[387] Tubule processing of glomerulofiltrate through selective metabolism and transport, may be essential in mitigating uremic toxicity. Cell-based therapies providing proximal tubule function are in development and have entered phase I human clinical trials in the treatment of patients with acute renal failure. Ultimately, partial or complete renal organogenesis may lead to successful renal replacement therapy without the allogenicity or xenogenicity associated with heterotopic transplantation.[522] We believe (and hope) that the future of renal replacement therapy is bright.

REFERENCES

1. Abel JJ, Rowntree LG, Turner BB: On the removal of diffusable substances from the circulating blood by means of dialysis. Transactions of the Association of American Physicians, 1913. Transfus Sci 11: 164-165, 1990.
2. Kolff W, Berek H: De kunstmatige nier, een dialysator met groot oppervlak. Ned Tijdschr Geneeskd 87:1684-1692, 1943.
3. Evans RW, Blagg CR, Bryan FA Jr: Implications for health care policy. A social and demographic profile of hemodialysis patients in the United States. JAMA 245:487-491, 1981.
4. United States Renal Data System (USRDS): Annual Data Report, N14. Bethesda, MD, USRDS, 470, 2001, p 470.
5. National Kidney Foundation: K/DOQI clinical practice guidelines for chronic kidney disease: Evaluation, classification and stratification. Am J Kidney Dis 39:S1-S266, 2002.
6. Kopple J, GTCCWHDMBMDSLSGWSZG: Modification of Diet in Renal Disease Study Group: Relationship between nutritional status and the glomerular filtration rate: Results from the MDRD Study. 57:1688-1703, 2000.
7. Collins AJ, Ma JZ, Xia A, Ebben J: Trends in anemia treatment with erythropoietin usage and patient outcomes. Am J Kidney Dis 32:133-141, 1998.
8. Parfrey PS, Foley RN, Harnett JD, et al: Outcome and risk factors for left ventricular disorders in chronic uraemia. Nephrol Dial Transplant 11:1277-1285, 1996.

9. Levin A, Foley RN: Cardiovascular disease in chronic renal insufficiency. Am J Kidney Dis 36:24-30, 2000.

10. Locatelli F, Conte F, Marcelli D: The impact of haematocrit levels and erythropoietin treatment on overall and cardiovascular mortality and morbidity—the experience of the Lombardy Dialysis Registry. Nephrol Dial Transplant 13:1642-4, 1998.

11. McClellan WM, Knight DF, Karp H, Brown WW: Early detection and treatment of renal disease in hospitalized diabetic and hypertensive patients: Important differences between practice and published guidelines. Am J Kidney Dis 29:368-375, 1997.

12. Ratcliffe PJ, Phillips RE, Oliver DO: Late referral for maintenance dialysis. Br Med J (Clin Res Ed) 288:441-443, 1984.

13. Eadington DW: Delayed referral for dialysis. Nephrol Dial Transplant 11:2124-2126, 1996.

14. Ifudu O, Dawood M, Homel P, Friedman EA: Excess morbidity in patients starting uremia therapy without prior care by a nephrologist. Am J Kidney Dis 28:841-845, 1996.

15. Schmidt RJ, Domico JR, Sorkin MI, Hobbs G: Early referral and its impact on emergent first dialyses, health care costs, and outcome. Am J Kidney Dis 32:278-283, 1998.

16. Roubicek C, Brunet P, Huiart L, et al: Timing of nephrology referral: Influence on mortality and morbidity. Am J Kidney Dis 36:35-41, 2000.

17. Kolff WJ, Berk HT: The artificial kidney: A dialyzer with a great area. Acta Med Scand 117:121-129, 1944.

18. Quinton W, Dillard D, Scribner BH: Cannulation of blood vessels for prolonged hemodialysis. ASAIO Trans 6:104-107, 1960.

19. Brescia MJ, Cimino JE, Appel K, Hurwich BJ: Chronic hemodialysis using venipuncture and a surgically recreated arteriovenous fistula. N Engl J Med 275:1089-1092, 1966.

20. Baker LD Jr, Johnson JM, Goldfarb D: Expanded polytetrafluoroethylene (PTFE) subcutaneous arteriovenous conduit: An improved vascular access for chronic hemodialysis. ASAIO Trans 22:382-387, 1976.

21. Kaplan MS, Mirahmadi KS, Winer RL, et al: Comparison of "PTFE" and bovine grafts for blood access in hemodialysis patients. ASAIO Trans 22:388-392, 1976.

22. Shaldon S, Chianussi L, Higgs B: Hemodialysis by percutaneous catheterization of the femoral artery and vein with regional heparinization. Lancet 2:75-81, 1961.

23. Uldall R, Dyke R, Woods F: A subclavian cannula for temporary vascular access for hemodialysis or plasmapheresis. Dialysis Transplantation 8:963-968, 1979.

24. Schwab SJ, Buller GL, McCann RL, et al: Prospective evaluation of a Dacron cuffed hemodialysis catheter for prolonged use. Am J Kidney Dis 11:166-169, 1988.

25. Schwab SJ, Weiss MA, Rushton F, et al: Multicenter clinical trial results with the LifeSite hemodialysis access system. Kidney Int 62:1026-1033, 2002.

26. Blake PG, Huraib S, Wu G, Uldall R: The use of dual-lumen jugular venous catheters as definitive long-term access for hemodialysis. Int J Artif Organs 13:26-31, 1990.

27. Hakim RM, Himmelfarb J: Hemodialysis access failure: A call to action. Kidney Int 54:1029-1040, 1998.

28. Pisoni RL, Young EW, Dykstra DM, et al: Vascular access use in Europe and the United States: Results from DOPPS. Kidney Int 61:305-316, 2002.

29. Rayner HC, Pisoni RL, Gillespie BW, et al: Creation, cannulation and survival of arteriovenous fistulae: Data from the Dialysis Outcomes and Practice Patterns Study. Kidney Int 63:323-330, 2003.

30. Dhingra RK, Young EW, Hulbert-Shearon TE, et al: Type of vascular access and mortality in US hemodialysis patients. Kidney Int 60:1443-1451, 2002.

31. End-Stage Renal Disease (ESRD) Clinical Performance Measures Project: Vascular access. Am J Kidney Dis 39:S23-S29, 2002.

32. Wedgwood KR, Wiggins PA, Guillou PJ: A prospective study of end-to-side vs. side-to-side arteriovenous fistulas for haemodialysis. Br J Surg 71:640-642, 1984.

33. Bonalumi U, Civalleri D, Rovida S, et al: Nine years' experience with end-to-end arteriovenous fistula at the "anatomic snuff box" for maintenance haemodialysis. Br J Surg 69:486-488, 1982.

34. Miller PE, Tolwani A, Luscy CP, et al: Predictors of adequacy of arteriovenous fistulas in hemodialysis patients. Kidney Int 56:275-280, 1999.

35. Rivers SP, Scher LA, Sheehan E, et al: Basilic vein transposition: An underused autologous alternative to prosthetic dialysis angioaccess. J Vasc Surg 18:391-396, 1993.

36. Gracz KC, Ing TS, Soung LS, et al: Proximal forearm fistula for maintenance hemodialysis. Kidney Int 11:71-74, 1977.

37. Oliver MJ, McCann RL, Indridason OS, et al: Comparison of transposed brachiobasilic fistulas to upper arm grafts and brachiocephalic fistulas. Kidney Int 60:1532-1539, 2001.

38. Dixon BS, Novak L, Fangman J: Hemodialysis vascular access survival: Upper-arm native arteriovenous fistula. Am J Kidney Dis 39:92-101, 2002.

39. Gibson KD, Caps MT, Kohler TR, et al: Assessment of a policy to reduce placement of prosthetic hemodialysis access. Kidney Int 59:2335-2345, 2002.

40. Silva MB, Hobson RW, Pappas PJ, et al: A strategy for increasing use of autogenous hemodialysis access procedures: Impact of preoperative noninvasive evaluation. J Vasc Surg 27:302-308, 1998.

41. Allon M, Lockhart ME, Lilly RZ, et al: Effect of preoperative sonographic mapping on vascular access outcomes in hemodialysis patients. Kidney Int 60:2013-2020, 2001.

42. Himmelfarb J, Saad T: Hemodialysis vascular access: Emerging concepts. Curr Opin Nephrol Hypertens 5:485-491, 1996.

43. Woods JD, Tureene MN, Strawderman RL, et al: Vascular access survival among incident hemodialysis patients in the United States. Am J Kidney Dis 30:50-57, 1997.

44. Kanterman RY, Vesely TM, Pilgram TK, et al: Dialysis access grafts: Anatomic location of venous stenosis and results of angioplasty. Radiology 195:135-139, 1995.

45. Swedberg SH, Brown BG, Sigley R, et al: Intimal fibromuscular hyperplasia at the venous anastomosis of PTFE grafts in hemodialysis patients. Circulation 80:1726-1736, 1989.

46. Roy-Chaudhury P, Kelly BS, Miller MA, et al: Venous intimal hyperplasia in polytetrafluoroethylene dialysis grafts. Kidney Int 59:2325-2334, 2002.

47. Weiss MF, Scivitarro V, Anderson JM: Oxidative stress and increased expression of growth factors in lesions of failed hemodialysis access. Am J Kidney Dis 37:970-980, 2001.

48. Himmelfarb J: Pharmacological prevention of vascular access stenosis. Curr Opin Nephrol Hypertens 8:569-572, 1999.

49. Schwab SJ, Raymond JR, Saeed M, et al: Prevention of hemodialysis fistula thrombosis: Early detection of various stenoses. Kidney Int 36:707-711, 1989.

50. Beathard GA: Physical examination of the dialysis vascular access. Semin Dial 11:231-236, 1998.

51. Besarab A, Sullivan KL, Ross RP, Moritz MJ: Utility of intra-access pressure monitoring in detecting and correcting venous outlet stenoses prior to thrombosis. Kidney Int 47:1364-1373, 1995.

52. McCarley P, Wingard RL, Shyr R, et al: Vascular access blood flow monitoring reduces access morbidity and costs. Kidney Int 60:1167-1172, 2001.

53. Neyra NR, Ikizler TA, May RE, et al: Change in access blood flow over time predicts vascular access thrombosis. Kidney Int 54:1714-1719, 1998.

54. Depner TA, Krivitsky NM: Clinical measurement of blood flow in hemodialysis access fistulae and grafts by ultrasound dilution. ASAIO J 41:M745-M749, 1995.

55. Depner TA: Analysis of new methods for vascular access monitoring. Semin Dial 12:376-381, 1999.

56. Krivitski NM: Theory and validation of access blood flow measurements by dilution technique during hemodialysis. Kidney Int 48:244-250, 1995.

57. Lindsay RM, Blake PG, Malek P, et al: Accuracy and precision of access recirculation measurements by the hemodynamic recirculation monitor. Am J Kidney Dis 31:242-249, 1998.

58. Bosman PJ, Boereboom FT, Eikelboom BC, et al: Graft flow as a predictor of thrombosis in hemodialysis grafts. Kidney Int 54:1726-1730, 1998.

59. Wang E, Schneditz D, Nepomuceno C, et al: Predictive value of access blood flow in detecting access thrombosis. ASAIO J 44:M555-M558, 1998.

60. Sands J, Glidden D, Miranda C: Access flow measured during hemodialysis. ASAIO J 42:M530-M532, 1996.

61. Bay WH, Henry ML, Lazarus JM, et al: Predicting hemodialysis access failure with color flow Doppler ultrasound. Am J Nephrol 18:296-340, 1998.

62. Strauch BS, O'Connell RS, Geoly KL, et al: Forecasting thrombosis of vascular access with Doppler color flow imaging. Am J Kidney Dis 19:554-557, 1992.

63. Tonelli M, Jindal K, Hirsch D, et al: Screening for subclinical stenosis in native vessel arteriovenous fistulae. J Am Soc Nephrol 12:1729-1733, 2001.

64. Schwab SJ, Beathard GA: The hemodialysis catheter conundrum: Hate living with them, but can't live without them. Kidney Int 56:1-17, 1999.

65. Sarnak MJ, Jaber BL: Mortality caused by sepsis in patients with end-stage renal disease compared with the general population. Kidney Int 58:1758-1764, 2000.

66. Marr KA, Sexton DJ, Conlon PJ, et al: Catheter-related bacteremia and outcome of attempted catheter salvage in patients undergoing hemodialysis. Ann Intern Med 127:275-280, 1997.

67. Krishnasami Z, Carlton D, Bimbo L, et al: Management of hemodialysis catheter-related bacteremia with an adjunctive antibiotic lock solution. Kidney Int 61:1136-1142, 2002.

68. Beathard GA: Management of bacteremia associated with tunneled-cuffed hemodialysis catheters. J Am Soc Nephrol 10:1045-1049, 1999.

69. Shaffer D: Catheter-related sepsis complicating long-term, tunneled central venous dialysis catheters: Management by guidewire exchange. Am J Kidney Dis 25:593-596, 1995.

70. Tanriover B, Carlton D, Saddekni S, et al: Bacteremia associated with tunneled dialysis catheters: Comparison of two treatment strategies. Kidney Int 57:2151-2155, 2000.

71. Mokrzycki MH, Jeane-Jerome K, Rush H, et al: A randomized trial of minidose warfarin for the prevention of late malfunction in tunneled, cuffed hemodialysis catheters. Kidney Int 59:1935-1942, 2001.

72. Bolz KD, Fjermeros G, Wideroe TE, Hatlinghus S: Catheter malfunction and thrombus formation on double-lumen hemodialysis catheters: An intravascular ultrasonographic study. Am J Kidney Dis 25:597-602, 1995.

73. Barrett N, Spenser S, McIvor J, Brown EA: Subclavian stenosis: A major complication of subclavian dialysis catheters. Nephrol Dial Transplant 3:423-425, 1988.

74. Cheung AK, Gregory MC: Subclavian vein thrombosis in hemodialysis patients. Trans ASAIO 31:131, 1985.

75. Fant GF, Dennis VW, Quarles D: Late vascular complications of the subclavian dialysis catheter. Am J Kidney Dis 7:225-228, 1986.

76. Hernandez D, Diaz F, Rufino M, et al: Subclavian vascular access stenosis in dialysis patients: Natural history and risk factors. J Am Soc Nephrol 9:1507-1510, 1998.

77. Khanna S, Sniderman K, Simons M, et al: Superior vena cava stenosis associated with hemodialysis catheters. Am J Kidney Dis 21:278-281, 1993.

78. Schwab SJ, Quarles D, Middleton JP, et al: Hemodialysis-associated subclavian vein stenosis. Kidney Int 33:1156-1159, 1988.

79. Beathard GA, Marston WA: Endovascular management of thrombosed dialysis grafts. Am J Kidney Dis 32:172-175, 1998.

80. Beathard GA: Percutaneous transvenous angioplasty in the treatment of vascular access stenosis. Kidney Int 42:1390-1397, 1992.

81. Beathard GA: Thrombolysis versus surgery for the treatment of thrombosed dialysis access grafts. J Am Soc Nephrol 6:1619-1624, 1995.

82. Valji K, Bookstein JJ, Roberts AC, Davis GB: Pharmacomechanical thrombolysis and angioplasty in the management of clotted hemodialysis grafts: Early and late clinical trials. Radiology 178:243-247, 1991.

83. Roberts AB, Kahn MB, Bradford S, et al: Graft surveillance and angioplasty prolongs dialysis graft patency. J Am Coll Surg 183:486-492, 1996.

84. Saeed M, Newman GE, McCann RL, et al: Stenoses in dialysis fistulas: Treatment with percutaneous angioplasty. Radiology 164:693-697, 1987.

85. Schwab SJ, Oliver MJ, Suhocki P, McCann R: Hemodialysis arteriovenous access: Detection of stenosis and response to treatment by vascular access blood flow. Kidney Int 59:358-362, 2001.

86. Sreedhara R, Himmelfarb J, Lazarus JM, Hakim RM: Antiplatelet therapy in graft thrombosis: Results of a prospective, randomized double-blind study. Kidney Int 45:1477-1483, 1994.

87. Schmitz PG, McCloud LK, Reikes ST, et al: Prophylaxis of hemodialysis graft thrombosis with fish oil: A double-blind, randomized, prospective trial. J Am Soc Nephrol 13:184-190, 2001.

88. Kaufman J, O'Connor T, Cronin R, et al: Combination aspirin plus clopidogrel in the prevention of hemodialysis access graft thrombosis. Abstract. J Am Soc Nephrol 12:219A, 2001.

89. Gradzki R, Dhingra RK, Port FK, et al: Use of ACE inhibitors is associated with prolonged survival of arteriovenous grafts. Am J Kidney Dis 38:1240-1244, 2001.

90. Saran R, Dykstra DM, Wolfe RA, et al: Association between vascular access failure and the use of specific drugs: The Dialysis Outcomes and Practice Patterns Study (DOPPS). Am J Kidney Dis 40:1255-1263, 2002.

91. Kaplow LS, Goffinet JA: Profound neutropenia during the early phase of hemodialysis. JAMA 203:1135-1137, 1968.

92. Mujais S, Schmidt B: Operating Characteristics of Hollow-Fiber Dialyzers, 3rd ed. Norwalk, Appleton & Lange, 1995, p 8.

93. Konstantin P, Bailey RM: Polycarbonate-polyether (PC-PE) flat sheet membrane: Manufacture, structure and performance. Blood Purif 4:6-12, 1986.

94. Gohl H, Raff M, Harttig H, Deppisch R: PC-PE hollow-fiber membrane: Structure, performance characteristics and manufacturing. Blood Purif 4:23-31, 1986.

95. Gohl H, Konstantin P: Membranes and filters for hemofiltration. In Henderson L, Quellhorst E, Baldamus C, Lysaght M (eds): Hemofiltration. Berlin, Springer-Verlag, 1986, pp 41-56.

96. Leypoldt JK, Frigon RP, Henderson LW: Macromolecular charge affects hemofilter solute sieving. Artif Intern Organs 32:384-387, 1986.

97. Kaplow LS, Goffinet JA: Profound neutropenia during the early phase of hemodialysis. JAMA 203:1135-1137, 1968.

98. Akizawa T, Kitaoka T, Koshikawa S, et al: Development of a regenerated cellulose non-complement activating membrane for hemodialysis. ASAIO Trans 32:76-80, 1986.

99. Cheung A: Interactions between Plasma Proteins and Hemodialysis Membranes, 22nd ed. Boston, Mosby–Year Book, 1993, pp 417-434.

100. Schulman G, Levin N: Membranes for hemodialyzers. Semin Dial 7:251-256, 1994.

101. Arbeit LA, Schulman G, Holmes T, et al: The binding of vasoactive substances to dialysis membranes is proportional to the negativity of the surface potential. Abstract. Kidney Int 31:122, 1987.

102. Lemke H, Fink E: Accumulation of bradykinin formed by the AN69 or PAN 17 DX-membrane is due to the presence of an ACE-inhibitor in vitro. Abstract. J Am Soc Nephrol 3:376, 1992.

103. Schulman G, Hakim R, Arias R, et al: Bradykinin generation by dialysis membranes: Possible role in anaphylactic reaction. J Am Soc Nephrol 3:1563-1569, 1993.

104. Parnes EL, Shapiro WB: Anaphylactoid reactions in hemodialysis patients treated with the AN69 dialyzer. Kidney Int 40:1148-1152, 1991.

105. Pegues DA, Beck-Sague CM, Woollen SW, et al: Anaphylactoid reactions associated with reuse of hollow-fiber hemodialyzers and ACE inhibitors. Kidney Int 42:1232-1237, 1992.

106. Horl WH, Schaefer RM, Heidland A: Effect of different dialyzers on proteinases and proteinase inhibitors during hemodialysis. Am J Nephrol 5:320-326, 1985.

107. Sawada K, Malchesky PS, Guidubaldi JM, et al: In vitro evaluation of a relationship between human serum- or plasma-material interaction and polymer bulk hydroxyl and surface oxygen content. ASAIO J 39:910-917, 1993.

108. Cheung AK, Chenoweth DE, Otsuka D, Henderson LW: Compartmental distribution of complement activation products in artificial kidneys. Kidney Int 30:74-80, 1986.

109. Schindler R, Linnenweber S, Schulze M, et al: Gene expression of interleukin-1 beta during hemodialysis. Kidney Int 43:712-721, 1993.

110. Greene WH, Ray C, Mauer SM, Quie PG: The effect of hemodialysis on neutrophil chemotactic responsiveness. J Lab Clin Med 88:971-974, 1976.

111. Bjorksten B, Mauer SM, Mills EL, Quie PG: The effect of hemodialysis on neutrophil chemotactic responsiveness. Acta Med Scand 203:67-70, 1978.

112. Vanholder R, Ringoir S, Dhondt A, Hakim RM: Phagocytosis in uremic and hemodialysis patients: A prospective and cross-sectional study. Kidney Int 39:320-327, 1991.

113. Friedlander MA, Hilbert CM, Wu YC, Rich EA: Role of dialysis modality in responses of blood monocytes and peritoneal macrophages to endotoxin stimulation. Am J Kidney Dis 22:11-23, 1993.

114. Pereira BJ, King AJ, Poutsiaka DD, et al: Comparison of first use and reuse of cuprophane membranes on interleukin-1 receptor antagonist and interleukin-1 beta production by blood mononuclear cells. Am J Kidney Dis 22:288-295, 1993.

115. Zaoui P, Green W, Hakim RM: Hemodialysis with cuprophane membrane modulates interleukin-2 receptor expression. Kidney Int 39:1020-1026, 1991.

116. Zaoui P, Hakim RM: Natural killer-cell function in hemodialysis patients: Effect of the dialysis membrane. Kidney Int 43:1298-1305, 1993.

117. Dinarello CA, Koch KM, Shaldon S: Interleukin-1 and its relevance in patients treated with hemodialysis. Kidney Int Suppl 24:21-26, 1988.

118. Hakim R: Personal communication, 1986.

119. Depner TA: Benefits of more frequent dialysis: Lower TAC at the same Kt/V. Nephrol Dial Transplant 13:20-24, 1998.

120. Ronco C, Brendolan A, Milan M, et al: Impact of biofeedback-induced cardiovascular stability on hemodialysis tolerance and efficiency. Kidney Int 58:800-808, 2000.

121. Ronco C, Ghezzi PM, La Greca G: The role of technology in hemodialysis. J Nephrol 12 Suppl 2:68-81, 1999.

122. Parker TF 3rd: Role of dialysis dose on morbidity and mortality in maintenance hemodialysis patients. Am J Kidney Dis 24:981-989, 1994.

123. Parker TF 3rd, Husni L, Huang W, et al: Survival of hemodialysis patients in the United States is improved with a greater quantity of dialysis. Am J Kidney Dis 23:670-680, 1994.

124. Keshaviah PR, Ebben JP, Emerson PF: On-line monitoring of the delivery of the hemodialysis prescription. Pediatr Nephrol 9(suppl):2-8, 1995.

125. Chauveau P, Naret C, Puget J, et al: Adequacy of haemodialysis and nutrition in maintenance haemodialysis patients: Clinical evaluation of a new on-line urea monitor. Nephrol Dial Transplant 11:1568-1573, 1996.

126. Krivitsky NM: Theory and validation of access flow measurement by dilution technique during hemodialysis. Kidney Int 48:244-250, 1995.

127. Leypoldt JK, Cheung AK, Steuer RR, et al: Determination of circulating blood volume by continuously monitoring hematocrit during hemodialysis. J Am Soc Nephrol 6:214-219, 1995.

128. Steuer RR, Germain MJ, Leypoldt JK, Cheung AK: Enhanced fluid removal guided by blood volume monitoring during chronic hemodialysis. Artif Organs 22:627-632, 1998.

129. Steuer RR, Leypoldt JK, Cheung AK, et al: Reducing symptoms during hemodialysis by continuously monitoring the hematocrit. Am J Kidney Dis 27:525-532, 1996.

130. Steuer RR, Leypoldt JK, Cheung AK, et al: Hematocrit as an indicator of blood volume and a predictor of intradialytic morbid events. ASAIO J 40:691-696, 1994.

131. Dunea G, Mahurkar SD, Mamdani B, Smith EC: Role of aluminum in dialysis dementia. Ann Intern Med 88:502-504, 1978.

132. Coburn JW, Norris KC, Sherrard DJ, et al: Toxic effects of aluminum in end-stage renal disease: Discussion of a case. Am J Kidney Dis 12:171-184, 1988.

133. Llach F, Felsenfeld AJ, Coleman MD, et al: The natural course of dialysis osteomalacia. Kidney Int Suppl 18:74-79, 1986.

134. Tokars JI, Alter MJ, Favero MS, et al: National surveillance of hemodialysis associated diseases in the United States, 1990. ASAIO J 39:71-80, 1993.

135. Alter MJ, Favero MS, Moyer LA, Bland LA: National surveillance of dialysis-associated diseases in the United States, 1989. ASAIO Trans 37:97-109, 1991.

136. Topple M, Bland L, Favero M, et al: Investigation of hemolytic anemia after chloramine exposure in a dialysis center. Letter. ASAIO J 34:1060, 1988.

137. Yawata Y, Kjellstrand C, Buselmeier T, et al: Hemolysis in dialyzed patients: Tap water–induced red blood cell metabolic deficiency. Trans Am Soc Artif Intern Organs 18:301-304, 1972.

138. Neilan BA, Ehlers SM, Kolpin CF, Eaton JW: Prevention of chloramine-induced hemolysis in dialyzed patients. Clin Nephrol 10:105-108, 1978.

139. Gordon SM, Drachman J, Bland LA, et al: Epidemic hypotension in a dialysis center caused by sodium azide. Kidney Int 37:110-115, 1990.

140. Lough J, Noonan R, Gagnon R, Kaye M: Effects of fluoride on bone in chronic renal failure. Arch Pathol 99:484-487, 1975.

141. National News. Dialysis patients in Chicago die from fluoride poisoning; FDA issues safety alert. Contemp Dial Nephrol 17:110-111, 1993.

142. Freeman RM, Lawton RL, Chamberlain MA: Hard-water syndrome. N Engl J Med 276:1113-1118, 1967.

143. Evans DB, Slapak M: Pancreatitis in the hard water syndrome. Br Med J 3:748-752, 1975.

144. Carlson DJ, Shapiro FL: Methemoglobinemia from well water nitrates: A complication of home dialysis. Ann Intern Med 73:757-759, 1970.

145. Manzler AD, Schreiner AW: Copper-induced acute hemolytic anemia: A new complication of hemodialysis. Ann Intern Med 73:409-412, 1970.

146. Matter BJ, Pederson J, Psimenos G, Lindeman RD: Lethal copper intoxication in hemodialysis. Trans Am Soc Artif Intern Organs 15:309-315, 1969.

147. Gallery E, Blomfield J, Dixon S: Acute zinc toxicity in haemodialysis. Br Med J 4:33, 1973.

148. Centers for Disease Control and Prevention (CDC): Formaldehyde Intoxication Associated with Hemodialysis. California Epidemic Investigation Report, EPI 81-733-2. Atlanta, CDC, May 7, 1984.

149. Orringer EP, Mattern WD: Formaldehyde-induced hemolysis during chronic hemodialysis. N Engl J Med 294:1416-20, 1976.

150. Johnson WJ, Taves DR: Exposure to excessive fluoride during hemodialysis. Kidney Int 5:451-4, 1974.

151. Favero MS, Petersen NJ, Carson LA, et al: Gram-negative water bacteria in hemodialysis systems. Health Lab Sci 12:321-34, 1975.

152. Bland L, Favero M: Microbiologic aspects of hemodialysis systems. *In* Association for the Advancement of Medical Instrumentation (eds): Dialysis, Vol 3. Arlington, VA, American National Standards, 1993, pp 257-265.

153. Lowry PW, Beck-Sague CM, Bland LA, et al: *Mycobacterium chelonei* infection among patients receiving high-flux dialysis in a hemodialysis clinic in California. J Infect Dis 161:85-90, 1990.

154. Carson LA, Bland LA, Cusick LB, et al: Prevalence of nontuberculous mycobacteria in water supplies of hemodialysis centers. Appl Environ Microbiol 54:3122-3125, 1988.

155. Carson LA, Petersen NJ, Favero MS, Aguero SM: Growth characteristics of atypical mycobacteria in water and their comparative resistance to disinfectants. Appl Environ Microbiol 36:839-846, 1978.

156. Bolan G, Reingold AL, Carson LA, et al: Infections with *Mycobacterium chelonei* in patients receiving dialysis and using processed hemodialyzers. J Infect Dis 152:1013-1019, 1985.

157. Favero M: Distinguishing between high-level disinfection, reprocessing and sterilization. *In* Association for the Advancement of Medical Instrumentation (eds): Reuse of Disposables: Implications for Quality Health Care and Cost Containment. Technical Assessment Report No. 6. Arlington, VA, American National Standards, 1983, pp 19-20.

158. Favero M, Bland L: Microbiologic principles applied to reprocessing hemodialyzers. *In* Deane N, Wineman R, Bemis J (eds): Guide to Reprocessing of Hemodialyzers. Boston, Martinus Nijhoff, 1986, pp 63-73.

159. Gordon SM, Oettinger CW, Bland LA, et al: Pyrogenic reactions in patients receiving conventional, high-efficiency, or high-flux hemodialysis treatments with bicarbonate dialysate containing high concentrations of bacteria and endotoxin. J Am Soc Nephrol 2:1436-1444, 1992.

160. Jones DM, Tobin BM, Harlow GR, Ralston AJ: Antibody production in patients on regular haemodialysis to organisms present in dialysate. Proc Eur Dial Transplant Assoc 9:575-576, 1972.

161. Hindman SH, Favero MS, Carson LA, et al: Pyrogenic reactions during haemodialysis caused by extramural endotoxin. Lancet 2:732-734, 1975.

162. Raij L, Shapiro FL, Michael AF: Endotoxemia in febrile reactions during hemodialysis. Kidney Int 4:57-60, 1973.

163. Passavanti G, Buongiorno E, De Fino G, et al: The permeability of dialytic membranes to endotoxins: Clinical and experimental findings. Int J Artif Organs 12:505-508, 1989.

164. Laurence RA, Lapierre ST: Quality of hemodialysis water: A 7-year multicenter study. Am J Kidney Dis 25:738-750, 1995.

165. Dinarello CA: Interleukin-1 and its biologically related cytokines. Adv Immunol 44:153-205, 1989.

166. Loppnow H, Brade H, Durrbaum I, et al: IL-1 induction-capacity of defined lipopolysaccharide partial structures. J Immunol 142:3229-3238, 1989.

167. Duff GW, Atkins E: The detection of endotoxin by in vitro production of endogenous pyrogen: Comparison with limulus amebocyte lysate gelation. J Immunol Methods 52:323-331, 1982.

168. Lonnemann G, Bingel M, Floege J, et al: Detection of endotoxin-like interleukin-1-inducing activity during in vitro dialysis. Kidney Int 33:29-35, 1988.

169. Evans RC, Holmes CJ: In vitro study of the transfer of cytokine-inducing substances across selected high-flux hemodialysis membranes. Blood Purif 9:92-101, 1991.

170. Favero M, Port F, Bernick J: In vivo studies of dialysis related endotoxemia and bacteremia. Nephron 37:307-312, 1981.

171. Klinkmann H, Falkenhagen D, Smollich BP: Investigation of the permeability of highly permeable polysulfone membranes for pyrogens. Contrib Nephrol 46:174-183, 1985.

172. Bingel M, Lonnemann G, Shaldon S, et al: Human interleukin-1 production during hemodialysis. Nephron 43:161-163, 1986.

173. Hakim RM, Breillatt J, Lazarus JM, Port FK: Complement activation and hypersensitivity reactions to dialysis membranes. N Engl J Med 311:878-882, 1984.

174. Cavallon J, Fitting C, Haeffner-Cavaillon N: Recombinant C5a enhances interleukin-1. Eur J Immunol 20:253-257, 1990.

175. Schindler R, Gelfand JA, Dinarello CA: Recombinant C5a stimulates transcription rather than translation of interleukin-1 (IL-1) and tumor necrosis factor: Translational signal provided by lipopolysaccharide or IL-1 itself. Blood 76:1631-1638, 1990.

176. Urena P, Herbelin A, Zingraff J, et al: Permeability of cellulosic and non-cellulosic membranes to endotoxin subunits and cytokine production during in-vitro haemodialysis. Nephrol Dial Transplant 7:16-28, 1992.

177. Gault MH, Duffett AL, Murphy JF, Purchase LH: In search of sterile, endotoxin-free dialysate. ASAIO J 38:431-435, 1992.

178. Centers for Disease Control and Prevention (CDC): Clusters of Bacteremia and Pyrogenic Reactions in Hemodialysis Patients: Georgia. Epidemic Investigation Report, EPI 86-65-2. Atlanta, CDC, April 22, 1987.

179. Centers for Disease Control and Prevention (CDC): Bacteremia associated with reuse of disposable hollow-fiber hemodialyzers. MMWR Morb Mortal Wkly Rep 35:417-418, 1986.

180. Centers for Disease Control and Prevention (CDC): Pyrogenic Reactions in Patients Undergoing High-Flux Hemodialysis: California. Epidemic Investigation Report, EPI 86-80-2. Atlanta, CDC, June 1, 1987, p 48.

181. Alter MJ, Favero MS, Miller JK, et al: Reuse of hemodialyzers. Results of nationwide surveillance for adverse effects. JAMA 260: 2073-2076, 1988.

182. Bland LA, Favero MS, Oxborrow GS, et al: Effect of chemical germicides on the integrity of hemodialyzer membranes. ASAIO Trans 34:172-175, 1988.

183. Jenkins S, Lin F, Lin R, et al: Pyrogenic reactions and *Pseudomonas* bacteremias in a hemodialysis center. Dial Transplant 16:192-197, 1987.

184. Oberle M, Favero M, Carson L, et al: Fatal endotoxemia in dialysis patients at a summer camp. Dial Transplant 9:549-550, 1980.

185. Bland L, Favero M: Microbiologic and endotoxin considerations in hemodialyzer reprocessing. *In* Association for the Advancement of Medical Instrumentation (eds): Dialysis, Vol 3. Arlington, VA, American National Standards, 1993, pp 45-52.

186. Gazenfield-Gazit E, Eliahou HE: Endotoxin antibodies in patients on maintenance hemodialysis. Isr J Med Sci 5:1032-1036, 1969.

187. Hakim RM, Friedrich RA, Lowrie EG: Formaldehyde kinetics and bacteriology in dialyzers. Kidney Int 28:936-943, 1985.

188. Kaufman AM, Frinak S, Godmere RO, Levin NW: Clinical experience with heat sterilization for reprocessing dialyzers. ASAIO J 38:338-340, 1992.

189. Vanholder R, Noens L, De Smet R, Ringoir S: Development of anti-N-like antibodies during formaldehyde reuse in spite of adequate predialysis rinsing. Am J Kidney Dis 11:477-480, 1988.

190. United States Department of Health and Human Services (USDHHS) and United States Food and Drug Administration (FDA): Paper T92-46. Atlanta, USDHHS & FDA, October 13, 1992.

191. Feldman HI, Kinosian M, Bilker WB, et al: Effect of dialyzer reuse on survival of patients treated with hemodialysis. JAMA 276: 620-625, 1996.

192. Chuang HY, Mohammad SF, Sharma NC, Mason RG: Interaction of human alpha-thrombin with artificial surfaces and reactivity of adsorbed alpha-thrombin. J Biomed Mater Res 14:467-476, 1980.

193. Cheung AK, Parker CJ, Janatova J, Brynda E: Modulation of complement activation on hemodialysis membranes by immobilized heparin. J Am Soc Nephrol 8:1328-1337, 1992.

194. Port FK, Wolfe RA, Hulbert-Shearon TE, et al: Mortality risk by hemodialyzer reuse practice and dialyzer membrane: Results from the USRDS Dialysis Morbidity and Mortality Study. Am J Kidney Dis 37:276-286, 2001.

195. Baris E, McGregor M: The reuse of hemodialyzers: An assessment of safety and potential savings. Can Med Assoc J 148:175-183, 1993.

196. Cazenave JP, Mulvilhill J: Interaction of blood with surfaces: Hemocompatibility and thromboresistance of biomaterials. Contrib Nephrol 62:118-127, 1988.

197. Ouseph R, Ward RA: Anticoagulation for intermittent hemodialysis. Semin Dial 13:181-187, 2000.

198. Gordon LA, Simon ER, Richards JM: Studies in regional heparinization. II. Artificial kidney hemodialysis without systemic heparinization—preliminary report of a method using simultaneous infusion of heparin and protamine. N Engl J Med 255:1063-1068, 1956.

199. Spencer P, Cozzi E, Easterling RE, Penner JA: Regional heparinization with hollow fiber artificial kidney. Proc Am Assoc Nephrol Nurses Technicians 4:69-72, 1977.

200. Lindholm DD, Murray JS: A simplified method of regional heparinization during hemodialysis according to a predetermined dosage formula. Trans Am Soc Artif Intern Organs 10:92-97, 1964.

201. Hampers CL, Blaufox MD, Merrill JP: Anticoagulation rebound after hemodialysis. N Engl J Med 275:776-781, 1966.

202. Blaufox MD, Hampers CL, Merrill JP: Heparinization for hemodialysis. Trans Am Soc Artif Intern Organs 12:207-209, 1966.

203. Schwab SJ, Onorato JJ, Sharar LR, Dennis PA: Hemodialysis without anticoagulation: One-year prospective trial in hospitalized patients at risk for bleeding. Am J Med 83:405-410, 1987.

204. Caruana R, Raja R, Bush J, et al: Heparin-free dialysis: Comparative data and results in high-risk patients. Kidney Int 31:1351-1355, 1987.

205. Charm S, Kurland G: Viscometry of human blood for shear rates 0-100,000 sec^{-1}. Nature 206:617-618, 1965.

206. Sigdell JE, Tersteegen B: Clearance of a dialyzer under varying operating conditions. Artif Organs 10:219-225, 1986.

207. Hootkins R, Bourgeois B: The effect of ultrafiltration on dialysance. Mathematical theory and experimental verification. Trans Am Soc Artif Intern Organs 37:M375-M377, 1991.

208. Waniewski J, Lucjanek P, Werynski A: Alternative descriptions of combined diffusive and convective mass transport in hemodialyzer. Artif Organs 17:3-7, 1993.

209. Tyagi VP, Abbas M: An exact analysis for solute transport, due to simultaneous dialysis and ultrafiltration in a hollow-fibre artificial kidney. Bull Math Biol 49:697-717, 1987.

210. Gupta BB, Jaffrin MY: In vitro study of the combined convection-diffusion mass transfer in hemodialysers. Int J Artif Organs 7: 263-268, 1984.

211. Sherman R, Levy SS: Rate-related recirculation: The effect of altering blood flow on dialyzer recirculation. Am J Kidney Dis 17: 170-173, 1991.

212. Sherman RA: Recirculation revisited. Semin Dial 4:221-223, 1991.

213. Schneditz D, Polaschegg HD, Levin NW, et al: Cardiopulmonary recirculation in dialysis—an underrecognized phenomenon. ASAIO J 38:M194-M196, 1992.

214. Schneditz D, Kaufman AM, Polaschegg HD, et al: Cardiopulmonary recirculation during hemodialysis. Kidney Int 42:1450-1456, 1992.

215. Depner TA, Rizwan S, Cheer A, Wagner J: Peripheral urea disequilibrium during hemodialysis is temperature-dependent. ASAIO Trans 37:141-143, 1991.

216. Sherman RA, Levy SS: Assessment of a two-needle technique for the measurement of recirculation during hemodialysis. Am J Kidney Dis 18:80-83, 1991.

217. Wang E, Schneditz D, Kaufman AM, Levin NW: Sensitivity and specificity of the thermodilution technique in detection of access recirculation. Nephron 85:134-141, 2000.

218. Magnasco A, Alloatti S, Bonfant G, et al: Glucose infusion test: A new screening test for vascular access recirculation. Kidney Int 57: 2123-2128, 2000.

219. Katzarski KS, Charra B, Luik AJ, et al: Fluid state and blood pressure control in patients treated with long and short haemodialysis. Nephrol Dial Transplant 14:369-375, 1999.

220. Charra B, Calemard E, Ruffet M, et al: Survival as an index of adequacy of dialysis. Kidney Int 41:1286-1291, 1992.

221. Alwall N: On the artificial kidney: I. Apparatus for dialysis of the blood in vivo. Acta Med Scand 128:317-323, 1947.

222. Wolf AV, Remp DG, Kiley JE, Currie GD: Artificial kidney function: Kinetics of hemodialysis. J Clin Invest 30:1062-1070, 1951.

223. Merrill JP, Schupak E, Cameron E, Hampers CL: Hemodialysis in the home. JAMA 190:466, 1964.

224. Boquin E, Parnell S, Grondin G, et al: Cross-over study of the effect of different dialysate sodium concentrations in large surface area short-term dialysis. Proc Clin Dial Transplant Forum 7:48-52, 1977.

225. Comty C, Rottka H, Shaldon S: Blood pressure control in patients with end-stage renal failure treated by intermittent hemodialysis. Proc Eur Dial Transplant Assoc 1:209-214, 1964.

226. Drukker W, Jungerius NA, Alberts C: Report on regular dialysis treatment in Europe. Proc Eur Dial Transplant Assoc 4:3, 1967.

227. Van Stone JC, Bauer J, Carey J: The effect of dialysate sodium concentration on body fluid distribution during hemodialysis. Trans Am Soc Artif Intern Organs 26:383-386, 1980.

228. Bosl R, Shideman JR, Meyer RM, et al: Effects and complications of high efficiency dialysis. Nephron 15:151-160, 1975.

229. Levine J, Falk B, Henriquez M, et al: Effects of varying dialysate sodium using large surface area dialyzers. Trans Am Soc Artif Intern Organs 24:139-141, 1978.

230. Henrich WL, Hunt JM, Nixon JV: Increased ionized calcium and left ventricular contractility during hemodialysis. N Engl J Med 310:19-23, 1984.

231. Bihaphala S, Bell AJ, Bennett CA, et al: Comparison of high-and low-sodium bicarbonate and acetate dialysis in stable chronic hemodialysis patients. Clin Nephrol 23:179-183, 1985.

232. Port FK, Johnson WJ, Klass DW: Prevention of dialysis disequilibrium syndrome by use of high sodium concentration in the dialysate. Kidney Int 3:327-333, 1973.

233. Flanigan MJ, Khairullah QT, Lim VS: Dialysate sodium delivery can alter chronic blood pressure management. Am J Kidney Dis 29:383-391, 1997.

234. Dumler F, Grondin G, Levin NW: Sequential high/low sodium hemodialysis: An alternative to ultrafiltration. Trans Am Soc Artif Intern Organs 25:351-353, 1979.

235. Raja R, Kramer M, Barber K, Chin S: Sequential changes in dialysate sodium (DNa) during hemodialysis. Trans Am Soc Artif Intern Organs 29:649-651, 1983.

236. Daugirdas JT, Al-Kudsi RR, Ing TS, Norusis MJ: A double-blind evaluation of sodium gradient hemodialysis. Am J Nephrol 5:163-168, 1985.

237. Song JH, Lee SW, Suh CK, Kim MJ: Time-averaged concentration of dialysate sodium relates with sodium load and interdialytic weight gain during sodium-profiling hemodialysis. Am J Kidney Dis 40:291-301, 2002.

238. Ketchersid TL, Van Stone JC: Dialysate potassium. Semin Dial 4:46-49, 1991.

239. Feig PU, Shook A, Sterns RH: Effect of potassium removal by hemodialysis. Nephron 27:25-30, 1981.

240. Sherman RA, Hwang ER, Bernholc AS, Eisinger RP: Variability in potassium removal by hemodialysis. Am J Nephrol 6:284-288, 1986.

241. Hou S, McElroy PA, Nootes S, Beach M: Safety and efficacy of low potassium dialysis. Am J Kidney Dis 13:137-143, 1989.

242. Karnik JA, Young BS, Lew NL, et al: Cardiac arrest and sudden death in dialysis units. Kidney Int 60:350-357, 2001.

243. Wing AJ: Optimum calcium concentration of dialysis fluid for hemodialysis. Br Med J 4:145-149, 1968.

244. Bone JM, Davison AM, Robson JS: Role of dialysate concentration on calcium mass transfer during maintenance hemodialysis. Lancet 1:1047-1048, 1972.

245. Fellner SK, Lang RM, Neumann A: Physiologic mechanisms for calcium-induced changes in systemic arterial pressure in stable dialysis patients. Hypertension 13:213-218, 1989.

246. Maynard JC, Cruz C, Kleerekoper M, Levin NW: Blood pressure response to changes in serum ionized calcium during hemodialysis. Ann Intern Med 104:358-361, 1986.

247. Sherman RA, Bialy GB, Gazinski B, et al: Th effect of dialysate calcium levels on blood pressure during hemodialysis. Am J Kidney Dis 8:244-247, 1986.

248. Wang CL, Lee WL, Wu MJ, et al: Increased QTc dispersion and mortality in uremic patients with acute myocardial infarction. Am J Kidney Dis 39:539-548, 2002.

249. Vaporean ML, Van Stone JC: Dialysate magnesium. Semin Dial 6:46-49, 1993.

250. Mion CM, Hegstrom RM, Boen ST, Scribner BH: Substitution of sodium acetate for bicarbonate in the bath fluid for hemodialysis. Trans Am Soc Artif Intern Organs 10:110-115, 1964.

251. Palmer BF: The effect of dialysate composition on systemic hemodynamics. Semin Dial 5:30-33, 1992.

252. Mendelssohn S, Swartz CD, Yudis M, et al: High glucose concentration dialysate in chronic hemodialysis. Trans Am Soc Artif Intern Organs 13:249-252, 1967.

253. Rosborough DC, Van Stone JC: Dialysis glucose. Semin Dial 6:260-263, 1993.

254. Berkes SL, Khan SI, Chazan JA, Garella S: Prolonged hemodialysis from overheated dialysate. Ann Intern Med 83:363-364, 1975.

255. Fortner RW, Nowakowski A, Carter CB, et al: Death due to overheated dialysate during dialysis. Ann Intern Med 73:443-444, 1970.

256. Maggiore Q, Pizzarelli F, Sisca S, et al: Blood temperature and vascular stability during hemodialysis and hemofiltration. ASAIO Trans 28:523-527, 1982.

257. Sherman RA, Rubin MP, Cody RP, Eisinger RP: Blood temperature and vascular stability during hemodialysis and hemofiltration. Am J Kidney Dis 5:124-127, 1985.

258. Sherman RA, Faustino EF, Bernholc AS, Eisinger RP: Effects of variations in dialysate temperature on blood pressure during hemodialysis. Am J Kidney Dis 4:66-68, 1984.

259. Coli U, Landinki S, Lucatello S, et al: Cold as cardiovascular stabilizing factor in hemodynamic evaluation. ASAIO Transactions 29:71-75, 1983.

260. Lindhold T, Thysell H, Yamamoto Y, et al: Temperature and vascular stability in hemodialysis. Nephron 39:130-133, 1985.

261. Kerr PG, van Bakel C, Dawborn JK: Assessment of the asymptomatic benefits of cool dialysate. Nephron 52:166-169, 1989.

262. Marcen R, Quereda C, Orfino L, et al: Hemodialysis with a low-temperature dialysate: A long-term experience. Nephron 49:29-32, 1988.

263. Orfino L, Marcen R, Quereda C, et al: Epidemiology of symptomatic hypotension in hemodialysis: Is cool dialysis beneficial for all patients? Am J Nephrol 10:177-180, 1990.

264. Rosales LM, Schneditz D, Morris AT, Rahmati S, Levin NW: Isothermic hemodialysis and ultrafiltration. Am J Kidney Dis 36:353-361, 2000.

265. Maggiore Q, Pizzarelli F, Santoro A, et al: The effects of control of thermal balance on vascular stability in hemodialysis patients: Results of the European randomized clinical trial. Am J Kidney Dis 40:280-290, 2002.

266. Shaldon S: Sequential ultrafiltration and dialysis. Proc Eur Dial Transplant Assoc 13:300-304, 1976.

267. Asaba H, Bergstrom J, Furst P, et al: Sequential ultrafiltration and diffusion as alternatives to conventional hemodialysis. Proc Clin Dial Transplant Forum 6:129-135, 1976.

268. Dheenan S, Henrich WL: Preventing dialysis hypotension: A comparison of usual protective maneuvers. Kidney Int 59:1175-1181, 2001.

269. Jaeger JQ, Mehta RL: Assessment of dry weight in hemodialysis: An overview. J Am Soc Nephrol 10:392-403, 1999.

270. Schneditz D, Roob J, Oswald M, et al: Nature and rate of vascular refilling during hemodialysis and ultrafiltration. Kidney Int 42:1425-1433, 1992.

271. Schneditz D, Pogglitsch H, Horina J, Binswanger U: A blood protein monitor for the continuous measurement of blood volume changes during hemodialysis. Kidney Int 38:342-346, 1990.

272. Leypoldt JK, Cheung AK, Steuer RR, et al: Determination of circulating blood volume by continuously monitoring hematocrit during hemodialysis. J Am Soc Nephrol 6:214-219, 1995.

273. Donauer J, Kölblin D, Bek M, et al: Ultrafiltration profiling and measurement of relative blood volume as strategies to reduce hemodialysis-related side effects. Am J Kidney Dis 36:115-123, 2000.

274. Oliver MJ, Edwards LJ, Churchill DN: Impact of sodium and ultrafiltration profiling on hemodialysis-related symptoms. J Am Soc Nephrol 12:151-156, 2001.

275. Santoro A, Mancini E, Paolini F, et al: Blood volume regulation during hemodialysis. Am J Kidney Dis 32:739-748, 1988.

276. United States Renal Data System (USRDS): USRDS 1999 Annual Data Report. Bethesda, MD, The National Institutes of Health, National Institute of Diabetes and Digestive and Kidney Disease, 1999.

277. Hakim RM: Assessing the adequacy of dialysis. Kidney Int 37:822-832, 1990.

278. Gotch FA, Yarian S, Keen M: A kinetic survey of US hemodialysis prescriptions. Am J Kidney Dis 15:511-515, 1990.

279. Sargent JA: Shortfalls in the delivery of dialysis. Am J Kidney Dis 15:500-510, 1990.

280. Hakim RM, Breyer J, Ismail N, Schulman G: Effects of dose of dialysis on morbidity and mortality. Am J Kidney Dis 23:661-669, 1994.

281. Collins AJ, Ma JZ, Umen A, Keshaviah P: Urea index and other predictors of hemodialysis patient survival. Am J Kidney Dis 23:272-282, 1994.

282. Dau P: Plasmapheresis therapy in myasthenia gravis. Muscle Nerve 3:468-482, 1980.
283. Babb AL, Farrell PC, Uvelli DA, Scribner BH: Hemodialyzer evaluation by examination of solute molecular spectra. Trans Am Soc Artif Intern Organs 18:98-105, 1972.
284. Schoots A, Mikkers F, Cramers C, et al: Uremic toxins and the elusive middle molecules. Nephron 38:1-8, 1984.
285. Vanholder R: Middle molecules as uremic toxins: Still a viable hypothesis. Semin Dial 7:65-68, 1994.
286. Malachi T, Bogin E, Gafter U, Levi J: Parathyroid hormone effect on the fragility of human young and old red blood cells in uremia. Nephron 42:52-57, 1986.
287. Bogin E, Massry SG, Harary I: Effect of parathyroid hormone on rat heart cells. J Clin Invest 67:1215-1227, 1981.
288. Hajjar SM, Fadda GZ, Thanakitcharu P, et al: Reduced activity of Na(+)-K+ ATPase of pancreatic islets in chronic renal failure: Role of secondary hyperparathyroidism. J Am Soc Nephrol 2:1355-1359, 1992.
289. Perna AF, Smogorzewski M, Massry SG: Effects of verapamil on the abnormalities in fatty acid oxidation of myocardium. Kidney Int 36:453-457, 1989.
290. Fadda GZ, Akmal M, Premdas FH, et al: Insulin release from pancreatic islets: Effects of CRF and excess PTH. Kidney Int 33:1066-1072, 1988.
291. Gejyo F, Brancaccio D: Beta-2-microglobulin: A possible new uremic toxin? Int J Artif Organs 11:3-5, 1988.
292. Eschbach JW, Abdulhadi MH, Browne JK, et al: Recombinant human erythropoietin in anemic patients with end-stage renal disease. Ann Intern Med 111:992-1000, 1989.
293. Lowrie EG, Laird NM, Parker TF, Sargent JA: Effect of the hemodialysis prescription on patient morbidity: Report from the National Cooperative Dialysis Study. N Engl J Med 305:1176-1181, 1981.
294. Sargent JA, Gotch FA: The analysis of concentration dependence of uremic lesions in clinical studies. Kidney Int Suppl Jan(2):35-44, 1975.
295. Lowrie EG, Lew NL: Death risk in hemodialysis patients: The predictive value of commonly measured variables and an evaluation of death rate differences between facilities. Am J Kidney Dis 15:458-482, 1990.
296. Gotch FA, Sargent JA: A mechanistic analysis of the National Cooperative Dialysis Study (NCDS). Kidney Int 28:526-534, 1985.
297. Keshaviah P: Urea kinetic and middle molecule approaches to assessing the adequacy of hemodialysis and CAPD. Kidney Int Suppl 40:28-38, 1993.
298. Charra B, Calemard E, Ruffet M, et al: Survival as an index of adequacy of dialysis. Kidney Int 41:1286-1291, 1992.
299. Canada–USA (CANUSA) Peritoneal Dialysis Study Group: Adequacy of dialysis and nutrition in continuous peritoneal dialysis: Association with clinical outcome. J Am Soc Nephrol 7:198-207, 1996.
300. National Kidney Foundation Dialysis Outcomes Quality Initiative (DOQI): Clinical practice guidelines for hemodialysis adequacy. V. Prescribed dose of hemodialysis. Am J Kidney Dis 30:S86, 1997.
301. National Kidney Foundation Dialysis Outcomes Quality Initiative (DOQI): Clinical practice guidelines for hemodialysis adequacy. V. Adequate dose of peritoneal dialysis. Am J Kidney Dis 30: 1997.
302. Eggers PW: Mortality rates among dialysis patients in Medicare's End-Stage Renal Disease Program. Am J Kidney Dis 15:414-421, 1990.
303. Owen WF, Lew NL, Liu Y, et al: The urea reduction ratio and serum albumin concentration as predictors of mortality in patients undergoing hemodialysis. N Engl J Med 329:1001-1006, 1993.
304. Pierratos A, Ouwendyk M, Francoeur R, Vet al: Nocturnal hemodialysis: Three-year experience. J Am Soc Nephrol 9:859-868, 1998.
305. Mucsi I, Hercz G, Uldall R, et al: Control of serum phosphate without any phosphate binders in patients treated with nocturnal hemodialysis. Kidney Int 53:1399-1404, 1998.
306. Schneditz D, Van Stone JC, Daugirdas JT: A regional blood circulation alternative to in-series two compartment urea kinetic modeling. ASAIO J 39:573-577, 1993.
307. Van Stone J, Daugirdas J: Physiologic principles. *In* Daugirdas J, Ing T (eds): Handbook of Dialysis, 2nd ed. Boston, Little, Brown, 1994, pp 13-29.
308. Shackman R, Chisholm G, Holden A, et al: Urea distribution in the body after hemodialysis. Br Med J 34:817-882, 1962.

309. Schleifer C, Snyder S, Jones K: The influence of urea kinetic modeling on gross mortality in haemodialysis. Abstract. J Am Soc Nephrol 2:349, 1991.
310. Frost TH, Kerr DN: Kinetics of hemodialysis: A theoretical study of the removal of solutes in chronic renal failure compared with normal health. Kidney Int 12:41-50, 1977.
311. Heineken F, Evans M, Keen M: Intercompartmental fluid shifts in hemodialysis patients. Biotechnol Prog 3:69-74, 1987.
312. Tsang H, Leonard E, Lefavour G, et al: Urea dynamics during and immediately after dialysis. ASAIO J 8:251-260, 1985.
313. Kjellstrand C, Kjellstrand P, Skroder R, et al: Dialysis kinetics using pre and post concentrations of BUN are not accurate. J Am Soc Nephrol 3:375, 1992.
314. Spiegel DM, Baker PL, Babcock S, et al: Hemodialysis urea rebound: The effect of increasing dialysis efficiency. Am J Kidney Dis 25:26-29, 1995.
315. Daugirdas JT, Schneditz D: Overestimation of hemodialysis dose depends on dialysis efficiency by regional blood flow but not by conventional two pool urea kinetic analysis. ASAIO J 41:719-724, 1995.
316. Eknoyan G, Beck GJ, Cheung AK, et al: Effect of dialysis dose and membrane flux in maintenance hemodialysis. N Engl J Med 347:2010-2019, 2002.
317. Eknoyan G, Levey A, Beck G, Schulman G: The hemodialysis (HEMO) study: Rationale for selection of interventions. Semin Dial 9:24-33, 1996.
318. Lindsay RM, Kortas C: Hemeral (daily) hemodialysis. Adv Ren Replace Ther 8:236-249, 2001.
319. Raj DS, Charra B, Pierratos A, Work J: In search of ideal hemodialysis: Is prolonged frequent dialysis the answer? Am J Kidney Dis 34:597-610, 1999.
320. Lindsay RM, Spanner E: A hypothesis: The protein catabolic rate is dependent upon the type and amount of treatment in dialyzed uremic patients. Am J Kidney Dis 13:382-389, 1989.
321. Lacson E, Diaz-Buxo JA: Daily and nocturnal hemodialysis: How do they stack up? Am J Kidney Dis 38:225-239, 2001.
322. Pierratos A, Ouwendyk M, Rassi M: Total body nitrogen increases on nocturnal hemodialysis. Abstract. J Am Soc Nephrol 10:299A, 1999.
323. O'Sullivan DA, McCarthy JT, Kumar R, Williams AW: Improved biochemical variables, nutrient intake, and hormonal factors in slow nocturnal hemodialysis: A pilot study. Mayo Clin Proc 73:1035-1045, 1998.
324. Raj DS, Ouwendyk M, Francoeur R, Pierratos A: Plasma amino acid profile on nocturnal hemodialysis. Blood Purif 18:97-102, 2000.
325. Andre MB, Rembold SM, Pereira CM, Lugon JR: Prospective evaluation of an in-center daily hemodialysis program: Results of two years of treatment. Am J Nephrol 22:473-479, 2002.
326. Simonsen O: Slow nocturnal dialysis (SND) as a rescue treatment for children and young patients with ESRD. Abstract. J Am Soc Nephrol 18:165A, 2002.
327. Chertow GM, Owen WF, Lazarus JM, et al: Exploring the reverse J-shaped curve between urea reduction ratio and mortality. Kidney Int 56:1872-1878, 1999.
328. Frankenfield DL, McClellan WM, Helgerson SD, et al: Relationship between urea reduction ratio, demographic characteristics, and body weight for patients in the 1996 National ESRD Core Indicators Project. Am J Kidney Dis 33:584-591, 1999.
329. Price DA, Owen WF Jr: African-Americans on maintenance dialysis: A review of racial differences in incidence, treatment, and survival. Adv Ren Replace Ther 4:3-12, 1997.
330. Owen WF Jr, Chertow GM, Lazarus JM, Lowrie EG: Dose of hemodialysis and survival: Differences by race and sex. JAMA 280:1764-1768, 1998.
331. Zhensheng L, Lew N, Lazarus M, et al: Comparing the urea reduction ratio and the urea product as outcome-based measures of hemodialysis dose. Am J Kidney Dis 35:598-605, 2000.
332. Lowrie EG, Zhu X, Lew NL: Primary associates of mortality among dialysis patients: Trends and reassessment of Kt/V and urea reduction ratio as outcome-based measures of dialysis dose. Am J Kidney Dis 32:16-31, 1998.
333. Kopple JD, Zhu X, Lew NL, Lowrie EG: Body weight-for-height relationships predict mortality in maintenance hemodialysis patients. Kidney Int 56:1136-1148, 1999.
334. Fleischmann E, Teal N, Dudley J, et al: Influence of excess weight on mortality and hospital stay in 1346 hemodialysis patients. Kidney Int 55:1560-1567, 1999.

335. Wolfe RA, Ashby VB, Daugirdas JT, et al: Body size, dose of hemodialysis, and mortality. Am J Kidney Dis 35:80-88, 2000.

336. Lowrie EG, Chertow GM, Lew NL, et al: The urea (clearance × dialysis time) product (Kt) as an outcome-based measure of hemodialysis dose. Kidney Int 56:729-737, 1999.

337. Gotch FA: Is Kt/V urea a satisfactory measure for dosing the newer dialysis regimens? Semin Dial 14:15-17, 2001.

338. Vanholder R, Argiles A, Baurmeister U, et al: Uremic toxicity: Present state of the art. Int J Artif Organs 24:695-725, 2001.

339. Erslev AJ: Humoral regulation of red cell production. Blood 8: 349-387, 1953.

340. Eschbach JW, Egrie JC, Downing MR, et al: Correction of anemia of end stage renal disease with recombinant human erythropoietin: Results of a combined phase I and II clinical trial. N Engl J Med 316:73-78, 1987.

341. Eschbach JW, Kelly MR, Haley NR, et al: Treatment of the anemia of progressive renal failure with recombinant human erythropoietin. N Engl J Med 321:158-163, 1989.

342. Verbeelen D, Bossuyt A, Smitz J, et al: Hemodynamics of patients with renal failure treated with recombinant human erythropoietin. Clin Nephrol 31:6-11, 1989.

343. Satoh K, Masuda T, Ikida Y, et al: Hemodynamic changes by recombinant erythropoietin therapy in hemodialyzed patients. Hypertension 15:262-266, 1990.

344. Mayer G, Cada EV, Watzinger U, et al: Hemodynamic effects of partial correction of chronic anemia by recombinant human erythropoietin in patients on dialysis. Am J Kidney Dis 17:286-289, 1991.

345. Low I, Grutzmacher P, Bergmann M, Schoeppe W: Echocardiographic findings in patients on maintenance hemodialysis substituted with recombinant human erythropoietin. Clin Nephrol 31:26-30, 1989.

346. Cannella G, La Canna G, Sandrini M, et al: Reversal of left ventricular hypertrophy following recombinant human erythropoietin treatment of anaemic dialysed uraemic patients. Nephrol Dial Transplant 6:31-37, 1991.

347. Pascual J, Teruel JL, Moya JL, et al: Regression of left ventricular hypertrophy after partial correction of anemia with erythropoietin in patients on hemodialysis: A prospective study. Clin Nephrol 35: 280-287, 1991.

348. Zehnder C, Zumer M, Sulzer M, et al: Influence of long-term amelioration of anemia and blood pressure control on left ventricular hypertrophy in hemodialyzed patients. Nephron 61:21-25, 1992.

349. Bommer J, Kugel M, Schwobel B, et al: Improved sexual function during recombinant human erythropoietin therapy. Nephrol Dial Transplant 5:204-207, 1990.

350. Shaefer RM, Kokot F, Wernze H, et al: Improved sexual function in hemodialysis patients on recombinant erythropoietin: A possible role for prolactin. Clin Nephrol 31:1-5, 1989.

351. Braumann KM, Nonnast DB, Boning D, Bocker A: Improved physical performance after treatment of renal anemia with recombinant human erythropoietin. Nephron 58:129-134, 1991.

352. Delano BG: Improvements in quality of life following treatment with r-HuEPO in anemic hemodialysis patients. Am J Kidney Dis 14:14-18, 1989.

353. Evans RW, Rader B, Manninen DL, et al: The quality of life of hemodialysis recipients treated with recombinant human erythropoietin. JAMA 263:825-830, 1990.

354. Evans RW: Recombinant human erythropoietin and the quality of life of end-stage renal disease patients: A comparative analysis. Am J Kidney Dis 18:62-70, 1991.

355. Ali M, Fayemi AO, Rigolosi R, et al: Hemosiderosis in hemodialysis patients: An autopsy study of 50 cases. JAMA 244:343-345, 1980.

356. Bregman H, Gelfand MC, Winchester JF, et al: HLA-linked iron overload and myopathy in maintenance hemodialysis patients. Trans Am Soc Artif Intern Organs 26:366-368, 1980.

357. Hakim RM, Stivelman JC, Schulman G, et al: Iron overload and mobilization in long-term hemodialysis patients. Am J Kidney Dis 10:293-299, 1987.

358. Kaufman JS, Reda DJ, Fye CL, et al: Subcutaneous compared with intravenous epoetin in patients receiving hemodialysis. N Engl J Med 339:578-583, 1998.

359. Besarab A, Reyes CM, Hornberger J: Meta-analysis of subcutaneous versus intravenous epoetin in maintenance treatment of anemia in hemodialysis patients. Am J Kidney Dis 40:439-446, 2002.

360. Besarab A, Bolton WK, Browne JK, et al: The effects of normal as compared with low hematocrit values in patients with cardiac disease who are receiving hemodialysis and erythropoietin. N Engl J Med 339:584-590, 1998.

361. Foley RN, Parfrey PS, Morgan J, et al: Effect of hemoglobin levels in hemodialysis patients with asymptomatic cardiomyopathy. Kidney Int 58:1325-1335, 2000.

362. Moreno F, Sanz-Guajardo D, Lopez-Gomez JM, et al: Increasing the hematocrit has a beneficial effect on quality of life and is safe in selected hemodialysis patients. J Am Soc Nephrol 11:335-342, 2000.

363. Collins AJ, Li S, St Peter W, et al: Death, hospitalization, and economic associations among incident hemodialysis patients with hematocrit values of 36 to 39%. J Am Soc Nephrol 12:2465-2473, 2001.

364. Radtke HW, Frei U, Erbes PM, et al: Improving anemia by hemodialysis: Effect on serum erythropoietin. Kidney Int 17: 382-387, 1980.

365. Santiago GC, Sreepada Rao TK, Laird NM: Effect of dialysis therapy on the hematopoietic system: The NCDS. Kidney Int Suppl 23:S95-S100, 1983.

366. Lindsay RM, Burton JA, Dargie HJ, et al: Dialyzer blood loss. Clin Nephrol 1:24-34, 1973.

367. Sweet SJ, McCarthy S, Steingart R, Callahan T: Hemolytic reactions mechanically induced by kinked hemodialysis lines. Am J Kidney Dis 27:262-266, 1996.

368. Hampers CL, Streiff R, Nathan DG, et al: Megaloblastic hematopoiesis in uremia and in patients on long-term dialysis. N Engl J Med 276:551-554, 1967.

369. Ibbotson T, Goa KL: Darbepoetin alfa. Review. Drugs 61:2097-2104, 2001.

370. Locatelli F, Olivares J, Walker R, et al: Novel erythropoiesis stimulating protein for treatment of anemia in chronic renal insufficiency. Kidney Int 60:741-747, 2001.

371. Macdougall IC, Gray SJ, Elston O, et al: Pharmacokinetics of novel erythropoiesis stimulating protein compared with epoetin alfa in dialysis patients. J Am Soc Nephrol 10:2392-2395, 1999.

372. Tang IY, Vrahnos D, Valaitis D, Lau A: Vascular access thrombosis during recombinant human erythropoietin therapy. ASAIO J 38: M528-M531, 1992.

373. Wingard RL, Parker RA, Ismail N, Hakim RM: Efficacy of oral iron therapy in patients receiving recombinant human erythropoietin. Am J Kidney Dis 25:433-439, 1995.

374. Besarab A, Amin N, Ahsan M, et al: Optimization of epoetin therapy with intravenous iron therapy in hemodialysis patients. J Am Soc Nephrol 11:530-538, 1999.

375. Fishbane S, Shapiro W, Dutka P, et al: A randomized trial of iron deficiency testing strategies in hemodialysis patients. Kidney Int 60:2406-2411, 2001.

376. Macdougall IC, Chandler G, Elston O, Harchowal J: Beneficial effects of adopting an aggressive intravenous iron policy in a hemodialysis unit. Am J Kidney Dis 23(suppl):S40-S46, 1999.

377. Feldman HI, Santanna J, Guo W, et al: Iron administration and clinical outcomes in hemodialysis patients. J Am Soc Nephrol 13: 734-744, 2002.

378. Salahudeen AK, Oliver B, Bower JD, Roberts LJ: Increase in plasma esterified F_2-isoprostanes following intravenous iron infusion in patients on hemodialysis. Kidney Int 60:1525-1531, 2001.

379. Roob JM, Khoschsorur G, Tiran A, et al: Vitamin E attenuates oxidative stress induced by intravenous iron in patients on hemodialysis. J Am Soc Nephrol 11:539-549, 2000.

380. Fishbane S, Ungureanu VD, Maesaka JK, et al: The safety of intravenous iron dextran in hemodialysis patients. Am J Kidney Dis 28:529-534, 1996.

381. Chandler G, Harchowal J, Macdougall IC: Intravenous iron sucrose: Establishing a safe dose. Am J Kidney Dis 38:988-991, 2001.

382. Michael B, Coyne DW, Fishbane S, et al, for the Ferlecit Publication Committee: Sodium ferric gluconate complex in hemodialysis patients: Adverse reactions compared with placebo and iron dextran. Kidney Int 61:1830-1839, 2002.

383. Van Wyck DB, Cavallo G, Spinowitz BS, et al: Safety and efficacy of iron sucrose in patients sensitive to iron dextran: North American Clinical Trial. Am J Kidney Dis 36:88-97, 2000.

384. Coyne DW, Adkinson NF, Nissenson AR, et al, for the Ferlecit Investigators: Sodium ferric gluconate complex in hemodialysis patients: II. Adverse reactions in iron dextran-sensitive and dextran tolerant patients. Kidney Int 63:217-224, 2003.

385. Foley RN, Parfrey PS, Sarnak MJ: Clinical epidemiology of cardiovascular disease in chronic renal disease. Am J Kidney Dis 32: S112-S119, 1998.

386. Lindner A, Charra B, Sherrard DJ, Scribner BH: Accelerated atherosclerosis and prolonged maintenance hemodialysis. N Engl J Med 290:697-701, 1974.

387. Scribner BH: The treatment of chronic uremia by means of intermittent hemodialysis: A preliminary report. Trans Am Soc Artif Intern Organs 6:114-122, 1960.

388. Goldsmith DJA, Covic A: Coronary artery disease in uremia: Etiology, diagnosis, and therapy. Kidney Int 60:2059-2078, 2001.

389. Sinha SK: Coronary angiography and coronary artery by-pass grafts in diabetics. Diabetes Res Clin Pract 30:89-92, 1996.

390. Schwarz U, Buzello M, Ritz E, et al: Morphology of coronary atherosclerotic lesions in patients with end-stage renal failure. Nephrol Dial Transplant 15:218-223, 2000.

391. Cheung AK, Wu LL, Kabitz C, Leypoldt JK: Atherogenic lipids and lipoproteins in hemodialysis patients. Am J Kidney Dis 11:271-276, 1993.

392. Cressman MD, Aboud D, O'Neil J, et al: Lp(a) and premature mortality during chronic hemodialysis treatment. Chem Phys Lipids 67-68:419-427, 1994.

393. Goldwasser P, Kaldas AI, Barth RH: Rise in serum albumin and creatinine in the first half year on hemodialysis. Kidney Int 56:2260-2268, 1999.

394. Kronenberg F, Neyer U, Lhotta K, et al: The low molecular weight apo(a) phenotype is an independent predictor for coronary artery disease in hemodialysis patients: A prospective follow-up. J Am Soc Nephrol 10:1027-1036, 1999.

395. Longenecker JC, Klag MJ, Marcovina SM, et al: Small apolipoprotein(a) size predicts mortality in end-stage renal disease—the CHOICE Study. Circulation 106:2812-2818, 2002.

396. Bostom AG, Lathrop L: Hyperhomocysteinemia in end-stage renal disease: Prevalence, etiology, and potential relationship to arteriosclerotic outcomes. Kidney Int 52:10-20, 1997.

397. Suliman ME, Qureshi AR, Barany P: Hyperhomocysteinemia, nutritional status, and cardiovascular disease in hemodialysis patients. Kidney Int 57:1727-1735, 2000.

398. Kaysen GA: The microinflammatory state in uremia: Causes and potential consequences. Abstract. J Am Soc Nephrol 12:1549-1557, 2001.

399. Arici M, Walls J: End-stage renal disease, atherosclerosis, and cardiovascular mortality: Is C-reactive protein the missing link? Kidney Int 59:407-414, 2001.

400. Cheung AK, Sarnak MJ, Yan G, et al, for the Hemodialysis (HEMO) Study: Atherosclerotic cardiovascular disease risks in chronic hemodialysis patients. Kidney Int 58:353-362, 2000.

401. Kaysen GA, Chertow GM, Adhikarla R, et al: Inflammation and dietary protein intake exert competing effects on serum albumin and creatinine in hemodialysis patients. Kidney Int 60:333-340, 2001.

402. Stenvinkel P, Heimburger O, Paultre F, et al: Strong association between malnutrition, inflammation, and atherosclerosis in chronic renal failure. Kidney Int 51:1899-1911, 1999.

403. Kato A, Odamaki M, Takita T, et al: Association between interleukin-6 and carotid atherosclerosis in hemodialysis patients. Kidney Int 61:1143-1152, 2002.

404. Pecoits-Filho R, Bárány P, Lindholm B, et al: Interleukin-6 is an independent predictor of mortality in patients starting dialysis treatment. Nephrol Dial Transplant 17:1684-1688, 2002.

405. Shlipak MG, Fried LF, Crump C, et al: Cardiovascular disease risk status in elderly persons with renal insufficiency. Kidney Int 62:997-1004, 2002.

406. Ayus JC, Sheikh-Hamad D: Silent infection in clotted hemodialysis access grafts. J Am Soc Nephrol 9:1314-1317, 1998.

407. Hakim RM: Clinical implications of hemodialysis membrane biocompatibility. Kidney Int 44:484-494, 1993.

408. Himmelfarb J, Ikizler TA, Stenvinkel P, Hakim RM: The elephant in uremia: Reflections on oxidant stress as a unifying concept. Kidney Int 62:1524-1538, 2002.

409. Boaz M, Smetana S, Weinstein T, et al: Secondary prevention with antioxidants of cardiovascular disease in end stage renal disease (SPACE): Randomised placebo-controlled trial. Lancet 356:1213-1218, 2000.

410. Tepel M, van der Giet M, Statz M, et al: The antioxidant acetylcysteine reduces cardiovascular events in patients with end-stage renal failure: A controlled trial. Abstract. Circulation 107:992, 2003.

411. Guerin AP, London GM, Marchais SJ, et al: Arterial stiffening and vascular calcifications in end-stage renal disease. Nephrol Dial Transplant 15:1014-1021, 2000.

412. Kassen PS, Lowrie EG, Reddan DN, et al: Association between pulse pressure and mortality in patients undergoing maintenance hemodialysis. JAMA 287:1548-1555, 2002.

413. Tozawa M, Iseki K, Iseki C, Takishita S: Pulse pressure and risk of total mortality and cardiovascular events in patients on chronic hemodialysis. Kidney Int 61:717-726, 2002.

414. Beaubien ER, Pylypchuk GB, Akhtar J, Biem HJ: Value of corrected QT interval dispersion in identifying patients initiating dialysis at increased risk of total and cardiovascular mortality. Am J Kidney Dis 39:834-842, 2002.

415. Zoccali C, Mallamaci F, Tripepi G: Nocturnal hypoxemia predicts incident cardiovascular complications in dialysis patients. J Am Soc Nephrol 13:729-733, 2002.

416. Zoccali C, Benedetto FA, Maas R, et al, for the CREED Investigators: Asymmetric dimethylarginine, C-reactive protein, and carotid intima-media thickness in end-stage renal disease. J Am Soc Nephrol 13:490-496, 2002.

417. Tornig J, Amann K, Ritz E, et al: Arteriolar wall thickening, capillary rarefaction and interstitial fibrosis in the heart of rats with renal failure: The effects of ramiprik, nifedipine, and moxonidine. J Am Soc Nephrol 7:667-675, 1996.

418. van Guldener C, Lambert J, Janssen MJ, et al: Endothelium-dependent vasodilatation and distensibility of large arteries in chronic haemodialysis patients. Nephrol Dial Transplant 12:14-18, 1997.

419. Narita M, Kurihara T, Sindoh T, et al: Characteristics of myocardial ischemia in patients with chronic renal failure and its relation to cardiac sympathetic activity. Kaku Igaku 36:979-987, 1999.

420. Amann K, Mall G, Ritz E: Myocardial interstitial fibrosis in uraemia: Is it relevant? Nephrol Dial Transplant 9:127-128, 1994.

421. Raine AE, Seymour AM, Roberts AF, et al: Impairment of cardiac function and energetics in experimental renal failure. J Clin Invest 92:2934-2940, 1993.

422. Pidgeon GB, Lynn KL, Bailey RR, Robson RA: Coronary angiography prior to renal transplantation. Nephrology 1:59-64, 1995.

423. Braun WE, Phillips DF, Vidt DG: Coronary artery disease in 100 diabetics with end-stage renal failure. Transplant Proc 16:603-607, 1984.

424. Kremastinos D, Paraskevaidis I, Voudiklari S, et al: Painless myocardial ischemia in chronic hemodialysed patients: A real event? Nephron 60:164-170, 1992.

425. Robinson TG, Carr SJ: Cardiovascular autonomic dysfunction in uremia. Kidney Int 62:1921-1932, 2002.

426. Murphy SW, Foley RN, Parfrey PS: Screening and treatment for cardiovascular disease in patients with chronic renal disease. Am J Kidney Dis 32(suppl 3):S184-S199, 1998.

427. Reis G, Marcovitz PA, Leichtman AB, et al: Usefulness of dobutamine stress-echocardiography in detecting coronary artery disease in end-stage renal disease. Am J Cardiol 75:707-710, 1995.

428. Herzog CA: Acute myocardial infarction in patients with end-stage renal disease. Kidney Int Suppl 56:S130-S133, 1999.

429. Herzog CA: Poor long-term survival of dialysis patients after acute myocardial infarction: Bad treatment or bad disease? Am J Kidney Dis 35:1217-1220, 2000.

430. Chertow GM, Normand SL, Silva LR, McNeill BJ: Survival after acute myocardial infarction in patients with end-stage renal disease: Results from the Cooperative Cardiovascular Project. Am J Kidney Dis 35:1044-1051, 2000.

431. Herzog MD, Ma JZ, Collins AJ: Poor long-term survival after acute myocardial infarction among patients on long-term dialysis. N Engl J Med 339:799-805, 1998.

432. Herzog MD, Ma JZ, Collins AJ: Comparative survival of dialysis patients in the United States after coronary angioplasty, coronary artery stenting, and coronary artery bypass surgery and impact of diabetes. Circulation 106:2207-2211, 2002.

433. Le Feuvre C: Angioplasty and stenting in patients with renal disease. Heart 83:7-8, 2000.

434. London GM, Pannier B, Guerin AP, et al: Alterations of left ventricular hypertrophy in and survival of patients receiving hemodialysis: Follow-up of an interventional study. J Am Soc Nephrol 12:2759-2767, 2001.

435. Silberberg JS, Barre PE, Prichard SS, Sniderman AD: Impact of left ventricular hypertrophy on survival in end-stage renal disease. Kidney Int 36:286-290, 1989.

436. Foley RN, Parfrey PS, Harnett JD, et al: Hypoalbuminemia, cardiac morbidity and mortality in end-stage renal disease. J Am Soc Nephrol 7:728-736, 1996.

437. Wanner C: C-reactive protein risk prediction: Adding cardiac hypertrophy to the list. Am J Kidney Dis 40:1340-1341, 2002.
438. Braun J, Oldendorf M, Moshage W, et al: Electron beam computed tomography in the evaluation of cardiac calcification in chronic dialysis patients. Am J Kidney Dis 27:394-401, 1996.
439. Goodman WG, Goldin J, Kuizon BD, et al: Coronary-artery calcification in young adults with end-stage renal disease who are undergoing dialysis. N Engl J Med 342:1478-1483, 2000.
440. Ahmed S, O'Neill KD, Hood AF, et al: Calciphylaxis is associated with hyperphosphatemia and increased osteopontin expression by vascular smooth muscle cells. Am J Kidney Dis 37:1267-1276, 2001.
441. Block GA, Hulbert-Shearon TE, Levin NW, Port FK: Association of serum phosphorus and calcium × phosphate product with mortality risk in hemodialysis patients. Am J Kidney Dis 31:601-617, 1998.
442. Davies MR, Hruska KA: Pathophysiological mechanisms of vascular calcification in end-stage renal disease. Kidney Int 60:472-479, 2001.
443. Ganesh SK, Stack AG, Levin NW, et al: Association of elevated serum CA × PO4 product, and parathyroid hormone with cardiac mortality risk in chronic hemodialysis patients. J Am Soc Nephrol 12:2131-2138, 2001.
444. Wang AYM, Woo J, Wang M, et al: Association of inflammation and malnutrition with cardiac valve calcification in continuous ambulatory peritoneal dialysis patients. J Am Soc Nephrol 12:1927-1936, 2001.
445. Chertow GM, Burke SK, Lazarus JM, et al: Poly(allylamine hydrochloride) (Rena Gel): A noncalcemic phosphate binder for the treatment of hyperphosphatemia in chronic renal failure. Am J Kidney Dis 29:66-71, 1997.
446. Chertow GM, Burke SK, Raggi P, for the Treat to Goal Working Group: Sevelamer attenuates the progression of coronary and aortic calcification in hemodialysis patients. Kidney Int 62:245-252, 2002.
447. Ilkani R, Gardezi S, Hedayati H, Schein M: Necrotizing mastopathy caused by calciphylaxis: A case report. Surgery 122:967-968, 1997.
448. Loynes JT: A rare cause of breast necrosis: Calciphylaxis. Postgrad Med 106:161-162, 1999.
449. Morris DG, Fisher AH, Abboud J: Breast infarction after internal mammary artery harvest in a patient with calciphylaxis. Ann Thorac Surg 64:1469-1471, 1997.
450. Patetsios P, Bernstein M, Kim S, et al: Severe necrotizing mastopathy caused by calciphylaxis alleviated by total parathyroidectomy. Am Surg 66:1056-1058, 2000.
451. Ruggian JC, Maesaka JK, Fishbane S: Proximal calciphylaxis in four insulin-requiring diabetic hemodialyis patients. Am J Kidney Dis 28:409-414, 1996.
452. Wilmer WA, Magro CM: Calciphylaxis: Emerging concepts in prevention, diagnosis, and treatment. Semin Dial 15:172-186, 2003.
453. Mazhar AR, Johnson RJ, Gillen D, et al: Risk factors and mortality associated with calciphylaxis in end-stage renal disease. Kidney Int 60:324-332, 2001.
454. Khafif RA, Delima C, Silverberg A, et al: Acute hyperparathyroidism with systemic calcinosis: Report of a case. Arch Intern Med 149:681-684, 1989.
455. Wilmer WA, Voroshilova O, Singh I, et al: Transcutaneous oxygen tension in patients with calciphylaxis. Am J Kidney Dis 37:797-806, 2001.
456. Selye H, Golie I, Strebel R: Calciphylaxis in relation to calcification in periarticular tissues. Clin Orthop 28:181-192, 1963.
457. Selye H, Somogyi A, Mecs I: Inhibition of local calcergy by topical application of calciphylactic challengers. Calcif Tissue Res 2:67-76, 1968.
458. Hakim RM, Levin NW: Malnutrition in hemodialysis patients. Am J Kidney Dis 21:125-137, 1993.
459. Kaysen GA, Dubin JA, Muller HG, et al, for the (HEMO) Study Group: The acute-phase response varies with time and predicts serum albumin levels in hemodialysis patients. Kidney Int 58:346-352, 2000.
460. Sreedhara R, Avram MM, Blanco M, et al: Prealbumin is the best nutritional predictor of survival in hemodialysis and peritoneal dialysis. Am J Kidney Dis 28:937-942, 1996.
461. Sanaka T, Shinobe M, Ando M, et al: IGF-I as an early indicator of malnutrition in patients with end-stage renal disease. Nephron 67:73-81, 1994.
462. Parker TF, Wingard RL, Husni L, et al: Effect of the membrane biocompatibility on nutritional parameters in chronic hemodialysis patients. Kidney Int 49:551-556, 1996.
463. Pollock CA, Ibels LS, Allen BJ: Nutritional markers and survival in maintenance dialysis patients. Nephron 74:625-641, 1996.
464. Stenver DI, Gotfredsen A, Hilsted J, Nielsen B: Body composition in hemodialysis patients measured by dual-energy x-ray absorptiometry. Am J Nephrol 15:105-110, 1995.
465. Chertow GM, Lowrie EG, Wilmore DW, et al: Nutritional assessment with bioelectrical impedance analysis in maintenance hemodialysis patients. J Am Soc Nephrol 6:75-81, 1995.
466. Borah MF, Schoenfeld PY, Gotch FA, et al: Nitrogen balance during intermittent dialysis therapy of uremia. Kidney Int 14:491-500, 1978.
467. Sargent J, Gotch F, Borah M, et al: Urea kinetics: A guide to nutritional management of renal failure. Am J Clin Nutr 31:1696-1702, 1978.
468. Schneeweiss B, Graninger W, Stockenhuber F, et al: Energy metabolism in acute and chronic renal failure. Am J Clin Nutr 52:596-601, 1990.
469. Ikizler TA, Wingard RL, Sun M, et al: Increased energy expenditure in hemodialysis patients. J Am Soc Nephrol 7:2646-2653, 1996.
470. Chanard J, Toupance O, Gillery P, Lavaud S: Evaluation of protein loss during hemofiltration. Kidney Int Suppl 33:S114-S116, 1988.
471. Graeber CW, Halley SE, Lapkin RA, et al: Protein losses with reused dialyzer. Abstract. J Am Soc Nephrol 4:349, 1993.
472. Guitierrez A, Alvestrand A, Wahren J, Bergstrom J: Effect of in vivo contact between blood and dialysis membranes on protein catabolism in humans. Kidney Int 38:487-494, 1990.
473. Guitierrez A: Protein catabolism in maintenance hemodialysis: The influence of the dialysis membrane. Nephrol Dial Transplant 11(suppl 2):108-112, 1996.
474. Caglar K, Peng Y, Pupim LB, et al: Inflammatory signals associated with hemodialysis. Kidney Int 62:1408-1416, 2002.
475. Jansen MAM, Korevaar JC, Dekker FW, et al, for the NECOSAD Study Group: Renal function and nutritional status at the start of chronic dialysis treatment. J Am Soc Nephrol 12:157-163, 2001.
476. Pupim LB, Kent P, Caglar K, et al: Improvement in nutritional parameters after initiation of chronic hemodialysis. Am J Kidney Dis 40:143-151, 2002.
477. Park JS, Kim SB, Park SK, et al: Effect of recombinant human erythropoietin on muscle energy metabolism in patients with end-stage renal disease: A ^{31}P-nuclear magnetic resonance spectroscopic study. Am J Kidney Dis 21:612-618, 1993.
478. Canaud B, Bouloux C, Rivory JP, et al: Erythropoietin-induced changes in protein nutrition: Quantitative assessment by urea kinetic modeling analysis. Blood Purif 8:301-308, 1990.
479. Caglar K, Fedje L, Dimmitt R, et al: Therapeutic effects of oral nutritional supplementation during hemodialysis. Kidney Int 62:1054-1059, 2002.
480. Eustace JA, Coresh J, Kutchey C, et al: Randomized double-blind trial of oral essential amino acids for dialysis-associated hypoalbuminemia. Kidney Int 57:2527-2538, 2000.
481. Heidland A, Kult J: Long-term effects of essential amino acids supplementation in patients on regular dialysis treatment. Clin Nephrol 3:234-239, 1975.
482. Leon JB, Majerle AD, Soinski JA, et al: Can a nutritional intervention improve albumin levels among hemodialysis patients? A pilot study. J Renal Nutr 11:9-15, 2001.
483. Ahmad S: L-Carnitine in dialysis patients. Semin Dial 14:209-217, 2001.
484. Golper TA, Wolfson M, Ahmad S, et al: Multicenter trial of L-carnitine in maintenance hemodialysis patients. I. Carnitine concentrations and lipid effects. Kidney Int 38:904-911, 1990.
485. Rodger RSC, Sheldon WL, Watson MJ, et al: Zinc deficiency and hyperprolactinaemia are not reversible causes of sexual dysfunction in uraemia. Nephrol Dial Transplant 4:888-892, 1989.
486. Stein G, Sperschneider H, Koppe S: Vitamin levels in chronic renal failure and need for supplementation. Blood Purif 3:52-62, 1985.
487. Descombes E, Hanck AB, Fellay G: Water-soluble vitamins in chronic hemodialysis patients and need for supplementation. Kidney Int 43:1319-1328, 1993.
488. Kopple JD, Swenseid ME: Vitamin nutrition in patients undergoing maintenance hemodialysis. Kidney Int Suppl 7:79-84, 1975.
489. Werb R, Clark WF, Lindsay RM, et al: Serum vitamin A levels and associated abnormalities in patients on regular dialysis treatments. Clin Nephrol 12:63-68, 1979.
490. Bloembergen BE, Port FK: Epidemiological perspective on infections in chronic dialysis patients. Adv Renal Replac Ther 3:201-207, 1996.

491. Carton JA, Maradona JA, Nuno FJ, et al: Diabetes mellitus and bacteraemia: A comparative study between diabetic and non-diabetic patients. Eur J Med 1:281-287, 1992.

492. Hoen B, Paul-Dauphin A, Hestin D, Kessler M: EPIBACDIAL: A multicenter prospective study of risk factors for bacteremia in chronic hemodialysis patients. J Am Soc Nephrol 9:869-976, 1998.

493. Keane WF, Shapiro FL, Raij L: Incidence and type of infections occurring in 445 chronic hemodialysis patients. Trans Am Soc Artif Intern Organs 23:41-47, 1977.

494. Mattern WD, Hak LJ, Lamana RW, et al: Malnutrition, altered immune function, and the risk of infection in maintenance hemodialysis patients. Am J Kidney Dis 1:206-218, 1982.

495. Dasgupta MK: Biofilms and infection in dialysis patients. Semin Dial 15:338-346, 2002.

496. Lewis SL, Van Epps DE: Neutrophil and monocyte alterations in chronic dialysis patients. Am J Kidney Dis 9:381-395, 1987.

497. Goldblum SE, Reed WP: Host defenses and immunologic alterations associated with chronic hemodialysis. Ann Intern Med 93:597-613, 1980.

498. Boelaert JR, Van Landuyt HW, Valcke YJ, et al: The role of iron overload in *Yersinia enterocolitica* and *Yersinia pseudotuberculosis* bacteremia in hemodialysis patients. J Infect Dis 156:384-387, 1987.

499. Bloembergen WE, Port FK, Hakim RM, et al: The relationship of dialysis membrane and cause-specific mortality in chronic hemodialysis patients. Am J Kidney Dis 33:217-220, 1999.

500. Tokars JI, Frank M, Alter MJ, Arduino MJ: National surveillance of dialysis-associated diseases in the United States, 2000. Semin Dial 15:162-171, 2002.

501. Edmond MB, Wallace SE, Pfeffer MA, et al: Surveillance of 49 US medical centers for VRE bacteremia. Paper presented at the 34th Annual Meeting of the Infectious Disease Society of America, September 1996, .

502. Knudsen F, Wantzin P, Rasmussen K, et al: Hepatitis C in dialysis patients: Relationship to blood transfusions, dialysis, and liver disease. Kidney Int 43:1353-1356, 1993.

503. Kuhns M, de Medina M, McNamara A, et al: Detection of hepatitis C virus RNA in hemodialysis. J Am Soc Nephrol 4:1491-1497, 1994.

504. Caramelo C, Ortiz A, Aguilera B, et al: Liver disease patterns in hemodialysis patients with antibodies to hepatitis C virus. Am J Kidney Dis 22:822-828, 1993.

505. Fabrizi F, Martin P, Dixit V, et al: Biological dynamics of viral load in hemodialysis patients with hepatitis C virus. Am J Kidney Dis 35:122-129, 2000.

506. Koenig P, Vogel W, Umlauft F, et al: Interferon treatment for chronic hepatitis C virus infection in uremic patients. Kidney Int 45:1507-1509, 1994.

507. Rangel MC, Coronado VG, Euler GL, Strikas RA: Vaccine recommendations for patients on chronic dialysis. Semin Dial 13:101-107, 2000.

508. Bregman H, Daugridas J, Ing T: Complications during hemodialysis. *In* Daugirdads J, Ing T (eds): Handbook of Dialysis, 2nd ed. Boston, Little, Brown, 1994, pp 13-29.

509. Wehle B: Factors affecting blood pressure in hemodialysis. Scand J Urol Nephrol Suppl 69:1-66, 1982.

510. Converse RL Jr, Jacobsen TN, Toto RD, et al: Sympathetic overactivity in patients with chronic renal failure. N Engl J Med 327:1912-1918, 1992.

511. Oe B, de Fijter CW, Oe PL, et al: Diameter of inferior caval vein (VCD) and bioelectrical impedance analysis (BIA) for the analysis of hydration status in patients on hemodialysis. Clin Nephrol 50:38-43, 1998.

512. Cruz DN, Mahnensmith RL, Brickel HM, Perazella MA: Midodrine and cool dialysate are effective therapies for symptomatic intradialytic hypotension. Am J Kidney Dis 33:920-926, 1999.

513. Roca AO, Jarjoura D, et al: Dialysis leg cramps. Efficacy of quinine versus vitamin E. ASAIO J 38:481-485, 1992.

514. Jansen PH, Veenhuizen KC, Wesseling AI, et al: Randomised controlled trial of hydroquinine in muscle cramps. Lancet 349:528-32, 1997.

515. Ahmad S, Robertson HT, Golper TA, et al: Multicenter trial of L-carnitine in maintenance hemodialysis patients. II. Clinical and biochemical effects. Kidney Int 38:912-918, 1990.

516. Zebe H: Atrial fibrillation in dialysis patients. Nephrol Dial Transplant 15:765-768, 2000.

517. Gehr T, Sica D: Antiarrhythmic medications: Practical guidelines for drug therapy in dialysis. Semin Dial 3:33-40, 1990.

518. Epstein A, Kay G, Plumb V: Considerations in the diagnosis and treatment of arrhythmias in patients with end-stage renal disease. Semin Dial 2:31-37, 1990.

519. De Backer WA, Verpooten GA, Borgonjon DJ, et al: Hypoxemia during hemodialysis: Effects of different membranes and dialysate compositions. Kidney Int 23:738-743, 1983.

520. Akl AI, Sobh MA, Enab YM, Tattersall J: Artificial intelligence: A new approach for prescription and monitoring of hemodialysis therapy. Am J Kidney Dis 38:1277-1283, 2001.

521. Chertow GM: "Wishing don't make it so"—why we need a randomized clinical trial of high-intensity dialysis. J Am Soc Nephrol 12:2850-2853, 2001.

522. Fissell WH, Lou L, Abrishami S, et al: Bioartificial kidney ameliorates gram-negative bacteria-induced septic shock in uremic animals. J Am Soc Nephrol 14:454-461, 2003.

CHAPTER 60

Peritoneal Dialysis

John M. Burkart, Pirouz Daeihagh, and Michael V. Rocco

At the end of the millennium, 275,053 patients were being treated by dialysis in the United States. Of this group, 87.9% were receiving in-center hemodialysis (HD); 0.5%, home HD; 5.2%, continuous ambulatory peritoneal dialysis (CAPD); and 4%, automated peritoneal dialysis (PD).[1] The percentage of patients using automated forms of PD has been increasing, now estimated to represent over 40% of all new patients versus the 22% who started on classic continuous cycling peritoneal dialysis (CCPD) in 1996. Estimates of percentages of dialysis patients receiving PD vary from county to country, with a range as low as 9% in Japan to as high as 58% in Mexico (Fig. 60-1).[1] The reasons for differences in

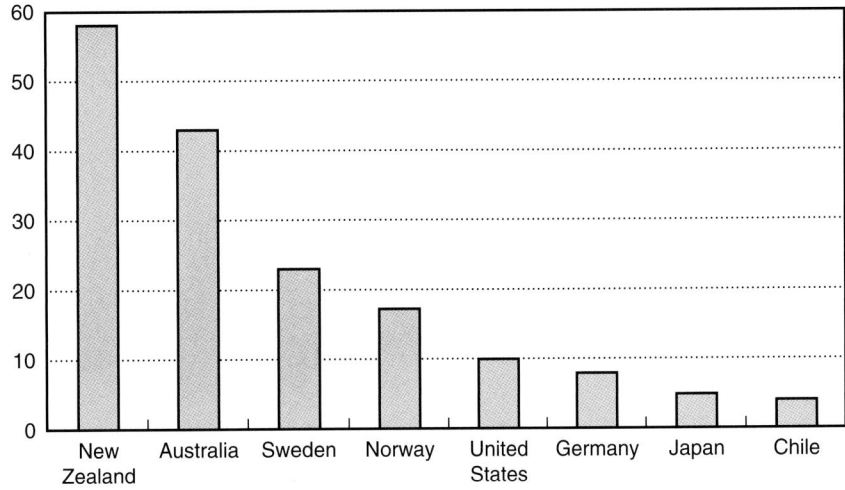

PERCENTAGE OF PREVALENT PATIENTS ON
PERITONEAL DIALYSIS BY COUNTRY

FIGURE 60-1. Percentage of all prevalent dialysis patients being treated by continuous ambulatory peritoneal dialysis or continuous cycling peritoneal dialysis in New Zealand, Australia, Japan, selected European countries, and the United States, end of December 2000. (From U.S. Renal Data System: USRDS 2002 Annual Data Report: Atlas of End-Stage Renal Disease in the United States. Bethesda, MD, National Institutes of Health, National Institute of Diabetes and Digestive and Kidney Diseases, 2002, pp 151-164.)

the use of PD around the world are multifactorial and include, but are not limited to access to PD, physician comfort/expertise with the therapy, and government reimbursement policies.[2, 3]

Ganter[4] described the first clinical use of PD in 1923. The clinical courses of most of the first 100 patients treated with PD were reviewed in 1950.[5] Of these patients, many were undergoing PD because of acute renal failure, and renal function was restored in 32 patients. Of the patients who died, three complications (uremia, peritonitis, and pulmonary edema) accounted for 88% of the deaths. Subsequent to that publication, clinical experience and many modifications of the initial procedure that addressed these initial complications were reported, but with little change in clinical outcome. It was not until 1976 that Popovich and colleagues[6] described the basic concept of CAPD as we know it today. An extensive review of the history of PD has been published in a previous edition of this book.[7] Since then, PD has continued to evolve. The U.S. Renal Data System (USRDS) 2000 report suggests that over the past 10 years, death rates for both PD and HD have fallen 38.5% overall, with the greatest decrease in death rate (63.7%) noted in patients receiving PD.[8] In fact, contemporary data from Canada[9] and the United States[10] suggest that over the first 1 to 2 years of end-stage renal disease (ESRD), patients maintained by PD have a survival advantage. As a result of recent outcome studies,[11] investigators have taken a new approach to the adequacy of PD in which special emphasis is placed on ultrafiltration and blood pressure control.[12] In addition, interest in the relationship between the dialysis solution used and chronic inflammation (a major predictor of outcome) has increased while research on infection prevention and catheter development continues.

COMPONENTS OF THE PERITONEAL DIALYSIS SYSTEM

Renal replacement therapy with PD requires three key components: the PD catheter, PD solutions, and the peritoneal membrane and its associated vascular supply. Each of these components has distinct differences from its counterparts in HD. First, optimal chronic PD access must traverse both a sterile (intraperitoneal portion) and a nonsterile (extraperitoneal portion) environment, as opposed to the sterile, subcutaneous optimal access in use for chronic HD, namely, the subcutaneous fistula or synthetic graft. Second, PD solutions must be sterile, and the containers must be amenable to self-care and easy home use. Third, the physician cannot pick and choose a dialyzer from a catalog of various membrane types or sizes for a particular PD patient. Patients are born with their "dialyzer." The physician must learn how to tailor the therapy for each patient's peritoneal membrane by adjusting dwell time and dialysis solutions.

Catheters

Access to the peritoneal cavity with a permanent indwelling catheter is at present one of the key factors determining the long-term success of PD. Palmer and co-workers[13] first introduced the silicone rubber catheter in 1963. Tenckhoff and Schechter[14] modified this catheter in 1968, and this version

of the catheter is still used by most nephrologists. Since the introduction of these original designs, most modifications have been directed toward improving subcutaneous anchorage of the catheter, preventing catheter migration, decreasing infectious complications, and addressing possible bioincompatibility issues, if any, related to the catheter.

Catheter Design

ACUTE USE CATHETERS. Introduced by Westin and Roberts[15] in 1965, acute PD catheters are straight, relatively rigid conduits about 3 mm in diameter and 25 to 30 mm in length that can be placed at the beside. With prolonged use, this catheter design, with bedside placement, is associated with a significant risk of peritonitis, malfunction, and bowel perforation. Therefore, it is recommended that these catheters not be left in place for longer than 3 days. For most patients with acute renal failure, the duration of therapy needed is unpredictable, and such patients usually require treatment for longer than 3 days. Therefore, use of the safer long-term catheter is recommended. However, in current practice, often because of the acuity and severity of illness in a patient with acute renal failure, most patients are treated with some form of HD.

CHRONIC USE CATHETERS. Standard chronic indwelling peritoneal catheters are constructed of soft materials such as silicone rubber or polyurethane. The most frequently used material is silicone rubber, a polymer of methylsilicate. It is relatively biocompatible and inert, has no leachable plasticizers, and is not traumatic to surrounding tissue. Polyurethane catheters have better wall strength and thus can have a smaller catheter wall,[16] larger internal lumen, and increased flow rates. However, cracking of the polyurethane catheter has been reported, especially after exit site care with polyethylene glycol, alcohol, or topical mupirocin. This catheter material is therefore not likely to be reliable for long-term use. The intraperitoneal portion of long-term catheters usually contains many 1-mm side holes for the passage of fluid, but it may also have modifications to facilitate fluid movement, alleviate symptoms associated with inflow or drainage, decrease catheter migration, and prevent trapping by omentum. Such modifications include a curled tip, two perpendicular disks (Oreopolulos-Zellerman), and a column disk (Lifecath). Extraperitoneal modifications include various means of external fixation and preformed angles in the subcutaneous portion designed to prevent catheter-related infection, migration, and dialysate leakage. Modifications include the use of one or two Dacron cuffs, one or two disk-bubble cuffs (Toronto), and arcuate (swan-neck), pail-handle (Cruz), or 90-degree (Lifecath) subcutaneous curves, as shown schematically in Figure 60-2.

DESIGN MODIFICATIONS. Because straight Tenckhoff catheters were associated with a high rate of external cuff extrusion and catheter migration (resulting in failure to drain), "swan-neck" catheters were developed.[17] This catheter type has a lateral or downward external exit site and a permanent bend in the subcutaneous portion of the catheter. This bend produces an arcuate tunnel that is convex upward so that both the internal (peritoneal) and external (skin) exits point downward. The bend and arc are designed to prevent catheter migration and cuff extrusion. The downwardly directed catheter exit and placement of the subcutaneous

CURRENTLY AVAILABLE CHRONIC PERITONEAL CATHETERS
COMBINATIONS OF IP AND EP DESIGNS

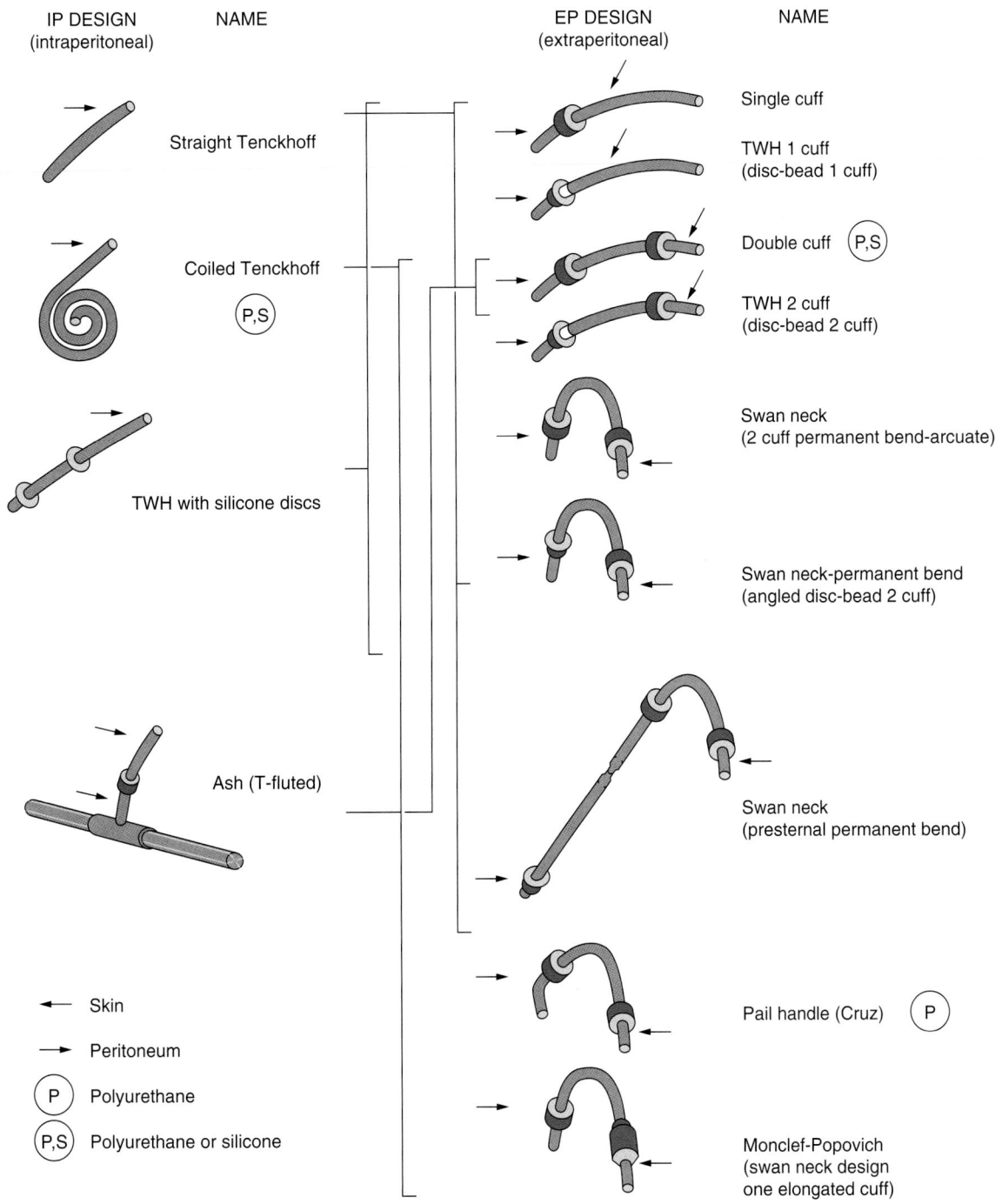

FIGURE 60-2. Currently available chronic peritoneal catheters showing combinations of intraperitoneal and extraperitoneal designs. (From Gokal R, Alexander S, Ash S, et al: Peritoneal catheters and exit site practices: Toward optimum peritoneal access: 1998 update. Perit Dial Int 18:11, 1998.)

cuffs are designed to decrease the likelihood of cuff extrusion and exit site infection. A description of the insertion technique is available elsewhere.[18] With these catheters, Twardowski and colleagues estimated a survival rate of 61% at 3 years, more than twice the historical survival rate at 3 years (30%) for the straight Tenckhoff and Toronto Western

Hospital catheters in use at their institution[19] and better than the results reported in the CAPD registry at that time.[20] These investigators have since made a further modification in their catheter in which the exit is located in the presternal area.[18] This modification is based on the theory that presternal exit sites would be subject to less trauma and chance of contamination. Another advantage of the presternal exit location is that it allows patients to "immerse" themselves in water (i.e., to use hot tubs and baths without immersing the exit site).

The Moncrief-Popovich catheter and insertion technique were developed to allow healing of the subcutaneous cuff in a sterile environment.[21] This catheter incorporates the swan-neck design and a novel insertion technique. The segment of the catheter that would normally be brought out through the skin is completely buried at the time of catheter insertion. At a subsequent date, optimally 4 to 6 weeks later, the distal segment of the catheter is exteriorized and dialysis is begun. During preliminary clinical trials, use of this catheter with the standard spike significantly reduced peritonitis rates, and when a disconnect technique was used, peritonitis rates were reduced even further.[22] During the period before exteriorization of the external end, no problems with omental wrapping were reported; in a study in dogs, Moncrief and colleagues demonstrated that omental wrapping does not occur without the instillation of fresh dialysis fluid,[23] thus suggesting that daily "flushing" of the peritoneal cavity after catheter placement is not needed. Another interesting preliminary finding in patients who have had catheters implanted with this technique is the absence of biofilm on subsequent electron microscopic evaluation of the subcutaneous portion of the catheter.[22] These data seem to demonstrate an improved bacteriologic barrier between the outside and the peritoneal cavity with this technique and confirm the significance of sources other than touch contamination as a cause of peritonitis. With this procedure, an incidence of one case of peritonitis per 29 patient-months was achieved versus a historical incidence of one case per 9 patient-months when the same type of spike-bag exchange system was used.[24] It was suggested that this difference was related to the development of less biofilm on the catheter during the subcutaneous rest period. However, in a unit where the overall baseline infection rates were low, a prospective randomized trial showed that this technique did not result in a reduction in peritonitis or exit site infection.[25] To date, this technique has gained minimal acceptance, in part because of the necessity for a second surgical procedure and the widespread use of prophylactic mupirocin at the exit site, which has markedly reduced exit site infections and *Staphylococcus aureus*–associated peritonitis.

Biofilm

Infections associated with implantable and indwelling devices are often persistent and refractory to medical therapy. Recurrent or relapsing peritonitis is a frequent cause of catheter loss in PD patients. It has been postulated that the presence of biofilm-containing microorganisms, or microbial biofilms, may be the cause.[26-28] Giangrande and co-workers[29] used scanning electron microscopy to analyze the surfaces of 18 silicone catheters removed from patients who had been receiving PD for between 2 and 77 months. All catheter surfaces were covered with protein-like granular deposits, six were covered with microbial biofilm, and culture of catheter segments was positive in six cases. Biofilms were found in some patients who had not had a recent bout of peritonitis. Structural defects and small linear tears were present on both the luminal and external surfaces of eight catheters and were

more frequent in those from patients with refractory or recurrent peritonitis, as were positive cultures. It has been shown that structural defects might provide a nidus for deposition of adherent exopolysaccharide matrix, which is crucial for biofilm formation and bacterial growth.[30] Previous studies have suggested that structural defects in the catheter predispose to peritonitis.[31] These studies are intriguing and suggest the need for further evaluation of the role of biofilm in disease, as well as the need for cuff maturation and improvements in the physicochemical characteristics and production of catheters.

Catheter Implantation Techniques

The technique of Tenckhoff catheter implantation has a significant influence on long-term catheter outcome. Sterile conditions are essential, and an experienced catheter insertion team is needed. An extensive review by Prowant and colleagues[32] of exit site maturation, histology, and morphology, as well as the relationship to infection and certain clinical problems such as exit site trauma, has better defined exit site care and Tenckhoff insertion practices. A panel of experts has agreed on five general standards for catheter placement: (1) the deep cuff should be in the anterior abdominal musculature, (2) the subcutaneous cuff should be near the skin surface and not less than 2 cm from the exit site to allow for drainage and provide a firm anchorage that prevents piston-like movements of the catheter,[33] (3) the catheter exit should be positioned laterally, (4) the exit site should be directed downward or laterally, and (5) the intra-abdominal portion of the catheter should be placed between the visceral and parietal peritoneum and in the middle of loops of bowel.[34]

Surgical insertion of catheters (placement by dissection) is the most commonly used placement procedure in clinical practice today. After surgical dissection through the rectus muscle, the catheter is placed in the pelvis under direct visualization.[35] According to the USRDS, before 1990, approximately 88% of catheters were inserted with this approach.[36] *Peritoneoscopic insertion* allows direct visualization of the course of the catheter, and in experienced hands, the results are good.[37, 38] Catheters inserted with this technique are placed by the surgeon or nephrologist. *Blind placement* does not allow direct visualization of the catheter or peritoneum. This procedure should not be used in markedly obese patients and in those who have had previous abdominal surgery because of the higher risk of complications such as bowel perforation in patients with unsuspected adhesions. Various devices have been developed to guide the clinician in blind insertion of the catheter. The *Moncrief-Popovich technique* incorporates two modifications of conventional implantation procedures. At time of implantation, the entire extraperitoneal portion of the catheter is placed subcutaneously, which theoretically allows the cuff to heal in a sterile environment and prevents bacterial colonization. At a subsequent date (4 to 6 weeks after implantation), the external portion of the catheter is exteriorized, and dialysis can be initiated immediately.[18] Placement techniques and their complication rates were recently reviewed by Gokal and colleagues[34] and by Ash.[39] These reviews suggest that in appropriate patients, outcome does not depend on the technique used for implantation as much as on the person (nephrologist or surgeon) who inserts the catheter. The most important requirement may be to have a trained, knowledgeable, and dedicated catheter-insertion team.

Pericatheter dialysate leaks are reduced by lateral catheter placement and positioning of the deep cuff on the posterior rectus fascia.[40, 41] Prophylactic partial omentectomy at the time of catheter placement is not recommended.[34] However, Nicholson and colleagues[42] reported a significant improvement in catheter outcome in patients who had undergone partial omentectomy at the time of surgical placement. Further studies are needed to confirm this finding, but if swan-neck catheters are used, this procedure is unlikely to add any benefit.

Catheter Break-In

It is normal to flush the peritoneal cavity with 500 to 1500 mL of dialysis fluid until clear immediately after placement. Heparin (500 to 1000 U/L) can be added in cases in which fibrin is present. Optimally, PD should not be initiated until 10 to 14 days after catheter placement to allow wound healing and cuff maturation and minimize the risk of leakage or infection. Experience in using the Moncrief-Popovich catheter and insertion technique suggests that the catheter does not need to be flushed during this period. Nevertheless, some investigators recommend periodic flushing, and if performed, once weekly seems reasonable. If PD must be started immediately after implantation or before optimal catheter break-in, it is recommended that intermittent dialysis with low dialysate volumes (i.e., less than 1500 mL) and the supine position be used. After catheter implantation, the exit site should be covered with sterile gauze and a nonocclusive dressing. The dressing should not be changed for several days unless excessive bleeding is evident. To ensure optimal tissue healing during this period, the catheter should be immobilized to prevent trauma to the exit site,[43] and exit site sutures should be avoided. In addition, patients should avoid submerging the exit site in water during this period.

Catheter Survival

Transfer from PD to HD is thought to be directly due to catheter-related problems in about 20% of cases,[34] usually a catheter-related infection but, occasionally, catheter migration and dialysate leaks. Early CAPD registry data (based on patients who were undergoing dialysis between January 1981 and August 1987) showed that the cumulative probability of a CAPD patient experiencing at least one catheter replacement was 32% at 2 years and 42% at 3 years.[44] These data were collected before the widespread use of swan-neck–type catheters, which have improved catheter survival. Catheter survival has been shown to correlate with the patient's weight, and weight at initiation of dialysis was predictive of catheter loss from infectious complications.[45] Outcomes of 213 curled catheters placed either surgically or percutaneously (63%) were analyzed over a 4-year period.[46] The actuarial catheter survival rate was 61% at 3 years and did not differ with the implantation technique used. Kaplan-Meier survival rates of 138 surgically placed, straight double-cuff catheters at one center were 87%, 69%, and 65%, at 1, 2, and 3 years, respectively.[47] At another center in which a mixture of straight Tenckhoff and swan-neck catheters was used, the proportion of patients who still had their original

catheter after 30 months of follow-up was 82%, and the need for catheter replacement was not related to the type of connection device used.[48] Once placed, catheters usually function well, although occasionally, failure to fill or drain occurs as a result of malposition, kinking, or omental wrapping. This problem can be treated surgically or by laparoscopic intervention.[49, 50]

Others[51] have reported a 3-year survival rate of 90% for swan-neck catheters versus 80% for Tenckhoff catheters; Lye and colleagues[52] reported a 1-year swan-neck catheter survival rate of 95%. All these results are encouraging and show that catheter survival is similar to that of natural arteriovenous fistulas in HD patients.

Indications for Catheter Removal

Indications for catheter removal include malfunction, relapsing or recurrent peritonitis, peritonitis that fails to resolve, chronic exit site or tunnel infection, fungal peritonitis, *Pseudomonas*-related peritonitis that is slow to respond to therapy, a perforated viscus, possibly multiorganism-related peritonitis, recovery of renal function, and permanent transfer to HD.[53]

Conclusions

At best, a 3-year catheter survival rate of 80% should be expected, with a minimally acceptable rate of 80% at 1 year.[34] Most centers achieve a better than 60% 3-year catheter survival rate. Catheter-related infections remain one of the major complications associated with PD. Recent developments in catheter technology have shown promise and have resulted in some improvement in the complication rate. Present data favor the use of two subcutaneous cuffs with a permanent arc in the subcutaneous portion of the catheter to prevent migration and infection. To reduce pain related to the "jet effect" from dialysate inflow and pressure of the catheter tip on the peritoneum, a curled tip is recommended. Further studies are needed to see whether burying the entire catheter in a subcutaneous tunnel at the time of implantation to allow cuff maturation in a sterile environment is advantageous. Emerging research topics include better fixation of cuffs to tissue by using fibrin glue or macroscopic and microscopic texturing. The use of more biocompatible materials for catheter construction and the introduction of antibiotic or bacteriostatic coatings are also being investigated, as is the need for a dual-lumen catheter if higher dialysate flow technologies are developed.

Dialysis Solutions

The first use of PD solutions in animals was described by Ganter.[4] Heusser and Werder[54] later reported using saline solutions and the addition of glucose to increase tonicity and achieve ultrafiltration. The next significant development was the substitution of lactate for acetate as a buffer. In 1959, the Don Baxter Company produced the first commercially available fluids in 1-L glass bottles. Maxwell and associates[55] reported using these fluids in clinical practice. Except for minor alterations, standard PD solutions have undergone little change until recent years despite concern about the concentration of certain cations[56] and the potential toxicity

TABLE 60-1

Standard Dialysate Composition

Dextrose, measured in g/dL as hydrous dextrose, available as 1.5%, 2.5%, and 4.25%
Sodium, available at 132 mEq/L
Chloride, available at 102, 96, and 95 mEq/L
Lactate, available at 35 and 40 mEq/L
Calcium, available at 2.5 and 3.5 mEq/L
Magnesium, available at 0.5 and 1.5 mEq/L
Bag volumes, available at 0.25, 0.5, 0.75, 1.0, 1.5, 2.0, 2.5, 3.0, and 5.0 L
Alternative solutions:
   7.5% polyglucose (in place of dextrose)
   1.1% amino acids (in place of dextrose)
   Combination lactate/bicarbonate or bicarbonate alone solutions

Modified from Golper TA, Burkart JM, Piraino B: Peritoneal dialysis. *In* Schrier RW, Gottschalk CW (eds): Diseases of the Kidney, 6th ed. Boston, Little, Brown, 1997, pp 2771-2805.

of these fluids as a result of bioincompatibility.[57] Typical dialysis fluid solute concentrations are found in Table 60-1. The early history of PD fluid development was reviewed in a previous edition of this text.[7]

Electrolytes

SODIUM. Na^+ has been added to the dialysis solution in varying concentrations ranging from 120 to 140 mEq/L. Early during the dwell period with glucose-containing fluids and crystalloid-induced ultrafiltration, Na^+ does not cross the peritoneal membrane as readily as water does. Therefore, because the concentration of Na^+ in the ultrafiltrate is lower than that in serum and may be as low as 70 mEq/L,[58-60] a transient decrease in dialysate Na^+ occurs during the dwell period as a result of aquaporin-mediated transcellular movement of water that is sodium free, a process called sodium sieving. It is most pronounced in patients who are slow transporters and when hypertonic dialysis fluids are used. After multiple rapid exchanges with hypertonic glucose, systemic hypernatremia has been described.[61] During long dwell periods, after transcellular water movement ceases, sodium moves from blood to the dialysate down its concentration gradient, and dialysate sodium concentrations increase. To avoid this problem, most commercially available dialysis fluids now have an Na^+ concentration of 132 mEq/L. To circumvent the development of hypernatremia, it may also be prudent to avoid repeated short dwell periods of exclusively hypertonic dialysis fluid unless the Na^+ concentration in the dialysis fluid is decreased.

Some studies have focused on the use of lower dialysate Na^+ concentrations to facilitate salt and water loss for better control of hypertension. With dialysate Na^+ concentrations of 98 to 120 mEq/L,[62] preliminary studies have shown an increase in net Na^+ loss and better volume and blood pressure control. Follow-up studies have adjusted glucose concentrations to keep ultrafiltration the same, but have lowered dialysate Na^+ levels to increase Na^+ loss.[63, 64] Further studies are needed to evaluate the role of lower dialysate Na^+ concentrations in blood pressure/volume control. It is acknowledged that ultrafiltration is of primary importance, and efforts involving the use of alternative osmotic agents to improve ultrafiltration may be of first priority.

POTASSIUM. K^+ is not usually added to chronic PD fluid.[65] In typical CAPD exchanges using dialysis fluid with no added K^+, dialysate K^+ approaches Gibbs-Donnan equilibrium. Patients tend to lose about 35 mEq/day in the dialysate while maintaining a serum K^+ concentration of approximately 4.0 mEq/L.[66] Net ultrafiltration increases K^+ removal. However, as with Na^+, ultrafiltrate concentrations are less than those in serum because of K^+ sieving across transcellular aquaporins. With rapid cycling, K^+ losses are augmented, but maximal rates are about 8 mEq/hr.[67] If needed, K^+ removal can be slowed by adding K^+ to the dialysate.

MAGNESIUM. Standard solutions used to have an Mg^{2+} concentration of 1.5 mEq/L, which resulted in serum Mg^{2+} concentrations that were slightly elevated in CAPD patients.[68, 69] However, toxic levels of hypermagnesemia have not been attributed to the use of standard PD fluids. Hypomagnesemia has been noted in HD patients after lowering dialysis fluid Mg^{2+}, an alteration that usually tends to normalize serum Mg^{2+} levels.[70] Dialysis solutions with an Mg^{2+} concentration of 0.5 mEq/L are now widely used and have been reported to normalize serum Mg^{2+} levels.[69] In addition, dialysis fluids with lower calcium and Mg^{2+} concentrations may allow the use of Mg^{2+} salts as a calcium-free phosphate binder. Solutions with a lower Mg^{2+} concentration have higher lactate concentrations.

CALCIUM. It is now recognized that the Ca^{2+} concentration of PD fluids needs to be tailored to different clinical situations.[71, 72] Control of Ca^{2+} and phosphate balance in ESRD is important to prevent the long-term complications of renal osteodystrophy. Unfortunately, phosphorus is only poorly removed by standard PD.[73] During the late 1970s and early 1980s, the standard of care was to use phosphate binders that contained aluminum along with dietary phosphate restriction to control serum PO_4^{3-} levels in PD patients. It was also common practice to treat the tendency for hypocalcemia by using a relatively high dialysis Ca^{2+} concentration (3.5 mEq/L) to facilitate mass transfer of Ca^{2+} from the dialysis fluid to blood. Now that aluminum's toxic effects are better recognized,[74, 75] most nephrologists have begun to use Ca^{2+} salts or resins such as Sevelamer as their primary phosphate binder.[76, 77] When Ca^{2+} salts are used, hypercalcemia (in 35% to 56% of patients) and metastatic calcification have been frequent complications with dialysis fluids containing Ca^{2+} concentrations of 3.5 mEq/L.[76-80] Because of these complications, dialysis fluids were developed with a lower, more nearly physiologic Ca^{2+} concentration (2.5 mEq/L).[81, 82] These concentrations are more physiologic than normal serum Ca^{2+} levels. Dialysate fluids with lower Ca^{2+} also have higher lactate and lower Mg^{2+} concentrations.

As shown in Figure 60-3A and B, clinical trials have demonstrated that the use of dialysis fluid with a lower Ca^{2+} concentration (2.3 mEq/L) has been associated with net Ca^{2+} flux from blood to the dialysate under most physiologic conditions.[83-86] Short-term use of these fluids in both established[87-91] and new[92, 93] patients has been associated with an improvement in biochemical parameters (serum Ca^{2+}, phosphorus, alkaline phosphatase, and parathyroid hormone [PTH] levels) in comparison to baseline. In some patients, improvement in bone histologic features[94, 95] and prevention of adynamic bone disease have been noted.[72] However, other patients have a risk of net Ca^{2+} loss with subsequent negative Ca^{2+} balance and an increase in PTH levels.[96, 97]

The estimated Ca^{2+} loss with a 2.3-mEq/L Ca^{2+} solution is presumably 100 mg/dL or 45 g/yr of Ca^{2+} (about 3% to 4% of total bone mineral content per year). A multicenter randomized trial of 103 CAPD patients in which standard dialysate calcium levels were compared with low levels showed that low-Ca^{2+} dialysate was successful with respect to the following three end points: reduction in hypercalcemic episodes, tolerance of higher doses of calcium-containing phosphate binders, and maintenance of stable PTH levels.[98] However, subgroup analysis demonstrated that in those with the highest baseline PTH level, PTH tended to increase even further. This tendency for increased PTH can be partially corrected by administering oral vitamin D metabolites,[99] and perhaps they should be used routinely. Similarly noted is the possibility of alkalosis and hypomagnesemia associated with the use of a low-Ca^{2+} solution.[100] Finally, some have suggested that dialysis solutions with lower calcium content may improve cardiac function by increasing cardiac relaxation.[101] Further long-term studies are needed.

Although individualization is necessary, it seems reasonable to use these fluids as the standard dialysis solution for most patients. Their usefulness lies in the ability to use them in combination with higher doses of Ca^{2+}-containing oral phosphate binders without inducing hypercalcemia or a progressive positive Ca^{2+} balance. Care must be taken to ensure that patients are given supplemental oral Ca^{2+} (the present standard phosphate binders) and that both serum (or ionized) Ca^{2+} and PTH[102] levels are closely monitored. The potential risk of loss of bone mineral content must be weighed against the risk of hyperphosphatemia and a resultant increase in hyperparathyroidism and metastatic calcification.

Buffers

Current standard PD fluids use lactate as the buffer; earlier formulations contained acetate. Even though no major difference has been noted in the relative control of chronic metabolic acidosis with the use of lactate or acetate buffer,[103]

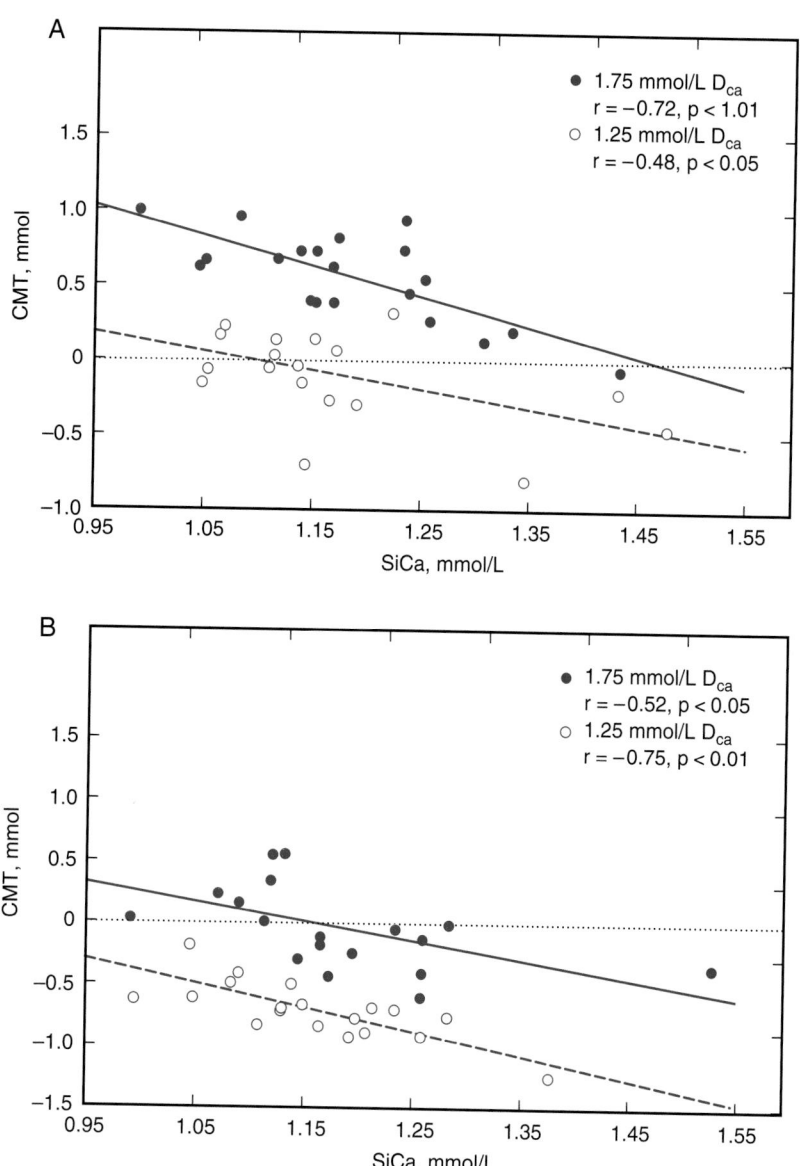

FIGURE 60-3. A and **B,** Ca^{2+} mean transfer values (CMT, mmol) plotted against serum Ca^{2+} levels (SiCa) with 1.25 and 1.75 mmol/L Ca^{2+} in 1.5 g/dL dextrose dialysate (**A**) and 4.25 g/dL dextrose dialysate (**B**). (From Bender FH, Bernardini J, Piraino B: Calcium mass transfer with dialysate containing 1.25 and 1.75 mmol/L calcium in peritoneal dialysis patients. Am J Kidney Dis 20:367-375, 1992.)

acetate has been implicated in the etiology of ultrafiltration failure caused by sclerosing peritonitis,[97, 104] and clinical observations suggest that it takes longer for acetate dialysis fluids to reach physiologic pH during the dwell period than it does for lactate.[105, 106] This delay in attaining physiologic pH may be associated with increased pain on inflow, but it may also be of importance when the biocompatibility of dialysis solutions is being considered.

Commercially available dialysis fluids contain a racemic mixture of both D- and L-lactate. The normal physiologic form of lactic acid is the L-form,[107] and the normal blood level of this isomer is about 300 times that of the D-form.[108] The D-isomer is metabolized at a much slower rate than the L-form is. Although both isomers are absorbed and supraphysiologic concentrations of either isomer have been associated with encephalopathy,[109] Nolph and co-workers[110] have shown that despite the high concentration of both isomers in standard dialysis preparations (35 to 40 mmol/L), even with rapid cycling such as with tidal dialysis, D-lactate levels are only minimally elevated. One significant drawback of lactate-based solutions is that the fluids have an unphysiologically low pH. Lactate-containing fluids are bioincompatible. Virtually all examined normal cellular functions of resident peritoneal cells are impaired with lactate-containing solutions.[111] The clinical significance of this impairment is uncertain.

A bicarbonate-based buffer system would be preferable for dialysis fluids, but many problems have been associated with bicarbonate-based PD solutions, including precipitation of Ca^{2+} and Mg^{2+} carbonates and caramelization of glucose at physiologic pH during sterilization (hence the acidic PD fluids). To avoid these problems, two methods of fluid preparation have been used: addition of acetate or glycylglycine[112, 113] at the time of manufacture or the use of a two-chamber bag in which the two solutions are combined at the time of use.[114, 115] Short-term studies using bicarbonate as a buffer in humans have been encouraging[116, 117]; the solutions have been well tolerated, and no significant changes in transport have been observed during short-term follow-up.[110] Long-term studies using a lactate/bicarbonate mixture (15 mmol/25 mmol/L) have been well tolerated, and when compared with standard solutions, no difference was noted in serum HCO_3^- levels at baseline and at the end of the study.[118] Furthermore, long-term (6 months to 1 year) use of 34 mmol/L bicarbonate did not induce any change in acid-base status over time or any difference from controls. A tendency for an increase in HCO_3^- levels in acidotic patients and a decrease in controls was noted. Also noted was an increased normalized protein catabolic rate.[119] These data show that bicarbonate is a well-tolerated "physiologic" buffer for PD fluids. Further studies are inevitable, and bicarbonate is likely to eventually replace lactate in some PD fluids in the near future.

Osmotic Agents

GLUCOSE. Standard dialysis solutions contain glucose as the osmotic agent. Glucose has been shown to be safe, effective, readily metabolized, and inexpensive. However, glucose is not an "ideal" osmotic agent because of the following properties or effects: rapid absorption, potential for metabolic derangements (such as hyperglycemia, hyperinsulinemia,[120]

TABLE 60-2

Alternative Osmotic Agents to Glucose and Their Potential Complications

OSMOTIC AGENT	COMPLICATIONS
Gelatin	Prolonged half-life and immunogenicity of some preparations
Xylitol	Peritoneal pain, lactic acidosis, hyperuricemia, carcinogenicity, and deterioration of liver function
Sorbitol	Metabolized through the polyol pathway, which may aggravate neuropathy, lactic acidosis, hyperuricemia, and hyperosmolality
Mannitol	Lactic acidosis, hyperuricemia
Fructose	Metabolized through the polyol pathway, which may aggravate neuropathy, hypernatremia, lactic acidosis, hyperuricemia, and hypertriglyceridemia
Dextrans	Risk of bleeding and systemic absorption
Glucose polymers	Prolonged half-life, impaired metabolism in uremia, and potential for high calorie loads
Polyanions	Damage to the peritoneum and cardiovascular instability
Glycerol	Retention, hypertriglyceridemia, sterile peritonitis, low ultrafiltration capacity, and hyperosmolality
Amino acids	Increased concentration of nitrogenous products in blood, increased H^+ generation, expensive optimal formulation not yet determined, and difficult to sterilize in combination with glucose

From Diaz-Buxo JA: Clinical use of peritoneal dialysis. *In* Nissenson AR, Fine RN, Gentile DE (eds): Clinical Dialysis, 2nd ed. Norwalk, CT, Appleton & Lange, 1990, pp 256-300.

hyperlipidemia,[121] obesity),[122] necessity for an acidic dialysis pH to prevent caramelization, and the potential nonenzymatic glycosylation of peritoneal tissue during periods of mesothelial cell loss.[123] Several other substances have been tried as osmotic agents, including both low-molecular-weight (glycerol, sorbitol, amino acids, xylitol, and fructose) and high-molecular-weight (glucose polymer, gelatin, polycations, dextrans, and polypeptides) agents. Despite theoretical advantages over glucose, significant problems have been associated with all these alternative agents (Table 60-2). At present, glucose remains the standard osmotic agent, but other osmotic agents (polyglucose and amino acids) are also used in clinical practice.

AMINO ACIDS. Emerging evidence suggests that protein malnutrition is a significant risk factor for morbidity and mortality in dialysis patients. Furthermore, because of an obligatory daily loss of protein and amino acids into the peritoneal effluent, a potential advantage of amino acid–containing fluids would be that the caloric source would be based on protein without the concomitant phosphorus load associated with oral protein sources. Since the original work by Oreopoulos and co-workers,[124] most[125, 126] but not all[127] studies have shown a benefit in nutritional parameters with amino acid–containing solutions. In a short-term (20-day) study in CAPD patients who were thought to be malnourished, significant increases in nitrogen balance, serum transferrin concentration, and total protein were achieved with the use of amino acid–containing PD fluids.[128] In addition, preliminary evidence indicates that these solutions may ameliorate some of the lipid abnormalities seen in PD patients.[129, 130] Complications include the development of metabolic acidosis and increased levels of serum urea nitrogen.

Possibly negating the benefit of amino acid absorption is the observation that intraperitoneal amino acids tend to cause vasodilatation, thus increasing the surface area and protein loss.[131] Douma and co-workers[132] did detect an increase in surface area and permeability with 1.1% amino acid–containing fluids, but no consistent increase in protein excretion, whereas in another study, a 20% increase in total protein loss was observed over the course of a 12-week trial with 1% amino acids.[133] Because of these concerns, a study was conducted to compare daily protein losses with amino acid absorption from one exchange per day of 1.1% amino acids. These data suggest that the amino acids absorbed more than adequately replaced the daily dialysate protein losses.[134]

Despite data showing that daily absorption of amino acids exceeds daily protein losses and that short-term balance studies suggest a benefit, the long-term usefulness of intraperitoneal amino acids has been controversial. The European experience has been favorable,[135] but in another study, no overall sustained positive effect on albumin over time was noted.[136] However, in subgroup analysis, those with the lower third of nutritional parameters had the best sustained response to intraperitoneal amino acids. It is likely that to prevent "uremic symptoms" from the increased protein load, total solute clearance will need to be carefully monitored and perhaps increased.

Ultrafiltration rates for 1.1% amino acid solutions are similar to those for 1.5% dextrose solutions.

POLYPEPTIDES AND OLIGOPEPTIDES. Klein and associates[137] first reported the use of peptides as osmotic agents for PD fluids in 1986. These peptides were derived from enzymatic hydrolysis of milk whey protein. Theoretical advantages of polypeptides over glucose include prolonged ultrafiltration because of a higher average molecular weight as a result of the presence of ionized branched chains that provide higher osmotic pressure on a molar basis, as well as the potential for providing protein-based calories. Polypeptides are rapidly metabolized to amino acids by plasma proteolytic enzymes after absorption. Preliminary studies have confirmed their superior ultrafiltration characteristics and transient increases in serum amino acid levels.[138] Polypeptides

are unlikely to cause any significant change in peritoneal transport. Oligopeptide use was reviewed by Wang and Lindholm.[139]

Traditionally, fluid moves across membranes driven by "crystalloid" osmotic differences between solutions. This process is valid only for "ideal" semipermeable membranes. For a membrane that is partially permeable to solutes, such as the peritoneal membrane, "colloid" osmosis is also possible. In this situation, the direction of the osmotic force is determined by differences in the sum of the products of the reflection coefficients and their molar concentration rather than the crystalloid osmotic gradient. If the number of macromolecules in one solution of similar osmolality is higher than in another, the solvent will move to the solution with the larger number of macromolecules (colloid osmotic force).[140] Thus, ultrafiltration is possible between iso-osmolar and hypo-osmolar solutions.[141]

Polymers of glucose can be used to bring about colloid-induced ultrafiltration. These polymers, such as the commercially prepared polymer icodextrin, are currently in clinical use. Polyglucose is manufactured by the enzymatic hydrolysis of corn starch first to maltodextrin, which is then further refined by membrane fractionation to polyglucose (icodextrin).[142] Whereas glucose induces transcapillary ultrafiltration across both small interendothelial and ultrasmall transcellular pores, glucose polymers induce ultrafiltration across interendothelial pores and the relatively few large pores.[143] Another difference is that glucose and polyglucose have markedly different transcapillary ultrafiltration profiles. Ultrafiltration with glucose is rapid, occurs early in the dwell period (because of the large crystalloid osmotic gradient), and decreases with time as glucose is absorbed, whereas with polyglucose, ultrafiltration increases linearly with time (Fig. 60-4). Once enough glucose is absorbed so that a crystalloid-induced osmotic gradient is no longer present, ultrafiltration ceases and lymphatic reabsorption of fluid predominates. In fact, during the long daytime dwell periods used with CCPD, it is not uncommon to drain out less than the instilled volume (net negative ultrafiltration). In contrast, polyglucose is slowly absorbed through the lymphatics.[144] Thus, polyglucose

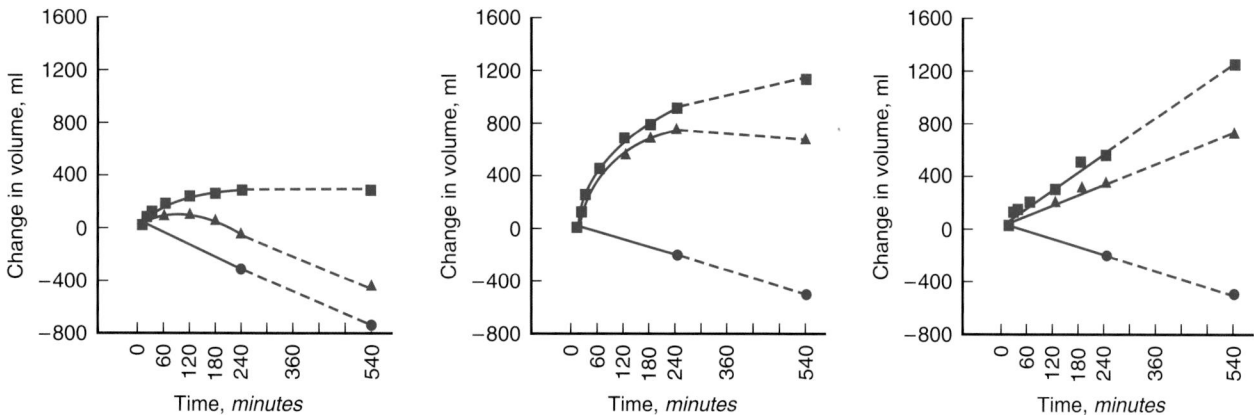

FIGURE 60-4. Time courses of intraperitoneal volume changes caused by transcapillary ultrafiltration *(square)* and lymphatic absorption *(bullet)* and that result in net ultrafiltration *(triangle)* during a 4-hour dwell with 1.36% glucose *(left)*, 3.86% glucose *(middle)*, and 7.5% icodextrin *(right)* in 10 stable continuous ambulatory peritoneal dialysis patients *(solid lines)*. Data were extrapolated to 9-hour values by using the Lineweaver-Burk plot for glucose and linear regression for icodextrin *(dashed lines)*. Median values are given. (Used with permission from Ho-dac-Pannekeet MM, Schouten N, Langendijk MJ, et al: Peritoneal transport characteristics with glucose polymer based dialysate. Kidney Int 50:979-986, 1996.)

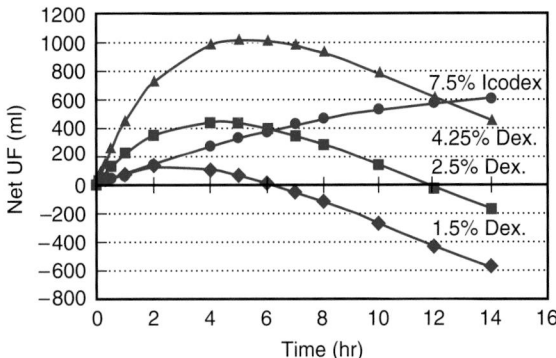

FIGURE 60-5. Representative net ultrafiltration curves for 4.25% dextrose *(triangles)*, 2.5% dextrose *(squares)*, 1.5% dextrose *(diamonds)*, and icodextrose (polyglucose—*circles*). (Modified from Ho-Dac-Pannekeet, Schouten N, Langendijk MJ, et al: Peritoneal transport characteristics with glucose polymer based dialysate. Kidney Int 50:979-986; and Douma CE, Hiralall JK, de Waart DR, et al: Kidney Int 53:1014-1021, 1998.)

solutions maintain a slow, but sustained colloid osmotic force and are ideal for producing sustained ultrafiltration over long dwell periods of up to 18 hours.[145-147] Furthermore, the rate of absorption is not influenced by the peritoneal transport type as is the absorption rate of glucose by diffusion. Hence, little difference in drain volume (ultrafiltration) after a 12-hour dwell period is noted in patients using icodextrin versus those using the less hypertonic dextrose-containing solutions (Fig. 60-5A and B).[148]

Initial studies have shown that these solutions are safe and well tolerated, with ultrafiltration rates similar to those of 2.5% dextrose and markedly better than those of 1.5% dextrose during overnight dwell.[149-152] Despite the potential for accumulation of metabolites such as maltose, little to no clinical toxicity has resulted from the prolonged use of these agents.[153] Icodextrin has been shown to lower cholesterol levels[154] and reduce serum insulin levels and insulin sensitivity[155] and can be used to increase ultrafiltration in patients with ultrafiltration failure so that they do not need to transfer to HD. In patients with ultrafiltration failure, 60% were still receiving the solution after 30 months. Ultrafiltration rates were maintained and the solution was well tolerated.[156]

The use of polyglucose is increasingly being indicated for long dwell periods (night CAPD, day CCPD) to avoid excessive glucose accumulation and achieve sustained ultrafiltration without hypertonic glucose. Another advantage of these solutions is the ability to combine osmotic agents (early ultrafiltration and late ultrafiltration) into "bimodal" solutions, such as amino acids and polyglucose.[157]

The safety of icodextrin use has been established. Rash is about twice as likely to occur with icodextrin as with glucose-containing fluids.[158] Although an exfoliative reaction is occasionally seen, no cases of Stevens-Johnson syndrome have ever been reported. Sterile peritonitis has been described but usually resolves with discontinuation of the product.[159, 160] Causes of sterile peritonitis in such cases are unclear and include, but are not limited to, the following[161]: (1) an allergy to dextrin itself—unlikely; (2) an allergy to dextran, although it has been shown that the occurrence of sterile peritonitis is not associated with presence or lack of dextran antibiodies[162]; and (3) the possibility that an impurity or allergen is somehow being introduced during the

manufacturing process. Maltose or other icodextrin metabolites may interfere with certain finger stick glucose estimations (tests that use the dehydrogenase pyrroloquinolinequinone reaction but not those using glucose oxidation or hexokinase testing).[163] Icodextrin and its metabolites may directly interfere with serum amylase determinations by slightly lowering values, thus suggesting that to make the diagnosis of pancreatitis, one may need to rely more on computed tomography (CT) or magnetic resonance imaging (MRI) than on serum amylase levels alone.[164]

Indications for the use of polyglycose include the long dwell times associated with CAPD (overnight) and CCPD (daytime), patients with loss of ultrafiltration (high transporters, those with loss of aquaporins), episodes of peritonitis, and patients with diabetes mellitus (to decrease the glucose load).[165]

Biocompatibility Issues

The peritoneal cavity is exposed to new dialysis fluids at least four times daily in the typical PD patient. At present, the PD solutions available exert biologically and chemically induced effects not only on the peritoneal membrane and mesothelial cell but also on the resident leukocytes, macrophages, and fibroblasts. This concept of biocompatibility (and the possible bioincompatibility of PD fluids) is the subject of extensive research. Peritoneal biopsy in patients undergoing long-term PD has revealed ultrastructural changes (e.g., glycosylation of capillary proteins), possibly induced in part by the dialysis solutions themselves.[123] Systemic toxic effects and morbidity have been associated with excessive absorption of glucose and Ca^{2+}. Over time, these long-term morphologic alterations seem to be associated with clinically relevant changes in peritoneal transport and ultrafiltration capability.[166] Several studies have identified increased vascularity and correlated it with changes in membrane function.[167] Occasionally, this increased vascularity is associated with the development of a debilitating, sclerosing process within the peritoneum. It has been suggested that this process may be due in part to the accumulation of advanced glycation end products (AGEs) within structures of the peritoneal membrane.[168] These and other concerns indicate that despite the documented long-term clinical safety and usefulness of the standard, currently available PD solutions, they are to some degree bioincompatible. The properties of an ideal dialysis solution are outlined in Table 60-3.

PERITONEAL MEMBRANE EFFECTS. Various morphologic changes in the peritoneal membrane have been observed

TABLE 60-3

Ideal Peritoneal Dialysis Solution

Good solute clearance and ultrafiltration capacity
Necessary solutes supplied and uremic toxins removed
Nutrition supplied or does not promote catabolism
Isosmolar solution, normal pH, bicarbonate as buffer
Minimal absorption of osmotic agent
Antibacterial and antifungal properties
Membrane biocompatible/does not promote chronic inflammation

From Balfe JW, Qamar I: The use of alternative peritoneal dialysis solutions in pediatric patients. Perit Dial Int 13(suppl 2):95-97, 1993.

in long-term PD patients.[169] When mesothelial cells were incubated with various concentrations of glucose, cell growth inhibition and cell damage were documented to occur in a dose-dependent manner.[170] The viability of human mesothelial cell monolayers was reduced after 3 hours of exposure to dialysis solutions.[171] Furthermore, mesothelial function may be altered by the indirect effects of dialysis solutions, such as the effect that these solutions have on the production of tumor necrosis factor (TNF), which causes injury to mesothelial monolayers.[172] Bicarbonate-containing fluids were less likely to inhibit cell growth, cause morphologic alterations, reduce phospholipid secretion, or induce interleukin-1 (IL-1) production than lactate-containing solutions were.[111, 173] Most historical studies were performed in a steady-state in vitro setting that simulates the effect of the initial dialysate composition on cellular function. In reality, during the dwell period, the composition and pH of the dialysis fluid become more physiologic, and thus it is possible that the in vitro findings may not mimic in vivo results.[174] To examine this possibility, Gotloib and colleagues[175] used mesothelial cell imprints and histochemical techniques to demonstrate that when the mesothelial cells of mice were exposed to effluent dialysate, the mesothelial cell injury was similar to that found in in vitro experiments.

In summary, it appears that long-term exposure of the peritoneal membrane to the currently available glucose-containing solutions results in minor, but progressive anatomic changes that produce alterations in structure and function. Mesothelial cells themselves not only produce surfactant (a lubricant that facilitates peristalsis) but also control the relative amount of inflammation and fibrinolysis within the peritoneal cavity. Therefore, a decrease in the number of functional mesothelial cells may predispose to unregulated inflammation with a predisposition to the formation of adhesions. Further studies are needed. It has been noted that adenovirus-mediated gene transfer is possible, and vectors to transfer genes coding for anti-inflammatory, antiangiogenic, and antifibrotic cytokines have been developed. The possible effects of these viral agents on peritoneal dynamics are currently undergoing study in a rat model of chronic peritoneal inflammation.[176]

HOST DEFENSE. PD patients are at constant risk for peritonitis. Therefore, to minimize risk and facilitate cure if peritonitis occurs, PD fluids must have minimal to no unwanted effects on resident peritoneal white blood cell viability or function. Unfortunately, such is not the case. First, peritoneal macrophages, neutrophils, lymphocytes, and opsonins are continually diluted and removed by the PD process. Second, the nonphysiologic pH, osmolality, and glucose concentrations of standard dialysis fluids have been shown to inhibit fundamental white blood cell functions both in vivo and in vitro. Finally, production and secretion of the various inflammatory mediators of host defense are altered by dialysis fluids. Detailed information on these effects of standard glucose-containing, lactate-buffered solutions is available elsewhere.[177] An important issue in biocompatibility, therefore, is the development of PD fluids that reduce these adverse affects on host defense.

Studies using polyglucose solutions have shown that phagocytic activity and the chemiluminescence of peritoneal macrophages is less impaired than with standard glucose-based solutions.[151] IL-6 is a 184–amino acid protein produced by peritoneal mesothelial cells in response to IL-1β and TNF-α. It is thus an indirect marker of the relative state of inflammation of the peritoneal cavity. Levels of IL-6 increase significantly during periods of inflammation.[178] Production of TNF and IL-6 was less suppressed when peripheral white blood cells were exposed to physiologic pH or glucose polymer–containing solutions than to standard low-pH, glucose-containing solutions.[179] Bicarbonate-based solutions were found to have a lower inhibitory effect on peripheral blood cytokine release than were lactate-containing solutions with a similar pH.[180] Even though the dialysate becomes more "physiologic" during the dwell period, data show that once cell function is altered, the effects can last for hours.[181] Further in vivo and ex vivo studies have confirmed that bicarbonate-based solutions are more biocompatible than conventional lactate-buffered solutions.[182] Recent studies have shown that a combined bicarbonate-lactate solution results in lower IL-6 levels than lactate alone does, perhaps because of the neutral pH of the solution and the presence of less glucose degradation products (GDPs) in the dialysis fluid.[183]

Some data suggest that the di(2-ethylhexyl)phthalate (DEHP), the most commonly used plasticizer for polyvinyl chloride, added to improve the flexibility of dialysate bag tubing may have adverse effects on macrophage function.[184] Furthermore, it has been shown that the GDPs produced during heat sterilization and storage of glucose-containing solutions participate in the nonenzymatic cross-linking of proteins leading to the formation of AGEs, which are thought to participate in the remodeling and fibrosis of the peritoneal membrane noted in long-term patients.[185] Solutions with less GDPs may be more biocompatible and result in improved mesothelial cell function.[186] It is unknown which intervention/improvement will ultimately be more beneficial: reducing GDPs or improving the pH. Will improvements in both be additive? Preliminary data suggest that newer fluids should address both issues.[187, 188]

Lowering the Ca^{2+} concentration of culture media has been shown to decrease macrophage function[189, 190] and may predispose to peritonitis,[191] although this finding has not been substantiated in other clinical trials.[192]

CONCLUSIONS. Although commercially available dialysis solutions based on lactate and glucose have provided adequate treatment of ESRD for thousands of patients, they do alter mesothelial cell and peritoneal macrophage function. Furthermore, pathologic alterations in the peritoneal membrane that may be related to components of the PD solutions have been described. It is not known whether the observed structural changes correlate with the observed functional changes. Long-term follow-up is needed to see whether more "biocompatible" solutions have any beneficial long-term effect. Newer solutions that address these needs have been developed and are in clinical use. However, the long-term outcomes and benefits of using such solutions for the patient are not yet fully understood.

Peritoneal Membrane

Anatomy

The peritoneal membrane is the primary interface between blood and the dialysate compartments. It is across this membrane that water and solute must be transported. The peritoneal membrane is composed of two principal parts: (1) the parietal peritoneum (about 10% of the total), which covers the inner surface of the abdominal and pelvic walls, including the diaphragm, and (2) the visceral peritoneum (about 90% of the total), which covers the visceral organs, including the intra-abdominal portion of the gastrointestinal tract, the liver, and the spleen, and forms the omentum and the visceral mesentery, where it reflects over and connects the loops of bowel. The total surface area of the peritoneal membrane (parietal and visceral) is thought to approximate the body surface area in most adults (i.e., 1 to 2 m^2).[193-195] Children have a disproportionately larger peritoneal surface area than most adults do.[196] The peritoneal membrane is continuous and forms a closed space in males. In females, it is continuous with the mucous membrane of the fallopian tubes. The intra-abdominal opening is normally collapsed, and hence no free communication usually exists between the peritoneal space and the exterior. However, this potential anatomic opening allows the possibility of communication between the intrauterine and intra-abdominal spaces in females. The peritoneal cavity generally contains about 100 mL or less of fluid, but a normal-sized adult can usually tolerate 2 L or more without discomfort or compromise of pulmonary function.

From the perspective of PD, important anatomic components of the peritoneal membrane include the mesothelial cells, the underlying basement membrane, the interstitium, the microcirculation, and the visceral lymphatics. A previous edition of this text includes a more detailed discussion of the peritoneal anatomy.[197]

MESOTHELIUM. The mesothelium is a continuous monolayer of flattened cells about 0.5 mm thick. The free surface area of the mesothelium is covered by countless microvilli that markedly increase the surface area.[198] The cells have tortuous boundaries, which increase the area of contact between them. These cells have several types of function that allow for adhesion and communication between cells,[199] including tight junctions,[200] which have an anchoring function that mechanically attaches cells to one another and the basement membrane, and gap junctions, which mediate the passage of chemical or electrical signals. The antiluminal surface has many open intercellular channels approximately 50 nm wide. In some areas, especially the subdiaphragmatic region, the absence of tight junctions results in the formation of stomas[201] that allow direct contact between the peritoneal cavity and the diaphragmatic lymphatics. Peritoneal fluid and its solutes are absorbed directly into the lymphatic system via the subdiaphragmatic stoma.

Anionic binding sites, which could theoretically influence the movement of charged ions, have been demonstrated on the luminal surface of peritoneal lymphatics after the injection of cationic ferritin in mice.[202] Ultrastructural examination of the peritoneum of normal rabbits after the intravenous injection of iron dextran, an electron-dense tracer, has revealed that dextran appears in intracellular vesicles. This observation supports the hypothesis that vesicular transport may play a role in the transport of high-molecular-weight substances across the peritoneum.[203]

Mesothelial cells are ultrastructurally similar to the type II pneumocytes found in the pulmonary alveoli[204]; they also contain lamellar bodies identical to those in type II pneumocytes.[205, 206] These cells may secrete a surfactant-like lubrication for the peritoneum.[207] In addition, mesothelial cells are active in modulating host defense[208] and have been shown to produce CA 125.[209] It has been suggested that CA 125 appearance rates in the dialysate effluent can be used to estimate mesothelial cell mass and possibly the effect that changing to more "biocompatible" solutions has on overall peritoneal membrane health.[210]

BASEMENT MEMBRANE. A homogeneous basement membrane underlies the mesothelial cells. In animals, it is between 25 and 40 mm thick. The basement membrane has some openings, particularly in the diaphragmatic peritoneum, and it may be absent under the omental mesothelium. It is believed to be formed by mesothelial cells and is composed of type IV collagen, proteoglycans, and glycoproteins. The basement membrane can act as a selective cellular barrier by preventing fibroblasts from contacting mesothelial cells while allowing macrophages and lymphocytes to pass through it. It may also play a role in tissue regeneration.

INTERSTITIUM. The interstitium is the primary supporting structure of the peritoneum and is composed primarily of a mucopolysaccharide matrix. It contains bundles of collagen fibers, blood vessels, the lymphatics, occasional macrophages, glycosaminoglycans, and fibroblasts. The interstitium has aqueous and lipophilic phases. The aqueous phase mediates the transport of water, electrolytes, protein, nutrients, and hormones. The distance between capillaries and the mesothelial surface may vary as the interstitium changes. One such glycosaminoglycan, hyaluronan, seems to play a role in influencing transport across the interstitium.[211] For a detailed discussion of the role of the extracellular matrix in transperitoneal transport, see work by Flessner and colleagues.[212]

BLOOD VESSELS. Total splanchnic blood flow in normal adult humans at rest ranges from 1000 to 2400 mL/min.[213] The blood supply to the visceral and parietal membranes arises from two different sources: the visceral peritoneal membrane is supplied by the celiac and mesenteric arteries, with venous drainage via the portal vein, whereas the parietal mesothelium is supplied by the circumflex, iliac, lumbar, intercostal, and epigastric arteries. Venous drainage from the parietal mesothelial surfaces empties directly into the systemic circulation, bypassing the hepatic portal system. An important clinical implication of this anatomy is that absorption of any drug from the visceral peritoneum results in rapid first-pass metabolism by the liver.

The number of perfused capillaries determines the so-called effective peritoneal surface area, that is, the functional area for exchange between blood and dialysate. The more perfused capillaries are, the more rapidly diffusion occurs. The density of the vascular bed varies in different parts of the peritoneum. Solute transport is also influenced by the number and size of pores present within these capillaries. The capillary walls are believed to contain at least two distinct pore sizes,[214] with the larger pores located primarily at the venular end and the smaller pores at the arteriolar end. Endothelial cells also appear to have intracellular pores or channels thought to be aquapores.[215]

PERITONEAL LYMPHATICS. As in most body tissues, a network of lymphatic vessels aid in the removal of fluids and solutes from the interstitium. They also function to maintain the relatively small volume of fluid (50 to 100 mL) normally found within the peritoneal cavity by returning excess intraperitoneal fluid, protein, and macromolecules to the circulation.[216] Fluid absorption occurs primarily through stomas in the subdiaphragmatic area,[217] where the lymphatic network is well developed and quite extensive.[218] In these areas the basement membrane is absent, so there is very little resistance to solute movement as fluid (solvent) is absorbed. The clinical significance of this observation is that as fluid is absorbed, solutes (urea, creatinine) and macromolecules (icodextrin) are returned to the circulation. Lymphatics are also present in the submucosal layers of most of the visceral and parietal mesothelium.[219] Many physiologic factors, including intraperitoneal hydrostatic pressure, body posture, and pharmacologic agents, notably alter the rate of lymphatic uptake.[220]

Anatomic Findings in Peritoneal Dialysis Patients

Clinical observations by surgeons with experience in treating CAPD patients suggest that diffuse opacification, at times with local accentuation, develops on the peritoneal surface and can progress to the "tanned" peritoneal syndrome or, in advanced stages, to sclerosing encapsulating peritoneal fibrosis.[221] A review of microscopic examination of randomly collected peritoneal tissue by the International Peritoneal Biopsy Registry indicates that the process of PD may induce significant ultrastructural deviations from normal in both the mesothelium and the underlying stroma.[169] Such abnormalities include loss of microvilli, hyperplasia of the rough endoplasmic reticulum, formation of unusual surface protuberances, disorganization of the normal collagen fibers, expansion of the underlying matrix ground substance,[222] and occasional reduplication of the basal lamina.[223] An increase in submesothelial thickening, often called fibrosis, tends to occur. When advanced, it turns a portion of the submesothelial area into a "cellular desert" where remesothelialization has failed to occur.[169, 224] The cytoplasmic inclusions characteristic of uremic patients before beginning PD[222] and in the pericardium of patients with uremic pericarditis are not found in long-term PD patients, thus suggesting that these inclusions are a marker of uremic serositis.[169]

In most patients, these changes are minimal, even in those who have been maintained on PD for up to 10 years.[222] However, the reaction of the peritoneal mesothelium and underlying stroma to the stress of continuous dialysis is likely to result in a spectrum of changes ranging from the minimal ones clinically associated with only peritoneal opacification to replacement of the peritoneal membrane with dense fibrous tissue that causes sclerosing peritonitis.[196] Marked changes are more likely in patients with a history of recurring or severe peritonitis. The diabetiform nature of capillary basement membrane lesions logically would incriminate dialysate glucose. This change could result from the peritonitis itself or from increased glucose flux during an episode of peritonitis. Surface microvilli are lost during episodes of peritonitis, and prominent intercellular gaps appear.[225, 226] However, in most patients, transport characteristics return to baseline after an episode of peritonitis. The hypothesis is that chronic uremia is associated with high levels of circulating reactive carbonyl compounds (RCCs) that initiate the formation of AGEs in the peritoneum. During PD, the RCCs in glucose-containing solutions (as a result of the sterilization process) will amplify AGE formation. RCCs and AGEs initiate a number of cellular responses, including vascular endothelial growth factor, which interacts with endothelial cells to stimulate angiogenesis and increase vascular permeability.[227] The use of more biocompatible solutions may slow or prevent this process.

Contribution of Peritoneal Structures to Dialysis

The relative contribution of each part (i.e., parietal versus visceral) of the peritoneal surface to overall solute clearance in humans is uncertain. If one were to take the product of the permeability and the area of the many different structures within the peritoneum and add up these products, the resultant overall mass transfer area coefficient (MTAC) of the peritoneum would be three to four times greater than the "effective" surface area that has been measured[228] and observed in clinical practice.[229] Supporting evidence is the finding of a threefold to fourfold increase in MTAC in rats after mixing with an orbital shaker.[230] Studies in animals have demonstrated that the absorption of glucose and other metabolites from the peritoneal cavity is only minimally reduced by omentectomy, mesenteriectomy, or evisceration.[231, 232] Experiments in rats using isolated chambers to determine the relative permeability of different parts of the peritoneal surface have shown that the liver is responsible for only a small part of the overall transport[228] and that drops in blood pressure that primarily affect blood flow to the liver, not the mesentery, have very little effect on overall solute transfer.[233] These experiments confirm earlier observations supporting the use of PD during conditions of shock.[234] Interestingly, in an anecdotal report, an infant with acute renal failure underwent successful PD after virtually complete resection of the small intestine.[235]

The reasons for these variable findings are unclear. Perhaps the visceral peritoneum may be the predominant transport surface in intact animals, and normally only a portion of all the surface area of the peritoneum is in contact with dialysate. Evisceration may expose a greater amount of parietal peritoneal surface area[231] to contact with dialysate. Alternatively, evisceration could change intra-abdominal pressure with a resultant change in transport.[236]

Taken together, these and other studies suggest that the parietal peritoneum may be more important than originally thought and that under usual circumstances, only about 25% of the total peritoneal surface area comes in contact with dialysis fluids.

The understanding of how each part of the peritoneal membrane contributes to dialysis is evolving and was recently reviewed.[237] The current view of transport developed by physiologists includes distribution of solute in individual capillaries, transport across capillaries, transport through the interstitium, and finally transport across the peritoneal membrane itself. The barrier properties of mesothelial cells remain controversial. It has been noted that a surface-active phospholipid is reversibly bound to the normal mesothelial cell surface.[238] The lining acts as a boundary lubricant and preserves the mechanical integrity of the epithelial surface.[239] Surface-active phospholipids are probably important for lubrication of the peritoneal surface, may play a role in host defense, and may also impart some of the semipermeability properties of the membrane that are important for maintaining ultrafiltration.[240] The absence of mesothelial cells results in a proliferation of fibroblasts, whereas an intact mesothelial surface prevents the scarring and fibrosis that could increase resistance to transport from blood to the peritoneal cavity.[241] A smoothly sliding surface may promote the distribution of peritoneal fluid. Thus, the mesothelium may not be significant in terms of resistance to transport, but it is important in keeping the system functional as a whole.

PERITONEUM AS A DIALYSIS SYSTEM

Resistance to Salt and Water Transport

If the effective surface area were the only factor limiting solute transport in PD, transport of solutes should be closely related to their free diffusion coefficients in water. Such is not the case, however, particularly for macromolecules.[242] Therefore, an additional barrier intrinsic to the peritoneal membrane itself must be present. In attempting to define this barrier, one must consider the potential resistance sites that solutes must cross as they move from the peritoneal capillaries into the peritoneal cavity. These potential resistance sites include (1) fluid films within the capillary lumen, (2) the endothelial layer (0.5 μm), (3) the capillary basement membrane (0.2 to 5 mm), (4) the interstitium (0.1 to 100 mm), (5) the mesothelial layer (0.9 mm), and (6) fluid films within the peritoneal cavity.[243]

The exact route taken by solutes as they pass from blood into the peritoneum has not been well established. It is known that solute transport occurs by both diffusive and convective forces (discussed later). The mass transport barrier appears to offer very little resistance to solute transport by diffusion but seems to offer significant resistance to solute transport by convection. The clinical significance of this finding is that solute removed by convection is not removed at the same concentration as it is in plasma. Resistance to the flow of solutes is greater than resistance to the flow of water. This greater resistance is especially evident when ultrafiltration is driven by small osmotic solutes, or "crystalloid osmosis," but it is less significant when ultrafiltration is driven by hydraulic pressure,[244, 245] or colloid osmosis.

Intracapillary fluid films are thought to exert little resistance, especially for low-molecular-weight solutes, because of the very short distance for molecules to pass through the fluid film.[246, 247] The capillary endothelium seems to serve as a selective barrier to solute transport. Experimentally, the endothelium acts as a low-resistance barrier to low-molecular-weight solutes with molecular weights up to the size of albumin, but they begin to offer significant resistance as the molecular weight increases further.[248] Grotte[249] first attempted to mathematically define solute transport and proposed a "two-pore" model of solute transport across the endothelium. This model suggested that transport of solute occurs through small pores with a diameter of 30 to 45 Å.[250] Transport of solute across the capillary endothelium is now better defined with a three-pore model.[251] Briefly, water channels, perhaps analogous to aquaporins,[252] permit only water to pass through them and thus approach the properties of an ideal semipermeable membrane. These channels are sensitive to crystalloid-driven (not colloid-induced) osmosis. They represent about 1% to 2% of the total pore number and have a radius smaller than 0.8 nm. Small pores, thought to be interendothelial clefts with a radius of 4 to 6 nm, account for 90% to 93% of the total pore area. They tend to be located along the arteriolar end of capillaries. These pores severely restrict the passage of protein but allow small molecules such as urea, creatinine, and water to flow freely. Small solutes move across these small pores via diffusion gradients and water via hydrostatic, colloid, and crystalloid osmotic pressure. Large pores, which have radii larger than 20 nm and are probably located in the venular side of capillaries, constitute between 5% and 7% of the overall pore area.[253] These pores allow the passage of macromolecules and water through hydrostatic forces (Fig. 60-6). Fox and co-workers[254] have shown that transport of macromolecules in vivo occurs through large gaps near the venules. Pappenheimer[255] has suggested that less than 0.2% of the luminal surface is made up of these large gaps.

Diffusion is postulated to occur through large pores located at the venular end of capillaries,[256] whereas convection occurs through small pores located primarily at the arteriolar end of capillaries. Two types of small pores have been identified. The first consists of transcellular aquaporins, which allow transport of water, but not solute. This type accounts for the sieving of solute during convection as a result of crystalloid-driven forces and the clinical observation that early in a dwell period with a crystalloid osmotic agent (glucose), dialysate sodium decreases. The second type consists of small pores located at the arteriolar end of capillaries, where some diffusion and most ultrafiltration occur (both via crystalloid- and colloid-driven forces).

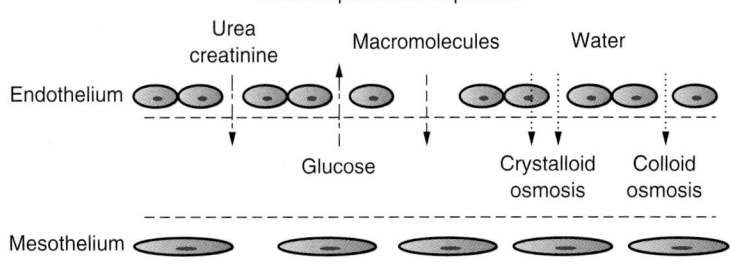

UNDERSTANDING FLUID MANAGEMENT
Pathways for solute and water transport

FIGURE 60-6. Various pore systems in the vascular wall. The small interendothelial pores are involved in the transport of low-molecular-weight solutes and in water transport. Large pores allow the passage of macromolecules. Crystalloid osmosis induces water transport partly across the small pores, but also through ultrasmall transcellular water channels. Colloid osmosis induces fluid transport only across the small pore system. The mesothelium is not an osmotic barrier. (From Andreucci VE, Fine LG: International Yearbook of Nephrology 1997. Oxford, Oxford University Press, 1998.)

Convection is confined to the small pores because it is hypothesized that the larger pores are so large that glucose does not exert sufficiently effective osmotic force across them. Hence, the membrane appears to be most permeable to diffusion through the large venular pores, where most diffusion occurs. It is less permeable for convective transport through the small arteriolar pores. Macromolecules are transported via large pores.

The capillary basement membrane seems to produce little effect on the diffusion of low-molecular-weight solutes,[257] although anionic sites predominantly composed of heparin sulfate and chondroitin sulfate, which could theoretically inhibit the transport of charged solutes, are regularly found in the basement membranes of the microvasculature.[258] These anionic sites are particularly abundant in fenestrated capillaries, some of which have been identified in human parietal and subdiaphragmatic peritoneum.[259]

The interstitium represents the longest distance that solutes must traverse. Increasing evidence suggests that the interstitium is one of the major resistance sites for urea and low-molecular-weight solute transport.[260, 261] The interstitium is thought to be represented by a two-phase system that contains a gelatinous mucopolysaccharide matrix interspersed with a water-rich, colloid-poor, free-fluid phase containing aqueous channels.[254] Small solutes may pass through these channels. Although these channels may normally offer little resistance to transport, hypertonic dialysis may dehydrate the interstitium, thus shortening the distance that the solute must traverse but making the channels more tortuous and thereby increasing resistance.[262] In addition, the fixed charges on the collagen or mucopolysaccharide molecules within the interstitium may influence the transport of charged solutes. These ionic charges are thought to restrict both diffusive and convective transport of charged solutes across the peritoneal membrane. For example, diffusive rates of transport for K^+, Li^+, and PO_4^{3-} are slower than the diffusive transport rates of uncharged, similarly sized solutes.[263] The larger the distance between the capillary wall and the peritoneal surface, the greater the resistance will become. For example, the proportion of resistance to diffusive transport of a small solute (e.g., sucrose) that is attributable to the interstitium increases from 29% if the capillary is located 50 μm from the peritoneum to 83% of the total if the capillary wall is located 600 μm from the peritoneum.[264] Thus, the interstitium can influence diffusion rates of the peritoneal membrane.

The mesothelium appears to be more permeable than the endothelium, possibly because of larger intercellular gaps.[265] It is thought that transport through the mesothelium occurs by way of these gaps and numerous intracellular vesicles. Therefore, it is believed to offer very little resistance to the transport of small and large solutes.[266] However, permeability is not uniform, and visceral mesothelium may be more permeable than parietal mesothelium.[267] Furthermore, it has been suggested that surface-active phospholipids adsorbed onto the mesothelial cell lining maintain the integrity of the "semipermeable" properties of the membrane.[268] Studies of transport across isolated mesentery suggest that mesothelial cells contribute some resistance to transport.[269] Other studies have shown that permeation of solutes into the isolated hemidiaphragm is less pronounced in areas covered by mesothelium than in bare areas.

Experimental data suggest that intraperitoneal fluid channels also limit solute transport. The many folds of the mesentery result in the formation of numerous relatively wide and stagnant intraperitoneal fluid films of dialysate during PD, which substantially limits transport.[270] This situation is unlike the conditions during conventional HD, in which the dialysate channels are small and dialysate flow is rapid.[271] In vitro experiments using hollow-fiber dialyzers that simulate the conditions of PD are unable to achieve the clearances obtained with conventional HD, further suggesting that fluid films limit the transport of solutes in PD.[247] Rapid cycling seems to have little influence on these fluid films,[272, 273] whereas abdominal compression in rats has been shown to increase clearance, perhaps by increasing the surface area that is in contact with dialysate.[274]

Summary of Resistance Sites for Small Solutes

Even with rapid cycling, the maximal urea clearance achieved clinically in most humans with the currently available PD technologies is about 40 mL/min.[270, 272] This maximal clearance is little changed (20%) even with the intraperitoneal use of potent vasodilators,[275, 276] which theoretically would increase both the number of capillaries perfused and capillary permeability, thus maximizing surface area and minimizing any endothelial resistance. Estimates of peritoneal capillary blood flow determined from the peritoneal clearance of carbon dioxide gas in humans and hydrogen gas in rabbits are two to three times the maximal urea clearance,[214] which suggests that small-solute clearance is not blood flow dependent[246, 277] and that even in severe shock, only a modest reduction in observed clearance would occur.[234] These data imply that the major resistance sites for small-solute clearance are the capillary endothelium, the interstitium, and intraperitoneal fluid films.

Summary of Resistance Sites for Large Solutes

Large solutes are thought to be transferred via large pores, which are predominately located at the venular end of capillaries. Hence, it appears that the major resistance site for large solutes is the peritoneal microcirculation, as postulated from the following indirect evidence. First, after the intravenous injection of fluorescent-tagged albumin, labeling of the interstitium occurs slowly unless agents are administered that increase vascular permeability. The increase in vascular permeability markedly enhances albumin uptake.[248] Second, the increase in inulin clearance is proportionally larger than that for urea after the intravenous injection of vasoactive drugs.[275] Third, peritoneal inflammation, which is associated with vasodilatation, is known to increase protein losses more than changes in small-solute transport.[278, 279] Finally, intraperitoneal nitroprusside, which enhances venular permeability, markedly increases protein loss.

Models of Peritoneal Transport

The peritoneal membrane and its vascular and lymphatic systems constitute a complex interactive and changing membrane for dialysis. Furthermore, this membrane is alive and likely to change with its environment. Various physiologic, pharmacologic, and morphologic studies described here and elsewhere in the literature have been able to define some, but not all the transport properties of the peritoneum. Despite this complexity, investigators have attempted to characterize peritoneal membrane transport properties in terms of classic membrane physiology by using mathematical models. These models can be of assistance to nephrologists in understanding peritoneal solute and water transport and can be used as a guide for individualizing prescriptions for patients.

These models describe transport by using various phenomenologic mathematical coefficients to describe known clinical and experimental observations, such as diffusive or convective transport. Virtually every element of experimental and clinical data taken separately can be defined by a simple semipermeable membrane model. However, when they are considered in total, the assembled clinical observations and laboratory findings cannot be explained in terms of simple membrane physiology. Modification of these models has allowed consideration of the effect of lymphatic flow, ultrafiltration, and the apparent heterogeneous nature of peritoneal membrane pores so that they closely approximate most, but not all transport properties of the membrane.

For any of these mathematical models to be valid, they must account for the following known properties of solute transport: (1) little to no resistance to solute transport by diffusion, (2) variable resistance to osmotically induced convective solute transport, and (3) little to no resistance to hydraulically induced convective solute transport.

The simplest models consider the peritoneum in terms of a homogeneous membrane that separates two well-mixed fluid compartments.[79, 280-282] As such, the peritoneal membrane represents both anatomic structures (e.g., the capillary endothelium, the interstitium, and the mesothelium) and the unstirred layers of fluid within both compartments. Any heterogeneities between tissues are ignored. Examples include the models of Randerson and Farrell,[283] Pyle,[284] Popovich and colleagues,[285] Garred and co-workers,[286] and Henderson and Nolph.[287] These models describe only certain aspects of membrane transport. In addition to the homogeneous membrane models, "distributed" models of peritoneal transport have been described.[288-290] These models assume that the barrier separating blood from dialysate is not homogeneous but is composed of distinct elements, including the capillaries and the interstitium, and that the blood phase is distributed within the peritoneal interstitium. Distributed models include the theory that transport is influenced by the distance between the capillary and mesothelial surface, as well as the number of capillaries. Other approaches include models of diffusive transport evaluated during periods of isovolemic dialysis, which eliminates the need to make any assumptions about the sieving properties of the membrane,[291, 292] the heteroporous model,[256] and triple-barrier models for solute transport.[293]

When reviewed, it was pointed out that none accurately modeled all aspects of transport.[294] The classic Pyle-Popovich model of transport and ultrafiltration, as modified by Vonesh and co-workers,[295] can be made to fit the observed data of patients when glucose is the osmotic agent. However, when higher-molecular-weight solutes are used as osmotic agents, ultrafiltration occurs even when using hypo-osmotic solutions, thus suggesting colloidal osmosis and the presence of a "third" pore.[296, 297] Hence, the most recent model,

the three-pore model,[296] yields the most realistic estimates of small-solute reflection coefficients, macromolecule transfer, and the effects of lymphatic absorption and ultrafiltration profiles observed clinically even when high-molecular-weight solutes are used as osmotic agents.

Physiology of Peritoneal Transport
Solute Transport by Diffusion

Diffusion, defined as a tendency for solutes to disperse themselves within the space available, is the most important mechanism responsible for solute transport into the peritoneum. The amount of solute that can pass through a membrane by diffusion per unit of time depends on the effective surface area of that membrane, its intrinsic permeability to that solute, and the volume of solvent (or rapidity of replacement) that the solute moves into. In PD, the diffusive clearance of any solute depends on the peritoneal membrane surface area, the intrinsic permeability of the membrane, dialysate flow, concentration gradients, and the time allowed for transport. Overall solute clearance can never exceed the lowest of these parameters.[298] The peritoneal surface area is estimated to be about 1 m² in adults.[193, 194] However, the "effective" peritoneal surface area is smaller than the measured surface[199, 299] and is primarily determined by the number of perfused capillaries. It is not a constant and is influenced by splanchnic blood volume[276, 300] and the presence of intraperitoneal dialysate.[301] Normally, only about 25% of the peritoneal capillaries are perfused.[302] Measurements of MTACs,[286] dialysance,[303] dialysate-plasma ratios of solutes,[304] and the standard peritoneal permeability analysis[305] are an attempt to classify differences in peritoneal membrane transport characteristics between individual patients.

Typical dialysate flow rates are markedly lower than those of capillary blood flow or membrane transport capabilities. Standard PD therapies are therefore limited by dialysate flow. As the clinician tries to increase dialysate flow rates by using standard technologies (CAPD < APD) while attempting to maintain a concentration gradient, the maximally effective dialysate flow rate is limited by loss of peritoneal membrane contact time during periods of inflow and drainage.[306] Thus, as dialysate flow rates increase to above 3.5 L/hr, small-solute clearance can decrease. Higher urea clearance rates have been achieved by the use of higher dialysate flow rates without increasing inflow or outflow times in a continuous flow system.[271, 307] Currently, continuous flow systems are not practical for use. Diffusion becomes more restricted as molecular weight increases (i.e., urea diffuses faster than creatinine). In fact, in contrast to what is observed for small-solute clearance, in which an increasing number of exchanges per day tends to increase daily clearance, even if the patient is already doing 24 hours of dwell time, once 24 hr/day of dwell time is instituted, further increases in the number of exchanges per day do not increase middle-molecule clearance rates.[308]

In conclusion, experimental data, clinical observations, and data from mathematical models suggest that the peritoneal membrane is very open to transport by diffusion. Such transport appears to occur mainly through large pores located near the venular end of capillaries.

Ultrafiltration

Ultrafiltration, or the transcapillary movement of fluids, has been reviewed by Renkin.[309] Attainment of a minimal daily amount of net ultrafiltration is an important clinical consideration because of the obvious necessity to maintain water balance and blood pressure control in patients with ESRD. Net ultrafiltration is achieved clinically by creating an osmotic pressure gradient (crystalloid or colloid) between blood and dialysate. Historically, dialysis fluids achieved this gradient via crystalloid osmosis by the addition of various concentrations of glucose to the solution. Newer fluids use polyglucose to induce colloid-driven ultrafiltration. The solutes present in body fluids can be swept along with the bulk solvent flow even in the absence of a concentration difference for net diffusion, thereby contributing to overall solute clearance. This contribution to net solute clearance has been termed "solvent drag" or "convection." Unfortunately, data suggest that in clinical practice, many PD patients are volume overloaded.[310-312]

KINETICS OF PERITONEAL ULTRAFILTRATION. In addition to ultrafiltration, absorption of fluid from the peritoneal cavity also occurs, mainly as a result of absorption by the peritoneal lymphatics. Intraperitoneal volume at any time is therefore determined by the relative magnitudes of transcapillary ultrafiltration and lymphatic absorption. Net ultrafiltration at the end of any dwell period is traditionally defined as the difference between drained volume and instilled volume.[313] This definition assumes that the residual volume in any patient is constant, which is often not the case.[314]

According to the law of Starling, transcapillary ultrafiltration depends on the hydraulic permeability of the peritoneal membrane, the surface area, and transmembrane pressure gradients. Capillary hydraulic pressure, colloid osmotic pressure, and crystalloid osmotic pressure all contribute to transmembrane pressure gradients.

Colloid osmotic pressure is exerted by macromolecules in solution. The average albumin concentration in dialysate is only about 1% of that in plasma, so with fluids using glucose as an osmotic agent, only a small osmotic pressure gradient is generated, and thus the plasma colloid osmotic pressure gradient opposes net ultrafiltration.[315] Hydraulic pressure differences in the peritoneal cavity vary, depending on posture and activities, and therefore could affect transcapillary ultrafiltration by affecting transmembrane pressure.[316, 317] Consequently, with glucose polymer, ultrafiltration can occur with iso-osmolar or hypo-osmolar solutions. The "force" is smaller, so the ultrafiltration rate is lower, but it is sustained during the dwell period because of slow absorption of the osmotic agent.[318]

Crystalloid osmotic pressure depends on the difference in the number of solutes in the solutions under consideration. For a given solution, the driving force for ultrafiltration is greatest across an ideal semipermeable membrane, that is, one that is impermeable to solute. The driving force for ultrafiltration decreases as the membrane becomes more permeable to solutes and the osmotic gradient diminishes as the solute moves down its concentration gradient from one compartment to the next. Therefore, because glucose is not completely rejected by the peritoneal membrane and is slowly reabsorbed from the dialysate, the driving force for ultrafiltration will change over time during a dwell period.

Net ultrafiltration is thus maximal during the first few minutes of the dwell period and progressively decreases over time as glucose is absorbed. With glucose-containing fluids, once osmotic equilibrium is approached, the crystalloid-induced transmembrane pressure becomes negligible and ultrafiltration ceases. After this time, there is net absorption of fluid and solutes through the subdiaphragmatic lymphatics and into the capillaries driven by other transcapillary osmotic pressure gradients (back-filtration).

MODELS OF ULTRAFILTRATION. To model mechanisms of ultrafiltration in PD, the clinician must first consider that solutes removed by convection are not always removed in amounts per volume of ultrafiltrate equal to their concentration in extracellular fluid.[319, 320] In other words, there is resistance to convection-driven ultrafiltration, and sieving occurs. Therefore, in attempting to define mathematical models of peritoneal ultrafiltration, a correction factor called the sieving coefficient or Staverman "reflection coefficient" must be considered for each solute in order to describe the sieving effect seen with solute transport by convection; such coefficients range between 0.0 and 1.0.[321] High-molecular-weight solutes such as dextran and albumin are almost completely rejected by the membrane and have reflection coefficients near unity. Other solutes such as glucose (molecular weight, 180) have minimal values for their reflection coefficient and therefore little to no membrane resistance to solute transport by convection.[322] Clinically, it is known that glucose is readily absorbed and that the osmotic force varies during the dwell period. This phenomenon is difficult to mathematically model so that ultrafiltration rates can be predicted accurately. Jaffrin and co-workers[323] modeled ultrafiltration with the assumption that glucose is the only osmotic solute whose concentration changes over the course of the dwell period. Nakanishi and colleagues[324] described a similar model in which three permeable solutes are assumed: urea, glucose, and Na^+. In this model, by using observed drain volumes and determining optimal values for peritoneal conductance, they found parameters for urea that were not physically realistic and concluded that urea was not an important osmotic solute for determining transperitoneal ultrafiltration, consistent with clinical observations. Predictive calculations using the distributed model of peritoneal transport are even more complex.[325] These models suggest that ultrafiltration takes place mainly in the proximal capillaries, where hydraulic pressure is the greatest and glucose is a relatively more effective generator of an osmotic pressure difference. In the distal capillaries, where hydraulic pressure is lower and plasma oncotic pressure higher, glucose is readily absorbed. Therefore, under normal conditions, absorption primarily of fluids would occur at the distal sites unless hypertonic solutions are used.

Blood flow rates were on average about six times greater than the maximal net ultrafiltration rates, thus suggesting that ultrafiltration is *not* limited by blood flow under usual clinical conditions.

CLINICAL FINDINGS. Ultrafiltration is an integral clinical component of PD for two reasons: to prevent volume overload and to allow solute clearance by convection. Ultrafiltration rates are highest at the beginning of the exchange and, as glucose is absorbed, decrease toward zero when osmotic equilibrium is reached.[326, 327] Depending on the concentration of instilled glucose, osmotic equilibrium is reached at different times in the dwell cycle. For 2-L solutions containing 1.5% dextrose (1.36% glucose), osmotic equilibrium and maximal drain volume are reached after about 2 hours of dwell time in most patients, whereas peak intraperitoneal volumes are not likely to occur until after a 3- or 4-hour dwell with 4.25% dextrose (3.86% glucose) (Fig. 60-7).[328] Transcapillary ultrafiltration ranged from a high of 7.4 mL/min after 10 minutes of dwell and fell to 1.3 mL/min after 345 minutes of dwell time when less of an osmotic gradient was available for net ultrafiltration.[329] For polyglucose solutions, ultrafiltration rates per minute are lower but are sustained during the dwell period because of slow uptake of the osmotic agent. However, the drain volume obtained after these dwell times is substantially lower than would be predicted from transcapillary ultrafiltration rates. Net drain volume, and therefore clearance, is a function of the relative rates of transcapillary ultrafiltration, lymphatic absorption, and transcapillary back-filtration, which is why patients seldom become acutely hypotensive during the dwell period despite ultrafiltration rates of up to 7.4 mL/min. The absorption rate ranges from 40 to 60 mL/hr and is attributable primarily to lymphatic drainage of the peritoneum (Fig. 60-8).[330] Lymphatic drainage can decrease net ultrafiltration by approximately 50%, with resultant reabsorption of approximately 15% of the metabolites in the peritoneal cavity, independent of molecular weight (see Fig. 60-8).

FACTORS THAT INFLUENCE ULTRAFILTRATION RATES. Net ultrafiltration can be modified with the use of hypertonic dialysis solutions, alternative osmotic agents such as polyglucose, shortening of the dwell time, drugs, and miscellaneous other mechanisms.[331] Intravenous dopamine is thought to increase ultrafiltration because of increased transcapillary hydrostatic pressure. Intravenous glucagon significantly increases mesenteric blood flow and solute transfer rates, whereas intravenous secretion increases ultrafiltration at any given osmotic stimulus, which suggests selective effects on solute and water transport.[332] Amphotericin B selectively increases peritoneal hydraulic permeability and thus increases ultrafiltration.[333] A mild increase in ultrafiltration is also seen with poly-L-lysine and furosemide, both of which promote Na^+ transport and limit early dialysate hyponatremia, thereby preventing a gradient for back-diffusion of water.[331] In patients with ultrafiltration failure, as well as in those with normal ultrafiltration rates, phosphatidylcholine has increased net ultrafiltration rates,[334, 335]

presumably through its surface-acting properties, which may help restore the semipermeability properties of the peritoneal membrane,[240] or via a decrease in lymphatic absorption. These topics are reviewed elsewhere.[309, 336]

Solute Transport by Convection

Solutes present in body fluids can be swept along with the bulk flow of water during ultrafiltration even in the absence of a concentration gradient for net diffusion. This solvent drag or "convective solute" transport does not always occur

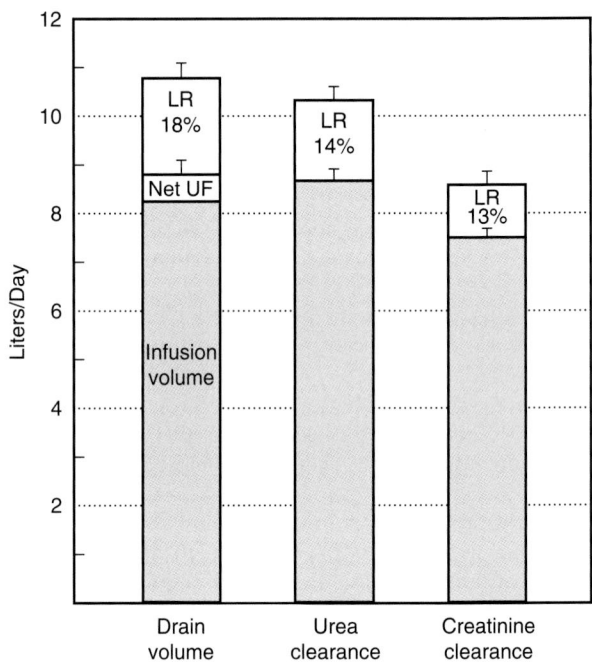

FIGURE 60-8. Contribution of back-filtration to loss of potential drain volume, urea clearance, and creatinine clearance (means ± SEM) in adult continuous ambulatory peritoneal dialysis patients (*n* = 18) receiving with four exchanges of 2.5% dextrose dialysis solution per day. (From Mactier RA: The Role of Lymphatic Absorption in Peritoneal Dialysis [thesis]. Glasgow, Scotland, University of Glasgow, 1988.)

RELATIONSHIP BETWEEN TIME, TRANSPORT TYPE & CLEARANCE

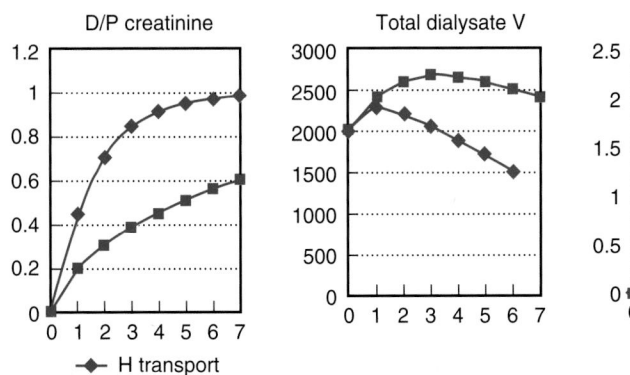

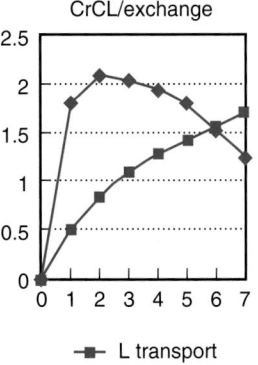

FIGURE 60-7. Theoretical relationships between dwell time, dialysate-plasma (D/P) ratio for creatinine, drain volume (V), and creatinine clearance (C_{cr}) in rapid and slow transporters. (From Twardowski ZJ: Nightly peritoneal dialysis. Why? who? how? and when? ASAIO Trans 36:8-16, 1990.)

in amounts per liter of ultrafiltrate equal to the physiologic concentration of solutes in body fluids. In other words, a sieving effect occurs that depends on resistance forces intrinsic to the membrane and solvents. This effect is most commonly observed during dwell cycles with solutions containing glucose as the osmotic agent and is mainly due to water movement across transcellular aquaporins.[337] The most important clinical consequences are those related to the transport of Na^+.[320, 338] The dialysate Na^+ concentration is reduced early in the dwell period because of Na^+ sieving during ultrafiltration. This relative hyponatremia in the dialysate tends to decrease later during the dwell period when less ultrafiltration is occurring, and the net effects on dialysate Na^+ concentration are now primarily due to diffusion of Na^+ down its concentration gradient from blood to the dialysate. Dialysate Na^+ concentrations are most strongly diminished by this mechanism in patients who are slow transporters because of their relatively higher ultrafiltration rates[338]; consequently, during a series of short dwell periods with hypertonic exchange, severe hypernatremia may develop in these patients.[339] Associated symptoms have included thirst and hypertension. These expected changes in dialysate Na^+ concentration during the dwell cycle can be helpful in evaluating a patient with loss of ultrafiltration.[340]

Lymphatic Absorption

The peritoneal lymphatics can be divided into two major systems. Lymphatics coursing through the mesentery convey solutes and water absorbed from the gastrointestinal tract to the systemic venous system. Some net transport from these lymphatics into the peritoneal cavity may occur, but it is thought to be minimal when compared with the diffusive and convective solute transport from the peritoneal capillaries. A second lymphatic system drains the parietal peritoneum, especially in the subdiaphragmatic area, and is thought to be the primary mechanism for net absorption of fluid and solutes from the peritoneal cavity.

PHYSIOLOGY OF LYMPHATIC REABSORPTION. Intraperitoneal fluid is continuously absorbed from the peritoneal cavity.[341] The fluid can be absorbed either directly into the subdiaphragmatic peritoneal lymphatics or through the interstitial tissue of the peritoneal membrane. Once in the interstitium, fluid and solutes can either be reabsorbed by the peritoneal capillaries (i.e., back-filtration) or be taken up by lymphatics that drain the interstitium. Experimental data suggest that absorption of isotonic fluid from the peritoneum occurs mainly by the subdiaphragmatic and interstitial lymphatics (60%) and to a lesser degree by visceral lymphatics and transcapillary back-diffusion (40%).[315, 342] Lymphatic drainage is primarily through specialized openings, or stomas,[343] located at the origin of the lymphatic channels, most of which are in the subdiaphragmatic area overlying the liver. These stomas may have diameters as large as 50 nm, which allows the movement of fluid, macromolecules, particulate matter, and even red blood cells along with the bulk flow of intraperitoneal fluid.

Hydraulic pressure effects when standing or when associated with activity may alter the relative amount of convective movement of fluids and solute into the subdiaphragmatic or other lymphatics. Twardowski and colleagues[344] have shown that there is a linear relationship between intraperitoneal

volume and intraperitoneal pressure in CAPD patients. Others have shown that lymphatic absorption rates are related to instilled volume[345] and external compression. These data seem to suggest that increases in intraperitoneal pressure are associated with an increase in lymphatic absorption rates.[237]

Lymphatic reabsorption rates also depend on diaphragmatic motion, which creates a pump-like mechanism for bulk fluid movement. During expiration, the diaphragm relaxes, as do the adjacent mesothelial and endothelial cells separating the lymphatic lacunae, thus creating a vacuum. Fluid then enters this vacuum through the stomas; during inspiration, with contraction of the diaphragm, the stomas close and the trapped fluid then flows into the upstream lymphatic channels.[346] Absorption rates decrease in the upright versus the supine position because of increased fluid contact with the subdiaphragmatic area in the supine position. Net absorption is also modified by the presence of any lymphatic obstruction.[347]

When hypertonic PD fluids are used, intraperitoneal volume begins to decrease before isosmolality is reached between the dialysate and plasma. This finding suggests that at a time when transcapillary ultrafiltration is still occurring and peritoneal volume should be increasing, fluid is being reabsorbed by some mechanism.[291, 327] Specifically, when transcapillary ultrafiltration rates are less than the lymphatic absorption rate, intraperitoneal volume will decrease despite the fact that some degree of ultrafiltration is still occurring. Eventually however, once the osmotic gradient is gone, the only activity that will be occurring is a slow but steady decrease in intraperitoneal volume as a result of the unopposed lymphatic reabsorption. Lindholm and colleagues[348] found that about 90% of total net ultrafiltration occurs during the first 90 minutes of the dwell cycle and that overall drain volume after 360 minutes is about 28% lower than the expected volume because of transcapillary ultrafiltration alone.[349] This net reduction in intraperitoneal volume after peak ultrafiltration is thought to represent the lymphatic reabsorption rate in excess of the net transcapillary ultrafiltration rate.

CLINICAL FINDINGS. Direct measurements of lymphatic flow from the peritoneum in CAPD patients are impossible. Therefore, indirect methods are used that measure the disappearance of macromolecules such as albumin from the peritoneum or their appearance in the circulation.[313] In a study in CAPD patients that correlated intraperitoneal fluid changes over time and manipulation of a mathematical model for peritoneal transport in which a three-pore model of membrane permeability was used, maximal peritoneal lymphatic flow rates were estimated to be 0.75 mL/min.[350] Measurements of lymphatic absorption rates in CAPD patients with intraperitoneal dextran used as a marker[330] ranged from 0.1 to 3.5 mL/min with a median value of 1.0 mL/min.

The average measured decrease in intraperitoneal volume after sequential dwell times in 29 CAPD patients was 39 mL/hr.[327, 351] Net reabsorption rates did not differ regardless of tonicity (1.5% versus 2.5% versus 4.25% dextrose)[327, 352] or instilled volumes.[353] Krediet and co-workers[354] have shown that the appearance of macromolecules in the peritoneal cavity, but not their disappearance, depended on molecular size. In related studies, these authors found that the MTAC for transport of inulin out of the peritoneal cavity was much higher than the MTAC for transfer of inulin into the peritoneal cavity.[355] Their explanation for this difference was uptake of inulin into the peritoneal lymphatics in addition to transport by diffusion. In another study, the rate of disappearance of sulfamethoxazole from the peritoneal cavity was not altered by albumin binding, and therefore its absorption was thought to be independent of size.[356] These data suggest that the primary mode of fluid and solute absorption from the peritoneum is convective in nature and that this fluid courses through the peritoneal lymphatics. There appears to be little sieving as seen with convective transport from blood to the peritoneum across the peritoneal membrane; therefore, most absorption seems to occur through stomas directly into the lymphatics. Polyglucose is absorbed via the lymphatics, although the absorption rate is slow.[144]

Extrapolation from these data suggests that in some CAPD patients, the average lymphatic absorption rate is about 2.2 L/day.[357] Such an absorption rate would reduce potential ultrafiltration after an average 4-hour dwell time by 343 ± 39 mL. Maneuvers that decrease lymphatic reabsorption would be beneficial to augment net ultrafiltration clearance. Attempts at pharmacologic manipulation of lymphatic reabsorption (such as the use of neostigmine and phosphatidylcholine) have had some clinical success to date and were reviewed elsewhere.[358]

CLINICAL OBSERVATIONS OF PERITONEAL MEMBRANE FUNCTION

Characterization of Peritoneal Membrane Transport

In the presence of infinite peritoneal capillary blood and dialysate flow, solute clearance is directly proportional to the peritoneal surface area and indirectly proportional to overall resistance. A measurement of clearance under these conditions is a measurement of the intrinsic transport properties of the peritoneal membrane. Ideally, these measurements are primarily a function of peritoneal diffusive permeability (centimeters per minute) and effective surface membrane area (square centimeters). MTAC measurements are thought to approximate this state.[359, 360]

A wide variation in MTAC values is observed in patients. Popovich and Moncrief[298] reported a mean MTAC for creatinine of 23.5 mL/min with a minimum of 5.1 mL/min, whereas others have reported a mean MTAC for creatinine of 10 mL/min with a range of 2.6 to 21.4 mL/min.[286] This variation between patients is also seen with other methods of classification of peritoneal membrane transport. Typical MTAC values for other solutes are found in Table 60-4. Because of the complexity of the initial MTAC calculations, simpler methods have been proposed.[361] An alternative method of classification of peritoneal transport based on dialysate-to-plasma (D/P) ratios[362] or the standardized peritoneal equilibration test (PET) has emerged.[304] When the PET was used for classification, the mean D/P for creatinine (D/P Cr) at 4 hours was 0.65; however, values ranged from 0.35 to 1.03. Teixido and associates[363] compared four simplified MTAC calculations and the PET with the standard complex calculation of MTAC. They found that the simplified MTAC calculations for urea and creatinine had an acceptable correlation with the complex MTAC calculation. Furthermore, D/P ratios at 240 minutes (by PET) also had

TABLE 60-4

Mass Transfer Urea Coefficients

SOLUTE (MOLECULAR WEIGHT)	MEAN VALUES
Blood urea nitrogen (60.1)	33.5
Creatinine (113)	23.5
Glucose (180)	18.1
Inulin (5500)	2.7
Dextran (70,000)	0.6

From Popovich RP, Moncrief JW, Pyle WK: Transport kinetics. *In* Nolph KD (ed): Peritoneal Dialysis, 3rd ed. Boston, Kluwer, 1989, p 96. Reprinted by permission of Kluwer Academic Publishers.

good correlation with complex MTAC calculations, and it was concluded that either could be used in clinical practice. However, D/P ratios are influenced by instilled volume, the rate of diffusion, net ultrafiltration, and solute transport by convection. Therefore, a change in a D/P value does not necessarily indicate that the patient's MTAC has changed.

To optimize an individual PD prescription, it is recommended that one characterize each patient's peritoneal membrane transport characteristics. In clinical practice, most nephrologists use D/P ratios from a standard PET to characterize an individual patient's peritoneal membrane and guide the prescription. On the basis of PET data, approximately 20% of patients are high transporters and another 15% are low transporters. It is important to identify patients at these extremes because to optimize their therapy, one may have to match dwell time to their transport type. The use of MTAC parameters requires the application of computer-assisted mathematics, but once obtained, these parameters offer a more precise mathematical modeling of the patient's prescription.[364] The "apex time," defined as the time required for the D/P ratio for urea to equal the ratio of dialysate glucose to the original dialysate glucose concentration, can also be used to characterize the membrane type.[365] The shorter this time, the more rapid peritoneal transport will be. Standard peritoneal permeability analysis[305] can also be used to assess transport but requires the use of dextran. A review of these tests can be found elsewhere.[366] These tests do not, however, measure the delivered dialysis dose. The dialysis dose can be estimated from PET data, but these estimates are not accurate.[367]

Stability of the Peritoneal Membrane over Time

Longitudinal observations in CAPD patients suggest that most patients have no significant change in small-solute clearance over time.[368-370, 371] However, in a retrospective analysis of long-term CAPD patients, the use of hyperosmolar bags increased with time on PD, thus suggesting that increased solute transport occurred.[372] In another study in which the transport characteristics of 20 long-term CAPD patients were compared with those of 20 matched patients just starting dialysis, MTAC values for low- and middle-molecular-weight solutes were higher and transport of beta$_2$-microglobulin was lower in the long-term group, whereas net ultrafiltration was lower.[373] The reasons for these changes are unclear. It is thought that continued exposure to nonphysiologic glucose-containing PD solutions increases vascularity and thus the "effective" surface area available for transport. Indirect evidence in support of this hypothesis is the observation that increased use of hypertonic glucose solutions preceded the change (increase) in peritoneal transport.[374] In the subgroup with no clinical need for increased use of hypertonic glucose exchange, peritoneal transport tended not to change.

In a retrospective analysis of a selected population, Lo and colleagues[375] found that initial high transporters tend to have a decrease in their 4-hour D/P Cr value over time whereas low and low-average transporters tend to increase their values over the first 2 years on CAPD. Ratios of dialysate glucose to the initial glucose concentration in the solution changed reciprocally. Note that this study did not monitor changes in transport in all patients over time.

In contrast to studies evaluating small-solute clearance, very few studies have looked at the change in macromolecule clearance over time. Over the first 2 to 3 years of PD, there tends to be no change in macromolecule clearance (measured as their restriction coefficients), but an increase in macromolecule restriction (decreased clearance) can be observed over time.[373, 376] The reasons for this change are unclear. It may be due to a reduction in the number or the radius of the large pores or, alternatively, an increase in the thickness of the submesothelial collagen layer.[377] Despite some day-to-day variation in protein clearance that increases as molecular weight increases, the intrinsic permeability of the peritoneal membrane, measured by comparing the clearance ratios of large and small proteins over time, was fairly constant over the short term. Day-to-day variations in protein transport were thought to be due to changes in effective surface area. Furthermore, no correlation was found between surface area and intrinsic permeability, which suggests that changes in surface area can occur independently of changes in intrinsic permeability.

Patients with diabetes mellitus have an abnormal microcirculation. Therefore, one might think that their peritoneal transport would be different from that of nondiabetics.[378, 379] However, most studies show no significant relationship between transport type and the cause of ESRD.[380, 381] Furthermore, there appears to be little difference in the distribution of transport types between countries.[382]

Conclusions

These studies suggest that for the average PD patient, peritoneal transport tends to be stable over time. The most commonly noted change is likely to be an increase in transport associated with a loss of ultrafiltration (formerly called type I membrane failure). It appears that day-to-day fluctuations in transport are due to changes in membrane surface area, whereas peritonitis and alterations in the production of various peritoneal cytokines can cause acute changes in intrinsic membrane permeability. The most common long-term changes in transport seem to reflect decreases in permeability coupled with increases in surface area. These studies are in agreement with the microscopic findings in long-term PD patients reported by the International Peritoneal Biopsy Registry, which show that although some changes occur in all patients, they are usually mild.[377] The most severe changes are seen in those who have had severe peritonitis. Possible approaches to PD in the next millennium with an emphasis on the development of solutions have been reviewed.[383, 384]

CLINICAL USE OF PERITONEAL DIALYSIS

Choice of Dialysis Modality

Most patients with ESRD are able to undergo either HD or PD. In choosing a dialysis modality, the nephrologist should first determine whether the individual patient has any potential indications or contraindications to PD.[385] Potential indications for PD include patients who have problematic vascular access or who prefer home dialysis but cannot perform home HD because of lack of a partner or suitable home environment. Absolute contraindications to PD include a documented loss of peritoneal function or extensive abdominal adhesions that limit dialysate flow. Under these conditions, it will not be possible to achieve an adequate dose of dialysis.[386, 387] Other absolute contraindications include uncorrectable mechanical defects that either increase the risk of infection or prevent access of the peritoneal dialysate to the vascular bed of the peritoneal membrane.[388, 389] Such defects can include large surgically irreparable hernias, diaphragmatic hernia, bladder extrophy, gastroschisis, and omphalocele. Finally, a patient who is physically or mentally incapable of performing PD and who does not have a suitable partner will not be able to identify and solve problems related to performing PD.

A number of relative contraindications to PD are recognized.[390] Body size limitations are probably the most common. When anuric, it is difficult, but not impossible to achieve current Dialysis Outcomes Quality Initiative (DOQI) targets for adequate dialysis in patients who weigh more than 100 kg (see adjustments to the dialysis prescription later). In addition, catheter placement is more challenging in the morbidly obese, and glucose adsorbed from the peritoneal dialysate may result in additional weight gain. Patients with bowel pathology, specifically diverticulitis, ischemic bowel disease, or inflammatory bowel disease, are at risk for peritonitis as a result of transmural contamination of the peritoneal cavity by enteric organisms.[391] Abdominal wall or skin infections increase the risk of catheter exit site infection and thus increase the risk for peritonitis.[388] It is possible, however, to perform PD in some patients who have either an ileostomy or a colostomy. The abdominal prosthesis should be in place for a minimum of 6 weeks, sometimes as long as 16 weeks, to allow sufficient time for complete healing before initiating PD. This waiting period should help minimize either leakage of peritoneal fluid or the spread of dialysis-related peritonitis to the prosthetic device. Although the presence of an abdominal aortic prosthetic graft is not a contraindication to PD, clinical experience in this area is limited. Six patients had an intra-abdominal vascular graft placed 3 to 32 months before beginning PD.[392] Two had peritonitis that responded to routine therapy. No patients had evidence of a graft infection or complications of the graft related to PD.[393]

Patients should receive education on the different dialysis modalities available when the glomerular filtration rate (GFR) is less than 25 mL/min. If the patient chooses HD, this timing will allow for placement and maturation of vascular access before starting HD. If the patient chooses PD, the timing will be appropriate for placement of a PD catheter before initiating dialysis therapy (see PD catheters later).

Peritoneal Dialysis Modalities

In the United States in the year 2000, approximately 55% of patients were receiving cycler PD, whereas the remaining patients were receiving CAPD.[394] These percentages have changed significantly since 1995, when 66% of patients were receiving CAPD and the remainder received cycler dialysis.[395]

CONTINUOUS AMBULATORY PERITONEAL DIALYSIS. Since the original description of this technique in the 1970s,[396] few changes have been made in the basic therapy. Most patients undergo four manual exchanges per day: three daytime exchanges of about 5 hours each and one overnight exchange of about 8 or 9 hours. Despite operating below the maximal peritoneal clearance rates for these solutes, one is able to achieve adequate daily small-solute clearance because of the continuous nature of the therapy. By adjusting the dwell volume appropriately (see the later section on adjusting the PD prescription), most CAPD patients can achieve an adequate dose of dialysis. A newer modification of CAPD incorporates one extra nighttime exchange with a simple nightly exchange device; that is, the patient receives a total of five exchanges per day: two overnight exchanges and three exchanges during the day.

CYCLER DIALYSIS. The technology for cycler dialysis has improved dramatically since the early 1990s. Cycler machines are much smaller and quieter than the versions developed in the 1970s and 1980s. These improvements have led to an increase in the percentage of PD patients who use the cycler in lieu of CAPD. All patients receiving cycler therapy use the cycler overnight to deliver three or more exchanges, typically over a 7- to 12-hour period. Most patients will also carry dialysate in the peritoneum for part or all of the day; these patients are considered to have a "wet day" or, alternatively, are described as performing CCPD. Patients undergoing CCPD will typically program the cycler machine to perform a "last bag fill"; that is, the machine will deliver a dialysate exchange at the end of the nighttime cycler dialysis. The patient will disconnect from the cycler with a full abdomen and carry this fluid for part or all of the day. In some cases, the patient will perform one or more manual exchanges during the day in addition to the last bag fill exchange. These additional exchanges are usually performed so that the patient can receive an adequate dose of dialysis (see "Adequacy of Peritoneal Dialysis" later).

A minority of patients will perform cycler dialysis overnight and not perform a last bag fill. Thus, these patients are dry; they do not carry any dialysate in their peritoneal cavity during the day. These patients are considered to have a "dry day" or, alternatively, are described as performing nightly intermittent peritoneal dialysis (NIPD).

TIDAL PERITONEAL DIALYSIS. Tidal PD (TPD) consists of the repeated instillation of small tidal volumes of dialysis fluid with the use of an automated cycler.[397] The procedure is usually performed nightly. Variables to be chosen include reserve volume, tidal outflow volume, tidal replacement volume, flow rates, and frequency of exchanges. Theoretically, maintaining an intraperitoneal reservoir by not attempting to completely drain the peritoneal cavity after each dwell results in more continuous contact of the dialysate with the peritoneal membrane. In addition, the more rapid cycling of dialysis may increase mixing and prevent the formation of stagnant fluid films within the abdomen. In most,[398, 399] but not all studies,[400] however, the use of TPD did not result in an increase in urea or creatinine clearance when compared with cycler PD. The differences in results among these studies are probably due to differences in the cycler and TPD prescriptions chosen for analysis. There is little evidence to suggest that TPD can provide clearance superior to that provided by cycler dialysis. It appears that TPD can decrease abdominal discomfort during inflow and outflow as a result of the continual presence of some dialysate in the peritoneal cavity during the cycling procedure.[401] A major disadvantage of TPD is the cost of the large volume of fluid needed.

Several CAPD and cycler prescriptions are shown in Figure 60-9. Typical clearances with the various modalities and specified dialysate flows are presented in Table 60-5.

INTERMITTENT PERITONEAL DIALYSIS. Intermittent PD (IPD) was commonly performed in the 1960s and 1970s, before the development of CAPD. Classically, IPD was a type of dialysis in which exchanges were not performed on a daily basis. The patient would typically use multiple short-dwell exchanges three or four times a week. Techniques included manual IPD, IPD with an automated cycler, IPD with a reverse osmosis machine, reciprocating IPD with an extracorporeal reconstituting circuit, and others. These techniques were described in detail in a previous edition.[7] IPD is rarely, if ever used in developed countries today.

Choice of Peritoneal Dialysis Modality

The patient's peritoneal membrane transport characteristics must be known to optimize the PD prescription. These characteristics are determined by using the PET. This equilibration test, first described by Twardowski in 1979,[66, 402] is a standardized method for categorizing patients into one of four transport categories by using the D/P Cr ratio at 4 hours: high (D/P Cr ratio >0.81), high-average (D/P Cr ratio between 0.81 and 0.65), low-average (D/P Cr ratio between 0.65 and 0.50), or low (D/P Cr ratio <0.50). After an overnight dwell, the PET is performed by instilling 2 L of 2.5% dextrose dialysis fluid, and the dialysate is allowed to dwell for 4 hours. Dialysate urea, creatinine, glucose, and Na^+ concentrations are measured at time 0 and after 2 and 4 hours of dwell time. Serum values are determined after 2 hours. In addition, 4-hour drain volume is also obtained. For each for these dwell times, D/P ratios are obtained for urea and creatinine. The ratio of glucose at the time of draining to the initial glucose concentration in dialysis fluid (D/D_0) is also obtained. On the basis of published data, the membrane type can be identified with this test (Fig. 60-10), and the PD prescription that would best match the patient's transport characteristics can be chosen (Table 60-6).

Several large retrospective studies have shown that most patients are either high-average or low-average transporters.[66, 403] Patients with these transport characteristics can usually perform either CAPD or CCPD and achieve both an adequate dose of dialysis and ultrafiltration. Patients who are low transporters have a slow increase in the D/P Cr ratio and therefore benefit from a longer dwell time (see Fig. 60-6).

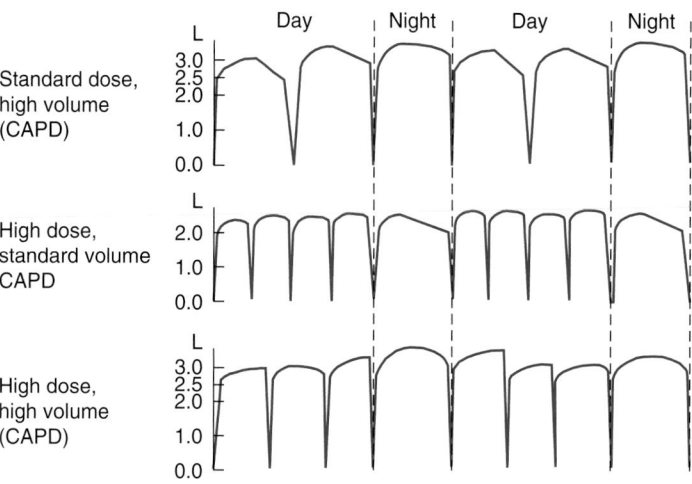

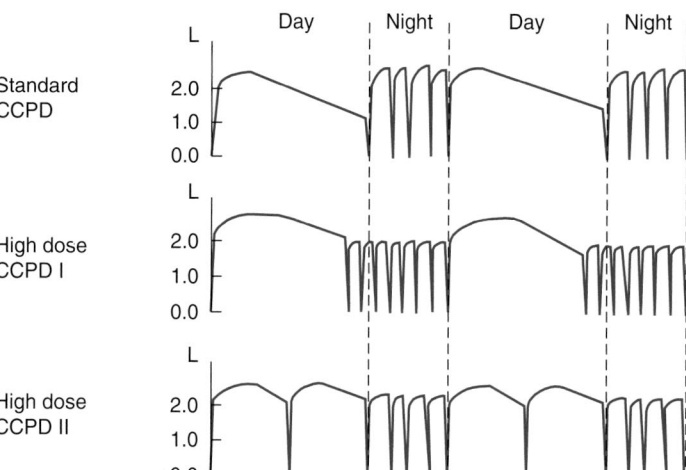

FIGURE 60-9. Alternative peritoneal dialysis prescriptions defined by varying dwell times, instilled volumes, and number of exchanges. CAPD, continuous ambulatory peritoneal dialysis; CCPD, continuous cycling peritoneal dialysis. (From Twardowski ZJ: Peritoneal dialysis glossary III. Perit Dial Int 10:173-175, 1990.)

TABLE 60-5

Clearances and Dialysis Solution Volumes with Different Dialysis Techniques

TECHNIQUE	TREATMENT TIME (HR/WK)	DIALYSATE FLOW L/hr	DIALYSATE FLOW L/wk	C_{urea} mL/min	C_{urea} L/wk
Manual PD	48	2	96	18	52
Rapid-cycling PD*	40	4	160	30	72
CAPD, CCPD	168	0.33	56	7	67
NIPD	56	3.25	182	6	59
TPD	56	3.38	189	7	73
Hemodialysis	15	30	450	150	135

*Cycler, reverse osmosis, reciprocating, recirculating.

CAPD, continuous ambulatory peritoneal dialysis; CCPD, continuous cyclic peritoneal dialysis; NIPD, nightly intermittent peritoneal dialysis; PD, peritoneal dialysis; TPD, tidal peritoneal dialysis.

From Nolph KD: Peritoneal dialysis. *In* Brenner BR, Rector FC (eds): The Kidney, Vol 1. Philadelphia, WB Saunders, 1989, p 2304.

Thus, these patients are more likely to achieve adequate dialysis with evenly spaced, long dwell periods (CAPD or CCPD with a last bag fill and midday exchange).[404] Patients who are high transporters have a rapid increase in the D/P ratio in the first 1 to 2 hours of dwell time, followed by a decline in the D/P value. These patients are more likely to achieve adequate dialysis when receiving cycler dialysis.[404] If these patients require daytime dwell periods to achieve adequate dialysis, they are most likely to benefit from dwell times less than 3 hours; they will derive little benefit from one daytime dwell that lasts the entire day.

ADEQUACY OF PERITONEAL DIALYSIS

The National Kidney Foundation Kidney Disease Outcomes Quality Initiative (NKF-K/DOQI) clinical practice guidelines, first published in 1997, provide evidence-based guidelines for the provision of adequate PD, specifically, about when to initiate dialysis, how and when to measure the

PERITONEAL EQUILIBRATION TEST

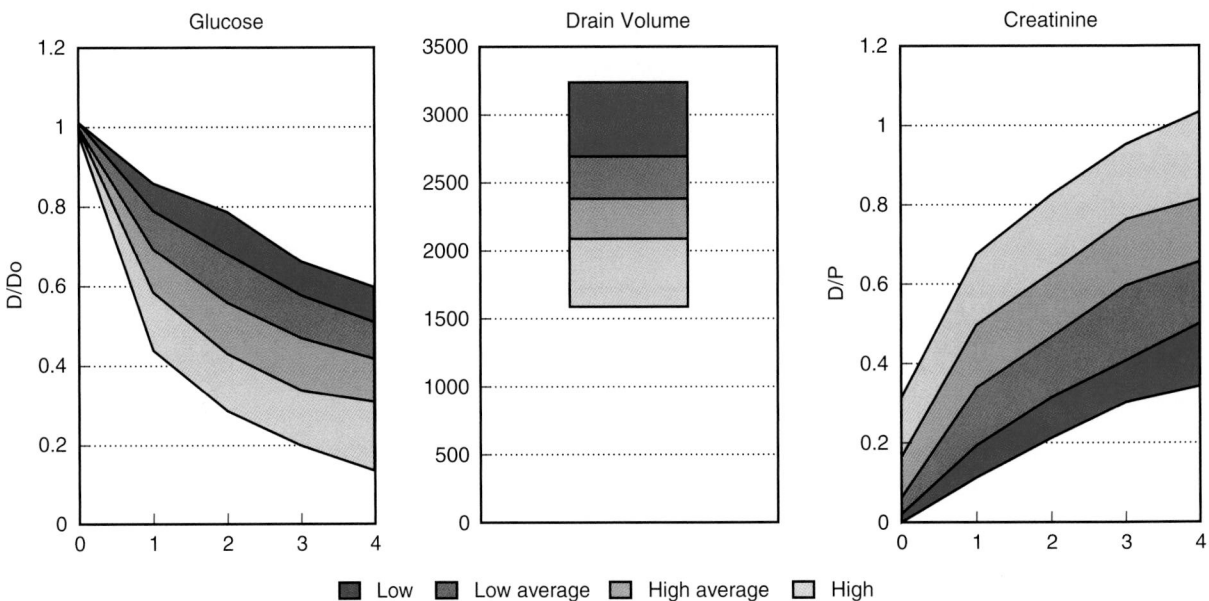

FIGURE 60-10. Dialysate-plasma (D/P) ratios for creatinine and ratios of glucose at the time of draining versus the initial dialysis, as well as expected drain volumes for various transport types after a timed 2-L 2.5% dextrose dwell period. (Modified from Twardowski ZJ: Clinical value of standard equilibration tests in CAPD patients. Blood Purif 7:95-108, 1989.)

TABLE 60-6

Baseline Peritoneal Equilibrium Test Prognostic Value

SOLUTE TRANSPORT	ULTRAFILTRATION	PREDICTED C_{cr}	PREFERRED PD MODALITY
High	Poor	Adequate	NPD, DAPD*
High-average	Adequate	Adequate	Standard-volume PD†
Low-average	Good	Adequate	High-volume PD‡
Low	Excellent	Inadequate	High-volume PD‡

*May need to do a midday exchange or a daytime polyglucose dwell to maintain ultrafiltration.

†CAPD with 8.0 to 10.0 or CCPD with a dialysis solution inflow of 6 to 8 L overnight and 2 L in the daytime for clearance, but may need a dry day, polyglucose, or midday exchange to maintain ultrafiltration.

‡CAPD with greater than 9.0 L/day, CAPD with a nightly exchange device, or CCPD with inflow greater than 8 L overnight and/or 2 L daytime and possible midday exchange.

CAPD, circulating ambulatory peritoneal dialysis; CCPD, continuous cycling peritoneal dialysis; DAPD, daytime ambulatory peritoneal dialysis; NPD, nightly peritoneal dialysis.

From Twardowski ZJ: Nightly peritoneal dialysis. Why? who? how? when? ASAIO Trans 36:8-16, 1990.

PD dose, and recommendations for an adequate dose of dialysis.

When to Initiate Dialysis

In most cases, PD is initiated once the weekly renal Kt/V for urea is less than 2.0 or the weekly creatinine clearance is less than the range of 9 to 14 mL/min.[405] Once kidney clearance falls below this level, patients are at increased risk for malnutrition and uremic complications.[406-408] When the GFR falls below 25 to 50 mL/min, patients often have a decline in dietary protein intake.[406, 409-411] In the Canadian-U.S. (CANUSA) study, patients who initiated dialysis at lower levels of residual renal function had worse nutritional status than did patients who started at higher levels of residual renal function.[408]

PD should be initiated at higher levels of kidney clearance (GFR up to 20 mL/min) if the patient shows signs of malnutrition, as defined by one of the following[412]:

1. A decrease in edema-free body weight of greater than 6% in less than 6 months or to an edema-free body weight that is less than 90% of the standard body weight
2. A reduction in serum albumin levels of greater than 0.3 g/dL to a level less than 4.0 g/dL in the absence of acute inflammation or infection
3. A decrease in the subjective global assessment (SGA) score of more than 1 point

Dialysis can be initiated at "full dose," that is, with a prescription of four 2-L exchanges per day, or it can be initiated at an "incremental dose," where the combination of kidney and peritoneal clearance meets the guidelines for adequate dialysis.[413-417] As noted later, if incremental dosing is chosen, monitoring for adequacy of dialysis must be performed on a more frequent basis (see the next section).

Measurement of the Peritoneal Dialysis Dose

When patients initiate PD, a good proportion of their total solute clearance is provided by residual renal function. Over a period of 24 to 36 months, this residual renal function will decline to zero. Thus, PD adequacy must be measured frequently and on a regular basis to ensure that the patient is receiving adequate dialysis. NKF-K/DOQI guidelines recommend that total solute clearance be measured at least twice during the first 6 months of PD. The first measurement of PD adequacy should be 2 to 4 weeks after starting PD or within 2 weeks if the patient is already undergoing PD and is transferring from another facility.[418] This measurement should include both the peritoneal component and the residual renal component, with calculations made to determine the weekly Kt/V, the total weekly creatinine clearance normalized to 1.73 m² body surface area (BSA),[419] and the protein equivalent of nitrogen appearance (with all its components). After the first 6 months of therapy, the aforementioned components of adequacy should be measured at least every 4 months.[420] Testing should be performed more frequently if either a significant change in clinical status has occurred or the PD prescription has changed.

Residual renal function is assessed by determining the renal component of Kt/V urea for the weekly Kt/V measure and determining the GFR for the weekly creatinine clearance measure. The patient's GFR is determined by taking the mean of urea and creatinine clearance.[421] If dialysis with the "incremental dose" method has been prescribed (see the previous section, "When to Initiate Dialysis"), residual kidney function is assessed every 2 months by collecting a 24-hour urine sample; otherwise, residual kidney function should be assessed every 4 months.[418] Measurements of residual renal function should continue on a routine basis until the weekly renal Kt/V urea is less than 0.1.[422]

Measurement of the PD dose should be performed in a standard and reproducible manner to allow for a comparison of the dose of dialysis over time in an individual patient and also across different dialysis facilities. Measurement of dialysis adequacy should be delayed for at least 4 weeks after a case of peritonitis has resolved.[423] For CAPD patients,

the serum sample can be obtained at any convenient time. For patients receiving automated therapy, the serum sample should be obtained at the midpoint of the daytime dry period for patients with a dry day and at the midpoint of the daytime dwell period or periods for patients with a wet day.[424] Specific formulas are used to calculate body water for Kt/V and BSA for creatinine clearance, as shown in Table 60-7.[431]

Adequate Dose of Peritoneal Dialysis

Based on the results of many clinical studies performed during the past 10 years, the NKF-K/DOQI work group has developed guidelines for an adequate dose of dialysis. For CAPD patients, the delivered PD dose for Kt/V urea should be at least 2.0. The recommended weekly creatinine clearance dose is based on the patient's transport characteristics. For patients who are high or high-average transporters, total creatinine clearance should be at least 60 L/wk/1.73 m². For patients who are low or low-average transporters, weekly creatinine clearance should be at least 50 L/wk/1.73 m².[432] The dosage recommendations for automated techniques are based on whether the patient also has daytime exchanges. For patients using the cycler who have a dry day, total Kt/V urea should be at least 2.2, and the weekly total creatinine clearance should be at least 66 L/1.73 m². For patients using the cycler who have at least one daytime dwell period, total Kt/V urea should be at least 2.1, and the total weekly creatinine clearance should be at least 63 L/1.73 m².[433] In malnourished patients, the estimate of body size is adjusted up to ideal body weight. Thus, for Kt/V urea, the target dose is increased by the ratio $V_{desired}/V_{actual}$, whereas for creatinine clearance, the target dose is increased by the ratio $BSA_{desired}/BSA_{actual}$.[434] An alternative method would be to use the patient's desired or target weight to calculate BSA or V.

The results of several large multicenter clinical studies were used to develop these dialysis dose adequacy guidelines. The CANUSA study enrolled 680 patients who were initiating PD. By multivariate analysis, the risk of death increased 5% for each 0.1-U decrease in the weekly Kt/V urea and increased 7% for each 5-L/wk/1.73 m² decrease in weekly creatinine clearance. The predicted 2-year survival rate associated with a Kt/V urea of 2.1 was 78%, with a corresponding creatinine clearance of 70 L/wk/1.73 m².[435] It is important to note, however, that the decline in dialysis dose over time that occurred in the CANUSA study was due to a decrease in residual renal function that was not compensated by a concomitant increase in the prescribed peritoneal component of clearance.[436]

A number of observational studies have also demonstrated an association of mortality with declining residual renal function. A study of 2686 patients in the United States demonstrated that although residual renal function was strongly associated with survival, no relationship was found between peritoneal clearance and survival.[437] Each 10-L/wk increase in residual renal function was associated with a 12% reduction in the odds ratio for death. Similar findings were reported by Rocco and colleagues with data from the 1996 survey conducted by ESRD Network Six[438] and with data from the Centers for Medicare and the Medicare Clinical Performance Measures Project.[439] Other smaller observational studies have also replicated these findings.[440-433]

TABLE 60-7

Estimating Total Body Water and Body Surface Area

V (total body water) should be estimated by using actual body weight and either the Watson[425] or the Hume[426] method in adults and the Mellitis-Cheek method[427] in children

Watson Method[425]

For men: $V (L) = 2.447 + 0.3362 \cdot Wt\,(kg) + 0.1074 \cdot Ht\,(cm) - 0.09516 \cdot Age\,(yr)$

For women: $V = 2.097 + 0.2466 \cdot Wt + 0.1069 \cdot Ht$

Hume Method[426]

For men: $V = -14.012934 + 0.296785 \cdot Wt + 0.194786 \cdot Ht$

For women: $V = -35.270121 + 0.183809 \cdot Wt + 0.344547 \cdot Ht$

Mellits-Cheek Method for Children[427]

For boys: $V (L) = -1.927 + 0.465 \cdot Wt\,(kg) + 0.045 \cdot Ht\,(cm)$, when Ht is ≤ 132.7 cm

   $V = -21.993 + 0.406 \cdot Wt + 0.209 \cdot Ht$, when height is >132.7 cm

For girls: $V = 0.076 + 0.507 \cdot Wt + 0.013 \cdot Ht$, when height is < 110.8 cm

   $V = -10.313 + 0.252 \cdot Wt + 0.154 \cdot Ht$, when height is ≥ 110.8 cm

Body surface area, BSA, should be estimated by using actual body weight and either the DuBois and DuBois method,[428] the Gehan and George method,[429] or the Haycock method[430]

For all formulas, Wt is in kg and Ht is in cm:

DuBois and Dubois method: $BSA\,(m^2) = 0.007184 \cdot Wt^{0.425} \cdot Ht^{0.725}$

Gehan and George method: $BSA\,(m^2) = 0.235 \cdot Wt^{0.51456} \cdot Ht^{0.42246}$

Haycock method: $BSA\,(m^2) = 0.024265 \cdot Wt^{0.5378} \cdot Ht^{0.3964}$

Several studies have evaluated the effect of peritoneal clearance on mortality in anuric patients. In a study of 140 anuric Chinese patients, a positive correlation was noted between peritoneal clearance and survival.[444] The mean weekly Kt/V urea was 1.72, and each 0.1-U decrease in Kt/V was associated with a 6% increase in mortality. Of note, 42.1% of patients were prescribed three 2-L exchanges per day, with 45.0% receiving four 2-L exchanges and 12.9% receiving 10 L/day. Bhaskaran and associates studied 122 PD patients who had been monitored for a median of 16.5 months before and 19.5 months after the development of anuria.[445] This analysis revealed that anuric patients with a weekly Kt/V greater than 1.8 had a significantly lower mortality rate (relative risk of 0.27, 95% confidence limit of 0.09 to 0.79) than did anuric patients with a weekly Kt/V less than 1.8. In addition, a weekly creatinine clearance of greater than 50 L/wk/1.73 m^2 was found to be associated with a 58% reduction in the risk of mortality; however, this decrease was not statistically significant because the 95% confidence limit was 0.14 to 1.31. The wide confidence interval reflects the low statistical power achieved in this study conducted with a relatively small number of patients.

After the last PD guidelines were revised by the NKF-K/DOQI work group, the ADAMEX trial was published.[11] A total of 965 subjects were randomized to either standard care, in which patients continued with their present PD prescriptions, or to an interventional group, in which dialysis prescriptions were modified to achieve a peritoneal creatinine clearance of 60 L/wk/1.73 m^2. All patients in the standard group received four 2-L exchanges, whereas the distribution of prescriptions in the interventional group was 10 L/day in 37% of patients, 11 L/day in 20%, 12 L/day in 21%, 12.5 L/day in 8%, and 15 L/day in 14%. The mean separation in peritoneal creatinine clearance in the two groups was approximately 10 L/wk/1.73 m^2. Residual renal function was similar in the two groups. Patient survival was also similar in the interventional and standard groups, even after adjustment for comorbid conditions such as age, the presence of diabetes mellitus, serum albumin levels, anuria, and the normalized protein equivalent of total nitrogen appearance. As noted in the observational studies cited earlier, residual renal function was also a predictor of mortality, with a 11% increase in mortality for each 10-L/wk/1.73 m^2 decrease in weekly renal creatinine clearance and a 6% increase in mortality for each 0.1-U decrease in weekly renal Kt/V urea clearance. These data are consistent with the magnitude of the effect of residual renal function on mortality cited in previous studies. Unfortunately, no data are provided on the effects of peritoneal clearance on mortality in the 55% of patients in this study who were anuric. A more in-depth analysis of the ADAMEX study has been published elsewhere.[446]

The revisions to the adequacy guidelines in 2001 reflected the observation that patients in different peritoneal transport groups achieved, on average, different weekly creatinine clearances at the same level of weekly Kt/v urea. This discrepancy is due to both the nonlinearity between V used for the calculation of weekly Kt/V and BSA used for the calculation of weekly creatinine clearance and to the different methods used to calculate residual renal function for weekly Kt/V urea and weekly creatinine clearance.[447, 448] Thus, it was thought that it would be difficult for an anuric low to low-average transport patient to be able to achieve a weekly creatinine clearance of 60 L/wk/1.73 m^2. This observation was coupled with data showing that low to low-average transporter patients have a higher survival rate than high-average or high transporter patients, even when controlling for the delivered dose of dialysis. Thus, the work group committee thought that the weekly creatinine clearance target in low to low-average transporters could be lowered from 60 to 50 L/wk/1.73 m^2 without jeopardizing patient outcomes.[420]

WRITING THE DIALYSIS PRESCRIPTION

Initial Prescription

The PD prescription can be developed either empirically or with the use of a computer modeling program.[449] Ideally, PD should not be started until the peritoneal catheter has been in place for at least 14 days. This 2-week rest period will help minimize the risk of both leakage about the catheter site and peritonitis.[450]

PD can be prescribed empirically by using data based on the patient's weight, residual renal function, and any lifestyle constraints that may be present. The guidelines in Table 60-8 are adapted from the NKF-K/DOQI clinical practice guidelines.[449]

Note that NIPD is not usually considered as a first therapy for PD patients unless the patient is being started on incremental dialysis, has significant residual kidney function, and is able to achieve significant diuresis from native kidney function.

If computer modeling is available, patient information on weight and residual renal function are entered into the program, and sample prescriptions are provided that should meet dialysis adequacy goals. For either empirical or computer-based dialysis prescriptions, patients should be monitored closely during the training period to ensure that the 4-hour drain volumes are those expected for the percent dextrose

TABLE 60-8

Recommended Prescriptions for Patients Starting CAPD or CCPD

	ESTIMATED GFR OF >2 mL/MIN	ESTIMATED GFR OF ≤2 mL/MIN
CAPD		
BSA <1.7 m^2	4 × 2.0-L exchanges/day	4 × 2.5-L exchanges/day
BSA 1.7-2.0 m^2	4 × 2.5-L exchanges/day	4 × 3.0-L exchanges/day
BSA ≥2.0 m^2	4 × 3.0-L exchanges/day	4 × 3.0-L exchanges/day
CCPD		
BSA <1.7 m^2	4 × 2.0 L (9 hr/night) + 2.0 L/day	4 × 2.5 L (9 hr/night) + 2.0 L/day
BSA 1.7-2.0 m^2	4 × 2.5 L (9 hr/night) + 2.0 L/day	4 × 3.0 L (9 hr/night) + 2.0 L/day
BSA ≥2.0 m^2	4 × 3.0 L (9 hr/night) + 3.0 L/day	4 × 3.0 L (9 hr/night) + 2 × 3.0 L/day

BSA, body surface area; CAPD, continuous ambulatory peritoneal dialysis; CCPD, continuous cycling peritoneal dialysis; GFR, glomerular filtration rate.

Modified from Burkart JM, Schreiber M, Korbet SM, et al: Solute clearance approach to adequacy of peritoneal dialysis. Perit Dial Int 16:457-470, 1996.

PD solution that is being used (see Fig. 60-10) and that no drainage is observed about the catheter exit site.

Adjustments to the Initial Dialysis Prescription

Two to 4 weeks after the initiation of PD, 24-hour collections of urine and dialysate should be performed, along with serum chemistry panels and a complete blood count, in order to calculate the weekly Kt/V urea and creatinine clearance.[418] The initial PET should be performed approximately 1 month after the initiation of dialysis. This waiting period is recommended because equilibrium test results can change during the first month of dialysis.[451] The PET is performed to rule out unexpected problems and also to identify patients who are either high or low transporters. High transporters will need short dwell prescriptions and may begin to have ultrafiltration problems as residual kidney function fails. Low transporters usually require high-dose CAPD or CCPD to maintain adequate dialysis as residual kidney function fails. If performance of the PET is not feasible, an approximation of the peritoneal transport rate can be made in CAPD patients by using the 24-hour D/P Cr ratio for characterizing the peritoneal membrane.[452, 453]

If clearances are at or above target, adequacy should be monitored at regular intervals as noted in the earlier section on measurement of the PD dose. If clearances are below target, the prescription should be modified and adequacy testing repeated.

Further Adjustments to the Dialysis Prescription

For CAPD patients, two methods can be used to increase dialysis adequacy. The most common approach is to increase the dwell volume in 500-mL increments. Accordingly, a patient receiving four 2-L exchanges per day would have the prescription increased to four 2.5-L exchanges per day.[454-457] Alternatively, a nocturnal exchange device is available that supplies an extra exchange overnight, thus providing the patient with a total of five exchanges per day.

For cycler patients, several methods are available for improving adequacy. These methods include increasing the dwell volume of an individual exchange, increasing the time spent overnight on the cycler, increasing the number of exchanges on the cycler, or increasing the number of daytime dwell periods. Sometimes a combination of these measures is used in an individual patient. A comparison of several different PD regimens demonstrated that increasing the number of 2-L overnight exchanges from five to seven to nine increased urea clearance from 7.5 to 8.6 to 9.1 L per night, respectively. In comparison, a 50% tidal prescription using 14 L of dialysate provided a urea clearance of 8.3 L per night.[398] Mean creatinine clearances also increased; however, the magnitude of this improvement will depend on the patient's peritoneal transport characteristics.[458] Other investigators have shown that an increase in fill volume is also effective in increasing urea and creatinine clearance.[459-461] For high transporters, both clearance and ultrafiltration can be optimized by the use of rapid-cycle, short-dwell exchanges.[404] Patients who are low or low-average transporters, however, will probably achieve higher clearances with the equally spaced dwells of CAPD than with classic cycler therapy.[404] Changes in the prescription should be made, if possible,

with the use of a computer modeling program, and patient lifestyle concerns should be taken into account.[449]

The distribution of PD prescriptions in the year 2000 for CAPD patients included a daily volume of 8000 to 9999 mL in 38%, 10,000 to 11,999 mL in 34%, and 12,000 mL or more in 18%.[394] For cycler patients, 90% of patients had at least one daytime dwell period. The mean nighttime dwell volume was 2000 mL in 27%, 2001 to 2499 mL in 15%, 2500 mL in 33%, and over 2500 mL in 17%. The number of nighttime exchanges was three in 13%, four in 41%, five in 25%, and six or more in 13%.[394] Although patients may be reluctant to increase the dwell volume and may note abdominal distention with a higher dwell volume, several randomized studies have shown that patients are not able to reliably determine the volume of a dwell that is infused into the peritoneal cavity.[459, 461-463] Abdominal symptoms that may be caused by the presence of intraperitoneal dialysate include delayed gastric emptying[464-466] and gastroesophageal reflux disease.[467] The former can be managed with either oral or intraperitoneal metoclopramide or erythromycin,[468-470] whereas the latter can be treated by elevating the head of the bed, antacids, H_2 receptor antagonists, or proton pump inhibitors.[471] Anuric patients who are either low transporters or are in excess of 100 kg will probably require a combination of CAPD and CCPD to achieve adequate dialysis.[472] Morbidly obese patients may be able to tolerate dwell volumes as large as 5 L.[473]

Success in Achieving Adequate Dialysis

In the United States, a random survey of PD adequacy has been conducted annually by the Centers for Medicare and Medicaid Services (CMS, formerly the Health Care Financing Administration [HCFA]) since 1994. For CAPD patients, the mean weekly Kt/V urea and creatinine clearance levels have increased from 2.0 ± 0.6 and 64.3 ± 23.6 L/wk/1.73 m², respectively, in 1995 to 2.31 ± 0.5 and 74.8 ± 26.3 L/wk/1.73 m² in 2001 (Fig. 60-11).[394] For cycler patients, the mean weekly Kt/V urea and creatinine clearance levels have increased from 2.12 ± 0.6 and 63.4 ± 23.5 L/wk/1.73 m², respectively, in 1995 to 2.33 ± 0.6 and 72.4 ± 26.1 L/wk/1.73 m² in 2001.[394]

The percentage of CAPD patients meeting the NKF-K/DOQI guidelines for weekly Kt/V has increased from 27% in 1995 to 67% in 2001, whereas for cycler patients, the percentage has increased from 28% to 58% over the same period. The percentage of CAPD patients meeting NKF-K/DOQI guidelines for weekly creatinine clearance has increased from 30% in 1995 to 61% in 2001, whereas for cycler patients, the percentage has increased from 26% to 52% over the same period.

A study using CMS clinical performance measures (CPM) data from 1999 indicates that 43% of CAPD patients and 54% of cycler patients who had an inadequate dose of dialysis had a change in the dialysis prescription.[474] Of the patients who received a new prescription, more than 75% had an improvement in weekly Kt/V urea and creatinine clearance values. In patients with improved adequacy values, the mean increase in weekly Kt/V urea was from 1.6 ± 0.3 to 2.1 ± 0.5, with an increase in peritoneal Kt/V urea from 1.5 ± 0.3 to 1.9 ± 0.4. Similarly, weekly creatinine clearance increased from 46.3 ± 7.5 to 59.1 ± 10.6 L/wk/1.73 m² with an increase in the peritoneal component of creatinine clearance from 42.0 ± 9.1 to 52.7 ± 9.9 L/wk/1.73 m².[474]

NUTRITION

Malnutrition

Malnutrition is a significant risk factor for mortality and hospitalization in chronic PD patients.[408, 475-478] Estimates of malnutrition in chronic PD patients range from 40% to 76%, with the variability in prevalence being due to differing definitions of malnutrition, as well as differences in the patient population studied.[478-481] This high incidence of malnutrition is not surprising because malnutrition is common even before the start of dialytic therapy.[482, 483]

Malnutrition can be reflective of poor nutritional intake, inflammation, or both.[484-486] It is well known from clinical and experimental observations that patients who are overtly uremic are anorectic and tend to have decreased protein intake,[487] whereas clinical observations in nondialyzed patients with renal failure suggest that anorexia or decreased protein intake could be a subtle sign of uremia. Therefore, the working hypothesis has been that underdialysis or uremia leads to a decreased appetite, malnutrition, and decreased albumin synthesis. Inflammation is also an important cause of malnutrition in PD patients. C-reactive protein (CRP) levels are abnormally high in most PD patients,[488, 489] and a direct association has been noted between elevated CRP levels and increased rates of mortality[488, 489] and cardiovascular disease.[489-491] Elevated levels of cytokines such as IL-6 and TNF-α can result in an increase in protein hydrolysis and muscle protein breakdown.[492, 493] Patients with anorexia have higher plasma levels of TNF-α than do patients who are not anorectic.[494]

Nutritional Parameters

Data from the CMS-CPM project for the year 2000 found that chronic PD patients had a mean body weight of 76 ± 19 kg and a body mass index (BMI) of 27.5 ± 6.4 kg/m². The normalized protein equivalent of nitrogen appearance (nPNA) of these patients was 0.95 ± 0.31 g/kg/day, and their normalized creatinine appearance rate (nCAR) was 17 ± 6.5 mg/kg/day, which resulted in a percent lean body mass (%LBM) of 64% ± 17% of actual body weight. Serum albumin correlated in a positive, but weak fashion with BMI, nPNA, nCAR, and %LBM, but not with weekly creatinine clearance.[495] Hypoalbuminemia was associated with older age, the presence of diabetes mellitus, female gender, the erythropoietin dose, the D/P Cr ratio, PET results, and a longer duration of dialysis.[495] Other investigators have demonstrated that older patients not only have lower serum albumin levels than younger patients do but also have higher peritoneal protein losses,[496, 497] lower nPNA values, lower LBM/weight ratios, and higher BMI values.[498] Metabolic acidosis is also correlated with higher serum albumin levels, with malnutrition being ascribed to low protein intake and decreased acid production.[499] Finally, in cross-sectional studies, high transporters have higher losses of peritoneal proteins and lower serum albumin levels than average or low-average transporters do.[500-502]

Few studies have provided data on longitudinal changes in nutritional parameters. A prospective study involving 118 patients who were started on PD found that mean serum albumin levels increased by approximately 0.2 g/dL over a 24-month period, nPNA declined by approximately 0.1 g/kg/24 hr, and BMI and body fat were essentially unchanged.[503] In a second prospective study of 235 CAPD patients, high-transport patients had slightly lower serum albumin, nPNA, and %LBM at baseline. No significant changes were observed in serum albumin, nPNA, or LBM over a 2-year period of follow-up, even in patients in the high-transport group.[504] A retrospective study of 303 PD patients found that patient weight increased during the first 12 months of dialysis and declined after 18 months of therapy. Similar changes were seen in mid-arm circumference.[166]

Nutrition Guidelines

The NKF-K/DOQI guidelines recently recommended dietary protein intake of 1.2 to 1.3 g/kg/day for chronic PD patients.[505]

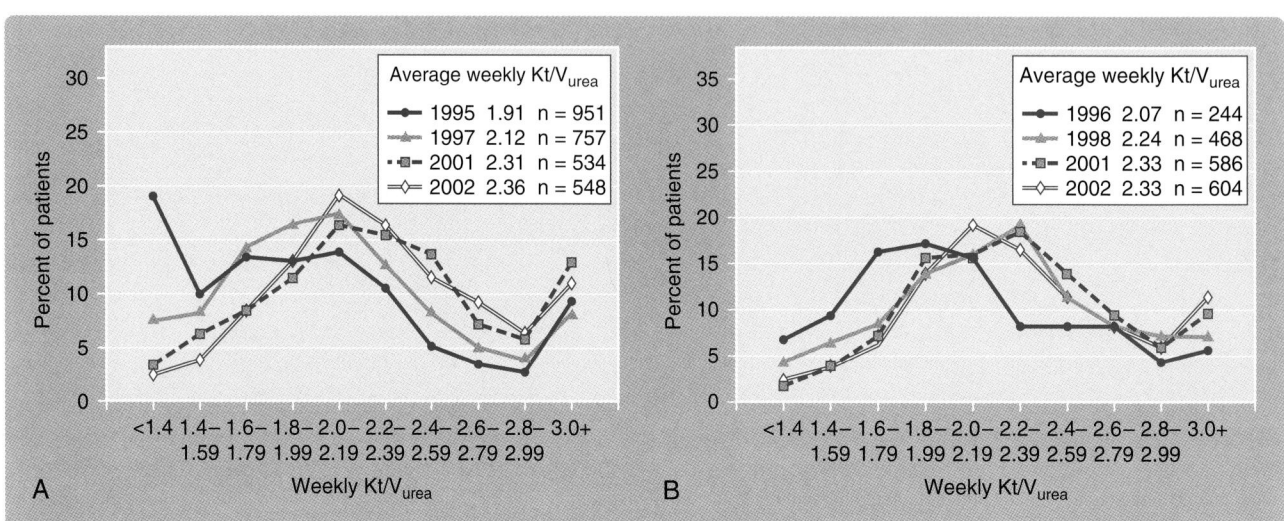

FIGURE 60-11. Distribution of mean weekly Kt/V$_{urea}$ values for adult circulating ambulatory peritoneal dialysis (CAPD) patients (**A**) and adult cycler patients with a daytime dwell (**B**), October 2000 to March 2001, compared with previous study periods. (From Centers for Medicare and Medicaid Services: 2002 Annual Report, End-Stage Renal Disease Clinical Performance Measures Project. Baltimore, Department of Health and Human Services, Centers for Medicare and Medicaid Services, Center for Beneficiary Choices, December 2002.)

Surveys of dietary intake, however, have shown that mean protein intake in patients without overt malnutrition is 0.9 to 1.2 g/kg/day.[506-508] Therefore, several investigators have proposed that the daily protein intake in these patients should be in the range of 0.9 to 1.1 g/kg/day.[509-511] Consideration also needs to be given to peritoneal protein losses, however, because these losses average 5 to 15 g/day but can be considerably higher with episodes of peritonitis.[512]

Patients undergoing chronic PD should have a total daily energy intake of 35 kcal/kg if younger than 60 years and 30 kcal/kg if 60 years or older.[513] This intake includes both dietary intake and the energy intake derived from glucose absorbed from the peritoneal dialysate. Surveys of energy intake have provided variable results, which are probably due to the patient population studied[508, 514-516] and the amount of residual renal function present.[508]

Interventions for Malnutrition

Cross-sectional studies have provided contradictory results regarding the potential association between nutrition and the dialysis dose in both PD[502, 508, 517-519] and HD patients.[506, 520, 521] Some investigators believe that mathematical coupling clouds the observed relationship between Kt/V urea and PNA levels.[522] Prospective studies, however, have demonstrated that increasing the dose of dialysis up to adequate levels results in an increase in nPNA values,[518, 523] energy intake,[524] and %LBM.[518] These findings are in accord with the observation that the relationship between the dose of dialysis and protein intake becomes flat at a Kt/V level greater than about 1.9.[502, 518, 519] Food supplements, enteral tube feedings, and both intradialytic and total parenteral nutrition have been used to treat malnutrition.[525] Percutaneous endoscopic gastrostomy tubes should be used cautiously, however, because they have been associated with a high rate of peritonitis.[526] In addition, bicarbonate supplementation can result in improvements in weight and BMI.[527, 528] Dietary modifications for other comorbid conditions need to be monitored, however, because patients prescribed a lipid-lowering diet had an average decrease in energy intake of 10%.[529]

PERITONEAL DIALYSIS IN SPECIAL POPULATIONS

Rapid Transporters

Data from several large databases suggest that approximately 10% to 15% of CAPD patients are high transporters when the PET is used to characterize the membrane type.

Patients who are high transporters have been shown to be at increased risk for mortality,[530-535] hypoalbuminemia, decreased LBM, and an increased incidence of weakness, fatigue, and hospitalization (Table 60-9).[501, 536, 537,538]

Reports on survival are contradictory, with some,[530, 525] but not all studies[532, 533] showing a higher mortality rate in high transporters. This increased rate of mortality and morbidity in high transporters has several possible etiologies, which were recently reviewed by Heaf.[538] First, these patients have a higher rate of hypoalbuminemia,[501, 531, 533, 539-544] and hypoalbuminemia is positively correlated with an increased rate of peritoneal loss of albumin (8 to 13 g/day versus 5 to 6 g/day in low transporters).[501, 531, 540, 545-549] Second, increased glucose absorption can lead to a variety of pathologic processes, including hyperlipidemia, hyperinsulinemia, obesity,[540] and increased peritoneal deposition of AGEs.[550, 551] High transporters are at increased risk of having elevated levels of low-density lipoprotein (LDL) cholesterol,[552] very low density lipoprotein (VLDL) cholesterol,[553] triglycerides,[500, 552, 554] plasma lipoprotein (a) [Lp(a)],[555] and depressed levels of high-density lipoprotein (HDL) cholesterol[549, 552] in most, but not all studies.[556] Third, loss of intraperitoneal osmotic pressure because of glucose absorption leads to reduced ultrafiltration, volume overload, and an increased requirement for antihypertensive drugs.[532, 539, 557] An alternative explanation is that high-transporter status is a marker of morbidity. Thus, patients who are malnourished or have chronic inflammation will have increased capillary permeability and as a result will be more likely to be a high transporter.[558]

Several possible modifications to the PD prescription may decrease glucose absorption and thus, at least theoretically, decrease the increased morbidity and mortality seen in these patients. First, the use of icodextrin can reduce glucose absorption by more than a third and thereby result in improved fluid control.[559] Second, cycler dialysis with rapid exchanges can be used to prevent glucose equilibrium and allow for preservation of ultrafiltration capacity. Unfortunately, the use of cycler therapy has resulted in either no decrease[560, 561] or little decrease[404] in peritoneal loss of protein. No clinical trials have evaluated the effectiveness of either of these two techniques in improving mortality and morbidity, however. Finally, patients with ultrafiltration failure or hypoalbuminemia can be switched to HD.

Elderly Patients

The percentage of PD patients who were older than 65 years was 28% in 1995 and 26% in 2001.[562] In the 2001 CMS-CPM

TABLE 60-9

Patient Survival by Solute Transport Group

AUTHOR (Ref)	NUMBER OF PATIENTS	FOLLOW-UP (YR)	PATIENT SURVIVAL (%) BY SOLUTE TRANSPORT GROUP			
			Low	Low-Average	High-Average	High Ref.
Churchill (531)	503	2	91	80	72	71
Fried (532)	123	3	100	89	91	71
Wang (533)	46	1	100	90	63	16
Davies (534)	303	5	70	57	46	42
Heaf (537)	202	3	72	66	60	31

Adapted from Heaf JG: Pathogenic effects of a high peritoneal transport rate. Semin Dial 13:188-193, 2000.

survey, 10% of PD patients were 65 to 69 years of age, 13% were 70 to 79 years old, and 3% were 80 years or older.[394] Data from the USRDS suggest that for the average 65-year-old patient who is starting dialysis, the average life expectancy is roughly 3.6 additional years.[1] Although this life expectancy is only a fifth of that for U.S. citizens aged 65 without renal disease, it is important to consider quality-of-life issues in these patients and to keep in perspective that these same USRDS data suggest that the average additional life expectancy for an ESRD patient 40 years old is about 8 years. Therefore, treatment of ESRD should not be denied on the basis of the patient's age alone.

Elderly patients may have a substantial number of comorbid medical conditions that may limit their ability to perform their own dialysis therapy. It is estimated that about 60% of patients older than 80 years need assistance with dialysis exchanges, exit site care, and medications.[563] If family support is not available, assistance can be provided by nursing home staff, daily care centers, or home care nurses.[564-566]

Mortality in patients older than 85 years in the first 90 days of ESRD therapy is 27%, and risk factors for mortality included not only the presence of comorbid medical conditions but also late referral to nephrology.[567] Thus, it is especially important to estimate the GFR in elderly patients on a regular basis to ensure that dialysis is initiated in accordance with national guidelines. Mortality rates among PD patients increase as age increases,[568-572] and the number of patients who withdraw from dialysis before death is twice as high in patients 65 years or older as in younger patients.[573] Hospitalization rates were also higher in elderly patients than younger patients.[563, 570, 574, 575] The most frequent cause of hospitalization was peritonitis.[563, 576, 577] Technique survival in elderly PD patients, however, is better than[574, 575, 578] or at least equal to[571, 576, 579] technique survival in younger patients. Finally, the nutritional status of elderly patients is worse than that of younger patients, as indicated by lower values for LBM-to-weight ratios,[498] creatinine and urea excretion,[496, 498] and serum albumin values[496] in the elderly.

Data are conflicting regarding the rate of peritonitis in elderly versus nonelderly PD patients.[569, 574, 579-581] Not surprisingly, bedridden patients have a higher rate of peritonitis, perhaps because of an increased frequency of bowel or bladder incontinence.[580] Exit site infections, however, appear to be less common in older patients than in younger patients, probably because of the decreased activity level of the older group.[576, 582]

Elderly patients are more likely to have problems related to bowel dysfunction. Constipation is most prevalent in the elderly. This problem can be due to decreased mobility, drug effects, altered diet, and concomitant diseases.[583] Constipation can be a cause of mechanical dysfunction of the Tenckhoff catheter. Thus, constipation must be assessed in all PD patients and treated appropriately. Colonic diverticula occur in 30% to 40% of individuals older than 50 years, and the frequency increases thereafter with each additional decade of life. Diverticula can cause peritonitis, although no evidence suggests that PD can aggravate diverticular disease.

Patients with Diabetes Mellitus

Patients with diabetes mellitus have both theoretical advantages and disadvantages for PD.[584] Potential advantages of PD include

1. Lack of anticoagulation and its possible benefit on diabetic retinopathy
2. Intraperitoneal administration of insulin, which should allow for more physiologic control of glucose metabolism
3. Increased removal of middle molecules, which may help prevent or minimize the complications of diabetic neuropathy

Potential disadvantages of PD include

1. Constant exposure to a hyperglycemic environment
2. Increased risk of peritonitis because of immunosuppression in diabetic patients

Survival data for diabetic patients by dialysis modality are contradictory,[9, 10, 585, 586] with the same caveats in terms of data analysis that are presented in the section on comparisons of PD and HD.

Although data from early reports suggested improvement or stabilization of diabetic nephropathy in patients undergoing PD versus HD,[587-592] more recent data show no difference in the natural history of this diabetic complication by dialysis modality.[593, 594] For diabetic neuropathy, more recent studies have again found no advantage of PD over HD.[593, 594] Data from the annual CMS survey have shown that in diabetic ESRD patients, the rate of retinopathy or lower extremity amputation was 8% in PD patients and 13% in HD patients. It is unclear, however, whether this variation was due to differences in patient comorbidity at the initiation of dialysis or due to the dialysis modality. Finally, most,[594, 595] but not all studies[596, 597] have shown no difference in the rates and severity of peritonitis between diabetic and nondiabetic patients.

Insulin may be administered to PD patients by either the subcutaneous or intraperitoneal route. Several regimens for intraperitoneal administration of insulin are available.[598-600] The use of intraperitoneal insulin results in glycemic control that is at least as good,[601] if not better[602, 603] than that achieved with subcutaneous injection; in addition, the frequency of hypoglycemic episodes is decreased.[603] Unfortunately, this improved glycemic control is also accompanied by a slightly higher rate of peritonitis[604, 605] because of the increased risk of contamination from the injection of insulin into bags containing PD fluid. In addition, absorption of intraperitoneal insulin is highly variable, with a range of 17% to 66%. This variability was not related to membrane transport characteristics and was not due to variability in the absorption of insulin onto the dialysate delivery system.[606] Finally, intraperitoneal insulin has been associated with subcapsular liver steatosis[607, 608] and malignant omentum syndrome.[609] This entity was found in seven of eight patients receiving intraperitoneal insulin and in none of eight patients receiving subcutaneous insulin. The amount of hepatic steatosis was directly correlated with both the peritoneal transport rate and body weight.

Black and Hispanic Patients

Black race is associated with an increased incidence of ESRD.[610, 611] Blacks are underrepresented among PD patients, however,[612, 613] the reasons for which are uncertain and probably multifactorial. Similarly, a smaller percentage of Hispanic patients receive PD than HD.[614, 615] A random sample of patients in the United States demonstrated that Hispanics were more likely to have diabetes mellitus as a cause of their ESRD than were either blacks or whites and that both blacks and Hispanics were younger than white patients.[615]

Most large databases show that black patients treated with PD are at increased risk for peritonitis, technique failure, and exit site infection[616] when compared with white patients.[44, 617, 618] The reason for the reported increased risk of peritonitis in black patients is unclear. When the subset of black patients in a study on disconnect devices was compared with white patients on disconnect devices, no difference was noted in peritonitis rates.[616] The increased risk of peritonitis in black patients may not be due to race but to a tendency toward a lower income and education level in this group. Others have shown that the risk of peritonitis is inversely correlated with the level of education at the time of initiating PD (patients with less than 8 years of formal education had the highest rates of peritonitis).[617, 618] Data are lacking on peritonitis rates in Hispanic patients.

Pediatric Patients

The introduction of long-term PD for the management of end-stage renal failure in children has been a major advance. The first reported use of PD in pediatric patients was by Bloxsum and Powell[619] in 1948. The use of standard CAPD was reported in 1979.[620] PD has widely been considered the treatment of choice for renal failure in infants and young children when transplantation is not an immediate option.[621] This therapy allows children of all ages to receive dialysis in their homes with no or minimal dietary restrictions. The use of CCPD in pediatric patients was first described in 1981 by Price and Suki.[622] A 1996 survey of the North American Pediatric Renal Transplant Cooperative Study showed that approximately two thirds of the pediatric dialysis population receives PD. Interestingly, a survey of adult and pediatric nephrologists indicated that the latter were 60% more likely to recommend PD instead of HD to identical patients in a case vignette scenario.[623] More PD patients attended school full-time than did HD patients at initiation of dialysis (77% versus 45%, respectively) and at 6, 12, and 24 months of follow-up.[624] An additional benefit of PD over HD is the well-documented increase in quality of life in both pediatric patients and their parents.[625, 626]

In a national survey of patients treated by dialysis in the United States, 1-year survival rates were 83% in infants starting dialysis before 3 months of age, 89% in 3- to 23-month-olds, and 95% in 2- to 5-year-olds.[627] Nonsurvivors were more likely to have pulmonary disease or hypoplasia (or both) than were survivors. Anuria was also a risk factor in patients younger than 2 years.[627] For pediatric patients receiving acute dialysis in intensive care units (ICUs), predictors of mortality in a multivariate model included age younger than 1 year and mechanical ventilation.[628] The mean PD catheter duration in infants less than 10 kg is 4.5 months, with a shorter duration in infants less than 5 kg at the start of dialysis therapy.[629] The mid-European survey of pediatric dialysis patients reported a technique survival rate of 95% at 2 years and 65% at 4 years.[630] The most common causes of treatment failure were recurrent peritonitis and ultrafiltration failure. Catheter survival was 82% at 1 year and

57% at 4 years.[630] Children with hypoalbuminemia or recurrent peritonitis are at increased risk for technique failure.[631]

Guidelines have been developed for levels of adequate PD in pediatric patients in both the United States[432, 433] and Europe,[632] as well as other countries. NKF-K/DOQI guidelines state that the target dose of PD in children should meet or exceed the adult standards but note that morbidity and mortality data regarding dose and outcomes are lacking. The European guidelines state that the weekly Kt/V urea should be at least 2.0, and these guidelines provide additional recommendations regarding the initial and subsequent PD prescription. Modification of the PD prescription has been successful in meeting adequacy guidelines, even in the face of declining residual renal function.[633] Detailed recommendations for improving dialysis adequacy in pediatric patients have been published.[634] Strategies to improve clearance include the use of continuous therapies and maximizing drain volume, especially by optimizing the exchange volume or by using either hypertonic dextrose solutions or icodextrin. Determination of adequacy values in children is complicated by the availability of several formulas to estimate the volume of urea distribution. Recent data using radiolabeled water suggest that new formulas from the Pediatric Peritoneal Dialysis Study Consortium are more accurate than the Mellits and Cheek formulas derived from healthy children.[635]

When traditional methods were used to calculate V, the mean weekly creatinine clearance in a European survey was 57 L/1.73 m^2 in both CAPD and cycler patients, and the total weekly Kt/v urea was 2.45 in cycler patients and 1.96 in CAPD patients.[630] The dialytic regimen for 110 patients receiving cycler therapy included a dry day in 58% of patients and TPD in 26%. The mean prescription parameters for cycler dialysis with a dry day included 13 ± 5.8 exchanges per day, a total duration of 10.0 ± 1.0 hours, and a dwell volume of 36.1 ± 5.9 mL/kg body weight. For patients with a wet day, these values were 13.0 ± 4.7, 10.1 ± 1.3 hours, and 37.7 ± 5.2 mL/kg body weight, respectively.[636] In children, the prescribed fill volume should be expressed per BSA. The optimal fill volume is thought to be less than 1400 mL/m^2.[637, 638] At fill volumes above this level, increasing signs of physical discomfort were noted, as well as an increase in intra-abdominal pressure.[637]

Guidelines have also been developed for choosing the appropriate dialysis solutions for children receiving PD.[639] The standard osmotic agent is glucose, and the lowest glucose concentration needed should be prescribed to decrease the risk of functional deterioration of the PD membrane.[640-643] In malnourished children, aggressive enteral nutrition is the preferred mode of therapy, but amino acid–based dialysate can also be considered. In one study conducted in eight children over a 6-month period, the use of an amino acid solution mixed with a glucose solution resulted in improvement in anthropometric parameters, but no change in serum albumin levels.[644] Polyglucose solutions are of definite benefit in patients who have difficulty with either ultrafiltration or solute removal. The very low absorption of these large-molecular-weight molecules allows for ultrafiltration for sustained periods.[645] In a study conducted in 11 children, the mean net ultrafiltration for a 12-hour dwell period with the icodextrin solution was similar to that obtained with a 3.86% dextrose solution. The use of icodextrin improved the weekly Kt/V urea by 0.52 ± 0.07.[646]

Several investigators have shown that the distribution of peritoneal transport types is similar in children and adults.[647] In patients without peritonitis, no change was reported in D/P Cr values during the first 24 months of PD therapy. After this period, the D/P Cr value increased from a mean of 0.66 ± 0.12 to 0.70 ± 0.09.[648] Pediatric patients with a history of peritonitis had higher D/P Cr values than did patients without a history of peritonitis.[649]

Consensus guidelines have also been developed for the diagnosis and treatment of peritonitis in pediatric patients receiving PD,[650] and these guidelines are reviewed in the section on peritonitis. Rates of peritonitis in multicenter surveys have improved from one episode per 5 to 8 patient-months[651, 652] to about one episode per 13 to 14 patient-months.[624, 653, 654] The risk of acquiring exit site infections or tunnel infections was not different with respect to patient age, patient race, or the type of PD catheter placed. The incidence of an exit site or tunnel infection was 11% at 30 days, 26% between 30 days and 6 months, and 30% between 6 months and 1 year. The rate of peritonitis was one episode per 13.2 patient-months. Patients with either an exit site infection or tunnel infection had a twofold higher risk of peritonitis and an almost threefold higher risk of requiring hospitalization for access infections or complications.[655] Peritonitis rates are lower in programs with more than 15 pediatric patients on PD and in programs that have longer training times dedicated to the theory and both the practical and technical skills of PD.[656]

Growth retardation is common in pediatric dialysis patients, and the prevalence of this problem has remained at about 50%.[630, 657] Although patients initiating PD are growth retarded, only infants show improvement in height after 2 years of dialysis (from −1.54 for the mean height standard deviation score [SDS] at initiation of dialysis to −1.21 SDS at 2 years).[658, 659] A variety of factors can cause growth retardation in these patients, including poor control of PTH levels, acidosis, and poor protein and caloric intake.[660-663] To minimize the development of growth retardation, all pediatric PD patients should receive at least 100% of the recommended daily allowance for energy intake.[664, 665] In addition, because protein losses are higher in young patients as a result of their larger peritoneal surface area, intake of adequate protein is crucial. Guidelines recommend an intake of 2.5 to 3.0 g/kg/day in infants up to 3 years of age, 2.0 to 2.5 g/kg/day for patients 3 years old to puberty, 2.0 g/kg/day in pubertal patients, and 1.5 g/kg/day in postpubertal patients.[665] Metabolic acidosis can contribute to growth retardation through disturbances in the growth hormone–insulin-like growth factor axis.[666-668] Therefore, metabolic acidosis should be aggressively treated in pediatric PD patients. Supplements of water-soluble vitamins,[669] the use of phosphate binders, and vitamin D analog therapy are also important.[659] Recombinant human growth hormone (rhGH) has become an important adjunct for the treatment of growth retardation in children when used either subcutaneously[670] or with intraperitoneal therapy.[671, 672] In a recent study, 20% of pediatric patients being treated with chronic PD were receiving growth hormone.[630] An rhGH dose of 0.05 mg/kg/day resulted in sustained catch-up growth for at least 2.5 years, whereas a dose of 0.025 mg/kg/day resulted in sustained catch-up growth for only the first 6 months of therapy.

Patients Infected with the Human Immunodeficiency Virus

Initial reports of the survival of human immunodeficiency virus (HIV)-infected patients with ESRD were much lower than those of ESRD patients without HIV, with median survival rates of 13 and 38 months, respectively.[673] More recent data have shown that the stage of HIV infection is more important than the presence of ESRD in determining survival,[674-677] with mean survival rates of up to 57 months reported.[678] Studies are contradictory with regard to an increased rate of peritonitis in HIV-infected versus non–HIV-infected patients.[675, 677, 679-682]

Most patients who are HIV positive will have PD cultures that are positive for HIV.[683] HIV can survive in PD effluent for up to 7 days and on PD tubing for up to 48 hours. Ten minutes of exposure to either 10% bleach or a 1:512 dilution of Amukin is effective in disinfecting dialysate effluent.[684] Therefore, infection control policies for such patients include universal body precautions, with use of bleach as a disinfectant, and then disposal of the dialysate down the sink or toilet; dialysis bags must be emptied into a biohazards bag.

The pharmacokinetics of most agents used to treat patients with HIV has been determined for those receiving PD.[685] The protease inhibitors amprenavir,[685] indinavir,[685] nelfinavir,[689] saquinavir,[685] and ritonavir[687] can be used in PD patients without dose adjustment. Zidovudine should be prescribed at 50% to 70% of the usual dose,[685] whereas stavudine and didanosine should be administered at one fourth the usual dose.[685, 688]

Pregnant Patients

Patients undergoing either HD or PD have been able to have successful pregnancies. A survey of 2299 dialysis units found that 2.0% of females aged 14 to 44 years became pregnant over a 4-year period (2.4% of HD patients and 1.1% of PD patients).[689] Premature infants were born to 84% of the women who conceived while receiving dialysis therapy. In the subset of these patients in whom the dialysis modality was known, no significant difference in infant survival was noted between PD and HD (37% versus 39.5%, respectively). In HD, increased time on dialysis was beneficial in increasing infant survival rates, but no evidence indicated that increasing the number of exchanges or the volume of the exchanges was beneficial in CAPD.[689, 690] Data on cycler prescriptions and infant survival are lacking, however. In the third trimester of pregnancy, it may become difficult for women to tolerate their usual exchange volume.[691] These patients may require a combination of CAPD and cycler dialysis to maintain an adequate dose of dialysis.[692] Bloody dialysate in a pregnant PD patient can be a sign of either placental separation or spontaneous abortion.[691] Peritonitis has been reported during pregnancy, and any obstetric infection can cause peritonitis.[692, 693] Cephalosporins and penicillin are generally considered safe in pregnancy, but data are more limited for vancomycin.[692, 694] Aminoglycosides can cause fetal ototoxicity, and ciprofloxacin can result in abnormal cartilage development; these agents should thus be avoided.[694]

Conception occurs in approximately 1 in every 200 women of childbearing age who receive chronic dialysis therapy.[689]

Therefore, family planning counseling should be offered to all women of childbearing age.[695] Dialysis patients planning for a pregnancy should receive folate supplementation to help prevent neural tube defects[696]; such supplementation is especially important because water-soluble vitamins are removed by the dialysis procedure. The average age of gestation when the diagnosis of pregnancy in chronic dialysis patients is made is 16 weeks,[697] probably because of the common occurrence of irregular menses and abdominal symptoms in dialysis patients.[692] If the patient sees her physician in the early stages of pregnancy, a thorough discussion of the maternal and fetal risks of pregnancy is recommended. Prenatal care is intensive in surveillance, with particular attention paid to preeclampsia, hypertension, preterm labor, intrauterine growth restriction, anemia, and infection. In one large survey, hypertension was present in 79% of women, and less than 6% of women were able to maintain a hematocrit greater than 30% throughout the pregnancy.[695] Hypertension is not usually more difficult to control in pregnant patients receiving erythropoietin[698]; however, erythropoietin therapy must be discontinued when severe hypertension is present. Antihypertensive agents that can be used safely in pregnancy have been reviewed by the Joint National Committee on Prevention, Detection, Evaluation, and Treatment of High Blood Pressure.[699]

About a third of patients conceive before the initiation of dialysis therapy. If these patients have preexisting renal insufficiency, it is estimated that 30% to 50% will have accelerated progression of kidney disease.[700-702] In particular, the elevated estrogen levels of pregnancy can cause lupus flares and acute renal failure.[703] Several authors have recommended that dialysis be initiated in pregnant patients with chronic kidney disease when the GFR is less than 20 mL/min.[692]

PERITONEAL DIALYSIS IN A NONCHRONIC SETTING

Acute Renal Failure

In resource-rich countries, the use of PD for the treatment of acute renal failure has declined while the use of continuous venovenous hemodialysis (CVVHD) and hemofiltration has increased. A survey of nephrologists in the United States indicated that 35% of nephrologists never used PD to treat acute renal failure and 48% used PD in less than 10% of cases of acute renal failure.[704-706] Nephrologists in private practice were more likely to use manual PD, whereas academic nephrologists were more likely to use automated PD. The major reasons for using PD were hemodynamic instability (56%) and absence of anticoagulation (18%). In the ICU, the HD nurse performed PD in about 50% of cases and the ICU nurse in about 30%.

The decrease in the use of PD in this setting is due to medical and technical reasons and has been reviewed by Van de Noortgate and colleagues.[707] First, PD has a lower efficiency than either HD or continuous extracorporeal therapies; hence, PD cannot often be used in patients who require significant volume or solute removal. Second, PD cannot be used in patients who have had intra-abdominal surgery. Third, because of respiratory compromise from increased intra-abdominal pressure, PD is often contraindicated in patients with adult respiratory distress syndrome. Finally, the use of fluid high in dextrose can lead to overfeeding with resultant hyperglycemia, hepatic steatosis, and increased CO_2 production with worsening respiratory failure.[708] Therefore, if supplemental nutrition is given, the glucose load from PD must be included in the calculation of daily energy supplementation.[708]

PD is still used commonly for the treatment of acute renal failure in developing countries because of a lower cost of the procedure in comparison to HD and continuous extracorporeal therapies.[706, 709] However, a recent study conducted in Vietnam in which PD was compared with pumped venovenous hemofiltration for acute renal failure (69% of cases were due to severe malaria) found that the odds ratio for death was 5.1 and the need for future dialysis was 4.7 in the group of patients randomized to PD versus patients randomized to hemofiltration. In addition, rates of resolution of acidosis and decline in the serum creatinine concentration were at least 50% lower in patients treated with PD than in those treated with hemofiltration.[710] Potential reasons for these differences included the estimate that creatinine clearance was 100% greater with venovenous hemofiltration than with PD and the use of acetate as the bicarbonate-generating base in the peritoneal dialysate.[711]

Several modifications of the technique of PD may be beneficial in the treatment of acute renal failure. A comparison of TPD with standard PD found that TPD provided higher clearances of creatinine and urea, as well as higher clearances of potassium and phosphorus.[712] In patients with acute renal failure and shock, the use of a bicarbonate solution that contains no calcium or magnesium in lieu of a standard lactate-based PD solution resulted in more rapid improvement and higher levels of blood pH, serum bicarbonate, systolic blood pressure, and mean arterial pressure.[713] In both the shock and nonshock groups, lactic acidosis was corrected more quickly when the bicarbonate solution was used. Therefore, bicarbonate solutions may be of particular benefit in patients with shock, lactic acidosis, and multiple organ failure. Finally, patients receiving PD instead of HD before transplantation had a lower incidence and severity of delayed recovery of renal function after renal transplantation,[714-716] possibly secondary to a higher likelihood of a well-hydrated state with PD versus HD.[717]

In infants and children, however, PD is still a commonly used modality to treat acute renal failure,[718-720] especially in neonates.[721] In one retrospective study of acute renal failure conducted over a 10-year period, complications were seen in 25% of patients receiving PD, with catheter malfunction being the most common complication.[720] In a second retrospective study, the complication rate was 20%, with catheter obstruction or dislocation (11%) and ultrafiltration problems (7%) being the most common complications.[722]

Nonuremic Uses of Peritoneal Dialysis

By design, both HD and PD are suited for blood purification and fluid removal. Thus, both modalities can be used for the treatment of conditions other than ESRD. Nonuremic uses of PD have been reviewed by several authors[723, 724] and are summarized in the following paragraphs.

CONGESTIVE HEART FAILURE. Numerous case reports have described the use of PD to treat patients with congestive heart failure.[725, 726] Potential benefits of this modality for congestive heart failure include improvements in functional status,[725, 727-729] ejection fraction,[730] and quality of life[727, 731] and a decrease in hospitalization rates.[727, 732] Patients have resolution of volume overload, including lower extremity edema and ascites.[727, 728, 732]

CHEMOTHERAPY. The intraperitoneal administration of antineoplastic agents has been found to be effective in treating malignancies of the peritoneal cavity.[733, 734] Protocols have been used for the treatment of colorectal cancer,[735-737] ovarian cancer,[738, 739] gastric cancer,[740] and mesothelioma.[741] Mathematical models have also been developed to describe key factors that influence drug delivery in intraperitoneal systems.[742] A modification of this technique, hyperthermic chemoperfusion, has been used for several intra-abdominal cancers.[743] With this technique, one or more PD catheters are placed for inflow, together with several outflow drains and a temperature probe. The perfusate, usually PD, is heated until a temperature of 41.5° C to 44° C is reached inside the abdomen. The chemotherapy is then added to the perfusate. The enhanced effect of chemotherapeutic agents with hyperthermia is thought to be secondary to several mechanisms, including an increase in cell membrane permeability, altered active drug transport, and altered cell metabolism.[744, 745]

HYPOTHERMIA. The use of PD for hypothermia was first reported in 1967.[746] Hypothermia can be managed in the field by removing wet garments, insulating the patient, and providing warm humidified air or oxygen. Patients who are severely hypothermic are treated in the hospital with heated (42° C to 46° C) humidified oxygen, intravenous fluids warmed to 43° C, and PD with dialysate warmed to 43° C.[747, 748]

LIVER DISEASE. Patients with liver disease and ascites can be successfully treated with PD.[749-754] In patients transferred for hemodynamic instability while on HD, stabilization of blood pressure can be achieved with PD.[754] Peritoneal losses of protein have been shown to decrease substantially over time, from greater than 30 g/day to less than 10 g/day.[755] PD has been used to treat Wilson disease, with the removal rate of copper increased by 5% to 20% when compared with urinary excretion alone.[756] Intraperitoneal deferoxamine has been used to treat hemochromatosis.[757]

NEPHROGENIC ASCITES. Nephrogenic ascites is defined as persistent ascites in a dialysis patient without evidence of an underlying etiology such as liver disease.[758] Possible causes of this entity include hypoalbuminemia,[759, 760] alterations in peritoneal membrane permeability,[761] and decreased lymphatic drainage.[762] Treatment of nephrogenic ascites has included daily HD, PD, peritoneovenous shunting, renal transplantation, intraperitoneal steroids, and bilateral nephrectomy (reviewed by Han and colleagues[761]). No controlled trials have compared the effectiveness of these therapies.

INBORN ERRORS OF METABOLISM. Despite much initial enthusiasm for the use of PD for the treatment of urea cycle disorders, propionicacidemia, and maple syrup urine disease, more recent data suggest that both CVVHD and continuous hemofiltration techniques are superior to PD with regard to reduction of plasma ammonia or plasma leucine levels.[763]

COMPLICATIONS OF PERITONEAL DIALYSIS

Cardiovascular Disease

Cardiovascular disease is the major cause of death in PD patients,[1] and rates of cardiovascular disease are higher in dialysis patients than in the general population.[764] Multifactorial atherosclerotic risk factors in PD patients include not only the traditional risk factors of smoking, hypertension, family history, obesity, diabetes mellitus, and hyperlipidemia, but also coronary calcification, hypoalbuminemia, hyperhomocysteinemia, and elevated levels of CRP and Lp(a).[765, 766]

Hypertension

Hypertension is very common and occurs in 50% to 90% of PD patients.[767, 768] Hypertension in PD patients may be explained in part by fluid retention as a result of impaired ultrafiltration.[769] Daytime blood pressure readings improve from the initiation of PD until the duration of dialysis is 6 to 12 months[770]; however, an improvement in nocturnal blood pressure is not seen.[771] Patients with an ambulatory nighttime systolic blood pressure load greater than 30% are at increased risk of having left ventricular hypertrophy (LVH).[772] In one study, severe LVH was found in a third of CAPD patients and was associated with significantly high cardiovascular morbidity and mortality.[773] Other studies have confirmed the association between LVH in PD patients and cardiac events, including cardiovascular death[774] and cardiac arrhythmias.[775] Finally, higher sodium and fluid removal was associated with both higher mortality and increased hospitalization rates.[776] Treatment of volume overload and hypertension in PD patients includes the prescription of loop diuretics, preservation of residual renal function, reduction of dietary salt intake and limitation of fluid intake, and prevention and treatment of peritoneal ultrafiltration failure.[777, 778]

Hyperlipidemia

The causes and magnitude of hyperlipidemia have been well summarized.[779] PD is associated with an increased glucose load because of constant absorption from the peritoneal cavity. The reported mean daily glucose absorption in CAPD patients varies from 100 to 200 g of glucose per day.[780-783] Because of this glucose load, PD patients have a constant susceptibility to the development of hyperglycemia and hyperinsulinemia.[784-786] Some patients even have frank diabetes that necessitates insulin therapy.[120, 787] This increase in insulin levels results in an increase in the synthesis of triglycerides in the liver.[788] In addition, dialysate protein loss of 5 to 15 g/day results in the loss of all lipoproteins, with preferential loss of small molecules such as HDL.[552] Therefore, it is not surprising that PD patients have a more atherogenic profile than HD patients do[788-793] and that elevated lipid and lipoprotein levels are associated with a higher risk of mortality.[545, 556, 794, 795]

Patients monitored after the initiation of PD therapy had a significant increase in both serum cholesterol and serum triglyceride levels,[786, 556] with elevated total cholesterol levels caused mainly by a rise in LDL-cholesterol.[796] The strongest predictors of worsening lipid profiles were weight gain, preexisting cardiovascular comorbidity,[556] and higher plasma glucose levels.[797] PD patients also have elevated levels of Lp(a)[798-802] and apolipoproteins, including individual apo A– and apo B–containing lipoproteins,[803] as well as apo C-III, apo B, and apo C.[804] The increased Lp(a) levels in PD patients are due to increased synthesis, not decreased clearance.[805]

Dietary modification was successful in lowering lipid levels in only 4 of 26 chronic PD patients, thus suggesting that most of these patients will require pharmacologic therapy for treatment of dyslipidemia.[529] In addition, a small study using one 1.1% amino acid dialysate exchange per day did not report any improvement in lipid parameters.[806] The use of polyglucose solutions has been associated with a decrease in lipid levels.[807, 808]

Hypercholesterolemia in PD patients has been successfully treated with atorvastatin[809-812] and gemfibrozil,[812] whereas hypertriglyceridemia has been successfully treated with atorvastatin,[778, 809] gemfibrozil,[812, 813] fibric acid analogs,[814] and fish oil supplementation.[815-818] The incidence of rhabdomyolysis in PD patients who were prescribed either hydroxymethylglutaryl–coenzyme A (HMG-CoA) reductase inhibitors or fibric acid analogs is not clearly known[814, 819, 820]; patients should be monitored closely. Although a number of clinical trials have shown that treatment of lipid abnormalities in the nondialysis population results in a reduction in cardiovascular mortality and morbidity, no evidence has been found for this reduction in cardiovascular events in the PD population.[779] Guidelines developed by the International Society for Peritoneal Dialysis recommend that LDL-cholesterol levels be less than 100 mg/dL and that HMG-CoA reductase inhibitors be used as first-line therapy. Liver function and creatinine phosphokinase should be routinely monitored.[779] Guidelines for the treatment of hyperlipidemia have also been developed by the NKF-K/DOQI lipid work group.[820a]

C-Reactive Protein

The relationship between inflammation and cardiovascular disease appears to be very strong in dialysis patients.[821, 822] PD patients have serologic evidence of an enhanced inflammatory response.[488, 489, 823, 824] Factors that can cause this enhanced inflammatory response include the decreased renal clearance of cytokines and AGEs,[825] the use of bioincompatible peritoneal dialysate solutions,[826] and comorbid medical conditions such as chronic heart failure and peritonitis. Both acute-phase reactants such as CRP,[827] Lp(a),[555, 828] and fibrinogen[828] and proinflammatory cytokines such as TNF-α[829, 830] and IL-6[831, 832] have direct atherogenic or thrombogenic properties (or both). Approximately 30% to 60% of PD patients have elevated CRP levels.[491, 823, 833] PD patients who have elevated CRP levels are at increased risk for atherosclerotic events and ischemic heart disease, cerebrovascular disease, and peripheral vascular disease.[490, 491, 823, 834] Some authors recommend that patients with persistently elevated CRP levels undergo a workup for ischemic heart disease or other atherosclerotic diseases such as carotid disease or peripheral vascular disease.[834]

Homocysteine

Most PD and HD patients have elevated homocysteine levels.[823, 835-839] In some,[835-837, 839] but not all studies,[840, 841] patients with low folate or vitamin B_{12} levels are at increased risk of having elevated homocysteine levels. Patients with the C677T transition polymorphism of the 5,10-methylenetetrahydrofolate reductase gene are at increased risk of having markedly elevated homocysteine levels.[836, 839]

Although homocysteine is removed by PD, the removal rate is not high enough to allow for the correction of hyperhomocysteinemia.[841, 842] Folic acid supplementation can decrease homocysteine levels in PD patients,[843-845] but it does not improve endothelial function.[845] Amino acid–based PD solutions that contain methionine cause an increase in homocysteine levels.[846] Although homocysteine levels have been correlated with atherosclerotic heart disease,[823, 847] no randomized clinical trials have been conducted to investigate the effect of folate supplementation on rates of cardiovascular events in PD patients with elevated homocysteine levels.

Treatment

Management of cardiovascular disease in PD patients has been reviewed recently.[848] Treatment is initiated with risk factor modification and medical therapy, including aspirin, β-blockers, angiotensin-converting enzyme inhibitors, and lipid-lowering agents. Revascularization can be performed with either percutaneous transluminal coronary angioplasty or coronary artery bypass grafting, with the latter procedure preferred in patients with multivessel disease, impaired left ventricular function, severe symptoms, or ischemia.[849, 850]

Comparison of Hemodialysis and Peritoneal Dialysis

The mortality and hospitalization rates of HD and PD have been compared in many studies. The results of these analyses have been contradictory, with some studies showing a survival advantage for HD,[585, 851, 852] other studies showing a survival advantage for PD,[9, 10, 853-855] and still other studies showing no difference in mortality rates.[586, 856-858] A number of reasons have been proposed for these discrepant results.[859] Selection bias occurs when patients who choose one modality are different from patients who choose the other modality; such differences include age, gender, race, and the presence and severity of comorbid conditions.[860, 861, 862] The use of different variables in multivariate models can result in different results.[863] Variation in the dose of dialysis delivered could also affect mortality rates.[586] Finally, the inadequate sample size of some studies may result in insufficient power to detect statistically significant results. Similar comments are applicable for comparing hospitalization rates in PD versus HD patients.[864]

Indications for Switching from Peritoneal Dialysis to Hemodialysis

In some situations a patient may not be able to continue PD and may need to switch to HD.[865] First, despite adjustment of the PD prescription, the patient may not be able to achieve adequate dialysis. A complete assessment of the possible causes for the inadequate dialysis should be undertaken, including patient noncompliance with the dialysis prescription and sampling and collection errors. Noncompliance with some part of the dialysis prescription is fairly common in PD patients. Sevick and associates compiled data from patient diaries and from an electronic monitoring device and found that approximately 20% of PD exchanges were missed and that 50% of patients were inconsistent with their exchange routine, either shortening treatments or missing exchanges altogether.[866] Several studies of noncompliance determined by assessment of inventory supplies have demonstrated a nonadherence rate between 12% (in Canadian patients)[867] and 40% (in American patients).[868, 869]

Inadequate ultrafiltration can be seen either in patients who are high transporters or in patients who have a mechanical defect that impairs outflow of dialysate from the peritoneal cavity.[557] High transporters are also at risk for excessive protein loss in the dialysate, which can lead to a significant decline in serum albumin levels. If malnutrition develops and cannot be rectified by aggressive nutritional supplementation and correction of underlying comorbid medical conditions, treatment should be switched to HD. Finally, patients who have frequent peritonitis, peritoneal access failure that cannot be readily corrected, or severe hypertriglyceridemia are also poor candidates for continuing with PD.

Noninfectious Complications
Mechanical Complications

INFLOW PAIN. If the catheter is correctly placed within the peritoneal cavity, inflow pain is typically due to positioning of the catheter tip adjacent to tissue that cannot move during fluid infusion. This type of pain tends to be minimized when curled tip catheters with multiple outflow pores are used. If this pain does not resolve over time, catheter repositioning may be required. Pain may also be related to the dialysate composition. An abnormally low dialysate pH may transiently cause pain in some patients. If low pH is the cause of the pain, it can be mitigated by adding 4 to 5 mEq/L of $NaHCO_3$ to the dialysis solution before infusion.[71] Other possible causes include the choice of buffer,[870] temperature, or any additives such as antibiotics and the introduction of air.

OUTFLOW FAILURE. Outflow failure is detected when the drained volume is substantially less than the instilled volume. If both outflow failure and inflow failure are present, it is probably secondary to either a kink in the catheter or catheter obstruction by fibrin or clots. If obstruction is suspected, the catheter can often be opened with an injection of urokinase or tissue plasminogen activator.[871, 872] Catheter kinking is usually treated by catheter replacement.

Once the possibility of ultrafiltration failure or dialysate leak has been ruled out, the differential diagnosis of isolated outflow failure is not long and includes catheter migration, omental wrapping, and adherence of bowel (as seen with constipation) or other tissue to the catheter. In these cases, the omentum or adherent tissue acts as a ball valve that allows the ingress of fluid but occludes the catheter pores when drainage is attempted. In such cases, the clinician should rule out constipation and then obtain a plain radiograph to determine the catheter's position. If the catheter has been malpositioned, repositioning can be attempted with

a malleable metal rod under fluoroscopic guidance,[873-875] with guidewires,[876] with channel cleaning brushes,[877] and as a last resort, via peritoneoscopy.[878] The alpha maneuver can also be used when the peritoneal catheter tip has migrated.[879] This procedure entails the introduction of a long metallic guide through the catheter to reposition the tip. The alpha maneuver was effective in 12 of 24 cases, with 7 failures caused by omental entrapment and 5 failures requiring catheter exchange.[880] Newer catheter designs have decreased the incidence of catheter malpositioning. Self-locating catheters are similar to Tenckhoff catheters, except for the addition of a small tungsten cylinder weighing 12 g that is located in the distal tip of the catheter.[881] Malfunction rates of self-locating catheters are lower than rates for other Tenckhoff catheter designs, with no increase in rates of peritonitis.[882] Catheters with a swan-neck configuration between the two cuffs also have a much lower rate of catheter migration than do catheters without the swan-neck configuration.[883] Laparoscopy has been successfully used for correction of catheter dysfunction caused by omental or small bowel wrapping with adhesions and catheter malposition.[878]

CATHETER DAMAGE. PD catheters can be damaged by exposure to antibacterial agents that are strong oxidants (alcohol and iodine), by accidental injury from sharp objects, and simply by wear from long-term use. Repair of damaged catheters by splicing the old catheter with extension tubing resulted in a mean increase in catheter life of 26 months (range, 1 to 87 months) without an increase in the rate of peritonitis.[884] Repairs should not usually be attempted if the breakage is less than 2 cm from the exit site.

Complications Related to Increased Intra-abdominal Pressure

The pressure in an empty peritoneal cavity is 0.5 to 2.2 cm H_2O.[885] Intra-abdominal pressure then increases linearly with increasing volume in routine PD. Typical pressures range from 2 to 10 cm H_2O and may be as high as 12 cm H_2O in patients receiving 3-L exchanges.[316, 344] Other factors that also influence net intra-abdominal pressure include weight, age, activity, and body position. During such activities as coughing or straining, intra-abdominal pressure can transiently reach values as high as 300 cm H_2O.[316] Therefore, excessive coughing or constipation should be avoided, especially in the period immediately after catheter implantation. According to the law of Laplace, these higher intra-abdominal pressures can increase tension on the wall of the abdomen as abdominal girth and pressure increase. This increased tension can result in undue stress on these structures and the possibility of an increased risk of hernia formation and dialysate leaks.

HERNIAS

In the 1980s, when many PD catheters were placed in the midline, the prevalence of hernias in CAPD populations was between 10% and 25%,[886, 887] but the prevalence in IPD patients was lower, presumably as a result of less elevated intra-abdominal pressure because such patients have a dry day and because pressures are lower in the supine position when the abdominal musculature is relaxed. With the change in placement of catheters to the paramedian approach, the incidence of hernias has decreased significantly. A retrospective study of hernias over a 15-year period determined that the risk of hernia formation was 5% in cycler patients and 13% in CAPD patients.[888] There does not appear to be a relationship between exchange volume and the rate of hernia formation.[888, 889]

Many different hernia types have been reported in PD patients, the most common being umbilical, inguinal, pericatheter, and at a previous surgical site.[890] Other rarer sites of hernia formation include paraesophageal hernias.[891] Risk factors for hernia formation include previous abdominal surgery and patient weight less than 60 kg.[890] Patients with hernias present in multiple ways. Findings include painless swelling, genital edema, peritonitis from incarcerated bowel, intestinal obstruction, or a hernia discovered on routine physical examination. Subclinical hernias have been detected by peritoneal scintigraphy.[892] A patent processus vaginalis is a common cause of indirect inguinal hernias, and they should be repaired if noted at the time of catheter implantation. Similarly, if other ventral or incisional hernias are noted, they should be repaired.

The natural course of these hernias is a tendency to enlarge over time. Any hernia, particularly a small one, carries a risk of bowel incarceration or strangulation. Earlier data suggest that incarceration or strangulation can occur in up to 15% of CAPD patients with hernias.[893] Pericatheter and incisional hernias were most likely to be associated with incarceration. Therefore, if one is noted in a PD patient, surgical repair should be strongly considered. Pericatheter hernias can be prevented by waiting 10 to 14 days after placement for catheter maturation before initiating ambulatory dialysis, by using low-volume dialysis in the supine position if dialysis is needed before catheter maturation, and by creating a paramedian or lateral exit[894-896] or using the swan-neck catheter design.[897] Hernias can be repaired by insertion of a polypropylene mesh and ligation of the hernia sac.[898] PD can be restarted several days after surgery, initially at a volume of 1.0 to 1.5 L and then with gradual reinstatement of the patient's original peritoneal prescription over the next 2 to 4 weeks.

DIALYSATE LEAKS, INCLUDING HYDROTHORAX

Dialysate leaks can occur at any location within the peritoneal cavity; this topic has been reviewed by LeBlanc and colleagues.[899] Leaks and hernias may occur concomitantly. Dialysate leaks are seen in about 5% to 10% of CAPD patients.[450, 899, 900] Studies have found an association between early leaks and immediate initiation of PD and possibly the median catheter insertion technique.[899] Leaks that occur within 30 days of PD catheter placement are called early leaks, and they are usually pericatheter leaks. These leaks are diagnosed by finding any dialysate around the peritoneal catheter exit site. Risk factors for early dialysate leaks include initiation of PD immediately after catheter placement and the use of nonstandard techniques for PD catheter placement.[450, 901, 902] Leaks that occur well after the initiation of dialysis are abdominal wall, genital, or pleural leaks. These leaks usually have a more subtle manifestation, which can include weight gain, peripheral or genital edema, subcutaneous swelling, edema, apparent ultrafiltration failure, and for pleural leaks, shortness of breath. Risk factors for

dialysate leaks include median placement of PD catheters instead of paramedian implantation, use of the dialysis catheter within 10 days of placement, and abdominal wall weakness caused by previous abdominal surgery, multiple pregnancies, hernias, heavy straining, abdominal obesity, and long-term steroid therapy.[450, 887, 903]

Hydrothorax probably occurs when peritoneal dialysate traverses the diaphragm through lymphatics or through defects in the diaphragm itself, most often through tendinous defects or diaphragmatic blebs.[904-909] The clinical manifestations of hydrothorax can vary from an asymptomatic finding on routine chest radiography to severe respiratory compromise. Often, patients first note minimal dyspnea. An attempt to treat this dyspnea with the use of hypertonic exchanges can result in the accumulation of additional fluid in the pleural space because of the increased intra-abdominal fluid and pressure. These leaks can occur any time during the course of PD and are more common on the right side.[887] One report described a PD patient in whom a large posterior mediastinal mass developed, which on surgical exploration was found to be a paraesophageal hernia sac filled with omentum and dialysis fluid.[891]

Genital edema can be caused by leakage of dialysate from a defect in the abdominal wall, an inguinal hernia, or a patent processus vaginalis.[910] Under the influence of increased abdominal pressure, dialysate can dissect through the peritoneal membrane into the soft tissues of the abdominal wall, especially in areas with a defect in the peritoneum, such as at previous surgical incisions or in the pericatheter area. These patients may or may not have an associated hernia. The extravasated fluid may then dissect along tissue planes to a more dependent position and result in genital edema. Another mechanism of genital edema formation is flow of dialysate through a patent processus vaginalis to the tunica vaginalis. From there, it can dissect through the tunica vaginalis into the scrotal or labial wall itself. Early reports suggested that the incidence of genital edema was 4% to 10%, but it is likely to be less common today.[910-912]

Vaginal leak of dialysate has also been reported.[913] Although the opening to the fallopian tubes represents a potential defect for leakage of dialysate, this mechanism has seldom been reported as the etiology for a vaginal leak. Potential treatment of this unusual problem would be tubal ligation. It appears more likely that vaginal leaks are caused by dissection through fascial planes with eventual progression to the vaginal vault.[914] Such dissection may explain the association of vaginal leaks with fungal peritonitis.[915, 916]

Peritoneal dialysate leaks can be diagnosed by one of several methods.[917] Imaging studies that can be used include abdominal CT with the addition of radiocontrast to the peritoneal dialysate,[918] peritoneography with technetium 99m added to the peritoneal dialysate,[892, 919, 920] and magnetic resonance peritoneography with gadodiamide added to the dialysate.[921] A pleural peritoneal leak can also be diagnosed by the presence of a high glucose concentration in pleural fluid.[922]

Treatment of dialysate leakage is initially conservative and entails withholding PD treatments for 1 to 2 weeks. If the leak recurs, surgical therapy is required. Treatment of hydrothorax includes open thoracotomy[923]; conventional pleurodesis with substances such as intrapleural talc, tetracycline,[903, 924-926] fibrinogen/thrombin adhesive,[905] or autologous blood[887, 927]; and thoracoscopic pleurodesis.[928-931]

ALTERATIONS IN RESPIRATORY FUNCTION

In seated patients, infusion of 2 L of dialysate results in a decrease in Po_2 and functional reserve,[932, 933] as well as a decrease in vital capacity of about 10% to 20%.[933, 934] At a dwell volume of either 2.5 L[353] or 3.0 L,[344] patients who were unable to tolerate these higher fill volumes had a significantly lower forced vital capacity in the sitting position than did patients who could tolerate these higher fill volumes. In the supine position, the decrease in forced vital capacity was as much as 42% less than in the upright position. These findings suggest that forced vital capacity in the supine position is the most sensitive predictor of tolerance to larger instilled volumes. Similar findings have been reported with pregnancy and obesity.[935, 936] Respiratory muscle strength is preserved in most PD patients without pulmonary disease. During CAPD, however, lung volumes and respiratory muscle function were decreased, but these alterations were not deemed to have a significant effect on respiratory function.[937]

Most patients with obstructive airway disease are able to tolerate CAPD without difficulty, perhaps because the "stretch" that the diaphragm undergoes with increased intra-abdominal volume improves the efficiency of its contractions.[887] If these patients have difficulty with respiratory symptoms while ambulatory, they may be able to tolerate exchanges while supine with cycler therapy.[938] Patients with restrictive lung disease, however, are likely to be symptomatic when receiving PD, with the most severe symptoms occurring while supine. An instillation test can be used to assess the potential for respiratory compromise in patients with severe pulmonary disease.[939]

BACK PAIN

Increased intra-abdominal pressure and volume tend to pull the lumbar vertebrae into a more lordotic position. The net effect is increased stress on the spine. Many ESRD patients already have degenerative disk disease, osteoporosis, or facet disease at initiation of dialysis, and their therapy may be complicated by the onset of renal osteodystrophy, which also has a predilection for symptomatology in this area. The addition of dialysate may lead to a new onset or worsening of back pain in these patients. Treatment is aimed at reducing intra-abdominal pressure, which may be achieved in some patients by decreasing instilled volumes or switching to cycler therapy.[881]

Volume-Overloaded Patients

Fluid management is one of the primary functions of native kidneys and is therefore a primary function of any renal replacement therapy. Because of its continuous nature, PD has the potential to be considered an optimal modality for achieving the therapeutic goal of maintaining euvolemia and blood pressure control and thus avoiding potential cardiovascular complications.[940] Not all volume-overloaded PD patients are volume overloaded as a result of membrane failure. Failure to maintain euvolemia can be the result of too much salt and water intake or too little salt and water removal.

Failure of ultrafiltration is not always due to an actual loss of peritoneal ultrafiltration capacity. Fluid overload that clinically mimics ultrafiltration failure may occur when urine volume decreases and fluid intake is excessive or when the patient is noncompliant with the prescribed salt and water

restrictions or the number and duration of exchanges. If dwell times with glucose-containing fluids are too long for an individual patient's transport type, more fluid may be absorbed during the dwell period than can be ultrafiltrated during the remaining dwell periods. Dialysate leaks from the intra-abdominal cavity into extra-abdominal tissue spaces may result in apparent loss of ultrafiltration. Other causes include loss of aquaporin-mediated water transport, excessive lymphatic reabsorption, and changes in peritoneal membrane transport not matched by a change in the prescription. The first steps in the evaluation of a patient with suspected ultrafiltration failure are to determine urine volume and establish whether net effluent drain volume or peritoneal transport, or both, have changed. Further workup can be directed by comparing these results with the patient's baseline values. Based on these results, the diagnostic approach to the workup of ultrafiltration failure can be completed. A rational approach to a patient with suspected ultrafiltration failure is found in Figure 60-12 and has been reviewed elsewhere.[941] As can be seen from this differential diagnosis, true membrane failure is seldom the cause of volume overload.

When a patient has signs or symptoms of fluid overload, it is important to obtain a good medial history and perform a thorough physical examination. Issues such as compliance with diet, salt, and water restrictions must be evaluated. Twenty-four-hour urine collections should be obtained to rule out loss of residual renal function as a cause. Historically, peritoneal ultrafiltration was considered inadequate when less than 5.5 mL of ultrafiltration was generated per gram of absorbed glucose.[942] Ultrafiltration failure may be defined clinically by the presence of fluid overload despite restriction of fluid intake and the use of three or more hypertonic (4.25% dextrose) exchanges per day.[340] The rest of the workup depends on comparing baseline with current PET results (including D/P ratios and dialysate sodium concentrations). Dialysate sodium should decrease early in the dwell period as a result of sodium sieving during crystalloid-induced ultrafiltration. Profiling the change in dialysate sodium at 0, 1, 2, and 4 hours during the dwell period requires little additional effort but can add a lot of helpful information to aid in the differential workup of a patient with ultrafiltration failure (Fig. 60-13). Most now recommend a modified PET in which 4.25% dextrose (3.86% glucose) is used to maximize the osmotic gradient and sodium profiling.[943] It has been noted that D/P Cr ratios in an individual patient with a 4.25% and the standard 2.5% PET are very similar.[944] With this equilibration test, the definition of true membrane failure is ultrafiltration of less than 400 mL after a 4-hour dwell period.

The prevalence and frequency of ultrafiltration failure are uncertain. At one center, the prevalence of ultrafiltration failure was 2.5% after 1 year of dialysis, 9.5% at 3 years, and 30.9% after 6 years. These authors also noted that the risk increased with time on PD.[352] Other authors have reported that ultrafiltration failure is responsible for up to 15% of withdrawals from PD[945, 946] and another 14% over an 18-month period.[947]

ULTRAFILTRATION FAILURE IN A PATIENT WITH HIGH SOLUTE TRANSPORT

Patients with loss of ultrafiltration and current 4-hour PET results showing D/D_0 glucose less than 0.3 and D/P Cr greater

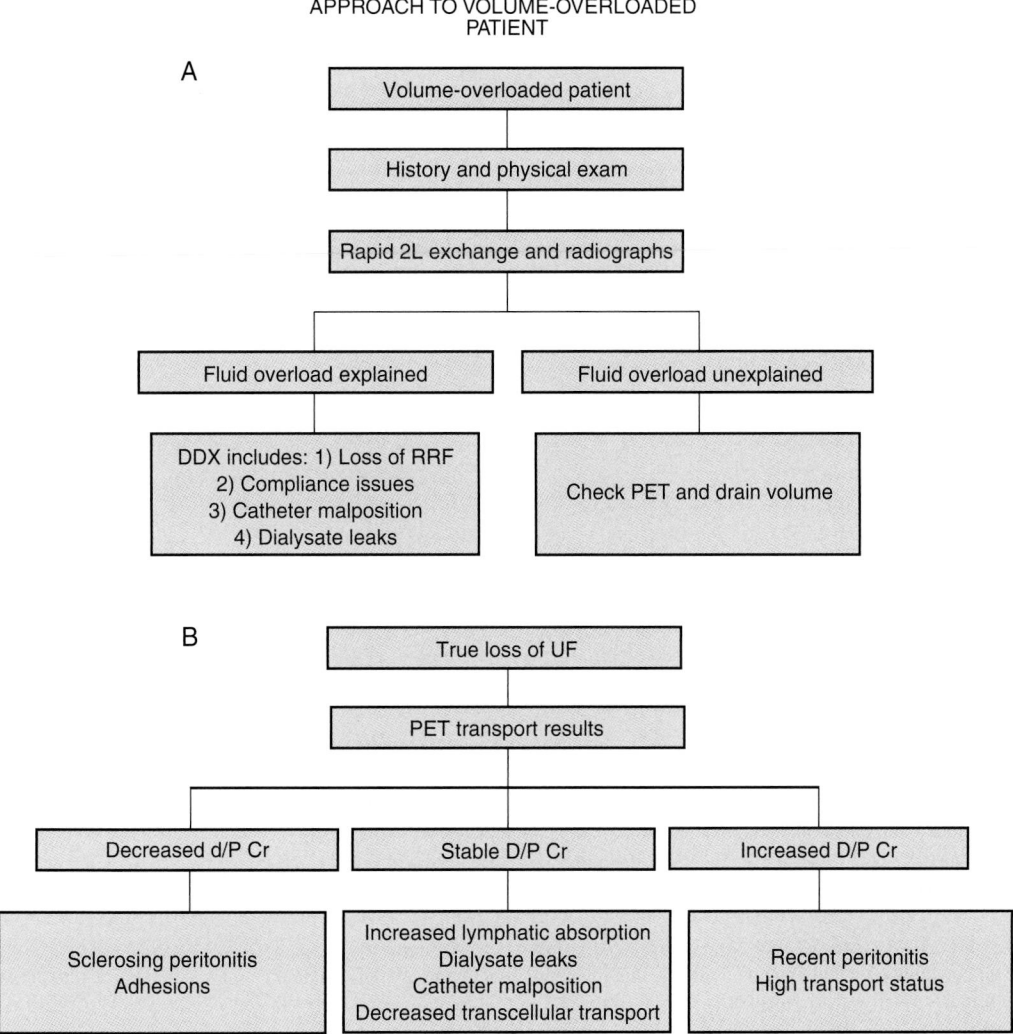

APPROACH TO VOLUME-OVERLOADED
PATIENT

FIGURE 60-12. Approach to a volume-overloaded patient. **A,** Formalized approach to the ongoing evaluation of unexplained fluid overload in a peritoneal dialysis patient. **B,** Differential diagnosis of the true loss of ultrafiltration (UF) based on peritoneal equilibration test (PET) results. DDX, differential diagnosis; RRF, residual renal function. (Modified from Korbet SM: Evaluation of ultrafiltration failure. Adv Ren Replace Ther 5:1-12, 1998.)

than 0.81 are characterized as high solute transporters. These patients tend to have poor ultrafiltration because of rapid glucose absorption and dissipation of the osmotic gradient. Some patients have these transport characteristics at baseline, and if their dwell times are mismatched for their membrane transport characteristics, they often appear to have ultrafiltration failure as they lose residual renal function and no longer have urine flow as a supplement to net daily fluid losses. In other patients, loss of ultrafiltration is due to a change in membrane transport (increase in transport) from baseline. Of patients in whom permanent loss of ultrafiltration develops, it is most commonly due to an increase in solute transport (historically called type I ultrafiltration failure). Because peritonitis leads to a similar, but transient increase in transport, this diagnosis cannot be made in patients with a recent episode of peritonitis.

RECENT PERITONITIS. It is a common clinical experience for PD patients to experience fluid retention during episodes of peritonitis. These patients often need a temporary change in their standard dialysis prescription (shortened dwell times or increased tonicity of fluids) to achieve net ultrafiltration. When compared with baseline, during peritonitis, PET data reveal an increase in the D/P ratio for creatinine and a decrease in the D/D_0 ratio for glucose. Peritonitis also results in increased protein loss and significantly decreased net ultrafiltration.[226] These changes associated with peritonitis are usually reversible, and after recovery, membrane transport returns to baseline. They are probably due to cytokine-mediated increases in vascularity. Microscopic findings in patients with acute peritonitis have revealed denudation of the mesothelial surface.[222, 225] However, in some patients, remesothelialization never occurs, even after recovery from peritonitis.[123] This persistent mesothelial denudation leads to chronic ultrafiltration loss and is often associated with an increase in transport.

HIGH TRANSPORT AS A RESULT OF LONG-TERM PERITONEAL DIALYSIS (FORMERLY TYPE I MEMBRANE FAILURE). The most common cause of chronic ultrafiltration failure in CAPD is high transport as a result of long-term PD, and it is thought to be due to an increase in

CHANGES IN DIALYSATE SODIUM DURING DWELL

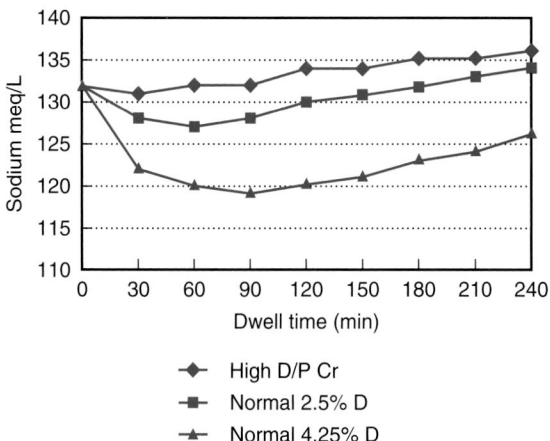

FIGURE 60-13. Dialysate sodium concentration over a 4-hour period. Two-liter dialysate volumes with 2.5% and 4.25% glucose concentrations were used in normal patients and a 2.5% glucose concentration in high transporters. The normal drop in sodium concentration is essentially lost in patients with markedly attenuated transcapillary ultrafiltration (i.e., high-transport patients and patients with impaired transcellular pore transport), but it is maintained in patients with ultrafiltration failure because of increased lymphatic absorption. (Modified from Korbet SM: Evaluation of ultrafiltration failure. Adv Ren Replace Ther 5:1-12, 1998.)

the "effective" peritoneal membrane surface area. Although the etiology is unclear, this increased surface area corresponds to neoangiogenesis in the peritoneal tissue of long-term patients.[948] Peritoneal equilibration testing confirms an increase in the D/P ratio and failure to see the expected decrease in dialysate sodium during the dwell period. (In reality, the dialysate sodium concentration does decrease, but in the first 60 minutes or so of the dwell time; by 1 to 2 hours, when sodium profiling is usually evaluated, these changes are no longer noted.) In contrast to the situation seen with peritonitis, in which transport changes are usually transient and protein loss is increased,[949] with high-transport status in a long-term patient, the small-solute transport changes are more permanent and protein mass transport is likely to not change or may even decrease.[340]

This problem was originally described with acetate-containing dialysis solutions[950] but has also been seen in patients who have used only lactate-containing solutions.[340] A history of recurrent peritonitis and the use of hypertonic exchanges[372, 951] have been observed in some, but not all studies.[340, 952] The incidence of ultrafiltration failure seems to increase with time on PD, thus implicating repeated exposure of the peritoneum to dialysate as a cause.[340, 953]

Therapy is directed toward improvement of ultrafiltration or attempts to reverse the membrane damage (or both). Clinically, most of these patients can be managed by shortening their dwell times, which will usually improve net ultrafiltration while maintaining total solute clearance. A better approach may be to shorten dwell times and use glucose polymers.[156, 954] Occasionally, resting the peritoneum for at least 4 weeks through a temporary transfer to HD has been associated with an improvement in ultrafiltration and normalization of transport characteristics.[362, 371, 954] It was postulated that these patients have a decrease in mesothelial cell

mass and associated surfactant production. Hence, the initial studies that used intraperitoneal phosphatidylcholine to treat patients with ultrafiltration failure yielded encouraging results.[334] Interestingly, increases in ultrafiltration were also seen in CAPD patients with no evidence of ultrafiltration failure after the use of intraperitoneal phosphatidylcholine.[955, 956] Further studies are needed. Although it is frequently possible to achieve adequate small-solute clearance in patients with type I membrane failure by these maneuvers, transfer to HD is often required for volume and blood pressure control. Concern has been expressed that continued membrane damage may result in eventual progression to peritoneal sclerosis or type II membrane failure, and if so, temporary or permanent transfer to HD may be indicated.[957, 958] It is uncertain which patients may be at risk for such progression. A possibility would be to monitor markers of peritoneal membrane function and viability. Peritoneal fluid CA 125 levels seem to be the most promising to date.[959] It may be that an increasing D/P Cr ratio in the presence of a decreasing CA 125 level indicates a patient at increased risk for type II failure.

ULTRAFILTRATION FAILURE AND NO CHANGE/AVERAGE SOLUTE TRANSPORT

Loss of ultrafiltration in patients with no change or average transport characteristics tends to be due to catheter malfunction, fluid leaks, excessive lymphatic reabsorption (formerly type III membrane failure), and a decrease in intracellular water transport. Other than the unusual case of a decrease in transcellular water transport, these conditions do not represent an intrinsic change in peritoneal membrane function.

EXCESSIVE LYMPHATIC ABSORPTION (FORMERLY TYPE III MEMBRANE FAILURE). Peritoneal fluid is continually removed via the peritoneal lymphatics and by back-filtration into the peritoneal capillaries. Absorption by the lymphatics has no significant effect on diffusive or convective transport. Therefore, dialysate Na^+ normally decreases (2 to 4 mEq/L) within 2 hours of the dwell period, thus suggesting normal transcapillary ultrafiltration. In these patients, the ultrafiltration failure is due to an increase in the rate of absorption by the lymphatics. Definite proof of this condition requires the identification of high rates of macromolecule clearance from the peritoneum.[960]

DIALYSATE LEAKS. Leak of dialysate from the peritoneal cavity into extra-abdominal tissue, such as the abdominal wall, results in decreased drain volume because of leakage of fluid and increased lymphatic absorption from abdominal tissues. This condition has no effect on diffusive or convective transport and tends to be associated with a normal decrease in dialysate Na^+ and unchanged PET values. Dialysate leaks are often diagnosed during the physical examination, when asymptomatic abdominal wall edema, genital edema, or hernia formation is noted. The diagnosis is then confirmed by using a radiologic technique that includes intraperitoneal infusion of radiographic contrast, usually CT. Dialysate leaks often respond by resting the peritoneum (decreasing intraperitoneal pressure) with a temporary transfer to HD or by using low-volume, supine, intermittent dialysis.

CATHETER MALPOSITION. Mechanical problems such as migration of the catheter from the pelvic space to a subdiaphragmatic position can result in an inability to drain, an increase in residual volume, and a decrease in drain volume. Again, no change in D/P Cr values or in sodium sieving is observed. Catheter position can easily be determined from a plane film radiograph. The catheter may be repositioned but often needs to be replaced.

DECREASED TRANSCELLULAR WATER TRANSPORT. Some patients have no change in D/P ratios, residual volume, or lymphatic absorption but do have a loss in the normal decrease in dialysate Na^+ that is thought to represent a loss of transcellular ultrafiltration.[961, 962] Only a small number of cases have been reported.[961] Decreased water transport is thought to be due to loss of aquaporin-1 water channels. One theory is that prolonged exposure of the peritoneum to glucose results in the formation of AGEs and abnormal transcellular pore function.[551] Treatment would entail the use of glucopolymers to maintain ultrafiltration. It is unknown whether patients with this type of membrane damage are likely to progress to any other type of membrane failure.

ULTRAFILTRATION FAILURE AND LOW SOLUTE TRANSPORT

Patients with ultrafiltration failure and low solute transport (D/D_0 glucose greater than 0.5 and D/P Cr less than 0.5) also tend to have inadequate small-solute clearance. Despite the slow diffusive properties (and therefore slow absorption of glucose), poor ultrafiltration occurs despite the maintenance of potential osmotic gradients. These patients are found to have loss of effective peritoneal surface area from either multiple peritoneal adhesions or peritoneal sclerosis (type II membrane failure). Such patients often require transfer to HD.

MULTIPLE ABDOMINAL ADHESIONS. Extensive intraabdominal adhesions may result after recurrent or severe peritonitis and after catastrophic intra-abdominal events. Adhesions limit dialysate flow throughout the abdomen, which results in fluid trapping, and they can decrease the amount of peritoneal membrane surface area that is in contact with dialysate. Although normal transport may occur in the membrane that is in contact with the dialysate, overall transport and net ultrafiltration decrease. The diagnosis can be made with plain radiographic films or CT with intraperitoneal infusion of radiocontrast material. Surgical lysis of adhesions may result in improvement, and patients may be able to continue PD if an adequate increase in surface area can be achieved. Occasionally, these patients present with pain during the dwell period or failure to drain.

PERITONEAL SCLEROSIS (TYPE II MEMBRANE FAILURE). An uncommon cause of ultrafiltration failure is sclerosing peritonitis, which is reported to affect less than 1% of all PD patients but a higher relative percentage of long-term patients. Patients present with both ultrafiltration and small-solute transport failure. Because of the association with intestinal adhesions, they may also have intestinal obstruction.[958]

The etiology of type II membrane failure is uncertain. Various peritoneal irritants have been implicated in its pathogenesis, including recurrent peritonitis, long-term use of PD, acetate-containing dialysate, chlorhexidine, β-blockers, and endotoxins. Extensive discussions of these and other agents are provided elsewhere.[958, 963] It appears that over time, patients have an increase in the fibrosis process associated with denudation of the mesothelial cell layer, angiogenesis, and increased formation of AGEs.[377]

These changes in lymphokine production are thought to be modulated by intracellular Ca^{2+} concentrations[964] and may be partially relieved with verapamil.[627] Tamoxifen, an antiestrogen agent that inhibits protein kinase C and is used to treat retroperitoneal sclerosis, has also been used to stabilize the process of peritoneal sclerosis.[965] A trial of tamoxifen may be reasonable in patients who are reluctant to switch to HD. Resting of the peritoneal membrane may allow remesothelialization to occur. The period of resting may need to be accompanied by occasional flushing of the peritoneal cavity to prevent extensive adhesion formation.

Sclerosing peritonitis may be an early stage of sclerosing encapsulating peritonitis (described in the next section).[966] Patients with type II membrane failure do not have the surgical findings associated with encapsulating fibrosis,[967] but they may have diffuse thickening and fibrosis of the parietal and visceral peritoneum.

SCLEROSING ENCAPSULATING PERITONITIS. Patients with this syndrome present with anorexia, weight loss, nausea, vomiting, intermittent bowel obstruction, ascites, bloody dialysate, malnutrition, and decreased peritoneal transport of solute and water. At laparotomy, patients are found to have a thick-walled, membranous cocoon entrapping loops of bowel.[968-970] It is unknown whether this condition is a disease process different from that of type II membrane failure (peritoneal sclerosis) or whether the two diseases are a spectrum of one disease. It has been mainly found in Europe, but sporadic cases have been reported in the United States.[971] The cause is uncertain, and as with sclerosing peritonitis, chemical irritants have been implicated. This syndrome has been the subject of three reviews.[972-974]

The exact etiology is unclear but is thought to be similar to the changes described for sclerosing peritonitis.[975] The overall incidence is uncertain, but the condition is believed to occur in 0.5% to 0.9% of the overall PD population, with the risk increasing with time on PD[976] such that it affects 15% to 20% of the subpopulation of PD patients receiving therapy for longer than 8 years.[974] In one report, 12 of 17 patients died of intestinal obstruction within 1 year of the diagnosis. The remaining five patients survived 1 to 5 years without intestinal obstruction. Four of five patients received a renal transplant and were treated with azathioprine and prednisone. One patient rejected the transplant and had a relapse of sclerosing peritonitis symptoms after the immunosuppression was stopped. The fifth patient did not receive a transplant, was treated empirically with immunosuppression, and was asymptomatic after 1 year of therapy.[977-979] Surgical intervention has been disappointing. In one review,[980] intestinal obstruction, small bowel necrosis, and enterocutaneous fistulas were common. Resection with primary anastomosis resulted in a high frequency of anastomotic failure.

Because of the poor outcome, prevention is the key. Fortunately, with the use of lactate-containing dialysis solutions, avoidance of intraperitoneal infusion of chemical irritants such as chlorhexidine, and prevention of severe prolonged episodes of peritonitis by early diagnosis, aggressive treatment, and early catheter removal when indicated, the frequency of encapsulating peritonitis may be minimized. The use of alternative osmotic agents[981] and identification of patients at risk by using peritoneal fluid markers such as CA 125 levels may also be helpful.[959]

Infectious Complications

Peritonitis and exit site infections are the major complications of PD. Infectious complications are one of the main reasons that a patient transfers to HD; they are a leading cause of hospitalization of PD patients,[982] and peritonitis is reported to be directly responsible for 1% to 6% of deaths.[983, 984] The PD catheter must traverse both a sterile and a nonsterile environment, and the exit site is on the abdominal wall, an area typically exposed to bacterial contamination and possible trauma. Hence, it would not be unexpected that exit sites are at risk for infection. The continuous introduction of nonphysiologic dialysis fluids into the peritoneal cavity significantly alters the normal host defense mechanisms and peritoneal environment. Additionally, every time that the dialysate is drained, resident macrophages and opsonins are removed. Consequently, a relatively small inoculum of bacteria could readily cause peritonitis in a PD patient, whereas similar small inoculations during surgical laparotomies seldom cause peritonitis. When compared with surgical peritonitis, PD-related bacterial peritonitis is usually due to a single pathogen, is generally confined to the peritoneum, and is seldom associated with positive blood cultures or abscess formation. Typically, these patients can be treated on an outpatient basis.

Host Defenses

Bacteria are cleared from the peritoneum by a process of opsonization, chemotaxis, phagocytosis, and intracellular killing. Lymphatic absorption of bacteria may play a role; however, because blood cultures are rarely positive in bacterial peritonitis, removal of bacteria by associated lymph nodes must be very efficient.[985] The likelihood of peritonitis developing depends on the balance between the number of bacteria introduced and the ability of the peritoneal defenses to eradicate them.[986] Bacterial contamination does not always result in peritonitis.[987, 988]

Peritoneal white blood cell counts from dialysate fluid in the absence of peritonitis are approximately 100- to 1000-fold less than the peritoneal fluid white blood cell counts from healthy individuals, in part because of dilution with dialysis solution. The white blood cell differential differs markedly among uninfected patients, with ranges of 20% to 95% for macrophages, 2% to 84% for lymphocytes, and 0% to 27% for neutrophils.[177] Although white blood cell counts tend to decrease with time on PD,[989] no significant differences in peritoneal effluent white blood cell counts are found in patients with a high or low frequency of peritonitis.[990] These data suggest that the absolute peritoneal fluid white blood cell count and differential are not the determining factors in the risk for peritonitis.

For phagocytosis to occur, recognition of bacteria by macrophages must first take place. Such recognition is achieved by opsonization of organisms with IgG, C3b, C4d, and fibronectin, given that opsonins are normally found in the peritoneal cavity. IgG is the primary immunoglobulin found in the peritoneal fluid of healthy individuals, usually at a concentration equal to that in blood. In contrast, levels in the dialysate of PD patients are only about 1% of the concentration in blood.[991, 992] However, dialysate IgG levels do not correlate with the frequency of peritonitis. It seems

likely that at the critical initial period immediately after an inoculum, the probability of contact between bacteria and white blood cells or opsonins is low, so bacterial growth can proceed unimpeded and peritonitis may occur.

NORMAL INFLAMMATORY RESPONSE. The normal peritoneal inflammatory response is a sequential, integrated response that is both vascular and cellular in nature. Regardless of whether the inciting event is traumatic or microbacterial in origin, the response is similar and often mediated by various chemical mediators and mesothelial cells.[993]

In the absence of peritonitis, the proportion of peritoneal lymphocytes is usually 20% to 40% of the total peritoneal leukocytes (range, 2% to 84%). Most of these cells (70% to 80%) are T lymphocytes. The first line of peritoneal defense is believed to be peritoneal macrophages, most of which are thought to be in peritoneal fluid as a result of inflammatory stimuli rather than as resident macrophages.[994] Peripheral blood monocytes are thought to be the precursor of these cells. Studies evaluating the functional capacity of peritoneal macrophages from PD patients yield conflicting results. Most studies show that phagocytosis is normal. However, some found that phagocytic activity was subnormal.[995]

Similarly, data are conflicting regarding the bactericidal activity of these macrophages. It appears that peritoneal macrophages from CAPD patients studied in dialysate-free media have intact bactericidal properties. However, some authors have suggested that a small subpopulation of patients may have reduced intracellular killing capabilities and a tendency for higher peritonitis rates.[996, 997] No difference in expression of complement receptors was seen when peritoneal macrophages were compared with peripheral macrophages. However, binding of C5a (a chemotactic factor) and Fc receptor (binds IgG) expression was increased in the peritoneal macrophages of uninfected patients,[998] thus suggesting that these cells are in a relative state of activation. This apparent state of activation can be the result of chronic exposure to small inocula of bacteria or chronic activation from dialysis fluid.

It has been demonstrated that mesothelial cells produce surfactant that can bind endotoxin and as a result may facilitate phagocytosis.[999] In response to other cytokines, mesothelial cells have also been shown to produce IL-8,[1000] which is chemotactic for neutrophils, thus suggesting that the mesothelial cell may be an important messenger cell in the host response to peritonitis.

Drainage of dialysate from the peritoneum is associated with the physical removal of bacteria and has been shown to be helpful, depending on the residual volume of fluid left in the peritoneal cavity.[1001] However, to eliminate *S. aureus*, a residual volume of less than 200 mL was needed. This volume is close to physiologic and can usually be achieved in a long-term PD patient after a period of abstinence from dialysis.

INFLAMMATORY RESPONSE DURING PERITONITIS. During episodes of peritonitis, peritoneal macrophages are primed to release increased amounts of IL-1β, which may increase permeability of the peritoneal membrane.[1002] Platelet-activating factor appears to be locally generated by neutrophils, macrophages, and endothelial cells during inflammation and may also contribute to the increased permeability noted during peritonitis.[1003] Furthermore, cytokines such as IL-6, an endogenous pyrogen that stimulates the secretion of acute-phase reactants by hepatocytes and also stimulates mucosal B lymphocytes, and IL-8, which is chemotactic and activates polymorphonuclear white blood cells, have been shown to increase acutely in the effluents of patients with peritonitis.[1004]

During peritonitis, peritoneal transport tends to increase. Under these conditions, patients may need to alter the dwell time or increase the tonicity of the infused solutions to prevent fluid absorption and maintain volume control. Increased peritoneal transport is associated with increased glucose absorption and a possible increased risk of damage to the peritoneal membrane. If available, one may consider using polyglucose solutions for the long dwell period to maintain ultrafiltration. It has been shown that such solutions are associated with preservation of the ultrafiltration profile during an episode of peritonitis.[1005]

Peritonitis is also associated with an increase in protein loss in the dialysate. Nitrogen losses were found to be 13.6 g/day in a group of patients with peritonitis. However, if oral intake is maintained, nitrogen balance tended to remain positive.

Prevention of Peritonitis

Presumed sources of bacterial peritonitis are intraluminal (touch contamination during the spike procedure), periluminal (related to catheter infection), transvisceral migration, hematogenous, vaginal leak, and intra-abdominal disease. In the early 1980s, the most common cause of peritonitis in PD patients was thought to be touch contamination during the spike procedure. Therefore, efforts to prevent peritonitis were initially directed toward preventing peritonitis as a result of spike contamination. The initial modifications of the classic spike technology are reviewed elsewhere.[1006] These attempts have been very successful in reducing peritonitis in some centers to as low as 0.22 episodes per year.[1007] Further attempts have focused on improving biocompatibility and host defense.

Y SYSTEMS. The first modification of the standard technique to result in a consistent reduction in peritonitis rates was the Y set introduced by Buoncristiani and associates.[1008] Y systems incorporate "flush-before-fill" technology, with any possible contamination of the spike flushed away from the peritoneum by draining after introduction of the spike. A further modification included a pre-attached bag of dialysate to eliminate the need to "spike" the bag of dialysate and further reduce peritonitis rates.[1009] These technologies are associated with peritonitis rates ranging from 0.7 to 1.7 episodes per year, mainly because of a decreased incidence of infections caused by skin organisms.[1010] In vitro evidence supporting these clinical findings of decreased peritonitis with Y systems includes the following: touch contamination was simulated by contaminating the spike with *Staphylococcus epidermidis, S. aureus,* and *Pseudomonas aeruginosa* immediately before an exchange.[1011] The dialysate was then cultured after an exchange incorporating the flush-before-fill technique. Despite the intentional contamination, 100% removal of *S. epidermidis* and partial removal of *S. aureus* and *P. aeruginosa* was accomplished with the flush alone if the exchanges were performed immediately. In other studies, flushing the tubing after touch contamination markedly reduced bacterial biofilm growth.[1012]

Most centers report a lower peritonitis rate in their patients on cyclers than in those in whom a standard spike is used.[1013] This finding would also be consistent with Y system data because the use of cycler therapy also incorporates the flush-before-fill technology. However, another reason may be that the peritoneum is left "dry" during the day, thereby allowing for restoration of host defense, or that during the long day dwell period, peritoneal immune function improves.[1014] However, some newer cycler technology does not allow flush-before-fill procedures, and peritonitis is therefore a possible risk with any contamination of the spike. In such cases, at some centers where overall peritonitis rates are low because of the use of pre-attached Y sets, patients on the cycler may have relatively higher peritonitis rates that at times will necessitate the use of assist devices to further reduce the risk of peritonitis.

DIALYSATE ADDITIVES. Keane and colleagues[1015] reported a reduced incidence of peritonitis with the use of intraperitoneal IgG, but only in a subgroup of patients found to have a low prestudy IgG level. Complete absence of IgG2 was detected in 11 of 12 children undergoing CAPD.[1016] These authors proposed that absence of IgG2 could explain the high peritonitis rates noted in children because most human antibodies to human carbohydrate antigens are in the IgG2 subclass. However, these data have not been confirmed in all studies. At present, clinical observations do not support the use of intraperitoneal IgG for prevention of peritonitis in the general PD patient population. However, its use may be indicated in the very small subgroup of patients with high rates of peritonitis and very low baseline IgG levels.

***STAPHYLOCOCCUS* NASAL CARRIAGE.** The annual probability of *S. aureus* peritonitis developing is about 15%.[1017] The probability that a CAPD patient will have a peritoneal catheter removed because of this infection is 3% to 7.5% (20% to 50% for each infection).[1006] Even if *S. epidermidis* peritonitis is completely eradicated by the use of Y systems, it should have little impact on catheter loss from severe peritonitis because *S. epidermidis*–related infections tend to be mild. Therefore, measures to reduce the incidence of *S. aureus* infection would be clinically important. Attempts to reduce *S. aureus* peritonitis by vaccination are inconclusive.

The primary reservoir for *S. aureus* is within the anterior nares.[1018] Nasal carriers of *S. aureus* have been shown to be at increased risk for the development of *S. aureus* exit site infections,[1019-1022] and they have an increased risk for peritonitis as well.[1021, 1023]

Historical trials using prophylactic antibiotics suggest that the frequency of peritonitis in carriers can be reduced.[1024] In one study, the effect of intermittent rifampin on the reduction of catheter-related infections was analyzed.[1025] Patients were randomly assigned to treatment (rifampin, 300 mg twice daily for 5 days every 3 months) or no treatment regardless of baseline carrier status. Rifampin-treated patients had a significant delay in the time to their first catheter infection and a lower overall catheter infection rate, but no reduction in overall peritonitis rates. Treatment of *S. aureus* carried nasally with intranasal mupirocin twice a day for 5 days has reduced the incidence of *S. aureus* catheter infections, but not *S. aureus* peritonitis or catheter loss in two studies.[1026, 1027] However, these studies were designed to show a reduction in catheter infection (which they did), not a reduction in peritonitis. Therefore, one cannot conclude from these studies that intranasal mupirocin will not reduce peritonitis. Topical daily mupirocin at the exit site has also been shown in three trials to reduce overall exit site infections and, at times, *S. aureus* peritonitis.[1028-1030] These and other studies using prophylactic antibiotics to reduce overall *S. aureus*–related infections were reviewed by Ritzau and co-workers, and the authors concluded that mupirocin ointment applied as part of routine exit site care or in the nares of carriers was the current method of choice to prevent infections.[1031] Although marginal evidence of resistance to mupirocin has been reported, its use is still recommended in the outpatient PD unit.[1032]

CATHETER-RELATED PERITONITIS. Peritonitis is often related to concomitant catheter infections. Therefore, prevention of peritonitis requires optimal catheter implantation and exit site care. The importance of catheter design and implantation techniques was reviewed by an expert panel.[34] Their findings are as follows: (1) double-cuff swan-neck catheters are preferred; (2) a laterally placed, downward- or sideward-directed exit is thought to be associated with fewer catheter infections; (3) most important, however, is catheter implantation, which must be performed by a competent and experienced catheter insertion team. Accuracy of placement of the cuffs is more important than the technique of placement used.

In summary, efforts to prevent peritonitis are imperative. With the use of Y systems, most centers can now achieve peritonitis rates of about 0.33 to 0.5 episode per patient-year. Y systems with pre-attached dialysis fluids are preferred. Efforts to reduce peritonitis also include efforts to reduce catheter infections. Such endeavors start at the time of catheter placement and include catheter design modifications. Epidemiologic data overwhelmingly support the association between *S. aureus* nasal carriage and exit site infections and peritonitis episodes. Therefore, efforts to reduce nasal carriage may also prevent peritonitis. A review of peritoneal infections, etiology, and prevention has been published.[1033]

Peritonitis

DIAGNOSIS. Peritonitis is often easily diagnosed on clinical grounds. Most patients present with abdominal pain and visibly cloudy fluid. In a review of 103 patients with peritonitis, fever (temperature above 37.5° C) was present in 53% of patients, abdominal pain in 79%, nausea in 31%, and diarrhea in 7%. In addition, 70% had abdominal tenderness and 50% had rebound pain.[1034] Patients rarely have other systemic signs and symptoms and are seldom hypotensive. Findings on physical examination are typical of those from any cause of peritonitis and include abdominal tenderness, decreased bowel sounds, guarding, and occasionally, rebound tenderness. Because of the increased frequency of hernias in PD patients, the possibility of peritonitis as a result of ischemic bowel from an incarcerated hernia must always be considered; therefore, ventral, incisional, and inguinal hernias must be looked for, and other intra-abdominal disease must be ruled out. Although most of the time that a PD patient presents with peritonitis it is due to bacterial contamination from a nonmalignant source, occasionally the patient has significant causative intra-abdominal disease. It is important to identify these patients because their treatment

and outcome may differ from those of patients with PD-related bacterial peritonitis.[984, 1035]

Standard laboratory investigation for the diagnosis of peritonitis includes peritoneal fluid cell counts with differential, Gram stain, and culture. Findings suggestive of peritonitis include a peritoneal fluid white blood cell count greater than 100 cells/mm^3, most of which are polymorphonuclear white blood cells. A predominance of lymphocytes may be seen with atypical infections such as tuberculosis,[1036] but such is not always the case. Gram stains of peritoneal fluid are seldom helpful, but if the response is positive, they are predictive of culture results 85% of the time. The peripheral white blood cell count may be increased. Blood cultures are rarely positive, which is one reason that PD has been recommended for patients with prosthetic valves or synthetic vascular grafts.[392, 1037]

Cultures of the dialysate should be obtained immediately, but the availability of culture results should not delay the onset of therapy. Sterile or aseptic peritonitis is usually due to inappropriate culture technique; the reported frequency varies from 2% to 20%, depending on the culture technique used. If proper culture technique is followed, peritoneal cultures should be positive in approximately 90% of cases of peritonitis.[1034] In the event of repeatedly sterile peritoneal fluid cultures and elevated peritoneal fluid white blood cell counts, other pathologic processes must be considered, including eosinophilic peritonitis. Atypical organisms, such as those that cause tuberculosis, should be looked for. Elevated neutrophil counts have been reported in association with well-differentiated hypernephroma of the kidney, perhaps from perinephric inflammation,[1038] and in a patient with lymphoma.[1039] One must also consider the possibility of sterile peritonitis (possibly caused by contamination during the manufacturing process) related to icodextrin use in patients in whom this alternative osmotic agent has been prescribed.[1040, 1041]

Intra-abdominal causes of peritonitis also may occur. No consistent difference in routine initial laboratory parameters and clinical findings has been reported in patients with PD-associated bacterial peritonitis and those with other intra-abdominal causes of peritonitis.[1042] In one review, intra-abdominal disease was the cause of less than 6% of cases of peritonitis in PD patients, but of the 26 patients with peritonitis related to intra-abdominal disease, 11 died.[1043] Mortality correlated not only with the disease process causing the peritonitis but also with time to surgical intervention, similar to the mortality rate reported in another review (46.3%).[1035] It appears as though the risk for abdominal catastrophe is 20 to 60 times higher in patients receiving PD than in other ESRD patients treated with HD,[1044] perhaps because of the reasons reviewed earlier related to host defense.

Peritoneal fluid amylase levels have been found to be helpful in the differential diagnosis of peritonitis.[1045] Elevated values were found in patients with peritonitis caused by intra-abdominal disease, such as pancreatitis or a perforated viscus (Fig. 60-14).[1046] In a subsequent review, it was suggested that any time that peritoneal fluid amylase levels are greater than 50 IU/L, peritonitis caused by an underlying intra-abdominal pathologic process should be considered.[1047] Therefore, it may be reasonable to obtain these levels routinely in all patients with peritonitis. In patients whose peritonitis fails to respond to therapy, peritoneal

PERITONEAL FLUID AMYLASE LEVELS

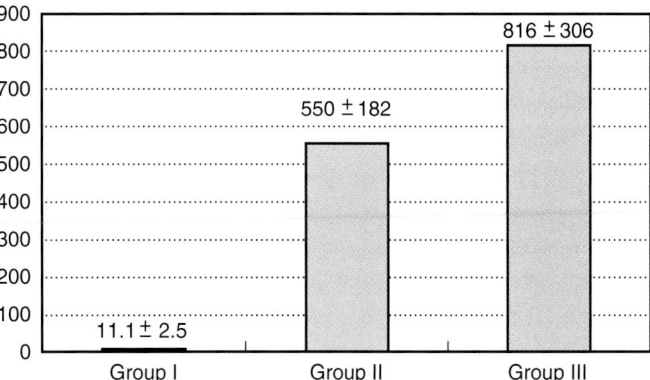

FIGURE 60-14. Comparison of peritoneal fluid amylase levels in peritoneal dialysis patients with various causes of peritonitis. Group I consists of 39 patients with infectious peritonitis; group II, 6 patients with pancreatitis; and group III, 5 patients with intra-abdominal disease. *P = .001. (From Burkart J, Haigler S, Caruana R, Hylander B: Usefulness of peritoneal fluid amylase levels in the differential diagnosis of peritonitis in peritoneal dialysis patients. J Am Soc Nephrol 1:1186-1190, 1991.)

TABLE 60-10

Reported Causes of Bloody Dialysate

After catheter implantation
Gynecologic
   Retrograde menstruation
   Ovulation
   Ruptured ovarian cyst
   Endometriosis
Traumatic
   Catheter related
   Blunt trauma
Anatomic
   Polycystic kidneys
   Intra-abdominal cancer
   Vascular disinfectant infusion
Status postcolonoscopy
Idiopathic thrombocytopenic purpura
Radiation therapy
Strenuous activity
Hemorrhagic pancreatitis
Vasculitis
Systemic bleeding
Sclerosing peritonitis

amylase levels do not increase when caused by routine bacterial-related peritonitis, but they often do when other abdominal pathology is present. Peritoneal fluid lipase levels are also helpful and, if elevated, suggest pancreatitis as the cause of peritonitis.[1047, 1048]

Occasionally, the dialysis effluent is bloody, the causes of which have been reviewed (Table 60-10).[1048] Bloody dialysate most commonly occurs after Tenckhoff placement, followed in frequency by that resulting from gynecologic causes; therefore, bloody dialysate does not always signify infection or disease.[1049]

Radiologic studies are occasionally indicated in the differential diagnosis of peritonitis and should be used with the same guidelines as in patients who are not undergoing PD. Free intraperitoneal air can occasionally be seen in patients treated by PD, and this finding on an acute abdominal series is not pathognomonic of a perforated viscus in these patients[1050]; however, free air should lead to consideration of perforation in the presence of peritonitis, especially with gram-negative rod or polymicrobial infections. CT is more sensitive than ultrasound in diagnosing pancreatitis, but findings are positive only in up to 60% of cases,[1051] hence the helpfulness of peritoneal fluid amylase levels. In patients with peritonitis caused by ischemic bowel secondary to incarcerated hernia, CT or radionucleotide scans to document the presence of extra-abdominal fluid may be helpful.

INFECTIOUS CAUSES OF PERITONITIS. Data on 3366 patients who started CAPD in the first 6 months of 1989 were reviewed by Port and associates.[1052] At the time of the first episode of peritonitis, 13% of the patients had a documented exit site infection. Peritoneal fluid leaks were found in 3%. The first peritonitis episode resulted in the hospitalization of 31% of patients, and cultures were sterile in 20%. Almost 50% of the infections were due to gram-positive organisms, followed next in frequency by gram-negative infections. Since then, the relative frequency of various pathogens has changed as a result of the introduction of prophylactic mupirocin at the exit site. In many units, overall peritonitis rates have decreased, as well as *S. aureus* peritonitis. The causative organisms in 399 episodes of peritonitis are noted in Table 60-11.[984] A small number of cases of peritonitis are caused by fungi, most of them *Candida* species. The role of viruses as a pathogen associated with peritonitis is uncertain, but anecdotal cases have been reported.[1053] More important is the possible role that viruses play in predisposing patients to peritonitis.[1054-1056]

GRAM-POSITIVE PERITONITIS. *S. epidermidis* was originally the most common causative agent of peritonitis, presumably as a result of touch contamination or pericatheter routes of infection.[1034] *S. epidermidis* typically causes mild cases of peritonitis that tend to respond rapidly to therapy. *S. aureus* is a more virulent pathogen and is likely to be more resistant to therapy. Patients with *S. aureus* peritonitis have presented with a toxic shock–like syndrome,[1057] and severe cases have been associated with progressive membrane damage. The relative percentage of peritonitis cases caused by these two organisms has changed recently because the frequency of peritonitis related to touch contamination has decreased with use of the Y systems.[1058] Consequently, overall peritonitis rates are decreasing, and most centers are experiencing fewer *S. epidermidis* infections because of the use of Y sets and fewer *S. aureus* infections because of the use of prophylactic antibiotics. Enterococci can cause peritonitis and, at times, may be resistant to vancomycin.

TABLE 60-11

Common Organisms Associated with Peritonitis in Patients Undergoing Peritoneal Dialysis

PATHOGEN	%*	EPISODES (n = 399)*	LITERATURE† (%)
Gram-positive bacteria			55–80
Coagulase-negative staphylococci	30.6	122	35–70
Staphyloccus aureus	17.5	70	10–25
Other gram-positive bacteria			
α-Hemolytic streptococci	9.0	36	3–15
Enterococci	3.5	14	3–10
Diphtheroids	2.0	8	NA
Others	2.5	10	0–4
Gram-negative bacteria			17–30
Escherichia coli	5.8	23	4–10
Pseudomonas spp.	3.5	14	5–10
Enterobacter spp.	3.3	13	0–3
Klebsiella spp.	2.7	11	1–5
Acinetobacter spp.	2.0	8	0–4
Serratia spp.	1.8	7	0–3
Other	5.8	23	
Polymicrobial	10.0	40	NA
Fungi			0–5
Mycobacteria			0–1
Total	100.0	399	

*From Krishnan M, Thodis E, Ikonomopoulos D, et al: Predictors of outcome following bacterial peritonitis in peritoneal dialysis. Perit Dial Int 22:573-581, 2002.

†Modified from Walshe JJ, Morse GD: Infectious complications of peritoneal dialysis. *In* Nissenson Ar, Fine RN, Gentile DE (eds): Clinical Dialysis, 2nd ed. Norwalk, CT, Appleton & Lange, 1990, pp 301-308; data from Golper TA, Burkart JM, Piraino B: Peritoneal dialysis. *In* Schrier RW, Gottschalk CW (eds): Diseases of the Kidney, 6th ed. Boston, Little, Brown, 1997, pp 2771-2805.

Three cases of peritonitis caused by group B streptococci have been reported in the literature. All three patients presented with severe systemic symptoms and septic shock within 24 hours after the onset of symptoms,[1059] one of whom died. These cases enforce the importance of having patients monitor their blood pressure and report symptoms of peritonitis early in the course of therapy when they are treated at home. Hypotension suggests the possibility of more severe disease and usually requires hospitalization.

GRAM-NEGATIVE PERITONITIS. Gram-negative organisms can cause peritonitis and produce a wide spectrum of clinical findings. Patients with gram-negative peritonitis typically respond to appropriate antibiotic therapy, but *Pseudomonas* infections are particularly difficult to eradicate. The bowel, skin, urinary tract, contaminated water, and animal contact have been implicated as sources of gram-negative peritonitis. In vitro studies have shown that human peritoneal macrophages are able to phagocytose *Escherichia coli* even in the absence of opsonins, which is perhaps the reason for the relative rarity of *E. coli* peritonitis in PD patients.[1060] Peritonitis associated with severe diarrhea has been caused by *Campylobacter* infection.[1061]

***Pseudomonas* Peritonitis.** *Pseudomonas* peritonitis was responsible for 4.8% of all peritonitis episodes over a 66-month period at a single center.[1062] Eighty percent of these episodes were treated successfully with the combination of an aminoglycoside and ceftazidime. In 5 of 25 episodes, the catheter was removed. Millikin and colleagues found that if *Pseudomonas* peritonitis was related to an exit site or catheter infection, the response rate was only 32%; when no clinical evidence of catheter-related infection was present, the reported response rate was 73%. *Pseudomonas* peritonitis can be associated with severe systemic manifestations such as white blood cell capillary margination and digital necrosis.[1063]

FUNGAL PERITONITIS. The initial signs and symptoms in patients with fungal peritonitis tend to be no different from those in patients with bacterial peritonitis and are most often due to *Candida* species.[1064] Fungal peritonitis is frequently preceded by a recent history of bacterial peritonitis and previous antibiotic therapy. The standard of antifungal therapy has been to treat with intravenous amphotericin B. Other antifungal agents have been used and include fluorocytosine, ketoconazole, miconazole, and econazole.[1065] All therapies have had successes and failures. In a recent retrospective review, it appeared that the combination of intraperitoneal fluorocytosine and oral ketoconazole seemed most efficacious.[512] Once-a-day oral fluconazole has been used to treat *Candida* peritonitis, but usually the catheter has to be removed.[1066, 1067] In a review of fungal peritonitis by Cheng and colleagues,[1064] three different catheter management approaches were described: immediate removal and antifungal therapy; delayed removal, usually after a period of failure to respond to antifungal therapy; and antifungal therapy without catheter removal. Mortality rates did not differ between groups. In the group of patients for whom the treatment strategy was antifungal therapy alone, 58 of 71 patients (82%) recovered from their infection without catheter removal. Given such limitations, these data suggest that catheter removal is not necessary in every case of fungal peritonitis. A reasonable therapeutic plan would be that if the patient is hemodynamically stable, the clinician ought to initiate appropriate antifungal therapy with close monitoring of the patient. If significant clinical improvement is not seen by day 4 or 5, the catheter should be removed. Therapy should be continued for a period of at least 10 days after catheter removal.

Fluconazole has no activity against filamentous fungi, for which intravenous amphotericin B is the antifungal agent of choice. Other causes of fungal peritonitis typically require antifungal agents and catheter removal. *Aspergillus* peritonitis has been treated with catheter removal and antifungal therapy.[1068]

TUBERCULOSIS. Except for its more insidious onset, tuberculous peritonitis is similar to other forms of peritonitis in clinical manifestations. In general, it represents reactivation of a latent peritoneal focus rather than primary infection. Tuberculous peritonitis is usually accompanied by a predominance of lymphocytes in the effluent, but such is not always the case. Occasionally, neutrophil predominance is observed.[1069] The diagnosis is often delayed and may require peritoneal biopsy. Peritonitis caused by *Mycobacterium tuberculosis, Mycobacterium kansasii,* and *Mycobacterium fortuitum* has been reported. No data exist on the optimal treatment and duration of therapy. In a review of five cases of tuberculous peritonitis, all patients responded to triple therapy (isoniazid, rifampin, and pyrazinamide), and three of five continued PD.[1070] Three cases of *M. tuberculosis* peritonitis seemed to have been treated with antibiotic therapy alone, and removal of the catheter was not needed.[1071] It appears that about a third of all cases of *M. tuberculosis* peritonitis can be treated without catheter removal, but in general, atypical infections require catheter removal.

BIOFILM. Although one large prospective study has demonstrated biofilms in peritoneal catheters removed from PD patients and although cultures of scrapings from these biofilms were often positive for *S. aureus* and *S. epidermidis*,[1072] no clear relationship with clinical peritonitis was noted.[27] Two other studies confirmed that biofilms could be present without any evidence of infection.[1073, 1074] Therefore, a firm relationship between biofilms and peritonitis has been lacking. In an in vivo rabbit model of peritonitis, skin bacteria of the animals routinely colonized the catheter through the exit site after placement, but before the onset of dialysis. Peritonitis did not occur until after the initiation of dialysis,[1075] possibly because the functions of host defense were altered by dialysis fluids and bacteria were no longer able to be contained in the biofilms. In vitro studies have demonstrated that biofilm growth is associated with antibiotic resistance[1076, 1077] and that significantly higher antibiotic levels are needed to eradicate biofilms in vitro. Dasgupta and co-workers[1078] described a way of culturing biofilm-forming bacteria in the dialysate effluents of PD patients with peritonitis by the use of a modified Robbins device. They found that patients with multiple episodes of peritonitis were likely to have stable biofilms, positive biofilm cultures, and a high frequency of catheter loss.[1079] Rifampin has been shown to have greater biofilm-penetrating capacity than most other antibiotics.[1080] Anecdotal reports have suggested the use of intracatheter urokinase or streptokinase to disrupt biofilm formation during episodes of refractory or relapsing peritonitis.

TREATMENT. Successful treatment of any episode of peritonitis not only has an impact on the patient's immediate well-being but also may influence the patient's long-term modality choice. Of patients with multiple episodes of peritonitis, more than 40% switched to another modality.[1081] Long-dwell exchanges are associated with larger numbers of macrophages in the effluent than short dwell periods are, and a higher percentage of these cells are found to be in a functional state.[1082] In addition, IgG concentrations in the effluent increase with increasing dwell time. Given these findings and the known effects that nonphysiologic dialysis fluids have on peritoneal white blood cell function initially, it is recommended that long dwell periods rather than rapid short dwell cycles be used to treat peritonitis. This recommendation must be weighed against the known problems with ultrafiltration associated with episodes of peritonitis. During peritonitis, prolonged dwell periods can be associated with fluid absorption from the peritoneum and even volume overload in some cases. It may be helpful to perform a few rapid exchanges initially if the patient is in pain or, if the patient has sepsis, to remove the endotoxin load and reduce the inflammation. Otherwise, rapid lavage is not indicated.[1083]

Millikin and co-workers[1084] published a retrospective review of data on the antimicrobial treatment of peritonitis before January 1990. These authors were quick to point out that although they estimated that 41,000 cases of peritonitis occurred yearly before their publication, the world literature at that time included reports of treatment for only 2037 cases of peritonitis. At about the same time, an ad hoc committee published a set of recommendations for the diagnosis and treatment of peritonitis.[1085] These recommendations were based on their clinical experience and the then current world literature on the treatment of peritonitis. They were meant to

be guidelines and by no means were intended to be the only acceptable therapy for peritonitis. Those recommendations were subsequently revised in 1993,[1086] 1996,[1087] and again in 2000.[1088] Pediatric antibiotic choices and dosage were reviewed by Lum.[1088a]

In the last few years, the prevalence of vancomycin resistance has been increasing, not only in *Staphylococcus* species[1089] but also in enterococci. This prevalence has increased from 0.4% to 14% in many university-affiliated hospitals. The change in vancomycin sensitivity has prompted worldwide agencies to discourage the routine use of vancomycin. However, vancomycin is still recommended for the treatment of patients with methicillin-resistant *S. aureus* and those who are allergic to other medications. Drugs such as clindamycin and rifampin, which suppress intracellular growth, may be beneficial in the treatment of *Staphylococcus* peritonitis. Ciprofloxacin has been shown in vitro to have substantial activity against most organisms that cause peritonitis in PD patients.[1090] Severe ototoxicity has been reported in PD patients treated with aminoglycosides.[1091] Because of concerns of ototoxicity and better understanding of the pharmacometrics of aminoglycoside therapy in PD patients, newer recommendations for aminoglycoside use include once-daily therapy. These and other reasons for this recommendation are outlined by Vas.[1092]

SUMMARY OF TREATMENT RECOMMENDATIONS. A summary of present antimicrobial recommendations and treatment algorithms can be found in the publication by the ad hoc committee on the treatment of peritonitis. Table 60-12 is an outline of initial treatment recommendations. Follow-up therapy for gram-positive peritonitis is outlined in Table 60-13.

Empirical initial therapy for peritonitis is now stratified for residual renal function. Recommendations are to start therapy with cefazolin or cephalothin (to cover gram-positives) *and* ceftazidime or an aminoglycoside (to cover gram-negatives) in most patients unless clinical conditions mandate another approach. In general, empirical vancomycin use is not recommended. The recommended duration of therapy for *S. aureus* is a total of 21 days. If *S. aureus* is identified and no clinical improvement is seen by 3 or 4 days, rifampin

---

TABLE 60-12

Empiric Initial Therapy For Peritoneal Dialysis–Related Peritonitis, Stratified for Residual Renal Function

ANTIBIOTIC	RESIDUAL RENAL VOLUME	
	<100 mL/day	>100 µL/day
Cefazolin or cephalothin	1 g/bag qd *or* 15 mg/kg BW/bag qd	20 mg/kg BW/bag qd
	And one of the following:	
Ceftazidime	1 g/bag qd	20 mg/kg BW/bag qd
Gentamicin, tobramycin, netilmicin	0.6 mg/kg BW/bag qd	Not recommended
Amikacin	2.0 mg/kg/bag qd	Not recommended

This dosing regimen is for intermittent dosing and is given once during the first day for at least a 6-hour dwell.

BW, body weight in kilograms; qd, once per day.

Modified from Keane WF, Bailie GR, Boeschoton E, et al: Adult peritoneal dialysis–related peritonitis treatment recommendations: 2000 update. Perit Dial Int 20:396-411, 2000.

TABLE 60-13

Treatment Strategies after the Causative Agent Is Known

Gram-Positive

Enterococcus	Stop cephalosporins
	Start ampicillin, 125 mg/L/each bag
	Consider adding an aminoglycoside
	Duration of therapy, 14 days
Staphylococcus aureus	Stop ceftazidime or aminoglycoside
	Continue cephalosporin
	Consider adding rifampin, 600 mg/day PO
	If MRSA, change to vancomycin or clindamycin
Other gram-positives	Stop ceftazidime or aminoglycoside
	Continue cephalosporin
	If MRSE, consider vancomycin or clindamycin

Gram-Negative

Single gram-negative	Adjust antibiotics to sensitivity:
	If <100 mL/day of urine, aminoglycoside
	If >100 mL/day of urine, ceftazidime
Pseudomonas	Continue ceftazidime and add:
	If <100 mL urine, aminoglycoside
	If >100 mL/day of urine, ciprofloxacin, 500 mg PO bid
	or piperacillin, 4 g IV q12h
	or aztreonam, load 1g/L; maintenance, 250 mg/L IP/bag
Multiple gram-negatives	Continue cefazolin and ceftazidime
	Add metronidazole, 500 mg q8h IV
	Consider surgical evaluation

MRSA, methicillin-resistant *Staphylococcus aureus*.

Modified from Keane WF, Bailie GR, Boeschoton E, et al: Adult peritoneal dialysis–related peritonitis treatment recommendations: 2000 update. Perit Dial Int 20:396-411, 2000.

is added. For other gram-positive organisms, final antibiotic therapy is guided by culture results, and the duration of therapy should be a total of 14 days.

After empirical therapy is initiated, if a gram-negative infection is identified, treatment should be directed by culture and sensitivity testing results. Continuation of an aminoglycoside or ceftazidime is recommended. Systemic levels do not need to be achieved, which should reduce the risk of ototoxicity. For single gram-negative infections, the length of therapy should be 14 days. If *P. aeruginosa* or *Xanthomonas* is identified, therapy should be extended for a total of 21 to 28 days, catheter removal is often required, and therapy with two antibiotics to which the organism is sensitive is recommended. For multiple gram-negatives or anaerobes (or for both), surgical evaluation should be considered, the initial empirical antibiotics should be continued with adjustments pending culture and sensitivity results, and metronidazole should be added.

For fungal peritonitis, the committee thought that a trial of antifungal agents was warranted but, if no obvious improvement was noted after 4 to 5 days, the catheter should be removed. It was thought that successful therapy should be continued for 4 to 6 weeks.

RELAPSING PERITONITIS. Relapsing peritonitis is arbitrarily defined as another episode of peritonitis caused by same organism associated with the preceding episode of peritonitis within 4 weeks of completion of the antibiotic course. In this situation, the clinician should first review the culture and sensitivity results. Noncompliance should always be considered. If *S. aureus* is cultured, because of the possibility of intracellular sequestration of bacteria, it is recommended that rifampin and another antibiotic guided by sensitivity results be used for a total of 4 weeks. Consideration should also be given to catheter infection or intra-abdominal abscess. Tunnel infections may contribute to relapsing peritonitis. An ultrasound or CT of the tunnel should be considered. Catheter removal is often necessary (in up to 80% of episodes of peritonitis associated with tunnel infections). The risk of tunnel infection seems to be greater early in the course of PD and in women with diabetes.

Anecdotal reports suggest that infusion of streptokinase or urokinase may be successful in treating relapsing or resistant peritonitis. The rationale behind this therapy is that it is possible that organisms may be protected in fibrin clots or in biofilms that may be exposed with the use of these drugs. Streptokinase is typically left in for an overnight dwell; urokinase is usually drained after a 2-hour dwell. These studies have no control groups but suggest that it may be useful in up to 50% of cases.

A more radical approach that has been suggested for the treatment of either acute peritonitis or relapsing peritonitis is to withhold PD in an attempt to allow restoration of normal host defenses. Two groups have had success in treating acute peritonitis in CAPD patients with a single dose of antibiotics and stopping therapy for 48 hours. These authors report an 85% cure rate for patients treated in this manner, similar to results with conventional therapy. This approach is more economical and has intellectual appeal, but it has not been widely adapted, primarily because it risks treating patients with more severe forms of peritonitis inappropriately. However, Cairns[986] has successfully treated 10 of 11 patients with recurrent coagulase-negative or persistent *S. aureus* infections with this technique, which suggests that short periods off PD may help restore normal host defenses.

INDICATIONS FOR CATHETER REMOVAL. The experience of a single center with peritonitis was reviewed. In 636 episodes of peritonitis in 440 patients, 16 deaths were associated with peritonitis (fatality rate of 2.5%). The catheter was removed between the 5th and 10th days in six patients and after 10 days in seven patients. The risk of death was increased in patients with delayed catheter removal. Peritonitis with sepsis was the cause of death in 13 patients. This experience points to the need for early catheter removal in patients with refractory peritonitis, not only to prevent sepsis-related death but also to avoid prolonged episodes of peritonitis that could potentially damage the peritoneal membrane.

Catheter removal is indicated for mechanical failure that does not respond to other maneuvers. Other indications for catheter removal include peritonitis associated with tunnel infections, some cases of chronic exit site or tunnel infection, *Pseudomonas* peritonitis unresponsive to appropriate antibiotic therapy, slowly improving fungal peritonitis, fecal peritonitis, significant intra-abdominal disease, and continually relapsing peritonitis with no obvious cause. Simultaneous catheter removal plus replacement is usually successful for noninfectious indications for catheter removal; however, one center also reported simultaneous replacement 83% of the time in patients with persistent or resistant infections.

EOSINOPHILIC PERITONITIS. This complication is usually observed early after catheter placement and is typically associated with sterile peritoneal cultures. Associated peripheral eosinophilia may or may not be present and is assumed to be due to chemical stimuli leached from the catheter. Fungal peritonitis and peritonitis resulting from other causes must be carefully excluded. Chemical peritonitis caused by hypersensitivity to drugs, most notably vancomycin, has been reported and may also be associated with eosinophilia. This condition originally seemed to occur only with large intraperitoneal loading doses of vancomycin, presumably because of impurities during the drug production process. Some authorities have expressed concern that the new peritonitis recommendations for large intraperitoneal loading doses of vancomycin will result in an increased frequency of chemical peritonitis. Most cases of eosinophilic peritonitis resolve spontaneously after 2 to 3 weeks.

STERILE PERITONITIS. At times, sterile peritonitis is seen in association with polyglycose (icodextrin) use and is a benign condition that usually resolves after discontinuation of the osmotic agent.[1040] When the patient is initially evaluated, one should treat as though the patient has bacterial peritonitis and perform a workup as described earlier. It is important to note that before the use of icodextrin, about 10% of cultures during episodes of peritonitis showed no growth; however, cultures may also be sterile when icodextrin is used. Unfortunately, no test can demonstrate whether the episode of peritonitis is icodextrin related or due to a bacterial pathogen. Icodextrin-associated sterile peritonitis tends to have lymphocytes rather than neutrophils, but overlap does occur and the differential is not always helpful. See further description in the earlier section on polyglucose.

Catheter Infections (Exit Site and Tunnel)

Unlike peritonitis, for which universally acknowledged criteria are available for its diagnosis, exit site infections currently have no singular or easily recognizable definition. Pierratos defined an exit site infection as "redness or skin induration or purulent discharge from the exit site."[1082] The formation of crust around the exit may not indicate infection. Positive cultures from the exit site in the absence of inflammation are not indicative of infection. This definition is not sufficiently precise, and therefore the definition of exit site infection varies from center to center. Although the percentage of "no growth" exit site infections must be low, they have been reported. Furthermore, a positive culture from a normal-appearing exit site represents colonization, not infection. Catheter infections may be confined to the exit site or may involve only the tunnel. Tunnel infections are often unsuspected and frequently only diagnosed with ultrasound or CT, but they should always be suspected in cases of relapsing peritonitis. Exit site infection rates as low as 0.05 to as high as 1.02 infections per patient-year have been reported, in part because of this difficulty with consistency in definition of the disease. At present, it is recommended that exit site infection be defined as the presence of marked pericatheter redness and wetness or exudate in the sinus tract, with or without a positive culture. Chronic infections often show exuberant granulation tissue in the sinus. Erythema or bleeding alone may simply indicate acute trauma. A tunnel infection can occur independently of an obvious exit infection and is thus defined as erythema, edema, or

TABLE 60-14

Microorganisms Causing Exit Site Infection in Continuous Ambulatory Peritoneal Dialysis

MICROORGANISM	RANGE (%) OF EXIT SITE INFECTION CAUSED BY ORGANISM
Staphylococcus aureus	25-85
Multiple organisms (includes *S. aureus* in mixed culture)	16-35
Enteric gram-negative bacteria	7-14
Staphylococcus epidermidis	5-14
Pseudomonas aeruginosa	8-12
Culture negative	7-11
Fungal agents	1-3

From Luzar MA: Exit-site infection in continuous ambulatory peritoneal dialysis: A review. Perit Dial Int 11:333-340, 1991.

tenderness of the subcutaneous tunnel, with or without discharge from the exit or a positive culture.

EXIT SITE INFECTIONS. Almost all healed exit sites are colonized by bacteria. Bacterial virulence is also important; the virulent pathogens *S. aureus* and *P. aeruginosa* are most likely to induce infection. Table 60-14 presents data on the causative microorganisms of exit site infections based on a literature review. In this review, which included reports on exit site infection rates from 11 centers, the mean exit site infection rate was 0.48 episode per patient-year. *S. aureus* has consistently been identified as the leading cause of exit site and tunnel infections. Although *Pseudomonas* infections are relatively infrequent, the severity of these infections, the difficulty in eradicating them, and the negative impact that they have on catheter survival warrant careful monitoring of this pathogen.

Defense mechanisms in a healed sinus are best in undamaged epidermis and granulation tissue. Trauma to these structures may tilt the balance toward bacteria overgrowth and allow infection to development.[33] Close examination of tunnel morphology by photography and magnifying lenses has allowed exit sites to be classified as perfect, good, equivocal, traumatized, acutely inflamed, and chronically inflamed. These observations suggest that a mature, healed external cuff does not function as a physical barrier per se against the spread of infection; rather, the external cuff functions in preventing infections by anchoring the catheter, which results in restriction of piston-like movements and possible trauma to the catheter exit site. These data suggest that efforts to reduce trauma at the exit would also reduce exit site infection rates. Catheter immobilization, especially in the immediate postoperative period, has been recommended.

TUNNEL INFECTIONS. The subcutaneous tunnel is the area between the two cuffs. After 2 months, this section of the catheter is covered with thick fibrous tissue (in silicon catheters) or thin fibrous tissue (in polyurethane catheters). Actual tunnel infections are rare. More commonly, they represent infection of the deep cuff. Although exit site infections can be treated successfully by antibiotics, deep cuff infections are rarely cured by antibiotics alone and usually require catheter removal. Catheter removal is strongly suggested in a patient with peritonitis and a known tunnel infection. Tunnel infections are often unsuspected and require ultrasound or CT to diagnose.

PREVENTION OF CATHETER INFECTIONS. The primary means of preventing catheter infections is to have a dedicated, knowledgeable catheter implantation team. As discussed earlier, in this situation no significant difference can be found in outcome between surgical and bedside placement or between insertion techniques.[34] Administration of prophylactic antibiotics before catheter placement has been documented to prevent subsequent infection. Postoperatively, it is important to immobilize the catheter and minimize handling. The exit should be covered with a sterile gauze dressing, which is not changed for several days unless excessive bleeding occurs. No clear consensus has emerged regarding when the patient should start daily exit site care. Recommendations vary from 2 to 8 weeks after placement. Swan-neck catheters, disconnect Y systems, eradication of *S. aureus* nasal carriage (discussed earlier), and possibly, use of the Moncrief-Popovich catheter implantation technique may prevent exit site infections, but definitive confirmatory studies are lacking.

In contrast to the general agreement regarding postoperative exit site care, there is marked variation in standard clinical practices for chronic exit site care and the effect that these different practices have on preventing infection. One study suggested that cleaning with soap and water is best, another study suggested that povidone-iodine results in fewer infections, whereas a third study found no difference in infection rates regardless of the cleansing agent. At present, no consensus has been reached regarding recommendations for the standard chronic care cleansing agent used. It may be that any cleansing agent that does not irritate the exit site is acceptable for chronic care, as long as the standard implantation and postimplantation practices are initially followed to allow for catheter maturation.

TREATMENT OF EXIT SITE INFECTIONS. Treatment of exit site/tunnel infections has been reviewed and guidelines published.[34] Few data are available on the therapeutic efficacy of the current methods for treatment of exit site or tunnel infections. Treatment recommendations include the use of hypertonic saline (3%), Na^+ hypochlorite, diluted hydrogen peroxide, or povidone-iodine to treat equivocal or mild exit site infections. Acutely inflamed, traumatized exits or chronic exit site infections require topical and parenteral antibiotics. Topical antibiotics include chlorhexidine, dilute hydrogen peroxide, and gentamicin eyedrops. Because of the high frequency of resistance, gram-positive infections may need to be treated parenterally with vancomycin. Oral cephalosporins or a penicillinase-resistant antibiotic can also be used if the organism is not resistant to these agents. Persistent infections can be treated with combined vancomycin and rifampin. For gram-negative infections, ciprofloxacin is usually appropriate, although some *Pseudomonas* infections may require other antipseudomonal agents. The recommended duration of therapy is 2 to 4 weeks. Occasionally, deroofing of the tunnel or exteriorizing the cuff may be helpful. Shaving the superficial cuff is also beneficial in about 50% of refractory exit infections.[1093]

FUTURE TRENDS IN PERITONEAL DIALYSIS

The purpose of renal replacement therapy is not only to keep the patient alive, but also maintain lifestyle and wellness.

PD can do both. It is a vibrant therapy practiced at home by patients and prescribed by the nephrology community. In the face of this success, peritoneal dialysis continues to evolve because of continued interest and the pursuit of excellence. As more is known about the physiology of the membrane and the use of peritoneal fluids, we have the opportunity to better individualize prescriptions and PD solutions in ways that should improve life expectancy, well-being, and quality of life for our patients.

ACKNOWLEDGMENT

Many thanks to Laura Furr, Sonya Ashburn, and Kim Hairston for their excellent secretarial assistance.

REFERENCES

1. U.S. Renal Data System: USRDS 2002 Annual Data Report: Atlas of End-Stage Renal Disease in the United States. Bethesda, MD, National Institutes of Health, National Institute of Diabetes and Digestive and Kidney Diseases, 2002, pp 151-164.
2. Lameire N, Biesen WM, Dombros N, et al: The referral pattern of patients with ESRD is a determinant in the choice of dialysis modality. Perit Dial Int 17(suppl 2):161, 1997.
3. Nissenson AR, Prichard SS, Cheng IKP, et al: Non-medical factors that impact on ESRD modality selection. Kidney Int Suppl 40:120, 1993.
4. Ganter G: Uber die Beseitigun giftiger Stoffe aus dem Blute durch Dialyse. Munch Med Wochenschr 70:1478, 1923.
5. Odel HM, Ferris DO, Power MH: Peritoneal lavage as an effective means of extrarenal excretion. Am J Med 9:63, 1950.
6. Popovich RP, Moncrief JW, Decherd JF, et al: The definition of a novel portable-wearable equilibrium peritoneal technique. ASAIO J 5:64, 1976.
7. Nolph KD: Peritoneal Dialysis. *In* Brenner BM, Rector FC (eds): The Kidney. Philadelphia, WB Saunders, 1986, p 1847.
8. U.S. Renal Data System, USRDS 2000 Annual Report: Atlas of End-Stage Renal Disease in the United States. Bethesda, MD, National Institutes of Health, National Institute of Diabetes and Digestive and Kidney Diseases, 2000.
9. Fenton SSA, Schaubel DE, Desmeules M, et al: Hemodialysis versus peritoneal dialysis: A comparison of adjusted mortality rates. Am J Kidney Dis 30:334-342, 1997.
10. Collins AJ, Hao W, Xia H, et al: Mortality risks of peritoneal dialysis and hemodialysis. Am J Kidney Dis 34:1065-1074, 1999.
11. Paniagua R, Amato D, Vonesh E, et al: Effects of increased peritoneal clearances on mortality rates in peritoneal dialysis: ADEMEX, a prospective, randomized, controlled trial. J Am Soc Nephrol 13:1307-1320, 2002.
12. Konings CJ, Kooman JP, Schonck M, et al: Fluid status, blood pressure, and cardiovascular abnormalities in patients on peritoneal dialysis. Perit Dial Int 22:477-487, 2002.
13. Palmer RA, Maybee TK, Henry EW, et al: Peritoneal dialysis in acute and chronic renal failure. Can Med Assoc J 88:920, 1963.
14. Tenckhoff H, Schechter H: A bacteriologically safe peritoneal access device. ASAIO J 14:181, 1968.
15. Westin RE, Roberts M: Clinical use of stylet catheter for peritoneal dialysis. Arch Intern Med 115:569, 1965.
16. Cruz C: Clinical experience with a new peritoneal access device (the Cruz catheter). *In* Ota K, Maher J, Winchester JF, et al (eds): Current Concepts in Peritoneal Dialysis. Tokyo, Excerpta Medica, 1992, p 164.
17. Twardowski ZJ, Nolph KD, Khanna R, et al: The need for a "swan neck" permanently bent, arcuate peritoneal dialysis catheter. Perit Dial Bull 5:219, 1985.
18. Twardowski ZJ, Khanna R: Swan neck peritoneal dialysis catheter. *In* Andreucci VE (ed): Vascular and Peritoneal Access for Dialysis. Dordrecht, The Netherlands, Kluwer Academic, 1989, p 271.
19. Twardowski ZJ, Prowant BF, Nichols WK, et al: Six-year experience with swan neck catheters. Perit Dial Int 12:384, 1992.
20. Lindblad AS, Hamilton RW, Novak JW: Complications of peritoneal catheters. *In* Lindblad AS, Novak JW, Nolph KD (eds): Continuous Ambulatory Peritoneal Dialysis in the USA—Final Report of the

National CAPD Registry. Dordrecht, The Netherlands, Kluwer Academic, 1989, p 157.

21. Moncrief JW, Popovich RP, Broadrick LJ, et al: The Moncrief-Popovich catheter: A new peritoneal access technique for patients on peritoneal dialysis. ASAIO J 39:62, 1993.

22. Moncrief JW, Popovich RP, Simmons E, et al: Peritoneal access technology. Perit Dial Int 13(suppl 2):121-123, 1993.

23. Moncrief JW, Popovich RP, Simmons E, et al: Catheter obstruction with omental wrap stimulated by dialysate exposure. Perit Dial Int 13(suppl):127-129, 1993.

24. Moncrief JW, Popovich RP, Dasgupta MK, et al: Reduction in peritonitis incidence in continuous ambulatory peritoneal dialysis with a new catheter and implantation technique. Perit Dial Int 13(suppl 2): 329-331, 1993.

25. Danielsson A, Blohme L, Traneaus A, et al: A prospective randomized study of the effect of a subcutaneously "buried" peritoneal dialysis catheter technique versus standard technique on the incidence of peritonitis and exit-site infection. Perit Dial Int 22:211-219, 2002.

26. Holmes CJ, Evans RE: Biofilm and foreign body infection—the significance to CAPD-associated peritonitis. Perit Dial Bull 6:168, 1986.

27. Dasgupta MK, Bettcher KB, Ulan RA, et al: Relationship of adherent bacterial biofilms to peritonitis in chronic ambulatory peritoneal dialysis. Perit Dial Bull 7:168, 1987.

28. Marrie TJ, Nobel MA, Costerton JW: Examination of the morphology of bacteria adhering to peritoneal dialysis catheter by scanning and transmission electron microscopy. J Clin Microsc 18:1388, 1983.

29. Giangrande A, Allaria P, Torpia R, et al: Ultrastructure analysis of Tenckhoff chronic peritoneal catheters used in continuous ambulatory peritoneal dialysis patients. Perit Dial Int 13(suppl 2):133-135, 1993.

30. Costerton JW, Cheng KJ, Gessy GG, et al: Bacterial biofilm in nature and disease. Annu Rev Microbiol 41:435, 1987.

31. Roxe DM, Santhanam S: Structural defects in chronic peritoneal dialysis catheter contributing to peritonitis. Nephron 34:267, 1983.

32. Prowant BF, Khanna R, Twardowski ZJ: Peritoneal catheter exit site morphology and pathology: Prevention, diagnosis, and treatment of exit site infections. Perit Dial Int 16(suppl 3):105-114, 1996.

33. Twardowski ZJ, Dobbie JW, Moore HL, et al: Morphology of peritoneal dialysis catheter tunnel. Perit Dial Int 11:237, 1991.

34. Gokal R, Alexander S, Ash S, et al: Peritoneal catheters and exit site practices: Toward optimum peritoneal access. Perit Dial Int 18:11, 1998.

35. Ash SR, Nichols WK: Placement, repair, and removal of chronic peritoneal catheters. *In* Gokal R, Nolph KD, (eds): Textbook of Peritoneal Dialysis. Dordrecht, The Netherlands, Kluwer Academic, 1994, p 315.

36. Centers for Medicare & Medicaid Services. 2001 Annual Report, End Stage Renal Disease Clinical Performance Measures Project. Baltimore, Department of Health and Human Services. Centers for Medicare & Medicaid Services, Center for Beneficiary Choices, 1992.

37. Maffei S, Bonello F, Stramignoni E, et al: Two years experience and 119 peritoneal dialysis catheters placed with peritoneoscopy control and Y-TEC system. Minerva Urol Nefrol 44:63, 1992.

38. Nahman NSJ, Middendorf DF, Bay WH, et al: Modification of the percutaneous approach to peritoneal dialysis catheter placement under peritoneoscopic visualization: Clinical results in 78 patients. J Am Soc Nephrol 3:103, 1992.

39. Ash S: Effects of catheter design, materials, and location. Semin Dial 3:39, 1990.

40. Helfrich GB, Pechan BWW, Alijani MR, et al: Reduced catheter complications with lateral placement. Perit Dial Bull 3(suppl 4):2, 1983.

41. Stegmayr B, Hedberg B, Sandzen B, et al: Absence of leakage by insertion of peritoneal dialysis catheter through the rectus muscle. Perit Dial Int 10:53, 1990.

42. Nicholson ML, Burton PR, Donnelly PK, et al: The role of omentectomy in continuous ambulatory peritoneal dialysis. Perit Dial Int 11:330, 1991

43. Gokoo CF, Lelah MD, Hauck W, et al: External catheter immobilization improves wound healing in micropigs. ASAIO J 35:412, 1990.

44. Lindblad AS, Novak JW, Nolph KD: The USA CAPD registry characteristics of participants and selected outcome measures for the period January 1, 1981 through August 31, 1987. *In* Nolph KD (ed): Peritoneal Dialysis. Dordrecht, The Netherlands, Kluwer Academic, 1990, p 389.

45. Piraino B, Bernardini J, Centa PK, et al: The effect of body weight on CAPD related infections and catheter loss. Perit Dial Int 11:64, 1991.

46. Swartz R, Messana JM, Rocher L, et al: The curled catheter: Dependable device for percutaneous access. Perit Dial Int 10:231, 1990.

47. Weber J, Mettang T, Hubel E, et al: Survival of 138 surgically placed straight double-cuff Tenckhoff catheters in patients on continuous ambulatory peritoneal dialysis. Perit Dial Int 13:224, 1993.

48. Burkart JM, Jordan JR, Durnell TA, et al: Comparison of exit-site infections in disconnect versus nondisconnect systems for peritoneal dialysis. Perit Dial Int 12:317, 1992.

49. Guner O: Malfunctioning peritoneal dialysis catheter and accompanying surgical pathology repaired by laparoscopic surgery. Perit Dial Int 22:454-462, 2002.

50. Zadronzy D, Niemierko ML, Draczkowski T, et al: Laparoscopic approach for dysfunctional Tenckhoff catheters. Perit Dial Int 19:170-171, 1999.

51. Eklund BH, Honkanen EO, Kalan AR, et al: Peritoneal dialysis access: Prospective randomized comparison of the swan neck and Tenckhoff catheters. Perit Dial Int 15:353, 1995.

52. Lye WC, Kour NW, van der Straaten JC, et al: A prospective randomized comparison of the swan neck, coiled and straight Tenckhoff catheters in patients on CAPD. Perit Dial Int 16(suppl 1):333, 1996.

53. Vas SI: Answers to what are the indications for removal of the permanent peritoneal catheter? Perit Dial Bull 1:145, 1981.

54. Heusser H, Werder H: Untersuchungen uber Peritonealdialyse. Bruns Beitr Klin Chir 141:38, 1927.

55. Maxwell M, Rockney R, Kleeman C, et al: Peritoneal dialysis. JAMA 170:917, 1959.

56. Parker A, Nolph KD: Magnesium and calcium transfer during continuous ambulatory peritoneal dialysis. ASAIO J 25:194, 1980.

57. Veech R: The untoward effects of the anions of dialysis fluids. Kidney Int 34:587, 1988.

58. Raja RM, Cantor RE, Boreyko C, et al: Sodium transport during ultrafiltration peritoneal dialysis. ASAIO J 18:429, 1972.

59. Daniel J, Ahearn DJ, Nolph KD: Controlled sodium removal with peritoneal dialysis. ASAIO J 18:423, 1972.

60. Nolph KD, Hano JE, Teschan PE: Peritoneal sodium transport during hypertonic peritoneal dialysis. Ann Intern Med 70:931-941, 1969.

61. Raja RM, Kramer MS, Rosenbaum JL, et al: Evaluation of hypertonic peritoneal dialysis solutions with low sodium. Nephron 11:342, 1973.

62. Nakayama N, Kawaguchi Y, Kubo H, et al: Clinical effects of low Na concentration dialysate (130 mg/L) for CAPD patients. Perit Dial Int 13(suppl 1):76, 1993.

63. Imholz ALT, Koomen GCM, Struijk DG, et al: Fluid and solute transport in CAPD patients using ultralow sodium dialysate. Kidney Int 46:333, 1994.

64. Leypolt JK, Charney DI, Cheung AK, et al: Ultrafiltration and solute kinetics using low sodium dialysate. Kidney Int 48:1959, 1995.

65. Nolph KD, Sorkin M, Gloor HJ: Considerations for dialysis solution modifications. *In* Atkins RC, Thomson NM, Farrell PC (eds): Peritoneal Dialysis. Edinburgh, Churchill Livingstone, 1981, p 236.

66. Nolph KD, Twardowski Z, Popovich RP, et al: Equilibration of peritoneal dialysis solutions during long-dwell exchanges. J Lab Clin Med 93:246-256, 1979.

67. Brown ST, Ahearn DJ, Nolph KD: Potassium removal with peritoneal dialysis. Kidney Int 4:67, 1973.

68. Mandelbaum JM, Heistand ML, Schardin KE: Six months' experience with PD-2 solution. Dial Transplant 12:259, 1983.

69. Nolph KD, Prowant B, Serkes KD, et al: Multicenter evaluation of a new peritoneal dialysis solution with a high lactate and a low magnesium concentration. Perit Dial Bull 3:63, 1983.

70. Gonella M, Ballanti P, Della Rocca C, et al: Improved bone morphology by normalizing serum magnesium in chronically hemodialyzed patients. Miner Electrolyte Metab 14:240, 1988.

71. Weinreich T, Rambausek M, Ritz E: Is control of secondary hyperparathyroidism optimal with the currently used calcium concentration in the CAPD fluid? Nephrol Dial Transplant 6:843, 1991.

72. Hutchison A, Boulton H, Freemont A, et al: Effective control of phosphate, intact PTH, and osteodystrophy by low calcium dialysate and oral CaCO$_3$ in CAPD. Perit Dial Int 12(suppl):35, 1992.

73. Delmez JA: Removal of phosphorus by peritoneal dialysis. Perit Dial Int 13(suppl):461, 1993.

74. DeBroe M, D'Hasse P, Elseviers M, et al: Aluminum and end stage renal failure. *In* Davidson A (ed): Nephrology: Proceedings of the Xth ICN. Cambridge, Ballière Tindall, 1988, p 1086.

75. Andreoli SP, Briggs JD, Junor B: Aluminium intoxication from aluminium-containing phosphate binders in children with azotemia not undergoing dialysis. N Engl J Med 310:1079, 1984.

76. Slatopolsky E, Weerts C, Lopez-Hilker S, et al: Calcium carbonate as a phosphate binder in patients with chronic renal failure undergoing dialysis. N Engl J Med 315:157, 1986.
77. Stein H, Yudis M, Sirota R: Calcium carbonate as a phosphate binder. N Engl J Med 316:109, 1987.
78. Slingeneyer A, Laroche B, Loupi G, et al: Calcium concentration in PD dialysate must be lowered. Exclusive use of $CaCO_3$ as a phosphate binder. Perit Dial Int 12(suppl 2):161, 1992.
79. Cunningham J, Sawyer N, Altmann P, et al: Mineral metabolism in CAPD patients treated with $CaCO_3$ as a phosphate binder. Kidney Int 141:455, 1992.
80. Salusky I, Coburn JW, Foley J, et al: Effects of oral calcium carbonate on control of serum phosphorus and changes in plasma albumin levels after discontinuation of aluminium-containing gels in children receiving dialysis. J Pediatr 108:767, 1986.
81. Martis L, Serkes KD, Nolph KD: Calcium carbonate as a phosphate binder: Is there a need to adjust peritoneal dialysate calcium concentrations for patients using $CaCO_3$? Perit Dial Int 9:325, 1989.
82. Brown CB, Hamdy N, Boletis J, et al: Rationale for the use of low calcium solution in CAPD. In La Greca G, Ronco C, Feriani M, et al (eds): Peritoneal Dialysis, Proceedings of the Fourth International Course on Peritoneal Dialysis. Milan, Wichtig Editore, 1991, p 125.
83. Bender FH, Bernardini J, Piraino B, et al: Calcium mass transfer with dialysate containing 2.5 and 3.5 mmol/L calcium in peritoneal dialysis patients. Am J Kidney Dis 20:367, 1992.
84. Brown CB, Hamdy N, Boletis J, et al: Osteodystrophy in continuous ambulatory peritoneal dialysis. Perit Dial Int 13(suppl):454, 1993.
85. Piraino B, Bernardini J, Holley JL, et al: Calcium mass transfer in peritoneal dialysis patients using 2.5 mEq/liter calcium dialysate. Clin Nephrol 37:48, 1992.
86. Hutchison AJ, Merchant M, Boulton HF, et al: Calcium and magnesium mass transfer in peritoneal dialysis patients using 1.25 mmol/l magnesium dialysis fluid. Perit Dial Int 13:219, 1993.
87. Piraino B, Perlmutter JA, Holley JL, et al: The use of dialysate containing 2.5 mEq/L calcium in peritoneal dialysis patients. Perit Dial Int 12:75, 1992.
88. Martis L, Zimmerman S, Delmez J, et al: Dianeal 2.5 mEq/L calcium and calcium carbonate in CAPD. Perit Dial Int 12(suppl 1):177, 1992.
89. Kawanishi H, Tsuchiya T, Namba S, et al: Clinical application of low calcium peritoneal dialysate. ASAIO J 37:M404, 1991.
90. Hutchison A, Gokal R: Towards tailored dialysis fluids in CAPD: The role of reduced calcium and magnesium dialysis fluids. ASAIO J 12:199, 1992.
91. Hutchison A, Freemont A, Lumb G, et al: Renal osteodystrophy in CAPD. Adv Perit dial 7:237-239, 1991.
92. Loschiavo C, Fabris A, Adami S, et al: Effects of continuous ambulatory peritoneal dialysis (CAPD) on renal osteodystrophy. Perit Dial Bull 5:53, 1985.
93. Hutchison AJ, Boulton H, Gokal R: Low calcium dialysate with oral $CaCO_3$ in CAPD. Perit Dial Int 11:116, 1991.
94. Hercz G, Pei Y, Manuel A, et al: Aplastic osteodystrophy without aluminium staining in dialysis patients [abstract]. Kidney Int 37:449, 1990.
95. Hutchison AJ, Gokal R: Improved solutions for peritoneal dialysis: Physiological calcium solutions, osmotic agents and buffers. Kidney Int Suppl 38:153, 1992.
96. Weinreich T, Colombi A, Echterhoff HH, et al: Transperitoneal calcium mass transfer using dialysate with a low calcium concentration (1.0 mm). Perit Dial Int 42(suppl 38):467, 1993.
97. Rotellar C, Kinsel V, Goggins M, et al: Does low calcium dialysate accelerate secondary hyperparathyroidism in continuous ambulatory peritoneal dialysis patients? Perit Dial Int 13(suppl):471, 1993.
98. Weinreich T, Passlick-Deetjen J, Ritz E: Low dialysate calcium in continuous ambulatory peritoneal dialysis: A randomized controlled multicenter trial. Am J Kidney Dis 25:452, 1995.
99. Johnson DW, Rigby R, McIntyre HD, et al: A randomized trial comparing 1.25 mmol/l calcium dialysate to 1.75 mmol/l calcium dialysate in CAPD patients. Nephrol Dial Transplant 11:88, 1996.
100. Tattersall JE, Dick C, Dolye S, et al: Alkalosis and hypomagnesaemia: Unwanted effects of a low-calcium CAPD solution. Nephrol Dial Transplant 10:258, 1995.
101. Tuncer M, Ermis C, Suleymanlar G, et al: Low calcium dialysate increases cardiac relaxation in CAPD patients. Perit Dial Int 22:714-718, 2002.

102. Ing TS, Daugirdas JT, Gandhi VC: Peritoneal sclerosis in peritoneal dialysis patients. Am J Nephrol 4:173, 1984.
103. Rossen B, Ladefoged J: A comparison between the effects of acetate and lactate in peritoneal dialysis solutions. Scand J Urol Nephrol 16:279, 1982.
104. Slingeneyer A, Mion C, Mourad G, et al: Progressive sclerosing peritonitis: A late and severe complication of maintenance peritoneal dialysis patients. ASAIO J 29:633, 1983.
105. Ing TS, Gandhi VC, Daugirdas JT, et al: Peritoneal dialysis using bicarbonate-buffered dialysate. Int J Artif Organs 7:166, 1984.
106. Kwong MBL, Wu GG, Rodella H, et al: Effect of the peritoneal dialysate buffer on ultrafiltration: Studies in normal rabbits. Perit Dial Bull 5:182, 1985.
107. Johnson R, Walton J, Krebs H, et al: Metabolic fuels during and after severe exercise in athletes and non-athletes. Lancet 2:452, 1969.
108. Brandt R, Siegel S, Waters M, et al: Spectroscopic assay for D(-) lactate in plasma. Anal Biochem 102:39, 1980.
109. Thurn J, Pierpont G, Ludvigsen C, et al: D-Lactate encephalopathy. Am J Med 79:717, 1985.
110. Nolph KD, Twardowski Z, Khanna R, et al: Tidal peritoneal dialysis with racemic or L-lactate solutions. Perit Dial Int 10:161, 1990.
111. Topley N, Kaur D, Petersen MM, et al: Biocompatibility of bicarbonate buffered peritoneal dialysis fluids: Influence on mesothelial cell and neutrophil function. Kidney Int 49:1447, 1996.
112. Yatzidis H: A new single bicarbonate CAPD solution. In La Graeca G, Ronco C, Feriani M, et al (eds): The Fourth International Course on Peritoneal Dialysis. Vincenza, Italy, Eichtig Editore, 1991, p 151.
113. Yatzidis H: A new stable bicarbonate dialysis solution for peritoneal dialysis: Preliminary report. Perit Dial Int 11:224, 1991.
114. Vaziri N, Ness R, Wellikson L, et al: Bicarbonate buffered peritoneal dialysis. An effective adjunct in the treatment of lactic acidosis. Am J Med 67:392, 1979.
115. Feriani M, Biasioli S, Bonn D, et al: Bicarbonate buffer for CAPD solution. ASAIO J 31:668, 1985.
116. Feriani M, Reinhardt B, La Graeca G: Calcium carbonate precipitation in oversaturated bicarbonate containing solution. In La Graeca G, Ronco C, Feriani M, et al (eds): The Fourth International Course on Peritoneal Dialysis. Vincenza, Italy, Wichtig Editore, 1991, p 1991.
117. Feriani M, Dissegna D, La Graeca G, et al: Continuous ambulatory peritoneal dialysis with bicarbonate buffer—a pilot study. Perit Dial Int 13(suppl):88, 1993.
118. Coles GA, Gokal R, Ogg C, et al: A randomized controlled trial of a bicarbonate and a bicarbonate/lactate containing dialysis solution in CAPD. Perit Dial Int 17:48, 1997.
119. Feriani M: Bicarbonate-buffered CAPD solutions: From clinical trails to clinical practice. Perit Dial Int 17(suppl 2):51, 1997.
120. Lindholm B, Bergstrom J: Nutritional aspects of CAPD. In Gokal R (ed): Continuous Ambulatory Peritoneal Dialysis. Edinburgh, Churchill Livingstone, 1986, p 228.
121. Gokal R, Ramos J, McGurk J, et al: Hyperlipidemia in patients on continuous ambulatory peritoneal dialysis. In Gahl GM, Kessel M, Nolph KD (eds): Advances in Peritoneal Dialysis. Amsterdam, Excerpta Medica, 1981, p 430.
122. Bouma S, Dwyer JT: Glucose absorption and weight exchange in 18 months of continuous ambulatory peritoneal dialysis. J Am Diet Assoc 84:194, 1984.
123. Dobbie JW: Pathogenesis of peritoneal fibrosing syndromes (sclerosing peritonitis) in peritoneal dialysis. Perit Dial Int 12:14, 1992.
124. Oreopoulos DG, Crassweller P, Kartirtzoglou A, et al: Amino acids as an osmotic agent (instead of glucose) in continuous ambulatory peritoneal dialysis. In Legrain M (ed): First International Symposium on CAPD. Paris, Excerpta Medica, 1979, p 335.
125. Williams PF, Marliss E, Anderson GH, et al: Amino acid absorption following intraperitoneal administration in CAPD patients. Perit Dial Bull 2:124, 1982.
126. Oren A, Wu G, Anderson GH, et al: Effective use of amino acid dialysate over four weeks in CAPD patients. Perit Dial Bull 3:66, 1983.
127. Dombros N, Prutis K, Tong M, et al: Six-month overnight intraperitoneal amino acid infusion in continuous ambulatory peritoneal dialysis patients—no effect on nutritional status. Perit Dial Int 10:79, 1990.
128. Kopple JD, Bernard D, Brunori G, et al: Nutritional effects of intraperitoneal (IP) amino acids (AA) in malnourished CAPD patients. J Am Soc Nephrol 2:362, 1991.

129. Bruno M, Bagnis C, Marangella M, et al: CAPD with an amino acid dialysis solution: A long-term cross-over study. Kidney Int 35:1189, 1989.

130. Prichard SS, Cianflone K, Zhang ZJ, et al: A novel mechanism to explain the dyslipidemia in CAPD and nephrotic patients. Perit Dial Int 12:150, 1992.

131. Steinhauer HB, Lubrick-Birkner I, Kluthe R, et al: Effect of amino acid based dialysis solution on peritoneal permeability and prostanoid generation in patients undergoing continuous ambulatory peritoneal dialysis. Am J Nephrol 12:61, 1992.

132. Douma CE, De Waart DR, Struijk DG, et al: Effect of amino acid based dialysate on peritoneal blood flow and permeability in stable CAPD patients: A potential role for nitric oxide? Clin Nephrol 5:302, 1996.

133. Young GA, Dibble JB, Taylor AE, et al: A longitudinal study on the effects of amino acid–based CAPD fluid on amino acid retention and protein loss. Nephrol Dial Transplant 4:900, 1989.

134. Jones MR, Gehr T, Burkart JM, et al: Replacement of amino acid and protein losses with 1.1% amino acid peritoneal dialysis solution. Perit Dial Int 18:210-216, 1998.

135. Faller B: Amino acid–based peritoneal dialysis solutions. Kidney Int Suppl 56:81-85, 1996.

136. Jones M, Hagen T, Boyle CA, et al: Treatment of malnutrition with 1.1% amino acid peritoneal dialysis solution: Results of a multicenter outpatient study. Am J Kidney Dis 32:761, 1998.

137. Klein E, Ward A, Williams TE, et al: Peptides as substitute osmotic agents for glucose in peritoneal dialysate. ASAIO J 32:550, 1986.

138. Martis L, Burke R, Klein E: Evaluation of a peptide-based solution for peritoneal dialysis. Perit Dial Int 13(suppl):92, 1993.

139. Wang T, Lindholm B: Oligopeptides as osmotic agents for peritoneal dialysis. Perit Dial Int 17(suppl 2):75, 1997.

140. Krediet RT: Osmotic agents in automated peritoneal dialysis solutions. Contrib Nephrol 50:979-986, 1999.

141. Mistry CD, Mallick VP, Gokal R: Ultrafiltration with an isosmotic solution during long peritoneal dialysis exchanges. Lancet 2:178, 1987.

142. Alsop RM: History, chemical and pharmaceutical development of icodextrin. Perit Dial Int 14(suppl 2):5-12, 1994.

143. Ho-dac-Pannekeet MM, Schouten N, Langedijk MJ, et al: Peritoneal transport characteristics with glucose polymer based dialysate. Kidney Int 50:979-986, 1996.

144. Moberly JB, Mujais S, Gehr T, et al: Pharmacokinetics of icodextrin in peritoneal dialysis patients. Kidney Int Suppl 81:23-33, 2002.

145. Plum J, Gentile S, Verger C, et al: Efficacy and safety of a 7.5% icodextrin peritoneal dialysis solution in patients treated with automated peritoneal dialysis; a prospective randomized multicenter trail. Am J Kidney Dis 39:862-871, 2002.

146. Wolfson M, Ogrinc FG, Mujais S: Review of clinical trial experience with icodextrin. Kidney Int Suppl 81:46-52, 2002.

147. Wolfson M, Piraino B, Hamburger RJ, et al: A randomized controlled trial to evaluate the safety and efficacy of icodextrin in peritoneal dialysis. Am J Kidney Dis 40:1055-1065, 2002.

148. Mujais S, Vonesh E: Profiling of peritoneal ultrafiltration. Kidney Int Suppl 81:17-22, 2002.

149. Woodrow G, Stables G, Oldroyd B, et al: Comparison of icodextrin and glucose solutions for the daytime dwell in automated peritoneal dialysis. Nephrol Dial Transplant 14:1530-1535, 1999.

150. Rubin J, Klein E, Jones Q, et al: Evaluation of a polymer dialysate. ASAIO J 29:62, 1983.

151. Higgins JT, Gross ML, Somani P, et al: Patient tolerance and dialysis effectiveness of a glucose polymer–containing peritoneal dialysis solution. Perit Dial Bull 4(suppl):131, 1984.

152. Gokal R, Mistry CD: Glucose polymer as an osmotic agent in CAPD. *In* La Graeca G, Ronco C, Feriani M, et al (eds): Fourth International Course on Peritoneal Dialysis. Vincenza, Italy, Wichtig Editore, 1991, p 119.

153. Mistry CD, Fox J, Mallick N, et al: Circulating maltose and isomaltose in chronic renal failure. Kidney Int Suppl 22:210, 1987.

154. Bredie SJH, Bosch FH, Demaacker PNM, et al: Effects of peritoneal dialysis with an overnight dwell on parameters of glucose and lipid metabolism. Perit Dial Int 21:275-281, 2001.

155. Amici G: Hyperinsulinemia reduction associated with icodextrin treatment in CAPD patients. Perit Dial Int 21(suppl):22, 2001.

156. Wilkie ME, Plant MJ, Edwards L, et al: Icodextrin 7.5% dialysate solution (glucose polymer) in patients with ultrafiltration failure: Extension of CAPD technique survival. Perit Dial Int 17:84, 1997.

157. Faller B, Shockley T, Genestier S, et al: Polyglucose and amino acids: Preliminary results. Perit Dial Int 27(suppl 2):63, 1997.

158. Wolfson M, Orginc F, Mujias S: Review of clinical trial experience with icodextrin. Kidney Int Suppl 81:46-52, 2002.

159. Pinerolo MC, Porri MT, D'Amico G: Recurrent sterile peritonitis at onset of treatment with icodextrin. Perit Dial Int 19:491-492, 1999.

160. William PF, Foggensteiner L: Sterile/allergic peritonitis with icodextrin in CAPD patients. Perit Dial Int 22:89-90, 2002.

161. Gokal R: Icodextrin-associated sterile peritonitis. Perit Dial Int 22:445-448, 2002.

162. Aanen MC, De Waart DR, Williams PF, et al: Dextran antibodies in peritoneal dialysis patients treated with icodextrin. Perit Dial Int 22:513-515, 2002.

163. Wens R, Taminne M, Devriendt J, et al: A previously undescribed side effect of icodextrin, an overestimation of glycemia by glucose analyzer. Perit Dial Int 18:603-609, 1998.

164. Schonicke G, Grabensee B, Plum J: Interference of icodextrin with serum amylase activity measurements [abstract]. J Am Soc Nephrol 10:229, 1999.

165. Gokal R: Newer peritoneal dialysis solutions. Adv Ren Replace Ther 7:302, 2000.

166. Davies SJ, Phillips L, Griffiths AM, et al: What really happens to people on long-term peritoneal dialysis. Kidney Int 54:2207-2217, 1998.

167. Plum J, Hermann S, Fussholler A, et al: Peritoneal sclerosis in peritoneal dialysis patients related to dialysis settings and peritoneal transport properties. Kidney Int Suppl 78:42-47, 2001.

168. Honda K, Nitta K, Horita S, et al: Accumulation of advanced glycation end products in the peritoneal vasculature of continuous ambulatory peritoneal dialysis patients with low ultrafiltration. Nephrol Dial Transplant 14:1541-1549, 1999.

169. Dobbie JW: The role of peritoneal biopsy in clinical and experimental peritoneal dialysis. Perit Dial Int 13(suppl 2):23, 1993.

170. Breborowicz A, Rodella H, Pagiamtzis J, et al: Glucose (G) toxicity to human mesothelial cells (MC) in vitro. Perit Dial Int 10(suppl 1):19, 1990.

171. Topley N, Mackenzie R, Petersen MM, et al: In vitro testing of a potentially biocompatible continuous ambulatory peritoneal dialysis fluid. Nephrol Dial Transplant 6:574, 1991.

172. Breborowicz A, Balaskas E, Diamandis E, et al: Effect of tumor necrosis factor on human mesothelial cells in in vitro culture. Perit Dial Int 12(suppl 2):6, 1992.

173. Di Paolo N, Garosi G, Traversari L, et al: Mesothelial biocompatibility of peritoneal dialysis solutions. Perit Dial Int 13(suppl 2):109, 1993.

174. Breborowicz A: In vitro study on the biocompatibility of the peritoneal dialysis solution. Perit Dial Int 13(suppl 2):105, 1993.

175. Gotloib L, Shostak A, Wajsbrot V, et al: Biocompatibility of dialysis solutions evaluated by histochemical techniques applied to mesothelial cell imprints. Perit Dial Int 13(suppl 2):113, 1993.

176. Margetts PJ, Kolb M, Hoff CM, Gauldie J: A chronic inflammatory infusion model of peritoneal dialysis in rats. Perit Dial Int 21(suppl 3):368-372, 2001.

177. Lewis S, Holmes CJ: Host defense mechanisms in the peritoneal cavity of continuous ambulatory peritoneal dialysis patients. Perit Dial Int 11:14, 1991.

178. Lai KN, Lai KB, Lam CW, et al: Changes of cytokine profiles during peritonitis in patients on continuous ambulatory peritoneal dialysis. Am J Kidney Dis 35:644-652, 2000.

179. Jorres A, Gahl GM, Muller C, et al: In vitro biocompatibility testing of a new glucose polymer dialysis fluid for CAPD. Nephrol Dial Transplant 7:774, 1992.

180. Jorres A, Gahl GM, Ludat K, et al: In vitro biocompatibility testing of a new bicarbonate-buffered dialysis fluid for CAPD. Perit Dial Int 12(suppl 2):26, 1992.

181. Jorres A, Williams JD, Topley N: Peritoneal dialysis solution biocompatibility: Inhibitory mechanisms and recent studies with bicarbonate-buffered solutions. Perit Dial Int 17(suppl 2):42, 1997.

182. Mackenzie R, Williams JD, Moseley A, et al: In vivo exposure to bicarbonate/lactate (TBL) and bicarbonate (TB) buffered dialysis fluids (PDF) improves peritoneal macrophage (PM) function. J Am Soc Nephrol 7:1342, 1996.

183. Cooker LA, Luneberg P, Holmes CJ, et al: Interleukin-6 levels decrease in effluent from patients dialyzing with bicarbonate-lactate based peritoneal dialysis solutions. Perit Dial Int 21(suppl 3):102-107, 2001.

184. Mettang T, Fischer FP, Dunst R, et al: Plasticizers in renal failure: Aspects of metabolism and toxicity. Perit Dial Int 17(suppl 2):31, 1997.

185. Krediet RT, Zweers MM, Ho-dac-Pannekeet MM: The effect of various dialysis solutions on peritoneal membrane viability. Perit Dial Int 19(suppl 2):257-266, 1999.

186. Wieslander A, Linden T, Musi B, et al: Biological significance of reducing glucose degradation products in peritoneal dialysis fluids. Perit Dial Int 20(suppl 5):23-27, 2000.

187. Wieczorowska-Tobis K, Polubinska A, Schaub TB, et al: Influence of neutral pH dialysis solutions on the peritoneal membrane: A long term investigation in rate. Perit Dial Int 21(suppl 3):108-113, 2001.

188. Wieslander A, Linden T, Kjellstrand P: Glucose degradation products in peritoneal dialysis fluids: How they can be avoided. Perit Dial Int 21(suppl 3):119-124, 2001.

189. Carozzi S, Nasini M, Schelotto C, et al: Peritoneal dialysis fluid (PDF) Ca^{++} and 1,25(OH)$_2$D$_3$ modulate peritoneal macrophage (PMO) antimicrobial activity in CAPD patients. Adv Perit Dial 6:110-113, 1990.

190. Suga H, Honda H, Naganuma S, et al: A low Ca^{++} level in effluent as a risk factor for the peritonitis in CAPD patients. Adv Perit Dial 6:102-105, 1990.

191. Piraino B, Bernardini J, Holley JL, et al: Increased risk of *Staphylococcus epidermidis* peritonitis in patients on dialysate containing 1.25 mmol/L calcium. Am J Kidney Dis 19:371, 1992.

192. Hutchison A, Turner K, Gokal R: Effect of long-term therapy with 1.25 mmol/L calcium peritoneal dialysis fluid on the incidence of peritonitis in CAPD. Perit Dial Int 12:321, 1992.

193. Wegner G: Chirurgische Bermekungen uber die peritonalhole, mit besonderer Berucksichtigung der Ovariotomie. Arch Klin Chir 20:51, 1877.

194. Hertzler AE: The Peritoneum. St. Louis, CV Mosby, 1919.

195. Knapowski J, Feder E, Simons ME, et al: Evaluation of the participation of parietal peritoneum in dialysis: Physiological, morphological, and pharmacological data. Proc Eur Dial Transplant Assoc 16:155, 1979.

196. Esperanca MJ, Collins DL: Peritoneal dialysis efficiency in relation to body weight. J Pediatr Surg 1:162, 1966.

197. Nolph KD: Peritoneal Dialysis. *In* Brenner BM, Rector FC (eds): The Kidney. Philadelphia, WB Saunders, 1991, p 2299.

198. Kolossow A: Ueber die Struktur des Endothels der Pleuroperitonealhole der Blut und Lymphgefasse. Biol Centralbl Erlang 12:87, 1892.

199. Nagy JA: Peritoneal membrane morphology and function. Kidney Int Suppl 56:2-11, 1996.

200. Baradi AF, Hope J: Observations on ultrastructure of rabbit mesothelium. Exp Cell Res 34:33, 1964.

201. Recklinhausen V: Zur Fettresorption. Arch Pathol Anat Physiol 26:172, 1863.

202. Leak LV: Distribution of cell surface charges on mesothelium and lymphatic endothelium. Microvasc Res 31:18-30, 1986.

203. Gotloib L, Digenis G: Ultrastructure of normal rabbit mesentery. Nephron 34:248, 1983.

204. Dobbie JW: Ultrastructural similarities between mesothelium and type II pneumocytes and their relevance to phospholipid surfactant production by the peritoneum. *In* Khanna R, Nolph KD, Prowant B, et al (eds): Advances in Peritoneal Dialysis. Toronto, University of Toronto Press, 1988, p 47.

205. Dobbie JW, Lloyd JK: Mesothelium secretes lamellar bodies in a similar manner to type II pneumocyte secretion of a surfactant. Perit Dial Int 9:215-219, 1989.

206. Dobbie JW: New concepts in molecular biology and ultrastructural pathology of the peritoneum. Am J Kidney Dis 15:97-109, 1990.

207. Dobbie JW: Surfactant protein A and lamellar bodies: A homologous secretory function of peritoneum, synovium, and lung. Perit Dial Int 16:574, 1996.

208. Valle MT, Deg'Innocenti ML, Bertelli R, et al: Antigen-presenting function of human peritoneum mesothelial cells. Clin Exp Immunol 101:172, 1995.

209. Zeillemaker AM, Verbrugh HA, Hoynck van Papendrecht AA, et al: CA125 secretion by peritoneal mesothelial cells. J Clin Pathol 47:263, 1994.

210. Visser CE, Brouwer-Steenbergen JJE, Betjes MGH, et al: Cancer antigen 125: A bulk marker for mesothelial mass in stable peritoneal dialysis patient. Nephrol Dial Transplant 10:64-69, 1995.

211. Wang T, Cheng HH, Heimburger O, et al: Hyaluronan decreases peritoneal fluid absorption: Effect of molecular weight and concentration of hyaluronan. Kidney Int 55:667-673, 1999.

212. Flessner MF: The role of extracellular matrix in transperitoneal transport of water and solutes. Perit Dial Int 21(suppl 3):24-29, 2001.

213. Wade OL, Combes B, Childs AW, et al: The effect of exercise on the splanchnic blood flow and splanchnic blood volume in normal man. Clin Sci 15:457, 1956.

214. Taylor AE, Granger DN: Exchange of macromolecules across the microcirculation. *In* Renkin EM, Michel CC (eds): Handbook of Physiology, Section 2, The Cardiovascular System, Vol IV, Microcirculation. Bethesda, MD, American Physiological Society, 1984, p 467.

215. Devuyst O, Nielsen S, Cosyus JP, et al: Aquaporin-1 and endothelial nitric oxide synthase expression in capillary endothelia of human peritoneum. Am J Physiol 275:H234-H242, 1998.

216. Casley-Smith JR: The passage of particles into and out of diaphragmatic lymphatics. Q J Exp Physiol 49:365, 1964.

217. Mactier RA, Khanna R: Peritoneal lymphatics. *In* Gokal R, Nolph KD, The Textbook of Peritoneal Dialysis edited by Dordrecht, The Netherlands, Kluwer Academic, 1994, p 115.

218. Allen L: The peritoneal stomata. Anat Rec 67:89, 1936.

219. Azzali G: Ultrastructure of small intestine, submucosal and serosal-muscular lymphatic vessels. Lymphology 15:106, 1982.

220. Hirsel P, Lameire N, Bogaert M: Pharmacologic alterations of peritoneal transport rates and pharmacokinetics of the peritoneum. *In* Gokal R, Nolph KD (eds): The Textbook of Peritoneal Dialysis. Dordrecht, The Netherlands, Kluwer Academic, 1994, p 1994.

221. Hauglustaine D, Monballyu J, van Meerbeek J, et al: Report of sclerotic alterations of the peritoneum in patients on CAPD. Lancet 1983.

222. Dobbie JW, Lloyd JK, Gall CA: Categorization of ultrastructural changes in peritoneal mesothelium, stroma and blood vessels in uremia and CAPD patients. Adv Perit Dial 6:3-12, 1990.

223. Karnovsky MJ: The ultrastructural basis of capillary permeability studied with peroxidase as a tracer. J Cell Biol 35:213, 1967.

224. Williams JD, Craig KJ, Topley N, et al: Morphologic changes in the peritoneal membrane of patients with renal disease. J Am Soc Nephrol 13:470-479, 2002.

225. Verger C, Luger A, Moore HL: Acute changes in peritoneal morphology and transport properties with infectious peritonitis and mechanical injury. Kidney Int 23:823, 1983.

226. Panasiuk E, Pietrzak B, Klos M, et al: Characteristics of peritoneum after peritonitis in peritonitis in CAPD patients. In Advances in Peritoneal Dialysis, Vol 4. Toronto, University of Toronto Press, 1988, p 42.

227. Devuyst O: New insights in the molecular mechanisms regulating peritoneal permeability. Nephrol Dial Transplant 17:548-551, 2002.

228. Flessner MF: Small-solute transport across specific peritoneal tissue surfaces in the rat. J Am Soc Nephrol 7:225, 1996.

229. Henderson LW: The problem of peritoneal membrane and permeability. Kidney Int 3:409, 1973.

230. Levitt MD, Kneip JM, Overdahl MC: Influence of shaking on peritoneal transfer in rats. Kidney Int 35:1145, 1989.

231. Rubin J, Jones Q, Planch A, et al: The minimal importance of the hollow viscera to peritoneal transport during peritoneal dialysis in a rat. ASAIO J 34:912, 1988.

232. Fox SD, Leypolt JK, Henderson LW: Visceral peritoneum is not essential for solute transport during peritoneal dialysis. Kidney Int 40:612, 1991.

233. Zakaria ER, Carlsson O, Sjunnession H, et al: Liver is not essential for solute transport during peritoneal dialysis. Kidney Int 50:298, 1996.

234. Erbe RW, Greene JA Jr, Weller JM: Peritoneal dialysis during hemorrhagic shock. J Appl Physiol 22:131, 1967.

235. Alon U, Bar-Maor JA, Bar-Joseph G: Effective peritoneal dialysis in an infant with extensive resection of the small intestine. Am J Nephrol 8:65, 1988.

236. Ored S: Experimental studies on protal circulation at increased intraabdominal pressure. Acta Physiol Scand 30(suppl 109):1, 1953.

237. Flessner MF: The peritoneal dialysis system: Importance of each component. Perit Dial Int 17(suppl 2):91, 1997.

238. Grahame GR, Torchia MG, Dankewich KA, Ferguson IA: Surface-active material in peritoneal effluent of CAPD patients. Perit Dial Bull 5:109-111, 1985.

239. Chen Y, Hills BA: Surgical adhesions: Evidence for adsorption of surfactant to the peritoneal mesothelium. Aust N Z J Surg 70:443-447, 2000.

240. Chen Y, Burke JR, Hills BA: Semipermeability imparted by surface-active phospholipid in peritoneal dialysis. Perit Dial Int 22:380-385, 2002.

241. DiZerega GS, Rodgers KE: The Peritoneum. New York, Springer-Verlag, 1992, p 8.

242. Krediet RT, Zuyderhoudt FMJ, Boeschoten EW, et al: Peritoneal permeability to proteins in diabetic and non-diabetic continuous ambulatory peritoneal dialysis patients. Nephron 42:133, 1986.

243. Nolph KD, Miller FN, Rubin J, et al: New directions in peritoneal dialysis concepts and applications. Kidney Int 18(suppl 10):111, 1980.

244. Bell JL, Leypolt JK, Firgon RP, et al: Heteroporosity model of peritoneal transport is not supported by hydraulically-driven convective transport. Kidney Int 33:243, 1988.

245. Lill SR, Parsons RH, Buhac I: Permeability of the diaphragm and fluid resorption from the peritoneal cavity in the rat. Gastroenterology 76:997, 1979.

246. Nolph KD, Popovich RP, Ghods AJ, Twardowski Z: Determinants of low clearances of small solutes during peritoneal dialysis. Kidney Int 13:117-123, 1978.

247. McGary TJ, Nolph KD, Rubin J: In vitro simulations of peritoneal dialysis: A technique for demonstrating limitations on solute clearances due to stagnant fluid films and poor mixing. J Lab Clin Med 96:148, 1980.

248. Wayland H: Transmural and interstitial molecular transport. *In* Legrain M (ed): Proceedings of an International Symposium, Paris. Amsterdam, Excerpta Medica, 1980, p 18.

249. Grotte G: Passage of dextran molecules across the blood-lymph barrier. Acta Chir Scand 211(suppl 1):1, 1956.

250. Pappenheimer JR, Renkin EM, Borrero LM: Filtration, diffusion, and molecular sieving through peripheral capillary membranes. A contribution to the pore theory of capillary permeability. Am J Physiol 167:13, 1951.

251. Rippe B, Stelin G, Haraldsson B: Computer simulations of peritoneal transport in CAPD. Kidney Int 40:315-325, 1991.

252. Agre P, Preston GM, Smith BL, et al: Aquaporin CHIP: The archetypal molecular water channel. Am J Physiol 265:F463, 1993.

253. Mayerson HS, Wolfram CG, Shirley HH Jr, et al: Regional differences in capillary permeability. Am J Physiol 198:155, 1960.

254. Fox J, Galey F, Wayland H: Action of histamine on the mesenteric microvasculature. Microvasc Res 19:108, 1980.

255. Papenheimer JR: Passage of molecules through capillary walls. Physiol Rev 33:387, 1953.

256. Nolph KD, Miller FN, Pyle WK, et al: An hypothesis to explain the ultrafiltration characteristics of peritoneal dialysis. Kidney Int 20:543, 1981.

257. Cotran RS: The Fine Structure of the Microvasculature in Relation to Normal and Altered Permeability. Philadelphia, WB Saunders, 1967.

258. Charonis AS, Wissig SL: Anionic sites in basement membranes. Differences in their electrostatic properties in continuous and fenestrated capillaries. Microvas Res 25:265, 1983.

259. Gotloib L: Anatomical basis for peritoneal permeability. *In* La Greca G, Chiaramonte S, Fabris A, et al (eds): Peritoneal Dialysis. Milan, Wichtig Editore, 1989, p 3.

260. Curry FE, Mason JC, Michel CC: Osmotic reflection coefficients of capillary walls to low molecular weight hydrophilic solutes measured in single perfused capillaries of the frog mesentery. J Physiol 261:319, 1976.

261. Michel CC: Filtration coefficients and osmotic reflection coefficients of the walls of single frog mesenteric capillaries. J Physiol 309:341, 1980.

262. Korten G: Measuring the thickness of the peritoneum as a dialysis membrane using various osmolar concentrations of dialysis fluid. Z Urol Nephrol 83:459, 1990.

263. Lasrich M, Maher M, Hirszel P, et al: Correlation of peritoneal transport rates with molecular weight: A method for predicting clearances. ASAIO J 2:107-113, 1979.

264. Flessner MF: The importance of the interstitium in peritoneal transport. Perit Dial Int 16(suppl 1):76, 1996.

265. Tsilibary EC, Wissig SL: Absorption from the peritoneal cavity: SEM study of the mesothelium covering the peritoneal surface of the muscular portion of the diaphragm. Am J Anat 149:127, 1977.

266. Flessner MF: Peritoneal transport physiology: Insights from basic research. J Am Soc Nephrol 2:122, 1991.

267. Cascarano J, Rubin AD, Chick WL, et al: Metabolically induced permeability changes across mesothelium and endothelium. Am J Physiol 206:373, 1964.

268. Hills BA: Role of surfactant in peritoneal dialysis. Perit Dial Int 20:503-515, 2000.

269. Breborowicz A, Knapowski J: Studies on the resistance of the peritoneal mesothelium to solute transport. Perit Dial Bull 4:37, 1984.

270. Goldschmidt ZH, Pote HH, Katz MA, et al: Effect of dialysate volume on peritoneal dialysis kinetics. Kidney Int 5:240, 1974.

271. Stephen RL, Atkin-Thor E, Kolff WJ: Recirculating peritoneal dialysis with subcutaneous catheter. Am Soc Artif Int Organs 22:575, 1976.

272. Tenckhoff H, Ward G, Boen ST: The influence of dialysate volume and flow rate on peritoneal clearance. Proc Eur Dial Transplant Assoc 2:113, 1965.

273. Lange K, Treser G, Mangalat J: Automatic continuous high flow rate peritoneal dialysis. Arch Klin Med 214:201, 1968.

274. Rubin J, Kirchner K, Bower J: Evaluation of stagnant fluid films during simulated peritoneal dialysis. Clin Exp Dial Apheresis 5:285, 1981.

275. Nolph KD, Ghods AJ, Van Stone J, et al: The effects of intraperitoneal vasodilators on peritoneal clearances. Trans Am Soc Artif Intern Organs 22:586, 1976.

276. Miller FN, Nolph KD, Harris PD, et al: Microvascular and clinical effects of altered peritoneal dialysis solutions. Kidney Int 15:630, 1979.

277. Aune S: Transperitoneal exchange 2. Peritoneal blood flow estimated by hydrogen gas clearance. Scand J Gastroenterol 5:99, 1970.

278. Blumenkrantz MJ, Roberts CE, Card B, et al: Nutritional management of the adult patient undergoing peritoneal dialysis. J Am Diet Assoc 73:251, 1978.

279. Giordano C, De Santo NG: Dietary management of patients on peritoneal dialysis. Contrib Nephrol 17:77, 1979.

280. Cunningham RS: The physiology of the serous membranes. Physiol Rev 6:242, 1926.

281. Clark AJ: Absorption from the peritoneal cavity. J Pharmacol Exp Ther 16:415, 1921.

282. Putnam TJ: The living peritoneum as a dialyzing membrane. Am J Physiol 63:548, 1922.

283. Randerson DH, Farrell PC: Mass transfer properties of the human peritoneum. ASAIO J 3:140, 1980.

284. Pyle WK: Mass Transfer in Peritoneal Dialysis. Ann Arbor, MI, University Microfilms International, 1992.

285. Pyle WK, Moncrief JW, Popovich RP: Peritoneal transport evaluation in CAPD. *In* Moncrief JW, Popovich RP (eds): Proceedings of the Second International Symposium on CAPD. New York, Masson, 1981, p 35.

286. Garred IJ, Canaud B, Farrell PC: A simple kinetic model for assessing peritoneal mass transfer in chronic ambulatory peritoneal dialysis. Trans Am Soc Artif Intern Organs 29:131, 1983.

287. Henderson LW, Nolph KD: Altered permeability of the peritoneal membrane after using hypertonic peritoneal dialysis fluid. J Clin Invest 48:992, 1969.

288. Dedrick RL, Flessner MF, Collins JM, et al: Is the peritoneum a membrane? ASAIO J 5:1, 1982.

289. Flessner MF, Dedrick RL, Schulz JS: A distributed model of peritoneal-plasma transport: Theoretical considerations. Am J Physiol 246:597, 1984.

290. Werynski A, Lindholm B: A model of solute transport in CAPD: Impact of peritoneal tissue and lymphatic flow. [Abstract]. Blood Purif 5:316, 1987.

291. Lindholm B, Werynski A, Bergstrom J: Kinetics of peritoneal dialysis with glycerol and glucose as osmotic agents. ASAIO J 33:19, 1987.

292. Lindholm B, Werynski A, Bergstrom J: Peritoneal dialysis with amino acid solutions: Fluid and solute transport kinetics. Artif Organs 12:2, 1988.

293. Henderson LW, Leypolt JK: Ultrafiltration with peritoneal dialysis. *In* Nolph KD (ed): Peritoneal Dialysis, 3rd ed. Boston, Kluwer Academic, 1990, p 117.

294. Waniewski J, Werynski AN: A comparative analysis of mass transport models in peritoneal dialysis. ASAIO J 37:65, 1991.

295. Vonesh EF, Lysaght MJ, Moran MJ, et al: Kinetic modeling as a prescription aid in peritoneal dialysis. Blood Purif 9:246, 1991.

296. Rippe B: A three-pore model of peritoneal transport. Perit Dial Int 13:S35, 1993.

297. Rippe B, Stelin G: Simulations of peritoneal solute transport during CAPD. Application of two-pore-formalism. Kidney Int 35:1234-1244, 1989.
298. Popovich RP, Moncrief JW: Kinetic modeling of peritoneal transport. Contrib Nephrol 17:59, 1979.
299. Nolph KD: The first hemodialyzer. ASAIO J 1:2, 1978.
300. Felt J, Richard C, McCaffrey C, et al: Peritoneal clearance of creatinine and inulin in dogs: Effect of splanchnic vasodilators. Kidney Int 16:459, 1979.
301. Granger DN, Ulrich M, Perry MA, Kvietys PR: Peritoneal dialysis solutions and feline splanchnic blood flow. Clin Exp Pharmacol Physiol 11:437, 1984.
302. Nolph KD, Ghods AJ, Brubaker PH, et al: Effects of nitroprusside on peritoneal mass transfer coefficients and microvascular physiology. ASAIO J 23:210, 1977.
303. Henderson LW, Cheung A, Chenoweth DE: Choosing a membrane. Am J Kidney Dis 3:5, 1983.
304. Twardowski Z, Nolph KD, Khanna R, et al: Peritoneal equilibration test. Perit Dial Bull 7:138, 1987.
305. Pannekeet NM, Imholz ALT, Struijk DG, et al: The standard peritoneal permeability analysis: A tool for the assessment of peritoneal permeability characteristics in CAPD patients. Kidney Int 48:866, 1995.
306. Boen ST: Kinetics of peritoneal dialysis. Medicine (Baltimore) 40:243, 1961.
307. Kablitz C, Stephen RL, Duff DP, et al: Technological augmentation of peritoneal urea clearance: Past, present, and future. Dial Transplant 9:741, 1980.
308. Kim DJ, Do JH, Huh W, et al: Dissociation between clearances of small and middle molecule in incremental peritoneal dialysis. Perit Dial Int 21:462-466, 2001.
309. Renkin EM: Relation of capillary morphology to transport of fluid and large molecules: A review. Acta Physiol Scand 463:81, 1979.
310. Tzamaoukas AH, Saddler MC, Murata GH, et al: Symptomatic fluid retention in patients on continuous ambulatory dialysis. J Am Soc Nephrol 6:198-206, 1995.
311. Frankenfield DL, Prowant BF, Flanigan MJ, et al: Trends in clinical indicators of care for adult peritoneal dialysis patients in the U.S. Kidney Int 55:1998-2010, 1999.
312. Cochi R, Esposti ED, Fabbri A, et al: Prevalence of hypertension in patients on peritoneal dialysis. Nephrol Dial Transplant 14:1536-1540, 1999.
313. Mactier RA, Khanna R, Twardowski Z, et al: Contribution of lymphatic absorption to loss of ultrafiltration and solute clearances in continuous ambulatory peritoneal dialysis. J Clin Invest 80:1311-1316, 1987.
314. Imholz ALT, Koomen GCM, Struijk DG: Residual volume measurements in CAPD patients with exogenous and endogenous solutes. Adv Perit Dial 8:33-38, 1992.
315. Krediet RT, Imholz ALT, Struijk DG, et al: Ultrafiltration failure in continuous ambulatory peritoneal dialysis. Perit Dial Int 13(suppl):59, 1993.
316. Twardowski Z, Khanna R, Nolph KD, et al: Intraabdominal pressures during natural activities in patients treated with continuous ambulatory peritoneal dialysis. Nephron 44:129-135, 1986.
317. Flessner MF, Schwab A: Pressure threshold for fluid loss from the peritoneal cavity. Am J Physiol 270:F377, 1996.
318. Mujais S, Vonesh E: Profiling of peritoneal ultrafiltration. Kidney Int Suppl 81:17-22, 2002.
319. Ahearn DJ, Nolph KD: Controlled sodium removal with peritoneal dialysis. ASAIO Trans 28:423, 1972.
320. Rubin J, Klein E, Bower JD: Investigation of the net sieving coefficient of the peritoneal membrane during peritoneal dialysis. ASAIO J 28:9, 1982.
321. Staverman AJ: The theory of measurement of osmotic pressure. Rec Trav Chim 70:344, 1951.
322. Rippe B, Perry MA, Granger DN: Permselectivity of the peritoneal membrane. Microvasc Res 29:89, 1985.
323. Jaffrin MY, Odell RA, Farrell PC: A model of ultrafiltration and glucose mass transfer kinetics in peritoneal dialysis. Artif Organs 11:198, 1987.
324. Nakanishi TY, Tanaka Y, Fuyjii M, et al: Nonequilibrium thermodynamics of glucose transport in continuous ambulatory peritoneal dialysis. In Maekawa M, Nolph KD, Kishimoto T, et al (eds): Machine Free Dialysis for Patient Convenience. Cleveland, OH, ISAO Press, 1984, pp 39-44.
325. Seames EL, Moncrief JW, Popovich RP: A distributed model of fluid and mass transfer in peritoneal dialysis. Am J Physiol 258:R958, 1990.
326. Popovich RP, Pyle WK: Kinetics of peritoneal transport. In Nolph KD (ed): Peritoneal Dialysis. The Hague, The Netherlands, Martinus Nijhoff, 1981, p 79.
327. Rubin J, Nolph KD, Popovich RP, et al: Drainage volumes during CAPD. ASAIO J 2:54, 1979.
328. Twardowski Z: Nightly peritoneal dialysis (why? who? how? and when?). ASAIO J 36:8, 1990.
329. Lysaght MJ, Moran J, Lysaght CB, et al: Plasma water filtration and lymphatic uptake during peritoneal dialysis. ASAIO J 37:M402, 1991.
330. Koomen GC, Krediet RT, Leegwater AC, et al: A fast reliable method for the measurement of intraperitoneal dextran 70, used to calculate lymphatic absorption. Adv Perit Dial 7:10-14, 1991.
331. Maher JF, Hirszel P: Learning peritoneal physiology by pharmacological manipulation. Perit Dial Int 13(suppl):27, 1993.
332. Maher JF, Hirszel P, Lasrich M: The effect of gastrointestinal hormones on transport by peritoneal dialysis. Kidney Int 16:130, 1979.
333. Maher JF, Hirszel P, Bennett RR, et al: Augmentation of peritoneal hydraulic permeability by amphotericin B: Locus of action. Perit Dial Bull 44:365, 1984.
334. Di Paolo N, Broncristiani U, Capotondo L, et al: Phosphatidylcholine and peritoneal transport during peritoneal dialysis. Nephron 44:365, 1986.
335. DiPaolo N, Capotondo L, Ciccoli L, et al: Phosphatidylcholine: A physiological modulator of the peritoneal membrane. In Avram MM, Giordano C (eds): Ambulatory Peritoneal Dialysis. New York, Plenum, 1990, p 44.
336. Mujais S, Nolph KD, Gokal R, et al: Evaluation and management of ultrafiltration problems in peritoneal dialysis. Perit Dial Int 20(suppl 4):5-21, 2000.
337. Feriani M, Biasioli S, Chiaramonte S, et al: Anatomical bases of peritoneal permeability: A reappraisal: Anatomy of peritoneum. Int J Artif Organs 5:345, 1982.
338. Nolph KD, Hano JE, Teschan PE: Peritoneal sodium transport during hypertonic peritoneal dialysis. Ann Intern Med 70:931, 1969.
339. Miller RB, Tassistro CR: Peritoneal dialysis. N Engl J Med 281:945, 1969.
340. Heimburger O, Waniewski J, Werynski A, et al: Peritoneal transport in CAPD patients with permanent loss of ultrafiltration capacity. Kidney Int 38:495-506, 1990.
341. Allen L: Lymphatics and lymphoid tissue. Annu Rev Physiol 29:197, 1967.
342. Rippe B, Zakaria EI, Riooe A: Transport of tracer albumin (RISA) from the peritoneal cavity to the blood in the rat. Role of diaphragmatic, visceral and parietal pathways. Perit Dial Int 14(suppl 1):7, 1994.
343. Olin T, Saldeen T: The lymphatic pathways from the peritoneal cavity: A lymphangiographic study in the rat. Cancer Res 24:1700, 1964.
344. Twardowski Z, Prowant BF, Nolph KD, et al: High volume, low frequency continuous ambulatory peritoneal dialysis. Kidney Int 23:64-70, 1983.
345. Krediet RT, Boeschoten EW, Struijk DG, et al: Differences in the peritoneal transport of water, solutes, and proteins between dialysis with two and with three liter exchanges. Nephrol Dial Transplant 2:198, 1988.
346. Morris B: The effect of diaphragmatic movement on the absorption of red cells and protein from the peritoneal cavity. Aust J Exp Biol Med Sci 31:239, 1953.
347. Courtice FC, Steinbeck AW: The effects of lymphatic obstruction and of posture on the absorption of protein from the peritoneal cavity. Aust J Exp Biol Med Sci 29:451, 1951.
348. Lindholm B, Heimburger O, Waniewski J, et al: Peritoneal ultrafiltration and fluid reabsorption during peritoneal dialysis. Nephrol Dial Transplant 4:805, 1989.
349. Lindholm B, Werynski A, Bergstrom J: Fluid transport in peritoneal dialysis. Int J Artif Organs 13:352, 1990.
350. Stelin G, Rippe B: A phenomenological interpretation of the variation in dialysate volume with dwell time in CAPD. Kidney Int 38:465-472, 1990.
351. Twardowski Z, Ksiazek A, Majdan M, et al: Kinetics of continuous ambulatory peritoneal dialysis (CAPD) with four exchanges per day. Clin Nephrol 15:119, 1981.

352. Heimburger O, Waniewski J, Werynski A, Lindholm B: A quantitative description of solute and fluid transport during peritoneal dialysis. Kidney Int 41:1320-1332, 1992.

353. Twardowski Z, Janicka L: Three exchanges with a 2.5 liter volume for continuous ambulatory peritoneal dialysis. Kidney Int 20:281, 1981.

354. Krediet RT, Struijk DG, Koomen GCM, et al: The disappearance of macromolecules from the peritoneal cavity during continuous ambulatory peritoneal dialysis (CAPD) is not dependent on molecular size. Perit Dial Int 10:147-152, 1990.

355. Struijk DG, Krediet RT, Koomen GCM, et al: Indirect measurement of lymphatic absorption with inulin in continuous ambulatory peritoneal dialysis (CAPD) patients. Perit Dial Int 10:141-146, 1990.

356. Rubin J, Planch A: Absorption of sulfamethoxazole and albumin from the peritoneal cavity. ASAIO J 36:834-837, 1990.

357. Mactier RA, Khanna R: Peritoneal cavity lymphatics. *In* Nolph KD (ed): Peritoneal Dialysis, 3rd ed. Boston, Kluwer Academic, 1990, pp 48-66.

358. Maher JF: Lubrication of the peritoneum. Perit Dial Int 12:346, 1992.

359. Farrell PC, Randerson DH: Mass transfer kinetics in continuous ambulatory peritoneal dialysis. *In* Legram M (ed): Proceedings of the First International Symposium on Continuous Ambulatory Peritoneal Dialysis. Amsterdam, Excerpta Medica, 1980, pp 34-41.

360. Pyle WK, Popovich RP: Mass transfer in peritoneal dialysis. *In* Gahl GM, Kessel M, Nolph KD (eds): Advances in Peritoneal Dialysis. Amsterdam, Excerpta Medica, 1981, p 46.

361. Krediet RT, Boeschoten EW, Zuyderhoudt MJ: Simple assessment of the efficacy of peritoneal transport in continuous peritoneal dialysis patients. Blood Purif 4:194, 1986.

362. Verger C, Larpen L, Dumontet M: Prognostic values of peritoneal equilibration curves in CAPD patients. In Frontiers in Peritoneal Dialysis. New York, Field, Rich, 1986, p 88.

363. Teixido J, Cofan F, Borras M, et al: Mass transfer coefficient: Comparison between methods. Perit Dial Int 13(suppl):47, 1993.

364. Vonesh E, Burkart JM, McMurray SD, et al: Peritoneal dialysis kinetic modeling: Validation in a multicenter clinical study. Perit Dial Int 16:471, 1996.

365. Verger C, Larpent L, Veniez G, et al: Monitoring of the peritoneal permeability in peritoneal dialysis. Rev Pract 41:1086, 1991.

366. Korbet S: Evaluation of ultrafiltration failure. Adv Ren Replace Ther 5:194, 1998.

367. Burkart JM, Jordan JR, Rocco MV: Assessment of dialysis dose by measured clearance versus extrapolated data. Perit Dial Int 13:184, 1993.

368. Krediet RT, Boeschoten EW, Zuyderhoudt FMJ, et al: Peritoneal transport characteristics of water, low-molecular weight solutes and proteins during long-term continuous ambulatory peritoneal dialysis. Perit Dial Bull 6:61-65, 1986.

369. Chan PCK, Chan CY, Wu PG, et al: Long-term peritoneal clearances in patients on continuous ambulatory peritoneal dialysis. Int J Artif Organs 13:707-708, 1990.

370. Lameire NH, Vanholder R, Veyt D, et al: A longitudinal, five-year survey of urea kinetic parameters in CAPD patients. Kidney Int 42:426, 1992.

371. Selgas R, Bajo MA, Paiva A, et al: Stability of the peritoneal membrane in long-term peritoneal dialysis patients. Adv Ren Replace Ther 5:168, 1998.

372. Ota K, Mineshima M, Watanabe N, et al: Functional deterioration of the peritoneum: Does it occur in the absence of peritonitis? Nephrol Dial Transplant 2:30, 1987.

373. Struijk DG, Krediet RT, Koomen GCM, et al: Functional characteristics of the peritoneal membrane in long-term continuous ambulatory peritoneal dialysis. Nephron 59:213, 1991.

374. Davies SJ, Phillips L, Naish PF, Gussel GI: Peritoneal glucose exposure and changes in membrane solute transport with time on peritoneal dialysis. J Am Soc Nephrol 12:1046-1051, 2001.

375. Lo W, Brendolan A, Prowant B, et al: Changes in the PET in selected CAPD patients. J Am Soc Nephrol 4:1466, 1994.

376. Ho-dac-Pannekeet MM, Koopmans JG, Struijk DG, Krediet RT: Restriction coefficients of low molecular weight solutes and macromolecules during peritoneal dialysis. Adv Perit Dial 13:17-22, 1997.

377. Coles GA, Toplet N: Long-term peritoneal membrane changes. Adv Ren Replace Ther 4:289-301, 2000.

378. Selgas R, Madero R, Munoz J, et al: Functional peculiarities of the peritoneum in diabetes mellitus. Dial Transplant 42:133, 1988.

379. Zimmerman AL, Sablay LB, Aynedjian HS, et al: Increased peritoneal permeability in rats with alloxan-induced diabetes mellitus. J Lab Clin Med 103:720, 1984.

380. Lee HB, Park MS, Chung SH: Peritoneal solute clearances in diabetes. Perit Dial Int 10:85, 1990.

381. Rubin J, Reed V, Adair C, et al: Effect of intraperitoneal insulin on solute kinetics in CAPD: Insulin kinetics on CAPD. Am J Med Sci 291:81, 1986.

382. Mujias S, Nolph KD, Gokal R, et al: Evaluation and management of ultrafiltration problems in peritoneal dialysis. Perit Dial Int 20(suppl 4): 5-21, 2000.

383. Gokal R: Newer peritoneal dialysis solutions. Adv Ren Replace Ther 7:302-309, 2000.

384. Oreopoulos DG, Tzamaloukas AH: Peritoneal dialysis in the next millennium. Adv Ren Replace Ther 7:338-346, 2000.

385. NKF-K/DOQI Clinical Practice Guidelines for Peritoneal Dialysis Adequacy. New York, National Kidney Foundation, 2000, pp 78-79.

386. Zawada EJ: Indications for dialysis. *In* Daugirdas J, Ing T (ed): Handbook of Dialysis. Toronto, Little, Brown, 1994, pp 6-7.

387. Korbet S, Rodby R: Peritoneal membrane failure: Differential diagnosis, evaluation, and treatment. Semin Dial 7:128-137, 1994.

388. Pritchard S: Treatment modality selection in 150 consecutive patients starting ESRD therapy. Perit Dial Int 16:69-72, 1996.

389. Charytan C, Spinowitz B: Dialysate leaks. *In* Nissenson AR, Fine R (eds): Dialysis Therapy. Philadelphia, Hanley & Belfus, 1993, pp 188-189.

390. NKF-K/DOQI Clinical Practice Guidelines for Peritoneal Dialysis Adequacy. New York, National Kidney Foundation, 2001, p 80.

391. Zappacosta A, Perras S: The process of prescribing CAPD. *In* Peritoneal Dialysis. Philadelphia, JB Lippincott, 1984, pp 4-23.

392. Gulanikar AC, Jindal KK, Hirsch DJ: Is chronic peritoneal dialysis safe in patients with intra-abdominal prosthetic vascular grafts? Nephrol Dial Transplant 6:215, 1991.

393. Schmidt RJ, Cruz C, Dumler F: Effective continuous ambulatory peritoneal dialysis following abdominal aortic aneurysm repair. Perit Dial Int 13:40, 1993.

394. Centers for Medicare & Medicaid Services: 2001 Annual Report, End-Stage Renal Disease Clinical Performance Measures Project. Baltimore, Department of Health and Human Services, Centers for Medicare & Medicaid Services, Center for Beneficiary Choices, December 2001.

395. Health Care Financing Administration: 1997 Annual Report, End Stage Renal Disease Core Indicators Project. Baltimore, Department of Health and Human Services, Health Care Financing Administration, Office of Clinical Standards and Quality, December 1996, 2002.

396. Popovich RP, Moncrief JW, Nolph KD, et al: Continuous ambulatory peritoneal dialysis. Ann Intern Med 88:449-456, 1978.

397. Twardowski Z, Prowant BF, Nolph KD, et al: Chronic nightly tidal peritoneal dialysis (NTDP). ASAIO J 36:M584-M588, 1990.

398. Perez RA, Blake PG, McMurray SD, et al: What is the optimal frequency of cycling in automated peritoneal dialysis? Perit Dial Int 20:548-556, 2000.

399. Juergensen PH, Murphy AL, Pherson KA, et al: Tidal peritoneal dialysis: Comparison of different tidal regimens and automated peritoneal dialysis. Kidney Int 57:2603-2607, 2000.

400. Fernandez RAM, Vega DN, Palop CL, et al: Adequacy of dialysis in automated peritoneal dialysis: A clinical experience. Perit Dial Int 17:435-439, 1997.

401. Juergensen PH, Murphy AL, Pherson KA, et al: Tidal peritoneal dialysis to achieve comfort in chronic peritoneal dialysis patients. Adv Perit Dial 15:125-126, 1999.

402. Twardowski ZJ: Clinical value of standardized equilibration tests in CAPD patients. Blood Purif 7:95-108, 1989.

403. Rodby RA, Firanek CA, Sarpolis AL: Re-evaluation of solute transport groups using the peritoneal equilibration test. Perit Dial Int 19:438-441, 1999.

404. Twardowski Z, Nolph KD, Khanna R, et al: Daily clearances with continuous ambulatory peritoneal dialysis and nightly peritoneal dialysis. ASAIO J 32:575-580, 1986.

405. Rose BD: Clinical Physiology of Acid-Base and Electrolyte Disorders, 2nd ed. New York, McGraw-Hill, 1984, p 33.

406. Ikizler TA, Greene JH, Wingard RL, et al: Spontaneous dietary protein intake during progression of chronic renal failure. J Am Soc Nephrol 6:1386-1391, 1995.

407. Pollack CA: Protein intake in renal disease. J Am Soc Nephrol 8:777-783, 1997.

408. McCusker FM, Teehan BP, Thrope K, et al: How much peritoneal dialysis is required for the maintenance of a good nutritional state? Canada-USA (CANUSA) Peritoneal Dialysis Study Group. Kidney Int Suppl 56:56-61, 1996.

409. Kopple JD, Chumlea WC, Gassman JJ, et al: Relationship between GFR and nutritional status—results from the MDRD study [abstract]. J Am Soc Nephrol 5:335, 1994.

410. Hakim RM, Lazarus JM: Initiation of dialysis. J Am Soc Nephrol 6:1319-1328, 1995.

411. Pollock CA, Ibels LS, Zhu FY, et al: Protein intake in renal disease. J Am Soc Nephrol 8:777-783, 1997.

412. NKF-K/DOQI Clinical Practice Guidelines for Peritoneal Dialysis Adequacy. New York, National Kidney Foundation, 2001, p 23.

413. Keshaviah P, Emerson P, Nolph KD: Timely initiation of dialysis: A urea kinetic approach. Am J Kidney Dis 33:344, 1999.

414. Golper T: Incremental dialysis [abstract]. J Am Soc Nephrol 9:107, 1998.

415. Burkart JM, Jordan J: Initial clinical experience with timely/incremental dialysis [abstract]. Perit Dial Int 19(suppl 1):51, 1999.

416. Williams PF: Timely initiation of dialysis [letter]. Am J Kidney Dis 34:594, 1999.

417. Gotch FA, Keen M: Kinetic modeling in peritoneal dialysis. In Nissenson AR, Fine RN, Gentile DE (eds): Clinical Dialysis. Norwalk, CT, Appleton & Lange, 1995, pp 343-375.

418. NKF/K/DOQI Clinical Practice Guidelines for Peritoneal Dialysis Adequacy. New York, National Kidney Foundation, 2001, p 26.

419. NKF-K/DOQI Clinical Practice Guidelines for Peritoneal Dialysis Adequacy. New York, National Kidney Foundation, 2001, p 28.

420. NKF-K/DOQI Clinical Practice Guidelines for Peritoneal Dialysis Adequacy. New York, National Kidney Foundation, 2001, p 29.

421. NKF-K/DOQI Clinical Practice Guidelines for Peritoneal Dialysis Adequacy. New York National Kidney Foundation, 2001, p 31.

422. NKF-K/DOQI Clinical Practice Guidelines for Peritoneal Dialysis Adequacy. New York, National Kidney Foundation, 2001, p 40.

423. NKF-K/DOQI Clinical Practice Guidelines for Peritoneal Dialysis Adequacy. New York, National Kidney Foundation, 2001, p 39.

424. NKF-K/DOQI Clinical Practice Guidelines for Peritoneal Dialysis Adequacy. New York, National Kidney Foundation, 2001, p 36.

425. Watson PE, Watson ID, Batt RD: Total body water volumes for adult makes and females estimated from simple anthropometric measurements. Am J Clin Nutr 33:27-39, 1980.

426. Hume R, Weyers E: Relationship between total body water and surface area in normal and obese subjects. J Clin Pathol 24:234-238, 1971.

427. Mellits ED, Cheek DB: The assessment of body water and fatness from infancy to adulthood. Monographs Soc Res Child Dev Series 140 35:12-26, 1970.

428. Du Bois D, Du Bois EF: A formula to estimate the approximate surface area if height and weight be known. Arch Intern Med 17:863-871, 1916.

429. Gehan E, George SL: Estimation of human body surface area from height and weight. Cancer Chemother Rep 5:225-235, 1970.

430. Haycock GB, Chir B, Schwartz GJ, Wisotsky DH: Geometric method for measuring body surface area: A height-weight formula validated in infants, children and adults. J Pediatr 93:62-66, 1978.

431. NKF-K/DOQI Clinical Practice Guidelines for Peritoneal Dialysis Adequacy. New York, National Kidney Foundation, 2001, p 37.

432. NKF-K/DOQI Clinical Practice Guidelines for Peritoneal Dialysis Adequacy. New York, National Kidney Foundation, 2001, p 47.

433. NKF-K/DOQI Clinical Practice Guidelines for Peritoneal Dialysis Adequacy. New York, National Kidney Foundation, 2001, p 50.

434. NKF-K/DOQI Clinical Practice Guidelines for Peritoneal Dialysis Adequacy. New York, National Kidney Foundation, 2001, p 51.

435. Churchill DN, Taylor DW, Keshaviah P: Adequacy of dialysis and nutrition in continuous peritoneal dialysis: Association with clinical outcomes. J Am Soc Nephrol 7:198-207, 1996.

436. Bargman JM, Thrope KE, Churchill DN: The importance of residual renal function for survival in patients on peritoneal dialysis. For the CANUSA Peritoneal Dialysis Study Group [abstract]. J Am Soc Nephrol 8:185, 1997.

437. Diaz-Buxo JA, Lowrie EG, Lew NL, et al: Associates of mortality among peritoneal dialysis patients with special reference to peritoneal transport rates and solute clearance. Am J Kidney Dis 33:523-534, 1999.

438. Rocco MV, Soucie JM, Pastan S, McClellan WM: Peritoneal dialysis adequacy and risk of death. Kidney Int 58:446-457, 2000.

439. Rocco MV, Frankenfield DL, Prowant B, et al: Risk factors for early mortality in U.S. peritoneal dialysis patients: Impact of residual renal function. Perit Dial Int 22:371-379, 2002.

440. Bargman JM, Thrope KE, Churchill DN: Relative contribution of residual renal function and peritoneal clearance to adequacy of dialysis: A reanalysis of the CANUSA study. J Am Soc Nephrol 12:2158-2162, 2001.

441. Szeto CC, Wong TYH, Leung CB, et al: Importance of dialysis adequacy in mortality and morbidity of Chinese CAPD patients. Kidney Int 58:400-407, 2000.

442. Jager KJ, Merkus MP, Dekker FW, et al: Mortality and technique failure in patients starting chronic peritoneal dialysis: Results of the Netherlands Cooperative Study on the Adequacy. Kidney Int 55:1476-1485, 1999.

443. Merkus MP, Jager KJ, Dekker FW, et al: Physical symptoms and quality of life in patients on chronic dialysis: Results of The Netherlands Cooperative Study on Adequacy of Dialysis (NECOSAD). Nephrol Dial Transplant 14:1163-1170, 1999.

444. Szeto CC, Wong TYH, Chow KM, et al: Impact of dialysis adequacy on the mortality and morbidity of anuric Chinese patients receiving continuous ambulatory peritoneal dialysis. J Am Soc Nephrol 12:255-260, 2001.

445. Bhaskaran S, Schaubel DE, Jassal SV, et al: The effect of small solute clearances on survival of anuric peritoneal dialysis patients. Perit Dial Int 20:181-187, 2000.

446. Churchill DN: The ADEMEX study: Make haste slowly. J Am Soc Nephrol 13:1415-1418, 2002.

447. Satko SG, Burkart JM, Bleyer AJ, et al: Frequency and causes of discrepancy between Kt/V and creatinine clearance. Perit Dial Int 19:31-37, 1999.

448. Tzamaloukas AH, Malhotra D, Murata GH: Gender, degree of obesity and discrepancy between urea and creatinine clearance in peritoneal dialysis. J Am Soc Nephrol 9:497-499, 1998.

449. NKF-K/DOQI Clinical Practice Guidelines for Peritoneal Dialysis Adequacy. New York, National Kidney Foundation, 2001, p 52.

450. Tzamaloukas AH, Gibel LJ, Eisenberg B, et al: Early and late peritoneal dialysate leaks in patients on CAPD. Adv Perit Dial 6:64-70, 1990.

451. Rocco MV, Jordan JR, Burkart JM: Changes in peritoneal transport during the first month of peritoneal dialysis. Perit Dial Int 15:12-17, 1995.

452. Rocco MV, Jordan JR, Burkart JM: Determination of peritoneal transport characteristics using 24 hour dialysate collections. J Am Soc Nephrol 5:1333-1338, 1994.

453. Rocco MV, Jordan JR, Burkart JM: 24 hour dialysate collection for the determination of peritoneal membrane transport characteristics: Longitudinal follow-up data for the dialysis adequacy and transport test (DATT). Perit Dial Int 16:593, 1996.

454. Diaz-Buxo JA, Gotch FA, Folden T, et al: Peritoneal dialysis adequacy: A model to assess feasibility with various modalities. Kidney Int 55:2493-2501, 1999.

455. Diaz-Buxo JA: Continuous cycling peritoneal dialysis, PD plus, and high-flow automated peritoneal dialysis: A spectrum of therapies. Perit Dial Int 20(suppl 2):93-97, 2000.

456. Rocco MV: Body surface areas limitations in achieving adequate therapy in peritoneal dialysis patients. Perit Dial Int 16:617-622, 1996.

457. Johnston JR, Bernardini J: Effect of increasing exchange volume or frequency on CAPD efficiency. Adv Perit Dial 11:97-100, 1995.

458. Harty J, Gokal R: The impact of peritoneal permeability and residual renal function on PD prescription. Perit Dial Int 16(suppl 1):147-152, 1996.

459. Fukatsu A, Komatsu Y, Senoh H, et al: Clinical benefits and tolerability of increased fill volumes in Japanese peritoneal dialysis patients. Perit Dial Int 21:455-461, 2001.

460. Harty J, Boulton H, Venning M, Gokal R: Impact of increasing dwell volume on adequacy targets: A prospective study. J Am Soc Nephrol 8:1304-1310, 1997.

461. Sarkar S, Bernardini J, Fried LF, et al: Tolerance of large exchange volumes by peritoneal dialysis patients. Am J Kidney Dis 33:1136-1141, 1999.

462. de Jesus Ventura M, Amato D, Correa-Rotter R, Paniagua R: Relationship between fill volume, intraperitoneal pressure, body size, and subjective discomfort perception in CAPD patients. Mexican Nephrology Collaborative Study Group. Perit Dial Int 20:188-193, 2000.

463. Gao H, Lew SQ, Bosch JP: The effects of increasing exchange volume and frequency on peritoneal dialysis adequacy. Clin Nephrol 50:375-380, 1998.

464. Brown-Cartwright D, Smith HJ, Feldman M: Gastric emptying of an indigestible solid in patients with end-stage renal disease on continuous ambulatory peritoneal dialysis. Gastroenterology 95:49, 1988.

465. Bird NJ, Streather CP, O'Doherty MJ, et al: Gastric emptying in patients with chronic renal failure on continuous ambulatory peritoneal dialysis. Nephrol Dial Transplant 9:287-290, 1994.

466. Fernstrom A, Hylander B, Gryback P, et al: Gastric emptying and electrogastrography in patients on CAPD. Perit Dial Int 19:429-437, 1999.

467. Kim MJ, Kwon KH, Lee SW: Gastroesophageal reflux disease in CAPD patients. Adv Perit Dial 14:98-101, 1998.

468. Seibert DG, Moss AH, Holley JL, Foulks CJ: Intraperitoneal metoclopramide improves symptoms of gastroparesis in a CAPD patient. Perit Dial Int 9:223-224, 1989.

469. Wadhwa NK, Atkins H, Cabralda T: Intraperitoneal erythromycin for gastroparesis. Ann Intern Med 114:912, 1991.

470. Gallar P, Oliet A, Vigil A, et al: Gastroparesis: An important cause of hospitalization in continuous ambulatory peritoneal dialysis patients and the role of erythromycin. Perit Dial Int 13(suppl 2):183-186, 1993.

471. Hunt RH: Importance of pH control in the management of GERD. Arch Intern Med 159:649-657, 1999.

472. Tzamaloukas AH, Dimitriadis A, Murata GH, et al: Continuous peritoneal dialysis in heavyweight individuals: Urea and creatinine clearances. Perit Dial Int 16:302-306, 1996.

473. DeMars S: CAPD with 5 liter exchanges. Perit Dial Int 19(suppl 1):52, 1999.

474. Rocco MV, Frankenfield DL, Prowant BF, et al: Response to inadequate dialysis in chronic peritoneal dialysis patients. Results from the 2000 Centers for Medicare and Medicaid (CMS) ESRD Peritoneal Dialysis Clinical Performance Measures (PD-CPM) Project. Am J Kidney Dis 41:840-848, 2003.

475. Young GA, Kopple JD, Lindholm B, et al: Nutritional assessment of CAPD patients: An international study. Am J Kidney Dis 17:462-471, 1991.

476. CANADA-USA (CANUSA) Peritoneal Dialysis Study Group: Adequacy of dialysis and nutrition in continuous peritoneal dialysis: Association with clinical outcomes. J Am Soc Nephrol 7:198-207, 1996.

477. Marckmann P: Nutritional status of patients on hemodialysis and peritoneal dialysis. Clin Nephrol 29:75-78, 1988.

478. Chung SH, Lindholm B, Lee HB: Influence of initial nutritional status on continuous ambulatory peritoneal dialysis patient survival. Perit Dial Int 20:19-26, 2000.

479. Tan SH, Lee EJ, Tay ME, Leo BK: Protein nutrition status of adult patients starting chronic ambulatory peritoneal dialysis. Adv Perit Dial 16:291-293, 2000.

480. Passadakis P, Thodis E, Vargemezis V, Oreopoulos DG: Nutrition in diabetic patients undergoing continuous ambulatory peritoneal dialysis. Perit Dial Int 19(suppl 2):248-254, 1999.

481. Mehrotra R, Kopple JD: Nutritional management of maintenance dialysis patients: Why aren't we doing better? Annu Rev Nutr 21:343-379, 2001.

482. Kopple JD, Greene T, Chumlea WC, et al: Relationship between GFR and nutritional status—results from the MDRD study. Kidney Int 57:1688-1703, 2000.

483. Stenvinkel P, Heimburger O, Paultre F, et al: Strong association between malnutrition, inflammation and atherosclerosis in chronic renal failure. Kidney Int 55:1899-1911, 1999.

484. Stenvinkel P, Heimburger O, Lindholm B, et al: Are there two types of malnutrition in chronic renal failure? Evidence for relationships between malnutrition, inflammation and atherosclerosis (MIA syndrome). Nephrol Dial Transplant 2000:953-960, 2000.

485. Kaysen GA, Stevenson FT, Depner T: Determinants of albumin concentration in hemodialysis patients. Am J Kidney Dis 29:658-668, 1997.

486. Kaysen GA, Rathore V, Shearer GC, Depter TA: Mechanism of hypoalbuminemia in hemodialysis patients. Kidney Int 48:510-516, 1995.

487. Gilbert R, Goyal RK: The gastrointestinal system. In Eknoyan G, Knochel JP (eds): The Systemic Consequences of Renal Failure. New York, Grune & Stratton, 1984, p 133.

488. Noh H, Lee SW, Kang SW, Shin SK, et al: Serum C-reactive protein: A predictor of mortality in continuous ambulatory peritoneal dialysis patients. Nephrol Dial Transplant 18:387-394, 1998.

489. Haubitz M, Brunkhorst R: C-reactive protein and chronic Chlamydia pneumoniae infection—long term predictors for cardiovascular disease survival in patients on peritoneal dialysis. Nephrol Dial Transplant 16:809-815, 2001.

490. Ducloux D, Bresson-Vautrin C, Kribs M, et al: C-reactive protein and cardiovascular disease in peritoneal dialysis patients. Kidney Int 62:1417-1422, 2002.

491. Herzig KA, Purdie DM, Chang W, et al: Is C-reactive protein a useful predictor of outcome in peritoneal dialysis patients? J Am Soc Nephrol 12:814-821, 2001.

492. Guttridge DC, Mayo MW, Madrid LV, et al: NF-κB–induced loss of MyoD messenger RNA: Possible role in muscle decay and cachexia. Science 289:2363-2365, 2000.

493. Mitch WE, Du J, Bailey JL, Price SR: Mechanisms causing muscle proteolysis in uremia: The influence of insulin and cytokines. Miner Electrolyte Metab 25:216-219, 1999.

494. Aguilera A, Codoceo R, Selgas R, et al: Anorexigen (TNF-alpha, cholecystokinin) and orexigen (neuropeptide Y) plasma levels in peritoneal dialysis (PD) patients. Their relationship with nutritional parameters. Nephrol Dial Transplant 13:1476-1483, 1998.

495. Flanigan MJ, Rocco MV, Prowant B, et al: Clinical performance measures: The changing status of peritoneal dialysis. Kidney Int 60:2377-2384, 2001.

496. Nakamoto H, Imai H, Kawanishi H, et al: Low serum albumin in elderly continuous ambulatory peritoneal dialysis patients is attributable to high permeability of peritoneum. Adv Perit Dial 17:238-243, 2001.

497. Sezer S, Ozdemir FN, Akman B, et al: Predictors of serum albumin level in patients receiving continuous ambulatory peritoneal dialysis. Adv Perit Dial 17:210-214, 2001.

498. Tzamaloukas AH, Oreopoulos DG, Murata GH, et al: The relation between nutrition indices and age in patients on continuous ambulatory peritoneal dialysis receiving similar small solute clearances. Int Urol Nephrol 32:449-458, 2001.

499. Kung SC, Morse SA, Bloom E, Raja RM: Acid-base balance and nutrition in peritoneal dialysis. Adv Perit Dial 17:235-237, 2001.

500. Kang DH, Yoon KI, Choi KB, et al: Relationship of peritoneal membrane transport characteristics to the nutritional status in CAPD patients. Nephrol Dial Transplant 14:1715-1722, 1999.

501. Nolph KD, Moore H, Prowant B, et al: Continuous ambulatory peritoneal dialysis with a high-flux membrane. ASAIO J 39:904-909, 1993.

502. Nolph KD, Moore HL, Prowant B, et al: Cross sectional assessment of weekly urea and creatinine clearances and indices of nutrition in continuous ambulatory peritoneal dialysis patients. Perit Dial Int 13:178-183, 1993.

503. Jager KJ, Merkus MP, Huisman RM, et al: Nutritional status over time in hemodialysis and peritoneal dialysis. J Am Soc Nephrol 12:1272-1279, 2001.

504. Szeto CC, Law MC, Wong TYH, et al: Peritoneal transport status correlates with morbidity but not longitudinal change of nutritional status of continuous ambulatory peritoneal dialysis patients: A 2-year prospective study. Am J Kidney Dis 37:329-336, 2001.

505. NKF-K/DOQI Clinical Practice Guidelines for Nutrition in Chronic Renal Failure. New York, National Kidney Foundation, 2001, p 43.

506. Bergstrom J, Lindholm B: Nutrition and adequacy of dialysis. How do hemodialysis and CAPD compare? Kidney Int Suppl 40:39-50, 1993.

507. Nolph KD: What's new in peritoneal dialysis—an overview. Kidney Int Suppl 38:148-152, 1992.

508. Wang AYM, Sea MM, Ip R, et al: Independent effects of residual renal function and dialysis adequacy on actual dietary protein, calorie and other nutrient intake in patients on continuous ambulatory peritoneal dialysis. J Am Soc Nephrol 12:2450-2457, 2001.

509. Lim VS, Flanigan MJ: Protein intake in patients with renal failure: Comments on the current NKF-DOQI guidelines for nutrition in chronic renal failure. Semin Dial 14:150-152, 2001.

510. Uribarri J: DOQI guidelines for nutrition in long-term peritoneal dialysis patients: A dissenting view. Am J Kidney Dis 37:1313-1318, 2001.

511. Uribarri J: The obsession with high dietary protein intake in ESRD patients on dialysis: Is it justified? Nephron 86:105-108, 2000.

512. Blumenkrantz M, Gahl GM, Kopple JD, et al: Protein losses during peritoneal dialysis. Kidney Int 19:593-602, 1981.

513. NKF-K/DOQI Clinical Practice Guidelines for Nutrition in Chronic Renal Failure. New York, National Kidney Foundation, 2001, p 45.

514. Uribarri J, Levin NW, Delmez J, et al: Association of acidosis and nutritional parameters in hemodialysis patients. Am J Kidney Dis 34:493-499, 1999.

515. Grzegorzewska AE, Dobrowolska-Zachwieja A, Chmurak A: Nutritional intake during continuous ambulatory peritoneal dialysis. Adv Perit Dial 13:150-154, 1997.

516. Fernstrom A, Hylander B, Rossner S: Energy intake in patients on continuous ambulatory peritoneal dialysis and haemodialysis. J Intern Med 240:211-218, 1996.

517. Lo WK, Tong KL, Li CS, et al: Relationship between adequacy of dialysis and nutritional status, and their impact on patient survival on CAPD in Hong Kong. Perit Dial Int 21:441-447, 2001.

518. Szeto CC, Wong TYH, Chow KM, et al: The impact of increasing the daytime dialysis exchange frequency on peritoneal dialysis adequacy and nutritional status of Chinese anuric patients. Perit Dial Int 22:197-203, 2002.

519. Harty J, Boulton H, Faragher B, et al: The influence of small solute clearance on dietary protein intake in continuous ambulatory peritoneal dialysis patients: A methodologic analysis based on cross-sectional and prospective studies. Am J Kidney Dis 28:553-560, 1996.

520. Lindsay RM, Spanner E: A hypothesis: The protein catabolic rate is dependent upon the type and amount of treatment in dialyzed uremic patients. Am J Kidney Dis 132:382-389, 1989.

521. Gotch FA: The application of urea kinetic modeling to CAPD. In La Greca G, Ronco C, Feriani M, et al (eds): Peritoneal Dialysis, Proceedings of the Fourth International Course on Peritoneal Dialysis. Milan, Wichtig Editore, 1991, p 47.

522. Harty JC, Farragher B, Boulton H, et al: Is the correlation between normalized protein catabolic rate and Kt/V due to mathematic coupling? J Am Soc Nephrol 4:407, 1993.

523. Mak SK, Wong PN, Lo KY, et al: Randomized prospective study of the effect of increased dialytic dose on nutritional and clinical outcome in continuous ambulatory peritoneal dialysis patients. Am J Kidney Dis 36:105-114, 2000.

524. Davies SJ, Phillips L, Griffiths AM, et al: Analysis of the effects of increasing delivered dialysis treatment to malnourished peritoneal dialysis patients. Kidney Int 57:1743-1754, 2000.

525. Kopple JD: Therapeutic approaches to malnutrition in chronic dialysis patients: The different modalities of nutritional support. Am J Kidney Dis 33:180-185, 1999.

526. Fein PA, Madane SJ, Jorden A, et al: Outcome of percutaneous endoscopic gastrostomy (PEG) feeding in patients on peritoneal dialysis. Adv Perit Dial 17:148-152, 2001.

527. Bansal VK, Popli S, Pickering J, et al: Protein-calorie malnutrition and cutaneous anergy in hemodialysis maintained patients. Am J Clin Nutr 33:1608-1611, 1980.

528. Pickering WP, Price SR, Bircher G, et al: Nutrition in CAPD: Serum bicarbonate and the ubiquitin-proteasome system in muscle. Kidney Int 61:1286-1292, 2002.

529. Saltissi D, Morgan C, Knight B, et al: Effect of lipid-lowering dietary recommendations on the nutritional intake and lipid profiles of chronic peritoneal dialysis and hemodialysis patients. Am J Kidney Dis 37:1209-1215, 2001.

530. Wu CH, Huang CC, Huang JY, et al: High flux peritoneal membrane is risk factor in survival of CAPD treatment. Adv Perit Dial 12:105-109, 1996.

531. Churchill DN, Thrope K, Nolph KD, et al: Increased peritoneal membrane transport is associated with decreased patient and technique survival for continuous peritoneal dialysis patients. J Am Soc Nephrol 9:1285-1292, 1998.

532. Fried LF: Higher membrane permeability predicts poorer patient survival. Perit Dial Int 17:387-389, 1996.

533. Wang T, Heimburger O, Waniewski J, et al: Increased peritoneal permeability is associated with decreased fluid and small solute removal and higher mortality in CAPD patients. Nephrol Dial Transplant 13:1242-1249, 1998.

534. Davies SJ, Phillips L, Russel GI: Peritoneal solute transport predicts survival on CAPD independently of residual renal function. Nephrol Dial Transplant 13:962-968, 1998.

535. Davies SJ, Phillips L, Griffiths AM, Russel GI: Impact of peritoneal membrane function on long-term clinical outcome in peritoneal dialysis patients. Perit Dial Int 19(suppl 2):91-94, 1999.

536. Blake PG, Sombolos K, Izatt S, Oreopoulos DG: Low serum albumin predicts poor outcome in CAPD and is related to high peritoneal permeability [abstract]. J Am Soc Nephrol 1:383, 1990.

537. Heaf JG: CAPD is contraindicated for patients with high peritoneal transport characteristics [abstract]. Nephrol Dial Transplant 14:234, 1999.

538. Heaf JG: Pathogenic effects of a high peritoneal transport rate. Semin Dial 13:188-193, 2000.

539. Heaf J: CAPD adequacy and dialysis morbidity: Detrimental effect of a high peritoneal equilibration rate. Ren Fail 17:575-587, 1995.

540. Blake PG, Flowerdew GF, Blake RM, Oreopoulos DG: Serum albumin in patients on continuous ambulatory peritoneal dialysis—prediction and correlations with outcomes. J Am Soc Nephrol 3:1501-1507, 1993.

541. Selgas R, Bajo MA, Fernandez-Reyes MJ, et al: An analysis of adequacy of dialysis in selected population on CAPD for over 3 years: The influence of urea and creatinine kinetics. Nephrol Dial Transplant 8:1244-1253, 1993.

542. Harty JC, Boulton H, Venning MC, Gokal R: Is peritoneal permeability an adverse risk factor for malnutrition in CAPD patients? Miner Electrolyte Metab 22:97-101, 1996.

543. Malhotra D, Tzamaloukas AH, Murata GH, et al: Serum albumin in continuous peritoneal dialysis: Its predictors and relationship to urea clearance. Kidney Int 50:243-249, 1996.

544. Cueto-Manzano AM, Espinosa S, Hernandez A, Correa-Rotter R: Peritoneal transport kinetics correlate with serum albumin but not with the overall nutritional status in CAPD patients. Am J Kidney Dis 30:229-236, 1997.

545. Pollock CA, Ibels LS, Caterson RJ, et al: Continuous ambulatory peritoneal dialysis. Eight years of experience at a single center. Medicine (Baltimore) 68:293-308, 1989.

546. Heimburger O, Bergstrom J, Lindholm B: Albumin and amino acid levels as markers of adequacy in continuous ambulatory peritoneal dialysis patients. Perit Dial Int 14(suppl 3):123-132, 1994.

547. Kagan A, Bar-Khayim Y: Role of peritoneal loss of albumin in the hypoalbuminemia of continuous ambulatory peritoneal dialysis: Relationship to peritoneal transport of solutes. Nephron 71:314-320, 1995.

548. Kang DH, Yoon KI, Choi KB, et al: Relationship of peritoneal membrane transport characteristics to the nutritional status in CAPD patients. Nephrol Dial Transplant 14:1715-1722, 1999.

549. Kaysen GA, Schoenfeld PY: Albumin homeostasis in patients undergoing continuous ambulatory peritoneal dialysis. Kidney Int 25:107-114, 1984.

550. Park MS, Lee HB: AGE accumulation in peritoneal membrane and cavity during peritoneal dialysis and its effect on peritoneal structure and function. Perit Dial Int 19(suppl 2):5357, 1999.

551. Nakayama M, Kubo H, Ogawa A, et al: Immunohistochemical detection of advanced glycation end products (AGEs) in the peritoneum and its possible pathophysiological role in CAPD. Kidney Int 51:182-186, 1997.

552. Kagan A, Bar-Khayim Y, Schafer Z, Fainaru M: Kinetics of peritoneal protein loss during CAPD. Part II: Lipoprotein leakage and its impact on plasma lipid levels. Kidney Int 37:980-990, 1990.

553. Kagan A, Bar-Khayim Y, Schafer Z, Fainaru M: Heterogeneity in peritoneal transport during continuous ambulatory peritoneal dialysis and its impact on ultrafiltration, loss of macromolecules and plasma level of proteins, lipids and lipoproteins. Nephron 63:32-42, 1993.

554. Lamiere N, Matthys D, Beheyt R: Effects of long-term CAPD on carbohydrate and lipid metabolism. Clin Nephrol 30(suppl 1):53-58, 1988.

555. Heimburger O, Stenvinkel P, Berglund L, et al: Increased plasma lipoprotein(a) in continuous ambulatory peritoneal dialysis is related to peritoneal transport of proteins and glucose. Nephron 72:135-144, 1996.

556. Little J, Phillips L, Russell L, et al: Longitudinal lipid profile on CAPD. Their relationship to weight gain, comorbidity and dialysis factors. J Am Soc Nephrol 9:1931-1939, 1998.

557. Tzamaloukas AH, Saddler MC, Murata GH, et al: Symptomatic fluid retention in patients on continuous peritoneal dialysis. J Am Soc Nephrol 6:198-206, 1995.

558. Blake PG: What is the problem with high transporters? Perit Dial Int 17:317-320, 1997.
559. Mistry CD, Gokal R, Peers E: A randomized multicenter clinical trial comparing isosmolar icodextrin and hyperosmolar glucose solutions in CAPD. MIDAS Study Group. Multicenter Investigation of Icodextrin in Ambulatory Dialysis. Kidney Int 46:496-503, 1994.
560. Burkart JM: Effect of peritoneal dialysis prescription and peritoneal membrane transport characteristics on nutritional status. Perit Dial Int 15(suppl):20-35, 1995.
561. Strauss FG, Holmes DL, Dennis RL: Dialysis adequacy indices in high transporters treated with short-dwell peritoneal dialysis. Perit Dial 15(suppl):47, 1995.
562. Health Care Financing Administration: 1997 Annual Report, End Stage Renal Disease Core Indicators Project. Baltimore, Department of Health and Human Services, Health Care Financing Administration, Office of Clinical Standards and Quality, January 1997.
563. Jagose JT, Afthentopoulos IE, Shetty A, Oreopoulos DG: Successful use of continuous ambulatory peritoneal dialysis in octogenarians. Geriatr Nephrol Urol 5:135-141, 1996.
564. Michel C, Bindi P, Viron B: CAPD with private home nurses: An alternative treatment for elderly and disabled patients. Adv Perit Dial 6(suppl):92-94, 1990.
565. Schleifer CR: Peritoneal dialysis in nursing homes. Adv Perit Dial 6(suppl):86-91, 1990.
566. Mattern WD: Adult day care centers and peritoneal dialysis. Adv Perit Dial 1990(suppl):95-96, 1990.
567. Mignon F, Siohan P, Legallicier B, et al: The management of uremia in the elderly: Treatment choices. Nephrol Dial Transplant 10(suppl 6): 55-59, 1995.
568. Stack AG, Messana JM: Renal replacement therapy in the elderly: Medical, ethical and psychosocial consideration. Adv Ren Replace Ther 7:52-62, 2000.
569. De Vecchi A, Maccario M, Braga M, et al: Peritoneal dialysis in non-diabetic patients older than 70 years: Comparison with patients aged 40 to 60 years. Am J Kidney Dis 31:479-490, 1998.
570. De Vecchi A, Maccario M, Ponticelli C: Peritoneal dialysis in the ninth decade of life: Experience in a single center. Geriatr Nephrol Urol 6:75-80, 1996.
571. Hung KY, Hsu WA, Tsai TJ, et al: Continuous ambulatory peritoneal dialysis in the elderly: A seven-up experience. Postgrad Med J 71:160-162, 1995.
572. Byrne C, Vernon P, Cohen JJ: Effect of age and diagnosis on survival of old patients beginning chronic dialysis. JAMA 271:34-36, 1994.
573. Tsakiris D, Jones EHP, Briggs JD, et al: Deaths within 90 days from starting renal replacement therapy in the ERA-EDTA Registry between 1990-1992. Nephrol Dial Transplant 14:2343-2350, 1999.
574. Gokal R: CAPD in the elderly—European and UK experience. Adv Perit Dial 6(suppl):38-40, 1990.
575. Gorban Brennan N, Kliger AS, Finkelstein FO: CAPD therapy for patients over 80 years of age. Perit Dial Int 13:140-141, 1993.
576. Nissenson AR, Gentile DE, Soderblom R: CAPD in the elderly: Southern California/southern Nevada experience. Adv Perit Dial 6(suppl):51-55, 1990.
577. Gentile DE, Geriatric Advisory Committee: Peritoneal dialysis in geriatric patients: A survey of clinical practices. Adv Perit Dial 6(suppl):29-32, 1990.
578. Segoloni GP, Salomone M, Piccoli G: CAPD in the elderly: Italian multicentric study experience. Adv Perit Dial 6(suppl):41-46, 1990.
579. Baek MY, Kwon TH, Kim YL, Cho DK: CAPD, an acceptable form of therapy in elderly ESRD patients: A comparative study. Adv Perit Dial 13:158-161, 1997.
580. Nolph KD, Lindblad AS, Novak JW, Steinberg SM: Experiences with the elderly in the National CAPD Registry. Adv Perit Dial 6:33-38, 1990.
581. Ross CJ, Rutsky EA: Dialysis modality in the elderly patients with end-stage renal disease: Advantages and disadvantages of peritoneal dialysis. Adv Perit Dial 6(suppl):11-17, 1990.
582. Holley JL, Bernardini J, Perlmutter JA, Piraino B: A comparison of infection rates among older and younger patients on continuous peritoneal dialysis. Perit Dial Int 14:66-69, 1994.
583. Adams PL, Rutsky EA, Rostand SG, Han SY: Lower gastrointestinal dysfunction in patients on chronic hemodialysis. Arch Intern Med 142:303-306, 1982.
584. Bertoli M, Bonfante L, Gambaro G, et al: Peritoneal dialysis in diabetic patients. Contrib Nephrol 131:51-60, 2001.
585. Bloembergen W, Port FK, Mauger E, Wolfe R: A comparison of mortality between patients treated with hemodialysis and peritoneal dialysis. J Am Soc Nephrol 6:177-183, 1995.
586. Keshaviah P, Collins AJ, Ma J, et al: Survival comparison between hemodialysis and peritoneal dialysis based on matched doses of delivered therapy. J Am Soc Nephrol 13(suppl 1):48-52, 2002.
587. Romagnoli GF, Di Landro D, Catalano C, et al: Short-term outcome of diabetic patients in renal replacement therapy. Nephrol Dial Transplant 13(suppl 8):30-34, 1998.
588. Chisholm L: Evolution of retinopathy in diabetics undergoing CAPD. Perit Dial Bull 3(suppl 2):42-47, 1982.
589. Diaz-Buxo JA: Influence of hypertension on vision in diabetics undergoing dialysis: Comparison of peritoneal and haemodialysis. *In* Maher F (ed): Frontiers in Peritoneal Dialysis. Manchester, Field, Rich & Associates, England, 1985, pp 457-468.
590. Rottembourg J: Visual function, blood pressure and blood glucose in diabetic patients undergoing CAPD. Proc Eur Dial Transplant Assoc 21:330-333, 1984.
591. Diaz-Buxo JA, Burgess WP, Greenman M, et al: Visual function in diabetic patients undergoing dialysis: Comparison of peritoneal and haemodialysis. Int J Artif Organs 5:257-262, 1984.
592. Khauli RB, Noviack AC, Steinmuller DR, et al: Comparison of renal transplantation and dialysis in rehabilitation of diabetic end-stage renal disease patients. Urology 6:521-525, 1986.
593. Coronel F, Hostal L, Horcajo P, et al: Complications in diabetic patients on dialysis: Experience in 10 years of treatment using three techniques. Rev Clin Esp 5:225-229, 1989.
594. Tzamaloukas AH, Yuan ZY, Balaskas E, Oreopoulos DG: CAPD in end-stage patients with renal disease due to diabetes mellitus—an update. Adv Perit Dial 8:185-191, 1992.
595. Troidke LK, Gorban Brennan N, Kliger AS, Finkelstein FO: Continuous cycler therapy, manual peritoneal dialysis therapy and peritonitis. Adv Perit Dial 14:137-141, 1998.
596. Lye WC, Leong SO, van der Straaten JC, Lee EJL: A prospective study of peritoneal-related infections in CAPD patients with diabetes mellitus. Adv Perit Dial 9:195-197, 1993.
597. Khanna R, Oreopoulos DG: CAPD in diabetics with end-stage renal disease: A combined experience of two North American centres. *In* Friedman EA (ed): Diabetic Renal Retinal Syndrome. New York, Grune & Stratton, 1986, p 363.
598. Tzamaloukas AH, Friedman EA: Diabetes. *In* Daugirdas JT, Blake PG, Ing TS (eds): Handbook of Dialysis, 3rd ed. Baltimore, Lippincott, Williams & Wilkins, 2001, pp 453-465.
599. Daniels ID, Markell MS: Blood glucose control in diabetics: II. Semin Dial 6:394, 1993.
600. Beardsworth SF: Intraperitoneal insulin: A protocol for administration during CAPD and review of published protocols. Perit Dial Int 8:145, 1988.
601. Scarpioni L, Ballocchi S, Castelli A, Scarpioni R: Insulin therapy in uraemic diabetic patients on CAPD: Comparison of intraperitoneal and subcutaneous administration. Perit Dial Int 14:127-131, 1994.
602. Nevalein PI, Lathela JT, Mustonen J, et al: The effect of insulin delivery route on lipoproteins in type I diabetic patients on CAPD. Perit Dial Int 19:148-153, 1999.
603. Bargman JM: The impact of intraperitoneal glucose and insulin on the liver. Perit Dial Int 16(suppl 1):211-214, 1996.
604. Scalamogna A, Castelnova C, Crepaldi M: Incidence of peritoneal in diabetic patients on CAPD: Intraperitoneal vs subcutaneous insulin therapy. *In* Khanna R (ed): Advances in CAPD. Toronto, Toronto University Press, 1987, pp 167-170.
605. Selgas R, Diez JJ, Munoz J, et al: Comparative study of two different routes for insulin administration in CAPD diabetic patients: A multicenter study. Adv Perit Dial 5:181-184, 1989.
606. Fine A, Parry D, Ariano R, Dent W: Marked variation in peritoneal insulin absorption in peritoneal dialysis. Perit Dial Int 20:652-655, 2000.
607. Wanless IR, Bargman JM, Oreopoulos DG, Vas SI: Subcapsular steatonecrosis in response to peritoneal insulin delivery: A clue to the pathogenesis of steatonecrocsis of obesity. Mod Pathol 2:69-74, 1989.
608. Nevalainen PI, Kallio T, Lahtela JT, et al: High peritoneal permeability predisposes to hepatic steatosis in diabetic continuous ambulatory peritoneal dialysis patients receiving intraperitoneal insulin. Perit Dial Int 20:637-642, 2000.
609. Harrison NA, Rainford DJ: Intraperitoneal insulin and the malignant omentum syndrome. Nephrol Dial Transplant 3:103, 1988.

610. Agodoa LY, Held PJ, Port FK: U.S Renal Data System 1991 Annual Data Report. Bethesda, MD, National Institutes of Health, National Institute of Diabetes and Digestive and Kidney Diseases, 1991.

611. Agodoa LY, Port FK, Held PJ: U.S. Renal Data System 1993 Annual Data Report. Bethesda, MD, National Institutes of Health, National Institute of Diabetes and Digestive and Kidney Diseases, 1993.

612. Xue JL, Chen SC, Ebben JP, et al: Peritoneal and hemodialysis: Differences in patient characteristics at initiation. Kidney Int 61:734-740, 2002.

613. Barker-Cummings C, McClellan W, Soucie JM, Krisher J: Ethnic differences in the use of peritoneal dialysis as initial treatment for end-stage renal disease. JAMA 274:1858-1862, 1995.

614. Frankenfield DL, Rocco MV, Roman SH, McClellan WM: Survival advantage for adult Hispanic hemodialysis patients? Findings from the end-stage renal disease (ESRD) clinical performance measures (CPM) project. J Am Soc Nephrol 14:180-186, 2003.

615. Rocco MV, Frankenfield DL, Frederick PR, et al: Intermediate outcomes by race and ethnicity in peritoneal dialysis patients: Results from the 1997 ESRD Core Indicators Project. National ESRD Core Indicators Workgroup. Perit Dial Int 20:328-335, 2000.

616. Holley JL, Bernardini J, Piraino B: A comparison of peritoneal dialysis–related infections in black and white patients. Perit Dial Int 13:45-49, 1993.

617. Korbet SM, Vonesh E, Firanek CA: A retrospective assessment of risk factors for peritonitis among an urban CAPD population. Perit Dial Int 13:126-131, 1993.

618. Rubin J, Ray R, Barnes T, et al: Peritonitis in continuous ambulatory peritoneal dialysis patients. Am J Kidney Dis 2:602-609, 1983.

619. Bloxsum A, Powell N: The treatment of acute temporary dysfunction of the kidneys by peritoneal irrigation. Pediatrics 1:52, 1948.

620. Oreopoulos DG, Katirtzoglou A, Arbus G: Dialysis and transplantation in young children. BMJ 1:1628, 1979.

621. Fine RN, Salusky IB, Ettenger RB: The therapeutic approach to the infant, child and adolescent with end-stage renal disease. Pediatr Clin North Am 34:789, 1987.

622. Price CG, Suki WN: Newer modifications of peritoneal dialysis: Options in the treatment of patients with renal failure. Am J Nephrol 1:97-104, 1981.

623. Furth SL, Hwang W, Yang C, et al: Relation between pediatric experience and treatment recommendations for children and adolescents with kidney failure. JAMA 285:1027-1033, 2001.

624. Lerner GR, Warady BA, Sullivan EK, et al: Chronic dialysis in children and adolescents. The 1996 annual report of the North American Pediatric Renal Transplant Cooperative Study. Pediatr Nephrol 14:404-417, 1999.

625. Alexander SR: Pediatric CAPD update. Perit Dial Bull 3(suppl):15, 1983.

626. Roscoe JM, Smith LF, Williams EA, et al: Medical and social outcome in adolescents with end-stage renal failure. Kidney Int 40:948-953, 1991.

627. Wood EG, Hand M, Briscoe DM, et al: Risk factors for mortality in infants and young children on dialysis. Am J Kidney Dis 37:573-579, 2001.

628. Gong WK, Tan TH, Foong PP, et al: Eighteen years experience in pediatric acute dialysis: Analysis of predictors of outcome. Pediatr Nephrol 16:212-215, 2001.

629. Beanes SR, Kling KM, Fonkalsrud EW, et al: Surgical aspects of dialysis in newborns and infants weighing less than ten kilograms. J Pediatr Surg 35:1543-1548, 2000.

630. Schaefer F, Klaus G, Muller-Wiefel DE, Mehls O: Current practice of peritoneal dialysis in children: Results of a longitudinal survey. Mid European Pediatric Peritoneal Dialysis Study Group (MEPPS). Perit Dial Int 19(suppl 2):445-449, 1999.

631. Gulati S, Stephens D, Balfe JA, et al: Children with hypoalbuminemia on continuous peritoneal dialysis are at risk for technique failure. Kidney Int 59:2361-2367, 2001.

632. Fischbach M, Stefanidis CJ, Watson AR: Guidelines by an ad hoc European committee on adequacy of the paediatric peritoneal dialysis prescription. Nephrol Dial Transplant 17:380-385, 2002.

633. Gong WK, Foong PP, Ramirez S, et al: Can dialysis adequacy be achieved by tailoring the dialysis prescription in an Asian pediatric population on nightly intermittent peritoneal dialysis? Adv Perit Dial 15:291-296, 1999.

634. Fischbach M, Terzic J, Bergere V, et al: The optimal approach to peritoneal dialysis prescription in children. Perit Dial Int 19(suppl 2):462-466, 1999.

635. Morgenstern B, Nair KS, Lerner G, et al: Impact of total body water errors on Kt/V estimates in children on peritoneal dialysis. Adv Perit Dial 17:260-263, 2001.

636. Verrina E, Zacchello G, Edefonti A, et al: A multicenter survey on automated peritoneal dialysis prescription in children. Adv Perit Dial 17:264-268, 2001.

637. Fischbach M, Terzic J, Gaugler C, et al: Impact of increased intraperitoneal fill volume on tolerance and dialysis effectiveness in children. Adv Perit Dial 14:258-264, 1998.

638. Fischbach M, Terzic J, Menouer S, et al: Impact of fill volume changes on peritoneal dialysis tolerance and effectiveness in children. Adv Perit Dial 16:321-333, 2000.

639. Schroder CH: The choice of dialysis solutions in pediatric chronic peritoneal dialysis: Guidelines by an ad hoc European committee. Perit Dial Int 21:568-574, 2001.

640. Linden T, Forsback G, Deppisch R, et al: 3-Deoxyglucosone, a promoter of advanced glycation end products in fluids for peritoneal dialysis. Perit Dial Int 18:290-293, 1998.

641. Schalkwijk CG, Posthuma N, ten Brink HJ, et al: Induction of 1,2-dicarbonyl compounds, intermediates in the formation of advanced glycation end-products, during heat-sterilization of glucose-based peritoneal dialysis fluids. Perit Dial Int 19:325-333, 1999.

642. Raj DSC, Choudhury D, Welbourne TC, Levi M: Advanced glycation end products: A nephrologist's perspective. Am J Kidney Dis 35:365-380, 2000.

643. Witowski J, Korybalska K, Wisniewska J, et al: Effect of glucose degradation products on human peritoneal mesothelial cell function. J Am Soc Nephrol 11:729-739, 2000.

644. Canepa A, Verrina E, Perfumo F, et al: Value of intraperitoneal amino acids in children treated with chronic peritoneal dialysis. Perit Dial Int 19(suppl 2):435-440, 1999.

645. Posthuma N, ter Wee PM, Donker AJM, et al: Assessment of the effectiveness, safety, and biocompatibility of icodextrin in automated peritoneal dialysis. Perit Dial Int 20(suppl 2):106-113, 2000.

646. De Boer AW, Schroder CH, Van Vliet R, et al: Clinical experiences with icodextrin in children: Ultrafiltration profiles and metabolism. Pediatr Nephrol 15:21-24, 2000.

647. Bouts AH, Davin JC, Groothoff JW, et al: Standard peritoneal permeability analysis in children. J Am Soc Nephrol 11:943-950, 2000.

648. Yoshino A, Honda M, Fukuda M, et al: Changes in peritoneal equilibration test values during long-term peritoneal dialysis in peritonitis-free children. Perit Dial Int 21:180-185, 2001.

649. Warady BA, Fivush B, Andreoli SP, et al: Longitudinal evaluation of transport kinetics in children receiving peritoneal dialysis. Pediatr Nephrol 13:571-576, 1999.

650. Warady BA, Schaefer F, Holloway M, et al: Consensus guidelines for the treatment of peritonitis in pediatric patients receiving peritoneal dialysis. Perit Dial Int 20:610-624, 2000.

651. Powell D, San Luis E, Calvin S, et al: Peritonitis in children undergoing continuous ambulatory peritoneal dialysis. Am J Dis Child 139:29-32, 1985.

652. Levy M, Balfe JW, Geary DF, et al: Peritonitis in children undergoing dialysis. 10 years experience. Child Nephrol Urol 9:253-258, 1988.

653. Furth SL, Donaldson LA, Sullivan EK, et al: Peritoneal dialysis catheter infections and peritonitis in children. Pediatr Nephrol 15:179-182, 2000.

654. Rinaldi S, Sera F, Verrina E, et al: The Italian registry of pediatric chronic peritoneal dialysis: A ten-year experience with chronic peritoneal dialysis catheters. Perit Dial Int 18:71-74, 1998.

655. Furth SL, Donaldson LA, Sullivan EK, Watkins SL: Peritoneal dialysis catheter infections and peritonitis in children: A report of the North American Pediatric Renal Transplant Cooperative Study. Pediatr Nephrol 15:179-182, 2000.

656. Holloway M, Mujais S, Kandert M, Warady BA: Pediatric peritoneal dialysis training: Characteristics and impact on peritonitis rates. Perit Dial Int 21:401-404, 2001.

657. Leichter HE, Slauski IB, Alliapoulos JC, et al: CAPD and CCPD in children: An experience of three and one-half years. J Pediatr 13:382, 1984.

658. North American Pediatric Renal Transplant Cooperative Study: 1999 Annual Report. Potomac, MD, Emmes Corp, 1991.

659. Flynn JT, Warady BA: Peritoneal dialysis in children: Challenges for the new millennium. Adv Ren Replace Ther 7:347-354, 2000.
660. Kohaut E: Growth in children treated with continuous ambulatory peritoneal dialysis. Int J Pediatr Nephrol 4:93-98, 1983.
661. Conley SB: Supplemental (NG) feedings of infants undergoing continuous peritoneal dialysis. *In* Fine RN (ed): Chronic and Ambulatory Peritoneal Dialysis (CAPD) and Chronic Cycling Peritoneal Dialysis (CCPD) in Children. Heidelberg, Germany, Springer-Verlag, 1987, p 263.
662. Fine RN: Growth in children undergoing continuous ambulatory peritoneal dialysis/continuous cycling peritoneal dialysis/automated peritoneal dialysis. Perit Dial Int 13(suppl 2):247-250, 1993.
663. Watkins SL: Growth failure in the pediatric ESRD patient. Perit Dial Int 17(suppl 3):12-14, 1997.
664. Salusky IB, Fine RN, Nelson P, et al: Nutritional status of children undergoing continuous ambulatory peritoneal dialysis. Am J Clin Nutr 38:599-611, 1983.
665. Alexander SR, Salusky IB, Warady BA, Watkins SL: Peritoneal dialysis workshop: Pediatrics recommendations. Perit Dial Int 17(suppl 3):25-27, 1998.
666. Challa A, Krieg RJ Jr, Thabet MA, et al: Metabolic acidosis inhibits growth hormone secretion in rats: Mechanism of growth retardation. Am J Physiol 265:E547-E553, 1993.
667. Challa A, Chan W, Krieg RJ Jr, et al: Effect of metabolic acidosis on the expression of insulin-like growth factor and growth hormone receptor. Kidney Int 44:1224-1227, 1993.
668. Brungger M, Hulter H, Krapf R: Effect of chronic metabolic acidosis on the growth hormone/IGF-1 endocrine axis: New cause of growth hormone insensitivity in humans. Kidney Int 51:216-221, 1997.
669. Pereira AM, Hamani N, Nogueira PC, Carvalhaes JT: Oral vitamin intake in children receiving long-term dialysis. J Renal Nutr 10:24-29, 2000.
670. Fine RN, Attie KM, Kuntze J, et al: Recombinant human growth hormone in infants and young children with chronic renal insufficiency. Genentech Collaborative Study Group. Pediatr Nephrol 9:451-457, 1995.
671. Watkins SL, Bliefeld C, Klee K, et al: Intraperitoneal somatotropin to improve the short stature associated with chronic renal failure in pediatric dialysis patients [abstract]. Pediatr Res 31:345, 1992.
672. Gipson DS, Kausz AT, Striegel JE, et al: Intraperitoneal administration of recombinant human growth hormone in children with end-stage renal disease. Pediatr Nephrol 16:29-34, 2001.
673. Kimmel PL, Phillips TM, Ferreira-Centeno A, et al: HIV-associated immune-mediated renal disease. Kidney Int 44:1327-1340, 1993.
674. Feinfeld DA, Kaplan R, Dressler R, Lynn RI: Survival of human immunodeficiency virus-I infected patients on maintenance hemodialysis. Clin Nephrol 32:221-224, 1989.
675. Tebben JA, Rigsby MO, Selwyn PA, et al: Outcome of HIV infected patients on continuous ambulatory peritoneal dialysis. Kidney Int 44:191-198, 1993.
676. Ortiz C, Meneses R, Jaffe D, et al: Outcome of patients with human immunodeficiency virus on maintenance hemodialysis. Kidney Int 34:248-253, 1988.
677. Kimmel PL, Umana WO, Simmens SJ, et al: Continuous ambulatory peritoneal dialysis and survival of HIV infected patients with end-stage renal disease. Kidney Int 44:373-378, 1993.
678. Ifudo O, Mayers JD, Matthew JJ, et al: Uremia therapy in patients with end-stage renal disease an human immunodeficiency virus infection: Has the outcome changed in the 1990s? Am J Kidney Dis 29:549-552, 1997.
679. Lewis M, Gorban Brennan N, Kliger AS, et al: Incidence and spectrum of organisms causing peritonitis in HIV positive patients on CAPD. Adv Perit Dial 6:136-138, 1990.
680. Dressler R, Peters AT, Lynn RI: Pseudomonal and candidal peritonitis as a complication of continuous ambulatory peritoneal dialysis in human immunodeficiency virus–infected patients. Am J Med 86:787-790, 1989.
681. Wasser WG, Boyle MJ, Brandon S: HIV positivity does not predispose peritoneal dialysis patients to peritonitis [abstract]. J Am Soc Nephrol 2:369, 1991.
682. Kiernan L, Finkelstein FO, Kliger AS, et al: Outcome of polymicrobial peritonitis in continuous ambulatory peritoneal dialysis patients. Am J Kidney Dis 25:461-464, 1995.
683. Scheel PJ Jr, Farzadegan H, Ford D, et al: Recovery of human immunodeficiency virus from peritoneal dialysis effluent. J Am Soc Nephrol 5:1926-1929, 1995.
684. Farzadegan H, Ford D, Malan M, et al: HIV-1 survival kinetics in peritoneal dialysis effluent. Kidney Int 50:1659-1662, 1996.
685. Bartlett JG, Gallant JE: 2000-2001 Medical Management of HIV Infection, 2000 ed. Baltimore, Johns Hopkins University, 2000.
686. Taylor S, Little J, Halifax K, et al: Pharmacokinetics of nelfinavir and nevirapine in a patient with end-stage renal failure on continuous ambulatory peritoneal dialysis. J Antimicrob Chemother 45:716-717, 2000.
687. Izzedine H, Launay-Vacher V, Deray G: Pharmacokinetics of ritonavir and nevirapine in peritoneal dialysis. Nephrol Dial Transplant 16:643, 2001.
688. Knupp CA, Hak LJ, Coakley DF, et al: Disposition of didanosine in HIV-seropositive patients with normal renal function or chronic renal failure: Influence of hemodialysis and continuous ambulatory peritoneal dialysis. Clin Pharmacol Ther 60:535-542, 1996.
689. Okundaye IB, Abrinko P, Hou SH: Registry of pregnancy in dialysis patients. Am J Kidney Dis 31:766-773, 1998.
690. Chan WS, Okun N, Kjellstrand CM: Pregnancy in chronic dialysis: A review and analysis of the literature. Int J Artif Organs 21:259-268, 1998.
691. Redrow M, Cherem L, Elliott J, et al: Dialysis in the management of pregnant patients with renal insufficiency. Medicine (Baltimore) 67:199-208, 1988.
692. Hou S, Firanek CA: Management of the pregnant dialysis patient. Adv Ren Replace Ther 5:24-30, 1998.
693. Tison A, Lozowy C, Benjamin A, et al: Successful pregnancy complicated by peritonitis in a 35 year old CAPD patient. Perit Dial Int 16(suppl):489-491, 1996.
694. Drugs in Pregnancy and Lactation. Baltimore, Williams & Wilkins, 1994.
695. Hussey MJ, Xavier P: Obstetric care for renal allograft recipients or for women treated with hemodialysis or peritoneal dialysis during pregnancy. Adv Ren Replace Ther 5:3-13, 1998.
696. Czeizel AE, Dudas I: Prevention of the first occurrence of neural-tube defects by periconceptional vitamin supplementation. N Engl J Med 327:1832-1835, 1992.
697. Hou S, Grossman SD: Pregnancy in chronic dialysis patients. Semin Dial 3:224-229, 1990.
698. Hou SH, Orlowski J, Pahl M, et al: Pregnancy in women with end stage renal disease: Treatment of anemia and premature labor. Am J Kidney Dis 21:16-22, 1993.
699. National Institutes of Health, National Heart, Lung, and Blood Institute: National High Blood Pressure Education Program. The Sixth Report of the Joint National Committee on Prevention, Detection, Evaluation and Treatment of High Blood Pressure (NIH Publication No. 98-4080). Bethesda, MD, National Institutes of Health, 1997.
700. Jones DC, Hayslett JP: Outcome of pregnancy in women with moderate or severe renal insufficiency. N Engl J Med 335:226-232, 1996.
701. Hou S, Grossman SD, Madias N: Pregnancy in women with moderate renal insufficiency. Am J Med 78:185-194, 1985.
702. Purdy LP, Hantch CE, Molitch ME, et al: Effects of pregnancy on renal function in patients with moderate to severe diabetic renal insufficiency. Diabetes Care 19:1067-1074, 1996.
703. Mintz G, Niz J, Gutierrez G, et al: Prospective study of pregnancy in systemic lupus erythematosus, results of a multidisciplinary approach. J Rheumatol 13:732-739, 1986.
704. Mehta RL, Letteri JM: Current status of renal replacement therapy for acute renal failure. Am J Nephrol 19:377-382, 1999.
705. Hyman A, Mendelssohn DC: Current Canadian approaches to dialysis for acute renal failure in the ICU. Am J Nephrol 22:29-34, 2002.
706. Ozdemir FN, Akcay A, Haberal M: Dialysis modalities in patients with acute renal failure. Nephrol Dial Transplant 16(suppl 6):18-20, 2001.
707. Van de Noortgate N, Verbeke F, Dhondt A, et al: The dialytic management of acute renal failure in the elderly. Semin Dial 15:127-132, 2002.
708. Manji S, Shikora S, McMahon M, et al: Peritoneal dialysis for acute renal failure: Overfeeding resulting from dextrose absorbed during dialysis. Crit Care Med 18:29-31, 1990.
709. Ash SR, Bever SL: Peritoneal dialysis for acute renal failure: The safe, effective and low-cost modality. Adv Ren Replace Ther 2:160-163, 1995.

710. Phu NH, Hien TT, Mai NT, et al: Hemofiltration and peritoneal dialysis in infection-associated acute renal failure in Vietnam. N Engl J Med 347:895-902, 2002.

711. Daugirdas J: Peritoneal dialysis in acute failure—why the bad outcome? N Engl J Med 347:933-935, 2002.

712. Chitalia VC, Almeida AF, Rai H, et al: Is peritoneal dialysis adequate for hypercatabolic acute renal failure in developing countries? Kidney Int 61:747-757, 2002.

713. Thongboonkerd V, Lumlertgul D, Supajatura V: Better correction of metabolic acidosis, blood pressure control, and phagocytosis with bicarbonate compared to lactate solution in acute peritoneal dialysis. Artif Organs 25:99-108, 2001.

714. Bleyer AJ, Burkart JM, Russell GB, Adams PL: PD patients have better outcomes in the first week after cadaveric renal transplantation than HD patients. Perit Dial Int 18(suppl 1):47, 1998.

715. Van Loo A, Heering P, Vanholder R, et al: Reduced incidence of acute renal graft failure in patients treated with peritoneal dialysis compared to haemodialysis. Nephrol Dial Transplant 13:831, 1998.

716. Van Biesen W, Vanholder R, Van Loo A, et al: Peritoneal dialysis favorably influences early graft function after renal transplantation compared to hemodialysis. Transplantation 69:508-514, 2000.

717. Rottembourg J: Residual renal function and recovery of renal function in patients treated by CAPD. Kidney Int Suppl 40:106-110, 1993.

718. Flynn JT: Choice of dialysis modality for management of pediatric acute renal failure. Pediatr Nephrol 17:61-69, 2002.

719. Bunchman TE, McBryde KD, Mottes TE, et al: Pediatric acute renal failure: Outcome by modality and disease. Pediatr Nephrol 16:1067-1071, 2001.

720. Flynn JT, Kershaw DB, Smoyer WE, et al: Peritoneal dialysis for management of pediatric acute renal failure. Perit Dial Int 21:390-394, 2001.

721. Gouyon JB, Guignard JP: Management of acute renal failure in newborns. Pediatr Nephrol 14:1037-1044, 2000.

722. Vande Walle J, Raes A, Castillo D, et al: New perspectives for PD in acute renal failure related to new catheter techniques and introduction of APD. Adv Perit Dial 13:190-194, 1997.

723. Bargman JM: Nonuremic indications for peritoneal dialysis. Perit Dial Int 13(suppl 2):159-164, 1993.

724. Mehrotra R: Peritoneal dialysis in adult patients without end-stage renal disease. Adv Perit Dial 16:67-72, 2000.

725. Parvathaneni LS, Guglelimi K, Silver MA: Difficult cases in heart failure: Role of continuous ambulatory peritoneal dialysis in refractory heart failure. Congest Heart Fail 5:283-285, 1999.

726. Mehrotra R, Khanna R: Peritoneal ultrafiltration for chronic congestive heart failure: Rationale, evidence and future. Cardiology 96:177-182, 2001.

727. Ryckelynck JP, Lobbedez T, Vallette B, et al: Peritoneal ultrafiltration and refractory congestive heart failure. Adv Perit Dial 13:93-97, 1997.

728. Tormey V, Conlon PJ, Farrell J, et al: Long-term successful management of refractory congestive cardiac failure by intermittent ambulatory peritoneal ultrafiltration. Q J Med 89:681-683, 1996.

729. Stegmayr BG, Banga R, Lundberg L, et al: PD treatment for severe congestive heart failure. Perit Dial Int 16(suppl 1):231-235, 1996.

730. Hebert MJ, Falardeau M, Pichette V, et al: Continuous ambulatory peritoneal dialysis for patients with severe left ventricular systolic dysfunction and end-stage renal disease. Am J Kidney Dis 25:761-768, 1995.

731. Elhalel-Dranitzki M, Rubinger D, Moscovici A, et al: CAPD to improve quality of life in patients with refractory heart failure. Nephrol Dial Transplant 13:3041-3042, 1998.

732. Bilora F, Petrobelli F, Boccioletti V, Pomerri F: Treatment of heart failure and ascites with ultrafiltration in patients with intractable alcoholic cardiomyopathy. Panminerva Med 44:23-25, 2002.

733. Markman M: Intraperitoneal chemotherapy in the management of malignant disease. Exp Rev Anticancer Ther 1:142-148, 2001.

734. Markman M: Intraperitoneal drug delivery of antineoplastics. Drugs 61:1057-1065, 2001.

735. de Bree E, Witkamp AJ, Zoetmulder FA: Intraperitoneal chemotherapy for colorectal cancer. J Surg Oncol 79:46-61, 2002.

736. Buecher B, Bleiberg H: Review article: Non-systemic chemotherapy in the treatment of colorectal cancer—portal vein, hepatic arterial and intraperitoneal approaches. Aliment Pharmacol Ther 15:1527-1541, 2001.

737. Markman M: Intraperitoneal chemotherapy in the management of colon cancer. Semin Oncol 26:536-539, 1999.

738. Ozols RF, Gore M, Trope C, Grenman S: Intraperitoneal treatment and dose-intense therapy in ovarian cancer. Ann Oncol 10(suppl 1):59-64, 1999.

739. Makhija S, Sabbatini P, Barakat RP: Intraperitoneal chemotherapy strategies in the treatment of epithelial ovarian carcinoma. Curr Opin Obstet Gynecol 11:23-27, 1999.

740. Bozzetti F, Vaglini M, Deraco M: Intraperitoneal hyperthermic chemotherapy in gastric cancer: Rationale for a new approach. Tumori 84:483-488, 1998.

741. Verschraegen CF: Intracavitary therapies for mesothelioma. Curr Treat Options Oncol 2:385-394, 2001.

742. el-Kareh AW, Secomb TW: Theoretical models for drug delivery to solid tumors. Crit Rev Biomed Eng 25:503-571, 1997.

743. Ceelen WP, Hesse U, de Hemptinne B, Pattyn P: Hyperthermic intraperitoneal chemoperfusion in the treatment of locally advanced intra-abdominal cancer. Br J Surg 87:1006-1015, 2000.

744. Hahn GM, Shiu EC: Effect of pH and elevated temperatures on the cytotoxicity of some chemotherapeutic agents on Chinese hamster cells in vitro. Cancer Res 43:5789-5791, 1983.

745. Hahn GM: Potential for therapy of drugs and hyperthermia. Cancer Res 39:2264-2268, 1979.

746. Lash RF, Burdette JA, Ozdil T: Accidental profound hypothermia and barbiturate intoxication. A report of rapid "core" rewarming by peritoneal dialysis. JAMA 201:269-270, 1967.

747. Weinberg AD: Hypothermia. Ann Emerg Med 22:370-377, 1993.

748. Zell S, Kurtz K: Severe exposure hypothermia: A resuscitation protocol. Ann Emerg Med 14:339-345, 1985.

749. Tse KC, Li FK, Tang S, et al: Peritoneal dialysis in patients with refractory ascites. Perit Dial Int 21:626-627, 2001.

750. Selgas R, Bajo MA, Jimenez C, et al: Peritoneal dialysis in liver disorders. Perit Dial Int 16(suppl 1):215-219, 1996.

751. Marcus RG, Messana JM, Swartz R: Peritoneal dialysis in end-stage renal disease patients with preexisting chronic liver disease and ascites. Am J Med 93:35-40, 1992.

752. Poulos AM, Howard L, Eisele G, Rodgers JB: Peritoneal dialysis therapy for patients with liver and renal failure with ascites. Am J Gastroenterol 88:109-112, 1993.

753. Durand PY, Freida P, Chanliau J, et al: Long-term follow-up in cirrhotic patients with chronic renal failure undergoing CAPD. Perit Dial Int 13(suppl 1):47, 1993.

754. Bajo MA, Selgas R, Jimenez C, et al: CAPD for treatment of ESRD patients with ascites secondary to liver cirrhosis. Adv Perit Dial 10:73-76, 1994.

755. Luca A, Feu F, Garcia Pagan JC, et al: Favorable effects of total paracentesis on splanchnic hemodynamics in cirrhotic patients with tense ascites. Hepatology 20:30-33, 1994.

756. Kuno T, Hitomi T, Zaitu M, et al: Severely decompensated abdominal Wilson disease treated with peritoneal dialysis: A case report. Acta Paediatr Jpn 40:85-87, 1998.

757. Swartz RD, Legault DJ: Long-term intraperitoneal deferoxamine for hemochromatosis. Am J Med 100:308-312, 1996.

758. Cintin C, Joffe P: Nephrogenic ascites: Case report and review of the literature. Scand J Urol Nephrol 28:311-314, 1994.

759. Gluck Z, Nolph KD: Ascites associated with end-stage renal disease. Am J Kidney Dis 10:9-18, 1987.

760. Rodriguez HJ, Walls J, Slatopolsky E, Klahr S: Recurrent ascites following peritoneal dialysis. Arch Intern Med 134:283-287, 1974.

761. Han SY, Reynolds TB, Fong TL: Nephrogenic ascites: Analysis of 16 cases and review of the literature. Medicine (Baltimore) 77:233-245, 1998.

762. Rubin J, Kiley J, Ray R, et al: Continuous ambulatory peritoneal dialysis: Treatment of dialysis related ascites. Arch Intern Med 141:1093-1095, 1981.

763. Schaefer F, Straube E, Oh J, et al: Dialysis in neonates with inborn errors of metabolism. Nephrol Dial Transplant 14:910-918, 1999.

764. Levey AS, Beto JA, Coronado BE, et al: Controlling the epidemic of cardiovascular disease in chronic renal disease: What do we know? What do we need to learn? Where do we go from here? National Kidney Foundation Task Force on Cardiovascular Disease. Am J Kidney Dis 32:853-905, 1998.

765. Prichard SS, Sniderman AD, Cianflone K, Marpole D: Cardiovascular disease in peritoneal dialysis. Perit Dial Int 16(suppl 1):19-22, 1996.

766. Rostand SG, Brunzell JD, Cannon IRC, Victor RG: Cardiovascular complications in renal failure. J Am Soc Nephrol 2:1053-1062, 1991.

767. Cocchi R, Esposti ED, Fabbri A, et al: Prevalence of hypertension in patients on peritoneal dialysis: Results of an Italian multicentre study. Nephrol Dial Transplant 14:1536-1540, 1999.

768. Health Care Financing Administration: 1997 Annual Report, End Stage Renal Disease Core Indicators Project. Baltimore, Department of Health and Human Services, Health Care Financing Administration, Office of Clinical Standards and Quality, 1997.

769. Bos WJ, Struijk DG, van Olden RW, et al: Elevated 24-hour blood pressure in peritoneal dialysis patients with ultrafiltration failure. Adv Perit Dial 14:108-110, 1998.

770. Menon MK, Naimark DM, Bargman JM, et al: Long-term blood pressure control in a cohort of peritoneal dialysis patients and its association with residual renal function. Nephrol Dial Transplant 16:2207-2213, 2001.

771. Shoda J, Nakamoto H, Okada H, Suzuki H: Impact of introduction of continuous ambulatory peritoneal dialysis on blood pressure: Analysis of 24-hour ambulatory blood pressure. Adv Perit Dial 16:97-101, 2000.

772. Wang T, Heimburger O, Bergstrom J, Lindholm B: Nutritional problems in peritoneal dialysis: An overview. Perit Dial Int 19(suppl 2): 297-303, 1999.

773. Silaruks S, Sirivongs D, Chunlertrith D: Left ventricular hypertrophy and clinical outcome in CAPD patients. Perit Dial Int 20:461-466, 2000.

774. Benedetto FA, Mallamaci F, Tripepi G, Zoccali C: Prognostic value of ultrasonographic measurement of carotid intima media thickness in dialysis patients. J Am Soc Nephrol 12:2458-2464, 2001.

775. Renke M, Zegrzda D, Liberek T, et al: Interrelationship between cardiac structure and function and incidence of arrhythmia in peritoneal dialysis patients. Int J Artif Organs 24:374-379, 2001.

776. Ates K, Nergizoglu G, Keven K, et al: Effect of fluid and sodium removal on mortality in peritoneal dialysis patients. Kidney Int 60:767-776, 2001.

777. Lameire N, Van Biesen W: Importance of blood pressure and volume control in peritoneal dialysis patients. Perit Dial Int 21:206-211, 2001.

778. Gunal AL, Duman S, Ozkahya M, et al: Strict volume control normalizes hypertension in peritoneal dialysis patients. Am J Kidney Dis 37:588-593, 2001.

779. Fried LF, Hutchison A, Stegmayr B, et al: ISPD guidelines/recommendations—recommendations for the treatment of lipid disorders in patients on peritoneal dialysis. Perit Dial Int 19:7-16, 1999.

780. De Santo NG, Capodicasa G, Denatore R, et al: Glucose utilization from dialysate in patients on continuous ambulatory peritoneal dialysis. Int J Artif Organs 2:119, 1979.

781. Lindholm B, Karlander SG, Norbeck HE, et al: Carbohydrate and lipid metabolism in CAPD patients. *In* Atkins RC, Thomson N, Farrell PC (eds): Peritoneal Dialysis. Edinburgh, Churchill Livingstone, 1981, p 198.

782. Splendiani G, Acitelli S, Albano V, et al: Metabolic aspects of CAPD. In Gahl GM, Kessel M, Nolph KD (eds): Advances in Peritoneal Dialysis. Amsterdam, Excerpta Medica, 1981, p 449.

783. Von Baeyer H, Gahl GM, Riedinger H, et al: Adaptation of CAPD patients to the continuous peritoneal energy uptake. Kidney Int 23:29, 1983.

784. Armstrong VW, Buschmann U, Ebert R, et al: Biochemical investigations of CAPD: Plasma levels of trace elements and amino acids and impaired glucose tolerance during the course of treatment. Int J Artif Organs 3:237, 1980.

785. Heaton A, Johnston DG, Burrin JM, et al: Carbohydrate and lipid metabolism during continuous ambulatory peritoneal dialysis (CAPD): The effect of a single dialysis cycle. Clin Sci 54:532, 1983.

786. Cheng SC, Chu TS, Huang KY, et al: Association of hypertriglyceridemia and insulin resistance in uremic patients undergoing CAPD. Perit Dial Int 21:282-289, 2001.

787. Kurtz SB, Wong VH, Anderson CF, et al: Continuous ambulatory peritoneal dialysis. Three years' experience at the Mayo Clinic. Mayo Clin Proc 58:633, 1983.

788. Lindholm B, Norbeck HE: Serum lipids and lipoproteins during continuous ambulatory peritoneal dialysis. Acta Med Scand 220:143-151, 1986.

789. Avram MM, Fein PA, Antignani A, et al: Cholesterol and lipid disturbances in renal disease: The natural history of uremic dyslipidemia and the impact of hemodialysis. Am J Med 87:55N-60N, 1989.

790. Horkko S, Huttunene K, Laara E, et al: Effects of three treatment modes on plasma lipids and lipoproteins in uremic patients. Ann Med 26:271-282, 1994.

791. Webb AT, Reaveley DA, O'Donnell M, et al: Lipids and lipoprotein(a) as risk factors for vascular disease in patients on renal replacement therapy. Nephrol Dial Transplant 10:354-357, 1995.

792. Siamopoulos KC, Elisaf MS, Bairaktari HT, et al: Lipid parameters including lipoprotein(a) in patients undergoing CAPD and hemodialysis. Perit Dial Int 15:342-347, 1995.

793. Llopart R, Donata T, Olivia JA, et al: Triglyceride-rich lipoprotein abnormalities in CAPD-treated patients. Nephrol Dial Transplant 10:537-540, 1995.

794. Gault MH, Longerich L, Prabhakaran V, Purchase L: Ischemic heart disease, serum cholesterol and apolipoproteins in CAPD. ASAIO Trans 37:M513-M314, 1991.

795. Gamba G, Mejia JL, Saldivar S, et al: Death risk in CAPD patients: The predictive value of the initial clinical and laboratory values. Nephron 65:23-27, 1993.

796. O'Riordan E, O'Donoghue DJ, Kalra PA, et al: Changes in lipid profiles in non diabetic, non nephrotic patients commencing continuous ambulatory peritoneal dialysis. Adv Perit Dial 16:313-316, 2000.

797. Cocchi R, Viglino G, Cancarini GC, et al: Prevalence of hyperlipidemia in a cohort of CAPD patients. Italian Cooperative Peritoneal Dialysis Study Group. Miner Electrolyte Metab 22:22-25, 1996.

798. Thomas ME, Moorhead JF: Lipids in CAPD: A review. Contrib Nephrol 85:92, 1990.

799. Gahl GM, Hain H: Nutrition and metabolism in continuous ambulatory peritoneal dialysis. Contrib Nephrol 84:36, 1990.

800. Chan MK: Sustained-release bezafibrate corrects lipid abnormalities in patients on continuous ambulatory peritoneal dialysis. Nephron 56:56, 1990.

801. Henriquez MA, Gonzalez A, Bemis JA: Body composition and lipid abnormalities in Hispanic and black patients on continuous ambulatory peritoneal dialysis. Perit Dial Int 13(suppl 2):424, 1993.

802. Shoji T, Nishizawa Y, Nishitani H, et al: High serum lipoprotein(a) concentrations in uremic patients treated with continuous ambulatory peritoneal dialysis. Clin Nephrol 38:271, 1992.

803. Johansson AC, Samuelsson O, Attman PO, et al: Dyslipidemia in peritoneal dialysis—relation to dialytic variables. Perit Dial Int 20:306-314, 2000.

804. Moberly J, Attman PO, Samuelsson O, et al: Apolipoprotein C-III, hypertriglyceridemia and triglyceride-rich lipoproteins in uremia. Miner Electrolyte Metab 25:258-262, 1999.

805. Misra M, Reaveley DA, Cooper C, et al: Mechanism for elevated plasma lipoprotein(a) concentrations in patients on dialysis: Turnover studies. Adv Perit Dial 14:223-227, 1998.

806. Misra M, Reaveley DA, Ashworth J, et al: Six-month prospective cross-over study to determine the effects of 1.1% amino acid dialysate on lipid metabolism in patients on continuous ambulatory peritoneal dialysis. Perit Dial Int 17:279-286, 1997.

807. Bredie SJH, Bosch FH, Demacker PNM, et al: Effects of peritoneal dialysis with an overnight icodextrin dwell on parameters of glucose and lipid metabolism. Perit Dial Int 3:275-281, 2001.

808. Gokal R, Moberly J, Ogrinc FG, et al: Improvement of hyperlipidemia with icodextrin use in CAPD patients. [Abstract]. J Am Soc Nephrol 9:283, 1998.

809. Hufnagel G, Michel C, Vrtovsnik F, et al: Effects of atorvastatin on dyslipidaemia in uraemic patients on peritoneal dialysis. Nephrol Dial Transplant 15:684-688, 2000.

810. Harris KP, Wheeler DC, Chong CC: A placebo-controlled trial examining atorvastatin in dyslipidemic patients undergoing CAPD. Kidney Int 61:1469-1474, 2002.

811. Saltissi D, Morgan C, Rigby R, Westhuyzen J: Safety and efficacy of simvastatin in hypercholesterolemic patients undergoing chronic renal dialysis. Am J Kidney Dis 39:283-290, 2002.

812. Akcicek F, Ok E, Duman S, et al: Lipid-lowering effects of simvastatin and gemfibrozil in CAPD patients: A prospective cross-over study. Adv Perit Dial 12:261-265, 1996.

813. Lee MS, Kim SM, Kim SB, et al: Effects of gemfibrozil on lipid and hemostatic factors in CAPD patients. Perit Dial Int 19:280-283, 1999.

814. Massy Z, Ma J, Louis T, Kasiske B: Lipid-lowering therapy in patients with renal disease. Kidney Int 48:188-198, 1995.

815. van Acker BAC, Bilo HJG, Popp-Snijders C, et al: The effect of fish oil on lipid profile and viscosity of erythrocyte suspensions in CAPD patients. Nephrol Dial Transplant 2:557-561, 1987.

816. Jones RG, Dibble JB, Gibson J, et al: Effect of dietary fish oil on lipid abnormalities in patients on continuous ambulatory peritoneal dialysis. Perit Dial Int 8:203-206, 1988.

817. Lempert KD, Rogers IJS, Albrink MJ: Effects of dietary fish oil on serum lipids and blood coagulation in peritoneal dialysis patients. Am J Kidney Dis 11:170-175, 1988.

818. Goren A, Stankiewicz H, Goldstein R, Drukker A: Fish oil treatment of hyperlipidemia in children and adolescents receiving renal replacement therapy. Pediatrics 88:265-268, 1991.

819. Dimitriadis A, Antonious S, Hatzisavvas N, et al: The effect of simvastatin on dyslipidemia in continuous ambulatory peritoneal dialysis patients. Perit Dial Int 13(suppl 2):434-436, 1993.

820. Balaskas E, Bamihas G, Tourkantonis A: Management of lipid abnormalities in patients on CAPD [letter]. Perit Dial Int 17:308-309, 1997.

820a. National Kidney Foundation: Clinical practice guidelines for managing dyslipidemias in chronic kidney disease. Am J Kidney Dis 41(suppl 3): S1-S91, 2003.

821. Zimmermann J, Herrlinger S, Pruy A, et al: Inflammation enhances cardiovascular risk and mortality in hemodialysis patients. Kidney Int 55:648-658, 1999.

822. Yeun JY, Levine RA, Mantadilok V, Kaysen GA: C-reactive protein predicts all-cause and cardiovascular mortality in hemodialysis patients. Am J Kidney Dis 35:469-476, 2000.

823. Zoccali C, Benedetto FA, Mallamaci F, et al: Inflammation is associated with carotid atherosclerosis in dialysis patients. J Hypertens 18:1207-1213, 2000.

824. Yeun JY, Kaysen GA: Acute phase proteins and peritoneal dialysate albumin loss are the main determinants of serum albumin and peritoneal dialysis patients. Am J Kidney Dis 30:923-927, 1997.

825. Stenvinkel P, Chung SH, Heimburger O, Lindholm B: Malnutrition, inflammation and atherosclerosis in peritoneal dialysis patients. Perit Dial Int 21(suppl 3):157-162, 2001.

826. Libetta C, Nicola L, Rampino T, et al: Inflammatory effects of peritoneal dialysis: Evidence of systemic monocyte activation. Kidney Int 49:506-511, 1996.

827. Pasceri V, Willerson JT, Yeh ETH: Direct proinflammatory effect of C-reactive protein on human endothelial cells. Circulation 102:2165-2168, 2001.

828. Bartens W, Nauck M, Schollmeyer P, Wanner C: Elevated lipoprotein(a) and fibrinogen levels [corrected] increase the cardiovascular risk in continuous ambulatory peritoneal dialysis patients. Perit Dial Int 16:27-33, 1996.

829. Bhagat K, Vallance P: Inflammatory cytokines impair endothelium-dependent dilatation in human veins in vivo. Circulation 96:3042-3047, 1997.

830. Tintut Y, Patel J, Parhami F, Demer LL: Tumor necrosis factor-α promotes in vitro calcification of vascular cells via the cAMP pathway. Circulation 102:2636-2642, 2000.

831. Huber SA, Sakkinen P, Conze D, et al: Interleukin-6 exacerbates early atherosclerosis in mice. Arterioscler Thromb Vasc Biol 19: 2364-2367, 1999.

832. Ridker PM, Rifai N, Stampfer MJ, Hennekens CH: Plasma concentration of interleukin-6 and the risk of future myocardial infarction among apparently healthy men. Circulation 101:1767-1772, 2000.

833. Fine A: Relevance of C-reactive protein levels in peritoneal dialysis patients. Kidney Int 61:615-620, 2002.

834. Kim SB, Min WK, Lee SK, et al: Persistent elevation of C-reactive protein and ischemic heart disease in patients with continuous ambulatory peritoneal dialysis. Am J Kidney Dis 39:342-346, 2002.

835. De Vecchi A, Bamonti-Catena F, Finazzi S, et al: Homocysteine, vitamin B_{12}, and serum and erythrocyte folate in peritoneal dialysis and hemodialysis patients. Perit Dial Int 20:169-173, 2000.

836. Vychytil A, Fodinger M, Wolfl G, et al: Major determinants of hyperhomocysteinemia in peritoneal dialysis patients. Kidney Int 53:1775-1782, 1998.

837. De Vecchi A, Bamonti-Catena F, Finazzi S, et al: Homocysteine, vitamin B_{12}, serum and erythrocyte folate in peritoneal dialysis patients. Clin Nephrol 55:313-317, 2001.

838. Holdt B, Korten G, Knippel M, et al: Increased serum level of total homocysteine in CAPD patients despite fish oil therapy. Perit Dial Int 16(suppl 1):246-249, 1996.

839. Fodinger M, Buchmayer H, Heinz G, et al Association of two MTHFR polymorphisms with total homocysteine plasma levels in dialysis patients. Am J Kidney Dis 38:77-84, 2001.

840. Moustapha A, Gupta A, Robinson K, et al: Prevalence and determinants of hyperhomocysteinemia in hemodialysis and peritoneal dialysis. Kidney Int 55:1470-1475, 1999.

841. Johnson DW, Kay TD, Vesey DA, et al: Peritoneal homocysteine clearance is inefficient in peritoneal dialysis patients. Perit Dial Int 20:766-771, 2000.

842. Vychytil A, Fodinger M, Papagiannopoulos M, et al: Peritoneal elimination of homocysteine moieties in continuous ambulatory peritoneal dialysis patients. Kidney Int 55:2054-2061, 1999.

843. De Vecchi A, Patrosso C, Novembrino C, et al: Folate supplementation in peritoneal dialysis patients with normal erythrocyte folate: Effect on plasma homocysteine. Nephron 89:297-302, 2001.

844. Janssen MJ, van Guldener C, de Jong GM, et al: Folic acid treatment of hyperhomocysteinemia in dialysis patients. Miner Electrolyte Metab 22:110-114, 1996.

845. van Guldener C, Janssen MJ, Lambert J, et al: Folic acid treatment of hyperhomocysteinemia in peritoneal dialysis patients: No change in endothelial function after long-term therapy. Perit Dial Int 18:282-289, 1998.

846. Brulez HF, van Guldener C, Donker AJ, ter Wee PM: The impact of an amino acid–based peritoneal dialysis fluid on plasma total homocysteine levels, lipid profile and body fat mass. Nephrol Dial Transplant 14:154-159, 1999.

847. Kim SS, Hirose S, Tamura H, et al: Hyperhomocysteinemia as a possible role for atherosclerosis in CAPD patients. Adv Perit Dial 10:282-285, 1994.

848. Burke SW, Solomon AJ: Cardiac complications of end-stage renal disease. Adv Ren Replace Ther 7:210-219, 2000.

849. Owen CH, Cummings RG, Sell TL, et al: Coronary artery bypass grafting in patients with dialysis-dependent renal failure. Ann Thorac Surg 58:1729-1733, 1994.

850. Simsir SA, Kohlman-Trigoboff D, Flood R, et al: A comparison of coronary artery bypass grafting and percutaneous transluminal coronary angioplasty in patients on hemodialysis. Cardiovasc Surg 6:500-505, 1998.

851. Winkelmayer WC, Glynn RJ, Mittleman MA, et al: Comparing mortality of elderly patients on hemodialysis versus peritoneal dialysis: A propensity score approach. J Am Soc Nephrol 13:2353-2362, 2002.

852. Collins AJ, Weinhandl E, Snyder JJ, et al: Comparison and survival of hemodialysis and peritoneal dialysis in the elderly. Semin Dial 15:98-102, 2002.

853. Heaf JG, Lokkegaard H, Madsen M: Initial survival advantage of peritoneal dialysis relative to haemodialysis. Nephrol Dial Transplant 17:112-117, 2002.

854. Avram MM, Sreedhara R, Fein P, et al: Survival on hemodialysis and peritoneal dialysis over 12 years with emphasis on nutritional parameters. Am J Kidney Dis 37(suppl 2):77-80, 2001.

855. Tanna MM, Vonesh E, Korbet SM: Patient survival among incident peritoneal dialysis and hemodialysis patients in an urban setting. Am J Kidney Dis 36:1175-1182, 2000.

856. Locatelli F, Marcelli D, Conte F, et al: Survival and development of cardiovascular disease by modality of treatment in patients with end-stage renal disease. J Am Soc Nephrol 12:2411-2417, 2001.

857. Selgas R, Cirugeda A, Fernandez-Perpen A, et al: Comparisons of hemodialysis and CAPD in patients over 65 years of age: A meta-analysis. Int Urol Nephrol 33:259-264, 2001.

858. Murphy SW, Foley RN, Barrett BJ, et al: Comparative mortality of hemodialysis and peritoneal dialysis in Canada. Kidney Int 57: 1720-1726, 2000.

859. Van Biesen W, Vanholder R, Debacquer D, et al: Comparison of survival on CAPD and haemodialysis: Statistical pitfalls. Nephrol Dial Transplant 15:307-311, 2000.

860. Miskulin DC, Meyer KB, Athienites NV, et al: Comorbidity and other factors associated with modality selection in incident dialysis patients: The CHOICE study. Am J Kidney Dis 39:324-336, 2002.

861. Vonesh E, Moran J: Mortality in end-stage renal disease: A reassessment of differences between patients treated with hemodialysis and peritoneal dialysis. J Am Soc Nephrol 10:354-365, 1999.

862. Port FK: Description and clinical outcomes of peritoneal dialysis: Analyses from the United States Renal Data System. Perit Dial Int 20(suppl 2):114-117, 2000.

863. Maiorca R, Cancarini GC, Zubani R, et al: CAPD viability: A long-term comparison with hemodialysis. Perit Dial Int 16:276-287, 1996.

864. Murphy SW, Foley RN, Barrett BJ, et al: Comparative hospitalization of hemodialysis and peritoneal dialysis patients in Canada. Kidney Int 57:2557-2563, 2000.

865. NKF-K/DOQI Clinical Practice Guidelines for Peritoneal Dialysis Adequacy. New York, National Kidney Foundation, 2001, p 82.

866. Sevick MA, Levine DW, Burkart JM, et al: Measurement of continuous ambulatory peritoneal dialysis prescription adherence using a novel approach. Perit Dial Int 19:23-30, 1999.

867. Fine A: Compliance with the CAPD regimen is good. Perit Dial Int 17:343-346, 1997.

868. Bernardini J, Piraino B: Measuring compliance with prescribed exchanges in CAPD and CCPD patients. Perit Dial Int 17:338-342, 1997.

869. Bernardini J, Nagy M, Piraino B: Patterns of noncompliance with dialysis exchanges in peritoneal dialysis patients. Am J Kidney Dis 35:1104-1110, 2000.

870. Ing TS, Gandhi VC, Daugirdas JT, et al: Peritoneal dialysis using bicarbonate-buffered dialysate. Int J Artif Organs 7:166, 1984.

871. Farooq MM, Freischlag JA: Peritoneal dialysis: An increasingly popular option. Semin Vasc Surg 10:144-150, 1997.

872. Sahani MM, Mukhtar KN, Boorgu R, et al: Tissue plasminogen activator can effectively declot peritoneal dialysis catheters. Am J Kidney Dis 36:675, 2000.

873. Moss JS, Minda SA, Newman GE, et al: Malpositioned peritoneal dialysis catheters: A critical reappraisal of correction by stiff-wire manipulation. Am J Kidney Dis 15:305-308, 1990.

874. Dobrashian RD, Conway B, Hutchison A, et al: The repositioning of migrated Tenckhoff continuous ambulatory peritoneal dialysis catheters under fluoroscopic control. Br J Radiol 72:452-456, 1999.

875. Simons ME, Pron G, Voros M, et al: Fluoroscopically-guided manipulation of malfunctioning peritoneal dialysis catheters. Perit Dial Int 19:544-549, 1999.

876. Jwo SC, Lee CM, Tsai CJ: Correction of a migrated Tenckhoff peritoneal dialysis catheter using a Lunderquist guidewire: Report of two cases. Changgeng Yi Xue Za Zhi 23:360-365, 2000.

877. Kumwenda MJ, Wright FK: The use of channel-cleaning brush for malfunctioning Tenckhoff catheters. Nephrol Dial Transplant 14:1254-1257, 1999.

878. Yilmazlar T, Yavuz M, Ceylan H: Laparoscopic management of malfunctioning peritoneal dialysis catheters. Surg Endosc 15:820-822, 2001.

879. Yoshihara K, Yoshi S, Miyagi S: Alpha replacement method for displaced swan neck catheters. Adv Perit Dial 9:227-230, 1993.

880. Hevia C, Bajo MA, Aguilera A, et al: Alpha replacement method for displaced peritoneal catheter: A simple and effective maneuver. Adv Perit Dial 17:138-141, 2001.

881. Di Paolo N, Broncristiani U, Capotondo L, et al: The self positioning catheter. *In* Proceedings of the VII Italian Congress on Peritoneal Dialysis. Milan, Wichtig Editore, 1993, pp 539-542.

882. Minguela I, Lanuza M, Ruiz de Gauna R, et al: Lower malfunction with self-locating catheters. Perit Dial Int 21(suppl 3):209-212, 2001.

883. Gadallah MF, Mignone J, Torres C, et al: The role of peritoneal dialysis catheter configuration in preventing catheter tip migration. Adv Perit Dial 16:47-50, 2000.

884. Usha K, Ponferrada L, Prowant BF, Twardowski Z: Repair of chronic peritoneal dialysis catheter. Perit Dial Int 18:419-423, 1998.

885. Gotloib L, Mines M, Garmizo L, et al: Hemodynamic effects of increasing intra-abdominal pressure in peritoneal dialysis. Perit Dial Bull 1:41, 1981.

886. Rocco MV, Stone WJ: Abdominal hernias in chronic peritoneal dialysis patients: A review. Perit Dial Bull 5:171, 1985.

887. Bargman JM: Complications of peritoneal dialysis related to increased intraabdominal pressure. Kidney Int Suppl 40:75-80, 1993.

888. Hussain SI, Bernardini J, Piraino B: The risk of hernia with large exchange volumes. Adv Perit Dial 14:105-107, 1998.

889. Bleyer AJ, Casey MJ, Russell GB, et al: Peritoneal dialysate fill-volume and hernia development in a cohort of peritoneal dialysis patients. Adv Perit Dial 14:102-104, 1998.

890. Afthentopoulos IE, Panduranga RS, Mathews R, Oreopoulos DG: Hernia development in CAPD patients and the effects of 2.51 dialysate volume in selected patients. Clin Nephrol 49:251-257, 1998.

891. Hughes GC, Ketchersid TL, Lenzen JM, Lowe JE: Thoracic complications of peritoneal dialysis. Ann Thorac Surg 67:1518-1522, 1999.

892. Canivet E, Lavaud S, Wampach H, et al: Detection of subclinical abdominal hernia by peritoneal scintigraphy. Adv Perit Dial 16:104-107, 2000.

893. Berman C, Velchik MG, Shusterman N, Alavi A: The clinical utility of the Tc-99m SC intraperitoneal scan in CAPD patients. Clin Nucl Med 14:405-409, 1989.

894. Helfrich GB, Pechan BWW, Alijani MR, et al: Reduced catheter complications with lateral placement. Perit Dial Bull 3(suppl4):2, 1983.

895. Spence PA, Mathews RE, Khanna R, et al: Improved results with a paramedian technique for the insertion of peritoneal dialysis catheters. Surg Gynecol Obstet 161:585, 1985.

896. Bernardini J: Peritoneal dialysis catheter complications. Perit Dial Int 16(suppl 1):468-471, 1996.

897. Twardowski Z, Prowant BF, Nichols WK, et al: Six-year experience with swan neck catheters. Perit Dial Int 12:384, 1992.

898. Mettang T, Stoeltzing H, Alscher DM, et al: Sustaining continuous ambulatory peritoneal dialysis after herniotomy. Adv Perit Dial 17:84-87, 2001.

898. Leblanc M, Ouimet D, Pichette V: Dialysate leaks in peritoneal dialysis. Semin Dial 14:50-54, 2001.

900. Balaskas EV, Ikonomopoulos D, Sioulis A, et al: Survival and complications of 225 catheters used in continuous ambulatory peritoneal dialysis: One-center experience in northern Greece. Perit Dial Int 19(suppl 2):167-171, 1999.

901. Ramon RG, Carrasco AM: Hydrothorax in peritoneal dialysis. Perit Dial Int 18:5-10, 1998.

902. Rodriguez-Perez JC: Late external peritoneal leakage in CAPD patients. Perit Dial Bull 5:255-256, 1985.

903. Nomoto Y, Suga T, Nakajima K, et al: Acute hydrothorax in continuous ambulatory peritoneal dialysis—a collaborative study in 161 centers. Am J Nephrol 9:363-367, 1989.

904. Lieberman FL, Hidermura R, Peters RL, et al: Pathogenesis and treatment of hydrothorax complicating cirrhosis with ascites. Ann Intern Med 64:341, 1966.

905. Okada H, Ryuzaki M, Kotaki S, et al: Thoracoscopic surgery and pleurodesis for pleuroperitoneal communication in patients on continuous ambulatory peritoneal dialysis. Am J Kidney Dis 34: 170-172, 1999.

906. Finn R, Jowett E: Acute hydrothorax complicating peritoneal dialysis. BMJ 2:94, 1970.

907. Townsend R, Fragula J: Hydrothorax in patient receiving CAPD. Arch Intern Med 142:1571-1572, 1982.

908. Green AN, Logan M, Medawar W, et al: The management of hydrothorax in continuous ambulatory peritoneal dialysis (CAPD). Perit Dial Int 10:271, 1990.

909. Le Veen H, Piccone V, Hutto R: Management of ascites with hydrothorax. Ann J Surg 148:210-213, 1984.

910. Kopecky R, Funk M, Kreitzer P: Localized genital edema in patients undergoing continuous ambulatory peritoneal dialysis. J Urol 134:880-884, 1985.

911. Khanna R, Oreopoulos DG, Dombros NV, et al: Continuous ambulatory peritoneal dialysis (CAPD) after three years: Still a promising treatment. Perit Dial Bull 1:24-34, 1981.

912. Abraham G, Blake PG, Mathews RE, et al: Genital swelling as a complication of continuous ambulatory peritoneal dialysis. Surg Gynecol Obstet 170:306-308, 1990.

913. Caporale N, Perez D, Alegre S: Vaginal leak of peritoneal dialysis liquid. Perit Dial Int 11:284-285, 1991.

914. Diaz-Buxo JD, Burgess P, Walker PJ: Peritoneovaginal fistula—unusual complication of peritoneal dialysis. Perit Dial Bull 3:142, 1983.

915. Coward RA, Gokal R, Mallick VP: Recurrent peritonitis associated with vaginal leak. Perit Dial Bull 3:164, 1983.

916. Wright CA, Moran J, Silk D: Is peritoneal-vaginal fistula the main cause of fungal peritonitis in female CAPD patients? Perit Dial Bull 4:51, 1984.

917. Galimberti E, Belluschi F, Bosaglia M, Bianchessi S: Radiology examinations in noninfectious complications of CAPD. EDTNA ERCA J 24:36-38, 1998.

918. Osborne TM: CT peritoneography in peritoneal dialysis patients. Australas Radiol 34:204-206, 1990.

919. Mandel P, Faegenburg MD, Imbraino LJ: The use of technetium-99m sulfur colloid in the detection of patient processus vaginalis in patients on continuous ambulatory peritoneal dialysis. Clin Nucl Med 10:553-555, 1985.

920. Juergensen PH, Rizvi H, Caride VJ, et al: Value of scintigraphy in chronic peritoneal dialysis patients. Kidney Int 55:1111-1119, 1999.

921. Prokesch RW, Schima W, Schober E, et al: Complications of continuous ambulatory peritoneal dialysis: Findings on MR peritoneography. AJR Am J Roentgenol 174:987-991, 2000.

922. Walker F, McAllister C, McKee P, et al: Intraperitoneal iopamidol, a new radiocontrast agent, in the diagnosis of a pleuroperitoneal communication. Perit Dial Bull 6:108, 1986.

923. Pattison C, Rodger R, Adu D, et al: Surgical treatment of hydrothorax complicating continuous ambulatory peritoneal dialysis. Clin Nephrol 21:191-193, 1984.

924. Benz R, Schleifer C: Hydrothorax in continuous ambulatory peritoneal dialysis: Successful treatment with intrapleural tetracycline and a review of the literature. Am J Kidney Dis 5:136-140, 1985.

925. Scheldewaert R, Bogaerts Y, Pauwels R, et al: Management of a massive hydrothorax in a CAPD patient: A case report and a review of the literature. Perit Dial Bull 2:69-72, 1982.

926. Vlachojannis J, Boettcher I, Brandt L, Schoeppe W: A new treatment of unilateral recurrent hydrothorax during CAPD. Perit Dial Bull 5:180-181, 1985.

927. Chao S, Tsai T: Recurrent hydrothorax following repeated pleurodesis using autologous blood. Perit Dial Int 13:321-322, 1993.

928. Mak SK, Chan M, Tai Y, et al: Thoracoscopic pleurodesis for massive hydrothorax complicating CAPD. Perit Dial Int 16:421-423, 1996.

929. Jagasia M, Cole F, Stegman M, et al: Video-assisted talc pleurodesis in the management of pleural effusion secondary to continuous ambulatory peritoneal dialysis: A report of three cases. Am J Kidney Dis 28:772-774, 1996.

930. Di Bisceglie M, Paladini P, Voltolini L, et al: Videothoracoscopic obliteration of pleuroperitoneal fistula in continuous peritoneal dialysis. Ann Thorac Surg 62:1509-1510, 1996.

931. Mak SK, Nyunt K, Wong PN, et al: Long-term follow-up of thoracoscopic pleurodesis for hydrothorax complicating peritoneal dialysis. Ann Thorac Surg 74:218-221, 2002.

932. Vladimirova NN, Darenkov AF, Pashkin IN, et al: A comparative evaluation of the central hemodynamic indices in patients with the terminal stage of kidney failure during dialysis therapy and allografting. Urol Nefrol 5:34, 1990.

933. O'Brien AA, Power J, O'Brien L, et al: The effect of peritoneal dialysate on pulmonary function and blood gases in CAPD patients. Ir J Med Sci 159:215-216, 1990.

934. Durand PY, Chanliau J, Gamberoni J, et al: Clinical measurement of the maximal acceptable intraperitoneal volume. Adv Perit Dial 10:63-67, 1994.

935. McAuliffe F, Kametas N, Costello J, et al: Respiratory function in singleton and twin pregnancy. Br J Obstet Gynaecol 109:765-769, 2002.

936. Unterborn J: Pulmonary function testing in obesity, pregnancy, and extremes of body habitus. Clin Chest Med 22:759-767, 2001.

937. Siafakas NM, Argyrakopoulos T, Andreopoulos K, et al: Respiratory muscle strength during continuous ambulatory peritoneal dialysis (CAPD). Eur Respir J 8:109-113, 1995.

938. Bhatla B, Satalowich R, Khanna R: Low-volume supine peritoneal dialysis in a chronic obstructive airway disease patient. Adv Perit Dial 10:120-123, 1994.

939. Leblanc M, Ouimet D, Tremblay C, Nolin L: Peritoneal instillation test before CAPD in a case of severe pulmonary disease. Perit Dial Int 15:384-387, 1995.

940. Gokal R: Fluid management and cardiovascular outcome in peritoneal dialysis patients. Semin Dial 12:126, 1999.

941. Abu-Alfa AK, Burkart JM, Piraino B, et al: Approach to fluid management in peritoneal dialysis. A practical algorithm. Kidney Int Suppl 81:8-16, 2002.

942. Twardowski ZJ, Nolph KD: Peritoneal dialysis: How much is enough? Semin Dial 2:75, 1988.

943. Ho-dac-Pannekeet MM, Atasever B, Struijk DG, Krediet RT: Analysis of ultrafiltration failure in peritoneal dialysis patients by means of the standard peritoneal permeability analysis. Perit Dial Int 17:144-150, 1997.

944. Pride ET, Gustafson J, Graham A, et al: Comparison of a 2.5% and a 4.25% dextrose peritoneal equilibration test. Perit Dial Int 22:365-370, 2002.

945. Faller B, Marichal JF: Loss of ultrafiltration in continuous ambulatory peritoneal dialysis. A role for acetate. Perit Dial Bull 4:10, 1984.

946. Bazzato G, Coli U, Landini S, et al: Restoration of ultrafiltration capacity of peritoneal membrane in patients on CAPD. Int J Artif Organs 7:93, 1984.

947. Davies SJ, Brown B, Bryer J, Russel GI: Clinical evaluation of the peritoneal equilibration test: A population-based study. Nephrol Dial Transplant 8:64-70, 1993.

948. Mateijsen MA, Van Der Wal AC, Hendriks PMEM, et al: Vascular and interstitial changes in the peritoneum of CAPD patients with peritoneal sclerosis [Abstract]. J Am Soc Nephol 8:268, 1997.

949. Krediet RT, Zuyderhoudt MJ, Boeschoten EW, Arisz L: Alterations in the peritoneal transport of water and solutes during peritonitis in continuous ambulatory peritoneal dialysis patients. Eur J Clin Invest 17:43-52, 1987.

950. Rottembourg J, Brouard R, Issad B, et al: Role of acetate in loss of ultrafiltration during CAPD. Contrib Nephrol 57:197, 1987.

951. Shaldon S, Koch KM, Quelhorst B, et al: Pathogenesis of sclerosing peritonitis in CAPD. ASAIO Trans 30:193, 1984.

952. Pollack CA, Ibels LS, Hallhagen MD, et al: Loss of ultrafiltration in continuous ambulatory peritoneal dialysis (CAPD). Perit Dial Int 9:107, 1989.

953. Miranda B, Selgas R, Celedilla O, et al: Peritoneal resting and heparinization as an effective treatment for ultrafiltration failure in patients on CAPD. Contrib Nephrol 89:199, 1991.

954. Johnson DW, Arndt M, O'Shea A, et al: Icodextrin as salvage therapy in peritoneal dialysis patients with refractory volume overload. Perit Dial Int 17:84-87, 2001.

955. Querques M, Procaccini DA, Pappani A, et al: Influence of phosphatidylcholine on ultrafiltration and solute transfer in CAPD patients. ASAIO J 36:M581, 1990.

956. Dombros N, Balaskas E, Savidis N, et al: Phosphatidylcholine increases ultrafiltration in continuous ambulatory peritoneal dialysis patients. In Avram MM, Giordano C (ed): Ambulatory Peritoneal Dialysis. New York, Plenum, 1990, p 39.

957. Huarte-Loza B, Selgas R, Carmona AR, et al: Peritoneal membrane failure as a determinant of the CAPD future. Contrib Nephrol 47:219, 1987.

958. Diaz-Buxo JA: Peritoneal sclerosis in a woman on continuous cyclic peritoneal dialysis. Semin Dial 5:317, 1992.

959. Ho-dac Pannekeet MM: Peritoneal fluid markers of mesothelial cells and function. Adv Ren Replace Ther 5:295, 1998.

960. Abensur H, Romao J, Prado E, et al: Use of dextran 70 to estimate peritoneal lymphatic absorption rate in CAPD. Adv Perit Dial 8:3-6, 1992.

961. Monquil MCJ, Imholz ALT, Struijk DG, et al: Does impaired transcellular water transport contribute to net ultrafiltration failure during CAPD? Perit Dial Int 15:42, 1995.

962. Dobbie JW, Krediet RT, Twardowski ZJ, et al: A 39-year-old man with loss of ultrafiltration. Perit Dial Int 14:384, 1994.

963. Afthentopoulos IE, Passadakis P, Oreopoulos DG: Sclerosing peritonitis in continuous ambulatory peritoneal dialysis patients: One center's experience and review of the literature. Adv Ren Replace Ther 5:157, 1998.

964. Lichtman AH, Segal GB, Lichtman MA: The role of calcium in lymphocyte proliferation: An interpretive review. Blood Purif 61:413, 1983.

965. Turner MW, Holleman JH: Successful therapy of sclerosing peritonitis. Semin Dial 5:316, 1992.

966. Bargman JM, Oreopoulos DG: Complications other than peritonitis or those related to the catheter and the fate of uremic organ dysfunction in patients receiving peritoneal dialysis. In Nolph KD (ed): Peritoneal Dialysis. Dordrecht, The Netherlands, Kluwer Academic, 1990, p 289.

967. Rottembourg J, Gahl GM, Poindexter P, et al: Severe abdominal complications in patients undergoing continuous ambulatory peritoneal dialysis. Eur Dial Transpl Assoc Proc 20:236, 1983.

968. Grefberg N, Nilsson P, Andreen T: Sclerosing obstructive peritonitis, beta blockers, and continuous ambulatory peritoneal dialysis. Lancet 2:733, 1983.

969. Bradley JA, McWhinnie DL, Hamilton DN, et al: Sclerosing obstructive peritonitis after continuous ambulatory peritoneal dialysis. Lancet 2:113-114, 1983.

970. Verger C, Celicout B, Larpent L, et al: Sclerosing encapsulating peritonitis during continuous ambulatory peritoneal dialysis. Presse Med 15:1311, 1986.

971. Pusateri R, Ross R, Marshall R, et al: Sclerosing encapsulating peritonitis: Report of a case with small bowel obstruction managed by long-term home parenteral hyperalimentation. Am J Kidney Dis 8:56, 1986.

972. Nomoto Y, Kawaguchi Y, Kubo H, et al: Sclerosing encapsulating peritonitis in patients undergoing CAPD: A report of the Japanese sclerosing encapsulating peritonitis study group. Am J Kidney Dis 28:420, 1996.

973. Yokota S, Kumano K, Sakai T: Prognosis for patients with sclerosing encapsulating peritonitis following CAPD. Adv Perit Dial 13:221-223, 1997.

974. Rigby RJ, Hawley CM: Sclerosing peritonitis: The experience in Australia. Nephrol Dial Transplant 13:154, 1998.

975. Namoto Y, Kawaguchi Y, Kubo H, et al: Sclerosing encapsulating peritonitis in patients undergoing continuous ambulatory peritoneal dialysis: A report on the Japanese sclerosing encapsulating peritonitis study group. Am J Kidney Dis 28:420-427, 1996.

976. Topley N, Craig JJ, Fallon M, et al: Morphologic changes in the peritoneal membrane of patients on peritoneal dialysis (PD) are related to time on treatment [Abstract]. J Am Soc Nephrol 10:324, 1999.

977. Junor BJR, McMillan MA: Immunosuppression in sclerosing peritonitis. *In* Khanna R, Nolph KD, Prowant BF (eds): Advances in Peritoneal Dialysis. Toronto, Peritoneal Dialysis Publications, 1993, p 187.

978. Hendriks PM, Ho-dac Pannekeet MM, Van Gulik TM, et al: Peritoneal sclerosis in chronic peritoneal dialysis patients: Analysis of clinical presentation, risk factors, and peritoneal transport kinetics. Perit Dial Int 17:136-143, 1997.

979. Mori Y, Matsuo S, Sutoh H, et al: A case of a dialysis patient with sclerosing peritonitis successfully treated with corticosteroid therapy alone. Am J Kidney Dis 30:275, 1997.

980. Kittur DS, Korpe SW, Raytch RE, et al: Surgical aspects of sclerosing encapsulating peritonitis. Arch Surg 125:1626, 1990.

981. Krediet RT: Prevention and treatment of peritoneal dialysis membrane failure. Adv Ren Replace Ther 5:212-217, 1998.

982. Fried LF, Abdi S, Bernardini J, et al: Hospitalization in peritoneal dialysis patients. Am J Kidney Dis 33:927-933, 1997.

983. Gokal R, Jakubowski C, King J, et al: Outcome in patients on continuous ambulatory peritoneal dialysis and haemodialysis: 4-year analysis of a prospective multicentre study. Lancet 1:105, 1987.

984. Krishnan MK, Thodis E, Ikonomopoulos D, et al: Predictors of outcome following bacterial peritonitis in peritoneal dialysis. Perit Dial Int 22:573-581, 2002.

985. Peterson PK, Keane WF: Infections in chronic peritoneal dialysis patients. Curr Clin Top Infect Dis 6:239, 1985.

986. Cairns HS: Continuous ambulatory peritoneal dialysis peritonitis: Role and treatment of impaired host defenses. Semin Dial 5:17, 1992.

987. Rubin J, Rogers WA, Taylor HM, et al: Peritonitis during continuous ambulatory dialysis. Ann Intern Med 92:7, 1980.

988. Holmes CJ, Lewis SL, Evans RC, et al: Periodic elevation of complement activation products in peritoneal dialysis effluent. ASAIO J 35:587, 1989.

989. McGregor SJ, Brock JH, Briggs JD, et al: Longitudinal study of peritoneal defense mechanisms in patients on continuous ambulatory peritoneal dialysis (CAPD). Perit Dial Int 9:115, 1989.

990. Holmes CJ, Lewis SL, Kubey WY, et al: Comparison of peritoneal white blood cell parameters from CAPD patients with a high or low incidence of peritonitis. Am J Kidney Dis 15:258, 1990.

991. De Veechi AF, Kopple JD, Young GA, et al: Plasma and dialysate immunoglobulin G in continuous ambulatory peritoneal dialysis patients: A multicenter study. Am J Nephrol 10:451, 1990.

992. Keane WF, Comty CM, Verbrugh HA, et al: Opsonic deficiency of peritoneal dialysis effluent in CAPD. Kidney Int 25:539, 1984.

993. Topley N, Williams JD: Role of the peritoneal membrane in the control of inflammation in the peritoneal cavity. Kidney Int Suppl 48:71, 1994.

994. Bos HJ, Van Bronswijk H, Helmerhorst TJM, et al: Distinct subpopulations of elicited human macrophages in peritoneal dialysis patients and women undergoing laparoscopy: A study of peroxidatic activity. J Leukoc Biol 43:172, 1988.

995. Brando B, Galato R, Seveso M, et al: Flow cytometric study of immunocompetent cell phenotypes and phagocytosis in CAPD effluent. ASAIO J 34:441, 1988.

996. McGregor SJ, Brock JH, Briggs JD, et al: Bactericidal activity of peritoneal macrophages from CAPD patients. Nephrol Dial Transplant 2:104, 1987.

997. Lamperi S, Carozzi S: Defective opsonic activity of peritoneal effluent during CAPD: Importance and prevention. Perit Dial Bull 6:87, 1986.

998. Goyert SM, Ferrero E, Rettig WJ, et al: The CD14 monocyte differentiation antigen maps to a region encoding growth factors and receptors. Science 239:497, 1988.

999. Kuan SF, Rust K, Crouch E: Interactions of surfactant protein D with bacterial lipopolysaccharides. J Clin Invest 90:97, 1992.

1000. Topley N, Brown Z, Jorres A, et al: Human peritoneal mesothelial cells (HPMC) synthesize interleukin-8 (IL-8): Introduction by cytokines. Perit Dial Int 12(suppl):21, 1992.

1001. Glancey GR, Cameron JS, Ogg CS: Peritoneal drainage: An important element in host defense against staphylococcal peritonitis in patients on CAPD. Nephrol Dial Transplant 7:627, 1992.

1002. Fieren MWJA, van den Bemd GJ, Bonta IL: Endotoxin-stimulated peritoneal macrophages obtained from continuous ambulatory peritoneal dialysis patients show an increased capacity to release interleukin-1 beta in vitro during infectious peritonitis. Eur J Clin Invest 20:453, 1990.

1003. Montrucchio G, Mariano F, Cavalli PL, et al: Platelet activating factor is produced during infectious peritonitis in CAPD patients. Kidney Int 36:1029-1036, 1989.

1004. Brauner A, Hylander B, Wretlind B: Interleukin-6 and interleukin-8 in dialysate and serum from patients on continuous ambulatory peritoneal dialysis. Am J Kidney Dis 22:430, 1993.

1005. Posthuma N, ter Wee PM, Donker AJM, et al: Icodextrin use in CCPD patients during peritonitis: Ultrafiltration and serum disaccharide concentrations. Nephrol Dial Transplant 13:2341-2344, 1998.

1006. Churchill DN: CAPD peritonitis: A critical appraisal of prophylactic strategies. Semin Dial 4:94, 1991.

1007. Imada A, Kawaguchi A, Kumano K, et al: The peritonitis study group in Japan and Baxter Healthcare. A multicenter study of CAPD related peritonitis in Japan [Abstract]. J Am Soc Nephrol 8:12216, 1997.

1008. Buoncristiani U, Cozzari M, Quintaliani G, et al: Abatement of exogenous peritonitis risk using the Perugia CAPD system. Dial Transplant 12:14, 1983.

1009. Balteau PR, Peluso FP, Coles GA, et al: Design and testing of the Baxter integrated disconnect system (IDS). Perit Dial Int 11:131, 1991.

1010. Honkanen E, Kala AR, Gronhagen-Riska C: Divergent etiologies of CAPD peritonitis in integrated double bag and traditional systems? Adv Perit Dial 7:129-132, 1991.

1011. Luzar MA, Slingeneyer A, Cantaluppi A, et al: In vitro study of the flush effect in two reusable continuous ambulatory peritoneal dialysis (CAPD) disconnect systems. Perit Dial Int 9:169, 1989.

1012. Dasgupta MK, Larabie M, Lam K, et al: Growth of bacterial biofilms on Tenckhoff catheter discs in vitro after simulated touch contamination of the Y-connecting set in continuous ambulatory peritoneal dialysis. Am J Nephrol 10:353, 1990.

1013. Holley JL, Bernardini J, Piraino B: Continuous cycling peritoneal dialysis is associated with lower rates of catheter infections than continuous ambulatory peritoneal dialysis. Am J Kidney Dis 16:133, 1990.

1014. de Fijter CWH, Verbrugh HA, Oe LP, et al: Peritoneal defense in continuous ambulatory versus continuous cyclic peritoneal dialysis. Kidney Int 42:947, 1992.

1015. Keane WF, Bergerson B, Pence T, et al: Challenges for continuous ambulatory peritoneal dialysis. *In* Davidson AM (ed): Nephrology: Proceedings of the Xth International Congress of Nephrology, Vol 2. London, Balliere Tindall, 1988, p 1225.

1016. Schroeder CH, Bakkeren JAJM, Weemaes CMR, et al: IgG2 deficiency in young children treated with continuous ambulatory peritoneal dialysis (CAPD). Perit Dial Int 9:201, 1989.

1017. Canadian CAPD Trial Group: Peritonitis in continuous ambulatory peritoneal dialysis (CAPD): A multicenter randomized clinical trial comparing the Y connector disinfectant system to standard system. Perit Dial Int 9:159, 1989.

1018. White A, Smith J: Nasal reservoir as the source of extranasal staphylococci. Antimicrob Agents Chemother 3:679, 1963.

1019. Sewell CM, Clarridge J, Lacke C, et al: Staphylococcal nasal carriage and subsequent infection in peritoneal dialysis patients. JAMA 248:1493, 1982.

1020. Sesso R, Draibe SA, Castelo A, et al: *Staphylococcus aureus* skin carriage and development of peritonitis in patients on continuous ambulatory peritoneal dialysis. Clin Nephrol 31:264, 1989.

1021. Luzar MA, Coles GA, Faller B, et al: *Staphylococcus aureus* nasal carriage and infection in patients on continuous ambulatory peritoneal dialysis. N Engl J Med 322:505, 1990.

1022. Davies SJ, Ogg CS, Cameron JS, et al: *Staphylococcus aureus* nasal carriage, exit site infection and catheter loss in patients treated with continuous ambulatory peritoneal dialysis. Perit Dial Int 9:61, 1989.

1023. Piraino B, Perlmutter JA, Holley JL, et al: *Staphylococcus aureus* peritonitis is associated with *Staphylococcus aureus* nasal carriage in peritoneal dialysis patients. Perit Dial Int 13:S332, 1993.

1024. Swartz R, Messana JM, Starmann B, et al: Preventing *Staphylococcus aureus* infection during chronic peritoneal dialysis. J Am Soc Nephrol 2:1085, 1991.

1025. Zimmerman SW, Ahrens B, Johnson CA, et al: Randomized controlled trail of prophylactic rifampin for peritoneal dialysis–related infections. Am J Kidney Dis 18:225, 1991.

1026. Perez-Fontan M, Garcia-Falcon T, Rosales M, et al: Treatment of *Staphylococcus aureus* nasal carriers in continuous ambulatory peritoneal dialysis with mupirocin: Long term results. Am J Kidney Dis 22:708, 1993.

1027. Nasal mupirocin prevents *Staphylococcus aureus* exit-site infection during peritoneal dialysis. Mupirocin Study Group. J Am Soc Nephrol 7:2403-2408, 1996.

1028. Bernardini J, Piraino B, Holley JL, et al: Randomized trial of *S. aureus* prophylaxis in PD patients: Mupirocin calcium ointment 2% applied to the exit site versus oral rifampin. Am J Kidney Dis 26:695, 1996.

1029. Thodis E, Bhaskaran S, Passadakis P, et al: Decrease in *Staphylococcus aureus* exit site infections and peritonitis in CAPD patients by local application of mupirocin ointment at the catheter exit site. Perit Dial Int 18:261-270, 1998.

1030. Casey MJ, Taylor J, Clinard P, et al: Application of mupirocin cream at the exit site reduces exit site infections and peritonitis in peritoneal dialysis patients. Perit Dial Int 20:566-568, 2000.

1031. Ritzau J, Hoffman RM, Tzamaloukas AH: Effect of preventing *Staphylococcus aureus* carriage on rates of peritoneal catheter related staphylococcal infections. Perit Dial Int 21:471-479, 2001.

1032. Conly JM, Vas SI: Increasing mupirocin resistance of *Staphylococcus aureus* in CAPD—should it continue to be used as prophylaxsis [editorial]? Perit Dial Int 22:649-652, 2002.

1033. Piraino B: Peritoneal infections. Adv Ren Replace Ther 7:281-288, 2000.

1034. Vas SI: Peritonitis. *In* Nolph KD (ed): Peritoneal Dialysis, 3rd ed. Dordrecht, The Netherlands, Kluwer Academic, 1989, p 261.

1035. Kern EO, Newman LN, Cacho C, et al: Abdominal catastrophe revisited: The risk and outcome of enteric peritoneal contamination. Perit Dial Int 22:323-324, 2002.

1036. Twardowski ZJ, Schreiber MJ, Burkart JM: Peritoneal dialysis forum: A 55-year-old man with hematuria and blood-tinged dialysate. Perit Dial Int 12:61, 1992.

1037. Charytan C: Continuous ambulatory peritoneal dialysis after abdominal aortic graft surgery. Perit Dial Int 12:227, 1992.

1038. Streather CP, Carr P, Barton IK: Carcinoma of the kidney presenting as sterile peritonitis in a patient on continuous ambulatory peritoneal dialysis. Nephron 58:121, 1991.

1039. Vlahakos D, Rudders R, Simon G, et al: Lymphoma-mimicking peritonitis in a patient on continuous ambulatory peritoneal dialysis (CAPD). Perit Dial Int 10:165, 1990.

1040. Tintillier M, Pochet JM, Christophe JL, et al: Transient sterile chemical peritonitis with icodextrin: Clinical presentation, prevalence, and literature review. Perit Dial Int 22:534-537, 2002.

1041. Williams PF, Foggensteiner L: Sterile/allergic peritonitis with icodextrin in CAPD patients. Perit Dial Int 22:89-90, 2002.

1042. Tzamaloukas AH, Obermiller LB, Gibel LJ, et al: Peritonitis associated with intra-abdominal pathology in continuous ambulatory peritoneal dialysis patients. Perit Dial Int 13:S335, 1993.

1043. Tzamaloukas AH, Murata GH, Fox L: Peritoneal catheter loss and death in continuous ambulatory peritoneal dialysis peritonitis: Correlation with clinical and biochemical parameters. Perit Dial Int 13:S338, 1993.

1044. Harwell C, Newman L, Cacho C, et al: Abdominal catastrophe: Visceral injury as a cause of peritonitis in patients treated by peritoneal dialysis. Perit Dial Int 17:586-594, 1997.

1045. Caruana RJ, Burkart JM, Segraves D, et al: Serum and peritoneal fluid amylase levels in CAPD. Am J Nephrol 7:169, 1987.

1046. Burkart JM, Haigler S, Caruana RJ, et al: Usefulness of peritoneal fluid amylase levels in the differential diagnosis of peritonitis in peritoneal dialysis patients. J Am Soc Nephrol 1:1186, 1991.

1047. Twardowski ZJ, Schrieber MJ, Burkart JM: A 69-year-old male with elevated amylase in bloody and cloudy dialysate. Perit Dial Int 13:142, 1993.

1048. Royse VL, Jensen DM, Corwin HL: Pancreatic enzymes in chronic renal failure. Arch Intern Med 147:537, 1987.

1049. Tse KC, Yip PS, Lam MF, et al: Recurrent hemoperitoneum complicating continuous ambulatory peritoneal dialysis. Perit Dial Int 22:488-491, 2002.

1050. Suresh KR, Port FK: Air under diaphragm in patients undergoing continuous ambulatory peritoneal dialysis (CAPD). Perit Dial Int 9:309, 1989.

1051. Silverstein W, Isikoff MB, Hill MC, et al: Diagnostic imaging of acute pancreatitis: Prospective study using CT and sonography. AJR Am J Roentgenol 137:497, 1981.

1052. Port FK, Held PJ, Nolph KD, et al: Risk of peritoneal and technique failure by CAPD connection technique: A national study. Kidney Int 42:967-974, 1992.

1053. Struijk RG, van Ketel RJ, Krediet RT, et al: Patient viral peritonitis in a continuous ambulatory peritoneal dialysis. Nephron 44:384, 1986.

1054. Lewis SL: Evidence of possible viral etiology. Am J Kidney Dis 17:343, 1991.

1055. Goodship THJ, Heaton A, Rodger RSC, et al: Factors affecting development of peritonitis in continuous ambulatory peritoneal dialysis. BMJ 289:1485, 1984.

1056. Lewis SL, Stephen AY, Wood BJ, et al: Relationship between frequent episodes of peritonitis and altered immune status. Am J Kidney Dis 22:456, 1993.

1057. Gregory MC, Duffy DP: Toxic shock following staphylococcal peritonitis. Clin Nephrol 20:101, 1983.

1058. Grutzmacher P, Tsobanelis T, Bruns M, et al: Decrease in peritonitis rate by integrated disconnect system in patients on continuous ambulatory peritoneal dialysis. Perit Dial Int 13(suppl):326, 1993.

1059. Borra SI, Chandarana J, Kleinfeld M: Fatal peritonitis due to group B β-hemolytic streptococcus in a patient receiving chronic ambulatory peritoneal dialysis. Am J Kidney Dis 19:375, 1992.

1060. Boner G, Mhashilkar AM, Rodriguez-Ortega M, et al: Lectin-mediated, nonopsonic phagocytosis of type 1 *Escherichia coli* by human peritoneal macrophages of uremic patients treated by peritoneal dialysis. J Leukoc Biol 46:239, 1989.

1061. Wood CJ, Fleming V, Turnidge J, et al: *Campylobacter* peritonitis in continuous ambulatory peritoneal dialysis: Report of eight cases and a review of the literature. Am J Kidney Dis 19:257, 1992.

1062. Chan MK, Chan PCK, Cheng IPK, et al: *Pseudomonas* peritonitis in CAPD patients: Characteristics and outcome of treatment. Nephrol Dial Transplant 4:814, 1989.

1063. Vassa N, Nolph KD, Khanna R: *Pseudomonas* peritonitis with white blood cell capillary margination and distal digital necrosis in a patient on CAPD. Perit Dial Int 12:323, 1992.

1064. Cheng IK, Fang GX, Chan TM, et al: Fungal peritonitis complicating peritoneal dialysis: Report of 27 cases and review of treatment. Q J Med 71:407, 1989.

1065. Bernard DB, Levine J, Idelson BA: A continuous ambulatory peritoneal dialysis patient with fungal peritonitis. Semin Dial 4:198, 1991.

1066. Brown E, Hendler E: *Rhodococcus* peritonitis in a patient treated with peritoneal dialysis. Am J Kidney Dis 14:417, 1989.

1067. Levine J, Bernard DB, Idelson BA, et al: Fungal peritonitis complicating continuous ambulatory peritoneal dialysis: Successful treatment with fluconazole, a new orally active antifungal agent. Am J Med 86:825, 1989.

1068. Stein M, Levine JF, Black W: Successful treatment of *Aspergillus* peritonitis in an adult on continuous ambulatory peritoneal dialysis. Nephron 59:145, 1991.

1069. Lye WC, Lee EJC: Tuberculous peritonitis in CAPD—a cause of hypercalcaemia. Perit Dial Int 10:307, 1990.

1070. Cheng IK, Chan PCK, Chan MK: Tuberculous peritonitis complicating long-term peritoneal dialysis. Report of 5 cases and review of the literature. Am J Nephrol 9:155, 1989.

1071. Keane WF, Bailie GR, Boeschoten EW, et al: ISPD guidelines/recommendations: Adult peritoneal dialysis–related peritonitis treatment recommendations. Perit Dial Int 4:396-411, 2000.

1072. Holley JL, Bernardini J, Piraino B: Risk factors for tunnel infections in continuous peritoneal dialysis. Am J Kidney Dis 18:344, 1991.

1073. Dasgupta MK: Use of streptokinase or urokinase in recurrent CAPD peritonitis. Adv Perit Dial 7:169-172, 1991.

1074. Domoto DT, Weindel ME, Blalock S, Ballal HS: Efficacy of streptokinase in resistant, relapsing, or recurrent CAPD peritonitis. Adv Perit Dial 7:173-175, 1991.

1075. Read RR, Dasgupta MK, Parker E, et al: Peritonitis in peritoneal dialysis: Bacterial colonization by biofilm spread along the catheter surface. Kidney Int 35:614, 1989.

1076. Murphy G, Tzamaloukas AH, Eisenberg B, et al: Intraperitoneal thrombolytic agents in relapsing or persistent peritonitis of patients on continuous ambulatory peritoneal dialysis. Int J Artif Organs 14:87, 1991.

1077. Guiberteau R, le Chapois D, Nony A, et al: Treatment of peritoneal infection of the natural defenses of the peritoneal cavity. Contrib Nephrol 57:92, 1987.

1078. Pagniez DC, MacNamara E, Fortin F, et al: Withdrawal of continuous ambulatory peritoneal dialysis to treat mild peritonitis. BMJ 297:1174, 1988.

1079. Digenis G, Abraham G, Savin B, et al: Peritoneal-related deaths in continuous ambulatory peritoneal dialysis (CAPD) patients. Perit Dial Int 10:45, 1990.

1080. Swartz R, Messana JM, Reynolds J, et al: Simultaneous catheter replacement and removal in refractory peritoneal dialysis infections. Kidney Int 40:1160, 1991.

1081. Johnson CA: Intraperitoneal vancomycin administration. Perit Dial Int 11:9, 1991.

1082. Pierratos A: Peritoneal dialysis glossary. Perit Dial Bull 1:2, 1984.

1083. Luzar MA, Brown CB, Balf D, et al: Exit-site care and exit-site infection in CAPD: Results of a randomized multicenter trial. Perit Dial Int 10:25, 1990.

1084. Millikin SP, Matzke GR, Geane WF: Antimicrobial treatment of peritonitis associated with continuous ambulatory peritoneal dialysis. Perit Dial Int 11:252, 1991.

1085. Piraino B, Bernardini J, Sorkin MI: A five-year study of the microbiologic results of exit-site infections and peritonitis in continuous ambulatory peritoneal dialysis. Am J Kidney Dis 10:281, 1987.

1086. Keane WF, Everett ED, Golper, TA, et al: Peritoneal dialysis-related peritonitis treatment recommendations: 1993 update. Perit Dial Int 13:14, 1993.

1087. Keane WF, Alexander SR, Bailie GR, et al: Peritoneal dialysis-related peritonitis treatment recommendations: 1996 update. Perit Dial Int 16:557, 1996.

1088. NKF-K/DOQI Clinical Practice Guidelines for Peritoneal Dialysis Adequacy. New York, National Kidney Foundation, 2000.

1088a. Lum GM: Peritonitis in infants and children on CAPD/CCPD. In Anderiotti VE, Fine RN (eds): Topics in Renal Medicine, Vol 4. Chronic Ambulatory Peritoneal Dialysis (CCPD) in Children. Amsterdam, Martinus Nijhoff, 1987, p 189.

1089. Twardowski ZJ: Exit-site infection. *In* La Greca G, Ronco C, Feriani M, et al (eds): Peritoneal Dialysis: Proceedings of the 4th International Course on Peritoneal Dialysis. Milan, Wichtig Editore, 1991, p 241.

1090. Pylypchuk GB, Conly J, Kappel JE, et al: Sensitivity of CAPD/IPD peritonitis organisms to ciprofloxacin. *In* Khanna R, Nolph KD, Prowant BF, et al (eds): Advances in Peritoneal Dialysis, Vol 7, Toronto, University of Toronto Press, 1991, p 135.

1091. Chong TK, Piraino B, Bernardini J: Vestibular toxicity due to gentamycin in peritoneal dialysis patients. Perit Dial Int 11:152, 1991.

1092. Vas SI: Single daily dose of aminoglycosides in the treatment of continuous ambulatory peritoneal dialysis peritonitis. Perit Dial Int 13:S355, 1993.

1093. Scalmogna A, Castelnovo C, De Vecchi A, et al: Exit site and tunnel infection in CAPD patients. Am J Kidney Dis 18:674, 1991.

CHAPTER 61

Intensive Care Nephrology

Matthew Dollins, Michael A. Kraus, and Bruce A. Molitoris

It is estimated that from 5% to 25% of critically ill patients will develop renal failure during the course of their illness,[1, 2] including between 9% and 40% of patients with sepsis,[3] 20% to 40% of patients with acute respiratory distress syndrome (ARDS),[4] 33% of patients with cardiogenic shock,[5] and 55% of patients with fulminant hepatic failure (FHF).[6] The nephrologist is a critical component in the care of these patients, and an understanding of the underlying pathophysiology of respiratory failure, shock, and management of mechanical ventilation is critical. The nephrologist should understand the literature behind the move to low tidal volume ventilation, as this will affect acid-base status, and has implications for bicarbonate prescriptions during renal replacement therapy (RRT). The management of shock is also a rapidly developing field, and nephrologists who are active in the care of many of these patients should have an understanding of this area.

ACUTE RESPIRATORY FAILURE

Acute respiratory failure can be defined as the inability of the respiratory system to meet the oxygenation, ventilation, or metabolic requirements of the patient.[7] This may occur in a previously healthy person with pneumonia or pulmonary embolism, or may complicate chronic respiratory failure in the setting of pulmonary fibrosis or chronic obstructive pulmonary disease (COPD). Respiratory failure can be divided into two main types: hypoxemic respiratory failure, which is failure to maintain adequate oxygenation, and hypercapnic respiratory failure, which is inadequate ventilation with CO_2 retention.

Respiratory failure is a common occurrence in the intensive care unit (ICU), and many of these patients develop renal failure during the course of their illness. Because nephrologists are often asked to assist with the acid-base

management of these patients, it is important that they have an understanding of mechanical ventilation and the newer treatment strategies for ARDS.

When patients with respiratory failure are unable to maintain their oxygenation or ventilation by noninvasive means such as supplemental oxygen, continuous positive airway pressure (CPAP), or bilateral positive airway pressure (BiPAP), they require intubation and mechanical ventilation. Several modes of mechanical ventilation are now available which differ in their indications. Synchronized intermittent mandatory ventilation (SIMV) allows the patient to breathe spontaneously between breaths assisted by the ventilator. The physician orders a set number of breaths, delivered every minute at a certain tidal volume, which is given in synchrony with inspiratory effort if the patient is able to generate inspiration. Any breaths beyond the set number must be generated by the patient. Assist control mode, or continuous mandatory ventilation (CMV), results in the ventilator delivering a breath every time the patient generates a negative inspiratory force, or at a set rate, whichever is the higher frequency. CMV minimizes the work of breathing done by the patient, and therefore should be used in the setting of myocardial ischemia or profound hypoxemia. One problem with CMV occurs in patients who are tachypneic or have obstructive lung disease. If there is inadequate time to exhale the full tidal volume, dynamic hyperinflation (breath stacking or "auto-PEEP" [positive end-expiratory pressure]) may occur, which can result in increased intrathoracic pressure, decreased cardiac output, and possibly barotrauma. Pressure control ventilation (PCV) differs from SIMV and CMV in that the physician sets an inspiratory pressure, not a tidal volume. During inspiration, a given pressure is imposed via the circuit, and the tidal volume delivered depends upon how much flow can be delivered prior to the airway pressure equilibrating with the inspiratory pressure. The tidal volume can vary from breath to breath, and thus the minute volume is variable.

CPAP is not a true form of mechanical ventilation, but provides a supply of fresh gas at a constant, specified pressure. It is most commonly used in weaning trials or in patients without respiratory failure who require an endotracheal tube to maintain an airway. Pressure support ventilation (PSV) is a patient-triggered mode of ventilation in which a preset pressure is maintained throughout inspiration. When inspiratory flow falls below a certain level, inspiration is terminated. PSV is commonly used in patients who require minimal support, or to assist the spontaneous breaths during SIMV. Airway pressure release ventilation (APRV) is used in a spontaneously breathing patient who is using CPAP. At the end of each ventilator cycle, the lungs are allowed to briefly deflate to ambient pressure, then rapidly reinflated to the baseline (CPAP) pressure with the next breath. The perceived advantage is that lung expansion during exhalation is maintained with CPAP, but the brief interruption of this pressure at the end of exhalation allows for further CO_2 elimination, as well as enhanced venous return.

In addition to the mode of ventilation, the physician prescribes the oxygen concentration to be delivered, the level of PEEP, the tidal volume, and the respiratory rate. When initially intubated, patients are typically placed on a high oxygen concentration and weaned down as quickly as possible. Multiple animal studies have supported the notion of oxygen toxicity, whereby higher oxygen concentrations lead to lung injury.[8-11] Studies of healthy volunteers have shown that after 6 hours on 100% oxygen, there is a change in whole-lung capacity and a decrease in vital capacity,[12] and after 24 hours, there is a reduction in lung compliance likely secondary to increased interstitial edema.[13] Although there are no conclusive studies showing the effects of high levels of inspired oxygen on the lungs during acute illness, most clinicians try to reduce the inspired oxygen concentration to 50% or less as quickly as possible.

PEEP provides a continuous airway pressure above atmospheric, preventing collapse of alveoli and small airways at end-expiration. By recruiting alveoli in this way, PEEP improves functional residual capacity and oxygenation. PEEP is most commonly set between 5 and 20 cm H_2O and titrated until adequate oxygenation is achieved. The level of PEEP directly increases airway pressures, so high levels of PEEP can result in barotrauma.

The tidal volume delivered during mechanical ventilation has recently undergone a dramatic change. Traditional tidal volumes were 12 to 15 mL/kg per breath, but as will be discussed in the ARDS section, recent studies support using lower tidal volumes in patients with lung injury. Patients who are felt to have acute lung injury or ARDS are now prescribed 4 to 8 mL/kg per breath with the goal of minimizing airway pressures. Some centers are now using this low tidal volume on all mechanically ventilated patients with the goal of preventing ventilator-induced lung injury from barotrauma.

The respiratory rate is set based on the patient's minute ventilation requirement. Patients who are septic or very metabolically active often require a high minute volume to adequately eliminate CO_2, and with the lower tidal volumes used now, respiratory rates are often increased. However, care must be taken in the patient with asthma or obstructive lung disease because a rate that is too high can lead to air trapping if the patient with prolonged expiratory phase requirements is not allowed to exhale the complete tidal volume before the next breath.

ADULT RESPIRATORY DISTRESS SYNDROME

The adult respiratory distress syndrome was first described in 1967 when Ashbaugh and colleagues described 12 patients with acute respiratory distress, hypoxia refractory to oxygen therapy, decreased lung compliance, and diffuse infiltrates on chest tomography.[14] This clinical entity is now referred to as the "acute respiratory distress syndrome" as it is recognized to occur in children as well as adults, affecting up to 150,000 patients per year in the United States.[15]

ARDS has historically had a high mortality rate, in some studies approaching 90%.[16-20] The lack of a uniform definition led to difficulty in designing studies and attempts at improving outcome, so in 1994 the American-European Consensus Conference developed a definition that is widely used today.[15] This conference established two categories, acute lung injury (ALI) and ARDS, depending on the severity of hypoxemia. The acute onset of hypoxemic respiratory failure with bilateral infiltrates on chest tomography, and a pulmonary artery wedge pressure of less than 18 mm Hg, or no clinical evidence of left atrial hypertension characterize both ALI and ARDS. ALI is present when the above criteria are present with arterial O_2, tension–fraction of inspired O_2 (Pa_{O_2}/F_{IO_2}) ratio of less than 300, and ARDS requires the above criteria with a Pa_{O_2}/F_{IO_2} ratio of less than 200. The syndromes represent two points on the same disease spectrum, and both appear to have similar outcomes.

Clinical Features

ALI and ARDS are usually diagnosed when a patient with a known risk factor develops acute dyspnea, hypoxemia, and tachypnea. Different stages are often apparent. The acute stage is characterized by the onset of acute respiratory failure, commonly associated with hypoxemia that is refractory to supplemental oxygen. Radiographic findings include bilateral infiltrates that may be indistinguishable from cardiogenic pulmonary edema,[21] and may be patchy or symmetrical Computed tomography shows the affected areas are primarily the dependant lung zones.[22] During this phase, patients previously requiring minimal oxygen often progress to requiring mechanical support as the work of breathing increases. Pathologic findings include damage to the capillary endothelial and alveolar epithelial cells.[23] This disruption of the normal barrier results in increased permeability and filling of the alveoli with protein-rich fluid and inflammatory cells.[24] There is also direct damage to type II pneumocytes, which are responsible for surfactant production. Reduction in surfactant production leads to increased surface tension within the alveoli and results in atelectasis. Interstitial edema also results in the collapse of small airways. As these nonventilated alveoli are perfused, severe, refractory hypoxemia develops, which accounts for the shunt physiology seen in this disorder. Mechanically ventilated ARDS patients often have very high airway pressures, a result of the reduction of ventilated alveoli and reduced compliance from the influx of inflammatory cells. This often necessitates a high minute ventilation to maintain an acceptable CO_2 tension (P_{CO_2}).

Following the acute phase, many patients recover completely, yet some develop a fibrotic phase characterized by fibrosing alveolitis, persistent hypoxemia, and further worsening of pulmonary complications.[24] Right ventricular failure can develop due to destruction of the pulmonary capillary bed. Even following the fibrotic phase, improvement in hypoxemia and lung compliance can occur gradually, with many patients returning to normal pulmonary function over 6 to 12 months.[25]

Risk Factors

ALI and ARDS can develop in association with several clinical conditions (Table 61-1), not all of which directly involve the pulmonary system. The most common condition associated with ARDS is sepsis, with up to 40% of septic patients developing ARDS.[20, 23]

Other common risk factors include shock, the systemic inflammatory response syndrome (SIRS), pneumonia, multiple transfusions, near drowning, aspiration, trauma, pancreatitis, burns, coronary artery bypass grafting, and disseminated intravascular coagulation (DIC).[13, 14, 26] Multiple risk factors increase the risk for ARDS synergistically.[23]

Pathophysiology

Several mediators contribute to the pathologic response seen in ARDS. Neutrophils play a prominent role in this process, as they are found in the alveoli as well as the interstitium during ARDS. They are recruited into the interstitium by cellular adhesion molecules such as selectins and β_2 integrins.[27] The neutrophils are activated by complement, interleukins-1 (IL-1), -6, -8, and -10, as well as tumor necrosis factor-α (TNF-α), and these activated neutrophils can then secrete other inflammatory mediators, as well as highly reactive oxidant species, proteolytic enzymes, and metabolites of arachidonic acid that can directly injure alveolar and capillary endothelial cells, allowing for fluid to leak into the alveoli with resultant edema.[28, 29] While neutrophils are a large component of the inflammatory response, they are not a requirement, as neutropenic patients can also develop ARDS. Alveolar macrophages are also involved in ARDS,

elaborating cytokines that contribute to the inflammatory process, as well as clearing neutrophils from the alveoli and aiding in the resolution of ARDS.

Thromboxane A$_2$ may interact with neutrophils to accentuate cell aggregation,[30] and lipoxygenase products are released in large quantities and may contribute to pulmonary vascular changes and permeability characteristics,[24] resulting in "leaky capillaries." Release of platelet-activating factor (PAF) leads to platelet aggregation in the microvasculature, which results in increased pulmonary vascular resistance and pulmonary hypertension. Infiltration of the interstitium with fibroblasts is seen during the late stage, resulting in the fibrosis seen in some cases.

Treatment

The treatment of ARDS has historically been one of support, but the high mortality rates prompted significant research into its cause and propagation. The underlying or predisposing factor should always be addressed promptly, and because sepsis is the most common cause of ARDS, a search for an undiagnosed infection should be undertaken if no clear etiology is present.

The primary mechanism of support is mechanical ventilation. The Acute Respiratory Distress Syndrome Network (ARDSNET) trial[31] recently showed that a "lung protective mechanism" of mechanical ventilation could improve survival. The goal is to provide adequate oxygenation while avoiding further trauma to the lung that can worsen existing injury.

Traditionally, tidal volumes used during mechanical ventilation were in the range of 12 to 15 mL/minute. Acute lung injury, similar to human ARDS, has been observed in animals mechanically ventilated with large tidal volumes.[32] It was reasoned that overdistention of the alveoli, leading to elevated airway pressure, was a primary element in this acute lung injury. Ventilation with high airway pressures has been shown to cause increased vascular permeability, acute inflammation, alveolar hemorrhage, and radiographic infiltrates.[33, 34] In persons with acute lung injury or ARDS, the large tidal volumes are shunted to the unaffected lung as they provide the least resistance, and overdistention results in damage to these previously unaffected segments.

The ARDSNET trial[31] was designed to assess if lower tidal volumes and hence lower airway pressures resulted in clinical benefit in ARDS. This trial compared traditional ventilation treatment, which was an initial tidal volume of 12 mL/kg ideal body weight (IBW), to a lower tidal volume group that started at 6 mL/kg IBW (IBW = 50 + 2.3 [height in inches −60] for males, 45.5 + 2.3 [height in inches −60] for females). In each group, the tidal volume was decreased in increments of 1 mL/kg to maintain the plateau pressure (the airway pressure measured after 0.5-second inspiratory pause) below 50 mm Hg for the traditional ventilation group, and below 30 mm Hg for the lower tidal volume group. The minimal tidal volume was 4 mL/kg. The level of PEEP and oxygen concentration was based on a sliding protocol (Table 61-2). This study was stopped early after 861 patients were enrolled because of a mortality benefit seen in the lower tidal volume group. The mortality rate was 39.8% in the group treated with traditional tidal volumes and 31% in the group treated with lower tidal volumes ($P = .007$). As expected, the group

TABLE 61-1

Risk Factors for Acute Respiratory Distress Syndrome

Pulmonary causes
  Pneumonia
  Aspiration
  Near-drowning

Nonpulmonary causes
  Sepsis
  Systemic inflammatory response syndrome
  Shock
  Trauma
  Multiple blood transfusions
  Pancreatitis
  Burns
  Coronary artery bypass grafting
  Disseminated intravascular coagulation

TABLE 61-2

Oxygen and PEEP Titration in the ARDSNET Trial (Goal:PaO$_2$ 55-80 mm Hg)

FIO$_2$	0.3	0.4	0.4	0.5	0.5	0.6	0.7
PEEP	5	5	8	8	10	10	10
FIO$_2$	0.7	0.7	0.8	0.9	0.9	1.0	
PEEP	12	14	14	16	18	20-24	

FIO$_2$, fraction of inspired oxygen; PEEP, positive end-expiratory pressure.
Data from the Acute Respiratory Distress Syndrome Network [ARDSNET]:
Ventilation with lower tidal volumes as compared with traditional tidal volumes
for acute lung injury and acute respiratory distress syndrome. N Engl J Med
342:1301, 2000.

receiving lower tidal volumes had a slightly higher PaCO$_2$ (43 vs. 36 at day 3) and lower pH (7.38 vs. 7.41 at day 3) than the traditional tidal volume group.

Because ARDS is a process that results in decreased lung compliance, patients can generally tolerate higher respiratory rates without the risk of air trapping that is seen in obstructive diseases such as asthma or COPD. The ARDSNET trial used a maximum respiratory rate of 35 breaths per minute. Despite this high rate, the low tidal volumes used to maintain plateau pressures below 30 mm Hg resulted in a minute ventilation too low to maintain acid-base balance in many patients, a result termed "permissive hypercapnia." When the arterial pH fell below 7.30 with a respiratory rate of 35 breaths per minute, an infusion of sodium bicarbonate was started.

Given that there have been no other studies in ARDS resulting in such an improvement in mortality, this mode of ventilation must be recommended for all patients with ARDS.

Low tidal volume ventilation clearly has an impact on the nephrologist caring for the ARDS patient with renal failure. Permissive hypercapnia may result in significant acidosis in a patient with renal failure who is unable to excrete the daily acid load. It also means that the nephrologist may have to use a higher bicarbonate bath during hemodialysis or continuous RRT, as increasing the minute volume to improve acid-base control is often not an option. In some patients with severe ARDS, large infusions of bicarbonate may not improve acidosis as CO$_2$ is produced, which the severely injured lungs may not be able to expel adequately. Tris(hydroxymethyl)-aminomethane (THAM) is a buffer that accepts one proton per molecule, generating HCO$_3^-$ but not CO$_2$. It has been shown to control arterial pH without increasing CO$_2$ in the setting of refractory respiratory acidosis.[35] THAM is excreted by the kidneys, so it is not recommended in renal failure.

How best to manage volume status in a patient with ALI or ARDS is controversial. There are substantial data from animal experiments indicating fluid restriction can reduce pulmonary edema in the setting of increased pulmonary vascular permeability, as in ALI or ARDS.[36] These data include an observational study where survival in ARDS was related to negative fluid balance,[37] a study in which patients with a 25% reduction in pulmonary capillary wedge pressure had a greater survival than other patients,[38] and a study where patients with less than 1 L of fluid gain after 36 hours of recruitment had a better survival than other patients.[39] Yet, there are other data suggesting patients with ALI or ARDS may do better with a strategy that increases oxygen delivery,

usually requiring volume expansion. Fluid restriction can reduce cardiac output and tissue perfusion, leading to worsening of the nonpulmonary organ dysfunction that is often seen in patients with ARDS. Several trials have assessed whether providing supranormal levels of oxygen delivery will improve outcome.[40-45] Some feel that in systemic inflammatory conditions, such as sepsis or trauma, normal cardiac output and tissue oxygen delivery may be inadequate to prevent organ dysfunction. In postoperative treatment of trauma patients, there was a trend toward decreased mortality with supranormal oxygen delivery,[40-42] but there has been no benefit in patients with ALI or ARDS,[43, 44] and one study showed an increased mortality in patients who received supranormal levels of oxygen delivery.[45] As there is no clear benefit to supranormal oxygen delivery, which requires volume expansion, and because fluid restriction can lead to worsening of nonpulmonary organ dysfunction, greatly increasing mortality, maintaining euvolemia (wedge pressure, 10-14 mm Hg, CVP 6-12 mm Hg) in patients with ARDS or ALI with use of fluids as guided by evidence of organ perfusion would be the most reasonable approach at this time.

The inflammatory nature of ARDS raises the possibility that glucocorticoids may be beneficial in treating this condition. High doses of glucocorticoids have not shown benefit when given to prevent ARDS in high-risk patients,[46-48] or when given early in the course of ARDS.[46, 49] However, the persistent inflammation and fibroproliferation seen in the late stage of ARDS may be improved by corticosteroids. One small study (32 patients)[50] evaluated prolonged methylprednisolone in ARDS patients who did not improve after 7 days of respiratory failure, and found an improvement in severity scores and mortality in those treated. Many physicians currently use glucocorticoids as a rescue therapy in prolonged ARDS, and the National Institutes of Health (NIH) ARDS network is currently conducting a trial to evaluate corticosteroids in late ARDS.

Prone positioning has been advocated as a means to ventilate the posterior lung regions that are more often atelectatic and flooded in ARDS. Once the patients is prone, these previously dependent lung regions open as the anterior lung regions become dependent. Several personnel are required to safely move a patient into the prone position to ensure that chest tubes, intravenous lines, and the endotracheal tube are not dislodged. Patients are rotated every 12 to 18 hours, and studies have shown improved gas exchange and oxygenation in the prone position,[51, 52] but recent studies have shown no improvement in outcomes with prone positioning.[53, 54]

Surfactant is normally produced by type II pneumocytes and allows patency of alveoli at lower airway pressures. In ARDS, surfactant production is decreased. Animal models of lung injury have shown a benefit from inhaled surfactant therapy,[55, 56] but a trial in 725 patients with ARDS showed no benefit from an artificial surfactant given by aerosol.[57] Newer surfactant preparations are currently being evaluated.

Nitric oxide is a vasodilator that when inhaled dilates pulmonary blood vessels perfusing aerated lung units, without systemic vasodilation. Inhaled NO has been found to improve the PaO$_2$/FIO$_2$ ratio,[58] but has not been found to lower mortality.[59, 60]

The inflammatory response seen in ALI or ARDS has led to many agents, in addition to corticosteroids, being evaluated as possible therapy. Prostaglandin E$_1$ (PGE$_1$),[61] ketoconazole[62] (an inhibitor of thromboxane and leukotriene synthesis), ibuprofen,[63] and oxothiazolidine carboxylate (Procysteine) or N-acetylcysteine[23] have all been evaluated and found to have no benefit. In addition, treatment of sepsis before, or early in the development of, ALI or ARDS with an antiendotoxin monoclonal antibody, anti-TNF-α, and anti-IL-1 have not shown benefit.[36] Studies using IL-10 and recombinant human platelet-activating factor are currently in the design stages.[64]

Extracorporeal CO_2 removal has been investigated and found to have no effect on mortality in one randomized controlled study.[65] Partial liquid ventilation with fluorocarbon liquids, which can dissolve 17 times more oxygen than water, has been evaluated with encouraging results, but more trials are needed before this therapy becomes widespread.[36]

Effects on Renal Function

Renal dysfunction is a common occurrence in patients with ARDS or ALI. In a retrospective study of 59 patients with ARDS, Valta and colleagues[4] found that 20% to 40% of patients had renal dysfunction. Although many patients with ARDS are also septic or hemodynamically unstable, mechanical ventilation itself has been found to be a predictor of need for dialysis.[66] Several studies have shown that mechanical ventilation can lead to reduced renal blood flow, decreased urine output, and sodium retention.[67-69] These changes in renal function are felt to be due to multiple factors. The first is the reduced cardiac output seen in the setting of positive pressure ventilation. Positive intrathoracic pressure from mechanical ventilation reduces venous return to the heart, resulting in decreased effective circulating volume, and increases pressure in the pulmonary vasculature, which results in elevated right ventricular afterload, factors that result in reduced cardiac output. The reduced airway compliance seen in ARDS leads to elevated intrathoracic pressures with even relatively small tidal volumes. In addition, the intrathoracic pressure increases linearly as the PEEP is increased. Because many patients with ARDS require a high PEEP to maintain patency of the alveoli and small airways for maintenance of oxygenation, this group of patients is particularly susceptible to the hemodynamic effects of mechanical ventilation.

Not all studies have shown a decrease in renal blood flow with positive pressure ventilation,[70] and it appears that volume status may play a role in the hemodynamic response to positive pressure ventilation. Those patients who are volume-depleted are more susceptible to reduced cardiac output.

As not all studies have shown a reduced cardiac output in association with renal dysfunction, it is likely that there are other factors involved. Hormonal changes during mechanical ventilation have been evaluated. Antidiuretic hormone (ADH) levels are elevated in mechanically ventilated patients, but may act primarily as a vasoconstrictor and have minimal effect on water retention.[70, 71] A sympathetically mediated increase in plasma renin activity results in a decline in the glomerular filtration rate (GFR) by reducing renal blood flow, and stimulating sodium retention via aldosterone.[72] Atrial natriuretic peptide may also be reduced as a consequence of the decreased venous return and lower atrial pressures, resulting in reduced urine output.[73] Other factors,

such as NO and endothelin, may also play a role, but their effect remains undetermined.

ARDS is a complex, inflammatory condition, and there appears to be more to its association with renal failure than changes induced by elevated intrathoracic pressures. ARDS is likely an early manifestation of a systemic inflammatory process that results in multiorgan dysfunction. Studies of bronchoalveolar fluid have shown increased TNF-α, IL-1β, and IL-6 concentrations during ARDS.[74, 75] It is possible that the lung produces cytokines, and ventilator-induced lung injury has been associated with increased pulmonary cytokine production that leads to elevations in systemic concentrations.[76] These cytokines have been shown to cause an ARDS-like condition in rats, but their role in human ARDS has not been fully unraveled.

TNF-α has been associated with the renal injury seen in ischemia-reperfusion models, as has IL-1, IL-2, IL-8, interferon-γ, and granulocyte-macrophage colony-stimulating factor.[77, 78] While the association between these cytokines, ARDS, and acute renal failure (ARF) has not been fully elucidated, it is likely ARDS represents an early stage in inflammation leading to multiorgan system failure, including ARF. Whether primary cytokine production by the injured lung leads to further organ dysfunction has yet to be established.

HYPOVOLEMIC SHOCK

Hypovolemic shock can be defined as a reduction in effective circulating blood volume, which leads to an oxygen deficit in the tissues, as oxygen supply is not able to meet oxygen demand. This imbalance in oxygen metabolism leads to cellular ischemia, and, if prolonged, cellular death. Hypovolemic shock occurs most commonly from trauma and hemorrhage,[79] but can also be seen in the setting of volume depletion from vomiting, diarrhea, burns, uncontrolled diabetes mellitus, pancreatitis, or addisonian crisis (Table 61-3).

TABLE 61-3

Etiology of Hypovolemic Shock

Blood loss
  External
    Trauma
    Gastrointestinal bleeding
    Massive hematuria
  Internal
    Aortic dissection/abdominal aortic aneurysm rupture
    Trauma
      Splenic laceration/rupture
      Hepatic laceration/rupture
      Pelvis/long bone fracture
    Ruptured ectopic pregnancy
Fluid loss
  Diabetic ketoacidosis
  Adrenal crisis
  Burns
  Diarrhea
  Vomiting
Lack of volume replacement
  Debilitation
  Coma/found down

Pathogenesis

Loss of circulating volume is the primary stimulus for the manifestation of shock. Once 10% of circulating volume has been lost, compensatory mechanisms are activated to maintain cardiac output despite the decreased ventricular filling pressures and stroke volume (Table 61-4).[80] Sympathetic discharge, as well as adrenal catecholamine release, leads to tachycardia, arterial vasoconstriction, and venoconstriction.[81, 82] As volume loss increases, the increase in heart rate is not able to overcome the loss of stroke volume, and cardiac output declines, which is initially detected as orthostatic hypotension and a fall in pulse pressure.[83] Once the loss of volume exceeds approximately 40%, or 20% to 25% if lost rapidly, hypotension and shock ensue.[84]

During hypovolemic shock, peripheral vascular resistance is elevated as a result of several responses. These include catecholamine secretion by the adrenal glands, activation of the sympathetic nervous system, the vasoconstrictive effects of angiotensin II via activation of the renin-angiotensin-aldosterone (RAA) system, and vasopressin released by the pituitary gland.[85-87] However, the rise in vascular resistance is not uniformly distributed throughout the organ systems.[82, 88] Although vasoconstriction increases vascular resistance, regional autoregulation to maintain blood flow can counteract this effect. NO is produced by endothelial cells which relaxes vascular smooth muscle cells,[89] and NO release may decrease responsiveness to endogenous and exogenous vasoconstrictors.[90, 91] Organs with reduced endothelium-dependent vasorelaxation have been found to have endothelial cell dysfunction,[92, 93] which may indicate that the NO-mediated relaxation provides protection against the response to shock. However, NO has been shown to inhibit mitochondrial respiration in vitro,[94] and one study[95] of 28 septic patients found an association between NO overproduction, antioxidant depletion, mitochondrial dysfunction, and decreased adenosine triphosphate (ATP) concentration that related to organ failure. CO_2[96] and adenosine[97] may also play a role in regional autoregulation, having been shown to produce

vasodilation. The end result of these competing interactions is that blood flow is reduced to the kidneys, skin, intestines, and skeletal muscle, and increased to the heart and brain.[84, 98, 99]

Blood flow through capillaries is slowed during hypovolemic shock, with evidence that this is secondary to reduction in perfusion pressure.[100] Endothelial cell swelling may contribute,[101] and expression of endothelial adhesion molecules has been found to be up-regulated during hypovolemic shock on both the neutrophil and endothelium,[102-104] suggesting neutrophil aggregation may also contribute to sluggish capillary flow. Responses to increase the circulating volume include reabsorption of interstitial fluid into the vascular space, a result of the decline in capillary hydrostatic pressure greater than the decline in interstitial hydrostatic pressure.[105] The transport of protein from blood to interstitium is decreased,[106] cellular water is mobilized to the extracellular space,[107] and activation of the RAA system, as well as increased levels of ADH, act to increase sodium and water reabsorption in the kidneys. Despite compensatory mechanisms to preserve the effective circulating volume and maintain blood pressure, hypotension and shock ensue if a large enough amount of fluid is lost. The reduction in perfusion to tissues results in an oxygen imbalance that is responsible for much of the organ failure seen in hypovolemic shock.

Oxygen Consumption and Delivery

Global oxygen delivery (Do_2) is the total amount of oxygen delivered to the tissues per minute, and under resting conditions it is more than adequate to meet the total oxygen requirements of the tissues.

Oxygen delivery is calculated by multiplying cardiac output by the oxygen content in blood, the latter of which is dependent on the amount of dissolved oxygen (Po_2), oxyhemoglobin saturation ($\%HbO_2$), and the hemoglobin (Hb) affinity for oxygen (typically expressed as 1.34):

$$Do_2 = \text{cardiac output} \times (1.34) \times (\text{grams of Hb}) \\ \times (\%HbO_2) + [Po_2 \text{ in mm Hg} \times (0.003)]$$

Oxygen consumption (Vo_2) can be measured directly from inspired and mixed expired oxygen concentrations and expired minute volume, or it may be derived from the cardiac output and arterial and venous oxygen contents:

$$Vo_2 = \text{cardiac output} \times (\text{arterial oxygen content} \\ - \text{mixed venous oxygen content})$$

The (Vo_2) as a fraction of Do_2 is the oxygen extraction ratio (O_2ER):

$$O_2ER = Vo_2/Do_2$$

In a normal adult performing routine activities, Vo_2 is approximately 250 mL/minute with an O_2ER of 25%, which can increase to 70% to 80% during maximal exercise.[108] In the setting of hypovolemic shock, a fall in hemoglobin or cardiac output can significantly reduce oxygen delivery to the tissues. It has been shown that below an oxygen delivery of approximately 8 mL/kg/minute, oxygen uptake is maximal (near 100%),[109] and a decrease in oxygen delivery below this level results in cellular ischemia as oxygen tissue demand is not being met.

Global oxygen delivery in shock may be normal, despite evidence of cellular ischemia.[110] This is often due to the

TABLE 61-4

Compensatory Responses to Shock

Maximization of intravascular volume
  Redistribution of fluid to intravascular space
    From interstitial compartments
    From intracellular compartments
  Renal adaptations
    Increased aldosterone
    Increased vasopressin
Maximization of blood pressure
  Increased sympathetic activity
  Increased catecholamines
  Increased angiotensin II production
  Increased vasopressin
Maximization of cardiac output
  Sympathetic stimulation
    Tachycardia
    Increased contractility
Maximization of oxygen delivery
  Metabolic acidosis
  Increased red blood cell 2,3-diphosphoglycerate
  Decreased tissue oxygen levels

regional differences in blood flow seen in hypovolemic shock, with some organs developing an oxygen debt despite normal global oxygen delivery.[108] Some authors have suggested that supranormal levels of oxygen delivery may be able to overcome these regional differences and improve outcome[111, 112]; this is discussed in the "Management" section. Cellular hypoxia is manifested in several ways. Once oxygen demands exceed oxygen delivery, anaerobic metabolism ensues, with the production of lactate. The blood lactate level has traditionally been used as an indicator of tissue hypoxia, representing a balance between the production of lactate and consumption by the liver, as well as cardiac and skeletal muscle.[113] However, a single level may be unreliable, and serial levels may be more reliable as an indicator of cellular hypoxia.[108]

Loss of function of cellular enzymes can occur during hypoxia, but there is a significant variation in sensitivity to hypoxia, with glucose oxidase being quite sensitive to hypoxia, whereas NADPH oxidase can function at 50%, and cytochrome-003 can function at 0.09% of the cellular oxygen required for glucose oxidase.[114]

Cellular ischemia in the gut may result in gastric ulcers, as well as disruption of the barrier function of the mucosa, which can result in translocation of bacteria from the bowel into the circulation.[115, 116] Hepatic ischemia can decrease the clearance of lactate[117] and drugs,[118] and centrilobular necrosis may result in elevated bilirubin and enzyme levels.[119] The spleen contracts during hypovolemic shock, releasing red blood cells into the circulation.[82] Myocardial ischemia can occur,[120] particularly in elderly patients who may have atherosclerotic coronary artery disease.

Reperfusion

Although restoration of flow to an ischemic organ is critical to restoring function, reperfusion itself may contribute to organ damage. Reactive oxygen species are formed once ischemic tissues are reperfused,[121] and these can cause direct cellular membrane damage by lipid peroxidation, as well as leukocyte activation and transmigration by stimulating leukocyte adhesion molecule expression.[122] The activated leukocytes contribute to cellular injury by releasing proteases and elastases, as well as cytokines that increase microvascular permeability, edema, and microthrombosis.[123] Ischemia-reperfusion also activates complement, which promotes leukocyte activation as well as altering vascular permeability, resulting in edema.[124] Data suggest that calcium influx into cells during reperfusion may contribute to injury by damaging cell organelles, inhibiting respiration, and activating protease and prostaglandin synthesis.[125, 126] Reperfusion injury can manifest as myocardial stunning, reperfusion arrhythmias, breakdown of the gut mucosal barrier, ARF, hepatic failure, or multiorgan dysfunction syndrome.[127-131]

Clinical Manifestations

Early in the course of hypovolemia or blood loss, the patient may not be hypotensive, and attention should be paid to other signs of fluid loss. Tachycardia is common, and tachypnea can occur early in the course. Orthostatic hypotension is a reliable sign; dry mucosal membranes and decreased skin turgor are less reliable, but indicative of hypovolemia.[132] If the patient is conscious, he or she may complain of thirst or

diaphoresis. Once volume losses become profound, hypotension ensues, confusion may occur, and the patient may develop oliguria and peripheral cyanosis as a result of diminished perfusion. Hypovolemic shock due to trauma or bleeding is usually apparent, but internal bleeding or the other causes listed in Table 61-3 may not be as obvious. The smell of acetone on the breath may point to uncontrolled diabetes mellitus, and adrenocortical insufficiency can result in brown discoloration of the mucous membranes.

Acidosis can occur, often from hypoperfusion of tissues resulting in lactate production. DIC can also occur during hypovolemic shock, resulting in microvascular thrombi formation, and may contribute to the multiple organ dysfunction often seen following traumatic or hypovolemic shock.[133]

Diagnosis

The initial evaluation of the patient in shock should include a determination of the cause of shock. In most cases of hypovolemic shock, it is readily apparent that trauma or blood loss is the primary cause, but care must be taken not to overlook septic, cardiogenic, or anaphylactic shock. Initial resuscitation should begin during the evaluation. In the case of external blood loss, crossmatching of blood should be done while fluids are infused for resuscitation. Gastrointestinal bleeding can be evaluated and potentially treated with upper or lower endoscopy once the patient is stabilized, as well as angiography. In the event of trauma, chest radiography should be performed to rule out tension pneumothorax or hemothorax. If abdominal trauma has occurred, peritoneal lavage can be performed to assess for hemorrhage, most commonly from splenic or hepatic lacerations.[134] If the patient is stabilized, computed tomography or ultrasound can also assess for intraabdominal hemorrhage as well as organ injury. Laboratory tests should include a complete blood count; a chemistry panel, including electrolytes, creatinine, glucose, and liver function tests; arterial blood gas; arterial lactate level; blood type and crossmatch; and urinalysis. In the event of trauma or bleeding, coagulation studies should include a platelet count, prothrombin time (PT), and partial thromboplastin time (PTT). If the cause of shock is not readily apparent, an electrocardiogram (ECG) should be performed to rule out myocardial infarction (MI).

Management

Resuscitation of the patient in shock should begin immediately, and not delayed while diagnostic procedures are undertaken. Fluid resuscitation should begin once large-bore intravenous catheters are placed. The primary goal in the treatment of hypovolemic shock is to return circulating volume to normal, and as a result, improve tissue perfusion, substrate delivery, and oxygen balance. Some authors have suggested that raising oxygen delivery and oxygen uptake to supranormal levels in the setting of trauma and hemorrhage may improve survival.[111, 112] Oxygen delivery can be maximized by increasing the cardiac output with either volume or dobutamine, increasing the oxygen saturation above 90%, and increasing the hemoglobin concentration. Care must be taken when transfusing, as a higher hematocrit can actually worsen oxygen balance by increasing viscosity and reducing capillary flow.[135] Although elderly patients with MI may benefit from transfusion to a hematocrit of 30%,[136] large transfusions of blood have been associated with multiple organ dysfunction,[137] and a liberal transfusion policy to a hemoglobin of 10 to 12 g/dL has been associated with increased mortality.[138] Measurement of oxygen delivery and consumption also requires pulmonary artery catheter placement, which may be an independent risk for mortality[139]; thus many physicians use improvement in blood pressure, metabolic acidosis, and serial lactate levels as markers that oxygen delivery and consumption are adequate. However, improvement of oxygen delivery in this setting may not improve cellular function. Tissue oxygen tension has been found to be increased in some studies of septic animals and patients with acidosis,[140, 141] indicating that dysoxia (inadequate utilization of oxygen), not hypoxia, may contribute to acidosis and organ failure.

Gastric tonometry has been proposed as a method to monitor a patient's perfusion status, and indirectly, oxygen delivery. The tonometer is inserted nasally or orally and advanced to the stomach, where it indirectly measures the pH of gastric mucosal cells. A low gastric mucosal pH (pH_i) may indicate two things. First, it may be an early indicator of reduced global oxygen delivery as the splanchnic bed is prone to hypoperfusion and hypoxia due to redistribution of blood flow. Second, intestinal mucosal hypoxia may result in increased permeability with increased translocation of bacteria and endotoxin, resulting in multiple organ system dysfunction. Low pH_i has been found to be a good indicator of poor outcome in the intensive care setting,[142-144] but no study has convincingly proved that therapy to improve pH_i has any effect on outcome.[145-148]

Further treatment depends on the cause of shock. Traumatic shock often requires surgical exploration to treat the source of bleeding. Upper gastrointestinal bleeding due to ulcers can be treated medically with intravenous proton pump inhibitors, or endoscopically by electrocautery, laser coagulation, or injection therapy. Esophageal varices can be treated with infusion of somatostatin, or interventionally with injection sclerotherapy, or a Sengstaken-Blakemore tube. Lower gastrointestinal bleeding can be treated with endoscopic therapies. Surgery is an option for recurrent bleeding. Diabetic ketoacidosis is treated with intravenous insulin, and adrenal crisis with intravenous hydrocortisone.

Fluid Resuscitation

Fluid resuscitation is the initial therapy in hypovolemic shock, as this helps restore circulating volume and oxygen delivery. The types of fluids used are quite varied (Table 61-5), and controversy exists as to which agent is the most efficacious. Both colloids (high-molecular-weight solutions) and crystalloids (electrolyte solutions) are used to treat shock.

Isotonic crystalloid solutions have traditionally been used as the primary fluid for volume expansion.[139] Normal saline (0.9%) and lactated Ringer's solution are both commonly used, although large volumes of lactated Ringer's solution should be avoided in the setting of renal failure, because of its potassium content, and possibly in hepatic failure as the damaged liver may not be able to convert lactate to bicarbonate. One advantage of isotonic crystalloids may be that they replace the interstitial fluid deficits seen after hypovolemic shock,[149] as 75% of the volume infused enters the interstitial space, while 25% remains intravascular.[150] However, the large volume of these fluids required leads to peripheral edema that may impair wound healing,[151] and has led to the study of hypertonic crystalloid and colloid solutions, which stay within the intravascular space to a greater degree, and thus require less total volume for a similar degree of resuscitation.

Hypertonic crystalloid solutions include 3%, 5% and 7.5% NaCl, and are considered plasma expanders as they act to increase the circulatory volume via movement of intracellular and interstitial water into the intravascular space.[139] The primary disadvantage of these agents is the risk of hypernatremia, and the safety of these agents depends partially on how much water can be shifted from the intracellular to extracellular space without resulting in cellular damage.

Colloids are also plasma expanders, as they are composed of macromolecules, and are retained in the intravascular space to a much greater extent than isotonic crystalloids. Albumin has a molecular weight of 69,000 Da, and a half-life of 15 to 20 days. Albumin may serve as a free radical scavenger,[152] and the increased intravascular oncotic pressure may protect the lungs and other organs from edema.[153] Dextran is a colloid agent prepared from glucose polymers. Dextran 40 has a molecular weight of 40,000 Da, and dextran 70 has a molecular weight of 70,000 Da. Dextran 70 has a longer intravascular retention time than dextran 40,[154] but either can cause histamine release from mast cells leading

TABLE 61-5

Fluids Used for Resuscitation

	SODIUM CHLORIDE (0.9%)	RINGER'S LACTATE	SODIUM CHLORIDE (3%)	ALBUMIN (5%)	HETASTARCH (6%)	DEXTRAN 70 + NaCl	UREA-GELATIN
Sodium (mEq/L)	154	130	513	130-160	154	154	145
Chloride (mEq/L)	154	109	513	130-160	154	154	145
Potassium (mEq/L)	0	4	0	0	0	0	5.1
Osmolarity (mOsm/L)	308	275	1025	310	310	310	391
Oncotic pressure (mm Hg)	0	0	0	20	30	60	26-30
Lactate (mEq/L)	0	28	0	0	0	0	0
Maximum dose (mL/kg/24 hr)	None	None	Limited by serum Na^+	None	20	20	20
Cost (L)	$1.26	$1.44	$1.28	$100	$27.30	$35.08	—

to anaphylactoid reactions.[155] Hetastarch is available in several different preparations (HES 200 or HES 450). Hetastarch is a natural starch of highly branched glucose polymers, similar in structure to glycogen, with a molecular weight of 200,000 or 450,000 Da, depending on the preparation, and a plasma half-life of approximately 17 days. Its volume expansion properties are almost identical to albumin.[154] Pentastarch has a molecular weight of 260,000 Da, but has a higher colloid oncotic pressure than hetastarch or albumin, thus producing more intravascular volume expansion than these agents.[156] There is recent evidence that the starches may be able to reduce capillary leak following ischemia or trauma, thereby decreasing edema formation.[157, 158] Both hetastarch and pentastarch may increase the amylase level in blood. Gelatins are polypeptides from bovine raw material, have a lower molecular weight than the starches or dextrans, and are poorly retained in the intravascular space. Their duration of effect is approximately 2 hours. Urea-gelatin 3.5% has a high concentration of potassium, which makes it unsuitable for patients with renal failure. The gelatins are not available in the United States at this time. Newer solutions consisting of hypertonic saline to which colloids have been added include NaCl 7.5% with dextran 70, NaCl 7.2% with dextran 60, and NaCl 7.5% with hetastarch.

CRYSTALLOID VERSUS COLLOID FOR RESUSCITATION

There has been much debate as to which type of fluid is best for resuscitation of shock. Colloids offer the theoretical advantage of expanding the intravascular space with less volume, and have been shown to increase blood pressure more rapidly than crystalloids.[159] One liter of dextran 70 increases intravascular volume by 800 mL; 1 L of hetastarch, by 750 mL; 1 L of 5% albumin, by 500 mL; and 1 L of saline, by 180 mL.[160] Yet in the setting of sepsis, where there is significant capillary leak, both albumin and normal saline were found to increase interstitial volume to the same extent.[161] Small studies have also found a lower incidence of pulmonary edema during resuscitation with colloids compared with crystalloids,[162] potentially less reperfusion injury to the myocardium after colloid resuscitation,[163] and better blood flow to the myocardium.[164] Yet there is also evidence that colloids can inhibit the coagulation system[165, 166] and cause anaphylactoid reactions.[167] Albumin has been shown in one study to have negative inotropic effects,[168] and another study found impaired salt and water excretion when albumin was used for resuscitation from shock.[169] Hetastarch may increase the risk of ARF when given for resuscitation of sepsis,[170] which may be due to inadequate free water replacement in the setting of a potent volume expander.

Meta-analyses of fluid administration and mortality have not supported a benefit for colloids over crystalloids.[171-176] In trauma patients, Wade and colleagues[171] found no difference in survival between those receiving hypertonic saline with dextran 60 or isotonic saline. Choi and colleagues[172] found crystalloids were associated with a significantly lower risk of death (relative risk [RR] 0.39; confidence interval [CI] 0.17-0.89). One meta-analysis[173] did find that hypertonic saline with dextran did improve survival compared to crystalloids in the setting of head injury. Several meta-analyses[174-176] have shown a trend toward increased mortality in heterogeneous groups of critically ill patients resuscitated with colloids; the Cochrane

Injuries Group Albumin Reviewers[177] found that the risk of death was significantly increased in critically ill patients who received albumin (RR 1.68; CI 1.26-2.23). Subgroup analysis of this study showed that the risk of death was increased in hypoalbuminemic patients (RR 1.69; CI 1.07-2.67), and a trend toward increased mortality was seen in the hypovolemic group (RR 1.46; CI 0.97-2.22). Given the large number of patients who receive albumin each year, and the potential for a small increase in mortality from albumin leading to thousands of deaths, the authors of this study stated that albumin should no longer be used in critically ill patients outside of randomized controlled trials. This viewpoint is refuted by some,[178] but no randomized clinical trial has been completed to assess the safety of albumin in critically ill patients.

Given the available data, and the potential risks of colloid solutions, crystalloids still remain the cornerstone of volume resuscitation, although patients with profound volume deficits may benefit from colloid solutions in addition to crystalloids to hasten restoration of circulating volume. Until more data are available on the safety of albumin, an alternative colloid agent should be used in this setting. A search is under way for red blood cell substitutes that can rapidly expand blood volume, as well as carry and deliver oxygen to tissues. Diaspirin cross-linked hemoglobin showed an increase in mortality when this agent was used in the treatment of severe traumatic shock.[179] No agent is currently in widespread use.

Vasopressors

The use of vasopressors in hypovolemic shock should be reserved for the setting in which adequate fluids are not yet available, or for the patient in whom adequate fluid infusion has not improved hypotension.[134] In this setting, a pulmonary artery catheter can help guide therapy, as persistent shock can be caused by either peripheral vasodilation or myocardial dysfunction. A wedge pressure of 12 to 16 mm Hg is indicative of adequate volume expansion. Animal studies have shown that vasopressin can reverse shock unresponsive to fluids and catecholamines,[180] and can improve survival after cardiac arrest in hypovolemic shock.[181] Although vasopressin has been shown in one small study[182] to improve blood pressure in septic shock, others have suggested it can cause a reduction in cardiac output,[183] and only case reports of improvement in hypovolemic shock are available.[180]

Treatment of Acidosis

Lactic acidosis due to tissue hypoperfusion is common in hypovolemic shock. Improvement of the effective circulating volume and restoring tissue oxygen balance will diminish the production of lactate, allowing for improvement of acidosis. Yet for cases of intractable shock, metabolic acidosis may persist despite aggressive therapy. Acidosis has been shown to decrease cardiac contractility in animal models,[184] and reduces the cardiac contractility response to catecholamines.[185] However, the effect of acidosis on cardiac function in the clinical setting is less well documented. Decreased cardiac contractility in the setting of lactic acidosis may be partially due to hypoxemia, hypoperfusion, or sepsis, and establishing the direct effects of the low pH is difficult.[186] In fact, many patients treated with permissive hypercapnia–low tidal volume ventilation develop acidosis that is well tolerated with minimal change in cardiac output.[187]

Treatment of acidosis with sodium bicarbonate has not been shown to be beneficial. Animal models of lactic acidosis fail to show improvement in hemodynamics from sodium bicarbonate compared with normal saline,[187-189] and human studies have shown no improvement in hemodynamics or catecholamine responsiveness.[190, 191] Furthermore, bicarbonate infusion has been theorized to cause worsening intracellular acidosis, as the CO_2, produced when bicarbonate reacts with acids can diffuse rapidly across the cell membrane, whereas bicarbonate cannot. Studies of intracellular pH changes have been mixed, with some showing an increase,[192] decrease,[193-195] or no change[185, 196, 197] in pH. Treatment of acidosis with bicarbonate has also been shown to increase hemoglobin affinity for oxygen in healthy volunteers, resulting in reduced oxygen delivery.[198]

As there is no documented benefit, and the potential for adverse effects appears real, treatment of lactic acidosis should not include administration of sodium bicarbonate unless further compelling evidence becomes available.

Effects on Renal Function

Acute renal failure is a common finding in a patient with shock. Diminished perfusion to the kidneys with resultant ischemia is a primary cause. Early in hypovolemia, renal perfusion can be maintained by intrarenal production of NO and prostaglandins that have vasodilating actions.[199, 200] However, once hypovolemia becomes severe and shock ensues, these mechanisms are not enough to prevent ischemia. Other factors seem to play a role as well. DIC can occur during traumatic or hypovolemic shock, and the resultant microvascular thrombi can cause renal ischemia.[133]

Hypovolemic shock has been shown to increase TNF-α and IL-1 release,[201, 202] and can activate the complement cascade.[203] These substances may contribute to acute renal failure. Their effects on renal function are discussed more fully in the following section on sepsis.

SEPSIS

It is estimated that sepsis accounts for up to 10% of admissions to the ICU.[204] There are 400,000 to 500,000 episodes of sepsis each year in the United States,[205] resulting in more than 100,000 deaths per year.[206] Sepsis and septic shock are common causes of ARF, and the nephrologist is frequently involved in the care of this disease. Despite improvements in our ability to monitor and treat patients in the ICU, the mortality rate for sepsis has increased.[205] A complete understanding of the pathophysiology and newer therapeutic approaches for sepsis is critical for any clinician involved in patient care.

Definition

The American College of Chest Physicians/Society of Critical Care Medicine Consensus Conference in 1991 led to a uniform definition of the systemic inflammatory response syndrome (SIRS), sepsis, severe sepsis, and septic shock[207] (Table 61-6 and Fig. 61-1). SIRS describes the

TABLE 61-6

Definition of Systemic Inflammatory Response Syndrome (SIRS), Sepsis, Severe Sepsis, Septic Shock

SIRS: presence of two or more of the following:
  Temperature > 38°C or < 36°C
  Heart rate > 90 beats/min
  Respiratory rate > 20 breaths/min
  White blood cell count > 12,000/mm³, < 4000/mm³, or >10% immature neutrophils
Sepsis: SIRS in the presence of documented infection
Severe Sepsis: Sepsis with hypotension, hypoperfusion, or organ dysfunction
Septic Shock: Sepsis with hypotension despite volume resuscitation and evidence of organ dysfunction or hypoperfusion

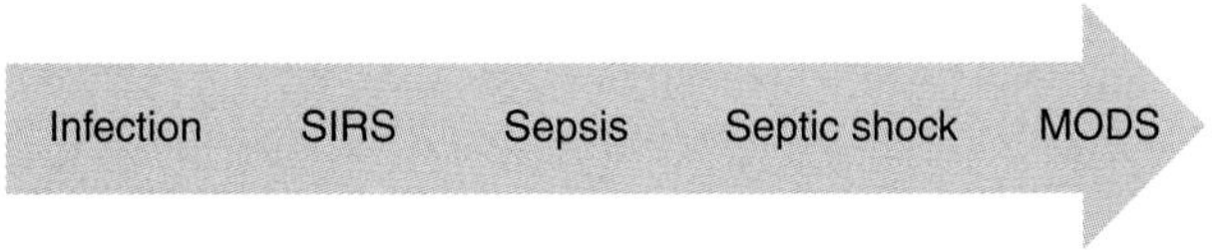

FIGURE 61-1. The spectrum of systemic inflammatory response syndrome (SIRS): sepsis, septic shock, and multiorgan dysfunction syndrome (MODS).

TABLE 61-7

Common Causes of Systemic Inflammatory Response Syndrome

Infections
  Bacterial
  Viral
  Protozoan
  Fungal
Trauma
Burns
Pancreatitis
Cirrhosis
Autoimmune disease

common systemic response to a wide variety of clinical insults (Table 61-7). It is characterized by two or more of the following: (1) temperature higher than 38° C or lower than 36° C; (2) heart rate greater than 90 beats per minute; (3) respiratory rate greater than 20 breaths per minute; and a (4) white blood cell count greater than 12,000/mm³, less than 4000/mm³, or more than 10% immature neutrophils. Sepsis is present when SIRS is diagnosed in the setting of a confirmed infection. Severe sepsis is defined as sepsis plus either organ dysfunction or evidence of hypoperfusion or hypotension. Septic shock is a subset of severe sepsis and is present when sepsis-induced hypotension persists despite fluid resuscitation, and is accompanied by hypoperfusion abnormalities or organ dysfunction. In a study of 2527 patients who met SIRS criteria in a single ICU, the mortality rate was found to increase as patients fulfilled more criteria and advanced along the spectrum. The mortality of patients with two SIRS criteria was 7%; three SIRS criteria, 10%; four SIRS, criteria 17%; sepsis, 16%; severe sepsis, 20%; and septic shock, 46%.[208]

Source of Infection and Microbiology

In the 1960s and 1970s, gram-negative organisms were the most common causes of septic shock,[209] but gram-positive organisms have now increased in prevalence. Gram-negative organisms are now estimated to be responsible for 25% of all cases of sepsis, with gram-positive organisms responsible for 25%, mixed gram-positive and gram-negative organisms for 20%, fungi for 3%, anaerobic organisms for 2%, and unknown organisms for 25%.[210] The most common gram-negative organisms are *Escherichia coli* (25%), *Klebsiella* (20%), and *Pseudomonas aeruginosa* (15%). The most common gram-positive organisms are *Staphylococcus aureus* (35%), *Enterococcus* (20%), and coagulase-negative staphylococcis (15)%.[210] The most common primary sites of infection in sepsis are the respiratory tract (50%), intra-abdominal and pelvic sites (20%), the urinary tract (10%), skin (5%), and intravascular catheters (5%).[210]

There has been a rise in the incidence of sepsis and septic shock over the last several decades.[210] Factors that are potentially responsible include the increasing number of immunocompromised people, from acquired immunodeficiency syndrome or cytotoxic and immunosuppressant therapy, and the increase in interventional procedures. Other risk factors for sepsis include malnutrition, alcoholism, malignancy, diabetes mellitus, advanced age, and chronic renal failure.[205]

Pathophysiology

While much has yet to be learned about the pathophysiology of sepsis, scientific advances have shed light on many of the factors that lead to the complex cascade that can result in septic shock and death. It has been hypothesized that the manifestations of sepsis result from excessive inflammatory response to bacterial organisms.[211] Gram-negative bacteria contain lipopolysaccharide (LPS) as a cell wall component, which can activate macrophages, as well as the complement cascade.[212] Gram-positive bacteria produce exotoxins, which can activate T cells and macrophages,[211] and release cell membrane components that can activate the inflammatory process.[213] Both proinflammatory and anti-inflammatory components are released in response to bacterial invasion, and these two systems are usually tightly controlled to destroy the infection while preventing damage to the host.[210] It is theorized now that sepsis is the result of an imbalance in these two processes, with the proinflammatory component overexpressed.[210, 214-216] Yet it has been shown that neutrophils in critically ill patients demonstrate functional abnormalities, including reduced migration, superoxide production, and bacterial killing, all factors that may impair host defense.[217, 218] Whether this neutrophil dysfunction leads to worsening of the sepsis syndrome is unknown.

Proinflammatory cytokines released in response to infectious stimuli include TNF-α, IL-1β, IL-6, and IL-8. Anti-inflammatory cytokines include IL-10, IL-13, and transforming growth factor-β (TGF-β). TNF-α and IL-1 have wide-ranging effects, including activation of macrophages, lymphocytes, and neutrophils; increased expression of adhesion molecules; and increased production of other proinflammatory cytokines.[210] Anti-inflammatory cytokines decrease production of IL-1 and TNF-α, and inhibit antigen presentation to T and B lymphocytes. Animal models have demonstrated that cytokines are a key component of sepsis, with infusions of TNF-α and IL-1 producing a state similar to septic shock,[219-221] and administration of antibodies to these cytokines resulting in attenuation of the shocklike state.[221-224]

Other mediators of sepsis include metabolites of the arachidonic cascade such as PGE_2, prostacyclin (PGI_2), and thromboxane A_2. PGE_2 causes vasodilation seen in septic shock[210]; thromboxane A_2 causes platelet and leukocyte aggregation and vasoconstriction.[225] PAF is produced by many cells in response to inflammatory stimuli,[226] amplifies many cytokines released in sepsis, and stimulates leukocyte activation and adherence to endothelial cells.[210]

Recently, interest has developed in the role of nuclear factor-κB (NF-κB) in multiple disease processes. NF-κB is a transcription factor located in the cytoplasm of most cell types.[227] Stimulation of the cells by cytokines or byproducts of bacterial and viral infection leads to translocation of NF-κB from the cytoplasm to the nucleus where it regulates transcription of target genes.[228] It appears that the genes affected by NF-κB activate and modulate cytokines, chemokines, and receptors involved in diseases such as sepsis, SIRS, ARDS, and multiorgan dysfunction.[229] Research is ongoing to ascertain the extent to which NF-κB is involved in these processes, and if its activation can be regulated.

The coagulation system also plays a role in the manifestation of sepsis. Levels of protein C are decreased,[220, 230] and its conversion to activated protein C, which inhibits thrombosis (Fig. 61-2), is down-regulated during sepsis.[231] Antithrombin III, (AT III), an inhibitor of thrombin and factor X, has been found to be dramatically reduced in septic shock.[232] Tissue factor pathway inhibitor, which inhibits the highly thrombogenic compound tissue factor, has also been found to be reduced in the setting of sepsis.[230] These factors contribute to the widespread microvascular thrombosis that occurs during sepsis, a result of which is reduction in perfusion to various tissues,[233] which may lead to the multiorgan dysfunction syndrome (MODS) seen in many patients with sepsis.

Clinical Features

Sepsis is a systemic process, and is defined by its clinical manifestations. Common clinical manifestations include changes in body temperature (fever or hypothermia), tachycardia, tachypnea, and leukocytosis or leukopenia. Many of the signs and symptoms of sepsis are induced by the inflammatory cytokines. Fever, for example, can be caused by TNF-α and IL-1,[205] and failure to develop fever has been associated with increased mortality.[234] Hypoglycemia, hyperglycemia, hypokalemia, hyponatremia, hypocalcemia, hypomagnesemia, and hypophosphatemia can also be seen. Tachycardia is a common, but nonspecific manifestation. Patients with severe sepsis and septic shock have hypotension, due in part to NO release,[235] as well as to decreased effective circulating volume. The intravascular volume depletion is related to several factors, including decreased systemic vascular resistance (SVR),[236] increased microvascular permeability, and increased insensible losses. Once

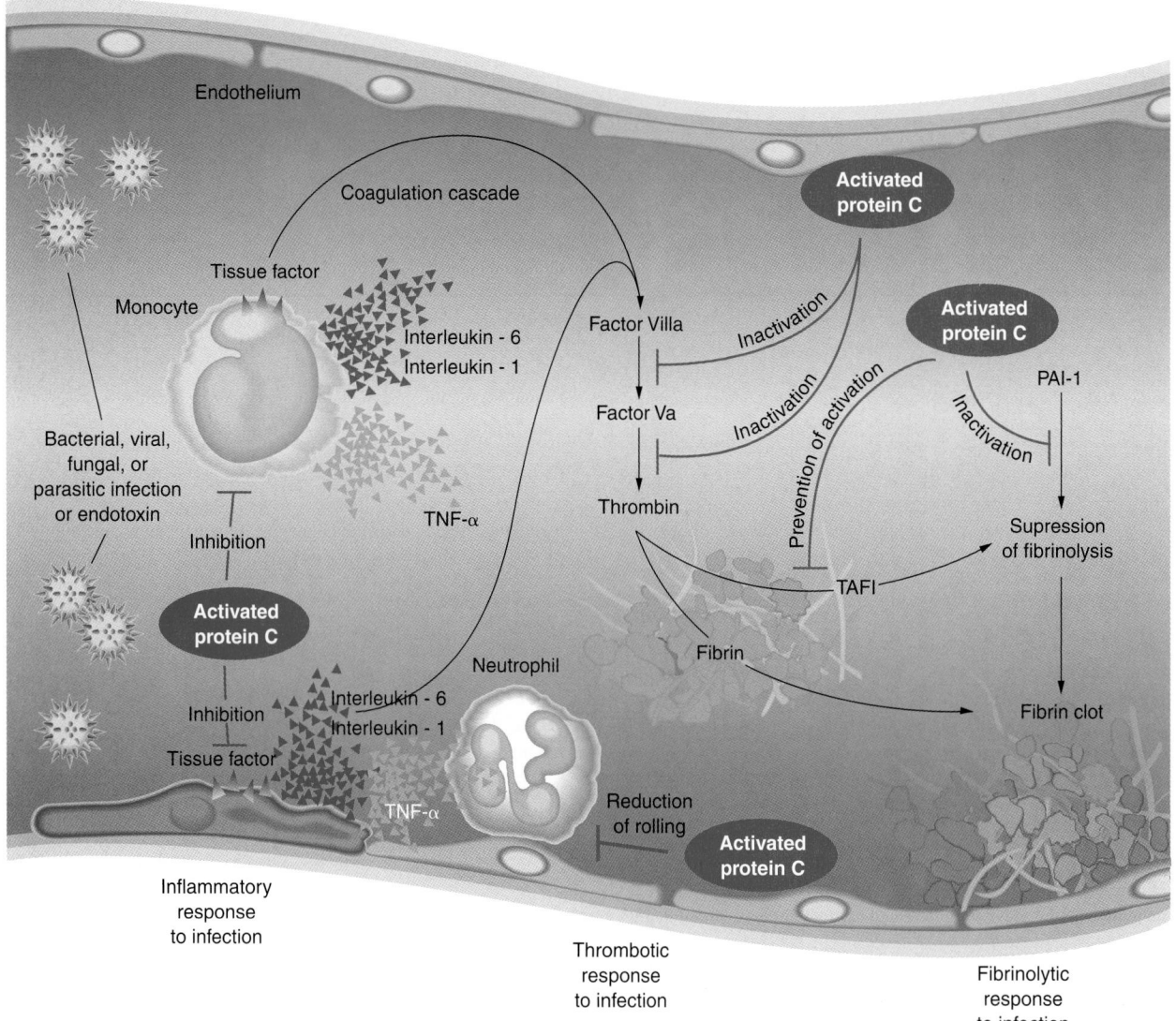

FIGURE 61-2. Proposed actions of activated protein C in modulating the systemic inflammatory, procoagulant, and fibrinolytic host responses to infection. The inflammatory and procoagulant host responses to infection are intricately linked. Infectious agents and inflammatory cytokines such as tumor necrosis factor-α (TNF-α) and interleukin-1 activate coagulation by stimulating the release of tissue factor from monocytes and the endothelium. The presentation of tissue factor leads to the formation of thrombin and fibrin clot. Plasminogen activator inhibitor-1 (PAI-1) is a potent inhibitor of tissue plasminogen activator, the endogenous pathway for lysing a fibrin clot. (From Bernard GR, Vincent JL, Laterre PF, et al: Efficacy and safety of recombinant human activated protein C for severe sepsis. N Engl J Med 344:699-709, 2001.)

volume-resuscitated, most patients with septic shock have evidence of hyperdynamic cardiovascular function with a normal or elevated cardiac output and decreased SVR.[236] Yet despite these findings from pulmonary artery catheterization, the heart may not be as hyperdynamic as it should be, given the clinical setting. Studies have shown that sepsis induces a depression in myocardial function,[237, 238] characterized by elevated left ventricular end-diastolic volume and decreased left ventricular systolic work index. This myocardial depression is believed to be caused by a myocardial depressant substance, which has not been fully identified, although TNF-α and IL-1 are leading candidates.[239]

Tachypnea and hypoxemia are common in sepsis, and ARDS has been reported to occur in up to 40% of patients

with sepsis.[18] Many view ARDS as an initial manifestation of multiorgan dysfunction syndrome, and believe it represents diffuse endothelial injury resulting from the exaggerated inflammatory response.[240-242]

Adrenal insufficiency is a common finding in septic shock, with a reported incidence of 25% to 40%.[243-245] Some authors now feel the threshold for diagnosing adrenal insufficiency should be a cortisol level of 25 to 30 μg/mL, instead of the usual 18 to 20 μg/mL, and low-dose (1-2 μg) adrenocorticotropic hormone (ACTH) stimulation should be used for diagnosis, as it represents physiologic stress levels of ACTH, in contrast to the standard ACTH stimulation test which uses doses that are 100- to 200-fold higher than maximal stress levels of ACTH.[246] It is also advocated that if a fluid-resuscitated patient is hypotensive and requires pressors, a baseline cortisol level of less than 25 μg/mL should be considered diagnostic of adrenal insufficiency.[247]

DIC is often seen in sepsis, and is characterized by enhanced activation of coagulation, with intravascular fibrin formation and deposition. The resulting microvascular thrombi can reduce blood flow to portions of organs, contributing to the onset of MODS. A reduction in circulating coagulation factors and platelets is often seen, as they are consumed in the production of microthrombi, and this can lead to bleeding episodes.[248] Laboratory studies in DIC typically show thrombocytopenia, with an elevation of the PT and activated partial PTT, as well as D dimer.

Central nervous system (CNS) alterations are frequently found in patients with sepsis,[249] and septic encephalopathy is the most common form of encephalopathy in ICUs.[250] Impaired mitochondrial function and oxygen extraction by the brain, increased permeability of the blood-brain barrier, and disruption of astrocyte end-feet, all caused by inflammatory mediators, contribute to the diffuse neuronal injury seen in septic encephalopathy.[251] Confusion, disorientation, lethargy, agitation, obtundation, and coma are the common clinical manifestations.

Critical illness polyneuropathy is a common occurrence in the setting of sepsis, and is often first recognized when the patient cannot be weaned from ventilatory support.[249] This illness is caused by axonal degeneration, is characterized by hyporeflexia, weakness distally greater than proximally, and normal or slightly elevated creatine kinase levels,[210] and may take up to 6 months for recovery.[249]

Renal dysfunction is found in 9% to 40% of patients with sepsis,[252] and the mortality rate in these patients is greater than 50%.[253] The clinical manifestations vary from acute tubular necrosis to bilateral cortical necrosis. Hypotension is commonly seen in sepsis, and renal hypoperfusion plays a major role in the incidence of ARF, as does the administration of nephrotoxic agents to treat sepsis. However, it is apparent that these are not the only factors involved in ARF induction. TNF-α released from mesangial cells causes leukocyte accumulation in the glomerulus, as well as apoptotic death of glomerular endothelial cells.[254] PAF levels, which are increased in sepsis and correlate with the severity of ARF,[255] increase both afferent and efferent arteriolar resistance, producing a decline in the GFR.[256] Endothelin-1 is secreted in response to septic mediators,[257, 258] and has been found to cause renal vasoconstriction,[259] as well as inhibition of sodium and water reabsorption by the collecting duct.[260, 261] Thromboxane A$_2$ decreases GFR and renal blood flow, and preferentially vasoconstricts the afferent arteriole.[262] Leukotrienes are released in endotoxemia[263] and also reduce GFR and renal blood flow.[262] Other mediators implicated in septic ARF include the renin-angiotensin system, atrial natriuretic factor, IL-1, adenosine, and catecholamines.[207] The role of DIC and diminished levels of activated protein C in the generation of microvascular thrombi has been discussed, and the diminished renal perfusion caused by the thrombi likely contributes to septic ARF.

As improvements in care of the critically ill patient have been developed, death from the initial disease process in sepsis has become less common, patients have lived longer, and the development of MODS has become more common. MODS is now the most common cause of death among patients with sepsis.[264] The exact pathophysiologic mechanism leading to MODS has not been fully defined, but mitochondrial dysfunction, microvascular thrombi, hypoperfusion, ischemia-reperfusion injury, circulating inflammatory factors, diffuse endothelial cell injury, bacterial toxin translocation, and increased tissue NO are all potential contributors.[253, 265, 266]

Management

The management of sepsis is primarily based on eradication of the infection and support of the patient's hemodynamics and other organ systems. Activated protein C has been approved for use in sepsis, and other immunomodulatory therapies are being evaluated.

Antibiotics

Identifying the source of sepsis should be one of the primary goals while treatment is being initiated. The choice of antibiotic often depends on the suspected site of infection. Initial antibiotic therapy usually requires multiple antibiotics to cover the likely pathogens,[210] and if culture results identify a source, coverage can be narrowed. Double antibiotic coverage is indicated in the treatment of *P. aeruginosa* infection, febrile neutropenic patients, and severe intraabdominal infections.[267] If no organism is isolated, initial broad-spectrum antibiotics can be continued so long as the patient is improving. Immediate institution of antibiotic therapy is critical, as there is a 10% to 15% higher mortality in patients not treated promptly.[267] A full discussion of antibiotic selection is beyond the scope of this chapter.

Hemodynamic Support

Intravascular volume depletion, peripheral vasodilation, and increased microvascular permeability all contribute to the hypotension seen in severe sepsis and septic shock,[210] and aggressive volume resuscitation should be the primary initial therapy.[268] The fluid requirements for resuscitation are very large, and often underestimated by the clinician. Up to 10 L of crystalloid are often required in the first 24 hours.[268] Boluses of fluid should be given until blood pressure, heart rate, or evidence of end-organ perfusion such as urine output have improved. Early therapy is crucial, and a recent study showed that early, goal-directed therapy, using central venous pressure, mean arterial pressure, hematocrit, and central venous oxygen saturation as end points, lowered mortality.[269] Crystalloids, such as normal saline, are the fluid of choice for volume resuscitation. Albumin is not recommended, as discussed in the "Hypovolemic Shock" section.

Despite adequate fluid resuscitation, many patients remain hypotensive,[210] and these patients require vasopressor agents. Dopamine is widely used, and the Society of Critical Care Medicine guidelines recommend dopamine as the agent of first choice.[270] However, chronotropic sensitivity to dopamine is increased in sepsis; thus tachycardia and arrhythmias may limit its use.[210] Norepinephrine is as effective in raising blood pressure as dopamine, but has less cardiac effect; it does not raise cardiac output as much as dopamine, and causes less tachycardia.[271] Phenylephrine has purely α-adrenergic effects, and fewer risks of tachyarrhythmias, but experience with it in septic shock is limited.[271]

Epinephrine can be used for refractory hypotension, but has been shown to cause a rise in serum lactate levels.[271] Dobutamine has been used in sepsis to improve oxygen delivery, but can potentiate hypotension due to β_2-adrenergic–mediated vasodilation. Dobutamine is recommended for patients with a low cardiac index (<2.5 L/minute/m^2) after volume resuscitation,[264] but if profound hypotension is present (systolic blood pressure < 80 mm Hg), it should be used in conjunction with an agent with more peripheral vasoconstrictor effects such as norepinephrine or phenylephrine.

Several studies have examined whether resuscitation of septic patients to predetermined end points of global oxygen delivery improves outcome. Earlier studies showed no benefit,[43, 45, 272] but enrolled patients up to 72 hours after admission. A more recent study showed early therapy to a predetermined central venous oxygen saturation level lowered mortality.[269] There is currently no consensus on treating septic patients to oxygen delivery end points.

Treatment of the Coagulation Cascade

DIC is a common finding, and treatment of the underlying condition will accelerate its resolution. No specific therapy is recommended for DIC unless severe or life-threatening hemorrhage occurs, at which time replacement with platelets, fresh-frozen plasma, and possibly cryoprecipitate is indicated.[230]

The finding that protein C levels are reduced in sepsis and are associated with an increased risk of death[74] led to the study of activated protein C (APC) in the treatment of sepsis. The PROWESS trial[273] was a randomized, controlled trial that evaluated APC in 1690 septic patients. Patients were eligible if they had known or suspected infection, three or more signs of SIRS, and at least one organ dysfunction. Patients were treated with placebo or a continuous infusion of APC for 96 hours. Patients treated with APC had a 19.4% reduction in the relative risk of death, and an absolute reduction in the risk of death of 6.1%. A post hoc analysis of this study by the Food and Drug Administration (FDA),[274] however, found that the benefit of APC seemed to be restricted to patients with more severe illness (an Acute Physiology and Chronic Health Evaluation [APACHE II] score of ≥ 25). A study is currently underway to assess the efficacy of APC in patients with an APACHE II score of less than 25. PROWESS was the first randomized controlled trial to show a survival benefit of a therapeutic intervention in sepsis. Because APC acts on the coagulation system, there is an increased risk of bleeding associated with its use, and the incidence of serious bleeding in the treated group in PROWESS was higher than in the controls (3.5% vs. 2.0%) despite fairly stringent criteria to exclude those at risk for bleeding. Activated protein C should be considered in all patients at high risk for death from sepsis: three SIRS criteria and at least one organ dysfunction. Patients with conditions that were exclusion criteria in the PROWESS trial, including pregnancy, breast-feeding, chronic renal failure requiring dialysis, acute pancreatitis without a known source of infection, cirrhosis, and human immunodeficiency virus (HIV) infection with a CD4$^+$ cell count less than 50/mm^3 should be evaluated carefully. Care should also be taken in the patient at risk for bleeding as this is the main side effect. Antithrombin (AT) III has been the subject of many clinical studies of sepsis,[275-277] and has shown improvement in DIC. However, AT III has only shown survival benefit in one study,[277] in a subgroup of patients with septic shock. These studies were all of small size, and a large multicenter study would better address the role of AT III. Recombinant tissue factor pathway inhibitor has been shown to be beneficial in animal models of septic shock,[278, 279] but has not shown survival benefit in human studies.[280] Site-inactivated factor VIIa, which competitively inhibits factor VIIa from binding to tissue factor and initiating coagulation, has been shown to prevent sepsis-induced acute lung injury and ARF in baboons,[281] but has not been evaluated in humans.

Immunomodulatory Therapy

Corticosteroids have long been the subject of studies in sepsis, the rationale being that minimization of the inflammatory cascade could improve outcome. Short-term therapy with glucocorticoids has not improved the outcome in sepsis,[282] and a meta-analysis of 10 studies showed no beneficial effect.[283] Yet two recent small studies (40 and 41 patients) did show an improvement in outcome.[284, 285] A large-scale, multicenter study is underway, but until more convincing data are available, steroid therapy is not recommended.

Antibodies to TNF have been studied in sepsis, and although most studies have found no benefit,[286-288] a recent study showed a risk-adjusted relative reduction in mortality of 14.3% for septic patients with an IL-6 level of greater than 1000 pg/mL when treated with anti-TNF antibody.[289]

Studies have been done to evaluate the benefit of antiendotoxin,[290] PAF antagonists,[291] bradykinin antagonists,[292] prostaglandin antagonists,[293, 294] IL-1 receptor antagonists,[295] nonselective NO synthase inhibitor,[296] N-acetylcysteine (NAC),[297] granulocyte colony-stimulating factor,[298] and intravenous immunoglobulin[299] in sepsis, and none have been shown to be beneficial. A recent study assessing C1 inhibitor in 40 patients found an improvement in serum creatinine values at days 3 and 4, but no survival benefit.[300]

Hemofiltration

The role of cytokines in sepsis and septic shock has led to the theory that removing them by hemofiltration may improve outcomes. Many studies have evaluated the effect of hemofiltration on cytokine levels and have shown clearance of cytokines, including TNF,[301, 302] IL-1,[301, 303, 304] IL-6,[215, 305] and IL-8,[305] by hemofiltration. Although a few studies have shown a reduction in the amount of cytokines in the plasma with hemofiltration,[306, 307] the preponderance of studies have shown no reduction in plasma cytokine levels.[308-313] The high production rate and rapid endogenous clearance of many cytokines[314] likely results in the amount being removed by hemofiltration to be too minor to change circulating levels. It also appears that a large percentage of the clearance of cytokines occurs as a result of adsorption to the dialysis membrane,[315] which becomes saturated after a short time, limiting the clearance.

In animal models, hemofiltration has improved survival in some studies,[316, 317] but these studies initiated hemofiltration before or shortly after the septic insult, which is generally not possible in clinical practice. Studies using a true infection model have not shown an effect on survival.[318, 319]

Prospective human studies to evaluate the benefit of hemofiltration in sepsis have generally been small. Reduction in the hyperdynamic response, including improved SVR,[320] improvement in APACHE II scores,[321] improvement in vasopressor requirement,[322] and beneficial hemostatic changes[323] has been obtained. One prospective uncontrolled study found that short-term (4-hour) high-volume hemofiltration, followed by conventional continuous venovenous hemofiltration, improved septic shock in 11 of 20 patients treated,[324] but no randomized controlled trial at this time has shown an improvement in survival when hemofiltration is used for sepsis. Recent studies have shown that adsorption coupled with hemofiltration,[325] and high-volume ultrafiltration with frequent membrane changes[315] may improve cytokine clearance, but currently there is no evidence to support the routine use of hemofiltration for sepsis.

CARDIOGENIC SHOCK

Cardiogenic shock is a state of decreased cardiac output in the setting of adequate intravascular volume, resulting in inadequate tissue perfusion. The diagnosis can be made clinically by the findings of poor tissue perfusion, such as oliguria or cool extremities, along with the hemodynamic criteria of sustained hypotension (systolic blood pressure < 90 mm Hg), reduced cardiac index (<2.2 L/minute/m^2), and congestion (pulmonary capillary wedge pressure >18 mm Hg).[326]

Cardiogenic shock occurs in 4.2% to 7.2% of MIs[327, 328] and is the most common cause of death among patients suffering from MI.[329] The first series, in 1967, evaluating the outcome of cardiogenic shock, found a mortality rate of 81%,[330] and a recent multicenter trial found a mortality rate of 60%.[331]

The most common cause of cardiogenic shock is massive MI,[332] but cardiogenic shock can also be caused by a smaller infarction in a patient with reduced left ventricular function, acute mitral regurgitation (from papillary muscle rupture), rupture of the interventricular septum, myocarditis, end-stage cardiomyopathy, valvular heart disease, or hypertrophic cardiomyopathy. In the SHOCK (*Sh*ould we emergently revascularize *o*ccluded coronaries in *c*ardiogenic shoc*k*?) Trial Registry,[331] of 1422 patients with cardiogenic shock, 79% of patients had left ventricular failure as the cause of shock, 6.9% had severe mitral regurgitation, 3.9% had ventricular septal rupture, 2.8% had isolated right ventricular shock, and 1.4% had cardiac tamponade. Shock may be found at presentation in patients with acute MI, but can be delayed. In the SHOCK trial, mean time to development of shock was 7 hours after infarction.[331]

Pathophysiology

In patients with MI or ischemia, cardiogenic shock may occur once 40% of the myocardium is lost.[332] The resultant clinical sequelae can potentiate the myocardial damage. Hypotension and tachycardia can increase ischemia in this setting. Coronary blood flow is dependent on the duration of diastole, which is significantly shortened in the tachycardic patient, resulting in reduced perfusion of the already ischemic myocardium.[332] The elevated wall stress resulting from left ventricular dilation and pump failure increases myocardial oxygen requirements, which also worsens ischemia.[332]

The cellular hypoxia seen in ischemia leads to a reduction in adenosine triphosphate (ATP) levels, and eventual myocyte swelling.[333] Apoptosis of myocytes occurs following MI,[334] and may contribute to the state of reduced cardiac output.

Clinical Features

Hypotension is universal in cardiogenic shock. Tachycardia is often present, but in the SHOCK Trial Registry, the mean heart rate was 96 beats per minute.[335] Arrhythmias may be present, and jugular venous distention, pulmonary rales, and a third heart sound are usually found. Signs of hypoperfusion may include confusion, mottling of the skin, and oliguria. In a study of 118 patients with cardiogenic shock, ARF occurred in 33% of patients within 24 hours, and increased mortality from 53% to 87%.[9] Multiple organ failure develops in many patients, primarily due to ischemia from decreased cardiac output. However, high plasma levels of IL-6 have been associated with multiple organ failure in this population,[336] indicating a possible role for systemic inflammation. Lactic acidosis may also occur from hypoperfusion.[337]

Evaluation

The primary goal in the evaluation of cardiogenic shock is to determine the primary cause. As stated previously, MI with reduced left ventricular systolic function is the most common cause,[330] and is often readily apparent on physical examination. However, other causes of shock, such as sepsis, hypovolemia, and pulmonary embolism, need to be considered. An ECG should be performed on arrival, and if an inferior MI is suspected, a right-sided ECG should be performed to evaluate for right-sided involvement. Routine blood tests, including cardiac enzymes, should be performed, a Foley catheter should be placed to monitor urine output, and a chest radiograph should be obtained.

Echocardiography is a valuable tool to confirm the diagnosis of cardiogenic shock, and can evaluate for potential mechanical causes that require surgical intervention, such as mitral regurgitation, papillary muscle rupture, tamponade, or left ventricular free wall rupture.

Although brain natriuretic peptide (BNP) has been found to be effective in the diagnosis of congestive heart failure (CHF), it is not typically used in the diagnosis of cardiogenic shock. BNP is a 32–amino acid polypeptide found in the cardiac ventricles. BNP release from the ventricles, and therefore serum levels, is indirectly proportional to ventricular volume expansion and pressure overload.[338] A BNP level greater than 100 pg/mL has a sensitivity of 82% for CHF, increasing to 99% for New York Heart Association (NYHA) class IV CHF.[339] BNP levels have been found to correlate closely with the NYHA classification, with mean levels in NYHA class IV greater than 900 pg/mL.[339] BNP levels have also been found to decline as pulmonary capillary wedge pressure decreases,[340] making it a possible monitoring tool in the treatment of severe CHF.

Management

Airway management and maintenance of adequate oxygenation should be the first concern during resuscitation. BiPAP or CPAP can improve oxygenation and prevent intubation in severe CHF,[341] although their use in cardiogenic shock has not been well studied. Intubation and mechanical ventilation may be required if supplemental oxygen or noninvasive ventilation cannot maintain adequate oxygenation with minimal work of breathing.

Patients treated with β-blockers, angiotensin-converting enzyme (ACE) inhibitors, and nitrates for MI who subsequently develop shock should have these agents discontinued as they may worsen the clinical state. Patients with mechanical causes of shock should be evaluated for surgical repair.

A minority of patients with cardiogenic shock may develop hypotension without evidence of pulmonary edema.[342] In these patients, a fluid challenge of 100 to 250 mL of normal saline should be given. In the patient who does not respond to fluids, or has pulmonary congestion, inotropic agents should be administered.

Dobutamine is primarily a β_1-adrenergic agonist, but a weak β_2- and α-adrenergic stimulator, and can improve myocardial contractility and cardiac output. Dobutamine is the drug of first choice when the systolic blood pressure (SBP) is greater than 80 mm Hg, but it can induce hypotension as a result of the β_2-adrenergic effect, so should either not be used when the SBP is less than 80 mm Hg, or used in conjunction with another vasopressor. Dobutamine may worsen tachycardia, and can cause arrhythmias.[343]

Dopamine should be used when the SBP is less than 80 mm Hg. At low doses (< 3 μg/kg/minute) β_1-adrenergic effects predominate, and as the dose is increased, α-adrenergic effects become more prevalent. Ischemia of the periphery, tachycardia, and arrhythmias can occur.[343] Norepinephrine is a pure α-adrenergic agonist and can be used when there is an inadequate response to dopamine.

Milrinone and amrinone are phosphodiesterase inhibitors that increase cyclic adenosine monophosphate levels in the myocardium. These agents increase inotropicity and cardiac output, without increasing myocardial oxygen consumption.[344] They do not induce direct tachycardia, but do cause a peripheral vasodilation, which can lead to hypotension and reflex tachycardia. Amrinone, as well as dopamine and dobutamine, may also improve myocardial mitochondrial function during shock.[345]

If hemodynamics have stabilized after the initiation of pressors, treatment of pulmonary edema with diuretics may be initiated. Direct vasodilator therapy can then be considered to decrease preload and afterload, which can improve ischemia. Sodium nitroprusside and nitroglycerin both have short half-lives, and can be carefully titrated, observing for worsening of the hemodynamic state.

Recombinant human BNP has been found to increase cardiac output, decrease pulmonary capillary wedge pressure and SVR, and improve natriuresis and diuresis in decompensated heart failure.[346, 347] It is FDA-approved for treatment of NYHA class IV CHF, but has not been evaluated in cardiogenic shock.

Intra-aortic balloon pumping (IABP) can improve diastolic blood pressure[348] and coronary perfusion,[349] and increase cardiac output.[348] In the Global Utilization of Streptokinase and TPA for Occluded Coronary Arteries (GUSTO-1) trial, patients who had early IABP placement had a trend toward improved survival,[350] and the SHOCK trial found a lower in-hospital mortality in patients who received IABP.[351] A recent study evaluated 23,180 patients with cardiogenic shock, 7268 of whom had IABP. IABP was associated with a significant

reduction in mortality among patients who received thrombolytic therapy (67% vs. 49%), but was of no benefit in patients treated with primary angioplasty (45% vs. 47%).[352] IABP has been shown to increase clot lysis when used in conjunction with thrombolytics in animal models,[353] likely owing to increased coronary blood flow, and this may explain the reduction in mortality when IABP and thrombolytics are used together.

IABP has been reported to have a complication rate between 2.6% and 15%, with a mortality rate of 0.05% to 0.4%.[354, 355] Most of the complications were vascular, with major bleeding occurring in 4.6%, and limb ischemia occurring in 3.3% of patients.[355] A study of 71 patients found a rate of bacteremia and sepsis to be 15% and 12%, respectively.[356] ARF was not reported as a complication in these studies, probably because the associated shock made attribution of ARF to IABP difficult.

The outcome of cardiogenic shock in the setting of MI is directly related to the patency of the involved coronary arteries.[357] Therefore, interventions to open occluded arteries are crucial. Thrombolytics have been shown to be able to reduce the incidence of shock when given for acute MI,[330] but once shock is established, the data are conflicting. The Gruppo Italiano per lo Studio-della Streptochinasi nell Infarto Miocardico (GISSI) trial[358] found a similar in-hospital mortality between patients treated with streptokinase (69.9%) and controls (70.1%). However, the SHOCK Trial Registry of 1190 patients found a lower in-hospital mortality among patients treated with thrombolytics (54%) compared to those who did not receive thrombolytic therapy (64%),[351] and a study of 23,180 patients in the National Registry of Myocardial Infarction 2 found a mortality rate of 59% for patients receiving only thrombolytic therapy compared with 77% in the group who received no reperfusion therapy.[354]

Despite the apparent benefit of thrombolytics, recent evidence has favored an even more aggressive approach to the treatment of cardiogenic shock. The SHOCK trial[359] randomized patients to early revascularization or initial medical stabilization, with 63% of the latter group receiving thrombolytics. The early revascularization group had a 30-day mortality similar to the medical therapy group (47% vs. 56%, $P = .11$), but 6-month mortality (50% vs. 63%, $P < .03$),[359] and 1-year mortality rates (53% vs. 66%, $P < .03$),[360] were improved. The choice of revascularization in the SHOCK trial was based on severity of coronary disease, with percutaneous intervention (64% of procedures) for one- or two-vessel disease, and surgery for left main stenosis or three-vessel disease. The mortality in the medical treatment group is lower than in many other studies, and may be related to the aggressive use of thrombloytics (63% of patients) and IABP (86% of patients). Other small studies suggest that administration of platelet glycoprotein IIb/IIIa inhibitor to coronary stenting may improve outcomes further.[361, 362]

Ventricular assist devices have been used in peri-infarction cardiogenic shock, acute myocarditis, and postcardiotomy shock to bridge patients to either recovery of adequate myocardial function or transplantation.[363]

As stated, ARF develops in one third of patients in cardiogenic shock, often necessitating a continuous renal replacement therapy (CRRT), given the hemodynamic instability. CRRT in the critically ill is discussed later.

Ultrafiltration by CRRT has also been proposed as a treatment for severe refractory heart failure in patients who do not have uremia. No studies have evaluated CRRT for treatment of cardiogenic shock without renal failure, but it has generated interest in the treatment of heart failure.

Chronic heart failure results in neuroendocrine activation that is initially a response to the decreased effective circulating volume, but eventually serves to worsen heart failure as volume overload progresses.[364, 365] The RAA system is activated, resulting in renal sodium and water retention as a result of increased aldosterone. The sympathetic nervous system is activated, and along with angiotensin II, results in peripheral vasoconstriction, which increases wall stress on the left ventricle, worsening heart failure. This increased wall stress due to volume and pressure overload results in ventricular remodeling, which potentiates heart failure,[361] worsening effective circulating volume and resulting in a further activation of the RAA system. In patients who are diuretic-resistant, there is no pharmacologic means to remove fluid and potentially shut down the cycle of neuroendocrine activation and worsening heart failure. Ultrafiltation, either by continuous or intermittent methods, has been proposed to accomplish this.[362, 366]

A study of 32 patients[367] found that circulating renin, aldosterone, and norepinephrine levels were highest in patients with the most advanced heart failure (NYHA class III-IV and urine output <1000 mL/24 hours), and treatment with ultrafiltration led to significant reductions in these values along with a nearly 500% increase in diuresis (from 379 to 2195 mL/24 hours), and a doubling of natriuresis (from 30 to 63 mEq/L). However, those patients with urine output greater than 1000 ml/day were found to have a reduction in diuresis and natriuresis.[367] In addition to improving the cycle of neuroendocrine activation, ultrafiltration has been proposed to improve refractory heart failure by removing the "myocardial depressant factor," which has been found in ultrafiltrate.[368]

Most studies have been retrospective or case reports. Studies that have been performed have shown that ultrafiltration can improve the hemodynamics in patients with acute heart failure,[369] and have shown that patients can respond to ultrafiltration with improved diuresis, reduced heart failure symptoms, and improved sensitivity to diuretics,[370-373] but there are conflicting data that hemofiltration may offer no benefit.[374] Unfortunately, all of the studies in this area are small.

Although hemofiltration may improve CHF in some patients, removal of intravascular volume may not be tolerated by all, and can clearly lead to permanent renal dysfunction. The choice of patients to undergo hemofiltration for refractory heart failure should be made very carefully, and the risks of permanent renal failure should be discussed with the patient in advance.

FULMINANT HEPATIC FAILURE

Fulminant hepatic failure is an acute and frequently fatal process that results in severe metabolic abnormalities, neurologic complications, and often multiorgan failure. Treatment in a critical care setting is required, and has helped improve the survival of many of these patients over the last several decades,[375] although mortality still remains high. Liver dialysis

has been investigated as a possible treatment for encephalopathic patients, and if it becomes widespread, may fall under the domain of the nephrologist.

Definition

Acute liver failure from hepatocyte dysfunction results in diminished synthesis of clotting factors, manifested by prolongation of the PT and a decrease in the level of factor V, protein, and often cerebral edema. *Fulminant hepatic failure* is defined as severe acute liver failure in a patient with no preexisting liver disease, with encephalopathy developing within 2 weeks of the first manifestation of liver disease, usually jaundice.[376] Liver failure that is complicated by encephalopathy between 3 and 12 weeks after the onset of jaundice has been termed *subfulminant hepatic failure* (SFHF).[376] Because the rate of onset of this disease process is an indicator of prognosis, with the patients having the most rapid onset of encephalopathy also having the best chance of recovery, a newer definition has been proposed to classify FHF and SFHF.[377] Hyperacute, acute, and subacute liver failure are defined by the time between the onset of jaundice and the development of encephalopathy (0-7 days, 8-28 days, and 29 days-12 weeks, respectively). The survival rate in hyperacute liver failure has been reported to be 36%; acute liver failure has a survival rate of 7% and subacute, 14%.[369] The most common cause of hyperacute liver failure is acetaminophen overdose, although hepatitis A and B can also result in this condition. Acute liver failure is predominantly caused by viral hepatitis and drug reactions[378]; subacute liver failure is most often caused by a hepatitis for which no viral cause can be found.[379]

Patients with chronic liver disease can also develop decompensation with complications similar to acute hepatic failure, except they typically do not develop brain edema.

Causes

There are many causes of FHF, and there are regional variations in the etiology. Acute viral hepatitis is the leading cause of FHF worldwide, although the vast majority of cases of viral hepatitis do not manifest as FHF.[380] Hepatitis A virus (HAV) is the most common cause of hepatitis worldwide, but accounts for less than 1% of all cases of FHF.[380] Of all the viral causes of FHF, HAV has the best prognosis with more than 60% of patients surviving without a transplant.[381] HAV does not lead to chronic hepatitis, and is diagnosed by the presence of HAV anti-IgM antibodies.

Hepatitis B virus (HBV) currently accounts for approximately 15% of cases of FHF in the United States,[378] and 23% in Europe.[380] Coinfection with hepatitis D virus (HDV; acquiring HBV and HDV simultaneously) is found in up to 30% of cases of FHF with hepatitis B.[382] Superinfection with HDV can occur in a patient known to have HBV, and can lead to FHF. Hepatitis C virus (HCV) coinfection with HBV may also precipitate FHF.[383] The diagnosis of acute HBV infection is based on the presence of anti-IgM antibodies to hepatitis B core antigen (HBcAg) because hepatitis B surface antigen (HBsAg) is often not detected in the acute setting.

HCV has traditionally not been felt to be a cause of FHF, but one recent study identified HCV RNA in 19% of patients with FHF.[384] A cause-and-effect relationship between HCV and FHF has not been fully established at this time.

Hepatitis E virus (HEV) is known to cause FHF, particularly in the third trimester of pregnancy, and is endemic to Asia and Africa. To date, no causes of FHF in the United States have been attributed to HEV,[383] but HEV should be considered in patients who have traveled to, or emigrated from, endemic areas. Herpes simplex virus and cytomegalovirus have been reported to cause FHF, but usually in the setting of immunosuppression or pregnancy. Adenovirus,[385] human herpes virus 6,[386] Epstein-Barr virus, and influenzavirus B have also been reported to cause FHF.[387] In patients with FHF that is suspected to be viral in origin, 10% to 20% of all cases cannot be identified, and these have been termed non-A, non-B, non-C FHF. This disease usually has a subacute presentation, and does not seem to recur after liver transplantation.[378]

Drug toxicity is the second most common cause of FHF, either by a direct hepatotoxic effect or by an idiosyncratic reaction. Acetaminophen is the most common drug to cause FHF in the United States and United Kingdom. Acetaminophen is partially converted to the toxic metabolite N-acetyl-p-benzoquinone-imine (NADQI), which is neutralized by reacting with glutathione. If the amount of acetaminophen ingested acutely or chronically overwhelms the ability of glutathione to inactivate NADQI, hepatotoxicity occurs. Persons with depleted glutathione stores from alcoholism or malnutrition are more susceptible to hepatotoxicity, as are persons taking cytochrome P-450 enzyme–inducing drugs. Single doses as low as 10 g can lead to FHF, but doses within the therapeutic range taken chronically by alcohol abusers can also lead to FHF. Halothane is known to be hepatotoxic, but is rarely used today in clinical practice. The newer halogenated agents enflurane, methoxyflurane, and isoflurane have a much lower risk of hepatotoxicity. Halothane hepatotoxicity is idiosyncratic, and there is cross-reactivity between the halogenated agents. Many other drugs have been associated with acute liver failure and FHF, including nonsteroidal anti-inflammatory drugs (NSAIDs), isoniazid, phenytoin, valproic acid, sulfonamides, propylthiouracil, amiodarone, and Ecstasy (3,4-methylenedioxymetamphetamine). A thorough history is critical for diagnosing drug-related FHF, which can be difficult in a profoundly encephalopathic patient.

Ingestion of the mushroom *Amanita phalloides* is a rare but well-recognized cause of FHF. Hepatic, pancreatic, renal, and cerebral damage can occur as a result of the toxin α-amantin.[388] Profuse watery diarrhea and abdominal pain develop within 24 hours of ingestion and last 1 to 6 days prior to the development of liver failure. As little as three mushrooms may lead to FHF.

Wilson disease presents as FHF in 10% of cases. This disease may be associated with hemolytic anemia secondary to massive copper release from the liver, and Kayser-Fleischer rings on slit-lamp examination of the cornea. Although no set of laboratory values can distinguish Wilson disease from other causes of FHF,[389] a low ceruloplasmin level and a low serum alkaline phosphatase are suggestive. Rapid recognition is key as this condition is 100% fatal without a liver transplantation.[377] Other conditions that can present as FHF are listed in Table 61-8.

Clinical Features

FHF presents with a variety of symptoms. Nausea and vomiting may be the first indicators, followed by jaundice.

Encephalopathy may develop rapidly. Several metabolic disorders result from the loss of hepatocyte function. Hypoglycemia results from impaired gluconeogenesis, high insulin levels, and inability to utilize stored glycogen. Metabolic acidosis is a consequence of poor tissue perfusion and inability to clear lactate. Hypokalemia and hyponatremia also occur frequently. By definition, FHF requires that encephalopathy be present, the etiology of which is felt to be multifactorial.[390] Ammonia, NO, manganese, and inhibition of the Na+,K+-ATPase pump in neuronal cells may all play a role in acute hepatic encephalopathy.[391] Increased production or diminished clearance of "endogenous" benzodiazepines may contribute to hepatic encephalopathy,[392, 393] and enhanced γ-aminobutyric acid (GABA)ergic inhibitory neurotransmission has also been postulated to have an effect.[394] Hepatic encephalopathy is graded on a scale of 1 to 4 as listed in Table 61-9. Strong consideration should be given to intubation for airway protection as encephalopathy progresses through stage 3.

Cerebral edema has been found in 40% of patients with FHF and advanced encephalopathy.[395] In patients dying with FHF, uncal or cerebellar herniation or both were found to be the cause of death in 80%.[396] The rapid increase in water content of the brain results from increased permeability of the blood-brain barrier.[397] The edematous brain is confined by the cranium, leading to increased intracranial pressure (ICP) and decreased cerebral perfusion.[398] Cerebral edema is manifested clinically by abnormal pupillary reflexes, systemic hypertension, and bradycardia. Decerebrate posturing and brainstem respiratory patterns are classic, but late, findings. Invasive monitoring by a subdural transducer does have a risk of bleeding and infection,[395, 399] but in the sedated and ventilated patient may be the only mechanism to assess ICP. Some authors have recommended ICP monitoring for all patients with grade 3 and 4 encephalopathy,[400, 401] and ICP monitoring has been shown to improve the outcome of liver transplantation by excluding those patients with low

TABLE 61-8

Additional Causes of Fulminant Hepatic Failure*

Autoimmune hepatitis	Metastatic tumor
Acute fatty liver of pregnancy	Budd-Chiari syndrome
HELLP syndrome	Portal vein thrombosis
Reye syndrome	Right-sided heart failure
Malignant hyperthermia	Acute rejection of liver transplantation

*After hepatitis, drug toxicity, mushroom poisoning, and Wilson disease.
HELLP, *h*emolysis, *e*levated *l*iver enzymes, *l*ow *p*latelet count.

TABLE 61-9

Stages of Hepatic Encephalopathy

Stage 1: euphoria, anxiety, disruption of sleep, shortened attention span, mild confusion, slight asterixis
Stage 2: slurred speech, lethargy, inappropriate behavior, asterixis, hypoactive reflexes, loss of continence
Stage 3: marked confusion, incoherent speech, hyperactive reflexes, somnolent but arousable
Stage 4: coma, unresponsive to pain, lacking asterixis

cerebral perfusion pressure (CPP = mean arterial pressure − ICP) who are likely to have permanent neurologic damage.[402, 403] However, there is currently no consensus as to which patients should receive ICP monitoring.[393] Most patients who recover from FHF with associated cerebral edema have full recovery of neurologic function, but permanent brain damage can occur.[404]

Patients with acute liver failure are often found to have profound circulatory changes. A reduction in the SVR, which manifests as hypotension, is common, and has been attributed to high levels of circulating endotoxin and TNF.[402] There is also microthrombi formation in small vessels, resulting in diminished perfusion of metabolically active tissues.[393] These two factors combine to reduce oxygen delivery and extraction, resulting in anaerobic metabolism, and contributing to the lactic acidosis and multiorgan failure seen in many patients. Coagulopathy is a common finding in FHF. Half of all patients develop thrombocytopenia,[405] caused by consumption, reduced bone marrow production, or, in a patient with preexisting liver disease, hypersplenism. Reduced production of factors I, II, V, VII, IX, and X lead to an increase in the PT. A reduction in factor V is seen rapidly because it has a short half-life. The level of factor V is often used as a marker for disease progression, and is considered an independent prognostic factor.[375] The synthesis of coagulation factors II, IX, and X may also be reduced, prolonging the PTT. DIC may be seen resulting from a combination of factors, including the release from necrotic hepatocytes of thromboplastic material, platelet activation from circulating bacterial endotoxins not cleared by the liver, and expression of tissue factor on activated endothelial cells stimulating the extrinsic coagulation cascade.[406] Although hemorrhage is uncommon, the gastrointestinal tract is the most common site of bleeding, and intracranial hemorrhage may rarely occur spontaneously.[407]

Bacterial infections may occur in up to 80% of patients with acute liver failure,[408] caused in part by diminished opsonic activity,[409] complement deficiency, and impaired neutrophil function.[410] Fungal infections are also common, the predominant organisms being *Candida albicans* or *Candida glabrata* and *Aspergillus*. There may be an absence of clinical signs of infection in FHF, so a high index of suspicion must be maintained, particularly when patients have a sudden deterioration. Prophylactic antibiotics have not been shown to be beneficial,[411] but are commonly used.

Renal dysfunction is present in up to 55% of all patients with FHF.[404] Direct toxicity can be a result of acetaminophen overdose, radiocontrast, or antibiotic use. The circulatory changes seen in FHF predispose patients to renal dysfunction as they have reduced renal blood flow.[393] Hepatorenal syndrome is a well-recognized occurrence and is discussed in Chapter 27. Intermittent hemodialysis has been reported to increase the ICP in patients with FHF[412]; studies comparing intermittent RRT with continuous modes found no increase in ICP with CRRT, but a significant increase with intermittent methods.[413, 414] CRRT should be considered first-line therapy in FHF, even in hemodynamically stable patients.

Evaluation

Initial laboratory tests should include chemistry profiles, coagulation studies, complete blood count, toxicology screen, viral serologies, ceruloplasmin (in patients <40 years old),

creatitine kinase, and urinalysis. Transaminases can be strikingly high, but the levels do not predict outcome. Increases in bilirubin, prothrombin, and a reduction in factor V have prognostic value and should be followed closely.

Signs of cardiac or renal failure should prompt consideration of Swan-Ganz catheter placement because the intravascular volume status can be difficult to determine otherwise in FHF. Sepsis must be looked for, including a search for fungal infections.

Intravenous H_2 blockers are considered routine to prevent gastric bleeding in the setting of coagulopathy. Liver biopsy is needed for diagnosis in a minority of cases, as the etiology is usually evident. Transjugular biopsy has become the favored method in the setting of coagulopathy as it has less risk of bleeding than the percutaneous approach.[415]

Management

There are few causes of FHF for which specific therapy is useful. Acetaminophen toxicity should be treated with NAC. NAC enhances the availability of glutathione, and administration up to 36 hours after an overdose of acetaminophen may improve outcome.[416] Therefore NAC should be given when acetaminophen overdose is suspected, even if levels are undetectable. The oral dose is 140 mg/kg initially, followed by 70 mg/kg every 4 hours for 17 doses. When given intravenously, the dose is a 150 mg/kg bolus followed by 70 mg/kg intravenously every 4 hours for 12 doses. Acyclovir should be used for herpes simplex infection and lamivudine has been proved to be of some benefit for hepatitis B infection.[417] Acute fatty liver of pregnancy and the HELLP (*h*emolysis, *e*levated *l*iver enzymes, and *l*ow *p*latelets) syndrome require immediate delivery of the fetus. *Amanita* poisoning should be treated with high-dose penicillin (300,000 to 1 million units/kg/day),[418] which has an antagonistic effect on the mushroom toxin amatoxin, and sylibin (20-48 mg/kg/day),[419] which blocks the hepatocellular uptake of amatoxin. The remainder of therapy for FHF is supportive. Fluid resuscitation is often required in the acute setting as there is hypotension from decreased SVR, as well as increased endothelial permeability, which leads to redistribution. Albumin and fresh-frozen plasma have traditionally been considered first-line agents for fluid resuscitation,[377, 420] as these patients often have renal sodium retention with ascites formation, and saline tends to lead to third-spacing. Recent studies[177, 178] suggesting that albumin may increase mortality in critically ill patients make this less attractive. FFP continues to be used as a first-line agent for volume resuscitation, although there are no studies to support its use over normal saline. Once volume resuscitation is complete, dextrose with 0.45% normal saline should be used for maintenance fluids, with careful monitoring of serum electrolytes.

Hypotension that persists after fluid resuscitation is adequate, as evidenced by a wedge pressure of 12 to 14 mm Hg, requires vasopressors. Norepinephrine is most commonly used for its preferential effect on peripheral α-adrenergic receptors.

In the seriously ill patient, intravenous NAC has been used to improve cardiac output and oxygen extraction, particularly in the setting of pressor use, which may increase tissue hypoxia due to vasoconstriction. Studies of NAC for this purpose have not been consistent, with some showing a benefit,[421] and others showing no improvement in oxygen extraction or markers for tissue hypoxia.[422] Epoprostenol, a prostacyclin that has microcirculatory vasodilation properties, has been studied in patients receiving vasopressors and found to improve oxygen delivery and the O_2ER,[423] but in a study of patients with renal failure, intravenous prostacyclin was found to decrease blood pressure and significantly reduce CPP.[424]

The treatment of hepatic encephalopathy is directed at limiting the production of ammonia and avoiding benzodiazepines. Most ammonia is derived from intestinal bacteria, and lactulose can help reduce the absorption of ammonia, although it has not been shown to increase survival in patients with advanced encephalopathy.[425] Neomycin has been used, but has not been shown to be useful in hepatic encephalopathy.[426] It also has the potential for ototoxicity and nephrotoxicity, and therefore should be avoided. Metronidazole (Flagyl) is used to reduce intestinal bacteria and decrease ammonia production. Flumazenil, a benzodiazepine antagonist, has been shown to offer short-term improvement in encephalopathy.[427]

Cerebral edema is a common cause of death in patients with FHF and should be treated aggressively. When ICP monitoring is performed, the CPP should be maintained above 50 mm Hg. An ICP greater than 30 mm Hg and a CPP of less than 40 mm Hg for 2 hours have been associated with permanent neurologic damage.[398, 425] Raising the head of the bed to 20 to 30 degrees may improve ICP. Fever can increase ICP and should be aggressively treated. Mannitol is commonly used in doses of 0.5 to 1.0 g/kg, and is effective in reducing ICP in patients with normal renal function. A diuresis of twice the volume of mannitol given should be expected in 1 hour. This dose can be repeated, but the serum osmolality must be monitored and mannitol stopped when the osmolality reaches 320 mOsm/kg. Mannitol can lead to intravascular volume depletion and ARF, and its use in patients with ongoing renal dysfunction will likely lead to ARF. In the setting of renal failure, mannitol can be coupled with hemofiltration to maintain the osmotic effect. Twice the volume of mannitol administered should be removed by ultrafiltration to ensure this effect.[393] Hyperventilation to a Pco_2 of 30 mm Hg is routinely used to transiently reduce ICP, but one study showed this had no benefit[428] and a Pco_2 below 24 mm Hg is associated with cerebral vasoconstriction.[429] Agitation should be kept to a minimum. If the above measures are inadequate to keep the CPP above 50 mm Hg, pentobarbital may be used to induce coma.

Most patients with FHF develop coagulopathy, but spontaneous hemorrhage is uncommon.[405] Parenteral vitamin K should be given for 3 days if coagulopathy develops, and fresh-frozen plasma should only be given for bleeding or in advance of invasive procedures. Other therapies, including insulin and glucagon,[430] corticosteroids,[431] and exchange transfusion,[432] have not been shown to be beneficial; plasmapheresis has had mixed results, and is not widely used.[433, 434]

Patients with acute liver failure are placed at the top of the liver transplant list, but the shortage of donor organs means that many will die waiting for transplantation. The King's College criteria (Table 61-10) are utilized to help decide when a patient should be listed for a transplant. Contraindications include uncontrolled intracranial hypertension, sepsis, ARDS, and dependence on pressors.[380] Transplantation of human hepatocytes into the splenic bed

TABLE 61-10

King's College Criteria for Liver Transplantation

Acetaminophen overdose patient
Arterial pH <7.3 with any degree of encephalopathy
INR >6.5
Creatinine >3.4 mg/dL in presence of grade III or IV encephalopathy

Non–acetaminophen-related liver failure
INR >6.5 with encephalopathy or any three of the following:
Age <10 or >40 yr
Etiology: idiopathic nonviral hepatitis, idiosyncratic drug reaction
Jaundice >7 days before onset of encephalopathy
Serum bilirubin >17.5 mg/dL
INR >3.5

INR, international normalized ratio.
Modified from Shakil AO, Kramer D, Mazariegos GV, et al: Acute liver failure: Clinical features, outcome analysis, and applicability of prognostic criteria. Liver Transpl 6:163-169, 2000.

has been tried with some success.[435] Living-related transplants have been used in Japan for FHF with a reported 1-year survival of 90% in a series of 14 patients,[436] and have been used successfully in the United States.[437]

Although the toxins that lead to hepatic encephalopathy, as well as other manifestations of FHF, have not been identified, extracorporeal detoxification has been examined as a way to remove these toxins, and potentially improve outcome. The liver dialysis unit utilizes hemodiabsorption (hemodialysis with a thick suspension of pulverized sorbents replacing the dialysate solution in the dialyzer) to remove potential toxins from the blood. The small particle size of the charcoal provides 300,000 m^2 of surface area, much more area for absorption than typical charcoal columns that only have a few thousand square meters.[438] Blood is pumped at a rate of 200 to 250 mL/minute, and toxins pass directly across the cellulose membrane where they bind to the small particles of charcoal or cation exchangers in the sorbent solution. Treatment of 6 hours daily for 5 days was studied in a trial of patients with either FHF or acute on chronic liver disease.[439] Fifty-six patients were enrolled: 31 treated with liver dialysis, 25 as controls. In the acute-on-chronic liver failure group, 72% of those treated with liver dialysis had recovery of liver function or improvement to transplantation, whereas only 36% of the control group had these outcomes (P = .036), but patients with FHF showed no benefit from treatment with liver dialysis. It is unclear why the difference was so striking between the acute-on-chronic liver failure group and the FHF group, but it has been postulated that the toxins in FHF are more protein-bound, such as the toxins of sepsis, and are not removed as effectively.[435] Both groups did show an improvement in neurologic outcomes following treatment, with over 50% of treated patients showing improvement in encephalopathy. The liver dialysis unit is currently not available for widespread use.

Another sorbent system that has been developed for treatment of hepatic failure is the molecular adsorbent recirculating system (MARS). In this system, a non–albumin-permeable polysulfone dialysis membrane is used, with blood perfused on one side and 20% albumin on the dialysate side. Albumin-bound substances such as bilirubin, bile acids, tryptophan, and fatty acids are cleared across the membrane to the dialysate albumin,[440] which is regenerated by passing through a charcoal column, followed by an anion exchange resin column, and finally dialyzed against a bicarbonate-buffered dialysate to remove the small toxins such as ammonium and aromatic amino acids. Results of trials are similar to liver dialysis, with improvement in outcomes in acute-on-chronic liver failure, but not FHF, and improved encephalopathy scores in both groups.[418] MARS was also found in one small study of 13 patients to improve survival in hepatorenal syndrome,[441] with none of five patients treated with hemodiafiltration alone alive at 7 days, whereas three of eight patients also treated with MARS were alive at 7 days and two of eight were alive at 30 days. MARS is currently available for investigational use only in the United States.

The high mortality rate in FHF patients awaiting liver transplant has made clear the need for a temporary support system that can act as a bridge until the failing liver regenerates, or until liver transplantation is available. A bioartificial liver (BAL) is a device in which hepatocytes are inoculated into one side of a semipermeable membrane. Blood is passed into a plasma separator, the plasma is warmed, oxygenated, and then passed through the device that houses the hepatocytes.[442] The membrane acts to prevent antibodies from entering the cell compartment from the plasma, but allows hepatocytes to extract oxygen, nutrients, and toxins from the plasma, and allows metabolites to pass from the hepatocytes into the plasma. The current BAL devices undergoing clinical trials are using either porcine hepatocytes or immortalized human hepatocytes. The BAL device using porcine hepatocytes was successful in a phase I trial in bridging 17 patients with FHF to orthotopic liver transplantation.[442] Further trials are underway. The BAL device utilizing immortalized human hepatocytes had similar positive results in an early evaluation,[443] but in a randomized, controlled trial of 24 patients demonstrated no survival benefit.[444] Further trials are needed to assess the efficacy of these devices.

RENAL REPLACEMENT THERAPY IN THE INTENSIVE CARE UNIT

ARF in the ICU is a grave situation. ICU patients suffer multiple organ failure concomitant with or before the onset of ARF. These patients are more likely to be septic, volume-overloaded, or profoundly acidotic. They often require blood pressure support and mechanical ventilation and they are twice as catabolic as patients with ARF outside the ICU setting. Secondary to these comorbidities, the ICU ARF patient is likely to require RRT. Those ICU patients who develop ARF and require RRT have significantly higher mortalities. Clermont and colleagues compared mortality in ICU patients without ARF, those with ARF not requiring RRT, those with end-stage renal disease (ESRD) on RRT, and those with ARF requiring RRT. The respective mortalities in these populations were respectively 5%, 23%, 11%, and 57%.[445] An increase in mortality clearly reflected a worse overall medical comorbid condition, but also suggested an effect on worsening mortality of renal failure.[445, 446] Whether the dose, timing, or type of RRT can have an effect on outcome has just recently become an area of intense research in the nephrology and ICU communities.[447]

Historically, the decision to initiate RRT was based on severe life-threatening complications of renal failure. Little attention had been placed on the nuances of the ICU patient with ARF. Hence RRT in the ICU had been administered with similar goals and techniques applied in the outpatient dialysis setting. Although a large body of literature exists for the outpatient end-stage renal disease (ESRD) population, it should not be assumed to apply to the ICU setting. There are marked differences in these populations: the principle of "steady-state" kinetics is not applicable to ARF. The protein catabolic rate in patients in the ICU is typically twice that of other populations.[448, 449] Furthermore, severe volume overload not only influences ultrafiltration requirements but also changes solute distribution volumes, and the use of vasopressors may decrease the efficiency of RRT. Finally, adequate therapy, including the timing of RRT initiation and dose, has not been defined for ARF.

Decisions regarding how to deliver RRT in the ICU should be made with every effort to improve the patients' mortality and morbidity. When approaching the patient who requires RRT the following questions should be asked: What access is best? When is it best to initiate RRT? Which RRT modality should be utilized? What degree of solute clearance is required?

Indications

Indications for initiation of RRT in the ICU should be expanded over those for initiation of RRT for ESRD. The presence of ARF requiring RRT is associated with a significant rise in ICU mortality. Mehta appropriately separated indications for RRT in the ICU into " renal replacement" and "renal support" therapy.[450] The indications for renal replacement are similar to those typically used for initiation of dialysis in ESRD patients, albeit expanded in the care of the ICU patient. The mnemonic *AEIOU* is useful when considering replacement therapy in the ICU.

*A*cidosis has historically been an indication for RRT when associated with azotemia. RRT is initiated as the serum bicarbonate declines and intravenous supplementation is inadequate or unacceptable due to sodium overload. However, with CRRT lactic acidosis can be controlled successfully and acidosis secondary to permissive hypercapnia can be modified.

*E*lectrolyte abnormalities are an indication for RRT in the ICU. Although hyperkalemia is the most common indication for intervention, all electrolyte abnormalities can be modified with RRT. Sodium can usually be modified with changes in free water intake or delivery but in rare instances RRT may be necessary. Calcium, phosphate, and uric acid abnormalities, such as are seen in tumor lysis syndrome and hypercalcemia from any cause, may require RRT to correct.

*I*ntoxications frequently require RRT—lithium, theophylline, ethylene glycol, methanol, aspirin, phenobarbitol, and cyclophosphamide (Cytoxan) overdoses may all be treated with RRT.

*V*olume overload is often and easily treated with RRT, but is usually reserved for patients, with oligoanuria unresponsive to diuretics. These patients are initiated on a form of RRT when they have pulmonary edema, severe hypertension, or significant edema.

*U*remia is also an indication for RRT. Unfortunately, no clear definition of uremia in the ICU patients exists. Certainly, mental status changes and pericarditis are easily defined complications of renal failure; they occur late in the course and likely should not be markers for initiation of therapy.

Renal support indications, as defined by Mehta,[450] represent a change in therapy from ameliorating the conditions directly resulting from lack of intrinsic renal function to one that supports the patient and the effects of the complications from other organ failure. The goal of therapy becomes increasing survival time to allow for recovery of multiple organ systems, including the recovery of renal function. Potential indications for renal support are extensions of renal replacement and novel approaches for care in the ICU. Volume overload without oligoanuria or even significant azotemia is an example of renal support. CRRT can be used in the patient with total body overload and with less than adequate urine output despite a response to diuretics. Renal support can allow for administration of total parenteral nutrition, fluid removal in CHF, and total fluid management in the patient with multiorgan failure. A patient in the ICU may require inputs of greater than 3 L/day if nutrition is maintained and antibiotics or blood products are required (Table 61-11). Continuous therapies allow for continuous fluid removal in excess of input despite hypotension or pressor requirements. Postoperative mortality rises with the percentage of body weight increase in the ICU[451] and CRRT allows for this fluid removal postoperatively, potentially reducing morbidity and mortality. In addition, fluid removal with continuous therapies has been shown by Manns and colleagues[452] to maintain urine output and GFR when compared to intermittent therapies. Finally, McDonald and Mehta have demonstrated better nutrition in the ICU patient on CRRT versus intermittent therapy.[453]

Knowing when to initiate RRT in the ICU is a complex decision. Traditionally, waiting for a life-threatening indication for renal replacement has dictated timing. However, as we consider renal support requirements, and the extremely high mortality in these patients, earlier intervention seems appropriate. Gettings and colleagues[454] retrospectively reviewed survival in two groups of trauma patients receiving CRRT in the ICU. Both groups received equivalent clearances and had similar characteristics. However, the group initiated on CRRT earlier, with a blood urea nitrogen (BUN) less than 60 mg/dL (mean, 42 mg/dL) had a survival of 39% compared to only 20% when CRRT was initiated after the BUN value exceeded 60 mg/dL (mean, 96 mg/dL).[454]

In the absence of controlled trials, definitive guidelines are not available. If the patient in the ICU is approached with consideration of renal support, as well as renal replacement as proposed by Mehta,[450] the patient should be initiated on

TABLE 61-11

Daily Fluid Requirements for a Typical Intensive Care Patient

SOURCE	VOLUME (L/DAY)
Medications (antibiotics/pressors)	1-2
Blood products	0.5-1.5
Alimentation (TPN, enteral feeds)	1.5-3.0
Total obligate input	**3-7 L/day**

TPN, total parenteral nutrition.

extracorporeal therapy when clinical judgment suggests an improvement that outweighs the risk can be obtained over the next 24 hours. Similarly, the decision to withhold RRT in the ICU should be based on the estimation that a lack of intervention with an extracorporeal therapy will not be detrimental to the patient. In other words, if return of renal function is likely or conservative management with furosemide, brain natriuretic factor, or another pharmacologic therapy is likely to succeed without harm to the patient, it is reasonable to observe the patient without extracorporeal therapy.

Vascular Access

Vascular access in the ICU is an important and often overlooked aspect of extracorporeal therapy. Poor access can lead to significant recirculation and inadequate flows, resulting in less efficient therapy and delivery of less than the prescribed Kt/V with intermittent hemodialysis. Poor access flow and high recirculation are also detrimental in continuous therapies. Increases in hematocrit in the system, resulting from recirculation rises, lead to clotting of the extracorporeal circuit. Factors determining catheter function include location of catheter placement and catheter design. Other factors of unstudied significance primarily include patient characteristics.

Most present-day noncuffed dialysis catheters are made of polyurethane. Polyurethane is fairly firm for easy insertion but relaxes at body temperature. The catheters are placed via the Seldinger technique. Some catheters are made of silicone; these are thicker-walled and more flexible. Placement of these catheters requires a peel-away sheath or stiffening stylet. Noncuffed catheters range in length from 15 to 24 cm. The 15-cm catheters are designed for placement via the right internal jugular vein. Although in most men and larger women, 19 to 20 cm may be required to reach the superior vena cava–right atrial junction. Catheters 20 cm and longer and designed for the left internal jugular and femoral approaches.

Cuffed catheters are designed for a tunneled placement. In general, these are placed when expected use of the catheter exceeds 2 to 3 weeks.[455] These catheters are silicone, hence more flexible than acute catheters, and longer. Placement is performed with a modified Seldinger technique using a peel-away sheath, and is more technically challenging. Cuffed hemodialysis catheters vary in length from 50 to 90 cm and are designed for internal jugular, femoral, transhepatic, or translumbar placement.

Catheter tip design varies by manufacturer. Designs include the step-tip (with or without side holes), single-lumen with a septum (various geometric designs), split-tip, or two separate single-lumen catheters. Studies comparing design variations have not been performed in patients with the acute catheters. At present all seem to have adequate initial flow and function when placed in the internal jugular vein. Cuffed dialysis catheters have been studied in patients. The blood flow achieved using either the split-tip catheter, larger step-tip catheters (15.5F), and twin catheters was similar to the blood pump setting measured with ultrasound dilution—100% of desired flow at blood pump speeds of 300 mL/minute and 93% to 95% of flow at 400 mL/minute. A 14.5F step-tip tunneled dialysis catheter had lower flows—97% of the desired flow at 300 mL/minute and only 82% at a blood pump speed of 400 mL/minute.[456-458]

Recirculation has been measured by catheter design and catheter placement. Recirculation in nontunneled dialysis catheters varies by location. Studies have demonstrated significantly higher recirculation values in femoral vein catheters than central—subclavian or internal jugular—veins. Most catheter recirculation is less than 5% in the subclavian or internal jugular vein.[458, 459] In the femoral vein, however, catheter recirculation may exceed 50% with a mean of 20% to 30% at blood pump speeds of 300 mL/minute. The amount of recirculation increases with blood pump speed and decreases when catheter length exceeds 19 cm.[455] Catheter design may also play a role in recirculation.

When catheter recirculation was studied in cuffed tunneled dialysis catheters, the recirculation in the split-tip catheter design was superior. At blood flows of 400 mL/minute the split-tip design had a mean recirculation of 1.3% to 4.9% compared to 5.2% with 14.5F step-tip catheters, 5.7% to 7.2% with 15.5F split-tip catheters, and 10.9% with twin catheters.[456-458]

In the acute dialysis unit, flow and recirculation can be measured with ultrasound dilution at varying pump speeds to maximize clearance with intermittent hemodialysis (IHD). Also, recirculation can be monitored with CRRT on a daily basis and the catheters changed or repositioned if recirculation rises. This, theoretically, could reduce or eliminate the degree of anticoagulation required and improve the circuit life of the CRRT system. However, to date, the value of this approach has not been evaluated.

Despite the improved flow and function of the subclavian placement versus femoral vein placement, subclavian access should be avoided whenever possible. Subclavian catheter insertion is associated with an unacceptable rate of central vein thrombosis and stenosis.[460] This damage to the vessels leads to loss of future arteriovenous fistula and graft sites, and frequently in patients with ARF it is difficult to determine who might need chronic RRT either at discharge or in the future. Despite the well-documented problems with subclavian catheters and clear guidelines,[455] a surprisingly high number of subclavian catheters are still used. According to the 2002 Dialysis Outcomes and Practice Patterns Study (DOPPS), 18% of European acute catheters and 46% of acute catheters in the United States are subclavian.[461] Dialysis catheters in the ICU should be placed in the internal jugular or the femoral position; the right internal jugular is usually preferred and femoral catheter length should exceed 19 cm.

Care of the Catheter

Catheter care is designed to prevent malfunction and infection. Malfunction is usually related to thrombus or fibrin sheath formation. Prevention with any particular type of locking solution has not been proved. Most institutions continue to use heparin or 4% citrate. When catheter dysfunction is present, line reversal may be successful and has acceptable recirculation characteristics, as demonstrated by Twardowski.[462] Alternatively, locking agents are used based on local preference, but no controlled data are available to demonstrate their effectiveness.

Infection is prevented by use of excellent local care and observation of Dialysis Outcome Quality Initiative (DOQI) guideline No. 15 (Table 61-12).[455] In addition, Oliver and colleagues,[463] have demonstrated improved infection rates in acute catheters with the use of local antibiotic ointment on a dry gauze at the exit site. Finally, the risk of bacteremia is associated with the development of an exit site infection and duration of catheter use. For femoral catheters, the risk of infection rises dramatically after 1 week and the risk of internal jugular vein catheter associated bacteremia rises after 3 weeks.[464] It is reasonable to try to limit catheter duration to within these periods. Once catheter exit site infection is recognized, the catheter should be removed as the risk of bacteremia rises within days—2% at 24 hours and 13% at 48 hours.[464] Catheter-associated bacteremia is treated with catheter removal and intravenous antibiotics.[455]

Modalities of Renal Replacement

Of the therapies of RRT available in the ICU, a superior modality has not been definitively demonstrated. CRRT offers recognized advantages in continuous fluid and solute control but has never been convincingly shown to improve mortality. IHD can be performed, and recently attention has shifted to increasing its frequency above the traditional thrice-weekly. Slow low-efficiency daily dialysis (SLEDD) increases volume control and solute clearance when compared to IHD and approaches CRRT. Peritoneal dialysis (PD) is also used in the ICU but requires an intact peritoneal cavity. A decision regarding which modality is selected is dependent on local preference, cost, and availability of therapies. However, ideally, the therapy should be tailored to the

TABLE 61-12

Recommendations for Catheter Care and Temporary Hemodialysis

CATHETER CARE ITEM	RECOMMENDATION
Catheter insertion site	*Femoral vein:* single use, severe CHF, use in bed-bound, use in ICU when other sites too risky. *Internal jugular vein:* preferred site when accessible (lowest recirculation and lowest risk of stenosis) *Subclavian vein:* avoid due to risk of stenosis
Catheter placement	*Femoral vein:* Use >19-cm catheter; consider monitoring recirculation to optimize efficiency *Internal jugular and subclavian veins:* right, use 15-20-cm catheters; left, 20-24-cm catheters; place tip at SVC-RA junction.
Exit site care	Dressing care and catheter manipulations to be performed by trained staff Examine catheter site each dialysis Dressing: dry gauze with skin disinfection; use povidone-iodine or mupirocin ointment with dressing changes Use sterile technique at all times; patient and nurse to wear mask; nurse to wear gloves
Duration of use	*Femoral vein:* < 1 wk *Internal jugular vein:* < 3 wk

CHF, congestive heart failure; SVC-RA, superior vena cava–right atrium.

needs of the ICU patient. Regardless of the RRT utilized, the goals should always be to improve the patient's fluid and electrolyte and acid-base balances, allowing for an optimal chance of renal and patient recovery.

Continuous Renal Replacement Therapies

With the advent of safe placement of double-lumen venous catheters, the CRRT options in general have developed into continuous venovenous modalities. Continuous arterial venous therapies, as initially described by Kramer in the 1970s, have the advantage of blood flow and filtration determined by blood pressure. This gives the theoretical advantage of fewer hypotensive episodes. Arterial venous circuitry also requires a simple, low-volume extracorporeal system with low resistance, thus obviating the need for expensive and complex pump-assisted devices. However, this therapy cannot obtain the higher volumes of ultrafiltration required for consistent metabolic control.[465] Arterial venous circuitry also requires a large-bore femoral artery catheter, with the risk of vascular complication estimated at up to 10%.[466] For these reasons arterial venous forms of CRRT are not widely used.

Pump-assisted circuits provide multiple options for fluid, electrolyte, and metabolic control (Figs. 61-3 and 61-4). In slow continuous ultrafiltration (SCUF), the extracorporeal system is simplified to include a blood system hooked inline with a high-efficiency or high-flux membrane. As blood passes through the filter, plasma water and solutes pass through the membrane to allow formation of an ultrafiltrate, which is discarded. No replacement fluids or dialysate fluids are required. Although SCUF is a purely convective modality, the ultrafiltrate volume is limited to inputs plus desired losses and hence not enough volume is generated to control azotemia or significant metabolic disorders. This therapy is reserved for patients with residual renal function with high volumes of input or significant fluid overload and a "relative" oliguria.

CRRT modalities designed for fluid and metabolic control require higher volumes of ultrafiltrate and hence require replacement fluid, dialysate fluid, or a combination of both. *Continuous venovenous hemofiltration* (CVVH) is an extracorporeal circuit using a double-lumen venous catheter hooked to an extracorporeal system with a blood pump, high-efficiency or high-flux dialysis membrane, and replacement fluid. As with SCUF, pure convection produces the ultrafiltrate, but, much greater volumes are generated. Volume status and metabolic improvements are maintained by the addition of replacement fluid in the circuit. Replacement fluid can be added pre-filter or post-filter. Pre-filter replacement carries a benefit of less hemoconcentration within the dialysis membrane but decreases clearances up to 15%.[467] Post-filter replacement maintains efficiency of the circuit but may be associated with an increase in thrombosis of the extracorporeal circuit. This latter point has been postulated but never demonstrated.

Continuous venovenous hemodialysis (CVVHD) is an extracorporeal circuit using a double-lumen venous catheter hooked to an extracorporeal system with a blood pump, high-efficiency or high-flux dialysis membrane, and dialysate fluid. As with IHD, the dialysate runs countercurrent to the blood pathway. As in other forms of CRRT, low efficiency is

maintained by limiting the dialysate volume to 1 to 3 L/hour. Although considered a diffusive therapy, convection may occur due to significant back-filtration. The degree of back-filtration and convective clearance is likely to vary by membrane and has not been studied to date. However, Brunet and colleagues[467] have shown significant middle molecule clearance with a polyacrylonitrile dialyzer (Gambro M100) and a dialysate rate of 2 L/hour. Beta$_2$-microglobulin clearance was 80% of that achieved with 2 L/hour of CVVH therapy.[467]

Continuous venovenous hemodiafiltration (CVVHDF) consists of an extracorporeal circuit using a double-lumen venous catheter hooked to an extracorporeal system with a blood pump, high-efficiency or high-flux dialysis membrane, and both replacement and dialysate fluid. In general, this combination is used to increase clearance; others utilize CVVHDF to simplify citrate delivery for anticoagulation.[468, 469] Clearly, both diffusive and convective forces determine solute clearances.

Intermittent Therapies

Conventional hemodialysis is typically delivered in the ICU setting three to four times a week with a standard Kt/V prescribed similar to that of ESRD.[470] Recently, Schiffl and colleagues demonstrated reduced mortality and increased renal recovery when the frequency was increased to daily.[471] Multiple studies have demonstrated an improvement in survival time with use of biocompatible membranes.[472] Conventional hemodialysis is diffusional, with ultrafiltration added as desired or tolerated to control fluid overload. Blood flow with intermittent therapies in the ICU ranges between 200 to 500 mL/minute. It may be varied to reduce recirculation or improve hemodynamic tolerance of therapy. Dialysate composition and flow are similar to ESRD therapy with dialysate flows of 500 to 800 mL/minute. Duration of therapy is typically 3 to 5 hours.

Slow low-efficiency daily dialysis (SLEDD) has been developed to be a hybrid therapy between continuous and intermittent therapy. Blood flows and dialysate flows are slowed to 200 to 300 mL/minute and 100 mL/minute respectively, and the therapy is prolonged to 8 to 12 hours/day.[465, 473] This slower form of dialysis theoretically allows for more hemodynamic stability with increased urea and creatinine clearances when compared to conventional hemodialysis. SLEDD also allows for time off the extracorporeal circuit, allowing time for the patient to travel to diagnostic studies. Because SLEDD utilizes standard hemodialysis machinery, the dialysate is generated online and the cost is potentially lower than that of CRRT, particularly if ICU personnel can be trained to monitor the dialysis session, obviating the need for dialysis nurses to be at bedside for the 8 to 12 hours of therapy.

Peritoneal dialysis, can also be utilized in the ICU. An intact peritoneum is required and a temporary or permanent PD catheter is placed. Standard PD solutions can be used. Clearance is convective and diffusive. Increasing the dextrose concentration in the dialysate and the frequency of exchanges adjusts the quantity of ultrafiltration. Transport kinetics are likely to be quite variable among patients and have not been studied in the setting of ARF. However, successful PD has been described in the ICU setting with adequate results,[474] but

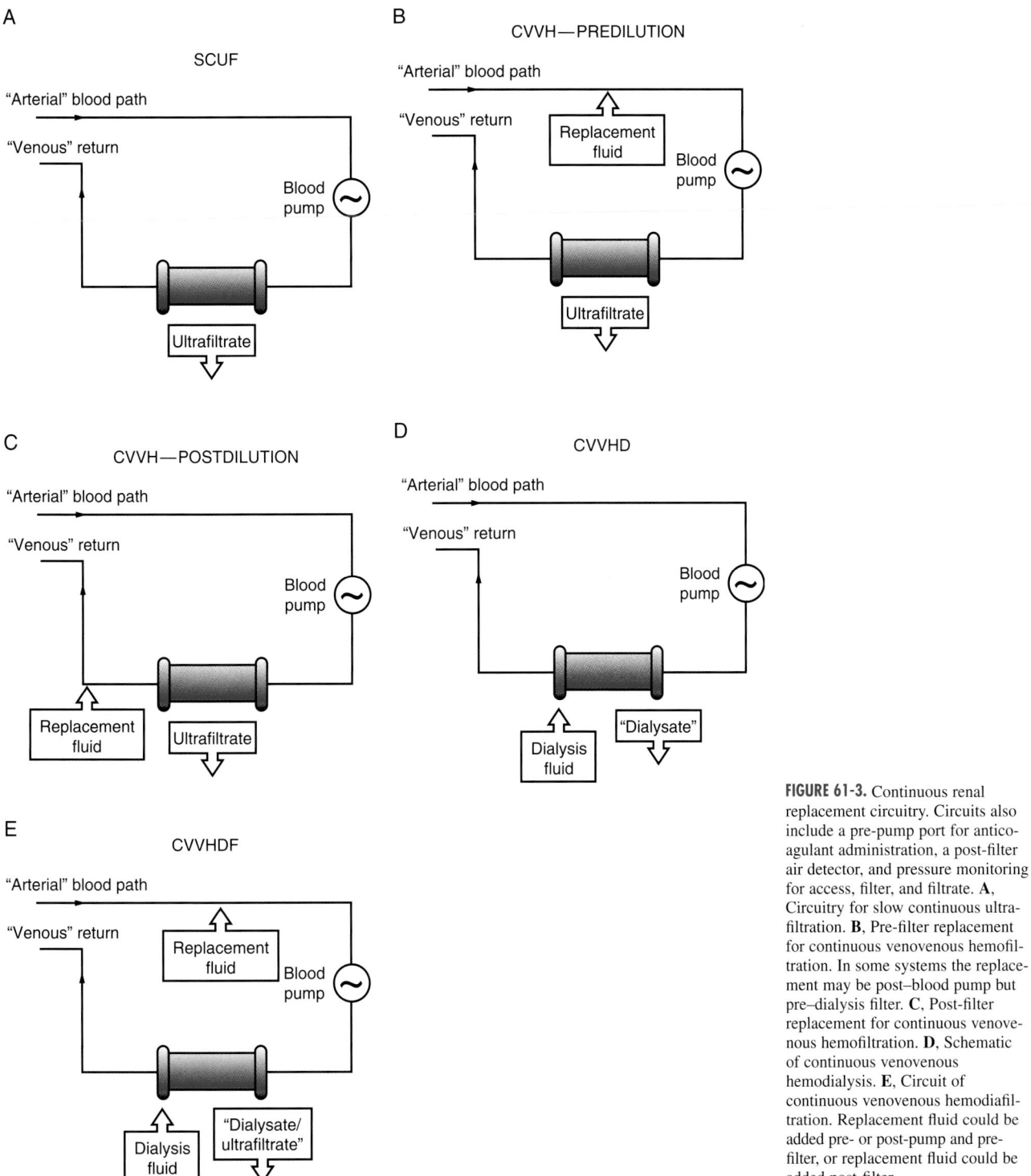

FIGURE 61-3. Continuous renal replacement circuitry. Circuits also include a pre-pump port for anticoagulant administration, a post-filter air detector, and pressure monitoring for access, filter, and filtrate. **A**, Circuitry for slow continuous ultrafiltration. **B**, Pre-filter replacement for continuous venovenous hemofiltration. In some systems the replacement may be post–blood pump but pre–dialysis filter. **C**, Post-filter replacement for continuous venovenous hemofiltration. **D**, Schematic of continuous venovenous hemodialysis. **E**, Circuit of continuous venovenous hemodiafiltration. Replacement fluid could be added pre- or post-pump and pre-filter, or replacement fluid could be added post-filter.

recently PD has been demonstrated to be inferior to CRRT in ARF due to sepsis and malaria.[475] PD offers the advantages of lack of anticoagulation and vascular problems, is hemodynamically stable, and is performed with relatively inexpensive and simple systems. The disadvantages include the need for an intact peritoneum, hyperglycemia, potential respiratory embarrassment due to increased abdominal pressure, the risk of peritonitis, and less clearance than can be obtained with SLEDD or CRRT.

Therapeutic Options

Unlike ESRD, there are no established standards of therapy in ARF. Absence of steady state, variable excesses of body water and variable frequency of therapies, and the potential lack of correlation of urea as a marker for toxins in ARF hamper quantification of the therapy delivered. An adequate dose of dialysis, the lowest clearance that maximizes survival and decreases morbidity, has not been established.

A

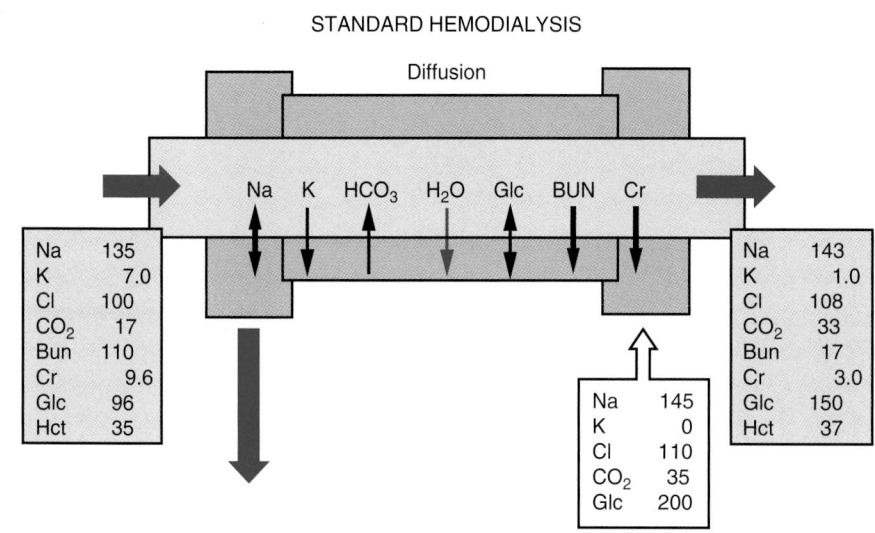

B

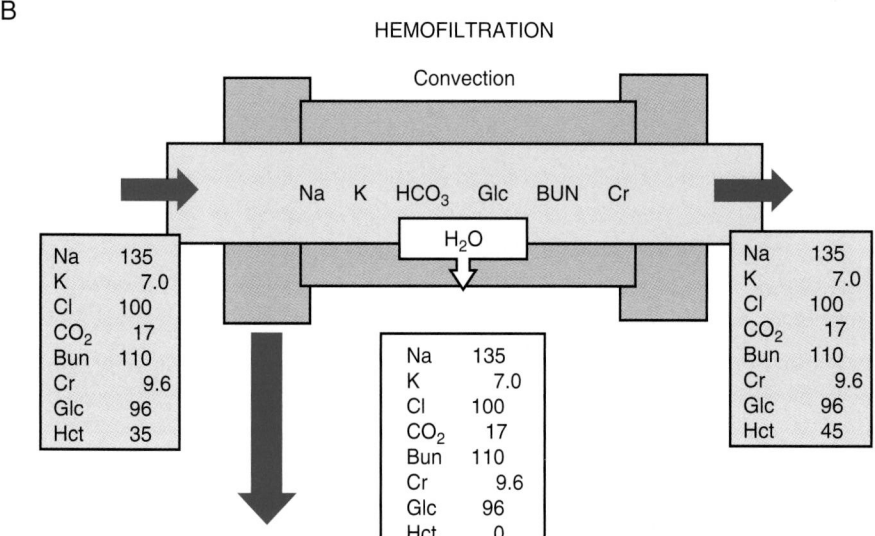

FIGURE 61-4. Pre- and post-blood composition as blood traverses a hemodialysis filter versus blood composition pre- and post-filter using hemofiltration. **A,** Note the significant clearance of small molecules by diffusion in hemodialysis. Comparatively, in hemofiltration there is little change in solute concentration except for a rise in hematocrit. The clearance in hemofiltration is solely convective. **B,** In hemofiltration a change in blood solute concentration is achieved by adding replacement fluid.

Liao and colleagues[476] modeled the dose capabilities of RRTs in ARF, allowing a comparison of removal of urea, inulin, and beta$_2$-microglobulin among the commonly used prescriptions of these extracorporeal therapies. The authors modeled clearances of IHD, SLEDD, and CVVH. Based on a 70-kg male with 10 kg of volume excess and an initial BUN of 90 mg/dL, comparisons were modeled with CVVH of 3 L/hour with pre-filter dilution, daily (six times a week) IHD of 4 hours' duration with a blood flow of 350 mL/minute and dialysate flow of 600 mL/minute, and SLEDD performed 7 days per week for 12 hours with a blood flow of 300 mL/minute and a dialysate flow of 100 mL/minute. Using these assumptions the equivalent renal clearances (EKRs) of urea, inulin, and beta$_2$-microglobulin were estimated with each therapy. Relative to SLEDD and daily IHD, the effective urea clearance was 8% and 60% higher in CVVH (the EKR of urea in mL/minute with CVVH was 33.7; SLEDD, 31.3; and IHD, 21.1). Differences in clearance of middle molecules were even more pronounced in CVVH (the EKR of inulin in mL/minute was 11.8 with

CVVH, 5.4 with IHD, and 3.0 with SLEDD; the EKR of beta$_2$-microglobulin was 18.2 in CVVH, 7.0 in IHD, and 4.2 in SLEDD). These superior middle molecule clearances achievable with CVVH are due to the combination of convective clearance and continuous operation.[476] This prescriptive model needs to be clinically substantiated.

Even if the adequate dose of dialysis were known, substantial barriers remain in obtaining this dose. With IHD Evanson and colleagues demonstrated that the delivered dose of dialysis was significantly below prescribed (Kt/V prescribed 1.25 ± 0.47 and delivered 1.04 ± 0.49).[470] Schiffl and co-workers also noted this in their comparison of daily versus thrice-weekly dialysis.[471] This difference between the prescribed and delivered dose of dialysis can be attributed to the difficulty in obtaining and maintaining blood flows, inability to achieve adequate ultrafiltration, shortened treatment times, and catheter malfunction. Venkataraman and colleagues[477] found similar differences between delivered and prescribed delivery in CRRT. In 110 patients the delivered CRRT dose was 68% of the prescribed dose.[477]

As opposed to IHD, no treatments were interrupted due to hemodynamic instability, but the authors attributed the low delivery of therapy to recurrent clotting of the CRRT system. Because SLEDD is low-flow and of shorter duration, prescribed therapy may be easier to obtain. Significant evidence is lacking, but one recent abstract evaluated delivered versus prescribed Kt/V in nine patients and found no significant difference between prescribed and delivered dose.[478]

Recently, an increasing body of evidence suggests that increasing the intensity and therapy dose of RRT in ARF influences outcome.[479] Dosing of intermittent dialysis has rendered some conflicting reports. An early study (1986) of 34 ICU patients by Gillum and co-workers[480] compared daily intensive therapy versus nonintensive therapy. In their small number of patients there was no difference in survival.[480]

Paganini and colleagues[481] reviewed the outcomes of 844 patients with ARF requiring RRT in the ICU between 1988 and 1994. The authors reported no difference in survival times in the most critically ill or those with low severity-of-illness scores based on dose of dialysis. However in the majority of patients, those with an intermediate severity-of-illness score, there was a significant improvement in survival with higher delivery of intermittent dialysis (Kt/V > 1.0).

Schiffl and associates[471] prospectively compared alternate-day to daily dialysis in the ICU. They described a decrease in mortality from 46% to 28% in patients who received daily dialysis compared to the alternate-day group. They also described a reduction in sepsis and an increased rate of renal function recovery in the daily group.

Similarly studies of CRRT also suggest a benefit in increasing the delivery of therapy. Storck and co-workers[482] compared survival in a nonrandomized prospective study of CAVH versus CVVH. Survival was significantly higher in the CVVH group and correlated with increasing volumes of ultrafiltration delivered (7.5 L/day in the CAVH group and 15.5 L/day in the CVVH group).

More recently, Ronco and colleagues[483] reported the results of a study comparing the dose of therapy in CVVH. Using a lactate-based post-filter CVVH system, the differences in outcome were reported in 420 ICU ARF patients randomized to receive replacement fluid rates of 20, 35, and 45 mL/kg/hour. Delivered ultrafiltration rates were 31, 56, and 68 L/day respectively. Survival was found to be significantly higher in the 35 mL/kg/hour and 45 mL/kg/hour groups (57% and 58%) when compared to the group of patients receiving 20 mL/kg/hour (survival of 41%; *P* <.001). Although not primary end points, this study noted a prolonged time to death with the higher therapies. BUN at the time of initiation was significantly lower in survivors versus nonsurvivors, and there was a tendency toward improved survival in the septic patients with 45 mL/kg/hour (although the number of septic patients was too small to be significant).

Comparisons of modalities of RRT with respect to ARF are few. Numerous historical controlled studies have suggested that CRRT may be superior to IHD. However, the data comparing CRRT to IHD are limited. Swartz and colleagues[484] did compare IHD to CRRT survival in 349 patients in the ICU at the University of Michigan. The study was not randomized and clearly comorbidities were higher in the group receiving CRRT. After adjusting for comorbidities, no difference in survival was seen.[484] Mehta and colleagues[485] performed a prospective randomized multicenter trial comparing CRRT to

IHD in 166 patients. Survival was actually higher in the group receiving IHD (58.5% survival in IHD vs. 40.5% in CRRT). This study excluded hemodynamically unstable patients and unfortunately the randomization was flawed as the patients in the CRRT group had significantly higher APACHE III scores and a greater percentage of liver failure.[485] Kellum and co-workers[486] tried to reconcile the differences in an excellent meta-analysis of studies comparing CRRT to IHD. Overall there was no difference in therapy, but when adjusting for studies with relative risk of death and of sufficient quality, the relative risk of death was substantially lower in CRRT. However, the authors concluded that given the quality of studies, there was insufficient evidence to draw strong conclusions.[486]

Although studies in the late 1970s and early 1980s demonstrated the efficacy of PD when compared to IHD, they were not randomized nor do they represent current methods of extracorporeal therapy.[474] Phu and associates[475] studied 70 adult patients with ARF from malaria (48 patients) or sepsis (22 patients) in Vietnam. The patients receiving PD had a mortality rate of 47% compared to 15% in the CVVH group (*P* < .005). PD was performed with 2-L exchanges and only 30-minute dwell times—thus limiting clearance significantly. The patients receiving CVVH were prescribed clearances of only 25 L/day. The study suggests that PD is inferior to CVVH in the treatment of ARF associated with malaria or sepsis.[475]

ARF in the ICU requiring RRT is associated with significant mortality and morbidity. Over time, the cause of death has changed from complications of uremia to complications of comorbidities. RRT needs to be prescribed based on individual patient needs, support of the patient, and allowing for time and other therapies to improve patient recovery. For the time being, local preferences and expertise in general determine the delivery of RRT. In the future, the ability to achieve goals of toxin clearance, fluid stabilization, and control of electrolyte and acid-base derangements may dictate the type, frequency, and duration of extracorporeal therapies.

REFERENCES

1. Hojs R, et al: Rhabdomyolysis and acute renal failure in intensive care unit. Ren Fail 21:675-684, 1999.
2. de Mendonca A, et al: Acute renal failure in the ICU: Risk factors and outcome evaluated by the SOFA score. Intensive Care Med 26:915-921, 2000.
3. Thijs A, Thijs LG: Pathogenesis of renal failure in sepsis. Kidney Int Suppl 66:S34-S37, 1998.
4. Valta P, et al: Acute respiratory distress syndrome: Frequency, clinical course, and costs of care. Crit Care Med 27:2367-2374, 1999.
5. Koreny M, et al: Prognosis of patients who develop acute renal failure during the first 24 hours of cardiogenic shock after myocardial infarction. Am J Med 112:115-119, 2002.
6. Ring-Larsen H, and Palazzo U: Renal failure in fulminant hepatic failure and terminal cirrhosis: A comparison between incidence, types, and prognosis. Gut 22:585-591, 1981.
7. Greene KE, Peters JI: Pathophysiology of acute respiratory failure. Clin Chest Med 15:1-12, 1994.
8. de los Santos R, et al: Hyperoxia exposure in mechanically ventilated primates with and without previous lung injury. Exp Lung Res 9:255-275, 1985.
9. Bryan CL, Jenkinson SG: Oxygen toxicity. Clin Chest Med 9:141-152, 1988.
10. Hayatdavoudi G, et al: Pulmonary injury in rats following continuous exposure to 60% O$_2$ for 7 days. J Appl Physiol 51:1220-1231, 1981.

11. Kistler D, et al: Development of fine structural damage to alveolar and capillary lining cells in oxygen poisoned rat lungs [abstract]. Am Rev Respir Dis 137:A78, 1988.

12. Comroe JJ, et al: Oxygen toxicity—the effects of inhalation of high concentration of oxygen for 24 hours on normal men at sea level and at simulated altitude of 18,000 feet. JAMA 128:710, 1945.

13. Pierce A: Oxygen toxicity. Basic Respir Dis 1:1, 1979.

14. Ashbaugh DG, et al: Acute respiratory distress in adults. Lancet 2:319-323, 1967.

15. Bernard GR, et al: The American-European Consensus Conference on ARDS. Definitions, mechanisms, relevant outcomes, and clinical trial coordination. Am J Respir Crit Care Med 149 (3 pt 1):818-824, 1994.

16. Suchyta MR, et al: The adult respiratory distress syndrome. A report of survival and modifying factors. Chest 101:1074-1079, 1992.

17. Zilberberg MD, Epstein SK: Acute lung injury in the medical ICU: Comorbid conditions, age, etiology, and hospital outcome. Am J Respir Crit Care Med 157 (4 pt 1):1159-1164, 1998.

18. Doyle RL, et al: Identification of patients with acute lung injury. Predictors of mortality. Am J Respir Crit Care Med 152 (6 pt 1): 1818-1824, 1995.

19. Montgomery AB, et al: Cause of mortality in patients with the adult, respiratory distress syndrome. Am Rev Respir Dis 132:485-489, 1985.

20. Hudson LD, et al: Clinical risks for development of the acute respiratory distress syndrome. Am J Respir Crit Care Med 151 (2 pt 1): 293-301.

21. Aberle DR, et al: Hydrostatic versus increased permeability pulmonary edema: Diagnosis based on radiographic criteria in critically ill patients. Radiology 168:73-79, 1988.

22. Gattinoni L, et al: Lung structure and function in different stage of severe adult respiratory distress syndrome. JAMA 271:1772-1779, 1999.

23. Ware LB, Matthay MA: The acute respiratory distress syndrome. N Engl J Med 342:1334-1349, 2000.

24. Fulkerson WJ, et al: Pathogenesis and treatment of the adult respiratory distress syndrome. Arch Intern Med 156:29-38, 1996.

25. McHugh LG, et al: Recovery of function in survivors of the acute respiratory distress syndrome. Am J Respir Crit Care Med 150:90-94, 1994.

26. Pepe PE, et al: Clinical predictors of the adult respiratory distress syndrome. Am J Surg 144:124-130, 1982.

27. Weinacker AB, Vaszar LT: Acute respiratory distress syndrome: Physiology and new management strategies. Annu Rev Med 52: 221-237, 2001.

28. Tate RM, Repine JE: Neutrophils and the adult respiratory distress syndrome. Am Rev Respir Dis 128:552-559, 1983.

29. Henderson WR Jr: Eicosanoids and lung inflammation. Am Rev Respir Dis 135:1176-1185, 1987.

30. Bernard GR, et al: Prostacyclin and thromboxane A_2 formation is increased in human sepsis syndrome. Effects of cyclooxygenase inhibition. Am Rev Respir Dis 144:1095-1101, 1991.

31. The Acute Respiratory Distress Syndrome Network: Ventilation with lower tidal volumes as compared with traditional tidal volumes for acute lung injury and acute respiratory distress syndrome. N Engl J Med 342:1301-1308, 2000.

32. Dreyfuss D, Saumon G: Ventilator-induced lung injury: Lessons from experimental studies. Am J Respir Crit Care Med 157:294-323, 1998.

33. Parker JC, et al: Lung edema caused by high peak inspiratory pressures in dogs. Role of increased microvascular filtration pressure and permeability. Am Rev Respir Dis 142:321-328, 1990.

34. Webb HH, Tierney DF: Experimental pulmonary edema due to intermittent positive pressure ventilation with high inflation pressures. Protection by positive end-expiratory pressure. Am Rev Respir Dis 110:556-565, 1974.

35. Kallet RH, et al: The treatment of acidosis in acute lung injury with trishydroxymethyl aminomethane (THAM). Am J Respir Crit Care Med 161 (4 pt 1): 1149-1153, 2000.

36. Brower RG et al: Treatment of ARDS. Chest 120:1347-1367, 2000.

37. Simmons RS, et al: Fluid balance and the adult respiratory distress syndrome. Am Rev Respir Dis 135:924-929, 1987.

38. Humphrey H, et al: Improved survival in ARDS patients associated with a reduction in pulmonary capillary wedge pressure. Chest 97:1176-1180, 1990.

39. Eisenberg PR, et al: A prospective study of lung water measurements during patient management in an intensive care unit. Am Rev Respir Dis 136:662-668, 1987.

40. Shoemaker WC, et al: Prospective trial of supranormal values of survivors as therapeutic goals in high-risk surgical patients. Chest 94:1176-1186, 1988.

41. Fleming A, et al: Prospective trial of supranormal values as goals of resuscitation in severe trauma. Arch Surg 127:1175-1179, 1992 [see discussion 1179-1181].

42. Boyd O, et al: A randomized clinical trial of the effect of deliberate perioperative increase of oxygen delivery on mortality in high-risk surgical patients. JAMA 270:2699-2707, 1993.

43. Yu M, et al: Effect of maximizing oxygen delivery on morbidity and mortality rates in critically ill patients: A prospective, randomized, controlled study. Crit Care Med 21:830-838, 1993.

44. Tuchschmidt J, et al: Elevation of cardiac output and oxygen delivery improves outcome in septic shock. Chest 102:216-220, 1992.

45. Hayes MA, et al: Elevation of systemic oxygen delivery in the treatment of critically ill patients. N Engl J Med 330:1717-1722, 1994.

46. Brower R, et al: Treatment of acute respiratory distress syndrome. Chest 120:1347, 2001.

47. Luce JM, et al: Ineffectiveness of high-dose methylprednisolone in preventing parenchymal lung injury and improving mortality in patients with septic shock. Am Rev Respir Dis 138:62-68, 1988.

48. Bone RC, et al: Early methylprednisolone treatment for septic syndrome and the adult respiratory distress syndrome. Chest 92: 1032-1036, 1987.

49. Bernard GR, et al: High-dose corticosteroids in patients with the adult respiratory distress syndrome.N Engl J Med 317:1565-1570, 1987.

50. Meduri GU, et al: Effect of prolonged methylprednisolone therapy in unresolving acute respiratory distress syndrome: A randomized controlled trial. JAMA 280:159-165, 1998.

51. Mure M, et al: Dramatic effect on oxygenation in patients with severe acute lung insufficiency treated in the prone position. Crit Care Med 25:1539-1544, 1997.

52. Fridrich P, et al: The effects of long-term prone positioning in patients with trauma-induced adult respiratory distress syndrome. Anesth Analg 83:1206-1211, 1996.

53. Gattinoni L, et al: Ventilation in the prone position. The Prone-Supine Study Collaborative Group. Lancet 350:815, 1997.

54. Gattinoni L, et al: Effect of prone positioning on the survival of patients with acute respiratory failure. N Engl J Med 345:568-573, 2001.

55. Loewen GM, et al: Alveolar hyperoxic injury in rabbits receiving exogenous surfactant. J Appl Physiol 66:1087-1092, 1989.

56. van Daal GJ, et al: Intratracheal surfactant administration restores gas exchange in experimental adult respiratory distress syndrome associated with viral pneumonia. Anesth Analg 72:589-595, 1991.

57. Anzueto A, et al: Aerosolized surfactant in adults with sepsis-induced acute respiratory distress syndrome. Exosurf Acute Respiratory Distress Syndrome Sepsis Study Group. N Engl J Med 334:1417-1421, 1996.

58. Rossaint R, et al: Inhaled nitric oxide for the adult respiratory distress syndrome. N Engl J Med 328:399-405, 1993.

59. Luhr O, et al: A retrospective analysis of nitric oxide inhalation in patients with severe acute lung injury in Sweden and Norway 1991-1994. Acta Anaesthesiol Scand 41:1238-1246, 1997.

60. Pagen V, et al: Results of the French prospective multicentric randomized double blind placebo controlled trial on inhaled nitric oxide in acute respiratory distress syndrome. Intensive Care Med 25:S166, 1999.

61. Bone RC, et al: Randomized double-blind, multicenter study of prostaglandin E_1 in patients with the adult respiratory distress syndrome. Prostaglandin E_1 Study Group. Chest 96:114-119, 1986.

62. The ARDS Network Authors: Ketoconazole for early treatment of acute lung injury and acute respiratory distress syndrome. JAMA 283:1995-2002, 2000.

63. Mathay M: Severe sepsis: A new treatment with both anticoagulant and anti-inflammatory properties. N Engl J Med 344:759-762, 2001.

64. Hite RD, Morris PE: Acute respiratory distress syndrome: Pharmacological treatment options in development. Drugs 61: 897-907, 2001.

65. Morris AH, et al: Randomized clinical trial of pressure-controlled inverse ratio ventilation and extracorporeal CO_2 removal for adult respiratory distress syndrome. Am J Respir Crit Care Med 149 (2 pt 1):295-305, 1994.

66. Chertow GM, et al: Predictors of mortality and the provision of dialysis in patients with acute tubular necrosis. The Auriculin Anaritide Acute Renal Failure Study Group. J Am Soc Nephrol 9:692-698, 1998.

67. Annat G, et al: Effect of PEEP ventilation on renal function, plasma renin, aldosterone, neurophysins and urinary ADH, and prostaglandins. Anesthesiology 58:136-141, 1983.

68. Jarnberg PO, et al: Effects of positive end-expiratory pressure on renal function. Acta Anaesthesiol Scand 22:508-514, 1978.

69. Hemmer M, Suter PM: Treatment of cardiac and renal effects of PEEP with dopamine in patients with acute respiratory failure. Anesthesiology 50:399-403, 1979.

70. Andrivet P, et al: Hormonal interactions and renal function during mechanical ventilation and ANF infusion in humans. J Appl Physiol 70:287-292, 1991.

71. Hemmer M, et al: Urinary antidiuretic hormone excretion during mechanical ventilation and weaning in man. Anesthesiology 52: 395-400, 1980.

72. Marquez J, et al: Renal function and renin secretion during high frequency jet ventilation at varying levels of airway pressure. Crit Care Med 11:930-932, 1983.

73. Pannu N, Mehta RL: Mechanical ventilation and renal function: An area for concern? Am J Kidney Dis 39:616-624, 2002.

74. Bellingan GJ: The pulmonary physician in critical care. 6: The pathogenesis of ALI/ARDS. Thorax 57:540-546, 2002.

75. Martin TR: Lung cytokines and ARDS: Roger S. Mitchell Lecture. Chest 116:(suppl) 2S-8S, 1999.

76. Ranieri VM, et al: Effect of mechanical ventilation on inflammatory mediators in patients with acute respiratory distress syndrome: A randomized controlled trial. JAMA 282:54-61, 1999.

77. Goes N, et al: Ischemic acute tubular necrosis induces an extensive local cytokine response. Evidence for induction of interferon-γ, transforming growth factor-β1, granulocyte-macrophage colony-stimulating factor, interleukin-2, and interleukin-10. Transplantation 59:565-572, 1995.

78. Chiao H, et al: Alpha-melanocyte-stimulating hormone protects against renal injury after ischemia in mice and rats. J Clin Invest 99: 1165-1172, 1997.

79. Heckbert SR, et al: Outcome after hemorrhagic shock in trauma patients. J Trauma 345:545-549, 1998.

80. Hosomi H, Sagawa K: Effect of pentobarbital anesthesia on hypotension after 10% hemorrhage in the dog. Am J Physiol 236:H607-H612, 1979.

81. Schwartz S, et al: Sequential hemodynamic and oxygen transport responses in hypovolemia, anemia, and hypoxia. Am J Physiol 241: H864-H871, 1981.

82. Koyama S, et al: Spatial and temporal differing control of sympathetic activities during hemorrhage. Am J Physiol 262(4 pt 2):R579-585, 1992.

83. Wong DH, et al: Changes in cardiac output after acute blood loss and position change in man. Crit Care Med 17:979-983, 1989.

84. Weil M, Rackow E: Hemmorrhagic shock. *In* Schwartz G (ed): Principles and Practices of Emergency Medicine, 4th ed. Baltimore, Williams & Wilkins, 1999, pp 36-45.

85. Forrest P: Vasopressin and shock. Anaesth Intensive Care 29:463-472, 2001.

86. Schadt JC, Ludbrook J: Hemodynamic and neurohumoral responses to acute hypovolemia in conscious mammals. Am J Physiol 260 (2 pt 2):H305-H318, 1991.

87. Bond RF, Johnson G 3rd: Vascular adrenergic interactions during hemorrhagic shock. Fed Proc 44:281-289, 1985.

88. Edouard AR, et al: Heterogeneous regional vascular responses to simulated transient hypovolemia in man. Intensive Care Med 20:414-420, 1994.

89. Alexander RW, Dzau VJ: Vascular biology: The past 50 years. Circulation 102(suppl 4): IV112-IV116, 2000.

90. Szabo C, Billiar TR: Novel roles of nitric oxide in hemorrhagic shock. Shock 12:1-9, 1999.

91. Pieber D, et al: Pressor and mesenteric arterial hyporesponsiveness to angiotensin II is an early event in haemorrhagic hypotension in anaesthetised rats. Cardiovasc Res 44:166-175, 1999.

92. Szabo C, et al: Hemorrhagic hypotension impairs endothelium-dependent relaxations in the renal artery of the cat. Circ Shock 36: 238-241, 1992.

93. Szabo C, et al: Role of the L-arginine-nitric oxide pathway in the changes in cerebrovascular reactivity following hemorrhagic hypotension and retransfusion. Circ Shock 4:37:307-316, 1992.

94. Clementi E, et al: Persistent inhibition of cell respiration by nitric oxide: Crucial role of S-nitrosylation of mitochondrial complex I and protective action of glutathione. Proc Natl Acad Sci USA 95: 7631-7636, 1998.

95. Brealey D, et al: Association between mitochondrial dysfunction and severity and outcome of septic shock. Lancet 360:219-223, 2002.

96. Stepp DW, et al: K⁺ATP channels and adenosine are not necessary for coronary autoregulation. Am J Physiol 273(3 pt 2):H1299-1308, 1997.

97. Marshall JM: Adenosine and muscle vasodilatation in acute systemic hypoxia. Acta Physiol Scand 168:561-573, 2000.

98. Fan FC, et al: Effects of hematocrit variations on regional hemodynamics and oxygen transport in the dog. Am J Physiol 238: H545-H522, 1980.

99. Maitra SR, et al: Alterations in renal gluconeogenesis and blood flow during hemorrhagic shock. Circ Shock 41:67-70, 1993.

100. Hansell P, et al: Pressure-related capillary leukostasis following ischemia-reperfusion and hemorrhagic shock. Am J Physiol 265 (1 pt 2):H381-388, 1993.

101. Botha AJ, et al: Early neutrophil sequestration after injury: A pathogenic mechanism for multiple organ failure. J Trauma 39:411-417, 1995.

102. Maekawa K, et al: Effects of trauma and sepsis on soluble L-selectin and cell surface expression of L-selectin and CD11b. J Trauma 44:460-468, 1998.

103. Boyd AJ, et al: A CD18 monoclonal antibody reduces multiple organ injury in a model of ruptured abdominal aortic aneurysm. Am J Physiol 277 (1 pt 2):H172-H182, 1999.

104. Mazzoni MC, et al: Amiloride-sensitive Na⁺ pathways in capillary endothelial cell swelling during hemorrhagic shock. J Appl Physiol 73:1467-1473, 1992.

105. Prist R, et al: A quantitative analysis of transcapillary refill in severe hemorrhagic hypotension in dogs. Shock 1:188-195, 1994.

106. Tucker VL, et al: Blood-to-tissue albumin transport in rats subjected to acute hemorrhage and resuscitation. Shock 3:189-195, 1995.

107. Bock JC, et al: Post-traumatic changes in, and effect of colloid osmotic pressure on the distribution of body water. Ann Surg 210: 395-403; discussion 403-395, 1989.

108. Leach RM, Treacher DF: The pulmonary physician in critical care. 2: Oxygen delivery and consumption in the critically ill. Thorax 57:170-177, 2002.

109. Ronco JJ, et al: Identification of the critical oxygen delivery for anaerobic metabolism in critically ill septic and nonseptic humans. JAMA 270:1724-1730, 1993.

110. Curtis SE, Cain SM: Regional and systemic oxygen delivery/uptake relations and lactate flux in hyperdynamic, endotoxin-treated dogs. Am Rev Respir Dis 145(2 pt 1):348-354, 1992.

111. Shoemaker WC, et al: Measurement of tissue perfusion by oxygen transport patterns in experimental shock and in high-risk surgical patients. Intensive Care Med; 16(suppl 2):S135-S144, 1990.

112. Girbes A, Groenveld A: Circulatory optimization in patients with or at risk for shock. Clin Intensive Care 11:77-81, 2000.

113. Vincent JL, et al: Oxygen uptake/supply dependency. Am Rev Respir Dis 142:2-7, 1990.

114. Robin ED: Of men and mitochondria: Coping with hypoxic dysoxia. The 1980 J. Burns Amberson Lecture. Am Rev Respir Dis 122: 517-531, 1980.

115. Xu D, et al: Calcium and phospholipase A₂ appear to be involved in the pathogenesis of hemorrhagic shock–induced mucosal injury and bacterial translocation. Crit Care Med 23:125-131, 1995.

116. Arden WA, et al: Scintigraphic evaluation of bacterial translocation during hemorrhagic shock. J Surg Res 54:102-106, 1993.

117. Tashkin DP, et al: Hepatic lactate uptake during decreased liver perfusion and hyposemia. Am J Physiol 223:968-974, 1972.

118. Chandel B, et al: MEGX (monoethylglycinexylidide): A novel in vivo test to measure early hepatic dysfunction after hypovolemic shock. Shock 3:51-53; discussion 54-55, 1995.

119. Fuchs S, et al: Ischemic hepatitis: Clinical and laboratory observations of 34 patients. J Clin Gastroenterol 26:183-186, 1998.

120. Miyazaki K, et al: Characterization of energy metabolism and blood flow distribution in myocardial ischemia in hemorrhagic shock. Am J Physiol 273(2 pt 2): H600-H607, 1997.

121. Collard CD, Gelman S: Pathophysiology, clinical manifestations, and prevention of ischemia-reperfusion injury. Anesthesiology 94: 1133-1138, 2001.

122. Toyokuni S: Reactive oxygen species–induced molecular damage and its application in pathology. Pathol Int 49:91-102, 1999.

123. Panes J, et al: Leukocyte-endothelial cell adhesion: Avenues for therapeutic intervention. Br J Pharmacol 126:537-550, 1999.

124. Collard CD, et al: Complement activation following oxidative stress. Mol Immunol 36:941-948, 1999.

125. Gunter TE, et al: Mitochondrial calcium transport: Physiological and pathological relevance. Am J Physiol 267(2 pt 1):C313-C339, 1994.

126. Murphy AN: Calcium mediated mitochondrial dysfunction and the protective effects of Bcl-2. Ann New York Acad Sci 893:19-32, 1999.

127. Carden DL, Granger DN: Pathophysiology of ischaemia-reperfusion injury. J Pathol 190:255-266, 2000.

128. Yamazaki S, et al: Effects of stages versus sudden reperfusion after acute coronary occlusion in the dog. J Am Coll Cardiol 7:564-572, 1986.

129. Weight SC, et al: Renal ischaemia—reperfusion injury. Br J Surg 83:162-170, 1996.

130. Delva E, et al: Vascular occlusions for liver resections. Operative management and tolerance to hepatic ischemia: 142 cases. Ann Surg 209:211-218, 1989.

131. Maxwell SR, Lip GY: Reperfusion injury: A review of the pathophysiology, clinical manifestations and therapeutic options. Int J Cardiol 58:95-117, 1997.

132. McGee S, et al: The rational clinical examination. Is this patient hypovolemic? JAMA 281:1022-1029, 1999.

133. Nast-Kolb D, et al: Indicators of the posttraumatic inflammatory response correlate with organ failure in patients with multiple injuries. J Trauma 42:446-454; discussion 454-445, 1997.

134. Canizaro PC, Pessa ME: Management of massive hemorrhage associated with abdominal trauma. Surg Clin North Am 70:621-634, 1990.

135. Voerman HJ, Groeneveld AB: Blood viscosity and circulatory shock. Intensive Care Med 15:72-78, 1989.

136. Wu W, et al: Blood transfusions in elderly patients with acute myocardial infarctions. N Engl J Med 345:1230-1236, 2002.

137. Sauaia A, et al: Early predictors of post injury multiple organ failure. Arch Surg 129:39-45, 1994.

138. Hebert PC, et al: A multicenter, randomized, controlled clinical trial of transfusion requirements in critical care. Transfusion Requirements in Critical Care Investigators, Canadian Critical Care Trials Group. N Engl J Med 340:409-417, 1999.

139. Gould SA, et al: Hypovolemic shock. Crit Care Clin 9:239-259, 1993.

140. Rossen DM, et al: Oxygen tension in the bladder epithelium rises in both high and low cardiac output endotoxemic sepsis. J Appl Physiol 79:1878-1882, 1995.

141. Boekstegers P, et al: Peripheral oxygen availability within skeletal muscle in sepsis and septic shock: Comparison to limited infection and cardiogenic shock. Infection 19:317-323, 1991.

142. Doglio GR, et al: Gastric mucosal pH as a prognostic index of mortality in critically ill patients. Crit Care Med 19:1037-1040, 1991.

143. Friedman G, et al: Combined measurements of blood lactate concentrations and gastric intramucosal pH in patients with severe sepsis. Crit Care Med 23:1184-1193, 1995.

144. Marik PE: Gastric intramucosal pH. A better predictor of multiorgan dysfunction syndrome and death than oxygen-derived variables in patients with sepsis. Chest 104:225-229, 1993.

145. Gutierrez G, et al: Gastric intramucosal pH as a therapeutic index of tissue oxygenation in critically ill patients. Lancet 339:195-199, 1992.

146. Ivatury RR, et al: A prospective randomized study of end points of resuscitation after major trauma: Global oxygen transport indices versus organ-specific gastric mucosal pH. J Am Coll Surg 183:145-154, 1996.

147. Pargger H, et al: Gastric intramucosal pH–guided therapy in patients after elective repair of infrarenal abdominal aneurysms: is it beneficial? Intensive Care Med 24:769-776, 1998.

148. Gomersall CD, et al: Resuscitation of critically ill patients based on the results of gastric tonometry: A prospective, randomized, controlled trial. Crit Care Med 28:607-614, 2000.

149. Shires GT, et al: Distributional changes in extracellular fluid during acute hemorrhagic shock. Surg Forum 11:115-150, 1960.

150. Waikar SS, Chertow GM: Crystalloids versus colloids for resuscitation in shock. Curr Opin Nephrol Hypertens 9:501-504, 2000.

151. Hauser CJ, et al: Oxygen transport responses to colloids and crystalloids in critically ill surgical patients. Surg Gynecol Obstet 150:811-816, 1980.

152. Holt ME, et al: Albumin inhibits human polymorphonuclear leucocyte luminol-dependent chemiluminescence: Evidence for oxygen radical scavenging. Br J Exp Pathol 65:231-241, 1984.

153. Demling RH: Effect of plasma and interstitial protein content on tissue edema formation. Curr Stud Hematol Blood Transfus 53:36-52, 1986.

154. Imm A, Carlson RW: Fluid resuscitation in circulatory shock. Crit Care Clin 9:313-333, 1993.

155. Thompson WL: Rational use of albumin and plasma substitutes. Johns Hopkins Med J 136:220-225, 1975.

156. Kohler H, et al: The effects of 500 ml 10% hydroxyethyl starch 200/0.5 and 10% dextran 40 on blood volume, colloid osmotic pressure and renal function in human volunteers [in German]. Anaesthesist 31:61-67, 1982.

157. Myers GA, et al: Effects of pentafraction and hetastarch plasma expansion on lung and soft tissue transvascular fluid filtration. Surgery 117:340-349, 1995.

158. Allison KP, et al: Randomized trial of hydroxyethyl starch versus gelatine for trauma resuscitation. J Trauma 47:1114-1121, 1999.

159. Wu JJ, et al: Hemodynamic response of modified fluid gelatin compared with lactated Ringer's solution for volume expansion in emergency resuscitation of hypovolemic shock patients: Preliminary report of a prospective, randomized trial. World J Surg 25:598-602, 2001.

160. Lamke LO, Liljedahl SO: Plasma volume changes after infusion of various plasma expanders. Resuscitation 5:93-102, 1976.

161. Ernest D, et al: Distribution of normal saline and 5% albumin infusions in septic patients. Crit Care Med 27:46-50, 1999.

162. Rackow EC, et al: Fluid resuscitation in circulatory shock: A comparison of the cardiorespiratory effects of albumin, hetastarch, and saline solutions in patients with hypovolemic and septic shock. Crit Care Med 11:839-850, 1983.

163. Dart RC, Sanders AB: Oxygen free radicals and myocardial reperfusion injury. Ann Emerg Med 17:53-58, 1988.

164. Tait AR, Larson LO: Resuscitation fluids for the treatment of hemorrhagic shock in dogs: Effects on myocardial blood flow and oxygen transport. Crit Care Med 19:1561-1565, 1991.

165. Tabuchi N, et al: Gelatin use impairs platelet adhesion during cardiac surgery. Thromb Haemost 74:1447-1451, 1995.

166. Messmer KF: The use of plasma substitutes with special attention to their side effects. World J Surg 11:69-74, 1987.

167. Laxenaire MC, et al: Anaphylactoid reactions to colloid plasma substitutes: Incidence, risk factors, mechanisms. A French multicenter prospective study. [in French]. Ann Fr Anesth Reanim 13:301-310, 1994.

168. Dahn MS, et al: Negative inotropic effect of albumin resuscitation for shock. Surgery 86:235-241, 1979.

169. Lucas CE, et al: Impaired salt and water excretion after albumin resuscitation for hypovolemic shock. Surgery 86:544-549, 1979.

170. Schorgen F, et al: Effects of hydroxyethylstarch and gelatin on renal function in severe sepsis: A multicentre randomised study. Lancet 357: 911-916, 2001.

171. Wade CE, et al: Efficacy of hypertonic 7.5% saline and 6% dextran-70 in treating trauma: A meta-analysis of controlled clinical studies. Surgery 122: 609-616, 1997.

172. Choi PT, et al: Crystalloids vs. colloids in fluid resuscitation: A systematic review. Crit Care Med 27:200-210, 1999.

173. Wade CE, et al: Individual patient cohort analysis of the efficacy of hypertonic saline/dextran in patients with traumatic brain injury and hypotension. J Trauma 42(suppl):S61-S65, 1997.

174. Velanovich V: Crystalloid versus colloid fluid resuscitation: A meta-analysis of mortality. Surgery 105: 65-71, 1989.

175. Bisonni RS, et al: Colloids versus crystalloids in fluid resuscitation: An analysis of randomized controlled trials. J Fam Pract 32:387-390, 1991.

176. Schierhout G, Roberts I: Fluid resuscitation with colloid or crystalloid solutions in critically ill patients: A systematic review of randomised trials. BMJ 316:961-964, 1998.

177. Human albumin administration in critically ill patients: Systematic review of randomized controlled trials. Cochrane Injuries Group Albumin Reviewers. BMJ 317:235-240, 1998.

178. Horsey P: Albumin and hypovolemia: Is the Cochrane evidence to be trusted? Lancet 359:70-72, 2002.

179. Sloan EP, et al: Diaspirin cross-linked hemoglobin (DCLHb) in the treatment of severe traumatic hemorrhagic shock: A randomized controlled efficacy trial. JAMA 282:1857-1864, 1999.

180. Morales D, et al: Reversal by vasopressin of intractable hypotension in the late phase of hemorrhagic shock. Circulation 100:226-229, 1999.

181. Voelckel WG, et al: Vasopressin improves survival after cardiac arrest in hypovolemic shock. Anesth Analg 91:627-634, 2000.

182. Malay MB, et al: Low-dose vasopressin in the treatment of vasodilatory septic shock. J Trauma 47:699-703, 1999 [see discussion 703-705].

183. Jackson WL Jr, Shorr AF: Vasopressin and cardiac performance. Chest 121:1723-1724, 2002 [see discussion 1724].

184. Poole-Wilson PA, Langer GA: Effect of pH on ionic exchange and function in rat and rabbit myocardium. Am J Physiol 229:570-581, 1975.

185. Shapiro JI: Functional and metabolic responses of isolated hearts to acidosis: Effects of sodium bicarbonate and Carbicarb. Am J Physiol; (6 pt 2):258:H1835-H1839, 1990.

186. Forsythe SM, Schmidt GA: Sodium bicarbonate for the treatment of lactic acidosis. Chest 117:260-267, 2000.

187. Arieff AI, et al: Systemic effects of $NaHCO_3$ in experimental lactic acidosis in dogs. Am J Physiol 242:F586-F591, 1982.

188. Graf H, et al: Metabolic effects of sodium bicarbonate in hypoxic lactic acidosis in dogs. Am J Physiol; (5 pt 2):249:F630-F635, 1985.

189. Tanaka M, Nishikawa T: Acute haemodynamic effects of sodium bicarbonate administration in respiratory and metabolic acidosis in anaesthetized dogs. Anaesth Intensive Care 25:615-620, 1997.

190. Cooper DJ, et al: Bicarbonate does not improve hemodynamics in critically ill patients who have lactic acidosis. A prospective, controlled clinical study. Ann Intern Med 112:492-498, 1990.

191. Mathieu D, et al: Effects of bicarbonate therapy on hemodynamics and tissue oxygenation in patients with lactic acidosis: A prospective, controlled clinical study. Crit Care Med 19:1352-1356, 1991.

192. Beech JS, et al: Haemodynamic and metabolic effects in diabetic ketoacidosis in rats of treatment with sodium bicarbonate or a mixture of sodium bicarbonate and sodium carbonate. Diabetologia 38:889-898, 1995.

193. Nakashima K, et al: The effect of sodium bicarbonate on CBF and intracellular pH in man: Stable Xe-CT and 31P-MRS. Acta Neurol Scand Suppl 166:96-98, 1996.

194. Bjerneroth G, et al: Effects of alkaline buffers on cytoplasmic pH in lymphocytes. Crit Care Med 22:1550-1556, 1994.

195. Ritten JM, et al: Paradoxical effect of bicarbonate on cytoplasmic pH. Lancet 335:1243-1246, 1990.

196. Thompson CH, et al: Effect of bicarbonate administration on skeletal muscle intracellular pH in the rat: Implications for acute administration of bicarbonate in man. Clin Sci (Colch) 82:559-564, 1992.

197. Bollaer PE, et al: Effects of sodium bicarbonate on striated muscle metabolism and intracellular pH during endotoxic shock. Shock 1:196-200, 1994.

198. Bellingham AJ, et al: Regulatory mechanisms of hemoglobin oxygen affinity in acidosis and alkalosis. J Clin Invest 50:700-706, 1971.

199. Vatner SF: Effects of hemorrhage on regional blood flow distribution in dogs and primates. J Clin Invest 54:225-235, 1974.

200. Lieberthal W, et al: Nitric oxide inhibition in rats improves blood pressure and renal function during hypovolemic shock. Am J Physiol 261(5 pt 2):F868-F872, 1991.

201. Bahrami S, et al: Significance of TNF in hemorrhage-related hemodynamic alterations, organ injury, and mortality in rats. Am J Physiol 272; (5 pt 2): H2219-H2226, 1997.

202. Chaudry IH, et al: Hemorrhage and resuscitation: Immunological aspects. Am J Physiol 259 (4 pt 2):R663-R678, 1990.

203. Spain DA, et al: Complement activation mediates intestinal injury after resuscitation from hemorrhagic shock. J Trauma 46:224-233, 1999.

204. Salvo I, et al: The Italian SEPSIS study: Preliminary results on the incidence and evolution of SIRS, sepsis, severe sepsis and septic shock. Intensive Care Med 21 (suppl 2):S244-S249, 1995.

205. Balk RA: Severe sepsis and septic shock. Definitions, epidemiology, and clinical manifestations. Crit Care Clin 16: 179-192, 2000.

206. Centers for Disease Control: Increase in national hospital discharge survey rates for septicemia—United States 1979-1987. JAMA 263: 937-938, 1990.

207. Bone RC, et al: Definitions for sepsis and organ failure and guidelines for the use of innovative therapies in sepsis. The ACCP/SCCM Consensus Conference Committee. American College of Chest Physicians/Society of Critical Care Medicine. Chest 101:1644-1655, 1992.

208. Rangel-Frausto MS, et al: The natural history of the systemic inflammatory response syndrome (SIRS). A prospective study. JAMA 273: 117-123, 1995.

209. Kreger BE, et al: Gram-negative bacteremia. III. Reassessment of etiology, epidemiology and ecology in 612 patients. Am J Med 68: 332-343, 1980.

210. Marik PE, Varon J: Sepsis: State of the art. Dis Mon 47:465-532, 2001.

211. Glauser MP: Pathophysiologic basis of sepsis: Considerations for future strategies of intervention. Crit Care Med (suppl):28 S4-S8, 2000.

212. Heumann D, Glauser MP: Pathogenesis of sepsis. Sci Am Sci Med 1:28-37, 1994.

213. Heumann D, et al: Molecular basis of host-pathogen interaction in septic shock. Curr Opin Microbiol 1:49-55, 1998.

214. Natanson C, et al: Selected treatment strategies for septic shock based on proposed mechanisms of pathogenesis. Ann Intern Med 120:771-783, 1994.

215. Freeman BD, Natanson C: Clinical trials in sepsis and septic shock. Curr Opin Crit Care 1:349, 1995.

216. Zeni F, et al: Anti-inflammatory therapies to treat sepsis and septic shock: A reassessment. Crit Care Med 25:1095-1100, 1997.

217. Tavares-Murta BM, et al: Failure of neutrophil chemotactic function in septic patients. Crit Care Med 30:1056-1061, 2002.

218. Manhart N, et al: Receptor and non-receptor mediated production of superoxide anion and hydrogen peroxide in neutrophils of intensive care patients. Wien Klini Wochenschr 110:796-801, 1998.

219. Natanson C, et al: Endotoxin and tumor necrosis factor challenges in dogs simulate the cardiovascular profile of human septic shock. J Exp Med 169:823-832, 1989.

220. Waage A, Espevik T: Interleukin-1 potentiates the lethal effects of tumor necrosis factor in mice. J Exp Med 169:823-832, 1988.

221. Okusawa S, et al: Interleukin 1 induces a shock-like state in rabbits. Synergism with tumor necrosis factor and the effect of cyclooxygenase inhibition. J Clin Invest 81:1162-1172, 1988.

222. Ohlsson K, et al: Interleukin-1 receptor antagonist reduces mortality from endotoxin shock. Nature 348:550-552, 1990.

223. Wakabayashi G, et al: A specific receptor antagonist for interleukin 1 prevents *Escherichia coli*–induced shock in rabbits. FASEB J 5:338-343, 1991.

224. Beutler B, et al: Passive immunization against cachectin/tumor necrosis factor protects mice from lethal effect of endotoxin. Science 229:869-871, 1985.

225. Petrak RA, et al: Prostaglandins, cyclo-oxygenase inhibitors, and thromboxane synthetase inhibitors in the pathogenesis of multiple systems organ failure. Crit Care Clin 5:303-314, 1989.

226. Mathiak G, et al: Platelet-activating factor (PAF) in experimental and clinical sepsis. Shock 7:391-404, 1997.

227. Siebenlist U, et al: Structure, regulation and function of NF-κB. Annu Rev Cell Biol 10:405-455, 1994.

228. Karin M: The beginning of the end: IκB kinase (IKK) and NF-κB activation. J Biol Chem 274:27339-27342, 1999.

229. Senftleben U, Karin M: The IKK/NF-κB pathway. Crit Care Med 30(suppl):S18-S26, 2002.

230. Lorente JA, et al: Time course of hemostatic abnormalities in sepsis and its relation to outcome. Chest 103:1536-1542, 1993.

231. Taylor FB Jr, et al: Protein C prevents the coagulopathic and lethal effects of *Escherichia coli* infusion in the baboon. J Clin Invest 79:918-925, 1987.

232. Fourrier F, et al: Septic shock, multiple organ failure, and disseminated intravascular coagulation. Compared patterns of antithrombin III, protein C, and protein S deficiencies. Chest 101: 816-823, 1992.

233. Ince C, Sinaasappel M: Microcirculatory oxygenation and shunting in sepsis and shock. Crit Care Med 27:1369-1377, 1999.

234. Kreger BE, et al: Gram-negative bacteremia. IV. Re-evaluation of clinical features and treatment in 612 patients. Am J Med 68: 344-355, 1980.

235. Kilbourn RG, et al: NG-methyl-L-arginine inhibits tumor necrosis factor–induced hypotension: Implications for the involvement of nitric oxide. Proc Natl Acad Sci U S A 87:3629-3632, 1990.

236. Parrillo JE, et al: Septic shock in humans. Advances in the understanding of pathogenesis, cardiovascular dysfunction, and therapy. Ann Intern Med 113:227-242, 1990.

237. Ellrodt AG, et al: Left ventricular performance in septic shock: Reversible segmental and global abnormalities. Am Heart J 110: 402-409, 1985.

238. Monsalve F, et al: Myocardial depression in septic shock caused by meningococcal infection. Crit Care Med 12:1021-1023, 1984.

239. Kumar A, et al: Myocardial dysfunction in septic shock. Crit Care Clin 16:251-287, 2000.
240. Balk RA, Bone RC: The septic syndrome. Definition and clinical implications. Crit Care Clin 5:1-8, 1989.
241. Pinsky MR, et al: Serum cytokine levels in human septic shock. Relation to multiple-system organ failure and mortality. Chest 103:565-575, 1993.
242. Meduri GU, et al: Persistent elevation of inflammatory cytokines predicts a poor outcome in ARDS. Plasma IL-1 β and IL-6 levels are consistent and efficient predictors of outcome over time. Chest 107:1062-1073, 1997.
243. Soni A, et al: Adrenal insufficiency occurring during septic shock: Incidence, outcome, and relationship to peripheral cytokine levels. Am J Med 98:266-271, 1995.
244. Bouachour G, et al: Adrenocortical function during septic shock. Intensive Care Med 21:57-62, 1995.
245. Marik PE, et al: Occult adrenal insufficiency in critically ill patients: An underdiagnosed entity [abstract]. Crit Care Med 27:A141, 1999.
246. Zaloga GP: Sepsis-induced adrenal deficiency syndrome. Crit Care Med 29:688-690, 2001.
247. Zaloga GP, Marik P: Hypothalamic-pituitary-adrenal insufficiency. Crit Care Clin 17:25-41, 2001.
248. Levi M: Pathogenesis and treatment of disseminated intravascular coagulation in the septic patient. J Crit Care 16:167-177, 2001.
249. Bolton CF: Sepsis and the systemic inflammatory response syndrome: Neuromuscular manifestations. Crit Care Med 24: 1408-1416, 1996.
250. Bleck TP, et al: Neurologic complications of critical medical illnesses. Crit Care Med 21:98-103, 1993.
251. Papadopoulos MC, et al: Pathophysiology of septic encephalopathy: A review. Crit Care Med 28:3019-3024, 2000.
252. Schor N: Acute renal failure and the sepsis syndrome. Kidney Int 61:764-776, 2002.
253. Groeneveld AB, et al: Acute renal failure in the medical intensive care unit: Predisposing, complicating factors and outcome. Nephron 59:602-610, 1991.
254. Messmer UK, et al: Tumor necrosis factor-α and lipopolysaccharide induce apoptotic cell death in bovine glomerular endothelial cells. Kidney Int 55:2322-2337, 1999.
255. Mariano F, et al: Production of platelet-activating factor in patients with sepsis-associated acute renal failure. Nephrol Dial Transplant 14:1150-1157, 1999.
256. Dos Santos OF, et al: Role of platelet activating factor in gentamicin and cisplatin nephrotoxicity. Kidney Int 40:742-747, 1991.
257. Kohan DE: Production of endothelin-1 by rat mesangial cells: Regulation by tumor necrosis factor. J Lab Clin Med 119:477-484, 1992.
258. Marsden PA, et al: Regulated expression of endothelin 1 in glomerular capillary endothelial cells. Am J Physiol 261 (1 pt 2): F117-F125, 1991.
259. Katoh T, et al: Direct effects of endothelin in the rat kidney. Am J Physiol 258 (2 pt 2):F397-F402, 1990.
260. Yoshitomi K, et al: Endothelin inhibits luminal sodium channel in rabbit cortical collecting duct. J Am Soc Nephrol 2:423, 1991.
261. Oishi R, et al: Endothelin-1 inhibits AVP-stimulated osmotic water permeability in rat inner medullary collecting duct. Am J Physiol 261(6 pt 2): F951-F956, 1991.
262. Klahr S: Role of arachidonic acid metabolites in acute renal failure and sepsis. Nephrol Dial Transplant (suppl)4:52-56, 1994.
263. Bremm KD, et al: Generation of slow-reacting substance (leukotrienes) by endotoxin and lipid A from human polymorphonuclear granulocytes. Immunology 53:299-305, 1984.
264. Balk RA: Pathogenesis and management of multiple organ dysfunction or failure in severe sepsis and septic shock. Crit Care Clin 16:vii, 337-352, 2000.
265. Fink MP, Evans TW: Mechanisms of organ dysfunction in critical illness: Report from a round table conference held in Brussels. Intensive Care Med 28:369-375, 2002.
266. Rybak MJ, McGrath BJ: Combination antimicrobial therapy for bacterial infections. Guidelines for the clinician. Drugs 52:390-405, 1996.
267. Wheeler AP, Bernard GR: Treating patients with severe sepsis. N Engl J Med 340:207-214, 1999.
268. Ognibene FP: Hemodynamic support during sepsis. Clin Chest Med 17:279-287, 1996.
269. Rivers E, et al: Early goal-directed therapy in the treatment of severe sepsis and septic shock. N Engl J Med 345:1368-1377, 2001.
270. Hollenberg S, et al: Practice parameters for hemodynamic support of sepsis in adult patients in sepsis. Task Force of the American College of Critical Care Medicine, Society of Critical Care Medicine. Crit Care Med 27:639-660, 1999.
271. Levy B, et al: Comparison of norepinephrine and dobutamine to epinephrine for hemodynamics, lactate metabolism, and gastric tonometric variables in septic shock: A prospective, randomized study. Intensive Care Med 23:283-287, 1997.
272. Gattinoni L, et al: A trial of goal-oriented hemodynamic therapy in critically ill patients. SvO_2 Collaborative Group. N Engl J Med 333:1025-1032, 1995.
273. Bernard GR, et al: Efficacy and safety of recombinant human activated protein C for severe sepsis. N Engl J Med 10:344 699-709, 2001.
274. Xigris: Drotrecogin alfa (activated): PV 3420 AMP. Rockville, MD, U.S. Food and Drug Administration, 2001.
275. Fourrier F, et al: Double-blind, placebo-controlled trial of antithrombin III concentrates in septic shock with disseminated intravascular coagulation. Chest 104:882-888, 1993.
276. Balk RA, et al: Prospective double blind placebo controlled trial of antithrombin III substitution in sepsis [abstract]. Intensive Care Med 21 (suppl 1): S17, 1995.
277. Baudo F, et al: Antithrombin III (ATIII) replacement therapy in patients with sepsis and/or postsurgical complications: A controlled double-blind, randomized, multicenter study. Intensive Care Med 24:336-342, 1998.
278. Creasey AA, et al: Tissue factor pathway inhibitor reduces mortality from *Escherichia coli* septic shock. J Clin Invest 91:2850-2856, 1993.
279. Carr C, et al: Recombinant *E. coli*–derived tissue factor pathway inhibitor reduces coagulopathic and lethal effects in the baboon gram-negative model of septic shock. Circ Shock 44: 126-137, 1994.
280. Creasey AA, Reinhart K: Tissue factor pathway inhibitor activity in severe sepsis. Crit Care Med 29(suppl):S126-S129, 2001.
281. Welty-Wolf KE, et al: Coagulation blockade prevents sepsis-induced respiratory and renal failure in baboons. Am J Respir Crit Care Med (10 pt 1): 164 1988-1996, 2001.
282. Bone RC, et al: A controlled clinical trial of high-dose methylprednisolone in the treatment of severe sepsis shock. N Engl J Med 317: 653-658, 1987.
283. Cronin L, et al: Corticosteroid treatment for sepsis: A critical appraisal and meta-analysis of the literature. Crit Care Med 23: 1430-1439, 1995.
284. Bollaert PE, et al: Reversal of late septic shock with supraphysiologic doses of hydrocortisone. Crit Care Med 26:645-650, 1998.
285. Briegel J, et al: Stress doses of hydrocortisone reverse hyperdynamic septic shock: A prospective, randomized, double-blind, single-center study. Crit Care Med 27:723-732, 1999.
286. Reinhart K, et al: Randomized, placebo-controlled trial of the anti-tumor necrosis factor antibody fragment afelimomab in hyperinflammatory response during severe sepsis: The RAMSES Study. Crit Care Med 29:765-769, 2001.
287. Clark MA, et al: Effect of a chimeric antibody to tumor necrosis factor-α on cytokine and physiologic response in patients with severe sepsis—a randomized, clinical trial. Crit Care Med 26:1650-1659, 1998.
288. Abraham E, et al: Double-blind randomised controlled trial of monoclonal antibody to human tumour necrosis factor in treatment of septic shock. NORASEPT II Study Group. Lancet 351:929-933, 1998.
289. Panacek E, et al: Neutralization of tumor necrosis factor by a monoclonal antibody improves survival and reduces organ dysfunction in human sepsis: Results of the MONARCS trial [abstract]. Chest 118(suppl 4):883, 2000.
290. Bone RC, et al: A second large controlled clinical study of E5, a monoclonal antibody to endotoxin: Results of a prospective, multicenter, controlled trial. The E5 Sepsis Study Group. Crit Care Med 23:994-1006, 1995.
291. Vincent JL, et al: Phase II multicenter, clinical study of the platelet-activating factor receptor antagonist BB-882 in the treatment of sepsis. Crit Care Med 28:638-642, 2000.
292. Fein AM, et al: Treatment of severe systemic inflammatory response syndrome and sepsis with a novel bradykinin antagonist, deltibant (CP-0127). Results of a randomized, double-blind, placebo-controlled trial. CP-0127 SIRS and Sepsis Study Group. JAMA 277: 482-487, 1997.

293. Bernard GR, et al: The effects of ibuprofen on the physiology and survival of patients with sepsis. The Ibuprofen in Sepsis Study Group. N Engl J Med 336:912-918, 1997.

294. Vincent JL, et al: A multi-centre, double-blind, placebo-controlled study of liposomal prostaglandin E_1 (TLC C-53) in patients with acute respiratory distress syndrome. Intensive Care Med 27:1578-1583, 2001.

295. Opal SM, et al: Confirmatory interleukin-1 receptor antagonist trial in severe sepsis: A phase III, randomized, double-blind, placebo-controlled, multicenter trial. The Interleukin-1 Receptor Antagonist Sepsis Investigator Group. Crit Care Med 25:1115-1124, 1997.

296. Grover R, et al: Multicenter, randomized, placebo-controlled, double blind study of the nitric oxide synthetase inhibitor 546C88: Effect on survival in patients with septic shock [abstract]. Crit Care Med 27(suppl 1):A33, 1999.

297. Peake SL, et al: N-acetyl-L-cysteine depresses cardiac performance in patients with septic shock. Crit Care Med 24:1302-1310, 1996.

298. Vincent JL, et al: Clinical trials of immunomodulatory therapies in severe sepsis and septic shock. Clin Infect Dis 34:1084-1093, 2002.

299. Werdan K: Supplemental immune globulins in sepsis. Clin Chem Lab Med 37:341-349, 1999.

300. Caliezi C, et al: C1-inhibitor in patients with severe sepsis and septic shock: Beneficial effect on renal dysfunction. Crit Care Med 30:1722-1728, 2002.

301. Elliott D, et al: Removal of cytokines in septic patients using continuous veno-venous hemodiafiltration. Crit Care Med 22:718-719, 1994 [see discussion 719-721].

302. Sander A, et al: The influence of continuous hemofiltration on cytokine elimination and the cardiovascular stability in the early phase of sepsis. Contrib Nephrol 116:99-103, 1995.

303. van Bommel EF, et al: Cytokine kinetics (TNF-α, IL-1 β, IL-6) during continuous hemofiltration: A laboratory and clinical study. Contrib Nephrol 116:62-75, 1995.

304. Barrera P, et al: Removal of interleukin-1β and tumor necrosis factor from human plasma by in vitro dialysis with polyacrylonitrile membranes. Lymphokine Cytokine Res 11:99-104, 1992.

305. Bellomo R, et al: Interleukin-6 and interleukin-8 extraction during continuous venovenous hemodiafiltration in septic acute renal failure. Ren Fail 17:457-466, 1995.

306. Kellum JA, et al: Diffusive vs. convective therapy: Effects on mediators of inflammation in patient with severe systemic inflammatory response syndrome. Crit Care Med 26:1995-2000, 1998.

307. Wakabayashi Y, et al: Removal of circulating cytokines by continuous haemofiltration in patients with systemic inflammatory response syndrome or multiple organ dysfunction syndrome. Br J Surg 83:393-394, 1996.

308. Sander A, et al: Hemofiltration increases IL-6 clearance in early systemic inflammatory response syndrome but does not alter IL-6 and TNF-α plasma concentrations. Intensive Care Med 23:878-884, 1997.

309. Hoffmann JN, et al: Effect of hemofiltration on hemodynamics and systemic concentrations of anaphylatoxins and cytokines in human sepsis. Intensive Care Med 22:1360-1367, 1996.

310. van Bommel EF, et al: Impact of continuous hemofiltration on cytokines and cytokine inhibitors in oliguric patients suffering from systemic inflammatory response syndrome. Ren Fail 19:443-454, 1997.

311. Heering P, et al: Cytokine removal and cardiovascular hemodynamics in septic patients with continuous venovenous hemofiltration. Intensive Care Med 23:288-296, 1997.

312. Hoffmann JN, et al: Hemofiltrate from patients with severe sepsis and depressed left ventricular contractility contains cardiotoxic compounds. Shock 12:174-180, 1999.

313. Cole L, et al: A phase II randomized, controlled trial of continuous hemofiltration in sepsis. Crit Care Med 30:100-106, 2002.

314. Kamijo Y, et al: The effect of a hemofilter during extracorporeal circulation on hemodynamics in patients with SIRS. Intensive Care Med 26:1355-1359, 2000.

315. De Vriese AS, et al: Cytokine removal during continuous hemofiltration in septic patients. J Am Soc Nephrol 10:846-853, 1999.

316. Grootendorst AF, et al: High volume hemofiltration improves hemodynamics and survival of pigs exposed to gut ischemia and reperfusion. Shock 2:72-78, 1994.

317. Lee PA, et al Continuous arteriovenous hemofiltration therapy for *Staphylococcus aureus*–induced septicemia in immature swine. Crit Care Med 21:914-924, 1993.

318. Heidemann SM, et al: Efficacy of continuous arteriovenous hemofiltration in endotoxic shock. Cric Shock 44:183-187, 1994.

319. Freeman BD, et al: Continuous arteriovenous hemofiltration does not improve survival in a canine model of septic shock. J Am Coll Surg 180:286-292, 1995.

320. Riegel W, et al: Influence of venovenous hemofiltration on posttraumatic inflammation and hemodynamics. Contrib Nephrol 116:56-61, 1995.

321. Braun N, et al: Effect of continuous hemodiafiltration on IL-6, TNF-α, C3a, and TCC in patients with SIRS/septic shock using two different membranes. Contrib Nephrol 116:89-98, 1995.

322. Bellomo R, et al: Preliminary experience with high-volume hemofiltration in human septic shock. Kidney Int Suppl 66:S182-S185, 1998.

323. Garcia-Fernandez N, et al: Haemostatic changes in systemic inflammatory response syndrome during continuous renal replacement therapy. J Nephrol 13:282-289, 2000.

324. Honore PM, et al: Prospective evaluation of short-term, high-volume isovolemic hemofiltration on the hemodynamic course and outcome in patients with intractable circulatory failure resulting from septic shock. Crit Care Med 28:3581-3587, 2000.

325. Tetta C, et al: Use of adsorptive mechanisms in continuous renal replacement therapies in the critically ill. Kidney Int Suppl 72:S15-S19, 1999.

326. Forrester JS, et al: Medical therapy of acute myocardial infarction by application of hemodynamic subsets (first of two parts). N Engl J Med 295:1356-1362, 1976.

327. Hasdai D, et al: Frequency and clinical outcome of cardiogenic shock during acute myocardial infarction among patients receiving reteplase or alteplase. Results from GUSTO-III. Global Use of Strategies to Open Occluded Coronary Arteries. Eur Heart J 20:128-135, 1999.

328. Holmes DR Jr, et al: Cardiogenic shock in patients with acute ischemic syndromes with and without ST-segment elevation. Circulation 100:2067-2073, 1999.

329. Holmes DR Jr, et al: Contemporary reperfusion therapy for cardiogenic shock: The GUSTO-I trial experience. The GUSTO-I Investigators. Global Utilization of Streptokinase and Tissue Plasminogen Activator for Occluded Coronary Arteries. J Am Coll Cardiol 26:668-674, 1995.

330. Killip T 3rd, Kimball JT: Treatment of myocardial infarction in a coronary care unit. A two year experience with 250 patients. Am J Cardiol 20:457-464, 1967.

331. Hochman JS, et al: Cardiogenic shock complicating acute myocardial infarction—etiologies, management and outcome: A report from the SHOCK Trial Registry. Should we emergently revascularize Occluded Coronaries for cardiogenic shocK? J Am Coll Cardiol 36 (suppl A): 1063-1070, 2000.

332. Hollenberg SM: Cardiogenic shock. Crit Care Clin 17:391-410, 2001.

333. Page DL, et al: Myocardial changes associated with cardiogenic shock. N Engl J Med 285:133-137, 1971.

334. Baliga RR: Apoptosis in myocardial ischemia, infarction, and altered myocardial states. Cardiol Clin 19:91-112, 2001.

335. Menon V, et al: The clinical profile of patients with suspected cardiogenic shock due to predominant left verntricular failure: A report from the SHOCK Trial Registry. SHould we emergently revascularize Occluded Coronaries in cardiogenic shocK? J Am Coll Cardiol 36(suppl A):1071-1076, 2000.

336. Geppert A, et al: Multiple organ failure in patients with cardiogenic shock is associated with high plasma levels of interleukin-6. Crit Care Med 30:1987-1994, 2002.

337. Chiolero RL, et al: Effects of cardiogenic shock on lactate and glucose metabolism after heart surgery. Crit Care Med 28:3784-3791, 2000.

338. Hama N, et al: Rapid ventricular induction of brain natriuretic peptide gene expression in experimental acute myocardial infarction. Circulation 92:1558-1564, 1995.

339. Maisel A: B-type natriuretic peptide in the diagnosis and management of congestive heart failure. Cardiol Clin 19:557-571, 2001.

340. Kazanegra R, et al: A rapid test for B-type natriuretic peptide correlates with falling wedge pressures in patients treated for decompensated heart failure: A pilot study. J Card Fail 7:21-29, 2001.

341. Bersten AD, et al: Treatment of severe cardiogenic pulmonary edema with continuous positive airway pressure delivered by face mask. N Engl J Med 325:1825-1830, 1991.

342. Shah PK, Francis GS: Pump failure, shock and cardiac rupture in acute myocardial infarction. *In* Francis GS, Alpert JS: Modern Coronary Care. Boston, Little, Brown, 1990, pp 295-315.

343. Tisdale JE, et al: Electrophysiologic and proarrhythmic effects of intravenous inotropic agents. Prog Cardiovasc Dis 38:167-180, 1995.
344. Baim DS: Effect of phosphodiesterase inhibition on myocardial oxygen consumption and coronary blood flow. Am J Cardiol 63:23A-26A, 1989.
345. Mukae S, et al: The effects of dopamine, dobutamine and amrinone on mitochondrial function in cardiogenic shock. Jpn Heart J 38:515-529, 1997.
346. Colucci WS, et al: Intravenous nesiritide, a natriuretic peptide, in the treatment of decompensated congestive heart failure. Nesiritide Study Group. N Engl J Med 343:246-253, 2000.
347. Marcus LS, et al: Hemodynamic and renal excretory effects of human brain natriuretic peptide infusion in patients with congestive heart failure. A double-blind, placebo-controlled, randomized crossover trial. Circulation 94:3184-3189, 1996.
348. Mueller H, et al: The effects of intra-aortic counterpulsation on cardiac performance and metabolism in shock associated with acute myocardial infarction. J Clin Invest 50:1885-1900, 1971.
349. Kern MJ, et al: Augmentation of coronary blood flow by intra-aortic balloon pumping in patients after coronary angioplasty. Circulation 87:500-511, 1993.
350. Anderson RD, et al: Use of intraaortic balloon counterpulsation in patients presenting with cardiogenic shock: Observations from the GUSTO-I Study. Global Utilization of Streptokinase and TPA for Occluded Coronary Arteries. J Am Coll Cardiol 30:708-715, 1997.
351. Sanborn TA, et al: Impact of thrombolysis, intra-aortic balloon pump counterpulsation, and their combination in cardiogenic shock complicating acute myocardial infarction: A report from the SHOCK Trial Registry. SHould we emergently revascularize Occluded Coronaries for cardiogenic shocK? J Am Coll Cardiol 36(suppl A):1123-1129, 2000.
352. Barron HV, et al: The use of intra-aortic balloon counterpulsation in patients with cardiogenic shock complicating acute myocardial infarction: Data from the National Registry of Myocardial Infarction 2. Am Heart J 141:933-939, 2001.
353. Prewitt RM, et al: Intraaortic balloon counterpulsation enhances coronary thrombolysis induced by intravenous administration of a thrombolytic agent. J Am Coll Cardiol 23:794-798, 1994.
354. Ferguson JJ 3rd, et al: The current practice of intra-aortic balloon counterpulsation: Results from the Benchmark Registry. J Am Coll Cardiol 38:1456-1462, 2001.
355. Cohen M, et al: Sex and other predictors of intra-aortic ballon counterpulsation–related complications: Prospective study of 1119 consecutive patients. Am Heart J 139(2 pt 1): 282-287, 2000.
356. Crystal E, et al: Incidence and clinical significance of bacteremia and sepsis among cardiac patients treated with intra-aortic balloon counterpulsation pump. Am J Cardiol 86:1281-1284, 2000.
357. Bengtson JR, et al: Prognosis in cardiogenic shock after acute myocardial infarction in the interventional era. J Am Coll Cardiol 20:1482-1489, 1992.
358. Gruppo Italiano per lo Studio della Streptochinasi nell Infarto Miocardico: Effectiveness of intravenous thrombolytic therapy after acute myocardial infarction. Drugs 52:589-605, 1996.
359. Hochman JS, et al: Early revascularization in acute myocardial infarction complicated by cardiogenic shock. SHOCK Investigators. Should We Emergently Revascularize Occluded Coronaries for Cardiogenic Shock? N Engl J Med 341:625-634, 1999.
360. Hochman JS, et al: One-year survival following early revascularization for cardiogenic shock. JAMA 285:190-192, 2001.
361. Chan AW, et al: Long-term mortality benefit with the combination of stents and abciximab for cardiogenic shock complicating acute myocardial infarction. Am J Cardiol 89:132-136, 2002.
362. Giri S, et al: Results of primary percutaneous transluminal coronary angioplasty plus abciximab with or without stenting for acute myocardial infarction complicated by cardiogenic shock. Am J Cardiol 89:126-131, 2002.
363. Young JB: Healing the heart with ventricular assist device therapy: Mechanisms of cardiac recovery. Ann Thorac Surg 71(suppl):S210-S219, 2001.
364. Sharma A, et al: Clinical benefit and approach of ultrafiltration in acute heart failure. Cardiology 96:144-154, 2001.
365. Packer M: Neurohormonal interactions and adaptations in congestive heart failure. Circulation 77:721-730, 1988.
366. Kumar A, et al: Congestive heart failure—can the nephrologist help? J R Coll Physicians Lond 34:36-37, 2000.
367. Marenzi G, et al: Interrelation of humoral factors, hemodynamics, and fluid and salt metabolism in congestive heart failure: Effects of extracorporeal ultrafiltration. Am J Med 94:49-56, 1993.
368. Blake P, et al: Isolation of "myocardial depressant factor(s)" from the ultrafiltrate of heart failure patients with acute renal failure. ASAIO J 42:M911-M915, 1996.
369. Marenzi G, et al: Circulatory response to fluid overload removal by extracorporeal ultrafiltration in refractory congestive heart failure. J Am Coll Cardiol 38:963-968, 2001.
370. Canaud B, et al: Slow continuous and daily ultrafiltration for refractory congestive heart failure. Nephrol Dial Transplant 13(suppl 4):51-55, 1998.
371. Susini G, et al: Isolated ultrafiltration in cardiogenic pulmonary edema. Crit Care Med 18:14-17, 1990.
372. Coraim FI, Wolner E: Continuous hemofiltration for the failing heart. New Horiz 3:725-731, 1995.
373. Agostoni PG, et al: Isolated ultrafiltration in moderate congestive heart failure. J Am Coll Cardiol 21:424-431, 1993.
374. Dormans TP, et al: Chronic intermittent haemofiltration and haemodialysis in end stage chronic heart failure with oedema refractory to high dose frusemide. Heart 75:349-351, 1996.
375. Bernuau J, et al: Multivariate analysis of prognostic factors in fulminant hepatitis B. Hepatology 6:648-651, 1986.
376. O'Grady JG, et al: Acute liver failure: Redefining the syndromes. Lancet 342:273-275, 1993.
377. Williams R: Classification, etiology, and considerations of outcome in acute liver failure. Semin Liver Dis 16:343-348, 1996.
378. Bernstein D, Tripodi J: Fulminant hepatic failure. Crit Care Clin 14:181-197, 1998.
379. Sinclair S, et al: Fulminant hepatitis. Springer Semin Immunopathol 12:33-45, 1990.
380. Sergi C, et al: The distribution of HBV, HCV and HGV among livers with fulminant hepatic failure of different aetiology. J Hepatol 29:861-871, 1998.
381. Williams R, Wendon J: Indications for orthotopic liver transplantation in fulminant liver failure. Hepatology (1 pt 2):20:S5-S10, 1994.
382. Feray C, et al: Hepatitis C virus RNA and hepatitis B virus DNA in serum and liver of patients with fulminant hepatitis. Gastroenterology 104:549-555, 1993.
383. Worm HC, et al: Hepatitis E: An overview. Microbes 4:657-666, 2002.
384. Saracco G, et al: Serologic markers with fulminant hepatitis in persons positive for hepatitis B surface antigen. A worldwide epidemiologic and clinical survey. Ann Intern Med 108:380-383, 1988.
385. Carmichael GP Jr, et al: Adenovirus hepatitis in an immunosuppressed adult patient. Am J Clin Pathol 71:352-355, 1979.
386. Sobue R, et al: Fulminant hepatitis in primary human herpesvirus-6 infection. N Engl J Med 18:324 1290, 1991.
387. Stanley TV: Acute liver failure following influenza B infection. NZ Med J 107(986 pt 1):382, 1994.
388. Wieland T, Faulstich H: Amatoxins, phallotoxins, phallolysin, and antamanide: The biologically active components of poisonous *Amanita* mushrooms. CRC Crit Rev Biochem 5:185-260, 1978.
389. Sallie R, et al: Failure of simple biochemical indexes to reliably differentiate fulminant Wilson's disease from other causes of fulminant liver failure. Hepatology 16:1206-1211, 1992.
390. Butterworth RF: The neurobiology of hepatic encephalopathy. Semin Liver Dis 16:235-244, 1996.
391. Colquhoun SD, et al: The pathophysiology, diagnosis, and management of acute hepatic encephalopathy. Adv Intern Med 46:155-176, 2001.
392. Jones EA, et al: Hepatic encephalopathy, GABA-ergic neurotransmission and benzodiazepine receptor ligands. Adv Exp Med Biol 272:121-134, 1990.
393. Ellis A, Wendon J: Circulatory, respiratory, cerebral, and renal derangements in acute liver failure: Pathophysiology and management. Semin Liver Dis 16:379-388, 1996.
394. Basile AS, et al: Relationship between plasma benzodiazepine receptor ligand concentrations and severity of hepatic encephalopathy. Hepatology 19:112-121, 1994.
395. Lidofsky SD, et al: Intracranial pressure monitoring and liver transplantation for fulminant hepatic failure. Hepatology 16:1-7, 1992.
396. Ede RJ, Williams RW: Hepatic encephalopathy and cerebral edema. Semin Liver Dis 6:107-118, 1986.
397. McClung HJ, et al: Early changes in the permeability of the blood-brain barrier produced by toxins associated with liver failure. Pediatr Res 28:227-231, 1990.

398. Blei AT: Cerebral edema and intracranial hypertension in acute liver failure: Distinct aspects of the same problem. Hepatology 13: 376-379, 1991.

399. Blei AT, et al: Complications of intracranial pressure monitoring in fulminant hepatic failure. Lancet 341:157-158, 1993.

400. Bass NM: Monitoring and treatment of intracranial hypertension. Liver Transpl Surg 6(suppl 1):S21-S26, 2000.

401. Inagaki M, et al: Advantages of intracranial pressure monitoring in patients with fulminant hepatic failure [abstract]. Gastroenterology 102:A826, 1992.

402. Herrera JL: Management of acute liver failure. Dig Dis 16:274-283, 1998.

403. Schafer DF, Shaw BW Jr: Fulminant hepatic failure and orthotopic liver transplantation. Semin Liver Dis 9:189-194, 1989.

404. O'Brien CJ, et al: Neurological sequelae in patients recovered from fulminant hepatic failure. Gut 28:93-95, 1987.

405. Ganger DR: Liver failure in critical care medicine: Principles of diagnosis and management in the adult. *In* Parillo, JE, Dillinger, RP (eds): Critical Care Medicine. Philadelphia, Mosby, 2001, 1355-1369.

406. Pereira SP, et al: The management of abnormalities of hemostasis in acute liver failure. Semin Liver Dis 16:403-414, 1996.

407. Gill RQ, Sterling RK: Acute liver failure. J Clin Gastroenterol 33:191-198, 2001.

408. Rolando N, et al: Prospective study of bacterial infection in acute liver failure: An analysis of fifty patients. Hepatology 11:49-53, 1990.

409. Almasio PL, et al: Characterization of the molecular forms of fibronectin in fulminant hepatic failure. Hepatology 6:1340-1345, 1986.

410. Bailey RJ, et al: Metabolic inhibition of polymorphonuclear leucocytes in fulminant hepatic failure. Lancet 1:1162-1163, 1976.

411. Rolando N, et al: Prospective controlled trial of selective parenteral and enteral antimicrobial regimen in fulminant liver failure. Hepatology 17:196-201, 1993.

412. Moore K: Renal failure in acute liver failure. Eur J Gastroenterol Hepatol 11:967-975, 1999.

413. Davenport A, et al: Early changes in intracranial pressure during haemofiltration treatment in patients with grade 4 hepatic encephalopathy and acute oliguric renal failure. Nephrol Dial Transplant 5:192-198, 1990.

414. Davenport A, et al: Continuous vs. intermittent forms of haemofiltration and/or dialysis in the management of acute renal failure in patients with defective cerebral autoregulation at risk of cerebral oedema. Contrib Nephrol 93:225-233, 1991.

415. Meng HC, et al: Transjugular liver biopsy: Comparison with percutaneous liver biopsy. J Gastroenterol Hepatol 9:457-461, 1994.

416. Harrison PM, et al: Improved outcome of paracetamol-induced fulminant hepatic failure by late administration of acetylcysteine. Lancet 335:1572-1573, 1990.

417. Santantonio T, et al: Lamivudine is safe and effective in fulminant hepatitis B. J Hepatol 30:551, 1999.

418. Broussard CN, et al: Mushroom poisoning—from diarrhea to liver transplantation. Am J Gastroenterol 96:3195-3198, 2001.

419. Wellington K, Jarvis B: Silymarin: A review of its clinical properties in the management of hepatic disorders. Biodrugs 15:465-489, 2001.

420. Lee WM: Management of acute liver failure. Semin Liver Dis 4: 369-378, 1996.

421. Harrison PM, et al: Improvement by acetylcysteine of hemodynamics and oxygen transport in fulminant hepatic failure. N Engl J Med 324:1852-1857, 1991.

422. Walsh TS, et al: The effect of *N*-acetylcysteine on oxygen transport and uptake in patients with fulminant hepatic failure. Hepatology 27:1332-1340, 1998.

423. Wendon JA, et al: Effects of vasopressor agents and epoprostenol on systemic hemodynamics and oxygen transport in fulminant hepatic failure. Hepatology 15:1067-1071, 1992.

424. Davenport A, et al: Adverse effects on cerebral perfusion of prostacyclin administered directly into patients with fulminant hepatic failure and acute renal failure. Nephron 59:449-454, 1991.

425. Munoz SJ: Difficult management problems in fulminant hepatic failure. Semin Liver Dis 13:395-413, 1993.

426. Strauss E, et al: Double-blind randomized clinical trial comparing neomycin and placebo in the treatment of exogenous hepatic encephalopathy. Hepatogastroenterology 39:542-545, 1992.

427. Sterling RK, et al: Flumazenil for hepatic coma: The elusive wake-up call? Gastroenterology 107:1204-1205, 1994.

428. Ede RJ, et al: Controlled hyperventilation in the prevention of cerebral oedema in fulminant hepatic failure. J Hepatol 2:43-51, 1986.

429. Wendon JA, et al: Cerebral blood flow and metabolism in fulminant liver failure. Hepatology 19:1407-1413, 1994.

430. Woolf GM, Redeker AG: Treatment of fulminant hepatic failure with insulin and glucagon. A randomized, controlled trial. Dig Dis Sci 36:92-96, 1991.

431. Rakela J, et al: A double-blinded, randomized trial of hydrocortisone in acute hepatic failure. The Acute Hepatic Failure Study Group. Dig Dis Sci 36:1223-1228, 1991.

432. Brunner G: Benefits and dangers of plasma exchange in patients with fulminant hepatic failure [abstract]. Artif Organs 12:165, 1988.

433. Lepore MJ, Martel AJ: Plasmapheresis in hepatic coma. Lancet 2:771-772, 1967.

434. Freeman JG, et al: Plasmapheresis in acute liver failure. Int J Artif Organs 9:433-438, 1986.

435. Strom SC, et al: Hepatocyte transplantation as a bridge to orthotopic liver transplantation in terminal liver failure. Transplantation 63: 559-569, 1997.

436. Miwa S, et al: Living-related liver transplantation for patients with fulminant and subfulminant hepatic failure. Hepatology 30: 1521-1526, 1999.

437. Marcos A, et al: Emergency adult to adult living donor liver transplantation for fluminant hepatic failure. Transplantation 69: 2202-2205, 2000.

438. Ash SR: Extracorporeal blood detoxification by sorbents in treatment of hepatic encephalopathy. Adv Ren Replace Ther 9: 3-18, 2002.

439. Ash SR, et al: Randomized clinical trial of liver dialysis in treatment of hepatic failure and hepatorenal failure. Ther Apheresis 4:421, 2000.

440. Stange J, et al: Molecular adsorbent recycling system (MARS): Clinical results of a new membrane-based blood purification system for bioartificial liver support. Artif Organs 23:319-330, 1999.

441. Mitzner SR, et al: Improvement of hepatorenal syndrome with extracorporeal albumin dialysis MARS: Results of a prospective, randomized, controlled clinical trial. Liver TransplSurg 6:277-286, 2000.

442. Watanabe FD, et al: Clinical experience with a bioartificial liver in the treatment of severe liver failure. A phase I clinical trial. Ann Surg 225:484-491; discussion 491-484, 1997.

443. Sussman NL, et al: Extracorporeal liver support. Application to fulminant hepatic failure. J Clin Gastroenterol 18:320-324, 1994.

444. Ellis AJ, et al: Pilot-controlled trial of the extracorporeal liver assist device in acute liver failure. Hepatology 24:1446-1451, 1996.

445. Clermont G, et al: Renal failure in the ICU: Comparison of the impact of acute renal failure and end-stage renal disease on ICU outcomes. Kidney Int 62:986-996, 2002.

446. Metnitz PG, et al: Effect of acute renal failure requiring renal replacement therapy on outcome in critically ill patients. Crit Care Med 30:2051-2058, 2002.

447. Kellum JA: The Acute Dialysis Quality Initiative: Methodology. Adv Ren Replace Ther 9:245-247, 2002.

448. Clark WR, et al: A comparison of metabolic control by continuous and intermittent therapies in acute renal failure. J Am Soc Nephrol 4:1413-1420, 1994.

449. Chima CS, et al: Protein catabolic rate in patients with acute renal failure on continuous arteriovenous hemofiltration and total parenteral nutrition. J Am Soc Nephrol 3:1516-1521, 1993.

450. Mehta RL: Indications for dialysis in the ICU: Renal replacement vs. renal support. Blood Purif 19:227-232, 2001.

451. Macias WL, et al: Continuous venovenous hemofiltration: An alternative to continuous arteriovenous hemofiltration and hemodiafiltration in acute renal failure. Am J Kidney Dis 18:451-458, 1991.

452. Manns M, et al: Intradialytic renal haemodynamics—potential consequences for the management of the patient with acute renal failure. Nephrol Dial Transplant 12:870-872, 1997.

453. McDonald BR, Mehta RL: Decreased mortality in patients with acute renal failure undergoing continuous arteriovenous hemodialysis. Contrib Nephrol 93:51-56, 1991.

454. Gettings LG, et al: Outcome in post-traumatic acute renal failure when continuous renal replacement therapy is applied early vs. late. Intensive Care Med 25:805-813, 1999.

455. III. NKF-K/DOQI Clinical Practice Guidelines for Vascular Access: Update 2000. Am J Kidney Dis 37(suppl 1):S137-S181, 2001.

456. Trerotola SO, et al: Randomized comparison of high-flow versus conventional hemodialysis catheters. J Vasc Interv Radiol 10:1032-1038, 1999.

457. Trerotola SO, et al: Randomized comparison of split tip versus step tip high-flow hemodialysis catheters. Kidney Int 62:282-289, 2002.

458. Leblanc M, et al: Effective blood flow and recirculation rates in internal jugular vein twin catheters: Measurement by ultrasound velocity dilution. Am J Kidney Dis 31:87-92, 1998.

459. Kraus MA, et al: Temporary hemodialysis catheter recirculation studies, a comparison of design and site selection. Blood Purif 13: 385-401, 1995.

460. G.E. Cimochowski, et al: Superiority of the internal jugular over the subclavian access for temporary dialysis. Nephron 2:54:154-161, 1990.

461. Pisoni RL, et al: Vascular access use in Europe and the United States: Results from the DOPPS. Kidney Int 61:305-316, 2002.

462. Twardowski ZJ, et al: Blood recirculation in intravenous catheters for hemodialysis. J Am Soc Nephrol 3:1978-1981, 1993.

463. Oliver MJ, et al: Randomized study of temporary hemodialysis catheters. Int J Artif Organs 25:40-44, 2002.

464. Oliver MJ, et al: Risk of bacteremia from temporary hemodialysis catheters by site of insertion and duration of use: A prospective study. Kidney Int 58:2543-2545, 2000.

465. Vanholder R, et al: What is the renal replacement method of first choice for intensive care patients? J Am Soc Nephrol 17(suppl): S40-S43, 2001.

466. Tominaga GT, et al: Vascular complications of continuous arteriovenous hemofiltration in trauma patients. J Trauma 35:285-288, 1993 [see discussion 288-289].

467. Brunet S, et al: Diffusive and convective solute clearances during continuous renal replacement therapy at various dialysate and ultrafiltration flow rates. Am J Kidney Dis 34:486-492, 1999.

468. Palsson R, Niles JL: Regional citrate anticoagulation in continuous venovenous hemofiltration in critically ill patients with a high risk of bleeding. Kidney Int 55:1991-1997, 1999.

469. Tolwani AJ, et al:Simplified citrate anticoagulation for continuous renal replacement therapy. Kidney Int 60:370-374, 2001.

470. Evanson JA, et al: Prescribed versus delivered dialysis in acute renal failure patients. Am J Kidney Dis 32:731-738, 1998.

471. Schiffl H, et al: Daily hemodialysis and the outcome of acute renal failure, N Engl J Med 346:305-310, 2002.

472. Hakim RM, et al: Effect of the dialysis membrane in the treatment of patients with acute renal failure. N Engl J Med 331:1338-1342, 1994.

473. Marshall MR, et al: Sustained low-efficiency dialysis for critically ill patients requiring renal replacement therapy. Kidney Int 60:777-785, 2001.

474. Ash SR: Peritoneal dialysis in acute renal failure of adults: The safe, effective, and low-cost modality. Contrib Nephrol 132:210-221, 2001.

475. Phu NH, et al: Hemofiltration and peritoneal dialysis in infection-associated acute renal failure in Vietnam. N Engl J Med 347:895-902, 2002.

476. Liao Z, et al: Dose capabilities of renal replacement therapies in acute renal failure (ARF) [abstract]. J Am Soc Nephrol 13:237A, 2002.

477. Venkataraman R, et al: Dosing patterns for continuous renal replacement therapy at a large academic medical center in the United States. J Crit Care 17:246-250, 2002.

478. Marshall MR, et al: Prescribed versus delivered dose of sustained low efficiency dialysis (SLED) [abstract]. J Am Soc Nephrol 11:324A, 2000.

479. Clark WR, Kraus MA: Dialysis in acute renal failure: Is more better? Int J Artif Organs 25:1119-1122, 2002.

480. Gillum DM, et al: The role of intensive dialysis in acute renal failure. Clin Nephrol 25:249-255, 1986.

481. Paganini EP, et al: Risk modeling in acute renal failure requiring dialysis: The introduction of a new model. Clin Nephrol 46:206-211, 1996.

482. Storck M, et al: Comparison of pump-driven and spontaneous continuous haemofiltration in postoperative acute renal failure. Lancet 337:452-455, 1991.

483. Ronco C, et al: Effects of different doses in continuous veno-venous haemofiltration on outcomes of acute renal failure: A prospective randomized trial. Lancet 356:26-30, 2000.

484. Swartz RD, et al: Comparing continuous hemofiltration with hemodialysis in patients with severe acute renal failure. Am J Kidney Dis 34:424-432, 1999.

485. Mehta RL, et al: A randomized clinical trial of continuous versus intermittent dialysis for acute renal failure. Kidney Int 60:1154-1163, 2001.

486. Kellum JA, et al: Continuous versus intermittent renal replacement therapy: A meta-analysis. Intensive Care Med 28:29-37, 2002.

CHAPTER 62

Extracorporeal Treatment of Poisoning

Ingrid J. Chang, Bernard V. Fischbach, Saba Silé, and Thomas A. Golper

Poisonings and toxic ingestions have been reported throughout history. Unfortunately, with the widespread use of recreational substances and the increase in prescription and over-the-counter medications, the incidence of toxic exposures has risen dramatically. The American Association of Poison Control Centers (AAPCC) compiles toxic exposure data on an annual basis. Sixty-four poison centers nationwide collect and submit individual exposure cases. The AAPCC database contains approximately 31.4 million toxic exposure cases. In 2001, a total of 2,267,979 cases was reported, a 4.6% increase from the year 2000 database.[1, 2]

Of the toxic exposures reported in 2001, approximately 92% occurred in a residence, and 2.4% occurred in the workplace. Children younger than 6 years accounted for 51.6% of cases. A male predominance was found for victims younger than 13 years. This gender distribution is reversed in teenagers and adults. Approximately 85% of the reported poison exposures were unintentional, and 7.4% were the result of therapeutic errors.

A total of 1074 fatal toxic exposures was reported in 2001. This represents a 17% increase over the number of fatalities reported in the prior year. For all ages, analgesics were the most common class of substances implicated in fatal toxic ingestions. Antidepressants were the second most common agent, followed by sedatives, street drugs or stimulants, and cardiovascular drugs.

Most exposure cases were manageable in a non–health care setting, although 22% of the poisonous ingestions required treatment in a health care facility. Table 62-1 inventories the different therapies used for the reported human exposures in 2001. Decontamination, specifically dilution with intravenous fluids and activated charcoal, were the two most frequently used therapeutic modalities. The use of ipecac

syrup has declined dramatically over the past 20 years and was used in only 0.7% of ingestions in 2001.[1]

Extracorporeal treatment of poisonings in 2001 was administered in 1351 of the reported human exposure cases. There are specific indications for the use of extracorporeal therapy in the setting of intoxications. Understanding the physiologic basis for these indications allows the clinician to effectively guide treatment of the overdose patient. This chapter discusses poisoning and management of the intoxicated patient. The specific focus of this section is to review

TABLE 62-1

Therapy Provided in Human Exposure Cases in 2001

THERAPY	NUMBER OF CASES
Decontamination	
Dilution or irrigation	1,055,129
Activated charcoal	149,442
Cathartic	56,784
Gastric lavage	29,798
Ipecac syrup	16,058
Whole-bowel irrigation	2,489
Extracorporeal Therapy	
Hemodialysis	1,280
Hemoperfusion	45
Other extracorporeal procedure	26
Specific Antidotes	44,772
Other Interventions	
Alkalinization	6,944
Transplantation	8

Adapted from Litovitz TL, Klein-Schwartz W, Rodgers GC Jr, et al: 2001 Annual Report of the American Association of Poison Control Centers Toxic Exposure Surveillance System. Am J Emerg Med 20:391-452, 2002.

fundamental concepts of the different extracorporeal techniques and their role in the treatment of acute poisonings.

GENERAL MANAGEMENT OF POISONING AND DRUG OVERDOSE

Toxic exposures may be local, systemic, or both. The distribution and absorption depends on the dose, route of exposure, and properties of the toxin. The molecular size, degree of protein binding, solubility in water versus lipids, and the degree of ionization affect the absorption and toxicity associated with the specific substance. These factors must be taken into account when determining the initial management of the poisoned patient.

Clinical History

The diagnosis of a toxic ingestion can often be established by the history, physical examination, and routine toxicology laboratory information. However, the overdose patient commonly presents to a health care facility in an obtunded state, making a thorough history difficult to obtain. In patients who are unable to give a history, questions regarding habits, hobbies, prescription medications, behavioral changes, and antecedent events should be directed to the family and friends. Discussions with emergency personnel also may reveal pertinent information. After initial airway and circulatory management, the clinician must gather data by means of physical examination and laboratory assessment to determine the cause of the toxic ingestion. The physician then must develop a treatment plan directed toward limiting the accumulation of toxin in the body.

Physical Examination

The physical examination findings of the poisoned patient are quite variable and often depend on the particular toxin ingested. Patients require close monitoring because they may deteriorate rapidly after the initial assessment. Frequent reevaluation of vital signs, cardiopulmonary condition, and neurologic status are essential for proper management. Specific clinical manifestations and physical findings are described in later sections of this chapter as they pertain to the individual toxins.

Laboratory Assessment

Laboratory assessment should be a routine procedure for the patient suspected of toxic exposure. A complete blood cell count, comprehensive metabolic panel, serum osmolality, arterial blood gas determinations, urinalysis, urine drug screen, and serum acetaminophen and salicylate levels should be part of the initial evaluation. An electrocardiogram (ECG) is also indicated, because conduction disturbances within the myocardium are common in patients presenting with toxic ingestions.[3-6]

Electrolyte disturbances are common in intoxications, and two key features that assist in determining the type of toxin ingested are the anion gap and osmolal gap. A *high–anion gap metabolic acidosis* is characteristic of salicylate, methanol, and ethylene glycol toxicity. Another cause

of an elevated anion gap acidosis in the setting of acute poisoning is lactic acidosis, which may be associated with hypoxia, hypotension, or seizures. A low-anion gap is observed with lithium, nitrate, iodine, and bromide poisoning. Ketosis may be present with acetone, isopropanol (i.e., isopropyl alcohol), and salicylate ingestion.

The *osmolal gap* is the difference between the measured serum osmolality and the calculated osmolality. The calculated osmolality is determined by the following formula:

$$\text{Osm}_{\text{calculated}}(\text{mOsm/kg}) = 2[\text{Na}] + \frac{[\text{glucose}]}{18} + \frac{[\text{BUN}]}{2.8}$$

The osmolal gap indicates the presence of an unmeasured solute and is considered elevated if the value is more than 10 to 12 mOsm/kg H_2O. An elevated osmolal gap is most commonly seen with ethanol, ethylene glycol, isopropanol, and methanol toxicity. To contribute to the serum osmolality, a substance must have a low molecular weight and be able to achieve high blood levels. The concept of the osmolal gap is discussed in detail in a later section (see "Ethylene Glycol: Diagnosis and Laboratory Data").

DECONTAMINATION AND FACILITATED REMOVAL

After the initial clinical and laboratory assessment, decontamination and facilitated removal of the toxin become the primary goals of therapy. The mode of decontamination depends on the route of exposure and on the specific properties of the poison. In the 2001 AAPC database, dilution and irrigation followed by the use of activated charcoal were the two most common treatment modalities.

Techniques That Prevent Further Absorption
Dilution and Whole-Bowel Irrigation

The ingestion of an alkaline or acidic agent is the main indication for *dilution*. Dilution should be performed immediately after exposure to decrease the concentration of the offending toxin and to minimize tissue damage. Approximately 5 mL/kg or 250 mL of water or milk are used. Dilution does not prevent absorption of the ingested toxin.

Whole-bowel irrigation (WBI) is performed with a solution containing electrolytes and iso-osmotic polyethylene glycol. The irrigating solution is given orally or through a nasogastric tube at a rate of 1 to 2 L/hour for adults until the rectal effluent is clear. WBI is indicated for toxins that are not well absorbed by activated charcoal (Table 62-2) and for

TABLE 62-2

Clinical Uses of Multiple-Dose Activated Charcoal

Agents effectively adsorbed	
Carbamazepine	Dapsone
Digoxin	Phenobarbital
Phenytoin	Salicylates
Theophylline	Quinine
Agents ineffectively adsorbed	
Aminoglycosides	Calcium channel blockers
Phenothiazines	Tricyclic antidepressants
Heavy metals (e.g., arsenic, lead)	Lithium

overdoses with sustained-release medications. It is contraindicated for patients with gastrointestinal bleeding, bowel obstruction, or perforation.[7]

Adsorbents

An adsorbent is an agent that binds to a toxic substance and prevents its absorption across the gastrointestinal membranes. Once bound, the toxin-adsorbent combination is excreted in the feces. The most commonly used adsorbent in clinical toxicology is *multiple-dose activated charcoal* (MDAC). Activated charcoal is a nonabsorbable carbon powder that is produced by the burning of organic material followed by treatment with steam and acid. This results in an extensive network of pores, which have a surface binding area of 900 to 1500 m^2/g. The absorptive capacity of activated charcoal depends on several characteristics of the ingested toxin, including the molecular size, structure, dose, and state of ionization. The activated charcoal is ineffective for toxins that bind poorly to it.[8, 9] Toxins that are not well absorbed by activated charcoal are listed in Table 62-2.

Preparations of commercially available activated charcoal include powder, tablet, or liquid form. Overall, the most efficacious and convenient preparation is the liquid form, which may be sweetened for improved palatability or instilled through a nasogastric tube. The recommended dose of activated charcoal is 1 g/kg or a dose of 25 to 100 g. Multiple doses can be given every 4 hours. The doses may be repeated until serum drug levels are reduced to nontoxic concentrations or clinical improvement has been documented. Treatment with MDAC should *not* be continued for longer than 24 hours. The efficacy of activated charcoal is greatest within 1 hour of ingestion but should be considered for all poisonings, unless the specific agent binds poorly to the adsorbent or there are contraindications to its use.[8, 10-12] Activated charcoal is contraindicated in patients with altered levels of consciousness, at least until airway protection is established. Other contraindications include bowel obstruction or perforation.

Another common adsorbent is *sodium polystyrene sulfonate* (Kayexalate), a cation exchange resin most often used in clinical nephrology for the treatment of hyperkalemia. Sodium polystyrene sulfonate may be given orally or as a retention enema. The typical dose is 50 to 150 g/day; 1 g of the resin is capable of removing 0.5 to 1.0 mEq of potassium. It is also used for the treatment of lithium overdose, although high doses of resin are required to diminish gastrointestinal absorption of the lithium.[13] *Cholestyramine*, another common adsorbent, enhances the elimination of the organochlorines (e.g., chlordecone, lindane) and digoxin.

Ipecac

The clinical use of ipecac has declined dramatically over the past 20 years. In 2001, ipecac was used in only 0.7% of exposures, compared with 13.4% in 1983. The emetic effects of ipecac are derived from its two alkaloid constituents: emetine and cephaline. Emetine acts locally in the gastrointestinal tract and systemically in the central nervous system (CNS). Cephaline causes emesis through its properties as a gastrointestinal irritant. Ipecac successfully induces emesis in more than 90% of patients.[14]

Although data regarding the role and efficacy of ipecac have been controversial, no study has convincingly demonstrated that the clinical outcome of poisoned patients improved with the use of ipecac.[14] Administration of this powerful emetic agent is not routinely advised. The primary role for ipecac is in the home, where it can be given within 1 hour of the toxic ingestion.

The dose of ipecac is 30 mL for adults and 15 mL for patients between the ages of 1 and 12 years. The use of ipecac is not recommended for patients younger than 6 months. Contraindications for the use of ipecac include patients who present with altered mental status, ingestion of corrosive agents, and loss of protective airway reflexes.[15]

Gastric Lavage

Gastric lavage was used in a total of 29,798 poisonings in 2001.[1] As with most methods of gastrointestinal decontamination, prompt administration of gastric lavage yields the highest efficacy. Gastric lavage can decrease the absorption of poisons by 10% to 25% if given within 30 to 60 minutes of the ingestion. However, gastric lavage is tedious to perform and time consuming.

Gastric lavage is performed with the patient in the left lateral decubitus position in a 15-degree Trendelenburg pose.[16] An orogastric tube is placed and its position confirmed by the aspiration of gastric contents or insufflation of air into the stomach. The stomach is drained of its contents and then filled with 100- to 200-mL aliquots of warm tap water or saline. The lavage fluid is then removed and the entire procedure repeated until the gastric contents are clear. Typically, 4 to 5 L of fluid are required for this technique.

Indications for gastric lavage include presentation to a health care facility within 1 hour of toxin ingestion or poisoning with a substance that is poorly absorbed by activated charcoal. Contraindications to gastric lavage include ingestion of a corrosive agent and history of esophageal or gastric pathology or surgery.[17, 18]

Complications associated with gastric lavage include placement of the orogastric tube into the trachea, esophageal perforation, aspiration, hypothermia, bleeding, cardiac arrhythmias, and hypoxia. Gastric lavage may also facilitate the movement of drug into the small intestine. Overall, gastric lavage may be a useful modality of decontamination if used within a narrow time period in appropriate patients.

Techniques That Enhance Elimination
Urinary Alkalinization and Acidification

Several normal physiologic mechanisms are involved in the elimination of drugs by the kidney. First, the drug may be filtered by the glomerulus. The principal determinant in the glomerular clearance of a drug is its degree of protein binding, because only unbound drug is available and readily filtered by the glomerulus. Second, the drug may be actively secreted into the tubule lumen through a variety of transport systems, which are commonly located within the proximal tubule. The third physiologic process that affects drug elimination by the kidney is passive distal tubule reabsorption.

This energy-independent process occurs more commonly during the elimination of lipid-soluble, nonionized drugs.

Several criteria determine whether a drug is amenable to urinary alkalinization. It must be (1) eliminated in a form unchanged by the kidney, (2) have extracellular distribution, (3) have a low level of protein binding, and (4) exist in a weakly acidic form with a dissociation constant (pK_a) of 3.0 to 7.5.

In the case of a toxic ingestion, urinary alkalinization and acidification are two processes used to enhance elimination. The goal of altering the urinary pH is to increase the ionized portion of the weak acid or weak base. By shifting the drug to its ionized form, passive reabsorption of the specific drug is inhibited. Depending on the type of replacement solution, the urinary pH can be altered. The dissociation of a weak acid or base into its ionized state is determined by its dissociation constant (pK_a). The pK_a is the pH at which the drug is 50% ionized and 50% nonionized. For example, the pK_a of salicylic acid is 3.0. When the urinary pH is 3.0, salicylate exists in a 1:1 ratio of ionized-to-nonionized drug. When urine is alkalinized to a pH of 7.4, the ratio is increased to approximately 20,000:1. The predominance of the ionized form allows enhanced elimination of the drug by decreasing its passive reabsorption.

Before initiating alkaline diuresis, a basic metabolic panel, urinary pH, arterial pH, and serum concentration of the ingested toxin should be obtained to establish baseline parameters. Urinary alkalinization can be achieved by using intravenous 5% dextrose in water (D_5W) or 0.2% or 0.45% saline with one to three ampules of sodium bicarbonate (i.e., 50 to 150 mEq) added to each liter. The rate of infusion should initially be based on the volume status of the patient. After volume expansion, the rate of fluid replacement should match the urine output, with a goal of 2 to 3 mL/kg/hour. In patients with altered sensorium, a urinary catheter may be placed for accurate monitoring of urinary output.

Serum electrolytes and urinary pH must be closely monitored every 2 to 3 hours during alkaline diuresis. The target range of urinary alkalinization is a pH value between 7.5 and 8.5. Urinary alkalinization effectively increases elimination of drugs such as phenobarbital, barbital, and salicylates. Complications of urinary alkalinization include hypokalemia, fluid overload, pulmonary edema, cerebral edema, hypernatremia (if free water restricted), and alkalemia. Alkalemia is of special concern in patients with renal dysfunction who are unable to excrete the bicarbonate load. Relative contraindications are congestive heart failure, renal failure, pulmonary edema, and cerebral edema. Intravenous diuretics may be used to enhance diuresis.

Acid diuresis is effective in the elimination of amphetamines, fenfluramine, phencyclidine, and quinine. To achieve an acid diuresis, intravenous arginine (10 g) or lysine hydrochloride (10 g) is administered in D_5 NS over 30 minutes, followed by oral ammonium chloride (4 g) every 2 hours. The goal of acid diuresis is a urinary pH of 5.5 to 6.5. However, acid diuresis has fallen out of favor due to its serious clinical sequelae of rhabdomyolysis and acute renal failure.[6, 19]

Antidotes

The management of certain poisonings requires the use of specific antidotes (Table 62-3). Although the use of antidotes

may markedly diminish the mortality rate associated with certain toxic exposures, most toxic ingestions have no specific antidote available.[4]

PRINCIPLES GOVERNING DRUG REMOVAL BY EXTRACORPOREAL TECHNIQUES

The clearance of a drug or toxin by extracorporeal therapy is determined by the pharmacokinetic and pharmacodynamic properties of the drug and by factors related to the extracorporeal technique itself (Table 62-4). The most important characteristics of the drug that influence its removal by dialysis include its molecular weight, the degree of protein binding, the volume of distribution, its lipid solubility and ionization, and rebound.[20, 21] Physical properties of dialysis that govern drug removal include the type of extracorporeal therapy used, properties of the specific dialysis membrane or cartridge, membrane surface area, blood flow rate, and dialysate flow rate.[22]

TABLE 62-3

Toxic Ingestions Treated with Specific Antidotes

POISON	ANTIDOTE
Acetaminophen	*N*-acetylcysteine
β-Blocking agents	Glucagon, atropine, isoproterenol
Carbon monoxide	Oxygen
Cyanide	Sodium nitrite, sodium thiosulfate, oxygen
Digoxin	Digoxin-specific Fab antibody fragment
Ethylene glycol and methyl alcohol	Ethanol, fomepizole
Isoniazid	Pyridoxine
Metallic poisons	
Arsenic	Dimercaprol
Iron	Deferoxamine
Lead	Dimercaprol, edetate disodium calcium, penicillamine
Mercury	Dimercaprol, penicillamine
Nitrates, nitrites, phenacetin	Methylene blue
Opioids	Naloxone
Codeine	
Heroin	
Meperidine	
Morphine	
Propoxyphene	
Organophosphates	Atropine, pralidoxime
Benzodiazepines	Flumazenil

TABLE 62-4

Factors That Enhance Drug Removal by Extracorporeal Therapy

DRUG-RELATED FACTORS	DIALYSIS-RELATED FACTORS
Low-molecular weight (<500 D)	Large surface area of dialysis membrane
Low protein binding (<80%)	High-flux dialyzer
Low volume of distribution (<1 L/kg)	High blood and dialysate flow
Water soluble	Increased ultrafiltration rate
Fast redistribution from peripheral compartments into blood	Increased time on dialysis

Drug-Related Factors

Molecular Weight

The molecular weight of a drug is a fundamental determinant in membrane transport. The larger the molecular weight, the slower is the rate of diffusion across a given membrane. Low-molecular-weight solutes (<500 daltons [D]) are readily filtered and diffuse easily through the pores of the membrane. The clearance of low-molecular-weight solutes depends primarily on the membrane surface area, blood-to-dialysate concentration gradient, and the blood and dialysate flow rates.[23] Middle-molecular-weight solutes (500 to 5000 D) and high-molecular-weight solutes (>5000 D) tend to diffuse more slowly across membranes. Because the larger solutes (>1000 D) have limited membrane permeability, their clearance is not determined by diffusion. The clearance of large solutes (>1000 D) depends on convection (or "solute drag" from ultrafiltration), membrane surface area, and time on dialysis.[23-25]

Protein Binding

The degree of protein binding by the toxin is another major determinant of drug clearance by extracorporeal therapy. Protein binding can occur in the plasma, most often to macromolecular proteins (albumin), or in the tissues to intracellular proteins. The degree of protein binding within the vascular space affects the mobility of the drug and limits the availability of unbound drug for transport into the peripheral tissues.

Protein binding in the plasma pharmacologically inactivates the drug and limits its clearance by glomerular filtration. Because the large size of the drug-protein complex also limits the ability of the drug to cross dialysis membranes, highly protein bound drugs are not easily removed by dialysis. It is only the unbound fraction of the drug that is pharmacologically active, metabolized, and available for removal by extracorporeal therapy.

Highly protein-bound drugs include arsenic, calcium channel blockers, diazepam, phenytoin, salicylate and other nonsteroidal anti-inflammatory drugs (NSAIDs), thyroxine, and tricyclic antidepressants. Compounds with minimal protein binding include the alcohols (e.g., methanol, ethylene glycol, isopropanol, ethanol), aminoglycosides, atenolol, and lithium.[26]

Many factors can affect the degree of protein binding, including the plasma protein concentration and toxin concentration.[21] In hypoalbuminemia (e.g., malnutrition, proteinuria), the decreased serum protein levels result in a decrease in available protein binding sites and an increase in the fraction of unbound, biologically active drug.[21] Certain pathologic states, including uremia,[27] acidosis, elevated free fatty acids,[28] temperature,[29] or the presence of displacing substances (e.g., organic acids, bilirubin, drugs[30]), can also alter protein binding and the fraction of unbound drug.

The uremic state is often associated with a reduction in drug-protein binding, resulting in an increase in the fraction of the unbound drug.[31, 32] This effect of uremia on drug-albumin affinity has been observed with several drugs such as penicillin, digitoxin, phenobarbital, phenytoin, warfarin, morphine, methotrexate, salicylate, theophylline, and sulfonamides.[27, 33-36]

Elevation in the levels of free fatty acids has a variable role in drug-protein binding. Certain antibiotics such as cefamandole are displaced from their albumin binding sites by the free fatty acids, but other cephalosporins such as cephalothin and cefoxitin have enhanced protein binding in the presence of free fatty acids.[28] Free fatty acids have also been shown to compete with other drugs for protein binding sites (e.g., tryptophan, sulfonamides, salicylates, phenylbutazone, phenytoin, valproic acid). In the setting of hemodialysis, administration of heparin activates lipoprotein lipase, releasing free fatty acids, which can then alter drug-protein binding.[30, 37, 38] Alterations in protein binding are especially clinically relevant in the setting of highly protein-bound drugs with a narrow therapeutic index (e.g., lithium, digoxin).

Volume of Distribution

The volume of distribution (V_d) is the apparent volume of water that a known amount of drug must be dissolved in to yield the observed steady-state plasma concentration. It is pharmacokinetically defined as follows:

$$V_d(L/kg) = \frac{Dose(mg/kg)}{Serum\,concentration(mg/L)}$$

It is a mathematical relationship that assumes the body is a single compartment of homogeneous water into which the drug is distributed. The V_d is one of the factors that determines the availability of a drug for removal by extracorporeal therapy. A low V_d implies that the drug is primarily restricted to the vascular space and is easily cleared by hemodialysis or hemoperfusion. Substances with a low V_d ($V_d < 0.5$ to 1.0 L/kg) include alcohols, salicylates, lithium, theophylline, atenolol, paracetamol, paraquat, sotalol, and aminoglycosides.

Substances that are highly bound in the peripheral tissues have a large V_d. These drugs are concentrated in the tissues, and the serum concentration therefore is low relative to the total body burden of the drug. These drugs are less accessible for clearance by extracorporeal techniques. Drugs with a large V_d ($V_d > 2$ L/kg) include calcium channel blockers, other β-blockers, chloroquine, colchicine, diazepam, digoxin, flecainide, quinidine, other antiarrhythmic drugs, organochlorine pesticides, phenothiazines, quinine, strychnine, metoclopramide, and tricyclic antidepressants.

The V_d of a drug can be altered by certain disease states, including renal failure.[31] In uremic patients, the V_d of digoxin is decreased compared with normal controls,[39] whereas the V_d of phenytoin is doubled in uremic patients compared with nonuremic patients.[40]

Lipid Solubility and Ionization

The degree of lipid solubility of a drug is a function of its partition coefficient, defined as the ratio between the concentration of the lipid, nonpolar phase, and the aqueous, polar phase of a nonionized drug at steady-state equilibrium.[23] The lipid solubility of a drug affects its transport across cell membranes and its accumulation throughout the body, especially to lipid-rich tissues (e.g., brain, fat). These lipophilic tissues serve as a reservoir, making the toxin inaccessible for removal by extracorporeal therapy.

The ionization state also affects the degree of lipid solubility. Nonionized drugs are more lipid soluble and can be easily transported across cell membranes. The ionized form does not readily cross cell membranes and is therefore more accessible for clearance by extracorporeal therapies. The degree of ionization of a drug is based on its pK_a, the pH at which the substance is 50% ionized and 50% nonionized. For a weak acid, as the pH increases above the pK_a, there is an increase in the ionized form. For a weak base, as the pH decreases below its pK_a, the ionized form increases. Because most drugs are weak acids or weak bases, their ionization state at physiologic pH affects their ability to transport across cell membranes and their availability in the vascular space for removal.

Rebound

Rebound refers to the movement of a drug from its peripheral tissues or cells into blood or plasma. If the redistribution of the drug from the tissues is slow, the total body clearance of the drug by extracorporeal therapy is hampered. The rebound phenomenon is seen in the elimination of drugs such as lithium,[41] methotrexate,[42] paraquat,[43] and digoxin.[44] Extracorporeal therapy removes the agent from the blood faster than it can be replaced from the peripheral compartment or tissue stores. In the case of lithium, hemodialysis effectively clears the lithium from the blood. After dialysis is discontinued, lithium slowly redistributes from the cells into the vascular space, resulting in the rebound of lithium a few hours after dialysis. In such cases, repeated dialysis or continuous therapy is required to eliminate the drug from the body.

Dialysis-Related Factors

Hemodialysis-related properties that influence drug elimination include the blood and dialysate flow rates, characteristics of the dialysis membrane (e.g., membrane type, surface area, porosity), the concentration gradient across the dialysis membrane, and the rate of ultrafiltration. The clearance of a drug by peritoneal dialysis depends on the transport characteristics of the peritoneal membrane, dialysate composition (e.g., pH, dextrose concentration, use of additives), frequency of exchanges, and dwell times. Hemofiltration depends on convective transport for solute removal. The rate of ultrafiltration, which depends on the blood flow rate, limits drug elimination in hemofiltration. These issues are discussed further in later sections as they pertain to each technique of extracorporeal therapy.

MEASUREMENTS OF DRUG REMOVAL EFFICIENCY: DIALYSANCE, CLEARANCE, AND EXTRACTION RATIO

Dialysance measures the efficiency of dialysis in the removal of solute. This is defined by the following equation:

$$D = Q_b \frac{(A - V)}{(A - D_b)}$$

In this equation, D is the dialysance, Q_b is the blood flow rate, A is the concentration of the drug entering the dialyzer, V is the concentration of the drug leaving the dialyzer, and D_b is the concentration of the drug in the dialysate. Dialysance takes

into account the decreasing blood-dialysate concentration gradient due to the increasing build-up of drug in the dialysate.[23] However, modern dialyzers use single-pass dialysis, in which the dialysate does not recirculate. When the concentration of a drug in the dialysate is negligible ($D_b = 0$), the dialysance is equivalent to the *dialysate clearance* (C). The clearance of solute is defined as follows:

$$C = Q_b \frac{A - V}{A} \quad \text{or} \quad Q_b \times \text{Extraction ratio}$$

The *extraction ratio* across a dialyzer is calculated as $(A - V)/A$. It represents the fraction of the drug removed from the plasma by the dialyzer. An extraction ratio of 1.0 represents complete elimination of a substance after a single pass through the extracorporeal circuit.

Although these measurements of solute removal assess the potential effectiveness of hemodialysis or hemoperfusion, they do not necessarily indicate that a clinically significant amount of drug is being removed from the body. The removal of the total burden of drug from the body relies on multiple factors, including the volume of distribution. For drugs with a large volume of distribution, the drug is primarily concentrated in the peripheral compartments and is not accessible for removal by extracorporeal therapy. Despite a high extraction ratio, only a minor fraction of the total body burden of the drug is eliminated after a single pass.

EXTRACORPOREAL TECHNIQUES FOR DRUG REMOVAL

After aggressive supportive therapy has failed in the setting of acute poisoning, extracorporeal treatment (i.e., hemodialysis, hemoperfusion, peritoneal dialysis, or hemofiltration) must be considered to increase clearance of the ingested toxin. The decision to initiate any form of extracorporeal therapy must take into account the patient's clinical status, drug-related factors, and dialysis-associated factors.[45]

There is no absolute drug level that indicates when dialysis must be initiated; instead, the decision is based on clinical judgment. Indications for extracorporeal therapy include progressive clinical deterioration despite aggressive supportive therapy, a drug or poison that can be removed at a rate that exceeds endogenous clearance, and ingestion of a dose that can cause toxicity or death for which supportive therapy is ineffective.

Hemodialysis

During hemodialysis, blood passes through an extracorporeal circuit that filters blood and toxins through a semipermeable membrane down a concentration gradient into dialysate. Hemodialysis is capable of correcting acute renal failure, pulmonary edema, and electrolyte disturbances (e.g., metabolic acidosis) that may accompany poisoning.

Features of the dialysis system that influence drug clearance include membrane type, surface area, and blood and dialysate flow rates. The newer, high-flux, biocompatible, more permeable membranes can remove high-molecular-weight substances. The larger the surface area of the dialyzer, the greater is the amount of the drug removed. Increasing the blood flow and dialysate flow rates helps to maintain an optimal concentration gradient between the blood and dialysate, resulting in greater diffusion and elimination of the drug.

Hemodialysis depends predominantly on diffusion, with a smaller contribution from convection for drug removal. As the molecular weight of a drug increases, its elimination is limited by the pore size of the dialyzer membrane. In this setting, clearance of the drug becomes more dependent on convection and the rate of ultrafiltration to increase solvent drag.

Characteristics of the ingested drug that make hemodialysis effective in toxin removal are low molecular weight (<500 D), small volume of distribution (<1 L/kg), low degree of protein binding, and a high level of water solubility. Drugs and chemicals that are removed by dialysis and hemoperfusion are listed in Table 62-5.[46]

It is also important to consider the rebound phenomenon after dialysis. Rebound occurs when the drug redistributes from tissues into the plasma after its removal from the plasma compartment. It is important to check drug concentration levels and provide continued renal replacement therapy or repeated dialysis sessions.

Acute hemodialysis requires cannulation of a large vessel and placement of a temporary double-lumen dialysis catheter. Femoral catheter insertions are quick and prone to fewer complications than subclavian lines. The extracorporeal circuit for hemodialysis consists of dialysis blood lines, a blood pump, and pressure devices. Systemic anticoagulation with heparin infused at approximately 2000 U/hour is also necessary to prevent clotting of the hemodialysis system. A blood flow rate of more than 300 mL/minute is considered efficient for drug removal. Pressure devices detect interior rises in pressure, which indicate clot formation within the device. The duration of the therapy is usually 4 to 8 hours but should be governed by the clinical response and serum drug concentrations. Complications of hemodialysis include laceration of the cannulated vessel, air embolus, hypotension, and bleeding due to anticoagulation. Relative contraindications of hemodialysis are active hemorrhage, coagulopathy, and hemodynamic instability.

There are no randomized, controlled studies to show that hemodialysis improves morbidity and mortality over supportive care or other modalities of therapy. The role of hemodialysis in acute poisoning is declining, which is attributed to improvements in aggressive supportive measures and the development of antidotes.

Hemoperfusion

Hemoperfusion is a procedure that involves the passage of blood through an extracorporeal circuit with a disposable, sorbent-containing cartridge.[47] There are various types of sorbent cartridges, and the most commonly available cartridges contain 100 to 300 g of activated charcoal or an exchange resin. The choice of cartridge depends on body size and properties of the drug involved. For example, a small cartridge is used for a child, and XAD-4 is used for lipid-soluble drugs such as glutethimide.[22] Activated charcoal originally consisted of uncoated granular carbon. Problems associated with the earlier cartridges included adsorption of platelets by charcoal, hypocalcemia, and complement release. The charcoal now is coated with albumin cellulose nitrate, which has improved its biocompatibility.

Charcoal hemoperfusion, which adsorbs polar and nonpolar drugs, has been used in the setting of various types of poisoning. Although certain exchange resins are highly effective in their removal of lipid-soluble drugs, they are no longer available in the United States. Available hemoperfusion devices are listed in Table 62-6.[46]

The extracorporeal circuit for hemoperfusion is similar to hemodialysis aside from the disposable adsorbent cartridges. The administration of hemoperfusion requires temporary vascular access through a double-lumen dialysis catheter. Blood is anticoagulated with heparin infusing at approximately 2000 U/hour to avoid clotting of the system. A blood flow rate maintained at more than 300 mL/minute is considered efficient for drug removal. Like hemodialysis, pressure devices detect interior rises in pressure caused by clot formation. Patients on hemoperfusion therapy must be monitored carefully for potential complications such as (1) mild thrombocytopenia and an average platelet loss of 30% caused by adsorption of platelets by the activated charcoal, with recovery of the platelet count within 24 to 48 hours; (2) transient leukopenia secondary to complement activation by surface contact and margination of leukocytes; (3) reduction of fibrinogen and fibronectin caused by charcoal adsorption; (4) hypothermia from the reinfusion of a large volume of unheated extracorporeal blood; (5) hypocalcemia due to absorption by charcoal; and (6) hypoglycemia. Most of these complications have been associated with the early charcoal devices. Coating the charcoal particles with a polymer solution has reduced such complications and has improved biocompatibility of these devices. Despite these newer cartridges, hemoperfusion still carries a higher risk for complications compared with hemodialysis. The decision to initiate hemoperfusion should be considered with caution.

Other considerations before starting hemoperfusion therapy are related to the properties of the drug ingested. Hemoperfusion is preferred when the toxin is lipid soluble or highly protein bound. However, if the toxin is eliminated equally well by hemodialysis and hemoperfusion, hemodialysis is the preferred treatment modality. Hemodialysis involves fewer complications, allows rapid correction of electrolyte disturbances, and is technically easier to perform. No randomized, controlled studies have compared hemodialysis with hemoperfusion and examined its range of indications, potential benefits, and cost effectiveness in the setting of acute poisoning. Consideration should be given to hemoperfusion in severe cases with specific toxins, especially if the extraction ratio is higher for hemoperfusion than hemodialysis or other modalities.

The principal disadvantage of hemoperfusion is the saturation of the adsorbent cartridge with time. Saturation, which occurs after 4 to 8 hours, results from the clotting and adherence of cellular debris and plasma proteins to the adsorbent.

Hemodialysis-Hemoperfusion

The concurrent use of hemodialysis and hemoperfusion is theoretically the optimal treatment in acute poisoning because it effectively removes toxin by adsorption and diffusion. However, hemodialysis-hemoperfusion is an expensive procedure, and the data on clinical outcomes are lacking. There are several case reports in which blood level

TABLE 62-5

Drugs and Chemicals Removed with Dialysis and Hemoperfusion

Antimicrobials or Anticancer Drugs

Cefaclor
Cefadroxil
Cefamandole
Cefazolin
Cefixime
Cefmenoxime
Cefmetazole
(Cefonicid)*
(Cefoperazone)*
Ceforanide
(Cefotaxime)*
Cefotetan
Cefotiam
Cefoxitin
Cefpirome
Cefroxadine
Cefsulodin
Ceftazidime
(Ceftriaxone)*
Cefuroxime
Cephacetrile
Cephalexin
Cephalothin
(Cephapirin)*
Cephradine
Moxalactam
Amikacin
Dibekacin
Fosfomycin
Gentamicin
Kanamycin
Neomycin
Netilmicin
Sisomicin
Streptomycin
Tobramycin
Bacitracin
Aztreonam
Cilastatin
Imipenem
(Chloramphenicol)*
(Amphotericin)†
Ciprofloxacin
(Enoxacin)*
Fleroxacin
(Norfloxacin)*
Ofloxacin
Isoniazid
(Vancomycin)*
Capreomycin
Periodic acid–Schiff
Pyrazinamide
(Rifampin)*
(Cycloserine)*
Ethambutol
5-Fluorocytosine
Acyclovir
(Amantadine)*
Didanosine
Foscarnet
Ganciclovir
(Ribavirin)*
Vidarabine
Zidovudine
(Pentamidine)*
(Praziquantel)*

(Fluconazole)*
(Itraconazole)*
(Ketoconazole)*
(Miconazole)*
(Chloroquine)*
(Quinine)*
(Azathioprine)*
Bredinin
Busulphan
Cyclophosphamide
(Diazepam)*
(Diphenylhydantoin)*
(Diphenylhydramine)*
Ethinamate
Ethchlorvynol
Ethosuximide
Gallamine
Glutethimide
(Heroin)*
Meprobamate
(Methaqualone)*
Methsuximide
Methyprylon
Paraldehyde
Primidone
Valproic acid

Cardiovascular Agents

Acebutolol
(Amiodarone)*
Amrinone
(Digoxin)*
Enalapril
Fosinopril
Lisinopril
Quinapril
Ramipril
(Encainide)*
(Flecainide)*
(Lidocaine)*
Metoprolol
Methyldopa
(Ouabain)*
N-Acetylprocainamide
Nadolol
(Pindolol)*
Practolol
Procainamide
Tranylcypromine
(Tricyclics)*

Solvents, Gases

Acetone
Camphor
Carbon monoxide
(Carbon tetrachloride)*
(Eucalyptus oil)*
Thiols
Toluene
Trichloroethylene

Plants, Animals, Herbicides, Insecticides

Alkyl phosphate
Amanitin
Demeton sulfoxide
Dimethoate
Diquat
Glufosinate

Methylmercury complex
(Organophosphates)*
Paraquat
Snake bite
Sodium chlorate
Potassium chlorate

Miscellaneous

Acipimox
Allopurinol
Aminophylline
Aniline
Borates
Boric acid
(Chlorpropamide)*
Chromic Acid
(Cimetidine)*
Colistin
Amoxicillin
Ampicillin
Azlocillin
Carbenicillin
Clavulanic acid
(Cloxacillin)*
(Dicloxacillin)*
(Floxacillin)*
Mecillinam
(Mezlocillin)*
(Methicillin)*
(Nafcillin)*
Penicillin
Piperacillin
Temocillin
Ticarcillin
(Clindamycin)*
(Erythromycin)*
(Azithromycin)*
(Clarithromycin)*
Metronidazole
Nitrofurantoin
Ornidazole
Sulfisoxazole
Sulfonamides
Tetracycline
(Doxycycline)*
(Minocycline)*
Tinidazole
Trimethoprim
5-Fluorouracil
(Methotrexate)*

Barbiturates

Amobarbital
Aprobarbital
Barbital
Butabarbital
Cyclobarbital
Pentobarbital
Phenobarbital
Quinalbital
(Secobarbital)*

Nonbarbiturate Hypnotics, Sedatives, Tranquilizers, Anticonvulsants

Carbamazepine
Atenolol
Betaxolol

(Bretylium)*
Clonidine
(Calcium channel blockers)*
Captopril
(Diazoxide)*
Carbromal
Chloral hydrate
(Chlordiazepoxide)*
Propranolol
(Quinidine)*
(Timolol)*
Sotalol
Tocainide

Alcohols

Ethanol
Ethylene glycol
Isopropanol
Methanol

Analgesics, Antirheumatics

Acetaminophen
Acetophenetidin
Acetylsalicylic acid
Colchicine
Methylsalicylate
(D-Propoxyphene)*
Salicyclic acid

Antidepressants

(Amitriptyline)*
Amphetamines
(Imipramine)*
Isocarboxazid
MAO inhibitors
Moclobemide
(Pargyline)*
(Phenelzine)*
Dinitro-O-cresol
Folic acid
Mannitol
Methylprednisolone
4-Methylpyrazole
Sodium citrate
Theophylline
Thiocyanate
Ranitidine

Metals, Inorganics

(Aluminum)†
Arsenic
Barium
Bromide
(Copper)†
(Iron)†
(Lead)†
Lithium
(Magnesium)*
(Mercury)†
Potassium
(Potassium dichromate)†
Phosphate
Sodium
Strontium
(Thallium)†
(Tin)*
(Zinc)*

*Poor removal.
†Removed with a chelating agent.
Adapted from Winchester JF: Dialysis and hemoperfusion in poisoning. Adv Ren Replace Ther 9:20-30, 2002.

TABLE 62-6

Available Hemoperfusion Devices

MANUFACTURER	DEVICE	SORBENT TYPE	AMOUNT OF SORBENT	POLYMER COATING
Asahi	Hemosorba	Petroleum-based spherical charcoal	170 g	Polyhema
Clark	Biocompatible system	Charcoal	50, 100, or 250 cc	Heparinized polymer
Gambro	Adsorba	Norit	100 or 300 g	Cellulose acetate
Organon-Teknika	Hemopur	Norit extruded charcoal	260 g	Cellulose acetate

From Winchester JF: Dialysis and hemoperfusion in poisoning. Adv Ren Replace Ther 9:20-30, 2002.

measurements demonstrated efficient clearance of toxins with hemodialysis-hemoperfusion.[48-50] However, the data comparing hemodialysis-hemoperfusion therapy to the various individual modalities are limited. Combination therapy is useful for toxins with a small volume of distribution. For drugs with larger volumes of distribution, the duration of treatment may be extended or the procedure repeated after the toxin redistributes back into the plasma.

Hemodialysis and hemoperfusion with chelating agents have been used in end-stage renal disease (ESRD) patients with aluminum (Al) and iron (Fe) intoxication.[51] The patients are treated with deferoxamine (DFO) in addition to dialysis or hemoperfusion. This therapy removes the DFO-Al or DFO-Fe complex and results in the clinical improvement of renal osteodystrophy, encephalopathy, iron overload, and anemia.

Hemofiltration

Hemofiltration is a process in which solutes are removed by convection. Drug elimination by hemofiltration depends on the rate of ultrafiltration, the drug protein binding, and the sieving coefficient of the membrane. The sieving coefficient is the mathematical expression of the ability of a solute to cross a membrane by convection. It is determined from the ratio of the solute concentration in the ultrafiltrate to the solute concentration in the plasma.[52] The process of hemofiltration efficiently eliminates high-molecular-weight toxins (40,000 D). Most poisons, however, are smaller, with a molecular size of less than 1000 D. Hemofiltration does not offer much advantage over hemodialysis. More important than size is the issue of protein binding, because hemofiltration removes only unbound drug from the vascular space.[53]

Continuous Renal Replacement Therapy

Continuous renal replacement therapy (CRRT) involves dialysis (i.e., diffusive transport) or filtration (i.e., convective transport) treatments that operate in a continuous mode. This form of treatment was developed for critically ill patients who were hypotensive and unable to tolerate conventional dialysis because of the rapid rate of solute and fluid loss. There are various types of CRRT, including continuous arteriovenous hemofiltration (CAVH), continuous

venovenous hemofiltration (CVVH), or CRRT combined with hemodialysis or hemoperfusion. During CAVH, blood exits the body from an artery and reenters through a vein. In CVVH, blood exits and enters through a vein with the assistance of a pump, which provides pressure to maintain adequate blood flow through the extracorporeal system.

CRRT is rarely used in patients with acute intoxication because of its low efficiency. However, CRRT is advantageous when the ingested drug has a large volume of distribution and slow rate of redistribution from the peripheral tissue. It has been used successfully to treat life-threatening lithium intoxication.[54] Extending treatment time and gradually removing intracellular lithium completely prevented postdialysis rebound.

Peritoneal Dialysis

There is little role for peritoneal dialysis in acute poisoning. It is a relatively inefficient method, achieving only 10 to 15 mL/minute of maximum drug clearance. The characteristics of the ingested drug that optimize elimination through peritoneal dialysis include low molecular weight, water solubility, low protein binding, and low volume of distribution. Solute removal also depends on the characteristics of the peritoneal membrane (i.e., low, average, or high transport status), dialysate composition, frequency of exchanges, and dwell time.

The composition of dialysate can be modified in several ways. By raising the dextrose concentration of the dialysate, ultrafiltration and convective transport are increased, resulting in enhanced elimination of water-soluble substances. Altering the dialysate pH above the pK_a for a weakly acidic drug can promote a shift to its ionized form, resulting in improved solute clearance from the body. The addition of albumin to the dialysate has been used to enhance the elimination of highly protein bound substances such as barbiturates.[55] Administration of preheated dialysate has been clinically effective in rapidly reversing hypothermia.[22]

Acute peritoneal access involves the placement of a semirigid catheter by the bedside, which is time consuming and often requires consultation with a surgeon. Approximately 2 L of sterile, preheated dialysate is placed in the peritoneal cavity, allowed to dwell for about 30 minutes, and then drained. Exchanges are usually performed hourly in the setting of acute intoxication.

Peritoneal dialysis is a less efficient method of detoxification than hemodialysis or hemoperfusion. Essentially, there are no advantages of peritoneal dialysis compared with hemodialysis in the setting of acute poisoning, unless other methods of extracorporeal therapy are unavailable.

Plasma Exchange

Plasma exchange is a process in which large quantities of plasma are removed from the patient and replaced with fresh frozen plasma or stored plasma. In acute poisoning, the role of plasma exchange is not well defined. Plasma exchange is used for toxins that are highly protein bound (>80%) and have low volumes of distribution (<0.2 L/kg of body weight).[56] Another indication for plasma exchange is in the management of sodium chlorate poisoning, which causes hemolytic anemia. Plasma exchange removes sodium chlorate and eliminates red cell fragments and free hemoglobin.[57] Adverse outcomes from plasma exchange involve complications associated with the insertion of vascular access, bleeding, and allergy to the replacement plasma proteins.

INTOXICATIONS RESPONSIVE TO EXTRACORPOREAL THERAPY

Alcohols: Ethylene Glycol, Methanol, and Isopropanol

Intoxications with ethylene glycol, methanol, or isopropanol are associated with significant morbidity and mortality. However, these ingestions are also treatable. If appropriate treatment is initiated early, the prognosis is excellent. These substances and their metabolites share several characteristics that make them ideal for removal by hemodialysis: low molecular weight, small volume of distribution, water solubility, and low levels of protein binding.

Ethylene Glycol
PHARMACOLOGY

Ethylene glycol is a colorless, odorless, sweet-tasting substance most commonly found in antifreeze. It is also used in solvents, hydraulic brake fluid, de-icing solutions, detergents, lacquers, and polishes. In adults, the ingestion is often intentional because ethylene glycol is an inexpensive substitute for ethanol or a means of suicide.

Ethylene glycol is rapidly absorbed by the gastrointestinal system. It reaches a peak serum concentration 1 to 4 hours after ingestion and has an elimination half-life of 3 hours. The molecular weight of ethylene glycol is 62 g/mol, and it is highly water soluble with a low volume of distribution of 0.5 to 0.8 L/kg.[58] The accepted minimum lethal dose of ethylene glycol for an adult is 1.0 to 1.5 mL/kg or 100 mL.

METABOLISM

Ethylene glycol itself is not toxic; instead, it is the accumulation of its metabolites that is responsible for its severe toxicity. Figure 62-1 illustrates the oxidative pathway of ethylene glycol metabolism. In the presence of the electron acceptor, nicotinamide adenine dinucleotide (NAD), ethylene glycol is oxidized to glycoaldehyde by alcohol dehydrogenase. Aldehyde dehydrogenase then rapidly converts glycoaldehyde to glycolic acid, followed by the slow conversion of glycolic acid to glyoxylic acid, which is the rate-limiting step in ethylene glycol metabolism. The final end products include oxalic acid, glycine, oxalomalic acid, and formic acid. Ethanol and fomepizole interfere with the breakdown of ethylene glycol by competitively inhibiting alcohol dehydrogenase.

PATHOPHYSIOLOGY

The underlying mechanisms of ethylene glycol toxicity are tissue destruction from calcium oxalate deposition and profound acidosis due to the accumulation of its metabolites (e.g., glycoaldehyde, glycolic acid, lactate). Systemic calcium oxalate deposition has been observed in the kidneys, heart and pericardium, meningeal vessels, brain, vasculature, spleen, and liver.[58, 59] In the kidney, reversible acute renal failure often develops. Acute tubular necrosis from calcium oxalate deposition in the proximal tubules, interstitial nephritis, focal hemorrhagic cortical necrosis, direct renal cytotoxicity, and obstruction are suggested mechanisms of renal toxicity in ethylene glycol poisoning.[58, 60, 61] The pathognomonic findings of ethylene glycol toxicity are the presence of calcium oxalate crystals in the kidney and acute tubular necrosis.[62] However, because the degree of renal injury does not correlate with the amount of calcium oxalate deposition in the kidney, it has been suggested that glycolic acid or its metabolites are primarily responsible for the renal failure.[63]

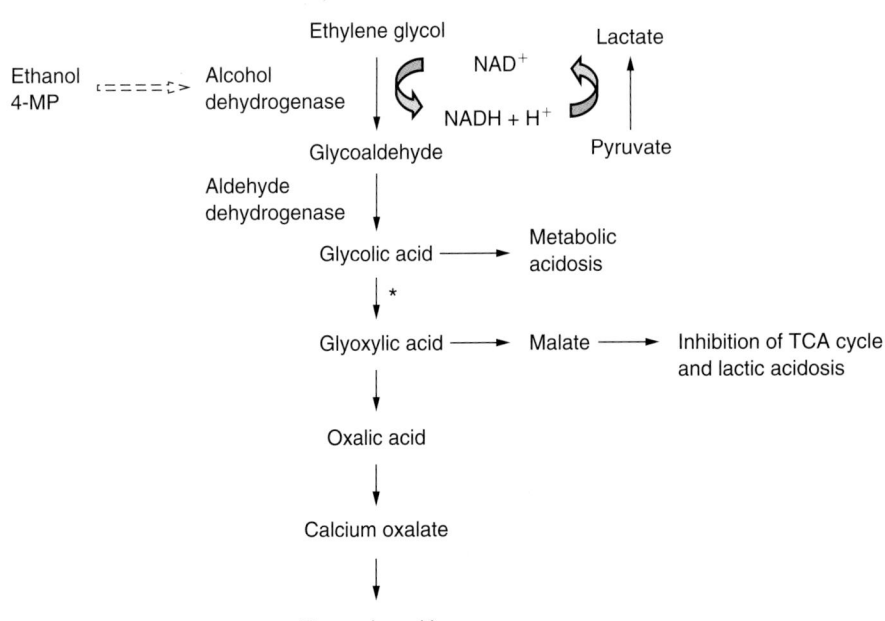

FIGURE 62-1. Metabolism of ethylene glycol. 4-MP, fomepizole; NAD⁺, nicotinamide adenine dinucleotide; NADH⁺, reduced form of nicotinamide adenine dinucleotide; TCA, tricarboxylic acid; *broken arrow*, inhibitors of alcohol dehydrogenase; *asterisk*, rate-limiting step.

The metabolic acidosis results from the formation of glycolic acid and increased lactic acid production. Because the rate-limiting step is the conversion of glycolic acid to glyoxylic acid, there is an accumulation of glycolic acid. Increases in glycolic acid levels correlate with increases in the anion gap and decreases in serum bicarbonate.[64] Glyoxylic acid and its byproducts inhibit the citric acid cycle, resulting in the accumulation of lactic acid.[65] A final contribution to the metabolic acidosis is the decrease in the NAD/NADH ratio during ethylene glycol metabolism. By changing the oxidation-to-reduction ratio of NAD/NADH, the reduction of pyruvate to lactate is favored. These mechanisms are responsible for the severe metabolic acidosis associated with ethylene glycol toxicity.

CLINICAL PRESENTATION

The clinical course of ethylene glycol toxicity occurs in three phases. The severity and progression of each stage depends on certain factors, such as the dose of ethylene glycol ingested, concurrent ingestion of ethanol, and timing of treatment.[66]

Phase 1 is the neurologic phase, occurring 0.5 to 12 hours after ingestion. Shortly after ethylene glycol ingestion, patients appear inebriated, similar to that observed with ethanol intoxication, but without the odor of alcohol on their breath. Because of the gastrointestinal irritation from ethylene glycol, they may develop nausea, vomiting, and hematemesis. As ethylene glycol undergoes oxidation to glycoaldehyde and glycolic acid (4 to 12 hours after ingestion), symptoms of CNS depression predominate. Altered consciousness may progress to coma and seizures in severe poisonings. Cerebral edema, nystagmus, ataxia, ophthalmoplegias, myoclonic jerks, and hyporeflexia may also occur.

Phase 2 is the cardiopulmonary phase, occurring 12 to 24 hours after ingestion. During the second phase of ethylene glycol intoxication, calcium oxalate crystals deposit in the vasculature, myocardium, and lungs. Patients may develop tachycardia, mild hypertension, congestive heart failure, acute respiratory distress syndrome, severe metabolic acidosis, and multiorgan failure. Most deaths occur during this phase.[1, 67]

Phase 3 is the renal phase, occurring 24 to 72 hours after ingestion. In this final stage, calcium oxalate precipitates in the kidney, resulting in flank pain, acute tubular necrosis, hypocalcemia, microscopic hematuria, and oliguric acute renal failure.

With early medical intervention, ethylene glycol toxicity tends to resolve completely. The removal of ethylene glycol and its toxic metabolites, as well as prevention of calcium oxalate formation, can reverse tissue destruction. Renal recovery is generally complete with proper supportive therapy, although permanent renal, CNS, and cranial nerve damage has been described.[59]

DIAGNOSIS AND LABORATORY DATA

The diagnosis of ethylene glycol toxicity should be suspected in patients who present with the following features: inebriation without the smell of alcohol on their breath, high–anion gap metabolic acidosis, altered mental status, osmolal gap, hypocalcemia, and calcium oxalate crystals in the urine.[58] The clinical utility of the osmolal gap is discussed in reference to ethylene glycol overdose, although its use may be applied to all the alcohol poisonings.

The *osmolal gap* is an extremely useful diagnostic tool in the various alcohol intoxications. The combination of a high–anion gap metabolic acidosis, osmolal gap, and hypocalcemia strongly suggests ethylene glycol intoxication. Because ethylene glycol is an osmotically active compound, it creates an osmolal gap. The osmolal gap is an estimation of the unmeasured, osmotically active substances in the serum. It is the difference between the measured osmolality, as determined by the freezing point depression method, and the calculated osmolality:

$$\Delta Osm_{gap} = Osm_{measured} - Osm_{calculated}$$

In this equation, ΔOsm_{gap} is the osmolal gap (mOsm/kg), $Osm_{measured}$ is the measured osmolality (mOsm/kg), and $Osm_{calculated}$ is the calculated osmolality (mOsm/kg). The calculated osmolality is based on the concentrations of sodium, glucose, and blood urea nitrogen in the serum. If coingestion of ethanol is suspected, the contribution of ethanol should be corrected for in the calculated osmolality as follows:

$$Osm_{calculated}(mOsm/kg) = 2[Na] + \frac{[glucose]}{18} + \frac{[BUN]}{2.8} + \left[\frac{[ethanol]}{4.6}\right]$$

In this equation, [Na] is the concentration of sodium in mEq/L, [glucose] is the concentration of glucose in mg/dL, and [BUN] is the concentration of blood urea nitrogen in mg/dL. The measured osmolality normally ranges between 270 and 290 mOsm/kg, and the normal osmolal gap is less than 10 to 12 mOsm/kg H_2O. An elevated osmolal gap suggests the presence of ethylene glycol, methanol, ethanol, isopropanol, propylene glycol, or acetone.

It is important to recognize that, although an elevated osmolal gap is a significant clinical finding, a normal osmolal gap does not exclude the diagnosis of ethylene glycol or methanol poisoning.[68, 69] In the case of ethylene glycol toxicity, glycolic acid does not contribute to the osmolal gap. As ethylene glycol is metabolized to glycolic acid, the osmolal gap may decrease to normal. Patients who present later in the course of their ethylene glycol intoxication may have a normal osmolal gap.[70]

The osmolal gap is also clinically useful in estimating the serum concentration of the toxin. The following equation can be used:

$$Concentration\ of\ toxin\ (mg/dL) = \Delta Osm_{gap} \times \frac{MW\ of\ toxin}{10}$$

In this equation, ΔOsm_{gap} is the osmolal gap, and MW is the molecular weight of the toxin: acetone (58 D), ethanol (46 D), ethylene glycol (62 D), isopropanol (60 D), and methanol (32 D). Using this calculation, serial measurements of the osmolal gap can be used to monitor changes in the ethylene glycol level during hemodialysis. This is especially useful if serum drug levels are not readily available to guide therapy during treatment. At a concentration of 100 mg/dL, the contribution to the osmolal gap is as follows: acetone (18 mOsm/kg H_2O), ethanol (22 mOsm/kg H_2O), ethylene glycol (16 mOsm/kg H_2O), isopropanol (17 mOsm/kg H_2O), and methanol (31 mOsm/kg H_2O).[59]

Urinalysis can often provide supporting evidence of ethylene glycol toxicity. Calcium oxalate crystals (monohydrate and dihydrate forms) may be present in the urine sediment and are birefringent when viewed under polarized light. Urinary calcium oxalate crystals appear 4 to 8 hours after ingestion[71, 72] and are found in approximately 50% of patients with ethylene glycol intoxication.[73] The presence in urine of the monohydrate form, described as prism or dumbbell shaped, is not specific for ethylene glycol toxicity because this can also normally be seen in individuals who ingest large amounts of vitamin C or high oxalate-containing foods (e.g., cocoa, garlic, tea, tomatoes, spinach, rhubarb). The dihydrate form, which is octahedral or tent shaped, is present only under high urinary calcium and oxalate conditions; therefore, the presence of the dihydrate form is more specific for ethylene glycol toxicity.

Urine that fluoresces under Wood lamp illumination is another unique feature of ethylene glycol ingestion. Many types of antifreeze contain sodium fluorescein, a fluorescent dye used as a marker to detect radiator leaks. For up to 6 hours after ingestion, sodium fluorescein can be detected in the urine. The presence of fluorescent urine by Wood lamp examination suggests ethylene glycol intoxication caused by antifreeze ingestion.[74]

In addition to the high–anion gap metabolic acidosis seen in ethylene glycol toxicity, other laboratory abnormalities may be observed. Hypocalcemia, caused by the formation of calcium oxalate complexes, can result in prolonged QT on ECG. Microscopic hematuria, leukocytosis, and an elevated protein level in cerebral spinal fluid may also be found.

Because the serum level of glycolic acid, which is primarily responsible for metabolic acidosis in ethylene glycol intoxication, correlates well with the increase in the anion gap and decrease in the serum bicarbonate level,[64] serial measurements of the anion gap can be used to monitor the improvement in metabolic acidosis during treatment.

TREATMENT

As with any intoxication, supportive therapy should be directed toward stabilization of the airway, breathing, and circulatory system. Intravenous glucose (50 mL of 50% glucose) should be administered in patients with altered mental status. If the patient is a suspected alcoholic or is malnourished, thiamine (100 mg every 6 hours), multivitamin supplementation, and pyridoxine (50 mg every 6 hours) should be given. Aggressive fluid resuscitation to maintain urine output, correct dehydration, and support circulatory shock should be initiated, although this must be done with caution to avoid volume overload in the setting of renal dysfunction. Metabolic acidosis should be treated with intravenous sodium bicarbonate therapy, especially if the serum bicarbonate concentration is less than 15 mEq/L or the arterial pH is less than 7.35.

Seizures, which may be caused by hypocalcemia, should be controlled with standard anticonvulsant therapy. In general, asymptomatic hypocalcemia is not routinely treated in the setting of ethylene glycol intoxication because this may potentially exacerbate calcium oxalate crystal formation and deposition. If seizures persist despite adequate anticonvulsant therapy, 10 to 20 mL of 10% calcium gluconate (0.2 to 0.3 mL/kg) can be infused slowly.

The antidotes for ethylene glycol toxicity are ethanol and fomepizole. Indications for use of an antidote in ethylene glycol toxicity according to the American Academy of Clinical Toxicology (AACT) guidelines are (1) a plasma ethylene glycol concentration of more than 20 mg/dL, (2) documented recent ingestion of toxic amounts of ethylene glycol and osmolal gap of more than 10 mOsm/L, or (3) a history or strong clinical suspicion of ethylene glycol poisoning and at least two of the following: arterial pH less than 7.3, serum bicarbonate level of less than 20 mEq/L, osmolal gap of more than 10 mOsm/L, or presence of oxalate crystals in the urine.[58]

Ethanol has been the traditional antidote for ethylene glycol and methanol intoxication. Because alcohol dehydrogenase has a 100-fold greater affinity for ethanol than ethylene glycol, the ethanol competitively inhibits alcohol dehydrogenase and prevents the metabolism of ethylene glycol to its toxic intermediates. At an ethanol serum concentration of 50 to 100 mg/dL, the active sites on alcohol dehydrogenase are saturated.[75]

Ethanol can be given intravenously as 10% ethanol diluted in D_5W. The loading dose of ethanol is 0.6 to 0.7 g ethanol/kg (7.6 mL 10% ethanol/kg), and the maintenance dose is 66 mg ethanol/kg/hour (0.83 mL 10% ethanol/kg/hour) for nondrinkers and 154 mg ethanol/kg/hour (1.96 mL 10% ethanol/kg/hour) for alcoholics. If hemodialysis is initiated, the ethanol dose must be adjusted to replace the ethanol removed during dialysis. The maintenance dose during dialysis is 169 mg ethanol/kg/hour (2.13 mL 10% ethanol/kg/hour) for nondrinkers and 257 mg ethanol/kg/hour (3.26 mL 10% ethanol/kg/hour) in alcoholics.[58, 76] Ethanol may also be added to the dialysate to give a concentration of 100 mg/dL using 95% ethanol instead.[77, 78] Serum ethanol concentrations should be monitored every 1 to 2 hours to ensure that blood levels remain therapeutic at 100 to 150 mg ethanol/dL.

The adverse side effects of ethanol are hypoglycemia, inebriation, CNS depression, emotional lability, poor coordination, and slurred speech. The altered mental status from ethanol therapy may mask the signs and symptoms of ethylene glycol toxicity. Use of ethanol requires close monitoring of serum ethanol levels to maintain therapeutic levels because its pharmacokinetic properties are erratic. Ethanol is not necessarily an ideal antidote.

Fomepizole (4-MP, 4-methylpyrazole) is a newer antidote that is a potent competitive inhibitor of alcohol dehydrogenase. By inhibiting alcohol dehydrogenase, fomepizole effectively blocks the formation of toxic metabolites and prevents end-organ damage in ethylene glycol and methanol ingestions. The U.S. Food and Drug Administration (FDA) has approved the use of fomepizole as first-line treatment for acute ethylene glycol intoxication (December 1997) and acute methanol toxicity (December 2000). There are several advantages of fomepizole compared with ethanol: (1) more potent inhibitor of alcohol dehydrogenase than ethanol, (2) ease of dosing, (3) predictable pharmacokinetics and no blood monitoring, (4) few adverse side effects with no CNS depression or hepatotoxicity, and (5) longer duration of action than ethanol.

The primary disadvantage of fomepizole is its cost. Adverse side effects include headache, nausea, dizziness, eosinophilia, rash, tachycardia or bradycardia, and mild but transient elevation of the hepatic transaminases. Most of these side effects were thought to be attributable to the toxic ingestion rather than fomepizole.[79]

Fomepizole is administered intravenously over 30 minutes. The loading dose of fomepizole is 15 mg/kg, followed by 10 mg/kg every 12 hours for 4 doses (i.e., 48 hours). After 48 hours, fomepizole is continued at 15 mg/kg every 12 hours until the ethylene glycol concentration is undetectable or less than 20 mg/dL *and* the patient is asymptomatic and has a normal arterial pH.[80] During hemodialysis, the dosing interval must be changed to every 4 hours, or a constant infusion of 1.0 to 1.5 mg/kg/hour can be used to maintain adequate therapeutic levels of fomepizole.[81]

Hemodialysis is an extremely effective method in the removal of ethylene glycol and its toxic metabolite, glycolic acid. The clearance of ethylene glycol ranges from 145 to 230 mL/minute and depends on the type of dialyzer and the blood flow rate. The elimination half-life of ethylene glycol on hemodialysis is 2.5 to 3.5 hours.[58, 78, 82] Glycolic acid is also easily eliminated by hemodialysis, with a clearance rate of 105 to 170 mL/minute and an elimination half-life of 2.5 hours.[58, 83]

Indications for hemodialysis are as follows: deteriorating clinical status despite supportive therapy, metabolic acidosis (arterial pH < 7.3), renal failure, or electrolyte abnormalities unresponsive to standard treatment. Traditionally, an ethylene glycol level of more than 50 mg/dL was an indication for hemodialysis. However, reports have described patients with normal renal function and no evidence of metabolic acidosis who have been effectively treated with fomepizole despite ethylene glycol levels of more than 50 mg/dL.[84, 85]

Hemodialysis should be continued until the ethylene glycol level is undetectable or until the ethylene glycol level is less than 20 mg/dL, no metabolic acidosis is present, and no evidence of systemic toxicity persists. Rebound distribution of ethylene glycol may occur within 12 hours of discontinuing hemodialysis; therefore, serum osmolality and electrolytes should be closely monitored every 2 to 4 hours for 12 to 24 hours after withdrawal of hemodialysis. Treatment with ethanol or fomepizole should be continued after hemodialysis for several hours to protect from possible rebound effects.

Methanol
PHARMACOLOGY

Methanol, or wood alcohol, is a clear, colorless liquid with a faint, slightly alcoholic scent. It is most often used as a solvent, an intermediate of chemical synthesis during various manufacturing processes, or as an octane booster in gasoline. The solvents that contain methanol include windshield or glass cleaning solutions, enamels, printing and duplicating solutions, stains, dyes, varnishes, thinners, paint removers, camp stove fuels, solid canned fuels, and antifreeze additives for gas. Most methanol poisonings result from ingestion, although there have been rare reported cases of methanol toxicity from inhalation or transdermal absorption.

Methanol is rapidly absorbed and distributed, with a mean absorption half-life of 5 minutes and mean distribution half-life of 8 minutes. Peak serum concentrations of methanol are reached within 30 to 60 minutes after ingestion, and the elimination half-life (untreated) is 12 to 20 hours. Methanol has a molecular weight of 32 g/mol, is water soluble, easily crosses the blood-brain barrier, and has a low volume of distribution (V_d = 0.60 to 0.77 L/kg) equivalent to water.[86] The estimated minimum lethal dose is 10 mL,[70] although this is highly variable.

METABOLISM

The parent compound, methanol, has low toxicity. It is the oxidation of methanol that produces the metabolites responsible for the toxicity seen in methanol poisoning. Figure 62-2 shows the metabolic pathway of methanol. In the liver,

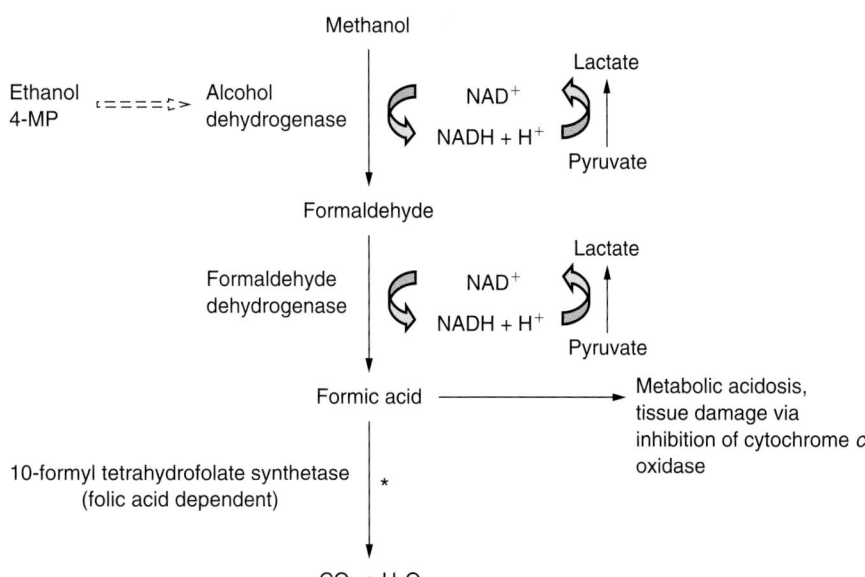

FIGURE 62-2. Metabolism of methanol. 4-MP, fomepizole; NAD^+, nicotinamide adenine dinucleotide; $NADH^+$, reduced form of nicotinamide adenine dinucleotide; *broken arrow,* inhibitors of alcohol dehydrogenase; *asterisk,* rate-limiting step.

methanol is oxidized by alcohol dehydrogenase to formaldehyde in the presence of NAD. Formaldehyde does not accumulate in the body because of its short half-life (1 to 2 minutes) and is rapidly oxidized by formaldehyde dehydrogenase to formic acid. The rate-limiting step, which depends on folic acid, involves the formation of 10-formyl tetrahydrofolate from folic acid and tetrahydrofolate. 10-Formyl tetrahydrofolate is then metabolized to its end products: carbon dioxide and water. Both antidotes for methanol poisoning, ethanol and fomepizole, competitively inhibit alcohol dehydrogenase and prevent the formation of the toxic metabolite, formic acid.

PATHOPHYSIOLOGY

The primary substance responsible for the toxicity of methanol poisoning is formic acid. Formic acid inhibits cytochrome c oxidase in the mitochondria of cells[87, 88] through its binding to the ferric moiety of cytochrome oxidase.[89] Cellular oxidative metabolism is interrupted, and this eventually leads to cell hypoxia and cell death. This mechanism of cellular injury is similar to that seen in cyanide or carbon monoxide poisoning, although formic acid is a weaker inhibitor of cytochrome oxidase.[90] It has been suggested that formic acid may also bind to the ferric part of hemoglobin, which may account for the rare cases of methemoglobinemia that have been observed in severe cases of methanol intoxication.

The cause of the metabolic acidosis in methanol poisoning is multifactorial. Evidence suggests that formic acid has direct and indirect roles in the development of acidosis. It has been shown that formic acid accumulation correlates with the severity of metabolic acidosis and the decrease in serum bicarbonate levels.[91, 92] Formic acid directly causes an acidosis by contributing a proton as it dissociates to formate and hydrogen ions.[86] An indirect mechanism of the formic acid-induced acidosis is the production of lactic acid. Because formic acid interferes with oxidative metabolism, mitochondrial respiration is shifted to anaerobic glycolysis. Lactic acid production and tissue hypoxia increase. As the cellular pH falls, inhibition of cytochrome oxidase by formic acid is increased,[93] exacerbating the acidosis and cellular injury. Another factor in the formation of lactate is the shift of the NAD/NADH ratio when methanol is converted to formaldehyde. The alteration in the NAD/NADH ratio promotes the metabolism of pyruvate to lactate.

Acidosis in the early stages of methanol poisoning primarily results from the accumulation of formic acid, whereas lactate (due to tissue hypoxia and the disruption of mitochondrial respiration) appears later in the course of intoxication.

The accumulation of formic acid in the eye has been implicated in the ocular toxicity that occurs with methanol ingestion. By binding to cytochrome oxidase in the optic nerve, formic acid disrupts the normal functioning of the nerve.[94-96] Because optic nerve cells possess few mitochondria and low cytochrome oxidase levels, the optic nerve is extremely susceptible to the toxic effects of formic acid.[93, 96] Clinical experience has shown that vision improves with the correction of the acidosis. Resolution of the acidosis results in an increase in the dissociated form of formic acid, which does not readily diffuse into the CNS.[89, 93] The accumulation of formic acid in the eye is decreased with resolution of the acidosis.

Methanol intoxication has been associated with hemorrhages within the subcortical white matter and edema or necrosis of the putamen. The suggested mechanisms of neurotoxicity involve direct toxicity by formic acid. Because of the targeted injury in the putamen, it has been proposed that the putamen may have a specific metabolic vulnerability to formic acid.

CLINICAL PRESENTATION

The principal sites of methanol toxicity are in the CNS, eyes, and gastrointestinal tract, and the most serious complications are blindness and death. As with ethylene glycol intoxication, the coingestion of ethanol with methanol can delay the onset of symptoms for more than 24 hours. The clinical presentation of methanol poisoning is distinguished by an early stage, latent interval, and delayed stage.

The *early stage* of methanol overdose is characterized by CNS depression in which the patient appears inebriated and drowsy. This phase is mild and transient and is followed by a *latent interval* lasting 6 to 30 hours. This period corresponds to the metabolism of methanol and the gradual accumulation of its toxic metabolite, formic acid. There is no altered mental status during the latent interval, and the only presenting symptom may be blurred vision. The length of the latent period depends on the dose of methanol ingested and the coingestion of ethanol; however, the duration of this period has no prognostic significance.[97] The latent interval is then followed by the *delayed stage* in which formic acid accumulates and systemic toxicity develops.

The visual changes associated with methanol poisonings tend to occur rapidly and symmetrically because formic acid is directly toxic to the retina. Ocular symptoms are highly variable and may include blurred vision, central scotoma, impaired pupillary response to light, decreased visual acuity, photophobia, visual field defects, or progression to complete blindness. Early findings on the ophthalmic examination are hyperemia of the optic disk and fixed, dilated pupils. Later manifestations of ocular toxicity include retinal edema, optic disk edema with loss of physiologic cupping, and optic atrophy.[98] Most often, the visual abnormalities resolve, although in 25% to 33% of patients with methanol poisoning, the visual changes are permanent.[86] Pupillary status and retinal edema correlate with the severity of methanol poisoning.[86]

The CNS effects of mild to moderate methanol toxicity are headache, vertigo, delirium, lethargy, restlessness, and confusion. In severe cases of methanol intoxication, the CNS symptoms may progress to coma and seizures from cerebral edema.[99] A Parkinson-like syndrome has also been observed and is associated with the neurotoxicity to the putamen and subcortical white matter.[100, 101]

Methanol toxicity commonly affects the gastrointestinal system. Typical symptoms during the delayed phase include nausea, vomiting, diarrhea, and abdominal pain from acute pancreatitis. There may also be mild elevations in the hepatic transaminases, but these findings are transient.

Rarely, myoglobinuric acute renal failure may develop. In such settings, the diagnosis may be complicated because methanol interferes with serum creatinine determinations.[102] Another uncommon complication of methanol toxicity is severe reversible cardiac failure.[103]

Poor prognostic signs include severe metabolic acidosis, elevated formic acid level, bradycardia, cardiovascular shock, anuria, and seizures or coma at presentation. The most common causes of death in methanol poisoning are respiratory failure or sudden respiratory arrest.[86]

DIAGNOSIS AND LABORATORY DATA

Methanol overdose should be considered in patients who present with visual changes, abdominal pain, high–anion gap metabolic acidosis, and elevated osmolal gap. Laboratory tests should include a complete blood cell count; assessments of electrolytes, serum calcium, lipase, amylase, creatine kinase, serum osmolality, and serum methanol and ethanol levels; urinalysis; and arterial blood gas determinations.

Formic acid and lactate accumulations in the body contribute to the development of an elevated–anion gap metabolic acidosis. Increases in serum formic acid and lactic acid levels correlate with the degree of acidosis and with clinical outcome.

Because methanol is an osmotically active compound, an osmolal gap is apparent during the early and latent phases of intoxication. For a serum level of 100 mg/dL, methanol contributes 31 mOsm/kg H_2O to the osmolal gap. During the delayed stage, as methanol is metabolized to formic acid, the osmolal gap may return to normal because formate is not osmotically active. A normal osmolal gap does not exclude the diagnosis of methanol poisoning. The specifics of the osmolal gap are described in greater detail in the previous section (see "Ethylene Glycol: Diagnosis and Laboratory Data").

Other laboratory abnormalities include increased serum amylase levels and mean corpuscular volumes. The serum amylase is typically elevated from inflammation of the salivary glands or acute necrotizing pancreatitis. The increased mean corpuscular volume is believed to result from the toxic effects of formaldehyde on cellular ion transport.[86]

TREATMENT

Initial management of methanol poisoning involves supportive care: stabilization of the airway, breathing, and circulation. The most serious sequelae of methanol overdose are metabolic acidosis, ocular toxicity, seizures, and coma. Treatment focuses on preventing these complications by limiting the accumulation of the toxic metabolites, formic acid and formaldehyde.

Metabolic acidosis (pH < 7.3) is treated aggressively with sodium bicarbonate therapy, because the severity of intoxication and clinical outcome correlate with the degree of acidosis.[86] Correction of the acidosis corrects the acid-base balance and improves pathophysiologic factors involved in methanol toxicity. The presence of acidosis increases the ratio of formic acid to formate. Formic acid inhibits cytochrome oxidase more effectively than its dissociated form (formate) resulting in increased anaerobic glycolysis and lactic acid production. By correcting the acidosis, the ratio of formic acid to formate is decreased, and inhibition of mitochondrial cytochrome oxidase is ameliorated.[90] It has been suggested that formate elimination may be pH dependent and correction of the acidosis may enhance its elimination.[104]

Folic acid supplementation plays a role in the treatment of methanol intoxication. The rate-limiting step of methanol metabolism is mediated by 10-formyl tetrahydrofolate synthetase, which is folic acid dependent. Although data are limited, folic acid has been shown to increase the metabolism of formic acid to carbon dioxide and water. The suggested dose of folic acid is 50 mg given intravenously every 4 hours for 5 doses and then once daily, although symptomatic patients should receive one intravenous dose of 1 mg/kg.[70] Thiamine and multivitamin supplementation should also be administered to patients suspected of ethanol abuse. Other measures include aggressive intravenous fluids to maintain adequate urine output and control of seizures with standard anticonvulsants.

Early recognition and rapid treatment are essential in the management of methanol toxicity. Similar to the treatment for ethylene glycol poisoning, the same inhibitors of alcohol dehydrogenase are used in methanol intoxications: ethanol and fomepizole. Ethanol or fomepizole should be quickly administered if methanol toxicity is suspected to prevent the formation of formic acid. The indications for the use of antidotes in methanol overdose are provided in the AACT guidelines: plasma methanol concentration of more than 20 mg/dL; documented recent ingestion of toxic amounts of methanol and osmolal gap of more than 10 mOsm/kg H_2O; or a history or strong clinical suspicion of methanol poisoning and at least two of the following: arterial pH less than 7.3, a serum bicarbonate level less than 20 mEq/L (mmol/L), or an osmolal gap more than 10 mOsm/kg H_2O.[86]

Ethanol binds to alcohol dehydrogenase with 10 to 20 times greater affinity than methanol.[105, 106] The loading dose of ethanol is 0.6 to 0.8 g ethanol/kg, with a maintenance dose that ranges from 66 mg ethanol/kg/hour (nondrinkers) to 154 mg ethanol/kg/hour (ethanol abusers). Dose adjustments are necessary during hemodialysis. The therapeutic target for serum ethanol concentration is 100 to 150 mg/dL. The loading dose of *fomepizole* is 15 mg/kg, followed by 10 mg/kg every 12 hours for 48 hours then 15 mg/kg every 12 hours until the methanol concentration is undetectable or symptoms *and* the metabolic acidosis resolves *and* the methanol level is less than 20 mg/dL. The use of ethanol and fomepizole in the treatment of methanol poisoning is similar to that of ethylene glycol and is described in detail in the previous section (see "Ethylene Glycol: Treatment").

Hemodialysis effectively removes methanol and formic acid, corrects metabolic acidosis, and shortens the course of hospitalization.[86] Because methanol overdose is associated with an increased frequency of intracerebral hemorrhage, the use of heparin during hemodialysis should be minimized. The clearance rates of methanol and formate are 125 to 215 mL/minute and 203 mL/minute, respectively, and the rate depends on blood flow and the type of membrane used.[86] Hemodialysis is indicated for the following: serum methanol levels higher than 50 mg/dL, metabolic acidosis (pH < 7.30), visual changes, dose of ingested methanol of more than 30 mL, seizures, deteriorating clinical status despite supportive therapy, renal failure, or electrolyte abnormalities not responsive to standard therapy.[86, 107] According to AACT guidelines, a methanol concentration of more than 50 mg/dL is no longer an absolute indication for hemodialysis because fomepizole may be used as first-line treatment of methanol poisoning.

Hemodialysis is continued until the serum methanol concentration is undetectable or until the methanol level is less than 25 mg/dL *and* the anion gap metabolic acidosis and osmolal gap are normal. The presence of visual changes is not an indication for continued dialysis because ophthalmologic abnormalities may be transient or permanent. Methanol redistributes after the discontinuation of hemodialysis and may result in rebound of the methanol levels. Close monitoring of the serum osmolality and electrolytes should be continued every 2 to 4 hours for 12 to 36 hours after hemodialysis. To protect the patient from the toxic effects of methanol rebound, fomepizole or ethanol therapy should be continued for several hours after withdrawal of hemodialysis, until methanol levels are undetectable or less than 20 mg/dL with resolution of acidosis and symptoms.[86]

Isopropanol
PHARMACOLOGY

Isopropanol (i.e., isopropyl alcohol) is a clear, colorless, bitter liquid. It is commonly found in "rubbing alcohol," skin lotion, hair tonics, aftershave lotion, denatured alcohol, solvents, cements, cleaning products, de-icers, and the manufacturing process of acetone and glycerin. Intoxication may occur through ingestion or inhalation of vapors, especially in infants.

Isopropanol is rapidly absorbed by the gastrointestinal system and reaches a peak serum concentration 15 to 30 minutes after ingestion with an elimination half-life of 3 to 7 hours. Isopropanol, which is water soluble, has a molecular weight of 60 g/mol and a volume of distribution equivalent to water ($V_d = 0.6$ L/kg). Unlike the other alcohols discussed previously, the parent compound isopropanol is responsible for the toxic effects observed in isopropanol intoxication. Delaying the metabolism of isopropanol therefore is not considered a beneficial method of treatment. The lethal dose ranges from 150 to 240 mL, although patients may become symptomatic with doses as low as 20 mL.[108]

METABOLISM

The metabolism of isopropanol is depicted in Figure 62-3. Isopropanol is oxidized to acetone by alcohol dehydrogenase in the presence of NAD. Acetone is then excreted in the breath and urine.[70]

CLINICAL PRESENTATION

The principal targets of isopropanol intoxication are the CNS, cardiovascular system, and gastrointestinal system.

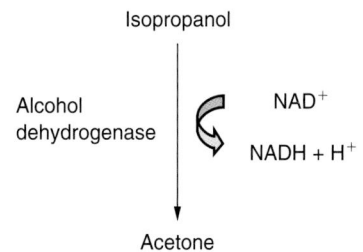

FIGURE 62-3. Metabolism of isopropanol. NAD$^+$, nicotinamide adenine dinucleotide; NADH$^+$, reduced form of nicotinamide adenine dinucleotide.

Clinical symptoms tend to appear within 1 hour of ingestion. Isopropanol is a potent CNS depressant, which is twice as effective as ethanol in its CNS toxicity.[20] Early effects of isopropanol overdose are therefore similar to those of ethanol: confusion, headache, poor coordination, lethargy, and dizziness. These symptoms may progress to ataxia, coma, and respiratory arrest in severe cases of poisoning.

Gastrointestinal effects include nausea, vomiting, and abdominal pain. Because isopropanol is a gastrointestinal irritant, hematemesis from severe gastritis or hemorrhage may develop. The combined effects of CNS depression and vomiting place the patient at risk for aspiration pneumonia. In animals, hepatotoxicity and fatty liver have also been described.[59]

Another unique feature of isopropanol intoxication is myocardial depression and myocyte toxicity. Hypotension is often severe and is caused by multiple factors, including cardiac depression, arrhythmias from cardiomyopathy, vasodilation, dehydration, and gastrointestinal bleeding. Hypotension is the strongest predictor of death in cases of isopropanol overdose.[108]

Acute renal failure may develop because of severe hypotension or myoglobinuria. Other systemic findings include hypoglycemia from impaired gluconeogenesis, hypothermia, and hemolytic anemia.

DIAGNOSIS AND LABORATORY DATA

The diagnosis of isopropanol overdose should be suspected in any patient presenting with altered sensorium, acetone on the breath, elevated osmolal gap, and acetonemia or acetonuria (i.e., positive sodium nitroprusside reaction in serum or urine) in the absence of hyperglycemia, glycosuria, or acidosis. Laboratory tests should include a complete blood cell count, electrolytes, serum osmolality, serum acetone, creatine kinase, urinalysis, and arterial blood gas determinations.

Because the end product of isopropanol metabolism, acetone, is not an organic acid, there is no elevated–anion gap metabolic acidosis. However, if hypotension is severe, poor tissue perfusion and hypoxia may result in lactic acid accumulation, and the development of metabolic acidosis may follow.

An osmolal gap is present because isopropanol is an osmotically active compound. For a serum level of 100 mg/dL, isopropanol contributes 17 mOsm/kg H_2O to the osmolal gap, and 100 mg/dL of acetone contributes an additional 18 mOsm/kg H_2O. The clinical utility of the osmolal gap is discussed in further detail in the previous section (see "Ethylene Glycol: Diagnosis and Laboratory Data").

Other laboratory abnormalities observed in isopropanol intoxication include hypoglycemia, elevated serum creatinine, elevated creatine kinase, and elevated protein in cerebral spinal fluid.

TREATMENT

Treatment for isopropanol toxicity focuses on appropriate supportive therapy. Because the oxidation of isopropanol does not produce toxic metabolites, agents that inhibit alcohol dehydrogenase are not used in the treatment of isopropanol poisoning. Intravenous fluids and pressors should be given in the setting of hypotension. Mechanical ventilation may be indicated for respiratory distress and airway protection.

Gastrointestinal lavage is effective in preventing systemic absorption of isopropanol. As much as 87% to 92% of isopropanol can be removed by activated charcoal when administered in a ratio of 20:1 (charcoal to alcohol).[109]

Hemodialysis effectively removes isopropanol and acetone. However, hemodialysis is usually unnecessary, except in severe cases of isopropanol intoxications. Indications for hemodialysis include an isopropanol level of more than 400 mg/dL, prolonged coma, hypotension, myocardial depression or tachyarrhythmias, and renal failure.[20] It has been suggested that early initiation of hemodialysis might benefit the clinical outcome by shortening the duration of coma and reversing hemodynamic instability.[110, 111]

Lithium Toxicity

PHARMACOLOGY

Lithium is an alkaline metal that since its discovery has found increasing use in the field of psychiatry. It is FDA approved for first-line therapy of bipolar affective disorder and has also been used to treat alcoholism, schizoaffective disorders, and cluster headaches.[112] Lithium has a narrow therapeutic index, with therapeutic levels between 0.6 and 1.5 mEq/L.[113] Lithium levels must be monitored carefully and frequently, with dose adjustments as needed. Patients who are especially susceptible to lithium toxicity include the elderly with a reduced glomerular filtration rate (GFR); patients on certain medications such as angiotensin-converting enzyme (ACE) inhibitors, thiazide diuretics and NSAIDs; and patients with lithium-induced diabetes insipidus from chronic lithium therapy.[41]

Lithium is rapidly and completely absorbed in the upper gastrointestinal tract. After a single oral dose, peak serum levels occur in 1 to 2 hours, and the drug is widely distributed in the body water. It is poorly bound to protein and has a low molecular weight (7 D) and small volume of distribution (0.6 L/kg).[112] Lithium is predominantly located intracellularly and diffuses slowly across cell membranes, making its removal by extracorporeal therapy a slow process. It is entirely eliminated by the kidneys,[113] and approximately 80% of the drug is reabsorbed in the proximal tubule by the same mechanism that promotes sodium reabsorption. Factors associated with reduced GFR or increased proximal tubule reabsorption (e.g., dehydration) increase the serum lithium level.

PATHOPHYSIOLOGY

Lithium can be exchanged for sodium or potassium on several transport proteins that normally transport those ions, providing a pathway for lithium entry into the cells. Because the transport systems out of the cell are limited, lithium accumulates intracellularly. Studies have shown that the transporters for lithium entry into cells include the amiloride-sensitive sodium channel (ENaC), Na^+/H^+ exchanger, and $Na^+/K^+/2Cl^-$ cotransporter.[114-116]

CLINICAL PRESENTATION

There are two types of lithium intoxication: acute (i.e., accidental ingestion or deliberate self-poisoning) and chronic. Acute intoxication usually occurs in the domestic setting, where a child accidentally ingests an adult household member's lithium. Acute overdose could also be a suicide attempt. Acute poisoning generally carries less risk of mortality, and patients have milder symptoms compared with that observed in chronic intoxication[112] because the elimination half-life is shorter in lithium-naïve individuals.[41] Chronic intoxication often develops during maintenance therapy when lithium reaches toxic levels because of increased-dose adjustments. Elevated lithium levels may occur in states of sodium retention (e.g., congestive heart failure, cirrhosis, gastrointestinal losses). The severity of chronic lithium intoxication correlates directly with the serum lithium concentration and may be categorized as mild (1.5 to 2.0 mEq/L), moderate (2.0 to 2.5 mEq/L), or severe (>2.5 mEq/L).[117]

Lithium intoxication often results in multiorgan dysfunction. In the kidneys, chronic lithium ingestion has been associated with several forms of renal injury such as nephrogenic diabetes insipidus, chronic interstitial nephritis, nephrotic syndrome, and renal failure. Lithium is concentrated within the thyroid and inhibits thyroid hormone (i.e., T_3 and T_4) secretion resulting in clinical hypothyroidism. Lithium overdose has also been associated with thyrotoxicosis, goiter, and chronic autoimmune thyroiditis. Bone marrow abnormalities have also been observed. Leukocytosis and aplastic anemia have been reported in acute and chronic poisoning, respectively. The most common manifestation of lithium toxicity is altered mental status. Symptoms of mild lithium poisoning include nausea, vomiting, and weakness. Severe toxicity, which can be life threatening, is associated with seizures, cardiac arrhythmias, hyperreflexia, coma, and death.

DIAGNOSIS AND TREATMENT

The best approach to lithium toxicity is anticipatory because of the narrow therapeutic index. Plasma levels should be monitored periodically with dose adjustments made accordingly. In clinical situations in which lithium excretion is decreased (e.g., volume depletion), the serum lithium concentration should be monitored closely to avoid toxic levels. Concurrent administration of NSAIDs or ACE inhibitors should also be avoided.

In the setting of lithium-induced nephrogenic diabetes insipidus, amiloride may be used to treat hypernatremia. Amiloride blocks the reabsorption of lithium by the collecting tubule cells. Amiloride significantly reduces urine volume in patients undergoing chronic lithium treatment.[118] The initial management of lithium intoxication involves supportive care, prevention of further absorption, and enhancement of lithium elimination. A serum lithium concentration, renal function tests, and electrolytes are necessary laboratory tests to immediately assess the degree of toxicity. Serum lithium levels correlate directly with the severity of chronic lithium intoxication. A nasogastric tube may be placed, followed by gastric lavage. Whole-bowel irrigation with polyethylene glycol solution has also been effective in removing unabsorbed lithium from the gastrointestinal tract and preventing its absorption.[112, 113] One of the major initial steps in lithium intoxication is volume resuscitation using half-normal saline. Administration of hypotonic fluid is especially important in patients with underlying lithium-induced diabetes insipidus because intravenous normal saline may precipitate hypernatremia.

After the patient is hemodynamically stable, treatment should focus on enhancing lithium elimination from the body. If renal function is preserved, the clearance rate of lithium by the kidneys is 10 to 40 mL/minute. Hemodialysis, the treatment of choice, removes lithium at a rate 70 to 170 mL/minute.[113] Because lithium is primarily intracellular, hemodialysis does not efficiently remove a significant amount of the total body burden of drug. Extending dialysis therapy to 8 to 12 hours prevents rebound of lithium levels.[119, 120] Theoretically, the advantage of CRRT is that postdialysis rebound of the lithium concentration is avoided. Lithium clearances of 60 to 85 L/day have been achieved with CAVHD or CVVHD.[54] There are a few reported cases of gradual and complete removal of lithium by CRRT without rebound of serum lithium concentration.[54]

In lithium toxicity, hemodialysis therapy should be initiated in the following circumstances: (1) serum lithium level of more than 4.0 mEq/L, regardless of the clinical status; (2) plasma lithium concentration of more than 2.5 mEq/L with neurologic symptoms or renal insufficiency; (3) plasma concentration of more than 2.5 mEq/L in asymptomatic patients with increasing lithium levels after admission; or (4) a plasma concentration of less than 2.5 mEq/L in ESRD patients.

Salicylates

PHARMACOLOGY

Salicylates are ubiquitous agents found in many over-the-counter medications and prescription drugs. The most common salicylate is aspirin (i.e., acetylsalicylic acid), although there are many different formulations such as methyl salicylate, salicylic acid, and bismuth subsalicylate. They frequently are prescribed for their anti-inflammatory, antipyretic, and analgesic properties. The volume of distribution of salicylate is 0.21 L/kg.

In the liver, acetylsalicylic acid is initially hydrolyzed to salicylic acid and then glycinated to salicyluric acid. Salicyluric acid, the less toxic metabolite, is then easily excreted by the kidneys. In salicylate intoxication, there are two principal alterations of the normal metabolic pathway that exacerbate and promote toxicity. At therapeutic levels (0.7 to 1.4 mmol/L), salicylate normally is 90% protein bound, with only 10% eliminated in the urine as the parent compound. At toxic doses, the excess salicylate overwhelms the protein binding capacity of albumin such that serum salicylate concentrations of 800 μg/mL result in a decrease in protein binding up to 50%.[121] The second mechanism that contributes to toxicity involves the delayed conversion to salicyluric acid. Saturation of this pathway results in excess plasma concentration of salicylate, which is poorly excreted by the kidneys. Both processes worsen salicylate toxicity.

Other factors contributing to toxicity are increased volume of distribution and prolonged half-life. With the decrease in protein binding in salicylate poisoning, there is more unbound drug available for distribution to the peripheral organs (i.e., CNS, lungs, liver, and kidneys). The renal clearance of salicylate is decreased because of this change in the volume of distribution, and the drug half-life is increased from 3 to 12 hours up to 15 to 36 hours.[20]

PATHOPHYSIOLOGY OF ACID-BASE ABNORMALITIES

Salicylate is a relatively strong acid and therefore contributes to the development of a high–anion gap metabolic acidosis. The cause of the metabolic acidosis is complex and poorly understood. The uncoupling of mitochondrial oxidative phosphorylation and inhibition of the tricarboxylic acid (TCA) cycle results in an increase in pyruvic acid and lactic acid production. Another pathophysiologic mechanism of the acidosis is increased lipid metabolism resulting in excess ketone body production (i.e., hydroxybutyric acid, acetoacetic acid, and acetone). Alterations in amino acid metabolism also contribute to the acidosis.

Salicylates directly stimulate the respiratory center of the brain resulting in hyperventilation. There is a fall in the Pco_2 and increase in the serum bicarbonate level. These events culminate in a second acid-base disorder, respiratory alkalosis.

When acid-base disturbances occur, a mixed respiratory alkalosis and metabolic acidosis predominate in 40% to 50% of the cases and an isolated metabolic alkalosis in 20% to 25% of cases.[122, 123] Rarely does salicylate toxicity induce isolated metabolic acidosis in adults, although this is a common finding in the pediatric population.[124]

CLINICAL PRESENTATION

Salicylate ingestion is a common cause of poisoning in children and adolescents. Because aspirin-containing analgesic products are readily available and found in virtually every household, they are common sources of accidental and suicidal ingestions. The symptoms of salicylate toxicity typically manifest 3 to 6 hours after ingestion. The clinical manifestations of salicylate intoxication involve disturbances of several organ systems, including the CNS, cardiovascular, pulmonary, hepatic, and renal systems. The global effects of salicylate poisoning are attributed to its uncoupling of oxidative phosphorylation, inhibition of TCA cycle enzymes, and disruption of amino acid synthesis.

In severe acute or chronic toxicity, CNS abnormalities such as agitation, confusion, seizures, stupor, and coma are common. Patients may also present with nausea, vomiting, fever, tinnitus, and hyperventilation. Noncardiogenic pulmonary edema results from increased capillary permeability and is observed in adult and elderly patients in chronic intoxication. Inhibition of prostaglandin synthesis can result in vasoconstriction within the kidney, resulting in oliguric acute renal failure. Direct hepatotoxicity has also been reported.

The overall severity of salicylate toxicity can be determined using three parameters: dose ingested, clinical presentation, and serum salicylate concentration. First, quantifying the amount of salicylate ingested may be beneficial because a dose of less than 150 mg/kg typically follows a benign clinical course. Second, the clinical signs and symptoms at presentation correspond with the severity of toxin exposure. Severe neurologic abnormalities, pulmonary edema, and acute renal failure are often observed in severe cases of salicylate overdose. Third, plasma salicylate levels correlate with the degree of toxicity. Mild toxicity is seen with serum salicylate levels of 300 to 500 mg/L 6 hours after ingestion, moderate toxicity with 500 to 700 mg/L, and severe toxicity with

750 mg/L or higher.[125] Frequent reassessment by the clinician is imperative because clinical deterioration may occur rapidly.

DIAGNOSIS AND LABORATORY DATA

The diagnosis of salicylate poisoning can often be obtained by means of a thorough history and physical examination. However, patients may be unwilling or unable to divulge information, making laboratory assessment beneficial in the diagnosis of salicylate intoxication. Salicylate poisoning should be suspected in patients presenting with hyperventilation, diaphoresis, tinnitus, and acid-base disturbances. An initial comprehensive metabolic panel, complete blood count, arterial blood gas, and salicylate level should be measured. Levels should be monitored every 3 to 4 hours until clinical improvement is observed or until a downward trend in the plasma level is documented. The ingestion of enteric-coated products may delay gastrointestinal absorption, thereby necessitating continuous monitoring of the patient and the plasma salicylate concentrations. The serum Phenistix or urine ferric chloride test may be used to rapidly diagnose salicylate poisoning. A positive Phenistix test result, or brown discoloration on exposure to serum, corresponds to a salicylate level of 700 µg/mL or higher.[20, 126] The purple discoloration observed with a positive urine ferric chloride test (performed by adding 4 drops of ferric chloride to 1 mL of urine) also suggests salicylate poisoning.[126]

The classic acid-base abnormalities in adults with salicylate poisoning are respiratory alkalosis or mixed high–anion gap metabolic acidosis and respiratory alkalosis. The metabolic acidosis tends to be more severe with chronic ingestions, pediatric patients, and worsening toxicity.[123, 127, 128] Electrolyte abnormalities are common in salicylate poisoning. Hypernatremia results from the insensible loss of free water due to increased metabolism, hyperpyrexia, and hyperventilation. Symptomatic hypokalemia, the consequence of intracellular shifting and urinary potassium wasting, is observed in severe toxicity.[129]

TREATMENT

The treatment of salicylate toxicity is variable and depends on the severity of exposure. The initial management should establish and maintain an adequate airway and circulation. The use of gastric lavage is controversial but may be beneficial if administered within 1 hour of ingestion. Activated charcoal (50 g or 1 g/kg) is effective in reducing gut absorption in mild or moderate toxicity. Another dose of activated charcoal 3 to 6 hours after ingestion may be beneficial if repeat salicylate levels continue to trend upward.[8, 130]

Salicylates are normally eliminated by glomerular filtration and tubule secretion by the proximal tubule. In mild or moderate toxicity, urinary alkalinization enhances renal excretion. An alkaline diuresis can be achieved by adding three ampules of sodium bicarbonate to 1 L of D_5W and infusing at a rate of 200 to 250 mL/hour, depending on the patient's volume status. Maintenance of a urinary pH of 7.5 or higher promotes renal clearance of the drug. Adequate renal function is necessary for urinary alkalinization to be effective in its elimination of the bicarbonate load.[6, 128] Frequent monitoring of electrolytes, volume status, and urinary pH is mandatory.

Extracorporeal therapy is indicated for moderate to severe salicylate toxicity, and the modality of choice is intermittent hemodialysis. Clinical signs of severe toxicity include seizures, coma, pulmonary edema, and acute renal failure. Several case reports have successfully used continuous venovenous hemodiafiltration (CVVHDF) for the treatment of severe salicylate toxicity.[131] Although this therapy may not be as efficient as hemodialysis, it is the treatment of choice in hemodynamically unstable patients and in patients who require prolonged therapy due to ingestion of delayed enteric formulations.[131, 132]

With toxic levels of salicylate, the level of protein binding decreases from 90% to approximately 50%, making the molecule more amenable for removal by hemodialysis. Hemoperfusion is not recommended for the treatment of salicylate toxicity because it does not correct the electrolyte and acid-base abnormalities.[20]

Theophylline
PHARMACOLOGY

Theophylline belongs to the group of pharmacologic compounds known as methylxanthines. Clinically, the use of theophylline as primary therapy for asthma and chronic obstructive pulmonary disease has been replaced by inhaled β-adrenergic agonists and inhaled corticosteroids. Although the use of theophylline has declined over the past decade, it continues to be used for patients with severe underlying disease or for those resistant to more standard therapy. The therapeutic index remains very narrow, with a range of 10 to 20 mg/L. The clinical manifestations of theophylline toxicity may be seen at levels as low as 15 mg/L but are most commonly observed at serum concentrations higher than 20 mg/L. The variability of theophylline absorption and metabolism and its narrow therapeutic index necessitate close monitoring of serum levels in all patients.

CLINICAL PRESENTATION

Theophylline intoxication can be divided into two clinical categories: acute (i.e., intentional overdose or accidental ingestion) and chronic. In chronic intoxication, several factors can decrease the metabolism of theophylline. Because theophylline undergoes biotransformation by the cytochrome P-450 system, drugs that interfere with cytochrome P-450 (e.g., erythromycin, cimetidine, allopurinol, diltiazem, propranolol) can reduce theophylline clearance. Cardiac and hepatic disease may also alter theophylline metabolism. Infants and adults older than 60 years are also susceptible to theophylline toxicity because of decreased clearance of the methylxanthines.[133, 134]

There is great variability in the clinical manifestations of theophylline poisoning, and it depends on the duration of therapy, dose of drug, comorbidities, and ability to metabolize the drug.[135, 136] Mild theophylline intoxication is characterized by nervousness, tremors, tachycardia, abdominal pain, vomiting, and diarrhea. In moderate toxicity, patients are often lethargic and disoriented and exhibit cardiovascular arrhythmias, such as supraventricular tachyarrhythmias and frequent premature ventricular contractions. Serious complications of severe intoxication include recurrent seizure activity and ventricular tachycardias. The seizures are typically generalized, although focal signs such as lip smacking and ocular deviation may occur. Seizure activity portends a poor prognosis and is frequently resistant to standard anticonvulsant therapy.

LABORATORY DATA

Hypokalemia resulting from a catecholamine-induced intracellular transport of potassium is the most common electrolyte abnormality associated with theophylline toxicity. Although the serum potassium may be profoundly low at the time of presentation, the total body stores of potassium are preserved. Serum potassium levels return to normal with a reduction in the theophylline concentration. Hyperglycemia, a consequence of increased catecholamine release, and hypomagnesemia, hypophosphatemia, and hypercalcemia are commonly observed. Respiratory alkalosis has also been reported and results from the direct stimulation of the central respiratory center.[134, 135, 137]

TREATMENT

The treatment of theophylline poisoning depends on the severity of intoxication. After hemodynamic stabilization, treatment focuses on the elimination of theophylline from the body. Use of multiple-dose activated charcoal decreases the serum elimination half-life from 7 to 20 hours to 1 to 3 hours. Activated charcoal (50 g or 1 g/kg) should be administered every 4 hours until the serum level is less than 20 mg/L. Addition of a cathartic, such as sorbitol, enhances elimination. For sustained-released preparations, the time to peak absorption may be delayed 15 to 24 hours.[138, 139]

The cardiac arrhythmias associated with theophylline are the result of excessive circulating catecholamines. Typically, the use of β-blockers slows the heart rate and controls the arrhythmia. If a patient is unable to tolerate the use of β-blockers, verapamil or diltiazem may be used.[140]

Seizures associated with theophylline toxicity are usually difficult to control. Benzodiazepines, phenytoin, and phenobarbital are the initial anticonvulsant agents. For recurrent seizures unresponsive to standard therapy, general anesthesia and neuromuscular paralysis may need to be implemented.[141]

Extracorporeal therapy is administered when the patient is clinically unstable with life-threatening cardiac arrhythmias or seizures. Although there is no definitive plasma theophylline level at which extracorporeal treatment should be initiated, a level of about 100 mg/L in acute intoxication or 40 mg/L in chronic poisoning is generally considered an indication for extracorporeal therapy. Other relative indications include an inability to tolerate activated charcoal, congestive heart failure, and liver disease because metabolism of theophylline is impaired in cardiac and hepatic disease.

Multiple studies have compared the efficacy of hemoperfusion with that of hemodialysis for the treatment of theophylline toxicity. Even with the use of high-flux dialysis, hemoperfusion is twice as effective as hemodialysis in the removal of theophylline from the systemic circulation. Hemoperfusion with activated charcoal cartridges can obtain extraction ratios of approximately 1.0. The hemoperfusion cartridges are easily saturated and need to be replaced after 2 hours of use.[140, 142-144]

It has been suggested that sequential and simultaneous "in series" hemodialysis and hemoperfusion may be even more advantageous for severe toxicity.[145] The added benefit of hemodialysis is its rapid correction of electrolyte and acid-base abnormalities. The use of simultaneous therapy delays the saturation of the activated charcoal membrane. Although hemoperfusion may be more effective in the removal of theophylline, its main disadvantage is the lack of availability in most medical centers. In this situation, hemodialysis may be initiated using high blood flow rates and high-flux membranes. High-flux hemodialysis achieves clearance rates of more than 200 mL/minute, which is equivalent to that of charcoal hemoperfusion. Extracorporeal therapy should be continued until clinical improvement and a plasma level of less than 25 mg/L is obtained.[145, 146]

Valproic Acid Toxicity

PHARMACOLOGY AND PATHOPHYSIOLOGY

Valproic acid (VPA), introduced in the late 1970s as an anticonvulsant drug, is used in several other neurologic conditions such as bipolar affective disorder and migraine headaches. Its mechanism of action involves blockade of the voltage-dependent sodium channels, which enhances postsynaptic γ-aminobutyric acid (GABA)–mediated inhibition. Acute VPA intoxication is usually self-limiting, although serious toxicity and deaths have been reported.

VPA is rapidly absorbed in the gastrointestinal tract and metabolized extensively by the liver through glucuronic acid conjugation and beta and omega oxidation. Only 1% of VPA is excreted unchanged in the urine.[147] VPA has a molecular weight of 144 D and a small volume of distribution (0.1 to 0.5 L/kg). At therapeutic levels (50 to 125 µg/mL), it is highly protein bound (90% to 95%).[147] At toxic concentrations, however, protein-binding sites become saturated, and the percentage of bound VPA decreases to as low as 15%.

CLINICAL PRESENTATION

VPA intoxication in adults typically occurs in the setting of an attempted suicide. Clinical manifestations of VPA toxicity include coma, severe respiratory depression, hypotension, tachycardia, and death. Common metabolic disorders in acute overdose include hypernatremia, hyperosmolality, hypocalcemia, high–anion gap metabolic acidosis, elevated serum aminotransferases, and hyperammonemia.[148]

DIAGNOSIS AND TREATMENT

Initial management of VPA toxicity consists of supportive care, prevention of further absorption, and enhancement of VPA removal. After hemodynamic stabilization, the mainstay of treatment includes gastrointestinal tract decontamination with activated charcoal. Charcoal is effective only if administered soon after VPA ingestion. Single-dose activated charcoal alone is usually sufficient for most VPA overdoses, and its administration is recommended for all patients. Multiple-dose activated charcoal use has not been clearly established in increasing effective drug removal.[149]

Because the excretion of VPA by the kidney is minor, forced diuresis is ineffective for increasing drug elimination.

There are several case reports recommending hemodialysis, hemoperfusion, or hemodialysis-hemoperfusion for VPA poisoning.[149, 150] Theoretically, VPA is a good candidate for removal by extracorporeal therapy because it is relatively small, water soluble, and has a low volume of distribution. However, the high degree of protein binding hinders its effective clearance by these treatment modalities. The data on overdose cases are controversial. Because neither hemodialysis nor hemoperfusion has been shown to be superior in efficacy, it is reasonable to select hemodialysis in treating severe VPA toxicity because hemodialysis is associated with fewer complications and easily corrects the associated metabolic abnormalities.

SPECIFIC POISONINGS LESS RESPONSIVE TO EXTRACORPOREAL THERAPY

Digoxin

PHARMACOLOGY

Digoxin is a cardiac glycoside that commonly is prescribed for elderly patients for the treatment of supraventricular arrhythmias or congestive heart failure. It has a narrow therapeutic index and tends to produce adverse effects, especially in the older populations.

Digoxin is a potent and highly selective inhibitor of Na^+K^+-ATPase. The net effect is the intracellular loss of potassium and the gain of sodium and calcium. The intracellular rise in calcium is largely responsible for the increase in cardiac contractility.[151] Digoxin has a large volume of distribution, and the principal target tissue is muscle. Dosing should be based on the estimated lean body mass. Digoxin is dosed once daily and has an elimination half-life of 36 to 48 hours in patients with normal or near-normal renal function.

PATHOPHYSIOLOGY

Digoxin toxicity occurs in the setting of chronic digoxin therapy, especially when the dosing is not adjusted for renal impairment. Several factors modify the sensitivity of the myocardium to digoxin and increase the potential for digoxin toxicity: hypokalemia, hypomagnesemia, hypocalcemia, other cardiac medications, certain antibiotics, and advanced age.[152] Impairment of renal function decreases digoxin excretion by the kidney and results in increased total body stores of digoxin and prolonged half-life.

CLINICAL PRESENTATION

The clinical diagnosis of digoxin intoxication is difficult because the symptoms and electrocardiographic changes are nonspecific. Symptoms of digoxin toxicity include fatigue, nausea, blurred vision, vomiting, dizziness, confusion, headaches, delirium, and hallucinations.[153] Cardiac arrhythmias, which account for the high mortality of digoxin overdoses, may take on any form. Diagnosis is often difficult because arrhythmias may be caused by underlying cardiac disease. It is possible that the only clinical clue to toxicity may be a change in the cardiac rhythm.[154] Among the common

electrocardiographic manifestations are atrioventricular node dysfunction, sinus bradycardia, junctional rhythm, and ectopic beats originating from the ventricle.

DIAGNOSIS AND TREATMENT

Serum digoxin levels do not always correlate with toxicity; therefore, the physician should not rely on the serum concentration but rather on clinical judgment. On early recognition of digoxin toxicity, initial therapy involves gastrointestinal decontamination because digoxin is effectively adsorbed by activated charcoal. Multiple-dose activated charcoal can be given to remove active metabolites as they are excreted by the biliary system. Cholestyramine is an alternative to activated charcoal but must be administered early to be effective. Electrolyte abnormalities should also be corrected. Most acute digoxin poisonings manifest with hyperkalemia and may be treated with insulin, glucose, and sodium bicarbonate. If these conservative measures fail and the patient also has renal dysfunction, hemodialysis should be considered. Symptomatic patients with arrhythmias such as bradycardia should receive atropine (0.5 to 2.0 mg), with electrical pacing reserved for refractory arrhythmias.

Patients with life-threatening digoxin toxicity require therapy with digoxin-specific antibody Fab fragments.[155] Fab fragments are purified from sheep IgG and rapidly bind to intravascular digoxin and digoxin within the interstitial space. Fab-bound digoxin is inactivated because it cannot reassociate with the inhibitory site of the α-subunit of Na^+K^+-ATPase.[151] The Fab fragments and the Fab-bound digoxin are then filtered by the glomeruli and rapidly excreted in the urine. In patients with ESRD, the Fab-digoxin complexes persist in the circulation and may dissociate, potentially resulting in rebound of free digoxin and recurrence of toxicity. To prevent this rebound phenomenon, plasmapheresis has been administered for the removal of Fab-digoxin complexes in patients with renal failure.[156] Although there have been no reported cases of severe anaphylactic reactions, Fab should be used with caution in patients with allergies to sheep protein. Other side effects of Fab fragment include exacerbation of congestive heart failure, rapid ventricular response in patients with atrial fibrillation, and hypokalemia.

Although hemodialysis or hemoperfusion can correct electrolyte disturbances, volume overload, and concurrent renal failure, their role in the treatment of digoxin toxicity is limited due to the extensive tissue binding and large volume of distribution of the drug.

Procainamide

PHARMACOLOGY

Procainamide is a class IA antiarrhythmic agent used for the treatment of supraventricular and ventricular arrhythmias. It is a small molecule that is minimally protein bound (14%). The aromatic amino group of procainamide is acetylated to form the major metabolite, *N*-acetylprocainamide (NAPA). Procainamide and NAPA are predominantly eliminated by the kidneys.

Procainamide toxicity is typically seen in patients with renal insufficiency or congestive heart failure. In this clinical setting, the procainamide and NAPA levels may be increased and need to be monitored closely. Therapeutic plasma concentrations of procainamide range from 4 to 10 mg/L. Toxic plasma levels are more than 30 mg/L, although clinical manifestations may be seen at levels as low as 15 mg/L.

CLINICAL PRESENTATION

Procainamide intoxication typically presents with nonspecific symptoms such as headache, dizziness, anorexia, nausea, and vomiting. Dermatologic manifestations include rash, digital vasculitis, and the Raynaud phenomenon. Severe pancytopenia and fever may result from hypersensitivity reactions and necessitate periodic monitoring of the white blood count and differential.[157] Cardiac arrhythmias such as torsade de pointes, conduction delays, and ventricular tachycardia are also observed.[158] A systemic lupus erythematosus (SLE)–like syndrome with arthralgias, fever, pleuritis, pericarditis, and hepatomegaly has been described with the use of procainamide. Approximately 60% to 70% of patients on chronic procainamide therapy develop antinuclear antibodies. This SLE-like syndrome occurs in 20% to 30% and resolves with the discontinuation of procainamide. It has been suggested that acetylation of the aromatic amino group in procainamide, resulting in NAPA formation, prevents the development of the SLE-like syndrome.[159, 160]

TREATMENT

The low molecular weight and minimal protein binding of procainamide makes it amenable to extracorporeal therapy in cases of intoxication. Several studies have looked at the relative efficacy of hemoperfusion versus hemodialysis in the treatment of procainamide and NAPA toxicity. The use of combined hemoperfusion and hemodialysis demonstrated effective plasma clearance of procainamide and NAPA.[161] Others have reported that hemoperfusion increased NAPA clearance by approximately 36% over hemodialysis, whereas combined hemoperfusion-hemodialysis was three times more effective than hemodialysis alone for the treatment of procainamide toxicity.[162]

Procainamide has a large volume of distribution, resulting in slow equilibration from the extravascular space into the vasculature. This results in rebound of the serum procainamide and NAPA concentrations, requiring continued monitoring and extracorporeal therapy. In the setting of severe toxicity, the use of continuous extracorporeal therapy after hemoperfusion and intermittent hemodialysis results in a more sustained decrease in the serum procainamide levels.

Procainamide toxicity is uncommon, but in older patients with renal insufficiency and congestive heart failure, this effective class IA antiarrhythmic must be used with caution. Frequent monitoring of serum procainamide and NAPA levels is mandatory.

REFERENCES

1. Litovitz TL, Klein-Schwartz W, Rodgers GC Jr, et al: 2001 Annual report of the American Association of Poison Control Centers Toxic Exposure Surveillance System. Am J Emerg Med 20:391-452, 2002.
2. Litovitz TL, Klein-Schwartz W, White S, et al: 2000 Annual report of the American Association of Poison Control Centers Toxic Exposure Surveillance System. Am J Emerg Med 19:337-395, 2001.
3. Shannon MW, Haddad LM: The emergency management of poisoning. In Haddad LM, Shannon MW, Winchester JF (eds): Clinical management of poisoning and drug overdose, 3rd ed. Philadelphia, WB Saunders, 1998, pp 2-31.
4. Goldberg MJ, Spector R, Park GD, et al: An approach to the management of the poisoned patient. Arch Intern Med 146:1381-1385, 1986.
5. Kulig K: Initial management of ingestions of toxic substances. N Engl J Med 326:1677-1681, 1992.
6. Vale A, Meredith T, Buckley B: ABC of poisoning. Eliminating poisons. Br Med J (Clin Res Ed) 289:366-369, 1984.
7. Tenenbein M, Cohen S, Sitar DS: Whole bowel irrigation as a decontamination procedure after acute drug overdose. Arch Intern Med 147:905-907, 1987.
8. Position statement and practice guidelines on the use of multi-dose activated charcoal in the treatment of acute poisoning. American Academy of Clinical Toxicology; European Association of Poisons Centres and Clinical Toxicologists. J Toxicol Clin Toxicol 37:731-751, 1999.
9. Tenenbein M: Multiple doses of activated charcoal: Time for reappraisal? Ann Emerg Med 20:529-531, 1991.
10. Bradberry SM, Vale JA: Multiple-dose activated charcoal: A review of relevant clinical studies. J Toxicol Clin Toxicol 33:407-416, 1995.
11. Chyka PA: Multiple-dose activated charcoal and enhancement of systemic drug clearance: Summary of studies in animals and human volunteers. J Toxicol Clin Toxicol 33:399-405, 1995.
12. Bond GR: The role of activated charcoal and gastric emptying in gastrointestinal decontamination: A state-of-the-art review. Ann Emerg Med 39:273-286, 2002.
13. Scharman EJ: Methods used to decrease lithium absorption or enhance elimination. J Toxicol Clin Toxicol 35:601-608, 1997.
14. Quang LS, Woolf AD: Past, present, and future role of ipecac syrup. Curr Opin Pediatr 12:153-162, 2000.
15. Krenzelok EP, McGuigan M, Lheur P: Position statement: Ipecac syrup. American Academy of Clinical Toxicology; European Association of Poisons Centres and Clinical Toxicologists. J Toxicol Clin Toxicol 35:699-709, 1997.
16. Lanphear WF: Gastric lavage. J Emerg Med 4:43-47, 1986.
17. Vale JA: Position statement: Gastric lavage. American Academy of Clinical Toxicology; European Association of Poisons Centres and Clinical Toxicologists. J Toxicol Clin Toxicol 35:711-719, 1997.
18. Perrone J, Hoffman RS, Goldfrank LR: Special considerations in gastrointestinal decontamination. Emerg Med Clin North Am 12:285-299, 1994.
19. Garrettson LK, Geller RJ: Acid and alkaline diuresis. When are they of value in the treatment of poisoning? Drug Saf 5:220-232, 1990.
20. Garella S: Extracorporeal techniques in the treatment of exogenous intoxications. Kidney Int 33:735-754, 1988.
21. Maher JF: Principles of dialysis and dialysis of drugs. Am J Med 62:475-481, 1977.
22. Winchester JF: Active methods for detoxification. In Haddad LM, Shannon MW, Winchester JF (eds): Clinical Management of Poisoning and Drug Overdose, 3rd ed. Philadelphia, WB Saunders, 1998, pp 175-188.
23. Blye E, Lorch J, Cortell S: Extracorporeal therapy in the treatment of intoxication. Am J Kidney Dis 3:321-338, 1984.
24. Babb AL, Popovich RP, Christopher TG, et al: The genesis of the square meter-hour hypothesis. Trans Am Soc Artif Intern Organs 17:81-91, 1971.
25. Keller F, Wilms H, Schultze G, et al: Effect of plasma protein binding, volume of distribution and molecular weight on the fraction of drugs eliminated by hemodialysis. Clin Nephrol 19:201-205, 1983.
26. Pond SM: Extracorporeal techniques in the treatment of poisoned patients. Med J Aust 154:617-622, 1991.
27. Gulyassy PF, Depner TA: Impaired binding of drugs and endogenous ligands in renal diseases. Am J Kidney Dis 2:578-601, 1983.
28. Suh B, Craig WA, England AC, et al: Effect of free fatty acids on protein binding of antimicrobial agents. J Infect Dis 143:609-616, 1981.
29. Lunde PK, Rane A, Yaffe SJ, et al: Plasma protein binding of diphenylhydantoin in man. Interaction with other drugs and the effect of temperature and plasma dilution. Clin Pharmacol Ther 11:846-855, 1970.
30. Storstein L, Janssen H: Studies on digitalis. VI. The effect of heparin on serum protein binding of digitoxin and digoxin. Clin Pharmacol Ther 20:15-23, 1976.

31. Gwilt PR, Perrier D: Plasma protein binding and distribution characteristics of drugs as indices of their hemodialyzability. Clin Pharmacol Ther 24:154-161, 1978.

32. Reidenberg MM: Effect of disease states on plasma protein binding of drugs. Med Clin North Am 58:1103-1109, 1974.

33. Reidenberg MM, Affrime M: Influence of disease on binding of drugs to plasma proteins. Ann N Y Acad Sci 226:115-126, 1973.

34. McNamara PJ, Lalka D, Gibaldi M: Endogenous accumulation products and serum protein binding in uremia. J Lab Clin Med 98:730-740, 1981.

35. Reidenberg MM: The binding of drugs to plasma proteins and the interpretation of measurements of plasma concentrations of drugs in patients with poor renal function. Am J Med 62:466-470, 1977.

36. Vanholder R, Van Landschoot N, De Smet R, et al: Drug protein binding in chronic renal failure: Evaluation of nine drugs. Kidney Int 33:996-1004, 1988.

37. Dromgoole SH: The effect of haemodialysis on the binding capacity of albumin. Clin Chim Acta 46:269-272, 1973.

38. Rutstein DD, Castelli WP, Nickerson RJ: Heparin and human lipid metabolism. Lancet 1:1003-1008, 1969.

39. Reuning RH, Sams RA, Notari RE: Role of pharmacokinetics in drug dosage adjustment. I. Pharmacologic effect kinetics and apparent volume of distribution of digoxin. J Clin Pharmacol New Drugs 13:127-141, 1973.

40. Odar-Cederlof I, Borga O: Kinetics of diphenylhydantoin in uraemic patients: Consequences of decreased plasma protein binding. Eur J Clin Pharmacol 7:31-37, 1974.

41. Timmer RT, Sands JM: Lithium intoxication. J Am Soc Nephrol 10:666-674, 1999.

42. Grimes DJ, Bowles MR, Buttsworth JA, et al: Survival after unexpected high serum methotrexate concentrations in a patient with osteogenic sarcoma. Drug Saf 5:447-454, 1990.

43. Hampson EC, Pond SM: Failure of hemoperfusion and haemodialysis to prevent death in paraquat poisoning: A retrospective review of 42 patients. Med Toxicol Adverse Drug Exp 3:64-71, 1988.

44. Gibson TP, Atkinson AJ Jr: Effect of changes in intercompartment rate constants on drug removal during hemoperfusion. J Pharm Sci 67:1178-1179, 1978.

45. Amir AR, Winchester JF: Hemodialysis and hemoperfusion in the managment of drug intoxication. In Glassock RJ (ed): Massry & Glassock's Textbook of Nephrology, 4th ed. Philadelphia, Lippincott Williams & Wilkins, 2001, pp 1729-1735.

46. Winchester JF: Dialysis and hemoperfusion in poisoning. Adv Ren Replace Ther 9:26-30, 2002.

47. Andrade JD, Van Wagenen R, Chen C, et al: Coated adsorbents for direct blood perfusion II. Trans Am Soc Artif Intern Organs 18:473-483, 485, 1972.

48. Nagler J, Braeckman RA, Willems JL, et al: Combined hemoperfusion-hemodialysis in organophosphate poisoning. J Appl Toxicol 1:199-201, 1981.

49. Frank RD, Kierdorf HP: Is there a role for hemoperfusion/hemodialysis as a treatment option in severe tricyclic antidepressant intoxication? Int J Artif Organs 23:618-623, 2000.

50. De Broe ME, Verpooten GA, Christiaens MA, et al: Clinical experience with prolonged combined hemoperfusion-hemodialysis treatment of severe poisoning. Artif Organs 5:59-66, 1981.

51. Vasilakakis DM, D'Haese PC, Lamberts LV, et al: Removal of aluminoxamine and ferrioxamine by charcoal hemoperfusion and hemodialysis. Kidney Int 41:1400-1407, 1992.

52. Colton CK, Henderson LW, Ford CA: Kinetics of hemodiafiltration: In vitro transport characteristics of a hollow fiber blood ultrafilter. J Lab Clin Med 85:355-360, 1975.

53. Golper TA, Bennett WM: Drug removal by continuous arteriovenous haemofiltration. A review of the evidence in poisoned patients. Med Toxicol Adverse Drug Exp 3:341-349, 1988.

54. Leblanc M, Raymond M, Bonnardeaux A, et al: Lithium poisoning treated by high-performance continuous arteriovenous and venovenous hemodiafiltration. Am J Kidney Dis 27:365-372, 1996.

55. Exaire E, Trevino-Becerra A, Monteon F: An overview of treatment with peritoneal dialysis in drug poisoning. Contrib Nephrol 17:39-43, 1979.

56. Choi JH, Oh JC, Kim KH, et al: Successful treatment of cisplatin overdose with plasma exchange. Yonsei Med J 43:128-132, 2002.

57. Meert KL, Ellis J, Aronow R, et al: Acute ammonium dichromate poisoning. Ann Emerg Med 24:748-750, 1994.

58. Barceloux DG, Krenzelok EP, Olson K, et al: American Academy of Clinical Toxicology practice guidelines on the treatment of ethylene glycol poisoning. Ad Hoc Committee. J Toxicol Clin Toxicol 37:537-560, 1999.

59. Winchester JF: Methanol, isopropyl alcohol, higher alcohols, ethylene glycol, cellosolves, acetone, and oxalate. In Haddad LM, Shannon MW, Winchester JF (eds): Clinical Management of Poisoning and Drug Overdose, 3rd ed. Philadelphia, WB Saunders, 1998, pp 491-504.

60. Walker JT, Keller MS, Katz SM: Computed tomographic and sonographic findings in acute ethylene glycol poisoning. J Ultrasound Med 2:429-431, 1983.

61. Bove KE: Ethylene glycol toxicity. Am J Clin Pathol 45:46-50, 1966.

62. Aquino HC, Leonard CD: Ethylene glycol poisoning: Report of three cases. J Ky Med Assoc 70:463-465, 1972.

63. Munro KM, Adams JH: Acute ethylene glycol poisoning: Report of a fatal case. Med Sci Law 7:181-184, 1967.

64. Clay KL, Murphy RC: On the metabolic acidosis of ethylene glycol intoxication. Toxicol Appl Pharmacol 39:39-49, 1977.

65. Bachmann E, Golberg L: Reappraisal of the toxicology of ethylene glycol. 3. Mitochondrial effects. Food Cosmet Toxicol 9:39-55, 1971.

66. Brown CG, Trumbull D, Klein-Schwartz W, et al: Ethylene glycol poisoning. Ann Emerg Med 12:501-506, 1983.

67. Gordon HL, Hunter JM: Ethylene glycol poisoning. A case report. Anaesthesia 37:332-338, 1982.

68. Glaser DS: Utility of the serum osmol gap in the diagnosis of methanol or ethylene glycol ingestion. Ann Emerg Med 27:343-346, 1996.

69. Church AS, Witting MD: Laboratory testing in ethanol, methanol, ethylene glycol, and isopropanol toxicities. J Emerg Med 15:687-692, 1997.

70. Abramson S, Singh AK: Treatment of the alcohol intoxications: Ethylene glycol, methanol and isopropanol. Curr Opin Nephrol Hypertens 9:695-701, 2000.

71. Saladino R, Shannon M: Accidental and intentional poisonings with ethylene glycol in infancy: Diagnostic clues and management. Pediatr Emerg Care 7:93-96, 1991.

72. Grauer GF, Thrall MA, Henre BA, et al: Early clinicopathologic findings in dogs ingesting ethylene glycol. Am J Vet Res 45:2299-2303, 1984.

73. Jacobsen D, Akesson I, Shefter E: Urinary calcium oxalate monohydrate crystals in ethylene glycol poisoning. Scand J Clin Lab Invest 42:231-234, 1982.

74. Winter ML, Ellis MD, Snodgrass WR: Urine fluorescence using a Wood's lamp to detect the antifreeze additive sodium fluorescein: A qualitative adjunctive test in suspected ethylene glycol ingestions. Ann Emerg Med 19:663-667, 1990.

75. Weiss B, Coen G: Effect of ethanol on ethylene glycol oxidation by mammalian liver enzymes. Enzymol Biol Clin (Basel) 6:297-304, 1966.

76. McCoy HG, Cipolle RJ, Ehlers SM, et al: Severe methanol poisoning. Application of a pharmacokinetic model for ethanol therapy and hemodialysis. Am J Med 67:804-807, 1979.

77. Nzerue CM, Harvey P, Volcy J, et al: Survival after massive ethylene glycol poisoning: Role of an ethanol enriched, bicarbonate-based dialysate. Int J Artif Organs 22:744-746, 1999.

78. Peterson CD, Collins AJ, Himes JM, et al: Ethylene glycol poisoning: Pharmacokinetics during therapy with ethanol and hemodialysis. N Engl J Med 304:21-23, 1981.

79. Chu J, Wang RY, Hill NS: Update in clinical toxicology. Am J Respir Crit Care Med 166:9-15, 2002.

80. Antizol (fomepizole) (injection product monograph). Minnesota, MN, Orphan Medical, December 2000.

81. Jobard E, Harry P, Turcant A, et al: 4-Methylpyrazole and hemodialysis in ethylene glycol poisoning. J Toxicol Clin Toxicol 34:373-377, 1996.

82. Cheng JT, Beysolow TD, Kaul B, et al: Clearance of ethylene glycol by kidneys and hemodialysis. J Toxicol Clin Toxicol 25:95-108, 1987.

83. Moreau CL, Kerns W 2nd, Tomaszewski CA, et al: Glycolate kinetics and hemodialysis clearance in ethylene glycol poisoning. META Study Group. J Toxicol Clin Toxicol 36:659-666, 1998.

84. Borron SW, Megarbane B, Baud FJ: Fomepizole in treatment of uncomplicated ethylene glycol poisoning. Lancet 354:831, 1999.

85. Hantson P, Hassoun A, Mahieu P: Ethylene glycol poisoning treated by intravenous 4-methylpyrazole. Intensive Care Med 24:736-739, 1998.

86. Barceloux DG, Bond GR, Krenzelok EP, et al: American Academy of Clinical Toxicology practice guidelines on the treatment of methanol poisoning. J Toxicol Clin Toxicol 40:415-446, 2002.

87. Nicholls P: The effect of formate on cytochrome *aa3* and on electron transport in the intact respiratory chain. Biochim Biophys Acta 430:13-29, 1976.

88. Keyhani J, Keyhani E: EPR study of the effect of formate on cytochrome C oxidase. Biochem Biophys Res Commun 92:327-333, 1980.

89. Roe O: Clinical investigations of methyl alcohol poisoning with special reference to the pathogenesis and treatment of amblyopia. Acta Med Scand 113:558-608, 1943.

90. Liesivuori J, Savolainen H: Methanol and formic acid toxicity: Biochemical mechanisms. Pharmacol Toxicol 69:157-163, 1991.

91. Sejersted OM, Jacobsen D, Ovrebo S, et al: Formate concentrations in plasma from patients poisoned with methanol. Acta Med Scand 213:105-110, 1983.

92. Hantson P, Haufroid V, Mahieu P: Determination of formic acid tissue and fluid concentrations in three fatalities due to methanol poisoning. Am J Forensic Med Pathol 21:335-338, 2000.

93. Jacobsen D, McMartin KE: Methanol and ethylene glycol poisonings. Mechanism of toxicity, clinical course, diagnosis and treatment. Med Toxicol 1:309-334, 1986.

94. Hayreh MS, Hayreh SS, Baumbach GL, et al: Methyl alcohol poisoning III. Ocular toxicity. Arch Ophthalmol 95:1851-1858, 1977.

95. Baumbach GL, Cancilla PA, Martin-Amat G, et al: Methyl alcohol poisoning. IV. Alterations of the morphological findings of the retina and optic nerve. Arch Ophthalmol 95:1859-1865, 1977.

96. Sharpe JA, Hostovsky M, Bilbao JM, et al: Methanol optic neuropathy: A histopathological study. Neurology 32:1093-1100, 1982.

97. Naraqi S, Dethlefs RF, Slobodniuk RA, et al: An outbreak of acute methyl alcohol intoxication. Aust N Z J Med 9:65-68, 1979.

98. Sullivan-Mee M, Solis K: Methanol-induced vision loss. J Am Optom Assoc 69:57-65, 1998.

99. Scrimgeour EM: Outbreak of methanol and isopropanol poisoning in New Britain, Papua New Guinea. Med J Aust 2:36-38, 1980.

100. McLean DR, Jacobs H, Mielke BW: Methanol poisoning: A clinical and pathological study. Ann Neurol 8:161-167, 1980.

101. Ley CO, Gali FG: Parkinsonian syndrome after methanol intoxication. Eur Neurol 22:405-409, 1983.

102. Grufferman S, Morris D, Alvarez J: Methanol poisoning complicated by myoglobinuric renal failure. Am J Emerg Med 3:24-26, 1985.

103. Cavalli A, Volpi A, Maggioni AP, et al: Severe reversible cardiac failure associated with methanol intoxication. Postgrad Med J 63:867-868, 1987.

104. Jacobsen D, Webb R, Collins TD, et al: Methanol and formate kinetics in late diagnosed methanol intoxication. Med Toxicol Adverse Drug Exp 3:418-423, 1988.

105. Peterson CD: Oral ethanol doses in patients with methanol poisoning. Am J Hosp Pharm 38:1024-1027, 1981.

106. Pappas SC, Silverman M: Treatment of methanol poisoning with ethanol and hemodialysis. Can Med Assoc J 126:1391-1394, 1982.

107. Wadgymar A, Wu GG: Treatment of acute methanol intoxication with hemodialysis. Am J Kidney Dis 31:897, 1998.

108. Lacouture PG, Wason S, Abrams A, et al: Acute isopropyl alcohol intoxication. Diagnosis and management. Am J Med 75:680-686, 1983.

109. Burkhart KK, Martinez MA: The adsorption of isopropanol and acetone by activated charcoal. J Toxicol Clin Toxicol 30:371-375, 1992.

110. Mecikalski MB, Depner TA: Peritoneal dialysis for isopropanol poisoning. West J Med 137:322-324, 1982.

111. King LH Jr, Bradley KP, Shires DL Jr: Hemodialysis for isopropyl alcohol poisoning. JAMA 211:1855, 1970.

112. Ellenhorn MJ, Schonwald S, Ordog G, et al: Lithium. *In* Wasserberger J (ed): Medical Toxicology: Diagnosis and Treatment of Human Poisoning. Baltimore, Williams & Wilkins, 1997, pp 1579.

113. Okusa MD, Crystal LJ: Clinical manifestations and management of acute lithium intoxication. Am J Med 97:383-389, 1994.

114. Greger R: Possible sites of lithium transport in the nephron. Kidney Int Suppl 28:S26-S30, 1990.

115. Lenox RH, McNamara RK, Papke RL, et al: Neurobiology of lithium: An update. J Clin Psychiatry 59(suppl 6):37-47, 1998.

116. Holstein-Rathlou NH: Lithium transport across biological membranes. Kidney Int Suppl 28:S4-S9, 1990.

117. Finley PR, Warner MD, Peabody CA: Clinical relevance of drug interactions with lithium. Clin Pharmacokinet 29:172-191, 1995.

118. Boton R, Gaviria M, Batlle DC: Prevalence, pathogenesis, and treatment of renal dysfunction associated with chronic lithium therapy. Am J Kidney Dis 10:329-345, 1987.

119. Hansen HE, Amdisen A: Lithium intoxication. Report of 23 cases and review of 100 cases from the literature. Q J Med 47:123-144, 1978.

120. Jacobsen D, Aasen G, Frederichsen P, et al: Lithium intoxication: Pharmacokinetics during and after terminated hemodialysis in acute intoxications. J Toxicol Clin Toxicol 25:81-94, 1987.

121. Wosilait WD: Theoretical analysis of the binding of salicylate by human serum albumin: The relationship between free and bound drug and therapeutic levels. Eur J Clin Pharmacol 9:285-290, 1976.

122. Gabow PA, Anderson RJ, Potts DE, et al: Acid-base disturbances in the salicylate-intoxicated adult. Arch Intern Med 138:1481-1484, 1978.

123. Hill JB: Salicylate intoxication. N Engl J Med 288:1110-1113, 1973.

124. Winters RW, White JS, Hughes MC: Disturbance of acid-base equilibrium in salicylate intoxication. Pediatrics 23:260, 1959.

125. Dargan PI, Wallace CI, Jones AL: An evidence based flowchart to guide the management of acute salicylate (aspirin) overdose. Emerg Med J 19:206-209, 2002.

126. Johnson PK, Free HM, Free AH: A simplified urine and serum screening test for salicylate intoxication. J Pediatr 63:949-953, 1963.

127. Proudfoot AT: Toxicity of salicylates. Am J Med 75(5A):99-103, 1983.

128. Prescott LF, Balali-Mood M, Critchley JA, et al: Diuresis or urinary alkalinisation for salicylate poisoning? Br Med J (Clin Res Ed) 285:1383-1386, 1982.

129. Robbin ED, Davis RP, Rees SB: Salicylate intoxication with special reference to the development of hypokalemia. Am J Med 26:869-882, 1959.

130. Barone JA, Raia JJ, Huang YC: Evaluation of the effects of multiple-dose activated charcoal on the absorption of orally administered salicylate in a simulated toxic ingestion model. Ann Emerg Med 17:34-37, 1988.

131. Wrathall G, Sinclair R, Moore A, et al: Three case reports of the use of haemodiafiltration in the treatment of salicylate overdose. Hum Exp Toxicol 20:491-495, 2001.

132. Higgins RM, Connolly JO, Hendry BM: Alkalinization and hemodialysis in severe salicylate poisoning: Comparison of elimination techniques in the same patient. Clin Nephrol 50:178-183, 1998.

133. Jacobs MH, Senior RM, Kessler G: Clinical experience with theophylline. Relationships between dosage, serum concentration, and toxicity. JAMA 235:1983-1986, 1976.

134. Shannon M: Predictors of major toxicity after theophylline overdose. Ann Intern Med 119:1161-1167, 1993.

135. Sessler CN: Theophylline toxicity: Clinical features of 116 consecutive cases. Am J Med 88:567-576, 1990.

136. Olson KR, Benowitz NL, Woo OF, et al: Theophylline overdose: Acute single ingestion versus chronic repeated overmedication. Am J Emerg Med 3:386-394, 1985.

137. Hall KW, Dobson KE, Dalton JG, et al: Metabolic abnormalities associated with intentional theophylline overdose. Ann Intern Med 101:457-462, 1984.

138. Goldberg MJ, Park GD, Berlinger WG: Treatment of theophylline intoxication. J Allergy Clin Immunol 78(Pt 2):811-817, 1986.

139. Radomski L, Park GD, Goldberg MJ, et al: Model for theophylline overdose treatment with oral activated charcoal. Clin Pharmacol Ther 35:402-408, 1984.

140. Greenberg A, Piraino BH, Kroboth PD, et al: Severe theophylline toxicity: Role of conservative measures, antiarrhythmic agents, and charcoal hemoperfusion. Am J Med 76:854-860, 1984.

141. Gaudreault P, Guay J: Theophylline poisoning: Pharmacological considerations and clinical management. Med Toxicol 1:169-191, 1986.

142. Park GD, Spector R, Roberts RJ, et al: Use of hemoperfusion for treatment of theophylline intoxication. Am J Med 74:961-966, 1983.

143. Ehlers SM, Zaske DE, Sawchuk RJ: Massive theophylline overdose. Rapid elimination by charcoal hemoperfusion. JAMA 240:474-475, 1978.

144. Russo ME: Management of theophylline intoxication with charcoal-column hemoperfusion. N Engl J Med 300:24-26, 1979.

145. Hootkins R Sr, Lerman MJ, Thompson JR: Sequential and simultaneous "in series" hemodialysis and hemoperfusion in the

management of theophylline intoxication. J Am Soc Nephrol 1: 923-926, 1990.

146. Benowitz NL, Toffelmin EB: The use of hemodialysis and hemoperfusion in the treatment of theophylline intoxication. Semin Dial 6:243-252, 1993.

147. Chadwick DW: Concentration-effect relationships of valproic acid. Clin Pharmacokinet 10:155-163, 1985.

148. Khoo SH, Leyland MJ: Cerebral edema following acute sodium valproate overdose. J Toxicol Clin Toxicol 30:209-214, 1992.

149. Graudins A, Aaron CK: Delayed peak serum valproic acid in massive divalproex overdose—treatment with charcoal hemoperfusion. J Toxicol Clin Toxicol 34:335-341, 1996.

150. Mortensen PB, Hansen HE, Pedersen B, et al: Acute valproate intoxication: Biochemical investigations and hemodialysis treatment. Int J Clin Pharmacol Ther Toxicol 21:64-68, 1983.

151. Smith TW: Digitalis: Mechanisms of action and clinical use. N Engl J Med 318:358-365, 1988.

152. Dick M, Curwin J, Tepper D: Digitalis intoxication recognition and management. J Clin Pharmacol 31:444-447, 1991.

153. Smith TW, Antman EM, Friedman PL, et al: Digitalis glycosides: Mechanisms and manifestations of toxicity. Part III. Prog Cardiovasc Dis 27:21-56, 1984.

154. Goodman LS: Digitalis. *In* Winchester JF (ed): Clinical Management of Poisoning and Drug Overdose, 3rd ed. Philadelphia, WB Saunders, 1998, pp 1001-1020.

155. Antman EM, Wenger TL, Butler VP Jr, et al: Treatment of 150 cases of life-threatening digitalis intoxication with digoxin-specific Fab antibody fragments: Final report of a multicenter study. Circulation 81:1744-1752, 1990.

156. Zdunek M, Mitra A, Mokrzycki MH: Plasma exchange for the removal of digoxin-specific antibody fragments in renal failure: Timing is important for maximizing clearance. Am J Kidney Dis 36:177-183, 2000.

157. Starkebaum G, Kenyon CM, Simrell CR, et al: Procainamide-induced agranulocytosis differs serologically and clinically from procainamide-induced lupus. Clin Immunol Immunopathol 78: 112-119, 1996.

158. Kim SY, Benowitz NL: Poisoning due to class IA antiarrhythmic drugs: Quinidine, procainamide and disopyramide. Drug Saf 5: 393-420, 1990.

159. Hopkins BE: Procainamide-induced lupus-like syndrome. Med J Aust 2:734-735, 1970.

160. Li GC, Greenberg CS, Currie MS: Procainamide-induced lupus anti-coagulants and thrombosis. South Med J 81:262-264, 1988.

161. Low CL, Phelps KR, Bailie GR: Relative efficacy of haemoperfusion, haemodialysis and CAPD in the removal of procainamide and NAPA in a patient with severe procainamide toxicity. Nephrol Dial Transplant 11:881-884, 1996.

162. Rosansky SJ, Brady ME: Procainamide toxicity in a patient with acute renal failure. Am J Kidney Dis 7:502-506, 1986.

CHAPTER 63

Transplantation Immunobiology

Anil Chandraker, David L. Perkins, Charles B. Carpenter, and Mohamed H. Sayegh

CHARACTERISTICS OF THE ALLOGENEIC IMMUNE RESPONSE

Allogeneic is the term that refers to the genetic relationship between two individuals of the same species, *xenogeneic* to that between two individuals of different species, and *syngeneic* to human monozygous twins or completely inbred animals of the same strain. The immune system evolved to protect us from invading microorganisms. It appears also to play a protective role in surveillance for altered normal cells, such as ones that have undergone malignant transformation. The components of the immune system that are recruited when a threat to body integrity occurs are multiple, and they vary according to the nature of the threat (e.g., viral versus bacterial) and the anatomic location of the insult (e.g., skin or gastrointestinal tract). Many important components of immunity that are ancient in evolutionary time are described as components of natural immunity. These include phagocytic cells, natural killer (NK) cells, complement, and some cytokines and chemokines. Tissue injury from any cause can activate the natural immune system. In contrast, immune reactants that specifically recognize regions called antigens on molecules from the microbial world produce adaptive immunity. The main components of such antigen-specific immunity are immunoglobulins, which are made by B cells and (thymus-dependent) T cells. Some investigators refer to an inflammatory response that involves only components of natural immunity as being "nonimmune." Most immunologists recognize natural immune reactants as being very important to the success of the overall immune response and do not limit immune phenomena to those that are antigen-specific. In transplantation immunity, recognition of donor antigens is crucial in developing antigen-specific clones of T and B cells, which then direct an even larger array of cellular and humoral responses, many of which do not utilize specific antigen receptors. Fundamentally, the "firestorm" of allograft rejection does not occur in the absence of cell-mediated responses initiated by specific T lymphocytes, but the full force of the rejection utilizes components of the natural immune system.

The first successful renal transplantation was performed at the Peter Bent Brigham Hospital in Boston, in 1954, between identical twins. In the 1960s, recognition of the immunosuppressive properties of azathioprine in combination with corticosteroids made possible successful transplants from nonidentical donors. With the development of newer immunosuppressive agents, including cyclosporine, tacrolimus, mycophenolate mofetil (MMF), as well as polyclonal and specific monoclonal antibodies, the incidence and intensity of acute rejection have been reduced, but the problem of chronic graft rejection remains a persistent obstacle. Since transplantation was a very rare event until modern times, the immune system clearly did not evolve to produce graft rejection. It was the investigation of the alloimmune response to transplanted tissues that led to the identification of major histocompatibility complex (MHC) molecules. This investigation, in turn, provided crucial insights into the process of immune recognition, because without the presentation of peptides by these molecules, T cells would be nonfunctional.

Although there are many similarities between immune recognition of conventional antigen and the recognition of allogeneic transplantation antigens, a major difference exists between the response to allogeneic and conventional antigens that has major implications for transplantation biology. The most striking difference is the markedly increased frequency of responding T cells in the allogeneic response. In addition, because recipient T cells recognize intact allogeneic

MHC molecules directly, they are stimulated maximally by the high density of MHC on the surfaces of transplanted cells. T cells do not contact allo-MHC molecules during development in the thymus and thus escape the deletion (negative selection) imposed by interaction with self-MHC. The molecular basis for the high frequency with which T cells respond to an allogeneic stimulus remains incompletely understood; however, the high frequency of alloantigen-specific T cells contributes to the vigorous nature of the immune response that causes graft rejection, and it is the major initial obstacle to successful organ transplantation.

Tolerance and Immunity: Self–Nonself Discrimination

The principal tenet of immune recognition is that the immune system must discriminate "self" from "nonself." This process has been viewed as being dependent on two components. First, the immune system must not respond to any self-antigens, which it does principally through the mechanisms of self-tolerance. Second, nonself (foreign)-antigens derived from numerous sources, including pathogens and tumor cells, must be effectively recognized to prevent infections and tumors. In this paradigm, the immune system simply recognizes transplanted tissues as nonself, causing graft rejection. In reality, it now seems that autorecognition of self-antigens is common and only rarely results in autoimmune disease. The key resides in an immune regulatory system that is more complex than was previously imagined. The ultimate goal of clinical transplantation is to develop protocols to induce specific tolerance to the graft so that the immune system is regulated to accept the graft as self without maintenance immunosuppression.

Antigen Recognition

Clearly, the immune system did not evolve to reject transplanted organs. It is commonly accepted that the major function of the immune response is to recognize foreign antigens derived from pathogens and tumors. However, we now know that the processes by which the immune system recognizes conventional and transplantation antigens have many similarities and involve the same antigen recognition molecules. Specifically, the antigen-specific receptors include the T cell receptor (TCR) on T lymphocytes and antibody molecules produced by B lymphocytes. As we discuss in more detail later, the TCR recognizes peptide fragments of processed antigen only when they are bound to MHC molecules expressed on the surface of antigen-presenting cells (APCs), whereas immunoglobulins can bind directly to peptide fragments or to the same peptide sequences in the intact native molecule.

In the early days of study of MHC antigens, investigators wondered why hematopoietic cells, especially B cells and monocyte-macrophages, have high expression of MHC molecules. It is now quite clear that the true role of the MHC is to present potentially immunogenic peptides of foreign antigens to T lymphocytes. Whereas the T cell response to a conventional antigen can be experimentally detected only after previous immunization, an allogeneic response, as assayed in a mixed lymphocyte culture (MLC) in vitro, can be readily detected in previously unimmunized (naïve) lymphocytes. At least part of the basis for the greater magnitude of the allogeneic response is the increased frequency of responding cells. For example, the frequency of specific T cells to conventional antigens is approximately 1 in 10^4 to 10^5, whereas the frequency responding during allogeneic stimulation can be as high as 1 in 10^1 to 10^2. The graft, which includes donor bone marrow–derived APCs, usually expresses several class I and class II MHC molecules that differ from the recipient's MHC molecules and that can directly stimulate recipient T cells (direct allorecognition).

Alternatively, donor antigens can be processed and peptide fragments presented by the host MHC molecules on self APCs, indirectly stimulating the recipient T cells (indirect allorecognition) via the same pathway that is used for responses to microbial antigens (see later). Relevant to clinical transplantation, the greater intensity of an allogeneic response can produce vigorous episodes of acute allograft rejection that can be difficult to control and may require large doses of immunosuppressive agents (see Chapter 65).

Immune Tolerance

Immune tolerance is a state of unresponsiveness to specific antigens derived from either self- or nonself-proteins. From numerous studies it is clear that maintenance of immune tolerance to self-antigens involves multiple mechanisms. First, tolerance can occur at the level of either T or B lymphocytes.[1, 2] Second, tolerance can be induced in either immature lymphocytes during the early steps of differentiation or in mature lymphocytes after they have migrated to the peripheral lymphoid tissues, including lymph nodes and spleen.[2-4] Third, tolerance, or immune unresponsiveness, can be mediated by several mechanisms, including clonal deletion of antigen-specific lymphocytes, anergy (inactivation of lymphocytes that nevertheless remain viable), and suppression involving regulatory processes between different subsets of lymphocytes.[5] Evidence from both human studies and animal models indicates that the maintenance of self-tolerance involves many, if not all, of these mechanisms.

The major mechanism of self-tolerance is the elimination of potentially autoreactive T cells at an immature stage of development during maturation in the thymus by a process called *negative selection*.[6] It is estimated that more than 95% of thymocytes die because of a high-affinity encounter with self-MHC before they migrate to the peripheral lymphoid organs.[7] Thymocyte clones that are positively selected for differentiation into mature peripheral T lymphocytes have receptors that are less avid for self-MHC[8] and possess the necessary repertoire to recognize a large number of peptide configurations when bound to self-MHC and, by cross-reaction (molecular mimicry), to the intact surfaces of allo-MHC. Although thymic selection is a major mechanism for maintaining self-tolerance, the main problem in clinical transplantation relates to preventing T cells that have already been selected in the thymus from rejecting an allograft. Thus, efforts to achieve donor-specific allograft tolerance must focus on mechanisms that regulate tolerance in mature peripheral T cells (see later discussion).

TRANSPLANTATION ANTIGENS

Normal persons maintain a state of self-tolerance to self-tissues. Allografts, however, express nonself-antigens to which the recipient is not tolerant, and they cause an antigraft immune response that initiates rejection. Several types of transplantation antigens have been characterized, including the MHC molecules, minor histocompatibility antigens, ABO blood group antigens, and monocyte–endothelial cell antigens.

The antigenic stimulus for initiation and progression of the rejection response to grafted tissue is provoked by cell-surface molecules that are polymorphic (i.e., that vary in structure from individual to individual and that are treated as foreign intruders that the body must recognize and destroy). The most important transplantation antigens are those of the MHC. In both animals and humans, this series of linked genes provides the strongest incompatibilities for any sort of tissue and organ transplant. The MHC antigens were originally discovered during tumor transplants between different inbred strains of mice, but their evolutionary conservation is based on defense against the microbial world. The MHC antigens are the strongest transplantation antigens and can stimulate a primary immune response without priming. The minor histocompatibility antigens are processed antigens in the form of small peptides that are presented by MHC molecules but are not derived from the MHC. T cells recognize a combination of the antigen and MHC molecule via a trimolecular interaction involving the TCR, MHC molecule, and processed antigen in the form of a short peptide. The minor histocompatibility antigens require priming and can be detected only in a secondary immune response. Understanding the roles of major and minor histocompatibility antigens is crucial to understanding transplantation biology.

The Major Histocompatibility Complex

Transplantation antigens are classified as either major or minor according to their relative potencies in eliciting rejection. The major antigens in all mammalian species studied are encoded by a closely linked series of genes in a chromosomal region called the MHC. The MHC was first defined in the mouse by Gorer[9] and Snell[10] as the agent of rapid rejection of tumor transplants between inbred strains of mice. This antigen system was called H-2 and was found to function in rejection of normal tissues as well. Rejection elicits serum antibodies that are used for typing of H-2 antigens. It was subsequently shown that cytotoxic T cells also arise in response to H-2 differences and that the H-2 genes are all clustered in a single region on chromosome 17.[11-13] Except for some details of the ordering of genes, the human (HLA) and rat (RT1) MHC regions are quite homologous to H-2 of the mouse. HLA is located on the short arm of chromosome 6.[14, 15] The species' chromosome numbers are different only because they have not been numbered in a manner that reflects the locations of actual genes.

Transplants compatible for the MHC antigens can still be rejected because of minor antigen (e.g., H-1, H-3, H-4) incompatibilities but not with the same intensity as with MHC-incompatible grafts. Modification of rejection by drugs or other means is more readily accomplished when the donor and recipient MHC antigens are matched. Extensive work in the mouse skin graft model with a large number of different major (H-2) and minor incompatibilities has shown that, in general, once the recipient has become immunized to such antigens, the total of multiple non–H-2 (minor) incompatibilities can be equal to the strength of the H-2 barrier alone in the unimmunized, or first-set, rejection response.[16] For both MHC and non-MHC barriers, placement of a second graft from the same donor is rejected at an accelerated rate (second-set rejection). The distinction of first- and second-set rejection phenomena in humans was first made by Holman in 1924 with skin grafts in burn patients.[17] During World War II, the problem of extensive burn injuries prompted fundamental studies of skin grafting by Medawar.[18]

Together with the emerging concept of a major transplantation antigen system,[9, 10] these studies laid the groundwork for the development of clinical transplantation in the second half of the 20th century. Although the initial discovery and definition of the MHC came from studies in transplantation, its central role in the initiation and expression of the immune response in general has become increasingly evident. The ability to produce an efficient immune response to many antigens is inherited in a mendelian autosomal-dominant fashion, and the controlling genes, called "Ir" (for immune response), are of the MHC. In fact, the failure to mount a response to a peptide antigen may now be attributed to a genetically determined inability to bind properly the antigenic fragment to MHC molecules.[19] The complex of antigen and MHC provides an efficient mode of presentation to clones of T lymphocytes that bear the appropriate antigen receptors. Indeed, it is clear that the TCR recognizes the total configuration of self-MHC plus the antigen fragment (peptide), and not antigen alone. Many experimental systems have demonstrated this MHC restriction phenomenon; that is, T cells, in order to respond, must share MHC antigens with the APCs.[20] The combined recognition of self-MHC plus antigen (self plus X hypothesis) is now being visualized at the molecular level (see later).

The HLA region on the short arm of chromosome 6 (Fig. 63-1) contains more than 3 million nucleotide base pairs. It encodes two structurally distinct classes of cell-surface molecules, termed *class I* and *class II* (Fig. 63-2). Traditionally, the term *MHC antigen* has been applied to the product of a given locus that displays polymorphism in a population of individuals. Now that the sequence and structure of molecules bearing MHC antigens have been extensively elucidated, it is known that the polymorphic, or antigenic, portions of MHC molecules are, indeed, quite small, often involving only one to four amino acid substitutions in regions of sequence hypervariability. In an MHC molecule, the specific substituted area that causes a change in antigenicity is called an *epitope*. Normal pregnancy induces antibodies against the HLA antigens of the fetus derived from the father's genes. Although blood from normal human pregnancies is the main source of antisera used for HLA typing, the first appreciation of the HLA system came from the studies of Dausset[14] on blood transfusion reactions due to antileukocyte antibodies. One such antibody from patient MAC proved to be a pregnancy-induced anti–HLA-2 response. Subsequent studies by Payne and co-workers[21] showed that such antibodies marked a codominantly expressed antileukocyte system that segregated in a mendelian distribution in families. International workshops on the HLA system began in 1962, and today they continue to accelerate progress in the definition and technical aspects of typing for the polymorphic antigens of this chromosome region.[22] The World Health Organization Nomenclature Committee has defined HLA as the "logo" for the human MHC. Although the individual

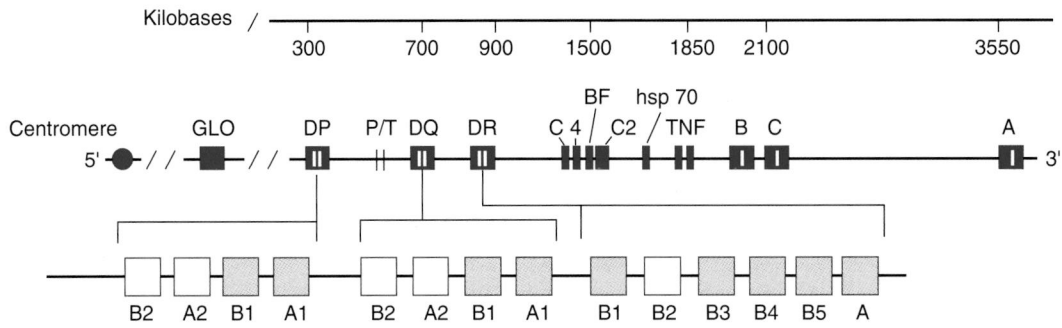

FIGURE 63-1. Schematic map of the *HLA* region on the short arm of chromosome 6. Distances are shown in kilobases derived from sequencing of DNA nucleotides. The centromere is to the left (5'). The boxes along the central line represent coding regions for the HLA polypeptides expressed on cell surfaces. *GLO* is a polymorphic red blood cell enzyme more than 4000 kilobases from *HLA*. On the right are the *HLA-A, HLA-B,* and *HLA-C* loci for the three sets of class I heavy chains, and on the left are the loci for the three sets of class II molecules, HLA-DP, HLA-DQ, and HLA-DR. The latter are composed of two chains, α and β, each the product of linked genes of the *DP, DQ,* or *DR* subregions. The *DRA* gene, for example, encodes the α-chain, and several *DRB* genes encode the β-chains of the heterodimeric HLA-DR molecules. In the case of DR, DRA is not polymorphic, so all the antigenicity lies with DRB. As shown in the expansion at the bottom, each subregion contains tandem sets of exons for one or more α- and β-chains. The gene for DR private specificities is *B1*; the more public DR51, DR52, and DR53 are encoded by the other B genes (see text). Pseudogenes, which are not expressed on the cell surface, are shown as white boxes. The HLA-DP and HLA-DQ molecules are also heterodimers, and both the α- and β-chains are polymorphic. Genes involved in proteolysis of proteins and the intracellular transport of peptides to meet up with class I molecules are in the class II region near DQ (shown as *P/T*). Between the class I and II loci are genes for the complement components C2, BF (factor B), and C4. Genes for 21OH (steroid 21-hydroxylase) are not shown but are between *C4* and *BF*. An expansion of the class III region would show that both *C4* and 21*OH* are reduplicated, so the order is this: -(*C4A-21OHA-C4B-21OHB-BF-C2*)-. The genes of this region are sometimes referred to as class III, although they bear little homology to class I and II, which do show homology for each other. The genes for TNF-α and TNF-β, and heat shock protein 70 (*hsp70*), have been mapped between the complement region and *HLA-B*. (From Carpenter CB: Histocompatibility systems in man. *In* Ginns LC, Cosimi AB, Morris PJ [eds]: Transplantation. Boston, Blackwell Science, 1999, p 61.)

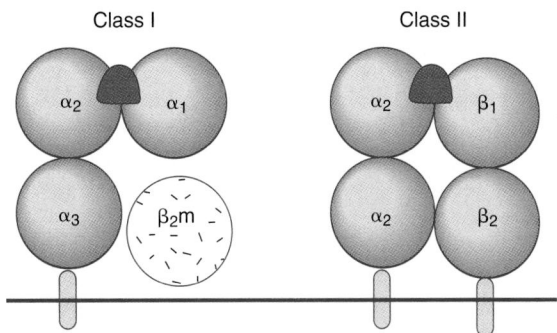

FIGURE 63-2. Diagrammatic view of class I and class II HLA molecules on a cell membrane as seen from the side of the molecules. The 44-kD α-chain is inserted through the lipid bilayer of the membrane and has three domains (α1, α2, α3), formed in part by disulfide bonding. β2-Microglobulin, encoded by a gene on chromosome 15, is noncovalently bound and is not membrane-inserted. The α2 and α1 domains form the β-strands and α-helices, which make up the base and sides, respectively, of the groove that binds a potentially immunogenic peptide. The variable amino acids that confer the antigenic differences between individual HLA types are arrayed along this groove. Class II molecules consist of one α-chain (34 kD) and one β-chain (28 kD), each having two domains, and each is membrane-inserted. A similar peptide-binding groove is formed by the α1 and β1 domains. (From Carpenter CB: Histocompatibility systems. *In* Ginns LC, Cosimi AB, Morris PJ [eds]: Transplantation. Boston, Blackwell Science, 1999, p 62.)

letters of the logo may have different colloquial meanings, such as human or histocompatibility; leukocyte, lymphocyte, or locus; antigen, for example, *HLA*, is to be used as the prefix to a locus or subregion designation that marks all that follows as a product of the human MHC chromosomal region (e.g., HLA-A2, HLA-DR4).[23] The term *human leukocyte*

antigen is to be avoided, because it has a broader meaning that includes cluster differentiation (CD) antigens, which are not histocompatibility antigens.

Class I and II molecules show some structural homology to immunoglobulins, to the T cell antigen receptor, and to molecules bearing the T cell differentiation antigens CD4 and CD8 (see later). The CD4 and CD8 antigens are part of the system whereby T cells interact preferentially with class II or class I molecules, respectively, on APCs or on cells that are targets for immune destruction. This family of cell-surface and extracellular recognition and interaction structures may have evolved from the same progenitor gene, diversifying by duplication and mutation, and in the process the new genes have moved to multiple chromosome sites. All mammalian species studied thus far have structural and functional representations of this "immunoglobulin supergene" family.[24]

HLA Molecules: Class I

Class I HLA molecules consist of two polypeptide chains in noncovalent association on cell surfaces. The heavy chain (44 kD) is inserted into the plasma membrane and contains the antigenic portions. The light chain (12 kD) is β2-microglobulin, encoded by a gene on chromosome 15.[15] There are three domains of the class I heavy chain, formed in part by disulfide bonding to make loops (see Fig. 63-2). The amino acid sequence variable regions are on the first (α1) and second (α2) domains. Class I molecules are expressed on almost all nucleated body cells, including the endothelium of blood vessels. Tissue typing is performed on peripheral blood, lymph node, or spleen lymphocytes, all of which strongly express HLA class I. Platelets are

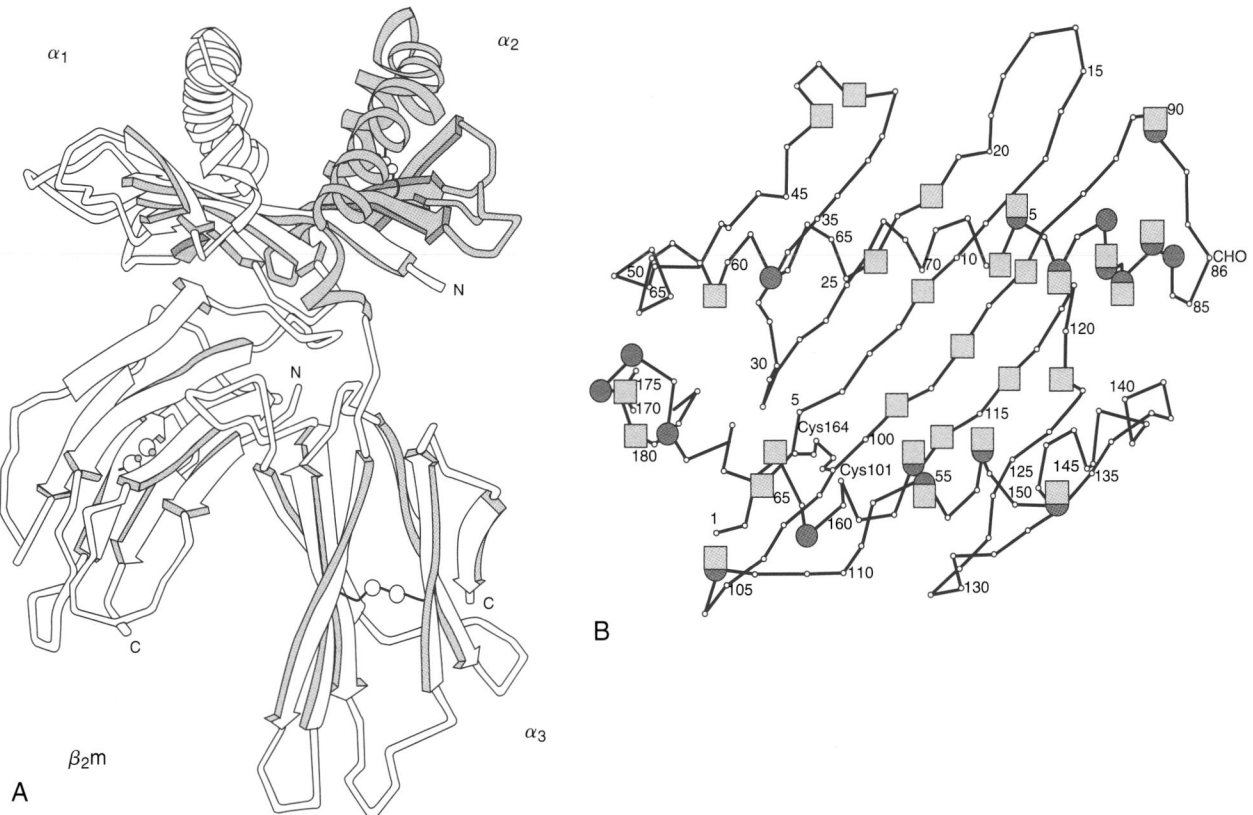

FIGURE 63-3. Diagram of the structure of the HLA-A2 molecule derived from x-ray crystallographic study. **A,** The flat ribbons represent the β-sheets or β-strands, and the spiral areas at the top (membrane distal) are the α-helices, which form the sides of a groove approximately 10 Å wide and 25 Å long. The floor of the groove is formed by eight parallel β-sheets. The COOH-terminal end of the α3 domain is inserted in the membrane. **B,** This view looks down on the top of the molecule, so that the groove goes from left to right. Diagrammed is the core structure of the amino acid sequence, consecutively numbered from 1 *(bottom left)* to 180 *(center left)*. The symbols show the variable amino acid substitutions that have been identified in different human or mouse haplotypes as relating to sites of reactivity to alloreactive T cells *(light blue squares)* or to monoclonal antibodies *(blue circles)*. Sites that relate to both are shown as dual symbols. Whereas the antibody sites are on the external surface of the helices, many of the T cell sites are at the base of the groove. The variable sites determine which peptide sequences can be bound by a given MHC allele (see text). (**A,** from Bjorkman P, Saper M, Samraoui B, et al: Structure of the human class I histocompatibility antigen, HLA-A2. Nature 329[6139]:506, 1987. **B,** modified from Bjorkman PJ, Saper MA, Samraoui B, et al: The foreign antigen binding site and T cell recognition regions of class I histocompatibility antigens. Nature 329[6139]:512, 1987.)

not commonly used for typing, but they are useful for absorbing anti–class I antibodies from serum, as they do not express class II antigens. Some organ-specific anatomic variations occur in endothelial expression, and in states of active inflammation the density of class I can be increased locally. There are three class I heavy chain loci: HLA-A, -B, and -C (see Fig. 63-1). Each locus product in a given individual bears a unique—so-called private—antigenic epitope plus additional "public" epitopes that are shared more widely among the population. There are more than 80 serologically defined A and B locus private antigens and 10 C locus ones, but more than 800 class I alleles have been defined by DNA techniques.[25] The independence of the HLA-A, -B, and -C molecules on the cell surface can be demonstrated by observing with fluorescent markers the separate aggregation and capping of each set of molecules when antibodies specific to each locus are added. When antibodies to β2-microglobulin are added, all class I molecules are capped.

The first MHC molecule to be crystallized was HLA-A2, and the structure of this class I allele was determined by x-ray diffraction studies to a resolution of 3.5 Å (Fig. 63-3).[26] This accomplishment afforded visualization of how the amino acid sequence relates to the folding of the chains into a three-dimensional structure. The two membrane distal domains, α1 and α2, form a groove along the top surface of the molecule facing away from the cell membrane. The margins of the groove are formed by α-helices, and the base is floored by a series of eight parallel β-strands, with the α1 and α2 domains contributing more or less equally to each side of the structure. In the crystallographic study, the groove, approximately 25 Å long and 10 Å wide, contained an unidentified molecule that in subsequent studies was shown to represent the bound peptide fragment, eight to nine amino acids long. These peptides have an extended linear core structure, and binding is to a large measure determined by side chain interactions. When the locations of amino acid variations, already known from the study of sequences and interactions with antibodies or cytotoxic T cells, are related to the crystal structure, it is remarkable that the HLA variable sites lie along the α-helical and β-strand surfaces that form the margins of the groove (see Fig. 63-3).[27] In other words, the polymorphisms serve to define the shape of the binding groove on MHC molecules and thus determine which peptides will be bound and recognized by T cells.

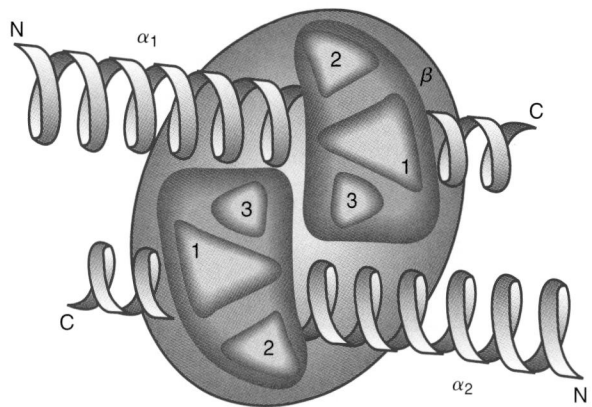

FIGURE 63-4. Illustration of the area of surface contact between the T cell receptor (TCR) and the major histocompatibility complex (MHC) peptide-binding groove of a class I molecule. The α-helices are shown from the same perspective as in Figure 63-3B. The footprint of the TCR, which consists of an α- and a β-chain, is shown to contact the α-helices and the peptide in the groove (not shown). Each chain has three hypervariable regions (CDRs), and they are aligned in such a way that the CDR3 regions of the TCR, the sites of greatest sequence variability, make contact with the peptide. (From Carpenter CB: Histocompatibility antigens and immune response genes. *In* Dale DC, Federman DD [eds]: Scientific American Medicine. New York, Scientific American, 1998.)

The sites that determine whether or not a given peptide binds may also confer a conformational change on the fragment. The result is that the TCR binds to the unique topography of the MHC surface formed by a given MHC and peptide combination.[28] The TCR has two chains, α and β, which form a heterodimer (Fig. 63-4). The membrane distal surface of the assembled TCR has six variable loops, called CDRα1, CDRα2, and CDRα3 and CDRβ1, CDRβ2, and CDRβ3, which provide the specificity of binding to the MHC α-helices and bound peptide antigen.[29] Additional human and mouse class I molecules have been crystallized, and the hypothesis that allelic polymorphisms determine binding of different peptide sequences has been confirmed. Peptides found in eluates from class I crystals or purified molecules are usually eight or nine residues in length.[30] Their origin is in the intracellular pool of polypeptides derived from metabolic turnover of housekeeping proteins or intracellular infections such as viruses. There is selective proteolysis and transmembrane transport from lysosomal compartments into the Golgi, where 8 to 9mer peptides are placed in class I binding sites before transport to the cell surface. Some of the genes that control this process are in the class II region of the MHC (see Fig. 63-1).[31, 32]

HLA Molecules: Class II

Class II HLA molecules consist of two membrane-inserted and non–covalently associated glycosylated polypeptides, called α (34 kD) and β (28 kD) (see Fig. 63-2). Each of these chains has two domains; again, the polymorphic regions are mostly on the outer, NH2-terminal, domains. The region of *HLA* encompassing class II genes is generally referred to as *HLA-D*. There are 21 *HLA-DR* alleles that have been defined serologically, but more than 320 alleles can be identified using DNA-typing techniques.[25] Although three class II molecules—HLA-DP, HLA-DQ, and HLA-DR—are generally

recognized on cell surfaces, the situation is not entirely analogous to that of class I, because the α- and β-chains of each class II molecule are encoded by separate, closely linked, genes (see Fig. 63-1). Although α- and β-chains of different parental haplotypes can associate, such hybrid associations are restricted to products of the same *DP, DQ,* or *DR* subregion.

The naming of *HLA-D*–region genes is based on knowledge of the biochemistry of expressed antigens and on the growing database of DNA nucleotide sequencing. The gene that encodes the HLA-DR α-chain, for example, is called *DRA*. It has no sequence variation (i.e., it is monomorphic). All the variability of different alleles lies in the DRB chains: *DRB1* encodes the private DR antigens 1 to 21, and *DRB3, DRB4,* and *DRB5* encode β-chains for DR52, DR53, and DR51. The *HLA-DQ* subregion contains the genes *DQA1, DQB1, DQA2,* and *DQB2*. The last two are nonexpressed pseudogenes; the products of the first two, DQ α and DQ β, are both polymorphic. *HLA-DP* is similarly organized and has polymorphisms on both chains. Study by the Southern blot technique to determine restriction fragment length polymorphisms (RFLPs) of DNA digested with various nucleases and hybridized to cDNA probes specific for the *HLA* genes has proved to be an alternative detection technique that has been particularly informative for class II genes.[33, 34] More rapid and precise detection of actual DNA sequences can now be accomplished by selective polymerase chain reaction amplification of polymorphic gene regions, followed by hybridization with short oligonucleotide probes specific for a given HLA sequence or by RFLP analysis of the amplified product.[35, 36] Comparative studies in ongoing workshops have demonstrated a strong correlation between serologically defined polymorphisms and those identified by T cell clones reactive to class II molecules.

Analysis of crystals of class II HLA-DR1 shows a remarkable similarity to class I molecules in the peptide-binding region (see Fig. 63-3). The α-helical and β-stranded core structures of class I and II are virtually superimposable. The main difference is at the ends of the groove, which in class II are more open, allowing for binding of longer peptides. Typically, the length of eluted peptides from class II molecules are 13 to 26 residues,[37] and the linearly arrayed peptide protrudes at both ends of the groove.[37, 38] Class II antigens are limited in expression to B lymphocytes, monocytes and macrophages, dendritic cells, and activated T lymphocytes. Human endothelium generally does not express class II, but this situation can change rapidly when inflammation is in the vicinity. In addition, epithelial cells of skin, intestine, and renal proximal tubule can synthesize and express class II molecules in response to injury and inflammation.[39]

Peptides bound to class II molecules are derived from proteolysis in acidic endosomal compartments and represent endocytosed proteins or microorganisms coming from outside the APC. Thus, the extracellular compartment, in contrast to the intracellular compartment for class I, is the responsibility of the typical class II–positive APC. When foreign polypeptide antigens are added to cultured APCs, peptide fragments appear on class II (but not on class I) molecules in a matter of minutes. Peptide fragments of self-MHC classes I and II are found in the eluates from class II molecules,[37] indicating that intracellularly synthesized products are represented on class II at the cell surface or that secreted molecules reenter the cell by the endocytic pathway.

Inheritance of HLA

Because chromosomes are paired, each person has two sets of HLA antigens, one set from each parent. The genetically linked antigens of the entire HLA region inherited from one parent collectively are called a *haplotype*, and, according to the rules of simple mendelian-dominant inheritance, any sibling pair has a 25% chance of inheriting the same two parental haplotypes, a 50% chance of sharing one haplotype, and a 25% chance of having two completely different haplotypes (Fig. 63-5). The main evidence that HLA is the major transplantation barrier in humans originally came from the observation that, in renal transplantation, HLA-identical sibling donor grafts provided the best long-term graft survival and required the least aggressive immunosuppression.[40-44] In the absence of a recombination (crossover), the entire *HLA-A to HLA-DP* region, including the specific electrophoretic polymorphisms of C4, BF, and C2, is expressed with each inherited haplotype. Recombination rates within the region are in the vicinity of less than 1%; thus, generally it is not necessary to "type" for the expressed products of all the loci to identify haplotypes within a family. Rarely, when recombination has occurred or when several common antigens are present on both sides of a family, complete molecular typing of HLA may be necessary.

The distribution of HLA antigens in the general population is not random. Some are more common than others, and racial and ethnic patterns are well known. Furthermore, within a given racial or ethnic group, certain HLA haplotypes or portions thereof are likely to be found with higher frequency than one would predict by random distribution. For example, HLA-A1, HLA-B8, and HLA-DR3 very often occur on the same haplotype in northern Europeans. These alleles are not in equilibrium, and, thus, are said to be in "linkage disequilibrium." When entire, so-called extended, haplotypes[42] are found in apparently unrelated persons, it is likely that they were inherited from a common and relatively recent ancestor. When alleles of adjacent loci of the HLA region (e.g., *B* and *DR*) are in linkage disequilibrium, the possibility exists that selective pressures were exerted over many generations to sustain the coexpression of a combination that favors defense against infectious diseases. Review of the associations of HLA alleles with a number of diseases is beyond the purpose of this chapter,[43] but the existence of linkage disequilibriums is relevant to considerations of HLA antigen distribution throughout the general population, a matter of direct concern when matching donors for transplantation.

HLA Typing

The main sources of antibodies for typing come from large-scale screenings of thousands of serum samples from multiparous women. Immunizations among humans yield the most highly specific antibodies to private HLA determinants. Anti–class I (HLA-A, HLA-B, HLA-C) antibodies react with both B and T lymphocytes, whereas anti–class II antibodies react with B, but not T, cells. Generally, a positive reaction is marked by cell lysis in the presence of rabbit complement. In addition, more broadly reactive antisera, originally thought to contain several antibodies in mixture, may have reactivity to the public determinants. For example, HLA-B molecules contain at least three immunogenic

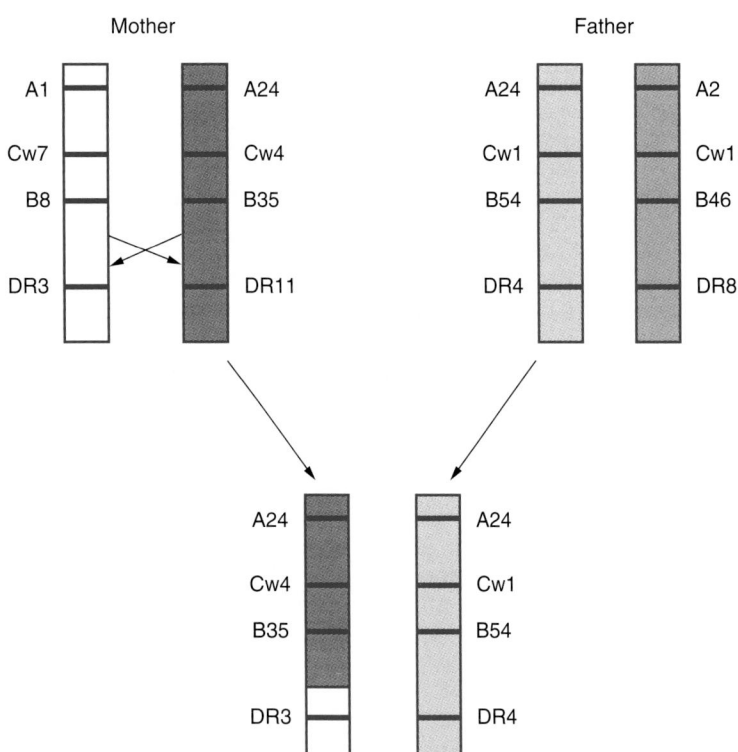

FIGURE 63-5. Inheritance of HLA haplotypes. The *HLA-A, HLA-Cw, HLA-B,* and *HLA-DR* genes are shown to represent the entire region. Children inherit one of each of the parental HLA haplotypes, and they are inherited as a block unless a recombination has occurred during meiosis of an ovum or sperm, shown here as an arrow between *B* and *DR* in the mother. Such events occur less than 1% of the time for HLA. The chances of an HLA-identical sibling or an entirely non-matching pair in a family is 1:4. Haploidentical siblings occur with odds of 1:2, and all children are haploidentical with each parent.

regions, one for private and two for public polymorphisms.[45] Monoclonal antibodies derived from the immunization of mice or rats with human lymphocytes only occasionally bind to the same antigenic sites defined by human antibodies. Although there are several examples of monoclonal antibodies that may substitute for human antisera, a large number of monoclonals react in a "public" fashion but not necessarily in the same patterns that human antisera do.

The mixed lymphocyte response (MLR) occurs when lymphocytes of one individual are cultured with those of another. Proliferation occurs over 5 to 7 days and is measured by the incorporation rate of 3H-thymidine into newly replicated DNA.[46] Usually, one population of cells is irradiated to prevent proliferation; then, the readout represents the response of nonirradiated helper T cells to the class II antigens present on stimulator B cells or macrophages or dendritic cells. Genetic identity for HLA yields a negative, nonproliferating MLR; similarity is revealed by weak proliferation. Before the HLA-DP, HLA-DQ, and HLA-DR subregions were clearly defined, incompatibility for the MLR was attributed entirely to "HLA-D." The MLR is rarely used now as a clinical test, because the complexity of HLA-D can be fully assessed by typing. HLA-DR determinants provide the strongest MLR stimulus, whereas HLA-DQ plays a lesser role. HLA-DP is recognized only by primed (i.e., previously immunized) cells. The MLR itself is a complex series of cellular responses. Helper cell clones are first activated to proliferate but then induce the proliferative burst of CD8+ cytotoxic T cells. The latter are generally directed to class I incompatibilities and injure appropriate target cells after direct cell-to-cell contact is initiated by T cell–antigen receptors. When cytotoxic T cells are tested against a large number of individuals typed by classic serologic techniques, a good, but not perfect, correlation is observed overall. Some antigenic sites, or epitopes, recognized by T cells are actually different from those on the same class I molecule that are recognized by antibodies.

This is explained by the fact that immunoglobulins can recognize small epitopes on intact whole molecules with tertiary structures, whereas T cells "see" only the complex surface made up of a peptide fragment bound in the MHC-binding groove. Further, more than one diversity site per HLA molecule provides targets for rejection. The private specificities are, by definition, most immunogenic in the human-antihuman alloresponse, but a given specificity usually involves a composite of small amino acid differences at more than one site in an HLA molecule.

The marked superiority of sibling donors with identical HLA haplotypes for organ and bone marrow transplantation has been demonstrable since the early 1970s.[40] When azathioprine and prednisone were used as standard therapy, initial graft loss rates were in the 5% to 10% range during the first year and graft survival half-lives in the 25- to 30-year range.[41] Now that HLA serologic typing is more reliable, a major question is whether similar results can be obtained if unrelated donors are matched for all, or most, of the HLA loci. The answer is evolving, as many other factors in clinical transplantation must be considered, but it is indisputable that both improved immunosuppression and reductions in histocompatibility barriers have contributed to better graft survival. In addition, management of infections and judicious attention to treatment of rejection activity contribute much to clinical success. Overall, patient and graft survival rates have been improving over the past decade—and had been improving even before use of cyclosporine became widespread.[47] One of the major problems in interpretation of any data relates to the fact that 1-year graft survival rates have been rising at the rate of 1.5% per year for more than two decades, and no single factor can explain this (Fig. 63-6). The technology of HLA typing need not be absolutely accurate for selection of sibling donors with identical HLA haplotypes, but, on the other hand, true definition of a zero-mismatched cadaver donor for HLA-A, HLA-B, and HLA-DR may require molecular DNA typing. It is fair to say that

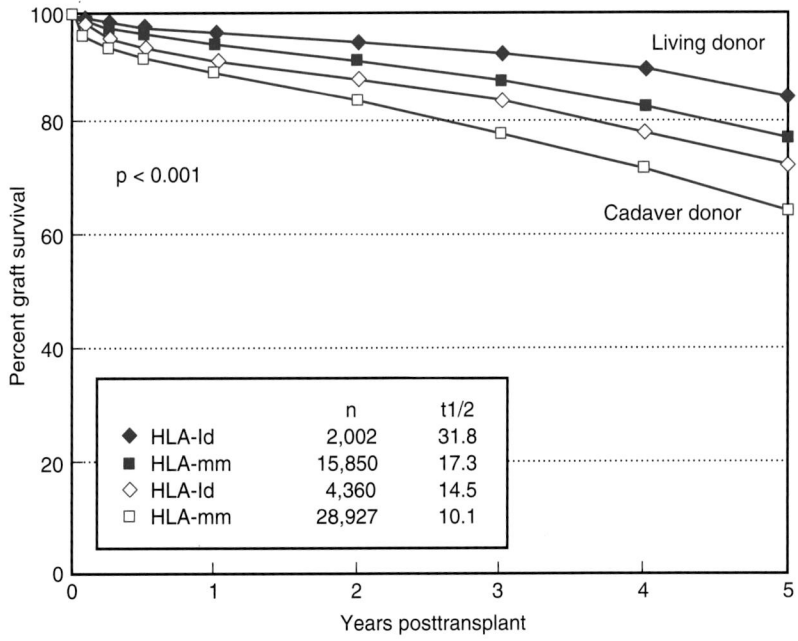

FIGURE 63-6. Long-term graft survival as a function of donor source and HLA matching. Data are from the UNOS registry, representing more than 50,000 renal transplants, typed by classic serologic methods. When HLA-identical sibs were donors, graft survival was superior: more than 80% were still functioning at 5 years (half-life > 30 years). The *middle curves* indicate the benefit of using a living donor, with HLA-incompatible living donors showing better 5-year survival than HLA-matched (HLA-A, HLA-B, and HLA-DR only) cadaver donors (first grafts only). The *bottom curve* is for randomly matched first cadaver cases. When this latter population is further subdivided according to numbers of HLA mismatches, there is a spread between those with one or two mismatches (12.5-year half-life and 70% survival at 5 years) and those with six mismatches (8.8-year half-life and 58% survival at 5 years) in recipients 50 years or younger (data not shown). (From Cecka JM, Terasaki PI [eds]: Clinical Transplants 2001. Los Angeles, UCLA Tissue Typing Laboratory, 2002, p 14.)

widespread competency in both class I and class II serologic typing has been achieved only in the past decade, but it is still imperfect. There is direct evidence that technical difficulties with HLA serologic methods can account for poor correlations with grafting results.[48] The most valuable databases now in existence are those that have pooled information from a large number of collaborating centers and that include tens of thousands of cases. Two registries in the world are particularly important: the UCLA studies of Cecka and Terasaki[49] and the Collaborative Transplant Study (CTS) of Opelz and colleagues.[50] Although such pooled data may suffer from variations in protocols and undocumented selection factors, the power of univariant analyses becomes compelling when several thousand patients are included. Furthermore, each of these studies provides a unique perspective, and each provides strong evidence of the role of HLA phenotypic matching in the success of cadaver renal transplantation. Cecka and Terasaki's registry[49] has functioned for many years, and it is the best source of information on the year-to-year changes in results related to donor source, blood transfusion, immunosuppression, and HLA matching and sensitization, mostly in cases from North America. It operates the United Network for Organ Sharing (UNOS) for transplants in the United States. In 1983 and 1984, Opelz and co-workers[51] organized a study related to the Ninth International Histocompatibility Workshop, utilizing data from experienced laboratories that had access to the best typing antisera. The CTS accepts only consecutive unselected cases and now has cases entered from more than 150,000 transplants.[50]

There is rather strong evidence that long-term graft survival is improved by avoiding HLA mismatches. Log-linear plots of graft survival always show a straight-line decline after the first year, which makes it possible to calculate a half-life and to project survival rates over time. Recent data (1996-2000) show that recipients of first cadaveric kidneys having no HLA-A, HLA-B, or HLA-DR antigen mismatches have graft half-lives of 14.5 years and a projected 73% chance of 5-year survival.[49] With one or two mismatches, the value is a 12.5-year half-life and 70% 5-year survival for recipients age 50 years or younger. These long-term results are to be compared with HLA-identical living related donors (32-year half-life) and all other living donors (17-year half-life) (see Fig. 63-6). Avoiding ischemic and storage injury of organs from living donors certainly enhances outcomes when compared with those predicted from the cadaver data. There is considerable opportunity both for matching more cases and for avoiding completely mismatched grafts. It is worth noting that current projections give the same, or better, 10-year graft survival rates to cadaver donor organs that are not mismatched with recipients for HLA-A, HLA-B, and HLA-DR and to family donors who have identical HLA haplotypes. It is for this reason that UNOS has a mandatory share policy for these cases. Because of the national pool available, about 15% to 20% of cadaver kidneys are now shared on this basis.

Relative Strengths of HLA Loci

Clinical data do not support the simple assumption that each mismatch for antigens of various loci has equal weight in causing graft loss. The major impact comes from the effects of B and DR antigens; little additional effect comes from the A locus.[51] Transplant data from the United Kingdom show that DR matching has a much greater effect than matching of A or B.[52] As compared with the results when no mismatches are present for A, B, or DR, the addition of a single mismatch for A, or B, or DR increases the chances of graft loss twofold for A, threefold for B, and fivefold for DR. The UNOS system uses as the mandatory sharing criterion of a zero mismatch for HLA-A, HLA-B, and HLA-DR (i.e., "six-antigen match").[53] An interesting finding from Eurotransplant indicates that time has an influence on the relative effects of HLA-A, HLA-B, and HLA-DR mismatches: DR is most important in the first 6 months after transplantation, B's effect emerges during the first 2 years, and A does not show an effect before 3 years.[54] These findings are similar to those of Opelz and associates, who found that during the first posttransplant year, the class II HLA-DR locus had a stronger impact than the class I HLA-A and HLA-B loci. In subsequent years, however, the influence on graft survival of the three loci was found to be equivalent and additive.[50] This would indicate that, in the absence of prior sensitization, HLA-A mismatches have a deleterious effect only on long-term graft survival.

The more effective immunosuppressive therapy in common use today produces 1-year cadaver graft survival rates as high as those associated with one–haplotype-matched living, related donors. The early results are approaching 95% graft survival for first grafts at 1 year (see Fig. 63-6). This is in keeping with the steady increase in early graft survival and late graft survival with newer and more powerful immunosuppressive agents. Data from the UNOS database show that from 1988 to 1996, the 1-year survival rate for grafts from living donors increased from 88.8% to 93.9%, and the rate for cadaveric grafts increased from 75.7% to 87.7% with the half-life for grafts from living donors increasing steadily from 12.7 to 21.6 years and for cadaveric grafts increasing from 7.9 to 13.8 years.[55] The effect of HLA matching was apparent on long-term allograft survival and was in part related to a lower impact of acute rejection in well-matched cases. Patients who experienced an acute rejection episode had shorter long-term allograft survival. Acute rejections were of less importance when donor and recipient were HLA matched. It should be noted that the degree of mismatch was not in itself directly predictive of early rejection, but it did predict the prognosis once a rejection episode had occurred. To a large extent, intrinsic responsiveness of individual patients may determine the rejection rate, but in those patients who do reject, the HLA barrier becomes important to short-term survival rates. Alternatively, the rejection tempo may be intrinsically more powerful when more antigens are mismatched. The question of defining intrinsic responsiveness remains open. Failure to reject may reflect the patient's susceptibility to immunosuppressive agents, or it may be related to different donor-recipient histocompatibility combinations. One example would be a patient who does well with a second transplant after vigorously rejecting a first graft, which bore different HLA antigens.

To improve the results for the 80% to 85% of patients who cannot be HLA-A, HLA-B, or HLA-DR matched, several schemes have been proposed for inclusion of racial and ethnic groups who do not "match" very well with the mostly white donor population.[56] One of these is to match for public antigens shared across certain antigen groups (i.e., a much broader cluster than a split). These have been called "CREGS" (for serologically cross-reacting groups), for which there are three somewhat different schemes.[57] Another approach is to count the total numbers of amino acid residue differences as mismatches.[58] Neither of these approaches seems useful. Finally, analysis of graft outcomes, in terms of tallying specific donor-recipient epitopes that did not impede graft success as "permissible mismatches,"[59-61] is an approach that seems to have some merit, but it is a work in progress.

Minor Histocompatibility Antigens

Minor histocompatibility antigens are fundamentally different from MHC antigens.[16, 44] They are recognized as peptides bound to self-MHC. Because most minor incompatibilities elicit class I–restricted CD8+ T cell responses, it seems likely that they are peptides derived from intracellular proteins of the same cell.[62-64] In mice, Y chromosome–encoded and mitochondrial gene-encoded minor antigens have been found. Many autosomal minor systems have also been identified. Minor antigenic peptides do not have sequence homologies with other sequences whose functions are known. It should be noted that these systems require that the recipient have the restricting MHC class I allele if a given antigen is to be operative as a transplantation antigen. This means that recipient T cells are capable of binding the minor donor peptide and that the donor cells express a shared MHC antigen that presents the same peptide. Although the targets for cytotoxic CD8+ T cells are class I molecules that bear the peptide, it is clear that a CD4+-mediated helper response is needed during immunization. Another feature of minor antigens is that they do not provoke an antibody response. Why the CD4 response does not characteristically help B cells to make immunoglobulins is not known.

It has been appreciated for several years that minor histocompatibility antigens can be immunogenic in humans, from observations based on organ graft rejections and bone marrow graft-versus-host reactions in cases of genetically matched HLA antigens. A few cases of donor-directed, HLA class I–restricted, cytotoxic T cell responses have been demonstrated in such cases.[65-67]

ABO Blood Group Antigens

The ABO blood group antigens were initially identified as the cause of transfusion reactions during red blood cell transfusions. The A and B groups are glycosylated differentially, whereas group O lacks the enzymes necessary for glycosylation. The antigens are readily recognized by natural antibodies, termed *hemagglutinins* because they cause red blood cell agglutination. They are relevant to transplantation because they are also expressed on other cell types, including the endothelium. Thus, they cause hyperacute rejection of vascular allografts owing to preformed natural antibodies. Specifically, individuals with group A or B types produce natural antibodies to the opposite type, and those with group O produce antibodies to both A and B. However, because group O does not express the glycosylated moiety, both A and B fail to produce antibodies to group O. Thus, group O grafts can be transplanted into recipients with blood types A, B, and AB. This is not commonly done, for ethical reasons, to prevent depletion of available grafts for type O recipients, who must receive an O organ.

Allograft rejection due to red blood cell type mismatching can be readily prevented by routine blood typing before transplantation. The rhesus (Rh) factor and other red blood cell antigens are of little concern, because they are not expressed on endothelial cells.

Monocyte and Endothelial Cell Antigens

Occasionally, allografts undergo hyperacute rejection, despite appropriate ABO matching. Some of these rejection episodes have been attributed to additional non-ABO antigens expressed on endothelial cells and monocytes.[68, 69] The characterization of these antigens has been an area of active research; however, these antigen systems remain poorly understood. Currently, pretransplant tissue typing does not evaluate the endothelial/monocyte antigens, owing to the apparent rarity of such antibodies and the lack of accurate reagents for typing.

Effects of Blood Transfusions

The historical data on the beneficial effects of blood transfusions are well known.[70] In recent years, the effect has been diminishing, until now it appears to have little impact on graft survival. Indeed, only in the nontransfused group is there some evidence of a detriment to graft survival. With the introduction of erythropoietin, the need for blood transfusions before transplantation has diminished dramatically, and transplant survival has increased enough to make the beneficial effects of transfusion less important. More important clinically is the need to minimize blood exposure to avoid transmission of viruses, and this can be accomplished with proper erythropoietin therapy.

THE IMMUNE RESPONSE TO ALLOGRAFTS

Acute allograft rejection in an unsensitized host is characterized by a lymphocytic infiltration into the allograft. The vast majority of these cells are T cells that are not alloantigen specific. As part of their immunosurveillance function, T cells pass from the circulatory system through the endothelium and into tissues before returning via the lymphatic system into the circulation. The inevitable tissue damage that occurs during transplantation results in a non–antigen-specific inflammatory response, which greatly increases leukocyte recruitment (including T cells). This is mediated through interactions between surface molecules (known as *adhesion molecules*) and their receptors on endothelial cells and leukocytes and also through the secretion and binding of small soluble proteins known as *chemokines*. Until recently, the site of alloantigen recognition had been believed to be the allograft itself, but recent data seem to indicate that antigen recognition may occur in lymphoid tissues.[71, 72] Regardless of the site, in the context of allograft rejection, T cells can recognize alloantigen through the usual pathway of recognition of foreign antigen, confusingly known as *the indirect pathway of allorecognition* (see below). Unique to the transplant setting, T cells may also recognize foreign

MHC and antigen through a process of "molecular mimicry," in which the foreign MHC and antigen complex resemble the intended receptor of the TCR and activate the T cell. After T cell interaction with APCs through the TCR, a number of other cellular interactions between the cells stabilize the interaction and lead to full T cell activation. The context of antigen presentation, most strongly defined by the type of cell that presents antigen is also increasingly recognized as important in whether the T cell mounts an aggressive or passive response to the antigen.

T CELL–ANTIGEN-PRESENTING CELL INTERACTIONS

In the MLR, allo-MHC molecules induce very strong primary immune responses in vitro.[73] It has long been recognized that the normal T cell repertoire contains a large cohort (1% to 10%) of total T cells, which are capable of responding to allo-MHC molecules.[74] This translates to a precursor frequency at least 100 times that of antigen-specific self-restricted T cells, which recognize conventional antigens as peptide fragments bound to self-MHC. The vigor of the primary alloimmune response has puzzled transplant immunologists for almost three decades.[75-77] The original hypothesis on the high frequency of alloreactive T cells[78] proposed that the repertoire of lymphocytes was preselected by evolutionary pressure to have specificity for the MHC molecules of the species. It was also proposed that the lymphocyte repertoire that recognizes conventional antigens was derived by somatic mutation of the TCR specific for self-MHC.[79] Today we know that TCRs do not undergo somatic mutations, and there is evidence from studies with T cell clones that the antigen-specific and alloreactive T cell repertoires may be contained in the same clones.[80-83]

The two fundamental questions in allorecognition are these: First, why is the frequency of alloreactive T cells so high? Second, how can positively selected (in the thymus) self-MHC–restricted T cells recognize foreign antigens as well as allo-MHC?

For one thing, it is apparent that there are at least two distinct, but not necessarily mutually exclusive, pathways of allorecognition.[71, 84, 85] In the so-called direct pathway, T cells recognize intact allo-MHC molecules on the surface of donor or stimulator cells. In the indirect pathway, T cells recognize processed alloantigen as peptides in the context of self-APCs, which is the normal route of T cell recognition of foreign antigens. Both pathways have been shown in experimental animals to contribute independently to allograft rejection.[86, 87] The relative contributions of the direct and indirect pathways of allorecognition to allograft rejection in humans are under investigation, although recent data in cardiac, renal, and lung transplant recipients suggest that indirect allorecognition of donor HLA peptides may play a key role in chronic rejection (Fig. 63-7).[88-90]

Direct recognition of intact MHC molecules, although focused on the polymorphic MHC epitopes, is strongly influenced by the presence of peptide in the MHC groove.[91] MHC molecules "empty" of peptide generally are not recognized unless the missing self-peptides are reconstituted.[92-96] It has also been shown that changing the bound peptide can alter the allorecognition of a given MHC molecule.[97] These observations have provided the rationale for studying the immunomodulatory functions of synthetic peptides, particularly MHC peptides in vitro and in vivo.[98]

The basic premise for indirect allorecognition as a mechanism for initiation or amplification of allograft rejection is that donor alloantigens are shed from the graft, taken up by recipient APCs, and presented to CD4+ T cells. Indeed, it has been demonstrated that intact HLA molecules are present in the circulation of renal transplant recipients.[99] Therefore, during transplantation, shed fragments of allo-MHC could be processed by host APCs and presented as allopeptides to T cells on self-MHC. This indirect pathway of allorecognition may lead to activation of helper T cells, which secrete lymphokines and provide the necessary signals for the growth and maturation of effector cytotoxic T lymphocytes, B cells, and monocytes or macrophages, leading to allograft rejection (see Fig. 63-7).[71, 85] Other important, yet poorly understood, mechanisms that may contribute to graft destruction include nonspecific tissue injury and repair and graft cell apoptosis. Ischemia plus reperfusion injury of the grafted organ leads to up-regulation of MHC class II and costimulatory molecules, which in turn increase the "immunogenicity of the graft" and amplify the immune response to it. The clinical syndromes of rejection are described in detail in Chapter 65.

FIGURE 63-7. Mechanisms of allorecognition and T cell response. T cells recognize antigen through direct and indirect pathways. The alloreactive T cell can undergo a number of different fates. They may provide help for macrophages, B cells, and monocytes by secreting cytokines and by cell-cell contact-dependent mechanisms or may kill graft cells in an antigen-specific manner through the release of toxic agents and by Fas-mediated apoptosis. As a process of activation, some T cells undergo cell death or become unresponsive (anergic) to antigenic stimulation either through regulation soluble factors or direct cell contact. Yet others may become memory T cells and await antigenic restimulation to provide a recall response. (From Salama AD, Remuzzi G, Harmon WE, Sayegh MH: Challenges to achieving clinical transplantation tolerance. J Clin Invest 108:943-948, 2001.)

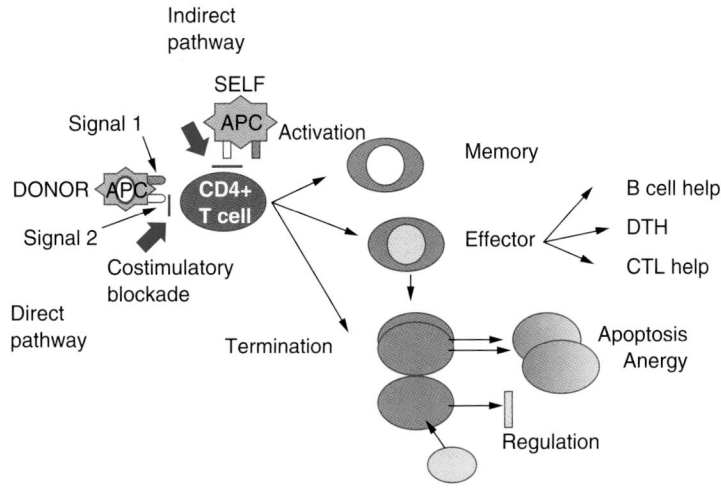

T Cell Receptor Complex

T cell recognition of alloantigens on APCs is the primary and central event that initiates allograft rejection.[84, 100] The interaction between T lymphocytes and APCs involves multiple T cell surface molecules and their counter-receptors expressed by APCs (Fig. 63-8).

Antigen specificity is determined by the TCR, which recognizes processed antigen in the form of short peptides bound to an MHC molecule. The specificity of antigen recognition is exquisitely precise; the alteration of a single amino acid in the peptide antigen or MHC molecule can alter recognition by the TCR. Thus, T cell recognition of antigen involves a trimolecular interaction affecting the TCR on the surface of the T cell, the MHC molecule on the surface of the APC, and the antigenic peptide bound to the MHC molecule. Although the T cell receptor is responsible for antigen recognition, the invariant proteins CD3 and ζ (which are noncovalently bound to the TCR) are responsible for signal transduction through the activation of protein tyrosine kinases associated with the cytoplasmic tails of CD3 and other TCR-associated receptors. This interaction provides "signal 1" of T cell activation (see later). Binding of the TCR to a peptide/MHC complex is of itself usually insufficient to cause T cell activation. Provision of signal 1 alone leads instead to a state of T cell unresponsiveness or "anergy."[101]

The OKT3 monoclonal antibody binds to the CD3 complex. OKT3 also induces signal transduction, including activation of specific kinases, activation of phospholipase C, and the increase in intracellular calcium and phosphoinositol metabolites.[102] The immunosuppressive effects of OKT3 are also dependent on signal transduction. The major immunosuppressive effect of OKT3 is the down-modulation of cell-surface expression of the TCR.[103] In addition, OKT3 causes the clearance of T cells from the circulation and their sequestration in the peripheral lymphoid organs, such as lymph nodes and spleen.[103] OKT3 is not cytotoxic and does not lyse peripheral T cells. Also, there is no convincing evidence that OKT3 directly interferes with antigen recognition by the TCR molecule. The side effects of OKT3 are also due to partial T cell activation causing the release of lymphokines, principally tumor necrosis factor-α (TNF-α), from large numbers of T cells.[104] For efficient T cell activation a number of other interactions between the APC and the T cell need to occur.[102]

CD4 and CD8 T Cell Receptor Coreceptors

The two major subsets of T cells, "cytotoxic" CD8+ T cells and "helper" CD4+ T cells, recognize processed antigen on MHC class I and II molecules, respectively. Although not directly involved in antigen recognition, the CD4 and CD8 coreceptors bind to nonpolymorphic regions of the MHC molecules. Thus, the specificity of class I versus class II recognition is determined by whether a T cell expresses CD4 or CD8 in conjunction with the specificity of the TCR. In addition, CD4 and CD8 promote and stabilize the immunologic synapse between the T cell and the APC. The cytoplasmic tails of CD4 and CD8 molecules are associated with the tyrosine kinase p56lck, which plays an important role in T cell activation.[105] Binding of the CD4 or CD8 coreceptor approximates the cytoplasmic tail to immunoreceptor tyrosine–based activation motifs on the CD3 complex. This, in turn, leads to the phosphorylation of a series of intracellular proteins, resulting in the activation of a variety of enzymes, including calcineurin (the target of the immunosuppressive drugs cyclosporine and tacrolimus), and the activation of transcription factors, such as nuclear factor of activated T cells (NFAT) and NF-κB. These transcription factors are responsible for the increased and in some cases decreased expression of a variety of gene products associated with T cell activation. This signaling process is also dependent on the binding of T cell costimulatory receptors with their specific ligands present on APCs.

Adhesion Molecules

Cells of the immune system infiltrate the graft from nearby lymphoid organs and the bloodstream by a three-step process. First, they roll along the vessel wall via interactions between selectins on the endothelium and receptors on immune cells. Second, they adhere to vessel endothelium. Third, chemoattractant cytokines (chemokines) are released. Adhesion molecules and chemokines are important regulators of rejection and appear to be targets for immunotherapy. Adhesion molecules on T cells include lymphocyte function–associated antigen (LFA)-1, which interacts with intercellular adhesion molecules (ICAM)-1 and ICAM-2; CD2, which interacts with CD58 (LFA-3); and VLA-4

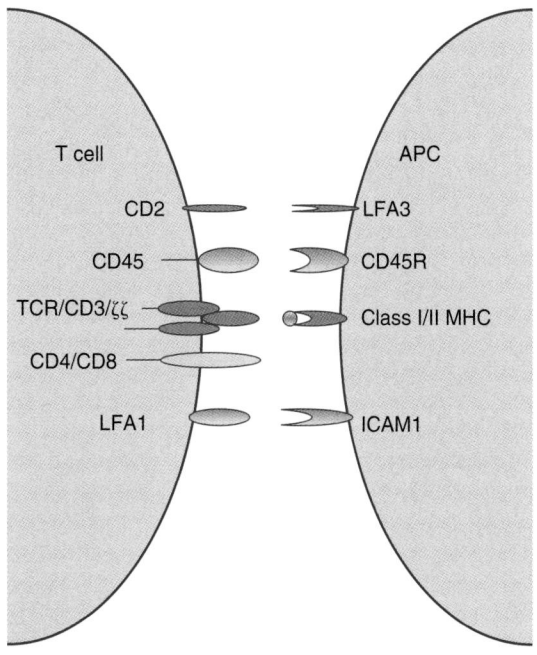

FIGURE 63-8. T cell interaction with an antigen-presenting cell (APC). Multiple receptors on the surface of T cells interact with counter-receptors on APCs. Binding of the T cell receptor (TCR) with major histocompatibility complex (MHC) class I or II provides specificity of T cell response. CD4 and CD8 act as co-receptors alongside the TCR and stabilize the interaction between the TCR and the MHC. Interaction of T cells and APCs is further strengthened by binding of adhesion molecules with their ligands (e.g., ICAM-1 and LFA-1). Although CD45 is thought to play a role in a memory response, its function is not well understood. T cells and APCs also interact through costimulatory molecules (see text).

(a4, b1 integrin, CDw49d, CD29), which interacts with vascular cell adhesion molecules (VCAM-1, CD106).[106]

These receptors are of two large structural families. The integrins, including LFA-1 and VLA-4, are made up of a, b heterodimers, whereas members of the immunoglobulin superfamily, including CD2, LFA-3, VCAM-1, and the ICAMs, are made up of disulfide-linked "receptor" domains. Some of these receptors have also been shown to transduce signals and, thus, are more appropriately called *accessory molecules*. The inhibition of adhesion/accessory cell function has been shown to be immunosuppressive.[106] Previous studies in a primate model showed increased graft survival with anti–ICAM-1 monoclonal antibodies, although recently completed clinical trials failed to show this in human renal transplant recipients.[107] Blockade of LFA-1, on the other hand, is being studied in the context of preventing delayed graft function after transplantation.[108]

Costimulatory Molecules

The classic understanding of T cell function is based on Bretscher and Cohn's two-signal hypothesis of T cell activation.[109] One signal is transduced by the antigen-specific TCR when it recognizes processed antigen bound to an MHC molecule on the surface of an APC. The second signal is mediated by a costimulatory molecule that is independent of antigen. The TCR and costimulatory signal transduction pathways are distinct and utilize different second messengers. At the level of the regulation of transcription, as shown for the interleukin-2 (IL-2) gene, the two pathways interact by poorly understood mechanisms to control gene expression. By controlling the level of expression of interleukin-2 (IL-2) and other genes, the TCR and costimulatory pathways can regulate T cell activation and function. The best-characterized costimulatory molecule is CD28, which is constitutively expressed on the surface of essentially all CD4+ and approximately 50% of CD8+ peripheral T lymphocytes.[110] CD28 binds a family of counter-receptors termed "B7" (B7-1 and B7-2 or CD80 and CD86, respectively), which are expressed by APCs. Costimulatory pathways may also down-regulate T cell responses.

Following activation, CTLA4, which also binds B7 but with greater affinity than does CD28, is expressed by the T cell. CTLA4 interaction with B7 transduces a "negative" signal to the T cell, resulting in physiologic termination of the immune response (Fig. 63-9).[84, 111] CTLA4 knockout mice die within a few weeks of birth from a disease process characterized by massive multiorgan lymphocytic infiltration, which emphasizes the importance of this pathway in turning off a lymphoproliferative response.[112]

Signaling via the TCR plus the CD28 costimulatory molecule is sufficient to activate T cells. In contrast, signaling via the TCR alone without costimulation induces long-term T cell unresponsiveness (i.e., anergy) or ignorance.[101, 113] Experimental analysis of the minimal signal transduction event necessary to induce anergy showed that an increase in intracellular calcium concentration was sufficient.[114] Because increased intracellular calcium is produced by signaling via the TCR, these results are consistent with the observation that anergy can be induced by monoclonal antibodies to the TCR or by APCs expressing the appropriate MHC molecule but lacking the costimulatory counter-receptor.[101, 113] In vivo, anergy is defined as failure of T cell clonal expansion after immunization with antigen.[101, 113] Anergic T cells remain viable but are unresponsive for at least several weeks in experimental murine models in vitro and in vivo.[101, 113-115] In vitro, some anergic states can be reversed by cytokines such as IL-2.[114] The fate and function of anergic T cells in vivo remain undetermined; however, evidence from experimental models suggests that anergic T cells can be reactivated by some processes (e.g., viral infections).[116]

These observations suggest that anergy is a reversible state, and that therapeutic use of anergy during clinical transplantation, although potentially very useful, requires thorough evaluation and careful monitoring. Certain anergic states may not be reversible and may be associated with T cell death by apoptosis.[117] Strategies targeted at inducing such states in vivo are clinically desirable. Inhibition of costimulation with soluble receptors to (e.g., CTLA4 Ig), or monoclonal antibodies against, the B7 molecules has been shown to prolong graft survival dramatically and to induce tolerance in some animal models.[84, 106] However, the fact that

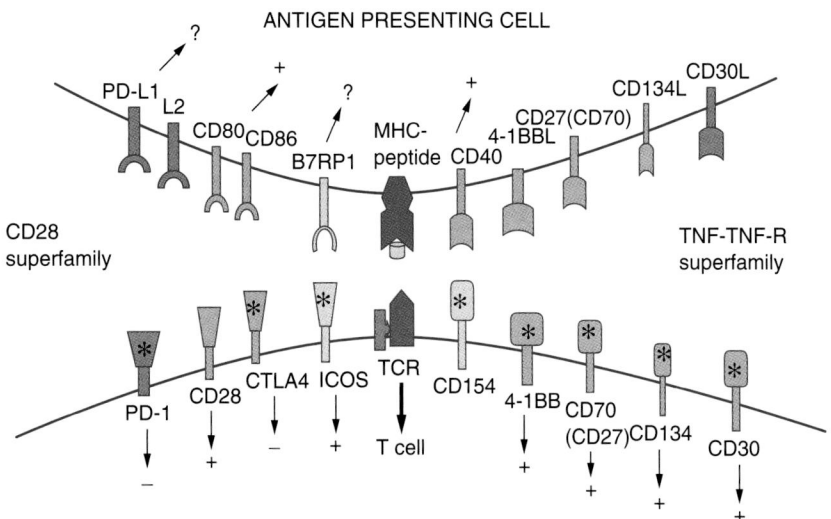

FIGURE 63-9. CD28-B7 and TNF–TNF-R T cell costimulatory superfamilies. Following ligation of the receptor-ligand pair, there is a net stimulatory (+) or inhibitory (−) signal transduced. In some cases there is bidirectional signaling, and for certain pairs both the ligand and the receptor are expressed on the same cell constitutively (in parenthesis) or more commonly following activation. Molecules that are induced on activated cells are shown by an asterisk. (From Salama AD, Sayegh MH: Alternative T cell costimulatory pathways in transplant rejection and tolerance induction: Hierarchy or redundancy? Am J Transplant 3:509-511, 2003.)

blockade of the CD28-B7 pathway alone does not appear to be effective at inducing tolerance in the more stringent models of transplantation, including primate models,[118, 119] and that CD28-deficient mice[120] are capable of rejecting allografts, albeit in a delayed fashion, has lead to speculation that other pathways are capable of providing T cell costimulation.

Additional members of the CD28 family with positive or negative costimulatory function have now been recognized. ICOS is a homologue of CD28 and binds to B7h.[121] It does not interact with B7-1 and B7-2, and, in contrast to CD28, it is not constitutively expressed but is up-regulated on activated T cells[122]; blocking this pathway leads to increased allograft survival in experimental models.[123] PD-1, which binds to its ligands PD-L1 and PD-L2, is the latest member of the CD28 family to be recognized.[124] Like CTLA4, it appears to be a negative regulator of T cell activation; however, knockout animals do not produce the same dramatic phenotype as the CTLA4 knockouts but do develop spontaneous autoimmune disease.[125]

A separate family of costimulatory molecules has now been recognized.[124] CD40 and its ligand CD40L (CD154) were the first members of this family to have demonstrable costimulatory function. CD40 is expressed on B cells and other APCs, including dendritic cells and endothelial cells, and belongs to the TNF superfamily of molecules. Its ligand, CD40L (CD154), is expressed early on activated T cells. CD40 is critical in providing cognate T cell help for B cell immunoglobulin production and class switching. A defect in CD154 expression is responsible for the hyper-IgM syndrome seen in humans. Blockade with anti-CD154 antibodies has been shown to be effective at prolonging allograft survival in rodent and primate models of transplantation.[124] Whether CD154 acts "directly" to transduce a costimulatory signal to the T cell or "indirectly" by ligation of CD40 on APCs, a strong inducer of B7 expression, is open to speculation. Therefore, CD40L on the T cell might serve merely to induce CD28 ligands or other costimulatory molecules on APCs. Other members of this group include the CD134-CD134L, CD30-CD30L, CD27-CD70, and the 4-1BB–4-1BBL pathways.[124]

Cytokines and Chemokines

In addition to cell-cell interactions, cell function can be directed through proteins produced by a variety of cell types. These cytokines can function as chemoattractants (chemokines) and as growth, activation, and differentiation factors. They can act locally or systemically through signaling cell-surface receptors, which results in changes in gene expression of the cell.

Cytokines are produced by cells that participate in the immune response, including T cells, B cells, and APCs. In addition, nonimmune cells such as endothelial cells also produce lymphokines that can modulate an immune response. Thus, complex regulatory networks of lymphokines that are incompletely understood modulate the antigraft immune response. In addition, it has been shown that different subsets of T cells can produce different patterns of cytokine secretion.[126] The two subsets of CD4+ T cells defined in terms of cytokine production are the Th1 and Th2 subsets. Both subsets produce some lymphokines such as IL-3, TNF-β, and granulocyte-macrophage colony-stimulating factor (GM-CSF),

whereas each subset produces a predominant set of lymphokines. The Th1 subset preferentially produces IL-2, gamma interferon (IFN-γ), and TNF-α. In contrast, the Th2 subset preferentially produces IL-4, IL-5, IL-10, and IL-13. The net effect of producing each cytokine profile is differential regulation of the immune response. The Th1 subset is considered proinflammatory, promoting delayed-type hypersensitivity (DTH) reactions and cytotoxic T lymphocyte expansion. The Th2 subset is considered a helper of B cells; however, the functional segregation between the Th1 and Th2 subsets remains incompletely understood. For example, IFN-γ secreted by Th1 cells regulates B cells by promoting antibody isotype switching to the IgG2a isotype. Also, secretion of IL-5 and IL-6 by Th2 cells increases eosinophil recruitment and expansion. In addition, some T cell clones analyzed in vitro express overlapping profiles of lymphokines.

Chemokines, chemoattractant cytokines,[127, 128] are structurally related by amino acid homologies, in particular the placement of cysteines. The nomenclature of chemokines is becoming increasingly complex. Four chemokine families are now recognized; the majority of members belong to the C-C chemokine family, represented by RANTES, or the C-X-C chemokine family, typified by IL-8. In general C-C chemokines attract monocytes and T lymphocytes, and C-X-C chemokines attract granulocytes.[127] Receptors on the surface of immune cells are named after the family of chemokines with which they interact, and the receptors can bind with a variety of chemokines in that family. For example, CCR1 and CCR5 can bind with the chemokines MCP-3 and MIP-1β, respectively, and both can bind RANTES and MIP-1α. They act to create a chemoattractant gradient across tissues to move cells into sites of inflammation. Detection of altered chemokine mRNA in experimental models of rejection suggests that they play an important role in this process; however, because of redundancy and differences between the function of chemokines in rodents and humans, the exact role individual chemokines play in an alloimmune response remains for the most part unclear.[127] Recent data may suggest that expression of CCR5 is associated with acute allograft rejection.[129]

In experimental models of transplantation, altering the T cell response from Th1 to Th2 has been shown to decrease acute graft rejection.[130] Except for blockade of the IL-2R,[131, 132] therapeutic strategies that modulate lymphokines have not proved highly effective. This may be due to the pleiotropic effects of each lymphokine and to the complex interactions exhibited by regulatory networks of multiple lymphokines. For example, IL-2 has been shown by several criteria to promote graft rejection, and blockade of the IL-2R has been shown to promote graft survival.[131, 132] However, knockout mice, which do not express any IL-2 owing to inactivation of the IL-2 gene by homologous recombination, reject grafts as easily as do normal mice.[133] Rejection in animals that lack IL-2 is likely mediated by other lymphokines that compensate for the IL-2 deficit by having overlapping functions. Furthermore, recent studies with specific Th1 or Th2 cytokine gene–knockout animals indicate the complexity of the Th1-Th2 paradigm in graft rejection and tolerance.[134-136] Recent data from animal and human studies have shown that Th2 clones propagated from patients with stable renal transplant function or animals tolerant to kidney transplants can regulate a proliferative response from Th1 clones isolated from patients or animals undergoing active rejection.[137, 138] Therefore, although manipulation of lymphokine functions may hold promise as a therapeutic modality, we will have to understand better the role of lymphokines in graft rejection and tolerance under physiologic conditions if we are to develop effective treatments.

In summary, cell-cell interactions between T cells and APCs can be mediated by five classes of receptors: the antigen-specific TCR, the CD4 or CD8 coreceptor, costimulatory molecules, accessory or adhesion molecules, and lymphokine receptors. Therapeutic or experimental manipulation of members of each class of receptors has been shown to prolong graft survival.[106] The most effective in clinical studies to date have been the anti-TCR monoclonal antibody OKT3 and antibodies targeted at the IL-2R complex.[106] Interaction of alloreactive T cells and alloantigen does not uniformly lead to an aggressive T cell response. Activated T cells may undergo a number of different "fates" after recognition of alloantigen. Some take on the role of effector cells and mediate an alloimmune B cell response, delayed-type hypersensitivity, or direct cell killing through a cytolytic T cell response. Others become memory cells awaiting antigenic restimulation at a later time to provide a rapid recall response. Alternatively, the T cell response may be terminated through anergy, activation-induced cell death, or active regulation by other cells or soluble factors.

EFFECTOR MECHANISMS OF ALLOGRAFT REJECTION

There are both cellular (DTH responses, cell-mediated cytotoxicity) and humoral components to transplant rejection. Once fully activated, CD4+ helper T cells produce cytokines that orchestrate various effector arms of the alloimmune response (see Fig. 63-7). Th1 cytokines activate macrophages,

and both CD4+ Th1 cells and activated macrophages effect DTH responses. Although initiated by a specific immune response, DTH results in nonspecific tissue injury and repair. Although the exact mechanisms by which DTH leads to graft destruction remain unclear, it is hypothesized that some of the cytokines produced by T cells and macrophages (TNF-α) mediate apoptosis of graft cells. It has been suggested that DTH responses, presumably initiated by indirect allorecognition, are particularly important in the pathogenesis of chronic rejection.

CD8+ precytolytic T lymphocytes recognize specific HLA class I antigens on the surface of donor cells, and, in the presence of helper T cytokines (IL-2, IL-4, and IL-5), differentiate and divide. Mature cytolytic T lymphocytes (CTL) damage target cells displaying foreign HLA class I by at least two mechanisms (Fig. 63-10).[19] A secretory pathway involves granule-mediated exocytosis of soluble factors, including granzymes (serine esterases), and a complement-like molecule, perforin. These proteins induce cell death via both DNA degradation and osmotic lysis secondary to pore formation in the target cell membrane. Detection of both perforin and granzyme mRNA from cells isolated from urine has been shown to predict whether acute rejection is ongoing within the allograft.[139, 140] A second cytolytic pathway involves interaction between Fas (CD95), a TNF-like protein, and Fas ligand. Fas ligand is induced on CTL via triggering of the TCR. Fas-expressing target cells undergo apoptosis when Fas ligand is engaged. The role in the rejection process of CD8+ T lymphocyte–mediated killing of graft cells remains controversial. It is possible to demonstrate ex vivo specific cytotoxicity against donor cells in graft-rejecting animals and humans. In addition, passive transfer of specific "killer" T cell clones to naive animals induces allograft rejection, particularly skin allografts. However, recent data using CD8 gene–knockout mice indicate that these animals are capable of rejecting skin and vascularized

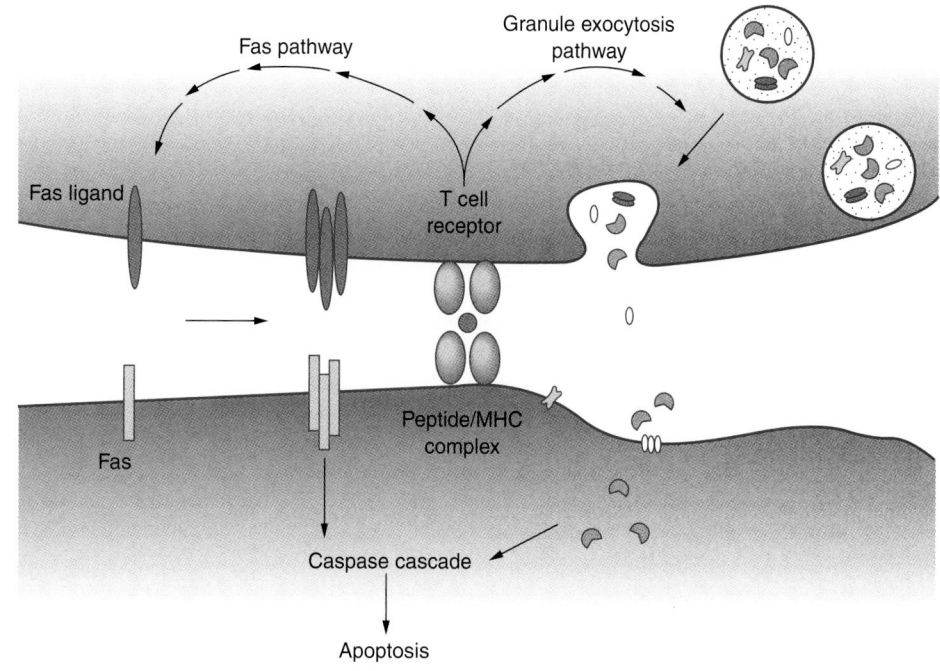

FIGURE 63-10. Mechanisms of CD8+ T cell–mediated killing. Cytotoxic T cells *(top)* activated via the class I major histocompatibility complex (MHC+) peptide complex can cause target cell killing by two pathways. One involves granule exocytosis, releasing perforin, granzymes, and granulysin, which in turn cause membrane damage and cell lysis by osmotic dysregulation and activation of caspase cascade, giving rise to programmed cell death (apoptosis). The second involves expression of Fas ligand on activated T cells. When Fas on target cells interacts with its ligand on activated T cells, the target cell undergoes apoptosis by activation of caspase cascade. (From Germain R: MHC-dependent antigen processing and peptide presentation: Providing ligands for T lymphocyte activation. Cell 76:288, 1994.)

allografts as easily as normal controls, whereas CD4 gene–knockout mice are incapable of rejecting an allograft, indicating that CD4+ helper T cells, but not CD8+ T cells, are essential to allograft rejection.[141] It is now thought that CD8+ T cells, which may contribute to acute allograft rejection through killer mechanisms, are not essential for allograft rejection to proceed. In addition, CD8+ killer lymphocytes may not play an important role in the process of chronic rejection.

B lymphocytes express clonally restricted antigen-specific cell-surface receptors, immunoglobulins. When cell-surface immunoglobulin binds specific antigen in the context of soluble helper factors such as IL-4, IL-6, and IL-8, B cells are activated. They differentiate, divide, and become plasma cells, which secrete soluble forms of antigen-specific antibodies that are displayed on their cell surfaces. These antibodies, in turn, can bind allogeneic target antigens and induce graft damage by binding complement or directing antibody-dependent cellular cytotoxicity. Both IgM and IgG alloantibodies can be detected in the serum and in the allografts (of animals and humans) that are being rejected. Preformed anti-HLA class I antibodies, and, occasionally, antiendothelial antibodies, play an important role in hyperacute rejection and accelerated vascular rejection observed in previously sensitized transplant recipients. In xenotransplantation, naturally occurring xenoreactive antibodies play a critical role in hyperacute rejection of grafts.[142] Finally, alloantibodies, particularly IgG, play important pathogenic roles in the development of chronic rejection and graft arteriosclerosis.

Other soluble factors induce additional effector mechanisms, including phagocytosis by granulocytes and macrophages and cell death via NK cells. NK cells express cell-surface receptors called *killer inhibitory receptors* (KIRs) that recognize HLA class I molecules.[143] Although the role of NK cell–mediated cytotoxicity in allograft rejection remains controversial, NK cells appear to play a key role in mediating delayed xenograft rejection.[142]

Recent completion of a draft of the sequence of the human genome,[144] in addition to concurrent technologic advances, has made the simultaneous analysis of tens of thousands of genes feasible. The application of DNA microarrays to the analysis of transplantation is in its infancy, but investigations in animal models and clinical studies are emerging. A study of rejection in human recipients of kidney allografts analyzed gene expression in biopsies of renal allografts from patients on triple immunosuppression with a confirmed diagnosis of acute rejection.[145] Transcripts of gene expression from seven renal biopsies with histopathologic evidence of acute cellular rejection were compared with transcripts of gene expression from tissue from three normal renal biopsies. Using a minimum threshold of fourfold induction, four genes were identified in each acute rejection sample: human monokine induced by interferon-γ (a C-X-C chemokine crucial for murine acute allograft rejection), TCR-active β-chain protein, IL-2–stimulated phosphoprotein (expressed predominantly in T cells), and RING4 (important in intracellular antigen processing). Murine cardiac allografts analyzed for the expression of approximately 6500 genes and expressed sequence tags (ESTs) following transplantation identified 181 genes with significantly modulated expression in at least one of the experimental groups

of ischemia, stress, innate, or adaptive immunity. In an additional study, differentially expressed genes were identified using self-organizing maps. Twenty-nine genes were up-regulated as early as 6 hours after transplantation.[146] These included IL-1 R, IL-6, and haptoglobin, which have all been associated with the acute phase response. In current clinical practice, acute rejection is typically diagnosed by histologic analysis of graft biopsies. The application of these newer technologies could produce a molecular profile of each biopsy specimen that would provide more precise diagnostic criteria.

CHRONIC REJECTION

The term *chronic rejection* is being replaced slowly by a variety of other terms, including *chronic allograft nephropathy* and *chronic allograft dysfunction*.[147, 148] The main reason for dissatisfaction with chronic rejection is that this term is a historical histologic description, which in kidney allografts consists of tubular atrophy, interstitial fibrosis, and fibrous neointimal thickening of arterial walls, and it does not differentiate among the multiple potential mechanisms of this disease entity. It was first described by Hume in one of the original transplants carried out at the Brigham and Women's Hospital in the 1950s.[149] In the case in question, the lesion occurred relatively quickly after transplantation and was likely related to an ongoing immune process. Since that time, chronic rejection has been increasingly recognized as a cause for late graft loss, and a number of different nonimmunologic factors have been associated with its progression.[148] These include some events that occur before transplantation, such as ischemia-reperfusion injury suffered by the kidney at the time of transplant, brain death in the donor, and nonspecific injury due to donor age, hypertension, and diabetes.

Post-transplant factors have also been shown to accelerate the course of chronic rejection, including reduced renal mass, calcineurin inhibitor toxicity, hypertension in the recipient, hyperlipidemia, and cytomegalovirus infection. However, in nearly every transplant a degree of tissue incompatibility is present, whether it is a mismatch of the minor histocompatibility antigens alone or one that occurs in combination with the MHC. The importance of this can been seen in Figure 63-6, where the half-life of kidney survival declines from 31.8 years in living HLA identical first allografts to 17.3 years in any degree of HLA mismatched living first allografts.

Although the immune response may be the prime driver (at least initially) of chronic rejection, the actual immune mechanisms responsible for it are still not clear. The same effector mechanisms that are responsible for acute rejection are thought to be active in chronic rejection, although the relative importance of each may be different. Indirect, as opposed to direct, allorecognition is thought to play an important role in the process. The evidence for this comes from a number of studies that have shown that donor MHC-derived peptides are capable of eliciting an immune response long after donor-derived APCs (the main target of the direct alloimmune response) have disappeared from the allograft.[147, 150] Alloantibodies have always been thought to be important in the development of chronic rejection, and recent studies have supported this hypothesis.[151, 152] Growth factors and, in particular, TGF-β are also thought to play an important role in the tissue remodeling and fibrosis that appear to take place in affected organs.[153] Despite these insights, our overall understanding of chronic rejection is still at a rudimentary level, and no model of chronic injury used to date has been shown to be perfect. If anything, the models indicate that a variety of different immune and non-immune responses can lead to lesions that are compatible with the histology of chronic rejection. This in itself illustrates the danger of making rigid assumptions about chronic rejection, as its pathogenesis clinically is likely to be as multifactorial as it is experimentally.

MECHANISMS OF IMMUNOSUPPRESSION

Corticosteroids

Most immunosuppressive drug regimens use an adrenocorticosteroid such as prednisone in combination with other immunosuppressive agents. Corticosteroids provide the most proximal block in the T cell activation cascade: they interfere indirectly with T cell proliferation, at least partially through their ability to block expression of the IL-1 and IL-6 genes.[106, 154] Macrophages treated with corticosteroids do not produce IL-1 or IL-6 mRNA, even after incubation with powerful macrophage stimulants. Because IL-2 release depends in part on IL-1–stimulated IL-6 release, corticosteroids also indirectly block IL-2. Corticosteroids modulate the immune response by regulating gene expression. The steroid molecule enters the cytosol, where it binds the steroid receptor, inducing a conformational change in the receptor. The complex then migrates to the nucleus and binds regulatory regions of DNA called *glucocorticoid response*

elements, which regulate the transcription of many genes. Thus, the many effects of corticosteroids on multiple cell types account for both their efficacy and their diverse array of complications (Fig. 63-11).

Conventional treatments for acute renal allograft rejection include high-dose pulses of glucocorticoids—drugs that have broad, nonspecific immunosuppressive and anti-inflammatory effects. In addition to their effects on lymphokines, glucocorticoids reduce the migration of monocytes to sites of inflammation. A major drawback to the use of glucocorticoids in the treatment of acute rejection is that they inhibit the entire immune and inflammatory systems and alter many other steroid-responsive systems. Large doses of glucocorticoids can thus produce undesirable side effects, including decreased inflammatory and phagocytic capacity, resulting in increased susceptibility to infection, hyperglycemia, hyperkalemia, osteoporosis, increased capillary fragility, and growth suppression in children.

Azathioprine

Azathioprine is a purine analog that is enzymatically converted to 6-mercaptopurine and other derivatives in vivo, molecules that function as antimetabolites.[155] After metabolic conversion, it has multiple activities, including incorporation into DNA, inhibition of purine nucleotide synthesis, and alteration of RNA synthesis. The major immunosuppressive effect is thought to be due to blocking of DNA replication, which prevents lymphocyte proliferation after antigenic stimulation. Although it is useful for inhibiting primary immune responses, azathioprine has little effect on secondary responses or on the reversal of acute allograft rejections, which are not dependent on lymphocyte proliferation. Azathioprine also decreases the number of migratory mononuclear and granulocytic cells while inhibiting proliferation of promyelocytes

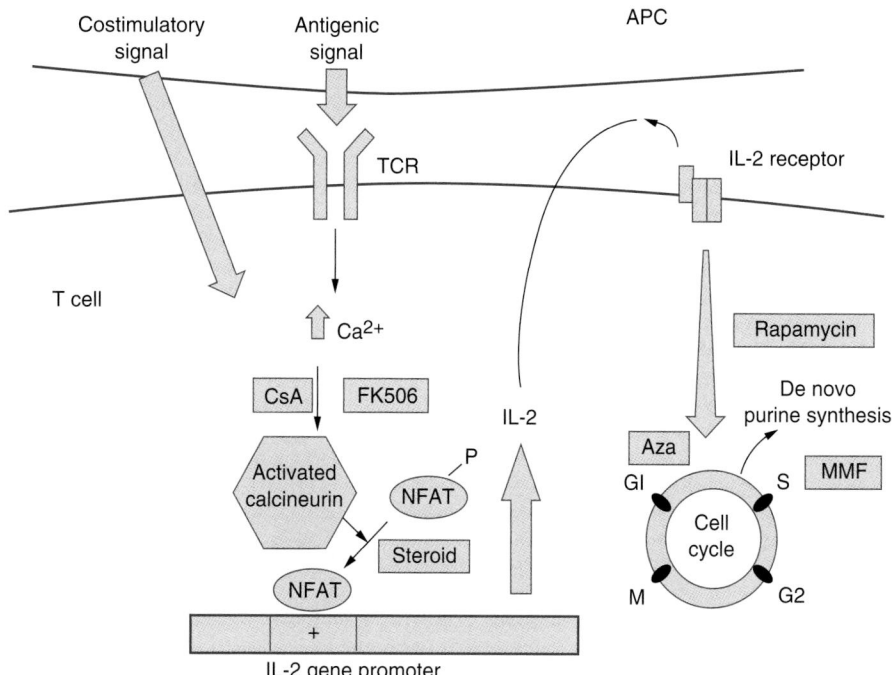

FIGURE 63-11. Mechanisms of action of immunosuppressive agents viewed as a function of inhibiting T cell activation. *Signal 1:* The calcium-dependent signal induced by T cell receptor (TCR) stimulation results in calcineurin activation, a process inhibited by cyclosporine and tacrolimus. Calcineurin dephosphorylates NFAT (nuclear factor of activated T cells), enabling it to enter the nucleus and bind to the IL-2 promoter. Corticosteroids bind to cytoplasmic receptors, enter the nucleus, and inhibit cytokine gene transcription in both T cells and the antigen-presenting cells (APCs). Corticosteroids also inhibit NF-κB activation (not shown). *Signal 2:* Costimulatory signals are necessary to optimize T cell IL-2 gene transcription, prevent T cell anergy, and inhibit T cell apoptosis. Experimental agents, but not current immunosuppressive agents, interrupt these intracellular signals. *Signal 3:* IL-2 receptor stimulation induces the cell to enter the cell cycle and proliferate. Signal 3 may be blocked by IL-2 receptor antibodies or by sirolimus, which inhibits S6 kinase activation. Following progression into the cell cycle, azathioprine and mycophenolate mofetil (MMF) interrupt DNA replication by inhibiting purine synthesis.

in bone marrow. As a result, the number of circulating monocytes capable of differentiating into macrophages is decreased. Among the possible deleterious effects of azathioprine administration are severe leukopenia and occasionally thrombocytopenia, gastrointestinal disturbances, hepatoxicity, and increased risk of neoplasia.

Mycophenolate Mofetil

In many centers, MMF is now replacing azathioprine in standard immunosuppression protocols for new kidney and pancreas-kidney transplants.[156] The rationale for this switch is that MMF is a selective inhibitor of the pathway of de novo purine synthesis. In the normal mammalian cell, guanine and adenine nucleotides are manufactured to form smaller precursors through two mechanisms, a de novo pathway or a salvage pathway (where purine bases are recycled). Mycophenolate is a reversible inhibitor of inosine monophosphate dehydrogenase (IMPDH), which is the rate-limiting enzyme in the de novo synthesis of guanosine nucleotide and nucleosides.[106] Inhibition of this enzyme results in the selective inhibition of T and B lymphocyte proliferation.

Mycophenolate has minimal effects on other cell populations because proliferation of T and B cells is dependent on the de novo pathway for purine synthesis, whereas other cells are capable of utilizing a salvage pathway. The main active metabolite of mycophenolate is glucuronidated mycophenolic acid (MPAG), which is excreted into bile and undergoes enterohepatic recirculation. Cyclosporine but not FK506 inhibits MPAG excretion into bile and thereby decreases circulating levels of mycophenolic acid,[157] which suggests that lower doses of mycophenolate are required when used in combination with FK506.

Three large multicenter trials have compared MMF to azathioprine or placebo in renal transplant patients receiving cyclosporin A and corticosteroids.[158] These studies show that MMF therapy is associated with a 50% reduction in the incidence of acute rejection in the first year after transplantation and less need for high-dose steroids and antilymphocyte antibody therapy to treat rejection.[159] In experimental animal models, MMF use prevents development of chronic rejection,[160] and most, but not all, studies have shown that there is some reduction in the rate of progression of chronic rejection if mycophenolate is substituted for azathioprine in renal transplant recipients. Side effects of MMF include gastrointestinal upset and diarrhea (which may be dose limiting) and some increased risk of tissue-invasive cytomegalovirus infection. MMF may also cause bone marrow suppression but less bone marrow suppression than is found with azathioprine use.

Cyclosporine

Cyclosporine, a small cyclic peptide of fungal origin, has played a major role in preventing graft rejection and has improved graft survival rates. Although highly effective in blocking the initiation of an immune response, cyclosporine, like azathioprine, is of limited value in treating acute allograft rejection.[106, 161] Its primary action is to block the expression of lymphokine genes produced by T cells, including IL-2, IL-3, IL-4, IFN-γ, and TNF-α[162, 163]; however, it does not interfere with IL-1, TNF-α, or transforming growth factor-β (TGF-β) produced by APCs, including macrophages. There is likewise no evidence that NK cells are affected by cyclosporine. In the presence of cyclosporine, T cell proliferation is indirectly inhibited owing to the absence of lymphokines; however, the addition of exogenous IL-2 has been shown to restore T cell proliferation.[164]

It is now understood that cyclosporine blocks the calcium-dependent component of the TCR signal transduction pathway (see Fig. 63-11). Previous work showed that cyclosporine binds to a family of cytoplasmic molecules termed *cyclophilins*, which have peptidyl-prolyl isomerase activity. After binding cyclophilin, cyclosporine inhibits the isomerase activity; however, it is now apparent that the immunosuppressive effects are not a result of this inhibition. This was shown by analogs of cyclosporine that bind cyclophilin and inhibit isomerase activity but do not cause immunosuppression.[165] More recent work has shown that the cyclophilin-cyclosporine complex binds to and inhibits calcineurin, which is a cytoplasmic serine threonine phosphatase.[166]

After T cell activation in the absence of cyclosporine, calcineurin dephosphorylates the cytosolic component of nuclear factor of activated T cells termed *NF-AT*. After dephosphorylation, NFAT is translocated from the cytosol to the nucleus, where it forms a complex with other DNA-binding proteins, including Fos and Jun.[167] The complex of DNA-binding proteins regulates gene transcription, including the IL-2 gene. During treatment with cyclosporine, the inhibition of the formation of the nuclear NF-AT complex has been shown to prevent transcription of the IL-2 gene,[168] and a similar complex has been shown to regulate TNF-α gene transcription. The net result is a reduction of IL-2 and resultant T cell activation. Clinically, a reduction in IL-2 concentrations minimizes the immune response associated with allograft rejection.

Patients maintained on therapeutic levels of cyclosporine experience approximately a 50% reduction in calcineurin activity, allowing the patient to retain a degree of immune responsiveness sufficient to maintain host defenses. It is likely that identical or similar DNA-binding complexes regulate the transcription of multiple lymphokine genes. The mechanism of action of cyclosporine in nonlymphocytes remains poorly understood; however, it has been shown that analogs of cyclosporine that lack toxicity also lack immunosuppressive effects.[169] These results suggest that the toxic and immunosuppressive effects are mediated by similar signal transduction mechanisms. The differential susceptibility to cyclosporine of lymphocytes, as compared with other cell types, may be due to different levels of expression of calcineurin and the cyclophilins.

FK506 (Tacrolimus)

FK506 is a potent immunosuppressive agent that inhibits T cell activation in vitro.[166, 170] FK506, in contrast to cyclosporine, is a macrolide antibiotic produced by fungi, yet the immunosuppressive effects on T cells are similar.[166, 170] Because of structural differences, FK506 binds a family of cytosolic proteins termed *FK506-binding proteins* (FKBP), which are different from the cyclosporine-binding cyclophilins. Interestingly, both FKBP and cyclophilin have peptidyl-prolyl isomerase activity and collectively are called *immunophilins*; however, the similar immunosuppressive properties of the two drugs are attributable to the fact that both agents inhibit the phosphatase activity of calcineurin.[171] Thus, although FK506 and cyclosporine have different structures, their immunosuppressive effects are mediated through a common final pathway. Thus, it is not surprising that both drugs block the induction of lymphokine mRNA, including IL-2, inhibit lymphokine production, and indirectly inhibit T cell proliferation.[166, 170] Owing to the similar mechanisms of action, the toxicities of FK506 and cyclosporine are also very similar. In experimental studies, the combination of FK506 and cyclosporine show additive increases in toxicity and in efficacy. Therefore, in clinical transplantation, immunosuppressive protocols involving multiple drugs utilize either cyclosporine or FK506.

Rapamycin (Sirolimus)

Rapamycin was first utilized as an immunosuppressive through a search for drugs with a similar structure to FK506. Like FK506, it is a macrolide antibiotic and binds to the same family of FKBP isomerase proteins.

However, whereas cyclosporine and FK506 inhibit calcineurin in the calcium-dependent component of the TCR signal transduction pathway, rapamycin binds to mTOR (mammalian target of rapamycin) and prevents phosphorylation of p70 S6 kinase in the CD28 costimulatory and IL-2R signal-transduction pathways (see Fig. 63-11).

In functional studies, activation of T cells by monoclonal antibodies to the TCR was inhibited by either cyclosporine or FK506 but not rapamycin.[172] Conversely, the activation of T cells by exogenous IL-2 plus protein kinase C stimulation with a phorbol ester was inhibited by rapamycin but not by cyclosporine or FK506. Similarly, T cell activation by monoclonal antibodies to the CD28 costimulatory molecule plus protein kinase costimulation with a phorbol ester was also inhibited by rapamycin but not by cyclosporine or FK506. Cell cycle analysis shows that rapamycin blocks T cell proliferation during late G_1 of the cell cycle and before S phase.[173-175] Thus, rapamycin inhibits late signals in T cell activation that are transduced by either the IL-2R or the CD28 costimulatory signal transduction pathways.[175] In contrast, cyclosporine and FK506 inhibit an early signal in T cell activation that is transduced by the TCR signal transduction pathway. Despite interacting with the same binding proteins as FK506, there is no competitive inhibition of these drugs, as the binding proteins are present in great excess compared with the FK506 and rapamycin. In experimental models the combination of rapamycin with a calcineurin inhibitor results in a synergistic effect.[106] This synergistic action has now been used with good effect in clinical studies.[176] Everolimus (RAD) is a rapamycin derivative and has a mode of action similar to that of sirolimus.

Polyclonal Immune Globulins

Polyclonal antilymphocyte globulin (ALG) or antithymocyte globulin (ATG) preparations have been available for approximately 2 decades and have proved to be more effective than steroids alone for reversing acute renal allograft rejection.[177] Polyclonal immune globulins are produced by injecting animals such as horses or rabbits with human lymphoid cells to obtain the purified γ-globulin fractions of the resulting immune sera. Cultured lymphoblasts (to produce ALG) and human thymocytes (to produce ATG) typically have been used. Because cultured lymphoblasts are B cells rather than T cells, one possible disadvantage of ALG is that the antiserum does not recognize the T cell molecules, including the TCR, CD28, and CD4 molecules, which are the ones most susceptible to immunosuppression. Human thymus tissue, an excellent source of T cell antigens, is not always available in adequate amounts. More important, polyclonal immune globulins represent a heterogeneous group of antibodies, only a minority of which are specific to T cells. Thus, the heterogeneous quality of these antisera makes the interpretations of clinical data and investigational findings on immunosuppressive mechanisms difficult to compare.

Polyclonal immune globulin may exert its immunosuppressive effect by several mechanisms, including classic complement-mediated lysis of lymphocytes, clearance of lymphocytes via reticuloendothelial uptake, masking of T cell antigens, and expansion of negative regulatory cells. Administration of immune globulins produces prompt and profound lymphopenia. It soon abates, however, and the number of circulating T cells gradually increases, even while treatment continues, but the proliferative response continues to be impaired. It has been suggested that suppressor cells may be responsible for the prolonged immunosuppressive effect that persists after the resolution of lymphopenia. Thus, the resolution of cell-mediated graft rejection results from elimination of circulating T cells, and the subsequent inhibition of proliferative responses sustains the immunosuppressive effect.

Each polyclonal immune globulin preparation has different constituent antibodies. Because of the unpredictable nature of the antibody mixtures, treatment is associated with variable efficacy and risks of adverse reactions. Batch standardization and assessments of immunosuppressive potency are, therefore, difficult. Unwanted antibodies can cause thrombocytopenia, granulocytopenia, serum sickness, or glomerulonephritis. Although polyclonal immune globulins are potent immunosuppressive agents, the major concern in their use is the potential for excessive immunosuppression, which not infrequently results in opportunistic infections. Therefore, caution is the rule when combining immune globulins with other immunosuppressive agents.

Monoclonal Antibodies

The development of monoclonal antibodies to T cell surface molecules offers the advantage of homogeneous preparations and more predictable therapeutic agents. A number of monoclonal antibodies have been shown in clinical trials to produce immunosuppression,[106] but the most effective monoclonal antibody tested to date is OKT3, which binds the CD3 of the TCR complex.[102, 178] The TCR is a complex of six or seven polypeptides, including the polymorphic α- and β-chains, which provide the antigen recognition component, and the γ-, δ-, and ε-chains, plus a ζζ-homodimer or ζη-heterodimer, which provide the signal transduction function of the receptor. OKT3 binds to the TCR ε-chain, which is a pan–T cell nonpolymorphic component of the antigen receptor.[102] Immunosuppression with OKT3 blocks both CD4+ and CD8+ T cell function.

Treatment with OKT3 produces multiple effects on T lymphocytes. The acute effect, which commences within minutes, is partial activation of T cells caused by signal transduction induced by the antibody.[106, 178] The activated T cells produce large amounts of lymphokines, among them TNF-α, which cause many of the acute side effects of treatment, including fever, chills, nausea, vomiting, diarrhea, headache, anorexia, and a capillary leak syndrome. In severe cases, patients can become hypotensive secondary to vasodilation and diarrhea. Alternatively, volume-overloaded patients are susceptible to pulmonary edema from the capillary leak syndrome. Therefore, patients should be within 3% of their estimated dry weight before commencing therapy. Later side effects include aseptic meningitis and serum sickness due to the development of antimouse antibodies. The development of antimouse antibodies results in rapid clearance of OKT3 from the serum and renders it ineffective. The presence of antimouse antibodies can be monitored by indirect immunofluorescence by flow cytometry. Owing to the profound immunosuppression, OKT3 treatment can be complicated by opportunistic infections, including an increased incidence of cytomegalovirus infection. Multiple courses of therapy have been associated with an increased incidence of malignancy, principally non-Hodgkin lymphoma.

There are at least two components to the mechanism of immunosuppression by OKT3.[102-104, 106, 178, 179] Within hours after administration, OKT3 causes profound depletion of peripheral T cells. Because OKT3 is not cytotoxic, the depletion is attributed to sequestration of the T cells. In addition, T cells down-modulate the expression of the TCR complex. Thus, after a few days of treatment by flow cytometry, circulating CD4[+] and CD8[+] cells can be shown to lack detectable TCR. It is thought that the TCR is internalized by endocytosis or shedding. The modulation of TCR expression is reversible, and, after elimination of OKT3, the TCR-CD3 complex is again expressed on the cell surface.[103, 179]

Chimeric and humanized antibodies targeted against the IL-2 receptor also have been developed. They are created by splicing together the DNA encoding the antigen recognition portion of the murine antibody with human immunoglobulin DNA. Humanized antibodies contain 90% human and 10% murine antibody sequences. Chimeric antibodies are composed of mouse light and heavy chains and the human Fc portion. Anti–IL-2R antibodies bind to the alpha subunit of the high affinity IL-2 receptor, which is only expressed on activated lymphocytes.[9] This agent competitively inhibits the IL-2 activation of lymphocytes. Therapy with IL-2 receptor antibodies results in a highly specific inhibition of the lymphocytic immune response of activated T cells, thus suppressing T cell activity against the allograft. However, in patients, 10% to 15% of T cells are IL-2Rα positive; therefore, use of IL-2R antibodies may also have more of a generalized anti-inflammatory effect. These antibodies are indicated for prophylaxis rather than for treatment of acute allograft rejection.

Experimental Immunosuppressive Drugs

A number of newer agents that have not been approved for use in clinical transplantation are currently undergoing evaluation in phase III studies. Campath 1H is a lymphocyte-depleting antibody (anti-CD52). It has been given at the time of transplantation in cadaveric renal transplantation with low-dose cyclosporine and no other immunosuppression. This regimen was well tolerated and had a low incidence of acute rejection. FTY-720, on the other hand, works by blocking chemokine-dependent lymphocyte homing into secondary lymphoid organs. It also has been shown to be an effective immunosuppressive agent in a primate kidney transplant model. T cell costimulatory blockade, in the form of CTLA4-Ig (LEA29Y), which blocks CD28 interaction with B7, is also being studied as a means of immunosuppression.

Donor-Specific Immune Tolerance

Although immunologists have induced tolerance successfully in experimental models for more than 3 decades, the mechanisms of tolerance remain incompletely understood.[162, 163, 180, 181] More important, physicians have been unable to induce organ-specific tolerance after transplantation, although some long-term patients have discontinued immunosuppressive therapy without consequences. The issue is one of developing strategies that will produce allograft tolerance. Initial studies from Billingham and co-workers demonstrated that it was possible to induce mice to accept skin grafts from donors of a different genetic background if the recipient mice were injected while still in utero (or neonatally) with hematopoietic cells of donor origin.[182] This was the first description of *acquired* tolerance. Neonatal tolerance is thought to be due largely to "clonal deletion": T cells reactive with alloantigen are deleted in the thymus, presumably by the same mechanisms that delete self-reactive T cells. Recently, other mechanisms (e.g., immune deviation to Th2 cells) have been described as possible mediators of neonatal tolerance, particularly to MHC class II antigens.[183] In adults, administration of donor alloantigen, with or without some form of brief induction immunosuppression regimen, has been shown to be effective in inducing tolerance to allografts in several experimental animal models. Several factors have been found to play a role in the induction and maintenance of the tolerance state: the type of donor cells, the route of administration, the dose of alloantigen, the timing of administration of alloantigen, and the accompanying induction immunosuppressive protocol. Tolerance strategies, including donor antigen, may utilize bone marrow infusion, augmentation or reconstitution, blood transfusions, and intrathymic injection of donor antigens.[162, 163, 180, 181, 183-187]

Recent advances in our understanding of T cell activation suggest novel strategies for inducing T cell tolerance. Specifically, CD28-B7 and CD40L-CD40 blockade have proved to be very effective in experimental animals, and clinical studies are being planned.[80, 81] Other experimental strategies include MHC peptides and gene therapy to deliver immunomodulatory cytokines.[162, 163, 180-182] The advantages of inducing donor-specific tolerance include prevention of immune-mediated graft destruction with no maintenance immunosuppression in an immunocompetent host.[180, 188] Development of novel clinical trials to induce tolerance depend not only on developing novel experimental strategies but also on understanding the mechanisms of tolerance[162, 163, 181, 182, 189-191] in humans and developing surrogate markers (the tolerance assay) to predict graft rejection or acceptance.

XENOTRANSPLANTATION

One of the most important problems currently encountered in kidney transplantation is the insufficiency of donor organs to satisfy the increasing recipient demand. In that regard, strategies targeted at expanding the donor pool without jeopardizing graft function and outcome are extremely important. The need to address this problem has stimulated research into xenotransplantation, organogenesis, and cellular transplantation to augment failing organs.

An area of obvious importance is xenotransplantation (i.e., transplantation across species). More than 25 years ago, baboon and chimpanzee organs were transplanted into humans, with short-term success. Currently, xenotransplantation studies are targeted at pig-to-primate xenografting as a preclinical model for developing pig-to-human transplantation. Several hurdles have yet to be overcome, however. They can be classified as immunologic and nonimmunologic.[142] The immunologic response to a xenotransplant can be envisaged as a series of waves consisting of hyperacute, acute vascular, cellular, and chronic rejection.[192] Hyperacute rejection is mediated by preformed complement-binding xenoreactive antibodies, which are present in primates and humans and are reactive to a carbohydrate epitope (Gal1α-3Gal) on endothelial cells of lower mammals, and occurs within hours of transplantation. Xenografts also express many other antigens that are unfamiliar to the host. These antigens can elicit a vigorous immune response that results in acute vascular rejection within days to weeks.[193] Experimental approaches to deal with these problems include development of transgenic pigs that express complement-regulatory proteins such as decay-accelerating factor (CD55)[194] and the generation of knockout animals that express lower levels of antigenic proteins.[195]

If it becomes possible to overcome the problems of hyperacute and acute vascular rejection, it is envisaged that xenotransplants would be susceptible to cellular and chronic rejection as well. These forms of immune response may also present major barriers to transplantation, as it is unlikely that immune regulatory responses that normally curb the immune response would work as efficiently across species. Nonimmunologic hurdles to xenotransplantation include risk of transmitting infections, physiologic compatibility, and ethical and religious issues related to using organs from animals in humans. These issues have also slowed down the development of xenotransplantation.

Organogenesis, or the growing of organs, is an exciting area. Research in this field remains rudimentary; however, the demonstration that rat metanephroi transplanted into the omentum of another rat are capable of growing, differentiating, becoming vascularized, and functioning has generated interest in this field.[196] As fetal tissue expresses lower levels of MHC and other antigens, organogenesis may have the advantage of stimulating less of a xenoimmune response when transplanted across species.[197]

Recently, it has been demonstrated that cellular transplantation of skeletal myoblasts appears to be able to augment cardiac function in a damaged heart.[198] The complexity of the kidney very likely precludes such straightforward replacement strategies, although it has been demonstrated clearly that recipient cells are capable of incorporating into donor kidneys and presumably function at some level.[199]

REFERENCES

1. Goodnow CC, Adelstein S, Basten A: The need for central and peripheral tolerance in the B cell repertoire. Science 248(4961):1373-1379, 1990.
2. Shevach EM: CD4+ CD25+ suppressor T cells: More questions than answers. Nat Rev Immunol 2:389-400, 2002.
3. Kappler JW, Roehm N, Marrack P: T cell tolerance by clonal elimination in the thymus. Cell 49:273-280, 1987.
4. Murphy KM, Weaver CT, Elish M, et al: Peripheral tolerance to allogeneic class II histocompatibility antigens expressed in transgenic mice: Evidence against a clonal-deletion mechanism. Proc Natl Acad Sci U S A 86(24):10034-10038, 1989.
5. Schwartz RH: Acquisition of immunologic self-tolerance. Cell 57:1073-1081, 1989.
6. Nossal GJ: Negative selection of lymphocytes. Cell 76:229-239, 1994.
7. Fry AM, Jones LA, Kruisbeek AM, Matis LA: Thymic requirement for clonal deletion during T cell development. Science 246(4933):1044-1046, 1989.
8. von Boehmer H: Positive selection of lymphocytes. Cell 76:219-228, 1994.
9. Gorer PA: The genetic and antigenic basis of tumor transplantation. J Pathol Bacteriol 44:691, 1937.
10. Snell GD: Methods for the study of histocompatibility genes. J Genetics 49:87, 1948.
11. Klein J: Evolution and function of the major histocompatibility system: Facts and speculations. *In* Goetze D (ed): The Major Histocompatibility System in Man and Animals. Berlin, Springer-Verlag, 1977, p 339.
12. Klein J: An attempt at an interpretation of the mouse H-2 complex. Contemp Top Immunobiol 5:297, 1976.
13. Shreffler DC, David CS: The H-2 major histocompatibility complex and the I immune response region: Genetic variation, function, and organization. Adv Immunol 20:125-195, 1975.
14. Dausset J: Iso-leuco anticorps. Acta Haematol 20:156, 1958.
15. Lamm LU, Friedrich U, Petersen CB, et al: Assignment of the major histocompatibility complex to chromosome No. 6 in a family with a pericentric inversion. Hum Hered 24:273-284, 1974.
16. Graff RJ, Silvers WK, Billingham RE, et al: The cumulative effect of histocompatibility antigens. Transplantation 4:605-617, 1966.
17. Holman E: Protein sensitization in iso-skin grafting. Is the latter of practical value? Surg Gynecol Obstet 38:100, 1924.
18. Medawar PB: The behaviour and fate of skin autografts and skin homografts in rabbits. J Anat 78:176, 1944.
19. Germain RN: MHC-dependent antigen processing and peptide presentation: Providing ligands for T lymphocyte activation. Cell 76:287-299, 1994.
20. Zinkernagel RM, Doherty PC: Restriction of in vitro T cell-mediated cytotoxicity in lymphocytic choriomeningitis within a syngeneic or semiallogeneic system. Nature 248(450):701-702, 1974.
21. Payne R, Tripp M, Weigle J, et al: A new leucocyte isoantigen system in man. Quant Biol 29:285, 1964.
22. Charron D: Genetic diversity of HLA: Functional and medical implication. Twelfth International Histocompatibility Workshop and Conference. Paris, EDK, 1997.
23. Bodmer JG, Marsh SG, Albert ED, et al: Nomenclature for factors of the HLA system, 1995. Tissue Antigens 46:1-18, 1995.
24. Williams AF: A year in the life of the immunoglobulin superfamily. Immunol Today 8:298, 1987.
25. Immunogenetics Data Base for HLA. http://www.ebi.ac.uk/imgt.
26. Bjorkman PJ, Saper MA, Samraoui B, et al: Structure of the human class I histocompatibility antigen, HLA-A2. Nature 329(6139):506-512, 1987.
27. Bjorkman PJ, Saper MA, Samraoui B, et al: The foreign antigen binding site and T cell recognition regions of class I histocompatibility antigens. Nature 329(6139):512-518, 1987.
28. Davis MM, Bjorkman PJ: T-cell antigen receptor genes and T-cell recognition. Nature 334(6181):395-402, 1988.
29. Garboczi DN, Ghosh P, Utz U, et al: Structure of the complex between human T-cell receptor, viral peptide and HLA-A2. Nature 384(6605):134-141, 1996.

30. Rotzschke O, Falk K: Naturally-occurring peptide antigens derived from the MHC class I–restricted processing pathway. Immunol Today 12:447-455, 1991.

31. Patel SD, Monaco JJ, McDevitt HO: Delineation of the subunit composition of human proteasomes using antisera against the major histocompatibility complex–encoded LMP2 and LMP7 subunits. Proc Natl Acad Sci U S A 91:296-300, 1994.

32. Powis SH, Rosenberg WM, Hall M, et al: TAP1 and TAP2 polymorphism in coeliac disease. Immunogenetics 38:345-350, 1993.

33. Marcadet A, Cohen D, Dausset J, et al: Genotyping with DNA probes in combined immunodeficiency syndrome with defective expression of HLA. N Engl J Med 312:1287-1292, 1985.

34. Bidwell J: DNA-RFLP analysis and genotyping of HLA-DR and DQ antigens. Immunol Today 9:18-23, 1988.

35. Higuchi R, von Beroldingen CH, Sensabaugh GF, Erlich HA: DNA typing from single hairs. Nature 332(6164):543-546, 1988.

36. Milford EL: HLA molecular typing. Curr Opin Nephrol Hypertens 2:892-897, 1993.

37. Chicz RM, Urban RG, Gorga JC, et al: Specificity and promiscuity among naturally processed peptides bound to HLA-DR alleles. J Exp Med 178:27-47, 1993.

38. Brown JH, Jardetsky TS, Gorga JC, et al: Three dimensional structure of the human class II histocompatibility antigen HLA-DR1. Nature 364:33, 1993.

39. Halloran PF, Wadgymar A, Autenried P: Inhibition of MHC product induction may contribute to the immunosuppressive action of ciclosporin. Prog Allergy 38:258-268, 1986.

40. Human Renal Transplant Registry: Report No. 12. JAMA 233:787, 1995.

41. Opelz G, Terasaki PI: Studies on the strength of HLA antigens in related donor kidney transplants. Transplantation 24:106-111, 1977.

42. Alper CA: Extended MHC haplotypes and disease markers. In ISI Atlas of Science: Immunology. Philadelphia, ISI, 1988.

43. Thorsby E: HLA-associated disease susceptibility. Which genes are involved? Immunologist 3:41, 1995.

44. Cook DJ, Terasaki PI, Iwaki Y, et al: An approach to reducing early kidney transplant failure by flow cytometry crossmatching. Clin Transplant 1:253, 1987.

45. Schwartz BD, Luehrman LK, Rodey GE: Public antigenic determinant on a family of HLA-B molecules. J Clin Invest 64:938-947, 1979.

46. Bach FH, van Rood JJ: The major histocompatibility complex– genetics and biology. (First of three parts.) N Engl J Med 295:806-813, 1976.

47. Terasaki PI: Overview. In Terasaki PI, Cecka M (eds): Clinical Transplantation. Los Angeles, UCLA Tissue Typing Laboratory, 1987, p 467.

48. Schreuder GM, Hendriks GF, D'Amaro J, Persijn GG: An eight-year study of HLA typing proficiency in Eurotransplant. Tissue Antigens 27:131-141, 1986.

49. Cecka JM, Terasaki PI: Clinical Transplantation 2001. Los Angeles, UCLA Tissue Typing Laboratory, 2002.

50. Opelz G, Wujciak T, Dohler B, et al: HLA compatibility and organ transplant survival. Collaborative Transplant Study. Rev Immunogenet 1:334-342, 1999.

51. Opelz G, Mytilineos J, Wujciak T, et al: Current status of HLA matching in renal transplantation. The Collaborative Transplant Study. Clin Invest 70:767, 1993.

52. Morris PJ, Johnson RJ, Fuggle SV, et al: Analysis of factors that affect outcome of primary cadaveric renal transplantation in the UK. HLA Task Force of the Kidney Advisory Group of the United Kingdom Transplant Support Service Authority (UKTSSA). Lancet 354(9185):1147-1152, 1999.

53. Takemoto SK, Terasaki PI, Gjertson DW, Cecka JM: Twelve years' experience with national sharing of HLA-matched cadaveric kidneys for transplantation. N Engl J Med 343:1078-1084, 2000.

54. Zantvoort FA, D'Amaro J, Persijn GG, et al: The impact of HLA-A matching on long-term survival of renal allografts. Transplantation 61:841-844, 1996.

55. Hariharan S, Johnson CP, Bresnahan BA, et al: Improved graft survival after renal transplantation in the United States, 1988 to 1996. N Engl J Med 342:605-612, 2000.

56. Takemoto S, Terasaki PI, Gjertson DW, Cecka JM: Equitable allocation of HLA-compatible kidneys for local pools and minorities. N Engl J Med 331:760-764, 1994.

57. Takemoto SK, Terasaki PI: Evaluation of the transplant recipient and donor: Molecular approach to tissue typing, flow cytometry and alternative approaches to distributing organs. Curr Opin Nephrol Hypertens 6:299-303, 1997.

58. Takemoto S: HLA amino acid residue matching. In Cecka JM, Terasaki PI (eds): Clinical Transplants 1997. Los Angeles, UCLA Tissue Typing Laboratory, 1997, p 397-424.

59. Vereerstraeten P, Dupont E, Andrien M, et al: Influence of donor-recipient HLA-DR mismatches and OKT3 prophylaxis on cadaver kidney graft survival. Transplantation 60:253-258, 1995.

60. Doxiadis II, Smits JM, Schreuder GM, et al: Association between specific HLA combinations and probability of kidney allograft loss: The taboo concept. Lancet 348(9031):850-853, 1996.

61. Takemoto S, Terasaki PI: Refinement of permissible HLA mismatches. In Cecka JM, Terasaki PI (eds): Clinical Transplants 1994. Los Angeles, UCLA Tissue Typing Laboratory, 1995, p 397-424.

62. Yard BA, Claas FH, Paape ME, et al: Recognition of a tissue-specific polymorphism by graft infiltrating T-cell clones isolated from a renal allograft with acute rejection. Nephrol Dial Transplant 9:805-810, 1994.

63. Yard BA, Kooymans-Couthino M, Reterink T, et al: Analysis of T cell lines from rejecting renal allografts. Kidney Int Suppl 39:S133-S138, 1993.

64. Roopenian DC, Christianson GJ, Davis AP, et al: The genetic origin of minor histocompatibility antigens. Immunogenetics 38:131-140, 1993.

65. Garovoy MR, Franco V, Zschaeck D, et al: Direct lymphocyte-mediated cytotoxicity as an assay of presensitisation. Lancet 1(7803):573-576, 1973.

66. Goulmy E, Termijtelen A, Bradley BA, van Rood JJ: Alloimmunity to human H-Y. Lancet 2(7996):1206, 1976.

67. Pfeffer PF, Thorsby E: HLA-restricted cytotoxicity against male-specific (H-Y) antigen after acute rejection of an HLA-identical sibling kidney: Clonal distribution of the cytotoxic cells. Transplantation 33:52-56, 1982.

68. Perrey C, Brenchley PE, Johnson RW, Martin S: An association between antibodies specific for endothelial cells and renal transplant failure. Transpl Immunol 6:101-106, 1998.

69. Lucchiari N, Panajotopoulos N, Xu C, et al: Antibodies eluted from acutely rejected renal allografts bind to and activate human endothelial cells. Hum Immunol 61:518-527, 2000.

70. Opelz G, Terasaki PI: Improvement of kidney-graft survival with increased numbers of blood transfusions. N Engl J Med 299:799-803, 1978.

71. Briscoe DM, Sayegh MH: A rendezvous before rejection: Where do T cells meet transplant antigens? Nat Med 8:220-222, 2002.

72. Lakkis FG, Arakelov A, Konieczny BT, Inoue Y: Immunologic "ignorance" of vascularized organ transplants in the absence of secondary lymphoid tissue. Nat Med 6:686-688, 2000.

73. Bach FH, Graupner K, Dan E, Klostermann H: Cell kinetic studies in mixed leukocyte cultures: An in vitro model of homograft reactivity. Proc Natl Acad Sci U S A 62:374, 1969.

74. Sherman LA, Chattopadhyay S: The molecular basis of allorecognition. Annu Rev Immunol 11:385-402, 1993.

75. Lechler RI, Lombardi G, Batchelor JR, et al: The molecular basis of alloreactivity. Immunol Today 11:83-88, 1990.

76. Lechler R, Batchelor R, Lombardi G: The relationship between MHC restricted and allospecific T cell recognition. Immunol Lett 29(1-2):41-50, 1991.

77. Eckels DD: Alloreactivity: Allogeneic presentation of endogenous peptide or direct recognition of MHC polymorphism? A review. Tissue Antigens 35:49-55, 1990.

78. Jerne NK: The somatic generation of immune recognition. Eur J Immunol 1(1), 1971.

79. von Boehmer H, Haas W, Jerne NK: Major histocompatibility complex–linked immune responsiveness is acquired by lymphocytes of low-responder mice differentiating in thymus of high-responder mice. Proc Natl Acad Sci U S A 75:2439-2442, 1978.

80. Srendni B, Schwartz RH: Alloreactivity of an antigen-specific T cell clone. Nature 287:855, 1980.

81. Braciale TJ, Andrew ME, Braciale VL: Simultaneous expression of H-2-restricted and alloreactive recognition by a cloned line of influenza virus-specific cytotoxic T lymphocytes. J Exp Med 153:1371-1376, 1981.

82. Finberg R, Burakoff SJ, Cantor H, Benacerraf B: Biological significance of alloreactivity: T cells stimulated by Sendai virus-coated

syngeneic cells specifically lyse allogeneic target cells. Proc Natl Acad Sci U S A 75:5145-5149, 1978.

83. Matis LA, Sorger SB, McElligott DL, et al: The molecular basis of alloreactivity in antigen-specific, major histocompatibility complex-restricted T cell clones. Cell 51:59-69, 1987.

84. Sayegh MH, Turka LA: The role of T-cell costimulatory activation pathways in transplant rejection. N Engl J Med 338:1813-1821, 1998.

85. Sayegh MH: Why do we reject a graft? Role of indirect allorecognition in graft rejection. Kidney Int 56:1967-1979, 1999.

86. Auchincloss H Jr, Lee R, Shea S, et al: The role of "indirect" recognition in initiating rejection of skin grafts from major histocompatibility complex class II–deficient mice. Proc Natl Acad Sci U S A 90:3373-3377, 1993.

87. Rogers NJ, Lechler RI: Allorecognition. Am J Transplant 1:97-102, 2001.

88. Vella JP, Spadafora-Ferreira M, Murphy B, et al: Indirect allorecognition of major histocompatibility complex allopeptides in human renal transplant recipients with chronic graft dysfunction. Transplantation 64:795-800, 1997.

89. Ciubotariu R, Liu Z, Colovai AI, et al: Persistent allopeptide reactivity and epitope spreading in chronic rejection of organ allografts. J Clin Invest 101:398-405, 1998.

90. SivaSai KS, Smith MA, Poindexter NJ, et al: Indirect recognition of donor HLA class I peptides in lung transplant recipients with bronchiolitis obliterans syndrome. Transplantation 67:1094-1098, 1999.

91. Lechler RI, Heaton T, Barber L, et al: Molecular mimicry by major histocompatibility complex molecules and peptides accounts for some alloresponses. Immunol Lett 34:63-69, 1992.

92. Heath WR, Hurd ME, Carbone FR, Sherman LA: Peptide-dependent recognition of H-2Kb by alloreactive cytotoxic T lymphocytes. Nature 341(6244):749-752, 1989.

93. Heath WR, Kane KP, Mescher MF, Sherman LA: Alloreactive T cells discriminate among a diverse set of endogenous peptides. Proc Natl Acad Sci U S A 88:5101-5105, 1991.

94. Elliott TJ, Eisen HN: Cytotoxic T lymphocytes recognize a reconstituted class I histocompatibility antigen (HLA-A2) as an allogeneic target molecule. Proc Natl Acad Sci U S A 87:5213-5217, 1990.

95. Ohlen C, Bastin J, Ljunggren HG, et al: Resistance to H-2–restricted but not to allo-H2–specific graft and cytotoxic T lymphocyte responses in lymphoma mutant. J Immunol 145:52-58, 1990.

96. Cotner T, Mellins E, Johnson AH, Pious D: Mutations affecting antigen processing impair class II–restricted allorecognition. J Immunol 146:414-417, 1991.

97. Bluestone JA, Kaliyaperumal A, Jameson S, et al: Peptide-induced changes in class I heavy chains alter allorecognition. J Immunol 151:3943-3953, 1993.

98. Magee CC, Sayegh MH: Peptide-mediated immunosuppression. Curr Opin Immunol 9:669-675, 1997.

99. Suciu-Foca N, Reed E, D'Agati VD, et al: Soluble HLA antigens, anti-HLA antibodies, and anti-idiotypic antibodies in the circulation of renal transplant recipients. Transplantation 51:593-601, 1991.

100. Krensky AM, Weiss A, Crabtree G, et al: T-lymphocyte–antigen interactions in transplant rejection. N Engl J Med 322:510-517, 1990.

101. Kearney ER, Walunas TL, Karr RW, et al: Antigen-dependent clonal expansion of a trace population of antigen-specific CD4+ T cells in vivo is dependent on CD28 costimulation and inhibited by CTLA-4. J Immunol 155:1032-1036, 1995.

102. Clevers H, Alarcon B, Wileman T, Terhorst C: The T cell receptor/CD3 complex: A dynamic protein ensemble. Annu Rev Immunol 6:629-662, 1988.

103. Caillat-Zucman S, Blumenfeld N, Legendre C, et al: The OKT3 immunosuppressive effect. In situ antigenic modulation of human graft-infiltrating T cells. Transplantation 49:156-160, 1990.

104. Gaston RS, Deierhoi MH, Patterson T, et al: OKT3 first-dose reaction: Association with T cell subsets and cytokine release. Kidney Int 39:141-148, 1991.

105. Shaw AS, Amrein KE, Hammond C, et al: The lck tyrosine protein kinase interacts with the cytoplasmic tail of the CD4 glycoprotein through its unique amino-terminal domain. Cell 59:627-636, 1989.

106. Denton MD, Magee CC, Sayegh MH: Immunosuppressive strategies in transplantation. Lancet 353(9158):1083-1091, 1999.

107. Haug CE, Colvin RB, Delmonico FL, et al: A phase I trial of immunosuppression with anti-ICAM-1 (CD54) mAb in renal

allograft recipients. Transplantation 55:766-772, 1993; discussion 772-773.

108. Hourmant M, Bedrossian J, Durand D, et al: A randomized multicenter trial comparing leukocyte function–associated antigen-1 monoclonal antibody with rabbit antithymocyte globulin as induction treatment in first kidney transplantations. Transplantation 62:1565-1570, 1996.

109. Bretscher P, Cohn M: A theory of self-nonself discrimination. Science 169(950):1042-1049, 1970.

110. Linsley PS, Greene JL, Tan P, et al: Coexpression and functional cooperation of CTLA-4 and CD28 on activated T lymphocytes. J Exp Med 176:1595-1604, 1992.

111. Bluestone JA: Is CTLA-4 a master switch for peripheral T cell tolerance? J Immunol 158:1989-1993, 1997.

112. Tivol EA, Borriello F, Schweitzer AN, et al: Loss of CTLA-4 leads to massive lymphoproliferation and fatal multiorgan tissue destruction, revealing a critical negative regulatory role of CTLA-4. Immunity 3:541-547, 1995.

113. Judge TA, Tang A, Spain LM, et al: The in vivo mechanism of action of CTLA4-Ig. J Immunol 156:2294-2299, 1996.

114. Schwartz RH: A cell culture model for T lymphocyte clonal anergy. Science 248(4961):1349-1356, 1990.

115. Perkins DL, Wang Y, Ho SS, et al: Superantigen-induced peripheral tolerance inhibits T cell responses to immunogenic peptides in TCR (beta-chain) transgenic mice. J Immunol 150:4284-4291, 1993.

116. Rocken M, Urban JF, Shevach EM: Infection breaks T-cell tolerance. Nature 359(6390):79-82, 1992.

117. Chen W, Sayegh MH, Khoury SJ: Mechanisms of acquired thymic tolerance in vivo: Intrathymic injection of antigen induces apoptosis of thymocytes and peripheral T cell anergy. J Immunol 160:1504-1508, 1998.

118. Kirk AD, Harlan DM, Armstrong NN, et al: CTLA4-Ig and anti-CD40 ligand prevent renal allograft rejection in primates. Proc Natl Acad Sci U S A 94:8789-8794, 1997.

119. Levisetti MG, Padrid PA, Szot GL, et al: Immunosuppressive effects of human CTLA4-Ig in a nonhuman primate model of allogeneic pancreatic islet transplantation. J Immunol 159:5187-5191, 1997.

120. Yamada A, Kishimoto K, Dong VM, et al: CD28-independent costimulation of T cells in alloimmune responses. J Immunol 167:140-146, 2001.

121. Sharpe AH, Freeman GJ: The B7-CD28 superfamily. Nat Rev Immunol 2:116-126, 2002.

122. Yoshinaga SK, Whoriskey JS, Khare SD, et al: T-cell co-stimulation through B7RP-1 and ICOS. Nature 402(6763):827-832, 1999.

123. Carreno BM, Collins M: The B7 family of ligands and its receptors: New pathways for costimulation and inhibition of immune responses. Annu Rev Immunol 20:29-53, 2002.

124. Yamada A, Salama AD, Sayegh MH: The role of novel T cell costimulatory pathways in autoimmunity and transplantation. J Am Soc Nephrol 13:559-575, 2002.

125. McAdam AJ, Greenwald RJ, Levin MA, et al: ICOS is critical for CD40-mediated antibody class switching. Nature 409(6816):102-105, 2001.

126. Mosmann TR, Cherwinski H, Bond MW, et al: Two types of murine helper T cell clone. I. Definition according to profiles of lymphokine activities and secreted proteins. J Immunol 136:2348-2357, 1986.

127. Hancock WW, Gao W, Faia KL, Csizmadia V: Chemokines and their receptors in allograft rejection. Curr Opin Immunol 12:511-516, 2000.

128. Nelson PJ, Krensky AM: Chemokines, lymphocytes and viruses: What goes around, comes around. Curr Opin Immunol 10:265-270, 1998.

129. Fischereder M, Luckow B, Hocher B, et al: CC chemokine receptor 5 and renal-transplant survival. Lancet 357(9270):1758-1761, 2001.

130. Sayegh MH, Akalin E, Hancock WW, et al: CD28-B7 blockade after alloantigenic challenge in vivo inhibits Th1 cytokines but spares Th2. J Exp Med 181:1869-1874, 1995.

131. Nashan B, Moore R, Amlot P, et al: Randomised trial of basiliximab versus placebo for control of acute cellular rejection in renal allograft recipients. CHIB 201 International Study Group. Lancet 350(9086):1193-1198, 1997.

132. Vincenti F, Kirkman R, Light S, et al: Interleukin-2–receptor blockade with daclizumab to prevent acute rejection in renal transplantation. Daclizumab Triple Therapy Study Group. N Engl J Med 338:161-165, 1998.

133. Steiger J, Nickerson PW, Steurer W, et al: IL-2 knockout recipient mice reject islet cell allografts. J Immunol 155:489-498, 1995.

134. Lakkis FG, Konieczny BT, Saleem S, et al: Blocking the CD28-B7 T cell costimulation pathway induces long term cardiac allograft acceptance in the absence of IL-4. J Immunol 158:2443-2448, 1997.

135. Konieczny BT, Dai Z, Elwood ET, et al: IFN-gamma is critical for long-term allograft survival induced by blocking the CD28 and CD40 ligand T cell costimulation pathways. J Immunol 160:2059-2064, 1998.

136. Dai Z, Konieczny BT, Baddoura FK, Lakkis FG: Impaired alloantigen-mediated T cell apoptosis and failure to induce long-term allograft survival in IL-2-deficient mice. J Immunol 161:1659-1663, 1998.

137. Waaga AM, Gasser M, Kist-van Holthe JE, et al: Regulatory functions of self-restricted MHC class II allopeptide-specific Th2 clones in vivo. J Clin Invest 107:909-916, 2001.

138. Kist-van Holthe JE, Gasser M, Womer K, et al: Regulatory functions of alloreactive Th2 clones in human renal transplant recipients. Kidney Int 62:627-631, 2002.

139. Li B, Hartono C, Ding R, et al: Noninvasive diagnosis of renal-allograft rejection by measurement of messenger RNA for perforin and granzyme B in urine. N Engl J Med 344:947-954, 2001.

140. Strehlau J, Pavlakis M, Lipman M, et al: Quantitative detection of immune activation transcripts as a diagnostic tool in kidney transplantation. Proc Natl Acad Sci U S A 94:695-700, 1997.

141. Krieger NR, Yin DP, Fathman CG: CD4+ but not CD8+ cells are essential for allorejection. J Exp Med 184:2013-2018, 1996.

142. Auchincloss H Jr, Sachs DH: Xenogeneic transplantation. Annu Rev Immunol 16:433-470, 1998.

143. Young NT, Bunce M, Morris PJ, Welsh KI: Killer cell inhibitory receptor interactions with HLA class I molecules: Implications for alloreactivity and transplantation. Hum Immunol 52:1-11, 1997.

144. Lander ES, Linton LM, Birren B, et al: Initial sequencing and analysis of the human genome. Nature 409(6822):860-921, 2001.

145. Akalin E, Hendrix RC, Polavarapu RG, et al: Gene expression analysis in human renal allograft biopsy samples using high-density oligoarray technology. Transplantation 72:948-953, 2001.

146. Christopher K, Mueller TF, Ma C, et al: Analysis of the innate and adaptive phases of allograft rejection by cluster analysis of transcriptional profiles. J Immunol 169:522-530, 2002.

147. Womer KL, Vella JP, Sayegh MH: Chronic allograft dysfunction: Mechanisms and new approaches to therapy. Semin Nephrol 20:126-147, 2000.

148. Halloran PF: Call for revolution: A new approach to describing allograft deterioration. Am J Transplant 2:195-200, 2002.

149. Hume DM, Merrill JP, Miller BF, Thorn GW: Experiences with renal homotransplantation in the human: Report of nine cases. J Clin Invest 34:327-382, 1955.

150. Baker RJ, Hernandez-Fuentes MP, Brookes PA, et al: Loss of direct and maintenance of indirect alloresponses in renal allograft recipients: Implications for the pathogenesis of chronic allograft nephropathy. J Immunol 167:7199-7206, 2001.

151. Mauiyyedi S, Pelle PD, Saidman S, et al: Chronic humoral rejection: Identification of antibody-mediated chronic renal allograft rejection by C4d deposits in peritubular capillaries. J Am Soc Nephrol 12:574-582, 2001.

152. Lee PC, Terasaki PI, Takemoto SK, et al: All chronic rejection failures of kidney transplants were preceded by the development of HLA antibodies. Transplantation 74:1192-1194, 2002.

153. Eddy AA: Molecular basis of renal fibrosis. Pediatr Nephrol 15:290-301, 2000.

154. Inaba K, Granelli-Piperno A, Steinman RM: Dendritic cells induce T lymphocytes to release B cell-stimulating factors by an interleukin 2-dependent mechanism. J Exp Med 158:2040-2057, 1983.

155. Bach JF: The Mode of Action of Immunosuppressive Agents: Thiopurines. Amsterdam, North-Holland Publishing Company, 1985.

156. Sievers TM, Rossi SJ, Ghobrial RM, et al: Mycophenolate mofetil. Pharmacotherapy 17:1178-1197, 1997.

157. van Gelder T, Klupp J, Barten MJ, et al: Comparison of the effects of tacrolimus and cyclosporine on the pharmacokinetics of mycophenolic acid. Ther Drug Monit 23:119-128, 2001.

158. Halloran P, Mathew T, Tomlanovich S, et al: Mycophenolate mofetil in renal allograft recipients: A pooled efficacy analysis of three randomized, double-blind, clinical studies in prevention of rejection. The International Mycophenolate Mofetil Renal Transplant Study Groups. Transplantation 63:39-47, 1997.

159. The Tricontinental Mycophenolate Mofetil Renal Transplantation Study Group: A blinded, randomized clinical trial of mycophenolate mofetil for the prevention of acute rejection in cadaveric renal transplantation. Transplantation 61:1029-1037, 1996.

160. Azuma H, Binder J, Heemann U, et al: Effects of RS61443 on functional and morphological changes in chronically rejecting rat kidney allografts. Transplantation 59:460-466, 1995.

161. Kronke M, Leonard WJ, Depper JM, et al: Cyclosporin A inhibits T-cell growth factor gene expression at the level of mRNA transcription. Proc Natl Acad Sci U S A 81:5214-5218, 1984.

162. Nickerson PW, Steurer W, Steiger J, Strom TB: In pursuit of the "holy grail": Allograft tolerance. Kidney Int Suppl 44:S40-S49, 1994.

163. Wood KJ: Transplantation tolerance. Curr Opin Immunol 3:710-714, 1991.

164. Emmel EA, Verweij CL, Durand DB, et al: Cyclosporin A specifically inhibits function of nuclear proteins involved in T cell activation. Science 246(4937):1617-1620, 1989.

165. Dumont FJ, Staruch MJ, Koprak SL, et al: Distinct mechanisms of suppression of murine T cell activation by the related macrolides FK-506 and rapamycin. J Immunol 144:251-258, 1990.

166. Schreiber SL, Crabtree GR: The mechanism of action of cyclosporin A and FK506. Immunol Today 13:136-142, 1992.

167. Liu J, Farmer JD Jr, Lane WS, et al: Calcineurin is a common target of cyclophilin-cyclosporin A and FKBP-FK506 complexes. Cell 66:807-815, 1991.

168. Jain J, McCaffrey PG, Valge-Archer VE, Rao A: Nuclear factor of activated T cells contains Fos and Jun. Nature 356(6372):801-804, 1992.

169. Bierer BE, Mattila PS, Standaert RF, et al: Two distinct signal transmission pathways in T lymphocytes are inhibited by complexes formed between an immunophilin and either FK506 or rapamycin. Proc Natl Acad Sci U S A 87:9231-9235, 1990.

170. Tocci MJ, Matkovich DA, Collier KA, et al: The immunosuppressant FK506 selectively inhibits expression of early T cell activation genes. J Immunol 143:718-726, 1989.

171. Clipstone NA, Crabtree GR: Identification of calcineurin as a key signalling enzyme in T-lymphocyte activation. Nature 357(6380):695-697, 1992.

172. Bierer BE, Schreiber SL, Burakoff SJ: The effect of the immunosuppressant FK-506 on alternate pathways of T cell activation. Eur J Immunol 21:439-445, 1991.

173. Kuo CJ, Chung J, Fiorentino DF, et al: Rapamycin selectively inhibits interleukin-2 activation of p70 S6 kinase. Nature 358(6381):70-73, 1992.

174. Calvo V, Crews CM, Vik TA, Bierer BE: Interleukin 2 stimulation of p70 S6 kinase activity is inhibited by the immunosuppressant rapamycin. Proc Natl Acad Sci U S A 89:7571-7575, 1992.

175. Morice WG, Wiederrecht G, Brunn GJ, et al: Rapamycin inhibition of interleukin-2-dependent p33cdk2 and p34cdc2 kinase activation in T lymphocytes. J Biol Chem 268:22737-22745, 1993.

176. MacDonald AS: A worldwide, phase III, randomized, controlled safety and efficacy study of a sirolimus/cyclosporine regimen for prevention of acute rejection in recipients of primary mismatched renal allografts. Transplantation 71:271-280, 2001.

177. Burdick JF: The biology of immunosuppression mediated by anti-lymphocyte antibodies. In Williams GM, Burdick JF, Solez K (eds): Kidney Transplant Rejection: Diagnosis and Treatment. New York, Marcel Dekker, 1986.

178. Norman DJ, Kahana L, Stuart FP Jr, et al: A randomized clinical trial of induction therapy with OKT3 in kidney transplantation. Transplantation 55:44-50, 1993.

179. Chatenoud L, Baudrihaye MF, Kreis H, et al: Human in vivo antigenic modulation induced by the anti–T cell OKT3 monoclonal antibody. Eur J Immunol 12:979-982, 1982.

180. Suthanthiran M: Transplantation tolerance: Fooling mother nature. Proc Natl Acad Sci U S A 93:12072-12075, 1996.

181. Charlton B, Auchincloss H Jr, Fathman CG: Mechanisms of transplantation tolerance. Annu Rev Immunol 12:707-734, 1994.

182. Billingham RE, Brent L, Medawar PB: Actively acquired tolerance to foreign cells, twin diagnosis and the Freemartin condition in cattle. Nature 172(603-606):33-39, 1953.

183. Field E, Gao Q, Chen NX, Rouse T: Balancing the immune system for tolerance: A case for regulatory CD4 cell. Transplantation 63:1-7, 1997.

184. Ildstad ST, Sachs DH: Reconstitution with syngeneic plus allogeneic or xenogeneic bone marrow leads to specific acceptance of allografts or xenografts. Nature 307(5947):168-170, 1984.

185. Starzl TE, Demetris AJ, Murase N, et al: Donor cell chimerism permitted by immunosuppressive drugs: A new view of organ transplantation. Immunol Today 14:326-332, 1993.

186. Fraser CC, Sykes M, Lee RS, et al: Specific unresponsiveness to a retrovirally-transferred class I antigen is controlled through the helper pathway. J Immunol 154:1587-1595, 1995.

187. Wekerle T, Sayegh MH, Hill J, et al: Extrathymic T cell deletion and allogeneic stem cell engraftment induced with costimulatory blockade is followed by central T cell tolerance. J Exp Med 187:2037-2044, 1998.

188. Sayegh MH, Carpenter CB: Tolerance and chronic rejection. Kidney Int Suppl 58:S11-S14, 1997.

189. Nickerson P, Steiger J, Zheng XX, et al: Manipulation of cytokine networks in transplantation: False hope or realistic opportunity for tolerance? Transplantation 63:489-494, 1997.

190. Piccotti JR, Chan SY, Van Buskirk AM, et al: Are Th2 helper T lymphocytes beneficial, deleterious, or irrelevant in promoting allograft survival? Transplantation 63:619-624, 1997.

191. Van Parijs L, Abbas AK: Homeostasis and self-tolerance in the immune system: Turning lymphocytes off. Science 280(5361):243-248, 1998.

192. Cascalho M, Platt JL: Xenotransplantation and other means of organ replacement. Nat Rev Immunol 1:154-160, 2001.

193. Leventhal JR, Matas AJ, Sun LH, et al: The immunopathology of cardiac xenograft rejection in the guinea pig-to-rat model. Transplantation 56:1-8, 1993.

194. Zaidi A, Schmoeckel M, Bhatti F, et al: Life-supporting pig-to-primate renal xenotransplantation using genetically modified donors. Transplantation 65:1584-1590, 1998.

195. Lin SS, Hanaway MJ, Gonzalez-Stawinski GV, et al: The role of anti-Galalpha1-3Gal antibodies in acute vascular rejection and accommodation of xenografts. Transplantation 70:1667-1674, 2000.

196. Hammerman MR: Growing kidneys. Curr Opin Nephrol Hypertens 10:13-17, 2001.

197. Hammerman MR: Xenotransplantation of developing kidneys. Am J Physiol Renal Physiol 283:F601-F606, 2002.

198. Menasche P, Hagege AA, Scorsin M, et al: Myoblast transplantation for heart failure. Lancet 357(9252):279-280, 2001.

199. Grimm PC, Nickerson P, Jeffery J, et al: Neointimal and tubulointerstitial infiltration by recipient mesenchymal cells in chronic renal allograft rejection. N Engl J Med 345:93-97, 2001.

CHAPTER 64

Donor and Recipient Issues in Renal Transplantation

Dianne B. McKay and Andrew J. King

ABSOLUTE CONTRAINDICATIONS TO TRANSPLANTATION

MEDICAL ISSUES THAT AFFECT CONSIDERATION FOR TRANSPLANTATION
Advanced Age
Obesity
Prior Kidney Transplant
Psychosocial Issues
Cardiovascular Diseases

Diabetes Mellitus
Infectious Diseases
Malignancy
Pulmonary Diseases
Gastrointestinal Diseases
Skeletal Diseases
Genitourinary Diseases
Evaluation of Renal Diseases with Potential for Recurrence in the Allograft

Intrinsic Renal Diseases
DONOR ISSUES
The Cadaver Organ Shortage
Cadaver Donor Procurement and Allocation
Live Donor
MATCHING POTENTIAL CANDIDATES TO DONORS

Transplant recipients and their donors must be thoroughly evaluated before transplantation. The purpose of the evaluation is to identify medical, surgical, and psychosocial issues that might adversely influence survival of the patient and graft. There is a profound shortage of donor organs, and careful pretransplantation management is needed to ensure optimal usage of this scarce resource. In all cases the potential benefits of transplantation must be weighed against immediate risks associated with the surgical procedure and the short- and long-term risks of immunosuppressive therapy.

The process of evaluating a patient's eligibility for transplantation incorporates experts from several disciplines. Ideally, the evaluation team includes transplant nephrologists, surgeons, transplant coordinators, social workers, and tissue typing experts who jointly make recommendations about the suitability of the recipient and donor. To prevent undue influence of the recipient's physician, many transplant centers mandate that a donor physician independently evaluate the live donor. During the evaluation there may be ethical or subjective issues that require consensus opinions of all the professionals involved. Because the evaluation process may involve complex ethical as well as medical issues, many transplant centers conduct a regular meeting of the transplant experts in order to agree upon the candidacy of all potential recipients.

Transplantation clearly improves the quality of life compared with other modalities of renal replacement therapy[1] and confers a survival benefit.[2] In an analysis of 46,164 patients who were listed for cadaveric renal transplantation, the patients who ultimately underwent transplantation had a lower mortality rate (48% to 82% lower) than patients who did not receive a transplant.[2] The survival benefit was most notable in patients who were younger (20 to 39 years old) and diabetic.[2]

This chapter reviews current guidelines for evaluating the eligibility of potential renal transplant candidates and their donors. These guidelines represent published views of transplant experts throughout the United States and are in agreement with clinical practice guidelines of the American Society of Transplantation.[3] As new immunosuppressive strategies and improvements in post-transplantation care of patients develop, the donor and recipient eligibility guidelines are likely to change.

ABSOLUTE CONTRAINDICATIONS TO TRANSPLANTATION

When evaluating the medical, surgical, and psychological conditions of a patient with end-stage renal disease (ESRD), there are several absolute contraindications to transplantation (Table 64-1). These include a short life expectancy (<1 year), untreatable malignancy that will lead to the patient's death, untreated acute or chronic infections, uncontrolled psychiatric disorders, active substance abuse, demonstrated recurrent noncompliance with medications, ABO blood group mismatch, and a positive crossmatch. Although the American Society of Transplantation[3] has published a list of absolute contraindications, some of the contraindications may be

TABLE 64-1

Exclusionary Conditions for Renal Transplantation

Patient will not live more than 1 year (even with a transplant)
Metastatic malignancy, not responsive to therapy
Acute or chronic infections that are not controlled
Severe psychiatric disease that impairs patient's consent and compliance
Recurrent and persistent noncompliance with medications
Substance abuse (includes tobacco abuse at some transplant centers)
Immunologic incompatibilities (ABP blood group mismatch and positive crossmatch)

modified by individual patients' circumstances. A patient with no dialysis access is an example of such an exception. Such a patient would die without renal replacement therapy and therefore may be accepted for transplantation despite problems that would otherwise be considered contraindications.

MEDICAL ISSUES THAT AFFECT CONSIDERATION FOR TRANSPLANTATION

Advanced Age

Advanced age itself is no longer a contraindication to renal transplantation. In fact, the ESRD population is approaching a majority of older patients. ESRD patients older than 65 years represented 49% of patients receiving dialysis in 1999.[4] This is reflected in a rise in older transplant recipients—in the year 2000, 46% of transplant recipients were older than 50[5] and 10.7% were older than 64.[6] Because the pool of potential transplant recipients is aging, most transplant centers now evaluate candidacy on the basis of the likelihood for excellent immediate and long-term outcome rather than the patient's chronologic age.

As the recipient population ages, unique immunologic features associated with aging need to be considered. Older patients more often lose their grafts because of death rather than acute or chronic rejection.[5] With age, the immune system appears to develop several deficiencies that lead to diminished alloresponsiveness.[7, 8] Immunologic alterations associated with immunosenescence may also explain the higher occurrence of infections and tumors with aging.[9, 10] Many transplant centers now advocate the use of lower doses of immunosuppressive medications in elderly patients.[5, 10] Other nonimmunologic explanations for superior graft survival in older patients exist, including better compliance with immunosuppressive medications and a selection bias in the choice of healthier older transplant candidates. Therefore, the lower risk of rejection in older patients may not be entirely associated with immunologic factors.

The pretransplantation history and physical examination of older patients with renal disease should be focused on uncovering naturally occurring age-related changes in extrarenal organ systems. Cardiac disease is the most frequent cause of morbidity in elderly transplant recipients,[11] and therefore thorough cardiovascular evaluation is needed in all older patients. Atherosclerotic disease may predispose to technical vascular anastomotic problems, and the peripheral vasculature should also be carefully screened before transplantation. Attention must also be paid to other common medical issues associated with the process of aging, such as increased rates of malignancy, and therefore screening for occult neoplasms is also mandated in this population of patients.

A reasonable approach to the older transplant candidate is to request screening examinations such as exercise stress thallium or dipyridamole thallium screening, stool for occult blood, or flexible sigmoidoscopies or barium enemas, or both, in all patients older than 50.[3] All men older than 50 should also have voiding cystourethrograms to be sure there is no evidence for urethral restriction. Attention to breast imaging and gynecologic examinations is mandated in all older women.

Obesity

The risk of postoperative complications and mortality after surgery may be increased in obese renal transplant recipients.[12] A retrospective analysis of 51,927 primary adult renal transplant recipients with an elevated body mass index (BMI) (>36 kg/m^2) suggested that an elevated BMI was significantly associated with worse graft survival independent of patients' survival.[13] Other studies have also shown that patients with a BMI greater than 30 kg/m^2 have a particularly bad outcome.[12, 14] There is some controversy regarding the impact of obesity in transplantation. In one large retrospective study at a single transplant center, there was no difference in outcomes related to BMI.[15] Yet another study of paired cadaver kidneys found that obesity was not a risk factor for delayed graft function, acute rejection, or 1-year graft survival, but it did affect medium- and long-term graft survival and reached statistical significance at 5 years.[16] The obese patient should be encouraged to achieve ideal body weight before transplantation. This often requires the assistance of a weight loss specialist.

Prior Kidney Transplant

Patients who have previously had a kidney transplant can safely undergo retransplantation. The pretransplantation evaluation for a second or even third allograft mandates careful attention to the reason the prior allograft failed. It is important to attend to any issues such as noncompliance with immunosuppressive medications, loss of the graft in association with recurrent renal disease, or high panel-reactive antibody (PRA) titers as well as any correctable factor that played a role in the loss of the previous graft. There is no difference in 1- to 3-year allograft survival between retransplant recipients and recipients of first transplants.[6] If recurrent renal disease is excluded from the analysis, there may be no difference even at 5 years.[17] Better long-term graft survival rates can be achieved by selecting for transplantation patients with low risk characteristics, such as first graft survival rates of greater than 3 months or negative flow cytometric crossmatches.[5] Patients who have been treated with immunosuppressive medications for a previous transplant may manifest infectious or malignant complications reflective of their prior immunosuppressive therapy. Therefore, aggressive pretransplantation screening is necessary before consideration of a second or third transplant.

Psychosocial Issues

The pretransplantation psychosocial evaluation should be conducted with the assistance of the transplant social worker and may require a formal psychiatric evaluation. The evaluation should be directed to assess the patient's ability to provide informed consent and to adhere to the post-transplantation immunosuppressive regimen.[3] It is also important to assess the potential for interactions of immunosuppressive medications with the patient's psychiatric medications.

Many studies have tried to identify characteristics of noncompliant patients, as noncompliance is a primary cause of allograft loss. Although a distinct profile of a noncompliant patient has not been made, high risk factors include low socioeconomic status and certain psychosocial profiles such as a history of substance abuse and history of noncompliance with dialysis treatments.[3, 18, 19] Therefore, the pretransplantation evaluation not only includes estimation of the risk of noncompliance but also assesses the patient's social supports. Because of the shortage of donor organs, it has been the policy at many transplant centers to approve patients with a history of substance abuse (including tobacco) or noncompliance only after a period of demonstrated compliance and avoidance of substance abuse.[3]

Cardiovascular Diseases

Cardiovascular disease is the most prevalent comorbid condition in patients with ESRD.[10, 11, 20-24] In fact, the National Kidney Foundation Task Force on Cardiovascular Disease has described cardiovascular disease as "epidemic" in the ESRD population.[11] The pretransplantation assessment for significant coronary artery disease should therefore be aggressively conducted in all candidates for renal transplantation. The ideal evaluation should be conducted by a cardiologist who has been designated to work with the transplant team.

Several traditional risk factors for atherosclerosis factor into the high incidence of cardiovascular disease in patients with ESRD, including hypertension, dyslipidemia, and diabetes mellitus.[11] In addition, there are nontraditional risk factors pertinent to this population such as hyperhomocysteinemia and as yet unidentified factors associated with uremia. The importance of nontraditional risk factors in atherogenesis is highlighted by the high prevalence of vascular pathology in pediatric transplant candidates. In a study of 39 patients (19 to 39 years old) with ESRD onset in childhood, 92% had evidence for coronary artery calcifications.[25] A correlation appears to exist between cumulative duration of ESRD and cumulative serum calcium-phosphate product.[25] Other investigators have suggested that disordered lipid metabolism[26] and hyperhomocysteinemia[27] play a role in the high incidence of coronary disease in the pediatric population, although the total length of ESRD is still considered the most important independent risk factor.[28]

One reason to screen for cardiovascular disease is to identify patients who may be at high cardiovascular risk for surgery. The groups of ESRD patients who appear to be at highest risk for postoperative cardiac complications include older patients (65 to 70 years old), patients with diabetes mellitus, and patients with a history of myocardial infarction or angina pectoris (Table 64-2).[11, 29] These patients should be aggressively screened for evidence of inducible ischemia and myocardial dysfunction. There are several methods of screening, and the best method is often determined by the expertise of the cardiology department at the transplant center.

TABLE 64-2

Characteristics of Patients with End-Stage Renal Disease at High Risk for Cardiovascular Disease*

Age >65
History of diabetes mellitus
History of myocardial infarction or myocardial dysfunction
History of angina pectoris
Long duration of end-stage renal disease

*All high-risk patients should be aggressively screened for inducible ischemia and myocardial dysfunction.

The optimal situation involves cardiovascular screening under the direction of a designated cardiologist who works closely with the transplant service.

Several algorithms have been developed by the American College of Cardiology, the American Heart Association, and the American College of Physicians in order to define cardiovascular risks of major noncardiac surgery.[30-32] Despite guidelines for the general population, there are no studies to date allowing the prediction of cardiovascular risks of renal transplant surgery. Therefore, the American Society of Transplantation has recommended aggressive screening of renal transplant candidates who are at high risk for cardiovascular disease.[3] Because the duration of ESRD also appears to be a factor in the development of cardiovascular pathology, it is probably important to consider duration of ESRD as another risk factor.

Screening for inducible ischemia and left ventricular dysfunction requires at least stress testing and echocardiography. Any patient with significant risk factors, symptoms of cardiac ischemia, or signs of congestive heart failure must undergo initial noninvasive screening for inducible ischemia and left ventricular dysfunction.[10] Many studies have tried to determine which noninvasive testing method (exercise electrocardiography, echocardiography, thallium scintigraphy [with exercise or dipyridamole], magnetic resonance imaging, single photon emission computed tomography, positron emission tomography, electron beam computed tomography) and which clinical risk factors offer the best predictive value for cardiovascular outcome after transplantation.[10, 33] The best method for cardiovascular screening depends on the expertise of the cardiology program at the individual transplant center. Because many patients with ESRD may not be able to complete exercise stress testing, it is important to be sure that the test adequately rules out inducible ischemia. Most high-risk patients eventually require angiography to define the extent of ischemic heart disease and need for revascularization.

If critical coronary lesions are demonstrated, the patient should ideally undergo revascularization before transplantation to avoid nephrotoxic insults.[3, 34] Revascularization, however, may be performed after transplantation with low risk to the patient and graft.[35, 36] Earlier clinical studies suggested that all necessary cardiac surgery should be conducted before transplantation to avoid the increased infection risk following transplantation.[37, 38] There was also thought to be an increased risk of restenosis after percutaneous angioplasty during dialysis, and therefore other investigators recommended delaying elective revascularization procedures to the post-transplantation period.[39, 40] A high rate of restenosis in dialysis patients has not been confirmed in other studies.[36, 37, 41] Although current studies suggest that cardiac surgery is safe after transplantation, the transplant center's experience and the patient's preference should guide the approach to revascularization in the patient with coronary artery disease that has not yet produced critical stenosis.

Potential transplant recipients may wait for years for an available cadaver organ. Therefore, an important part of pretransplantation screening for cardiovascular disease is reevaluation of the cardiac status at regular intervals, especially in patients with diabetes and those with increased risk factors for coronary ischemia. Given the consensus that ESRD promotes atherosclerosis, there should be a low threshold for retesting. Some centers mandate yearly rescreening for all high-risk patients and screening every other year for lower risk patients. Because the status of older patients may change within a short period of time before transplantation, they should be screened at least on a yearly basis.

Other causes of cardiac dysfunction may include amyloidosis, constrictive or restrictive pericarditis, thyroid dysfunction, and valvular heart disease.[3] Therefore, although many patients with ESRD have underlying coronary artery disease, other etiologies for myocardial dysfunction must also be considered in the pretransplantation evaluation of patients with ESRD.

Diabetes Mellitus

More than 17 million people living in the United States have diabetes, making this disease a modern epidemic.[42] The reason for the epidemic is not known, but the prevalence of the disease is increasing. Patients with diabetic nephropathy now represent the majority of ESRD patients needing renal replacement therapy.[43] Diabetics are also the group of patients who are likely to experience the greatest survival benefit from transplantation.[44]

The pretransplantation evaluation of the diabetic patient should include an aggressive search for evidence of atherosclerosis and cardiovascular disease. Atherosclerotic vascular disease results in the death of half of all diabetic transplant recipients by 3 years after transplantation,[45] and patients with type 1 diabetes with significant coronary artery disease have a less than 50% survival rate 2 years after transplantation.[34] Therefore, cardiovascular disease represents the primary barrier to successful post-transplantation outcome in diabetic patients.[34] The high incidence of silent coronary disease[46] and the unreliable nature of dipyridamole thallium and exercise thallium tests[34, 47] have led some transplant centers to mandate pretransplantation coronary angiography, with subsequent revascularization if necessary, in all high-risk patients with diabetes. The American Society of Transplantation has not advocated mandatory angiography in asymptomatic diabetic patients but rather suggests reserving invasive imaging for the symptomatic patient.[3]

A useful screening algorithm was originally developed by Manske and colleagues[48] to identify diabetic patients with low risk characteristics who do not need to undergo catheterization before transplantation. The characteristics that place a patient in the lower risk category include age younger than 45, no history of smoking, no ST-T wave changes on electrocardiography, and duration of diabetes mellitus less than 25 years.[48] Patients with type 1 diabetes older than 45 are viewed as at high risk with or without symptoms and angiography is recommended for these patients.[48]

Diabetic patients are also at high risk for other noncardiac vascular complications such as cerebral vascular accidents, peripheral vascular disease, and amputation. Carotid bruits or symptoms suggesting cerebrovascular disease require evaluation of the degree of carotid stenosis and risk for cerebral ischemia. If peripheral pulses are not palpable, a noninvasive vascular evaluation and referral to a vascular surgeon are required. All active foot ulcers must be healed without evidence of infection before transplantation. If the patient has had limb amputation, a vascular surgery consultation is recommended for a more aggressive evaluation.

Diabetic patients have been reported to have better long-term survival with transplantation than with dialysis, although there is a higher early post-transplantation mortality related to cardiovascular complications.[44] Therefore, many transplant physicians have acknowledged that transplantation may offer a survival advantage for diabetic patients. One caution with this interpretation is that high-risk diabetic patients are not offered transplantation and are therefore not included in the data analysis. Therefore, comparing survival of diabetic patients receiving dialysis and those receiving transplantation may not be valid. The population of diabetic patients requiring renal replacement therapy is growing, however, and many transplant physicians are suggesting that it is prudent to offer diabetic patients transplantation before initiation of dialysis to improve their survival advantage. Furthermore, aggressive management of blood glucose and lipids and use of angiotensin-converting enzyme inhibitors or angiotensin receptor blockers should be the standard of care both before and after transplantation.

Infectious Diseases

It is impossible to screen for all infectious diseases before transplantation. Therefore, the pretransplantation evaluation process focuses on the infectious diseases that have the greatest impact on survival of the patient and graft. Untreated bacterial or fungal infections can be particularly dangerous in the early post-transplantation period because of suppression of host defenses by immunosuppressive medications. Therefore, one important part of the pretransplantation evaluation is to detect and eliminate all active infections before surgery. Careful screening is mandated to detect occult dental abscess, urinary tract infections, or infections of dialysis accesses. The patient should be free of infection for at least 1 month before transplantation.[3] Patients should also receive standard vaccinations before transplantation as prophylaxis for influenza, pneumococcus, and hepatitis B as they are more likely to develop a protective antibody response before initiation of immunosuppressive therapy.[3] Protective antibody titers may decline after transplantation, however, and pretransplantation vaccination may have to be repeated.[49, 50]

Cytomegalovirus

Cytomegalovirus (CMV) infection is a major cause of morbidity after renal transplantation. CMV is a large virus that resides within monocytes and can be transmitted with the donor organ or through blood transfused at the time of transplantation. Because of the high risk for invasive CMV disease, seronegative patients on the waiting list for transplantation should be transfused only with blood that is irradiated to remove all white blood cells.

Screening for CMV antibody is performed before transplantation in all potential transplant recipients. A patient who has evidence of prior CMV exposure on the basis of antibody titer should be informed of the potential for post-transplantation CMV infection, including the possibility of death, graft loss, and significant morbidity.[3]

Immediately before transplantation, all cadaver donors are screened for antibodies to CMV and the screening result is communicated to the organ bank and the transplant physicians.

A living donor is screened upon initial evaluation and, if negative, the screening is repeated immediately before transplantation. If a donor is found to be seropositive, the recipient must be given pharmacologic prophylaxis.[51] Several therapeutic agents are available for prophylaxis for CMV disease, and these are discussed in Chapter 65.

The patients who are at the highest risk for clinically significant CMV disease are seronegative patients who receive a seropositive organ.[52, 53] Therefore, patients without antibody titers to CMV should receive either preemptive CMV immune globulin or ganciclovir.[51] Several large clinical trials have shown that preemptive ganciclovir therapy, acyclovir, valacyclovir, and intravenous CMV immune globulin diminish the occurrence of CMV disease.[54] A short course of intravenous ganciclovir followed by longer oral ganciclovir prophylaxis has also been found to be effective in preventing CMV disease in seronegative patients who are exposed to CMV through the donor organ.[51] Patients should not receive therapy while on the waiting list for transplantation.

Hepatitis Viruses

There are six hepatitis viruses—hepatitis A, B, C, D, E, and G. Of these, only B and C cause significant morbidity after transplantation. Coinfection with hepatitis D and hepatitis B viruses causes rapid progression of liver disease in immunosuppressed patients.[55] Hepatitis B–infected renal transplant patients may fare worse than infected dialysis patients,[56] although the exact risk cannot be determined for any individual patient.[3] Therapy for hepatitis B is limited for renal transplant recipients. Interferon therapy may increase the risk of graft loss,[56] and lamivudine may not be effective against all serotypes or mutations of the virus.[56] Newer nucleoside analogs may change the post-transplantation approach to therapy. The pretransplantation evaluation of patients infected with hepatitis B and clinical trials should clarify the role of the newer approaches.

It is not clear which hepatitis B–infected patients progress to chronic liver disease. Some hepatitis B surface antigen–positive (HBsAg+) transplant recipients manifest chronic liver disease that causes fulminant hepatic failure,[57, 58] whereas others remain asymptomatic carriers.[59, 60] In fact, there is controversy about the rate of hepatic damage and progression to hepatic failure when patients receiving dialysis are compared with transplant recipients.[57, 58] Several features characterize a subset of HBsAg+ patients who have a poorer outcome: (1) serologic evidence of active viral replication (hepatitis B early antibody [HBeAg] or hepatitis B virus DNA),[5] (2) antibodies to hepatitis D[55] or hepatitis C,[61, 62] and (3) persistent transaminitis.[63]

The detection of antibody to HBsAg is not itself a contraindication for transplantation, but it does mandate a careful pretransplantation evaluation for significant liver disease. Significant hepatic disease may occur with only mild transaminitis. Therefore, in order to stratify their risk of progression, a liver biopsy is often performed in HBsAg+ patients with even mildly elevated liver enzymes. The histologic evaluation is important from a prognostic standpoint as patients with chronic active hepatitis experience a higher risk of disease progression, although those with chronic persistent hepatitis appear not to progress.[64] Data to date suggest that all HBsAg+ patients should undergo evaluation for evidence of active liver disease (defined histologically by chronic active hepatitis or serologically by the presence of HBeAb or hepatitis B virus DNA, indicating increased viral load).[3] Evidence of hepatitis D and HCV virus should also be sought, and this information is critical in offering the patient an informed opinion regarding the possibility of progression of liver disease after transplantation. Patients with histologic evidence of chronic active hepatitis should be informed of a high risk for the development of hepatic failure after transplantation. All HBsAg antibody–negative patients should receive antibody prophylaxis before transplantation as they are more likely to have a protective antibody response during dialysis than after transplantation. Additional booster doses may be needed if the patient remains on the waiting list for a lengthy period of time.[3]

Hepatitis C virus (HCV) infection occurs frequently in patients with ESRD.[65] The Centers for Disease Control and Prevention (CDC) have reported an HCV infection prevalence of 8.9% nationwide in hemodialysis patients and a higher rate in other countries (e.g., 80% in Egypt[66]). Among renal transplant recipients, 10% to 41% have already been infected with the virus.[67]

All patients receiving hemodialysis should be considered at high risk for HCV infection because nosocomial transmission of HCV occurs within dialysis units.[68] The CDC has recommended screening patients every 6 months during dialysis.[69] Biyearly HCV screening results should therefore be reported to the transplant center for all renal transplant candidates.[3] After transplantation, the diagnosis of HCV infection can be difficult to make because of depressed antibody production.[70] Therefore, it is critical to make the diagnosis of HCV infection before transplantation.

Although reliable third-generation screening tests have improved detection, a 0.23% false-negative rate of detection has been reported in a study of 2576 hemodialysis patients.[71] If anti-HCV antibody is detected, the patient should also be tested for evidence of active infection (viremia) by polymerase chain reaction (HCV RNA).

Although methods of HCV detection have advanced over the years, the natural history of the disease in dialysis patients remains unclear. The course of HCV extends over years, exceeding the life span of most dialysis patients, and therefore the long-term consequences of HCV infection are impossible to determine. Several studies have suggested that the overall survival of patients with ESRD infected with HCV is improved with renal transplantation.[72] In an evaluation of patients awaiting transplantation with the New England Organ Bank, 287 anti-HCV–positive patients were compared with 286 anti-HCV–negative patients over a 73-month time span.[73] The majority of these patients underwent transplantation (61%). The anti-HCV–positive patients who underwent transplantation had a higher mortality rate initially but appeared to have better long-term survival than the anti-HCV–positive patients who continued dialysis.[73] Liver biopsy reports were not available, and the perception of improved life expectancy may reflect incomplete data rather than reality. Therefore, the natural history of HCV infection in transplant recipients is still not clear, leaving uncertainty with regard to recommendations for transplantation in HCV-infected patients.

A problem with comparing anti-HCV–positive hemodialysis patients and renal transplant patients is that patients with clinically overt liver disease are usually excluded from renal transplant evaluation, leading to underestimation of the consequences of HCV in the transplanted population. It is not known whether therapeutic immunosuppression after renal transplantation may accelerate the course of HCV infection. The other problem is that transplantation may improve the life span of patients and therefore the overall survival advantage of transplantation may outweigh the risks for progressive liver disease, particularly if liver disease is mild initially. Therefore, it is mandatory to inform anti-HCV–positive patients that the long-term effects of immunosuppression on progression of HCV liver disease are not known. Furthermore, there are extrahepatic consequences of HCV infection including the development of de novo HCV-related renal disease, and patients should be informed of this possibility.

Acute infection with HCV may be accompanied by only mild elevations in serum alanine aminotransferase (ALT), and normal ALT levels do not exclude the presence of significant liver disease.[70] Because liver enzymes cannot be used to detect the presence of significant hepatic disease, the pretransplantation evaluation of patients who are anti-HCV virus positive should include a liver biopsy.[3, 70] The severity of liver disease guides the approach to transplantation. Patients with chronic persistent hepatitis or mild active hepatitis may proceed with transplantation under informed consent.[3, 70] Patients with advanced chronic active hepatitis or early cirrhosis may progress to hepatic failure at a faster rate.[70] The presence of bridging fibrosis or frank cirrhosis is considered a contraindication to transplantation because of the risk of progressive liver disease.[70] In patients with decompensated cirrhosis, combined transplantation (orthotopic liver and kidney) may be an option. If patients with more advanced disease proceed with transplantation, it should be with informed consent. Many transplant physicians would discourage transplantation in patients with advanced liver disease.

If patients with HCV undergo transplantation, special considerations are needed regarding the post-transplantation immunosuppressive regimen. Azathioprine has been associated with increased hepatotoxicity in renal transplant recipients with concurrent hepatotropic viral infections. Mycophenolate mofetil was shown to increase significantly plasma HCV RNA levels. It is also known that coinfection with other hepatotropic viruses is associated with poor clinical outcomes and that alcohol use promotes the progression of chronic HCV-induced liver disease.

Mycobacterium

Immunosuppressive medications diminish host responses, increasing the risk for reactivation of latent tuberculosis and disseminated disease. There is an increased prevalence of mycobacterial disease in patients with ESRD (9% of hemodialysis patients have a positive purified protein derivative [PPD] test and 16% have a history of exposure to tuberculosis).[3, 74-76] The evaluation of a potential renal transplant candidate should include a chest radiograph and PPD skin testing if the patient has not had a positive test or bacille Calmette-Guérin vaccine in the past. Controversy exists in transplant centers regarding whether to treat PPD-positive patients with isoniazid before transplantation. Transplant physicians have been reluctant to treat ESRD patients with isoniazid prophylactically because of a greater potential for

hepatotoxicity.[56] Patients with active disease, however, should be treated for at least 6 months before transplantation.[3] Patients with a history of positive PPD or treated active tuberculosis should not be excluded from listing for kidney transplantation and should also receive chemoprophylaxis while awaiting either cadaveric or living donor transplantation.[3]

Human Immunodeficiency Virus and Acquired Immunodeficiency Syndrome

Patients infected with human immunodeficiency virus (HIV) were previously excluded from transplantation because of risks associated with immunosuppression and difficult ethical considerations.[77, 78] Potent antiretroviral therapy (i.e., highly active antiretroviral therapy [HAART]) has significantly prolonged the life of HIV-positive patients, causing transplant physicians to reconsider prior recommendations to avoid transplantation. Patients with HIV may tolerate immunosuppression[79] and may have allograft survival comparable to that of HIV-negative patients.[80, 81] There are advocates who argue that HIV infection is analogous to other chronic illnesses and HIV infection itself should not be a reason to exclude a patient from transplantation.[81]

The American Society of Transplantation has recommended that transplantation in HIV-infected individuals be considered an experimental procedure.[3] If transplantation is to be undertaken, the patient needs to understand the associated risks of morbidity and mortality. The current recommendations for transplantation in HIV patients include that transplantation should be undertaken only in HIV-infected patients who have been shown to be compliant with a HAART regimen and have no evidence for acute or chronic opportunistic infection.[3] Furthermore, the CD4 T cell count must be greater than 300 mm^3 and there must be no detectable viral load.[3] If any detectable viral load develops, the patients are removed from the transplant waiting list until the viral load has become reliably undetectable.

BK Virus

Transplant physicians have become keenly aware of an emerging syndrome of renal dysfunction associated with infection with polyomaviruses. There are three polyomaviruses that appear to infect humans: BK virus, which causes nephropathy; polyoma virus JC, which causes multifocal leukoencephalopathy; and simian virus 40 (SV40), which is thought to infect millions of people worldwide because of SV40-infected polio vaccines.[82] On the basis of serologic evidence, approximately 85% of people in the United States have been exposed to BK virus.[83] Despite a high rate of seropositivity, details regarding infectivity of the virus are not known. In the case of BK virus, several factors appear to predispose to BK nephropathy. These include tissue injury from donor ischemia, rejection, and a high number of human leukocyte antigen (HLA) mismatches.[83] The absence of BK virus nephropathy in most recipients of nonrenal organs suggests that renal injury is a cofactor for the development of disease.[84] Whether extrarenal diseases are promoted by infection with the polyomaviruses is not known at this time, but transplant physicians are concerned about the possibility of post-transplantation malignancies.

Although it is not current practice, in the future it may be considered reasonable to screen patients on the waiting list for evidence of active BK infection and to offer transplantation only to patients with latent infection. A case report suggests that patients who have lost a graft to BK nephropathy may undergo retransplantation if there is no evidence of active virus on screening for viral replication.[85]

Malignancy

Patients with ESRD are at increased risk for malignancy, and the risk increases after transplantation because of interference with immunosurveillance.[86] A retrospective analysis of 831,804 dialysis patients from 1980 to 1994 revealed that patients with ESRD have an increased risk for renal, bladder, thyroid, and other endocrine organ malignancies.[87] The risk for malignancy was associated with chronic infection, relative immunodeficiency, prior treatment with immunosuppressive or cytotoxic drugs, nutritional deficiency, and altered DNA repair.[87] Although widespread cancer screening of all dialysis patients has not been advocated,[88] the ESRD patients who undergo renal transplantation evaluation should be carefully evaluated for occult malignancy. The malignancies that are most common in the ESRD population include cancers of the kidney, bladder, thyroid, and other endocrine organs as well as virally induced cancers. Virus-associated cancers include hepatocellular carcinomas (hepatitis B and C); human papillomavirus–linked cancers of the tongue, cervix, vagina, vulva, and penis; and Epstein-Barr virus–associated lymphomas. The increased risk of cancer in ESRD patients appears to be related not to dialysis modality but rather the state of uremia, although carcinogenic uremic toxins have not been identified.

After transplantation, immunosuppressive therapy increases the risk of de novo malignancies and recurrent cancers because immune surveillance mechanisms are impaired. Therefore, careful pretransplantation screening for occult malignancy is mandatory. Several groups of patients may be considered at high risk for malignancy in the pretransplantation evaluation. These include patients with a prior transplant (or patients previously treated with immunosuppressive medications or cytotoxic agents) and older patients.

The Cincinnati Transplant Tumor Registry (CTTR) has provided an invaluable service by collecting data from all U.S. transplant centers on post-transplantation malignancies. Data from this registry have guided the approach to pretransplantation malignancy screening. The American Society of Transplantation has used data from the CTTR to make suggestions regarding waiting time before transplantation on the basis of type of cancer. In general, a 2- to 3-year waiting period is suggested for most types of cancer. An exception is made for cancers with a high rate of recurrence, for which a longer period of time may be suggested.

General guidelines for waiting times provided by Penn[89] were based on data from the CTTR. The reported risk of tumor recurrences was derived from a large series of transplant recipients. Low recurrence rates (<10%) were found for renal tumors, lymphomas, and testicular, uterine, cervical, and thyroid cancers; intermediate recurrence rates (11% to 25%) were found for carcinomas of the uterine body, Wilms tumors, and carcinomas of the colon, prostate, and breast. High recurrence rates (26% or higher) occurred with carcinomas of the

TABLE 64-3

Prediction of Risk of Recurrent Malignancy*

LOW RISK	INTERMEDIATE RISK	HIGH RISK
Encapsulated renal cancer	Carcinoma of uterine body	Bladder cancer
Basal cell cancer	Wilms tumor	Sarcoma
Testicular cancer	Colon cancer	Malignant melanoma
Uterine cervical cancer	Prostate cancer	Invasive renal cancers
Thyroid cancer	Breast cancer	Invasive skin cancer
Well-resected cancer in situ		Myeloma

*All patients with intermediate or high risk of recurrence should wait for 2 to 5 years before transplantation.

bladder, sarcomas, malignant melanomas, symptomatic renal carcinomas, nonmelanomatous skin cancers, and myelomas. It is recommended that transplantation be avoided in patients whose tumor recurrence rate is intermediate or high. If after 2 to 5 years there is no evidence of tumor recurrence, renal transplantation can be reconsidered. A waiting period may not be necessary for neoplasms with a low likelihood of metastasis, such as well-resected in situ carcinomas, basal cell carcinomas, renal cell carcinomas not metastasized beyond the capsule, and primary tumors of the central nervous system (Table 64-3).[89] The decision to offer transplantation to a patient with a prior history of malignancy needs to be considered with the assistance of an oncologist and in consideration of the histologic type of tumor and the staging of the tumor.

Although recurrence rates are high for patients with multiple myeloma and other paraproteinemias, including Waldenström macroglobulinemia, light-chain deposition disease, and primary amyloidosis, the post-transplantation course is often complicated by infections.[90] Patients with multiple myelomas are especially susceptible to recurrent globulinemia and plasmacytic interstitial infiltration.[3] Kaposi sarcoma recurs frequently after renal transplantation, probably because of reactivation of a herpesvirus.[91, 92] The incidence of melanoma is rising in the general population, and Penn[93] reviewed the recurrence rates of patients who had melanomas before transplantation and recommended that patients be tumor free for at least 5 years before transplantation. This is particularly relevant as Penn's study of 31 patients revealed a recurrence rate of 19% with a universally fatal outcome from recurrent malignancy. Therefore, a high recurrence rate of malignant melanoma and unpredictable behavior mandate extending the tumor-free time substantially beyond the 2 years recommended for most other types of cancer. An exception is made for melanoma in situ, which requires no waiting period. Also, patients with very small, well-resected melanomas may require only a 2-year waiting period.[93]

Pulmonary Diseases

Only scant information is available regarding the preoperative pulmonary risk assessment for renal transplant surgery. The best guidelines are derived from data on the pulmonary complications of surgery in the general population.[94] Any patient, including potential renal transplant recipients, with intrinsic pulmonary disease may be at higher risk for perioperative complications after surgery. The surgical site appears to be the most important predictor of pulmonary risk, with the risk increasing as the incision approaches the diaphragm.[94] The pulmonary risk factors that place patients at the highest risk for postoperative infections and ventilator dependence include chronic obstructive pulmonary disease, chronic interstitial pulmonary disease such as pulmonary fibrosis, extensive bronchiectasis, or a forced expiratory volume in 1 second less than 25% predicted.[3, 94] Patients with asthma may undergo surgery with little risk as long as their asthma is under control.[94] Evaluation of the pulmonary function of high-risk pretransplant patients should include spirometry in order to prepare the patient optimally for surgery. A screening chest radiograph is standard before transplantation, and if there are suspicious pulmonary lesions they need to be further evaluated.[3, 94] The risk of post-transplantation malignancies and cardiovascular disease is increased in smokers, and patients are told to discontinue smoking before transplantation at many centers.

Gastrointestinal Diseases

Patients with ESRD experience a high incidence of upper gastrointestinal disease. Active peptic ulcer disease is a relative contraindication to transplantation at many transplant centers because there is a high risk of perforation during treatment with the routine large post-transplantation doses of steroids. In fact, it was usual in the past to perform antiulcer surgery prophylactically before transplantation in all dialysis patients with documented hyperacidity. The trend now is toward conservative medical management[3, 95] unless surgical therapy is necessary because of failure to respond.

Other gastrointestinal disorders commonly seen in the pretransplantation workup include acute pancreatitis and cholelithiasis-cholecystitis. High post-transplantation morbidity and mortality are associated with acute pancreatitis.[10] Pancreatitis is commonly associated with immunosuppressive medications, CMV infections, hypercalcemia, and hypertriglyceridemia, and therefore any active pretransplantation disease should delay transplantation.[3] Many transplant centers mandate that patients have no clinical or biochemical signs of pancreatitis for 6 to 8 weeks before transplantation. Patients with gallstones do not necessarily need to undergo a cholecystectomy before transplantation if they have been asymptomatic.[96] If there are any episodes of acute or chronic cholecystitis, however, a pretransplantation cholecystectomy should be performed to avoid the high risk of life-threatening cholecystitis after transplantation.[96]

There is a high prevalence of diverticulosis in patients with ESRD related to constipation caused by the use of phosphate binders, low-fiber diet, and lower oral fluid intake. It is no longer routine to examine the lower gastrointestinal tract in all patients for the presence of diverticulosis. Now, only symptomatic patients are evaluated. Colonic rupture related to diverticulitis, however, results in severe morbidity and mortality after transplantation, and for this reason many transplant centers advocate elective partial colectomy for patients with preexisting diverticulitis.[3]

Skeletal Diseases

Transplantation may result in improved bone metabolism and marked clinical improvement. Osteodystrophy,

aluminum-associated bone disease, and hyperparathyroidism are improved after successful transplantation. Immediately after transplantation, there is an increase in osteopenia and bone fractures that seems to be correlated with cumulative steroid dose.[97, 98] Therefore, it is recommended that secondary hyperparathyroidism or aluminum-associated bone disease, or both, be minimized before transplantation by treatment with both vitamin D and phosphate binders, in the case of the former, or chelation in the case of the latter. Active parathyroid bone disease may require parathyroidectomy to avoid acute post-transplantation hypercalcemia.[3, 99] Pretransplantation screening for preexisting skeletal disease should be performed in all patients at high risk for osteopenia. This is especially important for patients with a long history of ESRD, a history of prior steroid use, or peri- and postmenopausal women.

Genitourinary Diseases

The workup for urologic disorders before transplantation is usually minimal. The high association of renal tumors with acquired renal cysts, however, has led many transplant centers to perform pretransplantation abdominal ultrasound screening of all patients with ESRD. If symptomatic cysts or questionable masses are identified, it is recommended that the patient be observed every 3 to 6 months while on the waiting list and after transplantation. Patients should also be screened for urinary tract infections or prostatic hypertrophy even though there is no prior urologic history or history of recurrent urinary tract infections. An extensive workup is mandated if there is a history of urologic disorders or if abnormalities are discovered on the initial screening. ESRD patients who require a urologic evaluation include those with recurrent urinary tract infections, pyelonephritis, vesicoureteral reflux, nephrolithiasis, renal malignancy, and neurogenic bladder. Any surgical corrections should be done before transplantation and all infections of the urinary tract must be eradicated, except in anuric patients with prostatic hypertrophy. In these patients, it is best to defer the operative procedure until after the patient has received the transplant and is making urine.

Most transplant centers require occasional monitoring of patients on the waiting list for urinary tract infections, especially high-risk patients such as those with polycystic kidney disease. Selected patients may require pretransplantation nephrectomy, including those with reflux associated with recurrent urinary tract infections, polycystic kidneys with infected cysts that cannot be cleared with antibiotics, severe nephrolithiasis and infected stones, or renal carcinoma.[3] The need for pretransplantation nephrectomy should be evaluated on an individual basis.

Evaluation of Renal Diseases with Potential for Recurrence in the Allograft

A complete discussion of risks and rate of recurrence of various causes of ESRD can be found in Chapter 65. Most renal disorders leading to ESRD can recur in the transplanted kidney, although they rarely cause renal dysfunction.[100] An important part of the pretransplantation evaluation is informing the potential recipient and live donor of the risk for recurrence and graft loss. Renal disorders with a high rate of recurrence need to be discussed with the patient.

For instance, patients with focal segmental glomerulosclerosis (FSGS) have a recurrence rate of 20% to 40% and a rate of graft loss of up to 40%.[100] Some patients may feel this risk is too high to consider live donation. Another important factor in the pretransplantation evaluation is to determine the activity of renal disorders caused by aberrant immunologic activity. Such disorders must be quiescent to minimize the risk of recurrence in the allograft.

Highlighted here are only the diseases with potential for recurrence that should be considered before transplant evaluation. To simplify the discussion, recurrent renal diseases have been divided into inherited disorders that cause renal disease, renal diseases associated with measurable immunologic activity, and intrinsic renal diseases.

Inherited Renal Disorders

Primary hyperoxalosis is due to an autosomal recessive deficiency of the hepatic enzyme peroxisomal alanine:glyoxylate aminotransferase (AGT). Deficiency of this enzyme is expressed to different degrees, and the severity of enzyme deficiency correlates directly with severity of disease. The disease is manifest as hyperoxaluria and hyperoxalemia that lead to nephrocalcinosis and urolithiasis. Most affected patients experience ESRD within the first two decades of life.[101] Renal transplantation has been contraindicated because of the high rate of recurrent oxalosis in the allograft. Some patients with residual AGT activity may do well after transplantation if treated with hydration, inhibitors of stone formation, and pyridoxine.[102] Early combined liver and kidney transplantation offers the optimal treatment for patients with complete absence of the enzyme.[103, 104] In patients who have not yet reached ESRD, aggressive preoperative or perioperative dialysis may decrease oxalate stores and reduce the risk of recurrent disease in the immediate post-transplantation period.[103] In these cases, live donors may be preferred as the timing of the transplant can be optimized to reduce the danger of the accumulated load of oxalate. Patients with oxalosis do well with dialysis, with a reported 30-month survival rate of 84%, and therefore many centers consider that dialysis is the preferred form of renal replacement therapy for these patients.[103, 105, 106]

Sickle cell disease is another inherited disorder that may lead to graft loss after transplantation if the patient continues to have frequent sickling crises. Graft survival rates have been variable with reports of 1-year survival rates of 25% to 67%.[107] Ojo and colleagues[108] reported survival data for patients and allografts from a large group of patients with sickle cell nephropathy who underwent renal transplantation. They found that there was no difference in 1-year cadaveric graft survival compared with that of patients with other causes of ESRD, but that 3-year graft survival rates were only 48% compared with 60% in patients with other causes of ESRD.[108] Generally, living donor transplantation has not been recommended for patients with sickle cell nephropathy.[107] One transplant center, however, reported successful living unrelated transplantation with prospective preparation of the patient.[109] The preparation regimen included preoperative transfusion until the sickle preparation was negative, use of induction immunosuppression with antithymocyte gamma globulin (ATGAM) rather than OKT3 to prevent potential hypoxic damage associated with the use

of OKT3, and modification of the postoperative immunosuppression by substitution of hydroxyurea for azathioprine to stimulate fetal hemoglobin production and decrease sickling events.[109] As there are only small numbers of patients with sickle cell disease who have received transplants at single centers, a cautious interpretation of data is recommended with regard to live donor transplantation.

Alport syndrome is an inherited disorder that affects type IV collagen–containing basement membranes. Patients with Alport syndrome do not experience recurrent disease, but they can have alloantibodies to antigens that are present in the donor kidney.[110] The risk for development of anti–glomerular basement membrane (anti-GBM) antibodies is small (1.9%), as reported for a group of 52 renal grafts transplanted into 41 patients.[111] A subset of patients with X-linked Alport syndrome at risk for anti-GBM disease are those who have a deletion in the *COL4A5* gene that encodes the alpha 5 chain of type IV collagen and develop antibodies to the NC1 domain of alpha 5 (IV) collagen.[110] Others have linked development of alloantibodies to the alpha 3 chain of type IV collagen to anti-GBM disease in the autosomal recessive form of Alport syndrome.[112] The recessive form of Alport syndrome is associated with defects in the *COL4A3* and *COL4A4* genes and has also been associated with post-transplantation anti-GBM disease.[113] Generally, it is considered that survival of patients and grafts is not different in Alport syndrome compared with other causes of ESRD and that Alport syndrome is not a contraindication to transplantation.[111]

Fabry disease is characterized by an X-linked deficiency of the lysosomal enzyme α-galactosidase resulting in accumulation of glycosphingolipids in the kidneys and other organs. Although histologic recurrences have been well documented, patients with Fabry disease appear to have excellent 3-year allograft survival, 80%.[114, 115] Patients with histologic findings of recurrent Fabry disease do not experience graft loss but may have microhematuria and a higher rate of post-transplantation infections.[106, 115] Through genetic engineering and enzyme replacement, therapy is becoming available in many countries and may postpone the need for renal transplantation in these patients.

Systemic Vasculitis

Patients with renal involvement of systemic vasculitis often have ongoing clinical or serologic activity that may predispose to post-transplantation allograft failure. Therefore, it is essential to evaluate both clinical and serologic markers to determine disease activity. In certain situations, active disease is manifest by both serologic and clinical markers, whereas in others, evidence of serologic activity alone precludes transplantation.

It is important when evaluating patients with *Goodpasture disease* (*anti-GBM disease*) to obtain current and historical anti-GBM antibody titers. These antibody titers should be absent for 6 months before transplantation to avoid recurrence of the disease in the allograft.[3] The presence of circulating antibodies in anti-GBM disease is considered a relative contraindication to transplantation because of reports from several centers of rapidly progressive allograft failure in patients with high circulating levels of these antibodies.[3] Others have reported that although all Alport patients develop anti-GBM antibodies, only a few develop nephritis, possibly because of genotypic differences in the ability to mount cellular immune responses.[112] Many transplant centers require patients to continue dialysis for 6 to 12 months after the disappearance of circulating anti-GBM antibodies to diminish the risk of recurrent disease.

Antineutrophil cytoplasmic autoantibodies (ANCAs) are developed against target neutrophil and monocyte proteins in a group of associated diseases that are characterized by renal involvement. *Wegener granulomatosis* is notable for antibodies to cytoplasmic ANCA (c-ANCA), and serum antibody titers generally reflect disease activity. Wegener granulomatosis can recur after transplantation and several case reports of recurrent disease have been published.[116-121] Renal transplantation is considered an acceptable treatment option for these patients.[122] Pauci-immune rapidly progressive glomerulonephritis and *microscopic polyarteritis* are characterized by perinuclear ANCA (p-ANCA) and there are case reports of recurrent p-ANCA–associated vasculitis after transplantation.[123-125] Most transplant centers suggest following ANCA titers before transplantation.[3] Whether ANCA titers are a reliable predictor of recurrent disease in asymptomatic patients is unknown.[125-127] In fact, there are reports of patients with high pretransplantation ANCA titers who have maintained excellent graft function using immunosuppression protocols that include cyclosporine.[126, 127] There are no reports yet of recurrence rates for newer immunosuppressive regimens.

Patients with ESRD related to *Schönlein-Henoch purpura* are more likely to experience recurrent disease if there is evidence of active disease within 18 months of the transplantation.[128] Up to 75% of patients may have histologic evidence of recurrence but only 10% manifest clinical evidence of disease.[3] The risk factors for recurrence of Schönlein-Henoch purpura are not known, although a short duration of original disease may suggest a more aggressive disease state with a higher risk of recurrence.[129]

A high rate of recurrence and graft loss (50%) has been reported in transplant patients with *mixed essential cryoglobulinemia*, especially when there is laboratory and clinical evidence of active disease.[130] Patients without active disease may experience recurrence without clinical manifestations[131] and therefore should be informed about the high risk for graft loss. Because there is a strong association between mixed essential cryoglobulinemia and HCV infection, patients should be screened for HCV infection.

Systemic Lupus Erythematosus

Systemic lupus erythematosus usually becomes quiescent after onset of dialysis and particularly after transplantation, probably because of the immunosuppressive medications used to suppress alloresponses. This is reflected in fewer clinical symptoms and diminished serologic parameters compared with those of patients receiving dialysis.[132] Patients who manifest symptoms of active clinical disease such as cerebritis, pericarditis, myocarditis, vasculitis, or recent (<6 months) nephritis should not be considered acceptable candidates for transplantation.[3] It is unclear what the role of serologic tests should be, but severely depressed serum complements or high anti-DNA antibodies may also be a relative contraindication.[10, 133] Patients with quiescent disease are considered good candidates for renal transplantation,

and when there is no serologic or clinical activity the disease rarely recurs.[3, 134] Anticardiolipin antibody should alert the transplant physician to the risk of thrombotic events, but its presence does not exclude lupus patients from transplantation.[133, 135] Whether there is an advantage to using live donor organs or cadaver organs with respect to recurrent lupus nephritis is unknown.

Thrombotic Microangiopathies

Patients with ESRD related to hemolytic-uremic syndrome (HUS) should be cautioned against living related transplantation because of the possibility of an inherited endothelial defect,[136, 137] especially if the patient lost a previous graft to recurrent HUS. Furthermore, patients with a family history of HUS should be advised against living related transplantation as there may be familial inheritance of various enzyme abnormalities.[136, 138] HUS has been shown to be associated with several conditions and medications: verocytotoxin-producing *Escherichia coli* (VTEC), viral infections, pregnancy, malignant hypertension, scleroderma, radiation nephritis, mitomycin C, cyclosporine, and oral contraceptives. Patients with HUS are at an especially high risk for graft loss after transplantation if the inciting condition has not resolved.[139, 140] Patients with so-called atypical HUS (i.e., not preceded by a diarrheal syndrome) may experience a higher risk of recurrent disease.[136] Cyclosporine, tacrolimus, antilymphocyte globulin, and OKT3 have each been reported to be associated with recurrence of HUS,[3] but others have reported that these agents may be used safely in patients with a history of HUS.[139, 141] Of those who ultimately experience recurrent HUS, one half lose their grafts.[136]

Paraproteinemias

Systemic amyloidosis (either AL or AA amyloid) is not a contraindication to transplantation provided the disease is not extensive or progressive. The extent of the disease is the primary determinant of poor outcome.[3] Patients with a particularly poor post-transplantation outlook include those with primarily amyloidosis and those with active infections and cardiovascular complications.[3, 142] If a patient has severe systemic manifestations, transplantation should be discouraged.[3, 142] In addition, patients with active disease must be informed that there is a 20% to 30% risk of recurrent disease.[3] Renal failure occurs commonly in patients with multiple myeloma. Transplantation may be an option for patients who have undergone successful tumor therapy, but there still remains a high risk for myeloma involvement of the allograft after transplantation and a high risk for infectious complications.[3] Dialysis-related (β_2-microglobulin–associated) amyloidosis has a good post-transplantation prognosis and there is risk of recurrence in the allograft. β_2-Microglobulin–associated amyloidosis can lead to debilitating joint involvement, but the joint disease does not progress after transplantation[143] and in fact may improve, although bone cysts are not reversed.[144]

Mixed Connective Tissue Diseases

Very few patients with mixed connective tissue diseases have undergone transplantation, and there are only scattered reports in the literature. In fact, most data derive from studies before the use of cyclosporine and angiotensin-converting enzyme inhibitors. Patients with scleroderma have undergone transplantation, although post-transplantation complications associated with uncontrolled hypertension or cardiovascular and gastrointestinal complications have been reported.[3] Unreliable absorption of immunosuppressive medications is particularly relevant in patients with gastrointestinal involvement.[3]

Diabetes Mellitus

Diabetic nephropathy recurs in 100% of transplanted allografts according to a histologic analysis.[145, 146] It does not produce alterations in renal function for many years, and the slowness of recurrence allows transplantation as a viable option for patients with ESRD related to diabetic nephropathy.[3] Given the survival advantage of transplantation over dialysis for diabetic patients with ESRD, histologic recurrence of diabetes should not be considered a deterrent to transplantation.

Intrinsic Renal Diseases

There are several risk factors for recurrence in patients with *primary focal segmental glomerulosclerosis*. These include early onset of disease and rapid progression from onset of disease to ESRD, a malignant clinical course, a time from initial diagnosis to ESRD less than 3 years, disease arising in children younger than 5 years, and histologic evidence of mesangial proliferation in the native kidney.[147-150] Patients without prior risk factors, however, have recurrence rates of about 10% to 30%.[150-152] In a multivariate analysis, the risk factors for recurrence were white recipient, younger recipient age, and treatment for rejection.[152] Of patients with recurrent disease, 40% to 50% lose their grafts.[148] If one graft has been lost to recurrent FSGS, the risk of recurrence in a second graft is as high as 60% to 80%.[10] Therefore, living donor grafts should not be used in patients who have previously lost a graft to recurrent disease. High-dose cyclosporine, plasmapheresis, or both have been reported to induce remission or stabilize graft function.[153, 154]

Patients with *membranoproliferative glomerulonephritis* (MPGN) type 1 have a risk of recurrence of about 20% to 30%.[154-156] About 40% of these patients with recurrent MPGN I experience graft loss,[154] whereas there is a risk of recurrence of about 80% with MPGN type II[154, 157] with a rate of graft loss of about 10% to 20%.[154, 155] MPGN has been found in association with several viral infections including HCV.[154, 158] Therefore, active viremia and subsequent immune complex deposition of viral antigen-antibody complexes may lead to glomerular injury in the allograft. All patients with MPGN should be screened for viral etiologies and informed of the potential for recurrent disease if they have active viremia.

Although there is a high likelihood of recurrent disease, patients with *immunoglobulin A (IgA) nephropathy* can safely receive transplants.[159, 160] Mesangial IgA deposits can be seen in up to 80% of cases in recipients.[160-163] Despite this high rate of recurrent IgA deposition, there is little clinical disease[154, 160] and there is no contraindication to use of live donors.[3]

DONOR ISSUES

The Cadaver Organ Shortage

The shortage of donor organs is the primary issue limiting success in the field of organ transplantation. More than 50,000 people are waiting for a kidney transplant in the United States, but fewer than 9000 cadaver kidneys are available.[164] The inadequate supply of organs is especially critical for heart, lung, and liver recipients, as these patients die without a replacement organ. In the case of renal transplantation, other forms of renal replacement therapy are available; however, transplantation clearly offers a survival benefit over dialysis,[2] especially for diabetic patients with ESRD.[2, 44]

If all potential donors were available, the available donor pool would increase by 60% to 80%.[165, 166] Therefore, several approaches have been taken to maximize donor organ capture, including promoting the use of marginal donors (by expanding the criteria that define a suitable organ donor) and increasing donor consent through public education efforts.

The United Network for Organ Sharing (UNOS) has defined expanded criteria donors (ECDs) as those whose kidneys have a 70% greater risk of graft failure than those of a reference group of nonhypertensive donors (age 10 to 39) who did not die of a cerebral vascular accident and whose terminal creatinine was less than or equal to 1.5 mg/dL (UNOS, www.unos.org, November 2002). Several donor factors have been associated with an increased rate of graft failure, including age 50 years or older, terminal creatinine greater than 1.5 mg/dL, cerebrovascular accident as a cause of death, and a history of hypertension. All donors 60 years of age or older automatically meet the criteria for ECDs.

Table 64-4 shows a matrix developed by UNOS that defines an ECD (UNOS, www.unos.org, November 2002). The ECD allocation system is now being implemented for patients on the waiting list who agree to accept offers of ECD kidneys. Transplant centers have been asked by UNOS to consider several criteria when agreeing to consider patients for ECD kidneys. For instance, it is recommended that ECD kidneys are procured and placed quickly to decrease the risk of delayed graft function. Therefore, it is UNOS policy that tissue typing and crossmatching are performed before organs

TABLE 64-4

Definition of Expanded Criteria Donor*

DONOR CONDITION	DONOR AGE CATEGORIES	
	50–59	>60
CVA + HTN + Creat > 1.5	X	X
CVA + HTN	X	X
CVA + Creat > 1.5	X	X
HTN + Creat > 1.5		X
CVA		X
HTN		X
Creatinine > 1.5		X
None of the above		X

Creat > 1.5, creatinine > 1.5 mg/dL; CVA, cerebrovascular accident was cause of death; HTN, history of hypertension at any time; X, expanded criteria donor.

Data from United Network for Organ Sharing web site UNOS, www.unos.org, November 2002.

are procured. ECD kidneys are first offered to candidates with zero antigen mismatch who have agreed in advance to accept an offer of an ECD kidney. If there are no candidates with zero antigen mismatch, the ECD kidneys are allocated by waiting time, first locally, then regionally, and then nationally (UNOS, www.unos.org, November 2002). The risk, however, of using suboptimal organs is a suboptimal outcome for the recipient. It is important to emphasize that the risk of using marginal organs must be weighed against the risk of remaining on the transplant list.[2, 167]

A significant proportion of marginal kidneys are harvested from older donors (>60 years old).[5, 168] The criteria used to determine whether an older organ is acceptable vary by transplant center, but it is generally agreed that donor renal function must be adequate (glomerular filtration rate GRF > 50 mL/min) and there should be minimal glomerulosclerosis on frozen histologic section.[169] The importance of glomerular sclerosis in the biopsy is debated. A point scoring system was developed on the basis of macroscopic evaluation of older kidneys in order to avoid a biopsy and potential graft damage.[170] One risk of using older donors is that there may be a higher incidence of delayed graft function[5] and early rejection.[5] Donors older than 60 are associated with a projected 21% 10-year survival rate versus 47% projected for donors aged 21 to 30.[171-173] Long-term graft survival is impaired by delayed graft function,[5] and older donors appear to experience a higher rate of delayed graft function. Therefore, many centers advocate that delayed graft function should be avoided in older donors. This may require a different allocation system for older donor organs. Because survival of patients has not been adversely affected by the use of older or marginal donors, the profound need for cadaver organs mandates the judicious use of marginal donors.

One way to improve use of marginal donors is to match functional nephron number between donors and recipients. Brenner and Milford[174] initially proposed the hypothesis of "nephron dosing" to diminish the risk of glomerular injury related to glomerular and systemic hypertension. This has led to nationwide interest in dual-kidney transplantation, and a registry has been developed to follow the clinical outcomes in patients who have received two kidneys from a single marginal donor.[175] The follow-up data to date suggest that short- and long-term survival of patients and grafts approaches that seen in recipients of a single kidney transplanted from younger donors.[175, 176] These kidneys would have been discarded, and it is important to realize that these marginal kidneys are a valuable resource. The single most important factor in long-term success appears to be avoidance of delayed graft function, which is dependent on length of cold storage time and warm ischemia.[175]

The public and health care professions need to be made aware of the importance of organ donation. About 50% of potential organs are not procured because of lack of consent.[177, 178] The reasons for lack of consent vary from inability to make a hasty decision in the presence of a great loss to religious and ethnic beliefs regarding organ harvesting and distribution.[179, 180] Verified consent must be obtained before the harvesting of any organ. Although patients have the right to offer this consent for themselves on the basis of the Uniform Anatomical Gift Act, in many cases the recently deceased has not discussed organ donation with the family or organ procurement organizations do not recognize this act

and feel they need to ask family members for consent. Health care professionals play an important role and need to be educated regarding policies on organ procurement and communication with family members at the time of death. One way to increase donation is through mandated choice for organ donation. Through the mandated choice proposal, a person's choice regarding organ donation would be listed with UNOS and upon death the patient's directive implemented.[166] A criticism of this approach is that patients may become even more reluctant to donate organs if the process appears to be regulated and not flexible in terms of family intervention.[177]

Cadaver Donor Procurement and Allocation

Acceptance of a cadaver organ for transplantation requires an efficient and accurate screening process. The donated kidney must be unimpaired or impaired within limits to be accepted as a marginal donation and must not be capable of transmitting infectious agents or malignancies. The local organ procurement agency is responsible for ensuring these safeguards through a series of mandated screening examinations that are performed on all donated organs. The laboratory examinations required include blood type; HLA screening; complete blood count; serum creatinine and electrolytes; blood, urine, and sputum cultures; urinalysis; and serologic tests for hepatitis viruses A, B, C, D, and E, human T cell lymphotropic virus type 1, the herpesviruses (CMV, herpes simplex virus, and Epstein-Barr virus), and HIV. In addition, the donor is screened for any history of high HIV risk behavior as defined by the CDC.

Generally, donors are not used if there is a history of malignancy because of a risk of transmission to the immunocompromised recipient. An exception exists in the case of a malignancy that originated in and is confined to the central nervous system or a malignancy that was considered cured for at least 2 years before the patient's death. In this case, an additional requirement would be no evidence of metastatic disease on autopsy.

Organ procurement agencies have adopted a policy to offer HCV+ organs only for lifesaving transplants (liver, heart, and lung).[181, 182] HCV+ organs are not offered to HCV-potential allograft recipients, although whether HCV+ organs should be offered to HCV+ recipients is debated. There are multiple serotypes of HCV, and antibody protection against one serotype does not necessarily confer protection against others in animal trials[183] or in human transplantation.[65] It is unlikely that all anti-HCV–positive donors have ongoing viremia, as detected by HCV RNA. Therefore, rapid assays to detect viremia are needed to allow more efficient use of these organs. It is also a general policy in most organ procurement organizations not to transplant kidneys from HBsAg+ donors because of the high risk of transmission of the hepatitis B virus.[3] The risks of transplanting organs from donors who are hepatitis B core antibody (HBcAb) positive have not been determined. In a single-center study of HBcAb-positive donors, it was found that transplants from donors who are HBcAb positive carried a small risk for hepatitis B surface antibody (3 of 27) and HBcAb (2 of 27) conversion, but there were no clinical signs of hepatitis.[184]

There has been concern regarding transmission of West Nile virus through blood transfusions and through transplanted tissue.[185] Although there is confirmatory evidence of blood-borne transmission, the risk of transmission through organ transplantation is not known. As screening tests become available for West Nile virus, the risk of transmission should become known.

The procurement and preparation of cadaver donor kidneys integrate the local organ procurement organization, the surgical harvest team, the surgical transplant team, and the tissue typing laboratory. Cadaver kidneys are harvested with a cuff of donor aorta, a procedure that has been shown to diminish the incidence of transplant renal artery stenosis. Before en bloc removal of the donor kidneys, the renal arteries are infused with a cold isotonic preservation solution. The solution most commonly used was developed at the University of Wisconsin (UW). The UW solution suppresses ischemia-induced cell membrane damage and maintains intracellular enzymes and normal intracellular adenosine triphosphate concentrations.[186] After infusion, the removed organs are placed in an ice bath, marking the beginning of cold ischemia time. Cold ischemia times greater than 24 hours are associated with higher rates of delayed graft function and lower long-term graft survival rates.[172] Warm ischemia (from donor asystole to harvest or from removal from cold storage to implantation) times greater than 20 minutes are also associated with poorer outcomes.[172] Most transplant centers preserve donor organs without mechanical perfusion, although there are reports of longer perfusion times using this method.[187] Mechanical perfusion has been associated with an increased incidence of endothelial cell damage and the development of a thrombotic microangiopathy.[188] Hypothermic pulsatile perfusion has been used to preserve organs from donors without heartbeats.[189]

Live Donor

By its very nature, kidney donation is an elective procedure. It is the ethical responsibility of the transplant center to provide donor candidates with an assessment of their personal risk and to ensure that the donated kidney is suitable and safe for the recipient. This process begins with an in-depth evaluation of the motivating factors of the donor, ensuring that there is not undue coercion. In general, donors are excluded when there is excessive surgical risk or evidence of preexisting renal disease or disorders that can cause renal disease (e.g., diabetes).

The standard donor evaluation utilizes a variety of laboratory and diagnostic tests to assess risk (Table 64-5). The transplant physician evaluating the donor must also take into consideration genetic factors that place the recipient at

TABLE 64-5

Criteria That Exclude a Live Donor

Age < 18 yr
Severe hypertension
Diabetes mellitus
Strong family history of diabetes mellitus
Impaired renal function
Family history of hereditary nephritis or polycystic kidney disease
History of nephrolithiasis
Hypercoagulability
Morbid obesity
Uncontrolled psychiatric disorders
Human immunodeficiency virus, hepatitis B, hepatitis C infection

higher risk for kidney disease in the future, such as a risk of type 2 diabetes if one or both parents have diabetes. Despite efforts to create guidelines, there are many factors that modulate the acceptance of risks for a donor. For example, two extremes would be a parent desiring to donate to a minor and a child desiring to donate to an elderly parent with multiple comorbid conditions and a short life expectancy. The former situation would allow higher risk tolerance than the latter. Ultimately, the determination of risk tolerance must be a joint decision of the candidate and the transplant committee.

Because of the shortage of cadaver organs, live organ donation is offered at most transplant centers and there are now more live than cadaver donors.[190] Since 1994, the total number of living donors has increased by 73% compared with an increase of only 9% in cadaver donors.[190] Because survival rates for patients and grafts are better after transplantation of a living versus a cadaver kidney,[190] live donation should be offered to all patients during the pretransplantation evaluation.

Several live donation options are now available at many transplant centers, including living related, living unrelated, paired kidney exchange (allowing a donor who is incompatible with the intended recipient to donate to a blood type–compatible recipient in exchange for that recipient's donor kidney), and nondirected live donation. Whether the donor and recipient are genetically related or unrelated, all potential live donors should be referred to a distinct donor physician to avoid undue influence of the recipient's physician and to ensure voluntary donation. It is important that the donation is voluntary and that any potential family or social pressures are carefully discussed in a complete psychosocial evaluation. Nondirected live donation has been the subject of considerable discussion, and it has been agreed by the transplant community that transplant centers performing nondirected live donation must carefully document informed consent detailing donor risks and take all safeguards to ensure donor safety.[191]

There are several criteria that, at most transplant centers, exclude a potential live donor, including age younger than 18 years; severe hypertension or end-organ damage associated with hypertension; diabetes mellitus or strong family history of diabetes; impaired renal function including proteinuria and pathologic hematuria or family history of hereditary nephritis or polycystic kidney disease; history of nephrolithiasis; hypercoagulability; morbid obesity; uncontrolled psychiatric disorders; and HIV, hepatitis B, or HCV infection (see Table 64-5).

An important consideration is the immediate and long-term risk of the donation. The immediate operative risks are low (0.1% to 0.4%) compared with those of similar surgical procedures and consist primarily of postoperative pulmonary and wound infections, myocardial infarction, and renal failure.[192, 193] Long-term risks in animal studies are glomerulosclerosis related to nephron hyperfiltration and impaired renal function.[100, 194] Although glomerulosclerosis has been demonstrated in rodent models, studies including over 600 living human donors have demonstrated no evidence for significant hypertension or renal insufficiency up to 20 years after donation.[100, 195-199] Approximately one third of patients who donate a kidney develop proteinuria, with an increase of 100 to 200 mg per 24 hours over baseline. This suggests that there is indeed an alteration in glomerular function associated with the reduction in nephron mass,[196, 198, 200] and therefore it is recommended that the potential donor be informed of this risk. Although there is no evidence for renal insufficiency based on a rise in serum creatinine for 20 years, longer term studies have not been performed to determine whether renal function and mild proteinuria remain stable beyond the first two decades after transplantation. Therefore, informed consent must include a recommendation that potential donors are closely observed for signs of renal impairment including regular urinalysis and 24-hour urine collections for creatinine and protein excretion.[100]

MATCHING POTENTIAL CANDIDATES TO DONORS

Immunologic matching of potential candidates to donors is an essential part of the pretransplantation evaluation. The immunologic evaluation process includes three primary components: ABO blood group typing, serum screening for PRAs, and pretransplantation crossmatching. Each component yields essential information that is used to minimize hyperacute and acute rejection episodes.

Allograft rejection is mediated through both humoral and cellular mechanisms that are activated by histocompatibility antigens expressed on the donor kidney. Histocompatibility antigens include HLA class I (A, B, or C) and HLA class II (DR and DQ, DP) histocompatibility antigens, non-HLA antigens,[201, 202] and ABO blood group antigens.[203] There are many different HLA A, B, C, and DR antigens that vary in structure and tissue distribution. Class I antigens are found on most nucleated cells, whereas class II antigens are found on B cells, antigen-presenting cells, activated endothelial cells, and some stromal cells and activated T cells. Every person has two A, B, C, and DR antigens, each inherited from one parent. Each set of A, B, C, and DR antigens is called a haplotype. There are therefore two HLA haplotypes per person. The reason that tissue typing is performed is that HLA antigens restrict and regulate the immune response in a highly specific way. Careful immunologic evaluation minimizes the likelihood of a recipient response to these antigenic targets.

The ABO blood group system is the most difficult antigen barrier to overcome. Therefore, donor organs are usually not offered to blood group–incompatible recipients except in emergency or experimental situations. Because the Rh antigen is not expressed in the kidney, the donor and recipient do not need to be Rh blood group matched. Although kidney donors need to be ABO compatible with their recipients, a small number of transplants have been mistakenly performed with ABO-mismatched kidneys and half of the grafts have lasted over 1 year.[204] Some grafts have been placed successfully into non-A_2 recipients from A_2 donors, although careful consideration of the titer of antibody against blood group A and DNA typing for A_2 antigen are needed before performing such transplantation.[205]

When a patient is on the transplant waiting list, a sample of blood is sent to the tissue typing laboratory each month. Technicians in the tissue typing laboratory centrifuge and separate red blood cells from serum of the sample and the serum is frozen for later antibody screening and crossmatching. Antibody screening of the serum detects preformed

antibodies that are specific for HLA antibodies. Although the majority of people in the general population do not have preexisting antibodies against HLA antigens, anti-HLA antibodies can develop after multiple blood transfusions, a previous allograft, or multiple pregnancies. To test for preexisting antibodies to HLA antigens, the serum is exposed to lymphocytes from a reference panel of normal individuals with a spectrum of HLA phenotypes. The most common method used is called the complement-dependent microcytotoxicity test.[206] Other methods utilize indirect immunofluorescence and enzyme-linked immunoassays to determine antibody reactivity toward cell panels or HLA antigens fixed to solid-state surfaces.[207-210]

Preexisting anti-HLA antibodies are quantitated by visual inspection and reported as the percent panel reactivity (or PRA). The PRA is a representation of the number of times a serum sample reacts with cells on the panel. The PRA is an important value because patients with a high percentage of panel reactivity reject a transplant by an antibody-mediated mechanism that is difficult to suppress, as indicated by a positive crossmatch.[211, 212] Therefore, patients with high PRAs generally wait for a long time for an immunologically compatible graft. The serum screening is also used to determine anti-HLA specificity of preexisting antibodies. This allows the avoidance of donors with antigens that increase the risk for rejection.

Tissue typing further identifies the HLA antigens of the donor and of the recipient. The ideal situation is to minimize the number of HLA antigen incompatibilities between the donor and recipient. In reality, this is rarely done except in the case of highly sensitized patients who are offered a zero antigen mismatch kidney. Tissue typing is performed in specialized laboratories that use standardized typing procedures. Minor histocompatibility antigens are not routinely screened. Of the HLA antigens, two HLA class I loci (A and B) and one HLA class II locus (DR) are typed before transplantation. Within each of the HLA antigens there are many serotypes, and new alleles are being identified by DNA typing that have not previously been detectable by serologic typing. DNA-based typing has been found to be more accurate and sensitive than serology and is gradually replacing the latter as a routine method.

The terms antigen matching and antigen mismatching are used by tissue typing laboratories to describe the degree of immunologic compatibility between a potential donor and recipient. These two terms mean different things, and therefore a table is provided to clarify the terminology. A donor and recipient can be matched for zero, one, or two antigens at each locus, and the matches are counted and the number of matches reported. The number of mismatched antigens can also be reported, and antigen mismatching gives a more complete picture of the immunologic compatibility between the donor and the recipient. The number of mismatches is not simply calculated from the number of matches. For example, a heterozygous recipient and a donor homozygous for one of the recipient HLA loci have only three or six antigens matched, yet no mismatched antigens are perceived at any of the three loci. Examples of matching and mismatching grades for some informative donor and recipient phenotypes are shown in Table 64-6. Graft survival is significantly increased in patients with zero mismatch at the A, B, and DR loci. But, because of the polymorphism of

TABLE 64-6

Relation between Degree of HLA Match and Mismatch*

RECIPIENT PHENOTYPE	DONOR PHENOTYPE	NUMBER OF MATCHES	NUMBER OF MISMATCHES
A1,A2,B7,B8,DR3,DR4	**A1,A2,B7,B8,DR3,DR4**	6	0
A1,**A2,B7,B8,DR3,DR4**	A3,**A2,B7,B8,DR3,DR4**	5	1
A1,A2,B7,B8,DR3,DR4	A3,A9,B45,B44,DR1,DR9	0	6
A1,A2,B7,**B8,DR3**,DR4	**A1**,A1,B8,**B8,DR3**,DR3	3	0

*This table illustrates the relation between degree of human leukocyte antigen (HLA) match and mismatch. The number of HLA mismatches usually equals 6 minus the number of matches for the A, B, and DR loci. The exception to this symmetry is in the case of recipients who are homozygous at one or more of the three loci. In the table, mismatched donor antigens are underlined and matched antigens are in boldface. Degree of mismatch is a more accurate measure of unidirectional recipient antidonor incompatibility.

the HLA system, cadaveric donors are rarely fully matched to the recipient.

Several national and international registries have shown that HLA matching improves renal allograft survival.[171] Allograft survival is better for HLA-identical siblings than for cadaver allografts with zero antigen mismatch. Proposed explanations for this survival advantage include shorter average cold and warm ischemia times and overall healthier living donor organs. Also, there is the immunologic advantage that the actual degree of compatibility for a zero HLA mismatch sibling is likely to be higher than for an apparently equivalent cadaver donor. The reason is that current HLA typing methods are not able to detect antigens at the level of the allele. Because of their common parentage, siblings with zero HLA mismatch share the same alleles, offering an immunologic advantage over cadaver donors.

The most important pretransplantation immunologic test is the recipient anti–donor HLA crossmatch. Crossmatching screens for preexisting anti–donor class I HLA antibodies immediately before transplantation using the most recent stored recipient sera. A positive crossmatch is correlated strongly with hyperacute rejection and therefore is an absolute contraindication to transplantation. The procedure for crossmatching requires donor T cells derived from spleen, lymph node, or blood. The donor T cells are exposed to the recipient serum and assayed for donor cell lysis. Lysis indicates the presence of preformed anti–donor class I HLA antibodies and defines a positive crossmatch. A positive B cell crossmatch is a relative contraindication to transplantation in patients who are highly sensitized or have received a prior transplant.[213, 214] Anti–donor HLA class II (HLA DR or DQ) antibodies are measured by performing a crossmatch with donor B lymphocytes as the target cells.[206] B cells express class I as well as class II antigens, and therefore the serum must be first absorbed with pooled platelets to remove anti–class I antibodies. This does not remove anti–class II antibodies and allows detection of preformed antibodies to HLA class II antigens. A complete description of the details of pretransplantation T and B cell crossmatching is provided in Chapter 65.

There are cases in which a positive crossmatch is not associated with allograft rejection. This occurs when antibodies are produced against non–HLA lymphocyte antigens. This situation arises particularly in patients with systemic lupus erythematosus and patients receiving α-methyldopa, procainamide, or hydralazine. In these cases, an autoantibody reacts with the patient's own lymphocytes and also with a variable proportion of individuals in the general population,

resulting in a high percent panel reactivity (PRA) on cytotoxic serum screening. Autoantibodies are usually of the IgM isotype and not directed against HLA antigens. Therefore, they are not a contraindication to successful kidney transplantation.

Transplantation offers improved quality and length of life for patients with ESRD. Consequently, many nephrologists consider all patients with ESRD as potential transplant candidates, leading to an enormous increase in transplant recipient evaluations. Improvements in immunosuppression and transplant recipient management have further eased the exclusionary criteria for transplantation. Now patients with chronic illness, such as HIV, are considered potential candidates at many transplant centers. Therefore, the transplant physician must carefully evaluate all potential candidates and donors in order to best utilize the scarce resource. Comorbid conditions such as cardiovascular disease, malignancies, bone disease, and infectious disease must be identified. In all cases, the benefits of transplantation need to be carefully considered against the short- and long-term risks of the surgical procedure and the immunosuppressive medications.

Unfortunately, there are no clear remedies for the deficit of transplantable organs. Therefore, many transplant centers consider live donation as the only potential solution for the near future. This is increasing the numbers of live donor transplants and has led to new options for live donation including living related donation, spousal donation, directed donation, and altruistic donation. The immediate risk to donors is considered low, but long-term follow-up of all donors for potential development of proteinuria and hypertension is mandatory. Despite the current lack of organs, the short- and long-term success of transplantation provides hope for patients with end-stage organ disease.

REFERENCES

1. Jofre R, Lopez-Gomez J, Moreno F, et al: Changes in quality of life after renal transplantation. Am J Kidney Dis 32:93-100, 1998.
2. Wolfe RA, Ashiby VB, Milford EL, et al: Comparison of mortality in all patients on dialysis, patients on dialysis awaiting transplantation, and recipients of a first cadaveric transplant. N Engl J Med 341:1725-1730, 1999.
3. Kasiske BL, Cangro CB, Hariharan S, et al: The evaluation of renal transplant candidates: Clinical practice guidelines. Am J Transplant 1(suppl 2):7-95, 2001.
4. System USRD: USRDS Annual Report: Atlas of End-Stage Renal Disease in the United States. Bethesda, MD, National Institutes of Health, National Institute of Diabetes and Digestive and Kidney Diseases, 2001.
5. Cecka JM: The UNOS renal transplant registry. Clin Transpl 1-18, 2001.

6. 2001 Annual Report of the U.S. Organ Procurement and Transplantation Network and the Scientific Registry for Transplant Recipients: Transplant Data 1991-2000. Rockville, MD, Department of Health and Human Services, Health Resources and Services Administration, Office of Special Programs, Division of Transplantation, United Network for Organ Sharing, University Renal Research and Education Association, 2001.

7. Miller RA: The aging immune system: Primer and prospectus. Science 273:70-74, 1996.

8. Venjatraman JT, Fernandes G: Exercise, immunity and aging. Aging 9:42-56, 1997.

9. Bradley BA: Rejection and recipient age. Transpl Immunol 10:125-132, 2002.

10. Kasiske B, Ramos EL, Gaston RS, et al: The evaluation of renal transplant candidates: Clinical practice guidelines. J Am Soc Nephrol 6:1-34, 1995.

11. Levey AS: Controlling the epidemic of cardiovascular disease in chronic renal disease: What do we know? What do we need to learn? Where do we go from here? Am J Kidney Dis 32:S1-S184, 1998.

12. Chertow GM, Milford EL, Mackenzie HS, et al: Antigen-independent determinants of cadaveric kidney transplant failure. JAMA 276:1732-1736, 1996.

13. Meier-Kriesche HU, Arndorfer JA, Kaplan B: The impact of body mass index on renal transplant outcomes: A significant independent risk factor for graft failure and patient death. Transplantation 73:70-74, 2002.

14. Gill IS, Hodge EE, Novick AC, et al: Impact of obesity on renal transplantation. Transplant Proc 25:1047-1048, 1993.

15. Howard RJ, Thai VB, Patton PR, et al: Obesity does not portend a bad outcome for kidney transplant recipients. Transplantation 73:53-55, 2002.

16. Yamamoto S, Hanley E, Hahn AB, et al: The impact of obesity in renal transplantation: An analysis of paired cadaver kidneys. Clin Transplant 16:252-256, 2002.

17. Matas A, Gillingham K, Payne W, et al: A third kidney transplant: Cost-effective treatment for end-stage renal disease. Clin Transplant 10:516-520, 1996.

18. Rovelli M, Paleri D, Vossler E, et al: Noncompliance in renal transplant recipients: Evaluation by socioeconomic groups. Transplant Proc 21:3979-3981, 1989.

19. Didlake RH, Dreyfus K, Kerman RH, et al: Patient noncompliance: A major cause of late graft failure in cyclosporine-treated renal transplants. Transplant Proc 20:63-69, 1988.

20. Foley RN, Parfrey PS, Harnett JD, et al: Clinical and echocardiographic disease in patients starting end-stage renal disease therapy. Kidney Int 47:186-192, 1995.

21. Kasiske BL: Risk factors for accelerated atherosclerosis in renal transplant recipients. Am J Med 1988:985-992, 1988.

22. Lemners MJ, Barry JM: Major role for arterial disease in morbidity and mortality after kidney transplantation in diabetic recipients. Diabetes Care 14:295-301, 1991.

23. Joki N, Hase H, Nakamura R, et al: Onset of coronary artery disease prior to initiation of haemodialysis in patients with end-stage renal disease. Nephrol Dial Transplant 12:718-723, 1997.

24. Wizemann V: Coronary artery disease in dialysis patients. Nephron 74:642-651, 1996.

25. Oh J, Wunsch R, Turzer M, et al: Advanced coronary and carotid arteriopathy in young adults with childhood-onset chronic renal failure. Circulation 106:100-105, 2002.

26. Saland JM, Ginsberg H, Fisher EA: Dyslipidemia in pediatric renal disease: Epidemiology, pathophysiology, and management. Curr Opin Pediatr 14:197-204, 2002.

27. Krmar RT, Ferraris JR, Ramirez JA, et al: Hyperhomocysteinemia in stable pediatric, adolescents, and young adult renal transplant recipients. Transplantation 71:1748-1751, 2001.

28. Nayir A, Bilge I, Kilicaslan I, et al: Arterial changes in paediatric haemodialysis patients undergoing renal transplantation. Nephrol Dial Transplant 16:2041-2047, 2001.

29. Eagle KA, Coley CM, Newell JB: Combining clinical and thallium data optimizes preoperative assessment of cardiac risk before major vascular surgery. Ann Intern Med 110:859-866, 1989.

30. Detsky AS, Abrams HB, Forbath N, et al: Cardiac assessment for patients undergoing noncardiac surgery. A multifactorial clinical risk index. Arch Intern Med 146:2131-2134, 1986.

31. Palda VA, Detsky AS: Perioperative assessment and management of risk from coronary artery disease. Ann Intern Med 127:313-328, 1997.

32. Eagle KA, Brundage BH, Chaitman BR, et al: Guidelines for perioperative cardiovascular evaluation for noncardiac surgery. Report of the American College of Cardiology/American Heart Association Task Force on Practice Guidelines. Committee on Perioperative Cardiovascular Evaluation for Noncardiac Surgery. Circulation 93:1278-1317, 1996.

33. Goodman WG, Goldin J, Kuizon BD, et al: Coronary-artery calcification in young adults with end-stage renal disease who are undergoing dialysis. N Engl J Med 342:1478-1483, 2000.

34. Manske CL, Wang Y, Rector T, et al: Coronary revascularisation in insulin-dependent diabetic patients with chronic renal failure. Lancet 340:998-1002, 1992.

35. Reddy VS, Chen AC, Johnson HK, et al: Cardiac surgery after renal transplantation. Am Surg 68:154-158, 2002.

36. Ono M, Wolf RK, Angouras DC, et al: Short- and long-term results of open heart surgery in patients with abdominal solid organ transplant. Eur J Cardiothorac Surg 21:1061-1072, 2002.

37. De Meyer M, Wyns W, Dion R, et al: Myocardial revascularization in patients on renal replacement therapy. Clin Nephrol 36:147-151, 1991.

38. Williams JS, Crawford FA, Kratz JM, et al: Cardiac surgery for patients maintained on chronic hemodialysis. J SC Med Assoc 87:569-573, 1991.

39. Kahn JK, Rutherford BD, McConahay DR, et al: Short- and long-term outcome of percutaneous transluminal coronary angioplasty in chronic dialysis patients. Am Heart J 119:484-489, 1990.

40. Rinehart AL, Herzog CA, Collins AJ, et al: A comparison of coronary angioplasty and coronary artery bypass grafting outcomes in chronic dialysis patients. Am J Kidney Dis 25:281-290, 1995.

41. Takeshita S, Yamaguchi T, Isshiki T, et al: Percutaneous transluminal coronary angioplasty and coronary bypass grafting for refractory angina in chronic dialysis patients. J Cardiol 22:383-390, 1992.

42. Howard BV, Rodriguez BL, Bennett PH, et al: Prevention Conference VI: Diabetes and Cardiovascular Disease: Writing Group I: Epidemiology. Circulation 105:e132-e137, 2002.

43. Friedlander M, Hricik D: Optimizing end-stage renal disease therapy for the patient with diabetes mellitus. Semin Nephrol 17:331-345, 1997.

44. Port FK, Wolfe RA, Mauger EA, et al: Comparison of survival probabilities for dialysis patients vs cadaveric renal transplant recipients. JAMA 270:1339-1343, 1993.

45. Manske CL, Wilson RF, Wang Y, et al: Atherosclerotic vascular complications in diabetic transplant patients. Am J Kidney Dis 29:601-607, 1997.

46. Manske CL: Coronary artery disease in diabetic patients with nephropathy. Am J Hypertens 6:367S-374S, 1993.

47. Redberg RF, Greenland P, Fuster V, et al: Prevention Conference VI: Diabetes and Cardiovascular Disease: Writing Group III: Risk assessment in persons with diabetes. Circulation 105:e144-e152, 2002.

48. Manske CL, Thomas W, Wang Y, et al: Screening diabetic transplant candidates for coronary artery disease: Identification of a low risk subgroup. Kidney Int 44:617-621, 1993.

49. Gunther M, Stark K, Neuhaus R, et al: Rapid decline of antibodies after hepatitis A immunization in liver and renal transplant recipients. Transplantation 71:477-479, 1991.

50. Sanchez-Fructuoso AI, Prats D, Naranjo P, et al: Influenza virus immunization effectivity in kidney transplant patients subjected to two different triple-drug therapy immunosuppression protocols: Mycophenolate versus azathioprine. Transplantation 69:436-439, 2000.

51. Rubin RH, Kemmerly SA, Conti D, et al: Prevention of primary cytomegalovirus disease in organ transplant recipients with oral ganciclovir or oral acyclovir prophylaxis. Transpl Infect Dis 2:112-117, 2000.

52. Weir MR, Irwin BC, Maters AW, et al: Incidence of cytomegalovirus disease in cyclosporine-treated renal transplant recipients based on donor-recipient pre-transplant immunity. Transplantation 43:187-193, 1987.

53. Balfour HH, Chace BA, Stapleton JT, et al: A randomized, placebo-controlled trial of oral acyclovir for the prevention of cytomegalovirus disease in recipients of renal allografts. N Engl J Med 320:1381-1387, 1989.

54. Hibberd PL, Tolkoff-Rubin NE, Conti D, et al: Preemptive ganciclovir therapy to prevent cytomegalovirus disease in cytomegalovirus antibody-positive renal transplant recipients. A randomized controlled trial. Ann Intern Med 123:18-26, 1995.

55. Huang CC, Lai MK, Fong MT: Hepatitis B liver disease in cyclosporine-treated renal allograft recipients. Transplantation 49:540-544, 1990.

56. Fabrizi F, Lunghi G, Poordad FF, et al: Management of hepatitis B after renal transplantation: An update. J Nephrol 15:113-122, 2002.

57. Harnett JD, Zeldis JB, Parfrey PA, et al: Hepatitis B disease in dialysis and transplant patients: Further epidemiologic and serologic studies. Transplantation 44:369-376, 1987.

58. Parfrey PS, Forbes RDC, Hytchinson TA, et al: The impact of renal transplantation on the course of hepatitis B liver disease. Transplantation 39:610-615, 1985.

59. Pol S, Debure A, Degott C, et al: Chronic hepatitis in kidney allograft recipients. Lancet 335:878-880, 1990.

60. Friedlaender MM, Kaspa RT, Rubinger D, et al: Renal transplantation is not contraindicated in asymptomatic carriers of hepatitis B surface antigen. Am J Kidney Dis 14:204-210, 1989.

61. Rostaing L, Izopet J, Cisterne JM, et al: Impact of hepatitis C virus duration and hepatitis C virus genotypes on renal transplant patients: Correlation with clinicopathological features. Transplantation 65:930-936, 1998.

62. Fornairon S, Pol S, Legendre C, et al: The long-term virologic and pathologic impact of renal transplantation on chronic hepatitis B virus infection. Transplantation 62:297-299, 1996.

63. Degos F, Lugassy C, Degott C, et al: Hepatitis B virus and hepatitis B–related viral infection in renal transplant recipients. Gastroenterology 94:151-156, 1988.

64. Rao KV, Kasiske BL, Anderson WR: Variability in the morphological spectrum and clinical outcome of chronic liver disease in hepatitis B-positive and B-negative renal transplant recipients. Transplantation 51:391-396, 1991.

65. Fabrizi F, Poordad FF, Martin P: Hepatitis C infection and the patient with end-stage renal disease. Hepatology 36:3-10, 2002.

66. Hepatitis C: Global prevalence. Wkly Epidemiol Rec 72:341-344, 1997.

67. Vosnides GG: Hepatitis C in renal transplantation. Kidney Int 52:843-861, 1997.

68. Fabrizi F, Martin P, Dixit V, et al: Acquisition of hepatitis C virus in hemodialysis patients: A prospective study by branched DNA signal amplification assay. Am J Kidney Dis 31:647-654, 1998.

69. Recommendations for prevention and control of hepatitis C virus (HCV) infection and HCV-related chronic disease. Centers for Disease Control and Prevention. MMWR Recomm Rep 47(RR-19):1-39, 1998.

70. Natov SN, Pereira BJ: Management of hepatitis C infection in renal transplant recipients. Am J Transplant 2:483-490, 2002.

71. Schneeberger PM, Keur I, van Loon AM, et al: The prevalence and incidence of hepatitis C virus infections among dialysis patients in the Netherlands: A nationwide prospective study. J Infect Dis 182:1291-1299, 2000.

72. Knoll GA, Tankersley MR, Lee JY, et al: The impact of renal transplantation on survival in hepatitis C–positive end-stage renal disease patients. Am J Kidney Dis 29:608-614, 1997.

73. Pereira BJ, Natov SN, Bouthot BA, et al: Effects of hepatitis C infection and renal transplantation on survival in end-stage renal disease. The New England Organ Bank Hepatitis C Study Group. Kidney Int 53:1374-1381, 1998.

74. John GT, Shankar V: Mycobacterial infections in organ transplant recipients. Semin Respir Infect 17:274-283, 2002.

75. Cavusoglu C, Cicek-Saydam C, Karasu Z, et al: *Mycobacterium tuberculosis* infection and laboratory diagnosis in solid-organ transplant recipients. Clin Transplant 16:257-261, 2002.

76. Niewczas M, Ziolkowski J, Rancewicz Z, et al: Tuberculosis in patients after renal transplantation remains still a clinical problem. Transplant Proc 34:677-679, 2002.

77. Ramos EL, Kasiske BL, Alexander SR: The evaluation of candidates for renal transplantation: The current practice of U.S. transplant centers. Transplantation 57:490-497, 1994.

78. Glassock RJ, Cohen AH, Danovitch G, et al: Human immunodeficiency virus infection and the kidney. Ann Intern Med 112:35-49, 1990.

79. Hogg RS, Heath KV, Yip B, et al: Improved survival among HIV-infected individuals following initiation of antiretroviral therapy. JAMA 279:450-454, 1998.

80. Ahuja TS, Zingman B, Glicklich D: Long-term survival in an HIV-infected renal transplant recipient. Am J Nephrol 17:480-482, 1997.

81. Halpern SD, Ubel PA, Caplan AL: Solid-organ transplantation in HIV-infected patients. N Engl J Med 347:284-287, 2002.

82. Ferber D: Public health. Creeping consensus on SV40 and polio vaccine. Science 298:725-727, 2002.

83. Fishman JA: BK virus nephropathy—Polyomavirus adding insult to injury. N Engl J Med 347:527-530, 2002.

84. Mylonakis E, Goes N, Rubin RH, et al: BK virus in solid organ transplant recipients: An emerging syndrome. Transplantation 72:1587-1592, 2001.

85. Poduval RD, Meehan SM, Woodle ES, et al: Successful retransplantation after renal allograft loss to polyoma virus interstitial nephritis. Transplantation 73:1166-1169, 2002.

86. Dunn GP, Bruce AT, Ikeda H, et al: Cancer immunoediting: From immunosurveillance to tumor escape. Nat Immunol 3:991-998, 2002.

87. Maisonneuve P, Agodoa L, Gellert R, et al: Cancer in patients on dialysis for end-stage renal disease: An international collaborative study. Lancet 354:93-98, 1999.

88. Chertow G, Paltiel A, Owen JW, et al: Cost-effectiveness of cancer screening in end-stage renal disease. Arch Intern Med 156:1345-1350, 1996.

89. Penn I: Tumors after renal and cardiac transplantation. Hematol Oncol Clin North Am 7:431-445, 1993.

90. Gerlag PGG, Koene RAP, Berden JHM: Renal transplantation in light chain nephropathy; case report and review of the literature. Clin Nephrol 25:101-104, 1986.

91. Chang Y, Cesarman E, Pessin MS, et al: Identification of herpesvirus-like DNA sequences in AIDS-associated Kaposi's sarcoma. Science 266:1865-1869, 1994.

92. Pellet C, Chevret S, Frances C, et al: Prognostic value of quantitative Kaposi sarcoma–associated herpesvirus load in posttransplantation Kaposi sarcoma. J Infect Dis 186:110-113, 2002.

93. Penn I: Evaluation of the candidate with a previous malignancy. Liver Transpl Surg 2:109-113, 1996.

94. Smethana GW: Preoperative pulmonary evaluation. N Engl J Med 340:937-944, 1999.

95. Barri YM, Ramos EL, Balagtas RS, et al: Cimetidine or ranitidine in renal transplant patients receiving cyclosporine. Clin Transplant 10:34-38, 1996.

96. Melvin WS, Meier DJ, Elkhammas EA, et al: Prophylactic cholecystectomy is not indicated following renal transplantation. Am J Surg 175:317-319, 1998.

97. Pichette V, Bonnardeaux A, Prudhomme L, et al: Long-term bone loss in kidney transplant recipients: A cross-sectional and longitudinal study. Am J Kidney Dis 28:105-114, 1996.

98. Wolpaw T, Deal CL, Fleming-Brooks S, et al: Factors influencing vertebral bone density after renal transplantation. Transplantation 58:1186-1189, 1994.

99. Nichol PF, Starling JR, Mack E, et al: Long-term follow-up of patients with tertiary hyperparathyroidism treated by resection of a single or double adenoma. Ann Surg 235:673-678; discussion 678-680, 2002.

100. Kasiske BL, Ma JZ, Louis TA, et al: Long-term effects of reduced renal mass in humans. Kidney Int 48:814-819, 1995.

101. Cochat P, Deloraine A, Rotily M, et al: Epidemiology of primary hyperoxaluria type 1. Nephrol Dial Transplant 10(suppl 8):3-7, 1995.

102. Allen AR, Thompson EM, Williams G, et al: Selective renal transplantation in primary hyperoxaluria type 1. Am J Kidney Dis 27:891-895, 1996.

103. Cibrik DM, Kaplan B, Arndorfer JA, et al: Renal allograft survival in patients with oxalosis. Transplantation 74:707-710, 2002.

104. Jamieson NV: The European Primary Hyperoxaluria Type 1 Transplant Registry report on the results of combined liver/kidney transplantation for primary hyperoxaluria 1984-1994. Nephrol Dial Transplant 10(suppl 8):33-37, 1995.

105. Gagnadoux MF, Lacaille F, Niaudet P, et al: Long term results of liver-kidney transplantation in children with primary hyperoxaluria. Pediatr Nephrol 16:946-950, 2001.

106. Nissenson AR, Port FK: Outcome of end-stage renal disease in patients with rare causes of renal failure. I. Inherited and metabolic disorders. Q J Med 73:1055-1062, 1989.

107. Barber WH, Deierhoi MH, Julian BA: Renal transplantation in sickle cell anemia and sickle disease. Clin Transplant 1:169-175, 1987.

108. Ojo AO, Govaerts TC, Schmouder RL, et al: Renal transplantation in end-stage sickle cell nephropathy. Transplantation 67:291-295, 1999.

109. Brennan DC, Lippman BJ, Shenoy S, et al: Living unrelated renal transplantation for sickle cell nephropathy. Transplantation 59:794-795, 1995.

110. Dehan P, Van den Heuvel L, Smeets H, et al: Identification of post-transplant anti-alpha 5 (IV) collagen alloantibodies in X-linked Alport syndrome. Nephrol Dial Transplant 11:1983-1988, 1996.

111. Byrne MC, Budisavljevic MN, Fan Z, et al: Renal transplant in patients with Alport's syndrome. Am J Kidney Dis 39:769-775, 2002.

112. Kalluri R, Torre A, Shield CF 3rd, et al: Identification of alpha3, alpha4, and alpha5 chains of type IV collagen as alloantigens for Alport posttransplant anti–glomerular basement membrane antibodies. Transplantation 69:679-683, 2000.

113. Ding J, Zhou J, Tryggvason K, et al: COL4A5 deletions in three patients with Alport syndrome and posttransplant antiglomerular basement membrane nephritis. J Am Soc Nephrol 5:161-168, 1994.

114. Obrador GT, Ojo A, Thadhani R: End-stage renal disease in patients with Fabry disease. J Am Soc Nephrol 13(suppl 2):S144-S146, 2002.

115. Ojo A, Meier-Kriesche HU, Friedman G, et al: Excellent outcome of renal transplantation in patients with Fabry's disease. Transplantation 69:2337-2339, 2000.

116. Haubitz M, Olbricht C, Maschek H, et al: Lethal relapse of Wegener's disease 4 years after successful kidney transplantation. Letter. Nephron 71:118-120, 1995.

117. Boubenider S, Akhtar M, Alfurayh O, et al: Late recurrence of Wegener's granulomatosis presenting as tracheal stenosis in a renal transplant patient. Clin Transplant 8:5-9, 1994.

118. Reaich D, Cooper N, Main J: Rapid catastrophic onset of Wegener's granulomatosis in a renal transplant. Nephron 67:354-357, 1994.

119. Rosenstein E, Ribot S, Ventresca E, et al: Recurrence of Wegener's granulomatosis following renal transplantation. Br J Rheumatol 33:869-871, 1994.

120. Rich L, Piering W: Ureteral stenosis due to recurrent Wegener's granulomatosis after kidney transplantation. J Am Soc Nephrol 4:1516-1521, 1994.

121. Fan SL, Lewis KE, Ball E, et al: Recurrence of Wegener's granulomatosis 13 years after renal transplantation. Am J Kidney Dis 38:E32, 2001.

122. Wrenger E, Pirsch JD, Cangro CB, et al: Single-center experience with renal transplantation in patients with Wegener's granulomatosis. Transpl Int 10:152-156, 1997.

123. Le Mao G, Rostaing L, Modesto A, et al: Recurrence of ANCA-associated microscopic polyangiitis after cadaveric renal transplant. Transplant Proc 28:2803-2804, 1996.

124. Grotz W, Wanner C, Rother E, et al: Clinical course of patients with antineutrophil cytoplasm antibody positive vasculitis after kidney transplantation. Nephron 69:234-236, 1995.

125. Nachman PH, Segelmark M, Westman K, et al: Recurrent ANCA-associated small vessel vasculitis after transplantation: A pooled analysis. Kidney Int 56:1544-1550, 1999.

126. Nyberg G, Akesson P, Norden G, et al: Systemic vasculitis in a kidney transplant population. Transplantation 63:1273-1277, 1997.

127. Rostaing L, Modesto A, Oksman F, et al: Outcome of patients with antineutrophil cytoplasmic autoantibody–associated vasculitis following cadaveric kidney transplantation. Am J Kidney Dis 29:96-102, 1997.

128. Nast CC, Ward HJ, Koyle MA, et al: Recurrent Henoch-Schönlein purpura following renal transplantation. Am J Kidney Dis 9:39-43, 1987.

129. Meulders Q, Pirson Y, Cosyns JP, et al: Course of Henoch-Schönlein nephritis after renal transplantation. Transplantation 58:1179-1186, 1994.

130. Hiesse C, Bastuji-Garin S, Santelli G, et al: Recurrent essential mixed cryoglobulinemia in renal allografts. Am J Nephrol 9:150-154, 1989.

131. Tarantino A, Moroni G, Banfi G, et al: Renal replacement therapy in cryoglobulinaemic nephritis. Nephrol Dial Transplant 9:1426-1430, 1994.

132. Mojcik CF, Klippel JH: End-stage renal disease and systemic lupus erythematosus. Am J Med 101:100-107, 1996.

133. Ward MM: Outcomes of renal transplantation among patients with end stage renal disease caused by lupus nephritis. Kidney Int 57:2136-2143, 2000.

134. Bartosh SM, Fine RN, Sullivan EK: Outcome after transplantation of young patients with systemic lupus erythematosus: A report of the North American pediatric renal transplant cooperative study. Transplantation 72:973-978, 2001.

135. Joseph RE, Radhakrishnan J, Appel GB: Antiphospholipid antibody syndrome and renal disease. Curr Opin Nephrol Hypertens 10:175-181, 2001.

136. Donne RL, Abbs I, Barany P, et al: Recurrence of hemolytic uremic syndrome after live related renal transplantation associated with subsequent de novo disease in the donor. Am J Kidney Dis 40:E22, 2002.

137. Hebert D, Sibley RK, Mauer SM: Recurrence of hemolytic uremic syndrome in renal transplant recipients. Kidney Int 30:S51-S58, 1986.

138. Remuzzi G, Marchesi D, Misiani R, et al: Familial deficiency of a plasma factor stimulating vascular prostacyclin activity. Thromb Res 16:517-525, 1979.

139. Conlon PJ, Brennan DC, Pfaf WW, et al: Renal transplantation in adults with thrombotic thrombocytopenic purpura/haemolytic-uraemic syndrome. Nephrol Dial Transplant 11:1810-1814, 1996.

140. Agarwal A, Mauer SM, Matas AJ, et al: Recurrent hemolytic uremic syndrome in an adult renal allograft recipient: Current concepts and management. J Am Soc Nephrol 6:1160-1169, 1995.

141. Miller RB, Burke BA, Schmidt WJ, et al: Recurrence of haemolytic-uraemic syndrome in renal transplants. Nephrol Dial Transplant 12:1425-1430, 1997.

142. Pasternack A, Ahonen J, Kuhlback B: Renal transplantation in 45 patients with amyloidosis. Transplantation 42:598-601, 1986.

143. Floege J, Ehlerding G: Beta-2-microglobulin–associated amyloidosis. Nephron 72:9-26, 1996.

144. Mourad G, Argiles A: Renal transplantation relieves the symptoms but does not reverse beta 2-microglobulin amyloidosis. JASN 7:798-804, 1996.

145. Bohman SO, Wilczek H, Tyden G, et al: Recurrent diabetic nephropathy in renal allografts placed in diabetic patients and protective effect of simultaneous pancreatic transplantation. Transplant Proc 19:2290-2293, 1985.

146. Lundgren G, Wilczek H, Bohman SO, et al: Development of diabetic nephropathy in renal allografts of diabetic patients. Transplant Proc 17:18-20, 1985.

147. Pinto J, Lacerda G, Cameron JS, et al: Recurrence of focal segmental glomerulosclerosis in renal allografts. Transplantation 32:83-89, 1981.

148. Artero M, Biava C, Amend W, et al: Recurrent focal glomerulosclerosis: Natural history and response to therapy. Am J Med 92:375-383, 1992.

149. Stephanian E, Matas AJ, Mauer SM, et al: Recurrence of disease in patients retransplanted for focal segmental glomerulosclerosis. Transplantation 53:755-757, 1992.

150. Dantal J, Baatard R, Hourmant M, et al: Recurrent nephrotic syndrome following renal transplantation in patients with focal glomerulosclerosis. A one-center study of plasma exchange effects. Transplantation 52:827-831, 1991.

151. Senggutuvan P, Cameron JS, Hartley RB, et al: Recurrence of focal segmental glomerulosclerosis in transplanted kidneys: Analysis of incidence and risk factors in 59 allografts. Pediatr Nephrol 4:21-28, 1990.

152. Abbott KC, Sawyers ES, Oliver JD 3rd, et al: Graft loss due to recurrent focal segmental glomerulosclerosis in renal transplant recipients in the United States. Am J Kidney Dis 37:366-373, 2001.

153. European best practice guidelines for renal transplantation: Section IV: Long-term management of the transplant recipient. IV.11 Paediatrics (specific problems). Nephrol Dial Transplant 17(suppl 4):55-58, 2002.

154. European best practice guidelines for renal transplantation: Section IV: Long-term management of the transplant recipient. IV.2.5. Chronic graft dysfunction. Late recurrence of primary glomerulonephritides. Nephrol Dial Transplant 17(suppl 4):16-18, 2002.

155. Cameron JS: Glomerulonephritis in renal transplants. Transplantation 34:237-245, 1982.

156. Curtis JJ, Wyatt RJ, Bhathena D, et al: Renal transplantation for patients with type I and type II membranoproliferative glomerulonephritis. Am J Med 66:216-225, 1979.

157. Eddy A, Sibley R, Mauer SM, et al: Renal allograft failure due to recurrent dense intramembranous deposit disease. Clin Nephrol 21:305-313, 1984.

158. Cruzado JM, Carrera M, Torras J, et al: Hepatitis C virus infection and de novo glomerular lesions in renal allografts. Am J Transplant 1:171-178, 2001.

159. Donadio JV, Grande JP: IgA nephropathy. N Engl J Med 347: 738-748, 2002.

160. Ponticelli C, Traversi L, Feliciani A, et al: Kidney transplantation in patients with IgA mesangial glomerulonephritis. Kidney Int 60: 1948-1954, 2001.

161. Bachman U, Biava C, Amend W, et al: The clinical course of IgA-nephropathy and Henoch-Schönlein purpura following renal transplantation. Transplantation 42:511-515, 1986.

162. Brensilver JM, Mallat S, Scholes J, et al: Recurrent IgA nephropathy in living-related donor transplantation: Recurrence or transmission of familial disease? Am J Kidney Dis 12:147-151, 1988.

163. Odum J, Peh CA, Clarkson AR, et al: Recurrent mesangial IgA nephritis following renal transplantation. Nephrol Dial Transplant 9:309-312, 1994.

164. Cecka JM: Donors without a heartbeat. N Engl J Med 347:281-283, 2002.

165. Evans RW, Orians CE, Ascher NL: The potential supply of organ donors. JAMA 267:239-246, 1992.

166. Spital A: Mandated choice for organ donation. Ann Intern Med 125:66-69, 1996.

167. Ojo AO, Hanson JA, Meier-Kriesche H, et al: Survival in recipients of marginal cadaveric donor kidneys compared with other recipients and wait-listed transplant candidates. J Am Soc Nephrol 12:589-597, 2001.

168. First MR: Expanding the donor pool. Semin Nephrol 17:373-380, 1997.

169. Alexander J, Zola J: Expanding the donor pool: Use of marginal donors for solid organ transplantation. Clin Transplant 10:1-19, 1996.

170. Berardinelli L, Beretta C, Raiteri M, et al: Early and long-term results using older kidneys from cadaver or living donors. Clin Transpl 157-166, 2001.

171. Terasaki PI: The HLA-matching effect in different cohorts of kidney transplant recipients. Clin Transpl 497-514, 2000.

172. Nishikawa K, Terasaki PI: Annual trends and triple therapy— 1991-2000. Clin Transpl 247-269, 2001.

173. Gjertson DW: A multi-factor analysis of kidney graft outcomes at one and five years posttransplantation. *In* Cecka JM, Terasaki PI (eds): Clinical Transplants 1996. Los Angeles, UCLA Tissue Typing Laboratory. 343-360, 1997.

174. Brenner BM, Milford EL: Nephron underdosing: A programmed cause of chronic renal allograft failure. Am J Kidney Dis 21:66-72, 1993.

175. Alfrey EJ, Lerner SM, Lu AD: The dual kidney transplant registry. Clin Transpl 107-111, 2001.

176. Remuzzi G, Grinyo J, Ruggenenti P, et al: Early experience with dual kidney transplantation in adults using expanded donor criteria. Double Kidney Transplant Group (DKG). J Am Soc Nephrol 10:2591-2598, 1999.

177. Klaussen AC, Klassen DK: Who are the donors in organ donation? The family's perspective in mandated choice. Ann Intern Med 125:70-73, 1996.

178. Coleman-Musser L: The physician's perspective: A survey of attitudes toward organ donor management. J Transpl Coord 7:55-58, 1997.

179. Durand-Zaleski I, Waissman R, Lang P, et al: Nonprocurement of transplantable organs in a tertiary care hospital: A focus on sociological causes. Transplantation 62:1224-1229, 1996.

180. Peters TG, Kittur DS, McGaw LJ, et al: Organ donors and nondonors. An American dilemma. Arch Intern Med 156:2419-2424, 1996.

181. Pereira BJ, Levey AS: Hepatitis C virus infection in dialysis and renal transplantation. Kidney Int 51:981-999, 1997.

182. Pereira BJG, Milford EL, Kirkman RL, et al: Prevalence of HCV RNA in hepatitis C antibody positive cadaver organ donors and their recipients. N Engl J Med 327:910-915, 1992.

183. Farci P, Alter HJ, Govindarajan S, et al: Lack of protective immunity against reinfection with hepatitis C virus. Science 258:135-140, 1992.

184. Satterthwaite R, Ozgu I, Shidban H, et al: Risks of transplanting kidneys from hepatitis B surface antigen–negative, hepatitis B core antibody–positive donors. Transplantation 64:432-435, 1997.

185. From the Centers for Disease Control and Prevention. West Nile virus activity—United States, September 26–October 2, 2002, and investigations of West Nile virus infections in recipients of blood transfusion and organ transplantation. JAMA 288:1975-1976, 2002.

186. Southard JH, Pienaar H, McAnulty JF, et al (eds): The University of Wisconsin Solution for Organ Preservation. Philadelphia, WB Saunders, 1989.

187. Barber WH, Deieirhoi MH, Phillips MG, et al: Preservation by pulsatile perfusion improves early renal allograft function. Transplant Proc 20:865-868, 1988.

188. Cerra FB, Raza S, Andres GA, et al: The endothelial damage of pulsatile renal preservation, and its relationship to perfusion pressure and colloid osmotic pressure. Surgery 81:534-541, 1977.

189. Polyak MM, Arrington BO, Stubenbord WT, et al: The influence of pulsatile preservation on renal transplantation in the 1990s. Transplantation 69:249-258, 2000.

190. Gjertson DW: Center and other factor effects in recipients of living-donor kidney transplants. Clin Transpl 2001:209-221.

191. Adams PL, Cohen DJ, Danovitch GM, et al: The nondirected live-kidney donor: Ethical considerations and practice guidelines: A National Conference Report. Transplantation 74:582-589, 2002.

192. Levey AS, Hou S, Bush HL: Kidney transplantation from unrelated living donors: Time to reclaim a discarded opportunity. N Engl J Med 314:914-916, 1986.

193. Bay WH, Hebert LA: The living donor in kidney transplantation. Ann Intern Med 106:719-727, 1987.

194. Brenner BM, Meyer TW, Hostetter TH: Dietary protein intake and the progressive nature of kidney disease. N Engl J Med 307:652-660, 1982.

195. Sutherland DE, Weiland D, Chavers B, et al: Information and long-term follow-up of a large number of related kidney donors at a single institution. Neth J Med 28:254-256, 1985.

196. Hakim RM, Goldszer RC, Brenner BM: Hypertension and proteinuria: Long-term sequelae of uninephrectomy in humans. Kidney Int 25:930-936, 1984.

197. Anderson CF, Velosa JA, Frohnert PP, et al: The risks of unilateral nephrectomy: Status of kidney donors 10 to 20 years postoperatively. Mayo Clin Proc 60:367-374, 1985.

198. Talseth T, Faucald P, Skrede S, et al: Long term blood pressure and renal function in kidney donors. Kidney Int 29:1072-1076, 1986.

199. Miller IJ, Suthanthiran M, Riggio RR, et al: Impact of renal donation. Long term clinical and biochemical follow-up of living donors in a single center. Am J Med 79:201-208, 1985.

200. Smith S, Laprad P, Grantham J: Long-term effect of uninephrectomy on serum creatinine concentration and arterial blood pressure. Am J Kidney Dis 6:143-148, 1985.

201. Colbaugh P, Stastny P: Antigens in human monocytes, III. Use of monocytes in typing for HLA-D related (DR) antigens. Transpl Proc 10:871-874, 1978.

202. Moraes JR, Stastny P: A new antigen system expressed in human endothelial cells. J Clin Invest 60:449-454, 1977.

203. Opelz G, Terasaki PI: Effect of blood group on relation between HLA match and outcome of cadaver kidney transplants. Lancet 1:220-222, 1977.

204. Toma H, Tanabe K, Tokumoto T: Long-term outcome of ABO-incompatible renal transplantation. Urol Clin North Am 28:769-780, 2001.

205. Rydberg L: ABO-incompatibility in solid organ transplantation. Transfus Med 11:325-342, 2001.

206. Noreen HJ: Interpretation of crossmatch tests. *In* Nikaein A, Phelan DL, Mickelson EM, et al (eds): American Society for Histocompatibility and Immunogenetics Laboratory Manual, 3rd ed. Lenexa, KS, ASHI, 1994, pp I.C.1.1-I.C.1.13.

207. Suthanthiran M, Garovoy MR: Immunologic monitoring of the renal transplant recipient. Urol Clin North Am 10:315-325, May 1983.

208. Iwaki Y, Cook DJ, Terasaki PI, et al: Flow cytometry crossmatching in human cadaver kidney transplantation. Transplant Proc 19:764-766, 1987.

209. Chapman JR, Taylor CJ, Ting A, Morris PJ: The positive crossmatch: Antibody class and specificity correlate with graft outcome. Transplant Proc 19(1 Pt 1):725-726, Feb 1987.

210. Thistlewaite JR, Buckingham MM, Stuart JK, et al: T cell immunofluorescence flow cytometry crossmatch results in cadaver donor renal transplantation. Transplant Proc 19:722-724, 1987.

211. Ting A: The lymphocytotoxic crossmatch test in clinical transplantation. Transplantation 35:403-407, 1983.

212. Ahern AT, Artruc SB, Della Pelle P, et al: Hyperacute rejection of HLA-AB identical renal allografts associated with B lymphocyte and endothelial reactive antibodies. Transplantation 33:103-106, 1982.

213. Buckingham JM, Geiss WP, Giacchino JL, et al: B-cell directed antibodies and delayed hyperacute rejection: A case report. J Surg Res 27:268-274, 1979.

214. Lobo PI: Nature of autolymphocytotoxins present in renal hemodialysis patients: Their possible role in controlling alloantibody formation. Transplantation 32:233-237, 1981.

CHAPTER 65

Clinical Aspects of Renal Transplantation

Colm C. Magee and Edgar Milford

THE RENAL TRANSPLANT SURGERY PROCEDURE

Cadaveric Kidney Transplantation

In adult recipients the donor kidney is transplanted into the extraperitoneal space of the right or left lower abdominal quadrant. The donor renal artery (or arteries) are usually excised in continuity with a small piece of aorta (a Carrel patch), which facilitates creation of an optimal vascular anastomosis. An end-to-side anastomosis to the external iliac, common iliac, or hypogastric artery is usually created. The renal vein(s) is usually anastomosed to the corresponding vein. The transplant ureter is either placed directly into the bladder wall using an antireflux technique or anastomosed to the recipient ureter. The latter method minimizes the risk of vesicoureteric reflux but usually requires ipsilateral nephrectomy. When there is a concern regarding the viability of the ureteric anastomosis, a temporary stent is inserted. Keeping the bladder catheter in situ for up to 5 days after surgery (depending on the type of urinary anastomosis) minimizes pressure in the urinary tract. Some surgeons place drains in the perinephric area; these should be removed as soon as drainage volumes are insignificant.

Living Donor Kidney Transplantation

The technique for living donor kidney transplantation is similar to that described for cadaveric donor transplantation except that a patch of donor aorta or vena cava cannot be used. Hence, creation of the vascular anastomoses can be more complicated. Laparoscopic retrieval of kidneys from donors is being increasingly employed; this method is not without drawbacks, however (Table 65-1). In particular, the incidence of early graft dysfunction is higher, probably because of the increased intra-abdominal pressure required during surgery, longer warm ischemia times, less experience with the technique, and more manipulation of the renal vessels.

Other Surgical Methods of Transplantation

Transplantation of kidneys into children and transplantation of two kidneys into one donor are more complicated and

TABLE 65-1

Donor and Recipient Outcomes in Living Donor Transplantation Using Open or Laparoscopic Nephrectomy

	OPEN NEPHRECTOMY	LAPAROSCOPIC NEPHRECTOMY
Donor		
Postoperative pain	++	+
Surgical scarring	++	+
Hospital stay	++	+
General recovery time	++	+
Long-term outcomes	Excellent	Unknown; probably excellent
Recipient		
Early graft dysfunction	0	+
Long-term outcomes	Excellent	Unknown; probably excellent

0, minimum; +, mild; ++, moderate; +++, severe.

beyond the scope of this chapter. Pancreas-kidney transplantation is associated with a higher incidence of technical complications (discussed later).

Surgical Complications of the Transplant Procedure

Surgical complications of renal transplantation have greatly decreased in incidence over the last 20 years, primarily due to improvements in surgical technique, in general medical and anesthesia care, and in immunosuppressive regimens. Major postoperative bleeding and wound infections are now relatively rare. Vascular and urologic complications are also less common but remain important causes of early allograft dysfunction (see later). Obesity and increased age are risk factors for postoperative complications.[1]

Perinephric lymphoceles have been reported to occur in up to 15% of transplant recipients.[2] They are formed by drainage from locally severed lymphatic vessels. The majority produce no symptoms and are noted incidentally on ultrasound. Some lymphoceles, particularly when large, can compress the ureter (causing obstruction) or the iliac veins (causing swelling and even thrombosis of the lower limb); some simply cause localized abdominal swelling. The differential diagnosis for a peritransplant fluid collection also includes seroma, hematoma, and urinoma. Often the clinical setting and the sonographic findings strongly suggest the collection is a lymphocele. Aspiration and analysis of fluid can confirm the diagnosis (but is rarely required): the creatinine concentration is equivalent to the plasma concentration, the protein content is high and the %lymphocytes is high. When graft excretory function is good, the fluid creatinine concentration will be much higher than the plasma concentration if the collection is a urinoma.

Treatment of lymphoceles is required only when they cause complications—the majority should be left alone. Percutaneous aspiration by strict aseptic technique is useful for the initial diagnosis and treatment, but recurrence is extremely common. To prevent recurrence, either external drainage with subsequent injection of a sclerosing agent or

internal drainage (marsupialization) is required. The latter can often be performed by laparoscopic technique. Management of lymphoceles is reviewed in an article by Odland.[2]

CURRENTLY USED IMMUNOSUPPRESSIVE AGENTS IN RENAL TRANSPLANTATION

Overview

Because the T lymphocyte plays a critical role in the rejection response, this cell is the primary target of immunosuppressive strategies.[3] Various steps in T cell activation and replication can be targeted, and these are shown in Figure 65-1. Many immunosuppressants, however, have additional effects on other immune cells such as B lymphocytes and mononuclear phagocytes. In broad terms, currently used agents can be classified as (1) antibodies that target receptors on the surface of the T cell; (2) calcineurin inhibitors (CNIs); (3) glucocorticoids; (4) inhibitors of purine synthesis; and (5) targets of rapamycin inhibitors.

Because the risk of rejection is greatest in the early post-transplant period, maximum immunosuppression is given at this time and progressively decreased in the weeks thereafter. Current initial immunosuppression usually consists of glucocorticoids plus CNIs plus mycophenolate mofetil (MMF); antibody preparations are sometimes added. Maintenance immunosuppression usually consists of lower doses of the first three agents. The rationale for such "triple therapy" is that adequate immunosuppression can be achieved without the need for toxic doses of any one agent. The availability of more antirejection medications has allowed more patient-specific immunosuppression. Unfortunately, accurate titration of total immunosuppressive dose is still not achievable. The properties of currently used maintenance agents are summarized in Table 65-2.

Nonspecific Antilymphocyte Antibodies

Two main preparations of nonspecific antilymphocyte antibodies are currently available: OKT3 and polyclonal antibodies. OKT3 is a mouse monoclonal antibody raised against the CD3-receptor complex on human T cells. Polyclonal antibody preparations such as antithymocyte globulin (ATG) or thymoglobulin are manufactured by immunizing horses or rabbits, respectively, with human lymphoid tissue. The harvested globulin fraction from the animals contains multiple antibodies directed against different leukocyte antigens.

Both OKT3 and the polyclonals are powerful, nonspecific immunosuppressive agents, with all the risks and benefits this property entails. They are prescribed in two situations: (1) as additional *initial* immunosuppression (usually for the first 5 to 14 days post-transplant) to patients with delayed graft function (DGF) or patients who are at high risk of acute rejection; and (2) for reversal of severe acute rejection. There are no large-scale studies comparing OKT3 and the polyclonals. Overall, their effectiveness is approximately equivalent; the polyclonals are probably better tolerated.[4-6] There is some evidence that rabbit thymoglobulin is more effective than other polyclonal preparations; this probably reflects more sustained depletion of recipient lymphocytes.

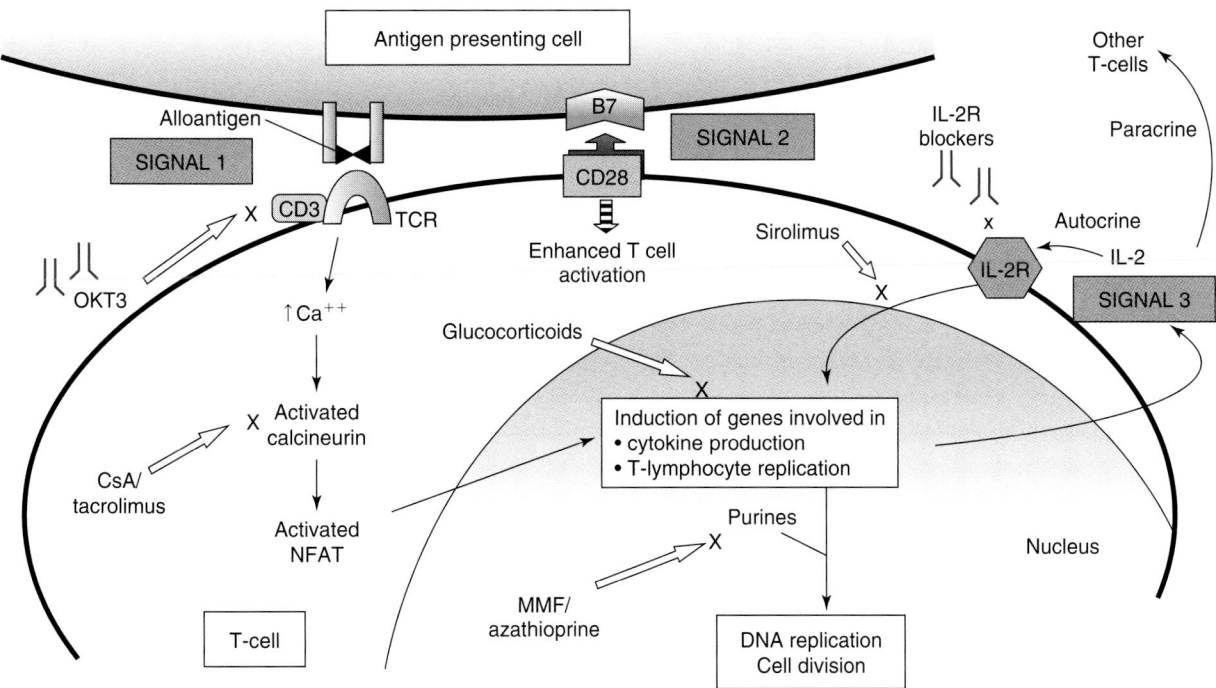

FIGURE 65-1. Stages of T cell activation: multiple targets for immunosuppressive agents. *Signal 1:* The Ca^{2+}-dependent signal induced by T-cell receptor stimulation results in calcineurin activation, a process inhibited by CsA and tacrolimus. Calcineurin dephosphorylates NFAT (nuclear factor of activated T cells), enabling it to enter the nucleus and bind to the interleukin 2 (IL-2) promoter. Glucocorticoids bind to cytoplasmic receptors, enter the nucleus, and inhibit cytokine gene transcription in both the T cell and antigen presenting cell (APC). Glucocorticoids also inhibit NF-kB activation (not shown). *Signal 2:* Costimulatory signals, such as those between CD28 on the T cell and B7 on the APC, are necessary to optimize T cell transcription of the IL-2 gene, prevent T cell anergy, and inhibit T cell apoptosis. Experimental agents interrupt these signals. *Signal 3:* IL-2 receptor stimulation induces the cell to enter the cell cycle and proliferate. IL-2 and related cytokines have both autocrine and paracrine effects. Signal 3 may be blocked by IL-2 receptor antibodies or by sirolimus. Further downstream, azathioprine and mycophenolate mofetil (MMF) inhibit progression into the cell cycle by inhibiting purine and therefore DNA synthesis.

TABLE 65-2

Drugs Used in Maintenance Immunosuppression

DRUG	MECHANISM OF ACTION	ADVERSE EFFECTS
Glucocorticoids	Block synthesis of several cytokines, including IL-2; multiple anti-inflammatory effects	Glucose intolerance, hypertension, hyperlipidemia, osteoporosis, osteonecrosis, myopathy, cosmetic defects; growth suppression in children
Cyclosporine	Inhibits calcineurin: synthesis of IL-2 and other molecules critical for T cell activation thereby inhibited	Nephrotoxicity (acute and chronic), hyperlipidemia, hypertension, glucose intolerance, cosmetic defects
Tacrolimus	Similar to cyclosporine, although binds to different cytoplasmic protein (FKBP)	Broadly similar to cyclosporine; diabetes mellitus more common; hypertension, hyperlipidemia and cosmetic defects less common
Azathioprine	Inhibits purine biosynthesis; lymphocyte replication therefore inhibited	Bone marrow suppression; rarely pancreatitis, hepatitis
MMF	Inhibits de novo pathway of purine biosynthesis (relatively lymphocyte selective); lymphocyte replication therefore inhibited	Bone marrow suppression, gastrointestinal upset; invasive CMV disease more common than with azathioprine
Sirolimus	Sirolimus-FKBP complex inhibits TOR; lymphocyte proliferation to cytokines thereby inhibited	Bone marrow suppression, hyperlipidemia, interstitial pneumonitis; enhances toxicity of cyclosporine

MMF, mycophenolate mofetil; FKBP, FK-binding protein; TOR, target of rapamycin; IL-2, interleukin-2; CMV, cytomegalovirus.

Humanized/Chimeric Anti–interleukin-2 Receptor Monoclonal Antibodies

Unlike OKT3 and the polyclonals, these have the potential for more specific immunosuppression because the full interleukin-2 (IL-2) receptor is only expressed on activated T cells. Humanization or chimerization of the antibody minimizes the problem of recipient generation of antimouse antibodies (a problem with repeat courses of OKT3), thus prolonging drug half-life and efficacy. Randomized, controlled trials have demonstrated an approximate one-third reduction in acute rejection rates with daclizumab or basiliximab compared with placebo, although the maintenance regimens used in these trials are not current standard of care.[7, 8]

Attempts to incorporate these agents into CNI-free regimens have led to high acute rejection rates. Ongoing studies are assessing the benefits of these agents in the setting of DGF.[9] These preparations are well tolerated with minimal toxic effects reported to date. They are indicated only for initial immunosuppression, not for the treatment of acute rejection. The role of the IL-2 receptor blockers in renal transplantation remains to be defined.

Calcineurin Inhibitors: Cyclosporine

Cyclosporine (formerly cyclosporin A) functions as an inhibitor of calcineurin, thereby reducing the synthesis of several critical T cell growth factors, including IL-2 (see Fig. 65-1). Acute rejection rates and 1-year graft outcomes have improved significantly since the introduction of cyclosporine. Important adverse effects include nephrotoxicity, hypertension, hyperlipidemia, glucose intolerance, hirsutism, and gum enlargement. Nephrotoxicity is troublesome because it may be difficult to clinically distinguish from other causes of acute and chronic dysfunction. Trough blood concentrations have traditionally been used to guide dosing, but retrospective and prospective studies have shown that lower C_2 concentrations (concentrations 2 hours after ingestion of cyclosporine) correlate well with the risk of acute rejection[10, 11]; to date, however, there are no studies showing better outcomes with C_2 monitoring.

A microemulsion formulation of cyclosporine with improved bioavailability and more consistent pharmacokinetics has replaced the standard preparation. There does appear to be a lower rate of acute rejection in de novo transplant recipients with the microemulsion compared with the standard formulation. The issue of converting stable patients from standard cyclosporine to cyclosporine microemulsion is a matter of center preference because no consistent benefits of such intervention have been shown. Generic versions of "improved bioavailability" cyclosporine are now available.

Because cyclosporine (and tacrolimus) are metabolized by the intestinal and hepatic cytochrome P450 systems, drugs that induce or inhibit these systems should be used with caution; more frequent monitoring of cyclosporine concentrations is required.

The contribution of long-term cyclosporine therapy to chronic renal allograft dysfunction is controversial. Although long-term deterioration in transplant or *native* kidney function in cyclosporine-treated patients is well documented, many clinicians think that chronic rejection—presumably reflecting inadequate immunosuppression—is a more important contributor to graft loss than is chronic cyclosporine nephrotoxicity (see later discussion).

Tacrolimus (FK-506)

Although tacrolimus is structurally distinct from cyclosporine, its mode of action, drug interactions, and side effects, including nephrotoxicity, are quite similar. Trough blood concentrations are also used to guide dosing. Its advantages over cyclosporine include lower rates of acute rejection, less hyperlipidemia, less hypertension, fewer cosmetic complications, and better reversal of refractory acute rejection. Steroid dosages can probably be lower with tacrolimus. Its disadvantages over cyclosporine include more neurotoxicity, more

nephrotoxicity, more gastrointestinal toxicity (particularly when combined with MMF), and more pancreatic toxicity (i.e., post-transplant diabetes mellitus is more common), although these problems are less common with the lower dosages currently employed. Thus, tacrolimus should be initially prescribed in patients at high risk of rejection or when cosmetic effects are a major concern. In general, patients on cyclosporine should be considered for conversion to tacrolimus if they have rejection, hyperlipidemia, or severe hypertension. Otherwise, the choice of cyclosporine or tacrolimus is mainly one of center preference. There is now some evidence that medium-term outcomes are better with tacrolimus than cyclosporine.[12]

Azathioprine

Azathioprine is a purine analog that inhibits DNA and RNA synthesis. It thereby inhibits proliferation of cells, including T and B lymphocytes. Bone marrow suppression is the most common side effect, but at doses of 1–2 mg/kg/day, azathioprine is usually well tolerated. It has been widely used in clinical transplantation for 30 years, but its role in maintenance therapy is being superseded by MMF. Azathioprine is inactivated by xanthine oxidase, the enzyme inhibited by allopurinol. If allopurinol therapy for recurrent gout is required (a relatively common problem in transplant patients), the dosage of azathioprine must be greatly reduced to avoid life-threatening bone marrow suppression.

Mycophenolate Mofetil

Mycophenolate mofetil (MMF) is a reversible inhibitor of inosine monophosphate dehydrogenase, the rate-limiting enzyme in de novo purine synthesis. Because B and T lymphocytes are mainly dependent on the de novo pathway for synthesis of guanosine nucleotides, the antiproliferative effect of MMF should be relatively lymphocyte specific. However, trials using doses of 2–3 g/day have not shown a lower incidence of bone marrow suppression compared to azathioprine.[13] A pooled analysis of three trials has shown that MMF (compared with placebo or azathioprine) halved the incidence of acute rejection in the first year post-transplant from 40% to 20%.[14] Registry and trial data also suggest better long-term graft outcomes.[15, 16] MMF is now the antiproliferative agent of choice in many centers. Blood concentrations are not monitored, although there is evidence of interpatient variability in its pharmacokinetics.[17] Higher doses of MMF may be required in black compared with nonblack recipients to effectively prevent acute rejection.[18]

The principal adverse effects are nausea, vomiting, and diarrhea—these usually respond to dose reduction. Tissue-invasive cytomegalovirus (CMV) infection may be more common; pneumocystosis is less common. MMF is not nephrotoxic. The combination of MMF and tacrolimus is highly effective in preventing acute rejection[19, 20] but is associated with a high incidence of adverse gastrointestinal effects. This probably reflects the higher MMF plasma concentrations obtained when the drug is prescribed with tacrolimus rather than cyclosporine.[21]

Glucocorticoids

Despite their well-known adverse effects, glucocorticoids remain a cornerstone of immunosuppression in most patients.

Their dosage is progressively decreased after transplantation to a maintenance regimen of prednisone 5 to 10 mg/day. The adverse effects of steroids are well known; of particular importance in the post-transplant setting are hyperlipidemia, hypertension, glucose intolerance, and osteoporosis. Unfortunately, even in stable transplant patients, complete withdrawal of steroids increases the risk of short-term and long-term graft dysfunction.[22] Newer "minimal-steroid" regimens incorporating various combinations of thymoglobulin, tacrolimus, MMF, and sirolimus are encouraging, but adequate long-term data are not yet available.[23, 24]

Sirolimus

Sirolimus (rapamycin) is the most recently licensed maintenance immunosuppressive agent in renal transplantation. Sirolimus blocks the proliferative responses of T and B lymphocytes—and probably other cell types—to cytokines. It binds to the same intracellular protein (FK-binding protein [FKBP]) as tacrolimus, but its mechanism of action is distinct; in particular, it does not directly inhibit calcineurin.[25] Instead, the sirolimus-FKBP complex binds to and inhibits a kinase called the *target of rapamycin*. Target of rapamycin is central to a pathway by which receptors for growth factors control the cell cycle.

The prolonged elimination half-life of sirolimus means that once-daily dosing is sufficient. Like the CNIs and many other drugs, it is metabolized via the cytochrome P450 system; thus, the potential for multiple drug interactions exists. Adverse effects of sirolimus include impaired wound healing, diarrhea, hyperlipidemia, anemia, thrombocytopenia, and interstitial pneumonitis.

In one major randomized, controlled trial, the combination of sirolimus, cyclosporine, and steroids was associated with a lower incidence of acute rejection compared to an azathioprine, cyclosporine, and steroid regimen.[26] Creatinine clearance was lower, however, in the sirolimus-treated patients, possibly reflecting enhanced cyclosporine nephrotoxicity (sirolimus has no intrinsic nephrotoxicity). Early data regarding the use of sirolimus in CNI-free regimens,[27] early CNI withdrawal regimens,[28] or low-dose tacrolimus regimens are somewhat encouraging.[29] Of potentially great clinical importance is the ability of sirolimus to impair proliferation of fibroblasts and other cells thought to be implicated in the pathophysiology of chronic allograft nephropathy (CAN). Data on long-term outcomes with sirolimus are not yet available. The role of this agent in routine maintenance therapy remains to be defined.

EVALUATION OF THE RECIPIENT IMMEDIATELY BEFORE THE TRANSPLANT

The general pretransplant workup is reviewed in Chapter 64.

Medical Status

The potential recipient of a renal transplant should be evaluated to ensure that there are no new contraindications to transplantation and general anesthesia. This is more relevant to recipients of cadaveric grafts, where the date of surgery cannot be planned. Occasionally, new medical problems such as chest pain, peritonitis, foot ulcers, and catheter-related

sepsis preclude or delay transplantation. A common question is whether hemodialysis, with its attendant delay of surgery and prolongation of cold ischemia time, is required. Preoperative hemodialysis is advisable if either a plasma K level higher than 5.5 mmol/L or severe volume overload are present. A short session of 1.5 to 2 hours of hemodialysis using minimal anticoagulation usually suffices. Patients on peritoneal dialysis need only drain out instilled fluid prior to surgery; if the patient is hyperkalemic, several rapid exchanges can be performed.

Immunologic Status

A pretransplant crossmatch of a recent donor serum against recipient lymphocytes must always be performed. The purpose of this is to detect preformed antibodies against the human leukocyte antigens (HLAs) of the donor. Prospective recipients should be specifically asked if they have recently received a red blood cell transfusion. For patients who are not high risk (Table 65-3), an enhanced antihuman globulin cytotoxicity assay is adequate screening for alloantibodies. The presence of cytotoxic donor IgG antibodies by this assay is a contraindication to immediate transplantation. Non-HLA autoantibodies (many of which are of the IgM isotype) can cause false-positive lymphocytotoxicity results; the serum can be treated to inactivate these antibodies. Not all IgM antibodies are benign, however.

For immunologically "high-risk" patients (see Table 65-3), many centers prefer to use the flow cytometry crossmatch (FCXM). This can detect very low concentrations of anti-donor antibodies. In high-risk patients, a negative antihuman globulin crossmatch but positive FCXM against donor T cells is a relative contraindication to transplantation. The clinical importance of an isolated positive B cell FCXM is less clear. Thus, the clinical significance of a positive crossmatch depends on the particular test used and the baseline immunologic status of the potential recipient. Close consultation with the tissue typing laboratory is essential.

CLINICAL APPROACH TO ALLOGRAFT DYSFUNCTION

Immediate Post-transplant Period
Evaluation of the Recipient Immediately after the Transplant

The nephrologist should carefully review the operating room notes with particular emphasis on the following: cold and warm ischemia times, technical difficulties encountered, intraoperative fluids administered, blood pressure, and urine output. Immediate excellent urine output, which should be

TABLE 65-3

Factors Suggesting a Recipient Is High Risk for Acute Rejection

Previous blood transfusions, particularly if recent
Previous pregnancies, particularly if multiple
Previous allograft, particularly if rejected early
History of high panel-reactive antigen (>50%)
Black race

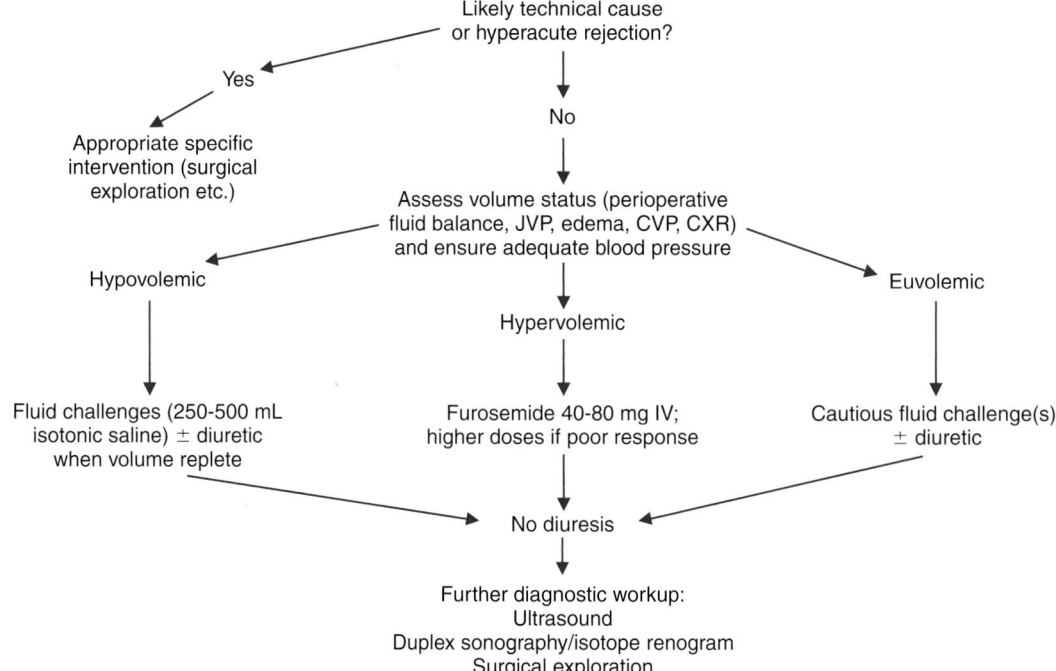

FIGURE 65-2. Management of renal allograft nonfunction or oliguria immediately after transplant. CVP, central venous pressure; CXR, chest x-ray; JVP, jugular venous pressure.

the norm with living donor transplants, greatly simplifies management. More complicated is the management of the oligoanuric recipient. This is discussed later, and an algorithm of management is shown in Figure 65-2.

Patients can be divided into three groups based on allograft function in the first post-transplant week: those with DGF, those with slow graft function (SGF), and those with excellent graft function. DGF is usually defined as failure of the renal allograft to function immediately post-transplant, with the need for one or more dialysis sessions within a specified period, usually 1 week. The management of DGF is discussed in detail later. Excellent graft function implies adequate urine output and rapidly falling plasma creatinine. Management of those with excellent function (almost all living donor recipients and a highly variable percentage of cadaveric kidney recipients) is relatively simple and includes adjustment of immunosuppression, maintenance of euvolemic state, and so forth. Routine imaging studies are not required. SGF defines a group of recipients with moderate early graft dysfunction. One definition is plasma creatinine level higher than 3 mg/dL and no dialysis at 1 week after transplant.[9] The causes, management, and outcomes of SGF are similar to DGF (see later). Interventions that simply convert SGF to DGF may have little effect on graft outcomes; more important but difficult is achieving immediate excellent function in most grafts.[9]

Delayed Graft Function

Delayed graft function (DGF) is a clinical diagnosis. Using requirement for dialysis as the sole criterion for diagnosis excludes some patients with residual native kidney function, however. Criteria for dialyzing patients post-transplant

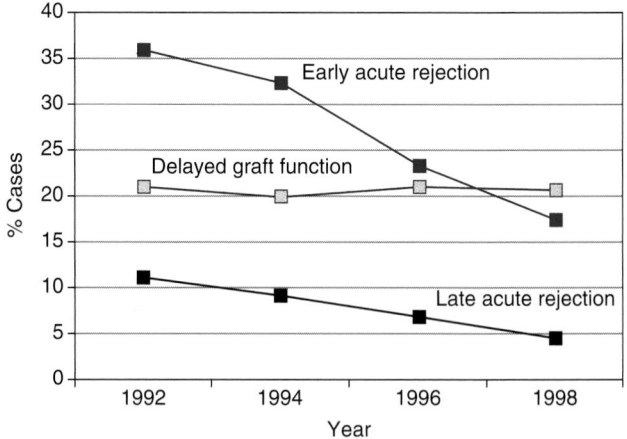

FIGURE 65-3. Annual incidences of early acute rejection, late acute rejection, and delayed graft function. Adapted from Gjertson DW: Impact of delayed graft function and acute rejection on kidney graft survival. Clin Transpl 467-480, 2000.

differ between centers. Recent United Network for Organ Sharing (UNOS) data show a 21% incidence of DGF, which is unchanged since 1991 (Fig. 65-3).[30]

Table 65-4 lists the causes of DGF, considered as prerenal, intrarenal, and postrenal insults. Frequently there is overlap of causes, in particular between ischemia and rejection. Ischemic acute tubular necrosis (ATN) is by far the most common cause of DGF; in fact, the two terms are often used interchangeably, although they are *not* equivalent.

Risk factors for DGF include recipient factors such as male sex, black race, longer duration on dialysis, higher panel-reactive antigen (PRA) status, and greater degree of HLA mismatching; donor factors such as use of cadaveric kidneys (especially if marginal), greater donor age, longer cold ischemia time, and nontraumatic death.[30] Most of these factors mediate their effects via ischemia reperfusion injury and immunologic mechanisms. Older studies suggested that CNIs prolonged and/or worsened DGF[31]; this is probably less of an issue with currently employed doses.

The diagnosis of the underlying cause of DGF is based on clinical, radiologic, and sometimes histologic findings. Figure 65-2 illustrates an algorithm for the diagnosis and management of transplant kidney nonfunction/oliguria immediately after surgery. Careful review of the donor history and of the harvesting and transplantation process provides clues as to the etiology of DGF. Note that interpretation of the urine output requires knowledge of the pre-transplant native kidney output. Prerenal and postrenal causes (including simple problems such as urinary catheter malposition or obstruction) should be excluded. A response to a fluid challenge implicates prerenal factors. If administration of fluids and diuretics fails to improve urine output,

further investigation is warranted, the urgency of which depends on the individual case. Persistent oliguria of a living donor kidney despite adequate volume expansion and administration of high-dose loop diuretics requires immediate radiologic evaluation of renal blood flow (by duplex study or isotope renography, or both) or immediate surgical re-exploration since the cause of impaired function is much more likely to be a major surgical complication than ATN. In contrast, a cadaveric kidney at high risk of ischemic ATN (e.g., elderly donor, prolonged ischemia time) would generally be less urgently investigated.

Radiologic evaluation of the graft is undertaken to assess perfusion and to rule out urinary obstruction or leakage. Standard ultrasonography is useful because it is inexpensive, noninvasive, and usually effective in excluding postrenal causes of renal failure. Duplex sonography is helpful in assessing renal arterial and venous blood flow but cannot reliably distinguish intrarenal causes based on changes in intrarenal vascular resistance. Isotope renography may provide additional information regarding renal perfusion and function. It is useful in confirming absent renal blood flow suggested by duplex studies. In rare cases, the presence of a urine leak or of urinary tract obstruction is detectable by renography but not by initial ultrasonography. Although intrarenal insults can result in typical renographic abnormalities, reliably distinguishing the causes (such as ATN or rejection) is again not possible.

In many cases of DGF, prerenal and postrenal causes can be excluded, and the clinical and radiologic findings are consistent with an intrarenal insult. Definitive diagnosis of the underlying cause requires allograft biopsy. The decision to biopsy depends mainly on the duration of DGF and the likelihood of the underlying cause being ATN as opposed to a more graft-threatening cause such as rejection. An algorithm for diagnostic biopsy and treatment of persistent DGF is shown in Figure 65-4. Specific treatment of DGF depends on the underlying cause and is discussed in the following sections.

TABLE 65-4

Causes of Delayed Graft Function

Prerenal

Severe hypovolemia/hypotension
Renal vessel thrombosis

Intrarenal

Ischemic ATN
Hyperacute rejection
Accelerated or acute rejection superimposed on ATN
Acute cyclosporine/tacrolimus nephrotoxicity (±ATN)

Postrenal

Urinary tract obstruction/leakage

ATN, acute tubular necrosis.

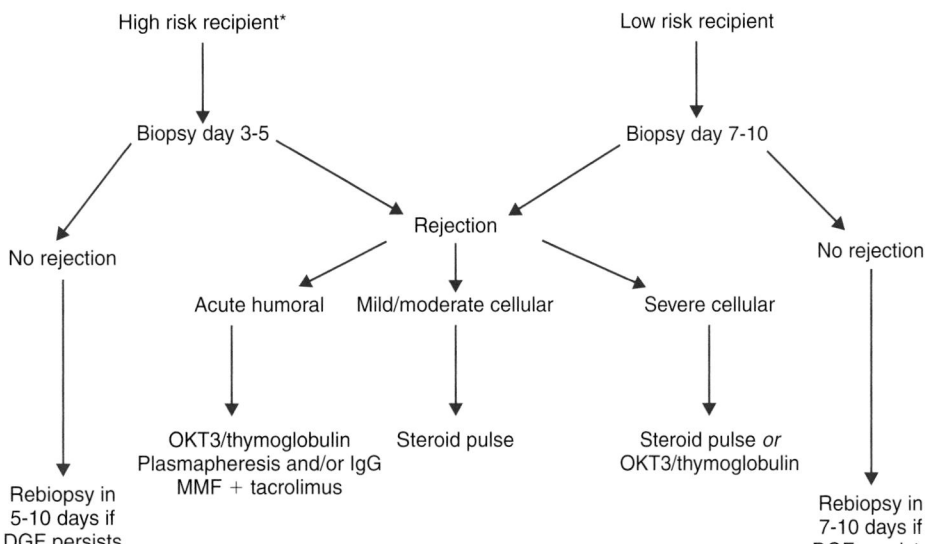

FIGURE 65-4. Algorithm for diagnostic biopsy of and treatment for persistent delayed graft function (DGF). *The presence of anti-donor HLA antibodies should prompt immediate biopsy in this setting.

CAUSES OF DELAYED GRAFT FUNCTION

Ischemic Acute Tubular Necrosis

Ischemic ATN is the most common cause of DGF in cadaveric kidney transplant recipients. The etiology of ATN in transplanted kidneys is presumed to be similar to that in native kidneys. At multiple steps during the surgical transplantation procedure, the cadaveric graft is at risk of ischemic damage (Table 65-5). Reperfusion injury via mechanisms such as direct endothelial trauma, oxygen free radical damage, and neutrophil activation also contribute to the development of this condition.[32]

There are no clinical or radiologic features unique to transplant ATN. As is the case with acute renal failure (ARF) in native kidneys, transplant ATN should be a diagnosis of exclusion. Several of the risk factors identified in Table 65-5 may be present. Radiologic studies confirm intact graft perfusion and are consistent with an intrarenal insult (i.e., a high resistive index by duplex or slow clearance of radiotracer in the kidney). Histology, if available, shows tubule cell damage and necrosis similar to that found in native kidneys with ATN, although transplant tubular necrosis is more overt. Patchy interstitial lymphocytic infiltrates but not tubulitis may be present. The natural history of uncomplicated ATN is one of spontaneous resolution. Usually improvements in urine output begin from 5 to 10 days post-transplant, but ATN may persist for weeks.

Management of the patient during this period is supportive, including avoidance of fluid overload and nutritional support and dialysis as needed. Glucose/insulin and albuterol are useful in controlling hyperkalemia and thus postponing the requirement for dialysis. Sorbitol-based ion exchange resins should be avoided in the early postoperative period because of the risk of colonic dilation and perforation. Although there are no randomized, controlled trials of the effects of frequent versus minimal hemodialysis in the setting of DGF, many centers try to minimize hemodialysis in the belief that it will exacerbate ischemic damage to the allograft. When hemodialysis is required, minimal anticoagulation should be used to reduce the risk of postsurgical bleeding. Intradialytic hypotension must be avoided. Although there is little direct evidence for the superiority of biocompatible over bioincompatible hemodialysis membranes in the setting of post-transplant ATN, biocompatible membranes are usually employed. In general, peritoneal dialysis is best avoided in the first week post-transplant because of the risk of peritonitis or leakage of dialysis fluid into the wound area.

A major concern in the management of the patient with post-transplant ATN is that the diagnosis of new-onset surgical or medical complications involving the graft is difficult. Rejection, for example, may be easily missed. In fact, acute rejection occurs more frequently in grafts with delayed as opposed to immediate function. The postulated mechanism is that ischemia and reperfusion injury increase the immunogenicity of the graft, thereby predisposing to acute rejection. Experimental animal models have demonstrated that ischemic ATN is associated with increased expression/production within the renal parenchyma of class I and II major histocompatibility complex (MHC) molecules, costimulatory molecules, proinflammatory cytokines, and adhesion molecules.[32] Such an altered local milieu could amplify alloimmune responses. A high degree of suspicion for additional complications related to the allograft must therefore be maintained. The possibility of accelerated acute rejection must be considered, particularly in the high-risk recipient. We recommend a low threshold for performing core kidney biopsies in patients with DGF (see Fig. 65-4). Radiologic evaluation of the graft should also be repeated to detect new urinary or vascular complications.

In the case of DGF secondary to ischemic ATN, an initial immunosuppression regimen incorporating antilymphocyte antibody preparations has been advocated. This has the potential benefit of avoiding CNI nephrotoxicity, which theoretically might prolong ATN, while reducing the chances of occult rejection in the nonfunctioning graft. Recipients are weaned from antibody therapy onto a CNI when graft function improves, such as when the plasma creatinine level falls below 5 mg/dL. Data from our own institution suggest that intraoperative thymoglobulin shortens the duration of DGF, possibly by blockade of multiple receptors on human leukocytes.[33] The advantages and disadvantages of antibody therapy in the setting of DGF are summarized in Table 65-6. Recent UNOS data suggest that antibody induction protocols slightly reduce the incidence of early acute rejection episodes in recipients with DGF and slightly improve graft survival.[34] There is speculation that IL-2 receptor blockers might be a less toxic and equally effective alternative to OKT3 or the polyclonals in delayed CNI introduction protocols, at least in patients at low risk of rejection.[9] This theory requires confirmation. The addition of sirolimus might maintain a low rate of acute rejection.[35] There is concern, however, that sirolimus may prolong ATN.

TABLE 65-5

Causes of Ischemic Damage to the Cadaveric Renal Allograft

Preharvest Donor State

Shock syndromes
Endogenous and exogenous catecholamines
?Brain injury
Nephrotoxic drugs

Organ Procurement Surgery

Hypotension
Trauma to renal vessels
Inadequate flushing

Organ Transport and Storage

Prolonged storage (cold ischemia time)
Pulsatile perfusion injury

Transplantation of Recipient

Prolonged second warm ischemia time
Trauma to renal vessels
Hypovolemia/hypotension

Postoperative Period

Cyclosporine/tacrolimus
Acute heart failure, myocardial infarction
?Hemodialysis

Hyperacute Rejection

Hyperacute rejection is now a rare cause of immediate renal allograft nonfunction. It is caused by preformed recipient antibodies reacting with antigens on the endothelial surface

TABLE 65-6

Advantages and Disadvantages of Various Induction Regimens in DGF

VARIABLE	POLYCLONALS	OKT3	IL-2 RECEPTOR BLOCKERS
Effectiveness in preventing early acute rejection	+++	+++	++
Effectiveness in reversing acute rejection	+++	+++	?
Increased risk of opportunistic infection	++	++	0
Increased risk of neoplasia	++	++	0
Cytokine release syndrome	+	++	0
Sensitization, affecting future use of product	+	++	0
Cost	+++	+++	+++

0, minimal; +, low; ++, medium; +++, high.

DGF, delayed graft function; IL-2, interleukin-2.

of the allograft, activating the complement and coagulation cascades. These antibodies can be directed against antigens of the ABO blood group system or against HLA class I antigens. Anti-HLA class I antibodies are formed in response to previous transplantation, blood transfusion, or pregnancy. Rarer causes are mediated by anti-HLA class II antibodies (associated with a positive B cell crossmatch) or antidonor endothelium/monocyte antibodies (these are not detected in the standard crossmatch). In classic hyperacute rejection, macroscopic changes are seen minutes after vascular anastomosis is established. Clinically, there is cyanosis and mottling of the kidney, anuria, and sometimes disseminated intravascular coagulopathy. Radiologic studies confirm absent or minimal renal perfusion, in contrast to ATN where blood supply is relatively well maintained. Histology shows widespread small vessel endothelial damage and thrombosis, usually with neutrophil polymorphs incorporated into the thrombus. There is no effective treatment, and transplant nephrectomy is indicated. Screening for recipient-donor ABO or class I MHC incompatibility (the presence of the latter is often referred to as a "positive T cell crossmatch") has ensured that hyperacute rejection is now uncommon. Rare cases occur because of clerical errors or due to the presence of the other preformed antibodies described earlier that are not detected by routine screening methods.

Several centers have described small series in which antidonor HLA antibodies have been removed by immunoadsorption prior to transplantation. Although this technique may allow transplantation of highly sensitized patients, rates of rejection and graft loss were relatively high. Recently, reports of pretransplant treatment with tacrolimus, MMF, plasmapheresis, and intravenous IgG have been more encouraging.[36, 37] In fact, repeat courses of intravenous IgG alone may adequately desensitize some patients.[38] Transplantation appears to be safe and well tolerated if the immediate pretransplant crossmatch is negative.

Accelerated Rejection Superimposed on Acute Tubular Necrosis

Accelerated acute rejection refers to rejection episodes occurring roughly between days 2 and 5 post-transplant. It is usually mediated by the humoral immune system. The cause is thought to be pretransplant sensitization of the recipient to donor alloantigens. Titers of alloantibody are too low to give a positive pretransplant lymphocytotoxicity crossmatch, but "second set" antibody production occurs rapidly after transplant. Patients who have a negative pretransplant

TABLE 65-7

Clinical, Flow Cytometric, and Histologic Differences between Pure Forms* of ACR and AHR

	ACR	AHR
Clinical onset	>5 days	>3 days
Donor-specific antibody	Usually absent	Present
Tubulitis	Present	Absent
Neutrophil polymorphs in glomerular and peritubular capillaries	Absent	Present
C4d staining of peritubular capillaries	Absent	Present
Primary therapy	Steroids	Plasmapheresis, IgG OKT3/polyclonals, tacrolimus, MMF

*There can be overlap.

ACR, acute cellular rejection; AHR, acute humoral rejection; MMF, mycophenolate mofetil.

lymphocytotoxicity crossmatch but a positive FCXM are at greater risk of developing this form of rejection.

Accelerated acute rejection may be superimposed on ischemic ATN, in which case there may be no signs of rejection, or it may occur in an initially functioning allograft. Diagnosis is made by renal biopsy and crossmatch findings. Histology usually shows evidence of predominantly antibody rather than cell-mediated immune damage. Typical features on light microscopy are the presence of thromboses in glomeruli and in small vessels and of neutrophil polymorphs in peritubular capillaries.[39] Immunofluorescence shows that the fibrinoid material contains immunoglobulin, complement, and fibrin. Recently, staining of the peritubular capillaries for C4d has been proposed as a reliable marker of acute humoral rejection.[40] In most cases, donor-specific antibody (DSA) is detectable against class I HLA antigens and less commonly against class I or II HLA antigens. Table 65-7 shows distinguishing features of acute cellular and humoral rejection.

Early diagnosis of this condition is crucial. Thus, high-risk patients with ongoing DGF should have biopsy and crossmatch studies performed 3 to 5 days after transplantation (see Fig. 65-4). Traditionally, reversing acute humoral rejection was difficult and the prognosis for the graft poor.

A regimen of plasmapheresis (to immediately remove DSA and possibly other humoral mediators of rejection) and enhanced immunosuppression (to suppress further production of DSA) is now yielding excellent results.[41] Single-center reports of using immunoadsorption rather than plasma exchange are also encouraging.[42]

Acute Cyclosporine or Tacrolimus Nephrotoxicity Superimposed on Acute Tubular Necrosis

Cyclosporine or tacrolimus, especially in high doses, causes an acute reversible decrease in glomerular filtration rate (GFR) by renal vasoconstriction, particularly of the afferent glomerular arteriole. Potentially, such vasomotor effects could exacerbate ischemic ATN. The clinical significance of these effects at currently employed doses of CNIs is unclear. Nevertheless, this is one reason thymoglobulin or OKT3 is substituted for CNIs in the setting of DGF (see previous). This is discussed in more detail later.

Vascular and Urologic Complications of Surgery

Renal vessel thrombosis, urinary leaks, and obstruction are rarer but important causes of DGF. These complications may also cause allograft dysfunction in the early postoperative period and are discussed later in this chapter.

OUTCOME AND SIGNIFICANCE OF DELAYED GRAFT FUNCTION

Patients with DGF require longer hospitalization and more investigations and are at higher risk of occult rejection. Postoperative fluid and electrolyte management are more difficult. In most cases, recovery of renal function is sufficient to become independent of dialysis. In less than 5% of cases do allografts with delayed function never recover: these are said to have *primary non-function.* However, although the majority become independent of dialysis, most studies have demonstrated that recipients with DGF have poorer long-term graft outcome compared to those without. Whether or not this effect is mediated by immune mechanisms (the increased risk of rejection), non-immune mechanisms or both is disputed. However, a recent multivariable analysis of UNOS data concerning renal transplants performed between 1985 and 1992 showed that DGF was an *independent* predictor of long-term graft loss, lowering half-lives by approximately 30%.[30] The additional presence of acute rejection further impacted on long-term survival. The importance of ischemic injury is further emphasized by the impressive graft survival outcomes in living nonrelated donor transplantation where ischemic times are very short and HLA matching is poor.

Measures to limit the incidence and duration of DGF are therefore very worthwhile. Obvious strategies include optimization of the hemodynamic status of the donor and recipient. As discussed in a recent review, donor management has traditionally been neglected.[43] Invasive vascular monitoring is useful in some patients for titrating fluid administration; in most cases, a central venous pressure line is sufficient. Intraoperative mean arterial pressure should be maintained higher than 70 mm Hg. Perioperative administration of high doses of mannitol, hetastarch, and similar high-osmolality compounds should be avoided because they have been associated with ARF in the non-transplant setting.[44] Meticulous surgical technique, rapid

transport of harvested grafts, and use of optimum preservation solutions are also of obvious extreme importance. Use of University of Wisconsin (UW) preservation solution during the cold ischemia period reduces the incidence of DGF, and its use is now standard practice in most centers. Whether machine perfusion of cadaveric renal allografts is more effective than simple cold storage in preventing DGF and improving long-term graft function remains controversial.[9] It is certainly more expensive and complex. Prospective, controlled trials where one kidney from each donor is allocated to machine perfusion and the other to cold storage (thus controlling for donor factors) have yielded conflicting results.[45, 46] There is some evidence that machine perfusion of grafts from non–heart-beating donors lowers the incidence of DGF.

The benefits and risks of induction therapy with anti-lymphocyte antibody preparations in the setting of DGF have been discussed briefly earlier. Calcium channel blockers have been shown in experimental models to prevent ischemic injury and attenuate CNI-mediated renal vasoconstriction. These properties suggested that administration of calcium channel blockers to cadaveric kidney transplant recipients in the perioperative period or to the donor before organ harvesting might reduce the incidence and duration of ischemic ATN. Unfortunately, studies have not provided definitive answers. Perioperative administration of dopamine to the recipient is of no benefit. Atrial natriuretic peptide has been of limited benefit in the setting of nontransplant ATN and is therefore unlikely to find use in the transplant situation. Attempts to prevent neutrophil-mediated reperfusion injury and adhesion molecule interaction have been of limited benefit.[47-49] Other strategies under investigation include the use of trimetazidine and prostaglandin E_1.[9] Unfortunately, DGF from ATN is likely to remain a significant problem in cadaveric kidney transplantation, particularly as the use of marginal donors continues to increase.

A national system that preferentially allocates cadaveric kidneys to zero HLA-mismatched recipients will result in prolongation of cold ischemia time in some cases. This is because of inevitable delays with matching of organs to recipients, transport of organs, and other reasons. Such a system operates in many countries, including the United States. Overall, national sharing of HLA-matched organs does has a benefit on allograft outcomes.[50, 51] Matas and Delmonico and others have recently advised several measures which should reduce cold ischemia times.[52, 53] These include faster identification of potential recipients and establishment of a list of patients in each transplant region who would quickly accept marginal kidneys.

Early Post-transplant Period

Table 65-8 shows the causes of allograft dysfunction during the early (1- to 12-week) post-transplant period. There is obviously some overlap in the causes of delayed and early allograft dysfunction. Despite its known limitations, the primary measure of early and late transplant function remains the plasma creatinine level. It is worthwhile to immediately recheck the plasma creatinine to confirm any increase and to determine its trend. Again, prerenal and postrenal failure should be systematically excluded.

TABLE 65-8

Causes of Allograft Dysfunction in the Early Postoperative Period

Prerenal

Hypovolemia/hypotension
Renal vessel thrombosis
Drugs: ACE inhibitors, NSAIDs
Transplant renal artery stenosis

Intrarenal

Acute rejection
Acute CNI nephrotoxicity
CNI-induced thrombotic microangiopathy
Recurrence of primary disease
Acute pyelonephritis
Acute interstitial nephritis

Postrenal

Urinary tract obstruction/leakage

ACE, angiotensin-converting enzyme; CNI, calcineurin inhibitor; NSAID, nonsteroidal anti-inflammatory drug.

TABLE 65-9

Risk Factors for Renal Vessel Thrombosis

RISK FACTOR	COMMENT
Pediatric recipient	Especially if < 6 years; reflects technical difficulties
Pediatric donor	Especially if < 6 years; reflects technical difficulties
History of thromboembolism or multiple-access thromboses	Should always be sought in the pretransplant evaluation
Antiphospholipid antibody syndrome and other thrombophilic states*	Presence of antiphospholipid antibodies or laboratory abnormalities alone does not necessarily increase risk

*Factor V Leiden, prothrombin gene mutations, and probably others.

Prerenal Dysfunction in the Early Post-transplant Period

HYPOVOLEMIA AND DRUGS

Hypovolemia may develop secondary to excessive diuresis from the transplanted kidney or from diarrhea. Diarrhea is a common adverse effect of the MMF plus tacrolimus combination. Patients accustomed to rigid fluid restriction on dialysis may have difficulty maintaining adequate fluid intake. Angiotensin-converting enzyme inhibitors (ACE-Is) and nonsteroidal anti-inflammatory drugs (NSAIDs) should be avoided in the early post-transplant period because of the risk of functional prerenal failure with the often fluctuating volume status; this risk is probably enhanced by the renal vasoconstrictive effects of CNIs.

RENAL VESSEL THROMBOSIS

Transplant renal artery or renal vein thrombosis usually occurs in the first 72 hours but may be delayed for up to 10 weeks post-transplant. Acute vascular thrombosis is the most common cause of graft loss in the first post-transplant week. Although poor surgical technique is undoubtedly a factor in some cases, there is now greater appreciation of the contributing role of hypercoagulable states.[54] Risk factors for renal vessel thrombosis are shown in Table 65-9.

Renal artery thrombosis presents with abrupt onset of anuria (unless there is a native urine output), rapidly rising plasma creatinine, but often little localized graft pain or discomfort. Duplex studies show absent arterial and venous blood flow. Renography shows absent perfusion and absent visualization of the transplanted kidney. Removal of the infarcted kidney is indicated.

Renal vein thrombosis also manifests with anuria and rapidly increasing plasma creatinine. Pain, tenderness, swelling in the graft, and hematuria are more pronounced than in renal artery thrombosis. Life-threatening complications such as embolization or graft rupture and hemorrhage may occur. Duplex studies show absent renal venous blood flow and characteristic highly abnormal renal arterial signals. Transplant nephrectomy is usually indicated. If the venous thrombosis extends beyond the renal vein, anticoagulation is necessary to reduce the risk of embolization. There are reports of salvaging renal function after early diagnosis of renal vessel thrombosis and its treatment with thrombolysis or thrombectomy. In almost all cases, however, infarction occurs too quickly to make this treatment worthwhile. Furthermore, thrombolysis is relatively contraindicated in the early post-transplant period because of the high risk of graft-related bleeding.

Meticulous surgical technique and avoidance of hypovolemia minimize the incidence of this devastating complication. Patients at high risk of renal vessel thrombosis should be anticoagulated immediately after surgery. Patients with a history of unexplained thromboembolic events should probably be tested before transplantation for the more common thrombophilic states such as antiphospholipid antibody syndrome (APS), activated protein C resistance, and mutations of the prothrombin gene. Readers are referred to recent reviews on this topic.[54] The duration and intensity of anticoagulation depend on the individual patient. For example, patients with known APS should be heparinized immediately after surgery and converted to lifelong warfarin with a target International Normalized Ratio (INR) greater than 3.0. The presence of antiphospholipid antibodies alone (i.e., without a history of thrombosis) does not warrant such aggressive anticoagulation. These antibodies are sometimes found in end-stage renal disease (ESRD) patients without pathologic sequelae.

Intrarenal Dysfunction in the Early Post-transplant Period

ACUTE REJECTION

Acute rejection is defined as an acute deterioration in renal allograft function associated with specific pathologic changes in the graft. Most cases of acute rejection occur in the first 6 months post-transplant, but this complication may occur at any time. With ongoing improvements in immunosuppression, the incidence of acute rejection continues to decrease. UNOS data show a decline in the reported incidence of early (0 to 6 months after transplant) acute rejection from 37% in 1991 to 18% in 1998 (see Fig. 65-3).[30]

Acute rejection is presumed to involve cellular and humoral immune mechanisms, but evidence of cell-mediated responses predominates on most biopsies. With current immunosuppression regimens, symptoms and signs of acute rejection are rarely pronounced, but fever, oliguria, and graft pain or tenderness may occur. Note that a raised plasma creatinine concentration is a relatively late marker of pathologic changes occurring within the graft, hence, the interest in developing markers of early immune system activation that precedes rejection. Renographic and sonographic studies are usually abnormal in acute rejection, but the changes are not specific enough to exclude other causes. Definitive diagnosis requires biopsy, but where there is a high likelihood of uncomplicated acute cellular rejection, empirical treatment is sometimes instituted.

The Banff classification (Table 65-10) is a widely used schema for classifying rejection. The classic histologic findings in acute cell-mediated rejection are (1) edema and mononuclear cell infiltration of the interstitium, mainly with CD4+ and CD8+ T lymphocytes but also with some macrophages and plasma cells, and (2) tubulitis (infiltration of tubule epithelium by lymphocytes). Glomerular involvement is rare. Vascular involvement (endothelialitis) is frequently a focal process and may be easily missed on biopsy. Here, mononuclear cells undermine endothelium and the endothelial cells are swollen and detached. Endothelialitis reflects more severe rejection. The term *vascular rejection* is best avoided because it fails to distinguish between cell-mediated vascular damage (endothelialitis) and humoral-mediated vascular damage (necrotizing arteritis). Whatever the predominant cause, vasculitis is associated with a poorer prognosis.[39] Adequate tissue is essential to avoid underdiagnosis of vasculitis.[39, 55]

Focal infiltrates of mononuclear cells without endothelialitis or tubulitis may occur in the presence of stable allograft function; treatment is not required. Conversely, histologic evidence of rejection can also be seen in the presence of stable allograft function, and there is evidence to support its treatment.[56] Infiltration of the interstitium with neutrophil polymorphs is unusual and should suggest the alternative diagnosis of infection. The presence of eosinophils in the cellular infiltrate suggests severe rejection, but allergic interstitial nephritis should also be considered. This is further discussed later. Differences between acute cellular and humoral

TABLE 65-10

Banff Classification of Renal Allograft Pathology

1. Normal
2. Antibody-mediated rejection
3. Borderline changes ("suspicious" for acute rejection); foci of mild tubulitis only
4. Acute/active rejection
   Type I: moderate or severe tubulitis
   Type II: mild, moderate, or severe intimal arteritis
   Type III: transmural arteritis and/or arterial fibrinoid change and necrosis of medial smooth muscle cells
5. Chronic sclerosing/allograft nephropathy; graded as mild (I), moderate (II), severe (III) based on degree of interstitial fibrosis and tubular atrophy
6. Other (changes not considered to be due to rejection)

Adapted from Racusen LC, Solez K, Colvin RB, et al: The Banff 97 working classification of renal allograft pathology. Kidney Int 55: 713-723, 1999.

rejection are summarized in Table 65-7. It should be noted that acute humoral rejection is being increasingly diagnosed—possibly because of more transplantation of high risk recipients and increased availability of better diagnostic tools, such as C4d staining. Note that polyoma virus infection may also be associated with tubulointerstitial nephritis.

Uncomplicated acute cellular rejection is generally treated with a short course of high-dose steroids, the so-called pulse treatment. Typically 500 to 1000 mg/day of methylprednisolone is given intravenously for 3 to 5 days. There is a 60% to 70% response rate to this regimen.[57] OKT3 and the polyclonals are highly effective in treating first rejection episodes, reversing them in more than 80% of cases.[57] Because of cost and toxicity, these agents are usually reserved for steroid-resistant cases or when there is severe rejection on the initial biopsy. After completion of pulse therapy, the maintenance oral steroid dose can be resumed immediately, although some centers prefer to taper back to the maintenance dose. An episode of acute rejection implies that prior immunosuppression has been inadequate. The patient's compliance with prescribed medications should be reviewed. If there are no contraindications, baseline immunosuppression should be increased, at least in the short term. Thus, patients on azathioprine should be converted to MMF. Patients on a CNI should probably have the dosage increased. In many centers, patients who reject while on cyclosporine are converted to tacrolimus.

Steroid-resistant acute rejection cases, defined somewhat arbitrarily as failure of improvement in urine output or plasma creatinine within 5 days of starting pulse treatment, are usually treated with OKT3 or polyclonal preparations. If steroid treatment was based on an empirical rather than a histologic diagnosis of acute rejection, a renal biopsy should be performed to confirm this diagnosis before starting treatment with these agents. The response rate to OKT3/polyclonals in these situations is higher than 80%.[58] Treatment of acute rejection with OKT3 may be associated with an increase in plasma creatinine 3 to 4 days into the course. This transient nephrotoxic effect is presumed to be mediated by increased release of cytokines such as tumor necrosis factor-α. OKT3 should be continued because this effect is transient and does not herald a poorer response to the drug. Rebound rejection may occur after OKT3 treatment, but this is usually mild and reversible with pulse steroids.

The most important adverse effects of OKT3/polyclonals—the increased risk of life-threatening infections and lymphoproliferative disease—are well known and should prompt careful analysis of the risks and benefits associated with their use in the treatment of aggressive rejection. There is limited evidence that OKT3 is more effective than ATG as primary therapy for acute rejection and for reversing steroid-resistant acute rejection. One randomized, controlled trial has shown rabbit thymoglobulin to be more effective than ATG as primary therapy for acute rejection.[59] There are no head-to-head comparisons of rabbit thymoglobulin to OKT3. Therefore, OKT3 or rabbit thymoglobulin is the preferred therapy. Finally, as discussed later, it is important to continue antimicrobial prophylaxis during and after the treatment of acute rejection, whatever the agents used.

REFRACTORY ACUTE REJECTION. Refractory acute rejection is generally defined as acute rejection resistant to a course of OKT3/polyclonals. By definition, the patient has already received aggressive immunosuppression; the risks and benefits of further amplifying immunosuppression should be carefully considered. Renal histology is helpful in this regard. A component of humoral rejection must be excluded. Therapeutic options include (1) continuing maintenance immunosuppression in the hope that renal function will slowly improve; (2) repeating a course of antilymphocyte antibody therapy; or (3) switching from cyclosporine to tacrolimus if the patient is on the former drug. Option No. 2 implies very aggressive immunosuppression and should rarely be used. Uncontrolled studies of tacrolimus rescue therapy have demonstrated improved renal function in more than 70% of such cases.[60] If repeat courses of OKT3 are used, the dosage may need to be increased in patients who produce neutralizing antimouse antibodies. One small study has suggested that sirolimus is more effective than MMF for "rescue" therapy.[60]

SIGNIFICANCE OF ACUTE REJECTION. Although acute rejection is frequently reversed (at least as assessed by plasma creatinine), retrospective studies show that it strongly associated with development of chronic rejection and poorer allograft survival. Poorer graft outcome also correlates with the severity of rejection, the number of rejection episodes, and with resistance to steroid therapy. Whatever the outcome is in terms of graft function, treatment involves exposing the patient to supplemental immunosuppression and its attendant risks. Reducing the incidence of acute rejection has been a major goal in renal transplantation. Fortunately, the incidence has steadily decreased over the last 20 years, mainly because of improvements in immunosuppression. The CNIs and MMF have been major factors in this regard.

ACUTE CALCINEURIN INHIBITOR NEPHROTOXICITY

The CNIs, especially in high doses, cause an acute reversible decrease in GFR by renal vasoconstriction, particularly of the afferent glomerular arteriole. This is manifested clinically as dose-dependent and blood concentration–dependent acute reversible increases in plasma creatinine concentration. Because acute CNI nephrotoxicity is mainly vasomotor/prerenal, histologic changes in this setting may be unimpressive. Histology may show tubule vacuolization; more prolonged toxicity is associated with hyaline thickening of arterioles[39]; these changes are not specific. Acute CNI nephrotoxicity responds to dosage reduction.

DISTINGUISHING ACUTE CNI NEPHROTOXICITY AND ACUTE REJECTION. Unfortunately, even with the aid of blood drug concentrations, distinguishing acute CNI nephrotoxicity and acute rejection clinically can be difficult. Low and high blood concentrations in the presence of deteriorating renal function suggest but do not imply rejection and drug nephrotoxicity, respectively. Both syndromes can coexist. Pointers toward a diagnosis of acute CNI nephrotoxicity are signs of extrarenal toxicity such as severe tremor, a moderate increase in plasma creatinine (<25% over baseline), and high CNI concentrations (e.g., cyclosporine > 350 ng/mL or tacrolimus levels > 20 ng/mL). Pointers toward a diagnosis of acute rejection are fever; allograft pain and tenderness (although with current drug regimens these symptoms or signs are uncommon); rapid, nonplateauing increases in plasma creatinine; and low drug concentrations (e.g., cyclosporine < 150 ng/mL). Fever and symptoms localized to the allograft do not occur with CNI

toxicity but by no means imply rejection; infections such as acute pyelonephritis must be considered.

The threshold for biopsy depends on the individual patient and perhaps on center practice. An algorithm for approaching this common clinical problem is shown in Figure 65-5. One common strategy is to institute a trial of therapy and, if the clinical response to this is unsatisfactory, to proceed to biopsy within 48 to 96 hours. For example, if acute CNI nephrotoxicity were suspected, the CNI dose would be reduced, which should improve renal function within 24 to 48 hours, were this diagnosis correct. A presumptive diagnosis of acute rejection would mean empirical treatment with a steroid pulse. Lack of response after several days of antirejection treatment because of resistant rejection, CNI nephrotoxicity, or another cause would be diagnosed by biopsy. The threshold for biopsy is lower in high-risk patients: those who are highly sensitized, have previously rejected a graft, or are at high risk of early recurrent primary renal disease (see later). In our center, we aim to minimize the use of empirical steroid pulses; with rapid biopsy (which is safe) and processing of tissue, basic histology is available within 6 to 8 hours. A delay of 6 to 8 hours in initiating specific therapy should not be detrimental to the graft. In addition to determining the degree of cellular and humoral rejection in the graft, histology also occasionally reveals unexpected pathology such as evidence of thrombotic microangiopathy (TMA) or polyomavirus infection. Biopsy results alone should not dictate management; rather, the constellation of clinical and histologic findings should be used to shape a treatment plan.

IMMUNE MONITORING

It has been suggested that measuring the serum or urine concentrations of cytokines, IL-2 receptor, adhesion molecules, or other inflammatory markers such as complement and acute-phase proteins could be useful in diagnosing acute allograft rejection. A serum or urine marker with high positive and negative predictive values might obviate the need for biopsy or aid the follow-up of treated rejection. Quantitative determination by reverse transcription–polymerase chain reaction (PCR) of certain gene transcripts within renal biopsy tissue was recently shown to be a sensitive and specific marker of acute rejection.[61] Combined analysis of Fas ligand, perforin, and granzyme B gene expression yielded the most accurate results. Preliminary data from the same group suggest that expression of these genes in peripheral blood leukocytes also correlates with acute rejection of the renal allograft.[62] Recently, Li and associates reported that quantification of messenger RNA transcripts of perforin and granzyme B in urinary cells was useful in predicting the presence or development of acute rejection.[63]

There are several concerns with regard to the applicability of these assays to clinical practice. First, these markers have not been validated in large-scale, multicenter human studies. Second, they cannot diagnose vascular involvement by rejection. Finally, infections due to CMV, polyomavirus, or other microbes could mimic acute rejection by elevating levels of inflammatory and immunologic markers. Thus, core kidney biopsy with appropriate histology remains the "gold standard" for diagnosing intrarenal causes of allograft dysfunction.

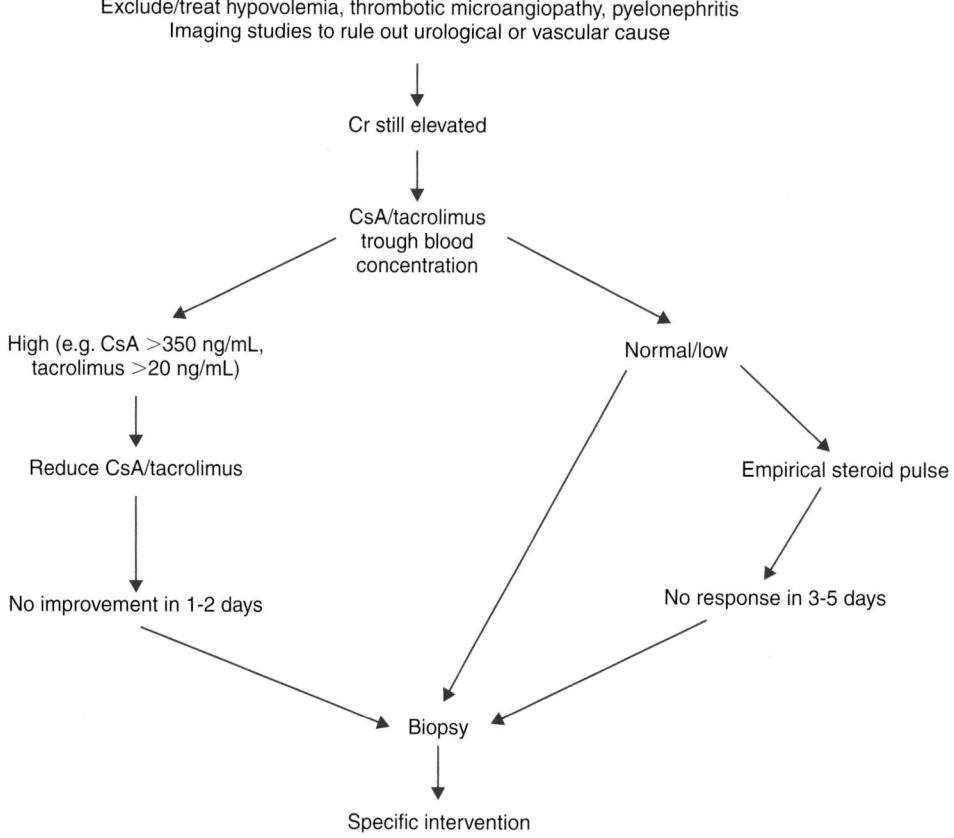

Exclude/treat hypovolemia, thrombotic microangiopathy, pyelonephritis
Imaging studies to rule out urological or vascular cause

↓

Cr still elevated

↓

CsA/tacrolimus trough blood concentration

High (e.g. CsA >350 ng/mL, tacrolimus >20 ng/mL)   Normal/low

↓

Reduce CsA/tacrolimus   Empirical steroid pulse

↓

No improvement in 1-2 days   No response in 3-5 days

Biopsy

↓

Specific intervention

FIGURE 65-5. Algorithm for management of allograft dysfunction in the early post-transplant period.

THROMBOTIC MICROANGIOPATHY

Thrombotic microangiopathy (TMA) after renal transplantation is a rare but serious complication.[64] CNIs and, to a lesser extent, other factors (non-CNI drugs such as OKT3, viral infection, APS) have been associated with development of this syndrome, which is presumed to be initiated by direct endothelial cell damage. Onset is usually in the early post-transplant period. The classic laboratory findings are increasing plasma creatinine and lactate dehydrogenase, thrombocytopenia, falling hemoglobin, and the presence of schistocytes on the blood film. The hematologic features of TMA may be easily missed, however. For example, other drugs such as thymoglobulin or MMF can depress platelet and red blood cell counts, although by different mechanisms. Renal biopsy shows damaged endothelium and thrombosis of glomerular capillaries and arterioles. Somewhat similar clinical and histologic changes may occur in cases of acute humoral rejection, malignant hypertension, recurrent hemolytic-uremic syndrome (HUS) and pulsatile perfusion injury.

The long-term prognosis for graft function is often poor. Early diagnosis of TMA is essential to salvage renal function. There are no controlled trials of therapy for TMA post-transplant. Suggested measures are cessation of CNIs and other implicated drugs and control of any hypertension present. The benefit of plasma exchange or administration of plasma is unclear. We advise avoiding CNIs long term because even switching from one to the other can induce a

second episode of TMA. Although data are lacking, it seems reasonable to treat such patients long term with a combination of MMF, steroids, and sirolimus. There is some evidence that post-transplant TMA may be associated with the presence of antiphospholipid antibodies and hepatitis C virus (HCV) infection.[65]

ACUTE PYELONEPHRITIS

Urinary tract infections (UTIs) may occur at any period but are most frequent shortly after transplantation because of catheterization, stenting, and aggressive immunosuppression. Other risk factors for UTI are anatomic abnormalities and neurogenic bladder. There is evidence that acute pyelonephritis in the early post-transplant period predisposes to acute rejection. Fortunately, acute pyelonephritis and urosepsis are much less common since the widespread use of prophylactic sulfamethoxazole-trimethoprim (SMX-TMP). Fever, allograft pain and tenderness, and raised peripheral blood white blood cell count are usually more pronounced in acute pyelonephritis than in acute rejection. Diagnosis requires urine culture, but empirical antibiotic treatment should be started immediately. The most commonly implicated microorganisms are gram-negative bacilli, coagulase-negative staphylococci, and enterococci—similar to nontransplant patients. Renal function usually returns to baseline quickly with antimicrobial therapy and volume expansion. Recurrent cases of pyelonephritis require investigation to rule out underlying urologic abnormalities.

ACUTE ALLERGIC INTERSTITIAL NEPHRITIS

Distinguishing acute allergic interstitial nephritis and acute rejection is very difficult. In fact, the pathogenesis is somewhat similar in both cases, involving mainly cell-mediated immunity. Fever and rash after ingestion of a new drug favor the former. These clinical features are rarely seen, however. Mononuclear cell and eosinophil infiltration of the transplanted kidney may occur with either condition, but endothelialitis implicates rejection. Polyomavirus infection must also be considered in the differential diagnosis. Both acute allergic interstitial nephritis and acute rejection usually respond to steroids; of course, the suspected drugs must be stopped. SMX-TMP is probably the drug most likely implicated in causing allergic interstitial nephritis in renal transplant patients. NSAIDs have also been reported to cause this syndrome.

RECURRENCE OF PRIMARY DISEASE

Several renal diseases may recur in the early post-transplant period and cause acute allograft dysfunction (diseases that recur later are discussed later) (Table 65-11). The conditions associated with early recurrence in transplanted kidneys may be classified into three groups: (1) glomerulonephritides, (2) metabolic diseases such as primary oxalosis, and (3) systemic diseases such as hemolytic-uremic syndrome/thrombotic thrombocytopenia purpura (HUS/TTP). The incidence of recurrence of primary kidney diseases is difficult to estimate: The original cause of ESRD is often unknown, and most relevant studies are small and retrospective and have variable follow-up periods. Randomized trials of treatment regimens for recurrent disease do not exist. Primary focal segmental glomerulosclerosis (FSGS) is considered in more detail in the following section because of its relatively high frequency of recurrence and its propensity to cause severe graft injury.

PRIMARY FOCAL SEGMENTAL GLOMERULOSCLEROSIS

Primary FSGS has a reported recurrence rate of 20% to 40% and causes graft loss in approximately 50% of recurrent cases.[66] Risk factors for graft loss from recurrence (by analysis of registry data) include white recipient, black donor, younger recipient, and treatment for rejection.[66] Other factors thought to predict recurrence and graft loss are rapidly progressive FSGS in the recipient's native kidneys, mesangial proliferation on the original biopsies, and, particularly, recurrence of disease in a previous allograft. Most cases become manifest hours to weeks post-transplant. This rapidity of recurrence suggests the presence of a pathogenic circulating plasma factor. There is now some experimental evidence for this conclusion. Proteinuria that may be massive is the main clinical feature. Early biopsy is indicated in those at risk who develop proteinuria. Early biopsy may not show FSGS lesions per se, but diffuse effacement of foot processes will be noted on electron microscopy. Treatment options include plasmapheresis[67] or immunoadsorption, high-dose glucocorticoids, high-dose CNIs, and cyclophosphamide, but controlled studies are lacking. ACE-Is help reduce proteinuria. Those at high risk of recurrence should probably be offered cadaveric rather than living donor kidneys.

ANTI–GLOMERULAR BASEMENT MEMBRANE DISEASE

Before transplantation, patients with ESRD due to anti–glomerular basement membrane (GBM) disease should be on dialysis for at least 6 months and have negative anti-GBM serology. If these criteria are fulfilled, post-transplant recurrence is rare. De novo anti-GBM disease can occur in recipients with Alport syndrome (see later).

DE NOVO GLOMERULONEPHRITIS

De novo anti-GBM disease may rarely arise in the early post-transplant period in grafts transplanted into recipients with Alport syndrome. Here the recipient with abnormal type IV collagen α chains produces antibodies against the previously "unseen" normal α chain in the basement membrane of the transplanted kidney. Patients with graft dysfunction should be treated with plasmapheresis and cyclophosphamide. Those with *only* immunofluorescence evidence of recurrence (i.e., linear staining of GBMs by IgG) do not require therapy.[68] Graft failure due to anti-GBM disease is more common in retransplants.

HEMOLYTIC-UREMIC SYNDROME/THROMBOTIC THROMBOCYTOPENIA PURPURA

As with native kidney disease, there are many causes of TMA after renal transplant. De novo TMAs were discussed earlier. Recurrence of classic (diarrhea-associated) HUS/TTP is uncommon. In contrast, recurrence of atypical (non–diarrhea-associated) HUS/TTP, particularly if inherited, is common. In one series of patients with an autosomal recessive form of HUS/TTP, there was recurrence in six of seven cases.[69] In general, the prognosis for the graft is poor if there is recurrence. Even when ESRD is due to the classic form, transplantation should be deferred until the disease is quiescent for at least 6 months.

There is a suggestion from retrospective studies that bilateral nephrectomy before transplantation reduces the risk of recurrence.[70] The prophylactic role of aspirin and other antiplatelet agents is unknown, but their use has been advocated.

Postrenal Dysfunction in the Early Post-transplant Period

The incidence of serious urologic complications and associated morbidity in transplant recipients has decreased significantly over the last 20 years to less than 10% in the first year post-transplant. Graft loss from urologic complications is now rare. Nevertheless, postrenal causes must always be considered in the differential diagnosis of ARF post-transplant. Most urologic complications are secondary to technical factors at the time of transplant and manifest themselves in the early postoperative period, but immunologic factors may play a role in some cases.

URINE LEAKS

Urine leaks usually occur in the first few weeks after transplantation. Leaks may occur at the level of the renal calyx, ureter, or bladder. Causes include infarction of the ureter

TABLE 65-1

Recurrent Disease after Renal Transplantation

DISEASE	APPROXIMATE CLINICAL RECURRENCE RATE IN GRAFT	TIME TO RECURRENCE AFTER TRANSPLANTATION	TREATMENT OF RECURRENCE	LIVING DONOR TRANSPLANTATION	COMMENTS
Glomerulonephritis					
Primary FSGS	40–50%	Hours to weeks	Plasmapheresis, steroids, ACE-I	No, if very high risk for recurrence	Increased risk in children, those with rapid progression to ESRD or previous allograft loss from this condition
IgA GN	35%	2 months onward	ACE-I;?fish oil; if crescentic GN: cytotoxics	Yes	Overall graft survival is equivalent to other renal diseases
Anti-GBM disease	Rare if appropriate delay before transplant	Immediately	Plasmapheresis, cyclophosphamide	Yes	Hold transplant until clinical remission and negative serology for 6-12 months
Metabolic Diseases					
Primary oxalosis	Was high; now much improved	Immediately onward	Prevention is achievable goal	Yes, but cadaveric liver + kidney transplantation often better	Early combined liver + kidney transplantation and intensive perioperative treatment to protect graft are best options
Systemic Diseases					
SLE	<10%	From 1st week	Increased steroids; MMF or cyclophosphamide	Yes	Severe recurrence is rare
Antiphospholipid antibody syndrome	30%	Immediately onward	Prevention with anticoagulation is best	Yes	Can be associated with large-vessel thrombosis and thrombotic microangiopathy
Wegener granulomatosis	10%	From 1st week	Cyclophosphamide	Yes	Avoid transplant if disease active, ? role of monitoring ANCA
HUS/TTP	Depends on cause: atypical > classic HUS	Immediately onward	Plasma exchange/infusion	Yes, if not familial HUS	Recurrence is associated with poor prognosis for graft; hold transplant until disease quiescent > 6 months

FSGS, focal segmental glomerulosclerosis; GN, glomerulonephritis; GBM, glomerular basement membrane; SLE, systemic lupus erythematosus; HUS/TTP, hemolytic-uremic syndrome/thrombotic thrombocytopenic purpura; ACEI, angiotensin-converting enzyme inhibitor; MMF, mycophenolate mofetil; ESRD, end-stage renal disease; ANCA, antineutrophil cytoplasmic antibody.

Adapted from Kotanko, et al: Recurrent GN after transplantation. Transplantation 63:1045-1050, 1997.

(usually the distal part) due to perioperative disruption of its blood supply and breakdown of the ureterovesical anastomosis. Severe obstruction may also result in rupture of the urinary tract with leakage. Clinical features include abdominal pain and swelling; the plasma urea and creatinine concentrations increase secondary to reabsorption of solutes across the peritoneal membrane. If a perirenal drain is being used, however, a urine leak may present with high-volume drainage of fluid. Ultrasound may demonstrate a fluid collection (urinoma); aspiration of fluid from the collection by sterile technique allows comparison of the fluid creatinine with plasma creatinine; this is useful if renal function is good. When renal excretory function is good, the creatinine concentration in the urinoma greatly exceeds that in the plasma.

In cases when ultrasound diagnosis is difficult, renal scintigraphy may be useful in demonstrating extravasation of tracer from the urinary system, provided there is adequate renal function. Rough localization of the site of the leak is sometimes possible by this technique. Antegrade pyelography allows precise diagnosis and localization of proximal urinary leaks. Cystography is the best test to demonstrate a bladder leak.

The clinical features may mimic those of acute rejection. Whenever urine leakage is suspected, a bladder catheter should be immediately inserted to decompress the urinary tract. Selected patients may do well with endourologic treatment. Most cases, however, require urgent surgical exploration and repair. The type of repair depends on the level of the leak and the viability of involved tissues.

URINARY TRACT OBSTRUCTION

Urinary tract obstruction can cause allograft dysfunction at any time after transplantation but is most common in the early postoperative period. The main intrinsic causes are poor implantation of the ureter into the bladder, intraluminal blood clots or slough material, and fibrosis of the ureter due to ischemia or rejection. The main extrinsic cause is an enlarged prostate in elderly men (causing bladder outlet obstruction); less common is compression by a lymphocele or other fluid collection. Rarely, calculi cause transplant urinary tract obstruction and renal dysfunction.

Typical clinical features of urinary tract obstruction are rising plasma creatinine concentration without localizing symptoms. In severe cases, high pressure within the urinary tract may result in rupture. Ultrasound usually demonstrates hydronephrosis. Because some dilation of the transplant urinary collecting system is often seen in the early postoperative period, serial scans showing worsening hydronephrosis may be needed to confirm the diagnosis. Renal scintiscan with diuretic washout is useful in equivocal cases. Percutaneous antegrade pyelography is the best radiologic technique for determining the site of obstruction and can be combined with interventional endourologic techniques. In expert hands, endourologic techniques (e.g., balloon dilation, stenting) may be effective in treating ureteric stenosis and stricture. More complicated cases require open surgical repair. Extrinsic compression requires specific intervention such as draining of the lymphocele. Obstruction in the early postoperative period due to an enlarged prostate should be

managed with bladder catheter drainage and drugs such as tamsulosin.

Late Acute Allograft Dysfunction

The causes and evaluation of *late* (>6 months post-transplant) acute renal allograft dysfunction are broadly similar to those of early acute dysfunction. Acute prerenal failure may occur at any time, and the causes are similar to those seen with native kidneys, such as shock syndromes and ACE-I or NSAID hemodynamic effects. Urinary tract obstruction must also be considered in the differential diagnosis. At this point, the causes of obstruction are similar to those associated with native kidney disease, including stones, bladder outlet obstruction, and neoplasia. Several causes of late acute allograft dysfunction are reviewed in more detail in the following sections.

LATE ACUTE REJECTION

With standard immunosuppressive protocols, acute rejection is uncommon after the first 6 months. Black patients appear to be at high risk of late acute rejection and graft loss. Late acute rejection should alert the physician to prescription of inadequate immunosuppression or patient noncompliance. Risk factors for noncompliance include younger age, more immunosuppressant side effects, lower socioeconomic status, minority status, and psychological stress or illness.[71] Transplant physicians should be alert to the possibilities of poor compliance in all their patients. Interventions that might reduce this problem include reiteration of the ongoing risk of rejection and the importance of daily intake of antirejection medication, simplification of the overall medicine regimen, and social worker assistance with high-risk cases.

Cessation of steroids is well known to increase the risk of deterioration of graft function over the long term. Acute rejection may also occur when steroids are stopped. Hence, patients must be carefully monitored for elevations in creatinine when maintenance steroids are stopped. Stopping CNIs may improve renal function but, again, some patients develop acute rejection.

Late acute rejection has a particularly deleterious effect on long-term graft outcome. Gjertson's recent analysis showed that late acute rejection had a more negative impact on graft survival than early acute rejection or DGF.[30] Late acute rejection reduced graft half-lives by approximately 50%.

The aggressiveness of antirejection therapy depends on the clinical situation and biopsy findings. The primary treatment is usually pulse steroids. If there is significant reversibility based on the graft histology and the time course of elevation in plasma creatinine, therapy in addition to pulse steroids can be used (see refractory acute rejection earlier). Some physicians are reluctant to use OKT3/polyclonals more than 6 months after transplantation, but reasonable outcomes have been reported.[72]

LATE ACUTE CALCINEURIN INHIBITOR NEPHROTOXICITY

Although lower doses of CNIs are generally prescribed after the first 6 to 12 months, acute CNI toxicity may occur at any

TABLE 65-12

Commonly Used Drugs Which May Induce Acute Renal Failure in Renal Transplant Recipients

DRUG	PATHOPHYSIOLOGY	COMMENT
NSAIDs	Functional prerenal failure, particularly if hypovolemia or renal artery stenosis present; rarely interstitial nephritis	Avoid in renal transplant patients
Acyclovir, foscarnet (high dose)	Crystal deposition in tubules causing obstruction and damage; also ATN	Hydration prevents crystal deposition
ACE-I, ARB	Functional prerenal failure, particularly if hypovolemia or renal artery stenosis present	Monitor renal function carefully after starting these drugs; avoid in early post-transplant period
SMX-TMP	High-dose SMX-TMP impairs tubular secretion of creatinine (no effect on GFR); rarely interstitial nephritis	In general, drug is well tolerated in transplant recipients
Amphotericin	Proximal and distal tubular damage; cumulative dose effect	Lysosomal preparation is less nephrotoxic but very expensive
Interferon-alfa	Immune stimulating effects promote acute rejection; other nephrotoxic effects reported	Risk/benefit of using interferon-alfa must be determined for individual patient
Erythromycin, verapamil, diltiazem, ketoconazole	Inhibit metabolism of cyclosporine/tacrolimus	Monitor cyclosporine/tacrolimus concentrations carefully
Statins (e.g., simvastatin)	Concentrations increased with concomitant cyclosporine therapy, increasing risk of rhabdomyolysis	Use lowest dose initially; monitor CK; pravastatin is the safest of this class
Radiocontrast	Hemodynamic effects; other effects	Hydration and use of minimum-volume nonionic contrast media reduce risk of contrast nephropathy; no data on acetylcysteine, but worth trying

NSAID, nonsteroidal anti-inflammatory drug; ACE-I, angiotensin-converting enzyme inhibitor; ARB, angiotensin receptor blocker; SMX-TMP, sulfamethoxazole-trimethoprim; ATN, acute tubular necrosis; GFR, glomerular filtration rate; CK, creatine kinase.

time after transplant. Intake of medications that impair metabolism of the CNIs (Table 65-12) may induce acute deterioration in renal function, but this should be reversible with appropriate drug adjustment.

TRANSPLANT RENAL ARTERY STENOSIS

Transplant renal artery stenosis can arise at any time after transplantation. The incidence is unclear: Retrospective studies report functionally significant stenosis in approximately 8% of transplanted patients. Luminal narrowing of 70% to 80% is probably required to render a stenosis functionally significant. The stenosis may occur in the donor or recipient artery or at the anastomotic site. Stenosis of the recipient iliac artery may also compromise renal arterial flow. Causes include operative trauma to these vessels, atheroma of the recipient vessels, and possibly immunologic factors. Suggestive signs of functionally significant stenoses are resistant hypertension, fluctuating renal function especially with hypovolemia or ACE inhibition, edema, new bruits over the kidney, and polycythemia.

The gold standard for diagnosis is renal angiography. Both magnetic resonance (MR) angiography and duplex sonography—in experienced hands—are highly sensitive in diagnosing transplant renal artery stenosis and are adequate screening tests. MR angiography has the advantage of better imaging the iliac arteries. Percutaneous transluminal angioplasty has been the treatment of choice. The clinical response rate to angioplasty is approximately 40% to 75%. Restenosis is relatively common and may require repeat intervention. Short- and medium-term results (albeit from small series) with angioplasty plus stenting have

been good. Surgical repair is sometimes performed when angioplasty has failed or is not possible. This is generally considered difficult and associated with a high frequency of graft loss, but good results have been reported from specialist centers.

To minimize radiocontrast toxicity from angiography, the following are advised: administration of normal saline before and after the procedure and use of minimum volume radiocontrast (the non-nephrotoxic agents, gadolinium or CO_2, can be substituted for much of the imaging). Although no data are available regarding the use of acetylcysteine in transplant recipients, it is reasonable to use this agent.

INFECTIONS CAUSING LATE ACUTE ALLOGRAFT DYSFUNCTION

Human Polyomavirus Infection

The polyomaviruses are DNA viruses, the best known of which are the BK virus, JC virus, and SV40 virus. Sixty percent to 80% of all adults have serologic evidence of past (usually subclinical) exposure. Reactivation of polyomavirus infection with shedding of infected urothelial cells (decoy cells) is estimated to occur in 10% to 60% of renal transplant recipients.[73] The clinical features associated with infection of renal transplant patients include asymptomatic infection (most common), acute graft dysfunction, and hemorrhagic cystitis. The acute graft dysfunction usually occurs secondary to interstitial nephritis, although ureteric stenosis has been described. Over the last 5 years polyomavirus has been increasingly recognized as an important cause of allograft interstitial nephritis. This probably reflects more recognition and reporting of the disease but also the effects of more powerful maintenance immunosuppression regimens incorporating MMF and tacrolimus.

Diagnosis of polyomavirus-associated interstitial nephritis obviously requires allograft biopsy. The presence of intranuclear tubule cell inclusions by light microscopy should raise suspicion of significant polyomavirus infection. This should be confirmed by immunohistochemistry. One retrospective study has found that testing for polyomavirus DNA in plasma samples by PCR is a useful marker of significant graft infection.[74] These interesting findings require confirmation in larger, prospective studies.

It is difficult to distinguish viral infection alone from infection plus superimposed rejection. Reduction in immunosuppression, in an attempt to augment host mechanisms of viral clearance, is the best option. Repeat biopsy is often required to monitor the status of infection and rejection. The long-term outlook for graft survival is often poor. There is very limited evidence that cidofovir has clinically important antipolyomavirus effects in patients with acquired immunodeficiency syndrome. Its efficacy in renal transplant recipients is unknown; it is potentially very nephrotoxic.

Hepatitis C and Interferon-α

HCV infection of the recipient may complicate all forms of solid-organ transplantation but is of particular importance in hepatic and renal transplantation. Infection of the recipient usually occurs pretransplant but may also arise from transplantation of HCV-infected kidneys. There is wide geographic variation in the prevalence of HCV infection in dialysis and transplant patients. Predictably, immunosuppression accelerates the progression of this systemic disease in some recipients. This does not mean that HCV-infected patients should forego transplantation. In fact, although

HCV-positive dialysis and transplant patients had poorer survival compared to HCV-negative controls, transplantation still conferred a survival benefit over dialysis in those with HCV infection.[75]

The purpose of investigating and treating HCV infection both pretransplant and post-transplant is to eliminate viral replication or, at least, slow progression to cirrhosis. The management of the pretransplant HCV-positive patient has not been standardized. Most experts recommend liver biopsy in all transplant candidates to guide prognosis and therapy.[76, 77] An algorithm for management of the HCV-positive pretransplant patient is shown in Figure 65-6. The response rates to interferon-alfa monotherapy are often higher in dialysis than in nondialysis patients. However, ribavirin is relatively contraindicated in the former group because of its accumulation in renal failure and associated risk of severe anemia.

Risk factors for progression of liver disease after transplant include use of OKT3/polyclonals, coinfection with hepatitis B, and alcohol abuse. The management of progressive HCV disease in renal transplant recipients remains unsatisfactory. Reduction in immunosuppression is the first step, and this obviously increases the risk of rejection. Treatment with interferon-alfa may induce temporary remission, but the rate of relapse is high. Furthermore, the risk of provoking acute graft dysfunction with this drug via rejection or other mechanisms is high.[78] Acute renal transplant failure associated with interstitial edema on biopsy has also been reported. There is speculation that the direct nephrotoxic effects of interferon-alfa may depend to some extent on the preparation used and its purity. In nontransplanted patients, better control of HCV infection is obtained with use of pegylated forms of interferon-alfa with or without ribavirin.

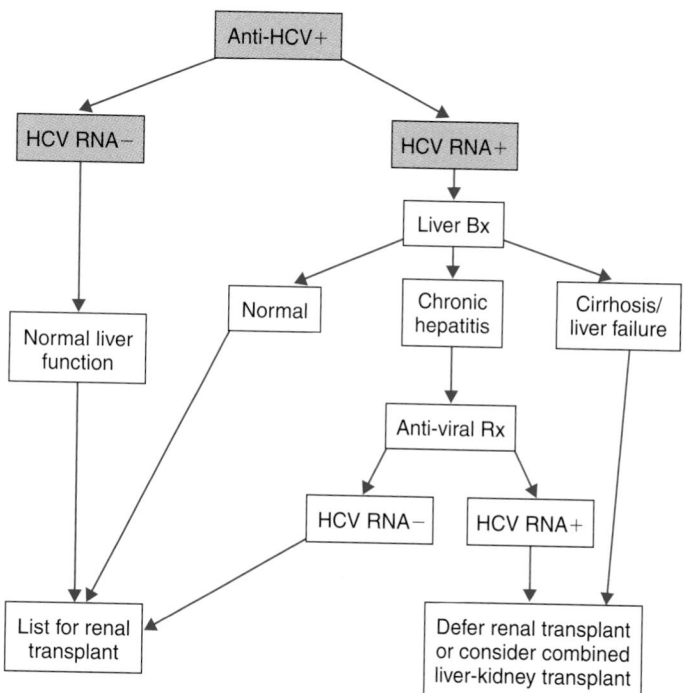

FIGURE 65-6. Management of the anti–hepatitis C virus (HCV) antibody-positive patient with early stage renal disease who is being considered for renal transplant. (Adapted from Morales JM, Campistol JM: Transplantation in the patient with hepatitis C. J Am Soc Nephrol 11:1343-1353, 2000.)

Although there are no data available regarding the use of these preparations in renal transplant patients, it seems reasonable to use them, provided that renal function is adequate in the case of ribavirin.

Both membranoproliferative glomerulonephritis (MPGN) and membranous nephropathy are more commonly found in HCV-positive compared to HCV-negative renal transplant recipients. The MPGN form can be associated with cryoglobulinemia, although systemic vasculitis is rare. An association of TMA with anticardiolipin antibodies in HCV-positive patients has also been reported.[65] Treatment of HCV-related glomerular lesions after renal transplant should involve supportive measures; antiviral therapy can be attempted, with these same caveats, based on limited data regarding the treatment of HCV-associated glomerulonephritis in liver transplant recipients.

Cytomegalovirus

One group has described a series of 21 patients with asymptomatic CMV infection and late acute allograft dysfunction who did not respond to conventional antirejection therapy. Treatment with ganciclovir resulted in stable improved renal function in 80% of cases.[79] This syndrome requires further confirmation. Foscarnet therapy for CMV in transplant patients has been associated with ARF; this is not a problem with ganciclovir. CMV infection is further discussed later.

DRUG AND RADIOCONTRAST-INDUCED ACUTE RENAL FAILURE IN SOLID-ORGAN TRANSPLANTATION

A variety of drugs can cause ARF of the renal allograft. In many cases, the offending agent (e.g., an aminoglycoside or amphotericin) is a well-recognized cause of ARF in native kidneys (see Chapter 27). However, a number of drug-related nephrotoxic effects are more common in the setting of transplantation (see Table 65-12). Many of these are due to interaction with the CNIs. Diltiazem, verapamil, ketoconazole, and the macrolide antibiotics, particularly erythromycin, impair CNI metabolism and may lead to acute CNI nephrotoxicity unless there is concomitant dose reduction of the CNI. There are reports implicating the newer antidepressants and some of the antiretroviral drugs in this regard.[80] High-dose SMX-TMP may cause an acute increase in plasma creatinine level by inhibiting tubule secretion of creatinine (in this case GFR per se is not compromised and serum creatinine level decreases within 5 days of stopping SMX-TMP). Rarely, SMX-TMP can provoke allergic interstitial nephritis; this is treated by cessation of the drug and administering high-dose steroids.

Not surprisingly, ACE-Is or angiotensin II receptor antagonists have been implicated in precipitating ARF in the presence of transplant renal artery stenosis. Overall, if carefully prescribed, these agents are well tolerated. The use of ACE-Is or angiotensin II antagonists in the immediate post-transplant period, when volume status and CNI dosages and concentrations are fluctuating, is not recommended.

Drugs with known nephrotoxic effects such as aminoglycosides or amphotericin probably have enhanced toxicity when used concomitantly with a CNI. Nevertheless, they are sometimes required in transplant recipients. Use of the lysosomal preparation of amphotericin is preferable because it is less nephrotoxic than the standard preparation.

NSAIDs have been implicated in several cases of acute interstitial nephritis in renal transplant recipients. Of more concern is their use when renal prostaglandins play a critical role in maintaining renal blood flow and GFR. This occurs in the setting of hypovolemia, heart failure, and probably CNI therapy. Administration of NSAIDs may block renal production of prostaglandins, resulting in functional ARF. Thus, the use of NSAIDs in all transplant recipients should be minimized.

Lipid-lowering agents are increasingly prescribed for solid-organ transplant recipients. The most commonly used agents are the hydroxymethylglutaryl–coenzyme A reductase inhibitors (statins). These drugs are generally well tolerated; however, there is an increased risk of rhabdomyolysis and ARF when they are used with cyclosporine. This is due mainly to cyclosporine-mediated impairment of statin metabolism. Coadministration of diltiazem or other drugs that also inhibit the cytochrome P450 system further increases plasma concentrations of statins.[81] These interactions have rarely been reported with tacrolimus, which could reflect less interaction with this particular CNI or less overall patient exposure to the tacrolimus plus statin combination. To minimize the risk of statin toxicity in renal transplant recipients, the following measures are advised: (1) usage of pravastatin or fluvastatin, which have less potential for interaction with cyclosporine; (2) starting with low doses of statins; (3) avoidance of other inhibitors of cytochrome P450 system metabolism; (4) avoidance of fibrates such as gemfibrozil; and (5) monitoring plasma creatine kinase (CK) and advising patients to seek medical attention if muscle symptoms occur.

The risk of developing ARF after administration of radiocontrast to renal transplant recipients has not been well defined. One study found an increase in plasma creatinine greater than 25% in 21% of cases.[82] Presumably, risk factors for postcontrast ARF are similar to those seen in nontransplanted patients (see Chapter 27). Thus, the same preventive measures should be used (see also Chapter 27).

LATE ALLOGRAFT DYSFUNCTION AND LATE ALLOGRAFT LOSS

By far, the most important cause of graft dysfunction and loss (excluding death) after the first 6 to 12 months is CAN. The causes of late dysfunction are summarized in Table 65-13 and

TABLE 65-13

Causes of Late Chronic Allograft Dysfunction

Prerenal
Transplant renal artery stenosis

Intrarenal
Chronic allograft nephropathy
Recurrence of primary disease
New disease

Postrenal
Urinary tract obstruction

further discussed in the following sections. Certain causes such as transplant renal artery stenosis and urinary tract obstruction have been discussed earlier.

Chronic Allograft Nephropathy

After censoring for death, chronic allograft nephropathy (CAN) is the most important cause of long-term graft loss. The term *CAN* is preferable to the older term *chronic rejection* because it encompasses the role of alloantigen-independent factors. Halloran and colleagues have defined CAN as a "state of impaired renal allograft function at least 3 months post-transplant, independent of acute rejection, overt drug toxicity, and recurrent or de novo specific disease entities, with typical features on biopsy."[83]

PATHOLOGY. Chronic changes occur in the tubulointerstitium, vessels, and glomeruli. These changes are not unique to CAN. Characteristic histologic findings are the following:

- Tubule atrophy and dropout with fibrosis and patchy mononuclear cell infiltration of the interstitium.
- Fibrointimal thickening of arterial walls. Certain vascular changes such as disruption of the elastica and the presence of inflammatory cells in the fibrotic intima suggest a significant component of chronic rejection.[39]
- Chronic transplant glomerulopathy (thickening and double contouring of capillary walls, segmental sclerosis, expansion of mesangial tissue, or mesangiolysis) is common.

Halloran and colleagues have emphasized the histologic overlap with aging or age-related diseases.[83]

PATHOGENESIS. The pathogenesis of CAN remains incompletely understood. Alloantigen-dependent and alloantigen-independent factors are considered to be important. Several of these factors probably interact in all patients with CAN. Figure 65-7 illustrates some of the postulated mechanisms through which these factors interact and lead to CAN.

CLINICAL FEATURES. Hypertension, proteinuria, and falling GFR occur. Onset is rarely less than 6 months post-transplant. Earlier onset or other atypical features should prompt a search for another diagnosis such as recurrent disease or primary donor renal disease. Often there is a history of overt acute rejection episodes that may have responded poorly to antirejection treatment. The rate of decrease in the GFR varies widely between patients but is usually progressive and irreversible. Proteinuria is usually in the range of 1 or 2 g/day but may be massive enough to cause nephrotic syndrome. Severe proteinuria and inadequately controlled hypertension are associated with more rapid deterioration in renal function.

DIAGNOSIS. The differential diagnosis of chronic allograft dysfunction is shown in Table 65-13. Renal ultrasound should be performed to rule out an obstructive cause. If there is suspicion of renal artery stenosis, further testing is indicated. Renal biopsy establishes the diagnosis of CAN, allows further estimation of disease severity, and occasionally yields unexpected information such as the presence of significant *acute* rejection or recurrent primary disease. In many cases, however, diagnosis is assumed without histologic support.

TREATMENT OF ESTABLISHED CHRONIC ALLOGRAFT NEPHROPATHY. Treatment options are very limited. If there is histologic evidence of significant acute rejection, a single course of pulse steroid therapy should be tried. If the clinical and histologic picture suggests predominantly chronic CNI nephrotoxicity, the CNI should be reduced in dosage or stopped (alternative agents such as MMF or sirolimus can be substituted). There is evidence that withdrawal or reduction in CNI dosages, on a background of MMF and steroid immunosuppression, is safe in many patients and can lead to a fall in plasma creatinine concentration.[84, 85]

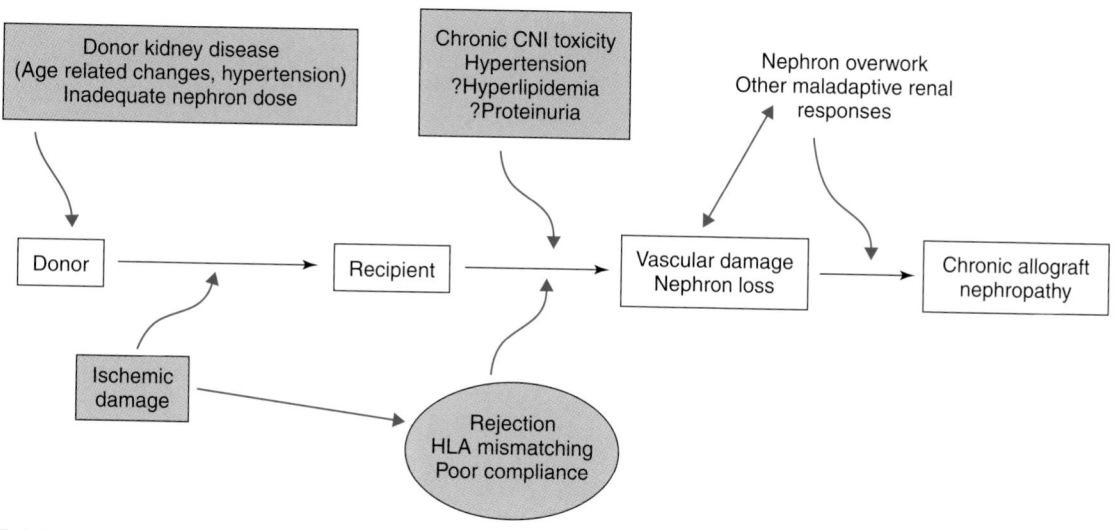

FIGURE 65-7. Alloantigen-dependent *(blue ovals)* and alloantigen-independent *(blue rectangles)* factors thought to be involved in the pathogenesis of chronic nephropathy. CNI, calcineurin inhibitor; HLA, human leukocyte antigen.

There is little role for dietary protein restriction in slowing the progression of transplant kidney disease, particularly because negative protein balance may occur secondary to steroids. Hypertension and hyperlipidemia should be rigorously controlled. As GFR deteriorates, preparations should be made for a return to dialysis. Erythropoietin, vitamin D analogs, and other supportive therapies often are required before dialysis resumes. CAN of itself is not a contraindication to subsequent transplantation.

In rat models (which resemble *to some extent* the human situation), ACE-I and angiotensin receptor blockers (ARBs) have been shown to slow the development of clinical and histologic signs of chronic rejection.[86, 87] This suggests a role of angiotensin II in the pathogenesis of chronic rejection. Long-term studies in humans are awaited.

PREVENTION OF CHRONIC ALLOGRAFT NEPHROPATHY. Prevention of CAN is obviously a major focus of current research. Strategies that may reduce the incidence of CAN include adequate "dosing" of functioning nephrons (including more use of living donors and perhaps dual kidney transplantation), minimizing ischemia-reperfusion injury, further reduction in the incidence of acute rejection, aggressive treatment of hyperlipidemia and hypertension, and interruption of pathways leading to fibrosis.

Although data from human studies are not yet available, sirolimus has the potential to slow the development and progression of CAN. Experimental models have shown that it can inhibit cytokine- and growth factor–induced proliferation of the various cells implicated in the pathophysiology of CAN. Furthermore, it permits use of low-dose CNIs, thus reducing CNI nephrotoxicity in the context of a low acute rejection rate.[88]

RECURRENCE OF PRIMARY DISEASE

Table 65-11 summarizes the conditions that recur at any time after transplantation. Diseases that recur early, such as FSGS, anti-GBM disease, and HUS/TTP have been discussed previously. Note that as renal allograft half-life continues to improve, recurrent disease is likely to be increasingly diagnosed (both clinically and histologically) and recognized as an important cause of late graft loss. The contribution of recurrent disease to allograft loss is discussed later.

IgA Glomerulonephritis

Studies with longer follow-up have shown that histologic recurrence of this condition is common. In one recent series it was at least 35%.[89] On multivariable analysis, recurrence was not associated with greater risk of graft failure. Although no prospective studies of treating recurrent IgA nephropathy are available, it seems reasonable to treat with fish oil and ACE-I.

Systemic Lupus Erythematosus Nephritis

Graft and patient survival overall are similar in patients with ESRD secondary to lupus nephritis compared to those with ESRD from other causes.[90] Recurrence of severe SLE,

systemically or within in the graft, is uncommon after transplant. This probably reflects the following: patient selection, disease activity "burning out" on chronic dialysis, and the effects of powerful post-transplant immunosuppression. After starting dialysis, patients should have clinically quiescent disease for 3 to 6 months before undergoing transplantation. Clinical criteria are a better guide to suitability for transplant than serologic criteria alone.

Note that SLE patients with APS probably have poorer graft and patient survival because of recurrent APS after transplant. These patients should resume full anticoagulation therapy immediately after surgery.

Wegener Granulomatosis and Microscopic Polyangiitis

Renal and extrarenal recurrence of these diseases have been described after renal transplantation. It is not yet known whether current regimens incorporating MMF or tacrolimus reduce that risk. In the largest reported series, with a mean follow-up time of 44 months, antineutrophil cytoplasmic antigen (ANCA)-associated small vessel vasculitis recurred in 17% of cases; renal involvement recurred in 10% of cases; the recurrence rate was not lower with cyclosporine therapy.[91] This and other studies have found that positive ANCA serology at the time of transplant does not predict later relapse. Of course, patients with ESRD secondary to ANCA vasculitis should not be transplanted until the disease is clinically in remission and "late" recovery of renal function has not occurred. Relapses usually respond to cyclophosphamide.

Membranoproliferative Glomerulonephritis

The primary forms of type I membranoproliferative glomerulonephritis (MPGN) and type II MPGN (dense deposit disease) can recur after transplant. The risk of recurrence is unclear because these are rare conditions and some cases of "primary" MPGN may in fact have been related to HCV infection (see later). Furthermore, type I MPGN is difficult to distinguish histologically from primary transplant glomerulopathy. One series found recurrence of type I MPGN in 33% of cases; graft survival was significantly poorer when this recurred.[92] Case reports have suggested a benefit of steroids, cyclophosphamide, and plasmapheresis.

Type II MPGN recurs, at least by histologic criteria, in most allografts.[93] Early reports suggested that associated graft failure was unusual. However, more recent series have documented allograft loss from recurrent type II MPGN in more than 20% of cases.[93]

Membranous Nephropathy

Membranous nephropathy may recur post-transplant, or more commonly, arise de novo. The associated clinical features vary from nonexistent (i.e., histologic evidence only) to nephrotic syndrome. In one series of 30 patients, the actuarial risk of recurrence at 3 years was 29% and recurrence was associated with poor graft survival.[94] De novo membranous nephropathy is often associated with CAN. As with native kidney disease, HCV infection and other causes of this glomerulopathy should be excluded. Management of membranous nephropathy post-transplant should include treatment of the underlying cause and supportive measures such as ACE-I. Intensification of immunosuppression solely to treat this lesion should probably be avoided.

Diabetes Mellitus

Recurrence of diabetic nephropathy in the allograft has not been well studied. This reflects the poor long-term survival of diabetic transplant recipients; the duration of exposure to the diabetic milieu is often insufficient to allow development of severe diabetic nephropathy. Kim and Cheigh performed a case control study of 78 patients with ESRD due to type I diabetes mellitus.[95] Overall graft survival was poorer in the diabetic group. If death was excluded as a cause of graft failure, however, graft survival was little different. Six of 16 patients who were biopsied had histologic evidence of recurrence, but this resulted in graft loss in only 1 case. It is likely that with better management of risk factors for cardiovascular disease, overall survival for diabetic patients will improve. Thus, recurrence of clinically significant diabetic nephropathy will probably become more common.

ASSESSING OUTCOMES IN RENAL TRANSPLANTATION

The most convenient and widely used method of assessing renal transplantation outcomes is measurement of allograft survival. Other important measures include allograft function (typically measured by plasma creatinine level), patient survival, number of rejection episodes, days of hospitalization, and quality-of-life indices.

Actual and Actuarial Allograft and Patient Survival

Allograft survival is calculated from the day of transplantation to the day of reaching a defined end point (either return to dialysis or retransplantation or death, whichever occurs first). In practice, survival is usually calculated by *actuarial* methods. These methods imply projection or estimation of survival because not all patients will have been followed for the same period. Also, because not all patients will have reached the defined end point, censoring of such patients is required. One year, 5-year, and 10-year actuarial survival rates are frequently presented. Another actuarial measure commonly used is graft half-life (median graft survival).

Traditionally, graft survival is assessed under two distinct time phases: early and late. Early graft loss refers to loss in the first 12 months; late loss to any time thereafter. This distinction is empirical but makes clinical sense. In the first 12 months, graft loss is *relatively* common, because of technical complications such as graft thrombosis and because of severe rejection. After 12 months, the incidence of graft loss is lower but remains quite stable over time. Usually, analysis of long-term survival is restricted to those allografts that have survived to 12 months post-transplant. The causes of late graft loss are also different and are discussed later. Note that using the earlier definition, patient death is equivalent to graft loss. Graft survival can also be calculated after censoring for patient death.

Survival Benefits of Renal Transplantation

Comparison of survival between the general dialysis population and transplanted patients is greatly affected by selection bias—only relatively healthy patients are referred for transplantation. Thus, comparisons between patients on the waiting list who do or do not receive a transplant are usually

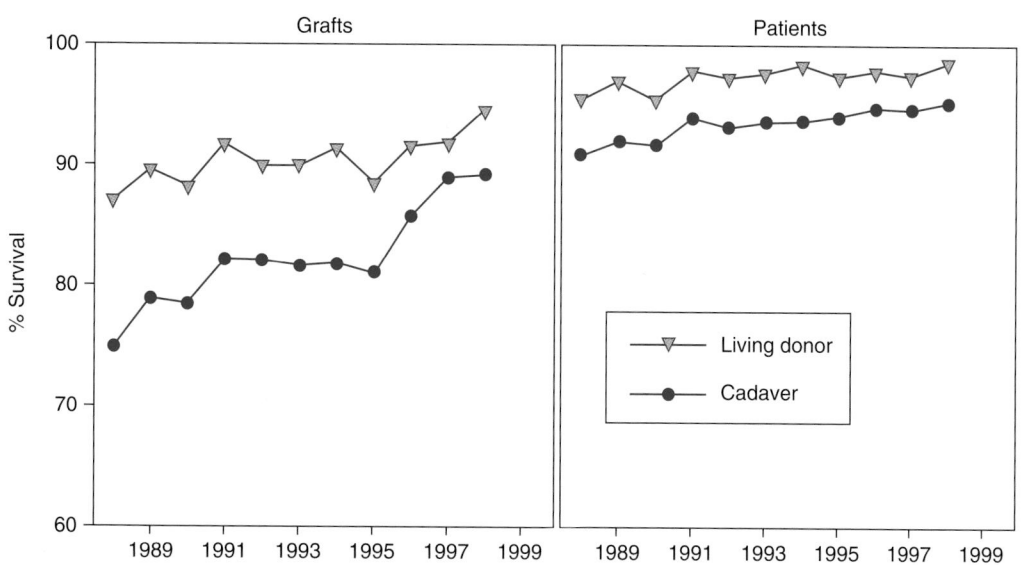

FIGURE 65-8. Trends in 1-year graft and patient survival rates in white recipients (adjusted for age, gender, primary diagnosis; standardized to 1997). (From USRDS: USRDS 2001 Annual Data Report: NIH and NIDDK, Bethesda, MD, 2002.)

TABLE 65-14

Causes of Allograft Loss after Year One

CAUSE	APPROXIMATE PERCENTAGE
Patient death	50
Chronic allograft nephropathy	35
Acute rejection/noncompliance	10
Recurrent disease	4

Data from Cecka JM: The UNOS Scientific Renal Transplant Registry, 2000. Clin Transpl 1-18, 2000.

performed instead. Of course, such analyses assume that the two groups (transplanted or still on the list) can otherwise be matched—this is not necessarily true.

One study of U.S. Renal Data Systems (USRDS) found that during the first 106 days after transplantation, the relative risk of death was greater than remaining on the waiting list (on dialysis). This mainly reflected the risks associated with the transplant procedure itself. Thereafter, however, transplantation conferred a survival benefit. On the basis of 3 to 4 years of follow-up, transplantation reduced the risk of death overall by 68%.[96] Transplantation was particularly life saving in diabetic patients.

Current Short-Term Outcomes in Renal Transplantation

For recipients of a first cadaveric kidney in the United States, current unadjusted 1-year patient and graft survival probabilities are 94.9% and 88.8%, respectively.[97] For recipients of a first living donor kidney, current unadjusted 1-year patient and graft survival probabilities are 98.0% and 94.1%, respectively. These outcomes have steadily improved over the last 25 years. This is illustrated in Figure 65-8. Similar outcomes have been reported from other registries.[98, 99] The principal causes of graft loss in the first post-transplant year are patient death, acute rejection, graft vessel thrombosis, and primary nonfunction. The principal causes of death during this period are cardiovascular disease (meaning cardiac and cerebrovascular disease), and infection.[100]

TABLE 65-15

Relative Influence of Various Factors on Long-Term Renal Allograft Survival

MORE INFLUENCE	LESS INFLUENCE
Donor age	Gender mismatch
Cadaver donor	Size mismatch
DGF	Donor race
Early acute rejection	Donor CMV-positive
Late acute rejection	Recipient age
HLA mismatching	Recipient race
Immunosuppression	Recipient hypertension
	Center effect

DGF, delayed graft function; HLA, human leukocyte antigen; CMV, cytomegalovirus.

Current Long-Term Outcomes in Renal Transplantation

Although static in the 1980s, long-term renal allograft survival has steadily increased over the last 10 years.[97, 98] For example, estimated cadaveric graft half-lives for the USRDS 1985–1989 (5-year) cohort were 7.7 years, for the 1990–1994 cohort 9.0 years, and for the 1995–1999 cohort 10.9 years.[100] This impressive improvement has occurred even in the setting of greater use of organs from older and less optimal donors.

Beyond the first post-transplant year, the principal causes of renal allograft loss are patient death and CAN; less common causes are late acute rejection and recurrent disease (Table 65-14).[100] The No. 1 cause of death remains cardiovascular disease, followed by infection and malignancy. Thus, the focus in renal transplantation is increasingly on methods to improve long-term outcomes by preventing and treating CAN, cardiovascular disease, and neoplasia.

Factors Affecting Renal Allograft Survival

Prospective studies and analyses of registry data have shown that many variables influence renal allograft survival. These variables are summarized in Table 65-15. These can be simplistically considered as *donor, recipient,* or *donor-recipient* factors. Many of them contribute to the development of CAN and have been discussed earlier.

Donor-Recipient Factors

DELAYED GRAFT FUNCTION

DGF, and probably SGF, is associated with poorer graft survival, poorer graft function, and greater risk of patient death.[9] Registry data show that DGF reduces graft half-lives by 30%, *a bigger effect than early acute rejection.*[30] Thus DGF is both an outcome and a predictor. The management of DGF has been discussed in detail earlier.

HUMAN LEUKOCYTE ANTIGEN MATCHING

Registry data clearly demonstrate that, even with current immunosuppression regimens, better HLA-matched allografts have better survival.[51, 100, 101] This benefit applies both to living donor and cadaveric donor grafts. Thus, the projected half-life varied from 13.0 years for first cadaveric renal allografts with zero HLA mismatches to 8.3 years for those with five or six HLA mismatches.[101] HLA-identical sibling grafts provide the best survival rates: a projected half-life in whites of over 41 years![100] The better outcomes are presumably related to fewer immunologic failures. A national strategy of preferentially performing zero HLA-mismatched transplants is worthwhile.[50, 51]

CYTOMEGALOVIRUS INFECTION

Registry data show a small but definite effect of donor and recipient CMV status on renal allograft survival. Donor negative–recipient negative pairings had the best outcomes, whereas donor positive–recipient positive pairings had the worst.[102] The reasons why donor positive–recipient positive pairings had worse outcomes than donor positive–recipient negative pairings are unclear. One theory is that two "hits" with two CMV virotypes is particularly deleterious. There is evidence that CMV infection up-regulates the immune response, thereby increasing the risk of rejection.

TIMING OF TRANSPLANTATION

In the case of living donor renal transplantation, there is evidence that preemptive (before initiation of dialysis) transplantation is associated with a lower risk of acute rejection and allograft failure.[103] Another multivariable analysis (of cadaveric and living donor recipients) showed that longer time on dialysis (compared to a reference group of < 12 months on dialysis) was independently associated with poorer graft survival.[30] Minimizing time on dialysis has many potential benefits; this strategy should thus be pursued whenever possible.

CENTER EFFECT

Not surprisingly, reported outcomes have varied widely from transplant center to center. This reflects normal statistical variance as well as center expertise. Outcomes are confounded by many donor and recipient factors that differ across centers. Thus, between-center comparisons are difficult. Recent UNOS data suggest minimal difference in outcomes between small and large transplant centers in the United States.[104]

YEAR OF TRANSPLANT

Long-term allograft survival is slowly but steadily increasing. This presumably reflects multiple factors: more effective (but not more toxic) immunosuppressive regimens, better pretransplant and post-transplant general medical care, more effective prevention, and treatment of opportunistic infections, particularly CMV.

GENETIC POLYMORPHISM

It has been hypothesized that genetic variation (with regard to the organ donor or recipient) may influence post-transplant outcomes such as susceptibility to infections, susceptibility to acute rejection, and allograft survival.[105] Candidate polymorphic genes are those encoding cytokines, chemokines, components of the angiotensin II system, adhesion molecules, and their relevant receptors. Some studies have suggested that polymorphisms of such molecules can influence outcomes. There are many caveats with regard to the current literature on this topic: Studies have been retrospective, usually single center, have not incorporated multivariable analysis, and, in some cases, have yielded contradictory results. Thus, it is premature to alter immunosuppression or other aspects of post-transplant care based on the data available. It is hoped that prospective, multicenter studies will be performed to assess the clinical importance of polymorphisms of immune molecules.

Donor Factors

The quality of the kidney immediately prior to transplantation has a major impact on long-term graft function and the risk of developing CAN.

DONOR SOURCE: CADAVER VERSUS LIVING DONOR

The donor source is one of the most important predictors of short- and long-term graft outcomes. In general, living donor grafts are superior to cadaveric grafts. Figure 65-8 illustrates how the survival of living donor allografts is clearly higher than for cadaveric grafts. This benefit applies across all degrees of HLA mismatching. The better outcomes reflect several factors: healthy living donors, avoidance of ischemia-reperfusion injury, high nephron mass, and probably the effects of a shorter waiting time (see earlier). Better compliance by the recipient may also play a role in improving outcome. Excellent results are now being demonstrated with living unrelated kidney transplantation where HLA matching is not optimum.[106] This further emphasizes the importance of the "healthy transplant kidney" effect.

DONOR AGE

Kidneys from those older than 45 years of age, and particularly older than 60 years, have poorer outcomes.[97] This effect is especially pronounced in cadaveric grafts. These results are thought to reflect a higher incidence of DGF and of nephron "underdosing." Grafts from older donors have fewer functioning nephrons because of the aging process and donor-related conditions such as hypertension and atherosclerosis. However, because of the organ donor shortage, elderly cadaveric kidneys are being increasingly used. Donor age younger than 5 years is also associated with poorer outcomes, reflecting relatively high rates of technical complications and probably nephron underdosing (see later). En bloc transplants from donors aged 0 to 5 years significantly improves survival, however.

DONOR RACE

In the United States, the survival of cadaveric grafts obtained from black donors is poorer than grafts from white donors.[30, 100, 107] This effect persists even in black recipients, implying that the poorer outcomes are not due to immunogenetic differences alone. Theories include kidneys from black donors being more susceptible to injury and having lower nephron number.

DONOR SEX

There is evidence that grafts from female donors have slightly poorer survival.[97, 107] Again, this probably reflects a nephron underdosing effect (see later), because females have smaller renal mass than males.

DONOR NEPHRON MASS

An imbalance between the metabolic/excretory demands of the recipient and the functional transplant mass has been postulated to play a causative role in the development and progression of CAN. Nephron underdosing exacerbated by perioperative ischemic damage and postoperative nephrotoxic drugs might lead to nephron overwork and eventual failure, similar to the mechanisms occurring in native kidney disease. Thus, kidneys from small or marginal donors and recipients of large body mass index would be at highest risk of this problem. There is increasing evidence to support this hypothesis.[107-109]

MARGINAL DONORS

The issue of nephron dosing has assumed greater importance because of the pressure to use cadaveric allografts from "expanded criteria" or marginal donors. Typically these kidneys have impaired *pretransplant* function because of advanced donor age (>60 years) and donor disease such as chronic hypertension. Not surprisingly, short- and long-term outcomes with such grafts have been somewhat inferior to grafts from "normal criteria" donors. However, transplantation with a marginal kidney confers a significant survival advantage compared to remaining on the transplant waiting list (on dialysis).[110]

Transplantation of both kidneys into one recipient would obviously double the functioning nephron number; limited medium-term data suggest that outcomes of this procedure are good. However, the number of recipients is obviously halved. Halloran and colleagues[83] have argued that dual-kidney transplantation should be performed only in the context of a randomized control trial comparing outcomes in recipients of two allografts to outcomes in the two recipients of single allografts. Otherwise, transplantation should be single kidney to single recipient (with informed consent), recognizing that long-term allograft function is more likely to be suboptimal.

Another group of marginal donors in which there has been renewed interest is non–heart-beating donors. The use of such donors has been controversial because short-term outcomes are inferior to those seen with heart-beating cadaveric donors. This reflects the longer period of warm ischemia. Reported rates of primary nonfunction are approximately 10% and of DGF, 45% to 80%. There is accumulating evidence, however, that long-term graft survival is similar to heart-beating cadaveric donors, although renal function may be inferior.[111]

Finally, the term "marginal donor" also encompasses cases where the transplant is considered to confer an increased risk (compared to a standard transplant) to the recipient.[52] DGF may not be the issue of concern. Typical examples are the use of kidneys from donors with central nervous system tumors or with HBV/HCV infection. Certain patients may benefit from such transplants.

Recipient Factors
RECIPIENT AGE

In general, graft survival rates are poorer in those at the extremes of age: younger than 18 and older than 60 years.[100] In the young, technical causes of graft loss such as vessel thrombosis are relatively more common. Acute rejection is also a more common cause of graft loss; conversely, death with a functioning graft is relatively rare.

Not surprisingly, compared to younger recipients, death with a functioning graft is a more common cause of graft loss (responsible for > 50% of graft failures) in the elderly, death being usually secondary to cardiovascular disease, infection, or neoplasia. Conversely, acute rejection is less common. Thus, although randomized, controlled trials are not available, it seems reasonable to use less aggressive immunosuppression in the elderly.

RECIPIENT RACE

In the United States, black recipients have poorer cadaveric and living donor graft survival compared to whites.[100] This probably reflects multiple factors including higher incidence of DGF, higher incidence of acute and late acute rejection, stronger immune responsiveness, a predominantly white donor pool (with resultant poorer matching of HLA and non-HLA antigens), altered pharmacokinetics of immuno-suppressive drugs, and a higher prevalence of hypertension. Socioeconomic factors associated with inability to pay for transplant medications (an issue in the United States where universal health coverage does not exist), poorer access to high-quality medical care, and noncompliance probably also play a role. There is some evidence to suggest that blacks also have inferior outcomes in Europe. Asian recipients have superior outcomes to whites; the reasons for this are unknown. These interracial differences in graft survival are shown in Figure 65-9.

In trials of recently introduced immunosuppressive drugs, rates of acute rejection were higher in blacks than whites. Post hoc analysis of one trial showed that, in black recipients, MMF 2 g/day was only partially effective in reducing acute rejection rates (compared to azathioprine); MMF 3 g/day was more effective. Conversely, MMF 2 g/day was adequate in whites.[18] Tacrolimus is also a very effective immunosuppressant in blacks. Thus, many American centers routinely use more aggressive immunosuppression, incorporating tacrolimus, in black recipients.

RECIPIENT GENDER

The impact of gender on transplant outcomes was recently assessed in a multivariable analysis of USRDS data.[112] Overall patient and graft survival was better in females compared to males, but graft survival was similar after censoring for death. Females were at higher risk of acute rejection but at lower risk of graft loss from chronic dysfunction. The higher rate of acute rejection could reflect unmeasured sensitizing effects of prior pregnancies (adjustment was made for PRA status). The reasons for the lower risk of graft loss from chronic dysfunction are unknown.

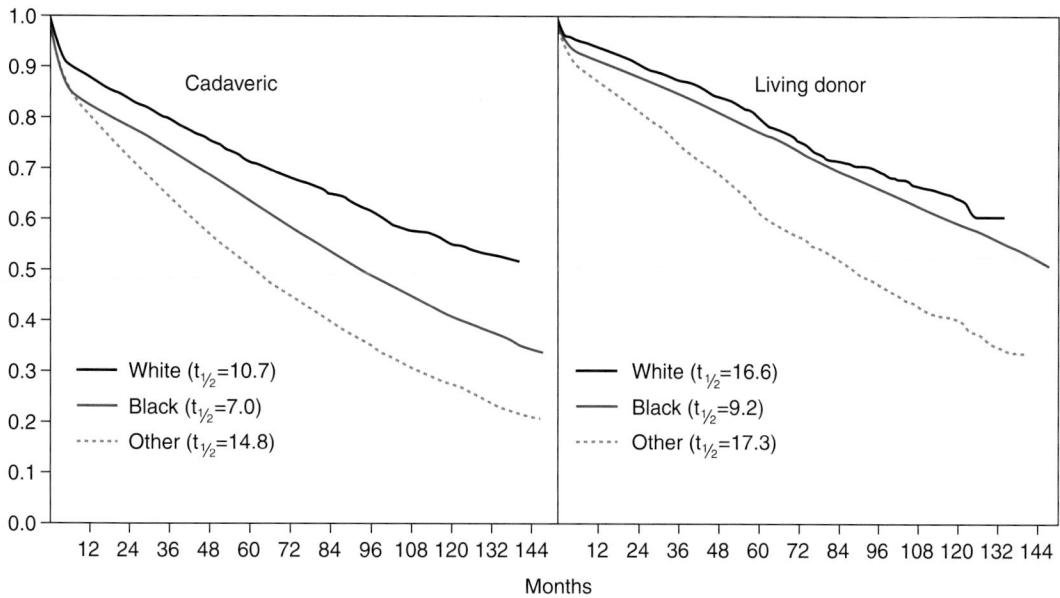

FIGURE 65-9. Effect of recipient race on allograft survival: Kaplan-Meier estimates in recipients of a first transplant between 1988 and 1998. Note: Other includes Asian. (From USRDS: USRDS 2001 Annual Data Report: NIH and NIDDK, Bethesda, MD, 2002.)

RECIPIENT SENSITIZATION

Patients who are highly sensitized (e.g., have a PRA status > 50%) generally have poorer early and late graft survival compared to nonsensitized recipients. This is mainly related to an increased incidence of complications in the early post-transplant period such as DGF and acute rejection. The principal reasons for sensitization are previous transplants, pregnancy, and previous blood transfusion. Thus, allograft survival is poorer in recipients of second or third transplants compared to recipients of a first transplant. In the 1995–1999 cohort of U.S. transplanted patients, graft half-life was 13.9 years in those with PRA less than 10% but 10.7 years in those with PRA higher than 50%.[101] Highly sensitized patients are thus usually given more intensive immunosuppression.

ACUTE REJECTION

Acute rejection has been consistently associated with an increased risk of graft loss. This is due to actual graft destruction at the time of acute rejection and probably ongoing subclinical immune-mediated injury. Such damage accentuates the effects of poor-quality donor tissue, perioperative ischemic injury, nephron underdosing, and so forth. Acute rejection refractory to steroids, acute rejection with a humoral component, and late acute rejection are particularly associated with poorer graft and patient outcomes. Gjertson's recent analysis of UNOS data showed that late acute rejection had a more negative impact on graft survival than early acute rejection or DGF, reducing graft half-lives by approximately 50%.[30] Fortunately, more effective immunosuppressive regimens have steadily decreased rates of acute rejection (see Fig. 65-3). This must be one of the primary reasons why

early and late renal allograft survival statistics have continued to improve.

RECIPIENT IMMUNOSUPPRESSION

Undoubtedly, the improvements in short- and long-term allograft survival reflect, in part, the effectiveness of the newer antirejection drugs such as the CNIs and MMF. The contribution of long-term CNI therapy, particularly with currently used maintenance doses, to chronic renal allograft dysfunction remains controversial. Traditionally, the CNIs have been thought to have greater beneficial effects on short-term compared to long-term renal graft survival. Certainly, in some non–renal transplant patients (e.g., those with cardiac allografts or autoimmune disease), prolonged intake of CNIs is associated with significant decreases in GFR and irreversible renal histopathologic changes. CNIs could contribute to chronic allograft dysfunction by induction of chronic renal ischemia, by stimulation of intragraft production of the fibrogenic cytokine transforming growth factor (TGF)-β, and by promotion of systemic hypertension. Balancing these effects, of course, is the high efficacy of CNIs in preventing acute rejection, one of the most important determinants of graft outcomes. The increases in short- and long-term graft survival in the CNI era (cyclosporine became widely used in the early 1980s) suggest that these antirejection effects override the nephrotoxic effects. Furthermore, lower dosages of cyclosporine (<5 mg/kg/day) have been associated with the development of CAN.[113]

There is accumulating evidence that MMF improves long-term graft survival both by preventing overt acute rejection and by other mechanisms.[16] No differences in survival with MMF compared to placebo were seen in the 3-year follow-up of the U.S. trial; the trial was not powered to detect such differences, however.

Although OKT3/polyclonals are widely used, particularly in the setting of DGF, their beneficial effect on long-term graft survival is controversial. Recent UNOS data suggest that antibody induction protocols slightly reduce early acute rejection episodes in recipients with DGF and slightly improve graft survival.[34]

RECIPIENT COMPLIANCE

Poor compliance with the immunosuppressive regimen is known to increase the risk of acute rejection (particularly late acute rejection) and CAN. The magnitude of this problem is difficult to define.

HIGH RECIPIENT BODY MASS INDEX

Pischon and Sharma recently reviewed the literature regarding obesity and outcomes in renal transplant recipients.[114] They concluded that obesity was associated with more transplant surgery–related complications, more DGF, higher mortality (related to cardiovascular complications), and poorer graft survival. Similar evidence of poorer patient and graft outcomes were found in a multivariable analysis of USRDS data.[115] Poorer long-term graft survival probably reflects the effects of DGF, nephron overwork, and more difficult dosing of immunosuppressive drugs. No data are available comparing survival outcomes of overweight dialysis patients remaining on the transplant waiting list with matched patients who receive a kidney transplant, but it is probable that transplantation is overall of benefit, as seen in other patient groups.[96]

However, transplantation brings the risk of further weight gain and worsening glucose intolerance. The question is: At what body mass index (BMI) are the risks of transplantation excessive? A reasonable approach is to enter all prospective recipients with BMI greater than 30 kg/m² into weight loss programs and, of course, to rigorously exclude or treat any cardiac disease. In those with persistent BMI greater than 30 kg/m² but without cardiac contraindications to surgery, eligibility for transplantation should be judged on a case-by-case basis. Dietary intervention after transplant can limit weight gain and hyperlipidemia.[116, 117] It is likely that pharmacologic treatment of obesity will be increasingly prescribed to transplant recipients. This subject has recently been reviewed.[118] Orlistat and similar compounds can reduce absorption of cyclosporine (and probably other immunosuppressives) and should be administered at least 2 hours separately; CNI concentrations should be closely monitored.[118]

RECIPIENT HYPERTENSION: THE RENIN-ANGIOTENSIN II SYSTEM

Retrospective studies have shown that the degree of hypertension correlates with the rate of deterioration in graft function and the severity of histologic change. Of course, hypertension could be a marker of deteriorating function rather than a cause. No prospective human studies of the effect of treating hypertension on allograft outcomes are available. Animal studies have shown that hypertension accelerates the development of CAN. Common sense dictates that aggressive treatment of hypertension should be the goal, to prevent both its renal and nonrenal complications.

Multiple studies have confirmed the ability of ACE-I and ARBs to slow the progression of both diabetic and nondiabetic proteinuric native kidney disease. Some have argued that ACE-I and ARBs should be similarly beneficial in transplant kidney disease and thus should be used more frequently.[119] Although several studies have shown that both classes of drugs are effective in treating post-transplant hypertension and in reducing proteinuria in the short term, no long-term studies of their effects on progression of transplant kidney dysfunction have been published.

RECIPIENT HYPERLIPIDEMIA

The prominence of the vascular lesions in CAN and the similarity of these lesions to atherosclerosis suggest that hyperlipidemia plays a role in the pathogenesis of CAN and graft failure. Some studies have suggested that hypercholesterolemia or hypertriglyceridemia, or both, are associated with poorer graft outcomes. Again, common sense dictates that hyperlipidemia should be treated aggressively to prevent both its renal and nonrenal complications.

Recurrence of Primary Disease

As discussed earlier, determining the incidence and prevalence of recurrent or de novo renal disease is difficult. A recent Australian study of patients with biopsy-proven glomerulonephritis found a 10-year incidence of graft loss from recurrence of 8.4%.[120] Overall allograft survival was not inferior, however, in patients whose primary renal disease had been biopsy-proven glomerulonephritis. It is likely that as renal allograft survival continues to improve, recurrent or de novo disease will be increasingly diagnosed (both clinically and histologically) and will become a more important cause of late graft loss.

To date, allograft failure from recurrence of diabetic nephropathy has not been a major problem. More important is the poor patient survival in this transplant population. It is likely that with better management of cardiovascular risk factors, overall survival for diabetic transplant recipients will improve. Thus, recurrence of clinically significant diabetic nephropathy will likely be more common. It should be emphasized that diabetic patients benefit greatly from renal transplantation.[96]

Proteinuria

The degree of proteinuria correlates with poorer renal outcome in both native and transplant kidney disease. Proteinuria may simply be a marker of renal damage, but there is speculation that proteinuria per se accelerates allograft loss from CAN. The role of ACE-I and ARBs in slowing the progression of proteinuric transplant renal diseases is discussed briefly earlier.

Improving Renal Allograft Outcomes

Measures that would likely further improve allograft survival are summarized in Table 65-16. Probably the most important (in terms of achievable impact) is increased use of living kidney donors. Ideally, most living donor kidneys would be transplanted before the recipient begins dialysis. It is critical, however, that donation should be allowed only when the risk of medical and psychological complications to the donor are minimal.

TABLE 65-16

Measures to Improve Renal Allograft Survival

MEASURE	COMMENT
Increased living donor donation: both related and nonrelated	Underutilized in many countries
Preemptive transplantation	Underutilized in many countries
Increased donation from younger, previously healthy cadaveric donors	Difficult to achieve; Spain best example of successful high donation rates
Zero HLA mismatching	Already practiced in many countries
Better donor preparation, improved organ preservation; faster matching and transplantation; reduced cold ischemia time	Somewhat neglected area of transplantation. Controversial if machine perfusion improves long-term graft function
ACE inhibitors, angiotensin receptor blockers	No data in transplant patients per se showing that renal function is better preserved; reasonable to extrapolate from native kidney disease
Nephron dosing (matching of donor-recipient sex, BMI, etc.)	No large randomized, controlled trials; complex to administer in practice
High-quality general medical care (aggressive control of hyperlipidemia, hypertension, etc.)	No randomized, controlled trials showing benefits in transplant patients, but benefits likely

HLA, human leukocyte antigen; ACE, angiotensin-converting enzyme; BMI, body mass index.

The criteria used for allocation of cadaveric allografts can have an important impact on *overall* allograft survival. A purely utilitarian approach would imply directing organs to those who possess certain demographic and clinical characteristics, are likely to live longer, and so forth. In practice, a balance must be struck between utility and equity (ensuring that anyone medically fit for a transplant has a reasonable chance of obtaining one). In many countries this balance is achieved by means of a points system—points being awarded for characteristics such as zero HLA mismatching and time on the waiting list.

MEDICAL MANAGEMENT OF THE TRANSPLANT RECIPIENT

With the current low acute rejection rates and improvements in long-term graft survival, more emphasis is being placed on the general medical management of transplant patients. The management of common electrolyte, endocrine, and cardiovascular complications post-transplant is discussed in the following sections. Readers are directed to several recent reviews for more information.[121-123]

Electrolyte Disorders

Hypophosphatemia

Hypophosphatemia is common in the early post-transplant period, particularly when graft function is excellent. This is mainly due to excess urinary excretion of phosphate. This hyperphosphaturia has several causes: residual hyperparathyroidism, glucocorticoids, low vitamin D state (relative to the degree of hypophosphatemia), and a putative humoral factor, phosphatonin.[124] Rarely, phosphate depletion is severe enough to cause profound muscle weakness, including respiratory muscle weakness. Because a persistent negative phosphate balance probably contributes to post-transplant bone disease, attempts should be made to increase the plasma phosphate level to 2.5 to 4.0 mg/dL.[124] Treatment involves high phosphate diet (e.g., low-fat dairy products), oral phosphate supplements, and vitamin D analogs. The plasma calcium

and phosphate levels should be closely monitored on such therapies.

Hyperkalemia

Mild hyperkalemia is common after renal transplant, even with good allograft function. The principal cause is CNI-induced impairment of tubule potassium secretion.[125] Hyperkalemia may be exacerbated by poor allograft function and ingestion of excess potassium (e.g., in phosphate compounds) and other medicines such as ACE-I and β-blockers. As the hyperkalemia is usually not severe and improves with reduction in CNI dosage, treatment is often not required; exacerbating factors should be minimized.

Metabolic Acidosis

Mild metabolic acidosis is also common and often associated with hyperkalemia. In most cases, it has the features of a distal (hyperchloremic) renal tubular acidosis (RTA). This reflects tubule dysfunction caused by CNIs, rejection, or residual hyperparathyroidism.[126, 127] Oral bicarbonate replacement is given in severe cases. Inappropriately low aldosterone concentrations or renal aldosterone resistance (believed to be an effect of the CNIs) can cause a type IV RTA. Fludrocortisone can be used to treat this, but the drug promotes sodium and water retention.

Hypercalcemia and Hyperparathyroidism

Hypercalcemia is common after renal transplantation and is due mainly to persistent hyperparathyroidism. Normalization of 1,25 vitamin D concentrations may also play a role. The management of post-transplant hyperparathyroidism is discussed below.

Other Electrolyte Abnormalities

Hypomagnesemia is common and due to a magnesuric effect of the CNIs. It is almost always asymptomatic. Magnesium supplements are sometimes prescribed when the plasma magnesium level is less than 1.5 mg/dL. However, their effectiveness is limited, they can cause diarrhea, and they add more complexity to the multidrug regimen of the transplant recipient.

Bone Disorders after Renal Transplantation

Bone disease in the ESRD patient is multifactorial and involves varying degree of hyperparathyroidism, vitamin D deficiency, aluminum intoxication, and amyloidosis (see Chapter 52). Successful renal transplantation offers the potential to reverse or at least prevent further progression of these conditions. Unfortunately, bone disease can be a major problem after renal transplantation due to persistence of the conditions discussed earlier and to the superimposed effects of immunosuppressants on bone.

Hyperparathyroidism

Hyperparathyroidism is very common in the first year after transplantation. Less obvious hyperparathyroidism may persist for years; one study found elevated parathyroid hormone concentrations in 23 (54%) of 42 normocalcemic patients who were more than 2 years after transplant and had plasma creatinine levels lower than 2 mg/dL.[128] Not surprisingly, the main risk factors for post-transplant hyperparathyroidism are the degree of pretransplant hyperparathyroidism and the duration of dialysis.[129] Inadequate 1,25 vitamin D_3 production and poor graft function probably contribute to persistence of the condition.[130]

Typically, post-transplant hyperparathyroidism is manifested by a low plasma phosphate level and a mild to moderate elevation in the plasma calcium level. Serum parathyroid hormone is inappropriately high for the degree of hypercalcemia. Post-transplant hyperparathyroidism is usually asymptomatic and tends to improve with time. Therefore, therapy in most cases involves cautious oral repletion of phosphate (see earlier) and administration of vitamin D analogs if 1,25 vitamin D concentrations are low.[128, 131] Of course, vitamin D analogs must be used with caution and stopped if the plasma calcium level exceeds 11.0 mg/dL or complications of hypercalcemia occur.

There are two main indications for post-transplant parathyroidectomy: (1) severe symptomatic hypercalcemia (usually in the early post-transplant period and now rare) and (2) persistent, moderately severe hypercalcemia (e.g., calcium > 12.0 mg/dL for 12 months). Subtotal parathyroidectomy is the procedure of choice.

Gout

The most important cause of hyperuricemia and gout after transplant is cyclosporine. Cyclosporine impairs renal urate clearance. The effects of tacrolimus are unclear, although there is a report of gout improving after switching from cyclosporine to tacrolimus.[132] Approximately 80% of cyclosporine-treated renal transplant recipients develop hyperuricemia, but only about 7% develop gout.[133]

Acute gout should be treated with colchicine or high-dose steroids; NSAIDs should generally be avoided. Colchicine-induced neuromyopathy is more common in cyclosporine-treated patients; therefore, lower doses should be used and patients should be monitored for muscle weakness and

rising plasma CK. For prevention of further gouty attacks, either allopurinol or uricosuric drugs (probenecid, benzbromarone) can be used. Note that the metabolism of azathioprine is greatly inhibited by allopurinol. If these drugs are coprescribed, the azathioprine dose should be reduced by 75% and the complete blood count closely monitored. A safer and easier alternative is to change azathioprine to MMF; no adjustment of MMF is required. Probenecid is effective only when the GFR is more than 30 mL/min. In cases of severe recurrent gout, it is worthwhile switching cyclosporine to tacrolimus or stopping CNIs altogether. Readers are directed to a recent review for further information.[134]

Calcineurin Inhibitor–Associated Bone Pain

A syndrome of severe bone pain in the lower limbs has been associated with CNI use. This is uncommon and thought to represent a vasomotor effect of the CNIs. Osteonecrosis and other common bone lesions should be excluded before the diagnosis is made. Symptoms usually respond to reduction in CNI dosage and administration of calcium channel blockers.

Osteonecrosis

Osteonecrosis (avascular necrosis) is the most serious bone complication of renal transplantation. The pathogenesis is not well understood, but high doses of steroids are one risk factor. Up to 8% of renal transplant patients develop osteonecrosis of the hips[135]; this figure may be falling with lower-dose steroid protocols. The most commonly affected site is the femoral head; other sites are the humeral head, femoral condyles, proximal tibia, vertebrae, and small bones of the hand and foot. Many patients have bilateral involvement at the time of diagnosis. The principal symptom is pain; signs are nonspecific. Diagnosis is made by imaging studies; MR imaging is the most sensitive, plain film is the least sensitive, and bone scan is intermediate. However, MR imaging abnormalities do not always imply clinically significant osteonecrosis. Treatment remains controversial. Options include resting the joint, core decompression, osteotomy, and joint replacement.

Osteoporosis

Osteoporosis is a common bone disorder characterized by a parallel reduction in bone mineral and bone matrix so that bone mass is decreased but is of normal composition. The most commonly used definition is that based on the World Health Organization scoring system. Bone density is accurately and easily measured by dual-energy x-ray analysis (DEXA). Osteoporosis is defined as bone density more than 2.5 SD below the mean of sex-matched, young adults (T score); osteopenia, as 1.0 to 2.5 SD below the T score. The greater the reduction in bone density in the nontransplant population, the greater the risk of fracture.

Reduction in bone mineral density is now recognized as a very common complication of solid-organ transplantation; one recent review estimated an incidence up to 60% in the first 18 months after renal transplant. The pathophysiology and treatment of osteoporosis may differ from those seen in the nontransplant population (Table 65-17). Most of the bone loss occurs in the first 6 months after transplant. The principal cause is steroids through direct inhibition of

TABLE 65-17

Differences between Postmenopausal and Post-transplant Osteoporosis

	POSTMENOPAUSAL OSTEOPOROSIS	POST-TRANSPLANT OSTEOPOROSIS
Pathophysiology		
Sex hormone deficiency	yes	sometimes
Increased osteoclast activity; accelerated bone breakdown	yes	sometimes
Decreased osteoblast activity; reduced bone synthesis	no	yes
Background of renal osteodystrophy	no	yes
Diagnosis		
DEXA predicts fracture risk	yes	unclear
Currently Advised Prevention and Treatment		
Weight-bearing exercise	yes	yes
Calcium	yes	yes
Vitamin D	yes	yes
Bisphosphonates	often used	reserve for highest risk patients

DEXA, dual-energy x-ray analysis.

osteoblastogenesis, induction of apoptosis in bone cells, inhibition of sex hormone production (in both men and women), decreased gut calcium absorption, and increased urinary calcium excretion.[136] Other factors that may play a role include cyclosporine, ongoing hyperparathyroidism, vitamin D deficiency or resistance, and phosphate depletion.

Low bone mineral density is presumed to be a risk factor for fracture in renal transplant recipients; this has not yet been proven. In fact, limited evidence suggests that DEXA-identified low bone mineral density is not a risk factor for future fracture.[137] There is no disputing, however, that pathologic fractures are very common after renal transplantation. Unlike nontransplant osteoporotic patients, fractures of the appendicular, rather than vertebral, skeleton are relatively more common.[138]

Diabetes mellitus and pancreas-kidney transplantation are associated with an increased risk of post-transplant fracture. The estimated total fracture rate in nondiabetic patients after renal transplantation is 2% per year, in preexisting diabetics 5% per year, and in pancreas-kidney recipients up to 12% per year.[138] Any interventions to minimize post-transplant bone loss must occur in the first 3 to 6 months. We recommend the following:

- Minimal steroid dosage: this is likely to be increasingly prescribed as more effective nonsteroid maintenance regimens become available.
- Unless contraindicated, all patients should receive 1000 mg/day of elemental calcium and 800 U/day of cholecalciferol. Certain patients may need more vitamin D to control hyperparathyroidism (see earlier). If GFR is less than 50 mL/min, then calcitriol should be substituted for standard vitamin D.
- Regular weight-bearing exercises should be instituted in all patients.
- DEXA should be performed in those at high risk of developing osteoporotic fractures (e.g., small stature, hypogonadism, history of fracture, history of diabetes mellitus, history of prior steroid use).

- Additional therapies such as sex hormone repletion or bisphosphonates should be used only after close consultation with an endocrinologist familiar with post-transplant bone disease. There are no data showing a reduction in fracture incidence in renal allograft recipients with these agents. Suppression of bone remodeling by bisphosphonates in patients who may have osteomalacia or adynamic bone, or both, could worsen the mechanical integrity of bone.[138] Furthermore, albeit at very high doses, bisphosphonates are highly nephrotoxic.[139] Thus, until more data become available, it is reasonable to reserve bisphosphonates only for the highest risk patients.

Cardiovascular Disease

Death with a functioning allograft is the most common cause of early and late graft loss. Data from both U.S. and European registries show that the leading cause of death is cardiovascular disease (30% to 40% of cases).[140, 141] The cumulative incidence of coronary heart disease, cerebrovascular disease, and peripheral vascular disease at 15 years after transplant has been estimated at 23%, 15%, and 15%, respectively.[121] The mechanisms by which this high incidence occurs are illustrated in Table 65-18. Addressing these mechanisms must now be an important component of standard management. All patients, of course, should be strongly encouraged to stop smoking.

Hypertension

The prevalence of hypertension in the CNI era is 60% to 80%.[121] Causes include steroids, CNIs, weight gain, allograft dysfunction, native kidney disease, and, less commonly, transplant renal artery stenosis. The complications of post-transplant hypertension are presumed to be a heightened risk of cardiovascular disease and of allograft failure,[142] although distinguishing cause and effect with regard to the latter is difficult. Hypertension should be aggressively managed in all patients. Joint National Committee (JNC) on Prevention, Detection, Evaluation, and Treatment of High Blood Pressure–VII guidelines are a useful aid in this regard; the target blood pressure should be less than 130/80.[143] Nonpharmacologic measures such as weight loss, moderation of sodium intake, moderation of alcohol intake, and increased exercise should be encouraged. The dosage of steroids and CNIs should be minimized. Antihypertensive drug therapy will still be required in most cases. Again, applying JNC-VI or JNC-VII guidelines, therapy should be started with one agent and the dose titrated up as needed; long-acting formulations are preferable; and diuretics should always be considered because they enhance the effects of other drugs. Table 65-19 shows the antihypertensive drugs commonly used in the post-transplant setting.

TABLE 65-18

Putative Pathogenesis of Cardiovascular Disease after Renal Transplant

ATHEROMA	LVH	VASCULAR CALCIFICATION
Older age	Hypertension	Hyperphosphatemia*
Male	Anemia*	Hyperparathyroidism
Smoking	Fluid overload*	
Obesity	DD genotype of ACE	
Hyperhomocystinemia		
DM		

*Mainly pretransplant.

DM, diabetes mellitus; LVH, left ventricular hypertrophy; ACE, angiotensin-converting enzyme.

Adapted from Reference 140.

Hyperlipidemia

The prevalence of hypercholesterolemia and hypertriglyceridemia after transplant has been estimated as 60% and 35%, respectively.[121] Steroids, CNIs—cyclosporine more than tacrolimus—and sirolimus are the principal causes. There is evidence that hyperlipidemia is associated with poorer graft outcomes, although no cause-effect relationship has been demonstrated.

Although data on the effects of lipid-lowering interventions on cardiovascular outcomes are not available, all transplant recipients should be managed according to the latest National Institutes of Health guidelines.[144] Because cardiovascular disease is so prevalent in these patients, it is reasonable to consider renal transplantation a "coronary heart disease risk equivalent" when applying the guidelines. This implies targeting low-density lipoprotein cholesterol to be lower than 100 mg/dL. Initial therapy is therapeutic lifestyle changes, including weight control, physical activity, low cholesterol levels, and low-saturated-fat diet. Minimizing steroid dosage and switching cyclosporine to tacrolimus are also worthwhile. Many patients still require pharmacologic treatment. Statins are the cholesterol-lowering drug of choice. Because metabolism of many statins is inhibited by cyclosporine (and probably tacrolimus), plasma concentrations of statins may be greatly increased in transplant recipients, thereby increasing the risk of rhabdomyolysis. This interaction is further potentiated if additional inhibitors of cytochrome P450 such as diltiazem are administered.[81]

Measures to minimize the risk of statin toxicity include the use of pravastatin or fluvastatin (which have the least interaction with CNIs), starting with low statin doses, avoidance of other inhibitors of the cytochrome P450 system, avoidance of fibrates, and periodic checking of plasma CK and liver function tests.[81] Rarely, nonstatin drugs are used to lower plasma lipids in transplant patients. Bile acid sequestrants, if used, should be taken separately from CNIs

TABLE 65-19

Commonly Used Antihypertensive Drugs in Renal Transplantation

DRUG	ADVANTAGES	DISADVANTAGES	COMMENTS
β-Blockers	Well proven to reduce complications of HTN and CHD; cheap	May exacerbate hyperkalemia	Diabetics have similar or greater reduction in complications of HTN with these agents
Loop diuretics	Treat hypervolemia; potentiate effects of other agents	Risk of hypovolemia, increased Cr	Use with caution in early post-transplant period
Thiazide diuretics	Well proven to reduce complications of HTN; cheap; potentiate effects of other agents	Risk of hypovolemia, increased Cr; worsen hyperuricemia	Low doses adequate: e.g., hydrochlorothiazide 12.5 mg qd
ACE-I/ARBs	Reduce proteinuria; many beneficial CV effects; ? slow progression of allograft dysfunction	Hyperkalemia, increased Cr	Use with caution in early post-transplant period; effective for post-transplant erythrocytosis; particularly useful if proteinuria or DM
CCBs	Well tolerated; suggestion of graft-protective effect (particularly if CNIs used)	Outcomes in general hypertensive population of concern	Caution with diltiazem, verapamil—impair CNI metabolism
α-Blockers	Well tolerated	Outcomes in general hypertensive population of concern	Reserve for resistant cases only

ACE-I, angiotensin-converting enzyme inhibitor; ARB, angiotensin receptor blocker; CCB, calcium channel blocker; HTN, hypertension; CHD, coronary heart disease; CV, cardiovascular; CNI, calcineurin inhibitor; Cr, creatinine; DM, diabetes mellitus.

because they impair absorption of these drugs. Fibrates should not be coprescribed with statins. Preliminary data suggested that statins had beneficial immunomodulatory effects in renal transplant recipients; this has not been confirmed in prospective trials.[145]

Hyperhomocystinemia

Plasma homocysteine concentrations typically fall after transplant but do not normalize. One prospective study found hyperhomocystinemia in 70% of renal transplant patients; hyperhomocystinemia was an independent risk factor for cardiovascular events.[146] Supplementation with B vitamins can reduce plasma homocysteine concentrations in transplant patients; the effects of such reduction are now being studied.[147] Until trial results are available, no firm recommendations can be made regarding B vitamin therapy for hyperhomocystinemia in transplant recipients.

Cancer after Renal Transplantation

Data on occurrence of malignancy after transplant are derived mainly from the Cincinnati Transplant Tumor Registry and the Australia–New Zealand Dialysis and Transplantation (ANZDATA) Registry.[148, 149] These data clearly show that the overall incidence of cancer in renal transplant recipients is greater than in dialysis patients and the general population. This increase in incidence applies to most cancers (at least in the ANZDATA Registry),[149] but certain "transplant-associated" ones are dramatically increased in risk (Table 65-20). The common nonskin cancers (breast, lung, and prostate) are little changed in incidence.

There are several reasons why reported cancer incidence is increased. First, immunosuppression allows uncontrolled proliferation of oncogenic viruses (Table 65-21). Second, immunosuppression may inhibit normal tumor surveillance mechanisms, allowing unchecked proliferation of "naturally occurring" neoplastic cells. There is also experimental

evidence that cyclosporine has tumor-promoting effects mediated by its effects on TGF-β production.[150] Third, factors related to the primary renal disease (analgesic abuse, HBV or HCV infection) or the ESRD milieu (acquired renal cystic disease) may promote neoplasia. Finally, an ascertainment bias may occur due to assiduous monitoring and reporting of transplant patients.

It is believed that the cumulative amount of immunosuppression rather than a specific drug is the most important factor increasing the cancer risk. However, there is evidence that the routine use of CNIs has increased the risk of skin cancers[149, 151, 152]; fortunately, these are usually not fatal. The long-term impact of currently employed powerful immunosuppression regimens on cancer incidence is unknown, but it is certainly of concern. The single most important measure to prevent cancers *is to minimize excess immunosuppression.* A general rule is that when cancer occurs, immunosuppression should be greatly decreased. In some cases, rejection of the graft may result, but the risks and benefits of immunosuppression must be judged on a case-by-case basis.

Readers are directed to a recently published review and to the guidelines of the American Society of Transplantation for more information.[121, 153] There is now experimental evidence that sirolimus has antineoplastic effects.[154]

Skin and Lip Cancers

Squamous cell carcinoma, basal cell carcinoma, and malignant melanoma are more common in renal transplant patients. Thirty years after transplant, an estimated 70% of Australian patients will have developed skin cancer.[149] Risk factors for skin cancer are time after transplant, cumulative immunosuppressive dose, exposure to ultraviolet light, fair skin and human papillomavirus (HPV) infection. Primary and secondary prevention is important: patients should be specifically counseled on minimizing exposure to ultraviolet light and to self-screen for skin lesions. Suspicious skin lesions should be surgically excised.

Anogenital Cancers

Cancers of the vulva, uterine cervix, penis, scrotum, anus, and perianal region are significantly more common, particularly in women. Infection with certain HPV strains is an important risk factor. These cancers tend to be multifocal and more aggressive than in the general population. Secondary prevention measures include yearly physical examination of the

TABLE 65-20

Relative Risk (RR) of Cancer following Primary Cadaveric and Living Unrelated Donor Kidney Transplantation, 1965–2000*

CANCER	RR
In situ carcinoma of uterine cervix	16.7
Invasive carcinoma of uterine cervix	3.1
Carcinoma of vulva or vagina	36.9
Kaposi's sarcoma (varies between ethnic groups)	73.9
Non-Hodgkin's lymphoma	8.3
CNS lymphoma	>1000
Liver	7.3
Renal carcinoma	6.2
Prostate	0.7
Breast	1.0
Malignant melanoma	3.5
Colon	2.4
Total (includes others not shown)	3.0

*N = 8554.

CNS, central nervous system.

Adapted from Reference 149.

TABLE 65-21

Viral Infections Associated with Development of Cancers in Renal Transplant Patients

VIRUS	NEOPLASM
HBV	Hepatocellular cancer
HCV	Hepatocellular cancer
EBV	PTLD
HPV	Squamous cell cancers of anogenital area and mouth
HHV-8	Kaposi's sarcoma

See text for abbreviations.

anogenital area and, in women, yearly pelvic examinations and cervical histology. Suspicious lesions should be excised, and patients should be closely followed for recurrence.

Kaposi's Sarcoma

The incidence of Kaposi's sarcoma in both transplant and nontransplant patients depends greatly on ethnic background. Those of Jewish, Arab, or Mediterranean ancestry are at much greater risk. Other risk factors are cumulative immunosuppressive dose and human herpes virus-8 infection.[121] Visceral (lymph nodes, lungs, gastrointestinal tract) and nonvisceral (skin, conjunctivae, oropharynx) involvement may occur. The prognosis for the former is poor, but for the latter it is good. Treatment involves various combinations of surgical excision, radiation therapy, chemotherapy, and immunotherapy (immunosuppression is, of course, reduced).

Post-transplant Lymphoproliferative Disorder

Post-transplant lymphoproliferative disorder (PTLD) is one of the most feared complications of transplantation because it can occur early after transplant and carries a high morbidity and mortality. The cumulative incidence in renal transplant patients overall is 1% to 5%.[121] The incidence has increased over the last 15 years, presumably reflecting more intense immunosuppression. More than 90% are non-Hodgkin's lymphomas, and most are of recipient B cell origin.[155] Most cases of PTLD occur in the first 24 months after transplant. Risk factors include (1) Epstein-Barr virus (EBV)-positive donor and EBV-negative recipient; (2) CMV-positive donor and CMV-negative recipient; (3) pediatric recipient (in part because children are more likely to be EBV negative); and (4) aggressive immunosuppression, especially with OKT3/polyclonals or tacrolimus.[156] Most important in the pathogenesis of PTLD is the infection and transformation of B cells by EBV; transformed B cells undergo proliferation that is initially polyclonal, but a malignant clone may evolve. Thus the clinical and histologic spectrum of PTLD at presentation and its treatment can vary greatly (Table 65-22). Extranodal, gastrointestinal tract, and

central nervous system involvement is much more common than in nontransplant lymphomas. The renal allograft may be involved in up to 20% of cases.[155]

The prognosis of severe forms of PTLD has traditionally been poor but will likely improve for several reasons. First, techniques for monitoring EBV viral load after transplantation are being developed. These could prove very useful in identifying patients who are at high risk of developing PTLD.[157] Second, new therapies are under investigation. Retrospective studies have shown very promising results with the use of the chimeric anti-CD20 monoclonal antibody, rituximab[158, 159]; prospective studies are underway. Early results of adoptive immunotherapy (using EBV-specific cytotoxic T lymphocytes) are promising.[160] Strategies such as antiviral therapy, intravenous immunoglobulin, and anticytokine therapy are also under investigation.[161]

To summarize, patients with cancer or those at high risk of cancer should be identified in the pretransplant evaluation (see Chapter 64). Excess immunosuppression should be avoided in all patients. Standard primary and secondary preventive strategies (e.g., smoking cessation, cervical smear) should be applied in all patients. If cancer occurs, immunosuppression should be greatly reduced.

Infectious Complications of Renal Transplantation

The transplant procedure itself and subsequent immunosuppression increase the risk of serious infection. The principal factors determining the type and severity of infection are the intensity of exposure (epidemiologic exposure) to potential pathogens and the overall state of immunosuppression.[162] Epidemiologic exposure occurs in the hospital and community. Factors affecting the net state of immunosuppression are shown in Table 65-23.

As outlined by Fishman and Rubin,[162] the patterns of infection after renal transplantation can be considered under three time periods: 0 to 1 month, 1 to 6 months, and more than 6 months after transplant. These divisions of time serve as guidelines only. Ongoing changes in overall transplant care may alter this "three-period" paradigm. Maintenance immunosuppressive regimens are becoming more powerful

TABLE 65-22

Clinical and Pathologic Spectrum of PTLD and Its Management

	EARLY DISEASE (50%)	POLYMORPHIC PTLD (30%)	MONOCLONAL PTLD (20%)
Clinical features	Infectious mononucleosis–type illness	Infectious mononucleosis–type illness ± weight loss, localizing symptoms	Fever, weight loss, localizing symptoms
Pathology	Preserved architecture; atypical cells infrequent	Intermediate	High-grade lymphoma with confluent transformed cells and marked atypia
Clonality	Polyclonal	Usually polyclonal	Monoclonal
Treatment	Reduce immunosuppression; acyclovir	Reduce immunosuppression; acyclovir; if poor response then treat as monoclonal PTLD	Reduce immunosuppression to low-dose steroids only; combination treatment: surgery, chemotherapy, radiation therapy, immunotherapy, rituximab. Acyclovir probably of little benefit
Prognosis	Good	Intermediate	Poor

PTLD, post-transplant lymphoproliferative disorder.

TABLE 65-23

Factors Affecting the Net State of Immunosuppression

Immunosuppressive agents: dose, type, duration
Comorbid illness (diabetes mellitus, malnutrition, etc.)
Infection with immune-modulating viruses: CMV, HIV
Integrity of mucocutaneous barriers

CMV, cytomegalovirus; HIV, human immunodeficiency virus.
Adapted from Reference 162.

and more elderly patients are likely to be transplanted; on the other hand, antimicrobial prophylaxis is becoming more effective.

A general point is that when life-threatening infection occurs—at any time—immunosuppression should be reduced to an absolute minimum or stopped altogether ("stress-dose" steroids often are required). Early aggressive diagnosis (e.g., by bronchoscopy in patients with pneumonitis) and therapy are essential.[162]

Infections in the First Month

The majority of infections in the first month are standard infections, as would be seen in nontransplant patients after surgery. Thus, infections of surgical wounds, the lungs, the urinary tract, and infections related to vascular catheters predominate. Bacterial infections are much more common than fungal ones. Preventive measures include ensuring that donor and recipient are free of overt infection before transplant, good surgical technique, and SMX-TMP prophylaxis to prevent UTIs.

Infections from One to Six Months after Transplant

Weeks of intensive immunosuppression now increase the risk of opportunistic infections. Infections with CMV, EBV, *Listeria monocytogenes*, *Pneumocystis carinii*, and *Nocardia* spp. are relatively common. Preventive measures include antiviral prophylaxis (for 3 to 6 months after transplant) and SMX-TMP prophylaxis (for 6 to 12 months after transplant).

Infections More than Six Months after Transplant

With gradual reduction in immunosuppression, the risk of infection long term generally diminishes. However, patients can be roughly divided into two groups based on risk. Group 1 patients (those with good ongoing allograft function and no need for late supplemental immunosuppression) rarely develop opportunistic infections unless exposure is intense (e.g., to *Nocardia* spp. from soil). Infection risk is quite similar to the background nontransplant population. Group 2 patients (those with poor graft function) remain at risk of opportunistic infection. This probably reflects both poor graft function and that many of these patients have received large cumulative doses of immunosuppression. Thus, the latter group should stay on long-term prophylaxis with SMX-TMP.

Late amplification of immunosuppression may increase the risk of opportunistic infection in *any* patient. Therefore, any patient receiving a "late" steroid pulse, tacrolimus rescue therapy, and so forth should be restarted on SMX-TMP and

anti-CMV prophylaxis (if donor or recipient were CMV positive). Readers are referred to recent reviews for a detailed discussion of specific infections after renal transplantation.[162, 163] Two are discussed here: CMV and *P. carinii* pneumonia (PCP). The role of EBV infection in causing PTLD has been discussed earlier.

Cytomegalovirus

Exposure to CMV (as evidenced by the presence in serum of anti-CMV IgG) increases with age; more than two thirds of donors and recipients are latently infected prior to renal transplantation. CMV infection after transplantation is taken to mean that there is only *laboratory* evidence of recent CMV exposure (e.g., a rise in IgG titers or demonstration of CMV in body fluids). Infection may arise from (1) reactivation of latent recipient virus; (2) primary infection with donor-derived virus (transmitted in the allograft or less commonly via blood products); or (3) reactivation of latent donor-derived virus.[164] CMV disease means that there is infection *with* symptoms or evidence of tissue invasion, or both. The risk of CMV infection or disease is highest in CMV-positive donor/CMV-negative recipient pairings, followed by CMV-positive donor/CMV-positive recipient pairings and then CMV-negative donor/CMV-positive recipient pairings. The risk is lowest with CMV-negative donor/CMV-negative recipient pairings. OKT3/polyclonal therapy, particularly when prescribed for treatment of rejection, significantly increases the risk of subsequent CMV disease.

CMV disease usually arises 1 to 6 months after transplantation, although gastrointestinal and retinal involvement often occur later. Typical clinical features are fever, malaise, and leukopenia; there may be symptomatic or laboratory evidence of specific organ involvement (Table 65-24). Urgent investigation and immediate empirical treatment are needed in severe cases. Confirmation of presumed CMV disease is by demonstration of the virus in body fluids or solid organs. Detection of CMV in blood or tissue fluids is best achieved by rapid shell-vial culture, CMV antigen assays, or PCR; the test used depends on local expertise. The virus is best identified in involved tissue by immunohistochemistry techniques. Low or negative CMV concentrations in peripheral blood do *not* exclude organ involvement (especially of the gastrointestinal tract); procedures such as bronchoscopy and endoscopy should be aggressively pursued according to symptoms and signs. A "tissue diagnosis" is also required to exclude coinfection with other microbes such as *P. carinii*.

CMV disease should be treated with reduction in immunosuppression and intravenous antiviral therapy for 2 to 4 weeks, followed by oral antiviral therapy for 2 to 3 months.[162] The intravenous antiviral agent of choice is ganciclovir. Dose adjustment is required in renal failure. Because of its nephrotoxicity, foscarnet should only be used in the rare CMV-resistant cases. Intravenous antiviral therapy should not be stopped until there is clinical improvement *and* documented clearance of viral antigen from peripheral blood. Although supportive data are unavailable, it is reasonable to add CMV hyperimmune globulin in severe cases.[102]

The prevention of CMV disease is of great clinical importance. One general strategy is to give prophylaxis to all patients at risk (i.e., where the donor or recipient is

TABLE 65-24

Manifestations of CMV Disease in the Renal Transplant Recipient

TISSUE AFFECTED	CLINICAL FEATURES	COMMENT
Systemic	Fever, malaise, myalgia	Nonspecific but very important clue to CMV disease
Marrow	Leukopenia	Usually not severe; reduce azathioprine or MMF. Ganciclovir can also cause leukopenia
Lungs	Pneumonitis	May be life threatening; exclude coinfection with other organisms
GI tract	Inflammation and ulceration of esophagus or colon	May be life threatening; often occurs late
Liver	Hepatitis	Rarely severe
Kidney	?	Unclear if direct renal allograft infection occurs
Eyes (retina)	Blurred vision, flashes, floaters	Rare in renal transplants; if occurs, usually late

CMV, cytomegalovirus; GI, gastrointestinal; MMF, mycophenolate mofetil.

TABLE 65-25

Prevention of CMV Disease after Renal Transplantation

DONOR	RECIPIENT	BASELINE RISK	ANTIVIRAL PROPHYLAXIS AFTER TRANSPLANT	DURATION OF PO THERAPY (MONTHS)	ADDITIONAL PROPHYLAXIS DURING OKT3/POLYCLONAL THERAPY AND AFTER	COMMENT
Neg.	Neg.	Very low	Acyclovir PO	3-6	None	Acyclovir given to prevent HSV infection
Neg.	Pos.	Moderate	Valganciclovir PO	3	Valganciclovir PO	Alternative, if no OKT3/polyclonals, is to use acyclovir with monitoring for antigenemia; positive test triggers course of valganciclovir
Pos.	Pos.	High	Valganciclovir PO	3	Valganciclovir PO	
Pos.	Neg.	Very high	Valganciclovir PO	4	Valganciclovir PO	When course of prophylaxis completed, consider monitoring for antigenemia

Partners' Protocol, courtesy of R. Rubin, MD.

CMV, cytomegalovirus; HSV, herpes simplex virus.

CMV positive. Another strategy is to target and intensify prophylaxis only to those at greatest risk. Both have advantages and disadvantages.[165] Table 65-25 shows the protocol, which combines elements of both strategies, currently used in our unit and some others. A limitation of oral ganciclovir is its low bioavailability, hence the need for intravenous administration during periods of intense immunosuppression. Its prodrug, valganciclovir, has greatly improved bioavailability and is currently under investigation in organ transplant recipients. It is likely that this drug will replace both intravenous and oral ganciclovir in many situations. CMV hyperimmune globulin is now less commonly used as a preventive agent because of its expense and variable efficacy.[102] One randomized, controlled trial found valacyclovir to be effective in preventing CMV disease,[166] but further studies are needed to confirm this.

There is accumulating evidence that CMV infection and disease are associated with adverse graft and patient outcomes, in addition to those described earlier. For example,

CMV donor positivity is associated with a small but persistent decrease in allograft survival[30] and, in some studies, with an increased risk of acute rejection,[166] PTLD,[167] and transplant renal artery stenosis.[168] In one series, late acute rejection associated with asymptomatic CMV infection responded to ganciclovir.[79] Putative mechanisms by which CMV could induce these effects include up-regulation of adhesion molecules and MHC products in graft tissue and systemic immunomodulatory effects.[102, 164, 169] Determining the independent effect of CMV infection in the context of rejection, amplified immunosuppression, and so forth is difficult. Other studies have not demonstrated these indirect effects.[170] The role of CMV in causing transplant glomerulopathy and TMA remains to be proven.

Pneumocystosis

Antimicrobial prophylaxis is very effective in preventing pneumonia due to *P. carinii*. The preventive agent of choice is SMX-TMP: It is cheap and generally well tolerated; furthermore, it prevents UTIs and opportunistic infections such as nocardiosis, toxoplasmosis, and listeriosis. Alternative preventive agents include dapsone and pyrimethamine, atovaquone, and aerosolized pentamadine.[171] Typical symptoms of pneumonia due to *P. carinii* are fever, shortness of breath, and nonproductive cough. Chest radiography characteristically shows bilateral interstitial-alveolar infiltrates. Diagnosis is dependent on detection of the organism in a clinical specimen by colorimetric or immunofluorescent stains. Because the organism burden is usually lower than in human immunodeficiency virus (HIV)-infected patients, the sensitivity of induced sputum or bronchoalveolar lavage specimens is lower in renal transplant recipients; tissue should be quickly obtained if these tests are negative and the clinical suspicion remains high.

The treatment of choice remains SMX-TMP.[171] High-dose SMX-TMP may increase the plasma creatinine without affecting GFR. There is no firm evidence to support the use of higher-dose steroids during the early treatment phase of pneumocystosis in renal transplant patients—unlike HIV-positive patients.

Immunization in Renal Transplant Recipients

Important general rules concerning immunization in renal transplant patients are the following: (1) immunizations should be completed at least 4 weeks before transplantation; (2) immunization should be avoided in the first 6 months after transplant because of ongoing high doses of immunosuppression and a risk of provoking graft dysfunction; and (3) live vaccines are generally contraindicated after transplantation. A comprehensive review of this issue has recently been published.[172] Household contacts of transplant recipients should receive yearly immunization against influenza.

Summary

Infections are a predictable complication of renal transplantation. Minimizing infection risk requires meticulous surgical technique, antiviral prophylaxis for the first 3 to 6 months, SMX-TMP prophylaxis for the first 6 to 12 months and, of course, avoidance of excess immunosuppression. The last point is particularly relevant to elderly recipients. A substantial increase in immunosuppression, no matter what the time period after transplant, should trigger resumption of antiviral prophylaxis and SMX-TMP.

TRANSPLANT ISSUES IN SPECIFIC PATIENT GROUPS

Transplantation in Diabetics

The quality of life and overall survival of ESRD patients with diabetes mellitus is significantly improved by renal transplantation compared to dialysis.[96] The best outcomes are achieved with living donor allografts.[173] Another major advantage of living donor transplantation is the potential to avoid dialysis altogether. Cardiovascular disease is highly prevalent in the diabetic ESRD population and must be rigorously excluded or addressed. This is discussed in more detail in Chapter 38. A subset of diabetic ESRD patients is also suitable for kidney-pancreas transplantation (see following discussion).

Kidney-Pancreas Transplantation

The two main goals of transplanting whole pancreas allografts or pancreatic islets are to (1) allow freedom from insulin therapy and the metabolic derangements of type I diabetes mellitus and (2) potentially slow or reverse the progression of end-organ damage from this condition. Transplantation of solid pancreas allografts is technically difficult and the recipient is exposed to high levels of immunosuppression. Thus, patients must be carefully selected for this procedure. Typical exclusion criteria for kidney-pancreas transplantation are cardiovascular disease and age older than 50 years. Common complications include graft thrombosis, graft infection, rejection, and problems related to drainage of the exocrine secretions. Drainage of exocrine secretions into the bladder affords the advantages of sterility and of serial measurement of urinary amylase concentrations that can aid in early detection of graft dysfunction. Important disadvantages include severe cystitis, hypovolemia, and acidosis (the last two due to large losses of bicarbonate-rich fluid). Because rates of technical complications from enteric drainage have decreased, this technique is becoming more popular.[174] Rates of DGF in kidney-pancreas transplantation have been relatively low, probably reflecting donor and recipient selection factors. In contrast, rates of acute renal rejection have generally been higher. The latter finding may reflect the greater antigen "load" of two transplanted organs and a lower threshold for diagnosing acute rejection.

For diabetic ESRD patients deemed suitable candidates for kidney *and* pancreas allografts, two main options are currently available: simultaneous kidney plus pancreas (SPK) transplantation or pancreas after kidney (PAK) transplantation. In the case of the latter, living donor kidneys are often used. In the United States in 1999, 75% of pancreas grafts were SPK, 18% were PAK, and 7% were pancreas alone.[174] Pancreatic allograft survival with PAK has been poorer than SPK transplantation, but this difference is narrowing.[174] In fact, PAK does offer several potential advantages: preemptive living donor kidney transplantation, better renal allograft outcomes, and fewer surgical complications.[175] Thus, the percentages of pancreas transplants performed as PAK have been recently increasing.[174] The improvements in PAK have recently been reviewed.[176]

Pancreas graft survival rates are steadily increasing, mainly due to fewer technical and immunologic failures. Recent registry data show a 1-year survival rate of 82% for SPK and 74% for PAK.[174] One-year renal allograft survival in SPK is well over 90%.[174] Because rejection has been a major problem in kidney-pancreas transplantation, immunosuppression tends to be more intense than for kidney alone. The majority of new kidney-pancreas recipients in the United States now receive either IL-2 receptor blockers or OKT3/polyclonals; MMF, tacrolimus, and steroids are often used as maintenance immunosuppressives. Greater use of MMF and tacrolimus is thought to be one of the principal reasons why rates of rejection have fallen.

Although successful kidney-pancreas transplantation undoubtedly improves the quality of life for previously uremic recipients, the effects of also transplanting the pancreas allograft on reversing or halting the complications of diabetes mellitus are less clear. There are no randomized, controlled trials of these outcomes, and none is likely to be performed. Overall, some benefit is likely,[177, 178] although in patients whose ESRD is due to diabetic nephropathy, other microvascular complications such as retinopathy are likely to be well established. Although there is evidence that pancreas transplantation can reverse the early pathologic changes of diabetic nephropathy in native kidneys,[179] the practical benefit of preventing diabetic nephropathy in renal allografts is currently limited because this is rarely a cause of allograft loss. There is accumulating evidence that, in selected patients, overall and cardiovascular mortality are reduced with combined kidney-pancreas transplantation compared to kidney alone.[173, 180]

Injection of isolated pancreatic islet allograft tissue into the portal venous system can potentially avoid many of the technical problems associated with whole-organ transplantation. This technique has had very limited success, probably because of difficulty in transplanting sufficient numbers of viable islet cells and because of the vulnerability of islets to rejection and other damage.[178] However, Shapiro and colleagues have reported excellent outcomes using a nonsteroidal regimen of daclizumab, tacrolimus, and sirolimus.[181] The Shapiro series did not include ESRD patients, but studies in this area are underway.

Renal Transplantation in the Elderly

In most western countries, the elderly are forming an increasing percentage of the incident and prevalent ESRD population. Many of these patients have significant comorbid disease, particularly cardiovascular disease and type II diabetes mellitus. Nevertheless, age per se is not a contraindication to transplantation: among elderly patients carefully screened and deemed fit for the procedure, long-term outcomes are clearly better with transplantation than dialysis.[96, 182, 183] The percentage of elderly ESRD patients in the United States who have received a kidney transplant is steadily increasing, from 3.7% in 1989 to 8.4% in 1998.[184] The same benefits of living donor allografts accrue to the elderly as to younger patients. Although matching older cadaveric kidneys to older recipients is a common practice (presumably in an attempt to allocate the best kidneys to younger recipients), recent analysis of USRDS data has shown that this does not improve overall graft survival.[185]

As discussed earlier, elderly recipients should receive less aggressive immunosuppression. In particular, avoidance of high-dose CNI or steroid protocols appears prudent because of the higher risk of post-transplant diabetes mellitus in this group.

Renal Transplantation in the Obese

This has been discussed above.

Renal Transplantation in Patients with Human Immunodeficiency Virus Infection

Until recently, HIV infection was considered an absolute contraindication to renal transplantation in most centers. This reflected fears that immunosuppression would facilitate progression of infection and that the short survival of HIV-positive transplanted patients would waste valuable allografts. With dramatic improvements in the survival of HIV-positive patients, these premises are being re-examined.[80, 186] These patients should be referred to centers specializing in the management of transplanted HIV-positive patients because their management is extremely complex. One difficulty is the potential for interactions between the multiple antiviral medicines, some of which inhibit and some of which induce the cytochrome P450 system.[80]

Pregnancy in the Renal Transplant Recipient

Female and male fertility improves after successful renal transplantation. Pregnancy is generally considered safe for the mother, fetus, and renal allograft if the following criteria are met before conception: good general health for more than 18 months before conception, stable allograft function with plasma creatinine less than 2.0 mg/dL (preferably <1.5 mg/dL), minimal hypertension, minimal proteinuria, immunosuppression at maintenance doses, and no dilation of the pelvicalyceal system on recent imaging studies. Of course, some pregnancies occur in less optimal conditions where the risk of permanent allograft damage will be higher.

The National Transplantation Pregnancy Registry is a useful source of information regarding pregnancy outcomes in renal transplant recipients.[187] The latest data show that hypertension occurs in approximately 63% of cases and preeclampsia in 30%. UTIs and asymptomatic bacteruria are also common. At least 20% of pregnancies are lost in the first trimester due to spontaneous or therapeutic abortion, but most of the remainder result in live birth. Prematurity and low birth weight are common. Data on allograft function are overall reassuring. However, the average plasma creatinine level does increase slightly (~0.2 mg/dL) after pregnancy. It is possible that pregnancy may affect long-term graft function by accentuating nephron hyperfiltration and overwork, but this has proved difficult to assess.

All pregnant renal allograft recipients should be managed as high-risk obstetric cases with nephrology involvement. Throughout the pregnancy, regular monitoring of blood pressure, proteinuria, renal function, and urine cultures is advised. Note that the plasma urate concentration may be difficult to interpret in patients on cyclosporine. Significant renal dysfunction occurs in a minority of cases; the principal causes are severe preeclampsia, acute rejection, acute pyelonephritis, and recurrent glomerulonephritis. Distinguishing these causes clinically may be difficult. Initial investigations of renal dysfunction should include plasma creatinine, creatinine clearance, 24-hour urinary protein excretion, urine microscopy, urine culture, and renal ultrasound. Acute rejection should be confirmed by allograft biopsy before instituting antirejection therapy. Pulse steroids are used to treat rejection.

There are no transplant-specific reasons to perform caesarean section; if it is performed (for obstetric reasons), care should be taken to avoid damaging the transplant ureter. Renal function should be monitored closely for 3 months postpartum because of the increased risk of HUS and possibly acute rejection.

Short-term and long-term data indicate that children born to transplant recipients using cyclosporine, steroids, or azathioprine do not have a significant increase in morbidity. Short-term data on tacrolimus are similarly reassuring. Dosages of cyclosporine and tacrolimus may need to be increased to maintain pre-pregnancy trough concentrations.

Because MMF is teratogenic in animals, it should not be used in women contemplating pregnancy. Nevertheless, successful outcomes have been reported.[187] Sirolimus should also be avoided. Limited data regarding paternal use of cyclosporine, steroids, azathioprine, tacrolimus, and MMF are reassuring.

Surgery in the Renal Transplant Recipient
Allograft Nephrectomy

Allograft nephrectomy is not commonly required. Indications include (1) allograft failure with ongoing symptomatic rejection causing fever, malaise, and graft pain; (2) infarction due to thrombosis; (3) severe infection of the allograft such as emphysematous pyelonephritis; and (4) graft rupture. The morbidity associated with allograft nephrectomy is relatively high. Ongoing rejection in a failed allograft can sometimes be controlled with steroids, but prolonged immunosuppression of a patient who is on dialysis is obviously not ideal. Rejection in this context is less likely to be controlled by small doses of steroids when it is acute and when the transplant is recent.

Nontransplant-Related Surgery or Hospitalization

Over time, many renal transplant recipients undergo nontransplant-related surgery or are hospitalized for nontransplant reasons. Common-sense measures such as maintenance of adequate volume status, avoidance of nephrotoxic medicines (including NSAIDs), and proper dosing of immunosuppressive drugs are usually all that are required to prevent dysfunction of the graft. Whenever possible, immunosuppressive drugs should be given by the enteral route; if this is not possible, a regimen of intravenous steroids and intravenous CNIs usually suffices. A simple way to dose intravenous steroids is to prescribe the same milligram-for-milligram dose of intravenous methylprednisolone as the maintenance prednisone dose; supplemental stress-dose hydrocortisone is then prescribed separately. Intravenous cyclosporine should be prescribed in slow infusion form at one third of the total daily oral dose, and intravenous tacrolimus should be at one fifth.

The Patient with the Failing Kidney

Over time, a high percentage of renal allografts ultimately fail. In most cases, patients resume dialysis and, if there are no contraindications, can be listed again for transplant. The waiting time for a second transplant may be prolonged, however, because of sensitization to alloantigens. As in the patient with native kidney disease, management of anemia, hyperparathyroidism, and hypertension and creation of appropriate dialysis access are important in the predialysis transplant patient.

TRANSPLANTATION/IMMUNOSUPPRESSION: THE FUTURE

Major areas of ongoing research and work are the following: expansion of the donor pool, optimization of immunosuppression regimens (with particular focus on individualizing immunosuppression), induction of tolerance, and xenotransplantation. There is also growing interest in therapies that modulate B cell and plasma cell function, thus preventing or treating humoral rejection.

New Immunosuppressive Drugs

Given the central role of the CD4[+] T cell in allograft rejection, most new strategies are targeting CD4+ T cell activation. These include blockade of T cell costimulation, blockade of T cell adhesion molecules, blockade of T cell accessory molecules, and gene therapy.[3] Obtaining tolerance remains an elusive goal in solid-organ transplantation. Tolerance is best defined as the absence of destructive antigraft immune responses in the presence of an otherwise competent immune system.[188] Tolerance to self-antigens is the norm in the healthy human being. This is thought to involve both thymic (central) and extrathymic (peripheral) mechanisms. Central tolerance involves clonal deletion and clonal abortion; peripheral tolerance involves clonal deletion, clonal abortion, clonal anergy, and the action of specific regulatory or suppressor cells. Manipulation of these physiologic mechanisms is a focus of ongoing research.[188]

New Drug Combinations

Of more immediate clinical interest are the ways in which presently available antirejection drugs can best be combined to minimize both rejection and adverse effects. Two areas of major focus have been the withdrawal, reduction, and nonuse of steroids or CNIs. A major limitation of such strategies is our current limited ability to measure an *individual* patient's degree of immunosuppression. A general guiding rule is that the risk of rejection on these low-dose regimens is greater in blacks, cadaveric kidney recipients, and those with a history of acute rejection.

Avoidance of CNIs altogether, even while using IL-2 receptor blockers and MMF, has been associated with unacceptably high rates of acute rejection[189, 190]; preliminary data with sirolimus are not very encouraging.[27] Late withdrawal of CNIs can improve GFR, but a significant minority, even of stable, white patients on MMF, develop acute rejection.[85] One recent meta-analysis found that withdrawal of cyclosporine in select patients was associated with an increased risk of acute rejection but not of graft failure.[191] However, the long-term effects of withdrawing CNIs are unclear. It is possible that "creatinine creep," as seen with steroid withdrawal, may still be problematic. Thus, the clinician is faced with the choice: Is it better to withdraw CNIs to potentially help the majority of patients while putting a minority at risk of late acute rejection? One strategy is to combine low-dose CNIs with sirolimus; short-term results are encouraging.[28, 29] More data are needed, however, before this strategy can be recommended outside clinical trials.

Enthusiasm for steroid withdrawal has been tempered by the associated risk of both acute and chronic graft dysfunction, at least with older cyclosporine plus azathioprine regimens.[191-193] With the availability of more powerful immunosuppressants such as tacrolimus and MMF, the issue is being revisited. Single-center results with various combinations of thymoglobulin, IL-2 receptor blockers, MMF, and CNIs are encouraging.[23, 24] Again, data from randomized, controlled trial are needed to confirm these observations. For now, routine steroid-free immunosuppression cannot be recommended.

Xenotransplantation

Transplantation of vital organs from other mammals may ultimately solve the organ donor shortage. However, aggressive immunologic responses to xenografts remain a significant obstacle.[194] Xenografts transplanted between closely related species are termed *concordant*; between distant species (e.g., swine to human) are referred to as *discordant*. Discordant xenotransplantation results in hyperacute rejection induced by preformed xenoreactive antibodies that bind mainly to carbohydrate antigens on the surface of graft endothelial cells and by activation of complement. Methods of depleting xenoreactive antibodies and of inactivating complement are being developed. Transgenic pigs, expressing human complement regulatory proteins, have been created; organs from such animals do not undergo hyperacute rejection. However, acute vascular rejection still occurs several days post-transplantation. This is thought to involve xenoreactive antibodies, complement, monocytes, and natural killer cells.[195] Currently, acute vascular rejection is the major immunologic obstacle to successful porcine-to-primate xenotransplantation. Even if both these processes are overcome, acute cellular rejection is likely to be a major problem. Less is known about this phenomenon in xenotransplantation, but available data suggest that the process is vigorous and involves both the direct and indirect pathways of allorecognition.[196]

Avoiding these immunologic complications may require very aggressive immunosuppression. Alternatives under study include immunoisolation of xenogeneic tissue in capsules or membranes or genetic alteration of xenogeneic tissue. There are other major concerns about xenotransplantation. First, the transmission of zoonotic diseases, particularly retroviruses, from animals to humans is a real risk.[197] Second, would the physiologic function of xenogeneic tissue be suboptimal (e.g., in its response to human hormones)? Would a porcine kidney respond correctly to human antidiuretic hormone? Would its vitamin D and erythropoietin be physiologically active? Finally, the ethics of xenotransplantation are still a matter of some controversy.

CONCLUSION

Improvements in short- and long-term renal allograft survival have been very encouraging. This reflects multiple influences, including more effective immunosuppression, more use of living donors, and better medical and surgical care. The focus is likely to shift somewhat toward improving other post-transplant outcomes such as complications of immunosuppression, allograft dysfunction, and morbidity from cardiovascular disease. Availability of adequate numbers of organs for transplantation remains an ongoing problem.

REFERENCES

1. Humar A, Ramcharan T, Denny R, et al: Are wound complications after a kidney transplant more common with modern immunosuppression? Transplantation 72:1920-1923, 2001.
2. Odland MD: Surgical technique/post-transplant surgical complications. Surg Clin North Am 78:55-60, 1998.
3. Denton MD, Magee CC, Sayegh MH: Immunosuppressive strategies in transplantation. Lancet 353:1083-1091, 1999.
4. Hanto DW, Jendrisak MD, So SK, et al: Induction immunosuppression with antilymphocyte globulin or OKT3 in cadaver kidney transplantation: Results of a single institution prospective randomized trial. Transplantation 57:377-384, 1994.
5. Bock HA, Gallati H, Zurcher RM, et al: A randomized prospective trial of prophylactic immunosuppression with ATG-Fresenius versus OKT3 after renal transplantation. Transplantation 59:830-840, 1995.
6. Cole EH, Cattran DC, Farewell VT, et al: A comparison of rabbit antithymocyte serum and OKT3 as prophylaxis against renal allograft rejection. Transplantation 57:60-67, 1994.
7. Vincenti F, Kirkman R, Light S, et al: Interleukin-2 receptor blockade with daclizumab to prevent acute rejection in renal transplantation. Daclizumab Triple-Therapy Study Group. N Engl J Med 338:161-165, 1998.
8. Nashan B, Moore R, Amlot P, et al: Randomised trial of basiliximab versus placebo for control of acute cellular rejection in renal allograft recipients. CHIB 201 International Study Group. Lancet 350:1193-1198, 1997.
9. Halloran P, Hunsicker L: Delayed graft function: State of the art. Am J Transplant 1:115-120, 2001.
10. Randomized, international study of cyclosporine microemulsion absorption profiling in renal transplantation with basiliximab immunoprophylaxis. Am J Transplant 2:157-166, 2002.
11. Nashan B, Cole E, Levy G, Thervet E: Clinical validation studies of Neoral C(2) monitoring: A review. Transplantation 73(9 Suppl):S3-S11, 2002.
12. Vincenti F, Jensik SC, Filo RS, et al: A long-term comparison of tacrolimus (FK506) and cyclosporine in kidney transplantation: Evidence for improved allograft survival at five years. Transplantation 73:775-782, 2002.
13. Fulton B, Markham A: Mycophenolate mofetil: A review of its pharmacodynamic and pharmacokinetic properties and clinical efficacy in renal transplantation. Drugs 51:278-298, 1996.
14. Halloran P, Mathew T, Tomlanovich S, et al: Mycophenolate mofetil in renal allograft recipients: A pooled efficacy analysis of three randomized, double-blind, clinical studies in prevention of rejection. The International Mycophenolate Mofetil Renal Transplant Study Groups. Transplantation 63:39-47, 1997.
15. Mycophenolate mofetil in renal transplantation: Three-year results from the placebo-controlled trial. European Mycophenolate Mofetil Cooperative Study Group. Transplantation 68:391-396, 1999.
16. Ojo AO, Meier-Kriesche HU, Hanson JA, et al: Mycophenolate mofetil reduces late renal allograft loss independent of acute rejection. Transplantation 69:2405-2409, 2000.
17. Cattaneo D, Gaspari F, Ferrari S, et al: Pharmacokinetics help optimizing mycophenolate mofetil dosing in kidney transplant patients. Clin Transplant 15:402-409, 2001.
18. Neylan JF: Immunosuppressive therapy in high-risk transplant patients: Dose-dependent efficacy of mycophenolate mofetil in African-American renal allograft recipients. U.S. Renal Transplant Mycophenolate Mofetil Study Group. Transplantation 64:1277-1282, 1997.
19. Ahsan N, Johnson C, Gonwa T, et al: Randomized trial of tacrolimus plus mycophenolate mofetil or azathioprine versus cyclosporine oral solution (modified) plus mycophenolate mofetil after cadaveric kidney transplantation: Results at two years. Transplantation 72:245-250, 2001.
20. Miller J, Mendez R, Pirsch JD, Jensik SC: Safety and efficacy of tacrolimus in combination with mycophenolate mofetil (MMF) in cadaveric renal transplant recipients. FK506/MMF Dose-Ranging Kidney Transplant Study Group. Transplantation 69:875-880, 2000.
21. Hubner GI, Eismann R, Sziegoleit W: Drug interaction between mycophenolate mofetil and tacrolimus detectable within therapeutic mycophenolic acid monitoring in renal transplant patients. Ther Drug Monit 21:536-539, 1999.
22. Hricik D: Steroid-free immunosuppression in kidney transplantation: An editorial review. Am J Transplant 2:19-24, 2002.
23. Birkeland SA: Steroid-free immunosuppression in renal transplantation: A long-term follow-up of 100 consecutive patients. Transplantation 71:1089-1090, 2001.
24. Matas A: Rapid discontinuation of steroids in living donor kidney transplantation: A pilot study. Am J Transplant 1:278-283, 2001.
25. Halloran PF: Sirolimus and cyclosporin for renal transplantation. Lancet 356:179-180, 2000.
26. Kahan BD: Efficacy of sirolimus compared with azathioprine for reduction of acute renal allograft rejection: A randomised multicentre study. Rapamune U.S. Study Group. Lancet 356:194-202, 2000.

27. Kreis H, Cisterne JM, Land W, et al: Sirolimus in association with mycophenolate mofetil induction for the prevention of acute graft rejection in renal allograft recipients. Transplantation 69:1252-1260, 2000.

28. Johnson RW, Kreis H, Oberbauer R, et al: Sirolimus allows early cyclosporine withdrawal in renal transplantation resulting in improved renal function and lower blood pressure. Transplantation 72:777-786, 2001.

29. McAlister VC, Gao Z, Peltekian K, et al: Sirolimus-tacrolimus combination immunosuppression. Lancet 355:376-377, 2000.

30. Gjertson DW: Impact of delayed graft function and acute rejection on kidney graft survival. Clin Transpl 467-480, 2000.

31. Novick AC, Hwei HH, Steinmuller D, et al: Detrimental effect of cyclosporine on initial function of cadaver renal allografts following extended preservation: Results of a randomized prospective study. Transplantation 42:154-158, 1986.

32. Shoskes DA: Nonimmunologic renal allograft injury and delayed graft function: Clinical strategies for prevention and treatment. Transplant Proc 32:766-768, 2000.

33. Goggins W, Pascual M, Farrell M, et al: Intraoperative versus postoperative thymoglobulin in cadaveric renal transplantation. Paper presented at a meeting of The International Congress of the Transplantation Society, Miami, FL, 2002.

34. Takemoto SK: Maintenance immunosuppression. Clin Transpl 481-495, 2000.

35. Chang GJ, Mahanty HD, Vincenti F, et al: A calcineurin inhibitor–sparing regimen with sirolimus, mycophenolate mofetil, and anti-CD25 mAb provides effective immunosuppression in kidney transplant recipients with delayed or impaired graft function. Clin Transplant 14:550-554, 2000.

36. Montgomery R, Zachary A, Racusen L, et al: Plasmapheresis and intravenous immune globulin provides effective rescue therapy for refractory humoral rejection and allows kidneys to be successfully transplanted into cross-match–positive recipients. Transplantation 70:887-895, 2000.

37. Schweitzer EJ, Wilson JS, Fernandez-Vina M, et al: A high panel-reactive antibody rescue protocol for cross-match–positive live donor kidney transplants. Transplantation 70:1531-1536, 2000.

38. Glotz D, Antoine C, Julia P, Suberbielle-Boissel C: Desensitization and subsequent kidney transplantation of patients using intravenous immunoglobulin. Am J Transplant 2:758-760, 2002.

39. Racusen LC, Solez K, Colvin RB, et al: The Banff 97 working classification of renal allograft pathology. Kidney Int 55:713-723, 1999.

40. Collins AB, Schneeberger EE, Pascual MA, et al: Complement activation in acute humoral renal allograft rejection: Diagnostic significance of C4d deposits in peritubular capillaries. J Am Soc Nephrol 10:2208-2214, 1999.

41. Pascual M, Saidman S, Tolkoff-Rubin N, et al: Plasma exchange and tacrolimus-mycophenolate rescue for acute humoral rejection in kidney transplantation. Transplantation 66:1460-1464, 1998.

42. Bohmig GA, Regele H, Exner M, et al: C4d-positive acute humoral renal allograft rejection: Effective treatment by immunoadsorption. J Am Soc Nephrol 12:2482-2489, 2001.

43. Valero R: Donor management: One step forward. Am J Transplant 2:693-694, 2002.

44. Balakrishnan P, DuBose T: Osmotic nephropathy. *In* Molitoris B, Finn W (eds): Acute Renal Failure: A Companion to Brenner and Rector's The Kidney. Philadelphia, WB Saunders, 2001.

45. Alijani MR, Cutler JA, DelValle CJ, et al: Single-donor cold storage versus machine perfusion in cadaver kidney preservation. Transplantation 40:659-661, 1985.

46. Merion RM, Oh HK, Port FK, et al: A prospective controlled trial of cold-storage versus machine-perfusion preservation in cadaveric renal transplantation. Transplantation 50:230-233, 1990.

47. Salmela K, Wramner L, Ekberg H, et al: A randomized multicenter trial of the anti-ICAM-1 monoclonal antibody (enlimomab) for the prevention of acute rejection and delayed onset of graft function in cadaveric renal transplantation: A report of the European Anti-ICAM-1 Renal Transplant Study Group. Transplantation 67:729-736, 1999.

48. Hourmant M, Bedrossian J, Durand D, et al: A randomized multicenter trial comparing leukocyte function–associated antigen-1 monoclonal antibody with rabbit antithymocyte globulin as induction treatment in first kidney transplantations. Transplantation 62:1565-1570, 1996.

49. Grino JM: BN 52021: A platelet-activating factor antagonist for preventing post-transplant renal failure—a double-blind, randomized study. The BN 52021 Study Group in Renal Transplantation. Ann Intern Med 121:345-347, 1994.

50. Takemoto SK, Terasaki PI, Gjertson DW, Cecka JM: Twelve years' experience with national sharing of HLA-matched cadaveric kidneys for transplantation. N Engl J Med 343:1078-1084, 2000.

51. Morris PJ, Johnson RJ, Fuggle SV, et al: Analysis of factors that affect outcome of primary cadaveric renal transplantation in the UK: HLA Task Force of the Kidney Advisory Group of the United Kingdom Transplant Support Service Authority (UKTSSA). Lancet 354:1147-1152, 1999.

52. Rosengard BR, Feng S, Alfrey EJ, et al: Report of the Crystal City meeting to maximize the use of organs recovered from the cadaver donor. Am J Transplant 2:701-711, 2002.

53. Matas A, Delmonico F: Transplant kidneys sooner: Discard fewer kidneys. Am J Transplant 1:301-304, 2001.

54. Morrissey P, Ramirez P, Gohh R, et al: Management of thrombophilia in renal transplant patients. Am J Transplant 2:872-876, 2002.

55. McCarthy GP, Roberts IS: Diagnosis of acute renal allograft rejection: Evaluation of the Banff 97 Guidelines for Slide Preparation. Transplantation 73:1518-1521, 2002.

56. Rush D, Nickerson P, Gough J, et al: Beneficial effects of treatment of early subclinical rejection: A randomized study. J Am Soc Nephrol 9:2129-2134, 1998.

57. Deierhoi MH, Barber WH, Curtis JJ, et al: A comparison of OKT3 monoclonal antibody and corticosteroids in the treatment of acute renal allograft rejection. Am J Kidney Dis 11:86-89, 1988.

58. Thistlethwaite JR Jr, Gaber AO, Haag BW, et al: OKT3 treatment of steroid-resistant renal allograft rejection. Transplantation 43:176-184, 1987.

59. Gaber AO, First MR, Tesi RJ, et al: Results of the double-blind, randomized, multicenter, phase III clinical trial of thymoglobulin versus Atgam in the treatment of acute graft rejection episodes after renal transplantation. Transplantation 66:29-37, 1998.

60. Hong JC, Kahan BD: Sirolimus rescue therapy for refractory rejection in renal transplantation. Transplantation 71:1579-1584, 2001.

61. Strehlau J, Pavlakis M, Lipman M, et al: Quantitative detection of immune activation transcripts as a diagnostic tool in kidney transplantation. Proc Natl Acad Sci U S A 94:695-700, 1997.

62. Vasconcellos LM, Schachter AD, Zheng XX, et al: Cytotoxic lymphocyte gene expression in peripheral blood leukocytes correlates with rejecting renal allografts. Transplantation 66:562-566, 1998.

63. Li B, Hartono C, Ding R, et al: Noninvasive diagnosis of renal-allograft rejection by measurement of messenger RNA for perforin and granzyme B in urine. N Engl J Med 344:947-954, 2001.

64. Ruggenenti P: Post-transplant hemolytic-uremic syndrome. Kidney Int 62:1093-1104, 2002.

65. Baid S, Pascual M, Williams WW Jr, et al: Renal thrombotic microangiopathy associated with anticardiolipin antibodies in hepatitis C–positive renal allograft recipients. J Am Soc Nephrol 10:146-153, 1999.

66. Abbott KC, Sawyers ES, Oliver JD III, et al: Graft loss due to recurrent focal segmental glomerulosclerosis in renal transplant recipients in the United States. Am J Kidney Dis 37:366-373, 2001.

67. Artero ML, Sharma R, Savin VJ, Vincenti F: Plasmapheresis reduces proteinuria and serum capacity to injure glomeruli in patients with recurrent focal glomerulosclerosis. Am J Kidney Dis 23:574-581, 1994.

68. Peten E, Pirson Y, Cosyns JP, et al: Outcome of thirty patients with Alport's syndrome after renal transplantation. Transplantation 52:823-826, 1991.

69. Kaplan BS, Papadimitriou M, Brezin JH, et al: Renal transplantation in adults with autosomal recessive inheritance of hemolytic uremic syndrome. Am J Kidney Dis 30:760-765, 1997.

70. Lahlou A, Lang P, Charpentier B, et al: Hemolytic-uremic syndrome: Recurrence after renal transplantation. Groupe Cooperatif de l'Ile-de-France (GCIF). Medicine (Baltimore) 79:90-102, 2000.

71. Gaston RS: Maintenance immunosuppression in the renal transplant recipient: An overview. Am J Kidney Dis 38(6 Suppl 6):S25-S35, 2001.

72. Butani L, Polinsky MS, Kaiser BA, Baluarte HJ: Anti-lymphocyte antibodies late in the course of pediatric renal transplantation. Pediatr Nephrol 13:192-194, 1999.

73. Randhawa PS, Demetris AJ: Nephropathy due to polyomavirus type BK. N Engl J Med 342:1361-1363, 2000.

74. Nickeleit V, Klimkait T, Binet IF, et al: Testing for polyomavirus type BK DNA in plasma to identify renal allograft recipients with viral nephropathy. N Engl J Med 342:1309-1315, 2000.

75. Pereira BJ, Natov SN, Bouthot BA, et al: Effects of hepatitis C infection and renal transplantation on survival in end-stage renal disease. The New England Organ Bank Hepatitis C Study Group. Kidney Int 53:1374-1381, 1998.

76. Fabrizi F, Martin P, Ponticelli C: Hepatitis C virus infection and renal transplantation. Am J Kidney Dis 38:919-934, 2001.

77. Morales JM, Campistol JM: Transplantation in the patient with hepatitis C. J Am Soc Nephrol 11:1343-1353, 2000.

78. Rostaing L, Modesto A, Baron E, et al: Acute renal failure in kidney transplant patients treated with interferon α2b for chronic hepatitis C. Nephron 74:512-516, 1996.

79. Reinke P, Fietze E, Ode-Hakim S, et al: Late-acute renal allograft rejection and symptomless cytomegalovirus infection. Lancet 344: 1737-1738, 1994.

80. Gow PJ, Pillay D, Mutimer D: Solid-organ transplantation in patients with HIV infection. Transplantation 72:177-181, 2001.

81. Bae J, Jarcho JA, Denton MD, Magee CC: Statin-specific toxicity in organ transplant recipients: Case report and review of the literature. J Nephrol 15:317-319, 2002.

82. Ahuja TS, Niaz N, Agraharkar M: Contrast-induced nephrotoxicity in renal allograft recipients. Clin Nephrol 54:11-14, 2000.

83. Halloran PF, Melk A, Barth C: Rethinking chronic allograft nephropathy: The concept of accelerated senescence. J Am Soc Nephrol 10: 167-181, 1999.

84. Weir MR, Ward MT, Blahut SA, et al: Long-term impact of discontinued or reduced calcineurin inhibitor in patients with chronic allograft nephropathy. Kidney Int 59:1567-1573, 2001.

85. Smak Gregoor PJ, van Gelder T, van Besouw NM, et al: Randomized study on the conversion of treatment with cyclosporine to azathioprine or mycophenolate mofetil followed by dose reduction. Transplantation 70:143-148, 2000.

86. Ziai F, Nagano H, Kusaka M, et al: Renal allograft protection with losartan in Fisher->Lewis rats: Hemodynamics, macrophages, and cytokines. Kidney Int 57:2618-2625, 2000.

87. Szabo A, Lutz J, Schleimer K, et al: Effect of angiotensin-converting enzyme inhibition on growth factor mRNA in chronic renal allograft rejection in the rat. Kidney Int 57:982-991, 2000.

88. Kahan BD: Potential therapeutic interventions to avoid or treat chronic allograft dysfunction. Transplantation 71(11 Suppl):S52-S57, 2001.

89. Ponticelli C, Traversi L, Feliciani A, et al: Kidney transplantation in patients with IgA mesangial glomerulonephritis. Kidney Int 60: 1948-1954, 2001.

90. Ward MM: Outcomes of renal transplantation among patients with end-stage renal disease caused by lupus nephritis. Kidney Int 57:2136-2143, 2000.

91. Nachman PH, Segelmark M, Westman K, et al: Recurrent ANCA-associated small vessel vasculitis after transplantation: A pooled analysis. Kidney Int 56:1544-1550, 1999.

92. Andresdottir MB, Assmann KJ, Hoitsma AJ, et al: Recurrence of type I membranoproliferative glomerulonephritis after renal transplantation: Analysis of the incidence, risk factors, and impact on graft survival. Transplantation 63:1628-1633, 1997.

93. Andresdottir MB, Assmann KJ, Hoitsma AJ, et al: Renal transplantation in patients with dense deposit disease: Morphological characteristics of recurrent disease and clinical outcome. Nephrol Dial Transplant 14:1723-1731, 1999.

94. Cosyns JP, Couchoud C, Pouteil-Noble C, et al: Recurrence of membranous nephropathy after renal transplantation: Probability, outcome, and risk factors. Clin Nephrol 50:144-153, 1998.

95. Kim H, Cheigh JS: Kidney transplantation in patients with type 1 diabetes mellitus: Long-term prognosis for patients and grafts. Korean J Intern Med 16:98-104, 2001.

96. Wolfe RA, Ashby VB, Milford EL, et al: Comparison of mortality in all patients on dialysis, patients on dialysis awaiting transplantation, and recipients of a first cadaveric transplant. N Engl J Med 341: 1725-1730, 1999.

97. USRDS: USRDS 2001 Annual Data Report: NIH and NIDDK, Bethesda, MD, 2002.

98. Russ GR: 2001 Report of the ANZDATA Registry. Chapter 8: Transplantation: Australia and New Zealand Dialysis and Transplant Registry (ANZDATA), 2002.

99. van Dijk PC, Jager KJ, de Charro F, et al: Renal replacement therapy in Europe: The results of a collaborative effort by the ERA-EDTA Registry and six national or regional registries. Nephrol Dial Transplant 16:1120-1129, 2001.

100. Cecka JM: The UNOS Scientific Renal Transplant Registry, 2000. Clin Transpl 1-18, 2000.

101. Terasaki PI: The HLA-matching effect in different cohorts of kidney transplant recipients. Clin Transpl 497-514, 2000.

102. Brennan DC: Cytomegalovirus in renal transplantation. J Am Soc Nephrol 12:848-855, 2001.

103. Mange KC, Joffe MM, Feldman HI: Effect of the use or nonuse of long-term dialysis on the subsequent survival of renal transplants from living donors. N Engl J Med 344:726-731, 2001.

104. Terasaki PI, Cecka JM: The center effect: Is bigger better? Clin Transpl 317-324, 1999.

105. Suthanthiran M: The importance of genetic polymorphisms in renal transplantation. Curr Opin Urol 10:71-75, 2000.

106. Gjertson DW, Cecka JM: Living unrelated donor kidney transplantation. Kidney Int 58:491-499, 2000.

107. Chertow GM, Milford EL, Mackenzie HS, Brenner BM: Antigen-independent determinants of cadaveric kidney transplant failure. JAMA 276:1732-1736, 1996.

108. Kasiske BL, Snyder JJ, Gilbertson D: Inadequate donor size in cadaver kidney transplantation. J Am Soc Nephrol 13:2152-2159, 2002.

109. Kim YS, Moon JI, Kim DK, et al: Ratio of donor kidney weight to recipient body weight as an index of graft function. Lancet 357: 1180-1181, 2001.

110. Ojo AO, Hanson JA, Meier-Kriesche H, et al: Survival in recipients of marginal cadaveric donor kidneys compared with other recipients and wait-listed transplant candidates. J Am Soc Nephrol 12:589-597, 2001.

111. Metcalfe MS, Butterworth PC, White SA, et al: A case-control comparison of the results of renal transplantation from heart-beating and non–heart-beating donors. Transplantation 71:1556-1559, 2001.

112. Meier-Kriesche HU, Ojo AO, Leavey SF, et al: Gender differences in the risk for chronic renal allograft failure. Transplantation 71: 429-432, 2001.

113. Almond PS, Matas A, Gillingham K, et al: Risk factors for chronic rejection in renal allograft recipients. Transplantation 55:752-757, 1993.

114. Pischon T, Sharma AM: Obesity as a risk factor in renal transplant patients. Nephrol Dial Transplant 16:14-17, 2001.

115. Meier-Kriesche HU, Arndorfer JA, Kaplan B: The impact of body mass index on renal transplant outcomes: A significant independent risk factor for graft failure and patient death. Transplantation 73: 70-74, 2002.

116. Patel MG: The effect of dietary intervention on weight gains after renal transplantation. J Renal Nutr 8:137-141, 1998.

117. Lopes IM, Martin M, Errasti P, Martinez JA: Benefits of a dietary intervention on weight loss, body composition, and lipid profile after renal transplantation. Nutrition 15:7-10, 1999.

118. Yanovski SZ, Yanovski JA: Obesity. N Engl J Med 346:591-602, 2002.

119. Remuzzi G, Perico N: Routine renin-angiotensin system blockade in renal transplantation? Curr Opin Nephrol Hypertens 11:1-10, 2002.

120. Briganti EM, Russ GR, McNeil JJ, et al: Risk of renal allograft loss from recurrent glomerulonephritis. N Engl J Med 347:103-109, 2002.

121. Kasiske BL, Vazquez MA, Harmon WE, et al: Recommendations for the outpatient surveillance of renal transplant recipients. American Society of Transplantation. J Am Soc Nephrol 11(Suppl 15):S1-S86, 2000.

122. Hariharan S: Long-term renal transplant management: Introduction. Am J Kidney Dis 38(6 Suppl 6):S1, 2001.

123. Howard AD: Long-term management of the renal transplant recipient: Optimizing the relationship between the transplant center and the community nephrologist. Am J Kidney Dis 38(6 Suppl 6): S51-S57, 2001.

124. Levi M: Post-transplant hypophosphatemia. Kidney Int 59:2377-2387, 2001.

125. Bantle JP, Nath KA, Sutherland DE, et al: Effects of cyclosporine on the renin-angiotensin-aldosterone system and potassium excretion in renal transplant recipients. Arch Intern Med 145:505-508, 1985.

126. Heering P, Degenhardt S, Grabensee B: Tubular dysfunction following kidney transplantation. Nephron 74:501-511, 1996.

127. Batlle DC, Mozes MF, Manaligod J, et al: The pathogenesis of hyperchloremic metabolic acidosis associated with kidney transplantation. Am J Med 70:786-796, 1981.

128. Lobo PI, Cortez MS, Stevenson W, Pruett TL: Normocalcemic hyperparathyroidism associated with relatively low 1:25 vitamin D

levels postrenal transplant can be successfully treated with oral calcitriol. Clin Transplant 9:277-281, 1995.

129. Messa P, Sindici C, Cannella G, et al: Persistent secondary hyperparathyroidism after renal transplantation. Kidney Int 54:1704-1713, 1998.

130. Caravaca F, Fernandez MA, Cubero J, et al: Are plasma 1,25-dihydroxyvitamin D_3 concentrations appropriate after successful kidney transplantation? Nephrol Dial Transplant 13(Suppl 3):91-93, 1998.

131. Steiner RW, Ziegler M, Halasz NA, et al: Effect of daily oral vitamin D and calcium therapy, hypophosphatemia, and endogenous 1-25 dihydrocholecalciferol on parathyroid hormone and phosphate wasting in renal transplant recipients. Transplantation 56:843-846, 1993.

132. Pilmore HL, Faire B, Dittmer I: Tacrolimus for the treatment of gout in renal transplantation: Two case reports and review of the literature. Transplantation 72:1703-1705, 2001.

133. Lin HY, Rocher LL, McQuillan MA, et al: Cyclosporine-induced hyperuricemia and gout. N Engl J Med 321:287-292, 1989.

134. Clive DM: Renal transplant–associated hyperuricemia and gout. J Am Soc Nephrol 11:974-979, 2000.

135. Braun WE, Richmond BJ, Protiva DA, et al: The incidence and management of osteoporosis, gout, and avascular necrosis in recipients of renal allografts functioning more than 20 years (level 5A) treated with prednisone and azathioprine. Transplant Proc 31:1366-1369, 1999.

136. Delmas PD: Osteoporosis in patients with organ transplants: A neglected problem. Lancet 357:325-326, 2001.

137. Grotz WH, Mundinger FA, Gugel B, et al: Bone fracture and osteodensitometry with dual energy X-ray absorptiometry in kidney transplant recipients. Transplantation 58:912-915, 1994.

138. Weber TJ, Quarles LD: Preventing bone loss after renal transplantation with bisphosphonates: We can... but should we? Kidney Int 57:735-737, 2000.

139. Markowitz GS, Appel GB, Fine PL, et al: Collapsing focal segmental glomerulosclerosis following treatment with high-dose pamidronate. J Am Soc Nephrol 12:1164-1172, 2001.

140. Briggs JD: Causes of death after renal transplantation. Nephrol Dial Transplant 16:1545-1549, 2001.

141. Cecka JM: The UNOS Scientific Renal Transplant Registry. Clin Transpl 1-21, 1999.

142. Opelz G, Wujciak T, Ritz E: Association of chronic kidney graft failure with recipient blood pressure. Collaborative Transplant Study. Kidney Int 53:217-222, 1998.

143. Chobanian AV, Bakris GL, Black HR et al: The seventh report of the Joint National Committee of prevention, detection, evaluation, and treatment of high blood pressure: the JNC–7 report. JAMA 289:2560-2572, 2003.

144. Detection, Evaluation, and Treatment of High Blood Cholesterol in Adults (Adult Treatment Panel III). Bethesda, MD, National Heart Lung and Blood Institute, 2001.

145. Holdaas H, Jardine AG, Wheeler DC, et al: Effect of fluvastatin on acute renal allograft rejection: A randomized multicenter trial. Kidney Int 60:1990-1997, 2001.

146. Ducloux D, Motte G, Challier B, et al: Serum total homocysteine and cardiovascular disease occurrence in chronic, stable renal transplant recipients: A prospective study. J Am Soc Nephrol 11:134-137, 2000.

147. Shemin D, Bostom AG, Selhub J: Treatment of hyperhomocysteinemia in end-stage renal disease. Am J Kidney Dis 38(4 Suppl 1):S91-S99, 2001.

148. Penn I: Posttransplant malignancies. Transplant Proc 31:1260-1262, 1999.

149. Sheil AG: 2001 Report of the ANZDATA Registry. Chapter 9: Cancer Report: Australia and New Zealand Dialysis and Transplant Registry (ANZDATA), 2002.

150. Hojo M, Morimoto T, Maluccio M, et al: Cyclosporine induces cancer progression by a cell-autonomous mechanism. Nature 397:530-534, 1999.

151. McGeown MG, Douglas JF, Middleton D: One thousand renal transplants at Belfast City Hospital: Postgraft neoplasia 1968-1999, comparing azathioprine only with cyclosporin-based regimes in a single centre. Clin Transpl 193-202, 1999.

152. Dantal J, Hourmant M, Cantarovich D, et al: Effect of long-term immunosuppression in kidney-graft recipients on cancer incidence: Randomised comparison of two cyclosporin regimens. Lancet 351:623-628, 1998.

153. Soulillou JP, Giral M: Controlling the incidence of infection and malignancy by modifying immunosuppression. Transplantation 72(12 Suppl):S89-S93, 2001.

154. Guba M, von Breitenbuch P, Steinbauer M, et al: Rapamycin inhibits primary and metastatic tumor growth by antiangiogenesis: Involvement of vascular endothelial growth factor. Nat Med 8:128-135, 2002.

155. Penn I: Neoplastic complications of transplantation. Semin Respir Infect 8:233-239, 1993.

156. Dharnidharka VR, Sullivan EK, Stablein DM, et al: Risk factors for post-transplant lymphoproliferative disorder (PTLD) in pediatric kidney transplantation: A report of the North American Pediatric Renal Transplant Cooperative Study (NAPRTCS). Transplantation 71:1065-1068, 2001.

157. Rowe DT, Webber S, Schauer EM, et al: Epstein-Barr virus load monitoring: Its role in the prevention and management of post-transplant lymphoproliferative disease. Transplant Infect Dis 3:79-87, 2001.

158. Cook RC, Connors JM, Gascoyne RD, et al: Treatment of post-transplant lymphoproliferative disease with rituximab monoclonal antibody after lung transplantation. Lancet 354:1698-1699, 1999.

159. Milpied N, Vasseur B, Parquet N, et al: Humanized anti-CD20 monoclonal antibody (rituximab) in post-transplant B-lymphoproliferative disorder: A retrospective analysis on 32 patients. Ann Oncol 11(Suppl 1):113-116, 2000.

160. Haque T, Taylor C, Wilkie GM, et al: Complete regression of post-transplant lymphoproliferative disease using partially HLA-matched Epstein Barr virus–specific cytotoxic T cells. Transplantation 72:1399-1402, 2001.

161. Preiksaitis JK: Epstein-Barr virus infection and malignancy in solid organ transplant recipients: Strategies for prevention and treatment. Transplant Infect Dis 3:56-59, 2001.

162. Fishman JA, Rubin RH: Infection in organ transplant recipients. N Engl J Med 338:1741-1751, 1998.

163. Patel R: Infections in recipients of kidney transplants. Infect Dis Clin North Am 15:901-952, xi, 2001.

164. Rubin RH: Cytomegalovirus in solid organ transplantation. Clin Infect Dis 3:S1-S5, 2001.

165. Kusne S, Shapiro R, Fung J: Prevention and treatment of cytomegalovirus infection in organ transplant recipients. Transplant Infect Dis 1:187-203, 1999.

166. Lowance D, Neumayer HH, Legendre CM, et al: Valacyclovir for the prevention of cytomegalovirus disease after renal transplantation. International Valacyclovir Cytomegalovirus Prophylaxis Transplantation Study Group. N Engl J Med 340:1462-1470, 1999.

167. Basgoz N, Preiksaitis JK: Post-transplant lymphoproliferative disorder. Infect Dis Clin North Am 9:901-923, 1995.

168. Pouria S, State OI, Wong W, Hendry BM: CMV infection is associated with transplant renal artery stenosis. Q J Med 91:185-189, 1998.

169. Soderberg-Naucler C, Emery VC: Viral infections and their impact on chronic renal allograft dysfunction. Transplantation 71(11 Suppl):S24-S30, 2001.

170. Dickenmann MJ, Cathomas G, Steiger J, et al: Cytomegalovirus infection and graft rejection in renal transplantation. Transplantation 71:764-767, 2001.

171. Kovacs JA, Gill VJ, Meshnick S, Masur H: New insights into transmission, diagnosis, and drug treatment of *Pneumocystis carinii* pneumonia. JAMA 286:2450-2460, 2001.

172. Stark K, Gunther M, Schonfeld C, et al: Immunisations in solid-organ transplant recipients. Lancet 359:957-965, 2002.

173. Ojo AO, Meier-Kriesche HU, Hanson JA, et al: The impact of simultaneous pancreas-kidney transplantation on long-term patient survival. Transplantation 71:82-90, 2001.

174. Gruessner AC, Sutherland DE: Pancreas transplant outcomes for United States (US) cases reported to the United Network for Organ Sharing (UNOS) and non-US cases reported to the International Pancreas Transplant Registry (IPTR) as of October 2000. Clin Transpl 45-72, 2000.

175. Humar A, Ramcharan T, Kandaswamy R, et al: Pancreas after kidney transplants. Am J Surg 182:155-161, 2001.

176. Hariharan S, Pirsch JD, Lu CY, et al: Pancreas after kidney transplantation. J Am Soc Nephrol 13:1109-1118, 2002.

177. Manske CL: Risks and benefits of kidney and pancreas transplantation for diabetic patients. Diabetes Care 22(Suppl 2):B114-B120, 1999.

178. Markmann JF, Campos L, Velidedeoglu E, et al: Annual literature review: Clinical transplants, 2000. Clin Transpl 411-465, 2000.

179. Fioretto P, Steffes MW, Sutherland DE, et al: Reversal of lesions of diabetic nephropathy after pancreas transplantation. N Engl J Med 339:69-75, 1998.

180. La Rocca E, Fiorina P, di Carlo V, et al: Cardiovascular outcomes after kidney-pancreas and kidney-alone transplantation. Kidney Int 60:1964-1971, 2001.

181. Shapiro AM, Lakey JR, Ryan EA, et al: Islet transplantation in seven patients with type 1 diabetes mellitus using a glucocorticoid-free immunosuppressive regimen. N Engl J Med 343:230-238, 2000.

182. Johnson DW, Herzig K, Purdie D, et al: A comparison of the effects of dialysis and renal transplantation on the survival of older uremic patients. Transplantation 69:794-799, 2000.

183. Cameron JS: Renal transplantation in the elderly. Int Urol Nephrol 32:193-201, 2000.

184. Kasiske BL, Snyder J, Matas A, Collins A: The impact of transplantation on survival with kidney failure. Clin Transpl 135-143, 2000.

185. Kasiske BL, Snyder J: Matching older kidneys with older patients does not improve allograft survival. J Am Soc Nephrol 13:1067-1072, 2002.

186. Halpern SD, Ubel PA, Caplan AL: Solid-organ transplantation in HIV-infected patients. N Engl J Med 347:284-287, 2002.

187. Armenti VT, Radomski JS, Moritz MJ, et al: Report from the National Transplantation Pregnancy Registry (NTPR): Outcomes of pregnancy after transplantation. Clin Transpl 123-134, 2000.

188. Salama AD, Remuzzi G, Harmon WE, Sayegh MH: Challenges to achieving clinical transplantation tolerance. J Clin Invest 108:943-948, 2001.

189. Tran HT, Acharya MK, McKay DB, et al: Avoidance of cyclosporine in renal transplantation: Effects of daclizumab, mycophenolate mofetil, and steroids. J Am Soc Nephrol 11:1903-1909, 2000.

190. Vincenti F, Ramos E, Brattstrom C, et al: Multicenter trial exploring calcineurin inhibitors avoidance in renal transplantation. Transplantation 71:1282-1287, 2001.

191. Kasiske BL, Chakkera HA, Louis TA, Ma JZ: A meta-analysis of immunosuppression withdrawal trials in renal transplantation. J Am Soc Nephrol 11:1910-1917, 2000.

192. Ratcliffe PJ, Dudley CR, Higgins RM, et al: Randomised controlled trial of steroid withdrawal in renal transplant recipients receiving triple immunosuppression. Lancet 348:643-648, 1996.

193. Sinclair NR: Low-dose steroid therapy in cyclosporine-treated renal transplant recipients with well-functioning grafts. The Canadian Multicentre Transplant Study Group. Can Med Assoc J 147:645-657, 1992.

194. Vanderpool HY: Xenotransplantation: Progress and promise. Interview by Clare Thompson. BMJ 319:1311, 1999.

195. Samstein B, Platt JL: Physiologic and immunologic hurdles to xenotransplantation. J Am Soc Nephrol 12:182-193, 2001.

196. Yamada K, Sachs DH, Der Simonian H: Human antiporcine xenogeneic T cell response: Evidence for allelic specificity of mixed leukocyte reaction and for both direct and indirect pathways of recognition. J Immunol 155:5249-5256, 1995.

197. Fishman JA: Infection in xenotransplantation. BMJ 321:717-718, 2000.

CHAPTER 66

Prescribing Drugs in Renal Disease

George R. Aronoff and Michael E. Brier

PHARMACOKINETICS
EFFECTS OF UREMIA ON DRUG
DISPOSITION
Bioavailability
Distribution
Metabolism

Renal Excretion
INITIAL PATIENT ASSESSMENT
FOR DRUG DOSING
CALCULATING DRUG DOSES IN
RENAL IMPAIRMENT

DRUG REMOVAL BY DIALYSIS
Factors Affecting Clearance
Dosing Considerations for Specific
  Drug Categories
DRUG LEVEL MONITORING

The number of patients with decreased kidney function has grown. Current estimates indicate approximately 10 million persons in the United States who are 12 years or older have impaired renal function.[1] Advances in the treatment of chronic diseases have permitted patients to live longer. Many of them develop decreased renal function over time. Kidney function also decreases with age, and when chronic renal failure occurs, age, diabetes mellitus, and coronary artery disease are no longer barriers to renal replacement strategies. The development of new dialysis membranes, the wide acceptance of chronic peritoneal dialysis, and the popularity of continuous renal replacement therapies add to the need for detailed understanding of drug transport across biologic and synthetic membranes. These factors combine to create a large patient group for which special understanding of drug disposition is important.

The kidney is the major regulator of the internal fluid environment, and uremia affects every organ system in the body. The physiologic changes associated with kidney disease have pronounced effects on the pharmacology of many drugs. Clinicians must take into account changes in the absorption, distribution, metabolism, and excretion of drugs and their active or toxic metabolites when dosing patients with decreased excretory ability or those on renal replacement therapy. The problems of kidney disease are often superimposed on underlying hypertension, diabetes mellitus, and heart disease, compounding the complexity of pharmacologic management.

At the same time that the number of patients with impaired renal function has grown, the number and complexity of new medications available have increased. The rapid development of complex, effective new drugs has added to the challenge of rational drug therapy in patients with impaired kidney function. Highly selective agonists or antagonists of cell receptors and specific enzyme inhibitors are routinely administered. Biosynthetic peptide hormones are available. These peptides have been modified to permit enhanced hormone function or block undesired hormone activity. The U.S. Food and Drug Administration approved for use in the United States more than 125 new molecular entities during the past 5 years.[2] More than one third of the antimicrobial agents in use were not available 5 years ago.

Physicians caring for patients with kidney disease must possess a basic understanding of the biochemical and physiologic effects of uremia on drug disposition and the effects of decreased kidney function and renal replacement therapies on drug and metabolite removal. This chapter considers these problems and offers suggestions on how to deal effectively with pharmacotherapy in patients with chronic kidney disease.

PHARMACOKINETICS

The ability to quantify drug bioavailability, distribution throughout the body, biotransformation to metabolites, and the elimination of drugs and metabolites from the body enhances practical therapeutics. *Pharmacokinetics* describes the time course of these events. However, pharmacologic effects are more than the sum of these processes. Pharmacodynamics involves the complex interaction of other pharmacologic factors, including drug concentrations, receptor-drug interactions, mechanism of action, and effect on body chemistry, as well as clinical factors, such as concurrent diseases and level of organ dysfunction. Knowledge of these aspects of drug disposition allows clinicians to predict drug behavior and clinical response, leading to rational dosimetry.

After a drug is given, it appears in the central circulation and distributes throughout the body. As shown in Figure 66-1, when given intravenously, a rapid decrease in the plasma level follows an initial high drug concentration. This fall occurs as the drug distributes from the plasma into the extravascular space. Concurrent with and after the distribution phase, the processes of metabolism and excretion eliminate the drug at a slower rate. During the elimination phase, drug concentrations in plasma are in equilibrium with concentrations in body tissues.

From graphical plots of plasma drug concentrations at different times after a dose is given, useful pharmacokinetic parameters may be determined. The rate and amount of drug absorption, the extent of drug distribution, and the rate of drug elimination may be measured. The *elimination half-life* of a drug is the time required for the plasma concentration to be decreased by one half and can also be determined from

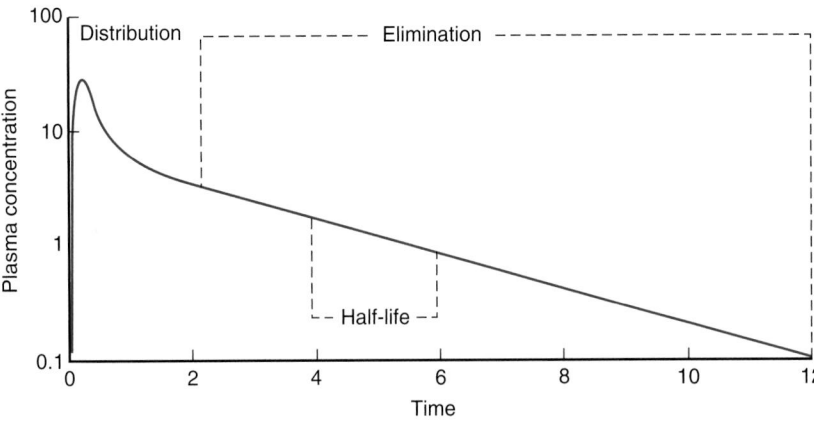

FIGURE 66-1. Distribution and elimination of a drug after intravenous administration.

the plot of plasma drug concentration versus time after the dose. It is calculated from the slope of the elimination phase and is a reflection of the drug's elimination rate from plasma. By comparing pharmacokinetic data obtained from patients with normal kidney function with data from patients with renal insufficiency, rational drug dosimetry may be determined for patients with impaired kidney function.

EFFECTS OF UREMIA ON DRUG DISPOSITION

Bioavailability

The relative amount of a drug that appears in the general circulation and the rate at which it appears are called *bioavailability*. The rate of absorption is reflected by a measure of time it takes to reach the maximum concentration, and the extent of drug absorption is often depicted as the area under the curve of the time after the dose and the plasma drug concentration.

Drugs given intravenously enter the central circulation directly and generally have a rapid onset of action. Drugs given by other routes must first traverse a series of membranes and may need to pass through important organs of elimination before entering the systemic circulation. Only a fraction of the administered dose may reach the circulation and become available at the site of drug action. Even drugs given intravenously and by inhalation must pass though the lungs before reaching arterial blood flow. Like other organs, the lungs remove substantial amounts of the agents. For example, Marik showed in the meta-analysis of 122 articles describing the effects of low-dose, intravenous dopamine in 970 subjects that the therapy has no renal protective effect.[3] Juste and colleagues previously demonstrated an explanation for the inefficacy of low-dose dopamine in improving renal function. They found it impossible to predict the plasma dopamine level from the infusion rate, probably because the compound is highly metabolized by the lungs before it gets into the systemic circulation and the kidneys.[4]

Most drugs are given orally. For these drugs, the rate and extent of gastrointestinal absorption are important considerations. After an orally administered drug is absorbed into the portal circulation, it must pass through the liver before reaching the systemic circulation. The bioavailability of a drug also depends on the extent of metabolism during its first pass through the liver.

First-pass biotransformation may also occur in the gut itself. For example, bioflavonoids in grapefruit juice can inhibit the isoenzyme cytochrome P-450 3A4 and noncompetitively inhibit the metabolism of drugs metabolized by this enzyme. This grapefruit juice–CYP 3A4 interaction was first noticed with the calcium channel blocker felodipine. Grapefruit juice increased felodipine bioavailability by 184% by inhibiting the enzyme present in gut mucosa.[5] This interaction also increases the bioavailability of cyclosporine and may increase the absorption of cyclosporine by as much as 20%.[6]

Generally, uremia decreases gastrointestinal absorption of drugs. Gastrointestinal symptoms are common in uremia, but little specific information about bowel function is available for patients with renal failure. When urea accumulates in the plasma, the salivary concentration of urea increases as well. Ammonia forms in the presence of gastric urease and buffers gastric acid, increasing gastric pH. The ammonia is absorbed and converted to urea again by the liver. The gastric alkalinizing effect of this internal urea-ammonia cycle decreases the absorption of drugs that are best absorbed in an acidic environment. For example, iron salts must be hydrolyzed by gastric acid for absorption. Uremic patients malabsorb these compounds if acid hydrolysis in the stomach is impaired. The dissolution of many tablet dosage forms requires the acid environment normally found in the stomach. Absorption of these products is incomplete and occurs more slowly in an alkaline environment.[7]

The ingestion of multivalent cations, frequently used in antacids, also diminishes drug absorption.[8, 9] Patients with renal impairment often ingest large quantities of antacids to bind dietary phosphate. Chelation and the formation of nonabsorbable complexes reduce bioavailability of some drugs. This effect is particularly important on the absorption of some antibiotics and digoxin.

Craig and colleagues demonstrated impaired gastrointestinal absorptive function. They showed that the absorption of the simple sugar, D-xylose, is reduced by nearly 30% in patients with renal failure requiring dialysis.[10] However, the processes of gastrointestinal drug absorption are complex, may be saturable and dose dependent, and are more variable in patients with renal failure than in those with normal renal function.[11] Gastroparesis, commonly observed in diabetic patients with renal failure, prolongs gastric emptying and delays drug absorption. Similarly, diarrhea decreases gut transit time and diminishes drug absorption by the small bowel.

Uremia alters first-pass hepatic metabolism. Decreased biotransformation leads to the appearance of increased amounts of active drug in the systemic circulation and enhanced bioavailability of some drugs. Conversely, impaired protein binding allows more unbound drug to be available at the site of hepatic metabolism, thereby increasing the amount of drug removed during the hepatic first pass. With the complex interaction of absorption and first-pass hepatic metabolism, it is not surprising that drug bioavailability is more variable in patients with renal impairment than in patients with normal renal function.

Distribution

After a drug is administered, it is dispersed throughout the body at a given rate. At equilibrium, the apparent volume of distribution is calculated by dividing the amount of the drug in the body by its plasma concentration. This apparent volume of distribution does not correspond to a specific anatomic space. Rather, the volume of distribution is a mathematical construct used to estimate the dose of a drug to be given to achieve a therapeutic plasma concentration. Agents that are highly protein bound or those that are water soluble tend to be restricted to the extracellular fluid space and have small volumes of distribution. Highly lipid-soluble drugs penetrate body tissues and exhibit large volumes of distribution.

Renal insufficiency frequently alters drug distribution volume. Edema and ascites increase the apparent volume of distribution of highly water-soluble or protein-bound drugs. Usual doses of such drugs given to edematous patients result in inadequate, low plasma levels. Conversely, dehydration or muscle wasting tends to decrease the volume of distribution. In these cases, usual doses result in unexpectedly high plasma concentrations. The distribution of drugs may be altered by fluid removal during dialysis.[12]

The alteration of plasma protein binding in patients with renal insufficiency is an important factor affecting eventual drug action. The volume of distribution of a drug, the quantity of unbound drug available for action, and the degree to which the agent can be eliminated by hepatic or renal excretion are all influenced by protein binding. Drugs that are protein bound attach reversibly to albumin or glycoprotein in plasma. Organic acids are thought to bind to a single binding site, whereas organic bases probably have multiple sites of attachment.[13, 14]

Protein-bound organic acids such as hippuric acid, indoxyl sulfate, and 3-carboxy-4-methyl-5-propyl-2-furan-propionic acid (CMPF) accumulate in renal failure and decrease protein binding of many acidic drugs.[15-17] Altered protein binding affects organic bases less than organic acids. A combination of decreased serum albumin concentration and a reduction in albumin affinity for the drug reduces protein binding in patients with uremia. Even when the plasma albumin concentration is normal, the protein-binding defect of some drugs correlates with the level of azotemia and may be corrected with dialysis.[18-21] As illustrated in Figure 66-2, affinity is influenced by uremia-induced changes in the structural orientation of the albumin molecule or by the accumulation of endogenous inhibitors of protein binding that compete with drugs for their binding sites.

The consequences of impaired plasma protein binding in uremia are important, because the unbound fraction of several

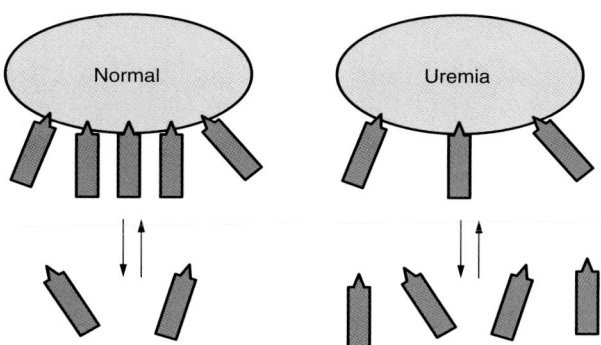

PROTEIN BINDING DEFECT IN UREMIA

FIGURE 66-2. Protein binding defect in uremia. Displacement of the drug from its binding site by an accumulation of undefined uremic toxin or a uremia-induced conformational change in the binding site geometry results in more free drug in the plasma.

acidic drugs is substantially increased. Serious toxicity can occur if the total plasma concentration of these drugs is pushed into the therapeutic range by increasing the dose. For such drugs, total and unbound plasma concentrations should be measured.

Predicting the clinical consequences of altered protein binding in uremia is difficult. Although decreased binding results in more unbound drug being available at the site of drug action or toxicity, the distribution volume is increased, resulting in lower plasma concentrations after a given dose. More unbound drug is available for metabolism and excretion, which decreases the half-life of the drug in the body. Drugs with decreased protein binding in dialysis patients are listed in Table 66-1.

Metabolism

Biotransformation is an important mechanism for drug elimination. Many compounds are highly lipid soluble, cross cell

TABLE 66-1

Drugs with Decreased Protein Binding in Dialysis Patients

Barbiturates
Cardiac glycosides
Dicloxacillin
Cephalosporins
Clofibrate
Doxepin
Loop diuretics
Oxazepam
Penicillins
Pentobarbital
Phenobarbital
Phenytoin
Sulfonamides
Salicylate
Temazepam
Theophylline
Valproic acid
Warfarin

membranes easily, and may have large volumes of distribution. Even when filtered by the glomerulus, these nonpolar molecules may diffuse from the tubule lumen and be reabsorbed into the circulation. Drug metabolism generally converts lipid-soluble compounds into more polar, water-soluble metabolites that have smaller distribution volumes and diffuse less readily across renal tubule cells. They are more easily excreted in the urine.

Although renal insufficiency is thought to affect primarily the renal elimination of drugs or metabolites, renal failure substantially affects drug biotransformation. Uremia slows the rate of reduction and hydrolysis reactions. For example, peptide and ester hydrolysis are substantially reduced. Microsomal oxidation may also be affected. In a model of uremic rats, Leblond and colleagues demonstrated up to a 50% decrease in the protein expression of several CYP450 isoforms and their mRNAs.[22]

Even glucuronidation to polar, water-soluble metabolites, once thought to occur normally in renal failure, is impaired in patients with decreased renal function. Formation of acyl-glucuronides is under the control of a feedback cycle in which plasma drug clearance is a function of the formation, hydrolysis, and renal clearance of the glucuronide conjugate. Impaired kidney function in rabbits decreased glucuronide formation by more than 20%, largely because of the decreased clearance of glucuronide from plasma.[23]

Uremia may also alter the disposition of drugs metabolized by the liver through changes in plasma protein binding. The systemic clearance of a highly protein bound drug with a low hepatic extraction ratio depends on the simultaneous effects of renal disease on protein binding and intrinsic metabolic drug clearance. Protein binding of such a drug is related to creatinine clearance in an inverse hyperbolic relationship, whereas the unbound intrinsic metabolic clearance declines linearly with creatinine clearance. Because the effects of renal failure on these two factors offset each other in terms of total systemic clearance, the lowest total systemic clearance is not seen in dialysis patients but rather occurs in those with moderate renal impairment. The systemic clearance of drugs with a high hepatic extraction ratio is not thought to be as susceptible to the effect of renal disease as that of drugs with a low extraction ratio.[24]

The production of active or toxic metabolites is an important aspect of drug metabolism in patients with renal failure. Many of these metabolites depend on the kidneys for their removal from the body. The accumulation of active metabolites can explain in part the high incidence of adverse drug reactions seen in renal failure. For example, propoxyphene is subject to extensive first-pass biotransformation after oral administration to its pharmacologically active metabolite norpropoxyphene, which is normally excreted in the urine. Norpropoxyphene substantially accumulates in renal failure and may result in oversedation.[25] Similarly, although the liver usually rapidly metabolizes morphine, it is excreted mainly in the urine as its active metabolites, morphine-3-glucuronide (M-3G) and morphine-6-glucuronide (M-6G). M-3G and M-6G readily cross the blood-brain barrier and bind with strong affinity to opiate receptors, exerting strong analgesic effects. In patients with renal failure, morphine itself is metabolized more slowly, and these active metabolites increase, making prolonged narcosis and respiratory depression more likely.[26]

The biotransformation of meperidine results in the production of normeperidine, a more polar metabolite that is rapidly excreted in the urine. Normeperidine has little narcotic effect, but it may lower the seizure threshold. In patients with renal impairment, frequently repeated doses of meperidine may result in the accumulation of this potentially toxic metabolite, with resultant seizures.[27] Table 66-2 lists some drugs that form active or toxic metabolites in patients with reduced kidney function.

Drug dosing guidelines for dialysis patients are usually derived from studies of patients with stable, chronic renal failure. However, these recommendations are often extrapolated to seriously ill patients with acutely decreased renal function. The preservation of nonrenal metabolic clearance has been demonstrated in patients with acute renal failure.[28] The preservation of metabolic clearance observed early in the course of acute renal failure suggests that drug dosing schemes extrapolated from individuals with stable chronic renal failure could result in potentially ineffectively low drug concentrations in patients with acute renal dysfunction.

TABLE 66-2

Drugs That Have Active or Toxic Metabolites in Dialysis Patients

Acetaminophen	Clofibrate	Nitrofurantoin
Angiotensin-converting enzyme inhibitors	Desipramine	Nitroprusside
	Diltiazem	Procainamide
Angiotensin receptor blockers	Encainide	Primidone
Adriamycin	Esmolol	Propoxyphene
Allopurinol	H_2-blockers	Pyrimethamine
Amiodarone	Hydroxyzine	Quinidine
Amoxapine	Imipramine	Serotonin reuptake inhibitors
Azathioprine	Isosorbide	Spironolactone
Benzodiazepines	Levodopa	Sulfonylureas
β-Blockers	Lorcainide	Sulindac
Bupropion	Meperidine	Thiazolidinediones
Buspirone	Metronidazole	Triamterene
Cardiac glycosides	Methyldopa	Trimethadione
Clorazepate	Miglitol	Verapamil
Cephalosporins	Minoxidil	Vidarabine
Chloral hydrate	Morphine	

Renal Excretion

The renal handling of drugs depends on the glomerular process of filtration and on the tubule processes of secretion and reabsorption. However, the rate of drug and metabolite elimination by the kidneys is proportional to the glomerular filtration rate (GFR). In addition to the GFR, the glomerular elimination of drugs depends on the molecular size and protein binding of the agent. Although protein binding decreases the filtration of drugs, it may increase the amount secreted by the renal tubule. When glomerular filtration is impaired by renal disease, the clearance of drugs eliminated primarily by this mechanism is decreased, and the plasma half-life of the drugs prolonged.

Although we do not clinically measure the tubule function of organic acid secretion, the excretion of drugs eliminated by active organic ion transport systems in the renal tubule is prolonged in patients with renal disease. As a patient's creatinine clearance decreases, her or his ability to eliminate many drugs is adversely affected. Because the proximal tubule secretion of some agents is carrier mediated and capacity limited, multiple drugs eliminated by tubule secretion may saturate the transport system if they are administered concurrently.

The rate of elimination of drugs excreted by the kidneys is proportional to the GFR. The serum creatinine or creatinine clearance is needed to determine renal function before prescribing any drug. The Cockroft and Gault[29] equation is useful for this purpose, as shown in this formula:

$$Clcr = \frac{(140 - age) \times (IBW)}{72 \times Scr} \times (0.85 \text{ if female})$$

In this equation, Clcr is the creatinine clearance (mL/min), Scr is the serum creatinine level (mg/dL), and IBW is the ideal body weight (kg), determined by the following equations:

IBW (men) = 50 kg + 2.3 kg per inch over 5 feet

IBW (women) = 45.5 kg + 2.3 kg per inch over 5 feet

For obese men (OM) and women (OW), the equation should be modified:

$$Clcr_{OM} = \frac{(137 - age) \times [(0.285 \times wgt) + (12.1 \times hgt^2)]}{51 \times Scr}$$

$$Clcr_{OW} = \frac{(146 - age) \times [(0.287 \times wgt) + (9.74 \times hgt^2)]}{60 \times Scr}$$

In this equation, wgt is the patient's weight (kg), and hgt is the patient's height (cm).

In cases of changing renal function, the serum creatinine level no longer reflects the true clearance rate. In these cases, a timed urine collection is needed to estimate renal function. The midpoint serum creatinine is useful to calculate the creatinine clearance for the collection period.

The serum creatinine level reflects muscle mass and the GFR. Serum creatinine measurements within the normal range are frequently used to establish normal renal function, but this erroneous assumption may cause serious overdose and resultant toxic drug accumulation in elderly or debilitated patients with decreased muscle mass. A 72-kg man with a serum creatinine level of 1 mg/dL has one half of the renal function at the age of 80 years as he did with the same body mass and serum creatinine at the age of 20 years. If the same doses of medications are given to the 80-year-old man as to the 20-year-old patient, adverse drug events are likely to result from drug and metabolite accumulation.

Some dialysis patients have residual renal function that substantially contributes to the elimination of drugs and their metabolites. Estimating residual renal function in dialysis patients still making urine is difficult, because the serum creatinine level reflects the adequacy of dialysis and muscle mass as well as residual GFR. Creatinine clearance measurements less accurately reflect the GFR in patients with such severe renal failure as to require dialysis. Changing serum creatinine levels over the duration of the clearance measurement, the contribution of tubule creatinine secretion, and the accumulation of chromogens contribute to the difficulty in measuring residual renal function. Serum creatinine measurements alone should not be used to estimate intrinsic renal function in dialysis patients. The plasma clearance rate of certain radioisotopes more accurately estimates residual renal function in these patients, although the use of radioisotopes is complicated by the need to dispose of radioactive materials.

Conventional quantification of residual renal function in hemodialysis patients is performed by measuring urea clearance, creatinine clearance, or a combination of both. This approach requires a 24-hour urine collection, which is often difficult to perform and inaccurate. It requires that serum urea and creatinine levels be measured before and after the urine collection to estimate the average values during the collection. Measuring the elimination of iohexol after an intravenous dose with a single blood measurement of iohexol has been reported to be an accurate and safe measure of residual renal function in dialysis patients and can potentially simplify drug dosing.[30] Residual renal function decreases over time and is usually less than 5 mL/minute after 1 year on hemodialysis.[31]

In addition to the process of filtration and secretion of drugs and metabolites into the urine, the kidney possesses enzymes capable of metabolizing drugs.[32] The kidney plays an important role in the metabolism of many proteins and small peptides. Clinically, the most important aspect of renal drug metabolism is the peptide hydrolysis of insulin. The kidney clears insulin by glomerular filtration and subsequent luminal reabsorption of insulin by proximal tubule cells. The second involves diffusion of insulin from peritubule capillaries and subsequent binding of insulin to the contraluminal membranes of tubule cells.[33] Impairment of the renal clearance of insulin prolongs the half-life of circulating insulin and often results in a decrease in the insulin requirement of diabetic patients with decreased renal function.[34]

INITIAL PATIENT ASSESSMENT FOR DRUG DOSING

Clinical evaluation always begins with a careful history and physical examination. Knowledge of previous medication history, drug-related allergy or toxicity, and concurrent medicines are important in the initial evaluation of patients on dialysis. Reviewing the possibility of drug interactions before choosing a drug regimen reduces potentially adverse drug effects. On average, dialysis patients routinely receive 11 different medications and have three times the incidence of adverse drug events as patients with normal renal function.[35-37] Focusing therapy on specific diagnoses allows the clinician to limit the number of drugs the patient is taking and lessens the chances of untoward drug interactions. When possible, drug therapy should be individualized to take advantage of the fact that one drug can be used to treat several conditions. For example, a calcium channel antagonist can be used to treat hypertension and angina.

Estimating extracellular fluid volume is necessary to determine the distribution volume of drugs. Edema or ascites increases the distribution volume of many drugs. Dehydration contracts this volume. Individualization of the drug regimen requires measurements of body height and weight. Many clinicians use the average of the measured body weight and the ideal body weight as the value on which to base drug doses.[38]

Evaluating functional impairment of other excretory organs is also important. The failure of other organs limits the possibilities for alternate pathways of drug and metabolite elimination. For instance, the stigmata of liver disease suggest the potential need to alter drug dosages further in patients with renal failure.

CALCULATING DRUG DOSES IN RENAL IMPAIRMENT

The goal of the initial drug dose is to achieve therapeutic drug concentrations rapidly. If no loading dose is prescribed, three to four half-lives of the drug must pass before the plasma levels are at steady state. The amount of the drug given affects how rapidly certain plasma levels are achieved and the magnitude of the steady-state plasma concentration. A loading dose equivalent to the dose given to a patient with normal renal function should always be given to patients with renal impairment if the drug's half-life is particularly long and if the physical examination suggests normal extracellular fluid volume. If the loading dose of a drug is not known, it can be calculated from the following expression:

Loading dose = $V_d \times IBW \times Cp$

In this equation, V_d is the drug's volume of distribution in L/kg, IBW is the patient's ideal body weight (kg), and Cp is the desired steady-state plasma drug concentration.

Several methods can be used to determine subsequent drug doses. The fraction of the normal dose recommended for a patient with renal failure can be calculated as follows:

Df = $t_{1/2}$ normal/$t_{1/2}$ renal failure

In this equation, Df is the fraction of the normal dose to be given, $t_{1/2}$ normal is the elimination half-life of the drug in a patient with normal renal function, and $t_{1/2}$ renal failure is the elimination half-life of the drug in a patient with renal failure. To maintain the normal dose interval in patients with renal impairment, the amount of each dose after the loading dose can be determined from the following relationship:

Dose in renal impairment = Normal dose $\times$ Df

The resulting dose is usually given at the same dose interval as that for patients with normal renal function. This method is effective for drugs with a narrow therapeutic range and short plasma half-life. Figure 66-3 illustrates plasma concentrations after an initial loading dose and reduction of the individual doses.

Prolonging the dose interval in dialysis patients is frequently a convenient method to reduce drug dosage. This method is particularly useful for drugs with a broad therapeutic range and long plasma half-life. If prolonging the dose interval, rather than decreasing the individual doses, is desirable, the dose interval in renal impairment can be estimated from the following expression, in which Df is the dose fraction:

Dose interval in renal impairment = Normal dose interval/Df

If the range between therapeutic and toxic levels is too narrow, potentially toxic or subtherapeutic plasma concentrations result. The resulting plasma concentrations from prolonging the dose interval in an individual with impaired renal function are shown in Figure 66-4.

A combined approach using the dose-reduction and interval-prolongation methods is often practical. Multiplying the

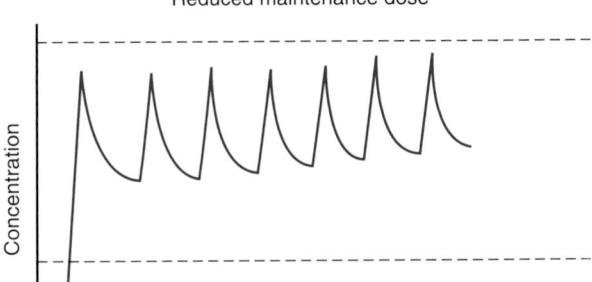

FIGURE 66-3. Plasma concentrations after a normal loading dose and reduced maintenance doses. This approach avoids high peak and low trough concentrations and is best for drugs with a narrow range between the therapeutic and toxic concentrations.

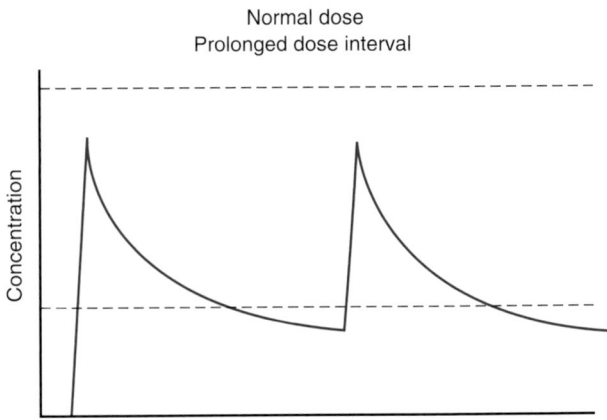

FIGURE 66-4. Plasma concentrations after a normal loading dose and repeated normal doses at a prolonged dose interval. Higher peak and lower trough concentrations result.

usual daily maintenance dose by the dose fraction modifies the dosage. After the average daily dose is calculated, it can be divided into convenient dosing intervals. The decision to extend the dosing interval beyond a 24-hour period should be based on the need to maintain therapeutic peak or trough levels. The dosing interval may be prolonged if the peak level is most important. When the minimum trough level must be maintained, it is preferable to modify the individual dose or use a combination of dose and interval methods to determine the correct dosing strategy. Drugs removed by dialysis given once daily should be given after the dialysis treatment.

DRUG REMOVAL BY DIALYSIS

Factors Affecting Clearance

Drug removal by conventional hemodialysis occurs primarily by the process of drug diffusion across the dialysis membrane. Diffusion proceeds down a concentration gradient from the plasma to the dialysate. Drug removal by conventional hemodialysis is most effective for drugs that are less than 500 daltons (D) and are less than 90% protein bound. Drugs that have small volumes of distribution are more effectively removed by dialysis than compounds that are distributed in adipose tissue or have extensive tissue binding. Removal of low-molecular-weight drugs is enhanced by increasing the blood and dialysate flow rates and by using large-surface-area dialyzers. Larger molecules require more porous membranes for increased removal. The hemodialysis clearance of a drug can be estimated from the following relationship:

$$Cl_{HD} = Cl_{urea} \times (60/MW_{drug})$$

In this equation, Cl_{HD} is the drug's clearance by hemodialysis, Cl_{urea} is the clearance of urea by the dialyzer, and MW_{drug} is the molecular weight of the drug.[39] The urea clearance for most standard dialyzers varies between 150 and 200 mL/minute.[40]

The use of porous dialysis membranes to perform high-flux dialysis decreases the importance of drug molecular mass in determining drug removal during extracorporeal circulation. During high-flux dialysis, the volume of distribution and percent of protein binding of the drug are more important determinants of drug clearance. Study results suggest that, for drugs that are not highly protein bound and have relatively small volumes of distribution, drug removal occurs by diffusion and parallels urea clearance, despite a very large molecular mass.[41, 42] The removal of drugs during high-flux dialysis depends more on treatment time, blood and dialysate flow rates, distribution volume, and binding of the drug to serum proteins. As a consequence, much more drug is removed during high-flux dialysis than previously estimated for conventional hemodialysis. Substantial amounts of drug may be removed if the agent is given during high-flux dialysis treatments.[43]

Peritoneal dialysis is much less efficient at removing drugs than hemodialysis.[44] As with conventional hemodialysis, drug removal by peritoneal dialysis is most effective for lower-molecular-weight drugs that are not extensively bound to serum proteins. Higher-molecular-weight drugs may be somewhat more removed by peritoneal dialysis

because of secretion into peritoneal lymphatic fluid. Similarly, drugs that have small volumes of distribution are more effectively removed than those that are distributed in adipose tissue or have extensive tissue binding. Removal of low-molecular-weight drugs depends on the number of peritoneal dialysis exchanges done daily. Peritoneal drug clearance can be estimated from the following relationship:

$$Cl_{PD} = Cl_{urea} \times \frac{\sqrt{60}}{\sqrt{MW_{drug}}}$$

In this equation, Cl_{PD} is the peritoneal drug clearance, Cl_{urea} is the peritoneal urea clearance, and MW_{drug} is the molecular weight of the drug. Peritoneal urea clearance is approximately 20 mL/minute. In general, if a drug is not removed by hemodialysis, it cannot be removed by peritoneal dialysis.

Drug transport by the peritoneal membrane is unidirectional.[45] Although peritoneal dialysis does not rapidly remove drugs, many are well absorbed when placed in peritoneal dialysate. Table 66-3 includes some commonly used antibiotics for patients on chronic ambulatory peritoneal dialysis and suggestions for dosages used to treat ambulatory peritonitis and systemic infections.

Molecular weight, membrane characteristics, blood flow rate, and the addition of dialysate determine the rate and extent of drug removal during continuous renal replacement therapies (CRRT). Molecular weight affects drug removal by diffusion during dialysis more than during convection during CRRT because of the large pore size of membranes used for CRRT. Because most drugs are less than 1500 D, drug removal by CRRT does not depend greatly on molecular weight.

The volume of distribution of a drug is the most important factor determining removal by CRRT. Drugs with a large volume of distribution are highly tissue bound and not accessible to extracorporeal circuit in quantities sufficient to result in substantial removal by CRRT. Even if the extraction across the artificial membrane is 100%, only a small amount of a

TABLE 66-3

Antibiotic Dosages for Patients on Chronic Ambulatory Peritoneal Dialysis

DRUG	LOADING DOSE	MAINTENANCE DOSE
Amikacin	7.5 mg/kg	25 mg/L
Ampicillin	1 g	60 mg/L
Aztreonam	15 mg/kg	250 mg/L
Carbenicillin	5 g	250 mg/L
Cefazolin	1 g	125 mg/L
Cefoperazone	—	2 g every other bag
Ceftazidime	1 g	125 mg/L
Ceftriaxone	—	1 g in one bag/day
Clindamycin	—	150 mg/L
Gentamicin	2 mg/kg	4 mg/L
Imipenem/cilastatin	500 mg	250 mg every other bag
Moxalactam	1 g	125 mg/L
Penicillin	500,000 U	100,000 U/L
Piperacillin	—	4 g every other bag
Ticarcillin/clavulanate	1.2 g	120 mg/L
Tobramycin	2 mg/kg	4 mg/L
Vancomycin	30 mg/kg	20 mg/L

drug with a large volume of distribution is removed. A volume of distribution greater than 0.7 L/kg substantially decreases CRRT drug removal.

Drug protein binding also determines how much is removed during CRRT. Only unbound drug is available for elimination by CRRT. Protein binding of more than 80% provides a substantial barrier to drug removal by convection or diffusion. During continuous hemofiltration, an ultrafiltration rate of 10 to 30 mL/minute is achieved. The addition of diffusion by continuous dialysis increases drug clearance, depending on blood and dialysate flow rates. As during high flux dialysis, drug removal parallels the removal of urea and creatinine. The simplest method for estimating drug removal during CRRT is to estimate urea or creatinine clearance during the procedure.[46]

Recommendations for dosing selected drugs in patients with impaired renal function are given in Table 66-4. These recommendations are meant only as a guide and do not imply efficacy or safety of a recommended dose in an individual patient. A loading dose equivalent to the usual dose in patients with normal renal function should be considered for drugs with a particularly long half-life. The table indicates potential methods for adjusting the dose by decreasing the individual doses or increasing the dose interval. In the table, when the dose method (D) is suggested, the percentage of the dose for normal renal function is given. When the interval method (I) is suggested, the actual dose interval is provided.

No controlled clinical trials have established the efficacy of these two methods of dose reduction. Prolonging the dose interval is often more convenient and less expensive. When the dose interval can safely be lengthened beyond 24 hours, extended parenteral therapy may be completed without prolonging hospitalization. In patients requiring chronic hemodialysis, many drugs need to be given only at the end of the dialysis treatment. Compliance with any drug regimen may be better when fewer doses can be taken at convenient times. In practice, a combination interval prolongation and dose-size reduction is often effective and convenient.

The effect of the standard clinical treatment on drug removal is shown for hemodialysis chronic ambulatory peritoneal dialysis, and continuous renal replacement therapy. Most of these recommendations were established before very-high-efficiency hemodialysis treatments were practical, continuous cycling nocturnal peritoneal dialysis was common, and diffusion was added to hemofiltration in continuous renal replacement therapies. Some drugs that have high dialysis clearance do not require supplemental doses after dialysis if the amount of the drug removed is not sufficient, as is the case if the volume of distribution is large. To ensure efficacy when information about dialysis loss is not available and to simplify dosimetry, maintenance doses of most drugs should be given after dialysis.

Peritonitis is a major complication of peritoneal dialysis, and treatment usually involves intraperitoneal administration of antibiotics. For some drugs, sophisticated pharmacokinetic studies are available, whereas for others, use is still based on empirical dosage recommendations. In general, there is excellent drug absorption after intraperitoneal administration of common antibiotics. Factors favoring absorption include inflamed membranes and high concentration

gradients. For many drugs, peritoneal fluid levels after intravenous or oral administration are inconsistent.

Dosing Considerations for Specific Drug Categories
Analgesics

Analgesic agents are frequently used for the management of pain in patients with impaired renal function. Most analgesics are eliminated by hepatic biotransformation. However, important changes in their metabolism and protein binding occur. The accumulation of active metabolites results in prolonged oversedation. The formation of toxic metabolites can cause CNS toxicity and seizures. Specifically, the disposition of morphine, meperidine, and dextropropoxyphene in patients with impaired renal function is complicated by the accumulation of active or toxic metabolites with prolonged use. Prolonged narcosis is associated with codeine and dihydrocodeine, whereas the use of fentanyl may lead to prolonged sedation.[47] Patient-controlled analgesia pumps should be used with caution by patients with decreased renal function.[48]

Saturable, nonlinear excretion complicates salicylate elimination kinetics. Because of the hemorrhagic diathesis in patients with severe renal failure and the variability of salicylate elimination, large doses of aspirin in patients with severe renal failure should be avoided.

Anticonvulsants

Generalized major motor seizures occur in patients with uremia, and phenytoin is one of the most frequently used drugs for such seizures. Phenytoin absorption is slow and erratic, hepatic metabolism is concentration dependent and saturable, and distribution and elimination vary.[49] Phenytoin protein binding is decreased and the distribution volume increased in renal failure.[50] With any given total serum phenytoin level, the concentration of active, free drug is higher in uremic patients than in patients with normal renal function. Most clinical laboratories measure the total serum drug concentration, and a low total phenytoin level in a patient with renal failure should not be misinterpreted as subtherapeutic.

Physical findings such as nystagmus may be helpful in deciding not to increase the dose. Seizures are also a manifestation of phenytoin excess, and small dosage increases may result in disproportionately large increases in the serum drug level. Dose increments should be small, sufficient time should be allowed for the patient to reach steady-state drug levels, and measurement of free serum phenytoin concentration should be done frequently in uremic patients who are not responding to therapy.

Antihypertensive and Cardiovascular Agents

Hypertension and cardiovascular disease are common in patients with renal insufficiency. Eighty percent of hemodialysis patients are hypertensive, and 75% have left ventricular hypertrophy.[51, 52] Antihypertensive and cardiovascular agents are the most commonly prescribed drugs for patients with renal disease. Despite the fact that the kidneys excrete many antihypertensive and cardiovascular drugs or their metabolites, most of the drugs are given by titrating the dose based on the clinical response. Long-acting drugs are

(text continued on page 2866)

TABLE 66-4

Drug Doses in Renal Failure

DRUG	DOSE METHOD	GFR > 50 (mL/min)	GFR 10–50 (mL/min)	GFR < 10 (mL/min)	SUPPLEMENTAL DOSE AFTER HEMODIALYSIS	CAPD	CRRT
Acarbose	D	50–100%	Avoid	Avoid	Unknown	Unknown	Avoid
Acebutolol	D	100%	50%	30–50%	None	None	Dose for GFR 10–50
Acetazolamide	I	q6h	q12h	Avoid	No data	No data	Avoid
Acetohexamide	I	Avoid	Avoid	Avoid	Unknown	None	Avoid
Acetohydroxamic acid	D	100%	100%	Avoid	Unknown	Unknown	Unknown
Acetaminophen	I	q4h	q6h	q8h	None	None	Dose for GFR 10–50
Acetylsalicylic acid	I	q4h	q4–6h	Avoid	Dose after dialysis	None	Dose for GFR 10–50
Acrivastine	D	Unknown	Unknown	Unknown	Unknown	Unknown	Unknown
Acyclovir	D, I	5 mg/kg q8h	5 mg/kg q12–24h	2.5 mg/kg q24h	Dose after dialysis	Dose for GFR < 10	3.5 mg/kg/day
Adenosine	D	100%	100%	100%	None	None	Dose for GFR 10–50
Albuterol	D	100%	75%	50%	Unknown	Unknown	Dose for GFR 10–50
Alcuronium	D	Avoid	Avoid	Avoid	Unknown	Unknown	Avoid
Alfentanil	D	100%	100%	100%	Unknown	Unknown	Dose for GFR 10–50
Allopurinol	D	75%	50%	25%	½ dose	Unknown	Dose for GFR 10–50
Alprazolam	D	100%	100%	100%	None	Unknown	NA
Altretamine	I	Unknown	Unknown	Unknown	No data	No data	Unknown
Amantadine	I	q24–48h	q48–72h	q7d	No data	No data	Dose for GFR 10–50
Amikacin	D, I	60% to 90% q12h	30–70% q12–18h	20–30% q24–48h	⅔ normal dose	15–20 mg/L/day	Dose for GFR 10–50
Amiloride	D	100%	50%	Avoid	NA	NA	NA
Amiodarone	D	100%	100%	100%	None	None	Dose for GFR 10–50
Amitriptyline	D	100%	100%	100%	None	Unknown	NA
Amlodipine	D	100%	100%	100%	None	None	Dose for GFR 10–50
Amoxapine	D	100%	100%	100%	Unknown	Unknown	NA
Amoxicillin	I	q8h	q8–12h	q24h	Dose after dialysis	250 mg q12h	Dose for GFR 10–50
Amphotericin	I	q24h	q24h	q24–36h	None	Dose for GFR < 10	Dose for GFR 10–50
Amphotericin B colloidal	I	q24h	q24h	q24–36h	None	Dose for GFR < 10	Dose for GFR 10–50
Amphotericin B lipid	I	q24h	q24h	q24–36h	None	Dose for GFR < 10	Dose for GFR 10–50
Ampicillin	I	q6h	q6–12h	q12–24h	Dose after dialysis	250 mg q12h	Dose for GFR 10–50
Amrinone	D	100%	100%	50–75%	No data	No data	Dose for GFR 10–50
Anistreplase	D	100%	100%	100%	Unknown	Unknown	Dose for GFR 10–50
Astemizole	D	100%	100%	100%	Unknown	Unknown	NA
Atenolol	D, I	100% q24h	50% q48h	30–50% q96h	25–50 mg	None	Dose for GFR 10–50
Atovaquone	D	100%	100%	100%	None	None	Dose for GFR 10–50
Atracurium	D	100%	100%	100%	Unknown	Unknown	Dose for GFR 10–50
Auranofin	D	50%	Avoid	Avoid	None	None	None
Azathioprine	D	100%	75%	50%	Yes	Unknown	Dose for GFR 10–50
Azithromycin	D	100%	100%	100%	None	None	None
Azlocillin	I	q4–6h	q6–8h	q8h	Dose after dialysis	Dose for GFR < 10	Dose for GFR 10–50
Aztreonam	D	100%	50–75%	25%	0.5 g after dialysis	Dose for GFR < 10	Dose for GFR 10–50
Benazepril	D	100%	50–75%	25–50%	None	None	Dose for GFR 10–50
Bepridil		Unknown	Unknown	Unknown	None	None	No data
Betamethasone	D	100%	100%	100%	Unknown	Unknown	Dose for GFR 10–50
Betaxolol	D	100%	100%	50%	None	None	Dose for GFR 10–50
Bezafibrate	D	70%	50%	25%	Unknown	Unknown	Dose for GFR 10–50
Bisoprolol	D	100%	75%	50%	Unknown	Unknown	Dose for GFR 10–50
Bleomycin	D	100%	75%	50%	None	Unknown	Dose for GFR 10–50
Bopindolol	D	100%	100%	100%	None	None	Dose for GFR 10–50

Continued

TABLE 66-4

Drug Doses in Renal Failure—cont'd

DRUG	DOSE METHOD	GFR > 50 (mL/min)	GFR 10-50 (mL/min)	GFR < 10 (mL/min)	SUPPLEMENTAL DOSE AFTER HEMODIALYSIS	CAPD	CRRT
Bretylium	D	100%	25-50%	25%	None	None	Dose for GFR 10-50
Bromocriptine	D	100%	100%	100%	Unknown	Unknown	Unknown
Brompheniramine	D	100%	100%	100%	Unknown	Unknown	NA
Budesonide	D	100%	100%	100%	Unknown	Unknown	Dose for GFR 10-50
Bumetanide	D	100%	100%	100%	None	None	NA
Bupropion	D	100%	100%	100%	Unknown	Unknown	NA
Buspirone	D	100%	100%	100%	None	Unknown	Dose for GFR 10-50
Busulfan	D	100%	100%	100%	Unknown	Unknown	Dose for GFR 10-50
Butorphanol	D	100%	75%	50%	Unknown	Unknown	NA
Capreomycin	I	q24h	q24h	q48h	Give dose after HD only	None	Dose for GFR 10-50
Captopril	D, I	100% q8-12h	75% q12-18h	50% q24h	25-30%	None	Dose for GFR 10-50
Carbamazepine	D	100%	100%	100%	None	None	None
Carbidopa	D	100%	100%	100%	Unknown	Unknown	Unknown
Carboplatin	D	100%	50%	25%	½ dose	Unknown	Dose for GFR 10-50
Carmustine	D	Unknown	Unknown	Unknown	Unknown	Unknown	Unknown
Carteolol	D	100%	50%	25%	Unknown	None	Dose for GFR 10-50
Carvedilol	D	100%	100%	100%	None	None	Dose for GFR 10-50
Cefaclor	D	100%	50-100%	50%	250 mg after dialysis	250 mg q8-12h	NA
Cefadroxil	I	q12h	q12-24h	q24-48h	0.5-1.0 g after dialysis	0.5 g/day	NA
Cefamandole	I	q6h	q6-8h	q12h	0.5-1.0 g after dialysis	0.5-1.0 g q12h	Dose for GFR 10-50
Cefazolin	I	q8h	q12h	q24-48h	0.5-1.0 g after dialysis	0.5 g q12h	Dose for GFR 10-50
Cefepime	I	q12h	q16-24h	q24-48h	1.0 g after dialysis	Dose for GFR < 10	Not recommended
Cefixime	D	100%	75%	50%	300 mg after dialysis	200 mg/day	Not recommended
Cefmenoxime	D, I	1.0 g q8h	0.75 g q8h	0.75 g q12h	0.75 g after dialysis	0.75 g q12h	Dose for GFR 10-50
Cefmetazole	I	q16h	q24h	q48h	Dose after dialysis	Dose for GFR < 10	Dose for GFR 10-50
Cefonicid	D, I	0.5 g/d	0.1 g-0.5 g/day	0.1 g/day	None	None	None
Cefoperazone	D	100%	100%	100%	1 g after dialysis	None	None
Ceforanide	I	q12h	q12-24h	q24-48h	0.5-1.0 g after dialysis	None	1.0 g/day
Cefotaxime	I	q6h	q8-12h	q24h	1 g after dialysis	1 g/day	1 g q12h
Cefotetan	D	100%	50%	25%	1 g after dialysis	1 g/day	750 mg q12h
Cefoxitin	I	q8h	q8-12h	q24-48h	1 g after dialysis	1 g/day	Dose for GFR 10-50
Cefpodoxime	I	q12h	q16h	q24-48h	200 mg after dialysis	Dose for GFR < 10	NA
Cefprozil	D, I	250 mg q12h	250 mg q12-16h	250 mg q24h	250 mg after dialysis	Dose for GFR < 10	Dose for GFR < 10
Ceftazidime	I	q8-12h	q24-48h	q48h	1 g after dialysis	0.5 g/day	Dose for GFR 10-50
Ceftibuten	D	100%	50%	25%	300 mg after dialysis	Dose for GFR < 10	Dose for GFR 10-50
Ceftizoxime	I	q8-12h	q12-24h	q24h	1 g after dialysis	0.5-1.0 g/day	Dose for GFR 10-50
Ceftriaxone	I	100%	100%	100%	Dose after dialysis	750 mg q12h	Dose for GFR 10-50
Cefuroxime axetil	D	100%	100%	100%	Dose after dialysis	Dose for GFR < 10	NA
Celiprolol	D	100%	100%	75%	Unknown	None	Dose for GFR 10-50
Cephalexin	I	q8h	q12h	q12h	Dose after dialysis	Dose for GFR < 10	NA
Cephalothin	I	q6h	q6-8h	q12h	Dose after dialysis	1 g q12h	1 g q8h
Cephapirin	I	q6h	q6-8h	q12h	Dose after dialysis	1 g q12h	1 g q8h
Cephradine	D	100%	50%	25%	Dose after dialysis	Dose for GFR < 10	NA
Cetirizine	D	100%	100%	30%	None	Unknown	NA
Chloralhydrate	D	100%	Avoid	Avoid	None	Unknown	NA
Chlorambucil	D	Unknown	Unknown	Unknown	Unknown	Unknown	Unknown
Chloramphenicol	D	100%	100%	100%	None	None	None
Chlorazepate	D	100%	100%	100%	Unknown	Unknown	NA

Drug	Method	GFR > 50	GFR 10–50	GFR < 10	Hemodialysis	CAPD	CAVH
Chlordiazepoxide	D	100%	100%	50%	None	Unknown	Dose for GFR 10–50
Chloroquine	D	100%	100%	50%	None	None	None
Chlorpheniramine	D	100%	100%	100%	None	Unknown	NA
Chlorpromazine	D	100%	100%	100%	Unknown	None	Dose for GFR 10–50
Chlorpropamide	D	50%	Avoid	Avoid	NA	NA	Avoid
Chlorthalidone	I	q24h	Avoid	Avoid	None	None	NA
Cholestyramine	D	100%	100%	100%	None	None	Dose for GFR 10–50
Cibenzoline	D, I	100% q12h	66% q24h	66% q24h	No data	No data	Dose for GFR 10–50
Cidofovir	D	Avoid	Avoid	Avoid	Avoid	Avoid	Avoid
Cilastatin	D	100%	50%	50%	None	None	Avoid
Cilazapril	D, I	75% q24h	50% q24–48h	10–25% q72h	Avoid	None	Dose for GFR 10–50
Cimetidine	D	100%	50%	25%	None	None	Dose for GFR 10–50
Cinoxacin	D	100%	50%	Avoid	Avoid	Avoid	Avoid
Ciprofloxacin	D	100%	50–75%	50%	250 mg q12h	250 mg q8h	200 mg IV q12h
Cisapride	D	100%	100%	50%	Unknown	Unknown	50–100%
Cisplatin	D	75%	75%	50%	Yes	Unknown	Dose for GFR 10–50
Cladribine	D	Unknown	Unknown	Unknown	Unknown	Unknown	Unknown
Clarithromycin	D	100%	75%	50% to 75%	Dose after dialysis	None	None
Clavulanic acid	D	100%	100%	50% to 75%	Dose after dialysis	Dose for GFR < 10	Dose for GFR 10–50
Clindamycin	D	100%	100%	100%	None	None	None
Clodronate	D	Unknown	Unknown	Avoid	Unknown	Unknown	Unknown
Clofazimine	D	100%	100%	100%	None	None	None
Clofibrate	I	q6–12h	q12–18h	Avoid	Unknown	Unknown	No data
Clomipramine	D	Unknown	Unknown	Unknown	Unknown	Unknown	NA
Clonazepam	D	100%	100%	100%	None	None	NA
Clonidine	D	100%	100%	100%	None	None	Dose for GFR 10–50
Codeine	D	100%	75%	50%	Unknown	Unknown	Dose for GFR 10–50
Colchicine	D	100%	100%	50%	None	Unknown	Dose for GFR 10–50
Colestipol	D	100%	100%	100%	None	None	Dose for GFR 10–50
Cortisone	D	100%	100%	100%	None	Unknown	Dose for GFR 10–50
Cyclophosphamide	D	100%	100%	75%	½ dose	None	Dose for GFR 10–50
Cycloserine	I	q12h	q12–24h	q24h	None	Unknown	Dose for GFR 10–50
Cyclosporine	D	100%	100%	100%	None	None	100%
Cytarabine	D	100%	100%	100%	Unknown	Unknown	Dose for GFR 10–50
Dapsone	D	No data	No data	No data	Dose for GFR < 10	Dose for GFR < 10	No data
Daunorubicin	D	100%	100%	100%	Unknown	Unknown	Unknown
Delavirdine	D	100%	100%	100%	None	No data	Dose for GFR 10–50
Desferoxamine	D	100%	100%	100%	Unknown	Unknown	Dose for GFR 10–50
Desipramine	D	100%	100%	100%	None	None	NA
Dexamethasone	D	100%	100%	100%	Unknown	Unknown	Dose for GFR 10–50
Diazepam	D	100%	100%	100%	None	Unknown	100%
Diazoxide	D	100%	100%	100%	None	None	Dose for GFR 10–50
Diclofenac	D	100%	100%	100%	None	None	Dose for GFR 10–50
Dicloxacillin	D	100%	100%	100%	None	None	NA
Didanosine	I	q12h	q24h	q24–48h	Dose after dialysis	Dose for GFR < 10	Dose for GFR < 10
Diflunisal	D	100%	50%	50%	None	None	Dose for GFR 10–50
Digitoxin	D	100%	100%	50–75%	None	None	Dose for GFR 10–50
Digoxin	D, I	100% q24h	25–75% q36h	10–25% q48h	None	None	Dose for GFR 10–50
Dilevalol	D	100%	100%	100%	None	None	Unknown
Diltiazem	D	100%	100%	100%	None	None	Dose for GFR 10–50
Diphenhydramine	D	100%	100%	100%	None	None	None
Dipyridamole	D	100%	100%	100%	Unknown	Unknown	NA
Dirithromycin	D	100%	100%	100%	None	None	Dose for GFR 10–50
Disopyramide	I	q8h	q12–24h	q24–40h	None	None	Dose for GFR 10–50
Dobutamine	D	100%	100%	100%	No data	No data	Dose for GFR 10–50

TABLE 66-4

Drug Doses in Renal Failure—cont'd

DRUG	DOSE METHOD	GFR >50 (mL/min)	GFR 10-50 (mL/min)	GFR <10 (mL/min)	SUPPLEMENTAL DOSE AFTER HEMODIALYSIS	CAPD	CRRT
Doxacurium	D	50%	50%	50%	Unknown	Unknown	Dose for GFR 10-50
Doxazosin	D	100%	100%	100%	None	None	Dose for GFR 10-50
Doxepin	D	100%	100%	100%	None	None	Dose for GFR 10-50
Doxorubicin	D	100%	100%	100%	None	Unknown	Dose for GFR 10-50
Doxycycline	D	100%	100%	100%	None	None	Dose for GFR 10-50
Dyphylline	D	75%	50%	25%	1/3 dose	Unknown	Dose for GFR 10-50
Ebastine	D	100%	50%	50%	Unknown	None	Dose for GFR 10-50
Enalapril	D	100%	75-100%	50%	20-25%	Unknown	Dose for GFR 10-50
Epirubicin	D	100%	100%	100%	None	None	Dose for GFR 10-50
Erythromycin	D	100%	100%	50-75%	None	None	None
Estazolam	D	100%	100%	100%	Unknown	Unknown	NA
Ethacrynic acid	I	q8-12h	q8-12h	Avoid	None	None	NA
Ethambutol	I	q24h	q24-36h	q48h	Dose after dialysis	Dose for GFR < 10	Dose for GFR 10-50
Ethchlorvynol	D	100%	Avoid	Avoid	None	None	NA
Ethionamide	D	100%	100%	50%	None	None	None
Ethosuximide	D	100%	100%	100%	None	Unknown	Unknown
Etodolac	D	100%	100%	100%	None	None	Dose for GFR 10-50
Etomidate	D	100%	100%	100%	Unknown	Unknown	Dose for GFR 10-50
Etoposide	D	100%	75%	50%	None	Unknown	Dose for GFR 10-50
Famciclovir	I	100%	q12-48h	50% q48h	Dose after dialysis	No data	Dose for GFR 10-50
Famotidine	D	50%	25%	10%	None	None	Dose for GFR 10-50
Fazadinium	D	100%	100%	100%	Unknown	Unknown	Dose for GFR 10-50
Felodipine	D	100%	100%	100%	None	None	Dose for GFR 10-50
Fenoprofen	D	100%	100%	100%	None	None	Dose for GFR 10-50
Fentanyl	D	100%	75%	50%	NA	NA	NA
Fexofenadine	I	q12h	q12-24h	q24h	Unknown	Unknown	Dose for GFR 10-50
Flecainide	D	100%	100%	50-75%	None	None	Dose for GFR 10-50
Fleroxacin	D	100%	50-75%	50%	400 mg after dialysis	400 mg/day	NA
Fluconazole	D	100%	100%	100%	200 mg after dialysis	Dose for GFR < 10	Dose for GFR 10-50
Flucytosine	I	q12h	q16h	q24h	Dose after dialysis	0.5-1.0 g/day	Dose for GFR 10-50
Fludarabine	D	100%	75%	50%	Unknown	Unknown	Dose for GFR 10-50
Flumazenil	D	100%	100%	100%	None	Unknown	NA
Flunarizine	D	100%	100%	100%	None	None	None
Fluorouracil	D	100%	100%	100%	Yes	Unknown	Dose for GFR 10-50
Fluoxetine	D	100%	100%	100%	Unknown	Unknown	NA
Flurazepam	D	100%	100%	100%	Unknown	Unknown	NA
Flurbiprofen	D	100%	100%	100%	None	None	Dose for GFR 10-50
Flutamide	D	100%	100%	100%	Unknown	Unknown	Unknown
Fluvastatin	D	100%	100%	100%	Unknown	Unknown	Dose for GFR 10-50
Fluvoxamine	D	100%	100%	100%	None	Unknown	NA
Foscarnet	D	28 mg/kg	15 mg/kg	6 mg/kg	Dose after dialysis	Dose for GFR < 10	Dose for GFR < 10
Fosinopril	D	100%	100%	75-100%	None	None	Dose for GFR 10-50
Furosemide	D	100%	100%	100%	None	None	NA
Gabapentin	D, I	400 mg tid	300 mg q12-24h	300 mg qd	300 mg load, then 200-300 mg		Dose for GFR 10-50
Gallamine	D	75%	Avoid	Avoid	Not applicable	NA	Dose for GFR 10-50
Ganciclovir	I	q12h	q24-48h	q48-96h	Dose after dialysis	Dose for GFR < 10	2.5 mg/kg/day
Gemfibrozil	D	100%	100%	100%	None	Unknown	Dose for GFR 10-50
Gentamicin	D, I	60-90% q8-12h	30-70% q12h	20-30% q24-48h	2/3 normal dose	3-4 mg/L/day	Dose for GFR 10-50

Glibornuride	D	Unknown	Unknown	Unknown	Unknown	Unknown	Avoid
Gliclazide	D	Unknown	Unknown	Unknown	Unknown	Unknown	Avoid
Glipizide	D	100%	100%	100%	None	None	Avoid
Glyburide	D	Unknown	Avoid	Avoid	None	None	Avoid
Gold sodium thiomalate	D	50%	Avoid	Avoid	None	None	Avoid
Griseofulvin	D	100%	100%	100%	None	None	None
Guanabenz	D	100%	100%	100%	Unknown	Unknown	Dose for GFR 10–50
Guanadrel	I	q12h	q12–24h	q24–48h	Unknown	Unknown	Dose for GFR 10–50
Guanethidine	I	q24h	q24h	q24–36h	Unknown	Unknown	Avoid
Guanfacine	D	100%	100%	100%	None	None	Dose for GFR 10–50
Haloperidol	D	100%	100%	100%	None	None	Dose for GFR 10–50
Heparin	D	100%	100%	100%	None	None	Dose for GFR 10–50
Hexobarbital	D	100%	100%	100%	Unknown	Unknown	NA
Hydralazine	I	q8h	q8h	q8–16h	None	None	Dose for GFR 10–50
Hydrocortisone	D	100%	100%	100%	Unknown	Unknown	Dose for GFR 10–50
Hydroxyurea	D	100%	100%	20%	Unknown	Unknown	Dose for GFR 10–50
Hydroxyzine	D	100%	100%	Unknown	100%	100%	100%
Ibuprofen	D	100%	100%	100%	None	None	Dose for GFR 10–50
Idarubicin	D	Unknown	Unknown	Unknown	Unknown	Unknown	Unknown
Ifosfamide	D	100%	100%	75%	Unknown	Unknown	Dose for GFR 10–50
Iloprost	D	100%	100%	50%	Unknown	Unknown	Dose for GFR 10–50
Imipenem	D	100%	100%	25%	Dose after dialysis	Dose for GFR < 10	Dose for GFR 10–50
Imipramine	D	100%	100%	100%	None	None	NA
Indapamide	D	100%	100%	Avoid	None	None	NA
Indinavir	D	100%	100%	100%	100%	Dose for GFR < 10	No data
Indobufen	D	100%	100%	25%	Unknown	Dose for GFR < 10	NA
Indomethacin	D	100%	100%	100%	None	None	Dose for GFR 10–50
Insulin	D	100%	75%	50%	None	None	Dose for GFR 10–50
Ipratropium	D	100%	100%	100%	None	None	Dose for GFR < 10
Isoniazid	D	100%	100%	50%	Dose after dialysis	Dose for GFR < 10	Dose for GFR 10–50
Isosorbide	D	100%	100%	100%	10–20 mg	None	Dose for GFR 10–50
Isradipine	D	100%	100%	100%	None	None	Dose for GFR 10–50
Itraconazole	D	100%	100%	50%	100%	100 mg q12–24h	100 mg q12–24h
Kanamycin	D, I	60–90% q8–12h	30–70% q12h	20–30% q24–48h	$\frac{2}{3}$ normal dose	15–20 mg/L/day	Dose for GFR 10–50
Ketamine	D	100%	100%	100%	Unknown	Unknown	Dose for GFR 10–50
Ketanserin	D	100%	100%	100%	None	None	None
Ketoconazole	D	100%	100%	100%	None	None	Dose for GFR 10–50
Ketoprofen	D	100%	100%	100%	None	None	Dose for GFR 10–50
Ketorolac	D	100%	100%	50%	None	None	Dose for GFR 10–50
Labetolol	D	100%	100%	100%	None	None	Dose for GFR 10–50
Lamivudine	D, I	100%	50–150 mg qd	25 mg qd	Dose after dialysis	dose for GFR < 10	Dose for GFR 10–50
Lamotrigine	D	100%	100%	100%	Unknown	Unknown	Dose for GFR 10–50
Lansoprazole	D	100%	100%	100%	Unknown	Unknown	Unknown
Levodopa	D	100%	100%	100%	Unknown	Unknown	Dose for GFR 10–50
Levofloxacin	D	50%	50%	25–50%	Dose for GFR < 10	Dose for GFR < 10	Dose for GFR 10–50
Lidocaine	D	100%	100%	100%	None	None	Dose for GFR 10–50
Lincomycin	I	q6h	q6–12h	q12–24h	None	None	NA
Lisinopril	D	100%	50–75%	25 to 50%	None	None	Dose for GFR 10–50
Lispro Insulin	D	100%	75%	50%	20%	None	None
Lithium carbonate	D	100%	50–75%	25 to 50%	Dose after dialysis	None	Dose for GFR 10–50
Lomefloxacin	D	100%	50–75%	50%	Dose For GFR < 10	Unknown	NA
Loracarbef	I	q12h	q24h	q3–5 d	Dose after dialysis	Dose For GFR < 10	Dose for GFR 10–50
Lorazepam	D	100%	100%	100%	Unknown	Unknown	Dose for GFR 10–50
Losartan	D	100%	100%	100%	Unknown	Unknown	Dose for GFR 10–50
Lovastatin	D	100%	100%	100%	Unknown	Unknown	Dose for GFR 10–50

TABLE 66-4

Drug Doses in Renal Failure—cont'd

DRUG	DOSE METHOD	GFR > 50 (mL/min)	GFR 10–50 (mL/min)	GFR < 10 (mL/min)	SUPPLEMENTAL DOSE AFTER HEMODIALYSIS	CAPD	CRRT
Low-molecular-weight heparin	D	100%	100%	50%	Unknown	Unknown	Dose for GFR 10-50
Maprotiline	D	100%	100%	100%	Unknown	Unknown	NA
Meclofenamic acid	D	100%	100%	100%	None	None	Dose for GFR 10-50
Mefenamic acid	D	100%	100%	100%	None	None	Dose for GFR 10-50
Mefloquine	D	100%	100%	100%	None	None	Dose for GFR 10-50
Melphalan	D	100%	75%	50%	Unknown	Unknown	Dose for GFR 10-50
Meperidine	D	100%	75%	50%	Avoid	None	Avoid
Meprobamate	I	q6h	q9-12h	q12-18h	None	Unknown	NA
Meropenem	D, I	500 mg q6h	250-500 mg q12h	250-500 mg q24h	Dose after dialysis	Dose For GFR < 10	Dose for GFR 10-50
Metaproterenol	D	100%	100%	100%	Unknown	Unknown	Dose for GFR 10-50
Metformin	D	50%	25%	Avoid	Unknown	Unknown	Avoid
Methadone	D	100%	100%	50-75%	None	None	NA
Methenamine mandelate	D	100%	Avoid	Avoid	NA	NA	NA
Methicillin	I	q4-6h	q6-8h	q8-12h	None	None	Dose for GFR 10-50
Methimazole	D	100%	100%	100%	Unknown	Unknown	Dose for GFR 10-50
Methotrexate	D	100%	50%	Avoid	Yes	None	Dose for GFR 10-50
Methyldopa	I	q8h	q8-12h	q12-24h	250 mg	None	Dose for GFR 10-50
Methylprednisolone	D	100%	100%	100%	Yes	Unknown	50-75%
Metoclopramide	D	100%	75%	50%	None	Unknown	50-75%
Metocurine	D	75%	50%	50%	Unknown	Unknown	Dose for GFR 10-50
Metolazone	D	100%	100%	100%	None	None	NA
Metoprolol	D	100%	100%	100%	50 mg	None	Dose for GFR 10-50
Metronidazole	D	100%	100%	50%	Dose after dialysis	Dose For GFR < 10	Dose for GFR 10-50
Mexiletine	D	100%	100%	50-75%	None	None	None
Mezlocillin	I	q4-6h	q6-8h	q8h	None	None	Dose for GFR 10-50
Miconazole	D	100%	100%	100%	None	None	Dose for GFR 10-50
Midazolam	D	100%	100%	50%	NA	NA	NA
Midodrine	D	5-10 mg q8h	5-10 mg q8h	Unknown	5 mg q8h	No data	Dose for GFR 10-50
Miglitol	D	50%	Avoid	Avoid	Unknown	Unknown	Avoid
Milrinone	D	100%	100%	50 to 75%	No data	No data	Dose for GFR 10-50
Minocycline	D	100%	100%	100%	None	None	Dose for GFR 10-50
Minoxidil	D	100%	100%	100%	None	None	Dose for GFR 10-50
Mitomycin C	D	100%	100%	75%	Unknown	Unknown	Unknown
Mitoxantrone	D	100%	100%	100%	Unknown	Unknown	Dose for GFR 10-50
Mivacurium	D	100%	50%	50%	Unknown	Unknown	Unknown
Moricizine	D	100%	100%	100%	None	None	Dose for GFR 10-50
Morphine	D	100%	75%	50%	None	None	Dose for GFR 10-50
Moxalactam	I	q8-12h	q12-24h	q24-48h	Dose after dialysis	Dose for GFR < 10	Dose for GFR 10-50
Nabumetone	D	100%	100%	100%	None	None	Dose for GFR 10-50
N-Acetylcysteine	D	100%	100%	75%	Unknown	Unknown	100%
Nadolol	D	100%	50%	25%	40 mg	None	Dose for GFR 10-50
Nafcillin	D	100%	100%	100%	None	None	Dose for GFR 10-50
Nalidixic acid	D	100%	Avoid	Avoid	Avoid	Avoid	NA
Naloxone	D	100%	100%	100%	NA	NA	NA
Naproxen	D	100%	100%	100%	None	None	Dose for GFR 10-50
Nefazodone	D	100%	100%	100%	Unknown	Unknown	Dose for GFR 10-50
Nelfinavir	D	No data	No data	No data	No data	No data	No data

Drug	Method	GFR >50	GFR 10–50	GFR <10	Supplement HD	Supplement CAPD	Supplement CVVH
Neostigmine	D	100%	50%	25%	Unknown	Unknown	Dose for GFR 10–50
Netilmicin	D, I	50–90% q8–12h	20–60% q12h	10–20% q24–48h	⅔ normal dose	3–4 mg/L/day	Dose for GFR 10–50
Nevirapine	D	100%	100%	100%	None	Dose for GFR < 10	Dose for GFR 10–50
Nicardipine	D	100%	100%	100%	None	None	Dose for GFR 10–50
Nicotinic acid	D	100%	50%	25%	Unknown	Unknown	Dose for GFR 10–50
Nifedipine	D	100%	100%	100%	None	None	Dose for GFR 10–50
Nimodipine	D	100%	100%	100%	None	None	Dose for GFR 10–50
Nisoldipine	D	100%	100%	100%	None	None	Dose for GFR 10–50
Nitrazepam	D	100%	100%	100%	Unknown	Unknown	NA
Nitrofurantoin	D	Avoid	Avoid	Avoid	NA	NA	NA
Nitroglycerine	D	100%	100%	100%	No data	No data	Dose for GFR 10–50
Nitroprusside	D	100%	100%	100%	None	None	Dose for GFR 10–50
Nitrosoureas	D	100%	75%	25–50%	None	Unknown	Unknown
Nizatidine	D	75%	50%	25%	Unknown	Unknown	Dose for GFR 10–50
Norfloxacin	I	q12h	q12–24h	Avoid	NA	NA	NA
Nortriptyline	D	100%	100%	100%	None	None	NA
Ofloxacin	D	100%	50%	25–50%	100 mg bid	Dose for GFR < 10	300 mg/day
Omeprazole	D	100%	100%	100%	Unknown	Unknown	Unknown
Ondansetron	D	100%	100%	100%	Unknown	Unknown	Dose for GFR 10–50
Orphenadrine	D	100%	100%	100%	Unknown	Unknown	NA
Ouabain	I	q12–24h	q24–36h	q36–48h	None	None	Dose for GFR 10–50
Oxaprozin	D	100%	100%	100%	None	None	Dose for GFR 10–50
Oxatomide	D	100%	100%	100%	None	None	NA
Oxazepam	D	100%	100%	100%	Unknown	Unknown	Dose for GFR 10–50
Oxcarbazepine	D	100%	100%	100%	Unknown	Unknown	Unknown
Paclitaxel	D	100%	100%	100%	Unknown	Unknown	Dose for GFR 10–50
Pancuronium	D	50%	50–75%	Avoid	Unknown	Unknown	Dose for GFR 10–50
Paroxetine	D	100%	50–75%	50%	Unknown	Unknown	NA
Paraamino salicylic acid (PAS)	D	100%	50–75%	50%	Dose after dialysis	Dose for GFR < 10	Dose for GFR 10–50
Penbutolol	D	100%	100%	100%	None	None	Dose for GFR 10–50
Penicillamine	D	100%	Avoid	Avoid	⅓ dose	Unknown	Dose for GFR 10–50
Penicillin G	D	100%	75%	20–50%	Dose after dialysis	Dose for GFR < 10	Dose for GFR 10–50
Penicillin VK	D	100%	100%	100%	Dose after dialysis	Dose for GFR < 10	NA
Pentamidine	I	q24h	q24–36h	q48h	None	None	None
Pentazocine	D	100%	75%	50%	50%	Unknown	Dose for GFR 10–50
Pentobarbital	D	100%	100%	100%	None	Unknown	Dose for GFR 10–50
Pentopril	D	100%	50–75%	50%	50%	Unknown	Dose for GFR 10–50
Pentoxifylline	D	100%	100%	100%	100%	Unknown	100%
Perfloxacin	D	100%	100%	100%	None	None	Dose for GFR 10–50
Perindopril	D	100%	75%	50%	25–50%	Unknown	Dose for GFR 10–50
Phenelzine	D	100%	100%	100%	Unknown	Unknown	NA
Phenobarbital	I	q8–12h	q8–12h	q12–16h	Dose after dialysis	½ normal dose	Dose for GFR 10–50
Phenylbutazone	D	100%	100%	100%	None	None	Dose for GFR 10–50
Phenytoin	D	100%	100%	100%	None	None	None
Pindolol	D	100%	100%	100%	Unknown	Unknown	Dose for GFR 10–50
Pipecuronium	D	100%	100%	50%	Unknown	Unknown	Dose for GFR 10–50
Piperacillin	I	q4–6h	q6–8h	q8h	Dose for GFR < 10	Dose for GFR < 10	Dose for GFR 10–50
Piretanide	D	100%	100%	100%	None	None	NA
Piroxicam	D	100%	100%	100%	None	None	Dose for GFR 10–50
Plicamycin	D	100%	75%	50%	Unknown	Unknown	Unknown
Pravastatin	D	100%	100%	100%	Unknown	Unknown	Dose for GFR 10–50
Prazepam	D	100%	100%	100%	Unknown	Unknown	NA
Prazosin	D	100%	100%	100%	None	None	Dose for GFR 10–50
Prednisolone	D	100%	100%	100%	Yes	Unknown	Dose for GFR 10–50

Continued

TABLE 66-4

Drug Doses in Renal Failure—cont'd

DRUG	DOSE METHOD	GFR > 50 (mL/min)	GFR 10–50 (mL/min)	GFR < 10 (mL/min)	SUPPLEMENTAL DOSE AFTER HEMODIALYSIS	CAPD	CRRT
Prednisone	D	100%	100%	100%	None	Unknown	Dose for GFR 10–50
Primaquine	I	100%	q8h	100%	None	None	Dose for GFR 10–50
Primidone	I	q8h	q8–12h	q12–24h	1/3 dose	Unknown	Unknown
Probenecid	D	100%	Avoid	Avoid	Avoid	Unknown	Avoid
Probucol	D	100%	100%	100%	Unknown	Unknown	Dose for GFR 10–50
Procainamide	I	q4h	q6–12h	q8–24h	200 mg	None	Dose for GFR 10–50
Promethazine	D	100%	100%	100%	Unknown	Unknown	Dose for GFR 10–50
Promethazine	D	100%	100%	100%	None	None	100%
Propafenone	D	100%	100%	100%	None	Unknown	Dose for GFR 10–50
Propofol	D	100%	100%	100%	None	None	Dose for GFR 10–50
Propoxyphene	D	100%	100%	Avoid	None	None	NA
Propranolol	D	100%	100%	100%	None	None	Dose for GFR 10–50
Propylthiouracil	D	100%	100%	100%	Unknown	Unknown	Dose for GFR 10–50
Protriptyline	D	100%	100%	100%	None	None	NA
Pyrazinimide	D	100%	Avoid	Avoid	Avoid	Avoid	Avoid
Pyridostigmine	D	50%	35%	20%	Unknown	Unknown	Dose for GFR 10–50
Pyrimethamine	D	100%	100%	100%	None	None	None
Quazepam	D	Unknown	Unknown	Unknown	Unknown	Unknown	NA
Quinapril	D	100%	75–100%	75%	25%	None	Dose for GFR 10–50
Quinidine	D	100%	100%	75%	100–200 mg	None	Dose for GFR 10–50
Quinine	I	q8h	q8–12h	q24h	Dose after dialysis	Dose for GFR < 10	Dose for GFR 10–50
Ramipril	D	100%	50–75%	25–50%	20%	None	Dose for GFR 10–50
Ranitidine	D	75%	50%	25%	1/2 dose	None	Dose for GFR 10–50
Reserpine	D	100%	100%	Avoid	None	None	Dose for GFR 10–50
Ribavirin	D	100%	100%	50%	Dose after dialysis	Dose for GFR < 10	Dose for GFR <10
Rifabutin	D	100%	100%	100%	None	None	Dose for GFR <10
Rifampin	D	100%	50–100%	50–100%	None	Dose for GFR < 10	Dose for GFR <10
Ritonavir	D	100%	100%	100%	None	Dose for GFR < 10	Dose for GFR 10–50
Saquinavir	D	100%	100%	100%	None	Dose for GFR < 10	Dose for GFR 10–50
Secobarbital	D	100%	100%	100%	None	None	NA
Sertraline	D	100%	100%	100%	Unknown	Unknown	NA
Simvastatin	D	100%	100%	100%	Unknown	Unknown	Dose for GFR 10–50
Sodium valproate	D	100%	100%	100%	None	None	None
Sotalol	D	100%	30%	15–30%	80 mg	None	Dose for GFR 10–50
Sparfloxacin	D, I	100%	50–75%	50% q48h	Dose for GFR < 10	No data	Dose for GFR 10–50
Spectinomycin	D	100%	100%	100%	None	None	None
Spironolactone	I	q6–12h	q12–24h	Avoid	None	NA	Avoid
Stavudine	D, I	100%	50% q12–24h	50% q24h	Dose after dialysis	No data	Dose for GFR 10–50
Streptokinase	D	100%	100%	100%	NA	NA	Dose for GFR 10–50
Streptomycin	I	q24h	q24–72h	q72–96h	1/2 normal dose	20–40 mg/L/day	Dose for GFR 10–50
Streptozotocin	D	100%	75%	50%	Unknown	Unknown	Unknown
Succinylcholine	D	100%	100%	100%	Unknown	Unknown	Dose for GFR 10–50
Sufentanil	D	100%	100%	100%	NA	Unknown	Dose for GFR 10–50
Sulbactam	I	q6–8h	q12–24h	q24–48h	Dose after dialysis	0.75–1.5 g/day	750 mg q12h
Sulfamethoxazole	I	q12h	q18h	q24h	1 g after dialysis	1 g/day	Dose for GFR 10–50
Sulfinpyrazone	D	100%	100%	Avoid	None	None	Dose for GFR 10–50
Sulfisoxazole	I	q6h	q8–12h	q12–24h	2 g after dialysis	3 g/day	NA
Sulindac	D	100%	100%	100%	None	None	Dose for GFR 10–50

Drug	Method	GFR >50	GFR 10–50	GFR <10	Hemodialysis	CAPD	CRRT
Sulotroban	D	50%	30%	10%	Unknown	Unknown	Unknown
Tamoxifen	D	100%	100%	100%	Unknown	Unknown	Dose for GFR 10–50
Tazobactam	D	100%	75%	50%	l/3 dose	Dose for GFR < 10	Dose for GFR 10–50
Teicoplanin	I	q24h	q48h	q72h	Dose for GFR < 10	Dose for GFR < 10	Dose for GFR 10–50
Temazepam	D	100%	100%	100%	None	None	NA
Teniposide	D	100%	100%	100%	None	None	Dose for GFR 10–50
Terazosin	D	100%	100%	100%	Unknown	Unknown	Dose for GFR 10–50
Terbutaline	D	100%	100%	Avoid	Unknown	Unknown	Dose for GFR 10–50
Terfenadine	D	100%	100%	100%	None	None	NA
Tetracycline	I	q8–12h	q12–24h	q24h	None	None	Dose for GFR 10–50
Theophylline	D	100%	100%	100%	l/2 dose	Unknown	Dose for GFR 10–50
Thiazides	D	100%	100%	Avoid	NA	NA	NA
Thiopental	D	100%	100%	75%	NA	NA	NA
Ticarcillin	D, I	1–2 g q4h	1–2 g q8h	1–2 g q12h	3 g after dialysis	Dose for GFR < 10	Dose for GFR 10–50
Ticlopidine	D	100%	100%	100%	Unknown	Unknown	Dose for GFR 10–50
Timolol	D	100%	100%	100%	None	None	Dose for GFR 10–50
Tobramycin	D, I	60–90% q8–12h	30–70% q12h	20–30% q24–48h	2/3 normal dose	3–4 mg/L/day	Dose for GFR 10–50
Tocainide	D	100%	100%	50%	200 mg	None	Dose for GFR 10–50
Tolazamide	D	100%	100%	100%	Unknown	None	Avoid
Tolbutamide	D	100%	100%	100%	None	None	Avoid
Tolmetin	D	100%	100%	100%	None	None	Dose for GFR 10–50
Topiramate	D	100%	50%	25%	Unknown	Unknown	Dose for GFR 10–50
Topotecan	D	75%	50%	25%	Unknown	Unknown	Dose for GFR 10–50
Torsemide	D	100%	100%	100%	None	None	NA
Tranexamic acid	D	50%	25%	10%	Unknown	Unknown	Unknown
Tranylcypromine	D	Unknown	Unknown	Unknown	Unknown	Unknown	NA
Trazodone	D	100%	Unknown	Unknown	Unknown	Unknown	NA
Triamcinolone	D	100%	100%	100%	Unknown	Unknown	Dose for GFR 10–50
Triamterene	I	q12h	q12h	Avoid	NA	NA	Avoid
Triazolam	D	100%	100%	100%	None	None	NA
Trihexyphenidyl	D	Unknown	Unknown	Unknown	Unknown	Unknown	Unknown
Trimethadione	I	q8h	q8–12h	q12–24h	Unknown	Unknown	Dose for GFR 10–50
Trimethoprim	I	q12h	q18h	q24h	Dose after dialysis	q24h	q18h
Trimetrexate	D	100%	50–100%	Avoid	No data	No data	No data
Trimipramine	D	100%	100%	100%	None	None	NA
Tripelennamine	D	Unknown	Unknown	Unknown	Unknown	Unknown	NA
Triprolidine	D	Unknown	Unknown	Unknown	Unknown	Unknown	NA
Tubocurarine	D	75%	50%	Avoid	Unknown	Unknown	Dose for GFR 10–50
Urokinase	D	Unknown	Unknown	Unknown	Unknown	Unknown	Dose for GFR 10–50
Vancomycin	D, I	500 mg q6–12h	500 mg q24–48h	500 mg q48–96h	Dose for GFR < 10	Dose for GFR < 10	Dose for GFR 10–50
Vecuronium	D	100%	100%	100%	Unknown	Unknown	Dose for GFR 10–50
Venlafaxine	D	75%	50%	50%	Unknown	Unknown	NA
Verapamil	D	100%	100%	100%	None	None	Dose for GFR 10–50
Vidarabine	D	100%	100%	75%	Infuse after dialysis	Dose for GFR < 10	Dose for GFR 10–50
Vigabatrin	D	100%	50%	25%	Unknown	Unknown	Dose for GFR 10–50
Vinblastine	D	100%	100%	100%	Unknown	Unknown	Dose for GFR 10–50
Vincristine	D	100%	100%	100%	Unknown	Unknown	Dose for GFR 10–50
Vinorelbine	D	100%	100%	100%	Unknown	Unknown	Dose for GFR 10–50
Warfarin	D	100%	100%	100%	None	None	None
Zafirlukast	D	100%	100%	100%	Unknown	Unknown	Dose for GFR 10–50
Zalcitabine	I	100%	q12h	q24h	Dose after dialysis	No data	Dose for GFR 10–50
Zidovudine (AZT)	D, I	200 mg q8h	200 mg q8h	100 mg q8h	Dose for GFR < 10	Dose for GFR < 10	100 mg q8h
Zileuton	D	100%	100%	100%	None	Unknown	Dose for GFR 10–50

CAPD, chronic ambulatory peritoneal dialysis; CRRT, continuous renal replacement therapies; D, decreasing individual doses; GFR, glomerular filtration rate; HD, hemodialysis; I, increasing individual doses; NA, not applicable.

preferred because of improved compliance. However, steady-state drug levels are usually not achieved until after the drug has been given for at least three or four half-lives. Narrow therapeutic range and individual variability in drug response complicate the use of these drugs.

Many cardiovascular drugs or their metabolites accumulate in patients with renal insufficiency. Abnormalities of drug binding to plasma proteins increase free drug at receptor sites, enhancing drug efficacy and toxicity.

Each of the antihypertensive drugs can be toxic. In general, the adverse effects are related to their pharmacologic effect and can be avoided by careful dose titration. The development of newer, effective antihypertensive agents allows more individualized pharmacotherapy. Choosing an antihypertensive agent should include understanding the altered homeostatic mechanisms in patients with impaired renal function.

The relation between renal drug elimination and the cardiovascular system is well established. Drugs may alter their own elimination rate or their effect on the kidneys by improving cardiac output and effective renal blood flow. For example, patients with decompensated congestive heart failure may be resistant to diuretics. If natriuresis can be initiated, subsequent improvement in cardiovascular function can increase response to the diuretic. The effect of cardiovascular drugs may also vary for individual patients as cardiac function changes.

The use of antiarrhythmic agents requires particular care. Because toxicity may appear as the arrhythmia the drug is intended to correct, recognition of toxicity may be delayed. Inappropriate increases in antiarrhythmic dose may be fatal. Monitoring other electrocardiographic evidence of toxicity such as a prolonged QT interval or widening of the QRS complex may be essential to proper diagnosis.

Diuretics may be helpful in patients with fluid overload and are as effective in lowering blood pressure as angiotensin-converting enzyme (ACE) inhibitors or calcium channel blockers.[53] However, the pharmacokinetics and pharmacodynamics of diuretics are altered in patients with proteinuria or renal impairment. Binding to proteins in tubule fluid decreases the diuretic efficacy of thiazide and loop diuretics. The natriuretic response to diuretics is limited by the counter-regulation of increased proximal tubule sodium reabsorption in response to hypovolemia and increased distal tubule sodium reabsorption in response to increased sodium load. Hypovolemia can result in a further decrease in renal function and should be carefully evaluated during diuretic therapy.

Diuretics can be grouped into two categories based on their clinical use. The potassium-sparing drugs (i.e., amiloride, spironolactone, and triamterene) may produce hyperkalemia in patients with creatinine clearances below 30 mL/minute and should be avoided in these patients. The remaining diuretics are organic acids and need to reach the tubule lumen to be active. In patients with impaired renal function, endogenous organic acids accumulate and compete with diuretics for secretion into the tubule lumen. Consequently, as renal function decreases, larger doses of diuretics are required. As glomerular filtration falls, the thiazides become ineffective. However, large doses of the loop diuretics (i.e., furosemide, bumetanide, torsemide, or ethacrynic acid) may still produce diuresis.

In patients with renal insufficiency, diuretic-induced dehydration may result in a further loss of renal function.

Unless patients require diuresis for substantial peripheral edema or congestive heart failure, hypertension in patients with decreased renal function should be managed to avoid unnecessary volume contraction.

Thiazides lose their diuretic efficacy when the GFR falls below about 30 mL/minute. Loop diuretics may remain effective at very low levels of renal function, although high doses may be required and a combination of loop diuretic with a thiazide may be required.[54]

Potassium-sparing diuretics are contraindicated in patients with impaired renal function and the decreased ability to excrete potassium because of the risk of life-threatening hyperkalemia. Clinical situations that increase the risk of hyperkalemia include the concurrent administration of potassium supplements, ACE inhibitors, and the use of non-steroidal anti-inflammatory drugs (NSAIDs).

ACE inhibitors and angiotensin receptor antagonists decrease the rate of progression of diabetic renal disease.[55, 56] However, these drugs must be given with caution in patients with decreased renal function and those on dialysis. The hemodynamic effects of decreased angiotensin II can result in a sudden decrease in renal function in patients with renal artery occlusion or severe, diffuse microvascular renal disease. The initial doses of ACE inhibitors and angiotensin receptor antagonists should be low and carefully titrated, and renal function should be monitored. Anaphylactoid reactions have been reported in hemodialysis patients taking ACE inhibitors during dialysis with polyacrylonitrile dialysis membranes.[57] Worsening anemia and erythropoietin resistance has also been reported in ACE-treated hemodialysis patients.[58]

When blood pressure is appropriately lowered in hypertensive patients with renal insufficiency, a transient decrease in renal function may occur. As hypertensive microvascular changes improve, renal function should again increase. In some cases, dialysis may be needed temporarily. If renal function decreases with antihypertensive therapy and does not improve, drug-related nephrotoxicity or another potentially reversible cause should be considered.

Antimicrobial Agents

The most important consideration in the use of antimicrobial drugs in patients with renal insufficiency is the early initiation of effective agents at doses that can achieve therapeutic drug concentrations quickly. Dose reduction that results in ineffectively low plasma concentration is the greatest danger in prescribing antimicrobial agents for patients with renal impairment. The initial drug choice may depend empirically on the source of the suspected infection. More specific treatment should follow an aggressive search for the pathogen. A single loading dose, equivalent to the usual maintenance dose for patients with normal renal function, should almost always be given to patients with impaired renal function. Although many antimicrobial drugs are excreted by the kidneys, the therapeutic range between efficacy and toxicity is generally wide, and the initial high doses used to achieve blood levels above the minimum inhibitory concentrations should be decreased, if necessary, in time to avoid toxicity from drug or metabolite accumulation. Therapeutic drug monitoring of drug levels and microbial sensitivities is the best guide to the use of many antimicrobial agents in patients with impaired drug excretion.

Antimicrobial therapy in patients with renal disease begins with an attempt to isolate the causative organism. Uremic patients with serious infections may not have elevated temperatures. Uremic symptoms or the effects of dialysis may mask nonspecific symptoms of infection. Because patients with renal insufficiency are more likely to have adverse effects from antimicrobial therapy than patients with normal renal function, culture documentation of bacterial infection is essential.

Adverse reactions to antimicrobial treatment in patients with impaired renal function are usually caused by the accumulation of drugs or their metabolites to toxic levels with repeated doses and may affect any organ system. Manian and colleagues divided the adverse effects of antibiotics due to drug or metabolite accumulation into six major categories, including neurologic toxicity, coagulopathy, nephrotoxicity, hypoglycemia, hematologic toxicity, and aminoglycoside inactivation by penicillins. They further considered neurologic toxicity according to central nervous system toxicity consisting primarily of encephalopathy and seizures, ototoxicity, peripheral neuropathy, or neuromuscular blockade with potential respiratory depression.[59] Drug toxicity should be considered in antibiotic-treated patients with renal insufficiency who develop new symptoms.

The choice of antimicrobial agents includes consideration of these potential toxicities and the consequences of inadvertent drug or metabolite accumulation. Side effects rarely seen in patients with normal renal function occur more frequently in patients with renal failure. For example, seizures from β-lactam accumulation are rare in patients with sufficient kidney function to prevent drug accumulation but may occur in patients with renal impairment when large doses are given.

Mild nephrotoxicity in patients with renal insufficiency may result in overt uremia. A decrease in renal function by as much as 50% from aminoglycoside nephrotoxicity may go unnoticed in patients with normal kidney function. A similar change in patients with creatinine clearances less than 20 mL/minute could precipitate the need for dialysis.

The accumulation of metabolic waste products in patients with impaired excretory capacity may cause symptoms. The anti-anabolic effects of tetracycline can cause an increase in the blood urea nitrogen. Drugs that increase metabolic load should be avoided in patients with decreased kidney function.

Nephrotoxicity of antimicrobial agents may be the result of direct, cellular toxicity or allergic interstitial nephritis. Although decreasing renal function during antimicrobial treatment may be the result of drug toxicity or the underlying infection, the suspicion of an adverse drug event should prompt careful evaluation. Drug level monitoring is particularly important in patients with unstable renal function.

Hypoglycemic Drugs

Nearly 46% of new dialysis patients have diabetes mellitus.[60] Careful consideration of hypoglycemic drug selection and dosage is important for patients with impaired renal function. The kidney accounts for almost 30% of the elimination of insulin from the body.[61] As renal function decreases, insulin clearance decreases because of impaired insulin filtration and decreased insulin uptake from the tubule lumen and peritubule surface.[62] As a result, insulin requirements often decrease in patients with decreasing renal function, and

hypoglycemia is more common in diabetics with impaired renal function.

The longer half-life of insulin in patients with impaired renal function may affect the use of drugs that enhance endogenous insulin secretion. For example, although glyburide pharmacokinetics do not differ after initial or chronic administration in patients with end-stage renal disease treated with hemodialysis compared with controls, hemodialysis patients treated with this oral hypoglycemic agent have increased C-peptide and insulin levels with chronic dosing.[63] Simply stated, patients with impaired renal function are at increased risk of hypoglycemia when they are treated with insulin or oral hypoglycemic drugs. Initial drug doses should be low and titrated carefully.

Lactic acidosis can result from metformin accumulation. Although a rare complication of the use of this drug, metformin plasma levels in excess of 5 μg/mL are generally found in patients with renal insufficiency, including intrinsic renal disease and renal hypoperfusion. The kidneys excrete metformin, and the risk of metformin accumulation and lactic acidosis increases with age and the degree of impairment of renal function. Consequently, metformin should not be used in patients with impaired renal function or in the elderly. Diabetic patients taking metformin should have their renal function measured frequently.

Nonsteroidal Anti-inflammatory Drugs

Adverse effects of NSAIDs can be the result of the pharmacologic action of prostaglandin synthesis inhibition or hypersensitivity. Prostaglandins are important in maintaining renal vasodilatation and ensuring adequate renal blood flow. NSAIDs are potent inhibitors of renal prostaglandin synthesis, resulting in renal arteriolar constriction, decreased renal blood flow, and a reduced GFR.

Prostaglandins are also important for maintaining fluid and electrolyte homeostasis. Reduction in glomerular filtration allows increased tubule reabsorption. Decreased prostaglandin production increases tubule chloride reabsorption in the loop of Henle and increases the effect of antidiuretic hormone on the distal tubule. These effects may lead to salt and water retention. Renin generation is also diminished. The resultant decrease in plasma aldosterone production can lead to potassium retention and hyperkalemia in patients with decreased renal function.

NSAIDs should be used cautiously in patients with decreased renal function. NSAIDs may cause a sudden decrease in renal function related to the hemodynamic effects of decreased renal prostaglandin production. Patients at greatest risk are those in whom renal vasoconstrictors are up-regulated and the renal vasodilatory properties of prostaglandins are the most important. Patients with congestive heart failure, volume contraction, and ascites or edema from liver failure are at greatest risk.[64] Hyperkalemia and sodium retention may also occur in patients with impaired renal function treated with NSAIDs. These drugs should not be used in patients with renal impairment without a specific indication, and when they are required, renal function and other signs of toxicity should be monitored.

The selective inhibition of certain cyclooxygenase (COX) isoforms, such as COX-2, was hoped to decrease toxicity of NSAIDs. However, it is now recognized that, because COX-2 is constitutively expressed in the kidney, it plays an important role in renal function.[65] The entire spectrum of NSAID effects on the kidney have also been observed with those NSAIDs that more specifically inhibit COX-2, and there appears to be no advantage in using these agents over less-expensive, nonselective inhibitors of prostaglandin synthesis.[66]

Acute renal failure characterized by proteinuria or the nephritic syndrome, hematuria, pyuria, and histologic evidence of immune glomerular injury or interstitial nephritis is consistent with a hypersensitivity reaction. Discontinuing treatment with the NSAID results in the gradual disappearance of proteinuria and a return toward normal renal function.[67]

Sedatives, Hypnotics, and Drugs Used in Psychiatry

Psychotherapeutic drugs are commonly given to patients with renal disease to relieve anxiety and depression. Excessive sedation is the most frequent adverse effect in patients with renal insufficiency. Because malaise, somnolence, and encephalopathy are also common uremic symptoms, recognition of adverse drug reactions may be delayed.

Benzodiazepines are often used to treat emotional stress associated with decreasing renal function in patients on dialysis, although the efficacy of chronic benzodiazepine treatment has been questioned. Members of this class are generally safer than other anxiolytic agents, and short-term administration is effective. Active polar metabolites of these compounds normally excreted by the kidneys are likely to accumulate in patients with renal impairment and produce enhanced, prolonged sedation. Diazepam, chlordiazepoxide, and flurazepam are examples of such compounds. Because of the potential for drug or metabolite accumulation, the chronic use of these agents and others in this drug class should be discouraged in patients with decreased renal function.

Phenothiazines, used to treat major psychoses, and tricyclic antidepressants, used for severe depression in patients with renal disease, can also produce excessive sedation. Patients taking these drugs may also exhibit anticholinergic effects, orthostatic hypotension, confusion, and extrapyramidal symptoms.

Lithium carbonate has become an increasingly prescribed antidepressant. The drug is excreted by the kidney and has a narrow therapeutic range. Careful dose reduction and plasma lithium level monitoring is required in patients with impaired or unstable renal function. Hemodialysis has been used in cases of lithium overdose. Although lithium is effectively removed by dialysis, a rebound increase in plasma levels is common after hemodialysis, and repeated treatments may be required.

DRUG LEVEL MONITORING

Measurement of plasma drug concentrations is helpful in assessing a particular dosage regimen when the relationship between drug levels and efficacy or toxicity has been established. These measurements are most important for drugs with a narrow therapeutic range or difficult-to-measure pharmacologic effects.

Serum levels are determined after an appropriate loading dose has been given. In the absence of a loading dose, 3 or 4 doses of the drug should be administered before serum

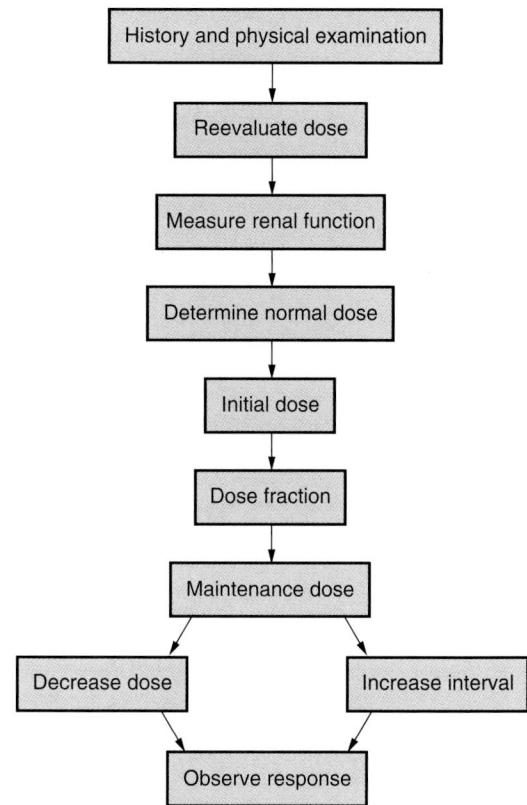

FIGURE 66-5. A practical scheme for drug dosing in dialysis patients.

levels are measured. This ensures that a steady-state serum concentration has been established. For some drugs, maximum and minimum concentrations are relevant. Peak levels are most meaningful when measured after rapid drug distribution has occurred. Conversely, minimum concentrations are usually measured just before giving the next scheduled dose. A practical schema for drug prescribing in patients with renal impairment is shown in Figure 66-5.

Adverse drug events are common and costly. Johnson and Bootman estimated the annual cost of drug-related morbidity and mortality in the U.S. ambulatory care population to be between $30.9 billion and $76.6 billion.[68] The heterogeneity of renal disease makes responses to drug therapy quite variable. Dosage nomograms, drug tables, and computer-assisted dosing recommendations provide guidelines for deriving an initial approach to drug administration in patients with decreased renal function. Continuing evaluation of the therapeutic response and modification of the regimen individualized for each patient and each clinical situation ensure effective clinical management of dialysis patients.

REFERENCES

1. Jones CA, McQuillan GM, Kusek JW, et al: Serum creatinine levels in the US population: Third National Health and Nutrition Examination Survey. Am J Kidney Dis 32:992-999, 1998.
2. U.S. Food and Drug Administration, Center for Drug Evaluation and Research: New Drug Approval Reports. October 7, 2002. Available at http://www.fda.gov/cder/rdmt/default.htm
3. Marik PE: Low-dose dopamine: A systematic review. Intensive Care Med 28:877-883, 2002.

4. Juste RN, Moran L, Hooper J, Soni N: Dopamine clearance in critically ill patients. Intensive Care Med 24:1217-1220, 1998.

5. Baily DG, Arnold JM, Munoz C, Spence JD: Grapefruit juice–felodipine interaction: Mechanism, predictability, and effect of naringin. Clin Pharmacol Ther 53:637-644, 1993.

6. Min DI, Ku YM, Perry PJ, et al: Effect of grapefruit juice on cyclosporine pharmacokinetics in renal transplant patients. Transplantation 62:123-125, 1996.

7. Anderson RJ, Gambertoglio JG, Schrier RW: Clinical Use of Drugs in Renal Failure. Springfield, IL, Charles C Thomas, 1976.

8. Hurwitz A: Antacid therapy and drug kinetics. Clin Pharmacokinet 2:269-280, 1977.

9. Maton PN, Burton ME: Antacids revisited: A review of their clinical pharmacology and recommended therapeutic use. Drugs 57:855-870, 1999.

10. Craig RM, Murphy P, Gibson TP, Quintanilla A: Kinetic analysis of D-xylose absorption in normal subjects and in patients with chronic renal failure. J Lab Clin Med 101:496-506, 1983.

11. Craig RM, Carlson S, Ehrenpreis ED: D-xylose kinetics and hydrogen breath tests in functionally anephric patients using the 15-gram dose. J Clin Gastroenterol 31:55-59, 2000.

12. Dahaba AA, Oettl K, von Klobucar F, et al: End-stage renal failure reduces central clearance and prolongs the elimination half life of remifentanil. Can J Anaesth 49:369-374, 2002.

13. Reidenberg MN: The binding of drugs to plasma proteins and the interpretation of measurements of plasma concentration of drugs in patients with poor renal function. Am J Med 62:482-485, 1977.

14. Piafsky KM, Borga O: Plasma protein binding of basic drugs. II. Importance of alpha 1-acid glycoprotein for interindividual variation. Clin Pharmacol Ther 22(Pt 1):545-549, 1977.

15. Dromgoole SH: The binding capacity of albumin and renal disease. J Pharmacol Exp Ther 191:318-323, 1974.

16. Niwa T: Organic acids and the uremic syndrome: Protein metabolite hypothesis in the progression of chronic renal failure. Semin Nephrol 16:167-182, 1996.

17. Mc Namara PJ, Lalka D, Gibaldi M: Endogenous accumulation products and serum protein binding in uremia. J Lab Clin Med 98:730-740, 1981.

18. Boobis SW: Alteration of plasma albumin in relation to decreased drug binding in uremia. Clin Pharmacol Ther 22:147-153, 1977.

19. Reidenberg MM, Affrime M: Influence of disease on binding of drugs to plasma proteins. Ann N Y Acad Sci 226:115-126, 1973.

20. Reidenberg MM, Odar-Cederlof I, Von Bahr C, et al: Protein binding of diphenylhydantoin and desmethylimipramine in plasma from patients with poor renal function. N Engl J Med 285:264-267, 1971.

21. Kovacs SJ, Tenero DM, Martin DE, et al: Pharmacokinetics and protein binding of eprosartan in hemodialysis-dependent patients with end-stage renal disease. Pharmacotherapy 19:612-619, 1999.

22. Leblond F, Guevin C, Demers C, et al: Downregulation of hepatic cytochrome P450 in chronic renal failure. J Am Soc Nephrol 12:326-332, 2001.

23. Sallustio BC, Purdie YJ, Birkett DJ, Meffin PJ: Effect of renal dysfunction on the individual components of the acyl-glucuronide futile cycle. J Pharmacol Exp Ther 251:288-294, 1989.

24. Yuan R, Venitz J: Effect of chronic renal failure on the disposition of highly hepatically metabolized drugs. Int J Clin Pharmacol Ther 38:245-253, 2000.

25. Gibson TP, Giacomini KM, Briggs WA, et al: Propoxyphene and norpropoxyphene plasma concentrations in the anephric patient. Clin Pharmacol Ther 27:665-670, 1980.

26. Osborne R, Joel S, Grebenik K, et al: The pharmacokinetics of morphine and morphine glucuronides in kidney failure. Clin Pharmacol Ther 54:158-167, 1993.

27. Szeto HH, Inturrisi CE, Houde R, et al: Accumulation of normeperidine, an active metabolite of meperidine, in patients with renal failure of cancer. Ann Intern Med 86:738-741, 1977.

28. Macias WL, Mueller BA, Scarim SK: Vancomycin pharmacokinetics in acute renal failure: Preservation of nonrenal clearance. Clin Pharmacol Ther 50:688-694, 1991.

29. Cockcroft DW, Gault MH: Prediction of creatinine clearance from serum creatinine. Nephron 16:31-41, 1976.

30. Swan SK, Halstenson CE, Kasiske BL, Collins AJ: Determination of residual renal function with iohexol clearance in hemodialysis patients. Kidney Int 49:232-235, 1996.

31. Lang SM, Bergner A, Topfer M, Schiffl H: Preservation of residual renal function in dialysis patients: Effects of dialysis-technique-related factors. Perit Dial Int 21:52-57, 2001.

32. Anders MW: Metabolism of drugs by the kidney. Kidney International 18:636-647, 1980.

33. Brier ME, Aronoff GR, Mayer PR: Effect of acute renal failure on insulin disposition in the isolated perfused rat kidney. Am J Physiol 253(Pt 2):F884-F888, 1987.

34. Rabkin R, Ryan MP, Duckworth WC: The renal metabolism of insulin. Diabetologia 27:351-357, 1984.

35. Manley HJ, Bailie GR, Grabe DW: Comparing medication use in two hemodialysis units against national dialysis databases. Am J Health Syst Pharm 57:902-906, 2000.

36. Jick H: Adverse drug effects in relation to renal function. Am J Med 62:514-517, 1977.

37. Pearson TF, Pittman DG, Longley JM, et al: Factors associated with preventable adverse drug reactions. Am J Hosp Pharm 51:2268-2272, 1994.

38. Aronoff GR, Abel SR: Principles of administering drugs to patients with renal failure. *In* Bennett WM, McCarron DA, Brenner BM, Stein JH (eds): Contemporary Issues in Nephrology. Pharmacotherapy of Renal Diseases and Hypertension. New York, Churchill-Livingstone 1987, p 1.

39. Maher JF: Pharmacokinetics in patients with renal failure. Clin Nephrol 21:39-46, 1984.

40. Oosterhuis WP, de Metz M, Wadham A, et al: In vivo evaluation of four hemodialysis membranes: Biocompatibility and clearances. Dial Transplant 24:450-454, 1995.

41. Scott MK, Mueller BA, Clark WR: Vancomycin mass transfer characteristics of high-flux cellulosic dialysers. Nephrol Dial Transplant 12:2647-2653, 1997.

42. Schaedeli F, Uehlinger DE: Urea kinetics and dialysis treatment time predict vancomycin elimination during high-flux hemodialysis. Clin Pharmacol Ther 63:26-38, 1998.

43. Scott MK, Macias WL, Kraus MA, et al: Effects of dialysis membrane on intradialytic vancomycin administration. Pharmacother 17:256-262, 1997.

44. Paton TW, Cornish WR, Manuel MA, Hardy BG: Drug therapy in patients undergoing peritoneal dialysis: Clinical pharmacokinetic considerations. Clin Pharmacokinet 10:404-426, 1985.

45. Bunke CM, Aronoff GR, Brier ME, et al: Cefazolin and cephalexin kinetics in continuous ambulatory peritoneal dialysis. Clin Pharmacol Ther 33:66-72, 1983.

46. Keller F, Bohler J, Czock D, et al: Individualized drug dosage in patients treated with continuous hemofiltration. Kidney Int Suppl 72:S29-S31, 1999.

47. Davies G, Kingswood C, Street M: Pharmacokinetics of opioids in renal dysfunction. Clin Pharmacokinet 31:410-422, 1996.

48. Hagmeyer KO, Mauro LS, Mauro VF: Meperidine-related seizures associated with patient-controlled analgesia pumps. Ann Pharmacother 27:29-32, 1993.

49. Browne TR: Pharmacokinetics of antiepileptic drugs. Neurology 51(suppl 4):S2-S7, 1998.

50. Vanholder R, Van Landschoot N, De Smet R, et al: Drug protein binding in chronic renal failure: Evaluation of nine drugs. Kidney Int 33:996-1004, 1988.

51. Levey AS, Beto JA, Coronado BE, et al: Controlling the epidemic of cardiovascular disease in chronic renal disease: What do we know? What do we need to learn? Where do we go from here? Am J Kidney Dis 32:853-906, 1998.

52. United States Renal Data System (USRDS): USRDS 1999 Annual Data Report. Comprehensive data analysis on Medicare eligible end-stage renal disease population. Bethesda, MD, National Institutes of Health, National Institute of Diabetes and Digestive and Kidney Diseases, 1999.

53. The Antihypertensive and Lipid-Lowering Treatment to Prevent Heart Attack Trial (ALLHAT) Officers and Coordinators for the ALLHAT Collaborative Research Group: Major outcomes in high-risk hypertensive patients randomized to angiotensin-converting enzyme inhibitor or calcium channel blocker vs diuretic: The Antihypertensive and Lipid-Lowering Treatment to Prevent Heart Attack Trial (ALLHAT). JAMA 288:2981-2997, 2002.

54. Sica DA, Gehr TWB: Diuretic combinations in refractory oedema states. Clin Pharmacokinet 30:229-249, 1996.

55. Lewis EJ, Hunsicker LG, Bain RP, Rohde RD: The effect of angiotensin-converting-enzyme inhibition on diabetic nephropathy. The Collaborative Study Group. N Engl J Med 329:1456-1462, 1993.

56. Brenner BM, Cooper ME, de Zeeuw D, et al: Effects of losartan on renal and cardiovascular outcomes in patients with type 2 diabetes and nephropathy. N Engl J Med 345:861-869, 2001.

57. Verresen L, Waer M, Vanrenterghem Y, Michielsen P: Angiotensin-converting-enzyme inhibitors and anaphylactoid reactions to high-flux membrane dialysis. Lancet 336:1360-1362, 1990.

58. Hatano M, Yoshida T, Mimuro T, Kimata N, et al: The effects of ACE inhibitor treatment and ACE gene polymorphism on erythropoiesis in chronic hemodialysis patients. Jpn J Nephrol 42:632-639, 2000.

59. Manian FA, Stone WJ, Alford RH: Adverse antibiotic effects associated with renal insufficiency. Rev Infect Dis 12:236-249, 1990.

60. United States Renal Data System (USRDS): USRDS 2002 Annual Data Report: Atlas of End-Stage Renal Disease in the United States. Bethesda, MD, National Institutes of Health, National Institute of Diabetes and Digestive and Kidney Diseases, 2002.

61. Herlitz H, Aurell M, Holm G, et al: Renal degradation of insulin in patients with renal hypertension. Scand J Urol Nephrol 17:109-113, 1983.

62. Brier ME, Aronoff GR, Mayer PR: Effect of acute renal failure on insulin disposition in the isolated perfused rat kidney. Am J Physiol 253(Pt 2):F884-F888, 1987.

63. Brier ME, Bays H, Sloan R, et al: Pharmacokinetics of oral glyburide in subjects with non–insulin-dependent diabetes mellitus and renal failure. Am J Kidney Dis 29:907-911, 1997.

64. Bennett WM, Henrich WL, Stoff JS: The renal effects of nonsteroidal anti-inflammatory drugs: Summary and recommendations. Am J Kidney Dis 28(suppl 1):S56-S62, 1996.

65. Harris RC, Breyer MD: Physiological regulation of cyclooxygenase-2 in the kidney. Am J Physiol Renal Physiol 281:F1-F11, 2001.

66. Brater DC: Effects of nonsteroidal anti-inflammatory drugs on renal function: Focus on cyclooxygenase-2-selective inhibition. Am J Med 107:65S-70S, 1999.

67. Henao J, Hisamuddin I, Nzerue CM, et al: Celecoxib-induced acute interstitial nephritis. Am J Kidney Dis 39:1313-1317, 2002.

68. Johnson JA, Bootman JL: Drug-related morbidity and mortality and the economic impact of pharmaceutical care. Am J Health Syst Pharm 54:554-558, 1997.

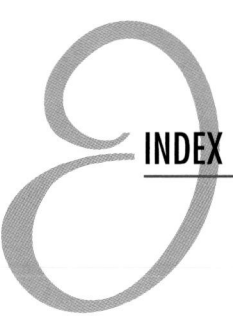

INDEX

Note: Page numbers followed by the letter f refer to figures, and those followed by t refer to tables.

A6 cell line, 144–145
ABC transporter, 233, 235–236
Abdominal adhesions, in peritoneal dialysis, 2665
Abdominal examination
  in acute renal failure, 1082–1083
  in chronic kidney disease, 1087
  in hypertension, 2051
Abdominal films (KUB), 1183
Abdominal mass, in renal cell carcinoma, 1898
Abdominal trauma, and renal artery thrombosis, 1571–1572, 1572f
ABO blood group antigens, 2768
ABO blood group matching, in renal transplantation, 2798
Abruptio placentae, 1678
Abscess, renal
  computed tomography in, 1199
  magnetic resonance imaging in, 1199f
Absorptiometry, dual x-ray, in renal osteodystrophy, 2279–2281
Acarbose, 2857t
ACE. *See* Angiotensin-converting enzyme (ACE).
ACE escape, 2385
ACE inhibitor. *See* Angiotensin-converting enzyme (ACE) inhibitors.
Acebutolol, 2395t, 2396t, 2397, 2857t
Acetaminophen
  and analgesic nephropathy, 1645
  and chronic interstitial nephritis, 1498
  and fulminant hepatic failure, 2714
  dosage modifications for, 2857t
Acetate, in dialysate
  for hemodialysis, 2588, 2609–2610
  for peritoneal dialysis, 2631–2632
Acetazolamide, 2345, 2346
  and phosphate transport, 561
  dosage modifications for, 2857t
Acetohexamide, 2857t
Acetohydroxamic acid
  dosage modifications for, 2857t
  for struvite stones, 1856
Acetyl coenzyme A transporter family (SLC33), 268t, 291
Acetylcholine, and glomerular filtration, 377–378, 390
Acetylcholine transporter family, 265t–266t, 284
N-Acetylcysteine
  dosage modifications for, 2862t
  for fulminant hepatic failure, 2715–2716

Acetylsalicyclic acid, 2857t
Acid(s)
  definition of, 922
  endogenous, sources of, 932
  impaired excretion of
    in acidosis of renal insufficiency, 960–961
    in aging, 2321, 2323f
    with hyperkalemia, 953–960. *See also* Renal tubular acidosis, distal (generalized).
    with hypokalemia, 950–953. *See also* Renal tubular acidosis, distal (classic).
  nonvolatile, systemic response to, 932–934, 932f–934f
  overproduction of, metabolic acidosis from, 1176
  renal excretion of, 933f, 934. *See also* Acidification; Hydrogen, secretion of.
  titratable, excretion of, 497
Acid disequilibrium pH, 498
Acid load
  distribution and cellular buffering of, 933–934, 933f, 934f
  hyperchloremic metabolic acidosis from, 946
Acid phosphatase, tartrate-resistant, in renal osteodystrophy, 2276
Acid-base balance, 921–924, 1171, 1173, 1173f
  and calcium transport, 544
  and distal nephron acidification, 515
  and magnesium transport, 551
  and phosphate transport, 558–559
  and potassium homeostasis, 999–1000
  and potassium transport, 479–482, 480f–482f
  and proximal tubule acidification, 504–505, 505f
  buffer systems in, 922–924
  disturbances of. *See* Acid-base disorder(s); Acidosis; Alkalosis.
  hepatic role in, 932–933, 932f
  in aging, 2321, 2323f
  renal regulation of, 497, 498f, 924–929, 932–933, 932f
Acid-base disorder(s)
  after nephron loss, 1965–1966
  and uric acid excretion, 649
  diagnosis of, 937–941
    anion gap in, 939t, 940–941, 941t
    clinical and laboratory parameters in, 939–940
    simple vs. mixed, 938–939, 939t

Acid-base disorder(s) *(Continued)*
    verification of laboratory values in, 937–938
  in salicylate intoxication, 2750
  limits of compensation in, 930t, 938–939
Acid-base nomogram, 938, 938f
Acid-base transporter(s), inherited disorders of, 1716–1719, 1717f
Acidemia
  neurorespiratory response to, 934
  potassium release in, 921
Acidic amino acid transporter(s), 419f, 420, 420t
Acidification. *See also* Hydrogen, secretion of.
  in distal nephron, 509–517, 925–929, 928f–929f
    ammonium excretion in, 927–929, 928f–929f
    cellular mechanisms in, 513–515
    hydrogen secretion in, 513–514, 925–927, 1175, 1175f
    regulation of, 515–517, 927, 927t
      acid-base balance in, 515
      endothelin-1 in, 516
      hormones in, 516–517
      luminal pH in, 515–516
      mineralocorticoids in, 516
      potassium depletion in, 516
      sodium delivery in, 516
      transepithelial voltage in, 516
  in loop of Henle and thick ascending limb, 507–508, 508f
  in proximal tubule, 500–509, 500f, 925, 926f
    bicarbonate transport in, 500f–503f, 501–504
    hydrogen transport in, 501–504, 501f–503f, 925, 926f, 1175
    regulation of, 504–507, 925, 927t
      acid-base balance in, 504–505, 505f
      hormones in, 506–507, 506f
      luminal bicarbonate concentration in, 505–506
      luminal flow rate in, 506
      peritubular pH in, 504–505, 505f
      potassium depletion in, 505
      signal transduction pathways in, 506, 506f, 507
      volume expansion in, 506
  renal mechanisms of, 497–519, 1716–1718, 1717f
  urinary
    and potassium transport, 479–482, 480f–482f

Adenoma
  parathyroid, hypercalcemia in, 1042–1043
  pituitary, and diabetes insipidus, 872
  villous, metabolic alkalosis in, 971
Adenosine
  and glomerular filtration, 384–385
  and mesangial cell contractility, 120
  and tubuloglomerular feedback, 18, 389
  dosage modifications for, 2857t
  in inner medullary collecting duct cell
      cultures, 158
  in renin secretion, 667
Adenosine diphosphate (ADP), and glomerular
    filtration, 385–386
Adenosine triphosphatase(s) (ATPases),
    232–236, 233t, 234f
  calcium, 235
    in basolateral calcium transport, 541f,
        542–543
    in connecting segment, 42
  calcium-magnesium, in distal convoluted
      tubule, 40–41
  chloride, 235
  hydrogen-potassium. See Hydrogen-
      potassium-ATPase.
  P-type, 232, 233–235
  sodium-potassium. See Sodium-
      potassium-ATPase.
  vacuolar hydrogen, 233, 235
    and coupling with glycolysis, 247
    in distal nephron acidification, 513
    in proximal tubule acidification, 502
Adenosine triphosphate (ATP)
  and active ion transport, 231–232, 232f
  and autoregulation of renal circulation, 342
  and glomerular filtration, 386
  depletion of
    in urinary tract obstruction, 1885
    necrosis and, 1227, 1229
  extracellular, and mesangial cell
      proliferation, 129
  in coupling between active sodium-
      potassium-ATPase and passive leak
      permeability, 461
  ion channels sensitive to, and coupling to
      cation transport, 246–247
  P2 purinergic receptors activated by, 247
  production of
    active solute transport and, coupling of,
        242–247, 243f–246f
    during hypoxia or ischemic conditions,
        252–253
    mitochondrial, 236–240, 237f, 239f, 240f
    sodium-potassium-ATPase dependence on,
        245, 245f
Adenosine triphosphate (ATP)–driven solute
    transport, 232–236, 233t, 234f
Adenosine triphosphate (ATP)–sensitive calcium
    channel, and coupling to cation transport,
    246–247
Adenosine triphosphate (ATP)–sensitive
    potassium channel (K-ATP), 246–247
Adenosine type 1 receptor antagonists, as
    diuretics, 2352
Adenovirus, in urinary tract infection, 1516
Adenylate cyclase system, activation of, in thick
    ascending limb, 38
ADH. See Vasopressin.
Adhesin(s), on *Escherichia coli*, and virulence,
    1525–1526
Adhesion molecule(s)
  in glomerular visceral epithelial cell cultures,
      133–134
  in immune response to allograft,
      2770–2771

Adhesion molecule(s) *(Continued)*
  matrix
    functions of, 201–203
    overview of, 199–200
Adiponectin, cardiovascular protective role of,
    2203
Adjuvant therapy, for renal cell carcinoma, 1912
ADP. *See* Adenosine diphosphate (ADP).
Adrenal enzymatic disorders, metabolic
    alkalosis in, 975
Adrenal hormones, in hypertrophic response to
    nephron loss, 1961
Adrenal hyperplasia, congenital
  11β-hydroxylase deficiency in, 1722
  17α-hydroxylase deficiency in, 1721–1722
  lipoid, hyperkalemia in, 1017–1018
Adrenal hypoplasia congenita, hyperkalemia in,
    1017
Adrenal insufficiency
  hyperkalemia in, 1017–1018
  hyponatremia in, 891
  in sepsis, 2708–2709
Adrenalectomy, for renal cell carcinoma, 1903
Adrenergic agonists, central
  antihypertensive efficacy and safety of, 2412
  dosage modifications for, 2388t
  for hypertensive emergencies, 2428t, 2429
  mechanisms of action of, 2410, 2410t
  pharmacodynamics of, 2411t
  pharmacokinetics of, 2410t
  receptor binding of, 2410t
  renal effects of, 2411–2412
  types of, 2410–2411
β-Adrenergic agonists
  for hyperkalemia, 1023–1024
  hypokalemia from, 1008
Adrenergic antagonists, central and peripheral,
    2412–2413
α₁-Adrenergic antagonists
  for hypertensive emergencies, 2429, 2430t
  moderately selective peripheral, 2414
  peripheral, 2414–2416, 2415t
  β- and, for hypertensive emergencies,
      2428–2429, 2428t
β-Adrenergic antagonists, 2394–2401
  α₁- and, for hypertensive emergencies,
      2428–2429, 2428t
  and diuretics, 2421t
  and impaired renin-aldosterone elaboration, 958
  antiproteinuric effects of, 2471
  classification of, 2395t
  dosage modifications for, 2388t
  efficacy and safety of, 2399–2401
  for hypertension, 2399
  hyperkalemia from, 1018
  in chronic kidney disease patient
    for heart failure, 2211
    for ischemic heart disease, 2211
  in hypertensive pregnant patient, 1675
  mechanisms of action of, 2394–2395
  nonselective, 2395–2396
    with α-adrenergic antagonism, 2397–2398
    with partial agonist activity, 2396–2397
  pharmacodynamics of, 2396t, 2398t
  pharmacokinetics of, 2396t, 2398t
  renal effects of, 2399
  renoprotective effects of, 2468
  β₁-selective, 2397
    for hypertensive emergencies, 2428, 2428t
    with partial adrenergic activity, 2397
  types of, 2395–2398
Adrenergic nervous system, in inner medullary
    collecting duct cell cultures, 158
α-Adrenergic responsiveness, in hypertension
    with renal disease, 2122

Adrenocortical hypertension, 2045–2046
Adrenocorticotropic hormone (ACTH),
    hypokalemia from, 1010–1011
Adrenomedullin
  and extracellular fluid volume control, 803
  and glomerular filtration, 386
  and mesangial cell proliferation, 127
  in edema formation, in congestive heart
      failure, 819–820
  in hypertension, 2119
Adsorbents, for poisoning, 2735
Adult respiratory distress syndrome. *See* Acute
    respiratory distress syndrome (ARDS).
Advanced glycation end products (AGEs)
  and chronic dialysis-dependent encephalopathy,
      2234
  as uremic toxins, 2146, 2236
  in aging kidney, 2311–2312, 2312f
  mesangial cell receptors for, 131
Adynamic bone disease
  histologic features of, 2282
  pathogenesis of, 2262–2263, 2263f
AE1 gene, in classical distal renal tubular
    acidosis, 951
Aerobactin, and *Escherichia coli* virulence, 1526
Afferent arteriole(s)
  anatomy of, 309–310, 310f, 311, 311f
  constriction of
    adenosine and, 385
    angiotensin II and, 364–365
    endothelin and, 368
    norepinephrine and, 367
    vasopressin and, 371
  dilation of
    atrial natriuretic peptide and, 383
    bradykinin and, 377
    nitric oxide and, 375
  vascular reactivity of, 338–339, 338f
Afferent limb of volume homeostasis, 777–783,
    778t
  in cirrhosis with ascites, 820–824
  in congestive heart failure, 805–807
AGEs (advanced glycation end products). *See*
    Advanced glycation end products (AGEs).
Aging. *See also* Elderly persons.
  and arterial stiffness, 2114
  and glomerular filtration, 391–392, 391f,
      2313–2316, 2314f, 2315f
  and graft survival, 2829, 2830
  and hypertension
    systolic, 2110–2111
    with renal deterioration, 2109–2110, 2110f
  and mineral and electrolyte balance,
      2321–2326
  and phosphate transport, 561
  and renal anatomy, 2305–2307, 2306f–2307f
  and renal failure, 2111
  and renal function, 2316–2321, 2316f–2323f,
      2493
  and renal plasma flow, 2313–2316, 2314f
  and renal transplantation, 2786
  and urinary tract infection, 1534–1535,
      1535f
  applications of tubule cell cultures to, 159
Agmatine, synthesis of, 253, 253f
AIDS. *See* Human immunodeficiency virus
    (HIV)–associated nephropathy (HIVAN);
    Human immunodeficiency virus (HIV)
    infection.
Air embolism, in hemodialysis, 2576
Airway pressure release ventilation (APRV), for
    acute respiratory failure, 2698
Alacepril, 2382, 2383t, 2384t
Alanine-glyoxylate aminotransferase deficiency,
    hyperoxaluria from, 1850, 1850f

β-Catenin, in nephrogenesis, 80t
Catheter(s)
  and bacteremia, in hemodialysis, 2570
  and peritonitis, 2668, 2673–2674, 2673t
  and urinary tract infection, treatment of, 1552–1553, 1553t
  for peritoneal dialysis, 2626–2629, 2627f. *See also* Peritoneal dialysis, catheters for.
  for vascular access
    care of, 2719, 2719t
    in renal replacement therapy, 2569–2570, 2718–2719
  subclavian, problems with, 2719
Cation(s), organic. *See* Organic cation(s).
Cation channel(s), amiloride-sensitive
  nonselective, in inner medullary collecting duct cell cultures, 157
Cation exchange resins, for hyperkalemia, 1024–1025
Cation-chloride cotransporter family (SLC12), 265t, 279–280
Cation-chloride cotransporter interacting protein (CIP), 265t, 280, 434
Cationic amino acid transporter(s) (CATs), 264t, 274–275
CCI-779, for renal cell carcinoma, 1912–1913
CD2-associated protein (CD2AP), in filtration slit diaphragm, 9, 206
CD4 cell(s), in immune response to allograft, 2770
CD8 cell(s), in immune response to allograft, 2770, 2773–2774, 2773f
CD11, in acute tubular necrosis, 1243
CD11a, monoclonal antibodies against, in acute renal failure, 218, 218t
CD11a/CD18
  characteristics of, 210t, 211f, 212
  expression of, in kidney, 215
  in tumor cell biology, 219
CD11b, monoclonal antibodies against, in acute renal failure, 218, 218t
CD11b/CD18
  characteristics of, 210t, 211f, 212
  expression of, in kidney, 215
  knockout mice for, 213
  monoclonal antibodies against, in renal inflammation, 216, 216t, 217
CD11c/CD18, characteristics of, 210t, 211f, 212
CD18
  in acute tubular necrosis, 1243
  monoclonal antibodies against, in acute renal failure, 217–218, 218t
CD28-B7, in immune response to allograft, 2771–2772, 2771f
CD34
  characteristics of, 210, 210t, 211f, 212
  expression of, in kidney, 215
CD40, in immune response to allograft, 2772
Cefaclor, 2858t
Cefadroxil, 2858t
Cefalothin, for peritonitis, 2671, 2671t
Cefamandole, 2858t
Cefazolin
  dosage modifications for, 2858t
  for peritonitis, 2671, 2671t
Cefepime, 2858t
Cefixime, 2858t
Cefmenoxime, 2858t
Cefmetazole, 2858t
Cefonicid, 2858t
Cefoperazone, 2858t
Ceforanide, 2858t
Cefotaxime, 2858t
Cefotetan, 2858t
Cefoxitin, 2858t

Cefpodoxime, 2858t
Cefprozil, 2858t
Ceftazidime
  dosage modifications for, 2858t
  for peritonitis, 2671, 2671t
Ceftibuten, 2858t
Ceftizoxime, 2858t
Ceftriaxone, 2858t
Cefuroxime, 2858t
Celecoxib, nephrotoxicity of, 1642
Celiprolol, 2395t, 2398, 2398t, 2858t
Cell cycle regulators
  and mesangial cell proliferation, 124, 125f
  in acute tubular necrosis, 1247
Cell injury, apoptosis from, 1236–1237
Cell polarity, loss of, in acute tubular necrosis, 1239
Cell-cell contact, loss of, apoptosis due to, 1236
Cell-cell interactions. *See also* Renal cell–leukocyte interactions.
  in tubule cell cultures, 108
Cell–crystal interactions, in calcium nephrolithiasis, 1824
Cell-matrix adhesion, loss of
  apoptosis due to, 1236
  sublethal injury due to, 1240
Cell-matrix interactions, 199–206, 204f–206f
  in renal injury, 206–208, 207f
Cell-mediated immunity
  in pyelonephritis, 1528
  in tubulointerstitial disease, 1487–1488
Cellulose dialysis membrane, 2573
Cellulose phosphate, for idiopathic hypercalciuria, 1840
Central core model, of axial osmolality gradient, 615–616, 615f
Central diabetes insipidus. *See* Diabetes insipidus, central.
Central nervous system
  disorders of
    and syndrome of inappropriate antidiuretic hormone, 898, 898t
    in hypermagnesemia, 1058
    in metabolic acidosis, 969
    in pre-eclampsia, 1670–1671
    uremic neurotoxins in, 2235–2236
Central nervous system control centers, in hypertension, 2116
Central nervous system sensors, and extracellular fluid volume control, 781
Central pontine myelinolysis, in hyponatremia, 901
Central venous thrombosis, postpartum, 1671
Cephadine, 2858t
Cephalexin, 2858t
Cephalosporins
  and organic anion transport, 653
  for urinary tract infection, in pregnant patient, 1551
  nephrotoxicity of, 1628
Cephalothin, 2858t
Cephapirin, 2858t
Cerebral aneurysm, in autosomal dominant polycystic kidney disease, 1754
Cerebral edema
  and hyponatremia, 900, 900f, 901
  in fulminant hepatic failure, 2714, 2716
Cerebral hemorrhage, in pre-eclampsia, 1670
Cerebral ischemia, molecular events initiated by, 2229f, 2243
Cerebral salt wasting, hyponatremia in, 891
Ceterizine, 2858t
Channel-activating protease 1 (CAP1), aldosterone induction of, and ENaC regulation, 1003, 1003f

Charcoal, activated, for poisoning, 2734t, 2735
Charcoal hemoperfusion, 2739
Chemokine(s)
  in atherosclerosis, 219
  in immune response to allograft, 2772–2773
  in leukocyte adhesion regulation, 213–214
  in mesangial cell cultures, 112t, 113
  in tubulointerstitial disease, 1488
Chemotherapy
  for renal cell carcinoma, 1907–1908, 1907t
  for Wilms tumor, 1915
  hyponatremia from, 896
  nephrotoxicity of, 1631–1635, 1633t
  peritoneal dialysis for, 2658
CHF (congestive heart failure). *See* Heart failure.
Children. *See also* Neonate(s).
  chronic renal failure in, protein restriction for, 2502
  glomerular filtration rate in, 2493, 2495
  peritoneal dialysis in, 2655–2656
  urinary tract infection in, 1551–1552
Chinese herb nephropathy, 1639
Chlamydia trachomatis, in urinary tract infection, 1516, 1548
Chloral hydrate, 2858t
Chlorambucil
  dosage modifications for, 2858t
  for membranous glomerulopathy, 1320–1321
  for minimal change glomerulopathy, 1306
Chloramines, in dialysis water, 2580
Chloramphenicol, 2858t
Chlorazepate, 2858t
Chlordiazepoxide, 2859t
Chloride
  conductance of
    basolateral
      in proximal tubule, 425–426
      in thick ascending limb, 435
    in collecting duct, 439–440
  deficiency of, in metabolic alkalosis, 936, 970–974
  exit of, in proximal tubule, and sodium chloride reabsorption, 424f, 425, 425f, 614
  fractional excretion of, 1162
  in dialysate, for hemodialysis, 2588–2589
  permeability of
    in medullary epithelia, 610–611
    in papillary surface epithelium, 609t, 611
  serum, in acid-base disorders, 940
  transport of
    in cortical collecting duct, 439–440
    in thin ascending limb, 431–432, 431f, 431t
    sodium-dependent. *See* Sodium-chloride co-transporter (NCCT).
Chloride channel(s)
  basolateral extrusion of, in distal nephron acidification, 515
  CIC-5, in Dent disease, 1699–1701, 1700f
  CLC-K1/KA, in thin ascending limb, 432
  CLC-K2/KB
    in thick ascending limb, 435
    mutations in, in Bartter syndrome, type III, 614
  in cortical collecting duct cell cultures, 155
Chloride-ATPase, 235
Chloride/base exchange
  apical, and sodium chloride reabsorption in proximal tubule, 423–425, 424f
  in proximal tubule acidification, 502
Chloride/bicarbonate exchanger
  apical
    in cortical collecting duct cell cultures, 155–156
    in distal nephron acidification, 514–515

Nephrotoxin(s) *(Continued)*
  chronic kidney disease from, 1086
  heavy metals as, 1636–1639
  hydrocarbons as, 1647
  hypomagnesemia from, 1053–1054
  intravenous immune globulin as, 1636
  nonsteroidal antiinflammatory drugs as, 733–735, 734f
  radiocontrast agents as, 1629–1630, 1630t
Nerve, renal. *See* Renal nerves.
Nerve growth factor, in mesangial cell cultures, 111
Nesiritide, for congestive heart failure, 817–818
Net acid excretion (NAE), calculation of, 497
Netlimicin, 2863t
Neural pathways, in atrial sensors, and extracellular fluid volume control, 778–779
Neurofibrillary tangles, in dialysis dementia, 2241
Neurohumoral factors, in hypertension with renal disease, 2116–2119
Neurohypophysis
  lesions of, in central diabetes insipidus, 871–872, 872f
  regulatory control of, 864, 864f
  vasopressin synthesis in, 860, 861f, 862
Neurokinin B, in pregnant patient, 1662
Neurologic abnormalities. *See also* Encephalopathy.
  from dialysis technical errors, 2242
  in acute renal failure, 2228
  in chronic renal failure, 2231–2233
  in end-stage renal disease, 2237–2244
  in hyponatremia, 900, 900f, 901–902, 902f
Neurologic examination, in hypertension, 2051
Neuromuscular abnormalities, in hypomagnesemia, 1055t, 1056
Neuropathy
  peripheral
    in diabetic nephropathy, 1792
    in uremia, 2245
  uremic, 2245–2246
Neuropeptide Y
  and glomerular filtration, 390
  in hypertension, in end-stage renal disease, 2119
  in uremia, 2153, 2153f
Neurophysin, types of, 862
Neuropsychiatric abnormalities, in acute renal failure, 1083
Neurotoxin(s), uremic. *See* Uremic toxin(s).
Neurotransmitter transporter(s), 263t–264t, 274
Neutral amino acid transporter(s), 419–420, 419f
Neutral endopeptidase (NEP, enkephalinase)
  and angiotensin-converting enzyme, dual inhibition of. *See* Vasopeptidase inhibitors.
  in angiotensin removal, 671
  in bradykinin breakdown, 688
  in natriuretic peptide degradation, 702
  inhibition of, 703–704
Neutrophil(s), in acute respiratory distress syndrome, 2699
Nevirapine, 2863t
NHE regulatory factor(s) (NHERFs), 264t, 276–277, 278f, 507
Niacin
  dosage modifications for, 2863t
  in uremia, 2519
Nicardipine, 2402t, 2403t, 2405
  dosage modifications for, 2863t
  for hypertensive emergencies, 2428t, 2429
Nicotinamide, for Hartnup disease, 1711
Nicotinate, excretion of, 639f

Nicotinic acid
  dosage modifications for, 2863t
  in uremia, 2519
Nifedipine, 2402t, 2403t, 2404–2405
  dosage modifications for, 2863t
  in hypertensive pregnant patient, 1675
  renoprotective effects of, 2467–2468
Nimodipine, 2863t
Nisoldipine, 2402t, 2403t, 2405–2406
  dosage modifications for, 2863t
  renoprotective effects of, 2468
Nitrate, in dialysis water, 2580
Nitrazepam, 2863t
Nitrendipine, renoprotective effects of, 2468
Nitric oxide
  and angiotensin II, 676
  and blood pressure, 2037
  and cytochrome p450 arachidonic acid metabolites, interaction between, 753
  and diuretic response, 2356
  and extracellular fluid volume control, 800–801
  and glomerular filtration, 373–376, 375f
  and mesangial cell apoptosis, 123
  and mesangial cell contractility, 121
  and mesangial cell proliferation, 129
  and mitochondrial respiration, 253–254
  and peripheral arterial vasodilation in cirrhosis, 823–824
  and pre-eclampsia, 1666
  and pressure natriuresis, 790–791, 2126
  and reactive oxygen species, interactions between, 2121
  and renal hemodynamics, 338–339
  and solute transport, 253
  and tubuloglomerular feedback, 18–19, 389–390
  and uremic bleeding, 2173–2174, 2174f
  as therapeutic target in renal inflammation, 217
  endothelial-derived, in acute tubular necrosis, 1241, 1242f
  for acute respiratory distress syndrome, 2700
  generation of, in L-arginine metabolism, 253, 253f
  in adaptation to nephron loss, 1958
  in aging kidney, 2311, 2311f, 2328, 2328f
  in anti–glomerular basement membrane disease, 1350
  in autoregulation of renal circulation, 343
  in edema formation, in congestive heart failure, 818–819
  in essential hypertension, 2039
  in hypertension, 2006, 2007–2008, 2007f
  in hypertension with renal disease, 2120–2121
  in ischemic nephropathy, 2072
  in mesangial cell cultures, 112t, 115
  in postobstructive vasoconstriction, 1880
  in pressure-natriuresis mechanism, 790–791
  in uremia, 2146
  inactivation of, 374
  isoforms of, 2120
  production of, acetylcholine and, 378
  release of, factors influencing, 373–374
  synthesis of
    factors influencing, 2007
    hemodialysis and, 2176, 2177f
    in glomerular endothelial cells, 7
Nitric oxide synthase
  in macula densa, 18
  inducible, in acute tubular necrosis, 1243
  subtypes of, 374
Nitrites, in urine, 1121–1122
Nitrofurantoin
  dosage modifications for, 2863t

Nitrofurantoin *(Continued)*
  for urinary tract infection
    in children, 1552
    in pregnant patient, 1551
  prophylactic, for recurrent urinary tract infections, in young women, 1548
Nitrogen
  excretion of, 2509–2510
  fecal, 2508–2509
  metabolism of, and metabolic acidosis, 2140–2141
  non-urea, excretion of, 2509, 2509f
  requirements for
    decreased, factors causing, 2518–2520
    in uremia, 2514–2516, 2515f–2516f
    increased, factors causing, 2516–2518
  skin losses of, 2509
  unmeasured, 2508
  urea. *See also* Blood urea nitrogen (BUN).
    appearance rate for, 2510–2511, 2511f
    reuse of, and decreased nitrogen requirements, 2518
Nitrogen conservation, in uremia, 2514–2516, 2515f–2516f
Nitrogen homeostasis, assessment of, 2509–2510
Nitroglycerine
  dosage modifications for, 2863t
  for hypertensive emergencies, 2427–2428, 2428t
Nitroprusside
  dosage modifications for, 2863t
  for hypertensive emergencies, 2427, 2428t
Nitrosoureas, 2863t
Nizatidine, 2863t
NKCC. *See* Sodium-potassium-chloride cotransporter(s) (NKCCs).
NO. *See* Nitric oxide.
Nocardiosis, glomerular involvement with, 1438
Nocturnal hemodialysis, 2594, 2596–2597
Nodular diabetic glomerulosclerosis, 1778, 1780f
Noggin, in nephrogenesis, 80t
Non–anion gap acidosis. *See* Metabolic acidosis, hyperchloremic.
Nonbiphenyl tetrazole derivatives, 2392
Nonheterocyclic derivatives, 2392
Nonmyeloablative allogeneic transplantation, for renal cell carcinoma, 1913
Nonprogressors, exclusion of, in determination of treatment effect, 2498
Nonsteroidal antiinflammatory drugs
  acute renal failure from, 734–735, 1640–1642, 1641t, 1642t
    after renal transplantation, 2822t, 2824
  and impaired renin-aldosterone elaboration, 958
  and sodium retention, 733–734, 734f, 1642–1643
  and water retention, 734, 734f, 1643
  antiproteinuric effects of, 2471
  chronic renal failure from, 1644–1645
  dosage considerations for, 2867–2868
  hyperkalemia from, 734, 1020–1021, 1643
  hypertension from, 734
  in hypertension with renal disease, 2126
  interstitial nephritis from, 735, 1492–1493
  nephropathy from, 733–735, 734f, 1446
  nephrotic syndrome from, 735
  nephrotoxicity of, 733–735, 734f, 1640–1645, 1640t–1643t
  papillary necrosis from, 734
  prerenal azotemia from, 1217
  renal dysgenesis from, 735
  tubulointerstitial disease from, 1643–1644, 1643t

Pressure-natriuresis relationships, 789–791, 790f, 2035, 2035f
and prostaglandin E receptors, 744
in essential hypertension, 2039
in hypertension with renal disease, 2125–2126
Pressure-volume homeostasis, in hypertension, 2115–2116
Primaquine, 2864t
Primidone, 2864t
Primitive duct, in renal dysplasia, 1767, 1767f
Principal cell(s)
in cortical collecting duct, 42–43, 43f, 44f
in inner medullary collecting duct, 50, 51f
in outer medullary collecting duct, 48
of collecting duct, 436f, 437–438, 438t
Probenecid
and uric acid nephrolithiasis, 1853
dosage modifications for, 2864t
Probucol, 2864t
Procainamide
dosage modifications for, 2864t
overdose of, 2753–2754
secretion of, 639f, 650
in pars recta, 30
systemic lupus erythematosus from, 1389
Procoagulant state, in sepsis-induced acute tubular necrosis, 1244–1245
Procollagen propeptides, in renal osteodystrophy, 2276
Progestational agents, for renal cell carcinoma, 1907, 1907t
Prolactin, secretion of, in pregnant patient, 1661
Proliferative glomerulonephritis
diffuse, acute, 1328
glomerular permselectivity in, 1933
in neoplasia, 1445–1446
in systemic lupus erythematosus, 1385, 1385f–1386f, 1388
mesangial
in HIV-infected patient, 1442
in temporal arteritis, 1410
Proline, transport of, 420
Prolylcarboxypeptidase, 686
Promethazine, 2864t
Prone positioning, for acute respiratory distress syndrome, 2700
Pronephros, 73, 74f
Propafenone, 2864t
Propofol, 2864t
Propoxyphene
dosage modifications for, 2864t
metabolism of, 2852
Propranolol, 2395, 2395t, 2396t
dosage modifications for, 2864t
for thyrotoxic periodic paralysis, 1009
Propylthiouracil, 2864t
Prorenin, 665, 668
and pre-eclampsia, 1666
in pregnant patient, 1661–1662
receptor for, in mesangial cell cultures, 110
uterine, 1662
Prostacyclin
as therapeutic target in renal inflammation, 217
during dialysis, and uremic bleeding, 2177
in hemolytic-uremic syndrome, 1605–1606
in pregnancy-induced hypertension, 749
in pregnant patient, 1660
receptors for, 740–741
synthesis of, 737
Prostacyclin synthase, 737
Prostaglandin(s)
and angiotensin II, 364f, 365, 366–367
and diuretic response, 2354–2355, 2355f
and extracellular fluid volume control, 793–796, 794t

Prostaglandin(s) (Continued)
and glomerular filtration, 376–377, 376f
and mesangial cell proliferation, 127–128
and sodium excretion, 795, 1642–1643
cyclopentenone, 746
in acute renal failure, 748
in adaptation to nephron loss, 1957–1958
in ascites formation, in cirrhosis, 827–828
in calcineurin nephrotoxicity, 748
in congestive heart failure, 819
in cortical collecting duct cell cultures, 156
in glomerular endothelial cell cultures, 142
in glomerular visceral epithelial cell cultures, 139
in hypertension with renal disease, 2123–2124
in inner medullary collecting duct cell cultures, 158
in ischemic nephropathy, 2074
in pressure-natriuresis mechanism, 790
in proximal tubule cell cultures, 153
in renal salt and water transport, 744–745
in renin secretion, 18–19, 667
in renomedullary interstitial cell cultures, 166–167
in urinary tract obstruction, 748
metabolism of, 745–746
production of
endothelin and, 368–369
vasopressin and, 370
renal, compartmentalization and functions of, 1640–1641, 1640t
renal excretion of, 644, 746
synthesis of, 735–738, 736f, 737–738
in mesangial cell cultures, 113–114
in mesangial cells, 13
in pregnant patient, 1662
in visceral epithelial cells, 9
inhibition of, consequences of, 1641
transport of, 746
Prostaglandin 9-ketoreductase, 737
Prostaglandin D synthase, 737
Prostaglandin D$_2$ receptor, 741
Prostaglandin E
receptors for
regulation of renal function by, 744
types of, 742–744
synthesis of, 737–738
Prostaglandin E$_2$
and mesangial cell contractility, 121
in diabetes mellitus, 749
in glomerular inflammatory injury, 746–747
in hepatorenal syndrome, 749
in regulation of salt and water excretion, 734f
in urinary tract obstruction, 1880, 1883
Prostaglandin F synthase, 737
Prostaglandin F2α receptor, 741–742
Prostaglandin synthase inhibitors, for diabetes insipidus, 885–886
Prostaglandin transporter (PGT), 266t, 285, 746
Prostanoid(s)
receptors for, 738–744, 738f–740f, 740t
synthesis of, 735–738, 736f
Prostanoid receptor knockout mice, phenotypes of, 740t
Prostasin, aldosterone induction of, and ENaC regulation, 1003, 1003f
Prostate cancer, and urinary tract obstruction, 1871
Prostatis
recurrent, 1540
treatment of, 1551
Protease activation, necrosis and, 1229
Protein(s)
absorption of, in proximal tubule, 27
clearance of, in glomerular disease, 1932–1933

Protein(s) (Continued)
degradation of. See Protein catabolism.
dietary. See Protein intake.
external losses of, and increased nitrogen requirements, 2517
function of, impact of DNA variation on, 1698t
intolerance of, lysinuric, 1710–1711
urinary, 1123–1128
in diagnosis and prognosis, 1127–1128
in screening for renal disease, 1126–1127
normal physiology of, 1123
tests for, 1123–1126, 1123f, 1125f
Protein binding
and extracorporeal drug removal, 2737
defects of, in uremia, 2851, 2851f, 2851t
Protein C
for sepsis, 1244, 2710
in nephrotic syndrome, 1946
in renal vein thrombosis, 1587
in sepsis, 2707, 2708f
Protein catabolism
and metabolic acidosis, 2140–2143, 2142f, 2142t
and urea generation, in dialysis patient, 2506, 2591f, 2592
osmotic diuresis from, 1154t, 1157, 1157f
toxic products of, 2143–2146, 2143f, 2143t, 2145f
Protein intake
acute effects of
on proteinuria, 2501
on renal hemodynamics, 2500–2501
and dialysis dose, 2592, 2592f
and glomerular filtration rate, 2493
and insulin resistance, 2499
and leucine turnover, 2514, 2515f
and nitrogen excretion, 2509, 2509f
and progression of chronic renal failure
mediators of effects of, 2502–2503
studies on, 2497f, 2501–2502
and renoprotective therapy, 2477
excessive, and progressive renal injury, 1976–1977
in hemodialysis patient
assessment of, 2606
recommendations for, 2606
in peritoneal dialysis patient, 2652–2653, 2656
in pregnant patient, 1685
in renal disease, 2500–2503
restriction of
and progression of chronic renal failure, 2501–2502
and progressive renal injury, 1977
compliance with, 2521
for acute renal failure, 1265
for diabetes mellitus, 1798
for nephrotic syndrome, 2505–2506
in children with chronic renal failure, 2502
in experimental renal failure, 2501
metabolic responses to, 2515–2516, 2516f
rationale for, 2520–2521
types of, comparison of, 2521–2523, 2522f–2523f, 2523t
variations in
and proteinuria/albuminuria, 2501
and renal hemodynamics, 2501
vegetable vs. animal, 2503
Protein kinase A
and mesangial cell proliferation, 125
phosphorylation by, and aquaporin-2 trafficking, 585
Protein kinase B, and mesangial cell proliferation, 125

Pyelonephritis, acute *(Continued)*
 and acute renal failure, 1255
 clinical presentations in, 1540
 in women, treatment of, 1550
 pathology of, 1530–1531
 and malakoplakia, 1555–1556, 1555f
 and tuberculosis, 1553–1554
 antibody production in, 1528
 autoimmune mechanisms in, 1528–1530
 cell-mediated immunity in, 1528
 chronic
  clinical presentations in, 1540–1541
  frequency of, 1533
  gross pathology of, 1532–1533,
   1532f–1533f
  hypertension in, 1542
  microscopic findings in, 1533–1534, 1534f
  terminology in, 1532–1533
  with obstruction, 1532
  with reflux. *See* Reflux nephropathy.
 computed tomography in, 1198f, 1199
 definition of, problems in, 1513
 evolution of renal lesion in, 1529–1530
 factors predisposing to, 1527
 in allograft, 2818
 in cortex vs. medulla, 1528
 in pregnant patient, 1676–1677
 magnetic resonance imaging in, 1199, 1199f
 natural history of, 1534–1538
 secondary, 1527–1528
 treatment of
  in children, 1551–1552
  in women, 1550
 ultrasonography in, 1198, 1199f
 urinalysis in, 1514
 xanthogranulomatous, 1554–1555, 1554f
Pyonephrosis, imaging of, 1201, 1201f
Pyrazinamide
 dosage modifications for, 2864t
 for renal tuberculosis, 1554
Pyridostigmine, 2864t
Pyridoxine, for hyperoxaluria, 1850
Pyrimethamine, 2864t
Pyrophosphate, as crystallization inhibitor, 1824
Pyruvate, metabolism of, 963
Pyuria, in urinary tract infection, 1515

Quality of life, hemoglobin normalization and, 2551
Quazepam, 2864t
Quinapril, 2383t, 2384, 2384t
 dosage modifications for, 2864t
Quinidine, 2864t
Quinine
 dosage modifications for, 2864t
 for cramps in hemodialysis patient, 2611
Quinton-Scribner shunt, for vascular access, 2568

Race
 and antihypertensive therapy, 2422–2423, 2423t
 and glomerulonephritis, 1333t
 and graft survival, 2829, 2830, 2831f
 and nephrotic syndrome, 1302t
 and peritoneal dialysis, 2654–2655
 and renal function, 2315, 2491–2492
Radial-cephalic fistula, 2569
Radiation nephritis, 1610–1612
 acute, 1610–1611
 and chronic interstitial nephritis, 1497–1498

Radiation nephritis *(Continued)*
 chronic, 1611
 clinical features of, 1610–1611
 pathogenesis of, 1611
 pathology of, 1611
 treatment of, 1611–1612
Radiation therapy
 for renal cell carcinoma, 1906
 for Wilms tumor, 1915
Radioactive microspheric measurement
 of cortical renal blood flow, 328
 of medullary blood flow, 332–333
 of total renal blood flow, 324
Radioactive tracer measurement
 of cortical renal blood flow, 326–328, 327f
 of medullary renal blood flow, 332t, 333–334
 of total renal blood flow, 324–325
Radiocontrast agents. *See* Contrast agents.
Radiofrequency ablation, of renal cell carcinoma, 1904
Radiography
 conventional, 1183–1184
 in essential hypertension, 2051
 in urinary tract obstruction, 1873, 1873f
Radiological assessment, 1183–1211. *See also specific modality, e.g.,* Computed tomography.
Radionuclide imaging
 in acute renal failure, 1085
 in renal cell carcinoma, 1900
 in vesicoureteral reflux, 1521
Radionuclide markers, for estimation of glomerular filtration rate, 1115–1117, 1116f
RAGE (AGE-receptor), in aging kidney, 2311
Ramipril, 2383t, 2384, 2384t
 dosage modifications for, 2864t
 in chronic kidney disease patient, for hypertension, 2214
 renoprotective effects of, 2466, 2466f, 2468
Randall plaque, 1824
Ranitidine, 2864t
RANTES, in mesangial cell cultures, 113
Rapamycin
 after renal transplantation, 2807t, 2809
 for immunosuppressive therapy, 2777
Rapidly progressive glomerulonephritis
 categorization of, 1344–1345, 1344t
 nomenclature in, 1344
 renal biopsy in, 1134–1135
Raynaud phenomenon, in systemic sclerosis, 1608
rBAT protein, model of, 1709f
rBAT/B0+AT transporter, 420–421, 420t
RBF. *See* Renal blood flow (RBF).
Reactive oxygen species. *See also* Oxidative stress.
 and chronic dialysis-dependent encephalopathy, 2234
 and mesangial cell apoptosis, 123
 and mesangial cell contractility, 120
 and nitric oxide, interactions between, 2121
 in chronic renal failure, 2119, 2120–2121
 in essential hypertension, 2040
 in hypertension with renal disease, 2119–2120, 2121
 in mesangial cell cultures, 112t, 115
 in necrosis, 1230, 1230f
 in tubule cell cultures, 161
Rebound phenomenon, and extracorporeal drug removal, 2738
Receiver-operating characteristic (ROC) curves, 1108
Receptor activator of NF-κB (RANK)
 as marker of bone resorption, 2278
 in osteoclast development, 2265, 2265f

Receptor activator of NF-κB ligand (RANKL)
 as marker of bone resorption, 2278
 in osteoclast development, 2264–2265, 2265f
Receptor tyrosine kinase, in nephrogenesis, 80t
Recipient factors, and graft survival, 2830–2832, 2831f
Recirculation, during dialysis, measurement of, 2585–2586
Recombinant erythropoietin (rHuEPO). *See* RHuEPO.
Red blood cell(s). *See* Erythrocytes.
Reduced folate transporter (RFT), 266t, 284
Refeeding, and hypophosphatemia, 1062
Reflux, vesicoureteral. *See* Vesicoureteral reflux.
Reflux nephropathy
 chronic, clinical presentations in, 1540–1541
 definition of, 1513
 gross pathology of, 1532–1533, 1532f–1533f
 hypertension in, 1542
 in pregnant patient, 1683
 natural history of, 1541–1543
 terminology in, 1532–1533
Rejection. *See* Allograft(s), rejection of.
Relaxin
 and glomerular filtration, 381–382, 381f
 in pregnant patient, 1662
Remnant kidney, cellular infiltration in, 1969–1970
Renal. *See also* Kidney.
Renal abscess
 computed tomography in, 1199
 magnetic resonance imaging in, 1199f
Renal angiography. *See also* Angiography.
 in acute renal failure, 1085
Renal angioplasty. *See* Percutaneous transluminal renal angioplasty (PTRA).
Renal aplasia, gene deletion experiments related to, 82t
Renal arteriography
 in renal artery thromboembolism, 1575, 1575f
 in renal cell carcinoma, 1899, 1901f
 in renal vein thrombosis, 1590
Renal arteriolar smooth muscle cell(s), in culture, 167–168
Renal artery
 accessory, 309
 anatomy of, 3, 3f, 5f
 magnetic resonance angiography of, 1189, 1190f
 occlusion of, and acute intrinsic renal azotemia, 1218
 reconstruction of, 2093–2095, 2094t–2095t, 2095f
 ultrasonography of, 1185
Renal artery aneurysm, 1576–1580
 anatomic and clinical characteristics of, 1576t
 clinical manifestations of, 1576t, 1577–1578
 dissecting, 1578–1580, 1579f
 fusiform, 1577, 1577f
 intraparenchymal, 1577
 rupture of, 1577–1578
 saccular, 1577
 treatment of, 1578, 1578t, 1579f
Renal artery stenosis
 after renal transplantation, 2815, 2815t
 and ischemic nephropathy, 2071–2075, 2072f, 2073f. *See also* Ischemic nephropathy.
 and renovascular hypertension, 2067, 2067t, 2068f. *See also* Renovascular hypertension.
 atherosclerotic, 2075–2076, 2076t, 2077, 2077f
  and concurrent diseases, 2081–2082
  angioplasty and stent placement for, 2096t, 2097–2099, 2098f–2099f

Urine, alkalinization of *(Continued)*
  for poisoning, 2735
  for salicylate intoxication, 967
antibacterial properties of, 1519
bilirubin in, 1121
blood in. *See* Hematuria.
casts in, 1131, 1132f
colony-forming units in, quantification of, 1514
color of, 1121
concentration of
    after nephron loss, 1965
    and urinary tract obstruction, 1883–1884
    countercurrent hypothesis for, 5–6,
        606–608, 607f
    disorders of, 870–888. *See also* Polyuria.
    and aquaporin-2 dysregulation, 589t,
        590f
    in aging, 2319–2320, 2319f
    in inner medulla, 615–623, 615f, 616t,
        618f, 618t, 620f
    and hyaluronan, 622
    external driving forces in, 622–623
    models of. *See* Osmolality, model(s) of.
    single effect in, 616–623, 616t
    in thin limbs of loop of Henle, 33–34
    long-term regulation of, 623–624
    mechanism of, 605–606, 605f
    medullary anatomy and, 5–6
    passive countercurrent multiplication model
        for, 617–618, 618f
    sites of, 603–604, 604
    vasopressin and, 606
crystals in, 1131, 1823, 1824–1826, 1825t
dilution of
    after nephron loss, 1964
    and urinary tract obstruction, 1883–1884
    disorders of, 888–903. *See also*
        Hyponatremia.
    in aging, 2320–2321
    mechanism of, 604–605
    normal determinants of, 889–890, 890f
    sites of, 603–604, 604f
fat in, 1131
glucose in, 1122
Griess nitrate reduction test for, 1544
hemoglobin in, 1122–1123
immunoglobulin light chains in, 1128
ketones in, 1122
leukocyte esterase test for, 1121–1122, 1515,
    1544
metastability of, limits of, 1822–1823, 1823f
microorganisms in, 1131
microscopic examination of, 1128
myoglobin in, 1122–1123
nitrites in, 1121–1122
pH of, 1121
    and ammonium excretion, 1174–1175, 1175f
    and cystine solubility, 1855, 1855f
    and uric acid nephrolithiasis, 1851
    factors influencing, 1851–1852
protein in. *See* Protein, urinary; Proteinuria.
specific gravity of, 1121
urobilinogen in, 1121
volume of, and polyuria, 1152–1153
white blood cells in. *See* Leukocyturia.
Urine anion gap (UAG)
  calculation of, 945
  in generalized distal renal tubular acidosis,
    955
  in hyperchloremic metabolic acidosis, 945
Urine flow
  calculation of, 1151, 1153–1154
  cessation of, in urinary tract obstruction, and
    sodium transport, 1882–1883
  in renal pelvis, 603, 604f

Urine leak, after renal transplantation, 2819,
    2821
Urine net charge, 1174, 1174f
Urine osmolal gap, 1174, 1174f
Urine osmolality, 1154
  aging and, 2319–2320, 2319f, 2320
  in acute renal failure, 1083t, 1084
  in pregnant patient, 1662–1663
Urine osmole(s), effective, 1151, 1154–1155
Urine output, in acute renal failure, 1084
Urine saturation, in calcium nephrolithiasis,
    1821–1822, 1822f, 1822t
Urine sediment
  in acute renal failure, 1083, 1083f, 1083t,
    1251–1252, 1251t
  in urinary tract obstruction, 1873
Urine specimen, collection of, 1120
Urine tests
  for urinary tract infection, 1543–1545
  in acute renal failure, 1083t
  in extracellular fluid volume abnormalities,
    1161–1162, 1161t
  in intracellular fluid volume abnormalities,
    1159–1160, 1160f
  in metabolic acidosis, 1173–1176,
    1174f–1175f
  in metabolic alkalosis, 1164–1165, 1166t
  in polyuria, 1153–1155, 1153t
Urobilinogen, in urine, 1121
Urodilatin, 702, 798–799
  and glomerular filtration, 382, 383–384
  in edema formation, in congestive heart
    failure, 818
  therapeutic uses of, 703
Urography
  intravenous. *See* Intravenous urography
    (IVU).
  magnetic resonance
    after renal transplantation, 1210
    in acute renal failure, 1191–1193, 1193f
    of calculi, 1202–1203
Uroguanylin, and extracellular fluid volume
    control, 783
Urokinase
  and mesangial cell proliferation, 127
  dosage modifications for, 2865t
  for relapsing peritonitis, 2672
  in glomerular visceral epithelial cell cultures,
    137–138
Uromodulin. *See* Tamm Horsfall protein.
Uropathy, obstructive, 1679
  definition of, 1867
  in elderly person, 2328–2329
  in pregnant patient, 1679
  renin-angiotensin system in, 682
Uropontin, as crystallization inhibitor, 1825,
    1825t
Urovirulence factors, 1524–1527
US. *See* Ultrasonography.
Uveitis, tubulointerstitial nephritis and, 1494

Vacuolar hydrogen-ATPase (V-ATPases), 233,
    235
  and coupling with glycolysis, 247
  in distal nephron acidification, 513
  in proximal tubule acidification, 502
Vacuolar-lysosomal system
  in pars convoluta, 25–26, 25f, 26f
  in pars recta, 29
Valerate, metabolism of, in proximal tubule, 249
Valproic acid
  dosage modifications for, 2864t
  intoxication from, 2752–2753

Valsartan, 2390t, 2391t, 2392
Valvular heart disease, in chronic kidney
    disease, 2199–2200, 2212
Vanadate, distal renal tubular acidosis from, 952
Vanadium, metabolism of, in uremia, 2143
Vancomycin
  dosage modifications for, 2865t
  for peritonitis, 2671
  nephrotoxicity of, 1628
Vasa recta, 602–603
  in medullary microcirculation, 333t, 334–335
  plasma, solute concentrations in, 625, 625t
  urea recycling through, 626–627
Vascular access
  for hemodialysis
    arteriovenous fistula as, 2569
    arteriovenous graft as, 2569
    cuffed venous catheter as, 2569–2570
    dysfunction of
      pharmacologic prevention of, 2570–2571
      treatment of, 2570
    epidemiology of, 2568
    history of, 2568
    monitoring and surveillance of, 2569
  for renal replacement therapy in intensive care
    unit, 2718–2719
  in diabetic nephropathy with end-stage renal
    disease, 1800
Vascular calcification
  in chronic kidney disease, 1093–1094, 2200
  in hemodialysis patient, 2604
Vascular cell(s), in culture, 167–169
Vascular cell adhesion molecule-1 (VCAM-1)
  characteristics of, 210t, 211f, 212
  expression of, in kidney, 215
  in mesangial cell cultures, 110
  knockout mice for, 213
Vascular congestion, in acute tubular necrosis,
    1241
Vascular disease
  in chronic kidney disease
    management of, 2212–2213
    pathophysiology of, 2200–2201
  in systemic lupus erythematosus, 1387–1388
Vascular endothelial growth factor(s), 92–93
  and mesangial cell proliferation, 126–127
  in glomerular endothelial cell regulation, 7
  in glomerular visceral epithelial cell cultures,
    137
  in mesangial cell cultures, 111
Vascular endothelial growth factor receptors,
    92–93
  in glomerular endothelial cells, 7
Vascular examination, in hypertension,
    2050–2051
Vascular factors, in hypertension with renal
    disease, 2121–2125
Vascular patterns
  in cortical postglomerular microcirculation,
    312–313, 313f–314f
  in medullary microcirculation, 319–322,
    320f–322f
Vascular remodeling, in essential hypertension,
    2038–2039
Vascular tone, control of, endothelial factors in,
    338–339
Vascular wall
  growth inhibitors in, 2011t
  in hypertension, 1999–2017. *See also*
    Hypertension, vascular wall in.
  peritoneal, pore systems in, 2638–2639, 2638f
Vascular-tubule relations
  in cortical postglomerular microcirculation,
    313f–316, 315f–316f
  in medullary microcirculation, 322–323, 323f

Set ISBN 0–7216–0164–2
Volume 2 P/N 9997637100

9 789997 637109